Rook's
Textbook of
Dermatology

EDITED BY

Tony Burns
MB, BS, FRCP, FRCP(Edin)
Emeritus Consultant Dermatologist, Leicester Royal Infirmary, Leicester

Stephen Breathnach
MA, MB, BChir, MD, PhD, FRCP
Consultant Dermatologist, St John's Institute of Dermatology, Guy's and St Thomas' NHS Foundation Trust, St Thomas'
Hospital, London, and Consultant Dermatologist, Epsom & St Helier University Hospitals NHS Trust, Epsom, Surrey

Neil Cox
BSc, MB, ChB, FRCP(Lond & Edin)
Consultant Dermatologist, Department of Dermatology, Cumberland Infirmary, and Visiting Professor, University of
Cumbria, Carlisle

Christopher Griffiths
BSc, MD, FRCP, FRCPath
Professor of Dermatology and Consultant Dermatologist, The Dermatology Centre, University of Manchester, Salford Royal
Hospital, Salford, Manchester

IN FOUR VOLUMES

VOLUME 3

EIGHTH EDITION

WILEY-BLACKWELL
A John Wiley & Sons, Ltd., Publication

Contents

VOLUME 3

VOLUME 4

The index to all four volumes can be found at the end of Volume 4.
The online version can be fully searched at www.rooksdermatology.com

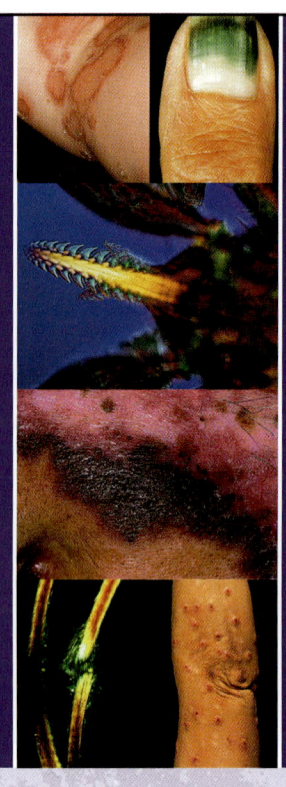
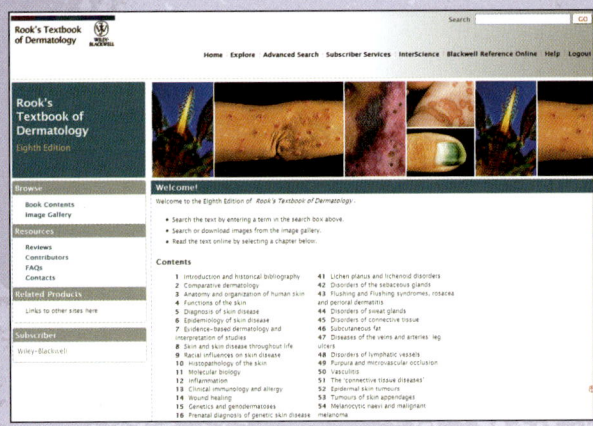
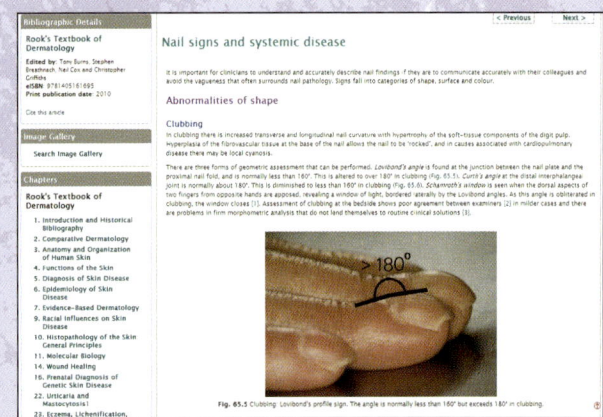
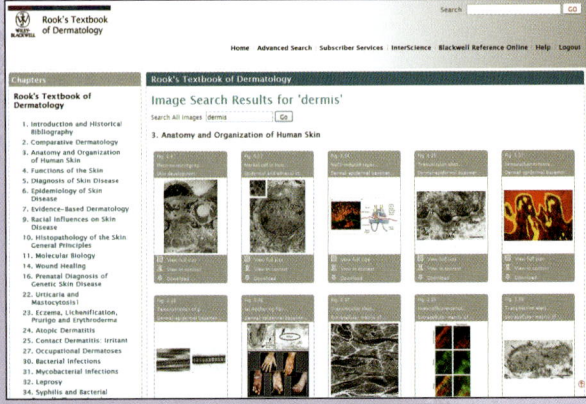
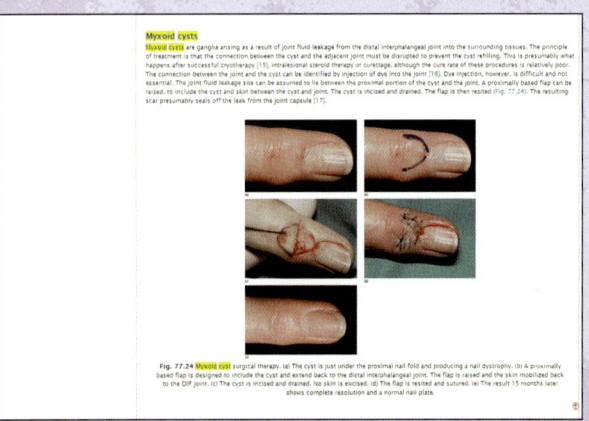

Contributors

Adriaans, Beverley M.
MD, FRCP
Consultant Dermatologist, Department of
Dermatology, Gloucestershire Royal Hospital,
Gloucester GL1 3NN
Co-author of
Chapter 30: Bacterial Infections

Anstey, Alexander V.
MD, FRCP
Consultant Dermatologist, Department of
Dermatology, Royal Gwent Hospital, Newport NP20
2UB
Author of
Chapter 58: Disorders of Skin Colour

Archer, Clive B.
BSc, MD, PhD, MSc Med Ed(Lond), FRCP (Edin, Lond)
Consultant Dermatologist, Honary Clinical Senior
Lecturer, Bristol Dermatology Centre, Bristol Royal
Infirmary, Bristol BS2 8HW
Author of
Chapter 4: Functions of the Skin
Co-author of
Chapter 63: The Skin and the Nervous System

Ardern-Jones, Michael R.
BSc, MRCP, DPhil
Senior Lecturer and Honorary Consultant in
Dermatology, Division of Infection, Inflammation and
Immunity, School of Medicine, University of
Southampton, Southampton General Hospital,
Southampton SO16 6YD
Co-author of
Chapter 24: Atopic Dermatitis

Ashbee, H. Ruth
BSc, PhD
Principal Clinical Scientist, Mycology Reference
Centre, Department of Microbiology, Leeds General
Infirmary, Leeds LS1 3EX
Co-author of
Chapter 36: Mycology

Baran, Robert
MD
Head of Nail Disease Centre, Le Grand Palais, 42 Rue
des Serbes, 06400 Cannes, and Consultant
Dermatologist, Gustave Roussy Cancer Institute,
94805 Villejuif, France
Co-author of
Chapter 65: Disorders of Nails

Barker, Jonathan N.W.N.
BSc, MD, FRCP, FRCPath
Professor of Clinical Dermatology, St John's Institute
of Dermatology, King's College London, Guy's
Hospital, London SE1 9RT
Co-author of
Chapter 20: Psoriasis

Barlow, Richard J.
MD, FRCP
Consultant Dermatologist, St John's Institute of
Dermatology, St Thomas' Hospital, Lambeth Palace
Road, London SE1 7EH
Author of
*Chapter 78: Lasers and Flashlamps in the Treatment of
Skin Disorders*

Beck, Michael H.
FRCP, MBchB
Honorary Clinical Lecturer Occupational and
Environmental Health Group, University of
Manchester and Retired Consultant Dermatologist
and Director of Contact Dermatitis Investigation Unit,
Department of Dermatology, Salford Royal Hospital,
Stott Lane, Salford M6 8HD
Co-author of
Chapter 25: Contact Dermatitis: Irritant
Chapter 26: Contact Dermatitis: Allergic

Berth-Jones, John
FRCP
Consultant Dermatologist, Department of
Dermatology, University Hospitals Coventry and
Warwickshire, Walsgrave, Coventry CV2 2DX
Author of
*Chapter 23: Eczema, Lichenification, Prurigo and
Erythroderma*
*Chapter 43: Rosacea, Perioral Dermatitis and Similar
Dermatoses, Flushing and Flushing Syndromes*
Chapter 73: Topical Therapy

Bigby, Michael
MD
Associate Professor of Dermatology, Harvard Medical
School and Beth Israel Deaconess Medical Center, 330
Brookline Avenue, Boston MA 02215, USA
Co-author of
Chapter 7: Evidence-Based Dermatology

Bourke, John F.
MD, FRCP(Ire)
Consultant Dermatologist, Department of
Dermatology, South Infirmary-Victoria Hospital, Old
Blackrock Road, Cork, Ireland
Co-author of
*Chapter 50: Vasculitis, Neutrophilic Dermatoses and
Related Disorders*

Breathnach, Stephen M.
MA, MD, PhD, FRCP
Consultant Dermatologist, St John's Institute of
Dermatology, Guy's and St Thomas' NHS Foundation
Trust, St Thomas' Hospital, Lambeth Palace Road,
London SE1 7EH
Editor
Author of
Chapter 41: Lichen Planus and Lichenoid Disorders
Chapter 75: Drug Reactions
*Chapter 76: Erythema Multiforme, Stevens–Johnson
Syndrome and Toxic Epidermal Necrolysis*
Co-author of
Chapter 59: Metabolic and Nutritional Disorders
Chapter 74: Systemic Therapy

Bunker, Christopher B.
MA, MD, FRCP
Consultant Dermatologist, Chelsea and Westminster
and Royal Marsden Hospitals, Professor of
Dermatology, Division and Faculty of Medicine,
Imperial College London, Department of
Dermatology, 369 Fulham Road, London SW10 9NH
Co-author of
Chapter 35: HIV and the Skin
Chapter 71: The Genital, Perianal and Umbilical Regions

Burd, D. Andrew R.

MBChB, FRCS, MD

Professor, The Chinese University of Hong Kong, Department of Surgery, 4/F Clinical Science Building, Prince of Wales Hospital, Shatin, New Territories, Hong Kong

Co-author of

Chapter 28: Mechanical and Thermal Injury

Burge, Susan M.

DM, FRCP

Consultant Dermatologist, Churchill Hospital, Old Road, Headington, Oxford OX3 7LJ

Co-author of

Chapter 39: Genetic Blistering Diseases

Burnand, Kevin G.

MBBS, FRCS, MS

Professor of Surgery, Academic Department of Surgery, St Thomas' Hospital, Lambeth Palace Road, London SE1 7EH

Co-author of

Chapter 47: Diseases of the Veins and Arteries: Leg Ulcers

Burns, David Anthony

MB BS FRCP

Emeritus Consultant Dermatologist, Leicester Royal Infirmary, Infirmary Square, Leicester LE1 5WW

Editor

Author of

Chapter 38: Diseases Caused by Arthropods and Other Noxious Animals

Chapter 60: Necrobiotic Disorders

Chapter 70: The Breast

Co-author of

Chapter 1: Introduction and Historical Bibliography

Chapter 2: Comparative Dermatology

Burrows, Nigel P.

MD, FRCP

Consultant Dermatologist and Associate Lecturer, Department of Dermatology, Addenbrooke's Hospital, Hills Road, Cambridge CB2 2QQ

Co-author of

Chapter 45: Disorders of Connective Tissue

Calonje, Eduardo

MD DipRCPath

Consultant Dermatologist, Department of Histopathology, St John's Institute of Dermatology, St Thomas' Hospital, Lambeth Palace Road, London SE1 7EH

Author of

Chapter 10: Histopathology of the Skin: General Principles

Chapter 53: Tumours of the Skin Appendages

Chapter 56: Soft-Tissue Tumours and Tumour-like Conditions

Cant, Andrew J.

BSc, MD, FRCP, FRCPCH

Consultant in Paediatric Immunology & Infectious Diseases, Children's BMT Unit, Newcastle General Hospital, Westgate Road, Newcastle upon Tyne NE4 6BE

Co-author of

Chapter 17: The Neonate

Chalmers, Robert J.G.

MB, FRCP

Consultant Dermatologist, Dermatology Centre, University of Manchester, Salford Royal Hospital, Stott Lane, Manchester M6 8HD

Co-author of

Chapter 74: Systemic Therapy

Chu, Anthony C.

FRCP

Professor of Dermatologic Oncology, Buckingham University and Consultant Dermatologist, Hammersmith Hospital, Du Cane Road, London W12 0HS

Author of

Chapter 55: Histiocytoses

Coulson, Ian H.

BSc, MB, BS, FRCP

Consultant Dermatologist, Dermatology Unit, Burnley General Hospital, Casterton Avenue, Burnley BB10 2PQ

Author of

Chapter 44: Disorders of Sweat Glands

Co-author of

Chapter 5: Diagnosis of Skin Disease

Chapter 62: Systemic Disease and the Skin

Cox, Neil H.

BSc, MB, ChB, FRCP

Consultant Dermatologist, Department of Dermatology, Cumberland Infirmary, Carlisle CA2 7HY and Visiting Professor, University of Cumbria, Carlisle CA1 2HH

Editor

Co-author of

Chapter 1: Introduction and Historical Bibliography

Chapter 2: Comparative Dermatology

Chapter 5: Diagnosis of Skin Disease

Chapter 49: Purpura and Microvascular Occlusion

Chapter 50: Vasculitis, Neutrophilic Dermatoses and Related Disorders

Chapter 62: Systemic Disease and the Skin

Creamer, Daniel

BSc, MD, FRCP

Consultant Dermatologist, Department of Dermatology, King's College Hospital, Denmark Hill, London SE5 9RS

Co-author of

Chapter 28: Mechanical and Thermal Injury

Dart, John K.G.

MA DM FRCS FRCOphth

Consultant Ophthalmologist, Moorfields Eye Hospital NHS Foundation Trust, 162 City Road, London EC1 2PD and Honorary Reader in Ophthalmology, University College London

Co-author of

Chapter 67: The Skin and the Eyes

de Berker, David A.R.

BA, MBBS, MRCP

Consultant Dermatologist, Bristol Dermatology Centre, Bristol Royal Infirmary, Marlborough Street, Bristol BS2 8HW

Co-author of

Chapter 65: Disorders of Nails

Chapter 66: Disorders of Hair

Eedy, David J.

MD, FRCP

Consultant Dermatologist, Department of Dermatology, Craigavon Area Hospital, 68 Lurgan Road, Portadown, Co Armagh BT63 5QQ

Co-author of

Chapter 63: The Skin and the Nervous System

English, John S.C.

FRCP

Consultant Dermatologist, Department of Dermatology, Queen's Medical Centre, Clifton Boulevard, Nottingham NG7 2UH

Author of

Chapter 27: Occupational Dermatoses

Ferguson, James

MD, FRCP

Professor and Consultant Dermatologist, Photobiology Unit, Department of Dermatology, Ninewells Hospital and Medical School, Dundee, Tayside DD1 9SY

Co-author of

Chapter 29: Cutaneous Photobiology

Fine, Jo-David

MD, MPH

Professor of Medicine (Dermatology) and Pediatrics, Vanderbilt University, School of Medicine, 1900 Patterson Street, Nashville, TN 37203, USA

Co-author of

Chapter 39: Genetic Blistering Diseases

Finlay, Andrew Y.

MBBS, FRCP (London & Glasgow)

Professor of Dermatology, Department of Dermatology, Cardiff University School of Medicine, Heath Park, Cardiff CF14 4XN

Co-author of

Chapter 72: General Aspects of Treatment

Flynn, Paul D.

PhD, FRCP, MRCPI
Consultant Physician, Acute and Metabolic Medicine,
Addenbrooke's Hospital, Cambridge CB2 2QQ and
Fellow and Director of Studies in Medical Science,
Sidney Sussex College, Cambridge
Co-author of
Chapter 59: Metabolic and Nutritional Disorders

Friedmann, Peter S.

MD, FRCP, FMedSci
Professor of Dermatology, Dermatopharmacology
Unit, Southampton General Hospital, Tremona Road,
Southampton SO16 6YD
Co-author of
Chapter 24: Atopic Dermatitis

Fuller, L. Claire

MA, FRCP
Consultant Dermatologist, Department of
Dermatology, Kent and Canterbury Hospital,
Ethelbert Road, Canterbury, Kent CT1 3NG
Co-author of
Chapter 9: Racial Influences on Skin Disease

Gawkrodger, David J.

MD, FRCP, FRCPE
Consultant Dermatologist and Honorary Professor of
Dermatology, Department of Dermatology, Royal
Hallamshire Hospital, Glossop Road, Sheffield S10
2JF
Author of
Chapter 61: Sarcoidosis

Gennery, Andrew R.

MD, MRCP, MRCPCH, DCH, DipMedSci
Reader, Paediatric Immunology, Children's BMT
Unit, Newcastle General Hospital, Westgate Road,
Newcastle upon Tyne NE4 6BE
Co-author of
Chapter 17: The Neonate

Goodfield, Mark J.D.

MD, FRCP
Consultant Dermatologist, Department of
Dermatology, Leeds General Infirmary, Great George
Street, Leeds LS1 3EX
Co-author of
Chapter 51: The 'Connective Tissue Diseases'

Gotch, Frances

PhD, FRCPath
Professor of Immunology, Department of
Immunology, Imperial College School of Medicine,
Chelsea and Westminster Hospital, 369 Fulham Road,
London SW10 9NH
Co-author of
Chapter 35: HIV and the Skin

Graham-Brown, Robin A.C.

BSc, MB, BS, FRCP, FRCPCH
Consultant Dermatologist and Honorary Senior
Lecturer, University Hospitals of Leicester, Leicester
LE1 5WW
Co-author of
Chapter 8: Skin and Skin Disease Throughout Life

Grattan, Clive E.H.

MA MD FRCP
Consultant Dermatologist, Department of
Dermatology, Norfolk and Norwich University
Hospital, Colney Lane, Norwich NR4 7UY
Co-author of
Chapter 22: Urticaria and Mastocytosis

Greaves, Malcolm W.

MD, PhD, FRCP, FAMS
Emeritus Professor of Dermatology, Cutaneous
Allergy Clinic, St John's Institute of Dermatology,
St Thomas' Hospital, Lambeth Palace Road, London
SEI 7EH
Author of
Chapter 21: Pruritus

Griffiths, Christopher E.M.

BSc, MD, FRCP, FRCPath
Professor of Dermatology and Consultant
Dermatologist, The Dermatology Centre, University
of Manchester, Salford Royal Hospital, Salford,
Manchester M6 8HD
Editor
Co-author of
Chapter 20: Psoriasis

Groves, Richard W.

MBBS, FRCP
Head, Clinical Immunodermatology, St John's
Institute of Dermatology, Guy's Hospital, Great Maze
Pond, London SE1 9RT
Co-author of
Chapter 12: Inflammation

Hawk, John L.M.

BSc, MD, FRACP, FRCP
Emeritus Professor of Dermatological Photobiology
and Honorary Consultant Dermatologist, St John's
Institute of Dermatology, St Thomas' Hospital,
Lambeth Palace Road, London SE1 7EH
Co-author of
Chapter 29: Cutaneous Photobiology

Hay, Roderick J.

DM, FRCP, FRCPath, FMedSci
Professor of Cutaneous Infection, Dermatology
Department, King's College Hospital, Denmark Hill,
Camberwell, London SE5 9RS
Co-author of
Chapter 30: Bacterial Infections
Chapter 36: Mycology
Chapter 37: Parasitic Worms and Protozoa
Chapter 74: Systemic Therapy

Hegarty, Anne

BA BDentSC, MSc, MFDRCSI, MBBS
Consultant in Oral Medicine, The Charles Clifford
Dental Hospital, Wellesley Road, Sheffield S10 2SZ
Co-author of
Chapter 69: The Oral Cavity and Lips

Higgins, Elisabeth M.

MA, FRCP
Consultant Dermatologist, Department of
Dermatology, King's College Hospital, Denmark Hill,
Camberwell, London SE5 9RS
Co-author of
Chapter 9: Racial Influences on Skin Disease

Hill, Peter B.

BVsc, PhD, DVD, DipACVD, DipECVD, MRCVS
Specialist in Veterinary Dermatology, Veterinary
Specialist Centre, North Ryde, Sydney, NSW 2113,
Australia
Co-author of
Chapter 2: Comparative Dermatology

Holden, Colin A.

BSc, MD, FRCP
Consultant Dermatologist, Department of
Dermatology, Epsom and St Helier NHS Trust,
Wrythe Lane, Carshalton, Surrey SM5 1AA
Co-author of
Chapter 24: Atopic Dermatitis

Irvine, Alan D.

MD, FRCPI, MRCP
Consultant Paediatric Dermatologist, Our Lady's
Hospital for Sick Children, Crumlin, Dublin 12,
Ireland
Co-author of
Chapter 15: Genetics and Genodermatoses

Jones, Stephen K.

BMedSci, BM, BS, FRCP (London & Edinburgh)
Consultant Dermatologist, Department of
Dermatology, Clatterbridge Hospital, Bebington,
Wirral CH63 4JY
Co-author of
Chapter 51: The 'Connective Tissue Diseases'

Jorizzo, Joseph L.

MD
Professor, Former and Founding Chair, Department
of Dermatology, Wake Forest University School of
Medicine, Winston-Salem, NC, USA
Co-author of
*Chapter 50: Vasculitis, Neutrophilic Dermatoses and
Related Disorders*

Judge, Mary R.

MD, FRCP, DCH
Consultant Dermatologist, Department of
Dermatology, Salford Royal Hospital, Greater
Manchester M6 8HD
Co-author of
Chapter 19: Disorders of Keratinization

Kelly, Charles G.

MSc, FRCP, FRCR

Consultant Clinical Oncologist, Northern Centre for
Cancer Treatment, Newcastle General Hospital,
Westgate Road, Newcastle upon Tyne NE4 6BE

Co-author of
*Chapter 79: Radiotherapy and Reactions to Ionizing
Radiation*

Kennedy, Cameron T.C.

MA, MB, BChir, FRCP

Consultant Dermatologist and Clinical Senior
Lecturer, Bristol Dermatology Centre, Bristol Royal
Infirmary, Marlborough Street, Bristol BS2 8HW

Author of
Chapter 68: The External Ear

Co-author of
Chapter 28: Mechanical and Thermal Injury

Kinghorn, George R.

MD, FRCP (London & Glasgow)

Consultant and Honorary Professor of Genitourinary
Medicine, Department of Genitourinary Medicine,
Royal Hallamshire Hospital, Glossop Road, Sheffield
S10 2JF

Author of
*Chapter 34: Syphilis and Bacterial Sexually Transmitted
Infections*

Kobza Black, Anne

MD, FRCP

Honorary Senior Lecturer, St John's Institute of
Dermatology, St Thomas' Hospital, London SE1 7EH

Co-author of
Chapter 22: Urticaria and Mastocytosis

Lawrence, Clifford M.

MD, FRCP

Consultant Dermatologist, Department of
Dermatology, Royal Victoria Infirmary, Queen
Victoria Road, Newcastle upon Tyne, Tyne and Wear
NE1 4LP

Co-author of
Chapter 77: Dermatological Surgery

Layton, Alison M.

MB, ChB, FRCP

Consultant Dermatologist, Harrogate and District
Hospital, Lancaster Park Road, Harrogate, North
Yorkshire HG2 2SX

Author of
Chapter 42: Disorders of the Sebaceous Glands

LeBoit, Philip E.

MD

Professor of Pathology and Dermatology, Division
Chief, Dermatopathology, University of California
San Francisco, 1701 Divisadero Street, San Francisco
CA94115, USA

Co-author of
Chapter 12: Inflammation

Leonard, Jonathan N.

BSc, MD, FRCP

Consultant Dermatologist, Department of
Dermatology, St Mary's Hospital, Praed Street,
London W2 1NY

Co-author of
Chapter 67: The Skin and the Eyes

Lockwood, Diana N.J.

MD, FRCP

Consultant Physician and Leprologist, Hospital for
Tropical Diseases, Mortimer Market, Capper Street,
London WC1E 6AU

Author of
Chapter 32: Leprosy

Lovell, Christopher R.

MD, FRCP

Consultant Dermatologist, Kinghorn Dermatology
Unit, Royal United Hospital, Combe Park, Bath, Avon
BA1 3NG

Co-author of
Chapter 45: Disorders of Connective Tissue

Lowe, Nicholas James

MD, FRCP, FACP

Consultant Dermatologist and Clinical Professor,
UCLA School of Medicine, Los Angeles, CA, USA
and The Cranley Clinic, Harcourt House, 19A
Cavendish Square, London W19 0PN

Author of
*Chapter 80: Minimally Invasive Treatments and
Procedures for Ageing Skin*

Luger, Thomas A.

MD

Professor and Chairman, Department of
Dermatology, University of Münster, Von
Esmarchstrasse 58, D-48149 Münster, Germany

Co-author of
Chapter 12: Inflammation

McGibbon, David H.

MB, ChB, FRCP

Consultant Dermatologist, St John's Institute of
Dermatology, St Thomas' Hospital, Lambeth Palace
Road, London SE1 7EH

Author of
Chapter 46: Subcutaneous Fat

McGrath, John A.

MD, FRCP

Professor of Molecular Dermatology, St. John's
Institute of Dermatology, King's College London,
London SE1 9RT

Author of
Chapter 16: Prenatal Diagnosis of Genetic Skin Disease

Co-author of
Chapter 3: Anatomy and Organization of Human Skin

McLean, W.H. Irwin

BSc (Hons), PhD, DSc, FRSE

Professor of Human Genetics, Human Genetics Unit,
Division of Pathology and Neuroscience, University
of Dundee, Ninewells Hospital and Medical School,
Dundee, Tayside DD1 9SY

Co-author of
Chapter 19: Disorders of Keratinization

Mellerio, Jemima E.

BSc, MD, FRCP

Consultant Dermatologist, St John's Institute of
Dermatology, St Thomas' Hospital, Lambeth Palace
Road, London SE1 7EH

Co-author of
Chapter 14: Wound Healing
Chapter 15: Genetics and Genodermatoses

Messenger, Andrew G.

MD, FRCP

Consultant Dermatologist, Department of
Dermatology, Royal Hallamshire Hospital, Sheffield,
UK

Co-author of
Chapter 66: Disorders of Hair

Millard Jonathan

MRCPsych

Consultant, The Becklin Centre, Alma Street, Leeds
LS9 7BE

Co-author of
Chapter 64: Psychocutaneous Disorders

Millard, Leslie G.

MD, FRCP

Consultant Dermatologist, Rotherham District
Hospitals Trust, Moorgate Road, Rotherham S60 2UD

Co-author of
Chapter 64: Psychocutaneous Disorders

Millington George W.M.

BSc, MB, PhD, MRCP

Consultant Dermatologist, Norfolk and Norwich
University Hospital, Norwich NR4 7UY

Co-author of
Chapter 8: Skin and Skin Disease Throughout Life

Morris, Andrew A.M.

BM, BCh, PhD, FRCPCH

Consultant Paediatrician with Special Interest in
Metabolic Diseases, Willink Biochemical Genetics
Unit, Department of Genetic Medicine, Royal
Manchester Children's Hospital, Oxford Road,
Manchester M13 9WL

Co-author of
Chapter 59: Metabolic and Nutritional Disorders

Mortimer, Peter S.

MD, FRCP

Professor of Dermatological Medicine, St George's, University of London, Cranmer Terrace, London SW17 ORE and Consultant Skin Physician, St George's Hospital London and the Royal Marsden Hospital, London SW3 6JJ

Author of
Chapter 48: Disorders of Lymphatic Vessels
Co-author of
Chapter 47: Diseases of the Veins and Arteries: Leg Ulcers

Moss, Celia

DM, FRCP, MRCPCH

Consultant Dermatologist and Honorary Professor of Paediatric Dermatology, Birmingham Children's Hospital, Steelhouse Lane, Birmingham B4 6NL

Co-author of
Chapter 18: Naevi and other Developmental Defects

Munro, Colin S.

MA, MD, FRCP

Professor of Dermatology, Alan Lyell Centre for Dermatology, Southern General Hospital, Glasgow G51 4TF

Co-author of
Chapter 19: Disorders of Keratinization

Neill, Sallie M.

FRCP

Consultant Dermatologist, St John's Institute of Dermatology, St Thomas' Hospital, Lambeth Palace Road, London SE1 7EH

Co-author of
Chapter 71: The Genital, Perianal and Umbilical Regions

Neumann, H.A. Martino

MD, PhD

Head of the Department of Dermatology and Venereology, Erasmus Medical Center, Rotterdam, The Netherlands

Co-author of
Chapter 47: Diseases of the Veins and Arteries: Leg Ulcers

Newton Bishop, Julia A.

MD, FRCP

Professor of Dermatology, Section of Epidemiology and Biostatistics, Leeds Institute of Molecular Medicine, St James's University Hospital, Leeds LS9 7TF

Author of
Chapter 54: Lentigos, Melanocytic Naevi and Melanoma

O'Toole, Edel A.

MB, BCh, PhD, FRCP(Ire), FRCP

Professor of Molecular Dermatology and Honorary Consultant Dermatologist, Centre for Cutaneous Research, Barts and The London School of Medicine & Dentistry, Queen Mary, University of London, 4 Newark Street, London E1 2AT

Author of
Chapter 11: Molecular Biology
Co-author of
Chapter 14: Wound Healing

Paige, David G.

MBBS, MA, FRCP

Consultant Dermatologist, Barts and the Royal London NHS Trust, Whitechapel, London E1 1BB

Co-author of
Chapter 17: The Neonate

Peat, Irene

FRCR, FRCP

Consultant Clinical Oncologist, Oncology Unit, Leicester Royal Infirmary, Leicester LE1 5WW

Co-author of
Chapter 79: Radiotherapy and Reactions to Ionizing Radiation

Perkins, William

MBBS, FRCP

Consultant Dermatologist, Nottingham University Hospital Queen's Medical Centre, Clifton Boulevard, Nottingham NG7 2UH

Co-author of
Chapter 52: Non-Melanoma Skin Cancer and Other Epidermal Skin Tumours

Piette, Warren W.

MD

Chair and Program Director of the Dermatology Training Program, John H Stroger Jr Hospital of Cook County, Division of Dermatology, 1900 W Polk St, Admin Bldg Rm 519, Chicago, Illinois 60612, USA

Co-author of
Chapter 49: Purpura and Microvascular Occlusion

Quinn, Anthony G.

BMSc, MBChB, PhD, FRCP

Senior Vice President and Chief Medical Officer, Synageva BioPharma Corporation, 60 Hickory Drive, Waltham, Massachusetts 02451, USA

Co-author of
Chapter 52: Non-Melanoma Skin Cancer and Other Epidermal Skin Tumours

Sarkany, Robert P.E.

FRCP, MD

Director of Photobiology, St John's Institute of Dermatology, St Thomas' Hospital, Lambeth Palace Road, London SE1 7EH

Co-author of
Chapter 59: Metabolic and Nutritional Disorders

Savage, Caroline O.S.

PhD, FRCP, FMedSci

Professor of Nephrology, Renal Immunobiology, School of Immunity and Infection, The College of Medical and Dental Sciences, University of Birmingham, Edgbaston, Birmingham B15 2TT

Co-author of
Chapter 50: Vasculitis, Neutrophilic Dermatoses and Related Disorders

Schwarz, Thomas

MD

Professor and Chairman, Department of Dermatology, Venereology and Allergology, University Hospital Schleswig-Holstein Campus, Kiel, Germany

Co-author of
Chapter 13: Clinical Immunology, Allergy and Photoimmunology

Scully, Crispian

CBE, MD, PhD, MDS, MRCS, BSc, FDSRCS, FDSRCPS, FFDRCSI, FDSRCSE, FRCPath, FMedSci, FHEA, FUCL, DSc, DChD, DMed(HC), Drh.c.

Director (Special Projects) and Professor UCL-EDI, 256 Gray's Inn Road, London WC1X 8LD

Co-author of
Chapter 69: The Oral Cavity and Lips

Shahidullah, Hossain

BMedSci, MD, FRCP Edin

Consultant Dermatologist, Department of Dermatology, Derbyshire Royal Infirmary, London Road, Derby DE1 2QY

Co-author of
Chapter 18: Naevi and other Developmental Defects

Sinclair, Rodney D.

MBBS, MD, FACD

Professor and Director of Dermatology, Department of Dermatology, St Vincent's Hospital, Fitzroy, Melbourne, Victoria 3065, Australia

Co-author of
Chapter 66: Disorders of Hair

Smith, Catherine H.

MD, FRCP

Consultant Dermatologist and Senior Lecturer, St John's Institute of Dermatology, St Thomas' Hospital, Lambeth Palace Road, London SE1 7EH

Co-author of
Chapter 72: General Aspects of Treatment
Chapter 74: Systemic Therapy

Spickett, Gavin P.

MA, DPhil, FRCPath. FRCP, FRCPE

Consultant Clinical Immunologist, Regional Department of Immunology, Royal Victoria Infirmary, Newcastle upon Tyne NE1 4LP

Co-author of
Chapter 13: Clinical Immunology, Allergy and Photoimmunology

Steinhoff, Martin

MD, PhD

Department of Dermatology, University of Münster, Von-Esmarch-Strasse 58D-48149, Münster, Germany

Co-author of
Chapter 12: Inflammation

Sterling, Jane C.

MB, BChir, MA, FRCP, PhD
Senior Lecturer, Department of Dermatology,
University of Cambridge, Addenbrooke's Hospital,
Hills Road, Cambridge CB2 2QQ
Author of
Chapter 33: Virus Infections

Telfer, Nicholas R.

FRCP
Consultant Dermatological Surgeon, Department of
Dermatology, Salford Royal Hospital, Stott Lane,
Salford, Lancs M6 8HD
Co-author of
Chapter 77: Dermatological Surgery

Uitto, Jouni

MD, PhD
Professor and Chair, Department of Dermatology and
Cutaneous Biology, Jefferson Institute of Molecular
Medicine, Thomas Jefferson University, 233 South
10th Street, Philadelphia PA19107, USA
Co-author of
Chapter 3: Anatomy and Organization of Human Skin

Veale, Douglas J.

MD, FRCFI, FRCP (Lon)
Consultant Rheumatologist, Department of
Rheumatology, Bone and Joint Unit, St Vincent's
University Hospital, Elm Park, Dublin 4, Republic of
Ireland
Co-author of
Chapter 51: The 'Connective Tissue Diseases'

Vega-López, Francisco

MD, MSc, PhD, MFTM, RCPSG, FRCP
Consultant Dermatologist, University College London
Hospitals NHS Foundation Trust and Honorary
Professor, London School of Hygiene and Tropical
Medicine, Keppel Street, London WC1E 7HT
Co-author of
Chapter 37: Parasitic Worms and Protozoa

Venning, Vanessa A.

DM, FRCP
Consultant Dermatologist, Department of
Dermatology, Churchill Hospital, Old Road,
Headington, Oxford OX3 7LJ
Co-author of
Chapter 40: Immunobullous Diseases

Weismann, Kaare

MD, PhD
Professor of Dermatology, Consultant Dermatologist,
The Skin Clinic, Privatehospital Hamlet, DK-2860
Søborg, Denmark
Co-author of
Chapter 59: Metabolic and Nutritional Disorders

Whittaker, Sean J.

MD, FRCP
Head of Clinical Services, St John's Institute of
Dermatology, St Thomas' Hospital, Lambeth Palace
Road, London SE1 7EH
Author of
*Chapter 57: Cutaneous Lymphomas and Lymphocytic
    Infiltrates*

Wilkinson, S. Mark

MD, FRCP
Department of Dermatology, Leeds General
Infirmary, Great George Street, Leeds LS1 3EX
Co-author of
Chapter 25: Contact Dermatitis: Irritant
Chapter 26: Contact Dermatitis: Allergic

Williams, Hywel C.

FRCP, MSc, PhD
Professor of Dermato-Epidemiology, Centre of
Evidence-Based Dermatology, Nottingham University
Hospitals NHS Trust, Derby Road, Nottingham NG7
2UH
Author of
Chapter 6: Epidemiology of Skin Disease
Co-author of
Chapter 7: Evidence-Based Dermatology

Wojnarowska, Fenella

BM, BCh, DM(Oxon), FRCP
Professor of Dermatology, Department of
Dermatology, Churchill Hospital, Old Road,
Headington, Oxford OX3 7LJ
Co-author of
Chapter 40: Immunobullous Diseases

Yates, Victoria M.

MBChB, FRCP
Honorary Consultant Dermatologist, The
Dermatology Centre, Salford Royal NHS Foundation
Trust, Greater Manchester and Department of
Dermatology, Royal Bolton NHS Trust, Minerva
Road, Bolton BL4 0JR
Author of
Chapter 31: Mycobacterial Infections

Young, Antony R.

PhD
Professor of Experimental Photobiology, St John's
Institute of Dermatology, Division of Genetics and
Molecular Medicine, King's College School of
Medicine, King's College London, Guy's Hospital,
London SE1 9RT
Co-author of
Chapter 29: Cutaneous Photobiology

Preface to the Eighth Edition

Just over forty years ago, the first edition of *Textbook of Dermatology* was published under the leadership of Arthur Rook, Darrell Wilkinson and John Ebling. Now designated *Rook's Textbook of Dermatology*, but known to many dermatologists as 'The Rook book', or simply 'Rook', it is in its eighth edition.

The editorial team that supervised compilation of the seventh edition has also been involved in preparation of the current edition. As always, we would like to express our gratitude to previous editors and contributors whose efforts have provided the framework upon which this book has expanded and continued to evolve over the years. We are also indebted to contributors to earlier editions who have generously allowed some of their material to be retained for the present edition, and to those colleagues who have donated colour photographs. The origin of these is given in the legend to each figure, and where no acknowledgement is given the figures have been provided by the authors of that chapter.

Our aim is to continue to provide an updated reference guide to dermatological diseases, and to encourage understanding of scientific aspects of dermatology, although the book is not intended to provide extensive details of research in the basic sciences. Nowadays there is electronic access to vast amounts of information, but we believe that a reference textbook, which can be readily accessed in the clinic or consulting room, or perused at leisure in an armchair, continues to be a valuable resource.

For this edition, every chapter has been updated, and several have been extensively modified and expanded, including the chapters on comparative dermatology and radiotherapy and reactions to ionizing radiation. There is also a separate chapter on the sexually transmitted diseases. Changes to chapters dealing with lasers and dermatological surgery reflect developments in recent years, and a new chapter describing skin rejuvenation procedures is indicative of the interest in this aspect of dermatology.

We thank our long-suffering wives and families for their tolerance and support over many years.

We should also like to thank the production team of Wiley-Blackwell for their efforts throughout the preparation of this edition, in particular Julie Elliott, Martin Sugden, Anne Bassett, the indexer Caroline Sheard, and the copy editor and proof reader.

D.A. Burns
S.M. Breathnach
N.H. Cox
C.E.M. Griffiths

Preface to the First Edition

No comprehensive reference book on dermatology has been published in the English language for ten years and none in England for over a quarter of a century. The recent literature of dermatology is rich in shorter texts and in specialist monographs but the English-speaking dermatologist has long felt the need for a substantial text for regular reference and as a guide to the immense monographic and periodical literature. The editors have therefore planned the present volume primarily for the dermatologist in practice or in training, but have also considered the requirements of the specialist in other fields of medicine and of the many research workers interested in the skin in relation to toxicology or cosmetic science.

An attempt has been made throughout the book to integrate our growing knowledge of the biology of skin and of fundamental pathological processes with practical clinical problems. Often the gap is still very wide but the trends of basic research at least indicate how it may eventually be bridged. In a clinical textbook the space devoted to the basic sciences must necessarily be restricted but a special effort has been made to ensure that the short accounts which open many chapters are easily understood by the physician whose interests and experience are exclusively clinical.

For the benefit of the student we have encouraged our contributors to make each chapter readable as an independent entity, and have accepted that this must involve the repetition of some material.

The classification employed is conventional and pragmatic. Until our knowledge of the mechanisms of disease is more profound no truly scientific classification is possible. In so many clinical syndromes multiple aetiological factors are implicated. To emphasize one at the expense of others is often misleading. Most diseases are to some extent influenced by genetic factors and a large proportion of common skin reactions are modified by the emotional state of the patient. Our knowledge is in no way advanced by classifying hundreds of diseases as genodermatoses and dozens as psychosomatic.

The true prevalence of a disease may throw light on its aetiology but reported incidence figures are often unreliable and incorrectly interpreted. The scientific approach to the evaluation of racial and environmental factors has therefore been considered in some detail.

The effectiveness of any physician in practice must ultimately depend on his ability to make an accurate clinical diagnosis. Clinical descriptions are detailed and differential diagnosis is fully discussed. Histopathology is here considered mainly as an aid to diagnosis but references to fuller accounts are provided.

The approach to treatment is critical but practical. Many empirical measures are of proven value and should not be abandoned merely because their efficacy cannot yet be scientifically explained. However, many familiar remedies old and new have been omitted either because properly controlled clinical trials have shown them to be of no value or because they have been supplanted by more effective and safer preparations.

There are over nine hundred photographs but no attempt has been made to provide an illustration of every disease. To have done so would have increased the bulk and price of the book without increasing proportionately its practical value. The conditions selected for illustrations are those in which a photograph significantly enhances the verbal description. There are a few conditions we wished to illustrate, but of which we could not obtain unpublished photographs of satisfactory quality.

The lists of references have been selected to provide a guide to the literature. Important articles now of largely historical interest have usually been omitted, except where a knowledge of the history of a disease simplifies the understanding of present concepts and terminology. Books and articles provided with a substantial bibliography are marked with an asterisk.

Many of the chapters have been read and criticized by several members of the team and by other colleagues. Professor Wilson Jones, Dr R.S. Wells and Dr W.E. Parish have given valuable assistance with histopathological, genetic and immunological problems respectively. Many advisers, whose services are acknowledged in the following pages, have helped us with individual chapters. Any errors which have not been eliminated are, however, the responsibility of the editors and authors.

The editors hope that this book will prove of value to all those who are interested in the skin either as physicians or as research workers. They will welcome readers' criticisms and suggestions which may help them to make the second edition the book they hope to produce.

CHAPTER 45

Disorders of Connective Tissue

N.P. Burrows[1] & C.R. Lovell[2]

[1]Department of Dermatology, Addenbrooke's Hospital, Cambridge, UK
[2]Kinghorn Dermatology Unit, Royal United Hospital, Bath, UK

Introduction

The connective tissue of the normal skin is discussed in Chapter 3.

Diseases that predominantly affect the cutaneous connective tissue (collagen, elastin and ground substance) can be divided into three main groups [1,2]:

1 Genetic abnormalities that affect connective tissue formation or metabolism. Examples include Ehlers–Danlos syndrome (EDS) (which affects collagen), pseudoxanthoma elasticum (PXE) (elastic tissue) and the mucopolysaccharidoses (ground substance).

2 Acquired metabolic or degenerative disorders, such as scurvy and solar elastosis, which are liable to affect people with no genetic defect if the environmental cause is present.

3 Inflammatory 'collagen vascular' or 'connective tissue' diseases, which damage connective tissue as a result of complex immunological reactions involving autogenous antigens. This group includes systemic lupus erythematosus, rheumatic fever, systemic sclerosis and dermatomyositis. Both genetic and acquired factors (including the possibility of infective agents) may play some part in producing these conditions, which are fully discussed in Chapter 51.

The attempt to classify the pathological changes according to whether ground substance, collagen, elastin or cellular components are mainly or wholly involved is not always easy, and may have been inaccurate in the past.

In this chapter, some of the genetic and acquired diseases that affect mainly collagen or elastin are discussed. Disorders of the ground substance are discussed elsewhere (see myxoedema, cutaneous mucinosis and mucopolysaccharidoses).

There are, in addition, many other disorders, including developmental defects, reactive or scarring conditions and benign or malignant neoplasms, that may involve the connective tissue.

References

1 Christiano AM, Uitto J. Molecular pathology of the elastic fibers. *J Invest Dermatol* 1994; **103**: S53–7.

2 Prockop DJ, Kivirikko KI. Collagens: molecular biology, diseases, and potentials for therapy. *Annu Rev Biochem* 1995; **64**: 403–34.

Rook's Textbook of Dermatology, 8th edition. Edited by DA Burns, SM Breathnach, NH Cox and CEM Griffiths. © 2010 Blackwell Publishing Ltd.

Cutaneous atrophy

Atrophy of the skin is a term that is applied to the clinical changes produced by a decrease in the dermal connective tissue. It is characterized by thinning and loss of elasticity. The skin usually appears smooth and finely wrinkled, and it feels soft and dry. Veins or other subcutaneous structures may be unduly conspicuous. There is often associated loss of hair follicles, and telangiectasia may also be present, due to the loss of connective tissue support of the capillaries. There may or may not be an associated atrophy of the epidermis.

Atrophy of the skin occurs in varying degree in a large number of skin conditions, and the underlying histological changes are also variable, because the several components of the connective tissue may be involved to a different degree. Atrophy that includes subcutaneous tissue or even deeper structures is referred to as *panatrophy*.

The main causes of cutaneous atrophy are as follows.
1 Generalized cutaneous thinning:
   (a) ageing
   (b) rheumatoid disease
   (c) glucocorticoids (exogenous or endogenous)
2 Poikiloderma
3 Atrophic scars (striae)
4 Anetoderma (see p. 45.17)
5 Chronic atrophic acrodermatitis (borreliosis)
6 Follicular atrophoderma
7 Vermiculate atrophoderma
8 Atrophoderma of Pasini and Pierini (probably morphoea)
9 Atrophic naevi
10 Panatrophy:
   (a) local panatrophy
   (b) facial hemiatrophy.

Generalized cutaneous atrophy

The skin becomes increasingly thin and atrophic in elderly people, and both the epidermis and the dermis are affected [1] (see Chapter 8 for further details). As a result, the aged skin becomes fragile, translucent, lax and wrinkled, with a tendency to easy bruising. Intrinsic ageing of skin may be compounded by environmental factors, such as chronic sun exposure and smoking. Dermal thickness is considerably decreased in the elderly [1]. Wound healing is delayed in the elderly because of a decrease in the numbers and synthetic capability of fibroblasts [2]. With increasing age, both keratinocytes and fibroblasts show a decreased response to various growth factors [3].

Ageing and wrinkles

Wrinkles may be defined as creases or furrows in the skin surface. They are generally distinguished from the lax pendulous folds of skin which occur in conditions such as PXE and cutis laxa, but the distinction is somewhat arbitrary, because loss of dermal elastic tissue is common to all these conditions. Deepening of the furrows occurs with advancing age [4]. Histologically, there is epidermal thinning, decrease in chondroitin sulphate and deposition of abnormal elastic tissue in the papillary dermis [5].

Wrinkles can be classified into three morphological types [6]:
1 **Crinkles.** This is a very fine wrinkling which occurs in aged skin, even in areas protected from sunlight. These fine wrinkles disappear when the skin is slightly stretched. They are caused by deterioration of elastin, especially the vertical subepidermal fine elastic fibres which keep the epidermis in tight apposition to the dermis [7,8]. Ultrastructural studies have shown that even in normal people the elastic fibres begin to deteriorate from the age of 30 years onwards, regardless of the amount of sun exposure, although sunlight undoubtedly increases the damage [9]. Crinkles are seen in a marked form in mid-dermal elastolysis (see below).
2 **Glyphic wrinkles.** These creases are an accentuation of the normal skin markings. They occur on skin which has been prematurely aged by elastotic degeneration caused by sunlight, for example on the sides and back of the neck (see actinic elastosis).
3 **Linear furrows.** These are long, straight or slightly curved grooves that are usually seen on the faces of elderly people. They include the horizontal frown lines along the forehead, the 'crows' feet' radiating from the lateral canthus of the eye and the creases from the nose to the corners of the mouth.

The facial skin has a remarkably complex and dense intradermal elastic tissue mesh. This sheath of elastin is unique to the face, not being found in such complexity elsewhere. In youth, the linear furrows caused by facial muscle contraction disappear due to elastic recoil, but in older people they become permanent. There is some controversy regarding the histology of these linear furrows. Several groups have claimed that the linear wrinkles cannot be distinguished by light or electron microscopy from the surrounding skin, and Kligman *et al.* [6] claim the furrow is merely a configurational change, like the crease in an old glove. Tsuji *et al.* [8], however, claim that the upper dermis in the furrow shows less elastotic change than the surrounding skin. Other authors [9,10], on the other hand, claim that the trabeculae of the retinacula cutis (which anchors the dermis to the underlying fascia) are broader and much shorter underneath the wrinkles than in the surrounding skin. The hypertrophy of these subcutaneous septa is probably related to repetitive mechanical stimuli generated by the facial muscles over the years.

Wrinkles are a characteristic feature of photodamaged skin (Chapter 29). Cigarette smoking is also a potent, independent cause of wrinkling. The so-called 'cigarette face' is characterized by pale, grey, wrinkled skin with rather gaunt features, so that heavy smokers can often be recognized from their facial appearance alone. Heavy smokers are five times more likely to be wrinkled than non-smokers of the same age, and cigarette smoking probably has at least as much effect on facial wrinkles as sun exposure [11,12]. The pathogenesis of these deleterious effects on facial skin is unknown, but causative factors might include ischaemia due to the vasoconstriction induced by nicotine or sympathetic nerve stimulation, decreased tissue oxygenation, increased tissue carboxyhaemoglobin, increased platelet aggregation, decreased prostacyclin formation and reduced collagen deposition [12]. Both UVA and tobacco smoke may cause wrinkling through additive induction of matrix metalloproteinase-1 (MMP-1) expression [13].

Treatment of wrinkles
See Chapter 80.

References

1 Kligman AM, Lavker RM. Cutaneous aging. The difference between intrinsic aging and photoaging. *J Cutaneous Aging Cosmetic Dermatol* 1988; **1**: 5–12.
2 Bolognia JL. Dermatologic and cosmetic concerns of the older woman. *Clin Geriatr Med* 1993; **9**: 209–29.
3 Gilchrest BA, Yaar M. Ageing and photoageing of the skin: observations at the cellular and molecular level. *Br J Dermatol* 1992; **127** (Suppl. 41): 25–30.
4 Akazaki S, Nakagawa H, Kazama H *et al.* Age-related changes in skin wrinkles assessed by a novel three-dimensional morphometric analysis. *Br J Dermatol* 2002; **147**: 689–95.
5 Contet-Audonneau JL, Jeanmaire C, Pauly G. A histological study of human wrinkle structures. Comparison between sun-exposed areas of the face, with or without wrinkles, and sun-protected areas. *Br J Dermatol* 1999; **140**: 1038–47.
6 Kligman AM, Zheng P, Lavker RM. The anatomy and pathogenesis of wrinkles. *Br J Dermatol* 1985; **113**: 37–42.
7 Lavker RM. Structural alterations in exposed and unexposed skin. *J Invest Dermatol* 1979; **73**: 59–69.
8 Tsuji T, Yorifuji T, Hamarta T *et al.* Light and scanning electron microscopic studies on wrinkles in aged person's skin. *Br J Dermatol* 1986; **114**: 329–35.
9 Braverman IM, Finferko E. Studies in cutaneous ageing. 1. The elastic fiber network. *J Invest Dermatol* 1982; **78**: 434–43.
10 Piérard GE, Lapière CM. The micro-anatomical basis of facial lines. *Arch Dermatol* 1989; **125**: 1090–2.
11 Davis BE, Koh HK. Faces going up in smoke. A dermatologic opportunity for cancer prevention. *Arch Dermatol* 1992; **128**: 1106–7.
12 Smith JB, Fenske NA. Cutaneous manifestations and consequences of smoking. *J Am Acad Dermatol* 1996; **34**: 717–32.
13 Yin L, Morita A, Tsuji T. Skin aging induced by ultraviolet exposure and tobacco smoking: evidence from epidemiological and molecular studies. *Photodermatol Photoimmunol Photomed* 2001; **17**: 178–83.

Atrophic skin with rheumatoid disease

In rheumatoid patients over the age of 60 years, especially women, the skin on the dorsa of the hands may become thin, loose, smooth, inelastic and transparent, so that the details of veins and tendons are clearly seen. The change is generalized but is seldom conspicuous, except on the hands and forearms. Histologically, the dermis is thinned but shows no distinctive changes.

There is a significant association between transparent skin, rheumatoid arthritis and osteoporosis, and it is assumed to form part of a general connective tissue defect [1]. Steroid therapy is not a factor but it will potentiate the problem [2]. Skin collagen is structurally abnormal [3]. A reported association with PXE may be coincidental [4].

References

1 McConkey B. Transparent skin and osteoporosis. A study of patients with rheumatoid disease. *Ann Rheum Dis* 1965; **24**: 219–23.
2 Shuster S, Raffle E, Bottoms E. Skin collagen in rheumatoid arthritis and the effect of corticosteroids. *Lancet* 1967; **i**: 525–7.
3 Adam M, Vitasek R, Deyl Z *et al.* Collagen in rheumatoid arthritis. *Clin Chim Acta* 1976; **70**: 61–9.
4 Praderio L, Marian JF, Baldini V. Pseudoxanthoma elasticum and rheumatoid arthritis. *Arch Intern Med* 1987; **147**: 206–7.

Glucocorticosteroid-induced atrophy [1]

Both systemic and topical steroid therapy can produce cutaneous atrophy by a dose-related pharmacological effect. The effect is more severe with the more potent steroids (as assessed by the vasoconstrictor assay test), but both fluorinated and non-fluorinated topical steroids can cause atrophy. The effect is most marked when potent steroids are applied topically under an occlusive dressing. The skin becomes thin, fragile and transparent, and striae may develop (see below) (Fig. 45.1).

Severe dermal atrophy can follow injection of intralesional steroids, such as triamcinolone acetonide (particularly if the higher concentration of 40 mg/mL is used, instead of the more usual 10 mg/mL, which is less likely to cause atrophy) (Fig. 45.2).

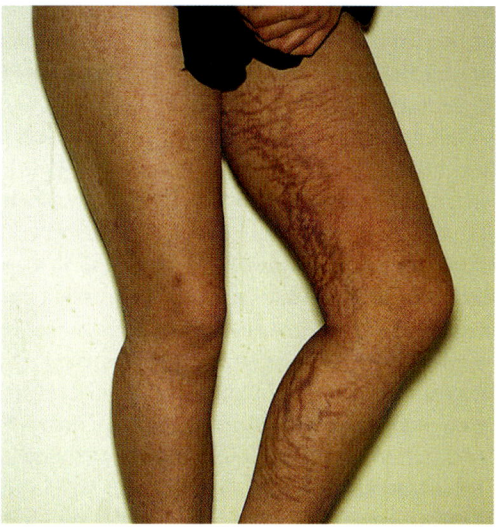

Fig. 45.1 Striae of the legs due to long-term application of a potent topical steroid in a young woman with psoriasis.

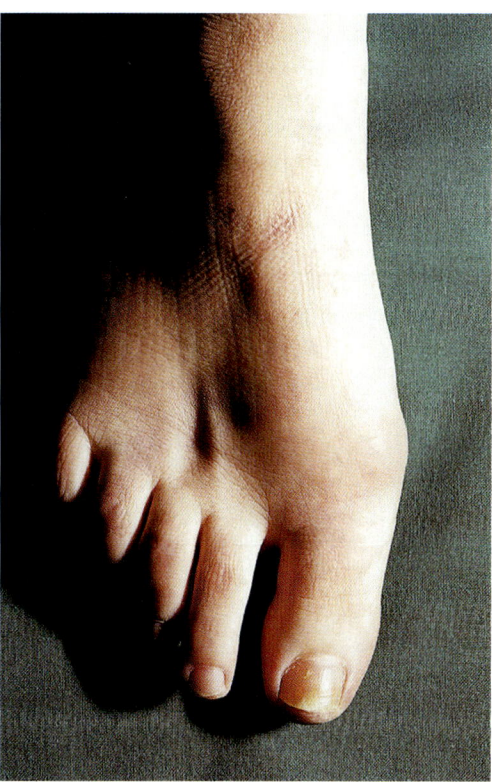

Fig. 45.2 Localized atrophy due to injection of a steroid (triamcinolone, 40 mg/mL) into the skin between the second and third metatarsals.

The earliest histological change is marked thinning of the epidermis, with flattening of the rete ridges and decreased corneocyte size [2]. This is followed a few weeks later by thinning of the dermis, which can be measured by skinfold callipers, ultrasonography or a radiographic technique [3–5].

The epidermal thinning probably results from a reduction of mitotic activity in the germinal layer [6], but the mechanism by which dermal thinning is produced is uncertain.

Loss of dermal ground substance leads to a reorganization of the dermal architecture. The spaces between the collagen and elastic fibres become smaller, so that the dermis becomes more compact but thinner [7]. Steroids are known to inhibit the formation of glycosaminoglycans, and hyaluronate and the major cell-surface hyaluronate receptor CD44 are depleted in atrophic skin [8,9]. The fibroblasts become shrunken, although their numbers do not decrease, but the number of mast cells is markedly reduced.

Topical steroids also inhibit the activity of enzymes involved in collagen biosynthesis [10], and they have been shown to depress synthesis of types I and III collagen *in vivo* [11–13]. Type III collagen synthesis is preferentially reduced in fibroblast cultures [14]. They can also depress collagenase production and collagen breakdown [15], and the rate of collagen turnover is probably decreased. Even a weak steroid, such as hydrocortisone, can suppress the stimulatory effect of cyclic nucleotides on collagenase production. Studies of the effect of topical steroids on collagen and elastic fibres *in vivo* have given conflicting results [7,16,17]. Collagen microfibrils may form globular microfibrillar bodies, although the changes are not specific for steroid atrophy [18]. These ultrastructural changes can develop in the early stages before there is clinical or histological evidence of atrophy. Digestion of collagen fibrils in the endocytic vesicles of fibroblasts may be involved in the production of steroid-induced atrophy [15].

Capillaroscopic studies have shown that steroid-induced vasoconstriction involves the superficial capillary network, and prolonged superficial ischaemia could also play a role in producing atrophy [10].

Treatment. It has been suggested that local and oral vitamin C therapy might help restore the normal skin thickness [19]. Concurrent application of retinoic acid may partially prevent the epidermal atrophy due to steroids [20]. Intralesional saline injections can restore surface contour [21]. Hyaluronate fragments are reported to induce skin thickening in corticosteroid-induced atrophy [9].

References
1 Henqqe VR, Ruzicka T, Schwartz RA *et al.* Adverse effects of topical corticosteroids. *J Am Acad Dermatol* 2006; **54**: 1–15.
2 Burton JL, Winter GD. Experimentally induced steroid atrophy in the domestic pig and man. *Br J Dermatol* 1976; **94** (Suppl. 12): 107–9.
3 Dykes PJ, Marks R. Measurements of skin thickness. A comparison of two *in vivo* techniques. *J Invest Dermatol* 1977; **69**: 275–8.
4 Dykes PF, Marks R. An appraisal of the methods used in the assessment of atrophy from topical corticosteroids. *Br J Dermatol* 1979; **101**: 599–609.
5 James MP, Black MH, Sparkes CG. Measurement of dermal atrophy induced by topical steroids using a radiographic technique. *Br J Dermatol* 1977; **96**: 303–5.
6 Marks R, Halprin K, Fukui K *et al.* Topically applied triamcinolone and macromolecular synthesis by human epidermis. *J Invest Dermatol* 1971; **56**: 470–3.
7 Lehmann P, Zheng P, Lavker RM *et al.* Corticosteroid atrophy in human skin. A study of light scanning and transmission electron microscopy. *J Invest Dermatol* 1983; **81**: 169–75.
8 Sarrni H, Hopsu-Havu BK. The decrease of hyaluronate synthesis by anti-inflammatory steroids *in vivo*. *Br J Dermatol* 1978; **98**: 445–9.
9 Kaya G, Tran C, Sorg O *et al.* Hyaluronate fragments reverse skin atrophy by a CD44-dependent mechanism. *PLoS Med* 2006; **3**: e493.
10 Risteli J. Effect of prednisolone on the activities of intracellular enzymes of collagen biosynthesis in rat skin. *Biochem Pharmacol* 1977; **26**: 1295–8.
11 Autio P, Oikarinen A, Melkko J *et al.* Systemic glucocorticoids decrease the synthesis of type I and type III collagen in human skin *in vivo*, whereas isotretinoin has little effect. *Br J Dermatol* 1994; **131**: 660–3.
12 Werth VP, Kligman AM, Shi X *et al.* Lack of correlation of skin thickness with bone density in patients receiving chronic glucocorticoid. *Arch Dermatol Res* 1998; **290**: 388–93.
13 Nuutinen P, Riekki R, Parikka M *et al.* Modulation of collagen synthesis and mRNA by continuous and intermittent use of topical hydrocortisone in human skin. *Br J Dermatol* 2003; **148**: 39–45.
14 Oishi Y, Fu ZW, Ohnuki Y *et al.* Molecular basis of the alteration in skin collagen metabolism in response to *in vivo* dexamethasone treatment: effects on the synthesis of collagen type I and III, collagenase, and tissue inhibitors of metalloproteinases. *Br J Dermatol* 2002; **147**: 859–68.
15 Koob TJ, Jeffrey JJ, Eisen AZ. Regulation of human skin collagenase activity by hydrocortisone and dexamethasone in organ culture. *Biochem Biophys Res Commun* 1974; **61**: 1083–8.
16 Jablonska S, Groniowska M, Dabrowski J. Comparative evaluation of skin atrophy in man produced by topical corticosteroids. *Br J Dermatol* 1979; **100**: 193–206.
17 Stevanovic DV. Corticosteroid-induced atrophy of the skin with telangiectasia. *Br J Dermatol* 1972; **87**: 548–56.
18 Holze E, Plewig G. Effects of dermatitis, stripping and steroids on the morphology of corneocytes. *J Invest Dermatol* 1977; **68**: 350–6.
19 Pinnell S. Management of cutaneous atrophy after corticosteroid injection. *J Am Acad Dermatol* 1987; **17**: 521.
20 McMichael AJ, Griffiths CEM, Talwar HS *et al.* Concurrent application of tretinoin (retinoic acid) partially protects against corticosteroid-induced epidermal atrophy. *Br J Dermatol* 1996; **135**: 60–4.
21 Shumaker PR, Rao J, Goldman MP. Treatment of local, persistent cutaneous atrophy following corticosteroid injection with normal saline infiltration. *Dermatol Surg* 2005; **31**: 1340–3.

Achenbach's syndrome [1–4]

Synonym
• Paroxysmal haematoma of the finger

This syndrome presents with the sudden spontaneous onset of one or more painful haematomas in the fingers, usually in a middle-aged female (Fig. 45.3). It may recur at intervals for several years. The cause is unknown—there is no evidence of vasculitis or amyloid on skin biopsy, and the condition, although troublesome, has a good prognosis. It may be mistaken for easy bruising due to steroid atrophy.

References
1 Achenbach W. Das paroxysmale Handhämatom. *Medizinische* 1958; **52**: 2138–40.
2 Stieler W, Heinze-Werlitz C. Paroxysmales Fingerhämatom (Achenbach Syndrom). *Hautarzt* 1990; **41**: 270–1.
3 Layton AM, Cotterill JA. A case of Achenbach's syndrome. *Clin Exp Dermatol* 1993; **18**: 60–1.
4 Parslew R, Verbov JL. Achenbach syndrome. *Br J Dermatol* 1995; **132**: 319.

Striae

Synonyms
• Striae atrophicans
• Striae distensae
• 'Stretch marks'

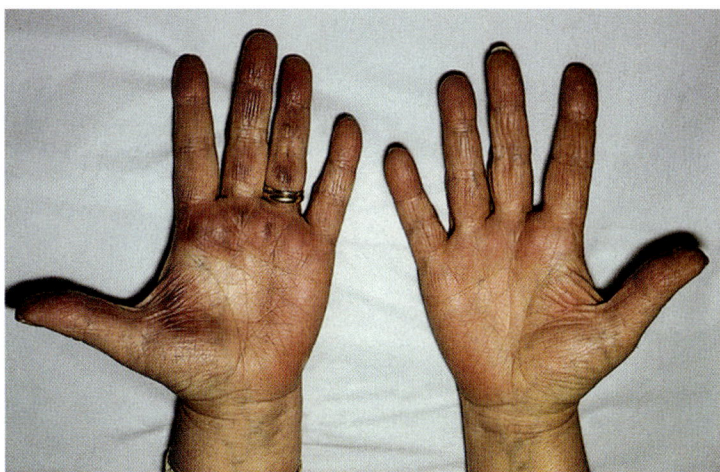

Fig. 45.3 Achenbach's syndrome. (Courtesy of Dr J. Verbov, Royal Liverpool University Hospitals, Liverpool, UK.)

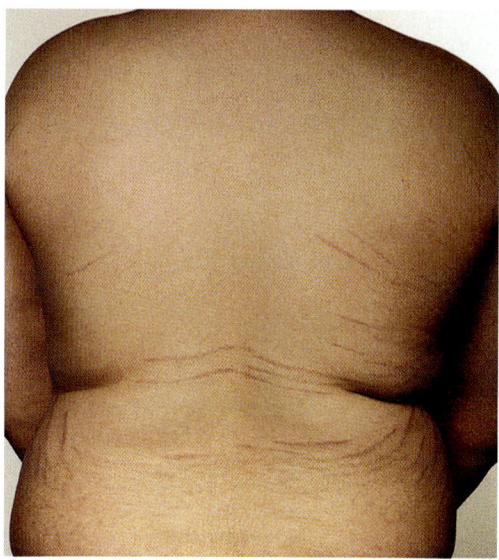

Fig. 45.4 Striae due to obesity in a young man.

Definition. Striae are visible, linear scars, which form in areas of dermal damage produced by stretching of the skin. They are characterized histologically by thinning of the overlying epidermis, with fine dermal collagen bundles arranged in straight lines parallel to the surface.

Aetiology. The factors that govern the development of striae are poorly understood. Many authors have suggested that striae develop as a result of stress rupture of the connective tissue framework [1], but others disagree. It has been suggested that they develop more easily in skin that has a critical proportion of rigid cross-linked collagen, as occurs in early adult life [2]. They are common during adolescence [3], and they seem to be associated with rapid increase in size of a particular region. They are very common over the abdomen and breasts in pregnancy, and they may develop on the shoulders in young male weightlifters when their muscle mass rapidly increases [4]. They are a feature of Cushing's disease, and they may be induced by local or systemic steroid therapy [2,5]. The effects of glucocorticoids on the dermal connective tissue are outlined above. Together with other steroid effects, striae have been reported in human immunodeficiency virus (HIV)-positive patients receiving the protease inhibitor, indinavir [6].

The importance of genetic factors in determining susceptibility of connective tissue is emphasized by their presence as one of the (minor) diagnostic criteria for Marfan's syndrome (MFS) [7], but they are commonly absent in pregnancy in EDS.

Pathology. In the early stages, inflammatory changes may be conspicuous; the dermis is oedematous and perivascular lymphocytic cuffing is present. In the later stages, the epidermis is thin and flattened [8]. The dermal collagen is layered in thin eosinophilic bundles, orientated in straight lines parallel to the surface in the direction of the presumed stress. Scanning electron microscopy shows amorphous, sheet-like structures [9,10]. With Luna's stain, the elastic fibres are numerous, close together, fine and straight, in the same direction as the collagen bundles [9]. On scanning electron microscopy, in collagen-free preparations there is an abundance of thin, curled and branched elastic fibres. The histology is that of a scar.

Clinical features. Striae are very common, and occur in most adult women, as they readily develop at puberty or during pregnancy. Adolescent striae may first develop soon after the appearance of pubic hair. The commonest sites are the outer aspect of the thighs and the lumbo-sacral region in boys (Fig. 45.4), and the thighs, buttocks and breasts in girls, but there is considerable variation, and other sites, including the outer aspect of the upper arm, are sometimes affected. Early lesions may be raised and irritable, but they soon become flat, smooth and livid red or bluish in colour. Their surface may be finely wrinkled. They are commonly irregularly linear, several centimetres long and 1–10 mm wide. After some years, they fade and become relatively inconspicuous.

The striae in Cushing's syndrome or those induced by steroid therapy may be larger and more widely distributed, and involve other regions, including sometimes the face. In pregnancy, the striae appear first and are most conspicuous on the abdominal wall, and later on the breasts, but may involve most or all of the pubertal sites [11].

The striae induced by topical steroid therapy occur particularly in the flexures, but may appear in other sites if occlusive plastic films increase absorption [12,13]. They may disappear or become less conspicuous when treatment is stopped.

Usually, striae are only a cosmetic problem, but occasionally, if extensive, they may ulcerate or tear easily should the patient be involved in an accident.

Diagnosis. The diagnosis of striae is usually simple. The possibility of Cushing's syndrome must be considered, although this is rarely the cause. In linear focal elastosis the lesions are yellow and palpable (p. 45.25).

Treatment. In the case of common adolescent striae, the patient may be reassured that in time they will become less conspicuous. Numerous unproven remedies are available from cosmetic companies.

Some cases appear to respond to treatment with topical tretinoin [14]. The erythema of 'younger' striae is claimed to respond to the 585 nm pulsed dye and Nd:YAG lasers [15,16]. Fractional photothermolysis has been used in chronic striae [17].

References

1 Stevanovic DV. Corticosteroid-induced atrophy of the skin with telangiectasia. A clinical and experimental study. *Br J Dermatol* 1972; **87**: 548–56.
2 Shuster S. The cause of striae distensae. *Acta Derm Venereol (Stockh)* 1979; **59** (Suppl. 85): 161–9.
3 Herxheimer H. Cutaneous striae in normal boys. *Lancet* 1953; **ii**: 204.
4 Carr RD, Hamilton JF. Transverse striae of the back. *Arch Dermatol* 1969; **99**: 26–30.
5 Thiers H, Moulin G, Larive M. Les vergetures de la corticothérapie locale. *Ann Dermatol Syphiligr (Paris)* 1969; **96**: 29–36.
6 Darvay A, Acland K, Lynn W *et al.* Striae formation in two HIV-positive persons receiving protease inhibitors. *J Am Acad Dermatol* 1999; **41**: 467–9.
7 De Paepe A, Devereux RB, Dietz HC *et al.* Revised diagnostic criteria for the Marfan syndrome. *Am J Med Genet* 1996; **62**: 417–26.
8 Zheng PS, Lauker RM, Lehmann P *et al.* Morphologic investigations on the rebound phenomenon after corticosteroid-induced atrophy in human skin. *J Invest Dermatol* 1984; **82**: 345–52.
9 Arem AJ, Kischer CW. Analyses of striae. *Plast Reconstr Surg* 1980; **65**: 22–9.
10 Zheng P, Lavker RM, Kligman AM. Anatomy of striae. *Br J Dermatol* 1985; **112**: 185–93.
11 Poidevin LOS. Striae gravidarum. Their relation to adrenal cortical hyperfunction. *Lancet* 1959; **ii**: 436–8.
12 Chernovsky ME, Knox JM. Atrophic striae after occlusive corticosteroid therapy. *Arch Dermatol* 1964; **90**: 15–9.
13 Kikuchi I, Horikawa S. Perilymphatic atrophy of the skin. A side effect of topical corticosteroid injection therapy. *Arch Dermatol* 1974; **109**: 558–9.
14 Elson ML. Treatment of striae distensae with topical tretinoin. *J Dermatol Surg Oncol* 1990; **16**: 267–70.
15 Alster TS. Laser treatment of hypertrophic scars, keloids and striae. *Dermatol Clin* 1997; **15**: 419–29.
16 Goldman A, Rossato F, Prati C. Stretch marks: treatment using the 1,064 nm Nd:YAG laser. *Dermatol Surg* 2008; **34**: 686–92.
17 Kou BJ, Lee DH, Kim MN *et al.* Fractional photothermolysis for the treatment of striae distensae in Asian skin. *Am J Clin Dermatol* 2008; **9**: 33–7.

Congenital reticulate scarring

Three children have been described who presented at birth with vesicles, deep erosions and erythematous patches. The vesicles were generalized, but spared the palms, soles and face, superficially resembling 'scalded skin syndrome'. Healing at around 3 months was followed by fragile reticulate scars; the affected areas were anhidrotic [1]. Two further children with this condition had epilepsy and delayed intellectual and motor milestones [2]. Histological examination showed that the reticular dermis was partially replaced by collagenous scar tissue, and eccrine glands were absent. The differential diagnosis includes Goltz syndrome, Rothmund–Thomson syndrome, acrodermatitis chronica atrophicans and aplasia cutis [1,2].

References

1 Cohen BA, Esterley NB, Nelson PF. Congenital erosive and vesicular dermatitis healing with reticulated supple scarring. *Arch Dermatol* 1985; **121**: 361–7.
2 Gupta AK, Rasmussen JE, Headington JT. Extensive congenital erosions and vesicles healing with reticulate scarring. *J Am Acad Dermatol* 1987; **17**: 369–76.

Localized cutaneous atrophy

Focal facial dermal dysplasia

Scar-like depressions on the face are a feature of this syndrome, which may be a variant of the Setleis syndrome (Chapters 15 & 18) [1,2].

References

1 Kowalski DC, Fenske NA. The focal facial dermal dysplasias: report of a kindred and a proposed new classification. *J Am Acad Dermatol* 1992; **27**: 575–82.
2 Ward KA, Moss C. Evidence for genetic homogeneity of Setleis' syndrome and focal facial dermal hypoplasia. *Br J Dermatol* 1994; **130**: 645–9.

Atrophic scars and pseudoscars

Atrophy may result from the destruction of connective tissue by trauma or by inflammatory changes. The distribution and character of the atrophic lesions may be so distinctive as to betray their origin, and is sometimes of considerable importance in diagnosis. Viral infections, such as varicella, can leave widespread, small, circular, atrophic scars [1]. The scars left by tertiary syphilis, certain tuberculides and some deep mycoses, especially sporotrichosis, are usually completely atrophic. Lupus erythematosus may also leave atrophy without clinical evidence of sclerosis. Lupus vulgaris and the chronic follicular pyodermas, and some cases of lupus erythematosus, leave a combination of atrophy and sclerosis, in which the latter predominates. Lesions that have been treated by intralesional steroid injections may also leave atrophic scars.

Exposure to ionizing radiation gives rise to a very striking combination of atrophy, pigmentation and telangiectasia (Chapter 79).

The wide atrophic scars which follow injuries in EDS (p. 45.31) emphasize the importance of constitutional factors in determining the pattern of dermal response to a known external injury.

Reference

1 Leung AKC, Pinkao C, Suave RS. Scarring resulting from chickenpox. *Pediatr Dermatol* 2001; **18**: 378–80.

Stellate and discoid pseudoscars [1,2]

Stellate pseudoscars are white, irregular or 'star-shaped' atrophic scars (Fig. 45.5). They are common on light-exposed skin, particularly on the extensor aspects of the forearms, often in association with senile purpura. These are seen in 20% of patients aged 70–90 years, and a much less common presenile form occasionally occurs before the age of 50 years. These pseudoscars are secondary to mild trauma, and are probably always preceded by haemorrhage into the dermis.

Stellate scars following trivial trauma can also occur in other conditions that cause fragile skin, for example porphyria cutanea tarda and prolonged use of potent topical steroids.

Brown pseudoscars may also develop over the shins of diabetic patients with no history of trauma (Fig. 45.6).

References

1 Colomb D. Stellate spontaneous pseudoscars. Senile and presenile forms: especially those forms caused by prolonged corticoid therapy. *Arch Dermatol* 1972; **105**: 551–4.
2 Zac FG, Pai SH, Kanshepolsky J. Stellate spontaneous pseudoscars (Colomb). *Arch Dermatol* 1968; **98**: 499–501.

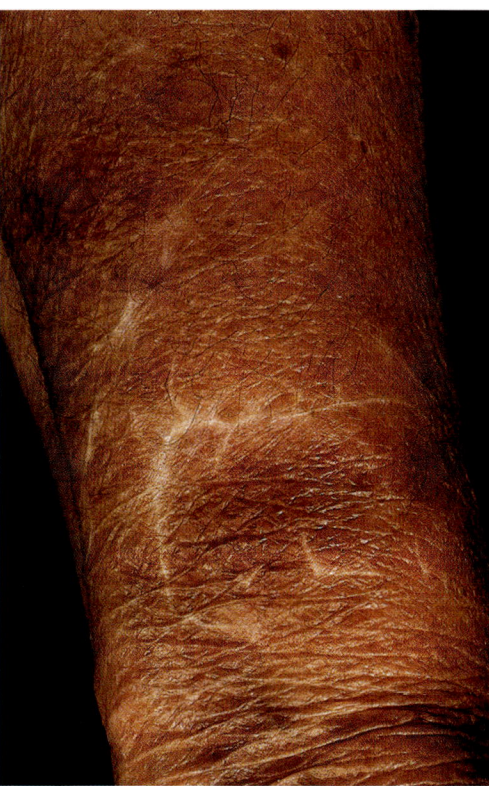

Fig. 45.5 Stellate pseudoscars on the forearm of an elderly woman. There was no history of trauma.

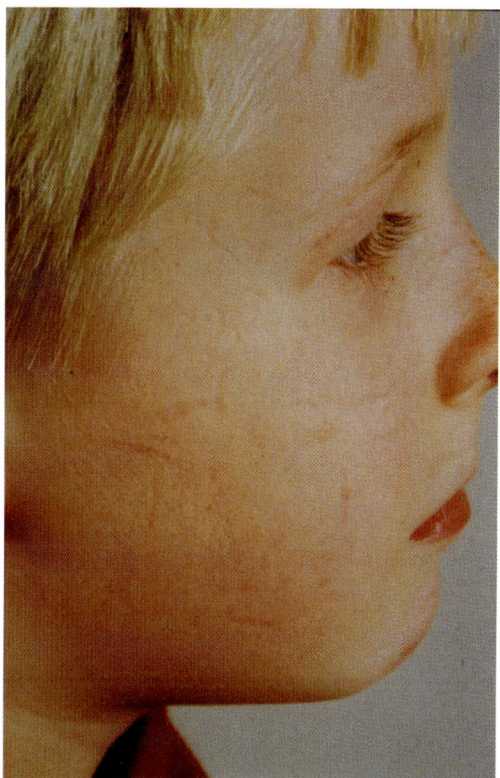

Fig. 45.7 Spontaneous atrophic scarring of the cheeks (varioliform atrophy). (Courtesy of Dr S. George, Amersham Hospital, Amersham, UK.)

This is a very rare condition in which spontaneous scars develop on the cheeks (Fig. 45.7) in young adults [1,2] or children [3]. The shallow atrophic lesions have sharp margins and may be linear, rectangular or varioliform. They may be preceded by slight erythema and scaling. Histology shows mild loss of collagen or elastic fibres; there may be thickening of the stratum corneum [4]. Familial cases are recorded [1,5]; inheritance is probably autosomal dominant [6]. The differential diagnosis includes vermiculate atrophoderma (p. 45.8), chickenpox scars and artefact.

References
1 Marks VJ, Miller OF. Atrophia maculosa varioliformis cutis. *Br J Dermatol* 1986; **115**: 105–9.
2 McCoriston LR, Roys HC. Atrophia maculosa varioliformis cutis. *Arch Dermatol* 1951; **64**: 59–61.
3 Paradisi M, Angelo C, Conti G *et al.* Atrophia maculosa varioliformis cutis: a pediatric case. *Pediatr Dermatol* 2001; **18**: 478–80.
4 Kolenik SA, Perez MI, Davidson DM *et al.* Atrophia maculosa varioliformis cutis. *J Am Acad Dermatol* 1994; **30**: 837–40.
5 Gordon PM, Doherty VR. Familial atrophia maculosa varioliformis cutis. *Br J Dermatol* 1996; **134**: 982–3.
6 Ou T, Wang B, Fang K. Familial atrophia maculosa varioliformis cutis: case report and pedigree analysis. *Br J Dermatol* 2005; **153**: 821–4.

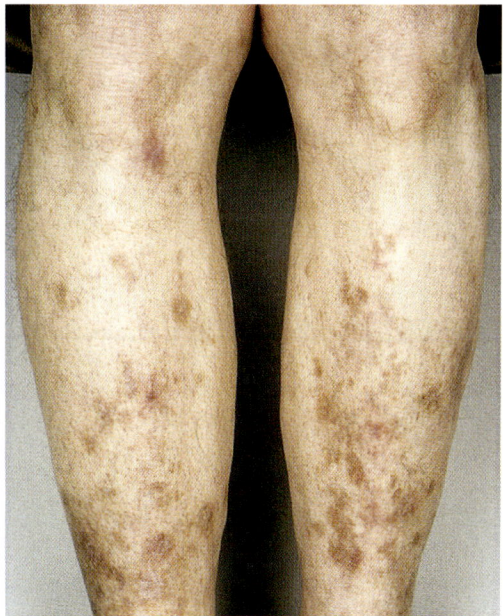

Fig. 45.6 Brown pseudoscars of the legs due to diabetic dermopathy. There was no history of trauma.

Spontaneous atrophic scarring of the cheeks

Synonyms
- Varioliform atrophy
- Atrophia maculosa varioliformis cutis

Atrophoderma
Follicular atrophoderma
In this distinctive syndrome dimple-like depressions at the follicular orifices are present from birth or early life, usually on the backs of hands (Fig. 45.8) and feet and sometimes in the elbow region.

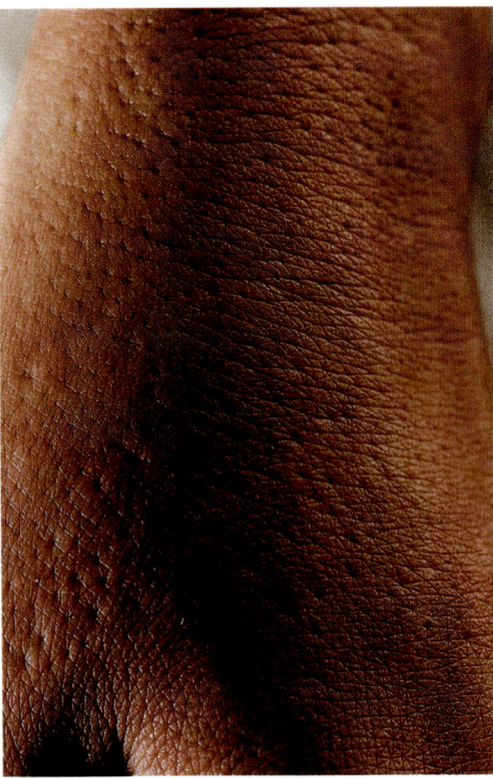

Fig. 45.8 Follicular atrophoderma in Conradi's syndrome. (Courtesy of Dr D.A. Burns, Leicester Royal Infirmary, Leicester, UK.)

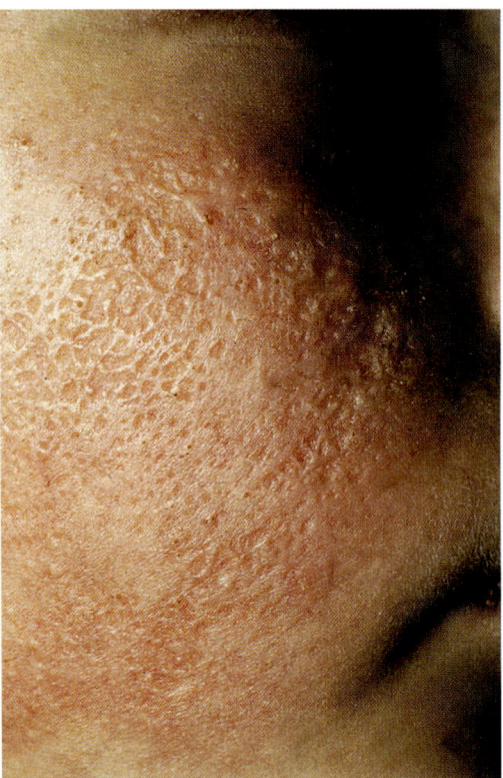

Fig. 45.9 Vermiculate atrophoderma on the cheek of a child. (Courtesy of Dr P. Frosch, Heidelberg, Germany.)

Histology shows widened follicular ostia with thickening of the connective tissue sheath of the follicle.

It appears to be due to a variety of genetic defects and it may be associated with the following conditions [1]:

1 Calcifying chondrodysplasia (Conradi's syndrome) (Chapter 19)
2 Bazex syndrome (Chapter 15) [2]
3 Hyperkeratosis palmoplantaris, follicular keratosis or palmo-plantar hyperhidrosis.

It may also occur as an isolated defect of limited extent.

References
1 Curth HO. The genetics of follicular atrophoderma. *Arch Dermatol* 1978; **114**: 1479–83.
2 Viksnins P, Berlin A. Follicular atrophoderma and basal cell carcinoma. The Bazex syndrome. *Arch Dermatol* 1977; **113**: 948–51.

Vermiculate atrophoderma

This rare condition has been described under a variety of other names, including atrophoderma reticulatum, folliculitis ulerythe-matosa reticulata and honeycomb atrophy. It is a characteristic reticulate or 'honeycomb' type of atrophy, which seems to develop as a late reaction to inflammation around horny follicular plugs on the cheeks (Fig. 45.9). The condition is now regarded as part of the keratosis pilaris syndrome, and is further discussed in Chapter 19.

Familial focal facial dermal dysplasia

Atrophic macules occur on the temples in this rare autosomal dominant disease (Chapters 15 & 18).

Hallermann–Streiff syndrome

There may be focal atrophy of the scalp skin in this condition (Chapter 18) [1].

Reference
1 Grattan CEH, Liddle BJ, Willshaw HE. Atrophic alopecia in the Hallermann–Streiff syndrome. *Clin Exp Dermatol* 1989; **14**: 250–2.

Atrophoderma of Pasini and Pierini

Definition. This condition appears to be an atrophic variant of morphoea (Chapter 51) in which one or more patches of skin become bluish and sharply depressed, with no surrounding ery-thema [1–3].

Aetiology. The cause is unknown. No genetic factor has been reliably incriminated, although familial cases have been reported [4], and morphoea and atrophoderma of Pasini have occurred in siblings with phenylketonuria [5].

Pathology [3]. The histological changes are slight. There may be increased pigmentation of the basal layer. During the earlier stages, the collagen in the lower dermis may be oedematous, and elastic tissue clumped and scanty. There may be a dermal perivas-cular infiltrate consisting of macrophages and T lymphocytes. Immunofluorescence studies may show IgM and C3 staining in the dermal blood vessels [6]. Later, the oedema subsides and there is some reduction in the total thickness of the dermis. Collagen

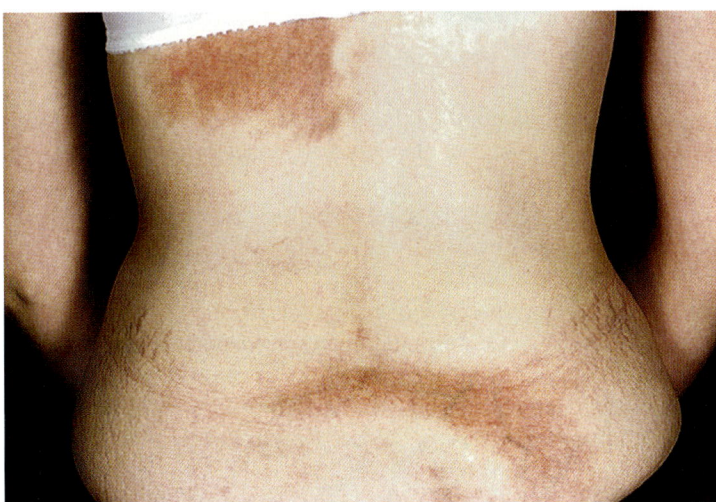

Fig. 45.10 Atrophoderma of Pasini and Pierini. (Courtesy of Dr D.A. Burns, Leicester Royal Infirmary, Leicester, UK.)

bundles appear homogeneous and clumped in the reticular dermis. Eventually there may also be some epidermal atrophy.

Clinical features [3,7,8]. The lesions, which may be single or multiple, range in size from 2 cm to many centimetres in diameter, and are round or oval in shape, but may become confluent to form irregular patches (Fig. 45.10). They are smooth, slate-coloured or violet brown, and are slightly depressed below the level of the entirely normal surrounding skin. The back is almost always involved, the chest and abdomen frequently, and the proximal parts of the limbs occasionally. The patches extend very slowly, increase in number for 10 years or more, and then usually persist unchanged. The eventual development of sclerodermatous changes within the patches has been observed, as has the presence in the same patient of lesions typical of atrophoderma and of morphoea.

Diagnosis. Clinical differentiation from morphoea, possibly an academic exercise, is based on the ivory-white, indurated plaque with an oedematous lilac ring so characteristic of the latter. Histologically, sclerosis may be prominent in morphoea and is usually absent in atrophoderma. Serological tests for *Borrelia burgdorferi* are negative [3].

Treatment. None is of proven efficacy, but psoralen and UVA (PUVA) has helped some patients. Hydroxychloroquine has been used [9].

References
1 Kee CE, Brothers WS, New W. Idiopathic atrophoderma of Pasini and Pierini with co-existent morphea. A case report. *Arch Dermatol* 1960; **82**: 154–7.
2 Miller RF. Idiopathic atrophoderma, report of a case and nosologic study. *Arch Dermatol* 1965; **92**: 653–60.
3 Beuchner SA, Rufli T. Atrophoderma of Pasini and Pierini. *J Am Acad Dermatol* 1994; **30**: 441–6.
4 Barsky S, Ke M. Congenital atrophoderma of the newborn. *Arch Dermatol* 1970; **101**: 374–5.
5 Lasser AE, Schultz BC, Beaff D *et al*. Phenylketonuria and scleroderma. *Arch Dermatol* 1978; **114**: 1215–7.
6 Berman A, Berman GD, Winkelmann RK. Atrophoderma (Pasini–Pierini) findings on direct immunofluorescent, monoclonal antibody and ultra-structural studies. *Int J Dermatol* 1988; **27**: 487–90.
7 Canizares O, Sachs PM, Jaimovich L *et al*. Idiopathic atrophoderma of Pasini and Pierini. *Arch Dermatol* 1958; **77**: 42–60.
8 Jablonska S, ed. *Scleroderma and Pseudoscleroderma*, 2nd edn. Warsaw: Polish Medical Publishers, 1975.
9 Carter JD, Valeriano J, Vasey FB. Hydroxychloroquine as a treatment for atrophoderma of Pasini and Pierini. *Int J Dermatol* 2006; **45**: 1255–6.

Linear atrophoderma

Pigmented atrophic bands follow Blaschko's lines [1] on the trunk, arms and legs. Histologically, collagen bundles are normal or thickened; the apparent atrophy may be due to loss of fat. Leukonychia has been associated [2]. The condition may reflect mosaicism for an autosomal lethal gene [3].

References
1 Moulin G, Hill MP, Guillaud V *et al*. Bandes pigmentées atrophiques acquises suivant les lignes de Blaschko. *Ann Dermatol Vénéréol* 1992; **119**: 729–36.
2 Atasoy M, Aliagaoglu C, Sahin O *et al*. Linear atrophoderma of Moulin together with leuconychia: a case report. *J Eur Acad Dermatol Venereol* 2006; **20**: 337–40.
3 Danarti R, Bittar M, Happle R *et al*. Linear atrophoderma of Moulin: postulation of mosaicism for a predisposing gene. *J Am Acad Dermatol* 2003; **49**: 492–8.

Acrodermatitis chronica atrophicans

Synonyms
- Chronic atrophic acrodermatitis
- Late-phase Lyme borreliosis

Definition. This is a late skin manifestation of Lyme borreliosis (Chapter 30). It is characterized by the insidious onset of painless, dull-red nodules or plaques on the extremities, which slowly extend centrifugally for several months or years, leaving central areas of atrophy.

Aetiology. The condition is due to infection with a spirochaete, *Borrelia burgdorferi sensu lato*, which is transmitted by ticks [1]. The disease occurs mainly in northern or central Europe, Italy and the Iberian Peninsula. Occasional cases occur in other parts of Europe and Africa, but it is very rare in the UK, America, Australia and Asia [2]. These geographical variations are related to different strains of the organism [3–5]. *Borrelia afzelii* is the predominant species associated with acrodermatitis chronica atrophicans. This species is transmitted by ticks in Western Europe, but is rare in the USA, where *Borrelia burgdorferi sensu stricto* predominates.

Pathology [6]. During the early stages, there is non-specific dermal oedema with perivascular inflammatory infiltration. Subsequently, the epidermis becomes atrophic and the epidermal appendages are destroyed. Beneath a subepidermal zone of degenerate connective tissue lies a dense, band-like infiltrate, predominantly consisting of lymphocytes, histiocytes and plasma cells. Ultimately, the infiltrate is reduced to narrow bands between collagen fibres. In some patients, scleroderma-like changes may develop [7,8]. *Borrelia afzelii* has been cultured from the atrophic skin [7] but culture is usually negative. *Borrelia afzelii* can be identified by polymerase chain reaction (PCR). The organism may be resistant to attack by the complement system and may lurk in immunologically protected areas such as fibroblasts and endothelial cells. Expression of cytokines, such as interferon-γ (IFN-γ), is impaired [9].

Clinical features

[10]. Most cases occur in country dwellers between the ages of 30 and 60 years.

The onset is usually insidious, and constitutional symptoms are exceptional. Painless, dull-red or bluish-red nodules or plaques, more or less infiltrated, develop on the feet or legs, and less often on the forearms and hands. The lesions themselves are typically painless, but there may be associated acral pain or paraesthesiae. Erythema chronicum migrans (Chapter 30) may have been present at the same site some years earlier. Extension to the trunk and the greater part of the body, including the face, is sometimes seen. Single or multiple lesions may be present. They slowly extend centrifugally, the active inflammatory stage persisting for months, years or even decades. Marginal extension may continue once the central areas have already entered the atrophic phase, in which the skin is smooth, hairless and tissue-paper-like, dull red, pigmented or poikilodermatous (Fig. 45.11).

Subcutaneous nodules may develop around the knees or elbows, and fibrous bands along the ulnar margin of the forearms. Gaiter-like sclerosis of the lower third of the legs, often accompanied by ulceration, is a further complication. Morphoea of the trunk and lichen sclerosus et atrophicus (both genital and extragenital) have also been reported as associated lesions [2,11], and it is interesting that *Borrelia* antibodies have been found in five of 10 patients with morphoea [12], although others have not confirmed this [13].

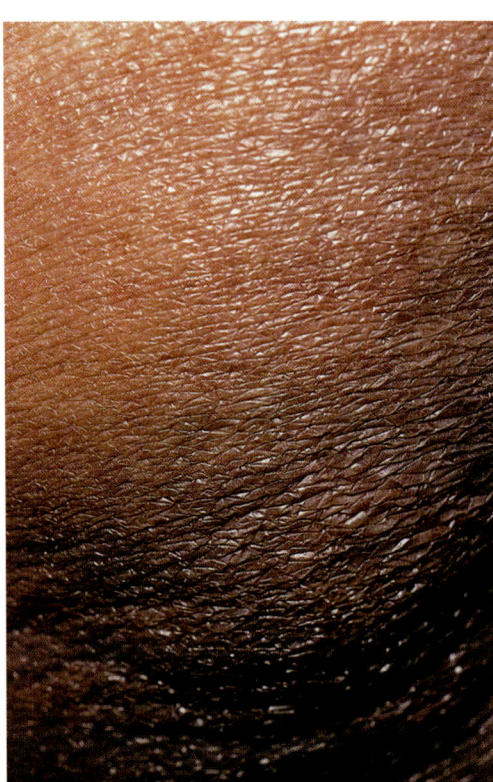

Fig. 45.11 Atrophic skin of the knee in acrodermatitis chronica atrophicans. (Courtesy of Dr T. Robinson, University College Hospital, London, UK.)

In some cases, involvement of the joint capsule or bone results in limitation of movement of the joints of the hands and feet, or of the shoulders.

Very rarely, squamous carcinoma has developed in the atrophic skin, and lymphoma has also been reported in the non-affected skin [14,15].

Other late syndromes of Lyme borreliosis (lymphocytoma, neurological, etc.) have been fully reviewed by Steere [1].

Diagnosis.

The appearance of erythema chronicum migrans may be similar, but the evolution of the annular lesions establishes the differentiation. In the atrophic stage, diagnosis is usually readily made, and can be confirmed histologically.

Immunoblotting, using *B. afzelii* flagellar antigen (41 kDa) is confirmatory [5]. Serology is used to confirm the diagnosis of Lyme disease, but false-negative and false-positive results are common. In chronic atrophic acrodermatitis, however, the antibody titre is very high. Serology may be positive on enzyme-linked immunosorbent assay (ELISA) but negative on immunoblotting, particularly in patients with neurological disease [16]. A high titre of antibodies may reflect occult central nervous system involvement, when the antibodies can also be demonstrated in colony-stimulating factor [17].

When it occurs on the lower legs, the condition can mimic venous insufficiency [18], with thick, cyanotic, itchy skin.

Treatment.

Oral antibiotics should be given for 1 month, for example doxycycline or amoxicillin in standard doses [1]. The improvement occurs gradually, several weeks after the course of treatment, but there may be no response if treatment is delayed until atrophy has developed. If the antibody titre is high, or there are clinical features of systemic disease (e.g. neuroborreliosis), intravenous penicillin G, ceftriaxone or cefotaxime should be given for 3 weeks [17]. There may be a case for chemoprophylaxis or even vaccine development in endemic areas [19].

References

1 Steere AC. Lyme disease. *N Engl J Med* 1989; **321**: 586–96.
2 Coulson IH. Acrodermatitis chronica atrophicans with coexisting morphoea. *Br J Dermatol* 1989; **121**: 263–9.
3 Aberer E, Kersten A, Klade H. Heterogeneity of *Borrelia burgdorferi* in the skin. *Am J Dermatopathol* 1996; **18**: 571–9.
4 Picken RN, Strle F, Picken MM. Identification of three species of *Borrelia burgdorferi sensu lato* among isolates from acrodermatitis chronica atrophicans lesions. *J Invest Dermatol* 1998; **110**: 211–4.
5 Flisiah I, Schwartz RA, Chodynicke B. Clinical features and specific immunological response against *Borrelia afzelii* in patients with acrodermatitis chronica atrophicans. *J Med* 1999; **30**: 267–78.
6 Boehmer-Andersson E, Hovmark A, Asbrink E. Acrodermatitis chronica atrophicans: histopathologic findings and clinical correlation in 111 cases. *Acta Derm Venereol* 1998; **78**: 207–13.
7 Asbrink E, Hovmark A. Successful cultivation of spirochaetes from the skin lesions of patients with erythema chronicum migrans and acrodermatitis chronicum atrophicans. *Acta Pathol Microbiol Immunol Scand (A)* 1985; **93**: 161–3.
8 Asbrink E, Hovmark A. Early and late cutaneous manifestations of *Ixodes* borne borreliosis (Lyme borreliosis). *Ann NY Acad Sci* 1988; **539**: 4–15.
9 Mullegger RR, McHugh G, Ruthazar R. Differential expression of cytokine mRNA in skin specimens from patients with erythema migrans or acrodermatitis chronica atrophicans. *J Invest Dermatol* 2000; **115**: 1115–23.
10 Burgdorf WHC, Worret W, Schultka O. Acrodermatitis chronica atrophicans. *Int J Dermatol* 1979; **18**: 595–601.

11 Ramelet AA. Association of acrodermatitis chronica atrophicans and morphoea. *Dermatologica* 1987; **175**: 253–6.

12 Aberer E, Neumann R, Stanek G. Is localised scleroderma a *Borrelia* infection? *Lancet* 1985; **ii**: 278.

13 Halkier-Sorensen L. Antibodies to the *Borrelia burgdorferi* in patients with scleroderma. *Acta Derm Venereol Suppl (Stockh)* 1989; **69**: 116–9.

14 Goos W, Schwarz-Speck M. Acrodermatitis chronica atrophicans. *Dermatologica* 1972; **145**: 287–90.

15 Garbe C, Stein H, Dienemann D, Orfanos CE. *Borrelia burgdorferi*-associated cutaneous B cell lymphoma. *J Am Acad Dermatol* 1991; **24**: 584–90.

16 Rees DHE, O'Connell S, Brown MM *et al.* The value of serological testing for Lyme disease in the UK. *Br J Rheumatol* 1995; **34**: 132–6.

17 Aberer E, Breier F, Stanek G. Success and failure in the treatment of acrodermatitis chronica atrophicans. *Infection* 1996; **24**: 85–7.

18 Fagrell B, Heiland RA, Howe TR. Acrodermatitis chronica atrophicans can mimic a peripheral vascular disorder. *Acta Med Scand* 1986; **20**: 485–8.

19 Stanek G, Strle F. Lyme borreliosis. *Lancet* 2003; **362**: 1639–47.

Local panatrophy

Definition and aetiology. Local panatrophy is a rare disorder involving partial or total loss of subcutaneous fat and atrophy of overlying skin, sometimes associated with atrophy or impaired growth of muscle or bone. A primary neurogenic disturbance has been postulated but not proved. The syndrome may represent the end result of more than one pathological process, but many cases may be due to a variant of morphoea.

The atrophic areas exhibit a reduced sympathetic response and aberrant production of non-esterified fatty acids after stimulation with norepinephrine (noradrenaline), and it has been suggested that there may be a primary abnormality of the sympathetic nervous system [1].

Two groups of cases can be differentiated:

1 **Panatrophy of Gower:** no scleroderma or other sclerotic process accompanies or follows the loss of subcutaneous tissue. Most cases have occurred in women, usually in the second to fourth decades.

2 **Sclerotic panatrophy:** either typical morphoea or similar sclerotic change in dermal collagen precedes the atrophy [2].

Clinical features of the two groups are as follows.

Panatrophy of Gower [3]. Sharply defined areas of atrophy, irregular in size, shape and distribution, develop over a period of a few weeks, without preceding inflammatory stages. In each affected area, the subcutaneous tissue disappears and the overlying skin appears atrophic but is otherwise normal. There may be a single area of atrophy or two or more. In size they range from 2 to 20 cm across, and in shape they are very variable but are sometimes triangular or quadrangular. Most lesions have occurred on the back, buttocks, thighs or upper arms, but some have involved forearms or lower legs. The atrophy reaches its maximum extent within a few months and then remains unchanged indefinitely.

Sclerotic panatrophy. Atrophy of the subcutis, and sometimes of underlying muscle and bone, may follow clinically and histologically typical morphoea, especially when the process begins in childhood and involves a limb (Chapter 51).

Sclerotic panatrophy may also occur in the absence of morphoea. The sclerosis involves subcutaneous tissue and muscle, and dense, sclerotic, scar-like, linear bands develop along a limb, or encircle the trunk in a metameric distribution, or encircle a limb. These lesions have also usually occurred in childhood. They cease to progress after a few months and, although new areas may be involved, most lesions have been solitary.

It is possible that Gower's panatrophy and linear morphoea are at the ends of a continuous disease spectrum. The histology of linear morphoea reveals thickened bundles of collagen, which appear to be intact on B-scan ultrasound imaging [4].

In the differential diagnosis of panatrophy, the various forms of panniculitis must be excluded. The preceding inflammatory changes are the single most distinctive feature, but they are not always easy to distinguish.

Facial hemiatrophy

> **Synonym**
> • Parry–Romberg syndrome

Definition and aetiology. Facial hemiatrophy is an atrophic dysplasia of the superficial facial tissues, but the underlying muscles, cartilage and bone may also be affected. The cause is unknown, but it may be a disorder of the sympathetic nervous system in some cases. Other cases have followed lupus panniculitis [5].

There is no evidence that it is usually genetically determined, but it appears to be hereditary in a few pedigrees. Some cases have been associated with syringomyelia, epilepsy or cerebrovascular disease, but in 90% of cases no such association is demonstrable. The sexes are equally affected.

Clinical features [6–8]. This rare disease usually starts within the first two decades. The first manifestation is usually increased or decreased pigmentation in irregular patches on cheeks, forehead or lower jaw. Occasionally, there may be premonitory muscle spasms or neuralgia. Progressive atrophy gradually develops in the affected sites, involving skin, subcutis, muscle and bone, and may extend in area—and sometimes in depth—for months or years with temporary remissions. The skin becomes dry, thin and atrophic, but may be scar-like and adherent in some areas. When the atrophy is fully developed, the contrast between the sunken, haggard, pigmented affected half of the face and the unaffected half is dramatic. The hair may be lost in the frontoparietal region on the affected side but is often normal; occasionally, localized canities is an early change. A variety of neurological signs have been reported, of which Horner's syndrome is the most frequent. Heterochromia of the iris has developed at the same time as the facial atrophy in about 5% of cases, and retinal changes may also be present [9]. There can be ipsilateral cerebral atrophy [10].

The atrophy may remain limited both in extent and depth. It may be confined to the distribution of one division of the trigeminal nerve or involve the whole of the side of the face, sharply demarcated at the midline. Rarely, it may be bilateral, and very rarely may involve half the body, usually on the same side as the face but exceptionally the opposite side—crossed hemiatrophy. The atrophy may, in such cases, begin on the trunk or a limb and only later involve the face.

The degree of bone atrophy as established radiologically is usually much less than the clinical appearance suggests, and is severe only in some cases of early onset. In such cases, the cerebral cortex may also be affected, and contralateral epilepsy may result.

Localized scleroderma of the 'coup de sabre' paramedian form may be associated with some degree of facial hemiatrophy, especially if it begins early in life. However, it is a more superficial process than progressive facial hemiatrophy. The skin in scleroderma is bound down and adherent, and loss of hair and pigmentary changes are conspicuous. In progressive facial hemiatrophy, the skin may remain mobile and grossly normal. The two processes have been confused frequently in the literature, and may coexist [11].

Diagnosis. When the cutaneous involvement is early and conspicuous, the diagnosis presents few difficulties. Hypoplasia following radiotherapy given in infancy, perhaps in treatment of a naevus in the region of the temporomandibular joint, could cause confusion. If the skin changes are slight, or of later onset, physiological asymmetry, unilateral mandibular agenesis, hemihypertrophy and atrophy secondary to facial paralysis must be excluded. Hemihypertrophy is always congenital. When the limbs are involved, infantile hemiplegia and lipodystrophy must also be considered.

Treatment. Plastic surgery using large, buried pediculated flaps of dermis and fat, or silicone implants, offers some cosmetic benefit [5,11–14].

References

1 Nakano R, Wakamatsu N, Tsujui S. Juvenile Sandhoff disease with local panatrophy. A case report. *Baillieres Clin Neurol* 1989; **29**: 1032–8.
2 Jablonska S, ed. *Scleroderma and Pseudoscleroderma*, 2nd edn. Warsaw: Polish Medical Publishers, 1975.
3 Barnes S. Gower's case of local panatrophy. *Br J Dermatol* 1939; **51**: 377–80.
4 Levy JJ, Gassmuller J, Anding H *et al.* Imaging subcutaneous atrophy in circumscribed scleroderma with 20 Mhz B-scan ultrasound. *Hautarzt* 1993; **44**: 446–51.
5 Moscona R, Bergman R, Friedman-Birnbaum R. Multiple dermal grafts for hemifacial atrophy caused by lupus panniculitis. *J Am Acad Dermatol* 1986; **14**: 840–3.
6 Bramley P, Forbes A. A case of progressive hemiatrophy presenting with spontaneous fractures of the lower jaw. *BMJ* 1960; **i**: 1476–8.
7 Ho KH. Hemifacial atrophy (Romberg's disease). *Br Dent J* 1971; **162**: 182–4.
8 Fry JA, Alvarellos A, Fink CW *et al.* Intracranial findings in progressive facial hemiatrophy. *J Rheumatol* 1992; **19**: 956–8.
9 Theodossiadis PG, Grigoropoulos VG, Emfietzoglou I *et al.* Parry–Romberg syndrome studied by optical coherence tomography. *Ophthalmic Surg Lasers Imaging* 2008; **39**: 78–80.
10 Chang S-E, Huh J, Choi J-H *et al.* Parry–Romberg syndrome with ipsilateral cerebral atrophy of neonatal onset. *Pediatr Dermatol* 1999; **16**: 487–8.
11 Handfield-Jones SE, Peachey RDG, Moss ACH *et al.* Ossification in linear morphoea with hemifacial atrophy—treatment by surgical excision. *Clin Exp Dermatol* 1988; **13**: 385–8.
12 Franz FP, Blocksma R, Brundage SR *et al.* Massive injection of liquid silicone for hemifacial atrophy. *Ann Plast Surg* 1988; **20**: 140–5.
13 Sakamoto T, Oku T, Takigawa M. Gower's local panatrophy. *Eur J Dermatol* 1998; **8**: 116–7.
14 Guerrerosantos JG, Guerrerosantos F, Orozco J. Classification and treatment of facial tissue atrophy in Parry-Romberg disease. *Aesthetic Plast Surg* 2007; **31**: 424–34.

Scleroatrophic syndrome of Huriez

This autosomal dominant congenital syndrome is discussed in more detail in Chapter 19. It comprises a triad of diffuse scleroatrophy of the hands, mild palmoplantar keratoderma and hypoplastic nail changes [1–4]. Scleroatrophy is accentuated on the palms and fingers, which are tapered as in sclerodactyly; however, Huriez syndrome is congenital, and Raynaud's phenomenon is absent. The acral hyperkeratosis is associated with dry skin, resulting in painful fissures in winter months. Nail changes include prominent lunulae, elongated cuticles, longitudinal and transverse ridging, increased longitudinal curvature [5] and V-shaped notches [6]. Squamous carcinoma may develop in the scleroatrophic skin, sometimes as early as the third or fourth decades of life [1,6]; fatal metastases may occur [7].

Histology shows marked orthokeratosis, acanthosis with a prominent granular cell layer, and mild fibrosis of the upper and mid-dermis. Elastic fibres are reduced. Epidermal Langerhans' cells are reduced in number, perhaps contributing to the risk of malignant change [6]. A gene has been identified which maps to chromosome 4q23 [7].

Patients should be followed throughout life, with early excision of suspected malignancies. Acitretin reduces the painful hyperkeratosis [8] and could reduce the incidence of skin cancer.

References

1 Huriez C, Agache P, Bombart M *et al.* Épithéliomes spinocellulaires sur atrophie cutanée congénitale dans deux familles à morbidité cancéreuse élevée. *Bull Soc Fr Dermatol Syphiligr* 1963; **70**: 24–8.
2 Huriez C, Agache P, Souillart F *et al.* Scléroatrophie familiale des extremités avec dégénérescences spinocellulaires multiples. *Bull Soc Fr Dermatol Syphiligr* 1963; **70**: 743–4.
3 Huriez C, Deminatti M, Agache P *et al.* Une Génodysplasie non encore individualisée; la génodermatose scléroatrophiante et kératodermique des extrémités fréquemment dégénérative. *Sem Hôp Paris* 1968; **44**: 481–8.
4 Downs AMR, Kennedy CTC. Scleroatrophic syndrome of Huriez in an infant. *Pediatr Dermatol* 1998; **15**: 207–9.
5 De Berker D, Kavanagh G. Distinctive nail changes in scleroatrophy of Huriez. *Br J Dermatol* 1993; **129** (Suppl. 42): 36 (Abstract).
6 Hamm H, Traupe H, Bröcker E-B *et al.* The scleroatrophic syndrome of Huriez: a cancer-prone genodermatosis. *Br J Dermatol* 1996; **134**: 512–8.
7 Lee YA, Stevens HP, Delaporte E *et al.* A gene for an autosomal scleroatrophic syndrome predisposing to skin cancer (Huriez syndrome) maps to chromosome 4q23. *Am J Hum Genet* 2000; **66**: 326–30.
8 Delaporte E, N'Guyen-Mailfer C, Janin A *et al.* Keratoderma with scleroatrophy of the extremities or sclerotylosis (Huriez syndrome): a reappraisal. *Br J Dermatol* 1995; **133**: 409–16.

Localized abdominal wall atrophy

Congenital cutis laxa (p. 45.14) may rarely be confined to an area such as the abdomen. There may be other associated defects, for example dysplasia of the abdominal muscles, deformity of the thorax or mediastinal hernia. This condition must be distinguished from centrifugal abdominal lipodystrophy (Chapter 46) and the prune belly syndrome, in which wrinkled abdominal skin due to underlying abdominal muscle deficiency is associated with malformation of the urogenital tract [1,2].

References

1 Orvis BR, Bottles K, Kogan BA. Testicular histology in the 'prune belly' syndrome. *J Urol* 1988; **139**: 335–7.

2 Pagon RA, Smith DW, Shepherd TH. Urethral obstruction malformation complex. A cause of abdominal muscle deficiency and the 'prune belly'. *J Pediatr* 1979; **94**: 900–6.

Poikiloderma

Poikiloderma is a descriptive term, often somewhat loosely applied. Atrophy, macular or reticulate pigmentation and telangiectasia are the essential features. Depigmentation, miliary lichenoid papules, fine scaling and small petechial haemorrhages are less constantly present.

Congenital poikiloderma

Poikiloderma may occur as an apparently primary abnormality in certain genetically determined syndromes, including the Rothmund–Thomson syndrome, dyskeratosis congenita (Chapter 15) and the Mendes da Costa syndrome (Chapter 19).

Several other syndromes have been described in which poikiloderma is a prominent feature [1].

Hereditary sclerosing poikiloderma of Weary [2]

This rare, autosomal dominant syndrome was described in a large black family. Generalized poikiloderma, which developed in early childhood, was accompanied by sclerosis of the palms and soles, and linear hyperkeratotic and sclerotic bands developed in the flexures of the arms and legs.

Kindler syndrome [3,4]

This is an autosomal recessive disorder characterized by acral blistering, which is usually present at birth, and early poikiloderma. The poikiloderma is progressive, resulting in thin, wrinkled skin without surface markings. Cutaneous atrophy is most pronounced on the hands and feet. Clinical overlap with epidermolysis bullosa and hereditary acrokeratotic poikiloderma may cause diagnostic confusion. Photosensitivity is common and, like other cutaneous features, tends to improve with time. However, recurrent acral blisters have been described in a 46-year-old Japanese male [5]. Kindler syndrome is caused by loss-of-function mutations in the *KIND1* gene, which encodes kindlin-1. This protein is involved in anchorage of the actin cytoskeleton to the extracellular matrix [6,7].

Hereditary acrokeratotic poikiloderma of Weary [1,8,9].

Weary described an autosomal dominant condition of vesicopustules of the hands and feet, which start at the age of 1–3 months and resolve in childhood. There is also a widespread eczema, and the gradual appearance of poikiloderma, which persists into adult life. Keratotic papules develop in childhood on the hands, feet, knees and elbows, and these also persist indefinitely. Mucosal involvement is frequent. Some cases do not fit clearly into either Weary's or Kindler's syndromes [10].

Diffuse and macular atrophic dermatosis [11]

This rare condition is characterized by the presence from birth of generalized poikilodermatous changes that give the appearance of prematurely sun-damaged skin. The facies, hair and skeleton are normal. Biopsy shows thinning of the epidermis, with large hyaline bodies in the superficial dermal collagen, and these stain positively with periodic acid–Schiff (PAS) and elastin stains. Electron microscopy shows that these globular structures consist of microfibrillar material, and the adjacent fibroblasts may be degenerative.

Degos–Touraine syndrome [12]

In this condition, incontinentia pigmenti is accompanied by poikiloderma of light-exposed areas, often with gastrointestinal symptoms. Both gastrointestinal and skin manifestations are said to disappear following treatment with diiodohydroxyquine. Small bullae on the extremities have been described, but the initial bullae appear on the face. Hyperpigmentation follows a chronic erythrodermatous phase.

Acquired poikiloderma

Poikiloderma may occur as a pattern of cutaneous response to injury by cold, heat or ionizing radiation [13]. So-called poikiloderma of Civatte (Chapter 58) is a similar reaction mediated by photosensitizing chemicals in cosmetics. Some inflammatory dermatoses, such as lichen planus, may also give rise to poikilodermatous changes.

Poikiloderma is also a feature of some inflammatory 'connective tissue' diseases, and is particularly characteristic of dermatomyositis. It is also seen in lupus erythematosus and rarely in systemic sclerosis. Poikiloderma occurs as a manifestation of some lymphomas, especially mycosis fungoides (Fig. 45.12).

References

1 Draznin MB, Esterly NB, Fretzin DF. Congenital poikiloderma with features of hereditary acrokeratotic poikiloderma. *Arch Dermatol* 1978; **114**: 1207–10.
2 Weary PE, Hsu YT, Richardson D. Hereditary sclerosing poikiloderma. Report of two families with an unusual and distinctive genodermatosis. *Arch Dermatol* 1969; **100**: 413–22.
3 Forman AB, Prendiville JS, Esterley NB *et al.* Kindler syndrome: report of two cases and review of the literature. *Pediatr Dermatol* 1989; **6**: 91–101.
4 Kindler T. Congenital poikiloderma with traumatic bulla formation and progressive cutaneous atrophy. *Br J Dermatol* 1954; **66**: 104–11.
5 Ban M, Hosoe H, Yamada T *et al.* Kindler's syndrome with recurrence of bullae in the fifth decade. *Br J Dermatol* 1996; **135**: 503–4.

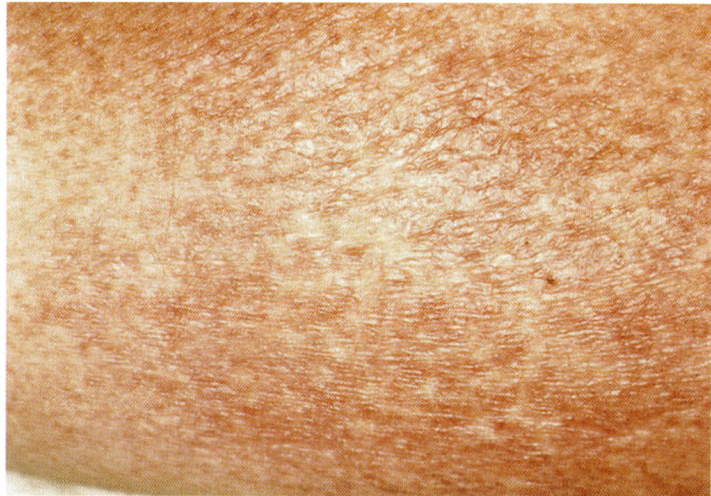

Fig. 45.12 Poikiloderma in a prelymphomatous eruption. The patient eventually developed cutaneous T-cell lymphoma.

6 Siegel DH, Ashton GH, Penagos HG *et al*. Loss of kindlin-1 a human homolog of the *Caenorhabditis elegans* actin-extracellular-matrix linker protein UNC-112, causes Kindler syndrome. *Am J Hum Genet* 2003; **73**: 174–87.

7 Arita K, Wessagowit V, Inamadar AC *et al*. Unusual molecular findings in Kindler syndrome. *Br J Dermatol* 2007; **157**: 1252–6.

8 Weary PE, Manley WF, Graham GF. Hereditary acrokeratotic poikiloderma. *Arch Dermatol* 1971; **103**: 409–22.

9 Larrègue M, Prigent F, Lorette G *et al*. Acrokeratose poikilodermique bulleuse et hereditaire de Weary–Kindler. *Ann Dermatol Syphiligr (Paris)* 1981; **108**: 69–76.

10 Person JR, Perry HO. Congenital poikiloderma with traumatic bulla formation, anhidrosis and keratoderma. *Acta Derm Venereol Suppl (Stockh)* 1959; **59**: 347–51.

11 Kirby JD. The diffuse and macular atrophic dermatosis. *Clin Exp Dermatol* 1980; **5**: 57–60.

12 Degos R, Touraine R. Incontinentia pigmenti avec état poikilodermique. *Bull Soc Fr Dermatol Syphiligr* 1961; **68**: 6–10.

13 Okazaki M, Kikuchi I. Radiodermatitis. An analysis of 43 cases. *J Dermatol* 1986; **13**: 356–65.

Disorders of elastic fibres

The capacity of the skin to adapt to local or general changes in body size and contour, and to allow for movement of head and limbs and a wide range of facial expression, depends upon its tension, elasticity and tensile strength. These properties may be congenitally defective or modified by ageing or disease [1–3]. Acquired disorders of elastic tissue have been reviewed in detail by Lewis *et al*. [4,5].

Elasticity. Elastic fibres are abundant in the skin, arteries, lungs and ligaments. They provide tissues with resilience and elasticity (the ability to resume its original shape after deforming forces have ceased to act). There is wide individual variation, but a tendency to decrease with age. Several diseases, such as cutis laxa, decrease cutaneous elasticity. Elastic fibres also provide adhesion for cells and play a role in regulating growth factors' (e.g. transforming growth factor-β) availability [2].

Tensile strength. The tensile strength of the skin is the degree to which it can be elongated before it tears. It is greatest in infancy and decreases with age, but is also abnormally low in diseases associated with collagen defects such as EDS and Cushing's syndrome [3].

References

1 Grahame R. A method for measuring human skin elasticity *in vivo* with observations on the effects of age, sex and pregnancy. *Clin Sci* 1970; **39**: 223–9.

2 Kielty CM. Elastic fibres in health and disease. *Expert Rev Mol Med* 2006; **8**: 1–23.

3 Uitto J. Biochemistry of collagen in diseases. *Ann Intern Med* 1986; **105**: 740–56.

4 Lewis KG, Bercovitch L, Dill SW *et al*. Acquired disorders of elastic tissue: Part 1. Increased elastic tissue and solar elastotic syndromes. *J Am Acad Dermatol* 2004; **51**: 1–21.

5 Lewis KG, Bercovitch L, Dill SW *et al*. Acquired disorders of elastic tissue: Part II. Decreased elastic tissue. *J Am Acad Dermatol* 2004; **51**: 165–85.

Lax skin

Increased laxity of the skin due to ageing (accelerated by dermal photodegradation) is of course extremely common, but cutaneous laxity can occasionally be due to marked weight loss (especially after gross obesity) or can follow recovery from severe oedema.

Less commonly, the skin may become lax due to localized or generalized defects in elastic tissue resulting from other causes, and these may be grouped as follows.

1 Generalized elastolysis (cutis laxa):
  (a) congenital
  (b) associated with other inherited disorders (PXE, SCARF syndrome (skeletal abnormalities, cutis laxa, craniostenosis, ambiguous genitalia, retardation and facial abnormalities), de Barsy syndrome, geroderma osteodysplastica)
  (c) acquired (numerous associated disorders, for example inflammatory skin disease, multiple myeloma, systemic lupus erythematosus, hypersensitivity reactions, complement deficiency, penicillamine therapy)
2 Localized elastolysis:
  (a) anetoderma
  (b) blepharochalasis
  (c) chronic atrophic acrodermatitis (due to *Borrelia*)
  (d) granulomatous slack skin (due to lymphoma)
  (e) other localized lesions, including mid-dermal elastolysis, post-inflammatory elastolysis and cutis laxa (PECL), elastic tissue naevi etc.

Generalized cutis laxa [1]

Synonyms
- Generalized elastolysis
- Generalized elastorrhexis
- Generalized dermatochalasis

Definition. Cutis laxa is characterized clinically by lax, pendulous skin and histologically by loss of elastic tissue in the dermis. It is a heterogeneous condition, with several causes and associations, and it may be inherited or acquired.

Aetiology. Cutis laxa may be *inherited*, either as an autosomal dominant or autosomal recessive trait [2]. Occipital horn syndrome was originally described as X-linked recessive cutis laxa and subsequently EDS type IX, but is now classified with Menkes' syndrome as a condition in which secondary changes in connective tissue are caused by abnormal copper metabolism [3–4] (p. 45.15 and Chapter 66).

Since the initial identification of mutations in the elastin gene in autosomal dominant cutis laxa [5,6] only a few similar families have been reported [7]. Abnormalities of the microfibrillary protein, fibulin-5, can also lead to autosomal dominant cutis laxa, indicating genetic heterogeneity [8]. Both fibulin-4 and some fibulin-5 mutations cause the more severe autosomal recessive phenotype [9,10]. Loss-of-function mutations in *ATP6V0A2*, encoding the α2 subunit of the V-type H^+ ATPase, have been identified in several families with autosomal recessive cutis laxa type II, resulting in abnormal glycosylation [11].

Cutis laxa may also be *acquired* following inflammatory skin disease [12], and it has occurred in babies born to women taking penicillamine [13]. An immunological pathogenesis has been suggested in some acquired cases because of the rare associations with drug hypersensitivity, complement deficiency, systemic lupus erythematosus, multiple myelomatosis and coeliac disease [14–18].

Amyloidosis seems to provoke cutis laxa in some cases [19], and it is known that amyloid can coat elastic fibres [20,21]. Cutis laxa may also accompany inherited disorders of connective tissue such as pseudoxanthoma elasticum and Ehlers–Danlos syndrome [22].

Pathology. The skin is of normal thickness, but the elastic fibres are sparse, short, fragmented and clumped, particularly in the upper dermis, and they show granular degeneration [23]. The elastic fibres are deficient in elastin, but their microfibrils appear normal [24,25]. Similar changes in elastic fibres may occur in the lungs and aorta.

Various ultrastructural changes have been described, including separation of the elastin microfibrils from the amorphous matrix, the presence of a 'wood-grain' pattern and aggregation, fragmentation and clumping of the elastic fibres [11,23,24].

Clinical features. In this rare condition, the skin becomes inelastic and hangs in redundant folds. The face and neck are often affected, which produces a 'bloodhound' appearance of premature ageing. The internal elastic tissues may also be affected, and emphysema and cardiovascular abnormalities occur in some types.

Hereditary forms [26] (Table 45.1)
Various clinical types have been described [27,28]. In the *autosomal dominant* form, the skin changes may develop at any age, but tend to present later than in the recessive form. Those presenting in adult life usually have no internal defects, and the life expectancy is normal [28]. When the condition presents in infancy there is intrauterine growth retardation, delayed fontanelle closure and ligamentous laxity [29]. The skin changes may be preceded by episodes of oedema, usually within the first 2 months of life, and the child may look aged by the end of the second year. Affected males may be impotent, with infantile genitalia and scanty body hair. Pulmonary emphysema due to a loss of elastic tissue in the lungs is common [2].

In the commoner, but more severe, *autosomal recessive* form there is a characteristic facies with downward slanting palpebral fissures, a broad flat nose, sagging cheeks and large ears. There are prominent skin folds around the knees, abdomen and thighs [28]. Herniae, diverticula, severe pulmonary emphysema and cor pulmonale are important complications. Death due to respiratory complications is common in the first few years of life. Dental caries, aortic aneurysm and osteoporosis may also occur.

The *de Barsey syndrome* is a rare type in which cutis laxa is accompanied by retarded psychomotor development and corneal clouding due to degeneration of the tunica elastica of the cornea [30–32]. Growth is retarded and there may be pseudoathetoid movements. Congenital cutis laxa has also been associated with SCARF syndrome [33], osteoporosis [34] and geroderma osteodysplastica, which is characterized by skeletal abnormalities, including joint hypermobility, Wormian bones and osteoporosis [35].

Although there are many similarities between the wrinkly skin syndrome and cutis laxa type II, the skin changes in the former are limited mainly to the abdomen, hands and feet. Facial dysmorphism is less pronounced in wrinkly skin syndrome and the large fontanelles have not been described [36].

Table 45.1 Cutis laxa syndromes.

Type	Molecular defect	Major clinical features
Autosomal dominant	*ELN*, *FBLN5*	Symptoms less severe than autosomal recessive types Onset usually childhood/early adult Cutis laxa, gastrointestinal diverticula, herniae, uterine prolapse, aortic dilatations
Autosomal recessive Type I	*FBLN4* and *FBLN5*	Cutis laxa, pulmonary emphysema, gastrointestinal and bladder diverticula, arterial aneurysms, pulmonary artery stenosis, herniae
Autosomal recessive Type II	Loss-of-function mutations *ATP6V0A2*	Cutis laxa, growth and developmental delay, skeletal abnormalities, large fontanelle with delayed closure, oxycephaly, herniae, hip dislocations
Autosomal recessive Type III (de Barsey syndrome)	Unknown	Cutis laxa, corneal opacities, mental retardation, pseudoathetoid movements
Other syndromes with cutis laxa		
X-linked (occipital horn syndrome)	*ATP7A* (allelic with Menkes syndrome)	Bladder diverticulae, inguinal hernias, slight skin laxity and hyperextensibility, joint laxity and coarse hair Skeletal abnormalities, including persistent open anterior fontanelle and occipital exostoses
SCARF syndrome	Unknown X-linked recessive	SCARF acronym: *s*keletal abnormalities, *c*utis laxa/craniostenosis, *a*mbiguous genitalia, *r*etardation, *f*acial abnormalities
Geroderma osteodysplastica	Unknown Autosomal recessive	Dwarfism with premature aged appearance, lax skin, osteoporosis, Wormian bones, mandibular prognathism, malar hypoplasia
Costello's syndrome	*HRAS*	Phenotypic overlap with cardiofaciocutaneous syndrome Characteristic coarse facies, short stature, cutis laxa particularly hands and feet, severe feeding difficulty and failure to thrive, cardiac anomalies, facial warts Often presents in childhood

Acquired forms [37]

Cutis laxa may rarely develop at any age following episodes of urticaria or angio-oedema, extensive inflammatory skin disease (such as systemic lupus erythematosus or erythema multiforme) or febrile illness. It may also follow hypersensitivity reactions such as penicillin allergy [14].

Cutis laxa has also been reported in association with complement deficiency, sarcoidosis, syphilis, multiple myeloma [15,17] and the Klippel–Trenaunay syndrome [24]. Focal elastolysis can also occur in association with lupus erythematosus [38], severe rheumatoid arthritis [39] and coeliac disease [18]. D-Penicillamine disrupts elastic fibre formation and may cause cutis laxa, elastosis perforans serpiginosa and pseudoxanthoma-like changes [40]. Congenital cutis laxa may also occur in offspring of mothers taking penicillamine [13].

There may be widespread, massive folds of lax skin, or the changes may be mild and confined to a limited area, in which case it cannot be distinguished from anetoderma. Purpura may follow slight trauma and fibrotic nodules may form over bony prominences. Organs other than the skin may also be involved. Emphysema, gastric fibromas and tracheobronchomegaly have been reported [41].

In acquired cutis laxa, dermal elastic tissue is markedly reduced, although collagen is normal. Fibroblasts express increased elastolytic activity (cathepsin G). Levels of serum α_1-antitrypsin and elastase inhibition are decreased [42].

Post-inflammatory elastolysis and cutis laxa also appears to develop as a distinctive syndrome in African children, with clinical features intermediate between anetoderma and cutis laxa [43] (p. 45.17). This condition might represent an unusual reaction to an arthropod bite, as the lesions are preceded by urticaria or multiple red papules, which slowly enlarge to form rings 2–10 cm in diameter.

Diagnosis. The diagnosis, which is suggested by finding loose skin that recoils only slowly after stretching, may be confirmed by histology.

In EDS, the skin is hyperextensible but not lax, and it recoils quickly. In PXE, the skin may be lax, but it is yellowish and the face is usually spared. It is distinguished histologically by the presence of calcification. There may be circumscribed folds of lax skin in neurofibromatosis, and loose folded skin may also occur in leprechaunism, Patterson syndrome and trisomy 18, but these conditions are distinguished by their associated features.

In Costello's syndrome there is skin laxity, especially on hands and feet, with joint hyperextensibility, but the elastin fibres are normal under both light and electron microscopy [44]. The other features of this rare syndrome include poor postnatal growth, developmental delay and a distinctive facies with macroglossia, bilateral ptosis, epicanthic folds and posterior rotation of the pinnae, with prominent helices and thickened lobes.

In severe actinic damage, there may be marked skin laxity due to damage to elastic fibres.

Treatment. Plastic surgery ('face-lift') may reduce the cosmetic disability. Investigations for emphysema are indicated, with referral to a pulmonary physician if necessary.

References

1 Goltz RH, Hult AM, Goldfarb M *et al*. Cutis laxa: a manifestation of generalized elastolysis. *Arch Dermatol* 1965; **92**: 373–87.

2 Agha A, Sakati NO, Higginbottom MC *et al*. Two forms of cutis laxa presenting in the newborn. *Acta Paediatr Scand* 1978; **67**: 775–80.

3 Byers PH, Siegel RC, Holbrook K *et al*. X-linked cutis laxa: defective cross-link formation in collagen. *N Engl J Med* 1980; **303**: 61–5.

4 Beighton P, de Paepe A, Hall JG *et al*. Molecular nosology of heritable disorders of connective tissue. *Am J Med Genet* 1992; **42**: 431–8.

5 Tassabehji M, Metcalfe K, Hurst J *et al*. An elastin gene mutation producing abnormal tropoelastin and abnormal elastic fibres in a patient with autosomal dominant cutis laxa. *Hum Mol Genet* 1998; **7**: 1021–8.

6 Zhang MC, He L, Giro M *et al*. Cutis laxa arising from frameshift mutations in exon 30 of the elastin gene (*ELN*). *J Biol Chem* 1999; **274**: 981–6.

7 Rodriguez-Revenga L, Iranzo P, Badenas C *et al*. A novel elastin gene mutation resulting in an autosomal dominant form of cutis laxa. *Arch Dermatol* 2004; **140**: 1135–9.

8 Markova D, Zou Y, Rinpfeil F *et al*. Genetic heterogeneity of cutis laxa: a heterozygous tandem duplication within the fibulin-5 (FBLN5) gene. *Am J Hum Genet* 2003; **72**: 998–1004.

9 Loeys B, Van Maldergem L, Mortier G *et al*. Homozygosity for a missense mutation in fibulin-5 (*FBLN5*) results in a severe form of cutis laxa. *Hum Mol Genet* 2002; **11**: 2113–8.

10 Hucthagowder V, Sausgruber N, Kim KH *et al*. Fibulin-4: a novel gene for an autosomal recessive cutis laxa syndrome. *Am J Hum Genet* 2006; **78**: 1075–80.

11 Kornak U, Reynders E, Dimopoulou A *et al*. Impaired glycosylation and cutis laxa caused by mutations in the vesicular H+-ATPase subunit ATP6V0A2. *Nat Genet* 2008; **40**: 32–4.

12 Nanko H, Jepson LV, Zachariae H *et al*. Acquired cutis laxa (generalised elastolysis): light and electron microscopic studies. *Acta Derm Venereol Suppl (Stockh)* 1979; **59**: 315–24.

13 Harpey J-P. Cutis laxa and low serum zinc after antenatal exposure to penicillamine. *Lancet* 1983; **ii**: 858–9.

14 Kerl H, Burg G. Fatal penicillin-induced generalized post-inflammatory elastolysis (cutis laxa). *Hautarzt* 1975; **26**: 191–8.

15 Tsuji T, Imajo Y, Sawabe M *et al*. Acquired cutis laxa concomitant with nephrotic syndrome. *Arch Dermatol* 1987; **123**: 1211–6.

16 Scott MA, Kauh YC, Luscombe HA. Acquired cutis laxa associated with multiple myelomatosis. *Arch Dermatol* 1976; **112**: 853–5.

17 Ting HC, Foo MH, Wang F. Acquired cutis laxa and multiple myelomatosis. *Br J Dermatol* 1984; **110**: 363–7.

18 García-Patos V, Pujol RM, Barnadas MA *et al*. Generalized acquired cutis laxa associated with coeliac disease: evidence of immunoglobulin A deposits on the dermal elastic fibres. *Br J Dermatol* 1996; **135**: 130–4.

19 Newton JA, McKee PH, Black MM. Cutis laxa associated with amyloidosis. *Clin Exp Dermatol* 1986; **11**: 87–91.

20 Winkelmann RK, Peters MS, Venencie PY. Amyloid elastosis. A new cutaneous and systemic pattern of amyloidosis. *Arch Dermatol* 1985; **121**: 498–502.

21 Yanagihara M, Kato F, Shikano Y. Intimate structural association of amyloid and elastic fibres in systemic and cutaneous amyloidoses. *J Cutan Pathol* 1985; **12**: 110–6.

22 Ostlere LS, Pope FM, Holden CA. Cutis laxa complicating Ehlers–Danlos syndrome type II. *Clin Exp Dermatol* 1996; **21**: 135–7.

23 Hashimoto K, Kanzaki T. Cutis laxa: ultrastructural and biochemical studies. *Arch Dermatol* 1975; **111**: 861–73.

24 Marchase P, Holbrook K, Pinnell SR. A familial cutis laxa syndrome with ultrastructural abnormalities of collagen and elastin. *J Invest Dermatol* 1980; **75**: 399–403.

25 Sephel GC, Byers PH, Holbrook KA *et al*. Heterogeneity of elastin expression in cutis laxa fibroblast strains. *J Invest Dermatol* 1989; **93**: 147–53.

26 Pope FM. Cutis laxa. In: Beighton P, ed. *McKusick's Heritable Disorders of Connective Tissue*, 5th edn. St Louis: Mosby, 1993: 253–79.

27 Fitzsimmons JS, Gilbert G. Variable clinical presentations of cutis laxa. *Clin Genet* 1985; **28**: 284–95.

28 Patton MA, Tolmie J, Ruthnum P *et al*. Congenital cutis laxa with retardation of growth and development. *J Med Genet* 1987; **24**: 556–61.

29 Gardner LI, Sanders-Fay K, Bifano EM *et al*. Congenital cutis laxa syndrome: relation of joint dislocations to oligohydramnios. *Arch Dermatol* 1987; **122**: 1241–3.

30 De Barsey AM. Dwarfism, oligophrenia and degeneration of the elastic tissue in skin and cornea. *Helv Paediatr Acta* 1968; **23**: 305–13.

31 Kunze J. De Barsey syndrome. *Eur J Pediatr* 1985; **144**: 348–54.

32 Pontz BF, Zepp F, Stöss H. Biochemical, morphological and immunological findings in a patient with a cutis laxa-associated inborn disorder (de Barsey syndrome). *Eur J Pediatr* 1986; **145**: 428–34.

33 Koppe R, Kaplan P, Hunter A, MacMurray B. Ambiguous genitalia associated with skeletal abnormalities, cutis laxa, craniostenosis, psychomotor retardation and facial abnormalities (SCARF syndrome). *Am J Med Genet* 1989; **34**: 305–12.

34 Sakati NO, Nyhan WL. Congenital cutis laxa and osteoporosis. *Am J Dis Child* 1983; **137**: 452–4.

35 Lisker R, Hernandez A, Martinez-Lavin M *et al.* Gerodermia osteodysplastica hereditaria: report of three affected brothers and literature review. *Am J Med Genet* 1979; **3**: 389–95.

36 Gupta N, Phadke SR. Cutis laxa type II and wrinkly skin syndrome: distinct phenotypes. *Pediatr Dermatol* 2006; **23**: 225–30.

37 Reed WB, Horowitz RE, Beighton P. Acquired cutis laxa. Primary generalized elastolysis. *Arch Dermatol* 1971; **103**: 661–9.

38 Randle EHW, Muller S. Generalised elastolysis associated with systemic lupus erythematosus. *J Am Acad Dermatol* 1983; **8**: 869–73.

39 Rongioletti F, Cutolo M, Bondavalli P, Rebora A. Acral localized acquired cutis laxa associated with rheumatoid arthritis. *J Am Acad Dermatol* 2002; **46**: 128–30.

40 Hill VA, Seymour CA, Mortimer PS. Penicillamine-induced elastosis perforans serpiginosa and cutis laxa in Wilson's disease. *Br J Dermatol* 2000; **142**: 560–1.

41 Wanderer AA, Ellis EF, Goltz RW *et al.* Tracheobronchomegaly and acquired cutis laxa in a child. *Pediatrics* 1969; **44**: 709–15.

42 Fornieri C, Quaglino D, Lungarella G *et al.* Elastin production and degradation in cutis laxa acquisita. *J Invest Dermatol* 1994; **103**: 583–8.

43 Verhagen AR, Woerdemann MJ. Post-inflammatory elastolysis and cutis laxa. *Br J Dermatol* 1975; **92**: 183–90.

44 Costello JM. A new syndrome. *NZ Med J* 1971; **74**: 397–40.

Anetoderma

Synonym
- Macular atrophy

Definition and nomenclature. The term anetoderma (*anetos* = slack) refers to a circumscribed area of slack skin associated with a loss of dermal substance on palpation and a loss of elastic tissue on histological examination.

'Primary' anetoderma implies that there is no associated, localized, underlying cutaneous disease, whereas 'secondary' anetoderma can be attributed to some associated condition.

In the past, cases of primary anetoderma were divided into the *Jadassohn–Pellizari* type, in which the lesions are preceded by erythema or urticaria, and the *Schweninger–Buzzi* type, in which there are no preceding inflammatory lesions. This is now of historical interest only, because in the same patient some lesions may be preceded by inflammation and others may not, and the prognosis and histology are identical in the two types [1–3].

Primary anetoderma

Aetiology. In a few cases there appears to be an underlying structural defect of connective tissue. Familial cases are reported [4,5] and there is an association with inherited bony or ocular abnormalities. The Blegvad–Haxthausen syndrome comprises anetoderma, blue sclerae and osteogenesis imperfecta (OI) (p. 45.14).

Recently, it has become apparent that 'primary' anetoderma is strongly associated with antiphospholipid antibodies, with or without a prothrombotic state [6,7]. It is probable that these anti-

bodies underlie the association historically noted with syphilis, and more recently with borreliosis [8] and systemic lupus.

The histology of anetoderma suggests that the basic abnormality is focal elastolysis [1,9,10]. This may be secondary to the release of elastase from the inflammatory cells, which are probably always present in the early stages. Metalloproteinases are increased in lesional skin [11].

Complement activation may be involved, as C3 is deposited on the remaining elastic fibres [12]. It has been suggested that decay-accelerating factor (DAF) and vitronectin (an inhibitor of the membrane-attack complex) may protect elastic fibres against this type of damage [13]. Abnormalities in the protective system could play a role in primary anetoderma.

Secondary anetoderma

This arises in association with another identifiable disease, but the atrophic areas do not always develop at the sites of the known inflammatory lesions. They are soft, round or oval areas which occur mainly on the trunk.

Lupus erythematosus. Anetoderma has occurred in association with systemic or chronic discoid lupus erythematosus, not always in relation to the lesions. Biopsy shows a focal loss of elastic tissue, and a perivascular infiltrate with prominent plasma cells [1,2]. Generalized elastolysis (cutis laxa) has also occurred [14]. Anetoderma is also associated with lupus profundus [15,16] and discoid lupus with hereditary complement (C2) deficiency [17].

Some cases of primary anetoderma have direct immunofluorescent findings similar to those of either chronic cutaneous or systemic lupus erythematosus, even though there may be no other features of lupus erythematosus [18,19].

No antibodies have been demonstrated against elastic fibres [19].

Other diseases [2]. Some of the other reported associations may be coincidental, but it is probable that many inflammatory diseases may occasionally be complicated by anetoderma. It has been reported in association with tuberculosis and leprosy [20], urticaria pigmentosa [21], pityriasis versicolor [22], granuloma annulare [23], and B- and T-cell lymphoma [24–26]. Localized anetoderma-like changes on histology have been reported in association with pilomatricoma [27], dermatofibroma [28], juvenile xanthogranuloma [29] and hamartomatous congenital naevi [30]. Penicillamine-induced anetoderma has also been reported [31].

Localized anetoderma may occur in premature infants, possibly due to the application of transcutaneous oxygen monitoring devices [32,33].

Lesions resembling anetoderma occur in post-inflammatory elastolysis and cutis laxa (p. 45.14).

Pathology [2,8]. During the early stages, the dermis is oedematous, and a lymphocytic infiltrate (predominantly helper T cells) surrounds the blood vessels and appendages [1,10]. Plasma cells and histiocytes, with some granuloma formation, may also be seen. Later, the oedema and perivascular infiltrate subside and elastic fibres become scanty. The persistence of fine, irregular or twisted elastic fibres is common. The dermal collagen may also be diminished, but the fragmentation and disappearance of elastic tissue is the essential change, beginning superficially in the sub-papillary zone and extending downwards. Electron microscopy shows phagocytosis of elastic fibres by macrophages [34,35].

Clinical features

[2]. This rare disorder occurs mainly in women aged 20–40 years, but is occasionally reported in younger and older patients of both sexes. It is perhaps more frequent in central Europe than elsewhere, which suggests a possible relationship to chronic atrophic acrodermatitis (due to *Borrelia* sp.) in some cases. In the most usual form, crops of round or oval, pink macules 0.5–1.0 cm in diameter develop on the trunk, thighs and upper arms, less commonly on the neck and face and rarely elsewhere. The scalp, palms and soles are usually spared. Each macule extends for a week or two to reach a size of 2–3 cm. Sometimes, there are larger plaques of erythema, and nodules have also been reported as a primary lesion [36]. Slowly, each lesion fades and flattens from the centre outwards to leave a macule of wrinkled, atrophic skin, which yields on pressure, admitting the finger through the surrounding ring of normal skin (Fig. 45.13). The colour varies from skin colour to grey, white or blue. The number of lesions varies widely, from less than five to 100 or more. The lesions remain unchanged throughout life, and new lesions often continue to develop for many years. If the lesions coalesce they form large atrophic areas, which are indistinguishable from acquired cutis laxa [2].

In some cases, the lesions are initially urticarial weals which, after a succession of exacerbations and remissions, perhaps continuing for many weeks, are succeeded by atrophy. They may become confluent, to cover large areas, especially at the roots of the limbs and on the neck.

Diagnosis.

The white cicatricial lesions of 'white spot disease' (extragenital lichen sclerosus) (Chapter 51) around the base of the neck and shoulders should not be confused with anetoderma.

Histological examination establishes the diagnosis. Focal dermal hypoplasia and atrophic scars (e.g. following varicella) must also be considered.

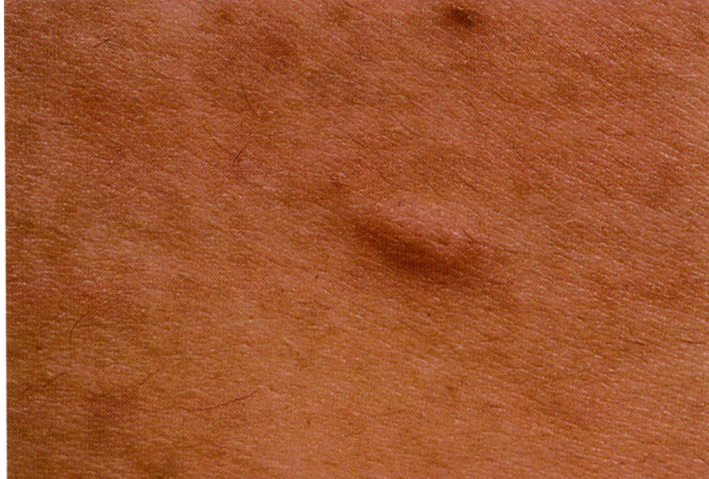

Fig. 45.13 Primary anetoderma. (Courtesy of Dr J. Ellis, Swindon, UK.)

Acquired cutis laxa is probably a variant of anetoderma.

The diagnosis of 'primary' anetoderma can be established only by excluding the presence of any of the diseases known to be associated with 'secondary' atrophy, for example perifollicular elastolysis (p. 45.20).

Treatment.

Penicillin and the antifibrinolytic drug ε-aminocaproic acid have been advocated [37], but Venencie *et al.* [2] studied 16 patients and found no treatment was beneficial once the atrophy had developed. Colchicine may prevent some atrophic changes [38]. In patients with primary anetoderma it is important to test for antiphospholipid syndrome and treat appropriately, for example with aspirin.

References

1 Venencie PY, Winkelmann RK. Histopathologic findings in anetoderma. *Arch Dermatol* 1984; **120**: 1040–4.

2 Venencie PY, Winkelmann RK, Moore BA. Anetoderma: clinical findings, associations, and long term follow-up evaluations. *Arch Dermatol* 1984; **120**: 1032–9.

3 Karrer S, Szeimies RM, Stoltz W, Landthaler M. Primary anetoderma in children: report of two cases and literature review. *Pediatr Dermatol* 1996; **13**: 382–5.

4 Peterman A, Scheel M, Sams WM Jr *et al*. Hereditary anetoderma. *J Am Acad Dermatol* 1996; **35**: 999–1000.

5 Zellman GL, Levy ML. Congenital anetoderma in twins. *J Am Acad Dermatol* 1997; **36**: 483–5.

6 Sparsa A, Piette JC, Wechsler B *et al*. Anetoderma and its prothrombotic abnormalities. *J Am Acad Dermatol* 2003; **49**: 1008–12.

7 Hodak E, David M. Primary anetoderma and antiphospholipid antibodies – review of the literature. *Clin Rev Allergy Immunol* 2007; **32**: 162–9.

8 Hofer T, Golderberger D, Itin PH. Anetoderma and borreliosis: is there a pathogenic relationship? *Eur J Dermatol* 2003; **13**: 399–401.

9 Venencie PY, Winkelmann RK, Moore BA. Ultrastructural findings in the skin lesions of patients with anetoderma. *Acta Derm Venereol Suppl (Stockh)* 1984; **64**: 112–20.

10 Venencie PY, Winkelmann RK. Monoclonal antibody studies in the skin lesions of patients with anetoderma. *Arch Dermatol* 1985; **121**: 747–9.

11 Ghomrasseni S, Dridi M, Gogly B *et al*. Anetoderma: an altered balance between metalloproteinases and tissue inhibitors of metalloproteinases. *Am J Dermatopathol* 2002; **24**: 118–29.

12 Kossard S, Kronman KR, Dicken CH *et al*. Inflammatory macular atrophy. Immunofluorescence and ultrastructural findings. *J Am Acad Dermatol* 1979; **1**: 325–34.

13 Werth VP. Decay-accelerating factor in human skin is associated with elastic fibers. *J Invest Dermatol* 1988; **91**: 511–6.

14 Randle HW, Muller S. Generalized elastolysis associated with systemic lupus erythematosus. *J Am Acad Dermatol* 1983; **8**: 869–73.

15 Ryll-Nardzewski C. Remarques sur le lupus érythémate profond et sur l'anetodermie érythématoide. *Ann Dermatol Syphiligr (Paris)* 1960; **87**: 627–36.

16 Schnitzler L, Sayag J. Pseudotumoral lupus anetoderma and infantile chorea. *Ann Dermatol Vénéréol* 1988; **115**: 679–85.

17 De Bracco MM, Bianchi CA, Bianchi O *et al*. Hereditary complement (C2) deficiency with discoid lupus erythematosus and idiopathic anetoderma. *Int J Dermatol* 1979; **18**: 713–5.

18 Bergman R, Friedman-Birnbaum R. An immunofluorescence study of primary anetoderma. *Clin Exp Dermatol* 1990; **15**: 124–30.

19 Hodak E, Shamai-Lubovitz O, David M *et al*. Primary anetoderma associated with a wide-spectrum of autoimmune abnormalities. *J Am Acad Dermatol* 1991; **25**: 415–8.

20 Inemadar AC, Palit A, Athanikar SB *et al*. Generalised anetoderma in a patient with HIV and dual mycobacterial infection. *Lepr Rev* 2003; **74**: 275–8.

21 Kalogeramitros D, Gregoriou S, Makris M *et al*. Secondary anetoderma associated with mastocytosis. *Int Arch Allergy Immunol* 2007; **142**: 86–8.

22 Tatnall F, Rycroft R. Pityriasis versicolor with cutaneous atrophy. *Clin Exp Dermatol* 1985; **10**: 258–61.

23 Ozkan S, Fetil E, Izler F *et al.* Anetoderma secondary to generalized granuloma annulare. *J Am Acad Dermatol* 2000; **42**: 335–8.

24 Jubert C, Cosnes A, Clerici T *et al.* Sjögren's syndrome and cutaneous B cell lymphoma revealed by anetoderma. *Arthritis Rheum* 1993; **36**: 133–4.

25 Sequrado M, Guerra-Tapia A, Zarco C *et al.* Anetoderma secondary to cutaneous B-cell lymphoma. *Clin Exp Dermatol* 2006; **31**: 130–1.

26 Requena L, González-Guerra E, Angulo J *et al.* Anetodermic mycosis fungoides; a new clinicopathological variant of mycosis fungoides. *Br J Dermatol* 2008; **158**: 157–62.

27 Shames BS, Nassif A, Bailey CS *et al.* Secondary anetoderma involving a pilomatrixoma. *Am J Dermatopathol* 1994; **16**: 557–60.

28 Page EH, Assaad M. Atrophic dermatofibroma and dermatofibrosarcoma protuberans. *J Am Acad Dermatol* 1987; **17**: 947–50.

29 Gamo R, Ortiz-Romero P, Sopeno J *et al.* Anetoderma developing in juvenile xanthogranuloma. *Int J Dermatol* 2005; **44**: 503–6.

30 Cockayne SE, Gawkrodger DJ. Hamartomatous congenital naevi showing secondary anetoderma-like changes. *J Am Acad Dermatol* 1998; **39**: 843–5.

31 Davis W. Wilson's disease and penicillamine-induced anetoderma. *Arch Dermatol* 1977; **113**: 976–7.

32 Prizant TL, Lucky AW, Frieden IJ *et al.* Spontaneous atrophic patches in extremely premature infants. Anetoderma of prematurity. *Arch Dermatol* 1996; **132**: 671–4.

33 Cartlidge PH, Fox PE, Rutter N. The scars of newborn intensive care. *Early Hum Dev* 1990; **21**: 1–10.

34 Oikarinen AK, Palatsi R, Adomian GE *et al.* Anetoderma: biochemical and ultrastructural demonstration of an elastin defect in the skin of three patients. *J Am Acad Dermatol* 1984; **11**: 64–72.

35 Zaki I, Scerri C, Nelson H. Primary anetoderma: phagocytosis of elastic fibres by macrophages. *Clin Exp Dermatol* 1994; **19**: 388–90.

36 Indianer L. Anetoderma of Jadassohn. *Arch Dermatol* 1970; **102**: 697–8.

37 Reiss F, Linn E. The therapeutic effect of ε-aminocaproic acid on anetoderma of Jadassohn. *Dermatologica* 1973; **146**: 357–60.

38 Braun RP, Borradori L, Chavaz P *et al.* Treatment of primary anetoderma with colchicine. *J Am Acad Dermatol* 1998; **38**: 1002–3.

Other localized forms of elastolysis

Idiopathic mid-dermal elastolysis

Several cases have been described in which idiopathic loss of the elastic fibres in the mid-dermis has led to widespread wrinkling of the crinkle type in an otherwise healthy, young or middle-aged woman (Fig. 45.14) [1,2]. The exact relationship between this condition and other elastolytic disorders, such as acquired cutis laxa (p. 45.16) and anetoderma (p. 45.17), is uncertain.

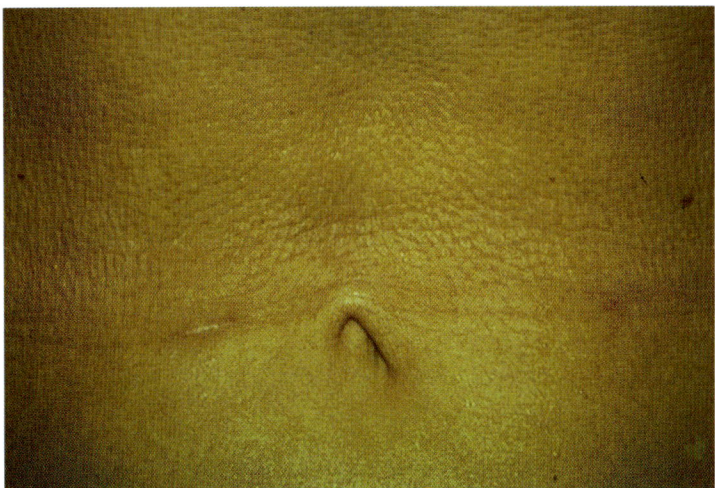

Fig. 45.14 Idiopathic mid-dermal elastolysis. (Courtesy of Dr L. Ostlere, St George's Hospital, London, UK.)

Maghraoui *et al.* [3] have distinguished post-inflammatory elastolysis, with or without features of cutis laxa, from non-inflammatory elastolysis. Inflammatory triggers may include UV radiation, insect bites, borreliosis and acute neutrophilic dermatosis [4]. Localized elastolysis adjacent to varicose veins has also been reported [5].

Ultrastructural studies of mid-dermal elastolysis demonstrate elastic fibres engulfed by macrophages [6]. Immunological studies of affected skin show a non-specific profile of immune activation [7]. Localized areas may clinically resemble PXE, although they are histologically distinct [8,9]. Cultured fibroblasts from lesional dermis exhibit increased elastolytic activity and reduced elastin mRNA compared with normal skin [10].

The histology of idiopathic mid-dermal elastolysis is similar to that of post-inflammatory elastolysis and cutis laxa (PECL), which occurs in young African girls (see below). Those lesions are preceded by inflammatory lesions, but the lesions of idiopathic mid-dermal elastolysis may also occasionally be preceded by erythema, urticaria or a burning sensation, and the two conditions are similar, if not identical.

No definite treatment exists but topical retinoic acid (0.01% gel) produced some cosmetic improvement in one patient [7].

References

1 Brenner W, Schmint FG, Konrad K *et al.* Non-inflammatory dermal elastolysis. *Br J Dermatol* 1978; **99**: 335–8.

2 Rae V, Falanga V. Wrinkling due to mid-dermal elastolysis. *Arch Dermatol* 1989; **125**: 950–1.

3 Maghraoui G, Grossin M, Crickx B *et al.* L'elastolyse acquise du derme moyen. *Ann Dermatol Vénéréol* 1994; **121**: 259–65.

4 Lewis KG, Dill SW, Wilkel CS *et al.* Mid-dermal elastolysis preceded by acute neutrophilic dermatosis. *J Cutan Pathol* 2004; **31**: 72–6.

5 Bayle-Lebey P, Periole B, Daste G *et al.* Acquired localized elastolysis associated with varicose veins. *Clin Exp Dermatol* 1995; **20**: 492–5.

6 Harmon CB, Su WPD, Gagne EJ *et al.* Ultra-structural evaluation of mid-dermal elastolysis. *J Cutan Pathol* 1994; **21**: 233–8.

7 Sterling JC, Coleman N, Pye RJ. Mid-dermal elastolysis. *Br J Dermatol* 1994; **130**: 502–6.

8 El-Charif M, Mousani AM, Rubeiz NG *et al.* Pseudoxanthoma elasticum-like papillary dermal elastolysis: a report of two cases. *J Cutan Pathol* 1994; **21**: 252–5.

9 Rongioletti F, Rebora A. Pseudoxanthoma elasticum-like papillary dermal elastolysis. *J Am Acad Dermatol* 1992; **26**: 648–50.

10 Tajima S, Imazumi T, Kojiya H *et al.* Elastin metabolism in skin fibroblasts explanted from a patient with mid-dermal elastolysis. *Br J Dermatol* 1999; **140**: 752–4.

Upper dermal elastolysis

Selective loss of elastic tissue in the papillary dermis has been described in an otherwise healthy 86-year-old woman, who presented with numerous yellowish papules on the neck and upper trunk, and associated coarse wrinkles [1].

Reference

1 Hashimoto K, Tye MJ. Upper dermal elastolysis: a comparative study with mid-dermal elastolysis. *J Cutan Pathol* 1994; **21**: 533–40.

Post-inflammatory elastolysis and cutis laxa

PECL is a distinctive severe variant of anetoderma (p. 45.17), which occurs predominantly in black girls living in a tropical climate [1–3]. It has a prolonged course, with relapsing inflammatory phases lasting for months or years. In the acute phase, there are firm, infiltrated plaques or rings, with a collarette of scale, and these progress to leave a diffuse, fine, wrinkled skin with the appearance of premature ageing. In some cases, most of the body surface may be involved. There is no internal involvement, and no preceding infection, such as syphilis or tuberculosis. Histological examination shows destruction of the elastic fibres in the upper and mid-dermis.

It is thought that PECL is a reaction to arthropod bites because some patients have eosinophilia, other family members may suffer from papular urticaria, the lesions show a predilection for exposed parts and no new lesions develop when the patient is in hospital. There is a resemblance to erythema chronicum migrans (Chapter 30).

References

1 O'Brien JP. Is actinic damage the provoking cause of postinflammatory elastolysis and cutis laxa? *Br J Dermatol* 1976; **95**: 105–6.
2 Lewis PG, Hood AF, Barnett NF. Post-inflammatory elastolysis and cutis laxa. *J Am Acad Dermatol* 1990; **22**: 40–8.
3 Verhagen AR, Woerdemann MJ. Post-inflammatory elastolysis and cutis laxa. *Br J Dermatol* 1975; **92**: 183–90.

Perifollicular elastolysis

Anetoderma-like changes in a perifollicular distribution have been described in three women aged 30–40 years [1]. The lesions were small, grey–white, finely wrinkled, round or oval areas, each with a central hair follicle. Some exhibited a balloon-like bulge above the surface. They occurred on the upper trunk, neck, earlobes and arms. Histology showed a non-inflammatory perifollicular loss of elastin fibres, and it was suggested that the lesions might have been caused by an elastase-producing strain of *Staphylococcus epidermidis* [2]. Similar changes are more commonly seen in acne scars (Chapter 42) [3].

References

1 Varadi DP, Saqueton AC. Perifollicular elastolysis. *Br J Dermatol* 1970; **83**: 143–50.
2 Dick GF. Elastolytic activity of *P. acnes* and *Staph. epidermidis* in acne and normal skin. *Acta Derm Venereol Suppl (Stockh)* 1976; **56**: 279–82.
3 Wilson BB, Dent CH, Cooper PH. Papular acne scars. A common cutaneous finding. *Arch Dermatol* 1990; **126**: 797–800.

Granulomatous slack skin

Granulomatous slack skin is a rare disease characterized by the slow development of pendulous folds of lax erythematous skin, which on histological examination contains a dense granulomatous dermal infiltrate, with destruction of dermal elastic tissue. It is now considered to be a type of lymphoma (Chapter 57).

Blepharochalasis [1–3]

Definition. Laxity of the eyelid skin due to a defect in the elastic tissue.

Aetiology. The cause is unknown. Most cases are sporadic, but some pedigrees show autosomal dominant inheritance. Some cases may be a localized form of post-inflammatory elastolysis or follow angio-oedema [4].

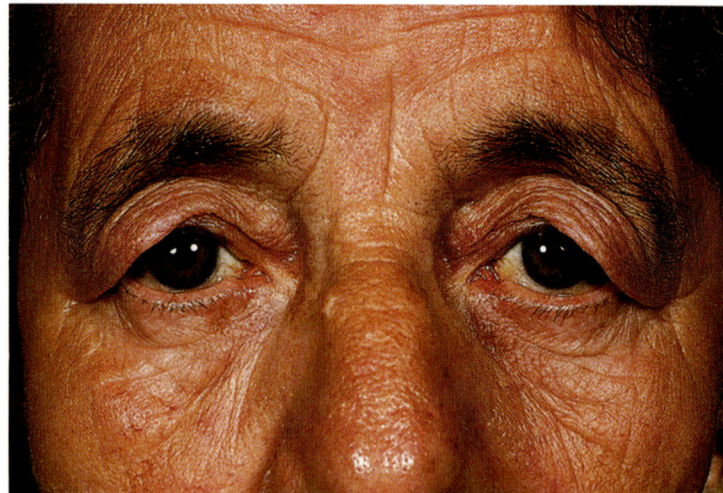

Fig. 45.15 Blepharochalasis. (Courtesy of Dr D.A. Burns, Leicester Royal Infirmary, Leicester, UK.)

Pathology [3]. In the early stages there may be a mild dermal lymphocytic infiltrate, and in the later stages the elastic fibres in the lids fragment and decrease. Normal elastin gene expression suggests other factors may be involved in elastic fibre loss [5]. IgA deposition may be detected on fibres, implying an immunopathogenic mechanism may be involved [6]. Disintegration of collagen fibres has also been observed in one case [7].

Clinical features. Blepharochalasis is an uncommon condition that usually develops insidiously around the time of puberty. Repeated, transient attacks of painless swelling of the eyelids lasting for 2 or 3 days are followed by laxity, atrophy, wrinkling and pigmentation, predominantly of the upper eyelids (Fig. 45.15). There may be multiple telangiectases. These changes produce an appearance of tiredness, debauchery or premature ageing.

Reduplication of the mucous membrane of the upper eyelid is associated with blepharochalasis in about 10% of cases, and this may make the eyelids appear thick.

Blepharochalasis is occasionally a manifestation of generalized cutis laxa, and it may form part of Ascher's syndrome (see below). Laxity of the eyelid skin also occurs in EDS, but other features of this syndrome will also be present. Occasionally, laxity particularly affecting the upper eyelid, occurs in otherwise healthy individuals [8].

Diagnosis. The many other causes of eyelid swelling must be excluded (Chapter 67). Ptosis is easily distinguished because the skin appears normal.

Treatment. Plastic surgery can be performed, but the condition may recur [2].

References

1 Brazin SA. Unilateral blepharochalasis. *Arch Dermatol* 1979; **115**: 479–81.
2 Harris WA, Dortzbach RK. Levator tuck. A simplified blepharoptosis procedure. *Ann Ophthalmol* 1975; **7**: 873–8.
3 Tepaszto I, Liszkay L, Vass Z. Some data on the pathogenesis of blepharochalasis. *Acta Ophthalmol (Copenh)* 1963; **41**: 167–75.

4 Jordan DR. Blepharochalasis syndrome: a proposed pathophysiologic mechanism. *Can J Ophthalmol* 1992; **27**: 10–5.
5 Kaneoya K, Momota Y, Hatamochi A *et al.* Elastin gene expression in blepharochalasis. *J Dermatol* 2005; **32**: 26–9.
6 Grasseger A, Romani N, Fritsch P *et al.* Immunoglobulin A (IgA) deposits in lesional skin of a patient with blepharochalasis. *Br J Dermatol* 1996; **135**: 791–5.
7 Dózsa A, Károlyi ZS, Degrell P. Bilateral blepharochalasis. *J Eur Acad Dermatol Venereol* 2005; **19**: 725–8.
8 Shah-Desai S, Sandy C, Collin R. Lax eyelid syndrome or "progeria" of eyelid tissues. *Orbit* 2004; **23**: 3–12.

Ascher's syndrome

Ascher's syndrome is the association of blepharochalasis with progressive enlargement of the upper lip due to hypertrophy and inflammation of the labial salivary glands [1–5]. The lip feels soft and lobulated and there may be excessive salivation. In some cases, the accessory lacrimal glands are also affected, with increased thickness of the eyelids. Enlargement of the thyroid has also been reported.

References

1 Findlay GH. Idiopathic enlargements of the lips: cheilitis granulomatosa, Ascher's syndrome and double lip. *Br J Dermatol* 1954; **66**: 129–38.
2 Papanayotou PH, Hatzoitis JC. Ascher's syndrome: report of a case. *Oral Surg Oral Med Oral Pathol* 1973; **35**: 467–71.
3 Pitanguy I. Ascher's syndrome. *Head Neck Surg* 1988; **10**: 309–10.
4 Halling F, Sandrock D, Merten HA *et al.* Das Ascher syndrome. *Dtsch Z Mund Kiefer Gesichtschir* 1991; **15**: 440–4.
5 Ali K. Ascher syndrome: a case report and review of the literature (epub). *Oral Surg Oral Med Oral Pathol Oral Radiol Endod* 2007; **103**: e26–8.

Pseudoxanthoma elasticum

Synonyms
- Systematized elastorrhexis
- Grönblad–Strandberg syndrome

Definition. PXE is an inherited disorder characterized by generalized fragmentation and progressive calcification of elastic tissue in the dermis, blood vessels and Bruch's membrane of the eye. This leads to laxity of the skin, arterial insufficiency and retinal haemorrhage.

Aetiology. Until recently the basic defect was unknown. Because the pathology affects elastic fibres the genes responsible for elastin and microfibrillary proteins were initially studied, but linkage analysis excluded these early candidate genes [1,2]. Positional cloning identified candidate genes on chromosome 16p13.1 and mutations have subsequently been identified in the *MRP6/ABCC6* gene [3–5]. This is a member of the ATP-binding cassette (ABC) family and acts as a transmembrane transporter. Mutations in the gene affect transport of anionic peptides [6]. *ABCC6* is expressed primarily, if not exclusively, in the liver and kidneys and absence of normal *ABCC6* may allow certain metabolic compounds to accumulate, resulting in progressive calcification of elastic fibres. This suggests that PXE may in fact be a primary metabolic disorder with secondary involvement of elastic fibres [7]. Genotype–phenotype analysis has failed to identify any correlation [8].

The inheritance of PXE has been controversial over the past few years, and historically at least five genetic groups have been described [9–11]. With molecular testing it is now apparent that familial inheritance is autosomal recessive and no confirmed autosomal dominant form has yet been shown [12]. Clinical features of PXE can be seen in unambiguously identified heterozygous carriers, and this, as well as pseudodominance, explains some earlier reports of different clinical types and modes of inheritance.

Pathology [13–19]. In the fully developed skin lesions, the elastic fibres in the mid-dermis are clumped, degenerate, fragmented and swollen, and the abnormal fibres stain positively for calcium. The collagen fibres are also abnormal, being split into small fibres.

Similar changes occur in the connective tissue of the media and intima of the blood vessels, Bruch's membrane of the eye, and in the endocardium and pericardium. The heart may occasionally be enlarged, with extensive calcification [20], and pulmonary calcification has been reported [21]. Calcification may occur in other viscera [22].

The vascular involvement may be generalized but may involve predominantly the larger arteries, the mesenteric and visceral arteries, or those of the extremities [23]. Calcification of the internal elastic lamina of the arteries leads to vascular occlusion. Hypertension, angina, myocardial infarction, cerebrovascular accidents and recurrent mucosal haemorrhages may result. The changes in Bruch's membrane give rise to angioid streaks, and rupture of the retinal vessels to haemorrhages and choroiditis.

The complete syndrome consists of the distinctive skin lesions, retinal changes (angioid streaks) and vascular disturbances. The characteristic skin changes and angioid streaks have also been reported as isolated findings, but this is unusual, and in ten patients with angioid streaks but no obvious skin abnormalities, a biopsy of scar tissue, regardless of site, was diagnostic of PXE in six patients, with three also having histological changes in elastic tissue in normal-appearing flexural skin [18]. The relatively low yield from biopsy of normal-looking axillary skin of patients with PXE at other skin sites has also been demonstrated [24].

Skin changes. The skin lesions are characteristic. They consist of small (1–3 mm), yellowish papules in a linear or reticular pattern, in confluent plaques, although the changes are sometimes very subtle. The skin is soft, lax and slightly wrinkled, and may hang in folds, especially in elderly people. There may be a slightly pebbly surface, which has been variously described as a 'cobblestone', 'Moroccan leather' or 'chicken skin' appearance (Fig. 45.16). The sites of predilection are the sides of the neck, below the clavicles, the axillae (Fig. 45.17), abdomen, groins, perineum and thighs. Reticulate pigmentation on the abdomen may occur [25]. Numerous acneiform lesions have been reported [26]. Although usually limited, the eruption may occasionally involve most of the body. It may develop in early childhood, and usually does so before the age of 30 years, but it may also first appear in old age. It usually persists unchanged indefinitely. Similar changes may occur in the soft palate, inside the lips and in the mucous membranes of stomach, rectum and vagina. In the mouth, the lesions may mimic sebaceous glands (Fordyce spots). Rarely, chronic granulomatous nodules have developed in the skin lesions [27].

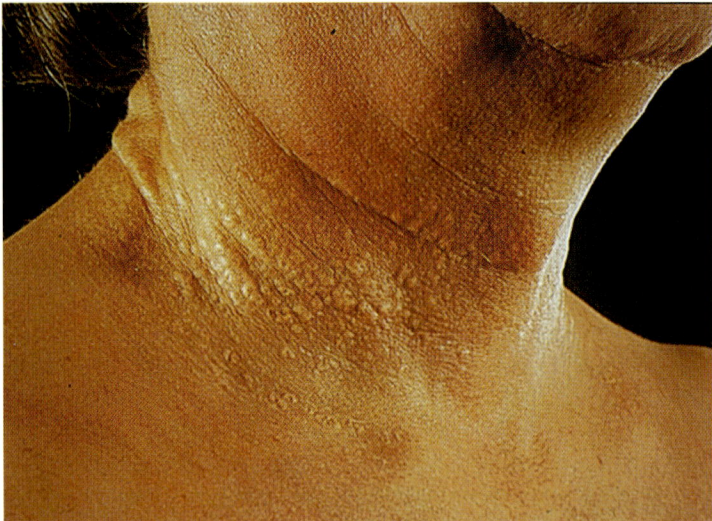

Fig. 45.16 Pseudoxanthoma elasticum, showing the typical 'chicken skin' appearance involving the neck.

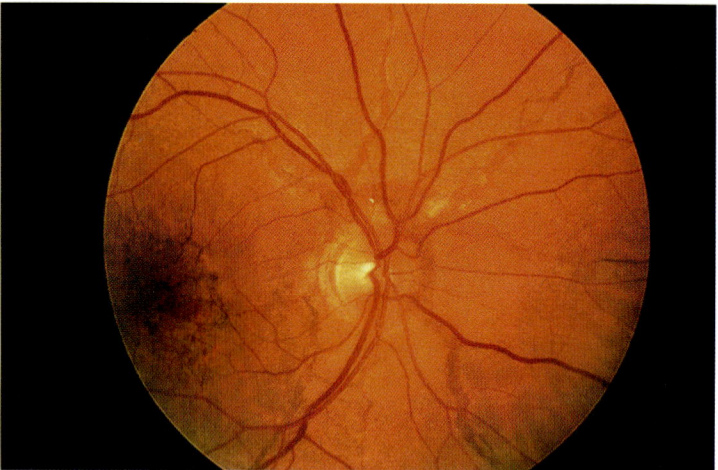

Fig. 45.18 Angioid streaks of the retina in pseudoxanthoma elasticum. (Courtesy of Professor D. Easty, Bristol Eye Hospital, Bristol, UK.)

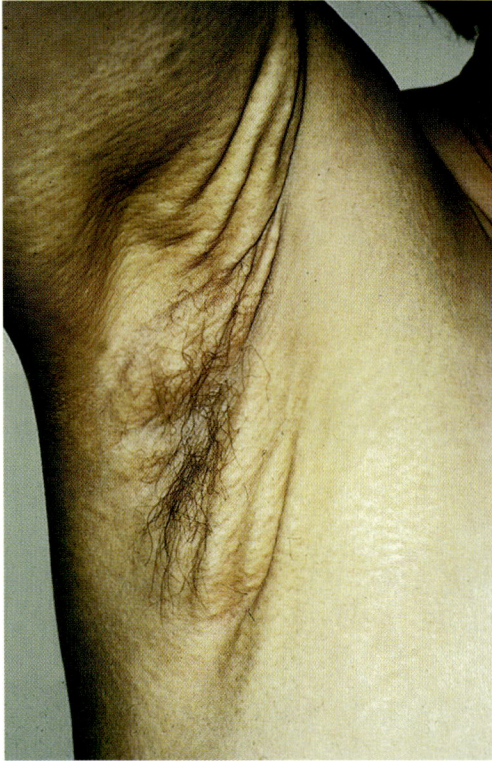

Fig. 45.17 Pseudoxanthoma elasticum of the axilla, showing the characteristic yellow discoloration of the skin and the loose folds. The changes in this condition are often much more subtle than in this patient.

Cardiovascular changes. The arteries throughout the body are affected. There may be intermittent claudication with diminished peripheral pulses, and there is accelerated atheroma, often with hypertension [29]. The circulatory disturbances are detectable by plethysmography or oscillometry, and angiography may show angiomatous malformations, aneurysmal dilatation, and narrowing or occlusion of peripheral or visceral arteries [30]. Signs of arterial degeneration may be seen by the age of 30 years, and death may result from cerebral haemorrhage, coronary occlusion or massive haemorrhage into the gut [31]. Cardiomyopathy has been reported [32,33].

Arterial involvement may not be clinically manifest until adult life, but intermittent claudication and angina have occurred in early childhood. Some patients, however, survive to old age.

Mitral valve prolapse occurs in about 5–8% of the normal population. In one series of 14 patients with PXE, 11 had mitral valve prolapse [34], but these individuals probably had an overlap with Marfanoid features [35].

Ocular changes. Angioid streaks [36,37] of the retina are seen as slate-grey, poorly defined streaks radiating from an incomplete greyish ring surrounding the nerve head (Fig. 45.18). They are bilaterally symmetrical, and usually first appear between the ages of 20 and 40 years. There may be no impairment of vision, but progressive visual failure may occur, and haemorrhages and choroiditis occasionally result in total blindness.

Other associated ocular findings include small, raised, pearly white *drusen*, or punched-out atrophic areas in focal areas of dehiscence of Bruch's membrane [38]. There may also be speckled yellowish mottling at the posterior pole, and this change, which has been called 'leopard spotting', may antedate the angioid streaks [39]. About 50% of patients also have a random scattering of small, round pigment dots throughout the macula and optic nerve [40]. These may resemble a string of pearls in some cases, and they are best seen on fluorescein angiography.

Abnormal visibility of the choroidal vessels has been present in some apparently unaffected members of some families with PXE [41].

Occasionally, there may be spontaneous perforating lesions, with transepidermal elimination of the fragmented elastic fibres. These present as hyperkeratotic papules, which leave a bleeding surface when dislodged.

The presence of an exaggerated mental (chin) crease has recently been shown to be a sensitive and highly specific finding in patients under the age of 30 years with PXE [28].

Obstetric risk. There is an increased risk of miscarriage in the first trimester, possibly related to failure of placental development [42], and abdominal striae develop during pregnancy in virtually all patients [43]. Opinions differ regarding the risk to the mother. Berde *et al.* [44] reviewed the literature and concluded that there was a serious risk of cardiovascular complications during pregnancy, but Viljoen *et al.* [43] reported 54 pregnancies in which there were no serious maternal complications. Subsequent reports also agree that although skin manifestations may worsen, the risks of pregnancy have been overstated [45].

Associated abnormalities. In most cases of PXE the serum calcium and phosphate levels are normal, but in a few patients the phosphate levels are increased, with mild hypercalcaemia and abnormalities of vitamin D metabolism [22,46]. The biochemical changes resemble those of tumoral calcinosis [47], although the clinical changes are those of PXE. This seems to be a distinctive, rare type of PXE which may be associated with renal failure in other members of the family. Some of these patients also have systemic sclerosis [48].

Other patients have been reported with multiple, calcified cutaneous nodules, with angioid streaks and hyperphosphataemia, but without pseudoxanthoma [49].

Skin changes of PXE and/or angioid streaks are occasionally seen in patients with osteitis deformans (Paget's disease). Pseudoxanthoma elasticum has also been reported in association with osteoectasia, which is characterized by dwarfism, bizarre radiographic changes and elevated serum alkaline phosphatase levels [50].

The development of both clinical and histopathological PXE-like changes, involving skin, eyes and vasculature, in sickle cell disease and β-thalassaemia has been well documented [51]. The abnormalities are most probably acquired and related to the consequences of the primary disease. The clinical features are of later onset and milder than in inherited PXE.

The typical features of PXE have been reported in a patient with true Marfan's syndrome, but it is likely that this is a chance association [52].

A group of patients with PXE-like phenotype with cutis laxa and deficiency of vitamin K-dependent clotting factors has been identified without causal mutations in *ABCC6* or *VKORC1* (vitamin K 2,3 epoxide reductase) [53]. This suggests a separate clinical and genetic entity.

Diagnosis. The clinical and histological changes of PXE are often distinctive, and the diagnosis is usually readily made when skin lesions are present. The disseminated form of dermatofibrosis lenticularis (Buschke–Ollendorff) can be clinically similar, and juvenile elastoma, which is a feature of this condition, shows thickened elastic fibres on histology. If laxity of the involved skin is extreme, other forms of dermatochalasis must be excluded.

In cases without skin lesions the diagnosis may be difficult, and attempts have been made to establish diagnostic criteria [1,19]. These are summarized in Table 45.2. It should be suspected in obliterative arterial disease of early onset and in unexplained gastrointestinal haemorrhage. The presence of angioid streaks or mucosal lesions should be sought. A skin biopsy from the side of

Table 45.2 Diagnostic criteria for pseudoxanthoma elasticum (PXE). (From Lebwohl *et al.* [19].)

Major criteria
1 Flexural yellow cobblestone lesions
2 Characteristic histological features of lesional skin, using elastic tissue and calcium stains (e.g. van Gieson and von Kossa)
3 Angioid streaks in the retina

Minor criteria
4 Characteristic histological changes in non-lesional skin
5 Family history of PXE in first-degree relatives

the neck may be helpful, even if there are no clinically evident changes, although the characteristic histological changes are not necessarily diagnostic [18,19]. The diagnosis can be difficult in the presence of marked solar elastosis and/or macular degeneration [54]. Soft-tissue or vascular calcification may be detectable radiologically [55], and angiography may be helpful [30]. Ultrasonography can detect early renal parenchymal calcification, although its prognostic significance remains uncertain [56].

Definitive diagnosis is made by molecular analysis of the *ABCC6* gene. This also provides a means for prenatal and presymptomatic testing in families at risk for recurrence [7,8]. Emerging evidence also suggests that heterozygosity for an *ABCC6* mutation (*R1141X*) confers a fourfold risk of developing coronary artery disease [57].

Treatment. It is important that the condition is accurately diagnosed so that appropriate genetic advice may be given. The most important aspect of treatment is to ensure that complications from vascular involvement are prevented or dealt with speedily by the appropriate specialist. Ophthalmologists will recommend that the patient learns to use an Amsler grid in the early detection of visual loss. Patients should avoid any activity that might cause sudden increase in blood pressure or contact injury to the eyes. Laser photocoagulation may be helpful in preventing further retinal haemorrhage. Cardiovascular risks should be minimized with control of blood pressure and serum lipids, and avoidance of smoking. The cosmetic appearance of the skin lesions may be improved by plastic surgery. Restriction of dietary calcium has been tried, with apparent benefit in some cases [47], but this treatment remains controversial.

References

1 Christiano AM, Lebwohl MG, Boyd CD *et al.* Workshop on pseudoxanthoma elasticum: molecular biology and pathology of the elastic fibres (Jefferson Medical College, Philadelphia). *J Invest Dermatol* 1992; **99**: 660–3.
2 Christiano AM, Uitto J. Molecular pathology of the elastic fibres. *J Invest Dermatol* 1994; **103**: S53–7.
3 Le Saux O, Urban Z, Tschuch C *et al.* Mutations in a gene encoding an ABC transporter cause pseudoxanthoma elasticum. *Nat Genet* 2000; **25**: 223–7.
4 Bergen AAB, Plomp AS, Schuurman EJ *et al.* Mutations in *ABCC6* cause pseudoxanthoma elasticum. *Nat Genet* 2000; **25**: 228–31.
5 Ringpfeil F, Lebwohl MG, Christiano AM *et al.* Pseudoxanthoma elasticum: mutations in the *MRP6* gene encoding a transmembrane ATP binding cassette (ABC) transporter. *Proc Natl Acad Sci USA* 2000; **97**: 6001–6.
6 Ilias A, Urban Z, Seidl TL *et al.* Loss of ATP-dependent transport actvitiy in pseudoxanthoma elasticum-associated mutants of human *ABCC6* (MRP6). *J Biol Chem* 2002; **277**: 16860–7.

7 Ringpfeil F, Pulkkinen L, Uitto J. Molecular genetics of pseudoxanthoma elasticum. *Exp Dermatol* 2001; **10**: 221–8.

8 Pfender EG, Vanakker O, Terry SF *et al*. Mutation detection in the *ABCC6* gene and genotype-phenotype analysis in a large international case series affected by pseudoxanthoma elasticum. *J Med Genet* 2007; **44**: 621–8.

9 Pope FM. Historical evidence for the genetic heterogeneity of pseudoxanthoma elasticum. *Br J Dermatol* 1975; **92**: 493–509.

10 Viljoen DL, Beighton P, Mabin T *et al*. Pseudoxanthoma elasticum in South Africa—genetic and clinical implications. *S Afr Med J* 1984; **66**: 813–6.

11 Viljoen DL, Pope FM, Beighton P *et al*. Heterogenicity of pseudoxanthoma elasticum: delineation of a new form? *Clin Genet* 1987; **32**: 100–5.

12 Ringpfeil F, McGuigan K, Fuchsel L *et al*. Pseudoxanthoma elasticum is a recessive disease characterized by compound heterozygosity. *J Invest Dermatol* 2006; **126**: 782–6.

13 Altman LK, Shenhav R, Schaudinischky L. Pseudoxanthoma elasticum. An underdiagnosed genetically heterogeneous disorder with protean manifestations. *Arch Intern Med* 1974; **134**: 1048–54.

14 Eddy DD, Farber EM. Pseudoxanthoma elasticum. Internal manifestations: case-reports and literature review. *Arch Dermatol* 1962; **86**: 729–40.

15 Goodman RM, Smith EW, Paton D *et al*. Pseudoxanthoma elasticum: a clinical and histopathological study. *Medicine* 1963; **42**: 297–334.

16 Gordon SG, Subryan VL, Solomons CC *et al*. *In vitro* uptake of calcium in dermis of patients with pseudoxanthoma elasticum. *J Lab Clin Med* 1975; **86**: 638–40.

17 Pasquali-Ronchetti I, Volpin D, Baccarani CM *et al*. Pseudoxanthoma elasticum. Biochemical and ultrastructural studies. *Dermatologica* 1981; **163**: 307–25.

18 Lebwohl M, Phelps RG, Yannuzzi L *et al*. Diagnosis of pseudoxanthoma elasticum in patients without characteristic skin lesions. *N Engl J Med* 1987; **317**: 347–50.

19 Lebwohl M, Nelder K, Pope FM *et al*. Classification of pseudoxanthoma elasticum. Report of a consensus conference. *J Am Acad Dermatol* 1994; **30**: 103–7.

20 Fang ML, Astarita RN, Steinman H. Cardiac calcifications and yellow papules in a young man. *Arch Dermatol* 1988; **124**: 1559–64.

21 Jackson A, Loh CL. Pulmonary calcification and elastic tissue damage in pseudoxanthoma elasticum. *Histopathology* 1980; **4**: 607–11.

22 Cnudde F, Muller P, Hajjar C *et al*. Pseudoxanthome élastique avec calcifications multiples et hyperphosphoremie. *Ann Dermatol Vénéréol* 1996; **123**: 563–6.

23 Bardsley JL, Ruben-Koehler P. Pseudoxanthoma elasticum: angiographic manifestations in abdominal vessels. *Radiology* 1969; **93**: 559–62.

24 Brown SJ, Talks SJ, Needham SJ *et al*. Pseudoxanthoma elasticum: biopsy of clinically normal skin in the investigation of patients with angioid streaks. *Br J Dermatol* 2007; **157**: 748–51.

25 Li T-H, Tseng C-R, Hsiao G-H. An unusual cutaneous manifestation of pseudoxanthoma elasticum mimicking reticulate pigmentary disorders. *Br J Dermatol* 1966; **134**: 1157–9.

26 Hartman A, Hartman-Visser SR. Pseudoxanthoma elasticum with extensive comedo formation. *Dermatologica* 1977; **154**: 318–9.

27 Heyl T. Pseudoxanthoma elasticum with granulomatous skin lesions. *Arch Dermatol* 1967; **96**: 528–31.

28 Lebwohl M, Lebwohl E, Bercovitch L. Prominent mental (chin) crease: a new sign of pseudoxanthoma elasticum. *J Am Acad Dermatol* 2003; **48**: 620–2.

29 Parker JC, Friedman-Kien AE, Levin S *et al*. Pseudoxanthoma elasticum and hypertension. *N Engl J Med* 1964; **271**: 1204–7.

30 Belli A, Cawthorne S. Visceral angiographic findings in pseudoxanthoma elasticum. *Br J Radiol* 1988; **61**: 368–71.

31 Kundrotas L, Novak J, Kremzier J *et al*. Gastric bleeding in pseudoxanthoma elasticum. *Am J Gastroenterol* 1988; **83**: 868–72.

32 Navarro-Lopez F, Llorian A, Ferrer-Roca O *et al*. Restrictive cardiomyopathy in pseudoxanthoma elasticum. *Chest* 1980; **78**: 113–5.

33 Przybojewski JZ, Hoffman H, de Graaf AS *et al*. Pseudoxanthoma elasticum with cardiac involvement. A case report and review of the literature. *S Afr Med J* 1981; **59**: 268–75.

34 Lebwohl MJ, Distefano D, Prioleau PG. Pseudoxanthoma elasticum and mitral-valve prolapse. *N Engl J Med* 1982; **307**: 228–31.

35 Pyeritz RE, Weiss JL, Rennie W *et al*. Pseudoxanthoma elasticum and mitral valve prolapse. *N Engl J Med* 1982; **307**: 1451–2.

36 Connor PJ, Juergeens JL, Perry HO *et al*. Pseudoxanthoma elasticum and angioid streaks. A review of 106 cases. *Am J Med* 1961; **30**: 537–43.

37 McWilliam RJ. Classification of angioid streaks. *Br J Ophthalmol* 1955; **39**: 298–300.

38 Clarkson JG, Altmann RD. Angioid streaks. *Surv Ophthalmol* 1982; **26**: 235–46.

39 Gills JP, Paton D. Mottled fundus oculi in pseudoxanthoma elasticum. *Arch Ophthalmol* 1963; **73**: 792–5.

40 McDonald HR, Schatz H, Aarberg TM. Reticular-like pigmentary patterns in pseudoxanthoma elasticum. *Ophthalmology* 1988; **95**: 306–11.

41 Berlyne GM, Bulmer MG, Platt R. The genetics of pseudoxanthoma elasticum. *QJM* 1961; **30**: 201–12.

42 Elejalda BR, de Elejalda MM, Samter T *et al*. Manifestations of pseudoxanthoma elasticum during pregnancy: a case report and review of the literature. *Am J Med Genet* 1984; **18**: 755–62.

43 Viljoen DL, Beatty S, Beighton P. The obstetric and gynaecological implications of pseudoxanthoma elasticum. *Br J Obstet Gynaecol* 1987; **94**: 884–8.

44 Berde C, Willis DC, Sandberg EC. Pregnancy in women with pseudoxanthoma elasticum. *Obstet Gynaecol Surg* 1983; **38**: 339–44.

45 Yoles A, Phelps R, Lebwohl M. Pseudoxanthoma elasticum and pregnancy. *Cutis* 1996; **58**: 161–4.

46 Mallette LE, Mechanick JI. Heritable syndrome of pseudoxanthoma elasticum with abnormal phosphorus and vitamin D metabolism. *Am J Med* 1987; **83**: 1157–62.

47 Prince MJ, Schaefer H, Goldsmith RS *et al*. Hyperphosphatemic tumoral calcinosis. *Ann Intern Med* 1982; **96**: 586–91.

48 Pai SH, Zak FG. Concurrence of pseudoxanthoma elasticum, elastosis perforans serpiginosa and systemic sclerosis. *Dermatologica* 1970; **140**: 54–9.

49 McPhaull JJ, Engel FL. Heterotopic calcification, hyperphosphataemia and angioid streaks of the retina. *Am J Med* 1961; **31**: 488–9.

50 Saxe N, Beighton P. Cutaneous manifestations of osteoectasia. *Clin Exp Dermatol* 1982; **7**: 605–9.

51 Aessopos A, Farmakis D, Loukopoulos D. Elastic tissue abnormalities resembling pseudoxanthoma elasticum in β thalassemia and the sickling syndromes. *Blood* 2002; **99**: 30–5.

52 Hidano A, Nakajima S, Shimizu T, Kimata Z. Pseudoxanthoma elasticum associated with Marfan syndrome. *Ann Dermatol Vénéréol* 1979; **106**: 503–5.

53 Vanakker OM, Martin L, Gheduzzi D *et al*. Pseudoxanthoma elasticum-like phenotype with cutis laxa and multiple coagulation factor deficiency represents a separate genetic entity. *J Invest Dermatol* 2007; **127**: 581–7.

54 Christen-Zäch S, Huber M, Lindpainter K *et al*. Pseudoxanthoma elasticum: evaluation of diagnostic criteria based on molecular data. *Br J Dermatol* 2006; **155**: 89–93.

55 James AE, Eaton SB, Blazek JV *et al*. Roentgen findings in pseudoxanthoma elasticum. *Am J Roentgenol* 1969; **106**: 642–4.

56 Crespi G, Derchi LE, Saffioti S. Sonographic detection of renal changes in pseudoxanthoma elasticum. *Urol Radiol* 1992; **13**: 223–5.

57 Trip MD, Smulders YM, Wegman JJ *et al*. Frequent mutation in the *ABCC6* gene (*R1141X*) is associated with a strong increase in the prevalence of coronary artery disease. *Circulation* 2002; **106**: 773–5.

Acquired PXE-like syndromes

Perforating PXE

Synonym
• Perforating calcific elastosis

Transepithelial elimination (TEE) of altered elastic fibres can occasionally occur in generalized hereditary forms of PXE (see above), but it can also occur as a localized, acquired defect in patients who do not have the other features of PXE [1]. These localized lesions usually occur in the periumbilical area in obese, multiparous black women, and it is possible that this represents a response to repeated cutaneous stretching, for example ascites or previous abdominal surgery [2,3]. Similar lesions on the breast have been reported in patients undergoing haemodialysis [4,5].

Clinically, asymptomatic yellow macules and papules coalesce into well-demarcated, hyperpigmented plaques which slowly enlarge. The surface may be atrophic, grooved, fissured or verrucous, and compression of the edge of the lesion may produce a liquid discharge.

It seems likely that most cases previously described as elastosis perforans serpiginosa in association with PXE were really examples of perforating PXE [6]. The histology of the two conditions is similar, but in perforating PXE there is TEE of altered basophilic, calcified, elastic fibres, which are short, fragmented, curled and predominantly in the mid-dermis, whereas in elastosis perforans serpiginosa the fibres are abnormally large, non-calcified, eosinophilic and straight.

Spontaneous resolution has been reported [7].

References

1 Premathala S, Yesudian P, Thambiah AS. Periumbilical pseudoxanthoma elasticum with transepithelial elimination. *Int J Dermatol* 1982; **10**: 604–5.
2 Kazakis AM, Parish WR. Periumbilical perforating pseudoxanthoma elasticum. *J Am Acad Dermatol* 1988; **19**: 384–8.
3 Somarsundaram V, Premathala S, Rao NR *et al.* Periumbilical perforating pseudoxanthoma elasticum. *Int J Dermatol* 1987; **26**: 536–7.
4 Nickoloff BJ, Noodleman FR, Abel EA. Perforating pseudoxanthoma elasticum associated with chronic renal failure and haemodialysis. *Arch Dermatol* 1985; **121**: 1321–2.
5 Kazakis AM, Parish WR. Periumbilical perforating pseudoxanthoma elasticum. *J Am Acad Dermatol* 1988; **19**: 384–8.
6 Lund HZ, Gilbert CF. Perforating pseudoxanthoma elasticum. Its distinction from elastosis perforans serpiginosa. *Arch Pathol Lab Med* 1976; **100**: 544–6.
7 Sueki H, Amemiya M, Watanaba H *et al.* Spontaneous resolution in a case of pseudo-pseudoxanthoma elasticum. *Br J Dermatol* 2001; **144**: 213–5.

Pseudo-PXE

Skin changes which are virtually identical to those of PXE can rarely be produced by penicillamine, although the systemic features do not occur [1]. The skin changes can be explained by the known effect of penicillamine in inhibiting collagen and elastin cross-linking, with the production of vastly increased amounts of abnormal elastin in the dermis [2]. Transepidermal extrusion of elastin has been reported in this condition [3]. Lesions clinically resembling PXE are reported in the eosinophilia–myalgia syndrome; dermal calcification is absent on histology [4]. Yellowish papules and plaques resembling PXE are seen in some patients with amyloidosis; amyloid deposits are seen and, again, dermal calcification is absent [5,6].

References

1 Burge S, Ryan T. Penicillamine-induced pseudo-pseudoxanthoma elasticum in a patient with rheumatoid arthritis. *Clin Exp Dermatol* 1988; **13**: 255–8.
2 Light N, Meyrick-Thomas RH, Stephens A *et al.* Collagen and elastin changes in D-penicillamine-induced pseudoxanthoma elasticum-like skin. *Br J Dermatol* 1986; **114**: 381–8.
3 Meyrick-Thomas RH, Kirby JDT. Elastosis perforans serpiginosa and pseudoxanthoma elasticum-like skin changes due to d-penicillamine. *Clin Exp Dermatol* 1985; **10**: 386–91.
4 Mainetti C, Masouye I, Saurat JH. Pseudoxanthoma elasticum-like lesions in the L-tryptophan- induced eosinophilia-myalgia syndrome. *J Am Acad Dermatol* 1991; **24**: 657–8.
5 Winkelmann RK, Peters MS, Venencie PY. Amyloid elastosis. A new cutaneous and systemic pattern of amyloidosis. *Arch Dermatol* 1985; **121**: 498–502.
6 Vecchietti G, Masouye I, Salomon D *et al.* An unusual form of primary systemic amyloidosis: amyloid elastosis—report of a case treated by haematopoietic cell transplantation. *Br J Dermatol* 2003: **145**: 154–9.

Saltpetre disease [1–3]

A condition which resembles the skin changes of PXE clinically, histologically and ultrastructurally has been described in a group of elderly farmers, who decades earlier had spread a fertilizer containing calcium-ammonium nitrate (Norwegian saltpetre). The patients developed cutaneous ulcers at sites of exposure (including antecubital fossae). These quickly healed to leave yellowish-white papules and plaques. None of the patients had a positive family history or other signs of PXE.

References

1 Christensen OB. An exogenous variety of pseudoxanthoma elasticum in old farmers. *Acta Derm Venereol Suppl (Stockh)* 1978; **58**: 319–22.
2 Neilson AO, Christensen OB, Hentzer B *et al.* Saltpetre-induced dermal changes electron microscopically indistinguishable from pseudoxanthoma elasticum. *Acta Derm Venereol Suppl (Stockh)* 1978; **58**: 323–7.
3 Neri I, Marzaduri S, Berdazzi F *et al.* Exogenous pseudoxanthoma elasticum: a new case in an old farmer. *Acta Derm Venereol* 1993; **78**: 153–4.

Williams–Beuren syndrome

The Williams–Beuren syndrome is a developmental disorder characterized by premature laxity of the skin, congenital heart disease (notably supravalvular aortic stenosis), metabolic abnormalities and dysmorphic facial features, which include baggy connective tissue around the eyes, full cheeks, prominent lips and dental malocclusion [1]. Delayed motor and perceptual development are sometimes masked by above-average language skills allied to a 'cocktail party' personality [2].

In situ hybridization techniques have revealed both inherited and new deletions at the elastin locus on chromosome 7q11.23 [3]. Size heterogeneity of the deletion exists, with multiorgan involvement as a consequence of contiguous gene deletions. At least 24 genes may be involved in the critical region [4]. Only the elastin gene deletion is associated with a specific phenotype (supravalvular aortic stenosis). An 'epidemic' of the Williams' syndrome was reported in the UK following the administration of excessive doses of vitamin D to prevent rickets in pregnant women [5]. Vitamin D is known to downregulate elastin gene expression [6].

References

1 Morris CA, Dilts C, Dempsey SA *et al.* The natural history of Williams syndrome: physical characteristics. *J Pediatr* 1988; **113**: 318–26.
2 Giddins NG, Finley JP, Nanton MA *et al.* The natural course of supravalvular aortic stenosis and peripheral pulmonary artery stenosis in Williams syndrome. *Br Heart J* 1989; **62**: 315–9.
3 Ewart AK, Morris CA, Atkinson D *et al.* Hemizygosity at the elastin locus in a developmental disorder: Williams syndrome. *Nat Genet* 1993; **5**: 11–6.
4 Tassabehji M. Williams-Beuren syndrome: a challenge for genotype-phenotype correlations. *Hum Mol Genet* 2003; **12**: R229–37.
5 Lightwood R, Sheldon W, Harris C *et al.* Hypercalcaemia in infants and vitamin D. *BMJ* 1965; **2**: 149.
6 Christiano AM, Uitto J. Molecular pathology of the elastic fibres. *J Invest Dermatol* 1994; **103** (Suppl.): S53–7.

Linear focal elastosis

Synonym
• Elastotic striae

This condition is characterized by asymptomatic, yellow, linear bands arranged horizontally on the lower back [1–4]. It less commonly occurs on the lower limbs and shoulders. Superficially, the lesions resemble striae distensae, but they are palpable rather than depressed and yellow rather than purplish or white. Although the two conditions are generally unrelated, linear focal elastosis has been reported adjacent to striae distensae [5], and in one case following potent topical corticosteroids [6]. The condition was originally described in elderly males [1], although it has been reported in a young black male whose father was similarly affected [7]. It may be commoner than is suggested by the paucity of reports. Ultrastructural studies reveal active elastogenesis. The middle and lower dermal collagen is separated by bluish grey, fine, fibrillar material, which is composed of thin, wavy elastic fibres and fragmented elastic fibre bundles. Early lesions may, in contrast, show elastolysis, with decreased elastin and microfibrillar proteins [8]. The elastic fibres are near to, or even in contact with, fibroblasts [9], and elastogenesis may occur in response to local trauma, ultraviolet light or perhaps following the development of striae distensae [10]. However, these mechanisms do not adequately explain the increasing number of cases reported, particularly in the young, and it may be that intrinsic defects of elastic fibre metabolism play a role [4].

References

1 Burket JM, Zelickson AS, Padilla RS. Linear focal elastosis (elastotic striae). *J Am Acad Dermatol* 1989; **20**: 633–6.
2 Vogel PS, Cardenas A, Ross EV *et al.* Linear focal elastosis. *Arch Dermatol* 1995; **131**: 855–6.
3 Kanitakis J, Chouvet B, Dupin M *et al.* Linear focal elastosis. *Eur J Dermatol* 1997; **7**: 300–2.
4 Péc J, Chromej I. Linear focal elastosis: what's new? *J Eur Acad Dermatol Venereol* 2004; **18**: 247–9.
5 White G. Linear focal elastosis: a degenerative or regenerative process of striae distensae. *J Am Acad Dermatol* 1992; **22**: 468.
6 Neve S, Kirtschig G. Elastotic striae associated with striae distensae after application of very potent topical corticosteroids. *Clin Exp Dermatol* 2006; **31**: 452–82.
7 Moiin A, Hashimoto K. Linear focal elastosis in a young black man: a new presentation. *J Am Acad Dermatol* 1994; **30**: 874–7.
8 Choi SW, Lee JH, Woo HJ *et al.* Two cases of linear focal elastosis: different histopathologic findings. *Int J Dermatol* 2000; **39**: 207–9.
9 Hagari Y, Mihara M, Morimura T *et al.* Linear focal elastosis: an ultrastructural study. *Arch Dermatol* 1991; **127**: 1365–8.
10 Hashimoto K. Linear focal elastosis: keloidal repair of striae distensae. *J Am Acad Dermatol* 1998; **39**: 309–13.

Late-onset focal dermal elastosis

Yellowish papules with a *peau d'orange* appearance appear on the flexures. Clinically and histologically the lesions resemble elastomas, but this rare condition has only been reported in elderly Japanese men [1,2].

References

1 Tajima S, Shimizu K, Izumi T *et al.* Late-onset focal dermal elastosis: clinical and histological features. *Br J Dermatol* 1995; **133**: 303–5.
2 Limas C. Late onset focal dermal elastosis: a distinct clinicopathologic entity? *Am J Dermatopathol* 1999; **21**: 381–3.

Actinic elastosis

Synonym
• Solar elastosis

Definition. This is a degenerative change in the dermis caused by prolonged exposure to electromagnetic (usually solar) radiation.

It is characterized clinically by yellowish discoloration and histologically by degeneration of elastic fibres.

Aetiology. Actinic elastosis usually results from prolonged exposure to sunlight, but it can also result from infrared (IR) radiation [1,2]. It is related to the cumulative dose of radiation, as it is more common in older people, outdoor workers and in sunny climates. There is, however, considerable variation in susceptibility between individuals. Fair-skinned people are the worst affected, although the condition can occur in black people [3,4]. Severe elastosis may occur in photosensitized skin, for example in porphyria cutanea tarda. UVB wavelengths are the most likely to cause solar elastosis, although UVA and PUVA therapy can also accentuate it [5,6].

Ageing normal skin becomes atrophic, with fewer elastic fibres [3]. In contrast, sun-damaged ('photo-aged') skin exhibits hypertrophy of elastic tissue, secondary to a prolonged inflammatory process [7]. Skin on the back of the neck exposed to chronic UV radiation shows partially degranulated mast cells in close apposition to fibroblasts. Metalloproteinases produced by mast cells and macrophages degrade skin collagen [8].

Pathology [9,10]. At an early stage, there is a perivenular lymphohistiocytic infiltrate, with degranulating mast cells [7,11]. The vessel walls become thickened due to deposition of a basement-membrane-like material [4]. The elastic fibres of the upper and middle dermis then become curled and fibrillar to form thick, irregular masses [12]. At a later stage, the elastotic degeneration becomes more diffuse, forming long, swollen bands of irregular texture, with finely granular elastin and dense microfibrillar masses. Actinic elastosis originates in elastic fibres rather than collagen, as shown by the findings that the abnormal fibres stain with antielastin antibody HB8, disappear with elastase but resist collagenolytic enzymes, and have a high desmosine content.

In the early stages of actinic elastosis, there is also an increase in collagen and in glycosaminoglycans, although ultimately fibrillar (types I and III) procollagens decrease. Anchoring fibrils (collagen type VII) and the fibrillin-rich microfibrils at the dermoepidermal junction are also reduced [13–15]. Collagenolytic enzymes, notably matrix metalloproteinase-I, are increased [16]. Eventually, the fibrous network degenerates into an amorphous, elastotic mass, and the dermal blood vessels become sparse and tortuous [3,4]. Increased dermal glycosaminoglycans are deposited on the elastotic material in the superficial dermis [17].

Clinical features. The condition is more common in later life. In temperate climates, it is rare before the fourth decade, but it starts earlier and is more severe in sunnier climates. The light-exposed areas are affected, particularly the forehead and the back of the neck. Mild degrees of elastosis may not be apparent until the skin is pinched up, when it may assume a wrinkled appearance. Elastosis is usually more advanced in the tissue than the clinical appearance would suggest.

The affected skin is diffusely thickened and yellowish (Fig. 45.19), and on the neck it may be divided by well-defined furrows into an irregular rhomboidal pattern (cutis rhomboidalis nuchae). There may also be more sharply marginated, thickened plaques on the face or neck. These are usually, but not always, symmetrical.

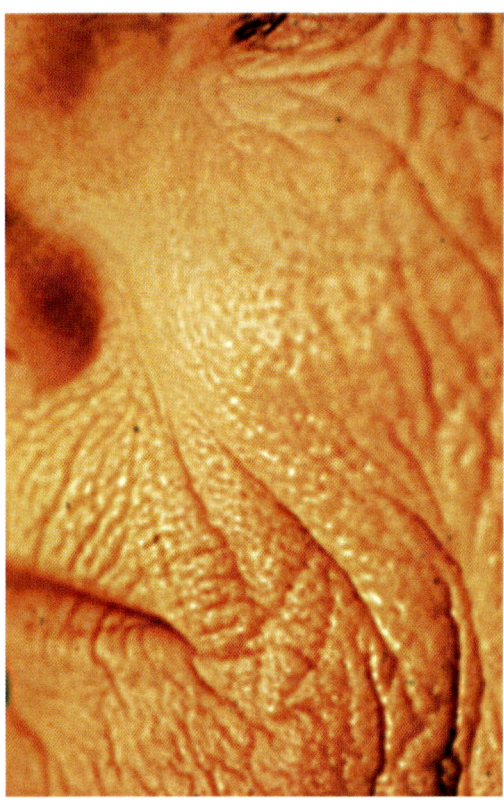

Fig. 45.19 Actinic (solar) elastosis, showing the characteristic yellowish discoloration, thickening and wrinkling of the facial skin.

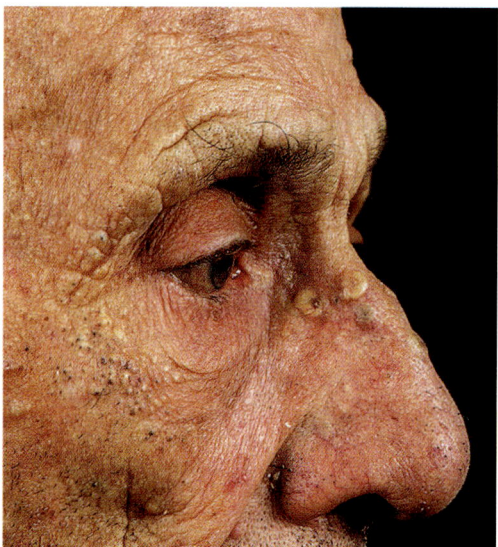

Fig. 45.20 Favre–Racouchot syndrome, showing comedones and actinic elastosis. (Courtesy of Professor R. Marks, St Vincent's Hospital, Melbourne, Victoria, Australia.)

When the skin around the orbits is affected, it is often studded with numerous comedones, and this has been called the *Favre–Racouchot syndrome* (Fig. 45.20). Favre–Racouchot syndrome is usually confined to facial skin and is bilaterally symmetrical, but unilateral and circumscribed forms have been reported [18]. The term actinic-comedonal plaque has been suggested for similar lesions which can rarely occur on other parts of the body, such as the forearm [19,20].

Skin which is affected by actinic elastosis is likely to develop other signs of sun damage, including irregular pigmentation, wrinkling, scaling, solar keratoses and malignancy. This range of changes due to chronic sun damage has been called *dermatoheliosis* [21].

Actinic elastosis may also be complicated by actinic granuloma (see below).

Photodamage is markedly exacerbated in smokers [22].

Diagnosis. Plane xanthoma, PXE and colloid milium may sometimes cause confusion, but the combination of the clinical and histological features is distinctive.

Treatment. Sunscreens protect against the development of photodamage both in humans and animals [23]. In hairless mice exposed to UVB radiation, synthesis of subepidermal collagen has been demonstrated in animals protected with a sunscreen [24]. Topical application of α-hydroxy acids ('fruit acids'), that is lactic, glycolic and citric acids, led to a modest improvement in photodamaged skin [25]. More impressive results have been obtained with topically applied tretinoin cream [26–28]. A double-blind study [29] demonstrated a decrease in papillary dermal collagen type I in photodamaged skin, and subsequent treatment with 0.1% tretinoin cream for 10–12 months resulted in an 80% increase in dermal collagen. Several studies have shown clinical and histological improvement after prolonged use [23]. Tretinoin may also repair skin changes due to intrinsic ageing [29,30]. Retinoids reduce MMP-1 expression *in vitro,* partially restoring levels of fibrillin-1 and collagens I and VII in the papillary dermis [27,31]. Similar results have been obtained in double-blind trials of topical isotretinoin [32] and tazarotene cream [33]. There has been interest in the use of so-called non-ablative lasers, including the 1320-nm Nd:YAG and 1540-nm erbium glass lasers, which are claimed to wound the upper dermis without epidermal damage [34]. Restoration of fibrillin-I in the microfibrillar network of the papillary dermis may prove a useful 'biomarker' for the efficacy of topical products used in the treatment of actinic elastosis [35,36].

References

1 Finlayson GR, Sams WM Jr, Smith JG. Erythema ab igne: a histopathological study. *J Invest Dermatol* 1966; **46**: 104–8.
2 Kligman AM. Early destructive effects of sunlight on human skin. *J Am Acad Dermatol* 1969; **210**: 2377–80.
3 Braverman IM, Fonferko E. Studies in cutaneous aging. I. The elastic fiber network. *J Invest Dermatol* 1982; **78**: 434–43.
4 Braverman IM, Fonferko E. Studies in cutaneous aging. II. The microvasculature. *J Invest Dermatol* 1982; **78**: 444–8.
5 Kumakiri M, Hashimoto K, Willis I. Biologic changes due to long-wave ultraviolet radiation in human skin. *J Invest Dermatol* 1977; **69**: 392–400.
6 Pfau RG, Hood AF, Morison WL. Photoageing: the role of UVB, solarsimulated UVB and psoralen PUVA. *Br J Dermatol* 1986; **114**: 319–27.
7 Lavker RM, Kligman AM. Chronic heliodermatitis: a morphologic evaluation of chronic actinic dermal damage with emphasis on the role of the mast cells. *J Invest Dermatol* 1988; **90**: 325–30.
8 Fisher GJ, Kang S, Varami J *et al.* Mechanisms of photoaging and chronological skin aging. *Arch Dermatol* 2002; **138**: 1467–70.
9 Carter VH, Constantine VS, Poole WL. Elastotic nodules of the antihelix. *Arch Dermatol* 1969; **100**: 282–5.

10 Mitchell RE. Chronic solar dermatosis: a light and electron microscopic study of the dermis. *J Invest Dermatol* 1967; **48**: 203–20.

11 Lavker RM. Structural alterations in exposed and unexposed aged skin. *J Invest Dermatol* 1979; **73**: 59–66.

12 Bouissou H, Pieraggi M-T, Julian M, Savit T. The elastic tissue of the skin. A comparison of spontaneous and actinic (solar) aging. *Int J Dermatol* 1988; **27**: 327–35.

13 Tolwar HS, Griffiths CEM, Fisher GJ *et al.* Reduced type I and type III procollagen in photodamaged adult human skin. *J Invest Dermatol* 1995; **105**: 285–90.

14 Craven NM, Watson REB, Jones CJP *et al.* Clinical features of photodamaged skin are associated with a reduction in collagen VII. *Br J Dermatol* 1997; **137**: 344–50.

15 Watson REB, Griffiths CEM, Craven NM *et al.* Fibrillin-rich microfibrils are reduced in photoaged skin distribution at the dermal-epidermal junction. *J Invest Dermatol* 1999; **112**: 782–7.

16 Brennan M, Bhatti H, Nerusu KC *et al.* Matrix metalloproteinase-1 is the major collagenolytic enzyme responsible for collagen damage in UV-irradiated human skin. *Photochem Photobiol* 2003; **78**: 43–8.

17 Bernstein EF, Underhill CB, Hahn PJ *et al.* Chronic sun exposure alters both the content and distribution of dermal glycosaminoglycans. *Br J Dermatol* 1996; **135**: 255–62.

18 Wojno T, Tenzel RR. Actinic comedonal plaque of the eye. *Am J Ophthalmol* 1983; **96**: 687–8.

19 Eastern JS, Martin S. Actinic comedonal plaque. *J Am Acad Dermatol* 1988; **3**: 633–6.

20 John SM, Hamm H. Actinic comedonal plaque. A rare ectopic form of the Favre–Racouchot syndrome. *Clin Exp Dermatol* 1993; **18**: 256–8.

21 Sams WM. Sun-induced aging. Clinical and laboratory observations in man. *Dermatol Clin* 1986; **4**: 509–16.

22 Davis BE, Koh HK. Faces going up in smoke. A dermatologic opportunity for cancer prevention. *Arch Dermatol* 1992; **128**: 255–62.

23 Gilchrest BA. A review of skin ageing and its medical therapy. *Br J Dermatol* 1996; **135**: 867–75.

24 Kligman LH. Connective tissue photo-damage in hairless mice is potentially reversible. *J Invest Dermatol* 1987; **88**: S12–7.

25 Moy LS, Murad H, Moy RL. Glycolic acid therapy, evaluation of efficacy and techniques in treatment of photodamaged lesions. *Am J Cosmetic Surg* 1993; **10**: 9–13.

26 Kligman AM, Grove GL, Hirose R *et al.* Topical tretinoin for photoaged skin. *J Am Acad Dermatol* 1986; **15**: 836–59.

27 Griffiths CEM, Russman AN, Majmuder G *et al.* Restoration of collagen formation in photodamaged human skin by tretinoin (retinoic acid). *N Engl J Med* 1993; **329**: 530–5.

28 Singh M, Griffiths CEM. The use of retinoids in the treatment of photoaging. *Dermatol Ther* 2006; **19**: 297–305.

29 Kligman AM, Dogadkina D, Lavker RM. Effects of topical tretinoin on non-sun-exposed protected skin of the elderly. *J Am Acad Dermatol* 1993; **29**: 25–33.

30 Gilchrest BA. Turning back the clock: retinoic acid modifies intrinsic aging changes. *J Clin Invest* 1994; **94**: 1711–2.

31 Lateef H, Stevens MJ, Varani J. All-*trans*-retinoic acid suppresses matrix metalloproteinase activity and increases collagen synthesis in diabetic human skin in organ culture. *Am J Pathol* 2004; **165**: 167–74.

32 Maddin S, Laurharanta J, Agache P *et al.* Isotretinoin improves the appearance of photodamaged skin: results of a 36-week, multicenter, double-blind, placebo-controlled trial. *J Am Acad Dermatol* 2000; **42**: 56–63.

33 Phillips TJ, Gottlieb AB, Leyden JJ *et al.* Efficacy of 0.1% tazarotene cream for the treatment of photodamage. *Arch Dermatol* 2002; **138**: 1486–93.

34 Ang P, Barlow RJ. Non-ablative laser resurfacing: a systematic review of the literature. *Clin Exp Dermatol* 2002; **27**: 630–5.

35 Watson REB, Craven NM, Kang S *et al.* A short-term screening assay, using fibrillin-1 as a reporter molecule for photoageing repair agents. *J Invest Dermatol* 2001; **116**: 672–8.

36 Watson REB, Long SP, Bowden JJ *et al.* Repair of photoaged dermal matrix by topical application of a cosmetic "antiageing" product. *Br J Dermatol* 2008; **158**: 472–7.

Elastotic nodules of the ear

In this variant of actinic elastosis, single or multiple firm papules occur on the anterior crus of the antihelix, usually in middle-aged or elderly males. Sometimes lesions have a pearly edge, clinically suggesting BCC, but histology reveals large aggregates of amorphous elastotic material, sometimes with degradation of underlying cartilage [1,2].

References

1 Carter VH, Constantine VS, Poole WC. Elastotic nodules of the antehelix. *Arch Dermatol* 1969; **100**: 282–5.

2 Weedon D. Elastotic nodules of the ear. *J Cutan Pathol* 1981; **8**: 429–33.

Digital papular calcific elastosis

Synonyms
- Keratoelastoidosis marginalis
- Collagenous and elastotic marginal plaques of the hands

Digital papular calcific elastosis (DPCE) is an acquired papular eruption in which keratoderma is associated with changes in dermal connective tissue. Predominantly it affects the radial aspect of the index finger, first web space and ulnar aspect of the thumb on the dominant hand [1,2]. Histologically there is hyperkeratosis, with sawtoothing of the rete ridges. The dermal collagen fibres are thickened and arranged haphazardly; there are basophilic elastotic masses, often containing calcium, in the upper reticular dermis [3]. Cases are sporadic, unlike the clinically similar disorders acrokeratoelastoidosis and focal acral hyperkeratosis (Chapter 19) [4]. Chronic friction and photodamage have been proposed as aetiological factors; the condition has been reported in manual workers and entirely from geographical areas with high solar irradiation. Digital papular calcific elastosis has been regarded as a variant of actinic elastosis [5], although actinic damage is not always observed clinically [6]. Furthermore, in DPCE, the elastotic process relatively spares the papillary dermis, and the basophilic areas containing calcium differ from the changes in actinic elastosis. Squamous carcinoma has been reported, arising from the lesion [7].

References

1 Burks JW, Wise LJ, Clark WH. Degenerative collagenous plaques of the hands. *Arch Dermatol* 1960; **82**: 362–6.

2 Jordaan HF, Rossouw DJ. Digital papular calcific elastosis: a histopathological, histochemical and ultrastructural study of 20 patients. *J Cutan Pathol* 1990; **17**: 358–70.

3 Menegesha YM, Kayal JD, Swerlick RA. Keratoelastoidosis marginalis. *J Cutan Med Surg* 2002; **6**: 23–5.

4 Rongioletti F, Betti R, Crosti C *et al.* Marginal papular acrokeratodermas: a unified nosology for focal acral hyperkeratosis, acrokeratoelastoidosis and related disorders. *Dermatology* 1994; **188**: 28–31.

5 Calderone DC, Fenske NA. The clinical spectrum of actinic elastotic. *J Am Acad Dermatol* 1995; **32**: 1016–24.

6 Mortimore RJ, Conrad RJ. Collagenous and elastoic marginal plaques of the hands. *Australas J Dermatol* 2001; **42**: 221–3.

7 Todd D, Al-Aboosi M, Hameed O *et al.* The role of UV light in the pathogenesis of digital papular calcific elastosis. *Arch Dermatol* 2001; **137**: 379–81.

Actinic granuloma

Synonym
- O'Brien's granuloma

Definition. This is an annular inflammatory reaction with a giant cell dermal infiltrate, which develops in an area of actinic elastosis. Some authors feel that this is not a specific entity, and the changes could be a feature of granuloma annulare or some other granulomatous disease that happens to occur on light-exposed skin [1]. Others point out that a similar granulomatous reaction to elastotic material can occur in pinguecula of the eye [2]. Histopathological studies support histological distinction of the two conditions [3–7]. There is minimal or no lysozyme activity in the histiocytes in the inflammatory area of actinic granuloma, in contrast with those of granuloma annulare, which exhibit abundant lysozyme activity [4].

The condition is more common in sunny countries, and fair-skinned or freckled subjects are particularly susceptible. It has been associated with doxycycline photosensitivity [8]. A similar condition has been described in dark-skinned people under the name of granuloma multiforme (Chapter 60).

Pathology [3–7]. A biopsy taken radially across the thickened edge of the lesion shows three distinct zones in the dermis. In the external 'normal' skin, there is actinic elastosis. In the thickened annulus, there is a histiocytic and giant cell inflammatory reaction in relation to elastotic fibres, and in the centre, within the annulus, little or no elastic tissue remains. The cellular infiltrate slowly expands outwards, leaving behind a central area from which elastic fibres have been removed by 'elastoclasis'.

The epidermis may be normal or it may show signs of actinic damage.

Clinical features. Lesions develop in the exposed 'weather-beaten' skin of patients after the third decade, particularly in fair-skinned or freckled subjects. They start insidiously as small, pink papules, which progress slowly to form an annulus of firm, superficial, dermal thickening. This is smooth, slightly raised and measures 0.2–0.5 cm in width. The ring may expand up to 6 cm in diameter. The centre may become slightly atrophic, and variable depigmentation may occur. The lesions are usually asymptomatic, but a sunburn reaction may provoke severe erythema and irritation.

Diagnosis. The condition must be distinguished from granuloma multiforme, granuloma annulare, serpiginous perforating elastosis, Miescher's disciform granuloma, sarcoidosis and necrobiosis lipoidica. The lesions of actinic granuloma are confined to light-exposed skin, and the infiltrate lacks the tidy palisaded arrangement that is normally seen with granuloma annulare. Rarely, granuloma annulare can occur in an actinic distribution [9].

Treatment. Infiltration of the annular edge of the lesions with triamcinolone may be effective. Sunscreens should be used to prevent further damage.

Isotretinoin (0.5 mg/kg/day) [10] and acitretin 25 mg/day [11] arrested the development of lesions in elderly males.

References
1 Ragaz A, Ackerman AB. Is actinic granuloma a specific condition? *Am J Dermatopathol* 1979; **1**: 43–50.
2 Dahl M. Is actinic granuloma really granuloma annulare? *Arch Dermatol* 1986; **122**: 39–40.
3 Al-Hoqail IA, Al-Ghamdi AM, Martinka M *et al.* Actinic granuloma is a unique and distinct entity: a comparative study with granuloma annulare. *Am J Dermatopathol* 2002; **24**: 209–12.
4 McGrae JD. Actinic granuloma: a clinical, histopathologic and immunocytochemical study. *Arch Dermatol* 1986; **122**: 43–8.
5 O'Brien JP. Actinic granuloma: an annular connective tissue disorder affecting sun and heat-damaged (elastotic) skin. *Arch Dermatol* 1975; **111**: 460–70.
6 Prendiville J, Griffiths WAD, Russell-Jones R. O'Brien's actinic granuloma. *Br J Dermatol* 1985; **113**: 353–8.
7 Limas C. The spectrum of primary cutaneous elastolytic granulomas and their distinction from granuloma annulare: a clinicopathological analysis. *Histopathology* 2004; **44**: 277–82.
8 Lim DS, Triscott J. O'Brien's granuloma associated with prolonged doxycycline photosensitivity. *Australas J Dermatol* 2003; **44**: 67–70.
9 Barker JNWN, Groves RW, MacDonald DM. Actinic granuloma annulare. *Br J Dermatol* 1991; **125** (Suppl. 38): 79–80.
10 Ratnavel RC, Grant JW, Handfield-Jones SE *et al.* O'Brien's actinic granuloma: response to isotretinoin. *J R Soc Med* 1995; **88**: P528–9.
11 Stefanaki C, Panagiotopoulos A, Kostakis P *et al.* Actinic granuloma successfully treated with acitretin. *Int J Dermatol* 2005; **44**: 163–6.

Elastofibroma [1–5]

Elastofibroma occurs predominantly in elderly women. Most cases are reported from Southern Japan. There may be a history of prolonged manual labour. The painless or slightly tender swelling situated beneath the lower angle of the scapula, and from 2 to 10 cm in diameter, is often discovered fortuitously. It may enlarge slowly, displacing neighbouring structures, and it can be clinically confused with a sarcoma. This is a benign lesion, however, despite the fact that it is poorly circumscribed. The growth is composed of mature fibrous tissue, containing fibres which stain as elastic fibres. The lesions may be solitary or multiple.

Histologically, the lesion contains abundant, large elastic fibres, some broken into irregular masses, and large amounts of relatively acellular collagen. The elastic fibres are composed of true elastin surrounded by a large amount of hydrophilic material forming an orderly array of tubules [4]. It is generally regarded either as a type of reactive hyperplasia, or as a hamartoma, arising either from dermis, subscapular connective tissue or periosteum [6]. It is cured by simple excision [7].

References
1 Nagamine N, Nohara Y, Ito E. Elastofibroma in Okinawa; a clinicopathologic study of 170 cases. *Cancer* 1982; **50**: 1794–805.
2 Fukuda Y. Histogenesis of the unique elastinophilic fibres of elastofibroma. *Hum Pathol* 1987; **18**: 424–9.
3 Kapff PD. Elastofibroma of hand. *J Bone Joint Surg* 1987; **69**: 468–9.
4 Govoni E. Elastofibroma: an *in vivo* model of abnormal elastoneogenesis. *Ultrastruct Pathol* 1988; **12**: 327–39.
5 Gartmann H, Groth W, Kuhn A. Elastofibroma dorsi. *Z Hautkr* 1988; **63**: 525–8.
6 Yamazaki K. An ultrastructural and immunohistochemical study of elastofibroma: CD 34, MEF-2, pronine 2 (CD33), and factor XIIIa- positive proliferating fibroblastic stromal cells connected by Cx43-type gap junctions. *Ultrastruct Pathol* 2007; **31**: 209–19.
7 Mortman KD, Hochheiser GM, Giblin EM *et al.* Elastofibroma dorsi: clinicopathologic review of 6 cases. *Ann Thorac Surg* 2007; **83**: 1894–7.

Elastoderma

Elastoderma is a very rare condition which is due to excessive elastogenesis, as distinct from acquired cutis laxa, where there is a loss of elastic tissue. A young woman developed a localized defect of the skin of one arm, which became pendulous and lax, but lost its elastic recoil. Histological and biochemical investigation showed this was due to accumulation of excessive elastin, with derangement of elastin fibrillogenesis [1].

In a further case, clinically uninvolved skin showed thin elastic fibres on haematoxylin and eosin staining [2].

References
1 Kornberg RL, Hendler SS, Oikarinen AI *et al.* Elastoderma—disease of elastin accumulation within the skin. *N Engl J Med* 1985; **312**: 771–2.
2 Yen A, Wen J, Grau M *et al.* Elastoderma. *J Am Acad Dermatol* 1995; **33**: 389–92.

Marfan's syndrome (MFS)

Definition. This is an autosomal dominant inherited disorder of connective tissue with variable clinical manifestations, both between and within families, and a prevalence of one in 5000–10 000 [1]. Up to 30% of cases are new mutations [2]. The full syndrome is characterized by aortic dilatation, ectopia lentis and skeletal abnormalities [3].

Aetiology. Mutations in the fibrillin-1 (*FBN1*) gene, located on chromosome 15q21.1, cause Marfan's syndrome [4]. Fibrillin is one component of the elastin-associated microfibrils, which are especially important in the ciliary zonule of the eye (the suspensory ligament of the lens). Patients with MFS show a striking lack of fibrillin in their skin and on culture of their dermal fibroblasts [5,6]. It has recently been recognized that changes in growth factor signalling are critical in MFS. As well as its structural role, fibrillin-1 also binds transforming growth factor β (TGF-β), and abnormal fibrillin leads to a detrimental increased expression of TGF-β [7]. In addition, a number of disorders with phenotypic overlap with MFS, for example Loeys–Dietz syndrome, are caused by mutations in the TGF-β receptor genes, *TGFBR1* and *TGFBR2* [8].

Pathology. The cardiovascular lesions are the most important. Fragmentation and sparsity of elastic fibres, with accumulation of mucinous material, occur in the media of the aorta [9–11]. These changes lead to aortic incompetence, dissecting aneurysm, or rupture of the aorta [12]. Mitral incompetence is common [13]. Dermal elastic fibres are narrower than normal and more resistant to neutrophil elastase [14]. Mild to severe degenerative changes in elastic tissue are also seen in the lungs [15].

Clinical features [3,10,16,17]. Despite recent advances in mutation detection, the diagnosis of MFS is primarily clinical and relies on the Ghent nosology [3]. The full syndrome comprises skeletal, ocular and cardiovascular defects. The patient is often, but not invariably, exceptionally tall, and the skeletal proportions are abnormal. The limbs are long, the excess being greatest distally, giving rise to arachnodactyly, and the length of the hallux is often particularly conspicuous. The skull is dolichocephalic, the paranasal sinuses are large and the palate high and arched [18]. Lax capsules result in unstable or hyperextensible joints, kyphoscoliosis, pectus excavatum and flat foot. Muscles may be underdeveloped and hypotonic, and subcutaneous fat is sparse.

The common ocular abnormalities [19] include ectopia lentis (usually upward), a trembling iris, myopia and retinal detachment; less frequent are blue sclerae and heterochromia of the iris.

Aneurysmal dilatation of the ascending aorta is the most important abnormality of the cardiovascular system, and aortic and mitral incompetence are common. Aortic dilatation may begin in childhood. Mitral valve prolapse occurs in 80% of cases [20].

Skin changes may be under-reported. Serpiginous perforating elastosis may occur [17]. In a recent study [21], striae atrophicae were observed in 7% of children and 35% of adults. Other features include papyraceous scars and skin hyperextensibility [22]. Several patients have been described with concomitant EDS and MFS [23].

Other abnormalities are frequent—nerve deafness occurs in 6%; pulmonary malformations are often reported at autopsy; renal abnormalities are manifest as proteinuria and raised blood urea [16].

The prognosis is related to the severity of the cardiac defects, the localization and progression of which are dependent on haemodynamic stresses [10,24]. Survival beyond the fifth decade is unusual, and some cases die in childhood. The average age at which dissection of the aorta develops is 30 years. Early death from cardiovascular disease may occur, even in apparently mild cases, and the correlation between cardiac and skeletal problems is poor [25–27].

Diagnosis [3,28]. The full syndrome is unmistakable, but diagnostic certainty is impossible in the partial forms. Clinical features are divided into major and minor according to their specificity. To make a diagnosis major criteria must be present in two organs and involvement in a third is required [3].

Simple screening tests that may be helpful include the thumb sign (positive if the thumb when completely opposed in the clenched hand projects beyond the ulnar border), the wrist sign (positive if the thumb and little finger overlap when wrapped around the opposite wrist) and the ratio of the lower segment (pubic ramus to floor) to the upper segment (height minus lower segment), but this ratio varies with age and sex.

Some tall people have high, arched palates and some degree of arachnodactyly. This is probably of no consequence in many cases, although a marfanoid habitus in women may be associated with mitral valve prolapse [20,29].

Joint hypermobility may also be associated with mitral valve prolapse [30]. Other causes of joint hypermobility, such as homocystinuria, may be confused with the partial forms of the syndrome. Homocystinuria should be considered in marfanoid patients with myopia or downward ectopia lentis. Urine screening is unreliable; blood levels of methionine and homocysteine should be measured. Prompt diagnosis and treatment reduce the risk of coronary artery or cerebrovascular thrombosis [31].

The marfanoid habitus has been reported in association with distal pigmentation, neuroma of the eyelids and tongue, medullary carcinoma of the thyroid and phaeochromocytoma [32] (see also multiple endocrine neoplasm syndrome (Chapter 62)).

Congenital contractural arachnodactyly is another fibrillinopathy, which is caused by mutations of the fibrillin-2 gene [33]. It is primarily an orthopaedic condition unrelated to MFS [34,35]. It produces multiple joint contractures, arachnodactyly, kyphoscoliosis, distorted pinnae and dolichostenomelia (long, thin limbs), but there are no cardiovascular complications.

Management [28]. Patients should be seen by an ophthalmologist and an orthopaedic surgeon, and they should be reviewed regularly by a cardiologist. Beta-blockers may be used to retard the development of aortic dilatation, and surgical replacement before the diameter exceeds 5.5–6.0 cm is recommended [11,36]. Losartan, an angiotensin II type I receptor antagonist has anti-TGF-β effects and, if administered postnatally to fibrillin-deficient mice, reverses aortic root dilatation [37]. Trials are underway to determine whether similar effects can be observed in young patients with Marfan's syndrome.

Oestrogen therapy has been used to prevent excessive stature in female patients [38].

Pregnancy is inadvisable, because of the 50% risk of inheritance in the fetus, and because of the risk of acceleration of aortic degeneration and vascular rupture. A pregnant patient with no cardiac signs needs monthly checks from the third month. Those with aortic or mitral valvular disease or dilatation of the aortic root are at high risk during pregnancy [39,40].

The majority of *FBN1* mutations are unique to one affected individual or family, but despite this and the presence of sporadic cases, prenatal and preimplantation diagnosis is feasible [2].

References

1 Pyeritz RE, Dietz HC. The Marfan syndrome and other microfibrillary disorders. In: Royce PM, Steinmann B, eds. *Connective Tissue and its Heritable Disorders: Molecular, Genetic and Medical Aspects*, 2nd edn. New York: Wiley–Liss, 2002: 585–626.

2 Toudjarska I, Kilpatrick MW, Lembessis P *et al.* Novel approach to the molecular diagnosis of Marfan syndrome: application to sporadic cases and in prenatal diagnosis. *Am J Med Genet* 2001; **99**: 294–302.

3 De Paepe A, Devereux RB, Dietz HC *et al.* Revised diagnostic criteria for the Marfan syndrome. *Am J Med Genet* 1996; **62**: 417–26.

4 Dietz HC, Cutting GR, Pyeritz RE *et al.* Marfan syndrome caused by a recurrent *de novo* missense mutation in the fibrillin gene. *Nature* 1991; **352**: 337–9.

5 Hollister DW, Godfrey MP, Keene DR *et al.* Immunohistologic abnormalities of the microfibrillar-fiber system in the Marfan syndrome. *N Engl J Med* 1990; **323**: 152–9.

6 Milewicz DM, Pyeritz R, Stanley Crawford E *et al.* Marfan syndrome: defective synthesis, secretion, and extracellular matrix formation of fibrillin by cultured dermal fibroblasts. *J Clin Invest* 1992; **89**: 79–86.

7 Neptune ER, Frischmeyer PA, Arking DE *et al.* Dysregulation of TGF-β activation contributes to pathogenesis in Marfan syndrome. *Nat Genet* 2003; **33**: 407–11.

8 Robinson PN, Arteaga-Solis E, Baldock C *et al.* The molecular genetics of Marfan syndrome and related disorders. *J Med Genet* 2006; **43**: 769–87.

9 Boucek RJ. The Marfan syndrome: a deficiency in chemically stable collagen cross-links. *N Engl J Med* 1981; **305**: 988–90.

10 Bruno L, Tredici S, Mangiavacchi M *et al.* Cardiac, skeletal and ocular abnormalities in patients with Marfan's syndrome and their relatives. *Br Heart J* 1984; **51**: 220–30.

11 Gott VL. Surgical treatment of aneurysms of the ascending aorta in the Marfan syndrome. *N Engl J Med* 1986; **314**: 1070–4.

12 Pyeritz RE. Marfan syndrome and other disorders of fibrillin. In: Rimoin DL, Connor JM, Pyeritz RE, Korf BR, eds. *Principles and Practice of Medical Genetics*, 4th edn. London: Churchill Livingstone, 2002: 3977–4020.

13 Roberts WC. The spectrum of cardiovascular disease in the Marfan syndrome. A clinico-morphologic study of 18 necropsy patients. *Am Heart J* 1982; **104**: 115–35.

14 Berteretche M-V, Hornebeck W, Pellat B *et al.* Histomorphometric parameters and susceptibility to neutrophil elastase degradation of skin elastic fibres from healthy individuals and patients with Marfan syndrome, Ehlers–Danlos type IV, and pseudoxanthoma elasticum. *Br J Dermatol* 1995; **133**: 836–41.

15 Soyers CP, Goltz RW, Mottiaz J. Pulmonary elastic tissue in generalized elastolysis (cutis laxa) and Marfan's syndrome: a light and electron microscopic study. *J Invest Dermatol* 1975; **65**: 451–7.

16 Loughridge LW. Renal abnormalities in the Marfan syndrome. *QJM* 1959; **28**: 531–43.

17 Loveman AB, Gordon AM, Fliegelmann MT. Marfan's syndrome. *Arch Dermatol* 1963; **87**: 428–33.

18 Wilner HJ, Finby N. Skeletal manifestations in Marfan's syndrome. *J Am Acad Dermatol* 1964; **187**: 490–5.

19 Wachtel JG. The ocular pathology of Marfan's syndrome including an explanation of ectopia lentis. *Arch Ophthalmol* 1966; **76**: 512–22.

20 Beighton P. Mitral valve prolapse and a Marfanoid habitus. *BMJ* 1982; **284**: 920.

21 Grahame R, Pyeritz RE. The Marfan syndrome. Joint and skin manifestations are prevalent and correlated. *Br J Rheumatol* 1995; **34**: 126–31.

22 Goodman RM, Allison ML. Observations on the heart in a case of combined Ehlers–Danlos and Marfan syndrome. *Am J Cardiol* 1969; **24**: 734–42.

23 Cunliffe WJ, Ead RD. A case of Marfan's syndrome occurring with Ehlers–Danlos syndrome. *Clin Exp Dermatol* 1977; **2**: 117–20.

24 Halpern B, Char F, Murdoch JL *et al.* A prospectus on the prevention of aortic rupture in the Marfan syndrome with data on survivorship without treatment. *Johns Hopkins Med J* 1971; **129**: 123–9.

25 Come PC. Echocardiographic recognition of silent aortic root dilatation in Marfan's syndrome. *Chest* 1977; **72**: 789–92.

26 Dalgleish R, Hawkins JR, Keston M. Exclusion of the α2 (I) and α1 (III) collagen genes as the mutant loci in a Marfan syndrome family. *J Med Genet* 1987; **24**: 148–51.

27 Marlow N, Gregg JEM, Qureshi SA. Mitral valve disease in Marfan's syndrome. *Arch Dis Child* 1987; **62**: 960–2.

28 Pyeritz RE, McKusick VA. The Marfan syndrome: diagnosis and management. *N Engl J Med* 1979; **300**: 772–7.

29 Schutte JE, Gaffney FA, Blend L *et al.* Distinctive anthropometric characteristics of women with mitral valve prolapse. *Am J Med* 1981; **71**: 533–8.

30 Grahame R, Edwards JC, Pitcher D *et al.* A clinical and echocardiograph study of patients with hypermobility syndrome. *Ann Rheum Dis* 1981; **40**: 451–6.

31 Cruysberg JRM, Boers GHJ, Frans Trijbels JM *et al.* Delay in diagnosis of homocystinuria: retrospective study of consecutive patients. *BMJ* 1996; **313**: 1037–40.

32 Cunliffe WJ, Hudgson P, Fulthorpe JJ *et al.* A calcitonin-secreting medullary thyroid carcinoma with mucosal neuromas, Marfanoid features, myopathy and pigmentation. *Am J Med* 1970; **48**: 121–6.

33 Putnam EA, Zhang H, Ramirez F, Milewicz DM. Fibrillin-2 (*FBN2*) mutations result in the Marfan-like disorder, congenital contractural arachnodactyly. *Nat Genet* 1995; **11**: 456–8.

34 Currarino G, Friedman JM. A severe form of congenital contractural arachnodactyly in two newborn infants. *Am J Med Genet* 1986; **25**: 763–73.

35 Travis RC, Shaw DG. Congenital contractural arachnodactyly. *Br J Radiol* 1985; **58**: 1115–7.

36 McDonald G, Schaff HV, Pyeritz RE. Surgical management of patients with Marfan syndrome and dilatation of the ascending aorta. *J Thorac Cardiovasc Surg* 1981; **81**: 180–6.

37 Habashi JP, Judge DP, Holm TM *et al.* Losartan, an AT1 antagonist, prevents aortic aneurysm in a mouse model of Marfan syndrome. *Science* 2006; **312**: 117–21.

38 Knudtzon J, Aarskog D. Estrogen treatment of excessively tall girls with Marfan's syndrome. *Acta Paediatr Scand* 1988; **77**: 537–41.

39 Mor-Yosef S, Younis J, Granat M *et al.* Marfan's syndrome in pregnancy. *Obstet Gyn Surv* 1988; **43**: 382–5.

40 Pyeritz RE. Maternal and fetal complications of pregnancy in the Marfan syndrome. *Am J Med* 1981; **71**: 784–90.

Disorders of collagen

Ehlers–Danlos syndrome

Synonym
- Cutis hyperelastica

Definition. Ehlers–Danlos syndrome (EDS) is a heterogeneous group of inherited disorders of connective tissue. Estimates of its prevalence vary between 1:560000 and 1:5000 [1]. For many patients the symptoms are so mild that they may not be recognized. The hallmarks of EDS are fragility of the skin and blood vessels, hyperextensibility of the skin and joint hypermobility [2]. The original classification divided EDS into 11 clinical types; however, in 1986, the International Nosology of Heritable Disorders of Connective Tissue redefined EDS into subtypes I–VIII and X [3]. It is now clear that certain phenotypic subtypes (EDS types I and II) overlap and some patients do not fit neatly into one category. Progress in molecular biology has been rapid in recent years, enabling further subdivision of some types [4].

Aetiology. Specific molecular and biochemical abnormalities have been identified in several types (Table 45.3) [5,6]. Attempts should be made to delineate the clinical, biochemical and, if possible, molecular abnormalities in a patient with EDS in view of the widely differing prognosis between different types. Defects predominantly involve collagen, although a fibronectin defect has been reported in type X [7], and most recently mutations in tenascin-X have been found to cause a newly recognized autosomal recessive form of EDS.

Pathology [8,9]. Skin histology is variable and often within normal limits. Typically, there is a loose, disordered dermal collagen network. Elastic fibres are usually increased and orientated irregularly. The 'pseudotumours' seen in classical EDS (type I) consist of fat and mucoid material in fibrous capsules; they may be calcified. Bone mineralization is decreased, and the collagen fibres are irregular. Adventitial defects of small arteries and inadequate support from the surrounding connective tissue account for the vascular vulnerability in vascular EDS (type IV) [10,11]. Although bruising can be explained on the basis of skin and blood vessel fragility, a few patients also exhibit both ultrastructural and functional platelet defects [12,13]. Clotting factor deficiencies have

Table 45.3 Clinical and molecular subtypes of Ehlers–Danlos syndrome.

EDS type	Synonym	Villefranche classification*	Mode of inheritance	Clinical features	Ultrastructural findings	Molecular defect
I II	Gravis Mitis	Classical	AD	Soft, velvety, hyperextensible skin; easy bruising; atrophic scars; hypermobile joints; pseudotumours	'Cauliflower' fibrils	COL5A1 & COL5A2 (& COL1A1) mutations
III	Hypermobile	Hypermobility	AD	Hypermobile joints; minimal skin abnormality	As above	?
IV	Acrogeric or ecchymotic	Vascular	AD	Thin skin; easy bruising; small joint hypermobility; vascular and bowel ruptures	Small variable fibrils	COL3A1 mutations
V	X-linked	Other form	XLR	Resembles mild classical type; bruising more pronounced	—	?
VI	Ocular-scoliotic	Kyphoscoliosis	AR	Soft, hyperextensible skin; hypermobile joints; scoliosis; ocular fragility; keratoconus	Small collagen bundles; fibrils normal or similar to classical type	Lysyl hydroxylase (PLOD) mutations
VIIA, B	Arthrochalasis multiplex congenita	Arthrochalasis	AD	Floppy infant; congenital hip dislocation; hypermobile joints; soft skin; normal scarring; short stature	Angular fibrils	A & B: COL1A1 & COL1A2 mutations, respectively, result in loss of exon 6 (procollagen N-proteinase/ADAMTS2 cleavage site)
VIIC	Dermatosparaxis	Dermatosparaxis	AR	Markedly hypermobile joints; very soft and extremely fragile skin; easy bruising	Hieroglyphic fibrils	Procollagen N-proteinase (ADAMTS2) mutations
VIII	Periodontal	Other form	AD	Severe periodontitis; pigmented pretibial plaques and scarring	Small fibrils in some patients	Occasionally collagen III deficient
X	Fibronectin	Other form	AR	Similar to mild classical type	Large, irregular fibrils	Fibronectin deficiency abnormality
—	Progeroid	Other form	AR	Atrophic scars; lax skin and joints; aged appearance; short stature; osteopenia; mental retardation	—	XGPT1 mutations
—	Tenascin-X	—	AR	Similar to mild classical type but no scarring	Normal fibrils but reduced density	Tenascin-X mutations

* The Villefranche classification simplifies EDS into six major types. The other types have been provisionally grouped under 'other forms' until more is known about their molecular basis.

AD, autosomal dominant; AR, autosomal recessive; EDS, Ehlers–Danlos syndrome; XLR, X-linked recessive.

been only rarely reported. Electron microscopy of dermal collagen consistently shows irregularities of fibril shape and size, although reliable subclassification of the more common subtypes is not possible [14]. Tenascin-X deficient patients have uniform collagen fibrils which are less densely packed and not as well aligned [15]. In contrast, arthrochalasia type EDS is characterized by angular fibrils in cross-section, and dermatosparaxis by grossly distorted, hieroglyphic fibrils. Biomechanical studies confirm increased skin elasticity and hyperextensibility, particularly in classical EDS (type I) [16,17].

Clinical features. These are summarized in Table 45.3. The india-rubber men and circus contortionists who are affected by EDS turn the syndrome to their advantage. More details are given in the accounts of each type.

Classical type (EDS I/II)

This subgroup, which is inherited as an autosomal dominant, includes both EDS type I (gravis) and II (mitis).

Pathology. Histology may be within normal limits; alternatively there may be thin, weakly polarized, dermal collagen bundles. Elastic fibres may be irregular and relatively increased [8,9]. At ultrastructural level, collagen bundles are of variable size with abnormally large, composite 'cauliflower' fibrils, reflecting abnormal fibrilogenesis [14,18,19]. Linkage to *COL5A1* was originally identified in a British family with EDS II, and analysis of further families subsequently showed that EDS I and II are allelic [20,21]. Up to half of all classical EDS patients have mutations in *COL5A1* or *COL5A2*, which encode the α_1 and α_2 chains of type V collagen, respectively. Although quantitatively minor (approximately 2–5% of dermal collagen), collagen V plays an important role in the regulation of type I collagen diameter [22]. Missense and exon skipping mutations with dominant-negative effects or mutations giving rise to haploinsufficiency may occur [15,23]. Genetic heterogeneity is apparent with reports of classical EDS caused by a mutation in the collagen I gene [24]. Furthermore, knock-out experiments with mice suggest other extracellular matrix components such as decorin, fibromodulin, thrombospondin-2, lumican and biglycan may be important [25,26].

Clinical features. The skin is soft, velvety and hyperextensible (Fig. 45.21) but retains its normal recoil. The skin on the palms and soles may be redundant, like a loose glove. The skin is not usually otherwise lax until later in life, when redundant folds occur on the eyelids (blepharochalasis), face and limbs. Secondary cutis laxa has been described on the lower back of a patient with mild classical EDS [27]. Striae do not develop during pregnancy. Trivial lacerations form gaping wounds that heal very slowly to leave broad, atrophic 'cigarette paper' scars (Figs 45.22 & 45.23). Sutures may tear out repeatedly. Blue-grey, spongy tumours (molluscoid pseudotumours), due to accumulation of connective tissue, may form on the skin, especially in scars or over pressure points. Smaller, firm, subcutaneous nodules (spheroids), which show calcification on X-ray, develop on the shins and forearms in up to a third of patients.

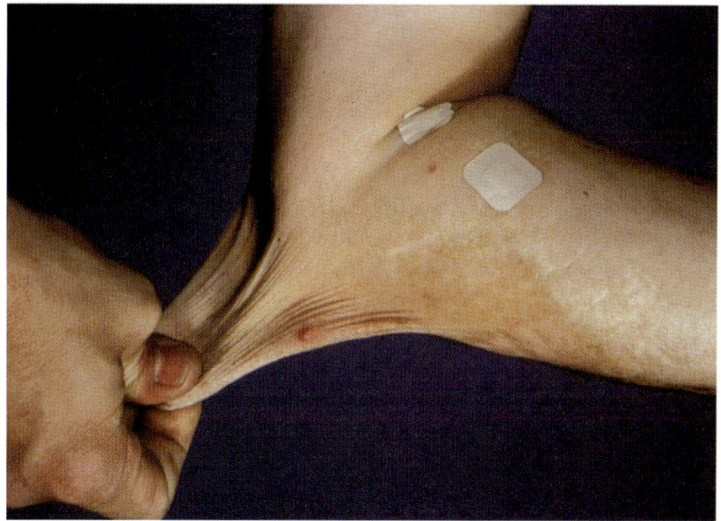

Fig. 45.21 Cutaneous hyperextensibililty in classical Ehlers–Danlos syndrome.

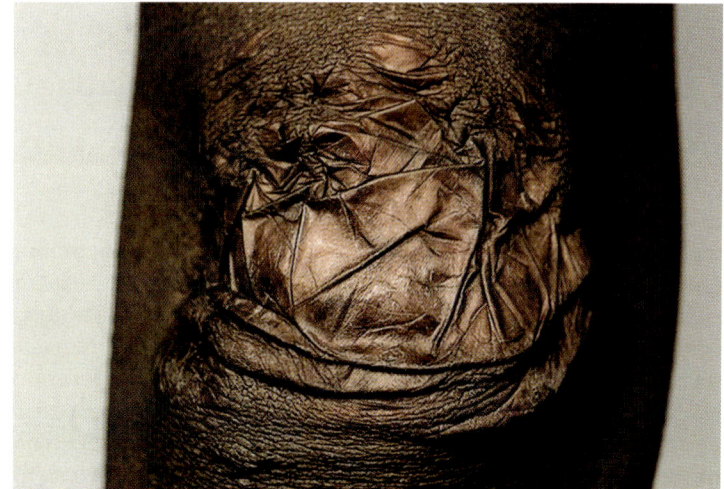

Fig. 45.22 Atrophic scarring of the elbow in classical Ehlers–Danlos syndrome.

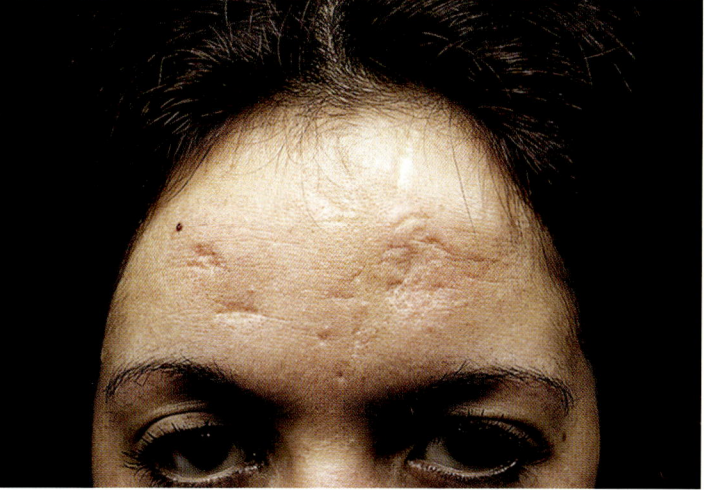

Fig. 45.23 Scarring of the forehead in classical Ehlers–Danlos syndrome.

Easy bruising may be the presenting symptom, and pigmentation due to haemosiderin deposition is often found on areas of repeated trauma.

The facies may be distinctive, with widely spaced eyes, a wide nasal bridge, and epicanthic folds. The sclerae are sometimes blue.

There is marked joint hypermobility, which can impair walking, especially during pregnancy. Subluxation of the large joints may occur, and genu recurvatum and kyphoscoliosis are frequent [28]. Muscle tone is often poor, and hernias develop. Pedal piezogenic papules are seen more frequently. Diaphragmatic eventration and gastric torsion have been reported [29]. Symptomatic bladder diverticula may develop [30]. Varicose veins may develop in early life. Prematurity due to ruptured fetal membranes is common.

As physical and mental development are normal, life expectancy is not reduced, hence large family pedigrees are not unusual. A mild variant of classical EDS has been described in 9% of a general dermatology population less than 50 years old, and merges with benign hypermobility syndrome and the normal spectrum [31]. A simple clinical scoring system, based on an assessment of joint hypermobility, skin extensibility and bruising might be useful in predicting which members of the general population are likely to produce poor scars following cutaneous surgery [32].

Hypermobility type (EDS III)

Hypermobile EDS and benign joint hypermobility syndrome (BJHS) are autosomal dominant and considered by some authors to be the same disorder. Revised criteria have been proposed for their diagnosis [33]. The Beighton score (Table 45.4) is a useful, quick method for assessing global joint hypermobility, and an adult score of four or more out of nine either currently or historically is considered hypermobile [34]. Ultimately, molecular analysis will determine whether these two groups are genetically heterogeneous. Haploinsufficiency of tenascin-X results in reduced dermal collagen and may account for 5–10% of hypermobile type EDS, although this has only been found in females [35]. There is one report of a family with hypermobile EDS phenotype due to collagen III deficiency, as occurs in vascular EDS [36]. The ultrastructural changes resemble those in classical EDS. The skin is only minimally affected by scarring and hyperextensibility, whereas joint mobility is markedly increased, and dislocation and joint pains are common [37,38]. A study of a small number of hypermobile patients showed they were resistant to the effects of intradermal or topical local anaesthetic compared with BJHS patients or controls, suggesting that the disorders are distinct [39]. However,

the criteria used to diagnose the hypermobile group were not clearly documented. In the authors' experience, patients with classical EDS may also rarely be resistant to local anaesthetic. Symptoms such as syncope, palpitations and fatigue suggest dysautonomia and are significantly more common in joint hypermobility patients, although the mechanisms remain unclear [40].

Vascular type (EDS IV)

This very severe form is inherited as an autosomal dominant. Cases previously reported as autosomal recessive inheritance were probably due to sporadic mutations [41–43]. It is rare, the prevalence being between one in 10^5 and one in 10^6 [41].

Pathology. The condition is characterized by an abnormality of the synthesis, secretion or structure of type III collagen due to an abnormality of the collagen III gene (*COL3A1*) [6,44]. Segregation studies using polymorphic restriction sites in the gene may be of use in prenatal diagnosis [45]. The syndrome is biochemically heterogeneous [5]. Several changes have been reported, the most common of which are point mutations (substituting other amino acids for glycine residues in the triple helical domain). Exon-skipping mutations are nearly as common; small genomic deletions within one exon and multiexon deletions have also been described [5,6,46]. It has been suggested that the region of the type III collagen molecule where mutation occurs may be linked with the clinical severity [6], although this has not been found in other studies [46].

These abnormalities all result in abnormal structure, synthesis or secretion of type III procollagen. Often, the skin is reduced to 25% of normal thickness, with small collagen fibre bundles. Fibril diameter is markedly variable in some patients [47]. In many patients, the fibroblasts contain prominent rough endoplasmic reticulum containing abnormal type III procollagen [47,48]. Cell strains from other individuals show markedly reduced extracellular accumulation of procollagen and collagen but without intracellular accumulation, perhaps due to rapid degradation of mutant chains [49]. Bizarre elastic fibres are often abundant.

The condition affects tissues rich in type III collagen, notably arterial media, bowel and uterus. Interestingly, type III collagen production by fibroblasts is decreased in some patients with ruptured cerebral aneurysm, even though they have no other stigmata of EDS [50]. The collagen deficiency in these patients does not appear to arise from *COL3A1* mutations, but may relate to abnormal post-translational modification or altered collagen metabolism [51].

Clinical features. The major clinical features are spontaneous rupture of large arteries, colon and gravid uterus. Dissecting aortic aneurysm is a common cause of sudden death [52]. Spontaneous carotid–cavernous fistula can also occur, resulting in unilateral exophthalmos [53]; it may respond to surgical repair or embolization [54]. Repair of rupture of the colon (usually sigmoid) is complicated by tissue friability and peritoneal contamination [55]. In one series complications of pregnancy led to death in the peripartum period in 12 of 81 women who had a total of 183 pregnancies [46]. Seven died following vessel rupture and five following uterine rupture.

Table 45.4 Beighton score [34].

Movement	Score
Dorsiflex L and R 5th finger >90°	2
Apposition L and R thumb to forearm	2
Hyperextend L and R elbow >10°	2
Hyperextend L and R knee >10°	2
Palms to floor	1
TOTAL	9

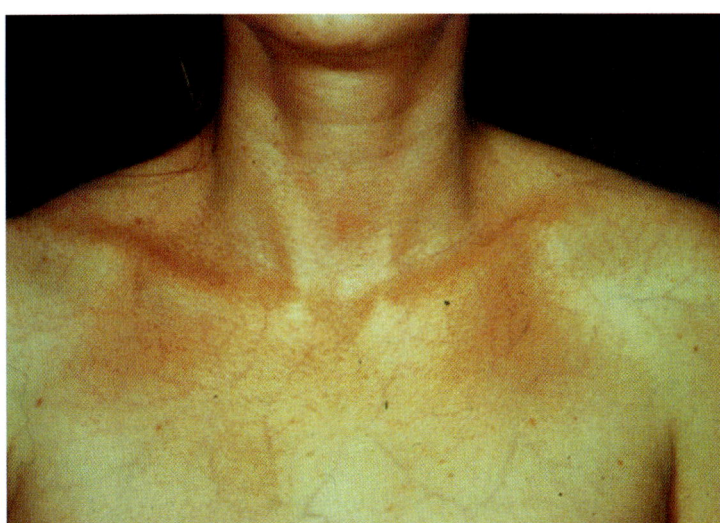

Fig. 45.24 Cutaneous atrophy in vascular (acrogeric) Ehlers–Danlos syndrome.

Other features include prematurity (due to rupture of friable placental membranes), low birth weight, short stature, easy bruising (which may lead to the mistaken accusation of child abuse) [56] and pneumothorax [57,58]. Elastosis perforans serpiginosa is seen more commonly in this EDS subtype.

Two phenotypic groups are recognizable. In the *acrogeric* type, individuals appear prematurely aged with thin, translucent, fragile skin (Fig. 45.24), a hollow-eyed appearance, thin, peaked nose and thin lips. Easy bruising predominates in the *ecchymotic* type, often falsely suggesting a primary disorder of coagulation [13]. Unlike other forms of EDS, the skin is not hyperextensible, and joint hypermobility is chiefly restricted to the small joints of the hands and feet. Surface veins are usually readily visible. There is a tendency to form keloid scars.

The largest case series to date of 220 index cases of vascular EDS patients and 199 affected relatives showed the median survival as 48 years, with 25% of index cases having their first significant complication by 20 years [46]. Most deaths follow arterial dissection or rupture, mainly of the thoracic and abdominal vessels. Milder variants may occur, presenting with cardiac features in later life [59].

Recently a new autosomal dominant aneurismal disorder, Loeys-Dietz syndrome, has been described. The major features of Loeys-Dietz syndrome type I patients overlap clinically with Marfan's syndrome whereas type II patients have a phenotype similar to vascular EDS. In a cohort of 40 patients with a presentation suggestive of vascular EDS, but normal type III collagen, Loeys and colleagues found mutations in the transforming growth factor-beta receptor genes *TGFBR1* and *TGFB2* [60]. Therefore Loeys-Dietz syndrome should be considered in any vascular EDS phenotype with normal collagen III.

X-linked type (EDS V)

Two families have been described as type V EDS. Clinically, it resembles mild classical EDS, but bruising is more marked. However, it is distinguished by X-linked inheritance [61]. The biochemical defect is unknown, and skin collagen cross-links are normal [62]. Lysyl oxidase activity has been reported to be reduced in one family [63], but these patients appear to form a clinically distinct subgroup. In other families, the lysyl oxidase levels have been normal [64]. Until a precise genetic or biochemical abnormality is found, the status of this type must remain in question [5].

Kyphoscoliosis type (EDS VI; ocular-scoliotic)

This autosomal recessive condition was the first true disorder of collagen structure to be described [64–66]. The biochemical abnormality in most, but not all, patients, is a deficiency of lysyl hydroxylase [65]. Different mutations in the lysyl hydroxylase gene (*PLOD*) have been identified in unrelated families. One is homozygous for a stop codon at residue 319 (R319X) [67]. In another, duplication of 180 base pairs in the coding sequence of the complementary DNA resulted in decreased enzyme function [68], and a further family revealed a compound heterozygote combining a three-base pair deletion and an amino acid substitution (G678A) [69].

Deficiency of the enzyme leads to reduced hydroxylation of lysyl residues in types I and III collagen in skin; hydroxylysine-containing cross-links are not formed [70]. Lysine-derived cross-links appear not to be as stable as those derived from hydroxylysine; the former do not mature as rapidly to stable intermolecular cross-links [71]. Types II, IV and V collagens are hydroxylated normally, which suggests that there may be different isoenzymes or different affinities of a single enzyme for specific collagen types [5]. Detection of abnormal pyridinoline cross-links in urine can be used as a diagnostic aid [72].

Clinical features include soft, velvety, hyperextensible skin and increased joint mobility. Scoliosis is common. Eye manifestations include microcornea, glaucoma, keratoconus and ocular fragility. Some patients have a marfanoid habitus. Bleeding may occur from major wounds, and there may be delayed motor development [73].

The kyphoscoliotic type of EDS appears to be rare, with less than two dozen cases reported in the literature [5]. Because it is inherited recessively, after the birth of an affected child there is a 25% risk of recurrence in each successive pregnancy. Measurement of lysyl hydroxylase activity in amniotic fluid enabled the prediction of a phenotypically normal heterozygous infant in a family at risk [74].

Some patients respond to treatment with ascorbic acid, which regulates collagen biosynthesis [75].

Arthrochalasia type (EDS VIIA and B; arthrochalasis multiplex congenita)

This rare autosomal dominant condition, like OI, results from mutations causing defects in type I collagen. Phenotypic overlap therefore occurs.

All or part of exon 6 of the *COL1A1* or *COL1A2* gene is deleted in types A and B, respectively, resulting in a defect in the cleavage sites of the substrate pro-α_1(I) or pro-α_2(I) chains [75–79]. Mutations appear to affect cross-link formation, decreasing tensile strength of tissues rich in type I collagen. Partially processed molecules accumulate in the dermis and other tissues, where they interfere with tissue function without much effect on fibrillar organization [76,80].

Arthrochalasis is characterized clinically by extreme joint hypermobility and multiple dislocations affecting both large and small

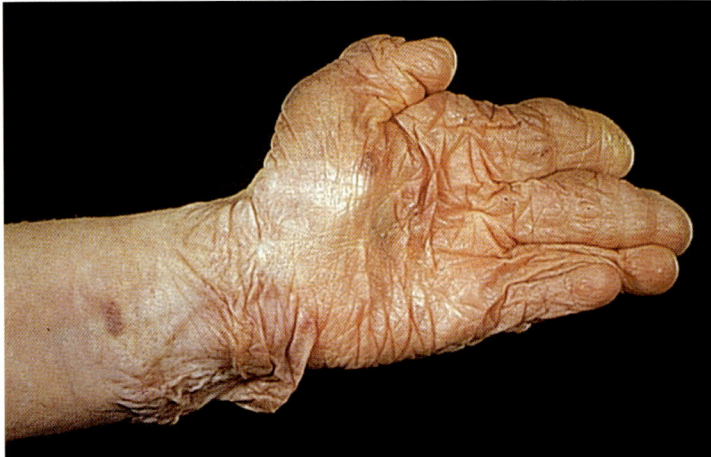

Fig. 45.25 Extreme cutaneous fragility and laxity in dermatosparaxis.

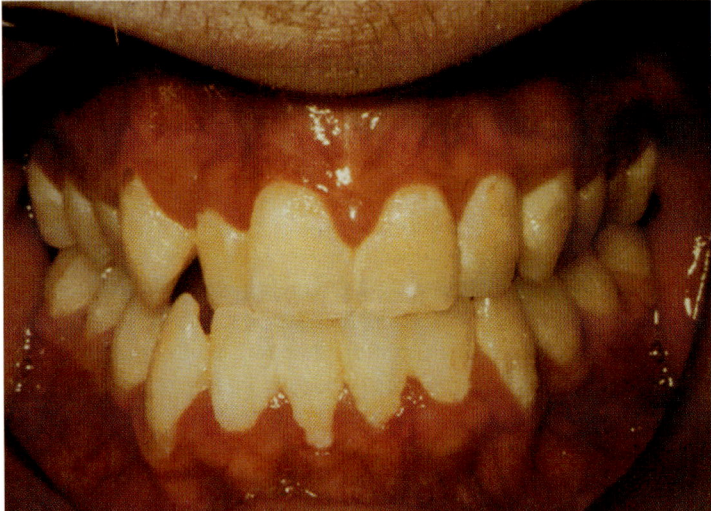

Fig. 45.26 Premature periodontal recession in periodontitis type Ehlers–Danlos syndrome (VIII).

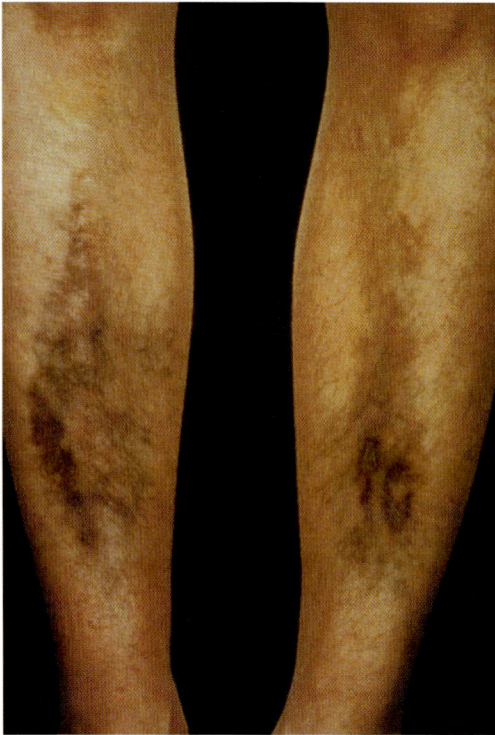

Fig. 45.27 Pigmented pretibial plaques in periodontitis type Ehlers–Danlos syndrome (VIII).

joints [27]. Bilateral hip dislocation presents a major surgical problem. Some individuals have a short stature. There may be a chubby facial appearance due to lax facial tissues, and a depressed nasal bridge [80].

Dermatosparaxis type (EDS VIIC)

This very rare autosomal recessive form is characterized by extreme skin fragility (Fig. 45.25), bruising, droopy skin, joint laxity, umbilical hernia and blue sclerae [81–84]. The condition is akin to dermatosparaxis, a disorder causing fragile skin in animals [85–86]. It is caused by homozygous mutations in the gene encoding procollagen I N-terminal proteinase (*ADAMTS2*), the enzyme that excises the N-propeptide of type I and II procollagens [87]. Collagen fibrils from affected children and animals are small, with a bizarre hieroglyphic-like appearance in cross-section; they are ribbon-like in longitudinal section [5].

Periodontitis type (EDS VIII)

This type has features similar to classical EDS but there is often only moderate small-joint hypermobility. The distinguishing clini-cal features are premature periodontal recession (Fig. 45.26), resulting in loss of teeth by the third decade, and heavily pigmented, pretibial plaques (Fig. 45.27) [88,89]. Little is known about the biochemical defect, although there is a reduced proportion of type III collagen in skin [89]. Some patients have small collagen fibrils [89]. It is inherited as an autosomal dominant and linkage has been shown to chromosome 12p13 in three out of five families, indicating genetic heterogeneity [91].

EDS IX (occipital horn syndrome)

This is an X-linked recessive disorder allelic to Menkes' syndrome and is no longer considered a variant of EDS [3]. It was formerly known as X-linked cutis laxa or 'occipital horn syndrome' and has been reclassified as a disorder of copper transport (p. 45.39).

Fibronectin-deficient type (EDS X)

Only one family has been identified to date with this autosomal recessive disorder. Skin and joint changes are mild, but bruising occurs readily due to defective platelet aggregation [7]. This defect is reversed *in vitro* by adding purified fibronectin to the assay. Some patients have composite fibrils in the dermal collagen, possibly due to a defect in fibronectin interactions [92].

Progeroid EDS

A rare association of EDS with progeroid facies, short stature, osteopenia and mental retardation is recognized [93]. Patients lack the full phenotype of progeria (p. 45.58) and do not fit in to the more well-defined progeroid syndromes. Galactosyltransferase I activity is reduced in patients' fibroblasts due to mutations in the *XGPT1* gene [94]. This enzyme is involved in the synthesis of glycosaminoglycans, suggesting that they may be involved in the process of senescence. The phenotype of decorin/biglycan double knock-out mice is similar to human progeroid EDS and occurs as the result of impaired binding of glycosaminoglycans to decorin and biglycan [25].

Tenascin-X-deficient type EDS

Tenascin-X deficiency causes a recently identified, clinically distinct, autosomal recessive form of EDS [95]. Patients have hyperextensible skin, bruising and joint laxity, but no scarring. The gene for tenascin-X (TNXB) overlaps the steroid 21-hydroxylase gene, and it was originally identified as a candidate gene for EDS in a patient with a contiguous-gene deletion giving rise to both 21-hydroxylase deficiency and EDS [96]. Tenascin-X is the first EDS gene that does not encode a fibrillar collagen or collagen-modifying enzyme. It is a large extracellular matrix protein that appears to be an essential regulator of collagen deposition by dermal fibroblasts [97].

Associated syndromes

Various unclassified forms of EDS overlap with other disorders, such as OI, PXE, MFS [98], renal tubular acidosis and medullary sponge kidney [99], and osteolysis of the terminal phalanges.

Diagnosis. The diagnosis is mainly clinical; a scoring system may be helpful in doubtful cases [100]. Confirmation of the subtype can require a combination of electron microscopy of dermal collagens, protein chemistry analysis from cultured fibroblasts and mutation detection. Immunofluorescent staining of fibroblasts for retained type III collagen may be a faster and cheaper method for the diagnosis of the important type IV EDS [101]. Similarly, the finding of reduced type III procollagen aminopropeptide in the serum of some, but not all, patients with EDS IV may help diagnosis [102]. Chorionic villus sampling may enable prenatal diagnosis of abnormalities of type I (and II) collagen [103]. Measurement of the ratio of urinary lysyl and hydroxylysyl pyridinolines is a non-invasive, reliable diagnostic test for kyphoscoliosis type EDS [72].

EDS should be distinguished from cutis laxa, in which the skin hangs in flaccid redundant folds. In EDS, redundant skin folds may develop in late adult life, but they are usually limited to the elbows and the skin around the eyes. Hyperelastic skin is a feature of Turner's syndrome (Chapter 15), but the dwarfism, cubitus valgus and webbed neck are distinctive. Hyperelastic skin with abnormal elastic fibres in the papillary dermis has been reported in the rare cartilage–hair hypoplasia syndrome [104].

Treatment. All patients should receive genetic counselling. Treatment is highly unsatisfactory, although some features of EDS VI may respond to oral ascorbic acid [74]. Patients with type IV EDS should be advised to avoid pregnancy and trauma, including physical contact sports, and to avoid activities, such as trumpet playing, which raise intracranial pressure by the Valsalva effect. Bleeding should be managed conservatively if at all possible. The fragility of blood vessels makes arteriography and surgical procedures dangerous and difficult. Surgeons must be made aware of the patient's diagnosis prior to surgery. Sutures should be buttressed, and tension avoided. Although re-excision of ugly scars can give a good cosmetic result it is not generally recommended [105].

References

1 Steinmann B, Royce PM, Superti-Furga A. The Ehlers–Danlos syndrome. In: Royce PM, Steinmann B, eds. *Connective Tissue and its Heritable Disorders: Molecular, Genetic and Medical Aspects*. New York: Wiley–Liss, 2002: 431–523.

2 Beighton P, ed. *The Ehlers–Danlos Syndrome*. London: Heinemann, 1970.

3 Beighton P, de Paepe A, Danks A *et al*. International nosology of heritable disorders of connective tissue, Berlin. *Am J Med Genet* 1988; **29**: 581–4.

4 Beighton P, de Paepe A, Steinmann B *et al*. Ehlers–Danlos syndromes: revised nosology, Villefranche, 1997. *Am J Med Genet* 1998; **77**: 31–7.

5 Byers PH. Ehlers–Danlos syndrome: recent advances and current understanding of the clinical and genetic heterogeneity. *J Invest Dermatol* 1994; **103**: S47–52.

6 Pope FM, Narcisi P, Nicholls AC *et al*. COL3A1 mutations cause variable clinical phenotypes including acrogeria and vascular rupture. *Br J Dermatol* 1996; **135**: 163–81.

7 Arneson MA, Hammerschmidt DE, Furcht LT *et al*. A new form of Ehlers–Danlos syndrome: fibronectin corrects defective platelet function. *JAMA* 1980; **244**: 144–7.

8 Sulica VI, Cooper PH, Pope M *et al*. Cutaneous histological features in Ehlers–Danlos syndrome: a study of 21 patients. *Arch Dermatol* 1979; **115**: 40–2.

9 Piérard GE, Piérard-Franchimont C, Lapière CM. Histopathological aid in the diagnosis of the Ehlers–Danlos syndrome, gravis and mitis types. *Int J Dermatol* 1993; **22**: 300–4.

10 Bopp P, Hatam K, Busat P *et al*. Cardiovascular aspects of the Ehlers–Danlos syndrome. *Circulation* 1965; **32**: 602–7.

11 Cikrit DF, Miles JH, Silver D. Spontaneous arterial perforation: the Ehlers–Danlos specter. *J Vasc Surg* 1987; **5**: 248–55.

12 Kashiwagi H, Riddle JM, Abraham JP. Functional and ultrastructural abnormalities of platelets in Ehlers–Danlos syndrome. *Ann Intern Med* 1965; **63**: 249–54.

13 Anstey A, Mayne K, Winter K *et al*. Platelet and coagulation studies in Ehlers–Danlos syndrome. *Br J Dermatol* 1991; **125**: 155–63.

14 Holbrook KA, Byers PH. Skin is a window on heritable disorders of connective tissue. *Am J Med Genet* 1989; **34**: 105–21.

15 Mao J-R, Bristow J. The Ehlers–Danlos syndrome. On beyond collagens. *J Clin Invest* 2001; **107**: 1063–9.

16 Grahame R, Beighton P. Physical properties of the Ehlers–Danlos syndrome. *Ann Rheum Dis* 1969; **28**: 246–51.

17 Henry F, Goffin V, Piérard-Franchimont CP *et al*. Mechanical properties of skin in Ehlers–Danlos syndrome types I, II and III. *Pediatr Dermatol* 1996; **13**: 464–7.

18 Piérard GE, Lê T, Piérard-Franchimont C *et al*. Morphometric study of 'cauliflower' fibrils in Ehlers–Danlos syndrome type I. *Coll Relat Res* 1988; **8**: 453–7.

19 Hausser I, Anton-Lamprecht I. Differential ultrastructural aberrations of collagen fibrils in Ehlers–Danlos syndrome type I–IV as a means of diagnostics and classification. *Hum Genet* 1994; **3**: 394–407.

20 Loughlin J, Irven C, Hardwick LJ *et al*. Linkage of the gene that encodes the α_1 chain of type V collagen (*COL5A1*) to type II Ehlers–Danlos syndrome (EDS II). *Hum Mol Genet* 1995; **4**: 1649–51.

21 Burrows NP, Nicholls AC, Yates JWR *et al*. The gene encoding α1 (V) (*COL5A1*) is linked to mixed Ehlers–Danlos syndrome type I/II. *J Invest Dermatol* 1996; **106**: 1273–6.

22 Fichard A, Kleman J-P, Ruggiero F. Another look at collagen V and XI molecules. *Matrix Biol* 1994; **14**: 515–31.

23 Burrows NP. The molecular genetics of the Ehlers–Danlos syndrome. *Clin Exp Dermatol* 1999; **24**: 99–106.

24 Nuytinck L, Freund M, Lagae L *et al*. Classical Ehlers–Danlos syndrome caused by a mutation in type I collagen. *Am J Hum Genet* 2000; **66**: 1398–402.

25 Corsi A, Xu T, Chen X-D *et al*. Phenotypic effects of biglycan deficiency are linked to collagen fibril abnormalities, are synergized by decorin deficiency, and mimic Ehlers–Danlos-like changes in bone and other connective tissues. *J Bone Miner Res* 2002; **17**: 1180–9.

26 Jepsen KJ, Wu F, Peragallo JH *et al*. A syndrome of joint laxity and impaired tendon integrity in lumican- and fibromodulin-deficient mice. *J Biol Chem* 2002; **277**: 532–40.

27 Ostlere LS, Pope FM, Holden CA. Cutis laxa complicating Ehlers–Danlos syndrome type II. *Clin Exp Dermatol* 1996; **21**: 135–7.

28 Beighton P, Grahame R, Bird H. *Hypermobility of Joints*, 3rd edn. London: Springer-Verlag, 1999: 147–77.

29 Phadke JG. Ehlers–Danlos syndrome with surgical repair of penetration of diaphragm and torsion of stomach. *J R Soc Med* 1979; **72**: 781–3.

30 Burrows NP, Monk BE, Harrison JB, Pope FM. Giant bladder diverticulum in Ehlers–Danlos syndrome type I causing outflow obstruction. *Clin Exp Dermatol* 1998; **23**: 109–12.

31 Holzberg M, Hewan-Lowe KO, Olansky AJ. The Ehlers–Danlos syndrome: recognition, characterization, and importance of a milder variant of the classic form. *J Am Acad Dermatol* 1998; **19**: 656–66.

32 Rebora A, Fiallo P, Muzio GF. Prediction of poor outcome of cutaneous surgery. *Lancet* 1989; **ii**: 1109.

33 Grahame R, Bird HA, Child A *et al.* The revised (Brighton 1998) criteria for the diagnosis of benign joint hypermobility syndrome (BJHS). *J Rheumatol* 2000; **27**: 1777–9.

34 Beighton PH, Solomon L, Soskolne CL. Articular mobility in an African population. *Ann Rheum Dis* 1973; **32**: 413–8.

35 Zweirs MC, Bristow J, Steijlen PM et al. Haploinsufficiency of TNXB is associated with hypermobility type of Ehlers-Danlos syndrome. *Am J Hum Genet* 2003; **73**: 214–7.

36 Narcisi P, Richards AJ, Ferguson SD *et al.* A family with Ehlers–Danlos syndrome type III/articular hypermobility syndrome has a glycine 637 to serine in type III collagen. *Hum Mol Genet* 1994; **3**: 1617–20.

37 Kaalund S, Høgsaa B, Grevy C. Coxa saltans in patients with Ehlers–Danlos syndrome type III. *Scand J Rheumatol* 1988; **17**: 229–30.

38 Sacheti A, Szemere J, Bernstein B *et al.* Chronic pain is a manifestation of the Ehlers–Danlos syndrome. *J Pain Symptom Manage* 1997; **14**: 88–93.

39 Arendt-Nielson L, Kaalund S, Hogsaa B *et al.* The response to local anaesthetics (EMLA®) as a clinical test to diagnose between hypermobility and Ehlers–Danlos III syndrome. *Scand J Rheumatol* 1991; **20**: 190–5.

40 Gazit Y, Nahir AM, Grahame R *et al.* Dysautonomia in the joint hypermobility syndrome. *Am J Med* 2003; **115**: 33–40.

41 Pope FM, Nicholls AC, Jones PM *et al.* EDS IV (acrogeria): new autosomal dominant and recessive types. *J R Soc Med* 1980; **73**: 180–6.

42 Sulh HMB, Steinmann B, Rao VH *et al.* Ehlers–Danlos syndrome type IVD. An autosomal recessive disorder. *Clin Genet* 1984; **25**: 278–87.

43 Superti-Furga A, Steinmann B, Byers PH. Type III collagen deficiency. *Lancet* 1989; **i**: 903–4.

44 Superti-Furga A, Gugler E, Gitzelmann R *et al.* Ehlers–Danlos syndrome type IV. A multi-exon deletion in one of the two COL3A1 alleles affecting structure, stability and processing of type III procollagen. *J Biol Chem* 1988; **263**: 6226–32.

45 Tsipouras P, Byers PH, Schwartz RC *et al.* Ehlers–Danlos syndrome type IV. Cosegregation of the phenotype to a COL3A1 allele of type III procollagen. *Hum Genet* 1986; **74**: 41–6.

46 Pepin M, Schwarze U, Superti-Furga A, Byers PH. Clinical and genetic features of Ehlers–Danlos syndrome type IV, the vascular type. *N Engl J Med* 2000; **342**: 673–80.

47 Byers PH, Holbrook KA, McGillivray B *et al.* Clinical and ultrastructural heterogeneity of type IV Ehlers–Danlos syndrome. *Hum Genet* 1979; **47**: 141–50.

48 Laurent R, Agache P. L'acrogéria est-elle une maladie du fibroblasts? *Dermatologica* 1974; **148**: 28–38.

49 Clark JG, Kuhn C III, Uitto J. Lung collagen in type IV Ehlers–Danlos syndrome: ultrastructural and biochemical studies. *Am Rev Respir Dis* 1980; **122**: 971–8.

50 Dwyer NG, Bartlett JR, Nicholls AC *et al.* Collagen deficiency and ruptured cerebral aneurysms. *J Neurosurg* 1983; **59**: 16–20.

51 Kuivaniemi H, Prockop DJ, Wu Y *et al.* Exclusion of mutations in the gene for type III collagen (*COL3A1*) as a common cause of intracranial aneurysms or cervical artery dissections: results from sequence analysis of the coding sequences of type III collagen from 55 unrelated patients. *Neurology* 1993; **43**: 2652–8.

52 Gertsch P, Loup PW, Lochman A *et al.* Changing patterns in the vascular form of Ehlers–Danlos syndrome. *Arch Surg* 1986; **121**: 1061–4.

53 Fox R, Pope FM, Narcisi P *et al.* Spontaneous carotid-cavernous fistula in Ehlers–Danlos syndrome. *J Neurol Neurosurg Psychiatry* 1988; **51**: 984–6.

54 Halbach VV, Higashida RT, Dowd CF *et al.* Treatment of carotid-cavernous fistula in Ehlers–Danlos syndrome. *Neurosurgery* 1990; **26**: 1021–7.

55 Pepin MG, Superti-Furga A, Byers PH. Natural history of Ehlers–Danlos syndrome type IV (EDS type IV): review of 137 cases. *Am J Hum Genet* 1992; **51**: A44.

56 Roberts DLL, Pope FM, Nicholls AL *et al.* Ehlers–Danlos type IV mimicking non-accidental injury in a child. *Br J Dermatol* 1984; **111**: 341–5.

57 Pope FM, Narcisi P, Nicholls AC *et al.* Clinical presentations of Ehlers–Danlos syndrome type IV. *Arch Dis Child* 1988; **63**: 1016–25.

58 Taylor DJ, Wilcox I, Russell JK. Ehlers–Danlos syndrome during pregnancy. A case report and review of the literature. *Obstet Gynecol Surv* 1981; **36**: 277–81.

59 Takahashi T, Koida T, Yamaguchi H *et al.* Ehlers–Danlos syndrome with aortic regurgitation, dilatation of the sinuses of Valsalva, and abnormal dermal collagen fibrils. *Am Heart J* 1992; **123**: 1709–12.

60 Loeys BL, Schwarze U, Holm T *et al.* Aneurysm syndromes caused by mutations in the TGF-beta receptor. *N Engl J Med* 2006; **355**: 788-98.

61 Beighton P, Curtis D. X-linked Ehlers–Danlos syndrome type V. The next generation. *Clin Genet* 1985; **27**: 472–8.

62 Siegel RC, Black CM, Bailey AJ. Cross-linking of collagen in the X-linked Ehlers–Danlos type V. *Biochem Biophys Res Commun* 1979; **88**: 281–7.

63 Di Ferrante N, Leachman RD, Angelini P *et al.* Lysyl oxidase deficiency in Ehlers–Danlos syndrome type V. *Connect Tissue Res* 1975; **3**: 38–53.

64 Ihme A, Krieg T, Nerlich A *et al.* Ehlers–Danlos syndrome type VI. Collagen type specificity of defective lysyl hydroxylation in various tissues. *J Invest Dermatol* 1984; **83**: 161–5.

65 Pinnell SR, Krane SM, Kenzora JE *et al.* A heritable disorder of connective tissue. Hydroxylysine-deficient collagen disease. *N Engl J Med* 1972; **266**: 1013–20.

66 Sussman M, Lichtenstein JR, Nigra TP *et al.* Hydroxylysine-deficient collagen in a patient with a form of the Ehlers–Danlos syndrome. *J Bone Joint Surg Am* 1974; **56**: 1228–34.

67 Hyland J, Ala-Kokko L, Royce P *et al.* A homozygous stop codon in the lysyl hydroxylase gene in two siblings with Ehlers–Danlos syndrome type VI. *Nat Genet* 1992; **2**: 228–31.

68 Hautala T, Keikkinen J, Kivirikko KI *et al.* A large duplication in the gene for lysyl hydroxylase accounts for the type VI variant of the Ehlers–Danlos syndrome in two siblings. *Genomics* 1993; **15**: 399–404.

69 Ha VT, Marshall MK, Elsas LJ *et al.* A patient with Ehlers–Danlos syndrome type VI is a compound heterozygote for mutations in the lysyl hydroxylase gene. *J Clin Invest* 1994; **93**: 1716–21.

70 Chamson A, Berbis P, Fabre JF *et al.* Collagen biosynthesis and isomorphism in a case of Ehlers–Danlos syndrome type VI. *Arch Dermatol Res* 1987; **279**: 303–7.

71 Eyre DR, Glimcher MJ. Reducible cross-links in hydroxylysine-deficient collagens of a heritable disorder of connective tissue. *Proc Natl Acad Sci USA* 1972; **69**: 2594–8.

72 Steinmann B, Eyre DR, Shao P. Urinary pyridinoline cross-links in Ehlers–Danlos syndrome type VI. *Am J Hum Genet* 1995; **57**: 1505–8.

73 Wenstrup RJ, Murad S, Pinnell SR. Ehlers–Danlos syndrome type VI; clinical manifestation of collagen lysyl hydroxylase deficiency. *J Pediatr* 1989; **115**: 405–9.

74 Dembure PP, Priest JH, Snoddy SC *et al.* Genotyping and prenatal assessment of collagen lysyl hydroxylase deficiency in a family with Ehlers–Danlos syndrome, type VI. *Am J Hum Genet* 1984; **36**: 783–90.

75 Dembure PP, Janko AR, Priest JH *et al.* Ascorbate regulation of collagen biosynthesis in Ehlers–Danlos syndrome type VI. *Metabolism* 1987; **36**: 687–91.

76 Steinmann B, Tuderman L, Peltonen L *et al.* Evidence for a structural mutation of procollagen type I in a patient with Ehlers–Danlos syndrome type VII. *J Biol Chem* 1980; **255**: 8887–93.

77 Wirtz MK, Glanville RW, Steinmann B *et al.* Ehlers–Danlos syndrome type VII B. Deletion of 18 amino acids comprising the N-telopeptide region of a proα2(I) chain. *J Biol Chem* 1987; **262**: 16 376–85.

78 Watson RB, Wallis GA, Holmes DF *et al.* Ehlers–Danlos syndrome type VII B. Incomplete cleavage of abnormal type I procollagen by N-proteinase *in vitro* results in the formation of copolymers of collagen and partially cleared pN collagen that are near circular in cross-section. *J Biol Chem* 1992; **267**: 9093–100.

79 D'Alessio M, Ramirez F, Blumberg BD *et al.* Characterization of a COL1A1 splicing defect in a case of Ehlers–Danlos syndrome type VII. Further evidence of molecular homogeneity. *Am J Hum Genet* 1991; **49**: 400–6.

80 Cole WG, Evans R, Sillence DO. The clinical features of Ehlers–Danlos syndrome type VII due to a deletion of 21 amino acids from the pro-α1(I) chain of type I procollagen. *J Med Genet* 1987; **24**: 698–701.

81 Smith LT, Wertelecki W, Milstone LM *et al.* Human dermatosparaxis: a form of Ehlers–Danlos syndrome that results from failure to remove the amino-terminal propeptide of type I procollagen. *Am J Hum Genet* 1992; **51**: 235–44.

82 Wertelecki W, Smith LT, Byers PH. Initial observations of human dermatosp-araxis: Ehlers–Danlos syndrome type VII C. *J Pediatr* 1992; **121**: 558–64.

83 Nusgens BV, Verellen-Dumoulin C, Hermanns Le T *et al.* Evidence for a rela-tionship between Ehlers–Danlos type VII C in humans and bovine dermatosp-araxis. *Nat Genet* 1992; **1**: 214–7.

84 Lehmann HW, Mundlos S, Winterpacht A *et al.* Ehlers–Danlos type VII. Pheno-type and genotype. *Arch Dermatol Res* 1994; **286**: 425–8.

85 Becker U, Timpl R. Amino-terminal extensions in skin collagen from sheep with a genetic defect in conversion of procollagen into collagen. *Biochemistry* 1976; **15**: 2853–62.

86 Counts DF, Byers PH, Holbrook KA *et al.* Dermatosparaxis in a Himalayan cat: biochemical studies on dermal collagen. *J Invest Dermatol* 1980; **74**: 96–9.

87 Colige A, Sieron AL, Li S-W *et al.* Human Ehlers–Danlos syndrome type VIIC and bovine dermatosparaxis are caused by mutations in the procollagen I N-proteinase gene. *Am J Hum Genet* 1999; **65**: 308–17.

88 Linch DC, Acton CH. Ehlers–Danlos syndrome presenting with juvenile destructive periodontitis. *Br Dent J* 1979; **147**: 95–6.

89 Stewart RD, Hollister DW, Rimoin DL. A new variant of the Ehlers–Danlos syndrome. An autosomal dominant disorder of fragile skin, abnormal scarring, and generalised periodontitis. *Birth Defects Orig Artic Ser* 1977; **13**: 85–93.

90 Lapière CM, Nusgens BV. Ehlers–Danlos type VIII skin has a reduced propor-tion of type III collagen. *J Invest Dermatol* 1981; **76**: 422 (Abstract).

91 Rahman N, Dunstan M, Teare MD *et al.* Ehlers-Danlos syndrome with severe early-onset periodontal disease (EDS-VIII) is a distinct, heterogeneous disorder with one predisposition gene at chromosome 12p13. *Am J Hum Genet* 2003; **73**: 198–204.

92 Holbrook KA, Byers PA. Ultrastructural characteristics of the skin in a form of Ehlers–Danlos syndrome. *Lab Invest* 1981; **44**: 342–9.

93 Hernandez A, Aguirre-Negrete MG, Ramirez-Soltero S *et al.* A distinct variant of the Ehlers–Danlos syndrome. *Clin Genet* 1979; **16**: 335–9.

94 Okajima T, Fukumoto S, Furukawa K *et al.* Molecular basis for the progeroid variant of Ehlers–Danlos syndrome. *J Biol Chem* 1999; **274**: 28 841–4.

95 Schalkwijk J, Zweere MC, Steijlen PM *et al.* A recessive form of the Ehlers–Danlos syndrome caused by tenascin-X deficiency. *N Engl J Med* 2001; **345**: 1167–75.

96 Burch GH, Gong Y, Liu W *et al.* Tenascin-X deficiency is associated with Ehlers–Danlos syndrome. *Nat Genet* 1997; **17**: 104–8.

97 Mao JR, Taylor G, Dean WB *et al.* Tenascin-X deficiency mimics Ehlers–Danlos syndrome in mice through alteration of collagen deposition. *Nat Genet* 2002; **30**: 421–5.

98 Cunliffe WJ, Ead RD. A case of Ehlers–Danlos syndrome occurring with Mar-fan's syndrome. *Clin Exp Dermatol* 1977; **2**: 117–20.

99 Levine AS, Michael AF Jr. Ehlers–Danlos syndrome with renal tubular acidosis and medullary sponge kidney. *J Pediatr* 1967; **71**: 107–13.

100 Holzberg M, Hewan-Lowe KO, Olansky AJ. The Ehlers–Danlos syndrome: recognition, characterization and importance of a milder variant of the classic form. A preliminary study. *J Am Acad Dermatol* 1988; **19**: 656–66.

101 Temple AS, Hinton P, Narcisi P *et al.* Detection of type III collagen in fibroblasts from patients with Ehlers–Danlos syndrome type IV by immunofluorescence. *Br J Dermatol* 1988; **118**: 17–26.

102 Steinmann B, Superti-Furga A, Joller-Jemelka HI *et al.* Ehlers–Danlos syndrome type IV. A subset of patients distinguished by low serum levels of the amino-terminal propeptide of type III procollagen. *Am J Med Genet* 1989; **34**: 68–71.

103 Raghunath M, Steinmann B, Delozier-Blanchet C *et al.* Prenatal diagnosis of collagen disorders by direct biochemical analysis of chorionic villus biopsies. *Pediatr Res* 1994; **36**: 441–8.

104 Brennan TE. Abnormal elastic tissue in cartilage hair hypoplasia. *Arch Dermatol* 1988; **124**: 1411–4.

105 Reidy JP. Cutis hyperelastica (Ehlers–Danlos) and cutis laxa. *Br J Plast Surg* 1963; **16**: 84–94.

Occipital horn syndrome

Synonyms
- X-linked cutis laxa
- Ehlers–Danlos syndrome type IX

In this rare, X-linked, recessive disorder, affected males have a defect in distribution of intracellular copper to copper-dependent enzymes, as in Menkes' syndrome [1]. Lysyl oxidase is a major copper-dependent enzyme, and its activity is markedly decreased in some patients [2], resulting in defective collagen cross-links. Serum copper and caeruloplasmin levels are low [1]. The disorder, like Menkes' syndrome, is caused by mutations in the gene (*ATP7A*) encoding for Cu^{2+}-transporting adenosine triphosphatase (ATPase) α-polypeptide [3,4].

Clinical manifestations include the development of bladder diverticula during childhood, inguinal herniae, mild laxity of skin and skeletal defects such as short humeri and clavicles. Bony occipital horns appear during adolescence [2]. Other features include mild chronic diarrhoea and orthostatic hypotension.

References
1 Peltonen L, Kuivaniemi H, Palotie A *et al.* Alterations in copper metabolism in the Menkes syndrome and a new subtype of Ehlers–Danlos syndrome. *Biochemistry* 1983; **22**: 6156–63.

2 Byers PH, Siegel RC, Holbrook KA *et al.* X-linked cutis laxa. Defective cross-linked formation in collagen due to decreased lysyl oxidase activity. *N Engl J Med* 1980; **303**: 61–5.

3 Levinson B, Gitschier J, Bulpe D *et al.* Are X-linked cutis laxa and Menkes disease allelic? *Nat Genet* 1993; **3**: 6.

4 Levinson B, Conant R, Schnur R *et al.* A repeated element in the regulatory region of the *MNK* gene and its deletion in a patient with occipital horn syndrome. *Hum Mol Genet* 1996; **5**: 1737–42.

Prolidase deficiency

Definition. Prolidase (peptidase D) is involved in the latter stages of degradation of endogenous and dietary proteins and is particu-larly important in collagen catabolism. Deficiency of prolidase is a rare inborn error of collagen metabolism, associated with chronic skin ulceration, mental retardation and recurrent respiratory infections.

Aetiology. The deficiency is inherited as an autosomal recessive [1,2]. Mutations in the prolidase gene (*PEPD*) result in loss of prolidase activity [3]. Some siblings of patients have the enzyme deficiency without clinical manifestations [4].

Pathology. Light and electron microscopy of cultured fibroblasts from affected patients suggest necrosis-like cell death with abnor-mal morphology and increased cytosolic vacuolization, and abnor-mal plasma membranes and mitochondria [3]. Large amounts of imidodipeptides are excreted in the urine [5,6], and the proline/hydroxyproline ratio in collagen is increased.

Abnormal laboratory findings include mild anaemia, thrombo-cytopenia and hypergammaglobulinaemia.

Clinical features [7]. Most patients are mentally defective, with an abnormal facies, but there is no characteristic or consistent pattern. Skin changes occur in about 85% of cases. The skin may feel spongy, with pitting and scarring, especially on the legs (Fig. 45.28). The skin is fragile and leg ulcers are common. Occasionally, there may be photosensitivity, telangiectasia, purpura, premature greying and lymphoedema.

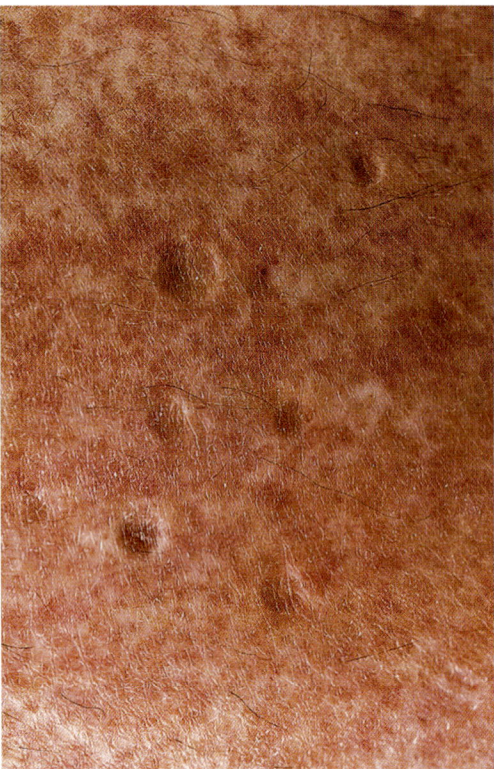

Fig. 45.28 Pitted skin in prolidase deficiency. (Courtesy of Dr D.A. Burns, Leicester Royal Infirmary, Leicester, UK.)

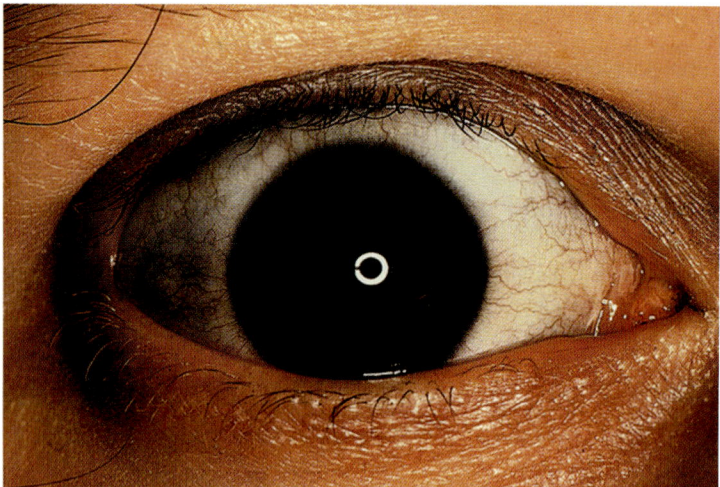

Fig. 45.29 Blue sclera in osteogenesis imperfecta.

Splenomegaly, recurrent infections and obesity or a protuberant abdomen occur in about 30% of cases. Families have been described with associated chronic lung disease, resembling cystic fibrosis [8].

Diagnosis. This is confirmed by the finding of massive imidodi-peptiduria with prolidase deficiency in the red cells, white cells or cultured fibroblasts. Mutations can be detected in the gene encoding for prolidase [3].

Treatment. Topical proline has been successfully applied to the leg ulcers [9]. Oral proline administration produces no clinical improvement. Enzyme replacement by transfusion of prolidase-containing red cells is a possibility, perhaps using manganese activation of the enzyme before transfusion [10]. Pulsed corticosteroids may help [11]. Apheresis exchange has improved skin ulceration in two patients [12].

References

1 Ogata A, Tanaka S, Tomoda T *et al.* Autosomal recessive prolidase deficiency. *Arch Dermatol* 1981; **117**: 689–97.
2 Powell GF, Kurosky A, Maniscalco RM. Prolidase deficiency: report of a second case with quantification of the excessively excreted amino-acids. *J Pediatr* 1977; **91**: 242–6.
3 Forlina A, Luupi A, Vaghi P *et al.* Mutation analysis of five new patients affected by prolidase deficiency; the lack of enzyme activity causes necrosis-like cell death in cultured fibroblasts. *Hum Genet* 2002; **111**: 3114–22.
4 Isemura M, Hanyu T, Gejyo F *et al.* Prolidase deficiency with imidodipeptiduria. *Clin Chim Acta* 1979; **93**: 401–7.
5 Arata J, Umemura S, Yamamoto Y *et al.* Prolidase deficiency. *Arch Dermatol* 1979; **114**: 62–7.
6 Sheffield LJ, Schlesinger P, Faull K *et al.* Imidopeptiduria, skin ulceration and edema in a boy with prolidase deficiency. *J Pediatr* 1977; **91**: 578–83.
7 Milligan A, Graham-Brown RAC, Burns DA *et al.* Prolidase deficiency. A case report and literature review. *Br J Dermatol* 1989; **121**: 405–9.
8 Luder AS, Mandel H, Khyat M *et al.* Chronic lung disease and cystic fibrosis phenotype in prolidase deficiency; a newly recognized association. *J Pediatr* 2007; **150**: 656–8.
9 Arata J, Hatakenaka K, Oono T. Effect of topical application of glycine and proline on recalcitrant leg ulcers of prolidase deficiency. *Arch Dermatol* 1986; **122**: 626–7.
10 Hechtman P, Richter A, Corman N *et al. In situ* activation of human erythrocyte prolidase. Potential for enzyme replacement therapy. *Pediatr Res* 1988; **24**: 709–12.
11 Yasuda K, Ogata K, Kodama H *et al.* Corticosteroid treatment of prolidase deficiency skin lesions by inhibiting iminodipeptide-primed neutrophil superoxide generation. *Br J Dermatol* 1999; **141**: 846–51.
12 Lupi A, Casado B, Soli M *et al.* Therapeutic apheresis exchange in two patients with prolidase deficiency. *Br J Dermatol* 2002; **147**: 1237–40.

Osteogenesis imperfecta (OI)

Definition. This term is applied to a heterogeneous group of heritable disorders characterized by osteoporosis with fractures, due predominantly to type I collagen abnormalities. Patients may also have blue sclerae (Fig. 45.29), deafness, skeletal deformity, abnormal dentine formation (dentinogenesis imperfecta), mild joint hypermobility, hernias, mitral valve prolapse, arterial fragility and thin, fragile skin [1,2].

Aetiology. Approximately 80–90% of patients with OI, who fit into types I–IV, have mutations in one of the type I collagen genes (*COL1A1, COL1A2*) [3]. The aetiology of the remainder is unclear. A variety of mutations are seen but very few families share the same mutation. Furthermore, considerable intrafamilial variation of phenotype occurs in type IA [4].

Pathology [5]. The bones are markedly collagen deficient, and often have a distorted architecture. The dermis is thin, with a relative increase of argyrophil and elastic fibres, and a deficiency of adult collagen [6].

Clinical features [1,2,5]. The following broad groups exist, although some patients are difficult to classify.

Type IA: Classic form. This is the commonest form. It is inherited as an autosomal dominant, although sporadic cases also occur [7]. Fractures are common in childhood. The sclerae are blue or grey, and easy bruising and early-onset deafness are common, but skeletal deformity is absent or mild. Joint laxity is common. The incidence of mitral valve prolapse is increased, and the aortic valves are thin and occasionally incompetent [8–10]. A few patients (type IB) have dentinogenesis imperfecta, but this is more common in the type IV group. Most patients have increased skin collagen, with an increased ratio of type I/type III [6]. Other patients have an abnormal α_2 chain, which is unduly susceptible to proteolysis by pepsin [11].

Type II: Lethal perinatal form. This is the rarest form. There are multiple fractures *in utero* and infants rarely survive for more than a few days after birth [12]. Avulsion of the limbs may occur during delivery due to a generalized connective tissue fragility. Radiography shows beaded ribs, crumpled femora and little skull calcification. This form has been subdivided on the basis of rib and limb bone abnormalities [6,13]. Inheritance is usually autosomal dominant. Multiple recurrence of gonadal mosaicism can mimic autosomal recessive inheritance [14].

Type III: Progressively deforming form. In this condition, there are fractures *in utero* or at birth, and the long bones are thin and occasionally cystic. As the child grows older, progressive scoliosis and bowing of long bones cause crippling deformities. The sclerae are blue in childhood but become normal in the adult. The inheritance is uncertain, but the disease may be genetically heterogeneous. Some patients with this form seem unable to synthesize α_2 chains [7,15].

Type IV: Mild form with normal sclerae. This condition is similar to type I in clinical features and inheritance, but the sclerae are not blue, dentinogenesis imperfecta is frequent and deafness is rare.

Diagnosis. Patients with short extremities and a large skull may be confused with achondroplasia, but bone fragility and thin skin do not occur in achondroplasia. Prenatal diagnosis of the more severe forms is possible, using ultrasonography from week 16 [16]. The skin of patients with OI is stiffer and less elastic than normal skin, and these differences in mechanical properties may prove useful in diagnosis and prognosis [17].

Treatment. This is essentially an orthopaedic problem, although many children die of respiratory infections [18]. Bisphosphonates have become standard care for patients with this condition although it is unclear how long therapy should be maintained [2]. Somatic cell therapy, using allogeneic bone marrow and mesenchymal stromal cell transplantation have been used [19,20].

References
1 Sillence DO, Senn A, Danks DM *et al.* Genetic heterogeneity in osteogenesis imperfecta. *J Med Genet* 1979; **16**: 101–16.
2 Glorieux FH. Experience with bisphosphonates in osteogenesis imperfecta. *Pediatrics* 2007; **119**: S163–5.
3 Byers PH, Wallis GA, Willing MC. Osteogenesis imperfecta: translation of mutation to phenotype. *J Med Genet* 1991; **28**: 433–42.
4 Willing MC, Deschenes SP, Scott DA *et al.* Osteogenesis imperfecta type I. Molecular heterogeneity for *COL1A1* null alleles of type I collagen. *Am J Hum Genet* 1994; **55**: 638–47.
5 Smith R. Osteogenesis imperfecta. *BMJ* 1984; **289**: 394–5.
6 Francis MJ, Williams KJ, Sykes BC, Smith R. The relative amounts of the collagen chains alpha 1 (I), alpha 2 and alpha 1 (III) in the skin of 31 patients with osteogenesis imperfecta. *Clin Sci (Lond)* 1981; **60**: 617–23.
7 Pope FM, Nicholls AC. Heterogeneity of osteogenesis imperfecta congenita. *Lancet* 1980; **i**: 820–1.
8 Pentinnen RP, Lichtenstein JR, Martin GR *et al.* Abnormal collagen metabolism in cultured cells in osteogenesis imperfecta. *Proc Natl Acad Sci USA* 1975; **72**: 586–9.
9 Pyeritz RE, Levin LS. Aortic root dilatation and vascular dysfunction in osteogenesis imperfecta. *Circulation* 1981; **64** (Suppl. 4): 311 (Abstract 1193).
10 White NJ, Winearls CG, Smith R *et al.* Cardiovascular abnormalities in osteogenesis imperfecta. *Am Heart J* 1983; **106**: 1416–20.
11 Nicholls AC, Pope FM, Craig D. An abnormal collagen α-chain containing cysteine in autosomal dominant osteogenesis imperfecta. *BMJ* 1983; **288**: 112–3.
12 Trelstad RL, Rubin D, Gross J. Osteogenesis imperfecta. Evidence for a generalized molecular disorder of collagen. *Lab Invest* 1977; **36**: 501–8.
13 Thompson EM, Young ID, Hall CM *et al.* Recurrence risks and prognosis in severe sporadic osteogenesis imperfecta. *J Med Genet* 1987; **24**: 390–405.
14 Byers PH. Brittle bones, fragile molecular disorders of collagen gene structure and expression. *Trends Genet* 1990; **6**: 293–300.
15 Nicholls AC, Pope FM, Schloon H *et al.* Biochemical heterogeneity of osteogenesis imperfecta: new variant. *Lancet* 1979; **i**: 1193–5.
16 Shapiro JE, Phillips JA, Byers PH *et al.* Prenatal diagnosis of lethal osteogenesis imperfecta (OI type II). *J Paediatr* 1982; **100**: 127–33.
17 Hansen B, Jemec GB. The mechanical properties of skin in osteogenesis imperfecta. *Arch Dermatol* 2002; **138**: 909–11.
18 Bleck EE. Non-operative treatment of osteogenesis imperfecta: orthotic and mobility management. *Clin Orthop* 1981; **159**: 111–22.
19 Horwitz EM, Prockop DJ, Gordon PL *et al.* Clinical responses to bone marrow transplantation in children with severe osteogenesis imperfecta. *Blood* 2001; **97**: 1227–31.
20 Horwitz EM, Prockop DJ, Fitzpatrick LA *et al.* Transplantability and therapeutic effects of bone-marrow derived mesenchymal cells in children with osteogenesis imperfecta. *Nat Med* 1999; **5**: 309–13.

Pachydermoperiostosis (see also Chapter 15)

Synonyms
- Primary (idiopathic) hypertrophic pulmonary osteoarthropathy
- Touraine–Solente–Golé syndrome

In this rare condition [1,2], inheritance is autosomal dominant, but autosomal recessive families probably also occur [3]. Digital clubbing is associated with cylindrical thickening of legs and forearms, hypohidrosis, seborrhoea, sebaceous gland hyperplasia and folliculitis. X-rays reveal symmetrical, irregular periosteal ossification, predominantly affecting the distal ends of long bones. Histology shows cutaneous sclerosis and hyalinosis, with perivascular infiltration by lymphoid cells in the dermis [2]. Additional clinical features include carpal and tarsal tunnel syndrome, chronic leg ulceration and calcification of the Achilles tendon [4]. Cultured dermal fibroblasts synthesize increased amounts of collagen and $\alpha_1(I)$ procollagen mRNA, and exhibit up-regulation of transcriptional activity of the $\alpha_1(I)$ procollagen gene promoter [5]. Proteoglycan synthesis is also affected [6].

When conventional treatments fail, intravenous pamidronate may help rheumatological manifestations [7].

References
1 Touraine A, Solente G, Golé L. Un syndrome osteodermopathique; la pachydermie plicaturée avec pachypériostose des extrémités. *Presse Med* 1958; **92**: 1820–4.

2 Matucci-Cerinic M, Lotti T, Jajic I *et al.* The clinical spectrum of primary hypertrophic osteoarthropathy. *Medicine* 1991; **70**: 208–14.

3 Castori M, Sinibaldi L, Mingarelli R *et al.* Pachydermoperiostosis: an update. *Clin Genet* 2005; **68**: 477–86.

4 Cantatore FP, Mancini L, Ingrosso AM *et al.* Pachydermoperiostosis. Dermatological, neurological and radiological observations. *Clin Rheumatol* 1995; **14**: 705–7.

5 Padula SJ, Broketa G, Sampieri A *et al.* Increased collagen synthesis in skin fibroblasts from patients with primary hypertrophic osteoarthropathy. Evidence for trans-activational regulation of collagen transcription. *Arthritis Rheum* 1994; **37**: 1386–94.

6 Wegrowski Y, Gillery P, Serpier H *et al.* Alteration of matrix molecule synthesis by fibroblasts from a patient with pachydermoperiostitis. *J Invest Dermatol* 1996; **106**: 70–4.

7 Guyot-Drouot MH, Solau-Gervais E, Cortet B *et al.* Rheumatologic manifestations of pachydermoperiostosis and preliminary experience with bisphosphonates. *J Rheumatol* 2002; **27**: 2418–23.

Relapsing polychondritis

Synonyms
- Atrophic polychondritis
- Systemic chondromalacia

Definition. In this non-infective condition, focal inflammatory destruction of cartilage is accompanied by fibroblastic regeneration. It is characterized by: (i) recurrent chondritis of the pinnae; (ii) chondritis of nasal cartilage; (iii) inflamed cartilage in the larynx, trachea or respiratory tract; (iv) ocular inflammation; (v) cochlear or vestibular lesions; and (vi) non-erosive arthritis. Three or more of these features are required for the diagnosis [1].

Aetiology. Relapsing polychondritis has been recorded as rare, but recent reports suggest that it is not so uncommon but is easily overlooked. The cause is unknown, but the association with rheumatoid arthritis, lupus erythematosus, vasculitis, Behçet's disease and Hashimoto's disease suggests that autoimmune mechanisms may be concerned (see also MAGIC syndrome, p. 45.44). Other reported associations include ulcerative colitis, Crohn's disease, psoriasis, glomerulonephritis, Sjögren's syndrome, thymoma, ankylosing spondylitis, myeloproliferative disorders and following intravenous injections [2–7]. Cutaneous manifestations have been reported in a patient treated for prostatic adenocarcinoma with goserelin, a luteinizing hormone releasing analogue [8].

Relapsing polychondritis probably overlaps with Wegener's syndrome. Auricular chondritis has been described in some patients with the latter [9], and cANCA, an antibody once regarded as specific for Wegener's syndrome, has been reported in patients with relapsing polychondritis [10].

Antibodies to type II collagen have been detected in the serum in acute polychondritis, and granular deposits of IgG, IgA, IgM and C3 at fibrochondral junctions have indicated a possible role of immune-complex deposits [11–15]. Antibody production is T-cell dependent and major histocompatibility complex (MHC) restricted; the arthritis in experimental animal models can be suppressed by synthetic type II collagen peptides [16]. The intravenous injection of papain into rabbits produces loss of cartilage rigidity, manifested by floppy ears [17], and it has been suggested that local protease activity may play some part in causing relapsing polychondritis [18]. Cartilage oligomeric matrix protein (COMP) is decreased and cartilage matrix protein (matrilin-1) increased. Both revert to normal levels during successful therapy [19].

Pathology [20]. Areas of damaged cartilage, which have lost the normal basophilic staining, are separated by areas of predominantly lymphocytic infiltration. Later, the fragments of cartilage are surrounded and replaced by abundant granulation tissue and even nascent cartilage. Occasionally there is evidence of vasculitis [21].

Clinical features [1,22–24]. The condition affects both sexes equally and usually begins between the ages of 30 and 50 years. Chondritis ultimately involves three or more sites in most patients but may be limited to one or two for long periods. The following tissues may be involved in decreasing order of frequency: auricular, joint, nasal, ocular, respiratory tract, heart valves and skin [25,26]. During the acute stage, the affected area is swollen, red and tender, and may be mistaken for cellulitis (Fig. 45.30). Sparing of the ear lobe is a useful differentiating sign. Serous otitis media can occur, and there may be loss of hearing even in the absence of chondritis [27]. Involvement of the nasal cartilage leads to obstruction and later to a saddle-nose deformity (Fig. 45.31). Cutaneous and systemic vasculitis, cerebral aneurysms, superficial thrombophlebitis and toxic erythema have been described [1,21,24,28,29].

The joint changes, usually affecting the smaller peripheral joints, may simulate rheumatoid arthritis [30]. Involvement of the larynx, trachea or bronchi produces respiratory embarrassment and recurrent infection. Permanent tracheostomy may be required

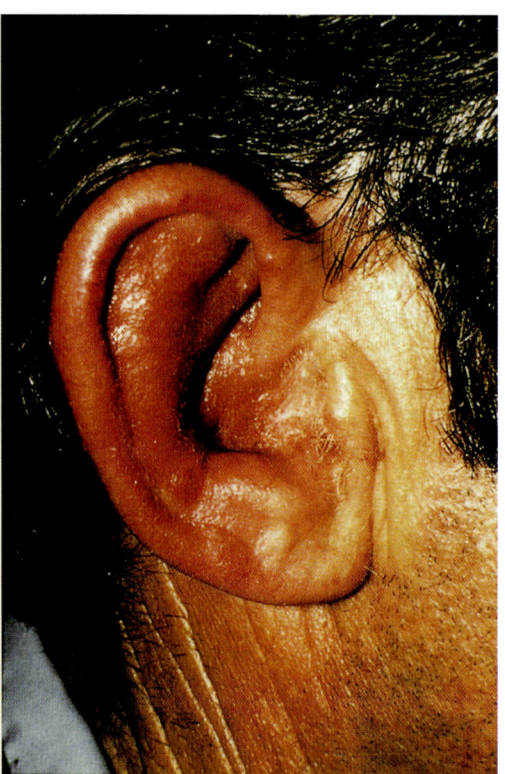

Fig. 45.30 Relapsing polychondritis, showing inflammation of the pinna.

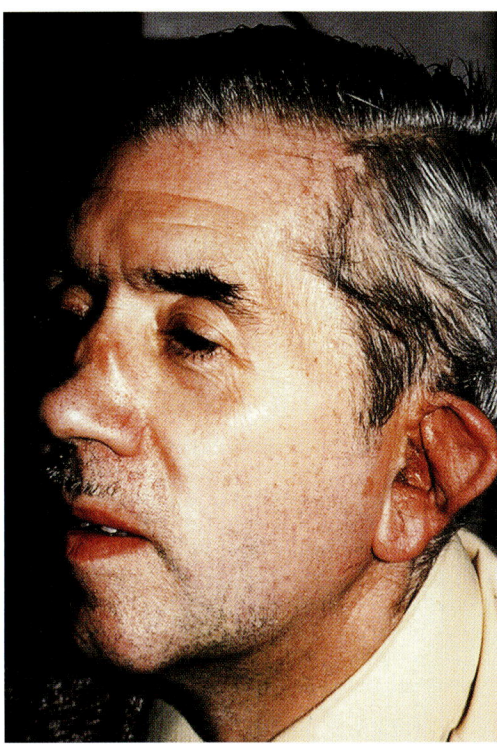

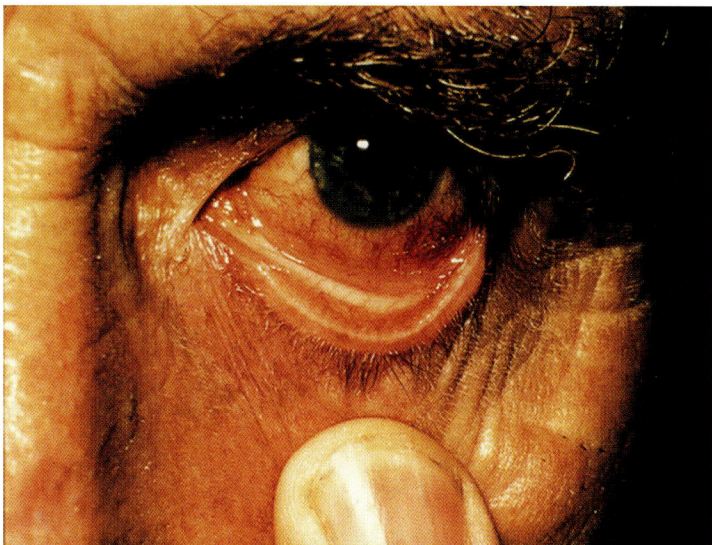

Fig. 45.32 Relapsing polychondritis, showing ocular involvement. (Courtesy of Dr N. Cox, Cumberland Royal Infirmary, Carlisle, UK.)

Fig. 45.31 Relapsing polychondritis: late stage, showing damage to the cartilage of the ear and nose. (Courtesy of Dr D.M. Wilkinson, Ackton Hospital, Pontefract, UK.)

[20,27]. An association with granulomatous lung disease has also been described. Ocular abnormalities are found in some cases—episcleritis, conjunctivitis and iritis (Fig. 45.32), or more rarely keratoconjunctivitis sicca or chorioretinitis. Proptosis occurs in 3% of cases [31,32]. Involvement of the heart valves may cause serious complications, including sudden valve rupture, even in a patient otherwise in remission [1,33,34].

The course of the disease is extremely variable [7]. Relapses are the rule, but they vary in frequency and severity. Some cases continue to relapse for over 20 years, but others become inactive within a short period. Pregnancy does not appear to affect the course of the disease, although complications are more frequent [35]. Deformity of the ears and nose is common, but in general the disease is a source of discomfort and disfigurement rather than a threat to life. Plasma viscosity or erythrocyte sedimentation rate is usually raised and anaemia is frequent. The rheumatoid factor and antinuclear factor are often positive. Leukocytosis is inconstant, but eosinophilia is found in 40% of cases. The characteristic biochemical finding is the increased urinary excretion of acid mucopolysaccharides during each relapse.

Radiological abnormalities are not pathognomonic, but evidence of extensive destruction of joint cartilage without changes in adjacent bone is suggestive. In some cases, the changes are indistinguishable from rheumatoid arthritis.

Diagnosis. Polychondritis may present to the dermatologist as 'chronic otitis externa with cellulitis of the pinna'. The diagnosis is established by biopsy, or by other associated changes, and by the examination of urine for acid mucopolysaccharides. Wegener's granulomatosis and lethal midline granuloma can produce a similar histology, but in these two conditions the involvement is more purely destructive.

Treatment. The progression of the acute relapse can be controlled with corticosteroids. An initial daily dose of 30 mg prednisone can be gradually reduced and finally discontinued as remission develops. Remissions may also be induced with indometacin or dapsone [13]. Colchicine is also helpful in some patients [36]. Immunosuppressive agents such as methotrexate and ciclosporin [15] may have a role. Pulsed intravenous cyclophosphamide has been used for renal disease [37]. Intravenous immunoglobulin [38] and anti-TNF therapies have been successful in a small number of patients [39]. Remission has followed autologous stem cell transplantation [40]. Surgical reconstruction of the nose or larynx is sometimes required.

References

1 McAdam LP, O'Hanlan MA, Bluestone R *et al.* Relapsing polychondritis: prospective review of 23 patients and review of the literature. *Medicine* 1976; **55**: 193–216.
2 Berger R. Polychondritis resulting from i.v. substance abuse. *Am J Med* 1988; **85**: 415–7.
3 Borbujo J, Balsa A, Aguado P *et al.* Relapsing polychondritis associated with psoriasis. *J Am Acad Dermatol* 1989; **20**: 130–2.
4 Conti JA, Colicchio AR, Howard LM *et al.* Thymoma, myasthenia gravis and relapsing polychondritis. *Ann Intern Med* 1988; **109**: 163–4.
5 Nield GH, Cameron JS, Lessof MH *et al.* Relapsing polychondritis with crescentic glomerulonephritis. *BMJ* 1978; **i**: 743–5.
6 Pazirandeh M, Ziran BH, Khandelwal BK *et al.* Relapsing polychondritis and spondyloarthropathies. *J Rheumatol* 1988; **15**: 630–2.
7 Michet CJ, McKenna CH, Luthra HS *et al.* Relapsing polychondritis: survival and predictive role of disease manifestation. *Ann Intern Med* 1986; **104**: 74–8.
8 Labarthe MP, Bayle-Lebey P, Bazex J. Cutaneous manifestations of relapsing polychondritis in a patient receiving goserelin for carcinoma of the prostate. *Dermatology* 1997; **195**: 391–4.
9 Small P, Black M, Davidman M *et al.* Wegener's granulomatosis and relapsing polychondritis: a case-report. *J Rheumatol* 1980; **7**: 915–8.
10 Papo T, Piette J-C, Le Thi Huong DU *et al.* Antineutrophil cytoplasmic antibodies in polychondritis. *Ann Rheum Dis* 1993; **52**: 384–5.

11 Ebringer R, Rook G, Swana GT *et al.* Autoantibodies to cartilage and type II collagen in relapsing polychondritis. *Ann Rheum Dis* 1981; **40**: 473–9.

12 Foidart JM, Abe S, Martin GR *et al.* Antibodies to type II collagen in relapsing polychondritis. *N Engl J Med* 1978; **299**: 1203–7.

13 Ridgeway HB, Hansotia PL, Schorr WF *et al.* Relapsing polychondritis. Unusual neurological features and therapeutic efficacy of dapsone. *Arch Dermatol* 1979; **115**: 43–5.

14 Ueno Y, Chai D, Barnatt EV. Relapsing polychondritis associated with ulcerative colitis: serial determinations of antibodies to cartilage and circulating immune complex by three assays. *J Rheumatol* 1981; **8**: 456–61.

15 Anstey A, Mayou S, Morgan K *et al.* Relapsing polychondritis: autoimmunity to type II collagen and treatment with cyclosporin A. *Br J Dermatol* 1991; **125**: 588–91.

16 Cremer MA, Rosloniec EF, Kang AH. The cartilage collagens: a review of their structure, organization and role in the pathogenesis of experimental arthritis in animals and in human rheumatic disease. *J Mol Med* 1998; **76**: 275–88.

17 McCluskey RT, Thomas L. The removal of cartilage matrix *in vivo* by papain. *J Exp Med* 1958; **108**: 371–84.

18 Gange RW. Relapsing polychondritis. Report of two cases with an immunopathological review. *Clin Exp Dermatol* 1976; **1**: 261–6.

19 Saxne T, Heinegard D. Serum concentrations of two cartilage matrix proteins reflecting different aspects of cartilage turnover in relapsing polychondritis. *Arthritis Rheum* 1995; **38**: 294–6.

20 Kaye RL, Sones DA. Relapsing polychondritis: clinical and pathological features in 14 cases. *Ann Intern Med* 1964; **60**: 653–64.

21 Michet CJ. Vasculitis and relapsing polychondritis. *Rheum Dis Clin North Am* 1990; **16**: 441–4.

22 Damiani J, Levine H. Relapsing polychondritis. Report of 10 cases. *Laryngoscope* 1979; **89**: 929–46.

23 Dolan DL, Lemmon GB, Teitelbaum SL. Relapsing polychondritis. Analytical literature review. *Am J Med* 1966; **41**: 285–99.

24 Hughes RAC, Berry CL, Seifert M *et al.* Relapsing polychondritis. Three cases with a clinicopathological study and literature review. *QJM* 1972; **41**: 363–80.

25 Balsa-Criada A, Garcia-Fernandez F, Roldan I *et al.* Cardiac involvement in relapsing polychondritis. *Int J Cardiol* 1987; **14**: 381–3.

26 Van Decker W, Panidis IP. Relapsing polychondritis and cardiac valvular involvement. *Ann Intern Med* 1988; **109**: 340–1.

27 Moloney JR. Relapsing polychondritis—its otolaryngological manifestations. *J Laryngol Otol* 1978; **92**: 9–14.

28 Meyrick-Thomas RH, Payne CMER, Black MM. Polychondritis as a concomitant feature of polyarteritis nodosa. *Clin Exp Dermatol* 1982; **7**: 519–22.

29 Stewart SS. Cerebral vasculitis in relapsing polychondritis. *Neurology* 1988; **38**: 150–2.

30 Franssen MJ, Boerbooms AM, van de Putt LB. Polychondritis and rheumatoid arthritis, case report and review of the literature. *Clin Rheumatol* 1987; **6**: 453–7.

31 McKay DA, Watson PG, Lyne AJ. Relapsing polychondritis and eye disease. *Br J Ophthalmol* 1974; **58**: 600–5.

32 Crovato F, Nigro A, de Marchi R *et al.* Exophthalmos in relapsing polychondritis. *Arch Dermatol* 1980; **116**: 383–4.

33 Marshall DAS, Jackson R, Rae AP *et al.* Early aortic valve cusp rupture in relapsing polychondritis. *Ann Rheum Dis* 1992; **51**: 413–5.

34 Buckley LM, Ades PA. Progressive aortic valve inflammation occurring despite apparent remission of relapsing polychondritis. *Arthritis Rheum* 1992; **35**: 812–4.

35 Papo T, Wechsler B, Bletry O *et al.* Pregnancy in relapsing polychondritis: twenty-five pregnancies in eleven patients. *Arthritis Rheum* 1997; **40**: 1245–9.

36 Mark KA, Franks AG. Colchicine and indomethacin for the treatment of relapsing polychondritis. *J Am Acad Dermatol* 2002; **46**: S22–4.

37 Stewart KA, Mazanec DJ. Pulsed intravenous cyclophosphamide for kidney disease in relapsing polychondritis. *J Rheumatol* 1992; **19**: 498–500.

38 Temier B, Aouba A, Bienvenu B *et al.* Complete remission in refractory relapsing polychondritis with intravenous immunoglobulin. *Clin Exp Rheumatol* 2008; **26**: 136–8.

39 Seymour MW, Home DM, Williams RO *et al.* Prolonged response to anti-tumour necrosis factor treatment with adalimumab (Humira) in relapsing polychondritis complicated by aortitis. *Rheumatology* 2007; **46**: 1738–9.

40 Rosen O, Thiel A, Massenkeil G *et al.* Autologous stem-cell transplantation in refractory auto-immune diseases after *in vivo* immunoablation and *ex vivo* depletion of mononuclear cells. *Arthritis Res* 2000; **2**: 327–36.

MAGIC syndrome

At least 13 patients have been described with features of both relapsing polychondritis and Behçet's syndrome [1]. The term MAGIC syndrome (*m*outh *a*nd *g*enital ulcers with *i*nflamed *c*artilage) has been used for this overlap syndrome. The underlying immunological defects are still unclear, but circulating immune complexes and autoantibodies to elastic tissue have been suggested as possible factors [1,2].

Aortic valve disease and aneurysmal aortitis have been associated with the syndrome [3,4], and features of the MAGIC syndrome have been described in an HIV-positive individual [5].

References

1 Orme RL, Nordlund JJ, Barich L *et al.* The MAGIC syndrome (mouth and genital ulcers with inflamed cartilage). *Arch Dermatol* 1990; **126**: 940–4.

2 Firestein GS, Gruber HE, Weisman MH *et al.* Mouth and genital ulcers with inflamed cartilage: MAGIC syndrome. *Am J Med* 1985; **79**: 69–72.

3 Le Thi Huong DU, Wechsler B, Piette J-C *et al.* Aortic insufficiency and recurrent valve prosthesis dehiscence in MAGIC syndrome. *J Rheumatol* 1993; **20**: 397–8.

4 Hidalgo Tenorio C, Sabio-Sánchez JM, Linares PJ *et al.* Magic syndrome and true aortic aneurysm. *Clin Rheumatol* 2008; **27**: 115–7.

5 Belzunegui J, Cancio J, Pego JM *et al.* Relapsing polychondritis and Behçet's syndrome in a patient with HIV infection. *Ann Rheum Dis* 1995; **54**: 780.

Fibromatoses

Fibrous overgrowth of dermal and subcutaneous connective tissue occurs most readily in certain sites and at certain ages, and some of the resulting syndromes are clinically and histologically distinctive and well defined. There are some cases, however, that defy precise classification, and others in which histological criteria may be a poor guide to prognosis. Invasiveness and a high local recurrence rate may or may not be associated with a tendency to metastasize. The borderline between simple overgrowth and a benign tumour may be equally difficult to define.

Fibromatosis is a benign, fibrous tissue proliferation, which is intermediate between benign fibroma and metastasizing fibrosarcoma. The lesions of fibromatosis tend to infiltrate and recur when removed, but they do not metastasize. The term should not be applied to reactive fibrous proliferation, or to keloid, which is usually secondary to injury. The lesions in fibromatosis may be single or multiple, and the likelihood of recurrence after surgical removal varies with the location of the lesion and the age of the patient. The fibromatoses occur in two major groups.

1 Superficial fibromatoses (fascial fibromatoses):
   (a) palmar (Dupuytren's)
   (b) plantar
   (c) penile (Peyronie's)
   (d) knuckle pads
2 Deep fibromatoses (non-metastasizing fibrosarcoma). These are rapidly growing tumours that usually involve the musculature or aponeuroses. Their tendon-like consistency accounts for their alternative name of desmoid tumours.

These conditions are discussed in more detail elsewhere (Chapter 56).

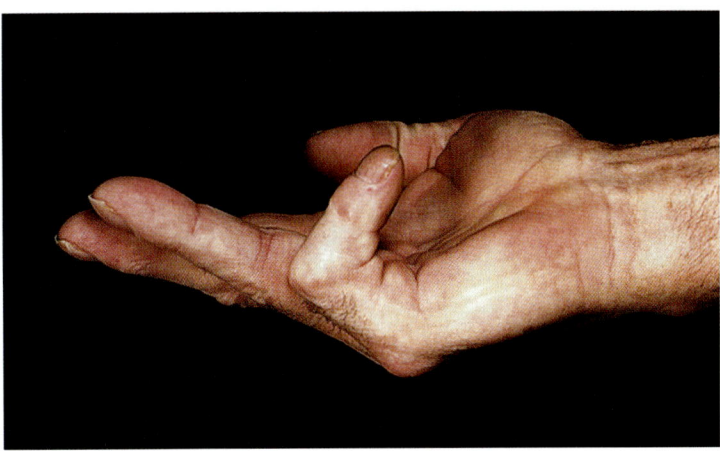

Fig. 45.33 Palmar fibromatosis (Dupuytren's contracture). (Courtesy of Dr D.A. Burns, Leicester Royal Infirmary, Leicester, UK.)

Palmar fibromatosis

Synonym
• Dupuytren's contracture

Definition. This is a fibromatous hyperplasia of the palmar aponeurosis, which is characterized by nodular thickening of the fascia with associated flexion contractures of one or more digits (Fig. 45.33).

Aetiology. The condition seems to be due to a reactive proliferation of fibroblasts with no inflammatory component, and the basic cause is obscure. Free radical production secondary to ischaemia may be involved, and the concentration of hypoxanthine substrate capable of releasing free radicals is greatly increased in the affected tissue [1]. Localized ischaemia has been thought to play a part, and in animal studies allopurinol (a competitive inhibitor of xanthine oxidase) has been shown to limit the damage associated with acute ischaemia [2]. High concentrations of free radicals are toxic, but in low concentration they stimulate fibroblast proliferation [1]. The contractures, which are a late complication, appear to follow the conversion of the fibroblasts to contractile myofibroblasts [3].

Palmar fibromatosis is often familial, and may be inherited as an autosomal dominant trait [4].

Some families are described in which there is a predominantly female expression [5]. The prevalence in the general adult population is around 2–6% [6], but it may approach 20% or more in elderly males [7–9], in diabetic patients and in patients with acquired immune deficiency syndrome (AIDS). It is relatively rare in black and oriental races.

Associated disorders. The condition occurs more commonly in patients with alcoholic cirrhosis, epilepsy [10] and diabetes mellitus [9,11], but the prevalence is decreased in rheumatoid arthritis [12].

Palmar fibromatosis is also associated in about 5% of patients with other fibrosing conditions, such as knuckle pads, Peyronie's disease, keloid scarring or plantar fibromatosis [13], and this has been termed the *polyfibromatosis syndrome*. Other conditions which have been less convincingly claimed to be associated with Dupuytren's contracture include periarthritis of the shoulder, chronic lung disease, gout, trauma and ulnar nerve damage [14]. Phenytoin appears to stimulate fibrosis in the polyfibromatosis syndrome [15] and it may also cause gingival hypertrophy by stimulating fibroblasts and increasing collagen production [10,16].

There is one case report of a girl aged 14 years who developed Dupuytren's contracture while receiving growth hormone therapy for hypopituitarism [17].

Pathology [18]. Fibroblasts in Dupuytren's contracture are identical to those in normal palmar fascia. However, there are more of them in Dupuytren's contracture and they tend to be clustered around narrowed microvessels [19]. In the early stages, there are nodules in the subcutaneous tissue, or within the fascia, composed of proliferating fibroblasts with irregular hyperchromatic nuclei, but with no excess of collagen. Later stages are characterized by the presence of myofibroblasts which have a fibrillary ultrastructure in the cytoplasm and seem to have some other properties of smooth muscle. The nuclei are deeply indented, and these constrictions may be related to the contractile properties of the cell. The cell also has surface membrane differentiations which provide attachment to neighbouring cells and stroma. Myofibroblasts have also been identified in the normal aorta and in granulation tissue, hypertrophic scars, keloids, liver fibrosis, dermatofibroma, etc. [3], in which their contractile properties may be important. The advanced stages of Dupuytren's contracture are characterized by dense, fibrous connective tissue with a few elongated cells. An increased concentration of type III collagen is present in the nodules [20]. This may be due to decreased degradation caused by increased levels of tissue inhibitors of metalloproteinases in the lesions [21]. Structural abnormalities of glycosaminoglycans, notably dermatan sulphate, may predispose to abnormal fibrillogenesis [22].

Clinical features. The age of onset is generally between 30 and 50 years, and the disease is less common and progresses more slowly in women [14]. The earliest sign is the development of a palmar nodule, usually in the ulnar half of the hand. There are usually no symptoms, but there may be a dull ache or tingling. Insidious progression of the fibrosis over several years causes flexion contractures of the affected fingers. There is often puckering of the overlying skin. Eventually, the function of the hand becomes impaired due to fixed flexion of one or more digits. If left untreated, there may be some improvement after many years.

Diagnosis. There are few diagnostic difficulties. There may be a histological resemblance to fibrosarcoma, but this is more pleomorphic, with larger nuclei and more mitoses. Juvenile aponeurotic fibroma may produce palmar or plantar nodules, but Dupuytren's contracture does not occur in young children.

Treatment. The advice of an orthopaedic or plastic surgeon should be sought. Complete removal of the palmar aponeurosis is generally recommended [23], although subtotal fasciectomy and direct closure may be an alternative approach [24].

Medical treatments are disappointing. Allopurinol may help by decreasing free-radical production [25], and it has been suggested that vitamin C might prevent progression of the disease by acting as a free-radical scavenger [7]. Many other non-surgical approaches have been tried, including continuous slow skeletal traction, radiotherapy, dimethyl sulfoxide, vitamin E, steroid injections and interferon, although none has been proven to be clinically useful [26]. However, placebo-controlled trials of collagenase injections look very promising [27].

Another suggestion, which has yet to be tested clinically, is the use of immunosuppressive therapy as an adjunct to surgery, on the grounds that the presence of CD3 lymphocytes and the expression of MHC class II proteins in the affected tissue imply that Dupuytren's disease is a T-cell-mediated autoimmune disorder [28].

References

1 Murrell GAC, Francis MJ, Bromley L et al. Free radicals and Dupuytren's contracture. *BMJ* 1987; **295**: 1373–5.

2 Granger DN. Superoxide radicals in feline intestinal ischaemia. *Gastroenterology* 1981; **81**: 22–9.

3 James WD, Odom RB. The role of the myofibroblast in Dupuytren's contracture. *Arch Dermatol* 1980; **116**: 807–11.

4 Ling RSM. The genetic factor of Dupuytren's disease. *J Bone Joint Surg* 1963; **45B**: 709–18.

5 Matthews P. Familial Dupuytren's contracture with predominant female expression. *Br J Plast Surg* 1979; **32**: 120–3.

6 Mikkelsen OA. The prevalence of Dupuytren's contracture in Norway. *Acta Chir Scand* 1972; **138**: 695–700.

7 Bower M, Nelson M, Gazzard BG. Dupuytren's contracture in patients infected with HIV. *BMJ* 1990; **300**: 164–5.

8 Evans RA. The aetiology of Dupuytren's disease. *Br J Hosp Med* 1986; **35**: 198–9.

9 Heathcote JG. Fibromatosis and diabetes mellitus. *Lancet* 1981; **i**: 1420.

10 Critchley EM, Vakil SD, Hayward HW et al. Dupuytren's disease in epilepsy: result of prolonged administration of anticonvulsants. *J Neurol Neurosurg Psychiatry* 1976; **39**: 498–50.

11 Larkin JG, Frier BM. Limited joint mobility and Dupuytren's contracture in diabetic, hypertensive and normal populations. *BMJ* 1986; **292**: 1494.

12 Arafa M, Steingold RF, Noble J et al. The incidence of Dupuytren's disease in patients with rheumatoid arthritis. *J Hand Surg (Am)* 1984; **9B**: 165–6.

13 Wolfe SJ, Summerskill WHJ, Davidson CS. Dupuytren's contracture associated with alcoholism and cirrhosis. *N Engl J Med* 1956; **255**: 559–63.

14 Allen PW. The fibromatoses. A clinicopathologic classification based on 140 cases. *Am J Surg Pathol* 1977; **1**: 255–70.

15 Piérard GE, Lapière CM. Phenytoin dependent fibrosis in polyfibromatosis syndrome. *Br J Dermatol* 1979; **100**: 335–41.

16 Hassell TM, Page RC, Narayanan AS et al. Diphenylhydantoin (Dilantin) gingival hyperplasia: drug-induced abnormality of connective tissue. *Proc Natl Acad Sci USA* 1976; **73**: 2909–12.

17 Kiess W, Butenandt O. Development of Dupuytren's contracture during growth hormone therapy. *Lancet* 1993; **342**: 181–2.

18 Gabbiani G, Manjo G. Dupuytren's contracture: fibroblast contraction. An ultrastructural study. *Am J Pathol* 1972; **66**: 131–46.

19 Murrell GA. The role of the fibroblast in Dupuytren's contracture. *Hand Clin* 1991; **7**: 669–80.

20 Bailey AJ, Sims TJ, Gabbiani G et al. Collagen of Dupuytren's disease. *Clin Sci Mol Med* 1977; **53**: 499–502.

21 Ulrich D, Hrynyschyn K, Pallua N. Matrix metalloproteinases and tissue inhibitors of metalloproteinases in sera and tissue of patients with Dupuytren's disease. *Plast Reconstr Surg* 2003; **112**: 1279–86.

22 Koźna EM, Glowacki A, Olazyk K et al. Dermatan sulphate remodeling associated with advanced Dupuytren's contracture. *Acta Biochim Pol* 2007; **54**: 821–30.

23 Rodrigo JJ, Niebauer JJ, Brown RL et al. Treatment of Dupuytren's contracture. Long-term result after fasciotomy and fascial excision. *J Bone Joint Surg Am* 1976; **58**: 380–7.

24 Shaw DL, Wise D, Holms W. Dupuytren's disease treated by palmar fasciectomy and an open palm technique. *J Hand Surg (Am)* 1996; **218**: 484–5.

25 Murrell GAC. Hypothesis for the resolution of Dupuytren's contracture with allopurinol. *Spec Sci Technol* 1987; **10**: 107–12.

26 Hurst LC, Badalamente MA. Nonoperative treatment of Dupuytren's disease. *Hand Clin* 1999; **15**: 97–107.

27 Badalamente MA, Hurst LC, Hentz VR. Collagen as a clinical target: Nonoperative treatment of Dupuytren's disease. *J Hand Surg (Am)* 2002; **27**: 788–98.

28 Baird KS, Alwan WH, Crossan JF, Wojciak B. T-cell mediated response in Dupuytren's disease. *Lancet* 1993; **341**: 1622–3.

Camptodactyly

Camptodactyly is a non-traumatic flexion deformity affecting the proximal interphalangeal joint of one or more fingers [1]. It may be a feature of a variety of syndromes; the molecular defects in several of these have been identified. Congenital camptodactyly is most notably associated with non-inflammatory arthropathy [2]. Additionally, other serous membranes undergo fibrosis, leading to constricting pericarditis and pleuritis (*CAP syndrome*) [3,4]. Familial camptodactyly of later onset has been described in association with an inflammatory arthritis with erosive changes [5]. *Blau's syndrome* encompasses familial camptodactyly, granulomatous arthritis, uveitis and an erythematous eruption with phenotypic overlap with early onset sarcoidosis [6]. Mutations in *NOD2/CARD15* have been shown to confer susceptibility to several chronic inflammatory disorders, including Crohn's disease, Blau syndrome and early-onset sarcoidosis [7]. In one family, taurinuria was associated [8]. Bilateral camptodactyly is also part of an autosomal recessive disorder (Crisponi syndrome) characterized by muscular contractions of the face, trismus, facial anomalies and death due to fevers. The syndrome is caused by *CRLF1* mutations and is allelic to cold-induced sweating syndrome type I [9].

Microdeletion of 1p36 is a relatively common syndrome, affecting 1 : 5000 neonates. Clinical features include camptodactyly, facial dysmorphism and low-set ears, cardiac and CNS defects; it is responsible for around 1% of idiopathic mental retardation [10]. Sporadic cases of camptodactyly have been linked with accelerated growth and osseous maturation, unusual facial appearance (including large ears, small mouth, broad forehead and hypertelorism), a hoarse, low-pitched cry and hypertonia (*Weaver's syndrome*) [11]. Other associated features include pectus excavatum and scoliosis.

Treatment, if required, is surgical [1,12,13].

References

1 Engbar WD, Flatt AF. Camptodactyly. An analysis of sixty-six patients and twenty-four operations. *J Hand Surg (Am)* 1977; **2A**: 216–24.

2 Jacobs JC, Downey JA. Juvenile rheumatoid arthritis. In: Downey JH, Low NC, eds. *The Child with Disabling Illness*. Philadelphia: Saunders, 1974: 5–24.

3 Martinez-Lavin M, Buendia A, Delgardo E et al. A familial syndrome of pericarditis, arthritis and camptodactyly. *N Engl J Med* 1983; **309**: 224–5.

4 Laxer RM, Cameron BJ, Chaisson D et al. The camptodactyly–arthropathy–pericarditis syndrome: case report and literature review. *Arthritis Rheum* 1986; **29**: 439–44.

5 Gigante MC, Santori FS, Zoppini A et al. Familial erosive arthritis associated with camptodactyly. *Scand J Rheumatol* 1970; **19**: 239–44.

6 Raphael SA, Blau EB, Zhang WH et al. Analysis of a large kindred with Blau syndrome for HLA, autoimmunity and sarcoidosis. *Am J Dis Child* 1993; **147**: 842–8.

7 Le Bourhis L, Benko S, Girardin SE. Nod1 and Nod2 in innate immunity and human inflammatory disorders. *Biochem Soc Trans* 2007; **35**: 1479–84.

8 Nevin NC, Hurwitz LJ, Neill DW. Familial camptodactyly with taurinuria. *J Med Genet* 1966; **3**: 265–8.
9 Dagoneau N, Bellais S, Blanchet P *et al*. Mutations in cytokine receptor-like factor 1 (CRLF1) account for both Crisponi and cold-induced sweating syndromes. *Am J Hum Genet* 2007; **80**: 966–70.
10 Battaglia A, Hayme HE, Dallapiccola B *et al*. Further delineation of deletion 1p36 syndrome in 60 patients: a recognizable phenotype and common cause of developmental delay and mental retardation. *Pediatrics* 2008; **121**: 404–10.
11 Weaver DD, Graham CB, Thomas IT *et al*. A new overgrowth syndrome with accelerated skeletal maturation, unusual facies and camptodactyly. *J Pediatr* 1974; **84**: 547–52.
12 Goffin D, Lenoble E, Marin-Braun F *et al*. Camptodactyly: classification and therapeutic results. *Ann Chir Main* 1994; **13**: 20–5.
13 Foucher G, Loréa P, Khouri RK *et al*. Camptodactyly as a spectrum of congenital deficiencies: a treatment algorithm based on clinical examination. *Plast Reconstr Surg* 2006; **117**; 1897–905.

Streblodactyly

Streblodactyly [1] is inherited as a sex-linked, autosomal, dominant character. The affected females show from birth a flexion deformity at the metacarpophalangeal joints of the thumbs and the proximal interphalangeal joints of the little fingers. Some fingers show swan-neck deformities and hyperextensible metacarpophalangeal joints. In one family there was an abnormal α-amino aciduria.

Reference

1 Parish JG, Horn DB, Thompson M *et al*. Familial streblodactyly with amino-aciduria. *BMJ* 1963; **ii**: 1247–50.

Plantar fibromatosis [1,2]

> **Synonym**
> • Ledderhose's disease

This is a much rarer condition than palmar fibromatosis. The lesions, which occur most often on the medial half of the mid-foot, present as one or more nodules, which may become painful and may ulcerate (Fig. 45.34). They rarely produce contractures, but they tend to be locally invasive and to recur. Total excision of the

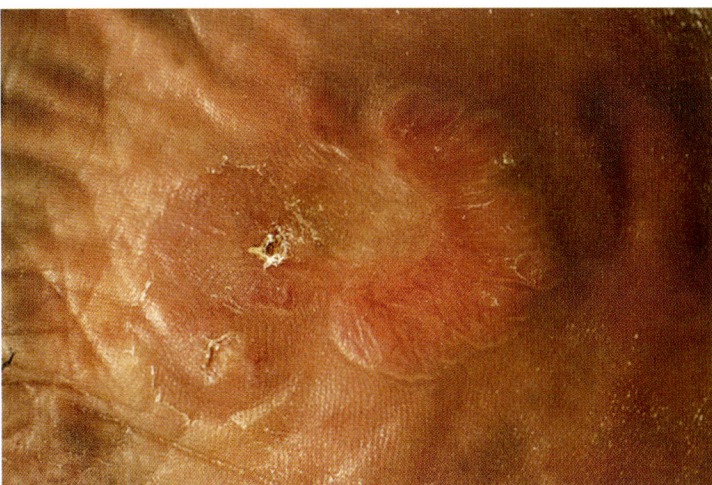

Fig. 45.34 Plantar fibromatosis. (Courtesy of Dr J. Ellis, Princess Margaret Hospital, Swindon, UK.)

lesion and the entire plantar fascia seems to give the best results, with the lowest incidence of recurrence. The differential diagnosis includes keloid and fibrosarcoma, and in younger patients aggressive infantile fibromatosis and aponeurotic fibroma must also be considered [3]. Similar nodules have been described symmetrically affecting the anteromedial heel pads in children. They are asymptomatic and may resolve spontaneously [4,5]. Surgery is contraindicated.

References

1 Allen RA, Woolner LB, Ghormley RK *et al*. Soft tissue tumours of the sole with special reference to plantar fibromatosis. *J Bone Joint Surg (Am)* 1995; **37**: 14–26.
2 Warthan TL, Rudolf RI, Gross PR *et al*. Isolated plantar fibromatosis. *Arch Dermatol* 1973; **108**: 823–5.
3 Fleischmajer R, Nedwich A, Reeves JR *et al*. Juvenile fibromatoses. *Arch Dermatol* 1973; **107**: 574–9.
4 Godette A, O'Sullivan M, Menelaus MB. Plantar fibromatosis of the heel in children: a report of 14 cases. *J Pediatr Orthop* 1997; **17**: 16–7.
5 Jacob CI, Kumm RC. Benign anteromedial plantar nodules of childhood: a distinct form of plantar fibromatosis. *Pediatr Dermatol* 2000; **17**: 472–4.

Penile fibromatosis

> **Synonyms**
> • Peyronie's disease
> • Plastic induration of the penis
> • Fibrous sclerosis of the penis

Definition. Penile fibromatosis is characterized by one or more irregular, dense fibrous plaques in the penile shaft.

Aetiology. Penile fibromatosis may occur as an isolated abnormality, or as one component of polyfibromatosis in association with palmoplantar fibromatosis, keloids and knuckle pads. Atheroma predisposes to the condition, and it is now thought that the association with the use of β-adrenoreceptor blocking drugs is probably attributable to concomitant atheroma [1,2]. There may be a genetic factor, but reliable studies of the mode of inheritance are lacking. The condition is rare below the age of 20 years, and the highest incidence is between 40 and 60 years. It is much less common than palmar or plantar fibromatosis.

Pathology [3]. The thickened plaque shows cellular fibroblastic proliferation surrounded by dense masses of collagen. Calcification and ossification may occur. The process appears to begin as a vasculitis in the areolar connective tissue beneath the tunica albuginea, whence it extends to adjacent structures.

Clinical features. The disease presents with painful erections and curvature of the erect penis due to a thickened subcutaneous plaque, rubbery or hard, usually on the dorsal aspect of the penis in its distal third. The erectile deformity may make vaginal penetration impossible, and pain or anxiety about performance may cause secondary impotence. Fibrosis of the underlying cavernous erectile tissue may lead to a constriction or 'waisting' of the penile shaft, leading to flaccidity of the distal portion.

The course is unpredictable [4]. The pain generally subsides within a few months, but the fibrous plaque may resolve, remain unchanged or progress [5].

The severity of the disease and the response to treatment can now be evaluated by high-resolution ultrasonography [6], computed tomography [7] or magnetic resonance imaging of the erect penis [8]. If necessary, an erection can be induced by the intracavernosal injection of papaverine [9].

Treatment. Many treatments have been tried, but there is little evidence that vitamin E, potassium aminobenzoate, orgotein, radiotherapy, ultrasonic therapy or intralesional steroids affect the long-term outcome, although they may relieve the pain [4]. Clostridial collagenase injections have given promising results [10]. Surgery is probably the treatment of choice, using Nisbet's operation, in which ellipses of normal tunica albuginea are excised from the side of the shaft, opposite the point of maximum curvature. An alternative is venous grafting, using the deep dorsal vein [11]. A semirigid penile prosthesis may also be inserted.

References

1 Chilton CP, Castle WM, Westwood CA *et al*. Factors associated in the aetiology of Peyronie's disease. *Br J Urol* 1982; **54**: 748–50.
2 Pryor JP. Association between Peyronie's disease and chronic degenerative arterial disease rather than β-adrenoreceptor blocking agents. *Prog Reprod Biol Med* 1983; **9**: 23–6.
3 Smith BH. Peyronie's disease. *Am J Clin Pathol* 1966; **45**: 670–8.
4 Gingell JC, Desai KM. Peyronie's disease. Treatment should always restore sexual function. *BMJ* 1988; **297**: 1489–90.
5 Williams JL, Thomas GG. The natural history of Peyronie's disease. *J Urol* 1970; **103**: 75–6.
6 Balconi G, Angeli E, Nessi R *et al*. Ultrasonic evaluation of Peyronie's disease. *Urol Radiol* 1988; **10**: 85–8.
7 Rollandi GA, Tentarelli T, Vespier M *et al*. Computed tomographic findings in Peyronie's disease. *Urol Radiol* 1985; **7**: 153–6.
8 Bystrom J, Johansson B, Edgren J *et al*. Induratio penis plastica (Peyronie's disease). Cavernosography in assessment of the disease process. *Scand J Urol Nephrol* 1974; **8**: 155–61.
9 Desai KM, Gingell JC. Outpatient assessment of penile curvature. *Br J Urol* 1987; **60**: 470–1.
10 Gelbard MK, Lindner A, Kaufman JJ *et al*. The use of collagenase in the treatment of Peyronie's disease. *J Urol* 1985; **134**: 280–3.
11 Hsu GC, Chen HS, Hsieh CH *et al*. Long term results of autologous venous grafts for penile morphological reconstruction. *J Androl* 2007; **28**: 186–93.

Knuckle pads [1–4]

> **Synonym**
> • Holoderma

Definition. Knuckle pads are circumscribed thickenings overlying the finger joints. The term is a misnomer as most lesions occur over the proximal interphalangeal rather than the metacarpophalangeal joints (knuckles).

Aetiology. The condition is usually sporadic but several pedigrees have shown an autosomal dominant inheritance. The age of onset and the distribution of the lesions tend to be more or less constant in each family, but show interfamily variation. The condition is not rare but the true prevalence is uncertain, as most patients ignore the lesions. Knuckle pads are thought to be idiopathic in children, although they occur at sites prone to picking, chewing or 'knuckle cracking' [4].

Pathology [1]. The epidermis is grossly hyperkeratotic and acanthotic. The dermal connective tissue is hyperplastic and individual collagen fibres may be obviously thickened. Histologically, the changes resemble those of palmar fibromatosis.

Clinical features [2,3]. Flat or convex, smooth, circumscribed keratoses develop slowly and almost imperceptibly over the course of months or years. In some patients they become very much raised and obviously indurated, but in others the dermal component is not clinically apparent. They are most commonly seen over the dorsa of the proximal interphalangeal joints, but occasionally develop over the knuckles or the distal interphalangeal joints. Any single site or combination of sites may be involved. Sites other than the hands are not often affected, but similar lesions on the knees were also present in one family [2].

The age of onset is variable but it is more common after the fourth decade. In some individuals, the lesions may not be conspicuous until they have been present for some years.

An association between Dupuytren's contracture and other fibromatous lesions has been recorded in some families. In one large family, knuckle pads were associated with sensorineural deafness and with leukonychia [5]. Knuckle pads have also been associated with epidermolytic palmoplantar keratoderma in a Chinese family due to keratin 9 mutations [6].

Another family has been described with knuckle pads in association with oesophageal cancer, hyperkeratosis and oral leukoplakia [7].

In differential diagnosis, occupational callosities, Heberden's nodes of osteoarthritis, pachydermodactyly, granuloma annulare, erythema elevatum diutinum and rheumatoid nodules must be excluded.

Treatment. There is no satisfactory treatment. Excision may be followed by keloidal scarring.

References

1 Lagier R, Meineke R. Pathology of knuckle pads. *Virchows Arch* 1975; **365**: 185–91.
2 Morginson WJ. Discrete keratodermas over the knuckle and finger articulations. *Arch Dermatol* 1955; **71**: 349–53.
3 Mikkelson OH. Knuckle pads in Dupuytren's disease. *Hand* 1977; **9**: 301.
4 Peterson CM, Barnes CJ, Davis LS. Knuckle pads: does knuckle cracking play an etiologic role? *Pediatr Dermatol* 2000; **17**: 450–2.
5 Bart RS, Pumphrey RE. Knuckle pads, leukonychia and deafness. *N Engl J Med* 1967; **276**: 202–7.
6 Lu Y, Guo C, Liu Q *et al*. A novel mutation of keratin 9 in epidermolytic palmoplantar keratoderma combined with knuckle pads. *Am J Med Genet* 2003; **120A**: 345–9.
7 Ritter SB, Peterson G. Esophageal cancer, hyperkeratosis and oral leukoplakia. *JAMA* 1976; **235**: 1723.

Pachydermodactyly [1–7]

This is a benign fibromatosis of the fingers that usually affects young adult males (Fig. 45.35). It produces a symmetrical, diffuse swelling of the skin around the dorsal and lateral aspects of the proximal phalanges of the index, ring and middle fingers. Pachydermodactyly has been recently reported in women [4,5] and two young girls, one of whom had tuberous sclerosis and the other EDS [6]. It may be associated with bilateral carpal tunnel

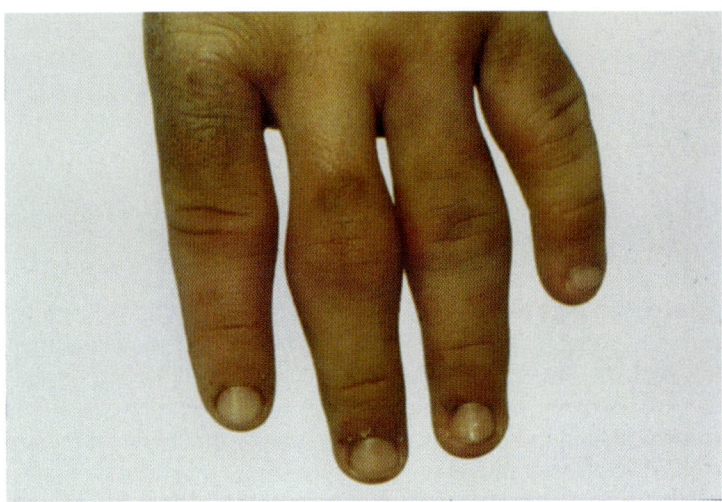

Fig. 45.35 Pachydermodactyly. (Courtesy of Dr A. Chamberlain, Churchill Hospital, Oxford, UK.)

syndrome [2] and varioliform atrophy [8]. A distal variant has been described in an elderly woman, who also presented with nodules over the extensor aspects of the elbows [9]. Affected families have been reported [10].

It has been suggested that repeated rubbing of the fingers or mechanical injury to the joints may contribute to the condition [3,6], but pachydermodactyly must be distinguished from occupational callosities, obsessive 'chewing pads' and true knuckle pads [11,12], although knuckle pads and pachydermodactyly coexisted in one family [13].

Histology shows epidermal hyperplasia and marked dermal thickening, with extension of collagenous fibres into the subcutaneous tissue. Types III and V collagen are increased, and electron microscopy shows increased numbers of fine-diameter collagen fibres.

References

1 Al Hammadi A, Hakim M. Pachydermodactyly: case report and review of the literature. *J Cutan Med Surg* 2007; **11**: 185–7.
2 Verbov J. Pachydermodactyly: a variant of the true knuckle pad. *Arch Dermatol* 1975; **111**: 524.
3 Meunier L, Pailler C, Barneon G, Meynadier J. Pachydermodactyly or acquired digital fibromatosis. *Br J Dermatol* 1994; **131**: 744–6.
4 Draluck JC, Kopf AU, Hodak E. Pachydermodactyly: first report in a woman. *J Am Acad Dermatol* 1992; **27**: 303–5.
5 Bardazzi F, Fanti PA, De Padova MP *et al.* Localized pachydermodactyly in a woman. *Acta Derm Venereol Suppl (Stockh)* 1994; **74**: 152–3.
6 Bardazzi F, Neri I, Fanti PA *et al.* Pachydermodactyly in two young girls. *Pediatr Dermatol* 1996; **13**: 288–91.
7 Curley RK, Hudson PM, Marsden RA. Pachydermodactyly: a rare form of digital fibromatosis—report of four cases. *Clin Exp Dermatol* 1991; **16**: 121–3.
8 Callot V, Wechsler J, Hovanian A *et al.* Pachydermodactyly and atrophia maculosa varioliformis cutis. *Dermatology* 1995; **190**: 56–8.
9 Tompkins SD, McNutt NS, Shea CR. Distal pachydermodactyly. *J Am Acad Dermatol* 1998; **38**: 359–62.
10 Russo F, Rodriguez-Picardo A, Camacho F. Familial pachydermodactyly. *Acta Derm Venereol* 1994; **74**: 386–7.
11 Kopera D, Soyer HP, Kerl H. An update on pachydermodactyly and a report of three additional cases. *Br J Dermatol* 1995; **133**: 433–7.
12 Lautenschlager S, Itin PH, Rufli T. Pachydermodactyly: reflecting obsessive-compulsive behavior? *Arch Dermatol* 1994; **130**: 387.
13 Chamberlain AJ, Venning VA, Wojnarowska F. Pachydermodactyly; a forme fruste of knuckle pads? *Australas J Dermatol* 2003; **44**: 140–3.

Juvenile fibromatoses

The term juvenile fibromatosis has been applied to a group of disorders occurring in infants and children, and characterized by proliferative activity of the fibroblasts [1–6]. There is a tendency to local recurrence but, unlike fibrosarcomas, they do not metastasize. The group includes a number of well-defined clinical entities that affect the skin:

1 infantile myofibromatosis
2 fibrous hamartoma of infancy
3 juvenile hyaline fibromatosis
4 infantile digital fibromatosis
5 calcifying aponeurotic fibroma
6 giant cell fibroblastoma.

These conditions are described in Chapter 56.

Juvenile hyaline fibromatosis

Synonyms
- Systemic hyalinosis
- Puretic syndrome

Definition. This is a disorder of glycosaminoglycan synthesis, which is characterized clinically by skin papules or tumours, gingival enlargement, osteolytic lesions and joint contractures, and histologically by deposition of amorphous hyaline material.

Aetiology. The cause is unknown, but increased chondroitin synthesis has been demonstrated in skin fibroblasts cultured from the tumour tissue [1]. The disease is very rare and occurs sporadically, but it has occurred in siblings.

Pathology [1–4]. The skin lesions contain 'chondroid' cells embedded in amorphous eosinophilic ground substance in the dermis. In the early lesions, this consists of glycosaminoglycans, but in the later lesions the matrix is mainly composed of chondroitin sulphate [5]. The dermal collagen is decreased and the collagen fibrils are fewer and thinner than in normal skin. The hyaline material may also be present in the muscles and bones. Absence of pro-α_2 chains and type III collagen has been demonstrated in affected skin [6].

Clinical features [4,7–10]. Skin lesions are present at birth or develop in early childhood. There may be small, pearly papules or nodules, particularly on the face or neck. Large subcutaneous tumours may also occur, particularly on the scalp. These may be hard or soft, fixed or mobile, and they may ulcerate. Gingival hypertrophy is commonly present, and flexion contractures of the fingers, elbows, hips and knees may develop. Osteolytic lesions can occur in the skull, long bones or phalanges. The musculature is poorly developed. The condition persists into adult life and the joint contractures are disabling. Infantile systemic hyalinosis is probably an extreme variant, leading to death in infancy.

Treatment. This is unsatisfactory. The tumours do not respond to radiotherapy, and they may recur after excision [11]. Joint contractures may respond to intralesional steroid injections in the early stages and they may also respond to systemic steroids and physiotherapy.

References

1 Iwata S, Horiuchi R, Maeda H *et al.* Systemic hyalinosis or juvenile fibromatosis. Ultrastructural and biochemical study of cultured skin fibroblasts. *Arch Dermatol Res* 1980; **267**: 115–21.

2 Chitale AR, Murthy AK, Maniar JK *et al.* Juvenile hyaline fibromatosis. *Ultrastruct Pathol* 1987; **11**: 771–5.

3 Ishikawa H, Maeda H, Takamatsu H *et al.* Systemic hyalinosis (juvenile hyaline fibromatosis). Ultrastructure of the hyaline with particular reference to the crossbanded structure. *Arch Dermatol Res* 1979; **265**: 195–206.

4 Finlay AY, Ferguson SD, Holt PJA *et al.* Juvenile hyaline fibromatosis. *Br J Dermatol* 1983; **108**: 609–16.

5 Mayer DA, Silva A. Juvenile hyaline fibromatosis. A histologic and histochemical study. *Arch Pathol Lab Med* 1988; **112**: 928–31.

6 Winik B, Boente M, Asail R. Juvenile hyaline fibromatosis: ultrastructural study. *Am J Dermatopathol* 1998; **20**: 372–8.

7 Camarasa JG, Moreno A. Juvenile hyaline fibromatosis. *J Am Acad Dermatol* 1987; **16**: 881–3.

8 Fayad MN, Yacoub A, Salman S *et al.* Juvenile hyaline fibromatosis. Two new cases and a review of the literature. *Am J Med Genet* 1987; **26**: 123–31.

9 Landing BH, Nadorra R. Infantile systemic hyalinosis. *Pediatr Pathol* 1986; **6**: 55–97.

10 Remberger K, Krieg J. Fibromatosis hyalinica multiplex (juvenile hyaline fibromatosis). *Cancer* 1985; **56**: 614–24.

11 Quintal D, Jackson R. Juvenile hyaline fibromatosis. A 15-year follow up. *Arch Dermatol* 1985; **121**: 1062–3.

Other benign fibrous cutaneous nodules

Nodular fasciitis

See Chapter 56. In this condition, there is fibroblastic proliferation of one or more nodules, usually on the limbs or trunk.

Collagenoma

Multiple fibrous dermal nodules with coarse, collagen fibres may develop as sporadic cases (*eruptive collagenoma*) or as a genetic disorder with a dominant inheritance (*familial cutaneous collagenoma*) (Chapter 18).

Collagen naevi

See Chapter 18.

Albopapuloid form of epidermolysis bullosa

Synonym
• Pasini's syndrome

This rare form of epidermolysis bullosa is characterized by the development of ivory-white papules on the trunk, which histologically show connective tissue hyperplasia. Epidermolysis bullosa is discussed in Chapter 39.

Buschke–Ollendorf syndrome

Extensive nodular fibrosis may occur in the Buschke–Ollendorf syndrome (Chapter 18), in association with juvenile elastoma and osteopoikilosis.

Fibrous digital nodules

In addition to giant cell synovioma and infantile digital fibromatosis, fibrous nodules in the digits may be due to acquired digital fibrokeratoma, fibrous papule of the finger, dermatofibroma (Chapter 56) or the Koenen tumour (Chapter 15).

Infantile stiff-skin syndromes

Several rare syndromes have been described in which hard, stiff skin and joint contractures develop in early life.

Systemic hyalinosis

Infantile systemic hyalinosis is an autosomal recessive condition in which the skin becomes diffusely thickened and hard in the first few weeks of life, with limited joint mobility. Other characteristic features include small nodular thickenings of the perianal region, ears or lips, and gingival hypertrophy. There may also be hyperpigmentation, painful swollen joints with contractures, osteopenia, diarrhoea, frequent severe infections and growth failure. The prognosis is poor, and survival beyond the age of 2 years is unlikely [1].

The tissues show widespread deposits of hyaline material with the general staining properties of collagen.

Clinically, this syndrome shares many similarities with juvenile hyaline fibromatosis (see p. 45.49) [2,3]. Mutations in capillary morphogenic protein 2 (*CMG2*) have been found in both conditions, indicating that they are allelic [4,5].

Winchester's syndrome

Diffusely stiff, thickened skin may also occur in Winchester's syndrome [6–8]. This is a rare, autosomal recessive disease of infancy characterized by joint contractures, gingival hypertrophy, dwarfism, osteolysis, arthralgia, corneal opacities and hypertrichosis. The prognosis is relatively good, and many patients survive into adult life.

Previously, similar cases have been described as *hereditary contractures with sclerodermatoid changes of skin* and *stiff-skin syndrome* [9], with increased mucopolysaccharides in the skin.

The skin changes resemble those of scleredema of Buschke but are distinguished by their early onset. The condition must also be distinguished from sclerema neonatorum, but this is a disorder of subcutaneous fat rather than the skin.

Winchester's syndrome is caused by mutations in the matrix metalloproteinase 2 (*MMP2*) gene. The clinical and molecular findings suggest that Winchester's syndrome, nodulosis–arthropathy–osteolysis (NAO) syndrome and Torg (hereditary multicentric osteolysis) syndrome are allelic disorders that form a clinical spectrum [10].

Congenital fascial dystrophy

Synonym
• Stiff-skin syndrome

This hereditary connective tissue disorder is characterized by mild hirsutism, limitation of joint mobility affecting gait and localized areas of stony-hard skin, which are otherwise normal in appearance [11]. It appears in early infancy, and is only slowly progressive. The condition affects the deeper skin and fascia, which is much thicker than normal, and tends to be most pronounced on the buttocks and legs, with a sharp demarcation of subcutaneous sclerosis at the inguinal canal. Unlike morphoea, no inflammatory changes are seen on histology. Electron microscopy of the skin shows large collagen fibres, and bundles of aggregated microfibrils [11]. Thickening of the thoracic fascia may cause hypoventilation due to thoracic underdevelopment, but there are no other systemic features of this disease.

The condition appears to be analogous to the tight-skin mouse [12].

Restrictive dermopathy

This very rare autosomal recessive laminopathy, also known as tight skin contracture syndrome, presents at birth with a taut, shiny skin, which restricts movement of the joints [13–15]. It is characterized by intrauterine growth retardation and premature birth, due to ruptured fetal membranes. The typical facies is a small, fixed, round, open mouth, micrognathia, small nose, low-set ears and widely spaced cranial sutures. The joints are all fixed in flexion, and gross restriction of the respiratory movements causes death within hours, or at most weeks. The epidermis shows hyperkeratosis and parakeratosis, and the keratohyaline granules are abnormal. The dermal–epidermal junction is flat, with a thin dermis, and a thick layer of subcutaneous fat. The eccrine and pilosebaceous glands are underdeveloped. The collagen bundles appear stretched, and orientated in parallel lines, as they are in a tendon [16].

Mutations have been found in the *LMNA* genes leading to synthesis of mutant prelamin A that cannot be processed into mature lamin A. Mutations in the prelamin A processing enzyme gene (*ZMPSTE24/FACE-1*) also cause abnormal accumulation of the precursor with deleterious effects on nuclear homeostasis [17,18].

References

1 Landing BH, Nadorra R. Infantile systemic hyalinosis: report of four cases of a disease, fatal in infancy, apparently different from juvenile systemic hyalinosis. *Pediatr Pathol* 1986; **6**: 55–79.

2 Nezelof C, Letourneux-Toromanoff B, Griscelli C *et al.* La fibromatose disseminée douloureuse (hyalinose systemique). *Arch Fr Pediatr* 1978; **35**: 1063–74.

3 Puretic S, Puretic B, Fiser-Herman M *et al.* A unique form of mesenchymal dysplasia. *Br J Dermatol* 1962; **74**: 8–19.

4 Dowling O, Difeo A, Ramirez MC *et al.* Mutations in capillary morphogenesis gene-2 result in the allelic disorders juvenile hyaline fibromatosis and infantile systemic hyalinosis. *Am J Hum Genet* 2003; **73**: 957–66.

5 Hanks S, Adams S, Douglas J *et al.* Mutations in the gene encoding capillary morphogenesis protein 2 cause juvenile hyaline fibromatosis and infantile systemic hyalinosis. *Am J Hum Genet* 2003; **73**: 791–800.

6 Winchester P, Grossman H, Lim WN *et al.* A new acid mucopolysaccharidosis with skeletal deformities simulating rheumatoid arthritis. *Am J Roentgenol* 1969; **106**: 121–8.

7 Cohen AH, Hollister DW, Reed WB. The skin in the Winchester syndrome. *Arch Dermatol* 1975; **111**: 230–6.

8 Prapanpoch S, Jorgensen RJ, Langlais RP *et al.* Winchester syndrome: a case report and literature review. *Oral Surg Oral Med Oral Pathol* 1992; **74**: 671–7.

9 Esterley NB, McKusick VA. Stiff skin syndrome. *Pediatrics* 1971; **47**: 360–9.

10 Zankl A, Bonafe L, Calcaterra V *et al.* Winchester syndrome caused by a homozygous mutation affecting the active site of matrix metalloproteinase 2. *Clin Genet* 2005; **67**: 261–6.

11 Jablonska S, Blaszczyk M. Scleroderma-like indurations involving fascias: an abortive form of congenital fascial dystrophy (stiff skin syndrome). *Pediatr Dermatol* 2000; **17**: 105–10.

12 Jiminez SA. Scleroderma-like alterations in collagen metabolism in the tight-skin mouse. *Arthritis Rheum* 1984; **27**: 180–5.

13 Witt DR, Hayden MR, Holbrook KA *et al.* Restrictive dermopathy: a newly recognised autosomal recessive skin dysplasia. *Am J Med Genet* 1986; **24**: 631–48.

14 Welsh KM, Smoller BR, Holbrook KA *et al.* Restrictive dermopathy. Report of two affected siblings and a review of the literature. *Arch Dermatol* 1992; **128**: 228–31.

15 Happle R, Stekhoven JHS, Hamel BCJ *et al.* Restrictive dermopathy in two brothers. *Arch Dermatol* 1992; **128**: 232–5.

16 Holbrook KA, Dale BA, Witt DR *et al.* Arrested epidermal morphogenesis in three newborn infants with a fatal genetic disorder (restrictive dermopathy). *J Invest Dermatol* 1987; **88**: 330–40.

17 Navarro CL, De Sandre-Giovannoli A, Bernard R *et al.* Lamina A and ZMPSTE24 (FACE-1) defects cause nuclear disorganization and identify restrictive dermopathy as a lethal neonatal laminopathy. *Hum Mol Genet* 2004; **13**: 2493–503.

18 Young SG, Meta M, Yang SH *et al.* Prelamin A farnesylaion and progeroid syndromes. *J Biol Chem* 2006; **281**: 39741–5.

Other causes of diffuse fibrosis

Environmental and drug-induced scleroderma
(see also Chapter 51)

A variety of environmental triggers may stimulate a localized or diffuse scleroderma-like reaction in a genetically susceptible host. Important causes are listed in Table 45.5. In most cases, the fibrotic process continues after withdrawal of the external stimulus. Sometimes, the ensuing clinical pattern resembles idiopathic forms of scleroderma (see Chapter 51).

Exposure to *vinyl chloride monomer* occurs in workers involved in polyvinyl chloride (PVC) production. One-third of male

Table 45.5 Cutaneous fibrosis due to chemical exposure.

Vinyl chloride
Silica dust
Organic solvents:
Aromatic hydrocarbons (e.g. toluene, benzene)
Aliphatic hydrocarbons:
Chlorinated (e.g. trichlorethylene, perchlorethylene)
Non-chlorinated (e.g. naphtha-*n*-hexane)
Epoxy resins
Toxic oil syndrome
Urea formaldehyde foam insulation
Breast augmentation (paraffin, silicone)
Drugs:
Reactions to local injection:
Phytomenadione
Pentazocine
Heparin
Reactions to systemic therapy:
Bleomycin
L-tryptophan (eosinophilia–myalgia syndrome)
Carbidopa and L-5-hydroxytryptophan
Penicillamine
Valproate sodium
Cocaine
Appetite suppressants (diethylpropion hydrochloride, amphetamine)
Diltiazem

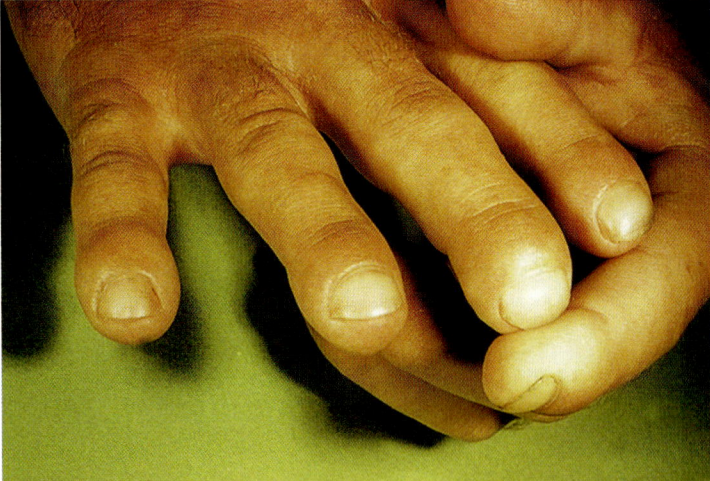

Fig. 45.36 Vinyl chloride-induced osteolysis affecting fingertips.

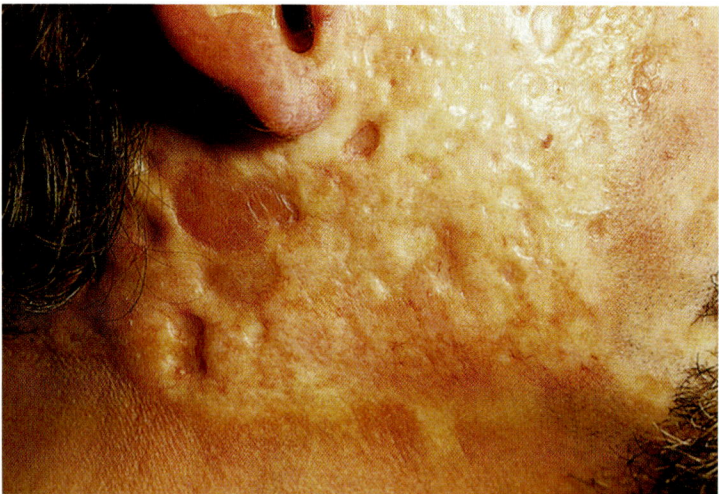

Fig. 45.37 Scleroderma and scarring of the face due to porphyria cutanea tarda. (Courtesy of Dr D.A. Burns, Leicester Royal Infirmary, Leicester, UK.)

operatives in a British factory developed a clinical syndrome that included Raynaud's phenomenon, dyspnoea, cutaneous sclerosis, pulp atrophy and radiological evidence of acro-osteolysis (Fig. 45.36) [1]. Genetic marker studies have demonstrated an increased incidence of human leukocyte antigen (HLA)-DR5 in affected individuals; severe disease is linked with B8 and DR3 [2]. A similar syndrome has been reported in gold miners exposed to silica dust [3], and in workers exposed to organic solvents, such as trichlorethylene [4] and perchlorethylene [5], which are structurally similar to vinyl chloride. Exposure to epoxy resin results in an acute syndrome of cutaneous sclerosis, muscle weakness, arthralgia, impotence, lung and oesophageal involvement [6]. The causative agent appears to be a cyclohexylamine. An increased prevalence of autoimmune disorders, including scleroderma, is reported in miners exposed to vermiculite contaminated with tremolite asbestos [7].

Toxic oil syndrome is a multisystem illness, reported in Spain in 1981. Acute fever, severe but transient pulmonary oedema, myalgia, and a pruritic exanthem and eosinophilia were followed after several months by widespread cutaneous sclerosis in 30% of cases [8,9]. The syndrome was probably due to ingestion of imported rapeseed oil mixed with an aniline denaturant, designed to make the oil unfit for human consumption. Toxic oil syndrome bears a striking resemblance to the *eosinophilia–myalgia syndrome* [10–12], linked with consumption of L-tryptophan; this is used as a 'food supplement' to treat insomnia and depression. The offending batches of L-tryptophan contained impurities similar to the contaminants in toxic oil [13,14].

In environmental fibrotic disorders, as in idiopathic scleroderma, subpopulations of fibroblasts appear to be activated to synthesize excess collagen; this property is perpetuated by fibroblasts *in vitro*, indicating that the elevated collagen gene expression is independent of extracellular stimuli [12]. Cytokines appear to stimulate the proliferation of these abnormal clones of fibroblasts; thus, transforming growth factor-β (TGF-β) and platelet-derived growth factor (PDGF) are elevated in the eosinophilia–myalgia syndrome [15].

Numerous drugs have been reported to induce cutaneous sclerosis. Lesions resembling morphoea may follow injections of pentaz-

ocine [16], heparin [17] and vitamin K_1 (phytomenadione) [18–20]; in the case of vitamin K_1, the trigger may be a solvent rather than vitamin K_1 itself [21]. Morphoea-like plaques have also been reported in patients taking penicillamine [22] and valproate [23].

Diffuse scleroderma-like changes have been reported following bleomycin therapy [24]. A combination of L-5-hydroxytryptophan and carbidopa induced lesions resembling eosinophilia–myalgia syndrome [25]. Phenytoin and diltiazem both induce gingival hypertrophy [26,27]. A patient on phenytoin developed florid hypertrophic retroauricular folds [28]. Thickened skin on the feet has been reported in a patient taking diltiazem [29].

Alcohol can provoke porphyria cutanea tarda, which can produce a sclerodermatous appearance (Fig. 45.37).

References

1 Ward AM, Udnoon S, Watkins J *et al.* Immunological mechanism in the pathogenesis of vinyl chloride disease. *BMJ* 1976; **i**: 936–8.

2 Black CM, Pereira S, McWhirter A *et al.* Genetic susceptibility to scleroderma-like syndrome in symptomatic and asymptomatic workers exposed to vinyl chloride. *J Rheumatol* 1986; **13**: 1059–62.

3 Sluis-Cremer GK, Hessel PA, Nizdo EH *et al.* Silica, silicosis and progressive systemic sclerosis. *Br J Ind Med* 1985; **42**: 838–43.

4 Saihan EM, Burton JL, Heaton KW. A new syndrome with pigmentation, scleroderma, gynaecomastia, Raynaud's phenomenon and peripheral neuropathy. *Br J Dermatol* 1978; **99**: 437–40.

5 Sparrow GP. A connective tissue disease similar to vinyl chloride disease in a patient exposed to perchlorethylene. *Clin Exp Dermatol* 1977; **2**: 17–22.

6 Yamakage A, Ishikawa H, Saito Y *et al.* Occupational scleroderma-like disorders occurring in men engaged in the polymerization of epoxy resins. *Dermatologica* 1980; **161**: 33–44.

7 Noonan CW, Pfau JC, Carson TC *et al.* Nested case-control study of autoimmune disease in an asbestos-exposed population. *Environ Health Perspect* 2006; **114**: 1243–7.

8 Iglesias JL, De Moragas JM. The cutaneous lesions of the Spanish toxic oil syndrome. *J Am Acad Dermatol* 1983; **9**: 159–60.

9 Phelps RG, Fleishmajer R. Clinical, pathologic, and immunological manifestations of the toxic oil syndrome. *J Am Acad Dermatol* 1988; **18**: 313–24.

10 Kaufman LD, Seidman RJ, Phillips ME *et al.* Cutaneous manifestations of the L-tryptophan-associated eosinophilia–myalgia syndrome: a spectrum of sclerodermatous disease. *J Am Acad Dermatol* 1990; **23**: 1063–9.

11 Kilbourne EM, Posada de la Paz M, Borda IA *et al.* Toxic oil syndrome: a current clinical and epidemiologic summary, including comparisons with the eosinophilia–myalgia syndrome. *J Am Coll Cardiol* 1991; **18**: 711–7.

12 Varga J, Jimenez SA. Chemical exposure-induced cutaneous fibrosis. Lessons from 'experiments of nature'. *Arch Dermatol* 1994; **130**: 97–100.

13 Slutsker L, Hoesly FC, Miller L *et al.* Eosinophilia–myalgia syndrome associated with exposure to tryptophan from a single manufacturer. *JAMA* 1990; **264**: 213–7.

14 Mayeno AN, Belongia EA, Lin F *et al.* 3-(Phenylamino) alanine, a novel aniline-derived amino acid associated with the eosinophilia–myalgia syndrome: a link to the toxic oil syndrome. *Mayo Clin Proc* 1992; **67**: 1134–9.

15 Kaufman LD, Gruber BL, Gomez-Reion JJ. Fibrogenic growth factors in the eosinophilia–myalgia syndrome and the toxic oil syndrome. *Arch Dermatol* 1994; **130**: 41–7.

16 Palestine RF, Millas JL, Spigel GT *et al.* Skin manifestations of pentazocine abuse. *J Am Acad Dermatol* 1980; **2**: 47–55.

17 Barthelemy H, Hermier C, Perrot H. Nécrose cutanée avec évolution scléroder-miforme aprés l'injection souscutanée d'heparinate de calcium. *Ann Dermatol Vénéréol* 1985; **112**: 245–7.

18 Brunskill NJ, Berth-Jones J, Graham-Brown RAC. Pseudosclerodermatous reaction to phytomenadione injection (Texier's syndrome). *Clin Exp Dermatol* 1988; **13**: 276–8.

19 Pujol RM, Puig L, Moreno A. Pseudoscleroderma secondary to phytomenadione (vitamin K_1) injections. *Cutis* 1989; **43**: 365–8.

20 Morel A, Betlloch I. Morphea-like reaction from vitamin K_1. *Int J Dermatol* 1995; **34**: 201–2.

21 Bourrat E, Moraillon I, Vignon-Pennamen MD. Placard sclérodermiforme de la cuisse de l'enfant aprés injection de vitamine K_1 à la naissance. *Ann Dermatol Vénéréol* 1996; **123**: 634–8.

22 Bernstein RM, Hall MA, Gostelow BE. Morphoea-like reaction to D-penicillamine therapy. *Ann Rheum Dis* 1981; **40**: 42–4.

23 Goihman-Yahr M, Leal G, Essenfeld-Yahr E. Generalised morphea: a side effect of valproate sodium? *Arch Dermatol* 1980; **116**: 621.

24 Finch WR, Rodnan GP, Buckingham RB *et al.* Bleomycin-induced scleroderma. *J Rheumatol* 1980; **7**: 651–9.

25 Sternberg EM, van Woert MH, Young SN *et al.* Development of a scleroderma-like illness during therapy with 1-5-hydroxytryptophan and carbidopa. *N Engl J Med* 1980; **303**: 782–7.

26 Hassell TM, Page RC, Narayanan AS *et al.* Diphenylhydantoin (Dilantin) gingival hyperplasia: drug-induced abnormality of connective tissue. *Proc Natl Acad Sci USA* 1976; **73**: 2909–12.

27 Guistiniani S, Robustelli F, Marieni M. Hyperplastic gingivitis during diltiazem therapy. *Int J Cardiol* 1987; **15**: 247–9.

28 Trunnell TN, Waisman M. Hypertrophic retroauricular folds attributable to diphenylhydantoin. *Cutis* 1982; **30**: 207–9.

29 Ilia R, Goldfarb B, Gueron M. Skin thickening and sensory loss of the feet during diltiazem therapy. *Int J Cardiol* 1992; **35**: 115.

Nephrogenic systemic fibrosis

Synonyms
- Scleromyxoedema-like illness of renal disease
- Nephrogenic fibrosing dermopathy

Acute onset of skin thickening has been reported in patients with renal disease undergoing haemodialysis or renal transplant [1]. Irregular erythematous or brownish indurated plaques, with amoeba-like projections and islands of sparing, occur chiefly on the lower trunk and legs. Sometimes the skin has a *peau d'orange* texture, which can mimic carcinoma erysipelatoides [2]. Dermal mucin is detected with Alcian-blue staining, and increased collagen is laid down in haphazard bundles; there are increased numbers of CD68+ histiocytes, dermal dendrocytes and fibroblasts. Inflammatory changes may predominate, including a septal panniculitis [3]. Although initially described as 'scleromyxoedema-like', the lesions have a different distribution and morphology, and there is no associated paraproteinaemia [4]. Initially thought to be restricted to the skin, there are several reports of involvement of internal organs including lungs, myocardium and striated muscle, which contribute to a high mortality [4].

The condition is strongly associated with the prior administration of gadolinium-based magnetic resonance contrast agents, particularly in patients with severe renal disease [5]. Gadolinium chelates stimulate fibroblast growth, synthesis and differentiation into myofibroblasts [6]. High-dose erythropoietin may also be implicated [7].

Usually, the condition is progressive, although it may remit spontaneously, particularly with the correction of renal abnormalities. No treatment is of proven benefit, but thalidomide [8], hydroxychloroquine [9], intravenous sodium thiosulphate and extracorporeal photopheresis [10] have been used empirically. Transient benefit has been reported with the use of the tyrosine kinase inhibitor imatinib mesylate [11].

References

1 Cowper S, Robin H, Steinberg S *et al.* Scleromyxedema-like cutaneous diseases in renal-dialysis patients. *Lancet* 2000; **356**: 1000–1.

2 Solomon GJ, Wu E, Rosen PP. Nephrogenic systemic fibrosis mimicking inflammatory breast carcinoma. *Arch Pathol Lab Med* 2007; **131**: 145–8.

3 Naylor E, Hu S, Robinson-Bostom L. Nephrogenic systemic fibrosis with septal panniculitis mimicking erythema nodosum. *J Am Acad Dermatol* 2008; **58**: 149–50.

4 Swaminathan S, High WA, Ranville J *et al.* Cardiac and vascular metal deposition with high mortality in nephrogenic systemic fibrosis. *Kidney Int* 2008; **73**: 1413–8.

5 Grobner T. Gadolinium—a specific trigger for the development of nephrogenic fibrosing dermopathy and nephrogenic systemic fibrosis? *Nephrol Dial Transplant* 2006; **21**: 1104–8.

6 Edward M, Quinn J, Mukherjee S *et al.* Gadodiamide contrast agent 'activates' fibroblasts: a possible cause for nephrogenic systemic fibrosis. *J Pathol* 2008; **214**: 584–93.

7 Swaminathan S, Ahmed I, McCarthy JT *et al.* Nephrogenic fibrosing dermopathy and high-dose erythropoietin therapy. *Ann Intern Med* 2006; **145**: 234–5.

8 Streams BN, Liu V, Liegois N *et al.* Clinical and pathologic features of nephrogenic fibrosing dermopathy: a report of two cases. *J Am Acad Dermatol* 2003; **48**: 42–7.

9 Kalb RE, Helm TN, Sperry H *et al.* Gadolinium-induced nephrogenic systemic fibrosis in a patient with an acute and transient kidney injury. *Br J Dermatol* 2007; **158**: 607–10.

10 Linfert DR, Schell JO, Fine DM. Treatment of nephrogenic systemic fibrosis: limited options but hope for the future. *Semin Dial* 2008; **21**: 155–9.

11 Kay J, High WA. Imatinib mesylate treatment of nephrogenic systemic fibrosis. *Arthritis Rheum* 2008; **58**: 2543–8.

GEMSS syndrome

This is an autosomal dominant condition, comprising *g*laucoma, lens *e*ctopia, *m*icrospherophakia (small, spherical lens), joint *s*tiffness and *s*hort stature [1]. Affected individuals have a stocky, 'pseudoathletic' build. Associated cutaneous sclerosis notably affects the upper back and limbs but spares the face. Skin histology is reminiscent of systemic sclerosis. Increased synthesis of collagen is reflected by markedly enhanced gene expression of $TGF\beta_1$ [2].

References

1 Verloes A, Hermia JP, Garland A *et al.* Glaucoma–lens ectopia–microspherophakia–stiffness–shortness (GEMSS) syndrome: a dominant disease with manifestations of Weill–Marchesani syndrome. *Am J Med Genet* 1992; **40**: 48–51.

2 Kunz M, Paulus W, Sollberg S *et al.* Sclerosis of skin in the GEMSS syndrome. *Arch Dermatol* 1995; **131**: 1170–4.

POEMS syndrome (see also Chapters 58 & 62)

This acronym is derived from *p*olyneuropathy, *o*rganomegaly (of liver, spleen or lymph nodes), *e*ndocrinopathy (often diabetes mellitus), *M* protein (a monoclonal gammopathy) and *s*kin lesions. The skin features include hyperpigmentation, hyperhidrosis, hypertrichosis and diffuse thickening resembling scleroderma [1–3]. Rarer features include angiomas, white fingernails and alopecia [3].

The syndrome appears to be a rare variant of myelomatosis [4], although skeletal X-rays show single or multiple osteosclerotic lesions with areas of bony proliferation rather than the lytic lesions that are more typical of myeloma [5].

Overproduction of vascular endothelial growth factor (VEGF) may explain the microangiopathy, neovascularization and accelerated vasopermeability that occur in this syndrome [6].

High-dose chemotherapy followed by autologous stem cell transplant is a successful treatment, although morbidity is high [7].

References
1 Shelley WB, Shelley ED. The skin changes in the Crow–Fukase (POEMS) syndrome. *Arch Dermatol* 1987; **123**: 85–7.
2 Manning WJ, Goldberger AL, Drews RE *et al.* POEMS syndrome with myocardial infarction: observations concerning pathogenesis and review of the literature. *Semin Arthritis Rheum* 1992; **22**: 151–61.
3 Amicha B, Giryes H, Ariad S *et al.* Alopecia as a rare cutaneous manifestation of the POEMS syndrome. *Br J Dermatol* 1994; **131**: 297–8.
4 Burton JL. Peripheral neuropathy associated with dysproteinaemia, skin changes and endocrinopathy. *BMJ* 1986; **292**: 1415–6.
5 Piette WW. Myeloma, paraproteinaemias and the skin. *Med Clin North Am* 1986; **70**: 155–76.
6 Watanabe O, Maruyama I, Arimura K *et al.* Overproduction of vascular endothelial growth factor/vascular permeability factor is causative in Crow–Fukase (POEMS) syndrome. *Muscle Nerve* 1998; **21**: 1390–7.
7 Dispenzieri A, Lacy MQ, Hayman SR *et al.* Peripheral blood stem cell transplant for POEMS syndrome is associated with high rates of engraftment syndrome. *Eur J Haematol* 2008; **80**: 397–406.

Keloids and hypertrophic scars

Both conditions represent an excessive connective tissue response to injury, which may be trivial. A keloid (cheloid, meaning 'crab claw') is a benign, well-demarcated area of fibrous tissue overgrowth that extends beyond the original defect. A hypertrophic scar is similar, but remains confined to the initial defect and tends to resolve with time [1].

Aetiology. The cause is unknown, although both local and constitutional factors are involved. A scar at any site has the potential to become hypertrophic or keloidal, although the earlobes, chin, neck, shoulders, upper trunk and lower legs are especially vulnerable. Ear piercing is an important cause of earlobe keloids. Burns or scalds and infected lesions predispose to hypertrophy. Another risk factor is the presence of foreign material, either exogenous (e.g. suture material) or endogenous (e.g. embedded hair). Some African tribes introduce foreign bodies into tribal marks to induce scar hypertrophy. Scarring acne, particularly on the trunk, may become keloid-like. Isotretinoin has been reported to delay wound healing and induce keloids in patients who received argon laser or dermabrasion for acne or rosacea [2,3].

Some races, notably Afro-Caribbeans, are more prone to develop keloids than others. A positive family history is obtained in 5–10% of Europeans with keloids, particularly severe lesions [4]. Family studies suggest an autosomal dominant inheritance with incomplete penetrance [5]. There is a genetic association with other 'fibromatoses' such as Dupuytren's contracture [6]. Keloids form readily in acromegalics, and after thyroidectomy in young patients. They have been reported in a boy with Dubowitz's syndrome [7]. Keloids are also recorded in association with EDS, pachydermoperiostosis and Rubinstein–Taybi syndrome [8]. Keloids are rare in infancy and old age, occurring chiefly between puberty and the age of 30 years. Women have a greater predisposition, and keloids may occur or enlarge during pregnancy [9].

Linear keloids have been reported to occur in athletes taking anabolic steroids [10].

Pathology [11–13]. Although the histology may be difficult to distinguish from normal wound healing in the early stages, hypertrophic scars and keloids typically exhibit increased cellularity. In keloids of recent onset, endothelial proliferation is surrounded by increased numbers of fibroblasts, which form large, irregular nodules or whorls of collagen with a peripheral capsule-like band [11]. Mast cells are increased in hypertrophic scars [12]. Mucinous material is deposited focally in keloids but not in hypertrophic scars. The epidermis is normal, or thinned by the underlying lesion.

On electron microscopy, the nodules contain stellate fibroblasts. It is uncertain whether these are [14] or are not [15] myofibroblasts. Scanning electron microscopy of keloids shows more haphazard organization of collagen bundles than in normal skin or mature scars. The collagen filaments are about half the diameter of those of normal skin.

Biochemical studies confirm that collagen and proteoglycan synthesis is increased in keloids and hypertrophic scars. Collagen degradation appears to be normal [16]. Synthesis of both types I and III collagen is increased [17], and hypertrophic scar collagen possesses the reducible keto cross-link, dehydrohydroxylysinonorleucine, normally associated with embryonic skin and granulation tissue [18]. Several growth factors have been studied using keloid fibroblasts *in vitro*. Keloid fibroblasts, unlike those from hypertrophic scar tissue, are hyperresponsive to both TGF-β, which is abundant in healing wounds [19], and PDGF [20]. Keloid fibroblasts also express increased levels of heat shock protein (HSP) 47, another stimulus to collagen synthesis [21].

Keloid fibroblasts secrete increased amounts of collagen and glycosaminoglycans for several passages in tissue culture [22]. It is unclear whether these cells represent a normal subgroup or have undergone transformation. Altered expression of proteoglycans in keloids may affect the three-dimensional organization of collagen fibres [23].

Immunohistochemical studies have shown that neuropeptide-containing nerves are present [24] and opioid receptors are upreg-

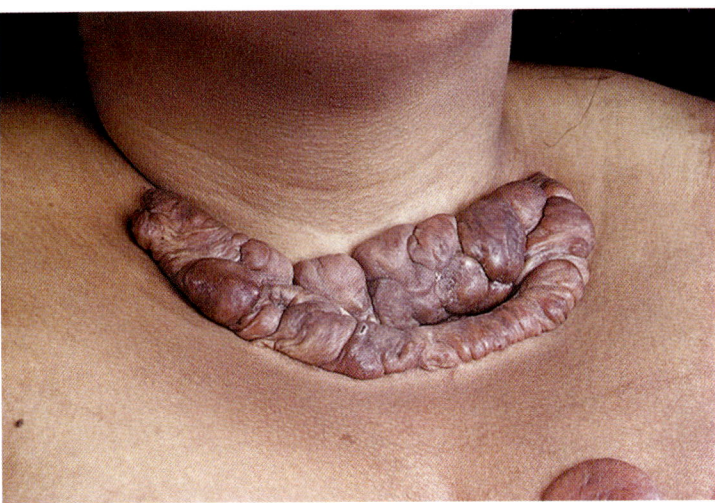

Fig. 45.38 Spontaneous keloids of the neck.

ulated [25] in hypertrophic scars but not in non-hypertrophic scars, and these may contribute to the symptoms of discomfort and itching in such scars.

Clinical features. Both hypertrophic scars and keloids become raised and thickened within 3–4 weeks of the provocative stimulus. The lesion becomes a firm, pink or red plaque, which may grow for months or years. Lesions often assume a 'dumb-bell' configuration, but sometimes become bizarre and irregular (Fig. 45.38). Usually, a hypertrophic scar shows signs of regression after a few months. The surface of a keloid becomes smoother and rounder, extending beyond the area of the original lesion. It is often irritable and hypersensitive, and sometimes exquisitely tender. Keloids tend to regress after several years; lesions on the beard area sometimes undergo central suppurative necrosis. Malignant degeneration has been reported [26], although a fibrosarcoma can mimic keloid clinically.

The diagnosis is usually simple if there is a history of trauma or an inflammatory skin lesion. Spontaneous keloids usually develop on the presternal region or upper chest. Lesions that can cause diagnostic difficulty include sclerotic basal cell carcinoma, scar sarcoid or malignancy developing in a scar, and dermatofibrosarcoma. In endemic areas, blastomycosis and lobomycosis cause keloidal reactions.

Prophylaxis and treatment. Although numerous treatments have been advocated with enthusiasm, a cure is rarely achieved [27]. Non-essential surgery should be avoided in the sites of predilection. If surgery is necessary, simple excision, ideally intralesional (core) excision, aiming to minimize skin tension and secondary infection, is preferable to electrocoagulation or caustic chemicals. In an individual at risk, preoperative radiotherapy to the excision site may be useful.

Keloids usually recur following simple excision, although adjuvant therapy, such as radiation, local compression with a custom-made pressure garment [28], particularly on the earlobe, or intralesional steroids may reduce the risk of recurrence. Some lesions respond to pressure alone, or to occlusion with a

hydrocolloid dressing. Small keloids can respond to self-adherent silicone sheeting/silicone gel [29,30]. Silicone gel treatment is also effective for hypertrophic scars [29]. Promising results have been obtained using a cream made of 20% silicone oil, applied under occlusion; this may be beneficial for sites where it is impracticable to apply gel-sheeting [31].

Radiotherapy, including superficial X-rays, implantation with iridium-192 wires, or more recently with electron beam may prevent recurrence following surgery [32,33], but electron-beam therapy offers no advantage over orthovoltage [34]. Intralesional triamcinolone (10 mg/mL) is useful, especially in early lesions. Several injections may be necessary at intervals of 3–6 weeks. Prior freezing with liquid nitrogen before the injection causes oedema, which allows the triamcinolone to be injected more readily. Acne keloids respond moderately well to either intralesional triamcinolone or cryotherapy, but the response to the latter is better in early vascular lesions [35].

Topical retinoic acid, applied daily, may be helpful [36,37], although systemic retinoids may enhance keloid formation [3]. Intralesional lathyrogens, such as β-aminoproprionitrile, have been used, but systemic penicillamine is ineffective [38]. Intralesional cytotoxic drugs may cause ulceration, but intralesional 5-fluorouracil and 585-nm flashlamp-pumped pulsed dye laser produced comparable improvement in one study [39]. Flattening and reduced pruritus is claimed to follow intralesional bleomycin, administered through multiple superficial punctures [40]. A preliminary study suggests that topical mitomycin C reduces the risk of recurrence after shave biopsy of keloids [41].

Inhibitory cytokines, such as IFN-α and IFN-γ [42–44] perhaps in conjunction with intralesional triamcinolone [45], and TGF-β analogues [46], show promise. Interferons appear to reduce fibroblast collagen synthesis and increase collagenase activity by reducing the steady-state levels of mRNA [44]. Imiquimod cream can prevent recurrence of earlobe keloids after excision but is of limited value for presternal lesions [47]. Studies of keloid fibroblasts *in vitro* suggest a possible future role for gene therapy [48].

Different modes of laser treatment, for example the pulsed dye, Nd : YAG and carbon dioxide lasers, have a high recurrence rate.

References

1 Köse O, Waseem A. Keloids and hypertrophic scars; are they two different sides of the same coin? *Dermatol Surg* 2008; **34**: 336–46.

2 Rubenstein R, Roenigk H, Stegmann S *et al.* Atypical keloids after dermabrasion of patients taking isotretinoin. *J Am Acad Dermatol* 1986; **15**: 280–5.

3 Zachariae H. Delayed wound healing and keloid formation following argon laser treatment or dermabrasion during isotretinoin treatment. *Br J Dermatol* 1988; **118**: 703–6.

4 Cosman B, Crikelair GF, Ju DMC *et al.* The surgical treatment of keloids. *Plast Reconstr Surg* 1961; **27**: 335–8.

5 Marneros AG, Norris JEC, Olsen BR *et al.* Clinical genetics of familial keloids. *Arch Dermatol* 2001; **137**: 1429–34.

6 González-Martínez R, Marín-Bertolín S, Amorrortu-Velayos J. Association between keloids and Dupuytren's disease: case report. *Br J Plast Surg* 1995; **48**: 47–8.

7 Paradisi M, Angelo C, Conti G *et al.* Dubowitz syndrome with keloidal lesions. *Clin Exp Dermatol* 1994; **19**: 425–7.

8 Kelly AP. Keloids: a review. *Dermatol Clin* 1988; **7**: 130–9.

9 Moustafa MFH, Abdul Fattah AF. Presumptive evidence of the effect of pregnancy oestrogens on keloid growth. *Plast Reconstr Surg* 1975; **56**: 450–3.

10 Scott MH Jr, Scott MJ, Scott AM. Linear keloids resulting from abuse of anabolic androgenic steroid drugs. *Cutis* 1994; **53**: 41–3.

11 Linares HA, Kischer CW, Dobrkovsky M *et al.* The histiotypic organization of the hypertrophic scar in humans. *J Invest Dermatol* 1972; **59**: 323–31.

12 Kischer CW, Bunce H III, Shetlar MR. Mast cell analyses in hypertrophic scars, hypertrophic scars treated with pressure and mature scars. *J Invest Dermatol* 1978; **70**: 355–7.

13 Herlich HP, Desmouliere A, Diegelmann RF *et al.* Morphological and immunochemical differences between keloid and hypertrophic scar. *Am J Pathol* 1994; **145**: 105–13.

14 James WD, Besanceney CD, Odom RB. The ultrastructure of a keloid. *J Am Acad Dermatol* 1980; **3**: 50–7.

15 Mutsuoka LY, Uitto J, Wortsman J *et al.* Ultrastructural characteristics of keloid fibroblasts. *Am J Dermatopathol* 1988; **10**: 505–8.

16 Milsom JP, Craig RDP. Collagen degradation in cultural keloid and hypertrophic scar tissue. *Br J Dermatol* 1973; **89**: 635–44.

17 Zhang K, Garner W, Cohen L *et al.* Increased types I and III collagen and transforming growth factor-β1 mRNA and protein in hypertrophic burn scar. *J Invest Dermatol* 1995; **104**: 750–4.

18 Bailey AJ, Bazin S, Sims TJ *et al.* Characterisation of the collagen of hypertrophic and normal human scars. *Biochem Biophys Acta* 1975; **405**: 412–21.

19 Younai S, Nichter LS, Wellisz T *et al.* Modulation of collagen synthesis by transforming growth factor-β in keloid and hypertrophic scar fibroblasts. *Ann Plast Surg* 1994; **33**: 148–51.

20 Haisa M, Okochi H, Grotendorst GR. Elevated levels of PDGF and receptors in keloid fibroblasts contribute to an enhanced response to PDGF. *J Invest Dermatol* 1994; **103**: 560–3.

21 Chen JJ, Zhao S, Cen Y *et al.* Effect of heat shock protein 47 on collagen accumulation in keloid fibroblast cells. *Br J Dermatol* 2007; **156**: 1188–95.

22 Duncan MR, Hasan A, Berman B. Oncostatin M stimulates collagen and glycosaminoglycan production by cultured normal dermal fibroblasts: insensitivity of sclerodermal and keloidal fibroblasts. *J Invest Dermatol* 1995; **104**: 128–33.

23 Hunzelmann N, Anders S, Sollberg S *et al.* Coordinate induction of collagen type I and biglycan expression in keloids. *Br J Dermatol* 1996; **135**: 394–9.

24 Crowe R, Parkhouse N, McGrouther D, Burnstock G. Neuropeptide-containing nerves in painful hypertrophic human scar tissue. *Br J Dermatol* 1994; **130**: 444–52.

25 Cheng B, Liu H-W, Fu XB *et al.* Coexistence and upregulation of three types of opioid receptor, mu, delta and kappa, in human hypertrophic scars. *Br J Dermatol* 2008; **158**: 713–20.

26 Kanaar P, Oort J. Fibrosarcomas developing in scar tissue. *Dermatologica* 1969; **138**: 312–9.

27 Leventhal D, Furr M, Reiter D. Treatment of keloids and hypertrophic scars: a meta-analysis and review of the literature. *Arch Facial Plast Surg* 2006; **8**: 362–8.

28 Kischer CW, Shetlar MR, Shetlar CL. Alteration of hypertrophic scars induced by mechanical pressure. *Arch Dermatol* 1975; **111**: 60–4.

29 Berman B, Flores F. Comparison of a silicone gel-filled cushion and silicone gel sheeting for the treatment of hypertrophic or keloid scars. *Dermatol Surg* 1999; **25**: 484–6.

30 Berman B, Perez OA, Konda S *et al.* A review of the biologic effects, clinical efficacy and safety of silicone elastomer sheeting for hypertrophic and keloid scar treatment and management. *Dermatol Surg* 2007; **33**: 1291–302.

31 Wong T-W, Chiu H-C, Chen J-S *et al.* Symptomatic keloids in two children: dramatic improvement with silicone cream occlusive dressing. *Arch Dermatol* 1995; **131**: 775–7.

32 Bischof M, Krempien R, Debus J *et al.* Postoperative electron beam radiotherapy for keloids: objective findings and patient satisfaction—self assessment. *Int J Dermatol* 2007; **46**: 971–5.

33 Ogawa R, Miyashita T, Hyakusoku H *et al.* Postoperative radiation protocol for keloids and hypertrophic scars: statistical analysis of 370 sites followed for over 18 months. *Ann Plast Surg* 2007; **59**: 668–91.

34 Klumpar DI, Murray JC, Anscher M. Keloids treated with excision followed by radiation therapy. *J Am Acad Dermatol* 1994; **31**: 225–31.

35 Layton AM, Yip J, Cunliffe WJ. A comparison of intralesional triamcinolone and cryosurgery in the treatment of acne keloids. *Br J Dermatol* 1994; **130**: 498–501.

36 De Limpens J. The local treatment of hypertrophic scars and keloid with topical retinoic acid. *Br J Dermatol* 1982; **103**: 319–23.

37 Panabiere-Castaings MH. Retinoic acid in the treatment of keloids. *J Dermatol Surg Oncol* 1988; **14**: 1275–6.

38 Mayou BJ. Treatment of keloids. *Br J Dermatol* 1981; **105**: 87–9.

39 Manuskiatli W, Fitzpatrick R. Treatment response of keloidal and hypertrophic sternotomy scars. Comparison among intralesional corticosteroid, 5-fluorouracil, and 585-nm flashlamp-pumped pulsed-dye laser treatments. *Arch Dermatol* 2002; **138**: 1149–55.

40 Aggarwal H, Saxena A, Lubana PS *et al.* Treatment of keloids and hypertrophic scars using bleomycin. *J Cosmetic Dermatol* 2008; **7**: 43–9.

41 Bailey JN, Waite AE, Clayton WJ *et al.* Application of topical mitomycin C to the base of shave-removed keloid scars to prevent their recurrence. *Br J Dermatol* 2007; **156**: 682–6.

42 Tredget EE, Shen YJ, Forsyth N *et al.* Regulation of collagen synthesis, intracellular degradation and mRNA levels by interferon α2β in hypertrophic scar fibroblasts. *Wound Repair Regen* 1993; **1**: 156–65.

43 Gransten RD, Rook A, Flotte TJ *et al.* A controlled trial of intralesional recombinant interferon-γ in the treatment of keloidal scarring. Clinical and histologic findings. *Arch Dermatol* 1990; **126**: 1295–302.

44 Harrop AR, Ghahary A, Scott PG *et al.* Regulation of collagen synthesis and mRNA expression in normal and hypertrophic scar fibroblasts *in vitro* by interferon-γ. *J Surg Res* 1995; **58**: 471–7.

45 Lee JH, Kim SE, Lee AY. Effects of interferon-alpha2b on keloid treatment with triamcinolone acetonide intralesional injection. *Int J Dermatol* 2008; **47**: 183–6.

46 Chu Y, Guo F, Li Y *et al.* A novel truncated TGF-beta receptor II down-regulates collagen synthesis and TGF beta 1 secretion of keloid fibroblasts. *Connect Tissue Res* 2008; **49**: 92–8.

47 Malhotra AK, Gupta S, Khaitan BK *et al.* Imiquimod 5% cream for the prevention of recurrence after excision of presternal keloids. *Dermatology* 2007; **215**: 63–5.

48 Xu B, Liu ZZ, Zhu GY *et al.* Efficacy of recombinant adenovirus mediated double suicide gene therapy in human keloid fibroblasts. *Clin Exp Dermatol* 2008; **33**: 322–8.

Premature ageing syndromes [1,2]

Increasing age appears to cause many anatomical and functional changes in human skin, but some of these may be the result of cumulative damage due to sun exposure, etc. To date, no disease has been found to cause a true acceleration of the rate of ageing in all tissues. More than 150 diseases manifest one or more features of apparent premature ageing, but there are discrepancies between this process and true ageing. All the premature ageing syndromes are probably inherited, although the defect may not be obvious in the first few years of life. Cutaneous changes that may be a sign of a premature ageing syndrome include atrophy, loss of cutaneous fat, wrinkling, canities, hair loss, nail dystrophy, defective pigmentation, poikiloderma, sclerosis and ulceration.

The conditions associated with cutaneous signs of premature ageing are shown below.

1 Classical inherited premature ageing syndromes:
   (a) pangeria (Werner's syndrome)
   (b) progeria (Hutchinson–Gilford syndrome)
   (c) acrogeria (Gottron's syndrome)
2 Other congenital progeroid syndromes:
   (a) trisomy 21 (Down's syndrome)
   (b) neonatal pseudohydrocephalic progeroid syndrome (Wiedemann–Rauchenstrauch)
   (c) osteodysplastic geroderma
   (d) wrinkly skin syndrome
   (e) familial mandibulo-acral dysplasia
   (f) progeroid EDS
3 Excessive exposure to irradiation (usually UV)
4 Photosensitivity, especially congenital, for example poikiloderma congenitale, xeroderma pigmentosum, Cockayne's syndrome

5 Diseases causing elastolysis, for example cutis laxa
6 Thickened immobile skin, for example diabetic cheiroarthropathy
7 Fragile skin, for example prolidase deficiency
8 Loss of subcutaneous fat, for example generalized lipodystrophy.

References

1 Beauregard S, Gilchrest BA. Syndromes of premature ageing. *Dermatol Clin* 1987; **5**: 109–21.
2 Martin GM. Syndromes of accelerated ageing. *NCI Monogr* 1982; **60**: 241–7.

Pangeria

> **Synonyms**
> - Werner's syndrome
> - Adult premature ageing syndrome

Definition. An inherited disorder in which the ageing process is accelerated, starting after puberty. It is characterized by short stature, senile appearance, cataracts, joint contractures, early menopause, premature arteriosclerosis, various skin changes (including scleroderma-like features, premature canities, baldness and ulceration) and an increased risk of malignancy [1]. Werner's syndrome is considered one of the genomic instability syndromes [2].

Aetiology. The syndrome is due to an autosomal recessive gene, with a calculated gene frequency of 1–5 per 1000 population [3].

Numerous abnormalities have been described in this syndrome, including chromosomal aberrations (most noticeably translocations, inversions and deletions), altered connective tissue metabolism, and abnormalities in the immune and endocrine systems [4–14].

Causal mutations have been identified in the RecQ type DNA helicase gene (*RECQL2, WRN* gene) [15,16]. Recent biochemical and genetic studies indicate that the *WRN* gene plays significant roles in DNA replication and repair and telomere maintenance [17].

Pathology. Many tissues show premature ageing, but the changes are not uniform. Microsplanchnia and generalized atheroma are usually present. The epidermis is atrophic and some appendages are sparse. The dermis is thickened, with replacement of subcutaneous fat by hyalinized collagen, increased glycosaminoglycans, abnormal elastic fibres, disorganized nerves and vessel changes, which resemble those seen in diabetes mellitus. These abnormalities are more marked in the acral skin than on the trunk [4].

Clinical features [1]. The earliest manifestation of the syndrome is greying at the temples, which usually develops between the ages of 14 and 18 years but may rarely be present as early as 8 years. The greying rapidly becomes uniform and is sometimes associated with progressive alopecia. The first significant changes are usually noticed between 18 and 30 years but may begin earlier. The lower legs, feet, forearms and hands are most severely involved, the face and neck less so; atrophy of the skin and loss of subcutaneous fat results in a tense, shining and adherent appear-

ance of the skin. Thin, spindly legs contrast with the normal or obese trunk, and there is a bird-like facies. The joints become fixed, and there may be sclerodactyly and acral gangrene. Mottled or diffuse pigmentation and telangiectasia are often conspicuous on the limbs, face and neck. Keratoses over pressure points on the feet and ankles separate to leave indolent ulcers. The voice may be high pitched and hoarse from thinning of the cords and fixation of the epiglottis. Intelligence is usually normal.

Most patients are of small stature and hypogonadal, with sparse or absent pubic and axillary hair, but some achieve normal stature and successful pregnancies. Other endocrine deficiencies are sometimes present; frank diabetes mellitus in at least 30% and abnormal glucose tolerance in many others. The diabetes is characterized by relatively low blood glucose levels and peripheral resistance to insulin [18,19].

Cataracts develop between the ages of 20 and 35 years in most cases and are usually posterior and subcapsular. Other ocular defects may occur [20].

The incidence of malignancy is high, especially fibrosarcomas, which occur in 10% of patients [21]. Carcinoma has developed in a chronic leg ulcer [22], but skin cancer is relatively rare. Generally, atheroma develops early. Abnormalities of metabolism are sometimes present but are not of uniform type. Death usually occurs in the fourth to sixth decade, due to myocardial infarction or malignancy [23].

The radiological changes [24] are often striking. There may be calcification of arteries, ligaments, tendons and subcutaneous tissues, with osteoporosis of the extremities, especially the legs.

Diagnosis. The prematurely aged appearance, the physical immaturity, the scleroderma-like changes and the cataracts, in combination, are unmistakable. In the Rothmund–Thomson syndrome, erythema, which is of early onset, is followed by poikilodermatous changes and, although the facies may be superficially similar, there is no sclerosis. In systemic sclerosis, the hands are involved more than the feet and there is no premature ageing; in some advanced cases, confusion is possible but can be resolved by biopsy.

Huriez syndrome may require exclusion (Chapter 19). The differentiation from some of the other ageing syndromes is indicated in Table 45.6.

Mutational analysis of the *WRN* gene is now possible, although diagnosis by immunoblot analysis using a monoclonal antibody directed against the *WRN* gene product is also feasible [25].

Treatment. Only symptomatic measures are available. The management of the recurrent, painful ulceration of the feet and legs is difficult, and amputation may be needed. Cataract surgery should be undertaken with special caution, for it is often complicated by severe degenerative changes of the cornea [20].

References

1 Furuichi Y. Premature aging and predisposition to cancers caused by mutations in RecQ family helicases. *Ann NY Acad Sci* 2001; **928**: 121–31.
2 Martin GM, Oshima J. Lessons from human progeroid syndromes. *Nature* 2000; **408**: 263–6.
3 Epstein CJ, Martin GM, Schultz AL *et al*. Werner's syndrome: a review. *Medicine* 1966; **45**: 177–221.

Table 45.6 Clinical features of the classical premature ageing syndromes.

	Pangeria (Werner's syndrome)	Progeria (Hutchinson-Gilford sndrome)	Acrogeria (Gottron's syndrome)
Stature	Small stature; cessation of growth at 12 years	Small stature	Normal
Facies	Beaked nose; skin of ears atrophic and tightly bound down	Mid-facial cyanosis; bird-like facies; glyphic nasal tip; prominent frontal tuberosities and scalp veins; chin recessed	Micrognathia; atrophy of skin on tip of nose
Skin	Dry atrophic skin; mottled hyperpigmentation; telangiectasia	Dry, thin and wrinkled with mottled pigmentation; may present with scleroderma-like changes on limbs	Atrophic with telangiectasia and mottled hyperpigmentation on extremities
Scalp hair	Premature greying at 20 years; loss of hair at 20–25 years	Hair lost in first 2 years of life	Normal
Eyes	Bilateral juvenile cataracts (20–30 years); keratopathy; glaucoma	Prominent eyes; otherwise normal	Normal
Nails	Normal	Thin and brittle	Dystrophic or thickened
Limbs	Lower limb ulcers; hyperkeratosis over bony prominences; generalized loss of subcutaneous fat	Prominent joints; coxa valga; generalized subcutaneous fat loss; poorly developed muscular system; no acrosclerosis or Raynaud's phenomenon	Atrophy of skin most marked on extremities; no leg ulcers

4 Bauer EA, Uitto J, Tan EM *et al.* Werner's syndrome. Evidence for preferential regional expression of a generalized mesenchymal cell defect. *Arch Dermatol* 1988; **124**: 90–101.

5 Gawkrodger DJ, Priestley GC, Vijayalaxmi *et al.* Werner's syndrome. Biochemical and cytogenetic studies. *Arch Dermatol* 1985; **121**: 636–41.

6 Kieras FJ, Brown WT, Houck GE *et al.* Elevation of urinary hyaluronic acid in Werner's syndrome and progeria. *Biochem Med Metab Biol* 1986; **36**: 276–82.

7 Muratta K. Urinary acidic glycosaminoglycans. *Experientia* 1982; **38**: 313–4.

8 Salk D. Werner's syndrome: a review of recent research. *Hum Genet* 1982; **62**: 1–15.

9 Salk D. *Werner's Syndrome and Human Ageing.* New York: Plenum Press, 1985.

10 Tao LC, Stecker E, Gardner HA *et al.* Werner's syndrome and acute myeloid leukemia. *Can Med Assoc J* 1971; **105**: 951–4.

11 Thompson KVA, Halliday R. Genetic effects on the longevity of human fibroblasts. I. Werner's syndrome. *Gerontology* 1983; **29**: 73–9.

12 Shannon-Danes B. Progeria: a cell culture study on aging. *J Clin Invest* 1971; **50**: 2000–3.

13 Higachi T, Ishikawa O, Hayashi H *et al.* Disaccharide analysis of skin glycosaminoglycans in patients with Werner's syndrome. *Clin Exp Dermatol* 1994; **19**: 487–91.

14 Fleischmajer R, Nedwich A. Werner's syndrome. *Am J Med* 1973; **54**: 111–8.

15 Yu C-E, Oshima J, Fu YH *et al.* Positional cloning of the Werner's syndrome gene. *Science* 1996; **272**: 258–62.

16 Yu C-E, Oshima J, Wijsman EM *et al.* Mutations in the consensus helicase domains of the Werner syndrome gene. *Am J Hum Genet* 1997; **60**: 330–41.

17 Cheng WH, Muftuoglu M, Bohr VA. Werner syndrome protein: functions in the response to DNA damage and replication stress in S-phase. *Exp Gerontol* 2007; **42**: 871–8.

18 Kuzuya H, Imura H. Insulin resistance associated with congenital disorders. Insulin receptors in Werner's syndrome, myotonic dystrophy and type A extreme insulin resistance. *Jpn J Med* 1988; **27**: 219–21.

19 Vannini P, Ciavarella A, Forlani G *et al.* Investigation of insulin resistance associated with Werner's syndrome. *Diabete Metab* 1987; **13**: 81–5.

20 Jonas JB, Ruprecht KW, Schmitz-Valckenbarg P. Ophthalmic surgical complications in Werner's syndrome. *Ophthalmic Surg* 1987; **18**: 760–4.

21 Bjornberg A. Werner's syndrome and malignancy. *Acta Derm Venereol Suppl (Stockh)* 1976; **56**: 149–50.

22 Revuz J, Abensour M, Clérici T *et al.* Squamous cell epithelioma on a leg ulcer in Werner's syndrome. *Ann Dermatol Vénéréol* 1987; **114**: 841–3.

23 Cohen JI, Arnett EN, Kolodny AL *et al.* Cardiovascular features of the Werner syndrome. *Am J Cardiol* 1987; **59**: 493–5.

24 Zucker FD, Rifkin H, Jacobson HG. Werner's syndrome: an analysis of 10 cases. *Geriatrics* 1968; **23**: 124–35.

25 Shimizu T, Tateishi Y, Furuichi Y *et al.* Diagnosis of Werner syndrome by immunoblot analysis. *Clin Exp Dermatol* 2002; **27**: 157–9.

Progeria

Synonym
• Hutchinson–Gilford syndrome

Definition. This is a rare disorder characterized by retarded physical development and abnormal facies, skeletal abnormalities and the onset in early childhood of scleroderma. Although progressive senile degeneration occurs, many of the more common features of ageing, such as cataracts, presbyacusis and presbyopia, are not seen.

Aetiology. It occurs due to *de novo* mutations of the lamin A gene (*LMNA*) which encodes for a major constituent of the inner membrane lamina [1]. Reduced cell proliferation and altered DNA-damage responses are common causal mechanisms in the pathogenesis of both Werner and Hutchinson--Gilford syndromes [2]. Affected families have a high risk of spontaneous abortion.

Various abnormalities of mesodermal tissue have been identified [3]. In tissue culture, progeria fibroblasts have a decreased survival time [4]. The fibroblasts show a threefold increase in the production of hyaluronic acid, and the urinary excretion of hyaluronic acid is increased [4–7]. Animal studies suggest that increased hyaluronic acid in the tissues might produce a reduction in vascularity [5,8]. Tropoelastin production is increased [9], and it has also been suggested that type IV collagen may accumulate due to an interaction between activated T lymphocytes and fibroblasts [10,11]. A preliminary study of cultured fibroblasts from two affected patients suggests mitotic instability [12]. A polymorphism in the galactosyltransferase gene (*B4GALT1*) has been identified in affected cell lines [13].

Fewer than 100 cases have been reported to date, and 97% of patients have been white [8].

Pathology [14]. The major changes are in the skin, bone and cardiovascular tissues.

The skin shows atrophy of epidermis and dermis. There may be progressive hyalinization of dermal collagen and loss of subcutaneous fat. Scanning electron microscopy of hairs from one patient showed unusual longitudinal depressions with minor cuticular defects [11].

The cardiovascular system shows extensive atheroma, and there may be extensive myocardial fibrosis, with extensive lipofuscin ('age pigment') deposition characteristic of elderly adults [15,16].

The bones show a variety of changes including osteolysis, osteoporosis, necrosis, dislocations and poorly healing fractures [17,18].

Clinical features [19]. Affected children usually appear normal at birth, and growth may be only slightly retarded in the first year, but during the second year there is profound growth failure, with reduced subcutaneous fat on the face and limbs [8]. The facial appearance is reminiscent of a fledgling bird, with a disproportionately large cranium with patent fontanelles and frontal bossing, prominent eyes and scalp veins, very sparse, downy scalp hair, sparse or absent eyebrows and eyelashes, centrofacial cyanosis, micrognathia, thin lips and a 'beaked' nose. By the second year, the skin has become thin, taut and shiny in some areas but lax and finely wrinkled in others. Eccrine sweating is decreased. The veins are prominent and there may be easy bruising. After several years, progressive mottled hyperpigmentation develops, most marked on exposed sites, but there is no photosensitivity. Thickened sclerotic areas may be present on the lower trunk or thighs, and in one case multiple keloids developed on the hands and arms [11]. The nails are usually small, thin and dystrophic, and koilonychia and onychogryphosis may occur. Generalized alopecia often begins in the first year of life and the few remaining hairs are pale, fine and 'fuzzy'. The nipples may be hypoplastic.

The dentition is abnormal and delayed, and there may be skeletal abnormalities such as dystrophic clavicles and coxa valga, with joint contractures and a 'horse-riding' stance. Progressive bone resorption may lead to frequent fractures [18]. Sexual maturation is absent but intelligence is normal.

Death usually occurs in the second decade as a result of severe, generalized atheroma.

Diagnosis. The large, bald head with conspicuous veins, the bird-like facies and the well-proportioned little body are distinctive. Bird-headed dwarfism (Chapter 15) is distinguished by the absence of skin atrophy.

Cockayne's syndrome may cause confusion, but progeria is distinguished by the loss of hair, the lack of photosensitivity and ocular changes, and the absence of disproportionately large extremities.

In metageria, sexual maturation and skeletal growth are normal [20].

References
1 Eriksson M, Brown WT, Gordon LB et al. Recurrent de novo mutations in lamin A cause Hutchinson–Gilford progeria syndrome. Nature 2003; **423**: 293–8.
2 Kudlow BA, Kennedy BK, Monnat RJ. Werner and Hutchinson-Gilford progeria syndromes: mechanistic basis of human progeroid diseases. Nat Rev Mol Cell Biol 2007; **8**: 394–404.
3 Gracy RW, Chapman ML, Cini JK et al. Molecular basis of the accumulation of abnormal proteins in progeria and aging fibroblasts. Basic Life Sci 1985; **35**: 427–42.
4 Danes BS. Progeria: a cell culture study of aging. J Clin Invest 1971; **50**: 2000–3.
5 Brown WT, Zebrower M, Kieras FJ et al. Progeria, a model disease for the study of premature ageing. Basic Life Sci 1985; **35**: 375–96.
6 Goldstein S, Moerman E. Heat-labile enzymes in skin fibroblasts in subjects with progeria. N Engl J Med 1975; **292**: 1305–9.
7 Zebrower M, Kieras FJ, Brown WT et al. Urinary hyaluronic acid elevation in Hutchinson–Gilford progeria syndrome. Mech Ageing Dev 1986; **35**: 39–46.
8 Badame AJ. Progeria. Arch Dermatol 1989; **125**: 540–4.
9 Sephel GC. Increased elastin production by progeria skin is controlled by steady-state levels of elastin mRNA. J Invest Dermatol 1988; **90**: 643–7.
10 Conover CA, Dollar LA, Rosenfeld RG et al. Somatomedin C-binding and action in fibroblasts from aged and progeric subjects. J Clin Endocrinol Metab 1985; **60**: 685–91.
11 Jimbow K, Kobayashi H, Ishii M et al. Scar and keloid like lesions in progeria. An electron microscopic and immunohistochemical study. Arch Dermatol 1988; **124**: 1261–6.
12 Ly DH, Lockhart DJ, Lerner RA, Schultz PG. Mitotic misregulation and human ageing. Science 2000; **287**: 2486–92.
13 O'Brien ME, Weiss AS. A novel β(1-4)galactosyltransferase gene silent mutation (594C > T) associated with Hutchinson–Gilford progeria. Hum Mutat 2001; **17**: 355–7.
14 Fleischmajer R, Nedwich A. Progeria (Hutchinson–Gilford). Arch Dermatol 1973; **107**: 253–8.
15 Baker PB, Baba N, Boesel CP. Cardiovascular abnormalities in progeria. Arch Pathol Lab Med 1981; **105**: 384–6.
16 Reichel W, Garcia-Bunuel R. Pathologic findings in progeria: myocardial fibrosis and lipofuscin pigment. Am J Clin Pathol 1970; **53**: 243–55.
17 Hamer L, Kaplan F, Fallon M et al. The musculoskeletal manifestations of progeria. A literature review. Orthopedics 1988; **11**: 763–9.
18 Moen C. Orthopedic aspects of progeria. J Bone Joint Surg Am 1982; **64**: 542–6.
19 De Busk FL. The Hutchinson–Gilford progeria syndrome. J Pediatr 1972; **80**: 697–724.
20 Gilkes JJH, Sharvill DE, Wells RS. The premature ageing syndromes. Br J Dermatol 1974; **91**: 243–62.

Acrogeria [1–4]

Synonym
- Gottron's syndrome

Definition. This disorder begins at birth or soon afterwards, and is characterized by cutaneous atrophy and loss of subcutaneous fat, particularly over the distal extremities, but with no tendency to atheroma, diabetes mellitus or decreased life expectancy. The term 'acrogeria' refers to premature ageing of the extremities.

Aetiology. Most cases occur without a family history, but presumed autosomal recessive as well as autosomal dominant inheritance has been reported [1,2]. Most patients have been female. COL3A1 mutations cause variable phenotype, including Gottron-type acrogeria and vascular EDS [5,6].

Pathology. The subcutaneous fat is absent in the most severely affected regions. The dermis is atrophic, with sparse, thin collagen bundles, but there is abundant elastin, which appears clumped due to the deficiency of collagen.

Clinical features. The changes develop at or soon after birth. The skin becomes dry, thin, transparent and wrinkled, especially over the hands and feet, although the trunk and face may be affected to a lesser extent. The veins are prominent, and there may be easy bruising, poikiloderma and telangiectasia. The nails may be atrophic or thickened. The face appears 'pinched', with a hollow-cheeked 'owl-eyed' appearance, a beaked nose and thin lips. Micrognathism may be present. The lack of subcutaneous fat accentuates the appearance of premature senility. Some patients have low birth weight and persistent short stature, but the general health and life expectancy are normal. The hands and feet may be very small.

Diagnosis. The normal hair and eyes help to distinguish the condition from progeria and pangeria. Cases are occasionally described which do not fit easily into any of the previously recognized categories and have been termed metageria and acrometageria [7,8]. It is not entirely clear whether these are separate entities.

References

1 Gottron H. Familiäre akrogeria. *Arch Dermatol Syphilol (Berlin)* 1941; **181**: 571–83.
2 De Groot WP, Tafelkruyer J, Woerdemann MJ *et al.* Familial acrogeria (Gottron). *Br J Dermatol* 1980; **103**: 213–23.
3 Venencie PY, Powell FC, Winkelmann RK *et al.* Acrogeria with perforating elastoma and bony abnormalities. *Acta Derm Venereol Suppl (Stockh)* 1984; **64**: 348–51.
4 Ho A, White SJ, Rasmussen JE *et al.* Skeletal abnormalities of acrogeria, a progeroid syndrome. *Skeletal Radiol* 1987; **16**: 463–8.
5 Jansen T, De Paepe A, Luytinck N, Plewig G. COL3A1 mutations leading to acrogeria (Gottron type). *Br J Dermatol* 2000; **142**: 178–9.
6 Pope FM, Narcisi P, Nicholls AC *et al.* COL3A1 mutations cause variable clinical phenotypes including acrogeria and vascular rupture. *Br J Dermatol* 1996; **135**: 163–81.
7 Gilkes JJH, Sharvill DE, Wells RS *et al.* The premature ageing syndromes. Reports of eight cases and description of a new entity named metageria. *Br J Dermatol* 1974; **91**: 243–62.
8 Greally JM, Boone LY, Lenkey SG *et al.* Acrometageria: a spectrum of 'premature aging' syndromes. *Am J Med Genet* 1992; **44**: 334–9.

Laboratory studies [1–3]

Fibroblasts from normal human skin have a limited lifespan in culture, which is inversely proportional to the age of the donor, and it seems that the *in vitro* ageing of fibroblasts may serve as a model for the *in vivo* ageing of the whole body. All the premature ageing syndromes studied to date have shown a marked reduction in fibroblast growth potential *in vitro*. These include Werner's syndrome, progeria, poikiloderma congenitale, trisomy 21 and diabetes mellitus. In addition, fibroblasts from progeria patients have shown a decrease in mitotic activity, rate of outgrowth from explants, DNA synthesis and cloning efficiency. Studies on fibroblasts from patients with progeria and Werner's syndrome have also shown enzyme changes consistent with an accelerated ageing process.

In the normal ageing process, there is a threefold increase in the affinity of surface insulin receptors for native insulin between the first and seventh decades. This accounts for the clinical finding of relative insulin resistance in the elderly. Patients with progeria also show increased insulin binding and relative insulin resistance.

Other cellular abnormalities in Werner's syndrome and progeria include a decrease in surface-membrane HLA antigens and a marked increase in the activity of a procoagulant, which may predispose to atheroma.

Post-irradiation DNA repair appears to be normal in progeria and pangeria, although the cultured fibroblasts may have reduced karyotype stability. A reduction in DNA stability might increase the rate of genomic deterioration, and this might accelerate cellular ageing.

References

1 Brown WT, Zebrower M, Kieras FJ *et al.* Progeria, a model disease for the study of accelerated aging. *Basic Life Sci* 1985; **35**: 375–96.
2 Martin GM. The biologic basis for aging: implications for medical genetics. In: Rimoin DC, Connor JM, Pyeritz RE, Korf BR, eds. *Principles and Practice of Medical Genetics*, 4th edn. London: Churchill Livingstone, 2002: 571–89.
3 Goldstein S. Studies on age-related diseases in cultured fibroblasts. *J Invest Dermatol* 1979; **73**: 19–23.

Other associated conditions

Premature ageing with short stature and pigmented naevi

Synonym
• Mulvihill–Smith syndrome

This rare syndrome [1] is characterized by low birth weight, short stature and moderate mental retardation, associated with multiple pigmented naevi and a distinctive bird-like facies. There is a small chin, with broad forehead, and the lack of facial subcutaneous fat gives an appearance of premature ageing. Other features include hypospadias, a high-pitched voice, irregular dentition, fine hair, hepatomegaly and low IgG. The clinical features tend to become more noticeable with increasing age.

Reference

1 de Silva DC, Wheatley DN, Herriot R *et al.* Mulvihill–Smith progeria-like syndrome: a further report with delineation of phenotype, immunologic deficits, and novel observation of fibroblast abnormalities. *Am J Med Genet* 1997; **69**: 56–64.

Neonatal pseudohydrocephalic progeroid syndrome of Wiedemann–Rautenstrauch [1–3]

This rare, autosomal recessive condition is characterized by mental and physical retardation and frontal and lateral bossing of the skull, with small facial bones, a small, beak-shaped nose, low-set ears, small mouth with dysodontia, and ectropion. The scalp hair and eyebrows are long and sparse, the extremities are thin, and the hands are large with long fingers and atrophic nails. The subcutaneous fat is decreased, the skin is thin and wrinkled, and the veins are prominent.

References

1 Devos EA, Leroy JG, Frijns JP *et al.* The Wiedemann–Rautenstrauch or neonatal progeroid syndrome. Report of a patient with consanguineous parents. *Eur J Pediatr* 1981; **136**: 245–8.
2 Snigula F, Rautenstrauch T. A new neonatal progeroid syndrome. *Eur J Pediatr* 1981; **136**: 325–4.
3 Pivnick EK, Angle B, Kaufman RA *et al.* Neonatal progeroid (Wiedemann–Rautenstrauch) syndrome: a report of five new cases and review. *Am J Med Genet* 2000; **90**: 131–40.

Gerodermia osteodysplastica [1]

Stunting of growth from early childhood is associated with senile changes in the skin, with normal scalp hair. Wrinkly, lax skin is most prominent on the dorsa of the hands and feet. Generalized osteoporosis, multiple fractures, joint laxity and skeletal malformations, including Wormian bones, occur. The face appears sad, with drooping eyelids and jowls, malar hypoplasia and mandibular prognathism. Relatives presenting partial forms of the syndrome showed cutaneous ageing and osteodysplasia without dwarfism. Skin biopsy may show fragmented elastic fibres. Two reports of consanguineous Arabian families showed features overlapping both gerodermia osteodysplastica and wrinkly skin syndrome, suggesting that they may represent variable manifestations of the same disorder [2,3].

References

1 Lisker R, Hernández A, Martinez-Lavin M. Gerodermia osteodysplastica hereditaria: report of three brothers and a literature review. *Am J Med Genet* 1979; **3**: 389–95.
2 Al-Gazali LI, Sztriha L, Skaff F, Haas D. Gerodermia osteodysplastica and wrinkly skin syndrome: are they the same? *Am J Med Genet* 2001; **101**: 213–20.
3 Nanda A, Alsaleh QA, Al-Sabah H *et al.* Gerodermia osteodysplastica/wrinkly skin syndrome: report of three patients and brief review of the literature. *Pediatr Dermatol* 2008; **25**: 66–71.

Wrinkly skin syndrome [1]

This rare, familial condition is characterized by the appearance at birth of dry, wrinkled skin of the hands, feet and ventral surfaces of the trunk. The veins are unduly prominent. There may also be mental retardation, ocular defects and poor muscle tone. The cause is unknown, and the dermal collagen and elastin appear normal on light microscopy. There is some phenotypic overlap with gerodermia osteodysplastica and autosomal recessive cutis laxa type II [2].

References

1 Gazit E, Goodman RM, Katznelson MB *et al.* Wrinkly skin syndrome. *Clin Genet* 1973; **4**: 186–7.
2 Gupta N, Phadke SR. Cutis laxa type II and wrinkly skin syndrome: distinct phenotypes. *Pediatr Dermatol* 2006; **23**: 225–30.

Poikiloderma congenitale

Synonym
• Rothmund–Thomson syndrome

This condition is fully described in Chapter 15. It may be considered as a premature ageing syndrome because of the atrophic hyperpigmented skin, the early onset of cataracts, and the premature greying and loss of hair. The striking poikiloderma is distinctive.

Cockayne's syndrome (Chapter 15)

The atrophic skin with mottled pigmentation and loss of subcutaneous fat on the face produce an appearance of premature senility, and the disease has often been confused with progeria.

Trisomy 21 (Chapter 15)

Synonym
• Down's syndrome

This disorder shows more features of true ageing than the classical premature ageing syndromes [1]. These features include progressive dementia with the neurofibrillary tangle seen in senile dementia, amyloid and lipofuscin deposition in many organs, diabetes mellitus, cataracts, cardiovascular disease, increased incidence of autoimmune disease and malignancy, and a decreased life expectancy [2].

The cutaneous features include dry, lax skin, and premature greying and loss of hair [2].

References

1 Martin GM. The biologic basis for aging: implications for medical genetics. In: Rimoin DC, Connor JM, Pyeritz RE, Korf BR, eds. *Principles and Practice of Medical Genetics*, 4th edn. London: Churchill Livingstone, 2002: 571–89.
2 Pueschel SM. Clinical aspects of Down syndrome from infancy to adulthood. *Am J Med Genet* 1990; **37** (Suppl.): 52–6.

Familial mandibulo-acral dysplasia

Synonym
• Craniomandibular dermatodysostosis

The main features of this rare syndrome are mandibular hypoplasia, delayed cranial suture closure, dysplastic clavicles, abbreviated club-shaped terminal phalanges associated with acro-osteolysis and atrophy of the skin over the hands and feet [1] (Fig. 45.39). Other characteristics may include short stature, multiple Wormian bones, prominent eyes and a sharp nose [2,3]. In one family, the condition was also associated with loss of the lower teeth and alopecia [4]. Two types of body fat distribution patterns, both of which are associated with insulin resistance and its metabolic complications, may be evident; partial lipodystrophy of the extremities (type A) and generalized loss of subcutaneous fat (type B) [5]. Both are autosomal recessive, with mutations in the gene encoding lamin A/C; *LMNA* underlie type A and mutations in the zinc metalloproteinase STE24 gene (*ZMPSTE24*) give rise to type B [6,7].

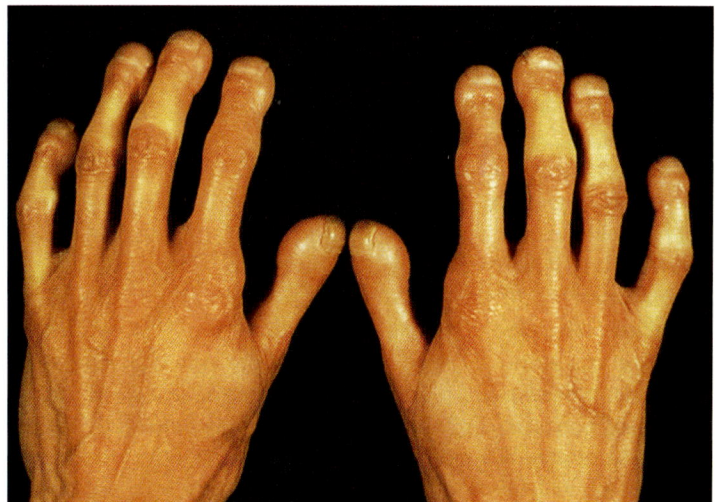

Fig. 45.39 Familial mandibulo-acral dysplasia, showing the short, club-shaped terminal phalanges, the so-called 'tree-frog' appearance. (Courtesy of Dr A.M. Zina, Turin University, Turin, Italy.)

The cutaneous changes are a milder phenotype of progeria and some cases have been mistakenly diagnosed in the past as acrogeria or Werner's syndrome.

References

1 Danks DM, Mayne V, Wettenhall NB *et al.* Craniomandibular dermato-dysostosis. *Birth Defects Orig Artic Ser* 1974; **X**: 99–105.
2 Tenconi R, Miotti F, Miotti A *et al.* Another Italian family with mandibulo-acral dysplasia. *Am J Med Genet* 1986; **24**: 357–64.
3 Zina AM, Cravario A, Bundino S. Familial mandibulo-acral dysplasia. *Br J Dermatol* 1981; **105**: 719–23.
4 Welsh O. Study of a family with a new progeroid syndrome. *Birth Defects Orig Artic Ser* 1975; **11**: 25–38.
5 Simha V, Garg A. Body fat distribution and metabolic derangements in patients with familial partial lipodystrophy associated with mandibuloacral dysplasia. *J Clin Endocrinol Metab* 2002; **87**: 776–85.
6 Novelli G, Muchir A, Sangiuolo F *et al.* Mandibuloacral dysplasia is caused by a mutation in LMNA-encoding lamin A/C. *Am J Hum Genet* 2002; **71**: 426–31.
7 Agarwal AK, Fryns J-P, Auchus RJ *et al.* Zinc metalloproteinase, ZMPSTE24, is mutated in mandibuloacral dysplasia. *Hum Mol Genet* 2003; **12**: 1995–2001.

Diabetic thick skin [1,2]

> **Synonym**
> • Cheiroarthropathy

Diabetes may be classified as a premature ageing syndrome because of the predisposition to cataracts and atheroma and the reduced life expectancy [1,3].

Some patients with diabetes mellitus have thick, tight, waxy skin and limited joint mobility. This combination has been called *cheiroarthropathy* [4]. Affected patients are unable to bring their palms completely together, and their fingers will not bend backwards. The 'prayer sign', in which the patient tries to oppose the two palms, provides an easy screening test [5]. Skin and tendon sheath thickness has also been measured by ultrasound [6,7].

Cheiroarthropathy is present in 30–40% of insulin-dependent diabetics, and in non-insulin-dependent diabetics the figures have varied widely, from 4% to 70%. The changes may even precede the diagnosis of diabetes [8]. The changes are important because affected patients have an increased risk of retinal and renal disease due to microvascular damage [9]. Patients with diabetic cheiroarthropathy also have an increased incidence of frozen shoulder and Dupuytren's contracture [10]. There is often associated thickening of the plantar fascia [11].

The biochemical change is not fully understood, but it seems likely that non-enzymatic glycosylation in diabetic subjects might alter collagen metabolism [1,3]. The lysines in collagen are slowly glycosylated with increasing age, and during this process the glucose attaches to the lysine and undergoes an Amadori rearrangement, thus making the process irreversible [12]. Enzymatic digestion of tendon collagen from young patients who died from diabetes showed that their collagen behaved as if it was from patients who were 50–65 years older than their actual age [13].

Studies of viscoelastic ratio and skin extensibility in patients with type 1 diabetes have shown subclinical stiffness and loss of skin elasticity [14].

The histology of the skin changes resembles systemic sclerosis, but there is a subtle difference, with a predominance of large collagen fibres, thickening of the capillary basement membrane and increased mucin [15].

In some diabetic patients with thick skin, the extensor surfaces of the fingers develop a characteristic, minutely pebbled appearance over or near the knuckles (Huntley's papules). On histology, this shows a papillated epidermal hyperplasia with hyperkeratosis [16].

Because biochemical studies suggest that collagen is 'aged' by increased binding with glucose, it is desirable to maintain tight control of blood glucose levels in diabetic patients [17]. A patient improved with aminobenzoic acid, colchicine and DMSO gel [18].

References

1 Burton JL. Skin and stiff joints in insulin dependent diabetes mellitus. *Br J Dermatol* 1982; **101**: 369–71.
2 Perez MI, Kohn SR. Cutaneous manifestations of diabetes mellitus. *J Am Acad Dermatol* 1994; **30**: 519–31.
3 Monnier VM, Sell DR, Nagaraj RH *et al.* Maillard reaction-mediated molecular damage to extracellular matrix and other tissue proteins in diabetes, aging and uraemia. *Diabetes* 1992; **41** (Suppl. 2): 36–41.
4 Editorial. Diabetic skin, joints and eyes—how are they related? *Lancet* 1987; **ii**: 313–4.
5 Starkman HS, Gleason RE, Rand LI *et al.* Limited joint mobility of the hands in patients with diabetes mellitus. *Ann Rheum Dis* 1986; **45**: 130–5.
6 Collier A, Matthews DM, Kellett HA *et al.* Change in skin thickness associated with cheiroarthropathy in insulin dependent diabetes mellitus. *BMJ* 1986; **292**: 936.
7 Ismail AA, Dasgupta B, Tanqueray AB *et al.* Ultrasonographic features of diabetic cheiroarthropathy. *Br J Rheumatol* 1996; **35**: 676–9.
8 Sherry DD, Rothstein RR, Petty RE *et al.* Joint contracture preceding insulin-dependent diabetes mellitus. *Arthritis Rheum* 1982; **25**: 1362–4.
9 Rosenbloom AL, Silverstein JH. Limited joint mobility in childhood diabetes mellitus. *N Engl J Med* 1981; **305**: 191–4.
10 Moren-Hybbinette I, Moritz U, Schersten B *et al.* The clinical picture of the painful diabetic shoulder. *Acta Med Scand* 1987; **221**: 73–82.
11 Duffin AC, Lam A, Kidd R *et al.* Ultrasonography of plantar soft tissues thickness in young people with diabetes. *Diabet Med* 2002; **19**: 1009–13.
12 Le Pape A, Muh JP, Bailey AJ. Characterisation of N-glycosylated type I collagen in streptozotocin-induced diabetes. *Biochem J* 1981; **197**: 405–12.
13 Hamlin CR, Kohn RR, Luschin JH *et al.* Apparent accelerated ageing of human collagen in diabetes mellitus. *Diabetes* 1975; **24**: 902–4.
14 Nikkels-Tassaudji N, Henry F, Letawe C *et al.* Mechanical properties of the diabetic waxy skin. *Dermatology* 1996; **192**: 19–22.
15 Hanna W, Friesen D, Bombardier C *et al.* Pathologic features of diabetic thick skin. *J Am Acad Dermatol* 1987; **16**: 546–53.
16 Huntley AC. Finger pebbles: a common finding in diabetes mellitus. *J Am Acad Dermatol* 1986; **14**: 612–7.
17 Lieberman LS, Rosenbloom AC, Riley WJ *et al.* Reduced skin thickness with pump administration of insulin. *N Engl J Med* 1980; **303**: 940–1.
18 Gruson LM, Franks A Jr. Scleredema and diabetic sclerodactyly. *Dermatol Online J* 2005; **30**: 3.

Leprechaunism

> **Synonym**
> • Donohue's syndrome

Definition. Leprechaunism is a rare and poorly defined syndrome characterized by severe intrauterine and postnatal growth retardation, decreased subcutaneous tissue and muscle mass, and a characteristic facies [1]. Tissue resistance to insulin appears to be an important feature, as hyperinsulinaemia and pancreatic β-cell hyperplasia are frequently present [2,3].

Aetiology. The condition is inherited as an autosomal recessive trait. The basis for the insulin resistance is homozygous or compound heterozygous mutations in the extracellular domain of the insulin receptor, which leads to markedly impaired insulin binding [4]. Mutations that retain significant insulin binding activity cause the less severe phenotype of Rabson–Mendenhall syndrome.

The fibroblasts have a prolonged doubling time *in vitro*. They respond poorly to the metabolic actions of insulin, and to the actions of several other growth factors, such as epidermal growth factor.

Pathology [5]. In the skin, the elastic and collagen fibres are few and fragmented. On the extremities, the horny layer is markedly thickened. The muscles show a proliferation of abnormal connective tissue. In some cases, the ovaries are large and cystic, and there is β-cell hyperplasia of the pancreatic islets.

Clinical features [5–8]. The child is abnormal at birth, with low birth weight. The nose is broad, the ears low set and large, the eyes widely spaced. There is hypertrichosis of the forehead and cheeks. The skin appears too large for the body, is loosely folded at the flexures and may be corrugated, with gyrate folds on the hands and feet, which may be disproportionately large. Muscle wasting, often progressive, is usually present. The breasts and the penis or clitoris may be slightly hypertrophic. The bone age is retarded and there may be metaphyseal and epiphyseal dystrophy.

Growth is generally retarded, the nutritional status remains poor and susceptibility to infection is high. Death by the age of 1 year is usual.

Diagnosis. The cutaneous changes could be confused with cutis laxa, but in leprechaunism the skin, although folded, is thickened and not lax. The diagnosis is confirmed by the associated features and the finding of raised plasma insulin levels.

References

1 Donohue WL, Uchida I. Leprechaunism: a euphemism for a rare familial disorder. *J Pediatr* 1954; **45**: 505–19.
2 Kaplowitz PB, D'Ercole J. Fibroblasts from a patient with leprechaunism are resistant to insulin, epidermal growth factor and somatomedin C. *J Clin Endocrinol Metab* 1982; **55**: 741–8.
3 Taylor SI, Hedo JA. Extreme insulin resistance in association with abnormally high binding affinity of insulin receptors from a patient with leprechaunism: evidence for a defect intrinsic to the receptor. *J Clin Endocrinol Metab* 1982; **55**: 1108–13.
4 Longo N, Wang Y, Smith SA *et al.* Genotype–phenotype correlation in inherited severe insulin resistance. *Hum Mol Genet* 2002; **11**: 1465–75.
5 Patterson JH, Watkins WL. Leprechaunism in a male infant. *J Pediatr* 1962; **60**: 730–9.
6 Kaloustian VM. Leprechaunism: a report of two new cases. *Am J Dis Child* 1971; **122**: 442–5.
7 Hartdegen RG, Dogliotti M, Rabinowitz L *et al.* Leprechaunism: case report in a black African child. *Br J Dermatol* 1975; **93**: 587–91.
8 Joan D, Dimitriu L, Belengeanu V *et al.* Leprechaunism: report of two cases and review. *Endocrinologie* 1988; **26**: 205–9.

Lipoatrophy

The absence of subcutaneous fat may give the appearance of premature ageing if the face is affected. Lipoatrophy is fully discussed in Chapter 46.

Perforating dermatoses

Many dermatoses occasionally exhibit the phenomenon of transepithelial elimination (TEE), in which material from the dermis is extruded through the epidermis to the exterior with little or no disruption of the surrounding structures [1]. The extruded material may include inflammatory cells, red cells, microorganisms and extracellular substances, such as mucin or altered connective tissue components [2,3]. In most of these conditions, the TEE is secondary to some underlying disease, such as granuloma annulare or PXE, but there are four conditions that are regarded as *primary perforating disorders*: Kyrle's disease (Chapter 19), perforating folliculitis (Chapter 30), reactive perforating collagenosis and perforating serpiginous elastosis. It is possible that these primary perforating disorders might be due to defects in the epidermal keratinocytes, hair follicle, collagen and elastic fibres, respectively, with TEE being the final common pathway [2,3].

In acquired reactive perforating dermatosis (see below), the bulk of the coarse granular basophilic material that is extruded by TEE appears to derive from the nuclei of polymorphonuclear leukocytes [4]. It has been suggested that lysosomal enzymes derived from leukocytes might be responsible for the altered staining of collagen fibres, the degradation of elastic fibres and the impairment of keratinocyte adhesion, which allows TEE of dermal components [4].

Acquired reactive perforating dermatosis

Until recently, the four conditions mentioned above were thought to be unrelated, but there have now been numerous reports of these perforating dermatoses occurring in diabetes mellitus or in patients with chronic renal failure, many of whom were undergoing haemodialysis [2,5–9]. An incidence of 11% has been reported, with a particular association with long-standing diabetes [9]. The keratotic lesions in this condition develop on the trunk and limbs, and are usually pruritic, dome-shaped papules with central crusts (Fig. 45.40). They are not related to trauma.

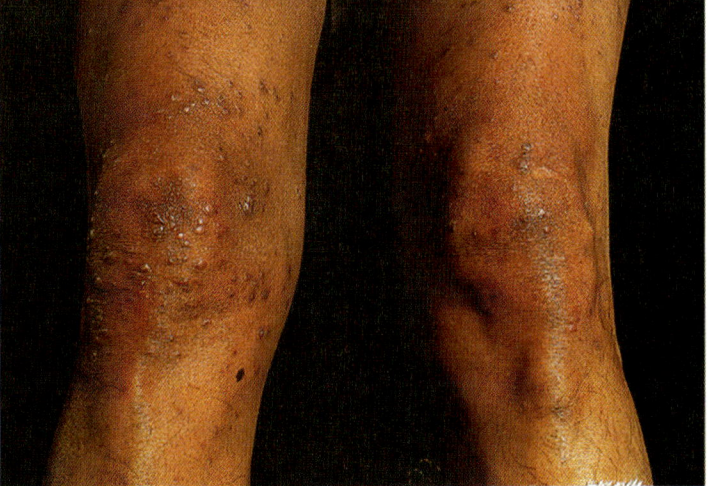

Fig. 45.40 Perforating dermatosis in a diabetic patient with renal failure. (Courtesy of Dr D.A. Burns, Leicester Royal Infirmary, Leicester, UK.)

The distinction between the four dermatoses has not always been clear-cut, and the presence or absence of the Koebner reaction, and the presence or absence of collagen fibres in the epidermis, are not reliable distinguishing features [2,3]. Both collagen and elastic fibres can be extruded in the same patient [7], and it seems likely that at least in the case of haemodialysis patients these conditions may overlap. The name *acquired reactive perforating dermatosis* has been suggested for this skin problem. These four conditions, however, appear to be separate entities when they occur outside the setting of renal failure or diabetes mellitus.

Topical or intralesional steroids or topical retinoids may be helpful, but some patients improve spontaneously [9]. Other reported treatments include rifampicin and allopurinol [10].

References

1 Mehregan RH. Transepithelial elimination. *Curr Probl Dermatol* 1970; **3**: 124–47.
2 Patterson JW. The perforating disorders. *J Am Acad Dermatol* 1984; **10**: 561–81.
3 Patterson JW. Progress in the perforating dermatoses. *Arch Dermatol* 1989; **125**: 1121–3.
4 Zelger B, Hintner H, Aubock J, Fritsch PO. Acquired perforating dermatosis. *Arch Dermatol* 1991; **127**: 695–700.
5 Cochran RJ, Tucker SB, Wilkin JK *et al.* Reactive perforating collagenosis of diabetes mellitus and renal failure. *Cutis* 1983; **31**: 55–8.
6 Poliak SC, Lebwohl MG, Parris A *et al.* Reactive perforating collagenosis associated with diabetes mellitus. *N Engl J Med* 1982; **306**: 81–4.
7 Rapini RP, Herbert AA, Drucker CR *et al.* Acquired perforating dermatosis: evidence of combined transepidermal elimination of both collagen and elastic fibres. *Arch Dermatol* 1989; **125**: 1074–8.
8 Stone RA. Kyrle-like lesions in two patients with renal failure undergoing dialysis. *J Am Acad Dermatol* 1981; **5**: 707–9.
9 Morton CA, Henderson IS, Jones MC *et al.* Acquired perforating dermatosis in a British dialysis population. *Br J Dermatol* 1996; **135**: 671–7.
10 Kruger K, Tebbe B, Krengel S *et al.* Acquired reactive perforating dermatosis. Successful treatment with allopurinol in two cases. *Hautzart* 1999; **50**: 115–20.

Perforating disease due to exogenous agents

Occasionally, a chemical that has been applied to the skin topically or by intradermal injection can be eliminated by the transepidermal route to produce a perforating disorder. Eight cases have been reported following occupational exposure to a caustic drilling fluid used in the petrochemical industry [1]. Each patient noted skin irritation following exposure to the fluid, and 1 or 2 days later developed tender papules with central umbilication, which ulcerated and crusted. Histological examination of the lesions revealed TEE of altered collagen and debris which stained for calcium.

It is possible that the lesions were due to follicular penetration by the calcium present in the drilling mud. The drilling fluids contain many additives, but calcium carbonate or calcium chloride are often present in high concentrations in the mud. Similar cases have been reported following the use of calcium-containing electroencephalography paste [2].

TEE of altered collagen has also been reported following the use of intradermal steroid injections [3,4].

References

1 Knox JM, Knox JM, Dinehart SM *et al.* Acquired perforating disease in oil field workers. *J Am Acad Dermatol* 1986; **14**: 605–11.
2 Shoenfeld RJ, Grekin JN, Mehregan A. Calcium deposition in the skin. A report of four cases following electroencephalography. *Neurology* 1965; **15**: 477–80.
3 Goette DK. Transepidermal elimination of altered collagen after intralesional adrenal steroid injections. *Arch Dermatol* 1984; **120**: 539–40.

4 Katz R, Hood AF. Transepidermal elimination following the use of a topical adrenal steroid. *Arch Dermatol* 1985; **121**: 412–3.

Reactive perforating collagenosis [1–4]

Definition. A rare inherited form of TEE in which collagen is extruded through the epidermis. It is usually precipitated by environmental cold or trauma. The commoner, acquired, form is often referred to as acquired perforating dermatosis (qv) which is typically associated with haemodialysis, although lesions have been recorded with internal neoplasia [4].

Aetiology. The cause is unknown, but the condition is often familial [5,6]. The basic defect seems to be a type of focal damage to collagen, which is then extruded as a result of necrolysis of the overlying epidermis [7].

Pathology [2,7,8]. The lesion originates in the papillary dermis, where collagen is surrounded and engulfed by focal epidermal proliferation. The collagen appears normal on electron microscopy, but gives an abnormal staining pattern with trichrome and phosphotungstic acid haematoxylin. The central crater which develops contains inflammatory cells and keratinous debris. Elastic tissue is typically absent, and the abnormal collagen is eliminated by transepithelial migration.

Clinical features [7]. The inherited form usually starts in early childhood as small papules on the extensor surface of the hands, the elbows and the knees following superficial trauma. Each skin-coloured papule increases to a size of about 6 mm over 3–5 weeks and then becomes umbilicated, with a keratinous plug. The lesions regress spontaneously in 6–8 weeks to leave a hypopigmented area or slight scar, but new lesions may appear. Lesions can be produced experimentally, and Koebner's phenomenon may be present, with linear lesions [9]. The papules can also be provoked by inflamed acne lesions, but deep incisions do not produce the lesions. The condition persists into adult life. In some cases, the disease is associated with intolerance to cold and improves in warm weather.

Diagnosis. The condition may be mistaken clinically for molluscum contagiosum, papular urticaria, perforating serpiginous elastoma, perforating folliculitis, perforating granuloma annulare and Kyrle's disease, but the histology is characteristic [6]. Verrucous perforating collagenoma must also be distinguished (see below). The nosological relationship between reactive perforating collagenosis and the acquired reactive perforating dermatosis of renal failure remains uncertain (see above) [4].

Treatment. Topical retinoic acid may reduce the number of lesions. Other treatments which may help include oral isotretinoin, methotrexate, emollient creams, topical steroids under occlusion [3,4] and PUVA [10].

References

1 Mehregan AH, Schwartz OD. Reactive perforating collagenosis. *Arch Dermatol* 1967; **96**: 277–82.

2 Fretzin DF, Beal DW, Jao W. Light and ultrastructural study of reactive perforating collagenosis. *Arch Dermatol* 1980; **116**: 1054–8.

3 Patterson JW. Progress in the perforating disorders. *Arch Dermatol* 1989; **125**: 1121–3.

4 Chae KS, Park YM, Cho SH *et al.* Reactive perforating collagenosis associated with periampullary carcinoma. *Br J Dermatol* 1998; **139**: 548–50.

5 Kanan MW. Familial reactive perforating collagenosis and intolerance to cold. *Br J Dermatol* 1974; **91**: 405–14.

6 Nair BKH, Sarojini PA, Basheer AM *et al.* Reactive perforating collagenosis. *Br J Dermatol* 1974; **91**: 399–403.

7 Cerio R, Calnan CD, Wilson-Jones E. A clinico-pathological study of reactive perforating collagenosis: report of 10 cases. *Br J Dermatol* 1987; **117** (Suppl. 32): 16–7 (Abstract).

8 Millard PR, Young E, Harrison DE *et al.* Reactive perforating collagenosis: light, ultrastructural and immunohistological studies. *Histopathology* 1986; **10**: 1047–56.

9 Bovenmeyer DA. Reactive perforating collagenosis. Experimental production of the lesion. *Arch Dermatol* 1970; **102**: 313–7.

10 Serrano G, Aliaga A, Lorente M *et al.* Reactive perforating collagenosis responsive to PUVA. *Int J Dermatol* 1988; **27**: 118–9.

Verrucous perforating collagenoma [1,2]

> **Synonym**
> - Collagenome perforant verruciforme

In this rare condition, severe (as opposed to superficial) trauma to the skin produces verrucous papules which show TEE of collagen. The eruption occurs as a single episode and is not familial.

References

1 Delacretaz J, Gattlen JM. Verrucous perforating collagenoma. *Dermatologica* 1976; **152**: 65–6.

2 Laugier P, Woringer F. Reflexions au sujet d'une collagenome perforant verruciforme. *Ann Dermatol Syphiligr (Paris)* 1963; **90**: 29–32.

Elastosis perforans serpiginosa

> **Synonyms**
> - Perforating elastoma
> - Elastoma intrapapillare perforans

Definition. In this reactive perforating dermatosis, the material extruded through the epidermis is derived from elastic fibres in the upper dermis.

Aetiology. The cause is unknown, but a genetically determined defect of elastic tissue may be involved [1]. The altered elastin resembles that seen in experimental animals subjected to lathyrogens or copper deficiency.

It is probable that the primary abnormality is in the dermal elastin, which provokes a cellular response that ultimately leads to extrusion of the abnormal elastic tissue. It may be significant that the lesions are commonly seen in areas subjected to wear and tear. The lesions may follow an abrasion.

Some 40% of reported cases have been associated with connective tissue disorders, such as PXE, EDS, MFS, OI and acrogeria [2,3]. It has also been reported in otherwise healthy individuals and in mental deficiency, especially Down's syndrome [4–6].

It sometimes occurs in patients taking penicillamine, which is known to cause the production of abnormal elastin [7–10].

The relationship to perforating PXE and pseudo-PXE due to penicillamine is discussed on p. 45.25.

Pathology [4,11–13]. The earliest detectable change is the focal development of elastotic staining tissue and basophilic debris in the dermis. This is followed by a reaction of the overlying epidermis, which grows down to engulf the elastotic material. The epidermis surrounding the fully developed lesion is acanthotic and hyperkeratotic. The papule consists of a circumscribed area of epidermal hyperplasia traversed by a channel communicating directly with the dermis and containing a mass of tissue, which projects above the surface. This plug consists of horny material in its upper third and of amorphous debris derived from elastin in its lower two-thirds [11]. In the dermis beneath and around the lesion, there is a foreign-body giant cell reaction. The elastotic material is finally extruded, to leave irregular scarring and warty thickening. Electron microscopy shows an increase in elastic fibres, with fine filaments on the surface similar to those seen in normal embryos. In penicillamine-induced cases the elastic fibres have a characteristic 'bramble bush' or 'lumpy bumpy' morphology [9]. The hydroxylation of dermal collagen is similar to that of newborn skin [12].

Clinical features [14,15]. The age of onset ranges from 6 to 20 years. Males are predominantly affected. Small, horny or umbilicated papules are characteristically arranged in lines, circles or segments of circles in a serpiginous pattern. The individual papules may remain small or may enlarge slightly to assume a crateriform appearance with an elevated edge and a central plug, or further to leave an area of atrophic skin surrounded by smaller papules, each with a horny plug. The rings may reach a diameter of 15–20 cm but are usually smaller (Fig. 45.41). The back and sides of the neck are most commonly affected, but the lesions may also occur on the cheeks or on the arms or thighs, and are sometimes bilaterally symmetrical. They may persist for several years, but eventually involute spontaneously to leave reticulate atrophic scars. Biopsy scars readily become keloidal.

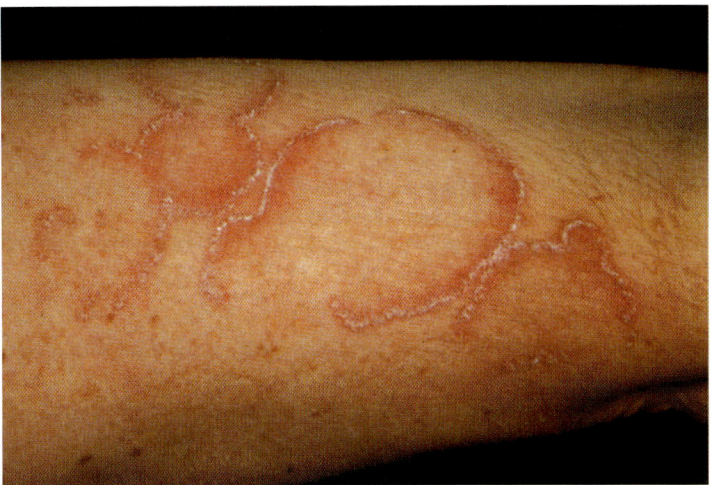

Fig. 45.41 Elastosis perforans serpiginosa in a patient with vascular Ehlers–Danlos syndrome.

Diagnosis. The annular or linear arrangements of the papules and their distribution suggest the diagnosis, which is confirmed by the characteristic histology. Conditions which may cause confusion include porokeratosis of Mibelli, reactive perforating collagenosis and perforating granuloma annulare.

A similar histological appearance can occur in the acquired reactive perforating dermatosis of renal failure (see above) [16].

Treatment. Careful removal of the nodules with a curette under local anaesthesia may give a reasonable cosmetic result. Freezing has been recommended [14,17]. Excision should be avoided, and dermabrasion may make the condition worse [4]. In a child with Down's syndrome and associated vitamin A deficiency, clinical improvement was observed with oral retinoid therapy, even though the treatment produced side effects [6]. Isotretinoin has been used successfully in a patient with penicillamine-induced disease [18]. There are reports of improvement following Sellotape stripping of the surface keratinous material [19], tazarotene [20], imiquimod [21], pulsed dye [22], ultrapulsed carbon dioxide [23] and Er : YAG [24] laser therapies.

References

1 Ayala F, Donofrio P. Elastosis perforans serpiginosa: report of a family. *Dermatologica* 1983; **166**: 32–4.
2 Reed WB, Pidgeon JW. Elastosis perforans serpiginosa with osteogenesis imperfecta. *Arch Dermatol* 1964; **89**: 342–4.
3 Mehta RK, Burrows NP, Payne CM *et al.* Elastosis perforans serpiginosa and associated disorders. *Clin Exp Dermatol* 2001; **26**: 521–4.
4 Patterson JW. The perforating disorders. *J Am Acad Dermatol* 1984; **10**: 561–81.
5 O'Donnell B, Kelly P, Dervan P *et al.* Generalized elastosis perforans serpiginosa in Down's syndrome. *Clin Exp Dermatol* 1992; **17**: 31–3.
6 Jan V, Saugier J, Arbeille B *et al.* Elastome perforant serpigineux avec hypovitaminose A chez une enfant ayant une trisomie 21. *Ann Dermatol Vénéréol* 1996; **123**: 188–90.
7 Pass F, Goldfischer S, Sternlieb I *et al.* Elastosis perforans serpiginosa during penicillamine therapy for Wilson's disease. *Arch Dermatol* 1973; **108**: 713–5.
8 Kirsch N, Hukill PB. Elastosis perforans serpiginosa induced by penicillamine. Electron microscopic observations. *Arch Dermatol* 1977; **113**: 630–5.
9 Bardach H, Gebhart W. Elastic fiber changes induced by penicillamine. *J Am Acad Dermatol* 1982; **6**: 398–9.
10 Light N, Meyrick-Thomas RH, Stephens A *et al.* Collagen and elastin changes in d-penicillamine-induced pseudoxanthoma elasticum-like skin. *Br J Dermatol* 1986; **114**: 381–8.
11 Hashimoto K, Hill WR. Elastosis perforans serpiginosa—histochemical and enzymic digestion studies. *J Invest Dermatol* 1960; **35**: 7–14.
12 Volpin D, Pasquali-Ronchetti I, Castellani I *et al.* Ultrastructural and biochemical studies on a case of elastosis perforans serpiginosa. *Dermatologica* 1978; **156**: 209–23.
13 Bergman R, Friedman-Burnbaum R, Hazaz B. A direct immunofluorescence study in elastosis perforans serpiginosa. *Br J Dermatol* 1985; **113**: 573–9.
14 Mehregan AH. Elastosis perforans serpiginosa. A review of the literature and report of 11 cases. *Arch Dermatol* 1968; **97**: 381–93.
15 Catterall MD, Padley NR. Elastosis perforans serpiginosa. *Clin Exp Dermatol* 1979; **4**: 119–22.
16 Schamroth JM. Elastosis perforans serpiginosa in a patient with renal disease. *Arch Dermatol* 1988; **122**: 82–4.
17 Whyte HJ, Winkelmann RK. Elastosis perforans—the association of congenital anomalies, and salient facts in histology. *J Invest Dermatol* 1960; **35**: 113–22.
18 Ratnavel RC, Norris PG. Penicillamine-induced elastosis perforans serpiginosa treated successfully with isotretinoin. *Dermatology* 1994; **189**: 81–3.
19 Langeveld-Wildschut EG, Toonstra J *et al.* Familial elastosis perforans serpiginosa. *Arch Dermatol* 1993; **129**: 205–7.
20 Outland JD, Brown TS, Callen JP. Tazarotene is an effective therapy for elastosis perforans serpiginosa. *Arch Dermatol* 2002; **138**: 169–71.
21 Kelly SC, Purcell SM. Imiquimod therapy for elastosis perforans serpiginosa. *Arch Dermatol* 2006; **142**: 829–30.
22 Kaufman AJ. Treatment of elastosis perforans serpiginosa with the flashlamp pulsed dye laser. *Dermatol Surg* 2000; **26**: 1060–2.
23 Abdullah A, Colloby PS, Foulds IS, Whitcroft I. Localized idiopathic elastosis perforans serpiginosa effectively treated by the Coherent Ultrapulse 5000°C aesthetic laser. *Int J Dermatol* 2002; **39**: 719–20.
24 Saxena M, Tope WD. Response of elastosis perforans serpiginosa to pulsed CO₂, Er:YAG, and dye lasers. *Dermatol Surg* 2003; **29**: 677–8.

Miscellaneous disorders

Colloid milium

Synonyms
• Colloid pseudomilium
• Colloid degeneration of the skin
• Elastosis colloidalis conglomerata

Definition. Colloid milium is a degenerative change characterized clinically by the development of yellowish, translucent papules or plaques on light-exposed skin, and histologically by the presence of colloid in the dermal papillae.

Aetiology. The cause is uncertain, and the condition may not represent a single entity. The rare juvenile form [1,2], beginning before puberty and often familial, can be distinguished from a non-familial form occurring in later life. Although light appears to play little part in provoking the lesions in the juvenile form, it is certainly implicated in older patients, among whom the incidence is highest in fair-skinned, outdoor workers in sunny climates [1,3,4]. Some authors consider the adult form to be a variant of actinic elastosis [5]. Cases among refinery workers in the tropics suggest that trauma and the photodynamic effects of phenols in oxide fuel (gas oil) may be contributory factors [6]. Cases have also been reported after the long-term application of strong hydroquinone bleaching creams. These patients also had ochronosis [7].

Pathology [7–13]. The earliest histological change is the appearance of colloid globules at the tips of the dermal papillae. Homogeneous fissured masses of colloid occupy the upper dermis, each surrounded by bands of collagen. The colloid is usually eosinophilic but may be basophilic. Within it, small blood vessels and the nuclei of fibroblasts are well preserved. In the larger, plaque-like lesions, the colloid change occurs diffusely throughout the dermis.

In the juvenile form, the colloid masses may also occur in the epidermis, and elastosis is not present, whereas in the adult form the colloid is separated from the epidermis by a band of elastin, and elastosis is present. In the juvenile form, 'immature' Civatte bodies occur in the epidermis.

The source of the colloid material is uncertain. It could be a protein synthesized by fibroblasts or it could be derived from degraded elastic fibres [1,3,9].

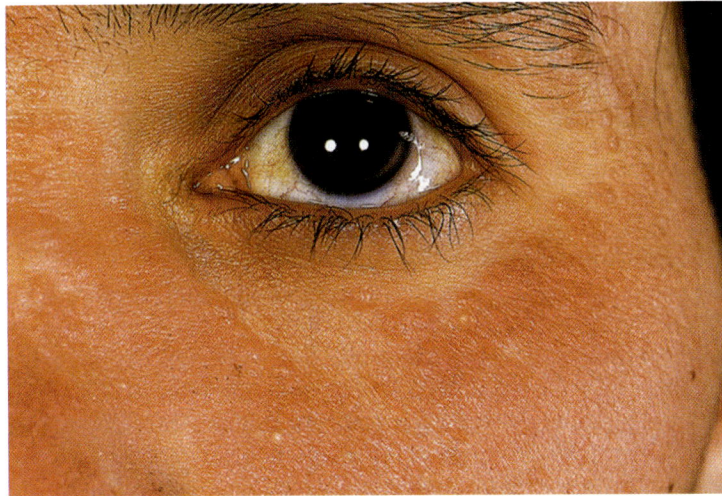

Fig. 45.42 Colloid milium of the infraorbital region. (Courtesy of Dr D.A. Burns, Leicester Royal Infirmary, Leicester, UK.)

The histological changes may be difficult to distinguish from those of amyloidosis, especially lichen amyloid. Electron microscopy may be needed for definitive diagnosis [7,9,13]. In adult colloid milium, the colloid is amorphous, with wavy, branching filaments. In the juvenile form, it is composed of closely packed filaments, which are often in parallel rows, forming whorled fascicles [1,13].

Clinical features. Small dermal papules 1–2 mm in diameter, yellowish brown and sometimes translucent, develop slowly and more or less symmetrically in irregular groups in areas exposed to sunlight (Fig. 45.42). They feel soft and may release their gelatinous contents when punctured. The most frequently involved sites are the face, especially around the orbits, the dorsa of the hands, the back and sides of the neck and the ears. There is some variation in the clinical features according to the age of onset. In young children, the lesions are often confined to the face, with diffuse infiltration surmounted by innumerable small papules, which may appear vesicular. In older patients, the papules are often fewer and larger, and their potential distribution is much wider, although often only one or two sites are involved in each individual. The changes induced by prolonged light exposure are associated to varying degrees. Although colloid milium may become more severe and more extensive over the years, most cases reach their maximum development within 3 years and then remain unchanged.

The juvenile form may be associated with conjunctival and gingival deposits of an amyloid-like homogeneous material [11].

A nodular form has been described in which lesions may be 5–50 mm in size and may be single or multiple [14].

Diagnosis. The histological and clinical findings together are unmistakable, although the former alone may be difficult to differentiate from amyloidosis. Similar papular lesions are seen in severe actinic elastosis [15]. Trichoepithelioma, tuberous sclerosis and hidrocystoma are distinguished by biopsy.

Treatment. Treatments for actinic elastosis have been used in adult patients, including topical retinoids [5]. Improvement has been reported following dermabrasion [15] and ablation with the Er:YAG laser [16]. Destruction of the lesions with the diathermy or with cryotherapy has also been advocated, but the cosmetic result is seldom satisfactory.

References
1 Handfield-Jones SE, Atherton D, Black M. Juvenile colloid milium. *Br J Dermatol* 1991; **125**: 80–1.
2 Chowdhury MMV, Blackford S, Williams S. Juvenile colloid milium. *Br J Dermatol* 1999; **141** (Suppl. 55): 102–7.
3 Innocenzi D, Barduagni F, Cerio R, Wolter M. UV-induced colloid milium. *Clin Exp Dermatol* 1993; **18**: 347–50.
4 Hashimoto K, Kumakiri M. Colloid-amyloid bodies in PUVA-treated human psoriatic patients. *J Invest Dermatol* 1979; **72**: 70–80.
5 Dummer R, Laetsch B, Stutz S *et al*. Elastosis colloidalis conglomerata (adult colloid milium, paracolloid of the skin) a maximal manifestation of actinic elastosis. *Eur J Dermatol* 2006; **16**: 163–6.
6 Findlay GH, Morrison JGL, Simson IW *et al*. Exogenous ochronosis and pigmented colloid milium from hydroquinone bleaching creams. *Br J Dermatol* 1975; **93**: 613–22.
7 Ebner H, Gebhart W. Colloid milium: light and electron microscopic investigations. *Clin Exp Dermatol* 1977; **2**: 217–26.
8 Hashimoto K, Miller F, Bereston ES. Colloid milium: histochemical and electron microscopic studies. *Arch Dermatol* 1972; **105**: 684–94.
9 Hashimoto K, Black M. Colloid milium: a final degeneration product of actinic elastoid. *J Cutan Pathol* 1985; **12**: 147–56.
10 Kobayashi H, Hashimoto K. Colloid and elastic fibre: ultrastructural study on the histogenesis of colloid milium. *J Cutan Pathol* 1983; **10**: 111–22.
11 Oskay T, Erdem C, Anadolu R *et al*. Juvenile colloid milium associated with conjunctival and gingival involvement. *J Am Acad Dermatol* 2003; **49**: 1185–8.
12 Patterson JW, Wilkin JK, Schatzki PF. Nodular colloid degeneration: distinctive histochemical and ultrastructural features. *Cutis* 1985; **10**: 355–8.
13 Hashimoto K, Nakayama H, Chimenti S *et al*. Juvenile colloid milium. Immunohistochemical and ultrastructural studies. *J Cutan Pathol* 1989; **16**: 164–74.
14 Kuittken J. Papular elastosis. *Cutis* 2000; **66**: 81–3.
15 Apfelberg DB, Druker D, Spence B *et al*. Treatment of colloid milium of the hand by dermabrasion. *J Hand Surg (Am)* 1978; **3**: 98–100.
16 Ammiraki CT, Granola JM, Hruza GJ. Adult-onset facial colloid milium successfully treated with the long-pulsed Er:YAG laser. *Dermatol Surg* 2002; **28**: 215–9.

White fibrous papulosis of the neck

Asymptomatic, small, white, fibrous papules around the neck have been described in several Japanese [1,2], Iranian and European patients [3,4]. The number of papules ranges from 10 to 100; middle-aged to elderly men are predominantly affected. The papules are round to oval, clearly marginated and non-follicular (Fig. 45.43). Histology is unremarkable, showing bundles of thickened collagen fibres in the mid-papillary dermis. Although lesions clinically resemble disorders of elastic tissue, such as anetoderma and dermatofibrosis lenticularis disseminata, elastic fibres are morphologically normal on histology. Acquired connective tissue naevi could exhibit similar features, although the late age of onset makes this diagnosis unlikely. The condition appears to have no prognostic significance, and may be under-reported. It may reflect intrinsic or photo-ageing [5].

Recently, it has been suggested that there may be a relationship between fibrous papulosis of the neck and acquired elastolysis of the papillary dermis [6]. These changes are attributed to ageing or photoageing [5,7].

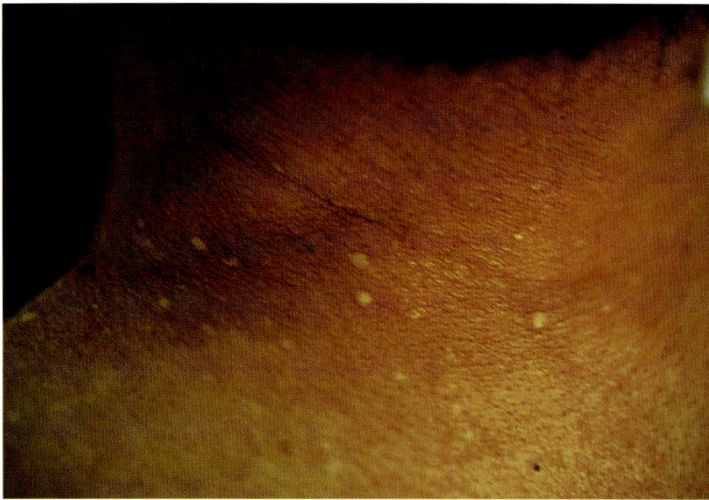

Fig. 45.43 White fibrous papulosis of the neck. (Courtesy of Professor H. Shimizu, Sapporo Hospital, Tokyo, Japan.)

References
1 Shimizu H, Nishikawa T, Kimura S. White fibrous papulosis of the neck: a review of 16 cases. *Jpn J Dermatol B* 1985; **95**: 1077–84.
2 Shimizu H, Kimura S, Harada T *et al.* White fibrous papulosis of the neck: a new clinicopathologic entity? *J Am Acad Dermatol* 1989; **20**: 1073–7.
3 Cerio R, Gold S, Wilson-Jones E. White fibrous papulosis of the neck. *Clin Exp Dermatol* 1991; **16**: 224–5.
4 Redondo P, Vázquez-Doval J, de Alava E. White fibrous papulosis of the neck. *Dermatology* 1993; **186**: 238–9.
5 Balus L, Amanthea A, Donati P *et al.* Fibroelastolytic papulosis of the neck: a report of 20 cases. *Br J Dermatol* 1997; **137**: 461–6.
6 Perrin CH, Castenet J, Lacour J-P *et al.* Papulose blanche du cou. Aspects cliniques de pseudoxanthoma elastique. *Ann Dermatol Vénéréol* 1996; **123**: 114–7.
7 Siragusa M, Schepis C, Palazzo R *et al.* Skin pathology findings in a cohort of 1500 adult and elderly subjects. *Int J Dermatol* 1999; **38**: 361–6.

Papular elastorrhexis

This is a rare variant of connective tissue naevus. Adolescents or young adults present with multiple, non-follicular oval white or yellowish papules on the trunk or limbs; dermal elastic fibres are decreased and fragmented on histology. Most reports are of sporadic cases, with no family history and no extracutaneous manifestations [1–3]. Similar lesions are seen in some patients with Buschke–Ollendorff syndrome (Chapter 18), in which osteopoikilosis is also a feature. To add to the confusion, abortive forms of Buschke–Ollendorff syndrome have been described, lacking osteopoikilosis [4]. A family has been described with this variant [5]. It is possible that papular elastorrhexis is not a separate entity [6]. Intralesional triamcinolone may be beneficial [7].

References
1 Bordas X, Ferrandiz C, Ribera M *et al.* Papular elastorrhexis: a variety of nevus anelasticus? *Arch Dermatol* 1987; **123**: 433–4.
2 Sears JK, Seabury Stone M, Argenyi Z. Papular elastorrhexis: a variant of connective tissue nevus. *J Am Acad Dermatol* 1988; **19**: 409–14.
3 Choonhakarn C, Jirarattanapochai K. Papular elastorrhexis. A distinct variant of connective tissue nevi or an incomplete form of Buschke–Ollendorff syndrome? *Clin Exp Dermatol* 2002; **27**: 454–7.
4 Schorr WF, Opitz JM, Reyes CN. The connective tissue nevus–osteopoikilosis syndrome. *Arch Dermatol* 1992; **106**: 208–14.

5 Schirren H, Schirren CG, Stolz W *et al.* Papular elastorrhexis: a variant of dermatofibrosis lenticularis disseminata (Buschke–Ollendorff syndrome). *Dermatology* 1994; **189**: 368–72.
6 Ryder HF, Antaya RJ. Nevus anelasticus, papular elastorrhexis and eruptive collagenoma: clinically similar entities with focal absence of elastic fibres in childhood. *Pediatr Dermatol* 2005; **22**: 153–7.
7 Lee SH, Park SH, Yoon TJ *et al.* Papular elastorrhexis improved by intralesional injection of triamcinolone. *J Dermatol* 2001; **28**: 569–71.

Progressive osseous heteroplasia [1,2]

This rare condition typically affects female infants and is characterized by ossification of skin and soft tissues. Ossification begins in the dermis, progressing to deeper tissues and to adjacent areas of skin. It is not associated with trauma or infection [3]. Skin lesions begin as groups of small, firm papules resembling rice grains; later, larger ossified nodules may develop. A skin biopsy should include subcutaneous fat. Cancellous and even mature intra-membranous bone is found in the dermis and subcutis. The differential diagnosis includes plate-like osteoma cutis (in which the lesion is solitary) (Chapter 56), Albright hereditary osteodystrophy (which is associated with dysmorphic features, including brachydactyly and short stature, and less severe ossification) and fibrodysplasia ossificans progressiva, in which ossification initially affects muscle or fascia and the great toes are malformed. The disorder is caused by a paternally inherited, inactivating *GNASI* mutation, which is also found in Albright hereditary osteodystrophy [4]. This gene encodes for guanine nucleotide-binding protein Gs alpha, which couples receptors to adenyl cyclases, generating cAMP. Studies in mice indicate that Gs alpha directly regulates the differentiation of growth plate cartilage and suppresses ectopic ossification, without affecting renal function [5,6].

The condition is progressive, and the morbidity depends on the site and the severity of the ossification. There is no effective treatment to prevent the ossification, but lesions that disrupt function or impair movement can sometimes be removed surgically.

References
1 Kaplan FS, Craver R, MacEwen GD *et al.* Progressive osseous heteroplasia: a distinct developmental disorder of heterotopic ossification. *J Bone Joint Surg Am* 1994; **76**: 425–36.
2 Miller ES, Esterly NB, Fairley JA. Progressive osseous heteroplasia. *Arch Dermatol* 1996; **132**: 787–91.
3 Kaplan FS, Shore EM. Progressive osseous heteroplasia. *J Bone Miner Res* 2000; **15**: 2084–94.
4 Shore EM, Ahn J, Jan de Beur S *et al.* Paternally inherited inactivating mutations of the *GNASI* gene in progressive osseous heteroplasia. *New Engl J Med* 2002; **346**: 99–106.
5 Bastepe M, Weinstein LS, Ogata N *et al.* Stimulatory G protein directly regulates hypertrophic differentiation of growth plate cartilage in vivo. *Proc Nat Acad Sci USA* 2004; **101**: 14794–9.
6 Castrop H, Oppermann M, Mizel D *et al.* Skeletal abnormalities and extra-skeletal ossification in mice with restricted Gs alpha deletion caused by a renin promoter–Cre transgene. *Cell Tissue Res* 2007; **330**: 487–501.

Fascial hernias of the legs [1,2]

Small fascial hernias of the lower legs are not uncommon in athletes and heavy manual workers, and may present a problem in differential diagnosis. Herniation of muscle takes place through the hiatus in the deep fascia where it is perforated by communicating veins.

The hernias develop suddenly as nodules on the anterolateral aspect of the lower leg and are usually about 15 cm above the lateral malleolus. The nodules are soft, compressible and 1.5–2.0 cm in diameter. If bilateral, they are strictly symmetrical. No treatment is required, although minimally invasive fasciotomy is claimed to give symptomatic benefit [3].

References
1 Kitchin ID, Richmond DA. Multiple muscle herniae. *BMJ* 1943; **i**: 602–3.
2 Obermayer ME, Wilson JW. Fascial hernias of the legs. *JAMA* 1951; **145**: 548–9.
3 deFijter WM, Scheltingen MB, Luiting MG. Minimally invasive fasciotomy in chronic exertional compartment syndrome and fascial hernias of the anterior lower leg: short and long-term results. *Mil Med* 2006; **171**: 399–403.

Constricting bands of the extremities

Synonym
- Ainhum and pseudo-ainhum

Definition. This is a constricting band around a digit or limb. The band may be shallow, involving only the skin, or it may be deeper, involving fascia or bone, and in some cases amputation may result. The term *ainhum* (an African word meaning 'to saw' [1]) is applied to a specific type in which a painful constriction of the fifth toe occurs in adults, with eventual spontaneous amputation. *Pseudo-ainhum* is the term applied to other constricting bands which are congenital or secondary to another disease.

Ainhum

Synonym
- Dactylolysis spontanea

Aetiology. The condition appears to be due to an abnormal blood supply to the foot in some patients, as arteriography has shown that in these patients the posterior tibial artery is attenuated at the ankle, and the plantar arch and its branches are absent [2]. Mechanical factors, including trauma from walking barefoot, may then precipitate the development of a groove in the ischaemic toe. Chronic fissuring in hyperkeratotic skin also seems to be an important factor. A family history is common, and the disease is more common in certain races. Ainhum is most common in black Africans, but many cases have been reported in black Americans, and it can also occur in other races.

Various tropical infections, including leprosy, tuberculosis and yaws, have been suggested as possible contributory factors, but these conditions are probably coexistent rather than causative [2,3].

Pathology [4]. Fissuring and hyperkeratosis on the medial aspect of the digit is followed by fibrosis, distal degeneration and osteoporosis, ultimately leading to spontaneous amputation. There may be secondary infection and osteomyelitis.

Clinical features. The condition is most common between the ages of 30 and 50 years, but the earliest stages may be seen in childhood. The presenting symptom is usually a painful fissure.

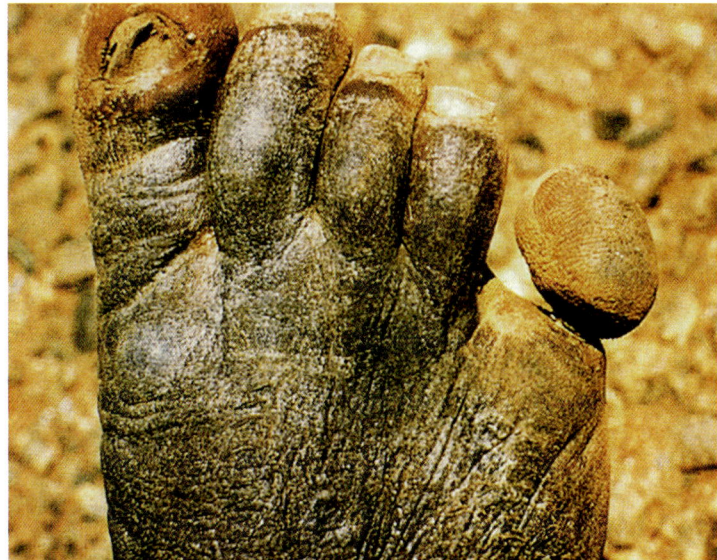

Fig. 45.44 Ainhum, just before shedding of the fifth digit. (Courtesy of Dr D. Burley, Princess Margaret Hospital, Swindon, UK.)

The toe is held dorsiflexed at the metatarsophalangeal joint, and gradually becomes clawed. Rest pain, coolness and cyanosis of the digit distal to the groove suggest that ischaemia is present. Once the constricting band has encircled the toe, the condition tends to progress rapidly. The toe becomes globular, hangs by a thread of fibrous tissue and is eventually shed (Fig. 45.44).

Diagnosis. The condition must be distinguished from pseudo-ainhum.

Treatment. Control of secondary infection and protection from trauma may prevent extension of the scarring process. If symptoms are severe, or the dangling digit is a disability, amputation is indicated.

Pseudo-ainhum

Congenital. Congenital pseudo-ainhum may involve a digit, a limb or even the trunk, and it ranges in severity from a superficial groove to amputation *in utero* [5–8]. The cause is unknown, but familial cases have been reported. Some cases of pseudo-ainhum may be due to amniotic bands [9] or adhesions *in utero*, which may arise as a result of tearing of the amnion some time after the 45th day of pregnancy [10]. Cases have occurred in EDS and after amniocentesis [10,11]. Several cases are reported where raised limb bands develop in the postnatal period, not always associated with amniotic tears; other possible causes include an early teratogenic insult [1,12].

Histology of the affected digit or limb reveals broad, finger-like projections of collagen, and coarse elastic bundles that penetrate deep into the subcutaneous fat [8].

Congenital pseudo-ainhum must be distinguished from: *aplasia* of the limbs with rudimentary digits; *acromelia* (in which part of the limb does not develop); and *hypoplasia* (in which the parts, although formed, are poorly developed).

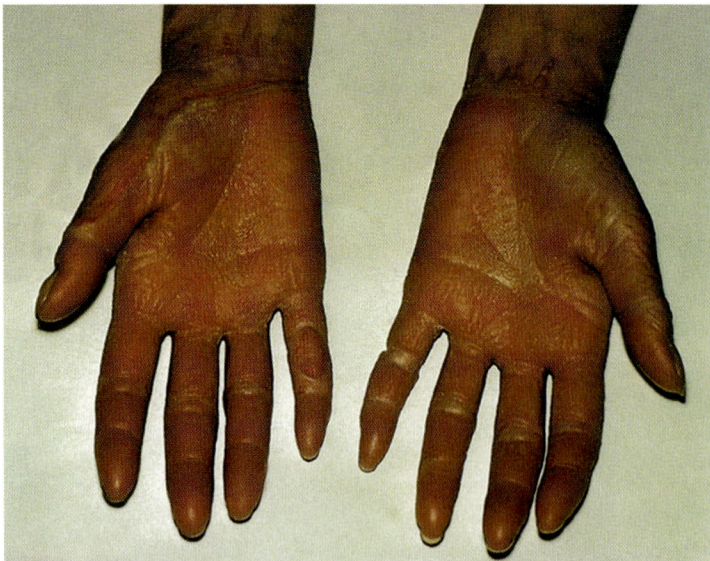

Fig. 45.45 Vohwinkel's disease with pseudo-ainhum of the fifth digit of the left hand. (Courtesy of Dr F.A. Ive, Durham, UK.)

Acquired. Pseudo-ainhum may be acquired as a result of infection (particularly leprosy), trauma, cold injury, neuropathy (especially congenital sensory neuropathy), systemic sclerosis, etc. [13] and chronic psoriasis [14], and it may occur in association with other hereditary diseases such as palmoplantar keratoderma (particularly Vohwinkel's disease) (Fig. 45.45), pachyonychia congenita, erythropoietic protoporphyria [15,16], and Olmsted's syndrome (Chapter 19). Factitial pseudo-ainhum has also been reported due to the self-application of a rubber tourniquet.

Multiple skin creases resembling constrictions may be seen in the Michelin baby syndrome (Chapter 18) and in 'multiple benign annular creases of the extremity' (Chapter 19).

Treatment. Staged Z-plasty sometimes gives an excellent result [17].

References

1 Meggitt ST, Harper J, Lacour M *et al*. Raised limb bands developing in infancy. *Br J Dermatol* 2002; **147**: 359–63.
2 Dent DM, Fataar S, Rose AG. Ainhum and angiodysplasia. *Lancet* 1981; **ii**: 396–7.
3 Editorial. Ainhum. *Lancet* 1975; **ii**: 19–20.
4 Browne SG. Ainhum. *Int J Dermatol* 1976; **15**: 348–50.
5 Glessner JR. Spontaneous intra-uterine amputation. *J Bone Joint Surg Am* 1963; **45**: 351–5.
6 Petereka ES, Karon IM. Congenital pseudo-ainhum of the finger. *Arch Dermatol* 1964; **90**: 12–4.
7 Raque CJ, Stein KM, Lane JM. Pseudo-ainhum constricting bands of the extremities. *Arch Dermatol* 1972; **105**: 434–8.
8 Rushton DI. Amniotic band syndrome. *BMJ* 1983; **286**: 919–20.
9 Young ID, Lindenbaum RH, Thompson EM *et al*. Amniotic bands in connective tissue disorders. *Arch Dis Child* 1985; **60**: 1061–3.
10 Lockwood C, Ghidini A, Romero R *et al*. Amniotic band syndrome: reevaluation of its pathogenesis. *Am J Obstet Gynecol* 1989; **160**: 1030–3.
11 Moessinger AC. Amniotic band syndrome associated with amniocentesis. *Am J Obstet Gynecol* 1981; **141**: 588–91.
12 Latteo SA, Taylor AE, Meggitt SJ. Raised limb bands developing in infancy. *Br J Dermatol* 2006; **154**: 791–2.
13 Bockers M, Benes P, Bork K *et al*. Persistent skin ulcers, mutilations and acro-osteolysis in hereditary sensory and autonomic neuropathy. *J Am Acad Dermatol* 1989; **21**: 736–9.
14 Almond SL, Curley RK, Feldberg L. Pseudoainhum in chronic psoriasis. *Br J Dermatol* 2003; **149**: 1064–6.
15 Christopher AP, Grattan CEH, Colvan MA. Pseudo-ainhum and erythropoietic protoporphyria. *Br J Dermatol* 1988; **118**: 113–6.
16 Schamroth JM. Mutilating keratoderma. *Int J Dermatol* 1986; **25**: 249–51.
17 Kamalan A. Ainhum trichosporosis Z-plasty. *Dermatologica* 1981; **162**: 372.

Heberden's and Bouchard's nodes

Heberden's nodes [1] are posterolateral bony outgrowths affecting one or more *distal* interphalangeal joints. Similar changes, affecting the *proximal* interphalangeal joints, are termed Bouchard's nodes. Both Heberden's and Bouchard's nodes are strongly associated with osteoarthritis, although they may be inherited independently as an autosomal dominant trait [2,3]. Characteristically, they are asymptomatic and of insidious onset, although tender nodes may develop acutely with a red, swollen joint. The association of multiple symmetrical nodes with distal interphalangeal joint arthritis has been termed 'primary generalized osteoarthritis'. Because this is associated with the tissue types HLA-A1 and B8 and shows a marked female preponderance, it has been postulated to be an autoimmune disorder; increased amounts of immune complexes can be detected in cartilage and synovium [4].

References

1 Kellgren JH, Moore R. Generalised osteoarthritis and Heberden's nodes. *BMJ* 1952; **i**: 181–7.
2 Stecker RM. Heberden's nodes. A clinical description of osteoarthritis of the finger joints. *Ann Rheum Dis* 1953; **48**: 523–7.
3 Irlenbusch U, Dominick G. Investigations into generalized osteoarthritis. Part 1: genetic study of Heberden's nodes. *Osteoarthritis Cartilage* 2006; **14**: 423–7.
4 Doherty M, Pattrick M, Powell RJ. Hypothesis—nodal generalised osteoarthritis is an auto-immune disease. *Ann Rheum Dis* 1990; **49**: 1017–20.

CHAPTER 46

Subcutaneous Fat

D.H. McGibbon

St John's Institute of Dermatology, St Thomas' Hospital, London, UK

Introduction

Subcutaneous fat (subcutis) occurs almost universally over the body surface between the skin and the deep fascia, but it is absent from the eyelids and the male genitalia. It varies in thickness with the race, age, sex, endocrine and nutritional status of the individual.

Subcutaneous fat acts as an insulating layer and a protective cushion; it also has an important role in thermogenesis, and as a store of readily available energy. In a normal person, fat constitutes about 10% of body weight, and provides about 40 days' reserve energy [1]. Brown fat has a very important thermoregulatory role and acts by increasing the basal metabolic rate [2]. This is particularly important in infancy, and heat production in response to cold exposure is maximal in neonates, who have large quantities of brown fat.

Fat also provides support and has a cosmetic function, for example in the contours of the face. It also has great social importance. Fat children may be bullied or ostracized at school [3], fat adults may find it harder to get certain jobs, and the contribution of fat to the shape of the breasts and buttocks as a secondary sexual development in the female has been known to influence social behaviour.

In addition to the above functions, the obesity epidemic and the metabolic consequences of abnormal fat distribution have underlined the fact that the subcutaneous fat, comprising as it does innumerable adipocytes secreting a large variety of enzymes, hormones and cytokines, is also a major endocrine organ [4].

Embryology [5,6]

The first fat-containing cell, the pre-adipocyte, appears in the mesenchyme around the 14th week of fetal life. The primitive mesenchymal cell that forms the determined pre-adipocyte is also capable of maturing to form a fibrocyte, a myocyte, a chondrocyte or an osteoblast. Pre-adipocytes can terminally differentiate into either brown adipocytes or white adipocytes.

Brown fat is a special type of granular fat that differs from white fat in its distribution, histology and function. It is multilocular and is metabolically very active with many mitochondria so that it is capable of transferring energy from food to produce heat. As it has a much greater capillary network surrounding it compared to white fat (which is partly responsible for the brown colour), heat can be rapidly transferred into the circulation. It is most prominent in the neck and upper thorax of the fetus, and it may be homologous to the hibernating gland fat found in some animals [7]. Brown fat is now known to persist into adult life [8], and it may have a role in preventing obesity [8]. Warm patches develop in the skin 1 hour after taking ephedrine orally, and these warm patches may indicate the site of thermogenic brown fat. Brown fat adipocyte mitochondria uniquely express uncoupling protein-1 (UCP-1), allowing confirmation that brown fat is present in adult white fat depots in variable amounts, and that transdifferentiation from white to brown adipocytes can occur. Development of brown fat begins at the 20th week of gestation, reaches its maximum at birth and then diminishes so that there are no large collections of brown fat in the adult, though fluorodeoxyglucose positron emission tomography (FDG PET) suggests that some adults have supraclavicular areas of brown fat [9]. Evidence for cold induction of brown fat as an adaptive response in humans is at present equivocal [9].

Histology

White fat adipocytes are the largest connective tissue cells in the body, with a diameter of up to 100 μm. Much of their differentiation occurs soon after birth. The mature fat cell has a characteristic signet-ring appearance, because the flat oval nucleus is displaced to the side by a single, large, intracellular, fat-containing vacuole,

Rook's Textbook of Dermatology, 8th edition. Edited by DA Burns, SM Breathnach, NH Cox and CEM Griffiths. © 2010 Blackwell Publishing Ltd.

which is surrounded by perilipin. Originally thought of as an inert store for emergency supplies of energy when necessary, it is now realized that the white adipocyte has a huge array of functions, secreting factors (adipokines) that affect lipid and glucose metabolism, endocrine functions, blood pressure control, coagulation, fibrinolysis, angiogenesis and inflammation. For a full review the reader is referred to Frühbeck [6]. Groups of lipocytes are arranged in lobules, which are separated by interlobular septa composed of collagen and reticulin fibres. The adipocytes may comprise only 25% of the total cell population of a lobule; the remainder, the stromavascular tissue, being macrophages, fibroblasts, mast cells, pericytes, endothelial cells and pre-adipocytes, allowing for considerable cross-talk between cells with even more factors being produced.

Fat tissue has an abundant blood supply, each individual lobule being supplied by a terminal arteriole from the vascular supply running along the septa, which then breaks up to form capillaries which come into close apposition with the individual fat cells. The subcutaneous fat also contains a rich lymphatic plexus, which receives vessels from the dermis. These lymph vessels traverse the subcutaneous layer parallel to the skin surface for some distance, before eventually penetrating the deep fascia and draining into the regional lymph nodes. The nature of the lipocyte and its relationship to blood vessels and lymphatics has been reviewed in detail by Ryan and Curri [10]. Both white fat and brown fat are innervated by noradrenergic fibres of the sympathetic nervous system and para-sympathetic fibres.

The fat tissue and the fat organ. All fat tissue is composed of lobules of fat cells with their supporting connective and stroma-vascular tissue. In addition to the subcutaneous fat, approximately 20% of fat tissue occurs internally, in the mediastinal and retroperitoneal tissues, the mesentery and the bone marrow and in and around individual organs, including blood vessels. This tissue, although it is widely scattered throughout the body, forms a true organ as regards both structure and function [1] but in which depot-specific differences occur [11]. For example, increases in subcutaneous upper body and visceral fat are associated with an increased cardiovascular and metabolic risk but increases in gluteofemoral subcutaneous fat are not [12]. In addition, perivascular adipose tissue shows increased angiogenesis compared to subcutaneous fat [13]. The fact that some genetic lipodystrophy patients lose peripheral fat but fat padding for absorption of mechanical pressure is maintained, is further evidence for depot-specific differences.

The combination of the obesity epidemic and the advent of liposuction has rekindled interest in the structure of subcutaneous fat with MRI scanning as the investigative tool [14]. Subcutaneous fat is divided by the superficial fascia into two compartments, superficial and deep. The fat mass in the superficial (areolar) layer is compartmentalized into lobules by vertical and oblique fibrous septal planes and bands, whilst that of the deeper (lamellar) layer has its septae more horizontally positioned. The superficial layer is fairly constant, but the deeper is more variable, with an increase in fat mass accumulating between split horizontal septae. In females, subcutaneous fat is most abundant in the gluteofemoral region and breasts, resulting in the so-called gynoid distribution,

whereas in males the android distribution of shoulders and upper arms, neck and lumbosacral area predominates.

Physiology [5,6,15–18]
Traditionally, adipose tissue was regarded as an inert energy store with insulating and padding properties. Whilst storage is still a major function, there is now an appreciation that adipocytes and their stromavascular tissue have many other highly complex and dynamic actions, including energy homeostasis, adipogenesis, insulin sensitivity and influences on immune and inflammatory responses.

Energy homeostasis. A major function of white adipose tissue is to store energy at times of calorie excess and release it when needed, such as during exercise or starvation. The synthesis (anabolism) and catabolism of fat in the subcutaneous depot depends on many factors, including nourishment, endocrine and nervous activity. The role of the autonomic nervous system in regulating fat metabolism is now well established [19], being particularly important for rapid energy need compared to the slower control exerted by neuroendocrine factors [20]. A decrease in parasympathetic activity results in increased lipolysis, as does an increase in sympathetic activity, with the opposites stimulating lipogenesis [21]. Hormones that may affect the energy metabolism of fat cells include insulin, cortisol, norepinephrine (noradrenaline) and several pituitary hormones, including somatotrophin, adrenocorticotrophic hormone (ACTH), thyrotrophin, lipotrophin and natruretic peptide [22].

The fats contained within the lipocytes are predominantly triglycerides (triacylglycerols), especially those of palmitic and stearic acids and the unsaturated oleic acid. All the fatty acids have an even number of carbon atoms, predominantly C16 and C18, with a few C14 and C12. Adipose tissue contains 10–30% of water with a small proportion of lipochromes, and less than 2% cholesterol. Fat-soluble substances are also present in varying amounts. These include fat-soluble vitamins and traces of chlorinated hydrocarbons (e.g. aldrin, dieldrin) ingested with the diet, as well as drugs such as acitretin. Adipose tissue *in vitro* has a metabolic rate similar to that of kidney tissue, and approximately half that of liver. Approximately half the triglyceride in the adipose tissue of rats and mice is catabolized and reconstituted in the course of a week or so.

The fat for storage enters the lipocyte as fatty acids, having been converted from lipoproteins by the extracellular enzyme lipoprotein lipase (Fig. 46.1). The fatty acids combine with coenzyme A, using the energy of adenosine triphosphate (ATP), to form the corresponding acyl coenzyme A compounds. Some of these are then oxidized to provide energy for the regeneration of ATP, but most are converted to triglyceride by combination with glycerol-3-phosphate derived from glucose.

The adipocyte is one of the few cells to express the insulin-dependent glucose transporter receptor 4 (GLUT-4), which mediates the passage of glucose into the cell, as well as leading to further triglyceride formation via *de novo* lipogenesis, the latter providing only a small contribution to the pool. At the same time, insulin inhibits hydrolysis and breakdown of triglyceride, conserving the energy store.

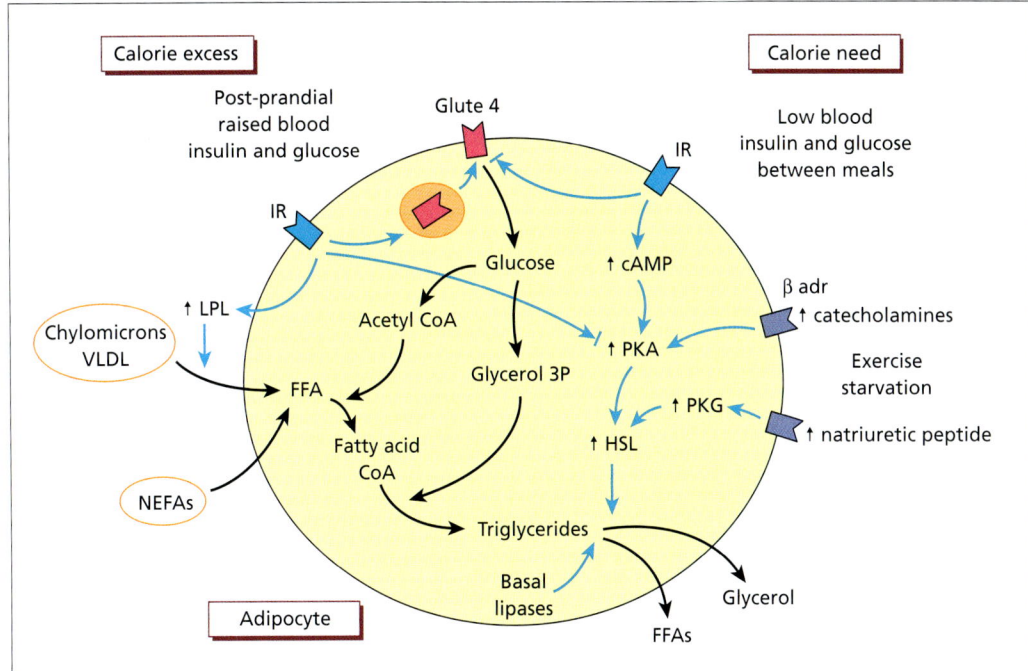

Fig. 46.1 Simplified outline of lipogenesis in an adipocyte during energy excess and lipolysis during calorie need. Effects of hormones and enzymes are in blue. β adr, β-adrenoceptor; cAMP, cyclic andenosine monophosphate; FFA, free fatty acid; Glute 4, insulin-sensitive glucose transporter; HSL, hormone-sensitive lipase; IR, insulin receptor; LPL, lipoprotein lipase; NEFAs, non-esterified fatty acids; PKA, protein kinase A; PKG, protein kinase G; VLDL, very low density lipoproteins.

When the body requires energy, lipolysis occurs. Triglyceride is hydrolysed in the adipocyte, converted to non-esterified fatty acids (NEFA) and glycerol, the rate-limiting enzyme being hormone-sensitive lipase (HSL). The NEFAs are conveyed in the blood to tissues such as liver and muscle, in which fatty acid oxidation readily takes place. In both tissues, the essential part of the process consists of the oxidation in the mitochondria of the long-chain fatty acids. The glycerol of the triglyceride molecule reacts with ATP to form glycerol phosphate, which is oxidized to glyceraldehyde-3-phosphate. This in turn may either be converted to glycogen by reversal of glycolysis, or it may be converted to pyruvate. Skeletal muscle readily oxidizes fatty acids but glucose, if available, is preferentially used. In cardiac muscle, fatty acids are a major source of energy. Lipolysis is regulated predominantly through insulin and catecholamines. The latter, elevated during a sudden energy demand, bind to β-adrenergic receptors on the adipocyte and activate HSL through the classic adenosine monophosphate-protein kinase A (AMP-PKA) pathway.

Leptin [23]. Leptin is an adipokine involved in energy homeostasis which may have evolved to help adaption from the starved to the adequately nourished state rather than to prevent obesity. Leptin, a product of the *ob* gene, is a 16-kDa polypeptide comprising 167 amino acids with a structural homology similar to other cytokine proteins such as TNF-α and interleukin-6. It is secreted by adipocytes predominantly, but also by the stomach, aiding immediate appetite control. Leptin receptors are present in the hypothalamus, on adipocytes, skeletal muscle, liver, pancreatic β-cells, ovary and endometrium. The main effect of leptin is via the satiety centres in the hypothalamus. If excess energy is being stored, rising leptin levels stimulate satiety centres to reduce appetite. Conversely, during starvation low leptin levels stimulate appetite. Circulating levels of leptin correlate with increasing

body mass index (BMI), but have little effect on satiety centres, indicating an apparent leptin resistance. Leptin also influences several other functions, including neuroendocrine and reproductive functions, insulin secretion and blood pressure. Patients with congenital leptin deficiency have gross obesity, hyperphagia, delayed pubertal development, abnormal T-cell number and function, and altered thyroid and growth hormone function [24]. In addition, leptin has a role in immune function and inflammation [25]. There is increased expression in chondrocytes and leptin may have a part to play in articular degenerative disease.

Adipogenesis. Adipogenesis refers to the recruitment from multipotent stem cells in the mesenchyme and stromavascular tissue, and proliferation of pre-adipocytes followed by their differentiation into mature fat cells. Culture of cell lines has led to the elucidation of many of the transcriptional factors involved in adipogenesis, the major ones being peroxisome proliferator-activated receptor-γ (PPARγ) and the CCAAT-enhancer-binding proteins (C/EBPs). The precise contribution of adipogenesis towards enlargement of the fat organ at different stages of human development and life changes is uncertain, but it seems maximal before and around birth before diminishing, then possibly continuing at a low rate throughout adult life. Glucocorticoids, growth hormone and insulin stimulate cells to terminal differentiation, but when mature fat cells reach a certain size, recruitment occurs so that the fat organ enlarges through hyperplasia (increased numbers of cells) rather than hypertrophy (increase in size of cells). Control of this hyperplastic response may come from the local adipocyte through paracrine effects involving local growth factors. During adipogenesis the local extracellular matrix also changes, the effects of which might play their own role in differentiation. This is supported by the fact that fat tissue repair is improved if elements of this matrix are included with the donor adipocytes.

Insulin sensitivity. Insulin secretion, stimulated by raised blood glucose levels after meals to reverse hyperglycaemia, has two major effects. It facilitates glucose uptake into most of the body's cells (liver, skeletal muscle and adipocytes) and it suppresses glucose output by the liver. Insulin resistance occurs when a target organ fails to respond normally to insulin, resulting in hyperinsulinaemia. The effect may be incomplete suppression of hepatic glucose output in the liver and/or impaired insulin-mediated glucose uptake in peripheral tissues, including adipocytes. If increased insulin secretion cannot prevent hyperglycaemia, type 2 diabetes mellitus results. Adipocytes secrete many factors, some of which have direct and indirect effects on insulin sensitivity. The effects of dysregulation of some of these factors are discussed under obesity, below.

Adiponectin [26–28]. Adiponectin is a 30-kDa protein comprised of 244 amino acids with some structural similarity to both collagen and complement C_1q. It is thought, at the moment, to be secreted exclusively by adipocytes and has autocrine/paracrine effects within the local adipose tissue and endocrine effects distantly. Locally, it can promote preadipocytes to become mature fat cells which, with increasing size, down-regulate their adiponectin secretion to exert some feedback control. Adiponectin receptors are present in many tissues as well as adipocytes. It is likely that adiponectin receptor-activated AMPK (AMP-activated protein kinase) leads to enhanced insulin signalling and therefore insulin sensitivity. Adiponectin expression is lower in visceral adipose tissue (VAT) adipocytes compared to subcutaneous depots (SAT) if BMI is increased. Serum adiponectin levels are lower with weight gain and higher with weight loss.

Adiponectin also exerts protective anti-inflammatory effects both locally, by inhibiting secretion of interleukin-6, interleukin-8, macrophage inflammatory protein-1 and monocyte chemotactic protein-1, and distantly on monocyte/macrophages, endothelial cells, hepatic and muscle cells directly, and via inhibition of TNF-α production and action. There is an, as yet unexplained, paradox concerning adiponectin and its anti-inflammatory effects. Obesity is associated with macrophages in the visceral adipose tissue that generate factors, particularly TNF-α, that suppress adiponectin secretion. However, low levels of adiponectin promote inflammation, generating a self-sustaining loop; thus in obesity low adiponectin levels negatively correlate with inflammatory markers. In autoimmune states, such as rheumatoid arthritis and systemic lupus erythematosus, adiponectin levels are raised, the level positively correlating with inflammatory markers. To explain this, it has been suggested that the adiponectin system has evolved as a mechanism for adaptation to starvation, a catabolic state [29]. It is therefore raised in other catabolic states such as autoimmune disease and inflammatory bowel disease, and it did not evolve as a protective device against insulin resistance.

Many other adipokines have been described [6,18] and most are still being evaluated for their relevance to human biology. The stromavascular tissue itself is also responsible for a variety of cytokines. Macrophages secrete TNF-α, interleukins 1, 6, 8 and 10, monocyte chemoattractant protein 1, macrophage migration inhibitory factor, angiotensinogen, and endothelial and vascular growth factors. Therefore, as well as affecting energy homeostasis,

insulin sensitivity and adipocyte differentiation, the fat organ has influences on inflammation, immune function, vascular inflammation and neo-angiogenesis. All of this lends credence to the concept of the fat organ being an endocrine organ in its own right. Whilst these discoveries are of the utmost importance for worldwide obesity-associated morbidity and mortality, except for lipodystrophy patients, their relevance has not provided much insight about the causation and treatment of classical skin panniculitides.

References

1 Lundgren H, Bengtsson C, Blohme E, Lapidus L. Adiposity and adipose tissue distribution in relation to incidence of diabetes in women. *Int J Obes* 1989; **13**: 413–8.

2 Heaton JM. The distribution of brown adipose tissue in the human. *Anatomy* 1972; **112**: 35–9.

3 Taitz LS. *The Obese Child*. Oxford: Blackwell Scientific Publications, 1983: 21.

4 Bays HE, González-Campoy JM, Henry RR *et al*. The Adiposopathy Working Group. Is adiposopathy (sick fat) an endocrine disease? *Int J Clin Pract* 2008; **62**: 1474–83.

5 Avram AS, Avram MM, James WD. Subcutaneous fat in normal and diseased states: 2. Anatomy and physiology of white and brown adipose tissue. *J Am Acad Dermatol* 2005; **53**: 671–83.

6 Frühbeck G. Overview of adipose tissue and its role in obesity and metabolic disorders. *Methods Mol Biol* 2008; **456**: 1–22.

7 Aherne W, Hull D. The site of heat production in the newborn infant. *Proc R Soc Med* 1964; **57**: 1172–3.

8 Jung RT, Shetty PS. Reduced thermogenesis in obesity. *Nature* 1979; **279**: 322–3.

9 Nedergaard J, Bengtsson T, Cannon B. Unexpected evidence for active brown adipose tissue in adult humans. *Am J Physiol Endocrinol Metab* 2007; **293**: E444–52.

10 Ryan TJ, Curri SB, eds. *Clinics in Dermatology*, Vol. 7. *The Cutaneous Adipose Tissue*. Philadelphia: JB Lippincott, 1989.

11 Giorgino F, Laviola L, Eriksson JW. Regional differences of insulin action in adipose tissue: insights from *in vivo* and *in vitro* studies. *Acta Physiol Scand* 2005; **183**: 13–30.

12 Lafontan M, Berlan M. Do regional differences in adipocyte biology provide new pathophysiological insights? *Trends Pharmacol Sci* 2003; **24**: 276–83.

13 Thalmann S, Meier CA. Local adipose tissue depots as cardiovascular risk factors. *Cardiovasc Res* 2007; **75**: 690–701.

14 Johnson D, Cormack GC, Abrahams PH *et al*. Computed tomographic observations on subcutaneous fat: implications for liposuction. *Plast Reconstr Surg* 1996; **97**: 387–96.

15 Bell GH. *Textbook of Physiology and Biochemistry*. Edinburgh: Churchill Livingstone, 1987.

16 Frayn KN. Adipose tissue metabolism. In: Ryan TJ, Curri SB, eds. *Clinics in Dermatology*, Vol. 7. *The Cutaneous Adipose Tissue*. Philadelphia: JB Lippincott, 1989: 48–61.

17 Avram MM, Avram AS, James WD. Subcutaneous fat in normal and diseased states 3. Adipogenesis: from stem cell to fat cell. *J Am Acad Dermatol* 2007; **56**: 472–92.

18 Wang P, Mariman E, Renes J, Keijer J. The secretory function of adipocytes in the physiology of white adipose tissue. *J Cell Physiol* 2008; **216**: 3–13.

19 Dalziel K. The nervous system and adipose tissue. In: Ryan TJ, Curri SB, eds. *Clinics in Dermatology*, Vol. 7. *The Cutaneous Adipose Tissue*. Philadelphia: JB Lippincott, 1989: 62–77.

20 Boden G, Hoeldtke RD. Nerves, fat, and insulin resistance. *N Engl J Med* 2003; **349**: 1966–7.

21 Romijn JA, Fliers E. Sympathetic and parasympathetic innervation of adipose tissue: metabolic implications. *Curr Opin Clin Nutr Metab Care* 2005; **8**: 440–4.

22 Langin D. Adipose tissue lipolysis as a metabolic pathway to define pharmacological strategies against obesity and the metabolic syndrome. *Pharmacol Res* 2006; **53**: 482–91.

23 Anubhuti, Arora S. Leptin and its metabolic interactions—an update. *Diabetes Obes Metab* 2008; **10**: 973–93.

24 Ranadive SA, Vaisse C. Lessons from extreme human obesity: monogenic disorders. *Endocrinol Metab Clin North Am* 2008; **38**: 733–51.

25 Lago R, Gómez R, Lago F *et al*. Leptin beyond body weight regulation—current concepts concerning its role in immune function and inflammation. *Cell Immunol* 2008; **252**: 139–45.

26 Lara-Castro C, Fu Y, Chung BH *et al*. Adiponectin and the metabolic syndrome: mechanisms mediating risk for metabolic and cardiovascular disease. *Curr Opin Lipidol* 2007; **18**: 263–70.

27 Fantuzzi G. Adiponectin and inflammation: consensus and controversy. *J Allergy Clin Immunol* 2008; **121**: 326–30.

28 Whitehead JP, Richards AA, Hickman IJ *et al*. Adiponectin—a key adipokine in the metabolic syndrome. *Diabetes Obes Metab* 2006; **8**: 264–80.

29 Behre CJ. Adiponectin: saving the starved and the overfed. *Med Hypotheses* 2007; **69**: 1290–2.

Obesity

Obesity is variously defined. Originally it was simply a condition in which there is excessive fat in the body. This has been modified slightly to the more subjective, an unhealthy excess of body fat that leads to an impaired quality of life, or the more specific, an unhealthy excess of body fat that increases the risk of morbidity and premature mortality.

Epidemiology. Body mass index (BMI: body weight in kilograms divided by height in metres squared) is used as a surrogate marker of adiposity. Both the World Health Organization (WHO) and the National Institutes of Health (NIH) classify adults with a BMI 25–29.9 kg/m^2 as overweight, above 30 kg/m^2 as obese and above 40 kg/m^2 as extremely obese [1,2]. For children and adolescents (under 20 years of age) the term obese is not used. 'At risk of overweight' is defined as a BMI for age at or above the sex-specific 85th centile and 'overweight' above the 95th centile. Being overweight as a child is of special significance, because many overweight children are obese as adults. Observations indicate that the prevalence of being overweight in childhood is high where adult obesity is common [3,4].

For adults, morbidity and mortality from hypertension, stroke, coronary artery disease and type 2 diabetes increase as the body mass index rises above 25 kg/m^2 [5], with more of an increase above 30 kg/m^2. These parameters were deduced from data on individuals under 50 years of age and they may not be true for individuals over 65 years with a BMI 25–27 kg/m^2 [6]. Nor does BMI take into account ethnicity [7]. BMI is an index of excess weight rather than excess body fat relative to height. More accurate measurements reveal that, for equivalent BMI levels, Asian people have more body fat, and Black people have less body fat, than do White people. To account for these differences in body fatness, it has been suggested that BMI cut-off points for overweight and obesity be lowered among Asian and increased among Black people. The same is true, but to a lesser extent, for children [7]. The other criticism of BMI is that it measures fatness as a whole and does not distinguish between visceral and subcutaneous adiposity. Visceral adiposity correlates better with morbidity and mortality and also correlates with body trunk measurements [8]. Waist circumference divided by hip circumference (WHR) can be used for this purpose. The waist is measured, after an overnight fast, halfway between the lower costal margin and the iliac crest, and hip circumference is measured over the widest part of the gluteal region [9]. WHR should not exceed 1.0 in men and 0.85 in women—cut-offs based on Scandinavian data [10]. Waist circumference is another reasonable way of assessing obesity. Circumference values that indicate a significant increased relative risk are more than 88 cm for women and more than 102 cm for men [10].

Measurement of skinfold thickness with callipers is another alternative technique, but there are possible variations in the distribution of fat between subcutaneous areas and deep body fat [11]. Computed tomography (CT), magnetic resonance imaging (MRI) and dual-energy X-ray absorptiometry (DEXA) are reserved for the more precise measurement during research rather than routine clinical practice.

The advantage of BMI is that it can be used easily for population screening. In the United States in 2003–4, among children and adolescents aged 2 to 19 years, 17.1% were overweight (above the 95th centile) and 32.2% of adults aged 20 years or older were obese. Sixty-five percent of all adults had a BMI above 25 kg/m^2. The prevalence of extreme obesity among adults was 4.8%. Between 1980 and 2002, obesity prevalence doubled in adults and overweight prevalence tripled in children and adolescents [12]. Between 1999 and 2004, the prevalence of overweight among children and adolescents and obesity among men continued to increase significantly, but no increase was observed among women over this 6-year period. Ethnicity differences remained. Among women, almost 58% of non-Hispanic black women aged 40 to 59 years were obese in 2003–2004 compared with about 38% of non-Hispanic white women of the same age. Among men, however, the prevalence of obesity did not differ by racial/ethnic group [12].

In England in 2006, 14% of 11 year olds were between the 85th and 95th centile and 17% were above the 95th centile [13]. In adults, the prevalence of obesity is much the same as the rest of Europe, with rates of around 20% [13]. Developing countries are now seeing serious increases in obesity, for example in the Caribbean, South America and South-East Asia [14,15], while in Australian Aborigines and Polynesia, figures approaching 80% have been recorded. China, except in poor rural areas, now has similar problems with childhood overweight and obesity approaching the epidemic levels of the USA [16]. It is estimated that globally there are 1 billion adults overweight of which 300 million are obese [17], a medical problem of a size beyond the capacity of even the best health-care system [1].

Obesity is accompanied by complications such as hypertension, non-insulin-dependent diabetes mellitus and atherosclerosis, which in turn cause ischaemic heart disease, stroke and premature death [18–20]. Other complications include hepatic steatosis, polycystic ovary syndrome, sleep apnoea, osteoarthritis, depression and certain malignancies such as prostate cancer. The alarming increase in diabetes is most probably a consequence of the current rapid rise in the prevalence of obesity.

Aetiology [21,22]. Very rarely obesity is monogenic [23]. It may be classified into three groups: due to gene mutations that affect the leptin–melanocortin system, mutations affecting hypothalamic development, or associated with a pleiotropic developmental syndrome such as Prader–Willi syndrome. Typically, these patients present with hyperphagia and very early onset obesity. Therapy

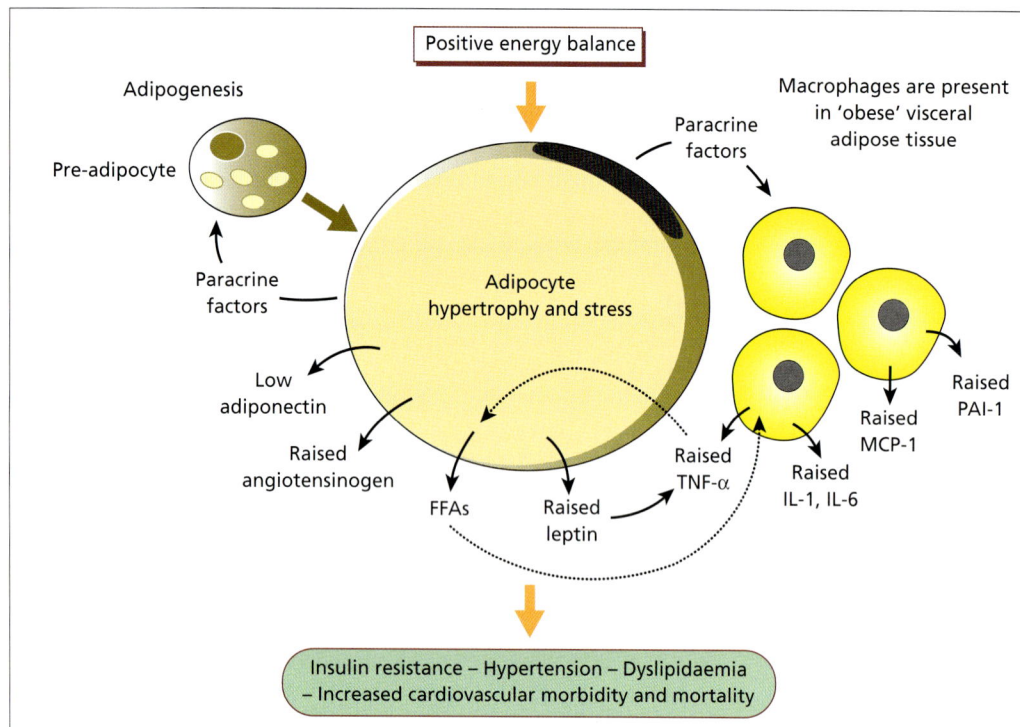

Fig. 46.2 Simplified outline of visceral adipocyte dysfunction in obesity leading to metabolic syndrome. FFAs, free fatty acids; IL-1, interleukin 1; IL-6, interleukin 6; MCP-1, monocyte chemoattractant protein-1; PAI-1, plasminogen activation inhibitor-1; TNF-α, tumour necrosis factor-α.

with leptin has transformed those with leptin deficiency. More frequently, obesity is associated with underlying disease such as polycystic ovary syndrome, hypothyroidism, Cushing's disease and hypothalamic injury, as well as corticosteroid and other drug therapy. By far and away the most frequent cause is common obesity—the result of genetic, behavioural, environmental, physiological, social, psychosocial and cultural factors that cause energy imbalance and promote excessive fat deposition. It has been suggested that inheritable factors contribute 45–75% to obesity. Bouchard *et al.* [24] demonstrated that the amount of body weight and fat gained, as well as the distribution of fat gained in response to overfeeding, had greater similarity within identical twin pairs. It is likely that genetic polymorphisms modify individual susceptibility to environmental factors [25,26]. Nutritional variability during fetal development is one such factor [27]. Maternal underweight before pregnancy [28], fetal under-nourishment and over-nourishment are all predictive of adult obesity, as is rapid weight gain in the first week of life. The pre-pubertal growth phase of early adolescence may be another susceptible time [29].

Obesity is the result of a positive energy balance input that exceeds output. The World Health Organization consultation on obesity [15] concluded that behavioural and environmental factors, such as sedentary lifestyles combined with excessive energy intake, are primarily responsible for the dramatic increase in obesity in the last 10–20 years. Food consumption has changed drastically over the last 30 years [30]. More calories are available to be consumed with a higher proportion of fats and sugar, often through increased snacking and soft drinks as well as increased portion sizes. Disordered eating behaviours, from missing meals such as breakfast, eating outside the home to binge eating, peer pressure and altered mental health may all contribute to an excessive intake. An increase in sedentary behaviour means

that this increase in energy intake is not burnt off. Only a small amount of excess daily calorie intake is needed to lead to obesity [31].

Chronic positive energy balance leads to increased storage of triglycerides into fat cells. The increase in fat mass occurs due to adipocyte hypertrophy and hyperplasia. It has been suggested that increased storage occurs at first in the superficial and deep components of subcutaneous tissue until the maximal capacity has been reached [32]. At that time the secondary fat depots, including visceral fat, are filled. The subcutaneous fat shows both hypertrophy and hyperplasia but the visceral depot shows hypertrophy alone [32].

In obese subjects, macrophages are present in subcutaneous fat and they diminish in number after surgery-induced weight loss [33]. They are more numerous in omental than subcutaneous fat [34]. Inflammation associated with these macrophages, whether triggered by dysregulated adipogenesis, excess adipocyte hypertrophy or adipocyte endoplasmic reticulum and mitochondrial stress [22], results in adipocyte insulin resistance and dysfunction (Fig. 46.2). Free fatty acids and triglycerides are released into the circulation, and there is an altered secreted adipokine profile and release of inflammatory mediators. Higher concentrations of circulating free fatty acids and triglycerides are associated with lipid accumulation in multiple tissues, including liver, skeletal muscle, heart, pancreatic β-cells and blood vessels. With the portal vein draining visceral fat tissue products directly into the liver, the effect is accentuated in this organ. Perivascular lipid deposits have a role in atherogenesis [35]. Although the adipocyte secretes many adipokines, leptin and adiponectin have been the best evaluated. Circulating leptin levels correlate with increasing BMI, but the chronic high levels in obesity seem to generate leptin resistance at the hypothalamic level, in that the satiety centres do not respond by diminishing appetite. Raised leptin levels contribute to hypertension as well as being independently moderately associated with coronary disease. In contrast, circulating adiponectin levels are low in obesity and therefore insulin sensitivity is blunted. TNF-α is an inflammatory marker associated with adiposity and cardiovascular risk factors. It inhibits lipoprotein lipase activity and increases lipolysis and also induces adipocyte apoptosis [36], as well as blunting insulin responsiveness. Increased angiotensinogen from the hypertrophied adipocyte contributes to hypertension. Monocyte chemoattractant protein 1 (MCP-1) plays an important role in atherogenesis, and plasminogen activation inhibitor-1 (PAI-1), a regulator of fibrinolysis, might be important in cardiac events [37]. Both MCP-1 and PAI-1 are produced by the stromavascular tissue.

Metabolic syndrome. The disease consequences of increasing amounts of fat tissue merits the fat being labelled as pathogenic. The traditional label for this has been the metabolic syndrome, though others prefer adiposopathy [38]. Adiposopathy is pathogenic adipose tissue that is promoted by a positive caloric balance and sedentary lifestyle in genetically and environmentally susceptible individuals. Diagnostic criteria for metabolic syndrome include glucose intolerance, elevated blood pressure, dyslipidaemia and measures of central obesity, and increased waist circumference or waist-to-hip ratio. Whilst metabolic syndrome is a convenient key for remembering its components, it may be no better as a predictor of future metabolic disease than assessment of its individual components. Also, there are five slightly different definitions of metabolic syndrome, of which three are given in Table 46.1; the use of these can blur the distinction between health and disease and exclude some individuals from preventive programmes [39,40]. Using the National Cholesterol Education Program (NCEP) metabolic syndrome criteria, the prevalence in adults in the USA is 35%, but it is 40% using criteria of the International Diabetes Federation (IDF) [41]. The prevalence in adolescents (with the IDF criteria) was 4.5% [42]. A global prevalence has been calculated at 16% [43].

Because obesity is associated with hyperinsulinaemia and diabetes, it is difficult to decide whether the skin manifestations seen in these conditions are due to obesity or its effects. Obesity impedes lymphatic flow with consequent lymphoedema. Acanthosis nigricans, the effects of hyperandrogenism, including hirsutism, hidradenitis suppurativa, striae distensae, venous hypertension, intertrigo and skin infections, are all seen more frequently in obese patients [44], as is plantar hyperkeratosis.

Prevention and treatment. The aim of obesity treatment is to achieve and then maintain clinically meaningful weight loss, with the ultimate aim of reducing the risk for, or severity of, obesity-related diseases. Measures directed at improving public health awareness should be given high priority in national efforts. They include: information campaigns, providing opportunities for exercise at school and in the community, making exercise-sparing devices such as escalators less readily available, and establishing bicycle and walking lanes in cities. Despite an increased focus on nutrition, an increased awareness of the energy and fat content of foods, and the availability of various reduced-fat, fat-free and sugar-free food and beverages, obesity continues to increase [45].

Effective therapeutic regimens for treating obesity should incorporate multiple approaches to encourage behavioural change or modification and create strategies to facilitate consistent and long-term follow-through [46]. Numerous options are available [46,47], including reduced-energy diets, physical activity and exercise, behavioural modification, pharmacotherapy and surgery.

The principle for treatment, self-evidently, is to induce a negative energy balance. Short-term weight loss is easy, but long-term weight maintenance after that is unusual [44,48]. The body weight itself is often not the most important problem, unless it is affecting mobility. It is the morbidity associated with the

Table 46.1 Three commonly used sets of criteria for the metabolic syndrome, showing differences.

	WHO	NCEP ATP III	IDF
Required criteria	Insulin resistance or impaired fasting glucose or impaired glucose tolerance or type 2 diabetes plus any 2 of the following:	3 or more of the following:	Central obesity and any 2 of the following:
Central obesity	BMI >30 kg/m² or waist to hip ratio >0.9 (men), >0.85 (women)	Waist circumference ≥102 cm (men), ≥88 cm (women)	Waist circumference ≥94 cm (European men), ≥90 cm (Asian men), ≥80 cm (women)
Insulin resistance	Insulin sensitivity < lowest quartile		
Glucose intolerance	Fasting glucose ≥110 mg/dL (6.1 mmol/L) or impaired glucose tolerance or previously diagnosed type 2 diabetes	Fasting glucose ≥110 mg/dL (6.1 mmol/L)	Fasting glucose ≥100 mg/dL (5.6 mmol/L), or previously diagnosed type 2 diabetes
Blood pressure	140/90 or above	130/85 or above	130/85 or above
Triglyceride	Triglyceride >150 mg/dL OR	Triglyceride ≥150 mg/dL (1.7 mmol/L)	Triglyceride ≥150 mg/dL (1.7 mmol/L), or specific treatment for this lipid abnormality
HDL cholesterol	HDLc <35 mg/dL (men), and <39 mg/dL (women)	HDLc <40 mg/dL (men), and <50 mg/dL (women)	HDLc <40 mg/dL (1.03 mmol/L) in men and <50 mg/dL (1.29 mmol/L) in women, or specific treatment for this lipid abnormality

WHO, World Health Organization; NCEP, National Cholesterol Education Program; IDF, International Diabetes Federation.

metabolic complications that is of major concern, and this can improve rapidly even after a limited loss of weight. A normal body weight is not necessary, and is often unrealistic in the long term.

Reduced energy intake must be individually tailored to allow normal activities. A deficit of 500–600 kcal (0.210–0.251 mJ) per day is usually well tolerated. Emphasis should be placed on fat intake and on the energy density of food. Involvement of the family is important [49]. A combination of exercise and diet is more effective than either alone [48], and long-term low-intensity exercise such as walking is as effective as high-intensity activities [50]. This is important because most obese patients are unaccustomed to sporting activities and will drop out of vigorous regimens.

Behaviour modification is an important component of all weight loss programmes [51,52]. Frequently, behavioural strategies are targeted toward identifying stimuli that signal unhealthy behaviours such as binge eating, learning about the role of readiness in initiating or continuing positive behaviours [53], and recognizing barriers that may compromise healthy pursuits.

Pharmacological agents may be used in conjunction with diet, exercise and behavioural strategies when non-pharmacological approaches have failed to produce a success. Several appetite-suppressant drugs are approved for weight loss and the reader is referred to authoritative sources on the subject [45]. In general, their use can achieve a weight loss of only 5 kg after 1 year [54]. For overweight children, medications and lifestyle interventions are similarly disappointing [55].

Surgery was once reserved for cases of extreme obesity (BMI over 40 kg/m^2) but is now also being recommended for a BMI over 35 kg/m^2 plus serious obesity-related co-morbid conditions [56]. Vertical gastric banding is the most common procedure. It is the best treatment for long-term weight loss and reduces mortality markedly for diabetes, heart disease and cancer [57].

An excellent review on the aetiology, prevalence and treatment of obesity is by Racette et al. [45] and on the particular problems for the adolescent by Jasik and Lustig [29]. With the elucidation of the neuroendocrine regulation of body weight it remains to be seen whether novel molecular compounds might become available in the future, but this should not be at the expense of simple dietary measures and exercise [58].

References

1 Bjorntorp P. Obesity. *Lancet* 1997; **350**: 423–5.

2 National Institutes of Health. Clinical guidelines on the identification, evaluation, and treatment of overweight and obesity in adults—the evidence report. *Obes Res* 1998; **6** (Suppl. 2): 51S–209S.

3 Chadwick DJ, Cardew G, eds. *The Origins and Consequences of Obesity.* London: Ciba Foundation/Wiley, 1996.

4 Guillaume M, Lapidus L, Beckers F et al. Cardiovascular risk factors in children from the Belgian Luxembourg Province: the Belgian Luxembourg Child Study. *Am J Epidemiol* 1996; **144**: 867–80.

5 Adams KF, Schatzkin A, Harris TB et al. Overweight, obesity, and mortality in a large prospective cohort of persons 50 to 71 years old. *N Engl J Med* 2006; **355**: 763–78.

6 Heiat A, Vaccarino V, Krumholz HM. An evidence-based assessment of federal guidelines for overweight and obesity as they apply to elderly persons. *Arch Intern Med* 2001; **161**: 1194–203.

7 Freedman DS, Wang J, Thornton JC et al. Racial/ethnic differences in body fatness among children and adolescents. *Obesity (Silver Spring)* 2008; **16**: 1105–11.

8 Bjorntrop P. Visceral obesity: a 'civilisation syndrome'. *Obes Res* 1993; **1**: 206–22.

9 World Health Organization. *Measuring Obesity: Classification and Description of Anthropometric Data* (EUR/ICP/Nut125). Copenhagen: WHO Regional Office for Europe, Nutrition Unit, 1988.

10 Iwao S, Iwao N, Muller DC et al. Does waist circumference add to the predictive power of the body mass index for coronary risk? *Obes Res* 2001; **9**: 685–95.

11 Womersley J, Durmin JVGA. A comparison of the skinfold method with extent of 'overweight' and various weight/height relationships in the assessment of obesity. *Br J Nutr* 1977; **38**: 271–84.

12 Ogden CL, Carroll MD, Curtin LR et al. Prevalence of overweight and obesity in the United States, 1999–2004. *JAMA* 2006; **295**: 1549–55.

13 Crowther R, Dinsdale H, Rutter H, Kyffin R (South East Public Health Observatory) on behalf of the Association of Public Health Observatories. *Analysis of the National Childhood Obesity Database 2005–06.* Department of Health. http://www.dh.gov.uk/en/Publicationsandstatistics/Publications/PublicationsStatistics/DH_063565.

14 International Association for the Study of Obesity. *Global prevalence of adult obesity.* http://www.iotf.org/database/documents/GlobalPrevalenceofAdultObesityMay2009pdf.pdf.

15 Prevention and management of the global epidemic of obesity. *Report of the WHO Consultation on Obesity, Geneva, 3–5 June 1997.* Geneva: World Health Organization, 1997.

16 Ji CY, Cheng TO. Prevalence and geographic distribution of childhood obesity in China in 2005. *Int J Cardiol* 2008; **131**: 1–8.

17 World Health Organization. *Global strategy on diet, physical activity and health 2008.* http://www.who.int/dietphysicalactivity/publications/facts/obesity/en/.

18 Flegal KM, Caroll MD, Kuczmarkski RJ et al. Over weight and obesity in the United States: prevalence and trends, 1960–94. *Int J Obes* 1998; **22**: 29–47.

19 Kaplan NM. The deadly quartet: upper-body obesity, glucose intolerance, hypertriglyceridemia and hypertension. *Arch Intern Med* 1989; **149**: 1514–20.

20 Bjorntorp P. Metabolic implications of body fat distribution. *Diabetes Care* 1991; **14**: 1132–43.

21 Bays HE, González-Campoy JM, Bray GA et al. Pathogenic potential of adipose tissue and metabolic consequences of adipocyte hypertrophy and increased visceral adiposity. *Expert Rev Cardiovasc Ther* 2008; **6**: 343–68.

22 de Ferranti S, Mozaffarian D. The perfect storm: obesity, adipocyte dysfunction, and metabolic consequences. *Clin Chem* 2008; **54**: 945–55.

23 Ranadive SA, Vaisse C. Lessons from extreme human obesity: monogenic disorders. *Endocrinol Metab Clin North Am* 2008; **37**: 733–51.

24 Bouchard C, Tremblay A, Despres JP et al. The response to long-term overfeeding in identical twins. *N Engl J Med* 1990; **322**: 1477–82.

25 Barsh GS, Farooqi IS, O'Rahilly S. Genetics of body-weight regulation. *Nature* 2000; **404**: 644–51.

26 Farooqi IS, O'Rahilly S. Genetic factors in human obesity. *Obes Rev* 2007; **8** (Suppl. 1): 37–40.

27 Kuzawa CW, Gluckman PD, Hanson MA. Development perspectives on the origins of obesity. In: Fantuzzi G, Mazzone T, eds. *Adipose Tissue and Adipokines in Health and Disease.* New Jersey: Humana Press, 2007: 207–19.

28 Stettler N, Stallings VA, Troxel AB et al. Weight gain in the first week of life and overweight in adulthood: a cohort study of European American subjects fed infant formula. *Circulation* 2005; **111**: 1897–903.

29 Jasik CB, Lustig RH. Adolescent obesity and puberty: the 'perfect storm'. *Ann N Y Acad Sci* 2008; **1135**: 265–79.

30 Diewald L, Dolan MS, Faith MS. Environmental aspects of obesity. In: Fantuzzi G, Mazzone T, eds. *Adipose Tissue and Adipokines in Health and Disease.* New Jersey: Humana Press, 2007: 197–206.

31 Ravussin E. Physiology: a NEAT way to control weight? *Science* 2005; **307**: 530–1.

32 Drolet R, Richard C, Sniderman AD et al. Hypertrophy and hyperplasia of abdominal adipose tissues in women. *Int J Obes (Lond)* 2008; **32**: 283–91.

33 Cancello R, Henegar C, Viguerie N et al. Reduction of macrophage infiltration and chemoattractant gene expression changes in white adipose tissue of mor-

bidly obese subjects after surgery-induced weight loss. *Diabetes* 2005; **54**: 2277–86.

34 Cancello R, Tordjman J, Poitou C *et al.* Increased infiltration of macrophages in omental adipose tissue is associated with marked hepatic lesions in morbid human obesity. *Diabetes* 2006; **55**: 1554–61.

35 Thalmann S, Meier CA. Local adipose tissue depots as cardiovascular risk factors. *Cardiovasc Res* 2007; **75**: 690–701.

36 Prins JB, Niesler CU, Winterford CM *et al.* Tumor necrosis factor-alpha induces apoptosis of human adipose cells. *Diabetes* 1997; **46**: 1939–44.

37 Sobel BE, Taatjes DJ, Schneider DJ. Intramural plasminogen activator inhibitor type-1 and coronary atherosclerosis. *Arterioscler Thromb Vasc Biol* 2003; **23**: 1979–89.

38 Bays HE, González-Campoy JM, Henry RR *et al.* The Adiposopathy Working Group. Is adiposopathy (sick fat) an endocrine disease? *Int J Clin Pract* 2008; **62**: 1474–83.

39 Sandhofer A, Iglseder B, Paulweber B *et al.* Comparison of different definitions of the metabolic syndrome. *Eur J Clin Invest* 2007; **37**: 109–16.

40 Lee CM, Huxley RR, Woodward M *et al.* Detect-2 Collaboration. Comparisons of metabolic syndrome definitions in four populations of the Asia-Pacific region. *Metab Syndr Relat Disord* 2008; **6**: 37–46.

41 Ford ES. Prevalence of the metabolic syndrome defined by the International Diabetes Federation among adults in the U.S. *Diabetes Care* 2005; **28**: 2745–9.

42 Ford ES, Li C, Zhao G *et al.* Prevalence of the metabolic syndrome among U.S. adolescents using the definition from the International Diabetes Federation. *Diabetes Care* 2008; **31**: 587–9.

43 Wild SH, Byrne CD. The global burden of the metabolic syndrome and its consequences for diabetes and cardiovascular disease. In: Byrne CD, Wild SH, eds. *The Metabolic Syndrome.* Chichester, England: John Wiley & Sons, 2005: 1–43.

44 Yosipovitch G, DeVore A, Dawn A. Obesity and the skin: skin physiology and skin manifestations of obesity. *J Am Acad Dermatol* 2007; **56**: 901–16.

45 Racette SB, Deusinger SS, Deusinger RH. Obesity: an overview of prevalence, etiology, and treatment. *Phys Ther* 2003; **83**: 276–88.

46 National Institute of Health, National Heart, Lung and Blood Institute, North American Association for the Study of Obesity. *The Practical Guide: Identification, Evaluation and Treatment of Overweight and Obesity in Adults.* Bethesda, MD: US Department of Health and Human Services, Public Health Service. National Institute of Health, National Heart, Lung and Blood Institute, 2000.

47 Rosenbaum M, Leibel RL, Hirsch J. Obesity. *N Engl J Med* 1997; **337**: 396–407.

48 Black DR, Threlfall WE. Partner weight status and subject weight loss: implications for cost-effective programs and public health. *Addict Behav* 1989; **14**: 279–89.

49 Skender ML. Comparison of a 2-year weight loss trends in behavioral treatments of obesity: diet, exercise and combination interventions. *J Am Diet Assoc* 1996; **96**: 342–6.

50 Despres JP, Lamarche B. Effects of diet and physical activity on adiposity and body fat distribution: implications for the prevention of cardiovascular disease. *Nutr Res Rev* 1993; **6**: 1–23.

51 Wadden TA, Foster GD. Behavioural treatment of obesity. *Med Clin North Am* 2000; **84**: 4441–61.

52 Brownell KD. Diet, exercise and behavioural intervention: the non-pharmacological approach. *Eur J Clin Invest* 1998; **28**: 19–22.

53 King AC, Frey-Hewitt B, Drecon DM *et al.* Diet against exercise in weight maintenance: effects of minimal intervention strategies and long-term outcomes in man. *Arch Intern Med* 1989; **149**: 2741–6.

54 Li Z, Maglione M, Tu W *et al.* Meta-analysis: pharmacologic treatment of obesity. *Ann Intern Med* 2005; **142**: 532–46.

55 McGovern L, Johnson JN, Paulo R *et al.* Clinical reviews: treatment of pediatric obesity: a systematic review and meta-analysis of randomized trials. *J Clin Endocrinol Metab* 2008; **93**: 4600–5.

56 Bult MJ, van Dalen T, Muller AF. Surgical treatment of obesity. *Eur J Endocrinol* 2008; **158**: 135–45.

57 Adams TD, Gress RE, Smith SC *et al.* Long-term mortality after gastric bypass surgery. *N Engl J Med* 2007; **357**: 753–61.

58 Foster-Schubert KE, Cummings DE. Emerging therapeutic strategies for obesity. *Endocr Rev* 2006; **27**: 779–93.

Cellulite

Cellulite is an alteration of the topography of the skin that occurs mainly in women in the pelvic region, the limbs and abdomen. It is characterized by a dimpled appearance if mild, and lumpy skin if severe, and affects 85% of post-pubescent females [1]. No formal quality of life study has been performed on this, probably normal, secondary sex characteristic but treatment improves self-esteem and the size of the anticellulite market attests to patients' concerns [2].

Many authors confuse cellulite with obesity. However, this is incorrect; in obesity only adipocyte hypertrophy and hyperplasia occurs [3], whereas in cellulite there are several structural alterations in the dermis, in the local microcirculation and within the adipocytes. These may result in further morphological, histochemical and biochemical modifications [4–7].

Cellulite may be classified in at least two ways. One classification divides cellulite into four stages according to the histopathological and clinical changes [3]:

Grade 1. The patient has no symptoms and there are no clinical alterations. Histologically, there may be an increased thickness of the areolar layer, increased capillary permeability and microhaemorrhages.

Grade 2. There are no obvious changes in the skin at rest, but after skin compression or muscular contraction small dimples, local pallor, decreased temperature and decreased elasticity may be evident.

Grade 3. A padded skin or an orange peel appearance is evident at rest, and there is a slight feeling of granularity in the deeper parts of the skin on palpation, which may be associated with some pain. At this stage, there is the beginning histologically of fatty tissue destruction and the formation of micronodules.

Grade 4. This stage is characterized by changes seen in grade 3 but with more visible palpable and painful nodules and an obvious wavy appearance of the skin surface. Histopathologically, the lobular structure of the fatty tissue has disappeared and some nodules are encapsulated by dense connective tissue and there may be much fibrosis.

Cellulite may also be classified by the consistency of the skin—being hard, flaccid, oedematous or mixed [8]. Hard cellulite is observed in young women who perform regular physical activity. The appearance is of compact, firm tissues and is not changed according to position. Flaccid cellulite is characteristically found in inactive women, especially if they have suddenly lost weight. In contrast, oedematous cellulite presents as an increased volume of the entire affected limb, and is associated with depression of the tissue to fingertip palpation, which persists when the finger is removed.

Aetiology. Just what precisely triggers the histopathological and clinical changes of cellulite is poorly understood. Hormonal factors may play a predisposing or aggravating part. Oestrogen is probably the most important hormone. Evidence for oestrogen involvement includes the fact that cellulite predominantly occurs in females, the onset of the disease after puberty, and aggravation of the condition during pregnancy, menstruation and with oestrogen therapy [9].

A genetic predisposition may also be important. White women tend to be more prone to cellulite than Asian or Black women and Latin women develop cellulite on the hips while Anglo-Saxon women develop cellulite on the abdomen.

Sedentary lifestyle contributes to the aggravation of cellulite as a consequence of a decrease in muscle mass, and the consequent decreased muscular pumping mechanism in the lower limbs inhibiting venous return. Obesity contributes to the problem by increasing the fatty mass. Factors that act as a mechanical barrier to the venous return are also likely to be important; tight clothes and pregnancy may be important in this context.

Traditionally, three major theories have been put forward to explain the abnormalities: oedema in the fat lobules; alterations in the fat microcirculation; and a structural conformation of the subcutaneous tissue that is different in women compared to men. Whilst there is evidence for all three, it is uncertain if these are the effects or the cause. MRI scanning has provided support for the anatomical case [10,11]. 'Pseudoherniation' of fat pushing into the lower layers of dermis is more prevalent in cellulite, perhaps due to a thinner dermis in women compared to men. Women appear to have a different fibrous septal structure in the upper layers of subcutaneous fat, tending to have more vertical bands and pillars than the oblique criss-crossing bands seen in men, which contain smaller fat chambers. In cellulite there would appear to be fewer vertical septal bands with some bands and pillars appearing thickened and some thinned. The histology of some of these thinner bands has appeared similar to the elastic tissue changes seen in cutaneous stretch marks [12]. What is unknown is what role the multifunctioning adipocyte has played in the development of this apparent remodelling process [13].

Treatment. Because of the multifactorial pathogenesis of cellulite, there are numerous therapeutic approaches—especially because many of the treatments are much less than optimal in their success. Treatments include reduction in aggravating factors, pharmacological agents, and the use of physical and mechanical methods, ultrasound and lasers.

Attempts to reduce weight, regular exercise and the use of non-hormonal contraceptives need to be encouraged, but weight loss improves the appearance of cellulite only in those with a high starting BMI and aggravates the appearance in those with a low BMI [14]. Several pharmacological agents have been tried, both topical and injectable (mesotherapy), but adequate double-blind, placebo-controlled studies are lacking [15]. Physical therapies, including thermotherapy, pressotherapy and lymphatic massage, have similar drawbacks. Local surgery, so-called subcision, seems effective and works by destroying the thicker fibrous septal bands using the cutting edge of a needle under local anaesthesia [16]. Focused ultrasound is helpful in dissolving fat in body-contouring and may prove useful for cellulite [17].

More recently, radiofrequency devices, such as low-energy diode laser and infra-red systems, have been reported to be of benefit [18–20]. A unipolar radiofrequency device with the capac-

ity to generate heat 15–20 mm into skin produced dermal fibrosis, which might be responsible for the observed good clinical benefit still present after 6 months [21].

References

1 Draelos ZD, Marenus KD. Cellulite. Etiology and purported treatment. *Dermatol Surg* 1997; **23**: 1177–81.

2 Hexsel D, Hexsel CL. Social impact of cellulite and its impact on quality of life. In: Goldman MP, Bacci PA, Leibaschoff G et al., eds. *Cellulite: Pathophysiology and Treatment*. New York: Taylor & Francis, 2006: 1–5.

3 Bray GA. Obesity: basic considerations and clinical approaches. *Disease-a-Month* 1989; **35**: 451–528.

4 Binazzi M, Papini M. Aspetti clinico histomorfologici. In: Ribuffo A, Bartoletti CA, eds. *La Cellulite*. Rome: Salus, 1983: 7–15.

5 Chimenti S, Pranteda G, Cantaresi F et al. Aspetti istochuimci. In: Ribuffo A, Bartoletti CA, eds. *La Cellulite*. Rome: Salus, 1983: 17–22.

6 Curri SB. Aspects morpho-histochimiques et biochimiques du tissue adipeux dans la dermo hypodermose cellulitique. *J Med Esth* 1976; **5**: 183.

7 Curri SB. Aspetti biochimici. In: Ribuffo A, Bartoletti CA, eds. *La Cellulite*. Rome: Salus, 1983: 29–36.

8 Bartoletti CA, Gualtierotti R, Rota M et al. Utilizzazione dell'estrato di centella asiatica nel trettomento della 'cellulite' edematosa degli arti inferiori. *La Med Est* 1983; **3**: 97–103.

9 Rossi AB, Vergnanini AL. Cellulite: a review. *J Eur Acad Dermatol Venereol* 2000; **14**: 251–62.

10 Querleux B, Cornillon C, Jolivet O et al. Anatomy and physiology of subcutaneous adipose tissue by *in vivo* magnetic resonance imaging and spectroscopy: relationships with sex and presence of cellulite. *Skin Res Technol* 2002; **8**: 118–24.

11 Mirrashed F, Sharp JC, Krause V et al. Pilot study of dermal and subcutaneous fat structures by MRI in individuals who differ in gender, BMI, and cellulite grading. *Skin Res Technol* 2004; **10**: 161–8.

12 Quatresooz P, Xhauflaire-Uhoda E, Piérard-Franchimont C et al. Cellulite histopathology and related mechanobiology. *Int J Cosmet Sci* 2006; **28**: 207–10.

13 Terranova F, Berardesca E, Maibach H. Cellulite: nature and aetiopathogenesis. *Int J Cosmetic Science* 2006; **28**: 157–67.

14 Smalls LK, Hicks M, Passeretti D et al. Effect of weight loss on cellulite: gynoid lipodystrophy. *Plast Reconstr Surg* 2006; **118**: 510–6.

15 Wanner M, Avram M. An evidence-based assessment of treatments for cellulite. *J Drugs Dermatol* 2008; **7**: 341–5.

16 Hexsel DM, Mazzuco R. Subcision: a treatment for cellulite. *Int J Dermatol* 2000; **39**: 539–44.

17 Moreno-Moraga J, Valero-Altés T, Riquelme AM et al. Body contouring by non-invasive transdermal focused ultrasound. *Lasers Surg Med* 2007; **39**: 315–23.

18 Alster T, Tanzi EL. Extended experience with a novel combination radiofrequency, infrared light and mechanical tissue manipulation device for the treatment of cellulite. *J Cosmetic Laser Ther* 2005; **7**: 81–5.

19 Sadick NS, Mulholland RS. A prospective clinical study to evaluate the efficacy and safety of cellulite treatment using the combination of optical and RF energies for subcutaneous tissue heating. *Journal Cosmetic Laser Ther* 2004; **6**: 187–90.

20 Nootheti PK, Magpantay A, Yosowitz G et al. A single center, randomized, comparative, prospective clinical study to determine the efficacy of the Velasmooth system versus the Triactive system for the treatment of cellulite. *Lasers Surg Med* 2006; **38**: 908–12.

21 Goldberg DJ, Fazeli A, Berlin AL. Clinical, laboratory, and MRI analysis of cellulite treatment with a unipolar radiofrequency device. *Dermatol Surg* 2008; **34**: 204–9.

General pathology of adipose tissue: panniculitis [1–11]

Inflammatory disorders of the subcutaneous fat present an important diagnostic challenge to the dermatologist, because the lesions often develop as subcutaneous nodules or plaques. An adequate diagnostic biopsy is essential as a prerequisite to accurate diagnosis in almost all instances. A larger scalpel incisional biopsy is preferred, which obviously should extend deeply through the subcutis. Conventional punch biopsies (4 mm or smaller) are totally inadequate, as the tissue tapers down to leave little, if any, subcutaneous tissue. However, trephine punches are adequate and provide acceptable cosmetic results [10]. The pathologist may well need to cut serial sections, as some of the panniculitides are characterized by rather focal or even scattered pathological changes, and to look for evidence of damage to larger blood vessels.

Most panniculitides are persistent, lasting for weeks or months. For diagnostic purposes, the biopsy should be taken from an active earlier lesion: erythematous, indurated and usually tender. Although the fat lobules have a rich capillary blood supply closely applied to fat cells, there are no lymphatics and very little intervening connective tissue [11]. Furthermore, the vasculature in the subcutis area is slow flowing. This renders the subcutaneous fat vulnerable to a variety of noxious insults [9]; for example, cold injury or enzymatic damage.

The sequence of cellular events following injury to the subcutis may take weeks or months to fully evolve, and is usually as follows [1,2]:

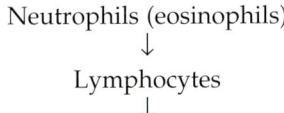

Neutrophils (eosinophils)
↓
Lymphocytes
↓
Histiocytes (granulomatous 'foamy macrophages')
↓
Fibroblasts (fibrosis)

The histological changes of the granulomatous stage are not necessarily diagnostic. When fat cells are damaged, the liberated lipid undergoes hydrolysis to glycerol and fatty acids, which usually provoke a foreign-body-type granulomatous reaction. Macrophages are attracted and foam cells are produced. After the phase of reaction to released lipocyte products, there is a period of reconstitution, the ease of repair depending on the extent of the initial lipocyte damage and the efficiency of the local circulation.

Atrophy of subcutaneous tissue (lipoatrophy) is a consequence of some types of inflammation in the fat lobules. In other instances, extensive fibrosis is inevitable after damage to subcutis, resulting in the formation of chronic subcutaneous fibrotic nodules.

In certain types of panniculitis, an ongoing slow chain reaction is set up, in which small foci of fat necrosis provoke a peripheral inflammatory reaction, which in itself leads to further peripheral fat necrosis, thus allowing the lesion to spread centrifugally. It is therefore clear that the histological findings will differ, depending on the age of the lesion biopsied.

In difficult cases of panniculitis, it is helpful to submit more than one biopsy from lesions at different stages of their clinical evolution. Polarization of sections should be routinely performed to look for crystalline material, and in certain clinical situations extra tissue should be submitted for bacterial or fungal culture.

Panniculitis may be classified histologically according to whether it is predominantly septal, mixed, or associated with vasculitis, as in the following [1–4]:

1 Septal panniculitis:
   (a) erythema nodosum (see Chapter 50)
   (b) erythema nodosum migrans (see Chapter 50); (subacute nodular migratory paniniculitis)
   (c) eosinophilic panniculitis (this condition may overlap with lobular or mixed panniculitis)
2 Lobular panniculitis:
   (a) relapsing febrile nodular panniculitis (Weber–Christian syndrome)
   (b) idiopathic nodular panniculitis
   (c) lipoatrophic panniculitis (formerly Rothman–Makai syndrome)
   (d) panniculitis associated with crystal deposition—sclerema neonatorum (see Chapter 17), subcutaneous fat necrosis of newborn (see Chapter 17), gout or factitial panniculitis, poststeroid panniculitis, calciphylaxis
   (e) enzymic (pancreatic) panniculitis
   (f) α_1-antitrypsin deficiency panniculitis
   (g) fat necrosis—cold injury, nodular cystic fat necrosis, lipomembranous
   (h) lymphomatous panniculitis
   (i) cytophagic histiocytic panniculitis
3 Mixed panniculitis:
   (a) lupus erythematosus profundus
   (b) scleroderma (fasciitis with eosinophilia, see Chapter 51)
   (c) connective-tissue panniculitis (overlaps with lipoatrophic panniculitis)
   (d) subcutaneous sarcoidosis (see Chapter 61)
   (e) subcutaneous granuloma annulare (see Chapter 60)
   (f) necrobiosis lipoidica (see Chapter 60)
   (g) infective panniculitis (e.g. opportunistic bacterial or fungal infections)
   (h) physical and factitious panniculitis (e.g. sclerosing lipogranuloma, oil granulomas, eosinophilic sclerosing lipogranuloma)
   (i) sclerosing panniculitis (lipodermatosclerosis)
   (j) fasciitis—panniculitis syndromes
4 Panniculitis with vasculitis (see Chapters 49 and 50):
   (a) small-vessel vasculitis—leukocytoclastic vasculitis
   (b) large-vessel vasculitis—polyarteritis nodosa, thrombophlebitis, nodular vasculitis (erythema induratum)
   (c) neutrophilic panniculitis
   (d) oedematous scarring vasculitic panniculitis: hydroa-like lymphoma.

References

1 Black MM. Panniculitis. *J Cutan Pathol* 1985; **12**: 366–80.
2 Black MM. Panniculitis: problems with diagnosis. *Australas J Dermatol* 1988; **29**: 79–84.
3 Requena L, Sánchez Yus E. Panniculitis. I. Mostly septal panniculitis. *J Am Acad Dermatol* 2001; **45**: 163–83.
4 Requena L, Sánchez Yus E. Panniculitis. II. Mostly lobular panniculitis. *J Am Acad Dermatol* 2001; **45**: 325–61.

5 Doyle IA, Connolly S, Winkelmann RK. Cutaneous and subcutaneous inflammatory sclerosis syndromes. *Arch Dermatol* 1982; **118**: 886–90.

6 Eng AM, Aronson JK. Dermatopathology of panniculitis. *Semin Dermatol* 1984; **3**: 1–9.

7 Patterson JW. New findings in the 'third compartment'. *Arch Dermatol* 1987; **123**: 1615–7.

8 Peters MS, Daniel Su WP. Panniculitis. *Dermatol Clin* 1992; **10**: 37–57.

9 Thiers BH. Panniculitis. *Dermatol Clin* 1983; **1**: 537–51.

10 Tok J, Abrahams I, Ravits MA *et al.* Surgical Pearl: the trephine punch for diagnosing panniculitis. *J Am Acad Dermatol* 1996; **35**: 980–1.

11 Ryan TJ. Panniculitis: its pathogenesis and management. In: Champion RH, Pye RJ, eds. *Recent Advances in Dermatology*, Vol. 9. Edinburgh: Churchill Livingstone, 1992: 17–32.

Inflammatory disorders of subcutaneous fat

Septal panniculitis

Erythema nodosum (see Chapter 50)

Although erythema nodosum is the prototype of a septal panniculitis, the inflammatory changes always involve the overlying dermis. In acute lesions, there is oedema of the septae with transudation of neutrophils, and sometimes eosinophils, into the septae and adjacent margin of fat lobules. In older lesions, the infiltrate becomes lymphohistiocytic and finally granulomatous, before the septae became thickened and finally fibrotic. Radial granulomas (Miescher) are often found in the interlobular septae in erythema nodosum [1]. There is still some debate as to whether *erythema nodosum migrans* (subacute nodular migratory panniculitis) [2–4] and the chronic and granulomatous forms of erythema nodosum [5] are variants of the same pathological process. Erythema nodosum migrans tends to be characterized by markedly thickened and fibrotic septae, marked capillary proliferation and a massive granulomatous reaction (with giant cells) along the borders of the widened septae [6].

Eosinophilic panniculitis

Eosinophilic panniculitis is characterized by a prominent infiltration of subcutaneous fat with eosinophils, and has been identified in patients presenting with a variety of associated clinical conditions [7–14].

The inflammatory infiltrate, including eosinophils, occurs principally within the septae but can involve the lobules. The overlying dermis is often involved, closely resembling eosinophilic cellulitis (Wells' syndrome) [9]. Fragmented eosinophilic granules (flame figures) are occasionally seen (Fig. 46.3). The current view of eosinophilic panniculitis is that it is not a disease entity, but it can be principally considered as a reactive process, often associated with a systemic condition [8].

More common causes of eosinophilic panniculitis include arthropod bites, atopic eczema, erythema nodosum, infectious causes (*Gnathostoma, Streptococcus, Toxocara*) and leukocytoclastic vasculitis [8]. The condition has also been associated with chronic recurrent parotitis [11], lupus panniculitis, morphoea profundus [12] and *Fasciola hepatica* infection [13]. Fortunately, only very rarely is eosinophilic panniculitis associated with malignancy, either leukaemia [14] or a solid tumour [9]. It has been seen in

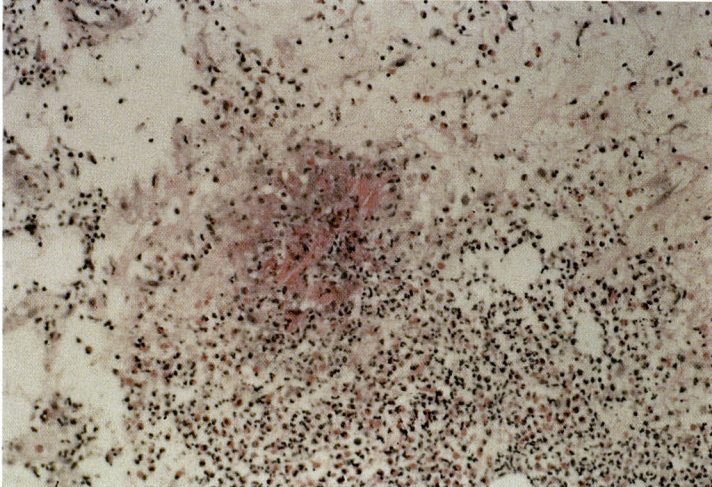

Fig. 46.3 Eosinophilic panniculitis. H&E, × 40.

association with trauma and autoinoculation with farm products [15] but may also arise spontaneously [16]. In a case of subcutaneous fat necrosis of the newborn, eosinophilic granules were seen inside giant cells [17].

References

1 Sánchez Yus E, Sanz Vico MD, de Diego V. Miescher's radial granuloma: a characteristic marker of erythema nodosum. *Am J Dermatopathol* 1989; **11**: 434–42.

2 Hannuksela M. Erythema nodosum migrans. *Acta Dermatol Venereol (Stockh)* 1973; **53**: 313–7.

3 Perry HO, Winkelmann RK. Subacute nodular migratory panniculitis. *Arch Dermatol* 1964; **89**: 170–9.

4 Vilanova X, Piñol Aguadé J. Subacute nodular migratory panniculitis. *Br J Dermatol* 1959; **71**: 45–50.

5 Forstrom L, Winkelmann RK. Granulomatous panniculitis in erythema nodosum. *Arch Dermatol* 1975; **111**: 335–46.

6 de Almeida Prestes C, Winkelmann RK, Su WPD. Septal granulomatous panniculitis: comparison of the pathology of erythema nodosum migrans (migratory panniculitis) and chronic erythema nodosum. *J Am Acad Dermatol* 1990; **22**: 477–83.

7 Burket JM, Burket BJ. Eosinophilic panniculitis. *J Am Acad Dermatol* 1985; **12**: 161–4.

8 Peters MS, Su WPD. Panniculitis. *Dermatol Clin* 1992; **10**: 37–57.

9 Winkelmann RK, Frigas E. Eosinophilic panniculitis: a clinicopathologic study. *J Cutan Pathol* 1986; **13**: 1–12.

10 Adame J, Cohen PR. Eosinophilic panniculitis: diagnostic considerations and evaluation. *J Am Acad Dermatol* 1996; **34**: 229–34.

11 Glass LA, Zaghloul AB, Solomon AR. Eosinophilic panniculitis associated with chronic recurrent parotitis. *Am J Dermatopathol* 1989; **11**: 555–9.

12 Peters MS, Su WPD. Eosinophils in lupus panniculitis and morphoea profunda. *J Cutan Pathol* 1991; **18**: 189–92.

13 Perez C, Vives R, Montes M *et al.* Recurrent eosinophilic panniculitis associated with *Fasciola hepatica* infection. *J Am Acad Dermatol* 2000; **42**: 900–2.

14 Marullo S, Dallot A, Carelier-Balloy B *et al.* Subcutaneous eosinophilic necrosis associated with refractory anaemia with an excess of myeloblasts. *J Am Acad Dermatol* 1989; **20**: 320–3.

15 Gómez Rodríguez N, Ortiz-Rey JA, de la Fuente Buceta A *et al.* Auto-induced eosinophilic panniculitis: a diagnostic dilemma. *Ann Med Interne* 2001; **18**: 635–7.

16 Liu Y, Xiao SX, Wang JM *et al.* Eosinophilic panniculitis: report of three cases. *Int J Dermatol* 2006; **45**: 1412–4.

17 Tajirian A, Ross R, Zeikus P *et al.* Subcutaneous fat necrosis of the newborn with eosinophilic granules. *J Cutan Pathol* 2007; **34**: 588–90.

Lobular panniculitis

Relapsing febrile nodular panniculitis

Synonym
- Weber–Christian syndrome

Relapsing febrile nodular panniculitis was first described by Pfeifer in 1892 [1]. The term Weber–Christian syndrome came to be used following the cases reported by Weber [2] and Christian [3]. Weber–Christian syndrome encompasses a febrile disease, characterized by the recurrent formation of single or multiple crops of tender inflammatory nodules in the subcutaneous fat. Because the range of clinical features differed, and the extent of systemic involvement varied, the concept of Weber–Christian syndrome never became popular and the view was put forward that it should not be considered to be a distinct entity [4–6]. The term nodular panniculitis was preferred [5]. Nodular panniculitis is essentially a lobular panniculitis in which fat necrosis develops in the absence of overt vasculitis.

Macrophages ingest fat released from damaged lipocytes, thus producing a characteristic foamy appearance. In some cases, liquefactive nodules appear, which ulcerate and discharge an oily yellow liquid [7]. In others, there is more systemic involvement, which may affect visceral fat or even the myocardium [8].

Nodular panniculitis can affect both adults and children, when it can occur in early infancy [9,10]. However, it must be stressed that nodular panniculitis or Weber–Christian syndrome may not be a distinct disease entity. On further investigation, many cases of nodular panniculitis can be subsequently reclassified depending on their cause; for example, pancreatic panniculitis, α_1-antitrypsin deficiency or cytophagic panniculitis. However, there are undoubtedly some cases of nodular panniculitis, in both children and adults, in which the aetiology remains to be determined.

References
1 Pfeifer V. Über einen Fall von Herdweiser: atrophie des subcutanen Fettgebewes. *Dtsch Arch Klin Med* 1892; **50**: 438–49.
2 Weber FP. A case of relapsing non-suppurative nodular panniculitis showing phagocytosis of subcutaneous fat cells by macrophages. *Br J Dermatol* 1925; **37**: 301–11.
3 Christian HA. Relapsing febrile nodular non-suppurative panniculitis. *Arch Intern Med* 1928; **42**: 338–51.
4 Förström L, Winkelmann RK. Acute panniculitis. *Arch Dermatol* 1977; **113**: 909–17.
5 Macdonald A, Feiwel M. A review of the concept of Weber–Christian panniculitis with a report of five cases. *Br J Dermatol* 1968; **80**: 355–61.
6 White JW, Winkelmann RK. Panniculitis: a review of 30 cases with this diagnosis. *J Am Acad Dermatol* 1998; **39**: 56–62.
7 Hoyas N, Schaffer B, Beerman H. Liquefying nodular panniculitis. *Arch Dermatol* 1965; **94**: 436–9.
8 Wilkinson PJ, Harman RRM, Tribe CR. Systemic nodular panniculitis with cardiac involvement. *J Clin Pathol* 1974; **27**: 808–12.
9 Aronson IK, Zeitz HJ, Variakojir D. Panniculitis in childhood. *Pediatr Dermatol* 1988; **5**: 216–30.
10 Randle SM, Richter MB, Palmer RG *et al.* Panniculitis: a report of four cases and literature review. *Arch Dis Child* 1991; **66**: 1057–60.

Idiopathic nodular panniculitis

An idiopathic condition characterized by recurrent crops of nodular panniculitis. Some cases are accompanied by fever,

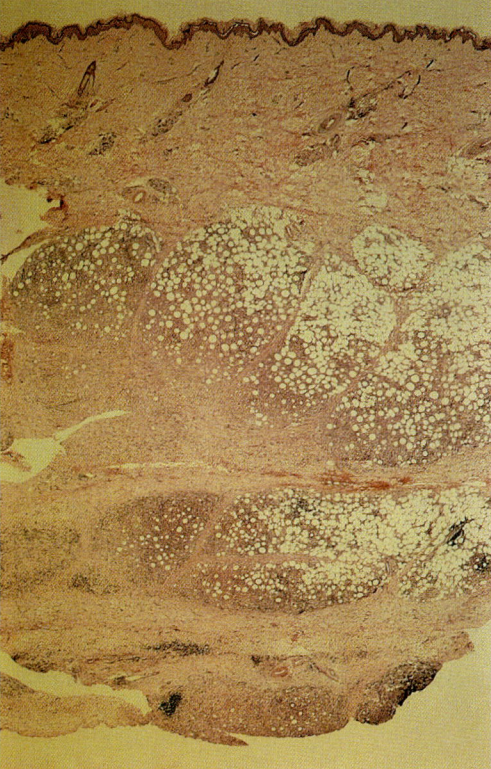

Fig. 46.4 Idiopathic nodular panniculitis. Low-power view showing lobular pattern of panniculitis. H&E, × 2.5.

malaise, abdominal pain and arthritis. As indicated above, the term Weber–Christian syndrome is best avoided. Many cases of nodular panniculitis can now be attributed to specific causes (see below).

Pathology. The histological changes are non-specific but the panniculitis is mainly lobular [1] (Fig. 46.4). In the early stages, the fat lobules are infiltrated with acute inflammatory cells, producing a pseudopyogenic reaction. Later, lymphocytes and macrophages appear to ingest the fat released from damaged lipocytes. These lipophages develop a characteristic foamy cytoplasm, producing the typical appearance of a lipophagic granuloma (Fig. 46.5). Healing is by fibrosis, the fibrocytes invading the lobules from the fibrous septae and ultimately producing complete lobular fibrosis.

Clinical features. Approximately 50% of cases of nodular panniculitis are idiopathic [2]. All ages may be affected, but the condition is very rare in childhood [3,4]. The majority of cases are young adult females who develop crops of dull-red, tender, subcutaneous nodules, usually about 1–2 cm in diameter. The lesions tend to be maximal on the lower limbs (Fig. 46.6), although the trunk and face can be affected.

Systemic features including fever, malaise, myalgia, arthralgia and weight loss are often present when there are multiple lesions. Many of the nodules eventually resolve, leaving a pigmented area or an atrophic depression. In a few cases, there may be overlying necrosis with drainage of oily, brownish, serous fluid (Fig. 46.7),

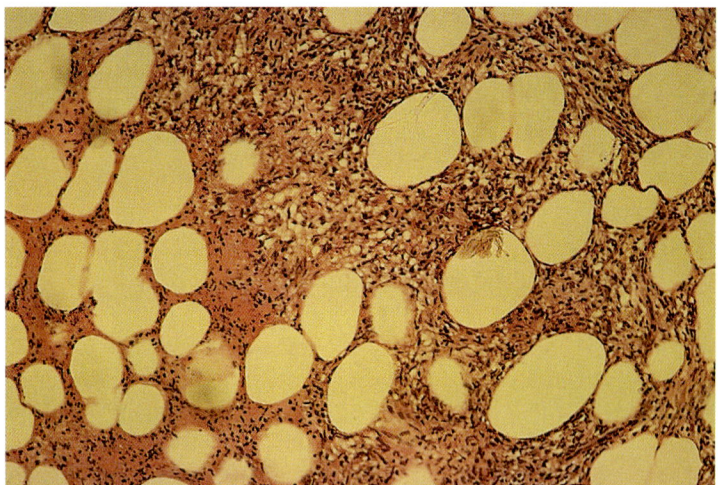

Fig. 46.5 Idiopathic nodular panniculitis: typical appearances of a lipophagic granuloma. H&E, × 40.

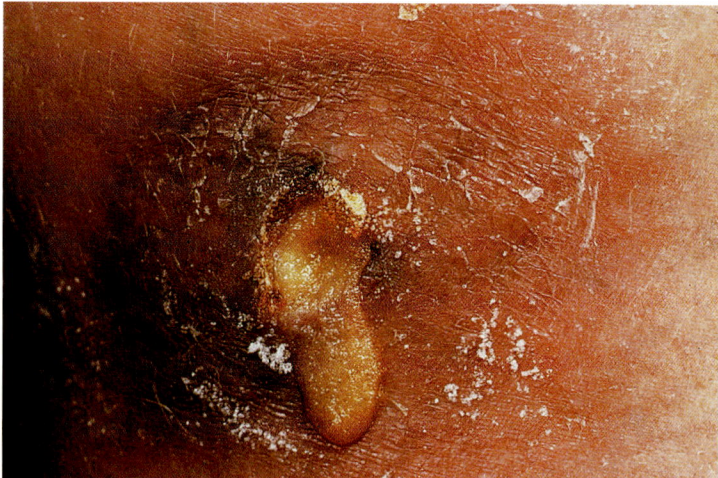

Fig. 46.7 Idiopathic nodular panniculitis: drainage of serous fluid.

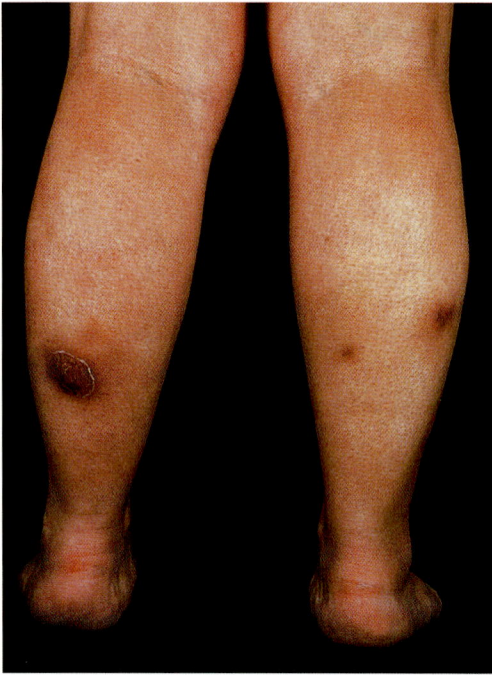

Fig. 46.6 Idiopathic nodular panniculitis.

eventually leading to scarring. Rarely, there may be involvement of visceral fat, including the heart, lungs, liver and kidneys, which may lead to death [5]. MRI scanning may disclose inflammation in an internal fat depot such as the retroperitoneum [6].

The laboratory features are non-specific, but there may be anaemia, leukocytosis or leukopenia, thrombocytopenia and a raised erythrocyte sedimentation rate.

Diagnosis. Idiopathic nodular panniculitis has to be distinguished from other forms of panniculitis (see below). It is important to perform repeated laboratory tests for pancreatic disease, autoimmune disease, complement deficiency, α_1-antitrypsin deficiency, and to exclude cytophagic histiocytic panniculitis. The possibility of factitial or infective panniculitis must also be considered.

Prognosis. When only subcutaneous fat is involved, the prognosis is good [2]. Some cases recover after a few months, and permanent remission within 2–5 years is usual. Rarely, recurrences may continue for 10 years or longer, but without serious deterioration of the general condition. Exceptionally, the condition can be fatal if there is visceral involvement [5].

Treatment. Once the possibility of systemic disease has been excluded, the treatment is mainly symptomatic. Analgesics may be needed to alleviate pain, and ulceration may need bland aseptic dressings. In severe cases, systemic corticosteroids may be effective, provided adequate dosage (up to 80 mg/day prednisolone) is used for 7–10 days. The dosage should then be slowly tapered over a period of 4–6 weeks. Other treatments that have helped in some cases include antimalarials [7] and thalidomide [8].

Unusual causes of lobular panniculitis resembling idiopathic nodular panniculitis

Increasing numbers of case reports, usually isolated, are appearing that link nodular panniculitis to other illnesses or events. Autoimmune diseases such as Sjögren's syndrome have been linked to a lobular plasma cell panniculitis [9], and ulcerative colitis and myopathy with nodular panniculitis [10].

Infections, for example hepatitis A [11], *Borrelia burgdorferi* [12,13] and brucellosis [14], have also been implicated in the causation of nodular panniculitis. Granulomatous panniculitis has been associated with crescentic glomerulonephritis [15]. Lobular panniculitis has been reported to develop at the site of interleukin-2 injections for treatment of metastatic carcinoma, and to be exacerbated by intravenous use of the same treatment [16]. Delayed expression of an octopus bite [17] and local reaction to glatiramer acetate injection for multiple sclerosis [18] are other causes. Oral administration of the low-calorie artificial sweetener aspartame (Nutra-Sweet®) has been implicated in the causation of lobular panniculitis [19].

References

1 Eng AM, Aronson IK. Dermatopathology of panniculitis. *Semin Dermatol* 1984; 3: 1–13.

2 Panush RS, Youker RA, Dlesk A *et al.* Weber–Christian disease: analysis of 15 cases and review of the literature. *Medicine* 1985; **64**: 181–91.

3 Aronson IK, Zeitz HJ, Variakojis D. Panniculitis in childhood. *Pediatr Dermatol* 1988; **5**: 216–30.

4 Randle SM, Richter MB, Palmer RG *et al.* Panniculitis: a report of four cases and literature review. *Arch Dis Child* 1991; **66**: 1057–60.

5 Aronson IK, West DP, Variakojis D *et al.* Fatal panniculitis. *J Am Acad Dermatol* 1985; **12**: 535–51.

6 Nakai M, Sato M, Sahara S *et al.* Weber–Christian disease presenting with retroperitoneal panniculitis. *Eur J Radiol Extra* 2006; **60**: 89–92.

7 Sorensen RU, Abramowsky C, Stern RC. Corticosteroid-sparing effect of hydroxychloroquin in a patient with early-onset Weber–Christian syndrome. *J Am Acad Dermatol* 1990; **22**: 1172–4.

8 Eravelly J, Waters MFR. Thalidomide in Weber–Christian disease. *Lancet* 1977; **i**: 251.

9 McGovern TW, Erickson AR, Fitzpatrick JE. Sjögren's syndrome, plasma cell panniculitis and hidradenitis. *J Cutan Pathol* 1996; **23**: 170–4.

10 Nozue M, Ono A, Goto N. Ulcerative colitis associated with Weber–Christian panniculitis and musculitis: a case report. *J Gastroenterol* 1994; **29**: 84–7.

11 Fowler JF Jr, Callen JP. Panniculitis associated with hepatitis. *Cutis* 1983; **32**: 543–7.

12 Haasler D, Zorn J, Zöller L *et al.* Noduläre Panniculitis: eine verlaufsform der Lyme Borreliose? *Hautarzt* 1992; **43**: 134–8.

13 Viljanen MK, Oksi J, Salomaa P *et al.* Cultivation of *Borrelia burgdorferi* from the blood and a subcutaneous lesion of a patient with relapsing febrile nodular nonsuppurative panniculitis. *J Infect Dis* 1992; **160**: 596–7.

14 Tanyel E, Fisgin NT, Yildiz L *et al.* Panniculitis as the initial manifestation of brucellosis: a case report. *Am J Dermatopathol* 2008; **30**: 169–71.

15 Thomashow DF, Huan Z, Sanchez MA *et al.* Granulomatous panniculitis associated with crescentic glomerulonephritis. *Nephron* 1994; **67**: 374–6.

16 Baars JW, Coenen JLLM, Wagstaff J *et al.* Lobular panniculitis after subcutaneous administration of interleukin-2 (IL-2) and its exacerbation during intravenous therapy with IL-2. *Br J Cancer* 1992; **66**: 698–9.

17 Misago N, Inoue T, Narisawa Y. Delayed reaction after an octopus bite showing a giant cell-rich granulomatous dermatitis/panniculitis. *J Cutan Pathol* 2008; **35**: 1068–72.

18 Ball NJ, Cowan BJ, Moore GR *et al.* Lobular panniculitis at the site of glatiramer acetate injections for the treatment of relapsing-remitting multiple sclerosis. A report of two cases. *J Cutan Pathol* 2008; **35**: 407–10.

19 McCauliffe DP, Poitras K. Aspartame-induced lobular panniculitis. *J Am Acad Dermatol* 1991; **24**: 298–300.

Lipoatrophic panniculitis

Synonyms
- Connective tissue panniculitis
- Autoimmune panniculitis

As the name implies, lipoatrophic panniculitis denotes the findings of prominent lipoatrophy. However, the development of lipoatrophy should be considered to be an 'end-stage' process, which is preceded by inflammation in the fat lobules and sometimes the fibrous septae. In the earlier literature, many cases of lipoatrophic panniculitis were considered to have Weber–Christian syndrome or Rothman–Makai syndrome [1]. As the aetiology of lipoatrophic panniculitis is unknown, it is perhaps not surprising that the nomenclature remains confused, and almost certainly there is considerable overlap in these clinical entities. 'Primary' lipophagic panniculitis has been described in adults (Fig. 46.8) [2] and children [3,4], either as an acute benign condition or as a chronic recurrent disabling disease. In children, a granulomatous histopathology can be seen prior to the development of lipoatrophy, for which the term lipophagic panniculitis is used [4]. Connective tissue panniculitis is a rare form of panniculitis, affecting septae and lobules, and leading to prominent lipoatrophy [5] (Fig. 46.9). The condition has been described in female adults and children [6]. Episodes of intense lymphocytic panniculitis lead to lipoatrophy. At various times in the illness, a circulating antinuclear antibody and/or SSB (La) antibodies may be detected [5,6]. The clinical spectrum of lipoatrophic panniculitis is thought to encompass connective tissue panniculitis [7]. Histologically, in connective tissue panniculitis there is no evidence of hyalinization of fat and collagen, which is typical of lupus erythematosus profundus [8]. Various other autoimmune diseases have been reported in association with lipoatrophic panniculitis, including diabetes mellitus, rheumatoid arthritis and Hashimoto's thyroiditis [3]. Lipoatrophic panniculitis has been reported in a very young child with a chromosomal abnormality on chromosome 10q26 [9].

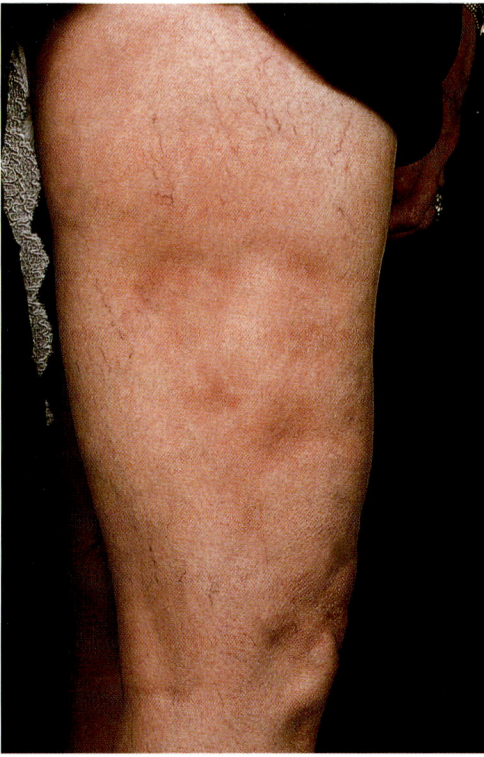

Fig. 46.8 Lipoatrophic panniculitis: recurrent episodes of panniculitis have resolved to leave prominent lipoatrophy on the outer thigh. (Courtesy of St John's Institute of Dermatology, King's College London, UK.)

Treatment. Systemic corticosteroids are effective, but usually only in higher doses. Antimalarial therapy, hydroxychloroquine or chloroquine, is the most effective acceptable treatment [10], but may not be sufficient alone [5,7]. Reconstructive surgery, in the form of vascular pedicles or alloplastic implants, has been successfully used in severe cases of lipoatrophic panniculitis [7].

References

1 Pierini LE, Abulafia J, Wainfeld S. Idiopathic lipogranulomatous hypodermatis. *Arch Dermatol* 1968; **98**: 290–8.

2 Umbert IJ, Winkelmann RK. Adult lipophagic atrophic panniculitis. *Br J Dermatol* 1991; **124**: 291–5.

3 Billings JK, Milgraum SS, Gupta AK *et al.* Lipoatrophic panniculitis: a possible autoimmune inflammatory disease of fat. *Arch Dermatol* 1987; **123**: 1662–6.

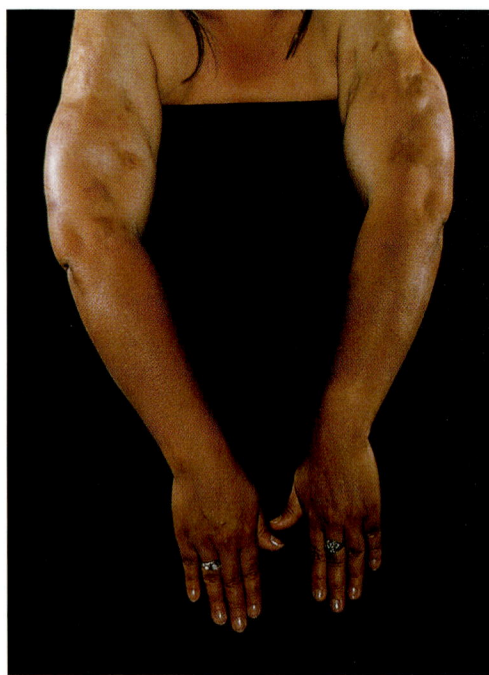

Fig. 46.9 Lipoatrophic (connective tissue) panniculitis: note the dimpled atrophic fat of the upper arms. (Courtesy of Dr M.R. Pittelkow, Mayo Clinic, Rochester, MN, USA.)

4 Winkelmann RK, McEvoy MT, Peters MS. Lipophagic panniculitis of childhood. *J Am Acad Dermatol* 1989; **21**: 971–8.
5 Winkelmann RK, Padilha-Goncalves A. Connective tissue panniculitis. *Arch Dermatol* 1980; **116**: 291–4.
6 Winkelmann RK. Panniculitis in connective tissue disease. *Arch Dermatol* 1983; **119**: 336–44.
7 Handfield-Jones SE, Stephens CJM, Mayou BJ *et al.* The clinical spectrum of lipoatrophic panniculitis encompasses connective tissue panniculitis. *Br J Dermatol* 1993; **129**: 619–24.
8 Sánchez NP, Peters MS, Winkelmann RK. The histopathology of lupus erythematosus panniculitis. *J Am Acad Dermatol* 1981; **5**: 673–80.
9 Martinez A, Malone M, Hoeger P *et al.* Lipoatrophic panniculitis and chromosome 10 abnormality. *Br J Dermatol* 2000; **142**: 1034–9.
10 Shelley WB. Chloroquine-induced remission of nodular panniculitis present for 15 years. *J Am Acad Dermatol* 1981; **5**: 168–70.

Panniculitis associated with crystal deposition

Polarization of skin histology is important in the assessment of any inflammatory or granulomatous type of panniculitis, as it may be the only way to identify crystals readily [1].

Lipid-containing crystals are dissolved out during formalin fixation, but usually leave cleft-like spaces, which often produce a characteristic histology. Needle-shaped clefts are characteristically seen in subcutaneous fat necrosis of the newborn (see Chapter 17), sclerema neonatorum (see Chapter 17) and post-steroid panniculitis. Cholesterol crystals may cause panniculitis, but the crystals are only found in the lumen of smaller blood vessels.

Post-steroid panniculitis [2–5]

Post-steroid panniculitis is now undoubtedly very rare. All the reported cases have been in children, in whom subcutaneous nodules developed 1–13 days after stopping high doses of systemic corticosteroids quickly. The nodules vary in size from 0.5 to 4 cm, and tend to localize in those areas where there is the greatest accumulation of fat from steroid therapy, but typically on the cheeks [6]. Although the nodules appear after the rapid discontinuation of steroids, they are not associated with systemic manifestations of the steroid-withdrawal syndrome. Resolution of the nodules is gradual, occurring over several weeks or months. There is no effective treatment.

The histology of post-steroid panniculitis is very similar to that of subcutaneous fat necrosis of the newborn, in that needle-shaped crystals may be found within lipocytes and histiocytes.

Calcifying panniculitis with renal failure [7]

In patients with chronic renal failure, a chronic alteration of calcium and phosphate metabolism often exists, and secondarily causes hyperparathyroidism. This combination leads to the processes of calciphylaxis and metastatic calcification [8,9]. Whilst calciphylaxis is almost always associated with chronic renal failure patients, many of whom are on long-term dialysis, it is seen in patients with normal renal function [10–12]. Some have, or have had, parathyroid problems, but it has also been reported in association with alcoholic cirrhosis [13] and malignancy, breast cancer and cholangiocarcinoma [14]. The calcification is principally present within smaller and medium-sized arteries. Weenig has suggested that vascular calcification results from the dysregulation of many factors, in particular nuclear factor κ-B (NFκ-B), a key transcription factor in bone mineral homeostasis, activation of which results in bone mineral loss [15]. If this local damage slows blood flow and contributes with other factors such as TNF-α to a local procoagulant state, the addition of a systemic hypercoagulable state, often present in these patients, would result in thrombosis.

Clinical features. The process begins with erythematous tender nodules or plaques that progress to violaceous livedo-like areas, usually located on the thighs (Fig. 46.10), abdomen or buttocks. These lesions tend to increase rapidly in size, progressing to large necrotic ulcers. In the acute stage a necrotic livedo pattern on the upper anterior thigh or lower abdomen in a patient with acute or chronic renal failure is a strong clinical pointer. Any long-term dialysis or chronic renal failure patient with a persisting leg ulcer should be assumed to have calciphylaxis until proved otherwise (Fig. 46.11). One clue is the really severe pain experienced, so extreme that patients cannot keep still. Parathyroid hormone levels are no different from dialysis patients without calciphylaxis, but are often high [16]. Sometimes repeated biopsy is required to find the calcified small vessels. Calcification in vessels is not pathognomonic, as it can be seen incidentally or in arteriopaths. Cutaneous necrosis mimicking calciphylaxis in renal failure has been reported, resulting from oxalate crystal deposition in the vessel wall [17]. Crystals from calcinosis in the fat induced by local heparin injection in renal patients and others are not in the vessel wall [18,19].

Treatment. Treatment should be aimed at preventing the hyperparathyroidism and secondary infection, but usually the disease has a high mortality, in one series only 46% surviving for a year [16]. Intravenous sodium thiosulphate [20] and biphosphonates

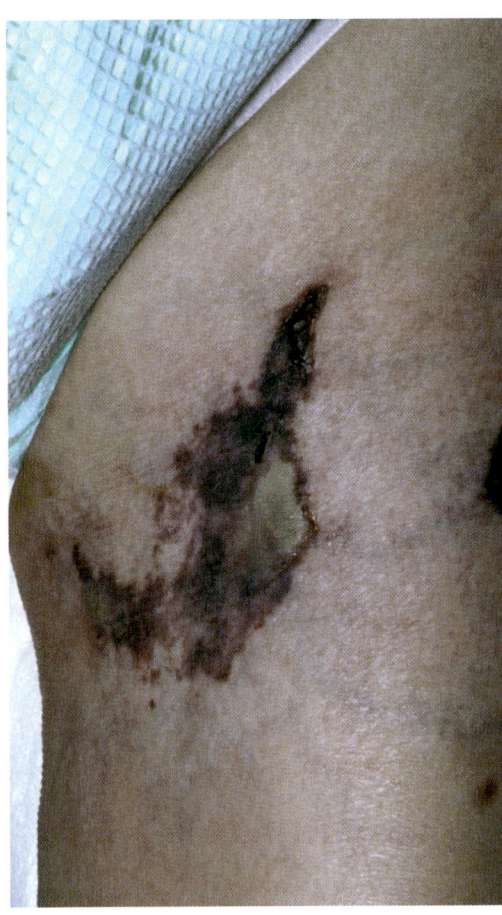

Fig. 46.10 Calciphylaxis of the upper thigh in a patient with renal failure.

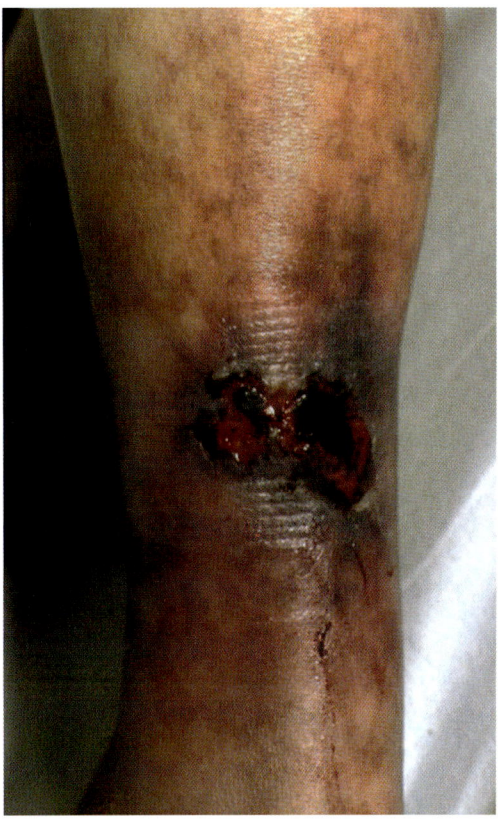

Fig. 46.11 Calciphylaxis of the lower leg in a patient on long-term dialysis.

have been used with success [21,22] and may prevent the need for parathyroidectomy, which is not always successful in reversing the skin changes.

Gout

Urate crystals are inflammatory, and occasionally lobular panniculitis can be caused by deposition of crystals secondary to hyperuricaemia [23–25] though a raised urate is not always present [26]. Painful, ulcerating nodules on the lower legs is the usual presentation, though only four cases have been described. Crystals may be sampled directly from the chalky ulcer exudate and polarized. Large, pink, amorphous deposits surrounded by a giant cell reaction with little other inflammatory response is seen in the subcutis on histology. One case showed a neutrophilic lobular panniculitis [24]. Urate crystals can be distinguished by their fine, needle-like shape and tendency to form sheaves, but are usually only visible in ethanol-fixed sections.

In a unique case [27] urate crystals were seen intracellularly in adipocytes, mimicking subcutaneous fat necrosis of the newborn and post-steroid panniculitis. They were only visible as tissue had been processed through alcohol. The 6-month-old immunosuppressed patient had a large subcutaneous fungal infection on the cheek caused by fungi of the class *Zygomycetes*. The crystals appeared concomitant with the infection, much as oxalate crystals are seen with *Aspergillus* infections.

Drugs

Lobular panniculitis with crystals can occur following injection of drugs such as meperidine and pentazocine (Fig. 46.12) [28,29].

Crystal-storing histiocytosis

Crystal-storing histiocytosis is a rare condition in which tumorous deposits of histiocytes containing crystalline immunoglobulins are deposited in soft tissue. The condition has been reported to cause panniculitis of Weber–Christian type in a patient with lymphoblastic lymphoma [30].

References

1 Black MM. Panniculitis. *J Cutan Pathol* 1985; **12**: 366–80.
2 Jaffe N, Hann HWL, Vauter GF. Post-steroid panniculitis in acute leukaemia. *N Engl J Med* 1971; **284**: 366–7.
3 Roenigk KH, Haserick JR, Arundell FD. Post-steroid panniculitis. *Arch Dermatol* 1964; **90**: 387–91.
4 Silverman RA, Newman AJ, Le Vine MJ. Post-steroid panniculitis: a case report. *Pediatr Dermatol* 1988; **5**: 92–3.
5 Spagnuolo M, Taranta A. Post-steroid panniculitis. *Ann Intern Med* 1961; **54**: 1181–90.
6 Kwon EJ, Emanuel PO, Gribetz CH *et al*. Poststeroid panniculitis. *J Cutan Pathol* 2007; **34** (Suppl. 1): 64–7.
7 Young DC, Cuozzo DW, Seidman AJ *et al*. Widespread livedo reticularis with painful ulcerations. *Arch Dermatol* 1995; **131**: 786–8.
8 Lowry LR, Tschen JA, Wolf JE *et al*. Calcifying panniculitis and systemic calciphylaxis in an end-stage renal patient. *Cutis* 1993; **51**: 245–7.
9 Lugo-Somolinos A, Sanchez JL, Mendez-Coll J *et al*. Calcifying panniculitis associated with polycystic kidney disease and chronic renal failure. *J Am Acad Dermatol* 1990; **22**: 743–7.
10 Pollock B, Cunliffe WJ, Merchant WJ. Calciphylaxis in the absence of renal failure. *Clin Exp Dermatol* 2000; **25**: 389–92.

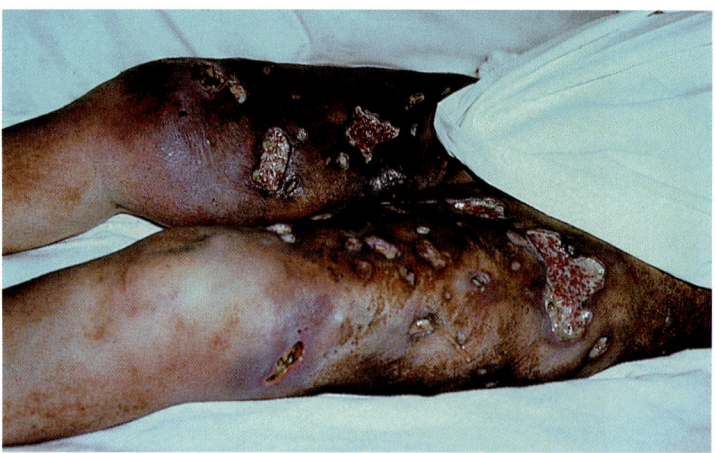

Fig. 46.12 Ulceration of the thighs secondary to panniculitis caused by injections of pentazocine. (Courtesy of Dr R.F. Palestine, Mayo Clinic, Rochester, MN, USA.)

11 Goyal S, Huhn KM, Provost TT. Calciphylaxis in a patient without renal failure or elevated parathyroid hormone: possible aetiological role of chemotherapy. *Br J Dermatol* 2000; **143**: 1087–90.

12 Couto FM, Chen H, Blank RD *et al*. Calciphylaxis in the absence of end-stage renal disease. *Endocr Pract* 2006; **12**: 406–10.

13 Ferreres JR, Marcoval J, Bordas X *et al*. Calciphylaxis associated with alcoholic cirrhosis. *J Eur Acad Dermatol Venereol* 2006; **20**: 599–601.

14 Riegert-Johnson DL, Kaur JS, Pfeifer EA. Calciphylaxis associated with cholangiocarcinoma treated with low-molecular-weight heparin and vitamin K. *Mayo Clin Proc* 2001; **76**: 749–52.

15 Weenig RH. Pathogenesis of calciphylaxis: Hans Selye to nuclear factor κ-B. *J Am Acad Derm* 2008; **58**: 458–71.

16 Weenig RH, Sewell LD, Davis MD *et al*. Calciphylaxis: natural history, risk factor analysis, and outcome. *J Am Acad Dermatol* 2007; **56**: 569–79.

17 Somach SC, Davis BR, Paras FA *et al*. Fatal cutaneous necrosis mimicking calciphylaxis in a patient with type I primary hyperoxaluria. *Arch Dermatol* 1995; **131**: 821–3.

18 van Haren FM, Ruiter DJ, Hilbrands LB. Nadroparin-induced calcinosis cutis in renal transplant recipients. *Nephron* 2001; **87**: 279–82.

19 Campanelli A, Kaya G, Masouyé I *et al*. Calcifying panniculitis following subcutaneous injections of nadroparin-calcium in a patient with osteomalacia. *Br J Dermatol* 2005; **153**: 657–60.

20 Subramaniam K, Wallace H, Sinniah R *et al*. Complete resolution of recurrent calciphylaxis with long-term intravenous sodium thiosulfate. *Australas J Dermatol* 2008; **49**: 30–4.

21 Rogers NM, Teubner DJ, Coates PT. Calcific uremic arteriolopathy: advances in pathogenesis and treatment. *Semin Dial* 2007; **20**: 150–7.

22 Hanafusa T, Yamaguchi Y, Tani M *et al*. Intractable wounds caused by calcific uremic arteriolopathy treated with bisphosphonates. *J Am Acad Dermatol* 2007; **57**: 1021–5.

23 Niemi KM. Panniculitis of the legs with urate crystal deposition. *Arch Dermatol* 1977; **113**: 655–6.

24 Le Boit PE, Schneider S. Gout presenting as lobular panniculitis. *Am J Dermatopathol* 1987; **9**: 334–8.

25 Snider AA, Barsky S. Gouty panniculitis: a case report and review of the literature. *Cutis* 2005; **76**: 54–6.

26 Dahiya A, Leach J, Levy H. Gouty panniculitis in a healthy male. *J Am Acad Derm* 2007; **57**: S52–S54.

27 Vernon SE, Dave SP. Cutaneous zygomycosis associated with urate panniculitis. *Am J Dermatopathol* 2006; **28**: 327–30.

28 Forström L, Winkelmann RK. Factitial panniculitis. *Arch Dermatol* 1974; **110**: 747–50.

29 Harisdangkul V. Factitial panniculitis. *Illinois Med J* 1978; **154**: 358–60.

30 Harada M, Shimada M, Fukayama M *et al*. Crystal-storing histiocytosis associated with lymphoplasmacytic lymphoma mimicking Weber–Christian disease: immunohistochemical, ultrastructural and gene-rearrangement studies. *Hum Pathol* 1996; **27**: 84–7.

Enzymic panniculitis

Synonym
- Pancreatic panniculitis [1]

Clinically, enzymic panniculitis overlaps closely with nodular panniculitis (Weber–Christian type) and leads to foci of subcutaneous fat necrosis. Systemic features are quite common, including arthritis, pleural effusions and ascites. The erythematous subcutaneous nodules tend to be present in the distal part of the extremities (often around periarticular areas). In milder cases, the nodule(s) can be single and resolve without ulcerating [2], mimicking erythema nodosum (Fig. 46.13), but usually they evolve into sterile necrotic abscesses, which spontaneously ulcerate and exude a thick, brown, oily material, which represents adipose tissue that has undergone liquefaction necrosis (Fig. 46.14).

Subcutaneous fat necrosis affects 2–3% of all patients with diseases of the pancreas [3]. It appears that all three pancreatic enzymes (lipase, trypsin and amylase) are needed to induce fat necrosis [4]. In 40% of cases associated with pancreatic-induced subcutaneous fat necrosis, the skin lesions were the presenting feature [5]. Monoarticular or oligoarticular arthritic symptoms are common, and may also precede diagnosis of pancreatic disease [6]. The nature of the pancreatic pathology can vary widely. Surgical correction of an anatomical ductal anomaly [7] or pancreatic pseudocyst [8] can result in complete resolution of panniculitis.

The syndrome has been described in post-traumatic pancreatitis [9], acute and chronic pancreatitis [10] and pancreatic carcinoma [1]. CT scanning can be useful in delineating the pancreatic lesion, as well as outlining areas of subcutaneous fat necrosis [11]. Rarely, acute panniculitis can be associated with a high urinary amylase excretion in the absence of overt pancreatic disease [12]. The association of subcutaneous fat necrosis with pancreatic disease has been reported in systemic lupus erythematosus [13].

Pancreatic panniculitis has been reported in association with primary human immunodeficiency virus (HIV) infection and a haemophagocytic syndrome [14], and in pancreatitis associated with hypertriglyceridaemia [15].

The histological changes of pancreatic panniculitis are unique but rarely encountered. Focal fat necrosis in the lobules occurs, which is probably initiated by circulating enzymes (Fig. 46.15). A characteristic coagulative necrosis of lipocytes ensues, which leads to ghosts of lipocytes and varying degrees of calcification [1]. In older lesions, fat necrosis and 'ghost' lipocytes become less prominent, and are replaced by a granulomatous infiltrate with Langhans' giant cells [1] (Fig. 46.16). In the very early stages of pancreatic panniculitis, a septal pattern of inflammatory involvement has been described [16].

The treatment of pancreatic panniculitis is primarily supportive and dependent on the underlying pancreatic pathology. Occasionally, complete resolution of symptoms occurs when gallstones are removed [17] or when an anatomical ductal anomaly has been divided [7]. Usually, the prognosis is gloomy. In a review of 27 patients with pancreatic panniculitis, all eight cases with pancreatic carcinoma and 42% of the 19 patients with pancreatitis died of their disease [18].

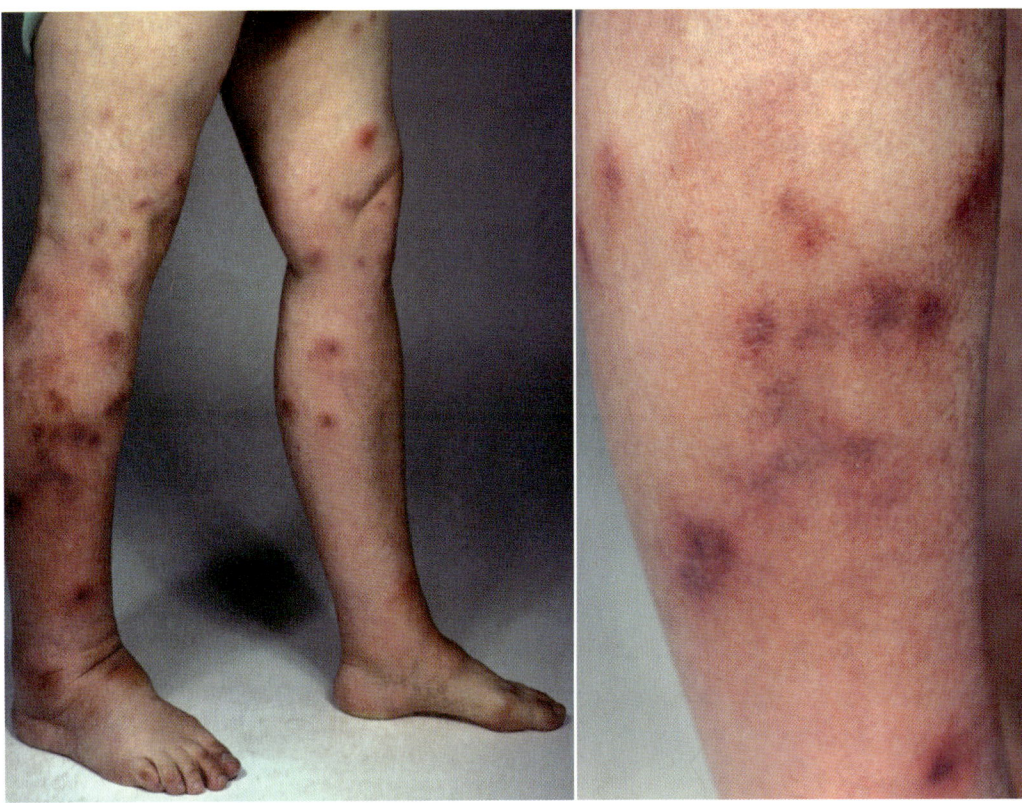

Fig. 46.13 Enzymic (pancreatic) panniculitis: transient nodules after cholecystitis mimicking erythema nodosum.

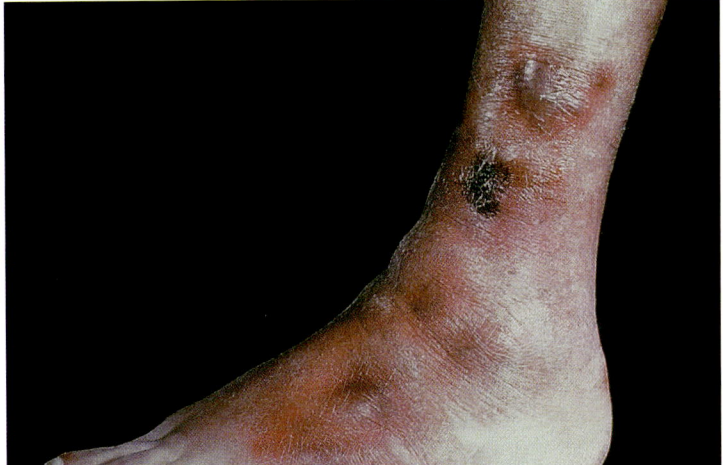

Fig. 46.14 Enzymic (pancreatic) panniculitis: suppurative nodules occurring around the ankles in a patient with pancreatic carcinoma.

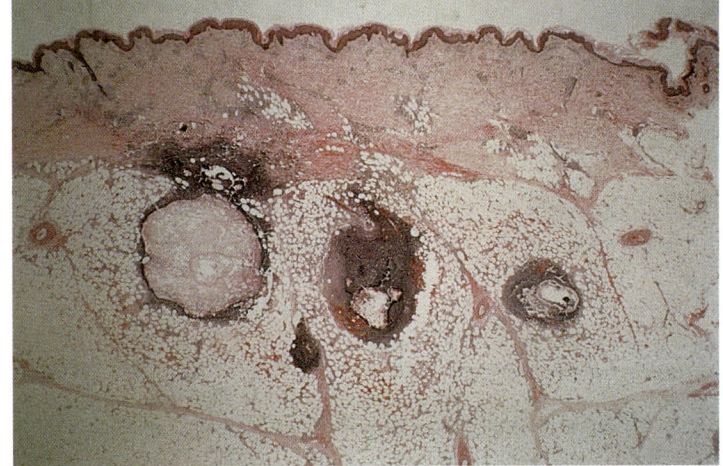

Fig. 46.15 Enzymic (pancreatic) panniculitis: low-power view showing foci of fat necrosis in lobules. H&E, × 4.

References

1 Dahl PR, Su WPD, Cullimore KC *et al.* Pancreatic panniculitis. *J Am Acad Dermatol* 1995; **33**: 413–7.

2 Herrera-Sanchez M, Suarez Fernandez R, Gomez Calcerrada MR. Single-nodule pancreatic panniculitis. *Dermatology* 1996; **193**: 269.

3 Sibrack LA, Goutermann IH. Cutaneous manifestations of pancreatic diseases. *Cutis* 1978; **21**: 763–8.

4 Panabokké RG. An experimental study of fat necrosis. *J Pathol Bacteriol* 1958; **75**: 319–31.

5 Hughes SH, Apisarnthanarax P, Mullins F. Subcutaneous fat necrosis associated with pancreatic disease. *Arch Dermatol* 1975; **111**: 506–10.

6 Saag KG, Niemann TH, Warner CA *et al.* Subcutaneous pancreatic fat necrosis associated with acute arthritis. *J Rheumatol* 1992; **19**: 630–2.

7 Haber RM, Assaad DM. Panniculitis associated with a pancreas division. *J Am Acad Dermatol* 1986; **14**: 331–4.

8 Millns JL, Evans HL, Winkelmann RK. Association of islet cell carcinoma of the pancreas with subcutaneous fat necrosis. *Am J Dermatopathol* 1979; **1**: 273–80.

9 Lee MS, Lowe PM, Nevell DF *et al.* Subcutaneous fat necrosis following traumatic panniculitis. *Australas J Dermatol* 1995; **36**: 196–8.

10 Cheng KS, Stansby G, Law N *et al.* Recurrent panniculitis as the first clinical manifestation of recurrent acute pancreatitis to cholelithiasis. *J R Soc Med* 1996; **89**: 106.

11 Patel JC, Robertson EM. Computed tomography appearances of acute pancreatitis presenting as polyarthropathy with subcutaneous fat necrosis. *Scot Med J* 1993; **38**: 183–4.

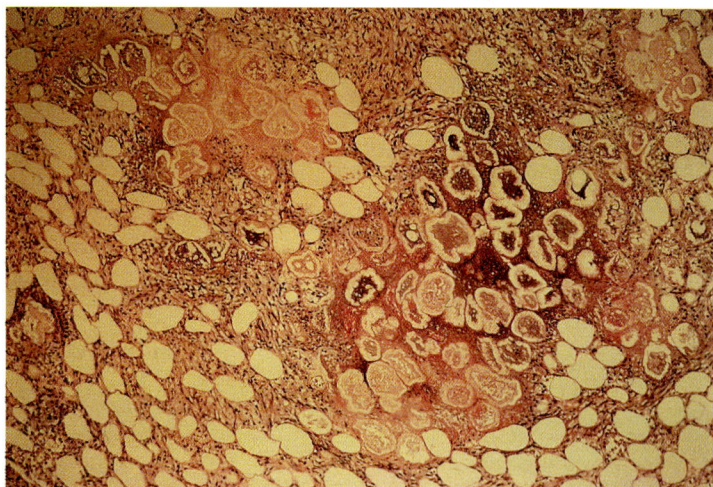

Fig. 46.16 Enzymic (pancreatic) panniculitis: coagulative necrosis of lipocytes, associated with ghosts of lipocytes and focal calcification. H&E, × 40.

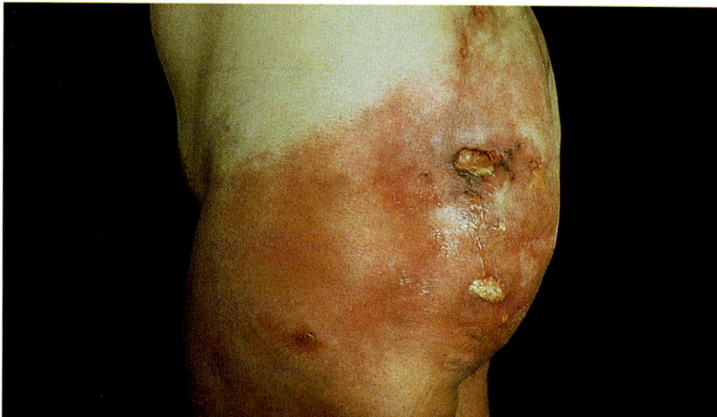

Fig. 46.17 Severe suppurative panniculitis secondary to deficiency of α₁-antitrypsin. (Courtesy of Dr M.R. Pittelkow, Mayo Clinic, Rochester, MN, USA.)

12 Förström L, Winkelmann RK. Acute, generalised panniculitis with amylase and lipase in the skin. *Arch Dermatol* 1975; **111**: 497–502.
13 Cutlan RT, Wesche WA, Jenkins SJ III *et al.* A fatal case of pancreatic panniculitis presenting in a young patient with systemic lupus. *J Cutan Pathol* 2000; **27**: 466–71.
14 Martinez-Escribano JA, Pedro F, Sabater V *et al.* Acute exanthem and pancreatic panniculitis in a patient with primary HIV infection and haemophagocytic syndrome. *Br J Dermatol* 1996; **134**: 804–7.
15 Suwattee P, Cham PM, Pope E *et al.* Pancreatic panniculitis in a 4-year-old child with nephrotic syndrome. *Pediatr Dermatol* 2007; **24**: 659–60.
16 Ball NJ, Adams SPA, Marx LH *et al.* Possible origin of pancreatic fat necrosis as a septal panniculitis. *J Am Acad Dermatol* 1996; **34**: 362–4.
17 Riaz AA, Smith F, Phylactides L *et al.* Panniculitis complicating gallstone pancreatitis with subsequent resolution after therapeutic endoscopic retrograde cholangiopancreatography. *Br J Dermatol* 2000; **143**: 1332–3.
18 Potts DE, Mass MF, Iseman MD. Syndrome of pancreatic disease, subcutaneous fat necrosis and polyserositis. *Am J Med* 1975; **58**: 417–23.

α₁-Antitrypsin-deficiency panniculitis (MIM +107400)

Subcutaneous panniculitis simulating Weber–Christian syndrome may be associated with deficiency of α₁-protease inhibitor (α₁-antitrypsin) [1].

Aetiology. Severe deficiency of this important inhibitor in the blood is inherited as the ZZ phenotype, which occurs in about 1 in 2500 people [2]. Severe deficiencies of α₁-antitrypsin can be associated with emphysema, hepatitis, cirrhosis, vasculitis, urticaria, angio-oedema and panniculitis.

The alleles of the gene involved are measured by electrophoretic ability and divided into medium (M), slow (S) and very slow (Z). MM is normal. Homozygous deficiency with phenotype ZZ is most commonly associated with panniculitis, although heterozygous deficiency with phenotype MZ has also been implicated [2,3] as has SS [4]. Patients with the MM phenotype have normal α₁-antitrypsin blood levels, whilst those with ZZ have the lowest.

α₁-Antitrypsin inhibits trypsin activity, but it is also active against neutrophil elastase, pancreatic elastase, serine proteases, collagenase, factor VIII and kallikrein [5].

The exact pathogenesis of the panniculitis is obscure, but deficiency of α₁-antitrypsin could accelerate the activation of lympho-cytes and phagocytes, thus producing severe inflammation as well as tissue necrosis secondary to protease action.

Pathology. Characteristically, the panniculitis is severely necrotic and suppurative, involving lobules and septae. Vasculitis, haemorrhage or phlebothrombosis can occur in areas of severe inflammation. The end result can be extensive liquefactive necrosis of the dermis and fibrous septae in the subcutis, leading to transepidermal elimination of necrotic material. Even so, large areas of normal fat can be found adjacent to necrotic lobular and septal areas, which contain abundant polymorphonuclear leukocytes and macrophages [6]. In the earliest stage of inflammation, splaying of neutrophils between collagen bundles in the reticular dermis has been noted [7].

Clinical features. The age of onset of the panniculitis ranges from infancy to old age. Early lesions may resemble a cellulitis, as has been described in Marshall's syndrome (Sweet's syndrome leading to acquired cutis laxa), which has been reported to be associated with α₁-antitrypsin deficiency, and may represent part of the disease spectrum [8]. A clue to the diagnosis of α₁-antitrypsin deficiency is that the ulcerative lesions occur predominantly on the trunk and proximal extremities [2] (Fig. 46.17). The clinical findings of ulcerative panniculitis, combined with the histological findings of acute inflammation, necrosis and haemorrhage, certainly justify investigation of α₁-antitrypsin blood levels. Some of the lesions may be precipitated by trauma, and can be exacerbated by surgical debridement [6]. Even cryosurgery has been implicated [9].

Treatment. Dapsone [10] or doxycycline [11] can be very effective in controlling panniculitis [2,10], while systemic steroids, antimalarials and immunosuppressive drugs often give an inconsistent response. For patients with more severe manifestations of disease (e.g. emphysema, lung fibrosis and liver failure), replacement with weekly intravenous α₁-antitrypsin (Prolastin®) offers a valuable treatment [2]. Each patient requires approximately 10 g/month; the treatment is expensive and not licensed everywhere [12], but may be life-saving even for patients with panniculitis [13].

References

1 Warter J, Storck D, Grosshans E *et al.* Syndrome de Weber–Christian associé à un déficit en α_1-antitrypsine: enquête familiale. *Ann Med Interne (Paris)* 1972; **123**: 877–82.
2 Smith KC, Pittelkow MR, Su WPD. Panniculitis associated with severe α_1-antitrypsin deficiency. *Arch Dermatol* 1987; **123**: 1655–61.
3 Hendrick SJ, Silvermann AK, Solomon AR *et al.* α_1-Antitrypsin deficiency associated with panniculitis. *J Am Acad Dermatol* 1988; **18**: 684–92.
4 Pinto AR, Maciel LS, Carneiro F *et al.* Systemic nodular panniculitis in a patient with alpha-1 antitrypsin deficiency (PiSS phenotype). *Clin Exp Dermatol* 1993; 18: 154–5.
5 Su WPD, Smith KC, Pittelkow MR *et al.* α_1-Antitrypsin deficiency panniculitis: a histopathologic and immunopathologic study of four cases. *Am J Dermatol* 1987; **9**: 483–90.
6 Smith KC, Su WPD, Pittelkow MR *et al.* Clinical and pathologic correlations in 96 patients with panniculitis, including 15 patients with deficient levels of α_1-antitrypsin. *J Am Acad Dermatol* 1989; **21**: 1192–6.
7 Geller JD, Su WPD. A subtle clue to the histopathologic diagnosis of early α_1-antitrypsin deficiency panniculitis. *J Am Acad Dermatol* 1994; **31**: 241–5.
8 Hwang ST, Williams ML, McCalmont TH *et al.* Sweet's syndrome leading to acquired cutis laxa (Marshall's syndrome) in an infant with α_1-antitrypsin deficiency. *Arch Dermatol* 1995; **131**: 1175–7.
9 Linares-Barnios M, Conejo-Min JS, Artola Igarza JL *et al.* Panniculitis due to α_1-antitrypsin deficiency induced by cryosurgery. *Br J Dermatol* 1998; **138**: 552–3.
10 Irvine C, Neild V, Stephens C *et al.* α_1-Antitrypsin deficiency panniculitis. *J R Soc Med* 1990; **83**: 743–4.
11 Chng WJ, Henderson CA. Suppurative panniculitis associated with α_1-antitrypsin deficiency (PiSZ phenotype) treated with doxycycline. *Br J Dermatol* 2001; **144**: 1282–3.
12 Ortiz PG, Skov BG, Benfeldt E. Alpha1-antitrypsin deficiency-associated panniculitis: case report and review of treatment options. *J Eur Acad Dermatol Venereol* 2005; **19**: 487–90.
13 Chowdhury MM, Williams EJ, Morris JS *et al.* Severe panniculitis caused by homozygous ZZ alpha1-antitrypsin deficiency treated successfully with human purified enzyme (Prolastin). *Br J Dermatol* 2002; **147**: 1258–61.

Fat necrosis

Fat necrosis is often an important accompanying feature in panniculitis, and can be prominent enough and sufficiently distinctive to merit separate description. Insults to the fat, including cold injury [1] or trauma [2], are well known to cause fat necrosis, often when there is accompanying venous insufficiency in the lower legs.

Cold panniculitis

Synonym
• Adiponecrosis e frigore (Haxthausen's disease) [1]

Cold panniculitis is a form of localized panniculitis that results from cold injury to subcutaneous fat.

Aetiology. The condition has been reported in neonates [2], children [1,3] and adults, notably as a consequence of ice cubes [4], ice packs [2] or exposure to mountain rivers [4,5] or freezing air temperatures, particularly in adults with a chilblain-type of circulation [6]. Cold panniculitis of the thighs or buttocks may occur in skiers or horse riders who wear inadequate clothing [6], although in this situation perniosis is more common than true panniculitis histologically [7]. Children sucking ice lollies (popsicles) can induce cold panniculitis in the facial subcutaneous tissues [8].

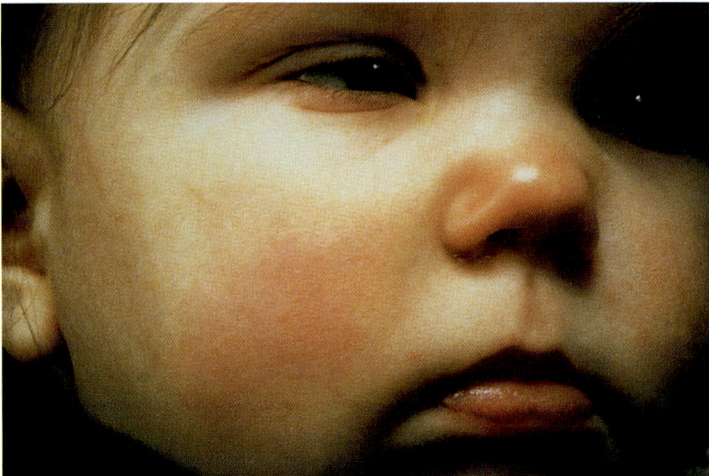

Fig. 46.18 Cold panniculitis: erythematous nodular area on the malar region of a 6-month-old infant which developed after exposure to a very cold wind. (Courtesy of Dr D.J. Atherton, St John's Institute of Dermatology, King's College London, UK.)

Pathology. The early features show a perivascular lymphohistiocytic infiltrate at the dermal–subcutaneous junction with established lesions showing a lobular panniculitis with a mixed infiltrate [5].

Clinical features. Some 48–72 h after cold exposure, the affected areas become indurated with an ill-defined margin. The inflamed skin may be red or bluish, but the diagnostic test is that the area is cold to the touch (Fig. 46.18). The subject may complain of a cold sensation or a dull ache. If the area is kept warm, the subcutaneous plaques slowly soften and resolve over weeks without scarring.

Differential diagnosis. The clinical appearances may resemble other forms of panniculitis (especially erythema induratum) but can usually be distinguished by the location, history of prior cold exposure and being cold to the touch.

Treatment. Cold panniculitis resolves spontaneously if further exposure to cold injury is avoided. In horse riders, tight jeans should be replaced by several layers of looser and thicker clothing. If the limb becomes thoroughly chilled, rapid rewarming should be avoided. Vasodilators tend not to be helpful [9]. One case had a dramatic response to tetracycline which was also effective prophylactically [10].

References

1 Haxthausen H. Adiponecrosis e frigore. *Br J Dermatol* 1941; **53**: 83–9.
2 Ter Poorten JC, Hebert AA, Ilkiw R. Cold panniculitis in a neonate. *J Am Acad Dermatol* 1995; **33**: 383–5.
3 Baruchin AM, Scharf S. Cold panniculitis in children (Haxthausen's disease). *Burns Incl Thermal Injury* 1988; **14**: 51–2.
4 Price RD, Murdoch DR. Perniosis (chilblains) of the thigh: report of five cases, including four following river crossings. *High Alt Med Biol* 2001; **2**: 535–8.
5 Solomon LM, Beerman H. Cold panniculitis. *Arch Dermatol* 1963; **88**: 897–900.
6 Beacham BE, Cooper PH, Buchanan S *et al.* Equestrian cold panniculitis in women. *Arch Dermatol* 1980; **116**: 1025–7.
7 Wall JM, Smith NP. Perniosis: a histopathological review. *Clin Exp Dermatol* 1981; **6**: 263–71.

8 Day S, Klein BL. Popsicle panniculitis. *Pediatr Emerg Care* 1992; **8**: 91–3.
9 Dowd PM. Cold-related disorders. *Prog Dermatol* 1986; **20**: 1–8.
10 Aroni K, Aivaliotis M, Tsele E *et al*. An unusual panniculitis appearing in the winter with good response to tetracycline. *J Dermatol* 1998; **25**: 677–81.

Nodular cystic fat necrosis [1]

> **Synonym**
> • Encapsulated fat necrosis [2]

The term denotes a characteristic form of encapsulated subcutaneous fat necrosis that presents as solitary or multiple subcutaneous nodules.

Aetiology. Early lesions begin as lobules of adipose tissue, which, because of compromised blood supply, often following trauma, become separated from the surrounding tissue [3]. These lobules subsequently become surrounded by thin fibrous tissue, and remain as encapsulated necrotic tissue or later undergo dystrophic calcification.

Pathology. The lesions are totally or nearly totally encapsulated, showing massive fat necrosis with preservation of the outlines of non-nucleated adipocytes, usually with little in the way of inflammatory changes. Fibrous septae within the lesion, and dystrophic calcification, tend to be seen in older lesions. Focal or extensive lipomembranous changes may coexist [4,5].

Clinical features. The painless lesions occur often on the lower legs of healthy adolescent boys or middle-aged women. The lesions can be solitary or multiple, often mobile, and varying from 2 to 35 mm in diameter, though 'giant-sized' cases 15–18 cm have been reported [4,6]. Multiple lesions have been described in both systemic lupus erythematosus and systemic sclerosis [7,8]. Preceding trauma is present in about 30% of cases. The nodules may be present for several weeks to years before excision. During surgical removal, a smooth-walled cyst within the subcutaneous fat containing solitary or multiple, free-floating or attached nodules is usually found. Nodular cystic fat necrosis is probably not uncommon, but not readily recognized. Similar changes in the fat have been reported within the abdominal cavity [9] or within the abdominal wall [10]. Some authors take the view that encapsulated angiolipomas and encapsulated lipomas are variants of nodular cystic fat necrosis, with a variable degree of vascularity [2,11].

Differential diagnosis. This includes lipoma, angiolipoma, pancreatic fat necrosis and membranous fat necrosis.

References

1 Przyjemski CJ, Schuster SR. Nodular-cystic fat necrosis. *J Pediatr* 1977; **91**: 605–7.
2 Kiryu H, Rikihisa W, Furue M. Encapsulated fat necrosis: a clinicopathological study of eight cases and a literature review. *J Cutan Pathol* 2000; **27**: 19–23.
3 Hurt MA, Santa Cruz DJ. Nodular-cystic fat necrosis. *J Am Acad Dermatol* 1989; **21**: 493–8.
4 Felipo F, Vaquero M, del Agua C. Pseudotumoral encapsulated fat necrosis with diffuse pseudomembranous degeneration. *J Cutan Pathol* 2004; **31**: 565–7.

5 Pujol RM, Wang CY, Gibson LE *et al*. Lipomembranous changes in nodular-cystic fat necrosis. *J Cutan Pathol* 1995; **22**: 551–5.
6 Sonmez E, Safak T, Kecik A. Giant nodular cystic fat necrosis: a report of a rare case. *J Plast Reconstr Aesthet Surg* 2009; **62**: 152–4.
7 Demitsu T, Yoneda K, Iida E *et al*. A case of nodular cystic fat necrosis with systemic lupus erythematosus presenting the multiple subcutaneous nodules on the extremities. *J Eur Acad Dermatol Venereol* 2008; **22**: 885–6.
8 Toritsugi M, Yamamoto T, Nishioka K. Nodular cystic fat necrosis with systemic sclerosis. *Eur J Dermatol* 2004; **14**: 353–5.
9 Lynn TE, Dockerty MB, Waugh JM. A clinicopathological study of the epiploic appendages. *Surg Gynecol Obstet* 1956; **103**: 423–33.
10 Herbert DC, DeGeus J. Post-traumatic lipomas on the abdominal wall. *Br J Plast Surg* 1975; **28**: 303–6.
11 Sahl WJ Jr. Mobile encapsulated lipomas: formerly called encapsulated angiolipomas. *Arch Dermatol* 1978; **114**: 1684–6.

Lipomembranous fat necrosis [1]

> **Synonym**
> • Membranocystic fat necrosis

Lipomembranous fat necrosis is a striking and distinctive alteration in adipose tissue that was first described in Nasu–Hakola disease, a genetic disorder characterized by profound membranocystic degeneration of long bones and systemic adipose tissue, with associated progressive sudanophilic leukodystrophy of the brain [2]. Cystic areas of fat necrosis are lined by wavy hyaline acidophilic membranes (Fig. 46.19). Convoluted projections and arabesques of the membranes into the interior of the cysts are prominent [3]. The membranous structures stain brightly with periodic acid–Schiff but are resistant to diastase. Ultrastructurally, the membranes consist of two layers [4].

Changes of lipomembranous fat necrosis can occur as a nonspecific reaction pattern in a wide range of autoimmune diseases, including lupus erythematosus [3], diabetes mellitus [3], morphoea [5] and dermatomyositis [6]. It may also be seen in panniculitis induced by chemotherapy [7]. In a clinical and pathological correlation of 1806 biopsies of panniculitis, lipomembranous fat necrosis was only identified in 13 cases [3]. It is now clear that venous stasis and ischaemia are important co-factors [1,3,8,9] in

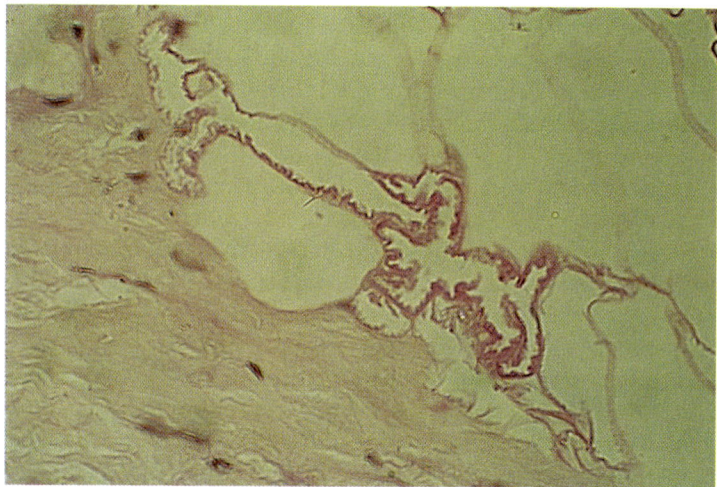

Fig. 46.19 Lipomembranous fat necrosis: the cystic areas are lined by wavy hyaline membranes. Periodic acid–Schiff (PAS) stain, × 25.

the development of lipomembranous fat necrosis. Most cases are seen in middle-aged, obese women who develop venous stasis-associated chronic sclerotic plaques on the lower legs and ankles [1]. The condition therefore overlaps with, or is a part of, sclerosing panniculitis [10], lipodermatosclerosis; some consider it to be a non-specific finding [11].

References

1 Snow JL, Su WPD. Lipomembranous (membrano-cystic) fat necrosis. *Am J Dermatopathol* 1996; **18**: 151–5.

2 Nasu T, Tsukahara Y, Terayama K. A lipid metabolic disease 'membranous lipodystrophy': an autopsy case demonstrating numerous peculiar membrane structures composed of compound lipid in bone and bone marrow and various adipose tissues. *Acta Pathol Jpn* 1973; **23**: 539–58.

3 Alegre VA, Winkelmann RK, Aliaga A. Lipomembranous changes in chronic panniculitis. *J Am Acad Dermatol* 1988; **19**: 39–46.

4 Sueki H, Shinura Y, Fujisawa R *et al.* Ultrastructural study of the histogenesis of membranocystic lesions (Nasu) in diabetes. *J Cutan Pathol* 1986; **13**: 390–401.

5 Snow JL, Su WPD, Gibson LE. Lipomembranous (membranocystic) changes associated with morphoea: a clinicopathologic study of three cases. *J Am Acad Dermatol* 1994; **31**: 246–50.

6 Ishikawa O, Tamura A, Ryuzaki K *et al.* Membranocystic changes in the panniculitis of dermatomyositis. *Br J Dermatol* 1996; **134**: 773–6.

7 Akay OM, Urer SM, Oner U *et al.* Lipomembranous panniculitis in a patient with acute leukemia induced by chemotherapy. *Leuk Res* 2008; **32**: 669–71.

8 Ahn S, Yoo M, Lee S. A clinical and histopathological study of 22 patients with membranous lipodystrophy. *Clin Exp Dermatol* 1996; **21**: 269–72.

9 Machinami R. Incidence of membranous lipodystrophy-like change among patients with limb necrosis caused by chronic arterial obstruction. *Arch Pathol Lab Med* 1984; **108**: 823–6.

10 Jorizzo JL, White WL, Zanolli MD *et al.* Sclerosing panniculitis: a clinico-pathologic assessment. *Arch Dermatol* 1991; **127**: 554–8.

11 Fernandoz-López E, Peñá-Peñabad C, Garcia Silva J *et al.* Membranous fat necrosis: a non-specific histological finding. *Eur J Dermatol* 2002; **12**: 82–4.

Panniculitis caused by cellular proliferative disease

Subcutaneous T-cell lymphoma is a rare type of peripheral T-cell lymphoma, which clinically and histologically may mimic benign forms of panniculitis [1]. Erythematous subcutaneous nodules localized to the extremities appear in crops, often accompanied by fever and malaise [1,2]. The lymphoma may behave indolently for months to years, but in most cases it enters an acute aggressive phase in which the majority of patients develop fatal haemophagocytic syndrome [3] or sometimes acute leukaemia [4].

Although low-power histological appearances may resemble benign panniculitis, high-power examination reveals cytological atypia of the malignant lymphoid cells, and immunochemistry studies confirm the T-cell lineage [5]. Angiocentric lymphoma can also cause lobular granulomatous panniculitis [6,7].

Cytophagic histiocytic panniculitis [1,2]

Cytophagic histiocytic panniculitis is the term commonly used to refer to the specific cutaneous manifestation of haemophagocytic syndrome (HPS) [3].

In HPS, there is a histiocytic proliferation throughout the reticuloendothelial system. The proliferation and phagocytic activity of histiocytes in HPS is associated with a proliferation of lymphocytes [3]. Indeed, the primary abnormality in cytophagic histiocytic panniculitis may be a clonal T-cell proliferation [8], though in familial HPS the genetic defect leads to an inability of natural killer cells to kill target cells, allowing lymphocytes and macrophages to proliferate [9].

Aetiology. The proliferation of lymphocytes and histiocytes in HPS may be secondary to microbial, particularly viral, infections (e.g. Epstein–Barr virus [10], cytomegalovirus), may be associated with autoimmune disease such as lupus erythematosus [11,12], or neoplastic in origin [2]. Cytophagic histiocytic panniculitis has been reported as a late complication of allogeneic bone marrow transplantation [13]. HPS has a higher rate of mortality when it is associated with a state of known immunosuppression, and has been reported in HIV-1 infections [2]. Indeed, lymphoma and infection may act as co-factors in the development of HPS. It has been postulated that in HPS cytokine production by the proliferating lymphocytes is important as a stimulus to activate macrophages [2]. In the light of a new classification of subcutaneous T-cell lymphoma [14], and case reviews [15], the histological picture of cytophagic histiocytic panniculitis may be thought of as occurring against a background of infection, in association with other diseases, particularly autoimmune, or in association with malignancy. Malignancy is further subdivided into subcutaneous panniculitis-like T-cell lymphoma of α/β T-cell phenotype (SPTL-AB) and SPTL with a γ/δ T-cell phenotype (SPTL-GD) [14]. Only 20% of SPTL-AB patients exhibit haemophagocytosis in the skin, compared to all SPTL-GD ones. Many SPTL-AB patients also have autoimmune diseases. SPTL-GD patients are now included in the cutaneous γ/δ T-cell lymphoma group (CGD-TCL) because of their poor prognosis.

Pathology [16]. Cytophagic histiocytic panniculitis may begin as a type of regional histiocytosis that primarily involves the subcutis. In most cases, the condition spreads to involve the bone marrow, lymph nodes and reticuloendothelial system. The affected tissues are gradually replaced by a syncytium of histiocytic cells with associated T lymphocytes and plasma cells. The histiocytes are actively cytophagic, so that they become stuffed with white blood cells, red cells, nuclear fragments and platelets, thus giving them a characteristic 'bean-bag' appearance (Fig. 46.20).

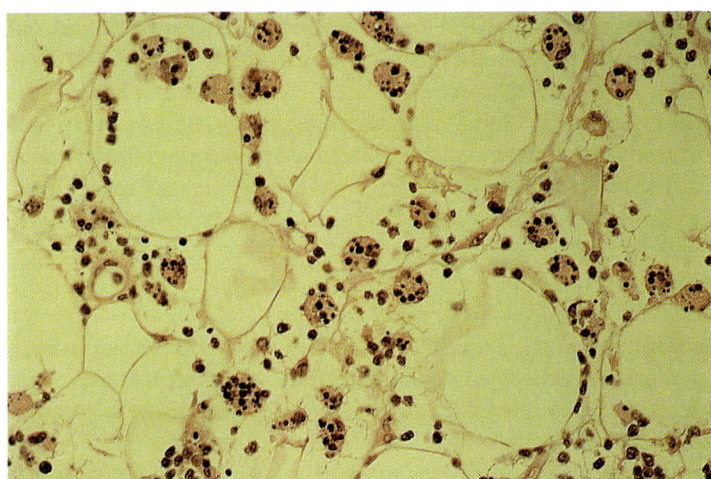

Fig. 46.20 Cytophagic histiocytic panniculitis: many histiocytes are present in the fat lobule, showing the characteristic 'bean-bag' appearance. H&E, × 25.

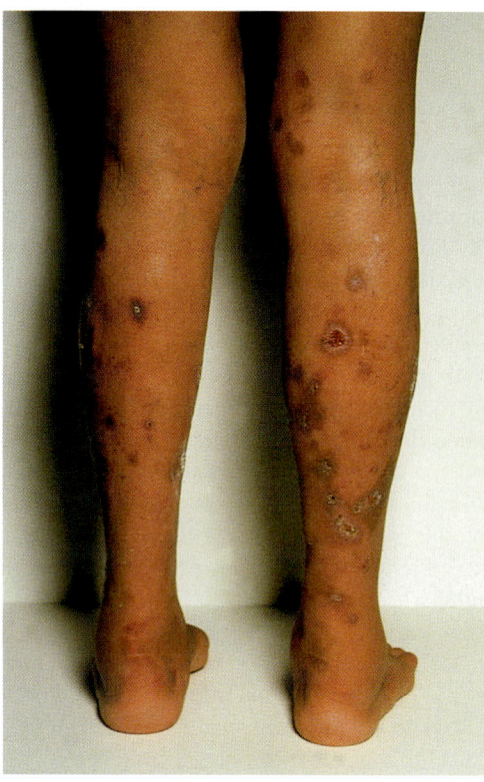

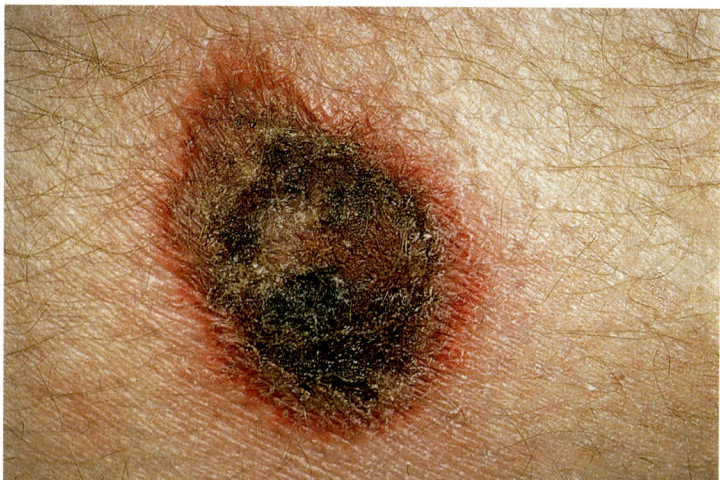

Fig. 46.22 Cytophagic histiocytic panniculitis: note the haemorrhagic nature of this early lesion on the thigh. (Courtesy of St John's Institute of Dermatology, King's College London, UK.)

Fig. 46.21 Cytophagic histiocytic panniculitis: early stage with recurrent crops of lesions. (Courtesy of the Mayo Clinic, Rochester, MN, USA.)

The histiocytic proliferation is accompanied by lobular panniculitis with areas of fat necrosis, together with massive hyaline necrosis, oedema and haemorrhage [16]. Immunohistochemical studies tend to show that the histiocytic population is benign, whereas the lymphoid element, whether benign or malignant, is composed primarily of T cells [2]. SPTL-AB lymphoma shows a lobular panniculitis with a lymphocytic infiltrate showing cells of variable size and irregularity. Rimming of individual adipocytes by neoplastic T cells is common. The presence of plasma cells points to the possibility of lupus erythematosus profundus being associated, whose gene rearrangement is polyclonal. The immunophenotype of SPTL-AB lymphoma is CD3+, CD8+ and CD4−. Conversely, the infiltrate in SPTL-GD is more extensive and diffuse, and involves the overlying dermis as well as the lobules; there is less rimming, it is more angioinvasive, and is comprised of more medium–large, irregular lymphocytes. The immunophenotype is CD3+, CD8− and CD4− and very often CD56+. *In-situ* hybridization for Epstein–Barr virus is negative in both. The diagnosis is confirmed by the presence of the appropriate clonal gene rearrangement [14].

Clinical features. This is a rare condition, which in the past has probably been labelled as systemic nodular panniculitis (Weber–Christian syndrome) [17,18]. The condition begins with crops of red tender nodules, associated with fever (Fig. 46.21). The nodules often develop a purpuric or bruised appearance (Fig. 46.22). The condition can be acute, or chronic with a febrile course associated with anaemia and pancytopenia. More severe cases tend to display

weight loss, thrombocytopenia, raised liver enzymes, serosal effusions and hepatosplenomegaly [17–19].

Most patients have a progressive form of the disease, which is ultimately fatal. The fatal progression is usually determined by the development of severe anaemia, thrombocytopenia and coagulation defects provoking bleeding, hypocalcaemia and liver failure [18,19]. At this stage, the development of terminal T-cell lymphoma [20,21], B-cell lymphoma [22,23], histiocytic lymphomas [24] or sinus histiocytosis with massive lymphadenopathy (Rosai–Dorfman) [25] may also be evident. The complex coagulation defects are not fully understood. There may be a combination of thrombocytopenia or thrombocytosis, decreased factor VIII and fibrinogen levels, and an increase in excretion of fibrin degradation products. It has been suggested that these abnormalities in coagulation may be caused by a circulating proteolytic enzyme other than thrombin, which may originate from proliferating lymphocytes [26].

However, prolonged survival after combination-type chemotherapy has been reported, even in cases where the clinical features indicate a poor prognosis [11,27]. Monitoring of phagocytic activity may be of value in assessing disease activity [11].

Treatment. Many cases are ultimately fatal, and for the progressive forms combination cytotoxic chemotherapy should be tried [10,19]. Prolonged survival or even complete remission have been reported with this type of treatment schedule [27,28]. Ciclosporin has been reported to be effective in cytophagic histiocytic panniculitis [29], presumably by suppression of the abnormal T-cell activation and proliferation. Combinations of systemic corticosteroids and azathioprine have been reported to be effective [30], as has the use of intravenous immunoglobulins [31]. The prognosis appears to depend on the presence or absence of systemic features of HPS and, if T-cell lymphoma is present, whether it is SPTL-AB or SPTL-GD in type. If systemic features of HPS are present (fever, unexplained cytopenia in two out of three lineages of the peripheral blood, hyperferritinaemia and histological evidence of haemophagocytosis in bone marrow or lymph node), then treatment should be directed there, but prognosis is poor [9]. SPTL-AB lymphoma may need only systemic steroids or immunosuppressive agents, whereas SPTL-GD lymphoma needs aggressive chemotherapy [14].

References

1 Marzano AV, Berti E, Paulli M et al. Cytophagic histiocytic panniculitis and subcutaneous panniculitis-like T-cell lymphoma. *Arch Dermatol* 2000; **136**: 889–96.

2 Wick MR, Patterson JW. Cytophagic histiocytic panniculitis: a critical reappraisal. *Arch Dermatol* 2000; **136**: 922–4.

3 Smith KJ, Skelton HG, Yeager J et al. Cutaneous histopathologic, immunohistochemical, and clinical manifestations in patients with haemophagocytic syndrome. *Arch Dermatol* 1992; **128**: 193–200.

4 Romero LS, Goltz RW, Nagi C et al. Subcutaneous T-cell lymphoma with associated haemophagocytic syndrome and terminal leukemic transformation. *J Am Acad Dermatol* 1996; **34**: 904–10.

5 Monterroso V, Bujan W, Jaramillo O. Subcutaneous tissue involvement by T-cell lymphoma. *Arch Dermatol* 1996; **132**: 1345–50.

6 Takeshita M, Akamatso M, Oshima K et al. Angiocentric immunoproliferative lesions of the skin show lobular panniculitis and are mainly disorders of large granular lymphocytes. *Hum Pathol* 1995; **26**: 1321–8.

7 Takeshita M, Kimura N, Suzumiya J et al. Angiocentric lymphoma with granulomatous panniculitis in the skin expressing natural killer cell and large granular T-cell phenotypes. *Virchows Arch* 1994; **425**: 499–504.

8 Hytiroglou P, Phelps RG, Wattenberg DJ et al. Histiocytic cytophagic panniculitis: molecular evidence for a clonal T-cell disorder. *J Am Acad Dermatol* 1992; **27**: 333–6.

9 Arceci RJ. When T cells and macrophages do not talk: the hemophagocytic syndromes. *Curr Opin Hematol* 2008; **15**: 359–67.

10 Harada H, Iwatsuki K, Kaneko F. Detection of Epstein–Barr virus genes in malignant lymphoma with clinical and histologic features of cytophagic histiocytic panniculitis. *J Am Acad Dermatol* 1994; **31**: 379–83.

11 Zollner TM, Podda M, Ochsendorf FR et al. Monitoring of phagocytic activity in histiocytic cytophagic panniculitis. *J Am Acad Dermatol* 2001; **44**: 120–3.

12 Tsukahara T, Horiuchi Y, Iidaka K. Cytophagic histiocytic panniculitis in systemic lupus erythematosus. *Hiroshima J Med Sci* 1995; **44**: 13–6.

13 Galande J, Vazquez ML, Almeida J et al. Histiocytic cytophagic panniculitis: a rare late complication of allogeneic bone marrow transplantation. *Bone Marrow Transplant* 1994; **14**: 637–9.

14 Willemze R, Jansen PM, Cerroni L et al; EORTC Cutaneous Lymphoma Group. Subcutaneous panniculitis-like T-cell lymphoma: definition, classification, and prognostic factors: an EORTC Cutaneous Lymphoma Group Study of 83 cases. *Blood* 2008; **111**: 838–45.

15 Craig AJ, Cualing H, Thomas G et al. Cytophagic histiocytic panniculitis – a syndrome associated with benign and malignant panniculitis: case comparison and review of the literature. *J Am Acad Dermatol* 1998; **39**: 721–36.

16 Alegre VA, Winkelmann RK. Histiocytic cytophagic panniculitis. *J Am Acad Dermatol* 1989; **20**: 177–85.

17 White JW Jr, Winkelmann RK. Cytophagic histiocytic panniculitis is not always fatal. *J Cutan Pathol* 1989; **16**: 137–44.

18 Crotty CP, Winkelmann RK. Cytophagic histiocytic panniculitis with fever, cytopenia, liver failure and terminal haemorrhagic diathesis. *J Am Acad Dermatol* 1981; **4**: 181–94.

19 Winkelmann RK, Walter Bowie EJ. Haemorrhagic diathesis associated with benign, histiocytic, cytophagic panniculitis and systemic histiocytosis. *Arch Intern Med* 1980; **140**: 1460–3.

20 Coupe M, Foroni L, Stamp G et al. Clonal rearrangement of the T-cell receptor γ gene associated with a bizarre lymphoproliferation syndrome. *Eur J Haematol* 1988; **41**: 289–94.

21 Avinoach I, Halery S, Argou S et al. Gamma/Delta T-cell lymphoma involving the subcutaneous tissue and associated with a haemophagocytic syndrome. *Am J Dermatopathol* 1994; **16**: 426–33.

22 Ando I, Okitsu H, Kukita A et al. A case of haemophagocytic syndrome associated with B-cell lymphoma. *J Eur Acad Dermatol Venereol* 1995; **4**: 77–81.

23 Peters MS, Winkelmann RK. Cytophagic panniculitis and B-cell lymphoma. *J Am Acad Dermatol* 1985; **13**: 882–5.

24 Jaffe ES, Costa J, Fauci AS et al. Malignant lymphoma and erythrophagocytosis simulating malignant histiocytosis. *Am J Med* 1983; **75**: 741–8.

25 Suster S, Cartagena N, Cabello-Inchausti B et al. Histiocytic lymphophagocytic panniculitis: an unusual extranodal presentation of sinus histiocytes with massive lymphadenopathy (Rosai–Dorfman disease). *Arch Dermatol* 1988; **124**: 1246–9.

26 Henriksson P. Generalised proteolysis in a young woman with Weber–Christian disease. *Scand J Haematol* 1975; **14**: 355–60.

27 Alegre VA, Fortea JM, Camps C et al. Cytophagic histiocytic panniculitis: case report with resolution after treatment. *J Am Acad Dermatol* 1989; **20**: 875–8.

28 Masue K, Itoh M, Tsukuda K et al. Successful treatment of cytophagic histiocytic panniculitis with modified CHOP-E. *Am J Clin Oncol* 1994; **17**: 470–4.

29 Royle G, Blacklock H, Miller M. Treatment of cytophagic panniculitis with cyclosporine A. *Am J Med* 1992; **92**: 704–5.

30 Pettersson T, Kariniemi AL, Tervonen S et al. Cytophagic histiocytic panniculitis: a report of four cases. *Br J Dermatol* 1992; **127**: 635–40.

31 Gill DS, Spencer A, Cobcroft RG. High-dose gammaglobulin therapy in the reactive haemophagocytic syndrome. *Br J Haematol* 1994; **88**: 204–6.

Mixed (septal and lobular) panniculitis

Lupus panniculitis

Synonym
• Le profundus

Lupus panniculitis is a rare condition in which the inflammatory changes primarily affect the deep dermis and subcutaneous fat. The overlying skin may be associated with discoid lupus erythematosus (LE) in 20% of cases [1,2]. The serum antinuclear antibody is usually positive in approximately 70% of cases, but only 25–50% fulfil the American Rheumatism Association criteria for systemic LE [1,2]. However, there are a significant number of cases of lupus panniculitis that never meet the criteria for systemic LE, and some have no extracutaneous manifestations [3]. Many patients with lupus panniculitis tend to have a relatively mild but usually chronic disease course [3]. Lupus panniculitis is seen predominantly in females [1–4], usually young adults, though childhood [5–7] and neonatal [8] cases do occur. It arises spontaneously but can be triggered by injury such as immunization [7] (Fig. 46.23). Local injections of glatiramer acetate for multiple sclerosis have induced lupus panniculitis-like histology in some instances [9]. Hepatitis B vaccination has reactivated old lesions of lupus profundus [10], whilst interferon-beta has induced new ones [11]. Some cases have been associated with complement deficiencies [7] which might have made the disease more extensive [12].

Clinical features. The lesions begin with subcutaneous nodules or plaques, where the overlying skin may appear normal, erythematous or may show changes characteristic of discoid LE [2]. The lesions can be painful and may ulcerate, leading to atrophy and scarring after healing [13], even giving an anetoderma-like appearance [14].

Common sites for nodules include thighs, buttocks, arms, breasts and face (Fig. 46.24). When breast tissue is involved (lupus mastitis), there may be difficulty in distinguishing lupus mastitis from breast carcinoma, even on mammography [15]. Indeed, lupus mastitis may account for 10% of all patients with lupus

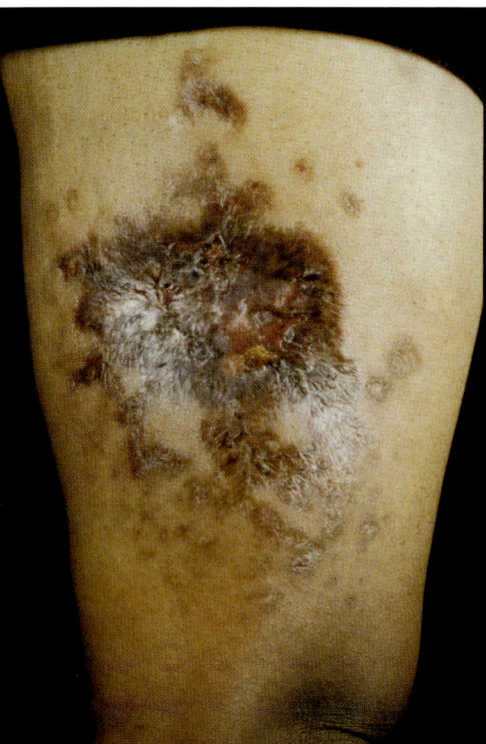

Fig. 46.23 Lupus panniculitis originally triggered by immunization. (Courtesy of St John's Institute of Dermatology, King's College London, UK.)

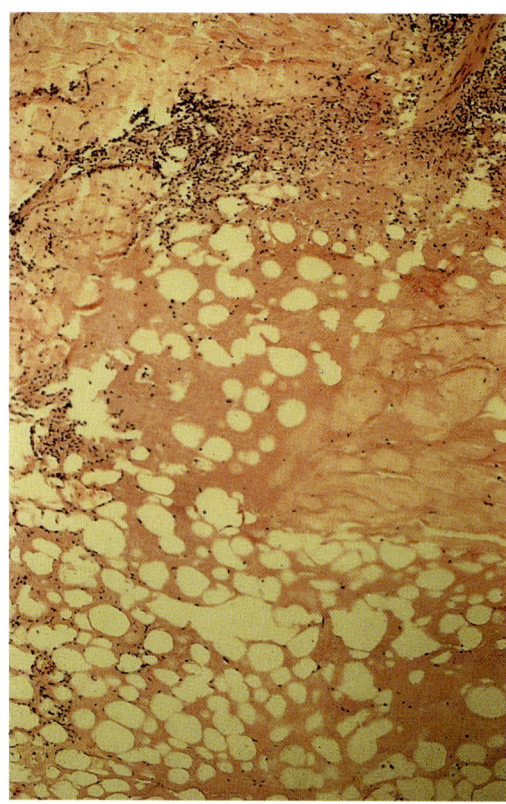

Fig. 46.25 Lupus panniculitis: extensive hyaline necrosis of fat with overlying lymphocytic aggregates are shown. H&E, × 4.

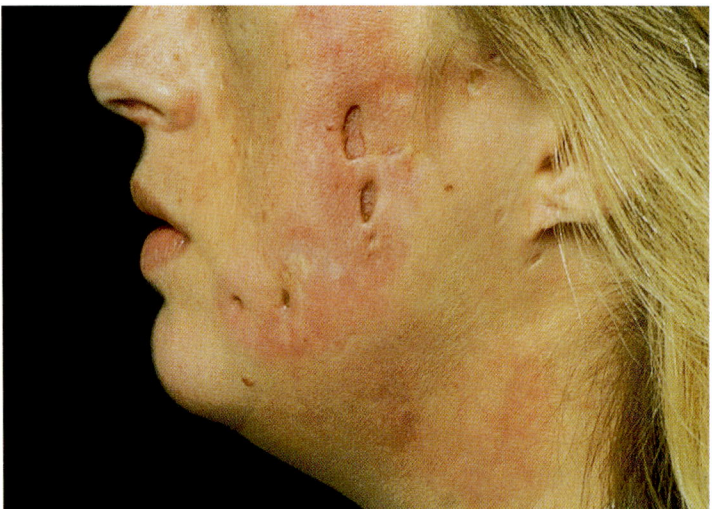

Fig. 46.24 Lupus panniculitis. (Courtesy of St John's Institute of Dermatology, King's College London, UK.)

panniculitis [16]. In black patients, peri-orbital oedema may be the initial presentation [4]. Many cases of lupus panniculitis may have only mild extracutaneous features, but the coexistence of photosensitivity, arthritis, pericarditis, renal involvement [3] and even neuropsychiatric manifestations has been reported [16].

Perhaps not surprisingly, lupus panniculitis can overlap with morphoea-like lesions [17], dermatomyositis [18] or other forms of connective tissue panniculitis [4]. Linear variants have been described [19,20].

Pathology. The major histological criteria needed for a diagnosis of lupus panniculitis include hyaline necrosis of fat, lymphocytic aggregates or lymphoid follicle formation, periseptal or lobular lymphocytic panniculitis, and calcification [1] (Fig. 46.25). Minor changes (not necessary for diagnosis) include overlying changes of discoid LE, hyalinization of the subepidermal zone, mucin deposition, lymphocytic vascular inflammation and collections of plasma cells and eosinophils [21]. Karyorrhexis from lymphocyte nuclear dust is common and a strong pointer [1,22]. The main differential diagnosis is subcutaneous panniculitis-like T-cell lymphoma (SPTL), where the presence of atypical CD8+ve T lymphocytes and the absence of septal fibrosis, B-cell follicles, and plasma cells are major clues [22]. Rimming of adipocytes by lymphocytes is common in lupus profundus and not diagnostic of SPTL. A lupus band on immunofluorescence is positive in most cases, even in the absence of epidermal changes on routine histopathology [1].

Treatment. Treatment can be difficult in chronic forms of lupus panniculitis. Local treatment in the form of potent corticosteroids under hydrocolloid dressings [23] or intralesional triamcinolone can be of benefit. Dapsone [24], oral hydroxychloroquine [4,5] and corticosteroids [4,15] can be effective in the management of lupus panniculitis. Low-dose thalidomide can be effective for antimalarial drug-resistant cases of discoid LE and LE profundus [7,25].

References

1 Sánchez NP, Peters MS, Winkelmann RK. The histopathology of lupus erythematosus panniculitis. *J Am Acad Dermatol* 1981; **5**: 673–80.

2 Tuffanelli DL. Lupus erythematosus panniculitis (profundus): clinical and immunologic studies. *Arch Dermatol* 1971; **103**: 231–42.

3 Watanabe T, Tsuchida T. Lupus erythematosus profundus: a cutaneous marker for a distinct clinical subset? *Br J Dermatol* 1996; **134**: 123–5.

4 Jacyk WK, Bhana KN. Lupus erythematosus profundus in black South Africans. *Int J Dermatol* 2006; **45**: 717–21.

5 Fox JN, Klapman MH, Rowe L. Lupus profundus in children: treatment with hydroxychloroquine. *J Am Acad Dermatol* 1987; **16**: 839–44.

6 Wimmershoff MB, Hohenleutner, M, Landthaler M. Discoid lupus erythematosus and lupus profundus in childhood: A report of two cases. *Pediatr Dermatol* 2003; **20**: 140–5.

7 Burrows NP, Walport MJ, Hammond AH *et al.* Lupus erythematosus profundus with partial C4 deficiency responding to thalidomide. *Br J Dermatol* 1991; **125**: 62–7.

8 Nitta Y. Lupus erythematosus profundus associated with neonatal lupus erythematosus. *Br J Dermatol* 1997; **136**: 112–4.

9 Ball NJ, Cowan BJ, Moore GR, Hashimoto SA. Lobular panniculitis at the site of glatiramer acetate injections for the treatment of relapsing-remitting multiple sclerosis. A report of two cases. *J Cutan Pathol* 2008; **35**: 407–10.

10 Choffray A, Pinquier L, Bachelez H. Exacerbation of lupus panniculitis following anti-hepatitis-B vaccination. *Dermatology* 2007; **215**: 152–4.

11 Gono T, Matsuda M, Shimojima Y *et al.* Lupus erythematosus profundus (lupus panniculitis) induced by interferon-beta in a multiple sclerosis patient. *J Clin Neurosci* 2007; **14**: 997–1000.

12 Nousari HC, Kimyai-Asadi A, Provost TT. Generalized lupus erythematosus profundus in a patient with genetic partial deficiency of C4. *J Am Acad Dermatol* 1999; **41**: 362–4.

13 Winkelmann RK. Panniculitis in connective tissue disease. *Arch Dermatol* 1983; **119**: 61–4.

14 Marzano A, Vanotti M, Alessi E. Anetodermic lupus panniculitis and antiphospholipid antibodies: report of three cases. *Acta Derm Venereol* 2004; **84**: 385–8.

15 Cernea SS, Kihara SM, Sotto MN *et al.* Lupus mastitis. *J Am Acad Dermatol* 1993; **29**: 343–6.

16 Biedermann T, Schirren CG, Meurer M *et al.* Lupus erythematosus profundus: Kaposi–Irgang. *Eur J Dermatol* 1996; **6**: 519–22.

17 Stork J, Vosmik F. Lupus erythematosus panniculitis with morphoea-like lesions. *Clin Exp Dermatol* 1994; **19**: 79–82.

18 Yoo JY, Jo SJ, Cho KH. Lupus panniculitis with combined features of dermatomyositis resulting in severe lipoatrophy. *J Dermatol* 2004; **31**: 552–5.

19 Tada J, Arata J, Katayama H. Linear lupus erythematosus in a child. *J Am Acad Dermatol* 1991; **24**: 871–4.

20 Marzano AV, Tanzi C, Caputo R *et al.* Sclerodermic linear lupus panniculitis: report of two cases. *Dermatology* 2005; **210**: 329–32.

21 Peters MS, Su WPD. Eosinophils in lupus panniculitis and morphoea profunda. *J Cutan Pathol* 1991; **18**: 189–92.

22 Massone C, Kodama K, Salmhofer W *et al.* Lupus erythematosus panniculitis (lupus profundus): clinical, histopathological, and molecular analysis of nine cases. *J Cutan Pathol* 2005; **32**: 396–404.

23 Yell JA, Burge SM. Lupus erythematosus profundus treated with clobetasol propionate under hydrocolloid dressings. *Br J Dermatol* 1993; **128**: 103.

24 Yamada Y, Dekio S, Jidai J *et al.* Lupus erythematosus profundus: report of a case treated with dapsone. *J Dermatol* 1989; **16**: 379–82.

25 Housman TS, Jorizzo JL, McCarty MA *et al.* Low dose thalidomide therapy for refractory cutaneous lesions of lupus erythematosus. *Arch Dermatol* 2003; **139**: 50–4.

Panniculitis with complement deficiency

Although complement deficiencies are perhaps better known for their association with lupus erythematosus and partial lipoatrophy syndromes [1], they have also been reported in lobular panniculitis. The association of an immunoglobulin E (IgE) paraproteinaemia and severe acquired depletion of C1-esterase inhibitor with episodes of nodular panniculitis and hepatitis has been reported [2]. Nodular panniculitis has also been associated with a low serum complement, together with a systemic LE-like disease and circulating IgM immune complexes [3].

References

1 Wayte J, Bird G, Wilkinson JD. The clinical significance of partial lipoatrophy and C3 hypocomplementaemia: a report of two cases. *Clin Exp Dermatol* 1996; **21**: 131–4.

2 Pascual M, Widmann JJ, Schifferli JA. Recurrent febrile panniculitis and hepatitis in two patients with acquired complement deficiency and paraproteinaemia. *Am J Med* 1987; **8**: 959–62.

3 Caldwell J, Cusumano C, Ludwig F. Circulating 7S IgM immune complexes and low serum complement in a patient with systemic Weber–Christian disease. *Clin Res* 1974; **22**: 416 (Abstract).

Infective panniculitis

Infective panniculitis (either through direct inoculation or as a manifestation of sepsis) is becoming an increasingly important cause of panniculitis [1]. This is particularly so for any immunocompromised patient, either as a result of steroid or immunosuppressive therapy [2] or brought about by HIV infection [3]. An association of acquired immune deficiency syndrome (AIDS) with cutaneous aspergillosis is developing, and some patients present with subcutaneous nodules [4].

Granulomatous panniculitis on the legs caused by *Candida albicans* has been reported in a diabetic who had not received immunosuppressive treatment [5]. Other occasional cases with infective panniculitis are not overtly immunosuppressed [1].

Clinical features [1]. Most cases of infectious panniculitis appear as inflamed subcutaneous nodules, plaques or ulcers [4] on the lower extremities. Other sites include the shoulders, arms, fingers, abdominal wall and gluteal region. The differential diagnosis includes erythema nodosum, abscess or other type of panniculitis.

A wide variety of organisms have been identified in infective panniculitis. These particularly include Gram-negative [3] and Gram-positive [1] bacteria, *Histoplasma* [2,6], *Mycobacterium tuberculosis* [7], atypical mycobacteria [8,9], *Actinomyces* and *Nocardia* species [1], *Candida* [4] and various fungi [1]. Occasionally, the diagnosis of infective panniculitis has been missed because the infection has occurred in a clinical setting where a non-infective panniculitis was expected [10]. Conversely the situation whereby the patient's clinical setting has suggested that the panniculitis should be infective but tissue staining, culture or PCR was not confirmatory has been labelled panniculitic bacterid [11].

Histology. Classically, in infective panniculitis there is a mixed pattern of septal and lobular involvement. Neutrophilic involvement of the fibrous septae can occur [1], a feature that can rarely overlap with acute erythema nodosum [12]. Indeed, neutrophilic involvement in infective panniculitis can also overlap with other neutrophilic dermatoses (neutrophilic vasculitis and panniculitis) [13]. Certain morphological changes are found in infective panniculitis, whatever the identity of the infective organism. Epidermal involvement is common, as is papillary dermal oedema with diffuse neutrophilic infiltrate, vascular proliferation and haemorrhage [1]. Focal necrosis of sweat glands and discrete microabscess formation may be noted [1].

It is important to stress that infection should be suspected in virtually any case of panniculitis when it is known that the patient is immunocompromised. Extra biopsy material submitted for tissue culture is highly desirable, if not essential [3], as special stains may fail to demonstrate the organisms [1].

References

1 Patterson JW, Brown PC, Broecker AH. Infection-induced panniculitis. *J Cutan Pathol* 1989; **16**: 183–93.

2 Silvermann AK, Gilbert SC, Watkins D *et al.* Panniculitis in an immunocompromised patient. *J Am Acad Dermatol* 1991; **24**: 912–4.

3 Smith RA, Ross JS, Branfoot C *et al.* Panniculitis with *Pseudomonas* septicaemia in AIDS. *J Eur Acad Dermatol Venereol* 1995; **4**: 166–9.

4 Murakawe GJ, Harvell JD, Lubitz P *et al.* Cutaneous aspergillosis and acquired immunodeficiency syndrome. *Arch Dermatol* 2000; **136**: 365–9.

5 Ginter G, Rieger E, Soyer P *et al.* Granulomatous panniculitis caused by *Candida albicans*: a case presenting with multiple leg ulcers. *J Am Acad Dermatol* 1993; **28**: 315–7.

6 Abildgaard WH, Hargrave RH, Kalivas J. *Histoplasma* panniculitis. *Arch Dermatol* 1985; **121**: 914–6.

7 Langenberg A, Egbert B. Neutrophilic tuberculosis panniculitis in a patient with polymyositis. *J Cutan Pathol* 1993; **20**: 177–9.

8 Drabick JJ, Duffy PE, Samlaska CP *et al.* Subspecies cheloniae infection with cutaneous and osseous manifestations. *Arch Dermatol* 1990; **126**: 1064–7.

9 Santa Cruz DJ, Strayer DS. The histologic spectrum of the cutaneous mycobacterioses. *Hum Pathol* 1982; **13**: 485–95.

10 Leung YY, Choi KW, Ho KM, Kun EW. Disseminated cutaneous infection with *Mycobacterium chelonae* mimicking panniculitis in a patient with dermatomyositis. *Hong Kong Med J* 2005; **11**: 515–9.

11 Magro CM, Dyrsen ME, Crowson AN. Acute infectious id panniculitis/panniculitic bacterid: a distinctive form of neutrophilic lobular panniculitis. *J Cutan Pathol* 2008; **35**: 941–6.

12 Forstrom L, Winkelmann RK. Acute panniculitis: a clinical and histopathologic study of 34 cases. *Arch Dermatol* 1977; **113**: 909–17.

13 Jorizzo JL, Solomon AR, Zanolli MD *et al.* Neutrophilic vascular reactions. *J Am Acad Dermatol* 1988; **19**: 983–1005.

Factitial panniculitis [1]

Factitial panniculitis is a rare condition in which the panniculitis is self-inflicted. Its importance lies in the fact that some cases may masquerade as systemic disease or idiopathic Weber–Christian syndrome. The causes and clinical features of factitial panniculitis may vary widely depending on the type of insult to the subcutaneous fat. Factitial panniculitis may result from blunt trauma to the skin, usually on the forearm and hand (l'oedème bleu) [2]. Histologically, such cases may show an organizing haematoma in the fat, together with haemosiderin and amorphous polysaccharide masses [2]. Cupping and acupuncture techniques for relief of pain may rarely lead to factitial panniculitis on the limbs [3]. More commonly, however, factitial panniculitis is induced by injected materials (e.g. drugs and silicone materials). Injected drugs such as morphine, pentazocine, meperidine or tetanus toxoid can all cause chronic ulcerative panniculitis on the thighs and buttocks, associated with 'woody-hard' fibrotic induration (see Fig. 46.12) [4,5]. Silicone injections (used by some patients to augment the size of breasts or genitalia) can cause panniculitis [6], as can the accidental injection of various oily vehicles for therapeutic agents. Povidine, a synthetic polymer used as a dispersing or suspending agent for drugs, has also been reported to cause panniculitis associated with fever [7]. The injection of mineral oil into tissues may induce a granulomatous foreign body reaction (sclerosing lipogranuloma) or 'paraffinoma' [8]. Histologically, paraffinomas show multiple 'Swiss-cheese-like' pseudocystic spaces (Fig. 46.26), which are surrounded by fibrosis and inflammation. Most paraf-

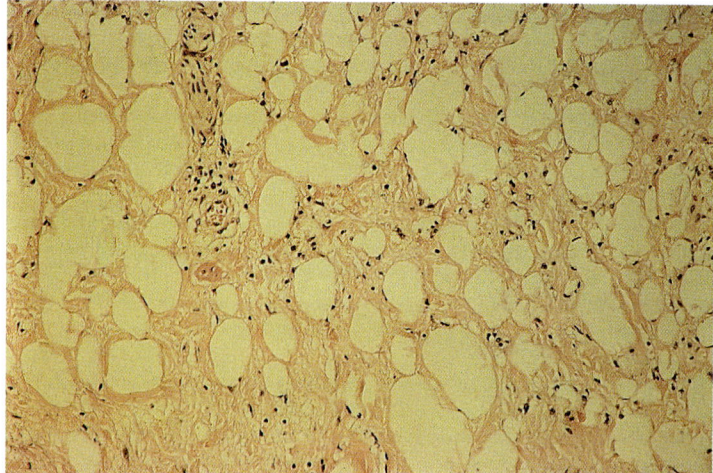

Fig. 46.26 Paraffinoma: showing typical 'Swiss-cheese'-like pseudocystic spaces. H&E, × 25.

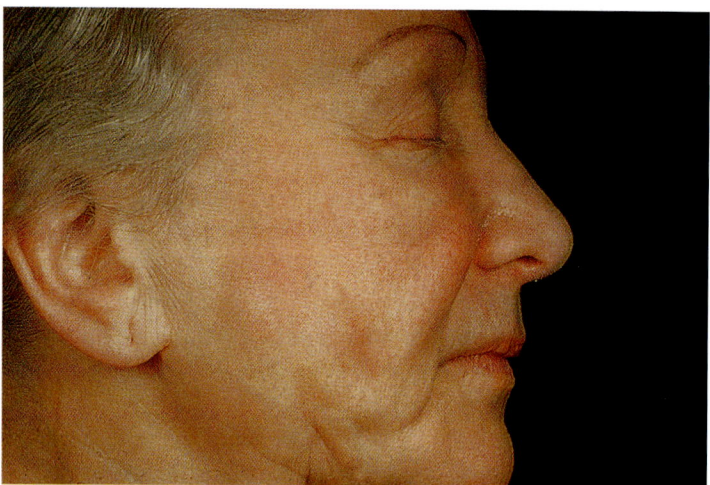

Fig. 46.27 Paraffinoma: firm indurated areas present on the malar areas, following paraffin oil injections many years before for cosmetic purposes. (Courtesy of St John's Institute of Dermatology, King's College London, UK.)

finomas occur on the head and neck area in women who have the injections for cosmetic reasons [9] (Fig. 46.27).

Rarely, however, paraffinomas are not factitial in origin. The development of orbital and palpebral paraffinoma has been reported to ensue after ethmoidectomy for chronic sinusitis, when the nasal cavity was packed with gauze containing a petrolatum-based antibiotic ointment [10]. Mentally disturbed patients have been known to inject milk or faeces, which produces a severe cellulitis or suppurative panniculitis.

Factitial panniculitis simulating pyoderma gangrenosum has also been reported in Münchausen syndrome [11] and eosinophilic panniculitis was triggered by autoinjection of several farming products [12].

Histology. The histology will obviously vary according to the type of noxious injury to the fat. Blunt trauma tends to produce deeper haematomas [2]. Polarization is essential to reveal the possibility of injected crystals [4,5]. The presence of vacuoles or pseudocystic spaces favours the injection of silicone [6] or paraffin [9,10].

The use of scanning electron microscopy or energy-dispersive spectroscopy techniques can aid in the identification of injected materials [6]. In general, factitial panniculitis is a mixed septal and lobular panniculitis that is associated with a prominent degree of inflammatory or granulomatous infiltrate, with fibrosis ensuing.

Differential diagnosis. The diagnosis may be suggested by the personality of the patient, the chronic and recurrent nature of the panniculitis and by its focal or bizarre site. In some cases, there may be fever or systemic symptoms and the condition may then be mistaken for systemic nodular panniculitis (Weber–Christian syndrome).

References

1 Forstrom L, Winkelmann RK. Factitial panniculitis. *Arch Dermatol* 1974; **110**: 747–50.
2 Winkelmann RK, Barker SM. Factitial traumatic panniculitis. *J Am Acad Dermatol* 1985; **13**: 988–94.
3 Lee JS, Ahn SK, Lee SH. Factitial panniculitis induced by cupping and acupuncture. *Cutis* 1995; **55**: 217–8.
4 Palestine RF, Millus JL, Spigel GT *et al.* Skin manifestations of pentazocine abuse. *J Am Acad Dermatol* 1980; **2**: 47–55.
5 Parks DL, Perry HO, Muller SA. Cutaneous complications of pentazocine injections. *Arch Dermatol* 1971; **104**: 231–5.
6 Rae V, Pardo RJ, Blackwelder PL, Falanga V. Leg ulcers following subcutaneous injection of a liquid silicone preparation. *Arch Dermatol* 1989; **125**: 1283–4.
7 Kossard S, Ecker RI, Dicken CH. Povidone panniculitis (polyvinylpyrrolidone panniculitis). *Arch Dermatol* 1980; **116**: 704–6.
8 Goldwyn RM. The paraffin story. *Plast Reconstr Surg* 1980; **65**: 517–24.
9 Bloem JJ, Van der Waal J. Paraffinoma of the face. *Oral Surg* 1974; **38**: 675–80.
10 Feldmann R, Harms M, Chavaz P *et al.* Orbital and palpebral paraffinoma. *J Am Acad Dermatol* 1992; **26**: 833–5.
11 Parent DJ, Krafft T, Noel JC *et al.* Cutaneous Münchausen syndrome with presentation simulating pyoderma gangrenosum. *J Am Acad Dermatol* 1994; **31**: 1072–4.
12 Gómez Rodríguez N, Ortiz-Rey JA, de la Fuente Buceta A *et al.* Auto-induced eosinophilic panniculitis: a diagnostic dilemma. *Ann Med Interne* 2001; **18**: 635–7.

Oil granuloma

Synonyms
- Oleogranuloma
- Oleoma
- Paraffinoma
- Sclerosing lipogranuloma

Definition. A granulomatous reaction to the injection of a relatively bulky oily fluid into the tissues. In many cases the condition overlaps with that of factitial panniculitis, but in some cases it may represent an industrial injury.

Aetiology. Many years ago, mineral oils, particularly liquid paraffin and soft paraffin, were in vogue for improving the contour of the body (breasts, face, genitalia) [1]. Oil granulomas are now less common since the development of less toxic silicones and bovine collagen for tissue replacement, or the use of liposuction techniques, but they still occur [2–4].

Grease-gun injuries can cause sclerosing lipogranulomas [5].

Histology. A massive injection of oil tends to provoke an initial acute inflammatory response, but some mineral oils will remain in the tissue for a considerable time without producing any marked inflammatory reaction. Larger oil droplets become encysted by fibrosis ('onion-skin cysts'). The classical 'paraffinoma' shows multiple, small cystic areas ('Swiss-cheese effect') associated with very little inflammatory change but a prominent degree of fibrosis. Certain animal fats produce a tuberculoid granuloma, whereas vegetable oils, by virtue of irritant substances liberated by hydrolysis, often provoke inflammatory changes and lipophagic granuloma.

Differential diagnosis of a mineral oil granuloma from idiopathic sclerosing lipogranuloma may be very difficult, although the use of scanning electron microscopy and energy-dispersive spectroscopy techniques can be of help [6].

Clinical features. The nodules or plaques usually appear several months after injection, but their onset can be delayed for up to 42 years [7]. Once initiated, the lesions tend to persist indefinitely. Firm, non-tender nodules or plaques form, which may be fixed to both skin and deeper fascia. Ulceration occasionally occurs. The common sites following cosmetic procedures are the face and breasts of women. Nodules on the thighs and buttocks are the result of injections of therapeutic agents in oily vehicles. It is not rare for some patients to strenuously deny any history of earlier injections for cosmetic or therapeutic purposes.

The grease-gun injury characteristically affects the dorsum of the left hand and appears as a nodule, plaque or sinus [2,8]. The onset is more rapid, the patient usually being unaware of the injury, but there may be an anaesthetic period before the gradual onset of swelling, pain and ischaemia. Rapid referral to a plastic surgeon or hand specialist is necessary. Perianal oil granulomas have been reported to follow injections for haemorrhoids [9]. Factitial panniculitis (dermatitis artefacta) can be caused by self-injection of mineral oils or silicones. An analysis of the lipid content in 23 cases of sclerosing lipogranuloma of the male genitalia demonstrated the presence of paraffin hydrocarbons in all specimens [10].

Prognosis. In chronic cases, the lesions remain essentially unchanged almost indefinitely, although the coexistence of squamous cell carcinoma [11,12] and sarcoma has been reported [13]. With acute grease-gun injuries, ischaemic changes may rapidly develop.

Treatment. MRI scanning can be diagnostic and show the extent of the problem [14]. Decompression and clearing of the affected area are needed in grease-gun injuries [2]. Tetanus toxoid may be needed along with high-dose systemic steroids if there has been a delay in diagnosis of grease-gun injuries [2]. If there is any doubt about the diagnosis of chronic oil granuloma, a deep surgical biopsy should be performed. No effective treatment exists other than complete excision.

Idiopathic sclerosing lipogranuloma (eosinophilic sclerosing lipogranuloma)

An idiopathic form of sclerosing lipogranuloma has also been reported [15]. Whilst it is possible that this really represents an oil granuloma in which the history is concealed [8,9], it is a real entity in Japan specifically involving the male genitalia [16,17] and other cases continue to be reported where there is no history of injury or injection [18,19]. Idiopathic lesions are more likely to involve the scrotum rather than penis and to be painless rather than painful. On examination there is usually a Y-shaped, string-like mass in the scrotum at the base of the penis. Peripheral eosinophilia is often present and the histology is also characterized by an eosinophil-rich granulomatous infiltrate with some lipid vacuoles and lipomembranous changes. MRI scanning can contribute to the diagnosis. Spontaneous remission does occur. Trauma and cold injury have been implicated in causation, but eosinophilic sclerosing lipogranuloma is often spontaneous. The diagnostic clue is the tissue and peripheral eosinophilia, which seems not to occur in secondary lipogranulomas.

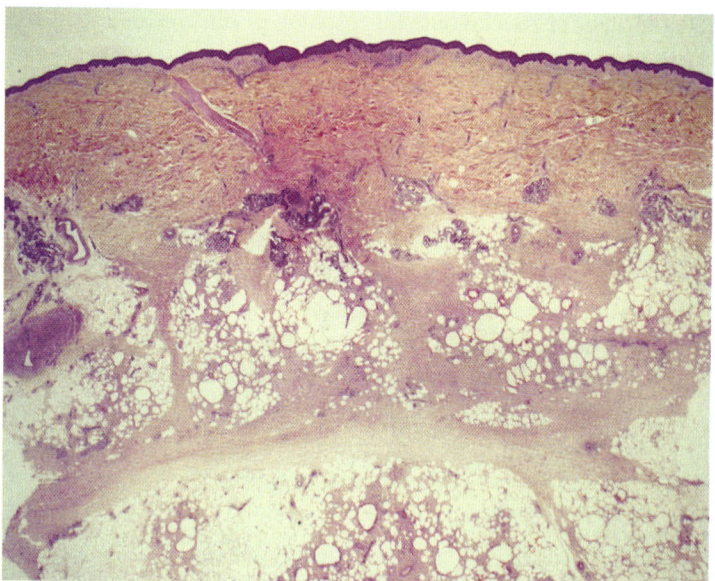

Fig. 46.28 Lipodermatosclerosis with thickened septa, lobular panniculitis and lipomembranous changes.

References

1 Goldwyn RM. The paraffin story. *Plast Reconstr Surg* 1980; **65**: 517–24.
2 D'costa GF, Hastak MS, Agale SV *et al.* Self-inflicted, bilateral oleogranuloma of the breast: report of a bizarre case. *Indian J Pathol Microbiol* 2007; **50**: 373–5.
3 Zickerman PM, Ratanawong C. Penile oleogranuloma among Wisconsin Hmong. *WMJ* 2007; **106**: 270–4.
4 De Gado F, Mazzocchi M, Chiummariello S *et al.* Johnson's baby oil, a new type of filler? *Acta Chir Plast* 2006; **48**: 123–6.
5 Macaulay JC. Occupational high-pressure injection injury. *Br J Dermatol* 1986; **115**: 379–81.
6 Rae V, Pardo RJ, Blackwelder PL *et al.* Leg ulcers following subcutaneous injection of a liquid silicone preparation. *Arch Dermatol* 1989; **125**: 670–3.
7 Klein JA, Cole G, Barr RJ *et al.* Paraffinomas of the scalp. *Arch Dermatol* 1985; **121**: 382–5.
8 Smith MGH. Grease-gun injury. *BMJ* 1964; **ii**: 918–20.
9 Symmers WC. Simulation of cancer by oil granulomas of therapeutic origin. *BMJ* 1955; **ii**: 1536–9.
10 Oertel YC, Johnson FB. Sclerosing lipogranuloma of male genitalia. *Arch Pathol Lab Med* 1977; **101**: 321–6.
11 Ciancio SJ, Coburn M. Penile salvage for squamous cell carcinoma associated with mineral oil injection. *J Urol* 2000; **164**: 1650.
12 Ko CJ, Sarantopoulos GP, Bhuta S *et al.* Scalp paraffinoma underlying squamous cell carcinoma. *Arch Pathol Lab Med* 2004; **128**: 1171–2.
13 Colomb D. L'avenir des paraffinomes. *Ann Dermatol Syphiligr* 1962; **89**: 36–46.
14 Motoori K, Takano H, Ueda T *et al.* Sclerosing lipogranuloma of male genitalia: CT and MR images. *J Comput Assist Tomogr* 2002; **26**: 138–40.
15 Smetana HF, Bernhard WG. Sclerosing lipogranuloma. *Am J Pathol* 1948; **24**: 675–7.
16 Matsuda T, Shichiri Y, Hida S *et al.* Eosinophilic sclerosing lipogranuloma of the male genitalia not caused by exogenous lipids. *J Urol* 1988; **140**: 1021–4.
17 Kojima Y, Inoue H, Adachi Y *et al.* Sclerosing lipogranuloma of the male genitalia: report of 2 cases–review of 72 cases reported in Japan. *Hinyokika Kiyo* 1992; **38**: 93–7.
18 Bussey LA, Norman RW, Gupta R. Sclerosing lipogranuloma: an unusual scrotal mass. *Can J Urol* 2002; **9**: 1464–9.
19 Lim HK, Byun JH, Yoon SE *et al.* Primary sclerosing lipogranuloma of the rectum: CT findings. *Br J Radiol* 2006; **79**: e190–2.

Sclerosing panniculitis [1–4]

Synonyms

• Lipodermatosclerosis [3]
• Hypodermatitis sclerodermaformis [3]

There is growing evidence that the term sclerosing panniculitis encompasses both lipodermatosclerosis and hypodermatitis sclerodermaformis, perhaps appearing in different stages [2]. The term lipodermatosclerosis was coined to describe the effects in the skin of chronic venous hypertension [5]. It is likely that its pathogenesis is multifactorial [6,7] but usually initiated by increased ambulatory venous pressure unrelieved by exercise. The original concept of physical obstruction to oxygen transport by pericapillary fibrin cuffs, slower capillary blood flow, white cell trapping and activation and highly convoluted capillaries, has been superseded by the realization that the changes probably result from highly complex interactions occurring in and around the endothelial cell, involving a huge variety of cytokines and growth factors [8] as well as matrix metalloproteinases [9]. The precise mechanism has yet to be elucidated. Not all cases are overtly associated with chronic venous hypertension [3]. It has been postulated that there may be overlap in the pathogenesis between lipodermatosclerosis and eosinophilic fasciitis [10] and that infective cellulitis may also have a role in exacerbating lipodermatosclerosis [11].

Histologically, there is a combination of fat necrosis and a lobular panniculitis, ultimately leading to fibrous thickening of the fascia and fibrous septae in the subcutis. Lipomembranous changes can coexist [12] (Fig. 46.28).

The patients, usually women in middle age with a high body mass index, gradually develop well-circumscribed, indurated plaques around the lower extremities, usually but not always on the medial aspect. In acute lipodermatosclerosis [3,13] (Fig. 46.29) the plaques are erythematous, painful and tender, simulating cellulitis. In the commoner chronic lipodermatosclerosis the indurated areas are skin coloured, with haemosiderin staining, eventually resulting in fibrotic narrowing of the lower leg.

Standard treatment is weight loss, elevation of legs and use of elastic compression stockings [2], but stockings cannot be tolerated in the acute situation. Stanazolol has been reported to be

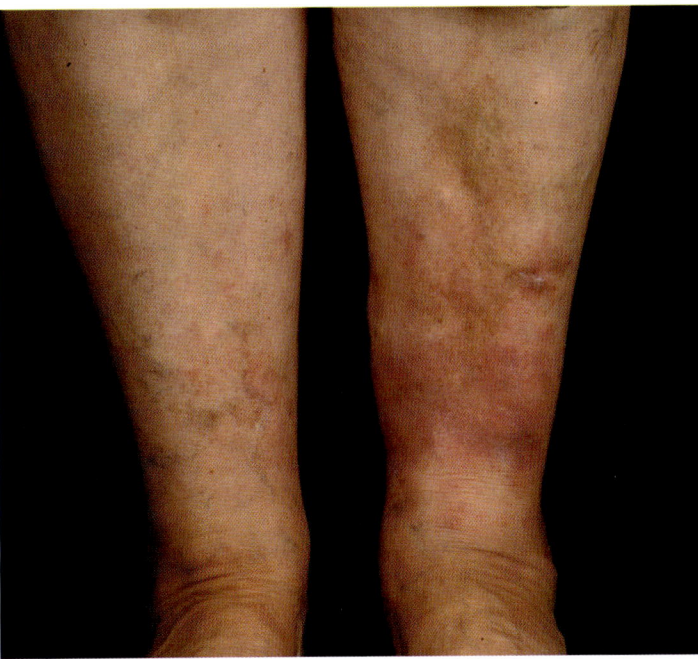

Fig. 46.29 Acute lipodermatosclerosis on the front of the left leg.

effective in both acute [14] and chronic stages [2]. Topical capsaicin is reported to have been of help in the acute stage [15].

References

1 Jorizzo JL, White WL, Zanolli MD *et al.* Sclerosing panniculitis: a clinico-pathologic assessment. *Arch Dermatol* 1991; **127**: 554–8.

2 Kirsner RS, Pardes JB, Eaglestein WH *et al.* The clinical spectrum of lipodermatosclerosis. *J Am Acad Dermatol* 1993; **28**: 623–7.

3 Bruce AJ, Bennett DD, Lohse CM *et al.* Lipodermatosclerosis: a review of cases evaluated at Mayo Clinic. *J Am Acad Dermatol* 2002; **46**: 187–92.

4 Huriez C, Legache G, Desmons F *et al.* Ulcères de jambes et troubles trophiques d'origine veineuse (donnés tirées de l'étude d'un millier d'ulcéreux hospitalisés). *Rev Pract* 1955; **5**: 2703–21.

5 Browse NL, Burnand KG. The cause of venous ulceration. *Lancet* 1982; **2**: 243–5.

6 Naschitz JE, Yeshurun D, Misselvrich I *et al.* The pathogenesis of lipodermatosclerosis: facts, uncertainties and theories. *J Eur Acad Dermatol Venereol* 1997; **9**: 209–14.

7 Valencia IC, Falabella A, Kirsner RS *et al.* Chronic venous insufficiency and venous leg ulceration. *J Am Acad Dermatol* 2001; **44**: 401–21.

8 Smith PC. The causes of skin damage and leg ulceration in chronic venous disease. *Int J Low Extrem Wounds* 2006; **5**: 160–8.

9 Herony Y, May AE, Pornschlegel G *et al.* Lipodermatosclerosis is characterised by elevated expression and activation of matrix metalloproteinases: implications for venous ulcer formation. *J Invest Dermatol* 1998; **111**: 822–7.

10 Naschitz JE, Yeshurun D, Schwartz H *et al.* Pathogenesis of lipodermato-sclerosis of venous disease: the lesson learned from eosinophilic fasciitis. *Cardiovasc Surg* 1993; **1**: 524–9.

11 Naschitz JE, Yeshurun D, Zuckermann E *et al.* The fasciitis–panniculitis syndrome: clinical spectrum and therapeutic response to treatment with cimetidine. *Semin Arthritis Rheum* 1992; **21**: 211–20.

12 Alegre VA, Winkelmann RK, Aliaga A. Lipomembranous changes in chronic panniculitis. *J Am Acad Dermatol* 1988; **19**: 39–46.

13 Greenberg AS, Hasan A, Montalvo BM *et al.* Acute lipodermatosclerosis is associated with venous insufficiency. *J Am Acad Dermatol* 1996; **35**: 566–8.

14 Vesić S, Vuković J, Medenica LJ *et al.* Acute lipodermatosclerosis: an open clinical trial of stanozolol in patients unable to sustain compression therapy. *Dermatol Online J* 2008; **14**: 1.

15 Yosipovitch G, Mengesha Y, Facliaru D *et al.* Topical capsaicin for the treatment of acute lipodermatosclerosis and lobular panniculitis. *J Dermatolog Treat* 2005; **16**: 178–80.

Fasciitis–panniculitis syndromes [1]

In eosinophilic fasciitis and related syndromes, the inflammation often extends to involve the fibrous septae and fat lobules, the subcutaneous fascia which becomes thickened, and the underlying perimysium, resulting in thickened fascia around smaller muscle bundles [1]. It has become increasingly recognized that a histological picture similar to eosinophilic fasciitis, involving the subcutaneous fat, can occur in a variety of diseases, including morphoea profunda [1], lupus panniculitis [1], toxic oil syndrome [2], L-tryptophan-induced eosinophilia–myalgia syndrome [3], graft-versus-host reaction [4], post-irradiation injury [5], infections [6] and cancer-related (paraneoplastic) syndromes [7,8]. The term fasciitis–panniculitis syndromes [1] was coined to draw attention to the fact that any of the above diseases might present with either a plaque or, if on a limb, a sleeve of indurated bound-down skin, unilateral or bilateral, and which had the histology of chronic inflammation with extensive scarring.

References

1 Naschitz JE, Boss JH, Misselvich I *et al.* The fasciitis–panniculitis syndromes: clinical and pathological features. *Medicine* 1996; **75**: 6–16.

2 Alonso-Ruiz A, Zea-Mendoza AC, Salazar-Vallines JM *et al.* Toxic oil syndrome: a syndrome with features overlapping those of various forms of scleroderma. *Semin Arthritis Rheum* 1986; **15**: 200–12.

3 Freundlich B, Werth VP, Rook AH *et al.* L-Tryptophane injection associated with eosinophilic fasciitis but not progressive systemic sclerosis. *Ann Intern Med* 1990; **112**: 758–62.

4 Janin A, Socie G, Devergie A *et al.* Fasciitis in chronic graft-versus-host disease. *Ann Intern Med* 1994; **120**: 993–8.

5 Winkelmann RK, Grado GL, Quimby SR. Pseudosclerodermatous panniculitis after irradiation: an unusual complication of megavoltage treatment of breast carcinoma. *Mayo Clin Proc* 1993; **68**: 122–7.

6 Zuckerman E, Naschitz J, Yeshurun D *et al.* Fasciitis–panniculitis in acute brucellosis. *Int J Dermatol* 1994; **33**: 57–9.

7 Cox NH, Ramsay B, Dobson C *et al.* Woody hands in a patient with pancreatic carcinoma: a variant of cancer-associated fasciitis–panniculitis syndrome. *Br J Dermatol* 1996; **135**: 995–8.

8 Naschitz JE, Yeshurun D, Zuckerman E *et al.* Cancer-associated fasciitis panniculitis. *Cancer* 1994; **73**: 231–5.

Panniculitis in other connective tissue diseases

As already indicated, panniculitis in connective tissue diseases may overlap with lupus panniculitis [1] and also lipoatrophic panniculitis [2]. Deep morphoea (morphoea profunda) may show lipoatrophy, scleroderma-like lesions and deeper subcutaneous nodules or plaques. They may also share some histological features, notably lymphocytic panniculitis, lymphoid nodular areas in the fat, widening of the fibrous septae and lymphocytic vasculitis [3–5].

The association of panniculitis with dermatomyositis is very rare but well documented [6–9]. The parallel course of panniculitis and muscular involvement, and their response to treatment, suggest that panniculitis may be an inherent part of dermatomyositis [6–9]. Subcutaneous nodules or plaques develop on the arms, buttocks, thighs and abdomen, or features of multifocal lipoatrophy may be present [10]. Partial lipoatrophy may also coexist with dermatomyositis [11,12]. The association of panniculitis and dermatomyositis has been reported to respond to a combination of low-dose methotrexate and prednisolone [10], or high-dose intravenous immunoglobulins [13].

References

1 Winkelmann RK. Panniculitis in connective tissue disease. *Arch Dermatol* 1993; **119**: 336–44.

2 Handfield-Jones SE, Stephens CJM, Mayou BJ *et al.* The clinical spectrum of lipoatrophic panniculitis encompasses connective tissue panniculitis. *Br J Dermatol* 1993; **129**: 619–24.

3 Person JR, Su WPD. Subcutaneous morphoea: a clinical study of 16 cases. *Br J Dermatol* 1979; **100**: 371–9.

4 Su WPD, Person JR. Morphoea profunda: a new concept and a histopathologic study of 23 cases. *Am J Dermatopathol* 1981; **3**: 251–60.

5 Whittaker SJ, Smith NP, Jones RR. Solitary morphoea profunda. *Br J Dermatol* 1989; **120**: 431–40.

6 Fusade T, Belanyi P, Joly P *et al.* Subcutaneous changes in dermatomyositis. *Br J Dermatol* 1993; **128**: 451–3.

7 Neidenbach PJ, Sahn EE, Helton J. Panniculitis in juvenile dermatomyositis. *J Am Acad Dermatol* 1995; **33**: 305–7.

8 Winkelmann WJ, Billick RC, Srolovitz H. Dermatomyositis presenting as panniculitis. *J Am Acad Dermatol* 1990; **23**: 127–8.

9 Chao YY, Yang LJ. Dermatomyositis presenting as panniculitis. *Int J Dermatol* 2000; **39**: 141–4.

10 Commens C, O'Neill P, Walker G. Dermatomyositis associated with multifocal lipoatrophy. *J Am Acad Dermatol* 1990; **22**: 966–9.

11 Kavanagh GM, Colaco CB, Kennedy CTC. Juvenile dermatomyositis associated with partial lipoatrophy. *J Am Acad Dermatol* 1993; **28**: 348–51.

12 Torrelo A, España A, Boixeda P *et al.* Partial lipodystrophy and dermatomyositis. *Arch Dermatol* 1991; **127**: 1846–7.

13 Sabroe RA, Wallington TB, Kennedy CTC. Dermatomyositis treated with high-dose intravenous immunoglobulins and associated with panniculitis. *Clin Exp Dermatol* 1995; **20**: 164–7.

Panniculitis with vasculitis

Because the vasculature of the subcutis is 'housed' in the fibrous septae that divide up fat lobules, it is obvious that most deep vasculitis syndromes (particularly large-vessel vasculitis) begin as a septal panniculitis and involve the fat lobules later.

Nearly all cases of leukocytoclastic vasculitis in the subcutis zone also affect the overlying dermis. Nodular forms of vasculitis affecting the fat are primarily dealt with in Chapter 50, together with larger vessel vasculitis syndromes (e.g. polyarteritis nodosa).

This section covers a series of miscellaneous entities that may overlap with vasculitis, or may in some way be associated with them.

Panniculitis has rarely been reported in association with relapsing polychondritis, and histologically was characterized by septal and lobular involvement with vasculitis [1,2]. The association of granulomatous lipophagic panniculitis with temporal arteritis and chronic active hepatitis has been reported, and perhaps represents three-organ manifestations of an underlying aberration of the immune defence mechanism [3].

Unusual forms of vasculitis-associated panniculitis include that resulting from the complications of jejunoileal bypass surgery for obesity (Fig. 46.30) [4,5].

Neutrophilic panniculitis

Subcutaneous neutrophilic infiltrates are a rare accompaniment in atypical Sweet's syndrome and bullous pyoderma gangrenosum

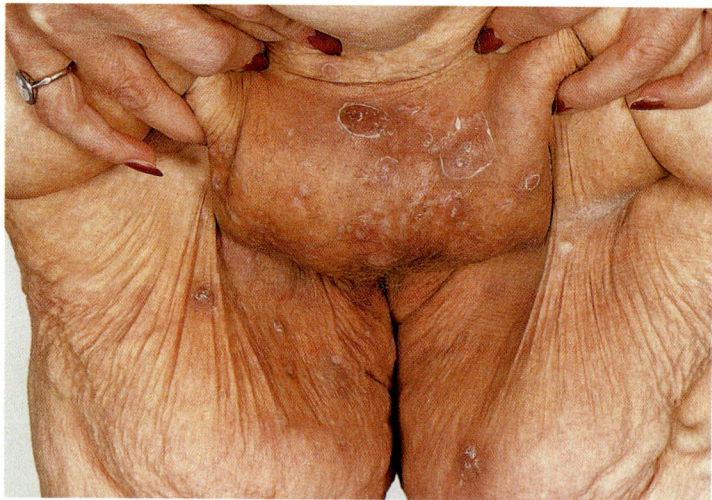

Fig. 46.30 Scarring of lower abdominal folds secondary to panniculitis and/or vasculitis following jejunoileal bypass for gross obesity.

[6]. Recent case reports have highlighted the association of neutrophilic panniculitis with myelodysplastic syndromes [7,8] and sometimes administration of granulocyte colony-stimulating factor (GCSF) [9]. The neutrophilic infiltrates spread out from the septa to the lobules, without evidence of necrotizing panniculitis. It has been postulated that neutrophilic panniculitis belongs to the spectrum of atypical neutrophilic dermatoses associated with myelodysplastic syndromes [7] and inflammatory bowel disease. Septal forms of neutrophilic panniculitis can occur in classical Sweet's syndrome, and may present as erythema nodosum-like eruptions [10]. All-*trans*-retinoic acid chemotherapy triggered a pure lobular neutrophilic panniculitis in a patient with acute promyelocytic leukaemia [11].

A pustular neutrophilic form of panniculitis has been associated with rheumatoid arthritis, both adult [12] and juvenile [13]. Neutrophilic panniculitis is also seen in α_1-antitrypsin deficiency and factitious panniculitis, and it is necessary to exclude an infective organism, particularly in an immunocompromised patient [14]. Occasionally, a neutrophilic panniculitis is seen where infection is expected from the clinical setting but nothing found from the tissue. The term acute infectious id panniculitis or panniculitic bacterid has been coined for this situation [15].

Oedematous scarring vasculitic panniculitis: hydroa-like lymphoma

A condition termed oedematous scarring vasculitic panniculitis has been identified in children, which is described as a novel multisystemic disease with a mortality rate of 35.7% [16]. The cutaneous lesions may initially resemble hydroa vacciniforme, but later disfiguring involvement affects both covered and sun-exposed areas. The lesions develop as oedematous vesicles, which progress to deep ulcerations and varicelliform scars. Histologically, panniculitis and vasculitis coexist with a heavy nodular lymphohistiocytic infiltrate. In cases with systemic involvement, malaise, fever, failure to thrive, leukopenia, thrombocytopenia, hepatosplenomegaly and increased levels of serum C3 have been frequently observed [16]. Several of the patients ultimately developed cutaneous lymphoma, after an interval of 5–8 years, though others wax and wane not unlike lymphomatoid papulosis. Other patients with 'hydroa vacciniforme' have also been reported to develop malignant lymphoma [17–19]. Thirty-one cases of this syndrome have now been reported, and it is likely that the entity is an evolutionary process in the development of malignant lymphoma in children, namely hydroa-like lymphoma. Most cases are CD4 or CD8 positive, but two cases with the natural killer cell phenotype CD56 have been reported [20].

References

1 Disdier P, Andrac L, Swiaden L *et al.* Cutaneous panniculitis and relapsing polychondritis: two cases. *Dermatology* 1996; **193**: 266–8.
2 Smith CR, Sawicka EH, Sheffield E *et al.* Relapsing polychondritis and Weber–Christian disease. *Br J Rheumatol* 1988; **27**: 486–9.
3 Naschitz JE, Yeshurun D, Barth J *et al.* Granulomatous lipophagic panniculitis and temporal arteritis in a patient with cryptogenic chronic active hepatitis. *Ann Rheum Dis* 1992; **51**: 812–4.
4 Kennedy CTC. The spectrum of inflammatory skin disease following jejuno-ileal bypass for morbid obesity. *Br J Dermatol* 1981; **105**: 425–35.
5 Williams HJ, Samuelson CO, Zone JJ. Nodular non-suppurative panniculitis associated with jejuno-ileal bypass surgery. *Arch Dermatol* 1979; **115**: 1091–3.
6 Cooper PH, Frierson HF, Greer KE. Subcutaneous neutrophilic infiltrates in acute febrile neutrophilic dermatosis. *Arch Dermatol* 1983; **119**: 610–1.
7 Matsumara Y, Tanabe H, Wada Y *et al.* Neutrophilic panniculitis associated with myelodysplastic syndromes. *Br J Dermatol* 1997; **136**: 142–4.
8 Suzuki Y, Kuroda K, Kojima T *et al.* Unusual cutaneous manifestations of myelodysplastic syndrome. *Br J Dermatol* 1995; **133**: 483–6.
9 Prendiville J, Thiessen P, Mallory SB. Neutrophilic dermatoses in two children with idiopathic neutropenia: association with granulocyte colony-stimulating factor (G-CSF) therapy. *Pediatr Dermatol* 2001; **18**: 417–21.
10 Blaustein A, Moreno A, Noguera J *et al.* Septal panniculitis in Sweet's disease. *Arch Dermatol* 1985; **121**: 785–8.
11 Jagdeo J, Campbell R, Long T *et al.* Sweet's syndrome-like neutrophilic lobular panniculitis associated with all-trans-retinoic acid chemotherapy in a patient with acute promyelocytic leukemia. *J Am Acad Dermatol* 2007; **56**: 690–3.
12 Anstey A, Wilkinson JD, Wojnarowska F *et al.* Pustular panniculitis in rheumatoid arthritis. *J R Soc Med* 1991; **84**: 307–8.
13 Dyer JA, Guitart J, Klein-Gitelman M *et al.* Neutrophilic panniculitis in infancy: a cutaneous manifestation of juvenile rheumatoid arthritis. *J Am Acad Dermatol* 2007; **57**: S65–8.
14 Patterson JW, Brown PC, Broecker AH. Infection-induced panniculitis. *J Cutan Pathol* 1989; **16**: 183–93.
15 Magro CM, Dyrsen ME, Crowson AN. Acute infectious id panniculitis/panniculitic bacterid: a distinctive form of neutrophilic lobular panniculitis. *J Cutan Pathol* 2008; **35**: 941–6.
16 Ruiz-Maldonado R, Parrilla FM, Orozco-Covarrubias ML *et al.* Oedematous, scarring vasculitic panniculitis: a new multisystemic disease with malignant potential. *J Am Acad Dermatol* 1995; **32**: 37–44.
17 Ibarra-Durán G, Rodriguez-Jurado R, Rodriguez-Moguel L *et al.* Linforma T cutáneo angiocèntrico en niña con hidroa vacciniforme. *Dermatol Rev Mex* 1991; **35**: 344–8.
18 Oono T, Arata J, Masuda T *et al.* Coexistence of hydroa vacciniforme and malignant lymphoma. *Arch Dermatol* 1986; **122**: 1306–9.
19 Steger GG, Dittrich C, Honigsmann H *et al.* Permanent cure of hydroa vacciniforme after chemotherapy for Hodgkin's disease (Letter). *Br J Dermatol* 1988; **119**: 684–5.
20 Doeden K, Molina-Kirsch H, Perez E *et al.* Hydroa-like lymphoma with CD56 expression. *J Cutan Pathol* 2008; **35**: 488–94.

Wells' syndrome [1–4]

Synonyms
- Eosinophilic cellulitis
- Recurrent granulomatous dermatitis with eosinophilia

Definition. This is a syndrome with an impressive and distinctive clinical picture resembling cellulitis, and with a typical histology characterized by tissue eosinophilia, oedema and 'flame' figures.

Aetiology. The syndrome can arise spontaneously or be apparently triggered by a particular stimulus, or be seen in association with other diseases. As such it may represent an allergic hypersensitivity response, with eosinophils playing a dominant role; the mechanism is unknown, but interleukin-5 may be involved [5,6]. Drugs [7] including cladribine for lymphoproliferative disease [8] and adalimumab [9], infection (HIV, herpetic, parasitic and fungal) and insect bites have all been incriminated. In one report, antiviral therapy led to a complete remission of the eosinophilic cellulitis associated with recurrent *Herpes simplex* virus type 2 infection [10]. Reactions to other triggers, such as thiomersal after immunization, can also occur [11]. More recently angioimmunoblastic lymphadenopathy, malignancy and inflammatory bowel disease have been added to the list [12–14]. Eosinophilic fasciitis [6], eosinophilic pustular folliculitis [15], Churg–Strauss syndrome [16] and immunobullous disease are other associations. Rarely, eosinophilic cellulitis is the first presentation of hypereosinophilic syndrome [17] and rarer still it is familial [18].

Pathology. Early on, there is an infiltrate of polymorphs and especially of eosinophils, with considerable oedema. Flame figures are noteworthy—clusters of eosinophils and histiocytes around a core of collagen and eosinophilic debris. The flame figures may disappear after the acute stage with the granulomatous infiltrate becoming more obvious. In bullous lesions, eosinophil-rich subepidermal and intraepidermal vesicles are found, but the dermal changes still dominate. Blood eosinophilia is usual but not invariable.

Clinical features. Wells' syndrome is rare. It can affect either sex, usually in adult life, but some congenital [18], neonatal [19] or childhood cases [20] have occurred. Any site may be involved, with single or multiple lesions. The disease evolves over a few weeks, and recurrences are common. Initially, the lesions are itchy erythematous plaques with features resembling both urticaria and cellulitis, sometimes evolving into a greenish morphoea-like plaque. Any pattern can occur, including unusual nodular variants [21] and lesions that follow the lines of Blaschko [22]. Vesicles and bullae may be dominant [15,16]. After a week or two, the lesions become flatter, and sometimes go through a greenish colour change before resolving without scarring. The general health is usually unimpaired, but fever has been reported, as has arthralgia and mild hepatic dysfunction.

Differential diagnosis. Clinically, erysipelas, cellulitis, urticaria and contact dermatitis are the main differential diagnoses. Multiple lesions in an atypical pattern far apart is a strong clinical pointer. *Toxocara* infections may be similar, both clinically and histologically. Infections such as ascariasis and onchocerciasis need to be excluded. Flame figures can be found in many other diseases, including insect-bite reactions, dermatophyte ide eruptions and pemphigoid; that is wherever the dermal infiltrate is eosinophil rich. The histology in Sweet's syndrome is neutrophil rich, and extra-facial Kimura's disease shows lymphoid follicles. In general, the presence of systemic features, especially if severe, makes the diagnosis of Wells' syndrome unlikely and drug eruption with eosinophilia and systemic symptoms (DRESS) should be excluded, as should hypereosinophilic syndrome or other associated disease.

Treatment. Often no specific treatment is needed. Low-dose systemic steroids can provide symptomatic relief in severe cases [23]. Cetirizine, interferon-α and ciclosporin have all proved effective [24–26].

References

1 Wells GC. Recurrent granulomatous dermatitis with eosinophilia. *Trans St John's Hosp Dermatol Soc* 1971; **57**: 46–56.
2 Wells GC, Smith NP. Eosinophilic cellulitis. *Br J Dermatol* 1979; **100**: 101–9.
3 Aberer W, Konrad K, Wolff K. Wells' syndrome is a distinctive disease entity and not a histological diagnosis. *J Am Acad Dermatol* 1988; **18**: 105–14.
4 Steffen C, Wells GC. Eosinophilic cellulitis (Wells' syndrome). *Am J Dermatopathol* 2002; **24**: 164–5.
5 Espana A, Sanz ML, Sola J et al. Wells' syndrome (eosinophilic cellulitis): correlation between clinical activity, eosinophil levels, eosinophil cation protein and interleukin-5. *Br J Dermatol* 1999; 140: 127–30.
6 French LE, Shapiro M, Junkins-Hopkins JM et al. Eosinophilic fasciitis and eosinophilic cellulitis in a patient with abnormal circulating clonal T cells: increased production of interleukin 5 and inhibition by interferon alfa. *J Am Acad Dermatol* 2003; **49**: 1170–4.
7 Seçkin D, Demirhan B. Drugs and Wells' syndrome: a possible causal relationship? *Int J Dermatol* 2001; **40**: 138–40.
8 Rossini MS, de Souza EM, Cintra ML et al. Cutaneous adverse reaction to 2-chlorodeoxyadenosine with histological flame figures in patients with chronic lymphocytic leukaemia. *J Eur Acad Dermatol Venereol* 2004; **18**: 538–42.
9 Boura P, Sarantopoulos A, Lefaki I, Skendros P et al. Eosinophilic cellulitis (Wells' syndrome) as a cutaneous reaction to the administration of adalimumab. *Ann Rheum Dis* 2006; **65**: 839–40.
10 Ludwig RJ, Grundmann-Kollmann M, Holtmeir W et al. Herpes simplex virus type 2-associated eosinophilic cellulitis (Wells' syndrome). *J Am Acad Dermatol* 2003; **48**: 560–1.
11 Koh KJ, Warren L, Moore L et al. Wells' syndrome following thiomersal-containing vaccinations. *Australas J Dermatol* 2003; **44**: 199–202.
12 Renner R, Kauer F, Treudler R et al. Eosinophilic cellulitis (Wells' syndrome) in association with angioimmunoblastic lymphadenopathy. *Acta Derm Venereol* 2007; **87**: 525–8.
13 Farrar CW, Guerin DM, Wilson NJE. Eosinophilic cellulitis associated with squamous cell carcinoma of the bronchus. *Br J Dermatol* 2001; **145**: 668–9.
14 Sakaria SS, Ravi A, Swerlick R et al. Wells' syndrome associated with ulcerative colitis: a case report and literature review. *J Gastroenterol* 2007; **42**: 250–2.
15 Arca E, Köse O, Karslioğlu Y et al. Bullous eosinophilic cellulitis succession with eosinophilic pustular folliculitis without eosinophilia. *J Dermatol* 2007; **34**: 80–5.
16 Schuttelaar ML, Jonkman MF. Bullous eosinophilic cellulitis (Wells' syndrome) associated with Churg–Strauss syndrome. *J Eur Acad Dermatol Venereol* 2003; **17**: 91–3.
17 Bogenrieder T, Griese DP, Schiffner R et al. Wells' syndrome associated with idiopathic hypereosinophilic syndrome. *Br J Dermatol* 1997; **137**: 978–82.
18 Davis MPD, Brown AC, Blackston RD et al. Familial eosinophilic cellulitis, dysmorphic habitus, and mental retardation. *J Am Acad Dermatol* 1998; **38**: 919–28.
19 Kuwahara RT, Randall MB, Eisner MG. Eosinophilic cellulitis in a newborn. *Pediatr Dermatol* 2001; **18**: 89–90.
20 Anderson CR, Jenkins D, Tron V et al. Wells' syndrome in childhood: case report and review of the literature. *J Am Acad Dermatol* 1995; **33**: 857–64.
21 Holme SA, McHenry P. Nodular presentation of eosinophilic cellulitis (Wells' syndrome). *Clin Exp Dermatol* 2001; **26**: 677–9.
22 Sommer S, Wilkinson SM, Merchant WJ. Eosinophilic cellulitis following the lines of Blaschko. *Clin Exp Dermatol* 1999; **24**: 449–51.
23 Coldiron BM, Robinson JK. Low dose alternate-day prednisone for persistent Wells' syndrome. *Arch Dermatol* 1989; **125**: 1625–6.
24 Aroni K, Aivaliotis M, Liossi A et al. Eosinophilic cellulitis in a child successfully treated with cetirizine. *Acta Derm Venereol* 1999; **79**: 332.
25 Husak R, Goerdt S, Orfanos CE. Interferon alfa treatment of a patient with eosinophilic cellulitis and HIV infection. *N Engl J Med* 1997; **337**: 641–2.
26 Karabudak O, Dogan B, Taskapan O et al. Eosinophilic cellulitis presented with semicircular pattern. *J Dermatol* 2006; **33**: 798–801.

Lipodystrophy

The terms lipoatrophy and lipodystrophy are sometimes used interchangeably and without precise definition. Perhaps it is best to define lipodystrophy as an abnormality of fat that is usually associated with atrophy (lipoatrophy), or infrequently hypertrophy of the adipose tissue. Lipoatrophy refers specifically to loss of fat. However, the lipoatrophy may be part of a local panatrophy affecting all mesodermal layers [1]. Lipodystrophies are a rare and heterogeneous group of disorders characterized by selective and variable reduction in and, more often, loss of adipose tissue from different parts of the body; in all but the more very localized varieties they are often associated with metabolic complications of insulin resistance, in particular insulin-resistant diabetes mellitus [2]. Over the last 5 years, there has been a much better understanding of the aetiology of these disorders. The loss of adipose tissue can have a genetic, immunological, infectious or drug-associated aetiology [3]. The age of onset may also determine the nomenclature of the disease. Some patients may develop the disease very early on in life—such patients are then sometimes referred to as having congenital lipodystrophy. In other patients, the disease occurs later on in life—so-called acquired lipodystrophy. The lipodystrophies can also be classified according to the extent of the disease into three major clinical entities: localized, partial-body and whole-body distribution. The atrophy may be localized (e.g. to the thighs); it can be widespread, involving the upper part of the trunk (partial lipodystrophy); or it may affect the whole body (generalized lipodystrophy).

Nevertheless, the aetiology and clinical presentation are not always clear-cut. For example, cases of partial lipoatrophy have been reported that have evolved into generalized lipoatrophy, suggesting some common link between these uncommon disorders.

References

1 Serup J, Weismann K, Kobayasi T et al. Local panatrophy with linear distribution. *Acta Derm Venereol (Stockh)* 1982; **62**: 101–5.
2 Reitman ML, Arioglu E, Gavrilova O, Taylor SI. Lipoatrophy revisited. *Trends Endocrinol Metab* 2000; **11**: 410–6.
3 Shalev A. Discovery of a lipodystrophy gene: one answer, 100 questions. *Eur J Endocrinol* 2000; **143**: 565–7.

Localized lipoatrophy

Localized atrophy may be seen following injection of medications, for example in insulin-dependent diabetics, induced by insulin [1–9]; following certain inflammatory conditions, such as panniculitis and morphoea; or as primary idiopathic lipoatrophy. The list of medications inducing atrophy includes corticosteroids, antibiotics, heparin, growth hormone and glatiramer [10]. The mechanism is uncertain and has been attributed directly to the medication, but localized lipoatrophy has been reported following acupuncture alone [11]. In many of these situations, spontaneous healing has occurred over the next month or two. Failure to perform a biopsy in the early phases of the atrophy may explain why some of the cases are labelled as idiopathic in origin. It has been suggested that many cases may be preceded by an inflammatory reaction in the fat (see also lipoatrophic panniculitis) [1].

Insulin lipodystrophies

This is a cosmetically distressing complication of insulin administration. Both atrophy and hypertrophy of the fat tissue can occur. It occurs in various degrees in up to 37% of insulin-dependent diabetics [2].

Aetiology. Insulin lipoatrophy is usually seen in women and children, rarely in men. The mechanism remains speculative but local changes induced by insulin or impurities are probably important [3] as are antibodies to insulin [4]. Most cases are associated with high levels of insulin requirement and/or an increased insulin-binding capacity.

Cross-reaction of insulin antibodies with cells thus changed could result in further damage [5]. It was thought that the introduction of highly purified insulin would make a significant impact in reducing the frequency of this disorder. There is evidence to support this view, because the subcutaneous damage is reduced if highly purified insulins are used, resulting in clinical improvement and a reduction in insulin requirements and insulin-binding capacity [5–7]. However, localized lipodystrophies in insulin-requiring patients are still very common, affecting up to 40% of patients.

A recent publication investigated a cross-sectional study of 112 children and adolescents with type 1 diabetes mellitus and related the presence of insulin antibodies to the clinical features of insulin lipodystrophies [4]. The antibodies against insulin increased significantly after diabetes manifestations and initiation of insulin treatment, while β-cell-specific antibodies did not. Severe lipohypertrophy was seen in four children, severe lipohypertrophy in 18 and moderate lipohypertrophy in 27 children. Among clinical and immunological parameters investigated, insulin antibodies were significantly associated with hypertrophy or atrophy of injection sites. It was concluded that lipodystrophies in diabetics are significantly associated with insulin antibodies, and that these may have a role in the development of the disease.

Histopathology. There is a loss of fat tissue and inflammatory changes are conspicuously absent. In lipohypertrophy, there may be replacement of mid-dermal collagen by hypertrophic fat cells.

Clinical features. Although both features can occur in the same patient, recent publications suggest that insulin fat hypertrophy is more common than atrophic changes [4]. Most cases present 6 months to 2 years after the start of insulin administration. Lesions may vary from only a small dimple to an extensive, disfiguring area with much local loss of fat or firm fatty induration. The changes are usually found only at the sites of injection, but loss of fat may occur elsewhere. There is a definite tendency to spontane-

ous recovery at the involved site when the site of injection is changed.

Treatment. A change to a purified insulin, particularly the new human insulin, is not necessarily curative [8]. Prevention is either by constant alteration of the site of injection, so that no two injections are given in exactly the same area more frequently than once a month, or by the use of the more purified insulins [5,9]. Alternatively, injection at the edge of the atrophy or combination with dexamethasone may help [12]. Liposuction may help the hypertrophic variety [13]. In one very resistant case of progressive lipoatrophy, continuous subcutaneous infusion with human insulin was required to control the atrophy [9] but continuous infusion itself may provoke the same reaction [14].

Localized lipohypertrophy has also been reported in a 51-year-old female patient with panhypopituitism during growth hormone replacement therapy [15].

References

1 Peters MS, Winkelmann RK. Localized lipoatrophy (atrophic connective tissue disease panniculitis). *Arch Dermatol* 1980; **116**: 1363–8.
2 Kakourou T, Dacou-Voutetakis C, Kavadias G *et al.* Limited joint mobility and lipodystrophy in children and adolescents with insulin-dependent diabetes mellitus. *Pediatr Dermatol* 1994; **11**: 310–4.
3 Eisert J. Diabetes and diseases of the skin. *Med Clin North Am* 1965; **49**: 621–32.
4 Raile K, Noelle V, Landgraf R, Schwarz HP. Insulin antibodies are associated with lipatrophy but also with lipohypertrophy in children and adolescents with type 1 diabetes. *Exp Clin Endocrinol Diabetes* 2001; **109**: 393–6.
5 Daggett P, Mustaffa BE, Nabarro JDN. Improvements in skin reactions to insulin produced by a highly purified preparation. *Br J Dermatol* 1977; **96**: 439–43.
6 Kristensen JS, Falhott K. Human monocomponent insulin in the treatment of insulin allergic diabetics. *Diabetes* 1983; **32** (Suppl. 1): 66.
7 Tantillo JJ, Karam JH, Burrill KC. Immunogenicity of 'single peak' beef–pork insulin in diabetic subjects. *Diabetes* 1974; **23**: 276–81.
8 Galloway JA, Bressler R. Insulin treatment in diabetes. *Med Clin North Am* 1978; **62**: 663–80.
9 Chantelau E, Reuter M, Scholes S *et al.* A case of lipoatrophy with human insulin therapy. *Exp Clin Endocrinol* 1993; **101**: 194–6.
10 Soos N, Shakery K, Mrowietz U. Localized panniculitis and subsequent lipoatrophy with subcutaneous glatiramer acetate (Copaxone) injection for the treatment of multiple sclerosis. *Am J Clin Dermatol* 2004; **5**: 357–9.
11 Drago F, Rongioletti F, Battifoglio ML, Rebora A. Localised lipoatrophy after acupuncture. *Lancet* 1996; **347**: 1484.
12 Richardson T, Kerr D. Skin-related complications of insulin therapy: epidemiology and emerging management strategies. *Am J Clin Dermatol* 2003; **4**: 661–7.
13 Field LM. Successful treatment of lipohypertrophic insulin lipodystrophy with liposuction surgery. *J Am Acad Dermatol* 1988; **19**: 570.
14 Radermecker RP, Piérard GE, Scheen AJ. Lipodystrophy reactions to insulin: effects of continuous insulin infusion and new insulin analogs. *Am J Clin Dermatol* 2007; **8**: 21–8.
15 Mersebach H, Feldt-Rasmussen UF. Localised liphypertrophy during growth hormone therapy. *Ugeskr Laeger* 2002; **164**: 1930–2.

Localized 'idiopathic' lipoatrophy

This group of disorders predominantly affects the thighs, ankles or abdomen, and all cases may possibly be variants of the same process.

Histopathology. Two histological subsets exist: involutional and inflammatory [1]. Sixty percent can be termed involutional; the adipocytes are small and embedded in hyaline connective tissue with many capillaries. Such patients usually have a single lesion,

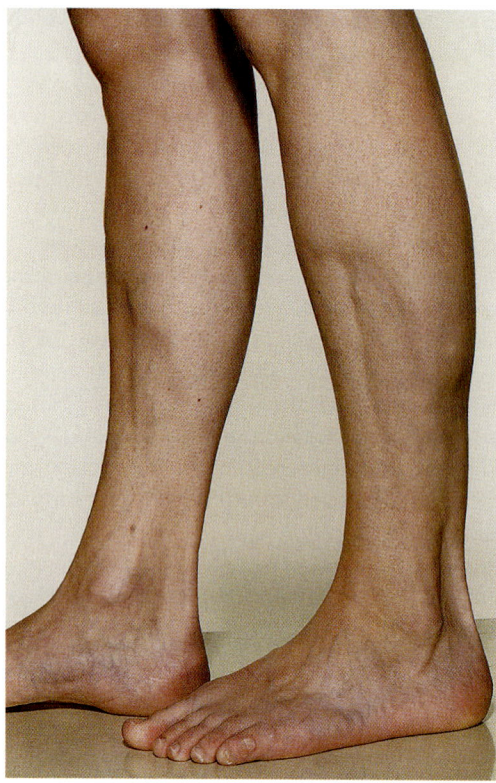

Fig. 46.31 Extensive lipoatrophy of the legs.

and only one-third show immunoreactants. Forty per cent can be classed as inflammatory [2]; the lipocytes are normal and there is a sparse infiltrate of lymphocytes, histiocytes and plasma cells; all show immunoreactants [1]. The epidermis is normal. The appearance should not be confused with the striking lipomembranous (membranocystic) changes seen occasionally in morphoea, panniculitis and other inflammatory dermatoses.

Clinical features. Two clinical groups, based on the localization of the atrophy, have been described.

Lipoatrophia semicircularis [3–5]. These patients show lesions on the anterolateral aspects of the thighs, characterized by a band-like circular depression, 2–4 cm in width. Patients have also been described with lipoatrophy of the ankles which can extend up the legs (Fig. 46.31) [6]. The overlying skin is normal. An association with osteodystrophy of the hands and feet has also been reported [7].

The loss of fat develops rapidly within several weeks, usually without associated symptoms, although rheumatic-like pains within the involved areas were reported by two women. Trauma is a possible triggering mechanism—a series of seven cases has been reported in individuals working in the same office. The exact position of the indentations corresponding to the height of the desks strongly supports the hypothesis that in some patients this condition is caused by repetitive trauma to the upper thighs [8].

Primary inflammatory vascular changes in the subcutaneous tissue have been demonstrated in these patients, and also during the early period of other lipoatrophies [9]. There is no treatment, but considerable improvement may occur after the activity of the disease settles.

Centrifugal lipodystrophy. Lipodystrophia centrifugalis abdominalis infantalis is rare, and has been seen predominantly in Japanese children [10–14], affecting the subcutaneous fat, usually of the abdomen and upper groin. Patients of Chinese and English ancestry have been reported [15]. The condition spreads in a centrifugal fashion, with a central, large, bluish depressed area and slight erythema of the edge. Further experience has shown that the original name is inappropriate, because the condition may affect other areas, and may occur outside infancy and not affecting the abdomen [16,17]. The condition may be strikingly unilateral [18,19]. One case is reported to have lasted over 40 years, and was associated with angioblastoma, which occurred at the same site at the age of 46 years [11]. Regional lymphadenopathy may occur [13]. A 10-year-old boy with a centrifugal lipodystrophy also developed serpiginous erythema of the scalp with scarring alopecia [20]. Ulceration may also be a complication [21].

Histology shows a decrease in the subcutaneous fat, with an inflammatory infiltrate in the lower dermis and subcutis. Immunocytochemistry has more recently suggested the possible involvement of apoptosis as a factor responsible for fatty tissue degeneration [22]. A patient has been reported who showed characteristics of both centrifugal and progressive lipodystrophy [17].

Treatment. Treatment is disappointing, although after the disease activity has ceased there seems to be regrowth of fat in 75% of cases. Some improvement has been reported in most cases treated with oral and topical corticosteroids [10].

References

1 Peters MS, Winkelmann RK. The histopathology of localized lipoatrophy. *Br J Dermatol* 1986; **114**: 27–36.
2 Rongioletti F, Rebora A. Annular and semicircular lipoatrophies: three cases and review of the literature. *J Am Acad Dermatol* 1989; **20**: 433–6.
3 Bloch PH, Runne U. Lipotrophia semicircularis beim Mann: Zusammentreffen von Arterienvariet und Mikrotraumata als mögliche Krankheitsursache. *Hautarzt* 1978; **29**: 270–2.
4 Gschwandter WR, Munzberger H. Lipoatrophia semicircularis. *Wien Klin Wochenschr* 1975; **87**: 164–8.
5 Karkaritas C, Miller JA, Kirby JD. Semicircular lipoatrophy. *Br J Dermatol* 1981; **105**: 591–3.
6 Jablonska S, Szczepanski A, Gorkiewicz A. Lipoatrophy of the ankles and its relation to other lipoatrophies. *Acta Derm Venereol (Stockh)* 1975; **55**: 135–40.
7 Masala MV, Tedde G, Cottoni F. Annular atrophy of the ankles: an unusual case associated with bone abnormality. *Dermatology* 2001; **203**: 81–2.
8 Gruber PC, Fuller LC. Lipoatrophy semicircularis induced by trauma. *Clin Exp Dermatol* 2001; **26**: 269–71.
9 Peters MS, Winkelmann RK. Localized lipoatrophy (atrophic connective tissue disease panniculitis). *Arch Dermatol* 1980; **116**: 1363–8.
10 Imamura S, Yamada M. Lipodystrophia centrifugalis abdominalis infantilis. *Br J Dermatol* 1977; **96**: 96.
11 Hiraiwa A, Takai K, Fukui Y *et al.* Non-regressing lipodystrophia centrifugalis abdominalis with angioblastoma (Nakagawa). *Arch Dermatol* 1990; **126**: 206–9.
12 Imamura S, Yamada M, Yamamoto K. Lipodystrophia centrifugalis abdominalis infantilis: a follow-up study. *J Am Acad Dermatol* 1984; **11**: 203–9.
13 Imamura S, Yamada M, Yamamoto K *et al.* Lipodystrophia centrifugalis abdominalis infantilis. *Hautarzt* 1979; **30**: 360–4.
14 Makino K, Inone T, Shimao S. Lipodystrophia centrifugalis abdominalis infantilis. *Arch Dermatol* 1972; **106**: 899–900.

15 Mak K-H, Ho H-F, Chan L-V, Chong L-Y. Lipodystrophia centrifugalis abdominalis infantalis: two cases from China. *J Dermatol* 2001; **28**: 320–3.

16 Hagari Y, Sasaoka R, Nishiura S *et al.* Centrifugal lipodystrophy of the face mimicking progressive lipodystrophy. *Br J Dermatol* 1992; **127**: 407–10.

17 Higuchi T, Yamakage A, Tamuea T *et al.* Lipodystrophia centrifugalis abdominalis infantilis occurring in the neck. *Dermatology* 1994; **188**: 142–4.

18 Franks A, Verbov JL. Unilateral localised idiopathic lipoatrophy. *Clin Exp Dermatol* 1993; **18**: 468–9.

19 Zachary CB, Wells RS. Centrifugal lipodystrophy. *Br J Dermatol* 1984; **110**: 107–10.

20 Hagari Y, Ikehara A, Nuno K, Mihara M. Centrifugal lipodystrophy presenting with serpiginous erythema and alopecia. *Cutis* 2002; **69**: 281–3.

21 Aoki E, Kawana S. Lipodystrophia centrifugalis abnominalis infantilis with ulceration. *Dermatology* 2000; **200**: 280–1.

22 Okita H, Ohtsuka T, Yamakage A, Yamazaki S. Lipodystrophia centrifugalis abdominalis infantilis: immunohistochemical demonstration of an apoptotic process in the degenerating fatty tissue. *Dermatology* 2000; **201**: 370–2.

Partial or generalized lipoatrophies [1–3]

HIV-associated lipodystrophy syndrome has become by far and away the commonest. The remainder are rare syndromes where there is extensive absence, or progressive loss, of subcutaneous fat. Several syndromes are described: congenital generalized lipodystrophy, acquired generalized lipodystrophy, partial (cephalothoracic) lipodystrophy and partial face-sparing lipodystrophy [4]. Genetic explanations for these diseases are increasingly being reported [5].

Congenital generalized lipodystrophy

Synonyms
- Lipoatrophic diabetes
- Berardinelli–Seip syndrome (MIM 608694; MIM269700)

A rare congenital generalized lipoatrophy, autosomal recessive, with loss of the subcutaneous and visceral fat, hepatomegaly, increased bone growth, hyperlipaemia and, later, diabetes mellitus [1,3,6–8].

Aetiology. Two gene abnormalities on different chromosomes have been described, but some phenotypically similar pedigrees have an as yet undetermined genetic abnormality [9]. Congenital generalized lipodystrophy type I (CGL1) was mapped to chromosome 9q34 and CGL2 to chromosome 11q13. CGL1 is caused by mutations in the *AGPAT2* gene [10]. AGPAT enzymes are involved in triglyceride and glycerophospholipid biosynthesis. How the abnormality is converted into lipoatrophy is undetermined. CGL2 is caused by mutations in the *BSCL2* gene encoding a protein, seipin, expressed in neural tissue as well as adipocytes [11]. Again the effect of the abnormality is unknown. The phenotypic expression of both types is much the same, but CGL2 would appear to cause more morbidity than CGL1, with a higher incidence of premature death, more severe fat loss, including that in mechanical areas, more severe cardiomyopathy and more severe intellectual impairment [12]. CGL2 patients have higher insulin levels and earlier onset diabetes [13]. Lipodystrophy with cystic angiomatosis (Brunzell syndrome) demonstrates an *AGPAT2* mutation [14].

Histopathology. There is complete loss of subcutaneous and visceral fat.

Clinical features. There is complete loss of subcutaneous and other fat, present at birth or before the age of 2 years. As such, the musculature appears more defined and prominent. The children have an elevated metabolic rate accompanied by an excessive appetite and accelerated growth, sometimes producing an acromegaloid appearance. They are tall for their age; the somatic musculature is increased and the abdomen markedly protuberant, often with an umbilical hernia. There is often generalized hypertrichosis, even at birth, and the scalp hair becomes abundant and often curly with the onset of disease. Acanthosis nigricans starts in childhood, becoming more severe through adolescence. There is precocious enlargement of the genitalia, and in females marked enlargement of the clitoris. Affected men have normal fertility, but females are prone to oligomenorrhoea, polycystic ovary and infertility. Hepatic steatosis leads to hepatomegaly, splenomegaly and cirrhosis. Younger patients show glycosuria only when given large amounts of glucose. Hyperglycaemia with excessive thirst and polyuria usually develop only after the age of 10 years, the evolving diabetes becoming markedly insulin resistant. Hypertriglyceridaemia, sometimes triggering pancreatitis, and low HDL cholesterol are other metabolic features.

Detailed metabolic and radiological studies have shown poor metabolically active adipose tissue, whereas mechanical adipose tissue may be well preserved [15]. X-rays show focal bone lesions which on MRI can be shown to be caused by absence of marrow fat [16].

Differential diagnosis. The main differential diagnosis of congenital generalized lipodystrophy is Donohue syndrome (leprechaunism) due to an insulin receptor defect [17]. Acanthosis nigricans and hypertrichosis may be present, as well as the generalized decrease in fat. However, the elfin facial appearance is a major difference. In SHORT syndrome (short stature, hyperextensibility of joints, ocular depression, Rieger anomaly and delay of dental eruption), an apparent autosomal dominant disorder, the lipodystrophy shows relative sparing on the legs [18]. Neonatal progeroid syndrome expresses fat loss confined to the face, distal extremities, and possibly the paravertebral and lateral gluteal regions [19]. Fat loss with mandibuloacral dysplasia is usually confined to the extremities though may be generalized [20].

Acquired generalized lipodystrophy [21]

Selective loss of body fat from large regions of the body occurs after birth, usually before adolescence.

Aetiology. The development of molecular genetics has allowed re-evaluation of the lipodystrophies, resulting in new diagnostic criteria for acquired generalized lipodystrophy (AGL), albeit still a heterogeneous mix. Individuals with a known or likely genetic abnormality are automatically excluded, as are patients with diminished subcutaneous fat in association with thyrotoxicosis, malabsorption, malnutrition and cachexia. Patients are then further divided into three groups: type 1, AGL with panniculitis

(25%); type 2, AGL with autoimmune disease (25%); and type 3, idiopathic (50%).

Histopathology. Type I AGL histology reveals a lobular panniculitis without vasculitis.

Clinical features. AGL is a disease of childhood and adolescence, with a female to male ratio of 3:1. The panniculitic type is expressed as a nodular inflammatory process occurring anywhere, but healing with a depressed area which might gradually enlarge without inflammation. More widespread, uninflamed fat loss might then occur, the whole evolving over several years. Some of these patients might have an autoimmune disease, but the true autoimmune AGL group do not have a clinical inflammatory panniculitis preceding the lipodystrophy. Juvenile dermatomyositis seems particularly associated with type 2 AGL [22]. The idiopathic group has neither of the features of type 1 or 2 AGL, and arises spontaneously or occasionally after a febrile illness. The degree of fat loss is less than the congenital counterpart; with variable preservation of visceral and mechanical fat pads but complete preservation of retro-orbital and bone marrow fat. Type 1 patients have less extensive fat loss, which may correlate with the less severe expression of anabolic and metabolic features. After fat loss, hepatomegaly from asteatosis is the commonest clinical feature, followed by acanthosis nigricans and hirsutism. Xanthomas are present in 50% of the type 3 group, but less in the other two. Excessive appetite and increased growth emphasize the overlap with the congenital type. Hyperinsulinaemia, diabetes mellitus, hypertriglyceridaemia, and low serum leptin and adiponectin levels are similarly present. Menstrual irregularities and polycystic ovary syndrome are less frequent than in the congenital type, as is hirsutism. Curly hair may still occur.

MRI imaging has provided a major advance in assessment of fat loss and fat hypertrophy, whether subcutaneous, visceral or mechanical [23]. Whether a simple MRI screening test of thigh fat will be a strong discriminator between normal and abnormal remains to be confirmed [23].

Patients with hepatomegaly may progress to cirrhosis, but the consequence of accelerated atherosclerosis seems a more important prognostic factor.

Differential diagnosis. In CGL fat loss is absent from birth. Other later-onset genetic lipodystrophies need to be excluded through clinical means, MRI scanning and confirmation of mutations. Cushing's syndrome, diabetes mellitus and thyrotoxicosis need to be excluded, as does any cachetic state such as HIV infection, malabsorption and malignancy. Localized lipoatrophy is focal and usually obvious from the history or distribution.

Treatment. Apart from genetic counselling, the management of CGL and AGL shows much overlap, with the emphasis placed on lessening the risk from glycaemic and dyslipidaemic metabolic consequences using standard management. If leptin deficiency and diabetes is present, CGL, AGL and partial lipodystrophic patients can have their insulin resistance and dyslipidaemia reversed if given continuing recombinant leptin therapy [24–27]. Diabetic complications and other features such as voracious appetite, hepatic steatosis, acanthosis nigricans and amenorrhoea can also be reversed, but not the subcutaneous fat loss. Surgical intervention for specific anatomical defects, such as the repair of severe buttock deformities with bilateral gluteus maximus muscle flap advancements [28], may be helpful.

References

1 Garg A. Acquired and inherited lipodystrophies. *N Engl J Med* 2004; **350**: 1220–34.

2 Hegele RA, Joy TR, Al-Attar SA *et al.* Thematic review series: adipocyte biology. Lipodystrophies: windows on adipose biology and metabolism. *J Lipid Res* 2007; **48**: 1433–44.

3 Seip M, Trygstad O. Generalized lipodystrophy. *Arch Dis Child* 1963; **38**: 447–53.

4 Mamalaki E, Katsantounis J, Papavasiliou S *et al.* A case of partial face sparing lipodystrophy combining features of generalised lipodystrophy. *J Am Acad Dermatol* 1995; **32**: 130–3.

5 Agarwal AK, Garg A. Genetic basis of lipodystrophies and management of metabolic complications. *Ann Rev Med* 2006; **57**: 297–311.

6 Berardinelli W. An undiagnosed endocrinometabolic syndrome: report of 2 cases. *J Clin Endocrinol Metab* 1954; **14**: 193–204.

7 Brunzell JD, Shankle SW, Bethune JE. Congenital generalized lipodystrophy accompanied by cystic angiomatosis. *Ann Intern Med* 1968; **69**: 501–16.

8 Reed WB, Dexter R, Corley C *et al.* Congenital lipodystrophic diabetes with acanthosis nigricans. *Arch Dermatol* 1965; **91**: 326–34.

9 Rajab A, Heathcote K, Joshi S *et al.* Heterogeneity for congenital generalized lipodystrophy in seventeen patients from Oman. *Am J Med Genet* 2002; **110**: 219–25.

10 Agarwal AK, Arioglu E, De Almeida S *et al.* AGPAT2 is mutated in congenital generalized lipodystrophy linked to chromosome 9q34. *Nat Genet* 2002; **31**: 21–3.

11 Magre J, Delepine M, Khallouf E *et al.* Identification of the gene altered in Berardinelli–Seip congenital lipodystrophy on chromosome 11q13. *Nat Genet* 2001; **28**: 365–70.

12 Van Maldergem L, Magre J, Khallouf TE *et al.* Genotype–phenotype relationships in Berardinelli–Seip congenital lipodystrophy. *J Med Genet* 2002; **39**: 722–33.

13 Fu M, Kazlauskaite R, Baracho Mde F *et al.* Mutations in Gng3lg and AGPAT2 in Berardinelli–Seip congenital lipodystrophy and Brunzell syndrome: phenotype variability suggests important modifier effects. *J Clin Endocrinol Metab* 2004; **89**: 2916–22.

14 Gomes KB, Pardini VC, Ferreira AC, Fernandes AP. Phenotypic heterogeneity in biochemical parameters correlates with mutations in AGPAT2 or Seipin genes among Berardinelli–Seip congenital lipodystrophy patients. *J Inherit Metab Dis* 2005; **28**: 1123–31.

15 Garg A, Fleckenstein JL, Peshock RM *et al.* Peculiar distribution of adipose tissue in patients with congenital generalized lipodystrophy. *J Clin Endocrinol Metab* 1992; **75**: 358–9.

16 Fleckenstein JL, Garg A, Bonte FJ *et al.* The skeleton in congenital, generalized lipodystrophy: evaluation using whole-body radiographic surveys, magnetic resonance imaging and technetium-99m bone scintigraphy. *Skeletal Radiol* 1992; **21**: 381–6.

17 Elsas LJ, Endo F, Strumlauf E *et al.* Leprechaunism: an inherited defect in a high-affinity insulin receptor. *Am J Hum Genet* 1985; **37**: 73–88.

18 Koenig R, Brendel L, Fuchs S. SHORT syndrome. *Clin Dysmorphol* 2003; **12**: 45–9.

19 O'Neill B, Simha V, Kotha V *et al.* Body fat distribution and metabolic variables in patients with neonatal progeroid syndrome. *Am J Med Genet A* 2007; **143A**: 1421–30.

20 Simha V, Garg A. Body fat distribution and metabolic derangements in patients with familial partial lipodystrophy associated with mandibuloacral dysplasia. *J Clin Endocrinol Metab* 2002; **87**: 776–85.

21 Misra A, Garg A. Clinical features and metabolic derangements in acquired generalized lipodystrophy: case reports and review of the literature. *Medicine (Baltimore)* 2003; **82**: 129–46.

22 Bingham A, Mamyrova G, Rother KI *et al.* Predictors of acquired lipodystrophy in juvenile-onset dermatomyositis and a gradient of severity. *Medicine (Baltimore)* 2008; **87**: 70–86.

23 Al-Attar SA, Pollex RL, Robinson JF *et al.* Quantitative and qualitative differences in subcutaneous adipose tissue stores across lipodystrophy types shown by magnetic resonance imaging. *BMC Med Imaging* 2007; **7**: 3.

24 Oral EA, Simha V, Ruiz E *et al.* Leptin-replacement therapy for lipodystrophy. *N Engl J Med* 2002; **346**: 570–8.

25 Moran SA, Patten N, Young JR *et al.* Changes in body composition in patients with severe lipodystrophy after leptin replacement therapy. *Metabolism* 2004; **53**: 513–9.

26 Ebihara K, Kusakabe T, Hirata M *et al.* Efficacy and safety of leptin-replacement therapy and possible mechanisms of leptin actions in patients with generalized lipodystrophy. *J Clin Endocrinol Metab* 2007; **92**: 532–41.

27 Park JY, Chong AY, Cochran EK *et al.* Type 1 diabetes associated with acquired generalized lipodystrophy and insulin resistance: the effect of long-term leptin therapy. *J Clin Endocrinol Metab* 2008; **93**: 26–31.

28 Okada E, Iwahira Y, Maruyama Y. Buttock deformity repair for congenital generalized lipodystrophy. *Plastic Reconstr Surg* 1995; **95**: 744–5.

Partial lipoatrophy [1,2]

Synonyms
- Partial lipodystrophy
- Barraquer–Simons disease
- Progressive lipodystrophy (MIM 608709)

This rare lipoatrophy occurs either in childhood or in young adults as an incidental part of a widespread mesodermal atrophy. The partial lipodystrophy locus has been mapped to chromosome 1q with no evidence of genetic heterogeneity [3].

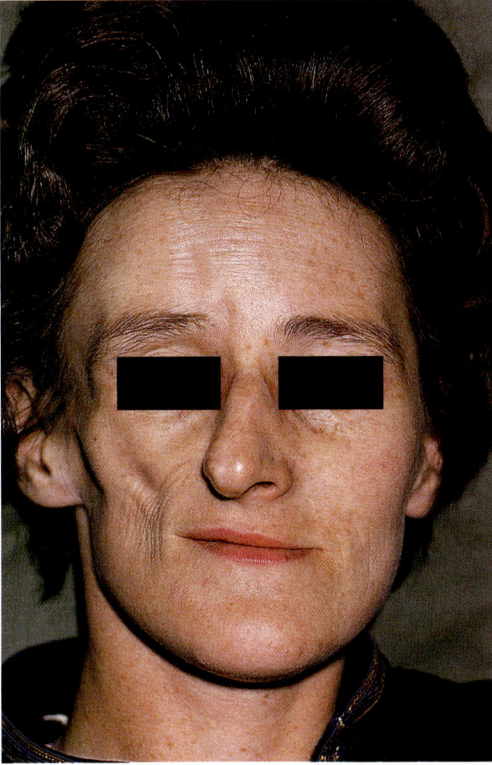

Fig. 46.32 The typical cadaveric facies of a patient with partial lipodystrophy. She also has melasma.

Aetiology. Most patients are children or young adults when the disorder begins, but onset in the first year and in middle age is reported. Females are affected four or five times more frequently than males [4], and the condition is sometimes familial. It may follow an acute specific fever such as measles, but the common occurrence of non-specific fevers makes proof of this observation difficult. Facial hemiatrophy associated with loss of subcutaneous fat in borreliosis has been reported [5]. Partial lipodystrophy has followed damage to the region of the mid-brain or diencephalon [6]. The association of lipodystrophy with immunologically related renal disease [4,7–10], systemic sclerosis [11], systemic lupus erythematosus [12] and high titres of thyroid antibodies, supports the view of lipodystrophy being an immunological disorder in some patients [13], but one that requires more investigation.

It is difficult to explain the abnormal distribution of adipose tissue in partial lipodystrophy. Fatty tissue autotransplanted to an atrophic site lost fat, while atrophic tissue autotransplanted to a fatty site accumulated it, suggesting that local factors determine the distributions of fat [14]. The local factor may be neuronally mediated, as suggested by observations that there may be symmetrical segmental loss of fat, and the line demarcating dystrophic and normal tissue in partial lipodystrophy may correspond to a dermatome. Jensen [15] described increased adrenergic activity in a patient with partial lipodystrophy, and proposed that this was of significance, as adipocytes in the upper body are sensitive to the lipolytic effects of epinephrine (adrenaline) and those in the lower body are not. Alternatively, the pattern of disease may be related to complement factor D expression, a serine protease expressed in the kidney, but also by adipocytes. Activation of the alternative complement pathway by C3 nephritic factor (see below) however, could lead to complement-dependent lysis of adipocytes [16]. But the finding of mutations in the *LMNB2* gene in some patients with acquired partial lipodystrophy [17] suggests that a simple autoimmune process involving C3 nephritic factor is only part of the story.

Histopathology. There is usually complete loss of adipose tissue over the affected areas.

Clinical features. The disease is characterized by the relatively slow, symmetrical disappearance of the facial fat, producing a cadaverous appearance (Fig. 46.32) and complete loss of the subcutaneous fat in the upper half of the body (Weir–Mitchell type). In some cases, there is a coincidental hypertrophy of the subcutaneous fat of the lower part of the body (Laignel–Lavastine and Viard type) [3]. Ten per cent may have 'hemilipodystrophy' involving half of the face or body. Up to 90% can develop progressive membranous mesangiocapillary glomerulonephritis [3,18,19] and this can be precipitated by the contraceptive pill, pregnancy (especially in the third trimester) or the use of ergot derivatives [4]. A successful outcome in pregnancy is uncommon [20]. Thus, such patients should be observed by a renal physician during pregnancy, and oral contraceptives are prohibited.

The association of hypocomplementaemia and mesangiocapillary glomerulonephritis is now well established [7,8]. Approximately half of the patients with this form of glomerulonephritis have a persistently low plasma concentration of the third component of complement (C3), while the concentration of the fourth component (C4) is normal. This is accompanied by the presence of a factor in serum that is capable of activating C3 without activation of the earlier components. This material has been termed 'C3 nephritic factor' or C3NeF [21,22]. Lupus, C3 nephritic factor and partial lipodystrophy are perhaps not as rare as previously thought [21,22]. Juvenile dermatomyositis is also a rare association [23].

The relationship between C3NeF, persistently low C3 and mesangiocapillary glomerulonephritis is not clear. It has been suggested that C3NeF predisposes the glomerulus to the development of mesangiocapillary glomerulonephritis in response to some other agent. In a series of 12 patients, four died from renal failure 10–25 years after the onset of the partial lipoatrophy [4]. Transplantation in one case resulted in normalization of C3 and the disappearance of C3NeF [18].

Insulin-dependent diabetes mellitus develops in one-third of patients with partial lipodystrophy. Retinitis pigmentosa, acanthosis nigricans and hepatomegaly are rare associated features [2]. Chronic purpura resulting from leukocytoclastic vasculitis has been reported [24]. This patient had extensive and moderate hypertrophy of the subcutaneous fatty tissue, macroglossia, polyarthralgia and mononeuritis. Myopathy associated with muscle weakness has rarely been reported, and is caused by fat droplets between the myofibrils [25]. Mammography in patients with partial lipodystrophy reveals unusually dense breasts with homogeneous opacities and ectopic fat depositions. These changes are possibly diagnostic, but confusing to the ill-informed radiologist [26]. Extrinsic allergic alveolitis has been reported in association with partial lipodystrophy, but with an acral distribution as opposed to the more usual facial involvement [27].

Treatment. There is little effective treatment, other than the prevention and treatment of kidney disease. New plastic surgical techniques, including free radial forearm adipofascial flaps, can markedly improve the facial appearance [28,29].

References

1 Poley JR, Stickler GB. Progressive lipodystrophy. *Am J Dis Child* 1963; **106**: 356–63.
2 Senior B, Gellis SS. The syndromes of total lipodystrophy and of partial lipodystrophy. *Pediatrics* 1964; **33**: 593–612.
3 Eisinger AJ, Shortland JR, Moorhead PJ. Renal disease in partial lipodystrophy. *QJM* 1972; **41**: 343–54.
4 Simpson NB, Cunliffe WJ, Davison A. Partial lipodystrophy, glomerulonephritis and hypocomplementaemia. *Br J Dermatol* 1979; **101** (Suppl. 17): 11.
5 Abele DC, Bedingfield RB, Chandler FW et al. Progressive facial hemiatrophy (Romberg syndrome) and borreliosis. *J Am Acad Dermatol* 1990; **22**: 531–5.
6 Hawes CR, Johnson FC, Palmer HD. Progressive hypothalamic dysfunction. *J Pediatr* 1954; **45**: 393–400.
7 Ipp MM, Minta JO, Gelfand EW. Disorders of the complement system in lipodystrophy. *Immunol Immunopathol* 1976; **7**: 281–7.
8 Sissons JGP, West RJ, Fallows J et al. The complement abnormalities of lipodystrophy. *N Engl J Med* 1976; **294**: 461–5.
9 Mehmet B, Ozlem E, Gulay D et al. Acute pancreatitis in a patient with partial lipodystrophy and membranoproliferative glomerulonephritis. *Nephrol Dial Transplant* 2001; **16**: 1930–1.
10 Levy Y, George J, Yona E, Shoenfeld Y. Partial lipodystrophy, mesangiocapillary glomerulonephritis, and complement dysregulation: an autoimmune phenomenon. *Immunol Res* 1998; **18**: 55–60.
11 Hall WS, Gillespie JJ, Tenczynski TE. Generalized lipodystrophy, scleroderma and Hodgkin's disease. *Arch Intern Med* 1978; **138**: 1303–4.
12 Ishiguro N, Kanazawa H, Ishibashi M, Kawashima M. Partial lipodystrophy in a patient with systemic lupus erythematosus. *Dermatology* 2002; **204**: 298–300.
13 Wilson WA, Sissons JGP, Morgan OS. Multiple autoimmune diseases with bilateral optic atrophy and lipodystrophy. *Ann Intern Med* 1978; **89**: 72–3.
14 Langhof H, Zabel R. Zür lipodystrophia progressiva. *Arch Klin Exp Dermatol* 1960; **210**: 313–21.
15 Jensen MD. Adrenergic regulation of lipolysis with lipoatrophy of the upper body. *Mayo Clin Proc* 1991; **66**: 704–10.
16 Mathieson PW, Peters DK. Lipodystrophy in MCGN type II: the clue to links between the adipocyte and the complement system. *Nephrol Dial Transplant* 1997; **12**: 1804–6.
17 Hegele RA, Cao H, Liu DM et al. Sequencing of the reannotated LMNB2 gene reveals novel mutations in patients with acquired partial lipodystrophy. *Am J Hum Genet* 2006; **79**: 383–9.
18 Ljunghall S, Fjellstrom KE, Wibell L. Partial lipodystrophy and chronic hypocomplementaemic glomerulonephritis. *Acta Med Scand* 1974; **195**: 493–7.
19 Peters DK, Charlesworth JA, Sissons JGP et al. Mesangiocapillary nephritis, partial lipodystrophy and hypocomplementaemia. *Lancet* 1973; **ii**: 535–8.
20 Akhter J, Quereshi R. Partial lipodystrophy and successful pregnancy outcome. *J Pak Med Assoc* 1995; **45**: 24–7.
21 Cronin CC, Higgins T, Molloy M. Lupus, C3 nephritic factor and partial lipodystrophy. *QJM* 1995; **88**: 298–9.
22 Walport MJ, Davies KA, Botto M et al. C3 nephritis factor and SLE: report of four cases and review of the literature. *QJM* 1994; **87**: 609–15.
23 Kavanagh GM, Colaco CB, Kennedy CTC. Juvenile dermatomyositis associated with partial lipoatrophy. *J Am Acad Dermatol* 1993; **28**: 348–51.
24 Perrot H, Delaup J-P, Chouvet B. Partial lipodystrophy, complement abnormalities and cutaneous leukocytoclastic vasculitis. *Ann Dermatol Vénéréol* 1987; **114**: 1083–91.
25 Orrell RW, Peatfield RC, Collins CE et al. Myopathy in acquired partial lipodystrophy. *Clin Neurol Neurosurg* 1995; **97**: 181–6.
26 Citagy OS, Benitez RP, Farzaneh NK et al. Unusual mammographic findings in a patient with partial lipodystrophy. *Am J Roentgen* 1993; **160**: 417–22.
27 Winhoven SM, Hafejee A, Coulson IH. An unusual case of an acquired acral partial lipodystrophy (Barraquer–Simons syndrome) in a patient with extrinsic allergic alveolitis. *Clin Exp Dermatol* 2006; **31**: 594–6.
28 Coessens BC, Van Geertrudyen JP. Simultaneous bilateral facial reconstruction of a Barraque–Simons lipodystrophy with free TRAM flaps. *Plast Reconstr Surg* 1995; **95**: 911–5.
29 Koshy CE, Evans J. Facial contour reconstruction in localised lipodystrophy using free radial forearm adipofascial flaps. *Br J Plast Surg* 1998; **51**: 499–502.

Partial face-sparing lipodystrophy

Synonym
- Kobberling–Dunnigan syndrome

This even rarer form is a genetically heterogeneous set of disorders characterized by a widespread but partial absence of subcutaneous fat usually sparing the face and neck; it can be easily missed because of the normal facial appearance [1]. Onset is usually during adolescence and the condition is often familial. With the development of molecular genetics this phenotype has been superseded by an evolving genetic classification into three groups: familial partial lipodystrophy (FPLD) one, two and three [2].

FPLD1. FPLD1 (Kobberling type; MIM 608600) at present has no known molecular genetic basis. Kobberling et al. described three patients [3], the proband, her mother and her sister, with the same clinical appearance of complete absence of subcutaneous fat of arms and legs but with well-developed adipose tissue on the trunk and face. His patient also had hyperlipidaemia, eruptive xanthoma and insulin-resistant diabetes. Herbst et al. [4] described a further 13 patients having this phenotype of peripheral lipodystrophy with normal or increased central obesity and absence of the FDLP1 and FDLP2 genotype, emphasizing the benefit of measuring the ratio of skinfold thickness from abdomen to thigh, which was significantly higher than normal. Patients also had components of the metabolic syndrome, including hypertension, insulin resistance and severe hypertriglyceridaemia resulting in pancreatitis. Premature coronary artery disease was present in 31%.

FPLD2. FPLD2 (Dunnigan type; MIM 151660) results from heterozygous mutations in the *LMNA* gene encoding nuclear lamin A/C usually of an autosomal dominant pattern, but rarely sex-linked recessive. Lamins are a class of intermediate filaments forming the inner membrane of a nucleus. The precise mechanism, structural or otherwise, whereby the gene defect leads to lipodystrophy is unknown, but as lamins are ubiquitous in human cells, different mutations allow lipodystrophy to be associated with other phenotypes, including Hutchinson–Gilford progeria syndrome (HGPS), atypical Werner syndrome, Emery–Dreifuss muscular dystrophy, limb-girdle muscular dystrophy, mandibuloacral dysplasia (MAD), cardiomyopathies, cardiac conduction defects and Charcot–Marie–Tooth disease [2].

Dunnigan [5] described two families with an autosomal dominant disorder appearing in adolescence, and manifesting as loss of subcutaneous fat on the limbs so that the underlying musculature and superficial veins were more defined. The face appeared fuller than normal and moderate genital hypertrophy was noted. Acanthosis nigricans, tuberoeruptive xanthomata and insulin resistance were commonly associated. With increasing numbers of mutations being described, phenotypic heterogeneity is becoming apparent [6]. Patients with abnormalities in the lamin A gene only may demonstrate mild loss of limb fat, no gluteal loss and little of the features of insulin resistance. Those patients with lamin A/C abnormalities are more likely to express more extensive loss of fat, hypertriglyceridaemia, diabetes mellitus, insulin resistance, acanthosis nigricans, hirsutism and polycystic ovary syndrome. Individuals with *LMNA* mutations are recognized as having premature atherosclerosis and early coronary heart disease [7].

FPLD3. FPLD3 (MIM 604637) is associated with many different heterozygous mutations in the *PPARG* gene encoding peroxisome proliferator-activated receptor-γ (PPARγ). The PPAR protein is a nuclear transcription factor important in adipocyte differentiation, and the precise mechanism of effect for the gene abnormality is uncertain [2]. The peripheral fat loss is not as pronounced as FPLD2, but metabolic changes may be more severe. Severe hypertension is a feature [8].

Because the overall distribution of fat loss in FLPD is peripheral with facial sparing, the differential diagnosis includes Cushing's syndrome. Some patients have increased fat deposition on the chin, face and neck, and a buffalo hump, to confuse things further. Truncal obesity, lipomatosis and HIV lipodystrophy also need to be excluded.

Treatment. Management involves genetic counselling, attention to metabolic consequences and exclusion of associated syndromes. Treatment of the metabolic effects with thiazolidinediones, which

attach to PPARγ, has been of some benefit in patients with and without defined gene defects [9]. They have increased subcutaneous fat in some subjects, but their use is of still uncertain benefit [10,11].

References

1 Mamalaki E, Katsantonis J, Papavasiliou S *et al.* A case of partial face-sparing lipodystrophy combining features of generalized lipodystrophy. *J Am Acad Dermatol* 1995; **32**: 130–3.

2 Hegele RA, Joy TR, Al-Attar SA *et al.* Thematic review series: adipocyte biology. Lipodystrophies: windows on adipose biology and metabolism. *J Lipid Res* 2007; **48**: 1433–44.

3 Kobberling J, Willms B, Kattermann R *et al.* Lipodystrophy of the extremities: a dominantly inherited syndrome associated with lipoatrophic diabetes. *Humangenetik* 1975; **29**: 111–20.

4 Herbst KL, Tannock LR, Deeb SS *et al.* Kobberling type of familial partial lipodystrophy: an underrecognized syndrome. *Diabetes Care* 2003; **26**: 1819–24.

5 Dunnigan MG, Cochrane M, Kelly A *et al.* Familial lipoatrophic diabetes with dominant transmission: a new syndrome. *QJM* 1974; **43**: 33–48.

6 Garg A, Vinaitheerthan M, Weatherall PT *et al.* Phenotypic heterogeneity in patients with familial partial lipodystrophy (Dunnigan variety) related to the site of missense mutations in lamin a/c gene. *J Clin Endocrinol Metab* 2001; **86**: 59–65.

7 Hegele RA. Premature atherosclerosis associated with monogenic insulin resistance. *Circulation* 2001; **103**: 2225–9.

8 Barroso I, Gurnell M, Crowley VEF *et al.* Dominant negative mutations in human PPAR-gamma associated with severe insulin resistance, diabetes mellitus and hypertension. *Nature* 1999; **402**: 880–3.

9 Sleilati GG, Leff T, Bonnett JW *et al.* Efficacy and safety of pioglitazone in treatment of a patient with an atypical partial lipodystrophy syndrome. *Endocr Pract* 2007; **13**: 656–61.

10 Arioglu E, Duncan-Morin J, Sebring N *et al.* Efficacy and safety of troglitazone in the treatment of lipodystrophy syndromes. *Ann Intern Med* 2000; **133**: 263–74.

11 Owen KR, Donohoe M, Ellard S *et al.* Response to treatment with rosiglitazone in familial partial lipodystrophy due to a mutation in the LMNA gene. *Diabet Med* 2003; **20**: 823–7.

HIV-associated lipodystrophy syndrome

Patterns of fat atrophy and hypertrophy with metabolic changes in HIV patients taking highly active antiretroviral therapy (HAART) are described below [1–3].

Aetiology. Since the syndrome was described in 1998 [1], evolving research continues to uncover different patterns, mechanisms and risk factors [4]. Three patterns are described: lipoatrophy, lipohypertrophy and mixed (lipoatrophy and lipohypertrophy), though one group has found no association between peripheral lipoatrophy and visceral hypertrophy [5,6]. Lipoatrophy may be peripheral subcutaneous (face, limbs and buttocks), central subcutaneous (trunk and neck) and/or visceral (omental, mesenteric and perinephric). Lipohypertrophy may occur at central subcutaneous sites, especially dorsocervical (buffalo hump) and chin, and/or viscerally. Intrathoracic fat may also be increased [7]. Patients with lipohypertrophy are at present classed as having the HIV-associated adipose redistribution syndrome (HARS), which may or may not be associated with lipoatrophy [8]. The prevalence of lipodystrophy in HIV is difficult to ascertain because of problems with diagnostic criteria, but may be 17% in adults treated with protease inhibitor-containing therapy for less than 1 year, and around 40% in those treated for 1 year or more [2,9] though it may be as high as 53% [10]. Significant risk factors include

CD4-positive count, viral load, duration of therapy and age. Patients with fat loss are more likely to have taken an older thymidine analogue nucleoside reverse transcriptase inhibitor (NRTI), particularly stavudine or zidovudine, and be of white race. Patients showing hypertrophy are more likely to have taken an older protease inhibitor (PI) (indinavir or nelfinavir), and be of female sex [11]. Rarely, lipoatrophy is seen in patients who have not been exposed to HAART. The syndrome also occurs in children but less so if they received a lower dose of the protease inhibitor [12]. Another childhood study showed a prevalence of lipodystrophy of 9%, 47% and 65% at 48, 96 and 144 weeks after HAART initiation respectively [13]. At week 144, central lipohypertrophy (46%) was most frequent, with peripheral lipoatrophy (20%), and combined type (34%) less frequent. This variety of patterns of fat atrophy and hypertrophy suggests different mechanisms dependent on drug combinations, viral effects and host factors, such as genetic polymorphisms, interacting to result in a particular phenotype [4].

Pathogenesis. The mechanisms of HIV lipodystrophy are complex [11,14]. Lipoatrophy is associated with impaired adipocyte differentiation and increased apoptosis, insulin resistance and increased lipolysis, altered adipocyte cytokine expression and mitochondrial toxicity. Both PIs and NRTIs can inhibit adipocyte differentiation. Both alter adipocytokine secretion (reduced adiponectin and normal or increased leptin) and adipocyte TNF-α secretion (increased). NRTIs seem mainly responsible for mitochondrial toxicity. Buffalo hump lipohypertrophy [15] shows unaltered expression of marker genes of adipogenesis, but altered gene expression for enhanced cell proliferation plus features of a brown-versus-white fat phenotype. TNF-α secretion is not increased. Cortisol-induced new adipogenesis may be responsible for visceral fat hypertrophy combined with a need for disposal of free fatty acids, generated by lipolysis [11].

Histopathology. There is a diminution in the volume of subcutaneous fat, with the lobules containing adipocytes of varying size, interspersed with increased capillaries. Foci of lymphoid infiltrates and lipogranulomas are seen [3]. Scattered apoptotic adipocytes may also be present [16]. Ultrastructurally, buffalo hump lipohypertrophy shows adipocytes intermediate between those in brown and white fat [17].

Clinical features. Females (28%) are affected by lipoatrophy less than males (38%) [5,6]. The loss is most apparent in the face. Loss of buccal, parotid and pre-auricular fat pads produces a prominent cheekbone, and melolabial folds emphasized by the sunken cheeks and sometimes enlarged parotid glands. Loss of retro-orbital fat produces sunken eyes. Limb fat loss allows superficial veins and muscle to appear more defined. Central subcutaneous fat accumulation may be present on the upper back, neck (buffalo hump), on the breasts, suprapubic area [18], below the jaw, in the supraclavicular region or as multiple lipomas. Omental fat accumulation produces a protuberant abdomen and an increased waist to hip circumference ratio, sometimes provoking symptomatology such as abdominal distension, gastroesophageal reflux and sleep disturbances.

Lipoatrophy of the face is so recognizable that the altered appearance, indicating potential HIV-positivity, can be devastating for the patient [19]. Erosion of self-esteem, diminished desirability, attractiveness and sexual function, anxiety and depression may lead to discontinuation of therapy, though non-adherence is disputed [20]. Patients' subjective reporting of lipodystrophy correlates better with diminished quality of life than physician evaluation [19], and the absence of universally accepted clinical measurement criteria for lipodystrophy is still a handicap. Objective measurement of body fat may be performed with ultrasonography, dual-energy X-ray absorptiometry (DEXA), CT and MRI scanning, though DEXA scans do not distinguish between visceral fat compartments [21]. Anthropometry, such as waist and hip circumference and ratio [22], perhaps combined with ultrasonography [23], may provide the simplest and cheapest clinical method of evaluation, particularly for metabolic risk factors, with MRI remaining the gold standard [24].

Metabolic changes do not appear to be as severe in the HIV lipodystrophy group as in CGL [25], with acanthosis nigricans, hypertrichosis and PCOS almost never being seen. This may be related to the fact that insulin resistance is less frequent. Abnormalities in glucose homeostasis occur in 23%, and in hyperlipidaemia in 74%, of patients [26]. In a study of 614 patients, 20 months after initiation of protease inhibitor therapy, a cross-sectional study demonstrated that 23% had abnormal glucose metabolism, 20% had hypertriglyceridaemia and 57% hypercholesterolaemia [27]. In children at 144 weeks, fasting hypertriglyceridaemia was detected in 12%, hypercholesterolaemia in 11%, and increased plasma glucose in 4% [13]. Insulin resistance is related to increased fat in the liver rather than visceral adiposity [28]. Hyperlactataemia may be seen. However, the prevalence of the metabolic syndrome in HIV patients without lipodystrophy is disputed. One study from the USA found a prevalence of 14–18%, compared to a control prevalence of 24% for a non-HIV-positive adult population [29]. In another study of female HIV-positive patients only, prevalence was 33% versus 22% in controls [30], while a third study found no difference between HIV positive and negative patients [31]. Where obvious lipoatrophy and an increased waist circumference is present, patients often have insulin resistance [25].

Differential diagnosis. HIV lipodystrophy can be differentiated from HIV-wasting syndrome in that it is seen in patients responding to HAART, and lean body mass is preserved.

Management. Prevention and delay of progression/reversal of lipodystrophy, treatment of metabolic effects, and surgical interventions provide the mainstay of treatment [32]. Choosing the right combination of newer HAART drugs, and avoiding stavudine and zidovudine, reduces the risk of developing lipoatrophy. Delaying the timing of treatment, employing treatment interruptions, and treatment switching may all help. The addition of a thiazolidinedione (pioglitazone) may be beneficial in lipoatrophy. Diet and exercise may reduce visceral adiposity, as may the use of growth hormone and metformin; possibly at the cost of aggravating subcutaneous lipoatrophy. Management of traditional risk factors, rather than HIV treatment-associated ones, may be more important for lessening cardiovascular disease from the metabolic syndrome [31]. Stopping smoking, diet and exercise to achieve an appropriate BMI should be the first line approaches. If lipid levels remain high after lifestyle changes and HAART switching, a statin, or fibrate if triglyceride levels are high as well as cholesterol, should be introduced. Likewise, if lifestyle changes have not achieved strict glycaemic control, metformin should be introduced for an overweight patient and pioglitazone for a lipoatrophic one. Hypertension, if present, should be addressed.

Surgical interventions for lipoatrophy include autologous fat injection, flaps and injection of fillers such as polylactic acid [33]. Fat injections may need to be repeated but can provide a satisfactory result [34], provided the source is not the brown fat in a buffalo hump. Polylactic acid, a synthetic polymer, may need to be injected repeatedly in severe facial wasting, but is safe, and effective, with good patient acceptance [35]. Liposuction is helpful for buffalo humps despite the fibrous septa and the high risk of recurrence [36]. Simple lipectomy treats gynaecomastia and lipomas.

References

1 Carr A, Samaras K, Burton S et al. A syndrome of peripheral lipodystrophy, hyperlipidaemia and insulin resistance in patients receiving HIV protease inhibitors. AIDS 1998; 12: F51–8.
2 Chen D, Misra A, Garg A. Clinical review 153: Lipodystrophy in human immunodeficiency virus-infected patients. J Clin Endocrinol Metab 2002; 87: 4845–56.
3 Pujol RM, Domingo P, Xavier-Matias-Guiu et al. HIV-1 protease inhibitor-associated partial lipodystrophy: clinicopathologic review of 14 cases. J Am Acad Dermatol 2000; 42: 193–8.
4 Lichtenstein KA. Redefining lipodystrophy syndrome: risks and impact on clinical decision making. J Acquir Immune Defic Syndr 2005; 39: 395–400.
5 Bacchetti P, Gripshover B, Grunfeld C et al. Study of fat redistribution and metabolic change in HIV infection (FRAM). Fat distribution in men with HIV infection. J Acquir Immune Defic Syndr 2005; 40: 121–31.
6 Study of Fat Redistribution and Metabolic Change in HIV Infection (FRAM). Fat distribution in women with HIV infection. J Acquir Immune Defic Syndr 2006; 42: 562–71.
7 Blanco JL, Biglia A, Martinez E et al. Intrathoracic fat in HIV-infected patients. HIV Med 2006; 7: 213–7.
8 Lichtenstein K, Balasubramanyam A, Sekhar R et al. HIV-associated adipose redistribution syndrome (HARS): definition, epidemiology and clinical impact. AIDS Res Ther 2007; 4: 16.
9 Thiébaut R, Daucourt V, Mercié P et al. Lipodystrophy, metabolic disorders, and human immunodeficiency virus infection: Aquitaine Cohort, France, 1999. Groupe d'Epidémiologie Clinique du Syndrome d'Immunodéficience Acquise en Aquitaine. Clin Infect Dis 2000; 31: 1482–7.
10 Miller J, Carr A, Emery S et al. HIV lipodystrophy: prevalence, severity and correlates of risk in Australia. HIV Med 2003; 4: 293–301.
11 Lichtenstein K, Balasubramanyam A, Sekhar R et al. HIV-associated adipose redistribution syndrome (HARS): etiology and pathophysiological mechanisms. AIDS Res Ther 2007; 4: 14.
12 Amaya RA, Kozinetz CA, McMeans A et al. Lipodystrophy syndrome in human immunodeficiency virus-infected children. Pediatr Infect Dis J 2002; 21: 405–10.
13 Aurpibul L, Puthanakit T, Lee B et al. Lipodystrophy and metabolic changes in HIV-infected children on non-nucleoside reverse transcriptase inhibitor-based antiretroviral therapy. Antivir Ther 2007; 12: 1247–54.
14 Mallewa JE, Wilkins E, Vilar J et al. HIV-associated lipodystrophy: a review of underlying mechanisms and therapeutic options. J Antimicrob Chemother 2008; 62: 648–60.
15 Guallar JP, Gallego-Escuredo JM, Domingo JC et al. Differential gene expression indicates that 'buffalo hump' is a distinct adipose tissue disturbance in HIV-1-associated lipodystrophy. AIDS 2008; 22: 575–84.
16 Domingo P, Matias-Guiu X, Pujol RM et al. Subcutaneous adipocyte apoptosis in HIV-1 protease inhibitor-associated lipodystrophy. AIDS 1999; 13: 2261–7.
17 Fessel WJ, Follansbee SB, Barker B. Ultrastructural findings consistent with brown adipocytes in buffalo humps of HIV-positive patients with fat redistribution syndrome. Antivir Ther 2000; 3 (Suppl. 5): 25.
18 Guaraldi G, Orlando G, Squillace N et al. Prevalence of and risk factors for pubic lipoma development in HIV-infected persons. J Acquir Immune Defic Syndr 2007; 45: 72–6.
19 Guaraldi G, Murri R, Orlando G et al. Severity of lipodystrophy is associated with decreased health-related quality of life. AIDS Patient Care STDS 2008; 22: 577–85.
20 Collins EJ, Burgoyne RW, Wagner CA et al. Lipodystrophy severity does not contribute to HAART nonadherence. AIDS Behav 2006; 10: 273–7.
21 Baril JG, Junod P, Leblanc R et al. HIV-associated lipodystrophy syndrome: A review of clinical aspects. Can J Infect Dis Med Microbiol 2005; 16: 233–43.
22 Scherzer R, Shen W, Bacchetti P et al. Study of Fat Redistribution Metabolic Change in HIV Infection (FRAM). Simple anthropometric measures correlate with metabolic risk indicators as strongly as magnetic resonance imaging-measured adipose tissue depots in both HIV-infected and control subjects. Am J Clin Nutr 2008; 87: 1809–17.
23 Padilla S, Gallego JA, Masiá M et al. Ultrasonography and anthropometry for measuring regional body fat in HIV-infected patients. Curr HIV Res 2007; 5: 459–66.
24 Dinges WL, Chen D, Snell PG et al. Regional body fat distribution in HIV-infected patients with lipodystrophy. J Investig Med 2005; 53: 15–25.
25 Leow MK, Addy CL, Mantzoros CS. Clinical review 159: Human immunodeficiency virus/highly active antiretroviral therapy-associated metabolic syndrome: clinical presentation, pathophysiology, and therapeutic strategies. J Clin Endocrinol Metab 2003; 88: 1961–76.
26 Carr A, Samaras K, Thorisdottir A et al. Diagnosis, prediction, and natural course of HIV-1 protease-inhibitor-associated lipodystrophy, hyperlipidaemia, and diabetes mellitus: a cohort study. Lancet 1999; 353: 2093–9.
27 Saves M, Raffi F, Capeau J et al. Factors related to lipodystrophy and metabolic alterations in patients with human immunodeficiency virus infection receiving highly active antiretroviral therapy. Clin Infect Dis 2002; 34: 1396–405.
28 Sutinen J, Hakkinen AM, Westerbacka J et al. Increased fat accumulation in the liver in HIV-infected patients with antiretroviral therapy-associated lipodystrophy. AIDS 2002; 16: 2183–93.
29 Samaras K, Wand H, Law M et al. Prevalence of metabolic syndrome in HIV-infected patients receiving highly active antiretroviral therapy using International Diabetes Foundation and Adult Treatment Panel III criteria: associations with insulin resistance, disturbed body fat compartmentalization, elevated C-reactive protein, and [corrected] hypoadiponectinemia. Diabetes Care 2007; 30: 113–9.
30 Sobieszczyk ME, Hoover DR, Anastos K et al. Prevalence and predictors of metabolic syndrome among HIV-infected and HIV-uninfected women in the Women's Interagency HIV Study. J Acquir Immune Defic Syndr 2008; 48: 272–80.
31 Mondy K, Overton ET, Grubb J et al. Metabolic syndrome in HIV-infected patients from an urban, midwestern US outpatient population. Clin Infect Dis 2007; 44: 726–34.
32 Lundgren JD, Battegay M, Behrens G et al. EACS Executive Committee. European AIDS Clinical Society (EACS) guidelines on the prevention and management of metabolic diseases in HIV. HIV Med 2008; 9: 72–81.
33 Nelson L, Stewart KJ. Plastic surgical options for HIV-associated lipodystrophy. J Plast Reconstr Aesthet Surg 2008; 61: 359–65.
34 Burnouf M, Buffet M, Schwarzinger M et al. Evaluation of Coleman lipostructure for treatment of facial lipoatrophy in patients with human immunodeficiency virus and parameters associated with the efficiency of this technique. Arch Dermatol 2005; 141: 1220–4.
35 Valantin MC, Aubron-Olivier C, Ghosn J et al. Polylactic acid implants (Newfill)® to correct facial lipoatrophy in HIV-infected patients: results of the open-label study VEGA. AIDS 2003; 17: 2471–7.
36 Davison SP, Timpone J Jr, Hannan CM. Surgical algorithm for management of HIV lipodystrophy. Plast Reconstr Surg 2007; 120: 1843–58.

Lipomas

Lipomas are benign tumours composed of mature fat cells. They are found in the subcutaneous tissue and less commonly in internal organs.

Aetiology. The metabolic changes associated with benign tumours are varied, but include fundamental defects responsible for the altered growth properties of the tumour. It has been demonstrated that loss of negative-feedback control regulatory enzymes (by citrate or phosphofructokinase) may be an early feature in the development of lipoma [1].

Histopathology. Fat cells in groups slightly larger than the normal lobule are typically enclosed within a capsule of connective tissue, but the capsule may be deficient and the tumour then appears locally invasive. Relatively large blood vessels are seen traversing the connective tissue septa. Primitive fat cells may be found in clinically benign lipomas in children [2]. Xanthomatous and mucinous changes appear in many lipomas. Lipomas exhibit, like many other solid tumours, distinctive cytogenic abnormalities (karyotypic aberrations affecting mainly 12q, 6p, 13q). Such distinctive changes may be of help in histologically borderline or difficult cases [3]. Variants of lipoma with large areas of normal fat cells such as spindle cell lipoma/pleomorphic lipoma and atypical lipomatous tumour are discussed in Chapter 56. For other rare lipomatous-like tumours the reader is referred to specialized texts [4].

Clinical features. A lipoma is a subcutaneous nodule, often lobulated, with a characteristic soft, putty-like consistency. The overlying skin is normal and moves freely over the tumour, and feels cooler than the surrounding skin. The tumour grows very slowly to reach a diameter that is usually between 2 and 10 cm but may be considerably greater. The most common sites are the neck, shoulders and upper arms, back and thighs. There are rarely any subjective symptoms, but pain from pressure on the nerves is sometimes experienced. Another rare event is infiltration of adjacent tissues, in a particular muscle [5]. In these patients, there is a high recurrence rate after surgical intervention because of its diffuse infiltration; thus complete surgical excision is often impossible [6]. Fat necrosis may cause enlargement, pain and tenderness. A large lipoma on the exposed skin of the lower legs is susceptible to nodular perniosis.

There may be only one lipoma, or large numbers [7] may develop at intervals over a period of years. Seven per cent of patients with lipoma have multiple lesions [8,9]. Such lipomas may be randomly distributed, or more or less confined to one region of the body. In most patients, the presence of multiple lipomas appears to have no special significance [2]. They may, however, be associated with neurofibromatosis, or with visceral lipomas in the respiratory, alimentary or genitourinary tract. Tendon sheath lipomas are rare and are usually associated with a mild discomfort [10]. They are an inconstant feature of Gardner's syndrome, in which they are associated with multiple sebaceous cysts, osteomas and polyposis of the colon. Multiple lipomas may also be a pointer to Proteus syndrome, Cowden's disease and Bannayan's syndrome. In addition to multiple lipomas, the latter exhibits macrocephaly, lymphangiomas and haemangiomas (see Congenital diffuse lipomatosis, below) [11].

Diagnosis. The diagnosis is usually easy, but in cases of doubt a biopsy should be performed. Angiolipomas are morphologically similar to lipomas, but are intermittently painful. Lipofascial herniae in the natal or perianal region simulate lipomas. Excision and suture are required to prevent recurrence. Mobile encapsulated lipomas are literally very mobile and can be moved from side to side over a range of up to 8 cm [12].

An epidermoid cyst can mimic a lipoma. However, the presence of the central punctum gives a clue to the correct diagnosis. The possibility of hibernoma should be considered when tumours appear in the thigh, neck and scapular region.

Treatment. This usually depends on the patient's desire for the lipoma to be surgically removed. Lipoma of the lumbar region may be associated with underlying spina bifida occulta, and removal of the tumour is dangerous without simultaneous exploration of the cauda equina. An MRI scan is essential in such patients; the spinal cord involvement is more frequent in girls than in boys, and is significantly associated with bladder dysfunction [13].

References

1 Atkinson JNC, Galton DJ, Gilbert C. Regulatory defect of glycolysis in human lipoma. *BMJ* 1974; **i**: 101–2.
2 Wakeley C, Somerville P. Lipomas. *Lancet* 1952; **ii**: 995–9.
3 Fletcher CDM, Akerman M, Dal Cin P *et al.* Correlation between clinicopathological features and karyotype in lipomatous tumours. *Am J Pathol* 1996; **148**: 623–6.
4 Mentzel T. Cutaneous lipomatous neoplasms. *Semin Diagn Pathol* 2001; **18**: 250–7.
5 Mattel SF, Persky MS. Infiltrating lipoma of the sternocleidomastoid muscle. *Laryngoscope* 1983; **93**: 205–7.
6 Chen CM, Lo LJ, Wong HF. Congenital infiltrating lipomatosis of the face: case report and literature review. *Chang Gung Med J* 2002; **25**: 194–200.
7 Adam BA, Chan YS. Congenital diffuse lipomatosis with diabetes mellitus. *Br J Clin Pract* 1974; **28**: 101–2.
8 Osment LS. Cutaneous lipomas and lipomatosis. *Surg Gynecol Obstet* 1968; **127**: 129–32.
9 Von Knoth W. Über Naevus lipomatosus cutaneous superficialis Hoffmann–Zurhelle und über Naevus naevocellularis partial lipomatoses. *Dermatologica* 1962; **125**: 161–73.
10 Sullivan CR, Dahlin DC, Bryan RS. Lipoma of the tendon sheath. *J Bone Joint Surg* 1956; **38**: 1275–80.
11 Bannayan GA. Lipomatosis, angiomatosis and macroencephalia. *Arch Pathol* 1971; **92**: 1–5.
12 Trapp CF, Baker EJ. Mobile encapsulated lipomas. *Cutis* 1992; **49**: 63–4.
13 Dorward NL, Scatliff JH, Hayward RD. Congenital lumbosacral lipomas: pitfalls in analysing the result of prophylactic surgery. *Childs Nerv Syst* 2002; **18**: 326–32.

Angiolipoma

Angiolipomas are benign encapsulated lobulated tumours, differing from a lipoma in the excessive degree of vascular (capillary) proliferation histologically and in the possession of a normal karyotype cytogenetically. Approximately 10% of all lipomatous lesions examined pathologically are angiolipomas [1]. The degree of vascularity varies and there is no agreed parameter to distinguish between a lipoma and a poorly-vascularized angiolipoma. Fibrin thrombi are common. The age of onset is relatively young, and in one series of 288 patients averaged 17 years. Clinically, the lesions are from 0.5 to 5 cm in diameter and closely resemble lipomas. They are usually painful and tender and are sometimes bluish in colour [2]. The degree of pain varies with the degree of vascularization. They occur most frequently on the arms, legs and abdomen, and are often multiple [3].

Angiolipomas are categorized into two groups: infiltrating and non-infiltrating [3]. The non-infiltrating angiolipoma is typically a soft, well-encapsulated, subcutaneous nodule. The non-infiltrating type occurs in younger individuals and is usually painful, often multiple and occasionally familial. Compression of nerve fibres that accompany the vascular channels may cause pain, which is usually dull. The infiltrating type, which is the less common type of angiolipoma, is solitary, has a more aggressive behaviour, and can infiltrate osseous, muscular, neural and fibro-collagenous tissues. It may cause signs and symptoms that can simulate malignant neoplasms. The infiltrating type has the propensity to recur following local surgical excision; therefore the treatment for infiltrating angiolipoma is wide excision to include normal tissue surrounding the tumour. Associated features are rare; the association of multiple angiolipomas, multiple cerebral aneurysms and multiple meningomas has been reported [4].

Three cases of HIV-1 infected patients have been described who developed symptomatic angiolipomas shortly after starting anti-retroviral therapy, including protease inhibitors [5].

Painful lesions can be excised if single. Conventional analgesics usually do not help. Multiple lesions have been shown to respond to β-blockade with atenolol (50 mg/day). Pain relief was evident after 24 h. Therapy should be continued for a pain-free period of 2–3 months [6]. A double-blind study proved the benefit of intra-venous lidocaine (lignocaine) (5 mg/kg) in saline given over 45 min. The pain disappeared after 1–2 days but reappeared 3 weeks later [7]. Infiltrating angiolipomas need wide excision [8]. Liposuction has been successfully used in one patient [9].

References

1 Howard WR, Helwig EB. Angiolipoma. *Arch Dermatol* 1960; **82**: 924–31.
2 Klem KK. Multiple angiolipomas. *Acta Chir* 1949; **97**: 527–32.
3 Dixon AY, McGregor DH, Lee SH. Angiolipomas: an ultrastructural and clinico-pathological study. *Hum Pathol* 1981; **12**: 739–47.
4 Stevenson JC, Choksey MS, McMahon J *et al*. Multiple cerebral aneurysms, multiple meningiomas and multiple subcutaneous angiolipomas: a case report. *Br J Neurosurg* 1994; **8**: 477–81.
5 Dank JP, Colven R. Protease inhibitor-associated angiolipomatosis. *J Am Acad Dermatol* 2000; **42**: 129–31.
6 Goodfield MJD, Rowell NR. The clinical presentation of cutaneous angio-lipomata and the response to β-blockade. *Clin Exp Dermatol* 1988; **13**: 190–2.
7 Fogh H, Agner T, Agner E. Multiple angiolipomata treated with intravenous infusions of lignocaine. *Clin Exp Dermatol* 1990; **15**: 63–4.
8 Tighe C, Lynn JA. Angiolipomas of the foot. *J Am Pediatr Med Assoc* 1994; **84**: 85–9.
9 Kaneko T, Tokushige H, Kimura N *et al*. Treatment of multiple angiolipomas by liposuction surgery. *J Dermatol Surg Oncol* 1994; **20**: 690–2.

Frontalis-associated lipoma [1,2]

This is a deeply placed lipoma of the forehead, which deserves special mention because it is often mistaken for an epidermoid cyst. The lipoma presents a smooth, doughy, dome-shaped mass, which appears relatively immobile and the skin glides over it. It arises either within the frontalis muscle or between the undersur-face of the muscle and its deep fascia, and its removal requires greater surgical skill than is required for removing an epidermoid cyst or lipoma. A layered closure is essential to repair the severed frontalis muscle, and a pressure dressing is advisable to close the 'dead space'.

References

1 Grosshams E, Fersing J, Marescaux J. Le lipome sous-aponeurotique frontal. *Ann Dermatol Vénéréol* 1987; **114**: 335–40.
2 Salasche SJ, McCollough ML, Angeloni VL *et al*. Frontalis-associated lipoma of the forehead. *J Am Acad Dermatol* 1989; **20**: 462–8.

Fat-storing hamartoma of dermal dendrocytes

One patient has been described with a congenital reddish-brown plaque over the lumbosacral area, which was composed of dermal dendrocytes that had phagocytosed lipid droplets [1]. There were no fat cells in the lesion and no associated metabolic abnormalities.

Reference

1 Bork K, Gabbert H, Knop K. Fat-storing hamartoma of dermal dendrocytes. *Arch Dermatol* 1990; **126**: 794–6.

Hibernoma [1–4]

> **Synonym**
> • Granular cell lipoma

This is a rare benign tumour, comprising primitive fetal brown fat cells in which an increasing variety of structural abnormalities for the chromosomal band 11q13 are being found [5]. In the Armed Forces Institute of Pathology series of 170 cases [4] the mean age was 38 years, with the site of predilection being the thigh, then the shoulder, back and neck. The average size was 9.3 cm. Whilst the histology is characteristic, showing masses of distinctive cells with fine granules and a solitary central nucleus [1–3], myxoid, spindle cell and lipoma-like variants are also seen [4]. Hibernoma presents as a firm, non-tender nodule, with vascular dilatation of the overlying skin. CT and MRI imaging may be helpful but is not diagnostic [6,7]. Surgical excision is the only treatment. Local recurrence at excision is unusual, the tumour being multilobular but encapsulated [4,8].

References

1 Angervall L, Nilsson L, Stener B. Microangiographic and histological studies in two cases of hibernoma. *Cancer* 1964; **17**: 685–92.
2 Jennings RC, Behr G. Hibernoma. *J Clin Pathol* 1955; **8**: 310–2.
3 Novy FG, Wilson JW. Hibernomas: brown fat tumors. *Arch Dermatol* 1956; **73**: 149–57.
4 Furlong MA, Fanburg-Smith JC, Miettinen M. The morphologic spectrum of hibernoma: a clinicopathologic study of 170 cases. *Am J Surg Pathol* 2001; **25**: 809–14.
5 Maire G, Forus A, Foa C *et al*. 11q13 alterations in two cases of hibernoma: large heterozygous deletions and rearrangement breakpoints near GARP in 11q13.5. *Genes Chromosomes Canc* 2003; **37**: 389–95.
6 Lee JC, Gupta A, Saifuddin A *et al*. Hibernoma: MRI features in eight consecutive cases. *Clinical Radiology* 2006; **61**: 1029–34.
7 Dursun M, Agayev A, Bakir B *et al*. CT and MR characteristics of hibernoma: six cases. *Clinical Imaging* 2008; **32**: 42–7.
8 Lele SM, Chundru S, Chaljub G *et al*. Hibernoma. *Arch Pathol Lab Med* 2002; **126**: 975–8.

Lipomatosis

Lipomatosis is diffuse infiltration of structures with non-encapsulated adipose tissue. Several different types of lipomatosis have been described.

1 Multiple symmetrical lipomatosis, characterized by a symmetric formation of fatty tumours, associated with signs of mediastinal location and neuropathy

2 Pelvic lipomatosis, characterized by fat accumulation in the pelvic cavity with vesical and ureteral displacement, compression and occlusion

3 Mediastinoabdominal lipomatosis, characterized by intrathoracic and intra-abdominal accumulation of fat, mimicking respiratory disease or ascites

4 Mediastinal lipomatosis, frequently associated with long-term oral steroid exposure

5 Renal sinus and perirenal lipomatosis, characterized by a tumour-like accumulation of fat in the renal and perirenal space inside the renal capsule

6 Adiposis dolorosa, or Dercum's disease, a disease affecting women, characterized by the formation of painful para-articular lipomatous masses.

The cutaneous lipomatoses [1,2] are well-defined but rare syndromes of which two major types are identified: the symmetrical and non-symmetrical varieties. Both produce marked disfigurement. Except in the rare cases when they compress a vital structure, they usually present no physical threat to the patient. Both are benign and non-encapsulated, and represent progressive growth and extension of mature adipose tissue far beyond its normal proportions. The fat accumulation is caused by an increase in cell number rather than cell size by a zonal differentiation of adipoblasts into mature adipocytes [3].

Non-symmetrical lipomatosis

The most common, albeit rare, form of localized lipomatosis is the non-symmetrical subcutaneous lipomatosis. It is a benign entity and normally has no clinical significance except for the cosmetic disability. A localized form affecting the shoulder girdle [4,5] may infiltrate the deeper structures and produce distal symptoms. A case has been reported with tuberous sclerosis, but the association may be fortuitous [6]. It is not usually the result of any metabolic disturbance, and is not usually associated with abnormalities of lipid metabolism; in one case there was familial hyperlipidaemia, the mode of inheritance suggesting an autosomal dominant trait [7]. Other associations include ipsilateral cranial and facial asymmetry, cranial and ocular manifestations, alopecia, spasticity and mental retardation. These associations occur with what is called encephalocraniocutaneous lipomatosis—a very rare syndrome [8,9]. It has been suggested that this syndrome is a variety of Proteus syndrome, in which such patients have hyperostoses of the skull, cutaneous lipomas outside the skull and visceral lipomatoses [10]. Co-occurrence with neurocutaneous melanosis has recently been described [11].

Multiple symmetrical lipomatosis

By contrast, multiple symmetrical lipomatosis (Fig. 46.33) is characterized by large, symmetrical masses of fat, mainly in the neck

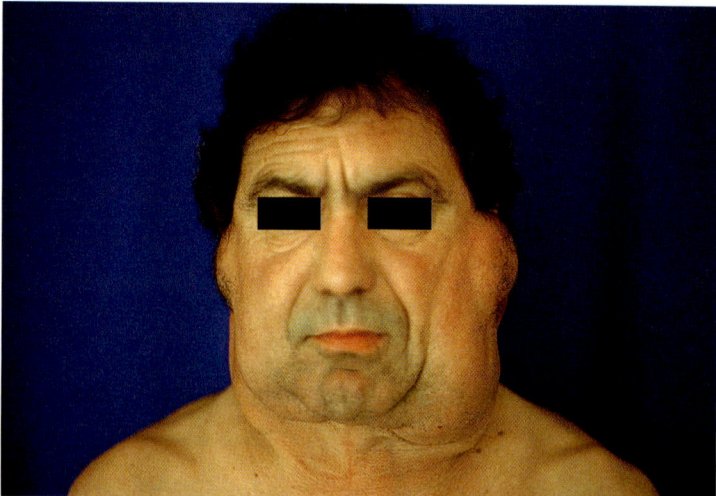

Fig. 46.33 Multiple symmetrical lipomatosis. (Courtesy of M.C. Rodrîguez-Cerdeira, R. Trillo and X.C. Brana, Meixoerio Hospital, Vigo, Spain.)

and shoulder region in a horse-collar distribution. MRI can be used to characterize the nature and extent of disease [12,13]. It may be associated with mild hypertriglyceridaemia, elevated high-density lipoprotein cholesterol [14], hyperuricaemia, impaired glucose tolerance and renal tubular acidosis. The lipomatous tissue in these patients has been shown to have enhanced lipoprotein lipase activity [15], a possible explanation for the elevated high-density lipoprotein cholesterol levels displayed by these patients. The inheritance in this type is autosomal dominant. Specific chromosomal abnormalities have been reported [16]. Mitochondrial dysfunction is common in multiple symmetrical lipomatosis and may be based on identifiable defects in the mitochondrial genome [17].

These patients may also have severe peripheral and autonomic neuropathies [18], often alcoholism, and mediastinal lipomas producing space-occupying symptoms [19]. Sebaceous naevus of Jadassohn has been reported in association with mediastinal lipomatosis [20]. Fifty per cent have a history of high alcohol intake with most of the remainder having a moderate intake or previous alcohol problems [2,21]. The male to female ratio is of the order of 6:1, with the distribution in female patients being proximal arms and legs and not the sub-mental neck pattern seen in men [21]. An unusual patient had benign symmetrical lipomatoses and giant rhinophyma producing a grotesque appearance [22]. Madelung's neck, probably the same condition, is a diffuse multilobular lipomatosis involving the back of the neck and the shoulders in a cape-like distribution. It classically afflicts wine porters and brewery workers. The disease may infrequently be sited in the upper thighs and lower abdomen [23]. Localization to the soles has been reported [24]. Localization of the symmetrical lipomatoses to the tongue results in macroglossia. Therapy is partial glossectomy [25].

The prominent fat deposits over the buttocks that constitute the steatopyga of the Bushmen and Hottentots may be regarded as a racial form of physiological lipomatosis. A distal form of acquired symmetrical lipomatosis of the hands has been reported in a chronic alcoholic Bantu male [26].

Treatment of lipomatosis is difficult. It includes classical lipectomy [27,28] but recurrence is common. Liposuction [29–31] has been reported to help considerably. Fenofibrate has been beneficial [32]. Unlike obesity there is no increase in cardiac mortality and the frequency of diabetes mellitus is the same as the normal population [33], but patients may have problems with autonomic neuropathy [34].

References

1 Shafar J, Behr G. Tumorous abnormalities of adipose tissue. *Postgrad Med J* 1965; **41**: 15–7.

2 Enzi G. Multiple symmetric lipomatosis: an updated clinical report. *Medicine* 1984; **63**: 56–64.

3 Anderson WAD. *Synopsis of Pathology*, 6th edn. New York: Mosby, 1964: 236–7.

4 Enzi G, Carraro R, Alfieri P *et al*. Shoulder girdle lipomatosis. *Ann Intern Med* 1992; **117**: 749–52.

5 McEachern A, Janzen DL, O'Connell JX. Shoulder girdle lipomatosis. *Skeletal Radiol* 1995; **24**: 471–3.

6 Klein JA, Barr RJ. Diffuse lipomatosis and tuberous sclerosis. *Arch Dermatol* 1986; **122**: 1298–302.

7 Rubinstein A, Goor Y, Gazit E *et al*. Non-symmetric subcutaneous lipomatosis associated with familial combined hyperlipidaemia. *Br J Dermatol* 1989; **120**: 689–94.

8 Nosti-Martinex D, del Castillo V, Duran-McKinster C *et al*. Encephalocraniocutaneous lipomatosis: an uncommon neurocutaneous syndrome. *J Am Acad Dermatol* 1995; **32**: 387–93.

9 Grimalt R, Ermacora D, Mistura L *et al*. Encephalocraniocutaneous lipomatosis: case report and review of literature. *Pediatr Dermatol* 1993; **10**: 164–8.

10 Rizzo R, Pavone L, Micali G *et al*. Encephalocraniocutaneous lipomatosis, Proteus syndrome and somatic mosaicism. *Am J Med Genet* 1993; **47**: 653–5.

11 Ahmed I, Tope WD, Young TL *et al*. Neurocutaneous melanosis in association with encephalocraniocutaneous lipomatosis. *J Am Acad Dermatol* 2002; **47**: S196–S200.

12 Martin DS, Sharafuddin M, Boozan J *et al*. Multiple symmetric lipomatosis (Madelung's disease). *Skeletal Radiol* 1995; **24**: 72–3.

13 Hermans R, Verellen S, Vergote G *et al*. Benign symmetric lipomatosis of the neck or Madelung–Launois–Bensaude syndrome, also known as Madelung's neck: CT findings in two cases. *Rofo-Fortschr Rontg* 1994; **161**: 248–50.

14 Deina L, Giovanni MP, Carru C *et al*. Extremely high HDL levels in a patient with multiple symmetric lipomatosis. *Clin Chim Acta* 1993; **223**: 143–7.

15 Enzi G, Favaretto L, Martini S *et al*. Metabolic abnormalities in multiple symmetric lipomatosis: elevated lipoprotein lipase activity in adipose tissue with hyper-alphalipoproteinemia. *J Lipid Res* 1983; **24**: 566–74.

16 Morelli A, Falchetti A, Weinstein L. RFLP analysis of human chromosome 11 region q13 in multiple symmetric lipomatosis and multiple endocrine neoplasia type-1 associated lipomas. *Biophys Res Comm* 1995; **207**: 363–8.

17 Klopstock T, Naumann M, Schalke B *et al*. Multiple symmetric lipomatosis: abnormalities in complex IV and multiple deletions in mitochondrial DNA. *Neurology* 1994; **44**: 862–9.

18 Teplitsky V, Huminer D, Dux S *et al*. Multiple symmetric lipomatosis presenting with polyneuropathy. *Israel J Med Sci* 1995; **31**: 693–5.

19 Munoz-Fernandez C, Aladro Y, Conde MA *et al*. Multiple symmetrical lipomatosis with familial polyneuropathy. *Rev Neurol* 2001; **32**: 1107–11.

20 Taboada E, Moledo E, Alvarez A *et al*. Sebaceous naevus of Jadassohn and primary mediastinal lipomatosis. *Br J Plast Surg* 1993; **46**: 264–5.

21 Busetto L, Strater D, Enzi G. Differential clinical expression of multiple symmetric lipomatosis in men and women. *Int J Obes* 2003; **27**: 1419–22.

22 Izu R, Gardeazabal J, Bejar J *et al*. A case of the elephant man phenotype with giant rhinophyma and benign symmetric lipomatosis. *Clin Exp Dermatol* 1994; **19**: 531–3.

23 Hacker SM, Ramos-Caro FA. An uncommon presentation of multiple symmetric lipomatosis. *Int J Dermatol* 1993; **32**: 594–7.

24 Requera L, Hasson A, Arias D *et al*. Acquired symmetric lipomatosis of the soles. *J Am Acad Dermatol* 1992; **26**: 860–2.

25 Katou F, Nabukazu S, Motegi K *et al*. Symmetrical lipomatosis of the tongue presenting as macroglossia. *J Cranio Maxillo Facial Surg* 1993; **21**: 298–301.

26 Findlay GH, Duvenage M. Acquired symmetrical lipomatosis of the hands: a distal form of the Madelung–Launois–Bensaude syndrome. *Clin Exp Dermatol* 1989; **14**: 58–9.

27 Boozan JA, Maves MD, Schuller DE. Surgical management of massive benign symmetric lipomatosis. *Laryngoscope* 1992; **102**: 94–7.

28 Ujpal M, Nemeth ZS, Reichwein A, Szabo GY. Long-term results following surgical treatment of benign symmetric lipomatosis (BSL). *Int J Oral Maxillofac Surg* 2001; **30**: 479–83.

29 Carlin MC, Ratz JL. Multiple symmetric lipomatosis: treatment with liposuction. *J Am Acad Dermatol* 1988; **18**: 359–62.

30 Basse P, Lohmann M, Hagard C *et al*. Multiple symmetric lipomatosis; combined surgical treatment and liposuction. *Scand J Plast Recons* 1992; **26**: 111–2.

31 Coleman WP, Glogau RG, Klein JA *et al*. Guidelines of care for liposuction. *Am Acad Dermatol* 2001; **45**: 438–47.

32 Heike Z, Gudrun UM, Frank RD *et al*. Multiple benign symmetric lipomatosis—a differential diagnosis of obesity: is there a rationale for fibrate treatment? *Obes Surg* 2008; **18**: 240–2.

33 Enzi G, Busetto L, Ceschin E *et al*. Multiple symmetric lipomatosis: clinical aspects and outcome in a long-term longitudinal study. *Int J Obes Relat Metab Disord* 2002; **26**: 253–61.

34 Nisoli E, Regianini L, Briscini L *et al*. Multiple symmetric lipomatosis may be the consequence of defective noradrenergic modulation of proliferation and differentiation of brown fat cells. *J Pathol* 2002; **198**: 378–87.

Congenital diffuse lipomatosis [1–4]

This has been infrequently recorded. Several syndromes that may involve a neuroectodermal defect have been described, in conjunction with various types of haemangioma or lymphangioma. Congenital lipomatosis may be associated with angiomatosis and macroencephalia (Bannayan's syndrome) [5]. The Proteus syndrome is very rare; the clinical features include hemihypertrophy, macrodactyly, exostoses, epidermal naevi, characteristic cerebriform masses involving the plantar or palmar surfaces, a variety of subcutaneous masses and scoliosis [6]. Histological examination of the subcutaneous masses has identified a variety of lipomatous and angiomatous tumours and hamartomas.

Treatment. Treatment is difficult but liposuction may help.

References

1 Baker AB, Adam JM. Lipomatosis of the central nervous system. *Am J Cancer* 1938; **34**: 214–9.

2 Cameron AH, McMillan DH. Lipomatosis of skeletal muscle in Maffucci's syndrome. *J Bone Joint Surg Br* 1956; **38**: 692–8.

3 Schlicht D. Recurrent lipomatosis in a child. *Med J Aust* 1965; **2**: 959–62.

4 Wising PJ. Hereditary multiple symmetric lipomatosis. *Nord Med* 1954; **51**: 279–81.

5 Bannayan GA. Lipomatosis, angiomatosis and macroencephalia. *Arch Pathol* 1971; **92**: 1–5.

6 Samlaska CP, Levin SW, James WD *et al*. Proteus syndrome. *Arch Dermatol* 1989; **125**: 1109–14.

Dercum's disease

Synonym
• Adiposis dolorosa

Dercum's disease is a rare, progressive disease characterized by localized overgrowth of fat with painful subcutaneous plaques and ecchymoses.

Aetiology. The mechanism of Dercum's disease is not known [1]. It most commonly affects menopausal women; they are usually

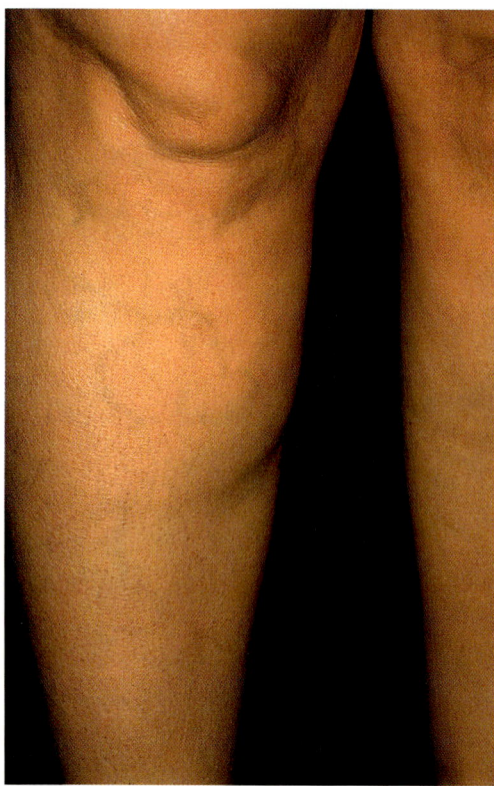

Fig. 46.34 Dercum's disease. (Courtesy of Dr R. Motley, University of Wales College of Medicine, Cardiff, UK.)

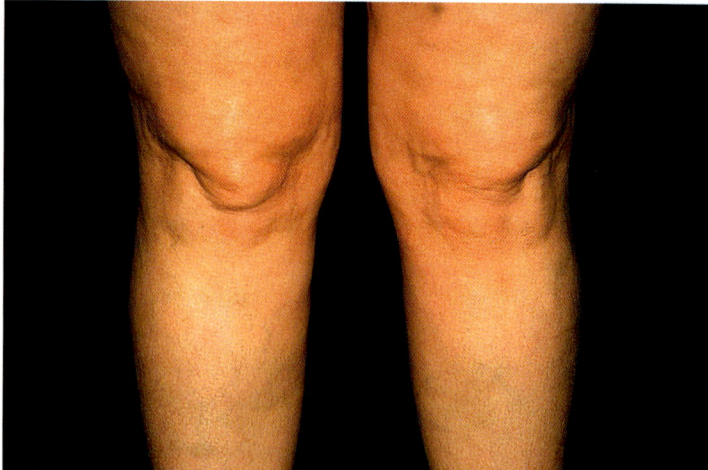

Fig. 46.35 Dercum's disease showing much improvement after liposuction. (Courtesy of Dr R. Motley, University of Wales College of Medicine, Cardiff, UK.)

obese at the time of onset of the disorder and severe emotional disturbance is common. A recent report implies that the disease is a severe expression of multiple painful lipomas [2] but clinical experience of patients in Sweden [3], where the disease appears to be more common, underlines the concept of, at present, a more heterogeneous group, divided into three types. In type I or juxta-articular type, painful folds of fat were seen on the inside of the knees and/or the hips. In type II, the diffuse type, there was widespread pain from increased fatty tissue. In type III, the nodular type, there was intense pain in and around multiple lipomas. In some families there is a dominant inheritance [4].

Histopathology. Histology in the nodular type reveals features of a lipoma or angiolipoma [1].

Clinical features [5,6]. Dercum [7] coined the term 'adiposis dolorosa' to describe three cases of a syndrome characterized by painful deposits of adipose tissue occurring over multiple areas of the body (Figs 46.34 & 46.35). Adiposis dolorosa occurs predominantly in postmenopausal women (female : male ratio of up to 30 : 1) and is associated with weakness, fatigue and, frequently, emotional disturbances. Obesity is almost always present initially, but patients may lose weight and become asthenic as the syndrome progresses. The painful areas of fat may occur as subcutaneous 'lumps', which feel like a 'bag of worms' on palpation, or may be diffuse in a localized or generalized pattern. The juxta-articular areas are the most commonly involved site [8], but painful areas have been described over virtually all areas of the body. The

pain occurs with palpation of the involved fat, but may also occur spontaneously, often with a fibromyalgia pattern and quality. The disease usually begins gradually with only mild discomfort, but may progress to exquisite pain, particularly with movement, so that the patient is effectively immobilized. The pain tends to be cyclical with constant mild to moderate discomfort punctuated by episodes of severe pain, which is unresponsive to many or all analgesic agents.

Psychiatric disturbances are frequently observed, ranging from mild irritability to dementia. Depression, failure of memory and hypochondriacal complaints are quite common.

Diagnosis. This is not difficult when the classical triad is present: painful plaques, ecchymoses and obesity, appearing in women with amenorrhoea and neurotic symptoms.

Cushing's disease with diffuse deposition of fat, plethora and hirsutes must be distinguished from Dercum's disease. Amenorrhoea and ecchymoses are common to both disorders.

Treatment. Weight reduction and surgical excision of individual tumours may be helpful [8]. The pain is usually unresponsive to conventional therapy but several cases have been shown to respond to intravenous lidocaine [5,9–13]. Two studies were placebo controlled. The pain relief was from 3 to 52 weeks, and repeat therapy was associated with increasing duration of benefit [5,12]. The lidocaine effect is very specific, as other types of pain (e.g. headaches) continued; the mechanism of action is unknown. Topical lidocaine may be an adequate alternative [14]. Some response to mexiletine 150–750 mg orally has been reported [15].

References

1 Wortham NC, Tomlinson IP. Dercum's disease. *Skinmed* 2005; **4**: 157–62.
2 Campen R, Mankin H, Louis DN *et al.* Familial occurrence of adiposis dolorosa. *J Am Acad Dermatol* 2001; **44**: 132–6.
3 Brorson H, Fagher B. Dercum's disease. Fatty tissue rheumatism caused by immune defense reaction? *Lakartidningen* 1996; **10**(93): 1433–6.
4 Lynch HT, Harlan WL. Hereditary factors in adiposis dolorosa (Dercum's disease). *Am J Hum Genet* 1963; **15**: 184–90.
5 Atkinson RL. Intravenous lidocaine for the treatment of intractable pain of adiposis dolorosa. *Int J Obesity* 1982; **6**: 351–7.

6 Palmer ED. Dercum's disease: adiposis dolorosa. *Am Fam Physician* 1981; **24**: 155–7.

7 Dercum FX. Three cases of a hitherto unclassified affliction resembling in its grosser aspects obesity, but associated with special nervous symptoms: adiposis dolorosa. *Am J Med Sci* 1892; **104**: 521–35.

8 Nahir AH, Schapira O, Scharf Y. Juxta-articular adiposis dolorosa: a neglected disease. *Isr J Med Sci* 1983; **19**: 858–9.

9 Juhlin L. Long-standing pain relief of adiposis dolorosa (Dercum's disease) after intravenous infusion of lidocaine. *J Am Acad Dermatol* 1986; **15**: 383–5.

10 Petersen P, Kastrup J. Treating the pain of Dercum's disease. *BMJ* 1984; **288**: 1880.

11 Petersen P, Kastrup J. Dercum's disease (adiposis dolorosa): treatment of the severe pain with intravenous lidocaine. *Pain* 1987; **28**: 77–80.

12 Atkinson RL. Intravenous lidocaine for the treatment of intractable pain of adiposis dolorosa. *Int J Obesity* 1982; **6**: 351–7.

13 Devillers AC, Oranje AP. Treatment of pain in adiposis dolorosa (Dercum's disease) with intravenous lidocaine: a case report with 10 year follow-up. *Clin Exp Dermatol* 1999; **24**: 240–1.

14 Desai MJ, Siriki R, Wang D. Treatment of pain in Dercum's disease with Lidoderm® (lidocaine 5% patch): A case report. *Pain Med* 2008; **9**: 1224–6.

15 Steiner J, Schiltz K, Heidenreich F, Weissenborn K. Lipomatosis dolorosa: a frequently overlooked disease picture. *Nervenarzt* 2002; **73**: 183–7.

CHAPTER 47

Diseases of the Veins and Arteries: Leg Ulcers

P.S. Mortimer[1], K.G. Burnand[2] & H.A.M. Neumann[3]

[1]St George's, University of London, London, UK
[2]Academic Department of Surgery, St Thomas' Hospital, London, UK
[3]Erasmus Medical Center, Rotterdam, The Netherlands

Arterial and arteriolar disorders

Vasculogenesis, angiogenesis and arteriogenesis

Vasculogenesis is the first step in the development of blood vessels and is the process by which endothelial cells differentiate from their mesodermal precursors. Vasculogenesis leads to the formation of a primary capillary plexus and occurs mainly in embryonal development [1]. Angiogenesis is the process by which new capillaries are formed from existing vessels by sprouting, expanding and remodelling [2]. Vasculogenesis precedes angiogenesis but the two processes continue in parallel during early development. The skin, being of ectodermal origin, is vascularized mainly by angiogenesis. The establishment and remodelling of blood vessels requires a complex orchestration of molecular regulators. First, the extracellular matrix is degraded by local tissue proteases. This permits migration of budding endothelial cells under the influence of angiogenic stimuli, particularly the family of vascular endothelial growth factors (vascular endothelial growth factors A, B, C, D and E (viral homologues) plus placental growth factor) and their tyrosine kinase receptors, VEGFR-1, VEGFR-2 and VEGFR-3. Stabilization and maintenance of newly formed vessels occur mainly as a consequence of the angiopoietins and the tie-receptors [3].

Differentiation into arteries, veins and capillaries is the responsibility of angiogenesis. Neoangiogenesis is an important cause of recurrent varicose veins after stripping [4]. Arteriogenesis produces rapid circumferential growth in the pre-existing collateral vessels, which are less perfused under normal flow conditions.

While local tissue ischaemia or hypoxia stimulates angiogenesis, arteriogenesis is mainly induced by inflammation and shear stress [5].

References

1 Risau W. Mechanisms of angiogenesis. *Nature* 1997; **386**: 671–4.
2 Carmeliet P. Angiogenesis in health and disease. *Nat Med* 2003; **9**: 677–84.
3 Cohen MM Jr. Vascular update: morphogenesis, tumors, malformations and molecular dimensions. *Am J Med Genet Part A* 2006; **140A**: 2013–38.
4 De Maeseneer MG, Vandenbroeck CP, Lauwers PR *et al*. Early and late complications of silicone patch saphenoplasty at the saphenofemoral junction. *J Vasc Surg* 2006; **44**: 1285–90.
5 Simons M. Angiogenesis. *Circulation* 2005; **111**: 1556–66.

Arterial disease and peripheral ischaemic disorders

Arterial disease

Current concepts on the aetiology of arterial disease, atherosclerosis and peripheral ischaemia

The mechanisms that initiate arterial disease are still poorly understood. Recent research has shown that inflammation plays a key role in atherosclerosis [1]. Early atherosclerotic lesions are dominated by immune cells (macrophages) and their effector molecules accelerate the progression of the lesions. Evidence suggests that cardiovascular risk factors induce endothelial injury and endothelial dysfunction. Endothelial progenitor cells derived from circulating mononuclear cells may protect against atherosclerosis and cardiovascular disease [2]. Atherosclerosis is a patchy accumulation of lipid, mostly in the form of cholesterol, within the intima of the vessel wall. Atheromatous plaques eventually ulcerate through the endothelial lining, exposing a highly thrombogenic surface [3]. Platelets adhere to the ulcerated plaque and platelet aggregates (platelet thrombi) may embolize distally or may initiate local thrombosis. Inadequate collaterals, or occlusion by thrombosis or embolism, will lead to tissue infarction (e.g. peripheral gangrene).

Atherosclerosis is responsible for more than 90% of all arterial disease in the Western world. It affects 5% of men over the age of 50 years, of which 10% may develop critical limb ischaemia; this increases to 20% if diabetic patients are included [4]. Apart from diabetes, tobacco smoking is one of the most important risk factors for arterial disease. A family history and hypercholesterolism are two other factors that are associated with atherosclerosis.

Atherosclerosis of the lower limb vessels

Many patients initially present with claudication (cramping pain on walking, which is usually experienced in the posterior calf muscles and is relieved by rest). The presence of persistent pain in the foot at night indicates the onset of critical ischaemia, which will lead to gangrene or ulceration if left untreated.

In the past, arteriosclerosis (hardening of the vessels) had been classified as a disease, but most authorities would now regard this as a physiological response to ageing. Thickening of the arterial wall, with an increase in collagen and calcium deposition, causes loss of elasticity and increased tortuosity of the vessels in the elderly [3]. Similar changes are seen in the vessels of younger patients with hypertension.

Clinical features [3–6]. All aspects of the patient's history and lifestyle are relevant, with particular attention being paid to risk factors such as cigarette smoking, hypertension, diabetes, diet, dyslipidaemia, hyperhomocysteinaemia, lack of exercise, obesity, occupation and a family history of cardiovascular disease [7]. In 1992, an examination of WHO epidemiological data from Toulouse (France) indicated that in spite of the population having a high saturated fat consumption, comparable serum cholesterol levels and other similar risks, there was a considerably lower incidence of death from coronary heart disease compared with other Western countries. Although the specific mechanism behind this 'French paradox' has not been identified, the flavonoid components in red wine are thought to have antioxidant activity which could contribute to cardiovascular benefits [8].

Most patients present with intermittent claudication, but ischaemic ulceration and skin infarction are more likely to be the presenting features in patients sent to the dermatologist (Fig. 47.1). Rest pain occurs if the disease progresses. This is experienced in the foot, and occurs predominantly at night. Altered skin colour (pallor or deep erythema) indicates ischaemia, and may be accompanied by other trophic skin changes such as dryness, scaling, loss of hair and thickened nails (Fig. 47.2).

A full general examination is essential. Particular attention should be paid to signs of anaemia, polycythaemia, xanthelasma and other xanthomatous deposits. Genetic disorders such as pseudoxanthoma elasticum, Ehlers–Danlos syndrome and Marfan's syndrome should be considered if an aneurysm is present. Cardiac examination should focus on dysrhythmias, particularly atrial fibrillation, murmurs and signs of heart failure.

Abdominal examination should detect the presence of a pulsatile mass, indicative of an abdominal aortic aneurysm. The fundi

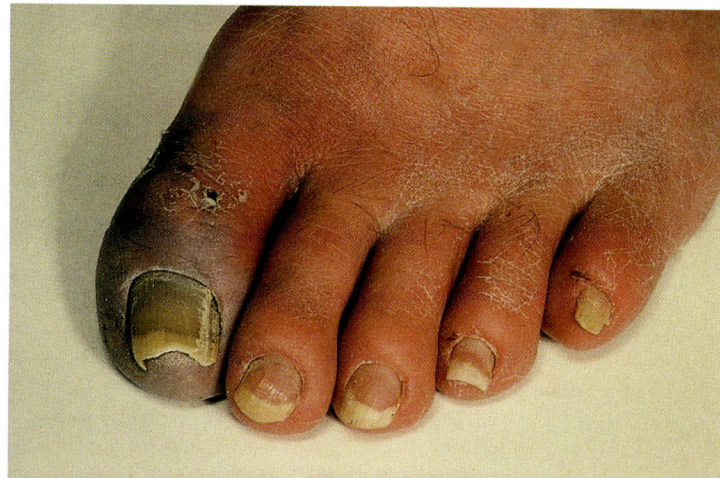

Fig. 47.1 An ischaemic hallux with pregangrene; the rest of the foot has an ischaemic erythema.

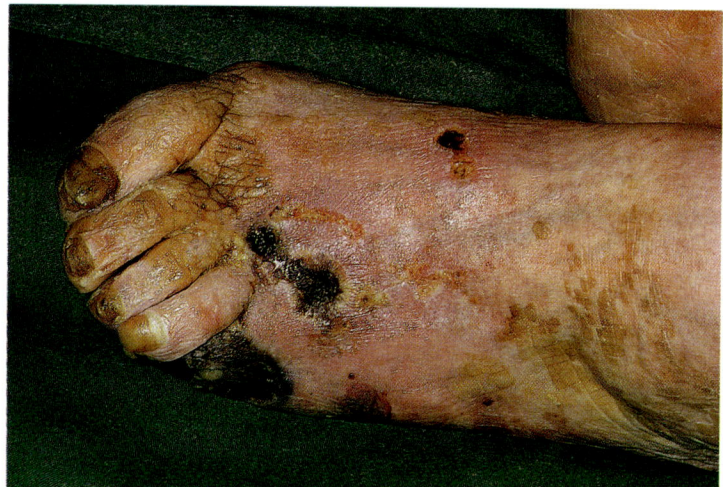

Fig. 47.2 An ischaemic foot showing patchy areas of gangrene and rubor. The skin is flaky and the nails are brittle.

should be examined for evidence of diabetic and hypertensive retinopathy. The blood pressure should be taken in both arms; a marked difference suggesting a stenosis or occlusion of the subclavian artery (although ischaemic disorders of the upper limbs are unusual).

The skin of the legs may have an erythematous or dusky mottled hue. When the ischaemia is marked, limb elevation causes pallor of the foot while dependency results in delayed but exaggerated hyperaemia, best observed on the dorsum of the foot (Buerger's sign) (Fig. 47.3) [9]. Inspection may reveal ulceration at sites of pressure (Fig. 47.4); small cracks may appear over the sole of the foot or heel (Fig. 47.5). Platelet emboli lodging in the plantar and digital vessels cause areas of discoloration, which are often present over many toes or on the sole of the foot (Fig. 47.6). They often look like ecchymoses initially and may be confused with vasculitis. The aortic, femoral, popliteal, dorsalis pedis and posterior tibial pulses must be carefully palpated. Abnormally situated pulsations may indicate a collateral circulation or a congenital arteriovenous fistula. Auscultation over the course of the arteries may reveal the presence of a bruit indicative of turbulent flow. This is

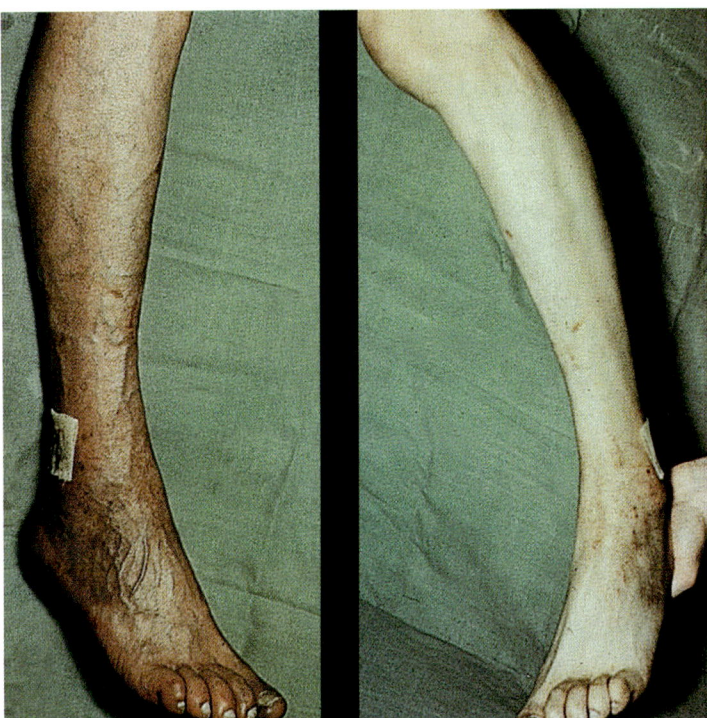

Fig. 47.3 Buerger's test showing postural colour change in an ischaemic foot—white when the foot is elevated (right) and red when lowered (left).

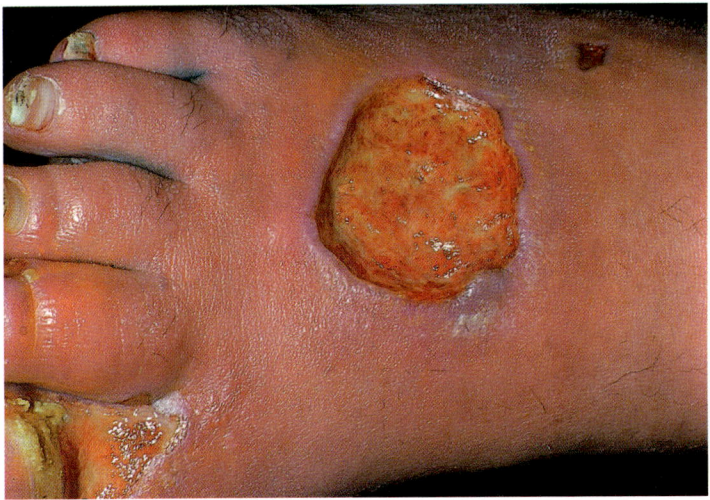

Fig. 47.4 An ischaemic ulcer on the dorsum of the foot with an ulcer arising in the first interdigital space. Pressure between the toes is a common consequence of tight bandages or footwear.

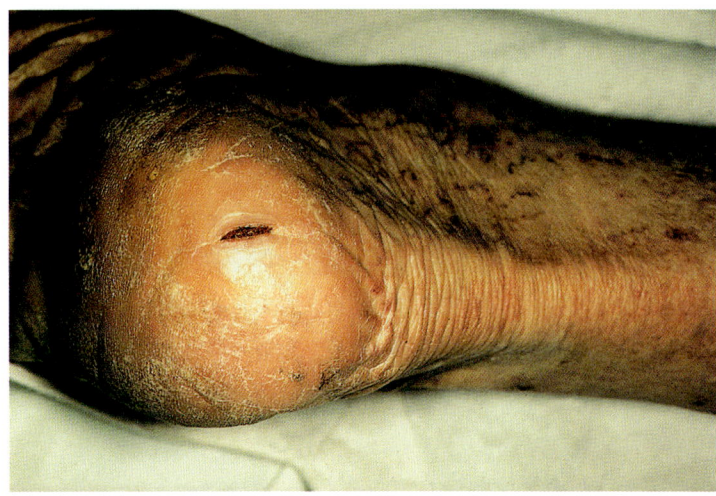

Fig. 47.5 An ischaemic 'crack' developing as a consequence of nutritional changes seen in hyperkeratosis and loss of suppleness of the skin of the heel.

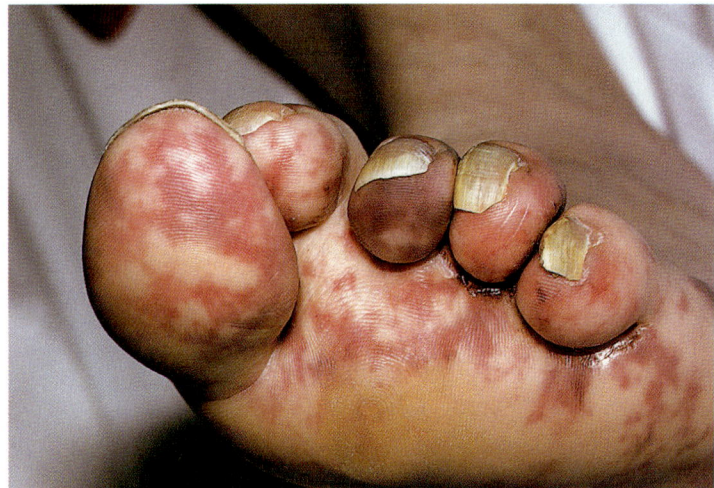

Fig. 47.6 Multiple platelet emboli into the skin of the foot.

commonly caused by an up-stream stenosis or by an arteriovenous fistula (which usually causes a 'machinery' murmur, present throughout systole and diastole). It should be noted that significant arterial disease demanding further investigation is uncommon when the foot pulses are easily palpable.

Investigations. Confirmation of the arterial disease of the lower limb can be obtained by measuring the ankle–brachial Doppler pressure index if peripheral pulses are reduced or absent or a bruit is heard [10]. After the Doppler ultrasound probe has been used to locate the dorsalis pedis or posterior tibial vessel a sphygmo-

manometer cuff is placed around the limb above the ankle and inflated (Fig. 47.7). The red cells flowing past the tip of the ultrasound probe deflect the beam, creating an audible noise. As the cuff is inflated above systolic pressure, flow in the artery ceases and the noise disappears. This ankle–brachial systolic gradient is normally unity, that is 1.0. A fall in ankle pressure results in a reduction of the pressure index: a ratio of 0.71 to 0.90 indicates the presence of mild peripheral arterial disease, an ankle–brachial index of 0.41 to 0.70 indicates moderate disease, and a ratio of 0.40 or less indicates severe disease. Pain at rest or severe occlusive disease typically occurs when an ankle–brachial index is less than 0.50. Ischaemic or gangrenous extremities are associated with an index of less than 0.20 [11]. Falsely high indices may be obtained in some limbs if the vessels are very calcified and fail to compress at systolic pressure. This is especially true for diabetic limbs. In such circumstances a more accurate means of assessment is to measure the Doppler pressures at the toe. Measurement of the transcutaneous Po_2 using a heated (Clark's) electrode applied to the skin of the lower limbs and compared with a reference site on

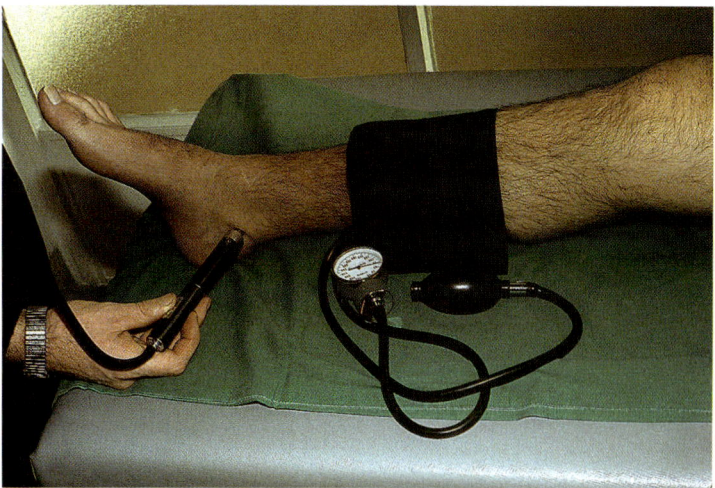

Fig. 47.7 Measurement of the ankle Doppler pressure using a sphygmomanometer cuff. The pressure at which the Doppler signal disappears in the leg is compared with the brachial pressure to give an index of blood supply.

the chest wall [12,13] can also be used to assess limb ischaemia. This usually fails to increase with inhalation of oxygen. Patients with severe venous incompetence can also have hypoxic extremities [14]. Isotope washout studies (which estimate clearance of an inert isotope from a tissue injection) can also be obtained [15].

Investigations in patients suspected of having peripheral arterial disease or critical leg ischaemia [4] should include: a full blood count to exclude anaemia or polycythaemia; electrolytes and creatinine to monitor renal function; and an electrocardiogram (often repeated after exercise) to detect rhythm abnormalities or cardiac ischaemia. A chest radiograph provides an assessment of cardiac size and excludes a coincidental bronchogenic carcinoma, which is common in smokers. Diabetes should be excluded, and plasma cholesterol, homocysteine and fasting triglycerides should be measured. Markers of inflammation, particularly C-reactive protein, have been associated with peripheral arterial disease. Raised haematocrit levels and hyperviscosity have all been reported in patients with peripheral arterial disease [7].

When surgery is contemplated, a detailed assessment of the anatomy of the arterial tree is also required. Duplex ultrasound scanning is often the initial investigation, and is used as a screening test to confirm the major sites of stenosis or occlusion in the vascular tree [16,17]. A duplex ultrasound scan provides both a B-mode image of the artery and a measurement of blood velocity; these can be combined to provide a map of stenoses and occlusions within the arterial tree from the aorta to the crural (calf) vessels. The greater the velocity, the tighter the stenosis. Most surgeons also obtain an arteriogram before angioplasty or bypass surgery is performed. Arteriography is performed by injection of non-ionic contrast media into the vascular tree, usually through a retrograde catheter inserted into the common femoral artery at the groin over a guide wire (Seldinger-type retrograde aortography), or from an intravenous or intra-arterial injection using digital subtraction equipment or computed tomography to enhance picture quality [18]. Each of these methods has its proponents, but retrograde aortography performed as an outpatient, or a combina-

tion of intravenous digital subtraction arteriography of the aorta, iliac and femoral vessels with femoral arteriography of the distal vessels, provide equivalent information. Thus invasive digital subtraction angiography remains the final investigation which is used if endovascular intervention is planned. Magnetic resonance angiography (MRA) of the extremities is sometimes useful to diagnose the anatomic location and degree of stenosis in peripheral arterial disease if patients are allergic to contrast. Computed tomography angiography is an alternative if patients have contraindications for MRA [7].

The further management of arterial disease is discussed under the heading of the individual diseases, and usually requires referral to an appropriately experienced surgeon and interventional radiologist.

References

1 Hansson GK. Mechanisms of disease: inflammation, atherosclerosis and coronary artery disease. *N Engl J Med* 2005; **352**: 1685–95.
2 Hill JM, Zalos G, Halcox JPJ *et al.* Circulating endothelial progenitor cells, vascular function and cardiovascular risk. *N Engl J Med* 2003; **348**: 593–600.
3 Woolf N, ed. *Pathology of Atherosclerosis.* London: Butterworth, 1982.
4 Dormandy JA, Stock G, eds. *Critical Leg Ischaemia: its Pathology and Management.* Berlin: Springer-Verlag, 1990.
5 Browse NL, Burnand KG, Irvine AJ, Wilson NM. *Diseases of the Veins,* 2nd edn. London: Arnold, 1999.
6 Rutherford RB, ed. *Vascular Surgery.* Philadelphia: Elsevier Saunders, 2005.
7 Norgren L, Hiatt WR *et al.* Inter-society consensus for the management of peripheral arterial disease (TASC II). *Eur J Endovasc Surg* 2007; **33** (Suppl.): 5–75.
8 Kar P, Laight D, Shaw KM, Cummings MH. Flavonoid-rich grapeseed extracts: a new approach in high cardiovascular rich patients? *Int J Clin Pract* 2006; **60**: 1484–92.
9 Insall RL, Davies RJ, Prout WG. Significance of Buerger's test in the assessment of lower limb ischaemia. *J R Soc Med* 1989; **82**: 729–31.
10 Summer SD, Strandness DE. The relationship between calf blood flow and ankle blood pressure in patients with intermittent claudication. *Surgery* 1969; **65**: 763–5.
11 Khan NA, Rahim SA, Anand SS, Simel DL, Panju A. Does the clinical examination predict lower extremity peripheral arterial disease? *JAMA* 2006; **295**: 536–46.
12 Clyne CAC, Ramsden WH, Chant ADB *et al.* Oxygen tension on the skin of the gaiter area of limbs with venous disease. *Br J Surg* 1985; **72**: 644–7.
13 Franzeck UK, Talke P, Bernstein EF *et al.* Transcutaneous *Po₂* measurements in health and peripheral arterial occlusive disease. *Surgery* 1982; **91**: 156–63.
14 Neumann HA, Van den Broek MJ, Boersma IH, Veraart JC. Transcutaneous oxygen tension in patients with and without pericapillary fibrin cuffs in chronic venous insufficiency, porphoria cutanea tarda and non-venous leg ulcers. *Vasa* 1996; **25**: 127–33.
15 Alpert JS, Garcia del Rio H, Lassen NA. Diagnostic use of radioactive xenon clearance and a standardised walking test in obliterative arterial disease of the legs. *Circulation* 1966; **34**: 849–55.
16 Koelemay MJW, Den Hartog D, Prins MH *et al.* Diagnosis of arterial disease of the lower extremities with duplex ultrasonography. *Br J Surg* 1996; **83**: 404–9.
17 Legemate DA, Teeuwen C, Hoeneveld H *et al.* The potential of duplex scanning to replace aorto-iliac and femoro-popliteal angiography. *Eur J Vasc Surg* 1989; **3**: 49–54.
18 Friedman SG, Moccio CG. A prospective comparison of intra-arterial digital subtraction and conventional angiography prior to lower extremity revascularisation. *J Cardiovasc Surg* 1989; **30**: 462–6.

Differential diagnosis. Thromboangiitis obliterans (Buerger's disease, p. 47.6–7) may be very difficult to distinguish from atherosclerosis. Preservation of the proximal femoral and popliteal pulses and the early age at first presentation usually indicates the possibility of this condition. Associated venous thromboses and characteristic histological changes on vessel biopsy make the diagnosis more secure. A skin biopsy can sometimes be helpful in diagnosing Buerger's disease [1]. Arteriography in Buerger's disease shows characteristic 'corkscrew collaterals' [1].

In patients with acute limb ischaemia it is important to exclude the possibility of embolism, which may be suggested by a recent myocardial infarction or the presence of atrial fibrillation. Transthoracic or transoesophageal echocardiography can demonstrate intracardiac thrombus and structural abnormalities, especially of the valves and, in the case of transoesophageal echocardiography, with great accuracy [2].

Rarer causes of ischaemia include external arterial compression (popliteal entrapment or a cervical rib), dissecting or thrombosed aneurysms, ergot alkaloid poisoning, intra-arterial injections of noxious substances, traumatic disruption of the arterial wall, coagulation disorders, particularly polycythaemia and thrombocytosis, and various forms of vasculitis. Diabetes must always be considered as a potentiating condition, even in patients with atherosclerotic disease.

Claudication pain may be mimicked by arthritic conditions of the hip, such as osteoarthritis or rheumatoid arthritis. Pain in the leg may also result from referred pain arising in the lumbosacral spine, and spinal claudication is sometimes very difficult to differentiate from arterial claudication. Occasionally, venous claudication may also be misdiagnosed. Ischaemic rest pain may have to be differentiated from other painful conditions of the feet and toes, such as gout, interdigital neuromas, glomangiomas, ingrowing toenails, flat feet, calcanial bursitis and plantar fasciitis. Other causes of gangrene may need to be excluded (e.g. clostridial infection, diabetes, other causes of vascular obstruction, vasculitis and coagulation disorders).

Prognosis. Patients with atherosclerotic disease of the lower limb vessels usually have other arteries affected. Coronary artery disease was found to be present in 90% of a group of patients with peripheral arterial disease [3]. The extent of the atheroma in the coronary and carotid arteries determines the life expectancy of the patient, although antiplatelet agents [4], lipid-lowering agents and bypass surgery may improve the patient's prognosis as well as their symptoms of ischaemia. Silent myocardial infarction is present in about one-third of those who presented with intermittent claudication.

Treatment. Treatment options differ for patients presenting with claudication, rest pain or gangrene and acute limb ischaemia.

Claudication. The indications for intervention in a patient with claudication are always relative and must be weighed against the risks of the procedure and the fact that the condition normally has a very benign course [5]. Only 5% of all patients with claudication progress each year to develop rest pain or gangrene; a far greater proportion die every year from other causes, such as myocardial infarction. Patients with intermittent claudication are therefore usually managed conservatively at first, as collateral vessels may develop with an associated improvement in the symptoms.

Smoking cessation has been shown to reduce the risk of progression in patients with lower extremity peripheral arterial disease presenting with claudication. Nicotine replacement has been shown to be a safe and effective method of aiding smoking cessation [6].

Patients should be encouraged to walk through the pain as this tends to stimulate the development of a collateral circulation, to recruit capillaries and to increase the claudication distance. There are a number of studies demonstrating that supervised exercise programmes are as effective as therapeutic intervention in alleviating claudication, although the benefits of supervised exercise may not persist [7].

Patients with peripheral arterial disease should have their blood pressure maintained below 130/85 mmHg [8], but antihypertensive treatment should not be instituted in patients with claudication whose lower limb systolic pressures are lower than 80 mmHg.

Pharmacological interventions comprise the following. Antiplatelet agents must be considered in patients with claudication. Based on the available evidence, the first-line antiplatelet therapy should be aspirin or clopidogrel [6]. Aspirin has not been shown to improve claudication itself, but patients with claudication treated by antiplatelet agents have a 25% reduction in subsequent serious cardiovascular events. Statins modify lipid levels and reduce the risks of disease progression. Statins reduce LDL-cholesterol levels causing a significant reduction in the all-cause mortality [6,8]. Diabetes mellitus is closely associated with peripheral arterial disease and its progression, and rigorous control of blood glucose in patients with diabetes reduces microvascular complications. Although intensive therapy (achieving a HbA_{1c} of below 7%) had no effect on the risk of death or amputation in patients with peripheral arterial disease, there was a trend in favour of a reduced risk of non-fatal cardiovascular events [6,8].

Further investigation is indicated if the claudication distance remains unacceptable despite the patient having stopped smoking and after a reasonable period of conservative treatment. Stenotic lesions confirmed by arteriography can be treated by balloon dilatation (angioplasty), using specially designed coaxial balloon catheters that are constructed to withstand high external pressures [9]. This technique works best on stenoses in large proximal vessels, and least well on long occlusions of the distal arterial tree. Potential complications include arterial rupture, aneurysm formation, thrombosis and dissection. Additionally, the results of angioplasty in the femoropopliteal segment remain disappointing with a 30% restenosis rate at 1 year. The role of primary stent placement in revascularization of the superficial femoral artery remains controversial, mainly because of the high restenosis rate. Chemically treated slow-release stents may overcome 'restenosis' in the future, although so far several randomized trials have failed to confirm this. Stents placed in the superficial femoral artery can undergo fracture, which has been linked to restenosis. A randomized trial by Schillinger et al., involving 104 patients with severe claudication, showed significantly higher patency rates at 1 year for lesions in the superficial femoral artery that were treated with stent placement than for lesions treated with angioplasty with a stent only being placed if there was a suboptimal result [10]. Long-term results are not, however, available.

Surgical endarterectomy or bypass remains the treatment of choice for extensive occlusions longer than 10 cm, or for occlusion of the popliteal or tibial–peroneal vessels [11]. Aortofemoral bypass has an excellent 5-year patency (90–95%), but the operative mortality varies between 1 and 5% [10]. Femoropopliteal vein bypass grafting has a lower 5-year patency (60–70%) but a lower operative mortality (usually less than 1%) [12]. Distal bypass surgery (the lower anastomoses being below the popliteal artery into one of the three crural vessels) has no part to play in the treatment of claudication, although this procedure is of considerable value in patients with rest pain and early gangrene (see below) [13]. Operative or chemical lumbar sympathectomy do not help to relieve claudication [14] and are mainly of value in patients with ischaemic ulcers or Buerger's disease.

Rest pain or gangrene. Once rest pain or early gangrene has developed the situation changes, for if this state is left untreated amputation will be necessary to relieve pain and preserve life. Patients with rest pain or gangrene must be rapidly admitted and investigated, because successful revascularization can avert limb loss [7]. Any anaemia or polycythaemia should be corrected, and if diabetes is found this should be brought under control. Dehydration and infection must be treated.

The increasing use of more distal surgery with bypasses to the dorsal pedis, posterior tibial, peroneal and even plantar vessels has saved many limbs that in the past would have been amputated [13,15]. Angioplasty, stenting and surgery to the proximal vessels are, of course, still of value as these arteries are the main sites of disease.

In patients without evidence of frank ischaemia, chemical sympathectomy may alleviate rest pain [16]. Prostacyclin, prostaglandin E_1 and prostacyclin analogues, such as iloprost, are being tried in patients in whom a bypass cannot be constructed. These compounds may preserve a small proportion of threatened limbs [17]. A meta-analysis of seven randomized trials involving 643 patients with ischaemic limbs showed a small but significant effect of prostaglandin E_1 on ulcer healing and/or pain reduction and on the combined end points of major amputation or death [18].

Therapeutic angiogenesis using gene therapy has been tried but clinical trials have not shown any benefit to date. A phase 1 study on plasmid transfer of vascular endothelial growth factor in nine patients with severe peripheral arterial disease has, however, shown that this technology is possible. Many other studies are under way to assess the utility of gene therapy in patients with severe peripheral arterial disease [18].

The immediate amputation rate can be lowered by a policy of aggressive reconstruction, but this probably comes at the cost of a few higher amputations and some increased loss of life when graft failure is associated with a continued ischaemia and consequent amputation [19].

Acute limb ischaemia. Patients presenting with acute limb ischaemia should be rapidly assessed and, unless there is unequivocal evidence of an embolus (suggested, for example, by normal vessels in the other limb, atrial fibrillation or recent myocardial infarction), the patient should have urgent angiography to confirm the diagnosis and to assess the cause of the occlusion. This should be followed by infusion of a tissue plasminogen activator into the thrombus or embolus via the catheter unless the state of the limb demands urgent revascularization or amputation [20]. Repeat angiography, to confirm continuing or successful thrombolysis, is required at frequent intervals, and residual stenoses responsible for the thrombosis may require angioplasty, stenting or surgery. When vessel patency has been restored by thrombolysis, patients must remain on anticoagulants.

Balloon-catheter embolectomy should be reserved for embolic occlusions. When platelet emboli are suspected, antiplatelet agents may be prescribed before a definitive surgical or radiological intervention to remove the source of the emboli.

Amputation remains the final option in all types of ischaemic disease of the lower limbs where revascularization is impossible or ineffective. The value of preserving the knee joint for subsequent mobility is well recognized. The mortality of amputation stays stubbornly high (15–20%).

References

1 Olin JW, Shih A. Thromboangiitis obliterans (Buerger's disease). *Curr Opin Rheumatol* 2006; **18**: 18–24.
2 Lagattolla NRF, Burnand KG, Stewart A. Role of transoesophageal echocardiography in determining the source of peripheral arterial embolism. *Br J Surg* 1995; **82**: 1651–4.
3 Golomb BA, Dang TT, Criqui MH. Peripheral arterial disease: morbidity and mortality implications. *Circulation* 2006; **114**: 688–99.
4 Canadian Cooperative Study Group. A randomised trial of aspirin and sulphin-pyrazone in threatened stroke. *N Engl J Med* 1978; **299**: 53–9.
5 Imparato AM, Kim GE, Davison T *et al.* Intermittent claudication: its natural course. *Surgery* 1975; **119**: 75–8.
6 Bendermacher BLW, Willigendael EM, Teijink JAW, Prins MH. Medical management of peripheral arterial disease. *J Thromb Haemost* 2005; **3**: 1628–37.
7 Dormandy JA, Stock G, eds. *Critical Leg Ischaemia: its Pathology and Management.* Berlin: Springer-Verlag, 1990.
8 Hankey GJ, Norman PE, Eikelboom JW. Medical treatment of peripheral arterial disease. *JAMA* 2006; **295**: 547–53.
9 Grüntzig A, Kumpe DA. Technique of percutaneous transluminal angioplasty with Grüntzig balloon catheter. *Am J Roentgenol* 1979; **132**: 547–52.
10 Schillinger M, Sabeti S, Loewe C *et al.* Balloon angioplasty versus implantation of nitinol stents in the superficial femoral artery. *N Eng J Med* 2006; **354**: 1879–88.
11 White C. Intermittent claudication. *N Engl J Med* 2007; **356**: 1241–50.
12 De Weese JA, Rob CG. Autogenous venous bypass grafts 5 years later. *Ann Surg* 1971; **174**: 346–56.
13 Tyson RR, Reichle FA. Femorotibial bypass. *Ann Surg* 1969; **170**: 429–34.
14 Haxton HA. Chemical sympathectomy. *BMJ* 1949; **1**: 1026–8.
15 Veith FJ, Gupta SK, Samson RH *et al.* Progress in limb salvage by reconstructive arterial surgery combined with new or improved adjunctive procedures. *Ann Surg* 1981; **194**: 386–401.
16 Cotton LT, Cross FW. Lumbar sympathectomy for arterial disease. *Br J Surg* 1985; **72**: 678–83.
17 Norgren L, Alwmark A, Angqvist KA *et al.* A stable prostacyclin analogue (iloprost) in the treatment of ischaemic ulcers of the lower limb: a Scandinavian-Polish placebo controlled randomised multicenter study. *Eur J Vasc Surg* 1990; **4**: 463–7.
18 Federman DG, Kravetz JD. Peripheral arterial disease: diagnosis, treatment, and systemic implications. *Clin Dermatol* 2007; **25**: 93–100.
19 Burnand KG, Layer G, Whitehead S *et al.* Critical ischaemia of the lower limb: can we save more limbs from amputation? *J Cardiovasc Surg* 1990; **31** (Suppl.): 77 (Abstract).
20 Ouriel K, Shortell CK, De Weese JA *et al.* A comparison of thrombolytic therapy with operative revascularization in the initial treatment of acute peripheral arterial ischaemia. *J Vasc Surg* 1994; **19**: 1021–30.

Thromboangiitis obliterans [1,2]

Synonym
• Buerger's disease

Definition. This appears to be a distinct condition separate from other forms of vascular occlusion [2,3], with differences in the pathological appearance of the vessel wall, and in the population affected, compared with other arterial diseases [2].

This condition was first recognized as an obliterative disorder of peripheral arteries of young males by Leo Buerger in New York [1]. The affected young men were all heavy smokers and the disorder involved the small vessels of the upper limb much more commonly than in atherosclerosis. While originally thought to occur only in men, there are increased reports of women with thromboangiitis obliterans, possibly as a consequence of the increasing use of cigarettes among women in the 20th century [4]. It is common in the Middle and Far East, and in the Indian subcontinent.

Aetiology [2]. The aetiology of the condition is unknown, although tobacco addiction is invariably a major contributing factor, and a failure to overcome this addiction is associated with progressive occlusion of the vessels. Autoantibodies have been found within the blood [5]. In particular, antiendothelial cell antibodies are present in high titre in active disease. They may be used to monitor disease activity and may have a pathogenic role [2].

Pathology [2,6]. The full thickness of the vessel wall is invaded by lymphocytes, eosinophils, plasma cells and monocytes, especially disrupting the internal elastic lamina, and there is luminal occlusion as a result of highly cellular thrombosis. Accompanying nerves and veins may become involved in the inflammatory process. All changes are segmental or focal. At a later stage in the disease, fibrosis occurs, which spreads to involve surrounding structures.

Clinical features. Pain is the main presenting symptom and may be of several types: intermittent claudication; rest pain, more severe at night; pain associated with ischaemic neuropathy, ulceration or superficial venous thrombosis. Sensitivity to cold is a frequent complaint. Claudication in the arch of the foot is especially characteristic [7].

Ulceration or gangrene may develop early in the disease, particularly following trauma, and often starts around the sides of the nails or tips of the digits (Fig. 47.8). Trophic changes, superficial venous thrombosis and oedema are also often present. Red or cyanotic acral colour changes are often unilateral, asymmetrical and may affect isolated digits.

Recurrent venous thrombosis is a frequent problem and may take the form of superficial red streaks and cords of 0.5–3 cm [2] or deep-vein thrombosis presenting with pain and swelling. Erythema nodosum may also develop.

Ischaemic areas are found on the tips of the fingers and toes and may initially present as chronic painful paronychia. The proximal pulses are usually present, but the dorsalis pedis, posterior tibial and brachial pulses are lost at an early stage.

Diagnosis. There are no specific laboratory tests to aid in the diagnosis of thromboangiitis obliterans [4]. The erythrocyte sedimentation rate (ESR) is often elevated and antiendothelial cell

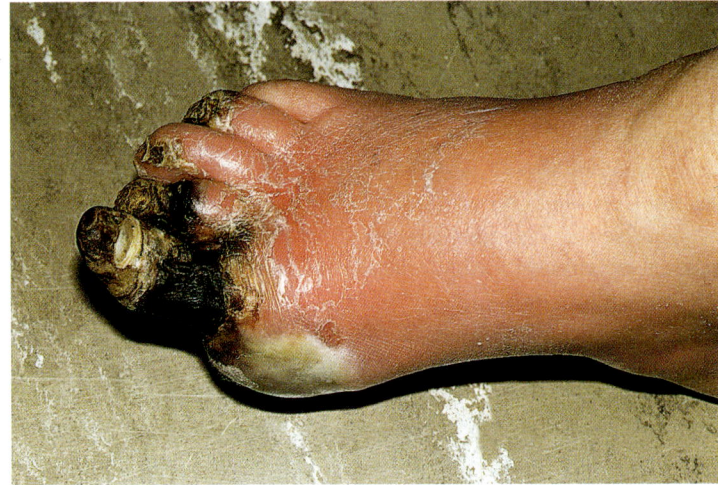

Fig. 47.8 Ischaemic toes in Buerger's disease.

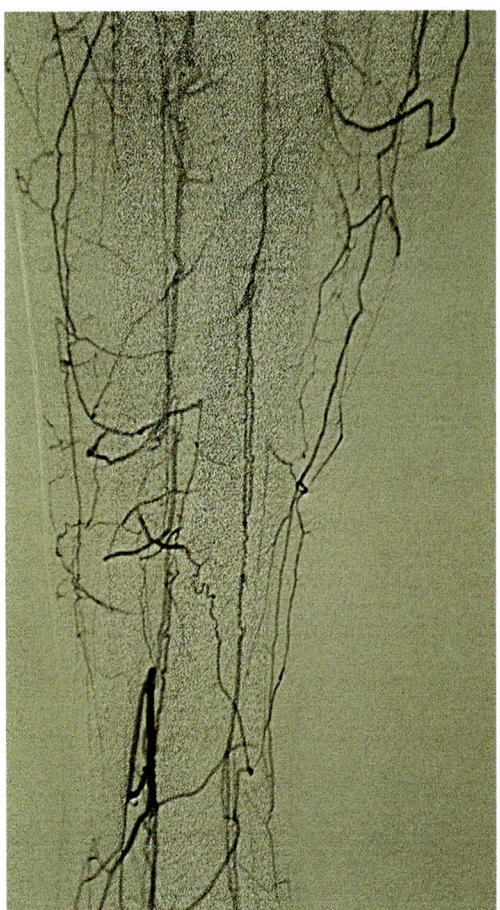

Fig. 47.9 An arteriogram in a patient with Buerger's disease. No major vessels are seen, just multiple collateral arteries.

autoantibodies may be detected. An arteriogram should be obtained and may suggest the diagnosis, if there are many 'corkscrew' collaterals [8] (Fig. 47.9). The proximal vessels are usually entirely normal while the distal arteries are diffusely affected with multiple stenoses and occlusions.

The differential diagnosis is wide. It includes atypical 'young onset' atherosclerosis, diabetic vasculopathy and rheumatoid arthritis. Collagen-vascular diseases, such as scleroderma and systemic lupus erythematosus, must also be considered in the differential diagnosis. Multiple emboli derived from a proximal source may pose real diagnostic difficulty, and ergotism, abuse of cocaine, amphetamines and cannabis must not be forgotten. Hypercoagulable states (Chapter 49) should be excluded. In mild cases, acrocyanosis, livedo reticularis and erythromelalgia may be considered.

Treatment and prognosis. The dermatologist may be faced with the problem of a patient referred for ulceration or erythema of the foot and toes. Once the diagnosis is established, the matter is best dealt with by the vascular surgeon, whose advice should be sought. Collateral development can be expected to occur during phases of inactivity of the disease. The essential requirement for successful outcome is the complete discontinuation of tobacco use. Bed rest and antibiotics are other facets of conservative treatment. Surgical or chemical sympathectomy is usually helpful and prostacyclin infusions may buy time and minimize ablative surgery [9]. In a double-blind study of a chemically stable prostacyclin analogue, 85% of patients treated showed ulcer healing or relief of pain compared with 17% of an aspirin-treated group [10].

Arterial reconstructive surgery has little part to play in the management of this condition because of the distal nature of the disease. After sympathectomy, every effort should be made to avoid major amputations by the use of antibiotics and, when necessary, toe excisions. Below-knee amputation may eventually be required, particularly if gangrene extends to the foot. It should not be unreasonably delayed. There are an increasing number of reports on the use of an implantable spinal cord stimulator in patients with Buerger's disease; this can produce a marked improvement in regional perfusion, thereby avoiding amputation. The limb survival rate was 93.1% [11].

The prognosis is poor in patients who continue to smoke; hands and feet may be lost.

References

1 Buerger L. Thromboangiitis obliterans: a study of the vascular lesions leading to presenile spontaneous gangrene. *Am J Med Sci* 1908; **136**: 567–80.

2 Totemchokchyakarn K. Thromboangiitis obliterans (Buerger's disease). In: Ball GV, Bridges SL, eds. *Vasculitis*. Oxford: Oxford University Press, 2002: 460–6.

3 Wessler S. Buerger's disease revisited. *Surg Clin North Am* 1969; **49**: 703–13.

4 Olin JW, Smith A. Thromboangiitis obliterans (Buerger's disease). *Curr Opin Rheumatol* 2006; **18**: 18–24.

5 Adar R, Papa MJ, Halpern Z *et al.* Cellular sensitivity to collagen in thromboangiitis obliterans. *N Engl J Med* 1983; **308**: 1113–6.

6 Shionoya S. Pathology of Buerger's disease, clinico-pathico-angiographic correlation. *Pathol Microbiol* 1975; **43**: 163–6.

7 Puéchal X, Fiessinger J-N. Thromboangiitis obliterans or Buerger's disease: challenges for the rheumatologist. *Rheumatology* 2007; **46**: 192–9.

8 Lazarides MK, Georgiadis GS, Papas TT, Nikolopoulos ES. Diagnostic criteria and treatment of Buerger's disease: a review. *Int J Low Extrem Wounds* 2006; **5**: 89–95.

9 Ohta T, Shionoya S. Fate of the ischaemic limb in Buerger's disease. *Br J Surg* 1988; **75**: 259–62.

10 Fiessinger JN, Schäfer M. Trial of iloprost versus aspirin treatment for critical limb ischaemia of thromboangiitis. *Lancet* 1990; **i**: 555–7.

11 Donas KP, Schulte S, Ktenidis K, Horsch S. The role of epidural spinal cord stimulation in the treatment of Buerger's disease. *J Vasc Surg* 2005; **41**: 830–6.

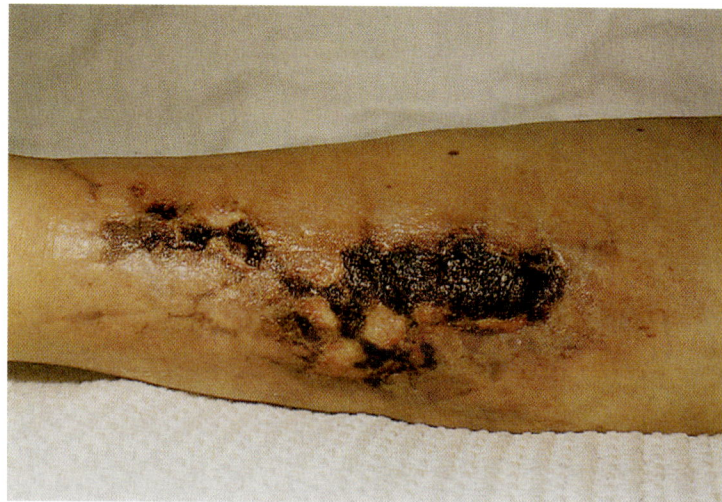

Fig. 47.10 Ulceration associated with calcification of arteries in secondary hyperparathyroidism.

Small vessel calcification and calcific uraemic arteriolopathy (calciphylaxis) [1,2]

Arterial calcification is a common and usually asymptomatic complication of chronic renal failure. Occasionally, especially when associated with hyperparathyroidism, it can cause complete vascular occlusion and infarction of the skin. This condition, calcific uraemic arteriolopathy (previously termed calciphylaxis), may begin as a small area of redness and tenderness or with a broad livedo reticularis pattern, evolving into intense erythema. This may progress to violaceous indurated plaques and nodules in the skin, attributable to fat necrosis [3]. The sites of predilection are the proximal extremities, especially the thighs, abdomen and buttocks (Fig. 47.10) [4]. Plain radiographs demonstrate small and large vessel calcification. The pathogenesis is unknown, and the condition is probably the result of a number of comorbid factors. The condition occurs in an estimated 1–4% of patients with terminal renal insufficiency and is much more common in women [3]. Uraemia and hyperphosphataemia are often more obvious than hypercalcaemia. The exact role of hyperparathyroidism is debated, but an elevated serum parathyroid hormone level is noted in most patients. The role of protein C and S remains to be determined, but a relative hypercoagulable state is present [3,4]. Histology usually confirms arterial medial calcification, intimal hyperplasia, fibrosis and vascular thrombosis and necrosis of the overlying epidermis [3].

The differential diagnosis of calcific uraemic arteriolopathy is extensive (Table 47.1) [3,4]. Treatment is unsatisfactory and the prognosis is poor, with sepsis as the main cause of death. Uraemia, and a raised serum calcium and phosphorus may be treated by dialysis; the mechanisms of the process, and medical treatments, are discussed in more detail in Chapter 49. Other important measures include pain control, wound management, sepsis prevention and avoidance of certain medications [3,4]. Parathyroidectomy is only indicated when there is evidence of hyperparathyroidism.

References

1 Chan YL, Mahony JF, Turner JJ, Posen S. The vascular lesions associated with skin necrosis in renal disease. *Br J Dermatol* 1983; **109**: 85–95.

Table 47.1 Differential diagnosis of calcific uraemic arteriolopathy (calciphylaxis).

Vascular causes
 Peripheral arterial occlusive disease
 Chronic venous insufficiency

Infections
 Subacute bacterial endocarditis
 Necrotizing fasciitis
 Deep fungal infections
 Erysipelas
 Cellulitis

Immune mediated
 Vasculitis
 Cryoglobulinaemia
 Lobular panniculitis (e.g. pancreatic)
 Connective tissue disorders
 Bullous pemphigoid
 Erythema nodosum

Coagulopathy
 Warfarin/coumarin necrosis
 Embolic phenomena
 Disseminated intravascular coagulation
 Antiphospholipid syndrome

Miscellaneous
 Porphyria cutanea tarda
 Neoplastic causes
 Calcinosis cutis

2 Ross CN, Cassidy MJD, Thompson M *et al.* Proximal cutaneous necrosis associated with small vessel calcification in renal failure. *QJM* 1991; **79**: 443–50.
3 Guldbakke KK, Khachemoune A. Calciphylaxis. *Int J Dermatol* 2007; **46**: 231–8.
4 Meissner M, Gille J, Kaufmann R. Calciphylaxis: no therapeutic concepts for a poorly understood syndrome? *J Dtsch Dermatol Ges* 2006; **4**: 1037–44.

Neurovascular disorders of the extremities

Erythromelalgia [1]

Definition [2]. This is a condition of painful, red extremities in which a sensation of burning is associated with small vessel vasodilatation in the affected skin. The synonyms erythermalgia [3] and erythralgia are confusing. There are three types of erythromelalgia:

Type 1: This is associated with thrombocythaemia and is relieved by aspirin.

Type 2 (Weir Mitchell's disease): This is a primary or idiopathic disorder which is usually congenital and is provoked by exercise or exposure to warmth.

Type 3: This is secondary to inflammatory or degenerative peripheral vascular disease.

However, the simpler division into primary (type 2) and secondary erythromelalgia may be preferred.

Pathogenesis. Type 1 is the result of thrombocythaemia and is seen in polycythaemia and myelofibrosis. It may be unilateral or even affect one finger or toe [4–7]. There is fibromuscular proliferation of the intima which leads to occlusive thrombosis of the digital arterioles and arteries [8].

Type 2 is confined to the lower legs and does not progress to ischaemia [9]. Primary erythromelalgia is often familial and is inherited in an autosomal dominant manner with the causative gene being located at chromosome 2q24 [10–12]. A prospective study by Davis *et al.* showed that most patients with erythromelalgia had a small-fibre neuropathy [13]. Primary erythromelalgia is the first inherited painful neuropathy to be understood at a molecular level, being due to mutations in the gene *SCN9A*, which encodes the voltage-gated channel Nav 1.7. *SCN9A* is preferentially expressed in most nocicepetive neurones and in sympathetic ganglia. Mutations cause a gain of function and a lower threshold for the influx of sodium ions in response to a stimulus such as increased temperature. Consequently, pain signalling increases in response to heat [14]. Families with erythromelalgia have been described in which inheritance is dominant although heterozygous mutations in Nav 1.7 are not always found. Mice homozygous for the mutation do not appear to feel pain. Nav 1.7 might not have a major role in post-traumatic neuropathic pain, but it does appear to have a role in inflammatory pain [12].

Pain has a direct relationship to the temperature of the limb; when this reaches a 'critical point', which normally lies between 32 and 36°C and which is constant for each individual, then pain will occur [14]. Pain is not a direct result of vasodilatation as it can be induced or maintained by warming the limb while its blood supply is occluded by a cuff. The pain is made worse by making the limb dependent, irrespective of its temperature. Pain may also be induced by obstructing the venous return. The involvement of small nerve fibres in primary erythromelalgia is likely as such manoeuvres do not cause pain or distress in normal subjects [15,16].

Type 3 erythromelalgia can occur in patients with connective tissue disorders and other inflammatory states. Certain drugs and peripheral vascular disease can also give rise to erythromelalgia and this can involve acral sites other than the hands and feet. Females are more often affected [17–22]. In types 1 and 3, the hands and feet are usually involved but sometimes only a part of one extremity is affected. The principal feature of erythromelalgia of all types is that attacks are precipitated by exercise or heat, such as a warm bed, and are relieved by rapid cooling, such as immersion in iced water. The patient complains of intense burning associated with erythema and increased warmth of the extremity. Attacks last from a few minutes to several hours. A warm climate and fever may increase the distress. Ulceration and trophic changes may result from cold immersion injury produced by attempts to relieve pain.

Diagnosis. The fully developed characteristics of the syndrome and the description given by the patient seldom leave doubt about the correct diagnosis. However, there are some important differential diagnoses and disease associations. Complex regional pain syndrome (reflex sympathetic dystrophy) following trauma can produce a similar clinical pattern. The effect of dependency, and the bizarre measures by which the patient may attempt to obtain relief, are also indicative of the diagnosis.

Disease associations include hypertension, diabetes, rheumatoid arthritis, lupus erythematosus, thromboangiitis obliterans, gout and vasculitis. The most important association of secondary erythromelalgia is with myeloproliferative disorders, for example polycythaemia rubra vera or thrombocythaemia. It may be a presenting and premonitory symptom of these conditions, often being present several years before they develop. Vasoactive drugs, such as nicardipine, have been incriminated as a cause [21].

Treatment and prognosis. No treatment is consistently effective and there is a dearth of adequate clinical trials. There is a significant decrease in survival compared to the general population, and most cases get worse over time [20].

Management consists of avoiding exacerbating factors, and controlling secondary and underlying factors [23]. Thrombocythaemia, or causes of inflammatory vascular disease, must be treated where possible. Small doses of aspirin give considerable relief in some patients—presumably by preventing platelet aggregation—and clopidogrel may be the most effective antiplatelet agent [5,24]. Patients with vasodilatation and warmth in their affected painful extremities prefer immersion in cold water. Elevation also provides some relief by decreasing oedema. Some have claimed relief of erythromelalgia with benoxybenzamine hydrochloride or propranolol [25]. Amitriptyline and neuropathic pain treatments such as gabapentin can help, and selective serotonin reuptake inhibitors have been used with success. Pain has been totally controlled by inserting an epidural block for up to 3 weeks, which allows healing of ulceration. The response of one family to pizotifen has been reported as spectacular [26]. Recombinant growth hormone therapy immediately relieved pain and healed cutaneous ulcers in a child with erythromelalgia and a growth hormone deficiency [27]. More recently, relief of pain was achieved in 18 out of 33 patients using a 5% lidocaine patch [28].

References

1 Brown GF. Erythromelalgia and other disturbances of the extremities accompanied by vasodilatation and burning. *Am J Med Sci* 1932; **183**: 468–85.
2 Mitchell SW. A rare vasomotor neurosis of the extremities and on maladies with which it may be confounded. *Am J Med Sci* 1878; **76**: 2–36.
3 Smith LA, Allen FV. Erythermalgia (erythromelalgia) of the extremities: a syndrome characterized by redness, heat and pain. *Am Heart J* 1938; **16**: 136–41.
4 Alarcon-Segovia D, Bag RR, Fairbain JF *et al.* Erythermalgia: a clue to early diagnosis of myeloproliferative disorders. *Arch Intern Med* 1966; **117**: 511–5.
5 Michiels JJ, Abels J, Steketee J *et al.* Erythromelalgia caused by platelet-mediated arteriolar inflammation and thrombosis. *Ann Intern Med* 1985; **102**: 466–71.
6 Michiels JJ, Van Joost T. Erythromelalgia and thrombocythemia: a causal relation. *J Am Acad Dermatol* 1990; **22**: 107–11.
7 Redding KG. Thrombocythaemia as a cause of erythermalgia. *Arch Dermatol* 1977; **113**: 448–71.
8 Michiels JJ, Van Joost TH, Vuzevski VD *et al.* Histopathology of erythromelalgia in thrombocythaemia. *Histopathology* 1984; **8**: 669–78.
9 Michiels JJ, Van Joost TH, Vuzevski VD. Idiopathic erythermalgia: a congenital disorder. *J Am Acad Dermatol* 1989; **21**: 1128–30.
10 Drenth JP, Finley WH, Breedveld GJ *et al.* The primary erythermalgia: susceptibility gene is located on chromosome 2q 31–2. *Am J Hum Genet* 2001; **68**: 1277–82.
11 Waxman SG, Dib-Hajj SD. Erythromelalgia: a hereditary pain syndrome enters the molecular era. *Ann Neurol* 2005; **57**: 785–8.
12 Waxman SG, Dib-Hajj SD. Molecular basis for an inherited pain syndrome. *Trends Mol Med* 2005; **11**: 555–62.
13 Davis MDP, Sandroni P, Rooke TW, Low PA. Erythromelalgia: vasculopathy, neuropathy, or both? A prospective study of vascular and neurophysiologic studies in erythromelalgia. *Arch Dermatol* 2003; **139**: 1337–43.
14 Han C, Lampert A, Rush AM *et al.* Temperature dependence of erythromelalgia mutation L858F in sodium channel Nav 1.7. *Mol Pain* 2007; **3**: 3.
15 Babb RR, Alarcon-Segovia D, Fairbain JF. Erythermalgia: review of 51 cases. *Circulation* 1964; **29**: 136–41.
16 Ørstavik K, Mørk C, Kvernebo K, Jørum E. Pain in primary erythromelalgia—a neuropathic component? *Pain* 2004; **110**: 531–8.
17 Davis MD, Fallon WM, Rogers RS III *et al.* Natural history of erythromelalgia: presentation and outcome of 168 patients. *Arch Dermatol* 2000; **136**: 330–6.
18 Alarcon-Segovia D, Diaz-Jouananen E. Erythermalgia in systemic lupus erythematosus. *Am J Med Sci* 1973; **266**: 149–51.
19 Ratz JI, Berfield WF, Steck WD. Erythermalgia with vasculitis. *J Am Acad Dermatol* 1979; **1**: 433–50.
20 Sandroni P, Davis MDP, Harper CM Jr *et al.* Neurophysiologic and vascular studies in erythromelalgia: a retrospective analysis. *J Clin Neuromusc Dis* 1999; **1**: 57–63.
21 Drenth JPH. Erythromelalgia induced by nicardipine. *BMJ* 1989; **298**: 1582.
22 Levesque H, Moore N, Wolf LM *et al.* Erythromelalgia induced by nicardipine (inverse Raynaud's phenomenon). *BMJ* 1989; **298**: 1252–3.
23 Davis MD, Rooke T. Erythromelalgia. *Curr Treat Options Cardiovasc Med* 2006; **8**: 153–65.
24 Michiels JJ, Lindemans J, Van Vliet HHDM *et al.* Survival kinetics of platelets and fibrinogen in thrombocythaemia related to erythromelalgia. *Br J Haematol* 1982; **50**: 690–1.
25 Bada SL. Treatment of erythromelalgia with propranolol. *Lancet* 1977; **ii**: 412.
26 Le Noach E, Guillet MH, Sassolas B *et al.* Erythromelalgie familiale; une observation traitée avec succes par pizotifene. *Ann Dermatol Vénéréol* 1994; **121** (Suppl. 1): 563.
27 Cimaz R, Rusconi R, Fossali E *et al.* Unexpected healing of cutaneous ulcers in a short child. *Lancet* 2001; **358**: 211–2.
28 Davis MDP, Sandroni P. Lidocaine patch for pain of erythromelalgia: follow-up of 34 patients. *Arch Dermatol* 2005; **141**: 1320–1.

Complex regional pain syndrome

Synonyms
• Complex regional pain syndrome types I and II
• Reflex sympathetic dystrophy
• Causalgia
• Sudeck's atrophy

Definition. Complex regional pain syndrome (CRPS) is the name now given to a syndrome of chronic pain and hyperalgesia, associated with sensory, motor, autonomic and dystrophic disturbances, usually in a limb. Two types can be distinguished:

CRPS 1: also known as reflex sympathetic dystrophy, typically develops after minor trauma with no obvious small nerve lesion

CRPS 2: also known as causalgia, in which there is clear evidence of nerve injury [1].

Pathogenesis. There is evidence to suggest that CRPS represents a spectrum of changes in the inflammatory, neural, vascular and musculoskeletal systems. Several mechanisms have been suggested, but none of them has so far explained the exact pathophysiology of this disease. Peripheral nerves or C and A-δ fibre terminals are injured in the autonomic and motor systems as well as in the pain fibres [2].

Clinical features. Patients typically describe pain, swelling and difficulty in using the affected limb. The pain has a burning or deep aching quality and is aggravated by movement. Consequently there is a tendency to avoid using the limb, and hyperalgesia encourages limb protection. The skin takes on a deep red to blue colour, suggesting that vasodilatation is occurring, and is initially warmer than the unaffected contralateral limb becoming cooler in the latter stages. Oedema may result from disuse and dependency, and the muscles atrophy (Sudeck's atrophy).

Diagnosis. CRPS is a clinical diagnosis and there is no simple diagnostic test. In 20% of the patients there are changes in the skin and less commonly in the nails and hair. There is a temperature and colour asymmetry in half the patients. Early hyperhidrosis, and later anhidrosis, may be demonstrated by starch-iodine testing. A decreased range of motion, weakness, dystonia and tremor may also be noted [3]. Increased blood flow is an important diagnostic feature of early CRPS [4]. It is clearly demonstrated by a three-phase bone scan [5]; the delayed phase of this scan is very sensitive, and a segmental diffuse increase in the uptake of radionuclide is very specific. Later the bone scan returns to normal and there are radiographic features of rapid bone loss including visible demineralization with patchy, subchondral or periosteal osteoporosis, metaphyseal banding and profound bone loss [6].

Treatment. The aim of treatment is to reduce pain and restore function of the affected limb as soon as possible. First-line treatment consists of physical therapy in combination with drugs. Medications that may improve neuropathic pain, including tricyclic antidepressants, anticonvulsants and opioid analgesia, are commonly used to treat patients with CRPS [7]. Although not well tolerated by most patients, compression bandaging is one of the mainstays of complex regional pain syndrome treatment, especially in reducing oedema and enhancing the circulation.

Free radical scavengers have been used in both the treatment and prevention of complex regional pain syndrome, based on the assumption that complex regional pain syndrome is induced by an exaggerated inflammatory response to tissue injury, mediated by excessive production of toxic oxygen radicals [8]. Promising results have been reported with dimethylsulfoxide and *N*-acetylcysteine [9].

Severe cases may require regional anaesthetic blockade. A meta-analysis by Hassantash *et al.* [10] found that 88% of 822 patients with CRPS 2 had a beneficial response to sympathetic blocks of the involved extremity. The same literature review demonstrated that 91% of 791 patients who were treated by sympathectomy had a relief of their symptoms after one procedure and 94% after a second procedure. In selected patients with severe chronic pain, electrical spinal cord stimulation can induce pain relief and improve the patient's quality of life.

References

1 Eisenberg E, Geller R, Brill S. Pharmacotherapy options for complex regional pain syndrome. *Expert Rev Neurother* 2007; **5**: 521–31.
2 Jänig W, Baron R. Complex regional pain syndrome: mystery explained? *Lancet Neurol* 2003; **2**: 687–97.
3 Harden RN, Bruehl SP. Diagnosis of complex regional pain syndrome: signs, symptoms, and new empirically derived diagnostic criteria. *Clin J Pain* 2006; **22**: 415–9.
4 Wasner G, Schattschneider J, Heckmann K *et al.* Vascular abnormalities in the reflex sympathetic dystrophy (CRPS 1): mechanisms and diagnostic value. *Brain* 2001; **124**: 587–99.
5 Driessens M, Dijs H, Verheyen G, Blockx P. What is reflex sympathetic dystrophy? *Acta Orthop Belg* 1999; **65**: 202–17.
6 Atkins RM. Aspects of current management: complex regional pain syndrome. *J Bone Joint Surg* 2003; **85-B**: 1100–6.
7 Sharma A, Williams K, Raja SN. Advances in treatment of complex regional pain syndrome: recent insights on a perplexing disease. *Curr Opin Anaesthesiol* 2006; **19**: 566–72.
8 Perez RSGM, Zuurmond WWA, Bezemer PD *et al.* The treatment of complex regional pain syndrome type I with free radical scavengers: a randomized controlled study. *Pain* 2003; **102**: 297–307.
9 Warltier DC. Preventing the development of complex regional pain syndrome after surgery. *Anesthesiology* 2004; **101**: 1215–24.
10 Hassantash SA, Afrakhteh M, Maier RV. Causalgia. A meta-analysis of the literature. *Arch Surg* 2003; **138**: 1226–31.

Angiodyskinesia

Paraesthesiae, painful burning sensations combined with redness or pallor of the legs after prolonged walking or dancing, has been described in young people [1,2] and it has been suggested that these were a consequence of abnormal functioning of the arteriovenous communications. The term 'angiodyskinesia' has been applied to this condition [3].

Under this title, Ryan and Wilkinson described a blotchy erythema of the legs in a 14-year-old boy [4]. His condition developed at the same time as osteochondritis dissecans. The erythematous areas were 2–3°C warmer than the adjoining skin, and disappeared when the patient was recumbent, reappearing and becoming uncomfortable when he was standing. These features suggest failure of the normal vasoconstriction that occurs when a limb is lowered. The condition was more marked in warmer conditions and after a bath.

References

1 Khobreh MT, Roy P. Functional circulatory disorders of the lower extremities due to regional hemokinetic imbalance: a new clinical and angiographic concept. *Surgery* 1967; **61**: 880–90.
2 Malan E. Vascular syndromes from dilatation of arteriovenous communications of the sole of the foot. *Arch Surg* 1958; **77**: 783–95.
3 Amir-Jahed AK. Angiodyskinesia. *Surg Gynaecol Obstet* 1968; **127**: 609–31.
4 Ryan TJ, Wilkinson DS. Angiodyskinesia and osteochondritis dissecans. *Proc R Soc Med* 1974; **67**: 1242–3.

Restless legs syndrome

Definition. Restless legs syndrome is a sensorimotor disorder characterized by an uncomfortable feeling in the legs that urges movement [1].

Pathophysiology. Restless legs syndrome can occur as a primary or a secondary disorder.

In the primary form there is no apparent cause other than a possible genetic predisposition [2]. Under the assumption of a recessive and dominant mode of inheritance, three loci for restless legs have been found on chromosomes 9p, 12q and 14q [3].

Restless legs syndrome occurring as a secondary condition is related to iron deficiency, pregnancy and end-stage renal disease. Clinical evidence suggests that restless legs syndrome is associated with decreased dopaminergic neurotransmission. The symptoms are worse at night when dopamine levels fall [2]. Restless legs syndrome is not associated with chronic venous insufficiency.

Clinical features. The core feature of this syndrome is a distressing, irresistible urge to move the legs (akathisia). This often coexists with an uncomfortable, hard to describe, sensation deep within the legs. The prevalence in the general population lies between 2.5–15%, increasing with age and being more common in women. A family history is often present in patients whose symptoms appear before 40 years of age [4].

Four essential criteria have been established for the diagnosis to be upheld:

1 An urge to move legs that is usually accompanied or caused by uncomfortable or unpleasant sensations in the legs
2 An urge to move or an unpleasant sensation that begins or worsens during periods of rest or inactivity
3 An urge to move or an unpleasant sensation that is partially or totally relieved by movement as long as the activity continues
4 An urge to move or an unpleasant sensation that is worse in the evening or at night rather than during the day or that only occurs during the evening or at night [1].

Diagnosis. The diagnosis is made from the criteria listed above; the most important aspect is to identify any treatable underlying cause and to exclude other disorders that have some clinical similarities. End-stage renal failure is probably the most obvious and best investigated secondary condition associated with restless legs syndrome. Several studies have shown an association between restless legs syndrome and pregnancy. After delivery, the prevalence of restless legs syndrome decreases to values found in the normal population. Disorders in iron regulation may be involved in primary forms of restless legs syndrome. Correcting iron status in patients with iron deficiency has been found to reduce symptoms in patients with restless legs syndrome. An association between Parkinson's disease and restless legs syndrome has been made because of the response to dopaminergic treatment in both disorders [5].

The differential diagnosis of restless legs syndrome includes both movement and sleep disorders. Most of these conditions typically do not have a circadian pattern, nor does movement relieve the symptoms [1]. Although restless legs syndrome may be triggered by radiculopathy, neuropathic pain syndromes or peripheral neuropathy, a distinction should be made between these conditions [6]. Restless legs syndrome should be differentiated from drug-induced akathisia (e.g. antiemetics, neuroleptics, antipsychotics, serotonin reuptake inhibitors and tricyclic antidepressants), positional discomfort and arthritis. Other disorders such as nocturnal leg cramps, restless insomnia and vascular insufficiency should also be distinguished from restless legs syndrome.

Treatment. Treatment of restless legs syndrome begins with an assessment of potential factors that may aggravate the symptoms.

Medications that can aggravate the symptoms of restless legs syndrome, such as dopamine-blocking agents, antiemetics, antihistamines and antidepressants, should be avoided. Other non-pharmacologic approaches consist of good sleep 'hygiene', behavioural interventions (for example a brief walk before bedtime and a hot bath) and avoidance of alcohol, nicotine and caffeine, especially in the evening [7].

Iron deficiency, confirmed by a low ferritin level, should be treated, as it has been reported that iron supplementation improves the symptoms of restless legs syndrome [4]. When drug management is required, dopaminergic agents are considered the first line of treatment in idiopathic restless legs syndrome. Other agents that have been shown to improve the symptoms of restless legs syndrome are opiates, benzodiazepines and anticonvulsant agents.

References

1 Kushida CA. Clinical presentation, diagnosis, and quality of life issues in restless legs syndrome. *Am J Med* 2007; **120** (Suppl. 1A): 4–12.
2 Allen RP. Controversies and challenges in defining the etiology and pathophysiology of restless legs syndrome. *Am J Med* 2007; **120** (Suppl. 1A): 13–21.
3 Winkelmann J, Ferini-Strambi L. Genetics of restless legs syndrome. *Sleep Med Rev* 2006; **10**: 179–83.
4 Earley CJ. Restless legs syndrome. *N Engl J Med* 2003; **348**: 2103–9.
5 Trenkwalder C, Paulus W, Walters AS. The restless legs syndrome. *Lancet Neurol* 2005; **4**: 464–75.
6 Garcia-Borreguero D, Egatz R, Winkelmann J, Berger K. Epidemiology of restless legs syndrome: the current status. *Sleep Med Rev* 2006; **10**: 153–67.
7 Hening WA. Current guidelines and strategies of practice for restless legs syndrome. *Am J Med* 2007; **120** (Suppl. 1A): 22–7.

Telangiectases

Definition. Telangiectases (Latin: tel, end + Greek: angos, vessel + ectasis from Greek: ektasis, expansion) are chronically dilated capillaries or venules. They appear on the skin and mucous membranes as small, dull red, linear, stellate or punctate markings. Telangiectases (telangiectasia) represent dilatations (expansion, stretching) of pre-existing vessels without any apparently new vessel growth (angiogenesis) occurring. As such, telangiectases can be bracketed with spider angioma (spider naevi) and capillary aneurysm–venous lakes, whereas vascular malformations represent anomalies of embryological development (disturbances in vasculogenesis or angiogenesis). Hamartomas include proliferation of other tissue elements, for example melanocytic or eccrine cells, and are not solely vascular [1].

Telangiectasia can also be part of chronic venous insufficiency. The red lesions have a higher oxygen content than the blue lesions, suggesting a different origin in the capillary bed [2].

Development of telangiectasia [3]

The common telangiectases can be explained by abnormalities in the organization and ultrastructure of the small vessels rather than by neovascularization (angiogenesis) or random anastomoses.

The *macular telangiectases* seen in scleroderma, generalized essential telangiectasia and naevus flammeus are produced by dilatation of the postcapillary venules of the upper horizontal (subpapillary) plexus.

Cherry angiomas are produced by spherical and tubular dilatations of capillary loops in the dermal papillae with tortuous cross-connections between individual loops.

Telangiectasia macularis eruptiva perstans is a rare form of cutaneous mastocytosis. Clinically, there are tan-to-brown macules with patchy erythema associated with telangiectases that usually involve the trunk. Histologically, there may be only subtle alterations in mast cell numbers. The cells tend to be fusiform and loosely arranged around the dilated vessels of the superficial plexus. Eosinophils are usually absent [4].

Angiokeratomas of Fabry and Fordyce have the ultrastructure of collecting venules that contain valves and appear to represent the ectopic development of small valve-containing collecting veins.

The cutaneous lesions of hereditary haemorrhagic telangiectasia (HHT) represent microvascular arteriovenous anastomoses.

The development of telangiectases is a complex dynamic process with different mechanisms likely to be involved. In HHT, for example, where arteriovenous anastomoses cause focal dilatations of postcapillary venules, different genetic mutations (discussed on p. 47.17) interfere with integral membrane proteins on vascular endothelial cells responsible for binding transforming growth factor-β (TGF-β). TGF-β signalling mediates vascular remodelling through effects on extracellular matrix production [5]. Disruption of this latter maturation phase of angiogenesis seems to be important in the development of HHT [6].

References

1 Requena L, Sangueza OP. Cutaneous vascular anomalies. Part I. Hamartomas, malformations and dilation of pre-existing vessels. *J Am Acad Dermatol* 1997; **37**: 523–49.

2 Sommer A, Van Mierlo PLHMJ, Kessels AGH, Neumann HAM. Red and blue telangiectasias. Differences in oxygenation? *Dermatol Surg* 1997; **23**: 55–9.

3 Braverman IM. Ultrastructure and organisation of the cutaneous microvasculature in normal and pathologic state. *J Invest Dermatol* 1989; **93** (Suppl. 2): 25–95.

4 Weedon D. Cutaneous infiltrates—non-lymphoid. In: Weedon D, ed. *Skin Pathology*, 2nd edn. London: Churchill Livingstone, 2002: 1057–93.

5 Fernàndez-L A, Sanz-Rodriguez F, Blanco FJ *et al*. Hereditary hemorrhagic telangiectasia, a vascular dysplasia affecting the TGF-β signaling pathway. *Clin Med Res* 2006; **1**: 66–78.

6 Lamouile S, Mallet C, Feige JJ, Bailly S. Activin receptor-like kinase 1 is implicated in the maturation phase of angiogenesis. *Blood* 2002; **100**: 4495–501.

Secondary telangiectasia and dilatation of pre-existing vessels

Telangiectases commonly represent the effect of wear and tear on the skin, and are particularly frequent in ageing, on light-exposed skin, or following trauma or X-irradiation, and in some skin diseases such as lupus erythematosus and dermatomyositis. In fact, they are found in most processes that cause atrophy of the skin, whatever their aetiology; they are prominent, for example, in poikiloderma. Smoking and UV-radiation are known to have a detrimental effect on human skin, characterized by elastosis and telangiectasia. The association between increasing age, sun exposure and the amount of telangiectasia is strong in men but less apparent in women. Similarly, smoking is associated with elastosis in both sexes but only with telangiectasia in men [1].

Prolonged vasodilatation may be followed by permanent telangiectases, for example, in rosacea. Varicose veins are frequently

Table 47.2 Vessel classification (Duffy, 1988 [3]).

Type I	Spider veins, 0.1–1 mm diameter
	telangiectatic matting <0.2 mm diameter
Type II	Venulectasia 1–2 mm
Type III	Reticular veins 2–4 mm diameter
	feeder veins
Type IV	Non-saphenous varicose veins, 3–8 mm
Type V	Saphenous varicose veins

Table 47.3 Some causes of telangiectasia.

Secondary telangiectasia
Prolonged vasodilatation (rosacea, varicose veins)
Prolonged exposure to sunlight, tar, etc.
Post-traumatic
Radiodermatitis
Xeroderma pigmentosum
Atrophy, e.g. poikiloderma, topical corticosteroids
Raynaud's disease
Lupus erythematosus
Dermatomyositis
Systemic sclerosis
Morphoea
Mastocytosis (telangiectasia macularis eruptiva perstans)
Acquired immune deficiency syndrome

Primary telangiectasia
Vascular naevi
Angiomas and angiokeratomas
Angioma serpiginosum
Hereditary haemorrhagic telangiectasia
Ataxia–telangiectasia
Generalized essential telangiectasia
Unilateral naevoid telangiectasia syndrome
Hereditary benign telangiectasia
Spider telangiectases
Bloom's syndrome
Morquio's syndrome
Angiotropic lymphoma
Mycosis fungoides
Naevus anaemicus with telangiectatic vessels
Cutis marmorata telangiectatica
Solitary plaque-like telangiectatic glomangioma

the cause of telangiectases on the legs, where they may produce a type of arborescent telangiectasia. Telangiectasias associated with chronic venous disease are assumed to be the result of a rise in venous pressure, which stretches the vulnerable venous end of the capillary or draining venule [2]. The significance of telangiectases of the lower limbs must not be underestimated. Considered a 'cosmetic' problem, their presence is often indicative of early or established abnormalities in the main leg veins. Telangiectases may be individual or they can arise in sheets or have an arborizing appearance. The colour of the telangiectasia depends on the calibre of the dilated venule. Large dilatations (<1 mm) are dark blue and often palpable. The smallest (0.1 mm), most superficial, telangiectases are red and barely empty when the leg is raised. Telangiectasias have been classified by Duffy (Table 47.2) [3]; some of the more important causes are listed in Table 47.3.

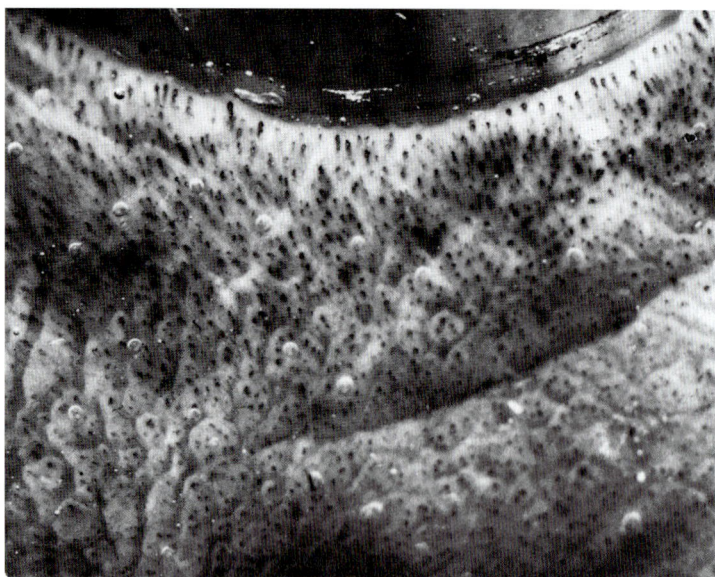

Fig. 47.11 Normal nail-fold capillaries. (Courtesy of Dr H.R. Maricq, Lyons, NJ, USA.)

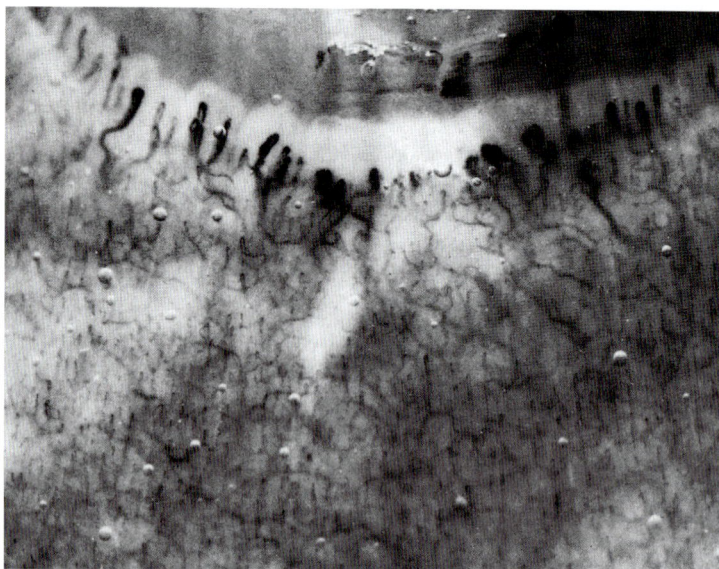

Fig. 47.12 Nail-fold capillaries in scleroderma. (Courtesy of Dr H.R. Maricq, Lyons, NJ, USA.)

The term *corona phlebectatica paraplantans* (venous ankle flare) [4] is used to describe perimalleolar and paraplantar venous telangiectasia that is always associated with venous hypertension. In contrast, telangiectases around the lower border of the ribs ('costal fringe') are virtually physiological in old age.

Telangiectases may be an important diagnostic sign in certain systemic disorders, especially in lupus erythematosus, dermatomyositis and scleroderma, or in association with Raynaud's phenomenon.

Capillary microscopy of nail-fold telangiectases may help in the differential diagnosis (Figs 47.11 & 47.12). Usually, the distribution and associated abnormalities leave little doubt about the diagnosis, but occasionally telangiectases may be the presenting or only sign, or may be the result of an otherwise burnt-out process. Patients with scleroderma, especially of the so-called Thibierge–Weissenbach or CREST type, may present with telangiectases that closely mimic HHT, and that may even cause severe bleeding. Patients with dermatomyositis may have telangiectases on the eyelids, hands or elsewhere. Localized areas of telangiectases on the face may be a manifestation of discoid lupus erythematosus. Telangiectases of the face and also of the mucous membranes are a common feature of Raynaud's phenomenon without other evidence of scleroderma. Telangiectases may be a manifestation of neonatal lupus erythematosus, with or without any other eruption [5].

Unusual mat-like telangiectases, especially on the upper back, have been reported in men working in an aluminium plant [6]. Telangiectases on the chest wall [7] and other sites [8] have been reported in patients with AIDS. Telangiectasias are also described in other conditions, including cutaneous mastocytosis (telangiectasia macularis eruptiva perstans) and angiotrophic (intravascular) lymphoma [9].

References

1 Kennedy C, Bastiaens MT, Bajdik CD *et al.* Effect of smoking and sun on the ageing skin. *J Invest Dermatol* 2003; **120**: 548–54.

2 Bergan JJ, Goldman MP. *Varicose Veins and Telangiectasias.* St. Louis: Quality Medical Publishing, 1993.

3 Duffy DM. Small vessel sclerotherapy: an overview. In: Callen JP. *et al.,* eds. *Advances in Dermatology*, Vol. 3. Chicago: Year Book Medical Publishers, 1988: 221.

4 Van der Molen HR. Die Corona Phlebectatica Paraplantaris. *Der Fuss*, 1982: 154–74.

5 Thornton CM, Eichenfield LF, Shinall EA *et al.* Cutaneous telangiectases in neonatal lupus erythematosus. *J Am Acad Dermatol* 1995; **33**: 19–25.

6 Thériault G, Cordier S, Harvey R. Skin telangiectases in workers at an aluminium plant. *N Engl J Med* 1980; **303**: 1278–81.

7 Fallo T, Abell E, Kingsley L *et al.* Telangiectasias of the anterior chest in homosexual men. *Ann Intern Med* 1986; **105**: 679–82.

8 Ruiz-Avila P, Tercedor J. Painful periungual telangiectasias in a patient with acquired immunodeficiency syndrome. *Int J Dermatol* 1995; **34**: 199–200.

9 Ozguroglu E, Buyulbabani N, Ozguroglu M *et al.* Generalised telangiectasia as the major manifestation of angiotropic (intravascular) lymphoma. *Br J Dermatol* 1997; **137**: 422–5.

Spider telangiectases

Synonyms
- Arterial spider
- Spider naevus
- Naevus araneus
- Spider angioma

Aetiology and pathology. Spider telangiectases occur in up to 15% of completely normal persons, and more frequently in children [1,2]. They occur in large numbers during pregnancy—one or more spider naevi are found in two-thirds of all pregnant women [1]. They may appear in the first few months, but tend to increase in number until term; they usually disappear within 6 weeks of delivery but may persist or recur in the same sites in subsequent pregnancies. They are also characteristically found in patients with liver disease, when they can be a presenting sign [3]. A relationship to oestrogens has been suggested on this clinical evidence. Palmar erythema may be associated with spider naevi, with or without liver disease or pregnancy.

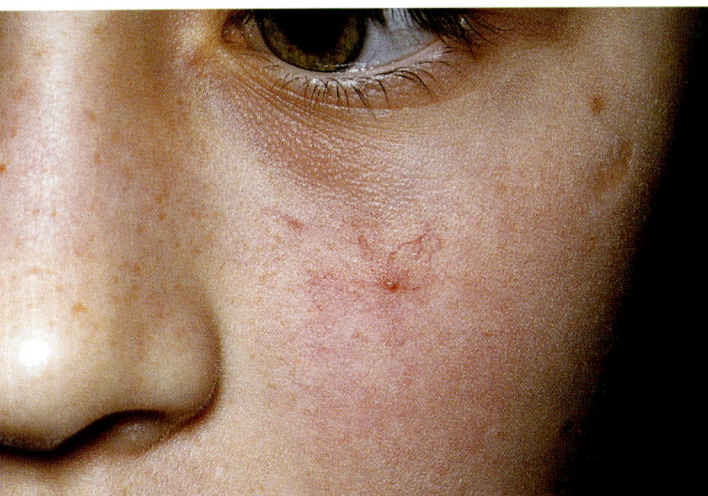

Fig. 47.13 Spider telangiectasis.

The main vessel of the spider telangiectasis is an arteriole. The blood flows from this to the periphery, and then passes into a capillary network [4]. The pressure in spider telangiectases rises to 40 mmHg. The lesions consist of a central, ascending, spiral, thick-walled arteriole which ends in a thin-walled ampulla just beneath the epidermis. From the ampulla, thin-walled branching channels radiate peripherally in the papillary dermis. Glomus cells have been described in the wall of the central arteriole [5]. Therefore these lesions actually resemble microarteriovenous malformations.

Clinical features. Spider naevi vary in size and shape, and may be up to 1.5 cm across. The central body may be raised, and is usually pulsatile on diascopy. The radiating vessels are just visible to the naked eye (Fig. 47.13). They occur on the upper half of the body, especially the face, neck and hands. They are frequently solitary, but may be multiple, even in health. Liver disease is seldom found, but should be suspected at any age when lesions are numerous. They may develop at sites of trauma and may be unilateral [6]. Similar lesions occur on the mucous membranes of the lips and nose. Here, the typical morphology is less apparent and the differentiation from HHT may be difficult.

The majority of lesions that occur in pregnancy disappear spontaneously, but some may persist. Lesions appearing in otherwise healthy children tend to persist indefinitely, but a small proportion regress spontaneously.

Diagnosis. The typical morphology, with a central pulsating vessel, does not occur in other conditions. In HHT, the telangiectases are macular, punctate or linear; when they are stellate they do not pulsate.

References

1 Bean WB. *Vascular Spiders and Related Lesions of the Skin.* Springfield: Thomas, 1958.
2 Wenzl JE, Burgess EO. The spider nevus in infancy and childhood. *Pediatrics* 1964; **33**: 227–32.
3 Whiting DA, Kallmeyer JC, Simson IW. Widespread arterial spiders in a case of latent hepatitis, with resolution after therapy. *Br J Dermatol* 1970; **82**: 32–6.
4 Martini GA, Staubesand J. Zur Morphologie des Gefässpinnen ('vascular spiders') in der Haut Leberkranker. *Virchows Arch Path Anat Physiol* 1953; **324**: 147–64.
5 Weedon D. Vascular tumors. In: Weedon D, ed. *Skin Pathology,* 2nd edn. London: Churchill Livingstone, 2002.
6 Cunliffe WJ, Dodman B, Butterworth MJ. Unilateral spider naevi. *Br J Dermatol* 1972; **87**: 51–2.

Cherry angiomas

Synonym
• Campbell de Morgan spots

These are particularly common on the trunk of middle-aged or elderly people. They disappear in extreme old age. Increased numbers have been recorded in diabetics [1], but this association is of doubtful significance. Ultrastructural examination has shown that they have reduplicated basement membranes with fenestrations of the endothelium [2,3].

When fully developed they are readily recognized. Tiny lesions, which may be very numerous (sometimes termed 'multiple minute Campbell de Morgan spots'), can resemble either petechiae or other types of telangiectases. They cannot always be made to blanch with pressure, and may need to be observed repeatedly to distinguish them from petechiae, although they are readily identifiable if magnified. Larger lesions can be excised or treated with a vascular laser under local anaesthetic if they are unsightly.

Angiokeratomas
Angiokeratomas are rare lesions that appear as dark red papules and plaques arranged either discretely or in clusters. Five different types can be distinguished from their morphology and location. Angiokeratomas are probably not vascular neoplasms but acquired telangiectases of pre-existing blood vessels of the papillary dermis, although some types of venular malformation cannot be excluded. All varieties of angiokeratomas are histologically similar and they possess the ultrastructure of collecting venules with valves [4].

References

1 Bean WB. *Vascular Spiders and Related Lesions of the Skin.* Springfield: Thomas, 1958.
2 Stehbens WE, Ludatscher RM. Fine structure of senile angiomas of human skin. *Angiology* 1968; **19**: 581–92.
3 Braverman IM. Ultrastructure and organisation of the cutaneous microvasculature in normal and pathologic states. *J Invest Dermatol* 1989; **93** (Suppl. 2): 25–95.
4 Mittal R, Aggarwal A, Srivastava G. Angiokeratoma circumscriptum: a case report and review of the literature. *Int J Dermatol* 2005; **44**: 1031–4.

Telangiectasia with calcium channel blocking drugs
There have been increasing numbers of reports associating telangiectasia with calcium channel blockers [1–3], particularly in sun-exposed sites. The aetiology of this disorder is not fully understood. Usually, the telangiectasias resolve within 3 to 6 months after discontinuation of the drug [4]. In a study of renal transplant recipients the grade of photodamage was strongly associated with the use of calcium channel blockers [5].

References

1 Basarab T, Yu R, Jones RR. Calcium antagonist-induced photo-exposed telangiectasia. *Br J Dermatol* 1997; **136**: 974–5.

2 Karonen T, Stubb S, Keski-Oja J. Truncal telangiectases coinciding with felodipine. *Dermatology* 1998; **196**: 272–3.

3 Grabczynska S, Cowley N. Amlodipine induced-photosensitivity presenting as telangiectasia. *Br J Dermatol* 2000; **142**: 1255–6.

4 Ioulios P, Charalampos M, Efrossini T. The spectrum of cutaneous reactions with calcium antagonists: a review of the literature and the possible etiopathogenic mechanisms. *Dermatology Online J* 2003; **5**: 6.

5 Cooper SM, Wojnarowska F. Photo-damage in Northern European renal transplant recipients is associated with use of calcium channel blockers. *Clin Exp Dermatol* 2003; **28**: 588–91.

Venous lakes [1]

A form of senile angioma found on the face, lips and ears of elderly patients. Histologically, they consist of greatly dilated, thin-walled venules without the proliferation of vascular tissue found in the true angioma. There is degeneration of the supporting connective tissue [2]. Treatment consists of primary excision of the lesion rather than laser therapy.

References

1 Bean WB, Walsh JR. Venous lakes. *Arch Dermatol* 1956; **74**: 459–63.

2 Kocsard E, Ofner F, D'Abrera VS *et al.* The phlebectasis of old age—incidence and diagnostic importance. *J Am Geriatr Soc* 1970; **18**: 31–8.

Hand varices

Small varicosities of the palms and fingers, particularly on the palmar phalangeal creases, are much more common than generally is known in elderly people [1]. They can be treated, like other varicose veins, with sclerotherapy [2] or with the Müller technique of phlebectomy [3].

References

1 Clark ANG, Melcher DH, Hall-Smith P. Palmar and finger varicosities of the aged. *Br J Dermatol* 1974; **91**: 305–14.

2 Duffy DM, Garcia C, Clark RE. The role of sclerotherapy in abnormal varicose hand veins. *Plast Reconstr Surg* 1999; **104**: 1474–9.

3 Ramelet AA. Phlebectomy. Technique, indications and complications. *Int Angiol* 2002; **21** (Suppl. 1): 46–51.

Primary telangiectasia

Angioma serpiginosum [1–4]

Angioma serpiginosum is a rare naevoid disorder affecting the small vessels of the upper dermis. Histology shows that the affected papillae are distended by a large, single, ectatic capillary, lined by flattened endothelial cells of normal appearance. Inflammatory changes are not present. The disease occurs predominantly in females (90%), and usually starts in childhood. Most cases are sporadic, but a family history suggesting X-linked dominant inheritance has been reported [5].

The commonly affected sites are the lower limbs and buttocks, but it can be more widespread (Fig. 47.14). It is often unilateral initially. Characteristically, there are red or purple puncta up to 1 mm in diameter. These are grouped in areas a few centimetres across, or sometimes form large sheets. Irregular lesions may arise, and commonly there is livedoid patterning of the puncta. Frequently, there is a background of more diffuse erythema. The lesions may not blanch completely on pressure, but, like multiple minute Campbell de Morgan angiomas, they have been confused with purpura [6]; that they consist of a cluster of small vessels

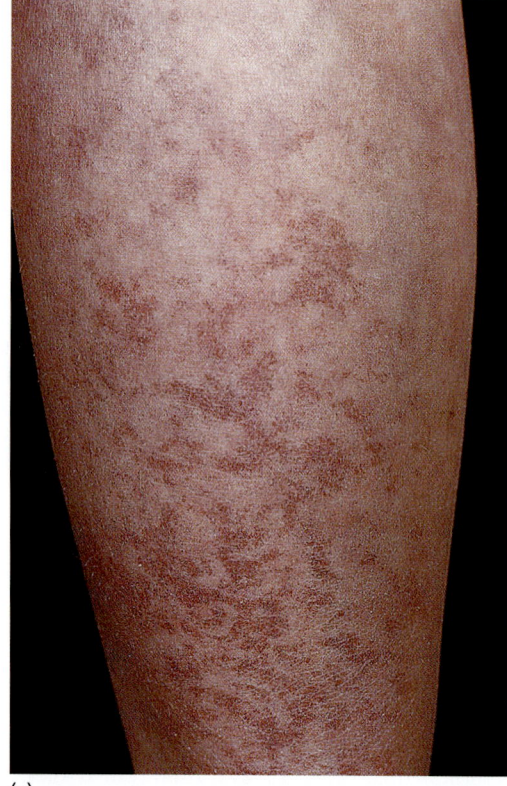

(a)

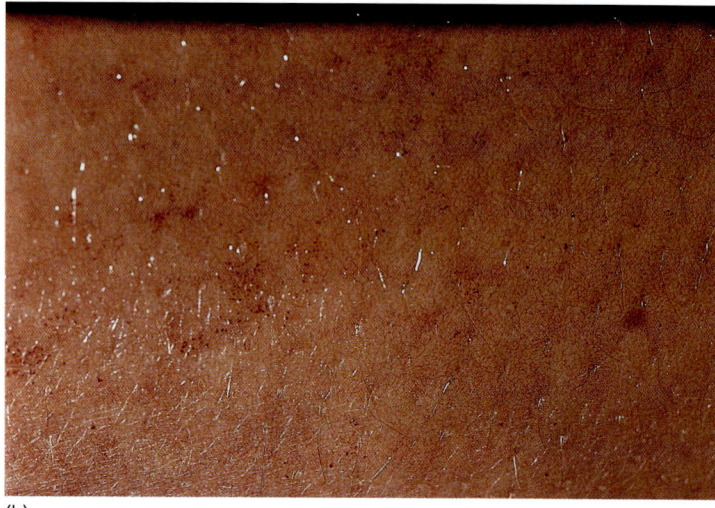

(b)

Fig. 47.14 Angioma serpiginosum. (a) Grouped lesions. (b) Close-up appearance.

rather than purpura can readily be distinguished by appropriate magnification [7].

The condition starts as one or more small lesions, and usually ceases, but may recommence in adult life. Individual puncta often disappear spontaneously, and complete regression of the eruption may occur, or traces may persist indefinitely. There are no symptoms, and no other changes in the skin, although slight atrophy has been reported [8].

The dilated capillaries are easy to see under the capillary microscope. The background erythema is the result of dilatation of the subpapillary venous plexus. Epiluminescence microscopy can be helpful in diagnosis by demonstrating 'red lagoons'. Histologically, dilated and tortuous capillaries are observed in the papillary dermis but without any inflammation or red cell extravasation.

The differential diagnosis includes angiokeratoma corporis diffusum, angiokeratoma circumscriptum naeviforme and forms of capillaritis. Treatment with vascular laser, such as pulsed dye laser and intense pulsed light source, improves the disorder, but is not always necessary [9].

References
1 Barker IP, Sachs PM. Angioma serpiginosum. *Arch Dermatol* 1965; **92**: 613–20.
2 Frain-Bell W. Angioma serpiginosum. *Br J Dermatol* 1957; **69**: 251–68.
3 Yaffee HS. Angioma serpiginosum. *Arch Dermatol* 1967; **95**: 667.
4 Kumakiri M, Katoh H, Mitura Y *et al.* Angioma serpiginosum. *J Cut Pathol* 1980; **7**: 410–21.
5 Marriott PJ, Munro DD, Ryan T. Angioma serpiginosum—familial incidence. *Br J Dermatol* 1975; **93**: 701–6.
6 Cox NH, Paterson WD. Angioma serpiginosum: a simulator of purpura. *Postgrad Medl J* 1991; **67**: 1065–6.
7 Ohnishi T, Nagayama T, Morita T *et al.* Angioma serpiginosum: a report of 2 cases identified using epiluminescence microscopy. *Arch Dermatol* 1999; **135**: 1366–8.
8 Gautier-Smith PC, Sanders MD, Sanderson KV. Ocular and nervous system involvement in angioma serpiginosum. *Br J Ophthalmol* 1971; **55**: 433–43.
9 Long CC. Treatment of angioma serpiginosum using a pulsed tunable dye laser. *Br J Dermatol* 1997; **136**: 631–2.

Hereditary haemorrhagic telangiectasia [1]

Synonym
• Osler–Rendu–Weber syndrome

Hereditary haemorrhagic telangiectasia (HHT) is an autosomal dominant disorder characterized by epistaxis, cutaneous telangiectasia and visceral arteriovenous malformations (AVMs). HHT is more prevalent than previously estimated [1]. The clinical diagnosis is made on the basis of: (i) epistaxis—spontaneous, recurrent nose bleeds; (ii) telangiectases—multiple, at characteristic sites (lips, oral cavity, fingers, nose); (iii) visceral lesions—such as gastrointestinal telangiectasia (with or without bleeding), pulmonary AVMs, hepatic AVMs, cerebral AVMs, spinal AVMs; and (iv) a family history—a first-degree relative with HHT. Three criteria indicate a definite diagnosis of the disorder; two a possible or suspected case [2].

Aetiology and pathogenesis. HHT has an autosomal dominant inheritance pattern associated with mutations in at least two genes. Mutations in the endoglin (*ENG*) gene on chromosome 9q34 are responsible for HHT1, while mutations in the activin receptor-like kinase 1 (*ACVRL1*) gene on chromosome 12q are responsible for HHT2. The corresponding proteins, endoglin and ALK-1, are specific endothelial receptors of transforming growth factor β (TGF-β) [3]. TGF-β signalling is essential during angiogenesis and can activate ALK-1 and ALK-5 in endothelial cells, each one leading to opposite effects on endothelial cell proliferation and migration [4]. In HHT there is decreased endoglin expression and impaired ALK-1. HHT1 families have a higher prevalence of pulmonary AVMs than HHT2 families, who generally have a milder phenotype and later onset. Mice lacking the *ENG* or *ACVRL1* genes develop age-dependent vascular lesions of the skin

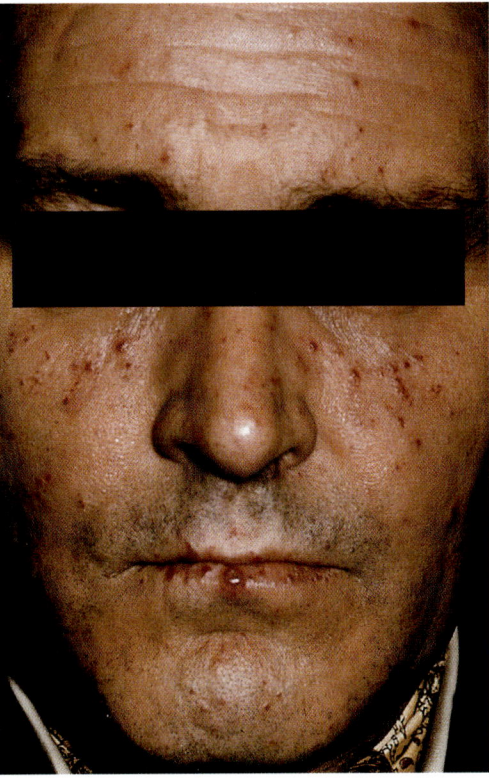

Fig. 47.15 Hereditary haemorrhagic telangiectasia.

of the extremities, oral cavity and internal organs in a phenotype very similar to the human condition [5].

Clinical features. Recurrent epistaxis is usually the presenting symptom. It may begin in childhood or even in infancy, but far more commonly begins at puberty or in early adult life. Telangiectasia of the skin is not often seen before puberty, and usually appears in the third or fourth decade, but it may be extensive in early childhood. The individual lesions are punctate or linear. On the rare occasions when they are spider naevus-like, they do not pulsate. Nodular lesions may be present but are sparse in comparison with the smaller lesions, which may be numerous. Lesions may occur anywhere, but especially on the upper half of the body—face, lips, ears, conjunctivae, trunk, forearms, hands and fingers (Fig. 47.15). They are often conspicuous in the nail beds. The soles and toes may also be affected. The skin lesions seldom bleed.

The mucous membranes are almost invariably involved. Lesions occur on the nasal septum, in the mouth, nasopharynx, and throughout the gastrointestinal tract [2,6,7], where they may be demonstrated by endoscopy or arteriography. They may also be found in many other organs, including the retina. The lesions on the tongue have a characteristic and perhaps diagnostic appearance on capillary microscopy. Within a fungiform papilla there is a single, very dilated vessel, which may cause the papilla to be expanded [8]. Haemorrhages may occur from any site, and their severity and frequency determine the clinical manifestations and course of the disorder. Pulmonary arteriovenous fistulae are present in some cases, and occur particularly in some families [9,10]. They reveal their presence by dyspnoea, cyanosis and clubbing of the fingers in adolescence. They can be demonstrated radiologically. Paradoxical embolization to the systemic circulation may occur. This disease is the commonest cause of pulmonary arteriovenous anastomoses. Cerebral vascular malformations occur in 10% of patients with HHT [11]. Hepatic arteriovenous anastomoses have been reported, and liver enlargement and cirrhosis also occur [9,11]. Aneurysms of other vessels, including the aortic arch and splenic artery [6], have been reported. Lesions of the eye [12] are uncommon.

Diagnosis. The history, family history and morphology of the individual lesions are usually sufficient to establish the diagnosis. The lesions do not have the characteristic morphology of a spider naevus. Other causes of telangiectasia have to be excluded. Epistaxis and the family history taken together usually permit the detection of patients potentially affected by HHT. The patients with known genetic mutations or clinically suspected familial HHT are then subjected to complete clinical screening. Screening programs are aimed at pre-symptomatic detection of AVMs in the brain or lung and should be recommended for all HHT patients and their relatives at risk [13].

It is recommended that patients with HHT have a complete blood count and haematocrit, evaluation of faeces for occult blood, brain MRI with and without gadolinium to screen for cerebral AVMs, and contrast echocardiography to screen for pulmonary shunting. Chest CT is done to characterize pulmonary AVMs if shunting is found. Screening for liver involvement is not currently performed on a routine basis [2].

Treatment. In mild cases, no treatment is needed. Anaemia from recurrent nosebleeds or gastrointestinal bleeding can be controlled with oral or parenteral iron, and sometimes blood transfusions are necessary for some patients. Laser therapy or intense pulsed light source (IPLS) treatment of telangiectasia of the skin and mucosae can be considered, if lesions bleed or for cosmetic reasons.

Epistaxis is the most common emergency, as it can be massive. Photocoagulation laser or septal mucosal dermoplasty is recommended if administration of tranexamic acid at high doses or combined oestrogen–progesterone preparations does not have any effect. Pulmonary AVMs are safely treated using transcatheter embolization. Although most neurological symptoms in HHT are treated by transcatheter embolization, stereotactic resection or stereotactic radiosurgery are occasionally necessary. Liver involvement may be silent, as the majority of patients remain symptomless throughout their lifetime. Organ transplant remains the treatment of choice when hepatic fistulae cause complications or if very severe liver insufficiency develops. Gastrointestinal bleeding can be treated medically by iron therapy and combined oestrogen–progesterone preparations [2,13].

The disease does not usually shorten life. The mortality rate is less than 10%.

References
1 Guttmacher AE, Marchuk DA, White RI Jr. Hereditary haemorrhagic telangiectasia. *N Engl J Med* 1995; **333**: 918–24.
2 Bayrak-Toydemir P, Mao R, Lewin S, McDonald J. Hereditary hemorrhagic telangiectasia: an overview of diagnosis and management in the molecular era for clinicians. *Genet Med* 2004; **6**: 175–91.
3 Abdalla SA, Letarte M. Hereditary haemorrhagic telangiectasia: current views on genetics and mechanisms of disease. *J Med Genet* 2006; **43**: 97–110.
4 Fernàndez LA, Sanz-Rodriquez F, Blanco FJ et al. Hereditary hemorrhagic telangiectasia, a vascular dysplasia affecting the TGF-β signaling pathway. *Clin Med Res* 2006; **4**: 66–78.
5 Urness LD, Sorensen LK, Li DY. Arteriovenous malformations in mice lacking activin receptor-like kinase-1. *Nat Gen* 2000; **26**: 328–31.
6 Muggia FM. Osler's disease with an aortic arch aneurysm. *Arch Intern Med* 1964; **114**: 307–10.
7 Williams GA, Brick IB. Gastrointestinal bleeding in hereditary hemorrhagic telangiectasia. *Arch Intern Med* 1955; **95**: 41–51.
8 Harders H. The micromorphology and biomicroscopical diagnosis of Osler's disease. *Bibl Anat* 1965; **7**: 523–9.
9 Peery WH. Clinical spectrum of hereditary hemorrhagic telangiectasia (Osler–Weber–Rendu disease). *Am J Med* 1987; **82**: 989–97.
10 Purriel P, Muras O. Aneurisms arteriovenosus de pulmòn. *Thorax* 1957; **6**: 101–58.
11 Begbie ME, Wallace GMF, Shovlin CL. Hereditary haemorrhagic telangiectasia (Osler–Weber–Rendu syndrome): a view from the 21st century. *Postgrad J Med* 2003; **79**: 18–24.
12 Landau J, Nelken E, Davis E. Hereditary haemorrhagic telangiectasia with retinal and conjunctival lesions. *Lancet* 1956; **ii**: 230–1.
13 Sabbà C. A rare and misdiagnosed bleeding disorder: hereditary hemorrhagic telangiectasia. *J Thromb Haemost* 2005; **3**: 2201–10.

Ataxia–telangiectasia

Synonym
- Louis–Bar syndrome

Ataxia–telangiectasia [1] is a rare, autosomal recessive disease with pleiotropic involvement of the nervous and lymphoid systems, caused by homozygous mutations in the ataxia–telangiectasia mutated (*ATM*) gene (OMIM: 208900, gene map locus 11q22.3) [2]. Defective repair of DNA damaged by UV-light, gamma or X-rays is responsible for its development. Most mutations are frameshift and nonsense mutations that are predicted to cause truncation of the ataxia–telangiectasia protein; the less common mutations are missense, splicing and there is one in-frame deletion [3]. Mutation of ATM causes defective cell cycle checkpoint activation, a reduced capacity for repair of DNA double strand breaks and abnormal apoptosis, all of which contribute to the major features of ataxia–telangiectasia, including genomic instability, increased cancer risk and neurodegeneration [4].

The syndrome manifests with telangiectases, progressive cerebellar ataxia, combined immunodeficiency and marked susceptibility to cancer, particularly lymphoma and leukaemia [2]. A diminished level of, or an absence of, IgA is characteristic of the condition but there may be a reduction in other immunoglobulins. Defects of T and B cell function may also be present.

Affected children, who are usually small, are apparently normal until the second year of life when they are noticed to be clumsy, and the ataxia becomes progressive, so that by the age of 12 years they are unable to walk without assistance. Other signs of cerebellar disease, such as nystagmus and slurred speech, and mental deterioration may be observed. Neurological symptoms may not begin before the age of 6 years. Telangiectases may be present as early as the second year of life, but usually develop between the ages of 3 and 5 years. They first appear on the bulbar conjunctiva, and subsequently involve the ears, eyelids and the butterfly area

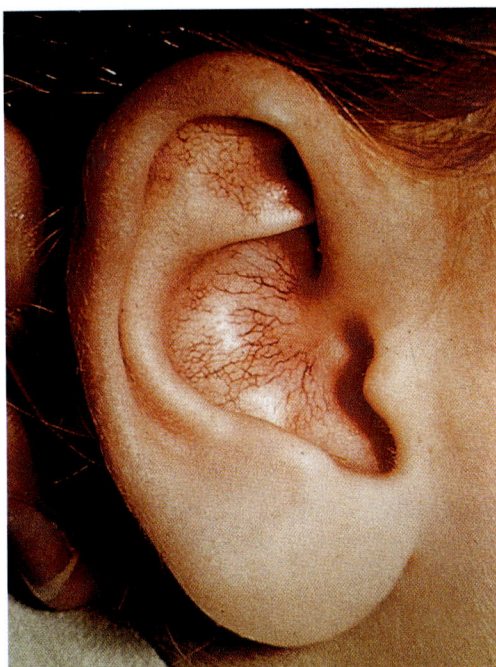

Fig. 47.16 Ataxia–telangiectasia. (Courtesy of Dr P.W.M. Copeman.)

of the cheeks and limbs (Fig. 47.16). Not all sites are affected in every case and bleeding is very uncommon. There may be some associated skin atrophy and dryness. The hair goes prematurely grey. Disturbances of pigmentation and eczematous lesions may also be present [5], as may granulomas [6]. Recurrent sinus and pulmonary infections are frequent, and may dominate the clinical picture; they are not infrequently fatal. Ovarian agenesis is not uncommon.

Ataxia–telangiectasia needs to be distinguished from other neurological disorders with similar features, including the ataxia–telangiectasia-like disorders ataxia oculomotor apraxia 1 and 2 [7].

The laboratory diagnosis currently relies on the measurement of serum alphafetoprotein (AFP), which is elevated in patients with ataxia–telangiectasia, and on demonstrating cellular sensitivity to ionizing radiation. Improved diagnostic testing by immunoblotting of nuclear lysates from lymphoid cell lines for ATM has been described [8]. After the age of 10 years, magnetic resonance imaging (MRI) shows cerebellar atrophy. These patients should have as few ionizing radiological investigations as possible.

Management is discussed in Chapter 15.

References
1 Perlman S, Becker-Catania S, Gatti RA. Ataxia-telangiectasia: diagnosis and treatment. *Semin Pediatr Neurol* 2003; **10**: 173–82.
2 McKinnon PJ. ATM and ataxia telangiectasia. *EMBO* 2004; **5**: 772–6.
3 Li A, Swift M. Mutations at the ataxia–telangiectasia locus and clinical phenotypes of A–T patients. *Am J Med Genet* 2000; **92**: 170–7.
4 Lavin MF, Kozlov S. ATM activation and DNA damage response. *Cell Cycle* 2007; **6**: 931–42.
5 Cohen LE, Tanner DJ, Schaeber HG *et al.* Common and uncommon cutaneous findings in patients with ataxia telangiectasia. *J Am Acad Dermatol* 1984; **10**: 431–8.
6 Joshi AK, Al Asiri RH, Haleem A *et al.* Cutaneous granuloma with ataxia telangiectasia—a case report and review of the literature. *Clin Exp Dermatol* 1993; **18**: 458–61.

7 Taylor AMR, Byrd PJ. Molecular pathology of ataxia telangiectasia. *J Clin Pathol* 2005; **58**: 1009–15.
8 Chun HH, Sun X, Nahas S *et al.* Improved diagnostic testing for ataxia telangiectasia by immunoblotting of nuclear lysates for ATM protein expression. *Mol Genet Metab* 2003; **80**: 437–43.

Generalized essential telangiectasia

Generalized essential telangiectasia [1–3] is a condition that is not as rare as the paucity of reported cases suggests. Many cases may be misdiagnosed as atypical HHT. The heading 'essential telangiectasia' probably includes more than one disease.

The condition occurs more frequently in females, and commonly starts in late childhood or early adult life. Generalized essential telangiectasia is characterized by a widespread cutaneous distribution with extensive sheets of telangiectases on the limbs or body (Fig. 47.17). The lesions may progress and become permanent when they are accentuated by dependency. There is an absence of coexisting epidermal or dermal changes [4]. The telangiectases are usually linear, but small angiomas may be present. Recurrent haemorrhages from the skin and mucous membranes or into the eye may produce incapacity, but in the majority of cases, the disease is only of cosmetic importance.

The diagnosis is made by excluding other causes of telangiectases. HHT is distinguished clinically by the distribution of the lesions, their presence in large and sometimes asymmetrical sheets, and by the absence of haemorrhages associated with generalized essential telangiectasia. High-energy, long-pulsed, frequency-doubled Nd:YAG laser treatment may be helpful but lesions tend to recur [5].

References
1 Bean WB, Rathe J. Universal angiomatosis. *Arch Int Med* 1963; **112**: 869–74.
2 Fox TC. A case of bilateral telangiectasis of the trunk, with a history of marked epistaxis in childhood and recent rectal haemorrhage. *Br J Dermatol* 1908; **20**: 145–62.
3 McGrae JD, Winkelmann RK. Generalised essential telangiectasia. *JAMA* 1963; **185**: 909–13.
4 Checketts SR, Burton PS, Bjorkman DJ, Kadunce DP. Generalized essential telangiectasia in the presence of gastrointestinal bleeding. *J Am Acad Dermatol* 1997; **37**: 321–5.
5 Gamblichler T, Avermaete A, Wilmert M *et al.* Generalised essential telangiectasia successfully treated with high-energy, long-pulse, frequency-doubled Nd:YAG laser. *Dermatol Surg* 2001; **27**: 355–7.

Unilateral naevoid telangiectasia syndrome

Unilateral naevoid telangiectasia can be congenital or acquired. There have been reports that suggest an increase in oestrogen and progesterone receptors in the skin. When this syndrome is acquired, it arises almost exclusively during periods of relatively increased oestrogen levels such as during pregnancy or puberty or in association with alcoholic cirrhosis or hepatitis C infection [1]. Polymorphic light eruption has been described confined to an area of acquired naevoid telangiectasia [2].

References
1 Hynes LR, Shenefelt PD. Unilateral nevoid telangiectasia: occurrence in two patients with hepatitis C. *J Am Acad Dermatol* 1997; **36**: 819–22.
2 Creamer D, Clement M, McGregor JM, Hawk JL. Polymorphic light eruption occurring solely on an area of naevoid telangiectasia. *Clin Exp Dermatol* 1999; **24**: 202–3.

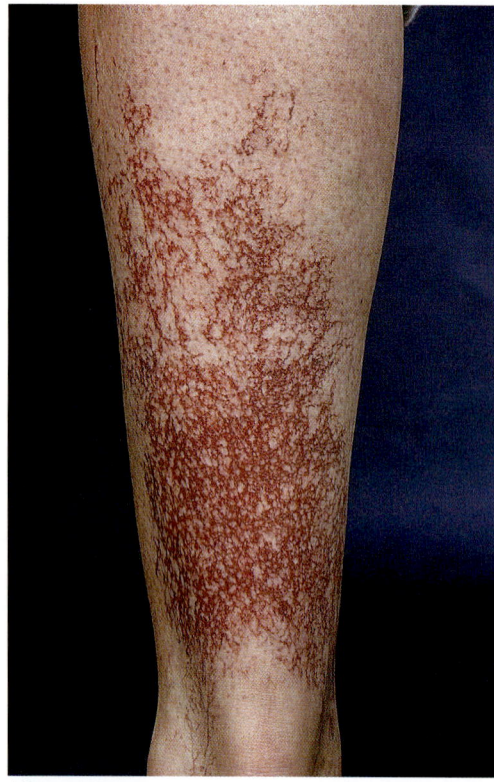

(a)

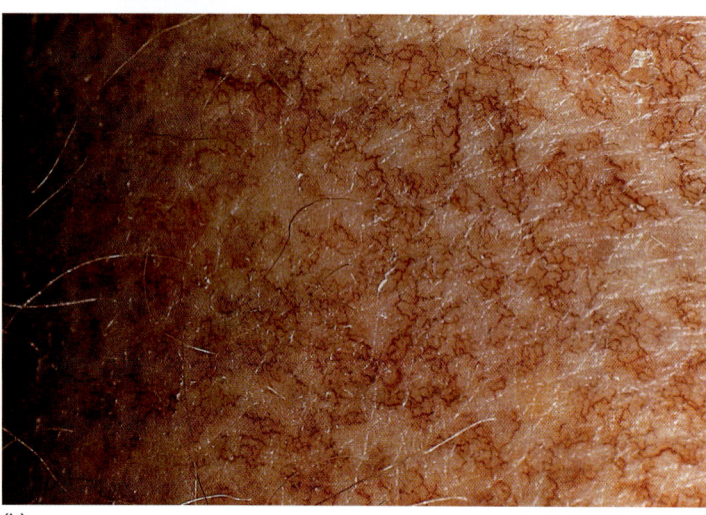

(b)

Fig. 47.17 Essential telangiectasia. (a) Arborizing pattern. (b) Close-up appearance.

Hereditary benign telangiectasia

This disorder probably has a dominant inheritance [1] and is characterized by the presence of extensive telangiectases resembling generalized essential telangiectasia, starting in childhood and without other systemic lesions [2,3]. Less commonly, the telangiectases may be present at birth [4]. They tend to occur more in light-exposed skin. Histology and electron microscopy have been used to distinguish this condition from HHT [5]. Distinction from HHT is dependent on the lack of bleeding, although lesions do appear related to arteriovenous anastomoses as in HHT [6].

References

1 Zahorcsek Z, Schneider I. Hereditary benign telangiectasia. *Dermatology* 1994; **189**: 286–8.

2 Gold MH, Eramo L, Prendiville JS. Hereditary benign telangiectasia. *Pediatr Dermatol* 1989; **6**: 194–7.

3 Ryan TJ, Wells RS. Hereditary benign telangiectasia. *Trans St John's Hospital Dermatol Soc* 1971; **57**: 148–56.

4 Watanebe M, Tomita, Y, Tagami H. Hereditary benign telangiectasia—a congenital type. *Dermatologica* 1990; **181**: 152–3.

5 Tsianakas P, Teillac-Hamel D, Fraitag S *et al*. Etude ultrastructurale des telangiectases héréditaires bénignes. *Ann Dermatol* 1995; **122**: 517–21.

6 Onishi Y, Ohara K, Shikida Y, Satomi H. Hereditary benign telangiectasia: image analysis of hitherto unknown association with arteriovenous malformation. *Br J Dermatol* 2001; **145**: 641–5.

Naevus anaemicus with telangiectatic vessels [1]

Following dermabrasion of the epidermis over a naevus anaemicus, enlarged telangiectatic vessels were observed within the previously pale area. The area was transplanted with thin epidermal grafts but 1 year later the naevus anaemicus looked the same as before grafting. The explanation proposed for a naevus anaemicus and port-wine stain coexisting was vascular twin spotting, but the primary abnormality could be telangiectasia with surrounding skin blanched through a 'steal' effect of blood flow.

Reference

1 Juhlin L, Olsson MJ. Naevus anaemicus with telangiectatic vessels. *Eur J Dermatol* 2001; **11**: 518–20.

Solitary plaque-like telangiectatic glomangioma [1]

A painful, solitary telangiectatic plaque revealed ectatic vascular lumens in the upper dermis surrounded by glomus cells on biopsy.

Reference

1 Requena L, Galvan C, Sanchez Yus E. Solitary plaque-like telangiectatic glomangioma. *Br J Dermatol* 1998; **139**: 902–5.

Treatment of telangiectasia [1,2]

The central vessel of a spider naevus can be destroyed with electrolysis or pin-point 'hyfrecation' without anaesthetic. A significant proportion of such lesions recur, which may be related to the origin of the lesions; that is mini-arteriolovenular malformations with relative high pressure. Larger, isolated angiomas can be treated by complete excision. Treatment of extensive small lesions is unsatisfactory. Various types of lasers have been recommended [3]. (Long-)pulsed Nd:YAG laser at 1064 nm, intense pulsed light source (IPLS) and the 585 nm flashlamp pulsed dye laser (PDL) all have shown a beneficial effect on telangiectasia [4–6]. IPLS is preferred because of the excellent cosmetic results without scarring. Spider naevi are also well treated by IPLS [5]. Cryotherapy is disappointing. Injection with sclerosants is a good treatment for venous telangiectasia [1–3,7]. Cosmetic camouflage is possible if no intervention is desired.

References

1 Goldman MP, Bennett RG. Treatment of telangiectases: a review. *J Am Acad Dermatol* 1987; **17**: 167–82.

2 Bergen JJ, Goldman MP. *Varicose Veins and Telangiectases*. St Louis: Quality Medical Publishing, 1993.

3 Gonzales E, Gange RW, Montaz KT. Treatment of telangiectases and other benign vascular lesions with the 577 nm pulsed dye laser. *J Am Acad Dermatol* 1992; **27**: 220–6.

4 Railan D, Parlatte EC, Uebelhoer NS, Rohrer TE. Laser treatment of vascular lesions. *Clin Dermatol* 2006; **24**: 8–15.

5 Landthaler M, Hohenleutner U. Laser therapy of vascular lesions. *Photodermatol Photoimmunol Photomed* 2006; **22**: 324–32.

6 Schroeter CA, Wilder D, Reineke T *et al*. Clincal significance of an Intense Pulsed Light Source on leg telangiectasias of up to 1 mm diameter. *Eur J Dermatol* 1997; **7**: 38–42.

7 Norris MJ, Carlin MC, Ratz JL. Treatment of essential telangiectasia: effect of increasing concentrations of polidocanol. *J Am Acad Dermatol* 1989; **20**: 683–9.

Malformations

It is convenient to consider the following separately:
1 Arteriovenous shunts
2 Arteriovenous aneurysms ('fistulae')
  i congenital
  ii acquired
3 Arteriovenous malformations.

Arteriovenous shunts

Arteriovenous shunts form an alternative peripheral system of blood flow and are an integral part of a compensating mechanism at times of capillary stress and injury. Although the pathophysiology of arteriovenous shunting has not been entirely elucidated, prolonged and diffuse patency of arteriovenous shunts may result in a syndrome of local venous dilatation and some degree of tissue ischaemia [1]. Their presence can be demonstrated by finding high oxygen saturation in venous blood and a reduced circulation time [2]. They are active in venous hypertension, varicose veins [3] and in leg ulcers [4]. They can be found in association with atherosclerosis [5] and perhaps with the hormonal changes of pregnancy [6]. Arteriovenous shunting in varicose veins appears to be a secondary rather than an initiating cause [7]. They are also active in psoriasis, in neoplasms [8] and in skin flaps. They may be responsible for the postural changes seen in angiodyskinesia, and are a feature of arborizing telangiectasia [8].

Arteriovenous fistulae

Arteriovenous fistulae [9] consist of direct connections between larger arteries and veins and are always pathological. Their various congenital and acquired forms have been given a large number of descriptive titles (cirsoid aneurysm, aneurysmal varix, pulsating angioma, etc.) but are best described here simply as congenital and acquired. Localized and pulsating, they may present as red nodules with overlying telangiectasis, like a giant spider naevus. While most common on acral sites, they also occur in the head and neck and on the trunk.

Congenital. These are discussed fully elsewhere (Chapter 18). They result from failure of embryological differentiation into an artery and vein [9]. The many clinical varieties that affect the skin and visceral organs have been grouped together under the term congenital dysplastic angiopathy [6]. When such congenital fistulae involve the limb vessels they often give rise to distinctive physical signs, described below.

Acquired. Apart from iatrogenic arteriovenous fistulae (usually for haemodialysis), acquired fistulae are almost always traumatic;

they are often large, and may therefore cause significant cardiovascular effects. Early diagnosis is important. Treatment is entirely within the province of the interventional surgeon or radiologist, who should be consulted if there is suspicion of the existence of such a fistula. Treatment is by inserting a covered stent to close off the opening from 'within', or by open surgical closure.

Signs and effects of arteriovenous fistulae [10,11]

Traumatic fistulae following penetrating wounds (classically a shell splinter, or occasionally an operation) can occur anywhere in the body. They should be suspected whenever venous varicosity is unilateral or when signs of venous insufficiency develop unexpectedly after an injury. Increased warmth of a limb and the finding of a machinery-like constant murmur or a palpable thrill establish the diagnosis.

Congenital fistulae commonly affect the limbs and are often multiple. They should be suspected when unilateral varicosities present early in life without a genetic background. The limb is warmer and may be larger than the contralateral limb. Slowing of the pulse produced by inflation of a proximal tourniquet at the root (Branham's sign) is indicative of a large shunt. Duplex ultrasound or arteriography confirms the site of the fistula and indicates the size of the communications.

The effects of arteriovenous aneurysms depend on their size and the volume of blood flow through the fistula rather than its site. No cardiovascular changes may be evident when small, although there will inevitably be some permanent diversion of blood from the capillary bed. Larger fistulae cause dilatation in the superficial veins distal to the site, with a varying degree of impairment of the arterial circulation. The cardiac output increases, often considerably; the heart is dilated and the diastolic blood pressure is reduced, increasing the pulse pressure.

Embolization under angiographic control is the most effective therapy. An alternative is to mobilize the vessel and ligate all the branches (skeletonization). It is also possible to insert a covered stent to block off a localized fistula and this is the treatment of choice in a traumatic fistula in an inaccessible location. Amputation may occasionally be necessary if congestive cardiac failure is a problem.

Arteriovenous malformations

Definition. Arteriovenous malformations are fast-flow vascular lesions composed of malformed arterial and venous vessels connected directly to one another without an intervening capillary bed [12].

Pathogenesis. Arteriovenous malformations may arise during early fetal development because of a failure of regression of arteriovenous channels in the primitive plexus. Although most cases of arteriovenous malformations are sporadic, there are a few inherited syndromes whose molecular genetics have been elucidated. A mutation in the gene *RASA1* has been identified on chromosome 5q in families with capillary malformations associated with arteriovenous malformations [13]. Although the pathogenesis of sporadic lesions still has to be clarified, it may involve an aberration in the TGF-β signalling pathway [14].

Clinical features. In patients with arteriovenous malformations, 40–60% are visible at birth and a further 30% become apparent during childhood. The lesions are more common in the head and neck area than in other locations. Excessive warmth, unusual pain and bleeding episodes provide clues but can occur in other conditions. Auscultation of the lesion should detect a machinery murmur. Duplex scans are helpful screening tools. Arteriovenous malformations may progress through four different stages [15,16].

Stage I. These lesions are in the quiescent phase, are asymptomatic and usually last from birth until adolescence. During this stage, the arteriovenous malformation may either not be apparent, or may have the appearance of a port-wine stain or involuting haemangioma.

Stage II. This is the progressive stage and most commonly begins during adolescence. In this stage, which is characterized by expansion, the vascular lesions enlarge, and darken, deforming the integument and invading deep structures. On examination, the local temperature is increased, a pulse or thrill can be palpated, and a continuous murmur is heard on auscultation. Puberty, trauma and pregnancy induce progression to this stage.

Stage III. This mimics stage II; deep destruction occurs with spontaneous necrosis, chronic ulceration, pain and haemorrhage.

Stage IV. This is defined by cardiac decompensation. High-output cardiac failure may result from increased blood flow through large arteriovenous malformations.

Diagnosis. Arteriovenous malformations are diagnosed by the clinical findings and confirmed by duplex ultrasound, which also allows assessment of the flow characteristics [12]. Other vascular malformations, vascular neoplasms and other neoplasms should be excluded. Radiological evaluation is needed to confirm the diagnosis, and angiography is used to assess the extent of the lesions.

Treatment. The treatment of arteriovenous malformations can be difficult. Extreme pain, ulceration, bleeding and extensive enlargement of the malformations are indications for treatment. Multimodal treatment, including preoperative embolization and complete surgical resection, is usually necessary for the management of localized arteriovenous malformations. Complete surgical resection of the lesions may be difficult, because of their widespread nature and the risk of bleeding. Palliative embolization may be used to treat symptomatic lesions when combination treatment cannot be performed [17]. This can be repeated on many occasions.

References
1 Haimovici H. Abnormal arteriovenous shunts associated with chronic venous insufficiency. *J Cardiovasc Surg* 1976; **17**: 473–82.
2 Piulachs P, Vidal-Barraquer F. Pathogenic study of varicose veins. *Angiology* 1953; **4**: 59–100.
3 Haimovici H, Steinman C, Caplan LH. Role of arteriovenous anastomoses in vascular diseases of the lower extremity. *Ann Surg* 1966; **164**: 990–1002.
4 Myers MB, Cherry C. Pathophysiology and treatment of stasis ulcers of the leg. *Am Surg* 1971; **37**: 167–74.
5 Ryan TJ. Arteriovenous pathways. In: Jarrett A, ed. *The Physiology and Pathophysiology of the Skin*. London: Academic Press, 1973: 586–91.
6 Bean WB, ed. *Vascular Spiders and Related Lesions of the Skin*. Springfield: Thomas, 1958.
7 Haimovici H. Role of A-V shunting in varicose veins: therapeutic implications. *J Cardiovasc Surg* 1995; **36**: 109–15.
8 Urbach F. The blood supply of tumors. In: Morgagna W, Ellis R, eds. *Advances in Biology of Skin*, Vol. 2. Oxford: Pergamon, 1961: 123–49.
9 Fairbairn JF II, Bernatz PF. Arteriovenous fistulas. In: Fairbairn JF II, Juergens JL, Spittell JA Jr, eds. *Peripheral Vascular Diseases,* 4th edn. Philadelphia: Saunders, 1972: 303–26.
10 Elkin DC, Warren JV. Arteriovenous fistulas: their effects on the circulation. *JAMA* 1947; **134**: 1524–8.
11 Holman E, ed. *Abnormal Arteriovenous Communications: Peripheral and Intracardiac, Acquired and Congenital*. Springfield: Thomas, 1968.
12 Garzon MC, Huang JT, Enjolras O, Frieden IJ. Vascular malformations: Part 1. *J Am Acad Dermatol* 2007; **56**: 353–62.
13 Eerola I, Boon LM, Mulliken JB *et al*. Capillary malformation-arteriovenous malformation, a new clinical and genetic disorder caused by RASA1 mutations. *Am J Hum Genet* 2003; **73**: 1240–9.
14 Vikkula M, Boon LM, Mulliken JB, Olsen BR. Molecular basis of vascular anomalies. *Trends Cardiovasc Med* 1998; **8**: 281–92.
15 Enjolras O, Logeart I, Gelbert F *et al*. Malformations artérioveineuses: étude de 200 cas. *Ann Dermatol Venereol* 1999; **127**: 17–22.
16 Kohout MP, Hansen M, Pribaz JJ, Mulliken JB. Arteriovenous malformations of the head and neck: natural history and management. *Plast Reconstr Surg* 1998; **102**: 643–54.
17 Komiyama M, Khosla VK, Yamamoto Y, Toyota N. Embolization in high-flow arteriovenous malformations of the face. *Ann Plast Surg* 1992; **28**: 575–83.

Acroangiodermatitis of Mali (pseudo-Kaposi's sarcoma)

A pigmented, purpuric eruption occurring around the malleolae and in the skin of the dorsal forefoot (particularly the base of the second toe) suggests acroangiodermatitis. Brown to plum-red papules coalescing into plaques resemble Kaposi's sarcoma clinically. The term acroangiodermatitis was introduced by Mali *et al*. in 1965 [1]. Histologically, there is marked benign capillary proliferation, plump endothelium and red cell extravasation. Rashkovsky *et al*. [2] described five possible causes:
1 Chronic venous hypertension
2 Arteriovenous malformations
3 Iatrogenic arteriovenous shunts in haemodialysis patients
4 Paralysed limbs
5 Amputation stumps.

Stewart–Bluefarb syndrome

In 1967, Stewart [3] and Bluefarb and Adams [4] independently described similar lesions on the legs of patients with arteriovenous malformations; in these cases the findings are usually unilateral and a palpable thrill may be noted. The condition can lead to ulceration of the toes and forefoot, in which case an arteriovenous shunt is the more likely underlying cause.

References
1 Mali JWH, Kuiper JP, Hamers AA. Acroangiodermatitis of the foot. *Arch Dermatol* 1965; **92**: 515–8.
2 Rashkovsky I, Gilead L, Schamroth J, Leibovici V. Acro-angiodermatitis: review of the literature and report of a case. *Acta Derm Venereol Suppl (Stockh)* 1995; **75**: 475–8.
3 Stewart WM. Fausse angiosarcomatose de Kaposi par fistules arteriovenulaire multiples. *Bull Soc Fr Dermatol Syphil* 1967; **74**: 664–5.

4 Bluefarb SM, Adams LA. Arteriovenous malformations with angiodermatitis. *Arch Dermatol* 1967; **96**: 176–81.

Venous malformations

Solitary venous malformations

Definition. Venous malformations are slow-flow, non-proliferating vascular birthmarks. They are composed of anomalous ectatic venous channels [1].

Pathogenesis. The histopathology of venous malformations reveals poorly circumscribed lesions composed of irregular, endothelial-lined vascular channels, with thin lumen walls that are deficient in smooth muscle cells [2]. This supports the theory that vascular malformations result from aberrant vascular development. Most cases of venous malformations are sporadic, but familial venous malformations can occur and are inherited in an autosomal dominant manner [3,4].

Clinical features. Venous malformations are present at birth, but typically become more prominent as the patient ages. The lesions usually present as soft, compressible blue masses that enlarge when the affected area is in a dependent position or with physical activity. The blue colour is pathognomonic and is caused by the presence of ectatic anomalous venous channels within the dermis. Venous malformations on the extremities are usually localized or segmental, although extensive deep involvement is common. Extensive, pure venous malformations of the extremities may extend into the skeletal muscles and joints and may be associated with either diminished girth or slight hypertrophy of the affected limb. Pain is a common complaint in extremity lesions and other complications include bleeding and phlebolith formation [1].

Diagnosis. The diagnosis of a venous malformation can be confirmed with MRI, which is also helpful in delineating the extent of the involvement of the lesion using the STIR sequence [5]. A coagulation profile, including D-dimer and fibrin, should be obtained to exclude an underlying coagulopathy. Localized intravascular coagulation within a venous malformation may result in abnormal coagulation profiles (consumptive coagulopathy) and may lead to episodes of bleeding and/or thrombosis.

Treatment. A multidisciplinary approach is essential for management of venous malformations. The general goals of therapy are to limit or avoid distortion of the facial features, limit bone deformation, preserve function and minimize painful swelling. Venous malformations may be treated with foam sclerotherapy [6] or surgery, or a combination of both. Large lesions, especially those extending into muscles and joints, are usually treated conservatively. Compression helps to decrease the discomfort caused by the venous malformations by reducing the volume, protecting the overlying skin, limiting swelling and improving localized intravascular coagulation.

Disorders associated with venous malformations
Klippel–Trenaunay syndrome

Definition. Klippel–Trenaunay syndrome (KTS) was first described in 1900, when Maurice Klippel and Paul Trenaunay reported two patients with a capillary malformation, varicosities and hypertrophy of soft tissue and bone in their lower limb [7]. In 1907, Frederick Parkes-Weber independently reported several cases similar to those described by Klippel and Trenaunay, though his cases were caused by multiple congenital arteriovenous malformations [7]. KTS is characterized by a capillary malformation (port-wine stain) of the skin associated with a soft tissue and bone overgrowth hypertrophy of the affected limb, in combination with varicose veins with or without deep venous and lymphatic abnormalities [8].

Pathogenesis. There are many theories on the aetiology of KTS and the genetic component is being defined. The disease may be best explained by either a paradominant disorder with autosomal lethal genes surviving only in the mosaic state, or as an autosomal dominant condition with incomplete penetrance (OMIM: gene map locus 8q22.3) [9,10]. KTS may be caused by a somatic mutation in a factor critical to vasculogenesis and angiogenesis during embryonic development [9].

Clinical features. The condition is characterized by the triad of: capillary malformations (port-wine stain/naevus flammeus), venous malformations (abnormal varicosities, persistent embryonal veins, and sometimes agenesis of deep veins or avalvulosis), with disproportionate limb growth of soft tissue and/or bone. It usually presents soon after birth. The naevus usually appears first; 95% of KTS patients exhibit a capillary malformation (port-wine stain), usually involving only the affected limb but sometimes extending beyond [11]. It usually has a metameric distribution. Limb hypertrophy develops later in childhood. Venous abnormalities may not be evident until adolescence. Lymphatic abnormalities frequently coexist, and affected children may present with a swollen limb. The surface veins are large and extensive with an abnormal distribution. A characteristic feature is a large ectatic 'primitive' vein in the lateral thigh. Varicosities may extend into the pelvis as well as down the leg. Superficial and deep-vein thrombosis is not uncommon, even in children. The bones may overgrow, resulting in increased leg length. Soft-tissue hypertrophy often occurs but may be difficult to distinguish from swelling caused by oedema or engorged veins or lymphatics. Pain is a significant and debilitating problem in KTS patients and has various causes [12].

Skin changes occur because of venous hypertension and abnormalities of lymphatic drainage. Other abnormalities associated with the syndrome include lymphangiectasia (cutaneous vesicles that leak lymph).

The abnormal veins (varicosity) lead to a significant increase in venous volume with age. As a consequence, the flow diminishes and the risk of deep and/or superficial thrombosis rises. There is also some evidence for a coexisting coagulopathy. These factors explain the high incidence of thrombosis in KTS patients. An acquired post-thrombotic syndrome aggravates the severity of KTS.

Diagnosis. The diagnosis is largely clinical. Physical examination should include auscultation and palpation of the involved area to assess for the presence of an arteriovenous malformation to rule out Parkes-Weber syndrome [8]. Duplex ultrasound scanning is the study of choice to evaluate for superficial and deep venous anomalies, and can also be used in differentiating vascular tumours from vascular malformations and arteriovenous fistulae [8,9]. MRI scans are effective for visualizing the extent of tissue overgrowth of lesions and infiltration of deeper tissues. X-rays may show increased thickness or abnormal density of the affected soft tissue as well as phleboliths [9]. Venograms may be required to delineate the venous abnormality and to exclude deep vein agenesis.

The differential diagnosis consists of other diseases associated with limb enlargement combined with a vascular lesion, for example Proteus syndrome, Parkes-Weber syndrome, Servelle–Martorell syndrome and hemihypertrophy with multiple lipomas. Other disorders that should be excluded are infantile haemangioma, kaposiform haemangioendothelioma and tufted angioma [8].

Treatment. Most patients with KTS can be managed conservatively with medical elastic compression stockings (MECS) to control venous hypertension, although patients with atresia of the deep venous system may complain of pain with compression [8]. Anticoagulants are administered to adults with thrombosis and anticoagulant prophylaxis is recommended after surgery, but long-term prophylaxis is not normally necessary, unless the patient is exposed to long periods of immobilization, for example long-term bed rest or air travel. Oral contraceptives should be avoided in women with KTS [9]. In treating varicose veins, (echo-guided) sclerotherapy is the treatment of first choice. Venous stripping, ligation or sclerosis can result in favourable outcomes in carefully evaluated and selected patients with symptomatic superficial varicose veins. If necessary, cutaneous lesions can be treated with vascular lasers or IPLS. Large limb-length discrepancies have been treated by osteotomy or epiphyseodesis as well as by epiphyseal stapling (which can be removed if further growth is required) [9,13].

Parkes-Weber syndrome

This syndrome was first described by Sir Fredrick Parkes-Weber in 1907. He reported a case involving arteriovenous fistula, together with varicosities and hypertrophy of the affected extremity. This syndrome is caused by congenital multiple arteriovenous fistulae, but can manifest with varicose veins and limb overgrowth as in KTS. There is no associated vascular naevus. Limb overgrowth gets progressively worse in Parkes-Weber syndrome, whereas in KTS leg-length disparity rarely increases after the age of 10 years [14]. Parkes-Weber syndrome more commonly affects the lower extremities, and lymphatic anomalies and lymphoedema can be present [8]. An obvious pulsatile swelling may be visible with discoloration of the overlying skin and large veins radiating from it. Duplex ultrasound demonstrates high blood flow and abnormal enlargement of the arteries [14]. During childhood, duplex ultrasound often shows enlarged arteries and patchy areas of hypervascularization; arteriovenous fistulae usually develop around puberty or after trauma. This disease may be complicated by cardiac enlargement and high-output congestive cardiac failure [8].

Conservative management consists of medical elastic compression stockings to prevent venous hypertension. Congestive cardiac failure requires active treatment. Repeated embolization under angiographic control is the most effective therapy. An alternative is to mobilize the vessel and ligate all the branches (skeletonization). Very occasionally, amputation may be necessary.

Genuine diffuse phlebectasia

Synonym
• Bockenheimer's syndrome

Phlebectasia is the term used to describe enlarged and irregular, superficial and deep veins. Histology of the phlebectasia shows a decrease in elastin in the wall of the ectatic veins. Thrombosis and calcification are often present [15]. Phlebangiomatosis involves cavernous angiomas, which manifest with cutaneous angiomas that extend into deeper layers including bone. Both conditions resemble KTS and Parkes-Weber syndrome but without an associated vascular naevus, bone overgrowth and arteriovenous fistula.

Servelle–Martorell syndrome [16]

This syndrome describes the association of a venous, and rarely arterial, malformation with skeletal abnormalities. Unlike KTS and Parkes-Weber syndrome, the intraosseous involvement leads to hypotrophy and therefore shortening of the limb bones. Deformation of the medullary cavity and thinning of the bone cortex can result in joint destruction. Otherwise the syndrome is similar, with ectasia and aneurysmal dilatation of superficial veins resulting in gross deformity of the extremity. The deep veins may be abnormally located or be hypoplastic with absent valves. Servelle–Martorell syndrome is considered to be an inverse form of KTS [17].

References

1 Garzon MC, Huang JT, Enjolras O, Frieden IJ. Vascular malformations: Part I. *J Am Ac Dermatol* 2007; **56**: 353–62.

2 Mulliken JB, Glowacki J. Hemangiomas and vascular malformations in infants and children: a classification based on endothelial characteristics. *Plast Reconstr Surg* 1982; **69**: 412–20.

3 Gallione CJ, Pasyk KA, Boon LM *et al*. A gene for familial venous malformations maps to chromosome 9p in a second large kindred. *Med Genet* 1995; **32**: 197–9.

4 Calvert JT, Riney TJ, Kontos CD *et al*. Allelic and locus heterogeneity in inherited venous malformations. *Hum Mol Genet* 1999; **8**: 1279–89.

5 Dubois J, Garel L. Imaging and therapeutic approach of hemangiomas and vascular malformations in the pediatric age group. *Pediatr Radiol* 1999; **29**: 879–93.

6 Pascarella L, Bergan JJ, Yamada C, Mekenas L. Venous angiomata: treatment with sclerosant foam. *Ann Vasc Surg* 2005; **19**: 457–64.

7 Parkes-Weber F. Angioma formation in connection with hypertrophy of limbs and hemihypertrophy. *Br J Dermatol* 1907; **19**: 231–5.

8 Garzon MC, Huang JT, Enjolras O, Frieden IJ. Vascular malformations: Part II. *J Am Acad Dermatol* 2007; **56**: 541–64.

9 Kihiczak GG, Meine JG, Schwartz RA, Janniger CK. Klippel–Trenaunay syndrome: a multisystem disorder possibly resulting from a pathogenic gene for vascular and tissue overgrowth. *Int J Dermatol* 2006; **45**: 883–90.

10 Tian X-L, Kadaba R, You S-A *et al.* Identification of an angiogenic factor that when mutated causes susceptibility to Klippel–Trenaunay syndrome. *Nature* 2004; **427**: 640–5.

11 Gloviczki P, Stanson AW, Stickler AW *et al.* Klippel–Trenaunay syndrome: the risks and benefits of vascular interventions. *Surgery* 1991; **110**: 469–79.

12 Lee A, Driscoll D, Gloviczki P *et al.* Evaluation and management of pain in patients with Klippel–Trenaunay syndrome: a review. *Pediatrics* 2005; **115**: 744–9.

13 Samuel M, Spitz L. Klippel–Trenaunay syndrome: clinical features, complications and management in children. *Br J Surg* 1995; **82**: 757–61.

14 Browse NL, Burnand KG, Irvine AT, Wilson NM, eds. *Diseases of the Veins*, 2nd edn. London: Arnold, 1999.

15 Van Geest AJ, Veraart JC, de Haan M, Neumann HA. Bockenheimer's syndrome. *J Eur Acad Dermatol Venereol* 1999; **12**: 165–8.

16 Weiss T, Madler U, Oberwittler H *et al.* Peripheral vascular malformation (Servelle–Martorell). *Circulation* 2000; **101**: e82–3.

17 Danarti R, Konig A, Bittar M, Happle R. Inverse Klippel–Trenaunay syndrome: review of cases showing deficient growth. *Dermatology* 2007; **214**: 130–2.

Capillary malformations

Capillary malformations are among the most common vascular malformations of the skin. They include telangiectases (p. 47.12) and port-wine stains (p. 47.23).

Venous disorders

Anatomy [1–7]

Most veins contain semilunar valves; these are usually in pairs, but some veins only contain one valve leaflet and sometimes three (tricuspid) valve leaflets are present. These valves are lined by endothelium and are found especially in the smaller veins and at the junction of these veins with larger branches. They prevent the reflux of blood and are particularly important in the leg, where their integrity, and that of the calf muscle pump (the venous heart), counters the gravitational hydrostatic pressure.

There are three systems: the deep veins, the superficial veins, and the perforating veins (or perforators). The perforating veins are numerous and inconstant, and connect the other two systems. During muscular activity, blood is directed from the superficial to the deep system, up from the foot to the thigh and thence to the abdomen, before venous blood returns towards the heart. Bicuspid valves are found in all three systems. The smallest veins to contain valves lie at the dermal subcutaneous junctions [4] and the valves are extremely variable. Valves may become damaged, thickened or degenerate with age [5]. Thrombosis also causes valvular destruction and a re-canalized post-thrombotic vein is valveless, anatomically distorted and functionally inefficient [5]. The most important perforating veins are considered to be on the medial side of the calf. Incompetence of the valves in these veins has been thought to be important in the causation of venous ulceration [5].

The superficial venous system of the leg begins from the veins on the dorsum of the foot, which join the greater saphenous vein (GSV) (originally called the long saphenous vein) and the short saphenous vein (SSV). They form a dorsal arch, which connects the territory of the SSV with that of the GSV. On the plantar side of the foot the same venous network joins to a plantar venous arch that also joins both saphenous veins [6,7].

References

1 Browse NL, Burnand KC, Irvine AT, Wilson NM, eds. *Diseases of the Veins*, 2nd edn. London: Arnold, 1999.

2 Tibbs D. *Varicose Veins and Related Disorders*. Oxford: Butterworth-Heinemann, 1992.

3 Gillot C. *Anatomical Atlas of the Lower Limb Superficial Venous Network*. St Gallen: Ganzoni & Cie AG, 2004.

4 Braverman IM, Keh-Yen A. Ultrastructure of the human dermal microcirculation. IV. Valve-containing collecting veins at the dermal-subcutaneous junction. *J Invest Dermatol* 1983; **81**: 438–42.

5 Chant ADB, Jones HO, Townsend JCF *et al.* Radiological demonstration of the relationship between calf varices and saphenofemoral incompetence. *Clin Radiol* 1972; **23**: 519–23.

6 Caggiati A, Bergan JJ, Glovicki P *et al.* Nomenclature of the veins of the lower limb: extensions, refinements and clinical application. *J Vasc Surg* 2005; **41**: 19–24.

7 Weiss MA, Weiss RA, Feied CF, eds. *Vein Diagnosis and Treatment: A Comprehensive Approach*. New York: McGraw-Hill Professional Publishing, 2001.

Physiology/pathophysiology

The venous macrocirculation [1,2]

Veins act as the capacitance vessels of the circulation. The 'venous return' is the blood returning to the heart via the great veins. Venous return from the lower limbs is achieved by the pumping action of the foot and calf muscles associated with competent valves that prevent backflow [1].

The venous system of the legs contains a volume of 300 to 350 mL in a healthy standing subject. The venous wall contracts in response to filling, and its function is called 'venous tone'. This acts as counter-pressure and automatically changes to attempt to maintain venous pressure at a constant level. The superficial veins drain through the communicating (perforating) veins into the deep system, and only 10% of the venous blood flow from the lower limb passes through the saphenofemoral junction (SFJ).

The deep veins are compressed by each muscle contraction shifting the blood column towards the heart against the pressure of gravity. The venous valves prevent backflow during muscle relaxation. This mechanism is the 'calf muscle pump'. Other muscle groups such as those of the foot also compress veins and aid venous return, but the calf muscle pump is the most important muscle pump of the leg.

References

1 Browse NL, Burnand KG, Lea Thomas M. Physiology and functional anatomy. In: Browse NL, Burnand KG, Lea Thomas M, eds. *Diseases of the Veins. Pathology, Diagnosis and Treatment*. London: Edward Arnold, 1988; 53–69.

2 Summer DS, Zierler RE. Vascular physiology: Essential hemodynamic principles. In: Rutherford RB, ed. *Vascular Surgery*. Philadelphia: Elsevier Saunders, 2005.

Venous reflux

Venous reflux is thought to be the major cause of venous disorders [1]. Reflux is the presence of retrograde flow in a vein in response to a stimulus such as a calf squeeze. It occurs during standing when the valves are incompetent [2]. It can occur in the superficial, deep and perforating veins of the lower extremity.

Venous pressure falls during calf muscle pump activity in healthy subjects and is known as normal lowering of ambulatory venous pressure [3,4]. An elevated and sustained ambulatory venous pressure (venous hypertension) is indicative of chronic venous insufficiency (CVI). This may be caused by valvular incompetence or venous outflow obstruction [5]. Venous outflow obstruction occurs in some patients after a deep-vein thrombosis (DVT), a situation known as the post-thrombotic leg. Obstruction is more serious than reflux and more difficult to treat. In this situation, when the leg muscles contract the venous pressure increases, rather than the usual lowering of venous pressure that occurs during ambulation when the vein is not obstructed. Such heightened pressure is transmitted distally as far as the capillary system of the skin, causing capillary hypertension, and eventually leading to destruction of the nutritive capillaries [6].

References

1 Reček Č. The venous reflux. *Angiology* 2004; **55**: 541–8.
2 Sarin S, Scurr JH, Coleridge Smith PD. Assessment of stripping the long saphenous vein in the treatment of primary varicose veins. *Br J Surg* 1992; **79**: 889–93.
3 Reček Č. Conception of the venous hemodynamics in the lower extremity. *Angiology* 2006; **57**: 556–63.
4 Summer DS, Zierler RE. Vascular physiology: essential hemodynamic principles. In: Rutherford RB, ed. *Vascular Surgery*. Philadelphia: Elsevier Saunders, 2005: 75–123.
5 Mendes RR, Marston WA. Physiologic assessment of the venous system. In: Rutherford RB, ed. *Vascular Surgery*. Philadelphia: Elsevier Saunders, 2005.
6 Jünger M, Hahn M, Klyscz T, Sterus A. Role of microangiopathy in the development of venous leg ulcers. *Prog Appl Microcirc* 1999; **23**: 180–3.

The venous microcirculation

Disturbances of the venous microcirculation account for almost all the clinical signs of chronic venous disease. The raised ambulatory venous pressure is transmitted directly to the venular side of the capillary bed. The capillaries in the skin of the lower leg are the most affected. Five theories have been developed to explain the mechanism for the microcirculatory disturbances in venous disease.

1 Capillary stasis. Homans postulated that 'stasis' of venous blood in patients with post-thrombotic syndrome gave rise to the development of anoxia which he thought caused venous ulcers [1]. Initially, when the oxygen content of blood samples taken from varicose veins was measured, lower values were found than in blood taken from healthy individuals [2]. One year later, however, Blalock produced completely different results. He reported that the oxygen content of the femoral venous blood of patients with varicose veins was higher than in healthy persons [3]. He concluded that the blood flow through the leg of patients with a venous ulcer was higher than that of healthy persons. Blalock's findings were subsequently confirmed by several investigators [4]. Only one study carried out in 1971 produced conflicting results [5].

When a contrast agent was injected into the femoral artery of patients with varicose veins it entered their veins faster than the veins of healthy controls [6,7]. The flow velocity may, however, be markedly decreased in certain locations in the venous system, for example in certain capillary beds. This decreased flow might be responsible for focal hypoxia [8], despite the overall increase in venous flow through the whole system.

It was shown that the transcutaneous oxygen tension (tcPo$_2$) was significantly lower in patients with CVI [9–11]. Low tcPo$_2$ values in patients with CVI cannot be fully explained at present. Morphological changes develop in the microcirculation in response

to prolonged CVI and these may also play a role in the lower tcPo$_2$ value.

Microangiopathy is a prominent sign of CVI [12] and was first reported by Bollinger *et al.*, who combined intravital capillaroscopy and fluorescence angiography with videodensitometry [13]. Bollinger's group measured the transcapillary and interstitial diffusion of a colorant (Na-fluorescein) into the skin of healthy volunteers. These results were then compared to results from patients with CVI. Reduced diffusion was present in the skin areas of patients with CVI that had a reduced capillary density. The density of fluorescein does not, of course, equate to oxygen diffusion. The capillary microscopy showed stagnant blood flow in some capillaries, leading to intracapillary coagulation. It was felt that capillary thrombosis might account for the disappearance of capillaries. The tcPo$_2$ value and cutaneous capillary density appear to be related [14]. The tcPo$_2$ value in capillary plexi with a low density approaches 0 mmHg at a distance of 100 μm or more between the capillaries.

References

1 Homans J. The etiology and treatment of varicose ulcer of the leg. *Surg Gynecol Obstet* 1917; **24**: 300–11.
2 De Takats G, Quint H, Tillotsen BI, Crittenden PJ. The impairment of the circulation in the varicose extremity. *Arch Surg* 1929; **18**: 671–86.
3 Blalock A. Oxygen content of blood in patients with varicose veins. *Arch Surg* 1929; **19**: 898–905.
4 Fagrell B. Local microcirculation in chronic venous incompetence and leg ulcers. *Vasc Surg* 1979; **13**: 217–25.
5 McEwan AJ, McArdle CS. Effect of hydroxyethylrutosides on blood oxygen levels and venous insufficiency symptoms in varicose veins. *BMJ* 1971; **2**: 138–41.
6 Piulachs P, Vidal-Barraquer F. Pathogenic study of varicose veins. *Angiology* 1953; **4**: 39.
7 Haimovici H. Abnormal arteriovenous shunts associated with chronic venous insufficiency. *J Cardiovasc Surg* 1976; **17**: 473–82.
8 Michiels C, Arnould T, Thibaut-Vercruyssen R *et al.* Perfused human saphenous veins for the study of the origin of varicose veins: role of the endothelium and of hypoxia. *Int Angiol* 1997; **16**: 134–41.
9 Neumann HAM, van Leeuwen M, van den Broek MJTB, Berretty PJM. Transcutaneous oxygen tension in chronic venous insufficiency syndrome. *VASA* 1984; **13**: 213–9.
10 Clyne CAC, Ramsden WH, Chant ADB, Webster JH. Oxygen tension of the skin of the gaiter area of limbs with venous disease. *Br J Surg* 1985; **72**: 644–7.
11 Stacey MC, Burnand KG, Layer GT, Pattison M. Transcutaneous oxygen tensions in assessing the treatment of venous ulcers. *Br J Surg* 1990; **97**: 1050–4.
12 Leu AJ, Yanar A, Pfister G *et al.* Mikroangiopathie bei chronischer venösen Insuffizienz. *Dtsch Med Wschr* 1991; **116**: 447–53.
13 Bollinger A, Jäger K, Geser A *et al.* Transcapillary and interstitial diffusion of NA-fluorescein in chronic venous insufficiency with atrophy. *Int J Microcirc Clin Exp* 1982; **1**: 5–17.
14 Huch A, Franzeck UK, Huch R, Bollinger A. A transparent transcutaneous electrode for simultaneous studies of skin capillary morphology, flow dynamics and oxygenation. *Int J Microcirc Clin Exp* 1983; **2**: 103–8.

2 Fibrin cuff-theory. Browse and Burnand postulated that venous ulceration could be the result of deposition of pericapillary fibrin [1]. This theory was later named the 'fibrin cuff-theory' [2]. The leakage of large molecules such as fibrinogen through the pericapillary space was caused by the high venous pressure associated with CVI. Fibrinogen was thought to polymerize to insoluble fibrin in the interstitium to form a pericapillary fibrin 'cuff'. This cuff might then function as a oxygen diffusion barrier. A significant increase in the collagen IV layer has also been found in and around the capillaries [3]. The authors suggested that fibrin could function as a matrix for collagen formation. The role of fibrin as a diffusion barrier was never conclusively proven and theoretical objections were put forward to its ability to reduce oxygen transfer [4]. In porphyria cutanea tarda (PCT) patients, where pericapillary fibrin deposits (cuffs) are present, normal $tcPo_2$ values exist [5]. The fibrin deposition appears to be an indicator of microcirculatory disturbance rather than the cause of a lower $tcPo_2$ value.

References

1 Burnand KG, Whimster I, Naidoo A, Browse NL. Pericapillary fibrin in the ulcer-bearing skin of the leg: the cause of lipodermatosclerosis and venous ulceration. *BJM* 1982; **285**: 1071–7.
2 Browse NL, Burnand KG. The cause of venous ulceration. *Lancet* 1982; **2**: 243–5.
3 Neumann HAM, van den Broek MJTB. Increased collagen IV layer in the basal membrane area of the capillaries in severe chronic venous insufficiency. *VASA* 1991; **20**: 26–9.
4 Michel CC. Oxygen diffusion in edematous tissue and through pericapillary cuffs. *Phlebology* 1990; **5**: 223–30.
5 Neumann HAM, van den Broek MJTB, Boersma IH, Veraart JCJM. Transcutaneous oxygen tension in patients with and without pericapillary fibrin cuffs in chronic venous insufficiency, porphyria cutanea tarda and non-venous leg ulcers. *VASA* 1996; **25**: 127–33.

3 White cell trapping.

In patients with lipodermatosclerosis, white blood cells disappear from the venous blood when the leg is in a dependent position [1]. Coleridge Smith *et al.* formulated a new theory for the aetiology of venous ulcers on the basis of these observations [2]. They suggested that the leukocytes may become trapped in the capillaries, obstructing flow and thereby leading to ischaemic ulceration. Adhesion molecules are over expressed and may play an important role by causing continuous leukocyte migration to the dermis [3,4].

References

1 Thomas PRS, Nash GB, Dormandy JA. White cell accumulation in the dependent legs of patients with venous hypertension. A possible mechanism for trophic changes in the skin. *BJM* 1988; **296**: 1693–5.
2 Coleridge Smith PD, Thomas P, Scurr JH, Dormandy JA. Causes of venous ulceration: a new hypothesis. *BJM* 1988; **296**: 1726–7.
3 Veraart JCJM, Verhaegh MEJM, Neumann HAM *et al.* Adhesion molecule expression in venous leg ulcers. *VASA* 1993; **22**: 213–8.
4 Peschen M, Lahaye T, Hennig B *et al.* Expression of the adhesion of molecules ICAM-1, VCAM-1, LFA-1 and VLA-4 in the skin is modulated in progressing stages of chronic venous insufficiency with and without atrophie blanche. In: Maessen-Visch MB. *Atrophie Blanche* (Thesis). Nijmegen: Drukkerij Hendrix Volharding, 1999: 77–87.

4 Trapping growth factors.

Falanga and Eaglestein hypothesized that the pericapillary fibrin cuffs, which included α2-macroglobulin, interfere with growth factor transport, making them biologically unavailable in patients with severe CVI. They felt that this might also account for delayed healing of ulcers [1]. The lack of availability of growth factors is controversial. Clinical research using topical epidermal growth factor (EGF), TGF-β and fibroblast growth factor (FGF) has failed to improve the healing of venous ulcers. The addition of a single growth factor has therefore not been able to restore the process of disturbed wound healing in patients with chronic venous ulcers.

Reference

1 Falanga V, Eaglestein WH. The 'trap' hypothesis of venous ulceration. *Lancet* 1993; **341**: 1006–8.

5 Multicausal model: the Maastricht model.

A dynamic conceptual model has been proposed by researchers at the University Hospital of Maastricht in the Netherlands [1,2]. They suggest that a raised pressure in the capillaries acts mainly on the venular side of the dermal microcirculation. The raised microcirculatory pressure is a consequence of elevated ambulatory venous pressure. The continuously elevated pressure leads to alterations in the structure of the capillary wall, in which the interendothelial space broadens and the collagen IV layer disintegrates. The capillary wall becomes thicker [3], and the structural changes interfere with capillary exchange [4]. Collagen IV disintegrates and the interendothelial space enlarges, in turn increasing the capillary filtration fraction.

In the first instance water diffusion is affected, causing oedema [5]; later, larger molecules escape into the tissues. Accumulation of these molecules leads to halo formation [6–8]. The fibrin/fibrinogen cuffs demonstrated by immunofluorescence studies are a sensitive sign of decompensating capillaries in the skin. The fibrin cuffs do not act simply as a diffusion barrier for oxygen; the presence of fibrin also serves as a stimulus for collagen formation. Collagen IV is laid down around the capillaries and collagens I and III in the dermis. α2-macroglobulin is also laid down and this binds molecules such as TGF-β, leading to decreased biological availability of various growth factors.

Widened capillaries have a lower flow velocity. White cells marginate and adhere to the capillary walls, sometimes blocking the circulation and leading to the formation of microthrombi. The escape of plasma proteins into the tissues enhances the inflammatory response, while the escape of leukocytes into the tissues releases proteolytic enzymes causing free radical damage. This is seen clinically as the changes of lipodermatosclerosis (LDS) [9].

There is evidence of continuous collagen degradation resulting from the increased action of the proteolytically active matrix metalloproteinase-1 (MMP-1) and matrix metalloproteinase-2 (MMP-2). Evidence of increased proteolytic activity has been found in patients with LDS who have decreased fibrinolytic activity [10]. It is attractive to assume that elevated proteolytic MMP-2 expression is a consequence of plasminogen activation in LDS which might cause an elevated matrix turnover [9]. This would be responsible for structural changes in the dermis and subcutaneous tissue which could then easily ulcerate.

Clotting and fibrinolytic disturbances play a role in the development of atrophie blanche [11]. The capillaries are obliterated in the affected areas leading to local hypoxia. Minimal trauma then leads to ulceration.

References

1 Neumann HAM, Tazelaar DJ. Compression therapy. In: Bergan JJ, Goldman MP, eds. *Varicose Veins and Telangiectasias, Diagnosis and Treatment*. St. Louis: Quality Medical Publishing Inc., 1993: 103–22.
2 Neumann HAM. Measurement of microcirculation. In: Altmeyer P. *et al.*, eds. *Wound Healing and Skin Physiology*. Berlin/Heidelberg: Springer Verlag, 1995: 115–26.
3 Neumann HAM, van den Broek MJTB. Increased collagen IV layer in the basal membrane area of the capillaries in severe chronic venous insufficiency. *VASA* 1991; **20**: 20–9.

4 Leu HJ. The prognostic significance of cutaneous and microvascular changes in venous leg ulcers. *Vasc Dis* 1965; **2**: 77–80.

5 Roztocil K, Prerovsky I, Olivia I. The effect of hydroxy-ethylrutosides on capillary filtration rate in the lower limb of man. *Eur J Clin Pharmacol* 1997; **11**: 435–8.

6 Neumann HAM, van den Broek MJTB, Boersma IH, Veraart JCJM. Transcutaneous oxygen tension in patients with and without pericapillary fibrin cuffs in chronic venous insufficiency, porphyria cutanea tarda and non-venous leg ulcers. *VASA* 1996; **25**: 127–33.

7 Fagrell B. Microcirculatory disturbances—the final cause for leg ulcers? *VASA* 1982; **11**: 101–3.

8 Burnand KG, Whimster I, Naidoo A, Browse NL. Pericapillary fibrin in the ulcer-bearing skin of the leg: the cause of lipodermatosclerosis and venous ulceration. *BJM* 1982; **285**: 1071–7.

9 Herouy Y, May AE, Pornschlegel G *et al*. Lipodermatosclerosis is characterized by elevated expression and activation of matrix metalloproteinases: implications for venous ulcer formation. *J Invest Dermatol* 1998; **111**: 822–7.

10 Jarrett PE, Burnand KG, Morland M, Browse NL. Fibrinolysis and fat necrosis in the lower leg. *Br J Surg* 1976; **63**: 157.

11 Maessen-Visch MB, Koedam MI, Hamulyák K, Neumann HAM. Atrophie blanche, a review. *Int J Dermatol* 1999; **38**: 161–72.

Venous thrombosis

Deep-vein thrombosis

Epidemiology. Deep-vein thrombosis (DVT) has an annual incidence of 0.2% in the urban population [1]. The disease is rare in children under 15 years old, but its frequency increases with age, with an incidence of 1.8 per 1000 person-years between 65 and 69 years and 3.1 per 1000 person-years between 85 and 89 years of age [2]. First episodes of DVT account for two-thirds of cases. The prevalence of DVT is highest in Caucasian adults and is low in Asian populations. The risk of a DVT seems to be slightly higher in men than in women, and the risk of recurrent venous thromboembolism is about 60% greater in men compared to women [3].

Aetiology and pathogenesis. In 1856, Virchow postulated that the main causes of thrombus formation were damage to the vessel wall, alterations in blood flow and hypercoagulability [2]. This is called 'Virchow's triad' and is still valid today. Risk factors for DVT include cancer, immobility, surgery and thrombophlebitis.

The maintenance of the fluidity and circulation of the blood and its ability to thrombose are essential for the maintenance of life and are governed by extremely complex homeostatic mechanisms. Thrombosis is a protective mechanism which prevents loss of blood and seals off damaged blood vessels. Fibrinolysis counteracts or stabilizes the thrombosis. Alterations in blood coagulability and platelet numbers, with associated changes in blood flow and endothelial damage, are the precursors of deep-vein thrombosis. The loss of normal vascular endothelial function is probably of primary importance [4].

Factor V Leiden, a pro-coagulant mutation, is present in 8% of patients with thrombosis. Anticardiolipin antibodies are also now recognized as an important cause of thrombosis [5,6]. A number of other hereditary and acquired conditions that predispose to thrombosis (thrombophilia) have also been recognized. These include protein C and S deficiency, antithrombin deficiency, the prothrombin 20210A gene mutation and activated protein C resis-

Table 47.4 Risk factors for deep-vein thrombosis [2,8].

Advancing age
Obesity
Previous venous thromboembolism
Family history of venous thromboembolism

Surgery, especially procedures lasting more than 30 min.
Trauma, especially of the spine or legs

Malignant tumours
Acute medical illnesses, e.g. acute myocardial infarction, heart failure, respiratory failure, infection
Inflammatory bowel disease
Antiphospholipid syndrome
Dyslipoproteinaemia
Nephrotic syndrome
Paroxysmal nocturnal haemoglobinuria
Myeloproliferative diseases
Behçet's syndrome

Varicose veins
Superficial vein thrombosis
Congenital venous malformation
Pulmonary embolism
May–Thurner syndrome
Long-distance travel
Prolonged bed rest or sitting
Immobilization
Hospitalization
Limb paralysis

Pregnancy/puerperium
Oral contraceptives
Hormone replacement therapy

Other drugs
Chemotherapy
Tamoxifen
Thalidomide
Antipsychotics

Central venous catheter
Vena cava filter
Intravenous drug use

tance (which is usually associated with the factor V Leiden genetic abnormality). Screening for thrombophilia, and for anticardiolipin antibodies, should be performed in patients presenting with a sporadic or recurrent thrombosis [7]. Surgical operations and pregnancy remain important triggers of thrombosis. Prolonged immobility (e.g. long-haul flights) and the contraceptive pill are also well-documented risk factors (Table 47.4).

Clinical features. The onset of a deep-vein thrombosis is often 'silent' and may remain so. It commonly occurs about 7 to 10 days after a surgical operation, childbirth or the onset of an acute infection. It is often associated with a rise in the platelet count and an increase in young 'sticky' platelets. Between one-third and two-thirds of patients complain of some swelling and pain in the leg, usually in the calf [4]. An iliac thrombosis should be suspected if the whole leg is swollen and dusky. There may be a pink or

Table 47.5 Clinical score list for predicting pretest probability for having a proximal deep vein thrombosis [11].

Clinical feature:
Active cancer treatment ongoing or within previous 6 months or palliative
Paralysis, paresis, or recent plaster immobilization of the lower leg(s)
Recent immobilization for more than 3 days or major surgery within last 4 weeks
Localized tenderness/pain along the distribution of the deep venous system
Entire leg swollen
Calf swelling by more than 2 cm when compared with the asymptomatic leg
   (measured 10 cm below tibial tuberosity)
Pitting oedema greater in the symptomatic leg
Collateral superficial veins (non-varicose)

Each factor scores 1; maximum score 8; see text for grading of risk according to score.

cyanotic hue to the leg and evidence of superficial venous dilation. The temperature of the leg may be raised, and pitting oedema of one ankle is an important physical sign.

Diagnosis. Pain and tenderness in the calf and popliteal fossa may occur in other conditions such as a ruptured Baker's cyst, a haematoma, or muscle tears or pulls. Infection (e.g. cellulitis) and lipodermatosclerosis should also be differentiated from a DVT. These can usually be distinguished clinically.

Assessment should include a clinical score and a D-dimer test, as a negative D-dimer test, in combination with a low-risk clinical score, avoids the need for compression ultrasound (CUS) in every patient with a painful or swollen leg [9]. The clinical score, based on medical history and physical examination, divides patients into low, moderate and high-risk categories for having a DVT (Table 47.5). A score of 0 (asymptomatic) means a low probability, a score of 1 or 2 a moderate probability, and a score of 3 or more a high probability, for DVT.

D-Dimer is a degradation product of a cross-linked fibrin clot. A negative test is useful for ruling out a DVT because the test has high sensitivity, but its specificity is low; it can be raised in various other conditions, such as post-surgery, inflammation of various causes, pregnancy and cancer. A moderate or high clinical probability, or a low clinical probability in combination with a high D-dimer, should therefore be followed by CUS of the legs (Fig. 47.18). The sensitivity of CUS is 97% for proximal and 73% for distal vein thrombosis compared with phlebography. CUS has many advantages over phlebography. It is non-invasive, simple, easy to repeat, relatively inexpensive and free of complications.

There are, however, two main disadvantages of CUS. Calf vein thrombosis can be missed, especially when the examination is limited to the popliteal and femoral veins, and small isolated thrombi in the iliac and superficial femoral veins or within the adductor canal can be difficult to detect and therefore easily overlooked [10].

CUS should be repeated after 1 week if the D-dimer is high and the CUS was negative but there is still a moderate or high probability of DVT on clinical grounds. The newer investigations of CT venography and MRI imaging appear to have advantages in certain circumstances, but at present their cost and availability limit their application.

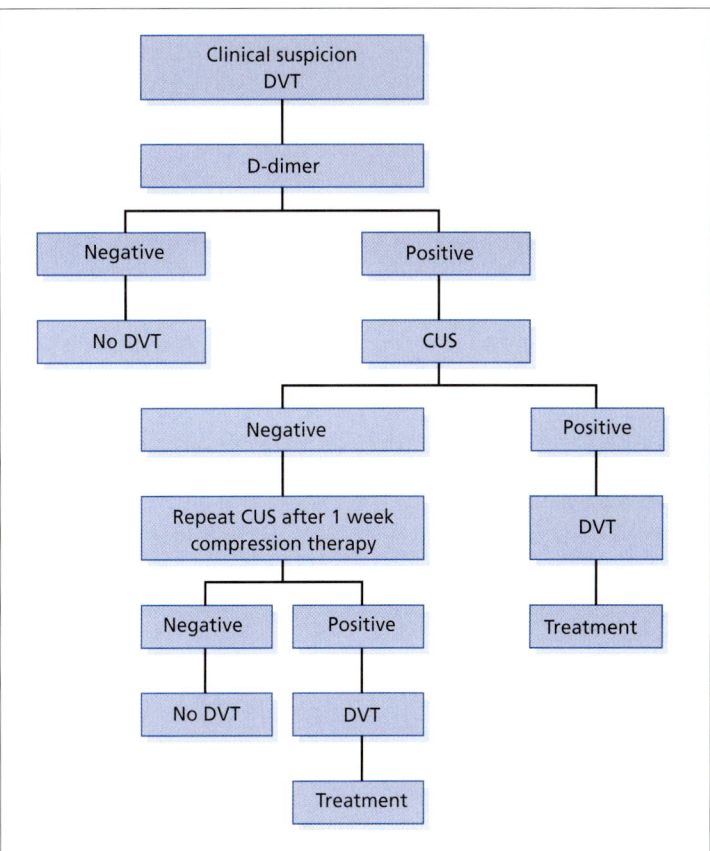

Fig. 47.18 Procedure to safely exclude deep vein thrombosis.

Treatment. Treatment includes the immediate therapy, awareness and prevention of complications and prevention of further episodes. Pulmonary embolism, post-thrombotic syndrome (PTS) and recurrent thrombosis are the main complications of DVT. About 10–30% of patients with DVT develop PTS. DVT has a recurrence rate of about 20% after 5 years, but the rate varies depending on the presence of risk factors [12]. Preventive measures should therefore be undertaken in every patient who has an increased risk of developing venous thromboembolism. Low-molecular-weight heparins (LMWH), intermittent pneumatic compression and medical elastic compression stockings (MECS) should be used as prophylaxis [13].

Active treatment is as follows. Initially a LMWH is given subcutaneously (150 to 200 IU/kg once daily). It can be given as an outpatient without the need for monitoring. It only needs to be given once daily and the risk of heparin-induced thrombocytopenia (Chapter 49) is negligible with LMWH compared with standard heparin preparations [2]. Vitamin K antagonists such as warfarin should be added to the LMWH at 24 or 48 hours unless contraindicated. Monitoring of anticoagulation is done by the prothrombin time, expressed in terms of the international normalized ratio (INR). A ratio between 2.0 and 3.0 should be achieved for adequate anticoagulation with a low risk of bleeding. LMWH can be discontinued when the correct INR has been attained [2]. Idiopathic venous thromboembolism is generally treated for 6 months, but anticoagulation may be for life if the condition recurs or a high risk exists [14].

LMWH and oral anticoagulants should be combined with compression stockings. Once oedema has reduced, class II MECS are prescribed to be worn for life. Class III MECS can be prescribed if the oedema remains a problem [15]. MECS significantly reduce the development of post-thrombotic syndrome.

References

1 Nordstrøm M, Lindblad B, Bergqvist D, Kjellstrom T. A prospective study of the incidence of deep-vein thrombosis within a defined urban population. *J Intern Med* 1992; **232**: 155–60.
2 Kyrle PA. Deep vein thrombosis. *Lancet* 2005; **365**: 1163–74.
3 McRae S, Tran H, Schulman S *et al.* Effect of patient's sex on risk of recurrent venous thromboembolism: a meta-analysis. *Lancet* 2006; **368**: 371–8.
4 Browse NL, Burnand KC, Irvine AT, Wilson NM, eds. *Disease of the Veins*, 2nd edn. London: Arnold, 1999.
5 Boey ML, Colaco CB, Chavari AE *et al.* Thrombosis in systemic lupus erythematosus: striking association with the presence of circulating antcoagulants. *BMJ* 1983; **287**: 289.
6 Mueh JR, Herbst KD, Rapaport SI. Thrombosis in patients with the lupus coagulant. *Ann Intern Med* 1980; **92**: 156–9.
7 Dahlback B. Physiological anticoagulation. *J Clin Invest* 1994; **94**: 923.
8 Cushman M. Epidemiology and risk factors for venous thrombosis. *Semin Hematol* 2007; **44**: 62–9.
9 Stein PD, Hull RD, Patel KC *et al.* D-Dimer for the exclusion of acute venous thromboembolism and pulmonary embolism. *Ann Intern Med* 2004; **140**: 589–602.
10 Michiels JJ, Gadisseur A, van der Planken M *et al.* A critical appraisal of non-invasive diagnosis and exclusion of deep vein thrombosis and pulmonary embolism in outpatients with suspected deep vein thrombosis or pulmonary embolism: how many tests do we need? *Int Angiol* 2005; **24**: 27–39.
11 Michiels JJ, Gadisseur A, van der Planken M *et al.* Screening for deep vein thrombosis and pulmonary embolism in outpatients with suspected DVT or PE by sequential use of clinical score: a sensitive quantitative D-dimer test and non-invasive diagnostic tools. *Semin Vasc Med* 2005; **5**: 351–64.
12 Segal JB, Streiff MB, Hofmann LV *et al.* Management of venous thromboembolism: a systematic review for a practice guideline. *Ann Intern Med* 2007; **146**: 211–22.
13 Pini M, Spyropoulos AC. Prevention of venous thromboemolism. *Semin Thromb Hemost* 2006; **32**: 755–66.
14 Blann AD, Lip GYH. Venous thromboembolism. *BMJ* 2006; **332**: 215–9.
15 Wentel TD, Neumann HAM. Management of the postthrombotic syndrome: the Rotterdam approach. *Semin Thromb Hemost* 2006; **32**: 814–21.

Superficial venous thrombosis

> **Synonym**
> • Superficial thrombophlebitis

Incidence. Most studies report a female preponderance (female proportion between 55 and 70%) and a mean age of onset of 60 years [1].

Aetiology and pathogenesis. Several studies have described an association between superficial venous thrombosis and venous thromboembolism. Superficial venous thrombosis located in the main trunk of the saphenous vein has the strongest association with venous thromboembolism [2,3].

Predisposing risk factors for superficial venous thrombosis are similar to those for deep-vein thrombosis [3]. Superficial venous thrombosis usually develops in the lower limbs. In 60–80% of cases the greater saphenous vein (GSV) system is involved, and in 10–20% the short saphenous (SSV) system [4]. The main cause of superficial venous thrombosis of the lower limbs is varicose veins, which are present in 70% of cases [5]. The main cause of superficial venous thrombosis in the upper limb is iatrogenic, for example intravenous catheters or infusion of drugs such as chemotherapy or heroin. Mondor's disease may also be a form of superficial venous thrombosis.

Clinical features. The patient usually presents with pain and a reddened, warm, tender cord extending along the vein. The overlying skin may show signs of erythema and oedema. The differential diagnosis includes cellulitis, panniculitis, erythema nodosum, insect bites and lymphangitis [5].

Diagnosis. Duplex ultrasound can be used to confirm the diagnosis [1,4,5], and to exclude a coexisting deep-vein thrombosis. Patients should be further investigated if they have idiopathic or recurrent superficial venous thrombosis or if they have a superficial venous thrombosis without varicose veins [5].

Treatment. LMWH and non-steroidal anti-inflammatory drugs (NSAIDs) appear to be the best treatments for superficial venous thrombosis of the leg veins [3]. Sclerotherapy and stripping of any varicose veins should only be performed some months after the acute superficial venous thrombosis has settled. When a thrombus is found in or near the saphenofemoral junction or saphenopopliteal junction, especially if it extends as free-floating thrombus extending into the common femoral vein or popliteal veins, it should be treated by surgical removal, combined with ligation and stripping. The patient can receive a 3-month therapeutic course of LMWH [4]. The thrombus can be squeezed out of the vein through a needle puncture. This should be followed by application of compression bandages or stockings.

References

1 Marchiori A, Mosena L, Prandoni P. Superficial vein thrombosis: risk factors, diagnosis, and treatment. *Semin Thromb Hemost* 2006; **32**: 737–43.
2 Wichers IM, Di Nisio M, Büller HR, Middelkoop S. Treatment of superficial vein thrombosis to prevent deep vein thrombosis and pulmonary embolism: a systematic review. *Haematologica* 2005; **90**: 672–7.
3 Di Nisio M, Wichers IM, Middelkoop S. Treatment for superficial thrombophlebitis of the leg. *Cochrane Database Syst Rev* 2007; **18**: CD004982.
4 Leon L, Giannoukas AD, Dodd D *et al.* Clinical significance of superficial vein thrombosis. *Eur J Vasc Endovasc Surg* 2005; **29**: 10–7.
5 Decousus H, Epinat M, Guillot K *et al.* Superficial venous thrombosis: risk factors, diagnosis, and treatment. *Curr Opin Pulm Med* 2003; **9**: 393–7.

Thrombophlebitis migrans [1–4]

Recurrent migratory thrombophlebitis is an uncommon condition that affects large and small veins throughout the body. The superficial veins of the lower extremities, abdominal wall, flank, arms or elsewhere undergo segmental thrombosis, causing crops of tender, linear or oval subcutaneous lumps or streaks. This is a pattern seen in Behçet's disease (Chapter 50) [5,6]. Fazeli *et al.* [7] also found an association between thrombophlebitis migrans and Buerger's disease in 65.4% of 86 patients, though others have put this percentage lower.

Much of the literature regarding migratory thrombophlebitis is concerned with the link with underlying malignancy, termed

Trousseau's syndrome (Chapter 62). This association was carefully reviewed by Sack *et al.* [8] and by Samlaska *et al.* [9], who suggested that migratory thrombophlebitis is a chronic disorder of disseminated intravascular coagulation.

Clues to a primary hypercoagulable state include a family history, recurrent thrombosis, an unusual anatomical site, an early age of onset and resistance to conventional anticoagulation. Secondary hypercoagulable states are a consequence of malignancy, infection, pregnancy, the contraceptive pill, nephritis or liver disease [3,4,9].

A follow-up study of 4399 patients who had venography for suspected DVT recorded that 150 of 1383 with proven DVT and 182 of 2412 without thrombosis developed cancer; although the overall difference was not significant, there were significantly more cancers in the DVT group (66 cancers) than in the non-DVT group (37 cancers) in the first 6 months after the venography [10]. A more severe type of thrombophlebitis is associated with malignant disease. In 1500 cases of thrombophlebitis, 31 of 77 occurring in association with malignancy were of a migratory type [2]. Carcinomas of the lung and pancreas were the most common sites for the primary tumours, although carcinomas of the breast, colon and stomach were also reported.

Treatment. Malignancy must be carefully excluded in patients with migratory thrombophlebitis. It may be difficult to locate, especially if the patient has a pancreatic carcinoma. Computed tomography (CT) scanning, ultrasound, MRI and even positron emission tomographic (PET) scans of the abdomen may be necessary. Treatment is generally conservative, and patients should be treated with adequate anticoagulation. Lowering triglycerides may be advisable and exercise is good prophylaxis. Medical elastic compression stockings or bandages may alleviate symptoms. Stripping of the saphenous system has been advocated [1]. Earlier observations on the good effects of oral fibrinolytic agents [11,12] in Behçet's disease have not been substantiated by some later case reports [13].

References
1 Cruikshrank AH. Venous thrombosis in the internal organs associated with thrombosis of the leg veins. *J Pathol Bacteriol* 1956; **71**: 383–6.
2 Lieberman JS, Borrero J, Urdanetta E *et al*. Thromboembolism associated with neoplasm: review of 77 cases. *Circulation* 1960; **22**: 780.
3 Samlaska CP, James WD. Superficial thrombophlebitis. I. Primary hypercoagulable states. *J Am Acad Dermatol* 1990; **22**: 974–89.
4 Samlaska CP, James WD. Superficial thrombophlebitis. II. Secondary hypercoagulable states. *J Am Acad Dermatol* 1990; **23**: 1–18.
5 Bollinger A, Leu HJ. Thrombophlebitis saltans. *Deutsch Med Wochenschr* 1974; **99**: 1433–6.
6 Forman L. Thrombophlebitis and arteritis in the pathology of Behçet's syndrome. *Hautarzt* 1960; **11**: 363–6.
7 Fazeli B, Modaghegh H, Ravrai H, Kazemzadeh G. Thrombophlebitis migrans as a footprint of Buerger's disease: a prospective-descriptive study in north-east of Iran. *Clin Rheumatol* 2008; **27**: 55–7
8 Sack C, Levin J, Bell WR. Trousseau's syndrome and other manifestations of chronic disseminated coagulopathy in patients with neoplasms: clinical, pathophysiologic and therapeutic features. *Medicine* 1977; **56**: 1–37.
9 Samlaska CP, Jones WD, Simel DL. Superficial migratory thrombophlebitis and factor XII deficiency. *J Am Acad Dermatol* 1990; **22**: 939–43.
10 Nordstrom M, Lindblad B, Anderson H *et al*. Deep vein thrombosis and occult malignancy: epidemiological study. *BMJ* 1994; **308**: 891–4.
11 Chajek T, Fainaru M. Behçet's disease with decreased fibrinolysis and superior vena cava occlusion. *BMJ* 1973; **1**: 782.
12 Cunliffe WJ, Roberts BE, Dodman B. Behçet's disease syndrome and oral fibrinolytic therapy. *BMJ* 1973; **2**: 486–7.
13 Graham-Brown RAC, Sarkany I. Failure of colchicine and fibrinolytic therapy in Behçet's disease. *Clin Exp Dermatol* 1980; **5**: 87–92.

Mondor's disease

The classic Mondor's disease is located in the chest wall and affects veins that include the lateral thoracic vein, the superior epigastric vein and the thoracoepigastric vein [1,2]. Similar cases have been reported in the antecubital fossa, inguinal area, axilla, penis [3], abdomen and lower limbs. The aetiology of the disorder is unknown.

Pathogenesis. A venous thrombosis which may partially or totally occlude the vein is followed by re-canalization. Fibromuscular hyperplasia develops in the vessel wall with infiltration and fibrosis of the surrounding subcutaneous cellular tissue [2]. Trauma or friction causes a sclerosing phlebitis of the affected vein and aggravates the course of the disease.

Clinical features. Women account for 75% of those affected, generally between the second and fifth decade of life [2]. Sudden, localized chest pain is the main presenting symptom, and is accompanied by the appearance of grooved, hardened 'cords' that are visible and palpable on the chest wall where they resemble wires. These cord-like structures attach to the overlying skin before retracting, with the formation of characteristic linear grooves. Patients may have fever and significant regional inflammation in the acute phase. As the disorder is self-limiting [2], relief of pain follows with complete resolution of the symptoms in about 2 to 8 weeks. Mondor's disease has been associated with primary or metastatic mammary carcinoma in up to 12% of cases [4].

Treatment. Mondor's disease is a self-limiting disease which nearly always resolves spontaneously. Anti-inflammatory agents (e.g. ibuprofen) and 75 mg salicylic acetic acid per day are recommended, plus local application of heat and physiotherapy involving gentle stretching of the cords where possible. Neither anticoagulation nor antibiotics are indicated. Resection of thrombotic vessels can be considered to treat the patient and confirm the diagnosis when symptoms are intractable.

References
1 Mondor H. Tronculite sous-cutanee subaigue de la paroi thoracigue antero-laterale. *Mem Acad Chir* 1939; **65**: 1271–8.
2 De Godoy JM, Godoy MF, Batigália F, Braile DM. The association of Mondor's disease with protein S deficiency: case report and review of literature. *J Thromb Thrombolysis* 2002; **93**: 187–9.
3 Al-Mwalad M, Loertzer H, Wicht A, Fornara P. Subcutaneous penile vein thrombosis (penile Mondor's disease): pathogenesis, diagnosis, and therapy. *Urology* 2006; **67**: 586–8.
4 Catania S, Zurrida S, Veronesi P *et al*. Mondor's disease and breast cancer. *Cancer* 1992; **69**: 2267–70.

Axillary web syndrome

Axillary web syndrome (AWS) follows axillary lymphadenectomy for breast cancer and manifests with palpable cords which 'bowstring' across the axilla, creating a web of skin [1,2]. The cords are painful and restrict shoulder movement. They can extend into the ipsilateral arm, even forearm, and can create a linear groove somewhat like those seen in Mondor's disease. Indeed, it is probably a site-specific variant of this condition, and probably has a traumatic cause; it has also been reported after skin surgery [3]. The cause is unclear but the condition usually resolves over 6 months.

References

1 Moskovitz AH, Anderson BO, Yeung RS *et al*. Axillary web syndrome after axillary dissection. *Am J Surg* 2001; **181**: 434–9.
2 Leidenius M, Leppänen E, Krogerus L, von Smitten K. Motion restriction and axillary web syndrome after sentinal node biopsy and axillary clearance in breast cancer. *Am J Surg* 2003; **185**: 127–30.
3 Craythorne EE, Roberts J, Higgins EM, Macfarlane CS. 'Axillary web syndrome' or 'cording': an unusual postsurgical complication and localized variant of Mondor's disease. *Br J Dermatol* 2008; **159** (Suppl. 1): 109.

Deep-vein obstruction [1]

The most common cause of chronic deep-vein obstruction is a previous DVT. Non-thrombotic causes include malignant disease or other pelvic masses compressing the iliac veins. Retroperitoneal fibrosis can obstruct the iliac veins and the inferior vena cava. The iliac compression syndrome (Cockett's or May–Thurner syndrome) is present when the left common iliac vein is compressed by the right common iliac artery crossing its course to the inferior vena cava [2]. Flow alterations do not usually cause problems unless thrombosis takes place. Large tumours (e.g. soft-tissue sarcomas) or aneurysms in the thigh may compress the deep femoral vein. In the popliteal fossa an aneurysm or a Baker's cyst can compress the popliteal vein. Primary tumours of the vein wall (leiomyosarcoma) are rare but are found more often in the lower limb. Ligation of deep veins may be unavoidable when removing a malignancy or when repairing vein damage from accidental trauma.

References

1 Browse NL, Burnand KG, Irvine NM. *Disease of the Veins,* 2nd edn. London: Arnold, 1999: 409–25.
2 Cockett FB, Thomas ML. The iliac compression syndrome. *Br J Surg* 1965; **52**: 816–21.

Chronic venous insufficiency

Classification

Several classifications have been used to describe the severity of chronic venous insufficiency (CVI), of which the classifications by Widmer *et al*. (Table 47.6) [1] and the CEAP classification (Clinical status, Etiology, Anatomy, Pathophysiology) (Table 47.7) [2,3] are the best known. The CEAP classification is a well-recognized classification for varicose veins, despite its deficiencies. In 2000, the Venous Clinical Severity Score (VCSS) was developed, which provides a slightly more detailed description of the factors contributing to CVI (Table 47.8) [4].

References

1 Widmer LK, Plechl SC, Leu HJ *et al*. Venenkrankungen bei 1800 Berufstätigen. Basel Studie II. *Schweiz Med Wochensch* 1967; **97**: 107–10.
2 Porter JM, Moneta GL. Reporting standard in venous disease: an update. International Consensus Committee on Chronic Venous Disease. *J Vasc Surg* 1995; **21**: 635–45.
3 Eklof B, Rutherford RB, Bergan J *et al*. Revision of the CEAP classification for chronic venous disorders: consensus statement. *J Vasc Surg* 2004; **40**: 1248–52.
4 Rutherford RB, Padberg FT Jr, Comerota AJ *et al*. Venous severity scoring: an adjunct to venous outcome assessment. *J Vasc Surg* 2000; **31**: 1307–12.

Chronic venous insufficiency/reflux

Chronic venous insufficiency may be classified anatomically into three categories (Fig. 47.19).

Superficial vein insufficiency. This is actually indicated by the presence of visible, tortuous, truncal varicose veins. It arises from

Table 47.6 The Widmer classification of chronic venous insufficiency [1].

Classification	Symptom
I	Corona phlebectatica paraplantaris, mild oedema
II	Hyperpigmentation, lipodermatosclerosis (LDS), atrophie blanche, oedema, eczema
III	Healed or active ulcer

Table 47.7 The CEAP (Clinical status, Etiology, Anatomy, Pathophysiology) classification [2,3].

C Clinical status	E Etiology	A Anatomy	P Pathophysiology
C0 no visible disorder			
C1 telangiectases or reticular veins	Ec congenital	As superficial	Pr reflux
C2 varicose veins	Ep primary	Ap perforating	Po obstruction
C3 oedema	Es secondary (post-thrombotic)	Ad deep	Pr,o combination
C4a pigmentation, oedema	En no known venous etiology	An no known venous location	Pn no known venous pathophysiology
C4b lipo- et dermatosclerosis, white atrophy			
C5 healed ulcer			
C6 active, venous ulcer			
S symptomatic			
A asymptomatic			

Table 47.8 The VCSS (Venous Clinical Severity Score) classification of factors contributing to chronic venous insufficiency [4].

Attribute	Absent = 0	Mild = 1	Moderate = 2	Severe = 3
Pain	None	Occasional, not restricting activity or requiring analgesics	Daily, moderate activity limitation, occasional analgesics	Daily, severe limiting activities or requiring regular use of analgesics
Varicose veins	None	Few, scattered: branch varicose veins	Multiple: GSV varicose veins confined to calf or thigh	Extensive: thigh and calf or GSV and SSV distribution
Venous oedema	None	Evening ankle oedema only	Afternoon oedema, above ankle	Morning oedema above ankle and requiring activity change, elevation
Skin pigmentation	None or focal, low intensity (tan)	Diffuse, but limited in area and old (brown)	Diffuse over most of gaiter distribution (lower 1/3) or recent pigmentation (purple)	Wider distribution (above lower 1/3) and recent pigmentation
Inflammation	None	Mild cellulitis, limited to marginal area around ulcer	Moderate cellulitis, involves most of gaiter area (lower 1/3)	Entire lower third of leg or more
No. of active ulcers	0	1	>2	>2
Active ulceration, duration	None	<3 months	>3 months, <1 year	Not healed >1 year
Active ulcer, size	None	<2 cm diameter	2 to 6 cm diameter	>6 cm diameter
Compressive therapy	Not used or not compliant	Intermittent use of stockings	Wears stockings most days	Full compliance: stockings + elevation

GSV, greater saphenous vein; SSV, short saphenous vein.

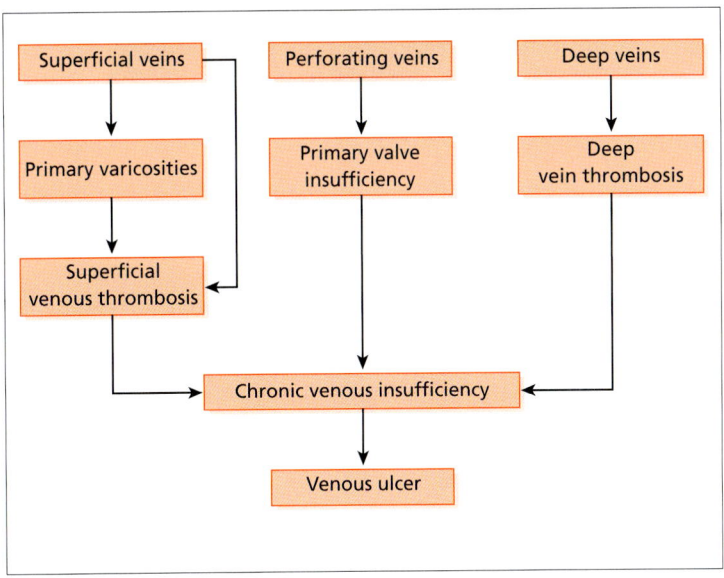

Fig. 47.19 Schematic presentation of the development of chronic venous insufficiency.

Reference

1 Mellor RH, Brice G, Stanton AW *et al*. Mutations in *FOXC2* are strongly associated with primary valve failure in veins of the lower limb. *Circulation* 2007; **115**: 1912–20.

Clinical signs of chronic venous insufficiency

Pitting oedema. Pitting oedema as a result of venous incompetence is worst at the end of the day and usually disappears at night. Patients may complain of a tight feeling in the oedematous leg and night cramps. The capillary filtration rate increases as a consequence of the increased ambulatory venous (and consequently capillary) pressure and overwhelms lymph drainage. This oedema always has a low protein content and pits easily, being mainly present around the ankle.

Corona phlebectatica paraplantaris (ankle flare). An ankle flare (the corona phlebectatica) is an early and important clinical sign of CVI and is a direct consequence of increased capillary pressure, which causes these vessels to expand.

Hyperpigmentation. Pigmentation in the 'gaiter skin' associated with CVI is invariably the result of haemosiderin accumulation after extravasation of erythrocytes (red cells). The pinpoint or patchy pigmentation may be minimal but may also extend over large indurated skin areas. In some cases pigmentation caused by melanin occurs as a secondary effect (post-inflammatory melanosis). Pigmentation begins modestly in the 'gaiter' area above the ankle and progresses to induration and inflammation, which indicates that lipodermatosclerosis has developed.

Pressure erythema. This is a direct result of elevated capillary pressure. Grouped, confluent, very small telangiectasiae develop. They are often found near incompetent perforating veins. Pressure erythema is often one of the first signs of evolving venous insufficiency.

primary valve failure or when the superficial veins become distended, causing the valves to become secondarily incompetent.

Perforating vein insufficiency. This is a rare condition in isolation, when it is caused by primary valve insufficiency. Secondary perforating vein insufficiency often occurs in combination with deep vein insufficiency (post-thrombotic limb).

Deep vein insufficiency. Reflux is the most common type of abnormality, but in about 10% of cases a functional obstruction from thrombosis (non-recanalized thrombosis) will be present, in which case it is likely to be associated with the post-thrombotic syndrome. Avalvulosis is rare unless associated with a mutation of the *FOXC2* gene [1].

Eczema. Several types can be recognized:

1 *Eczema as a result of venous disturbances* (synonyms: stasis dermatitis, hypostatic eczema, venous eczema, dermatitis veineuse). Usually this type of eczema starts round varicosities at the medial ankle, in the region of the Cockett perforating veins in the lower one-third of the leg. The eczema is relatively sharply demarcated and somewhat infiltrated with papules and vesicles, which may also extend beyond the main area of eczematous skin. Scaling and itching develops. Chronic lichenified eczema may develop with time. The aetiology is not completely clear. Homing of activated T-lymphocytes appears to be the most reasonable explanation.

2 *Allergic contact dermatitis.* This form of eczema is typically well demarcated but often with secondary involvement of adjacent or even distant non-contact sites. The most common sensitizing agents are locally applied drugs. Patch testing should be performed to exclude a contact allergic dermatitis. Patients with leg ulcers become more easily sensitized than healthy individuals [1,2], and therefore potential sensitizing agents should be avoided in these patients. Patients treated by MECS may develop an allergic contact dermatitis from the rubber constituents that provide elasticity, or from dyes that are used to give the stockings their colour.

3 *Asteatotic dermatitis* (synonym: eczema craquelé). Frequent washing may cause extreme dehydration of the skin. A morphologically similar eczema with a 'crazy paving' appearance occurs in some patients who develop rapid, lower leg oedema [3]. Patients who routinely wear MECS may develop an itching, dry and desquamating eczema. Application of a bland emollient at night will usually improve their symptoms.

4 *Impetiginization of eczematous dermatitis* (synonym: infected dermatitis). Wet eczema of the lower leg is often extensively colonized with bacteria, yeasts and fungi. Even after the infectious agent has been treated, an eczematous dermatitis may persist.

5 *Secondary spread ('id' eruption, 'autosensitization' eczema).* Varicose dermatitis and allergic contact dermatitis may cause secondary spread onto adjacent and distant non-contact sites. Itching may develop at any site including the palms and soles.

Lipodermatosclerosis (LDS). This is a specific skin disorder that is pathognomonic of venous and lymphatic hypertension. It is a consequence of an increased matrix turnover caused by a chronic inflammatory reaction in response to escaped plasma constituents. LDS is known to be associated with an increased risk of leg ulcer development [4]. As a rule, the skin and subcutaneous tissues feel hard on palpation. At an early stage LDS may feel a little indurated and often has an inflamed, erythematous appearance. It is also quite often tender and painful. It is often confused with erysipelas, superficial venous thrombosis or even deep-vein thrombosis. In long-standing LDS the skin surface becomes pigmented (Fig. 47.20). It is often found just above the medial malleolus, at the level of the Cockett perforating veins, which are usually incompetent, as is the great saphenous vein. When the small saphenous vein is incompetent, the lipodermatosclerosis often affects the lateral side of the calf. The most characteristic histological findings are dermal and subcutaneous fibrosis, with fat degeneration.

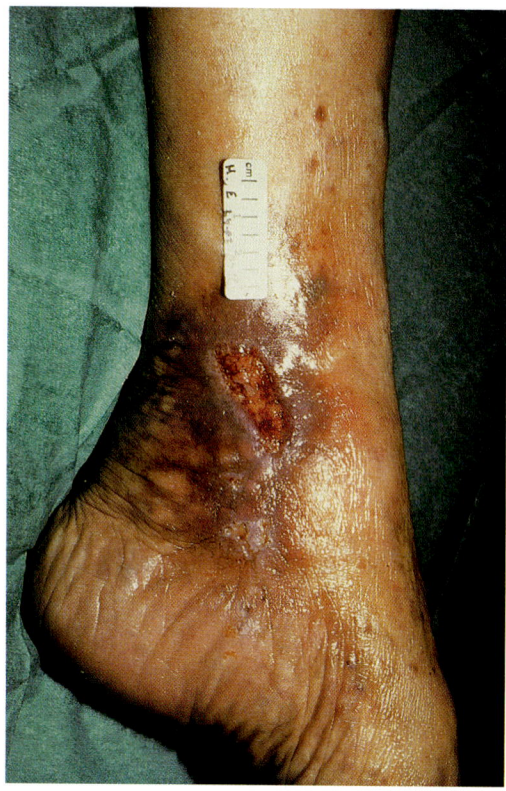

Fig. 47.20 A venous ulcer on the medial side of the leg surrounded by pigmented sclerotic skin (lipodermatosclerosis).

White atrophy (atrophie blanche). This is the result of decreased capillary density caused by microthrombi and matrix degradation causing hypoxia. White atrophy is seen as an atrophic, ivory-white, depressed skin lesion often located on the lower legs (Fig. 47.21). The lesions have a diameter that varies from 0.5 to 15 cm and are almost always multiple. The lesions often contain many centrally enlarged capillaries that are visible as red dots. White atrophy is characterized histologically by an atrophic epidermis and a thickened and scleroderma-like dermis with proliferative, dilated capillaries. One or more capillaries are often occluded with fibrinoid material [5]. White atrophy does not cause clinical symptoms, but the associated ulcers are very painful. White atrophy does not respond well to treatment but antiplatelet agents and fibrinolytic-enhancing drugs have been tried with some success. White atrophy may also be seen in association with other disorders including lupus erythematosus, scleroderma, vasculitides, cryoglobulinaemia, polycythaemia and leukaemia. Summer ulceration is an idiopathic form of white atrophy in which ulcers develop on legs that show no evidence of chronic venous disease. The pathogenesis is largely unknown. Probably, the capillaries occlude as a consequence of microthrombosis during the 'summer' months.

Livedoid vasculopathy (livedo vasculitis). Livedoid vasculopathy is an occlusive thrombotic disease that affects superficial small blood vessels of the lower extremities (see also p. 47.55 and Chapter 49).

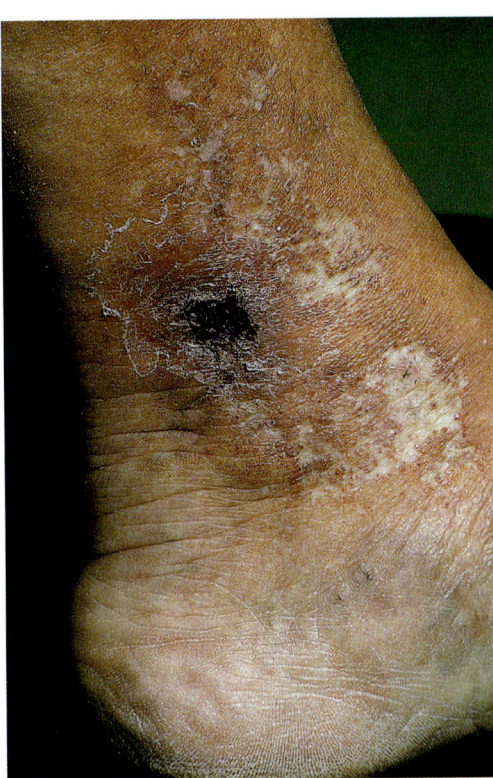

Fig. 47.21 Atrophie blanche: white scars with a central ischaemic ulcer and telangiectasia at the edge of the white areas.

Varicosities. Varicosities represent dilated and tortuous veins. In about the half of the patients CVI is the result of primary varicosities. In the 'post-thrombotic syndrome', venous hypertension often induces incompetence of the superficial venous system, and may lead to secondary varicosities [6].

Venous ulcer (ulcus cruris). This is an end stage of CVI.

Secondary (high output) lymphoedema. This may develop in patients with long-lasting CVI. Secondary lymphoedema develops when the previously healthy local lymphatic system fails in the face of an overwhelming filtration load, with eventual structural obliteration of lymphatic routes.

References
1 Malten LE, Kuiper JP, van der Staak WBJM. Contact allergic investigations in 100 patients with ulcus cruris. *Dermatologica* 1973; **147**: 241–5.
2 Perrenoud D, Ramelet AA. Chronic leg ulcers and eczema. *Curr Probl Dermatol* 1999; **27**: 165–9.
3 Bhushan M, Cox NH, Chalmers R. Eczema craquele due to oedema. *Br J Dermatol* 2001; **145**: 355–7.
4 Burnand KG, Whimster I, Naidoo A, Browse NL. Pericapillary fibrin in the ulcer-bearing skin of the leg: the cause of lipodermatosclerosis and venous ulceration. *BMJ* 1982; **285**: 1071–7.
5 Maessen-Visch MB, Koedam MI, Hamulyak K, Neumann HAM. Atrophie blanche, a review. *Int J Dermatol* 1999; **38**: 161–72.
6 Janssen MC, Haenen JH, Asten WN *et al.* Clinical and haemodynamic sequelae of deep venous thrombosis: retrospective evaluation after 7–13 years. *Clin Sci* 1997; **93**: 7–12.

Investigations of chronic venous insufficiency
Duplex ultrasound
Colour Doppler duplex ultrasound has become the first choice investigation for most venous problems. Duplex gives excellent information on venous anatomy and reflux. Reflux does not always indicate a functional defect, because muscle pump capacity can compensate for reflux. It is not easy to diagnose venous obstruction with Duplex scanning. Colour imaging allows the direction of flow to be clearly seen. Duplex ultrasound is very 'operator dependent' and requires considerable experience and a detailed knowledge of venous anatomy.

Technique. A 7.5-MHz high-frequency linear array transducer (probe) is usually satisfactory for venous examination. A probe of 7.5 to 13 MHz is appropriate to obtain good quality images of the superficial veins of the lower limbs. For very large or oedematous legs a curvilinear array transducer of 3.5 to 5 MHz may be useful [1].

Examination of the superficial veins should be performed with the patient standing erect as the detection of reflux and assessment of the vein diameter is inaccurate when the patient is supine. Both transverse and longitudinal views of the veins should be obtained. The investigation should be performed in a warm environment, to encourage venous dilatation.

When compression is applied distal to the probe antegrade (forward) flow is elicited. Reflux (backward or retrograde flow) may subsequently occur when the manual compression is abruptly released. This retrograde flow (reflux) is the result of gravity. A small amount of retrograde flow occurs in normal veins to produce valve closure. Venous reflux is considered to be normal when it lasts less than 0.5 s [2]. Reflux may be elicited by manual compression of varices, of the saphenous trunks or by squeezing the feet. It can also be stimulated by pneumatic calf cuff deflation [3], the Valsalva manoeuvre or by active foot dorsiflexion and relaxation.

Duplex ultrasound allows the communications between the deep and superficial veins to be directly assessed [4].

Indications. The most important indications for venous duplex are: (recurrent) varicose veins, signs of deep vein pathology, analyzing the veins of the popliteal fossa, analyzing the perforating veins, preoperative marking of varicose veins, assessing venous malformations, surveillance after treatment, duplex-guided sclerotherapy, evaluation before endovenous interventions, diagnosing (deep-vein) thrombosis and follow-up after treatment [2].

References
1 Coleridge-Smith P, Labropoulos N, Partsch H *et al*. Duplex ultrasound investigation of veins in chronic venous disease of the lower limbs—UIP consensus document. Part I. Basic principles. *Eur J Vasc Endovasc Surg* 2006; **31**: 83–92.
2 Lagatolla NR, Donald A, Lockhart S, Burnand K. Retrograde flow in the deep veins of subjects with normal venous function. *Br J Surg* 1997; **84**: 36–9.
3 van Bemmelen PS, Mattos MA, Hogdson KJ *et al*. Does air plethysmography correlate with duplex scanning in patients with chronic venous insufficiency? *J Vasc Surg* 1993; **18**: 796–807.
4 Ricci S, Georgiev M. Ultrasound anatomy of the superficial veins of the lower limb. *J Vasc Technol* 2002; **26**: 183–99.

Venous pressure measurement

At the beginning of the 20th century, Von Recklinghausen (1906) measured the venous pressure, followed by Roulson (1911) and Beecher (1936) [1]. The technique that is still used, and remains the gold standard for investigation of venous hypertension, was introduced in 1925 by Barber and Shatara [2], who demonstrated that venous pressure decreases during calf movement. The venous pressure drop during walking is less in patients with varicosities than in healthy individuals [3,4]. Arnoldi demonstrated that the pressure in the superficial venous system and the deep venous system was similar [4]. A correlation exists between calf muscle function and venous pressure [5].

Technique. A vein in the foot is cannulated and the patient stands on tiptoe 10 times. The venous pressure drops and the pressure drop is measured. This is defined as the ambulatory venous pressure. The patient stands still until the pressure returns; the time taken for the pressure to return is defined as the venous refill time.

Interpretation. The venous pressure is between 5 and 10 mmHg in the supine position. During standing the venous pressure is defined by the hydrostatic pressure being dependent on the subject's height. The distance between the right atrium and the puncture location determine the standing venous pressure. This value is between 80 and 100 mmHg in the average European. During the exercise, the pressure should drop to below 40 mmHg (or reach at least 50% of the standing venous pressure). Healthy individuals usually reach an ambulant venous pressure of around 20 mmHg, with a venous refill time of over 25 s.

References

1 Beecher HK, Field ME, Krogh A. Effect of walking on venous pressure at the ankle. *Skand Arch Physiol* 1936; **73**: 133–9.
2 Barber RF, Shatara FI. The varicose disease. *NY State J Med* 1925; **31**: 574–80.
3 Pollack AA, Wood EH. Venous pressure in the saphenous vein in ankle in men during exercise and changes in posture. *J Appl Physiol* 1949; **1**: 649–53.
4 Arnoldi CC. Venous pressure: the function of the venous pump in chronic venous insufficiency. *J Cardiovasc Surg (Torino)* 1961; **2**: 116–27.
5 Kuiper JP. Venous pressure determination (direct method). *Dermatologica* 1966; **132**: 206–17.

Plethysmography

Plethysmography records volume changes in the limb. It was first described by Brodie and Russel in 1905 [1].

Photoplethysmography. Photoplethysmography (PPG) is the most commonly used non-invasive technique. Hertzman in 1938 [2] was the first to describe a photoelectric plethysmographic method of measuring the skin circulation. The intensity of light reflected from the skin red cells correlated with the blood volume in the skin [3]. Venous refill time after a standardized exercise is obtained with the PPG. The venous refill time should not be confused with venous pressure, although there is a relationship between the two [4]. Bays *et al.* found a positive predictive value of venous refill time examined with PPG of 77% and a negative predictive value of 100% [5].

References

1 Brodie TG, Russel AE. On the determination of the rate of blood flow through an organ. *J Physiol* 1905; **32**: 47.
2 Hertzman AB. The blood supply of various skin areas as estimated by the photoelectric plethysmography. *Am J Physiol* 1938; **124**: 328–40.
3 Abramowitz HB, Queral LA, Flinn WR. The use of photoplethysmography in the assessment of venous insufficiency. A comparison to venous pressure measurements. *Surgery* 1979; **86**: 434–41.
4 Wienert V, Blazek V. New method for non-invasive measurement of venous pressure. *Hautarzt* 1982; **33**: 498–9.
5 Bays RA, Healy DA, Atnip RG, Neumyer M, Thiele BL. Validation of air plethysmography, photoplethysmography, and duplex ultrasonography in the evaluation of severe venous stasis. *J Vasc Surg* 1994; **20**: 721–7.

Light reflection rheography and digital photopleuthysmography. The technique of light-reflection rheography (LRR) is based on the technique of PPG and was developed by Wienert and Blazek in the 1980s [1]. Digital photoplethysmography (DPPG) is a further development of LRR (second generation LRR) [2]. The results of LRR and DPPG have been compared and show a high degree of correlation, particularly in patients with venous disorders [3,4]. The correlation from LRR to ambulatory venous pressure is 0.73 for venous return and 0.93 for expelled volume [5].

References

1 Wienert V, Blazek V. Eine neue Methode zur unblutigen dynamischen Venendruckmessung. *Hautarzt* 1982; **33**: 498–9.
2 Blazek V, Schmitt HJ, Schultz-Ehrenberg U. Digitale Photoplethysmographie: Ein neues mikroprozessorgesteuertes Messsystem für die Beinvenendiagnostik. *Biomed Tch* 1988; **33**: 307–8.
3 Kerner J, Schultz-Ehrenberg U, Blazek V. Digitale Photoplethysmographie (D-PPG)—klinische Eignung der neuen Messmethode zur venosen Funktionsdiagnostik. *Phlebol Proktol* 1989; **18**: 98–103.
4 Veraart JCJM, van der Kley AMJ, Neumann HAM. Digital photoplethysmography and light reflection rheography. *J Dermatol Surg Oncol* 1994; **20**: 470–3.
5 O'Donnell TF, McEnroe CS, Heggerick P. Chronic venous insufficiency. *Surg Clin North Am* 1990; **70**: 159–80.

Phlebography

Water-soluble contrast media have lowered the risk of causing DVT to nearly zero.

Ascending phlebography. The objective of the examination is to visualize the deep venous system from the foot to the lower inferior vena cava. Contrast injected into a foot vein is driven into the deep veins by an ankle tourniquet.

Varicography. This is a variant of ascending phlebography. Varicography is performed by directly injecting contrast into a varicose vein or veins. It determines the route of 'drainage' from the varicose veins through communicating veins in the deep venous system and defines the anatomical extent of the varicosities [1]. It indicates the major point of the origin of the reflux, and is very useful for investigating patients with recurrent varicose veins.

Descending phlebography. This has nowadays been replaced by duplex ultrasound.

Reference

1 Lea Thomas M, ed. *Phlebography of the Lower Limbs*. New York: Churchill Livingstone, 1982.

Varicose veins

Synonym
• Venous varicosity

This is the name given when there is visible, tortuous elongation and dilatation of the larger superficial venous trunks and their tributaries. Leg varicosities seldom develop before adolescence in women. Other types of venous dilatation are often incorrectly included within the category of 'varicose veins'. Capillary telangiectasias (diameter 0.1–0.4 mm) are predominantly red and intradermal. The colour of telangiectasias depends upon the calibre of the dilated venule; large dilatations are dark blue and often palpable (although still less than 1 mm in diameter). Reticular varicose veins are subcutaneous (2–4 mm in diameter) and arise from a blue leash of small veins.

Prevalence. The prevalence of varicose veins in the Western population is estimated to be between 10 and 50% although the higher figure is of dubious validity. The prevalence of varicose veins increases with age. By 20 years it is 10%; by the age of 40 years it is 40% in women and 25% in men, and varicose veins are present in about 70% of 80-year-old women and 60% of 80-year-old men. Women that give birth to several children have an increased risk of developing varicose veins [1]. A population-based cross-sectional survey in Germany of 3072 participants found that the prevalence of varicose veins was twice as high in an urban population as in a rural population [2].

Classification. Varicose veins are either primary or secondary.

Primary varicose veins have no obvious underlying cause. The superficial veins dilate and become tortuous with an associated valvular incompetence. The mechanisms for these changes are still not clearly defined. Biochemical abnormalities in the vein wall, genetic predisposition and haemodynamic factors may all affect the development of varicose veins. Haemodynamic changes do not seem to be of major importance in reticular and branch varicosities. Disorders of the endothelium and the extracellular matrix may account for the development of these minor varicosities. The recent report of venous reflux in 100% of patients with mutations in the *FOXC2* gene strongly suggests that at least some forms of varicose veins have a genetic basis which is the result of primary venous valve failure [3]. Similarly, the presence of varicose veins in congenital syndromes such as Klippel–Trenaunay syndrome indicate a genetic basis, although the fault may be in the vein wall as much as the valve.

Secondary varicose veins are the result of raised endoluminal venous pressure (venous hypertension) for which post-thrombotic damage is the most important cause. The deep venous system should be evaluated in all patients in whom secondary varicose veins are suspected to avoid operating on surface veins unnecessarily when prescription of elastic support stockings would be preferable.

References
1 Krijnen RMA, de Boer EM, Bruyunzeel DP. Epidemiology of venous disorders in the general and occupational population. *Epidemiol Rev* 1997; **19**: 294–309.

2 Rabe E, Pannier-Fischer F, Bromen K *et al*. Bonner Venenstudie der Deutschen Gesellschaft für Phlebologie—epidemiologische Untersuchung zur Frage der Häufigkeit und Ausprägung von chronischen Venenkrankheiten in der städtischen und ländlichen Wohnbevölkerung. *Phlebologie* 2003; **32**: 1–14.
3 Mellor RH, Brice G, Stanton AW *et al*. Mutations in *FOXC2* are strongly associated with primary valve failure in veins of the lower limb. *Circulation* 2007; **115**: 1912–20.

Clinical features. Varicose veins may be a purely cosmetic problem but many patients also complain of aching pain, which tends to be worse on prolonged standing at the end of the day, and which is relieved by leg elevation or compression. Symptoms such as itching, ankle swelling, and ultimately the development of lipodermatosclerosis or ulceration indicate haemodynamic failure and the need for investigation.

Complications of varicose veins, such as haemorrhage and thrombophlebitis, result from the varicose veins themselves whereas oedema, haemosiderin pigmentation, varicose eczema, atrophie blanche, lipodermatosclerosis and venous ulceration result from venous hypertension.

Diagnosis. Colour duplex Doppler ultrasound scanning is increasingly being used to investigate all patients with varicose veins, and is the investigation of choice for detecting deep-vein reflux. Duplex scanning is also essential to investigate patients with skin changes attributed to venous hypertension. There is some evidence that the incidence of recurrent varicose veins is lower after duplex assessment has been used to plan surgery.

Treatment of truncal varicose veins. The recognition of the skin changes which are associated with varicose veins is important because of the likely risk of progression to venous ulceration. Causes of secondary varicose veins should be sought, including DVT and intra-abdominal pathology.

Only varicose veins (superficial venous reflux) that are associated with cutaneous complications demand treatment. Many patients, especially women, present for treatment of varicose veins or telangiectases for cosmetic reasons. At present there is no means of assessing which limbs will progress to develop chronic venous insufficiency.

Several types of treatment for varicose veins are discussed [1–7] and the most common complications of these treatments are shown in Table 47.9.

References
1 Munavalli GS, Weiss RA. Complications of sclerotherapy. *Semin Cutan Med Surg* 2007; **26**: 22–8.
2 van den Bos R, Arends L, Kockaert M *et al*. Endovenous therapies of lower extremity varicosities: a meta-analysis. *J Vasc Surg* 2009; **49**: 230–9.
3 Iafrati MD. Subfascial endoscopic perforator vein surgery. *Semin Cutan Med Surg* 2005; **24**: 209–15.
4 De Roos KP, Nieman FHM, Neumann HAM. Ambulatory phlebectomy versus compression sclerotherapy: results of a randomized controlled trial. *Dermatol Surg* 2003; **29**: 221–6.
5 van den Bos RR, Kockaert MA, Neumann HAM, Nijsten T. Technical review of endovenous laser therapy for varicose veins. *Eur J Vasc Endovasc Surg* 2008; **35**: 88–95.
6 Mussa FF, Peden EK, Zhou W, Lin PH *et al*. Iliac vein stenting for chronic venous insufficiency. *Tex Heart Inst J* 2007; **34**: 60–6.
7 Apfelberg DB, Smith T, Maser MR. Study of three laser systems for treatment of superficial varicosities of the lower extremity. *Lasers Surg Med* 1987; **7**: 219–23.

Table 47.9 Important complications of the treatment of varicose veins [1–7].

Treatment	Complications
Sclerotherapy	Skin necrosis, hyperpigmentation, DVT (rare), superficial venous thrombosis, arterial thrombosis (very rare), allergic reactions [1]
Surgical therapy	
Stripping	Nerve damage, haematoma, infection, DVT, lymphocele, hypertrophic scarring, lymphoedema
SEPS	DVT, haematoma [2]
Phlebectomy	DVT, neuralgia, haematoma, infection [3]
	Haematoma, phlebitis [4]
Endovascular treatment	
Laser	Vein perforation, DVT, ecchymoses, skin burns, superficial venous thrombosis [5]
Foam sclerosant	DVT, allergic reactions, stroke, transient blindness
Stenting	Thrombosis [6]
Lasers	
IPLS	(Temporary) hyperpigmentation [7]
Nd : YAG	(Temporary) hyperpigmentation, scar formation [7]

DVT, deep vein thrombosis. IPLS, intense pulsed light source. SEPS, subfascial endoscopic perforator surgery.

Sclerotherapy

Sclero (compression) therapy is indicated for leg telangiectasias (thread veins), reticular veins, minor tributary veins, varicosities, and recurrent varicose veins following surgery (see Telangiectasia, p. 47.20). The aim of treatment is to obliterate the lumen of the injected veins. The most frequently used sclerosants are sodium tetradecyl sulphate (STD), polidocanol (aethoxysclerol), 23.4% saline, and a combination of 25% dextrose with 10% saline [1]. Several randomized controlled trials have shown that sclerosant choice, dose, local pressure dressing, degree and length of compression have no significant effect on the efficacy of sclerotherapy for varicose veins [2].

References

1 Zimmet SE. Sclerotherapy treatment of telangiectasias and varicose veins. *Tech Vasc Interv Radiol* 2003; **6**: 116–20.
2 Tisi PV, Beverley C, Rees A. Injection sclerotherapy for varicose veins. *Cochrane Database Syst Rev* 2006; **4**: CD001732.

Compression therapy

Graduated elastic compression stockings are classified by the European Standardization Commission into four categories, which have different uses [1,2]:
Class I, 15–21 mmHg: thrombosis prophylaxis
Class II, 23–32 mmHg: mild/moderate oedema, mild CVI, after sclerotherapy, pregnancy
Class III, 34–46 mmHg: severe CVI, severe oedema, lymphoedema, post-thrombotic syndrome
Class IV, >46 mmHg: severe lymphoedema.

Class II or III should be chosen, depending on the severity of the venous hypertension. It is of the utmost importance that stockings are carefully fitted and that patients are instructed about how to put them on and take them off. An applicator may need to be purchased. Hosiery is not usually worn overnight, but this may be ignored if patients find stockings difficult to apply. At least two pairs of stockings should be provided, to allow for daily changing and washing. Washing is necessary to retain the elastic property of Lycra-containing hosiery. Two stockings per leg should last 6 months before compression is lost and replacements are required [3]. Patients should be encouraged to wear elastic compression stockings for the rest of their lives. A healthy lifestyle with regular daily exercise, for example walking, and maintaining an ideal weight is to be encouraged.

Stockings can be below-knee (A–D stockings), thigh length (also named A–F), or tights. Graduated compression stockings may improve the short-term haemodynamics in patients with varicose veins, thereby relieving symptoms [4,5]. There are no data on their long-term benefits. Wearing class II stockings may reduce venous reflux but they do not appear to prevent the development of superficial varicose veins [6]. Wearing class II below-knee stockings is an alternative treatment for patients with severe varicose veins who do not wish to have invasive treatment.

References

1 Neumann HAM. Compression therapy with medical elastic compression stockings for venous diseases. *Dermatol Surg* 1998; **24**: 765–70.
2 Comité European de Normalisation, adopted European prestandard. *Medical Compression Hosiery*. ENV 12718. Brussels: Comité Européen de Normalisation, 2001.
3 Veraart JC, Daamen E, de Vet HC *et al*. Elastic compression stockings: durability of pressure in daily practice. *Vasa* 1997; **26**: 282–6.
4 Anderson JA *et al*. Paroven and graduated compression hosiery for superficial venous insufficiency. *Phlebology* 1990; **5**: 271–6.
5 Labropoulos N, Leon M, Volteas N, Nicolaides AN. Acute and long-term effects of elastic stockings in patients with varicose veins. *Int Angiol* 1994; **13**: 119–23.
6 Thaler E, Huch R, Huch A, Zimmermann R. Compression stockings prophylaxis of emergent varicose veins in pregnancy: a prospective randomised controlled study. *Swiss Med Wkly* 2001; **131**: 659–62.

Surgical therapy

Venous surgery is potentially curative for refluxing superficial veins when the deep veins are competent. Conversely, surgery should be avoided in patients in whom the superficial veins may be acting as collaterals, which are the major route for venous return, in a severely post-thrombotic limb.

Flush ligation and stripping. For more than 100 years saphenous incompetence has been treated by flush ligation and stripping [1]. Although the technique varies, the results are the same. Most surgeons no longer strip the great saphenous vein (GSV) to the ankle. Damage to the saphenous nerve is avoided if the vein is stripped to the knee The short strip appears to be as effective as the long strip, but it does not influence the venous haemodynamics in the lower leg. Veins in the calf can be subsequently treated with foam sclerotherapy [2]. The results of surgical stripping are slightly disappointing, with a success rate of only 79.7% 1 year after treatment [3]. The recurrence of varicose veins is often the result of neovascularization, which will occur in 20 to 30% [4]. However, high saphenous ligation with stripping of the GSV remains the most commonly performed intervention for varicose veins in the world.

Ligation and stripping of the short saphenous vein (SSV) is technically more demanding than stripping of the GSV, which explains why more and more incompetent SSVs are treated by endovenous techniques or by foam sclerotherapy.

References
1 Keller WL. A new method of extirpating the internal saphenous and similar veins in varicose conditions: a preliminary report. *NY Med J* 1905; **82**: 385–6.
2 Ceulen RPM, Kessels A, Veraart JCJM, van Neer PAFA. Lateral venous ulceration and incompetence of the small saphenous vein. *Dermatol Surg* 2007; **33**: 727–30.
3 van den Bos R, Arends L, Kockaert M *et al*. Endovenous therapies of lower extremity varicosities: a meta-analysis. *J Vasc Surg* 2009; **49**: 230–9.
4 De Maeseneer MG, Van Schil PE, Philippe MM *et al*. Is recurrence of varicose veins after surgery unavoidable? *Acta Chir Belg* 1995; **95**: 21–6.

Subfascial endoscopic perforator surgery (SEPS). Incompetent perforating veins of the lower limb have been correlated with leg ulceration. Linton's and Cockett's operations to ligate these veins became discredited partly because the post-operative complication rate was high [1], and there was little evidence that this form of surgery was efficacious in preventing recurrent ulceration. A minimally invasive approach (SEPS) was introduced by Hauer in 1985 [2], but in a prospective randomized controlled trial Van Gent *et al.* showed that this procedure did not prevent recurrent venous ulceration [3].

References
1 Kalra M, Gloviczki P. Subfascial endoscopic perforator vein surgery: who benefits? *Semin Vasc Surg* 2002; **15**: 39–49.
2 Hauer G. The endoscopic subfascial division of the perforating veins—preliminary report. *Vasa* 1985; **14**: 59–61.
3 Van Gent WB, Hop WC, Van Praag MC *et al*. Conservative versus surgical treatment of venous leg ulcers: a prospective, randomized, multicenter trial. *J Vasc Surg* 2006; **44**: 563–71.

Phlebectomy (Muller technique). Removing tributary veins through small incisions has been around for many years, but in 1966 Robert Muller re-described a minimal invasive surgical technique [1]. He used stab avulsions (microincisions) and fine hooks to extract the varicose vein tributaries. This technique is time-consuming but gives excellent cosmetic results. This means of treating varicose tributaries is significantly better than sclerotherapy [2].

References
1 Muller R. Traitement des varices par la phlébectomie ambulatoire. *Phlébologie* 1966; **19**: 277–9.
2 De Roos KP, Nieman FH, Neumann HAM. Ambulatory phlebectomy versus compression sclerotherapy: results of a randomized controlled trial. *Dermatol Surg* 2003; **29**: 221–6.

Endovascular treatment [1,2]
Endovascular treatments do not disconnect the GSV from the femoral vein, which may explain the absence of neovascularization. Endovascular laser treatment (EVLT) was introduced in the late 1990s and has become tremendously popular, especially for the treatment of GSV incompetence. Radiofrequency ablation (RFA) is probably equivalent to EVLT and both types of endovenous treatment appear to have early benefits in pain and return to work. The wavelengths of the laser can be varied in absorption spectra of haemoglobin (e.g. 840 or 940 nm) or water (1320 or 1499 nm). It is not yet known which is the best wavelength. Damage to the vein wall and surrounding tissues may lead to pain and pigmentation.

References
1 van den Bos R, Arends L, Kockaert M *et al*. Endovenous therapies of lower extremity varicosities: a meta-analysis and meta-regression of case series and randomized clinical trials. *J Vasc Surg* 2009; **49**: 230–9.
2 Van den Bos RR, Kockaert MA, Neumann HAM, Nijsten T. Technical review of endovenous laser therapy for varicose veins. *Eur J Vasc Endovasc Surg* 2008; **35**: 88–95.

Foam sclerosant treatment. Tessari introduced a technique in which air and a sclerosing agent are mixed [1]. Both polidocanol and sodium tetradecyl sulphate (STD) are detergents, and mixing them with air results in a firm foam. This foam is stable for a couple of minutes and can be injected directly into the vein under Duplex imaging. The foam allows this to be visualized [2]. This is now being used to obliterate saphenous systems. Comparisons against other techniques are, however, essential.

References
1 Tessari L, Cavezzi A, Frullini A. Preliminary experience with a new sclerosing foam in the treatment of varicose veins. *Dermatol Surg* 2001; **27**: 58–60.
2 O'Hare JL, Earnshaw JJ. The use of foam sclerotherapy for varicose veins: a survey of the members of the Vascular Society of Great Britain and Ireland. *Eur J Vasc Endovasc Surg* 2007; **34**: 232–5.

Stenting. A small group of patients with post-thrombotic syndrome may benefit from this treatment when the iliac vein compression syndrome is present [1,2].

References
1 Neglén P, Berry MA, Raju S. Endovascular surgery in the treatment of chronic primary and post-thrombotic iliac vein obstruction. *Eur J Vasc Endovasc Surg* 2000; **20**: 560–71.
2 Neglén P, Raju S. Proximal lower extremity chronic venous outflow obstruction: recognition and treatment. *J Vasc Surg* 2002; **15**: 57–64.

Lasers for treatment of cosmetic reticular veins and venous telangiectasia. The neodymium : YAG laser (1064 nm, long pulses >40 msec, high energy system) or an intense pulsed light source (IPLS) may be used to treat reticular veins or telangiectases (Fig. 47.22). Several studies have shown that IPLS is more effective in the treatment of veins with a diameter up to 1 mm, while 1064 nm Nd:YAG is more effective in veins from 1 to 4 mm in diameter [1–3].

References
1 Schroeter CA, Wilder D, Reineke T *et al*. Clinical significance of an Intense Pulsed Light Source on leg telangiectasias of up to 1 mm diameter. *Eur J Dermatol* 1997; **7**: 38–42.
2 Sadick NS. A dual wavelength approach for laser/intense pulsed light source treatment of lower extremity veins. *J Am Acad Dermatol* 2002; **46**: 66–72.
3 Fodor L, Ramon Y, Fodor A *et al*. A side-by-side prospective study of intense pulsed light and Nd: YAG laser treatment for vascular lesions. *Ann Plast Surg* 2006; **56**: 164–70.

Pharmacological treatment. There is little to no place for drugs in treating varicose veins, although some drugs may relieve the symptoms of chronic venous insufficiency [1]. Rutoside

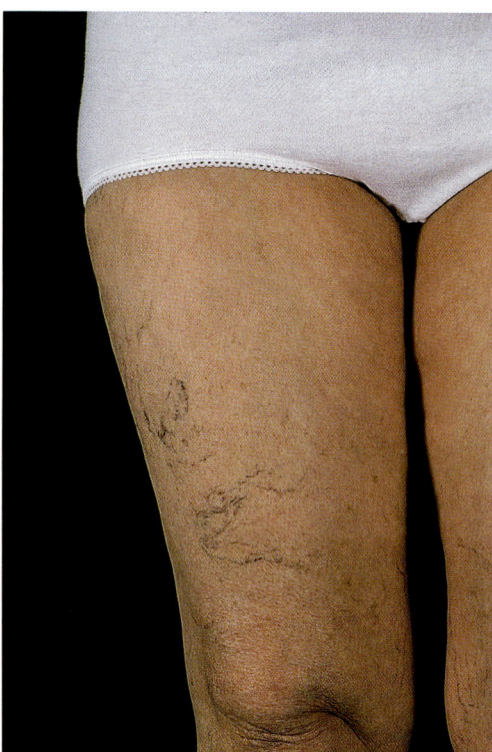

Fig. 47.22 'Sunburst veins'.

derivatives diminish capillary filtration rate and may improve aching pain, although there is a marked placebo effect [2].

References

1 Martinez MJ, Bonfill X, Moreno RM, Vargas E, Capellà D. Phlebotonics for venous insufficiency. *Cochrane Database Syst Rev* 2005; CD003229.
2 Pulvertaft TB. General practice treatment of symptoms of venous insufficiency with oxerutins. Results of a 660 patients multicentre study in the UK. *Vasa* 1983; **12**: 373–6.

Post-thrombotic syndrome

Synonym
• Post-phlebitic syndrome

Definition. The post-thrombotic syndrome (PTS) is a chronic condition of the deep venous system in patients with a documented history of deep-vein thrombosis (DVT) [1].

Incidence. DVT has an annual incidence of 0.2% and about one-third of affected patients develop PTS within 5 years [2,3]. The incidence of PTS is about 10% 1 year after an episode of DVT, and increases to about 50% over a period of 5 to 8 years. The only clear, identified risk factor is recurrent DVT, which increases the risk of PTS as much as six-fold [4].

Pathophysiology. Venous hypertension plays a key role in the pathophysiology of PTS [1,5] and is the result of valvular incompetence, outflow obstruction and dysfunction of the calf muscle pump. After the initial thrombosis, resolution of the thrombus

may start but propagation of the thrombus can also occur. The two processes can also occur simultaneously.

Loss of valve function leads to overloading of the venous system, which in turn leads to dilatation of the veins and to an increase in the venous volume. If this surpasses the capacity of the calf muscle pump, ambulatory venous hypertension results; this in turn causes further distension of the veins, leading to more valvular incompetence and the development of secondary varicose veins. When there is residual venous obstruction, the venous resistance and the venous pressure increases, which also leads to an increase in venous volume. In general, reflux causes more problems if it occurs in the distal part of the venous system and obstruction causes more problems when it occurs proximally.

Clinical features. The clinical symptoms of PTS are similar to those of CVI. They are, however, often more pronounced but may vary considerably from scarcely visible skin changes to pigmentation, lipodermatosclerosis, venous dilatation, oedema and ulceration. In the early stages of PTS, clinical signs do not correlate with the severity of disturbed venous haemodynamics [1]. Patients experience pain, heaviness, swelling, cramps, itching or tingling in the affected limb. Symptoms may be present in various combinations and may be persistent or intermittent. Typically, symptoms are aggravated by standing or walking and improve with rest and leg elevation, particularly lying down [4,6].

Diagnosis. The severity of PTS is often scored by the Villalta–Prandoni scale [7], which combines objective and subjective assessments. The simple Widmer score is also useful for PTS [8]. Duplex ultrasound provides information on reflux in both the deep and superficial venous systems. Non- or partially recanalized veins can usually be detected using this technique, although considerable interobserver variability is present. Phlebography is still necessary when the duplex scan is equivocal or direct deep venous surgery is being considered.

The range of movement in the ankle and knee joints should be tested because impaired movement in the lower leg reduces the effectiveness of the calf muscle pump [1].

Treatment. Prevention is an important part of treatment. Patients diagnosed with a DVT should be treated with a LMWH and oral anticoagulants. Once the oedema has settled, class II graduated elastic compression stockings are prescribed [3,9]. Patients should be reviewed annually after a DVT. A stent [10] or a Palma procedure [11] can be considered when there is evidence of venous obstruction. Graduated compression stockings should be worn for life.

References

1 Wentel TD, Neumann HAM. Management of the postthrombotic syndrome: the Rotterdam approach. *Semin Thromb Hemost* 2006; **32**: 814–21.
2 Kolbach DN, Sandbrink MWC, Neumann HAM, Prins MH. Compression therapy for treating stage I and II (Widmer) post-thrombotic syndrome. *Cochrane Database Syst Rev* 2003; **4**: CD004177.
3 Kolbach DN, Sandbrink MWC, Hamulyak K *et al.* Non-pharmaceutical management for prevention of post-thrombotic syndrome. *Cochrane Database Syst Rev* 2004; **1**: CD004174.
4 Kahn SR. The post-thrombotic syndrome: The forgotten morbidity of deep venous thrombosis. *J Thromb Thrombolysis* 2006; **21**: 41–8.

5 Neumann HAM, Veraart JCJM. Morphological and functional skin changes in postthrombotic syndrome. *Wien Med Wschr* 1994; **144**: 204–6.

6 Kahn SR. The post-thrombotic syndrome: progress and pitfalls. *Br J Haematol* 2006; **134**: 357–65.

7 Villalta S, Bagatella P, Piccioli A *et al.* Assessment of validity and reproducibility of a clinical scale for the post-thrombotic syndrome. *Haemostasis* 1994; **24** (Suppl. 1): 57a (abstract).

8 Kolbach DN, Neumann HAM, Prins MH. Definition of the post-thrombotic syndrome, differences between existing classifications. *Eur J Vasc Endovasc Surg* 2005; **30**: 404–14.

9 Prandoni P, Lensing AWA, Prins MH *et al.* Below-knee elastic compression stockings to prevent the post-thrombotic syndrome. A randomized controlled trial. *Ann Intern Med* 2004; **141**: 249–56.

10 Neglén P, Raju S. Proximal lower extremity chronic venous outflow obstruction: recognition and treatment. *Semin Vasc Surg* 2002; **15**: 57–64.

11 Palma EC, Esperon R. Vein transplants and grafts in the surgical treatment of the postphlebitic syndrome. *J Cardiovasc Surg* 1960; **1**: 94–107.

Deep vein incompetence

Secondary venous incompetence

All patients with varicose veins should have a colour Doppler duplex ultrasound of their deep venous system. DVT often permanently damages deep veins and their valves leading to deep vein incompetence with the superficial veins then acting as collateral drainage routes; for example, when the popliteal vein is occluded the superficial veins are the major outflow tracts from the limb. Because superficial varicose veins serve as necessary collateral drainage in these circumstances, surgery to ablate varicose veins is contraindicated and graduated compression stockings should be worn instead.

Primary deep vein incompetence

Congenital absence of venous valves is extremely rare [1]. It can affect only the lower limb veins or the whole body. Kistner has described a group of patients with floppy valves [2]. This abnormality is an enlarged valve cusp with a long, free edge that allows the cusp to prolapse when subjected to retrograde flow. Whether this is a congenital or an acquired abnormality is not known.

Mutations in the *FOXC2* gene, the cause of lymphoedema–distichiasis syndrome, has been shown to cause deep venous reflux in one-third of cases [3].

References

1 Basmajian JW. The distribution of valves in the femoral, external iliac and common iliac vein and their relationship to varicose veins. *Surg Gynec Obstet* 1952; **95**: 537.

2 Kistner RL. Surgical repair of the incompetent femoral vein valve. *Arch Surg* 1975; **110**: 1336.

3 Mellor RH, Brice G, Stanton AW *et al.* Mutations in *FOXC2* are strongly associated with primary valve failure in veins of the lower limb. *Circulation* 2007; **115**: 1912–20.

Leg ulcers

Leg ulceration

Definitions and epidemiology. Leg ulcers represent a break of the skin, sometimes extending through the dermis or deeper. Causes are listed in Table 47.10. A chronic ulcer is defined as one

Table 47.10 Causes of lower limb ulceration.

Venous hypertension	Varicose veins, deep-vein thrombosis, venous obstruction, congenital vascular malformations, Klippel–Trenaunay syndrome
Arterial disease	Atherosclerosis, diabetes, hypertension, embolism, calcific uraemic arteriolopathy (calciphylaxis)
Skin cancer	Basal and squamous cell carcinoma, melanoma or any fungating tumour
Vasculitis	Connective tissue diseases, e.g. systemic lupus erythematosus, rheumatoid disease, progressive systemic sclerosis, necrotizing leukocytoclastic vasculitis, ANCA-associated disorders, polyarteritis nodosa
	Livedoid vasculopathy, cryoglobulinaemia
Haematological disorders	Coagulation states, e.g. factor V Leiden, protein S or C deficiency, hyperhomocysteinaemia, antithrombin III deficiency, sickle cell disease, thalassaemia, spherocytosis, antiphospholipid syndrome, myeloproliferative disorders, e.g. polycythaemia rubra vera, thrombocythaemia
Emboli	Cholesterol, platelets, tumour cells, infective
Loss of sensation	Leprosy, diabetes, spina bifida
Infections	Diabetes, osteomyelitis, Buruli ulcer, fungal infections, syphilis, mycobacteria, leishmaniasis, acute 'desert' sore, necrotizing fasciitis and cellulitis
Trauma	Physical, e.g. pressure sore, chemical or thermal (e.g. burns or cold injury)
	Self-harm
	Intravenous drug use
Drugs/therapy	Radiation
	Hydroxycarbamide, ergotamine
	Iododerma
Skin conditions	Pyoderma gangrenosum
	Necrobiosis lipoidica
	Scleroderma
	Graft-versus-host disease
	Blistering disorders (e.g. pemphigoid)
	Bites and stings: insects, snake, scorpion
Genetic	Prolidase deficiency
	Klinefelter's syndrome

lasting more than 6 weeks [1]. Healed and active ulcers of the lower limb affect 1% of the adult population and 3.6% of people older than 65 years [2]. The main causes are venous hypertension, arterial disease and diabetes, but many factors may contribute (Table 47.10). Venous disease is the single most common cause, but gravitational and venous influences may contribute to the development of other pathologies in the lower leg (e.g. vasculitis).

Venous ulceration of the leg [3,4]

Definition. Ulceration of the lower leg occurring as the result of persistently elevated venous pressure and its secondary effects on the microvascular system. Nearly half of all venous ulcers are associated with deep-vein valvular incompetence or post-thrombotic damage, while the remainder result from incompetence of the superficial or communicating veins.

Epidemiology [5–7]. Community surveys suggest an overall incidence of about 0.2% [5]. It is an age-related disease, mainly affecting older women. Women are two to three times more often affected than men; 2% of all those over the age of 80 years suffer with ulceration. About half of the ulcers heal within 4 months but approximately 20% have not healed after 1 year and about 8% have not healed after 5 years. The annual recurrence rate is 6 to 15% and most ulcers recur more than once.

Venous ulceration is a common disease of all Western communities [7]. It appears to be associated with a sedentary and physiologically unnatural mode of life and is comparatively rare in African people, although the incidence may be underrated [8–10].

A study of 4422 healthy working adults in Basle found 'chronic venous insufficiency' in 19% of men and in 25% of women [11]. Ulceration was present in 1.1 and 1.4%, respectively. Figures from other surveys are similar. It has been emphasized that up to one-third of ulcers in elderly people have coexisting arterial insufficiency as one factor contributing to their failure to heal. A family history of leg ulcers is found in over half of those affected [12]; this applies about equally to those who have suffered a known thrombosis and to those who have not. The significance of this is not known, although inheritance of coagulation defects may be one factor.

Venous disease accounts for 1–2% of the health-care budgets of European countries [13].

Pathogenesis. Venous ulcers are the end result of superficial venous insufficiency or the post-thrombotic syndrome (PTS) described above. The consequent ambulatory venous hypertension causes alterations in the microvasculature and interstitium which make the skin more liable to break down, or to fail to repair, following minor episodes of trauma. The fundamental fault is a sustained capillary hypertension resulting from persistently raised venous pressure. A failure to reduce venous pressure satisfactorily when the lower limb is dependent is consequent upon a failure of venous valves (allowing reflux) and poor calf muscle pump function. The lack of skin viability must reflect local hypoxia but the exact mechanism is not understood. The pathogenesis of the microvascular damage from the venous hypertension is discussed on p. 47.26.

A history of deep leg-vein thrombosis is obtained from a significant proportion of patients. In Anning's carefully documented series [12], a story of prior thrombosis was obtained in 75% of the patients. Leg injuries, particularly fractures, are frequently followed by thrombosis [14]. Other relatively common causes include hip replacements, pelvic and lower abdominal operations, medical illnesses and prolonged recumbency from any cause. In one study, 12 of 46 patients admitted to hospital with leg ulcers demonstrated resistance to activated protein C [15], a finding that has been observed in 20–40% of patients known to have had a previous DVT. Patients with chronic venous ulcers have a 41% prevalence rate of thrombophilia, which is 30 times higher than the general population [16]. Interestingly, thrombophilia does not necessarily appear to be related to past DVT [17]. Subjects with Klinefelter's syndrome have an increased risk of leg ulceration through an abnormality in platelet aggregability and fibrinolysis associated with elevated levels of plasminogen activator inhibitor-1 [18].

Up to 60% of patients with venous ulcers have isolated superficial vein incompetence with normal deep veins [19]. The concept of a primary defect in collagen or elastic tissue has been revised by the recognition of ulceration consequent on prolidase deficiency (p. 47.54). Congenital absence of venous valves as a cause of leg ulcers is probably rare [20].

Clinical features. The ulcer may be preceded by patchy erythema or discoloration of an intense bluish red colour, in which ischaemia of the skin finally leads to necrosis, often following a minor episode of trauma. This intense bluish colour can be seen by capillary microscopy to be caused by capillary congestion [21].

The ulcer is characteristically situated on the medial lower aspect of the leg, the 'gaiter' region, which is drained on the medial side by three large pairs of perforating veins. Venous ulcers do not usually develop initially below the level of the malleoli or in the foot unless complicated by livedoid vasculitis or arterial disease.

Two events may lead to a break in the continuity of surface epithelium. The first is capillary thrombosis, when the complete outline of the capillary can be seen to be filled with broken-up thrombus, which does not disperse on pressure. The second is a small bleed from the peak of the capillary; this separates the epidermis from its blood supply. These changes in the capillaries supplying the epidermis are frequently induced by small knocks, scratching or epidermal pathology such as dermatitis. The skin around an ulcer is frequently irritated by exudate, and inflamed varicose or medicament dermatitis may contribute to preventing healing and extending the ulcer size. Other signs of venous hypertension are usually present, for example lipodermatosclerosis, varicose veins (corona phlebectasia), varicose eczema or oedema; sometimes a nearby perforator vein may be evident by a palpable depression in the subcutaneous fat.

Ulcers often show pseudoepitheliomatous hyperplasia at their edge, which may be mistaken for a squamous cell carcinoma. The ulcer is covered with yellowish exudate over granulation tissue [22].

Healing ulcers have a shallow sloping edge with healthy granulation in their base and little slough. Epithelial islands may become scattered over the surface of a well-vascularized bed, and quickly enlarge (Fig. 47.23). The pink lip of the epithelium at the edge of an ulcer is uniform and supplied by relatively uncongested capillaries. The overall appearance is like a normal nail fold and cuticle. By contrast, a non-healing ulcer resembles a severe paronychia, being boggy, undermined and congested from oedema. The base is often white and very fibrous.

The coexistence of arterial disease can contribute to the progression of a venous ulcer, so symptoms and signs of peripheral ischaemia should be sought in all patients with leg ulceration. Rest pain can occur in the absence of arterial disease. Patients develop typical ischaemic pain on elevation of the ulcerated leg, which is oedematous. To relieve this pain, the patient keeps the leg in a dependent position, especially at night; this exacerbates the underlying pathogenesis.

After excluding arterial disease, a period of enforced elevation, necessitating strong analgesia, results in disappearance of the oedema with subsequent relief of the venous rest pain. Occasion-

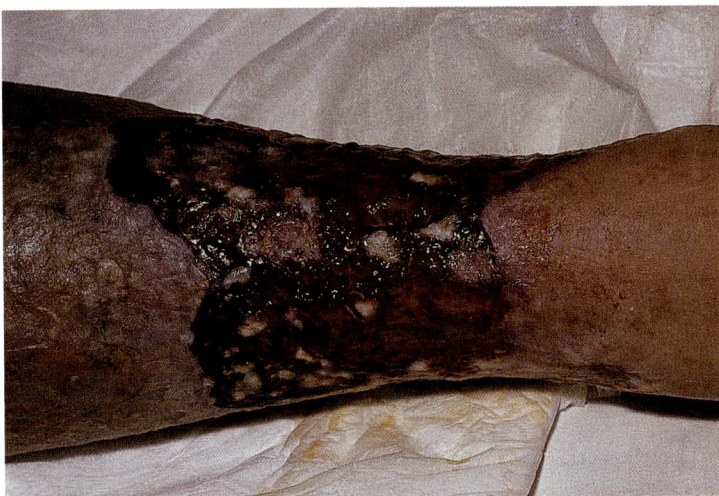

Fig. 47.23 A healing venous ulcer. There are multiple islands of reforming epithelium spreading over healthy granulation tissue.

ally, venous ulceration occurs at other sites in the limb, but other aetiologies should be suspected in such instances, especially if ulcers are present over the foot or just below the knee. Hyperkeratosis and papillomatosis around an ulcerated area or along the border of the foot, particularly below the malleoli, is a result of impaired local lymphatic drainage.

References

1 Reichenberg J, Davis M. Venous ulcers. *Semin Cutan Surg* 2005; **24**: 216–61.
2 Ruckley CV. Caring for patients with chronic leg ulcer. *BMJ* 1998; **3316**: 407–8.
3 Valencia IC, Falabella A, Kirsner RS *et al*. Chronic venous insufficiency and venous leg ulceration. *J Am Acad Dermatol* 2001; **44**: 401–21.
4 Bergan JJ, Schmid-Schonbein GW, Coleridge Smith PD *et al*. Mechanisms of disease: chronic venous disease. *N Eng J Med* 2006; **355**: 288–98.
5 Cornwall JV, Dore CJ, Lewis JD. Leg ulcers: epidemiology and aetiology. *Br J Surg* 1986; **73**: 693–6.
6 Callum MJ, Ruckley CV, Harper DR *et al*. Chronic ulceration of the leg: extent of the problem and provision of care. *BMJ* 1985; **290**: 1855–6.
7 Nelzen O, Bergquist D, Lindhagen A. Venous and non-venous leg ulcers: clinical history and appearance in a population study. *Br J Surg* 1994; **81**: 182–7.
8 Schulz EJ, Findlay GH, Scott FP. Skin disease in the Bantu: a survey of 4000 cases from the Transvaal and Orange Free State. *S Afr Med J* 1962; **36**: 199–202.
9 Shrank AB, Harman RRM. The incidence of skin disease in a Nigerian teaching hospital dermatological clinic. *Br J Dermatol* 1966; **78**: 235–41.
10 Doglietti M. Skin disorders in the Bantu: a survey of 2000 cases from Baragwanath Hospital. *S Afr Med J* 1970; **44**: 670–2.
11 Borschberg E, ed. *The Prevalence of Varicose Veins of the Lower Extremities*. Basle: Karger, 1967.
12 Anning ST, ed. *Leg Ulcers: Their Causes and Treatment*. London: Churchill, 1954.
13 Ruckley CV. Socioeconomic impact of chronic venous insufficiency and leg ulcers. *Angiology* 1997; **48**: 67–9.
14 Hjelmstedt A, Bergvall U. Incidence of thrombosis in patients with tibial fractures. *Acta Chir Scand* 1967; **134**: 1–10.
15 Munkvad S, Jørgensen M. Resistance to activated protein C: a common anticoagulant deficiency in patients with venous leg ulceration. *Br J Dermatol* 1996; **134**: 296–8.
16 Maessen-Visch MB, Hamulyak K, Tazelaar DJ *et al*. The prevalence of factor V Leiden mutation in patients with leg ulcers and venous insufficiency. *Arch Dermatol* 1999; **135**: 41–4.
17 Mackenzie RK, Ludlam CA, Ruckley CV *et al*. The prevalence of thrombophilia in patients with chronic venous ulceration. *J Vasc Surg* 2002; **35**: 718–22.
18 Zollner TM, Veraart JC, Wolter M *et al*. Leg ulcers in Klinefelter's syndrome—further evidence for an involvement of plasminogen activator inhibitor-1. *Br J Dermatol* 1997; **136**: 341–4.
19 Scriven JM, Hartshorne T, Bell PRF *et al*. Single visit venous ulcer assessment clinic: the first year. *Br J Surg* 1997; **84**: 334–6.
20 Lodin A, Lindvall N, Gentele H. Congenital absence of venous valves as a cause of leg ulcers. *Acta Chir Scand* 1959; **116**: 256–70.
21 Ryan TJ. The epidermis and its blood supply in venous disorders of the leg. *Trans St John's Hosp Dermatol Soc* 1969; **55**: 51–65.
22 Grey JE, Enoch S, Harding KG. Venous and arterial leg ulceration. *BMJ* 2006; **52**: 593–603.

Associations and complications of venous leg ulcers

The main conditions associated with venous ulceration are anaemia and malnutrition (especially in elderly people living alone), and these must be assessed and corrected as far as possible.

General disease [1–3]. Coincidental obesity and hypertension are common. The relationship of these to the presence of the ulcer is uncertain, but they are undoubtedly perpetuating causes. Increased intra-abdominal pressure, for example from obesity, can increase cardiac filling pressures, femoral venous pressures, renal vein pressure, systemic blood pressure and vascular resistance [4]. Cardiovascular disease is common and heart failure can be a major contributor to venous ulceration through its effect on: (i) further raising venous pressure; (ii) creating peripheral oedema; and (iii) encouraging long periods of sitting. Joint disease, peripheral arterial disease and neurological disease can obviously impair the already precarious nutrition of the skin and the action of the muscle pump. Severe rheumatoid disease or long-standing poliomyelitis also reduce the effectiveness of the muscle pump and encourage recurrence.

Anaemia and hypoproteinaemia. Sickle cell anaemia [5] can cause ulceration, and the presence of marked anaemia, for example due to iron-deficiency anaemia or thalassaemia, may prevent other ulcers from healing by reducing peripheral oxygenation. Repeated infection or chronic inflammation arising from the ulcer may itself cause a normochromic normocytic anaemia. A poor diet, combined with continuous seepage of protein and blood from an untreated ulcer, relatively commonly leads to anaemia and hypoalbuminaemia.

Diabetes. Diabetes is common, and will compound any venous ulcer through arterial disease, infection and neuropathy.

Personal attitudes and habits: sociology [6]. Patients with long-standing ulcers commonly develop a number of complications that stem from the personality, domestic and social situation of the patient. Walking has long been abandoned and substituted by more damaging motionless sitting. The ankle can become fixed in equinus and the foot inverted leading to an irreversible condition. The leg becomes transformed into a useless and deformed peg and the calf muscles atrophy. Apathy, often with depression and apparent acceptance of the condition, is frequent. Affected patients may become chairbound with decreasing mobility and malnourishment, but potentially receiving much attention and sympathy from family members. Many such patients never go to bed but sit motionless in the chair all night. In a few cases, it is clear that any real attempt to cure the ulcer will be resisted unless this can be accompanied by a vigorous social and psychological rehabilitation. Lonely patients may find that an ulcer is their only means of obtaining a visitor, be it district nurse or doctor.

Zinc depletion. This has received considerable attention [7–14], following the observation that zinc deficiency in rats impairs wound healing. Low plasma zinc levels have been found in patients with venous ulceration, and accelerated healing of such ulcers after oral zinc sulphate therapy has been reported. It is, however, the tissue levels of zinc that are of most importance in ulcer healing, and these have never been shown to be low in patients with leg ulcers. Analysis of six randomized trials indicates that oral zinc does not aid healing of leg ulcers, except possibly in patients with low serum zinc [15].

References

1 Browse NL, Burnand K, Irvine AT, Wilson NM. *Diseases of the Veins*, 2nd edn. London: Arnold, 1999.
2 Ryan TJ, ed. *Management of Leg Ulcers*. Oxford: Oxford University Press, 1987.
3 Stevens AE, Ball KP. General disease among leg ulcer patients. *Trans St John's Hosp Dermatol Soc* 1964; **50**: 43–7.
4 Sugerman HJ. Effects of increased abdominal pressure in severe obesity. *Surg Clin North Am* 2001; **81**: 1063–75.
5 Koshy M, Entsuah R, Koranda A *et al*. Leg ulcers in patients with sickle cell disease. *Blood* 1989; **74**: 1403–8.
6 Wilkinson DS. *Nursing and Management of Skin Diseases*, 4th edn. London: Faber and Faber, 1977.
7 Greaves M, Boyde TRC. Plasma-zinc concentrations in patients with psoriasis, other dermatoses and venous leg ulceration. *Lancet* 1967; **ii**: 1019–20.
8 Greaves MW, Ive FA. Double-blind trial of zinc sulphate in the treatment of chronic venous leg ulceration. *Br J Dermatol* 1972; **87**: 632–4.
9 Greaves MW, Skillen AW. Effects of long-continued ingestion of zinc sulphate in patients with venous leg ulceration. *Lancet* 1970; **ii**: 889–91.
10 Myers MB, Cherry G. Zinc and the healing of chronic leg ulcers. *Am J Surg* 1970; **120**: 77–81.
11 Serjeant GR, Galloway RE, Gueri MC. Oral zinc sulphate in sickle-cell ulcers. *Lancet* 1970; **ii**: 891–2.
12 Pories WJ, Henzel JH, Rob CG *et al*. Acceleration of wound healing in man with zinc sulphate given by mouth. *Lancet* 1967; **i**: 121–4.
13 Hallböök T, Lanner E. Serum-zinc and healing of venous ulcers. *Lancet* 1972; **ii**: 780–2.
14 Husain SL. Oral zinc sulphate in leg ulcers. *Lancet* 1969; **i**: 1069–71.
15 Wilkinson EA, Hawke CI. Oral zinc for arterial and venous leg ulcers. *Cochrane Database Syst Rev* 2000; CD001273.

Infection [1]. The role of antisepsis in the healing of leg ulcers is much debated [2–4]. Pathogenic organisms are commonly found in leg ulcers of all types [3]. The bacterial flora is often profuse and usually mixed, but *Staphylococcus aureus* predominates. There is still insufficient evidence to determine to what extent such a flora influences the rate of healing, but quantitative bacteriology has indicated that fewer than 100 000 organisms per square centimetre of surface area or per gram of tissue does not delay repair [5]. Certain pathogens are, however, traditionally taken seriously; for example, the group A β-haemolytic *Streptococcus* or a heavy growth of *Pseudomonas* spp. Unimpeded resolution of uncomplicated leg ulcers under occlusive compressive bandaging is frequently accompanied by considerable pus formation, but healing is not necessarily impaired. Sometimes lakes of pus develop in an atrophic skin that readily breaks down. Referred to as erosive pustular dermatosis of the leg, the pus is sterile and

the condition responds to intermittent use of potent topical steroids [6].

Fungi vary in extent and importance. Some authors have found *Candida albicans* only rarely [7], but it can be a common commensal organism, perhaps because of the widespread use of specific antibiotics. Ointment-impregnated bandages without preservatives were blamed for candidal overgrowth in one study [8]. Moist wound healing using contemporary occlusive dressings seems not to encourage infection [9].

Penicillin- and tetracycline-resistant staphylococci, and *Pseudomonas aeruginosa*, are very common in hospital-treated patients, and cross-contamination is very common in leg ulcer clinics [10]. *Proteus vulgaris* and other Gram-negative organisms are probably of little importance. The role of non-clostridial anaerobic organisms such as *Bacteroides* spp. in delaying ulcer healing has probably been underestimated. As with other types of infection, large controlled trials are required to measure healing after the ulcer surface has been sterilized. This information is not currently available to provide advice on the value of infection control. Venous ulcers are less likely to develop infection than arterial or diabetic ulcers [11]. All the antibiotic trials on ulcer healing that have been carried out have failed to show benefit.

Contact dermatitis. The skin around an ulcer frequently becomes red and sore, caused predominantly by the irritant effect of exudate (Fig. 47.24). Small pustules and superficial ulcers may develop, especially in the presence of β-haemolytic streptococci. Eczema may be responsible for further compromising skin viability, and

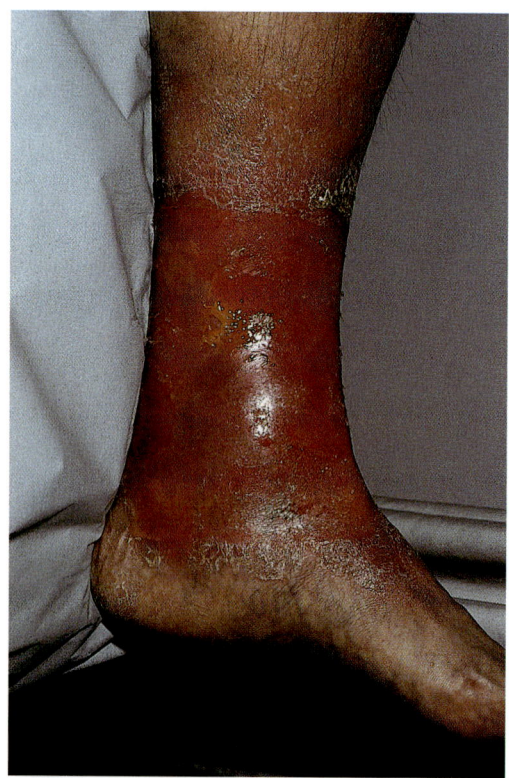

Fig. 47.24 Redness caused by exudate localized to the site of an overlying dressing, often confused with a contact allergy to the dressing.

Table 47.11 Leg ulcer allergens.

Ointment bases and preservatives
Wool alcohols (lanolins)
Parabens
Propylene glycol
Chlorocresol
Ethylenediamine
Cetostearyl alcohols

Additives in bandages
Ester gum resin
Azo disperse (dyes)
Colophony (adhesives)
Additives that prevent rubber and elastic from perishing

Antibacterial agents
Sodium fusidate
Gentamicin sulphate
Neomycin
Framycetin
Quinoline mix (Vioform, Chinoform)

Self-medication
Caine mix (local anaesthetics)
Antihistamine creams
Chlorxylenol (Dettol)
Germolene

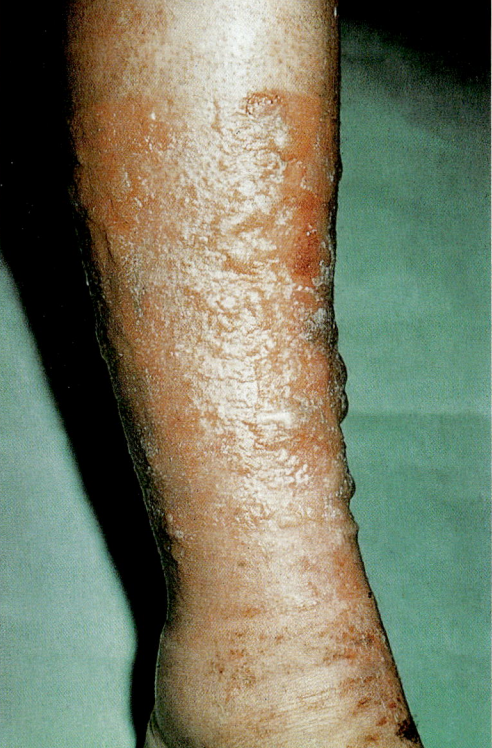

Fig. 47.25 A sensitivity reaction to strapping showing blistering.

so increasing the size of an ulcer. In most cases, the eczema is the result of local treatment (Table 47.11) and sensitivity can be demonstrated by patch testing. Patients with venous ulcers appear to become sensitized easily (Fig. 47.25) [12], often to several medicaments including lanolin and rubber [13–15]. The components of paste bandages may be responsible [16]. True medicament sensitivity is a frequent complication of therapy (Fig. 47.26) [17].

It is unfortunately not widely appreciated that the effect of potent topical corticosteroids on leg ulcers may inhibit healing for several weeks by producing an indolent 'arterial-type' ulcer with a deep adherent slough, 'steroid ulcer' (p. 47.56).

Haemorrhage [18,19]. Spontaneous haemorrhage occasionally occurs, especially from large ulcers [19]. This may be severe and can cause death if the patient faints and is held in the vertical position. First-aid measures include immediately lying the patient on the floor and elevating the limb while applying firm direct pressure to the bleeding point in the base of the ulcer. Occasionally, a suture will be required, but a tight bandage and elevation usually prevents further bleeding.

Lymphoedema (Chapter 48). The superficial lymphatics are absent in and around ulcers and their distortion or obliteration contributes to hyperkeratosis, papillomatosis, dermal fibrosis and oedema. An inadequacy of the lymphatic drainage predisposes to attacks of cellulitis [20], and with each episode of infection damage is compounded and chronic lymphoedema delays ulcer healing.

Malignant change [21]. Primary malignancies of the leg presenting as ulcers are increasingly common in an ageing population or

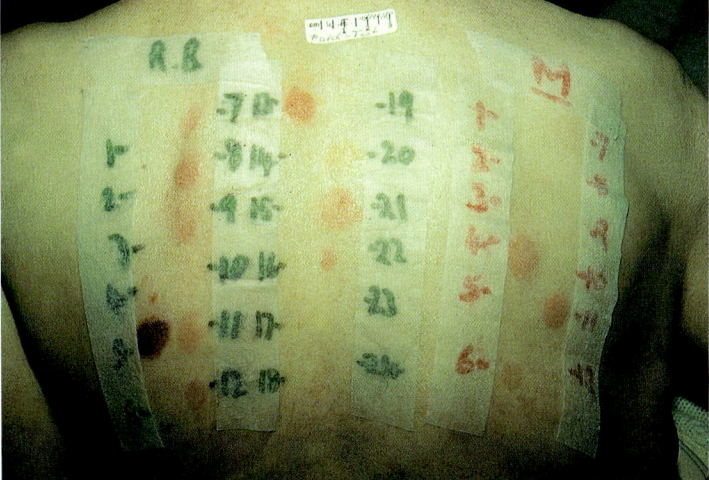

Fig. 47.26 Patch testing: 72-h reading showing multiple sensitivities, typical of patients with a long history of ulcer therapy.

those with sun exposure or transplantation-associated immunosuppression. Malignant change in an established ulcer is much rarer but carries a worse prognosis. Squamous epitheliomas may be difficult to distinguish from pseudoepitheliomatous hyperplasia, but if missed because of a failed diagnosis will often metastasize [22]. Biopsy should be considered if the diagnosis is in doubt [23]; multiple biopsies have been recommended as features may vary throughout the ulcer-associated tumour [24]. The edge becomes progressively heaped up (Fig. 47.27), vegetating and cauliflower-like and does not flatten with compressive therapy. Basal cell carcinomas may remain quite flat and undetected (Fig. 47.28).

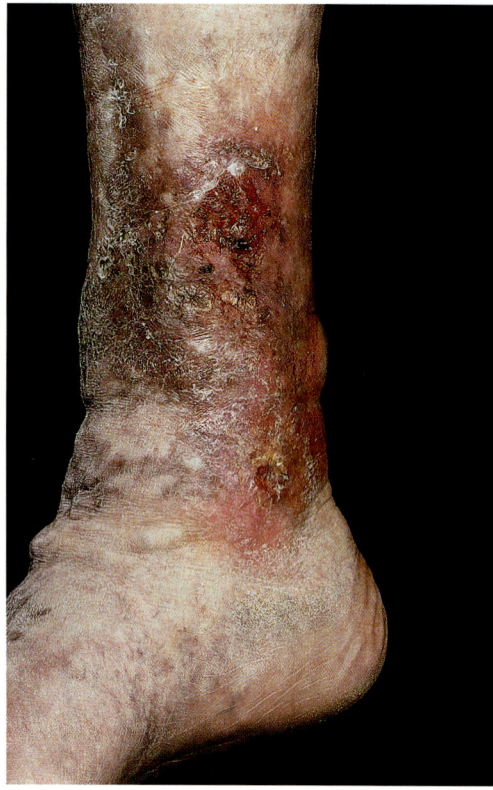

Fig. 47.27 Heaped-up squamous epithelioma.

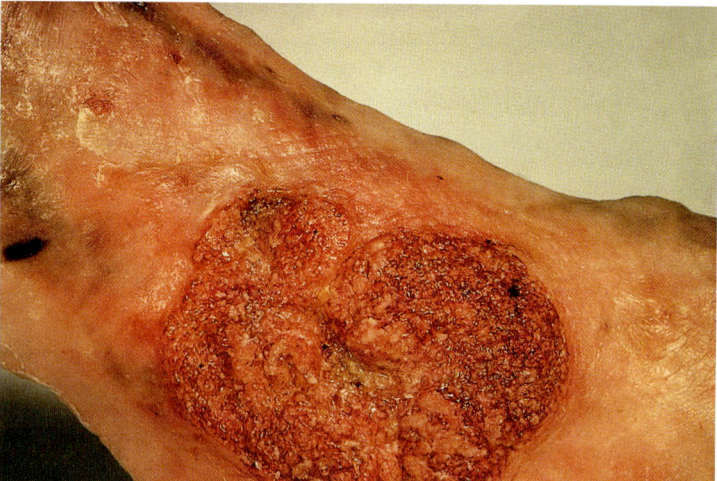

Fig. 47.28 A flat basal cell carcinoma complicating lipodermatosclerosis.

Suspicion may be aroused when the ulcer fails to respond to compression therapy. A distinction should be made between the rarity of malignant change in a chronic ulcer associated with disorders of the venous system, and the common primary malignancy occurring in the skin of legs that have had prolonged exposure to sunlight.

Subcutaneous calcification (post-phlebitis subcutaneous calcinosis) [25]. This is often widespread. It occurs in up to 10% of patients with chronic venous insufficiency [25]. It may cause non-healing of an ulcer or be found incidentally. The calcification, which is sometimes osteoid, occurs around areas of fat necrosis and fibrosis [26]. Radiography reveals a coarse network of calcification, the edges of individual plaques impinging on the dermis. Other causes of calcification include phleboliths, atherosclerotic calcification, cysticercosis and a heterotopic form of dystrophic calcification (in which the serum calcium and phosphorus levels are normal). Calcium deposits act as a foreign body nidus for organisms and delay healing, particularly when they are extruded through the skin as a foreign body.

Bone changes. Periostitis is commonly seen beneath a chronic ulcer. Osteoporosis is often present in the later stages because of disuse atrophy. Osteoarthritis is a common concomitant condition in the affected or unaffected leg, especially the knee. Fibrous ankylosis of the ankle occurs also from disuse.

References

1 Kontiainen S, Rinne E. Bacteria in ulcera crurum. *Acta Derm Venereol (Stockh)* 1988; **68**: 240–4.

2 Alinovi A, Bassini P, Pini M. Systemic administration of antibiotics in the management of venous ulcers. *J Am Acad Dermatol* 1986; **15**: 186–91.

3 Phillips TJ, Dover JS. Leg ulcers. *J Am Acad Dermatol* 1991; **25**: 965–89.

4 Rodehaver G. Controversies in topical wound management. *Wounds* 1989; **1**: 19–27.

5 Lookingbill DP, Miller SH, Knowles RC. Bacteriology of chronic leg ulcers. *Arch Dermatol* 1978; **114**: 1765–8.

6 Bull RH, Mortimer PS. Erosive pustular dermatosis of the leg. *Br J Dermatol* 1995; **132**: 279–82.

7 English MP, Smith RJ, Harman RRM. The fungal flora of ulcerated legs. *Br J Dermatol* 1971; **84**: 567–81.

8 Hanson C, Faergemann J, Swanbeck E. Fungal infections occurring under bandages in leg ulcer patients. *Acta Derm Venereol (Stockh)* 1987; **67**: 341–5.

9 Mertz PM, Eaglstein WH. The effect of occlusive dressing on the microbial population in superficial wounds. *Arch Surg* 1984; **119**: 287–9.

10 Mitchell AAB, Pettigrew JB, MacGillvray D. Varicose ulcers as reservoirs of hospital strains of *Staph. aureus* and *Pseudomonas pyocyanea*. *Br J Clin Pract* 1970; **24**: 223–6.

11 Schmidt K, Debus ES, Jessberger ST *et al*. Bacterial population of chronic crural ulcers: is there a difference between the diabetic, the venous and the arterial ulcer? *Vasa* 2000; **29**: 62–70.

12 Tavadia S, Bianchi J, Dawe RS *et al*. Allergic contact dermatitis in venous leg ulcer patients. *Contact Dermatitis* 2003; **48**: 261–5.

13 Angelini G, Rantuccio F, Meneghini CL. Contact dermatitis in patients with leg ulcers. *Contact Dermatitis* 1975; **1**: 81–7.

14 Kulozik M, Powell S, Cherry GW *et al*. Contact sensitivity in community-based leg ulcers. *Clin Exp Dermatol* 1988; **13**: 82–4.

15 Wilson CL, Cameron J, Powell SM *et al*. High incidence of contact dermatitis in leg ulcer patients: implications for management. *Clin Exp Dermatol* 1991; **16**: 250–3.

16 Hardie RA, Benton EC, Hunter JAA. Adverse reactions to paste bandages. *Clin Exp Dermatol* 1982; **7**: 135–42.

17 Jankićević J, Vesić S, Vukićević J *et al*. Contact sensitivity in patients with venous leg ulcers in Serbia: comparison with contact dermatitis patients and relationship to ulcer duration. *Contact Dermatitis* 2008; **58**: 32–6.

18 Harman RRM. Haemorrhage from varicose veins. *Lancet* 1974; **i**: 363.

19 Evans CA, Evans DMD, Seal RME *et al*. Spontaneous fatal haemorrhage caused by varicose veins. *Lancet* 1973; **ii**: 1359–61.

20 Dupuy A, Benchikhi H, Roujeau JC *et al*. Risk factors for erysipelas of the leg (cellulitis): case–control study. *BMJ* 1999; **318**: 1591–4.

21 Pennel TC, Hightower F. Malignant changes in post-phlebitic ulcers. *South Med J* 1965; **58**: 779–81.

22 Baldursson BT, Hedblad MA, Beitner H *et al*. Squamous cell carcinoma complicating chronic venous leg ulceration: a study of the histopathology, course and survival in 25 patients. *Br J Dermatol* 1999; **140**: 1148–52.

23 Lagattolla NRF, Burnand KG. Chronic venous disease may delay the diagnosis of malignant ulceration of the leg. *Phlebology* 1994; **9**: 167–9.

24 Cox NH, Long ED. Pseudoangiosarcomatous squamous cell carcinoma of skin. *Histopathology* 1993; **22**: 295–6.
25 Sarkany I, Kreel L. Subcutaneous ossification of the legs in chronic venous statis. *BMJ* 1966; **ii**: 27–8.
26 Lippman HI, Goldin RR. Subcutaneous ossification of the legs in chronic venous insufficiency. *Radiology* 1960; **74**: 279–81.

Diagnosis of venous ulceration. This is essentially clinical; based on finding ulceration in the gaiter area with the presence of signs of venous hypertension (p. 47.33). A past history of venous thrombosis, treatment for varicose veins or a family history of venous disease is supportive evidence. Arterial disease must be excluded and the ulcer should respond to compression therapy. Colour Doppler duplex ultrasound should be performed, not just to confirm venous reflux but also to see if superficial venous incompetence is responsible, in which case venous surgery may be an option if the deep veins are competent [1]. The preference is to wait for ulceration to heal before fully assessing the venous system. Plethysmography may be useful to investigate calf muscle pump function when venous duplex ultrasound is normal [2].

An ankle–brachial pressure index should be performed if foot pulses are not easily palpable, although the diagnosis of arterial disease does not exclude the possibility of an ulcer predominantly caused by venous disease (mixed origin). Arterial duplex Doppler scanning or arteriography should be undertaken if doubts remain regarding the presence of arterial ischaemia. A skin biopsy does not help in the diagnosis and may not heal in the presence of venous hypertension but is indicated if alternative causes such as skin malignancy [3] or vasculitis are possibilities. Signs of a peripheral neuropathy should be excluded and the range of hip, knee and particularly ankle movement should be tested.

References
1 Grabs AJ, Wakely MC, Nyamekye I *et al*. Colour duplex ultrasonography in the rational management of chronic venous leg ulcers. *Br J Surg* 1996; **83**: 1380–2.
2 Reichenberg J, Davis M. Venous ulcers. *Semin Cutan Med Surg* 2005; **24**: 216–26.
3 Lagattolla NRF, Burnard KG. Chronic venous disease may delay the diagnosis of malignant ulceration of the leg. *Phlebology* 1994; **9**: 167–9.

Management of venous ulcers [1–4]

General management

Most venous ulcers are cared for in the community by appropriately trained nurses and general practitioners. First-line therapy for venous ulcers is compression bandaging. The concept is to reduce venous pressure, particularly during walking, by improving calf muscle pump function and by opposing gravitational venous reflux. Exercise and movement are to be encouraged, while long periods spent sitting and standing should be discouraged. When resting, the legs should be elevated, ideally with the ulcer just above the level of the heart to ensure the maximum reduction in venous pressure. Thus, lying is always preferable to sitting with the leg elevated. Patients should always be instructed to sleep in a bed; this might sound obvious but it is remarkable how many patients with venous ulcers fall asleep and remain in chairs with dependent legs both day and night, so exacerbating venous ulcers (despite bandaging) because of limited reduction in venous pressure.

Obesity is often a problem that becomes worse with immobility, boredom and social isolation. Weight control is therefore essential, but malnourishment with anaemia and poor protein intake can coexist with obesity. Frail, elderly patients are at risk of malnutrition. Adequate intake of essential vitamins and minerals in a balanced diet is essential for wound healing [5]. The contribution of other medical conditions, particularly heart and chest problems, needs to be considered. Heart failure exacerbates venous hypertension, while the need to sit upright in bed or in a chair to alleviate dyspnoea will fail to reduce leg venous pressures. Smoking should be stopped and excessive alcohol intake should be curtailed as both compromise wound healing [6,7].

Intravenous drug users that have used lower limb veins are at increased risk of venous leg ulcers. Management must consider any HIV or hepatitis risk to both the patient and the health-care professional (through wound fluids).

Assessment. After taking a full and detailed history clinical examination should include identifying signs of venous disease, palpation of the peripheral pulses, testing for any loss of cutaneous sensation and for the range of hip, knee and particularly ankle movement. The patient should be observed walking to identify any reasons preventing a normal heel to toe gait. Signs of heart failure should be carefully looked for and any sleep-apnoea syndrome considered, particularly in the obese.

Investigations. Blood tests should seek to exclude significant anaemia (a mild normochromic normocytic anaemia is to expected secondary to the ulcer), infection (indicated by neutrophilia and raised CRP), and hypoalbuminaemia (which will discourage healing and exacerbate oedema). A fasting glucose (plus a HbA_{1c} level in known diabetic individuals), as well as renal and liver function, should be measured [8]. A sickle cell test should be undertaken when sickle cell disease is a possibility. Patients with a history of recurrent thrombosis or family history of thrombosis should be investigated for a thrombophilia [9].

An ankle–brachial pressure index should be performed if foot pulses are not easily palpable. Arterial duplex Doppler scanning or arteriography should be undertaken if doubts remain regarding the presence of arterial ischaemia. Colour duplex Doppler ultrasound should be performed at some stage to see if superficial venous incompetence is responsible, in which case surgery may be indicated.

Compression therapy [10]. Compression therapy is the mainstay of treatment. In addition to stimulating fibrinolytic activity and reducing discomfort and oedema, compression therapy counteracts venous hypertension by facilitating venous return, improving calf muscle pump function and lymph drainage [11]. Many methods of compression are available, for example non-elastic (short stretch) wraps, elastic (long stretch) wraps and pneumatic compression devices. Compression may be administered in the form of single layer bandages, multilayer bandages, compression stockings or a combination of stockings and bandages. Any of these should exert 30–40 mm Hg of pressure at the ankle for effective compression. Compression increases ulcer healing rates compared with no compression. Multilayered systems are more effective than single-layered systems. High compression is more effective than low compression but there are no clear differences in the effectiveness of different types of high compression. Graduated multilayer high compression bandage regimens capable of sustaining compression for a week at a time should be the first line of treatment for uncomplicated venous ulcers with an ankle–brachial pressure index above 0.8 [12].

When leg ulcer clinics have promoted compression treatment, healing rates have generally improved when compared with usual care given by community nurses [13]. Enthusiasm by professionals and a defined strategy, however, may explain the improvement.

In the UK, elastic (long-stretch) bandages are mainly used, whereas in Europe short-stretch bandages are preferred. Elastic bandages sustain compression for longer, whereas short-stretch bandages produce high 'venous' pumping pressures during exercise but lower resting pressures [14]. Multilayer bandaging has gained popularity owing to the high healing rate success reported in one study [15]. Unfortunately, all large ulcers were excluded and grafted in this study, and others have had difficulty in reproducing these results. Nevertheless, multilayer bandaging provides good conforming properties for a graduated distribution and sustainability of pressures.

Adequate training is essential for good results [16]. Incorrectly applied bandages can be harmful. Although compression therapy for the treatment of leg ulcers is in general performed with bandages, new medical elastic compression stockings were recently introduced for this treatment. A comparative study shows that this type of medical elastic compression stocking is more effective in daily practice than standard compression therapy with bandages [17].

Dermatological assessment. The condition of the ulcer and of the surrounding skin influences treatment outcome. If eczema is present, exudation and scratching will jeopardize the integrity of the surrounding skin. Consideration must be given to the underlying cause of the eczema which may be: (i) varicose; (ii) contact allergy; or (iii) contact irritant (e.g. caused by maceration from soaked dressings, see p. 47.44). A topical steroid is indicated to treat eczema, whereas emollients alone are sufficient for non-inflamed skin. Fragile oedematous skin needs careful application of compression bandages (but not necessarily less compression).

Cleansing and debridement. Management of the leg ulcer itself is important but should only be addressed once the patient's general health and venous hypertension have been considered. Cleansing of the ulcer should be kept simple [17,18]. Irrigation of the ulcer with warmed tap water or sterile saline is usually sufficient [19,20].

Any dressing technique should be clean and aimed at preventing cross-infection. Strict antisepsis is unnecessary. It is customary to remove slough, eschar and bacterial biofilms from the ulcer bed by debridement, as this improves wound healing [21]. Sharp debridement using scalpel, scissors or curette is most rapid and precise [22–23]. Autolytic or enzymatic debridement can be undertaken using moisture-donating dressings or protease preparations, respectively, but both are slow [24]. Debridement can also be achieved by topical negative pressure or vacuum-assisted closure (V.A.C.®) [25]. Maggots are used in some clinics for debridement

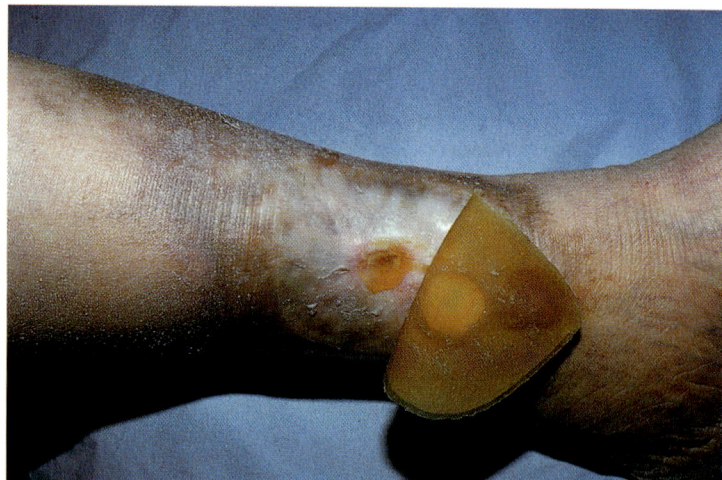

Fig. 47.29 A hydrocolloid dressing applied to an ulcer provides comfort and stimulus to healing. The centre of the dressing dissolves and contributes to odour and exudates on removal.

but have never been compared with surgical debridement [26]. An ultrasound debriding instrument was very acceptable to patients and has provided some promising early results [27].

Dressings and topical therapies [28–30]. Dressings should keep the ulcers moist but not wet. Dressings should be simple, low adherent, inexpensive and safe. There is no evidence that any particular dressing or dressing type is more effective in healing venous leg ulcers. 'It's not what you do with the ulcer that is important, it is what you do with the leg' is a good axiom, reflecting the fact that the most important aspect of treatment is reversing the venous hypertension, not the choice of wound dressing.

Ideally, a dressing should be left undisturbed for as long as possible so the ulcer can get on with the job of healing. Changes of dressing only disrupt new fragile epithelium. Conversely, a wet, soaked dressing and bandage tends to produce maceration of surrounding skin and encourage infection. 'Strike-through' of exudate to the outside of a bandage is usually an indication for a dressing change.

First-line primary dressings include a knitted viscose primary dressing (e.g. N-A Dressing®) with a superimposed absorbent pad (secondary dressing). Tulle dressings impregnated with paraffin (e.g. Jelonet®) can increase maceration; medicated tulle dressings are not generally recommended unless infection is likely [31]. An absorptive dressing may be valuable in a highly exuding wound (e.g. foam, alginate or hydrofibre). Hydrocolloid dressings can be helpful in dry, sloughy wounds to reduce pain but are not recommended if there is much exudate (Fig. 47.29). In malodorous wounds foam, alginate, hydrocolloid and charcoal are recommended [9]. Zinc paste bandages (e.g. Steripaste®) can be applied directly to the wound base and to the intact skin from the base of toes to knee, with a covering compression bandage in one or two layers (Fig. 47.30). These dressings have been shown to increase the speed of ulcer healing in one controlled study where four-layer bandages were used as the comparator [32]. Patients can develop allergies after using a product for some time [33]. Patch testing should be considered if dermatitis develops or is difficult to control.

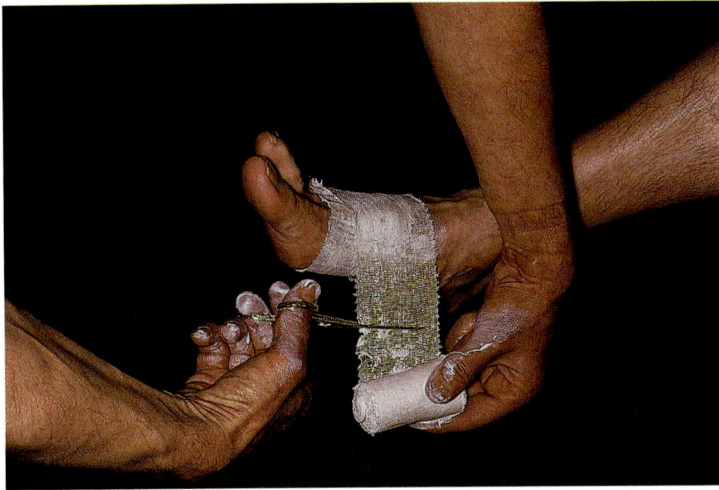

(a)

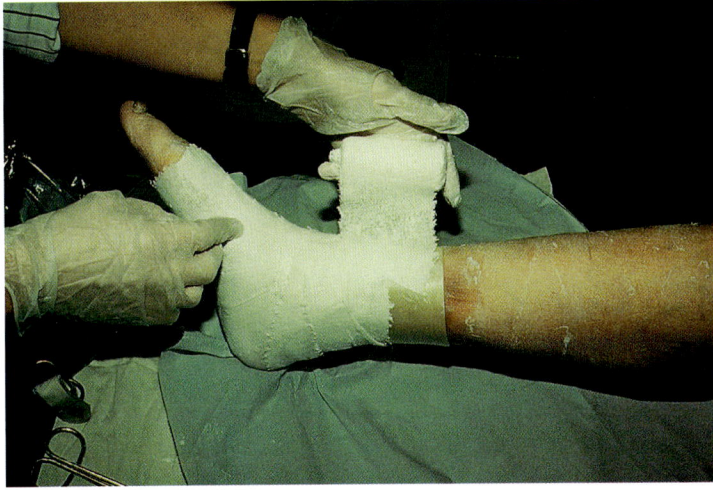

(b)

Fig. 47.30 Applying a past bandage to an ulcer, avoiding a tourniquet effect by frequent: (a) cutting; (b) folding.

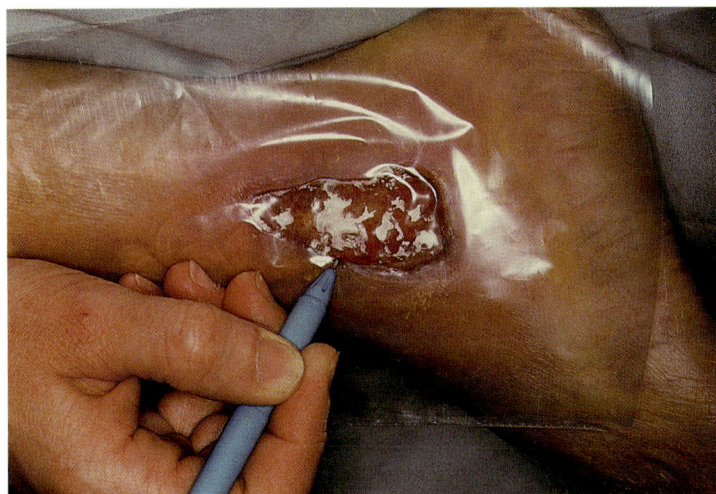

Fig. 47.31 Tracing around the margins of an ulcer to ensure the healing is occurring.

Skin and substitutes. Three different types of transplants can be used in ulcer management; these are autologous, donor skin and allogeneic transplants. The autologous transplants consist of three main techniques, namely split-skin grafts, punch grafts and cultured autologous keratinocytes. Donor skin may be cadaver or pig skin. Allogeneic techniques involve a bilayered skin substitute, which consists of allogeneic keratinocytes and fibroblasts in a collagen gel. The disadvantage of this technique is that it is expensive and has shown only minor improvements in healing in certain subgroups [34].

Microbiology [35]. Chronic leg ulcers are usually colonized by microorganisms but whether this affects healing is debatable [36,37]. Routine wound swabs for bacteriology are unnecessary unless there is evidence of clinical infection such as: (i) surrounding inflammation; (ii) increased pain; (iii) heavy or purulent exudate; (iv) a rapid deterioration of the ulcer; or (v) fever. The identification of group A haemolytic *Streptococcus* should prompt use of a course of penicillin, but otherwise antibiotics should not be used too readily. The use of topical antibiotics is discouraged because of the risks of contact allergy and antibiotic resistance.

Pain relief. Most patients with venous ulcers suffer moderate to severe pain [33]. Pain can result in reduced mobility, particularly of the range of joint movement, leading to a poor calf muscle pump. Pain may also indicate other pathology such as arterial insufficiency, malignancy or infection. Analgesia is recommended if compression and elevation fail to resolve pain from a venous ulcer. Opioids may be necessary in some cases. Some deep pain is mediated by the autonomic nervous system and may be helped by amitriptyline, gabapentin or a guanethidine block [38,39]. Quinine is a useful therapy for night cramp [40].

Measurement [41]. It is unwise to recommend any agent for the healing of ulcers that has not been subjected to a properly controlled trial. The only measurement that matters is the time taken for total healing of a large number of ulcers, which would, if possible, be stratified by initial ulcer size. The size influences the time taken for total healing to occur [42]. Large ulcers generally take significantly longer to heal than small ones. The healing rate is a poor measure; however, it is of value in monitoring the progress of individual ulcers (Fig. 47.31).

Systemic therapy. Systemic antibiotics have not been shown to improve the healing rates of venous ulcers and should be reserved for ulcers with clear evidence of infection [43].

The effectiveness of pentoxifylline in healing venous leg ulcers may be because of its fibrinolytic action and a reduction in leukocyte adhesion. Although randomized trials have reported both positive and negative results, a systematic review was positive [44]. A dose of 800 mg three times daily may be better than 400 mg three times daily as conventionally used.

An increased rate of venous ulcer healing with the use of oral enteric-coated aspirin (300 mg) daily was reported in one randomized trial [45]. Mixtures of flavonoid drugs (e.g. oxerutins) are licensed for use in venous disease. Daflon 500 accelerated healing of small ulcers in a randomized trial [46].

Stanozolol, an androgenic steroid with fibrinolytic properties, is helpful in improving lipodermatosclerosis [47] but no studies have demonstrated improved ulcer healing.

Complications. Cellulitis (erysipelas) frequently complicates leg ulcers and in deep, long-standing ulcers osteomyelitis has to be considered [48]. Malignant transformation in a non-healing ulcer is significant, with a relative risk of 5.80 in one study [49].

References

1 Browse NL, Burnand KG, Irvine AT, Wilson NM. *Diseases of the Veins*, 2nd edn. London: Arnold, 1999.

2 Ryan TJ, ed. *The Management of Leg Ulcers*, 2nd edn. Oxford: Oxford University Press, 1987.

3 Callam MJ, Ruckley CV, Harper DR, Dale JJ. Chronic ulceration of the leg: extent and provision of care. *BMJ* 1985; **290**: 1855–6.

4 Freak L, Simon D, Kinsella A *et al.* Leg ulcer care: an audit of cost effectiveness. *Health Trends* 1995; **27**: 133–6.

5 Mathus-Vliegen EM. Old age, malnutrition and pressure sores; an ill-fated alliance. *J Gerontol A Biol Sci Med Sci* 2004; **59**: 355–60.

6 Freiman A, Bird G, Metelitsa AL *et al.* Cutaneous effects of smoking. *J Cutan Med Surg* 2004; **8**: 415–23.

7 Benveniste K, Thut P. The effect of chronic alcoholism on wound healing. *Proc Soc Exp Biol Med* 1981; **166**: 568–75.

8 Hess CT, Trent JT. Incorporating laboratory values in chronic wound management. *Adv Skin Wound Care* 2004; **17**: 378–86.

9 Etufugh CN, Philips TJ. Venous ulcers. *Clin Dermatol* 2007; **25**: 121–30.

10 Fletcher A, Cullum N, Sheldon TA. A systematic review of compression treatment for venous leg ulcers. *BMJ* 1997; **325**: 576–80.

11 Cullum N, Fletcher A, Nelson E, Sheldon T. Compression for venous leg ulcers. *Cochrane Database Syst Rev* 2001; **2**: CD000265.

12 Van Gent WB, Hop WC, van Praag MC *et al.* Conservative versus surgical treatment of venous leg ulcers: a prospective, randomized, multicenter trial. *J Vasc Surg* 2006; **44**: 563–71.

13 Morrell CJ, Walters SJ, Dixon S *et al.* Cost effectiveness of community leg ulcer clinics: randomised controlled trial. *BMJ* 1998; **316**: 1487–91.

14 Thomas S. Bandages and bandaging: the science behind the art. *Care Sci Pract* 1990; **8**: 61–2.

15 Blair SD, Wright DDT, Backhouse CM *et al.* Sustained compression and healing of chronic venous ulcers. *BMJ* 1988; **297**: 1159–61.

16 Nelson EA, Ruckley CV, Barbenel JC. Improvements in bandaging technique following training. *J Wound Care* 1995; **4**: 181–4.

17 Jünger M, Wollina U, Kohnen R, Rabe E. Efficacy and tolerability of an ulcer compression stocking for the therapy of chronic venous ulcer compared with a below-knee compression bandage: results from a prospective, randomized, multicentre trial. *Curr Med Res Opin* 2004; **20**: 1613–23.

18 Lucaroth ME, Morgan AP, Leaper DT. The effect of antiseptics and the moist wound environment on ulcer healing: an experimental and biochemical study. *Phlebology* 1990; **5**: 173–9.

19 Svedman P. Irrigation treatment of leg ulcers. *Lancet* 1983; **ii**: 532–4.

20 Angeras HM, Brandberg A, Falk A, Seeman T. Comparison between sterile saline and tap water for the cleansing of acute soft tissue wounds. *Eur J Surg* 1992; **158**: 347–50.

21 Bradley M, Cullum N, Sheldon T. The debridement of chronic wounds: a systematic review. *Health Technol Assess* 1999; **3**: 1–78.

22 Steed DL. Debridement. *Am J Surg* 2004; **187**: S71–4.

23 Williams D, Enoch S, Miller D *et al.* Effect of sharp debridement using curette on recalcitrant venous ulcers: a concurrently controlled, prospective cohort study. *Wound Rep Reg* 2005; **13**: 131–7.

24 Konig M, Vanscheidt W, Augustin M *et al.* Enzymatic versus autolytic debridement of chronic leg ulcers: a prospective randomized trial. *J Wound Care* 2005; **14**: 320–3

25 Vuerstaek JD, Vainas T, Wuite J *et al.* State-of-the-art treatment of chronic leg ulcers: a randomized controlled trial comparing vacuum-assisted closure (V.A.C.) with modern wound dressings. *J Vasc Surg* 2006; **44**: 1029–37.

26 Sherman RA, Tran JM, Sullivan R. Maggot therapy for venous stasis ulcers. *Arch Dermatol* 1996; **132**: 254–6.

27 Tan J, Abisi S, Smith A, Burnand KG. A painless method of ultrasonically assisted debridement of chronic leg ulcers: a pilot study. *Eur J Vasc Endovasc Surg* 2007; **33**: 234–8.

28 Thomas S. *Wound Management and Dressings*. London: Pharmaceutical Press, 1990.

29 Fonder MA, Lazarus GS, Cowan DA *et al.* Treating the chronic wound: a practical approach to the care of non-healing wounds and wound care dressings. *J Am Acad Dermatol* 2008; **58**: 185–206.

30 Palfreyman S, Nelson EA, Michaels JA. Dressings for venous leg ulcers: systematic review and meta-analysis. *BMJ* 2007; **335**: 244.

31 British Medical Association and Royal Pharmaceutical Society of Great Britain. *British National Formulary* 2002; **44**: 745–57.

32 Mayer W, Jochmann W, Partsch H. Varicose ulcer: healing in conservative therapy. A prospective study. *Wien Med Wochenschr* 1994; **144**: 250–2.

33 Siegel DM. Contact sensitivity and recalcitrant wounds. *Ostomy Wound Manage* 2000; **46**: S65–74.

34 Falanga V, Margolis D, Alvarez O *et al.* Rapid healing of venous ulcers and lack of clinical rejection with an allogeneic cultured human skin equivalent. *Arch Dermatol* 1998; **134**: 293–300.

35 O'Meara S, Al-Kurdi D, Ovington L. Antibiotics and antiseptics for venous leg ulcers. *Cochrane Database Syst Rev* 2008; **1**: CD003557.

36 Skene AI, Smith JM, Dore CJ *et al.* Venous leg ulcers: a prognostic index to predict time to healing. *BMJ* 1992; **305**: 1119–21.

37 Trengove NJ, Stacey MC, McGechie DF *et al.* Qualitative bacteriology and leg ulcer healing. *J Wound Care* 1996; **5**: 277–80.

38 Hofman D, Ryan TJ, Arnold F *et al.* Pain in venous leg ulcers. *J Wound Care* 1997; **6**: 222–4.

39 Hannington-Kiff JG. Pharmacological target blocks in painful dystrophic limbs. In: Wall PD, Melzack R, eds. *Textbook of Pain*. Edinburgh: Churchill Livingstone, 1989: 754–66.

40 Young JB, Javid M, George J. Rest cramps in the elderly. *J R Coll Phys (Lond)* 1989; **23**: 103–5.

41 Eriksson G, Eklund A, Liden S *et al.* Comparison of different treatments of venous leg ulcers: a controlled study using stereophotogrammetry. *Curr Ther Res* 1984; **35**: 678–84.

42 Stacey MC, Burnand KG, Layer FT *et al.* Measurement of the healing of venous ulcers. *Aust N Z J Surg* 1991; **61**: 844–8.

43 Alinovi A, Bassissi P, Pini M. Systemic administration of antibiotics in the management of venous ulcers: a randomized clinical trial. *J Am Acad Dermatol* 1986; **15**: 186–91.

44 Jull A, Arroll B, Parag V, Waters J. Pentoxifylline for treating venous leg ulcer. *Cochrane Database Syst Rev* 2007; **3**: CD001733.

45 Layton AM, Ibbotson SH, Davies JA *et al.* Randomised trial of oral aspirin for chronic venous leg ulcers. *Lancet* 1994; **344**: 164–5.

46 Guilhou JJ, Dereure O, Marzin L *et al.* Efficacy of Daflon 500 mg in venous leg ulcer healing: a double blind randomized controlled versus placebo trial in 107 patients. *Angiology* 1997; **48**: 77–85.

47 Burnand K, Clemenson S, Morland M *et al.* Venous lipodermatosclerosis: treatment by fibrinolytic enhancement and elastic compression. *BMJ* 1980; **280**: 7–11.

48 Fernandes Abbade LP, Lastoria S. Venous ulcer: epidemiology, physiopathology, diagnosis and treatment. *Int J Dermatol* 2005; **44**: 449–56.

49 Baldursson B, Sigurgeirsson B, Lindelof B. Venous leg ulcers and squamous cell carcinoma: a large-scale epidemiological study. *Br J Dermatol* 1995; **133**: 571–4.

Recurrent ulcers and their prevention

Once their ulcer is healed, patients should be transferred from a bandage regimen to compression hosiery [1,2].

Many recurrences are the result of poor follow-up and inadequate or worn-out elastic stockings. Indeed, the 50% overall recurrence rate over 5–7 years has been shown to be higher in those prescribed stockings and is an indication of poor supervision [3]. Some recurrences are the result of superimposed arterial disease causing tissue ischaemia and skin necrosis. Many ulcers are precipitated by minor trauma, in which case a foam or felt pad should be worn over or under the stocking over vulnerable areas. Despite this, a considerable proportion of well-treated, formerly ulcerated limbs develop recurrences from time to time, often for no obvious

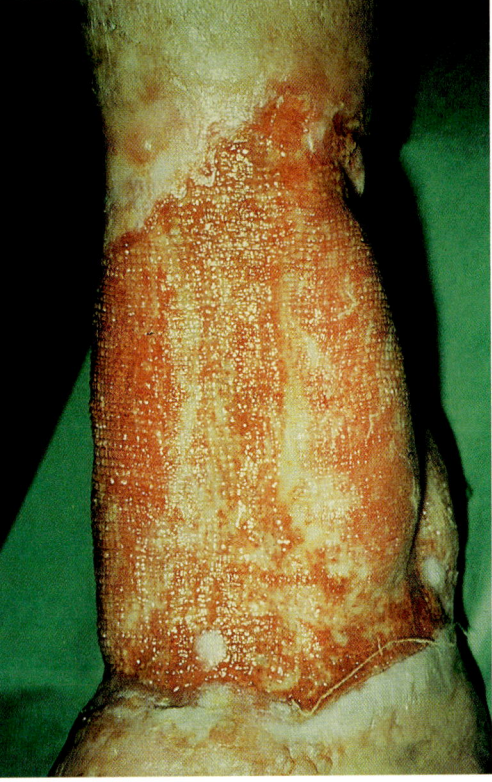
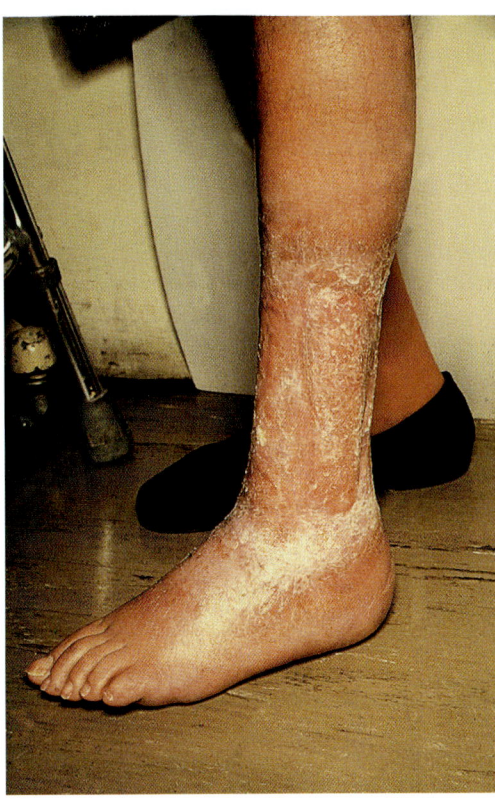

Fig. 47.32 A large ulcer (a) before and (b) after skin grafting.

(a)

(b)

reason. These recurrences are more likely in post-thrombotic limbs. Obsessional attention to detail in stocking use, avoidance of minor trauma and early vigorous treatment of any breakdown should reduce the period of re-ulceration to a minimum.

Surgical ligation of the saphenous veins and of incompetent communicating veins appears no better than stanozolol and stockings in preventing ulcer breakdown. Ablation of venous reflux by conventional surgery or endovenous treatment (plus compression hosiery) can reduce the risk of ulcer recurrence [4].

References
1 Anon. Compression hosiery for stasis disorders. *Drug Ther Bull* 1982; **20**: 81–4.
2 Thomas S. Bandages and bandaging: the science behind the art. *Care Sci Pract* 1990; **8**: 61–2.
3 Browse NL, Burnand KG, Irvine AT *et al.*, eds. *Diseases of the Veins: Pathology, Diagnosis and Treatment*, 2nd edn. London: Arnold, 1999.
4 Neumann HAM Compression therapy with medical elastic stockings for venous disease. *Dermatol Surg* 1998; **24**: 765–70.

Surgical treatment [1]
Surgical removal of the superficial incompetent varicose veins in patients with normal deep veins does not improve ulcer healing but significantly reduces the incidence of ulcer recurrence (Effects of Surgery and Compression on Healing and Recurrence (ESCHAR) trial) [2]. Recurrence rates of 30–50% after different surgical manoeuvres have been reported within 5 years [3–5]. Ligation and stripping of the saphenous veins and compressive sclerotherapy are the procedures most frequently undertaken, although with endovenous treatments the same results should be obtained. Complete extirpation of the communicating veins

'feeding' the ulcer is a logical approach but has failed to show any benefit in the only controlled trial that has been reported [6].

It would appear that surgical eradication of superficial incompetent veins is effective in preventing recurrence in patients without post-thrombotic damage but has little place in preventing recurrent ulceration in patients with damage to the deep venous system [7]. The newer procedures of deep-vein bypass, valvuloplasty and brachial valve transplant have still not been subjected to rigorous assessment by independent centres concerned with treating large numbers of patients with post-thrombotic limbs and venous ulcers. The value of these techniques in preventing ulcer recurrence in post-thrombotic limbs is therefore unknown. Elastic stockings must be worn for life and renewed at 6-monthly intervals if recurrence is to be prevented, and even these are not totally effective [8].

Shave therapy, a method of excision of ulcer and surrounding lipodermatosclerosis followed by meshed split-skin graft, healed 88% of ulcers in 18 patients [9]. The long-term results of this therapy show that 50% of the ulcers remain healed at 5 years [10].

Skin grafting on the lower legs is a means of considerably reducing the time taken for the ulcers to heal. It is usually performed on in-patients but can be carried out as an outpatient ambulatory procedure [11]. Pinch grafting provides small quantities of dermis as well as epidermis but leaves unsightly donor sites; large ulcers usually require split-skin grafts, which must be placed on surgically debrided beds. The application of mesh grafts has proved very effective when combined with ulcer excision (Fig. 47.32) [12,13]. Recurrence rates depend on patient selection. Those with many underlying medical or social problems are likely to have ulcer recurrence within a few weeks or months of grafting. Many studies of skin grown *in vitro* have indicated that keratinocytes will stimulate healing with the repopulation of host tissues even though the grafts may not themselves survive. Mechanisms underlying growth stimulation by cytokines have led to a growth-factor industry [12]. No cytokine, however, can be relied upon to promote healing unless most of the above-mentioned management factors are first attended to. If the underlying causes of ulceration are well managed, healing rates are excellent and added cytokines are not necessary [14].

Surgical options to correct venous reflux, such as endovenous procedures (foam sclerotherapy and endovenous laser), perforator interruption (SEPS), deep venous reconstruction and ligation and stripping of incompetent superficial veins, have not been shown to improve ulcer healing [15,16]. A randomized, controlled trial demonstrated that compression therapy alone did not differ from surgical correction of superficial venous reflux in combination with compression therapy in healing of venous ulcers [2]. Correction of confirmed superficial vein incompetence should be considered once healing is complete.

References

1 Tibbs D. *Varicose Veins and Related Disorders*, 2nd edn. Oxford: Butterworth–Heinemann, 1997.

2 Gohel MS, Barwell JR, Taylor M *et al.* Long term results of compression therapy alone versus compression plus surgery in chronic venous ulceration (ESCHAR): randomised controlled trial. *BMJ* 2007; **335**: 83–8.

3 Fegan WG. *Varicose Veins and Compression Sclerotherapy*. London: Heinemann, 1971.

4 Lofgren KA, Lauvstad WA, Bonnemaison MFE. Surgical treatment of large stasis ulcer: review of 129 cases. *Mayo Clin Proc* 1965; **40**: 560–3.

5 Silver D, Gileysteen JJ, Rhodes GR *et al.* Surgical treatment of refractory postphlebitic ulcer. *Arch Surg* 1971; **103**: 554–60.

6 Padberg FT Jr. Surgical intervention in venous ulceration. *Cardiovasc Surg* 1999; **7**: 83–90.

7 Burnand K, Thomas ML, O'Donnell T *et al.* Relation between post-phlebitic changes in the deep veins and results of surgical treatment of venous ulcers. *Lancet* 1976; **i**: 936–8.

8 Anon. Compression hosiery for stasis disorders. *Drug Ther Bull* 1982; **20**: 81–4.

9 Schmeller W, Gaber Y, Gehl HB. Shave therapy is a simple effective treatment of persistent venous ulcers. *J Am Acad Dermatol* 1998; **39**: 232–8.

10 Abisi S, Tan J, Burnand KG. Excision and meshed skin grafting for leg ulcers resistant to compression therapy. *Br J Surg* 2007; **94**: 194–7

11 Dahl MGC. Skin grafting on the lower leg as an outpatient ambulatory procedure. *Br J Dermatol* 1985; **113** (Suppl. 29): 14.

12 Harrison PV. Split skin grafting of varicose leg ulcers: a survey and the importance of assessment of risk factors in predicting outcome from the procedure. *Clin Exp Dermatol* 1987; **13**: 4–6.

13 Phillips TJ, Bhawan J, Leigh IM *et al.* Cultured epidermal autografts and allografts: a study of differentiation and allograft survival. *J Am Acad Dermatol* 1990; **23**: 189–98.

14 Nanninga PB, Mekkes JR, De Vries HJC *et al.* Grafting techniques. In: Westerhoff W, ed. *Leg Ulcers: Diagnosis and Management*. Amsterdam: Elsevier, 1993: 335–55.

15 Welch HJ. Surgical options for the treatment of venous ulcers. *Vasc Endovasc Surg* 2004; **38**: 195–202.

16 Van Gent WB, Hop WC, Van Praag *et al.* Conservative versus surgical treatment of venous leg ulcers: a prospective, randomized, multicentre trial. *J Vasc Surg* 2006; **44**: 563–71.

Arterial ulceration

Death of the skin automatically follows occlusion of its arterial blood supply unless this occurs slowly enough to allow a collateral circulation to be established. Arterial or arteriolar occlusion, if present, also complicates the treatment and prognosis of ulcers that are primarily venous in origin. A study of 600 patients with leg ulcers in the Lothian and Forth Valley, Scotland, revealed evidence of arterial disease in slightly less than one-quarter of those affected [1].

Atheroma of the abdominal and limb vessels is the single most common cause of ischaemic ulceration likely to be seen by the dermatologist involved in the care of patients with leg ulcers. Many other pathological states may, however, cause arterial occlusion, and not all can be defined with accuracy on clinical grounds. A useful empirical approach to the diagnosis of clinically ischaemic ulcers is to consider the causes in three main groups:

1 Extramural 'strangulation'
2 Mural thickening or accretion
3 Intramural restriction of blood flow.

There is often considerable overlap, and the exact pathology cannot always be well defined.

Extramural causes. Scar tissue and radiodermatitis cause a fibrotic strangulation of the arterioles and may give rise to small but persistent ulcers. Ulceration occurs in a number of diseases associated with dermal sclerosis, including scleroderma and progeria (Werner's syndrome; Chapter 15). Compression by tumours may also obstruct arterial flow.

Mural causes. Ulceration depends on the speed with which changes take place in the vessel wall. In vasculitis this is often sudden, but in hypertension it is slower and is preceded by pain, erythema and tenderness. In atherosclerosis the accretion of intimal plaques may proceed with a reduced flow until thrombosis, embolism or infection precipitate complete closure.

Intramural causes. Microvascular occlusion caused by changes in blood viscosity and clotting mechanisms is discussed in Chapter 49.

Clinical features [2]. The general symptoms and signs exhibited by the patient with advancing ischaemic disease of the limbs have already been described (p. 47.1). Arterial ulcers frequently arise in the pretibial area, the foot or on the toes, whereas venous ulcers favour the gaiter region.

Severe pain is usual, but is not a reliable discriminator from venous ulceration, which can also be very painful. Pain is as marked in small ischaemic ulcers as in large ulcers. The edges of the ulcers are sharply defined and the ulcer itself is often punched out.

There is often no pigmentation or lipodermatosclerosis in the surrounding skin, unlike the changes around venous ulcers, but the two can coexist. Usually, exudation from arterial ulcers is minimal. The base is often pale and covered with a slough which may have bare tendons in its base (Fig. 47.33). When smaller arteries and arterioles are occluded, the ulceration may have an irregular outline with strands of infarction extending along a vascular pattern in the skin. The condition is often indolent, healing only when the blood supply is improved and the ulcer base is excised and grafted.

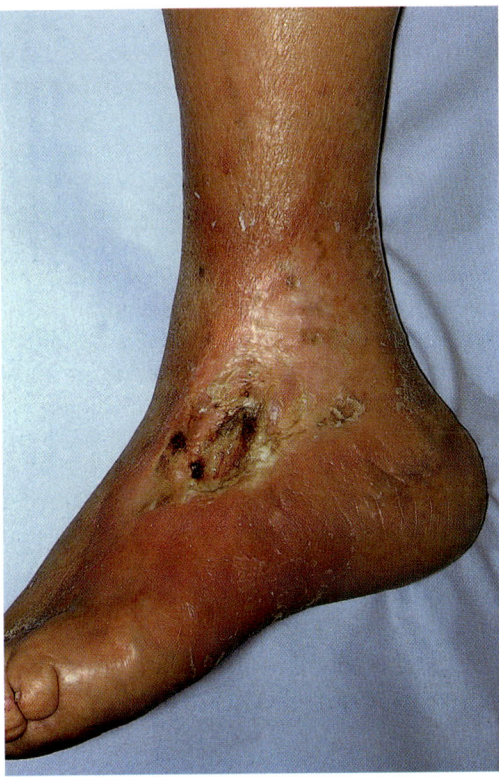

Fig. 47.33 An ischaemic ulcer with slough and exposed tendons.

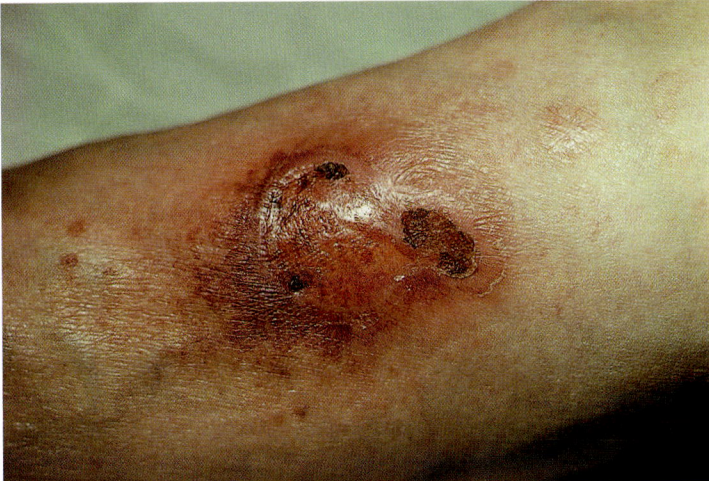

Fig. 47.34 A Martorell ulcer. High blood pressure causes vessel wall hypertrophy or vasospasm. Pain and ulceration with a livid reticulate edge but no lipodermatosclerosis is diagnostic. It is usually more proximal than a venous ulcer.

Hypertensive ulcer

Synonym
- Martorell's ulcer

Hypertensive leg ulcers are a unique form of lower extremity ischaemic leg ulcer. First described by Martorell, and by Hines and Farber in the 1940s [1,2], these ulcers are defined by pain disproportionate to the size of the ulcer, specific location on the lower extremity, female-to-male predominance, association with long-standing, often poorly controlled, hypertension, and healing response to specific antihypertensive agents [3].

Hypertensive ulceration tends to be bilateral and produces superficial ulceration yet the peripheral pulses are always present, distinguishing the condition from atherosclerosis. It is often initiated by trauma, and the ischaemia may be a consequence of a failure to meet the demands for repair. Whether it truly represents a specific disease has been questioned [4].

On biopsy there is increased thickening of the arteriolar walls with luminal narrowing by subendothelial hyalin degeneration. Smooth-muscle hyperplasia is most marked in the media and is most easily recognized by an increase in the number of smooth-muscle nuclei. It is later replaced by collagen fibres.

The ulcer is initially preceded by a small macular cyanotic lesion present on the anterior external aspect of the leg at a point between the middle and lower thirds of the limb. It is usually extremely painful, and this may be alleviated by holding the leg in the dependent position. The livid edge is a characteristic feature (Fig. 47.34).

The blood pressure should be controlled, and the leg should be placed in a position to prevent oedema but not so high as to promote further ischaemia. A firm non-elastic (short stretch) support bandage, without compression, is the most helpful treatment. At this site on the leg, the blood supply is difficult to re-establish, and several weeks may pass before the ischaemic necrotic tissue separates and granulation tissue begins to form. Smoking should be stopped and β-blockers avoided. Excision of the ulcerated area with grafting has been advised.

Treatment. Legs with severe arterial disease (APBI < 0.5) should be considered for immediate revascularization after assessment by arterial duplex ultrasound or angiography. Those with moderate arterial compromise (APBI > 0.5 but < 0.85) should be treated with modified compression, for example short stretch bandages that convey low resting pressures. Revascularization should be considered in ulcers that do not heal [3,4]. Limb salvage can be achieved in most patients but those failing the interventions described above, or who are unsuitable for revascularization, may require amputation. There is weak evidence that intermittent pneumatic compression is of benefit [5]. There is insufficient evidence to determine whether the choice of a topical agent or dressing affects the healing of arterial leg ulcers [6].

References
1 Callam MJ, Harper DR, Dale JJ *et al*. Arterial disease in chronic leg ulceration: an underestimated hazard? Lothian and Forth Valley leg ulcer study. *BMJ* 1987; **294**: 929–31.
2 Browse NL. Diseases of the heart and blood vessels: ischaemia of the lower limbs. *BMJ* 1996; **ii**: 157–9.
3 Humphreys ML, Stewart AH, Gohel MS *et al*. Management of mixed arterial and venous ulcers *Br J Surg* 2007; **94**: 1104–7.
4 Hafner J, Schaad I, Schneider E *et al*. Leg ulcers in peripheral arterial disease (arterial leg ulcers): impaired wound healing above the threshold of chronic critical limb ischemia. *J Am Acad Dermatol* 2000; **43**: 1001–8.
5 Kavros SJ, Delis KT, Turner NS *et al*. Improving limb salvage in critical ischaemia with intermittent pneumatic compression: a controlled study with 18-month follow-up. *J Vasc Surg* 2008; **47**: 543–9.
6 Nelson EA, Bradley MD. Dressings and topical agents for arterial leg ulcers. *Cochrane Database Sys Rev* 2007; CD001836.

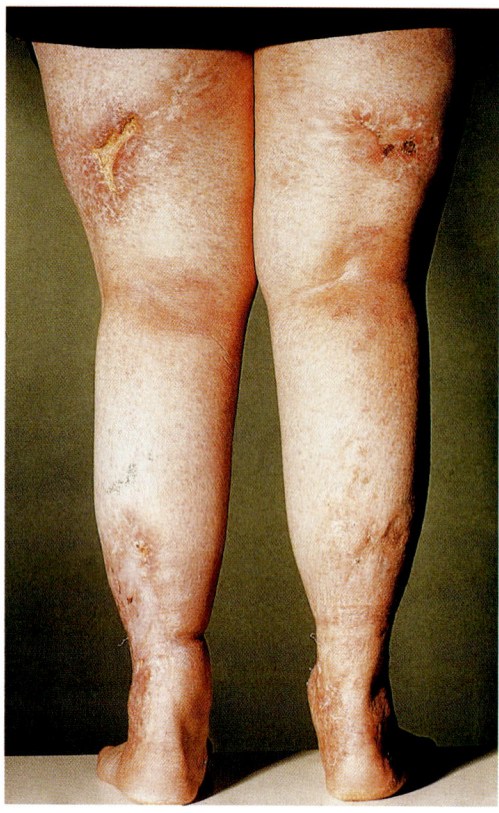

Fig. 47.35 Multiple ulcers with unusual distribution associated with prolidase deficiency.

References

1 Martorell F. Hypertensive ulcer of the leg. *Angiology* 1950; **1**: 133–40.
2 Alberti JMZ. Hypertensive ulcers: Martorell's ulcer. *Phlebology* 1988; **3**: 139–42.
3 Graves JW, Morris JC, Sheps SG. Martorell's hypertensive leg ulcer: case report and concise review of the literature. *J Hum Hypertens* 2001; **15**: 279–83.
4 Leu HJ. Hypertensive ischaemic leg ulcer (Martorell's ulcer): a specific disease entity? *Int Angiol* 1992; **11**: 132–6.

Other causes of leg ulceration

Prolidase deficiency

Prolidase deficiency is transmitted as an autosomal recessive condition and has a European incidence of less than 5 : 10 000 people [1]. This rare disease is caused by a defect in the prolidase (PEPD, iminodipeptidase) gene on chromosome 19cen-q13.11. Prolidase is one of the enzymes that degrade collagen to iminodipeptides, it cleaves dipeptides with hydroxyproline or proline at the C-terminus [2]. Decreased activity of prolidase causes excretion of large amounts of proline and hydroxyproline, bound to amino acids as iminodipeptides in the urine, resulting in a depletion of the total pool of proline [3].

Prolidase deficiency is a multisystem disorder and the skin is its primary target organ. Clinical symptoms commence before the age of 12 years [3]. Ninety per cent of patients have dermatological features. Recurrent, multiple ulcers of the lower extremities are seen in over 50% of patients (Fig. 47.35). The development of a squamous cell carcinoma in the ulcer is an uncommon complication. Fragility of the skin, resulting in breakdown at the site of injury, is often preceded by purpura or bruising. Fine scarring, telangiectasia and eczematous lesions may be a feature. The facies

are characteristic, consisting of hypertelorism with a saddle nose, and patients are mentally retarded. Other associations, not present in all cases, are dental caries, splenomegaly, hyperextensibility of ligaments, osteoporosis, respiratory infections, corneal opacities, amblyopia and optic atrophy. The skin may have a doughy consistency as in other collagen diseases [4].

The diagnosis is ascertained by iminodipeptiduria greater than 5 mmol/24 h [5]. In the blood a decreased prolidase activity is found. Laboratory abnormalities associated with prolidase deficiency consist of thrombocytopenia, hypergammaglobulinaemia and iron-deficiency anaemia [2]. Skin biopsy is almost normal in prolidase deficiency, although fragmentation of collagen fibres with impaired aggregation or a decrease in the size of collagen fibres may be found.

A characteristic feature of the disorder is absolute resistance to all forms of treatment, including rejection of skin grafts. Using topical antibiotics may control infections, and developing infections should be treated with oral or intravenous antibiotics [2]. Because co-factors of prolidase are ascorbic acid and manganese, these have been recommended therapies, as has diphenylhydantoin [6]. Japanese investigators recommend an ointment containing 5% glycine and 5% proline [7], and this was confirmed to be effective by Jemec and Moe [6]. Apheresis exchange was successful in two patients [8] and the combination of topical and systemic growth hormone resulted in transient healed recalcitrant leg ulcers in a 13-year-old boy [9].

References

1 Viglio S, Annovazzi L, Conti B *et al*. The role of emerging techniques in the investigation of prolidase deficiency: from diagnosis to the development of a possible therapeutical approach. *J Chromatogr B* 2006; **832**: 1–8.
2 Trent J, Kirsner RS. Leg ulcers secondary to prolidase deficiency. *Adv Skin Wound Care* 2004; **17**: 468–72.
3 Kokturk A, Kaya TI, Ikizoglu G, Koca A. Prolidase deficiency. *Int J Dermatol* 2002; **41**: 46–8.
4 Milligan A, Graham-Brown RAC, Burns DA *et al*. Prolidase deficiency: a case report and literature review. *Br J Dermatol* 1989; **121**: 405–9.
5 Buist NRM, Strandholm JJ, Bellinger JF *et al*. Further studies on a patient with iminodipeptiduria: a probable case of prolidase deficiency. *Metabolism* 1972; **21**: 1113–23.
6 Jemec, GBE, Moe ATT. Topical treatment of skin ulcers in prolidase deficiency. *Pediatr Dermatol* 1996; **13**: 58–60.
7 Arata J, Hatakenaka K, Oono T. Effect of topical application of glycine and proline on recalcitrant leg ulcers of prolidase deficiency. *Arch Dermatol* 1986; **122**: 626–7.
8 Lupi A, Casado B, Soli M *et al*. Therapeutic apheresis exchange in two patients with prolidase deficiency. *Br J Dermatol* 2002; **147**: 1237–40.
9 Monafo V, Marseglia GL, Maghnie M *et al*. Transient beneficial effect of GH replacement therapy and topical GH application on skin ulcers in a boy with prolidase deficiency. *Pediatr Dermatol* 2000; **17**: 227–30.

Hydroxycarbamide (hydroxyurea) therapy

Hydroxycarbamide (formerly hydroxyurea) is a chemotherapeutic agent that acts during cellular replication and inhibits DNA synthesis without affecting RNA synthesis [1]. It is currently the drug of choice for treatment of chronic myelo- and certain lymphoproliferative disorders, for example chronic myeloid leukaemia, chronic lymphocytic leukaemia, polycythaemia vera and essential thrombocythaemia [2]. It is also used in the treatment of sickle cell anaemia. Dermatological adverse effects have been well documented. In a study by Vassallo *et al.*, all 158 patients using hydroxycarbamide for the treatment of chronic myeloid leukaemia suffered cutaneous xerosis and mild stomatitis [3]. Other adverse effects include hyperpigmentation, brown nail discoloration, acral erythema, scaling of the face, hands and feet, dermatomyositis-like eruptions, partial alopecia, atrophy of the skin and subcutaneous tissue, and leg ulcers.

In a prospective study, leg ulceration was reported to occur in 9% of patients taking hydroxycarbamide [4]. In three-quarters of patients, the ulcers are located on or near the malleoli [2]. The ulcers usually develop after at least 1 year of treatment. The lesions are generally very painful and resemble atrophie blanche. Hydroxycarbamide therapy is associated with leg ulceration in a dose-dependent fashion; with higher doses, wound size increases and healing is usually observed after withdrawal of hydroxycarbamide.

Several pathogenetic mechanisms have been postulated, but currently it is unclear how hydroxycarbamide induces leg ulcers. Histological examination shows non-specific changes [5].

Differential diagnosis includes cutaneous leukocytoclastic vasculitis, cryoglobulinaemia and pyoderma gangrenosum, and these diseases should be ruled out.

After withdrawal of hydroxycarbamide, 85% of ulcers spontaneously heal in 1–9 months [2]. In most other patients, a reduction in ulcer size is observed. A split skin graft, preceded by surgical debridement, may be performed in cases without spontaneous resolution. Many patients will develop new ulcers after restarting hydroxycarbamide therapy, so this should be avoided if an alternate agent can be prescribed.

References

1 Sirieix M-E, Debure C, Baudot N et al. Leg ulcers and hydroxyurea. Arch Dermatol 1999; **135**: 818–20.

2 Bader U, Banyai M, Burg G, Hafner J. Leg ulcers in patients with myeloproliferative disorders: disease- or treatment-related? Dermatology 2000; **200**: 45–8.

3 Vassallo C, Passamonti F, Merante S et al. Mucocutaneous changes during long-term therapy with hydroxyurea in chronic myeloid leukemia. Clin Exp Dermatol 2001; **26**: 141–8.

4 Najean Y, Rain JD. Treatment of polycythemia vera: the use of hydroxyurea and pipobroman in 292 patients under the age of 65 years. Blood 1997; **90**: 3370–7.

5 Best PJ, Daoud MS, Pittelkow MR, Petitt RM. Hydroxyurea-induced leg ulceration in 14 patients. Ann Intern Med 1998; **128**: 29–32.

Vasculitis/vasculopathy

Most acute forms of vasculitis, and some subacute and chronic forms, are likely to cause ulceration. Vasculitic lesions are usually, but not always, multiple. Palpable purpura is characteristic but vasculitis may be polymorphous, even pustular.

Rheumatoid disease [1].

Leg ulceration in rheumatoid arthritis is common and the causes can be multifactorial. Poor joint movement impairs the calf muscle pump and immobility increases the risk of DVT. True 'rheumatoid ulcers' occur as a manifestation of rheumatoid arteritis. Ulcers are often situated in the gaiter region and have a sloughy base with poor granulation. The absence of surrounding lipodermatosclerosis or of other signs of venous disease, the presence of a positive rheumatoid factor (particularly if at high titre) and demonstration of normal Doppler pressures and venous duplex studies suggest that the ulcer is truly 'rheumatoid'. Biopsy may be helpful but is not always con-firmatory and the site may not heal. Ulceration of rheumatoid nodules is uncommon except at pressure sites in bedridden patients. Thinned skin because of long-term corticosteroid treatment, and the use of methotrexate, both increase the risk of ulceration. Healing can be very impaired, particularly in the presence of muscle atrophy, immobility and oedema but patients should be treated with immunosuppression to control the vasculitic component.

Other autoimmune disease.

Leg ulceration in patients with lupus erythematosus is well recognized [2]. In Felty's syndrome and Still's disease, multiple painful ulcers occur on the legs and feet and are difficult to heal. Ulcers also occur in polyostotic fibrous dysplasia (Jaffe–Lichtenstein disease), in which a diffuse mesenchymal abnormality is present. Ulceration occurs over large areas of subcutaneous or muscular calcinosis, especially around the knee.

Sarcoidosis.

Sarcoidosis can rarely result in leg ulceration due to granulomatous vasculitis [3].

Livedo reticularis.

Livedo reticularis, a fixed but broken pattern of mottling, may result from vasculitis but also occurs with intravascular thrombosis caused by cryoproteinaemias [4], antiphospholipid syndrome and Sneddon's syndrome (Chapter 49).

Livedoid vasculopathy (livedo vasculitis).

This condition is a more specific form of occlusive vasculopathy limited to the gaiter skin and often extending onto the dorsum of the foot. Ulcers are small, painful and heal with ivory-white scars (atrophie blanche). The mechanism appears to be more to do with hyalinization and thrombosis of the microvasculature with scarce inflammatory infiltrate unlike a leukocytoclastic vasculitis; therefore immunosuppression treatment is not so effective and consideration needs to be given to hypercoagulable states and their treatment [5]. Livedo with summer ulceration is a variant of the same condition (Chapter 49).

Cutaneous polyarteritis nodosa may rarely present with ulcerating atrophie blanche. Associated sensory loss (mononeuritis multiplex) and medium vessel vasculitis may be the only positive findings [6].

Treatment of leg ulceration secondary to vasculitis or vasculopathy involves control of any underlying condition combined with compression, as gravitational forces largely determine the localization of ulceration to the gaiter region.

References

1 Allison JH, Bettley FR. Rheumatoid arthritis with chronic leg ulceration. Lancet 1957; **i**: 288–90.

2 Goslen JB. Autoimmune ulceration of the leg. Clin Dermatol 1990; **8**: 92–117.

3 Poonawalla T, Colome-Grimmer MI, Kelly B. Ulcerative sarcoidosis in the legs with granulomatous vasculitis. Clin Exp Dermatol 2008; **33**: 282–6.

4 Williamson AE, Cone LA, Huard GS. Spontaneous necrosis of the skin associated with cryofibrinogenaemia, cryoglobulinaemia and homocysteinaemia. Ann Vasc Surg 1996; **10**: 365–9.

5 Hairston BR, Davis MD, Pittelkow MR, Ahmed I. Livedoid vasculopathy: further evidence for procoagulant pathogenesis. Arch Dermatol 2006; **142**: 1413–8.

6 Mimouni D, Ng PP, Rencic A et al. Cutaneous polyarteritis nodosa in patients presenting with atrophie blanche. Br J Dermatol 2003; **148**: 789–94.

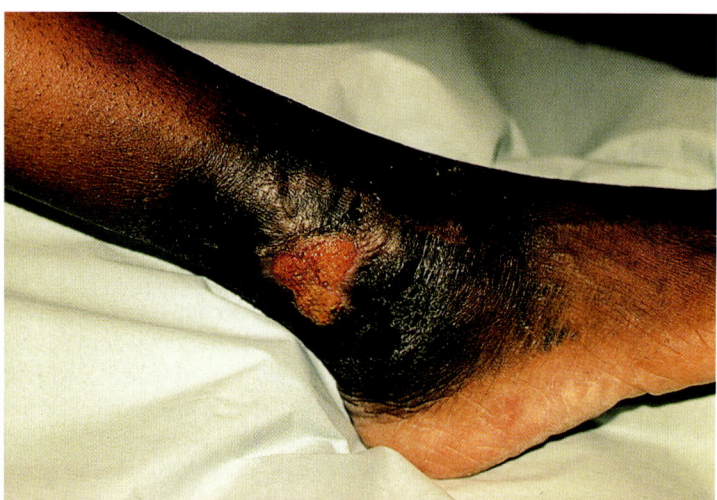

Fig. 47.36 Sickle cell ulcer.

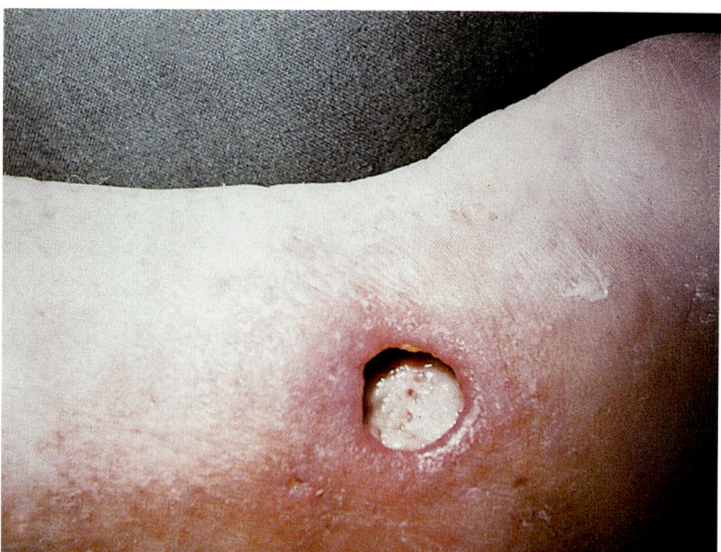

Fig. 47.37 'Steroid ulcer' with totally suppressed granulation tissue.

Haematological disorders

Indolent non-healing ulcers on the leg are a feature of sickle cell anaemia (Fig. 47.36), hereditary spherocytosis and other haemolytic anaemias [1]. Sickle cell ulcers were reported in 2.5% of over 2000 patients with sickle cell anaemia aged 10 or over and were more common in patients with sickle cell anaemia and thalassaemia genotypes [2]. There is a high incidence of venous reflux in sickle cell disease, indicating the need for compression therapy as well as treatment for the sickle cell anaemia itself [3]. Other haemolytic anaemias also predispose to leg ulceration [4].

Myeloproliferative disorders may contribute to leg ulceration if cell size compromises capillary perfusion or if thrombosis develops, but it can be difficult to distinguish between disease-related and treatment-related (e.g. hydroxycarbamide) ulceration.

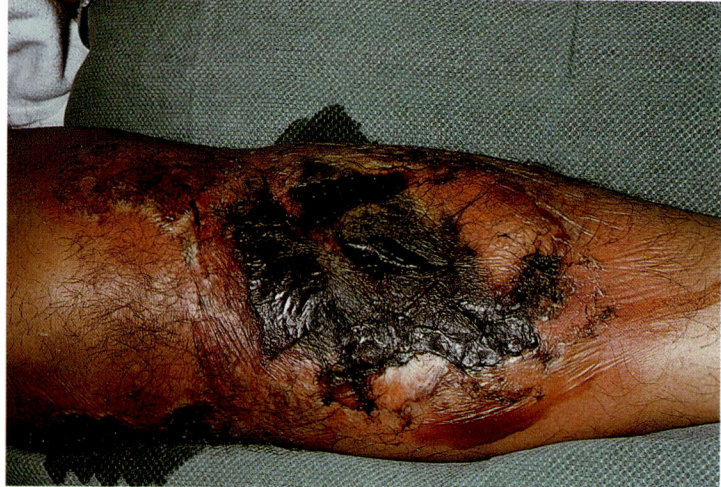

Fig. 47.38 Meleny's spreading gangrene.

References
1 Pascher F, Keen R. Ulcers of the leg in Cooley's anemia. *N Engl J Med* 1957; **256**: 1220–2.
2 Koshy M, Entsuah R, Koranda A *et al.* Leg ulcers in patients with sickle cell disease. *Blood* 1989; **74**: 1403–8.
3 Clare A, Fitzhenley M, Harris J *et al.* Chronic leg ulceration in homozygous sickle cell disease: the role of venous incompetence. *Br J Haematol* 2002; **119**: 567–71.
4 Sawhney H, Weedon J, Gillette P *et al.* Predilection of haemolytic anaemia-associated leg ulcers for the medial malleolus. *Vasa* 2002; **31**: 191–3.

'Steroid ulcers'

Intralesional steroid injections, especially if made in areas with an already impoverished blood supply, may cause an indolent ulcer with a characteristic greyish slough (Fig. 47.37) [1]. This condition is most commonly seen when strong topical corticosteroids are applied to venous or other ulcers of the lower leg and ankle. Long-term use of potent topical steroids on the shins can also lead to poor wound healing after traumatic injury.

Reference
1 Bjornberg A, Hellgren L. Necrosis in leg ulcers: probable role of fluocinolone acetonide. *Arch Dermatol* 1965; **92**: 52–3.

Infection

Infection may lead to ulceration, which is often slow to heal because of associated oedema, cellulitis, thrombophlebitis, diabetes or underlying vascular disease. Primary uncomplicated pyococcal ulceration is rare; ecthyma is an example. Meleney's ulcer (bacterial synergistic gangrene) extends rapidly and has a burrowing, bluish, undermined and painful edge (Fig. 47.38). Tuberculous ulcers occur in erythema induratum (Bazin's disease) and are chronic, often on the back of the calves. They usually have undermined edges and considerable surrounding inflammation (Chapter 31). Other mycobacterial infections may be more common than suspected (Chapter 31). Ulcers in leprosy are usually on the foot, especially the dorsum, and on the proximal phalanx of the great toe, but can occur occasionally on the leg. The 'classical' appearances of the ulceronodular form of tertiary syphilis are well known, but this is extremely rare. Multiple tissue-paper scars on the legs occur typically in yaws (Chapter 34). The so-called 'desert' or 'veldt' sore is shallow and crusted; the role of *Corynebacterium diphtheriae* is uncertain. The 'tropical' ulcer is a variety of phagedenic ulcer with a mixed symbiotic infection and rapid spread. Leishmaniasis, relatively uncommon on the legs, should be remembered as a possible cause of an indolent granulomatous ulcer. Among other uncommon infective causes of ulceration are glanders, tularaemia, brucellosis and cat scratch fever.

Pyoderma gangrenosum (Chapter 50)

This causes rapidly spreading and often bizarre and extensive ulceration, which may mimic an artefact, particularly when it precedes obvious ulcerative colitis. Underlying systemic disease such as inflammatory bowel disease, rheumatoid arthritis and haematological malignancies are found in some 70% of cases [1,2].

References
1 Callen JP. Pyoderma gangrenosum. *Lancet* 1998; **351**: 581–5.
2 Su WP, Davis MD, Weenig RH *et al*. Pyoderma gangrenosum: clinicopathologic correlation and proposed diagnostic criteria. *Int J Dermatol* 2004; **30**: 790–800.

Necrobiosis lipoidica and granulomatous diseases

Necrobiosis lipoidica may ulcerate following trauma, is extremely indolent, and should be regarded as ischaemic. Similarly, any granulomatous lesion may ulcerate if its blood supply is inadequate or if the vessels are involved in the granulomatous process, as may occur in sarcoidosis.

Decubitus and neuropathic ulceration

Pressure sores occur easily and with little warning on the heels and ankles of elderly people, especially in those who are comatose or have neurological disease. Pressure, including from bandages, may cause ulceration in those with compromised blood supply or reduced cutaneous sensation. In all cases where ulceration is protracted in the absence of venous, arterial or other obvious disease, artefact must be considered; interference with ulcers already present may also occur, even through bandages [1].

Neuropathic ulceration of the foot benefits from protection from shearing forces [2] by the use of a plaster cast or 'Scotchcast boot'. If this fails to achieve healing, the pressure must be taken off the foot and the base of the ulcer excised before being grafted. Split skin, rotation flaps or pedicle flaps may be used to cure the defect. It may be simpler to excise the toe and most of the first metatarsal to achieve rapid healing if the ulcer is situated over the ball of the foot. Patient education is of prime importance to avoid recurrent, inadvertent self-trauma.

References
1 Chan CL, Meyer FJ, Hay RJ *et al*. The ulceration associated with compression bandaging: observational study. *BMJ* 2001; **323**: 1099.
2 Burden AC, Jones CR, Jones R *et al*. Use of the 'Scotchcast boot' in treating diabetic foot ulcers. *BMJ* 1983; **286**: 1555–7.

Diabetic foot ulcers

Diabetic foot ulceration is a common, yet in many cases an eminently preventable, complication that affects 1 in 20 patients with diabetes. Risk factors for ulceration include reduced sensation (secondary to somatic neuropathy), high foot pressures, callus formation (a consequence of sympathetic neuropathy and high foot pressures), deformities (such as claw feet, prominent meta-

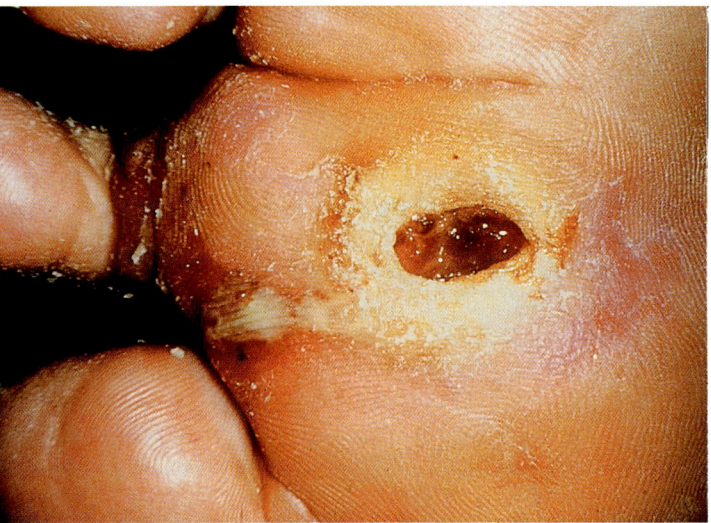

Fig. 47.39 Neuropathic–ischaemic ulcers over the base of the foot (diabetic).

tarsal heads, etc.), peripheral vascular disease, and, most importantly, a past history of ulceration [1].

The natural history in the development of the diabetic foot can be divided into five stages: stage 1, a normal foot; stage 2, a high risk foot; stage 3, an ulcerated foot; stage 4, an infected foot; and stage 5, a necrotic foot. This covers the entire spectrum of foot disease but emphasizes the development of the foot ulcer as a pivotal event in stage 3, which demands urgent and aggressive management. An important prelude to diabetic foot treatment is the differing diagnosis of neuropathic and neuroischaemic foot. In the neuropathic foot, ulcers commonly develop on the plantar surface of the foot and the toes (Fig. 47.39), and are associated with neglected callus and high plantar pressures. In the neuroischaemic foot, ulcers are commonly seen around the edges of the foot, including the tips of the toes and the back of the heel, and are associated with trauma or wearing unsuitable shoes. Ulcers in stage 3 need relief of pressure (mechanical control), sharp debridement and dressings (wound control), and neuroischaemic foot ulcers may need vascular intervention (vascular control). In stage 4, microbiological control is crucial; severe infections need intravenous antibacterial therapy, and urgent assessment of the need for surgical drainage and debridement. Without urgent treatment, severe infections will progress to necrosis. In stage 5, necrosis can be divided into wet and dry necrosis. Wet necrosis in neuropathic feet requires intravenous antibacterials and surgical debridement, and wet necrosis in neuroischaemic feet also needs vascular reconstruction [2].

Infection is most often a consequence of foot ulcerations, which typically follows trauma to a neuropathic foot. Tissue specimens are strongly preferred to wound swabs for wound cultures. Gram-positive bacteria are the sole causative pathogens for most mild and moderate infections. These infections can usually be treated with culture-based narrow-spectrum antibacterials along with appropriate surgical debridement in an outpatient setting. In contrast, severe infections are often polymicrobial, requiring hospitalization and treatment with broad-spectrum antibacterials along with appropriate medical and surgical interventions. The initial empirical antibacterial regimen may be tailored based on the results of culture and sensitivity tests from properly obtained specimens [3].

Diabetic foot care in all stages needs multidisciplinary management to control mechanical, wound, microbiological, vascular, metabolic and educational aspects. Achieving good metabolic control of blood glucose, lipids and blood pressure is important in each stage, as is education to teach proper foot care appropriate for each stage. In the management of neuropathic ulcers, pressure relief is of the utmost importance, and total contact casting remains the 'gold standard' means of achieving such pressure redistribution. Alleviation of the mechanical load on ulcers (off-loading) should always be a part of treatment. Neuropathic ulcers typically heal in 6 weeks with total contact casting, because it effectively relieves pressure at the ulcer site and enforces patient compliance [4].

An ulcer that does not heal for many months has a high probability of leading to osteomyelitis, for which treatment with antibiotics is not useful and which usually requires a surgical procedure. Charcot neuroarthropathy is a particular complication of neuropathy, which may lead to fragmentation or destruction of joints and bones.

Osteomyelitic bones in the foot must be excised and diabetic ischaemic ulceration treated by revascularization and split skin grafting with mesh where appropriate.

References
1 Boulton AJ. Pressure and the diabetic foot: clinical science and offloading techniques. *Am J Surg* 2004; **187**: 17S–24S.
2 Edmonds M. Diabetic foot ulcers: practical treatment recommendations. *Drugs* 2006; **66**: 913–29.
3 Rao N, Lipsky BA. Optimising antimicrobial therapy in diabetic foot infections. *Drugs* 2007; **67**: 195–214.
4 Cavanagh PR, Lipsky BA, Bradbury AW, Botek G. Treatment for diabetic foot ulcers. *Lancet* 2005; **366**: 1725–35.

CHAPTER 48

Disorders of Lymphatic Vessels

P.S. Mortimer

St George's Hospital, University of London, London, UK

Introduction

The lymphatic system comprises the lymph, lymphatic vessels, lymph nodes and other organs containing lymphoid tissue, especially the spleen and bone marrow. A close developmental and working relationship exists between the lymphatic vessels and the blood circulation, particularly the veins. Although not a true circulation like the blood vascular system, the lymphatic system does provide an important 'limb' to the microcirculation, particularly in the skin, and, with the blood vessels, caters for the constant recirculation of protein and cells. While lymph drainage serves a predominantly 'plumbing' role, the lymphatic system does possess important immunological responsibilities. The lymphatic vessels are essential for the continual drainage from the tissues of the body of both plasma proteins and lymph-borne cells, for example lymphocytes and macrophages [1].

While technology has advanced our knowledge of the lymphatic system at the cellular and molecular level, our understanding of whole-body physiology lags behind. Nevertheless, the importance of the lymphatic vessel in disease is demonstrated by recent evidence implicating it in the pathogenesis of several conditions including cancer metastasis [2], asthma and airways obstruction [3], atherosclerosis [4], Crohn's disease [5], arthritis [6] and renal transplant rejection [7].

Rook's Textbook of Dermatology, 8th edition. Edited by DA Burns, SM Breathnach, NH Cox and CEM Griffiths. © 2010 Blackwell Publishing Ltd.

References

1 Yoffey JM, Courtice JM. *Lymphatics, Lymph and the Lymphomyeloid Complex*. New York: Academic Press, 1970.

2 Harrell MI, Iritani BM, Ruddell A. Tumor-induced sentinel lymph node lymphangiogenesis and increased lymph flow precede melanoma metastasis. *Am J Pathol* 2007; **170**: 774–86.

3 Baluk P, Tammela T, Ator E *et al.* Pathogenesis of persistent lymphatic vessel hyperplasia in chronic airway inflammation. *J Clin Invest* 2005; **115**: 247–57.

4 Xu X, Lin H, Lv H *et al.* Adventitial lymphatic vessels—an important role in atherosclerosis. *Med Hypotheses* 2007; **69**: 1238–41.

5 Pedica F, Ligorio C, Tonelli P *et al.* Lymphangiogenesis in Crohn's disease: an immunohistochemical study using monoclonal antibody D2-40. *Virchows Arch* 2008; **452**: 57–63.

6 Polzer K, Baeten D, Soleiman A *et al.* TNF blockade increases lymphangiogenesis in murine and human arthritic joints. *Ann Rheum Dis* 2008; **67**: 1610–6.

7 Kerjaschki D, Huttary N, Raab I *et al.* Lymphatic endothelial progenitor cells contribute to de novo lymphangiogenesis in human renal transplants. *Nat Med* 2006; **12**: 230–4.

Lymphatic development

The embryonic origin of the lymphatic system has long been uncertain, but its close development with the venous system is not in doubt. In 1902, Sabin proposed that early in fetal development isolated primitive lymph sacs originate by endothelial cell budding from embryonic veins [1,2] and that the skin lymphatic vessels develop by endothelial sprouting from these primary lymph sacs (centrifugal development). Alternatively, it has been suggested that initial lymph sacs develop from precursor cells, 'lymphangioblasts', in the mesenchyme (centripetal development)

[3]. Recent work indicates that lymphangioblasts are located in the confluence of the cranial and caudal cardinal veins, where the jugular lymph sac (JLS) forms. Cell lineage studies show that the JLS is of venous origin. In contrast, the lymphatic vessels of the dermis are derived from mesenchymal lymphangioblasts, suggesting a dual origin of lymphatic endothelial cells (LECs), both central and peripheral, although the primary source of embryonic LECs probably resides in specific embryonic veins [4].

Lymphvasculogenesis and lymphangiogenesis

Lymphvasculogenesis is the *de novo* production of LECs. It may occur in the embryo from specific veins and possibly in the adult from bone-marrow derived progenitor cells [5]. It is essential for establishing the lymphatic system initially.

Lymphangiogenesis is the production of new lymphatic vessels by splitting and splicing of existing LECs, and occurs both in the embryo and the adult.

Vascular endothelial growth factor (VEGF)

In 1995, the first specific growth factor receptor of lymphatic vessels was identified and termed FLT-4 [6]. It is now termed vascular endothelial growth factor receptor-3 (VEGFR-3). The family of vascular endothelial growth factor receptors and their ligands are central to the development of blood and lymph vessels [6]. In embryos, VEGFR-3 is initially expressed in all vasculature, but during development its expression in blood vessels (veins not arteries) becomes restricted to the developing lymphatic vessels. In embryos, therefore, VEGFR-3 is important for cardiovascular development, but in adults it is responsible for the regulation of the lymphatic vessels [7].

Lymphatic development requires the activation of the transcription factor PROX1 [8], which acts as the LEC master control gene and then regulates the expression of VEGFR-3, a receptor for VEGF-C and -D. LECs expressing VEGFR-3 bud off and migrate away from the embryonic cardinal vein in response to a gradient of VEGF-C produced by the nearby mesenchymal cells [9]. The migrating LECs assemble into lymph sacs which extend through sprouting to lay down the lymphatic network.

Post-natal lymphangiogenesis

Lymphatic vessel growth is regulated by several lymphangiogenic factors, including members of the vascular endothelial growth factor (VEGF), platelet-derived growth factor (PDGF), fibroblast growth factor (FGF), hepatocyte growth factor (HGF) and angiopoietin families. VEGF-C and -D are the main ligands for VEGFR-3, which is lymphatic-specific, and therefore specific for lymphangiogenesis. The most potent inducer of lymphatic sprouting is VEGF-C. Over-expression of VEGF-C in skin keratinocytes leads to dermal lymphatic hyperplasia [10].

While lymphangiogenesis is mediated mainly via VEGF-C and -D binding to VEGFR-3, lymphangiogenic responses can occur through VEGFR-2 and VEGFR-3. In addition to VEGF-C and -D, VEGF-A (also called vascular permeability factor) is able to stimulate lymphangiogenesis. VEGFR-2 has been detected on endothelial cells of the lymphatic vessels, suggesting its direct role in the stimulation of lymphangiogenesis [11]. Alternatively, VEGF-A might recruit inflammatory cells that indirectly stimulate lym-

phangiogenesis through the secretion of cytokines and growth factors [12].

Recently, VEGFR-1, in response to VEGF-A binding, has been shown to promote lymphangiogenesis, as well as angiogenesis, via bone marrow-derived macrophage recruitment, but probably only in pathological states. For example, progenitor cells have been shown to participate in lymphangiogenesis in chronic renal transplant rejection [13]. VEGFR-1 is expressed not only on vascular and lymphatic endothelium but also on monocytes/macrophages. VEGFR-1 could be involved in lymphangiogenesis in one of three ways: firstly, VEGFR-1 contributes to vascular permeability, and resulting exudates induce lymph vessel dilatation and lymphangiogenesis; secondly, VEGF-A recruits bone marrow-derived macrophages in a VEGFR-1 signal-dependent manner; and thirdly, recruited macrophages express VEGF-C which binds to VEGFR-3 [14]. It is still unclear how physiological lymphangiogenesis is regulated.

Vascular separation

The separation of lymphatic vessels from blood vessels is important for their independent functioning. Syk and SLP-76 deficiency leads to arteriovenous shunting and lymphovenous connections [15]. These proteins and those of the Spred/Sprouty family may have implications in mixed vascular malformations where blood-filled lymphatic vessels can occur.

Lymphatic remodelling

After the initial lymphatic vasculature is established, it is then remodelled into a functioning network comprising lymphatic capillaries/initial lymphatics and collecting lymphatics possessing smooth muscle. FOXC2, EphrinB2 and Angiopoietin-2 play important roles in the remodelling process, including recruitment of smooth muscle cells and formation of valves [16].

References

1 Sabin FR. On the origin of the lymphatic system from the veins and the development of lymph hearts and thoracic duct in the pig. *Am J Anat* 1902; **i**: 3671.

2 Sabin FR. On the development of the superficial lymphatics in the skin of the pig. *Am J Anat* 1904; **9**: 43–91.

3 Huntington GS, McClure CFW. The anatomy and development of the jugular lymph sacs in the domestic cat. *Am J Anat* 1908; **22**: 1–19.

4 Buttler K, Ezaki T, Wilting J. Proliferating mesodermal cells in murine embryos exhibiting macrophage and lymphendothelial characteristics. *BMC Dev Biol* 2008; **8**: 43.

5 Religa P, Cao R, Bjorndahl M *et al*. Presence of bone marrow-derived circulating progenitor endothelial cells in the newly formed lymphatic vessels. *Blood* 2005; **106**: 4184–90.

6 Kaipainen A, Korhonen J, Mustonen T *et al*. Expression of the fms-like tyrosine kinase FLT4 gene becomes restricted to lymphatic endothelium during development. *Proc Natl Acad Sci* 1995; **92**: 3566–70.

7 Jussila L, Alitalo K. Vascular growth factors and lymphangiogenesis. *Physiol Rev* 2002; **82**: 673–700.

8 Wigle JT, Oliver G. Prox-1 function is required for the development of the murine lymphatic system. *Cell* 1999; **98**: 769–78.

9 Olsson AK, Dimberg A, Kreuger J, Claesson-Welsh L. VEGF receptor signaling-in control of vascular function. *Nat Rev Mol Cell Biol* 2006; **7**: 359–71.

10 Saaristo A, Veikkola T, Tammela T *et al*. Lymphangiogenic gene therapy with minimal blood vascular side effects. *J Exp Med* 2002; **196**: 719–30.

11 Nagy JA, Vasile E, Feng D *et al*. Vascular permeability factor/vascular endothelial growth factor induces lymphangiogenesis as well as angiogenesis. *J Exp Med* 2002; **196**: 1497–506.

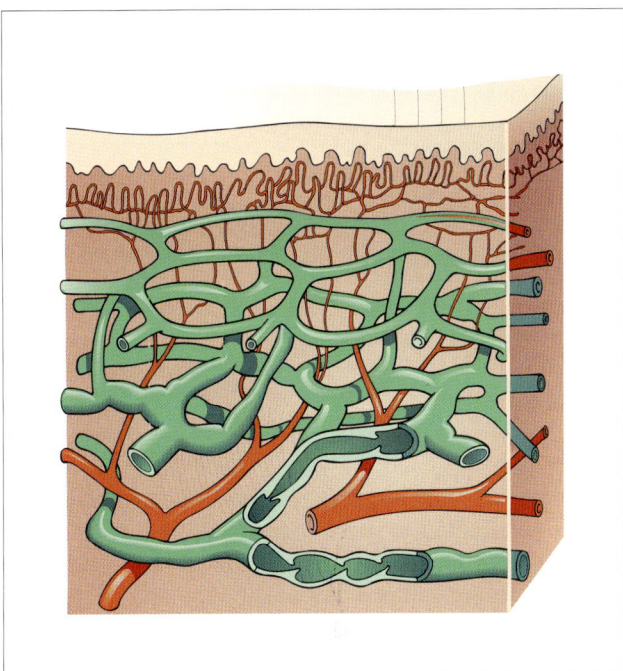

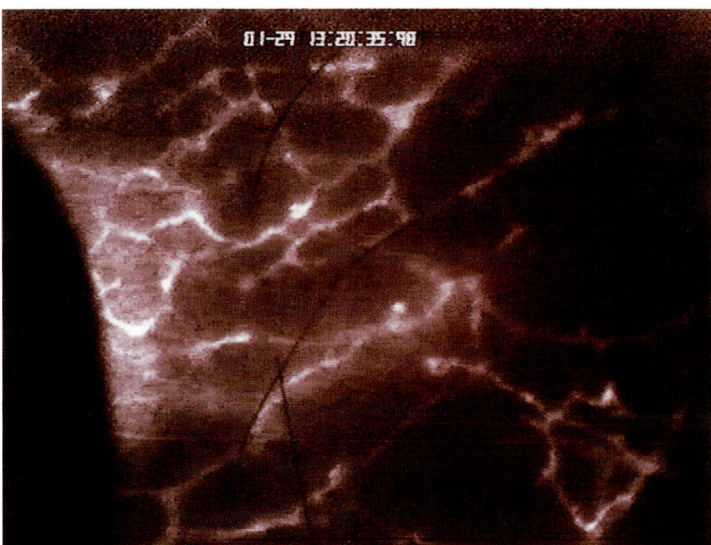

Fig. 48.2 Superficial network of dermal lymphatic vessels as viewed *in vivo* using fluorescence microlymphography.

Fig. 48.1 Diagram of superficial and deep initial lymphatic vessels in the skin. Lymph vessels are coloured green, blood vessels are coloured red. (From Kubik and Manestar [1], with permission.)

12 Cursiefen C, Chen L, Borges LP *et al*. VEGF-A stimulates lymphangiogenesis and hemangiogenesis in inflammatory neovascularization via macrophage recruitment. *J Clin Invest* 2004; **113**: 1040–50.

13 Kerjaschki D, Huttary N, Raab I *et al*. Lymphatic endothelial progenitor cells contribute to de novo lymphangiogenesis in human renal transplants. *Nat Med* 2006; **12**: 230–4.

14 Murakami M, Zheng Y, Hirashima M *et al*. VEGFR1 tyrosine kinase signaling promotes lymphangiogenesis as well as angiogenesis indirectly via macrophage recruitment. *Arterioscler Thromb Vasc Biol* 2008; **28**: 658–64.

15 Abtahian F, Guerriero A, Sebzda E *et al*. Regulation of blood and lymphatic vascular separation by signaling proteins SLP-76 and Syk. *Science* 2003; **299**: 247–51.

16 Hosking B, Makinen T. Lymphatic vasculature: a molecular perspective. *Bioessays* 2007; **29**: 1192–202.

Anatomy

In the skin, lymphatic vessels form two horizontally running networks, a narrow-meshed, superficial network lying subepidermally and a deeper, wide-meshed network. The networks are connected to each other through obliquely-running vessels (Fig. 48.1). Although fewer in number than blood vessels, lymphatics are potentially larger at capillary level. Lymphatics are essentially of two types:

1 Smaller, non-contractile, initial lymphatics (these used to be called terminal lymphatics), which commence or 'initiate' the drainage process within the tissues

2 Larger, contractile, lymphatic collectors, into which the initial lymphatics drain [1].

Afferent collectors drain to lymph nodes and efferent collectors (trunks) drain from lymph nodes. Lymphatic capillaries originate as blind-ending, endothelial-lined tubes in the subpapillary region, and are rarely seen within dermal papillae except in certain disease states—for example, in psoriasis [2,3]. From the superficial lymphatic plexus in the upper dermis, lymph drains through a series of enlarging precollectors into the contractile collecting trunks close to the dermosubcutaneous junction [1]. The lobules of adipose tissue have lymphatics only in their periphery, and clearance of lymph from the centre of the lobule is slow [4].

Initial lymphatics in the skin are arranged in loosely constructed polygonal meshes (Fig. 48.2) high in the dermis [1,5]. Territories of skin are drained by these meshes into the vertically draining precollectors. A series of luminal valves ensure that flow is unidirectional. Such is the capacity of initial lymphatics for dilatation that the valves can become incompetent. Obstruction to deeper lymphatic routes leads to re-routing of lymph and results in 'dermal backflow', as witnessed both on conventional X-ray lymphography and lymphoscintigraphy. In this way, the initial lymphatic network of the skin provides collateralization by which lymph can escape to other (more) normally draining areas [6].

References

1 Kubik S, Manestar M. Anatomy of the lymph capillaries and precollectors of the skin. In: Bollinger A, Partsch H, Wolfe JJN, eds. *The Initial Lymphatics*. Stuttgart: Thieme, 1985: 66–74.

2 Braverman I. The role of blood vessels and lymphatics in cutaneous inflammatory processes: an overview. *Br J Dermatol* 1983; **109** (Suppl. 25): 89–98.

3 Braverman IM. Ultrastructure and organisation of the cutaneous microvasculature in normal and pathologic states. *J Invest Dermatol* 1989; **93**: 25–95.

4 Ryan TJ. Lymphatics and adipose tissue. *Clin Dermatol* 1995; **13**: 493–8.

5 Bollinger A, Jager K, Spier F, Seglias J. Fluorescence microlymphography. *Circulation* 1981; **64**: 1195–200.

6 Tiedjen KU, Knorz S, Heimann KD. The skin: lymphatic collateral organ? *Scope Phlebol Lymphol* 1994; **1**: 7–12.

Structure and function

Description

Initial lymphatics/lymphatic capillaries

The lymphatic capillary is lined by a fine endothelium which is more attenuated than that of blood capillaries (Fig. 48.3). Potentially larger than blood capillaries, lymphatics are frequently not visualized in histological sections, because they are collapsed. A

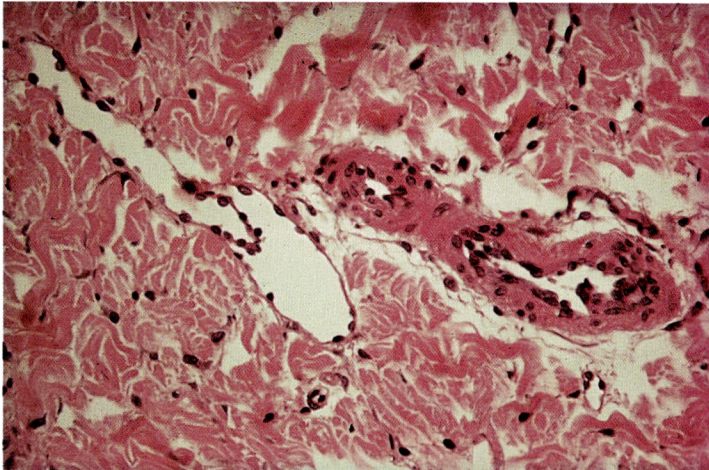

Fig. 48.3 Mid-dermal vessels showing the typical appearance of a mid-dermal blood capillary with plump endothelium compared with adjacent lymphatic vessels with attenuated endothelium and a valve. Such valves are not present in blood vessels high in the dermis.

distended lymphatic exhibits characteristically thin, attenuated walls with nuclei bulging into the lumen. On electron microscopy, the gaps between overlapping endothelial cells are much larger than in the blood capillary. These 'open junctions' act as primary (mural) valves and serve as the entry point for macromolecules [1]. Initial (dermal) lymphatics have little in the way of a basement membrane or pericytes [2]. The lymphatic endothelium contains very few pinocytotic vesicles and lacks Weibel–Palade bodies and fenestrae [3]. Attached to the outside of the endothelium are anchoring filaments which attach the lymphatic to surrounding collagen and elastic fibres [4]. The main molecular component of the anchoring filaments is fibrillin [5]. The elastic fibres form a partial envelope around the dermal lymphatics [6]. In addition to the flap valves in the lymphatic wall are bileaflet intraluminal valves [7].

Lymphatic–vasculature function critically depends on extracellular matrix (ECM) and on its connections with LECs. EMILIN1, an elastic microfibril-associated protein, is highly expressed by LECs *in vitro* and colocalizes with lymphatic vessels in several mouse tissues. The phenotype displayed by *Emilin1*(−/−) mice is the first abnormal lymphatic phenotype associated with the deficiency of an ECM protein and identifies EMILIN1 as a novel local regulator of lymphangiogenesis [8].

Contractile collecting lymphatics

Contractile lymphatics are endowed with a basement membrane and are covered by mural cells, both pericytes and smooth muscle cells. They contain a regularly spaced chain of lumenal valves that prevent retrograde flow even at high pressures. Segments of lymphatic collecting vessel, between one valve and the next, act as active pumps called lymphangions. They are innervated and respond to vasoactive mediators including nitric oxide [9].

References

1 Trzewik J, Mallipattu SK, Artmann GM *et al.* Evidence for a second valve system in lymphatics: endothelial microvalves. *FASEB* 200; **15**: 1711–7.
2 Barsky SH, Baker A, Siegal GP *et al.* Use of anti-basement membrane antibodies to distinguish blood vessel capillaries from lymphatic capillaries. *Am J Surg Pathol* 1983; **7**: 667–77.
3 Ryan TJ. Structure and function of lymphatics. *J Invest Dermatol* 1989; **93**: 18–24.
4 Leak LV, Burke JF. Ultrastructural studies on the lymphatic anchoring filaments. *J Cell Biol* 1968; **36**: 129–49.
5 Weber E, Rossi A, Solito R *et al.* The pattern of fibrillin deposition correlates with microfibril-associated glycoprotein 1 (MAGP-1) expression in cultured blood and lymphatic endothelial cells. *Lymphology* 2004; **37**: 116–26.
6 Mortimer PS, Cherry GW, Jones RL *et al.* The importance of elastic fibres in skin lymphatics. *Br J Dermatol* 1983; **108**: 561–6.
7 Daroczy J. *The Dermal Lymphatic Capillaries*. Berlin: Springer, 1988.
8 Danussi C, Spessotto P, Petrucco A *et al.* Emilin1 deficiency causes structural and functional defects of lymphatic vasculature. *Mol Cell Biol* 2008; **28**: 4026–39.
9 Hagendoorn J, Padera TP, Kashiwagi S. Endothelial nitric oxide synthase regulates microlymphatic flow via collecting lymphatics. *Circ Res* 2004; **95**: 204–9.

Identification of skin lymphatics—molecular markers

The recent discovery of specific markers for lymphatic endothelium has contributed greatly to the identification of skin lymphatics in tissue sections. Previously, the only certain way of distinguishing a lymphatic from a blood vessel was by electron microscopy. Intramural valves between overlapping endothelial cells are pathognomonic of skin lymphatic vessels [1]. If large skin biopsies are fixed in an expanded condition by stretching the specimen in different directions, as would be the case *in vivo*, lymphatic vessels become visible for both light and transmission electron microscopy [2].

A number of markers are available for labelling endothelial cells, but the majority stain both blood and lymph vessels (e.g. factor VIII-related antigen, CD31 (PECAM-1)). Because initial lymphatics lack a continuous basement membrane, immunocytochemistry for the extracellular matrix components type IV collagen and laminin has been used to distinguish them from blood capillaries [3]. Pal-E monoclonal antibody is consistently negative in lymphatic vessels but positive in venules and small veins, the vessels most likely to be mistaken for lymphatics [4].

Of the newer molecular markers, VEGFR-3 was the first to be documented to be expressed in lymphatic endothelium, but it can also be found in a subset of blood vessels and in angiogenic vessels in certain pathological conditions. LYVE-1 (lymphatic vessel hyaluronan receptor-1) is a homolog of hyaluronan receptor CD44 [5] (Fig. 48.4). It is present in initial lymphatics but not in the larger contractile lymphatics. LYVE-1 is also present in activated macrophages in skin and is frequently down-regulated on lymphatics in inflammation.

Podoplanin is a glomerular podocyte membrane mucoprotein which is highly expressed in lymphatic endothelial cells [6]. It is also expressed in keratinocytes but is very specific for dermal lymphatics. Studies in cultured endothelial cells indicate that T1α/podoplanin promotes cell adhesion, migration and tube formation, whereas small interfering RNA-mediated inhibition of T1α/podoplanin expression decreased lymphatic endothelial cell adhesion [7].

Other markers reported to be positive in lymphatic, but not in blood, vessels include Prox-1 which is a nuclear stain [8]. CCL21 is produced by lymphatic endothelium and directs homing of cells such as lymphocytes possessing CC receptors [9]. It is unlikely that any one marker will be totally specific, particularly

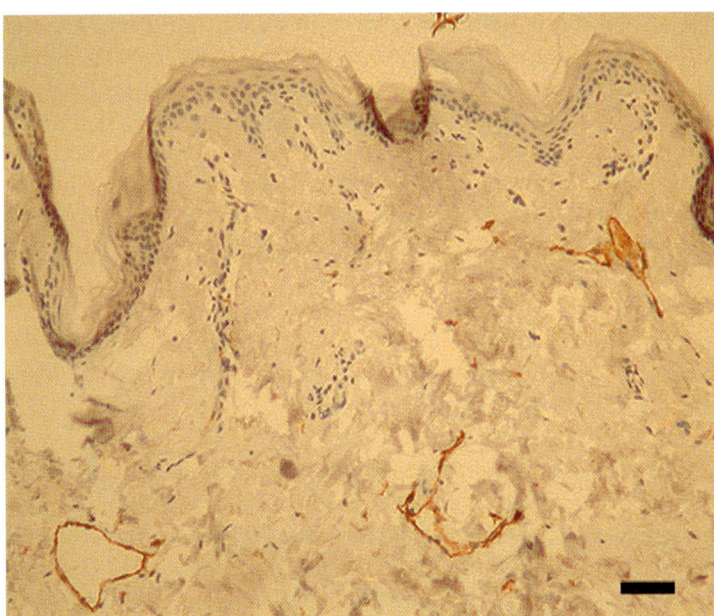

Fig. 48.4 LYVE-1 antibody marker for lymphatic endothelium. (Courtesy of Dr D.G. Jackson.)

Table 48.1 Markers for lymphatic vessels. (Adapted from [10].)

Molecule	Protein class	Biological effect
VEGFR-3	Receptor tyrosine kinase on endothelial cell	Lymphangiogenesis
LYVE-1	Receptor for extracellular matrix glycosaminoglycan	Transport of HA from tissues to lymph nodes
Prox-1	Transcription factor	Lymphvasculogenesis
Podoplanin (D2-40)	Integral membrane protein	Lymphatic morphogenesis
CCL21	Chemokine	T-cell trafficking

HA, hyaluronan; LYVE-1, lymphatic vessel endothelial HA receptor; VEGFR-3, vascular endothelial growth factor receptor-3; CC, chemokine with two adjacent cysteine residues.

in disease states, and the use of several markers is recommended (Table 48.1).

References
1 Braverman IM. Ultrastructure and organization of the cutaneous micro-vasculature in normal and pathologic states. *J Invest Dermatol* 1989; **93**: 25–9S.
2 Lubach D, Wawrzyniak-Schulz A, Neukam D, Nissen S. The extension technique: a new method of demonstrating initial lymph vessels in excised human skin. *Br J Dermatol* 1990; **123**: 179–85.
3 Barsky SH, Baker A, Siegal GP *et al*. Use of anti-basement membrane antibodies to distinguish blood vessel capillaries from lymphatic capillaries. *Am J Surg Pathol* 1983; **7**: 667–77.
4 Schlingemann RO, Rietweld FJ, Kwaspen F *et al*. Differential expression of markers for endothelial cells, pericytes and basal lamina in the microvasculature of tumours and granulation tissue. *Am J Pathol* 1991; **138**: 1335–42.
5 Banerji S, Ni J, Wang SX *et al*. LYVE-1, a new homologue of the CD44 glycoprotein, is a lymph specific receptor for hyaluronan. *J Cell Biol* 1999; **144**: 789–801.
6 Breiteneder-Geleff S, Soleman A, Kowalski H *et al*. Angiosarcomas express mixed endothelial phenotypes of blood and lymphatic capillaries: podoplanin as a specific marker for lymphatic endothelium. *Am J Pathol* 1999; **154**: 385–94.
7 Schacht V, Ramirez MI, Hong YK *et al*. T1alpha/podoplanin deficiency disrupts normal lymphatic vasculature formation and causes lymphedema. *EMBO J* 2003; **22**: 3546–56.
8 Wigle JT, Oliver G. Prox-1 function is required for the development of the murine lymphatic system. *Cell* 1999; **98**: 769–78.
9 Shields JD, Emmett MS, Dunn DB *et al*. Chemokine-mediated migration of melanoma cells towards lymphatics—a mechanism contributing to metastasis. *Oncogene* 2007; **26**: 2997–3005.
10 Jussila L, Alitalo K. Vascular growth factors and lymphangiogenesis. *Physiol Rev* 2002; **82**: 673–700.

Purpose of lymphatics

Lymphatic vessels are primarily concerned with draining, from the tissue spaces, materials which cannot directly return to the bloodstream. While the bloodstream essentially supplies the tissues, the lymphatic system essentially drains them. This includes proteins as well as cells—extravasated erythrocytes, dendritic cells, macrophages, lymphocytes and, of course, malignant cells.

Contrary to traditional teaching, the lymphatic is the main drainage route for fluid. Only transiently is fluid reabsorbed by venous capillaries. It is important to understand this role of the lymphatic acting as a 'safety valve' or buffer against fluid overload, because it means that every form of oedema indicates some degree of lymphatic failure [1].

Lymphatics carry foreign material that has penetrated the dermis, including microorganisms, injected vaccines, solvents of skin cosmetics, inorganic material such as silica and stains from tattoos [2]. Bacterial and other microorganisms are channelled through lymphatics as a protective mechanism to prevent noxious agents from directly entering the bloodstream. Presumably this failure to 'police' infection is the reason why cellulitis/erysipelas can cause rapid systemic illness in lymphoedema before local signs are evident.

Snake envenomation causes a dose-dependent contraction of collecting lymphatic vessels, resulting in a reduction of their lumen and in a halting of lymph flow so venom remains contained within the lymphatics following a bite [3].

References
1 Mortimer PS, Levick JR. Chronic peripheral oedema: the critical role of the lymphatic system. *Clin Med* 2004; **4**: 448–53.
2 Ikomi F, Schmid-Schonbein GW. Lymph transport in the skin. *Clin Dermatol* 1995; **13**: 419–27.
3 Mora J, Mora R, Lomonte B, Gutiérrez JM. Effects of *Bothrops asper* snake venom on lymphatic vessels: insights into a hidden aspect of envenomation. *PLoS Negl Trop Dis* 2008; **2**: e318.

Lymph transport

After filtration from the microvasculature, interstitial fluid enters a series of passive initial lymphatics and is then propelled within the collecting trunks through a series of intervalvular pumping segments (lymph hearts) to the lymph nodes before eventually returning to the venous system at the thoracic duct. Transport of fluid and other materials (prelymph) across the interstitial space towards initial lymphatics is a passive process, dependent upon changes in local pressures (convective flow) [1,2]. Deformation or movement of the dermis by surface pressure and underlying muscle contractions and by dermal components, such as arterioles, causes expansion or compression of the initial lymphatics. The process of expansion is likely to result from pulling of the anchoring filaments on the abluminal surface of the lymphatic [3]. These probably act to prevent lymphatic collapse when interstitial pressure is high, as in oedema [4]. Negative fluid pressure inside the initial lymphatics serves to open the interendothelial junctions (flap valves) and to permit inflow of interstitial fluid. After filling and equilibration of pressure the flap valves close. Compression of the filled lymphatic then moves lymph downstream, that is towards bigger lymphatics; the valves within the lymphatic vessels ensure that flow is in one direction. Recoil of the initial lymphatic occurs when the compression wave (squeezing) of the lymphatic ceases and the cycle repeats itself. Cardiac arrest leads to cessation of lymph flow, but lymph flow can be maintained with active skin massage even after the arrest of the heart.

Lymph does not passively 'drain downstream' through the collecting lymphatic vessels because the net pressure gradients oppose flow. Instead, the collecting vessels must act as both the conduits, that direct and regulate lymph flow, and the pumps that generate the lymph flow. The regulation of lymphatic muscle contractions is thought to occur via the interaction of cell calcium with regulatory and contractile proteins. This is almost certainly one of the mechanisms whereby calcium channel blocking agents cause peripheral oedema. However, our knowledge of this regulation of lymphatic contractile function is far from complete [5].

References

1 Ikomi F, Schmid-Schonbein GW. Lymph transport in the skin. *Clin Dermatol* 1995; **13**: 419–27.
2 Levick JR, McHale N. The physiology of lymph production and propulsion. In: Browse NL, Burnand KG, Mortimer PS, eds. *Diseases of the Lymphatics*. London: Arnold, 2003: 44–64.
3 Leak LV. Ultrastructure and function of the interstitial–lymphatic interface. In: Staub NC, Hogg JC, Hargens ASR, eds. *Interstitial–Lymphatic Liquid and Solute Movement*. Basel: Karger, 1986: 1–14.
4 Castenholz A. Functional microanatomy of initial lymphatics with special consideration of the extracellular matrix. *Lymphology* 1998; **31**: 101–18.
5 Muthuchamy M, Zawieja D. Molecular regulation of lymphatic contractility. *Ann N Y Acad Sci* 2008; **1131**: 89–99.

Immune functions

The principal immune function of the afferent lymphatics is to bear antigens and leukocytes from peripheral tissues to the draining lymph nodes. Recent research has shown that passage of leukocytes into the afferent lymphatic capillaries is far from an indolent process; rather it is carefully orchestrated by an array of adhesion molecules, as well as by chemokines and their receptors [1].

Lymphocytes and mononuclear phagocytes constantly patrol the skin, leaving via the afferent lymphatic vessels for the lymph nodes. Epidermal (e.g. Langerhans' cells) and dermal dendritic cells screen the skin for invading antigens. They migrate from the skin to regional nodes where a primary immune response is initiated [2]. Dendritic cells enter dermal lymphatics by transmigration through intercellular spaces of adjacent endothelial cells, frequently carrying material such as melanosomes and apoptotic bodies [3].

Under normal physiological conditions immature dendritic cells migrate constitutively and continuously from skin to lymph nodes via afferent lymphatics, undertaking immune surveillance [4]. Subsequent to inflammation the number of dendritic cells increases dramatically and they change from phagocytes into professional antigen-presenting cells [5]. Receptors on lymphatic endothelial cells facilitate migration of proteins and cells to, and within, lymphatics. CCL21 is a chemokine that is produced constitutively by lymphatic endothelial cells in the skin [6]. Disruption of the CCR7 gene, which prevents expression of CCL21, thereby prevents migration of dendritic cells from tissue to regional nodes. CCR7-deficient mice lack contact sensitivity due to a failure of translymphatic migration of epidermal dendritic cells [7]. CCR7 and its ligands (CCL21 and 19) are also important in regulating lymphatic trafficking of T cells [8].

Without intact lymphatics a primary immune response cannot develop. In the case of allogeneic skin grafts, removal of the lymph drainage channels causes cessation of the cellular reactions in the lymph nodes until lymphatic pathways are re-established [9,10]. Rejection is delayed in grafted skin sites where all draining lymphatics are severed [11]. Studies in lymphoedema following curative breast cancer treatment demonstrated an impaired response to dinitrochlorobenzene testing in the swollen limb but not in the contralateral control limb [12]. Similar results were reported in lymphoedema associated with Kaposi's sarcoma [13].

Bacteria, viruses, fungi and toxins which penetrate the skin are absorbed by lymphatics and not by blood capillaries [14,15]. Virulent haemolytic streptococci, tubercle bacilli and many types of soluble or particulate antigens injected intradermally readily reach the regional lymph node [9].

References

1 Johnson LA, Jackson DG. Cell traffic and the lymphatic endothelium. *Ann N Y Acad Sci* 2008; **1131**: 119–33.
2 Silverberg-Sinakin I, Thorbecke GJ, Baer RL et al. Antigen-bearing Langerhans cells in skin, dermal lymphatics and in lymph nodes. *Cell Immunol* 1976; **25**: 137–51.
3 Stoitzner P, Pfaller K, Stossel H, Romani N. A close-up view of migrating Langerhans cells in the skin. *J Invest Dermatol* 2002; **118**: 117–25.
4 Smith JB, McIntosh GH, Morris B. The traffic of cells through tissues; a study of peripheral lymph in sheep. *J Anat* 1970; **107**: 87–100.
5 Steinman RM, Hawiger D, Nussenzweig MC. Tolerogenic dendritic cells. *Annu Rev Immunol* 2003; **21**: 685–711.
6 Saeki H, Moore AM, Brown MJ, Hwang ST. Cutting edge: secondary lymphoid tissue chemokine (SLC) and cc chemokine receptor 7 (CCR7) participate in the emigration pathway of mature dendritic cells from the skin to regional lymph nodes. *J Immunol* 1999; **162**: 2472–5.
7 Ohl L, Mohaupt M, Czeloth N et al. CCR7 governs skin dendritic cell migration under inflammatory and steady-state conditions. *Immunity* 2004; **21**: 279–88.
8 Worbs T, Mempel TR, Bölter J et al. CCR7 ligands stimulate the intranodal motility of T lymphocytes in vivo. *J Exp Med* 2007; **204**: 489–95.
9 Yoffey JM, Courtice JM. *Lymphatics, Lymph and the Lymphomyeloid Complex*. New York: Academic Press, 1970.
10 Lambert PB, Frank HA, Bellman S, Farnsworth D. The role of the lymph trunks in the response to allogeneic skin transplants. *Transplantation* 1965; **3**: 62–73.
11 Tilney NL, Gowans JL. The sensitisation of rats by allografts transplanted to alymphatic pedicles of skin. *J Exp Med* 1971; **133**: 951–62.
12 Mallon E, Powell S, Mortimer PS, Ryan TJ. Evidence for altered cell mediated immunity in postmastectomy lymphoedema. *Br J Dermatol* 1997; **137**: 928–33.
13 Ruocco V, Satriano RA, Astarita C. Anomalies régionales des voies lymphatiques et de la réponse au DNCB dans le sarcome de Kaposi classique. *Ann Dermatol Vénéréol* 1985; **112**: 283–6.
14 Barnes JM, Trueta J. Absorption of bacteria, toxins and snake venoms from the tissues. *Lancet* 1941; **i**: 623–6.
15 De Long TG, Simmons RL. Role of lymphatic vessels in bacterial clearance from early soft tissue infection. *Arch Surg* 1982; **117**: 123–8.

Table 48.2 Causes of oedema.

Increased capillary filtration
Increased capillary pressure
  Increased venous pressure, e.g. right heart failure, DVT, obstructing malignancy,
    overtransfusion
  Increased blood flow, e.g. inflammation, arteriovenous fistula
Reduced plasma proteins
  Increased loss, e.g. nephrotic syndrome, protein-losing enteropathy
  Reduced synthesis, e.g. cirrhosis, advanced cancer
  Malabsorption, malnutrition
Increased capillary permeability
  Inflammation, e.g. varicose eczema, psoriasis, urticaria and angioedema

Reduced lymph drainage
Primary lymphatic insufficiency
  Genetic (and inherited)
  Milroy's disease (onset at or soon after birth)
  Lymphoedema, distichiasis (postpubertal)
  Meige's disease (postpubertal)
  Constitutive (presumed genetic)
Secondary lymphatic insufficiency
  Iatrogenic interruption to drainage routes, e.g. surgery, radiotherapy
  Cancer (particularly relapsed)
  Infection, e.g. filariasis, cellulitis
  Accidental trauma
Dysfunctional lymphatics
  Dependency syndrome
  Loss of mobility
  High output failure, e.g. venous disease
  Deep-vein thrombosis

Chronic oedema

Oedema is an excess of interstitial fluid. Interstitial fluid volume must increase by over 100% before oedema is clinically detectable. Dermal oedema manifests as 'peau d'orange' due to expansion of the interfollicular dermis, whereas subcutaneous oedema gives rise to pitting.

Any oedema, whatever the cause, is due to capillary filtration overwhelming the lymph drainage for a sufficient period of time [1]. Interstitial fluid is reabsorbed almost entirely by the lymphatics. Contrary to popular belief, venous reabsorption of interstitial fluid cannot be maintained for any length of time except in certain vascular beds, for example that of the kidney [1]. The causes of oedema formation are listed in Table 48.2. Most chronic oedemas arise from increased capillary filtration overwhelming lymph drainage. To some extent, therefore, any chronic oedema incriminates the lymphatic system through its failure to keep up with demand. Lymphoedema, however, is oedema arising principally from a failure in lymph drainage.

Therefore any chronic oedema indicates lymphatic failure. It is best not to approach a lower limb chronic oedema clinically by trying to pigeon-hole the diagnosis into 'heart failure', 'venous oedema', 'lymphoedema' etc. A far better approach is to consider if the oedema represents pure lymphatic failure, or, as is most common, lymphatic failure due to lymph drainage being overwhelmed by increased capillary filtration. Most cases of chronic oedema have more than one factor contributing to impaired lymph drainage and increased capillary filtration. Therefore terms such as lymphoedema (predominantly lymph drainage failure) or a filtration oedema (predominantly increased capillary filtration) are suggested [2] (Table 48.2).

References

1 Levick JR. *An Introduction to Cardiovascular Physiology*, 4th edn. London: Arnold, 2003.
2 Mortimer PS, Levick JR. Chronic peripheral oedema: the critical role of the lymphatic system. *Clin Med* 2004; **4**: 448–53.

Lymphoedema

Definition. Swelling due to the excess accumulation of lymph in the tissues caused by inadequate lymph drainage. Lymphoedema differs clinically from other forms of chronic oedema by its altered skin texture and the brawny quality of the subcutaneous tissues, which limit pitting. There may be no distinguishing features, particularly in the early stages of swelling. A more precise definition would be 'a swelling of soft tissues which is the result of accumulation of protein-rich interstitial fluid caused by a low output failure of lymph' [1].

Primary lymphoedema implies a genetic or constitutive cause whereby there is an intrinsic fault in lymph drainage determined by a lymphatic maldevelopment or functional weakness. Secondary lymphoedema implies an acquired failure of previously normal lymph drainage due to an identifiable cause extrinsic to the lymphatic system.

Epidemiology

Lymphoedema *per se* is perceived as uncommon, yet lymphatic insufficiency is a major contributing cause of chronic ankle oedema, which is considered common (particularly in the elderly) [2]. Because lymphoedema can be a difficult diagnosis, particularly if mild or in the early stages, it is frequently underdiagnosed. One survey, which determined the problem of chronic oedema (as a surrogate for lymphoedema) in the community, ascertained 823 patients in a catchment area of 619 000 in south-west London. This estimated the overall prevalence of chronic oedema as 1.33/1000 population; the prevalence increased with age and was 5.4/1000 in subjects aged over 65 years. In only a quarter did the oedema arise from cancer treatment. Twenty-nine per cent had experienced at least one attack of cellulitis over the previous year. Ten per cent of subjects had lost, or had had to change, employment as a result of their chronic oedema. Chronic oedema that was likely to be lymphatic in origin is common in the community and often goes unrecognized [3].

Primary types of lymphoedema tend to affect females more frequently (70–80% of patients are female). In less than 10% of cases is swelling present at birth; most cases present at or soon after puberty. It is estimated that 80% will present before the age of 35 years (lymphoedema praecox) and 10% after the age of 35 years (lymphoedema tarda) [4]. Data on prevalence of lymphoedema are few, and a figure for overall prevalence of primary lymphoedema is not available. However, a study of 1000 young adults showed that 8% of women demonstrated signs of lymph-oedema in the lower limb [5].

Secondary types of lymphoedema are more common than primary. In developed countries cancer treatment dominates as a cause whereas in tropical climates infection dominates [6].

Breast cancer-related lymphoedema (BCRL). The cumulative prevalence of swelling following breast cancer treatment in women is 28% [7]. The introduction of sentinel lymph node biopsy (SLNB), used as a staging investigation for cancer, has not necessarily reduced the incidence of lymphoedema as was hoped. While the incidence of BCRL following SLNB has reduced to 5–7%, the need for axillary clearance in the 30% who are node-positive can lead to an incidence of up to 45% in that group.

Pelvic malignancy. The incidence of lower limb lymphoedema following radical hysterectomy alone is estimated at 5–10% [8] but can be as high as 49% by 10 years of follow up in patients who have also received adjuvant radiation treatment [9]. The incidence after vulval cancer is reported at 28% [10]. Following prostate cancer the incidence has been reported at 3–8% [6], and after penile cancer 23–33% [11].

Melanoma. The incidence after lymphadenectomy can be up to 44% after therapeutic groin dissection for palpable disease [12], but the incidence following sentinel lymph node biopsy is much less [13]. Patients undergoing an inguinal lymph node dissection (ILND) for a positive SLN have a significantly lower risk of post-operative complication or lymphoedema than do patients undergoing ILND for clinically palpable disease [14].

Pathophysiology

Physiologically, there are only a limited number of ways lymphatics may fail. They may be reduced in number, obliterated, obstructed or simply fail to function. A lack of sensitive methods for investigation makes it difficult to distinguish between these mechanisms (Table 48.3).

A reduction in lymphatics may be due to hypoplasia such as the reduction of skin lymphatics in Milroy's disease. In the commonest form of primary lymphoedema, that presenting at or soon after puberty with distal leg swelling, lymphangiograms usually

Table 48.3 Possible causes of lymph drainage failure.

Mechanism	Causes
Reduced lymph-conducting pathways	Hypoplasia of whole vessel, reduced numbers of vessels (initial or collecting)
	May be developmental failure or acquired obliteration of lymphatic lumen (e.g. lymphangiothrombosis, lymphangitis)
Poorly functioning lymphatics	May be physiological due to lack of movement or structural, e.g. pump (contractility) failure
Obstructed lymphatics	'Scarring' from lymphadenectomy, radiotherapy or infection
Lymph reflux	Megalymphatics, lymph vessel hyperplasia

demonstrate a reduction in the size and number of superficial leg lymphatic collectors. It is often assumed that the lymphatics have been abnormal since birth but it is always possible that the lymph vessels have undergone an accelerated atrophy or ageing process. The congenitally determined abnormality may not therefore be an underdevelopment of lymphatics from birth, but rather a failure of growth/regeneration or function following damage or injury. This would explain the latent period before swelling manifests, particularly in those forms presenting later in life (lymphoedema tarda). In truth, we do not know and these possibilities are speculative.

An obliterative process, where there is permanent obliteration of the lymphatic lumen and consequently of the vessel itself, probably develops through lymphangiothrombosis or lymphangitis in the same way as for veins. Obliterative lymphangitis is probably the mechanism following infection or longstanding hand eczema.

Obstruction will cause increased outflow or downstream resistance and lead to re-routing via collateral pathways. Whether lymphoedema develops is dependent on the efficiency of such collaterals to accommodate the lymph load.

Reflux results from incompetence of intraluminal lymphatic valves. This is seen in lymphoedema–distichiasis syndrome, where there appears to be genetically-determined valve maldevelopment affecting both lymphatic and venous valves [15].

Pathology. Decreased transport of lymph from the skin leads to an increase in protein-rich interstitial fluid. In circumstances other than where dermal lymphatics are congenitally absent (for example, Milroy's disease) or are destroyed (for example, post-erysipelas/cellulitis), interstitial pressure consequently rises and lymphatics dilate. Temporal changes observed in experimental lymphoedema indicate that the collagen fibres initially become swollen and separated [16]. Mononuclear cells are seen around the lymphatic and blood vessels [17]. Lymphatic walls thicken and fibrose. The muscular elements of the collecting trunks atrophy. Macrophages, fibroblasts and lymphocytes accumulate. Overgrowth of the interstitial connective tissue gradually transforms the soft stage of lymphoedema into the hard late-stage form [18]. The simple excess of protein seems to be the cause of the fibrosis [19,20]. The number of blood vessels greatly increases.

In human skin, the epidermis overlying an area of lymphoedema becomes acanthotic, with reduplication of the epidermodermal basement membrane. In the dermis, there is an increase in collagen, but the elastic fibres, including anchoring filaments, disappear. Ultrastructurally, the basal lamina of the dermal lymphatics thickens, but remains discontinuous, connective tissue microfilaments are increased, myofibroblasts appear and the connective tissue ground substance becomes hyalinized [21]. Inflammatory cells are conspicuous in the dermis. In the infiltrate, mast cells, macrophages, plasma cells and lymphocytes can be observed. Extravasated erythrocytes are often seen and large amounts of fibrin become deposited. Well-characterized morphological changes develop in the blood vessels (lymphostatic vasculopathy). In the upper dermis, numerous newly formed vessels can be seen. Angiogenesis results in a highly vascularized dermis.

Table 48.4 Causes of primary lymphoedema.

Congenital onset		Postpubertal onset	
Familial	**Sporadic**	**Familial**	**Sporadic**
Milroy's disease: below knee and bilateral	Turner's syndrome, Noonan's syndrome: can be transient; other phenotype abnormalities Neurofibromatosis, Proteus syndrome Pure or mixed vascular lymphatic malformations, lymphangiomatosis, Klippel–Trenaunay syndrome, Maffucci's syndrome: usually unilateral Amniotic bands: associated with autoamputation	Distichiasis–lymphoedema, Meige's disease: below knee and bilateral	Distal hypoplasia, lymph reflux: bilateral foot and lower leg swelling Ilioinguinal node sclerosis: whole limb and unilateral Yellow nail syndrome: bilateral, widespread oedema

References

1 Földi M. Insufficiency of lymph flow. In: Földi M, Casley-Smith JR, eds. *Lymphangiology*. Stuttgart: Schattauer, 1983: 195–213.

2 Bull RH, Gane JN, Evans J *et al.* Abnormal lymph drainage in patients with chronic venous leg ulcers. *J Am Acad Dermatol* 1993; **28**: 585–90.

3 Moffatt CJ, Franks PJ, Doherty DC *et al.* Lymphoedema: an underestimated health problem [abstract]. *Br J Dermatol* 2002; **147** (Suppl. 62): 8.

4 Dale RF. The inheritance of primary lymphoedema. *J Med Genet* 1985; **22**: 274–8.

5 Scharz U. Die Häufigkeit des primären Lymphödems. Eine epidemiologische Studie an über 1000 Probanden. *Med Lymph* 1990; **1**: 29–34.

6 Rockson SG, Rivera KK. Estimating the population burden of lymphedema. *Ann N Y Acad Sci* 2008; **1131**: 147–54.

7 Mortimer PS, Bates DO, Brassington HD *et al.* The prevalence of arm swelling following breast cancer treatment. *QJM* 1996; **89**: 377–80.

8 Snijders-Keilholz A, Hellebrekers BW, Zwinderman AH *et al.* Adjuvant radiotherapy following radical hysterectomy for patients with early-stage cervical carcinoma (1984–1996). *Radiother Oncol* 1999; **51**: 161–7.

9 Chatani M, Nose T, Masaki N, Inoue T. Adjuvant radiotherapy after radical hysterectomy of the cervical cancer. Prognostic factors and complications. *Strahlenther Onkol* 1998; **174**: 504–9.

10 Gaarenstroom KN, Kenter GG, Trimbos JB *et al.* Postoperative complications after vulvectomy and inguinofemoral lymphadenectomy using separate groin incisions. *Int J Gynecol Cancer* 2003; **13**: 522–7.

11 Bevan-Thomas R, Slaton JW, Pettaway CA. Contemporary morbidity from lymphadenectomy for penile squamous cell carcinoma: the M.D. Anderson Cancer Center Experience. *J Urol* 2002; **167**: 1638–42.

12 Allan CP, Hayes AJ, Thomas JM. Ilioinguinal lymph node dissection for palpable metastatic melanoma to the groin. *Aust NZ J Surg* 2008; **78**: 982–6.

13 Wrone DA, Tanabe KK, Cosimi AB *et al.* Lymphedema after sentinel lymph node biopsy for cutaneous melanoma: a report of 5 cases. *Arch Dermatol* 2000; **136**: 511–4.

14 Sabel MS, Griffith KA, Arora A *et al.* Inguinal node dissection for melanoma in the era of sentinel lymph node biopsy. *Surgery* 2007; **141**: 728–35.

15 Mellor RH, Brice G, Stanton AW *et al.* Lymphoedema Research Consortium. Mutations in FOXC2 are strongly associated with primary valve failure in veins of the lower limb. *Circulation* 2007; **115**: 1912–20.

16 Altorfer JL, Clodius L. Chronic experimental lymphedema of the extremities: pathological changes. *Experientia* 1976; **32**: 823–5.

17 Olszewski WL. Pathophysiological and clinical observations of obstructive lymphedema of the limbs. In: Clodius L, ed. *Lymphedema*. Stuttgart: Thieme, 1977: 79–102.

18 Drinker CK, Field ME, Homans J. The experimental production of oedema and elephantiasis as a result of lymphatic obstruction. *Am J Physiol* 1934; **108**: 509–20.

19 Willoughby DA, DiRosa M. A unifying concept for inflammation: a new appraisal of some old mediators. *Excerpta Med* 1970; **229**: 28–38.

20 Casley-Smith JR, Gaffney RM. Excess plasma proteins as a cause of chronic inflammation. *J Pathol* 1981; **133**: 227–72.

21 Daroczy J. Pathology of lymphedema. *Clin Dermatol* 1995; **13**: 433–44.

Aetiology and classification

Lymphoedema may be primary (see Table 48.4), secondary (see Table 48.5), dysfunctional or cancer-related.

Primary lymphoedema

Lymphoedema arising from an intrinsic abnormality of the lymph-conducting pathways is referred to as primary lymphoedema [1] (Table 48.4). A simple classification by age of onset without reference to aetiology or other clinical features is into the following subdivisions: congenital (present at or very soon after birth), praecox (presenting before age 35 years) and tarda (presenting after age 35 years). The development of lymphangiography in the 1950s resulted in a radiological classification: aplasia (no formed lymph pathways found), hypoplasia (lymphatics smaller or fewer than normal) and hyperplasia (lymphatics larger and more numerous). Aplasia, hypoplasia and hyperplasia refer to abnormalities in the main (leg) conducting lymph vessels as opacified on lymphangiography, and not to the initial lymphatics, which are not imaged with this method. Further investigation revealed types of lymphoedema where few, if any, lymph conducting vessels could be identified in the foot, but vessels were found to be normal further up the limb [2].

An increasing understanding of the genetic basis of primary lymphoedema has further changed classification and to some extent made the praecox and tarda categories redundant. For example in lymphoedema–distichiasis syndrome (LDS), the onset of lower-limb oedema can range from puberty to 40 years old despite the same cause, namely a mutation in the *FOXC2* gene [3]. Conversely, LDS and Meige forms of primary lymphoedema can both present at puberty with similar lower lymphoedema but have different genotypes and different mechanisms; LDS is associated with hyperplasia and valve reflux of collecting lymphatics whereas Meige's disease is associated with hypoplasia of collecting vessels. In the future, classification of lymphoedema is likely to be based on phenotype, unless the genotype is known.

Inherited forms of lymphoedema where the gene is known

1 *Milroy's disease* (primary congenital lymphoedema, hereditary lymphoedema type 1; MIM 153100). Milroy first described the disease in 1892 but published definitively on it in 1928. He

described a large pedigree with lymphoedema beginning at or soon after birth [4]. Although the same condition was described earlier by Nonne [5], it was Milroy who gave the most complete description, and the eponym 'Milroy's disease' is universally accepted. Milroy's disease is often considered synonymous with primary lymphoedema, but the term should be restricted to cases of congenital lymphoedema with linkage to chromosome 5 or mutations in the *VEGFR-3* gene [6–8]. A failure of lymphangiogenesis due to inactivation of *VEGFR-3* appears to be responsible for the autosomal dominant inheritance of Milroy's disease [8]. Genotype–phenotype correlation demonstrates swelling which is confined to below the knee, and which is often brawny in the extreme with little pitting. Hydrocoele can be an additional feature, as can superficial vein incompetence but, much as Milroy described, there appear to be no other manifestations.

2 *Lymphoedema–distichiasis syndrome* (LDS; MIM 153400). Distichiasis is a congenital anomaly in which accessory eyelashes occur along the posterior border of the lid margins in the position of the Meibomian glands. It causes symptoms of corneal irritation, conjunctivitis and photophobia and occurs from birth. Lymphoedema in this syndrome, however, does not develop before puberty and may be delayed in onset until the fifth decade. Other features of this syndrome include ptosis, congenital heart defects and varicose veins [3]. The lymphatic abnormality appears to be lymph reflux with an increased number of lower-limb lymph vessels [9]. LDS shows an autosomal-dominant pattern of inheritance with variable expression and has been mapped to 16q24.3 [10]. Mutations in *FOXC2* (*MFH-1*), a forkhead family transcription factor, are now known to be responsible for this condition [11].

3 *Hypotrichosis–lymphoedema–telangiectasia syndrome* is a rare inherited disorder caused by mutations in *SOX18* transcription factor and manifesting with bilateral lymphoedema of the legs, hypotrichosis, telangiectases and angiomata limited to acral regions [12]. SOX18 acts as a molecular switch to induce differentiation of lymphatic endothelial cells early in development [13].

4 *Incontentia pigmenti* (MIM 308300). Incontentia pigmenti (IP) is not usually associated with lymphoedema in surviving females. The second liveborn male to be reported recently led to the identification of a *NEMO* (NFκB essential modulator) stop codon mutation in the affected child and in his mother, who had classical IP [14]. He had features of hypohidrotic ectodermal dysplasia with immune deficiency, recurrent infections and lower-limb lymphoedema which developed at a few weeks of age. A lymphoscintigram showed severe lymphatic obstruction. MRI suggested a lymphangiomatous malformation. Cutaneous capillary angiomas and possible mixed vascular/lymphatic malformations coexisted in the gut [15].

Other germline forms of lymphoedema

1 *Meige's disease* (Kinmonth's lymphoedema praecox, hereditary lymphoedema type II; MIM #153200). In 1898, Meige described the pedigree of a family with a distinct history of lymphoedema appearing at puberty [16]. The eponym Meige's disease has therefore come to be associated with this, the commonest variety of primary lymphoedema, which predominantly affects adolescent females. Swelling is usually mild, rarely extends above the knee and is generally bilateral. Lymphography demonstrates a reduced number of distal lymphatics (hypoplasia) with proximal collectors remaining patent. The term Meige's disease should be reserved for familial lymphoedema developing at or soon after puberty in which there are no associated abnormalities, for example distichiasis.

2 *Turner's syndrome*. This well-known abnormality is due to the absence of one X chromosome. Early spontaneous abortion occurs in over 95% of fetuses. Severely affected fetuses who survive to the second trimester can be detected on ultrasonography, which may reveal cystic hygroma, chylothorax, ascites and hydrops fetalis. The diagnosis may be suggested in the newborn by redundant neck skin and peripheral oedema. Surviving children have webbed necks and may exhibit peripheral oedema which often diminishes with age. Conversely oedema may present later in life. Chromosomal testing should always be undertaken in neonates or young children with primary lymphoedema.

3 *Noonan's syndrome* (MIM #163950). Noonan's syndrome is a multiple congenital anomaly syndrome for which mutations in *PTPN11* have been discovered to be the cause [17]. Lymphoedema is usually present at birth but the age of onset may vary from the prenatal period to adulthood. Phenotypic characteristics include short stature, ptosis, low-set ears and posterior hairline, neck webbing and congenital cardiac anomalies (typically pulmonary stenosis).

4 *Hennekam lymphangiectasia–lymphoedema syndrome* (MIM *235510). A syndrome of intestinal lymphangiectasia with severe lymphoedema of the limbs, genitalia and face, with mental retardation [18]. The intestinal lymphangiectasia causes hypoproteinaemia, hypogammaglobulinaemia and lymphopenia. Facial anomalies are characteristic and look somewhat oriental, with flat face, flat nasal bridge, epicanthic folds, hypertelorism, tooth abnormalities and small ears. Onset of lymphoedema is between birth and 12 years, with probable autosomal-recessive inheritance.

5 *Cholestasis–lymphoedema syndrome* (Aagenaes's syndrome; MIM *214900). Jaundice becomes evident soon after birth and recurs throughout life. Oedema of the leg, due to hypoplasia of the lymph vessels, begins at school age and progresses [19].

6 *Microcephaly lymphoedema–chorioretinal dysplasia* (MIM *152950). An autosomal dominant syndrome [20] in which microcephaly and lymphoedema are linked to chorioretinopathy.

7 *Pes cavus and lymphoedema*. Lymphangiography has revealed hypoplasia of leg lymphatics in this disease association [21].

8 *Yellow nail syndrome* (YNS; MIM #153300). The evidence that YNS is inherited is unsubstantiated, only one report describing YNS with familial primary hypoplasia of leg lymphatics [22].

Other genetic forms of lymphoedema

A number of sporadic forms of lymphoedema occur, usually presenting at birth or during childhood. The defect in such cases is likely to be due to a somatic rather than a germ-line mutation.

Klippel–Trenaunay syndrome (MIM 149000) is the commonest type, in which lymphoedema may be the presenting abnormality.

Subsequently, more characteristic features such as limb overgrowth, cutaneous angiomas and venous disease may develop.

Proteus syndrome (MIM 176920) is a very rare syndrome manifesting with many varied (protean) abnormalities. Characteristic features are asymmetrical overgrowth of almost any part of the body, macrodactyly, and rugose or cerebriform overgrowth of the palmar and plantar soft tissue. Verrucous epidermal naevi, angiomas and lymphangiomatous swelling also occur. Germ-line mutations in *PTEN* have been proposed but are not often found [23].

Amniotic bands: another poorly understood form of congenital lymphoedema is that associated with amniotic bands. These bands, which allegedly wrap around digits or limbs, cause circumferential fibrosis and scarring. This can lead to amputation of digits or lymphoedema distal to the band [24].

Maffucci's syndrome (dyschondroplasia with haemangioma, MIM #166000) usually manifests with venous cavernous malformations in infancy, but cavernous lymphangiomas are also often seen, and may be the sole manifestation, giving rise to limb swelling. Hard nodules arise from the bones, especially of the fingers and toes; these are pathologically enchondromas and are radiologically translucent. The malignant potential of the syndrome is high [25].

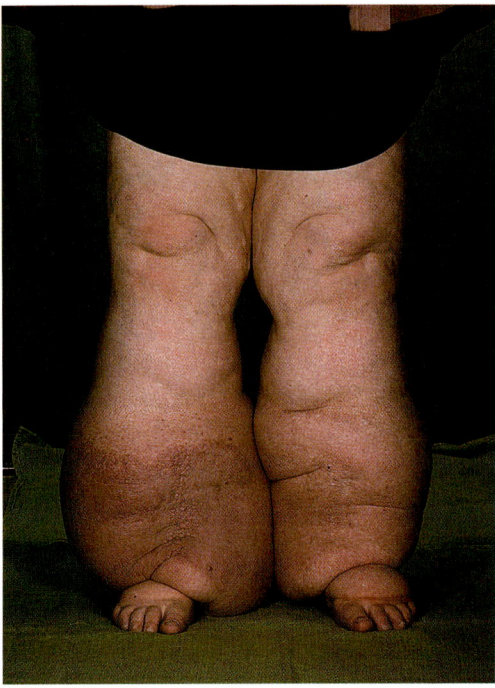

Fig. 48.5 The commonest form of primary lymphoedema: distal hypoplasia of peripheral lymphatic vessels presenting with asymmetrical but usually bilateral swelling of feet and lower legs.

References

1 Browse NL, Stewart G. Lymphoedema: pathophysiology and classification. *J Cardiovasc Surg* 1985; **6**: 91–106.

2 Browse NL. The diagnosis and management of primary lymphoedema. *J Vasc Surg* 1996; **3**: 181–4.

3 Brice G, Mansour S, Bell R *et al*. Analysis of the phenotypic abnormalities in lymphoedema distichiasis syndrome in 74 patients with FOXC-2 mutations or linkage to 16q.24. *J Med Genet* 2002; **39**: 478–83.

4 Milroy WF. Chronic hereditary oedema: Milroy's disease. *JAMA* 1928; **91**: 1172–5.

5 Nonne M. Vier Fälle von Elephantiasis congenita hereditaria. *Virchows Arch* 1891; **125**: 189–96.

6 Ferrell RE, Levinson KL, Esman JH *et al*. Hereditary lymphoedema: evidence for linkage and genetic heterogeneity. *Hum Mol Genet* 1998; **7**: 2073–8.

7 Evans AL, Brice G, Sotirova V *et al*. Mapping of primary congenital lymphoedema to the 5q.35.3 region. *Am J Hum Genet* 1999; **64**: 547–55.

8 Karkkainen MJ, Ferrell RE, Lawrence EC *et al*. Missense mutations interfere with VEGFR-3 signalling in primary lymphoedema. *Nat Genet* 2000; **25**: 153–9.

9 Dale RF. Primary lymphoedema when found with distichiasis is of the type defined as bilateral hyperplasia by lymphography. *J Med Genet* 1987; **24**: 170–1.

10 Mangion J, Rahman N, Mansour S *et al*. A gene for lymphedema-distichiasis maps to 16q 24.3. *Am J Hum Genet* 1999; **65**: 427–32.

11 Fang J, Dagenais SL, Erickson RP *et al*. Mutations in FOXC-2 (MFH-1) a forkhead family transcription factor are responsible for hereditary lymphedema–distichiasis syndrome. *Am J Hum Genet* 2000; **67**: 1382–8.

12 François M, Caprini A, Hosking B *et al*. Sox18 induces development of the lymphatic vasculature in mice. *Nature* 2008; **456**: 643–7.

13 Irrthum A, Devriendt K, Chitayat D *et al*. Mutations in the transcription factor gene SOX18 underlie recessive and dominant forms of hypotrichosis-lymphedema-telangiectasia. *Am J Hum Genet* 2003; **72**: 1470–8.

14 Smahi A, Courtois G, Vabres P *et al*. Genomic rearrangement in NEMO impairs NFκB activation and is a cause of incontinentia pigmenti. *Nature* 2000; **405**: 466–72.

15 Mansour S, Woffendin H, Mitton S *et al*. Incontentia pigmenti in a surviving male is accompanied by hypohidrotic ectodermal dysplasia and recurrent infection. *Am J Med Genet* 2001; **99**: 172–7.

16 Meige H. Dystrophie oedemateuse héréditaire. *Presse Méd* 1898; **6**: 341–3.

17 Tartaglia M, Mehler EL, Godberg R *et al*. Mutations in PTPN11, encoding the protein tyrosine phosphatase SHP-2, cause Noonan syndrome. *Nat Genet* 2001; **29**: 465–8.

18 Hennekam RCM, Geerdink RA, Hamel BCJ *et al*. Autosomal recessive intestinal lymphangiectasia and lymphedema with facial anomalies and mental retardation. *Am J Med Genet* 1989; **34**: 593–600.

19 Aagenaes O. Hereditary cholestasis with lymphoedema (Aagenaes syndrome): new cases and follow-up from infancy to adult age. *Scand J Gastroent* 1998; **33**: 335–45.

20 Jarmas AL, Weaver DD, Ellis FD, Davis A. Microcephaly, microphthalmia, falciform retinal folds and blindness: a new syndrome. *Am J Dis Child* 1981; **135**: 930–3.

21 Jackson BT, Kinmonth JB. Pes cavus and lymphoedema. *J Bone Joint Surg* 1970; **52**: 518–20.

22 Wells GC. Yellow nail syndrome with familial primary hypoplasia of lymphatics, manifest late in life. *Proc R Soc Med* 1966; **59**: 447.

23 Zhou XP, Hampel H, Thiele H *et al*. Association of germline mutation in the PTEN tumour suppressor gene and Proteus and Proteus-like syndrome. *Lancet* 2001; **358**: 210–1.

24 Coady MS, Moore MH, Wallis K. Amniotic band syndrome: the association between rare facial clefts and limb ring constrictions. *Plast Reconstr Surg* 1998; **101**: 640–9.

25 Carlton A, St. Elkington JC, Greenfield JG *et al*. Maffucci's syndrome. *QJM* 1942; **11**: 203–8.

Phenotypes of primary lymphoedema

Lower limb

1 *Distal hypoplasia.* The most common presentation, contributing about 80% of all cases of primary lymphoedema, is that of mild oedema of both feet and ankles. Patients are usually female with onset at puberty. The swelling is often asymmetrical and deteriorates slowly. Extension above the knee is uncommon and mild (Fig. 48.5). The cause is a paucity of distal lymph vessels.

2 *Proximal obstruction.* This variety is unilateral in 85% of cases. It usually involves the whole limb and develops rapidly. There is no family history. It is of paramount importance to exclude pelvic causes of venous or lymphatic obstruction—for example, tumour or thrombosis. The cause in primary lymphoedema is

fibrosis within ilioinguinal lymph nodes or obliteration of proximal lymph vessels [1].

3 *Bilateral whole-limb swelling*. Reflux of lymph due to gravitational forces and gross incompetence of valves leads to huge dilatation of lymphatic collectors (megalymphatics) in a manner similar to venous reflux and varicose veins. Chylous reflux may coexist. Progressive distal failure of lymphatic collectors, the so-called 'die-back' phenomenon, occurs with time as a result of proximal obstruction or reflux [2].

Upper limb

Upper limb lymphoedema, if primary in type, usually presents at birth. It may be unisegmental, affecting one limb and the root of that limb, or may be multisegmental in which case it can be associated with lower limb, facial, genital or systemic involvement. Upper limb lymphoedema may form part of a syndrome with overgrowth, for example in Klippel–Trenaunay syndrome.

Genital lymphoedema

Lymphoedema is rarely confined just to the genitalia and is usually associated with intestinal lymphangiectasia/chylous reflux or lower limb swelling.

Facial lymphoedema

If primary facial lymphoedema occurs it is invariably present at birth and improves over time. It is usually asymmetrical and associated with lymphoedema elsewhere. Head and neck oedema occurring *in utero* may regress by birth but leave signs such as prominent medial epicanthic folds or neck webbing.

Secondary lymphoedema

Secondary lymphoedema refers to those forms of lymphoedema resulting from acquired obstruction or obliteration of lymph-conducting pathways due to some identifiable pathological process arising extrinsic to the lymphatic system (Table 48.5). These processes include infection, inflammation, trauma (including surgery and radiation) and malignant disease. No form of lymphoedema is mutually exclusive, and frequently a number of factors combine to produce swelling. For example, lymphoedema may become clinically obvious only when the lymphatic load is increased through higher fluid filtration exhausting lymph drainage capacity.

Lymphoedema associated with infection

Infection may cause progressive damage to lymph drainage routes by intraluminal obliteration of lymphatic vessels through processes such as lymphangitis and lymphangiothrombosis.

In recurrent cellulitis or erysipelas, the damage to lymphatics may ultimately lead to formation of lymphoedema, which itself predisposes to further episodes of infection, so exacerbating the lymphoedema [3,4].

Lymphatic filariasis is concentrated in the tropics and subtropics and is the most common cause of lymphoedema worldwide, with an estimated 90 million people affected [5]. Infection is transmitted by mosquitoes, which introduce microfilariae into the skin. These larvae migrate to the lymphatics, where they mature into adult worms. Progressive and permanent damage to the infested lymphatics causes lymphoedema. It has been established in animal

Table 48.5 Causes of secondary lymphoedema.

Cancer
Treatment
Surgery
Radiotherapy
Tumour
Kaposi's sarcoma
Infiltrative cancer
Lymphoma
Relapsed tumour
Infection
Filariasis
Lymphangitis, lymphadenitis
Cellulitis
Tuberculosis
Lymphogranuloma inguinale
Lice
Inflammation
Lymphatic occlusion
Podoconiosis
Pretibial myxoedema
Dermatitis, e.g. hand eczema
Rheumatoid arthritis
Psoriasis
Rosacea/acne
Granulomatous disease
Orofacial granulomatosis
Crohn's disease
Sarcoidosis
Vascular
Venous disease
Post-thrombotic syndrome
Venous leg ulcers
Trauma
Surgery
Lymphadenectomy
Vein harvesting
Femoropopliteal bypass
Self-harm
Tourniquet application
Intravenous drug abuse
Accident
Degloving injury
Burns

studies that, within days of infection, vigorous movement by adult worms directly impacts on the endothelial lining of the lymphatic trunks and indirectly distorts the local lymph-node architecture. Dilated lymphatics with thickened walls and valves, thrombus formation and perilymphangitis result [6].

Lymphogranuloma inguinale and tuberculous node infection can cause lower limb lymphoedema [7]. Lymphoedema of the ear lobe has been described following infestation with head lice [8].

Lymphoedema associated with inflammation

Circumstances exist in which chronic inflammation without evidence of infection is associated with the development of lymphoedema. It is assumed that the inflammation progressively damages lymph drainage routes.

Facial lymphoedema may result from rosacea or even acne vulgaris. Skin or subcutaneous initial lymphatics fail rather than main regional collecting trunks. Telangiectasia and inflammation contribute to oedema through increased fluid filtration. In rosacea (Morbihan's disease, solid facial oedema) epithelioid granulomas are often seen with dilated dermal lymphatics [9].

Upper limb swelling may occur following chronic hand dermatitis, with or without documented episodes of lymphangitis [10]. Like other forms of lymphoedema, once established it tends to be permanent, irrespective of remission of the skin disease.

Podoconiosis (non-filarial elephantiasis) is a form of lymphoedema caused by particles of silica dust, present in certain soils, which penetrate the skin of the foot during barefoot walking. The microparticles are taken up by the lymphatics, causing damage. Soils rich in these substances determine the geographical distribution of the condition [11].

Studies with quantitative lymphoscintigraphy and fluorescence microlymphography have confirmed functional and structural changes to lymph drainage in pretibial myxoedema. It is likely that mucin deposition in the dermis impairs initial lymphatic function, resulting in the clinical appearance which resembles lymphoedema [12].

A small number of patients with rheumatoid arthritis develop lymphoedema, predominantly of the upper limbs. A study in rheumatoid arthritis found impaired lymph drainage only in patients with lymphoedema [13]. This suggested that inflammatory arthritis alone does not directly impair lymphatic drainage. Similar findings have been described in psoriatic arthritis [14].

Granulomatous diseases such as Crohn's disease, sarcoidosis, orofacial and anogenital granulomatosis and foreign body reactions from cosmetic procedures [15,16] cause inflammatory changes in local skin and subcutaneous lymphatics, leading to lymphoedematous swelling.

Panniculitis that is extensive enough to cause severe fibrosis may produce lymphoedema. This has been described following idiopathic retroperitoneal fibrosis [17].

Lymphoedema secondary to trauma

Trauma to lymphatics, either from elective surgery or by accident, usually needs to be extensive to induce lymphoedema. Indeed, the experimental production of lymphoedema is extremely difficult to achieve owing to the excellent regenerative powers of lymphatics [18]. It is possibly the failure of lymphatics to regenerate and re-anastomose satisfactorily through scarred or irradiated tissue which is responsible for lymphoedema following cancer treatment. Surgical excision of axillary or ilioinguinal lymph nodes will not uncommonly produce limb lymphoedema. The puzzles are why such intervention in animal models rarely produces chronic swelling and why there can be such a delay—up to 20 years—before lymphoedema manifests [19]. Radiotherapy to lymph nodes can be as much a risk factor towards lymphoedema as surgery [20]. The incidence of lymphoedema following varicose vein surgery is estimated to be 0.5% [21].

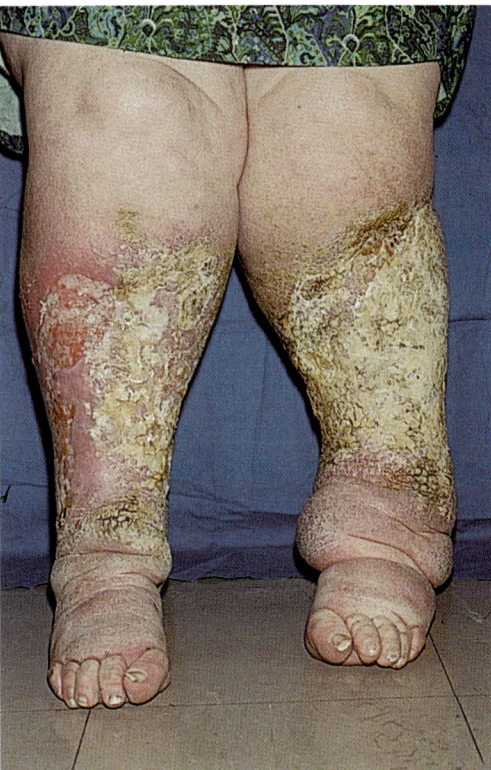

Fig. 48.6 Lymphoedema associated with chronic venous disease.

Accidental trauma, such as a degloving injury to a limb, will produce lymphoedema distal to the injury if widespread circumferential scarring occurs.

Self-inflicted injury, such as the repeated application of a tourniquet, will eventually cause permanent lymphatic damage and chronic swelling (Secrétan's syndrome) [22]. The abrupt termination of the swelling often coincides with a depression due to subcutaneous atrophy caused by a tight constricting band. Skin pigmentation may also coexist at the site.

Intravenous drug abuse may cause lymphoedema due to a combination of infection and associated venous damage.

Lymphoedema and venous disease (phlebolymphoedema)

Oedema is a common complication of venous insufficiency. It is assumed that venous oedema is the sole consequence of increased capillary filtration from venous hypertension. As lymph drainage is the main buffer against oedema, it is in fact the failure of local lymphatics to compensate for the increased lymph load from filtration that leads to oedema. Thrombosis of the major veins and deep vein incompetence does not generally affect the main collecting lymphatics but the small initial and precollecting lymphatics of the skin and subcutaneous tissues of the lower leg are damaged by prolonged venous hypertension. Lymphoedema develops with chronic lipodermatosclerosis, with or without venous ulceration. Lymphoscintigraphy has shown impaired limb lymph drainage [23] while fluorescence microlymphography has revealed damaged skin lymphatics [24]. Lymphoedema associated with venous disease can give rise to the most gross swelling and skin changes owing to the combined effect of impaired lymph drainage in the face of increased lymph load (capillary filtration) (Fig. 48.6).

Malignancy-related lymphoedema

Lymph flow is remarkably well maintained through malignant nodes, therefore cancer does not usually present with swelling. The few exceptions to this general rule are lymphophilic tumours, such as malignant eccrine poroma or Kaposi's sarcoma, as well as advanced cancers where other factors such as venous obstruction and hypoproteinaemia will contribute to oedema formation. Recurrent cancer, however, should always be considered as a cause of limb swelling, particularly if associated with pain. Full staging investigations should always be undertaken in such circumstances. Therefore, in general, malignancy-related lymphoedema usually results from cancer therapy, that is surgery, radiotherapy or a combination of the two, or from recurrent tumour directly infiltrating collateral drainage routes.

Kaposi's sarcoma may present with lymphoedema, sometimes years before tumour is evident. The association with lymphoedema [25] supports the view that in Kaposi's sarcoma the endothelial cell phenotype is lymphatic [26].

Lymphoedema arising from dysfunctional lymphatics

Lymph drainage, unlike blood flow, requires intermittent changes in local tissue pressure generated by movement and exercise in order to produce initial lymphatic transport. Consequently, immobility tends to encourage swelling, particularly if gravitational forces (dependency syndrome) encourage ongoing fluid filtration. A common scenario is 'armchair legs', a term coined by Sneddon and Church [27], where patients sit in a chair day and night with their legs dependent (otherwise known as elephantiasis verrucosis nostras, because of the severe lymphoedema skin changes that ensue). No premorbid abnormalities of lymphatics exist, but the immobility results in minimal lymph drainage and a functional lymphoedema due to a lack of movement or exercise to stimulate normal lymph drainage. Dependency of the limb compounds the problem by increasing capillary filtration. The syndrome is not confined to the legs, but can affect any chronically dependent and immobile part, as demonstrated in the pendulous abdomen [28]. With time, pathological changes within the failing lymphatics occur and an irreversible lymphoedema develops.

References

1 Kinmonth JB, Wolfe JH. Fibrosis of the lymph nodes in primary lymphoedema. *Br J Surg* 1966; **53**: 917–25.
2 Fyfe NCM, Wolfe JHN, Kinmonth JB. 'Die-back' in primary lymphoedema. *Lymphology* 1982; **15**: 66–9.
3 Damstra RJ, van Steensel MA, Boomsma JH *et al.* Erysipelas as a sign of subclinical primary lymphoedema: a prospective quantitative scintigraphic study of 40 patients with unilateral erysipelas of the leg. *Br J Dermatol* 2008; **158**: 1210–5.
4 Cox NH. Oedema as a risk factor for multiple episodes of cellulitis/erysipelas of the lower leg: a series with community follow-up. *Br J Dermatol* 2006; **155**: 947–50.
5 Jamal S. Dramatic manifestations of filarial infection. *Lymphology* 1985; **18**: 148–68.
6 Case T, Leis B, Witte M *et al.* Vascular abnormalities in experimental and human lymphatic filariasis. *Lymphology* 1991; **24**: 174–83.
7 Ngu V, Konstam PG. Chronic lymphoedema in Western Nigeria. *Br J Surg* 1964; **51**: 101–10.
8 Manzoon S, Azadeh B. Elephantiasis of external ear: a rare manifestation of pediculosis capitis. *Acta Derm Venereol (Stockh)* 1983; **63**: 363–5.
9 Nagasaka T, Koyama T, Matsumura K, Chen KR. Persistent lymphoedema in Morbihan disease: formation of perilymphatic epithelioid cell granulomas as a possible pathogenesis. *Clin Exp Dermatol* 2008; **33**: 764–7.
10 Worm AM, Staberg B, Thomsen K. Persistent oedema in allergic contact dermatitis. *Contact Dermatitis* 1983; **9**: 517–8.
11 Price EW. *Podoconiosis, Non-Filarial Elephantiasis.* Oxford: Oxford University Press, 1990.
12 Bull RH, Coburn PR, Mortimer PS. Pre-tibial myxoedema: a manifestation of lymphoedema? *Lancet* 1993; **341**: 403–4.
13 Kiely PD, Bland JM, Joseph AE *et al.* Upper limb lymphatic function in inflammatory arthritis. *J Rheumatol* 1995; **22**: 214–7.
14 Mulherin DM, Fitzgerald O, Bresnihan B. Lymphoedema of the upper limb in patients with psoriatic arthritis. *Semin Arthritis Rheum* 1993; **22**: 350–6.
15 Murphy MJ, Kogan B, Carlson JA. Granulomatous lymphangitis of the scrotum and penis. Report of a case and review of the literature of genital swelling with sarcoidal granulomatous inflammation. *J Cutan Pathol* 2001; **28**: 419–24.
16 Salles AG, Lotierzo PH, Gemperli R *et al.* Complications after polymethylmethacrylate injections: report of 32 cases. *Plast Reconstr Surg* 2008; **121**: 1811–20.
17 Mahoney EM, Edwards EA. Spontaneous regression of leg edema and hydronephrosis following idiopathic retroperitoneal fibrosis. *Am J Surg* 1962; **103**: 514–7.
18 Danese C, Bower R, Howard JM. Experimental anastomoses of lymphatics. *Arch Surg* 1962; **84**: 6–9.
19 Stanton AW, Modi S, Bennett Britton TM *et al.* Lymphatic drainage in the muscle and subcutis of the arm after breast cancer treatment. *Breast Cancer Res Treat* 2009; **7**: 29–45.
20 Kissin MW, della Rovere GQ, Easton D *et al.* Risk of lymphoedema following the treatment of breast cancer. *Br J Surg* 1986; **73**: 580–4.
21 Ouvry PA, Guenneguez H. Lymphatic complications from variceal surgery. *Phlebologie* 1993; **46**: 563–8.
22 Reading G. Secrétan's syndrome: hard edema of the dorsum of the hand. *Plast Reconstr Surg* 1980; **65**: 182–7.
23 Bull RH, Gane JN, Evans J *et al.* Abnormal lymph drainage in patients with chronic venous leg ulcers. *J Am Acad Dermatol* 1993; **28**: 585–90.
24 Bollinger A, Isrensing G, Franzeck U. Lymphatic microangiopathy: a complication of chronic venous insufficiency. *Lymphology* 1982; **15**: 60–5.
25 Bossuyt L, Van Den Oord JJ, Degreef H. Lymphangioma like variant of AIDS-associated Kaposi's sarcoma with pronounced oedema formation. *Dermatology* 1995; **190**: 324–6.
26 Cueni LN, Detmar M. New insights into the molecular control of the lymphatic vascular system and its role in disease. *J Invest Dermatol* 2006; **126**: 2167–77 [Review].
27 Sneddon I, Church R. *Practical Dermatology*, 4th edn. London: Arnold, 1983: 166.
28 Bull RH, Mortimer PS. Acute lipodermatosclerosis in a pendulous abdomen. *Clin Exp Dermatol* 1993; **18**: 164–6.

Clinical diagnosis of lymphoedema

Lymphoedema most commonly affects the extremities. This predilection for the limbs is due, at least in part, to the limited collateral drainage available at the root of a limb. Careful examination often reveals extension of the swelling to the associated quadrant of the trunk because the lymph drainage routes are shared with the limb.

The major clinical changes of lymphoedema take place in the skin and subcutaneous tissues; such changes are of value in diagnosis. Lymphoedema differs from all other oedemas (in which increased capillary filtration is the major factor) in that cells, proteins, lipids and debris accumulate in addition to water. This results in a 'solid' as well as a 'fluid' component to the swelling, so giving rise to the brawny nature of the oedema which does not readily pit [1]. The lack of pitting is an unreliable sign in lymphoedema, however, because easy displacement of tissue fluid on pressure can often be demonstrated, particularly in the early stages.

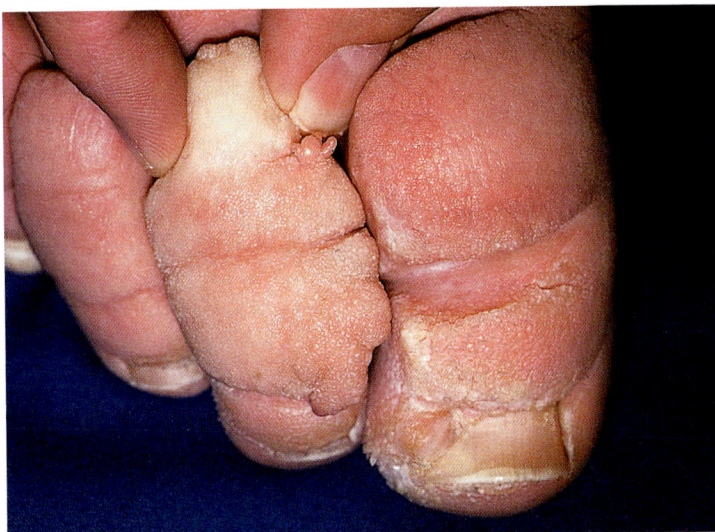

Fig. 48.7 The Kaposi–Stemmer sign: inability to pinch or pick up a fold of skin at the base of the second toe indicates lymphoedema.

Lymphoedema does not usually respond to elevation or diuretics, except in the early stages or when it is compounded by increased capillary filtration. Chronic oedema that does not reduce significantly after overnight elevation is likely to be lymphatic in origin. The symptoms accompanying uncomplicated lymphoedema are few. Swelling frequently develops rapidly, for example overnight. In the distal hypoplastic type, one ankle may swell. Pain may feature initially, prompting diagnoses including deepvein thrombosis or soft-tissue injury. Oedema is often intermittent before becoming permanent, and is often painless although discomfort, aching and tightness are commonly reported symptoms. Eventually both legs swell. In proximal obstructive lymphoedema, swelling usually develops in the thigh and progresses distally.

Although swelling occurs most in the subcutaneous layer, the skin exhibits most changes. It becomes thicker, as demonstrated by the Kaposi–Stemmer sign (inability to pick or pinch a fold of skin at the base of the second toe) (Fig. 48.7) [2]. Skin creases become enhanced and hyperkeratosis develops. Dilatation of upper dermal lymphatics with consequent organization and fibrosis gives rise to papillomatosis. As dermal lymph stasis progresses these skin changes become more marked and are referred to as elephantiasis. Occasionally, the tissue fibrosis and thickening may become so marked in the later stages of lymphoedema that pitting is absent.

Complications

Complications of lymphoedema are mainly due to swelling and infection.

Swelling. Limb swelling leads to discomfort, limb heaviness, reduced mobility and, on occasions, impaired function. The size and weight of affected limbs can result in secondary musculoskeletal complications such as back pain and joint problems. Thickening of the skin causes pseudoscleroderma and consequently impairs small-joint mobility. The difficulty in finding clothes or shoes to fit creates social problems. Poor footwear will further compound the swelling by discouraging a normal gait or enough exercise.

Leakage of lymph through the skin (lymphorrhoea) may occur from engorged dermal lymphatics (lymphangiectasia).

Infection. Episodes of secondary infection, particularly cellulitis or erysipelas, are a characteristic feature of lymphoedema. Patients with lymphoedema irrespective of cause are liable to these attacks, which reflect a failure of immune surveillance. Constitutional symptoms such as fever, rigors, headache or vomiting can be profound and sudden in onset. Within 24 h, redness appears within the lymphoedematous area but without the advancing border. Pain and heat also feature. Recurrent episodes may be frequent and further impair lymph drainage, so exacerbating the lymphoedema. Thus, a vicious cycle is established. Haemolytic streptococci of group A, B or G have been demonstrated [3], although the bacterial aetiology has been brought into question [4]. Indeed, it is not unusual for patients to comment that attacks of cellulitis can be induced by strenuous exercise or long car journeys. This suggests a mechanism not dissimilar to herpes simplex where the microorganism is always present but becomes reactivated.

Fungal infections, particularly tinea pedis, are difficult to avoid because of web-space skin maceration from swollen toes. Local immune deficiency is likely to be a contributing factor, as illustrated by a case of cryptococcosis complicating congenital lymphoedema [5].

Malignancy. A rare but important complication of chronic lymphoedema is the development of cutaneous malignancy. Although the best-known associated malignancy is lymphangiosarcoma [6], other tumours have been recorded and include basal cell carcinoma [7], squamous cell carcinoma, lymphoma [8–11], melanoma [12,13], malignant fibrous histiocytoma [14] and Kaposi's sarcoma [15]. The Stewart–Treves syndrome describes lymphangiosarcoma developing from well-established postmastectomy oedema. However, lymphangiosarcoma is now described as occurring with lymphoedema of any cause. The favoured theory for these associations is altered immune surveillance in the lymphoedematous region [16].

Miscellaneous conditions. A range of other cutaneous conditions have been reported as occurring preferentially at sites of lymphoedematous involvement. These include xanthomatous deposits [17], atypical pemphigoid [18], toxic epidermal necrolysis [19], atypical neutrophilic dermatosis [20] and severe necrotizing fasciitis [21].

References

1 Mortimer PS. Managing lymphoedema. *Clin Exp Dermatol* 1995; **20**: 98–106.
2 Stemmer R. Ein klinisches Zeichen zur Früh- und Differentialdiagnose des Lymphödems. *Vasa* 1976; **5**: 261–2.
3 Baddour LM, Bisno AL. Non-group A β-haemolytic streptococcal cellulitis: association with venous and lymphatic compromise. *Am J Med* 1985; **79**: 155–9.
4 Edwards EA. Recurrent febrile episodes and lymphoedema. *JAMA* 1963; **184**: 858–62.
5 Krywonis N, Kaye VN, Lynch PJ. Cryptococcal cellulitis in congenital lymphoedema. *Int J Dermatol* 1990; **29**: 41–4.

6 Stewart FW, Treves N. Lymphangiosarcoma in postmastectomy lymphoedema. *Cancer* 1948; **1**: 64–81.

7 Benson PM, Pessoa CM, Lupton GP *et al.* Basal cell carcinomas arising in chronic lymphoedema. *J Dermatol Surg Oncol* 1988; **14**: 781–3.

8 Epstein JL, Mendelsohn G. Squamous carcinoma of the foot arising in association with longstanding verrucous hyperplasia in a patient with congenital lymphoedema. *Cancer* 1984; **54**: 943–7.

9 Waxman M, Fatteh S, Elias JM *et al.* Malignant lymphoma of skin associated with postmastectomy lymphoedema. *Arch Pathol Laboratory Med* 1984; **108**: 206–8.

10 Tatnall FM, Mann BS. Non-Hodgkin's lymphoma of the skin associated with chronic limb lymphoedema. *Br J Dermatol* 1985; **113**: 751–6.

11 Hills RJ, Ive FA. Cutaneous secondary follicular centre cell lymphoma in association with lymphoedema praecox. *Br J Dermatol* 1993; **129**: 186–9.

12 Sarkany I. Malignant melanomas in lymphoedematous arm following radical mastectomy for breast carcinoma. *J R Soc Med* 1972; **65**: 253–4.

13 Bartal AH, Pinsky CM. Malignant melanoma appearing in a postmastectomy lymphoedematous arm: a novel association of double primary tumours. *J Surg Oncol* 1985; **30**: 16–8.

14 Fergusson CM, Copeland SA, Horton L. Unusual sarcoma arising in lymphoedema. *J R Soc Med* 1985; **78**: 1497–8.

15 Merimsky O, Chaitchik S. Kaposi's sarcoma on a lymphoedematous arm following radical mastectomy. *Tumori* 1992; **78**: 407–8.

16 Shreiber H, Barry FM, Russell WC *et al.* Stewart–Treves syndrome: a lethal complication of post mastectomy lymphoedema and regional immune deficiency. *Arch Surg* 1979; **114**: 82.

17 Tatnall FM, Sarkany I. Primary focal lymphoedema with xanthoma. *J R Soc Med* 1988; **81**: 113–4.

18 Callens A, Vaillant L, Machet MC *et al.* Localized atypical pemphigoid on lymphoedema following radiotherapy. *Acta Derm Venereol (Stockh)* 1993; **73**: 461–4.

19 Wilkinson SM, Heagarty AH, Smith AG. Toxic epidermal necrolysis localized to an area of lymphoedema. *Clin Exp Dermatol* 1991; **17**: 456–7.

20 Demitsu T, Tadaki T. Atypical neutrophilic dermatosis on the upper extremity affected by post-mastectomy lymphoedema: report of 2 cases. *Dermatologica* 1991; **183**: 230–3.

21 Kaier T, Larsen J. Necrotizing fasciitis in congenital lymphoedema. *Int J Dermatol* 1990; **29**: 41–4.

Midline lymphoedema

Lymphoedema localized to central regions such as the head and neck, trunk or external genitalia is uncommon, presumably because bilateral drainage routes operate and cross-flow from one region to another prevents swelling. Midline lymphoedema therefore usually develops when the lymphatics of the skin or subcutaneous tissue rather than the regional lymphatics fail.

Head and neck lymphoedema

Facial swelling can coexist with obvious primary lymphoedema of one or more limbs, suggesting that there is widespread congenitally determined lymphatic insufficiency. More commonly, the problem occurs later in life secondary to a variety of inflammatory or traumatic mechanisms. Rosacea, and less commonly acne [1,2], are the commonest causes of facial lymphoedema when it is known as Morbihan's disease or solid facial oedema. Swelling affects the central forehead, periocular skin and cheeks where it may be surprisingly asymmetrical. In rosacea, erythema is always present, but inflammatory pustules and papules may be conspicuous by their absence.

Chronic oedema of the eyelids is common and may be quite simply due to acquired lax skin from photo-ageing and other processes which have undermined tissue compliance, such as blepharochalasis [3]. Congenital eyelid lymphoedema may be associated with conjunctival oedema. Medical conditions to be considered with periocular oedema are dermatomyositis, thyroid or renal disease. Contact allergy or angio-oedema, if persistent or recurrent, may slowly compromise lymphatic function. Equally, one severe attack of facial erysipelas or cellulitis may damage lymphatics sufficiently to cause lymphoedema. Angiosarcoma or Kaposi's sarcoma may infiltrate local lymph drainage, and manifest with eyelid oedema.

Redness and swelling of one or both ears may indicate lymphoedema. Rosacea is the most frequent cause [4] but eczema, psoriasis, infection, pediculosis, trauma (cauliflower ears), pediculosis or congenital lymphoedema may also be responsible.

Oedema of the upper or lower lip (or both) may be congenital or result from recurrent angioedema, orofacial granulomatosis (OFG) or from administration of lip fillers for cosmetic purposes. OFG starts with intermittent bouts of swelling resembling angio-oedema, but with time the condition may become persistent. Extension of oedema within the mouth is common and is the reason for the rugose changes on buccal mucosae and tongue (scrotal tongue). Biopsy may or may not reveal the presence of granulomas. If present, a diagnosis of orofacial granulomatosis (granulomatous cheilitis, Melkersson–Rosenthal syndrome) is made, but it remains unclear if the granulomas are cause or effect [5]. It is possible that granulomatous inflammation in isolation can cause orofacial granulomatosis but a thorough search for gastrointestinal Crohn's or systemic sarcoidosis should be made. Despite negative investigations, Crohn's disease of the bowel can become apparent some time later.

Genital lymphoedema

Genital lymphoedema is more common in the male and may develop from lymphatic obstruction due to advanced pelvic/abdominal cancer or its treatment. Bilateral inguinal lymph node biopsy or infiltration of dermal lymphatics from tumour may also cause genital lymphoedema. Genital swelling may be precipitated by compression therapy to one or both lymphoedematous legs by forcing fluid into the adjoining trunk.

Infection may compromise local lymphatics. Recurrent cellulitis is frequently associated and may antedate the swelling.

Granulomatous inflammation from Crohn's disease, hidradenitis suppurativa or sarcoidosis may manifest only with oedema of the penis or scrotum. As with orofacial granulomatosis, anogenital granulomatosis may occur in isolation without associated granulomatous disease elsewhere.

Primary lymphoedema may involve the genitalia but usually in association with leg swelling. In these circumstances vulval lymphoedema may develop into a swollen fold which can extend from a pedicle and become a polyp [6].

References

1 Connelly MG, Winkelmann RK. Solid facial edema as a complication of acne vulgaris. *Arch Dermatol* 1985; **121**: 87–90.

2 Nagasaka T, Koyama T, Matsumura K, Chen KR. Persistent lymphoedema in Morbihan disease: formation of perilymphatic epithelioid cell granulomas as a possible pathogenesis. *Clin Exp Dermatol* 2008; **33**: 764–7.

3 Dozsa A, Karoli ZS, Degrell P. Bilateral blepharochalasis. *J Eur Acad Dermatol Venereol* 2005; **19**: 725–8.

4 Carlson JA, Mazza J, Kircher K, Tran TA. Otophyma: a case report and review of the literature of lymphoedema (elephantiasis) of the ear. *Am J Dermatopathol* 2008; **30**: 67–72.

5 Nozicka Z. Endovasal granulomatous lymphangitis as a pathogenetic factor in cheilitis granulomatosa. *J Oral Pathol* 1985; **14**: 363–5.

6 Orosz Z, Lehoczky O, Szoke J, Pulay T. Recurrent giant fibroepithelial stromal polyp of the vulva associated with congenital lymphedema. *Gynecol Oncol* 2005; **98**: 168–71.

Localized lymphoedema

Breast lymphoedema

As changes to breast cancer treatment have led to more breast-conserving surgery and increased use of therapeutic radiation, so the incidence of lymphoedema localized to the breast has risen [1]. The risk is higher in the obese and in women with larger breasts; the more pendulous the breast, the greater the risk. Inflammation is generally present, resulting in a red, painful swollen breast. Pitting and peau d'orange are most noticeable on the undersurface of the breast. Cellulitis can coexist and is difficult to distinguish from post-radiation changes, as often the only systemic sign of chronic infection is tiredness. Low-dose antibiotics, for example phenoxymethylpenicillin 1 g/day for 6 weeks, may be the only means of proving infection.

Massive localized lymphoedema

Lymphoedema typically affects a region such as a limb but uncommonly it can present as a localized mass resembling a tumour. It is not unusual for an area of lymphoedema on the lower inner thigh or inguinal region to hypertrophy into an enlarged fold and then, under the influence of gravity, progress into a pendulous swelling (Fig. 48.8). Solid or papillomatous plaques can mimic tumours but biopsy will reveal typical features of lymphoedema

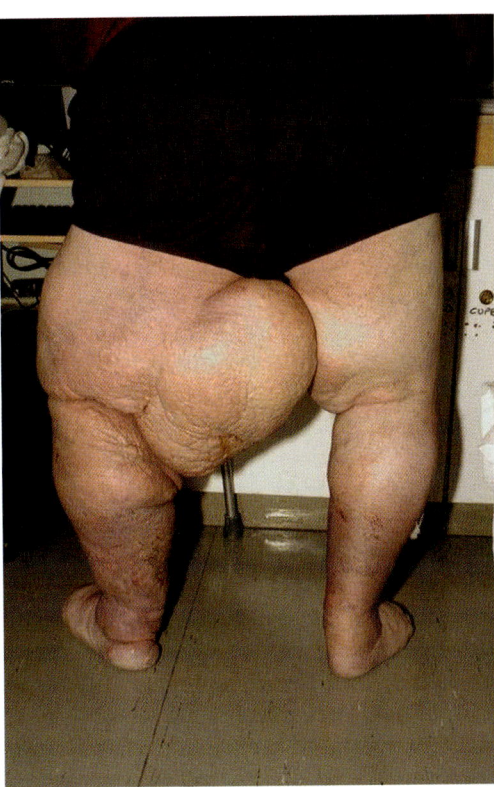

Fig. 48.8 Massive localized lymphoedema.

Scar lymphoedema

Swelling within a scar and adjacent tissues, such as a flap, is common. Impaired lymph drainage contributes to raised and swollen tissues abutting a U-shaped scar because lymphatic pathways do not always re-establish drainage across scars [4].

References

1 Goffman TE, Laronga C, Wilson L, Elkins D. Lymphedema of the arm and breast in irradiated breast cancer patients: risks in an era of dramatically changing axillary surgery. *Breast J* 2004; **10**: 405–11.

2 Farshid G, Weiss SW. Massive localized lymphedema in the morbidly obese: a histologically distinct reactive lesion simulating liposarcoma. *Am J Surg Pathol* 1998; **22**: 1277–83.

3 Lu S, Tran Ta, Jones DM *et al.* Localized lymphedema (elephantiasis): a case series and review of the literature. *J Cutan Pathol* 2008; **36**: 1–20.

4 Warren Ag, Slavin SA. Scar lymphedema: fact or fiction? *Ann Plast Surg* 2007; **59**: 41–5.

(elephantiasis), namely: oedema, dilated lymphatics, fibrosis, fat, epidermal acanthosis and hyperkeratosis, and inflammatory dermal infiltrate. Obesity and localized tissue damage increase risk [2,3].

Investigations

Swollen limb

There are limited methods available that permit reliable investigation of lymphatics. Lymphoscintigraphy (isotope lymphography) involves the interstitial (dermis or subcutis) injection of a radio-labelled protein or colloid. Radioactivity, measured using a wide field-of-view γ-camera, is determined over the injection site depot and at regions of interest over vessels or nodes. Measurement of transit times and time activity curves permit quantitative analysis of lymph drainage [1]. Measurement of tracer uptake within axillary or inguinofemoral lymph nodes at a specified time following a standardized exercise routine will discriminate lymphoedema from oedema of non-lymphatic origin [2] (Fig. 48.9).

Computed tomography (CT) of lymphoedematous limbs has demonstrated a characteristic 'honeycomb' pattern in the subcutaneous compartment which other oedemas do not show [3]. CT not only provides information through cross-sectional area of volume change to a limb, but will also identify the compartment in which that change takes place. Whereas in post-thrombotic syndrome the muscle compartment deep to the fascia is enlarged, in lymphoedema it is unchanged or may even show some reduction in size. Thickening of the skin is also a characteristic feature of lymphoedema, although not specific. Magnetic resonance imaging (MRI) is potentially better than CT for distinguishing types of oedema [4].

X-ray contrast lymphography remains the gold standard for demonstrating lymphatic collecting trunks and nodes [5]. The technique is invasive and difficult to perform in the presence of oedema. It involves first of all the interstitial subcutaneous injection of a vital dye—for example, patent blue—to visualize the lymphatic for cannulation. The oily contrast medium Lipiodol is then administered directly into the peripheral lymphatic identified, usually on the dorsum of the foot. The failure to opacify subcutaneous collectors with the vital dye and its persistence in

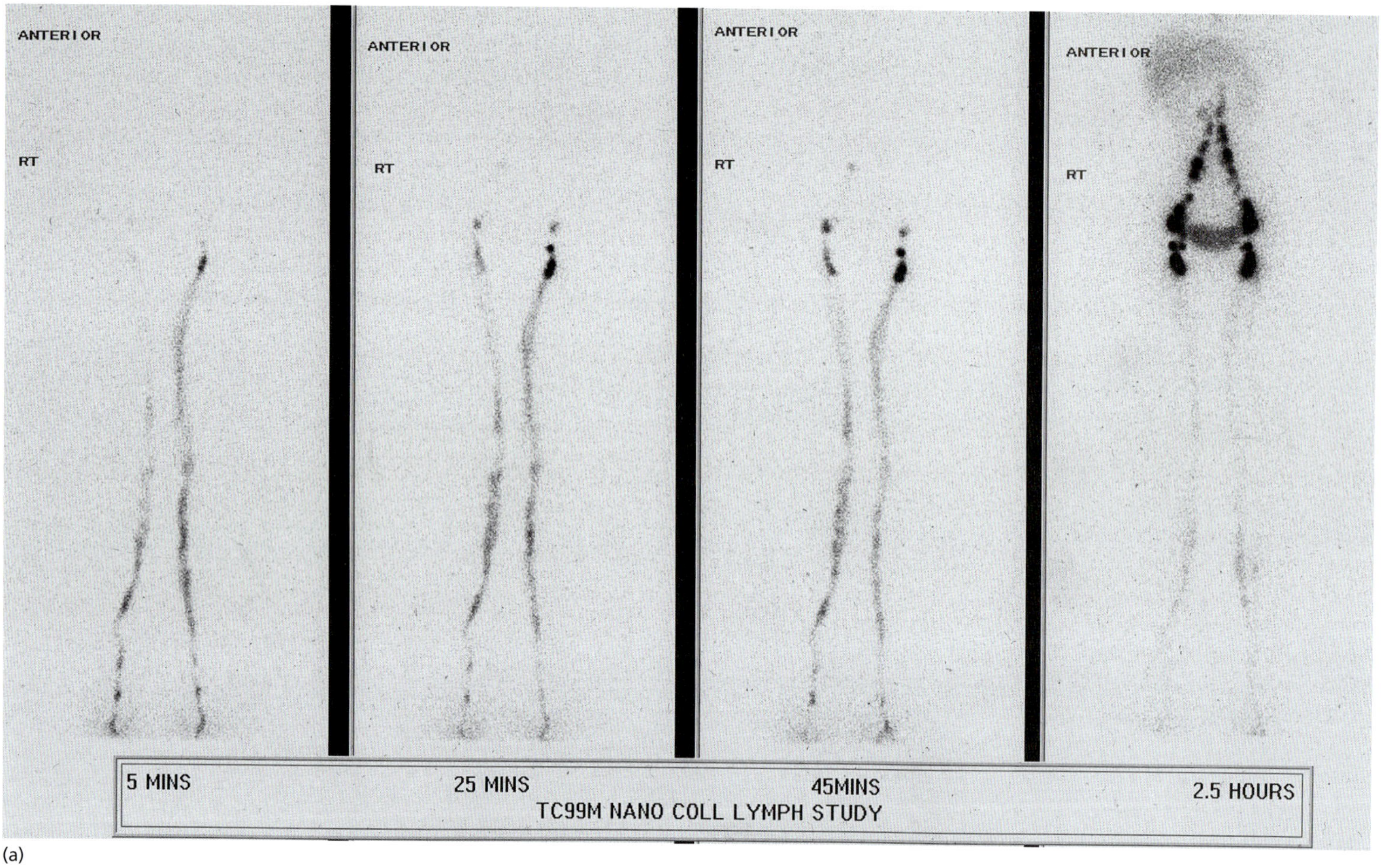

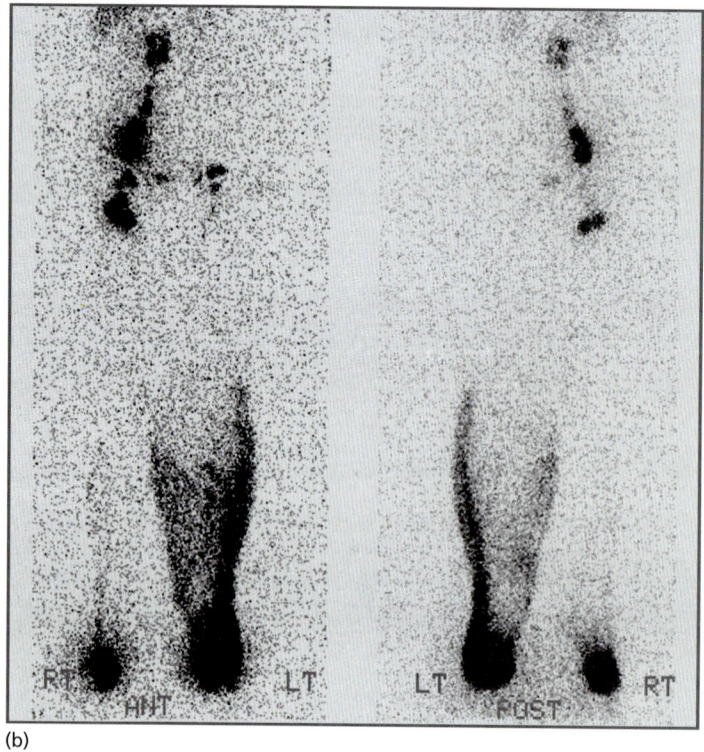

Fig. 48.9 (a) Normal lymphoscintigraphy. Images show patent lymph routes draining tracer from feet to ilio-inguinal nodes. (Courtesy of Professor A.M. Peters.) (b) Obstruction of lymph drainage at the groin leads to re-routing of tracer through skin collaterals (dermal backflow).

the tissues for days afterwards are sufficient evidence for a diagnosis of lymphoedema. If there is lymphatic obstruction, the dye will often flow retrogradely into the dermal network—so-called 'dermal backflow'. Lymphography has been used to confirm lymphoedema less often since the advent of lymphoscintigraphy.

MR lymphangiography (MRL) has recently been introduced to overcome the invasive nature of X-ray lymphography. MRL involves the interstitial injection of paramagnetic contrast agent which delineates the collecting lymphatic vessels of the limb as well as regional lymph nodes and any re-routing such as collateral dermal backflow [6,7].

Initial lymphatics

In vivo visualization of lymphatic vessels (lymphangiography) was first achieved using vital dyes—for example, patent blue—to delineate intradermal and subcutaneous lymphatics. Some classic studies were undertaken in this way [8]. Fluorescence micro-lymphangiography enables the superficial lymphatic network of the skin to be seen under the vital microscope by means of fluo-rescing molecules (FITC-Dextran, Sigma) which, when injected subepidermally, are taken up by the initial lymphatics. Informa-tion regarding the morphology of functional initial lymphatics and the extent of tracer propagation within the dermal lymphatic network can be recorded on video for analysis [9].

Indirect lymphography involves the intracutaneous injection of a water-soluble contrast medium. Using an infusion pump, the contrast medium is administered over 10 min to create a depot of approximately 3 mL. Intradermal and subcutaneous lymphatics can be opacified by X-ray using the mammography film method, sometimes as far as the first lymph node [10,11]. The advantages over conventional lymphography are the convenience of the inter-stitial injection without recourse to direct access into the lymphat-ics, and the ease of application to multiple sites.

Skin biopsy

The distinction between lymphatic and blood vessels in skin biopsy sections has been made more straightforward by specific lymphatic markers. D2-40 (Podoplanin) is considered the most robust as it stains initial lymphatics, pre-collectors and collecting vessels but not blood vessels. LYVE-1 stains initial lymphatics but also macrophages and is down-regulated by inflammation. Prox-1 and VEGFR3 are also lymphatic-specific and stain larger vessels. A panel of markers is recommended, particularly in vascular mal-formations where differentiation between venous and lymphatic phenotypes may not be clear-cut [12].

CD31 and CD34 stain both lymphatic and blood vascular endothelium.

References

1 Stewart G, Gaunt J, Croft DN *et al.* Isotope lymphography: a new method of investigating the role of lymphatics. *Br J Surg* 1985; **72**: 906–9.
2 Proby CM, Gane JN, Joseph AE *et al.* Investigation of the swollen limb with isotope lymphography. *Br J Dermatol* 1990; **123**: 29–38.
3 Vaughan BF. CT of swollen legs. *Clin Rad* 1990; **41**: 24–30.
4 Duewell S, Hagspiel KD, Zuber J *et al.* Swollen limb extremity: role of MR imaging. *Radiology* 1992; **184**: 227–31.
5 Kinmonth JB. Lymphangiography in man. *Clin Sci* 1952; **11**: 13–20.
6 Lohrmann C, Felmerer G, Foeldi E *et al.* MR lymphangiography for the assess-ment of the lymphatic system in patients undergoing microsurgical reconstruc-tion of lymphatic vessels. *Microvasc Res* 2008; **76**: 42–5.
7 Lu Q, Xu J, Liu N. Chronic lower extremity lymphedema: a comparative study of high-resolution interstitial MR lymphangiography and heavily T2-weighted MRI. *Eur J Radiol* 2008. (Epub ahead of print.)
8 Hudack SS, McMaster PD. Lymphatic participation in human cutaneous phe-nomena. *J Exp Med* 1933; **57**: 751–74.
9 Bollinger A, Jager K, Spier F, Seglias J. Fluorescence microlymphography. *Cir-culation* 1981; **64**: 1195–200.
10 Partsch HT, Urbanek A, Wenzel-Hora B. The dermal lymphatics in lymphoe-dema visualized by indirect lymphography. *Br J Dermatol* 1984; **110**: 431–8.
11 Partsch H, Stoberl CL, Urbanek A *et al.* Clinical use of indirect lymphography in different forms of leg oedema. *Lymphology* 1988; **21**: 152–60.
12 Costa da Cunha Castro E, Galambos C. Prox-1 and VEGFR3 antibodies are superior to D2-40 in identifying endothelial cells of lymphatic malformations—a proposal of a new immunohistochemical panel to differentiate lymphatic from other vascular malformations. *Pediatr Dev Pathol* 2009; **12**: 187–94.

Differential diagnosis of the swollen limb (Table 48.6)

Swelling of a limb may be caused by oedema, in which case pitting should be evident to some degree, or it may be caused by an increase in volume of other tissue elements, for example bone, muscle or fat. MRI scanning is useful in circumstances where the nature of the swelling is uncertain. One must remember also that a patient may perceive one leg to be swollen when in fact the other leg has become smaller, for example through atrophy of muscle or fat.

Obvious lymphoedema with characteristic skin changes is not usually a difficult diagnosis but such cases are relatively uncom-mon. Milder cases frequently go unrecognized. Chronic non-inflammatory, and in particular asymmetrical, limb oedema should always suggest lymphoedema. In such cases lymphoscin-tigraphy is the investigation of choice.

Systemic causes of oedema including cardiac disease, renal disease or hypoproteinaemia should always be considered, par-ticularly if bilateral leg swelling is present. Calcium channel block-ing agents cause peripheral oedema in 50% of cases.

Lipoedema

A condition frequently misdiagnosed as lymphoedema is lipo-edema (lipidosis, lipodystrophy) in which a 'fatty', non-pitting swelling is confined to the legs, thighs, hips and sometimes arms overlying the triceps [1,2]. Lipoedema is peculiar to females and is usually dismissed as a variant of normality in women with chunky legs and a 'bottom-heavy' weight distribution. Features of importance in recognition include: (i) onset at puberty or times of hormonal change, for example oral contraception, pregnancy or menopause; (ii) bilateral and symmetrical involvement of the lower limbs with sparing of the feet resulting in an 'inverse shoul-dering' effect at the malleoli (Fig. 48.10); (iii) tenderness and easy bruising; (iv) absence of pitting and lack of benefit from elevation; and (v) lack of benefit from dieting (dieting tends to result in weight loss from body sites other than those affected by lipoe-dema). Lymph drainage within main leg lymphatics is relatively normal [3] until the later stages when foot oedema develops—the so-called lipoedema–lymphoedema syndrome.

Table 48.6 Causes of a swollen limb.

Congenitally determined
Vascular
    Vascular malformation
    Diffuse phlebectasia
    Klippel–Trenaunay syndrome
    Parkes-Weber syndrome
    Maffucci's syndrome
Lymphatic
    Lymphoedema
    Lymphatic malformation (Lymphangioma)
Other
    Fat hypertrophy
    Lipoedema
    Plexiform neurofibroma
    Proteus syndrome
    Muscle hamartoma
    Gigantism
    Tissue hypertrophy/hemihypertrophy

Acquired
Vascular
    Deep venous thrombosis
    Post-thrombotic syndrome
    Chronic venous reflux
    Venous outflow obstruction
    Thrombophlebitis
    Venous injury, e.g. intravenous drug abuse
    Idiopathic oedema of women
    Acute arterial ischaemia
    Reflex sympathetic dystrophy
Lymphatic
    Lymphoedema
    Dependency syndrome/elephantiasis/armchair legs
    Trauma
    Reconstructive surgery
    Femoropopliteal bypass
    Vein harvesting
    Factitial (tourniquet)
    Pretibial myxoedema
Inflammatory
    Cellulitis/erysipelas
    Varicose eczema
    Asteatotic eczema
    Psoriasis
Musculoskeletal
    Rheumatoid arthritis
    Joint effusion
    Ruptured Baker's cyst
    Haematoma
    Torn muscle
    Pathological fracture
    Achilles tendonitis
    Myositis ossificans
    Paget's disease
Tumours
    Lymphoma
    Sarcoma
    Metastases

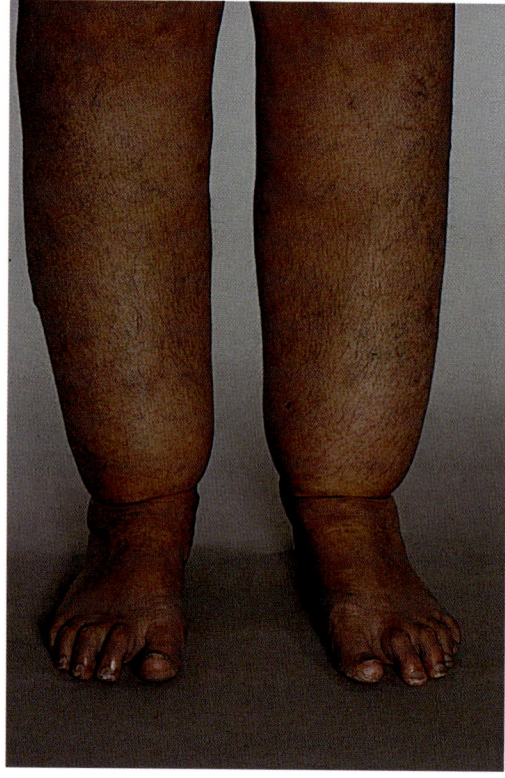

Fig. 48.10 Lipoedema.

Patients with lipoedema gain weight easily and often prefer to be fat than to diet furiously and suffer the embarrassment of thin torso, face and neck while retaining huge legs.

Liposuction performed with tumescent local anaesthesia and using vibrating microcannulae has proved to be a new effective treatment. A targeted and permanent reduction of the fat tissue leads to an increased quality of life due to an improved appearance, reduced tendency to swelling and less pain [4].

Males are very rarely involved and only when there is an underlying hormonal problem such as testosterone deficiency or oestrogen excess with chronic liver disease.

Dercum's disease (adiposis dolorosa, lipomatosis dolorosa, morbus Dercum) is a rare disorder resulting in painful fatty deposits around the upper legs, trunk and upper arms [5]. When pain is a significant symptom with lipoedema it is known as the painful fat syndrome and indistinguishable from Dercum's disease.

Obesity and lymphoedema

Obesity is a significant risk factor for lymphoedema in the arms as well as the legs. Obesity increases the risk of breast cancer-related lymphoedema [6]. Furthermore, dieting improves arm swelling beyond that possible through loss of subcutaneous fat from weight loss [7], irrespective of the diet used [8].

The pathophysiology of lower-limb lymphoedema can be complex. Increased abdominal girth and intra-abdominal pressure impair venous return, particularly when sitting, with the abdominal apron compressing the thighs. Higher venous pressures will increase fluid filtration into the legs so increasing lymph load. However, lymph drainage may also be compromised in the same sitting position, and is certainly decreased as a result of the reduced exercise associated with obesity [9]. Severely obese patients suffering from sleep apnoea will tend to retain fluid for complex hormonal and autonomic reasons, while sleeping in a chair causes 'armchair legs' as described earlier.

Limb overgrowth (hypertrophy)

Limb hypertrophy (overgrowth) may be mistaken for lymphoedema but also be associated with it. Occasionally, lymphoedema coexists with complete hemihypertrophy, Klippel–Trenaunay syndrome, Parkes-Weber syndrome (multiple arteriovenous anastomoses) or proteus syndrome. Elephantiasis neurofibromatosa is a diffuse neurofibromatosis of nerve trunks with overgrowth of the subcutaneous tissue and of the skin, producing considerable enlargement of that region.

Yellow nail syndrome

YNS is associated with peripheral oedema, but the clinical features rarely resemble classical lymphoedema. Lymphangiogram abnormalities have been described [10], although a lymphoscintigraphic study demonstrated that a primary lymphatic abnormality is unlikely [11].

References

1 Wold LE, Hines EA, Allen EV. Lipoedema of the legs. *Ann Intern Med* 1949; **34**: 1243–50.
2 Kröger K. Lymphoedema and lipoedema of the extremities. *VASA* 2008; **37**: 39–51.
3 Harwood CA, Bull RH, Evans J *et al.* Lymphatic and venous function in lipoedema. *Br J Dermatol* 1996; **134**: 1–6.
4 Schmeller W, Meier-Vollrath I. Tumescent liposuction: a new and successful therapy for lipedema. *J Cutan Med Surg* 2006; **10**: 7–10.
5 Wortham NC, Tomlinson IP. Dercum's disease. *Skinmed* 2005; **4**: 157–62.
6 Hayes SB, Freedman GM, Li T *et al.* Does axillary boost increase lymphedema compared with supraclavicular radiation alone after breast conservation? *Int J Radiat Oncol Biol Phys* 2008; **72**: 1449–55.
7 Shaw C, Mortimer P, Judd PA. A randomized controlled trial of weight reduction as a treatment for breast cancer-related lymphedema. *Cancer* 2007; **110**: 1868–74.
8 Shaw C, Mortimer P, Judd PA. Randomized controlled trial comparing a low-fat diet with a weight-reduction diet in breast cancer-related lymphedema. *Cancer* 2007; **109**: 1949–56.
9 Mortimer PS, Levick JR. Chronic peripheral oedema: the critical role of the lymphatic system. *Clin Med* 2004; **4**: 448–53.
10 Emerson PA. Yellow nails, lymphoedema and pleural effusions. *Thorax* 1966; **21**: 247–53.
11 Bull RH, Fenton DA, Mortimer PS. Lymphatic function in the yellow nail syndrome. *Br J Dermatol* 1996; **134**: 307–12.

Management of lymphoedema

Lymphatic failure results in the accumulation of protein as well as water within the swollen tissues. Treatment is difficult because of the presence of the 'solid' component in the swelling. The management of lymphoedema varies greatly around the world. In developed countries, the emphasis is more on physical forms of therapy involving massage, exercise and compression designed to stimulate lymph drainage, whereas in poorer, hotter countries where hosiery and appropriate bandages are too costly and uncomfortable, surgery may be the mainstay of treatment. Two particular problems need to be overcome with lymphoedema: the

swelling and the predisposition to infections, particularly recurrent cellulitis.

There is limited research to inform evidence-based guidelines on the treatment of lymphoedema. Nevertheless, robust guidelines developed through consensus by experts do exist [1, 2].

References

1 Medical Education Partnership. *Best Practice for the Management of Lymphoedema: International Consensus.* London: MEP Ltd, 2006. www.library.nhs.uk
2 Clinical Resource Efficiency Support Team. *Guidelines on the Diagnosis, Assessment and Management of Lymphoedema,* 2008. www.crestni.org.uk

Assessment

Medical

Medical assessment aims to identify and exclude other causes of peripheral oedema. In circumstances where systemic causes for peripheral oedema, for example heart failure, have led to, or coexist with, the lymphoedema, then treatment of the internal medical condition must be undertaken before embarking on specific lymphoedema therapy. Where necessary, appropriate investigations should be performed to confirm lymphoedema and to identify treatable underlying causes (e.g. active cancer) or co-morbidities (e.g. superficial venous incompetence).

Lymphoedema therapy

All patients with a diagnosis of lymphoedema should be referred to the local trained lymphoedema therapist. A list of trained therapists can usually be accessed through the national professional body for lymphoedema, for example the British Lymphology Society (http://www.thebls.com/directory); the National Lymphedema Network (USA) (http://www.lymphnet.org); and the Lymphoedema Association of Australia (http://www.lymphoedema.org.au).

Best practice for management will focus on the needs of each individual patient. This may include: (i) risk reduction, for example breast cancer patients; (ii) swelling reduction and improvement of shape; (iii) treatment and prevention of infection; (iv) treating skin problems such as elephantiasis, lymphorrhoea and wounds as well as discouraging tissue fibrosis; (v) restoring functional independence and correcting posture imbalance; and (vi) pain and psychosocial management. Therapy assessment will also include setting the benchmarks against which improvement can be judged, for example limb volume measurement, mobility and functional assessments. A treatment plan will depend on the site and severity of the lymphoedema and the need to engage other services, for example leg ulcer, oncology, vascular etc.

Physical therapy (decongestive lymphatic therapy, combined decongestive treatment)

Physical methods of treating lymphoedema have been practised in Europe for many years [1]. Therapy essentially aims to control lymph formation (capillary filtration), including treatment of inflammatory causes or of venous hypertension, and to improve lymph drainage through existing lymphatics and collateral routes by applying normal physiological procedures that stimulate lymph flow. Physical treatment can, in the majority of cases,

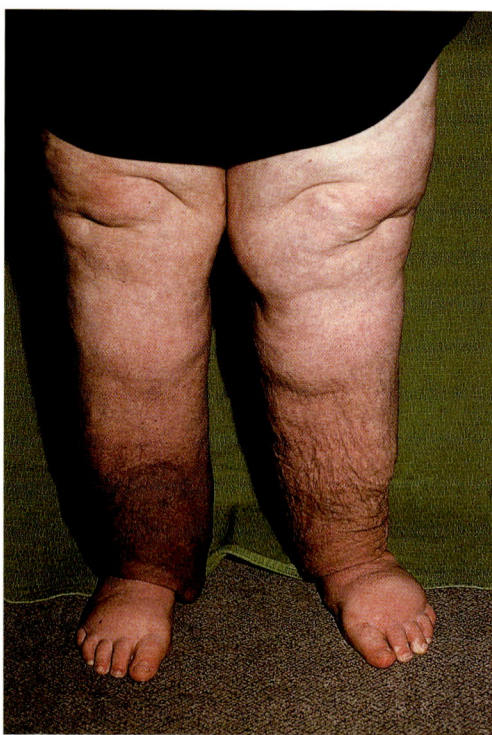

Fig. 48.11 Reduction of swelling in lymphoedema following 3 weeks' intensive therapy with multilayer bandaging and an exercise programme (the same patient as in Fig. 48.5).

improve quality of life considerably (Fig. 48.11). Central to management is getting patients to understand their condition and know what they can do for themselves [2]. Only then can a high level of motivation and compliance with treatment be generated.

It is important to explain to patients that, unlike the blood, which is propelled by the heart, lymph drainage relies on local changes in tissue pressure generated by exercise and movement. Physical treatment exploits these principles, enhancing lymph flow as much as possible within the limits of a compromised drainage. It should be appreciated that lymph flow still exists in lymphoedema, otherwise swelling would be a relentlessly progressive process.

Cornerstones of physical therapy

1 Care of the skin and prevention of infection
   Elephantiasis skin changes are not only unsightly but lead to problems including infection, odour, lymphorrhoea, restricted movement from fibrosis (pseudoscleroderma) and possibly poor wound healing. Such problems can be particularly troublesome where fibrosis has become excessive—for example after trauma or surgery. Regular application of an emollient is important for hydrating the hardened skin so making it more supple and discouraging hyperkeratosis. Tinea pedis is almost invariable because of the closely apposed swollen toes, circumstances not improved by elastic hosiery. Modern antifungal creams unfortunately macerate skin further and therefore it is suggested that terbinafine cream is applied for 2 weeks followed by an alcohol wipe (assuming the skin is not broken). For deep cracks and crevices which bacteria may readily colonize, regular

toilet is necessary followed by an antiseptic soak, for example potassium permanganate. Hyperkeratosis can often be improved through the regular application of 5% salicylic acid ointment, but the best treatment to reverse elephantiasis skin changes is long-term compression. Areas that constantly seep lymph should also respond to sustained compression.

Prevention of infection, particularly lymphangitis/cellulitis, is crucial to the control of lymphoedema. Care of the skin, good hygiene, control of tinea pedis and good antisepsis following abrasions and minor wounds are important to reduce risk of cellulitis.

2 Exercise
   Exercise and movement are crucial to lymph drainage [3,4]. Dynamic muscle contractions (isotonic exercises) encourage both passive (movement of lymph along tissue planes or through non-contractile lymphatics) and active (increased contractility and therefore propulsion of lymph within contractile lymphatics) phases of lymph drainage. Overexertion and excessive static (isometric, e.g. gripping) exercise increase blood flow, which therefore tends to increase oedema.

3 External compression (hosiery, bandage or pneumatic compression)
   External compression complements the exercise programme. Such compression is not intended to 'squeeze' oedema but to act as a counterforce to striated muscle activity and so generate higher tissue pressures during contractions. This provides the most powerful stimulus to lymph drainage. Compression also limits capillary filtration by opposing capillary pressure. Without exercise compression is much less effective.

Multilayer bandaging can be used for limb reduction, but also has the advantage of restoring limb shape so that subsequent use of compression garments (hosiery) is more effective at controlling swelling [5]. Bandaging may be the only method suitable for huge misshapen limbs and for controlling lymphorrhoea. Layers of strong, non-elastic (short-stretch) bandages are applied to generate a high pressure during muscular contractions but low pressure at rest. The use of foam or soft padding helps to distribute pressure more evenly and to protect the skin. The digits are also bandaged to control swelling of fingers and toes. The strategic positioning of rubber pads 'irons out' pockets of swelling and deep skin folds. Multilayer bandaging is a skill that takes time to learn and should not be undertaken by any professional without appropriate training. The compression administered may have to be modified in circumstances such as cancer requiring palliative treatment, moderate limb ischaemia, or if there is any neurological deficit.

Hosiery (below-knee or full-length stockings, half or full tights, sleeves) usually requires high compression and double hoses may occasionally be required. Most garments last no more than 6 months. Two garments (or pairs) should be provided, one to wear and one for the wash. Washing is necessary to maintain the compression properties of the garment. The patient's technique for application, removal and care of garments are crucial for a successful outcome.

Pneumatic compression therapy (intermittent/sequential pneumatic compression) should not be used in preference to exercise and compression but can be useful in mixed lymphovenous oedema and in infirm patients [6]. An inflatable boot, legging or sleeve is connected to a motor-driven pump and lymph is displaced towards the root of the limb. If hosiery is not fitted immediately following compression therapy, the swelling readily recurs. Pneumatic compression softens the tissues and reduces limb volume during treatment, but it is doubtful that any long-term benefit is gained over hosiery and exercise alone.

4 Massage (manual lymphatic drainage therapy)
Massage is an important component of treatment, particularly for midline lymphoedema where there are few alternatives [1]. The problem is that there are different forms of massage, used mostly for increasing blood flow and therefore of vigorous nature. Tissue movement, if gentle, is a stimulus to lymph flow without increasing blood flow [7]. Indeed, in the absence of lymphatic contractility, massaging of filled lymphatics by muscle exercise or surface massage may be the major stimulus to lymph flow, just as it is with blood flow during cardiac arrest [4]. The skin lymphatic network is the likely route for collateral drainage to areas which have normal lymph drainage [8]. The practice that encourages such flow, referred to as manual lymphatic drainage therapy (MLD), is directed at normally draining lymph node regions; this 'siphons' or 'milks' lymph away from congested lymphoedematous areas, so complementing attempts to improve drainage 'upstream' by exercise and external compression. Continuous MLD delivered by a therapist is expensive and few health care providers will fund this long term. Simple lymphatic drainage (SLD) is a best alternative to MLD, and can be delivered by a partner or carer trained in the technique.

5 Breathing, postural exercise, elevation and rest
Breathing and postural exercises are also important, particularly for clearance of lymph from the thorax and abdomen. Without the dispersal of truncal lymph, more peripheral limb oedema will not drain. Elevation *per se* does nothing to improve lymph drainage, but lowering venous pressure (and therefore filtration) can help to reduce swelling. Rest and elevation alone, however, are not the correct treatment for lymphoedema!

Additional therapies

1 Weight loss. Many patients with lymphoedema are overweight, because of morbid obesity as well as fluid retention. Excessive weight gain is likely to impair lymph drainage in the same way as it impairs venous drainage, and obesity reduces mobility (and therefore exercise). Control of weight in combination with physical treatment may be sufficient to resolve oedema completely in some patients. Weight loss irrespective of type of diet has been shown to reduce arm volume over and above what would be expected from fat loss alone in breast cancer related lymphoedema [9,10].

2 Hyperbaric oxygen (HBO), low-level laser therapy (LLLT) and Kinesiotaping. There are some data recommending the use of HBO and LLLT independently in breast cancer related lymphoedema [11–13]. Kinesiotaping has been shown to increase lymph flow [14].

Intensive and maintenance treatment

Patients with mild limb lymphoedema, no fibrosis and no shape distortion can be started on maintenance treatment with compression hosiery. Intensive therapy, comprising a 2- to 4-week course of daily skin care, MLD, multi-layer bandaging and exercises, is indicated for patients with moderate to severe limb swelling, poor limb shape or tissue changes such as fibrosis, elephantiasis or lymphorrhoea. Once intensive treatment is complete, maintenance treatment is started.

Evidence of efficacy

While decongestive lymphatic therapy has become accepted first-line therapy [15], evidence for best treatment is weak. Using limb volume change as the main outcome measure, bandaging plus hosiery was significantly more effective at 6 months than hosiery alone [5]; hosiery was more effective than no hosiery [16]; MLD was more effective than SLD [17], although effects on total arm volume can be small [18]. Pneumatic compression therapy was no better than no treatment [19].

Management of midline lymphoedema

Management of lymphoedema of the head and neck, trunk, breast or genitalia can be challenging.

Truncal lymphoedema implies involvement of a body quadrant, for example a forequarter or hindquarter, and is usually associated with swelling of the adjoining limb. Lymphatic obstruction at the root of the limb, for example from tumour, should always be considered with truncal oedema. Clearance of the trunk, usually with MLD, is necessary before improvement of the limb can be expected.

Breast lymphoedema generally follows cancer treatment and is usually associated with inflammation from radiation or infection. Infection may be extremely difficult to control in these circumstances, requiring low-dose antibiotics, for example phenoxymethylpenicillin 500 mg twice daily for many weeks. Dependency is a contributing factor to oedema formation, particularly in a large breast, and a firm supportive bra, day and night, is recommended. Only then should MLD be introduced.

Genital lymphoedema can occur in the male or female but is more severe in the penis and scrotum due to a combination of dependency and limited drainage outlet routes. Genital lymphoedema is associated with lower-limb swelling when oedema creeps up to involve the lower trunk, such as following surgery or radiotherapy to ilioinguinal lymph nodes, in heart failure and sometimes with genetic forms of lymphoedema. Sadly, genital swelling may appear for the first time when lower limb oedema is forced up into the trunk by over-vigorous leg compression. When lymphoedema is limited to the male genitalia then underlying inflammation from granulomatous disease (Crohn's disease, sarcoidosis, hidradenitis suppurativa or anogenital granulomatosis) or due to infection have to be considered before embarking on specific lymphoedema treatment. MLD and innovative ways of applying compression [20] are most widely used but surgery can be considered at an early stage.

Lymphoedema of the head and neck is often a complication of cancer or its treatment. Facial lymphoedema (solid facial oedema) is most frequently caused by rosacea or acne but a differential diagnosis includes dermatomyositis, thyroid disease, lymphoma and (lymph)angiosarcoma. Periorbital oedema may result from loose eyelid skin, for example blepharochalasia (floppy eyelid syndrome), where low compliance encourages oedema [21]. Once underlying conditions have been treated or excluded, MLD and SLD are introduced. Raising the head of the bed with blocks can be invaluable for preventing reaccumulation of oedema overnight.

References

1 Foldi E, Foldi M, Weissleder H. Conservative treatment of lymphoedema of the limbs. *Angiology* 1985; **36**: 171–80.

2 Mortimer P, Todd J. *Lymphoedema: Advice on Self-management and Treatment*, 3rd edn. Beaconsfield: Beaconsfield Publishers, 2007.

3 Ikomi F, Schmid-Schonbein GW. Lymph transport in skin. *Clin Dermatol* 1995; **13**: 419–27.

4 Roddie IC. Lymph transport mechanisms in peripheral lymphatics. *News Physiol Sci* 1990; **5**: 85–9.

5 Badger CMA, Peacock JL, Mortimer PS. A randomized, controlled, parallel group clinical trial comparing multi-layer bandaging followed by hosiery versus hosiery alone in the treatment of patients with lymphedema of the limb. *Cancer* 2000; **88**: 2832–7.

6 Anonymous. Compression for lymphoedema. *Lancet* 1986; **i**: 896.

7 Mortimer PS, Simmonds R, Rezvani M *et al*. Measurement of skin lymph flow by an isotope clearance technique: reliability, reproducibility effect of injection dynamics and lymph flow enhancement. *J Invest Dermatol* 1990; **95**: 677–82.

8 Tiedjen KU, Knorz S, Heimann KD. The skin: lymphatic collateral organ? *Scope Phlebol Lymphol* 1994; **1**: 7–12.

9 Shaw C, Mortimer P, Judd PA. A randomised controlled trial of weight reduction as a treatment for breast cancer-related lymphedema. *Cancer* 2007; **110**: 1868–74.

10 Shaw C, Mortimer P, Judd PA. Randomised controlled trial comparing a low-fat diet with a weight-reduction diet in breast cancer-related lymphedema. *Cancer* 2007; **109**: 1949–56.

11 Gothard L, Stanton A, MacLaren J *et al*. Non-randomised phase II trial of hyperbaric oxygen therapy in patients with chronic arm lymphoedema and tissue fibrosis after radiotherapy for early breast cancer. *Radiother Oncol* 2004; **70**: 217–24.

12 Carati CJ, Anderson SN, Gannon BJ, Piller NB. Treatment of postmastectomy lymphedema with low-level laser therapy: a double blind, placebo-controlled trial. *Cancer* 2003; **98**: 1114–22. [Erratum *Cancer* 2003; **98**: 2742.]

13 Kozanoglu E, Basaran S, Paydas S, Sarpel T. Efficacy of pneumatic compression and low-level laser therapy in the treatment of postmastectomy lymphedema: a randomized controlled trial. *Clin Rehabil* 2009; **23**: 117–24.

14 Tsai HJ, Hung HC, Yang JL *et al*. Could Kinesio tape replace the bandage in decongestive lymphatic therapy for breast-cancer-related lymphedema? A pilot study. *Support Care Cancer* 2009. [Epub ahead of print.]

15 Rockson S, Miller L, Senie R. Workshop III: diagnosis and management of lymphedema. *Cancer* 1998; **83** (Suppl.): 282–5.

16 Hornsby R. The use of compression to treat lymphedema. *Prof Nurse* 1995; **11**: 127–8.

17 Williams AF, Vadgama A, Franks P, Mortimer PS. A randomized controlled cross-over study of manual lymphatic drainage therapy in women with breast cancer-related lympoedema. *Eur J Cancer Care* 2002; **11**: 254–61.

18 Andersen L, Hojris I, Erlandsen M, Andersen J. Treatment of breast-cancer related lymphoedema with or without manual lymph drainage: a randomized study. *Acta Oncol* 2000; **39**: 399–405.

19 Dini D, Del Mastro L, Gozza A *et al*. The role of pneumatic compression in the treatment of postmastectomy lymphedema: a randomized phase III study. *Ann Oncol* 1998; **9**: 187–90.

20 Whitaker J. Best practice in managing scrotal lymphoedema. *Br J Community Nurs* 2007; **12** (Suppl.): S17–21.

21 Collin JR. Blepharochalasis. A review of 30 cases. *Ophthal Plast Reconstr Surg* 1991; **7**: 153–7.

Prevention and treatment of infection

Infections are common with lymphoedema because of the compromised immune status of the swollen tissues. The recommendations for management are born more out of consensus than robust research [1,2]. Skin care is the first priority as maintenance of skin integrity and an effective barrier will reduce entry of microorganisms.

Acute cellulitis (erysipelas)

Cellulitis is probably more likely to result from a pre-existent lymphatic insufficiency than to be a primary cause of lymphoedema. Nevertheless, it is not unusual for cellulitis to manifest lymphoedema without any prior knowledge of a lymph drainage weakness.

Administration of antibiotics at the time of an attack of cellulitis must be prompt, otherwise they do not significantly influence the course of the illness. Therefore, patients need to carry a supply of antibiotics—for example, co-amoxiclav or amoxicillin—with them at all times [3].

Recurrent cellulitis

For attacks recurring more than once a year, prophylactic antibiotics are the recommended treatment [3]. Phenoxymethyl penicillin 500 mg daily is as effective as any broad-spectrum antibiotic. Long-term prophylaxis is often necessary [4]. Control of the oedema and diabetic-type skin care may help reduce antibiotic requirements.

The only trials investigating prophylaxis against infection in lymphoedema were undertaken in filarial lymphoedema and compared the efficacy of diethylcarbamazine (DEC), ivermectin and skin care in preventing lymphangitis/adenitis [5]. The authors concluded that a foot care programme alone can drastically reduce the number of attacks of acute adenolymphangitis. In a second study [6], the same group compared oral penicillin, diethylcarbamazine and antibiotic cream. Both the penicillin group and the DEC group had significantly reduced frequency of attacks of lymphangitis compared with patients treated with placebo. The authors concluded that antifilarial drugs do not have a role in reducing acute inflammatory attacks (lymphangitis, cellulitis), but that penicillin does contribute significantly to a reduction in attacks when combined with foot care.

References

1 Medical Education Partnership. *Best Practice for the Management of Lymphoedema: International Consensus*. London: MEP Ltd, 2006. http://www.library.nhs.uk

2 Clinical Resource Efficiency Support Team. *Guidelines on the Diagnosis, Assessment and Management of Lymphoedema*, 2008. http://www.crestni.org.uk

3 British Lymphology Society. *Consensus Document on the Management of Cellulitis in Lymphoedema*. http://www.thebls.com/concensus.php

4 Vignes S, Dupuy A. Recurrence of lymphoedema-associated cellulitis (erysipelas) under prophylactic antibiotherapy: a retrospective cohort study. *J Eur Acad Dermatol Venereol* 2006; **20**: 818–22.

5 Shenoy RK, Suma TK, Rajan K *et al*. Prevention of acute adenolymphangitis in brugian filariasis: comparison of the efficacy of ivermectin and diethylcarbamazine each combined with local treatment of the affected limb. *Ann Trop Med Parasit* 1998; **92**: 587–94.

6 Shenoy RK, Kumaraswami V, Suma TK *et al*. A double blind placebo controlled study of the efficacy of oral penicillin, diethylcarbamazine or local treatment of the affected limb in preventing acute adenolymphangitis in lymphoedema caused by brugian filariasis. *Ann Trop Med Parasit* 1999; **93**: 367–77.

Drug therapy

Drug therapy is generally disappointing. Diuretics remain the most commonly used treatment because most doctors consider oedema to be an indication for such drugs. Diuretics alone have little benefit in lymphoedema because their main mode of action is to limit capillary filtration by reducing circulating blood volume. Improvement with diuretics suggests that the predominant cause of the oedema is not lymphatic.

The benzopyrone group of drugs have been advocated as treatment for lymphoedema, but their clinical effect seems to be small. In the UK, the only available oral prescription medication in this class (although only actually licensed for venous disease) is oxerutins (Paroven®). Three randomized and placebo-controlled trials have been published, all demonstrating a marginal significant effect on limb volume but of little clinical benefit [1]. Other benzopyrone drugs investigated include Daflon® and coumarin (5,6-benzo-α-pyrone) and, while most trials claim significant volume reduction, the poor reporting means a meta-analysis is not possible. One robust trial concluded that there was no difference in effect between coumarin and placebo, and reported serious liver toxicity from coumarin [2].

References

1 Mortimer PS, Badger C, Clarke I, Pallett J. A double blind, randomized, parallel group, placebo-controlled trial of O-(-β hydroxyethyl)-rutosides in chronic arm oedema resulting from breast cancer treatment. *Phlebology* 1995; **10**: 51–5.
2 Loprinzi CL, Kugler JW, Sloan JA *et al*. Lack of effect of coumarin in women with lymphoedema after treatment for breast cancer. *N Eng J Med* 1999; **340**: 346–50.

Surgery

Surgery has a specific role in the management of lymphoedema [1]. It is of value in limb lymphoedema in a few patients in whom, even after conservative treatment, the size and weight of a limb inhibit its use or interfere with mobility. Surgery involves either removing excessive tissue or bypassing local lymphatic defects. Lifelong non-surgical measures—for example, hosiery—must be continued postoperatively.

Reduction (excisional) operations remove a longitudinal ellipse of skin and the underlying abnormal subcutaneous tissue down to the deep fascia in a 'melon slice' that permits primary closure of skin edges (Sistrunk procedure). Undercutting of the skin allows removal of additional tissue (Homans' procedure). This procedure is preferred to circumferential excision and skin grafting (Charles' procedure) or to the addition of in-rolling of a skin flap (Thompson buried dermis flap operation). Procedures involving surgery both above and below the knee or the elbow are usually undertaken one region at a time, because blood loss can be extensive.

A new, less invasive, form of debulking has been successfully employed using liposuction but necessitates compression garments 24 hours a day [2].

Reduction/debulking surgery is used sooner rather than later for genital [3] and eyelid lymphoedema.

Bypass operations involve either bridging an area of defective lymphatics with tissue containing lymphatics or with a vessel graft. If the lymphoedema results from excision of, or damage to, a local group of lymph nodes (e.g. in the axilla or groin) the area can be bridged with omentum or with an isolated and opened-out segment of gut. Lymph node-to-venous and direct lymph vessel-to-venous shunts have been undertaken but long-term patency is doubtful [4]. Lymph vessel transplantation, where autologous lymphatics are removed from an unaffected part of the body and anastomosed end-to-end with other unaffected collectors proximal and distal to the obstruction, has been shown to improve lymph transport [5]. Two to three microsurgical lymphatico-venous anastomoses (small subdermal venules joined to local lymphatics) are claimed to be sufficient to reduce limb volume [6].

References

1 Browse NL, Burnand KG, Mortimer PS. *Diseases of the Lymphatics*. London, Arnold, 2003.
2 Brorson H, Ohlin K, Olsson G *et al*. Controlled compression and liposuction treatment for lower extremity lymphedema. *Lymphology* 2008; **41**: 52–63.
3 Garaffa G, Christopher N, Ralph DJ. The management of genital lymphoedema. *BJU Int* 2008; **102**: 480–4.
4 Campisi C. Use of autologous interposition vein graft in management of lymphedema: preliminary experimental and clinical observations. *Lymphology* 1991; **24**: 71–6.
5 Baumeister RG, Siuda S. Treatment of lymphedema by microsurgical lymphatic grafting: what is proved? *Plast Reconstr Surg* 1990; **85**: 75–6.
6 Nagase T, Gonda K, Inoue K *et al*. Treatment of lymphedema with lymphaticovenular anastomoses. *Int J Clin Oncol* 2005; **10**: 304–10.

Lymphatic malformations, lymphangioma and lymphangiectasia

The reclassification of vascular anomalies into vascular tumours and vascular malformations should apply to lymphangioma and lymphatic disorders [1].

Lymphatic malformations represent a failure of lymphatic development and often exist in isolation with no communication with otherwise normal lymph drainage pathways (extratruncular) or with some sort of communication as seen on lymphoscintigraphy (truncular) [2]. It is best to consider lymphatic malformations as genetically determined structural anomalies with normal endothelial cell turnover, rather than as tumours which are proliferative with endothelial hyperplasia. Malformations increase in size by distension or hypertrophy, not through increased cell division.

The term lymphangioma should only be used if progression through proliferation occurs, otherwise lymphatic malformation is to be preferred. Unfortunately, like haemangioma, the term lymphangioma, implying tumour, is often inappropriately used in clinical dermatology. Nevertheless some lymphatic malformations progress on a lethal, inexorably expanding, unalleviated course making distinction from lymphangioma (tumour process) impossible [1].

Acquired simple sustained dilatation of otherwise normal lymphatic vessels is referred to as lymphangiectasia [3].

References

1 Enjolras O, Wassef M, Chapot R. *Color Atlas of Vascular Tumors and Vascular Malformations*. Cambridge: Cambridge University Press, 2007.
2 Lee BB, Kim YW, Seo JM *et al*. Current concepts in lymphatic malformation. *Vasc Endovasc Surg* 2005; **39**: 67–81.
3 Blei F. Congenital lymphatic malformations. *Ann N Y Acad Sci* 2008; **1131**: 185–94.

Lymphatic malformations (lymphangioma)

Localized congenital lymphatic malformations (LMs) are frequently referred to as 'lymphangioma' and can be divided into macrocystic, or deep, and microcystic, or superficial, lesions. Lymphatic malformations that appear microcystic, localized and superficial within the skin are called 'lymphangioma circumscriptum', but the term is a misnomer because there is frequently communication with a more extensive deeper malformation (particularly if the lesion is at the root of a limb). Macrocystic LMs are usually visible at birth in the neck and are referred to as cystic hygroma. Distinction between the two types is important because treatment and prognosis can differ [1]. Nevertheless, LMs can have both microcystic and macrocystic components.

The most important feature of congenital LMs is that they can be isolated from the normal lymph conducting system (extratruncal). When connected to the main collecting system they are referred to as truncal lymphatic malformations and can then be associated with lymphoedema. There have been attempts to classify LMs into localized or diffuse, with diffuse indicating that there will be associated lymphoedema, but lymphoedema in general is not due to LMs.

LMs are usually congenital but may not be apparent at birth. They may enlarge if infected or traumatized and only then become symptomatic. No evidence for inheritance exists, suggesting a somatic mutation in a restricted area of the lymphatic network as the mechanism for development [2].

LMs/lymphangiomas are classified according to their morphology as seen histologically or by imaging (e.g. using ultrasound), into macrocystic, microcystic and combined lymphangioma [3]. LMs/lymphangiomas have to be distinguished from true lymphatic neoplasms such as acquired progressive lymphangioma (lymphangioendothelioma) and lymphangiomatosis. LMs/lymphangiomas at least partially and temporarily depend on active lymphangiogenesis, and possibly on active angiogenesis, during the course of development or progression [4].

References

1 Garzon M, Huang J, Enjolras O, Frieden I. Vascular malformations, part I. *J Am Acad Dermatol* 2007; **56**: 353–70.
2 Brouillard P, Vikkula M. Genetic causes of vascular malformations. *Hum Mol Genet* 2007; **16**: 140–9.
3 Marler J, Mulliken J. Current management of hemangiomas and vascular malformations. *Clin Plast Surg* 2005; **32**: 99–116.
4 Wiegand S, Eivazi B, Barth P *et al*. Pathogenesis of lymphangioma. *Virchows Arch* 2008; **453**: 1–8.

Lymphangioma circumscriptum

Lymphangioma circumscriptum is a term best reserved for a lymphatic malformation that is localized to an area of skin, subcutaneous tissue and sometimes muscle [1]. Clinically, the condition manifests with fluid-filled vesicles ('lymph blisters') which bulge on the skin surface (Fig. 48.12). The vesicles may be well defined and discrete, or may be grouped into structures resembling frogspawn. They may be translucent when the overlying epidermis is very thin, or they may vary in colour from red to blue-black when they contain blood, a frequent occurrence. The most common symptom is recurrent oozing, usually of clear fluid (lymph), known as lymphorrhoea. Alternatively, the surface of the lymphangiomas may appear extremely warty and the lesions may be mistaken for viral warts. Complications include ulceration, bleeding and secondary infection. Squamous cell carcinoma is described arising within lymphangioma circumscriptum [2].

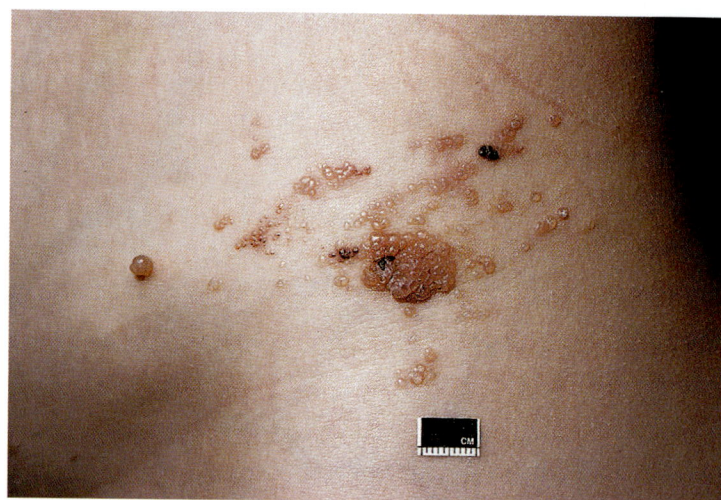

Fig. 48.12 Lymphangioma circumscriptum: fluid-filled vesicles resembling frogspawn. At times the vesicles can contain blood, weep clear fluid (lymphorrhoea) or become warty.

There may or may not be swelling of the underlying tissues, depending on the presence and size of enlarged, abnormal, anastomosing lymphatic channels beneath the skin or how compromised lymph drainage is, that is where there is a contribution of lymphoedema. It has been postulated that the original malformation arises from deep contractile lymphatics which are malformed and not in continuity with the normal lymph-conducting pathways. Tissue drainage into these abnormal lymphatics results in their gradual dilatation into lymphatic cisterns, contraction of which results in retrograde flow into the skin initial lymphatics [3]. Only by identifying the limits of the subcutaneous cisterns prior to wide excision will there be any chance of cure.

Lymphangioma circumscriptum may present at any age but is usually noted at birth or appears during childhood. The commonest sites are the axillary folds, shoulders, flanks, proximal parts of the limbs and perineum. Doppler ultrasound will distinguish macrocystic from microcystic lesions as well as excluding any high flow and therefore vascular component. MRI is the best for delineating the extent of the lesion [4].

The treatment of choice for lymphangioma circumscriptum is radical surgery [5]. However, inadequate surgical excision of the visible lymphangioma frequently results in further development of surface vesicles, indicating the presence of a more widespread subcutaneous malformation. Therefore a stable, asymptomatic 'lymphangioma' may be better left alone. Bacterial superinfection is common, particularly with weeping lesions, and manifests with pain, systemic upset or cellulitis. Palliation for lymphorrhoea or to improve the appearance of vesicles can be achieved through intralesional administration of a sclerosant—for example, doxycycline [6], picibanil (OK-432) [7] or hypertonic saline [8]. Simple electrocautery and vaporization with carbon dioxide laser can be of palliative benefit, and superficial X-rays have been used successfully [9].

Macrocystic lymphatic malformations

Lymphangiomas with few but large macrocystic swellings containing clear lymph are called cystic hygromas (hygroma = moist or watery tumour). Most occur in the neck, but they frequently extend into the upper mediastinum. The term tends to be reserved for those congenital lymphatic malformations that present at birth or are diagnosed by prenatal ultrasound. In the neck they presumably arise from an embryonic jugular lymph sac. Individuals with Turner's syndrome are particularly prone to both hydrops and cystic hygroma. Exceptionally, a cystic hygroma occurs in the groin, presumably from an embryonic iliac lymph sac. Fetal cystic hygroma can give rise to severe abnormalities, leading to fetal death [10].

Deeper, larger and cavernous lymphangiomas (LMs) are best called macrocystic LMs. Surface pressure with a digit will result in an indentation but a cavernous LM will rapidly refill, unlike the situation in pitting oedema where it takes many seconds for the interstitial fluid to redistribute when the pressure is released (like a sponge). They may be an isolated entity, part of a mixed vascular malformation (combined lymphatic–venous or capillary malformation) or associated with vascular syndromes such as Klippel–Trenaunay or proteus syndromes [11,12]. Cervicofacial LMs may cause airways obstruction, difficulty with feeding and speech development. Periorbital and skeletal hypertrophy are other complications of head and neck LMs [13].

References

1 Peachey RC, Lim CC, Whimster IM. Lymphangiomas of the skin. *Br J Dermatol* 1970; **83**: 519–27.
2 Wilson GR, Cox NH, McLean NR *et al.* Squamous cell carcinoma arising within lymphangioma circumscriptum. *Br J Dermatol* 1993; **129**: 337–9.
3 Whimster I. The pathology of lymphangioma circumscriptum. *Br J Dermatol* 1976; **94**: 473–86.
4 McAlvanny JP, Jorizzo JL, Zanoll D *et al.* Magnetic resonance imaging in the evaluation of lymphangioma circumscriptum. *Arch Dermatol* 1993; **129**: 194–7.
5 Browse NL, Whimster I, Stewart G *et al.* Surgical management of 'lymphangioma circumscriptum'. *Br J Surg* 1986; **73**: 585–8.
6 Molitch HL, Unger ES, Witte CL *et al.* Percutaneous sclerotherapy of lymphangiomas. *Radiology* 1995; **194**: 343–7.
7 Mikhail M, Kennedy R, Cramer B *et al.* Sclerosing of recurrent lymphangioma using OK-432. *J Pediatr Surg* 1995; **30**: 1159–60.
8 Bikowski J, Dumont M. Lymphangioma circumscriptum: treatment with hypertonic saline sclerotherapy. *J Am Acad Dermatol* 2005; **53**: 442–4.
9 O'Cathail S, Rostom AY, Johnson ML. Successful control of lymphangioma circumscriptum by superficial x-rays. *Br J Dermatol* 1985; **113**: 611–5.
10 Chervanak FA, Isaacson G, Blakemore KJ *et al.* Fetal cystic hygroma, cause and natural history. *N Engl J Med* 1983; **309**: 822–5.
11 Irvine AD, Sweeney L, Corbett J. Lymphangioma circumscriptum associated with paravesical cystic retroperitoneal lymphangioma. *Br J Dermatol* 1996; **134**: 1135–7.
12 Blei F. Congenital lymphatic malformations. *Ann N Y Acad Sci* 2008; **1131**: 185–94.
13 Greene A, Burrows P, Smith L, Mulliken J. Periorbital lymphatic malformation: clinical course and management in 42 patients. *Plast Reconstr Surg* 2005; **115**: 22–30.

Diffuse lymphangiomatosis

There is no clear distinction between lymphatic malformations and lymphangiomatosis. The difference may depend solely on the extent of the malformation. Most LMs are stable and run a completely benign course. Conversely, some visceral thoracic and abdominal LMs can relentlessly progress, infiltrating vital organs with fatal outcome and making distinction from frank neoplasia difficult; for example multifocal lymphangioendotheliomatosis with thrombocytopenia [1]. The CNS seems to be spared, presumably because of its lack of lymphatic vessels. Thoracic involvement leads to pleural and pericardial effusions and severe pulmonary infections [2]. Disseminated intravascular coagulation can give rise to thrombosis and haemorrhage [3]. Gorham's disease (Gorham–Stout disease; disappearing/vanishing bone disease) is characterized by proliferation of lymphatic vessels resulting in progressive destruction and resorption of osseous matrix. Skin 'lymphangiomas' may be the clue to the underlying diagnosis [1,4]. The outcome in diffuse lymphangiomatosis is poor, despite reports of successful use of interferon [5].

References

1 North P, Kahn T, Cordisco M *et al.* Multifocal lymphangioendotheliomatosis with thrombocytopenia: a newly recognized clinico-pathological entity. *Arch Dermatol* 2004; **140**: 599–606.
2 Alvarez O, Kjellin I, Zuppan C. Thoracic lymphangiomatosis in a child. *J Pediatr Hematol Oncol* 2004; **26**: 136–41.
3 Mazreeuw-Hautier J, Syed S, Leisner R, Harper J. Extensive venous/lymphatic malformations causing life-threatening haematological complications. *Br J Dermatol* 2007; **157**: 558–63.
4 Bruch-Gerharz D, Gerharz C, Stege H *et al.* Cutaneous lymphatic malformations in disappearing bone (Gorham-Stout) disease: a novel clue to the pathogenesis of a rare syndrome. *J Am Acad Dermatol* 2007; **56** (Suppl. 2): S21–5.
5 Ozeki M, Ito M, Teramoto T *et al.* Clinical improvement of diffuse lymphangiomatosis with pegylated interferon alpha-2b therapy. *J Pediatr Hematol Oncol* 2007; **24**: 513–24.

Chylous reflux, intestinal lymphangiectasia

Chyle is a 'milky lymph' which flows from the lacteals of the gut through the cisterna chyli and even through the thoracic duct. Incompetence of valves within main abdominal lymphatic trunks results in gross reflux of chyle. This can include reflux to the skin below the waist [1]; the most commonly affected sites are the genitalia, perineum and thigh. Chylous reflux is often associated with truncular lymphatic malformations in which case lymphoedema may be present, but the characteristic symptom is oozing of milky fluid through the skin, usually from visibly dilated chylous vesicles (chylous lymphangiectasia or 'lymphangioma'). Rupture of such vesicles may result in a spurt of chyle under pressure, or chronic leakage may give rise to warty plaques of a cream-yellow colour.

Chylous reflux is often associated with intestinal lymphangiectasia, which can lead to hypoalbuminaemia, hypogammaglobulinaemia and lymphopenia due to protein and cell loss through the gut. Capsule endoscopy is the investigation of choice [2]. Dietary replacement of fat with medium chain triglycerides (MCTs) is recommended as MCTs are absorbed and directed to the portal venous system rather than to the intestinal lacteals [3].

While intestinal lymphangiectasia is usually considered primary and therefore genetic in origin, for example Hennekam's syndrome [4], it can occur secondary to a range of gut pathologies where intestinal lymph drainage is altered [5].

References

1 Browse NL. Management of lymph and chyle reflux. In: Browse NL, Burnand KG, Mortimer PS, eds. *Diseases of the Lymphatics*. London: Arnold, 2003: 259–92.
2 Lee J, Kong MS. Primary intestinal lymphangiectasia diagnosed by endoscopy following the intake of a high-fat meal. *Eur J Pediatr* 2008; **167**: 237–9.

3 Bliss CM, Schroy PC III. Primary intestinal lymphangiectasia. *Curr Treat Options Gastroenterol* 2004; **7**: 3–6.

4 Van Balkom ID, Alders M, Allanson J *et al.* Lymphedema-lymphangiectasia-mental retardation (Hennekam) syndrome: a review. *Am J Med Genet* 2002; **112**: 412–21.

5 Safatle-Ribeiro AV, Iriya K, Couto DS *et al.* Secondary lymphangiectasia of the small bowel: utility of double balloon enteroscopy for diagnosis and management. *Dig Dis* 2008; **26**: 383–6.

Cutaneous lymphangiectasia (lymphangiectasis, acquired lymphangioma, benign lymphangiomatous papules)

The surface 'lymph blisters' seen in cutaneous lymphangiectasia are not necessarily structurally or histologically any different from those seen in 'lymphangioma'; both represent distended, otherwise normal, dermal lymphatics engorged with lymph due to a failure of downstream drainage.

Lymphangiectasia can be seen as translucent, almost flat, papules or vesicles in the skin, which may ooze lymph spontaneously or after trauma. Acquired or secondary lymphangioma is an alternative term, but confusing as there is no tumour or proliferative component. Benign lymphangiomatous papules represent the same process [1,2].

The clinical appearance of lymphangiectases/acquired lymphangiomas may vary greatly, ranging from clear fluid-filled blisters to smooth flesh-coloured papules or nodules.

Histologically, the latter show oedematous polypoid nodules within which are dilated lymphatics. Lesions may be solitary but scattered throughout a lymphoedematous limb, or they may be grouped, as seen in lymphangioma circumscriptum.

Lymphangiectases arise following damage to previously normal, deep lymphatic vessels [3]. The mechanism by which they form is identical to congenitally determined lymphatic malformations (lymphangiomas), that is obstruction to drainage leads to back-pressure and dermal backflow, with subsequent dilatation of upper dermal lymphatics. Lymphangiectases are not true neoplasms or hamartomas, but represent simple expansion and engorgement (lymphangiectasia) of lymphatic vessels.

Lower-limb lesions usually arise in association with lymphoedema following either ilioinguinal block dissection or pelvic surgery and radiotherapy for gynaecological cancer. Lymphangiectasias/acquired lymphangiomas have been described in association with scarring processes, including recurrent or chronic infections (such as the scrofuloderma variant of tuberculosis), radiotherapy, scleroderma, keloid, tumour and repeated trauma [4]. They may also occur as a consequence of defective collagen or elastin, as documented in a report of penicillamine dermopathy [5].

Genital skin is particularly prone to lymphangiectasia. Lymph blisters of the penis or scrotum (and less commonly vulva), leaking lymph or chyle, may be seen in primary lymphoedema. In such circumstances the lymphangiectasia represents reflux of lymph or chyle from incompetent pelvic lymphatics and is usually associated with lymphoedema of one or both lower limbs.

Lymphangiectasia/acquired lymphangioma of the vulva or scrotum is described following cancer treatment, tuberculous inguinal lymphadenitis and genital involvement with Crohn's disease. Clinically, the most common pattern is that of circum-

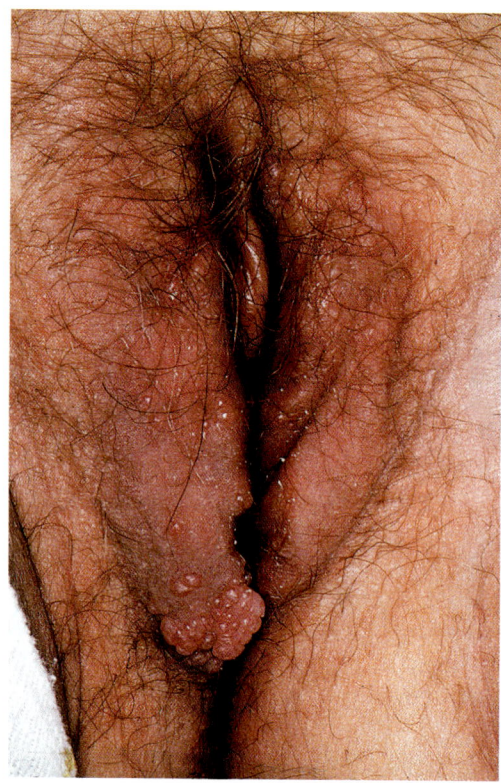

Fig. 48.13 Acquired lymphangiomas (lymphangiectasias) following cervical cancer treatment. The lymphangiomas were mistaken for genital warts.

scribed groups of tense, thin-walled vesicles. However, a hyperkeratotic appearance may make distinction from viral warts difficult [6] (Fig. 48.13). Recognition and appropriate treatment of vulval lymphangiectasia is important primarily because the lesions may act as portals of entry for infection. In addition, persistent leakage of lymphatic fluid may be mistaken for urinary incontinence.

Treatment of lymphangiectasia/acquired lymphangiomas is essentially the reduction of underlying lymphoedema and control of infection. This may be relatively straightforward on the leg, but is not so easy on the genitalia, where compression is not possible. Destruction of the 'lymph blisters' by laser or diathermy is helpful palliative treatment [7].

Lymphangiectasia/acquired lymphangiomas may be widespread and problematic in palliative circumstances where advanced cancer produces profound oedema of lower limbs, genitalia and lower trunk. In these circumstances copious lymph may weep. Opposing intralymphatic pressure with equivalent surface compression is the only way of controlling the lymphorrhoea unless the lymphatic obstruction can be relieved.

References

1 Diaz-Cascajo C, Borghi S, Weyers W *et al.* Benign lymphangiomatous papules of the skin following radiotherapy: a report of five new cases and review of the literature. *Histopathology* 1999; **35**: 319–27.

2 Gengler C, Coindre JM, Leroux A *et al.* Vascular proliferations of the skin after radiation therapy for breast cancer: clinicopathologic analysis of a series in favor of a benign process: a study from the French Sarcoma Group. *Cancer* 2007; **109**: 1584–98.

3 Mallett RB, Curley RK, Mortimer PS. Acquired lymphangiomata: report of four cases and a discussion of the pathogenesis. *Br J Dermatol* 1992; **126**: 380–2.

4 El Sayed F, Basex J, Bouissou X *et al.* Acquired cutaneous lymphangiectasia mimicking plantar warts. *Br J Dermatol* 1996; **132**: 1014–6.

5 Goldstein JB, McNatt NS, Hambrick GW. Penicillamine dermopathy with lymphangiectases. *Arch Dermatol* 1989; **125**: 92–7.

6 Harwood CA, Mortimer PS. Acquired vulval lymphangiomata mimicking genital warts. *Br J Dermatol* 1993; **129**: 334–6.

7 Makh DS, Mortimer P, Powell B. A review of the surgical treatment of vulval lymphangioma and lymphangiectasia: four case reviews. *J Plast Reconstr Aesthet Surg* 2006; **59**: 1442–5.

Acquired lymphatic abnormalities

Lymphangitis

In theory, the lymphatic system has evolved in humans as a host defence mechanism. Noxious agents and predators such as bacteria, if not dealt with at the point of entry to the host, access the lymphatic system. Lymphatic vessels, together with adjoining lymph nodes, effectively act as the second line of defence, hopefully preventing further onward spread and so limiting systemic involvement. In some circumstances, the inflammatory response may be profound, perhaps due to a heavy infection load, and either an overt lymphangitis or lymphadenitis, or both, arise. Lymphangitis represents inflammation of the lymphatic collectors and is clinically seen as tender red streaks up the limb corresponding to the inflamed vessels. In the lower limb, oedema is so often an accompanying feature that red streaks, such as are seen with lymphangitis of the arm, are rarely seen. A more diffuse erythema is seen extending up the medial side of the leg and thigh. Distinction from an ascending cellulitis becomes difficult.

Infection is usually limited by the lymph nodes, and in the lower limb lymphadenitis may give rise to painful swelling in the groin. Occasionally, infection bypasses a group of lymph nodes and affects those at a higher level. Constitutional upset can be severe and is greater the more proximally the infection has extended.

Lymphangitis may occur without any demonstrable inflammation or may be recurrent, for example following relapsing herpes simplex infection. Permanent obliteration of lymphatic collectors may follow severe or recurrent lymphangitis. In such cases, if reserve lymphatic capacity is limited, permanent swelling (lymphoedema) can result.

Recurrent cellulitis

Synonyms
- Recurrent inflammatory episodes
- Erysipelas
- Lymphangitis

Where lymphatic insufficiency exists and the local lymphoid tissue/lymphatic system fails in its host defence duty, recurrent infection can occur. Clinically, this manifests as recurrent cellulitis/erysipelas. Indeed, any patient who presents with even one attack of cellulitis in one leg may have a compromised lymph drainage in that leg, whether overt lymphoedema is present or not [1]. In most cases, however, subtle signs of lymphoedema are evident, particularly in the skin over the toes and forefoot. Because there is no localization of infection by the lymphatics, the first sign of illness will be constitutional upset with fever, rigors or vomiting. Only later may redness and tenderness appear in the leg and the diagnosis become clear.

Lymphangitis, as witnessed by red streaks up the leg, is generally not seen, presumably because the infection, uncontrolled by the lymphatic system, has spread through tissue planes (cellulitis) with rapid dissemination into the circulation. However, inflammation following the line of lymphatic channels can sometimes be apparent at the proximal border of a cellulitic area in patients with lymphoedema [2].

Treatment for recurrent cellulitis should first of all address predisposing factors such as tinea pedis, foot dermatitis, leg ulcers, etc. [3]. If no portal of entry or cause can be identified, then long-term prophylactic antibiotics may be necessary if the debilitating attacks are to be controlled but even that may fail to control attacks [4].

References

1 Damstra RJ, van Steensel MA, Boomsma JH *et al.* Erysipelas as a sign of subclinical primary lymphoedema: a prospective quantitative scintigraphic study of 40 patients with unilateral erysipelas of the leg. *Br J Dermatol* 2008; **158**: 1210–5.

2 Cox NH. Streptococcal cellulitis in reticulate lymphoedema selectively affects the lymphoedematous herniations. *Br J Dermatol* 1998; **139**: 358–9.

3 British Lymphology Society. *Consensus Document on the Management of Cellulitis in Lymphoedema.* http://www.thebls.com/concensus.php

4 Vignes S, Dupuy A. Recurrence of lymphoedema-associated cellulitis (erysipelas) under prophylactic antibiotherapy: a retrospective cohort study. *J Eur Acad Dermatol Venereol* 2006; **20**: 818–22.

Lymphangiothrombosis

Lymph is capable of clotting, but the circumstances in which this happens, and what pathological effect lymph thrombosis has, are totally unknown. Extrapolating from knowledge about venous thrombosis would suggest that lymph thrombosis is likely to impair the function of lymphatic valves and the contractility of lymph-collecting vessels.

Mondor's disease, axillary web syndrome

Mondor's disease is alleged to be a superficial thrombophlebitis of the breast and chest wall [1] (see Chapter 47). A similar process, whereby cords or threads like violin strings extend down the inner arm, is frequently seen following axillary lymphadenectomy [2]. The manner in which the cords 'bowstring' across the axilla with the arm abducted, their diameter and the fact that the cords can snap between finger and thumb suggests that lymph thrombosis may be a more likely explanation than phlebothrombosis/thrombophlebitis. An equivalent condition may well exist in the lower limb but be mistaken for thrombophlebitis.

'Seroma'

Synonyms
- Lymphocoele
- Lymphocyst

Following lymphadenectomy, it is not unusual for a localized swelling containing clear fluid to develop. Often referred to as a 'seroma', the fluid is not serum, but lymph which has drained from the cut ends of the lymphatic collectors, so filling the space originally occupied by the nodes. The wall of lymphocoeles is 'false', in that no endothelial lining exists and instead a dense network of fibrin with lymphocytes is present [3]. Aspirated fluid is indistinguishable from lymph. Repeat aspiration is often necessary until a collateral lymph drainage forms. A 'seroma', particularly if infected, may herald the onset of lymphoedema if alternative drainage routes are not established.

References

1 Marsch W, Haas N, Stuttgen G. Mondor's phlebitis: a lymphovascular process. *Dermatologica* 1986; **172**: 133–8.
2 Moskovitz AH, Anderson BO, Yeung RS *et al*. Axillary web syndrome after axillary dissection. *Am J Surg* 2001; **181**: 434–9.
3 Ferguson JH, Maclure JG. Lymphocele following lymphadenectomy. *Am J Obstet Gynecol* 1961; **82**: 783–92.

Lymphatic tumours

Tumours of lymphatic vessels allegedly make up only a small group of vascular neoplasms but the use of specific lymphatic markers may change this view or make us realize that venous and lymphatic phenotypes can coexist within one tumour type, for example Kaposi's sarcoma and papillary intralymphatic angioendothelioma (Dabska's tumour) [1].

Reference

1 Goh S, Calonje E. Cutaneous vascular tumours: an update. *Histopathology* 2008; **52**: 661–73.

Acquired progressive lymphangioma

Synonym
• Benign lymphangioendothelioma

This benign tumour differs from simple 'acquired lymphangioma' or simple cutaneous lymphangiectasia by its clinical behaviour and histopathology [1]. Acquired progressive lymphangioma presents as reddish or bruise-like plaques which are usually located on the abdominal wall, thigh or calf. Typically, the condition affects young adolescents but may also arise in adults. It is usually localized, flat and grows slowly. Considered to originate from lymphatic endothelium, the histopathological appearance can mimic a low-grade sarcoma or Kaposi's sarcoma [2]. Anastomosing dilated channels, with a tendency to dissect the collagen bundles, are lined by swollen endothelial cells but without cellular atypia. It usually runs a long and benign course.

References

1 Wilson Jones E, Winkelmann RK, Zachary CB *et al*. Benign lymphangio-endothelioma. *J Am Acad Dermatol* 1990; **23**: 229–34.
2 Guillou L, Fletcher CD. Benign lymphangioendothelioma (acquired progressive lymphangioma): a lesion not to be confused with well-differentiated angiosarcoma and patch stage Kaposi's sarcoma: clinicopathologic analysis of a series. *Am J Surg Pathol* 2000; **24**: 1047–57.

Lymphangiomyomatosis

Synonym
• Lymphangiopericytoma

This condition affects primarily pre-menopausal women, and presents with central lymphatic problems, typically progressive dyspnoea associated with chylous effusions and a chest X-ray which reveals honeycombing of the lungs [1]. Masses of spindle cells proliferate in and around the walls of lymph vessels, particularly in retroperitoneal tissues and in the mediastinum. These cells (lymphangiomyomatosis cells, LAMs) have a smooth muscle phenotype and have mutations in one of the tuberous sclerosis complex genes (*TSC1* or *TCS2*). Skin involvement, with facial angiofibromas, forehead plaques and periungual fibromas, can occur in lymphangiomyomatosis [2]. Lymphoedema of one or both legs can develop due to infiltration of LAM cells in the walls of main lymphatic trunks, and sometimes beyond this into surrounding adipose tissue. Suppression of mTOR signalling might constitute an ameliorative treatment in patients with the tuberous sclerosis complex or sporadic lymphangioleiomyomatosis [3].

References

1 Joliat G, Stalder H, Kapanci Y. Lymphangiomyomatosis: a clinico-anatomical entity. *Cancer* 1973; **31**: 455–61.
2 Glasgow C, Taveiro-Dasilva A, Darling T, Moss J. Lymphatic involvement in lymphangiomyomatosis. *Ann N Y Acad Sci* 2008; **1131**: 206–14.
3 Bissler JJ, McCormack FX, Young LR *et al*. Sirolimus for angiomyolipoma in tuberous sclerosis complex or lymphangioleiomyomatosis. *N Engl J Med* 2008; **358**: 140–51.

Kaposi's sarcoma

There is increasing evidence that Kaposi's sarcoma (KS) may arise from lymphatic rather than from vascular endothelium, although its origins may lie with transdifferentiation from blood vascular to lymphatic phenotype [1,2].

The classical form of the disease, as described by Kaposi, presents with dark-blue or purple lesions, usually on the feet. Initially, lesions may be flat; when they become tumid, diascopy may produce partial blanching to reveal a brown tinge from extravasated blood. Individual tumours enlarge to a diameter of 10–30 mm and stop growing, whereupon adjacent areas fuse to form a plaque or tumour. New lesions appear proximally alongside a superficial vessel. Unlike the situation in patients with lymphangiosarcoma, lymphoedema may not be evident at the time the first lesions appear, but otherwise the morphology is similar. KS, however, is characteristically multifocal and, in time, symmetrical, affecting both lower limbs. Brawny oedema resembling lymphoedema develops with advanced KS.

In the African and Mediterranean types of KS, oedema is often the first sign with lymph nodes as the main tissue involved.

KS associated with immunodeficiency, whether HIV-induced or not, produces subtle lesions which are often widely scattered and quite dissimilar from the classical type.

KS can cause lymphoedema but can also follow lymphoedema. Presumably the local immunodeficiency derived from the lymphatic insufficiency promotes the development and progression of KS in the same way that lymphoedema encourages infection and skin cancer.

Treatment is dependent on the type of KS. In AIDS-related KS, treatment of HIV is paramount and both KS and lymphoedema may regress. In endemic African-type KS, staging of nodal involvement is necessary before consideration of chemotherapy with or without radiotherapy. For localized disease, radiotherapy is the treatment of choice.

References

1 Skobe M, Brown LF, Tognazzi K *et al.* Vascular endothelial growth factor (VEGF-C) and its receptor KDR and flt-4 are expressed in AIDS-associated Kaposi's sarcoma. *J Invest Dermatol* 1999; **113**: 1047–53.
2 Cueni LN, Detmar M. New insights into the molecular control of the lymphatic vascular system and its role in disease. *J Invest Dermatol* 2006; **126**: 2167–77.

Maffucci's syndrome

Maffucci's syndrome consists of diffuse haemolymphangiomatosis accompanied by severe, widespread deformities of bone and cartilage, notably enchondromas of the digits [1]. The lymphangiomas do not appear, on lymphography, to communicate with the main lymphatic pathways and often possess both blood vascular and lymphatic elements. Bony deformity may be gross and slowly uniting pathological fractures are common. The disease has high malignant potential including lymphangiosarcoma.

Reference

1 Carlton A, St Elkington JC, Greenfield JG *et al.* Maffucci's syndrome. *QJM* 1942; **11**: 203–28.

Atypical post-radiation vascular proliferation

Cutaneous vascular proliferations that occur within the field of prior radiotherapy include angiosarcoma and small cutaneous solitary or multiple papules with a pseudosarcomatous pattern which resemble angiosarcoma (post-radiotherapy vascular proliferations, post-radiotherapy atypical vascular lesions). Clinical and histological distinction can be difficult but atypical vascular proliferations appear to have a benign prognosis [1].

Reference

1 Gengler C, Coindre J-M, Leroux A. Vascular proliferations of the skin after radiation therapy for breast cancer: clinicopathologic analysis of a series in favor of a benign process. *Cancer* 2007; **109**: 1584–98.

Lymphangiosarcoma

This is a rare but well-recognized complication of any chronic lymphoedema, irrespective of cause. Red–brown or purple discoloration, like a bruise, appears in the skin of the lymphoedematous limb. Nodules or raised plaques may appear later. As the tumours proliferate, the oedema may increase and older lesions may ulcerate. The tumour metastasizes early and has a poor prognosis.

The tumour is best described in the upper limb following breast cancer treatment (Stewart–Treves syndrome) [1], but it is well reported in the lower limb in association with lymphoedema, usually of many years' duration [2]. Radical amputation, if performed early enough, may offer hope of cure. Isolated limb perfusion has been reported for non-resectable limb tumour [3].

References

1 Stewart FW, Treves N. Lymphangiosarcoma in postmastectomy lymphoedema. *Cancer* 1948; **1**: 64–81.
2 Eby CS, Brennan MJ, Fine G. Lymphangiosarcoma: lethal complication of chronic lymphedema: report of two cases and review of the literature. *Arch Surg* 1967; **94**: 223–30.
3 Lans TE, de Wilt JH, van Geel AN, Eggermont AM. Isolated limb perfusion with tumor necrosis factor and melphalan for nonresectable Sewart-Treves lymphangiosarcoma. *Ann Surg Oncol* 2002; **9**: 1004–9.

Carcinoma erysipeloides

Synonym

• Carcinoma telangiectatica

Carcinoma erysipeloides manifests clinically with a fixed erythematous patch or plaque resembling cellulitis/erysipelas, but without fever [1]. The inflamed area may show a distinct raised periphery and oedema secondary to lymphatic obstruction. Histology reveals plugging of superficial and deep dermal lymphatics by adenocarcinoma, usually carcinoma of the breast, but the condition has been described with melanoma, lung, ovarian, colonic and pancreatic tumours [2]. The redness appears to be a consequence of the dermal lymphatic plugging with tumour, presumably through the release of cytokines. The term carcinoma telangiectatica refers to the presence of purpuric plaques, papules and vesicles where only the more superficial lymphatics are involved. 'Inflammatory breast carcinoma' has been suggested as an alternative term to 'carcinoma erysipeloides', but oncologists already classify inflammatory breast carcinoma as a subtype of cancer within the breast.

References

1 Finkel LJ, Griffiths CEM. Inflammatory breast carcinoma (carcinoma erysipeloides), an easily overlooked diagnosis. *Br J Dermatol* 1993; **129**: 324–6.
2 Marneros AG, Blanco F, Husain S *et al.* Classification of cutaneous intravascular breast cancer metastases based on immunolabeling for blood and lymph vessels. *J Am Acad Dermatol* 2009; **60**: 633–8.

CHAPTER 49
Purpura and Microvascular Occlusion

N.H. Cox¹ & W.W. Piette²

¹Department of Dermatology, Cumberland Infirmary, Carlisle, UK
²John H Stroger Jr Hospital of Cook County, Division of Dermatology, Chicago, IL, USA

Introduction

Purpura and bruising, the main terms used to describe bleeding into the skin, may occur as isolated phenomena or as part of a systemic disorder. Purpura is the hallmark of vasculitis affecting the (usually smaller vessels of the) skin, and may be the dominant feature or a minor part of a systemic vasculitis (see Chapter 50). However, it may occur as a result of other non-vasculitic abnormalities of the blood vessel wall and, overall, much the commonest causes (although largely not seen by dermatologists) are haematological conditions due to platelet and coagulation disorders. Vasculitis typically causes other cutaneous lesions, including urticarial lesions, nodules, ulcers, livedo and frank necrosis, which have a purpuric component due to vessel wall damage. Several of these also occur in disorders in which vessels are occluded, as discussed later in this chapter. An appreciation of the morphology and associated features is of great value in the diagnostic approach [1].

Patients with purpura may require management involving one or more of several disciplines, including haematology, general medicine, nephrology and rheumatology, as well as dermatology; multidisciplinary management is often appropriate as each specialty sees a different range of clinical manifestations and has different areas of expertise.

Classification of purpura is difficult, as no single approach is satisfactory. The same clinical pattern may arise from many different causes, both vasculitic and non-vasculitic, and the aetiology of either purpura or vasculitis may be impossible to determine. Classifications based on morphology or aetiology therefore have limitations. For example, clinically non-specific capillaritis may be idiopathic, drug-induced or a manifestation of cutaneous T-cell lymphoma. Even within frank haematological causes of purpura, idiopathic thrombocytopenic purpura is not only viewed as a mixture of diseases but varies in its definitions and clinical descriptions [2]. Furthermore, intravascular events such as microvascular occlusion may give rise to palpable lesions and inflammation as a secondary component, thereby mimicking vasculitis and confusing both the clinical and histopathological picture.

Despite these limitations, as a practical matter the initial approach to a patient with purpura must typically start with a

Rook's Textbook of Dermatology, 8th edition. Edited by DA Burns, SM Breathnach, NH Cox and CEM Griffiths. © 2010 Blackwell Publishing Ltd.

differential diagnosis based on morphology [1], as few patients present with a known aetiology of their lesions. In practice, overt haematological causes (thrombocytopenia and clotting factor abnormalities) can be rapidly and easily evaluated by full blood count and laboratory measures of clotting times. Beyond this, diagnostically more complex haematological disorders (e.g. thrombophilias or abnormal platelet function), vessel wall defects (both structural and others) [3], infections, immunological disorders and thrombotic microvascular occlusion disorders may all need to be considered. The importance of trying to differentiate between disorders causing primarily inflammatory or non-inflammatory lesions is clear [4,5].

This chapter addresses purpura that is not primarily of vasculitic causation; Chapter 50 deals with disorders in which a primary vasculitis is involved.

References

1 Piette WW. The differential diagnosis of purpura from a morphologic perspective. *Adv Dermatol* 1994; **9**: 3–23.

2 Marco R, Fortuna S, Rodeghiero F. Heterogeneity of terminology and clinical definitions in adult idiopathic thrombocytopenic purpura: a critical appraisal from a systematic review of the literature. *Haematologica* 2008; **93**: 98–103.

3 Bick R. Vascular thrombohemorrhagic disorders: hereditary and acquired. *Clin Appl Thrombosis Hemostasis* 2001; **7**: 178–94.

4 Piette WW. Primary systemic vasculitis. In: Sontheimer RD, Provost TT, eds. *Cutaneous Manifestations of Rheumatic Diseases*. Baltimore: Williams & Wilkins, 1996: 177–232.

5 Jones A, Walling H. Retiform purpura in plaques: a morphological approach to diagnosis. *Clin Exp Dermatol* 2007; **32**: 596–602.

Definition of purpura

Purpura is discoloration of the skin or mucous membranes due to extravasation of red blood cells. *Petechiae* are small purpuric lesions usually 1–2 mm (occasionally up to 4 mm) across, often occurring in crops. *Ecchymoses* or *bruises* are larger extravasations of blood. The many causes of petechiae and ecchymoses overlap, for example thrombocytopenia usually causes petechiae but more extensive bleeding may occur at lower levels of platelet count. In contrast, coagulation disorders usually cause ecchymoses rather than petechiae [1–4]. For example, haemophilias usually present as bleeding from the umbilical cord or gingivae, or as haematomas or haemarthroses—although dermatologists need to be aware that haemorrhagic subcutaneous nodules may be the first sign of an inherited haemophilia [5]. Gingival bleeding, epistaxis or internal bleeding may occur with platelet or coagulation disorders.

The sequence of colour changes in a bruise can help to identify it as such, should doubt exist, and can also help to establish its duration. Extravasated blood is broken down to various other pigments derived from haem, usually within 2 or 3 weeks. The characteristic colour changes [6–8] include red, blue and purple in the first 5 days (although these colours can occur at other times, particularly red), green after 5–7 days and yellow after 7–14 days (never less than 18 h). Many factors, both intrinsic to the individual (age, sex, skin colour, body site) and related to the injury (amount of blood extravasated, depth of bruising, medications that alter bruise dispersion), influence the timescale of colour changes [9]. In smaller and more superficial purpuric lesions,

orange or brown colours due to residual haemosiderin may predominate. Assessment of traumatic ecchymotic lesions is not a major part of routine dermatological practice, but may be important in suspected child abuse [9].

Unlike purpura, increased intravascular blood in the skin, whether as diffuse erythema or within telangiectatic vessels, can be blanched by pressure, typically using the technique of diascopy (see Chapter 5). However, not all telangiectatic lesions can be emptied in this way. Small angiomas (e.g. in angioma serpiginosum or the multiple minute variant of Campbell de Morgan spots) and angiokeratomas may cause particular confusion [10]. Sometimes, observation over several days is necessary. Capillary microscopy or, more recently, dermoscopy may also be helpful in determining whether blood is intravascular or extravascular.

References

1 Lichtman MA, Buetler E, Kaushansky K *et al.*, eds. *Williams' Hematology*, 7th edn. New York: McGraw-Hill, 2005.

2 Greer JP, Foerster J, Lukens JN *et al.*, eds. *Wintrobe's Clinical Hematology*, 12th edn. Philadelphia: Lippincott, Williams & Wilkins, 2008.

3 Hoffbrand AV, Catovsky D, Tuddenham EGD, eds. *Postgraduate Haematology*, 5th edn. Oxford: John Wiley and Sons Ltd, 2008.

4 Harmening DM, ed. *Clinical Hematology and Fundamentals of Hemostasis*, 5th edn. Philadelphia: F.A. Davis Company, 2008.

5 Davis G, Butler DF, Greene J. Hemorrhagic subcutaneous nodules: an initial sign of hemophilia A. *Pediatr Dermatol* 2007; **24**: 121–4.

6 Schwartz AJ, Ricci LR. How accurately can bruises be aged in abused children? Literature review and synthesis. *Pediatrics* 1996; **97**: 254–7.

7 Langlois NE, Gresham GA. The ageing of bruises: a review and study of the colour changes with time. *Forensic Sci Int* 1991; **50**: 227–38.

8 Stephenson T. Ageing of bruising in children. *J R Soc Med* 1997; **90**: 312–4.

9 Pride HB. Child abuse and mimickers of child abuse. *Adv Dermatol* 1999; **14**: 417–55.

10 Cox NH, Paterson WD. Angioma serpiginosum: a simulator of purpura. *Postgrad Med J* 1991; **67**: 1065–6.

Classification and investigation of purpura

An aetiological classification of purpura is provided in Table 49.1. However, for clinical purposes, correlations can be made between the clinical features and the mechanism of purpura. Purpura occurs as a result of one or more of the following main mechanisms in cutaneous vessels:

1 Simple haemorrhage
2 Inflammatory haemorrhage
3 Occlusion/ischaemia.

Characteristics of lesions, including size, number, distribution pattern, and presence or absence of palpability and erythema, can be very useful in focusing on the most likely mechanisms of haemorrhage within these subsets.

In general, simple haemorrhage presents as macules without erythema (Table 49.2), although sufficient haemorrhage into subcutaneous tissue becomes palpable as a haematoma. The size of the macules has diagnostic importance. Inflammatory causes of haemorrhagic lesions usually evolve with increasing erythema in the first 24–36 h, along with increasing purpura. Such lesions are frequently, but not invariably, palpable. A subset of palpable purpura syndromes may uncommonly also produce lesions with retiform or stellate patterning, with accompanying early erythema

Table 49.1 Causes of purpura and ecchymosis.

Platelet disorders (see also Table 49.3)
Thrombocytopenia
Abnormal platelet function
Thrombocytosis

Coagulation disorders
Inherited, e.g. haemophilia or acquired factor deficiency or dysfunction (e.g.
  antibody inhibitor)
Drugs, e.g. anticoagulants
Localized, e.g. heparin injection sites, some insect bites
Metabolic, e.g. vitamin K deficiency, hepatic failure (decreased synthesis of clotting
  factors)
Thrombophilias, e.g. protein C deficiency, protein S deficiency
Disseminated intravascular coagulopathy and purpura fulminans
Secondary to systemic disease (often multifactorial, e.g. macrophage activation
  syndrome)

Other intravascular causes of purpura/microvascular occlusion
Dysproteinaemias, e.g. hypergammaglobulinaemic purpura (Waldenström), Sjögren's
  syndrome
Cryoproteinaemias
Emboli: crystal, fat, myxoma, infective

Mechanical vascular causes of purpura
Raised intravascular pressure
  Coughing, vomiting, Valsalva manoeuvre, tourniquet
  Stasis
Decreased support
  Actinic ('senile') purpura
  Corticosteroid purpura
  Scurvy
  Amyloidosis
Inherited disorders of connective tissue (pseudoxanthoma elasticum, Ehlers–Danlos
  syndromes)
Abnormal vasculature
Purpura around vascular lesions, e.g. targetoid haemosiderotic haemangioma, tufted
  angioma, aneurysmal fibrous histiocytoma

Purpura with inflammation
Non-thrombocytopenic toxin- and drug-induced purpura
Contact purpura
Purpura associated with infections
Capillaritis (pigmented purpuric dermatoses)
  Idiopathic
  Drug-induced
  Pre-mycotic
Inflammatory purpura/vasculitis (see Chapter 50), e.g. Henoch–Schönlein purpura,
  acute haemorrhagic oedema
Associated with other inflammatory dermatoses that are not usually purpuric
Solar purpura

External and other causes of purpura or ecchymosis
Physical and artefactual causes
Easy bruising syndrome and purpura simplex
Paroxysmal finger haematoma (Achenbach's syndrome)
Painful bruising (autoerythrocyte sensitization, Gardner–Diamond) syndrome
Stigmata

Table 49.2 Diagnosis of macular non-retiform haemorrhage/petechiae/ecchymosis
by size.

Lesions <4 mm
  Thrombocytopenia
    Immune thrombocytopenic purpura
    Thrombotic thrombocytopenic purpura
    Disseminated intravascular coagulation (DIC)
    Other causes (see Table 49.3)
  Abnormal platelet function
    Congenital/hereditary
    Acquired: drug, systemic disease
    In myeloproliferative disease
    Other causes (see Table 49.3)
  With normal platelets
    Raised intravascular pressure
    Trauma
    Scurvy (perifollicular pattern)
    Hypergammaglobulinaemic purpura (Waldenström)

Intermediate-sized lesions
  Hypergammaglobulinaemic purpura (Waldenström)
  Infection in patients with thrombocytopenia or immune compromise
  Early lesions of vasculitis (sometimes)

Lesions >1 cm (all causes involve a degree of minor trauma)
  Procoagulant defect
    Anticoagulation
    Liver failure
    Vitamin K deficiency
    DIC (some)
  Poor dermal support
    Actinic and corticosteroid purpura
    Scurvy
    Hereditary: Ehlers–Danlos syndrome
    Amyloidosis
  Platelet deficiency or functional defect
  Other causes
    Hypergammaglobulinaemic purpura (Waldenström)
    Capillaritis
    Easy bruising syndrome; purpura simplex
    Physical and artefactual causes
    Gardner–Diamond syndrome
    Stigmata

and palpability (inflammatory retiform purpura). By 48 h, erythema and palpability begin fading in both types of lesions, although the purpura may persist for several days. In contrast, lesions of occlusion/ischaemia usually begin with minimal or no erythema, and may show minimal palpability unless eschar forms, but may develop erythema if sufficient necrosis occurs to induce a wound healing response. Occlusive syndromes tend to manifest retiform or branching patterns of purpura (non-inflammatory retiform purpura), sometimes with accompanying localized livedo reticularis, or as necrotic plaques with minimal erythema.

Non-inflammatory purpura is generally due to haematological causes and detailed discussion is outside the remit of this chapter; specialized haematology texts [1–7] and online review resources [8] can be consulted. Similarly, structural and non-inflammatory vessel wall changes that allow extravasation of blood are discussed in other chapters of this text, and reviewed elsewhere [9].

References

1 Lichtman MA, Buetler E, Kaushansky K *et al.*, eds. *Williams' Hematology*, 7th edn. New York: McGraw-Hill, 2005.
2 Hoffman R, Furie B, McGlave P *et al.*, eds. *Haematology. Basic Principles and Practice*, 5th edn. Edinburgh: Churchill Livingstone, 2008.
3 Greer JP, Foerster J, Lukens JN *et al.*, eds. *Wintrobe's Clinical Hematology*, 12th edn. Philadelphia: Lippincott, Williams & Wilkins, 2008.
4 Hoffbrand AV, Catovsky D, Tuddenham EGD, eds. *Postgraduate Haematology*, 5th edn. Oxford: John Wiley and Sons Ltd, 2008.
5 Colman RW, Marder VJ, Clowes AW *et al.*, eds. *Hemostasis and Thrombosis: Basic Principles and Clinical Practice*, 5th edn. Philadelphia: Lippincott, 2005.
6 Harmening DM, ed. *Clinical Hematology and Fundamentals of Hemostasis*, 5th edn. Philadelphia: F.A. Davis Company, 2008.
7 O'Shaughnessy D, Makris M, Lillicrap D, eds. *Practical Hemostasis and Thrombosis*. Oxford: Wiley Blackwell, 2005.
8 http://asheducationbook.hematologylibrary.org
9 Bick R. Vascular thrombohemorrhagic disorders: hereditary and acquired. *Clin Appl Thrombosis Hemostasis* 2001; 7: 178–94.

Diagnosis and pathophysiology of simple macular haemorrhage [1–6]

Purpura due to simple haemorrhage is suggested by the presence of purpura that is macular (non-palpable) and that has no blanching component in newly developed lesions (Table 49.2). Palpable lesions, or a blanching component, suggest that there is associated inflammation (which may occur as a secondary effect, hence the emphasis that evaluation must concentrate on new lesions). It should be noted that pale (not blanching) areas often appear in a perifollicular or blotchy pattern in older ecchymosis as extravasated blood is resorbed. The size of lesions, clinical patterns and body sites affected may all be diagnostically useful.

Size of lesions

Petechiae are often defined as lesions of 2 mm or less in diameter, although non-palpable, non-blanching lesions up to 4 mm usually suggest the same process. The main mechanisms of simple haemorrhage are:

1 Thrombocytopenia (platelet count always $<50 \times 10^9$/L, usually $<10 \times 10^9$/L)
2 Platelet dysfunction (uncommonly a cause of clinical purpura, although some degree of platelet dysfunction occurs in many systemic diseases or due to a variety of drugs)
3 Regional or localized increased intravascular pressure
4 Abnormal vascular support/vessel fragility
5 Many forms of capillaritis (pigmented purpura).

In contrast, macular lesions of 1 cm or greater in diameter (ecchymoses) usually result from disorders of the cascade coagulation system (especially acquired), platelet dysfunction or poor dermal vascular support. Such lesions are usually provoked by minor trauma. This results in two important clinical clues. The first is that lesions tend to localize to areas prone to frequent minor trauma, such as the extensor forearm and dorsal hand, lateral thigh and anterior lower leg. The second finding is a linear or geometric shape of individual lesions, because such lesions typically result from a frictional injury or extension of blunt trauma. Finally, as photodamage of fair skin is a very common cause of poor dermal support, ecchymotic haemorrhage is very commonly

found on areas with chronic exposure to both sun and trauma, for example the extensor forearm and dorsal hand.

It is evident that some aetiologies can cause purpuric lesions of variable size. For example, scurvy (a disorder in which the collagen of vessels and dermis is altered) may cause small perifollicular petechiae or large sheets of bruising with significant induration. Drug-induced platelet dysfunction may cause small petechiae, capillaritis-type areas of discoloration, or frank bleeding. Moderately severe thrombocytopenia (platelet count around 10–20×10^9/L) may cause petechiae or broad ecchymoses.

Clinical patterns of purpura

The clinical pattern may help to determine which patients require investigation, and may suggest the most likely major pathophysiological mechanisms. Tiny purpuric spots on the lower legs, for example, are not uncommon in the elderly, in patients taking antiplatelet drugs, or in the context of an inflammatory dermatosis; investigation of such lesions in these settings is seldom needed. Similarly, larger lesions that are macular, purple, stellate or blotchy, and confined to photo-aged skin on the dorsum of hands or forearms are generally diagnosed clinically as a consequence of actinic damage (although the same process on the face may produce smaller or more linear lesions, clinically resembling amyloidosis, and more widely distributed lesions of this morphology occur in Cushing's syndrome). Some degree of purpura is not uncommon in inflammatory skin disease of several types, but investigation is likely to be aimed at the disease process rather than the purpuric component *per se*.

Features that suggest a need for further investigation include:

- Larger or variably sized lesions, particularly when not in sun-damaged skin
- Numerous or widespread lesions
- Lesions occurring in crops
- Palpable lesions
- Lesions forming reticulate patterns (livedo, retiform pattern)
- Associated features such as pustules, necrosis, nodules, splinter haemorrhages, etc.
- Evidence of bleeding from other sites, e.g. haematuria
- Associated general symptoms, e.g. fever, malaise, arthralgia.

Diagnosis of purpura at various body sites

Gravitational change has a major influence on the distribution of purpuric lesions, as discussed elsewhere in this section. Other body sites of specific importance include the following.

- Eyelids: purpura due to increased venous pressure—classically due to performing the Valsalva manoeuvre, but in practice more likely after severe coughing or vomiting, and also described after endoscopy, etc. (also affects the cheeks; Fig. 49.1); purpura or ecchymosis in amyloidosis (panda sign), due to abnormal vessels and supporting dermis; ecchymosis related to neuroblastoma.
- Ears: purpura due to cryoglobulinaemia and other hyperviscosity disorders; purpura due to some drugs, e.g. antineutrophil cytoplasm antibody (ANCA)-positive propylthiouracil reaction, levamisole
- Face, ears and acral: acute haemorrhagic oedema of childhood (Chapter 50); cryoglobulinaemia

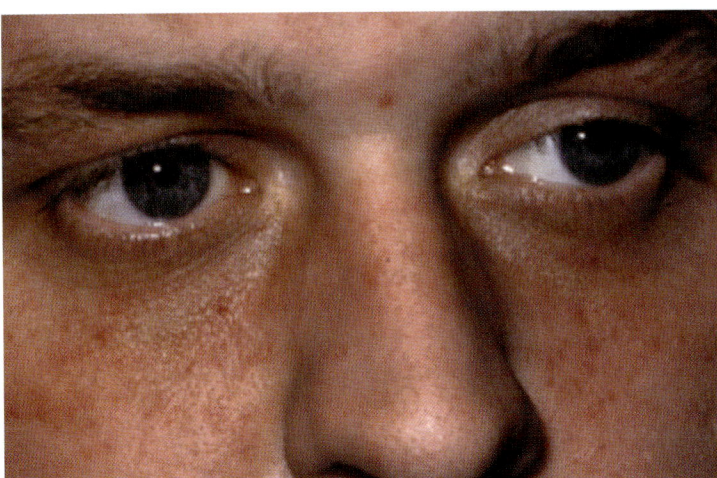

Fig. 49.1 Purpura on the face due to the raised intravascular pressure that occurs during vomiting. The lesions are small, non-palpable and all of the same age.

- Acral: purpura due to cryoglobulinaemia and other hyperviscosity disorders; embolic causes of purpura; rickettsial infection
- Friction sites: clothing contact purpura; some cases of capillaritis; Henoch–Schönlein purpura and other small-vessel vasculitis; ecchymosis of Ehlers–Danlos syndrome
- Intraoral: thrombocytopenia; amyloidosis; myelomonocytic leukaemia; angina bullosa haemorrhagica.

Laboratory tests

Platelet count and function [1–4,7–9]

This is the most important investigation in patients with non-palpable petechiae. The normal count is $150–400 \times 10^9$/L. It varies greatly from person to person, and from time to time in the same person. It may be affected by numerous exogenous factors such as infections, and by internal factors such as hormonal changes. Purpura due to thrombocytopenia seldom occurs with a platelet count above 50×10^9/L, and significant spontaneous bleeding is unlikely unless the count is less than 20×10^9/L. Thrombocytosis may also be a cause of bleeding. As well as variation in number, variation in function of platelets may need to be assessed by specialized *in vitro* tests. A full blood count should always be undertaken in the investigation of purpura; in general, especially for milder bleeding problems, a staged approach to diagnostic testing is appropriate depending on the results of initial tests and the clinical suspicions [10].

Tests of occult bleeding

Simple tests to detect other sites of bleeding, whether in vasculitis or in haematological causes of purpura, include fundoscopy, urinalysis and faecal occult blood tests. Haematuria may occasionally occur in disorders that are felt to be essentially dermatological but non-vasculitic, such as drug-induced pigmented purpuric dermatoses [11,12].

Histology

Histological examination of non-palpable, non-blanching, small purpuric lesions is usually unhelpful; it is essential, however, to consider whether lesions are palpable or partially blanching. If there are palpable or partially blanching lesions, then vasculitis should be considered and biopsy is likely to be informative. If lesions are larger but not palpable, and platelet parameters are normal, then biopsy of the skin is appropriate, for example to assess disease of the vessel wall or surrounding tissues.

Capillary resistance and fragility [13–16]

If the pressure difference between the tissues and the capillaries is sufficiently increased, leakage of blood cells occurs. This is the basis of a variety of semi-quantitative tests for capillary fragility. However, the integrity of the capillary endothelium itself, and also the ability of platelets to fill any gaps which may arise in it, contribute to this type of bleeding. Abnormal results may therefore occur in conditions where there is thrombocytopenia, abnormal platelet function or intravascular coagulopathy, as well as in conditions where there is a vessel wall defect. Indeed, the precise aetiology may be mixed; for example, some types of Ehlers–Danlos syndrome (EDS IV) have abnormal vessel wall collagen, abnormal perivascular support, and may occasionally have associated platelet dysfunction, and several defects of haemostasis occur in hereditary haemorrhagic telangiectasia (HHT) as well as the vascular abnormalities [16].

Sometimes capillary leakage is discovered accidentally due to development of a shower of purpura on the arm distal to a blood pressure cuff immediately after the pressure has been released (Rumpel–Leede sign). More commonly, tests are performed to provoke purpura; the simplest clinical test, which essentially performs the same process, is the Hess test. A standardized increase in capillary pressure is produced by inflating a sphygmomanometer cuff around the upper arm to a constant pressure of 80 mmHg (or less if this approaches the systolic blood pressure) for 5 min. Petechiae develop over the next few minutes and can be counted in a measured area of 5 cm diameter just below the antecubital fossa; up to five may be considered normal. However, our experience is that the greatest density of purpura provoked by a Hess test is usually in the 'snuff-box' area over the space between the thumb and index finger metacarpals on the dorsum of the hand.

'Negative-pressure' tests require some simple apparatus to apply negative pressure to an area of skin usually 1–2 cm across. This technique is suitable for repeated tests in the same subject. The application of such a negative pressure at the rim of a cup may only be acting as a local venous tourniquet. Using these techniques capillary resistance is found to vary greatly, as does the platelet count, from individual to individual and with site and numerous other factors.

Bleeding time [4,17–20]

This is the time taken for bleeding to cease after a standardized tiny incision, usually in the skin of the forearm. This type of bleeding normally ceases because of contraction of the small vessels aided by production of a platelet plug. Techniques can be standardized in various ways, for example with a sphygmomanometer cuff at 40 mmHg the bleeding time is usually 4–10 min. The bleeding time is usually prolonged in thrombocytopenia where the platelet count is below 80×10^9/L and becomes progressively prolonged as the count falls, being 30 min at counts less than

$10 \times 10^9/L$. It may be prolonged in von Willebrand's disease, other disorders of platelet function, severe anaemia, and in patients taking aspirin or receiving heparin, as well as being affected by age and skin laxity. Although often stated to be normal in disorders of coagulation, it may be prolonged in severe haemophilia. It is a rather insensitive test whose wide range of normal values makes it of limited use, even as a screening test. The bleeding time does not accurately predict internal surgical bleeding [19], although it has been used to investigate the effect of aspirin and non-steroidal anti-inflammatory drugs (NSAIDs), which may be relevant as a cause of bleeding during skin surgery [20].

Platelet function analysers (PFA), measuring the PFA closure time, may be more useful, but may vary in sensitivity and specificity according to the disorder being examined, the PFA being more accurate than the bleeding time for diagnosis of type I von Willebrand disease [21]. A study of the combined PFA closure times for ADP and epinephrine in normal subjects (the PFA-100) showed a false-positive rate of almost 16% and, of those who did have a platelet function abnormality, the specificity was 79% compared with 91% for the bleeding time [22]. Current techniques such as the PFA-100, even if less specific, do have the advantage of simplicity, are *in vitro* and therefore less invasive, and are more reproducible than the bleeding time. Although clinical experience with this technique is recent, this and similar methods (such as the Thrombostat 4000) are largely replacing the bleeding time in many clinical haematology laboratories.

Coagulation screen

Major coagulation defects can be excluded by a clotting screen including measurement of prothrombin time, kaolin cephalin clotting time, thrombin clotting time and fibrinogen levels. Clinical considerations and the results of the screening tests may suggest further laboratory tests, for example levels of individual clotting factors [10] or antiphospholipid antibodies. Discussion of how these tests are performed is beyond the scope of this book, but they are described in detail in other publications [23–25].

Capillary microscopy

Direct microscopic examination of capillaries is disappointing in the elucidation of haemorrhagic and purpuric diseases, although it is useful to determine whether small punctate lesions are actually petechial or small convoluted but intact capillaries. Purpura may at times be seen in the nail fold capillaries when not present elsewhere in the skin. Extravasation of blood may occur at the junction of the precapillary arteriole with the capillary, at the tip of the capillary or more usually at the venous end. Capillary microscopy is discussed further in Chapter 47 and, in relation to nailfolds in collagen vascular diseases, in Chapter 51.

Other haematological, biochemical and immunological tests

A number of other haematological tests may be indicated, depending on the likely diagnostic area. As a simple example, a blood film, bone marrow examination, and tests for antiplatelet antibodies may all contribute in distinguishing between thrombocytopenia due to decreased production versus peripheral destruction. This is the province of the haematologist, and is addressed in

major haematological texts [1,2]. It is worth being aware that abnormalities predisposing to bleeding may coexist, and may require a wider range of tests than usual for the presumed diagnosis; examples include abnormal platelet function (relatively common), fibrinolytic defects and low-grade disseminated intravascular coagulopathy (DIC) (possibly in 50% of patients) in HHT [16], platelet dysfunction in Ehlers–Danlos syndrome [16], acquired factor X (sometimes IX and X) in systemic amyloidosis [16], bone marrow necrosis in antiphospholipid syndrome [26], thrombocythaemia with antiphospholipid syndrome [27], heparin-induced thrombocytopenia with the antiphospholipid syndrome [28], and the multiple causes of bleeding in acute promyelocytic leukaemia (DIC, fibrinolysis, and proteolysis of fibrinogen and von Willebrand factor) [29]. Some of these are discussed in more detail later in the chapter.

Hyperferritinaemia is a well documented feature of some inflammatory disorders. Ferritin is produced by phagocytic macrophages, and high levels occur in disorders where there is histiocytic proliferation and haemophagocytosis. This occurs in a little known disorder termed the *macrophage activation syndrome* (also termed autoimmune disease-associated reactive haemophagocytic lymphohistiocytosis), a complication mainly occurring in systemic onset juvenile idiopathic arthritis (Still's disease) and sometimes in juvenile systemic lupus erythematosus; it has also been documented in adult-onset Still's disease, and may be triggered by infections or by drugs. Purpura, bruising and mucosal bleeding occur due to a combination of thrombocytopenia and coagulopathy (prolonged prothrombin time and partial thromboplastin time, with fibrin degradation products and hypofibrinogenaemia) [30,31]. Other biochemical abnormalities include low sodium levels, and elevation of triglycerides, lactose dehydrogenase and transaminases.

Although not routinely performed, a variety of serological tests can give an indication of vascular damage; these include levels of thromboxane, endothelin, prostacyclin, soluble thrombomodulin, platelet activating factor, e-selectin and von Willebrand factor. Antibodies against platelets, clotting factors and others are sometimes measured. Emergent antibodies, but still of uncertain clinical application, include those against annexins II and V, which are important in fibrinolysis in acute promyelocytic leukaemia and in the antiphospholipid syndrome, respectively [32]. β_2-glycoprotein I is discussed later in relation to antiphospholipid syndrome.

Genetic tests

Although rarely the first approach, many causes of bleeding and thrombosis are now well characterized at a genetic level; appropriate tests may be used to confirm a diagnosis, and in some cases to estimate prognosis or suitability for specific treatment options. Some examples of relevance in evaluation of purpura and bleeding include cytogenetic testing (for example, demonstrating a high risk of bleeding in patients with acute promyelocytic leukaemia who have t(15:17) translocation), documentation of activated protein C resistance (factor V Leiden; pp. 49.38–39) and genetic tests such as identifying different types of Ehlers–Danlos syndrome (type IV, associated with severe bleeding due to vascular rupture, being due to mutations in the *COL3A1* gene), confirming different types and zygosity in homocystinaemia, distinguishing between HHT I (endogulin gene mutations) versus HHT II (*ALK1* gene) in hereditary haemorrhagic telangiectasia, and demonstrating ADAMTS13 deficiency in thrombotic thrombocytopenic purpura [33].

Summary

To avoid performing every type of investigation in all cases of purpura, the following broad generalizations may be made.

1 Purpura of mild degree on the lower legs alone is commonly hydrostatic, especially in the elderly, in those with other evidence of venous disease, or in the distribution of other skin diseases, and seldom requires extensive investigation.

2 Coagulation defects usually present as large ecchymoses and external or internal bleeding but not as petechiae; inherited types may present as gingival bleeding. Capillary fragility tests are normal unless there is severe deficiency of clotting factors.

3 Thrombocytopenia is often associated with petechiae but there may also be external or internal haemorrhages and bruising.

4 External bleeding and large ecchymoses are due to coagulation or platelet defects, or to diseases of connective tissue such as Ehlers–Danlos syndrome.

5 Petechiae are due to platelet defects or capillary changes.

6 Dysproteinaemias may cause lesions of simple haemorrhage, inflammatory haemorrhage or occlusion, depending on the properties of individual abnormal proteins.

7 Thrombophilias may present with livedoid change, retiform purpura or usually non-inflammatory cutaneous necrosis.

8 An initial retiform pattern without blanchable erythema or palpable lesions is generally indicative of microvascular occlusion.

9 Inflammatory lesions of the vessels are seldom the cause of external bleeding or ecchymoses, but are the most common cause of persistent and localized purpura. A blanchable erythematous inflammatory component is often present in early lesions.

10 Inflammatory purpuric lesions are due to vascular changes rather than simple haemorrhage.

11 Splinter haemorrhages of the nails are due to purpura of the nail bed, are most commonly due to trauma and are not diagnostic of any one condition (see Chapter 65).

References

1 Lichtman MA, Buetler E, Kaushansky K *et al.*, eds. *Williams' Hematology*, 7th edn. New York: McGraw-Hill, 2005.

2 Greer JP, Foerster J, Lukens JN *et al.*, eds. *Wintrobe's Clinical Hematology*, 12th edn. Philadelphia: Lippincott, Williams & Wilkins, 2008.

3 Taylor RE, Blatt PM. Clinical evaluation of the patient with bruising and bleeding. *J Am Acad Dermatol* 1981; **4**: 348–68.

4 Hardisty RM. Platelet disorders. In: Hoffbrand AV, Lewis SM, eds. *Postgraduate Haematology*, 3rd edn. Oxford: Heinemann, 1989: 598–626.

5 Lowe GDO. Vascular disease and vasculitis. In: Ratnoff OD, Forbes CD, eds. *Disorders of Haemostasis*, 3rd edn. London: Saunders, 1996.

6 Piette WW. The differential diagnosis of purpura from a morphologic perspective. *Adv Dermatol* 1994; **9**: 3–23.

7 Seegmiller A, Sarode R. Laboratory evaluation of platelet function. *Haematol Oncol Clin North Am* 2007; **21**: 731–42.

8 Shen-Yu MP, Frenkel EP. Acquired platelet dysfunction. *Haematol Oncol Clin North Am* 2007; **21**: 647–71.

9 Visentin GP, Liu CY. Drug-induced thrombocytopenia. *Haematol Oncol Clin North Am* 2007; **21**: 685–96.

10 Hayward CPM. Diagnosis and management of mild bleeding disorders. *Hematology Am Soc Hematol Educ Program* 2005: 423–8.

11 Crowson AN, Magro CM, Zahorchak R. Atypical pigmentary purpura: a clinical, histopathologic, and genotypic study. *Hum Pathol* 1999; **30**: 1004–12.

12 Cox NH, Walsh ML, Robson RH. Purpura and bleeding due to calcium channel blockers: an underestimated problem? Case reports and a pilot study. *Clin Exp Dermatol* 2009; **34**: 487–91.

13 Gough KR. Capillary resistance to suction in hypertension. *BMJ* 1962; **i**: 21–4.

14 Kramar J. The determination and evaluation of capillary resistance. *Blood* 1962; **20**: 83–93.

15 Peck SM. Diagnosis and treatment of skin manifestations of capillary fragility. *N Engl J Med* 1946; **235**: 900–6.

16 Bick R. Vascular thrombohemorrhagic disorders: hereditary and acquired. *Clin Appl Thrombosis Hemostasis* 2001; **7**: 178–94.

17 Anonymous. What about the bleeding time? *BMJ* 1985; **291**: 91.

18 Lind SE. Prolonged bleeding time. *Am J Med* 1984; **77**: 305–12.

19 Lind SE. The bleeding time does not predict surgical bleeding. *Blood* 1991; **77**: 2547–52.

20 Lawrence C, Sakuntabhai A, Tiling-Grosse S. Effect of aspirin and nonsteroidal antiinflammatory drug therapy on bleeding complications in dermatologic surgical patients. *J Am Acad Dermatol* 1994; **31**: 988–92.

21 Hassan AA, Kroll MH. Acquired disorders of platelet function. *Hematology Am Soc Hematol Educ Program* 2005: 403–8.

22 Posan E, McBane RD, Grill DE *et al.* Comparison of PFA-100 testing and bleeding time for detecting platelet hypofunction and von Willebrand disease in clinical practice. *Thromb Haemost* 2003; **90**: 892–8.

23 Helbert M, Bodger S, Cavenagh J *et al.* Optimising testing for phospholipid antibodies. *J Clin Pathol* 2001; **54**: 693–8.

24 Pierangeli SS, Harris EN. Clinical laboratory testing for the antiphospholipid syndrome. *Clin Chim Acta* 2005; **357**: 17–33.

25 Hoppensteadt DA, Fabbrini N, Bick RL *et al.* Laboratory evaluation of the antiphospholipid syndrome. *Haematol Oncol Clin North Am* 2008; **22**: 19–32.

26 Paydas S, Koçak R, Zorludemir S, Baslamisli F. Bone marrow necrosis in antiphospholipid syndrome. *J Clin Pathol* 1997; **50**: 261–2.

27 Harrison CN, Machin SJ. Antiphospholipid antibodies and essential thrombocythemia. *Am J Med* 1997; **102**: 317–8.

28 Hoppensteadt DA, Walenga JM. The relationship between the antiphospholipid syndrome and heparin-induced thrombocytopenia. *Haematol Oncol Clin North Am* 2008; **22**: 1–18.

29 Tallman MS, Abutalib SA, Altman JK. The double hazard of thrombophilia and bleeding in acute promyelocytic leukaemia. *Semin Thromb Hemost* 2007; **33**: 330–8.

30 Kelly A, Ramanan AV. Recognition and management of macrophage activation syndrome I juvenile arthritis. *Curr Opin Rheumatol* 2007; **19**: 477–81.

31 Castillo L, Carcillo J. Secondary hemophagocytic lymphohistiocytosis and severe sepsis/systemic inflammatory response syndrome/multiorgan dysfunction syndrome/macrophage activation syndrome share common intermediate phenotypes on a spectrum of inflammation. *Pediatr Crit Care Med* 2009; **10**: 387–92.

32 Rand JH. 'Annexinopathies'—a new class of diseases. *N Engl J Med* 1999; **340**: 1035–6.

33 Kobaashi T, Wada H, Nishioka N *et al.* ADAMTS13 related markers and von Willebrand factor in plasma from patients with thrombotic microangiopathy (TMA). *Thromb Res* 2007; **121**: 849–54.

Purpura due to thrombocytopenia or platelet defects

Platelets are an essential component of the haemostatic process. Thrombocytopenia or abnormal platelet function from any cause may therefore produce purpura or a bleeding tendency, as discussed in the general haematology texts previously listed and in references listed below [1–7].

Table 49.3 Platelet disorders causing purpura.

Thrombocytopenia	*Abnormal platelet function*
Defective platelet production	Inherited and congenital
Bone marrow abnormality	Von Willebrand disease and defects of the platelet von Willebrand factor receptor
Aplasia: toxic, immunological, idiopathic	Hereditary haemorrhagic telangiectasia (often have platelet dysfunction also)
Neoplasia: leukaemia, myeloma, carcinomatosis	Bernard–Soulier disease (GpIb/IX/V receptor defect with low platelet count)
Replacement: myelofibrosis, radiation damage, sarcoidosis	GpIa deficiency
Other impaired production: Wiskott–Aldrich syndrome, vitamin B_{12} or folate	Glanzmann's thrombasthenia (GpIIb/IIIa deficiency)
deficiency	MYH9-related disorders (e.g. May–Hegglin abnormality)
Metabolic: uraemia, alcohol, drugs	α-granule disorders
Infections	Dense granule (δ-granule) disorders (Hermansky–Pudlak syndrome, Chediak–
Diminished platelet survival	Higashi syndrome, storage pool disease)
Platelet alloantibodies	Abnormalities of signal-transduction pathways
Neonatal	Membrane phospholipids abnormalities (e.g. Scott syndrome)
Post-transfusion	Wiskott–Aldrich syndrome (δ-granule abnormality) and X-linked thrombocytopenia
Antilymphocyte globulin	(WASP gene mutations)
Platelet autoantibodies	Drug-induced
Idiopathic (immune) thrombocytopenic purpura	Uraemia
Marrow transplant	Cardiac bypass
Antiphospholipid antibodies	Platelet antibodies
Systemic lupus erythematosus	Idiopathic (immune) thrombocytopenic purpura
Mechanical: prosthetic heart valves	Systemic lupus erythematosus/antiphospholipid syndrome
Drugs and vaccines	Myeloproliferative disorders
Infections, sepsis syndrome	Dysproteinaemias (especially IgA myeloma and macroglobulinaemia)
Excessive platelet consumption	Cold-stored (blood bank) platelets
Disseminated intravascular coagulation	
Haemangioma (Kasabach–Merritt)	*Thrombocytosis*
Hereditary haemorrhagic telangiectasia ('mini-Kasabach–Merritt')	Essential thrombocythaemia
Thrombotic microangiopathies	Other myeloproliferative syndromes
Haemolytic–uraemic syndrome	Medical diseases and other causes
Thrombotic thrombocytopenic purpura	Blood loss, trauma, burns
Sequestration	Post-splenectomy
Splenomegaly	Malignant disease
Hypothermia	Tuberculosis
	Sarcoidosis

Platelets exposed to damaged endothelium adhere to one another and to collagen and other subendothelial components. Numerous complex interactions occur, involving von Willebrand factor and its glycoprotein receptor, various integrin adhesion molecules, thrombospondin, fibronectin, laminin, phospholipases and ADP released from damaged cells, as well as collagen and platelets. Platelet activation causes release of serotonin and thromboxane A_2, both of which cause vasoconstriction, and increase platelet adhesiveness and aggregation leading to formation of a platelet plug. This process is aided further by the presence of plasma fibrinogen and by thrombin. Production of prostacyclin, a powerful vasodilator and inhibitor of platelet aggregation, is decreased as a result of endothelial damage. Developing platelet plugs are reinforced by fibrin strands formed as a result of activation of the plasma clotting system by platelet factor 3, when this is exposed by alterations in the surface characteristics of the aggregated platelets.

Purpura due to platelet defects can be divided into three groups:

- Thrombocytopenia, i.e. decreased platelet numbers
- Abnormalities of platelet function
- Thrombocytosis, i.e. increased platelet numbers

Thrombocytopenia

The platelet count at which purpura occurs is extremely variable. Purpura due to platelet deficiency usually occurs with a count below $20 \times 10^9/L$ and is seldom observed with a count above $50 \times 10^9/L$. The main causes of thrombocytopenia are listed in Table 49.3.

References

1 McCrae KR, Bussel JB, Mannucci PM *et al*. Platelets: an update on diagnosis and management of thrombocytopenic disorders. *Hematology Am Soc Hematol Educ Program* 2001: 282–305.

2 Handin RI. Inherited platelet disorders. *Hematology Am Soc Hematol Educ Program* 2005: 396–402.

3 Cines DB, Bussel JB, McMillan RB, Zehnder JL. Congenital and acquired thrombocytopenia. *Hematology Am Soc Hematol Educ Program* 2004: 390–406.

4 Hayward CPM. Diagnosis and management of mild bleeding disorders. *Hematology Am Soc Hematol Educ Program* 2005: 423–8.

5 Bussel JB, Kunicki TJ, Michelson AD. Platelets: new understanding of platelet glycoproteins and their role in disease. *Hematology Am Soc Hematol Educ Program* 2000: 222–40.

6 George JN, Shattil SJ. The clinical importance of acquired abnormalities of platelet function. *N Engl J Med* 1991; **324**: 27–39.

7 Hassan AA, Kroll MH. Acquired disorders of platelet function. *Hematology Am Soc Hematol Educ Program* 2005: 403–8.

Idiopathic (immune) thrombocytopenic purpura [1–9]

Idiopathic immune thrombocytopenic purpura (ITP) results from immune destruction of platelets; transient ITP has been documented in children born to affected mothers, and passive transfer has been demonstrated. The prevalence is about 1/10 000 population per year, and it is about twice as common in women, except in childhood where males predominate [10]. Half of cases occur in children [4] (two-thirds before age 21 years), and it may occur in 0.1–0.2% of pregnancies. Familial and twin cases have occurred, some populations show an association with HLA-DRw2 or DRB1*0410 alleles, and a genetic predisposition appears likely [11]. There is an association with other autoimmune diseases, such as celiac disease [12] and thyroid disease [13]; other predisposing factors include certain immunodeficiencies, complement C2 or C4 deficiency, and abnormalities of the Fas pathway [1]. The onset may be gradual or, especially in children, acute, and the overall course may be self-limiting (especially in children) or long-term. Chronic ITP is usually autoimmune and apparently idiopathic.

The autoantibodies often show specificity for the platelet membrane glycoproteins IIb/IIIa (integrin αIIbβ3) and Ib/IX [5], and less often for Ia/IIa, IV or V. It is unclear why these develop but there is a Th1 cytokine profile and T cells may drive the process by stimulating antibody synthesis after being exposed to fragments of glycoprotein IIb/IIIa, but not to the intact native protein; such fragments may arise from destruction of platelets within antigen-presenting cells or by other mechanisms [5,8]. A current theory suggests that there is upregulation of CD40 ligand (CD40L, CD154) on T cells, which causes co-stimulatory B cell activation and ongoing antibody production. Viral antigen–antibody reactions may be demonstrated in acute forms of the disease, usually in children following an acute viral illness such as rubella, varicella, parvovirus B19, Epstein–Barr virus, echoviruses and others. Vaccines to prevent viral illness have also been implicated, including recently the combined measles, mumps and rubella (MMR) vaccine. Chronic infections that can provoke chronic (mainly adult) ITP include HIV, hepatitis C virus and possibly *Helicobacter pylori* [1,13].

Some cases are drug-induced (see later) or are associated with systemic lupus erythematosus (SLE) and other autoimmune connective tissue diseases, with agammaglobulinaemia, or with lymphoproliferative disease (e.g. chronic lymphocytic leukaemia, lymphomas) or with myelodysplasia. ITP may also coexist with other haematological abnormalities, for example the combination of ATP and neutrophilia, which presents as mucosal bleeding with infections; the platelet deficiency tends to be chronic. Of greater dermatological importance is Evans' syndrome, which comprises Coombs-positive haemolytic anaemia with ITP; this is also associated with collagen vascular disorders, usually SLE or scleroderma but occasionally dermatomyositis [14,15].

From the haematology perspective, the platelet count falls below 50×10^9/L and may even be zero. Usually the only symptom is a tendency to bleed from gingivae after brushing teeth, or into

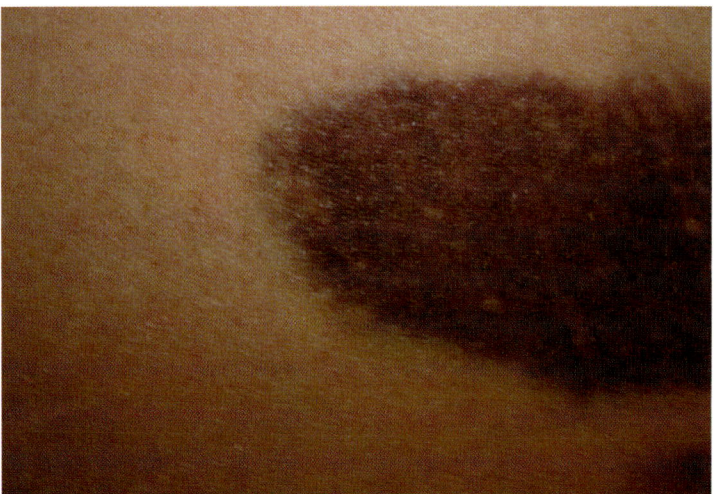

Fig. 49.2 Spontaneous bruising in drug-induced idiopathic thrombocytopenic purpura.

the skin to produce crops of petechiae or larger haemorrhages (Fig. 49.2). Bleeding may occur in any organ but joint involvement is unusual. The spleen may be slightly enlarged but gross splenomegaly should suggest an alternative diagnosis. Intracranial haemorrhage occurs in about 0.2% of children and is often fatal, but is very unlikely unless the platelet count is less than 10×10^9/L.

Lupus erythematosus develops in a small proportion of cases [16], although there are differences in immunopathogenesis between the thrombocytopenia of SLE and that of ITP [17]. About 20% of adult patients with immune thrombocytopenia have associated features of the primary antiphospholipid antibody syndrome (APLS), with a prolonged activated partial thromboplastin time (aPTT), lupus anticoagulant and anticardiolipin antibodies. The immune thrombocytopenia associated with APLS is rarely severe [18].

The diagnosis is established by the clinical picture, low platelet count, exclusion of other causes of thrombocytopenia and the mainly negative bone marrow findings (megakaryocytes are present in normal or increased numbers in the bone marrow, but bone marrow examination is not routinely performed, especially in younger subjects without other abnormal findings); ITP has historically been largely a diagnosis of exclusion. Various methods of demonstrating platelet antibodies have been used, but are largely of little help; they are sensitive but non-specific as they detect non-pathological antibodies. Antibodies bound to platelet glycoproteins have been felt to be pathological and more suitable for assay [19], with a positive predictive value of about 80% [4]. Their lack of specificity, and the variability of commercial assays, means that they are of limited value [1,8], although patients with antiplatelet glycoprotein antibodies tend to need more intensive therapy [8]. Elevated levels of caeruloplasmin may help to identify chronic ITP compared with other causes of thrombocytopenia [20]. New biomarkers of the autoimmune reaction (leptin, cell-bound antiplatelet antibodies, specific B cells) and of thrombopoiesis (thrombopoietin, glycocalicin, reticulated platelets) may advance diagnosis in the future [21]. The differential diagnosis is wide but especially includes SLE, drug-induced purpura, disseminated intravascular coagulation (DIC) and renal failure.

Spontaneous remission often occurs in acute attacks (most children have spontaneous improvement within a month or two, and the disorder resolves in about two-thirds within 2–4 months [9]), but spontaneous remission is rare in chronic cases of more than 3 months' duration, where a continuous or fluctuating course may occur. A variety of treatments have been used [1,3–6,8,9,22–25], the aim being prevention of serious bleeding rather than normalization of the platelet count. In children, observation alone is often satisfactory unless there is bleeding, but in adults severe thrombocytopenia is an indication for treatment even in the absence of serious bleeding. A platelet count of below $30 \times 10^9/L$ is usually the threshold for intervention. Corticosteroid therapy (prednisolone 1 mg/kg/day) is most commonly used but other regimens, such as a 4-day course of high-dose dexamethasone, may achieve better remission rates; about 50% of adults treated with corticosteroids achieve complete remission but platelet counts often fall as the treatment is tapered. Splenectomy is beneficial in at least two-thirds of chronic cases and in acute cases in which a spontaneous or steroid-induced remission cannot be achieved, but carries some risk. After splenectomy the platelet count tends to remain low but the purpura tends to cease. Immunosuppressive therapy or other treatments are indicated in cases that fail to respond to splenectomy and steroids, or where splenectomy is contraindicated; treatments that have been used in patients with refractory ITP include danazol, azathioprine, vincristine, interferon-α, ciclosporin, mycophenolate mofetil, Fc receptor blockade using intravenous immunoglobulin (IVIG) or intravenous anti-D antiserum (antiD), plasma exchange, various monoclonal antibodies and biological agents such as rituximab (anti-CD20), Campath-1-H (anti-CD52), second generation thrombopoietic agents [24,26,27], pegylated recombinant megakaryocyte-derived growth factor [8], and, rarely, autologous stem cell transplantation. AntiD only works in patients who are Rhesus D-positive and who have a spleen, but in such individuals there is typically a very rapid improvement in platelet count; IVIG is useful in achieving rapid responses, although its mechanism involves upregulation of FcRIIb rather than the competitive binding to FcRIII that occurs with antiD [1], and it also appears to be active in ITP caused by viruses such as parvovirus B19 and Epstein–Barr virus. In view of the possible link between *H. pylori* and ITP (especially in adults), appropriate testing and eradication, if indicated, would appear appropriate before using more toxic therapies. Similarly, hepatitis C infection should be treated if present. Beyond the standards of steroids and splenectomy, for rapid response, IVIG may be the best current agent, for remission rituximab (33% durable remission) and for the future non-thrombopoietin-like thrombopoietic agents and anti-CD154 antibodies.

Various measures have been used to predict and monitor outcome and treatment response in ITP, in addition to the platelet count [4,28–30]. Other than young age, which is associated with a shorter disease course (but which does not predict response to corticosteroids if used), the most useful clinical aspect is that splenectomy is most successful in those who responded initially to steroids, and who get a rapid improvement in platelet count after splenectomy. HLA-DRB1*14 and DRB1*0410 are associated with good prognosis and good response to common interventions, and HLA-DRB1*13 and DR4 with poor prognosis or therapeutic resistance. Serum IL-2 is a good prognostic marker in ITP, relapse is lower in children treated with corticosteroids, and platelet-associated IgGs are a useful monitoring parameter.

References

1 McCrae KR, Bussel JB, Mannucci PM *et al.* Platelets: an update on diagnosis and management of thrombocytopenic disorders. *Hematology Am Soc Hematol Educ Program* 2001: 282–305.

2 Cines DB, Bussel JB, McMillan RB, Zehnder JL. Congenital and acquired thrombocytopenia. *Hematology Am Soc Hematol Educ Program* 2004: 390–406.

3 Kelton JG, Bussel JB, eds. Idiopathic thrombocytopenic purpura. *Semin Hematol* 2000; **37**: 219–314.

4 Cines DB, Blanchette VS. Immune thrombocytopenic purpura. *N Engl J Med* 2002; **346**: 995–1008.

5 McMillan R. The pathogenesis of chronic immune thrombocytopenic purpura. *Semin Hematol* 2007; **44** (Suppl. 5): S3–11.

6 Psaila B, Bussel JB. Immune thrombocytopenic purpura. *Haematol Oncol Clin North Am* 2007; **21**: 743–59.

7 Bussel JB, Kunicki TJ, Michelson AD. Platelets: new understanding of platelet glycoproteins and their role in disease. *Hematology Am Soc Hematol Educ Program* 2000: 222–40.

8 Beardsley DS. ITP in the 21st century. *Hematology Am Soc Hematol Educ Program* 2006: 402–7.

9 Nugent DJ. Immune thrombocytopenic purpura of childhood. *Hematology Am Soc Hematol Educ Program* 2006: 97–103.

10 Segal JB, Powe NR. Prevalence of immune thrombocytopenia: analyses of administrative data. *J Thromb Haemost* 2006; **4**: 2377–83.

11 Rischewski JR, Imbach P, Paulussen M, Kühne T. Idiopathic thrombocytopenic purpura (ITP): is there a genetic predisposition? *Pediatr Blood Cancer* 2006; **47** (5 Suppl.): 678–80.

12 Olén O, Montgomery SM, Elinder G *et al.* Increased risk of immune thrombocytopenic purpura among patients with celiac disease. *Scand J Gastroenterol* 2008; **43**: 416–22.

13 Liebman H. Other immune thrombocytopenias. *Semin Hematol* 2007; **44** (Suppl. 5): S24–34.

14 Fong KY, Loizou S, Boey ML, Walport MJ. Anticardiolipin antibodies, haemolytic anaemia and thrombocytopenia in systemic lupus erythematosus. *Br J Rheumatol* 1992; **31**: 453–5.

15 Chang DK, Yoo DH, Kim TH *et al.* Induction of remission with intravenous immunoglobulin and cyclophosphamide in steroid-resistant Evans' syndrome associated with dermatomyositis. *Clin Rheumatol* 2001; **20**: 63–6.

16 Hepburn MJ, English JC, Keeling JH. Autoimmune idiopathic thrombocytopenic purpura with the subsequent occurrence of systemic lupus erythematosus. *Cutis* 1997; **60**: 185–7.

17 Lazarus AH, Ellis J, Semple JW *et al.* Comparison of platelet immunity in patients with SLE and ITP. *Transfusion Sci* 2000; **22**: 19–27.

18 Cuadrado MJ, Hughes GRV. Hughes (antiphospholipid) syndrome. Clinical features. *Rheum Dis Clin N Am* 2001; **27**: 507–24.

19 Warner M, Kelton JG. Laboratory investigation of immune thrombocytopenia. *J Clin Pathol* 1997; **50**: 5–12.

20 Chousa M, Hiroyasu I, Kuniaki S *et al.* The measurement of serum ceruloplasmin is useful for diagnostic differentiation of immune thrombocytopenic purpura. *Clin Chim Acta* 2008; **389**: 132–8.

21 Sachs UJH. Diagnosis of idiopathic thrombocytopenic purpura. *Haemostaseologie* 2008; **28**: 72–6.

22 Stasi R, Provan D. Management of immune thrombocytopenic purpura in adults. *Mayo Clin Proc* 2004; **79**: 504–22.

23 George JN, Vesely SK. Immune thrombocytopenic purpura—let the treatment fit the patient. *N Engl J Med* 2003; **349**: 903–5.

24 Bromberg ME. Immune thrombocytopenic purpura—the changing therapeutic landscape. *N Engl J Med* 2006; **355**: 1643–5.

25 Arnold DM, Kelton JG. Current options for the treatment of idiopathic thrombocytopenic purpura. *Semin Hematol* 2007; **44** (Suppl. 5): S12–23.

26 Andemariam B, Psaila B, Bussel JB. Novel thrombopoietic agents. *Hematology Am Soc Hematol Educ Program* 2007: 106–13.

27 Newland A. Thrombopoietin mimetic agents in the management of immune thrombocytopenic purpura. *Semin Hematol* 2007; **44** (Suppl. 5): S35–45.

28 Leung AY, Chim CS, Kwong YL *et al.* Clinicopathologic and prognostic features of chronic idiopathic thrombocytopenic purpura in adult Chinese patients: an analysis of 220 cases. *Ann Haematol* 2001; **80**: 384–6.

29 Syed-Naveen N, Adil-Salman N, Sajid S *et al.* Chronic ITP: analysis of various factors at presentation which predict failure to first line treatment and the response to second line therapy. *J Pak Med Assoc* 2007; **57**: 126–9.

30 Tag LM, Ezz-Eldeen AM, Mahmoud MS *et al.* Serum IL-2 and platelet-associated immunoglobulins are good prognostic markers in immune thrombocytopenic purpura. *Egypt J Immunol* 2004; **1**: 121–32.

Secondary or symptomatic thrombocytopenia

Drugs and toxins [1]

Drug- or toxin-induced purpura may occur as a result of thrombocytopenia, altered platelet function or vascular damage. Each of these may be caused by many different mechanisms. The last two are considered later. The main causes of drug- or toxin-induced thrombocytopenia are:

- Direct bone marrow toxicity, e.g. benzol, nitrogen mustard, or general myelotoxicity (e.g. chemotherapeutic agents)
- Immunological bone marrow damage, e.g. chloramphenicol
- Destruction of formed platelets, via either immunological (e.g. apronalide (Sedormid), quinidine, quinine, sulphonamides) or non-immunological mechanisms (e.g. bleomycin).

The immunological mechanisms have been divided into [1]:

- Hapten-induced antibody (e.g. penicillins)
- Drug-dependent (compound or conformational) antibody (e.g. quinine, quinidine, NSAIDs, anticonvulsants, antibiotics and many others)
- Inhibitors of the platelet glycoprotein GIIb/IIIa—further divided into four known or probable mechanisms (ligand mimetic, drug-specific antibody, drug-induced antibody and immune complex-mediated).

Some of these are of interest as they relate to new types of drug, for example the chimeric Fab fragment of abciximab induces antibody specific for murine sequences that control GIIb/IIIa (with onset sometimes within hours of exposure). However, the most important mechanism, in that it is pertinent to most drug-induced thrombocytopenia, is that where a drug-specific antibody is created by the drug (or metabolite) binding to a platelet glycoprotein to create either an antibody-inducing drug–glycoprotein epitope or a conformational change elsewhere in the target glycoprotein for which the antibody is specific. The mechanisms for many drugs, and certainly the binding sites, are often uncertain; some drugs may cause thrombocytopenia by more than one mechanism (e.g. thiazides may cause selective inhibition of megakaryocyte production as well as immunological peripheral destruction).

It has been suggested that at least 200 drugs cause thrombocytopenia. The most common are cytotoxic/chemotherapeutic drugs, quinine, quinidine, gold salts, heparin, sulphonamides, penicillins, thiazides and furosemide (frusemide), procainamide, indometacin (indomethacin) and other NSAIDs, thiouracils and carbimazole, bismuth, arsenicals, rifampicin and isoniazid, acetazolamide, acetylsalicylic acid, imipramine, interferon, various sedatives, and anticonvulsants such as phenytoin, carbamazepine and sodium valproate [2–4]. Recently implicated drugs include tirofiban, roxifiban, eptifibatide and abciximab. Various biological agents used in dermatology, such as efalizumab [5], have also been implicated as a cause of drug-induced thrombocytopenia.

Onset of thrombocytopenia is usually after a week with first exposure but can be within 2–3 days on re-exposure [1]; improvement is usually within 10 days of stopping the culprit drug. However, the duration of thrombocytopenia after stopping the drug is too long to be explained on the basis of either drug clearance or platelet lifespan in some cases, particularly with quinidine or quinine, suggesting that true autoantibodies may be produced [6]. The severity of thrombocytopenia does not necessarily correlate with the implicated drug, mechanism, or specific glycoprotein to which the drug may bind.

Heparin-induced thrombocytopenia (HIT) [7–13] is discussed in more detail later. It may present as isolated thrombocytopenia (which may be severe but can be of modest severity compared with other drug-induced causes), but may also cause platelet-rich clot formation leading to venous thrombosis, limb ischaemia, injection site necrosis, adrenal crisis due to adrenal vein necrosis, and severe systemic post-bolus injection reactions. The risks are greater in females, in surgical settings and with unfractionated heparins; it occurs in about 2% of subjects exposed to heparin, but in up to 40% after cardiac surgery. It is important as it can be confused with post-transfusion purpura in early stages, but the greatest importance (which also helps to distinguish it from other drug-induced thrombocytopenias) is the association with arterial or venous thrombosis (heparin-associated thrombocytopenia and thrombosis syndrome), which occurs in about a third of patients with HIT, and with heparin-induced skin necrosis, as discussed later. A crucial issue in such instances is to avoid coumarins, which will not work (they may in fact worsen thrombosis by depleting protein C, and coumarin-induced thrombosis is about 100-fold more likely if HIT is present than if it is not). Treatment is therefore with agents that directly inhibit thrombin or its generation [11]. It is due to formation of antibodies against an immunogenic complex involving heparin and platelet factor 4 (PF4), the antibody reaction causing platelet aggregation; there are also high levels of thrombin–antithrombin complexes.

Other toxic causes of thrombocytopenia include alcohol, snake venoms and, rarely, foods and food additives.

Infections

Thrombocytopenia may occur with a wide variety of infections, often with associated capillary damage. Infections that may be associated with thrombocytopenia include septicaemia of many aetiologies, typhoid, typhus, tuberculosis, smallpox, chickenpox, vaccinia, scarlet fever, influenza, measles, rubella, cat-scratch disease, infective hepatitis, subacute bacterial endocarditis, glandular fever, malaria, dengue fever, human immunodeficiency virus (HIV), hepatitis C and other virus infections.

Bone marrow diseases

Bone marrow diseases, for example leukaemia or aplastic anaemia, are the commonest causes of thrombocytopenia (see Table 49.3). In addition to the abnormal platelet production, there may be platelet antibodies formed in patients with lymphoma or leukaemia. Splenomegaly of many different aetiologies causes sequestration of platelets in the splenic sinuses but rarely produces a platelet count low enough to cause purpura. Purpura and ecchymosis are among the commoner cutaneous features of the haemophagocytic syndrome.

Pregnancy

Numerous reasons may explain thrombocytopenia in pregnancy [13]. The commonest cause is termed gestational or incidental thrombocytopenia, and accounts for three-quarters of cases, but does not cause platelet counts low enough to cause purpura. Thus, if purpura is present, other more significant disorders should be considered. ITP accounts for 5% of cases, occurring in 0.1% of pregnancies, and thrombotic thrombocytopenic purpura, drug-induced and infection-induced thrombocytopenia may all occur. The last-mentioned is of dermatological importance, as the likely infections include HIV and cytomegalovirus, both of which may cause congenital infection in the neonate. Pregnancy-specific thrombocytopenias include those due to pre-eclampsia, HELLP (haemolysis, elevated liver function tests, low platelets; discussed on p. 49.31) or fatty liver. There are also potential systemic disease associations, including SLE, antiphospholipid syndrome and disseminated intravascular coagulation, as well as various conditions of bone marrow failure and nutritional deficiencies.

Platelet consumption and the thrombotic microangiopathies (thrombotic thrombocytopenic purpura and haemolytic–uraemic syndrome)

Thrombocytopenia may be associated with haemangiomas (Kasabach–Merritt syndrome, see Chapter 18). This is caused by ongoing chronic consumption and there is often compensated subacute or chronic DIC. Relevant haemangiomas are usually large and have undergone an increase in size and become tender when the thrombocytopenia develops, but a low-grade version can occur in hereditary haemorrhagic telangiectasia.

Thrombotic thrombocytopenic purpura (TTP, Moschowitz's syndrome) [13–20] in adults and haemolytic–uraemic syndrome (HUS) in children are rare forms of thrombotic microangiopathy in which thrombocytopenic purpura and bleeding are associated with fever, haemolytic anaemia and renal and neurological symptoms. HUS has recently been shown to involve a severe prothrombotic coagulation disturbance before onset of clinical features; the main clinically apparent feature is bloody diarrhoea due to Shiga toxin from *Escherichia coli* (mainly serotype 0157:H7). TTP is multifactorial, and may occur due to neoplasia, drugs, infections or organ transplantation, but many cases are due to an acquired autoimmune deficiency of ADAMTS13 (a metalloprotease). Platelets adhere to 'ultra-large' von Willebrand factor (ULVWF) multimers that are secreted from endothelial cells, and are normally cleaved by ADAMTS13; failure of this control mechanism leads to platelet-rich thrombotic microvascular plugging. Schistocytes (fragmented erythrocytes) are seen on blood films. Microvascular injury and intraluminal platelet thrombosis, and platelet plugging in myeloproliferative disorders, are discussed in more detail on p. 49.27.

References

1 Visentin GP, Liu CY. Drug-induced thrombocytopenia. *Haematol Oncol Clin N Am* 2007; **21**: 685–96.

2 George JN, Shattil SJ. The clinical importance of acquired abnormalities of platelet function. *N Engl J Med* 1991; **324**: 27–39.

3 Bruinsma W. *A Guide to Drug Eruptions*. Amsterdam: Excerpta Medica, 1973: 55–8.

4 Bork K. *Cutaneous Side-effects of Drugs*. Philadelphia: Saunders, 1988: 191.

5 Hostetler SG, Zirwas M, Bechtel MA. Efalizumab-associated thrombocytopenia. *J Am Acad Dermatol* 2007; **57**: 707–10.

6 Aster RH. Can drugs cause autoimmune thrombocytopenic purpura? *Semin Hematol* 2000; **37**: 229–38.

7 Fabris F, Luzzatto G, Stefani PM *et al*. Heparin-induced thrombocytopenia. *Haematologica* 2000; **85**: 72–81.

8 Warkentin TE. Heparin-induced thrombocytopenia. *Haematol Oncol Clin N Am* 2007; **21**: 589–607.

9 Stricker H, Lämmle B, Furlan M, Sulzer I. Heparin-dependent in vitro aggregation of normal platelets by plasma of a patient with heparin-induced skin necrosis: specific diagnostic test for a rare side-effect. *Am J Med* 1988; **85**: 721–4.

10 Arnold DM, Kelton JG. Heparin-induced thrombocytopenia: an iceberg rising. *Mayo Clin Proc* 2005; **80**: 988–90.

11 Warkentin TE. Think of HIT. *Hematology Am Soc Hematol Educ Program* 2006: 408–14.

12 Hoppensteadt DA, Walenga JM. The relationship between the antiphospholipid syndrome and heparin-induced thrombocytopenia. *Haematol Oncol Clin N Am* 2007; **21**: 1–18.

13 McCrae KR, Bussel JB, Mannucci PM *et al*. Platelets: an update on diagnosis and management of thrombocytopenic disorders. *Hematology Am Soc Hematol Educ Program* 2001: 282–305.

14 Moake JL. Thrombotic microangiopathies. *N Engl J Med* 2002; **347**: 589–600.

15 Elliott MA, Nichols WL. Thrombotic thrombocytopenic purpura and hemolytic uremic syndrome. *Mayo Clin Proc* 2001; **76**: 1154–62.

16 Grabowski EF. The hemolytic-uremic syndrome—toxin, thrombin and thrombosis. *N Engl J Med* 2002; **346**: 58–61.

17 Chandler WL, Jelacic S, Boster DR *et al*. Prothrombotic coagulation abnormalities preceding the hemolytic–uremic syndrome. *N Engl J Med* 2002; **346**: 23–32.

18 Sadler JE, Moake JL, Miyata T, George JN. Recent advances in thrombotic thrombocytopenic purpura. *Hematology Am Soc Hematol Educ Program* 2004: 407–23.

19 Sadler JE. Thrombotic thrombocytopenic purpura: a moving target. *Hematology Am Soc Hematol Educ Program* 2006: 415–20.

20 Tsai H-M. Thrombotic thrombocytopenic purpura: a thrombotic disorder caused by ADAMTS13 deficiency. *Hematol Oncol Clin N Am* 2007; **21**: 1773–7.

Abnormalities of platelet function

Several haemorrhagic syndromes have become recognized in which platelet function is abnormal although the total count may be normal [1–5] (Table 49.3). Such changes may be inherited, idiopathic or secondary to drugs or many other illnesses. These syndromes include thrombopathia, thrombasthenia, von Willebrand's disease, severe anaemia, chronic renal failure and fibrinogen defects. Hermansky–Pudlak syndrome consists of a bleeding disorder due to storage pool disorder, with oculocutaneous albinism and pigment-containing cells in the bone marrow (see Chapter 58). Laboratory testing of platelet function is of limited direct relevance to dermatologists but is reviewed in [6].

Drugs that may cause abnormal platelet function with clinical bleeding include aspirin, NSAIDs, some penicillin and β-lactam antibiotics (especially high-dose penicillin), alteplase and other antifibrinolytic drugs, prostacyclin, thienopyridines (ticlopidine and clopidogrel), glycoprotein IIb/IIIa antagonists (see below), cardiovascular drugs (nitrates, calcium channel blockers and quinidine), antidepressants and phenothiazines, and some chemotherapeutic agents such as mitomycin and daunorubicin [3–5]. Volume expanders such as dextran or hydroxyethylstarch, and radiocontrast media, are often forgotten as a cause of platelet dysfunction but can be particularly important in intensive care

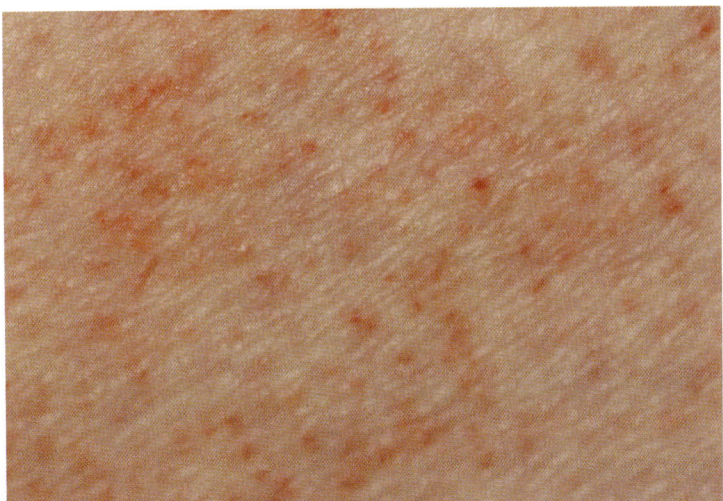

Fig. 49.3 Purpura due to a calcium channel antagonist, an effect probably caused by platelet dysfunction.

situations, as can fibrinolytic agents such as streptokinase, and agents that increase platelet cAMP levels such as iloprost or prostacyclin. Natural and herbal remedy agents that can cause platelet dysfunction include fish oil, garlic, cumin, turmeric, *Gingko biloba* and black tree fungus [5]. In some instances, the mechanisms are well-understood but in others they are obscure. Aspirin causes irreversible acetylation of platelet cyclo-oxygenase-1 (COX-1), thereby inhibiting thromboxane A_2 (TXA$_2$) synthesis. NSAIDs also inhibit COX-1 but reversibly, such that platelet function recovers quickly once the agents are stopped [2]. COX-II inhibitors have no direct effect on platelets, which do not express COX-II; they may in fact increase thrombosis by an indirect effect as they block prostacyclin production, and prostacyclin has an inhibitory effect on platelet function. Clopidogrel (like ticlopidine) irreversibly binds to platelet purinergic receptor P2Y$_{12}$, blocking response to intrinsic platelet-generated and extrinsic ADP, with a biological half-life of about 3 days. Antagonists of the platelet glycoprotein IIb/IIIa (integrin αIIβ3), such as abciximab, tirofiban and eptifibatide, are strong inhibitors of platelet function, used in coronary artery surgery. Purpura, as provoked by Hess testing, sometimes with clinical bleeding but with normal platelet numbers, appears to be a class effect of calcium channel blockers [7] (Fig. 49.3); although the vasodilating action of such drugs cannot be excluded as a contributory cause, a platelet function abnormality seems most likely. Many other drugs may cause abnormal platelet aggregation *in vitro*, sometimes with abnormal bleeding time, but not necessarily with clinical bleeding [3–5].

Drug-induced platelet function abnormalities are of potential relevance to dermatologists because of issues regarding bleeding during skin surgery. Aspirin, NSAIDs, clopidogrel and calcium channel blockers have all been implicated in bleeding related to skin (and other) surgery, and whether to transiently discontinue such medications needs to be considered, as well as considering anticoagulant monitoring results, as part of the pre-operative management [7–11]. A questionnaire study suggested that stopping warfarin or aspirin before dermatological surgery might cause a thrombotic risk (1/6219 operations for warfarin and 1/21448 operations for aspirin), but only a third of surveyed sur-

geons responded, there was no control population considered and no contemporaneous estimate of recalled significant bleeding [12]. Recent studies still conflict to some extent; some feel that the risks of operative bleeding due to aspirin [13], warfarin (with an international normalized ratio (INR) below 3.5) [14], or either drug [15], does not warrant stopping these treatments provided that careful attention is paid to haemostasis. However, there is some evidence that being on two or more different antithrombotic agents does increase the risk of bleeding after skin surgery [16], warfarin has been shown to increase risk of surgical bleeding in dermatology, an INR in the normal range being a poor predictor of this complication [17], and the combination of diltiazem and aspirin in normal subjects has a partially additive effect on platelet function (causing a bleeding time of over 15 min in two of five patients in one study [18]). These medications should probably be continued, but the risk of postoperative bleeding needs to be explained, particularly for difficult closures and body sites where application of pressure is awkward; the need for antithrombotic therapy (especially multiple therapies) and the risk to the patient of stopping treatment may need to be considered, and careful peroperative haemostasis should be performed.

Causes of abnormal platelet function may overlap with causes of thrombocytopenia. For example, both may occur in chronic renal failure (in which the abnormality of function is most important) or in myeloproliferative disorders (in which thrombocytopenia is usually paramount). Patients with Waldenström's macroglobulinaemia often have abnormal platelet function, less commonly those with IgA myeloma or benign monoclonal gammopathy, but bleeding in these conditions is usually due to hyperviscosity rather than to the platelet function defect. The platelet function defect is usually due to non-specific binding of immunoglobulin to platelets, but in some of these disorders other mechanisms may also be pertinent, including thrombocytopenia, inhibition or increased clearance of clotting factors and the hyperviscosity component.

Skin diseases in themselves may also alter platelet function in diverse ways, for example in eczemas, urticaria and psoriasis, potentially influencing expression of immune system inflammatory mediators [19].

References

1 Handin RI. Inherited platelet disorders. *Hematology Am Soc Hematol Educ Program* 2005: 396–402.
2 Neunert CE, Journeycake JM. Congenital platelet disorders. *Hematol Oncol Clin N Am* 2007; **21**: 663–84.
3 George JN, Shattil SJ. The clinical importance of acquired abnormalities of platelet function. *N Engl J Med* 1991; **324**: 27–39.
4 Hassan AA, Kroll MH. Acquired disorders of platelet function. *Hematology Am Soc Hematol Educ Program* 2005: 403–8.
5 Shen Y-MP, Frenkel EP. Acquired platelet dysfunction. *Hematol Oncol Clin N Am* 2007; **21**: 647–61.
6 Seegmiller A, Sarode R. Laboratory evaluation of platelet function. *Hematol Oncol Clin N Am* 2007; **21**: 731–42.
7 Cox NH, Walsh ML, Robson RH. Purpura and bleeding due to calcium channel blockers: an underestimated problem? Case reports and a pilot study. *Clin Exp Dermatol* 2009; **34**: 487–91.
8 Wagenknecht LE, Furberg CD, Hammon JW *et al*. Surgical bleeding: unexpected effect of a calcium antagonist. *BMJ* 1995; **310**: 776–7.
9 Yesudian PD, Velangi SS, Velangi MR *et al*. Postoperative bleeding in a patient on diltiazem. *Br J Dermatol* 2001; **145** (Suppl. 59): 87.

10 Stables G, Lawrence CM. Management of patients taking anticoagulant, non-steroidal anti-inflammatory and other anti-platelet drugs undergoing dermatological surgery. *Clin Exp Dermatol* 2002; **27**: 632–5.

11 Lawrence C, Sakuntabhai A, Tiling-Grosse S. Effect of aspirin and nonsteroidal antiinflammatory drug therapy on bleeding complications in dermatologic surgical patients. *J Am Acad Dermatol* 1994; **31**: 988–92.

12 Kovich O, Otley OC. Thrombotic complications related to discontinuation of warfarin and aspirin therapy perioperatively for cutaneous operation. *J Am Acad Dermatol* 2003; **48**: 233–7.

13 Fijnheer R, Urbanus RT, Nieuwenhuis HK. Withdrawing the use of acetylsalicylic acid prior to an operation is usually not necessary. *Ned Tijdschr Geneeskd* 2003; **147**: 31–5.

14 Ah-Weng A, Natarajan S, Velangi S, Langtry JAA. Preoperative monitoring of warfarin in cutaneous surgery. *Br J Dermatol* 2003; **149**: 386–9.

15 Shalom A, Klein D, Friedman T, Westreich M. Lack of complications in minor skin lesion excisions in patients taking aspirin or warfarin products. *Am Surg* 2008; **74**: 354–7.

16 Shimizu I, Jellinek NJ, Dufresne RG *et al.* Multiple antithrombotic agents increase the risk of postoperative hemorrhage in dermatologic surgery. *J Am Acad Dermatol* 2008; **58**: 810–6.

17 Blasdale C, Lawrence CM. Perioperative international normalized ratio level is a poor predictor of postoperative bleeding complications in dermatological surgery patients taking warfarin. *Br J Dermatol* 2008; **158**: 522–6.

18 Ring ME, Corrigan JJ Jr, Fenster PE. Effects of oral diltiazem on platelet function: alone and in combination with 'low dose' aspirin. *Thromb Res* 1986; **44**: 391–400.

19 Kasperska-Zajac A, Brzoza Z, Rogala B. Platelet function in cutaneous diseases. *Platelets* 2008; **19**: 317–21.

Thrombocytosis

Abnormally high platelet counts may occur as a result of essential thrombocythaemia or other myeloproliferative disorders, or secondary to a variety of other disease processes (see Table 49.3). This may lead to a tendency to platelet plugging and thrombosis or, paradoxically, to a bleeding tendency (particularly when the platelet count exceeds 1000×10^9/L with a clonal platelet defect such as an acquired form of storage pool disease). Many cases of thrombocytosis do not achieve this high platelet count and are unlikely to cause purpura unless there are additional reasons related to the causative disorder (such as lymphoma or other malignant disease).

Dermatological manifestations and associations of thrombocythaemia include purpura with or without necrosis, livedo reticularis, acrocyanosis, purple (blue) toe syndrome, Raynaud's phenomenon, erythromelalgia, other vascular symptoms including gangrene, and associated disorders such as pyoderma gangrenosum [1–9]. The last-mentioned is relatively uncommon in pure thrombocythaemia [7] (the patient described in [7] subsequently developed further myeloproliferative features; cited in [8]). In one large study, 22% of patients with essential thrombocythaemia had skin lesions; 41% of these had haematomas, ecchymosis, petechiae or purpura, and 26% had erythromelalgia [9]. Many of these presentations are also seen in other hyperviscosity and dysproteinaemic conditions.

Platelet hyper-reactivity is not usually a dermatological consideration, but it is a factor in peripheral arterial disease and thrombotic emboli [10]. It is more common in females, linked with higher mean platelet volume and higher fibrinogen levels, and is partly genetically determined (especially associated with integrin α2 and β3 mutations that lead to high platelet glycoprotein IIb/IIIa levels).

References

1 Champion RH, Rook A. Idiopathic thrombocythemia: cutaneous manifestations. *Arch Dermatol* 1963; **87**: 302–5.

2 Amblard P, Lèques B, Seigneurin D *et al.* Manifestations cutanées des thrombocytémies. *Ann Dermatol Vénéréol* 1977; **104**: 115–20.

3 Singh AK, Wetherley-Mein G. Microvascular lesions in primary thrombocythaemia. *Br J Haematol* 1977; **36**: 553–64.

4 Preston FE, Emmanuel IG, Winfield DA, Malia RG. Essential thrombocythaemia and peripheral gangrene. *BMJ* 1974; **ii**: 548–52.

5 Martin EA, Lavin PJ, Thompson AJ. Painful extremities and neurological disorder in essential thrombocythaemia. *J R Soc Med* 1984; **77**: 372–4.

6 Hachulla E, Rose C, Trillot N *et al.* What vascular events suggest a myeloproliferative disorder? *J Mal Vasc* 2000; **25**: 382–7.

7 Shepherd P, Liddell K. Pyoderma gangrenosum associated with primary thrombocythaemia. *BMJ* 1982; **285**: 837–8.

8 Cox NH, White SI, Walton S *et al.* Pyoderma gangrenosum associated with polycythaemia rubra vera. *Clin Exp Dermatol* 1987; **12**: 375–7.

9 Itin PH, Winkelmann RK. Cutaneous manifestations in patients with essential thrombocythemia. *J Am Acad Dermatol* 1991; **24**: 59–63.

10 Bray PF. Platelet hyperreactivity: predictive and intrinsic properties. *Hematol Oncol Clin N Am* 2007; **21**: 633–45.

Non-thrombocytopenic vascular causes of purpura and syndromes of primarily ecchymotic haemorrhage

A number of disorders cause purpura or ecchymosis due to vascular fragility/poor dermal support, intravascular pressure increase, platelet dysfunction (see also earlier), thrombocytosis (above) or coagulation cascade defects (Table 49.4). Minor trauma is often the precipitant of lesions. Disorders in which inflammation around vessels leads to purpura are discussed separately; these include the pigmented purpuric dermatoses and several conditions in which there is non-specific inflammation.

Purpura due to raised intravascular pressure

Raised intravascular pressure may cause purpura in the absence of any other disease. Crops of petechiae after prolonged coughing or vomiting occur, especially on the relatively loose tissues of the face and neck (see Fig. 49.1). They are of no significance other than causing concern if their cause is not appreciated.

Gravity and venous stasis are the most important causes of this type of purpura. Many purpuric eruptions are maximal on, or even restricted to, the lower leg. Likewise, many erythematous eruptions on the lower legs, especially in the elderly or those with leg oedema, show some degree of purpura that can usually be ignored. Bizarre patterns of purpura should always suggest the possibility of artefact.

Deaths from asphyxia are said to be associated with facial and conjunctival petechiae but the mechanism is probably due to vascular occlusion causing raised intravascular pressure rather than to hypoxia *per se* [1].

Purpura due to abnormal blood vessels or decreased support of blood vessels

Several disorders are associated with abnormal collagen, elastic or other structural proteins, leading to abnormal vessels or poor dermal support or both (Table 49.4). Conditions such as Ehlers–Danlos syndrome (collagen), pseudoxanthoma elasticum (elastic)

Table 49.4 Some dermatologically-relevant non-thrombocytopenic causes of purpura, easy bruising or cutaneous bleeding.

Type of disorder	Examples
Inherited defects affecting structural components of the dermis and/or vascular wall	Ehlers–Danlos syndrome* Marfan syndrome* Osteogenesis imperfecta Pseudoxanthoma elasticum
Acquired defects affecting structural components of the dermis and/or vascular wall	Deposition disorders, e.g. amyloidosis† Solar damage (solar/actinic purpura) Scurvy
Haemangiomatous disorders	Cavernous haemangioma† Hereditary haemorrhagic telangiectasia*†
Clotting factor and related inherited or acquired deficiencies	Haemophilias Von Willebrand disease Vitamin K deficiency Other nutritional deficiencies (often mixed)
Non-thrombocytopenic platelet abnormalities	See Table 49.3
Biochemical (congenital or acquired)	Homocystinuria Hyperhomocystinaemia*† Diabetes mellitus Cushing's syndrome
Collagen vascular disorders	Systemic sclerosis Dermatomyositis
Paraproteinaemias and hyperviscosity	Waldenström's macroglobulinaemia* Other paraproteinaemias*
Intra- or perivascular inflammation	Capillaropathies (see p. 49.22) Vasculitides (Chapter 50) Behçet's disease (Chapter 50) Many inflammatory dermatoses
Microvascular occlusion	See p. 49.26
Infection	See p. 49.20
Increased pressure within vessels	Valsalva manoeuvre Cough purpura Distal to a sphygmomanometer cuff
Physical	Simple trauma Venous rupture (Achenbach's syndrome) Artefactual Chemical and mechanical contact irritants (p. 49.21)
Drugs	Drugs altering vascular permeability or causing direct endothelial damage (p. 49.21) Antiangiogenic drugs
Others	Malignant hypertension Autoerythrocyte sensitization

* May also have platelet dysfunction.

† May also have clotting factor abnormalities.

and amyloidosis (abnormal protein) are discussed in more detail elsewhere. Facial or periorbital purpura ('panda sign') occurs in 15% of patients with primary amyloidosis [2]. In osteogenesis imperfecta, bruising tends to occur rather than purpura; both occur in Ehlers–Danlos and Marfan syndromes and in osteogenesis imperfecta [3] (as well as frank bleeding in Ehlers–Danlos syndrome and osteogenesis imperfecta). In hereditary haemorrhagic telangiectasia (Chapter 47) there may be bleeding from telangiectasias; the structural vascular defects may be accompanied by platelet and other haemostatic defects. Paraproteins act in various ways, causing coating of endothelial cells, occlusion of vasa vasora, and also causing platelet dysfunction as discussed earlier. In Cushing's syndrome, loss of dermal mucopolysaccharides that normally support the vessels, and of elastic tissue from the dermis and from vessels, may be the explanation for purpura; deposition of fibrin leading to thrombosis and 'downstream' capillary stasis is thought to explain purpura in malignant hypertension, diabetes mellitus and chronological ageing.

Scurvy is discussed in more detail in Chapter 59. Altered collagenous support for the blood vessels is manifest by either petechiae, especially on the legs, or by small or large bruises on the limbs following mild or inapparent trauma. Large deep bruises may lead to woody induration, usually of the legs. Perifollicular purpura is typical but is not diagnostic and is frequently absent. Diagnosis is established by the associated symptoms and signs (twisted 'corkscrew' hairs, gingival bleeding), dietary history, laboratory tests and therapeutic response.

Actinic purpura (*Bateman's purpura*, *'senile' purpura*) and *corticosteroid purpura* [4,5] are the commonest patterns of purpura due to lack of support of the blood vessels. They occur most commonly in skin altered by both age and solar radiation, but may occur in premature ageing syndromes. Corticosteroid purpura has the same pattern whether due to topical, oral, endogenous (Cushing's syndrome) or even inhaled [6] corticosteroids. The precipitating factor is a shearing stress. Patients who develop this type of purpura with ageing, in association with rheumatoid arthritis or with corticosteroids, are more liable to develop osteoporosis of the spine than patients without this sign [7]. The purpura occurs mainly in atrophic skin on exposed parts of the hands and forearms, or on the legs. Lesions appear after minor trauma or apparently spontaneously. They are usually asymptomatic and vary in size from a few millimetres to several centimetres across. They are often arranged linearly, and may show a linear or geometric shape. The appearance of the lesions is characteristic, with irregular areas, usually not palpable, that show little inflammatory reaction and which are usually dark purple rather than having the sequential colour changes of a normal bruise. They may persist for several weeks. Treatment is usually not necessary or possible.

References

1 Ely SF, Hirsch CS. Asphyxial deaths and petechiae: a review. *J Forensic Sci* 2000; **45**: 1274–7.
2 Kyle RA, Gertz MA. Primary systemic amyloidosis: clinical and laboratory features in 474 cases. *Semin Hematol* 1995; **32**: 45–59.
3 Bick R. Vascular thrombohemorrhagic disorders: hereditary and acquired. *Clin Appl Thrombosis Hemostasis* 2001; **7**: 178–94.
4 Feinstein RJ, Halprin KM, Penneys NS *et al.* Senile purpura. *Arch Dermatol* 1973; **108**: 229–32.
5 Shuster S, Scarborough H. Senile purpura. *QJM* 1961; **30**: 33–40.
6 Capewell S, Reynolds S, Shuttleworth D *et al.* Purpura and dermal thinning associated with high dose inhaled corticosteroids. *BMJ* 1990; **300**: 1548–51.
7 McConkey B, Fraser GM, Bligh AS. Osteoporosis and purpura in rheumatoid disease: prevalence and relation to treatment with corticosteroids. *QJM* 1962; **31**: 419–27.

Easy bruising syndrome and purpura simplex

The term 'easy bruising syndrome' has been used in various ways, usually for a mild purpura for which no cause has been detected, especially on the thighs of women ('devil's pinches'). It has been used to include those cases of a mild bleeding tendency in which changes in the morphology of capillaries may be seen by capillary microscopy, and in some of which variable but slight changes in coagulation factors have also been found. There are significant limitations in deciding what constitutes 'abnormal' or excessive bleeding [1]. The term 'purpura simplex' has also been used for any inflammatory purpura without vasculitis, including disorders with the morphology of the pigmented purpuric dermatoses [2,3], and this term is therefore also of uncertain value. Autosomal dominant inheritance of purpura simplex has been reported [4] and presumably represents a subtle haemostatic defect; in one family, purpura simplex was coinherited with ptosis [5].

References

1 George JN, Shattil SJ. The clinical importance of acquired abnormalities of platelet function. *N Engl J Med* 1991; **324**: 27–39.
2 Lee GR, Bithell TC, Foerster J *et al.*, eds. *Wintrobe's Clinical Hematology*, 9th edn. Philadelphia: Lea & Febiger, 1993.
3 Ratnam KV, Daniel Su WP. Purpura simplex (inflammatory purpura without vasculitis): a clinicopathologic study of 174 cases. *J Am Acad Dermatol* 1991; **25**: 642–7.
4 Davis E. Hereditary familial purpura simplex. *Lancet* 1941; **i**: 145–6.
5 Fisher B, Zuckerman GH, Douglas RC. Combined inheritance of purpura simplex and ptosis in 4 generations of one family. *Blood* 1954; **9**: 1199–204.

Physical and artefactual causes of purpura

Bruising due to trauma seldom causes diagnostic problems, as there is usually a clear history, except when it occurs as an artefact or in child abuse. Bizarre patterns of purpura may be caused by suction, for example vacuum extractors in the neonate, electrocardiogram leads or around the mouth after sucking out the air from a glass [1]. Cultural remedies such as cupping, coin rubbing (Cao Gio) and spooning (Quat sha) may also produce unusual patterns of purpura that are usually obviously extrinsic in causation [2]. Black heel (talon noire) is a form of purpura due to frictional shearing of vessels, and is considered in Chapter 28.

Paroxysmal finger haematoma [3–5]

Synonym
- Achenbach's syndrome

In this syndrome there are recurrent episodes of painful bruising on the palms and palmar aspects of the fingers (Fig. 49.4). It seems likely that it represents venous rupture, as frictional trauma may be reported, such as turning on a tap or twisting the top off a jar. It is probably more common than the number of reported cases would suggest. Its importance is that it may be confused with Raynaud's phenomenon or acute connective tissue diseases and investigated unnecessarily.

Autoerythrocyte sensitization syndrome [6–9]

Synonyms
- Painful bruising syndrome
- Gardner–Diamond syndrome

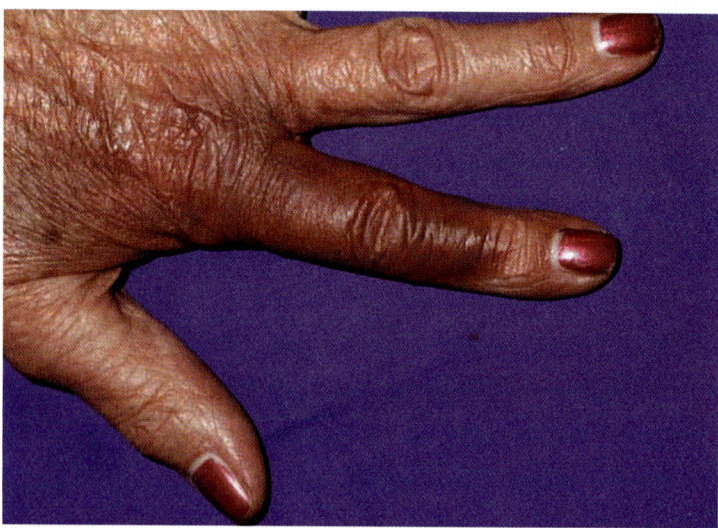

Fig. 49.4 Achenbach's syndrome; acute bruising of the entire finger, presumably due to venous rupture after minor trauma.

This is a distinctive but rare clinical entity apparently due, in many cases, to allergic sensitivity to red cells in the tissues. Minor extravasations of blood, for example those so common on the thighs of women, are followed by an intense inflammatory reaction. The disease occurs most frequently in young adult and middle-aged females, who are nearly always psychiatrically abnormal. They present with recurrent, painful erythematous and purpuric lesions on the thighs and elsewhere. The diagnosis may be confirmed by intradermal injections of red cells or their washed stroma, or of phosphatidylcholine. This reaction occurs even in some subjects in whom a psychological cause is suspected and whose disease responds to psychological intervention [10,11].

Sensitivity to DNA [12,13] or to exogenous antigens attached to red cells [14] may present a similar picture. The condition is usually chronic, seldom disabling or associated with other abnormalities and is unresponsive to treatment. Plasmapheresis has been used successfully in isolated cases [15] and antimalarials are said to be effective in DNA sensitivity [16]. Dermatitis artefacta may produce a similar clinical picture, and is believed by some to account for all such cases [8,11,17].

Stigmata

In this very rare disorder there is exudation of apparently fresh blood through the unbroken skin of the hands, feet and side. The mechanism is obscure but, as with the previous syndrome, many if not all cases may have a traumatic origin [8,18].

References

1 Metzker A, Merlob P. Suction purpura. *Arch Dermatol* 1992; **128**: 822–4.
2 Pride HB. Child abuse and mimickers of child abuse. *Adv Dermatol* 1999; **14**: 417–55.
3 Layton AM, Cotterill JA. A case of Achenbach's syndrome. *Clin Exp Dermatol* 1993; **18**: 60–1.
4 Parslew R, Verbov JL. Achenbach syndrome. *Br J Dermatol* 1995; **132**: 319.
5 Stieler W, Heinze-Werlitz C. Paroxysmal finger hematoma (Achenbach syndrome). *Hautarzt* 1990; **41**: 270–1.
6 Gardner FH, Diamond LK. Auto-erythrocyte sensitisation. *Blood* 1955; **10**: 675–90.
7 Hersle K, Mobacken H. Auto-erythrocyte sensitisation syndrome (painful bruising syndrome). *Br J Dermatol* 1969; **81**: 574–87.

8 Ratnoff OD. The psychogenic purpuras: a review of autoerythrocyte sensitisation, autosensitisation to DNA, 'hysterical' and factitial bleeding and the religious stigmata. *Semin Hematol* 1980; **17**: 192–213.

9 Berman DA, Roenigk HH, Green D. Autoerythrocyte sensitization syndrome (psychogenic purpura). *J Am Acad Dermatol* 1992; **27**: 829–32.

10 Uthman IW, Moukarbel GV, Salman SM *et al.* Autoerythrocyte sensitization (Gardner–Diamond) syndrome. *Eur J Haematol* 2000; **65**: 144–7.

11 Cox NH, Wilkinson DS. Dermatitis artefacta as the presenting feature of autoerythrocyte sensitization syndrome and naproxen-induced pseudoporphyria in a single patient. *Br J Dermatol* 1992; **126**: 86–9.

12 Little AS, Bell HE. Painful subcutaneous haemorrhages of the extremities with unusual reaction to injected deoxyribonucleic acid. *Ann Intern Med* 1964; **60**: 886–91.

13 Chandler D, Nalbandian RM. DNA autosensitivity. *Am J Med Sci* 1966; **251**: 145–9.

14 Shelley WB, Florence R. Chronic urticaria due to mold hypersensitivity. *Arch Dermatol* 1961; **83**: 549–58.

15 Hamblin TJ, Hart S, Mufti GJ. Plasmapheresis and a placebo procedure in autoerythrocyte sensitisation. *BMJ* 1981; **81**: 1575–6.

16 Sams WM Jr. Macular purpuras. In: Sams WM Jr, Lynch P, eds. *Principles and Practice of Dermatology*, 2nd edn. New York: Churchill Livingstone, 1996: 559–64.

17 Stefanini M, Blumgart ET. Purpura factitia. *Arch Dermatol* 1972; **106**: 238–41.

18 Simpson CJ. The stigmata: pathology or miracle? *BMJ* 1984; **289**: 1746–8.

Purpura in other dermatoses

Many eruptions on the lower leg, especially in the elderly, tend to become purpuric due to a combination of gravitational changes with vascular damage caused by the dermatosis. Rapid development of lower leg oedema may cause an eczematous eruption in which purpura may be prominent [1].

Even without the gravitational component, many dermatoses may be sufficiently intense to cause purpura. Sometimes this is physically due to scratching, but some disorders such as lichen planus, lichen nitidus and Langerhans' cell histiocytosis are not infrequently purpuric. Purpuric erythema annulare centrifugum, dermatitis herpetiformis, pemphigoid, pityriasis rosea and eczemas (especially of discoid type) may all occur. Purpura may be present in lymphomas and lupus erythematosus, either because of platelet deficiency or, more commonly, because of vascular abnormalities.

Lichen sclerosus often has a haemorrhagic component due to loss of collagenous support for the vessels.

Some insect bite reactions have a purpuric centre due to inoculation of the skin with anticoagulant chemicals in the bite (purpura pulicosa, maculae ceruleae).

Purpura may also occur around localized lesions with a strong vascular component if there are fragile vessels, for example targetoid haemosiderotic haemangioma or aneurysmal fibrous histiocytoma.

A rather characteristic disorder of children under the age of 1 year has been termed the *persistent acrovasculopathy syndrome*. Lesions occur on the ears, cheeks and extremities and are scaly and erosive; they may be purpuric, and there may be local lipoatrophy and distal phalangeal osteopenia.

Most of these conditions are discussed in more detail in other chapters; two disorders are specifically described here.

Solar purpura [2–5]

This condition is distinct from the actinic purpura discussed previously which is a manifestation of cumulative sunlight-induced

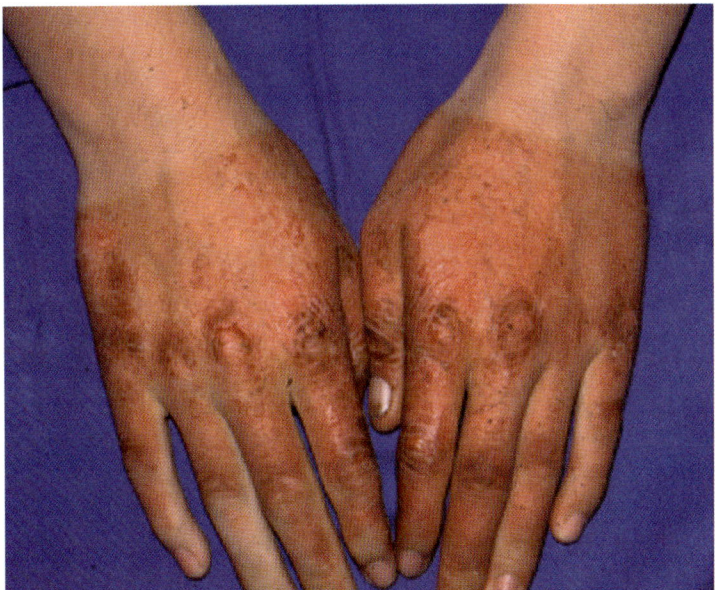

Fig. 49.5 Erythropoietic protoporphyria: marked purpura with sharp cut-off after sunlight exposure.

ageing of the skin. The term 'solar purpura' is used to describe rapid development of purpuric lesions after exposure to sunlight. The precise nature of this disorder is uncertain. Some view it as a variant of polymorphic light eruption. It is distinct from erythropoietic protoporphyria, although purpura clearly occurs in this dermatosis in some patients (Fig. 49.5). Some cases may simply be a variation of purpura in dermatoses that are not usually purpuric, but where profound inflammation has allowed purpura to develop.

Acroangiodermatitis (of Mali) [6–8]

Synonyms
- Dermite ocre of Favre
- Gravitational purpura
- Pseudo-Kaposi's sarcoma

This chronic dermatosis is associated with venous insufficiency or with vascular anomalies such as Klippel–Trenaunay syndrome [9], and there are several reports of it occurring as a stump dermatosis in amputees [10]. It has been reported in a patient with a thrombophilic prothrombin mutation [11]. It may mimic a pigmented purpuric dermatosis (p. 49.22) but is discussed here as the purpura is due to abnormal vasculature rather than to capillaritis. It occurs more often in men than in women.

The lesions occur especially on the lower legs but may extend on to the dorsa of the feet and toes, and up the leg, especially over dilated varicosities. Individual lesions are minute purpuric macules that coalesce to form irregular plaques, which may be several centimetres in diameter. Follicular lesions may occur. The colour of the lesions is not usually the purple colour of fresh purpura but varying shades of yellow (ochre) and brown from haemosiderin and other breakdown products. The epidermis may be normal or show mild eczematous changes. Oedema, sclerosis, ulceration and other signs of venous insufficiency may be associated, but may be entirely absent even in cases of long duration.

Differential diagnosis includes ordinary gravitational dermatitis, Schamberg's disease and Kaposi's sarcoma; the last mentioned can be distinguished by the staining pattern with CD34 antigen, which stains perivascular spindle cells in Kaposi's sarcoma but only the endothelial cells in acroangiodermatitis [12]. Treatment is unsatisfactory but support hosiery seems logical.

References

1 Bhushan M, Cox NH, Chalmers R. Eczema craquelé due to oedema. *Br J Dermatol* 2001; **145**: 355–7.
2 Leung AKC. Purpura associated with exposure to sunlight. *J R Soc Med* 1986; **79**: 423–4.
3 Kalivas J, Kalivas L. Solar purpura appearing in a patient with polymorphous light reaction. *Photodermatol Photoimmunol Photomed* 1995; **11**: 31–2.
4 Guarrera M, Parodi A, Rebora A. Solar purpura is not related to polymorphous light eruption. *Photodermatol* 1989; **6**: 293–4.
5 Torinuki W, Miura T. Erythropoietic protoporphyria showing solar purpura. *Dermatologica* 1983; **167**: 220–2.
6 Favre M. Angiodermite pigmentée et purpurique des membres inferieurs. In: Darier J, Sabouraud R, Gougerot H *et al. Nouvelle Pratique Dermatologie*, Vol. 5. Paris: Masson, 1936: 413–40.
7 Mali JWH, Kuiper JP, Hamers AA. Acro-angiodermatitis of the foot. *Arch Dermatol* 1965; **92**: 515–8.
8 Rao B, Unis M, Poulos E. Acroangiodermatitis: a study of ten cases. *Int J Dermatol* 1994; **33**: 179–83.
9 Lyle WG, Given KS. Acroangiodermatitis (pseudo-Kaposi's sarcoma) associated with Klippel–Trenaunay syndrome. *Ann Plast Surg* 1996; **37**: 654–6.
10 Badell A, Marcoval J, Graells J *et al.* Kaposi-like acroangiodermatitis induced by a suction-socket prosthesis. *Br J Dermatol* 1994; **131**: 915–7.
11 Martin L, MacHet L, Michalak S *et al.* Acroangiodermatitis in a carrier of the thrombophilic 20210A mutation in the prothrombin gene. *Br J Dermatol* 1999; **141**: 752.
12 Kanitakis J, Narvaez D, Claudy A. Expression of the CD34 antigen distinguishes Kaposi's sarcoma from pseudo-Kaposi's sarcoma (acroangiodermatitis). *Br J Dermatol* 1996; **134**: 44–6.

Multifactorial purpura associated with systemic diseases

Non-thrombocytopenic purpura may be caused by a variety of systemic diseases. Many of these have already been discussed, but in some cases there may be mixed mechanisms of purpura or easy bruising. Of these, renal disease is perhaps the most important; petechiae, ecchymoses or mucosal bleeding are common in end-stage renal failure [1]. Platelet dysfunction is probably the major factor [2], but there may also be frank thrombocytopenia. Diabetes, severe anaemia, liver disease, haemochromatosis and carcinomatosis may also cause purpura.

In amyloidosis, with or without myelomatosis, purpura may be due to infiltration of the capillaries and perivascular tissue with amyloid, but platelet changes and liver disease may also contribute.

Purpura occurs in patients with malnutrition. It seems probable that changes in coagulation, platelets and capillaries all play their part. For example, in cystic fibrosis there may be dysproteinaemia, vasculitis and vitamin K deficiency.

Purpura has been associated with ovarian and other endocrine abnormalities [3], for example Cushing's disease, and may vary with the menstrual cycle.

References

1 Remazzi G. Bleeding in renal failure. *Lancet* 1988; **i**: 1205–8.
2 George JN, Shattil SJ. The clinical importance of acquired abnormalities of platelet function. *N Engl J Med* 1991; **324**: 27–39.
3 Wells R. Haemorrhagic diathesis due to increased capillary fragility secondary to ovarian deficiency. *Lancet* 1958; **i**: 886–7.

Exercise-induced purpura/vasculitis

This is probably an underestimated condition, and histologically is a form of leukocytoclastic vasculitis [1,2]. It is therefore discussed in more detail in Chapter 50. The typical presentation is with purpuric lesions on the lower legs after prolonged walking (many descriptions are in golfers, marathon runners or long-distance walkers), usually in hot weather. Lesions may be urticarial. Patients are generally middle-aged, and otherwise well with no evidence of venous disease. Compression stockings may reduce its occurrence. It is discussed here as it can present as a pigmented purpuric dermatosis related to exercise [3], and has also been described in a child with recurrent purpura on the trunk after vigorous exercise [4].

References

1 Prins M, Veraart JC, Vermeulen AH *et al.* Leucocytoclastic vasculitis induced by prolonged exercise. *Br J Dermatol* 1996; **134**: 915–8.
2 Ramelet AA. Exercise-induced purpura. *Dermatology (Basel)* 2004; **208**: 293–6.
3 Allan SJR, Humphreys F, Buxton PK. Annular purpura and step aerobics. *Clin Exp Dermatol* 1994; **19**: 418.
4 Leung AK, Grant RM, Truscott R. Exercise-induced purpura. *J Sports Med Phys Fitness* 1990; **30**: 329–30.

Inflammatory haemorrhage: Henoch–Schönlein purpura and acute haemorrhagic oedema of childhood

Vessel damage with inflammation may lead to haemorrhage, typically manifest as palpable purpuric lesions. This is usually caused by one of the types of antigen–antibody reaction discussed in Chapter 13 but may be due to a direct toxic effect. The antigen in the allergic mechanism may be a component of the vessel itself or of surrounding tissues or, more commonly, an exogenous substance bound to the blood vessel or other tissues. Such substances include drugs, bacterial products and food additives; they may reach the blood vessel via the bloodstream or from the skin surface. The antigen–antibody reaction may occur on the surface of the endothelial cells or in adjacent tissues, or the vessels may be damaged by soluble complexes. The localization of many such lesions will be determined by local factors, for example changes due to gravity, cold and trauma. This inflammatory process is therefore a vasculitis, and is discussed in Chapter 50. Two conditions of this type are briefly discussed here, one because it carries the name purpura (Henoch–Schönlein purpura) and the other because it may present with striking haemorrhagic lesions (acute haemorrhagic oedema of childhood).

Henoch–Schönlein purpura (HSP, anaphylactoid purpura) is a vasculitic process due to IgA-immune complex deposition in the walls of arterioles and venules that gives rise to palpable inflammatory lesions; these are often purpuric as well as erythematous and may vary in size from 0.5 to 1 cm or more. However, minor lesions of HSP may sometimes be confused clinically with other types of purpura.

Acute haemorrhagic oedema of childhood is a small vessel cutaneous vasculitis; it has been proposed to be a variant of HSP, but IgA immune complexes often cannot be demonstrated. It has also been described as cocarde purpura, Seidlmayer's syndrome and Finkel-stein's disease. Most cases have been reported from continental Europe [1,2], but English [3] and American [4] cases are also reported. It may be overtly haemorrhagic, but can present as arci-form or annular brown lesions that are of acute onset but which have some morphological similarity to pigmented purpuric dermatoses.

References

1 Lambert D, Laurent R, Bouilly D *et al.* Oedème aigu hémorrhagique du nourisson. Données immunologiques et ultrastructurales. *Ann Dermatol Vénéréol* 1979; **106**: 975–87.
2 Legrain V, Lejean S, Täieb A *et al.* Infantile acute haemorrhagic edema of the skin: study of ten cases. *J Am Acad Dermatol* 1991; **24**: 17–22.
3 Cox NH. Seidlmayer's syndrome: postinfectious cockade purpura of early child-hood. *J Am Acad Dermatol* 1992; **26**: 275.
4 Cunningham BB, Caro WA, Eramo LR. Neonatal acute hemorrhagic edema of childhood: case report and review of the English-language literature. *Pediatr Dermatol* 1996; **13**: 39–44.

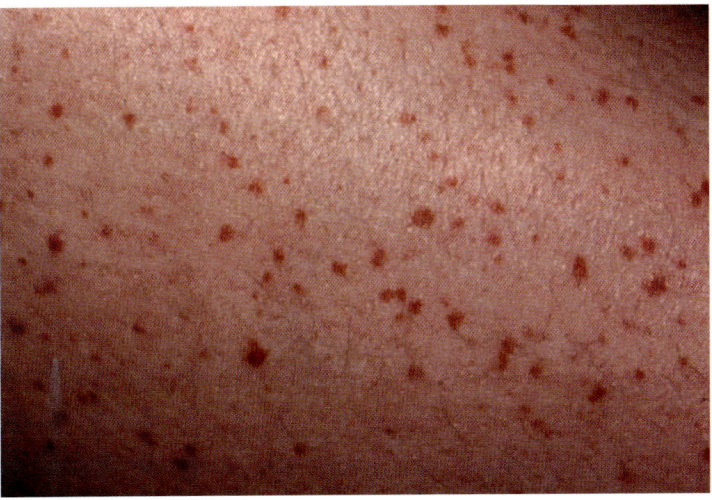

Fig. 49.6 Waldenström's hypergammaglobulinaemic purpura: lower leg lesions, in this patient usually provoked by prolonged standing or heat.

Dysproteinaemic purpura and Waldenström's hypergammaglobulinaemic purpura

Purpura may be the presenting and sometimes the only symptom of disturbances in plasma proteins. It may occur at exposed skin sites in cryoproteinaemia (see Chapter 28 and p. 49.32) and may occur due to monoclonal hypergammaglobulinaemia in myeloma. In such instances there may be platelet dysfunction, but clinical bleeding is usually related to the hyperviscosity syndrome rather than to the altered platelet function. Cutaneous features of para-proteinaemia include various patterns of vasculitis and neutro-philic dermatosis (see Chapter 50), cryoglobulinaemia (see below), urticaria and systemic capillary leak syndrome, abnormalities of lipid metabolism (notably diffuse plane xanthomatosis), subcor-neal pustular dermatosis, lichen myxoedematosus and sclero-myxoedema, amyloidosis, and features due to hyperviscosity (purpura, mucous membrane bleeding, retinopathy and neuro-logical disturbance) [1,2]. Haemorrhagic features are particularly seen in Waldenström's macroglobulinaemia.

Waldenström's hypergammaglobulinaemic purpura is generally taken to imply an idiopathic phenomenon but in fact two of Waldenström's three cases had sicca symptoms, one with sarcoid-osis [3]. Hypergammaglobulinaemic purpura is usually a poly-clonal disorder most commonly linked with sarcoidosis, lupus erythematosus, Sjögren's syndrome and other autoimmune condi-tions [4–10]. The majority of patients have positive antinuclear antibody and anti-SSA (Ro) or anti-SSB (La) antibodies [6–10]. Other features that have been associated include arthropathy (not uncommon), renal tubular acidosis, chest infections, lymphopenia and immune hypersensitivity pneumonitis. Most patients are female [11].

Clinically the pattern of purpura is often non-specific, usually consisting of crops of small erythematous macular or palpable purpuric spots on the lower leg (Fig. 49.6) [3–10], but unusual patterns with reticulate lesions may occur [12]. Prolonged walking, standing or sitting with the legs dependent, or other increase in venous pressure, may be an obvious provocative factor [9,10]. Itch or a burning sensation may occur. It is likely that this disorder is an immune complex vasculitis: immune complexes can be detected, histology may show vasculitic change, and direct immu-nofluorescence may show immunoglobulin in blood vessel walls [8,12,13]. Hyperviscosity leading to stasis and endothelial damage plays some part. There may be an abnormal ratio of IgG sub-classes, with low IgG1/IgG2 ratio [14].

Lesions usually resolve in about a week but may become con-fluent and permanent. Treatment is often not required, although prednisolone, NSAIDs, hydroxychloroquine and etamsylate (ethamsylate) have been used.

A similar pattern has been reported in association with cystic fibrosis, due to either hypergammaglobulinaemia or cryoglobu-linaemia [15,16]. It may appear suddenly, affects the lower legs mainly, and is exacerbated by prolonged standing or by tight gar-ments or footwear. It is associated with severe lung disease and poor prognosis; a high antigenic load due to chronic lung infection may be the cause.

References

1 Russell Jones R. The cutaneous manifestations of paraproteinaemia. I. *Br J Dermatol* 1980; **103**: 335–45.
2 Russell Jones R. The cutaneous manifestations of paraproteinaemia. II. *Br J Dermatol* 1981; **104**: 209–20.
3 Waldenström J. Three new cases of purpura hyperglobulinaemica. A study of a long-standing benign increase in serum globulin. *Acta Med Scand* 1952; **266** (Suppl.): 931–46.
4 Carr RD, Heisel EB. Purpura hyperglobulinemia. *Arch Dermatol* 1966; **94**: 536–41.
5 Kyle RA, Gleich GJ, Bayrd ED *et al.* Benign hypergammaglobulinemic purpura of Waldenström. *Medicine (Baltimore)* 1971; **50**: 113–23.
6 Finder KA, McCollough ML, Dixon SL *et al.* Hyperglobulinemic purpura of Waldenström. *J Am Acad Dermatol* 1990; **23**: 669–76.
7 Miyagawa S, Fukumoto T, Kanauchi M *et al.* Hypergammaglobulinaemic purpura of Waldenström and Ro/SSA autoantibodies. *Br J Dermatol* 1996; **134**: 919–23.
8 Sugai S, Shimizu S, Tachibana J *et al.* Hypergammaglobulinemic purpura in patients with Sjögren's syndrome: a report of nine cases and a review of the Japanese literature. *Jpn J Med* 1989; **28**: 148–55.
9 Malaviya AN, Kaushik P, Budhiraja S *et al.* Hypergammaglobulinaemic purpura of Waldenström: report of 3 cases with a short review. *Clin Exp Rheumatol* 2000; **18**: 518–22.
10 Senecal JL, Chartier S, Rothfield N. Hypergammaglobulinaemic purpura in sys-temic autoimmune rheumatic disease: predictive value of anti-Ro (SSA) and

anti-La (SSB) antibodies and treatment with indomethacin and hydroxychloroquine. *J Rheumatol* 1995; **22**: 868–75.

11 Olmstead AD, Zone JJ, La Salle B *et al.* Immune complexes in the pathogenesis of hypergammaglobulinemic purpura. *J Am Acad Dermatol* 1980; **3**: 174–9.

12 Tan E, Ng SK, Tan SH, Wong GC. Hypergammaglobulinaemic purpura presenting as reticulate purpura. *Clin Exp Dermatol* 1999; **24**: 469–72.

13 Lopez LR, Schocket AL, Carr RI, Kohler PF. Lymphocytotoxic antibodies and intermediate immune complexes in hypergammaglobulinaemic purpura of Waldenström. *Ann Allergy* 1988; **61**: 93–6.

14 Eriksson P, Almroth G, Denneberg T, Lindstrom FD. IgG2 deficiency in primary Sjögren's syndrome and hypergammaglobulinaemic purpura. *Clin Immunol Immunopathol* 1994; **70**: 60–5.

15 Garty BZ, Scanlin T, Goldsmith DP *et al.* Cutaneous manifestations of cystic fibrosis: possible role of cryoglobulins. *Br J Dermatol* 1989; **121**: 655–8.

16 Schidlow DV, Panitch HB, Zaeri N *et al.* Purpuric rashes in cystic fibrosis. *Am J Dis Child* 1989; **143**: 1030–2.

Purpura associated with infection

Purpuric skin lesions associated with infection [1] may be due to numerous mechanisms, more than one of which may be operative, including:

- Thrombocytopenia (discussed above)
- Localized or disseminated intravascular coagulation (discussed above)
- Direct vascular damage (invasion or occlusion by organisms)
- Vascular effects of toxins
- Immunological vascular damage (vasculitis, immune complex deposition)
- Emboli.

Purpura is a characteristic feature of certain bacterial infections, for example meningococcal or other septicaemias and bacterial endocarditis, and of many viral and rickettsial infections, for example typhus, Rocky Mountain spotted fever, dengue fever and the viral haemorrhagic fevers (see Chapters 30 and 33) [2–9]. Acral purpuric lesions are typical of Rocky Mountain spotted fever [3]; the histological features include a lymphohistiocytic capillaritis and venulitis with variable leukocytoclastic vasculitis, fibrin thrombi, capillary wall necrosis and immunofluorescent evidence of organisms within endothelial cells, suggesting that it is therefore a type of septic vasculitis. In typhus, however, acral sites are generally spared. Dengue fever has three subtypes, dengue fever, dengue haemorrhagic fever (DHF) and dengue septic shock (DSS); in DHF there may be petechiae of acral sites, face, soft palate and axillae, with larger purpuric lesions, epistaxis, gingival bleeding and more serious bleeding (gastrointestinal bleeding, menorrhagia) in some subjects, due to thrombocytopenia. Haemoconcentration is also a feature in DHS and DSS. In hantavirus infection, thrombocytopenia is a typical part of the hantavirus pulmonary syndrome (HPS); skin haemorrhages, gingival bleeding, epistaxis, haematuria and gastrointestinal bleeding are mainly due to thrombocytopenia, but coagulopathy can occur.

Skin lesions are the presenting feature in 70–90% of patients with meningococcaemia and are purpuric in 50%, often stellate in shape and tender. In some cases of meningococcal septicaemia, organisms can be seen on blood smears taken from scraped skin lesions [10]. There may be a leukocytoclastic vasculitis with thrombi and meningococci within endothelial cells or leukocytes, typically resulting in a clinical lesion of classical palpable purpura, ranging in size from 2 to 8 mm in diameter. Lesions may progress to purpura fulminans due to microvascular occlusion, with lesions typically enlarging and often developing stellate or retiform features with minimal to no erythema (discussed above). The mechanism of coagulopathy in severe meningococcal sepsis is probably multifactorial, sharing some features with other conditions of severe sepsis and potentially leading to large vessel thrombosis with digital or limb infarction. Levels of protein C, protein S and antithrombin antigen are reduced, thrombocytopenia and haemophagocytosis occur, and fibrinolysis is reduced. Critically, there is dysfunction of the protein C activation pathway such that the prothrombotic activity of thrombin escapes its usual regulation, and a procoagulant state results [11]; it is now routine for patients with severe sepsis, including that due to meningococcal disease, to be treated with activated protein C [12].

Various congenital infections may cause neonatal purpura (p. 49.49). Purpura may appear in the prodromal period of many infections, for example measles, in which case it is often a sign of a severe infection. When it occurs at the height of the infection it is of less serious importance. A large number of infections may cause purpuric lesions in children [13]. In neonates, congenital infections may cause 'blueberry muffin syndrome' with dermal erythropoiesis, originally described in congenital rubella with thrombocytopenia. There are several non-infectious causes, but the most important infections are those covered by the acronym TORCH (toxoplasmosis, other infections, rubella, cytomegalovirus and herpesviruses). The 'other infection' group that should be screened includes syphilis, coxsackieviruses (especially B2) and HIV [14].

The petechial gloves and socks syndrome, or papular–purpuric gloves and socks syndrome, is a distinctive syndrome that has been attributed to parvovirus B19 infection [15,16] or to other viruses such as measles, hepatitis B, coxsackievirus B6 and cytomegalovirus [13,17] (see also Chapter 33). Purpura may also occur in the laterothoracic eruption, which may have an infectious aetiology (often parvovirus B19), and a genital or 'bathing trunk' distribution of purpura has also been described due to parvovirus B19 [18].

Other infections may be associated with characteristic distributions of purpura, for example *Strongyloides* causes 'thumb-print' periumbilical purpuric lesions [19]. Based on six patients with cancer, immunosuppressed by disease or treatment, this feature was felt to be associated with septic shock and death [20].

References

1 Kingston ME, Mackey D. Skin clues in the diagnosis of life-threatening infections. *Rev Infect Dis* 1986; **8**: 1–11.

2 Anonymous. Viral haemorrhagic fevers. *Lancet* 1981; **ii**: 182–3.

3 Kao GF, Evancho CD, Ioffe O *et al.* Cutaneous histopathology of Rocky Mountain spotted fever. *J Cutan Pathol* 1997; **24**: 604–10.

4 Suresh V. The enigmatic haemorrhagic fevers. *J R Soc Med* 1997; **90**: 622–4.

5 Lupi O, Tyring SK. Old-World haemorrhagic fevers. In: Tyring SK, Lupi O, Hengge UR. *Tropical Dermatology*. London: Elsevier, 2006: 125–32.

6 Glass GE. Hantaviruses. *Curr Opin Infect Dis* 1997; **10**: 362–6.

7 Lupi O, Semenovitch I. New-World haemorrhagic fevers. In: Tyring SK, Lupi O, Hengge UR. *Tropical Dermatology*. London: Elsevier, 2006: 133–6.

8 World Health Organization. *Dengue Haemorrhagic Fever. Diagnosis, Treatment, Prevention and Control*, 2nd edn. Geneva: WHO, 1997.

9 Lupi O, Kouri G, Guzman MG. Dengue. In: Tyring SK, Lupi O, Hengge UR. *Tropical Dermatology*. London: Elsevier, 2006: 136–41.

10 Taylor MR, Keane CT, Periappuram M. Skin scraping is a useful investigation in meningococcal disease. *BMJ* 1997; **314**: 831–2.

11 Faust SN, Levin M, Harrison OB *et al.* Dysfunction of endothelial protein C activation in severe meningococcal sepsis. *N Engl J Med* 2001; **345**: 408–16.

12 Parillo JE. Severe sepsis and therapy with activated protein C. *N Engl J Med* 2005; **353**: 1398–400.

13 Baselga E, Drolet BA, Esterley NB. Purpura in infants and children. *J Am Acad Dermatol* 1997; **37**: 673–705.

14 Hoeger PH. Cutaneous manifestations of congenital infections. In: Harper J, Oranje A, Prose N. *Textbook of Pediatric Dermatology,* 2nd edn. Oxford: Blackwell Publishing, 2006: 72–8.

15 Harmes M, Feldman R, Saurat JH. Papulo-purpuric 'gloves and socks syndrome'. *J Am Acad Dermatol* 1990; **23**: 850–4.

16 Halasz CLG, Den Cormier DM. Petechial glove and sock syndrome caused by parvovirus B19. *J Am Acad Dermatol* 1992; **27**: 835–8.

17 Vargas-Diez E, Buezo GF. Papular–purpuric glove-and-sock syndrome. *Int J Dermatol* 1996; **35**: 626–32.

18 Krankimel N, LeClerc-Mercier S, Rozenberg F *et al.* An adult presenting with a bathing-trunk eruption associated with primary infection to human parvovirus B19. *Br J Dermatol* 2007; **158**: 407.

19 Bank DE, Grossman ME, Kohn SR, Rabinowitz AD. The thumbprint sign: rapid diagnosis of disseminated strongyloidiasis. *J Am Acad Dermatol* 1990; **23**: 324–6.

20 Salluh JIF, Bozza FA, Pinto TS *et al.* Cutaneous periumbilical purpura in disseminated strongyloidiasis in cancer patients: a pathognomonic feature of potentially lethal disease? *Braz J Infect Dis* 2006; **9**: 419–24.

Non-thrombocytopenic toxin- and drug-induced purpura [1–6]

Many agents may lead to purpura by causing thrombocytopenia (discussed above). There are also many substances capable of causing capillary damage with or without any change in platelets, either by direct toxicity or through an allergic reaction. The purpura varies in degree from a few petechiae to massive extravasation of blood. Sometimes there is obvious evidence of inflammatory lesions, as well as purpura, implying a frankly vasculitic process [7]. Exposure may be industrial, accidental or therapeutic. Some drugs may cause thrombocytopenia and either vascular purpura and/or frank vasculitis; the thrombocytopenia in such cases may be caused by a direct effect on platelets or by endothelial damage leading to platelet aggregation.

Substances capable of causing capillary damage include acetylsalicylic acid, allopurinol, *p*-aminosalicylic acid, arsenic, atropine, barbiturates, bismuth, carbimazole, carbromal, chloramphenicol, chlordiazepoxide, chlorothiazide, chlorpromazine, diethylstilbestrol, furosemide, gold, hair dye, indometacin, iodides, isoniazid, menthol, meprobamate, methyldopa, piperazine, quinidine, quinine, reserpine, snake venoms, sodium salicylate, sulphonamides, tartrazine and other food additives, thiouracil, tolbutamide and glyceryl trinitrate.

Carbromal is one of the few drugs that caused a rather distinctive pattern of purpura. The widespread areas of capillary leakage combined with erythema produced a picture which resembled itching purpura and Schamberg's disease. Drug-induced pigmented purpuric dermatoses are considered elsewhere.

Trimethoprim–sulfamethoxazole has been reported to cause an acral purpuric eruption, proven by rechallenge, that resembled the purpuric 'gloves and socks' syndrome more commonly caused by parvovirus B19 [8].

A diagnosis of toxin- and drug-induced purpura usually depends on circumstantial evidence. Unfortunately, laboratory tests are mainly unhelpful, although some drugs that cause purpuric reactions will produce a purpuric reaction when patch tested. Rechallenge may be dangerous; generally the diagnosis is made by careful history taking.

Drug-induced vasculitis or livedo are also discussed in Chapter 75; drugs that cause skin necrosis are considered later in the present chapter (see Table 49.9, p. 49.50).

References

1 Bruinsma W. *A Guide to Drug Eruptions.* Amsterdam: Excerpta Medica, 1973: 55–8.

2 Lee GR, Bithell TC, Foerster J *et al.*, eds. *Wintrobe's Clinical Hematology*, 9th edn. Philadelphia: Lea & Febiger, 1993.

3 Breathnach SB, Hintner H. *Adverse Drug Reactions and the Skin.* London: Blackwell Scientific Publications, 1992: 45–7.

4 Litt JZ. *Drug Eruption Reference Manual 2001.* New York: Parthenon Publishing, 2001.

5 Dowd PM, Champion RH. Purpura. In: Champion RH, Burton JL, Burns DA, Breathnach SM, eds. *Textbook of Dermatology*, 6th edn. Oxford: Blackwell Science, 1998: 2141–54.

6 Michaelsson G, Petterson L, Juhlin L. Purpura caused by food and drug additives. *Arch Dermatol* 1974; **109**: 49–52.

7 Dubost J-J, Souteyrand P, Sauvezie B. Drug-induced vasculitides. *Bailliere's Clin Rheumatol* 1991; **5**: 119–38.

8 van Rooijen MM, Brand CU, Ballmer-Weber BK *et al.* Drug-induced papular–purpuric gloves and socks syndrome. *Hautarzt* 1999; **50**: 280–3.

Contact purpura [1]

Purpura may occur as an irritant reaction to mechanical friction from abrasive agents such as woollen clothing or fibreglass. Some topical medications may rarely cause purpura that appears to be of irritant or toxic causation, such as clioquinol (at flexural sites), benzoyl peroxide or EMLA local anaesthetic [2,3]. Textile and rubber chemicals [4–6] are particular causes of contact purpura that may have little or no eczematous component, although itch or lichenoid morphology may be prominent in some instances. Such reactions may be widespread, the distribution corresponding only approximately with the distribution of contact, and may therefore be confused with idiopathic pigmented purpuras.

Purpura around the acrosyringium may occur at patch-test sites to cobalt, and purpuric patch tests to apronalide and quinidine have been reported in subjects with a purpuric rash after systemic administration of these agents.

The main groups of chemicals that have been reported to cause contact purpura are:
- Dyes and textile agents: azo dyes, paraphenylenediamine, optical whiteners
- Rubber antioxidants: IPPD, isopropylaminodiphenylamine
- Resins: urea formaldehyde compounds, epoxy resin
- Plants: *Rhus*, *Agave*
- Others: topical medicaments, balsam of Peru, mercury.

References

1 Rietschel RL, Fowlet JF. *Fisher's Contact Dermatitis.* Philadelphia: Lippincott, Williams & Wilkins, 2001: 73–5.

2 van Joost T, van Ulsen J, Vuzevski VD *et al.* Purpuric contact dermatitis to benzoyl peroxide. *J Am Acad Dermatol* 1990; **22**: 358–61.

3 de Waard-van der Spek FB, Oranje JP. Purpura caused by EMLA is of toxic origin. *Contact Dermatitis* 1997; **36**: 11–3.

4 Calnan CD, Peachey RDG. Allergic contact purpura. *Clin Allergy* 1971; **1**: 287–90.

5 Roed-Petersen J, Clemmensen OJ, Menne T, Larsen E. Purpuric contact dermatitis from black rubber chemicals. *Contact Dermatitis* 1988; **18**: 166–8.

6 Lazarov A, Cordoba M. Purpuric contact dermatitis in patients with allergic reaction to textile dyes and resins. *J Eur Acad Dermatol Venereol* 2000; **14**: 101–5.

Pigmented purpuric dermatoses

Synonyms
• Capillaritis
• Purpura progressiva pigmentosa

Capillaritis is the generic term for a variety of chronic conditions that share certain histological features. The term 'purpura simplex' has also been applied to this group of disorders, on the basis of the common histological aspects. However, the same term has been applied to other mild and unexplained but morphologically different patterns of purpura such as easy bruising, and it is therefore potentially confusing. The term 'pigmented purpuric dermatoses' may be preferred, at least at present, as it conveys the message of a component beyond simple transient purpura.

The sometimes striking morphological patterns of the pigmented purpuric dermatoses have given rise to a wide range of descriptive and eponymous names [1–8]. Typical examples of the various eponymous diseases are sufficiently distinctive to warrant separate description but in many cases the clinical features may not be characteristic of any one of the eponymous variants. As their aetiology is unknown, and no clear distinction has been established between the different patterns other than on clinical morphological grounds, classification remains clinical. Identification of pigmented purpuric dermatoses secondary to a systemic cause is potentially important and is discussed below. Gravity and increased venous pressure are important localizing factors in many cases. Exercise may be a provoking factor. Most are chronic but two-thirds may improve or clear eventually [5]. Adults are mainly affected but there are several series of cases in childhood [9,10].

Most authors would accept five different morphological variants of idiopathic pigmented purpuric dermatosis, each of which will be discussed separately, namely:

1 Schamberg's disease (about half of cases)
2 Itching purpura (eczematid-like purpura of Doucas and Kapetanakis) (about 10%)
3 Pigmented purpuric lichenoid dermatosis of Gougerot and Blum (about 5%)
4 Lichen aureus (about 10%)
5 Purpura annularis telangiectodes (Majocchi's disease) (about 5%).

A further variant, termed Favre-Chaix's purpura, occurs on the lower leg and comprises purpura and pigmentation associated with oedema, cyanosis and sclerosis; it would appear to be simply a manifestation of venous disease and is not considered further here. However, additional types (such as granulomatous), or subtypes (e.g. segmental variants of the above list) also warrant mention as they may in time prove to be aetiologically distinct; furthermore, about 20% of cases are unclassifiable [5] and many drugs, systemic diseases or local conditions of the skin may lead to localized, mild purpura with haemosiderin deposition and secondary melanin pigmentation [11]. These are summarized briefly before considering the idiopathic variants, and will be discussed in differential diagnosis of the named disorders in this group.

Pathologically, these disorders are characterized by narrowing of the lumen and endothelial swelling of superficial small vessels, accompanied by perivascular T-lymphocytic infiltration, extravasation of erythrocytes and haemosiderin deposits in macrophages. An appearance termed 'ectasizing endocapillaritis' has been reported, in a study in which the authors divided 22 cases into those that were papular (with an upper dermal band-like infiltrate), macular (with a perivascular infiltrate) or eczematous (with exocytosis and spongiosis) [11], but this has not led to any fundamental advance in understanding these diseases. The cellular infiltrate in all types contains CD4+ T cells in close contact with CD1a+ Langerhans' cells [12,13], suggesting that a cell-mediated immune reaction is operative. Strong expression of endothelial cell adhesion receptors ICAM-1 and ELAM-1 may determine the pattern of the infiltrate [13]. Immune complex deposition has also been reported but direct immunofluorescence is often negative. An IgA-associated lymphocytic vasculopathy has been described in eight patients, in six of whom the clinical and histological features were those of a pigmented purpuric dermatosis [14]; the significance of this is unclear but it is notable that many of the subjects had a preceding or associated condition, including viral infection, Henoch–Schönlein purpura, undifferentiated connective tissue disease, lupus erythematosus profundus, Degos' disease and Buerger's disease.

References

1 Randall SJ, Kierland RR, Montgomery H. Pigmented purpuric eruptions. *Arch Dermatol Syphilol* 1951; **64**: 177–91.

2 Farrokhzad S, Champion RH. Pigmented purpuric dermatoses. *Dermatologica* 1970; **140**: 45–53.

3 Touraine A. Le purpura annulaire telangiectasique de Majocchi et ses parentés. *Presse Med* 1949; **57**: 934–6.

4 Tristani-Firouzi P, Meadows KP, Vanderhooft S. Pigmented purpuric eruptions of childhood: a series of cases and review of literature. *Pediatr Dermatol* 2001; **18**: 299–304.

5 Ratnam KV, Su WPD, Peters MS. Purpura simplex (inflammatory purpura without vasculitis): a clinicopathologic study of 174 cases. *J Am Acad Dermatol* 1991; **25**: 642–7.

6 Rabinowitz LG. Pigmented purpuras. In: Harper J, Oranje AP, Prose N, eds. *Textbook of Pediatric Dermatology*, 2nd edn. Oxford: Blackwell Science, 2006: 1927–32.

7 Baselga E, Drolet BA, Esterley NB. Purpura in infants and children. *J Am Acad Dermatol* 1997; **37**: 673–705.

8 Sardana K, Sarkar R, Seghal VN. Pigmented purpuric dermatoses: an overview. *Int J Dermatol* 2004; **43**: 482–8.

9 Tristani FP, Meadows KP, Vanderhooft S. Pigmented purpuric eruptions of childhood: a series of cases and review of literature. *Pediatr Dermatol* 2001; **18**: 299–304.

10 Torrel A, Requena C, Mediero IG, Zambrano A. Schamberg's purpura in children: a review of 13 cases. *J Am Acad Dermatol* 2003; **48**: 31–3.

11 Petruzzellis V, Vadala' P, Inverardi D et al. Idiopathic chronic pigmentary purpura. Findings in 22 cases and proposal of a new classification. *VASA* 1994; **23**: 114–9.

12 Aiba S, Takami H. Immunohistological studies in Schamberg's disease. *Arch Dermatol* 1988; **124**: 1058–62.

13 Ghersetich I, Lotti T, Bacci S et al. Cell infiltrate in progressive pigmented purpura (Schamberg's disease): immunophenotype, adhesion receptors and intercellular relationships. *Int J Dermatol* 1995; **34**: 846–50.

14 Crowson AN, Magro CM, Usmani A, McNutt NS. Immunoglobulin A-associated lymphocytic vasculopathy: a clinicopathologic study of eight patients. *J Cutan Pathol* 2002; **29**: 596–601.

Secondary pigmented purpuric dermatoses and systemic causes

Many underlying causes have been proven or suggested for the various patterns of pigmented purpuric dermatosis, although with limited specificity [1,2]. Most cases in which a cause is found either resemble Schamberg's disease or are unclassifiable (similar to 70% of idiopathic cases) and drugs have been documented as a cause in all of the main clinical patterns. The apparently idiopathic variants of pigmented purpuric dermatosis, while much the commonest cause, are therefore a diagnosis made by exclusion. The most important underlying conditions are listed below.

Drugs and food additives [1,3–6]. Drugs caused 14% of cases in one large series [1]. Drugs reported to cause capillaritis resembling a pigmented purpuric dermatosis include calcium channel antagonists [6], β-blockers, angiotensin-converting enzyme inhibitors, nitrites, furosemide and other diuretics, antihistamines, antidepressants, chlordiazepoxide, carbamazepine, analgesics such as paracetamol, non-steroidal anti-inflammatory agents, glipizide, bezafibrate, medroxyprogesterone acetate, raloxifene, pseudoephedrine, vitamin B_1 derivatives, interferon-α (in hepatitis C infection), antibiotics including ampicillin and cotrimoxazole, polyvinyl pyrrolidone and topical 5-fluorouracil [2–6]. Amongst food additives and related agents, tartrazine and creatine supplements have been implicated. Minocycline has been reported to selectively pigment areas of pre-existing capillaritis [7], and minocycline-induced ITP has mimicked Schamberg's disease, but it does not seem to be a specific cause of pigmented purpuric dermatoses.

External contact agents. Both contact irritants and allergens, especially clothing dyes, have been implicated as a cause of pigmented purpuric dermatoses [8–10]; these are discussed separately above (p. 49.21). Patch testing at the lesional site has been suggested.

Infections. β-haemolytic streptococci, toxoplasma and rickettsiae have been linked to development of pigmented purpuric dermatoses. More recently, a case has been made for hepatitis viruses being associated with pigmented purpuric dermatoses; in a series of 10 patients, five had hepatitis C antibodies and two had hepatitis B antibodies, although no random controls were tested [11]. One case was reported in association with cryoglobulinaemia, hepatitis C and rheumatoid arthritis (which itself has been linked with pigmented purpuric dermatoses, below) and one with interferon treatment for hepatitis C (above). In five patients, a chronic pigmented purpuric dermatosis (Schamberg pattern in four and itching purpura in one) resolved after treatment of dental infections, either periodontitis or pulpitis [12].

Neoplasia. There are many reported instances in which an apparent pigmented purpuric dermatosis has been a manifestation (sometimes the only manifestation) of mycosis fungoides [4,13–

15]. In one instance, pigmented purpuric dermatosis preceded the diagnosis of mycosis fungoides by 24 years [16]. Some have linked this subtle presentation of mycosis fungoides predominantly with the lichenoid patterns of pigmented purpuric dermatosis [17,18], but many cases are of lichen aureus, Schamberg or non-specific capillaritis pattern. Monoclonality, demonstrated by T-cell receptor-gamma [17,18] or beta [19,20] gene rearrangement studies, has been demonstrated in some cases, occurring in almost half of cases in one series [19], although it may also occur in collagen vascular disease and drug reactions as well as representing cutaneous T-cell lymphoma, and some reported cases with clonality have had a benign behaviour [18]. In one series of 23 cases of lichen aureus, half had T-cell monoclonality but none showed progression to mycosis fungoides and over half had no evidence of skin disease after a mean follow-up of over 8 years [21]. Cases with monoclonality thus account for a small minority of pigmented purpuric dermatoses, but it seems prudent to suggest a skin biopsy in cases that are atypical in age-group, site, extent or morphology, or that are progressive or recurrent in behaviour. Other malignancies have been linked with development of pigmented purpuric dermatoses, including neoplasms of breast, bladder, intestine and lung, as well as leukaemia and Hodgkin's disease, but the strength of such associations is unclear.

Collagen vascular disorders. Both lupus erythematosus and rheumatoid disease [22] have been reported in association with pigmented purpuric dermatoses.

Vascular and haematological diseases. Stasis dermatitis commonly includes a component of pigmented purpuric dermatosis, either around the ankle or overlying varicosities. There is a single case of association with spherocytosis. Apparent 'venous' pigmented purpuric dermatosis in younger patients, without overt varicosities, should raise suspicion of a thrombophilia (Fig. 49.7).

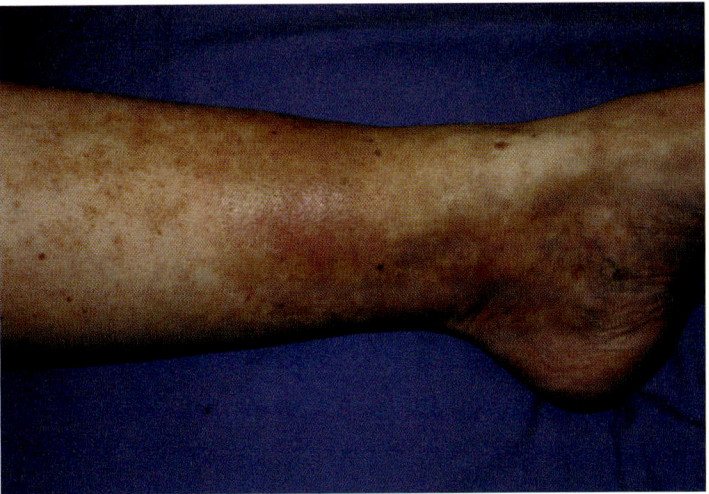

Fig. 49.7 A pigmented purpuric dermatosis suggestive of venous disease but occurring in a young male without varicose veins; thrombophilia screening documented a lupus anticoagulant.

Miscellaneous. Diabetes, thyroid disease, liver disease and obesity have all been reported in association with pigmented purpuric dermatoses although causative relationships are not clear in these cases.

References

1 Ratnam KV, Su WPD, Peters MS. Purpura simplex (inflammatory purpura without vasculitis): a clinicopathologic study of 174 cases. *J Am Acad Dermatol* 1991; **25**: 642–7.

2 Petruzzellis V, Vadala' P, Inverardi D *et al*. Idiopathic chronic pigmentary purpura. Findings in 22 cases and proposal of a new classification. *VASA* 1994; **23**: 114–9.

3 Nishioka K, Katayama I, Masuzawa M *et al*. Drug-induced chronic pigmented purpura. *J Dermatol* 1989; **16**: 220–2.

4 Crowson AN, Magro CM, Zahorchak R. Atypical pigmentary purpura: a clinical, histopathologic, and genotypic study. *Hum Pathol* 1999; **30**: 1004–12.

5 Kalinke DU, Wuthrich B. Purpura pigmentosa progressiva in type III cryoglobulinaemia and tartrazine intolerance. A follow-up over 20 years. *Hautarzt* 1999; **50**: 47–51.

6 Cox NH, Walsh ML, Robson RH. Purpura and bleeding due to calcium channel blockers: an underestimated problem? Case reports and a pilot study. *Clin Exp Dermatol* 2009; **34**: 487–91.

7 Madan V, Lear JT. Minocycline-induced pigmentation of pre-existing capillaritis. *Br J Dermatol* 2007; **156**: 590–1.

8 Shah SA, Ormerod AD. Pigmented purpuric clothing dermatitis due to disperse dyes. *Contact Dermatitis* 2000; **43**: 360.

9 Komericki P, Aberer W, Arbab E, Kovacevic Z, Kränke B. Pigmented purpuric contact dermatitis from Disperse Blue 106 and 124 dyes. *J Am Acad Dermatol* 2001; **45**: 456–8.

10 Engin B, Ozdemir M, Kaplan M, Mevlitoglu I. Patch test results in patients with progressive pigmented purpuric dermatosis. *J Eur Acad Dermatol Venereol* 2009; **23**: 209.

11 Dessoukey MW, Abdel-Dayem H, Omar MF, Al-Suweidi NE. Pigmented purpuric dermatosis and hepatitis profile: a report on 10 patients. *Int J Dermatol* 2005; **44**: 486–8.

12 Satoh T, Yokozeki H, Nishioka K. Chronic pigmented purpura associated with odontogenic infection. *J Am Acad Dermatol* 2002; **46**: 942–4.

13 Barnhill RL, Braverman IM. Progression of pigmented purpura-like eruptions to mycosis fungoides: report of three cases. *J Am Acad Dermatol* 1988; **19**: 25–31.

14 Lipsker D, Cribier B, Heid E, Grosshans E. Cutaneous lymphoma masquerading as pigmented purpuric capillaritis. *Acta Derm Venereol (Stockh)* 1999; **126**: 321–6.

15 Ameen M, Darvay A, Black MM *et al*. CD8-positive mycosis fungoides presenting as capillaritis. *Br J Dermatol* 2000; **142**: 564–7.

16 Viseux V, Schoenlaub P, Cnudde F *et al*. Pigmented purpuric dermatitis preceding the diagnosis of mycosis fungoides by 24 years. *Dermatology Basel* 2003; **207**: 331–2.

17 Toro JR, Sander CA, LeBoit PE. Persistent pigmented purpuric dermatitis and mycosis fungoides: stimulant, precursor, or both? A study by light microscopy and molecular methods. *Am J Dermatopathol* 1997; **19**: 108–18.

18 Lor P, Krueger U, Kempf W, Burg G, Nestle FO. Monoclonal rearrangement ot the T cell receptor gamma-chain in lichenoid pigmented purpuric dermatitis of Gougerot-Blum responding to topical corticosteroid therapy. *Dermatology Basel* 2002; **205**: 191–3.

19 Magro CM, Schaefer JT, Crowson NA *et al*. Pigmented purpuric dermatosis: classification by phenotypic and molecular profiles. *Am J Clin Pathol* 2007; **128**: 218–29.

20 Plaza JA, Morrison C, Magro CM. Assessment of TCR-beta clonality in a diverse group of cutaneous T-cell infiltrates. *J Cutan Pathol* 2008; **35**: 358–65.

21 Fink-Puches R, Wolf P, Kerl H, Cerroni L. Lichen aureus. Clinicopathologic features, natural history, and relationship to mycosis fungoides. *Arch Dermatol* 2008; **144**: 1169–73.

22 Wilkinson SM, Smith AG, Davis M, Dawes PT. Capillaritis: a manifestation of rheumatoid disease. *Clin Rheumatol* 1993; **12**: 53–6.

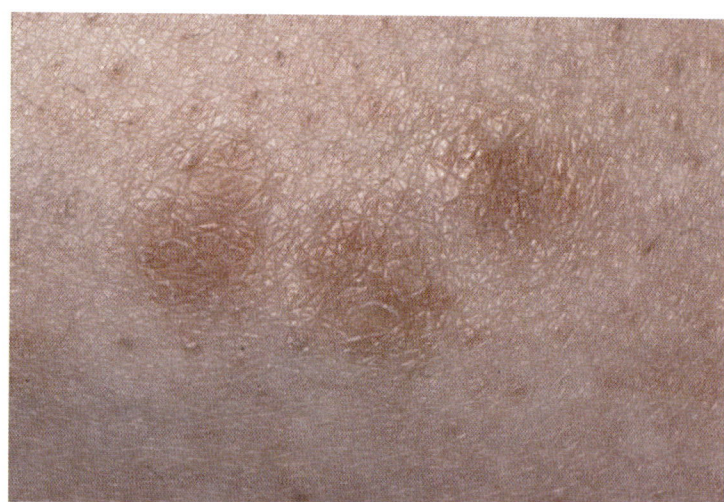

Fig. 49.8 Schamberg's disease.

Schamberg's disease [1,2]

> **Synonym**
> • Progressive pigmented purpuric dermatosis

This uncommon eruption is most common in young adult males but may occur at any age including childhood. Familial incidence has been reported [3]. The lesions are most frequent on the legs but may occur anywhere on the body, including the palms [4], and may be few in number or very extensive. They consist of irregular plaques of orange or brown pigmentation due to haemosiderin, with characteristic 'cayenne pepper' spots appearing within and at the edge of old lesions (Fig. 49.8). Slight changes in the epidermis may occur. There are usually no symptoms, although there may be some slight itching. The eruption is characteristically very chronic and may persist for many years. The pattern of the eruption changes, with slow extension and often some clearing of the original lesions. Spontaneous cure may occur eventually. Many patients have an eruption with features both of this disease and of the other pigmented purpuric dermatoses. An annular configuration may occur and there may be small lichenoid papules.

Itching purpura is a disorder that may be similar to Schamberg's disease, but the intensity of itch serves to distinguish the two.

Itching purpura [5–7]

> **Synonyms**
> • Eczematide-like purpura (of Doucas and Kapetanakis)
> • Disseminated pruriginous angiodermatitis

This condition has many similarities to Schamberg's disease but is generally more extensive, develops more rapidly and is characterized by persistent, intense itch. It occurs most frequently in adult men and is of unknown aetiology. Purpuric lesions usually commence around the ankles and in a few weeks spread to involve the whole legs, sometimes the lower part of the body, and even elsewhere. They are more pronounced at sites of friction with clothing. The lesions consist of erythematous and purpuric macules that may become confluent. The eruption often has a rather characteristic orange colour. The dermal perivascular changes are those seen generally in the pigmented purpuric dermatoses and there are variable changes in the overlying epidermis, including spongiosis. Spontaneous improvement after a few months is usual, but recurrences may occur and a fluctuating but chronic course is frequent. The itching may respond to topical corticosteroids and oral antihistamines.

An almost identical picture occurs with carbromal sensitivity, and less commonly with other drugs such as meprobamate, carbamazepine and perhaps even some foods. Clothing or rubber dermatitis may produce a similar picture, and may explain many cases of itching purpura.

Pigmented purpuric lichenoid dermatosis of Gougerot and Blum [8]

This eruption occurs especially in men aged between 40 and 60 years. It usually affects the legs, but lesions may occur elsewhere. The characteristic clinical feature of the dermatosis is the presence of lichenoid papules in association with purpuric lesions similar to those of Schamberg's disease, and this may simply be a variation of the same disorder. This clinical pattern has been found in association with porphyria [9] and a similar pattern of eruption may occur in the oral mucosa [10].

Lichen aureus [11,12]

> **Synonym**
> • Lichen purpuricus

This is a more localized, more intensely purpuric but often asymptomatic eruption that may have rather lichenoid morphology. Young adults and children are often affected, on body, limbs or even face. The lesions are often solitary and may be yellowish, golden, rust-coloured or purple. They may resemble a bruise, and hence must be distinguished from non-accidental injury in children, but may persist for a few years. Histologically, lichen aureus is distinguished from other pigmented purpuric dermatoses by a lack of epidermal component and in some cases a Grenz zone.

Purpura annularis telangiectodes [13,14]

> **Synonym**
> • Majocchi's disease

This eruption occurs especially in adolescents and young adults of either sex but may occur at any age, and may be familial [15]. Exercise may have been a provoking factor in one case [16]. The clinical features are distinctive and described in its name. Lesions occur at any site, often in the absence of venous stasis, and may be few in number or very numerous. They consist of small plaques 1–3 cm across that are usually annular from their onset (Fig. 49.9). Lesions consist of telangiectases and haemosiderin staining of the skin. They may be purple, yellow or brown, and may contain 'cayenne pepper' spots. Individual lesions persist unchanged for many months or years, or there may be slow centrifugal extension with development of slight central atrophy. Sometimes the lesions disappear and are replaced by similar lesions nearby. Treatment

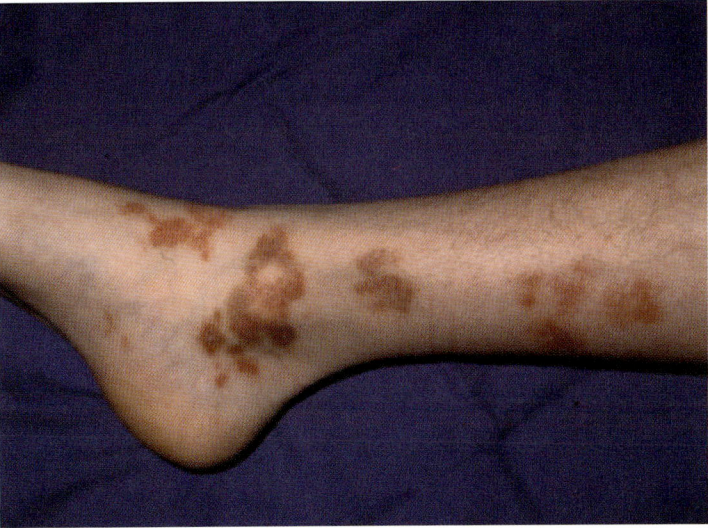

Fig. 49.9 Majocchi's purpura annularis telangiectodes.

is usually ineffective. A variant termed *purpura telangiectatica arciformis (Touraine)* consists of fewer, larger and irregularly arciform lesions [17].

Granulomatous pigmented purpuric dermatosis

An uncommon variant of pigmented purpuric dermatosis has been reported in which there is granulomatous histology [18,19]. In a series of four Asian cases, three had hyperlipidaemia, suggesting that this is worthy of evaluation in this rare variant of pigmented purpuric dermatosis [20].

Familial pigmented purpuric eruption

There are rare reported instances of the familial occurrence of Schamberg's disease [3,21] and of purpura annularis telangiectodes [14]. A distinctive pigmented purpuric eruption has been observed in several members of a family in which it was probably determined by an autosomal dominant gene [22]. Discrete reddish-brown spots developed in childhood or adolescence. The individual macules were larger than in Schamberg's disease and were arranged in a mosaic pattern. The lesions gradually covered a larger area and involved new sites, mainly on the limbs and in the larger flexures, but without any symptoms. Another family has been reported in which three generations were affected, supporting an autosomal dominant inheritance pattern [23].

Linear and quadrantic pigmented purpuric dermatoses

Various morphological types of pigmented purpuric eruption may occur in a linear or zosteriform distribution [24–28], or less commonly may diffusely involve a single quadrant of the body [29]. Linear lesions affect the legs more often than the arms. Individual lesions usually resemble lichen aureus or Schamberg's disease. In one case, trauma-induced linear pigmented purpuric dermatosis evolved into linear morphoea [30].

References

1 Schamberg JF. A peculiar progressive pigmentary disease of the skin. *Br J Dermatol* 1901; **13**: 1–5.

2 Schamberg JF. Report of 3 cases of progressive pigmentary dermatosis with particular reference to the blood cholesterol. *Br J Dermatol* 1927; **39**: 389–93.

3 Baden HP. Familial Schamberg's disease. *Arch Dermatol* 1964; **90**: 400.

4 Moyer DG, Chernita SA. Capillaritis of the palms. *Arch Dermatol* 1969; **99**: 591–2.

5 Doucas C, Kapetanakis J. Eczematid-like purpura. *Dermatologica* 1953; **106**: 86–95.

6 Loewenthal LJA. Itching purpura. *Br J Dermatol* 1954; **66**: 95–103.

7 Mosto SJ, Casala AM. Disseminated pruriginous angiodermatitis (itching purpura). *Arch Dermatol* 1965; **91**: 351–6.

8 Gougerot H, Blum P. Purpura angioscereux prurigineux aux elements lichen-oides. *Bull Soc Fr Dermatol Syphiligr* 1925; **32**: 161.

9 Ippen H, Goerz G, Bruster H. Purpura porphyrica. *Arch Klin Exp Derm* 1965; **223**: 128–35.

10 Scully C, Eveson JW. Pigmented purpuric stomatitis. *Oral Surg Oral Med Oral Pathol* 1992; **74**: 780–2.

11 Kanitakis C, Tsoitis G. Lichen purpurique. *Ann Dermatol Vénéréol* 1982; **109**: 445–52.

12 Price ML, Wilson Jones E, Calnan CD *et al.* Lichen aureus: a localised persistent form of pigmented purpuric dermatosis. *Br J Dermatol* 1984; **112**: 307–14.

13 Majocchi D. Sopra una dermatosi telangiectode non ancora descritta: purpura annularis. *G Ital Mal Vener Pelle* 1896; **31**: 263–4.

14 Mackee GM. Purpura annularis telangiectodes. *J Cutan Genitourin Dis* 1915; **33**: 129–41.

15 Borelli G. Purpura annularis teleangectoides: tre casi familiari. *Arch Ital Derm Sif Vener* 1953; **25**: 259–71.

16 Allan SJR, Humphreys F, Buxton PK. Annular purpura and step aerobics. *Clin Exp Dermatol* 1994; **19**: 418.

17 Brehm G. Zur purpura telangiectatica arciformis (Touraine). *Z Haut Geschlechtskr* 1957; **17**: 331–6.

18 Wong WR, Kuo TT, Chen MJ, Chan HL. Granulomatous variant of chronic pigmented purpuric dermatosis: report of two cases. *Br J Dermatol* 2001; **145**: 162–4.

19 Saito R, Matsuoka Y. Granulomatous pigmented purpuric dermatosis. *J Dermatol* 1996; **23**: 551–5.

20 Li WL, Kuo TT, Shih PY *et al.* Granulomatous variant of chronic pigmented purpuric dermatosis: report of four new cases and an association with hyper-lipidaemia. *Clin Exp Dermatol* 2007; **32**: 513–5.

21 Kanwar AJ, Thami GP. Familial Schamberg's disease. *Dermatology* 1999; **198**: 175–6.

22 Gould WM, Farber EM. A familial pigmented purpuric eruption. *Dermatologica* 1966; **132**: 400–8.

23 Sethuraman G, Sugandhan S, Bansal A *et al.* Familial pigmented purpuric der-matoses. *J Dermatol* 2006; **33**: 639–41.

24 Braun-Falco O, Abeck O, Betke M *et al.* Lichen aureus zosteriformis. *Hautarzt* 1989; **40**: 373–5.

25 Riordan CA, Darley C, Markey AC *et al.* Unilateral linear capillaritis. *Clin Exp Dermatol* 1992; **17**: 182–5.

26 Filo V, Galbavy S, Filova A *et al.* Unilateral progressive pigmented capillaropa-thy (Schamberg's disease) of the arm. *Br J Dermatol* 2001; **144**: 190–1.

27 Hamada T, Inoue Y, Nakama T, Hashimoto T. A case of zosteriform pigmented purpuric dermatosis. *Arch Dermatol* 2007; **143**: 1599–600.

28 Ma-Hui JZhao G, Liu W, Dang YP, Li-Dong G. Unilateral linear capillaritis: two unusual Chinese cases. *Eur J Dermatol* 2007; **17**: 160–3.

29 Higgins EM, Cox NH. A case of quadrantic capillaropathy. *Dermatologica* 1990; **180**: 93–5.

30 Bell HK, Dobson CM, Jackson SP, King CM. Localized morphoea preceded by a pigmented purpuric dermatosis. *Clin Exp Dermatol* 2003; **28**: 369–71.

Treatment of pigmented purpuric dermatoses

These disorders may persist for many years [1–3] and are very resistant to any form of therapy; explanation without active inter-vention, or simply support hosiery, is often the most appropriate approach. Topical steroids may be of some help, especially for itch, but very prolonged use is best avoided. Emollients can be used as necessary. A rapid response of lichen aureus to topical pimecrolimus has been reported [4]. Psoralen and UVA (PUVA) [5–7] has proven effective in treating capillaritis of Schamberg, Gougerot–Blum and lichen aureus patterns, and TL01 UVB has been reported as effective in Schamberg's disease [8] and in Goug-erot–Blum pigmented purpuric lichenoid dermatitis [9]. Ciclospo-rin [10] and griseofulvin [11] have also been effective in individual reports; calcium dobesilate has been suggested as first-line therapy as nine treated patients stopped developing new lesions within 2 weeks, but as the improvement at 12 months was graded as mod-erate in one patient, mild in six and none in two, it is not clear that this agent has much useful benefit [12].

References

1 Ratnam KV, Su WPD, Peters MS. Purpura simplex (inflammatory purpura without vasculitis): a clinicopathologic study of 174 cases. *J Am Acad Dermatol* 1991; **25**: 642–7.

2 Rabinowitz LG. Pigmented purpuras. In: Harper J, Oranje AP, Prose N, eds. *Textbook of Pediatric Dermatology*, 2nd edn. Oxford: Blackwell Science, 2006: 1927–32.

3 Price ML, Wilson Jones E, Calnan CD *et al.* Lichen aureus: a localised persistent form of pigmented purpuric dermatosis. *Br J Dermatol* 1984; **112**: 307–14.

4 Böhm M, Bonsmann G, Luger T. Resolution of lichen aureus in a 10-year-old child after topical pimecrolimus. *Br J Dermatol* 2004; **150**: 519–20.

5 Wong WK, Ratnam KV. A report of two cases of pigmented purpuric dermatosis treated with PUVA therapy. *Acta Derm Venereol (Stockh)* 1991; **71**: 68–70.

6 Ling TC, Goulden V, Goodfield MJD. PUVA therapy in lichen aureus. *J Am Acad Dermatol* 2001; **45**: 145–6.

7 Seckin D, Yazici Z, Senol A, Demircay Z. A case of Schamberg's disease respond-ing dramatically to PUVA treatment. *Photodermatol Photoimmunol Photomed* 2008; **24**: 95–6.

8 Gudi VS, White GI. Progressive pigmented purpura (Schamberg's disease) responding to TL-01 ultraviolet B therapy. *Clin Exp Dermatol* 2004; **29**: 683–4.

9 Kocaturk E, Kavala M, Zindanci I *et al.* Narrowband UVB treatment of pig-mented purpuric lichenoid dermatitis (Gougerot-Blum). *Photodermatol Photoim-munol Photomed* 2009; **25**: 55–6.

10 Okada K, Ishikawa O, Miyachi Y. Purpura pigmentosa chronica successfully treated with oral cyclosporin A. *Br J Dermatol* 1995; **134**: 180–1.

11 Tamaki K, Yasaka N, Osada A *et al.* Successful treatment of pigmented purpuric dermatosis with griseofulvin. *Br J Dermatol* 1995; **132**: 159–60.

12 Agrawal SK, Gandhi V, Bhattacharya SN. Calcium dobesilate in pigmented purpuric dermatosis (PPD): a pilot evaluation. *J Dermatol* 2004; **31**: 98–103.

Disorders of cutaneous microvascular occlusion

Numerous conditions may cause microvascular occlusion (Table 49.5). This process may involve abnormal coagulation (e.g. DIC, APLS), platelet plugging (e.g. heparin necrosis), emboli or crystal deposition (e.g. cholesterol emboli), abnormal eryth-rocytes (e.g. sickle cell disease) or abnormal proteins (e.g. cryo-proteinaemia). Many of these conditions may cause purpura as one of their manifestations; many cause an initial non-inflamma-tory purpuric process that can be diagnostically helpful in dif-ferentiation from vasculitis. Morphological features that suggest this category of disease as an aetiology for early lesions include purpura without erythema, eschar without erythema, branching or fingering extension of the margins, or lesions that show purpuric, non-erythematous retiform, branching, or stellate configurations.

Table 49.5 Disorders of cutaneous microvascular occlusion: differential diagnosis by pathophysiological mechanism.*

Occlusion due to platelet plugs
Heparin-induced thrombocytopenia
Myeloproliferative disorders
Paroxysmal nocturnal haemoglobinuria
Thrombotic thrombocytopenic purpura (TTP)/haemolytic–uraemic syndrome (HUS)†

Occlusion due to cryogelling
Cryoglobulinaemia
Cryofibrinogenaemia
Cold-agglutinin-related occlusion

Occlusion due to vessel-invasive organisms
Ecthyma gangrenosum
Lucio phenomenon
Vessel-invasive fungi
Disseminated strongyloidiasis

Occlusion due to embolus
Cholesterol embolus
Oxalate crystal embolus
Atrial myxoma
Cardiac sterile thrombi
Septic emboli
Fat emboli‡

Occlusion due to systemic coagulopathies with cutaneous manifestations
Protein C/S/thrombomodulin pathway anomalies
   Neonatal purpura fulminans
   Coumadin necrosis
   Sepsis-related purpura fulminans
   Post-infectious purpura fulminans
Antiphospholipid antibody syndrome

Occlusion due to vascular coagulopathies§
Sneddon's syndrome
Livedoid vasculopathy/atrophie blanche
Malignant atrophic papulosis

Occlusion due to reticulocyte occlusion¶
Sickle cell disease
Other severe haemolytic anaemias

Occlusion due to unknown or controversial mechanisms
Cutaneous calciphylaxis
Some insect bites, especially *Loxosceles* (brown recluse spider)
Some snake bite syndromes**

* Most of these disorders present with purpura or necrosis with minimal inflammation, and frequently show retiform (stellate, branching) morphologies.
† TTP/HUS is usually occlusive in visceral vessels, but skin lesions are most often non-palpable petechiae, and not due to occlusion.
‡ Fat emboli typically cause occlusion in viscera, especially lungs; cutaneous lesions are rare and typically petechial, due to minute fat particle occlusion.
§ Sneddon's syndrome typically presents with pathological livedo reticularis; livedoid vasculopathy may have retiform purpura morphologies, however, atrophie blanche and malignant atrophic papulosis are often not purpuric, but heal with a characteristic atrophic scar with surrounding telangiectasia.
¶ Syndromes involving reticulocyte occlusion often heal with lesions mimicking atrophie blanche, and are seldom purpuric or retiform.
** Most snake bites cause haemorrhage; if fulminant disseminated intravascular coagulation results, some lesions might be occlusive.

Occlusion due to platelet plugs

Heparin-induced thrombocytopenia and heparin necrosis [1,2]

Aetiology and pathogenesis. The syndrome of heparin-induced thrombocytopenia (HIT) is an uncommon paradoxical response to heparin, with some female predominance [1]. This syndrome can be defined as any clinical event best explained by PF4/heparin-reactive antibodies (HIT antibodies) in a patient who is receiving, or who has recently received, heparin [1]. Although IgA and IgM class antibodies may play a role, IgG antibody is most closely associated with this syndrome [3]. The antibody that causes HIT is not simply an antiheparin antibody. Heparin and certain other polyanions, when bound to PF4, can induce conformational changes in tetrameric PF4, exposing new epitopes on PF4. This may trigger antibody production to these newly exposed regions. When antiheparin/PF4 antibody binds with heparin/PF4 complexes on the surface of platelets, platelet activation and aggregation results. Not all heparin/PF4 antibodies appear to be pathogenic, and some antibodies responsible for HIT do not bind to heparin/PF4 complexes but to chemokines or cytokines, such as neutrophil activating peptide-2 (NAP-2) and interleukin-8, somehow activating platelets [1–3].

Unfractionated heparin is three times more likely to be associated with HIT following orthopaedic surgery compared with low-molecular-weight heparin [1]. HIT is more likely to be induced by bovine-derived unfractionated heparin than the porcine-derived variety, consistent with the hypothesis that longer and more flexible heparins bind to PF4 tetramers in ways that induce more conformational change and more exposure of neoepitopes. This may also explain the lower risk of HIT with low-molecular-weight heparins. HIT is even less likely to be triggered by fondaparinux, a pentasaccharide anticoagulant modelled after the antithrombin binding region of heparin [1]. The risk of HIT is highest in post-surgical patients, less so in medical patients requiring heparin and lowest in obstetric settings [1].

Clinical features. Patients with HIT usually develop absolute or relative thrombocytopenia (90%), often followed by evidence of venous or arterial thromboses or of heparin necrosis in the skin [1]. A proportional drop of over 50% in platelet number from the pre-treatment count may be a better indication of early heparin-induced platelet aggregation than an absolute thrombocytopenia of $100–150 \times 10^9$/L [1]. This may occur immediately after heparin administration if the patient has been previously sensitized and has received heparin within the past 100 days. In two-thirds of patients, the fall in platelet count begins between days 5 and 10 of heparin administration, although significant thrombocytopenia may take 7–14 days to develop [1,4,5]. Uncommonly, patients may develop HIT several days after stopping heparin (delayed-onset HIT); this is attributed to the presence of high-titre antibodies that can recognize PF4 neoepitopes even in the absence of heparin binding, perhaps binding instead to chondroitin sulphate [1]. A history of HIT is not predictive of a second episode if the patient last received heparin more than 100 days previously. Although essential to thrombosis, HIT-IgG antibodies are not sufficient alone to produce thrombosis. Only 5–30% of patients who form HIT-IgG will develop clinical HIT [1]. Only half of antibody-positive patients produce IgG class antibodies, and only half of the IgG class group show biological activity.

Accumulating reports of catastrophic thrombotic episodes, typically venous limb gangrene, suggest that there may be a synergistic thrombophilic state in patients with HIT also treated with warfarin, presumably through both HIT and protein C-depletion pathways [1].

Heparin administration commonly induces cutaneous findings of simple haemorrhage with ecchymoses, and occasionally triggers urticaria or infiltrated plaques [6–8]. Uncommonly, the syndrome of heparin necrosis results as a cutaneous microvascular occlusion subset of HIT. Purpuric, tender, sharply demarcated plaques develop; retiform extensions that sometimes develop at the lesional margins are characteristic of heparin necrosis. Erythema may sometimes accompany such lesions, and necrosis is frequent. Lesions are most common at subcutaneous injection sites but can occur elsewhere [9–11] (Fig. 49.10). Interestingly, as few as one-third of patients with skin lesions of heparin necrosis may develop absolute thrombocytopenia, even when HIT antibodies are detected [1]. Haemorrhagic adrenal infarction has been reported in such cases. Histological examination of lesions reveals 'white clots', representing platelet–fibrin thrombi, in the cutaneous microvasculature [5,12].

Treatment. Treatment of HIT and heparin necrosis continues to evolve. The correct diagnosis is important, because many patients on heparin develop thrombocytopenia for reasons other than the development of HIT antibodies; conversely, patients may develop the arterial or venous thromboses, or especially heparin necrosis, without manifesting thrombocytopenia [1]. Stopping heparin is important, although some patients do not worsen if heparin is continued whereas others may progress despite stopping heparin. Although replacing heparin with coumadin was previously thought to be effective in treating HIT and heparin necrosis, coumadin substitution is not only ineffective but may in fact induce venous limb gangrene [1]. Low-molecular-weight heparin is much less likely to cause HIT, but it is contraindicated for treatment of patients with HIT due to other types of heparin. Surprisingly, heparin is the appropriate treatment for cardiac surgery patients with a previous history of HIT, but whose antibodies have disappeared (beyond 100 days). The anticoagulants currently used to treat patients with HIT are danaparoid (a heparinoid) and two thrombin inhibitors, lepirudin and argatroban [1]. Even with treatment with one of these agents, there is a 5–20% frequency of new thromboses. Major bleeding in HIT patients has occurred in 3.1% of those treated with argatroban, and in 5.9–14.4% of those treated with lepirudin. Danaparoid is available in many countries, including the UK, but not currently in the United States.

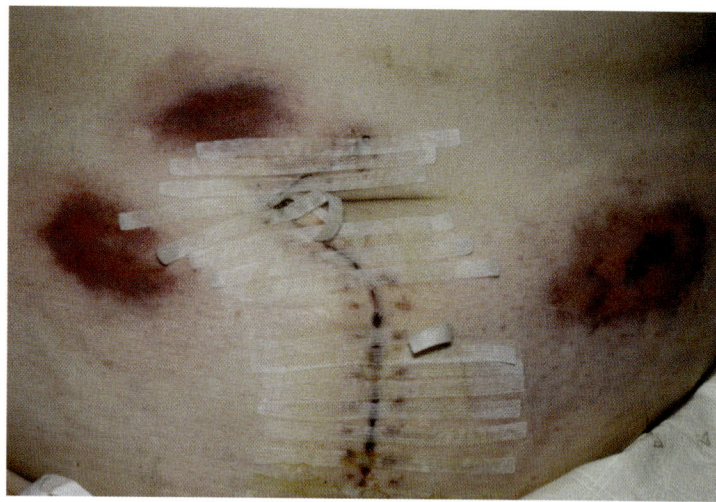

(a)

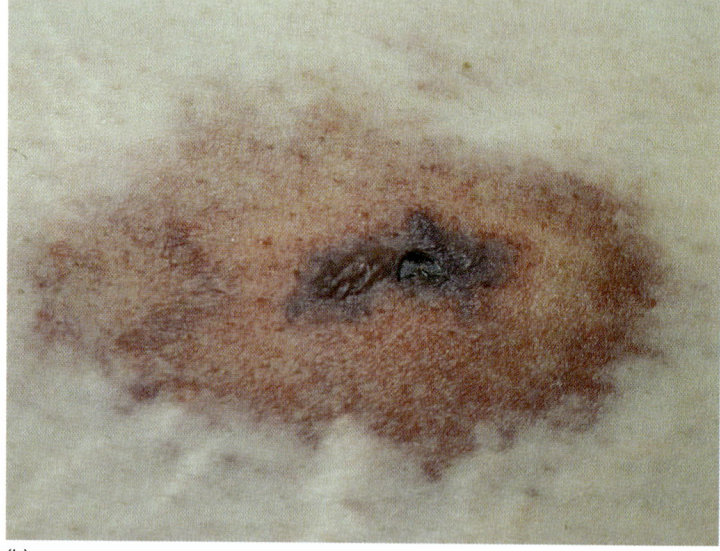

(b)

Fig. 49.10 (a) Heparin necrosis at sites of subcutaneous heparin injection. (b) Close-up of a 15-cm lesion on left abdomen. Lesion is a non-palpable haemorrhage with retiform margins, minimal erythema and central retiform intense haemorrhage, early necrosis and bullae formation. (From Robson K, Piette W. The presentation and differential diagnosis of cutaneous vascular occlusion syndromes. *Adv Dermatol* 1999; **15**: 153–82, with permission from Mosby.)

References

1 Kelton JG, Warkentin TE. Heparin-induced thrombocytopenia: a historical perspective. *Blood* 2008; **112**: 2607–15.

2 Arepally GM, Ortel TL. Heparin-induced thrombocytopenia. *N Engl J Med* 2006; **355**: 809–17.

3 Untch B, Ahmad S, Jeske W *et al.* Prevalence, isotype, and functionality of antiheparin–platelet factor 4 antibodies in patients treated with heparin and clinically suspected for heparin-induced thrombocytopenia. The pathogenic role of IgG. *Thromb Res* 2002; **105**: 117–23.

4 Sallah S, Thomas D, Roberts H. Warfarin and heparin-induced skin necrosis and the purple toe syndrome: infrequent complications of anticoagulant treatment. *Thromb Haemost* 1997; **78**: 785–90.

5 Gross A, Thompson F, Arzbiaga M *et al.* Heparin-associated thrombocytopenia and thrombosis (HATT) presenting with livedo reticularis. *Int J Dermatol* 1993; **32**: 276–9.

6 Tuneu A, Moreno A, de Moragas J. Cutaneous reactions secondary to heparin injections. *J Am Acad Dermatol* 1985; **12**: 1072–7.

7 Klein G, Kofler H, Wolf H *et al.* Eczema-like, erythematous, infiltrated plaques: a common side effect of subcutaneous heparin therapy. *J Am Acad Dermatol* 1989; **21**: 703–7.

8 Rose GA, Spencer H. Polyarteritis nodosa. *QJM* 1957; **27**: 43.

9 Levine L, Bernstein J, Soltani K *et al.* Heparin-induced cutaneous necrosis unrelated to injection sites: a sign of potentially lethal complications. *Arch Dermatol* 1983; **7**: 674–7.

10 Santamaria A, Romani J, Souto J *et al.* Skin necrosis at the injection site induced by low-molecular-weight heparin: case report and review. *Dermatology* 1998; **196**: 264–5.

11 Tietge U, Schmidt H, Jackel E *et al.* Low molecular weight heparin-induced skin necrosis occurring distant from injection sites and without thrombocytopenia. *J Intern Med* 1998; **243**: 313–5.

12 Chang J. White clot syndrome associated with heparin-induced thrombocytopenia: a review of 23 cases. *Heart Lung* 1987; **16**: 403–7.

Myeloproliferative disorders

Cutaneous lesions are common in thrombocythaemia and other myeloproliferative disorders (see also Chapter 62). Paradoxically, patients with myeloproliferative thrombocytosis may both bleed and clot abnormally. Skin lesions were documented in 22% of 268 patients with essential thrombocythaemia [1], and included urticaria, livedo reticularis, petechiae, ecchymoses, haematomas, erythromelalgia, Raynaud's phenomenon, recurrent superficial thrombophlebitis, necrotizing vasculitis, leg ulceration and gangrene. Biopsy findings were variable, but some livedo reticularis and acral infarcts were associated with evidence of microvascular occlusion. Additionally, tender erythematous facial plaques and palmar violet macules and papules were reported as manifestations of platelet plugging in a patient with atypical chronic myeloproliferative disease and a history of Budd–Chiari syndrome, another known thrombotic complication of myeloproliferative disease [2]. This patient's cutaneous lesions were unresponsive to coumadin, but cleared within 24 h of aspirin administration following identification of platelet plugs as the cause of previously identified microvascular occlusion.

Essential thrombocytosis and polycythaemia vera, although rare, are the first and second most common causes of elevated platelet counts, with an increased frequency of thrombotic events and of erythromelalgia [3]. A recent study of 605 patients with essential thrombocythaemia found a 10-year risk of thrombosis of 14% [4]. These diseases are more common at younger ages and in women. However, reactive or post-splenectomy thrombocytosis at any level is not associated with occlusion, suggesting that thrombosis in the setting of myeloproliferative disease is not a function of thrombocytosis alone. Multiple studies have shown that a specific mutation in the JAK2 tyrosine kinase (JAK2V617F) is found in many patients with essential thrombocytosis, polycythaemia vera, and primary myelofibrosis, and a gain-of-function mutation in the thrombopoietin receptor (MPL) in a subset of patients with essential thrombocytosis but who are JAK2V617-negative [5]. The mechanisms for ischaemic or occlusive syndromes in myeloproliferative disease must therefore depend on more than platelet number alone; the following factors may be relevant. Acquired von Willebrand factors in myeloproliferative disease have been associated with both bleeding and thrombotic complications. Anticardiolipin antibodies, factor V Leiden mutations, abnormal endothelial cell function, and decreased levels of protein C and protein S may be synergistic for thrombosis in chronic myeloproliferative diseases [6,7]. In addition to high platelet counts, abnormal platelet function occurs in myeloproliferative or myelodysplastic disease, although whether this can lead to vascular occlusion at platelet counts less than 1000×10^9/L is controversial. Thrombotic events have been reported at platelet counts below 600×10^9/L in patients with essential thrombocyto-

sis, including some events at normal platelet counts [8]. In a study of 56 consecutive patients with essential thrombocytosis, 46 developed complications mostly related to thrombosis [8]. In these 46 patients, severe complications occurred in 22% at platelet counts lower than 600×10^9/L, in 15% at counts lower than 500×10^9/L, and in 4% at counts lower than 400×10^9/L. In a cohort of 1063 patients with essential thrombocythaemia, a paradoxical finding reported was that a platelet count greater than 1000×10^9/L was associated with a lower risk of thrombocytosis, and if combined with a leukocyte count less than 11×10^9/L pointed to a 'low-risk' category of thrombosis [9].

Erythromelalgia (erythralgia) can occur as a primary or secondary syndrome. This intensely uncomfortable burning associated with paroxysmal erythema of the distal extremities is frequently triggered by skin contact with a warm surface. Although erythromelalgia has been seen in many different settings, the association of purpuric or necrotic areas on hands and feet with the dysaesthetic erythema is exclusively seen with myeloproliferative or myelodysplastic thrombocytosis [10]. Because of the platelet origin of occlusion and vascular symptoms in the myeloproliferative subset of erythromelalgia, aspirin administration is notably effective in clearing lesions and alleviating symptoms, whereas it is much less effective in primary and other secondary forms of erythromelalgia.

Splenomegaly may be seen in all forms of myeloproliferative syndromes. Ruddy cyanosis is characteristic of polycythaemia vera, as is elevation of haemoglobin, haematocrit and red cell mass. All syndromes may show elevations in white count, but this is most characteristic of chronic granulocytic leukaemia, especially in association with elevated eosinophil and basophil counts. Anaemia and altered red cell morphology can occur over time in all patients, and all these diseases have some risk of transition to dyspoiesis and severe anaemia, leukaemia or myelofibrosis.

Many therapies previously used for myeloproliferative thrombocytosis increase the risk of leukaemic transformation and of complications in fertility and pregnancy. Low-dose aspirin has been widely accepted as effective thrombosis prophylaxis, although definitive proof of its efficacy is lacking. Its dramatic reversal of signs and symptoms in erythromelalgia provides some clinical evidence for its usefulness in thrombocythaemic complications. Hydroxycarbamide is the drug of choice for prevention of transient ischaemic attacks, but may not be effective in preventing venous thrombosis, and anagrelide treatment may reduce the risk of venous thrombosis but appears to dramatically increase the risk for arterial thrombosis and haemorrhage. Anagrelide has become an important therapeutic agent, acting to both inhibit platelet activity and decrease the platelet count [11,12]. The JAK2 mutations seem to correlate with leukocyte and platelet proliferation, but the role for the JAK2 and MPL mutations in enhancing thromboses is less clear [5,13]. Multiple studies suggest that the presence of the JAK2V617F mutation translates into activation of haemostasis, at least in part through increase in platelet-associated tissue factor microparticles and increased platelet–neutrophil aggregates [14].

References

1 Itin P, Winkelmann R. Cutaneous manifestations in patients with essential thrombocythemia. *J Am Acad Dermatol* 1991; **24**: 59–63.

2 Stone M, Robson K, Piette W. Erythematous plaques due to platelet plugging: a clue to underlying myeloproliferative disorder. *J Am Acad Dermatol* 2000; **43**: 355–7.

3 Tefferi A, La S, Silverstein M. A clinical update in polycythemia vera and essential thrombocythemia. *Am J Med* 2000; **109**: 141–9.

4 Passominti F, Rumi E, Arcaini L *et al.* Prognostic factors for thrombosis, myelofibrosis, and leukemia in essential thrombocythemia: a study of 605 patients. *Haematologica* 2008; **93**: 1645–51.

5 Levine RL, Heaney M. New advances in the pathogenesis and therapy of essential thrombocythemia. *Hematology Am Soc Hematol Educ Program* 2008: 76–82.

6 Sanchez-Luceros A, Meschengieser S, Woods A *et al.* Acquired von Willebrand factor abnormalities in myeloproliferative disorders and other hematologic diseases: a retrospective analysis by a single institution. *Haematologica* 2002; **87**: 264–70.

7 Jensen M, Brown P, Thorsen S, Hasselbalch H. Frequent occurrence of anticardiolipin antibodies, Factor V Leiden mutation, and perturbed endothelial function in chronic myeloproliferative disorders. *Am J Hematol* 2002; **69**: 185–91.

8 Regev A, Stark P, Blickstein D, Lahav M. Thrombotic complications in essential thrombocythemia with relatively low platelet counts. *Am J Hematol* 1997; **56**: 168–72.

9 Carrobio A, Finazzi G, Antioneli E *et al.* Thrombocytosis and leukocytosis interaction in vascular complications of essential thrombocythemia. *Blood* 2008; **112**: 3134–7. (Comment in *Blood* 2008; **112**: 3526; author reply 3526–7.)

10 Michiels J, ten Kate F. Erythromelalgia in thrombocythemia of various myeloproliferative disorders. *Am J Hematol* 1992; **39**: 131–6.

11 Tefferi A, Silverstein M, Petitt R *et al.* Anagrelide as a new platelet-lowering agent in essential thrombocythemia: mechanism of action, efficacy, toxicity, current indications. *Sem Thromb Hemost* 1997; **23**: 379–83.

12 Emadi A, Spivak JL. Anagrelide: 20 years later. *Expert Rev Anticancer Ther* 2009; **9**: 37–50.

13 Austin SK, Lambert JR. The JAK2 617F mutation and thrombosis. *Br J Haematol* 2008; **143**: 307–20.

14 Falanga A, Barbui T, Rickles FR. Hypercoagulability and tissue factor gene upregulation in hematologic malignancies. *Semin Thromb Hemost* 2008; **34**: 204–10.

Paroxysmal nocturnal haemoglobinuria

Paroxysmal nocturnal haemoglobinuria (PNH) is an acquired clonal blood disorder associated with deficient haematopoiesis, intravascular haemolysis and venous thrombosis [1,2]. Episodic haemoglobinuria is the characteristic result of nocturnal haemolysis, although it is the presenting feature in only 26% of patients [1,2]. The sleep-associated haemoglobinuria is secondary to an abnormally increased sensitivity of red blood cells to lysis by serum complement [1]. This increased sensitivity to complement lysis is related to abnormal regulation at two different points of the complement cascade, and this abnormal regulation is due in turn to the partial to complete deficiency of two membrane-associated inhibitors of the complement cascade, decay-accelerating factor (DAF) and membrane inhibitor of reactive lysis (MIRL, also known as CD59). DAF inhibits the activity of classic complement pathway C3 convertase and of alternative pathway C3 convertase, and MIRL/CD59 regulates the activity of the complement membrane attack complex on red cells. These two inhibitors are part of a group of roughly 20 red cell membrane proteins that share a common post-translational modification in the glycosylphosphatidylinositol (GPI) anchor. In PNH, a somatic mutation in the phosphatidylinositol glycan class A gene (*PIG-A*) on the X chromosome alters the ability of proteins sharing the GPI anchor to bind to the membrane [1–3]. Whereas previous diagnostic tests for PNH relied on the haemolytic sensitivity of PNH red blood cells, current tests rely on detection of loss of CD59 and/or CD55 on red cells, loss of CD59, CD24, CD16, or other GPI-anchored proteins on granulocytes, or lack of FLAER (Fluorescently Labelled inactive toxin AERolysin) binding to granulocytes, which also depends on binding to GPI anchors [4].

This complex pathophysiology explains the haemolysis and haemoglobinuria in PNH, but does not yet completely explain other manifestations of this disease such as thrombosis. Although 10–15% of patients may show spontaneous remission, the median survival is 10–15 years [4]. Thrombosis is a major morbidity; 40% of patients develop venous thrombosis [2], and this is the most frequent cause of death [4]. At least some of the thrombotic tendency may be related to complement-mediated activation of platelets or to platelet–leukocyte complexes, which share the defect in GPI-anchored proteins. Budd–Chiari syndrome (hepatic vein thrombosis) is common, as are thromboses in unusual sites such as cerebral, dermal, hepatic and portal, mesenteric and splanchnic veins [1]. This unusual localization may also favour a role of platelets in the thrombophilic state. The most likely pathway for this appears to be the development of microparticles from complement-damaged red cells and platelets, leading to an increase of phospholipid membrane surface area in blood. Episodes of thrombosis often follow haemolytic episodes, also suggesting that haemolysis-associated changes, such as nitric oxide depletion by released haemoglobin, may play an important role in thrombogenesis [4]. This same pathway is implicated in the vascular occlusion seen in sickle cell disease, another haemolytic anaemia. Clinical dermatological features of PNH include pyoderma gangrenosum, haemorrhagic bullae, cutaneous venous thrombosis and DIC [4,5].

Anticoagulants, corticosteroids and thrombolytic therapy may be effective in treating thrombotic episodes; the role of antiplatelet therapy is unclear [6]. More recently, the use of the humanized monoclonal antibody eculizumab, directed against the C5 component of complement, to reduce haemolysis, has also resulted in reduction in thromboses from 7.37 per 100 patient years to 1.07 per hundred patient years in PNH. This supports the hypothesis that haemolysis induces a thrombophilic state, either through nitric oxide reduction by free haemoglobin or inhibition of membrane damage which might otherwise lead to microparticle formation [7,8]. The only observed risk for infection from this therapy appears to be an increase in the risk of infection by *Neisseria meningitidis* or by *N. gonorrhoeae* (0.5 cases per 100 patient years with eculizumab). Although the antibody-induced equivalent of a late complement component deficiency may lead to an increased risk of infection, the complications from such an infection appear to be less than anticipated, as in patients with inherited terminal complement deficiency. The risk of infection can also be reduced by vaccination with tetravalent meningococcal vaccine, and by counselling of patients to promote early recognition and treatment of possible meningococcal infection [7].

References

1 Parker CJ. Historical aspects of paroxysmal nocturnal haemoglobinuria: 'defining the disease'. *Br J Haematol* 2002; **117**: 3–22.

2 Rosse W, Bunn H. Hemolytic anemias and acute blood loss. In: Fauci A, Braunwald E, Isselbacher K *et al.*, eds. *Harrison's Principles of Internal Medicine*. New York: McGraw-Hill, 1998: 659–71.

3 Maceijewski J, Young N, Yu M *et al.* Analysis of the expression of glycosylphosphatidylinositol anchored proteins on platelets from patients with paroxysmal nocturnal hemoglobinuria. *Thromb Res* 1996; **83**: 433–47.

4 Bessler M, Hiken J. The pathophysiology of disease in patients with paroxysmal nocturnal hemoglobinuria. *Hematology Am Soc Hematol Education Program* 2008: 104–10.

5 Rietschel RL, Lewis CW, Simmons RA, Phyliky RL. Skin lesions in paroxysmal nocturnal hemoglobinuria. *Arch Dermatol* 1978; **114**: 560–3.

6 Beutler E. Paroxysmal nocturnal hemoglobinuria. In: Beutler E, Coller B, Lichtman M *et al.*, eds. *Williams' Hematology*, 6th edn. New York: McGraw-Hill, 2001: 419–24.

7 Hillmen P. The role of complement inhibition in PNH. *Hematology Am Soc Hematol Educ Program* 2008: 116–23.

8 Hillmen P, Muus P, Duhrsen U *et al.* Effect of the complement inhibitor eculizumab on thromboembolism in patients with paroxysmal nocturnal hemoglobinuria. *Blood* 2007; **110**: 4123–8.

Thrombotic thrombocytopenic purpura/haemolytic–uraemic syndrome

Thrombotic thrombocytopenic purpura (TTP) was first reported by Moschowitz in 1924 as an acquired syndrome, and subsequently as a congenital syndrome by Schulman (Upshaw–Schulman syndrome) in 1960 [1]. For many years, criteria for the diagnosis of TTP included thrombocytopenic purpura, microangiopathic haemolytic anaemia, renal dysfunction or failure, neurological abnormalities and fever, with a fatal outcome in 90% of patients [2]. Once plasma exchange proved at least sometimes effective in treating this disorder, criteria for diagnosis were pared to include only thrombocytopenia and microangiopathic haemolytic anaemia. Haemolytic–uraemic syndrome (HUS) was originally described in children with acute renal failure, microangiopathic haemolytic anaemia and, usually, thrombocytopenia, but no purpura, neurological findings or fever. Current diagnostic criteria do not distinguish between TTP and HUS. However, childhood HUS is distinguished clinically because most cases are related to enteric infection with *Escherichia coli* O157:H7, HUS developing about 1 week after diarrhoea due to this agent; most children survive without plasma exchange [2]. Epidemic forms of HUS are most common, associated with prodromal diarrhoea and with verotoxin (shigatoxin S1 or S2)-producing organisms, usually the *E. coli* strain mentioned previously, or enterococcus [3]. *Mycoplasma* can also provoke TTP. Pregnancy can induce TTP/HUS, as well as *HELLP* syndrome (haemolysis, elevated liver enzymes, low platelet count), as a complication of pre-eclampsia and eclampsia, and these may be difficult to distinguish [3]. TTP/HUS has been reported secondary to drugs (especially mitomycin C, ciclosporin, ticlopidine and quinine), after allogeneic bone marrow transplantation, and associated with autoimmune connective tissue disease (lupus erythematosus, scleroderma), vasculitis (polyarteritis nodosa), APLS [4], Sjögren's syndrome or metastatic carcinoma.

The molecular basis of TTP is a severe deficiency of a protease (ADAMTS13, 'A Disintegrin-like And Metalloprotease with Thrombospondin repeats' family of metalloproteases) that cleaves von Willebrand factor, resulting in persistence in plasma of ultra-large von Willebrand multimers secreted by endothelial cells [1–3]. Persistence of such large multimers in the circulation leads to formation of microvascular platelet thrombi. Congenital deficiency of ADAMTS13 leads to lifelong, recurrent episodes of TTP; mechanisms for acquired ADAMTS13 are still unclear, but can

include acquired autoantibody. Some regard ADAMTS13 deficiency as a diagnostic feature of TTP (congenital and idiopathic), although ADAMTS13 levels are reported to be normal in most patients with secondary TTP/HUS [1,5,6]. Von Willebrand factor protease is deficient in hereditary, intermittent relapsing, intermittent acute, ticlodipine-induced and clopidogrel-induced TTP, but is normal in HUS and in transplantation-related thrombotic microangiopathy. However, not all patients with deficient von Willebrand factor protease have active TTP. ADAMTS13 deficiency rarely if ever occurs in the diarrhoea-associated HUS (D+ HUS) caused by shigatoxin-producing *E. coli*. HUS without antecedent diarrhoea is termed 'atypical HUS'; it also is typically not associated with ADAMTS13 deficiency, but frequently has alternate complement pathway abnormalities due to mutations in complement factor H, I, B, or in membrane cofactor protein [1].

Treatment options include plasma exchange with fresh frozen whole plasma or parts of plasma (e.g. cryoprecipitate-reduced plasma, high-molecular-weight fraction); corticosteroids, vincristine and antiplatelet drugs may also have a role. Outcome is usually good in childhood but less so in familial forms. As a practical matter, the response of patients to plasma exchange treatment in TTP or HUS is independent of whether they have deficient or normal levels of ADAMTS13 [7].

Microvascular platelet thrombi are characteristically seen in patients with TTP, especially in the renal and cerebral circulation [2]. Some have reported that HUS patients more often have fibrin-rich thrombi and more limited visceral vessel involvement [8]. Purpuric skin lesions are frequently mentioned in reports and reviews of TTP, but histological characterization of such cutaneous lesions is very sparse. Hyaline microthrombi composed of platelets and fibrin have been reported [9]. It seems likely from evaluation of lesional photographs that many, if not most, of the skin lesions in TTP are related to thrombocytopenia and simple haemorrhage rather than to microvascular platelet plugs as seen in the cerebral and renal vessels.

References

1 Sadler JE. Von Willebrand factor, ADAMTS13, and thrombotic thrombocytopenic purpura. *Blood* 2008; **112**: 11–8.

2 George J, Vesely S. Thrombotic thrombocytopenic purpura: from the bench to the bedside, but not yet to the community. *Ann Intern Med* 2003; **138**: 152–4.

3 Allford S, Hunt B, Rose P, Machin S. Guidelines on the diagnosis and management of the thrombotic microangiopathic haemolytic anaemias. *Br J Haematol* 2003; **120**: 556–73.

4 George J, Rizvi M. Thrombocytopenia. In: Beutler E, Lichtman M, Coller B *et al.*, eds. *Williams' Hematology*, 6th edn. New York: McGraw-Hill, 2001: 1495–539.

5 Moake J. Thrombotic microangiopathies. *N Engl J Med* 2002; **347**: 589–600.

6 Veyradier A, Obert B, Houllier A *et al.* Specific von Willebrand factor-cleaving protease in thrombotic microangiopathies: a study of 111 cases. *Blood* 2001; **98**: 1765–72.

7 Vesely S, George J, Lammle B *et al.* ADAMTS13 activity in thrombotic thrombocytopenic purpura–hemolytic uremic syndrome: relation to presenting features and clinical outcomes in a prospective cohort of 142 patients. *Blood* 2003; **102**: 60–8.

8 Hosler G, Cusumano A, Hutchins G. Thrombotic thrombocytopenic purpura and hemolytic uremic syndrome are distinct pathologic entities: a review of 56 autopsy cases. *Arch Pathol Lab Med* 2003; **127**: 834–9.

9 Zucker-Franklin D. Cutaneous manifestations of hematologic disorders. In: Fitzpatrick J, Eisen A, Wolff K *et al.*, eds. *Dermatology in General Medicine*. New York: McGraw-Hill, 1993: 1993–2003.

Occlusion due to cryogelling

Common clinical features

Occlusion syndromes triggered by cold exposure are suggested by an acral distribution of lesions of necrosis or purpura, often with retiform features, and sometimes associated with acral livedo reticularis. An acral distribution must be distinguished from a dependent distribution of lesions. Both patterns may involve hands and feet, but with a dependent pattern there are typically many more lesions on the feet and legs than on the hands. A dependent distribution of lesions suggests immune complex-mediated disease, and usually presents as classical palpable purpura or occasionally as inflammatory retiform purpura, not as bland or non-inflammatory purpura or pauci-erythematous necrosis. An acral distribution of lesions is also characteristic of erythema multiforme. However, erythema multiforme presents with target lesions, atypical target lesions or classical palpable purpura, rather than non-inflammatory retiform purpura or necrosis, and it is not associated with livedo reticularis. In addition, the acral distribution of cryo-occlusion syndromes often includes the ears and nose, sites usually unaffected by erythema multiforme. Although ill patients with immune complex vasculitis may develop dependent lesions on the posterior portions of the ears if supine due to their illness, their other lesions are typically in dependent areas as well, and there is usually no history of cold exposure as the precipitating factor. A biopsy of early lesions, before necrosis has had time to trigger a secondary vasculitic histology, should show non-inflammatory occlusion of dermal vessels with cryoprotein or agglutinated red cells.

Careful handling of serum and plasma is necessary to allow identification of cryogelling proteins, because those most likely to cause disease are those that gel at temperatures very close to normal body temperature. Likewise, identification of cryoproteins or cryoagglutinins does not prove a cryo-occlusion syndrome, because these may either gel at temperatures that are not relevant to typical cold exposure or may simply represent incidental findings. The latter is especially true of cryofibrinogens and cold agglutinins.

Cryoglobulins

Cryoglobulins, immunoglobulins that reversibly precipitate or gel in the cold, were first reported in 1933 and were named cryoglobulins in 1947 [1–4]. In 1974, Brouet et al. [1] proposed the now standard subset classification of cryoglobulins into types I, II and III. In the 1990s, a large proportion of cases were found to be associated with hepatitis C. Although precipitation of cryoglobulins is primarily related to reversible cold-induced denaturation of protein, other factors such as cryoglobulin concentration in the microvascular environment, pH and non-covalent binding factors also influence the likelihood and intensity of precipitation.

Type I (single molecule) cryoglobulins are single monoclonal immunoglobulins, usually IgG or IgM, less commonly IgA, and rarely Bence–Jones protein. Accounting for 10–15% of cryoglobulins, they are often associated with an underlying lymphoproliferative disorder, especially multiple myeloma or Waldenström's macroglobulinaemia [5]. As type I cryoglobulins are single proteins and are neither immune complexes nor proven to activate complement, if they are to cause vascular injury or occlusion they can do so only by cryogelling and not by immune complex vasculitis.

Types II and III, termed mixed cryoglobulins, are multiple molecule proteins, typically immune complexes, that gel under laboratory conditions (2–4°C). Unless they gel at temperatures close to body temperature, they are much more likely to cause disease as immune complexes than as cryoproteins, but they can cause disease through either or both mechanisms in any given patient. Rheumatoid factor activity (defined by anti-Fc binding) is detectable in the sera of 87–100% of patients with mixed cryoglobulinaemia [3]. Type II cryoglobulins are composed of monoclonal proteins of IgM, IgG or occasionally IgA class that bind to an antigen present in the blood, most commonly the Fc portion of polyclonal IgG molecules. Those that bind immunoglobulin (usually IgG) by anti-Fc affinity are also, by definition, rheumatoid factors, although only the IgM/anti-IgG rheumatoid factors are recognized by standard rheumatoid factor testing. In up to 95% of type II cryoglobulins with IgM as the antirheumatoid factor immunoglobulin, the IgM contains a κ light chain, which would not be expected by chance alone [3,6]. Type III mixed cryoglobulins are also most commonly rheumatoid factors, but the IgM, IgG or IgA anti-Fc antibodies in this group are polyclonal rather than monoclonal. In patients with mixed type II or III cryoglobulins, complement levels are usually reduced, especially the C4 component.

Antibodies to hepatitis C virus (HCV) have been found in more than 50% (42–98%) of patients with type II and III cryoglobulins [2–4]. Conversely, 13–54% of patients with HCV have mixed cryoglobulins detected in the laboratory, and the majority of these are type III cryoglobulins (67–91%). Of HCV-infected individuals with cryoglobulins, only 27% had clinical signs consistent with the syndrome of cryoglobulinaemia [2]. The reasons why only a fraction of HCV-infected and cryoglobulin-positive patients develop symptomatic cryoglobulinaemia are unknown.

In a multicentre Italian cooperative study of 913 patients with cryoglobulinaemia, 8.9% of all patients with symptomatic cryoglobulinaemia had lymphoproliferative disease at diagnosis [2]. Of this subset of patients, 27% had type I, 68% had type II and 5% had type III cryoglobulins. Although type I cryoglobulinaemia is usually associated with lymphoproliferative disease, it is a much less common type than types II and III; the latter two types therefore accounted for the majority of cryoglobulinaemia-associated lymphoproliferative disease in this study from a region with a high endemic rate of HCV and mixed cryoglobulinaemia.

Other syndromes are also associated with cryoglobulins detectable in serum. Patients with connective tissue disease also have higher rates of cryoglobulinaemia: it occurs in up to 25% of patients with SLE, 12.5% of patients with systemic sclerosis, 46% of patients with active rheumatoid arthritis and 17–37% of patients with Sjögren's syndrome [2]. In addition to HCV, other chronic infections such as Lyme disease, subacute bacterial endocarditis (up to 90%), Q fever, hepatitis A and B, hantavirus, cytomegalovirus, human T-cell leukaemia virus I and HIV have been reported [2,7]. Chronic inflammatory disease, such as liver cirrhosis from any cause, is also associated with a higher than expected rate of detectable cryoglobulins. The presence of cryoglobulins in serum does not invariably predict disease; cryoglobulins were present at low titre in as high as 51% of normal individuals in one study [8]. In fact, despite detectable serum cryoglobulins in the patient groups mentioned, most will not develop symptomatic cryoglobulinaemia [2].

There are only two known ways in which cryoglobulins can result in disease. The first is by precipitation within the vascular lumen, typically cold-induced, with hyaline plug formation and minimal early-phase inflammation. Typical clinical lesions would be minimally inflammatory cutaneous infarction with or without associated livedo reticularis, or non-inflammatory retiform purpura. Since there is little evidence that cryogelling of monoclonal antibody induces complement activation, cryogelling is the only known mechanism for vascular lesions for type I cryoglobulins [5]. The second mechanism is that of immune complex vasculitis. As nearly all type II and III cryoglobulins are immune complexes, they should all be capable of inducing an immune complex vasculitis, although many do not. If they cryoprecipitate near body temperature, they could also cause vascular injury by simple occlusion, although most appear to gel at temperatures well below 37°C.

The median age at diagnosis of cryoglobulinaemia is early to middle sixth decade, with a female to male ratio of 2:1 [2]. Recurrent showers of dependent palpable purpura, sometimes with burning or itching, frequently associated with arthritis or arthralgia, is the classic presentation of mixed (type II and III) cryoglobulinaemia (the combination of purpura, asthenia and arthralgia has been termed Meltzer's triad). Patients with symptomatic cryoglobulinaemia of any type most often present with cutaneous lesions, usually purpura (in 55–100%, especially if HCV-associated) [2–4,9]. Ulceration, haemorrhagic crusts or cutaneous infarction are seen in 10–25% of patients, most often with type I cryoglobulins. Cold-induced acrocyanosis of acral areas, and non-inflammatory retiform purpura are also more typical of type I cryoglobulinaemia. Other reported cutaneous findings include acral cyanosis, Raynaud's phenomenon, urticarial lesions, ulceration and livedo reticularis [4,10,11]. Histological demonstration of non-inflammatory hyaline thrombosis is more common in patients with type I cryoglobulinaemia, but some such patients have also been reported to have cutaneous vasculitis [9]. A prospective study of biopsies of only new lesions (duration <48 h) of purpura in type I cryoglobulin patients has not been published. This leaves unresolved the issue of whether all reports of vasculitis in type I disease are those of vasculitis secondary to occlusive necrosis or ulceration. Non-cutaneous clinical findings most frequently include involvement of the joints (35–92%), peripheral nerves (17–56%), kidneys (21–29%) and liver [2–4].

Confirmation of cryoglobulins in sera requires careful handling of specimens to prevent cryoprecipitation before they can be detected. Collection of 10–20 mL of blood is suggested, and this must be kept warm and allowed to clot at 37°C for 30–60 min before centrifugation. The serum supernatant is left at 4°C for up to 7 days, with types I and II most likely to precipitate by 24 h [2,3,12]. A true cryoglobulin should once again be soluble if the sample is reheated to 37°C. Cryocrit measurements represent the percentage of the precipitate compared with the serum supernatant. Despite the presence of monoclonal protein, polyclonal gam-

mopathy is the most frequent finding on serum protein electrophoresis of serum samples (not cryoprecipitate specimens) in patients with type II cryoglobulinaemia [2]. A more sensitive technique, such as immunofixation, is needed to identify the presence of a clonal protein.

Treatment of cryoglobulinaemia is often problematic, and prospective or controlled trials are rare [3,4]. If symptoms are mild, no treatment may be needed. If symptoms of acral lesions are precipitated by cold, then protection of affected areas may be sufficient. Measures to reduce the concentration of a type I cryoglobulin, such as plasmapheresis, plasma exchange or cytotoxic therapy, are occasionally effective, although unfortunately usually only in the short term. For immune complex-related disease, corticosteroids, cytotoxic agents or plasmapheresis may be effective, but relapse is typical once therapy is stopped. Interferon-α has been used to treat HCV-associated cryoglobulinaemia, with or without ribavarin [3,4,11]. Treatment with these agents has resulted in partial or complete remissions of vasculitic findings, but relapse often follows cessation of therapy. The therapy itself has occasionally been implicated in triggering the onset of vasculitis. In patients with mixed cryoglobulinaemia troubled primarily by recurrent cutaneous vasculitic lesions, colchicine or dapsone therapy may be of some help in reducing the frequency and severity of episodes.

Cryofibrinogenaemia

Cryofibrinogen deposits consist of a complex of fibrinogen, fibrin and fibronectin that forms on cold exposure [13]. Since cryofibrinogens can be cleaved to form fibrin, plasma rather than serum must be tested to detect these cryogelling proteins. Cryoglobulins should be present in both plasma and sera [13,14].

Cryofibrinogenaemia is common as a laboratory abnormality but is a rare cause of symptomatic clinical disease. One study found an incidence of 3% in a random sample of hospital patients, usually as an incidental finding [15]. Therefore, clinicopathological correlation is important. Cryofibrinogenaemia may be idiopathic or can be associated with malignant disorders (especially haematological), thromboembolic disease, IgA nephropathy or various inflammatory, connective tissue or infectious syndromes [16,17].

Acquired dysfibrinogenaemia very rarely may mimic a cryofibrinogen syndrome by acral occlusion, including gangrene. Interestingly, this subset of dysfibrinogenaemia appears to act by greatly increasing red cell aggregation, mimicking occlusion-inducing cold agglutinins. Blood smear preparations show marked rouleaux formation.

The most common cutaneous findings are cold intolerance, purpura, necrosis, livedo reticularis, gangrene and ulceration (Fig. 49.11) [14,16,17]. The purpura or necrosis typically has a non-inflammatory retiform purpura morphology. Biopsy specimens from skin lesions typically show thrombi in small vessels with dermal necrosis [16]. Leukocytoclastic vasculitis has been reported, but is probably due to ischaemic necrosis rather than being a cause [17]. Fibronectin may be a major component of vascular plugs in patients with cryofibrinogenaemia alone, whereas vascular occlusion in patients with both cryofibrinogens and cryoglobulins shows a predominance of cryoglobulin deposition [17]. Treatment

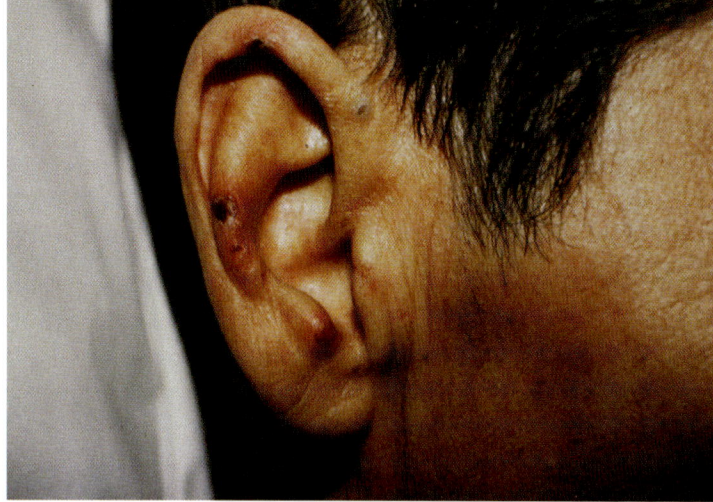

(a)

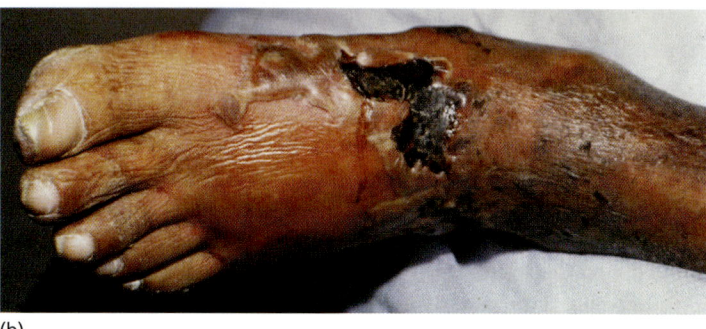

(b)

Fig. 49.11 Cold-induced lesions due to cryofibrinogenaemia, (a) on the ear and (b) on the foot. Acral location is typical for cryogelling. Foot lesion shows minimal erythema, retiform bullae and haemorrhage with necrosis.

of cryofibrinogenaemia should be aimed at the underlying disease, where possible, and at protecting areas from cold exposure [18]. Stanozolol, an androgenic steroid with fibrinolysis-enhancing effects, has also been used for treatment of cryofibrinogenaemia, as have other fibrinolytic agents [19].

Cold agglutinin-related cutaneous occlusion

Cold agglutinins are immunoglobulins that are able to agglutinate red blood cells below normal body temperatures. As agglutination of red blood cells depends on binding of antibody to more than one cell at a time, pentavalent IgM is almost exclusively responsible for this phenomenon. Just as with cryoglobulins, there are both monoclonal and polyclonal cold agglutinins, usually directed at I, i or Pr antigens of erythrocytes [20,21]. Monoclonal cold agglutinins are idiopathic or secondary to malignant lymphoproliferative diseases. Polyclonal cold agglutinins are usually associated with infection, especially due to *Mycoplasma pneumoniae*, less often HCV, parvovirus B19 or leptospiral infections.

Just as with many cryoglobulins and most cryofibrinogens, cold agglutinins are most likely to be asymptomatic. When responsible for disease, reversible acrocyanosis secondary to cold-induced acral agglutination is most common. Livedo reticularis, Raynaud's phenomenon, cold urticaria and rarely cutaneous necrosis may occur. In addition to acral lesions on environmental cold exposure,

cold intravenous infusions can also trigger localized cutaneous necrosis [20]. Cold agglutinins can induce complement activation after cold-induced binding to red blood cells, followed by lysis and haemolytic anaemia, independent of occlusive syndromes from agglutination.

Patients with cold-induced agglutination syndromes must avoid cold exposure. Therapies such as corticosteroids, cytotoxic agents, danazol, rituxan or interferon-α have been occasionally beneficial [21].

References

1 Brouet JC, Clauvel JP, Danon F *et al.* Biologic and clinical significance of cryoglobulins: a report of 86 cases. *Am J Med* 1974; **57**: 775–88.
2 Dispenzieri A, Gorevic P. Cryoglobulinemia. *Hematol Oncol Clin North Am* 1999; **13**: 1315–49.
3 Dammacco F, Sansonno D, Piccoli C *et al.* The cryoglobulins: an overview. *Eur J Clin Invest* 2001; **31**: 628–38.
4 Rieu V, Cohen P, Andre M *et al.* Characteristics and outcome of 49 patients with symptomatic cryoglobulinaemia. *Rheumatology* 2002; **41**: 290–300.
5 Davis M, Su W. Cryoglobulinemia: recent findings in cutaneous and extracutaneous manifestations. *Int J Dermatol* 1996; **35**: 240–8.
6 Grey H, Kohler P. Cryoimmunoglobulins. *Semin Hematol* 1973; **10**: 87.
7 Bonnet F, Pineau J, Taupin J *et al.* Prevalence of cryoglobulinemia and serological markers of autoimmunity in human immunodeficiency virus infected individuals: a cross-sectional study of 97 patients. *J Rheumatol* 2003; **30**: 2005–10.
8 Cream J. Cryoglobulins in vasculitis. *Clin Exp Immunol* 1972; **10**: 117.
9 Cohen SJ, Pittelkow MR, Su WPD. Cutaneous manifestations of cryoglobulinemia: clinical and histopathologic study of seventy-two patients. *J Am Acad Dermatol* 1991; **25**: 21–7.
10 Speight E, Lawrence C. Reticulate purpura, cryoglobulinaemia and livedo reticularis. *Br J Dermatol* 1993; **129**: 319–23.
11 Burke E, Humphrey R, Horn T. Nonhealing ulcers on the extremities: cryoglobulinemia. *Arch Dermatol* 1997; **133**: 911–4.
12 Kallemuchikkal U, Gorevic P. Evaluation of cryoglobulins. *Arch Pathol Lab Med* 1999; **123**: 119–25.
13 Beightler E, Diven D, Sanchez R *et al.* Thrombotic vasculopathy associated with cryofibrinogenemia. *J Am Acad Dermatol* 1991; **24**: 342–5.
14 Williamson A, Cone L, Huard G. Spontaneous necrosis of the skin associated with cryofibrinogenemia, cryoglobulinemia, and homocystinuria. *Ann Vasc Surg* 1996; **10**: 365–9.
15 Smith A, Arkin C. Cryofibrinogenemia: incidence, clinical correlations, and a review of the literature. *Am J Clin Pathol* 1972; **58**: 524–30.
16 Jantunen E, Soppi E, Neittaanmaki H *et al.* Essential cryofibrinogenaemia, leukocytoclastic vasculitis and chronic purpura. *J Intern Med* 1993; **234**: 331–4.
17 Blain H, Cacoub P, Musset L *et al.* Cryofibrinogenaemia: a study of 49 patients. *Clin Exp Immunol* 2000; **120**: 253–60.
18 Kwaan H, Bongu A. The hyperviscosity syndromes. *Semin Thromb Hemost* 1999; **25**: 199–208.
19 Falanga V, Kirsner R, Eaglstein W *et al.* Stanozolol in treatment of leg ulcers due to cryofibrinogenaemia. *Lancet* 1991; **338**: 347–8.
20 Stone MS, Piette WW, Davey WP. Cutaneous necrosis at sites of transfusion: cold agglutinin disease (letter). *J Am Acad Dermatol* 1988; **19**: 356–7.
21 Lauchli S, Widmer L, Lautenschlager S. Cold agglutinin disease: the importance of cutaneous signs. *Dermatology* 2001; **202**: 356–8.

Occlusion due to vessel-invasive organisms

Ecthyma gangrenosum

Ecthyma gangrenosum is a cutaneous syndrome characterized by usually painless, minimally erythematous macules or thin papules or plaques that typically progress to bullous lesions, followed by haemorrhage and necrosis, often with retiform extensions from lesional margins [1]. The anogenital area is a frequent site of involvement, but lesions can develop anywhere and at widespread cutaneous sites [2,3]. Patients are almost invariably immunocompromised, and the infectious agent is usually *Pseudomonas aeruginosa*.

In a small series of cases of ecythma gangrenosum, all eight patients had haematological disease and were receiving immunosuppressive medications [4]. All had positive blood cultures, seven of which were *Ps. aeruginosa*. Biopsies of ecthyma gangrenosum reveal minimal vascular neutrophilic infiltration despite necrotizing vessel injury, and special stains show extensive bacillary infiltration of the perivascular region, the adventitia and the media of larger subcutaneous arterioles, with sparing of the lumen and intima [3–5]. Other bacterial-induced vasculitides tend to show bacterial invasion of the vessel lumen and fibrin thrombi.

Prompt recognition of this syndrome is critical, because prognosis correlates partly with delay in instituting effective intravenous antipseudomonal therapy. Other factors correlating with poor prognosis include multiple lesions and neutropenia [4]. Other organisms that may induce ecthyma gangrenosum-like lesions include *Ps. cepacia* and *Ps. maltophilia*, *Serratia marcescens*, *Aeromonas hydrophila*, *Klebsiella pneumoniae*, *E. coli*, *Vibrio vulnificus*, *Morganella morganii*, *Staphylococcus aureus*, *Mucor*, *Aspergillus fumigatus*, *Fusarium*, *Scytalidium dimidiatum*, *Candida albicans* and *Moraxella* [6,7].

Lucio's phenomenon

Lucio's phenomenon (erythema necroticans) is a rare syndrome almost exclusively limited to leprosy patients from Mexico and Central America, but is rarely reported from Cuba, South America, the USA, India, Polynesia, South Africa and South-East Asia [8–10]. It is a type 2 reaction that may be fatal, despite being the presenting feature of leprosy for many patients who develop this reaction. Lesions may be recurrent and sometimes cyclical over periods of 2 months to 10 years, most often on the legs, but occasionally on the arms and trunk [9]. Lesions usually begin as painful purpuric macules, plaques or vesicles, often ulcerate and heal with atrophic scars. Unlike erythema nodosum leprosum, it is restricted to patients with diffuse non-nodular lepromatous leprosy, is not associated with fever, leukocytosis or tenderness, and fails to respond to thalidomide.

At least in some reports, some lesions appear to induce non-inflammatory retiform purpura, eschar or ulceration [8,9]. Ulceration of lesions is common. Histological findings include either leukocytoclastic vasculitis or endothelial proliferation and thrombus formation in dermal or subcutaneous vessels, with a sparse lymphocytic infiltrate [8–10]. How often vasculitic change is secondary to necrosis or ulceration is unclear, but at least in some cases an occlusive mechanism for purpura and necrosis seems likely. Aggregates of bacilli within proliferating cells are evident on acid-fast stain of biopsy material [9,10].

Treatment includes the standard multidrug therapy for lepromatous leprosy (rifampicin, clofazimine and dapsone). Control of infection and attention to fluid and electrolyte balance are important. Prednisone, thalidomide and clofazimine may all be required to control the reaction. Response to treatment is often reported as poor, with severe morbidity and frequent deaths, but numbers of reported cases are small.

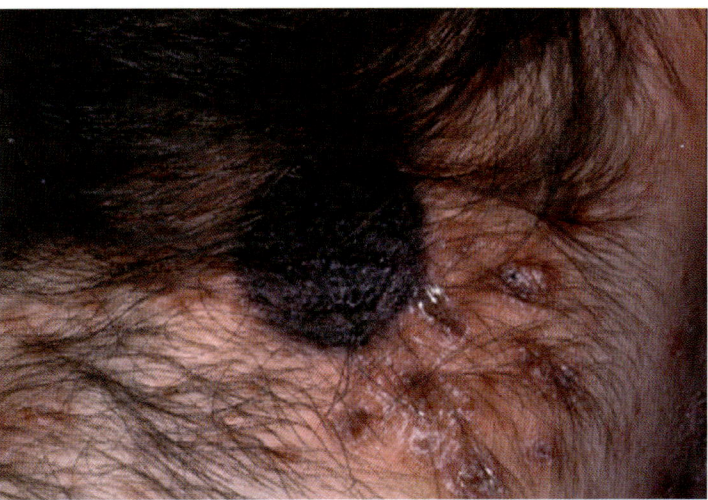

Fig. 49.12 Necrotic cutaneous lesion due to zygomycosis: invasion of vessel walls was apparent histologically.

Vessel-invasive fungi

As alluded to in the ecthema gangrenosum section, fungi may cause overwhelming infections in immunocompromised patients, often with cutaneous lesions, some of which may become purpuric or necrotic due to vessel-invasive organisms and thrombosis. *Aspergillus* and *Mucor* are two of the most commonly reported fungal groups to cause such vessel-invasive lesions.

Cutaneous lesions of *Aspergillus* may be either primary or secondary from haematogenous dissemination. Primary lesions typically occur at intravenous infusion sites, tubing sites secured by tape, or in skin in chronic contact with a colonized intravenous board [11,12]. Primary cutaneous aspergillosis can occur in immunocompetent patients, as well as in patients with burns or surgical wounds. Cutaneous lesions from systemic involvement have been divided into five categories: (i) a solitary necrotizing plaque; (ii) a subcutaneous abscess or granuloma; (iii) eruptive maculopapules with suppurative, vegetating or necrobiotic features; (iv) erythematous or exanthem-like reactions; and (v) progressive confluent granulomas [12,13]. Organisms in lesions appear as septate hyphae with acute-angle branching, invading blood vessels and surrounding tissues, often with minimal inflammation [13]. *Aspergillus fumigatus* is the most common cause of colonization and of disseminated infection by the *Aspergillus* group of fungi. *Fusarium* infections are increasing in frequency in patients with haematological malignancy; 72–91% of patients with this infection have skin lesions, which may be either metastatic or primary [14]. Metastatic skin lesions are described as either subcutaneous nodules, usually painful, or ecthyma gangrenosum-like.

The class Zygomycetes includes *Mucor*, *Absidia* and *Rhizopus* organisms, which can cause identical clinical manifestations (Fig. 49.12) [11]. Lesions may be either primary or secondary to disseminated disease, and include superficial vesiculopustules, ulcerating gangrenous lesions, purpuric nodules, cellulitis and necrotic ulcers. These organisms easily invade the epidermis and spread rapidly in the dermis, with vessel invasion by very large and long non-septate hyphae, resulting in thrombosis and infarction [15].

Response to therapy in these types of infection is relatively refractory. With *Fusarium* infections, for example, response rates are 30–48% with current therapies and support measures [14].

Disseminated strongyloidiasis

Strongyloides stercoralis is the nematode responsible for the human parasitic infestation known as strongyloidiasis. Affecting 100 million people worldwide, it is endemic in tropical or subtropical soil that is contaminated by faeces, in some temperate-zone areas such as the rural south-east and Appalachia of the USA, or in closed communities such as immigrant populations, close-quartered military personnel or institutions [16]. Filiform larvae from contaminated soil penetrate the skin, enter the blood vessels, exit through the lungs and migrate to the glottis, where they are swallowed [16–18]. They mature and reproduce in the upper small bowel, with hatching of non-infective (rhabditiform) larvae. Transformation of these into infective larvae can lead to autoinfection through penetration of intestinal mucosa or perianal skin [18]. Skin lesions with simple infection include papules or erythematous serpiginous tracts, which can extend several centimetres per hour and represent cutaneous migration of the larvae (larva currens).

In immunocompromised patients, including those on corticosteroids, hyperinfection and dissemination of organisms can occur [16]. In this setting, the diagnosis is usually made through examination of stool samples, and skin lesions are uncommon. However, with such overwhelming infection, petechiae, purpura and reticulated purpuric skin lesions have been described [16,17,19,20]. These lesions may be widespread but may cluster, particularly in the periumbilical region where they are said to have a thumb-print appearance. Biopsy of purpuric lesions has shown larvae within capillaries and between collagen bundles in the dermis, with extravasated red cells [20].

Mortality in disseminated strongyloidiasis is high, up to 70–90% [16]. Treatment is with oral thiabendazole, and may need to be prolonged in immunocompromised patients [17,18].

References

1 Robson K, Piette W. The presentation and differential diagnosis of cutaneous vascular occlusion syndromes. *Adv Dermatol* 1999; **15**: 153–82.

2 Boisseau A, Sarlangue J, Perel Y et al. Perineal ecthyma gangrenosum in infancy and early childhood: septicemic and nonsepticemic forms. *J Am Acad Dermatol* 1992; **27**: 415–8.

3 Song W, Kim Y, Park H, Cinn Y. Ecthyma gangrenosum without bacteremia in a leukemic patient. *Clin Exp Dermatol* 2001; **26**: 395–7.

4 Greene S, Su W, Muller S. Ecthyma gangrenosum: report of clinical, histopathologic, and bacteriologic aspects of eight cases. *J Am Acad Dermatol* 1984; **11**: 781–7.

5 Lucas S. Bacterial disease. In: Elder D, Elenitsas R, Jaworsky C, Johnson B Jr, eds. *Lever's Histopathology of the Skin*, 8th edn. Philadelphia: Lippincott-Raven, 1997: 465.

6 Prins C, Chavaz P, Tamm K et al. Ecthyma gangrenosum-like lesions: a sign of disseminated *Fusarium* infection in the neutropenic patient. *Clin Exp Immunol* 1995; **20**: 428–30.

7 Del Pozo J, Garcia-Silva J, Almagro M et al. Ecthyma gangrenosum-like eruption associated with *Morganella morganii* infection. *Br J Dermatol* 1998; **139**: 520–1.

8 Ang P, Tay Y, Ng S, Seow C. Fatal Lucio's phenomenon in 2 patients with previously undiagnosed leprosy. *J Am Acad Dermatol* 2003; **48**: 958–61.

9 Rea T, Levan N. Lucio's phenomenon and diffuse nonnodular lepromatous leprosy. *Arch Dermatol* 1978; **114**: 1023–8.

10 Pursley T, Jacobson R, Apisarnthanarax P. Lucio's phenomenon. *Arch Dermatol* 1980; **116**: 201–4.

11 Elewski B, Radentz W, Gupta A. Opportunistic mycoses. In: Elewski B, ed. *Cutaneous Fungal Infections*. Malden, MA: Blackwell Science, 1998: 225–59.

12 Prystowsky S, Vogelstein B, Ettinger D et al. Invasive aspergillosis. *N Engl J Med* 1976; **295**: 655–8.

13 Galimberti R, Kowalczuk A, Hidalgo Parra I et al. Cutaneous aspergillosis: a report of six cases. *Br J Dermatol* 1998; **139**: 522–6.

14 Boutati E, Anaissie E. *Fusarium*, a significant emerging pathogen in patients with hematological malignancy. Ten years' experience at a cancer center and implications for management. *Blood* 1997; **90**: 999–1008.

15 Meyer R, Kaplan M, Ong M et al. Cutaneous lesions in disseminated mucormycosis. *JAMA* 1973; **225**: 737–8.

16 Ly M, Bethel S, Usmani A, Lambert D. Cutaneous *Strongyloides stercoralis* infection: an unusual presentation. *J Am Acad Dermatol* 2003; **49**: S157–S160.

17 Kalb R, Grossman M. Periumbilical purpura in disseminated strongyloidiasis. *JAMA* 1986; **256**: 1170–1.

18 Kalter D, Meinking T, Garcia E et al. Parasitic diseases. In: Arndt K, Leboit P, Robinson J et al., eds. *Cutaneous Medicine and Surgery: an Integrated Program in Dermatology*. Philadelphia: Saunders, 1996: 1172–89.

19 Purvis R, Beightler E, Diven D et al. *Strongyloides* hyperinfection presenting with petechiae and purpura. *Int J Dermatol* 1992; **31**: 169–71.

20 Ronan S, Reddy R, Manaligod J et al. Disseminated strongyloidiasis presenting as purpura. *J Am Acad Dermatol* 1989; **21**: 1123–5.

Occlusion due to embolus

Cholesterol embolus

Aetiology. The most commonly diagnosed cutaneous embolic syndrome is cholesterol embolus, which occurs secondary to fragmentation of ulcerated arteriosclerotic plaques, with distal cutaneous and visceral vessel obstruction. As it occurs secondary to atheromatous plaques, it is no surprise that cholesterol embolus is a syndrome reported primarily in men aged 50 years or older, and is associated with peripheral vascular disease and the known risk factors for atherosclerosis such as diabetes, hypertension and smoking [1,2]. Although cholesterol embolus may be spontaneous, known triggers include angiography, angioplasty, vascular surgery, intra-aortic pump placement, cardiopulmonary resuscitation (all inducing traumatic rupture of plaques, usually within hours or days), thrombolytic therapy (acute clot lysis in plaque with release of friable plaque within hours or days) and anticoagulation (slow reduction of clot with release of plaque fragments, usually after at least 2 months of therapy) [2,3]. Blue toe syndrome associated with coumadin use is a syndrome of cholesterol embolus and not of coumadin necrosis.

Clinical features. There are two 'classic' clinical triads of cholesterol embolus. The first comprises leg or foot pain, livedo reticularis and preservation of good peripheral pulses [3]. The second comprises livedo reticularis, renal insufficiency and eosinophilia [4]. Cutaneous findings are frequent in patients recognized as experiencing episodes of cholesterol embolus. Reported in 35% of patients in one series, findings include livedo reticularis (49%), gangrene (35%), cyanosis (28%), ulceration (17%), nodules (10%) and purpura (9%) [1]. Additional clinical findings include fever, myalgia, altered mental status, sudden-onset arterial hypertension, gastrointestinal ulceration and renal insufficiency that may progress to renal failure [3,4].

The incidence of cholesterol embolization syndrome (CES) following vascular procedures has ranged from 0.15% to 30%, with large retrospective studies reporting figures of 0.6–0.9% [5–7]. Autopsy studies have shown cholesterol emboli in 77% of patients who underwent aortic aneurysm resection [6]. A prospective study of 1786 consecutive patients aged over 40 years who underwent left-heart catheterization found an incidence of cholesterol embolus of 1.4%, with nearly half having definite CES and the remainder having possible CES with primarily renal abnormalities [5]. Patients with cutaneous findings (livedo reticularis, blue toe syndrome or digital gangrene) were considered to have definite CES and comprised 48% of the total. In-hospital mortality was 16% and was associated with progressive renal dysfunction.

Investigation. Eosinophilia is a frequent finding in CES, occurring in up to 80% of patients, and may be related to generation of the C5 component of complement [5,8]. Pre-procedure elevation in serum levels of C-reactive protein has been associated with an increased risk of post-procedure CES [5]. Additional laboratory findings may include leukocytosis, thrombocytopenia, pyuria, eosinophiluria, blood-positive urine or stool, elevated values of red cell sedimentation rate, creatinine, urea and amylase, and decreased serum levels of complement [1,2,8].

The traditional recommendation for cutaneous biopsy of livedo reticularis has been elliptical excisions centred on normal skin areas within rings of livedo reticularis, deep enough to include an ample specimen of subcutaneous fat. However, our experience is that careful examination of the livedo reticularis reveals that many patients will have retiform purpura, and such areas are high-yield biopsy sites for demonstrating the diagnostic cholesterol crystals on histological examination. On histological examination, the arteriole involved in the skin is usually at the dermosubcutaneous junction, with elongated clefts within small-vessel lumina along with thrombi [9]. The clefts result from fixation-related dissolving of cholesterol crystals. In experimentally produced cholesterol embolus, a mixed inflammatory infiltrate may be seen in arterial walls within 24–48 h, followed by multinucleated histiocytes within 3–6 days, and subsequent occasional intimal fibrosis.

Treatment. Treatment of cholesterol emboli involves trying to minimize the risk of further embolization (removal of remaining plaque or perhaps stenting of an atheromatous segment of a major vessel), minimizing damage to end organs, and preventive therapies aimed at slowing progression of atheromatous disease. Statins, iloprost (prostacyclin analogue), pentoxifylline (oxpentifylline) and steroids have been reported as having limited success in therapeutic interventions to minimize organ damage [6,10]. As anticoagulant use may precipitate cholesterol emboli, avoidance of these agents in patients with known CES seems prudent [3,7]. However, some types of cardiac surgery that may precipitate CES may also require post-operative anticoagulation, for example valvular prostheses [3,7].

Oxalate crystal embolus

Oxalate crystals are a rare cause of symptomatic emboli, but can mimic the cutaneous findings of cholesterol embolism. Although primary hyperoxaluria is rare, it is the most common cause of oxalate crystal embolus. Two enzyme defects are associated with primary hyperoxaluria: type I hyperoxaluria (glycolic aciduria) is due to deficiency of the hepatic peroxisomal enzyme alanine: glyoxylate aminotransferase; type II hyperoxaluria (L-glyceric aciduria) is due to diminished activity of D-glyceric acid dehydrogenase [11,12]. Absorptive hyperoxaluria is also reported due to idiopathic intestinal hyperabsorption of oxalate. Secondary hyperoxaluria can be due to excessive intake of oxalate or its precursors (ethylene glycol, methoxyflurane anaesthesia, very-high-dose ascorbic acid), pyridoxine deficiency, ileal resection, some intestinal diseases or long-term haemodialysis [11,13].

Type I hyperoxaluria is the most common and has three forms. The infantile form has no history of nephrolithiasis but has rapidly progressive renal failure. The juvenile form is the common type I subset. In this group, recurrent calcium oxalate nephrolithiasis precedes renal failure. Patients with the adult form typically present with renal failure and later develop complications of oxalate tissue deposition.

Cutaneous manifestations of primary hyperoxaluria are primarily those of oxalate crystal embolization: livedo reticularis, acrocyanosis, and peripheral gangrene, purpura or ulcerations [12,13]. Secondary hyperoxaluria, especially when due to long-term dialysis, is more likely to lead to extravascular cutaneous deposits of oxalate, producing calcified cutaneous nodules, or firm miliary papules that tend to form on the palmar aspect of the fingers [14].

Cardiac sources of embolization

Atrial myxomas, marantic endocarditis and septic endocarditis can be associated with cutaneous embolic phenomena. Although rare, atrial myxomas are the most common benign cardiac tumour, with an estimated incidence of 0.03% [15] and onset usually between the third and sixth decades [16]. The left atrium is the most frequent tumour site. Symptoms may partly mimic those of infectious endocarditis, connective tissue disease, vasculitis or rheumatic fever, with constitutional symptoms such as fever, malaise, arthralgia or weight loss. Obstruction of intracardiac blood flow mimicking valvular disease or embolic phenomena may also occur. Lentigines may be a cutaneous finding in the hereditary NAME or LAMB syndrome, which is associated with cardiac myxomas. Cutaneous findings of myxomatous emboli include livedo reticularis, splinter haemorrhages, Raynaud's phenomenon, an acral papular eruption with claudication, serpiginous or annular purpuric lesions of the fingertips, red–violet malar flush, petechiae of hands and feet, or toe necrosis [16–18]. Histology can confirm myxomatous emboli, but finding the emboli may require serial sectioning and multiple biopsies [16,19]. An echocardiogram is useful in evaluating patients with a history or physical examination compatible with emboli. Atrial myxomas require surgical treatment.

Marantic endocarditis results in the attachment of fibrin vegetations to heart valve leaflets, similar to those seen in acute rheumatic endocarditis and Libman–Sacks (APLS) valve disease, and these vegetations can embolize [19]. Infective endocarditis can also produce emboli from vegetations, but these are usually associated with acute bacterial endocarditis. Lesions in subacute bacterial endocarditis may be from either emboli or immune complex-related vasculitis. Idiopathic hypereosinophilic syndrome is associated with intracardiac mural thrombi, which can also produce emboli [20,21]. Documentation of cutaneous emboli is limited, with clinical lesions described as splinter haemorrhages, non-blanching livedoid discoloration, or necrotic, blistering or purpuric lesions [22–24].

Crystal globulin vasculopathy is a rare syndrome, usually associated with IgG or light-chain paraproteins, that can produce intravascular occlusion by spontaneous crystallization [25,26]. This syndrome results in rapidly progressive renal failure, polyarthropathy, peripheral neuropathy and skin lesions. Cutaneous lesions include ulcerations, petechiae and ecchymoses, with intravascular thrombus and crystalline deposits [27].

Other emboli

Petechiae, which may be few or very numerous, are an important sign of fat embolism [28,29]. They occur particularly on the upper part of the body 2–3 days after a major injury and are an important clue to this diagnosis. Minute fat emboli have been found within the vessels at the sites of the petechiae.

Emboli may also occur from tumours at sites other than the cardiac myxomas discussed above.

References

1 Falanga V, Fine M, Kapoor W. The cutaneous manifestations of cholesterol crystal embolization. *Arch Dermatol* 1986; **122**: 1194–8.

2 Chandrashekariah R, Fresko O, Lynfield Y. Cholesterol embolism: a case report and review of the literature. *Cutis* 2001; **68**: 263–7.

3 Pennington M, Yeager J, Skelton H, Smith K. Cholesterol embolization syndrome: cutaneous histopathological features and the variable onset of symptoms in patients with different risk factors. *Br J Dermatol* 2002; **146**: 511–7.

4 Mieszczanska H, Lazar J, Marzo K, Cunha B. Cholesterol emboli mimicking acute bacterial endocarditis. *Heart Lung J Acute Crit Care* 2002; **31**: 452–4.

5 Fukumoto Y, Tsutsui H, Tsuchihashi M et al. The incidence and risk factors of cholesterol embolization syndrome, a complication of cardiac catheterization: a prospective study. *J Am Coll Cardiol* 2003; **42**: 211–6.

6 Bashore T, Gehrig T. Cholesterol emboli after invasive cardiac procedures. *J Am Coll Cardiol* 2003; **42**: 217–8.

7 Doty J, Wilentz R, Salazar J et al. Atheroembolism in cardiac surgery. *Ann Thorac Surg* 2003; **75**: 1221–6.

8 Lawson J. Cholesterol crystal embolization: more common than we thought? *Am J Gastroenterol* 2001; **96**: 3230–2.

9 Kang K, Botella R, White C Jr. Subtle clues to the diagnosis of cholesterol embolism. *Am J Dermatopathol* 1996; **18**: 380–4.

10 Elinav E, Chajek-Shaul T, Stern M. Improvement in cholesterol emboli syndrome after iloprost therapy. *BMJ* 2002; **324**: 268–9.

11 Bogle M, Teller C, Tschen J et al. Primary hyperoxaluria in a 27-year-old woman. *J Am Acad Dermatol* 2003; **49**: 725–8.

12 Marconi V, Mofid M, McCall C et al. Primary hyperoxaluria: report of a patient with livedo reticularis and digital infarcts. *J Am Acad Dermatol* 2002; **46**: S16–S18.

13 Greer KE, Cooper PH, Campbell F et al. Primary oxalosis with livedo reticularis. *Arch Dermatol* 1980; **116**: 213–4.

14 Ohtake N, Uchiyama H, Furue M, Tamaki K. Secondary cutaneous oxalosis: cutaneous deposition of calcium oxalate dihydrate after long-term hemodialysis. *J Am Acad Dermatol* 1994; **31**: 368–72.

15 Reed R, Utz M, Terezakis N. Embolic and metastatic cardiac myxoma. *Am J Dermatopathol* 1989; **11**: 157–65.

16 Greeson D, Wright J, Zanolli M. Cutaneous findings associated with cardiac myxomas. *Cutis* 1998; **62**: 275–80.

17 Feldman A, Keeling J. Cutaneous manifestation of atrial myxoma. *J Am Acad Dermatol* 1989; **21**: 1080–4.

18 Abraham Z, Rozenbaum M, Rosner I et al. Cutaneous eruption in a patient with cardiac myxoma. *J Dermatol* 1995; **22**: 276–8.

19 Young R, Zalneraitis E. Marantic endocarditis in children and young adults: clinical and pathological findings. *Stroke* 1981; **12**: 635–9.

20 Ommen S, Seward J, Tajik A. Clinical and echocardiographic features of hypereosinophilic syndromes. *Am J Cardiol* 2000; **86**: 110–3.

21 Bishop G, Bergin J, Kramer C. Hypereosinophilic syndrome and restrictive cardiomyopathy due to apical thrombi. *Circulation* 2001; **104**: E3–E4.

22 Fitzpatrick J, Johnson C, Simon P, Owenby J. Cutaneous microthrombi: a histologic clue to the diagnosis of hypereosinophilic syndrome. *Am J Dermatopathol* 1987; **9**: 419–22.

23 Sanchez J, Padilla M. Hypereosinophilic syndrome. *Cutis* 1982; **29**: 490–4.

24 Weller P, Bubley G. The idiopathic hypereosinophilic syndrome. *Blood* 1994; **83**: 2759–79.

25 Stone G, Wall B, Oppliger I et al. A vasculopathy with deposition of lambda light chain crystals. *Ann Intern Med* 1989; **110**: 275–8.

26 Hasegawa H, Ozawa T, Tada N et al. Multiple myeloma-associated systemic vasculopathy due to crystalglobulin or polyarteritis nodosa. *Arthritis Rheum* 1996; **39**: 330–4.

27 Ball N, Wickert W, Marx L et al. Crystalglobulinemia syndrome: a manifestation of multiple myeloma. *Cancer* 1993; **71**: 1231–4.

28 Sevitt S. The significance and classification of fat-embolism. *Lancet* 1960; **ii**: 825–8.

29 Mellor A, Soni N. Fat embolism. *Anaesthesia* 2001; **56**: 145–54.

Systemic coagulopathies with cutaneous predilection

There are several systemic coagulopathies that have a predilection for the cutaneous microvasculature. Cutaneous lesions may occasionally be a minor feature of a multiorgan syndrome, the most prominent findings of multiorgan involvement or sometimes the sole target of occlusion. The importance of recognizing these syndromes is critical in order to begin early, and sometimes syndrome-specific, therapy. There are two natural anticoagulant pathways that exist in humans. The most well known, the antithrombin III–heparin/heparan pathway, is important for primarily venous large-vessel thrombosis. The only cutaneous lesions related to antithrombin III disorders are stasis ulcers secondary to recurrent venous thrombosis with venous insufficiency. In contrast, disorders of the thrombomodulin–protein C/S anticoagulant pathway are important causes of severe cutaneous occlusion syndromes.

An understanding of this pathway is important in diagnosing and treating these syndromes. The end point of the coagulation cascade is conversion of prothrombin to thrombin, which rapidly catalyses the conversion of fibrinogen to fibrin and clot formation. The procoagulant role of thrombin is well known; less well known is its critical role in anticoagulation. When thrombin fails to bind to procoagulant sites on membranes and binds instead to the membrane protein receptor thrombomodulin, this powerful prothrombotic molecule undergoes a remarkable transformation. Bound to thrombomodulin, thrombin becomes ineffective at binding and activating clotting factors, and instead rapidly converts protein C in the plasma to activated protein C. Activated protein C, stabilized by certain phospholipids and by protein S, down-regulates clotting by cleaving circulating activated clotting factors, including factor VIIIa and most importantly factor Va. It thus exerts an anticoagulant effect; deficiency of protein C, or of its co-factor protein S, therefore creates a procoagulant tendency. The factor V Leiden mutation renders the factor V Leiden molecule much less sensitive to cleavage by activated protein C (APC resistance); about 5% of the UK and Caucasian North American population are heterozygous for this mutation (reported incidence is highest in Cyprus, Sweden and Turkey at 10–15%, and lowest incidence in Asia and Africa, and in populations of those ethnicities). This protection from cleavage means that activated factor V Leiden remains longer in the plasma and continues to enhance coagulation. It would be expected then that factor V Leiden mutation should be synergistic with deficiencies in the thrombomodulin–protein C pathway. In fact, in some kindreds of protein C-deficient families, the presence of the factor V Leiden mutation appears to be an important predictor for who will develop large-vessel thrombosis in individuals with similar levels of protein C deficiency.

Another major cluster of systemic coagulopathies with cutaneous microvascular occlusion are those related to lupus anticoagulant activity and APLS. The mechanisms for clotting in this group are less well understood, and will be addressed following discussion of protein C/S-related syndromes.

Protein C/protein S-related disease

Neonatal purpura fulminans: homozygous protein C or protein S deficiency

Protein C and S deficiencies can be inherited autosomally with variable penetrance. Patients who are heterozygous for deficiency may develop repeated venous thrombosis or pulmonary embolism early in adult life, or may be asymptomatic [1,2]. One variable affecting the likelihood of thrombosis in these individuals is known—the previously mentioned co-inheritance of homozygous or heterozygous factor V Leiden mutations [3,4]. The frequency of homozygous protein C deficiency is estimated at 1 in 250 000–500 000 births [1]. Homozygous deficiency of either protein C or protein S is associated with neonatal purpura fulminans as well as with cerebral and ophthalmic vessel thrombosis. Retiform (stellate) purpura and necrosis is the most typical cutaneous finding that results from thrombosis within the cutaneous microvasculature. Skin lesions typically begin within a few hours to 5 days after birth, and are most commonly distributed on the extremities, abdomen, buttocks and scalp; they may localize to sites of pressure or previous trauma [1,5,6]. Laboratory findings are consistent with DIC, with evidence of consumption of clotting factors (prolonged partial thromboplastin time, PTT), clot lysis (elevated fibrin split products) and often thrombocytopenia. In the absence of appropriate therapy, lesions invariably progress to full-thickness cutaneous necrosis.

Traditional treatment included fresh frozen plasma to try to replace deficient protein C or S, or oral anticoagulants to reduce procoagulant factors. More recently, protein C and activated protein C concentrates have been used for treatment of both acute disease and as prophylaxis against subsequent episodes [7,8].

Coumadin (coumarin, warfarin) necrosis: severe acquired protein C dysfunction

Coumadin necrosis usually presents as the sudden onset of pain within affected areas 3–5 days after beginning coumadin therapy, followed by well-demarcated erythema progressing to haemorrhage, necrosis and often haemorrhagic bullae or eschar [9]. Although coumadin necrosis may rarely involve acral areas, acral cutaneous purpura in patients on coumadin is more likely to be due to cholesterol embolus—so-called purple (blue) toe syndrome. The risk of coumadin necrosis is increased if loading doses (10 mg or more) of warfarin are used and if a second form of anticoagulation such as heparin therapy is not used to cover the initial phase of anticoagulant therapy [10,11]. Warfarin (coumadin) necrosis is more likely to occur in areas with abundant fatty subcutis, such as breast, hip, buttocks and thigh [9,10]. The peak incidence is between the sixth and seventh decades, and is four times higher in women.

The therapeutic effect of coumadin is due to inhibition of γ-carboxylation of the vitamin K-dependent coagulant factors II, VII, IX and X. Although these factors are still produced and may be antigenically detected within the plasma, without γ-carboxylation they are dysfunctional. Importantly, protein C and protein S are also vitamin K-dependent plasma factors, and their inhibition can lead to a prothrombotic state. Protein C and factor VII, with half-lives of roughly 5 h, are particularly vulnerable to early inhibition, whereas protein S and the remaining procoagulant factors with much longer half-lives remain active for a considerably longer period [11,12]. There is thus a period, after the early inhibition phase, when the anticoagulant effect of protein C has been inhibited but there is an excess of uninhibited procoagulant clotting factors. Although up to one-third of patients with coumadin-induced skin necrosis may have partial protein C deficiency, the majority of cases appear unrelated to inherited deficiencies of protein C [10]. As coumadin action mimics that of vitamin K deficiency, it would be expected that depletion of vitamin K should result in coumadin necrosis-like findings, but this has not been documented.

Restoration of protein C activity can be accomplished through protein C concentrates, and presumably also through the use of activated protein C. If these are not available, heparin therapy has been recommended.

Sepsis-related purpura fulminans (bland retiform purpura) with DIC: acquired severe protein C deficiency

The term 'purpura fulminans' is used by physicians for many different situations. It was originally coined in 1887 to describe a syndrome occurring days to a few weeks after some preceding infection, especially varicella zoster or streptococcal infections (now termed 'post-infectious purpura fulminans') [13]. The term 'purpura fulminans' has subsequently been used for widespread cutaneous haemorrhage in patients with sepsis, including infection with Neisseria meningitidis, Staphylococcus aureus, groups A and B β-haemolytic streptococci, Streptococcus pneumoniae, Haemophilus influenzae and Haemophilus aegyptius [14]. However, haemorrhage in patients with DIC may be due to septic vasculitis, simple bleeding or microvascular thrombosis. The patterns of cutaneous haemorrhage for each of these different mechanisms are distinctive, and can be a guide to pathophysiology and therapy [15]. Cutaneous microvascular occlusion in sepsis with DIC presents clinically as non-inflammatory (bland) haemorrhage, usually with a retiform, stellate or branching configuration, with rapid transition to necrosis and eschar [16,17]. In a small study, early biopsy of retiform purpuric lesions showed microvascular occlusion with fibrin, and perivascular haemorrhage with minimal to no inflammation; these findings correlated with severe protein C deficiency [17]. This was not true of other forms of purpura in sepsis with DIC. The protein C pathway is increasingly recognized as critically important in bacterial sepsis, acting to inhibit both coagulation and inflammation [18]. The use of activated protein C concentrate in sepsis appears to be beneficial, especially in severe cases, although whether all patients with sepsis should receive this is not clear [19–22]. In patients with sepsis, DIC and retiform (occlusion) purpura, it seems reasonable to assume severe protein C deficiency in the acute setting and to treat appropriately. Protein C concentrates and plasma exchange have also been successfully used to replace protein C in purpura fulminans [23].

Post-infectious purpura fulminans: acquired severe protein S dysfunction

As mentioned previously, post-infectious purpura fulminans occurs primarily in children as rapidly progressive purpura a few days to weeks after a febrile illness [14,24,25]. The most common associated infections are varicella zoster and streptococci. This syndrome has been associated with lupus anticoagulant activity and with autoantibodies to protein S [14,25,26]. Replacement of protein S activity is difficult, presumably because this condition is not due to simple clearing of protein S but rather to inhibition of protein S function by an antibody. Such antibody-mediated dysfunction is difficult to overcome by replacement of factor, and concentrated sources of protein S are unavailable.

Antiphospholipid antibody/lupus anticoagulant syndrome

From the original description as recurrent venous or arterial thrombosis, repeated fetal loss and thrombocytopenia to consensus statement criteria, APLS continues to be redefined [27–29], most recently by the addition of β_2-glycoprotein I (β_2-GPI) antibodies to the laboratory criteria for diagnosis (Table 49.6) [30].

A variety of serological markers exist, usually detected as antibody against phospholipids (especially cardiolipin) in combination with antigens from a co-factor molecule (e.g. β_2-GPI,

Table 49.6 International consensus statement preliminary criteria for antiphospholipid antibody syndrome (definitive diagnosis requires at least one clinical and one laboratory criterion) [30].

Clinical criteria
Vascular thrombosis
  One or more clinical episodes of arterial, venous or small-vessel thrombosis
Complications of pregnancy
  One or more unexplained deaths of morphologically normal fetuses at or after 10
    weeks of pregnancy or
  One or more premature births of morphologically normal neonates at or before
    34 weeks of gestation or
  Three or more unexplained consecutive spontaneous abortions before 10 weeks
    of gestation

Laboratory criteria
Anticardiolipin antibodies, IgG or IgM, present at moderate or high levels on two or
  more occasions at least 6 weeks apart
Lupus anticoagulant antibodies on two or more occasions at least 6 weeks apart
β_2-Glycoprotein I antibodies on two or more occasions at least 6 weeks apart

prothrombin, annexin V, plasmin, tissue plasminogen activator, thrombin), or as an inhibitor of an *in vitro* coagulation test. Detection of antiphospholipid antibodies is roughly five times more common than detection of lupus anticoagulant [31].

APLS may occur as a primary or secondary disorder. In one large study, primary APLS comprised 53% of cases, lupus-associated APLS 36%, lupus-like APLS 5% and other disease associations with APLS 6%, with catastrophic APLS occurring in 0.8% [32]. Compared with primary syndrome patients, lupus patients with APLS were more likely to have arthritis, livedo reticularis, thrombocytopenia or leukopenia. The mean age was 42 ± 14 years at study entry, onset of symptoms was most often in young to middle-aged patients (2.8% before age 15 years, 12.7% after age 50), and there was a strong female predominance (82%).

Mechanisms of coagulation in APLS are only partially understood. These antibodies were first detected in 1906 in patients with syphilis, and measured as false-positive serological tests for syphilis in 1952 [29]. However, today they are most often detected as β_2-GPI antibodies, lupus anticoagulants or antiphospholipid antibodies. The lupus anticoagulant activity is detected, often incidentally, by prolongation of the activated partial thromboplastin time (aPTT), the dilute Russell's viper venom time (dRVVT), or the kaolin clotting time [33]. Both a test of activation of the intrinsic pathway (either aPTT or kaolin clotting time) and direct activation of Factor X (dRVVT) is recommended. The presence of an inhibitor is determined by 1:1 mixing studies with normal plasma. As such mixing guarantees at least 50% levels of all clotting factors, failure to correct the clotting test indicates the presence of an inhibitor. The proof of phospholipid dependency for this inhibitor is often done by the platelet neutralization procedure, in which washed platelets are used to provide enough phospholipid surface to bind the interfering antibodies while still providing excess phospholipid to support the clotting reaction. Although prolongation of these tests would seem to predict a tendency towards bleeding, individuals with lupus anticoagulant activity very rarely bleed abnormally, but may be paradoxically predisposed to clot formation.

Antiphospholipid antibody activity is detected by one of several antibody assays, the most common being ELISA screens for IgG or IgM antibody affinity for cardiolipin, a negatively charged phospholipid molecule found in mitochondrial membranes. Although anticardiolipin antibodies can be detected in the absence of binding to a co-factor such as β_2-GPI, antiphospholipid antibodies which bind to phospholipid alone without a coactor molecule are not usually physiologically relevant in inducing thrombosis. Studies have shown that in patients with both lupus anticoagulant activity and anticardiolipin activity, there may be little or no cross-reaction between antibodies which bind to each. Both the lupus anticoagulant test and the various antiphospholipid antibody assays can be positive in a great many patients who never develop any thrombosis. Likewise, until the mechanisms responsible for thrombosis in patients with these antibodies are understood, it is possible that some patients with thrombosis may test negative with current assays, and yet ultimately be found to have disease mediated by antibodies interfering with physiological pathways responsible for clinical APLS.

The most important autoantigen in APLS appears to be β_2-GPI (apolipoprotein H), which binds anionic phospholipids as part of physiological disposal of apoptotic cells [34]. β_2-GPI is composed of five complement control modules, domains I to V. Infections may trigger β_2-GPI antibodies (e.g. leprosy, leishmaniasis and leptospirosis), as may childhood atopic dermatitis. These antibodies may differ from those that trigger thrombosis by binding to domain V of the β_2-GPI molecule, rather than to the domain I region which appears to be characteristic of the thrombogenic subset [35]. Infection-related antibodies, especially in leprosy, are more often IgM than IgG type. In general, IgM β_2-GPI antibodies are seldom implicated in thrombotic events, except perhaps in cerebral stroke. IgG antibodies to β_2-GPI, especially the IgG_2 subset, are the most likely to be thrombogenic [33]. The binding of the glycoprotein to negatively-charged phospholipid or *in vitro* to an irradiated negatively-charged plastic plate induces a conformational change in β_2-GPI, leading to exposure of a cryptic epitope in domain I and, in some cases, to autoantibody formation. *In vivo*, the usual binding sites for β_2-GPI which induce the conformational change are membrane phospholipids, especially phosphatidyl serine, which is expressed by agonist stimulation of platelets, for example, with flipping of membrane bilayer phospholipids that are normally on the inner surface to the outer membrane layer [35].

Multiple pathways have been implicated by which antiphospholipid antibodies may promote thrombosis: promotion of procoagulant reactions (interfering with protective membrane proteins such as β_2-GPI or annexin V), interference with anticoagulant pathways (inhibition of protein C/S and antithrombin III pathways), activation of platelets by membrane binding, interference with prostacyclin production and release by endothelium, or interference with fibrinolytic pathways (inhibition of endothelial plasminogen activator or kallikrein activation) [29,36–38]. However, current investigation points to β_2-GPI antibodies being the likely prothrombotic pathway in most patients. The mechanism of thrombosis with antibody-bound β_2-GPI is thought to occur predominantly through disruption of a crystal shield of annexin V which covers the membrane and ordinarily prevents binding of procoagulant molecules [39]. An important physiological role for β_2-GPI is believed to be inhibition of atherosclerosis by preventing scavenger receptor-mediated uptake of oxLDL by macrophages, but β_2-GPI antibodies binding to β_2-GPI-oxLDL mediates atherosclerosis by promoting phagocytosis of the oxLDL complex by macrophages via Fc receptors. This suggests that in addition to potential thrombogenesis, β_2-GPI antibody complexes may also be atherogenic.

Although thrombocytopenia was frequently mentioned in early descriptions of the APLS, this is no longer a diagnostic criterion for the syndrome. Mechanisms for thrombocytopenia or a role for APL antibodies have been difficult to find, but recently it has been shown that β_2-GPI may inhibit both von Willebrand factor-mediated platelet aggregation and binding of platelets to a von Willebrand factor-coated surface, and that antibodies to β_2-GPI reduce the ability of β_2-GPI to inhibit these activities [40]. If this is true, then a role for platelet-mediated vascular occlusion may exist in some patients with antibodies to β_2-GPI.

Investigators have shown that β_2-GPI-oxLDL complexes can frequently be detected in sera from patients with APLS and/or

Table 49.7 Cutaneous findings in antiphospholipid antibody syndrome.

Livedo reticularis, with or without retiform purpura or retiform necrosis
Sneddon's syndrome
Livedoid vasculopathy/atrophie blanche
Raynaud's phenomenon
Anetoderma-like lesions with thrombosis
Behçet's-like lesions
Nailfold ulcers
Widespread cutaneous necrosis (catastrophic antiphospholipid antibody syndrome)
Leg ulcers, secondary to recurrent thrombosis with stasis, or from conditions in this table
Cholesterol embolus-like proximal livedo reticularis, with or without distal retiform purpura
Acral livedo
Degos (malignant atrophic papulosis)-like lesions
Pseudo-Kaposi's sarcoma
Vasculitis-like lesions
Pyoderma gangrenosum-like ulcers
Splinter haemorrhages
Superficial thrombophlebitis migrans

systemic lupus erythematosus, but not in healthy individuals [41]. Furthermore, patients with APS have been shown to have autoreactive CD4$^+$ T cells responsive to β_2-GPI in patients with APLS, and which can promote pathogenic IgG anti-β_2-GPI antibody production by autologous B cells. These T cells do not respond to native β_2-GPI, but will respond to chemically reduced or bacterially expressed recombinant β_2-GPI, further supporting the hypothesis that it is a cryptic epitope that is responsible for pathological β_2-GPI antibodies. This insight leads to the possibility of future therapies targeted at depleting or blocking binding domain I-directed β_2-GPI antibodies, or inhibiting their production through elimination or inhibition of the pathological autoreactive CD4$^+$ T-cell subset [41].

Clinically, APLS can present with a variety of cutaneous findings (Table 49.7) [42]. Livedo is one of the most common, but least specific as this and retiform purpura or necrosis occur in other microvascular occlusion disorders [42]. In one large study the frequency of these findings was livedo reticularis 24%, leg ulcers 5.5%, pseudovasculitis 3.9%, digital gangrene 3.3%, cutaneous necrosis 2.1% and splinter haemorrhages 0.7% [32]. Catastrophic APLS is an uncommon but disastrous variant in which patients typically present with widespread cutaneous necrosis and multi-organ failure, especially renal and pulmonary. Precipitating factors include infections, surgical procedures, drugs and discontinuation of anticoagulation. The most common extracutaneous manifestations of non-catastrophic APLS include deep-vein thrombosis, pulmonary embolus and central nervous system abnormalities.

Specific therapy in APLS awaits an understanding of the mechanism by which thrombosis occurs in individual patients, and thus the capability to use tailored therapies to specifically oppose that pathway in a particular individual. As alluded to previously, investigation of the role of autoreactive CD4$^+$ T cells driving B-cell production of pathogenic β_2-GPI antibodies may provide more effective therapies in the future. For now, treatment is empirical. Antiplatelet therapy is of uncertain benefit; most therapy depends on acute and often chronic anticoagulation, either with standard or low-molecular-weight heparin initially followed by coumadin [34]. Antimalarial therapy may be of some benefit for atrophie blanche-like or Degos-like syndromes in lupus patients; evidence suggests a protective effect in lupus patients against arterial or venous thromboses [29]. There is evidence that hydroxychloroquine may interfere with the binding of IgG-β_2-GPI complexes on phospholipid bilayers or to a line of cultured human monocytic leukaemia cells, which may provide some rationale for possible prophylactic benefit in APLS patients [43].

References

1 Marlar RA, Montgomery RR, Broekmans AW. Diagnosis and treatment of homozygous protein C deficiency. Report of the Working Party on homozygous protein C deficiency of the subcommittee on protein C and protein S, International Committee on Thrombosis and Haemostasis. *J Pediatr* 1989; **114**: 528–34.

2 Comp P, Nixon R, Cooper M *et al.* Familial protein S deficiency is associated with recurrent thrombosis. *J Clin Invest* 1984; **74**: 2082–8.

3 Koeleman BP, van Rumpt D, Hamulyák K *et al.* Factor V Leiden: an additional risk factor for thrombosis in protein S deficient families? *Thromb Haemost* 1995; **74**: 580–3.

4 Simioni P, Sanson B, Prandoni P *et al.* Incidence of venous thromboembolism in families with inherited thrombophilia. *Thromb Haemost* 1999; **81**: 198–202.

5 Marlar RA, Neumann A. Neonatal purpura fulminans due to homozygous protein C or protein S deficiencies. *Semin Thromb Hemost* 1990; **16**: 333–40.

6 Ezer U, Misirlioglu E, Colba V *et al.* Neonatal purpura fulminans due to homozygous protein C deficiency. *Pediatr Hematol Oncol* 2001; **18**: 453–8.

7 Dreyfus M, Magny JF, Bridey F *et al.* Treatment of homozygous protein C deficiency and neonatal purpura fulminans with a purified protein C concentrate. *N Engl J Med* 1991; **325**: 1565–8.

8 Nakayama T, Matsushita T, Hidano H *et al.* A case of purpura fulminans is caused by homozygous delta8857 mutation (protein C-nagoya) and successfully treated with activated protein C concentrate. *Br J Haematol* 2000; **110**: 727–30.

9 Comp P, Elrod J, Karzenski S. Warfarin-induced skin necrosis. *Semin Thromb Hemost* 1990; **16**: 293–8.

10 Griffin J. Anticoagulants and skin necrosis. *Adverse Drug React Toxicol Rev* 1994; **13**: 157–67.

11 Sallah S, Thomas D, Roberts H. Warfarin and heparin-induced skin necrosis and the purple toe syndrome: infrequent complications of anticoagulant treatment. *Thromb Haemost* 1997; **78**: 785–90.

12 O'Brien A, Tate G, Shiach C. Evaluation of protein C and protein S levels during oral anticoagulant therapy. *Clin Lab Haematol* 1998; **20**: 245–52.

13 Hjort PF, Rapaport SI, Jorgensen I. Purpura fulminans: report of a case successfully treated with heparin and hydrocortisone. Review of 50 cases from the literature. *Scand J Haematol* 1964; **1**: 169.

14 Levin M, Eley B, Louis J *et al.* Postinfectious purpura fulminans caused by an autoantibody directed against protein S. *J Pediatr* 1995; **127**: 355–63.

15 Piette WW. The differential diagnosis of purpura from a morphologic perspective. *Adv Dermatol* 1994; **9**: 3–24.

16 Robson K, Piette W. The presentation and differential diagnosis of cutaneous vascular occlusion syndromes. *Adv Dermatol* 1999; **15**: 153–82.

17 Piette W, Shasby DM, Kealey P, Olson J. Retiform purpura is a sign of severe acquired protein C deficiency and risk of progression to purpura fulminans in sepsis and disseminated intravascular coagulation. *Clin Res* 1993; **41**: 253A.

18 Esmon C. Protein C pathways in sepsis. *Ann Med* 2002; **34**: 598–605.

19 Warren H, Suffredini A, Eichacker P, Munford R. Risks and benefits of activated protein C treatment for severe sepsis. *N Engl J Med* 2002; **347**: 1027–30.

20 Manns B, Lee H, Doig C *et al.* An economic evaluation of activated protein C treatment for severe sepsis. *N Engl J Med* 2002; **347**: 993–1000.

21 Siegel J. Assessing the use of activated protein C in the treatment of severe sepsis. *N Engl J Med* 2002; **347**: 1030–4.

22 Ely E, Bernard G, Vincent J. Activated protein C for severe sepsis. *N Engl J Med* 2002; **347**: 1035–6.

23 Hodgson A, Ryan T, Moriarty J *et al.* Plasma exchange as a source of protein C for acute onset protein C pathway failure. *Br J Haematol* 2002; **116**: 905–8.

24 Frances RB Jr. Acquired purpura fulminans. *Semin Thromb Hemost* 1990; **16**: 310–25.

25 Manco-Johnson M, Nuss R, Key N *et al.* Lupus anticoagulant and protein S deficiency in children with postvaricella purpura fulminans or thrombosis. *J Pediatr* 1996; **128**: 319–23.

26 van Ommen C, van Wijnen M, de Groot F *et al.* Postvaricella purpura fulminans caused by acquired protein S deficiency resulting from antiprotein S antibodies: search for the epitopes. *J Pediatr Hematol Oncol* 2002; **24**: 413–6.

27 Lockshin M. Antiphospholipid antibody syndrome. *JAMA* 1992; **268**: 1451–3.

28 Kampe C. Clinical syndromes associated with lupus anticoagulants. *Semin Thromb Hemost* 1994; **20**: 16–26.

29 Levine J, Branch D, Rauch J. The antiphospholipid syndrome. *N Engl J Med* 2002; **346**: 752–63.

30 Miyakis S, Lockshin MD, Atsumi T *et al.* International consensus statement on an update of the classification criteria for definite antiphospholipid syndrome (APS). *J Thromb Haemost* 2006; **4**: 295–306.

31 Gibson G, Su P, Pittelkow M. Antiphospholipid syndrome and the skin. *J Am Acad Dermatol* 1997; **36**: 970–82.

32 Cervera R, Piette J, Font J *et al.* Antiphospholipid syndrome: clinical and immunologic manifestations and patterns of disease expression in a cohort of 1,000 patients. *Arthritis Rheum* 2002; **46**: 1019–27.

33 Giannakopoulos B, Passam F, Ioannou Y, Krilis SA. How we diagnose the antiphospholipid syndrome. *Blood* 2009; **113**: 985–94.

34 Lockshin M, Erkan D. Treatment of the antiphospholipid syndrome. *N Engl J Med* 2003; **349**: 1177–9.

35 Giannakopoulo B, Passam F, Rahgozar S, Krilis SA. Current concepts on the pathogenesis of the antiphospholipid syndrome. *Blood* 2007; **109**: 422–30.

36 Angles-Cano E, Guillin M. Antiphospholipid antibodies and the coagulation cascade. *Rheum Dis Clin North Am* 2001; **27**: 573–86.

37 Nojima J, Kuratsune H, Suehisa E *et al.* Acquired activated protein C resistance is associated with the co-existence of anti-prothrombin antibodies and lupus anticoagulant activity in patients with systemic lupus erythematosus. *Br J Haematol* 2002; **118**: 577–83.

38 Izumi T, Pound M, Su Z *et al.* Anti-beta$_2$-glycoprotein I antibody-mediated inhibition of activated protein C requires binding of beta$_2$-glycoprotein I to phospholipids. *Thromb Haemost* 2002; **88**: 620–6.

39 De Laat B, Wu XX, van Lummerl M *et al.* Correlation between antiphospholipid antibodies that recognize domain I of β2-glycoprotein I and a reduction in the anticoagulant activity of annexin A5. *Blood* 2007; **109**: 1490–4.

40 Hulstein JJ, Lenting PJ, de Laat B *et al.* β2-glycoprotein I inhibits von Willebrand factor dependent platelet adhesion and aggregation. *Blood* 2007; **110**: 1483–91.

41 Yamaguchi Y, Seta N, Kaburaki J *et al.* Excessive exposure to anionic surfaces maintains autoantibody response to β2-glycoprotein I in patients with antiphospholipid syndrome. *Blood* 2007; **110**: 4312–8.

42 Weinstein S, Piette WW. Cutaneous manifestations of antiphospholipid antibody syndrome. *Haematol Oncol Clin North Am* 2008; **22**: 67–77.

43 Rand JH, Wu XX, Quinn AS *et al.* Hydroxychloroquine directly reduces the binding of antiphospholipid antibody-β2-glycoprotein I complexes to phospholipid bilayers. *Blood* 2008; **112**: 1687–95.

Occlusion due to vascular coagulopathies

Sneddon's syndrome

Definition. This syndrome comprises generalized livedo racemosa or livedo reticularis with cerebrovascular lesions that cause focal neurological symptoms or signs [1–5]. Livedo racemosa is usually the first manifestation, initially affecting the lower trunk and proximal part of the legs but becoming more generalized. It typically has a broad network pattern (Fig. 49.13). Associated Raynaud's phenomenon or acrocyanosis may occur, and may be the presenting feature.

Incidence. This has been estimated as four cases per million population per year [5]. Sneddon's syndrome is twice as common in

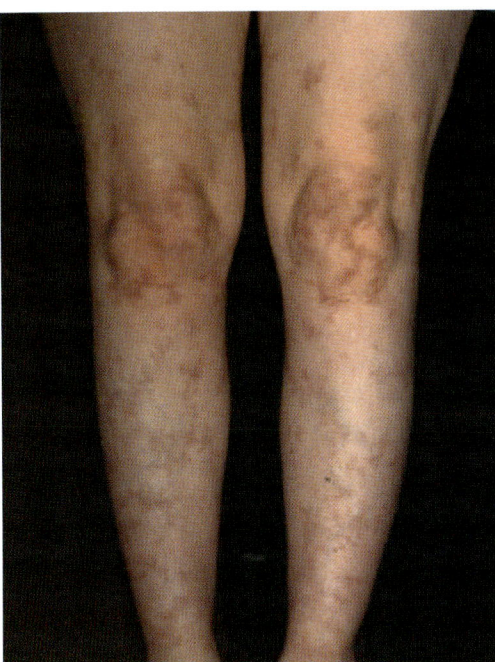

Fig. 49.13 Sneddon's syndrome showing a typical broad racemose livedo patterning.

women as in men, and typically presents in the fourth or fifth decade of life. It is usually sporadic, although familial Sneddon's syndrome has been reported.

Pathogenesis. Several authors have reported the presence of anti-nuclear antibodies or of antiphospholipid antibodies/lupus anti-coagulant (reviewed in [6]), but others would only accept the diagnosis of Sneddon's syndrome if these antibodies were absent. Differences have been documented between the clinical features of patients with Sneddon's syndrome depending on the presence or absence of antiphospholipid antibodies; those without antiphospholipid antibodies typically have a larger-sized livedo pattern, whereas those with antiphospholipid antibodies have a higher risk of seizures, mitral regurgitation and thrombocytopenia [7]. It is likely that there is a spectrum of disease from APLS to SLE that includes the preferential arteriolar pattern of Sneddon's syndrome. Antiprothrombin antibodies were demonstrated in 57% of 46 patients in one series [8], and there are reports of platelet activation in a patient with persistently elevated levels of circulating PF4 [9], of increased levels of antithrombin III [10], of factor V Leiden mutation [11] and of activated protein C resistance [12].

Histopathology. Biopsies may show an endarteritis of dermal arterioles. It has been demonstrated that the most informative biopsies are from the clinically normal centre of any network area rather than from the peripheral 'watershed' area of livedo, and that taking multiple biopsies increases the sensitivity [13]. Initial changes are endothelial swelling with a mixed inflammatory infiltrate, progressing to vascular plugging, subendothelial proliferation and eventual vascular occlusion, fibrosis and disappearance of the inflammatory component [14]. It is possible, if not likely, that the histological findings in patients with antiphospholipid antibodies, especially in association with lupus or lupus-like disease, would be more typical of non-inflammatory occlusion.

Clinical features. In addition to the cutaneous livedo, there may be non-specific neurological prodromal symptoms such as headache, migraine, dizziness or vertigo. Later neurological features include focal paresis or hemiparesis, focal sensory or hemisensory symptoms, fits and visual defects, and later cognitive changes. Transient ischaemic attacks are commoner than completed stroke [15]. Peripheral nerves may also be affected. Hypertension may be present and confers a worse prognosis if untreated; hypertension and the neurological aspects are sometimes aggravated by pregnancy or use of oral contraceptives. There may be renal or cardiac involvement, including valve defects such as mitral regurgitation, although internal organ involvement other than neurological is often asymptomatic [5]. Other features such as shortened digits have rarely been reported.

The differential diagnosis is wide, from both the cutaneous and the neurological perspective. In particular, other causes of livedo and microvascular occlusion syndromes discussed in this chapter need to be considered as well as vasculitic causes (e.g. polyarteritis nodosa). However, it should be noted that other patterns of livedo with anticardiolipin antibodies may be associated with evidence of cerebral microthrombosis, for example livedo with summer ulceration or livedo with pyoderma gangrenosum-like lesions [16].

Magnetic resonance imaging (MRI), electroencephalography and arteriography may help to confirm the neurological component; skin biopsy (as above) and exclusion of other causes of livedo are necessary. Patients with positive antiphospholipid antibodies more commonly have infarcts in the distribution of the main cerebral arteries on MRI, whereas those with negative antibodies have small lacunar infarcts [17] and progressive leukoencephalopathy [15].

Treatment. There is generally no very effective treatment, reflecting the non-inflammatory nature of the disease. Corticosteroids may have some benefit but this is variable and often difficult to assess due to the intermittent nature of the neurological disease; other immunosuppressive agents are often disappointing. Avoidance of smoking and oral contraceptives, and treatment of hypertension and hyperlipidaemia (both of which are commonly present), are important. Thrombolytic agents and vasodilators have been used in the acute situation, and antiplatelet agents appear to be effective in the longer term [7]. In patients with antiphospholipid antibodies or lupus anticoagulants, maintenance of anticoagulation at an international normalized ratio (INR) of 2–3 seems warranted.

References

1 Sneddon IB. Cerebro-vascular lesions and livedo reticularis. *Br J Dermatol* 1965; **77**: 180–5.
2 Daoud MS, Wilmoth GJ, Su WPD, Pittelkow MR. Sneddon syndrome. *Semin Dermatol* 1995; **14**: 166–72.
3 Alegre VA, Winkelmann RK, Gastineau DA. Cutaneous thrombosis, cerebrovascular thrombosis, and lupus anticoagulant: the Sneddon syndrome. Report of 10 cases. *Int J Dermatol* 1990; **29**: 45–9.
4 Lubach D, Schwabe C, Weissenborn K *et al.* Livedo racemosa generalisata: an evaluation of thirty-four cases. *J Am Acad Dermatol* 1990; **22**: 633–9.
5 Zelger B, Sepp N, Stockhammer G *et al.* Sneddon's syndrome: a long-term follow-up of 21 patients. *Arch Dermatol* 1993; **129**: 437–47.

6 Frances C, Piette JC. The mystery of Sneddon syndrome: relationship with antiphospholipid syndrome and systemic lupus erythematosus. *J Autoimmun* 2000; **15**: 139–43.

7 Frances C, Papo T, Wechsler B *et al.* Sneddon syndrome with or without antiphospholipid antibodies. A comparative study in 46 patients. *Medicine (Baltimore)* 1999; **78**: 209–19.

8 Kalashnikova LA, Korczyn AD, Shavit S *et al.* Antibodies to prothrombin in patients with Sneddon's syndrome. *Neurology* 1999; **53**: 223–5.

9 Matsumura Y, Tomimoto H, Yamamoto M *et al.* Sneddon syndrome with multiple cerebral infarctions 12 years after the onset of livedo vasculitis: a possible involvement of platelet activation. *J Dermatol* 2001; **28**: 508–10.

10 Bolayir E, Kececi H, Akyol M *et al.* Sneddon's syndrome and antithrombin III. *J Dermatol* 1999; **26**: 532–4.

11 Besnier R, Francès C, Ankri A *et al.* Factor V Leiden mutation in Sneddon syndrome. *Lupus* 2003; **12**: 406–8.

12 Gualtieri RJ, Walton GD. Activated protein C resistance and Sneddon's syndrome. *Am J Med* 1999; **107**: 293.

13 Wohlrab J, Fischer M, Wolter M, Marsch WC. Diagnostic impact and sensitivity of skin biopsies in Sneddon's syndrome: a report of 15 cases. *Br J Dermatol* 2001; **145**: 285–8.

14 Zelger B, Sepp N, Schmid KW *et al.* Life history of cutaneous vascular lesions in Sneddon's syndrome. *Hum Pathol* 1992; **23**: 668–75.

15 Boesch SM, Plörer AL, Auer AJ *et al.* The natural course of Sneddon syndrome: clinical and magnetic resonance imaging findings in a prospective six year observation study. *J Neurol Neurosurg Psychiatry* 2003; **74**: 542–4.

16 Suzuki Y, Otoyama K, Katayama I *et al.* Livedo with cerebrovascular thrombosis: correlation between clinical features, anti-cardiolipin antibodies, and cerebral microinfarction. *Jpn J Dermatol* 1990; **100**: 1437–44.

17 Fetoni V, Grisoli M, Salmaggi A *et al.* Clinical and neuroradiological aspects of Sneddon's syndrome and primary antiphospholipid antibody syndrome: a follow-up study. *Neurol Sci* 2000; **21**: 157–64.

Livedoid vasculopathy; atrophie blanche

Synonyms
- Livedo reticularis with summer ulceration
- Segmental hyalinizing vasculitis

This syndrome is most common in young to middle-aged women as either an idiopathic or secondary syndrome [1]. One of the most commonly noted associations is with chronic venous hypertension and varicosities, although the atrophic scarring in this setting is not usually preceded by small painful ulcerations, nor with surrounding livedo reticularis. It would seem appropriate to separate venous stasis-related atrophie blanche from more typical forms of the syndrome.

Pathogenesis. The pathogenesis of livedoid vasculopathy is unknown. Clearly, APLS, with or without a lupus association, can produce this clinical syndrome [2]. Multiple pathophysiological abnormalities have been implicated, including platelet activation, factor V Leiden, altered fibrinolysis, antiphospholipid antibodies and hyperhomocystinaemia [1–4]. In one series of 32 patients, heterozygous factor V Leiden mutation was found in two of nine tested (22%), decreased protein C or protein S activity in two of 15 (13%), prothrombin G20210A mutation in one of 12 (8%), lupus anticoagulant in five of 28 (18%), anticardiolipin antibodies in eight of 29 (29%) and elevated homocysteine levels in three of 21 (14%) [5].

Histology. The most characteristic histological findings in this syndrome are some thickening or hyaline changes in the walls of superficial dermal vessels, and luminal fibrin deposition [1,6]. Red cell extravasation and perivascular lymphocytic infiltrates are expected findings. In a series of 45 skin biopsies from 32 patients, all but one showed intraluminal thrombus and direct immunofluorescence was positive in 86% [5].

Clinical features. Persistent, very painful and often punched-out ulcerations of the legs, especially around the malleoli, in women are typical of atrophie blanche [6]. The disease is bilateral in most cases. When accompanied by surrounding livedo reticularis, the term 'livedoid vasculitis' is more likely to be applied. Retiform or stellate purpura or ulcer extension can occur; healing results in a porcelain-white scar, frequently surrounded by telangiectasia. Besides venous hypertension and antiphospholipid antibody-related syndromes, sickle cell ulcers can show the same porcelain-white scar of atrophie blanche.

Treatment. Antiplatelet, anticoagulant and fibrinolytic therapies have been reported to be helpful in this syndrome, as well as anabolic steroids such as danazol and stanozolol [2]. PUVA therapy has been reported as effective in some cases [7]. In patients with lupus and atrophie blanche-like lesions, antimalarial therapy may be effective. Rapid relief of pain has been reported with use of intravenous immunoglobulins [8], postulated to be due to inhibition of the vasoconstrictor chemicals thromboxane A_2 and endothelin which thereby improves perfusion. Lipoprostaglandin E_1 has been used with good response in a patient with livedoid vasculitis and essential cryoglobulinaemia [9], but this may have been mediated by an effect on the cryoprotein levels, which fell dramatically; there are anecdotal reports of response to tetracyclines [10], and dapsone has also been used in patients with underlying myeloproliferative syndromes.

References
1 Maessen-Visch M, Koedam M, Hamulyak K, Neumann H. Atrophie blanche. *Int J Dermatol* 1999; **38**: 161–72.

2 Acland K, Darvay A, Wakelin S, Russell-Jones R. Livedoid vasculitis: a manifestation of the antiphospholipid syndrome? *Br J Dermatol* 1999; **140**: 131–5.

3 Calamia K, Balabanova M, Perniciaro C, Walsh J. Livedo (livedoid) vasculitis and the factor V Leiden mutation: additional evidence for abnormal coagulation. *J Am Acad Dermatol* 2002; **46**: 133–7.

4 Anavekar NS, Kelly R. Heterozygous prothrombin gene mutation associated with livedoid vasculopathy. *Australas J Dermatol* 2007; **48**: 120–5.

5 Hairston BR, Davis MPD, Pittelkow MR, Ahmed I. Livedoid vasculopathy: further evidence for procoagulant pathogenesis. *Arch Dermatol* 2006; **142**: 1413–8.

6 Robson K, Piette W. The presentation and differential diagnosis of cutaneous vascular occlusion syndromes. *Adv Dermatol* 1999; **15**: 153–82.

7 Lee J, Choi H, Kim S *et al.* Livedoid vasculitis responding to PUVA therapy. *Int J Dermatol* 2001; **40**: 153–7.

8 Kreuter A, Gambichler T, Breukermann F *et al.* Pulsed intravenous immunoglobulin therapy in livedoid vasculitis: an open trial evaluating 9 consecutive patients. *J Am Acad Dermatol* 2004; **51**: 574–9.

9 Kawakami T, Kawasaki K, Mizoguchi M, Soma Y. Therapeutic effect of lipoprostaglandin E_1 on livedoid vasculitis associated with essential cryoglobulinaemia. *Br J Dermatol* 2007; **157**: 1051–3.

10 Webster G, del Rosso JQ. Anti-inflammatory activity of tetracyclines. *Dermatol Clin* 2007; **25**: 133–5.

Malignant atrophic papulosis

Definition. Malignant atrophic papulosis is a progressive vasculopathy causing occlusion of small and medium-sized arteries [1–6]. Originally reported separately by Kohlmeier [7] and Degos [8], it was also described as lethal cutaneous and gastrointestinal arteriolar thrombosis [9]. It is characterized by skin and gastrointestinal lesions, but neurological features are also frequent and post-mortem studies show widespread organ involvement. The skin lesions are usually the first feature, and may be the only manifestation over many years [2]; whether this represents a truly 'benign' variant is uncertain.

Incidence. It is rare; a review in 1995 suggested that about 120 cases had been reported [4]. It is mainly reported in white people, has a slight male predominance and is mainly a disease that presents in young adults, although it can affect any age group [3,5]. Familial cases have been reported [10].

Pathogenesis [3,5]. The pathogenesis probably involves abnormal coagulation, although the precise mechanism is uncertain. Platelet and fibrin thrombi are apparent in dermal, mesenteric and nervous system blood vessels, and both abnormal platelet aggregation and inhibition of fibrinolysis have been reported [3,5,11–14]. However, most patients have no clear evidence of a systemic coagulopathy, suggesting that the thrombotic tendency is at the microvascular level. Antiphospholipid antibodies have been documented in a small number of patients, usually in the context of SLE, although they may also occur even in the benign cutaneous variant [15].

There is also some support for a mechanism involving vascular inflammation. An autoimmune mechanism is suggested by the occurrence of lesions resembling malignant atrophic papulosis in some patients with SLE, rheumatoid arthritis, scleroderma or dermatomyositis [16–19]; antiendothelial antibodies have also been demonstrated but are probably not the cause of the disease [5]. Circulating immune complexes, or deposition of immune complexes or complement, are not usually demonstrated [2,20]. Although there can be a prominent lymphocytic infiltrate in later lesions, especially around venules, true arteritis and leukocytoclasis are not found [3,5,21].

Abnormal mucin deposits, which may be thrombogenic, occur even in early lesions although they tend to be more apparent in later lesions [3,5,21]. It is possible that they may be induced by activated T cells.

A viral aetiology was proposed on the basis of electron microscopic demonstration of interwoven tuboreticular structures resembling viral inclusions within endothelial cells [22], but these are seen in other disorders, including SLE, and can be induced by interferon [5]. Cases have been reported with HIV infection but a causal association is unproven.

Histopathology [2–6]. The histological picture in Degos' disease depends upon the duration of the lesion biopsied. Early lesions show a superficial and deep perivascular, perineural and periappendageal chronic inflammatory cell infiltrate [21]. Deep dermal vessels show endovascular inflammation, proliferation and thickening with thrombosis [23]. Mucin deposition is seen at all stages [2–4,21,24], and fibrin deposition may be demonstrated; fibrinoid necrosis of vessel walls may occur [23]. Immunofluorescence is occasionally positive for IgG or C3. From a histopathological perspective, the presence of lymphocytes, which may be seen within the damaged vessel wall, is viewed as abnormal and has led to classification of Degos' disease as a lymphocytic vasculitis [25] although it is not documented that this is a primary abnormality. Later lesions show a classical 'wedge-shaped' pattern of sclerotic change in the dermis, which is usually only sparsely cellular. Between these stages there is a phase with neutrophilic and eosinophilic infiltrate around adnexae and a dense perivascular lymphocytic infiltrate [21]. The epidermis, initially showing a mild vacuolar reaction, becomes atrophic with slight scaling, resembling that seen in lichen sclerosus and corresponding with the typical 'porcelain-white' colour seen clinically. There may be some associated pigmentary incontinence.

Panniculitis resembling that seen in lupus profundus has recently been reported [26]. Similar changes occur in the intestinal wall, particularly the submucosa. The muscularis mucosae is intact. Blood vessels are thickened and disorganized, with fibrinoid degeneration; platelet–fibrin thrombi are more prominent than in skin biopsy material.

Microaneurysms of the bulbar conjunctival vessels have been described. Renal changes include thickening of the afferent glomerular arterioles and of the capillary basement membrane.

Clinical features [1–8]. Cutaneous lesions usually precede systemic manifestations by months to years. They develop as crops over a period of time and are usually asymptomatic, although they may be preceded by slight burning. Skin lesions affect any site, mainly the trunk and proximal limbs; the face, palms and soles are generally spared. Although they may evolve gradually, and the number of lesions may vary considerably, about 30–40 active lesions are usually present [4]. Oral mucosal lesions are rare but penile lesions may occur [27]; the bulbar conjunctiva is often affected by lesions, which appear as sharply demarcated avascular areas [4]. Peristomal lesions have been reported.

Early skin lesions are pink or red, dome-shaped papules, usually 2–5 mm in size but sometimes up to about 15 mm. Papules soon become necrotic and umbilicated with central 'porcelain-white' pallor and scaling, and the pink oedematous border becomes telangiectatic. Most heal rather slowly to leave a small white scar, often surrounded by telangiectases as in atrophie blanche. Urticaria-like, ulceropustular and gumma-like nodules have been reported. New crops of lesions may continue for several years.

Similar lesions occur in many organs. Gastrointestinal lesions are the most important, as perforation of the gut is a cause of death. Neurological symptoms are also relatively common. The features in different systems include the following [4].

- Gastrointestinal: dyspepsia, abdominal pain or distension, bleeding, perforation, peritonitis, fistulae (enteroenteral or enterocutaneous), obstruction, pancreatitis
- Neurological: cerebral infarction (causing headache, aphasia, dementia, focal epilepsy, hemiparesis, pseudobulbar palsy), cord infarction (paraplegia/quadriplegia, transverse myelopathy), peripheral nerve (cauda equina syndrome, mononeuritis multiplex), various sites (sensory disturbance)
- Ocular: ptosis, diplopia, nystagmus, ophthalmoplegia, optic neuritis, papilloedema, visual field loss, pupillary reaction defects, conjunctival avascular lesions, posterior subcapsular cataract
- Cardiovascular: renal artery occlusion, pericardial effusion, constrictive pericarditis, ventricular wall defects
- Pulmonary: pleuritis.

Differential diagnosis. There is sometimes a resemblance to atrophie blanche or to guttate lichen sclerosus, although the evolution of lesions is different. Identical lesions have been described in cases of various connective tissue diseases [16–19] and in a patient with Crohn's disease [28]. The characteristic features can scarcely be confused. A disorder termed 'cutaneous–intestinal syndrome with oropharyngeal ulceration' [29] included a combination of macular, blistering and crusting lesions of the skin, with oropharyngeal ulceration and death from perforation of one of many intestinal ulcers. This differed both clinically and histologically from Degos' disease. Patients in whom systemic disease precedes skin lesions may cause particular diagnostic problems.

Prognosis [4]. Although possibly overestimated by reporting bias, and acknowledging that there does appear to be a benign cutaneous ('skin-limited') variant, mortality of 50–60% within 2–5 years is anticipated. Prognosis in males appears to be worse than in females.

Treatment. There is no consistently effective treatment [2–4]. Steroids do not help, although some benefit in neurological symptoms has been suggested. Aspirin, antiplatelet agents, fibrinolytic agents and pentoxifylline, alone or in combination, may lead to remission and are perhaps most effective in the cutaneous disease [2–6,11,15,30–32]; phenylbutazone has been reported to be effective. Heparin may produce short-term benefit. There is one report of a good response to transdermal nicotine patches [33]. Warfarin, dextrans, chloroquine, immunosuppressive agents and plasma exchange have all been tried. Surgery to treat intestinal perforation may resolve the acute situation but is difficult as there are usually multiple lesions, and there is no long-term benefit from this approach.

References

1 Degos R. Malignant atrophic papulosis. *Br J Dermatol* 1979; **100**: 21–36.
2 Su WPD, Schroeter AL, Lee DA *et al.* Clinical and histologic findings in Degos' syndrome (malignant atrophic papulosis). *Cutis* 1985; **35**: 131–8.
3 Magrinat G, Kerwin KS, Gabriel DA. The clinical manifestations of Degos' syndrome. *Arch Pathol Lab Med* 1989; **113**: 354–62.
4 Snow JL, Muller SA. Degos syndrome: malignant atrophic papulosis. *Semin Dermatol* 1995; **14**: 99–105.
5 Chatham WW. Miscellaneous forms of vasculitis. In: Ball GV, Bridges SL Jr, eds. *Vasculitis*. Oxford: Oxford University Press, 2002: 513–32.
6 Assier-Bonnet H, Chosidow O, Frances C. Degos disease. *Ann Dermatol Vénéréol* 1997; **124**: 273–9.
7 Kohlmeier W. Multiple Hautnelnosen bei Thromboangiitis obliterans. *Arch Dermatol Syphilol* 1941; **181**: 783–4.
8 Degos R, Delort J, Tricot R. Dermatite papulosquamose atrophiante. *Bull Soc Fr Dermatol Syphil* 1942; **49**: 148–50.
9 Sidi E, Reinberg A, Spinasse JB *et al.* Lethal cutaneous and gastrointestinal arteriolar thrombosis. *JAMA* 1960; **174**: 1170–3.
10 Katz SK, Mudd LJ, Roenigk HH Jr. Malignant atrophic papulosis (Degos' disease) involving three generations of a family. *J Am Acad Dermatol* 1997; **37**: 480–4.
11 Drucker CR. Malignant atrophic papulosis: response to antiplatelet therapy. *Dermatologica* 1990; **180**: 90–2.
12 Aizawa H, Takase Y, Inoue K *et al.* An autopsy case of Degos disease with neurological symptoms: neuropathological observations and increased platelet aggregation. *Rinsho Shinkeigaku* 1992; **32**: 23–9.
13 Black MM, Nishioka K, Levene GM. The role of dermal blood vessels in the pathogenesis of malignant atrophic papulosis (Degos' disease). *Br J Dermatol* 1973; **88**: 213–9.
14 Caux F, Aractingi S, Scrobohaci ML *et al.* Abnormal fibrinolysis in Degos disease. A study of 3 cases. *Ann Dermatol Vénéréol* 1994; **121**: 537–42.
15 Farrell AM, Moss J, Costello C *et al.* Benign cutaneous Degos' disease. *Br J Dermatol* 1998; **139**: 708–12.
16 Black MM, Hudson PM. Atrophie blanche lesions closely resembling malignant atrophic papulosis (Degos' disease) in systemic lupus erythematosus. *Br J Dermatol* 1976; **95**: 649–52.
17 Durie BGM, Stroud JD, Kahn JA. Progressive systemic sclerosis with malignant atrophic papulosis. *Arch Dermatol* 1969; **100**: 575–81.
18 Demitsu T, Kakurai M, Marata S *et al.* Degos' disease associated with rheumatoid arthritis. *J Dermatol* 1997; **24**: 488–90.
19 Tsao H, Busam K, Barnhill RL, Haynes HA. Lesions resembling malignant atrophic papulosis in a patient with dermatomyositis. *J Am Acad Dermatol* 1997; **36**: 317–9.
20 Tribble K, Archer ME, Jorizzo JL *et al.* Malignant atrophic papulosis: absence of circulating immune complexes or vasculosis. *J Am Acad Dermatol* 1986; **15**: 365–9.
21 Harvell JD, Williford PL, White WL. Benign cutaneous Degos' disease: a case report with emphasis on histopathology as papules chronologically evolve. *Am J Dermatopathol* 2001; **23**: 116–23.
22 Bleehen SS. Intraendothelial tubular aggregates in malignant atrophic papulosis (Degos' disease). *Clin Exp Dermatol* 1977; **2**: 73–4.
23 Soter NA, Murphy GF, Mihm MC Jr. Lymphocytes and necrosis of the cutaneous microvasculature in malignant atrophic papulosis. A refined light microscopy study. *J Am Acad Dermatol* 1982; **7**: 620–30.
24 Feuerman EJ, Dollberg L, Salvador O. Malignant atrophic papulosis with mucin in the dermis. *Arch Pathol* 1970; **90**: 310–5.
25 Carlson JA, Chen K-R. Cutaneous vasculitis update: neutrophilic muscular vessel and eosinophilic, granulomatous, and lymphocytic vasculitis syndromes. *Am J Dermatopathol* 2007; **29**: 32–43.
26 Grilli R, Soriano ML, Izquierdo MJ *et al.* Panniculitis mimicking lupus erythematosus profundus: a new histopathologic finding in malignant atrophic papulosis (Degos disease). *Am J Dermatopathol* 1999; **21**: 365–8.
27 Thomson KF, Highet AS. Penile ulceration in fatal malignant atrophic papulosis (Degos' disease). *Br J Dermatol* 2000; **143**: 1320–2.
28 Castenet J, Lacour J-P, Perrin C *et al.* Cutaneous vasculitis with lesions mimicking Degos' disease and revealing Crohn's disease. *Acta Derm Venereol (Stockh)* 1995; **75**: 408–9.
29 Bettley FR. A fatal cutaneo-intestinal syndrome. *Br J Dermatol* 1960; **72**: 423–6.
30 Stahl D, Thomsen K, Hou-Jensen K. Malignant atrophic papulosis. *Arch Dermatol* 1978; **114**: 1687–9.
31 Torrelo A, Sevilla J, Medeiro IG *et al.* Malignant atrophic papulosis in an infant. *Br J Dermatol* 2002; **146**: 916–8.

32 Vicktor C, Schultz-Ehrenburg U. Malignant atrophic papulosis (Kohlmeier–Degos): diagnosis, therapy and course. *Hautarzt* 2001; **52**: 734–7.

33 Kanekura T, Uchino Y, Kanzaki T. A case of malignant atrophic papulosis successfully treated with nicotine patches. *Br J Dermatol* 2003; **149**: 660–2.

Occlusion due to reticulocytes

Patients with sickle cell anaemia may develop leg ulcers, which in tropical climates typically progress rapidly due to secondary bacterial infection [1]. However, in temperate climates the lesions are often perimalleolar, quite painful, and may heal with a porcelain-white scar, often mimicking atrophie blanche. Although this ulceration might be attributed solely to sickling of erythrocytes with microvascular occlusion, similar ulcers have been reported in other instances of severe chronic haemolytic anaemia, such as thalassaemia or antibody-mediated haemolysis, where sickling is not possible [2]. Multiple studies of possible occlusive mechanisms in sickle cell disease have shown that both young and old red cells have abnormally sticky membranes. In addition, abnormal leukocyte adhesion may initiate occlusion episodes, followed by adhesion of erythrocytes to these leukocytes, with a drop in tissue perfusion, followed by hypoxia and sickling with propagation of occlusion [3]. A number of platelet, procoagulant, anticoagulant and fibrinolytic abnormalities have been noted in sickle cell disease [3–5]. These might more properly be considered consequences of sickle cell disease vasculopathy [6]. A central mechanism for this vasculopathy seems to be haemolysis-associated reduction in the bioavailability of nitric oxide. Consequences of this reduction include endothelial cell activation, upregulation of the vasoconstrictor endothelin-1, vasoconstriction, platelet activation, increased tissue factor, and coagulation activation. Some of these mechanisms may be operative in other haemolytic anaemias, such as paroxysmal nocturnal haemoglobinuria (see previously) and thalassaemia [7]. Patients with sickle cell disease who are treated with hydroxycarbamide (hydroxyurea) appear to have a higher rate of ulcer development than other patients treated with hydroxycarbamide [7]. Although the mechanism is unclear, macroerythrocytes may play a role in initiation of hydoxyurea-induced leg ulcers and also in syndromes of severe haemolytic anaemia with high reticulocyte count and very early reticulocytes, but without sickling [2]. Whatever studies eventually prove, it seems that erythrocytes or their lysis may play an active role in some occlusive syndromes.

References

1 Piette W. Hematologic associations of leg ulcers. *Clin Dermatol* 1990; **8**: 66–85.

2 Velez A, Garcia-Aranda J, Moreno J. Hydroxyurea-induced leg ulcers: is macroerythrocytosis a pathogenic factor? *J Eur Acad Dermatol Venereol* 1999; **12**: 243–4.

3 Ataga K, Orringer E. Hypercoagulability in sickle cell disease: a curious paradox. *Am J Med* 2003; **115**: 721–8.

4 Shet A, Aras O, Gupta K *et al.* Sickle blood contains tissue factor-positive microparticles derived from endothelial cells and monocytes. *Blood* 2003; **102**: 2678–83.

5 Okpala I. The intriguing contribution of white blood cells to sickle cell disease, a red cell disorder. *Blood Rev* 2004; **18**: 65–73.

6 Morris CM. Mechanisms of vasculopathy in sickle cell disease and thalassemia. *Hematology Am Soc Hematol Education Program* 2008: 177–85.

7 Chaine B, Neonato M, Girot R, Aractingi S. Cutaneous adverse reactions to hydroxyurea in patients with sickle cell disease. *Arch Dermatol* 2001; **137**: 467–70.

Occlusion due to other mechanisms

Calcific uraemic arteriolopathy

Synonym
• Cutaneous calciphylaxis

Calcific uraemic arteriolopathy is a rare, but increasingly frequent, complication of renal failure and dialysis [1–4]. It may very rarely occur in other situations, such as alcoholic liver disease, and occasionally after chemotherapy, in patients with normal renal function. Women are most at risk, accounting for over 80% of cases, mainly in the sixth decade, and even in non-dialysed subjects about a third have diabetes [2]. One large institutional study showed that, compared with other patients on dialysis, risk factors included obesity, liver disease, corticosteroid use, elevated calcium-phosphate product and elevated aluminium levels [2]. Hypoalbuminuria (or albumin infusions), recent rapid weight loss, protein C or protein S deficiency, warfarin treatment and hypotension have also been implicated as risk factors. The original term 'calciphylaxis' referred to an experimental situation of systemic necrosis in rats that were hypercalcaemic due to treatment with vitamin D or with parathyroid hormone, but did not specifically relate to vascular calcification, hence the change in terminology [3].

Early lesions tend to present as painful plaques, often with a retiform or stellate pattern, and may show central necrosis. They may resemble the lesions of hyperoxaluria. Some may become semiconfluent as a 'broken' livedo. The abdomen, thigh and hips are typical sites but the breasts may be involved, in some patients the disease is mainly acral, and uncommon sites include the penis and the tongue [5,6] as well as muscles and internal organs [3]. Woody induration with extending ulcer and eschar formation typically develops.

Pathologically, there is calcification in the medial layer of the wall of small subcutaneous vessels, with necrosis of overlying tissue [1–4]. Some calcification may occur in dermal vessels, in septae within the subcutaneous fat, and in adipocytes themselves. Thrombosed vessels are seen occasionally, presumably as a secondary effect as the calcification of small-vessel walls extends more widely than the thrombotic change or the extravascular calcification [4]. Dermal inflammation may occur without ulceration, and bullae sometimes occur.

Most patients have secondary or tertiary hyperparathyroidism, although the disorder can rarely occur in some with primary hyperparathyroidism. An elevated calcium–phosphorus product is generally expected, but some authors have suggested that this may be present in only a third of cases. Use of vitamin D, or of calcium carbonate (used as a phosphate binder in chronic renal failure), are risk factors. Relevant aspects of calcium homeostasis are discussed in [3]. Vascular calcification induces a phenotypic switch of the vascular myofibroblast to one of an osteoprogenitor. Local (paracrine) pro-mineralization chemicals that are involved include osteopontin (itself stimulated by high glucose levels), bone morphogenetic protein-2 (BMP-2) and Pit-1, as well as matrix metalloproteinases that are stimulated by a catabolic state.

Inhibitors of mineralization include parathormone-related peptide (which is inhibited by vitamin D) and matrix Gla protein (which is inhibited by warfarin); fetuin A inhibits calcification but is inhibited by vitamin D. Thus vitamin D, a commonly used treatment (often as the precursor alpha-calcidol) in chronic renal failure, and warfarin, may both provoke this process, although vitamin D is also used as therapy in patients with hyperparathyroidism who are not considered suitable for parathyroidectomy. It is felt that tensile stress and vascular stasis within calcified areas may also play a part by creating tissue ischaemia.

Parathyroidectomy has been cited as effective, but there is clearly bias in patient selection for this procedure towards those who can tolerate the procedure and are therefore a relatively healthy subgroup. Reduction of the calcium–phosphorus product when elevated is recommended (using low calcium dialysate fluids, and non-calcium oral phosphate binders), as is good wound care and attention to possible accompanying infection, which is a common cause of death. Hyperbaric oxygen, pamidronate, and tissue plasminogen activator have all been used in treatment. Newer treatments that may influence the outcome of this disorder include sodium thiosulphate [7,8], which increases solubility of calcium deposits and has an antioxidant function that may improve endothelial cell function, and cinacalcet hydrochloride [9], which is a calcimimetic therapy that suppresses levels of parathyroid hormone. Logically, cinacalcet should be most useful in patients with hyperparathyroidism and sodium thiosulphate in those without (or in whom it is controlled). Insufficient numbers of patients have been treated with these agents to determine their overall effect on outcome; the prognosis is generally considered poor, with mortality of 50–80%, although there are occasional reports of a more benign course [1,10].

References

1 Oh D, Eulau D, Tokugawa D et al. Five cases of calciphylaxis and a review of the literature. *J Am Acad Dermatol* 2000; **40**: 979–87.

2 Weenig RH, Sewell LD, Davis MPD et al. Calciphylaxis: natural history, risk factor analysis, and outcome. *J Am Acad Dermatol* 2007; **56**: 569–79.

3 Somach SC. Calciphylaxis (calcific uremic arteriolopathy). In: Morgan MB, Smoller BR, Somach SC, eds. *Deadly Dermatologic Diseases. Clinicopathologic Atlas and Text.* New York: Springer, 2007: 167–72.

4 Au S, Crawford R. Three-dimensional analysis of a calciphylaxis plaque: clues to pathogenesis. *J Am Acad Dermatol* 2002; **47**: 53–7.

5 Rifkin BS, Perazella MA. Calcific uremic arteriolopathy (calciphylaxis). *Mayo Clin Proc* 2006; **81**: 9.

6 Bedoya RM, Gutierrez JL, Mayorga F. Calciphylaxis causing localized tongue necrosis: a case report. *J Oral Maxillofac Surg* 1997; **55**: 193–6.

7 Baker BL, Fitzgibbons CA, Buescher LS. Calciphylaxis responding to sodium thiosulphate therapy. *Arch Dermatol* 2007; **143**: 269–70.

8 Ackerman F, Levy A, Daugas E et al. Sodium thiosulphate as first-line treatment for calciphylaxis. *Arch Dermatol* 2007; **143**: 1336–7.

9 Robinson MR, Augustine JJ, Korman NJ. Cinacalcet for the treatment of calciphylaxis. *Arch Dermatol* 2007; **143**: 152–4.

10 Kalajian AH, Malhotra PS, Callen JP, Parker LP. Calciphylaxis with normal renal and parathyroid function: not as rare as previously believed. *Arch Dermatol* 2009; **145**: 451–8.

Specific clinical presentations

This section briefly discusses clinical presentations that are common to a number of occlusive, embolic or vasculitis disorders, in order to allow an approach to the differential diagnosis.

Livedo [1,2]

Livedo describes a reticulate pattern of slow blood flow, with resultant desaturation of blood and bluish discoloration of the skin, which should be completely blanchable if vessels and the blood are normal. Livedo has been divided into two patterns.

Livedo reticularis tends to develop as a tight, net-like pattern of discoloration, often symmetrically distributed, and is more likely to be associated with general disturbances of blood flow such as cold-induced cutaneous vasoconstriction or vascular flow disturbances such as seen in polycythaemia or some cryogelling syndromes. Cutis marmorata in infancy is a perfect example of this pattern. Cutis marmorata telangiectatica congenita is a condition that causes a similar livid reticulate pattern because of telangiectasia.

Livedo racemosa typically has breaks in the tight, net-like pattern, resulting in larger, irregular rings ('broken livedo') than seen in livedo reticularis. It is seldom symmetrical. Livedo racemosa may be more indicative of focal impairment of blood flow, such as with vasculitis, and seems to be the pattern of livedo most often described in European cases of Sneddon's syndrome. The distinction between livedo reticularis and racemosa may be important, but frequently the term 'livedo reticularis' is used to describe both patterns, so careful documentation of the clinical usefulness of this distinction is limited. Finally, lesions of a variety of vascular occlusion syndromes have sometimes been described as lesions of livedo (as discussed above). Although livedo reticularis or racemosa may accompany or surround lesions of retiform purpura, the presence of purpura provides a more specific finding to aid in diagnosis. Whether such conditions frequently present with livedo alone is unclear as these terms have often been used interchangeably in the dermatological literature, and also because semiconfluent retiform lesions may sometimes resemble a broken livedo.

Localized lower extremity livedo (livedoid vasculopathy) is discussed further on p. 49.44.

Conditions that may present as livedo are listed in Table 49.8. It should be noted that more than one factor may apply in some patients, suggesting that a background abnormality has been 'exposed' by an additional event; examples include a patient with antiphospholipid syndrome and fibromuscular dysplasia of peripheral arteries, who developed livedo racemosa and digital necrosis [3]. The same applies in other retiform purpuras, such as phenylephedrine treatment causing microvascular occlusion syndrome in a patient with factor V Leiden [4], and the same applies in purpura fulminans (p. 49.39) in which, for example, meningococcal septicaemia causing thrombosis is strongly linked with background protein C or protein S abnormalities.

References

1 Fleischer AB Jr, Resnick SD. Livedo reticularis. *Dermatol Clin* 1990; **8**: 347–54.

2 Picascia DD, Pellegrini JR. Livedo reticularis. *Cutis* 1987; **39**: 429–32.

3 Eisendle K, Jaschke W, Sepp N. Livedo racemosa and digital necrosis in a patient with primary seronegative antiphospholipid syndrome and fibromuscular dysplasia of peripheral arteries. *Br J Dermatol* 2007; **157**: 389–91.

4 Kalajian AH, Turpen KB, Donovan KO et al. Phenylephedrine-induced microvascular occlusion syndrome in a patient with a heterozygous factor V Leiden mutation. *Arch Dermatol* 2007; **143**: 1314–7.

Table 49.8 Acquired livedo reticularis, non-physiological.

Vascular disease-associated
Vasculitis, especially microscopic polyangiitis, cutaneous periarteritis nodosa, rheumatic vasculitides, mixed cryoglobulinaemia, temporal arteritis, Sneddon's syndrome, livedoid vasculitis, arteriosclerosis

Rheumatic diseases
Lupus erythematosus, dermatomyositis, scleroderma, Sjögren's syndrome, antiphospholipid syndrome

Increased blood viscosity, decreased blood flow
Polycythaemia rubra vera, thrombocytosis, cryoglobulinaemia, cryofibrinogenaemia, cold agglutinaemia, monoclonal gammopathy, hypergammaglobulinaemia

Embolic and hypercoagulable disorders
Cholesterol emboli, thrombotic emboli (secondary to cardiac valvular disease, vascular stenosis or aneurysms, etc.), oxalate emboli, decompression sickness with nitrogen bubble embolization, ventilator gas embolization, antiphospholipid antibody syndrome, thrombophilias

Infection
Some reports of livedo with infection may be secondary to emboli (e.g. endocarditis), angiitis (rickettsial) or purpura fulminans-related occlusion (meningococcal); syphilis, tuberculosis and viral diseases are also important

Endocrine
Hyperparathyroidism, pseudohyperparathyroidism, hypothyroidism, Cushing's disease, carcinoid syndrome, phaeochromocytoma

Nutritional
Pellagra

Iatrogenic
Bismuth (intra-arterial), catecholamines/phenylephedrine, amantadine, quinidine (with drug-induced lupus syndrome), arsphenamine

Cutaneous necrosis

Necrosis of the skin occurs in numerous diverse conditions and may present a diagnostic and therapeutic dilemma. Many of the conditions leading to skin necrosis are discussed elsewhere in this chapter or in Chapter 50; vasculitis and vascular occlusion disorders comprise a significant proportion of such cases, but other disorders are briefly considered here [1–9]. Table 49.9 lists some of the more important causes of cutaneous necrosis. It is not intended to be comprehensive, and the disorders listed are those that either commonly cause cutaneous necrosis or in which cutaneous necrosis is a significant risk. The table therefore lists the most important diagnoses to consider, such as vasculitides or sepsis (Fig. 49.14). Not uncommonly, more than one cause may be present, for example in patients with HIV treated for HCV infection with interferon, or use of anticoagulants or chemotherapy in patients subsequently found to have protein C deficiency.

In some instances, the cause is uncertain; localized skin necrosis at injection or vaccination sites (embolia cutis medicamentosa, Nicolau syndrome) may in different cases be due to arterial spasm, thrombosis due to intra-arterial injection of the drug or arterial occlusion due to inflammation.

In some cases cutaneous necrosis may have predictive value, for example it has been suggested to be linked with the presence of underlying malignancy in patients with dermatomyositis [2].

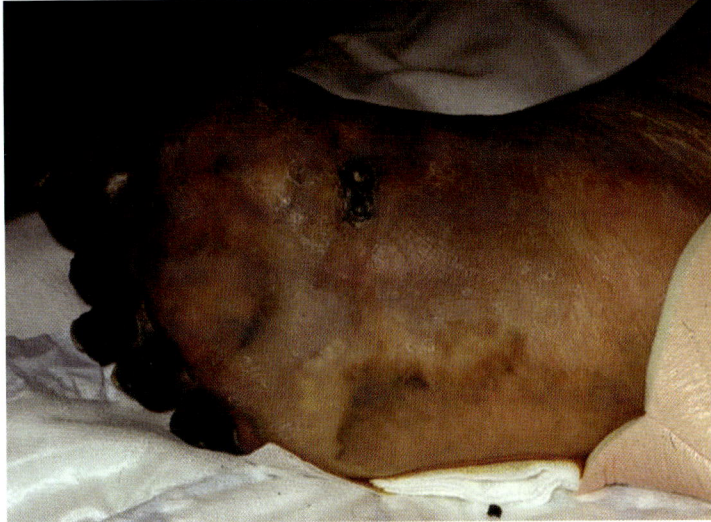

Fig. 49.14 Acral necrosis due to sepsis; treatment with activated protein C may prevent vascular thrombosis in some patients.

References
1 Baker WF Jr, Bick RL. Treatment of hereditary and acquired thrombophilic disorders. *Semin Thromb Hemost* 1999; **25**: 387–406.
2 Basset-Seguin N, Roujeau JC, Gherardi R *et al*. Prognostic factors and predictive signs of malignancy in adult dermatomyositis. A study of 32 cases. *Arch Dermatol* 1990; **126**: 633–7.
3 Bronza JP. Shwartzmann reaction. *Semin Thromb Hemost* 1990; **16**: 326–32.
4 Oh DH, Eulau D, Tokugawa DA *et al*. Five cases of calciphylaxis and a review of the literature. *J Am Acad Dermatol* 1999; **40**: 979–87.
5 Dubost J-J, Souteyrand P, Suavezie B. Drug-induced vasculitides. *Baillière's Clin Rheumatol* 1991; **5**: 119–38.
6 Clark SM, Lanigan SW. Acute necrotic skin reaction to intramuscular Depo-Provera. *Br J Dermatol* 2000; **143**: 1356–7.
7 Merkel PA. Drugs associated with vasculitis. *Curr Opin Rheumatol* 1998; **10**: 45–50.
8 Chan YC, Valenti D, Mansfield AO, Stansby G. Warfarin induced skin necrosis. *Br J Surg* 2000; **87**: 266–72.
9 Allee JE, Saria EA, Rosenblum D *et al*. Intrauterine epidermal necrosis. *J Cutan Pathol* 2001; **28**: 383–6.

Neonatal purpura [1]

The differential diagnosis of purpura or bleeding in neonates includes most of the causes of purpura. However, it is discussed as a separate entity due to the diagnostic dilemmas that may arise. The main causes are listed below.
- Deficiency of clotting factors and coagulation disorders (including purpura fulminans and vitamin K deficiency)
- Thrombocytopenia: congenital, maternal antibodies (ITP, SLE, others)
- Extramedullary erythropoiesis ('blueberry muffin' baby)
- Infections, e.g. TORCH syndrome, which comprises *t*oxoplasmosis, *o*ther infections (syphilis and viral), *r*ubella, *c*ytomegalovirus and *h*erpes simplex, may cause blueberry muffin baby; other infectious causes include HIV, parvovirus B19 and sepsis
- Congenital/inherited conditions, e.g. Wiskott–Aldrich syndrome
- Maternal antibody-mediated: autoimmune (ITP, SLE, drug) or alloimmune (isoimmune) due to fetomaternal incompatibility
- Associated with haemangiomas

Table 49.9 Some causes of cutaneous necrosis.

Coagulation defects [1]

Purpura fulminans, disseminated intravascular coagulopathy

Protein C or S deficiency, antithrombin III deficiency, prothrombin 20210A mutations

Vasculitis

Most vasculitides may cause skin necrosis, e.g. polyarteritis nodosa, Behçet's disease, Wegener's granulomatosis, Churg–Strauss disease, Henoch–Schönlein purpura (see Chapter 50)

Connective tissue disease (see Chapter 51)

Antiphospholipid syndrome/lupus anticoagulant, dermatomyositis [2], relapsing polychondritis, systemic lupus erythematosus, systemic sclerosis

Immunological

Shwartzmann reaction [3]

Hyperviscosity

Cryoglobulinaemia, cryofibrinogenaemia, cold agglutinins, paraproteinaemia, POEMS syndrome

Embolic

Cholesterol emboli, cardiac myxoma, bacterial endocarditis/septic emboli, emboli from arterial aneurysms, neoplasms, emboli through patent foramen ovale (thrombus, infective) from venous cannulae

Metabolic (see Chapter 59)

Diabetes, hyperhomocystinaemia, oxalosis, calciphylaxis [4], subcutaneous calcification

Arterial occlusion or spasm, neurovascular disease

Arteritis (e.g. temporal arteritis, Buerger's disease), Degos' disease, thrombosis, intra-arterial cocaine, aneurysm, anastomosis, compartment syndrome, embolia cutis medicamentosa (Nicolau syndrome), complex regional pain syndrome (reflex sympathetic dystrophy)

Infections (see Chapters 30–36)

Bacterial, e.g. necrotizing fasciitis, cellulitis, streptococci, clostridia, meningococcus, pseudomonas (ecthyma gangrenosum), leprosy (Lucio's reaction), sepsis (any cause) (Fig. 49.14)

Viral, e.g. HIV, cytomegalovirus, hepatitis B or C, herpes zoster

Fungal, e.g. deep/disseminated fungal infection (especially *Aspergillus, Mucor, Rhizopus, Histoplasma*)

Venoms

Snake bites, spider bites, stings (e.g. scorpion, stingray)

Drugs and toxins (see also Chapter 75) [5–8]

Systemic

   Anticoagulants, e.g. warfarin (coumadin), heparin

   Vasoactive drugs, e.g. vasopressin, norepinephrine, dopamine, metaraminol, β-blockers

   Chemotherapeutic drugs, e.g. methotrexate, bleomycin, cyclophosphamide, vincristine

   Cytokines and growth factors, e.g. tumour necrosis factor, interferons, interleukin-3, G-CSF, GM-CSF

   Antimicrobials, e.g. penicillins, sulphonamides, aciclovir, levamisole

   Antithyroid, e.g. thiouracils, carbimazole

   Toxins, e.g. carbon monoxide poisoning

   Illicit drugs, e.g. cocaine

   Miscellaneous, e.g. penicillamine, iodides, bromides, phenytoin

Topical

   Glutaraldehyde, cetrimide, calcium chloride, mustard gas, hydrofluoric acid, phosphorus

Injection sites

   Calcium salts, interferon, aminoglycosides, collagen, silicone, hydrocarbons, vaccines (DTP, BCG), iron dextran, chemotherapy extravasation, Depo-Provera, several illicit drugs, intra-arterial injections

Malignant disease

Leukaemia, lymphoma (especially angiotropic types), mycosis fungoides, lymphomatoid granulomatosis, hypereosinophilic syndrome, myelodysplastic syndrome, Langerhans' cell histiocytosis

Phaeochromocytoma (localized or acral necrosis)

Paraneoplastic thrombosis, paraneoplastic acral vasculopathy (Chapter 62)

Physical damage

Burns, radiation, trauma, factitious ulcer, sclerotherapy, liposuction

Inflammatory dermatoses

Sarcoidosis, pityriasis lichenoides acuta, febrile necrotic Mucha–Haberman disease, pyoderma gangrenosum and neutrophilic dermatoses, panniculitides

Miscellaneous

Intrauterine epidermal necrosis [9]

BCG, bacillus Calmette–Guérin; DTP, diphtheria–tetanus–pertussis; G-CSF, granulocyte colony-stimulating factor; GM-CSF, granulocyte–macrophage colony-stimulating factor; HIV, human immunodeficiency virus; POEMS, polyneuropathy, organomegaly, endocrinopathy, M protein, skin changes

- Traumatic: caput succedaneum and facial petechiae (prolonged vertex delivery)
- Others, e.g. vascular purpura, non-accidental injury (both rare in this age group).

The three most important groups for dermatologists are purpura fulminans, blueberry muffin baby and infections [1]. Purpura fulminans in the neonate is an important manifestation of protein S or protein C deficiency (discussed on p. 49.39). Skin lesions in blueberry muffin baby are distinguished from purpura as they are palpably firm and elevated, but non-palpable purpura may coexist. The TORCH group of infections may cause this condition, but haemolysis (such as rhesus incompatibility), hereditary spherocytosis and twin transfusion syndrome may also be associated with extramedullary erythropoiesis.

Haemorrhagic disease of the newborn is due to accentuation of the normal fall of prothrombin within the first week of life but is now uncommon due to routine vitamin K prophylaxis. An early form, within the first 24 h of life, may occur if there is maternal intake of drugs that interfere with vitamin K (such as oral anticoagulants), and a late form (1–12 months) occurs in children with impaired gastrointestinal absorption and may cause deep nodular ecchymoses. Haemophilia and other coagulation factor deficiencies only rarely cause bleeding at this age.

Of the many causes of purpura fulminans [2], the following are most likely in neonates or young infants:

- Acute infectious: usually bacterial sepsis [3], including meningococcus, streptococcus, *Haemophilus* and other infections
- Post-infectious: varicella, streptococcus and others (usually 7–10 days post-infection)
- Congenital protein C or S deficiency; factor V Leiden mutation
- Acquired protein C or S deficiency: coumarins, hepatic cholestasis, nephrotic syndrome, renal dialysis, marrow transplantation
- Heparin-induced skin necrosis (most cases are related to local skin injection).

In older children, additional causes include:

- Antiphospholipid syndrome
- Vasculitis: polyarteritis nodosa, Henoch–Schönlein purpura, others
- Thrombotic thrombocytopenic purpura/haemolytic uraemic syndrome, paroxysmal nocturnal haemoglobinuria
- Toxins and poisons: snake and spider bites (usually maximal purpura at the inoculation site).

Antiphospholipid syndrome (APLS) is rare in children although low-titre antiphospholipid antibodies, possibly provoked by infection, are relatively frequent (being found in about 10% of healthy children) [4]. Transplacental transfer of anticardiolipin antibodies occurs in neonates born to mothers with APLS but does not appear to result in thrombotic complications, despite the fact that antithrombin III levels are low in neonates and theoretically would represent a further risk factor. When APLS is associated with purpura fulminans, this is termed the 'catastrophic antiphospholipid antibody syndrome'; patients may have a preceding infection, rarely associated SLE, but do not tend to have protein C or protein S abnormalities [5].

It should be noted that the term purpura fulminans has been used either as a broad term for widespread cutaneous purpura of any type, or more specifically for disorders in which cutaneous microvascular occlusion is the known cause of widespread cutaneous purpura. Especially in neonates, in whom (in the absence of a clotting factor deficiency) infection and/or congenital thrombophilic states are the most likely associated causes of widespread purpura, it is prudent to assume that there may be a protein C or protein S abnormality.

References

1 Baselga E, Drolet BA, Esterley NB. Purpura in infants and children. *J Am Acad Dermatol* 1997; **37**: 673–705.
2 Levin M, Eley B, Faust SN. Purpura fulminans. In: Harper J, Oranje AP, Prose N, eds. *Textbook of Pediatric Dermatology*, 2nd edn. Oxford: Blackwell Science, 2006: 1902–16.
3 Hotchkiss RS, Karl IE. The pathophysiology and treatment of sepsis. *N Engl J Med* 2003; **348**: 138–50.
4 Cimaz R, Descloux E. Pediatric antiphospholipid syndrome. *Rheum Dis Clin N Am* 2006; **32**: 559–73.
5 Cervera R, Asherson RA, Font J. Catastrophic antiphospholipid syndrome. *Rheum Dis Clin N Am* 2006; **32**: 575–90.

CHAPTER 50

Vasculitis, Neutrophilic Dermatoses and Related Disorders

N.H. Cox[1], J.L. Jorizzo[2], J.F. Bourke[3] & C.O.S. Savage[4]

[1]Department of Dermatology, Cumberland Infirmary, Carlisle, UK
[2]Department of Dermatology, Wake Forest University School of Medicine, Winston-Salem, NC, USA
[3]Department of Dermatology, South Infirmary–Victoria Hospital, Cork, Ireland
[4]Division of Immunity and Infection, University of Birmingham, UK

Vasculitis

Introduction

Vasculitis is a term applied to inflammation and necrosis of blood vessels, whether they be arteries, veins or both. Vasculitis may be local or systemic, and may be primary or secondary to another disease process. Small vessels (such as capillaries, arterioles and venules), medium-sized vessels (such as visceral vasculature, including renal, coronary or hepatic arteries) and large vessels (the aorta and its great vessels) may be affected. Many vasculitides have a cutaneous component. A dermatologist can provide invaluable assistance in the clinicopathological diagnosis of vasculitis and by guiding patient evaluation and treatment.

Because of the wide range of organ systems affected by vasculitis of blood vessels of various sizes, the clinical presentation of the many vasculitides is varied. However, classic cutaneous manifestations, such as palpable purpura in dependent areas, typically the ankles and lower legs, characterizes smaller vessel involvement, whereas necrotizing livedo reticularis or multiple sites of peripheral gangrene characterize larger vessel vasculitis. It is also important to note that vasculitides may be present without any cutaneous signs or symptoms, especially in the case of cerebral vasculitis.

Infiltration of inflammatory cells with subsequent destruction of blood vessel walls is classically demonstrated in nearly all vasculitides. However, specific histopathological features are dependent on the type and size of the affected blood vessel.

Many vasculitides are triggered by various antigenic agents, such as infection or medication, or are related to underlying disease such as connective tissue, vascular or inflammatory bowel disease, myelodysplastic or other malignancies. However, a single trigger may be associated with several distinct vasculitides, implying that different and more specific mechanisms of inflammation apply in different disorders. Pathogenetic factors in vasculitis are discussed below.

Classification and nomenclature

The classification of vasculitides has been a confusing and debate-provoking topic over the last half century. The first attempt at a

Rook's Textbook of Dermatology, 8th edition. Edited by DA Burns, SM Breathnach, NH Cox and CEM Griffiths. © 2010 Blackwell Publishing Ltd.

Table 50.1 1990 American College of Rheumatology criteria for hypersensitivity vasculitis (traditional format) [5].

1 Age at disease onset >16 years
2 Medication at disease onset
3 Palpable purpura
4 Maculopapular rash
5 Biopsy including arteriole and venule with histological changes showing granulocytes in a perivascular or extravascular location

At least three of the five criteria must be present. The presence of three criteria was associated with a specificity of 83.9% and a sensitivity of 71.0% [5].

classification was by Zeek in 1952 [1]. In her classification of necrotizing vasculitis, she incorporated a clinicopathological evaluation based on the size of the blood vessel involved in the inflammatory process. Zeek differentiated five types of necrotizing angiitis: periarteritis nodosa, hypersensitivity arteritis, rheumatic arteritis, allergic granulomatous angiitis and temporal arteritis [2].

Other factors that may be considered in the classification of vasculitis were discussed by Winkelmann [3]. He incorporated clinical classification, systemic versus cutaneous involvement, muscular vessel versus small vessel disease, and histopathological features in his schema. He also discussed 'laboratory vasculitis', which reviewed the laboratory findings of patients with vasculitis as part of a classification scheme, as well as aetiological factors of various vasculitides [3].

In 1976, James Gilliam [4] proposed a classification of necrotizing vasculitis as part of Medical Grand Rounds at the University of Texas Southwestern Medical Center.

The American College of Rheumatology published classification criteria for vasculitis in 1990 [5]. However, several problems exist with this classification scheme, which is shown in Table 50.1. Particular problems with the criteria include an attempt to codify histological findings of small vessel ('hypersensitivity') vasculitis using 14 biopsy criteria. Furthermore, the use of such terms as 'maculopapular rash', 'medication at onset' and 'eosinophils on biopsy', as well as the separate classification of Henoch–Schönlein purpura, seem inappropriate to most dermatologists.

In 1994, the Chapel Hill Consensus Conference [6] addressed the nomenclature problems relating to primary systemic vasculitides, aiming to create a standardized nomenclature (which is depicted in Table 50.2). This system divided the vasculitides into small, medium and large vessel types, but specifically did not aim to determine clinical criteria for classification or diagnosis of individual patients.

A further attempt to classify vasculitides based on an updated version of Gilliam's 1976 scheme is presented in Table 50.3.

Classifications based on histopathology features are described in [7,8]. Additional classifications have been proposed but have yet to stand the test of time; examples are described in [9–11] and discussed in [12]. Classifications that include, or are based on, serological markers such as antineutrophil cytoplasm antibodies (ANCA) are increasingly important, but the emphasis is often on primary systemic vasculitides and not all suggested classifications translate easily to understanding vasculitis of the skin. Thus, despite numerous attempts over 50 years, the development of a

Table 50.2 Chapel Hill Consensus Conference classification of vasculitis [6].

I   *Large vessel vasculitis*
A   Giant cell arteritis
B   Takayasu's arteritis
II   *Medium-sized vessel vasculitis*
A   Classic polyarteritis nodosa
B   Kawasaki disease
III *Small vessel vasculitis*
A   Wegener's granulomatosis
B   Churg–Strauss syndrome
C   Microscopic polyangiitis (polyarteritis)
D   Henoch–Schönlein purpura
E   Essential cryoglobulinaemia
F   Cutaneous leukocytoclastic vasculitis

Table 50.3 Proposed working classification of vasculitis.

Small vessel vasculitis
Cutaneous small vessel vasculitis—not further classified
Henoch–Schönlein purpura
Essential mixed cryoglobulinaemia (Chapter 49)
Waldenström's hypergammaglobulinaemic purpura (Chapter 49)
Associated with collagen vascular disease (Chapter 51)
Urticarial vasculitis
Erythema elevatum diutinum
Eosinophilic vasculitis
Rheumatoid nodules (Chapter 51)
Reactive leprosy (Chapter 32)
Septic vasculitis

Larger vessel vasculitis
Polyarteritis nodosa
• Microscopic polyarteritis
• Cutaneous form
• Systemic form
Granulomatous vasculitis
• Wegener's granulomatosis
• Allergic granulomatosis of Churg and Strauss
• Lymphomatoid granulomatosis (Chapter 57)
Giant cell arteritis
• Temporal arteritis
• Takayasu's arteritis
Larger vessel vasculitis with collagen vascular disease
Nodular vasculitis

clinically relevant and easy-to-use classification system for vasculitis that incorporates clinical features, vessel size, histopathological and laboratory features, and aetiologies, is a goal that has not yet been fully achieved.

Despite the obstacles, various groups continue to incorporate current knowledge into revised classifications. As an example, the recent consensus criteria for the classification of childhood vasculitides produced by the European League against Rheumatism (EULAR) and the Paediatric Rheumatology European Society (PReS) have deleted the ACR age criterion for diagnosis of HSP, and have added the fact that skin or renal biopsy should show predominant IgA deposition [9] (the criteria state that there must be palpable purpura with at least one of four other criteria—

diffuse abdominal pain, biopsy with predominant IgA deposition, acute arthritis or arthralgia and renal involvement).

The situation is further complicated by a number of disorders that appear to overlap with vasculitis, in that they may, in at least some cases, include vasculitis. A large group of 'neutrophilic dermatoses' come into this category; although we previously considered these as neutrophilic vascular reactions, the accepted spectrum of such disorders has widened, and histological evidence of vasculitis has been reported sufficiently often that, even though it may be a secondary effect, it is appropriate to discuss this group of conditions here (although epidermal neutrophilic dermatoses, such as neutrophilic IgA pemphigus, are discussed elsewhere). Indeed, in the case of Sweet's syndrome, one of the best accepted neutrophilic dermatoses, histological evidence of vasculitis was once considered inconsistent with the diagnosis but has recently been described as being present in 74% of 31 cases studied [13].

Similarly, the more aggressive forms of pityriasis lichenoides have a vasculitic component and are included here.

Between the extremes of pure vasculitis and pure neutrophilic dermatoses or vascular reactions, Behçet's disease may have pustules similar to bowel-associated dermatitis–arthritis syndrome, pathergy similar to pyoderma gangrenosum, and vasculitis of various sizes and types of blood vessel. The vasculitis of Behçet's disease arguably has features that separate it from other vasculitides, the associated aphthous ulceration of mucosae differs from the main vasculitides or neutrophilic dermatoses, and we have therefore discussed this as a separate entity with mixed features between vasculitis and neutrophilic dermatoses.

References

1 Zeek PM. Periarteritis nodosa: a critical review. *Am J Clin Path* 1952; **22**: 777–90.
2 Zeek PM. Periarteritis nodosa and other forms of necrotizing angiitis. *N Engl J Med* 1953; **248**: 764–72.
3 Winkelmann RK. Classification of vasculitis. In: Wolff K, Winkelmann RK, eds. *Vasculitis*. Philadelphia: Saunders, 1980: 322–32.
4 Gilliam JN, Smiley JD. Cutaneous necrotizing vasculitis and related disorders. *Ann Allergy* 1976; **37**: 328–9.
5 Hunder GG, Arend WP, Block DA *et al*. The American College of Rheumatology 1990 Criteria for the Classification of Vasculitis. *Arthritis Rheum* 1990; **33**: 1065–136.
6 Jennette JC, Falk RG, Andrassy K *et al*. Nomenclature of systemic vasculitides: proposal of an international consensus conference. *Arthritis Rheum* 1994; **37**: 187–92.
7 Carlson JA, Chen K-R. Cutaneous vasculitis update: small vessel neutrophilic vasculitis syndromes. *Am J Dermatopathol* 2006; **28**: 486–506.
8 Carlson JA, Chen K-R. Cutaneous vasculitis update: neutrophilic muscular vessel and eosinophilic, granulomatous, and lymphocytic vasculitis syndromes. *Am J Dermatopathol* 2007; **29**: 32–43.
9 Ozen S, Ruperto N, Dillon MJ *et al*. EULAR/PReS endorsed consensus criteria for the classification of childhood vasculitides. *Ann Rheum Dis* 2006; **65**: 936–41.
10 Watts R, Lane S, Hanslik T *et al*. Development and validation of a consensus methodology for the classification of the ANCA-associated vasculitides and polyarteritis nodosa for epidemiological studies. *Ann Rheum Dis* 2006; **66**: 222–7.
11 Hogan SL, Falk RJ, Nachman PH, Jennette JC. Various forms of life in antineutrophil cytoplasmic antibody-associated vasculitis. *Ann Intern Med* 2006; **144**: 377–8.
12 Jenette JC, Falk RJ. Nosology of primary vasculitis. *Curr Opin Rheumatol* 2007; **19**: 10–16.
13 Ratzinger G, Burgdorf W, Zelger BG, Zelger B. Acute febrile neutrophilic dermatosis: a histopathologic study of 31 cases with review of literature. *Am J Dermatopathol* 2007; **29**: 125–33.

Pathogenesis of vasculitis

The pathogenesis of vasculitis is a complex subject, not least because there are likely to be many different pathogeneses reflecting the many different causes and pathological entities. This brief overview describes some of the major mechanisms and systems involved, with emphasis on those that have clinical importance (such as the diagnostic potential of ANCA). More detailed recent reviews can be consulted [1–9]; factors pertaining to specific vasculitides are summarized, with more specific references, in the relevant sections discussing specific types of vasculitis.

Histopathologically, cutaneous necrotizing vasculitis may be leukocytoclastic with a neutrophilic infiltrate and a presumed immune complex pathogenesis, or may be lymphomonocytic and pauci-immune; however, this is not always helpful diagnostically as the change from the former to the latter occurs as part of a dynamic sequence, leukocytoclastic vasculitis generating a secondary cell-mediated immune response. Factors that play a part in the pathogenesis of vasculitis include antigen–antibody related mechanisms (including autoantibodies and immune complex diseases), inflammatory cells and their lysosomal content, complement, cytokines, chemokines, adhesion molecules, vascular and cellular growth factors, genetic influences, pro-coagulant factors and the fibrinolytic system, as well as direct vessel wall damage (e.g. by some infectious organisms). Local blood flow influences the development of the vasculitis lesion, as evidenced by lesions occurring at areas of constriction by tight clothing, and local release of histamine also has a role. It is apparent that none of these factors operates in isolation—for example, endothelial damage will cause expression of cell-surface adhesion molecules, production of cytokines and influx of pro-inflammatory cells—so there is inevitably some overlap between the following sections, which address some of the more important and better documented factors involved in vasculitic inflammation.

References

1 Ball GV, Bridges SL. Pathogenesis of vasculitis. In: Ball GV, Bridges SL, eds. *Vasculitis*. Oxford: Oxford University Press, 2002: 34–52.
2 Piette WW. Primary systemic vasculitis. In: Sontheimer RD, Provost TT, eds. *Cutaneous Manifestations of Rheumatic Diseases*. Baltimore: Williams & Wilkins, 1995: 177–232.
3 Kallenberg CGM. Laboratory findings in the vasculitides. *Baillières Clin Rheumatol* 1997; **11**: 395–421.
4 Nowack R, Flores-Suárez LF, van der Woude FJ. New developments in pathogenesis of systemic vasculitis. *Curr Opin Rheumatol* 1998; **10**: 3–11.
5 Savage COS. The evolving pathogenesis of systemic vasculitis. *Clin Med* 2002; **2**: 458–64.
6 Lotti T, Ghersetich I, Comacchi C, Jorizzo JL. Cutaneous small-vessel vasculitis. *J Am Acad Dermatol* 1998; **39**: 667–87.
7 Klippel JH, Dieppe PA. *Rheumatology*, 2nd edn. London: Mosby, 1998: 7.19.1–8.
8 Sneller MC, Fauci AS. Pathogenesis of vasculitis syndromes. *Med Clin N Am* 1997; **81**: 221–42.
9 Jenette JC, Falk RJ. New insight into the pathogenesis of vasculitis associated with antineutrophil cytoplasmic antibodies. *Curr Opin Rheumatol* 2008; **20**: 55–60.

Table 50.4 Theory of pathogenesis of cutaneous small vessel vasculitis. (Modified from [4].)

- Immune complexes interact with the complement system to generate C3a and C5a anaphylatoxins, which stimulate:
  production of chemotactic factors which initiate chemotaxis of neutrophils
  release of vasoactive amines (such as histamine), which cause endothelial cell retraction
  release of proinflammatory cytokines (e.g. IL-1, TNF-α) which induce the expression of adhesion molecules (ICAM-1, VCAM-1, P- and E-selectin) in endothelial cells
  adhesion molecules (ICAM-1, VCAM-1, P- and E-selectin) in endothelial cells
- Activation of the membrane attack complex of complement directly damages membrane integrity of endothelial cells
- Immune complexes deposit in vascular walls after histamine-induced endothelial retraction which increases selectin expression in endothelial cells
- Attracted neutrophils produce lysosomal enzymes in an attempt to engulf deposited immune complexes
- Neutrophils are activated through Fc binding and degranulate, and also produce reactive oxygen species
- Ultimate inflammation and 'bystander' fibrinoid necrosis of blood vessel wall

---

Antigens, immune complexes and complement

Antigenic triggers of immunological responses targeted at components of blood vessel walls elicit most vasculitides. The importance of circulating immune complexes has long been recognized in studies of serum sickness [1], and the deposition of immune complexes in blood vessel walls is the best characterized mechanism for the vascular injury associated with vasculitis [2]. This mechanism appears to be particularly important in leukocytoclastic necrotizing cutaneous small vessel vasculitis; potential antigens of relevance include bacteria, viruses, drugs and other chemicals. Most evidence for an immune complex-mediated pathogenesis is circumstantial (e.g. the demonstration of immunoglobulins in skin lesions) and is better documented for cutaneous small vessel vasculitis than for systemic vasculitides. It is generally accepted that immune complexes have a role in Henoch–Schönlein purpura (HSP), serum sickness, hepatitis B and C virus-induced vasculitis, urticarial vasculitis and cryoglobulinaemic vasculitis.

A theory about the pathogenesis of cutaneous small vessel vasculitis is described below and depicted in Table 50.4 [3,4]. The circulating immune complexes mediating vasculitis interact with the complement system to generate C3a and C5a anaphylatoxins which degranulate mast cells. They stimulate the production of chemotactic factors and subsequent chemotaxis, the release of vasoactive amines (such as histamine) and the release of proinflammatory cytokines which induce the subsequent expression of adhesion molecules. Circulating immune complexes may also be bound by myelomonocytic cells (via the Fcγ receptor) and by endothelial cells (via FcγRIIa (CD32)) [5]. Immune complexes with a sedimentation coefficient greater than 19S are deposited in vessel walls, a process that is strongly influenced by platelet-derived vasoactive amines. Endothelial cell retraction and detachment occur due to altered membrane integrity that is induced by vasoactive amines and probably by the membrane attack complex of complement [6]. Secreted cytokines, including interleukin-1

(IL-1), gamma-interferon (IFN-γ) and tumour necrosis factor-alpha (TNF-α), cause increased expression of adhesion molecules (ICAM-1, E-selectin and VCAM-1) and HLA-DR (the 'adhesion cascade') by endothelial cells, which recruit neutrophils [5]. The CD40 ligand, which is structurally similar to TNF-α and which is present on stimulated CD4+ T cells, mast cells and platelets, may also activate secretion of cytokines and expression of adhesion molecules by endothelial cells. Neutrophils that are attracted to the site of immune complex deposition are activated *in situ* through binding of the fragment crystallizable (Fc) portion of the antibody, and release lysosomal enzymes in a teleological attempt to engulf the deposited immune complexes. This causes degranulation and destruction of the neutrophils (visible histologically as leukocytoclasis) with release of collagenase and elastase, and generation of reactive oxygen species, ultimately resulting in inflammation and 'bystander' fibrinoid necrosis of vessel walls. It is of practical importance to appreciate that neutrophils degrade immune complexes within 24–48 h after they are deposited [7], usually within 24 h; hence, direct immunofluorescence of vasculitis lesions older than 3–12 h will generally yield negative results [3,8]. Eosinophils are also attracted in some situations, and also contain cytotoxic lysosomal enzymes. Survival of neutrophils or eosinophils at sites of inflammation may be aided by the antiapoptotic effect of colony stimulating factors (this is discussed with relation to TNF-related apoptosis-induced ligand-3 (TRAIL3) and death receptors in the section on Churg–Strauss syndrome).

Immune complexes may also activate endothelial cells to produce tissue plasminogen activator (t-PA) and thus alter local fibrinolysis and vascular permeability [3]. There are therefore many complex and dynamic changes that occur.

Paraneoplastic vasculitis is thought to be caused by tumour antigens stimulating cell-mediated immunity or forming tumour antigen immune complexes, although direct vessel wall damage or occlusion can occur as a result of emboli. Haematological malignancies are the most common to be associated with vasculitis [9].

Antiphospholipid antibodies are important as a cause of microvascular thrombosis (Chapter 49). However, they also bind to endothelial cells and have numerous effects; they are proinflammatory, induce monocyte activation, stimulate cytokine and vascular adhesion factor expression, and result in a thrombophilic state [10]. In autoimmune conditions, binding requires plasma β2glycoprotein-I (β2-GP-I), which itself binds to endothelial cells and complexes with phospholipids.

Superantigens have also been implicated in development of vasculitis; this is discussed in more detail in the next section.

Complement activation leads to the adherence of C3b to immune complexes, such that they remain soluble and are cleared by macrophages. Immune complexes that have bound C3b also bind to erythrocytes via the complement receptor type 1 (CR1), about 90–95% of which is located on the surface of erythrocytes, leading to clearance of immune complexes from the reticuloendothelial system and preventing interaction with endothelial cells and other structures. Complement deposition is documented in skin lesions (e.g. in HSP) and genetic deficiency of complement is associated with immune complex diseases. However, IgA immune complexes in patients with HSP do not appear to activate the classical complement pathway, although activation of the alternative pathway by IgA1 (the main IgA subclass in HSP) may allow complexes to be made soluble.

References
1 Lawley TJ, Bielory L, Gascon P et al. Prospective clinical and immunologic analysis of patients with serum sickness. N Engl J Med 1984; **311**: 1407–13.
2 Dixon FJ, Cochrane CG. The pathogenicity of antigen–antibody complexes. Pathol Annu 1970; **5**: 355–79.
3 Lotti T, Ghersetich I, Comacchi C, Jorizzo JL. Cutaneous small-vessel vasculitis. J Am Acad Dermatol 1998; **39**: 667–87.
4 Klippel JH, Dieppe PA. Rheumatology, 2nd edn. London: Mosby, 1998: 7.19.1–8.
5 Witort-Serraglini E, del Rosso M, Lotti TM, Matucci-Cerinic M. Endothelial injury in vasculitides. Clin Dermatol 1999; **17**: 587–90.
6 Kawana S. The membrane attack complex of complement alters the membrane integrity of cultured endothelial cells: a possible pathophysiology for immune complex vasculitis. Acta Derm Venereol (Stockh) 1996; **76**: 13–6.
7 Cochrane CG, Weigle WO, Dixon FJ. The role of polymorphonuclear leukocytes in the initiation and cessation of the Arthus vasculitis. J Exp Med 1959; **110**: 481–94.
8 Yancey KB, Lawley TJ. Circulating immune complexes: their immunochemistry, biology and detection in selected dermatologic and systemic diseases. J Am Acad Dermatol 1984; **10**: 711–31.
9 Paydas S, Zorludemir S, Sabin B. Vasculitis and leukaemia. Leuk Lymphoma 2000; **40**: 105–12.
10 Meroni PL, Raschi E, Testoni C et al. Antiphospholipid antibodies and the endothelium. Rheum Dis Clin North Am 2001; **27**: 587–602.

The role of infections [1–4]

Infections appear to provoke some vasculitides, particularly those relevant to dermatologists; the role of specific infections and the strength of such associations is discussed in sections relating to specific entities such as Henoch–Schönlein purpura (HSP) (in which a role for infective triggers is well documented) and large vessel vasculitides. Vaccinations have also been implicated in some vasculitides, notably acute haemorrhagic oedema of childhood and occasionally in cutaneous small vessel vasculitis. Conditions that mimic vasculitis, such as bacterial or fungal emboli, are not discussed here other than in terms of their potential to damage vessels. This section discusses mechanisms by which infections may be involved in pathogenesis of vasculitis, some of which may apply to other causes as well. There is evidence in most of the 'primary' vasculitides that at least some cases can be linked to one or another form of action of infective organisms [3]; the problems are that studies have produced conflicting evidence, that more than one infection may be linked with any particular pattern of vasculitis, and that the pathogenetic mechanisms have often not been elucidated. Several potential mechanisms, one or more of which may apply in some situations, have been proposed, as below. It must be stressed that this attempt to explain possible mechanisms is probably over-simplistic as they may not occur in isolation—for example, immune complexes may be formed in relation to an antigenic component of a circulating organism, to exposed antigens of an organism that has become intracellular, or to self antigens exposed by cellular infection. Equally, activation of cytokines may be a response to pathogens themselves, or be triggered by cellular damage consequent to an infection. Pathogens themselves may provoke a variety of different responses—for example, cytomegalovirus (a major cause of vascular morbidity in immunosuppressed individuals) infects and damages endothelial cells, causes ischaemia and thrombosis, and expresses antigens that may stimulate an immune response [5]. Thus, one or more of the following may occur as a result of infection:

1 Immune complex reactions (Gell and Coombs type 3 reaction): this has been discussed above as a major mechanism in vasculitis, due to several triggers (e.g. drugs) as well as in response to infections. Immune complexes may be formed between antibodies and an entire organism or specific antigenic components, and may become trapped in vessels, stimulating a cascade of reactions as described above. The pustular vasculitis of gonococcal infection and much of the vasculitis in subacute bacterial endocarditis probably occur due to immune complex formation, and circulating or tissue deposits of immune complexes have been found in hepatitis B, hepatitis C and human immunodeficiency virus (HIV) infections. Immune complexes related to infectious agents may be formed in the circulation or in situ in infected vascular cells.

2 Direct activation of complement by infectious organisms: as well as activating the classical complement pathway via formation of immune complexes, some microbial products directly activate the alternative pathway of complement. These include polysaccharides (e.g. from Candida spp.) as well as various parts of both Gram-positive and Gram-negative bacteria [1].

3 Direct activation of other pro-inflammatory mechanisms: bacterial lipopolysaccharides, as well as heat shock proteins from several organisms, induce tumour necrosis factor-alpha (TNF-α) production by macrophages, which in turn stimulates vascular endothelial cells to express cell adhesion molecules. Lipopolysaccharides and heat shock proteins also stimulate production of interleukins IL-1 and IL-6 from endothelial cells, and may directly stimulate secretion of matrix metalloproteinases.

4 Molecular mimicry hypothesis: if endothelial cells or other cells comprising vessel walls share epitopes with an infective organism, then humoral and cell-mediated responses to infection will also target the host cells that carry the same epitope. There is some evidence for this mechanism in, for example, renal involvement in HSP; group A β-haemolytic streptococci are implicated as a trigger in about a third of affected subjects, and renal glomerular vessels express nephritis-associated plasmin receptor (NAPlr) which is a streptococcal antigen [6]. Heat shock proteins, which are expressed by endothelial cells following stress, and which have considerable homology with some antigens of infective organisms, have been implicated in such a process but this is not a proven mechanism of autoimmunity in humans.

5 Superantigen hypothesis: superantigens directly activate T cells, without the need for antigen-presenting cells, by interaction with Vβ segments of the T cell receptor (TCR); they may also stimulate B cells. Analysis of Vβ sequences of the TCR of circulating T cells, or the V_H repertoire of B cells in lesional biopsies can be used to demonstrate patterns consistent with superantigen-induced proliferation. A role for superantigens of Staphylococcus aureus is a factor in atopic dermatitis (Chapter 24); in the vasculitides, most evidence for a role of staphylococcal superantigens has been documented in Kawasaki disease and in Wegener's granulomatosis (WG) [3]. In Kawasaki disease,

strains of *S. aureus* expressing the toxic shock syndrome toxin-1 (TSST-1) antigen have been implicated in causation. In WG, the evidence for a role of staphylococcal superantigens in disease perpetuation is better than for disease causation (and is supported by benefit from prophylactic treatment with cotrimoxazole). However, other infections have also been linked with both of these conditions [3], such as New Haven coronavirus in Kawasaki disease, so this hypothesis may not be the only pathogenetic factor.

6 Direct non-specific vessel wall or perivascular invasion and damage (also termed the bystander activation hypothesis), especially by vasculotropic viruses such as cytomegalovirus and human herpes-virus HHV-6; this causes both direct and indirect mechanisms of damage:

   i Direct damage: the infection may cause endothelial cell dysfunction, as well as generating cytokines and chemoattractants that augment the initial damage and attract proinflammatory cells that further extend the damage. Infected endothelial cells may express cell wall molecules that make them more procoagulant, more prone to oxidative damage, more able to bind inflammatory cells and less able to vasodilate. Infection may also alter other cells of the vessel wall, as discussed below.

   ii Indirect damage: it has been suggested that an additional effect of damage to the vascular cells is that it exposes sequestered autoantigens, thereby generating an autoimmune response. Additionally, some infections, via increased production of TNF-α and IL-1, may cause upregulation of cell surface expression of proteinase 3 (PR3) and myeloperoxidase (MPO) on endothelial cells and inflammatory cells. These proteins are the main targets for antineutrophil cytoplasm antibodies (ANCA), which, when bound to the PR3 or MPO, produce degranulation of neutrophils and a sequence of ongoing vascular damage and cytokine production. ANCA are discussed further below.

7 Altered self hypothesis: in this hypothesis the infective organism interacts directly with vessel proteins to create neo-antigens that in turn will activate the immune system.

8 Alterations of vessel wall components: various organisms may produce an increase in smooth muscle cells of the vessel walls, both by stimulation of the proliferation and migration of these cells and by inhibiting normal apoptosis [4]. Such processes may be important in medium and large vessel vasculitides.

9 Autoantigen complementarity hypothesis: this hypothesis has particularly been proposed in relation to ANCA-associated vasculitides [3,7]. In this hypothesis, the proposed immunogens are 'complementary' to parts of the PR3 and MPO ANCA autoantigens, that is are homologous with the amino acid sequence of the antisense RNA of the non-coding strand of the ANCA autoantigen gene. Such proteins could induce production of antibodies which react with the autoantigen. In support of this, many microbial and fungal proteins have sequences that show homology with the protein product of the middle portion of the antisense RNA of PR3. Thus, these infective agents could trigger production of ANCA-associated vasculitis.

Specific infections that have been implicated in individual vasculitis patterns or syndromes are discussed where appropriate

in the relevant disease sections later, and a list of infections that have been documented as causes of vasculitis is provided on p. 50.55.

References
1 Millikan LE, Flynn TC. Infectious etiologies of cutaneous vasculitis. *Clin Dermatol* 1999; **17**: 509–14.
2 Mandell BF, Calabrese LH. Infections and systemic vasculitis. *Curr Opin Rheumatol* 1998; **10**: 51–7.
3 Rodríguez-Pla A, Stone JH. Vasculitis and systemic infections. *Curr Opin Rheumatol* 2006; **18**: 39–47.
4 Yang Y-H, Chuang Y-H, Wang L-C *et al*. The immunobiology of Henoch–Schönlein purpura. *Autoimm Rev* 2008; **7**: 179–84.
5 Golden MP, Hammer SM, Wanke CA, Albrecht MA. Cytomegalovirus vasculitis. *Medicine (Baltimore)* 1994; **73**: 246–55.
6 Masuda M, Nakanishi K, Yoshizawa N *et al*. Group A streptococcal antigen in the glomeruli of children with Henoch-Schönlein nephritis. *Am J Kidney Dis* 2003; **41**: 366–70.
7 Pendergraft WF III, Pressler BM, Jenette JC *et al*. Autoantigen complementarity: a new theory implicating complementary proteins as initiators of autoimmune disease. *J Mol Med* 2005; **83**: 12–25.

Effector cells: T lymphocytes and polymorphonuclear leukocytes

T lymphocytes are found in the inflammatory infiltrate in all vasculitis. In some types of vasculitis, lymphocytes and monocytes appear to be predominant, but this may also relate to the stage at which a biopsy is taken, many vasculitides characterized by neutrophils developing an increase in the proportion of mononuclears with the passage of time. $CD4^+$ T helper (T_H) cells secrete cytokines, notably IL-1, INF-γ and TNF-α, and cause recruitment of $CD8^+$ (cytotoxic) T cells, B cells and natural killer (NK) cells. The cytokines produced not only induce expression of major histocompatibility MHC 1 antigens, which can be presented to $CD8^+$ cells, but also upregulate expression of adhesion molecules by endothelial cells.

A role for γ/δ T lymphocytes ($CD3^+$, $CD4^-$, $CD8^-$) has been proposed in vasculitis. These cells are cytotoxic against various cells but also exhibit some T_H functions; they secrete many cytokines, including interleukins IL-2 and IL-4, granulocyte–monocyte colony stimulating factor (GMCSF) and INF-γ. They are thought to recognize portions of the major histocompatibility complex and peptide antigens within these structures, without the full antigen processing that is required to cause proliferation of α/β T cells, and also recognize human heat shock proteins, notably HSP65. They are found in significant numbers in the later stages of leukocytoclastic vasculitis, and are especially associated with infective causes of vasculitis [1,2].

A population of T lymphocytes that express CXCL8 appear to be important in chemoattraction of neutrophils in Behçet's disease and in pustular drug eruptions; their role in leukocytoclastic vasculitis and neutrophilic dermatoses is less certain [3].

Neutrophils and eosinophils are the predominant cells in many vasculitides, including most that are related to infections, drugs, foods, collagen vascular diseases, type II or III cryoglobulins, IgA-mediated, and many others [4,5]. They are recruited in response to infection; the other main pathogenetic processes that attract them to the skin have been summarized as vasculitis, antibody and complement, mast cell release and T-cell-mediated neutrophil activation [6]. Neutrophil adhesion mainly occurs in small vessels, in a process that is induced by several factors, including stimulation by TNF-α or ANCA (MPO-ANCA being more potent than PR3-ANCA), although ANCA also accelerate polymorphonuclear cell apoptosis. The role of immune complexes has been discussed, but is still not fully understood. The interaction between ANCA, their antigens, and endothelial cells, in binding polymorphonuclear cells is discussed later, as ANCA play an important role in leukocyte–endothelial interaction. Binding and activation of neutrophils or eosinophils causes release of toxic enzymes and generation of reactive oxygen species, leading to tissue damage. This process seems to require the presence of CD18, as injected polymorphonuclear cells in CD18-deficient mice will gather around perivascular immune complexes but without causing vessel damage [7]. Interestingly, several single nucleotide polymorphisms (SNP) have been associated with MPO–ANCA+ vasculitis [8]. This suggests that some CD18 polymorphisms may facilitate polymorphonuclear cell adhesion, degranulation and respiratory burst, predisposing to vasculitis.

The mechanism by which leukocytoclasis occurs in vasculitis is also not fully understood; it also occurs in neutrophilic dermatoses in which vasculitis is an inconstant feature. The usual expectation would be for late apoptotic polymorphonuclear cells to be phagocytosed by macrophages; electron microscopy immuno-gold methods in anaphylactoid purpura have demonstrated that apoptotic polymorphonuclear cell removal may be incomplete, many polymorphonuclear cells in fully developed leukocytoclastic vasculitis having relatively intact nuclei but disintegration of plasma organelles and cell membrane [9]. One explanation for this relates to the prototypical tissue pentraxin PTX3, which inhibits the anticipated phagocytosis of late-stage apoptotic polymorphonuclear cells by macrophages. This has been demonstrated to be upregulated at sites of leukocytoclastic vasculitis infiltrates, with levels paralleling vasculitis activity; it may therefore permit accumulation of leukocytoclastic debris by inhibition of phagocytosis [10].

References

1 Lotti T, Ghersetich I, Comacchi C, Jorizzo JL. Cutaneous small-vessel vasculitis. *J Am Acad Dermatol* 1998; **39**: 667–87.

2 Comacchi C, Ghersetich I, Katsambas A, Lotti TM. γ/δ T lymphocytes and infection: pathogenesis of cutaneous necrotizing vasculitis. *Clin Dermatol* 1999; **17**: 603–7.

3 Keller M, Spanou Z, Schaerli P *et al*. T cell-regulated neutrophilic inflammation in autoinflammatory diseases. *J Immunol* 2005; **175**: 7678–86.

4 Magro CM, Crowson NA. The cutaneous neutrophilic vascular injury syndromes: a review. *Semin Diag Pathol* 2001; **18**: 47–58.

5 Carlson JA, Chen K-R. Cutaneous vasculitis update: small vessel neutrophilic vasculitis syndromes. *Am J Dermatopathol* 2006; **28**: 486–506.

6 von den Driesch P. Polymorphonuclears: structure, function and mechanisms of involvement in skin diseases. *Clin Dermatol* 2000; **18**: 233–44.

7 Sindrilaru A, Seeliger S, Ehrchen JM *et al*. Site of blood vessel damage and relevance of CD18 in a murine model of immune complex-mediated vasculitis. *J Invest Dermatol* 2006; **127**: 447–54.

8 Meller S, Jagiello P, Borgmann S *et al*. Novel SNPs in the CD18 gene validate the association with MPO–ANCA+ vasculitis. *Genes Immun* 2001; **2**: 269–72.

9 Yamamoto T, Kaburagi T, Izaki S *et al*. Leukocytoclasis: ultrastructural in situ nick end labeling study in anaphylactoid purpura. *J Dermatol Sci* 2000; **24**: 158–65.

10 van Rossum AP, Pas HH, Fazzini F *et al*. Abundance of the long pentraxin PTX3 at sites of leukocytoclastic lesions in patients with small-vessel vasculitis. *Arthritis Rheum* 2006; **54**: 986–91.

Antiendothelial cell antibodies and endothelial cell dysfunction in vessel wall injury

Antiendothelial cell antibodies (AECA) are of uncertain importance in the pathogenesis of vasculitis [1–4]. They can be identified at high titre in most patients with Takayasu's arteritis or with active thromboangiitis obliterans, and are variably demonstrated in patients with Wegener's granulomatosis (WG), microscopic polyangiitis, Kawasaki disease, hepatitis B-associated polyarteritis nodosa, Henoch–Schönlein purpura, Behçet's disease and systemic lupus erythematosus (SLE)-associated vasculitis. They are also found in several other connective tissue diseases and in haemolytic uraemic syndrome/thrombotic thrombocytopenic purpura, IgA nephropathy, ulcerative colitis and diabetes mellitus, as well as in some normal individuals. Some studies correlate their titre with disease activity in medium or large vessel arteritis, but whether this reflects a pathogenic role or vascular damage is unclear. The fact that they bind preferentially to endothelium of mesenteric vessels supports the possibility of a pathogenetic role in visceral arteritis [5].

Mechanisms by which AECA might have a pathogenetic role in vasculitis include those listed below [4], although it should be acknowledged that no target antigens of AECA are specifically expressed by endothelial cells, and also that endothelial cell-specific target antigens of AECA remain unidentified in systemic vasculitides [4]:

1 Direct activation, or indirect induction of activation, of endothelial cells: activation of endothelial cells leads to up-regulation of adhesion molecules such as intercellular adhesion molecule-1 (ICAM-1), vascular cell adhesion molecule-1 (VCAM-1) and E-selectin [6,7]; this may be mediated by nuclear factor (NF)-κB [8]. Increased neutrophil cytotoxicity results. E-selectin is a promoter of endothelial cell activation and of leukocyte–endothelial cell interaction, being expressed on cytokine-activated endothelial cells, and might therefore have an active role in the pathogenesis of vasculitis; however, E-selectin levels in a variety of systemic vasculitides do not correlate with disease activity [9]. Identification of AECA with specificity for α-enolase, expressed by endothelial cells, and the possibility of this having an infectious trigger, is discussed in the section on pathogenesis of Behçet's disease. More recently, it has been shown that AECA upregulated expression of two inflammatory molecules, vascular adhesion protein-1 (VAP-1) and MHC class I-related antigen A (MICA) on renal endothelial cells in Wegener's granulomatosis, in turn leading to phosphorylation of stress activated protein kinase (SAPK)/c-Jun N-terminal kinase (JNK), activation of NFκB, and production of the chemoattractant cytokines monocyte chemoattractant protein-1 and granulocyte chemotactic protein-2; blocking SAPK/JNK significantly reduced the chemokine production and decreased expression of MICA, confirming that AECA have a role in generating pro-inflammatory endothelial cell responses [10].

2 Cytotoxicity, which may be direct, complement-dependent or indirect due to complement-independent antibody-dependent cytotoxicity: such cytotoxicity has been demonstrated in mice immunized with purified IgG AECA from a patient with Wegener's granulomatosis, and which subsequently developed

endogenous AECA with renal and pulmonary lymphoid infiltrates [11].

3 Induction of coagulation: von Willebrand factor, factor VIII and soluble thrombomodulin levels may all be increased in vasculitis, possibly due to AECA, although other evidence suggests that these changes are probably a secondary effect resulting from vascular damage. Soluble thrombomodulin levels have been shown to be related to disease activity in WG [9], although this is also increased in disseminated intravascular coagulopathy, thrombotic thrombocytopenic purpura, sepsis, malaria, diabetic microangiopathy and various other disorders in which there is damage to vessels.

4 Induction of apoptosis, for example by binding of phospholipids or of heat shock protein 60.

Several cytokines that may be involved in vasculitis are discussed later. Some cytokine events that are related to the interaction of endothelial cells and AECA have also been discussed above. Again, many of these effects are probably non-specific. For example, high levels of soluble VCAM-1 are found in Kawasaki disease but were even higher in febrile controls [6], and this finding is therefore presumably also a non-specific result of vascular injury. Similarly, nitric oxide production is also increased in some vasculitides but is not specific to an individual vasculitis syndrome; neutrophil-derived nitric oxide is known to be damaging to endothelial cells [12] (see above for a discussion of neutrophils).

Endothelial cell dysfunction has been recognized as a common event and active contributor in systemic vasculitis and connective tissue disease-associated vasculitis, rather than purely occurring as an uninvolved consequence of injury [13]. Endothelial cell dysfunction occurs at sites distant from active vasculitis in several primary small and medium vasculitides, independent of ANCA status or renal involvement (itself a cause of endothelial cell dysfunction), and with improvement correlating with disease suppression in some instances [13]. In Kawasaki disease, impaired endothelial cell function appears to persist for years after the clinical disease, with impaired fibrinolytic activity, and abnormal coronary blood flow, unrelated to the presence or absence of early-stage coronary artery aneurysms, after cold pressor testing [14]. Although this abnormality is prolonged in nature, it can be reversed by ascorbate. Circulating endothelial cell microparticles that can cause endothelial cell injury and apoptosis have been demonstrated in Kawasaki disease, as well as in some primary vasculitides, correlating with other markers of disease activity, and supporting a role of endothelial cell damage in the pathogenesis of these disorders [15]. Endothelial cell dysfunction has been related to either depressed release, or increased breakdown, of nitric oxide; polymorphisms of endothelial nitric oxide synthase (eNOS) have been related to risk of giant cell arteritis and Behçet's disease (discussed further in the section on Behçet's disease).

References

1 Ball GV, Bridges SL. Pathogenesis of vasculitis. In: Ball GV, Bridges SL, eds. *Vasculitis*. Oxford: Oxford University Press, 2002: 34–52.
2 Piette WW. Primary systemic vasculitis. In: Sontheimer RD, Provost TT, eds. *Cutaneous Manifestations of Rheumatic Diseases*. Baltimore: Williams & Wilkins, 1995: 177–232.
3 Goeken JA. Antineutrophil cytoplasmic and antiendothelial cell antibodies: new mechanisms for vasculitis. *Curr Opin Dermatol* 1995; **2**: 75–82.
4 Guilpain P, Mouthon L. Antiendothelial cell antibodies in vasculitis-associated systemic diseases. *Clin Rev Allergy Immunol* 2008; **35**: 59–65.
5 Brasile L, Kremer JM, Clarke JL, Cerilli J. Identification of an autoantibody to vascular endothelial cell-specific antigens in patients with systemic vasculitis. *Am J Med* 1989; **87**: 74–80.
6 Kallenberg CGM. Laboratory findings in the vasculitides. *Baillières Clin Rheumatol* 1997; **11**: 395–421.
7 Carvalho D, Savage CO, Isenberg D, Pearson JD. IgG anti-endothelial cell autoantibodies from patients with systemic lupus erythematosus or systemic vasculitis stimulate the release of two endothelial cell-derived mediators, which enhance adhesion molecule expression and leukocyte adhesion in an autocrine fashion. *Arthritis Rheum* 1999; **42**: 631–40.
8 Blank M, Krause I, Goldkorn T et al. Monoclonal anti-endothelial cell antibodies from a patient with Takayasu arteritis activate endothelial cells from large vessels. *Arthritis Rheum* 1999; **42**: 1421–32.
9 Boehme MWJ, Schmitt WH, Youinou P et al. Clinical relevance of elevated serum thrombomodulin and soluble E-selectin in patients with Wegener's granulomatosis and other systemic vasculitides. *Am J Med* 1996; **101**: 387–94.
10 Holmén C, Elsheikh E, Christensson M et al. Anti-endothelial cell autoantibodies selectively activate SAPK/JNK signaling in Wegener's granulomatosis. *J Am Soc Nephrol* 2007; **18**: 2424–6.
11 Davianovich M, Gilburd B, George J et al. Pathogenic role of antiendothelial cell antibodies in vasculitis: an idiotypic experimental model. *J Immunol* 1996; **156**: 4946–51.
12 Bratt J, Palmblad J. Cytokine-induced neutrophil-mediated injury of human endothelial cells. *J Immunol* 1997; **159**: 912–8.
13 Bacon PA. Endothelial cell dysfunction in systemic vasculitis: new developments and therapeutic prospects. *Curr Opin Rheumatol* 2004; **17**: 49–55.
14 Furuyama H, Odagawa Y, Katoh C et al. Altered myocardial flow reserve and endothelial function late after Kawasaki disease. *J Pediatr* 2003; **142**: 149–52.
15 Brogan PA, Shah V, Brachet C et al. Endothelial and platelet microparticles in vasculitis of the young. *Arthritis Rheum* 2004; **50**: 927–36.

Antineutrophil cytoplasm antibodies

In comparison with other pathogenetic factors, many of which are either not routinely measurable or are of uncertain relevance to pathogenesis, antineutrophil cytoplasm antibodies (ANCA) have diagnostic value as well as an important role in the pathogenesis of vasculitis [1–13].

ANCA are classified, according to their indirect immunofluorescence (IIF) pattern on ethanol-fixed neutrophils, into C-ANCA (granular cytoplasmic staining with accentuation between the nuclear lobes), P-ANCA (perinuclear and/or nuclear staining) and atypical ANCA (various patterns, including diffuse cytoplasmic and 'very perinuclear'; atypical ANCA are also termed X-ANCA, snowdrift-ANCA or more recently a-ANCA) [3,7,9]. These patterns correlate with varying degrees of specificity to specific neutrophil granule contents (Table 50.5). ANCA are usually of IgG type but may be IgM or IgA. In addition to systemic vasculitides, ANCA may be positive in various infections (malaria, human immunodeficiency virus infection; HIV), connective tissue disorders (SLE, rheumatoid arthritis) and gastrointestinal diseases (inflammatory bowel disease, chronic autoimmune liver and biliary tract disease), as well as occasionally in some apparently healthy individuals.

In most disorders other than vasculitides, the types of ANCA identified are of P-ANCA or atypical ANCA type, and in most of these disorders there is no consistent ANCA specificity or correlation with disease activity. However, there are some exceptions, such as the association of cathepsin G-ANCA with malaria [14].

Table 50.5 Antigenic specificity and clinical correlates of antineutrophil cytoplasm antibodies.

Antigen	Usual ANCA pattern on IIF	Most commonly associated diseases
PR3	C-ANCA	WG, MPA, CSS, necrotizing and crescentic GN
MPO	P-ANCA	Idiopathic progressive GN, MPA, CSS, WG, SLE, ANCA-positive drug-induced systemic vasculitis, thromboangiitis obliterans
Cathepsin G	P-ANCA	IBD, especially ulcerative colitis, PSC, malaria
BPI (= CAP 57)	C-ANCA	Systemic vasculitis, SLE, IBD, PSC, cystic fibrosis, chronic airway infections, other chronic infections
Azurocidin (= CAP 37)	P-ANCA or C-ANCA	Systemic vasculitis, drug-induced systemic vasculitis
Lactoferrin	P-ANCA or atypical ANCA	Rheumatoid arthritis, SLE especially with serositis or livedo reticularis, systemic vasculitis, ulcerative colitis, PSC, hydralazine-related vasculitis, thromboangiitis obliterans
HLE	P-ANCA	WG, propylthiouracil-related systemic vasculitis, some other drug-induced vasculitides, HIV infection
β-glucuronidase	P-ANCA	IBD
Lysozyme	P-ANCA	SLE, IBD, HIV infection
h-lamp-2	P-ANCA	Necrotizing and crescentic GN, pyoderma gangrenosum
Others: actin, catalase, α-enolase, high mobility group protein	Anti-actin is C-ANCA, others P-ANCA or atypical	Mainly present in autoimmune hepatitis, primary biliary cirrhosis, inflammatory bowel disease

BPI, bactericidal permeability-increasing protein; C-ANCA, cytoplasmic antineutrophil cytoplasm antibody; CSS, Churg–Strauss syndrome; GN, glomerulonephritis; HIV, human immunodeficiency virus; h-lamp-2, human lysosome-associated membrane protein-2; HLE, human leukocyte elastase (also termed human neutrophil elastase, or simply elastase); IBD, inflammatory bowel disease; MPA, microscopic polyangiitis; MPO, myeloperoxidase; P-ANCA, perinuclear antineutrophil cytoplasm antibody; PBC, primary biliary cirrhosis; PR3, proteinase-3; PSC, primary sclerosing cholangitis; SLE, systemic lupus erythematosus; WG, Wegener's granulomatosis.

The presence of P-ANCA in SLE, although originally felt not to have any particular link with disease pattern [15], has been associated with serositis, livedo reticularis, venous thrombosis, anticardiolipin and anti-SSA/Ro positivity, and periodontal disease [16,17]; in particular, lactoferrin-ANCA is strongly linked with livedo reticularis [14]. Bactericidal/permeability increasing protein (BPI) ANCA and proteinase 3 (PR3) ANCA have also been linked with serositis in patients with SLE. Anti-dsDNA and anti-SSA/Ro antibodies may resemble P-ANCA, depending on fixation methods [18]. Human lysosome-associated membrane protein-2 (h-lamp-2) ANCA has been linked with pyoderma gangrenosum.

Generally, the P-ANCA pattern is relatively non-specific, having various (often undetermined) antigen specificities and often no link with disease activity. In contrast, the C-ANCA pattern almost always corresponds with antibodies against PR3, a 29-kDa neutral serine protease, and clinically with WG or other systemic vasculitis. In the context of systemic vasculitis, the important P-ANCA groups are those with antibodies against myeloperoxidase (MPO). It is therefore important to confirm MPO or PR3 antibodies, usually by enzyme-linked immunosorbent assay (ELISA), in the context of a positive ANCA test identified by IIF screening, and to refer to the more specific result where possible (e.g. as PR3-ANCA) [9]. Immunofluorescence is more sensitive, and ELISA more specific, so combining the two tests is most useful if clinical suspicion of an ANCA-associated systemic vasculitis is high. Other solid-phase assays such as immunodot and multiplex assay are also used.

A positive C-ANCA has a sensitivity of 66% (91% if only considering active disease) and specificity of 98% for WG [19], but may be positive in about one-third of patients with microscopic polyangiitis or with necrotizing crescentic glomerulonephritis, and in about 20% with Churg–Strauss syndrome (CSS). Patients with WG who are negative for C-ANCA/anti-PR3 usually have positive P-ANCA/anti-MPO. In addition, anti-MPO are found in about 65% with progressive idiopathic glomerulonephritis, in about 50% with microscopic polyangiitis or CSS, and may be found in SLE or in ANCA-associated drug reactions (notably to propylthiouracil or hydralazine). If ANCA are present in drug-induced systemic vasculitis the pattern is usually P-ANCA or atypical ANCA. It is important to be aware that 10–20% of patients with Wegener's granulomatosis, and 40–50% with Churg–Strauss syndrome, will have negative tests for ANCA (or may develop a positive test later in the disease). Of interest, patients with Churg–Strauss syndrome who are ANCA-positive are much more likely to have associated necrotizing vasculitis and, particularly, necrotizing and crescentic glomerulonephritis, than those who are ANCA-negative [20], suggesting the possibility that the vasculitic component of the disease may be ANCA mediated but that other manifestations may have a different pathogenesis [12]. A pathogenetic role for drug-induced ANCA is best documented in relation to propylthiouracil, but the ANCA response may be heterogeneous in comparison with the situation in primary vasculitides; of 19 patients with propylthiouracil-induced ANCA-positive vasculitis, all 15 with renal disease had MPO-ANCA but many other specificities were demonstrated in this group, over half of them having ANCA directed against cathepsin G and/or leukocyte elastase, and between a quarter and half having ANCA against one or more of lactoferrin, azurocidin and PR3 [21]. Production of ANCA requires competent T-cell and B-cell function; this may explain why anti-B cell treatments (such as the monoclonal antibody rituximab) can be effective in ANCA-associated systemic vasculitis such as Wegener's granulomatosis.

Numerous studies suggest a pathogenetic role for at least anti-PR3 and anti-MPO antibodies in systemic vasculitides. Both clinical and *in vitro* evidence for pathogenicity have been reviewed [12]. In particular, the IgG3 subclass of PR3 is implicated, a rise in titres in WG being predictive of relapse [3]; this subclass is a particularly strong activator of neutrophils. The role of ANCA in the pathogenesis of vasculitis is multifactorial. ANCA cause activation of neutrophils primed by TNF-α (or by lipopolysaccharide), leading to production of reactive oxygen species, nitric oxide and cytokines such as IL-1 and IL-8 (a neutrophil chemoattractant), as well as enhancing degranulation with release of proteolytic enzymes. Neutrophils activated by ANCA up-regulate adhesion molecules, adhere to platelet monolayers or to TNF-activated endothelial cells *in vitro* rather than their usual behaviour of 'rolling', and develop pseudopodia [5]. ANCA also up-regulate expression of adhesion molecules (ICAM-1, E-selectin and VCAM-1; the adhesion cascade) and IL-6 production by endothelial cells, which in turn causes neutrophil adhesion, transmigration and tissue damage. The subject of endothelial cell adhesion and recruitment of neutrophils is discussed in detail in [22]. ANCA also stimulate monocytes to produce reactive oxygen species and to produce IL-8; monocyte activation may also be important in non-ANCA-associated vasculitides such as Behçet's disease [4].

Elastase is one of the main tissue-damaging enzymes released by neutrophil degranulation. It is potentially important that elastase stimulates release of tissue factor from cultured endothelial cells (human umbilical vein endothelial cells; HUVEC), as this may be relevant in development of microthrombi *in vivo* (PR3, but not MPO, also stimulates production of tissue factor from HUVEC) [23]. It is also of interest that autoantibodies to elastase enhance rather than decrease elastase activity, thus leading to tissue damage [24]; this might be a pathogenetic mechanism of injury by human leukocyte elastase (HLE)-ANCA.

References

1 Ball GV, Bridges SL. Pathogenesis of vasculitis. In: Ball GV, Bridges SL, eds. *Vasculitis*. Oxford: Oxford University Press, 2002: 34–52.
2 Piette WW. Primary systemic vasculitis. In: Sontheimer RD, Provost TT, eds. *Cutaneous Manifestations of Rheumatic Diseases*. Baltimore: Williams & Wilkins, 1995: 177–232.
3 Kallenberg CGM. Laboratory findings in the vasculitides. *Baillières Clin Rheumatol* 1997; **11**: 395–421.
4 Nowack R, Flores-Suárez LF, van der Woude FJ. New developments in pathogenesis of systemic vasculitis. *Curr Opin Rheumatol* 1998; **10**: 3–11.
5 Savage COS. The evolving pathogenesis of systemic vasculitis. *Clin Med* 2002; **2**: 458–64.
6 Lotti T, Ghersetich I, Comacchi C, Jorizzo JL. Cutaneous small-vessel vasculitis. *J Am Acad Dermatol* 1998; **39**: 667–87.
7 Radice A, Sinico RA. Antineutrophil cytoplasmic antibodies. *Autoimmunity* 2005; **38**: 93–103.
8 Goeken JA. Antineutrophil cytoplasmic and antiendothelial cell antibodies: new mechanisms for vasculitis. *Curr Opin Dermatol* 1995; **2**: 75–82.
9 Bajema IM, Hagen EC. Evolving concepts about the role of antineutrophil cytoplasm autoantibodies in systemic vasculitis. *Curr Opin Rheumatol* 1999; **11**: 34–40.
10 Salama AD. Pathogenesis and treatment of ANCA-associated systemic vasculitis. *J R Soc Med* 1999; **92**: 456–91.
11 Savage COS, Harper L, Holland M. New findings in pathogenesis of antineutrophil cytoplasm antibody-associated vasculitis. *Curr Opin Rheumatol* 2002; **14**: 15–22.
12 Jennette JC, Falk RJ. New insight into the pathogenesis of vasculitis associated with antineutrophil cytoplasmic autoantibodies. *Curr Opin Rheumatol* 2008; **20**: 55–60.
13 Kluth DC, Hughes J. ANCA-associated systemic vasculitis (AASV). *J R Coll Physicians Edin* 2007; **37**: 128–34.
14 Yahya TM, Benedict S, Shalabi A, Bayoumi R. Anti-neutrophil cytoplasmic antibody (ANCA) in malaria is directed against cathepsin G. *Clin Exp Immunol* 1997; **110**: 41–4.
15 Schnabel A, Csernok E, Isenberg DA *et al.* Antineutrophil cytoplasmic antibodies in systemic lupus erythematosus: prevalence, specificities and clinical significance. *Arthritis Rheum* 1995; **38**: 633–7.
16 Galeazzi M, Morrozi G, Sebastiani GD *et al.* Anti-neutrophil cytoplasmic antibodies in 566 European patients with systemic lupus erythematosus: prevalence, clinical associations and correlation with other autoantibodies. *Clin Exp Rheumatol* 1998; **16**: 541–6.
17 Novo E, Garcia-McGregor E, Viera N *et al.* Periodontitis and anti-neutrophil cytoplasmic antibodies in systemic lupus erythematosus and rheumatoid arthritis: a comparative study. *J Periodontol* 1999; **70**: 185–8.
18 Savige JA, Paspaliaris B, Silvestrini R *et al.* A review of immunofluorescent patterns associated with antineutrophil cytoplasmic antibodies (ANCA) and their differentiation from other antibodies. *J Clin Pathol* 1998; **51**: 568–75.
19 Rao JK, Weinberger M, Oddone EZ *et al.* The role of antineutrophil cytoplasmic antibody testing in the diagnosis of Wegener granulomatosis. *Ann Intern Med* 1995; **123**: 925–32.
20 Sinico RA, Di Toma L, Maggiore U *et al.* Renal involvement in Churg–Strauss syndrome. *Am J Kidney Dis* 2006; **47**: 770–9.
21 Yu F, Chen M, Gao Y *et al.* Clinical and pathological features of renal involvement in propylthiouracil-associated ANCA-positive vasculitis. *Am J Kidney Dis* 2007; **49**: 607–14.
22 Kluger MS. Vascular endothelial cell adhesion and signaling during leukocyte recruitment. *Adv Dermatol* 2004; **20**: 163–94.
23 Haubitz M, Gerlach M, Kruse HJ, Brunkhorst R. Endothelial tissue factor stimulation by proteinase 3 and elastase. *Clin Exp Immunol* 2001; **126**: 584–8.
24 Morcos M, Zimmermann F, Radsak M *et al.* Autoantibodies to polymorphonuclear neutrophil elastase do not inhibit but enhance elastase activity. *Am J Kidney Dis Online* 1998; **31**: 978–85.

Other cytokines and chemokines, and the cellular response [1–3]

Numerous cytokines have been implicated in vasculitis; some have already been discussed. Many are released as part of an acute phase response or because of upregulation of production by peripheral blood neutrophils or monocytes, such as IL-1, IL-2, IL-6, IL-8, interferon (IFN) and TNF-α. These may therefore be non-specifically elevated in vasculitis, but may play a part in ongoing damage. TNF-α is important for priming endothelial cells to express E- and P-selectin, ICAM-1 and 2, and VCAM-1 (see above), and also primes neutrophils to produce reactive oxygen species and to degranulate after exposure to ANCA. IL-8 is a potent neutrophil chemoattractant that is expressed by endothelial cells after stimulation by ANCA, and after non-cytotoxic binding of AECA. IL-6 has been studied especially in giant cell arteritis and Takayasu's arteritis, in which it appears to reflect disease activity. Increased levels of soluble TNF receptor have been demonstrated in ANCA-positive vasculitides.

Other chemokines that have enhanced tissue expression in vasculitis include monocyte chemotactic protein-1 (MCP-1), macrophage inflammatory protein-1α and -1β and RANTES (regulated upon activation, normal T-cell expressed and secreted) [4]. Expression of MAC-1 by neutrophils is up-regulated by ANCA.

Based on a mouse model in which genetic deficiency of IL-1 receptor antagonist (IL-1Ra) is associated with arterial inflammation, it has been suggested that IL-1Ra has a significant role in vasculitis and that a recombinant IL-1Ra might be a useful treatment [5].

T cells, monocytes and macrophages play a part in vasculitis injury, in addition to the role of neutrophils discussed above. Both CD4+ and CD8+ T cells accumulate at the site of injury. In WG there is a Th1 cytokine profile, with increased IFN-γ, TNF and IL-12 but not IL-4, IL-5 or IL-10 [4], and CD28 expression; however, some studies have suggested a Th2 response in nasal mucosa, which may be of importance as nasal staphylococcal infection is associated with relapses in WG. Monocytes from patients with systemic necrotizing vasculitis produce more superoxide and MPO than monocytes from controls, and they can also be induced to express PR3 and to release IL-8 when exposed to ANCA [6]. However, monocyte activation also occurs in Behçet's disease, which is not ANCA-related. Defective macrophage apoptosis may lead to persistence and ongoing damage at the vasculitic site, as occurs with neutrophils [3].

References

1 Ball GV, Bridges SL. Pathogenesis of vasculitis. In: Ball GV, Bridges SL, eds. *Vasculitis*. Oxford: Oxford University Press, 2002: 34–52.

2 Kallenberg CGM. Laboratory findings in the vasculitides. *Baillières Clin Rheumatol* 1997; **11**: 395–421.

3 Nowack R, Flores-Suárez LF, van der Woude FJ. New developments in pathogenesis of systemic vasculitis. *Curr Opin Rheumatol* 1998; **10**: 3–11.

4 Savage COS, Harper L, Holland M. New findings in pathogenesis of antineutrophil cytoplasm antibody-associated vasculitis. *Curr Opin Rheumatol* 2002; **14**: 15–22.

5 Nicklin MJ, Hughes DE, Barton JL, Ure JM, Duff GW. Arterial inflammation in mice lacking the interleukin 1 receptor antagonist gene. *J Exp Med* 2000; **191**: 303–12.

6 Savage COS. The evolving pathogenesis of systemic vasculitis. *Clin Med* 2002; **2**: 458–64.

Genetic factors

Familial clustering has been documented in some vasculitides such as WG, although this is uncommon [1,2]. Various explanations have been proposed, including the occurrence of TNF gene polymorphisms, genetic heterogeneity of ANCA antigens or their expression, and neutrophil Fcγ receptor polymorphisms. For example, expression of PR3 on resting neutrophils shows marked individual variation, the proportion of neutrophils expressing PR3 varying from approximately 10 to 80%, but being quite stable in any individual [1,3] This is now known to be genetically determined [4], and high expression has been associated with a higher risk of WG. Severe renal disease in WG has been linked with expression of the neutrophil receptor FcγRIIIb-NA1, although this is disputed [2,5]. The genetic region for elastase, azurocidin and PR3 is highly polymorphous, but no apparent associations with clinical disease have been identified [1]. Further polymorphisms are increasingly being documented; the association between some CD18 polymorphisms and Wegener's granulomatosis has been referred to earlier, and numerous polymorphisms have been linked with Behçet's disease (and are discussed in the relevant disease section). In particular, a predilection associated with various cytokine and inflammatory mediator alleles and polymorphisms, including polymorphisms in endothelial nitric oxide synthase (eNOS), in interleukin-10 (IL-10), IL-8, and CD28 genes, and presence of the antitumour necrosis factor-alpha (TNF-α) 1031C allele, are all associated with Behçet's disease susceptibility [6].

α_1-Antitrypsin (α_1AT) is a natural inhibitor of PR3 and elastase in neutrophil alpha-granules (as is caeruloplasmin for MPO). Deficiency of α_1AT may be genetic or may be acquired by the formation of α_1AT–PR3 complexes by anti-PR3 ANCA. An association between the α_1AT-deficient PiZZ phenotype and ANCA-positive vasculitis has been described, and PiZ heterozygosity has been linked with poor prognosis in ANCA-positive systemic vasculitis [7,8]. However, a large study of PiZZ-deficient sera showed an association with antibodies against elastase but not against PR3, MPO or lactoferrin, and α_1AT deficiency is not in itself sufficient to induce ANCA-associated vasculitis [5,9]. An α_1 protease inhibitor has been used with dramatic response in the treatment of chronic vasculitis in a patient with α_1AT deficiency [10].

In Kawasaki disease, the G2350A polymorphism in the angiotensin converting enzyme (ACE) gene has been associated with risk of the condition (but not with risk of coronary artery aneurysms) [11]; however, the itpkc_3 polymorphism in the inositol 1,4,5-triphosphate 3-kinase C (*IKPKC*) gene (a negative regulator of T cell activation) seems to be linked to immune hyper-reactivity and is associated with increased risk of Kawasaki disease itself and of coronary artery aneurysms [12]. There are also reported polymorphisms in chemokine receptor genes within the *CCR3-CCR2-CCR5* gene cluster, and polymorphisms in genes for some matrix metalloproteinases (a possible explanation for the variable risk of development of aneurysms).

In Henoch–Schönlein purpura (HSP), there have been reported associations with HLA class 1 alleles; HLA A2, A11 and B35 having an association with increased risk of HSP and HLA A1, B49 and B50 being associated with decreased risk [13]. These alleles did not appear to alter risk of renal disease, whereas some vascular endothelial growth factor polymorphisms may increase, or protect against, the risk of nephritis in HSP [14].

It is likely that advances in genetics will identify many polymorphisms that may alter susceptibility, severity or specific features of different vasculitides, quite possibly in a hierarchical or polygenic fashion [15].

References

1 Nowack R, Flores-Suárez LF, van der Woude FJ. New developments in pathogenesis of systemic vasculitis. *Curr Opin Rheumatol* 1998; **10**: 3–11.

2 Gross WL, Csernok E, Trabandt A. Wegener's granulomatosis: pathogenesis. In: Ball GV, Bridges SL, eds. *Vasculitis*. Oxford: Oxford University Press, 2002: 340–56.

3 Halbwachs-Mecarelli L, Bessou G, Lesavre P *et al*. Bimodal distribution of proteinase 3 (Pr3) surface expression reflects a constitutive heterogeneity in the polymorphonuclear neutrophil pool. *FEBS Lett* 1995; **374**: 29–33.

4 Schreiber A, Busjahn A, Luft FC, Kettritz R. Membrane expression of proteinase 3 is genetically determined. *J Am Soc Nephrol* 2003; **14**: 68–75.

5 Savage COS, Harper L, Holland M. New findings in pathogenesis of antineutrophil cytoplasm antibody-associated vasculitis. *Curr Opin Rheumatol* 2002; **14**: 15–22.

6 Krause I, Weinberger A. Behçet's disease. *Curr Opin Rheumatol* 2008; **20**: 82–7.

7 Ball GV, Bridges SL. Pathogenesis of vasculitis. In: Ball GV, Bridges SL, eds. *Vasculitis*. Oxford: Oxford University Press, 2002: 34–52.

8 Griffith ME, Lovegrove JU, Gaskin G *et al*. C-antineutrophil cytoplasmic antibody positivity in vasculitis patients is associated with the Z phenotype of alpha-1-antitrypsin, and P-antineutrophil cytoplasmic antibody positivity with the S allele. *Nephrol Dial Transplant* 1996; **11**: 438–43.

9 Audrain MAP, Sesboüé R, Baranger TAR *et al*. Analysis of anti-neutrophil cytoplasmic antibodies (ANCA): frequency and specificity in a sample of 191 homozygous (PiZZ) alpha-1-antitrypsin-deficient subjects. *Nephrol Dial Transplant* 2001; **16**: 39–44.

10 Dowd SK, Rodgers GC, Callen JP. Effective treatment with α_1 protease inhibitor of chronic cutaneous vasculitis associated with α_1-antitrypsin deficiency. *J Am Acad Dermatol* 1995; **33**: 913–6.

11 Wu SF, Chang JS, Peng CT *et al*. Polymorphism of angiotensin-1 converting enzyme gene and Kawasaki disease. *Pediatr Cardiol* 2004; **25**: 529–33.

12 Yoshihiro O, Tomohiko G, Burns JC *et al*. ITPKC functional polymorphism associated with Kawasaki disease susceptibility and formation of coronary artery aneurysms. *Nat Genet* 2008; **40**: 35–42.

13 Peru H, Soylemezoglu O, Gonen S *et al*. HLA class 1 associations in Henoch Schönlein purpura: increased and decreased frequencies. *Clin Rheumatol* 2008; **27**: 5–10.

14 Blanca R, Perez AC, Lopez SL *et al*. Association between functional haplotypes of vascular endothelial growth factor and renal complications in Henoch-Schönlein purpura. *J Rheumatol* 2006; **33**: 69–73.

15 Nose M. A proposal concept of a polygene network in systemic vasculitis: lessons from MRL mouse models. *Allergy Int* 2007; **56**: 79–86.

Evaluation of the patient with suspected vasculitis

The essential aspects in the approach to a patient with suspected vasculitis, from a clinical dermatological perspective, have been described in various publications [1–14], some providing either flowchart [2,3,5,8,12] or algorithm approaches [7,11]. Additional approaches and classifications directed by histopathological features are also useful [15–17].

In broad terms, the evaluation of a patient with suspected vasculitis involves histopathological confirmation of the clinical diagnosis, an assessment of the extent of the disease (both the degree of skin damage, and the involvement of internal organs) and an attempt to establish an underlying aetiology. Clinical patterns that may suggest a vasculitis, other than the overtly vasculitic lesions discussed in this chapter, include cutaneous livedo, cutaneous necrosis, non-specific purpura and purple (blue) toe syndrome; these patterns can also occur in non-vasculitic microvascular occlusion disorders, and their significance and likely causes are discussed in Chapter 49.

Histopathological confirmation of suspected small vessel vasculitides is best performed by taking a punch biopsy of the lesions at the appropriate stage, recognizing that lesions represent various chronological stages of the disease process. Deeper, elliptical incisional biopsies should be performed for suspected larger vessel vasculitides. Processing part of the biopsy, or a separate biopsy, for direct immunofluorescence is potentially important. This initial investigative step usually confirms the presence of a vasculitis (or may show evidence of a vasculitis mimic, such as a vasculopathy). It also helps to define the type of vasculitis, based on vessel type and size, type of reaction (e.g. segmental arteritis in polyarteritis nodosa), infiltrating cells (e.g. prominently eosinophilic infiltrate in some drug-induced vasculitides), extent of infiltrate (e.g. pan-dermal small vessel disease in a patient with fever suggests possible sepsis) and may define a specific vasculitis process (e.g. CSVV with vascular IgA deposits in Henoch–Schönlein purpura).

In attempting to assess the extent of the disease, it is important to consider where circulating immune complexes may deposit. Specifically, the following systems should be evaluated, especially but not exclusively for the features listed:

- **General.** Myalgia, arthralgia, fever
- **Renal.** Proteinuria, haematuria
- **Nervous system.** Central or peripheral, diffuse or localized findings
- **Musculoskeletal.** Non-erosive polyarthritis
- **Gastrointestinal.** Abdominal pain, gastrointestinal bleeding

- **Pulmonary.** Pleural effusion, pleuritis, pneumonitis
- **Cardiac.** Pericardial effusion, pericarditis
- **Other systems.** Upper respiratory tract (larger vessel vasculitides), eyes (Behçet's disease, larger vessel vasculitides), larger vessels

The overall clinical pattern needs to be taken into account when evaluating internal disease, for example the combination of respiratory symptoms and mononeuritis multiplex would suggest possible Churg–Strauss syndrome.

Additional investigations should be performed to try to determine the aetiology of the vasculitis. It may be helpful to screen for medications, infections or diseases associated with immune complexes (connective tissue vascular diseases, malignancy, inflammatory bowel disease, etc.). Although 'directed' sequential blood tests are ideal, depending on the clinical picture and results of simpler tests, from a pragmatic perspective it is often the case that a 'vasculitis screen' is performed. Reasonable initial tests might include:

- Full blood count with differential white cell count
- Markers of inflammation: erythrocyte sedimentation rate (ESR), C-reactive protein (CRP)
- Electrolytes and hepatic transaminases, glucose
- Urinalysis for protein and blood
- Blood cultures (if pyrexial)
- Serology—ANA (+/− antibodies to extractable nuclear antigens; dsDNA if ANA positive), ANCA, complement C3 and C4, antistreptolysin-O titre, viral titres (e.g. hepatitis B and hepatitis C, possibly HIV, CMV, parvovirus B19 and others if recent infection), others if indicated or to exclude differentials (e.g. rheumatoid factor, electrophoresis, immune complexes)
- cryoglobulins
- chest radiograph (if symptoms, signs, ANCA-positive or suspected larger vessel disease)
- additional organ-directed investigations as necessary (renal, nerve, bone marrow biopsy; arteriography; etc.).

As well as being important for investigation of causes of vasculitis, blood tests requested should also include markers of severity (e.g. C-reactive protein, erythrocyte sedimentation rate), tests to determine the systemic effect of vasculitis (e.g. renal function) and baseline tests for possible corticosteroid or immunosuppressive therapy (glucose, thiopurine methylytransferase (azathioprine), G-6-PD status (dapsone), etc.).

The extent of additional investigation may depend on initial findings, severity of vasculitis and of general symptoms, and on response to therapy. It is important to remember, for example, that investigations for cutaneous small vessel vasculitis fail to demonstrate a cause in up to 50% of cases, and to consider the need for further investigation in a patient in whom the disorder is resolving. It is also often helpful to work with a colleague in internal medicine or paediatrics when evaluating the patient, particularly if larger vessel disease is suspected, as additional investigations might include biopsies of artery, kidney, lung or nerve, radiology studies such as arteriography of aortic arch or visceral vessels, etc. Even if the cutaneous vasculitis has resolved, it is appropriate to perform urinalysis and blood pressure monitoring subsequently (perhaps monthly and 3-monthly respectively, for 6 months) as delayed effects of concurrent renal involvement may become apparent. In those who do have renal involvement, this may persist as renal impairment later in life [18] so there is an argument for annual tests of renal function in such individuals.

The information in the following sections discusses the definition, history, aetiology, pathogenesis, histopathology, clinical features, diagnosis and treatment of various vasculitides affecting small, medium and large blood vessels.

References

1 Lotti T, Ghersetich I, Comacchi C, Jorizzo JL. Cutaneous small-vessel vasculitis. *J Am Acad Dermatol* 1998; **39**: 667–87.

2 Callen JP. A clinical approach to the vasculitis patient in the dermatologic office. *Clin Dermatol* 1999; **17**: 549–53.

3 Gibson LE. Cutaneous vasculitis update. *Dermatol Clin* 2001; **19**: 603–15.

4 Stone JH, Nousari HC. 'Essential' cutaneous vasculitis: what every rheumatologist should know about vasculitis of the skin. *Curr Opin Rheumatol* 2001; **13**: 23–34.

5 Cohen MD, Conn DL. An approach to the adult with suspected vasculitis. In: Ball GV, Bridges SL, eds. *Vasculitis*. Oxford: Oxford University Press, 2002: 227–33.

6 Goldmuntz EA, White PH. An approach to the child with suspected vasculitis. In: Ball GV, Bridges SL, eds. *Vasculitis*. Oxford: Oxford University Press, 2002: 234–45.

7 Fiorentino DF. Cutaneous vasculitis. *J Am Acad Dermatol* 2003; **48**: 311–40.

8 Gonzalez-Gay MA, Garcia-Porrua C, Pujol RM. Clinical approach to cutaneous vasculitis. *Curr Opin Rheumatol* 2005; **17**: 56–61.

9 Schmidt WA, Gromnica-Ihle E. What is the best approach to diagnosing large-vessel vasculitis? *Clin Rheumatol* 2005; **19**: 223–42.

10 Ozen S, Ruperto N, Dillon MJ et al. EULAR/PReS endorsed consensus criteria for the classification of childhood vasculitides. *Ann Rheum Dis* 2006; **65**: 936–41.

11 Watts R, Lane S, Hanslik T et al. Development and validation of a consensus methodology for the classification of the ANCA-associated vasculitides and polyarteritis nodosa for epidemiological studies. *Ann Rheum Dis* 2006; **66**: 222–7.

12 Jenette JC, Falk RJ. Nosology of primary vasculitis. *Curr Opin Rheumatol* 2007; **19**: 10–16.

13 Chen K-R, Carlson AJ. Clinical approach to cutaneous vasculitis. *Am J Clin Dermatol* 2008; **9**: 71–92.

14 Russell JP, Gibson LE. Primary cutaneous small vessel vasculitis: approach to diagnosis and management. *Int J Dermatol* 2006; **45**: 3–13.

15 Crowson AN, Mihm MC Jr, Magro CM. Cutaneous vasculitis: a review. *J Cutan Pathol* 2003; **30**: 161–73.

16 Carlson JA, Chen K-R. Cutaneous vasculitis update: small vessel neutrophilic vasculitis syndromes. *Am J Dermatopathol* 2006; **28**: 486–506.

17 Carlson JA, Chen K-R. Cutaneous vasculitis update: neutrophilic muscular vessel and eosinophilic, granulomatous, and lymphocytic vasculitis syndromes. *Am J Dermatopathol* 2007; **29**: 32–43.

18 Ronkainen J, Nuutinen M, Koskimies O. The adult kidney 24 years after childhood Henoch-Schönlein purpura: a retrospective cohort study. *Lancet* 2002; **360**: 666–70.

Cutaneous small vessel vasculitis

Synonyms
- Cutaneous leukocytoclastic vasculitis
- Hypersensitivity angiitis/vasculitis variants confined to skin
- Cutaneous necrotizing venulitis (necrotizing variant involving predominantly venules)

Definition. Affecting mainly cutaneous post-capillary venules, cutaneous small vessel vasculitis (CSVV) is the most common type of vasculitis in dermatology. Features of CSVV include palpable purpura, urticaria or ulcers on the legs. It affects both children and adults, and is seen more commonly in women. Extracutaneous manifestations of CSVV are by definition relatively uncommon and should prompt a search for other pathology such as Henoch–Schönlein purpura (HSP).

History and nomenclature. In the 1950s, Zeek described small vessel vasculitis related to drug exposure as a separate entity from large vessel vasculitis, and termed the small vessel vasculitis 'hypersensitivity angiitis'. Because of ambiguity, the term hypersensitivity angiitis was redefined by the Chapel Hill Consensus Conference in 1994 to describe patients with a small vessel vasculitis with primarily cutaneous involvement [1].

Aetiology and pathogenesis. A history of drug exposure or recent infection is frequently present in cases of CSVV, and circulating immune complexes can be identified in a large percentage of patients. It is important to be aware that CSVV can occur as part of microscopic polyangiitis or Wegener's granulomatosis, and that some patients with HSP may be erroneously thought to have 'simple' CSVV if renal involvement is delayed or if skin biopsy fails to show IgA deposits (as occurs in biopsy of older lesions). A detailed review suggested that about 50% of cases of cutaneous vasculitis are 'idiopathic', 15–20% due to infection, 15–20% related to inflammatory diseases (such as collagen vascular disorders), 10–15% due to medications and other drugs, and less than 5% are associated with malignancy [2]. CSVV is therefore a term delineating the extent of vasculitis, usually of leukocytoclastic type, but is really a diagnosis of exclusion, as discussed in more detail below.

Histopathology. Leukocytoclastic vasculitis with segmental inflammation in an angiocentric pattern, swelling of the endothelium, fibrinoid necrosis of vessel walls, extravasation of erythrocytes, and an infiltrate of neutrophils with karyorrhexis of nuclei (i.e. leukocytoclasia) are major features of CSVV (Figs 50.1 & 50.2).

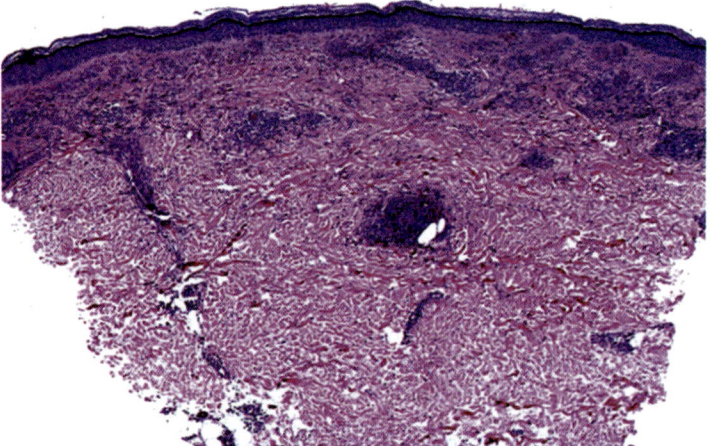

Fig. 50.1 Leukocytoclastic vasculitis. Low power photomicrograph showing perivascular infiltrates and fibrinoid deposits within the vessels of the upper dermis. (Courtesy of Dr Omar Sangueza, Wake Forest University School of Medicine, Winston-Salem, NC, USA.)

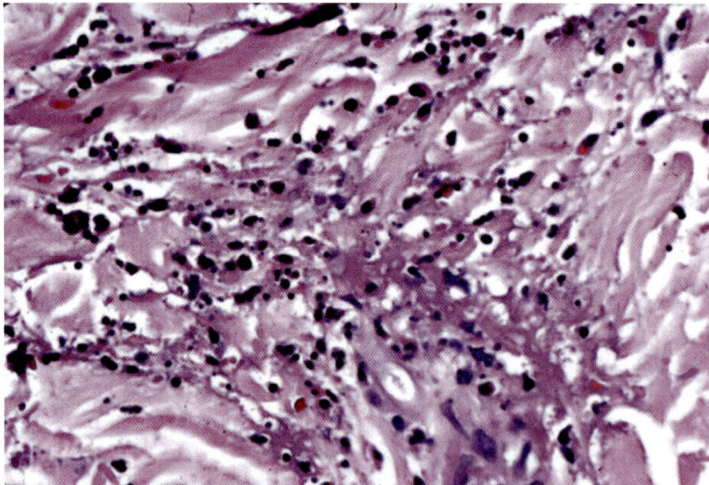

Fig. 50.2 Leukocytoclastic vasculitis. Higher magnification demonstrates nuclear dust, fibrinoid deposits, vascular alteration and collagen degeneration. (Courtesy of Dr Omar Sangueza, Wake Forest University School of Medicine, Winston-Salem, NC, USA.)

In superficial dermal papillary vessels, IgM or complement C3 perivascular deposits are demonstrated in over 80% of fresh lesions [3]. Some studies state lower proportions, but this may depend on timing of biopsy and also because IgM is relatively poor at fixing complement. IgG is found less often.

Clinical features [2,4–13]. The skin lesions of CSVV typically arise as a simultaneous 'crop', resulting from the exposure to an inciting stimulus. They usually resolve within several weeks or a few months although, anecdotally, approximately 10% of patients will have recurrent disease at intervals up to years. In one retrospective analysis, a quarter of patients with cutaneous leukocytoclastic vasculitis had either a chronic course (over 3 months) or recurrent symptoms, including all those with hepatitis C-associated vasculitis and five of nine with a streptococcal aetiology [11]. The major cutaneous manifestation of CSVV is palpable purpura, ranging in size from 1 mm to several centimetres (Figs 50.3–50.5). Sometimes macular in the early stages, such purpura may progress to a wide array of lesions including papules, nodules, vesicles, plaques, bullae or pustules, with secondary findings of ulceration, necrosis and post-inflammatory hyperpigmentation. Other cutaneous findings include oedema, livedo reticularis and urticaria. The presence of the latter two should prompt consideration of cutaneous polyarteritis nodosa and urticarial vasculitis, respectively (see pp. 50.33 and 50.21). Lesions typically occur in areas prone to stasis, commonly including the ankles and lower legs [2,4–10], and typically sparing intertriginous regions. Although often asymptomatic, pruritus, pain or burning may be experienced, as well as systemic symptoms including fever, arthralgia, myalgia and anorexia. The presence of symptoms affecting other organ systems should raise the suspicion of other vasculitides such as HSP, mixed cryoglobulinaemia, or CSVV associated with polyarteritis nodosa (PAN) or with WG.

Diagnosis. A thorough history and physical examination is essential for correct diagnosis of CSVV, with screening for

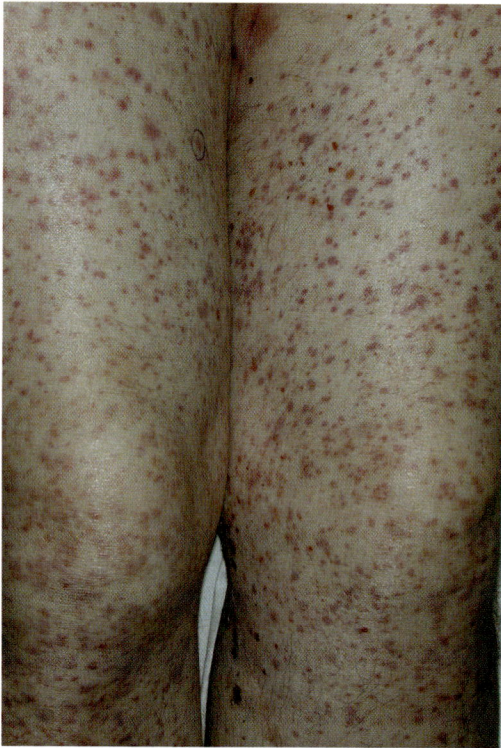

Fig. 50.3 Cutaneous small vessel vasculitis on the thighs. There was similar involvement on the lower legs.

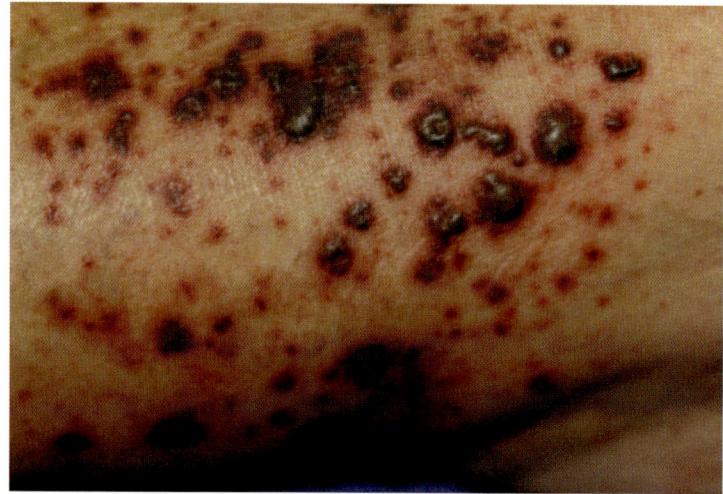

Fig. 50.4 Cutaneous small vessel vasculitis progressing to blistering.

infections, connective tissue disease, medication usage and cancer. Vasculitides with systemic manifestations must be ruled out, as CSVV is diagnosed by exclusion. Table 50.6 describes the evaluation of a patient with a suspected CSVV (see also the preceding section 'Evaluation of the patient with suspected vasculitis', p. 50.12, and [2,8–10]). The differential diagnosis of CSVV includes many more specifically defined disorders, which are discussed in this chapter and listed in [2,3,9–13].

As indicated, a diagnosis of CSVV should be treated with some caution, not only because of the extensive differential diagnosis of the pathological features but also because other features may become apparent and make the diagnosis of CSVV, or of

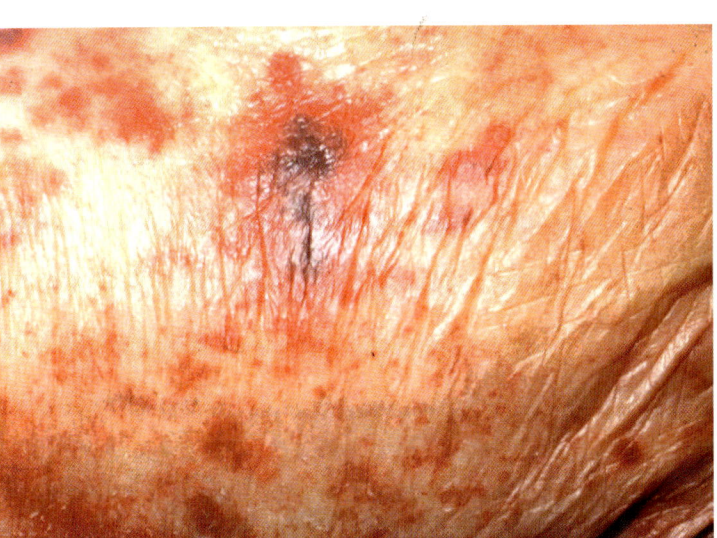

(a)

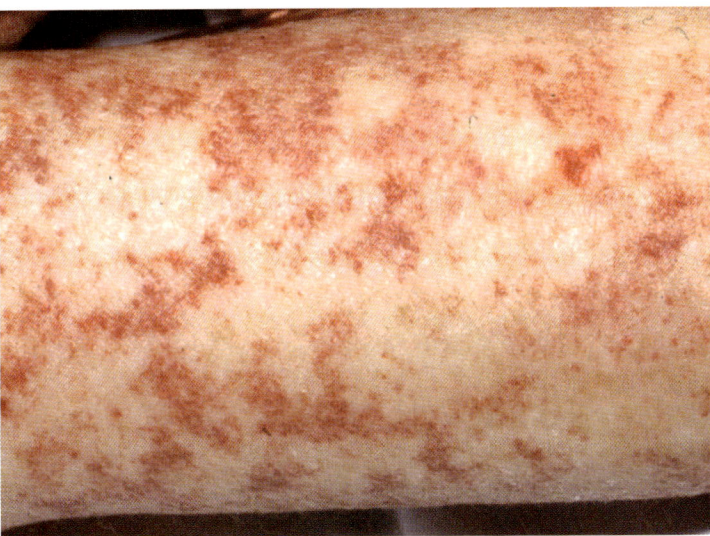

(b)

Fig. 50.5 Vasculitis due to sepsis, in a patient with impaired level of consciousness. The necrotic lesion in (a) and the reticulate pattern on the leg in (b) are clues to involvement of deeper vessels. Histologically, vasculitis due to infection may involve vessels at all levels of the dermis.

Table 50.6 Evaluation of a patient with suspected cutaneous small vessel vasculitis.

Confirm the clinical diagnosis histopathologically
   Punch biopsy of lesion at the appropriate stage
   Direct immunofluorescence
   Incisional biopsy for suspected larger vessel vasculitis

Assess the extent of the disease
   General
   • Myalgia
   • Arthralgia
   • Fever
   Renal involvement
   • Proteinuria
   • Haematuria
   Nervous system
   • Central or peripheral
   • Diffuse or local findings
   Musculoskeletal involvement
   • Non-erosive polyarthritis
   Gastrointestinal system
   • Abdominal pain
   • Gastrointestinal bleeding
   Pulmonary involvement
   • Pleural effusion
   • Pleuritis
   Pericardial involvement
   • Pericardial effusion

Attempt to establish the aetiology (idiopathic in 50%)
   Drugs
   Infections
   Diseases associated with immune complexes
   • Connective tissue vascular diseases
   • Malignancy
   • Inflammatory bowel disease
   • Chronic active hepatitis
   Idiopathic (50%)

idiopathic CSVV, insecure. The frequency of this occurrence is difficult to ascertain as some retrospective analyses exclude patients with associated collagen vascular disease, infection, etc. Two retrospective reviews of patients diagnosed as having cutaneous vasculitis or CSVV suggest that about a third of patients may have a more specific diagnosis or evidence of internal disease. In one study of 90 patients with CSVV, renal involvement was documented in 39 (43%); in 29 of these, renal biopsy was performed and led to reclassification as HSP (10 patients), microscopic polyangiitis (MPA) (13 patients) or WG (six patients) [14]. In a review of 93 patients, 57 were felt to have 'hypersensitivity vasculitis', the remainder having more specific diagnoses including HSP (11), urticarial vasculitis (six), types of polyangiitis (microscopic polyangiitis, five; classic PAN, one; cutaneous PAN, three), WG (two) and others; 20/93 had renal involvement, comprising six each with hypersensitivity vasculitis and HSP, and four each with microscopic polyangitis and septic vasculitis [11]. In this study, 44% were classed as idiopathic.

Treatment. Treatment of CSVV is typically unnecessary, as the disease is usually self-limiting. The evidence for efficacy of any therapy in the management of vasculitis is derived from clinical experience rather than controlled trials. However, if any triggering agents are identified, such as a drug or infection, they should be removed or treated. Efforts to minimize stasis, such as use of compression hosiery and elevation of dependent areas, as well as the use of non-steroidal anti-inflammatory drugs (NSAIDs) and antihistamines, typically produce a decrease in symptoms [10], although there is little reason to suppose that they alter the course of the disease. Furthermore, oral corticosteroids at a dosage of 30–80 mg once daily, tapered over 2–3 weeks, often give effective symptom control, although no controlled trials have been carried out to evaluate the treatment of CSVV with oral corticosteroids. Corticosteroid use may be of particular benefit in cases with painful progressive cutaneous lesions, and they prevent glomerulonephritis in patients who actually have HSP. No data support

Table 50.7 Therapeutic ladder for patients with cutaneous small vessel vasculitis.

Symptomatic relief
  Supportive therapy (3)
  Antihistamines (3)
  Non-steroidal anti-inflammatory drugs (2)

Skin lesions alone
  Pentoxiphylline (3)
  Colchicine (2)
  Dapsone (2)

Ulcerative skin lesions alone
  Thalidomide (3)
  Low-dose weekly methotrexate (3)
  Prednisolone (2)

Systemic disease
  Prednisolone (2)
  Azathioprine (2)
  Cyclophosphamide (2)
  Mycophenolate mofetil (3)
  Ciclosporin (3)
  Interferon-α (if hepatitis C-associated) (1)
  Intravenous gammaglobulin (3)
  Extracorporeal immunomodulation (3)
  Infliximab (3)
  Rituximab (3)

1, double-blind studies; 2, case series; 3, case reports.

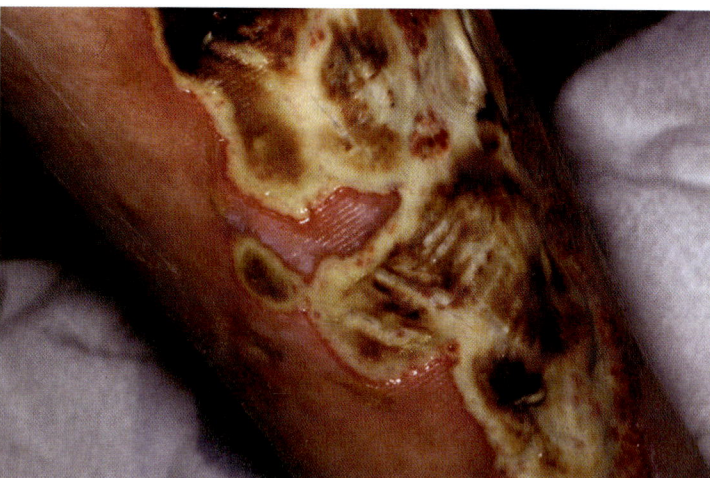

Fig. 50.6 Prolonged leg ulceration in a patient with cutaneous small vessel vasculitis, without systemic involvement; the main factor impairing healing was diabetic arterial disease.

the use of topical corticosteroids or antibiotics in CSVV, although such therapies are commonly used. Colchicine given at a dose of 0.6 mg twice daily has been shown to be of benefit by anecdotal evidence and open-label studies [15–17]. Similarly, the use of dapsone is based only on anecdotal or small case series, yet some believe that the use of dapsone along with colchicine may be advantageous in the treatment of CSVV [18–21]. In patients with disease refractory to the above therapies, cytotoxic agents may be considered. Such agents include azathioprine (typically at a dosage of 2 mg/kg/day; see also Chapter 74), methotrexate at a low dose of less than 25 mg/week, ciclosporin and cyclophosphamide [22–26]. Table 50.7 describes a therapeutic ladder for patients with CSVV. A therapeutic ladder based on individual diagnostic entities is provided in [2].

More recently, biological agents have shown some promise in the treatment of vasculitis, although they are rarely required for CSVV; infliximab, which blocks TNF-α, and rituximab, by blocking CD20 and thus inhibiting B-cell antibody production, appear to be the most promising [27,28]. Paradoxically, both of these agents have also been reported to cause vasculitis [29,30].

In some cases, ulceration, particularly of the lower legs, may prove difficult to heal despite apparently appropriate interventions. Although the cause(s) may be those that impair healing of the lower leg in any situation, such as obesity, diabetes, arterial disease, etc. (Chapter 47) (Fig. 50.6) it is also pertinent to note that hypercoagulability conditions (Chapter 49) may also impair healing; in a study of 13 patients with refractory leg ulcers following leukocytoclastic vasculitis, seven (53%) had either factor V Leiden or a lupus anticoagulant [31].

References

1 Jennette JC, Falk RG, Andrassy K *et al*. Nomenclature of systemic vasculitides. Proposal of an international consensus conference. *Arthritis Rheum* 1994; **37**: 187–92.
2 Fiorentino DF. Cutaneous vasculitis. *J Am Acad Dermatol* 2003; **48**: 311–40.
3 Carlson JA, Chen K-R. Cutaneous vasculitis update: small vessel neutrophilic vasculitis syndromes. *Am J Dermatopathol* 2006; **28**: 486–506.
4 Blanco R, Martinez-Taboada VM, Rodriguez-Valverde V, Garcia-Fuentes M. Cutaneous vasculitis in children and adults: associated diseases and aetiologic factors in 303 patients. *Medicine* 1998; **77**: 403–18.
5 Ekenstam E, Callen JP. Cutaneous leukocytoclastic vasculitis: clinical and laboratory features of 82 patients seen in private practice. *Arch Dermatol* 1984; **120**: 484–9.
6 Martinez-Taboada VM, Blanco R, Garcia-Fuentes M, Rodriguez-Valverde V. Clinical features and outcome of 95 patients with hypersensitivity vasculitis. *Am J Med* 1997; **102**: 186–91.
7 Sais G, Vidaller A, Jucgla A *et al*. Prognostic factors in leukocytoclastic vasculitis: a clinicopathologic study of 160 patients. *Arch Dermatol* 1998; **134**: 309–15.
8 Gonzalez-Gay MA, Garcia-Porrua C, Pujol RM. Clinical approach to cutaneous vasculitis. *Curr Opin Rheumatol* 2005; **17**: 56–61.
9 Chen K-R, Carlson AJ. Clinical approach to cutaneous vasculitis. *Am J Clin Dermatol* 2008; **9**: 71–92.
10 Lotti T, Ghersetich I, Comacchi C, Jorizzo JL. Cutaneous small-vessel vasculitis. *J Am Acad Dermatol* 1998; **39**: 667–87; quiz 688–90.
11 Tai YJ, Chong AH, Williams RA *et al*. Retrospective analysis of adult patients with cutaneous leukocytoclastic vasculitis. *Australas J Dermatol* 2006; **47**: 92–6.
12 Magro CM, Crowson AN. The cutaneous neutrophilic vascular injury syndromes: a review. *Semin Diag Pathol* 2001; **18**: 47–58.
13 Crowson AN, Mihm MC Jr, Magro CM. Cutaneous vasculitis: a review. *J Cutan Pathol* 2003; **30**: 161–73.
14 Ioannidou DJ, Krasagakis Sotsiou F, Tosca AD. Cutaneous small vessel vasculitis: an entity with frequent renal involvement. *Arch Dermatol* 2002; **138**: 413–4.
15 Hazen PG, Michel B. Management of necrotizing vasculitis with colchicine: improvement in patients with cutaneous lesions and Behçet's syndrome. *Arch Dermatol* 1979; **115**: 1303–6.
16 Plotnick S, Huppert AS, Kantor G. Colchicine and leukocytoclastic vasculitis. *Arthritis Rheum* 1989; **32**: 1489–90.
17 Callen JP. Colchicine is effective in controlling chronic cutaneous leukocytoclastic vasculitis. *J Am Acad Dermatol* 1985; **13**: 193–200.
18 Callen JP. A clinical approach to the vasculitis patient in the dermatologic office. *Clin Dermatol* 1999; **17**: 549–53.
19 Wells GC. Allergic vasculitis (tri-symptom of Gougerot) treated with dapsone. *Proc R Soc Med* 1969; **62**: 665–6.
20 Asghar SS, Westerhof W, Das PK *et al*. Treatment of vasculitis with chlorpromazine and dapsone. *Arch Dermatol Res* 1985; **277**: 504–6.

21 Fredenberg MF, Malkinson FD. Sulfone therapy in the treatment of leukocytoclastic vasculitis: report of three cases. *J Am Acad Dermatol* 1987; **16**: 772–8.

22 Jorizzo JL, White WL, Wise CM *et al*. Low-dose weekly methotrexate for unusual neutrophilic vascular reactions: cutaneous polyarteritis nodosa and Behçet's disease. *J Am Acad Dermatol* 1991; **24**: 973–8.

23 Heurkens AH, Westedt ML, Breedveld FC. Prednisone plus azathioprine treatment in patients with rheumatoid arthritis complicated by vasculitis. *Arch Intern Med* 1991; **151**: 2249–54.

24 Boehm I, Bauer R. Low dose methotrexate controls a severe form of polyarteritis nodosa. *Arch Dermatol* 2000; **136**: 167–9.

25 Vena GA, Cassano N. Immunosuppressive therapy in cutaneous vasculitis. *Clin Dermatol* 1999; **17**: 633–40.

26 Callen JP, Spencer LV, Burruss JB, Holtman J. Azathioprine: an effective, corticosteroid-sparing therapy for patients with recalcitrant cutaneous lupus erythematosus or with recalcitrant cutaneous leukocytoclastic vasculitis. *Arch Dermatol* 1991; **127**: 515–22.

27 Uthman IW, Touma Z, Sayyad J, Salman S. Response of deep cutaneous vasculitis to infliximab. *J Am Acad Dermatol* 2005; **53**: 353–4.

28 Chung L, Funke AA, Chakravarty EF *et al*. Successful use of rituximab for cutaneous vasculitis. *Arch Dermatol* 2006; **142**: 1407–10.

29 Anandacoomarasamy A, Kannangara S, Barnsley L. Cutaneous vasculitis associated with infliximab in the treatment of rheumatoid arthritis. *Intern Med J* 2005; **35**: 638–40.

30 Kandula P, Kouides PA. Rituximab-induced leukocytoclastic vasculitis: a case report. *Arch Dermatol* 2006; **142**: 246–7.

31 Mekkes JR, Loots MA, van der Wal AC, Bos JD. Increased incidence of hypercoagulability in patients with leg ulcers caused by leukocytoclastic vasculitis. *J Am Acad Dermatol* 2004; **50**: 104–7.

Drug-induced vasculitis

Definition. Vasculitis of various morphological types can be caused by drug ingestion. This is briefly discussed as a discrete topic as it is always important to consider medications and other ingested drugs as a possible cause of vasculitis. The clinical pattern is usually that of a superficial small vessel cutaneous leukocytoclastic vasculitis but other patterns, including systemic vasculitis, occur. Drug-induced vasculitis is also considered in Chapter 75 with emphasis on causative agents.

Causes. Many drugs may cause vasculitis, and are listed in several reference sources [1–6]. The validity and importance of some reports of drug-induced vasculitis is uncertain as not all are histologically confirmed, the frequency in relation to the number of patients treated with any specific causative drug is often unknown, and most surveillance systems rely on spontaneous reporting. About 200 drug causes of vasculitis are listed by Litt [5]; even allowing for uncertainty in some cases, it seems likely that over 100 drugs are implicated as causes of drug-induced vasculitis or the closely related drug-induced lupus-like syndrome [7], although the actual frequency of drug-induced vasculitis is very low [6], possibly 1/100 000 people. However, it is also clear that, for any drug, vasculitis is one of the rarer reaction patterns that occurs (typically accounting for <1% of reactions to any individual drug). Some of the more important drugs that can cause vasculitis are also listed in Table 50.8. Those most frequently implicated are penicillins, sulphonamides, quinolones, analgesics (including non-steroidal anti-inflammatory drugs), thiazides and other diuretics, anticonvulsants, phenothiazines, allopurinol, and colony-stimulating factors [1–9]. Less commonly used drugs, but

with a significant risk of causing vasculitis, include hydralazine, quinidine, thiouracils and various biological agents.

Drugs that may cause skin necrosis or drug-induced purpura are discussed in Chapter 49. It is important to be aware that illicit drugs (especially cocaine and sympathomimetics, such as ephedrine or amphetamines), drug excipients, vaccines (especially influenza and hepatitis B), herbal remedies [10] and food additives can all cause vasculitis, as these may otherwise be overlooked as possible triggers. Cannabis tends to cause an atherosclerosis-like arterial occlusion, mimicking severe peripheral arterial disease [11]. It has been suggested that routine influenza vaccination may lead to an increased number of cases of vasculitis in the target groups for immunization; when this does occur, the vasculitis may be cutaneous or systemic, usually occurs about 2 weeks after the vaccination, and is usually in patients who have had a previous uneventful influenza vaccination [12].

It is always important to consider the possibility of vasculitis in relation to newer drugs, as such reactions may only become apparent during wider use than in clinical trials. This is particularly difficult as some are used for systemic diseases where it may be difficult to distinguish drug-induced vasculitis from vasculitis due to the underlying disease or to other mechanisms (such as infection). Relatively new, or increasingly used, classes of drugs that can cause vasculitis include interferons, retinoids (mainly isotretinoin), leukotriene inhibitors, anti-TNF agents and other monoclonals, and colony stimulating factors. Bortezomib, a proteosome inhibitor used in treatment of haematological malignancies, has been associated with both a Sweet's syndrome-like neutrophilic dermatosis and with leukocytoclastic vasculitis [13]; occurrence of this eruption appears to be associated with a better treatment outcome than in patients who do not develop a rash. Dermatologists need to be aware that anti-TNF agents are not an uncommon cause of skin or systemic vasculitis; one study reported 39 cases during 1 year in France [14].

Mechanisms. Most drug-induced vasculitis is of hypersensitivity type and presumed to be immune complex-mediated; it probably accounts for 10–20% of small vessel cutaneous vasculitis [4]. The evidence for this assumption is often indirect, although sulphonamide crystals have been observed in blood vessel walls [15]. This pattern is provoked by various antibiotics, diuretics, NSAIDs, anticonvulsants, antipsychotics, cardiac drugs such as diltiazem, and others [3,4]. Relatively recent drugs that can cause this pattern include zidovudine, various haemopoietic growth factors and etanercept.

True serum sickness, originally related to use of hyperimmune sera, is rarely seen, although it does occur with protein drugs such as streptokinase and antithymocyte globulin; a serum sickness-like pattern of eruption is more commonly seen, occurring in relation to penicillins or sulphonamides, and less commonly with drugs such as thiouracil, phenytoin (hydantoin) or phenylbutazone.

Any of the other classical Gell and Coombs mechanisms for vasculitis may occur, although the mechanism by which drugs provoke systemic vasculitis is often less clear than in the immune complex pattern. In some instances, such as leukotriene antagonists administered for asthma 'causing' CSS (Chapter 62), there is

Table 50.8 Some causes of drug-induced vasculitis and the patterns of vasculitis they most commonly provoke.

Type of drug or organ targeted	Examples
Antibiotics/anti-infection	Penicillins, sulphonamides, quinolones, cephalosporins, minocycline, clindamycin, vancomycin, macrolides, rifampicin, isoniazid, imidazoles, griseofulvin, zidovudine, didanosine, efavirenz, mefloquine
	(all usually cause CLV ± SV; penicillins are also the commonest cause of SSLR; cephalosporins may also cause HSP or AASV; ciprofloxacin may also cause AASV; minocycline can cause CLV, AASV/C-PAN and LELS)
Antithyroid	Propylthiouracil; less frequently carbimazole or methimazole (LCV, AASV/MPA)
Rheumatological	NSAIDs (including cycloxygenase-2 inhibitors) (CLV, SV)
	Allopurinol (CLV, AASV)
	Penicillamine (AASV); sulphasalazine (CLV, AASV)
Cardiac	Anticoagulant/antiplatelet: aspirin (CLV); streptokinase (SS, CLV); warfarin (coumadin)(CLV ± SV); heparin (CLV)
	Diuretics (thiazides, furosemide, metolazone) (CLV ± SV; thiazides can cause AASV)
	Antiarrhythmics: amiodarone (CLV), quinidine (CLV ± SV)
	Antihypertensives: hydralazine (CLV, AASV, LELS); calcium channel blockers (CLV, SV); beta-blockers (CLV ± SV)
Neurological and psychiatry	Anticonvulsants: hydantoins, carbamazepine, most others (CLV ± SV; phenytoin reported to cause AASV)
	Phenothiazines, several antidepressants (CLV ± SV)
Oncology	Cytarabine, dacarbazine, gemcitabine, others (CLV ± SV)
Immunosuppressives and related agents	Ciclosporin (AASV, CV); azathioprine, methotrexate, busulphan, cyclophosphamide, melphalan, gold, tacrolimus, dapsone (all CLV ± SV)
Monoclonals	Anti-TNF agents (CLV, SV, HSP, AASV); rituximab (CVL,SV), bortezomib (CLV); colony stimulating factors (CLV); interferons (CLV, AASV, LELS); omalizumab (CSS)
Illicit drugs	Amphetamines/ecstasy, ephedrine, cocaine, heroin (CLV; cocaine causes AASV; cannabis causes atherosclerosis-like arterial occlusion; many may cause cerebral vasospasm or frank CV also)
Vaccines	Influenza (most cases), hepatitis B, hepatitis A, rubella, measles, MMR, pneumococcus, BCG, tetanus/DPT, rabies, smallpox (mostly CLV ± SV; influenza vaccine may also cause MPA; rabies vaccine may cause SS; hepatitis B vaccine may cause AASV/PAN/C-PAN, HSP, UV, CryoV, KD)
Miscellaneous	Warfarin (coumadin), quinine, potassium iodide and iodinated radiocontrast media (all CLV ± SV)
	Leukotriene inhibitors (AASV, CSS)
	Retinoids (CLV ± SV; PAN; AASV; pulmonary capillaritis)

AASV, ANCA-associated systemic vasculitis; CLV, cutaneous leukocytoclastic vasculitis; C-PAN, cutaneous polyarteritis nodosa; CryoV, cryoglobulinaemic vasculitis; CSS, Churg–Strauss syndrome; CV, cerebral vasculitis; DPT, diphtheria–pertussis–tetanus; HSP, Henoch–Schönlein purpura; KD, Kawasaki disease; LELS, LE-like syndrome; MMR, mumps–measles–rubella; MPA, microscopic polyangiitis; NSAIDs, non-steroidal anti-inflammatory drugs; PAN, polyarteritis nodosa; SS, serum sickness; SSLR, serum sickness-like reaction; SV, systemic vasculitis.

an argument that the asthma may simply have been an early feature of CSS and that the drug is not relevant. However, ANCA-positive (particularly MPO-positive) vasculitis has been convincingly linked with drugs such as hydralazine (which may also cause small vessel leukocytoclastic vasculitis) and thiouracils, and less commonly with penicillamine, allopurinol, minocycline and sulfasalazine [16–18]. Glomerulonephritis may occur related to propylthiouracil-induced ANCA-positive vasculitis, although in general internal involvement is relatively mild in ANCA-positive drug-induced vasculitis.

Drug-induced lupus erythematosus is discussed in Chapter 51; drug-induced neutrophilic dermatoses are discussed later in this chapter.

Pathology. A small vessel vasculitis with a lymphocytic infiltrate and little leukocytoclasia, or the presence of some degree of tissue eosinophilia, are suggestive of the possibility of drug-induced vasculitis. Although none of these is sensitive or specific, tissue eosinophilia was significantly greater in drug-induced cases of CSVV than in non-drug-related cases [19] and should arouse suspicion of a drug-induced vasculitis, especially in the absence of systemic symptoms and if ANCA are negative. Serum com-

plement levels are generally normal. ANCA may be positive (see above).

Clinical features. Drug-induced leukocytoclastic vasculitis presents with palpable purpura, petechiae, necrosis and urticarial lesions, indistinguishable from other causes of this pattern of vasculitis.

In the serum sickness-like reaction, the initial rash may be acral, with urticaria or purpura, followed by more generalized annular urticarial lesions. There may be fever, arthralgia, haematuria or proteinuria, lymphadenopathy and decreased complement levels.

Medium and large vessel vasculitides mimic the patterns described elsewhere in this chapter, although there may be atypical features such as eosinophilia or the fact that all lesions appear to be of similar duration. Some drug-induced cases resembling CSS have relatively minor respiratory symptoms compared with the idiopathic condition.

Diagnosis. Generally, drug-induced vasculitis is indistinguishable clinically from the same clinical picture occurring due to other causes. This is particularly the case in CSVV or leukocytoclastic vasculitis with systemic involvement. Timing of the eruption in relation to starting a new drug may be informative, especially if the drug is only administered once (such as vasculitis due to streptokinase, which occurs early after administration). However, in some instances, such as vasculitis due to diuretics, onset may be delayed for several months.

Eosinophilia may be a useful guide. Blood eosinophilia is found in almost 80% of patients with drug-induced systemic vasculitis, but in less than a quarter in whom the reaction is CSVV alone [20]; tissue eosinophilia is also more likely in drug-induced CSVV [19].

ANCA-associated vasculitides generally mimic the primary disease but with less systemic disease, although the differential diagnosis may be difficult, particularly if the cause is concealed, for example when illicit drugs are involved. Cocaine, in particular, is recognized as a cause of systemic vasculitis (notably including cerebral vasculitis), but may also cause facial midline destructive lesions that mimic WG and that cause particular diagnostic problems as over 80% have a positive ANCA (usually P-ANCA, but the pattern may vary even within one individual); a useful distinction is that most ANCA in Wegener's granulomatosis is directed against PR3 and sometimes MPO, whereas patients with cocaine-induced midline destructive lesions do not have MPO-ANCA, and even if they also have a PR3-ANCA, they have ANCA against human neutrophil elastase (human leukocyte elastase, HLE) which is not a specificity seen in WG [21,22]. Drug causes for ANCA-associated systemic vasculitides should be considered if there are multiple ANCA specificities or anti-HLE, rather than the more usual anti-MPO or anti-PR3 ANCA of the main differential diagnoses; for example, minocycline has been linked with MPO, HLE, cathepsin G, bactericidal permeability-increasing protein ANCA as well as with antihistone and anticardiolipin antibodies [7].

Treatment. Stopping any suspect drug is important and may be all that is required for cutaneous vasculitis. In cases with systemic disease, corticosteroids and even other immunosuppressive agents may be necessary. Supportive treatment such as compression hosiery may be required as in other forms of small vessel vasculitis. Renal function and urinalysis should be monitored.

In most instances, the causative drug should not be used again. It is also important to be aware of possible cross-reactions (notably between diuretics) when substituting a different drug.

References

1 Bruinsma W. *A Guide to Drug Eruptions*. Amsterdam: Excerpta Medica, 1973: 51–4.
2 Bork K. *Cutaneous Side-Effects of Drugs*. Philadelphia: Saunders, 1988: 152–5.
3 Ball GV, Bridges SL. Pathogenesis of vasculitis. In: Ball GV, Bridges SL, eds. *Vasculitis*. Oxford: Oxford University Press, 2002: 34–52.
4 Dubost JJ, Souteyrand P, Sauvezie B. Drug-induced vasculitides. *Baillières Clin Rheumatol* 1991; **5**: 119–38.
5 Litt JZ. *Drug Eruption Reference Manual*, 12th edn. London: Taylor and Francis, 2006: 655–6.
6 Merkel PA. Drug-induced vasculitis. *Rheum Dis Clin N Am* 2001; **27**: 849–62.
7 Wiik A. Drug-induced vasculitis. *Curr Opin Rheumatol* 2008; **20**: 35–9.
8 Doyle MK, Cuellar ML. Drug-induced vasculitis. *Expert Opin Drug Saf* 2003; **2**: 401–9.
9 Del Rosso A, Generini S, Pignone A, Matucci-Cerinic M. Vasculitides secondary to systemic diseases. *Clin Dermatol* 1999; **17**: 533–47.
10 Ingraffea A, Donohue K, Wilkel C, Falanga V. Cutaneous vasculitis in two patients taking an herbal supplement containing black cohosh. *J Am Acad Dermatol* 2007; **56**: S124–6.
11 Noel B, Ruf I, Pannizon RG. Cannabis arteritis. *J Am Acad Dermatol* 2008; **58** (Suppl. 1): S65–7.
12 Tavadia S, Drummond A, Evans CD, Wainwright HJ. Leukocytoclastic vasculitis and influenza vaccination. *Clin Exp Dermatol*; **28**: 154–6.
13 Garcia-Navarro X, Puig L, Fernández-Figueras MT *et al.* Bortezomib-associated cutaneous vasculitis. *Br J Dermatol* 2007; **157**: 799–801.
14 Saint Marcoux B, de Bandt M. Vasculitides induced by TNF alpha antagonists: a study in 39 patients in France. *Joint Bone Spine* 2006; **73**: 710–3.
15 Mullick FG, McAllister HA, Wagner BM, Fenoglio JJ. Drug related vasculitis: clinicopathologic correlations in 30 patients. *Hum Pathol* 1979; **10**: 313–25.
16 Choi HK, Merkel PA, Walker AM, Niles JL. Drug-associated antineutrophil cytoplasmic antibody-positive vasculitis: prevalence among patients with high titers of antimyeloperoxidase antibodies. *Arthritis Rheum* 2000; **43**: 405–13.
17 Merkel PA. Drugs associated with vasculitis. *Curr Opin Rheumatol* 1998; **10**: 45–50.
18 Aloush V, Litinsky I, Caspi D, Elkayam O. Propylthiouracil-induced autoimmune syndromes: two distinct clinical presentations with different course and management. *Semin Arthritis Rheum* 2006; **36**: 4–9.
19 Bahrami S, Malone JC, Webb KG, Callen JP. Tissue eosinophilia as an indicator of drug-induced cutaneous small-vessel vasculitis. *Arch Dermatol* 2006; **142**: 155–61.
20 Fiorentino DF. Cutaneous vasculitis. *J Am Acad Dermatol* 2003; **48**: 311–40.
21 Molloy ES, Langford CA. Vasculitis mimics. *Curr Opin Rheumatol* 2008; **20**: 29–34.
22 Wiesner O, Russell KA, Lee AS *et al.* Antineutrophil cytoplasmic antibodies reacting with human neutrophil elastase as a diagnostic marker for cocaine-induced midline destructive lesions but not autoimmune vasculitis. *Arthritis Rheum* 2004; **50**: 2954–65.

Henoch–Schönlein purpura

Synonyms
- IgA immune complex vasculitis
- Anaphylactoid purpura
- Purpura rheumatoide

Definition. Originally described as a tetrad of palpable purpura, arthritis, gastrointestinal involvement and renal glomerular involvement [1,2], HSP is defined by the Chapel Hill Consensus Conference as a vasculitis affecting small vessels, involving deposition of IgA immune complexes, that characteristically involves the skin, gastrointestinal system and glomeruli with or without arthralgia or arthritis [3]. Unfortunately, many literature reports have previously assumed that all cutaneous small vessel vasculitis in children is HSP, rather than insisting on confirmed presence of IgA immune complexes, which causes great confusion. This has been addressed by the EULAR/PReS consensus [4], although some cases are acceptable in which IgA is not demonstrated (presumed to reflect delayed biopsy with destruction of immunoreactants). Although it can occur in adults, HSP is much more common in childhood; 75% of cases occur in children under 6 years old and 90% in children under 10 years old [5–9]. Furthermore, HSP occurs in various racial and ethnic groups [9–11].

History and nomenclature. Heberden first described HSP in 1801, in a young boy with abdominal pain, emesis, bloody stools, arthritis and a purpuric eruption. The eponymous term Henoch–Schönlein purpura was later applied after Johann Schönlein and Eduard Henoch described features of the vasculitis in the mid-19th century.

Aetiology and pathogenesis [9,12]. Some infections, such as those caused by Group A β-haemolytic streptococci, are implicated in the cause of HSP, although evidence for streptococcal infection is only found in approximately 30% of children [8] (the range from different studies is about 20–50% [12]). Additionally, although other pathogens have been implicated (including *Bartonella henselae*, parvovirus B19, *Staphylococcus aureus*, coxsackieviruses, adenovirus, hepatitis A and B viruses), a triggering pathogen is not found in the majority of cases. Seasonal outbreaks have been described. The demonstration of nephritis-associated plasmin receptor NAPlr, a Group A streptococcal antigen, in renal mesangial vessels of children with HSP-associated nephritis (discussed earlier, p. 50.5) suggests a causative role for streptococci in at least some cases.

IgA is thought to play a pivotal part in the pathogenesis of HSP, as increased levels of IgA in the serum (in 50% with active disease), increased circulating immune complexes containing IgA, and increased deposition of IgA in blood vessel walls and in the renal mesangium are associated with HSP. In patients with HSP, IgA1 rather than IgA2 is the main IgA subclass deposited in the skin lesions [12,13]. Diminished glycosylation of the proline-rich hinge region of the IgA1 heavy chain is thought to be an important factor in allowing the IgA to be deposited in the mesangium and to activate the alternative pathway of complement in IgA, as it makes such IgA1 molecules more prone to forming macromolecular complexes [8,9].

Other IgA antibodies that occur in HSP include IgA ANCA, although this finding is very variable between studies. IgA rheumatoid factor and IgA anticardiolipin antibodies are also sometimes present, as are IgA AECA.

Activation of several cytokines is documented, although it is difficult to determine if any are a primary cause. TNF-α levels are increased, and TNF-α can be detected in skin lesions; IL-6, IL-8, transforming growth factor-beta (TGF-β) and vascular endothelial growth factor (VEGF) levels are all increased in active HSP. TGF-β is of particular interest as blood levels of T cells that produce this cytokine are increased in HSP, and it is known to enhance IgA1 responses. Neutrophil activation, elevated nitric oxide levels, reactive oxygen species and increased urinary leukotriene are all documented.

Familial clustering has been reported, which may support an infectious aetiology; however, various polymorphisms that either increase risk of HSP or are associated with more severe renal disease have been described and would also explain familial HSP (examples include polymorphisms in TGF-β, IL-1β, IL-8 and VEGF).

Histopathology. Biopsy specimens of the purpuric lesions demonstrate leukocytoclastic vasculitis affecting capillaries and post-capillary venules. Direct immunofluorescence microscopy of lesional and perilesional skin reveals deposition of IgA, C3 and fibrin in dermal blood vessel walls.

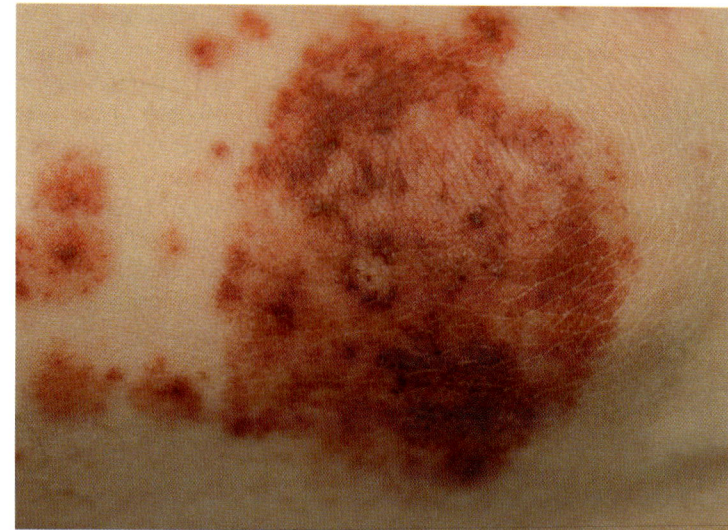

Fig. 50.7 Henoch-Schönlein purpura, with typical retiform pattern.

Clinical features. Most commonly, HSP manifests at the outset with the classic findings of purpura, arthralgia and abdominal pain [8–10]. The cutaneous findings are typically erythematous urticarial papules, which may evolve within 24 h into palpable purpura with haemorrhage. Furthermore, urticaria, vesicles, bullae and necrotic ulcers may develop. A retiform pattern within lesions is characteristic, but not necessarily present (Fig. 50.7). Typically involving the extensor aspects of the limbs (especially elbows and knees) and buttocks in a symmetrical fashion, HSP may also affect the trunk and face. Usually fading within 5–7 days, crops of lesions can recur for a few weeks to several months. Although HSP is chronic in 5–10% of patients, the cutaneous involvement usually lasts between 6 and 16 weeks and then subsides. Rarely, gastrointestinal involvement and arthritis can occur in the absence of skin disease. Renal involvement with HSP is common, occurring in approximately 40–50% of patients; 25% have gross haematuria and the remainder microscopic haematuria [9]. Proteinuria occurs in 60% of these, but is uncommon in the absence of haematuria. Only 1–3% of these patients progress to end-stage renal disease, although one-third to half of patients have renal abnormalities on long-term follow-up [9,14]. Furthermore, gastrointestinal involvement is common (65%), with frank gastrointestinal bleeding in 30% of patients with HSP [9]. Painful arthritis is seen in about 75% of patients, most frequently affecting the knees and ankles. Less common manifestations of HSP include orchitis (in 10–20% of boys), intussusception, pancreatitis, neurological abnormalities, uveitis, carditis and pulmonary haemorrhage [9].

Diagnosis. HSP is a clinical diagnosis, with confirmation by direct immunofluorescence and routine histology. Perivascular IgA deposits are characteristic of HSP and can help to distinguish it from other vasculitides including CSVV, WG, CSS and MPA. IgA immune complexes are not specific to HSP, but can be seen in a variety of patients including those with SLE, endocarditis, dermatitis herpetiformis, alcoholism, IgA nephropathy, inflammatory bowel disease, ankylosing spondylitis, Sjögren's syndrome, rheumatoid arthritis, some cancers and in some drug hypersensitivity reactions [15–18]. No laboratory tests are specific for HSP.

Treatment. HSP is frequently self-limiting, the majority of patients fully recovering within several weeks or months, so treatment is mainly supportive. Although no data demonstrate the effectiveness of systemic corticosteroids in treating purpura, shortening the duration of HSP or decreasing the frequency of recurrences, they have been shown in a randomized controlled study to be effective in the treatment of abdominal pain and arthritis, and accelerated resolution of mild nephritis [19] (the dose was 1 mg/kg/day for 2 weeks, tapering over a further 2 weeks).

Dapsone (100 mg once daily) seems to shorten the duration of HSP as well as having a beneficial effect on the cutaneous lesions [6]. One trial proposed that factor XIII replacement may be useful in the treatment of abdominal pain and gastrointestinal bleeding associated with HSP [20], and another small trial demonstrated a decrease in the duration and severity of abdominal pain, as well as a decreased bleeding risk, with the use of ranitidine [21].

The presence of renal disease is the major factor determining the long-term morbidity and mortality associated with HSP [7,9]. Although no controlled trials have been conducted, data from several studies, as well as a case series, suggest a benefit from high-dose corticosteroids, either alone [19,22] or with cyclophosphamide and dipyridamole [23–25] in patients with progressive renal involvement associated with HSP. Ciclosporin and azathioprine have both been used [9], and case reports suggest that gastrointestinal involvement and cutaneous disease may be lessened, and rapidly progressive nephritis may be halted, by the use of intravenous immunoglobulin [26,27]. Patients with severe nephritis, including nephritic syndrome, have poor short-term and long-term outlook compared with those with milder disease; severe nephritis is typically treated with high-dose methylprednisolone at a dosage of 30 mg/kg once daily for 3 days followed by oral corticosteroids and an immunosuppressive drug such as azathioprine or cyclophosphamide [6]. NSAIDs have minimal, if any, benefit in the treatment of HSP, and should not be used in patients with renal involvement. For the cutaneous lesions, the therapeutic ladder presented for cutaneous small vessel vasculitis is also applicable for patients with HSP.

References

1 Henoch E. Uber ein eigentümliche Form von Purpura. *Berl Munch Tierarztl Wochenschr* 1874; **11**: 641–3.

2 Schönlein H. *Allgemeine und Specielle Pathologie und Therapie*, 3rd edn. Wurzburg: Herisau, 1837.

3 Jennette JC, Falk RG, Andrassy K *et al*. Nomenclature of systemic vasculitides. Proposal of an international consensus conference. *Arthritis Rheum* 1994; **37**: 187–92.

4 Ozen S, Ruperto N, Dillon MJ *et al*. EULAR/PReS endorsed consensus criteria for the classification of childhood vasculitides. *Ann Rheum Dis* 2006; **65**: 936–41.

5 Blanco R, Martinez-Taboada VM, Rodriguez-Valverde V, Garcia-Fuentes M. Cutaneous vasculitis in children and adults: associated diseases and aetiologic factors in 303 patients. *Medicine* 1998; **77**: 403–18.

6 Saulsbury FT. Henoch–Schönlein purpura in children: report of 100 patients and review of the literature. *Medicine* 1999; **78**: 395–409.

7 Calvino MC, Llorca J, Garcia-Porrua C *et al*. Henoch–Schönlein purpura in children from northwestern Spain: a 20-year epidemiologic and clinical study. *Medicine* 2001; **80**: 279–90.

8 Trapani S, Micheli A, Grisolia F *et al*. Henoch–Schonlein purpura in childhood: epidemiological and clinical analysis of 150 cases over a 5-year period and review of literature. *Semin Arthritis Rheum* 2005; **35**: 143–53.

9 Saulsbury FT. Clinical update: Henoch–Schönlein purpura. *Lancet* 2007; **369**: 976–8.

10 Blanco R, Martinez-Taboada VM, Rodriguez-Valverde V *et al*. Henoch–Schönlein purpura in adulthood and childhood: two different expressions of the same syndrome. *Arthritis Rheum* 1997; **40**: 859–64.

11 Mills JA, Michel BA, Bloch DA *et al*. The American College of Rheumatology 1990 criteria for the classification of Henoch–Schönlein purpura. *Arthritis Rheum* 1990; **33**: 1114–21.

12 Yang Y-H, Chuang Y-H, Wang L-C *et al*. The immunobiology of Henoch–Schönlein purpura. *Autoimm Rev* 2008; **7**: 179–84.

13 Egan CA, Taylor TB, Meyer LJ *et al*. IgA1 is the major IgA subclass in cutaneous blood vessels in Henoch–Schönlein purpura. *Br J Dermatol* 1999; **141**: 859–62.

14 Ronkainen J, Nuutinen M, Koskimies O. The adult kidney 24 years after childhood Henoch-Schönlein purpura: a retrospective cohort study. *Lancet* 2002; **360**: 666–70.

15 Saklayen MG, Schroeter AL, Nafz MA, Jalil K. IgA deposition in the skin of patients with alcoholic liver disease. *J Cutan Pathol* 1996; **23**: 12–8.

16 Swerdlow MA, Chowdhury LN, Mishra V, Kavin H. IgA deposits in the skin in alcoholic liver disease. *J Am Acad Dermatol* 1983; **9**: 232–6.

17 Thompson AJ, Chan YL, Woodroffe AJ *et al*. Vascular IgA deposits in clinically normal skin of patients with renal disease. *Pathology* 1980; **12**: 407–13.

18 Magro CM, Crowson AN. The cutaneous neutrophilic vascular injury syndromes: a review. *Semin Diagn Pathol* 2001; **18**: 47–58.

19 Ronkainen J, Koskimies O, Ala-Houhala M *et al*. Early prednisone therapy in Henoch-Schönlein purpura: a randomized, double–blind, placebo-controlled trial. *J Pediatr* 2006; **149**: 241–7.

20 Fukui H, Kamitsuji H, Nagao T *et al*. Clinical evaluation of a pasteurized factor XIII concentrate administration in Henoch–Schönlein purpura. *Jpn Pediatr Group* 1989; **56**: 667–75.

21 Narin N, Akcoral A, Aslin MI, Elmastas H. Ranitidine administration in Henoch–Schönlein vasculitis. *Acta Paediatr Jpn* 1995; **37**: 37–9.

22 Niaudet P, Habib R. Methylprednisolone pulse therapy in the treatment of severe forms of Schönlein–Henoch purpura nephritis. *Pediatr Nephrol* 1995; **12**: 238–43.

23 Oner A, Tinaztepe K, Erdogan O. The effect of triple therapy on rapidly progressive type of Henoch–Schönlein nephritis. *Pediatr Nephrol* 1995; **9**: 6–10.

24 Iijima K, Ito-Kariya S, Nakamura H, Yoshikawa N. Multiple combined therapy for severe Henoch–Schönlein nephritis in children. *Pediatr Nephrol* 1998; **12**: 244–8.

25 Flynn JT, Smoyer WE, Bunchman TE *et al*. Treatment of Henoch–Schönlein purpura glomerulonephritis in children with high-dose corticosteroids plus cyclophosphamide. *Am J Nephrol* 2001; **21**: 128–33.

26 Lamireau T, Rebouissoux L, Hehunstre JP. Intravenous immunoglobulin therapy for severe digestive manifestations of Henoch–Schönlein purpura. *Acta Paediatr* 2001; **90**: 1081–2.

27 Rostoker G, Desvaux-Belghiti D, Pilatte Y *et al*. High dose immunoglobulin therapy for severe IgA nephropathy and Henoch–Schönlein purpura. *Ann Intern Med* 1994; **120**: 476–84.

Urticarial vasculitis

Synonyms
- Chronic urticarial lesions as a manifestation of venulitis
- Unusual systemic lupus erythematosus-like syndrome
- Hypocomplementaemic vasculitis
- Hypocomplementaemic–urticaria–vasculitis syndrome (HUVS)

Definition. Of patients with chronic urticaria, roughly 5–10% have urticarial vasculitis (UV) [1,2]. This is a chronic disease, which presents as urticarial lesions that most often occur on the trunk or proximal limbs, frequently with associated angio-oedema

[3]. Lesions differ from those of simple urticaria in that individual lesions persist for greater than 24 h, often demonstrate purpura and post-inflammatory pigmentation, and cause symptoms of burning. Two types of UV have been described: UV associated with hypocomplementaemia, and UV without associated hypo-complementaemia (normocomplementaemic UV). Hypocomplementaemic UV is defined by the presence of anti-C1q precipitin and/or a decrease in the level of C1 [2,4]. Although all patients with hypocomplementaemic UV have these antibodies, this process must be distinguished from SLE, which can show similar laboratory findings [5,6]. Urticarial vasculitis may be described as a continuum starting with patients who have only skin lesions, progressing to patients with skin lesions and hypocomplementae-mia, and finally to those who meet the criteria for SLE. UV without hypocomplementaemia has a slight female predominance, whereas hypocomplementaemic UV is seen almost exclusively in female patients.

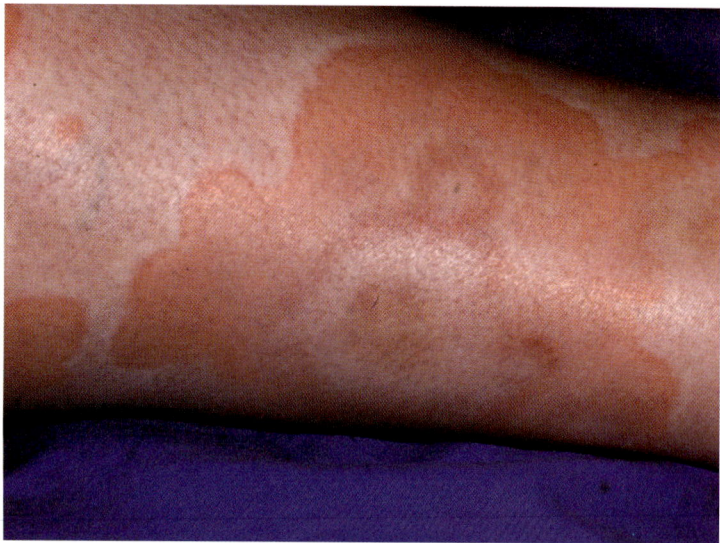

Fig. 50.8 Urticarial vasculitis.

History and nomenclature. Agnello *et al.* [7] first discussed UV, which was later described as a syndrome consisting of hypocom-plementaemia, cutaneous vasculitis and arthritis by McDuffie *et al.* [8].

Aetiology and pathogenesis. UV is strongly associated with some connective tissue diseases, having a prevalence of 32% in patients with Sjögren's syndrome and 20% in patients with SLE [1]. Other associations include physical urticarias, hepatitis B or C, IgM or IgA gammopathies, serum sickness, colonic cancer and drug ingestion. Some cases of UV have been reported in association with exercise or with exposure to ultraviolet light and cold. UV is thought to represent a type III hypersensitivity reaction, as circulating immune complexes may be demonstrated in up to 75% of patients [9]. Complement and immunoreactant deposition in vessel walls, with complement cascade activation in patients with UV [10], further supports this theory. Additionally, removal of immune complexes via plasmapheresis has been shown to briefly alleviate some symptoms of UV [11]. In hypocomplementaemic UV, autoantibodies are directed against the collagen-like region of C1q, resulting in a reduction of C1q in the serum with subsequent activation of the complement pathway [12].

Histopathology [13–16]. Lesions of UV are typically viewed as showing a leukocytoclastic vasculitis; hypocomplementaemic UV shows a large number of interstitial neutrophils, rather than eosinophils, and may therefore be distinguished from normocom-plementaemic UV [13,14]. However, a recent prospective study of 22 patients suggested that a leukocytoclastic vasculitis was only present in the minority, most having a lymphocyte-predominant infiltrate with an admixture of eosinophils [17]. The neutrophilic group had more resistant disease, and had a statistical association with leukocytoclasis, fibrin deposition, hypocomplementaemia and anaemia. The significance of this is uncertain—many collagen vascular diseases (with which UV is associated) may cause cutane-ous lymphocytic vasculitis (p. 50.47), and the general view that UV is characterized by leukocytoclastic vasculitis may reflect a group of patients with more systemic features and greater likelihood of having a skin biopsy. However, it appears that some

cases, especially of normocomplementaemic type, may have a lymphocytic vasculitis.

Clinical features. Cutaneous lesions of both the hypocomplemen-taemic and normocomplementaemic forms of UV are erythema-tous indurated weals that may contain purpuric foci (Fig. 50.8). Angio-oedema and macular erythema may also occur; livedo reticularis, nodules and bullae may be evident, and may also contain purpuric foci. Patients with the hypocomplementaemic form may have constitutional symptoms such as fever, malaise and myalgia, as well as other symptoms and signs including lymphadenopathy, hepatosplenomegaly, abdominal pain with or without nausea and/or diarrhoea, laryngeal oedema, dyspnoea, chronic obstructive pulmonary disease (COPD), glomerulonephri-tis, conjunctivitis, uveitis and episcleritis. Although hypocomple-mentaemic UV has features similar to SLE, signs such as ocular inflammation, angio-oedema and COPD distinguish the two processes.

Diagnosis. If urticarial lesions last for longer than 24 h (which can be determined by drawing around their margin), then by defini-tion they are not ordinary urticaria and a skin biopsy should be performed. Pain rather than itch, or the presence of purpura, also suggest UV. History, physical examination and laboratory studies, including C3, C4 and antinuclear antibody (ANA), should help to establish the extent of disease and to exclude underlying disease (e.g. hepatitis C), and to evaluate for SLE. Some patients may demonstrate an elevated erythrocyte sedimentation rate (ESR), hypocomplementaemia, a low-titre positive ANA and haematuria. A biopsy must be performed to confirm the diagnosis and to exclude other disorders such as atypical erythema multiforme.

Treatment. Although no single treatment is effective for all cases of UV, the majority of patients respond to systemic corticosteroids. However, other agents should be considered as steroid-sparing therapies [15,16,18]. Drugs that have been shown to be effective for the treatment of UV include dapsone (100–200 mg once daily), colchicine (0.6 mg twice to three times daily) and hydroxychloroquine (200 mg once to twice daily) [19–23]. Dapsone plus pentoxifylline (400 mg three times daily) has been used in one patient [24], and mycophenolate mofetil (2 g once daily) has been successfully tried as a maintenance therapy in two other patients [25]. Some patients require oral antihistamines for control of angio-oedema and urticaria-like lesions, in addition to the aforementioned therapies directed at the vasculitis.

References

1 Black AK. Urticarial vasculitis. *Clin Dermatol* 1999; **17**: 565–9.
2 Wisnieski JJ. Urticarial vasculitis. *Curr Opin Rheumatol* 2000; **12**: 24–31.
3 Stone JH, Nousari HC. 'Essential' cutaneous vasculitis: what every rheumatologist should know about vasculitis of the skin. *Curr Opin Rheumatol* 2001; **13**: 23–34.
4 Wisnieski JJ, Baer AN, Christensen J *et al*. Hypocomplementemic urticarial vasculitis syndrome: clinical and serologic findings in 18 patients. *Medicine* 1995; **74**: 24–41.
5 Wisnieski JJ, Jones SM. IgG autoantibody to the collagen-like region of C1q in hypocomplementemic urticarial vasculitis syndrome, systemic lupus erythematosus, and six other musculoskeletal or rheumatic diseases. *J Rheumatol* 1992; **19**: 884–8.
6 Wener MH, Uwatoko S, Mannik M. Antibodies to the collagen-like region of C1q in sera of patients with autoimmune rheumatic diseases. *Arthritis Rheum* 1989; **32**: 544–51.
7 Agnello B, Koffler D, Eisenberg JW *et al*. C1q precipitins in the sera of patients with systemic lupus erythematosus and other hypocomplementemic states: characterization of high and low molecular weight types. *J Exp Med* 1971; **134** (Suppl.): 228S.
8 McDuffie FC, Sams WM Jr, Maldonado JE. Hypocomplementemia with cutaneous vasculitis and arthritis: possible immune complex syndrome. *Mayo Clin Proc* 1973; **48**: 340–8.
9 Berg RE, Kantor GR, Bergfeld WF. Urticarial vasculitis. *Int J Dermatol* 1988; **27**: 468–72.
10 Mehregan DR, Gibson LE. Pathophysiology of urticarial vasculitis. *Arch Dermatol* 1998; **134**: 88–9.
11 Russell Jones R, Bhogal B, Dash A, Schifferli J. Urticaria and vasculitis: a continuum of histopathological and immunological changes. *Br J Dermatol* 1983; **108**: 695–703.
12 Wisnieski JJ, Jones SM. Comparison of autoantibodies to the collagen-like region of C1q in hypocomplementemic urticarial vasculitis syndrome and systemic lupus erythematosus. *J Immunol* 1992; **148**: 1396–403.
13 Sanchez NP, Van Hale HM, Su WP. Clinical and histopathologic spectrum of necrotizing vasculitis: report of findings in 101 cases. *Arch Dermatol* 1985; **121**: 220–4.
14 Davis MD, Daoud MS, Kirby B, Gibson LE, Rogers RS III. Clinicopathologic correlation of hypocomplementemic and normocomplementaemic urticarial vasculitis. *J Am Acad Dermatol* 1998; **38**: 899–905.
15 Mehregan DR, Hall MJ, Gibson LE. Urticarial vasculitis: a histopathologic and clinical review of 72 cases. *J Am Acad Dermatol* 1992; **26**: 441–8.
16 Sanchez NP, Winkelmann RK, Schroeter AL, Dicken CH. The clinical and histopathologic spectrums of urticarial vasculitis: study of 40 cases. *J Am Acad Dermatol* 1982; **7**: 599–605.
17 Lee JSS, Loh TH, Seow SC, Tat SH. Prolonged urticaria with purpura: the spectrum of clinical and histopathologic features in a prospective series of 22 patients exhibiting the clinical features of urticarial vasculitis. *J Am Acad Dermatol* 2007; **56**: 994–1005.
18 Worm M, Muche M, Schulze P *et al*. Hypocomplementaemic urticarial vasculitis: successful treatment with cyclophosphamide-dexamethasone pulse therapy. *Br J Dermatol* 1998; **139**: 704–7.
19 Fortson JS, Zone JJ, Hammond ME, Groggel GC. Hypocomplementemic urticarial vasculitis syndrome response to dapsone. *J Am Acad Dermatol* 1986; **15**: 1137–42.
20 Eiser AR, Singh P, Shanies HM. Sustained dapsone-induced remission of hypocomplementemic urticarial vasculitis: a case report. *Angiology* 1997; **48**: 1019–22.
21 Wiles JC, Hansen RC, Lynch PJ. Urticarial vasculitis treated with colchicine. *Arch Dermatol* 1985; **121**: 802–5.
22 Werni R, Schwarz T, Gschnait G. Colchicine treatment of urticarial vasculitis. *Dermatologica* 1986; **172**: 36–40.
23 Lopez LR, Davis KC, Kohler PF, Schocket AL. The hypocomplementemic urticarial–vasculitis syndrome: therapeutic response to hydroxychloroquine. *J Allergy Clin Immunol* 1984; **73**: 600–3.
24 Nurnberg W, Grabbe J, Czarnetzki BM. Urticarial vasculitis syndrome effectively treated with dapsone and pentoxifylline. *Acta Derm Venereol* 1995; **75**: 54–6.
25 Worm M, Sterry W, Kolde G. Mycophenolate mofetil is effective for maintenance therapy of hypocomplementaemic urticarial vasculitis [letter; comment]. *Br J Dermatol* 2000; **143**: 1324.

Exercise-induced vasculitis

This is probably an underestimated condition, several series of ten or more cases having been reported [1–3]. Although also described as exercise-induced purpura [4], the histological features are those of a leukocytoclastic vasculitis with variable deposition of IgM and complement C3 [1]. The typical presentation is with purpuric lesions on the lower legs after prolonged walking (many descriptions are in golfers, marathon runners or long-distance walkers), usually in hot weather. Lesions may be urticarial, plaques, palpable purpura or petechial. Compressed areas, such as the tops of socks, may be spared [4]. Patients are generally middle-aged, and otherwise well with no evidence of venous disease; there is a strong female predominance.

Extrinsic causes such as insect bites, reactions to socks or allergies to grass or ground plants may be suspected if the condition is not known. The disorder has a relapsing course, but patients may prevent it occurring as some know how much walking is likely to provoke the eruption. Treatments have included compression hosiery, manual lymphatic drainage, diuretics, or steroids (local or systemic) [4].

In cases with urticarial vasculitis provoked by exercise, eosinophils predominate in early lesions, with a neutrophilic infiltrate and leukocytoclastic vasculitis subsequently [5]. As CSVV of several aetiologies, and HSP, are often aggravated by exercise, it has been suggested that the pathogenesis of exercise-induced urticarial vasculitis lesions might be extrapolated to other leukocytoclastic vasculitides [6].

References

1 Prins M, Veraart JC, Vermeulen AH *et al*. Leucocytoclastic vasculitis induced by prolonged exercise. *Br J Dermatol* 1996; **134**: 915–8.
2 Kelly RI, Opie J, Nixon R. Golfer's vasculitis. *Australas J Dermatol* 2005; **46**: 11–4.
3 Ramelet AA. Exercise-induced vasculitis. *J Eur Acad Dermatol Venereol* 2006; **20**: 423–7.
4 Ramelet AA. Exercise-induced purpura. *Dermatology (Basel)* 2004; **208**: 293–6.
5 Kano Y, Orihara M, Shiohara T. Cellular and molecular dynamics in exercise-induced urticarial vasculitis lesions. *Arch Dermatol* 1998; **134**: 62–7.
6 Sais G, Vidaller A. Pathogenesis of exercise-induced urticarial vasculitis lesions: can the changes be extrapolated to all leukocytoclastic vasculitis lesions? *Arch Dermatol* 1999; **135**: 87–9.

Cryoglobulinaemic vasculitis

Definition. A form of vasculitis due to cryoglobulins deposited as immune complexes in types II and III cryoglobulinaemia. Small and medium sized vessels are affected, mainly in skin and kidneys. Not all cryoglobulinaemia is associated with symptoms. Type I cryoglobulinaemia is monoclonal rather than forming immune complexes (therefore causes cryogelling rather than vasculitis), and types II and III cryoglobulinaemia may cause cryogelling as well as an immune complex vasculitis; details of the history, aetiology and pathogenesis of cryoglobulin-associated disease are therefore provided in Chapter 49 and only a brief outline of these aspects is provided here.

Aetiology and pathogenesis. Cryoglobulinaemia as a cause of vasculitis and vascular occlusion is an increasingly recognized condition, largely due to the association between types II and III cryoglobulinaemia with hepatitis C virus infection. Cryoglobulins may be divided into three main subtypes:

I   Monoclonal immunoglobulin, usually IgG or IgM, and usually associated with lymphoproliferative disease, especially multiple myeloma or Waldenström's macroglobulinaemia; accounts for about 10–25% of cases. This is discussed in Chapter 49 and is not considered further here.

II Mixed polyclonal (usually IgG) immunoglobulin and monoclonal (usually IgMκ) immunoglobulin, the latter having rheumatoid factor activity; accounts for about 25% of cases.

III Polyclonal IgM with rheumatoid factor activity and polyclonal IgG with antigenic activity; accounts for about 50–65% of cases.

The causes of cryoglobulinaemia include myeloproliferative disorders, systemic lupus erythematosus and chronic infections; all disease associations are discussed in more detail in Chapter 49, and a more detailed summary of the pathogenesis is provided in [1]. Immune complex vasculitis is limited to types II and III (together termed 'mixed' cryoglobulinaemia). The strongest aetiological factor in mixed cryoglobulinaemia is hepatitis C virus (HCV) infection, which accounts for about 80–90% of cases of what was previously termed 'essential' mixed cryoglobulinaemia; hepatitis G may coexist in about 30% of such cases [2]. However, although mixed cryoglobulinaemia can be detected in about 50% of subjects with HCV, immune complex vasculitis occurs in less than 5% [3]. There is also a strong link between mixed cryoglobulinaemia and connective tissue disorders, especially Sjögren's syndrome, in which cryocrit measurements of cryoglobulins may be indistinguishable from those of patients with HCV [1], and a 35-fold increased frequency of non-Hodgkin's lymphoma [3]. Chronic antigenic stimulation (by hepatitis C or other antigens) is felt to lead to B-cell proliferation, production of IgM with rheumatoid factor activity, mainly monoclonal cryoglobulin production and, in some cases, progression to B-cell non-Hodgkin's lymphoma [1–5]. Various factors are involved in the B-cell stimulation [1]. Especially in type II cryoglobulinaemia there may be t(14:18) translocations in peripheral blood lymphocytes; these activate the proto-oncogene Bcl-2, which increases B-cell survival by inhibiting apoptosis. Additionally, the E2 protein of the HCV envelope binds to CD81 on lymphocytes (and hepatocytes), complexing with CD21, CD19 and Leu 13, again causing B-cell activation [1].

HCV causes both cytotoxic and autoimmune hepatitis, and clonal B-cell expansion occurs in both blood and liver. HCV virions bind to IgG and are then complexed with monoclonal IgM which are deposited in vessel walls as an immune complex, causing complement-mediated vascular damage; HCV RNA sequences have been detected in vessel walls [2]. HCV-related mixed cryoglobulinaemia and/or vasculitis has been linked with HLA-B8, DR3 and DRB1*11 [1,4], and some HCV genotypes are predominant (1, 2, 2A/III) [2].

Histopathology [6]. Mixed cryoglobulinaemia affects capillaries, arterioles and venules, producing a pan-dermal leukocytoclastic vasculitis that may extend into the subcutis. Eosinophilic, PAS-positive, globular cryoglobulin deposits are seen, as well as (PAS-negative) intraluminal and fibrin deposition. More chronic lesions develop a mononuclear-predominant infiltrate and may become granulomatous. Changes in other organs include membranoproliferative glomerulonephritis (in a third of cases), and deposition of immune complexes in lung alveolar vessels (leading to lung fibrosis) and in vasa vasora of nerves (causing peripheral neuropathy).

In the liver, chronic HCV is one of several infections that cause a histological pattern termed a fibrin ring granuloma; it has been suggested that this may be a manifestation of endothelial injury related to immune complex deposition [7].

Clinical features [1,7,8]. Features of immune complex vasculitis predominate over those that relate mainly to cryogelling. Palpable purpura, especially of the lower legs but potentially including the buttocks and trunk, occurs in 60–90% and urticated lesions are common, reminiscent of the skin vasculitis seen in HSP. Worsening of skin lesions after prolonged standing is common, and symptoms are often intermittent initially. Polyarteritis-like dermal nodules may occur in 20%. Raynaud's phenomenon, and cold-aggravation of the vasculitis lesions, are each present in about a third of subjects. Livedo, bullae, necrosis and ulceration are all less common.

Associated glomerulonephritis is common and important. Arthralgia, or migratory myalgia, occurs in most patients. Overt lung involvement is uncommon, but may present as dyspnoea or haemoptysis. Peripheral neuropathy, if present, is predominantly sensory and usually mild.

Diagnosis. It is important to distinguish cryoglobulinaemic vasculitis from other causes of CSVV because corticosteroid therapy, although sometimes necessary short-term, will in the longer term worsen the underlying infection that is present in the majority of cases. Most other causes of leukocytoclastic vasculitis cause a more superficial vasculitis on biopsy specimens, and if cryoglobulin deposits are seen histologically then the diagnosis is usually suspected (although this is much commoner in type I cryoglobulinaemia).

Clinically, head and neck involvement, significant livedo, acrocyanosis, Raynaud's phenomenon or larger vessel occlusion, are all more suggestive of type I cryoglobulinaemia.

Blood tests may be helpful in suggesting this diagnosis [9]. A low complement C4 level is found in 90%, rheumatoid factor is positive in 70% and ANA in 20%, elevated transaminases are found in a third, and some patients (with type II cryoglobulinaemia) will have a monoclonal band on electrophoresis. Obtaining samples for identification of cryoproteins is discussed in Chapter 49. Testing for antibodies to HCV should always be performed.

These factors combined with the clinical picture have been gathered to create possible diagnostic criteria [1]; major criteria include mixed cryoglobulins, purpura and leukocytoclastic vasculitis, with minor clinical features including chronic hepatitis, membranoproliferative glomerulonephritis, peripheral neuropathy and skin ulcers, and minor pathology/serology features including positive rheumatoid factor, HCV or HBV, and clonal B-cell infiltrate of liver or bone marrow.

Treatment. Treatment will depend on the underlying cause. Although most cases of mixed cryoglobulinaemia are HCV-associated, SLE and other autoimmune conditions need to be considered and treated appropriately, and other infections need to be considered as alternative (or, especially in the case of HIV, as coexisting) infections that may also require specific therapy.

The treatment of HCV-associated mixed cryoglobulinaemic vasculitis has recently been reviewed [1,3]. Pegylated interferon-α with ribavirin is the usual initial choice for patients with relatively mild symptoms (purpura, arthralgia, proteinuria without haematuria or casts or abnormal renal function, mild neuropathy); in such patients, immunosuppressive agents can be avoided, or relatively non-aggressive therapy can be used (low-dose corticosteroids, or colchicine). There is some logic in also adding rituximab, as this combination targets the causative HCV infection and the cryoglobulin-producing B cells; using rituximab with antiviral therapy is recommended for those with more severe disease or those with an associated B-cell non-Hodgkin's lymphoma [1]. Treatments with corticosteroids, other immunosuppressive agents (cyclophosphamide, azathioprine, mycophenolate mofetil) and plasmapheresis all have a role in patients with severe membranoproliferative glomerulonephritis, severe (especially motor) neuropathy, significant skin necrosis, lung disease or, as occurs in some cases, widespread multiorgan life-threatening vasculitis. Plasmapheresis is recommended if there are features of hyperviscosity, although it also produces rapid response of other complications by removal of immune complexes and inflammatory mediators; if used for its speed of action in severe disease, it must be combined with immunosuppression in order to prevent a rebound flare of activity. Ciclosporin, melphalan and intravenous immunoglobulin have all been used with anecdotal success.

In general, the response of cutaneous vasculitis and arthralgia is quicker than that of renal or neurological disease, where (despite a rapid reduction in viral load) the response to antiviral therapy is slow; thus, immunosuppressives may need to be used whilst awaiting response to the antiviral regimen. Older age (especially age over 60 years), long duration of infection, high cryoglobulinaemia level and renal involvement all infer a poor prognosis, although the response of cryoglobulin levels does not always correlate with overall therapeutic benefit. Response of skin and joint symptoms is expected in over 80%, whereas response of nephropathy and cryoglobulinaemia may be less than 50% and 65% respectively, and mortality at 5 years may be as high as 50% in those with severe renal involvement. Antiviral treatment should be continued for at least 12 months [3]; some genotypes of HCV may be relatively resistant, but an early (3 months) complete virological response is associated with a better prognosis.

References
1 Ferri C, Mascia MT. Cryoglobulinemic vasculitis. *Curr Opin Rheumatol* 2006; **18**: 1854–63.
2 Del Rosso A, Generini S, Pignone A, Matucci-Cerinic M. Vasculitides secondary to systemic diseases. *Clin Dermatol* 1999; **17**: 533–47.
3 Saadoun D, Delluc A, Piette JC, Cacoub P. Treatment of hepatitis C-associated mixed cryoglobulinaemic vasculitis. *Curr Opin Rheumatol* 2008; **20**: 23–8.
4 Saadoun D, Sellam J, Ghillani-Dalbin P et al. Increased risks of lymphoma and death among patients with nonhepatitis C virus-related mixed cryoglobulinaemia. *Arch Intern Med* 2006; **166**: 2101–8.
5 González-Gay MA, García-Porrúa C. Epidemiology of the vasculitides. *Rheum Dis Clin N Am* 2001; **27**: 729–46.
6 Magro CM, Crowson AN. The cutaneous neutrophilic vascular injury syndromes: a review. *Semin Diagn Pathol* 2001; **18**: 47–58.
7 Glazer E, Ejaz A, Coley CJ 2nd et al. Fibrin ring granuloma in chronic hepatitis C: virus-related vasculitis and/or immune complex disease? *Semin Liver Dis* 2007; **27**: 227–30.
8 Trejo O, Ramos-Casals M, Garcia-Carrasco M et al. Cryoglobulinaemia: study of etiologic factors and clinical and immunological features in 443 patients from a single center. *Medicine* 2001; **80**: 252–62.
9 Fiorentino DF. Cutaneous vasculitis. *J Am Acad Dermatol* 2003; **48**: 311–40.

Erythema elevatum diutinum

Definition. Erythema elevatum diutinum (EED) is a rare, chronic, cutaneous eruption that is most commonly seen in the adult population. The first description of EED was by Hutchinson and Bury in the 1880s, and the condition was later named in 1894 by Radcliffe-Crocker and Williams. EED is characterized by fibrosing plaques with histological evidence of leukocytoclastic vasculitis. In addition to the characteristic polymorphonuclear fragmentation, endothelial swelling, extravasation of erythrocytes and fibrinoid necrosis of vessel walls, dermal nodules of EED contain spindle cells and fibrosis [1].

Aetiology and pathogenesis. Although EED is thought to be related to an Arthus-type reaction with immune complex deposition and subsequent inflammation, the exact aetiology is unknown. It has been associated with autoimmune diseases such as rheumatoid arthritis, coeliac disease, inflammatory bowel disease, and type I diabetes mellitus. Associations with infections, including streptococcus, hepatitis and syphilis, have also been suggested [2–11]. Lesions characteristic of EED have been induced by injection of streptococcal antigen into the dermis [12–15], and have occurred at sites of mosquito bites [10]. Erythema elevatum diutinum has also been associated with human immunodeficiency virus (HIV) infection, as lesions of EED have responded to antiretroviral and dapsone treatment in HIV-positive patients [16–22]. EED is now recognized as one of the defined reactive dermatoses associated with HIV [23]. In addition, EED has been associated with hypergammaglobulinaemia and IgA monoclonal gammopathies, as well as with myelodysplasia, pyoderma gangrenosum, and relapsing polychondritis. The association with haematological abnormalities, such as multiple myeloma, is strong; however, EED may precede the haematological disease by several years [24].

Histopathology (Figs 50.9 & 50.10). Acutely, lesions of EED demonstrate leukocytoclastic vasculitis, with little fibrin deposition. Eosinophils may also be present in the upper and mid-dermis.

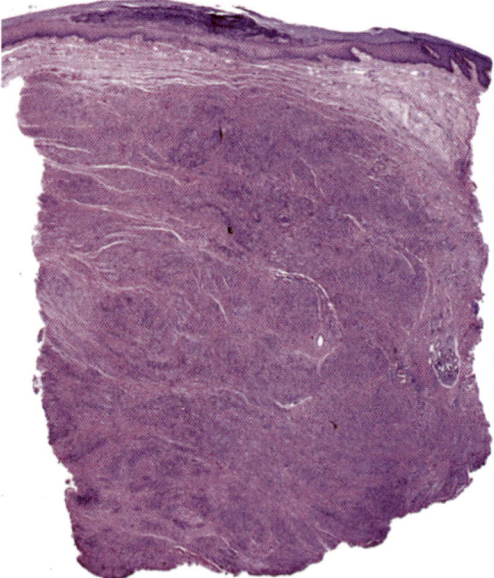

Fig. 50.9 Erythema elevatum diutinum. Low-power photomicrograph shows diffuse infiltrates throughout the entire dermis and areas of fibrosis. (Courtesy of Dr Omar Sangueza, Wake Forest University School of Medicine, Winston-Salem, NC, USA.)

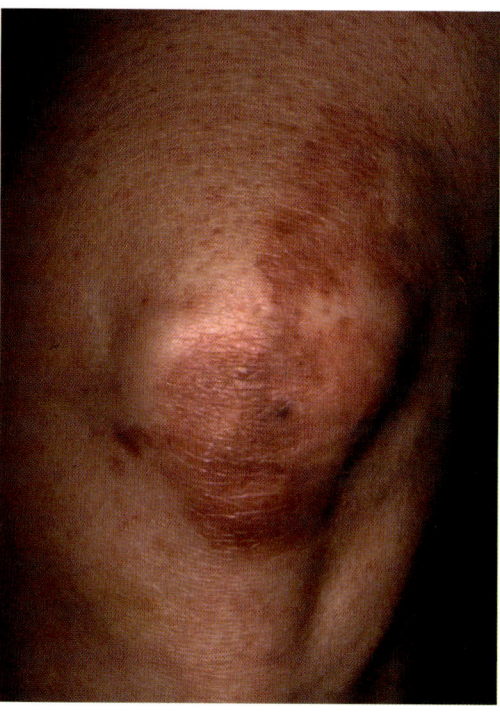

Fig. 50.11 Early non-fibrotic lesions of erythema elevatum diutinum at a typical site on the knee. This patient also had EED on the hands, and pyoderma gangrenosum.

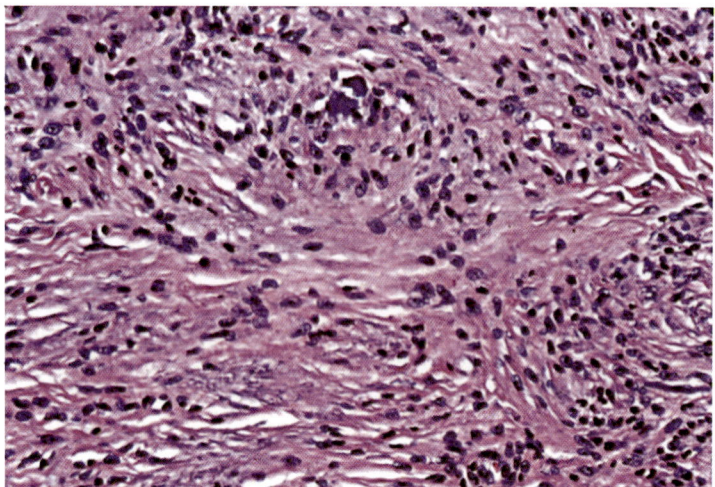

Fig. 50.10 Erythema elevatum diutinum. At higher magnification there is evidence of marked fibrosis and an inflammatory infiltrate composed of lymphocytes, histiocytes, neutrophils and nuclear dust. (Courtesy of Dr Omar Sangueza, Wake Forest University School of Medicine, Winston-Salem, NC, USA.)

Depending on the degree of oedema and infiltration into the dermis, unaffected collagen may be present just under the epidermis. Chronically, lesions demonstrate angiocentric eosinophilic fibrosis, capillary proliferation, and infiltration of macrophages, plasma cells, and lymphocytes. Cholesterol deposits in histiocytes and in the extracellular tissue (the latter corresponding to a pattern that has been termed 'extracellular cholesterolosis') may be present in older lesions [25].

Clinical features. Patients are usually adult, although occasional childhood cases are reported [26]. Lesions of EED most commonly appear chronically in a symmetrical fashion over the dorsa of the hands, the knees, buttocks and Achilles tendons (Fig. 50.11). They

are red-violaceous, red-brown or yellowish papules, plaques or nodules. Occasionally, the face and ears are also affected by EED. Initially, the lesions are soft, but eventually they fibrose, and later leave atrophic scars. Although they may be asymptomatic, the lesions of EED may also be painful. EED may last from 5 to 35 years, with crops of new lesions developing every few weeks to months.

Diagnosis. Although EED may be difficult to distinguish from cutaneous small vessel vasculitis histologically, the clinical presentation differs from that of other chronic small vessel vasculitis syndromes, allowing for an accurate diagnosis. EED and Sweet's syndrome are both described as neutrophilic dermatoses. However, EED differs from Sweet's syndrome by the character of the lesions and their distribution, as well as by histopathological features. The classic assumption that lesions from patients with Sweet's syndrome universally lack histopathological fibrinoid necrosis of vessel walls has been challenged; in one series, 29% of patients had biopsy specimens showing leukocytoclastic vasculitis [27], although it was felt that frank vasculitis was a consequence of neutrophil metabolites and occurred in older lesions. Clinically, the lesions in Sweet's syndrome are acute, more often asymmetrical and located on the arms, face and neck [28]. In contrast, EED lesions are chronic, symmetrical and classically located over the dorsum of the hands and knees, buttocks, and Achilles tendon. Although leukocytoclastic vasculitis has now been reported as a possible feature of Sweet's lesions [2], it is not always present and the fibrosis seen in lesions of EED correlates with the clinical chronicity.

The demonstration of IgA ANCA (with various specificities) in 6/10 cases of EED has been suggested to be of some diagnostic value [29]; in this series, seven of the ten patients had raised IgA levels (monoclonal in three).

Treatment. Several medications have been used in the treatment of EED. Dapsone has a remarkable effect on EED [15], although stopping it is often followed by swift return of the lesions. Niacinamide has also been used with good effect [30]. High potency topical, or intralesional, corticosteroids may minimize the size of lesions in patients with limited disease. Treatment of an associated disorder such as HIV infection or paraproteinaemia [31] may be effective. Other therapies used for cutaneous small vessel vasculitis may also be effective in treating patients with EED.

References

1 Shanks JH, Banerjee SS, Bishop PW *et al*. Nodular erythema elevatum diutinum mimicking cutaneous neoplasms. *Histopathology* 1997; **31**: 91–6.

2 Collier PM, Neill SM, Branfoot AC *et al*. Erythema elevatum diutinum—a solitary lesion in a patient with rheumatoid arthritis. *Clin Exp Dermatol* 1990; **15**: 394–5.

3 Buahene K, Hudson M, Mowat A *et al*. Erythema elevatum diutinum—an unusual association with ulcerative colitis. *Clin Exp Dermatol* 1991; **16**: 204–6.

4 Walker KD, Badame AJ. Erythema elevatum diutinum in a patient with Crohn's disease. *J Am Acad Dermatol* 1990; **22**: 948–52.

5 Bernard P, Bedane C, Delrous JL *et al*. Erythema elevatum diutinum in a patient with relapsing polychondritis. *J Am Acad Dermatol* 1992; **26**: 312–5.

6 Planagumá M, Puig L, Alomar A *et al*. Pyoderma gangrenosum in association with erythema elevatum diutinum: report of two cases. *Cutis* 1992; **49**: 201–6.

7 Cordier JF, Faure M, Hermier C *et al*. Pleural effusions in an overlap syndrome of idiopathic hypereosinophilic syndrome and erythema elevatum diutinum. *Eur Respir J* 1990; **3**: 115–8.

8 Creus L, Salleras M, Sola MA *et al*. Erythema elevatum diutinum associated with pulmonary infiltrate. *Br J Dermatol* 1997; **137**: 652–3.

9 Tasanen K, Raudasoja R, Kallioinen M *et al*. Erythema elevatum diutinum in association with coeliac disease. *Br J Dermatol* 1997; **136**: 624–7.

10 Sangüeza OP, Pilcher B, Sangüeza JM. Erythema elevatum diutinum: a clinicopathological study of eight cases. *Am J Dermatopathol* 1997; **19**: 214–22.

11 Orteu C, McGregor JM, Whittaker SJ *et al*. Erythema elevatum diutinum and Crohn disease: a common pathogenic role for measles virus? *Arch Dermatol* 1996; **132**: 1523–5.

12 Weidman FD, Bensaççon JH. Erythema elevatum diutinum. Role of streptococci and relationship to other rheumatic dermatoses. *Arch Dermatol Syphilol* 1929; **20**: 593–620.

13 Wolff HH, Scherer R, Maciejewski W *et al*. Erythema elevatum diutinum. II. Immunelekroneumikroskopische Untersuchung der leukocytocklastishew vaskulitis in einer Intrakutanreaktion mit Streptokokkenantigen. *Arch Dermatol Res* 1978; **261**: 17–26.

14 Cream JJ, Leven GM, Calnan CD. Erythema elevatum diutinum: an unusual reaction to streptococcal antigen and response to dapsone. *Br J Dermatol* 1971; **84**: 393–9.

15 Katz SI, Gallin JI, Hertz KC *et al*. Erythema elevatum diutinum: skin and systemic manifestation, immunologic studies, and successful treatment with dapsone. *Medicine* 1977; **56**: 443–55.

16 Cockerell CJ. Noninfectious inflammatory skin diseases in HIV-infected individuals. *Dermatol Clin* 1991; **9**: 531–41.

17 Da Cunha Bang F, Weismann K, Ralfkiaer E *et al*. Erythema elevatum diutinum and pre-AIDS. *Acta Derm Venereol* (Stockh) 1986; **66**: 272–4.

18 Dronda F, González-López A, Lecona M *et al*. Erythema elevatum diutinum in human immunodeficiency virus-infected patients—report of a case and review of the literature. *Clin Exp Dermatol* 1996; **21**: 222–5.

19 Shanks JH, Banerjee SS, Bishop PW *et al*. Nodular erythema elevatum diutinum mimicking cutaneous neoplasms. *Histopathology* 1997; **31**: 91–6.

20 Revenga FM, Vera A, Munoz A *et al*. Erythema elevatum diutinum and AIDS: are they related? *Clin Exp Dermatol* 1997; **22**: 250–6.

21 Suárez J, Miguélez M, Villalba R. Nodular erythema elevatum diutinum in an HIV-1 infected woman: response to dapsone and antiretroviral therapy. *Br J Dermatol* 1998; **138**: 706–23.

22 Hon Pak CPT, Montemarano AD, Berger T. Purpuric nodules and macules on the extremities of a young woman. *Arch Dermatol* 1998; **134**: 232–3.

23 Rover PA, Bittencourt C, Discacciati MP *et al*. Erythema elevatum diutinum as a first clinical manifestation for diagnosing HIV infection: case history. *Sao Paulo Med J* 2005; **123**: 201–3.

24 Yiannias JA, el-Azhary RA, Gibson LE. Erythema elevatum diutinum: a clinical and histopathologic study of 13 patients. *J Am Acad Dermatol* 1992; **26**: 38–44.

25 LeBoit PE, Yen TS, Wintroub B. The evolution of lesions in erythema elevatum diutinum. *Am J Dermatopathol* 1986; **8**: 392–402.

26 Tomasini C, Seia Z, Dapavo P *et al*. Infantile erythema elevatum diutinum: report of a vesiculo-bullous case. *Eur J Dermatol* 2006; **16**: 683–6.

27 Malone JC, Slone SP, Wills-Frank LA *et al*. Vascular inflammation (vasculitis) in Sweet syndrome: a clinicopathologic study of 28 biopsy specimens from 21 patients. *Arch Dermatol* 2002; **138**: 345–9.

28 Cohen PR. Sweet's syndrome—a comprehensive review of an acute febrile neutrophilic dermatosis. *Orphanet J Rare Dis* 2007; **2**: 34.

29 Ayoub N, Charuel J-L, Diemerte M-C *et al*. Antineutrophil cytoplasmic antibodies of IgA class in neutrophilic dermatoses with emphasis on erythema elevatum diutinum. *Arch Dermatol* 2004; **140**: 931–6.

30 Kohler IK, Lorincz AL. Erythema elevatum diutinum treated with niacinamide and tetracycline. *Arch Dermatol* 1980; **116**: 693–5.

31 Chow RKP, Benny WB, Coupe RL *et al*. Erythema elevatum diutinum associated with IgA paraproteinaemia successfully controlled with intermittent plasma exchange. *Arch Dermatol* 1996; **132**: 1360–4.

Eosinophilic vasculitis

> **Synonym**
> • Recurrent cutaneous eosinophilic necrotizing vasculitis [1,2]

Definition. A relatively recently described and rare vasculitis consisting of a predominantly centripetal purpuric papular rash, angio-oedema, peripheral blood eosinophilia and an eosinophilic necrotizing vasculitis of small vessels.

History. This condition was recently distinguished from other eosinophilic vasculitides that affect medium to large vessels (CSS; see later in this chapter) and from eosinophilic disorders in which pruritic papules and/or angio-oedema may occur, such as hypereosinophilic syndrome, episodic angio-oedema with eosinophilia, dermatitis herpetiformis, Wells' syndrome, polymorphic eruption of pregnancy or drug eruptions. Association with connective tissue diseases and with rheumatoid arthritis has been reported [3,4].

Aetiology and pathogenesis. The cause is unknown. As in other strongly eosinophilic disorders, eosinophil cytokines such as IL-5, and toxic eosinophil granule proteins such as the major basic protein, have been demonstrated in serum and tissues, respectively, and presumably play a part in the tissue damage. Neutrophil elastase is prominent around vessels, and mast cell degranulation occurs. Eosinophilic vasculitis has also been reported in a patient with the hypereosinophilic syndrome; in this patient, CD40 (a glycoprotein of the TNF receptor family) was considered to be important in pathogenesis [5].

Histopathology. Shows fibrinoid deposition and necrosis of small dermal vessels with an infiltrate of eosinophils and absent or minimal leukoclasis. Small epidermal vesicles containing eosinophils may be present. Immunoglobulin deposition is not a feature. This eosinophilic small vessel vasculitis is distinct from other vasculitides such as CSS, in which medium to large vessels are affected, and from most drug-induced vasculitis in which eosinophils are generally less prominent.

Clinical features. Recurrent pruritic papules and urticarial lesions occur at any site, especially the head and neck, with angio-oedema of the face and extremities. Either sex and any age group may be affected. The course is long and recurrent but fever, arthralgia and visceral involvement are absent. Digital occlusions manifest as Raynaud's phenomenon or digital gangrene have been reported in patients with cutaneous eosinophilic vasculitis associated with the hypereosinophilic syndrome [5,6], but they can also occur in the hypereosinophilic syndrome in the absence of cutaneous eosinophilic vasculitis [7,8].

An eosinophilic vasculitis, typically with hypocomplementaemia, also occurs in connective tissue diseases [9].

Treatment. Oral corticosteroids, intermittently or as prolonged maintenance therapy depending on response, appear to be effective.

References

1 Chen K-R, Su WPD, Pittelkow MR, Leiferman KM. Eosinophilic vasculitis syndrome: recurrent cutaneous eosinophilic necrotizing vasculitis. *Semin Dermatol* 1995; **14**: 106–10.
2 Chen KR, Pittelkow MR, Su D *et al*. Recurrent cutaneous eosinophilic necrotizing vasculitis: a novel eosinophil-mediated syndrome. *Arch Dermatol* 1994; **130**: 1159–66.
3 Chen K-R, Su WPD, Pittelkow MR *et al*. Eosinophilic vasculitis in connective tissue disease. *J Am Acad Dermatol* 1996; **35**: 173–82.
4 Yomoda M, Inoue M, Nakama T *et al*. Cutaneous eosinophilic vasculitis associated with rheumatoid arthritis. *Br J Dermatol* 1999; **140**: 754–5.
5 Jang KA, Lim YS, Choi JH *et al*. Hypereosinophilic syndrome presenting as cutaneous necrotizing eosinophilic vasculitis and Raynaud's phenomenon complicated by digital gangrene. *Br J Dermatol* 2000; **143**: 641–4.
6 Kim SH, Kim TB, Yun YS *et al*. Hypereosinophilia presenting as eosinophilic vasculitis and multiple peripheral artery occlusions without organ involvement. *J Korean Med Sci* 2005; **20**: 677–9.
7 Oppliger R, Gay-Crosier F, Dayer E, Hauser C. Digital necrosis in a patient with hypereosinophilic syndrome in the absence of cutaneous eosinophilic vasculitis. *Br J Dermatol* 2001; **144**: 1087–90.
8 Hamada T, Kimura Y, Hayashi S *et al*. Hypereosinophilic syndrome with peripheral circulatory insufficiency and cutaneous microthrombi. *Arch Dermatol* 2007; **143**: 812–3.
9 Chen KR, Su WP, Pittelko MR *et al*. Eosinophilic vasculitis in connective tissue disease. *J Am Acad Dermatol* 1996; **35**: 173–82.

Granuloma faciale

Definition. Granuloma faciale (GF) is an uncommon condition typified by asymptomatic cutaneous nodules occurring primarily on the face, with occasional extrafacial involvement. Granuloma faciale is limited to the skin, without any systemic manifestations. It is most common in males [1], typically in white people, although cases have been observed in populations of African or oriental ancestry [1,2]. Wigley [3] first described GF in 1945 as a type of eosinophilic granuloma, although it was distinguished from other

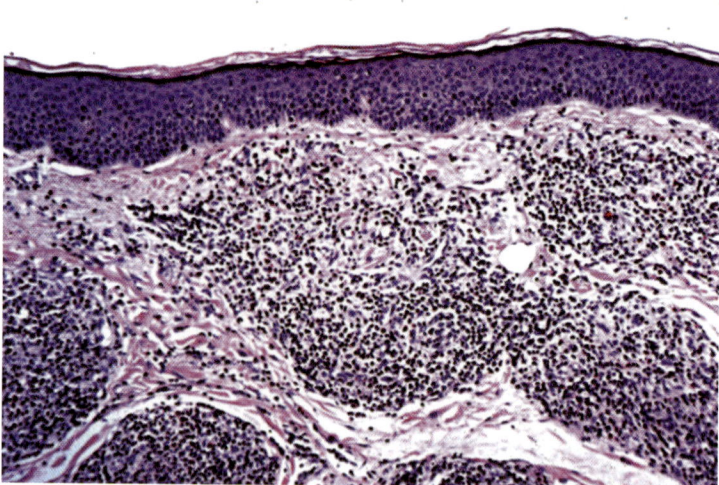

Fig. 50.12 Granuloma faciale. Low-power view shows perivascular nodular infiltrates within the dermis. (Courtesy of Dr Omar Sangueza, Wake Forest University School of Medicine, Winston-Salem, NC, USA.)

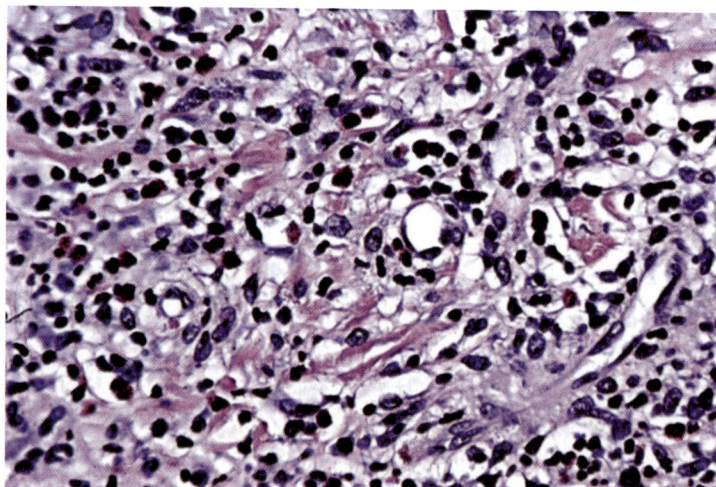

Fig. 50.13 Granuloma faciale. At higher magnification the infiltrate shows lymphocytes, eosinophils and a few neutrophils. (Courtesy of Dr Omar Sangueza, Wake Forest University School of Medicine, Winston-Salem, NC, USA.)

eosinophilic granulomas by Lever and Leeper in 1950 [4]. Pinkus recommended the present name in 1952 [5].

Aetiology and pathogenesis. Although the aetiology is somewhat unclear, GF is considered to be a histological variant of leukocytoclastic vasculitis with a prominent eosinophilic infiltrate, and confined to the skin [6]. Deposition of IgG in and around dermal vasculature has been demonstrated, lending some support to the idea that GF is immune complex-mediated [7]. Clonal expansion of T cells producing IL-5, a powerful eosinophil chemoattractant, has been described within GF lesions [8].

Histopathology [9,10]. GF is characterized by a mixed inflammatory infiltrate with a predominance of neutrophils and eosinophils, although the latter is not constant [10], mainly in the upper half of the dermis but with occasional spread into the lower dermis and subcutaneous tissue (Figs 50.12 & 50.13). A band of normal

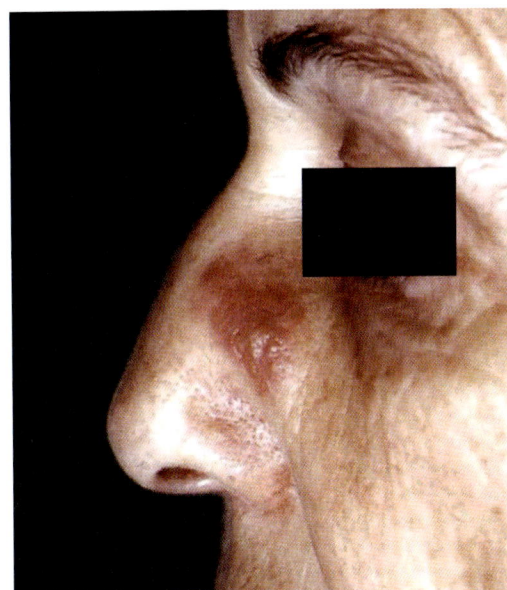

Fig. 50.14 Granuloma faciale. A reddish-brown plaque on the nose. (Courtesy of Dr G. Dawn, Monklands Hospital, UK.)

Table 50.9 Therapeutic ladder for granuloma faciale.

Topical corticosteroids
Topical tacrolimus (3)
Intralesional corticosteroids (3)
Cryosurgery ± intralesional corticosteroids (3)
Clofazimine (3)
Dapsone (3)
Surgery (3)
Laser (3)

1, double-blind studies; 2, case series; 3, case reports.

collagen referred to as a 'Grenz' zone typically separates the inflammatory infiltrate from the epidermis and pilosebaceous appendages. Nuclear dust (fragmented neutrophil nuclei) may be observed near capillaries. Vasculitis, with fibrinoid deposits near and within vessel walls, as well as haemorrhage, may be noted, and even frank vascular necrosis. Immune complexes have been documented either around vessels or at the dermoepidermal junction in several studies, but were lacking in many cases in a large series of patients [10].

Clinical features [10]. Lesions of GF are soft, brown-red nodules or plaques that most commonly occur on the face (Fig. 50.14); multiple lesions are present in about a third of cases but extrafacial involvement is uncommon, occurring in five of 66 patients in one study [10]. The nodules or plaques are smooth, with prominent follicular orifices and telangiectatic surface changes or scaling. Lesions of GF never ulcerate. They are almost always asymptomatic, although some patients may describe itching, burning or pain associated with the lesions [11].

In a review of 14 patients with extrafacial GF, nearly all lesions coexisted with facial lesions, mainly occurring after the facial lesions, and there was a male predominance [12].

An additional rare diagnosis in this category is eosinophilic angiocentric fibrosis, which is a mucosal variant of GF that may occur in nasal passages or upper airways, and which may be associated with skin lesions of GF [13,14].

Diagnosis. A definitive diagnosis of GF requires clinically consistent lesions and a confirmatory biopsy. Although most laboratory studies are normal, mild peripheral blood eosinophilia may be present [10].

Treatment. GF typically follows a chronic course with intermittent acute flares, and is often refractory to treatment. As a result, a wide variety of treatment methods, both surgical and medical,

have been used to treat this condition. Examples include topical, intralesional or systemic corticosteroid, dermabrasion [15], laser treatments of various types [15–17], electrosurgery [15], cryosurgery [18], psoralen with ultraviolet A (PUVA) [19], and other systemic treatments including dapsone [11,20], clofazimine [21] and antimalarials [22]. Some cases have been treated with surgical excision [22]. More recently, topical tacrolimus has been reported to be effective, but in reports to date has required regular use for 2 months, then gradual reduction with ongoing once weekly use for many months to maintain remission [17,23]. A therapeutic ladder for GF is depicted in Table 50.9.

References

1 Black C. Granuloma faciale. *Cutis* 1977; **20**: 66–8.
2 Koplon BS, Wood MG. Granuloma faciale: first reported case in a negro. *Arch Dermatol* 1967; **96**: 188–92.
3 Wigley JEM. Sarcoid of Boeck? Eosinophilic granuloma. *Br J Dermatol* 1945; **57**: 68–9.
4 Lever WF, Leeper RW. Eosinophilic granuloma of the skin: report of cases representing two different diseases described as eosinophilic granuloma. *Arch Derm Syph* 1950; **62**: 85–96.
5 Pinkus H. Granuloma faciale. *Dermatologica* 1952; **105**: 85–8.
6 Lever WF, Schaumburg-Lever G, eds. Granuloma faciale. In: *Histopathology of the Skin*. New York: Lippincott, 1990: 193–5.
7 Nieboer C, Kalsbeek GL. Immunofluorescence studies in granuloma eosinophilicum faciale. *J Cutan Pathol* 1978; **5**: 68–75.
8 Gauger A, Ronet C, Schnopp C *et al*. High local interleukin 5 production in granuloma faciale (eosinophilicum): role of clonally expanded skin-specific CD4⁺ cells. *Br J Dermatol* 2005; **153**: 454–7.
9 Crowson AN, Mihm MC Jr, Magro CM. Cutaneous vasculitis: a review. *J Cutan Pathol* 2003; **30**: 161–73.
10 Ortonne N, Wechsler J, Bagot M *et al*. Granuloma faciale: a clinicopathologic study of 66 patients. *J Am Acad Dermatol* 2005; **53**: 1002–9.
11 Guill MA, Aton JK. Facial granuloma responsive to dapsone therapy. *Arch Dermatol* 1982; **118**: 332–5.
12 Inanir I, Alvur Y. Granuloma faciale with extrafacial lesions. *Br J Dermatol* 2001; **145**: 360–1.
13 Yung A, Wachsmuth R, Ramnath R *et al*. Eosinophilic angiocentric fibrosis – a rare mucosal variant of granuloma faciale which may present to the dermatologist. *Br J Dermatol* 2005; **152**: 574–6.
14 Holme SA, Laidler P, Holt PJA. Concurrent granuloma faciale and eosinophilic angiocentric fibrosis. *Br J Dermatol* 2005; **153**: 851–3.
15 Dinehart SM, Gross DJ, Davis CM, Herzberg AJ. Granuloma faciale: comparison of different treatment modalities. *Arch Otolaryngol Head Neck Surg* 1990; **116**: 849–51.
16 Apfelberg DB, Maser MR, Lash H *et al*. Expanded role of the argon laser in plastic surgery. *J Dermatol Surg Oncol* 1983; **9**: 145–51.
17 Ludwig E, Allam J-P, Bieber T, Noval N. New treatment modalities for granuloma faciale. *Br J Dermatol* 2003; **149**: 634–7.
18 Zacarian S. Cryosurgery effective for granuloma faciale. *J Dermatol Surg Oncol* 1985; **11**: 11–2.

19 Hudson LD. Granuloma faciale: treatment with topical psoralen and UVA. *J Am Acad Dermatol* 1983; **8**: 559–61.

20 Van de Kerkhof PC. On the efficacy of dapsone in granuloma faciale. *Acta Derm Venereol* 1994; **74**: 61–2.

21 Jacyk WK. Facial granuloma in a patient treated with clofazimine. *Arch Dermatol* 1981; **117**: 597–8.

22 Phillips DK, Hymes SR. Recurrent facial plaques following full-thickness grafting: granuloma faciale. *Arch Dermatol* 1994; **130**: 1436–7.

23 Marcoval J, Moreno A, Bordas X, Peyri J. Granuloma faciale: treatment with topical tacrolimus. *J Am Acad Dermatol* 2006; **55** (Suppl.): S110–1.

Acute haemorrhagic oedema of childhood [1]

Synonyms
- Haemorrhagic oedema of childhood
- Acute haemorrhagic oedema of infancy
- Finkelstein's disease
- Seidlmayer's syndrome
- Purpura en cocarde avec oedeme
- Post-infectious cockade purpura

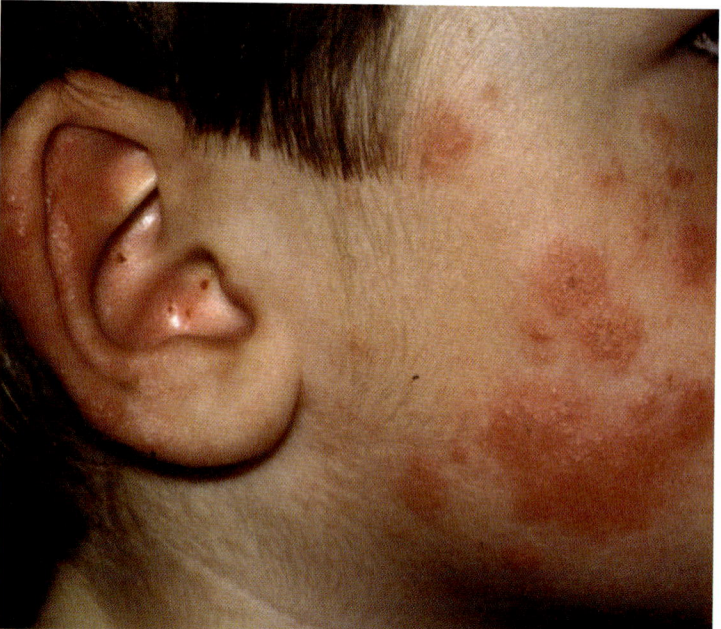

Fig. 50.15 Early discoid erythematosus lesions in acute haemorrhagic oedema of childhood.

Definition. Acute haemorrhagic oedema of childhood (AHEC) is a rare disorder, whose manifestations are almost exclusively cutaneous. It occurs in children under 2 years old, and rarely outside this age group. There is often a history of a recent upper respiratory infection and/or treatment with antibiotics. Clinical features include petechiae and ecchymoses of the head and distal extremities. Snow first described AHEC in 1913 in the United States. In 1938 in Europe, Finkelstein published his paper on the disease.

Aetiology and pathogenesis. Infections (usually respiratory tract or urinary, e.g. streptococcal, staphylococcal, *Escherichia coli*, cytomegalovirus, adenovirus, coxsackievirus, or rotavirus infections), drugs, or vaccines may trigger AHEC, which may be a variant of childhood cutaneous small vessel vasculitis [1–4]. The age group, body sites affected, lesion morphology, rare renal or gastrointestinal involvement, and inconstant demonstration of IgA deposition in biopsies all serve to distinguish AHEC from HSP.

Histopathology. Leukocytoclastic vasculitis is evident in lesions of AHEC. As in cutaneous small vessel vasculitis (CSVV), the features include: karyorrhexis of neutrophils, endothelial swelling and extravasation of erythrocytes. Lesions of AHEC may show more prominent dermal oedema than lesions of CSVV.

Clinical features. Non-tender facial oedema may be the presenting sign of AHEC lesions, which are often asymmetrical. AHEC is characterized by sudden development of tender, oedematous lesions with petechiae and ecchymoses on the head and distal extremities. Large annular, arciform, coin-shaped or targetoid lesions (Fig. 50.15), that may later develop into bullae or necrotizing lesions, are typical. Lesions of AHEC start distally and progress proximally, sometimes involving the scrotum in males. Clinically, patients with AHEC are typically medically stable, although they may be febrile. Less dramatic presentations, in which the preceding infection and post-inflammatory pigmentation of annular and arciform skin lesions are dominant, may be mistaken for a drug rash or exanthem [5]. Although AHEC may rarely involve joints, the gastrointestinal tract, or the kidneys with vasculitic manifestations, it typically follows a benign course, lasting 1 to 3 weeks and with no persistent adverse effects following resolution [1–3]. Intussusception, classically associated with HSP, has also been reported with AHEC [6].

Diagnosis. AHEC may be diagnosed only after meningococcaemia, erythema multiforme, UV, Sweet's syndrome, cutaneous small vessel vasculitis and Kawasaki disease have been ruled out.

Treatment. Supportive care is the only treatment usually necessary for patients with AHEC, although other treatments used in infants with CSVV or HSP may be appropriate in more severely affected patients.

References

1 Taïeb A, Legrain V. Acute haemorrhagic oedema of the skin in infancy. In: Harper J, Oranje A, Prose N. *Textbook of Pediatric Dermatology*, 2nd edn. Oxford: Blackwell Publishing, 2006: 1897–901.

2 Cunningham BB, Caro WA, Eramo LR. Neonatal acute hemorrhagic edema of childhood: case report and review of the English-language literature. *Pediatr Dermatol* 1996; **13**: 39–44.

3 Legrain B, Lejean S, Taïeb A *et al.* Infantile acute hemorrhagic edema of the skin: study of ten cases. *J Am Acad Dermatol* 1991; **24**: 17–22.

4 Kuroda K, Yabunami H, Hisanaga Y. Acute haemorrhagic oedema of infancy associated with cytomegalovirus infection. *Br J Dermatol* 2002; **147**: 1254–7.

5 Cox NH. Seidlmayer's syndrome: post-infectious cockade purpura. *J Am Acad Dermatol* 1992; **26**: 275.

6 Yu JE, Mancini AJ, Miller ML. Intussusception in an infant with acute hemorrhagic edema of infancy. *Pediatr Dermatol* 2007; **24**: 61–4.

Nodular vasculitis

Synonyms
- Lobular panniculitis with vasculitis
- Erythema induratum of Bazin and of Whitfield

Definition. Nodular vasculitis (NV) is a chronic relapsing lobular panniculitis with septal vasculitis. It is characterized by a vasculitis of subcutaneous arteries and veins, with subsequent ischaemia of subcutaneous tissue, which results in clinical suppuration. The cause may be a hypersensitivity reaction to an antigenic trigger such as a bacterial infection. It occurs primarily in middle-aged women, and is manifest as tender nodules or plaques on the legs that may later progress to ulceration.

History and nomenclature. Erythema induratum of Bazin was initially described by Bazin in 1861 as indurated plaques on the legs of women of middle age [1]. In 1900, French dermatologists described an association between erythema induratum and tuberculosis [2], although British physicians reported similar patients without evidence of tuberculosis at approximately the same time, a pattern which was later designated 'Whitfield's erythema induratum' [3–5]. In the middle of the 20th century, American physicians suggested the term nodular vasculitis for Whitfield's erythema induratum, which was thought to be distinct from erythema induratum of Bazin [6]. There remains controversy about whether erythema induratum of Bazin and nodular vasculitis should viewed as distinct, or as the same entity but with tuberculosis as just one cause. Many authors combine these entities [7], some view them as simply different names for the same condition [8], whereas others refer to them as nodular vasculitis/ erythema induratum (or vice versa) [9,10], reflecting some uncertainty. Others have used the term erythema induratum, but qualify it as Bazin-type if due to tuberculosis and Whitfield type if not [11]. A similar debate surrounds the putative role of tuberculosis as the cause; hyperreactivity to purified protein derivative, *Mycobacterium tuberculosis* DNA sequences in lesions, and response to antituberculous therapy all suggest that tuberculosis has a causal role in some cases, yet other convincing causative associations (medications, other infections) are recorded and negative results on investigation for tuberculosis in other cases. Even in terms of detection of *M. tuberculosis* DNA, studies differ; in one study 77% of 50 biopsy specimens were positive (with no obvious clinical or histopathological differences between those with positive or negative results) [10], whereas a more recent study found no positive results in 10 cases [9]. The latter study also had negative PCR results for DNA of several non-tuberculosis mycobacteria. Both studies used retrospective cases, so it is uncertain whether the archived diagnosis might have been influenced by the nosology of nodular vasculitis at the time the specimens were reported. We recommend using the term nodular vasculitis, as it then does not presuppose a single aetiology, but being aware that tuberculosis must be excluded in patients with lesions that fit this clinicopathological pattern, and that there are no histological features that reliably distinguish a tuberculous from a non-tuberculous aetiology.

Aetiology and pathogenesis. Several antigenic triggers have been implicated as the source for the hypersensitivity reactions with resultant subcutaneous vasculitis and lobular panniculitis in NV, as alluded to above. These include bacterial infections, such as streptococcal or mycobacterial infections, viral infections such as hepatitis C virus [12], and drugs such as propylthiouracil. NV has also been reported as occurring repeatedly in association with flares of autoimmune colitis [13], and related to colonic carcinoma [14]. The pathogenesis may be similar to that of cutaneous small vessel vasculitis, probably being immune complex-mediated, but causing a persistent delayed hypersensitivity or Arthus-type reaction [11] and with septal vessels in the panniculus as the target. Similar lesions may occur in rheumatoid disease.

Histopathology. Controversy exists as to whether arteries, veins or both are affected in NV. Regardless of the type of vessel involved, the early changes are of leukocytoclastic (sometimes lymphocytic or granulomatous [8]) vasculitis of vessels in the subcutaneous tissue leading to ischaemic changes, followed by inflammation and injury to lipocytes [7–11]. It has been suggested that the lesions can be classified on pathological grounds into type I (focal panniculitis with central neutrophilic muscular vasculitis, resembling PAN), and type II (diffuse panniculitis with multiple foci of neutrophilic small and muscular vessel vasculitis) [8]. C-PAN can usually be distinguished, as inflammation does not extend beyond the adventitia of arteries. In both histopathological types, there is coagulation and some caseation necrosis, the resulting occlusion leading to ischaemia and necrosis of fat lobules that may eventually involve the overlying dermis. Early in the disease process, the necrotic subcutaneous fat demonstrates fat cysts bordered by a finely granular eosinophilic substance with pyknotic nuclei. Later, foamy histiocytes encircle the necrotic areas, creating granulomatous inflammation (consistent with an additional name that has been used, lobular granulomatous panniculitis) (Figs 50.16 & 50.17).

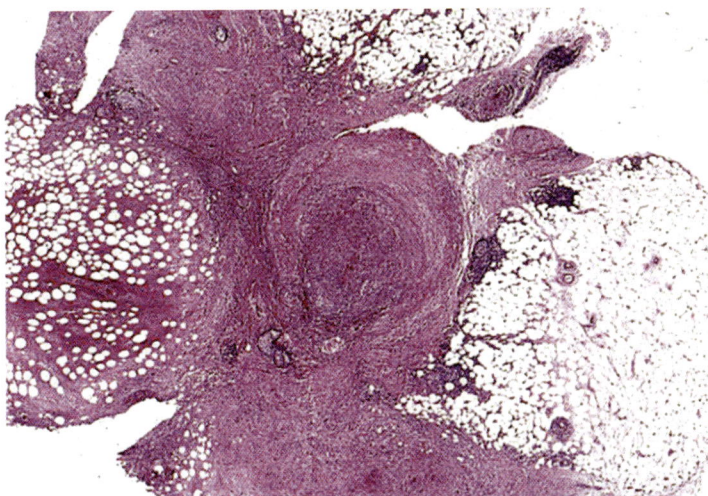

Fig. 50.16 Nodular vasculitis. Lobular panniculitis with prominent inflammation. Note the alteration of a vascular structure in the middle of the photograph. (Courtesy of Dr Omar Sangueza, Wake Forest University School of Medicine, Winston-Salem, NC, USA.)

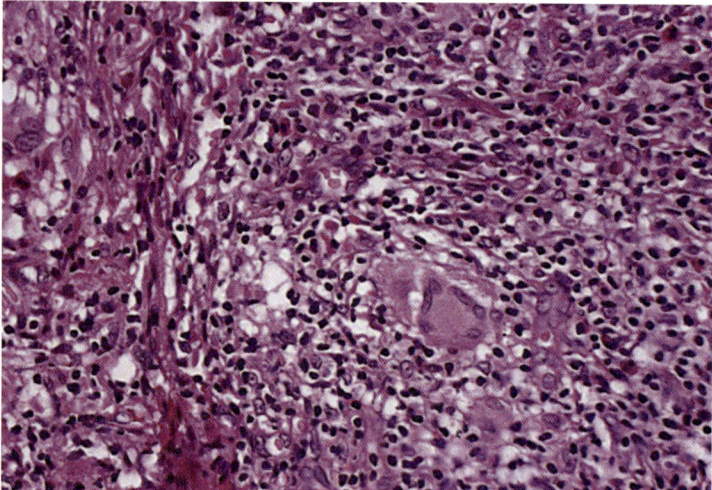

Fig. 50.17 Nodular vasculitis: the inflammatory infiltrate within the vessel wall is composed of lymphocytes and histiocytes, some of them multinucleated. (Courtesy of Dr Omar Sangueza, Wake Forest University School of Medicine, Winston-Salem, NC, USA.)

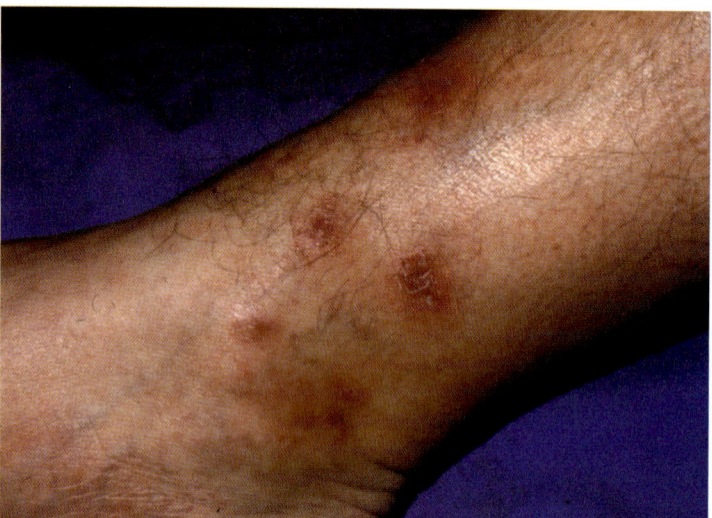

Fig. 50.18 Bazin's disease on the lower legs.

Clinical features. NV is manifest as tender, dusky, often suppurative, nodules or plaques on the posterolateral aspect of the legs (Fig. 50.18). It is typically seen in healthy, middle-aged, sometimes obese, women who may have venous stasis. Patients often have 'thick' calves with erythrocyanosis and perifollicular erythema. Lesions may be unilateral, are often inflamed and may progress to ulceration. The lesions of NV heal slowly, sometimes leaving an atrophic scar. The course of NV is chronic, with relapses typically occurring over several years. Nodular vasculitis may sometimes be seen in men, with unilateral nodules or plaques involving the anterior aspect of the thighs and legs, and other locations.

Lesions that have previously been termed 'erythrocyanosis with nodules' may have been examples of NV, or alternatively a pattern of perniosis.

Diagnosis. NV is a clinicopathological diagnosis, which requires deep incisional biopsy of active lesions. Lesions may resemble

Table 50.10 Treatment of nodular vasculitis.

Tuberculosis present
Triple-agent antituberculosis therapy for a minimum of 9 months

Tuberculosis not present
Palliative treatments
• Compression hosiery
• Bed rest
• Non-steroidal anti-inflammatory drugs
Systemic corticosteroids
Potassium iodide
Other treatments used to treat patients with small vessel vasculitis (Table 50.7)

other panniculitides, erythema nodosum, perniosis, pyoderma gangrenosum, skin infections and the cutaneous lesions of polyarteritis nodosa (p. 50.33) or Takayasu's arteritis (p. 50.44). In cases where a tuberculous aetiology is suspected, a tuberculin skin test and chest X-ray should be performed. The recently developed ELISpot, which detects peripheral blood IFN-γ-secreting T cells, may also be useful [15]. Other tests for tuberculosis are discussed in Chapter 31. Evaluation is otherwise similar to that for patients with cutaneous small vessel vasculitis.

Treatment. In patients in whom tuberculosis is demonstrated, at least a 9-month course of triple-agent antituberculosis therapy should be given (Chapter 31) [16,17]. In non-tubercular cases, supportive measures, such as compression hosiery, bed rest and NSAIDs are recommended. Systemic corticosteroids may also be considered, as well as potassium iodide, which has been reported as an effective treatment of NV [18,19]. Other treatments outlined for patients with small vessel vasculitis might also be appropriate for patients with NV. Mycophenolate mofetil has been used in one case [20]. The treatment of NV is shown in Table 50.10.

References

1 Bazin E. *Leçons Théoriques et Cliniques Sur la Scrofule*, 2nd edn. Paris: Delahaye, 1861: 146.
2 Cribier B, Grosshans E. Erythéme induré de Bazin: concept et terminologie obsolétes. *Ann Dermatol Venereol* 1990; **117**: 937–43.
3 Galloway J. A probable case of Bazin's disease. *Br J Dermatol* 1899; **11**: 206–7.
4 Whitfield A. On the nature of the disease known as erythema induratum scrofulosorum. *Br J Dermatol* 1901; **13**: 386–7.
5 Whitfield A. A further contribution to our knowledge of erythema induratum. *Br J Dermatol* 1905; **15**: 241–7.
6 Montgomery H, O'Leary PA, Barker NW. Nodular vascular diseases of the legs: erythema induratum and allied conditions. *JAMA* 1945; **128**: 335–45.
7 Requena L, Sánchez Yus E. Panniculitis, Part II. Mostly lobular panniculitis. *J Am Acad Dermatol* 2001; **45**: 325–61.
8 Carlsson AJ, Chen K-R. Cutaneous vasculitis update: neutrophilic muscular vessel and eosinophilic, granulomatous and lymphocytic vasculitis. *Am J Dermatopathol* 2007; **29**: 32–43.
9 Bayer-Garner IB, Cox MD, Scott MA, Smoller BR. Mycobacteria other than *Mycobacterium tuberculosis* are not present in erythema induratum / nodular vasculitis: a case series and literature review of the clinical and histologic findings. *J Cutan Pathol* 2005; **32**: 220–6.
10 Baselga E, Margall N, Barnadas MA *et al*. Detection of *Mycobacterium tuberculosis* DNA in lobular granulomatous panniculitis (erythema induratum–nodular vasculitis). *Arch Dermatol* 1997; **133**: 457–62.
11 Weedon D. *Skin Pathology*, 2nd edn. London: Churchill Livingstone, 2002: 521–41.

12 Ural I, Erel A, Ozenirler S *et al.* Nodular vasculitis associated with chronic hepatitis C. *J Eur Acad Dermatol Venereol* 2002; **16**: 298–9.

13 Pozdnyakova O, Garg A, Mahalingam M. Nodular vasculitis—a new cutaneous manifestation of autoimmune colitis. *J Cutan Pathol* 2008; **35**: 315–9.

14 Khachemoune A, Longo MI, Phillips TJ. Nodular vasculitis as a paraneoplastic presentation? *Int J Dermatol* 2003; **42**: 639–42.

15 Clayton R, Grabczynska S, Wilkinson JD. Nodular vasculitis: an indicator for ELISpot screening for tuberculosis? *Clin Exp Dermatol* 2007; **32**: 761–2.

16 Anderson S. Erythema indutatum (Bazin) treated with isoniazid. *Acta Derm Venereol (Stockh)* 1970; **50**: 65–8.

17 Rademaker M, Lowe DG, Munro DD. Erythema induratum (Bazin's disease). *J Am Acad Dermatol* 1989; **21**: 740–5.

18 Schulz EJ, Whiting DA. Treatment of erythema nodosum and nodular vasculitis with potassium iodide. *Br J Dermatol* 1976; **94**: 75–8.

19 Hoti H, Imamura S, Danno K, Ofuji S. Potassium iodide in the treatment of erythema nodosum and nodular vasculitis. *Arch Dermatol* 1981; **117**: 29–31.

20 Taverna JA, Radfar A, Pentland A *et al.* Case reports: nodular vasculitis responsive to mycophenolate mofetil. *J Drugs Dermatol* 2006; **5**: 992–3.

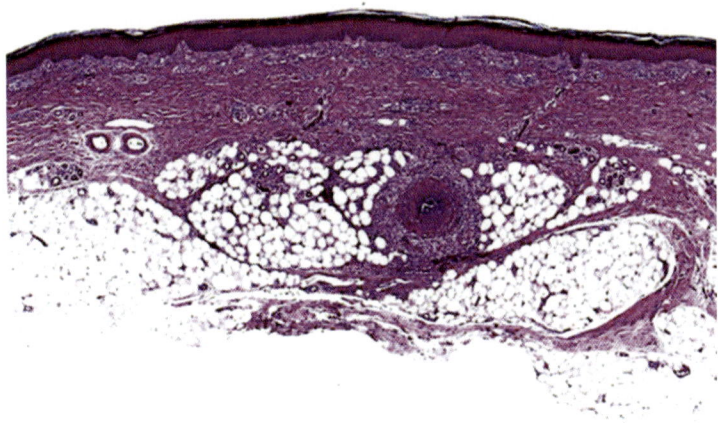

Fig. 50.19 Polyarteritis nodosa. Note the characteristic targetoid alteration of a vascular structure within the subcutaneous tissue. (Courtesy of Dr Omar Sangueza, Wake Forest University School of Medicine, Winston-Salem, NC, USA.)

Polyarteritis nodosa

Synonyms
- Classic polyarteritis nodosa
- Periarteritis nodosa

Definition. Polyarteritis nodosa (PAN) constitutes a necrotizing inflammation of medium-sized or small arteries without glomerulonephritis or vasculitis in arterioles, capillaries or venules [1]. It was originally described by Kussmaul and Maier in 1866 [2] as 'periarteritis nodosa', and was renamed 'polyarteritis nodosa' in 1903 after Ferrari recognized its multivessel involvement as well as its transmural inflammation. Segmental involvement of medium-sized arteries is usual. Affected patients may have several signs and symptoms involving multiple organ systems. Ischaemia, infarcts and haemorrhage result from the vasculitis and lead to end-organ damage in patients with PAN. It has been described in all racial groups [3–5], with an incidence of 4.6–9 per million per year [6]; in populations with a low incidence of hepatitis B, its incidence is less than 5 per million population, but where hepatitis B is hyperendemic, the incidence rises dramatically (for example 77 per million in an Alaskan Eskimo population [7]). There may be an equal sex incidence or male predominance.

Aetiology and pathogenesis. Immune complexes are most commonly implicated in development of PAN. Immune complexes may activate complement with subsequent recruitment of neutrophils to the vessel wall. Progression of the inflammatory and immune response leads to recruitment of T lymphocytes, particularly CD8+ T cells, and macrophages. Antiendothelial cell antibodies have also been proposed as a pathogenic mechanism, but specific antigens have not been identified and such antibodies are not specific to PAN [8]. The occurrence of nodose lesions and aneurysms at arterial branch points has also led to theories that the increased shear stress at these areas causes up-regulation of endothelial inflammatory factors [9–12], and that there may also be a greater number of macrophages in the tunica intima at these stress points [13,14], adding to the susceptibility of endothelial cells to inflammatory activity.

In cases of PAN associated with hepatitis B virus infection, HbsAg is thought to be the triggering antigen; typically this applies to 5–7% of patients with PAN, although incidences of associated hepatitis B as high as 10–54% have been reported [6]. Rarely, other viruses have been associated with PAN, including hepatitis C, parvovirus B19, human immunodeficiency virus and herpes zoster virus, as well as streptococcal infection. PAN has been described in association with malignancies, particularly hairy cell leukaemia [15], as well as with inflammatory conditions such as SLE, inflammatory bowel disease, familial Mediterranean fever and Cogan's syndrome. Minocycline has been implicated in a minority of individuals [16].

Histopathology. PAN affects small and medium-size muscular arteries and sometimes arterioles [6,17]. Lesions often develop at branch points, where there is a focal necrotizing arteritis; the inflammatory infiltrate is neutrophil-rich initially but subsequently mononuclear cells are predominant. There may be focal panniculitis; granulomata are absent. The vasculitis causes nodose swellings and may cause development of microaneurysms as blood vessel walls become weak and potentially necrotic. The most severely affected arterial branch points of vessels may rupture, leading to luminal thrombosis and obliteration, thus resulting in widespread distal tissue ischaemia and ultimately necrosis (Figs 50.19 & 50.20). Lesions heal by fibrosis. In patients with hepatitis B-associated PAN, HbsAg may be present within the lesions.

Clinical features. Patients with PAN usually have constitutional upset, including fever, weight loss, arthralgia and malaise. Organs commonly targeted comprise kidneys (infarctions and ischaemic nephropathy lead to hypertension and renal failure), heart (angina, myocardial infarction), gut (ischaemia, bleeding, perforation or infarction, presenting as abdominal pain) and peripheral nerves (mononeuritis multiplex) [8]. Rupture of an aneurysm may cause acute haemorrhage within the affected organ. In males, orchitis is a characteristic feature. Importantly for differential diagnosis, PAN does not affect the lung parenchyma and does not cause glomerulonephritis—patients in whom glomerulonephritis is a

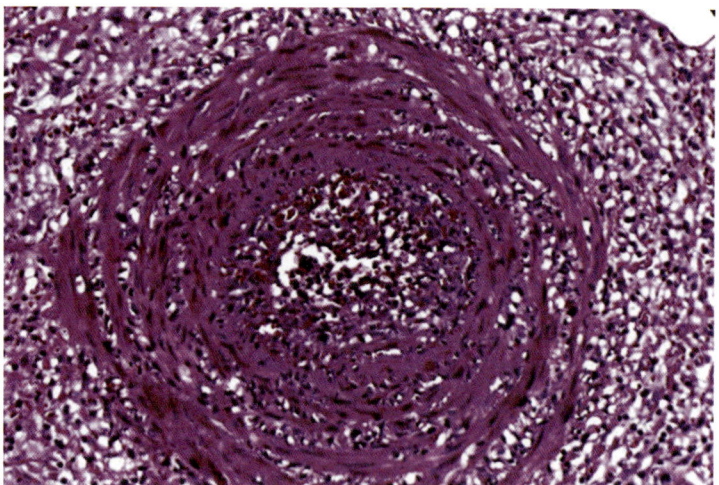

Fig. 50.20 Polyarteritis nodosa. Higher magnification demonstrates the partial destruction of the vessel wall and the inflammatory infiltrate composed of lymphocytes and neutrophils. (Courtesy of Dr Omar Sangueza, Wake Forest University School of Medicine, Winston-Salem, NC, USA.)

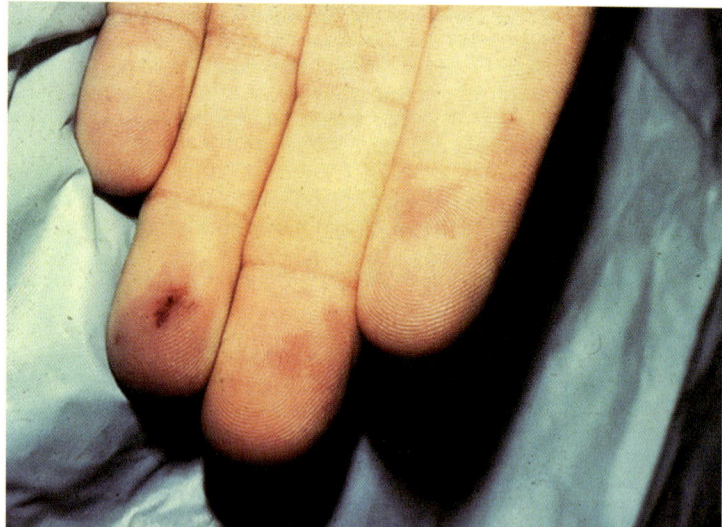

Fig. 50.22 Polyarteritis nodosa. Multiple lesions on the fingers.

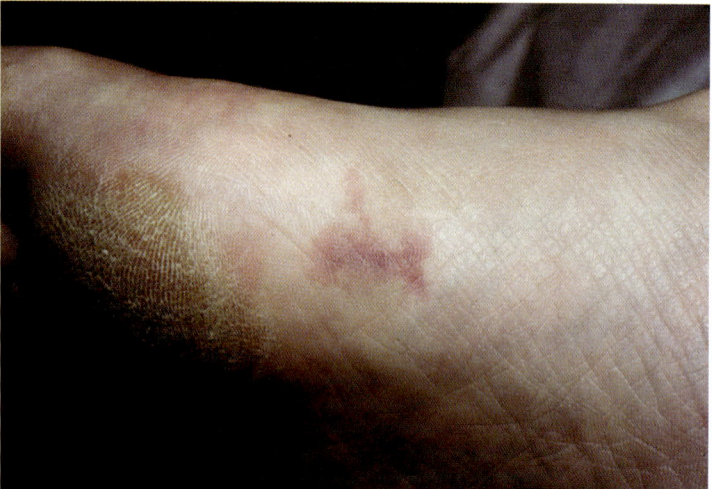

Fig. 50.21 Polyarteritis nodosa. Note the location of the lesion on the patient's foot.

dominant feature are more likely to have microscopic polyangiitis. Patients with hepatitis B virus-associated PAN may have features of hepatitis.

Skin features of PAN are common, occurring in about half of patients depending on the series, although early reports included patients with microscopic polyangiitis where small vessel involvement with purpuric manifestations may have confused the picture [8]. In PAN, a subcutaneous nodule or group of nodules ranging from 0.5–2 cm (mostly 5–10 mm) may develop, predominantly on the lower limbs and often in proximity to vessels. Typical sites are around the knee, anterior lower leg and dorsum of the foot. Nodules may be tender, pulsatile or secondarily ulcerated, with either normal or erythematous overlying skin. Livedo reticularis may occur, with or without ulceration. Ulcers have a 'punched-out' appearance. Ulceration and gangrene of the digits or penis may develop. Cutaneous lesions in patients with PAN are depicted in Figs 50.21 and 50.22.

Diagnosis. Conventional angiography of hepatitic, renal, splanchnic and splenic circulations remains the most reliable method of demonstrating the aneurysms, stenoses and abnormal vessels in PAN [18], although they are not specific to this disorder. Tissue biopsy of affected muscle or nerve may confirm the presence of vasculitic lesions [19]; sensitivities of muscle and sural nerve biopsy specimens are 60% and 70%, respectively, in cases of symptomatic muscle involvement and nerve involvement demonstrated electrophysiologically [20,21]. Renal biopsy specimens (when urinalysis is abnormal) and angiography and/or aortography demonstrating pathognomonic aneurysmal dilatation of vessel walls may also be used to help establish a diagnosis of PAN. Although very sensitive, skin biopsy is not specific, and is usually not sufficient to establish the diagnosis of PAN. A study of 29 patients with skin ulcers due to PAN (fulfilling both American College of Rheumatology and Chapel Hill Consensus Conference criteria) showed that the highest yield was achieved by biopsying both the peripheral area of the ulcer and the central area (the rationale being that the central area would represent the apex of a wedge-shaped infarct); 26 diagnoses were confirmed but biopsies needed to contain subcutaneous tissue, 9/26 confirmed cases required multiple biopsies and diagnosis could not be achieved from the skin ulcers in the other three [22].

During acute disease, the ESR and CRP will be elevated and there may be other non-specific laboratory abnormalities such as leukocytosis with neutrophilia, thrombocytosis, normocytic anaemia, hypergammaglobulinaemia and cryoglobulinaemia, as well as haematuria, proteinuria. Antineutrophil cytoplasm antibodies are negative; although P-ANCA has been said to be positive in 20% of cases of PAN, it is more commonly seen in MPA or CSS (suggesting that some cases may have been misclassified), whereas a positive C-ANCA is typically associated with WG, CSS or MPA but not with PAN. Patients who test positive for hepatitis B will all be HbsAg-positive and most will be hepatitis B early antigen-positive.

Treatment. Patients who do not have hepatitis B-associated disease benefit from high-dose corticosteroids, commencing at 1 mg/kg/day and tapering over 1 year to 5–10 mg/day; the ESR is useful for monitoring disease activity. Such treatment has improved the 5-year survival from about 10% to over 50% [23]. In patients with severe disease, three daily pulses of methylprednisolone, 500–1000 mg, may be considered although there is no evidence to suggest that this is any better than daily oral prednisolone. Severe disease is indicated by the presence of renal (renal insufficiency, proteinuria >1 g/day), gut, cardiac or central nervous system involvement [24].

It is possible that cyclophosphamide may be useful in achieving remission in patients with severe disease [22]; one recommendation is for 12 pulses of cyclophosphamide, given at 0.6 g/m^2 every 2 weeks for the first three pulses and thereafter monthly [25], although it is worth pointing out that the trial from which these recommendations stem included patients with both PAN and microscopic polyangiitis; patients with PAN were in the minority. Plasma exchange does not appear to have any additional benefit in patients with non-hepatitis B-associated PAN.

Patients with hepatitis B-associated PAN appear to benefit from a combination of antiviral and immune suppressing drugs [26]. Corticosteroids should only be used short-term because of the possibility of increased viral replication; one regimen involves corticosteroids for 2 weeks, followed by the antiviral lamivudine combined with plasma exchanges. Relapses are rare and do not occur once viral replication has ceased and seroconversion has been obtained.

Treatment for hypertension and pain are important. Surgery may be needed for complications.

References

1 Jennette JC, Falk RJ, Andrassy K *et al.* Nomenclature of systemic vasculitides: the proposal of an International Consensus Conference. *Arthritis Rheum* 1994; **37**: 187–92.

2 Kussmaul AMR. Uber eine bisher beschreinbene eigentumliche Arterienenerkrankung (perarteritis nodosa) die mit Morbus Birghitii un rapid fortschreitender allgemeinen Muskellahmung einhergeht. *Arch Klin Med* 1866; **1**: 484–518.

3 Watts RA, Gonzalez-Gay MA, Lane SE *et al.* Geoepidemiology of systemic vasculitis: comparison of the incidence in two regions of Europe. *Ann Rheum Dis* 2001; **60**: 170–2.

4 Watts RA, Lane SE, Bentham G. Epidemiology of systemic vasculitis: a 10-year study in the United Kingdom. *Arthritis Rheum* 2000; **43**: 414–9.

5 Bonsib SM. Polyarteritis nodosa. *Semin Diag Pathol* 2001; **18**: 14–23.

6 Lhote F, Cohen P, Guillevin L. Polyarteritis nodosa, microscopic polyangiitis and Churg–Strauss syndrome. *Lupus* 1998; **7**: 238–58.

7 McMahon BJ, Heyward WL, Templin DW *et al.* Hepatitis B-associated polyarteritis nodosa in Alaskan Eskimos: clinical and epidemiologic features and long-term follow-up. *Hepatology* 1989; **9**: 97–101.

8 Guillevin L. Polyarteritis nodosa and microscopic polyangiitis. In: Ball GV, Bridges SL, eds, *Vasculitis.* Oxford: Oxford University Press, 2002: 300–20.

9 Morigi M, Zoja C, Figliuzzi M *et al.* Fluid shear stress modulates surface expression of adhesion molecules by endothelial cells. *Blood* 1995; **85**: 1696–703.

10 Nagel T, Resnick N, Dewey CF, Gimbrone MA. Vascular endothelial cells respond to spatial gradients in fluid shear stress by enhanced activation of transcription factors. *Arterioscler Thromb Vasc Biol* 1999; **19**: 1825–34.

11 Iiyama K, Hajra L, Iiyama M *et al.* Patterns of vascular cell adhesion molecule-1 and intercellular adhesion molecule-1 expression in rabbit and mouse atherosclerotic lesions and at sites predisposed to lesion formation. *Circ Res* 1999; **85**: 199–207.

12 Cybulsky MI, Lichtman AH, Hajra L, Iiyama K. Leukocyte adhesion molecules in atherogenesis. *Clin Chim Acta* 1999; **286**: 207–18.

13 Malinauskas RA, Herrmann RA, Truskey GA. The distribution of intimal white blood cells in the normal rabbit aorta. *Atherosclerosis* 1995; **115**: 147–63.

14 Stary HC. Macrophages, macrophage foam cells, and eccentric intimal thickening in the coronary arteries of young children. *Atherosclerosis* 1987; **64**: 91–108.

15 Hasler P, Kistler H, Gerber H. Vasculitides in hairy cell leukemia. *Semin Arthritis Rheum* 1995; **25**: 134–42.

16 Schrodt BJ, Callen JP. Polyarteritis nodosa attributable to minocycline treatment of acne vulgaris. *Pediatrics* 1999; **103**: 503–4.

17 Churg J, Churg A. Idiopathic and secondary vasculitis: a review. *Modern Pathol* 1989; **2**: 144–60.

18 Stanson AW, Friese JL, Johnson CM *et al.* Polyarteritis nodosa: spectrum of angiographic findings. *Radiographics* 2001; **21**: 151–9.

19 Churg A, Churg J. *Systemic Vasculitides.* New York: Igaku-Shoin, 1991.

20 Albert DA, Rimon D, Silverstein MD. The diagnosis of polyarteritis nodosa. I. A literature-based decision analysis approach. *Arthritis Rheum* 1988; **31**: 1117–27.

21 Lightfoot RW Jr, Michel BA, Bloch DA *et al.* The American College of Rheumatology 1990 criteria for the classification of polyarteritis nodosa. *Arthritis Rheum* 1990; **33**: 1088–93.

22 Ricotti C, Kowalcyzk JP, Gherst M, Nousari CH. The diagnostic yield of histopathologic sampling techniques in PAN-associated cutaneous ulcers. *Arch Dermatol* 2007; **143**: 1335–6.

23 Gayraud M, Guillevin L, le Toumelin P *et al.* Long-term follow up of polyarteritis nodosa, microscopic polyangiitis, and Churg–Strauss syndrome: analysis of four prospective trials including 278 patients. *Arthritis Rheum* 2001; **44**: 666–75.

24 Guillevin L, Lhote F, Gayraud M *et al.* Prognostic factors in polyarteritis nodosa and Churg-Strauss syndrome. *Medicine* 1996; **75**: 17–28.

25 Guillevin L, Cohen P, Mahr A *et al.* Treatment of polyarteritis nodosa and microscopic polyangiitis with poor prognosis factors: a prospective trial comparing glucocorticoids and six or twelve cyclophosphamide pulses in sixty-five patients. *Arthritis Rheum* 2003; **49**: 93–100.

26 Guillevin L, Mahr A, Callard P *et al.* Hepatitis B virus-associated polyarteritis nodosa: clinical characteristics, outcome, and impact of treatment in 115 patients. *Medicine (Baltimore)* 2005; **84**: 313–22.

Microscopic polyangiitis

Synonyms
- Microscopic polyarteritis nodosa
- Microscopic polyarteritis

Definition. Microscopic polyangiitis (MPA) is a systemic vasculitis affecting blood vessels ranging in size from capillaries to medium-sized arteries. In some instances, there is only venous involvement in histopathological specimens from lesions in patients with MPA. MPA is strongly associated with lung involvement (primarily alveolar haemorrhage) and with crescentic glomerulonephritis [1]. The incidence of MPA is six to eight per million per year [2].

Patients demonstrating signs of PAN without cutaneous nodules were first described by Wohlwill in 1923, and then by Arkin in 1930. In 1948, articles were published that distinguished MPA from PAN. In 1994, MPA was termed microscopic polyangiitis instead of microscopic polyarteritis by a consensus conference because of the lack of arterial involvement in some patients and the involvement of vessels other than arteries [1].

Aetiology and pathogenesis. The exact pathogenesis of MPA is poorly understood, although it is considered a pauci-immune vasculitis because of the relative absence of immunoglobulins or complement in affected vessel walls [3–7]. P-ANCA may have a role in the aetiology by activating neutrophils and monocytes via interactions with enzymes on the surface of or directly around endothelial cells [8], initially causing direct injury to the vessel endothelium. This is demonstrated in early findings of pauci-immune small vessel vasculitides in which there is fibrin accumulation in the subendothelium [7,9] as well as lysis of leukocytes within the vascular space [9] associated with endothelial injury. Products from neutrophils and monocytes (such as serine proteinases and metalloproteinases) may be inactivated at distant sites [10], accounting for the large degree of local tissue injury in lesions of MPA. Direct interactions between these cells and the endothelium may also explain the predilection of the disease for small rather than larger sized vessels. In some patients, there is a relationship between MPA and infection with either hepatitis B or C viruses [11,12]. Recent evidence suggests that antimyeloperoxidase (MPO) antibodies, present in 70% of MPA patients, may play a role in the damage to blood vessels by activating an oxidative burst [13].

Histopathology. Histological specimens from MPA lesions demonstrate segmental vascular necrosis. Neutrophils and monocytes permeate vessel walls, causing leukocytoclasia, accumulation of fibrin and haemorrhage. Biopsy specimens from lesions of palpable purpura demonstrate leukocytoclastic vasculitis.

Clinical features. Many patients with MPA initially experience constitutional symptoms, including fever, weight loss, myalgia and arthralgia. These may be present for several years before the onset of the pulmonary and renal disease that often occurs in patients with MPA. Between 79 and 90% of patients with MPA have necrotizing glomerulonephritis, and 25–50% have lung involvement, sometimes leading to pulmonary–renal syndrome [14], and leading to pulmonary haemorrhage in up to 29% of patients [15–17]. Although less common than in patients with PAN, symmetrical peripheral neuropathies or mononeuritis multiplex may occur in patients with MPA. Gastrointestinal (GI) manifestations are present in half of MPA patients. Although GI disease in MPA is usually mild at presentation, there has been a report of initial presentation with extensive colonic ulcerations and haemorrhage, characterized by a crypt abscess [18]. Nearly half of patients have palpable purpura on dependent skin sites upon presentation [19], but the presence of nodules should raise the suspicion of PAN, Wegener's granulomatosis (WG), or Churg–Strauss syndrome (CSS).

Diagnosis. MPA must be clinically distinguished from other vasculitides such as WG, CSS, CSVV, or PAN. In patients with MPA, positive P-ANCA and rheumatoid factor tests are common, unlike in patients with PAN. Some authors claim that small vessel vasculitis in the skin can distinguish MPA from PAN, stating that cutaneous small vessel vasculitis lesions do not typically occur in patients with PAN, although this is controversial. When palpable purpuric lesions are present in the absence of constitutional symptoms or the systemic features of MPA, patients most probably have CSVV rather than MPA. Small vessel vasculitis in the absence of granulomatous inflammation or asthma suggests MPA instead of CSS or WG [1].

Treatment. The management of MPA has recently been reviewed [20]. The approaches needed for induction, maintenance and long-term follow-up all differ. A preceding 'identification' phase may be associated with delay in treatment, especially if renal disease is absent or ANCA is negative. Initially, patients with MPA should be treated with high-dose corticosteroids and immunosuppressive treatment; cyclophosphamide has been used for some decades and, although strong evidence-based support, such as that supporting its use in patients with WG, is lacking, this combination leads to remission in 75–90% of patients at 6 months [20]. This regimen remains the mainstay of treatment for MPA associated with pulmonary haemorrhage or rapidly progressive glomerulonephritis. Methotrexate achieves similar early results but with a much higher relapse rate. Plasma exchange, or plasma filtration, are used for those with severe renal disease and, although associated with high early disease-related mortality, does appear to reduce longer-term need for dialysis. Intravenous immunoglobulin has also been used with benefit. For those who may not tolerate a steroid–cyclophosphamide regimen, such as the elderly, gabexate mesilate has been employed as an alternative treatment [21]. Based on evidence of an anti-MPO antibody-mediated oxidative burst, a compound such as N-acetylcysteine (NAC) may show promise for future therapy; NAC is an antioxidant that blocks HOCl production during the oxidative burst and thus avoids endothelial lysis [13]. Anti-TNF agents have been used but have given rise to concerns about malignancy in the context of vasculitis; additionally, other damaging cytokines (such as IL-18) are not affected by TNF blockade [20]. Selective blockade of different TNF receptors in glomerular vessels may be future targets for therapy. Rituximab has been used in a small number of cases with good results, especially as those treated had refractory disease [20].

The course of MPA is characterized by relapses, in contrast with that of PAN [20,22]. The prognosis is worst in older age, in those with low glomerular filtration rate, and in those with more glomeruli affected, or with extra-glomerular arteritis, on renal biopsy. Long-term follow-up is necessary, with monitoring of renal parameters and ANCA.

References

1 Jennette JC, Thomas DB, Falk RJ. Microscopic polyangiitis (microscopic polyarteritis). *Semin Diag Pathol* 2001; **18**: 3–13.

2 Scott DG, Watts RA. Systemic vasculitis: epidemiology, classification and environmental factors. *Ann Rheum Dis* 2000; **59**: 161–3.

3 Jennette JC, Falk RG, Andrassy K *et al*. Nomenclature of systemic vasculitides. Proposal of an international consensus conference. *Arthritis Rheum* 1994; **37**: 187–92.

4 Savage CO, Winearls CG, Evans DG *et al*. Microscopic polyarteritis: presentation, pathology and prognosis. *QJM* 1985; **56**: 467–83.

5 Jennette JC, Falk RJ. Small vessel vasculitis. *N Engl J Med* 1997; **337**: 1512–23.

6 Jennette JC, Falk RJ. The pathology of vasculitis involving the kidney. *Am J Kidney Dis* 1994; **24**: 130–41.

7 D'Agati V, Chander P, Nash M *et al*. Idiopathic microscopic polyarteritis nodosa: ultrastructural observations on the renal vascular and glomerular lesions. *Am J Kidney Dis* 1986; **7**: 95–110.

8 Jennette JC, Falk RJ. Pathogenesis of the vascular and glomerular damage in ANCA-positive vasculitis. *Nephrol Dial Transplant* 1998; **13** (Suppl. 1): 16–20.

9 Donald KJ, Edwards RL, McEvoy JDS. An ultrastructural study of the pathogenesis of tissue injury in limited Wegener's granulomatosis. *Pathology* 1976; **8**: 161–9.

10 Weiss SJ. Tissue destruction by neutrophils. *N Engl J Med* 1989; **320**: 365–76.

11 Harper L, Savage CO. Pathogenesis of ANCA-associated systemic vasculitis. *J Pathol* 2000; **190**: 349–59.

12 Franssen CF, Stegeman CA, Kallenberg CG *et al*. Antiproteinase 3- and antimyeloperoxidase-associated vasculitis. *Kidney Int* 2000; **57**: 2195–206.

13 Guilpain P, Servettaz A, Goulvestre C *et al*. Pathogenic effects of antimyeloperoxidase antibodies in patients with microscopic polyangiitis. *Arthritis Rheum* 2007; **56**: 2455–63.

14 Niles J, Bottinger E, Saurina G *et al*. The syndrome of lung hemorrhage and nephritis is usually an ANCA-associated condition. *Arch Intern Med* 1996; **156**: 440.

15 Savige J, Davies D, Falk RJ *et al*. Antineutrophil cytoplasmic antibodies and associated diseases: a review of the clinical and laboratory features. *Kidney Int* 2000; **57**: 846–62.

16 Guillevin L, Lhote F. Treatment of polyarteritis nodosa and microscopic polyangiitis. *Arthritis Rheum* 1998; **41**: 2100–5.

17 Lauque D, Cadranel J, Lazor R *et al*. Microscopic polyangiitis with alveolar hemorrhage. A study of 20 cases and review of the literature. Groupe d'Etudes et de Recherche sur les Maladies 'Orphelines' Pulmonaires (GERM'O'P). *Medicine (Baltimore)* 2000; **79**: 222–33.

18 Tsai C-N, Chang C-M, Chuang C-H *et al*. Extended colonic ulcerations in a patient with microscopic polyangiitis. *Ann Rheum Dis* 2004; **63**: 1521–2.

19 Burrows NP, Lockwood CM. Antineutrophil cytoplasmic antibodies and their relevance to the dermatologist. *Br J Dermatol* 1995; **132**: 173–81.

20 Jayne D. Challenges in the management of microscopic polyangiitis: past, present and future. *Curr Opin Rheumatol* 2008; **20**: 3–9.

21 Miyawaki K, Shiraishi J, Tsutsumi Y *et al*. Beneficial effect of gabexate mesilate on microscopic polyangiitis with renal dysfunction and pulmonary hemorrhage: a case report. *Angiology* 2006; **57**: 522–5.

22 Gayraud M, Guillevin L, le Toumelin P *et al*. Long-term follow-up of polyarteritis nodosa, microscopic polyangiitis, and Churg-Strauss syndrome: analysis of four prospective trials including 278 patients. *Arthritis Rheum* 2001; **44**: 666–75.

Cutaneous polyarteritis nodosa

Synonym
- Benign cutaneous periarteritis nodosa

Definition. Cutaneous polyarteritis nodosa (C-PAN) is a variant of PAN that is limited primarily to the skin. It was first described by Lindberg in 1931 [1] as a more benign variant of systemic PAN that did not have visceral involvement, although controversy exists over whether or not it simply represents an early or more limited form of PAN [2,3]. Thus, C-PAN can only be diagnosed by exclusion of findings that would alter the diagnosis to that of classic PAN. The course of C-PAN is typically benign and relapsing, despite the presence of moderate constitutional symptoms and mild nerve and muscle involvement in some patients [4,5].

Aetiology and pathogenesis. Infections such as streptococcus (particularly in children), parvovirus B19, HIV, and hepatitis B, as well as inflammatory bowel disease (IBD), have been associated with C-PAN [6], although the exact aetiology is unknown. Medications including minocycline, prescribed for acne, have also been reported to induce C-PAN [7–9]. Immunological mechanisms are thought by some authors to be involved only in the pathogenesis of systemic polyarteritis nodosa, and not in the development of C-PAN [10]. Whether C-PAN is part of the disease progression of systemic polyarteritis nodosa or should remain a separate clinical

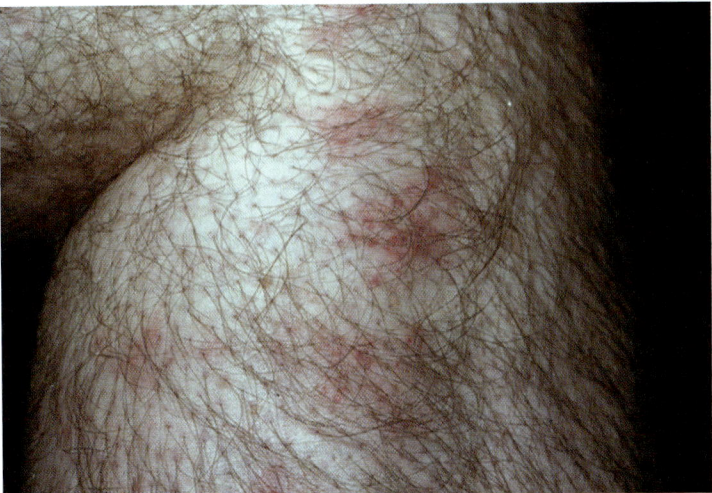

Fig. 50.23 Cutaneous polyarteritis nodosa. Erythematous lesions on the leg.

clinical entity remains a topic of debate. Evidence suggests that C-PAN should remain separate from PAN as it rarely progresses into PAN and, unlike PAN, it rarely exhibits systemic involvement and has a good prognosis [10–14].

Histopathology. Early in the course of C-PAN, there is a predominantly neutrophilic inflammatory infiltrate in the walls of medium-sized arteries and arterioles of septae in the upper portions of the subcutaneous fat. The involved vessels classically demonstrate a target-like appearance resulting from an eosinophilic ring of fibrinoid necrosis. Later in the disease process the infiltrate becomes less neutrophilic, consisting predominantly of lymphocytes and histiocytes. Complement and IgM deposits in vessel walls of lesions of C-PAN from some patients may be demonstrated by direct immunofluorescence [15]. Unlike those of systemic PAN, lesions of C-PAN do not typically involve arterial bifurcations.

Clinical features. Although some patients with C-PAN may report constitutional symptoms as well as chronic, mild involvement of both muscles and nerves [4,5], cutaneous manifestations are the most striking feature of the disease. Dermal or subcutaneous nodules are most commonly located on the distal lower extremities near the malleoli (Fig. 50.23) and may extend proximally to the thighs, buttock, arms or hands. Patients may report tenderness associated with the nodules, which may ulcerate (Fig. 50.24) or more commonly demonstrate necrotizing livedo reticularis, also referred to as retiform purpura. Gangrene of the digits can ultimately occur, most commonly in children with C-PAN, but this finding should trigger an aggressive search to exclude systemic PAN [16,17]. Recurrent spiking fevers, polyarthralgia and macular upper extremity cutaneous eruption, symptoms shared by both C-PAN and adult-onset Still's disease (AOSD), sometimes create a challenge when diagnosing C-PAN. The presence of livedo reticularis (Fig. 50.25) and the finding of a characteristic skin biopsy appearance with C-PAN help to differentiate it from AOSD [18].

Diagnosis. Patients with necrotizing lesions of livedo reticularis must be evaluated for vasculitis or vasculopathy (e.g.

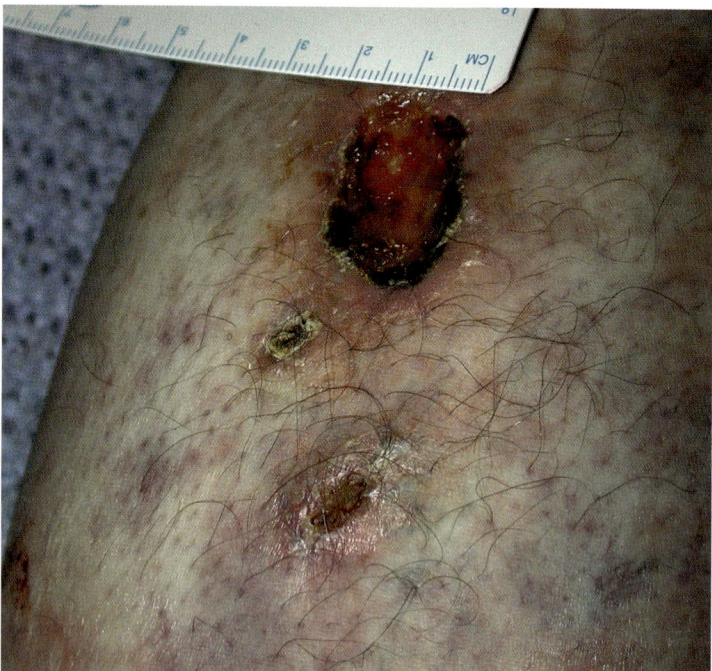

Fig. 50.24 Cutaneous polyarteritis nodosa. Nodules and ulceration.

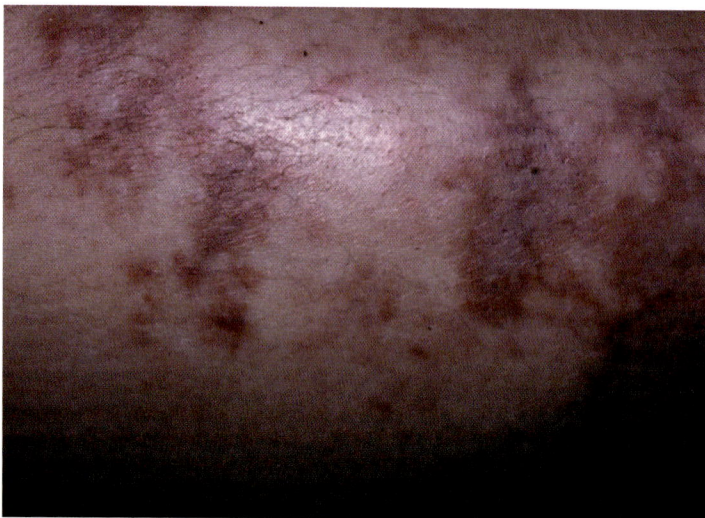

Fig. 50.25 Cutaneous polyarteritis nodosa. Livedo of legs.

antiphospholipid antibody syndrome, cholesterol emboli or other factors that can produce non-vasculitic vessel occlusion; see Chapter 49). If nodules are present, they should be biopsied by incisional biopsy methods to assess for a panarteritis of muscular arteries which would confirm a diagnosis of C-PAN. The distinction from systemic PAN requires patient evaluation by history, physical examination, screening laboratory tests and ongoing follow-up. In addition, rheumatological consultation is often appropriate.

Treatment. Although no double-blind prospective trials have been performed, several reports suggest that non-steroidal anti-inflammatory drugs and salicylates can be an effective treatment for symptoms of C-PAN [19]. High-dose corticosteroids followed by tapering of the dosage may occasionally be necessary for some patients [20,21]. Also without evidence from controlled trials, but based on the strong association with streptococcal infection, penicillin is often used for treatment and prophylaxis in children with C-PAN. Screening for recent streptococcal infection with anti-DNAse B or other tests may guide this decision. Other treatments documented in anecdotal reports include dipyridamole, sulfapyridine, pentoxifylline and dapsone in patients with C-PAN. Low-dose weekly methotrexate (7.5–20 mg/week) has been successful in some patients with skin lesions unresponsive to corticosteroids given topically, intralesionally and orally [22]. In addition, chronic leg ulcers resistant to treatment with high-dose corticosteroids have recently been successfully treated with granulocyte-macrophage colony stimulating factor (GM-CSF) which has been shown to improve wound healing [23]. GM-CSF improves the clearance of bacteria and debris through the local attraction of neutrophils, promotes neovascularization and enhancement of keratinization, and induces acceleration of the formation of new tissue [23]. However, low-dose weekly methotrexate therapy and gradient support hosiery are anecdotally adequate therapy for the majority of patients with C-PAN [22].

References

1 Lindberg K. Ein Beitrag zur Kenntnis der Periarteritis nodosa. *Acta Med Scan* 1931; **76**: 183–225.
2 Thomas RH, Black MM. The wide clinical spectrum of polyarteritis nodosa with cutaneous involvement. *Clin Exp Dermatol* 1983; **8**: 47–59.
3 Minkowitz G, Smoller BR, McNutt NS. Benign cutaneous polyarteritis nodosa. Relationship to systemic polyarteritis nodosa and to hepatitis B infection. *Arch Dermatol* 1991; **127**: 1520–3.
4 Borrie P. Cutaneous polyarteritis nodosa. *Br J Dermatol* 1972; **87**: 87–95.
5 Khoo BP, Ng SK. Cutaneous polyarteritis nodosa: a case report and literature review. *Ann Med Assoc Singapore* 1998; **27**: 868–72.
6 Mat C, Yurdakul S, Tuzuner N, Tuzun Y. Small vessel vasculitis and vasculitis confined to skin. *Baillières Clin Rheumatol* 1997; **11**: 237–57.
7 Tehrani R, Nash-Goelitz A, Adams E *et al.* Minocycline-induced cutaneous polyarteritis nodosa. *J Clin Rheumatol* 2007; **13**: 146–9.
8 Culver B, Itkin A, Pischel K. Case report and review of minocycline-induced cutaneous polyarteritis nodosa. *Arthritis Rheum* 2005; **53**: 468–70.
9 Abad S, Kambouchner M, Nejjari M *et al.* Additional case of minocycline-induced cutaneous polyarteritis nodosa: comment on the article by Culver *et al. Arthritis Rheum* 2006; **55**: 831, author reply 832.
10 Daoud MS, Hutton KP, Gibson LE. Cutaneous periarteritis nodosa: a clinico-pathological study of 79 cases. *Br J Dermatol* 1997; **136**: 706–13.
11 Choi SW, Lew S, Cho SD *et al.* Cutaneous polyarteritis nodosa presented with digital gangrene: a case report. *J Korean Med Sci* 2006; **21**: 371–3.
12 Gushi A, Hashiguchi T, Fukumaru K *et al.* Three cases of polyarteritis nodosa cutanea and a review of the literature. *J Dermatol* 2000; **27**: 778–81.
13 Bauza A, Espana A, Idoate M. Cutaneous polyarteritis nodosa. *Br J Dermatol* 2002; **146**: 694–9.
14 Misago N, Mochizuki Y, Sekiyama-Kodera H *et al.* Cutaneous polyarteritis nodosa: therapy and clinical course in four cases. *J Dermatol* 2001; **28**: 719–27.
15 Diaz Perez JL, Schroeter AL, Winkelmann RK. Cutaneous periarteritis nodosa: immunofluorescence studies. *Arch Dermatol* 1980; **116**: 56–8.
16 Kumar L, Thapa BR, Sarkar B. Benign cutaneous polyarteritis nodosa in children below 10 years of age—a clinical experience. *Ann Rheum Dis* 1995; **54**: 134–6.
17 Stone MS, Olson RR, Weismann DN *et al.* Cutaneous vasculitis in the newborn of a mother with cutaneous polyarteritis nodosa. *J Am Acad Dermatol* 1993; **28**: 101–5.
18 Kato T, Fujii K, Wakabayashi T *et al.* A case of cutaneous polyarteritis nodosa manifested by spiking high fever, arthralgia and macular eruption like adult-onset Still's disease. *Clin Rheumatol* 2006; **25**: 419–21.
19 Diaz Perez JL, Winkelmann RK. Cutaneous periarteritis nodosa: a study of 33 cases. In: Wolff K, Winkelmann RK, eds. *Vasculitis.* London: Lloyd-Luke, 1980: 273–84.

20 Sheth AP, Olson JC, Esterly NB. Cutaneous polyarteritis nodosa of childhood. *J Am Acad Dermatol* 1994; **31**: 561–6.

21 Siberry GK, Cohen BA, Johnson B. Cutaneous polyarteritis nodosa. Reports of two cases in children and review of the literature. *Arch Dermatol* 1994; **130**: 884–9.

22 Jorizzo JL, White WL, Wise CM *et al*. Low-dose weekly methotrexate for unusual neutrophilic vascular reactions: cutaneous polyarteritis nodosa and Behçet's disease. *J Am Acad Dermatol* 1991; **24**: 973–8.

23 Tursen U, Api H, Kaya TI *et al*. Rapid healing of chronic leg ulcers during peri-lesional injections of granulocyte-macrophage colony-stimulating factor therapy in a patient with cutaneous polyarteritis nodosa. *J Eur Acad Dermatol Venereol* 2006; **20**: 1341–3.

Wegener's granulomatosis

Definition. WG is classically described as a triad consisting of systemic small vessel vasculitis, necrotizing granulomatous inflammation of both the upper and lower respiratory tracts, and glomerulonephritis. The first description of a patient with WG was by Klinger in 1931, but the disease was later defined in 1936 by Wegener who described three patients. It is a potentially severe disease which, if not treated, can lead to end-organ damage and/or death. Affecting males and females equally, the incidence of WG is 5–10 per million per year, with the majority of cases occurring in Caucasians [1–3]. The average age at onset is 40 years [4].

Aetiology and pathogenesis. Although the pathogenesis of WG is not well understood, it is believed that it may involve an amplified immune response to an antigenic stimulus, such as an infection. Clinical observation points to *Staphylococcus aureus* as a potential trigger in some patients. The incidence of chronic nasal carriage of *S. aureus* is significantly higher in patients with Wegener's granulomatosis compared with healthy individuals [5]. One theory regarding the pathogenesis of WG is that neutrophils are activated via cytokines or apoptosis and degranulate, expressing cytosolic proteins on their surfaces and releasing harmful oxygen radicals as well as chemoattractants [6–9]. This enables ANCA to form against complementary peptide sequences to proteinase-3, otherwise known as the 'Wegener's autoantigen' [10,11]. Wegener's autoantigen may be introduced by a pathogen, specifically *S. aureus*, which exhibits a protein with a peptide sequence that mimics that of antisense PR3 [11]. The cytoplasmic antinuclear cytoplasmic antibodies (C-ANCA) are directed at antisense PR3 sequences which then cross-react with PR3 peptide sequences, thereby functioning as autoantibodies [11]. The perinuclear antineutrophil cytoplasmic antibodies (P-ANCA) are directed at myeloperoxidase (MPO). PR3 induces dendritic cell maturation via the protease activated receptor (PAR)-2, which in turn induces a strong Th1-type T-cell response. The PR3-induced T-cell response in WG is stronger than in healthy and disease controls [10,12]. In addition, activated neutrophils then attract additional neutrophils and damage vascular endothelium by attaching to blood vessel walls [13–15]. Another theory about the role of ANCA in the pathogenesis of WG is that activated neutrophils located at damaged blood vessels release antigens, causing a secondary ANCA response [16].

Histopathology. Although most biopsy specimens taken from patients with WG show perivascular lymphocytic infiltrates, such

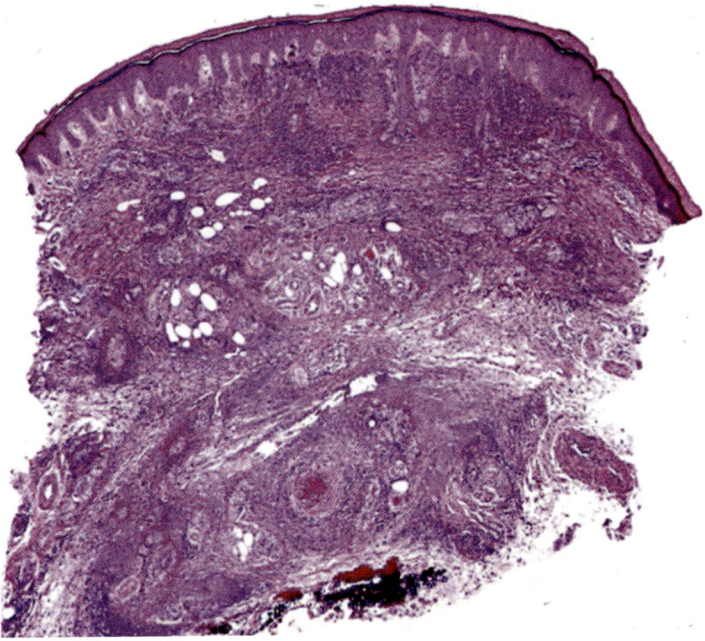

Fig. 50.26 Wegener's granulomatosis. There is extensive leukocytoclastic vasculitis involving the entire dermis. (Courtesy of Dr Omar Sangueza, Wake Forest University School of Medicine, Winston-Salem, NC, USA.)

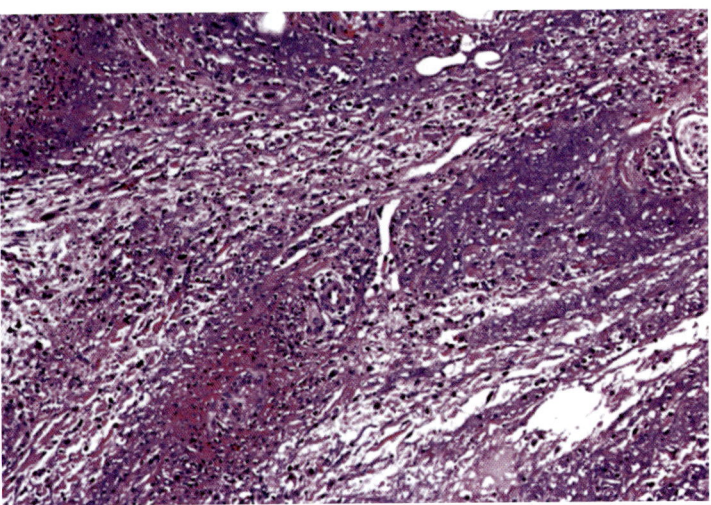

Fig. 50.27 Wegener's granulomatosis. Note the extensive area of collagen degeneration, destruction of vessels and mixed inflammatory infiltrate. (Courtesy of Dr Omar Sangueza, Wake Forest University School of Medicine, Winston-Salem, NC, USA.)

non-specific infiltrates may not be related to the pathogenesis of the disease [17]. More specific findings such as leukocytoclastic vasculitis and/or granulomatous inflammation may be present in up to 50% of skin biopsy specimens (Figs 50.26 & 50.27), although granulomatous inflammation around vessels or palisading necrotizing granulomas are uncommonly demonstrated in skin lesions.

Clinical features. Features of the classic triad of WG are not always present early in the course of the disease, making the diagnosis sometimes difficult. Furthermore, presentation without involvement of the classical sites, including skin, respiratory tract

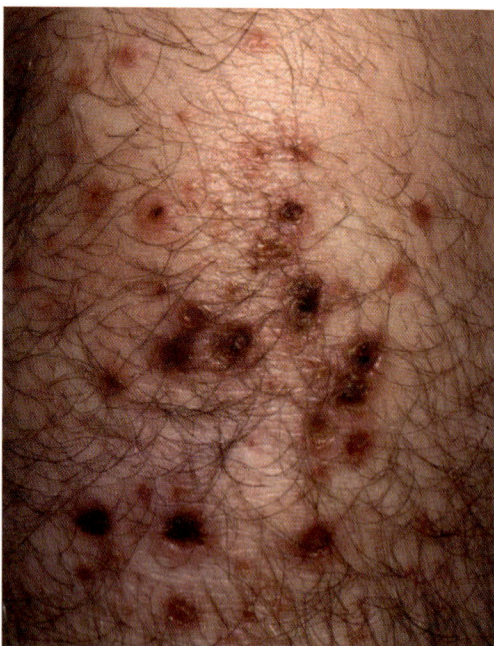

Fig. 50.28 Wegener's granulomatosis. Ulcerated lesions of cutaneous small vessel vasculitis.

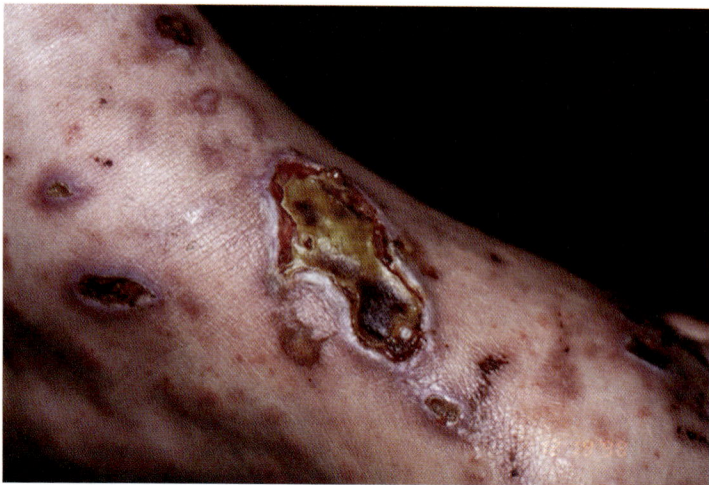

Fig. 50.29 Wegener's granulomatosis. Larger ulcerated lesions with background vasculitis.

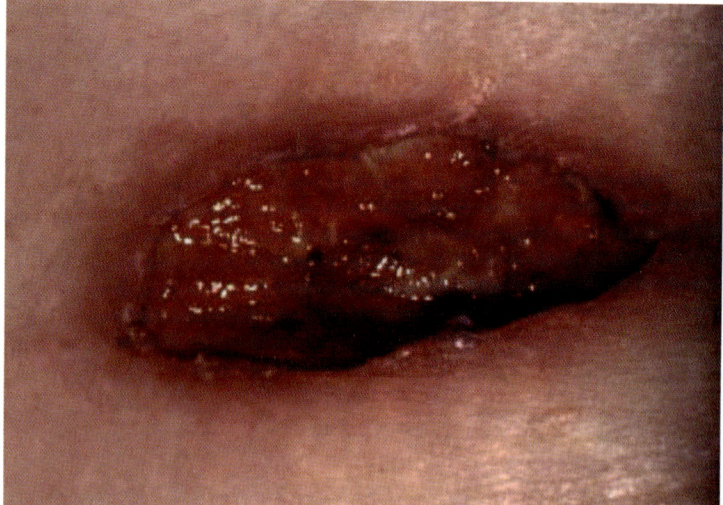

Fig. 50.30 Wegener's granulomatosis, presenting with two deep skin ulcers and nasal symptoms.

having 'malignant pyoderma' may actually have had lesions secondary to WG. Nodular, or even papulonecrotic, lesions most commonly occur on the extremities but may also occur on the face and scalp. These non-specific lesions (also found in patients with CSS, rheumatoid arthritis, SLE, inflammatory bowel disease and some infectious states) may be differentiated from rheumatoid nodules in that they ulcerate, whereas rheumatoid nodules do not [20–22]. Oral ulcers are the second most common mucocutaneous sign of WG. The upper respiratory tract is most commonly affected by WG, with otitis, epistaxis, rhinorrhea and sinusitis as common presenting signs and symptoms. A saddle nose deformity may result from necrotizing granulomas of the nasal mucosa. Lower respiratory signs and symptoms include cough, dyspnoea, chest pain and haemoptysis. Ulcerative lesions in WG are shown in Figs 50.28–50.30.

Diagnosis. Wegener's granulomatosis must be differentiated from CSS. Important differences in these vasculitis syndromes are the lack of upper respiratory involvement and lack of severe glomerulonephritis in CSS, as well as the presence of asthma and eosinophilia in CSS but not in WG. Laboratory findings in WG include elevated ESR and CRP, anaemia, leukocytosis and positive rheumatoid factor [2,3]. Although a small percentage of patients will have a positive P-ANCA, or no ANCA reactivity, up to 80% of patients will have a positive C-ANCA (with anti-PR3 specificity) [23]. Those few patients with no ANCA reactivity may well have localized WG and a better prognosis when compared with those who are ANCA-positive [24,25]. Nodular densities from necrotizing granulomatous inflammation of lung tissue and pulmonary haemorrhage may be present on chest radiography; almost any chest X-ray change may represent WG, with the exception of hilar adenopathy [26].

Treatment. Inducing remission in patients with Wegener's granulomatosis is most successfully accomplished using a combination of corticosteroids and cytotoxic agents, such as cyclophosphamide. This combination of therapy results in a significant resolu-

and kidneys, can occur. However, in up to 80% of patients, symptoms involving the upper or lower respiratory tract are present [18], and at presentation approximately 73% of patients will have nasal, sinus, tracheal or ear involvement. Less than half of all patients with WG present with pulmonary infiltrates or nodules. Renal disease is initially present in only 18% of patients, although approximately 77% will eventually develop glomerulonephritis [19]. Although 40% of patients with WG will eventually manifest skin findings, cutaneous manifestations and oral ulcers are only found in 13% and 6% of patients at initial presentation, respectively [19]. The most common cutaneous manifestation of WG is palpable purpura on dependent skin sites; other skin lesions include tender subcutaneous nodules, papules, vesicles and petechiae, as well as non-specific ulcers or pyoderma gangrenosum-like lesions. It is thought that patients previously diagnosed as tion of symptoms in greater than 90% of patients, with remission in 75%, and 87% surviving between 6 months and 24 years [19]. However, oral cyclophosphamide has significant toxicity and therefore other drugs, such as methotrexate, have been studied. Recent data suggest that, in patients with normal renal function, a methotrexate and prednisone regimen shows remission rates similar to the traditional cyclophosphamide and prednisone regimen. However, preliminary data suggest that the methotrexate plus prednisone regimen shows higher relapse rates, and therefore this regimen is suggested for inducing remission in a milder form of WG, such as head- and neck-limited disease [27]. The median survival for untreated WG remains only 5 months, and this prognosis is not appreciably altered by treatment with corticosteroids given as a monotherapy. Long-term treatment with trimethoprim–sulfamethoxazole (co-trimoxazole) has been documented to reduce the incidence of relapses, although side effects are relatively common [5]. Treatment options for refractory WG include anti-TNF-α agents such as infliximab or etanercept, and antilymphocyte antibodies such as rituximab. Rituximab is a monoclonal antibody that targets $CD20^+$ B-cells. It is currently used in the treatment of non-Hodgkin's lymphoma and rheumatoid arthritis but is also under investigation as a treatment option for refractory WG and other autoimmune diseases [28]. Impressive results can be seen, but development of antibodies to rituximab (due to its murine component) may limit long-term use.

References

1 Scott DG, Watts RA. Systemic vasculitis: epidemiology, classification and environmental factors. *Ann Rheum Dis* 2000; **59**: 161–3.

2 Stegeman CA, Kallenberg CG. Clinical aspects of primary vasculitis. *Springer Semin Immunopathol* 2001; **23**: 231–51.

3 Yi ES, Colby TV. Wegener's granulomatosis. *Semin Diag Pathol* 2001; **18**: 34–46.

4 Cotch MF, Hoffman GS, Yerg DE *et al*. The epidemiology of Wegener's granulomatosis. Estimates of the five-year period prevalence, annual mortality, and geographic diseases distribution from population-based data sources. *Arthritis Rheum* 1996; **39**: 87–92.

5 Popa ER, Tervaert JW. The relation between *Staphylococcus aureus* and Wegener's granulomatosis: current knowledge and future directions. *Intern Med* 2003; **42**: 771–80.

6 Falk RJ, Terrell RS, Charles LA, Jennette JC. Anti-neutrophil cytoplasmic autoantibodies induce neutrophils to degranulate and produce oxygen radicals in vitro. *Proc Natl Acad Sci USA* 1990; **87**: 4115–9.

7 Brouwer E, Huitema MG, Mulder L *et al*. Neutrophil activation in vitro and in vivo in Wegener's granulomatosis. *Kidney Int* 1994; **45**: 1120–31.

8 Cockwell P, Brooks CJ, Adu D, Savage CO. Interleukin-8: a pathogenetic role in antineutrophil cytoplasmic autoantibody-associated glomerulonephritis. *Kidney Int* 1999; **55**: 852–63.

9 Kettritz R, Choi M, Butt W *et al*. Phosphatidylinositol 3-kinase controls antineutrophil cytoplasmic antibodies-induced respiratory burst in human neutrophils. *J Am Soc Nephrol* 2002; **13**: 1740–9.

10 Lamprecht P, Gross WL, Kabelitz D. T cell alterations and lymphoid neogenesis favoring autoimmunity in Wegener's granulomatosis. *Arthritis Rheum* 2007; **56**: 1725–7.

11 Erickson VR, Hwang PH. Wegener's granulomatosis: current trends in diagnosis and management. *Curr Opin Otolaryngol Head Neck Surg* 2007; **15**: 170–6.

12 Csernok E, Ai M, Gross WL *et al*. Wegener autoantigen induces maturation of dendritic cells and licenses them for Th1 priming via the protease-activated receptor-2 pathway. *Blood* 2006; **107**: 4440–8.

13 Ewert BH, Jennette JC, Falk RJ. Anti-myeloperoxidase antibodies stimulate neutrophils to damage human endothelial cell. *Kidney Int* 1992; **41**: 375–83.

14 Yang JJ, Falk RJ, Jennette JC, Preston GA. Apoptosis of human endothelial cells induced by the neutrophil serine proteases proteinase 3 and elastase. *J Am Soc Nephrol* 1997; **8**: 431A.

15 Salant DJ. ANCA: Fuel for the fire or the spark that ignites the flame (editorial)? *Kidney Int* 1999; **55**: 1125–7.

16 Johnson RJ. The mystery of the antineutrophil cytoplasmic antibodies (editorial). *Am J Dis* 1995; **26**: 57.

17 Lie JT. Wegener's granulomatosis: histological documentation of common and uncommon manifestations in 216 patients. *Vasa* 1997; **26**: 261–70.

18 Lauque D, Cadranel J, Lazor R *et al*. Microscopic polyangiitis with alveolar hemorrhage. A study of 20 cases and review of the literature. Groupe d'Etudes et de Recherche sur les Maladies 'Orphelines' Pulmonaires (GERM'O'P). *Medicine (Baltimore)* 2000; **79**: 222–33.

19 Hoffman GS, Kerr GS, Leavitt RY *et al*. Wegener granulomatosis: an analysis of 158 patients. *Ann Intern Med* 1992; **116**: 488–98.

20 Magro CM, Crowson AN. The cutaneous neutrophilic vascular injury syndromes: a review. *Semin Diagn Pathol* 2001; **18**: 47–58.

21 Finan M. Rheumatoid papule, cutaneous extravascular necrotizing granuloma, and Churg–Strauss granuloma: are they the same entity? *J Am Acad Dermatol* 1990; **22**: 142–3.

22 Finan M, Winkelmann R. The cutaneous extravascular necrotizing granuloma (Churg–Strauss granuloma) and systemic disease: a review of 27 cases. *Medicine (Baltimore)* 1983; **62**: 142–58.

23 Jennette JC, Falk RJ. Small vessel vasculitis. *N Engl J Med* 1997; **337**: 1512–23.

24 Homer RJ. Antineutrophil cytoplasmic antibodies as markers for systemic autoimmune disease. *Clin Chest Med* 1998; **19**: 627–39.

25 Specks U, Wheatley C, McDonald T *et al*. Anticytoplasmic autoantibodies in the diagnosis and follow-up of Wegener's granulomatosis. *Mayo Clin Proc* 1989; **64**: 28–36.

26 Stone JH, Calabrese LH, Hoffman GS *et al*. Vasculitis. A collection of pearls and myths. *Rheum Dis Clin North Am* 2001; **27**: 677–728.

27 Belmont HM. Treatment of ANCA-associated systemic vasculitis. *Bull NYU Hosp Jt Dis* 2006; **64**: 60–6.

28 Antoniu SA. Treatment options for refractory Wegener's granulomatosis: a role for rituximab? *Curr Opin Investig Drugs* 2007; **8**: 927–32.

Churg–Strauss syndrome

Synonyms

- Allergic granulomatosis
- Vasculitis of Churg and Strauss

Definition. CSS is a rare vasculitis affecting multiple organ systems. The majority of patients demonstrate cutaneous findings while in the active phase of the disease. The disease is characterized by asthma, peripheral blood eosinophilia and necrotizing vasculitis with extravascular granulomas. Originally described by Rackermann and Greene in 1939, as an allergic disease not classified as periarteritis nodosa, Churg and Strauss later described the syndrome and its histopathological characteristics in 1951.

Aetiology and pathogenesis. The aetiology of CSS is unknown, although vaccination, desensitization and rapid discontinuation of corticosteroids have been associated with the onset of symptoms of CSS [1]. In the past it was believed that leukotriene antagonists were associated with the onset of CSS; however, new research suggests that, after adjustment for other asthma drugs, there is not a strong association [2]. Leukotriene antagonists are a marker for more severe asthma and severe asthma is thought to be a risk factor for CSS [3]. The pathogenesis of CSS is not completely understood. Immune complex deposition was once thought to be the mechanism of vasculitis in CSS, although eosinophils, mediated by a Th-2 response, are now thought to be the effector cells in the disease [4].

There is growing evidence for increased eosinophil survival in blood and tissues in CSS [5], possibly due to decreased apoptosis. Recent research has documented increased expression of TRAIL receptor 3 on eosinophils in patients with CSS [6]. TRAIL is a member of the tumour necrosis factor superfamily (TNF-Related Apoptosis-Induced Ligand) that normally binds to two 'death receptors' and two decoy receptors (TRAIL receptors 3 and 4); these decoy receptors are expressed on eosinophils and have an antiapoptotic function, as they cannot transduce the death signal that is activated when TRAIL binds to death receptors. Thus increased expression of TRAIL receptor 3 would be expected to compete with death receptors for TRAIL binding, leading to prolonged eosinophil survival. Eosinophils secrete several highly toxic cytokines such as eosinophil major basic protein, eosinophil cationic protein (ECP), and eosinophil-derived neurotoxin, all of which cause tissue damage. Serum levels of ECP, which is a marker of eosinophil activation, often correspond with disease activity in CSS [7] and may be used to predict relapse [8].

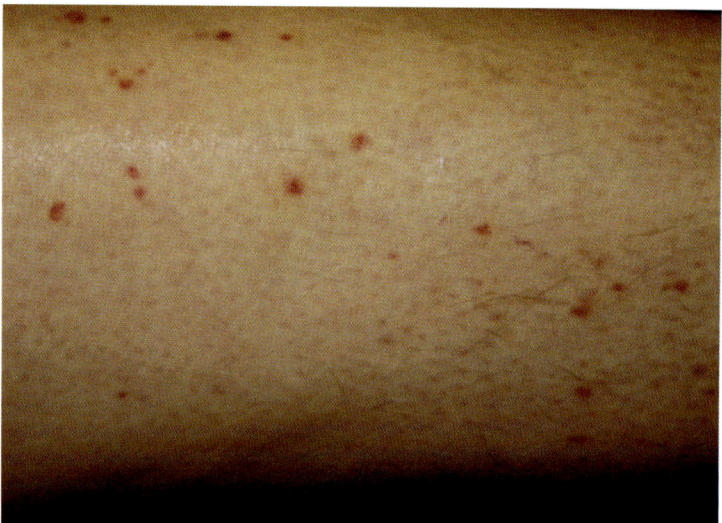

Fig. 50.31 Relatively subtle vasculitis on the legs in Churg–Strauss syndrome; the patient also had eosinophilia and rapidly developed mononeuritis multiplex.

Histopathology. Churg–Strauss syndrome is characterized by three key histopathological features: eosinophilic infiltration of tissue, formation of extravascular granulomas of the visceral and cutaneous tissue and vasculitis involving both arteries and veins. A biopsy specimen of a cutaneous lesion from a patient with CSS may demonstrate any one, if not all, of these features [9]. The granulomas of CSS contain necrotic polymorphonuclear leukocytes, eosinophils, severe fibrinoid and fibrillar collagen degeneration, and a proliferation of granulomatous tissue.

Clinical features [1,5,9]. Three phases of CSS have been described. The first phase, which may continue for years, consists of allergic rhinitis, nasal polyps, asthma and peripheral blood eosinophilia. The asthma component of this phase typically begins in adulthood, in contrast with allergic asthma. The second phase of CSS is vasculitis; this phase is characterized by disease affecting almost all organ systems, including cardiac, pulmonary, nervous, gastrointestinal, renal, genitourinary and musculoskeletal systems. Cardiac involvement is the primary cause of death in patients who do not respond to conventional corticosteroid therapy [10]. In this vasculitic phase, 70% of patients have skin lesions (Fig. 50.31). The third stage of CSS is characterized by allergic rhinitis, asthma, hypertension due to damage to the kidneys that occurred in the second phase, and peripheral neuropathies. There is typically complete resolution of damage to other organ systems. Nearly half of patients in all phases of the disease have cutaneous manifestations of the disease [1,9], with approximately 5% demonstrating cutaneous vasculitis [9]. Palpable purpura and infiltrated nodules (typically located on the scalp or limbs) [11] are the most common skin manifestations, but livedo reticularis, necrotizing livedo (i.e. retiform purpura), migratory erythema, new-onset Raynaud's phenomenon, aseptic pustules or vesicles, or infiltrated papules may also be present.

Diagnosis. The American College of Rheumatology 1990 criteria for the classification of Churg–Strauss syndrome are as follows: asthma, eosinophilia greater than 10% on differential white blood cell count, mononeuropathy (including multiplex) or polyneuropathy, non-fixed pulmonary infiltrates on roentgenography, paranasal sinus abnormality, and biopsy containing a blood vessel with extravascular eosinophils [12]. The manifestations of CSS may be easily confused with lesions of Wegener's granulomatosis (WG), although CSS is strongly associated with both asthma and involvement of the gastrointestinal tract, spleen and heart, in contrast with the strong association with renal disease in patients with WG. The triad of asthma, eosinophilia and extravascular granulomas may also be used to distinguish CSS from other disease processes.

Treatment. Corticosteroids alone have been shown to be an effective treatment of CSS [5], with clinical remission achieved in over 90% of patients. However, the addition of cytotoxic agents, especially cyclophosphamide in severely affected patients, or therapy such as intravenous immunoglobulin (IVIG), may be useful in patients with recalcitrant disease or those with poor prognostic factors such as cardiac, GI, renal or CNS involvement [10], although no double-blind, prospective trials have been done to establish their use.

References

1 Guillevin L, Cohen P, Gayraud M *et al*. Churg–Strauss syndrome. Clinical study and long-term follow-up of 96 patients. *Medicine (Baltimore)* 1999; **78**: 26–37.
2 Harrold LR, Patterson MK, Andrade SE *et al*. Asthma drug use and the development of Churg–Strauss syndrome. *Pharmacoepidemiol Drug Saf* 2007; **16**: 620–6.
3 Lilly CM, Churg A, Lazarovich M *et al*. Asthma therapies and Churg–Strauss syndrome. *J Allergy Clin Immunol* 2002; **109**: S1–19.
4 Kiene M, Csernok E, Muller A *et al*. Elevated interleukin-4 and interleukin-13 production by T cell lines from patients with Churg–Strauss syndrome. *Arthritis Rheum* 2001; **44**: 469–73.
5 Noth I, Strek ME, Leff AR. Churg–Strauss syndrome. *Lancet* 2003; **361**: 587–94.
6 Mitsuyama H, Matsuyama W, Watanabe M *et al*. Increased expression of TRAIL receptor 3 on eosinophils in Churg–Strauss syndrome. *Arthritis Rheum* 2007; **56**: 662–73.
7 Schmitt WH, Csernok E, Kobayashi S *et al*. Churg–Strauss syndrome: serum markers of lymphocyte activation and endothelial damage. *Arthritis Rheum* 1998; **41**: 445–52.

8 Hurst S, Chizzolini C, Dayer JM *et al*. Usefulness of serum eosinophil cationic protein (ECP) in predicting relapse of Churg and Strauss vasculitis. *Clin Exp Rheumatol* 2000; **18**: 784–5.

9 Davis MD, Daoud MS, McEvoy MT, Su WP. Cutaneous manifestations of Churg–Strauss syndrome: a clinicopathologic correlation. *J Am Acad Dermatol* 1997; **37**: 199–203.

10 Taniguchi M, Tsurikisawa N, Higashi N *et al*. Treatment for Churg–Strauss syndrome: induction of remission and efficacy of intravenous immunoglobulin therapy. *Allergol Int* 2007; **56**: 97–103.

11 Lhote F, Cohen P, Guillevin L. Polyarteritis nodosa, microscopic polyangiitis and Churg–Strauss syndrome. *Lupus* 1998; **7**: 238–58.

12 Masi AT, Hunder GG, Lie JT *et al*. The American College of Rheumatology 1990 criteria for the classification of Churg–Strauss syndrome (allergic granulomatosis and angiitis). *Arthritis Rheum* 1990; **33**: 1094–100.

Giant cell arteritis

Synonyms
- Temporal arteritis
- Cranial arteritis

Definition. The definition provided by an International Consensus Conference for giant cell arteritis (GCA) was of a granulomatous arteritis of the aorta and its major branches, with a predilection for the extracranial branches of the carotid artery [1]. It often involves the temporal artery, usually occurs in patients older than 50 years and is often associated with polymyalgia rheumatica (PMR), a syndrome comprising aching and morning stiffness of the shoulder or pelvic girdle muscles that may precede or accompany GCA. However, the similar histopathological findings between GCA, PMR and Takayasu's arteritis have led some investigators to question whether they are separate entities or represent a continuum of disease [2,3]. The matter is not wholly settled.

Epidemiology. GCA is considered a disease that particularly targets Caucasians of European origin, being less common in African Americans, native Americans and Asians. The disease is about three times more common in women than men. The incidence appears to differ with geographical area, being commoner in more northern climes, but overall the worldwide incidence is about 1/50000/year. The incidence may be increasing, particularly amongst women.

Aetiology and pathogenesis. Ethnic and geographical observations suggest that genetic factors probably contribute to development of GCA. Several studies have indicated an over-representation of HLA-DR4; recent associations have included HLA-class I and MICA and HLA-B polymorphisms [4]. It is suggested that the pathogenesis of GCA, as with many diseases, represents an aberrant response to an infectious agent and that the immune system appears to have a central role in the pathogenesis. The arterial adventitia contains dendritic cells, in close proximity with vasa vasorum, that are in an immature state in normal arterioles but that have a mature and activated phenotype in GCA, so that they are capable of triggering antigen-specific T cells [5]. Activated CD4+ T cells that have undergone clonal expansion are also present in the adventitia and produce large quantities of IFN-γ [6]. In turn, IFN-γ can modify effector functions of macrophages and multi-

nucleated giant cells that locate at the junction between the tunica intima and tunica media, setting up a vicious cycle with further production of proliferative and pro-inflammatory mediators. Distinct subsets of macrophages are present with non-overlapping functions that lead to production of proinflammatory cytokines, the release of reactive oxygen radicals, production of growth and angiogenic factors such as platelet-derived growth factor (PDGF) and vascular endothelial cell growth factor (VEGF), and production of nitric oxide synthase. The intimal hyperplasia and neovascularization that occurs in GCA, and which is largely responsible for the vascular occlusion and ischaemia, is probably driven by oxidative and nitrosactive stress within the medial smooth muscle cell layer. Intimal hyperplasia is also associated with the increased production of IFN-γ and formation of multinucleate giant cells.

Interestingly, in PMR, the arterial wall dendritic cells are in an activated state but there is aborted recruitment of CD4+ T cells and macrophages, suggesting that PMR may be a *forme fruste* of GCA [6].

Histopathology. Almost any artery can be affected in GCA. Indeed, an exhaustive autopsy study by Ostberg in 1972, in which the entire aorta and its major branches were removed and sectioned, suggested that involvement of aortic branch vessels was common [7]. The affected artery demonstrates lymphocytic and macrophage infiltrates in the tunica media that can extend from the tunica intima to the adventitia. The internal elastic lamina is fragmented and concentric intimal thickening develops, leading to occlusion of the vessel lumen. Giant cells can be present but are not required for the diagnosis. Granulomas and fibrinoid necrosis are seen infrequently.

Clinical features. The symptoms and signs of GCA result from the inflammation and occlusion of affected arteries. The disease appears to target those arteries that contain an internal elastic lamina, that is extracranial vessels, sparing intracranial vessels.

Constitutional upset occurs in many patients with fever and weight loss, and GCA is associated with PMR in about half of individuals. Headache is common and may be localized to the area of the affected artery, that is temporal with temporal arteritis, or occipital with vertebrobasilar arteritis. The headache may start abruptly and may be associated with tender arteries that may be pulseless or nodular. Facial pain may occur on chewing due to claudication of jaw muscles. A feared complication is sudden, permanent visual loss related to ocular or orbital artery involvement. Transient monocular loss of vision (amaurosis fugax) may precede permanent loss in some individuals. Vertebrobasilar artery involvement may cause ataxia, vertigo or deafness.

Involvement of the aorta or of its main branches is common. In one longitudinal cohort study that used vascular imaging, 72% of patients had large artery involvement, usually of the aorta, axillary and subclavian arteries [8]. Aortic involvement can cause aortic arch syndrome with absent pulses and upper arm claudication, and aortic aneurysms can lead to life-threatening dissection.

Less common features include cerebrovascular accidents, neuropsychiatric manifestations, angina or myocardial infarction, bowel angina or infarction, leg claudication and renal involvement. Unilateral or bilateral scalp ulceration, with or without necrosis, may occur. Rarely, tongue ulceration or infarction, or corneal ulceration, develops.

Diagnosis. The gold standard is histological diagnosis following biopsy of an affected artery, usually a temporal artery. The biopsy should ideally comprise a 2 cm length of vessel and, for the greatest chance of obtaining a tissue diagnosis, the biopsy should be performed within 24 h of commencing corticosteroid therapy. A negative biopsy does not exclude the diagnosis, because timing is important and the disease may be quite focal.

Imaging is playing an increasing role in diagnosis. Superficial temporal arteries and axillary arteries may be amenable to duplex ultrasound, and fluorodeoxy-glucose-positron emission tomography and magnetic resonance angiography are increasingly being used for evaluation of disease activity and extent [9,10].

The acute inflammatory response can be measured by C-reactive protein (CRP) levels and erythrocyte sedimentation rate (ESR). Interleukin-6 levels may be a more sensitive biomarker of disease activity than the ESR [11]. A normochromic, normocytic anaemia, thrombocytosis and raised alkaline phosphatase may all be present.

Treatment. Suspected PMR responds well to oral corticosteroids such as prednisolone, 15–20 mg daily. The dose can usually be reduced slowly in small steps every month, providing that the CRP/ESR levels remain controlled. Treatment is usually for 2–3 years. Higher doses of corticosteroids, for example prednisolone 40–60 mg daily, are needed for GCA. Treatment should be started as soon as the diagnosis is suspected in order to avoid the potential for the complications discussed earlier; if the diagnosis turns out to be incorrect, the corticosteroids can be quickly withdrawn. There is some evidence that initial high-dose methylprednisolone may allow for more rapid tapering of oral corticosteroids and may be associated with a greater number of patients experiencing long-term remission after discontinuation of treatment [12]. Intravenous methylprednisolone 500–1000 mg daily for 3 days, followed by oral prednisolone, may be particularly beneficial in those with visual loss. Unfortunately, if visual loss has already occurred, this may be permanent, but it is important to preserve residual vision and prevent further strokes. The dose of prednisolone can be reduced to 10–20 mg/day by 6 months, and then in small increments with discontinuation by 2–3 years, depending on ESR/CRP/interleukin-6 responses. Sometimes additional immunosuppressive therapy, such as azathioprine, mycophenolate mofetil or methotrexate, is required; some patients require treatment for many years. Aspirin is recommended providing there are no contraindications. Carotid artery stenoses may require angioplasty to improve perfusion.

References

1 Jennette JC, Falk RJ, Andrassy K et al. Nomenclature of systemic vasculitides: the proposal of an International Consensus Conference. *Arthritis Rheum* 1994; **37**: 187–92.
2 Gonzalez-Gay MA. Giant cell arteritis and polymyalgia rheumatica: two different but often overlapping conditions. *Semin Arthritis Rheum* 2004; **33**: 289–93.
3 Maksimowicz-McKinnon K, Hoffman GS. Large vessel vasculitis. *Clin Exp Rheumatol* 2007; **25** (Suppl. 44): S58–9.
4 Gonzalez-Gay MA, Rueda B, Vilchez JR et al. Contribution of MHC class I region to genetic susceptibility for giant cell arteritis. *Rheumatology (Oxford)* 2007; **46**: 431–4.
5 Ma-Krupa W, Jeon MS, Spoerl S et al. Activation of arterial wall dendritic cells and breakdown of self tolerance in giant cell arteritis. *J Exp Med* 2004; **199**: 173–83.
6 Weyand CM, Ma-Krupa W, Goronzy JJ. Immunopathways in giant cell arteritis and polymyalgia rheumatica. *Autoimmun Rev* 2004; **3**: 46–53.
7 Ostberg G. Morphological changes in the large arteries in polymyalgia arteritica. *Acta Med Scand* 1972; Suppl. 533: 135–59.
8 Maksimowicz-McKinnon K, Clark T, Hoffman GS. The prevalence of signs and symptoms of polymyalgia rheumatica (PMR) and giant cell arteritis (GCA) in Takayasu's arteritis. *Arthritis Rheum* 2004; **50**: S1072.
9 Dasgupta B, Hassan N. Giant cell arteritis: recent advances and guidelines for management. *Clin Exp Rheumatol* 2007; **25** (Suppl.): S62–3.
10 Bley TA. Imaging studies in the diagnosis of large vessel vasculitis. *Clin Exp Rheumatol* 2007; **25** (Suppl.): S60–1.
11 Weyand CM, Fulbright JW, Hunder GG et al. Treatment of giant cell arteritis: interleukin-6 as a biologic marker of disease activity. *Arthritis Rheum* 2000; **43**: 1041–8.
12 Mazlumzadeh M, Hunder GG, Easley KA et al. Treatment of giant cell arteritis using induction therapy with high-dose glucocorticoids: a double-blind, placebo-controlled, randomized prospective clinical trial. *Arthritis Rheum* 2006; **54**: 3310–8.

Takayasu's arteritis

Synonyms
- Takayasu's disease
- Takayasu's syndrome
- Aortic arch syndrome
- Pulseless disease
- Occlusive thromboarteriopathy
- Aortitis syndrome

Definition. Takayasu's arteritis (TA) is a granulomatous inflammation of the aorta and its major branches that usually occurs in patients aged younger than 50 years [1]. Although it is most common in individuals less than 40–50 years of age, it may occasionally be diagnosed in older people.

Epidemiology. The disorder is often described as affecting young females of Oriental origin and, indeed, it appears to be a relatively common cause of renovascular hypertension in the Far East, although it does have a worldwide distribution and racial heterogeneity.

Aetiology and pathogenesis. TA is associated with an acute inflammatory response, and the histopathology of acute lesions is similar to that described in GCA, so inflammatory and immune mechanisms appear to be necessary for pathogenesis. Genetic, infectious and environmental triggers have been sought but none has been associated conclusively with the disease. Various HLA associations have been described depending on the population under study, and susceptibility has been linked to polymorphisms around the HLA-B and MICA genes [2]. Tubercle bacilli have been scrutinized as a possible precipitant, but patients generally respond to immunosuppression without development of overt tuberculosis.

Histopathology. The aorta and its branches are targeted and skip lesions can occur [3]. During the acute phase, a pan-arteritis is present. The inflammatory infiltrate may be predominantly around the vasa vasorum. Fibrosis gradually replaces inflammatory infiltrates. The vessel lumen may be narrowed secondary to the fibrosing stenotic lesions and/or by intraluminal thrombosis. In older patients there may be superimposed atherosclerosis, and calcification in the wall may occur as a late feature.

Clinical features. The symptoms and signs of TA result from inflammation, ischaemia and aneurysm formation within the aorta and its branches [4]. There may be overlap in features of TA with those of GCA [5]. Hypertension is a common presenting feature in Asian and Far Eastern patients and the blood pressure should be recorded in all four limbs. Renal artery stenosis, increased arterial stiffness and increased sensitivity of the carotid sinus reflex, all contribute to hypertension. Involvement of the renal arteries can also cause renal dysfunction, and abdominal pain, bleeding or perforation may result from ischaemia or infarction of a viscus. Involvement of the aortic arch and its branches can lead to 'aortic arch syndrome' with arm claudication, absent radial or brachial pulses (hence 'pulseless disease') or subclavian artery bruits. Aortic regurgitation, coronary artery ischaemia with angina or myocardial infarction, pulmonary hypertension, stroke, syncope and visual disturbances can occur.

Skin lesions have been reported in up to a third of cases and may comprise erythema nodosum, erythema induratum and pyoderma gangrenosum [6], as well as ulcerated subacute nodular lesions, papulonecrotic eruptions, papular erythematous lesions of the hands and fingers, facial lupus-like rashes and panniculitis [7]. Cutaneous necrotizing vasculitis has been described resembling nodular vasculitis/erythema induratum, suggesting that Takayasu's arteritis may occasionally involve small blood vessels [8]. The skin lesions do not appear to relate to the distribution of vascular involvement in any way.

Diagnosis. TA is best diagnosed using imaging techniques [9]. Angiography and magnetic resonance angiography may demonstrate stenotic lesions of the aorta or its branches. Increasingly, enhanced magnetic resonance perfusion imaging, duplex ultrasonography and positron emission tomography are being used [10].

In the early stages of the disease, inflammatory markers such as CRP and ESR may be elevated. However, if disease presentation occurs late, features of an acute inflammatory response may be absent. A normochromic normocytic anaemia is often present.

Treatment. The acute phase of TA is managed in a similar way to GCA. The response is usually less dramatic than in GCA and secondary immunosuppressant medication is often required. However, once arterial damage has occurred and the inflammatory component has settled, immunosuppression is unlikely to be helpful. Stenotic lesions may require treatment with angioplasty or stenting. Hypertension requires aggressive management. Smoking should be discouraged and, as there is an increased risk of premature atherosclerosis, cardiac risk factors should be sought and dealt with.

References

1 Jennette JC, Falk RJ, Andrassy K et al. Nomenclature of systemic vasculitides: the proposal of an International Consensus Conference. *Arthritis Rheum* 1994; **37**: 187–92.
2 Kimura A, Ota M, Katsuyama Y et al. Mapping of the HLA-linked genes controlling the susceptibility to Takayasu's arteritis. *Int J Cardiol* 2000; **75** (Suppl. 1): S105–10.
3 Lie JT. Takayasu's arteritis. In: Churg A, Churg J, eds. *Systemic Vasculitides*. New York: Igaku-Shoin, 1991: 159–79.
4 Sharma BK, Jain S. Takayasu's arteritis. In: Ball GV, Bridges SL, eds. *Vasculitis*. Oxford: Oxford University Press, 2002: 278–89.
5 Maksimowicz-McKinnon K, Clark T, Hoffman GS. The prevalence of signs and symptoms of polymyalgia rheumatica (PMR) and giant cell arteritis (GCA) in Takayasu's arteritis. *Arthritis Rheum* 2004; **50**: S1072.
6 Pascual-Lopez M, Hernandez-Nunez A, Aragues-Montanes M et al. Takayasu's disease with cutaneous involvement. *Dermatology* 2004; **208**: 10–15.
7 Boisnic F, Bletry O, Dallot A et al. Cutaneous manifestations of Takayasu arteritis. A retrospective study of 80 patients. *Dermatologica* 1990; **181**: 266–72.
8 Skaria AM, Ruffieux P, Piletta P et al. Takayasu arteritis and cutaneous necrotizing vasculitis. *Dermatology* 2000; **200**: 139–43.
9 Rizzi R, Bruno S, Stellaci C, Dammacco R. Takayasu's arteritis: a cell-mediated large-vessel vasculitis. *Int J Clin Res* 1999; **29**: 8–13.
10 Bley TA. Imaging studies in the diagnosis of large vessel vasculitis. *Clin Exp Rheumatol* 2007; **25** (Suppl.): S60–1.

Other vasculitides and mimics of vasculitis

Kawasaki disease [1]

This eponymous disease is a mucocutaneous lymph node syndrome, predominantly affecting young children, although recurrent disease in adults and adult-onset disease can occur. It is discussed briefly here as the systemic component includes a multisystem vasculitis; however, the exanthem it causes is not vasculitic. It is discussed in more detail in Chapter 30 (Bacterial infections) because it occurs in epidemics and there is some evidence to suggest an infective aetiology, possibly involving *Staphylococcus aureus*, *Streptococcus pyogenes* or *Yersinia pseudotuberculosis*. Bacterial superantigens, notably staphylococcal toxic shock syndrome toxin type-1 (STSS-1) and streptococcal pyrogenic exotoxins B and C, have particularly been implicated, although evidence to support this is poor [2]. More recently, an IgA response to cytoplasmic inclusion bodies has been documented as a possible cause [3].

At a pathogenetic level, many factors common to medium and larger vessel vasculitides can be found, including activated T cells, B cells and monocyte/macrophages, as well as elevated TNF-α, IFN-γ, IL-1, IL-2, IL-6, IL-12 and ICAM-1 [1]; antiendothelial cell antibodies are also present. Elevated levels of anti-α-enolase antibodies have been demonstrated and suggested to have a pathogenetic role [4]. The elastolytic role of matrix metalloproteinases is also thought to be involved; MMP-1, MMP-2, MMP-9 and MMP-13 have all been implicated, but high circulating levels of MMP-2 and MMP-9 were shown not to be significantly associated with coronary outcome after adjusting for demographic, clinical and laboratory features in patients or in a mouse model [5]. However, a genetic polymorphism in MMP-13 has been proven to occur with a significant difference in frequency in patients with Kawasaki disease with coronary artery lesions than in those without such lesions [6].

The angiitis of Kawasaki disease affects nearly all organs, with a very high frequency of cardiac involvement, which follows four stages [1]. Initially, there is perivasculitis and vasculitis of small vessels (capillaries, small veins and arteries, including those of the vasa vasora of the main coronary arteries); as the stages progress there is a gradual decrease in the small vessel vasculitis but development of focal panvasculitis of medium-size arteries, especially of the heart, with a mixed inflammatory infiltrate. During this phase (stage 2), aneurysms, thrombosis and stenoses of medium-size arteries develop, with gradual scarring and loss of acute vasculitis by stage 4. Deaths may occur due to myocarditis, dysrhythmias, pericarditis, rupture of aneurysms and occlusion of coronary arteries; there is also an increased risk of atherosclerosis due to endothelial cell dysfunction. Coronary aneurysms are demonstrated in almost 20% of patients (and in 90% of those who die); some will regress (potentially with stenosis) but giant aneurysms (>8 mm) rarely regress, carry a high risk of death and may require bypass surgery. Clinical factors that predict a higher risk of coronary artery arteritic lesions or aneurysms, or that predict a poor response to treatment, include age below 1 year, low serum albumin, low haemoglobin, high CRP, abnormal liver function and, especially, duration of fever before treatment [7–10]; peripheral blood eosinophilia (>4%) after treatment is also associated with treatment resistance [10].

The angiitis of Kawasaki disease can be divided into that which affects medium- and large-size arteries outside organs (mainly the coronary arteries, in 90%, also the iliac and other arteries), arteritis within organs (also mainly cardiac, but also the skin, kidneys, gastrointestinal tract and others), and venulitis. Thrombotic disease, which may be triggered by tissue factor [11], is probably important as a cause of morbidity and mortality; gangrene of the legs and disseminated intravascular coagulopathy (DIC) have both been reported [12,13]. Clinically, the skin lesions are polymorphous, including urticarial, morbilliform, maculopapular, erythema-multiforme-like patterns, and less commonly aseptic pustules on knees or buttocks, or a scarlatina-like erythroderma. Hands and feet become swollen, with palmoplantar erythema and subsequent desquamation.

Treatment is with intravenous immunoglobulin (IVIG) and aspirin, which reduce fever and development of aneurysms. There is conflicting evidence regarding the benefits of additionally using pulsed corticosteroid therapy. Other cardiac medications or surgery may be required; formal high-dose anticoagulation is needed for those with large coronary aneurysms. In those in whom IVIG fails (based on echocardiological assessment for aneurysms), re-treatment may be tried, plasma exchange may be successful, and infliximab has also been used. Diagnosis and treatment, with an emphasis on long-term treatment and cardiac disease, have been documented in detail by an expert consensus committee [14].

References

1 Kawasaki T. Kawasaki disease. In: Harper J, Oranje A, Prose N, eds. *Textbook of Pediatric Dermatology*, 2nd edn. Oxford: Blackwell Publishing, 2006: 1953–63.

2 Komatsu H, Fujisawa T. Kawasaki disease and infection. *Nippon Rinsho* 2008; **66**: 278–82.

3 Rowley AH, Baker SC, Orenstein JM, Shulman ST. Searching for the cause of Kawasaki disease—cytoplasmic inclusion bodies provide new insight. *Nat Rev Microbiol* 2008; **6**: 394–401.

4 Chun JK, Lee TJ, Choi KM *et al*. Elevated anti-alpha-enolase antibody levels in Kawasaki disease. *Scand J Rheumatol* 2008; **37**: 48–52.

5 Lau AC, Rosenberg H, Duong TT *et al*. Elastolytic matrix metalloproteinases and coronary outcome in children with Kawasaki disease. *Pediatr Res* 2007; **61**: 710–5.

6 Ikeda K, Ihara K, Yamaguchi K *et al*. Genetic analysis of MMP gene polymorphisms in patients with Kawasaki disease. *Pediatr Res* 2008; **63**: 182–5.

7 Honkanen VEA, McCrindle BW, Laxer RM *et al*. Clinical relevance of the risk factors for coronary artery inflammation in Kawasaki disease. *Pediatr Cardiol* 2003; **24**: 122–6.

8 Zhan W, Li Q, Zhao X-D *et al*. Clinical analysis of 942 cases of Kawasaki disease. *Zhonghua Er Ke Za Zhi* 2006; **44**: 324–8.

9 Sano T, Kurotobi K, Kouji M *et al*. Prediction of non-responsiveness to standard high-dose gamma-globulin therapy in patients with Kawasaki disease before starting initial treatment. *Eur J Pediatr* 2007; **166**: 131–7.

10 Kuo-Ho C, Yang KD, Liang CD *et al*. The relationship of eosinophilia to intravenous immunoglobulin treatment failure in Kawasaki disease. *Pediatr Allergy Immunol* 2007; **18**: 354–9.

11 Pucci A, Martino S, Celeste A *et al*. Angiogenesis, tumor necrosis factor-alpha and procoagulant factors in coronary artery giant aneurysm of a fatal infantile Kawasaki disease. *Cardiovasc Pathol* 2008; **17**: 186–9.

12 Dogan OF, Kara A, Devrim I *et al*. Peripheral gangrene associated with Kawasaki disease and successful management using prostacycline analogue: a case report. *Heart Surg Forum* 2007; **10**: E70–2.

13 Parvathy VK, Manuel AD, Criton S, Rajesh G. Kawasaki disease with DIC as a complication. *Indian J Pediatr* 2007; **74**: 1049.

14 Newburger JW, Takahashi M, Gerber MA *et al*. Diagnosis, treatment, and long-term management of Kawasaki disease: a statement for health professionals from the committee on rheumatic fever, endocarditis, and Kawasaki disease, Council on Cardiovascular Disease in the Young, American Heart Association. *Pediatr* 2004; **114**: 1708–33.

Cerebral vasculitis and mimics

Some of the primary vasculitides discussed earlier have cerebral vasculitis as a possible component. There are also various infections, tumours, autoimmune disorders (such as antiphospholipid syndrome), collagen vascular disorders and other systemic diseases (such as sarcoidosis) that may combine neurological and cutaneous lesions and for which vasculitis might be considered in the differential diagnosis. Hypercoagulable states, sickle cell disease, thrombi (e.g. myxoma), Sneddon's syndrome (Chapter 49) and Fabry disease (Chapter 59) may all have both central nervous system and cutaneous features. Although vasculitides with predominantly cerebral features will not present to dermatologists, a few disorders warrant specific mention in the differential diagnosis of cerebral vasculitis as they may have skin manifestations that might suggest a vasculitis, thrombotic or microvascular occlusive process.

Intravascular lymphoma (intravascular lymphomatosis, angiotropic lymphoma, malignant angioendotheliomatosis) is caused by proliferation of clonal lymphocytes (usually B cells) within small vessels, and most commonly affects the central nervous system (CNS) and the skin. Cerebral vasculitis is often in the differential diagnosis of CNS involvement, both clinically and radiologically, and some of the cerebral pathology is due to thrombosis. Skin lesions occur in 40%, and may be the only site affected in 25%; they include localized or generalized telangiectasia, and tender indurated dermal or subcutaneous plaques or nodules with a blue to red colour, mainly on the lower legs, with associated painful swelling. The physical signs may mimic erythema nodosum, thrombophlebitis, adult Still's disease or cellulitis [1,2]. Gangrene of the lower extremities has been reported, and a vasculitis-like illness with dementia [3]. One case has been reported with systemic lupus erythematosus (SLE) [4]; however, significantly raised serum ANA levels may be found in the absence of other features of SLE [3,5,6], erroneously suggesting a possible diagnosis of connective tissue disease-related vasculitis.

CADASIL (cerebral autosomal dominant arteriopathy with subcortical infarcts and leukoencephalopathy) is a rare disorder that often presents as a form of dementia. It is due to a mutation in *NOTCH3* on chromosome 19 and is characterized histologically by granular osmiophilic material in the media of arterioles and small arteries, although this also occurs in non-muscular vessels including veins and capillaries [7]. Although the skin is not usually involved clinically, it is at a microscopic level, vessel walls being thickened by PAS-positive material. Additionally, haemorrhagic macular lesions with strong positive direct immunofluorescence for immunoglobulins, complement and fibrin, have been reported in CADASIL [8]. The neurological presentations include transient ischaemic attacks, which, if occurring in combination with haemorrhagic skin lesions, would mean that embolic or vasculitic processes might easily be suspected. Electron microscopy or NOTCH3 immunostaining [9] of skin biopsies may be useful, but gene analysis is more precise.

Leukoencephalopathies [10]. Two such disorders have particular relevance to dermatologists. *Progressive multifocal leukoencephalopathy* is caused by reactivation of the JC polyoma virus. It is particularly linked with systemic lupus erythematosus (SLE) and other collagen vascular diseases or vasculitides, even in patients on mild immunosuppressive regimens, suggesting that immune dysregulation may play a part in viral reactivation. It should be considered if cerebral symptoms are thought to be due to the underlying connective tissue disorder but fail to respond to increased immunosuppression; the importance is that it is progressive and usually fatal, and immunosuppressive treatment should be discontinued rather than increased. *Reversible posterior leukoencephalopathy syndrome* has also been associated with immunosuppressive therapy, usually more intensive treatment of renal disease or accelerated hypertension in SLE or Wegener's granulomatosis.

In tertiary referral practice, cerebral vasculitis occurs as a primary disorder (about 10% of cases), or is part of PAN (15%), MPA (10%), adult HSP (10–15%), WG (15–20%), SLE (15%) or cutaneous vasculitis (4%) [11]. The course and outcome of primary angiitis of the central nervous system (PACNS) appears to be related to the size of vessel involved, small-vessel disease being responsive to immunosuppression but having a relapsing recurrent course with severe brain injury, whereas medium-vessel disease tends to occur as isolated episodes with few relapses after treatment is discontinued. Therapy is recommended for at least 5 years for those with small-vessel disease, which may represent a limited form of PAN [11].

References

1 Röglin J, Böer A. Skin manifestations of intravascular lymphoma mimic inflammatory diseases of the skin. *Br J Dermatol* 2007; **157**: 16–25.
2 Kiyohara T, Kumakiri M, Kobayashi H *et al*. A case of intravascular large B-cell lymphoma mimicking erythema nodosum: the importance of multiple skin biopsies. *J Cutan Pathol* 2000; **27**: 413–8.
3 Demirer T, Dail DH, Aboulafia DM. Four varied cases of intravascular lymphomatosis and a literature review. *Cancer* 1994; **73**: 1338–45.
4 Sánchez CD, Callejas RJL, Vilanova MA *et al*. Intravascular lymphoma in a patient with systemic lupus erythematosus: a case report. *Lupus* 2007; **16**: 525–8.
5 Carter DK, Batts KP, de Groen PC, Kurtin PJ. Angiotropic large cell lymphoma (intravascular lymphomatosis) occurring after follicular small cleaved cell lymphoma. *Mayo Clin Proc* 1996; **71**: 869–73.
6 Scully RE, Mark EJ, McNeely WF, Ebeling SH. Case records of the Massachusetts General Hospital. Case 30–1996. *N Engl J Med* 1996; **335**: 952–9.
7 Rafalowska J, Fidzianska A, Dziewulska D *et al*. CADASIL or CADVaSIL? *Neuropathology* 2004; **24**: 16–20.
8 Ratzinger G, Ramsmayr G, Romani N, Zelger B. CADaSIL—an unusual manifestation with prominent cutaneous involvement. *Br J Dermatol* 2005; **152**: 346–9.
9 Lesnik-Oberstein SAJ, van Duinen SG, van den Boom R *et al*. Evaluation of diagnostic NOTCH3 immunostaining in CADASIL. *Acta Neuropathol (Berlin)* 2003; **106**: 107–11.
10 Molloy ES, Langford CA. Vasculitis mimics. *Curr Opin Rheumatol* 2008; **20**: 29–34.
11 MacLaren K, Gillespie J, Shestha S *et al*. Primary angiitis of the central nervous system: emerging variants. *QJM* 2005; **98**: 643–54.

Lymphocytic vasculitis

Lymphocytic vasculitis does not neatly fit into classifications of vasculitis, except perhaps those based mainly on histopathological features [1–4]. Suggested classifications [3] have never really crossed from pathological to clinical practice, even though some skin disorders (e.g. graft-versus-host disease, Chapter 62) are good examples of lymphocytic vascular damage. To aid understanding of this area, the optimum terminology for lymphocytic vasculitis may need to be slightly different from that of leukocytoclastic vasculitides; for example, the use of terms such as lymphocytic endovasculitis, angiodestructive lymphocytic vasculitis, lichenoid lymphocytic vasculitis, lymphocytic granulomatous vasculitis and lichenoid dermatitis with granulomatous lymphocytic vasculitis, has been proposed [1,4].

It has been suggested that clinicians may try to adapt lymphocytic vasculitis into their working concept of neutrophilic vasculitis and its causes, possibly to the detriment of understanding of lymphocytic vasculitis. This perhaps occurs in part because many of the disorders already discussed may have a lymphocyte-predominant infiltrate at some point in their evolution (typically in more chronic lesions, thereby detracting from the possibility of acute lymphocytic vasculitis), partly because karyhorrhexis (nuclear fragmentation) is more associated with polymorphonuclear cells (leukocytoclasis) than with lymphocytes, and also because other identifying features of vasculitis, such as fibrin deposition, are less constant in lymphocytic disease. Probably, some lymphocytic 'vasculopathies' actually represent lymphocytic vasculitis. Additionally, for the clinician, a histopathology report of a lymphocytic vasculitis often indicates that finding a cause will be difficult and that treatment may be difficult, even though lymphocytic vasculitis confined to the skin is often more indolent than its leukocytoclastic counterpart. An additional issue that makes lymphocytic vasculitis more difficult to understand is that, whereas neutrophils in vessel walls may be innocent (undergoing diapedesis) or harmful, lymphocytes in the wall of a muscular vessel are abnormal [3]. Fibrin deposition does occur, as with leukocytoclastic vasculitis, but in many respects the histopathological techniques necessary to understand lymphocytic vasculitis are less advanced than for leukocytoclastic disease. The benefits of anti-TNF agents and of rituximab in vasculitides point to an important role of both T and B lymphocytes.

This section discusses some of the causes of vasculitis that are particularly associated with a lymphocyte-predominant (but not granulomatous) infiltrate. A histopathological classification (noting that different pathological patterns may coexist) can be summarized as [4]:

1 angiodestructive lymphocytic vasculitis—rare, usually seen in angiodestructive lymphomas or lymphomatoid granulomatosis, but occurs in some patterns of lupus erythematosus and in Behçet's disease

2 lichenoid lymphocytic vasculitis—the most common pattern, which may occur in viral infections, drug reactions, erythema multiforme, lupus erythematosus, graft-versus-host disease, pityriasis lichenoides, lymphomatoid papulosis, lichenoid mycosis fungoides and Degos' disease; a granulomatous component may also occur in some cases of lichenoid and granulomatous mycosis fungoides [5], as well as in mycobacterial infection and in patients with associated hepatobiliary disease [6]

3 lymphocytic endovasculitis—this affects medium size vessels causing intimal hyperplasia and vessel wall mucinosis, or causes segmental hyalinization of smaller vessels with thrombosis; examples include chronic graft-versus-host disease, scleroderma, lupus erythematosus profundus, some livedoid vasculopathy and Degos' disease.

A clinically orientated summary, based on aetiology, is suggested in Table 50.11; disorders discussed elsewhere in this section are cross-referenced from the table.

Leukocytoclastic vasculitis of many types may, in older lesions, have lymphocyte predominance. Examples include GF (in which the mononuclear infiltrate may appear pseudolymphomatous in late lesions, although plasma cells are also present as well as angiocentric fibrosis [1]), EED (although the infiltrate of older lesions also usually contains lipid-laden histiocytes and plasma cells, and exhibits fibrosis), C-PAN (histiocytes also present) and GCA (mixed infiltrate). In *urticarial vasculitis*, a recent study has suggested that the majority of cases have a lymphocyte-predominant infiltrate with an admixture of eosinophils, and that a neutrophilic infiltrate with leukocytoclasis is present in the minority [7], although in the past a leukocytoclastic vasculitis has usually been described; this issue is discussed on p. 50.22. *Macular arteritis* is discussed below (p. 50.51); its infiltrate is typically lymphocytic.

Collagen vascular disorders such as *systemic lupus erythematosus* (SLE), *rheumatoid disease*, *dermatomyositis* and *sclerodermas* may exhibit a type II immune response leading to either a pauci-inflammatory thrombogenic vasculopathy and/or a lymphocytic vasculitis [1], although SLE and rheumatoid disease in particular can also be associated with neutrophilic leukocytoclastic vasculitis. In rheumatoid disease, this may vary from superficial neutrophilic lesions (occasionally pustular or Sweet's syndrome-like) to pallisaded neutrophilic granulomatous dermatitis (discussed below, p. 50.52). SLE is associated predominantly with thrombotic infarction, but a lymphocytic vasculitis may affect any organ; in the skin it is often pan-dermal rather than the more superficial leukocytoclastic pattern. Numerous skin lesions are associated with

Table 50.11 An aetiological classification of lymphocytic vasculitis*.

Type of process	Examples
Inherited	X-linked lymphoproliferative syndrome
	Autosomal dominant cutaneous small vessel lymphocytic vasculitis
Collagen vascular diseases	Systemic lupus erythematosus
	Rheumatoid disease
	Sclerodermas
	Dermatomyositis
	Sjögren's syndrome
Other autoimmune conditions	Lichen sclerosus
	Diabetic mastopathy
Vasculitides, vasculopathies and microvascular occlusion disorders	Older lesions of several leukocytoclastic vasculitides (see text)
	Urticarial vasculitis (some cases) (p. 50.21)
	Polyarteritis nodosa (classic and cutaneous types)
	Nodular vasculitis
	Behçet's disease (some lesions) (p. 50.56)
	Pyoderma gangrenosum (some cases)
	Degos' disease and Sneddon's syndrome (Chapter 49)
	Buerger's disease and Mondor's disease
	Macular arteritis (p. 50.51)
	Lymphocytic thrombophilic arteritis (p. 50.51)
	Pityriasis lichenoides et varioliformis acuta (p. 50.50)
	IgA-associated lymphocytic vasculitis
	Pigmented purpuric dermatosis (some)
	Kawasaki disease
Infections	Viral, especially:
	Epstein-Barr virus
	varicella-zoster virus (may also be granulomatous)
	cytomegalovirus
	Rickettsial
Drugs and vaccinations	Anti-TNF monoclonals
	Interferon
	Bortezomib
	Other systemic drugs, various
	Topical NSAIDs
	Imiquimod
	Various vaccines
Malignancy and paraneoplastic	Chronic lymphocytic leukaemia
	Lymphomas (especially angiocentric T-cell lymphomas)
	Myeloproliferative disorders and leukaemia (some)
	Paraneoplastic vasculitis (some)
Miscellaneous	Perniosis
	Graft-versus-host disease
	Some arthropod bites

* Note that other patterns of vasculitis, or thrombotic vasculopathy, may also occur in many of the disorders listed.

rheumatoid disease (Chapter 51), including various forms of vasculitis, but a thrombotic and lymphocytic vasculitis may affect vessels of all sizes. Less commonly, an eosinophilic vasculitis may also occur in collagen vascular diseases [8]. Vasculitis occurring with *relapsing polychondritis* is usually leukocytoclastic but in a small proportion of cases it may be lymphocytic. The vasculitis that may occur in *Sjögren's syndrome* is immune complex mediated, due to increased immunoglobulin production as a result of B-cell hyperreactivity, and is almost always neutrophilic.

Lupus erythematosus panniculitis may have features of lymphocytic vasculitis in a third of cases [9]; this, combined with the demographics (usually young females), site (usually upper arm or trunk), hyalinization of fat [4] and deposition of mucin in many cases, help to distinguish it from other causes of panniculitis. Similarly, scleroderma profunda is associated with a lymphocytic pattern of vasculitis [4,10].

Behçet's disease is discussed in detail later (p. 50.56). Numerous patterns of vascular injury occur including neutrophilic infiltrates with or without vasculitis, lymphocytic vasculitis, thrombotic lesions which may cause secondary vascular injury, histiocytic panniculitis (erythema nodosum-like lesions), and others [1,11]. Lymphocytic vasculitis is common in the erythema nodosum-like lesions [1,12,13], occurs in acral papular lesions, and is even present in nearly 30% of pustular lesions [14]. Lymphocytic vasculitis has also occasionally been reported in some cases of *pyoderma gangrenosum* [15,16], although leukocytoclastic vasculitis is more common in those cases that have a vasculitic component.

Viral and occasionally other infections are an important cause of lymphocytic vasculitis. Those most commonly implicated are Epstein–Barr virus (EBV), varicella-zoster virus and cytomegalovirus [17–21]. These viruses all have an affinity for endothelial cells, and can all generate clonal T-cell expansion, although the relationship between cutaneous and peripheral T-cell expansion does not appear to be straightforward [16]. EBV may also play a role in the lymphocytic vasculitis of X-linked lymphoproliferative disorder (discussed below). In some cases, viral inclusion bodies are seen in endothelial cells, but in others there is no PCR evidence of viral DNA in the infiltrating cells, so the precise mechanisms of the lymphocytic vasculitis are not fully explained. A lymphocytic vasculitis and perineuritis was documented in a case of parvovirus B19 infection [22]. Rickettsiae also infect endothelial cells and may cause lymphocytic vasculitis [2], and lymphocytic vasculitis has also been reported in dengue fever.

Drugs of many types may cause vasculitis of different types (see p. 50.17). Amongst the most important to recognize is the lymphocytic vasculitis that occurs due to *anti-TNF agents* [23,24]. This may be diagnostically difficult if the drugs are being used in patients with a vasculitis-prone disorder (such as rheumatoid disease), or indeed to treat vasculitis; notable features are that the vasculitis due to these drugs may be aggravated by a change to a different agent, and may relapse at intervals for several years after exposure [24]. Another new drug that can cause a cutaneous lymphocytic vasculitis is *bortezomib*, a proteosome inhibitor used in treatment of non-Hodgkin's lymphoma; patients who develop vasculitis also appear to have a better response to treatment [25]. Several drug causes of lichenoid and granulomatous dermatitis are listed in [6]; in some cases, granulomatous lymphocytic vasculitis was documented.

Topical drugs may also be associated with vasculitis; cases due to non-steroidal anti-inflammatory drugs may have a leukocytoclastic or a lymphocytic vasculitis [26], and lymphocytic vasculitis has been reported due to imiquimod [27]. Vaccination reactions may also cause lymphocytic vasculitis. This has been reported with anthrax vaccine [28] and with tetanus toxoid, the latter case progressing to membranous fat necrosis [29].

Vasculitis mimics such as Degos' disease (a form of microvascular occlusion; Chapter 49) [4] and pityriasis lichenoides may exhibit an element of lymphocytic vasculitis (in the latter case, in its pityriasis lichenoides et varioliformis acuta form; p. 50.50) [4]. Pigmented purpuric dermatoses typically have a mild capillaritis (Chapter 49) but in some instances a lymphocytic vasculitis has been suggested; one possible variant which clinically resembled a pigmented purpuric dermatosis was documented as *IgA-associated lymphocytic vasculitis* [30]. In the cases reported, preceding diseases included HSP, undifferentiated connective tissue disease (known to be associated with lymphocytic vasculitis [31]), lupus erythematosus profundus (see above), Degos' disease, Buerger's disease and viral infection. An immune complex pathogenesis was proposed.

Paraneoplastic vasculitis may sometimes cause a vasculitis of lymphocytic type. The most frequent is that associated with chronic lymphocytic leukaemia (CLL) [32,33] although other lymphomas, hairy cell leukaemia and myeloproliferative disorders may all be associated with a lymphocytic pattern of vasculitis. Rarely, CLL has been associated with an ANCA-positive systemic vasculitis.

Lichen sclerosus (LS; Chapters 51 and 71) is generally viewed as an autoimmune condition with a lymphocytic lichenoid infiltrate histologically. However, a large study of both vulval and penile LS biopsies found that both a perivascular lymphocytic infiltrate without vascular damage and a frank lymphocytic vasculitis were common; the latter had a concentric pattern around vascular adventitiae mainly in penile LS, and subendothelial infiltration with occasional fibrin deposition which was most common in vulval LS [34]. Larger muscular vessel wall infiltration was also documented in some cases, and a granulomatous component in some cases (including one patient with LS and hepatitis C, although the changes in this patient were superficial and lichenoid and not documented as prominently vasculitic [6]).

Diabetic mastopathy [35] is a rare condition but could present to dermatologists. It occurs mostly in type I diabetes, and presents as a unilateral (about 75%) or bilateral (25%) discrete mass or diffuse nodularity, predominantly of the subareolar region. Histologically there is a lymphocytic ductitis and lobulitis, with vasculitis in some cases. Recurrence, or involvement of the contralateral breast, occurs in a third of cases. The specificity of this disorder is uncertain as it also occurs in type 2 diabetes, occasionally in non-diabetic subjects, and in males.

Inherited lymphocytic vasculitis is rare [36,37]. In X-linked lymphoproliferative syndrome, the cause has been felt to be an abnormal response to EBV infection; however, a recent study failed to demonstrate EBV genomic sequences in lesions, so this pathogenetic mechanism is uncertain.

References
1 Crowson AN, Mihm MC, Magro CM. Cutaneous vasculitis: a review. *J Cutan Pathol* 2003; **30**: 161–73.
2 Carlson JA, Chen K-R. Cutaneous vasculitis update: neutrophilic muscular vessel and eosinophilic, granulomatous, and lymphocytic vasculitis syndromes. *Am J Dermatopathol* 2007; **29**: 32–43.

3 Carlson JA, Mihm MC Jr, LeBoit PE. Cutaneous lymphocytic vasculitis: a definition, a review, and a proposed classification. *Semin Diagn Pathol* 1996; **13**: 72–90.

4 Kossard S. Defining lymphocytic vasculitis. *Australas J Dermatol* 2000; **41**: 149–55.

5 Shapiro PE, Pinto FJ. The histologic spectrum of mycosis fungoides / Sézary syndrome (cutaneous T-cell lymphoma): a review of 222 biopsies, including newly described patterns and the earliest pathologic changes. *Am J Surg Pathol* 1994; **18**: 645–67.

6 Magro CM, Crowson AN. Lichenoid and granulomatous dermatitis. *Int J Dermatol* 2000; **39**: 126–33.

7 Lee JSS, Loh TH, Seow SC, Tat SH. Prolonged urticaria with purpura: the spectrum of clinical and histopathologic features in a prospective series of 22 patients exhibiting the clinical features of urticarial vasculitis. *J Am Acad Dermatol* 2007; **56**: 994–1005.

8 Chen KR, Su WP, Pittelkow MR *et al.* Eosinophilic vasculitis in connective tissue disease. *J Am Acad Dermatol* 1996; **35**: 173–82.

9 Ng PPL, Tat SH, Tan T. Lupus erythematosus panniculitis: a clinicopathologic study. *Int J Dermatol* 2002; **41**: 488–90.

10 Balabanova M, Obreshkova E. Scleroderma profunda. Clinicopathological studies. *Adv Exp Med Biol* 1999; **455**: 105–9.

11 Chen K-R, Kawahara Y, Miyakawa S, Nishikawa T. Cutaneous vasculitis in Behçet's disease: a clinical and histopathologic study of 20 patients. *J Am Acad Dermatol* 1997; **36**: 689–96.

12 Kim B, LeBoit PE. Histopathologic features of erythema nodosum-like lesions in Behçet's disease: a comparison with erythema nodosum focusing on the role of vasculitis. *Am J Dermatopathol* 2000; **22**: 379–90.

13 Yi SW, Kim EH, Kang HY *et al.* Erythema nodosum: clinicopathologic correlations and their use in differential diagnosis. *Yonsei Med J* 2007; **48**: 601–8.

14 Ilknur T, Pabuçcuogle U, Akin C *et al.* Histopathologic and direct immunofluorescence findings in the papulopustular lesions in Behçet's disease. *Eur J Dermatol* 2006; **16**: 146–50.

15 Mika RB, Riahi I, Fenniche S *et al.* Pyoderma gangrenosum: a report of 21 cases. *Int J Dermatol* 2002; **41**: 65–8.

16 von den Driesch P. Pyoderma gangrenosum: a report of 44 cases with follow-up. *Br J Dermatol* 1997; **137**: 1000–5.

17 Nakagawa A, Ito M, Saga S. Fatal T-cell proliferation in chronic active Epstein-Barr virus infection in childhood. *Am J Clin Pathol* 2002; **117**: 283–90.

18 Gallot G, Hamidou MA, Clémeceau B *et al.* T cell repertoire and Epstein-Barr virus-specific T cell response in chronic active Epstein-Barr virus infection: a case study. *Clin Immunol* 2006; **119**: 79–86.

19 Aram G, Rohwedder A, Nazeer T *et al.* Varicella-zoster-virus folliculitis promoted clonal cutaneous lymphoid hyperplasia. *Am J Dermatopathol* 2005; **27**: 411–7.

20 Uhoda I, Piérard-Franchimont C, Piérard G. Varicella-zoster virus vasculitis: a case of recurrent varicella without epidermal involvement. *Dermatology (Basel)* 2000; **200**: 173–5.

21 Golden MP, Hammer SM, Wanke CA, Albrecht MA. Cytomegalovirus vasculitis. Case reports and review of the literature. *Medicine (Baltimore)* 1994; **73**: 246–55.

22 Aquilar BM, Bassa VJ, Torné-Gutiérrez JI *et al.* Presence of perineuritis in a case of papular purpuric gloves and socks syndrome associated with mononeuritis multiplex attributable to B19 parvovirus. *J Am Acad Dermatol* 2006; **54**: 896–9.

23 Srivastava MD, Alexander F, Tuthill RJ. Immunology of cutaneous vasculitis associated with both etanercept and infliximab. *Scand J Immunol* 2005; **61**: 329–36.

24 Clemente RE. Demyelinating disease and cutaneous lymphocytic vasculitis after etanercept therapy in a patient with rheumatoid arthritis. *Scand J Rheumatol* 2007; **36**: 244–5.

25 Gerecitano J, Goy A, Wright J *et al.* Drug-induced cutaneous vasculitis in patients with non-Hodgkin lymphoma treated with the novel proteosome inhibitor bortezomib: a possible surrogate marker of response? *Br J Haematol* 2006; **134**: 391–8.

26 Delbarre M, Joly P, Balguerie X *et al.* Contact vasculitis caused by topical agents with non-steroidal anti-inflammatory agents or analgesics. *Ann Dermatol Venereol* 1997; **124**: 841–4.

27 Treviño J, Prieto VG, Hearne R *et al.* Atypical lymphocytic reaction with epidermotropism and lymphocytic vasculopathic reaction (lymphocytic vasculitis) after treatment with imiquimod. *J Am Acad Dermatol* 2006; **55** (Suppl.): S123–5.

28 Muñiz AE. Lymphocytic vasculitis associated with anthrax vaccine: case report and review of anthrax vaccination. *J Emerg Med* 2003; **25**: 271–6.

29 Ramdial PK, Chetty R. Vasculitis-induced membranous fat necrosis. *J Cutan Pathol* 1999; **26**: 405–10.

30 Crowson NA, Magro CM, Usmani A, McNutt NS. Immunoglobulin A-associated lymphocytic vasculopathy: a clinicopathologic study of eight patients. *J Cutan Pathol* 2002; **29**: 596–601.

31 Oh C-W, Lee S-H, Heo-Eun P. A case suggesting lymphocytic vasculitis as a presenting sign of early undifferentiated connective tissue disease. *Am J Dermatopathol* 2003; **25**: 423–7.

32 Robak E, Robak T. Skin lesions in chronic lymphocytic leukaemia. *Leuk Lymphoma* 2007; **48**: 855–65.

33 Cabuk M, Inanir I, Türkdogan P *et al.* Cyclic lymphocytic vasculitis associated with chronic lymphocytic leukaemia. *Leuk Lymphoma* 2004; **45**: 811–3.

34 Regauer S, Liegl B, Reich O, Beham-Schmid C. Vasculitis in lichen sclerosus: an under-recognized feature? *Histopathology* 2004; **45**: 237–44.

35 Ely KA, Tse G, Simpson JF *et al.* Diabetic mastopathy. A clinicopathologic review. *Am J Clin Pathol* 2000; **113**: 541–5.

36 Sellick GS, Coleman RJ, Webb EL *et al.* Dominantly inherited cutaneous small vessel lymphocytic vasculitis maps to chromosome 6q26-q27. *Hum Genet* 2005; **118**: 82–6.

37 Kanegane H, Ito Y, Ohshima K *et al.* X-linked lymphoproliferative syndrome presenting with systemic lymphocytic vasculitis. *Am J Hematol* 2005; **78**: 130–3.

Pityriasis lichenoides (Chapter 57)

Although an overlap with vasculitis and an immune complex-mediated pathogenesis has been suggested, there is increasing evidence that the three entities that make up pityriasis lichenoides represent a cytotoxic CD8+ T cell proliferation that may occur in different settings [1,2], at least some cases having convincing evidence of an infective trigger [3,4]. The clinically milder and smaller lesions of pityriasis lichenoides chronica (PLC) are unlikely to be confused with a vasculitis, but the more severe and sometimes necrotic lesions of pityriasis lichenoides et varioliformis acuta (PLEVA, Mucha–Habermann disease) may resemble a vasculitis, pyoderma gangrenosum or lymphomatoid papulosis. Vasculitic features are prominent in the much rarer and aggressive form, febrile ulceronecrotic Mucha–Habermann disease (FUMHD) [3–8] (Fig. 50.32). In contrast with PLC and PLEVA, which occur mainly in childhood and which may coexist, FUMHD usually occurs in

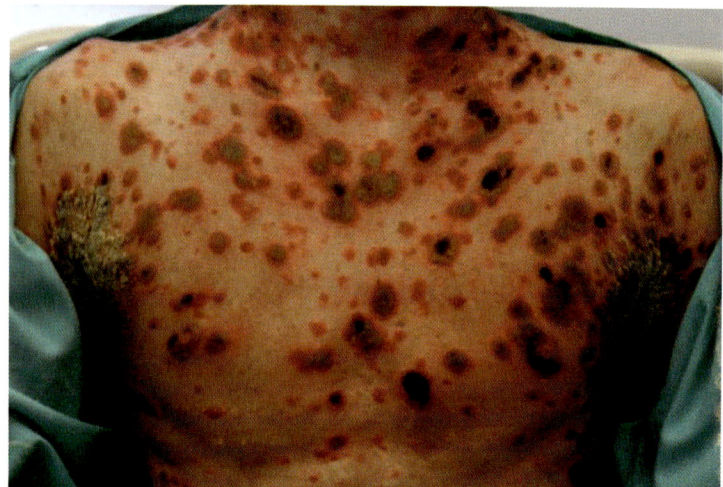

Fig. 50.32 Febrile ulcerative Mucha–Habermann disease, a disorder with pronounced systemic features that may mimic a vasculitis. (Courtesy of Drs I. Helbling and V. Yates, Hope Hospital, Salford, UK).

males in the second or third decade of life [3], and, although it can evolve from PLC or PLEVA [4], it usually occurs in isolation without more recognizable, milder pityriasis lichenoides lesions.

The lesions of PLEVA are oedematous papules and nodules that undergo central vesiculation (sometimes forming larger bullae) and haemorrhagic necrosis, eventually healing with varioliform scarring. In FUMHD, there are abundant, large necrotic lesions. Additional clinical features that might suggest a vasculitis include constitutional symptoms such as fever, headache, malaise and arthralgia that may precede or accompany the onset of PLEVA; in FUHMD there is high fever, general malaise, weakness, myalgia, neuropsychiatric symptoms and lymphadenopathy, with non-specific serological markers of inflammation such as raised ESR and C-reactive protein, and a fulminating course that may even be fatal [8].

Histological features that may suggest vasculitis in inflammatory or necrotic lesions include extravasation of erythrocytes and endothelial proliferation, although in PLEVA the infiltrate (comprised mainly of CD8 lymphocytes) may be deep, dense and wedge-shaped rather than predominantly perivascular. Immunofluorescence studies have variably demonstrated IgM, C3 or fibrin in vessel walls of fresh (usually purpuric) lesions, or at the dermoepidermal junction, and some studies have documented circulating immune complexes, all features that might be consistent with an immune complex-mediated vasculitic pathogenesis [3]. Indeed, in FUMHD there may be marked fibrinoid necrosis of deep vessels with luminal thrombi, partial necrosis of follicles and complete necrosis of eccrine glands [5], which may not be histologically distinguishable from other forms of acute necrosis of the skin.

Treatment options in aggressive PLEVA or FUMHD include systemic corticosteroids, methotrexate, dapsone, ciclosporin and intravenous immunoglobulin. Investigation for possible infection, with appropriate treatment, is also potentially important; serological evidence of associated herpes varicella-zoster [2] and cytomegalovirus [9] infections has been recorded in FUMHD.

References

1 Wenzel J, Gütgemann I, Distelmaier U et al. The role of cytotoxic skin-homing CD8+ lymphocytes in cutaneous cytotoxic T-cell lymphoma and pityriasis lichenoides. J Am Acad Dermatol 2005; **53**: 422–7.

2 Helmbold P, Gaisbauer G, Fielder E et al. Self-limited variant of febrile ulceronecrotic Mucha–Habermann disease with polyclonal T-cell receptor rearrangement. J Am Acad Dermatol 2006; **54**: 1113–4.

3 Bowers S, Warshaw EM. Pityriasis lichenoides and its subtypes. J Am Acad Dermatol 2006; **55**: 557–72.

4 Khachemoune A, Blyumin ML. Pityriasis lichenoides. Pathophysiology, classification, and treatment. Am J Clin Dermatol 2007; **8**: 29–36.

5 Tsuji T, Kasamatsu M, Yokota M et al. Mucha–Habermann disease and its febrile ulceronecrotic variant. Cutis 1996; **58**: 123–31.

6 Degos R, Duperrat B, Daniel F. Le parapsoriasis ulcero-necrotique hyperthermique. Ann Dermatol Syphiligr 1966; **93**: 481–96.

7 De Cuyper C, Hindryckx P, Deroo N. Febrile ulceronecrotic pityriasis lichenoides et varioliformis acuta. Dermatology 1994; **189** (Suppl. 2): 50–3.

8 Puddu P, Cianchini G, Colonna L et al. Febrile ulceronecrotic Mucha–Habermann's disease with fatal outcome. Int J Dermatol 1997; **36**: 691–4.

9 Tsai KS, Hsieh HJ, Chow KC et al. Detection of cytomegalovirus infection in a patient with febrile ulceronecrotic Mucha–Habermann's disease. Int J Dermatol 2001; **40**: 694–8.

Macular arteritis [1–3]

This recently described disorder is of uncertain causation. The clinical presentation is development of multiple asymptomatic or mildly pruritic, hyperpigmented macules on the trunk or, most commonly, the limbs; the lesions may have slight induration and sometimes have a degree of linearity or reticulation. Histology shows a deeply situated perivascular lymphocytic infiltrate or lymphocytic vasculitis affecting small arteries, which may be in the subcutaneous fat. An admixture of plasma cells is present in some cases. Fibrinoid necrosis of the vascular adventitia may occur, with luminal narrowing and eventual obliteration, but the tunica elastica is intact. There is no leukocytoclasis, no granuloma formation and no haemosiderin or melanin incontinence to explain the pigmentation (which is presumed to be epidermal). Patients are systemically well, do not have renal involvement, have negative ANCA and usually have no other serological abnormality.

Although earlier descriptions distinguished this disorder from C-PAN because the primary lesion is a pigmented macule, and there is no associated livedo, no ulceration, no non-pigmented dermal nodules and no tenderness of lesions [1,2], a recent pathological evaluation of biopsies from a patient with lesions on the instep of one foot led to the suggestion that this might be a latent, non-nodule forming variant of C-PAN [3].

References

1 Fein H, Sheth AP, Mutasim DF. Cutaneous arteritis presenting with hyperpigmented macules: macular arteritis. J Am Acad Dermatol 2003; **49**: 519–22.

2 Matsuoka Y, Takai I, Noda M, Kubota Y. Macular arteritis in Japanese patients. J Am Acad Dermatol 2005; **52**: 364–6.

3 Al Daraji W, Gregory AN, Carlson JA. Macular arteritis: a latent form of cutaneous polyarteritis nodosa? Am J Dermatopathol 2008; **30**: 145–9.

Lymphocytic thrombophilic arteritis [1,2]

This is a very recently described, medium-size vessel arteritis, reported in five young women; all had gradually progressing patchy and reticulate pigmentation, subtle (more marked in one case) subcutaneous indurated areas, with livedo racemosa of the lower limbs [1]. Pain was a feature in one patient, and Raynaud's phenomenon in another. Histologically, there was a predominantly lymphocytic infiltrate in the muscular wall of small arteries of the deep dermis and superficial subcutis, with a ring of fibrin deposition concentrically situated at the periphery of all affected vascular lumina. Granulocytes were scanty or absent, and inflammation was tightly confined within the panniculus in the vicinity of affected vessels. Four of the patients had antiphospholipid antibodies, one also having factor V Leiden; three had positive antinuclear antibodies (but this was negative in two cases on retesting) and three had modestly elevated erythrocyte sedimentation rate. The combined features of lymphocytic vascular inflammation and thrombophilic endovasculitis suggested that the term lymphocytic thrombophilic arteritis was appropriate.

The nosology of this condition has been discussed by LeBoit [2], and it may represent the same condition as the macular arteritis described above. Clinically, polyarteritis nodosa is probably the most likely differential diagnosis, or collagen vascular diseases with livedo and antiphospholipid antibodies.

References

1 Lee JS-S, Kossard S, McGrath MA. Lymphocytic thrombophilic arteritis. A newly described medium-sized vessel arteritis of the skin. *Arch Dermatol* 2008; **144**: 1175–82.
2 LeBoit PE. The enigma of lymphocytic vasculitis. *Arch Dermatol* 2008; **144**: 1215–6.

Palisaded neutrophilic and granulomatous dermatitis [1–4]

Churg–Strauss granulomas were originally described by Churg and Strauss as a histological feature of skin lesions in allergic granulomatosis, later known as Churg–Strauss syndrome. Winkelmann and colleagues described similar lesions in Wegener's granulomatosis, rheumatoid disease and systemic lupus erythematosus, and further delineated the histological features of what they termed the *cutaneous extravascular necrotizing granuloma* [2]. These lesions combine: (1) an interstitial (and variably perivascular) granuloma annulare-like or necrotizing extravascular granulomatous process with basophilic degenerate collagen; (2) intense tissue neutrophilia, leukocytoclasis, small vessel leukocytoclastic vasculitis (in about 50%) and sometimes an admixture with eosinophils; (3) positive direct immunofluorescence for complement, fibrin and immunoglobulins in vessel walls; and (4) associated circulating immune complexes in some cases [1–4]. Similar lesions were subsequently described as *rheumatoid papules*, and have also been documented in Behçet's disease, Takayasu's aortitis and other vasculitides, connective tissue, autoimmune and inflammatory disorders (including inflammatory bowel disease). LeBoit's group suggested that these features could be grouped together as '*palisaded neutrophilic and granulomatous dermatitis of immune complex diseases*' [3]. Other terms that have been applied include *interstitial granulomatous dermatitis with plaques*, *linear rheumatoid nodule*, and *interstitial granulomatous dermatitis with cutaneous cords and arthritis* [1,5–7]. Although it has been suggested that *palisaded neutrophilic granulomatous dermatitis* (PNGD) and interstitial granulomatous dermatitis (IGD) are separate, it is increasingly generally accepted that these are part of a spectrum (at least when associated with a connective tissue or immune complex-mediated disease); drug-induced IGD should probably be distinguished.

Clinical features include: erythematous urticated plaques or papules; firm, violaceous or waxy plaques; skin-coloured or erythematous papular or nodular lesions, sometimes annular and sometimes with ulceration or crusting; tender subcutaneous nodules; and firm linear subcutaneous cords or bands. The most typical presentation is as smooth, asymptomatic or tender papules, nodules or plaques on the forearms and dorsal hands, or on the buttocks and lower legs. Later lesions are usually more centripetal; cord-like lesions may be flexural. Sangueza and colleagues demonstrated a spectrum of clinical disease; earlier lesions are more urticated, whereas older lesions comprise firmer nodules and bands [7]. This would be consistent with the suggestion that the lesions start as leukocytoclastic vasculitis but progress to form palisaded granulomas and dermal fibrosis [1].

Treatment options may be dictated in part by the background disease (most commonly rheumatoid arthritis, in 40%), and include corticosteroids (topical or oral), colchicine, hydroxychloroquine, dapsone, ciclosporin and cyclophosphamide. It is important to be aware that TNF-α inhibitors, increasingly used in treatment of rheumatoid disease, can cause IGD [8]; distinction between disease-associated and drug-induced lesions may be difficult other than by withdrawal of treatment.

Other conditions that may rarely produce a cutaneous granulomatous vasculitis are herpes virus infections (herpes simplex and herpes varicella-zoster) and hepatitis C virus infection [9].

References

1 Draft KS, Wiser EB, Elenitsas R. Dermatopathology update of newer manifestations of systemic disease. *Adv Dermatol* 2001; **21**: 101–32.
2 Finan MC, Winkelmann RK. The cutaneous extravascular necrotizing granuloma (Churg–Strauss granuloma) and systemic disease: a review of 27 cases. *Medicine* 1983; **62**: 142–58.
3 Chu P, Connolly MK, LeBoit PE. The histopathologic spectrum of palisaded neutrophilic and granulomatous dermatitis in patients with collagen vascular disease. *Arch Dermatol* 1994; **130**: 1278–83.
4 Magro CM, Crowson AN. The spectrum of cutaneous lesions in rheumatoid vasculitis: a clinical and pathological study of 43 patients. *J Cutan Pathol* 2003; **30**: 1–10.
5 Gottlieb GB, Duve RS, Ackerman AB. Interstitial granulomatous dermatitis with cutaneous cords and arthritis: linear subcutaneous bands in rheumatoid arthritis revisited. *Dermatopathol: Pract Concept* 1995; **1**: 3–6.
6 Tomasini C, Pippione M. Interstitial granulomatous dermatitis with plaques. *J Am Acad Dermatol* 2002; **46**: 892–9.
7 Sangueza OP, Caudell MD, Mengesha YM *et al.* Palisaded neutrophilic granulomatous dermatitis in rheumatoid arthritis. *J Am Acad Dermatol* 2002; **47**: 251–7.
8 Deng A, Harvey V, Sina B *et al.* Interstitial granulomatous dermatitis associated with use of tumor necrosis factor α inhibitors. *Arch Dermatol* 2006; **142**: 198–202.
9 Pagnoux C, Kluger N, Francès C, Guillevin L. Cutaneous granulomatous vasculitis and extravascular granulomas. *Expert Rev Dermatol* 2006; **1**: 315–26.

Vasculitis as a component of other systemic diseases

Vasculitis is a feature of many systemic diseases that are mainly discussed in other chapters; a representative list is given in Table 50.12. They include collagen vascular diseases (Chapter 51) and disorders such as sarcoidosis (Chapter 61) in which there may be either a large vessel granulomatous vasculitis or an immune complex-associated small vessel cutaneous vasculitis. *Necrotizing sarcoid granulomatosis* is a variant of nodular sarcoidosis that is in the differential diagnosis of Wegener's granulomatosis of the lung [1]; although it is unlikely to present to dermatologists, the occurrence of extrapulmonary lesions is common, and skin involvement has been reported [2].

Sjögren's syndrome is associated with purpuric lesions similar to those of Waldenström's hypergammaglobulinaemic purpura, and with vasculitis that often has an urticarial or urticated component and predominantly affects the lower limbs [3–5]. Pathologically, the vasculitis covers a wide spectrum; one study of 558 patients with Sjögren's syndrome documented 52 patients (51 being female) with vasculitis that was classified as urticarial in 11, cryoglobulinaemic in 14 and CSSV in the remainder. Of 38 patients biopsied, 36 had a leukocytoclastic vasculitis and two had a medium-size vessel necrotizing vasculitis [5]. Vasculitis in these patients had a statistically significant association with the presence of arthritis (occurring in 50%), peripheral neuropathy (31%), Raynaud's phenomenon (40%), renal involvement (10%), antinuclear antibodies (88%), anti-Ro/SSA antibodies (70%) and rheumatoid factor (78%) [5]. Cutaneous livedo, subacute cutaneous lupus erythematosus, erythema nodosum and cytopenias also occur; 10–20% have

Table 50.12 Some systemic diseases in which vasculitis may occur (excluding those in this chapter).

Type of disease	Examples
Collagen vascular and rheumatological diseases	Lupus erythematosus (including drug-induced) Rheumatoid disease Sjögren's disease Dermatomyositis Scleroderma/progressive systemic sclerosis Mixed connective tissue disease Relapsing polychondritis Still's disease Reiter's disease
Gastrointestinal	Inflammatory bowel disease Bowel bypass (see p. 50.87) Primary biliary cirrhosis Peritoneal fibrosis
Granulomatous	Sarcoidosis
Periodic fevers/ autoinflammatory syndromes	Familial Mediterranean fever Hyper-IgD syndrome PFAPA syndrome
Haematological and malignancy	Lymphomas Hairy cell leukaemia Other leukaemias and myeloproliferative disorders Myeloma Hypereosinophilic syndrome Autoerythrocyte sensitization syndrome Wiskott–Aldrich syndrome Solid organ-specific tumours (Chapter 62)
Miscellaneous	Goodpasture's syndrome Cystic fibrosis α_1-antitrypsin deficiency Kikuchi disease (necrotizing lymphadenitis)

PFAPA, periodic fever, aphthous stomatitis, pharyngitis, adenitis.

positive antiphospholipid antibodies or ANCA, but less than 10% of these have vasculitis [4]. High parotid scintigraphy scores and low complement C4 levels are both associated with vasculitis and are predictive that it is likely to occur [6]. Vasculitis, cryoglobulinaemia and hypocomplementaemia are all independently associated with risk of death [6]; 70% with Sjögren's syndrome and cutaneous vasculitis develop peripheral or central nervous system involvement, which is felt to be due to vasculopathy [3]. Hypocomplementaemia is associated with cryoglobulinaemia, systemic disease, lymphoma and death [7]. Less dramatic but of direct dermatological interest, dry skin is also a feature of Sjögren's syndrome; in one patient with cryoglobulinaemia, cutaneous vasculitis and generalized hypohidrosis, a skin biopsy showed dense peri-eccrine lymphocytic infiltration with glandular shrinkage [8], which was presumably distinct from the vasculitis process.

Cystic fibrosis is a cause of episodic vasculitis, especially in more severe cases; purpuric and vasculitis lesions may occur, most commonly on the lower limbs. Bullae and urticarial vasculitis have been reported, but the overall pattern in most cases suggests an immune complex-mediated leukocytoclastic vasculitis [9]. There is often associated arthralgia, and neurological and renal involvement occur. Immune complexes have been demonstrated in the circulation; skin biopsies show leukocytoclastic vasculitis, fibrin deposition and may have positive direct immunofluorescence for complement C3. The episodic nature (usually lasting about 2 weeks) and the link with respiratory symptoms suggests that the antigen in many cases may be from bacteria (or antibiotic treatments). However, cryoglobulins and positive rheumatoid factor have also been documented in some cases.

Hypereosinophilic syndrome (HES; Gleich syndrome; Chapter 62) is an uncommon entity, which may include more than one form of haematological malignancy [10]. In some instances, there is a clonal T-cell production of interleukin IL-5, a major controlling cytokine in production, release and differentiation of eosinophils. In other cases, there is clonal expansion of eosinophils with hepatosplenomegaly and thrombocytopenia; this condition appears to be due to a cytogenetic defect t(9;22)(q34;q11) in which there is chromosomal breakage and reciprocal exchange of chromosomal fragments that leads to formation of a fusion tyrosine kinase FIP1L1–PDGFRα. Various skin lesions have been reported in HES, including eosinophilic vasculitis with gangrene [11] and thrombotic damage with dense perivascular eosinophilic infiltrate but without vasculitis [12,13]. Although these cases were treated with steroids, newer treatments combined with identification of the causative abnormality may allow targeted therapy; imatinib mesylate, used mainly in treatment of chronic myelogenous leukaemia, targets the platelet-derived growth factor receptor (PDGFR) in the fusion tyrosine kinase of HES [14], described above, and mepolizumab, an anti-IL-5 monoclonal antibody, has also been used recently to treat HES [15].

Alpha$_1$-antitrypsin (AAT) deficiency is discussed in Chapter 46 in relation to panniculitis. It may also be associated with systemic necrotizing vasculitis; in a series of eight patients, six had an MPA pattern of vasculitis, one had WG and one had HSP [16]. These authors reviewed additional cases; all had cutaneous vasculitis and either renal or joint involvement, and two-thirds died (mainly due to renal failure).

Autoinflammatory diseases (including the disorders previously termed hereditary fever syndromes or periodic fevers, such as *familial Mediterranean fever* (FMF), *hyperimmunoglobulinaemia D with periodic fever syndrome* and others), are also a potential cause of vasculitis, as well as causing multiple other symptoms (see also Chapter 62). The evolution of understanding of this group of disorders, which also includes cryopyrin-associated periodic syndromes (CAPS), tumour necrosis factor receptor-associated periodic syndrome (TRAPS), PAPA (pyogenic arthritis, pyoderma gangrenosum and acne), Schnitzler syndrome (Chapter 22) and CINCA syndrome (chronic infantile neurologic, cutaneous, articular syndrome; also termed neonatal-onset multisystem inflammatory disease, NOMID), is summarized in recent reviews [17–19]. It is important to consider FMF as a cause of vasculitis in children with apparent HSP in areas where FMF is prevalent, as HSP is much more common in families with FMF compared with the general population [20]; diagnostic delay is common. Tests for faecal occult blood are often positive during acute attacks of FMF. Other vasculitic features in FMF include purpura, subcutaneous nodules and associated PAN (which occurs in about 1% of patients);

in particular, perirenal haematoma is usually associated with PAN secondary to FMF [20]. Both circulating IgD immune complexes and IgD deposits on direct immunofluorescence of the skin have been identified in hyperimmunoglobulinaemia D syndrome [21], and HSP has been reported in this condition [22]. Lymphocytic vasculitis was reported in a child with *PFAPA syndrome* (Periodic Fever, Aphthous stomatitis, Pharyngitis, Adenitis) [23].

Paraneoplastic vasculitis (Chapter 62) is particularly associated with haematological malignancies; mechanisms include vasculitis related to paraproteins, cryoglobulins or to the presence of antinuclear antibodies. Hairy cell leukaemia appears to be especially associated with vasculitis, which may be of leukocytoclastic, lymphocytic or polyarteritis nodosa pattern.

Vasculitis may also be a feature of *Wiskott–Aldrich syndrome* (Chapter 15), usually leukocytoclastic small vessel vasculitis but aortitis and mesenteric or renal arteritis may occur [24].

Several forms of vasculitis have been associated with *relapsing polychondritis*, discussed on p. 50.91.

Autoerythrocyte sensitization syndrome (Chapters 49 and 64) has also been reported with cutaneous vasculitis [25].

References

1 Quaden C, Tillie-Leblond I, Delobbe A *et al*. Necrotising sarcoid granulomatosis: clinical, functional, endoscopical and radiographical evaluations. *Eur Respir J* 2005; **26**: 778–85.

2 Shirodaria CC, Nicholson AG, Hansell DM *et al*. Lesson of the month: Necrotising sarcoid granulomatosis with skin involvement. *Histopathology* 2003; **43**: 91–3.

3 Alexander E, Provost TT. Sjögren's syndrome. Association of cutaneous vasculitis with central nervous system disease. *Arch Dermatol* 1987; **123**: 801–10.

4 Ramos-Casals M, Brito-Zerón P, Font J. The overlap of Sjögren's syndrome with other systemic autoimmune diseases. *Semin Arthritis Rheum* 2007; **36**: 246–55.

5 Ramos-Casals M, Anaya JM, García-Carrasco M *et al*. Cutaneous vasculitis in primary Sjögren syndrome: classification and clinical significance of 52 patients. *Medicine (Baltimore)* 2004; **83**: 96–106.

6 Brito-Zerón P, Ramos-Casals M, Bove A *et al*. Predicting adverse outcomes in Sjögren's syndrome: identification of prognostic factors. *Rheumatology (Oxford)* 2007; **46**: 1359–62.

7 Ramos-Casals M, Brito-Zerón P, Yägue J *et al*. Hypocomplementaemia as an immunological marker of morbidity and mortality in patients with primary Sjögren's syndrome. *Rheumatology (Oxford)* 2005; **44**: 89–94.

8 Sais G, Admella C, Fantova MJ, Montero JC. Lymphocytic autoimmune hidradenitis, cutaneous leukocytoclastic vasculitis and primary Sjögren's syndrome. *Br J Dermatol* 1998; **139**: 1073–6.

9 Bernstein ML, McCusker MM, Grant-Kels JM. Cutaneous manifestations of cystic fibrosis. *Pediatr Dermatol* 2008; **25**: 150–7.

10 Schwartz RS. The hypereosinophilic syndrome and the biology of cancer. *N Engl J Med* 2003; **348**: 1199–200.

11 Jang K-A, Lim Y-S, Choi J-H *et al*. Hypereosinophilic syndrome presenting as cutaneous necrotizing eosinophilic vasculitis and Raynaud's phenomenon complicated by digital gangrene. *Br J Dermatol* 2000; **143**: 641–4.

12 Hamada T, Kimura Y, Hayashi S *et al*. Hypereosinophilic syndrome with peripheral circulatory insufficiency and cutaneous microthrombi. *Arch Dermatol* 2007; **143**: 812–3.

13 Oppliger R, Gay-Crosier F, Dayer E, Hauser C. Digital necrosis in a patient with hypereosinophilic syndrome in the absence of cutaneous eosinophilic vasculitis. *Br J Dermatol* 2001; **144**: 1087–90.

14 Cools J, DeAngelo DJ, Gotlib J *et al*. A tyrosine kinase created by fusion of the PDGFRA and FIP1L1 genes as a therapeutic target of imatinib in idiopathic hypereosinophilic syndrome. *N Engl J Med* 2003; **348**: 1201–14.

15 Rothenberg ME, Klion AD, Roufosse FE *et al*. Treatment of patients with the hypereosinophilic syndrome with mepolizumab. *N Engl J Med* 2008; **358**: 1215–28.

16 Mazodier P, Elzouki A-NY, Segelmark M, Eriksson S. Systemic necrotizing vasculitides in severe alpha$_1$-antitrypsin deficiency. *QJM* 1996; **89**: 599–611.

17 Rose CD, Martin TM. Caspase recruitment domain 15 mutations and rheumatic diseases. *Curr Opin Rheumatol* 2005; **17**: 579–85.

18 Shinkai K, Kilcline C, Connolly MK, Frieden IJ. The pyrin family of fever genes. Unmasking genetic determinants of autoinflammatory disease. *Arch Dermatol* 2005; **141**: 242–7.

19 Ryan JG, Goldbach-Mansky R. The spectrum of autoinflammatory diseases: recent bench to bedside observations. *Curr Opin Rheumatol* 2008; **20**: 66–75.

20 Hamuryudan V, Özdogun H, Yazici H. Other forms of vasculitis and pseudovasculitis. *Baillières Clin Rheumatol* 1997; **11**: 335–55.

21 Boom BW, Daha MR, Vermeer BJ, van der Meer JW. IgD immune complex vasculitis in a patient with hyperimmunoglobulinaemia D and periodic fever. *Arch Dermatol* 1990; **126**: 1621–4.

22 Wickiser J, Saulsbury FT. Henoch-Schönlein purpura in a child with hyperimmunoglobulinemia D and periodic fever syndrome. *Pediatr Dermatol* 2005; **22**: 138–41.

23 Lee WI, Yang MH, Lee KF *et al*. PFAPA syndrome (Periodic Fever, Aphthous stomatitis, Pharyngitis, Adenitis). *Clin Rheumatol* 1999; **18**: 207–13.

24 McCluggage WG, Armstrong DJ, Maxwell RJ *et al*. Systemic vasculitis and aneurysm formation in the Wiskott-Aldrich syndrome. *J Clin Pathol* 1999; **52**: 390–2.

25 Cansu D, Kasifoglu T, Pasaoglu O, Korkmaz C. Autoerythrocyte sensitization syndrome (Gardner-Diamond syndrome) associated with cutaneous vasculitis. *Joint Bone Spine* 2008; **75**: 721–4.

Microvascular occlusion disorders (Chapter 49)

It is important in the differential diagnosis of vasculitis to be aware of disorders that may present with livedo or infarcted lesions, such as *cryoglobulinaemic vasculitis, cholesterol embolization, cardiac myxoma emboli, Sneddon's disease* and *malignant atrophic papulosis* (*Degos' disease*). The major pathology in these is either initially occlusive, or is probably mediated by antiphospholipid antibodies (in Sneddon's syndrome), and so they are all discussed in the section on microvascular occlusion in Chapter 49. Other disorders associated with antiphospholipid antibodies are also discussed. In *calcific uraemic arteriolopathy* (*calciphylaxis*) (Chapter 49), the earliest event is vessel wall calcification [1], therefore this also is discussed in the section on microvascular occlusion rather than as a primarily vasculitic disorder. *Hyperoxaluria* may cause acrocyanosis, gangrene and livedo reticularis. *Hyperhomocysteinaemia*, typically in homozygotes for methyl tetrahydrofolate reductase mutation C677T, also predisposes to endothelial damage and vasculopathy. Vessel wall deposition disorders such as *amyloidosis*, or vessel leakage in *scurvy* or some *pigmented purpuric dermatoses*, may also mimic vasculitis, but histology demonstrates erythrocyte leakage without vasculitis. Thrombotic thrombocytopenic purpura, leukaemias and lymphomas may all occasionally mimic vasculitis.

Thromboangiitis obliterans (*Buerger's disease*) [2] is a disorder of small or medium-sized arteries (less commonly veins) in which there is an inflammatory non-suppurative panarteritis or panphlebitis with thrombosis. Antiendothelial cell antibodies may be significantly elevated in active disease and have a role in monitoring the disease [3]. This disorder is discussed in more detail in Chapter 47.

Other arterial thrombotic disorders that may mimic vasculitis include hypothenar hammer syndrome (Chapter 28), thrombosis resulting from polyvinyl chloride haemodialysis tubing [4], vessel wall invasion by tumour or organisms and sickle cell anaemia. Amyloid infiltration of the vessel wall may cause occlusion. Drugs such as ergot, amphetamines or epinephrine (adrenaline) typically cause vasospasm but there may be histological evidence of vasculitis.

References

1 Au S, Crawford RI. Three-dimensional analysis of a calciphylaxis plaque: clues to pathogenesis. *J Am Acad Dermatol* 2002; **47**: 53–7.
2 Totemchokchyakarn K. Thromboangiitis obliterans (Buerger's disease). In: Ball GV, Bridges SL, eds. *Vasculitis*. Oxford: Oxford University Press, 2002: 460–6.
3 Eichhorn J, Sima D, Lindschau C, Turowski A. Antiendothelial cell antibodies in thromboangiitis obliterans. *Am J Med Sci* 1998; **315**: 17–23.
4 Bommer J, Ritz E, Andrassay K. Necrotizing dermatitis resulting from haemodialysis with polyvinylchloride tubing. *Ann Intern Med* 1979; **91**: 869–70.

Infections [1–4]

Mechanisms by which infections may cause vasculitis have been discussed on p. 50.5. Several infections are implicated in the pathogenesis of vasculitides, such as streptococci in HSP, hepatitis C in mixed cryoglobulinaemic vasculitis (an immune complex-mediated process p. 50.23) or hepatitis B in PAN. These have been discussed in relation to specific vasculitides earlier. This brief section summarizes some of the preceding discussion of infections, and notes some infections that mimic vasculitis. Lists of infections linked with vasculitis are provided in many texts and references [3,4]; a summary of the most important is provided in Table 50.13.

Table 50.13 Some infections that have been documented to cause vasculitis.

Type of infection	Examples
Bacteria	Streptococci
	Staphylococci
	Neisseria spp.: *N. meningitidis*, *N. gonorrhoea*
	Spirochaetes: *Borrelia burgdorferi*, *Treponema pallidum*
	Yersinia
	Salmonella
	Helicobacter pylori
	Pseudomonas spp.
	Mycobacterium spp.
Viruses	Herpesviruses: herpes simplex, varicella-zoster, cytomegalovirus
	Hepatitis viruses: A, B and C
	Epstein–Barr virus
	Immune deficiency: HIV, HTLV-1
	Parvovirus B19
	Influenza and parainfluenza
	Other common viruses: adenovirus, rubella
	Hantavirus
Fungi	*Candida*
	Aspergillus
Others	Rickettsia
	Mycoplasma spp.
	Toxoplasma
	Pneumocystis carinii (in HIV infection)
Vaccinations (see Table 50.8)	Influenza
	Hepatitis B, hepatitis A
	Rubella/measles/mumps–measles–rubella (MMR)
	BCG

Kawasaki disease is discussed in Chapter 30, but a brief summary of the vasculitis-related aspects is provided below.

Vasculitis in patients with subacute bacterial endocarditis or with gonococcal infection is mainly immune complex-mediated, although bacterial emboli can also occur; this may also be a feature of mycotic aneurysms, which potentially mimic medium vessel vasculitis. Other infections may cause a vasculitis by direct infection of endothelial cells, notably in rickettsial or cytomegalovirus (CMV) infection. CMV has a particular affinity for endothelial cells, especially those of allografts, and may also provoke thrombosis; infections in immunocompromised patients may respond to intravenous ganciclovir but there is still significant mortality [5].

Some apparent associations, such as that of *Staphylococcus aureus* with Wegener's granulomatosis (p. 50.39) are less well understood. Herpesvirus infections and HIV may also cause or mimic vasculitis. HIV has been associated with numerous patterns of vasculitis including leukocytoclastic and necrotizing vasculitides, HSP, EED, C-PAN, CSS and eosinophilic vasculitis, cerebral vasculitis and others; however, in some instances, HIV-associated vasculitis may be due to therapy (especially zidovudine and didanosine) or to secondary infections such as cytomegalovirus [4].

Vaccines have been implicated as causes of vasculitis. The two that are most frequently reported as causes of different vasculitis syndromes are influenza and hepatitis B. Influenza vaccine has been linked with CSVV, systemic leukocytoclastic vasculitis (LCV), and MPA; hepatitis B vaccine has been linked with development of CSVV, LCV with systemic involvement, Kawasaki disease, HSP, CSS and Takayasu's arteritis.

However, infections may also mimic vasculitis, particularly by embolization or by direct invasion of vessel walls. Zygomycosis is an important cause, occurring especially in immunosuppressed subjects; cutaneous infarction by zygomycosis has been described as having a targetoid 'bull's-eye' appearance [6] but may just cause a necrotic discoid lesion (Chapter 49). Other important examples are *Salmonella* spp. causing aortitis, embolic lesions of *S. aureus* infections, and *Nocardia* infections mimicking Wegener's granulomatosis [7]. Disseminated candidosis has been reported as resembling leukocytoclastic vasculitis [8]. Such infections may occur in subjects who are being treated with immunosuppressive agents, and may be mistaken for a disease flare with the consequent risk of immunosuppressive treatment being increased. Even serological tests may be misleading in such situations—ANCA positivity has been documented in endocarditis, septic shock and others [9,10]. It is important to consider infection in the differential diagnosis of vasculitis (especially if clinically atypical) or as a cause of unexpected disease flares, to ensure that any pustular lesions are sterile, and to carefully investigate fever in patients with vasculitis.

References

1 Somer T, Finegold SM. Vasculitides associated with infections, immunization, and antimicrobial drugs. *Clin Infect Dis* 1995; **20**: 1010–36.
2 Mandell BF, Calabrese LH. Infections and systemic vasculitis. *Curr Opin Rheumatol* 1998; **10**: 51–7.
3 Chatham WW. Miscellaneous forms of vasculitis. In: Ball GV, Bridges SL, eds. *Vasculitis*. Oxford: Oxford University Press, 2002: 513–32.

4 Del Rosso A, Generini S, Pignone A, Matucci-Cerinic M. Vasculitides secondary to systemic diseases. *Clin Dermatol* 1999; **17**: 533–47.

5 Golden MP, Hammer SM, Wanke CA, Albrecht MA. Cytomegalovirus vasculitis. Case reports and review of the literature. *Medicine (Baltimore)* 1994; **73**: 246–55.

6 Rubin AI, Grossman ME. Bull's-eye cutaneous infarct of zygomycosis: a bedside diagnosis confirmed by touch preparation. *J Am Acad Dermatol* 2004; **51**: 996–1001.

7 Gibb W, Williams A. Nocardiosis mimicking Wegener's granulomatosis. *Scand J Infect Dis* 1986; **18**: 583–5.

8 Glaich AS, Krathen RA, Smith MJ, Hsu S. Disseminated candidiasis mimicking leukocytoclastic vasculitis. *J Am Acad Dermatol* 2005; **53**: 544–6.

9 Sato A, Jorgensen C, Oksman F et al. Endocarditis accociated with ANCA. *Clin Exp Rheumatol* 1994; **12**: 203–4.

10 Mege JL, Escallier JC, Capo C et al. Anti-neutrophil cytoplasmic antibodies (ANCA) and infection. In: Gross WL, ed. *ANCA-Associated Vasculitides: Immunological and Clinical Aspects*. New York: Plenum Press, 1993: 353–6.

Behçet's disease

Synonym
• Adamantiades–Behçet's disease

Definition. Behçet's disease, named after the Turkish dermatologist who first described the condition, is a multisystem disease that is defined by the presence of oral aphthosis with at least two of the following: genital aphthae, synovitis, posterior uveitis, cutaneous pustular vasculitis or meningoencephalitis, in the absence of IBD or autoimmune diseases [1–3]. With respect to classification, it is something of an enigma; it is viewed by some as a neutrophilic dermatosis [4], or as a neutrophilic dermatosis that can be associated with leukocytoclastic vasculitis [5], but by others as a true neutrophilic [6,7] or lymphocytic [8] vasculitis. It is also associated with thrombotic arterial or venous disease [9], and has been described as a pauci-inflammatory thrombogenic vasculopathy. Indeed, it has been suggested that it is unique in being a primary vasculitis with predominant venous involvement [10]. However, it has also been reported to occur in association with other 'classical' neutrophilic dermatoses such as pyoderma gangrenosum and Sweet's syndrome. These apparently conflicting or overlapping features are discussed in subsequent sections, but all of the above processes occur in different lesion types and stages.

Because of these classification difficulties, we have specifically discussed this entity between the sections on vasculitis and neutrophilic dermatoses, the two main groups of disorders comprising this chapter. As a generalization, skin and mucous membrane lesions in Behçet's disease mainly represent a neutrophilic dermatosis, cerebral involvement also represents a vasculopathy rather than vasculitis, but other lesions are vasculitic or thrombotic.

It typically affects young adults, but can occur in children [11]. It is uncommon in northern Europe and the USA, but is common in Middle Eastern and Japanese (i.e. 'silk route') populations [12]. In Arab populations, males are affected about four times as often as females, but in many other populations the sex ratio is approximately equal.

Aetiology and pathogenesis. Although the exact cause of Behçet's disease is unknown, a genetic component of the disease is suggested by its association with HLA-B51 [2,13]. However, this only accounts for a minority of sibling risk, and at least 16 genetic loci have been linked with Behçet's disease [10]. The HLA-B51 association is less strong in populations with a lower frequency of Behçet's disease, where a link with HLA-C*15 and HLA-C*16 may be more apparent. More recent studies have also shown a predilection associated with various cytokine and inflammatory mediator alleles and polymorphisms, including polymorphisms in endothelial nitric oxide synthase (eNOS), in interleukin-10 (IL-10), IL-8, and CD28 genes, and presence of the antitumour necrosis factor-alpha (TNF-α) 1031C allele are all associated with Behçet's disease susceptibility [14]. Several of these have only been found in certain ethnic groups, for example Glu298Asp polymorphisms of eNOS in Turks.

At least during disease flares, there is a Th1-predominant immune reaction. Specific triggering of certain subsets of γδT cells has been documented [15,16], for example Vγ9Vδ2 T cells in the intraocular fluid of patients with uveitis. The cytokine IL-12, serum levels of which correlate with disease activity, not only promotes a Th1 response, but also causes proliferation of γδT cells, suggesting that this is important in pathogenesis.

The possibility that infections may stimulate an abnormal immune response in persons susceptible to Behçet's disease has some support; IL-12B heterozygosity is associated with susceptibility, and plays a part in Th1 antistreptococcal activity [14], and demonstration of altered expression and function of Toll-like receptor 6 on granulocytes and monocytes in Behçet's disease (lower than in controls at basal levels, but enhanced after stimulation with heat shock protein or streptococcal extracts) support a role for microorganisms in the pathogenesis [17]. Further, antibodies to heat shock protein 60 (a streptococcal protein) have been demonstrated, increased serum levels of HSP60 occur but do not seem to correlate with disease activity [18], and the 336–351 sequence of HSP60 induces uveitis in a rat model. Antibodies against *Saccharomyces cerevisiae*, also found in Crohn's disease, are significantly more common in patients with intestinal Behçet's disease (and in their relatives) compared with those without gastrointestinal involvement [14], but a causal relationship has not been established. Parvovirus B19 DNA was detected significantly more often in skin of 40 patients with Behçet's disease than in controls [19].

Altered expression of various adhesion molecules, such as VCAM-1, CD44, CD86, CD58 and CD54, as well as changes in various cytokines and apoptotic markers, has been demonstrated in the oral ulcers in Behçet's disease [20], but, although relevant to cell and matrix interactions at the site of lesions, has not elucidated the pathogenesis. Serum VEGF is elevated, and may be a risk factor for ocular disease [18]. Increased levels of IL-23 p19 subunit (measured by RNA expression) have been demonstrated in the erythema nodosum-like lesions of Behçet's disease [21], but its role is unclear. Acting via CXCR-1 and CXCR-2 receptors, IL-8 is a neutrophil chemoattractant whose serum levels have some correlation with Behçet's disease activity [16]. IL-8 also activates endothelium, creating a pro-thrombotic environment [16].

Homozygosity of the T allele of the methylenetetrahydrofolate reductase (MTHFR) gene is more common in Behçet's disease; it is associated with low thiolactonase activity and high homocysteine levels, creating a pro-thrombotic situation [22]. Increased platelet activation has also been suggested as an explanation for the thrombotic component of the disease. Neutrophil chemotaxis, activation and production of reactive oxygen species is also a feature; recent studies have shown that a subset of T cells producing CXCL8 may be relevant in this and other neutrophilic dermatoses [23], and also that patients with active Behçet's disease (and those with Sweet's syndrome) have elevated levels of granulocyte colony-stimulating factor (GCSF), which suppresses neutrophil apoptosis [24].

Autoantibodies such as ANCA and anticardiolipin antibodies do not appear to have a pathogenic role in Behçet's disease. Although anticardiolipin/antiphospholipid antibodies have been described in up to 50% of cases, most studies suggest that they are not present, or only in a small proportion, and their presence does not appear to correlate with specific events or overall disease activity [25], although higher serum levels have been reported in patients with thromboses [18]. Other antibodies that have been demonstrated include antiribosomal phosphoprotein and antiphosphatidylserine antibodies; the latter have a role in apoptosis and may be implicated in the development of vasculitis [26]. Antiendothelial cell antibodies (AECA), as in many vasculitides, are found but are of uncertain relevance; a more specific role is suggested by the identification of IgM AECA directed against α-enolase in the vascular wall [27]. Further supporting the possibility that an immune response to microorganisms may be involved in the aetiopathogenesis of Behçet's disease, α-enolase-like molecules are found in the cell wall of streptococci and many fungi [16]. Thus several microorganisms, rather than one specific infection, might cause the same complex immune response, generating anti-α-enolase antibodies that can bind to endothelium, thereby increasing IL-8 production and activating neutrophils.

High prevalences of procoagulant mutations such as factor V Leiden (factor V gene mutation G1691A) [28] and prothrombin gene mutation G20210A [29] have been reported in patients with Behçet's disease in whom thrombotic events occur; each was found in a third of patients with Behçet's disease and thrombosis, compared with those without thrombosis in whom the expected background prevalence (each about 1–5%) is observed. In a study of 64 patients with Behçet's disease (32 with thrombosis and 32 without), over half of those with thrombosis had one or both mutations [29]. Other prothrombotic tendencies therefore seem to augment the thrombotic tendency in this disease.

References

1 Jorizzo JL, Hudson RD, Schmalstieg FC *et al.* Behçet's syndrome: immune regulation, circulating immune complexes, neutrophil migration, and colchicine therapy. *J Am Acad Dermatol* 1984; **10**: 205–14.

2 Jorizzo JL. Behçet's disease: an update based on the 1985 international conference in London. *Arch Dermatol* 1986; **122**: 556–8.

3 O'Duffy JD, Carney JA, Deodhar S. Behçet's disease: report of 10 cases, three with new manifestation. *Ann Intern Med* 1971; **75**: 561–70.

4 Callen JP. Neutrophilic dermatoses. *Dermatol Clin* 2002; **20**: 409–19.

5 Fiorentino D. Cutaneous vasculitis. *J Am Acad Dermatol* 2003; **48**: 311–40.

6 Sams HH, Sams WM. Cutaneous leukocytoclastic vasculitis. In: Ball GV, Bridges SL, eds. *Vasculitis*. Oxford: Oxford University Press, 2002: 467–75.

7 Carlson JA, Chen KR. Cutaneous vasculitis update: small vessel neutrophilic vasculitis syndromes. *Am J Dermatopathol* 2006; **28**: 486–506.

8 Gibson LE. Cutaneous vasculitis update. *Dermatol Clin* 2002; **19**: 603–15.

9 Fessler BJ. Thrombotic syndromes and autoimmune disease. *Rheum Dis Clin N Am* 1997; **23**: 461–79.

10 Melikoglu M, Kural-Seyahi E, Tascilar K, Yaziei I. The unique features of vasculitis in Behçet's syndrome. *Clin Rev Allerg Immunol* 2008; **35**: 40–6.

11 Amman AJ, Johnson A, Fyfe GA *et al.* Behçet's syndrome. *J Pediatr* 1985; **107**: 41–3.

12 James DG. Silk route disease. *Postgrad Med J* 1986; **62**: 151–3.

13 Baricordi OR, Sensi A, Pivetti-Pezzi P *et al.* Behçet's disease associated with HLA-B51 and DRw52 antigens in Italians. *Hum Immunol* 1986; **17**: 297–301.

14 Krause I, Weinberger A. Behçet's disease. *Curr Opin Rheumatol* 2008; **20**: 82–7.

15 Yurdakul S, Hamuryudan V, Yazici H. Behçet's disease. *Curr Opin Rheumatol* 2003; **16**: 38–42.

16 Kalayciyan A, Zouboulis CC. An update on Behçet's disease. *J Eur Acad Dermatol Venereol* 2007; **21**: 1–10.

17 Yavuz S, Elbir Y, Tulunay A *et al.* Differential expression of toll-like receptor 6 on granulocytes and monocytes in Behçet's disease etiopathogenesis. *Rheumatol Int* 2008; **28**: 401–6.

18 Shaker O, Ay El-Deen MA, El Haddidi H *et al.* The role of heat shock protein 60, vascular endothelial growth factor and antiphospholipid antibodies in Behçet disease. *Br J Dermatol* 2007; **156**: 32–7.

19 Baskan EB, Yilmaz E, Saricaoglu H *et al.* Detection of parvovirus B19 DNA in the lesional skin of patients with Behçet's disease. *Clin Exp Dermatol* 2007; **32**: 186–90.

20 Kose O, Stewart J, Waseem A *et al.* Expression of cytokeratins, adhesion and activation molecules in oral ulcers of Behçet's disease. *Clin Exp Dermatol* 2007; **33**: 62–9.

21 Lew W, Chang JY, Jung JY, Bang D. Increased expression of interleukin-23 p19 mRNA in erythema nodosum-like lesions of Behçet's disease. *Br J Dermatol* 2008; **158**: 505–11.

22 Koubaa N, Hammami S, Nakbi A *et al.* Relationship between thiolactonase activity and hyperhomocysteinaemia according to MTHFR gene polymorphism in Tunisian Behçet's disease patients. *Clin Chem Lab Med* 2008; **46**: 187–92.

23 Keller M, Spanou Z, Schaerli P *et al.* T cell-regulated neutrophilic inflammation in autoinflammatory disease. *J Immunol* 2005; **175**: 7678–86.

24 Kawakami T, Ohashi S, Kawa Y *et al.* Elevated serum granulocyte colony-stimulating factor levels in patients with active phase of Sweet syndrome and patients with active Behçet's disease. Implication in neutrophil apoptosis dysfunction. *Arch Dermatol* 2004; **140**: 570–4.

25 Fessler BJ. Thrombotic syndromes and autoimmune diseases. *Rheum Dis Clin N Am* 1997; **23**: 461–79.

26 Berlit P, Stueper B, Fink I *et al.* Behçet's disease is associated with increased concentrations of antibodies against phosphatidylserine and ribosomal phosphoproteins. *VASA* 2005; **34**: 176–80.

27 Lee KH, Chung HS, Kim HS *et al.* Human alpha-enolase from endothelial cells as a target antigen of the anti-endothelial cell antibody in Behçet's disease. *Arthritis Rheum* 2003; **48**: 2025–35.

28 Gül A, Özbek U, Öztürk C *et al.* Coagulation factor V gene mutation increases the risk of venous thrombosis in Behçet's disease. *Br J Rheumatol* 1996; **35**: 1178–80.

29 Gül A, Aslantas AB, Tekinay T *et al.* Procoagulant mutations and venous thrombosis in Behçet's disease. *Rheumatology (Oxford)* 1999; **38**: 1298–9.

Histopathology. As discussed above, the type of reaction (vasculitic or not) and infiltrate (neutrophilic, lymphocytic or pauci-inflammatory) viewed as most characteristic of Behçet's disease is controversial. Even the predominant size of vessels involved (a frequently applied method to classify vasculitides) varies between authors, some classifying Behçet's disease as a primary vasculitis affecting predominantly large vessels (but may also involve small and medium vessels) [1], and others viewing it as predominantly a disease of small and medium-sized vessels [2].

It is probably best viewed as a systemic vasculitis that can affect any vessel size, any organ, and in which individual lesions may have vasculopathic/vasculitic or thrombogenic aetiology, with variable cellular infiltrate in both type and degree [3,4]. As a general rule, larger vessel involvement tends to be thrombotic or aneurysmal [3]. The mucosal and some skin lesions often have features of a neutrophilic vascular reaction rather than of frank vasculitis, although a leukocytoclastic vasculitis can occur [3–9]; later lesions are lymphocytic, and primary lymphocytic vasculitis occurs in erythema nodosum-like lesions (described below). Pustular lesions are sterile and, even though they may be inflammatory and appear to have clinical features of pustular vasculitis, histologically they may have a neutrophilic infiltrate and leukocytoclasis without vasculitis, resembling the lesions of Sweet's syndrome, bowel-associated dermatitis-arthritis syndrome or rheumatoid neutrophilic dermatosis. Erythema nodosum-like lesions usually contain at least focal lymphocytic or neutrophilic vasculitis, unlike erythema nodosum from other causes, and may have microabscesses, phlebitis or arteriolitis [10]. The tendency of erythema nodosum-like lesions to develop necrosis may reflect a component of thrombophlebitis, coexistence with small vessel vasculitis, or indicate that the panniculitis is occurring due to a medium-size vessel vasculitis; these lesions also tend to scar or heal with hyperpigmentation; neither ulceration, pigmentation nor scarring are typical of 'ordinary' erythema nodosum.

Using pathergy reactions, the initial inflammatory response consists of neutrophils, monocyte/macrophages and CD11c$^+$ dendritic cells followed by an exaggerated Th1 immune response [11].

A review of the pathological features of vasculitides described three main types of reaction in Behçet's disease [4], namely:

1 Vascular, including:
   (a) a lymphocytic or granulomatous vasculitis with or without thrombosis, necrosis and fibrinoid deposition
   (b) a pauci-cellular thrombogenic vasculopathy
   (c) a neutrophilic vascular reaction that may affect capillaries as well as arteries or veins of any size, and that includes a leukocytoclastic vasculitis and a Sweet's syndrome-like reaction

2 Extravascular with or without vasculopathy, including a mononuclear cell- or neutrophil-predominant inflammation of the dermis and/or panniculus, or a histiocytic panniculitis

3 A suppurative or mixed suppurative/granulomatous folliculitis comprising acneiform lesions

According to these authors [4], additional patterns include acral purpuric papulonodules characterized by a lymphocytic interface and perivascular reaction, and the oral or genital aphthae which have a central dense neutrophilic infiltrate with necrosis, but a dense lymphocytic infiltrate in the submucosa.

The acneiform lesions are debated; other authors have described pustules as non-follicular and representing a neutrophilic pustular vasculitis. Non-follicular papulopustular lesions are useful for diagnosis, as they usually have features of a leukocytoclastic vasculitis (sometimes a neutrophilic infiltrate without vasculitis, occasionally a lymphocytic vasculitis), often with positive direct immunofluorescence (especially IgM in vessels) [12].

References

1 Saleh A, Stone JA. Classification and diagnostic criteria in systemic vasculitis. *Clin Rheumatol* 2005; **19**: 209–21.

2 Carlson JA, Chen KR. Cutaneous vasculitis update: small vessel neutrophilic vasculitis syndromes. *Am J Dermatopathol* 2006; **28**: 486–506.

3 Melikoglu M, Kural-Seyahi E, Tascilar K, Yaziei I. The unique features of vasculitis in Behçet's syndrome. *Clin Rev Allerg Immunol* 2008; **35**: 40–6.

4 Crowson AN, Mihm MC, Magro CM. Cutaneous vasculitis: a review. *J Cutan Pathol* 2003; **30**: 161–73.

5 Jorizzo JL, Hudson RD, Schmalstieg FC *et al*. Behçet's syndrome: immune regulation, circulating immune complexes, neutrophil migration, and colchicine therapy. *J Am Acad Dermatol* 1984; **10**: 205–14.

6 Chajek T, Fainaru M. Behçet's disease: report of 41 cases and a review of the literature. *Medicine* 1975; **54**: 179–96.

7 Nazzaro P. Cutaneous manifestations of Behçet's disease. In: Monacelli M, Nazzaro P, eds. *International Symposium on Behçet's Disease in Rome*. Basel: Karger, 1966: 15–41.

8 Jorizzo JL, Solomon AR, Cavallo T. Behçet's syndrome: immunopathologic and histopathologic assessment of pathergy lesions is useful in diagnosis and follow-up. *Arch Pathol Lab Med* 1985; **109**: 747–51.

9 Muller W, Lehner T. Quantitative electron microscopical analysis of leukocyte infiltration in oral ulcers of Behçet's syndrome. *Br J Dermatol* 1982; **106**: 535–44.

10 Kim B, LeBoit PE. Histopathologic features of erythema nodosum-like lesions in Behçet disease: a comparison with erythema nodosum focusing on the role of vasculitis. *Am J Dermatopathol* 2000; **22**: 379–90.

11 Melikoglu M, Uysal S, Kreuger JG *et al*. Characterization of the divergent wound-healing responses occurring in the pathergy reaction and normal healthy volunteers. *J Immunol* 2006; **177**: 6415–21.

12 Alpsoy E, Uzun S, Akman A *et al*. Histological and immunofluorescence findings of non-follicular papulopustular lesions in patients with Behçet's disease. *J Eur Acad Dermatol Venereol* 2003; **17**: 521–4.

Clinical features. The clinical course of Behçet's disease is highly variable, although patients typically have oral aphthae with any combination of genital aphthae, cutaneous pustular vasculitis, ocular lesions or arthritis. The International Study Group criteria for the diagnosis of Behçet's disease [1] are depicted in Table 50.14. Two large series of 387 and 661 patients provide a basis for giving an approximate frequency of the various findings [2,3], although it should be noted that both were from areas with a high frequency of Behçet's disease, and some features may have a different incidence in other parts of the world.

Oral and genital lesions (Figs 50.33 & 50.34). Oral ulceration is a defining criterion for Behçet's disease, and therefore is present in 100%, but is not a very sensitive feature for diagnosis as it is common in the general population. Genital ulcers, present in about 90% of subjects [2,3], are possibly slightly more common in

Table 50.14 International Study Group criteria for the diagnosis of Behçet's disease [1] (applicable only in the absence of other explanations for the clinical findings).

Recurrent oral ulceration	Minor aphthous, major aphthous, or herpetiform ulceration observed by physician or patient that recurred at least 3 times in one 12-month period
Plus two of the following criteria:	
Recurrent genital ulceration	Aphthous ulceration or scarring observed by physician or patient
Eye lesions	Anterior uveitis, posterior uveitis, or cells in vitreous on slit-lamp examination; *or* retinal vasculitis observed by ophthalmologist
Skin lesions	Erythema nodosum observed by physician or patient, pseudofolliculitis or papulopustular lesions; *or* acneiform nodules observed by physician in post-adolescent patients not receiving corticosteroid treatment
Positive pathergy test	Read by physician at 24–48 h

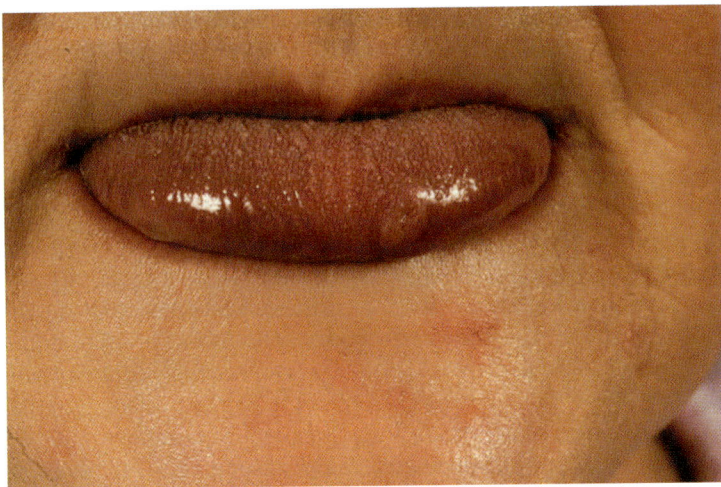

Fig. 50.33 Behçet's disease. This patient demonstrates oral aphthosis.

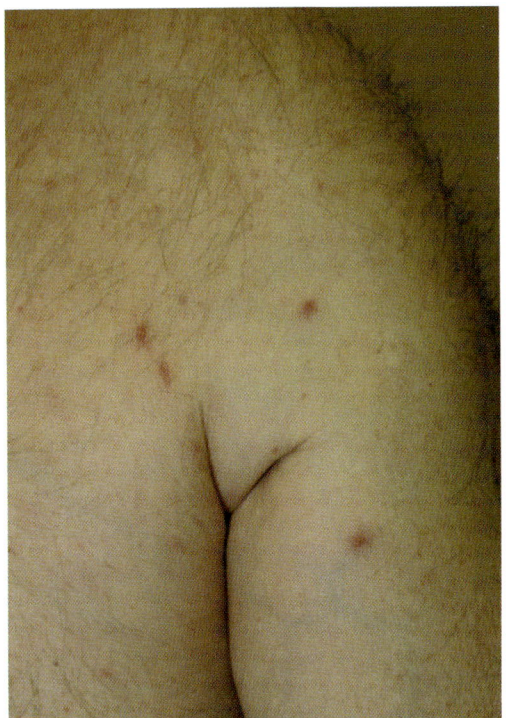

Fig. 50.35 Behçet's disease. Non-follicular pustules on the upper arm.

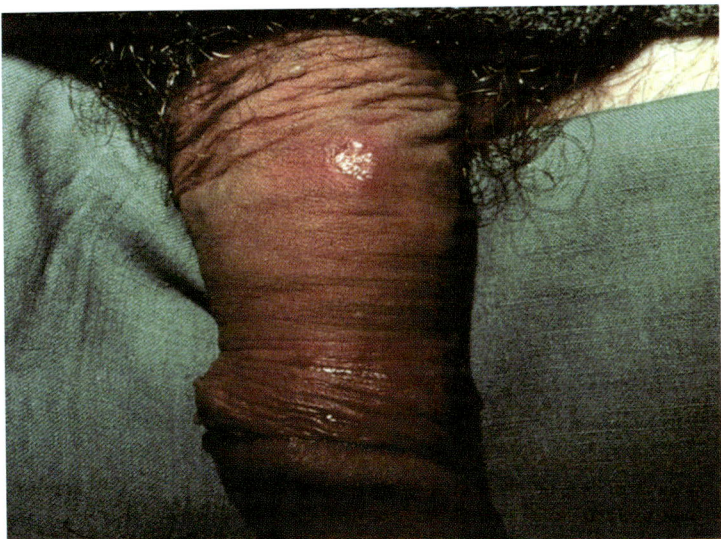

Fig. 50.34 Behçet's disease. An aphtha is present on the penis.

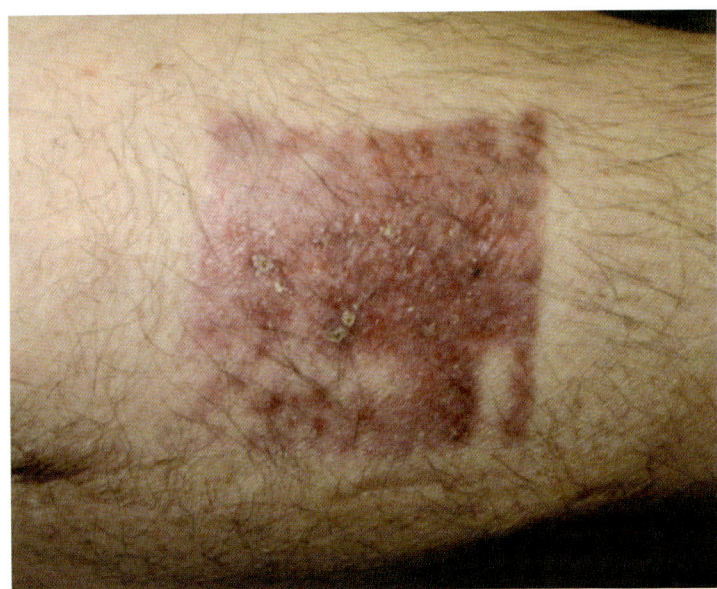

Fig. 50.36 Behçet's disease. An unusual manifestation—the patient had a skin graft site that had failed to heal after 9 months (pathergic pyoderma gangrenosum).

males than in females; they usually occur on the shaft of the penis or on the scrotum in males, and on the labia majora or minora in females. Residual scarring is common.

Skin lesions (Figs 50.35 & 50.36). Other than mucosal ulcers, skin lesions are the most common manifestation of Behçet's disease. Of the possible skin lesions, only pustular vasculitis (present in 55–83% of subjects, more often in males than in females [2,3]) and erythema nodosum-like nodules (44–62% of subjects, more common in females) should be used to satisfy diagnostic criteria when considering Behçet's disease. A wide range of additional cutaneous findings includes Sweet's syndrome-like and pyoderma gangrenosum-like lesions, abscesses, palpable purpura/leukocytoclastic vasculitis, acral purpuric papulonodules, and panniculitis [4–9].

Pathergy, the triggering of a significant inflammatory response by minor injuries such as venepuncture, is a feature of Behçet's disease that is sufficiently specific and frequent (occurring in about 40%, more often in males than females [3]) that it is considered to be a diagnostic criterion; however, it also occurs in several neutro-philic dermatoses, such as pyoderma gangrenosum. Several mechanisms may be involved, including HLA-B51-related hyper-reactivity of neutrophils. It typically develops within 48 h, either after specific provocation by needle-prick [6] or following vene-puncture or other venous access, and may evolve to form larger lesions inseparable from pyoderma gangrenosum [10].

Other organ systems. Uveitis (usually posterior or pan-uveitis) is the main ocular feature of Behçet's disease, occurring in about 30–45% of subjects, rather more common in males than in females.

The posterior uveitis observed in Behçet's disease is a consequence of retinal vasculitis and may result in blindness, a feared complication of Behçet's disease. Hypopyon uveitis is associated with severe retinal vasculitis and is very suggestive of Behçet's disease, although it is rare [6]. Episcleritis may occur but is not very specific.

Vascular involvement in Behçet's disease may affect arteries and veins, leading to aneurysms or occlusions that are sometimes fatal [6,11,12]. The frequency of vascular disease rises from about 30% at initial presentation, to approaching 50% during the course of the disease, and is most common in males. Venous thromboses are most frequent (seven times more common than arterial occlusion [13]), especially lower limb deep vein thrombosis or superficial thrombophlebitis of extremities. Patients with thrombophlebitis are at greater risk of developing deep venous thrombosis. Other sites of venous thrombosis include the vena cava, hepatic veins (Budd–Chiari syndrome), and cerebral venous sinuses. Arterial lesions include inflammatory stenoses, thrombosis, and, especially, true or false aneurysms of the abdominal aorta, pulmonary or peripheral arteries (with a strong male predominance), in contrast with large vessel vasculitides which tend to affect the aortic arch, renal or mesenteric vessels [6]. Vascular complications should always be borne in mind in patients with known Behçet's disease, particularly pulmonary artery aneurysm as a cause of haemoptysis (the presence of haemoptysis and deep-vein thrombosis may erroneously suggest pulmonary embolism, which is relatively uncommon in Behçet's disease); pulmonary artery aneurysm may occur in isolation (described as the Hughes–Stovin syndrome, but probably part of the spectrum of Behçet's disease). Vessels may show an arteritis, particularly of the vasa vasora, but the aneurysms and thrombosis are not necessarily a consequence of vasculitis, and therefore may not respond to medical therapies for vasculitis. Endovascular control of bleeding aneurysms has been described [13].

Many neurological manifestations may be present in patients with Behçet's disease, including parenchymal and dural sinus thromboses and meningoencephalitis [6,14], but only occur in about 3% of patients. A particular problem of this 'neuro-Behçet's disease' is distinguishing it from central nervous system involvement in Sweet's syndrome (neuro-Sweet's syndrome). Peripheral neuropathies are rare, although brainstem or spinal cord involvement may occur. An asymmetrical, migratory, non-erosive oligoarthritis that may mimic rheumatoid arthritis occurs in 30–40% [3,4,6,15]. Gastrointestinal involvement is uncommon; when it occurs, it consists of mucosal ulceration, especially in the terminal ileum or colon, mimicking inflammatory bowel disease. In contrast with Crohn's disease, which is the most frequent differential diagnosis, anal lesions are rare, and inflammatory markers such as CRP are usually modestly elevated in comparison with active Crohn's disease. Renal involvement is rare, a useful distinction from many vasculitides.

Diagnosis. The diagnosis of Behçet's disease should be suspected in any patient with recurrent and extensive oral aphthosis. However, in these persons, other causes of aphthosis such as inflammatory bowel disease, as well as lesions that mimic aphthae such as herpes simplex infection, must be excluded before a diagnosis of Behçet's disease can be made. Papulopustular lesions, especially outside the normal body site distribution for acne, and with a neutrophilic vascular reaction histologically, suggest Behçet's disease, as do erythema nodosum-like lesions with ulceration, scarring, residual pigmentation or a medium-size vessel vasculitis histologically. The diagnosis should be considered in young patients with deep-vein thrombosis, especially in males or in the absence of other risk factors or thrombophilia. Anterior chamber uveitis with severe retinal vasculitis is not a feature of other vasculitides [6] and therefore suggests a diagnosis of Behçet's disease; similarly, dural sinus thrombosis, aortic or peripheral arterial aneurysms in a young male, or aneurysm(s) of the pulmonary artery or its main branches, strongly suggest this diagnosis. A clinical picture suggesting a medium or large vessel vasculitis, but lacking supporting features such as renal or mesenteric involvement, a positive ANCA, peripheral neuropathy or granulomatous histology, suggests the possibility of Behçet's disease. A positive pathergy provocation test may further support the diagnosis. Ophthalmology, neurology and rheumatology consultations may be beneficial when evaluating a patient with suspected Behçet's disease.

Some patients are encountered in whom recurrent, severe aphthous ulceration dominates the clinical picture; although not fulfilling diagnostic criteria for Behçet's disease they may represent a *forme fruste* of the disorder [16]. Along similar lines, clinical experience also reveals some individuals with severe, non-infective genital ulceration, either in isolation or sometimes with a neutrophilic dermatosis or other features of Behçet's disease, but who deny oral ulceration, and in whom classification is difficult as they appear to have Behçet's disease but in the absence of the main disease-defining criterion. In general, the diagnostic criteria are most reliable in areas of higher prevalence.

References

1 International Study Group for Behçet's disease. Criteria for diagnosis of Behçet's disease. *Lancet* 1990; **335**: 1078–80.
2 Kural-Seyahi E, Fresko I, Seyahi N *et al*. The long-term mortality and morbidity of Behçet syndrome: a 2-decade outcome survey of 387 patients followed at a dedicated center. *Medicine (Baltimore)* 2003; **82**: 60–76.
3 Alpsoy E, Donmez L, Onder M *et al*. Clinical features and natural course of Behçet's disease in 661 cases: a multicentre study. *Br J Dermatol* 2007; **157**: 901–6.
4 Jorizzo JL. Behçet's disease: an update based on the 1985 international conference in London. *Arch Dermatol* 1986; **122**: 556–8.
5 Nazarro P. Cutaneous manifestations of Behçet's disease. In: Monacelli M, Nazzaro P, eds. *International Symposium on Behçet's Disease in Rome*. Basel: Karger, 1966: 15–41.
6 Melikoglu M, Kural-Seyahi E, Tascilar K, Yaziei I. The unique features of vasculitis in Behçet's syndrome. *Clin Rev Allerg Immunol* 2008; **35**: 40–6.
7 Callen JP. Pustular eruptions in systemic disease. *Clin Dermatol* 2000; **18**: 349–53.
8 Jorizzo JL, Solomon AR, Zanolli MD, Leshin B. Neutrophilic vascular reactions. *J Am Acad Dermatol* 1988; **19**: 983–1005.
9 Crowson AN, Mihm MC, Magro CM. Cutaneous vasculitis: a review. *J Cutan Pathol* 2003; **30**: 161–73.
10 Munro CS, Cox NH. Pyoderma gangrenosum associated with Behçet's syndrome—response to thalidomide. *Clin Exp Dermatol* 1988; **13**: 408–10.
11 Shimizu T, Ehrlich GE, Goro I *et al*. Behçet's disease. *Semin Arthritis Rheum* 1979; **8**: 223–60.
12 Shimizu T. Vascular lesions in Behçet's disease. *Cardioangiology* 1977; **1**: 124–9.
13 Cantasdemir M, Kantarci F, Adaletli I *et al*. Emergency intravascular management of pulmonary artery aneurysms in Behçet's disease: report of 2 cases and review of the literature. *Cardiovasc Intervent Radiol* 2002; **25**: 533–7.

Table 50.15 Medical treatments for Behçet's disease.

Palliative treatment of aphthae
Topical corticosteroids/corticosteroid mouthwash
Intralesional corticosteroids
Topical sucralfate
Topical tacrolimus
Nicotine patches
Topical viscous lidocaine (lignocaine)
Topical granulocyte colony-stimulating factor

Mucocutaneous manifestations
Colchicine
Dapsone
Dapsone and colchicine

Systemic involvement
Systemic corticosteroids
Immunosuppressants, cytokines and related agents for most severe disease

- Azathioprine
- Methotrexate
- Ciclosporin
- Cyclophosphamide
- Chlorambucil
- Thalidomide
- Interferon-α
- Anti-TNF agents (infliximab, etanercept)

14 O'Duffy JD, Goldstein NP. Neurologic involvement in seven patients with Behçet's disease. *Am J Med* 1976; **61**: 171–8.
15 Yurkakul S, Yuzici H, Tuzun Y *et al*. The arthritis of Behçet's disease: a prospective study. *Ann Rheum Dis* 1983; **42**: 505–15.
16 Jorizzo JL, Taylor RS, Schmalstieg FC *et al*. Complex aphthosis: a forme fruste of Behçet's syndrome? *J Am Acad Dermatol* 1985; **13**: 80–4.

Treatment (Table 50.15). Oral or genital ulcers may be treated symptomatically with topical or intralesional corticosteroids, topical sucralfate gel, topical tacrolimus and/or viscous lidocaine (lignocaine) applied to individual lesions [1,2]. Nicotine patches applied to oral aphthae have been reported to have rapid benefit [3]. Topical application of granulocyte colony-stimulating factor has been demonstrated to be effective but is expensive [4]. Betamethasone used as a mouthwash is a practical treatment if there are several ulcers. Rebamipide (a mucosal protective agent used in some countries) may also be useful for oral aphthae [5]. Colchicine (0.6 mg two to three times daily) may also be used to treat mucocutaneous manifestations, including aphthae, papulopustules and erythema nodosum-like lesions, although this treatment option is limited by gastrointestinal intolerance and requires monitoring for neutropenia [6–8]. Dapsone alone has demonstrated efficacy in treating Behçet's disease [9], and anecdotally has been effective in combination with colchicine.

Behçet's disease that has manifestations other than mucocutaneous involvement may be treated with systemic corticosteroids, although such treatment may not control severe ocular, neurological or non-vasculitic vascular disease [10–14]. Immunosuppressive agents such as azathioprine, methotrexate or ciclosporin may be used in the treatment of patients with severe Behçet's disease [10,15]. There is a potential concern that ciclosporin can cause neurotoxicity that appears very similar to neuro-Behçet's disease

(some feel that it actually provokes neuro-Behçet's disease), so, although useful for treating uveitis, a degree of caution is warranted. Cytokines such as interferon-α are useful (alone or with azathioprine) [5,16], and thalidomide can be effective [1,17] but requires careful monitoring for neurological toxicity. Anecdotal reports suggest use of intravenous immunoglobulin (IVIG) with aspirin, and granulocyte and monocyte adsorption apheresis.

Increasingly, anti-TNF agents such as infliximab or etanercept have been documented to be effective [5,16], especially for uveitis or for severe oral aphthae (although dapsone is a more effective inhibitor of the pathergic response than is etanercept). Novel treatments under investigation for Behçet's disease include induction of tolerance using oral administration of the 336–351 sequence of HSP60 linked to recombinant cholera B-toxin B-subunit [16]. Surgical treatments for large-vessel disease are outside the remit of dermatologists but are summarized in [18].

There is an increasing case for early and aggressive treatment of Behçet's disease, especially in those with, or at risk of, severe symptoms. The highest risk of serious ocular, pulmonary artery or neurological involvement is in males, especially those with disease onset below age 40 years [19]. In general, the risk of complications gradually decreases with increasing age.

References

1 Ghate JV, Jorizzo JL. Behçet's disease and complex aphthosis. *J Am Acad Dermatol* 1999; **40**: 1–18.
2 Alpsoy E, Er H, Durusoy C, Yilmaz E. The use of sucralfate suspension in the treatment of oral and genital ulceration of Behçet disease. *Arch Dermatol* 1999; **135**: 529–32.
3 Scheid P, Bohadana A, Martinet Y. Nicotine patches for aphthous ulcers due to Behçet's syndrome. *N Engl J Med* 2000; **343**: 1816–7.
4 Bacanli A, Yerebakan Dicle O, Parmaksizoglu B *et al*. Topical granulocyte colony-stimulating factor for the treatment of oral and genital ulcers of patients with Behçet's disease. *J Eur Acad Dermatol Venereol* 2006; **20**: 931–5.
5 Yurdakul S, Hamuryudan V, Yazici H. Behçet's disease. *Curr Opin Rheumatol* 2003; **16**: 38–42.
6 Jorizzo JL, Hudson RD, Schmalstieg FC *et al*. Behçet's syndrome: immune regulation, circulating immune complexes, neutrophil migration, and colchicine therapy. *J Am Acad Dermatol* 1984; **10**: 205–14.
7 Mizushima Y, Matsumura N, Mori M. Chemotaxis of leukocytes and colchicine treatment in Behçet's disease. *J Rheumatol* 1979; **6**: 108–10.
8 Miyachi Y, Taniguchi S, Ozaki M, Horio T. Colchicine in the treatment of the cutaneous manifestations of Behçet's disease. *Br J Dermatol* 1981; **104**: 67–9.
9 Sharquie KE, Najim RA, Abu-Raghif AR. Dapsone in Behçet's disease: a double-blind, placebo-controlled, cross-over study. *J Dermatol* 2002; **29**: 267–79.
10 Jorizzo JL. Behçet's disease: an update based on the 1985 international conference in London. *Arch Dermatol* 1986; **122**: 556–8.
11 O'Duffy JD, Carney JA, Deodhar S. Behçet's disease: report of 10 cases, three with new manifestation. *Ann Intern Med* 1971; **75**: 561–70.
12 Chajek T, Fainaru M. Behçet's disease: report of 41 cases and a review of the literature. *Medicine* 1975; **54**: 179–96.
13 Chamberlain MA. Behçet's syndrome in 32 patients in Yorkshire. *Ann Rheum Dis* 1977; **36**: 491–9.
14 Oshima Y, Shimuzu T, Yokohari R *et al*. Clinical studies on Behçet's syndrome. *Ann Rheum Dis* 1963; **22**: 36–45.
15 Wong VG. Immunosuppressive therapy of ocular inflammatory disease. *Arch Ophthalmol* 1969; **81**: 628–37.
16 Pipitone N, Olivien I, Cantini F *et al*. New approaches in the treatment of Adamantiades-Behçet's disease. *Curr Opin Rheumatol* 2006; **18**: 3–9.
17 Munro CS, Cox NH. Pyoderma gangrenosum associated with Behçet's syndrome—response to thalidomide. *Clin Exp Dermatol* 1988; **13**: 408–10.
18 Calamia KT, Schirmer M, Melikoglu M. Major vessel involvement in Behçet disease. *Curr Opin Rheumatol* 2004; **17**: 1–8.

19 Alpsoy E, Donmez L, Onder M *et al*. Clinical features and natural course of Behçet's disease in 661 cases: a multicentre study. *Br J Dermatol* 2007; **157**: 901–6.

Neutrophilic dermatoses

Introduction

The spectrum of disorders currently considered as 'neutrophilic dermatoses' has widened hugely over the last two decades [1–6]. The common features in most of these entities can be summarized as follows:

1 the histological features are dominated by a neutrophilic vascular reaction that typically (although variably) falls short of vasculitis

2 within any diagnostic entity a significant proportion of cases can be demonstrated to have a reactive cause or systemic association (mainly haematological or gastrointestinal diseases, or drug-induced aetiology)

3 many of these disorders may coexist or occur in sequence in an affected individual, and

4 the neutrophilic process itself may in some cases cause systemic disease.

Epidermal neutrophilic dermatoses are not discussed here, other than where they are part of a disease overlap spectrum or where they share a common aetiology with neutrophilic dermatoses affecting the dermis or subcutaneous fat.

The following sections define and discuss the history, aetiology, pathogenesis, histopathology, clinical features, diagnosis and treatment of the major neutrophilic dermatoses, as well as briefly addressing histopathological overlaps, internal (systemic) neutrophilic dermatoses, and identifying areas of controversy. The conditions discussed are characterized by a neutrophilic infiltrate and blood vessel damage, probably as a result of immune complex deposition as well as involving neutrophil-induced injury. Increasingly, different types of infiltrate (lymphocytic, or early myeloid cells), and the presence of at least some features of vasculitis, are being accepted within the spectrum of neutrophilic dermatoses, although in some instances these variations may be secondary and reflect the timing of obtaining histopathology specimens. Some mechanisms of involvement of neutrophils in this group of dermatoses, and of their chemoattraction to tissues, have been discussed in [7–10].

References

1 Jorizzo J, Solomon AR, Zanolli MD, Leshin B. Neutrophilic vascular reactions. *J Am Acad Dermatol* 1988; **19**: 983–1005.

2 de Moragos JM, Pujol RM. Neutrophilic dermatoses. *Curr Opin Dermatol* 1997; **4**: 13–20.

3 Huang W, McNeely MC. Neutrophilic tissue reactions. *Adv Dermatol* 1998; **13**: 33–63.

4 Wallach D. Neutrophilic dermatoses: an overview. *Clin Dermatol* 2000; **18**: 229–31.

5 Callen JP. Neutrophilic dermatoses. *Dermatol Clin* 2002; **20**: 409–19.

6 Wallach D, Vignon-Pennamen M-D. From acute febrile neutrophilic dermatosis to neutrophilic disease: forty years of clinical research. *J Am Acad Dermatol* 2006; **55**: 1066–71.

7 von den Driesch P. Polymorphonuclears: structure, function, and mechanisms of involvement in skin diseases. *Clin Dermatol* 2000; **18**: 233–44.

8 Schröder J-M. Chemoattractants as mediators of neutrophilic tissue recruitment. *Clin Dermatol* 2000; **18**: 245–63.

9 Kluger MS. Vascular endothelial cell adhesion and signaling during leukocyte recruitment. *Adv Dermatol* 2004; **20**: 163–94.

10 Schaerli P, Britschgi M, Keller M *et al*. Characterization of human T cells that regulate neutrophilic skin inflammation. *J Immunol* 2004; **173**: 2151–8.

Classification

A suggested classification of neutrophilic dermatoses is shown in Table 50.16. It should be noted that frank vasculitides, neutrophilic vascular reactions secondary to primary microvascular occlusion (Chapter 49), and infective causes of neutrophilic vasculopathy are not normally included in such classifications.

We have not included, or have listed but will not discuss, additional disorders in which the neutrophilic infiltrate is primarily epidermal such as *subcorneal pustular dermatosis, pustular psoriasis, Reiter's syndrome, intraepidermal neutrophilic IgA dermatosis, infantile acropustulosis* and *drug-induced pustular eruptions*, although one might also term these neutrophilic in type of infiltrate. Some authors have also suggested the inclusion of *Rosai–Dorfman disease with neutrophilic predominance* and of *congenital erosive and vesicular dermatosis with reticulated supple scarring*, based on histopathological similarity, but these conditions do not share the disease associations or behaviour of more accepted dermal neutrophilic dermatoses. All of these are discussed in other chapters.

There remain some areas of overlap or uncertainty. Some disorders, notably *Behçet's disease*, have features of vasculitis, pustular vasculitis and thrombosis, and therefore exhibit overlap between neutrophilic dermatosis and vasculitis, as discussed earlier (p. 50.56). *Erythema elevatum diutinum* (EED) is variably classified as a vasculitis or as a neutrophilic dermatosis; we have elected to discuss it as a vasculitis (p. 50.25). *Neutrophilic eccrine hidradenitis* (NEH) appears to have different aetiologies (physical/cold in children, often related to cytotoxic or other drugs and/or haematological malignancies in adults) and is neutrophilic but not primarily vascular; it is also discussed in Chapter 44. *Subcorneal pustular dermatosis* is not a vascular reaction but does share aetiological factors (notably monoclonal gammopathy) with disorders such as pyoderma gangrenosum and EED, and may coexist with them (especially in patients with myelodysplastic disorders), so is included in the classification but is discussed in Chapter 40. Some histological issues that influence classification (e.g. early lymphocytic rather than neutrophilic infiltrates) are discussed in relation to specific conditions below.

Neutrophilic sebaceous adenitis [1,2] is very rare, and how to classify it is unclear. Clinically it presents as annular plaques and papules, spreading from the face to the body and having some resemblance to Sweet's syndrome; histologically it is characterized by a sterile, neutrophilic and sometimes suppurative infiltrate around sebaceous lobules (although cases with a myelomonocytic [3] or granulomatous infiltrate are also reported [2]). It usually has a short, self-limiting course or responds to topical corticosteroids. An autoimmune aetiology has been proposed but it is tempting to suggest that this could be a sebaceous equivalent of neutrophilic eccrine hidradenitis (NEH), as the distribution, morphology, duration and neutrophilic infiltrate, in the presence of necrotic sebocytes without infection, would parallel several aspects of NEH. We have therefore very tentatively suggested that it may belong

Table 50.16 Neutrophilic dermatoses: an aetiological classification.

'Classical' neutrophilic dermatoses
- Pyoderma gangrenosum (various subtypes)
- Sweet's syndrome/acute febrile neutrophilic dermatosis (and possible variants: neutrophilic dermatosis of the dorsal hands; chronic recurrent [annular] neutrophilic dermatosis)

Overlap with vasculitis
- Behçet's disease
- Erythema elevatum diutinum

Specific link with gastrointestinal disease*
- Neutrophilic vascular reaction in bowel-associated dermatosis arthritis syndrome (BADAS)
- Pustular vasculitis/neutrophilic pustulosis (many cases represent pustular pyoderma gangrenosum)
- Aseptic abscesses in Crohn's disease
- Pyodermatitis–pyostomatitis vegetans (?)
- Peristomal pyoderma gangrenosum

Associated with acne or pustulosis†
- Synovitis, acne, pustulosis, hyperostosis, osteomyelitis (SAPHO)
- Pyogenic arthritis, pyoderma gangrenosum, acne (PAPA)

Associated with connective tissue disease or immune complex disease
- Rheumatoid neutrophilic dermatitis/dermatosis
- Palisaded neutrophilic and granulomatous dermatitis
- Relapsing polychondritis
- Sweet's syndrome-like, erythema gyratum repens-like, and figurate neutrophilic infiltrate, in systemic lupus erythematosus

Paraneoplastic or typically chemotherapy-associated
- Paraneoplastic neutrophilic figurate erythema
- Neutrophilic eccrine hidradenitis

Systemic neutrophilic dermatoses
- Neuro-Sweet's syndrome
- Other internal sites: myositis, pulmonary, pericarditis, osteitis (deep to pyoderma gangrenosum, or distant), lymph nodes, other sites of aseptic neutrophilic abscesses (often splenic or visceral), etc.

Other extra-cutaneous neutrophilic disease
- Peripheral ulcerative keratitis
- Neutrophilic panniculitis

Autoinflammatory diseases‡
- Familial Mediterranean fever
- Hyper-IgD syndrome

Non-vessel centred and miscellaneous
- Subcorneal pustular dermatosis (Sneddon–Wilkinson disease)
- Intraepidermal neutrophilic IgA dermatosis
- Neutrophilic urticaria
- Neutrophilic spongiosis?
- Neutrophilic sebaceous adenitis?

---

* Many of the neutrophilic dermatoses have a strong association with gastrointestinal disease, but this link is especially strong in the disorders listed.
† Pustules are also a feature in many of the other patterns listed, such as Behçet's disease, Sweet's syndrome, BADAS and others.
‡ Autoinflammatory diseases are increasingly classified on the basis of genetic findings, but Sweet's syndrome-like lesions and aseptic pustules, with leukocytosis, are often described.

in the neutrophilic dermatosis spectrum. *Neutrophilic spongiosis*, a disorder of uncertain classification, is discussed in the section on neutrophilic pustular disorders.

Aseptic and TORCH-screen negative pustular eruptions in children, with some features reminiscent of Sweet's syndrome, should be viewed with some suspicion. Paediatric Sweet's syndrome and PG may both occur, but a perforating neutrophilic and granulomatous dermatitis of the newborn was described in two children with immunodeficiency [4], and children with Down's syndrome are prone to transient myeloproliferative disorders, leukaemoid reactions and leukaemia cutis; the lesions may contain immature blast-like immature haemopoietic cells and, like neutrophilic dermatoses, may exhibit pathergy [5,6].

Lupus erythematosus has also been linked with Sweet's syndrome or other neutrophilic dermatoses; earlier reports were those in which hydralazine was implicated [7], but there are other reports where this was not the case [8] and there are increasing reports of neutrophilic dermatoses as the presenting feature of lupus erythematosus [9,10]. Sweet's syndrome, PG (8 years before lupus erythematosus [11]), and figurate and erythema gyratum repens-like patterns [12] of neutrophilic dermatosis have all been reported, as well as other potentially related conditions such as neutrophilic urticaria/urticarial erythema with neutrophilic infiltration [13,14], neutrophilic eccrine hidradenitis (after cyclophosphamide treatment [15]) and palisaded neutrophilic and granulomatous dermatitis. It has been recommended that lupus erythematosus should be considered in the differential diagnosis of neutrophilic dermatoses [10].

References

1 Renfro L, Kopf AW, Gutterman A *et al.* Neutrophilic sebaceous adenitis. *Arch Dermatol* 1993; **129**: 910–1.
2 Newman J, Jacobsom M, Sicari M, Hayman R. Neutrophilic sebaceous adenitis: a report of two cases. *J Clin Pathol* 2007; **34**: 78 [Abstract].
3 Martins C, Tellechea O, Mariano A, Baptista AP. Sebaceous adenitis. *J Am Acad Dermatol* 1997; **36**: 845–6.
4 Torrelo A, Vera A, Portugués M *et al.* Perforating neutrophilic and granulomatous dermatitis of the newborn—a clue to immunodeficiency. *Pediatr Dermatol* 2007; **24**: 211–5.
5 Burch JM, Weston WL, Rogers M, Morelli JG. Cutaneous pustular leukaemoid reactions in trisomy 21. *Pediatr Dermatol* 2003; **20**: 232–7.
6 Nijhawan A, Baselga E, Gonzalez-Ensenat A *et al.* Vesicopustular eruptions in Down syndrome neonates with myeloproliferative disorders. *Arch Dermatol* 2001; **137**: 760–3.
7 Ramsay-Goldman R, Franz T, Solano FX, Medsger TA Jr. Hydralazine induced lupus and Sweet's syndrome. Report and review of the literature. *J Rheumatol* 1990; **17**: 682–4.
8 Goette DK. Sweet's syndrome in subacute cutaneous lupus erythematosus. *Arch Dermatol* 1985; **121**: 789–91.
9 Hou TY, Chang DM, Gao HW *et al.* Sweet's syndrome as an initial presentation in systemic lupus erythematosus: a case report and review of the literature. *Lupus* 2005; **14**: 399–402.
10 Gleason BC, Zembowicz A, Granter SR. Non-bullous neutrophilic dermatosis: an uncommon dermatologic manifestation in patients with lupus erythematosus. *J Cutan Pathol* 2006; **33**: 721–5.
11 Waldman MA, Callen JP. Pyoderma gangrenosum preceding the diagnosis of systemic lupus erythematosus. *Dermatology (Basel)* 2005; **210**: 64–7.
12 Khan DB, Andrassy K, Hartschuh W. Neutrophilic dermatosis with an erythema gyratum repens-like pattern in systemic lupus erythematosus. *Acta Derm Venereol* 2005; **85**: 455–6.
13 Kawana S, Nishioka K, Nishiyama S. Urticarial erythema with neutrophilic infiltration—correlation of cutaneous vascular changes with clinical severity. *Nippon Hifuka Gakkai Zasshi* 1991; **101**: 951–7.

14 Davis MD, Daoud MS, Kirby B *et al*. Clinicopathologic correlation of hypocomplementemic and normocomplementemic urticarial vasculitis. *J Am Acad Dermatol* 1998; **38**: 899–905.

15 Lienesch DW, Mutasin DF, Singh RR. Neutrophilic eccrine hidradenitis mimicking cutaneous vasculitis in a lupus patient: a complication of cyclophosphamide. *Lupus* 2003; **12**: 707–9.

Pyoderma gangrenosum

Definition. Pyoderma gangrenosum (PG) is a rare, non-infectious neutrophilic dermatosis commonly associated with underlying systemic disease. Diagnosis is based on typical clinical features and exclusion of other cutaneous ulcerating diseases, as described in several reviews [1–10].

History and nomenclature. Brocq first described PG in 1916 [11]. It was later described in 1930 by Brunsting *et al*. [12]. The prevalence of PG in inflammatory bowel disease (IBD) was discussed by Greenstein *et al*. in 1976 [13]. Several clinical variants of PG have been described (Table 50.17), diagnostic criteria have been published [3], and PG at unusual sites or with specific triggers, such as pathergy, have also been reviewed [4]. The significance of the different variants described is unclear. There is some evidence that the pustular type may be mainly associated with IBD, the bullous type with haematological malignancies, and that the vegetative type is usually not associated with underlying disease [2,3]. Others describe lesions on the hands, arms and face as being associated with haematological diseases (and thus potentially overlapping with Sweet's syndrome, and with neutrophilic dermatosis of the dorsal hands) [8]. The peristomal pattern, unsurprisingly, is mainly but not exclusively associated with IBD. However, different morphologies may coexist with each other or with other neutrophilic dermatoses or pustular vasculitis [14] (although the vegetative pattern of PG is usually not accompanied by other lesions), or may evolve from one form to another [15], and none of the morphologies is consistently or exclusively associated with any specific cause; such classifications are, however, convenient for discussion and for initiation of the potentially most rewarding investigations. The different patterns are discussed in more detail below. As a guide, about 50–70% of patients will have an underlying disease, approximately equally divided between IBD, arthritides and haematological causes; conversely, about 2% of patients with IBD will develop PG.

Table 50.17 The main variants of pyoderma gangrenosum in selected reviews.

Authors (reference)	Main variants
Powell *et al*. [2,3]	Ulcerative
Wollina [9]	Pustular
De Moragas & Pujol [16]	Bullous
	Vegetative (= superficial granulomatous pyoderma)
Callen [4]	Typical (classical)
	Atypical (more superficial)
	Pustular eruption of ulcerative colitis
	Peristomal
	Vulvar
	Pyostomatitis vegetans
	Malignant pyoderma
	Bullous
Ahmadi & Powell [6]	*Main classification*:
	Ulcerative
	Pustular
	Bullous
	Vegetative
	Unusual presentations:
	Pathergic
	Peristomal
	Dorsal hand
	Head and neck (malignant pyoderma)
	Multisystem
	Paraneoplastic
Callen & Jackson [8,10]	Classic (usually on the legs)
	Atypical (hands, arms, face)
	Peristomal
	Other sites not specifically viewed as distinct (vulva, penis and oropharynx [pyostomatitis vegetans])
Present text (an arbitrary division according to morphology and/or site, where these factors influence diagnostic aspects, likely disease associations or therapy)	Classic/ulcerative
	Atypical forms:
	Pustular
	Bullous
	Upper limbs/trunk
	Superficial (vegetative)
	Peristomal
	Other specific sites that influence diagnostic aspects, disease associations or therapy (face/scalp, breast, genital, mucosal, etc)
	Pyostomatitis vegetans (?)
	Neutrophilic dermatosis of dorsal hands (? Sweet's syndrome or pyoderma gangrenosum)

References

1 Callen JP. Pyoderma gangrenosum and related disorders. *Dermatol Clin* 1990; **7**: 1249–59.

2 Powell FC, Su WPD. Pyoderma gangrenosum: classification and management. *J Am Acad Dermatol* 1996; **34**: 395–409.

3 Powell FC, Collins C. Pyoderma gangrenosum. *Clin Dermatol* 2000; **18**: 283–93.

4 Callen JP. Neutrophilic dermatoses. *Dermatol Clin* 2002; **20**: 409–19.

5 Su WPD, Davis MD, Weenig RH *et al*. Pyoderma gangrenosum: clinicopathologic correlation and proposed diagnostic criteria. *Int J Dermatol* 2004; **43**: 790–800.

6 Ahmadi S, Powell FC. Pyoderma gangrenosum: uncommon presentations. *Clin Dermatol* 2005; **23**: 612–20.

7 Provost TT, Harris ML. Pyoderma gangrenosum. In: Provost TT, Flynn JA, eds. *Cutaneous Medicine: Cutaneous Manifestations of Systemic Disease*. Hamilton, Ontario: Decker, 2001: 464–72.

8 Jackson JM, Callen JP. Pyoderma gangrenosum: an expert commentary. *Expert Rev Dermatol* 2006; **1**: 391–400.

9 Wollina U. Pyoderma gangrenosum—a review. *Orphanet J Rare Dis* 2007; **2**: 19.

10 Callen JP, Jackson JM. Pyoderma gangrenosum: an update. *Rheum Dis Clin N Am* 2007; **33**: 787–802.

11 Brocq L. Nouvelle contribution à l'étude du phagedeniome geometrique. *Ann Dermatol Syphiligr (Paris)* 1916; **6**: 1–39.

12 Brunsting LA, Goeckerman WH, O'Leary PA. Pyoderma gangrenosum: clinical and experimental observations in five cases occurring in adults. *Arch Dermatol* 1930; **22**: 655–80.

13 Greenstein AJ, Janowitz HD, Sachar DB. The extra-intestinal complications of Crohn's disease and ulcerative colitis: a study of 700 patients. *Medicine (Baltimore)* 1976; **55**: 401–12.

Table 50.18 Diseases associated with pyoderma gangrenosum.

Category	Examples*
Gastrointestinal	Ulcerative colitis, Crohn's disease, collagenous colitis, gastritis, gastroduodenal ulcers, intestinal polyps
Arthritides	Rheumatoid arthritis, seronegative arthritis (sometimes with IBD), osteoarthritis
Haematological	Leukaemias (especially myelogenous, hairy cell), myelofibrosis, myelodysplastic syndromes/polycythaemia vera, paraproteinaemia including (usually IgA) monoclonal gammopathy, Waldenström's macroglobulinaemia, paroxysmal nocturnal haemoglobinuria, splenomegaly, T-cell lymphomas (less commonly)
Hepatic	Chronic active hepatitis, primary biliary cirrhosis, sclerosing cholangitis
Other vasculitides, collagen vascular and related disorders	Wegener's granulomatosis, Takayasu's arteritis, Behçet's disease, systemic lupus erythematosus, systemic sclerosis
Acne and related disorders	Acne conglobata, acne fulminans, hidradenitis suppurativa, PAPA (recurrent familial arthritis)
Other dermatoses	Many other neutrophilic dermatoses, relapsing polychondritis, pustular vasculitis (this chapter) Psoriasis
Autoimmune	Thyroid disease, diabetes mellitus
Drugs	Colony-stimulating factors† (several), gefinib (epidermal growth factor receptor inhibitor), interferon†, propylthiouracil, isotretinoin, several others (with apparently unrelated structures/activities)
Solid organ tumours	Colon, pancreas, breast, bronchus, carcinoid
Miscellaneous	Sarcoidosis Infections, including HIV, hepatitis C Chronic lung disease Immunological: congenital hypergammaglobulinaemia, autoimmune neutropenia in infancy, immunosuppression, complement deficiencies (C2, C4, C7 deficiency all described) Familial

PAPA: pyogenic arthritis, pyoderma gangrenosum, acne.

* It is not certain that all conditions listed represent true or causal associations.

† Have also been used therapeutically.

14 Wilson DM, John GR, Callen JP. Peripheral ulcerative keratitis—an extracutaneous neutrophilic disorder: report of a patient with rheumatoid arthritis, pustular vasculitis, pyoderma gangrenosum, and Sweet's syndrome with an excellent response to cyclosporine therapy. *J Am Acad Dermatol* 1999; **40**: 331–4.

15 Marzano AV, Tourlaki A, Alessi E, Caputo R. Widespread idiopathic pyoderma gangrenosum evolved from ulcerative to vegetative type: a 10-year history with a recent response to infliximab. *Clin Exp Dermatol* 2007; **33**: 156–9.

16 de Moragos JM, Pujol RM. Neutrophilic dermatoses. *Curr Opin Dermatol* 1997; **4**: 13–20.

Aetiology and pathogenesis. Although the pathogenesis of PG is not fully understood, an immune-mediated process is thought to have an important role. Rather more than 50% of patients with PG have an associated systemic disease [1–3]. Common associations include IBD (in about 15–20% of cases with an associated disease), arthritis of several types, haematological malignancies and monoclonal gammopathies (Table 50.18). The strength of the different associations shows some variation with clinical pattern (see Clinical features section), but some associations may have pathogenetic importance (discussed below).

Both humoral and cell-mediated abnormalities have been associated with PG. Humoral defects reported include autoantibodies against skin and bowel, a dermonecrotic factor present in the serum that produces necrosis when injected into the subject's own skin, and a serum factor present in patients with PG that produces PG-like lesions when injected into guinea pigs [4,5]. Other studies have suggested the mechanism underlying PG is consistent with the Arthus and Schwartzmann reactions in which circulating immune complexes are deposited in vessels leading to activation of the classical and alternative complement pathways [4,6,7]. Direct immunofluorescence staining studies to detect immunoglobulins, complement and fibrin deposits in post-capillary venules have yielded inconsistent results [8,9]. The possibility of cross-reactivity between bacterial and cutaneous antigens has been suspected for many years [10], and treatment to decrease bowel bacteria has shown some benefit in therapy of PG [11], with *Escherichia coli* particularly implicated. Recent support for this possibility was documented in a study in which heat-killed *E. coli* were injected subcutaneously into clinically normal skin; in normal volunteers inflammation peaks at 24 h and fades by 48 h, but in some patients with ulcerative colitis (although in none with Crohn's disease) the inflammation persists; one patient went on to develop PG-like bullous lesions with very high IL-8 levels [12,13] (IL-8 being a very potent neutrophil chemoattractant, discussed further below). The patient had had a previous florid response to an infected wound on the foot, but did not have pathergy at needle injury sites. The authors suggest that this represents an abnormal reaction to bacteria, rather than being a form of pathergy, and suggest a local failure to terminate IL-8 production, resulting in marked neutrophilic infiltration. However, a study of Crohn's disease lesions found intracellular consensus bacterial 16S rRNA in most bowel biopsies but in no lesions of PG, neutrophilic folliculitis and other skin lesions, including skin lesions from three patients with Crohn's disease and associated skin lesions [14]. The role of bacterial antigens warrants further study.

Cell-mediated defects found include cutaneous anergy to *Candida*, streptokinase and purified protein derivative, as well as altered production of macrophage inhibition factor by lymphocytes [15]. The association with inflammatory bowel disease and various arthritides, in which T cells play a part in the pathogenesis, prompted investigation of clonal T-cell responses in patients with PG. In five patients (three with classical and two with peristomal PG), all patients had evidence of expanded T-cell clones in peripheral blood, and four of them also had clonality identified in the skin at the leading edge of the PG lesions, some of the clones in each of these cases being shared between the skin and the blood (including one patient without underlying IBD) [16]. These results were interpreted as confirming an oligoclonal T-cell response due to an antigenic stimulus, and trafficking between the skin and blood (and, therefore, potentially to other organs also). Clonal gamma and beta T-cell receptor rearrangements have also been demonstrated in PG associated with haematological disease (including splenomegaly) [17], but a recent study (including patients with Sweet's syndrome or PG) found that clonal restriction of neutrophils was present not only in over half of patients with myeloid disorders but also in a rather higher proportion of controls (one of whom later developed myelodysplasia) [18]. Thus, clonality of both T cells and of neutrophils has been demonstrated in different studies, and neither appears to be specifically related to any particular associated disease entity.

Additional reports have described decreased neutrophil chemotaxis and impaired monocyte phagocytosis in association with PG [19]. These leukocyte abnormalities may contribute to the pathergic phenomenon that occurs in up to 50% of PG patients, whereby new lesions can be induced at sites of minor skin trauma including venepuncture, vaccination and surgical procedures [1–3], and also for occurrence of the Koebner reaction in some patients with PG [20]. Various studies support the importance of IL-8 as a neutrophil chemoattractant involved in the pathogenesis of PG. Overexpression of IL-8 induced in immunodeficient mice bearing human skin xenografts caused PG-like ulceration [21], high IL-8 levels in blood have been documented in PG [22], and high IL-8 levels have been demonstrated in fibroblasts from PG ulcers [21,22]; in cultured PG ulcer fibroblasts from one patient, the initially elevated IL-8 production fell over a few weeks to the same undetectable levels as demonstrated throughout the culture period in fibroblasts from normal skin in the same patient [22]. Thus the IL-8 production (which also occurs in IBD) is induced rather than constitutive, suggesting a potential role for cytokines that stimulate its production, such as IL-1 or TNF-α.

Early reports of PG emphasized the association with ulcerative colitis (UC) but, although UC remains more commonly associated with PG than is Crohn's disease, the latter became increasingly recognized as having an association with PG; both classic and peristomal PG have been reported with UC, Crohn's disease and collagenous colitis. Three areas of interest regarding the associa-

tion of IBD with PG are the different immunopathogenesis of the UC (a Th2-type enteritis) and Crohn's disease (Th1-type), the role of cigarette smoking, and the role of bacteria, especially *E. coli* (discussed above). The possible protective role of smoking in UC has been uncertain, but a recent meta-analysis documented that smoking is protective against UC, is associated with less complications once UC has developed and with disease flares if smoking is discontinued, whereas the opposite (for all these aspects) applies to Crohn's disease [23]. A possible mechanism for the benefit of smoking on UC is that nicotine upregulates the lamina propria nicotinic acetylcholine receptor and could alter the bowel mucosal immune balance towards a Th1 pattern [24]. However, smoking is a significant factor favouring development of extraintestinal manifestations of UC, including PG and erythema nodosum [25]. Combined with the fact that PG may develop up to a decade after panproctocolectomy for UC [26], this dissociation of effect of smoking on the bowel and skin lesions suggests that the UC phenotype may be more important than the presence of colonic mucosa.

PG is not usually associated with vasculitis, but cases with positive tests for either C-ANCA or P-ANCA are occasionally reported (some in the context of drug-induced PG, typically with thiouracils). Patients with PG and other ANCA specificities are of some interest with regard to possible disease mechanisms. A patient who clinically had bullous and ulcerative PG on the legs, with polyarthritis, was found to have lung cysts and a novel ANCA to azurocidin [26]; the patient later developed a lesion on the ankle resembling blastomycosis-like pyoderma that was associated with autoantibodies to BPI. Azurocidin and BPI are antimicrobial components of neutrophil azurophilic granules (see discussion of ANCA in vasculitis, p. 50.8); antibodies to these proteins could potentially interfere with their antibacterial activity, thereby reducing innate immunity. Autoantibodies to azurocidin have also been associated with systemic and cutaneous vasculitis as well as with hydralazine-induced vasculitis [27]. More recently, a patient with PG and C-ANCA specific for h-lamp-2 has been reported [28].

Despite the evidence for cellular and cytokine responses being induced (presumably by antigenic stimuli), some cases may have a constitutive component. Several families with inherited PG have been described [29,30]; although cases have presented at any age in some kindreds, this should be noted as a possible explanation for neonatal PG which is generally rare [31]. There is also a predisposition to PG in patients with a mutation in caspase recruitment domain 15, leading to the autosomal dominant autoinflammatory syndrome of pyogenic arthritis, pyoderma gangrenosum and acne (PAPA); the relevant mutations affect CD2-binding protein 1 (CD2BP1, also known as PSTPIP1), a protein that is involved in cytoskeletal organization and that also reacts with pyrin, mutations in PAPA being predominantly expressed in granulocytes [32]. Other mutations in the same gene are the cause of some of the autoinflammatory (periodic fever) syndromes, some cases of Crohn's disease, familial granulomatous arthritis, and others [33,34].

References

1 Von den Driesch P. Pyoderma gangrenosum: a report of 44 cases with follow-up. *Br J Dermatol* 1997; **137**: 1000–5.

2 Jackson JM, Callen JP. Pyoderma gangrenosum: an expert commentary. *Expert Rev Dermatol* 2006; **1**: 391–400.

3 Wollina U. Pyoderma gangrenosum—a review. *Orphanet J Rare Dis* 2007; **2**: 19.

4 Samitz MH. Cutaneous vasculitis in association with ulcerative colitis. *Cutis* 1966; **2**: 383–7.

5 Ebringer A, Doyles AE, Harris GS. Dermonecrotic factor I: nature and properties of a dermonecrotic factor to guinea pig skin found in human serum. *Br J Exp Pathol* 1969; **50**: 559–65.

6 Samitz MH, Dana AS, Rosemberg P. Cutaneous vasculitis in association with Crohn's disease: review of statistics of skin complications. *Cutis* 1970; **6**: 51–6.

7 Lotti T, Ghersetich I, Comacchi C *et al*. Cutaneous small-vessel vasculitis. *J Am Acad Dermatol* 1998; **39**: 667–87.

8 Ullman S, Halberg P, Howitz J. Deposits of complement and immunoglobulins in vessel walls in pyoderma gangrenosum. *Acta Derm Venereol (Stockh)* 1982; **62**: 340–1.

9 Powell FC, Schroeter AL, Perry HO *et al*. Direct immunofluorescence in pyoderma gangrenosum. *Br J Dermatol* 1983; **108**: 287–93.

10 Samitz MH. Cutaneous vasculitis in association with ulcerative colitis. *Cutis* 1966; **2**: 383–7.

11 Driessen LHHM, Van Saene HKF. A novel treatment of pyoderma gangrenosum by intestinal decontamination. *Br J Dermatol* 1983; **108**: 108 [Abstract].

12 Marks DJ, Harbord MW, MacAllister R *et al*. Defective acute inflammation in Crohn's disease: a clinical investigation. *Lancet* 2006; **367**: 668–78.

13 Marks DJB, Rahman FZ, Novelli M *et al*. An exuberant inflammatory response to *E. coli*: implications for the pathogenesis of ulcerative colitis and pyoderma gangrenosum. *Gut* 2006; **55**: 1662–3.

14 Crowson NA, Nuovo GJ, Mihm MC Jr, Magro C. Cutaneous manifestations of Crohn's disease, its spectrum, and its pathogenesis: intracellular consensus bacterial 16S rRNA is associated with the gastrointestinal but not the cutaneous manifestations of Crohn's disease. *Hum Pathol* 2003; **34**: 1185–92.

15 Lazarus GS, Goldsmith LA, Rocklin RE *et al*. Pyoderma gangrenosum, altered delayed hypersensitivity, and polyarthritis. *Arch Dermatol* 1972; **105**: 46–51.

16 Brooklyn TN, Williams AN, Dunnill MGS, Probert CS. T-cell receptor repertoire in pyoderma gangrenosum: evidence for clonal expansions and trafficking. *Br J Dermatol* 2007; **157**: 960–6.

17 Mittal S, Milner BJ, Vickers MA. Pyoderma gangrenosum as a cause of splenomegaly and association with a T-cell clone. *Clin Lab Haematol* 2005; **6**: 402–4.

18 Magro CM, Kiani B, Li J, Crowson AN. Clonality in the setting of Sweet's syndrome and pyoderma gangrenosum is not limited to underlying myeloproliferative disease. *J Cutan Pathol* 2007; **34**: 526–34.

19 Nerella P, Daniela A, Guido M *et al*. Leukocyte chemotaxis and pyoderma gangrenosum. *Int J Dermatol* 1985; **24**: 45–7.

20 Papi M, Didona B, Chinni LM *et al*. Koebner phenomenon in an ANCA-positive patient with pyoderma gangrenosum. *J Dermatol* 1997; **9**: 583–6.

21 Oka M, Berking C, Nesbit M *et al*. Interleukin-8 overexpression is present in pyoderma gangrenosum ulcers and leads to ulcer formation in human skin xenografts. *Lab Invest* 2000; **80**: 595–604.

22 Oka M. Pyoderma gangrenosum and interleukin-8. *Br J Dermatol* 2007; **157**: 1279–81.

23 Latakos PL, Szamosi T, Latakos L. Smoking in inflammatory bowel disease: good, bad or ugly? *World J Gastroenterol* 2007; **13**: 6134–9.

24 Kikuchi H, Itoh J, Fukada S. Chronic nicotine stimulation modulates the immune response of mucosal T cells to Th1-dominant pattern by upregulation of Th1-specific transcriptional factor. *Neurosci Lett* 2008; **432**: 217–21.

25 Manguso F, Sanges M, Staiano T *et al*. Cigarette smoking and appendectomy are risk factors for extraintestinal manifestations in ulcerative colitis. *Am J Gastroenterol* 2004; **99**: 327–34.

26 Grattan CEH, McCann BG, Lockwood CM. Pyoderma gangrenosum, polyarthritis and lung cysts with novel antineutrophil cytoplasmic antibodies to azurocidin. *Br J Dermatol* 1998; **139**: 340–61.

27 Zhao MH, Lockwood CM. Azurocidin is a novel antigen for anti-neutrophil cytoplasmic autoantibodies (ANCA) in systemic vasculitis. *Clin Exp Immunol* 1996; **103**: 397–402.

28 Hoffman MD. Pyoderma gangrenosum associated with c-ANCA (h-lamp-2). *Int J Dermatol* 2001; **40**: 135–7.

29 Alberts JH, Sams HH, Miller JL. Familial ulcerative pyoderma gangrenosum: a report of two kindreds. *Cutis* 2002; **69**: 427–30.

30 Khandpur S, Mehta S, Reddy BS. Pyoderma gangrenosum in two siblings: a familial predisposition. *Pediatr Dermatol* 2001; **18**: 308–12.

31 al Rimawi HS, Abuekteish FM, Daoud AS, Oboosi MM. Familial pyoderma gangrenosum presenting in infancy. *Eur J Pediatr* 1996; **155**: 759–62.

32 Shoham NG, Centola M, Mansfield E *et al*. Pyrin binds the PSTPIP1/CD2BP1 protein, defining familial Mediterranean fever and PAPA syndrome as disorders in the same pathway. *Proc Natl Acad Sci USA* 2003; **100**: 13501–6.

33 Rose CD, Martin TM. Caspase recruitment domain 15 mutations and rheumatic diseases. *Curr Opin Rheum* 2005; **17**: 579–85.

34 Farasat S, Aksentijevich I, Toro JR. Autoinflammatory diseases: clinical and genetic advances. *Arch Dermatol* 2008; **144**: 392–402.

Histopathology. Although the histopathological findings of PG are often variable and non-specific, they can be useful in excluding other possible aetiologies. Several variables must be considered when evaluating the histopathology, including the type of lesion, the site of the lesion from which the biopsy is obtained, the site within the lesion (biopsy of the edge reduces potentially misleading features that may occur in any chronic ulcerating lesions), the stage of evolution of the lesion, and therapy [1]. Typical findings include central necrosis and ulceration of the epidermis and dermis surrounded by an intense, acute inflammatory cell infiltrate, with a more peripheral mixed to chronic inflammatory cell infiltrate [2–4]. Each clinical variant has additional, more specific, histopathological findings. In the ulcerative variant of PG, there is massive dermal–epidermal neutrophilic infiltrate with suppuration/abscess formation; in pustular PG, a perifollicular neutrophilic infiltrate with subcorneal pustule formation; the bullous variant shows a neutrophilic infiltrate with intraepidermal vesicle formation; and in vegetative PG, there is a granulomatous reaction with peripheral palisading histiocytes and giant cells [4,5]. Otherwise, the presence of giant cells appears to be linked with IBD, especially Crohn's disease (and thus with peristomal PG, but distinct from stomal involvement by Crohn's disease) [6]. Although of different importance between countries, and depending on immune status/associated haematological malignancy, culture and staining of biopsy tissue for fungi, mycobacteria and other organisms is advisable—especially if any granulomas are present in the absence of IBD.

The presence of vasculitis in PG is an area of debate. Many investigators have reported findings consistent with a neutrophilic vascular reaction or leukocytoclastic vasculitis, fibrinoid necrosis, segmental necrotizing vasculitis, granulomatous vasculitis and lymphocytic vasculitis [2–4,7–10], although this is not supported by all studies [11]. True vasculitides and infective causes should be carefully excluded if vasculitis is evident.

References

1 Powell FC, Su WPD. Pyoderma gangrenosum: classification and management. *J Am Acad Dermatol* 1996; **34**: 395–409.

2 Su WPD, Schoeter AL, Perry AL *et al*. Histopathologic and immunopathologic study of pyoderma gangrenosum. *J Cutan Pathol* 1996; **13**: 323–30.

3 Crowson NA, Mihm MC Jr, Magro C. Pyoderma gangrenosum: a review. *J Cutan Pathol* 2003; **30**: 97–107.

4 Benci M, Menchini G, Lotti TM. Pyoderma gangrenosum, an unusual aspect of cutaneous vasculitis. *Clin Dermatol* 1999; **17**: 581–5.

5 Callen JP. Pyoderma gangrenosum. *Lancet* 1998; **351**: 581–5.

6 Sanders S, Tahan SR, Kwan T, Magro CM. Giant cells in pyoderma gangrenosum. *J Cutan Pathol* 2001; **28**: 97–100.

7 Stolman LP, Rosenthal D, Yaworsky R *et al.* Pyoderma gangrenosum and rheumatoid arthritis. *Arch Dermatol* 1975; **111**: 1020–3.

8 Bishopric GA, Bracken JS. Pyoderma gangrenosum as the presenting sign of regional enteritis. *South Med J* 1964; **57**: 675.

9 Dantzig PI. Pyoderma gangrenosum. *N Engl J Med* 1975; **292**: 47–8.

10 Meler F, Berner D, Scherwitz C *et al.* An unusual case of pyoderma gangrenosum with necrotizing granulomatous dermatitis. *J Dtsch Dermatol Ges* 2003; **1**: 302–5.

11 Bennett ML, Jackson JM, Jorizzo JL *et al.* Pyoderma gangrenosum: a comparison of typical and atypical forms with an emphasis on time to remission. *Medicine* 2000; **79**: 37–46.

Clinical features. PG can have a variety of clinical presentations. Extracutaneous involvement is discussed separately later. Diagnostic criteria have been proposed for the cutaneous lesions of classic ulcerative PG [1], with various amendments suggested [2,8], and, although not formally validated, can be summarized as:

Major criteria (both required)

1 Rapid (usually >1 cm/day) progression of painful, necrolytic ulceration with an irregular, undermined, violaceous border—usually with a preceding papule, pustule or bulla, and pain out of proportion to the size of the ulcerated area

2 Exclusion of other causes of ulceration.

Minor criteria (at least two required)

1 (a) history of pathergy, or (b) presence of cribriform scarring

2 Presence of a disease known to be associated with PG (usually listed as IBD, polyarthritis, myelodysplasia or leukaemia, but monoclonal gammopathy should be added to this list; overall about 50% have an associated systemic disease)

3 Appropriate histopathological findings (again, specifically excluding infective causes)

4 Rapid response to oral corticosteroid therapy (usually interpreted as at least 50% reduction in size using 1–2 mg/kg/day).

As described above, for pragmatic reasons of diagnosis, disease association or therapy (below) we have divided the types of PG as follows:

Classic/ulcerative PG [2–9]. This is the commonest and best recognized variant of PG, presenting with small, tender, red–blue papules, plaques or pustules that evolve into painful ulcers with characteristic violaceous undermined edges (Fig. 50.37). There may be granulation tissue, necrosis or purulent exudate at the ulcer base. Lesions may be solitary or multiple, and occur most commonly on the legs (in 70%), but may affect any body site. Pathergy occurs in 25% (usually defined as following minor injuries such as venesection, but numerous reports of PG at operation sites, especially after breast surgery, are also reported, and other forms of skin injury such as scalds or varicella may also act as a pathergic trigger). Healing usually occurs with an atrophic cribriform scar. Associated symptoms include fever, malaise, myalgia and arthralgia. Frequent disease associations include IBD, arthritis, monoclonal gammopathy or internal malignancy; over 70% have one of these [4]. Genital and mucosal involvement (other than pyostomatitis vegetans) are generally considered to be within this category, but are discussed separately below as they raise additional diagnostic issues.

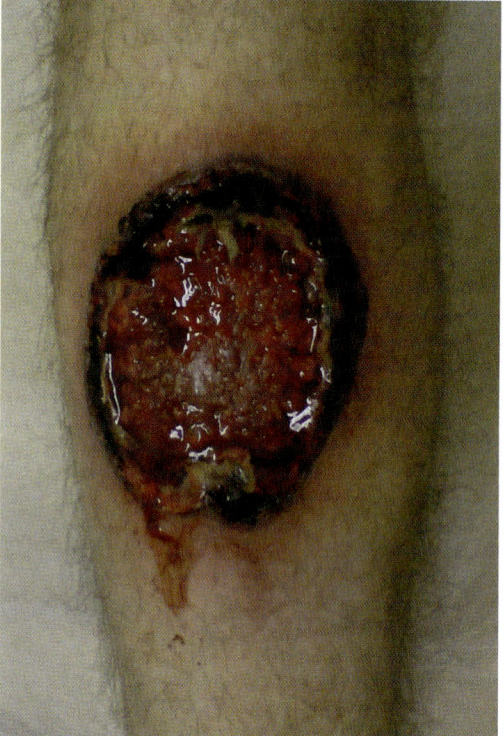

Fig. 50.37 Pyoderma gangrenosum. Classic type, showing a deep ulcer with inflammatory border.

Atypical forms. The term 'atypical PG' has been used in several rather different contexts, and it may be useful to subdivide them. At one time bullous PG, possibly overlapping with bullous Sweet's disease (and being strongly linked with haematological malignancy), was the main 'atypical' form. It is now more common for atypical PG to mean a pattern that is relatively superficial, may be pustular and Sweet's syndrome-like or may be ulcerated, tends to occur on hands, arms and face or upper trunk, and is linked with myeloproliferative disorders and gammopathies (usually IgA) [2,8]; it overlaps with neutrophilic dermatosis of the dorsal hands, discussed separately later. However, others view peristomal or genital PG as also being 'atypical'—to bridge this gap between terminologies, and to help explain the patterns, we have subdivided the 'atypical' forms of PG into three morphological types and some site-specific variants.

Atypical form: (a) pustular PG. Pustular PG is a variant, noted two decades ago [4], that often occurs during acute exacerbations of IBD. Discrete painful pustules, with a surrounding halo of erythema, develop on normal skin [4,9]. These pustules commonly arise with a scattered distribution on the extensor aspects of the limbs. Nomenclature for these lesions varies somewhat, including pustular vasculitis and neutrophilic pustules, as well as pustular PG. This diagnostic area is discussed later with some other pustular neutrophilic dermatoses. Pustular PG lesions often resolve with control of IBD (in some cases using treatments appropriate for both PG and for IBD, discussed later) but some may evolve to form ulcerated classic PG.

Atypical form: (b) bullous PG. This pattern has also traditionally been termed 'atypical' PG. It presents with rapidly arising, superficial, haemorrhagic bullae, often located on the arms [4,6].

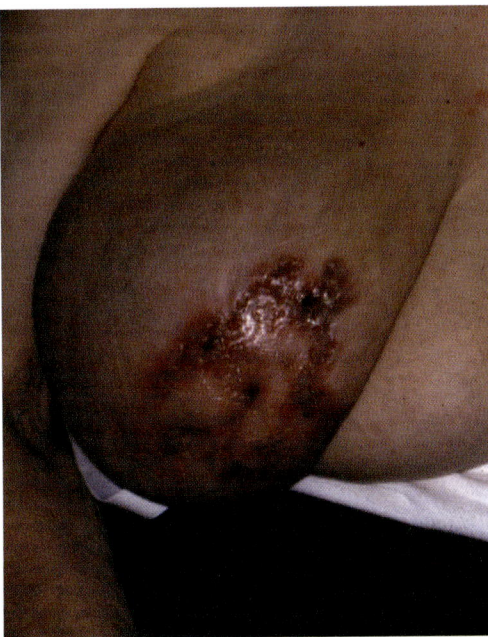

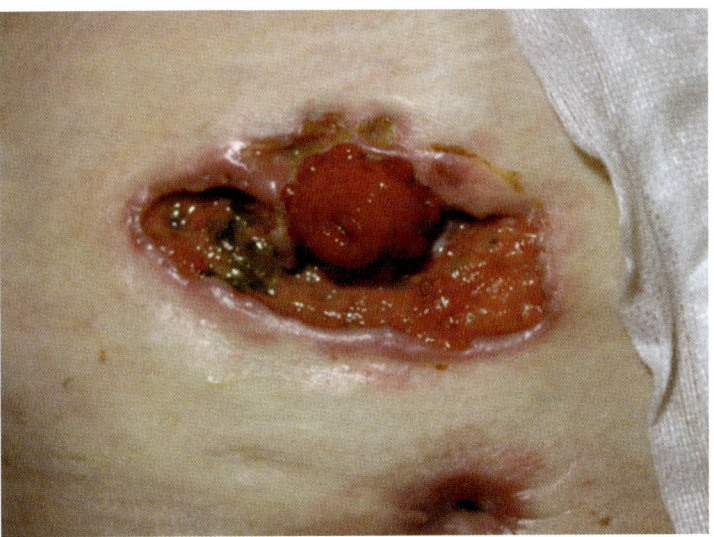

Fig. 50.38 Pyoderma gangrenosum. Superficial granulomatous type; the breast is a common site.

Fig 50.39 Pyoderma gangrenosum. Peristomal type, with additional pathergic involvement of surgical wounds. Systemic therapy was contraindicated by pelvic sepsis but the lesion healed with very potent topical corticosteroid treatment. Opiate analgesia and nitrous oxide for severe local pain was able to be discontinued by using topical instillation of amethocaine-prilocaine cream for an hour before dressing changes.

It shares clinical and histopathological findings with Sweet's syndrome, but typically ulcerates and heals with scarring. Bullous PG is especially associated with myeloproliferative disorders [1,4,7,9,10]; if it occurs with IBD it is usually in patients with a significant disease flare.

Atypical form: (c) upper limbs/trunk/face. The pattern of PG that is now often simply referred to as 'atypical PG' [2,8] is a more superficial variant than classic PG. It can occur at any site but most commonly on the arms or face. It can be bullous, and it may be difficult to differentiate from Sweet's syndrome. It is viewed as including neutrophilic dermatosis of the dorsal hands (discussed separately below to explain nomenclature and histological features in more detail; p. 50.80 and Fig. 50.42). The importance of this pattern is that the strongest link with internal disease is with myelogenous leukaemias, myeloproliferative disorders or IgA gammopathies.

Superficial (vegetative) PG (synonym superficial granulomatous pyoderma) presents as a superficial ulcer, usually on the trunk (Fig. 50.38) or sometimes the face, although it can occur at other sites. It has a non-purulent base and generally lacks the violaceous, undermined border of classic PG [4,9,11]. It is often a solitary, slowly progressing, relatively non-painful, variant that resolves with less aggressive treatment [12] and is not usually associated with any systemic disease [13]. Infections are the commonest differential diagnosis. The confusingly similarly-named, morphologically similar, but pathogenetically quite different disorder pyoderma vegetans is discussed on p. 50.89.

Peristomal PG [2,7–9,14] is currently a relatively common pattern of PG, perhaps accounting for about 15% of cases, and sometimes coexisting with pustular vasculitis or PG at other sites (Fig. 50.39).

It has several notable features: it is almost always associated with IBD, biopsy may show giant cells or bacteria (the latter mainly due to contamination/colonization of ulcerated skin), there is a significant risk of the area being treated as an infected or broken-down surgical wound, and therapy may be very difficult (see later). Other associations of peristomal PG include diverticular disease, bowel carcinoma, perforated bowel and neurogenic bladder in one series [14], as well as recent reports of collagenous colitis [15] and systemic sclerosis [16].

Other specific sites of PG that influence diagnostic aspects, disease associations or therapy

(a) **PG of the face, lips, orbital adnexae or upper trunk** has already been discussed as these are sites that should give rise to suspicion of associated myeloproliferative disease. However, PG at these areas also causes differential diagnostic problems that may be a lesser consideration at other sites; orbital cellulitis, destructive lymphomas and factitious disease (discussed later) cause particular problems. Ulcerated neoplasms that have been concealed also need to be considered. Another difficult differential diagnosis is a condition termed malignant pyoderma (MP), first described by Perry *et al.* in 1968 [17] as a rapidly progressive ulcerative disease localized to the head, neck and upper trunk. Controversy exists as to whether MP represents a head and neck variant of PG or a cutaneous manifestation of WG. PG and WG may have similar clinical and histopathological findings, and both have been the reported cause of MP in some cases [18–22]. Interestingly, two of the original three reported cases of MP are now believed to represent WG. The presence of C-ANCA, which is highly specific for WG, should mean that it is now easier to distinguish PG from WG. However, some patients with WG may have negative C-ANCA test results, and thus close follow-up is warranted for possible pulmonary or renal lesions that may develop in WG [21–23]. Because of the uncertainty regarding the nosology of MP, it has been suggested that this term should not be used as a final diagnosis [21].

(b) **PG of the genitalia** includes both penile [24] and vulval involvement. There is no reason to suppose that these sites of involvement represent a different form of PG (except perhaps in children, as perianal and genital involvement appears to be over-represented in the first decade of life [25]), or have specific disease associations, but differential diagnosis (below) may be difficult and PG may not be suspected.

(c) **PG of the breast** is also not a specific entity—most cases are either vegetative PG, or the breast is affected with the face or arms in the haematological disease-associated atypical variety. However, there are again specific differential diagnosis issues, one that has caused some problems in recent publications being that of factitial disease (discussed below). PG after breast surgery has been reported on many occasions [26,27].

(d) **PG of oral, pharyngeal, laryngeal, nasal, respiratory tract and ocular mucosae** [28–34] does have some reasons to be discussed separately. Diagnosis and treatment may be difficult, and respiratory involvement may have a predilection for children [33,34]. Ocular lesions are documented in Table 50.18, the most specific being peripheral ulcerative keratitis [28] and possibly nodular episcleritis. Pyostomatitis vegetans is an oral mucosal disease that in some instances appears to be related to PG, having a very strong link with IBD, but is less certain in other instances—it is briefly discussed separately below. Other oral lesions may be aphthous, pustular, frank extensive PG [29,30] or occur within the spectrum of Behçet's disease [31]. Nasal mucosal involvement may occur [29,32], even septal perforation [32], as well as tracheal [33] or respiratory tract involvement [34], either of these having a differential diagnosis of WG as discussed above for 'malignant pyoderma'.

(e) Systemic disease (affecting lung, bone, etc.) is discussed separately on p. 50.81.

Pyostomatitis vegetans [35–38] is nosologically an enigmatic disorder. It is a disorder in which there is oral mucosal thickening with multiple pustules and 'snail track' ulcers on an erythematous base (at any site, although the tongue is less affected). The oral lesions have a very strong link with IBD, especially active ulcerative colitis; this, combined with the presence of Sweet's syndrome-like or PG-like skin lesions in some cases, has led several reviewers to consider this disorder as a manifestation of PG. However, several factors argue against this. Although deeper tissues have a mixed infiltrate including neutrophils, early and superficial lesions have a preponderance of eosinophils and often associated peripheral blood eosinophilia. The skin lesions (perhaps best termed pyodermatitis vegetans, and discussed later in the differential diagnosis of pustular eruptions, p. 50.89) are often flexural and (although clearly distinguished by histology and direct immunofluorescence) are clinically more suggestive of pemphigus vegetans. The various terminologies are used interchangeably, which does not enhance understanding. On present evidence, it is probably best to view this as a predominantly IBD-associated eruption but not as a form of PG.

Diagnosis. There are two facets to diagnosis in PG; one is distinguishing PG from several possible alternatives, and the other is evaluation for underlying causes (of which arthritis and IBD are generally apparent, but haematological causes may not be). PG is often a diagnosis of exclusion as laboratory and histopathological findings are variable and non-specific; some of the more important differential diagnoses are enumerated in Table 50.19 [7–9,39,40]. Patient evaluation should include a detailed history, physical examination and skin biopsies for histopathology and culture (including unusual fungi, atypical mycobacteria and opportunistic infections, in the majority of cases), as well as appropriate laboratory tests to help rule out other possible aetiologies. Sweet's syndrome can often be distinguished by its rather sudden onset of non-ulcerating lesions that generally heal without scarring, although both share some aetiologies, both may coexist, and (especially associated with haematological malignancy) a clinical picture with features of both may occur (typically bullous, and variably termed atypical Sweet's syndrome or atypical PG). Syndromes with vasculitis such as WG, Behçet's disease and SLE can also be confused with PG; however, leukocytoclastic vasculitis is not a feature of PG.

There are examples of both factitious disease or other causes of ulceration being erroneously diagnosed as PG [40,41], and PG has also been misdiagnosed as factitial [42]; both situations are hugely important due to the extensive tissue destruction that may occur, so, provided infection is excluded, a trial of corticosteroid therapy is appropriate as PG is likely to respond. However, this should be limited in duration and other diagnoses considered if response is poor. In one study of 95 patients with ulcers resembling PG, 64 had been treated on this basis for 3–180 (median 10) months, 23 (36%) without response and eight (12%) with deterioration; final diagnoses included vascular occlusion, venous disease, vasculitis, neoplasia, various forms of tissue injury (five had factitial disease) and other inflammatory disorders [40].

In evaluation of associated diseases, it should be noted that the course of PG does not necessarily parallel that of IBD, but that PG in haematological disorders (unless provoked by a neutrophil-increasing therapy, such as colony-stimulating factors) may be an indicator of transformation to a higher grade malignancy [43–45]. Thus careful re-evaluation is appropriate. It is also worth considering re-evaluation of patients with ulcerative colitis who develop peristomal PG, as some will prove to have Crohn's disease.

References

1 Su WPD, Davis MD, Weenig RH *et al.* Pyoderma gangrenosum: clinicopathologic correlation and proposed diagnostic criteria. *Int J Dermatol* 2004; **43**: 790–800.
2 Callen JP, Jackson JM. Pyoderma gangrenosum: an update. *Rheum Dis Clin N Am* 2007; **33**: 787–802.
3 Callen JP. Pyoderma gangrenosum and related disorders. *Dermatol Clin* 1990; **7**: 1249–59.
4 Powell FC, Su WPD. Pyoderma gangrenosum: classification and management. *J Am Acad Dermatol* 1996; **34**: 395–409.
5 Powell FC, Schroeter AL, Su WPD *et al.* Pyoderma gangrenosum: a review of 86 patients. *QJM* 1985; **55**: 173–86.
6 Bennett ML, Jackson JM, Jorizzo JL *et al.* Pyoderma gangrenosum: a comparison of typical and atypical forms with an emphasis on time to remission. *Medicine* 2000; **79**: 37–46.
7 Wollina U. Pyoderma gangrenosum—a review. *Orphanet J Rare Dis* 2007; **2**: 19.

Table 50.19 Some differential diagnoses of pyoderma gangrenosum.

Category	Examples	Comment
Infection	Bacterial: ecthyma, mycobacteria, syphilis, tropical ulcer, necrotizing fasciitis; folliculitis, gonococcaemia and other pustular infections may also mimic pustular PG Fungi: blastomycosis, sporotrichosis, cryptococcosis, zygomycoses, alternaria, *Penicillium marneffei* Viral: herpes simplex Other: amoebiasis	Consider infections especially in instances where 'pathergy' may have actually represented inoculation, and in immunosuppressed subjects (including therapeutic immunosuppression for IBD or arthritis, haematology disease-related immune compromise)
Vascular disease	Arterial disease, venous disease Occlusive angiopathic disorders (cryogelling, livedoid vasculopathy, antiphospholipid syndrome, calcific uraemic arteriolopathy, etc. (Chapter 49) Others: sickle cell disease, thalassaemia/haemoglobinopathies	
Vasculitis	Wegener's granulomatosis (WG), leukocytoclastic vasculitis, polyarteritis nodosa, mixed cryoglobulinaemia, Takayasu's arteritis	The differential diagnosis of WG may be difficult at head and neck sites, or if there is internal neutrophilic dermatosis
Neoplasia	Lymphoma (especially aggressive angiocentric T-cell lymphomas, anaplastic large cell lymphoma, bullous mycosis fungoides) Leukaemia cutis Langerhans' cell histiocytosis	Both a differential diagnosis and a possible cause of PG
Drugs	Halides: e.g. bromoderma Ulceration due to hydroxycarbamide Drug-induced lupus erythematosus	Check ANCA, often positive in thiouracil-induced PG or vasculitis; note that drugs may cause true PG rather than simulators Ulceration due to hydroxycarbamide particularly needs to be considered in patients being treated with this for a known haematological disorder
Other tissue injury	Necrotic bite reations: spiders, others Factitious injury (including panniculitis due to infective or toxic agents); intravenous drug abuse (± secondary infection); cocaine ulceration	Beware of cases without a response to corticosteroids
Medical disorders	Amyloidosis (especially bullous) Ulcerative sarcoidosis Cutaneous (metastatic) Crohn's disease Other neutrophilic disorders Necrobiosis lipoidica Pyodermatitis–pyostomatitis vegetans (see text)	Many of these have also been described as causes of PG

8 Jackson JM, Callen JP. Pyoderma gangrenosum: an expert commentary. *Expert Rev Dermatol* 2006; **1**: 391–400.

9 Ahmadi S, Powell FC. Pyoderma gangrenosum: uncommon presentations. *Clin Dermatol* 2005; **23**: 612–20.

10 Perry HO, Winkelmann RK. Bullous pyoderma gangrenosum and leukaemia. *Arch Dermatol* 1972; **106**: 901–5.

11 Wilson-Jones E, Winkelmann RK. Superficial granulomatous pyoderma: a localized vegetative form of pyoderma gangrenosum. *J Am Acad Dermatol* 1988; **18**: 511–21.

12 Lichter MD, Welykyj SE, Gradini R *et al*. Superficial granulomatous pyoderma. *Int J Dermatol* 1991; **30**: 418–21.

13 Quimby SR, Gibson LE, Winkelmann RK. Superficial granulomatous pyoderma: clinicopathologic spectrum. *Mayo Clin Proc* 1989; **64**: 37–43.

14 Lyon CC, Smith AJ, Beck MH *et al*. Parastomal pyoderma gangrenosum: clinical features and management. *J Am Acad Dermatol* 2000; **42**: 992–1002.

15 Davis MPD, Holderness Nakamura KJ. Peristomal pyoderma gangrenosum associated with collagenous colitis. *Arch Dermatol* 2007; **143**: 669–70.

16 Fujikura M, Ohtsuka T, Oyamada Y. Systemic sclerosis in association with peristomal pyoderma gangrenosum. *Br J Dermatol* 2007; **157**: 618–9.

17 Perry HO, Winkelmann RK, Muller SA *et al*. Malignant pyodermas. *Arch Dermatol* 1968; **98**: 561–74.

18 Malkinson FD. Pyoderma gangrenosum vs. malignant pyoderma: lumpers vs. splitters. *Arch Dermatol* 1987; **123**: 333–7.

19 Erdi H, Anadolu R, Piskin G *et al*. Malignant pyoderma: a clinical variant of pyoderma gangrenosum. *Int J Dermatol* 1996; **35**: 811–3.

20 Spenatto N, Viraben R. Malignant pyoderma. *J Eur Acad Dermatol Venereol* 1999; **12**: 275–6.

21 Gibson LE, Daoud MS, Perry HO. Malignant pyodermas revisited. *Mayo Clin Proc* 1997; **72**: 734–6.

22 Cone LA, Annunsiata GM, Gebhart RN *et al*. Malignant pyoderma and Wegener's granulomatosis. *Mayo Clin Proc* 1998; **73**: 390–1.

23 Jayne DRW, Rasmussen N (European Community Systemic Vasculitis Clinical Trials Study Group (ECSYSVASTRIAL)). Treatment of antineutrophil cytoplasm autoantibody-associated systemic vasculitis: initiatives of the European Community Systemic Vasculitis Trials Study Group. *Mayo Clin Proc* 1997; **72**: 737–47.

24 OLally A, Hollowood K, Bunker CB, Turner R. Penile pyoderma gangrenosum treated with topical tacrolimus. *Arch Dermatol* 2005; **141**: 1175–6.

25 Graham JA, Hansen KK, Rabinowitz LG, Esterley NB. Pyoderma gangrenosum in infants and children. *Pediatr Dermatol* 1994; **11**: 10–17.

26 van Pouke S, Jorens PG, Peeters R *et al*. Pyoderma gangrenosum: a challenging complication of bilateral mastopexy. *Int Wound J* 2004; **1**: 207–13.

27 Davis MPD, Alexander JL, Prawer SE. Pyoderma gangrenosum of the breasts precipitated by breast surgery. *J Am Acad Dermatol* 2006; **55**: 317–20.

28 Wilson DM, John JR, Callen PR. Peripheral ulcerative keratitis: an extracutaneous neutrophilic disorder. Report of a patient with rheumatoid arthritis, pustular

vasculitis, pyoderma gangrenosum, and Sweet's syndrome with an excellent response to cyclosporine therapy. *J Am Acad Dermatol* 1999; **40**: 331–4.

29 Kennedy KS, Prendergast ML, Sooy CD. Pyoderma gangrenosum of the oral cavity, nose and larynx. *Otolaryngology* 1987; **97**: 487–90.

30 Setterfield JF, Shirlaw PJ, Challacombe SJ, Black MM. Pyoderma gangrenosum associated with severe oropharyngeal involvement and IgA paraproteinaemia. *Br J Dermatol* 2001; **144**: 402–5.

31 Munro CS, Cox NH. Pyoderma gangrenosum associated with Behçet's syndrome: response to thalidomide. *Clin Exp Dermatol* 1988; **13**: 408–10.

32 Somura I, Miyawaki S, Morita A. Pyoderma gangrenosum associated with nasal septal perforation, oropharyngeal ulcers and IgA paraproteinaemia. *J Dermatol* 2005; **32**: 193–8.

33 Merke DP, Honig PJ, Potsic WP. Pyoderma gangrenosum of the skin and trachea in a 9-month-old boy. *J Am Acad Dermatol* 1996; **34**: 681–2.

34 Takeuchi K, Kyoko H, Hachiya M et al. Pyoderma gangrenosum of the skin and respiratory tract in a 5-year-old girl. *Eur J Pediatr* 2003; **162**: 344–5.

35 Storwick GS, Prihoda MB, Fulton RJ, Wood WS. Pyoderma—pyostomatitis vegetans: a specific marker for inflammatory bowel disease. *J Am Acad Dermatol* 1994; **31**: 336–41.

36 Mehravaran M, Kemény L, Husz S et al. Pyoderma–pyostomatitis vegetans. *Br J Dermatol* 1997; **137**: 266–9.

37 Nigen S, Poulin Y, Rochette L et al. Pyoderma–pyostomatitis vegetans. Two cases and a review of the literature. *J Cutan Med Surg* 2003; **7**: 250–5.

38 Hegarty AM, Barrett AW, Scully C. Pyostomatitis vegetans. *Clin Exp Dermatol* 2003; **29**: 1–7.

39 Powell FC, Collins S. Pyoderma gangrenosum. *Clin Dermatol* 2000; **18**: 283–93.

40 Weenig RH, Davis MPD, Dahl PR, Su WPD. Skin ulcers misdiagnosed as pyoderma gangrenosum. *N Engl J Med* 2002; **347**: 1412–8.

41 Oh CCY, McKenna DB, McLaren KM, Tidman MJ. Factitious panniculitis masquerading as pyoderma gangrenosum. *Clin Exp Dermatol* 2005; **30**: 253–5.

42 Harries MJ, McMullen E, Griffiths CEM. Pyoderma gangrenosum masquerading as dermatitis artefacta. *Arch Dermatol* 2006; **142**: 1509–10.

43 Sheps M, Shapero H, Ramsay C. Bullous pyoderma gangrenosum and acute leukaemia. *Arch Dermatol* 1978; **114**: 1842–3.

44 Cox NH, White SI, Walton S et al. Pyoderma gangrenosum associated with polycythaemia rubra vera. *Clin Exp Dermatol* 1987; **12**: 375–7.

45 Grob JJ, Mege JL, Frax AM et al. Disseminated pustular dermatosis in polycythemia vera. *J Am Acad Dermatol* 1988; **18**: 1212–8.

Treatment. Many effective treatment strategies have been reported, and have been the subject of extensive review articles [1–6], some evidence-based from literature on large numbers of patients [5], some giving doses and hints for use [4] and others addressing specific patterns of PG [6].

Choice of treatment generally depends on disease severity as well as on the presence of associated disease. For early or mild lesions, topical therapy may be sufficient [1]. This includes wet compresses, hydrophilic occlusive dressings, antimicrobial agents and topical corticosteroids. Topical tacrolimus is also useful for treatment of early PG lesions [7], and intralesional corticosteroids are another therapeutic option of reported benefit [8]. Indeed there may be situations, for example if there is a post-surgical infection which precludes use of systemic immunosuppressive therapy, where analgesia and topical treatment of PG is the most appropriate option (Fig. 50.39). Other topical agents, such as benzoyl peroxide, 5-aminosalicylic acid, nitrogen mustard (20% aqueous), cromoglycate preparations, platelet-derived growth factor, and intralesional therapy with ciclosporin, all have only anecdotal or small series data [5]. Topical nicotine cream was not considered in [5], but a recent (two patient) report supported previous suggestions of efficacy [9].

For more severe disease, or for PG resistant to topical therapy, oral corticosteroids have been the mainstay of therapy. Pulsed intravenous corticosteroid therapy has been reported to be effective in some cases refractory to oral corticosteroids; it has been recommended in PG refractory to other forms of treatment [10]. Evidence for benefit from sulphones and other antimicrobials such as dapsone, clofazimine and minocycline, which may have anti-inflammatory effects or modulate neutrophil function, is anecdotal [5]; however, these are widely used alone or with corticosteroids. Dapsone is probably most frequently used, although low-dose colchicine was recently advocated in a report of two patients [11]. Various immunosuppressant agents (Table 50.20) have been found to be useful in corticosteroid-unresponsive PG, either alone or as corticosteroid-sparing agents. Assessing their individual benefit is difficult as many have been used with other therapy, such as corticosteroids; because of the risk of severe adverse effects such as bone marrow suppression, use of these agents has usually been limited to severe or refractory PG. Ciclosporin was widely used due to rapid action [2] and several case series were published [5], but is not ideal long term. Cyclophosphamide, chlorambucil, intravenous tacrolimus, mycophenolate mofetil and thalidomide have all been effective in a limited number of patients reported [1–6,12–20]; although not providing high-quality evidence, use of these agents has often been in patients refractory to less complex therapies. Ideally, it is best to choose a treatment that will also address any underlying disease, such as melphalan in the case of patients with paraproteinaemia [21], or methotrexate in those with underlying arthritis or IBD [22]. In peristomal PG [6], there are two main issues that are slightly different from treatment of PG at other sites; one of these is that topical therapies (typically corticosteroids or tacrolimus) need to be formulated in a way that neither irritates unduly nor interferes with adhesion of appliances, the other is that, because of the strong link with IBD, there may be a lower threshold to consider systemic therapies (especially those that may be beneficial for both the PG and the bowel disease). Intralesional corticosteroids may avoid some of these problems. Achieving analgesia at this site, where activity of the stoma and need for adhesive appliances in close proximity to the PG both potentially add to discomfort, may be difficult.

In many of these situations, biologically engineered TNF-α inhibitors are now being used in preference to older agents, especially where there is associated IBD or inflammatory arthritis which is also likely to respond; there are several reports of benefit to etanercept, adalimumab and infliximab [23–29]. These reports include one randomized, controlled trial of infliximab (with benefit unrelated to underlying disease) [25], a report of benefit from adalimumab after failure of etanercept [24], reports of benefit of infliximab in vegetative PG [26] and in PG as part of PAPA syndrome [27], and a report of use of infliximab and adalimumab in systemic PG (aseptic abscesses of psoas muscle and spleen) [28]. However, these agents are expensive, and are contraindicated in the presence of malignancy or infection, but may be the most appropriate choice for severe PG with associated active IBD [29].

Other treatments that have been effective in small studies include plasmapheresis [14], leukocytapheresis/granulocytapheresis [30,31] and intravenous immunoglobulin (IVIG) [32–34]. In a retrospective review of ten therapy-resistant patients treated with IVIG, seven cleared, six maintaining benefit with ongoing

Table 50.20 Therapeutic ladder for pyoderma gangrenosum.

Topical:
Topical or intralesional corticosteroids (2)
Tacrolimus (2)
Nicotine (3)
Cromolyn sodium/disodium cromoglycate (3)
Platelet-derived growth factor (3)

Systemic:
Prednisolone (oral or pulsed intravenous) (2)
Dapsone (2), sulphapyridine (3), sulphamethoxypyridazine (3)
Minocycline (3)
Clofazimine (2)
Colchicine (3)
Potassium iodide (3)
Sulfasalazine (2)
Infliximab (1)
Etanercept (3)
Adalimumab (3)
Thalidomide (3)
Methotrexate (weekly pulse) (3)
Ciclosporin (2)
Azathioprine (3)
Cyclophosphamide (3)
Mycophenolate mofetil (3)
Intravenous immunoglobulins (2)
Colony-stimulating factors (perilesional injection) (3)
Interferon-α (3; a patient with hepatitis C)

Other (physical and non-drug therapies):
Skin grafting, flap repairs etc. (3)
Bioengineered skin equivalents, cultured keratinocyte sheets and other keratinocyte
    delivery systems (3)
Hyperbaric oxygen (3)
Low pressure dressings (3)
Leukocytapheresis/granulocytapheresis (3)
Radiotherapy (3; probably not beneficial)

1, double-blind studies; 2, case series (> just 2 or 3 cases); 3, case reports.

intermittent infusions [33]; one study reported rapid relief of pain after IVIG [34]. Aggressive surgical debridement is contraindicated because of possible exacerbation of PG by the pathergic response. However, split-skin grafts and cultured keratinocyte autografting have been demonstrated to be effective if performed while the pathergic response is minimized using prolonged courses of immunosuppressants, and a variety of bioengineered dressings or keratinocyte delivery systems have been tried [5,35–37]. Low-pressure dressings, and hyperbaric oxygen therapy, have been reported as beneficial in single cases. Gradient support hosiery is probably beneficial for leg lesions.

Therapy decisions depend on an assessment of the degree of active inflammation as opposed to simple wound healing requirements in refractory ulcers. Treatment of PG is usually discontinued after complete healing of lesions. Recurrences may occur but are unpredictable and therefore do not justify prolonged maintenance therapy [2]. A summary of therapeutic options for PG is depicted in Table 50.20; in general, initial treatment for localized disease comprises topical or intralesional corticosteroid or topical tacrolimus, for resistant localized or more widespread PG comprises systemic corticosteroids with possible addition of one of the less toxic steroid-sparing agents (usually dapsone, mycophenolate mofetil, medium-term ciclosporin), and for more severe disease, or where there is an associated disease requiring concurrent therapy, an appropriate systemic agent (increasingly, an anti-TNF monoclonal agent).

References

1 Powell FC, Su WPD. Pyoderma gangrenosum: classification and management. *J Am Acad Dermatol* 1996; **34**: 395–409.
2 Chow RKP, Ho VC. Treatment of pyoderma gangrenosum. *J Am Acad Dermatol* 1996; **34**: 1047–60.
3 Ahmadi S, Powell FC. Pyoderma gangrenosum: uncommon presentations. *Clin Dermatol* 2005; **23**: 612–20.
4 Jackson JM, Callen JP. Pyoderma gangrenosum: an expert commentary. *Expert Rev Dermatol* 2006; **1**: 391–400.
5 Reichrath J, Bens G, Bonowitz A, Tilgen W. Treatment recommendations for pyoderma gangrenosum: an evidence-based review of the literature based on more than 350 patients. *J Am Acad Dermatol* 2005; **53**: 273–83.
6 Lyon CC, Smith AJ, Beck MH *et al*. Parastomal pyoderma gangrenosum: clinical features and management. *J Am Acad Dermatol* 2000; **42**: 992–1002.
7 Petering H, Kiehl P, Breuer C *et al*. Pyoderma gangrenosum: successful topical therapy with tacrolimus (FK506). *Hautarzt* 2001; **52**: 47–50.
8 Gardner LW, Acker DW. Triamcinolone and pyoderma gangrenosum. *Arch Dermatol* 1972; **106**: 559–60.
9 Patel GK, Rhodes JR, Evans B, Holt PJA. Successful treatment of pyoderma gangrenosum with topical 0.5% nicotine cream. *J Dermatol Treat* 2004; **15**: 122–5.
10 Johnson RB, Lazarus GS. Pulse therapy: therapeutic efficacy in the treatment of pyoderma gangrenosum. *Arch Dermatol* 1982; **118**: 76–84.
11 Kontochristopoulos GJ, Stavropoulos PG, Gregoriou S *et al*. Treatment of pyoderma gangrenosum with low-dose colchicine. *Dermatology* 2004; **209**: 233–6.
12 Callen JP, Case JD, Sager D. Chlorambucil: an effective corticosteroid sparing therapy for pyoderma gangrenosum. *J Am Acad Dermatol* 1989; **21**: 515–9.
13 Newell LM, Malkinson FD. Pyoderma gangrenosum: response to cyclophosphamide therapy. *Arch Dermatol* 1983; **119**: 495–7.
14 Kaminska R, Ikaheimo R, Hollmen A. Plasmapheresis and cyclophosphamide as successful treatments for pyoderma gangrenosum. *Clin Exp Dermatol* 1999; **24**: 81–5.
15 Ackerman D, Abu-Elmagd K, Venkataramanan K *et al*. Recalcitrant psoriasis and pyoderma gangrenosum treated with FK506. *J Invest Dermatol* 1991; **96**: 536.
16 Munro CS, Cox NH. Pyoderma gangrenosum associated with Behçet's syndrome: response to thalidomide. *Clin Exp Dermatol* 1988; **13**: 408–10.
17 Federman GL, Federman DG. Recalcitrant pyoderma gangrenosum treated with thalidomide. *Mayo Clin Proc* 2000; **75**: 842–4.
18 Daniels LH, Callen JP. Mycophenolate mofetil is an effective treatment for peristomal pyoderma gangrenosum. *Arch Dermatol* 2004; **140**: 1427–9.
19 Cox NH, Palmer JG. Bowel-associated dermatitis-arthritis syndrome associated with ileo-anal pouch anastamosis, and treatment with mycophenolate mofetil. *Br J Dermatol* 2003; **149**: 1296–7.
20 Lee MR, Cooper MJ. Mycophenolate mofetil in pyoderma gangrenosum. *J Dermatol Treat* 2004; **15**: 303–7.
21 Moller H, Waldenstrom JG, Kettervall O. Pyoderma gangrenosum (dermatitis ulcerosa) and monoclonal (IgA) globulin healed after melphalan treatment. *Acta Med Scand* 1978; **203**: 293–6.
22 Bennett ML, Jackson JM, Jorizzo JL *et al*. Pyoderma gangrenosum: a comparison of typical and atypical forms with an emphasis on time to remission. *Medicine* 2000; **79**: 37–46.
23 Pastor N, Betlloch I, Pascua JC *et al*. Pyoderma gangrenosum treated with anti-TNF alpha therapy (etanercept). *Clin Exp Dermatol* 2005; **31**: 152–3.
24 Pomerantz RG, Husni ME, Mody E, Qureshi AA. Adalimumab for treatment of pyoderma gangrenosum. *Br J Dermatol* 2007; **157**: 1274–5.
25 Brooklyn TN, Dunnill MSG, Shetty A *et al*. Infliximab for the treatment of pyoderma gangrenosum: a randomized, double blind, placebo controlled trial. *Gut* 2006; **55**: 505–9.

26 Marzano AV, Tourlaki A, Alessi E, Caputo R. Widespread idiopathic pyoderma gangrenosum evolved from ulcerative to vegetative type: a 10-year history with a recent response to infliximab. *Clin Exp Dermatol* 2007; **33**: 156–9.

27 Stichweh DS, Punaro M, Pascual V. Dramatic improvement of pyoderma gangrenosum with infliximab in a patient with PAPA syndrome. *Pediatr Dermatol* 2005; **22**: 262–5.

28 Hubbard VG, Friedmann AC, Goldsmith P. Systemic pyoderma gangrenosum responding to infliximab and adalimumab. *Br J Dermatol* 2005; **152**: 1059–61.

29 Reguiaï Z, Grange F. The role of anti-tumor necrosis factor-alpha therapy in pyoderma gangrenosum associated with inflammatory bowel disease. *Am J Clin Dermatol* 2007; **8**: 767–77.

30 Fujimoto E, Fujimoto N, Kuroda K, Tajima S. Leukocytapheresis treatment for pyoderma gangrenosum. *Br J Dermatol* 2004; **151**: 1090–2.

31 Okuma K, Mitsuishi K, Hasegawa T et al. A case report of steroid and immunosuppressant-resistant pyoderma gangrenosum successfully treated by granulocytapheresis. *Therap Apher Dial* 2007; **11**: 387–90.

32 Dirschka T, Kastner U, Behrens S et al. Successful treatment of pyoderma gangrenosum with intravenous human immunoglobulin. *J Am Acad Dermatol* 1998; **39**: 789–90.

33 Cummins DL, Anhalt GJ, Monahan T, Meyerle JH. Treatment of pyoderma gangrenosum with intravenous immunoglobulin. *Br J Dermatol* 2007; **157**: 1235–9.

34 Kreuter A, Reich-Schupke S, Stücker M et al. Intravenous immunoglobulin for pyoderma gangrenosum. *Br J Dermatol* 2008; **158**: 856–7.

35 Cliff S, Holden CA, Thomas PR et al. Split skin grafts in the treatment of pyoderma gangrenosum. *Ann Plast Surg* 2001; **46**: 23–8.

36 Limova M, Mauro T. Treatment of pyoderma gangrenosum with cultured keratinocyte autografts. *J Dermatol Surg Oncol* 1994; **20**: 833–6.

37 de Imus G, Golomb C, Wilkel C et al. Accelerated healing of pyoderma gangrenosum treated with bioengineered skin and concomitant immunosuppression. *J Am Acad Dermatol* 2001; **44**: 61–6.

Sweet's syndrome

Synonyms
- Acute febrile neutrophilic dermatosis
- Gomm–Button disease

Definition. Sweet's syndrome is characterized by fever, peripheral neutrophil leukocytosis, acute onset of painful, erythematous papules, plaques or nodules and histological findings of a dense neutrophilic infiltrate without evidence of primary vasculitis [1]. Sweet's syndrome can be subdivided into three groups, depending on the clinical setting:

1 classical or idiopathic (classical may be the better term, as upper respiratory and other infections, IBD and pregnancy are all well documented triggers; thus the condition is not really idiopathic in such cases)
2 malignancy-associated
3 drug-induced [2].

Diagnostic criteria have been proposed for Sweet's syndrome [3,4] and also specifically for drug-induced cases [5]. The subject has been reviewed on many occasions, including two recent and comprehensive reviews [6,7]. It is also now acknowledged to have systemic manifestations, discussed separately (p. 50.81).

History and nomenclature. Sweet first described eight women with a 'distinctive and fairly severe illness' in 1964 [1]. The name Gomm–Button disease referred to initial patients with the condition. In retrospect, a patient described by Costello [8] probably had the same condition and was thus the first malignancy-associated case, having acute myelogenous leukaemia [8]. Sweet's syndrome is now considered the prototype of the wider spectrum of neutrophilic dermatoses discussed earlier.

References
1 Sweet RD. An acute febrile neutrophilic dermatosis. *Br J Dermatol* 1964; **76**: 349–56.
2 Cohen PR, Kurzrock R. Sweet's syndrome: a neutrophilic dermatosis classically associated with acute onset and fever. *Clin Dermatol* 2000; **18**: 265–82.
3 Su WPD, Liu H-NH. Diagnostic criteria for Sweet's syndrome. *Cutis* 1986; **37**: 167–74.
4 von den Driesch P. Sweet's syndrome: acute febrile neutrophilic dermatosis. *J Am Acad Dermatol* 1994; **31**: 535–56.
5 Walker DC, Cohen PR. Trimethoprim-sulfamethoxazole-associated acute febrile neutrophilic dermatosis: case report and review of drug induced Sweet's syndrome. *J Am Acad Dermatol* 1996; **34**: 918–23.
6 Cohen PR, Kurzrock R. Sweet's syndrome revisited: a review of disease concepts. *Int J Dermatol* 2003; **42**: 761–78.
7 Cohen PR. Sweet's syndrome—a comprehensive review of an acute febrile neutrophilic dermatosis. *Orphanet J Rare Dis* 2007; **2**: 34.
8 Costello MJ, Canizares O, Montague M III et al. Cutaneous manifestations of myelogenous leukaemia. *Arch Dermatol* 1955; **71**: 605–14.

Aetiology and pathogenesis. Sweet's syndrome is associated with underlying disease in approximately 50% of cases (Table 50.21) [1–6].

Classical or idiopathic Sweet's syndrome typically affects women in the third to fifth decade and has been associated with infection (streptococcal upper respiratory infections and yersinial gastrointestinal infections), IBD (ulcerative colitis and Crohn's disease) [1–6] and pregnancy [7].

Malignancy-associated Sweet's syndrome is estimated to comprise 20–25% [1,3,4,8–10]; in this situation, men and women are equally affected [3,10]. Most tumours are haematological malignancies, especially acute myelogenous leukaemia. However, solid tumours, most commonly of genitourinary organs, breast and gastrointestinal tract, are present in about 15% [8,9]. Sweet's syndrome may be the initial manifestation of malignancy or may precede the diagnosis by months to years, making close follow-up essential. In addition, recurrent episodes of Sweet's syndrome may be an indication of cancer recurrence [2,10].

Drug-induced Sweet's syndrome most commonly occurs in patients receiving granulocyte colony-stimulating factor (G-CSF) therapy [11,12], including recent pegylated types and other newer preparations [13,14]. Additional drugs implicated include all-*trans*-retinoic acid [15,16], minocycline [17,18], trimethoprim–sulfamethoxazole [19], carbamazepine [5] and oral contraceptives [20]; other drug associations (some possibly being coincidental) are listed in [3,21].

Other conditions reported in association with Sweet's syndrome include Behçet's disease [22], erythema nodosum [23], sarcoidosis [24–26], rheumatoid arthritis [4,27] and thyroid disease [28]; again, some reports may represent coincidental occurrences rather than true disease associations. The most reported, or most logical, are listed in Table 50.21. Triggering by various different types of trauma, although possibly only relevant if there is an existing systemic stimulus, are discussed in the section on clinical features. There may be some familial tendency; sibling cases have been described [29] and an association with HLA-type Bw54 (discussed

Table 50.21 Conditions that have been associated with Sweet's syndrome/neutrophilic dermatosis.

Category	Examples	Comment
Infections	Streptococcal and upper respiratory tract Gastrointestinal (especially *Salmonella*, *Yersinia*) Mycobacterial infections (including vaccinations) Many others	Upper respiratory tract infections; *Salmonella* and *Yersinia* are well documented causes of 'classical' Sweet's syndrome See also text for discussion of human granulocytic anaplasmosis
Inflammatory bowel disease	Ulcerative colitis Crohn's disease	Well documented causes of 'classical' Sweet's syndrome
Endocrine	Pregnancy Autoimmune thyroid disease	Pregnancy and thyroid disease are relatively well documented
Immunological disorders	Collagen vascular disorders: lupus erythematosus, Sjögren's syndrome, others Others: autoimmune thrombocytopenic purpura, pemphigus	
Haematological malignancy and related conditions, immunodeficiencies	Acute myelogenous leukaemias Myelodysplastic conditions, polycythaemia Aplastic anaemia Fanconi's anaemia Monoclonal gammopathy Lymphomas (various, less common) Chronic granulomatous disease Congenital deficiencies: neutropenia, T-cell immunodeficiency, complement deficiency	Strong evidence linking leukaemias and myelodysplastic disorders Some series suggest a significant association with paraproteinaemias; chronic granulomatous disease, see text
Other malignancies	Genitourinary Breast Gastrointestinal Prostate Larynx Many others	No specific site-association apparent other than the haematological group
Other medical conditions	Sarcoidosis Rheumatoid arthritis Still's disease SAPHO	Many reports of sarcoidosis
Medications	Numerous; the most consistently associated agents are: • Colony-stimulating factors (including recent pegylated types) • Neutrophil-maturation drugs (all-*trans* retinoic acid) • Other haematological treatments (imatinib mesylate, bortezomib) • contraceptives • propylthiouracil Physical treatments for haematological malignancy have also been implicated, in a patient having splenic irradiation	Although most colony-stimulating factor-related Sweet's syndrome has been reported in patients with haematological malignancy, there are also several reports of the same phenomenon in other contexts (e.g. congenital immunodeficiencies) As with vasculitis, there may be positive ANCA with thiouracils
Other neutrophilic dermatoses and related conditions	Pyoderma gangrenosum Neutrophilic dermatosis of the dorsal hands Erythema elevatum diutinum Relapsing polychondritis Neutrophilic eccrine hidradenitis Subcorneal pustular dermatosis Erythema nodosum Behçet's disease Vasculitis (various)	In some cases, several are associated either concurrently or sequentially
Mucosal manifestations of Sweet's syndrome	Oral or genital mucosa ulceration Ocular inflammation especially conjunctivitis, also nodular episcleritis	Oral lesions especially in cases with haematological malignancy; conjunctivitis mainly in classical Sweet's syndrome
Systemic manifestations of neutrophilic dermatoses, and deeper variants	Bone, muscle, tendons, neuro-Sweet's, heart, lung, liver, intestine, spleen, kidney, subcutaneous (Sweet's panniculitis)	Summarized on p. 50.80
Unusual consequences of Sweet's syndrome	Acquired cutis laxa, mid-dermal elastolysis, elastophagocytosis	Several cases of acquired cutis laxa

SAPHO: synovitis, acne, pustulosis, hyperostosis, osteomyelitis.

in more detail in the differentiation between neuro-Sweet's syndrome and neuro-Behçet's disease, p. 50.82).

As with the other neutrophilic dermatoses, the pathogenesis of Sweet's syndrome is unknown, but it is thought to be related to altered immunological reactivity. A hypersensitivity reaction to bacterial, viral, drug or tumour antigens has been suggested as a possible aetiology. This hypothesis is supported by the frequent association of Sweet's syndrome with infection, drugs or malignancy, along with the clinical improvement of symptoms and lesions with corticosteroid treatment. Circulating autoantibodies [30], immune complexes [31] and cytokines have also been proposed to play a part in the pathogenesis of Sweet's syndrome. Atypical ANCA have been found in a few cases of Sweet's syndrome but not in others [30]; in ten patients with Sweet's syndrome, two had C-ANCA of IgA class (both with BPI specificity) but these could only be demonstrated on ethanol-fixed neutrophils, and formaldehyde fixation gave uniformly negative results [32]. Interleukin IL-1 has been suspected of playing a role for some years [33], but IL-3, IL-6, IL-8 and colony stimulating factors are also probably relevant [4]. Cytokine dysregulation has been a favoured theory in the pathogenesis of Sweet's syndrome, an imbalance of cytokine secretion from helper T cells (Th) being implicated. Th1 cytokines (IL-2 and IFN-γ) rather than Th2 cytokines (IL-4) are the proposed mediators, which in turn may stimulate the cytokine cascade leading to activation of neutrophils and release of toxic metabolites [34]; however, an integral role for colony-stimulating factors would appear to have more support.

Elevated serum levels of granulocyte colony-stimulating factor were demonstrated in patients with active Sweet's syndrome, and were associated with reduced neutrophil apoptosis; furthermore, incubation of autologous neutrophils with patient serum caused reduced apoptosis [35], and would account for accumulation of neutrophils which are the hallmark of this condition. Increased superoxide anion generation, a potential consequence of tissue neutrophilia (and for which prednisolone is a potent inhibitor), has been documented in leukaemia- and myelodysplasia-associated Sweet's syndrome [36], and various diverse tumours produce granulocyte colony-stimulating factor [4,37].

There are some issues of interest in relation to the involvement of neutrophils in Sweet's syndrome, that extend the recognized fact that neutrophilic dermatoses can occur during granulocytopenia [38]. The occurrence of other cell types is discussed in the section on histology. First, Sweet's syndrome has been reported in a patient with *chronic granulomatous disease*, a condition in which defects in NADPH-oxidase lead to failure of neutrophil intracellular oxidative killing; thus, this mechanism does not have to be functional in order to develop Sweet's syndrome [39]. Second, there is an interesting case of Sweet's syndrome in a patient with *human granulocytic anaplasmosis* (formerly human granulocytotropic ehrlichiosis) [40]. The causative organism, *Anaplasma phagocytophilum*, is an intracellular infection that infects, multiplies in and disrupts neutrophil function. Whether this means that human granulocytic anaplasmosis is a true cause of Sweet's syndrome is uncertain but, again, it documents that Sweet's syndrome can occur when there is impairment of normal neutrophil function. Third, a patient with congenital neutropenia developed Sweet's syndrome when he was treated with *pegfilgrastim*, a pegylated granulocyte colony-stimulating factor, despite many uneventful treatments both before and subsequently with standard granulocyte colony-stimulating factor [14]. The observation was made that pegfilgrastim has a half-life of 33 h in comparison with 3.4 h for the parent drug, filgrastim; furthermore, filgrastim is largely renally-excreted whereas pegfilgrastim is too large to be eliminated in this fashion, and it is actually removed from the circulation by neutrophil receptor-mediated clearance (binding to the neutrophil G-CSF receptor ligand) and therefore stimulating production of (potentially abnormally functional) neutrophils. Finally, there are reported cases of Sweet's syndrome associated with specific (6:9) translocations in myelodysplastic syndromes [41,42]; it has been suggested that these patients may have clonal neutrophils that could perhaps be more susceptible to the stimuli such as colony-stimulating factors, or exhibit an enhanced skin tropism to account for associated Sweet's syndrome.

Other aspects relating to pathogenesis that have been examined include immunohistochemical studies to detect immune complex deposition in blood vessels. These have yielded inconsistent results, some investigators reporting immunoglobulins and complement within vessel walls [43–45] but others not confirming this [1,46]. Additional studies have found perivascular IgG, IgM, C3 and fibrin, thought to represent non-specific leakage from damaged vessels [47].

References

1 von den Driesch P. Sweet's syndrome: acute febrile neutrophilic dermatosis. *J Am Acad Dermatol* 1994; **31**: 535–56.

2 Su WPD, Liu H-NH. Diagnostic criteria for Sweet's syndrome. *Cutis* 1986; **37**: 167–74.

3 Cohen PR, Kurzrock R. Sweet's syndrome revisited: a review of disease concepts. *Int J Dermatol* 2003; **42**: 761–78.

4 Cohen PR. Sweet's syndrome—a comprehensive review of an acute febrile neutrophilic dermatosis. *Orphanet J Rare Dis* 2007; **2**: 34.

5 Cohen PR, Kurzrock R. Sweet's syndrome: a neutrophilic dermatosis classically associated with acute onset and fever. *Clin Dermatol* 2000; **18**: 265–82.

6 Kemmett D, Hunter JAA. Sweet's syndrome: a clinicopathologic review of 29 cases. *J Am Acad Dermatol* 1990; **23**: 503–7.

7 Cohen PR. Pregnancy-associated Sweet's syndrome: world literature review. *Obstet Gynecol Surv* 1993; **48**: 584–7.

8 Cohen PR, Talpaz M, Kurzrock R. Malignancy-associated Sweet's syndrome: review of the world literature. *J Clin Oncol* 1988; **6**: 1887–97.

9 Cohen PR, Holder WR, Tucker SB *et al*. Sweet syndrome in patients with solid tumors. *Cancer* 1993; **72**: 2723–31.

10 Cohen PR, Kurzrock R. Sweet's syndrome and cancer. *Clin Dermatol* 1993; **11**: 149–57.

11 Paydas S, Berksoy S, Seyrek E *et al*. Sweet's syndrome associated with G-CSF. *Br J Haematol* 1993; **85**: 191–2.

12 Park JW, Mehrotra B, Barnett BO *et al*. The Sweet syndrome during therapy with granulocyte-colony stimulating factor. *Ann Intern Med* 1992; **116**: 996–8.

13 Kumar G, Bernstein JM, Waibel JS, Baumann MA. Sweet's syndrome associated with sargramostin (granulocyte-macrophage colony-stimulating factor). *Am J Hematol* 2004; **76**: 283–5.

14 Draper BK, Robbins JB, Stricklin PG. Bullous Sweet's syndrome in congenital neutropenia: association with pegfilgrastim. *J Am Acad Dermatol* 2005; **52**: 901–5.

15 Cox NH, O'Brien HAW. Sweet's syndrome associated with *trans*-retinoic acid treatment in acute promyelocytic leukemia. *Clin Exp Dermatol* 1994; **19**: 51–2.

16 Piette WW, Trapp JF, O'Donnell MJ *et al*. Acute neutrophilic dermatosis with myeloblastic infiltrate in a leukemia patient receiving all-*trans*-retinoic acid therapy. *J Am Acad Dermatol* 1994; **30**: 293–7.

17 Mensing H, Kowalzick L. Acute febrile neutrophilic dermatosis (Sweet's syndrome) caused by minocycline. *Dermatologica* 1991; **182**: 43–6.

18 Thibault MJ, Billick RC, Srolovitz H. Minocycline-induced Sweet's syndrome. *J Am Acad Dermatol* 1992; **27**: 801–4.

19 Walker DC, Cohen PR. Trimethoprim-sulfamethoxazole-associated acute febrile neutrophilic dermatosis: case report and review of drug-induced Sweet's syndrome. *J Am Acad Dermatol* 1996; **34**: 918–23.

20 Tefany FJ, Georgouras K. A neutrophilic reaction of Sweet's syndrome type associated with the oral contraceptive. *Australas J Dermatol* 1991; **32**: 55–9.

21 Thompson DF, Montarella KE. Drug-induced Sweet's syndrome. *Ann Pharmacother* 2007; **41**: 802–11.

22 Lee MS, Barnetson R. Sweet's syndrome associated with Behçet's disease. *Australas J Dermatol* 1996; **37**: 99–101.

23 Waltz KM, Long D, Marks JG *et al.* Sweet's syndrome and erythema nodosum: the simultaneous occurrence of two reactive dermatoses. *Arch Dermatol* 1999; **135**: 62–6.

24 Gillott TJ, Whallett AJ, Struthers GR *et al.* Concurrent Sweet's syndrome (acute febrile neutrophilic dermatosis), erythema nodosum, and sarcoidosis (letter). *Clin Exp Dermatol* 1996; **22**: 54–6.

25 Pouchot J, Bourgeots-Droin C, Vinceneu P *et al.* Sweet's syndrome and mediastinal lymphadenopathy due to sarcoidosis: three cases of a new association. *Arch Dermatol* 1993; **129**: 1062–4.

26 Wilkinson SM, Heagerty AHM, English JSC. Acute febrile neutrophilic dermatosis in association with erythema nodosum and sarcoidosis. *Clin Exp Dermatol* 1993; **18**: 47–9.

27 Wilson DM, John JR, Callen PR. Peripheral ulcerative keratitis: an extracutaneous neutrophilic disorder. Report of a patient with rheumatoid arthritis, pustular vasculitis, pyoderma gangrenosum, and Sweet's syndrome with an excellent response to cyclosporine therapy. *J Am Acad Dermatol* 1999; **40**: 331–4.

28 O'Brien TJ, Darling JA. Sweet's syndrome and hypothyroidism. *Australas J Dermatol* 1994; **35**: 91–2.

29 Parsapour K, Reep MD, Gohar K *et al.* Familial Sweet's syndrome in 2 brothers, both seen in the first 2 weeks of life. *J Am Acad Dermatol* 2003; **49**: 132–8.

30 Kemmett D, Harrison DJ, Hunter JAA. Antibodies to neutrophil cytoplasmic antigens: a serologic marker for Sweet's syndrome. *J Am Acad Dermatol* 1991; **24**: 967–9.

31 Behm FG, Kay S, Aportela R. Febrile neutrophilic dermatoses associated with acute leukemia. *Am J Clin Pathol* 1981; **76**: 344–7.

32 Ayoub N, Charuel J-L, Diemerte M-C *et al.* Antineutrophil cytoplasmic antibodies of IgA class in neutrophilic dermatoses with emphasis on erythema elevatum diutinum. *Arch Dermatol* 2004; **140**: 931–6.

33 Bourke JF, Jones JL, Fletcher A, Graham-Brown RAC. An immunohistochemical study of the dermal infiltrate and epidermal staining for interleukin-1 in 12 cases of Sweet's syndrome. *Br J Dermatol* 1996; **134**: 705–9.

34 Giasuddin ASM, El-Orfi AHAM, Ziu MM, El-Barnawi NY. Sweet's syndrome: is the pathogenesis mediated by helper T cell type 1 cytokines? *J Am Acad Dermatol* 1998; **39**: 940–3.

35 Kawakami T, Ohashi S, Kawa Y *et al.* Elevated serum granulocyte colony-stimulating factor levels in patients with active phase of Sweet syndrome and patients with active Behçet disease. Implication in neutrophil apoptosis dysfunction. *Arch Dermatol* 2004; **140**: 570–4.

36 Komiya I, Tanoue K, Kakinuma K *et al.* Superoxide anion hyperproduction by neutrophils in a case of myelodysplastic syndrome. Association with Sweet's syndrome and interstitial pneumonia. *Cancer* 1991; **67**: 237–41.

37 Shinojima Y, Toma Y, Terui T. Sweet syndrome associated with intrahepatic cholangiocarcinoma producing granulocyte colony-stimulating factor. *Br J Dermatol* 2006; **154**: 1103–4.

38 Aractingi S, Mallet V, Pnquier L *et al.* Neutrophilic dermatoses during granulocytopenia. *Arch Dermatol* 1995; **131**: 1141–5.

39 Lyon CC, Griffiths CEM. Chronic granulomatous disease and acute neutrophilic dermatosis. *Clin Exp Dermatol* 1999; **24**: 368–71.

40 Halasz CLG, Niedt GW, Kurtz CP *et al.* A case of Sweet syndrome associated with human granulocytic anaplasmosis. *Arch Dermatol* 2005; **141**: 887–90.

41 Soekarman M, Von Lindern M, Daenen S *et al.* The translocation (6:9) (p23:q34) shows consistent rearrangement of two genes and defines a myeloproliferative disorder with specific clinical features. *Blood* 1992; **79**: 2990–7.

42 Mégarbane B, Bodemer C, Valensi F *et al.* Association of acute neutrophilic dermatosis and myelodysplastic syndrome with (6:9) chromosome translocation: a case report and review of the literature. *Br J Dermatol* 2000; **143**: 1327–9.

43 Nunzi E, Crovato F, Dallegri R *et al.* Immunopathological studies on a case of Sweet's syndrome. *Dermatologica* 1981; **163**: 393–400.

44 Takeuchi S, Mashiko T, Ingarashi M. A case of Sweet's disease with deposition of immunoglobulins and complement. *Rinsho Hifuka* 1982; **36**: 557–62.

45 Maekawa Y, Kageshita T, Nagata T. A case of acute febrile neutrophilic dermatosis (Sweet's syndrome): a demonstration of IgM and C3 deposits. *J Dermatol* 1984; **11**: 560–4.

46 Malone JC, Slone SP, Wills-Frank LA *et al.* Vascular inflammation (vasculitis) in Sweet syndrome. *Arch Dermatol* 2002; **138**: 345–9.

47 Going JJ, Going SM, Myskow MW *et al.* Sweet's syndrome: histological and immunohistochemical study of 15 cases. *J Clin Pathol* 1987; **40**: 175–9.

Histopathology. The diagnostic histopathological features of Sweet's syndrome include a dense, predominantly neutrophilic, infiltrate located in the superficial dermis, and prominent papillary dermal oedema which may occasionally lead to subepidermal vesiculation [1–4]. Lymphocytes, eosinophils and 'histiocytes' may be present (discussed below). The infiltrate often occurs in a diffuse pattern, but may be perivascular or have an upper dermal band-like distribution [5]. Neutrophil karyorrhexis (fragmented neutrophil nuclei; nuclear dust) is a common finding [2]. The epidermis is often normal, but spongiosis may be present, and rarely neutrophils may extend into the epidermis to form subcorneal pustules [6]. There are two major histopathological controversies in Sweet's syndrome, one being the role of different cell types in the infiltrate, and the other being whether or not vasculitis occurs; these will be briefly discussed.

In most instances, the main cell type present is the neutrophil. Several studies suggest that there may be an admixture of lymphocytes and/or eosinophils, either of which can be prominent in some cases [2,3]. Several small case series have documented a lymphocytic infiltrate over many months, typically in patients who then develop a haematological malignancy [7,8]. There has been debate about whether frankly malignant myeloid cells might be present in some cases, but it seems unreasonable that a skin infiltrate in a patient with circulating leukaemic cells might not have some abnormal myeloid series cells present [9–11], as documented in some reports [9] prior to the claimed 'first' demonstration of this feature [10]. It has also now been clearly documented that 'histiocytoid' cells in the infiltrate actually represent myeloblast-like immature neutrophil granulocytes [12]; although the histiocytoid cells in 41 patients stained positively with monocyte-histiocyte markers, they also stained strongly with myeloperoxidase, and a variety of measures, including fluorescent *in situ* hybridization studies in 14 patients to exclude *bcr/abl* gene fusion, confirmed that these cells did not represent a leukaemic infiltrate.

Historically, the presence of vasculitis excluded the diagnosis of Sweet's syndrome, but recent studies have reported histopathological features consistent with leukocytoclastic vasculitis. These findings include fibrinoid necrosis along with the presence of inflammatory cells within vessel walls. Additional evidence of vessel wall damage includes extravasated erythrocytes and intraluminal thrombi. However, multiple immunofluorescence studies have failed to consistently demonstrate immune complex-mediated injury, further supporting the theory of secondary vessel damage rather than a primary vasculitis. It has been proposed that toxic metabolites released by activated neutrophils may have a role in the secondary vessel wall injury [1–3,5,13,14]. In a recent study, 74% of biopsies showed all criteria for a diagnosis of leukocytoclastic vasculitis (vessel disruption by neutrophils, leukocytoclasis and fibrin in or around vessels walls [2]), and nearly two-thirds also had erythrocyte extravasation.

References

1 von den Driesch P. Sweet's syndrome: acute febrile neutrophilic dermatosis. *J Am Acad Dermatol* 1994; **31**: 535–56.

2 Ratzinger G, Burgdorf W, Zelger BG, Zelger B. Acute febrile neutrophilic dermatosis: a histopathologic study of 31 cases with review of literature. *Am J Dermatopathol* 2007; **29**: 125–33.

3 Jordaan HF. Acute febrile neutrophilic dermatosis: a histopathological study of 37 cases and a review of the literature. *Am J Dermatopathol* 1989; **11**: 99–111.

4 Kemmett D, Hunter JAA. Sweet's syndrome: a clinicopathologic review of 29 cases. *J Am Acad Dermatol* 1990; **23**: 503–7.

5 Malone JC, Slone SP, Wills-Frank LA *et al.* Vascular inflammation (vasculitis) in Sweet syndrome. A clinicopathologic study of 28 biopsy specimens from 21 patients. *Arch Dermatol* 2002; **138**: 345–9.

6 Wallach D. Maladie neutrophilique. *Rev Prat* 1999; **49**: 356–8.

7 Evans AV, Sabroe RA, Liddell K, Russell-Jones R. Lymphocytic infiltrates as a presenting feature of Sweet's syndrome with myelodysplasia and response to cyclophosphamide. *Br J Dermatol* 2002; **146**: 1087–90.

8 Vignon-Pennamen M-D, Juillard C, Rybojad M *et al.* Chronic recurrent lymphocytic Sweet syndrome as a predictive marker of myelodysplasia. A report of 9 cases. *Arch Dermatol* 2006; **142**: 1170–6.

9 Cox NH, O'Brien HAW. Sweet's syndrome associated with *trans*-retinoic acid treatment in acute promyelocytic leukemia. *Clin Exp Dermatol* 1994; **19**: 51–2.

10 Urano Y, Miyaoka Y, Kosaka M *et al.* Sweet's syndrome associated with chronic myelogenous leukaemia: demonstration of leukaemic cells within a skin lesion. *J Am Acad Dermatol* 1999; **40**: 275–9.

11 Morgan KW, Callen JP. Sweet's syndrome in acute myelogenous leukaemia presenting as periorbital cellulitis with an infiltrate of leukaemic cells. *J Am Acad Dermatol* 2001; **45**: 590–5.

12 Requena L, Kutzner H, Palmedo G *et al.* Histiocytoid Sweet syndrome. A dermal infiltration of immature neutrophil granulocytes. *Arch Dermatol* 2005; **141**: 834–42.

13 Malone JC, Slone SP. Sweet syndrome. A disease in histologic evolution? *Arch Dermatol* 2005; **141**: 893–5.

14 von den Driesch P. Sweet's syndrome and vasculitis. *J Am Acad Dermatol* 1996; **34**: 539.

Clinical features. The clinical presentation of Sweet's syndrome is usually distinctive. The patient typically appears ill, with a persistent high fever, neutrophilia and an elevated ESR. The cutaneous manifestations consist of erythematous to violaceous tender papules or nodules that often coalesce to form irregular plaques (Figs 50.40 & 50.41) [1–6]. The lesions typically involve the arms, face and neck, but may occur anywhere, and are usually multiple but may be solitary. Later lesions may appear pseudovesicular because of the prominent dermal oedema [1,2,7], and may be studded with tiny pustules resulting from neutrophil migration into the epidermis; in some cases frank bullae develop [8]. The plaques may develop central yellowish discoloration, producing a targetoid appearance [1]. The distribution may be localized, particularly on the face [1–6], or widespread, as may occur in malignancy-associated cases [9]. Several unusual body site distributions have been reported, including localization to recent wounds (Koebner response) [10], localization to old scars [11], localization to an area of lymphoedema (in a patient receiving colony-stimulating factor) [12] and localization to an area of radiotherapy [13]. Photoaggravated and photoinduced Sweet's

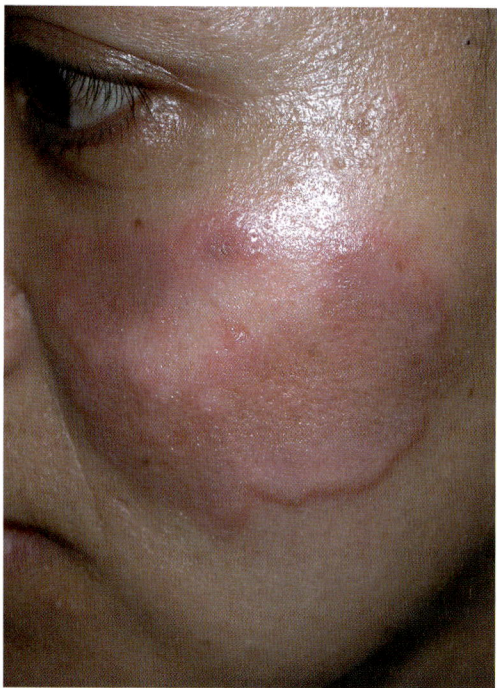

Fig. 50.40 Sweet's syndrome. The face is often affected.

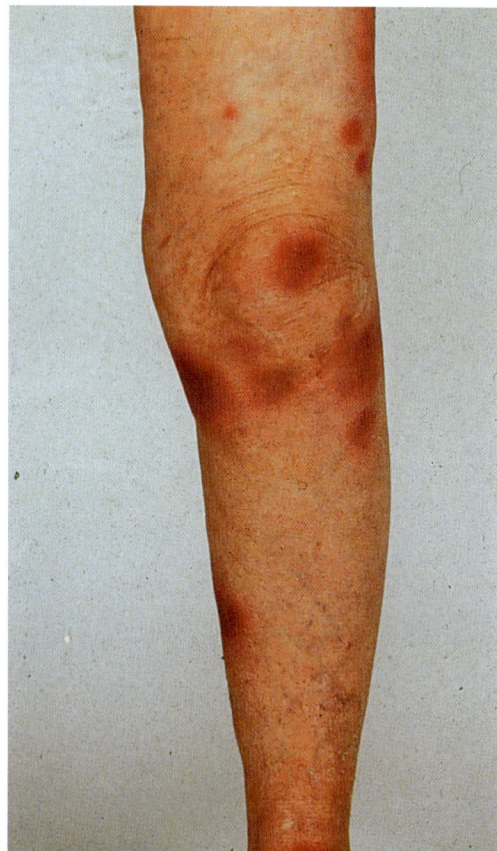

Fig. 50.41 Sweet's syndrome. Multiple, large erythematous lesions on the legs.

syndrome have also been reported [14]. Healing usually occurs without scarring, although this can occur, particularly on the hands where it may have a reticulated appearance (see Fig. 50.43).

Associated features typically, but not always, include fever and malaise; fever is the most common but may be absent, especially in malignancy-associated Sweet's syndrome [9]. Ocular manifestations are often found, most commonly conjunctivitis or episcleritis. Oral lesions are uncommon in the classical pattern but are more strongly linked with underlying haematological disorders [9]; genital lesions also occur. Subungual erythema has been reported [15]. A variety of systemic manifestations can occur, arthralgia, myalgia and arthritis also occurring frequently. Systemic manifestations of neutrophilic dermatoses are discussed on p. 50.80.

Diagnosis. The proposed diagnostic criteria for Sweet's syndrome state that patients must meet both of the two major criteria and two of the four minor criteria for the diagnosis [16,17].
Major criteria:
1 Acute onset of typical skin lesions
2 Histopathological findings consistent with Sweet's syndrome
Minor criteria:
1 Fever >38°C or general malaise
2 Association with malignancy, inflammatory disorder or pregnancy, or antecedent respiratory or gastrointestinal infection
3 Excellent response to systemic corticosteroids or potassium iodide (KI)
4 Abnormal laboratory values at presentation (three of four required: ESR >20 mm; leukocytes >8000; neutrophils >70%; positive C-reactive protein).

For drug-induced Sweet's syndrome, both major criteria and fever >38°C are required, together with two proposed additional criteria: (i) a temporal relationship between drug administration and clinical presentation; and (ii) a temporal relationship between drug withdrawal and disease resolution [18].

Otherwise, the differential diagnosis is wide. It includes infections (cellulitis/erysipelas, herpes virus infections, viral and bacterial exanthems), inflammatory dermatoses (erythema multiforme, urticaria, erythema nodosum, rosacea, pyoderma faciale, lupus erythematosus, drug eruptions, halogenodermas), tumours (especially leukaemia cutis), and other neutrophilic dermatoses and vasculitides.

References
1 von den Driesch P. Sweet's syndrome: acute febrile neutrophilic dermatosis. *J Am Acad Dermatol* 1994; **31**: 535–56.
2 Cohen PR. Sweet's syndrome—a comprehensive review of an acute febrile neutrophilic dermatosis. *Orphanet J Rare Dis* 2007; **2**: 34.
3 Cohen PR, Kurzrock R. Sweet's syndrome: a neutrophilic dermatosis classically associated with acute onset and fever. *Clin Dermatol* 2000; **18**: 265–82.
4 Callen JP. Neutrophilic dermatoses. *Dermatol Clin* 2002; **20**: 409–19.
5 Whittle CH, Beck GA, Champion RH. Recurrent neutrophilic dermatosis of the face: a variant of Sweet's syndrome. *Br J Dermatol* 1968; **80**: 806–10.
6 Bulengo-Ransby SM, Brown MD, Dubin HV *et al*. Sweet's syndrome presenting as an unusual periorbital eruption. *J Am Acad Dermatol* 1991; **24**: 140–1.
7 Honigsmann H, Kempter R, Wolff K. Acute febrile neutrophile dermatose. *Wien Klin Wochenschr* 1979; **91**: 842–7.
8 Neoh CY, Tan AWH, Ng SK. Sweet's syndrome: a spectrum of unusual clinical presentations and associations. *Br J Dermatol* 2007; **156**: 480–5.
9 Cohen PR, Kurzrock R. Sweet's syndrome and cancer. *Clin Dermatol* 1993; **11**: 149–57.
10 Tavadia SMB, Smith G, Herd RM, Zuk RJ. Sweet's syndrome associated with oral squamous cell carcinoma and exhibiting the Koebner phenomenon. *Br J Dermatol* 1999; **141**: 169–70.
11 Atzori L, Ferreli C, Pinna AL *et al*. P07.16. Sweet's syndrome lesions within pre-existing scars. *J Eur Acad Dermatol Venereol* 2004; **18** (Suppl.): 363.
12 Petit T, Francès C, Marinho E *et al*. Lymphoedema-area-restricted Sweet syndrome during G-CSF treatment. *Lancet* 1996; **347**: 690.
13 Vergara G, Vargas-Machuca I, Pastor MA *et al*. Localization of Sweet's syndrome in radiation-induced locus minoris resistentae. *J Am Acad Dermatol* 2003; **49**: 907–9.
14 Bessis D, Dereure O, Peyron J-L *et al*. Photoinduced Sweet syndrome. *Arch Dermatol* 2003; **137**: 1106–8.
15 Viseux V, Boulenger A, Jestin B, Plantin P. Transient subungual erythema in a patient with idiopathic Sweet's syndrome. *J Am Acad Dermatol* 2003; **49**: 554–5.
16 Su WPD, Liu H-NH. Diagnostic criteria for Sweet's syndrome. *Cutis* 1986; **37**: 167–74.
17 von den Driesch P. Sweet's syndrome: acute febrile neutrophilic dermatosis. *J Am Acad Dermatol* 1994; **31**: 535–56.
18 Walker DC, Cohen PR. Trimethoprim-sulfamethoxazole-associated acute febrile neutrophilic dermatosis: case report and review of drug-induced Sweet's syndrome. *J Am Acad Dermatol* 1996; **34**: 918–23.

Treatment. Treatments used in Sweet's syndrome have been summarized in [1–3]; further comprehensive details of the therapies discussed below are provided. Therapies for Sweet's syndrome are depicted in Table 50.22.

Systemic corticosteroids are a standard and effective therapy for Sweet's syndrome. A 4- to 6-week course of prednisone is generally sufficient to resolve cutaneous and systemic symptoms and signs, but occasionally prolonged low-dosage treatment may be required to prevent recurrences. In addition, topical and intralesional corticosteroids may be used alone or as adjuvant therapy for localized lesions [4].

Many corticosteroid-sparing agents have been reported to be effective in the treatment of Sweet's syndrome. Oral therapy with potassium iodide and colchicine has led to rapid regression of lesions and symptoms. These agents may be reasonable first-line therapy in patients with milder disease [5–9]. Indometacin and clofazimine have been used with success but appear to be less effective than corticosteroids, potassium iodide and colchicine [1–3,10]. Dapsone and ciclosporin have also been reported to be effective therapeutic agents, but require laboratory monitoring because of their potentially serious adverse effects [1–3,11–15].

Table 50.22 Treatment of Sweet's syndrome.

Corticosteroids
Systemic for 4–6 weeks
Adjuvant therapy for localized lesions
Topical
Intralesional
Corticosteroid-sparing agents
Potassium iodide
Colchicine
Dapsone
Indometacin
Clofazimine
Ciclosporin
Cyclophosphamide
Acitretin
Thalidomide
Intravenous immunoglobulin
Interferon-α

Small studies have reported clinical improvement in Sweet's syndrome using etretinate or IFN-γ [4,16,17]. Thalidomide [18], cyclophosphamide [19] and intravenous immunoglobulins [20] have also been used; more toxic agents obviously have a greater place if treatment of an underlying haematological disorder is needed. In one patient, with Sweet's syndrome due to myelodysplasia, and refractory to numerous therapies (including several of the above, plus azathioprine, mycophenolate mofetil and plasmapheresis), use of rabbit-antithymocyte-globulin caused remission of the myelodysplasia and the associated skin lesions. Looking forward, it will be interesting to see the effect of repertaxin, which inhibits chemokine receptors CXCR1 and CXCR2 [21], thereby inhibiting responses of IL-8 (CXCL8) which is a major activator of neutrophils; such approaches may be particularly valuable in those with systemic neutrophilic dermatoses. Other avenues of exploration include development of further inhibitors of IL-8 activated neutrophil chemotaxis, such as thapsigargin [22].

References

1 Cohen PR. Sweet's syndrome—a comprehensive review of an acute febrile neutrophilic dermatosis. *Orphanet J Rare Dis* 2007; **2**: 34.

2 Cohen PR, Kurzrock R. Sweet's syndrome. A review of current treatment options. *Am J Clin Dermatol* 2002; **3**: 117–31.

3 Cohen PR, Kurzrock R. Sweet's syndrome revisited: a review of disease concepts. *Int J Dermatol* 2003; **42**: 761–78.

4 Brodkin RH, Schwartz RA. Sweet's syndrome with myelofibrosis and leukemia: partial response to interferon. *Dermatology* 1995; **190**: 160–3.

5 Hommel L, Harms M, Saurat JH. The incidence of Sweet's syndrome in Geneva: a retrospective study of 29 cases. *Dermatology* 1993; **187**: 303–5.

6 Myatt AE, Baker DJ, Byfield DM. Sweet's syndrome: a report on the use of potassium iodide. *Clin Exp Dermatol* 1987; **12**: 345–9.

7 Smith HR, Ashton RE, Beer TW *et al*. Neutrophil-poor Sweet's syndrome with response to potassium iodide. *Br J Dermatol* 1998; **139**: 555–6.

8 Maillard H, Leclech C, Peria P *et al*. Colchicine for Sweet's syndrome: a study of 20 cases. *Br J Dermatol* 1999; **140**: 565–6.

9 Ritter S, George R, Serwatka LM *et al*. Long-term suppression of chronic Sweet's syndrome with colchicine. *J Am Acad Dermatol* 2002; **47**: 323–4.

10 Jeanfils S, Joly P, Young P *et al*. Indomethacin treatment of 18 patients with Sweet's syndrome. *J Am Acad Dermatol* 1997; **36**: 436–9.

11 Aram H. Acute febrile neutrophilic dermatosis (Sweet's syndrome): response to dapsone. *Arch Dermatol* 1984; **120**: 245–7.

12 Sharpe GR, Leggat HM. A case of Sweet's syndrome and myelodysplasia: response to cyclosporin. *Br J Dermatol* 1992; **127**: 538–9.

13 von den Driesch P, Steffan C, Zobe A *et al*. Sweet's syndrome: therapy with cyclosporin. *Clin Exp Dermatol* 1994; **19**: 274–7.

14 Bourke JF, Berth-Jones J, Graham-Brown RA. Sweet's syndrome responding to cyclosporine. *Br J Dermatol* 1992; **127**: 36–8.

15 Wilson DM, John JR, Callen PR. Peripheral ulcerative keratitis: an extracutaneous neutrophilic disorder. Report of a patient with rheumatoid arthritis, pustular vasculitis, pyoderma gangrenosum, and Sweet's syndrome with an excellent response to cyclosporine therapy. *J Am Acad Dermatol* 1999; **40**: 331–4.

16 Altomare G, Capella GL, Frigerio E. Sweet's syndrome in a patient with idiopathic myelofibrosis and thymoma–myasthenia gravis immunodeficiency complex: efficacy of treatment with etretinate. *Haematologica (Pavia)* 1996; **81**: 54–8.

17 Bianchi L, Masi M, Hagman JH *et al*. Systemic interferon-γ treatment for idiopathic Sweet's syndrome. *Clin Exp Dermatol* 1999; **24**: 443–5.

18 Browning CE, Dixon JE, Malone JC, Callen JP. Thalidomide in the treatment of recalcitrant Sweet's syndrome associated with myelodysplasia. *J Am Acad Dermatol* 2005; **53**: S135–8.

19 Evans AV, Sabroe RA, Liddell K, Russell-Jones R. Lymphocytic infiltrates as a presenting feature of Sweet's syndrome with myelodysplasia and response to cyclophosphamide. *Br J Dermatol* 2002; **146**: 1087–90.

20 Haliasos E, Soder B, Rubenstein DS *et al*. Pediatric Sweet syndrome and immunodeficiency successfully treated with intravenous immunoglobulin. *Pediatr Dermatol* 2005; **22**: 530–5.

21 Casilli F, Bianchini A, Gloaguen I *et al*. Inhibition of interleukin-8 (CXCL8 / IL-8) responses by repertaxin, a new inhibitor of the chemokine receptors CXCR1 and CXCR2. *Biochem Pharmacol* 2005; **69**: 385–94.

22 Elferik JG, de Koster BM. Inhibition of interleukin-8-activated human neutrophil chemotaxis by thapsigargin in a calcium- and cyclic AMP-dependent way. *Biochem Pharmacol* 2000; **59**: 369–75.

Neutrophilic dermatosis of the (dorsal) hands

Synonyms
- Pustular vasculitis of the (dorsal) hands
- Acral Sweet's syndrome
- Atypical pyoderma gangrenosum

Several case series [1–5] and individual reports have helped to define this disorder (Figs 50.42 & 50.43). An early case series described lesions that morphologically and histologically resembled Sweet's syndrome, but had additional histological features of vessel wall necrosis and deposition of fibrin around vessels, thereby constituting a vasculitis [1]. The presence of vasculitic change in this pattern of disease has varied in subsequent reports [2,6], but most reports do not suggest a primarily angiocentric angiodestructive process [7] and, as in Sweet's syndrome [8], the presence of vasculitis in neutrophilic dermatosis of the dorsal hands is probably a consequence of intense inflammation [9].

Thus, although it has been suggested that this entity might be a vasculitic process in the spectrum of EED [10], a site-variant of Sweet's syndrome, or a, usually superficial, variant of pyoderma gangrenosum, maintaining the term 'neutrophilic dermatosis of the dorsal hands' acknowledges the disease spectrum in a way that pustular vasculitis does not. Reviewing the disease associations of this entity reveals a very similar list to that of Sweet's syndrome, including streptococcal infections/pharyngitis [5], gastroenteritis [5], monoclonal gammopathy [5], IBD [4], myelodysplasia [3], lymphoma [4] or solid organ cancers [3,4]. Additional causes include other infections [11], sarcoidosis [11], medications [12] and SAPHO [13], all associated with Sweet's

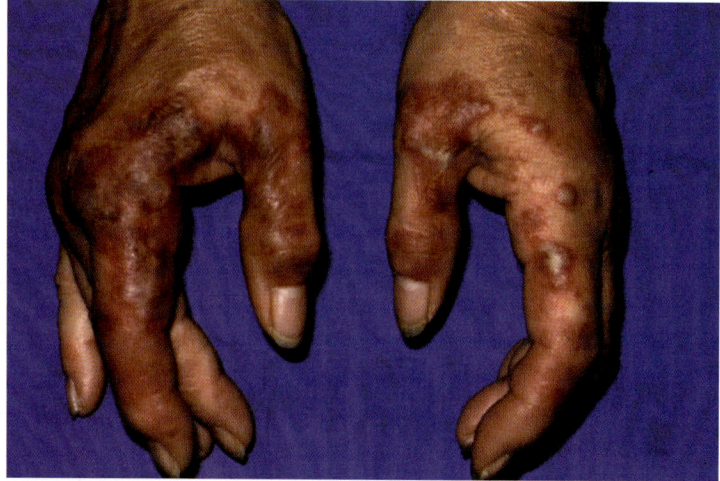

Fig. 50.42 Neutrophilic dermatosis of the dorsal hands.

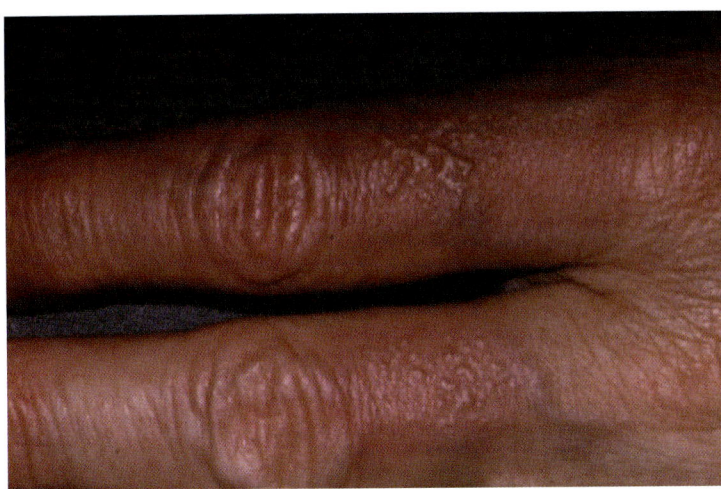

Fig. 50.43 Healing of neutrophilic dermatosis of the dorsal hands (without any associated disease) with reticulated scarring.

syndrome. Additionally, nearly 50% have lesions of Sweet's syndrome at other body sites [9], fever and leukocytosis occur in about 50% [1,2], the disorder can occur as an isolated event [5] or as a recurrent process [2], and treatments with corticosteroids or dapsone are usually effective [9].

In the review of Weenig *et al.* in 2004 [3], 25% of reported cases had had a myelodysplastic syndrome or leukaemia, supporting the view that this is an important association with neutrophilic dermatosis/atypical PG of the dorsal hands [7,14] (and often only becoming apparent after the cutaneous eruption). Indeed, review of dorsal hand lesions published earlier as either Sweet's syndrome or PG [15–18] reveals, for example, cases of newly diagnosed polycythaemia as a result of the dorsal hand lesion (termed PG) [15], of worsening myelofibrosis requiring splenectomy (PG) [16], of postpolycythaemic myeloid metaplasia progressing to leukaemia (Sweet's syndrome) [17] and of leukaemia diagnosed due to the hand lesions (Case 2; neutrophilic dermatosis) [18]. The term neutrophilic dermatosis of the dorsal hands thus lies closest to Sweet's syndrome nosologically, but includes lesions indistinguishable from PG, and has a stronger link with haematological malignancy than does 'ordinary' Sweet's syndrome, justifying retention of this terminology.

Streptococcal infection [19], other infections, neutrophilic eccrine hidradenitis, EED and other differential diagnoses for Sweet's syndrome are all in the clinical differential diagnosis; treatment is as for Sweet's syndrome or as determined by an underlying disorder.

References

1 Strutton G, Weedon D, Robertson I. Pustular vasculitis of the hands. *J Am Acad Dermatol* 1995; **32**: 192–8.
2 DiCaudo DJ, Connolly SM. Neutrophilic dermatosis (pustular vasculitis) of the dorsal hands: a report of seven cases and review of the literature. *Arch Dermatol* 2002; **138**: 361–5.
3 Weenig RH, Bruce AJ, McEvoy MT *et al.* Neutrophilic dermatosis of the hands: four new cases and review of the literature. *Int J Dermatol* 2004; **43**: 95–102.
4 Walling HW, Snipes CJ, Gerami P, Piette WW. The relationship between neutrophilic dermatosis (pustular vasculitis) of the dorsal hands and Sweet syndrome. Report of 9 cases and comparison to atypical pyoderma gangrenosum. *Arch Dermatol* 2006; **142**: 57–63.
5 Del Pozo J, Sácristan F, Martínez W *et al.* Neutrophilic dermatosis of the hands: presentation of eight cases and review of the literature. *J Dermatol* 2007; **34**: 243–7.
6 Galaria NA, Junkins-Hopkins JM, Kligman D, James WD. Neutrophilic dermatosis of the dorsal hands: pustular vasculitis revisited. *J Am Acad Dermatol* 2000; **43**: 870–4.
7 James WD. Newer neutrophilic dermatoses. *Arch Dermatol* 2003; **139**: 101–2.
8 Malone JC, Slone SP, Wills-Frank LA *et al.* Vascular inflammation (vasculitis) in Sweet syndrome: a clinicopathologic study of 28 biopsy specimens from 21 patients. *Arch Dermatol* 2002; **138**: 345–9.
9 Cohen PR. Skin lesions of Sweet syndrome and its dorsal hand variant contain vasculitis: an oxymoron or an epiphenomenon? *Arch Dermatol* 2002; **138**: 400–3.
10 Ayoub N, Tomb R. Neutrophilic dermatosis of the dorsal hands: a variant of erythema elevatum diutinum? *Arch Dermatol* 2003; **139**: 102.
11 Baz K, Yazici AC, Kaya TI *et al.* Neutrophilic dermatosis of the hands (localized Sweet's syndrome) in association with chronic hepatitis C and sarcoidosis. *Clin Exp Dermatol* 2003; **28**: 377–9.
12 Hoverson AR, Davis MPD, Weenig RH, Wolanskyj AP. Neutrophilic dermatosis (Sweet syndrome) of the hands associated with lenalidomide. *Arch Dermatol* 2006; **142**: 1070–1.
13 Bachmeyer C, Begon E, Blum L *et al.* Overlapping neutrophilic dermatosis in a patient with SAPHO syndrome. *Arch Dermatol* 2007; **143**: 275–6.
14 Callen JP, Jackson JM. Pyoderma gangrenosum: an update. *Rheum Dis Clin N Am* 2007; **33**: 787–802.
15 Cox NH, Leggat H. Sweet's syndrome associated with polycythaemia rubra vera. *J Am Acad Dermatol* 1990; **23**: 1171–2.
16 Young VL, Fernando B, Tabas M *et al.* A case study of pyoderma gangrenosum. *J Hand Surg* 1988; **13A**: 259–62.
17 Horan MP, Redmond J, Gehle D *et al.* Postpolycythemic myeloid metaplasia, Sweet's syndrome, and acute myeloid leukaemia. *J Am Acad Dermatol* 1987; **16**: 458–62.
18 Gibson LE, Dicken CH, Flach DB. Neutrophilic dermatoses and myeloproliferative disease; report of two cases. *Mayo Clin Proc* 1985; **60**: 735–40.
19 Yung A, Merchant W, Sheehan-Dare R. *Streptococcus* induced pustular vasculitis affecting the hands resembling pustular vasculitis of the hands—first reported case. *Clin Exp Dermatol* 2005; **30**: 366–8.

Extracutaneous neutrophilic dermatoses

A number of extracutaneous internal manifestations of neutrophilic dermatoses have been described, separate from internal features of an underlying cause (haematological, inflammatory bowel disease, etc.). These are different from the systemic features (fever, malaise, myalgia, arthralgia, conjunctivitis, scleritis, etc.) that commonly occur in patients with Sweet's syndrome, in that they affect a small minority of patients. Inevitably, they all cause diagnostic problems; most will require involvement of other relevant disciplines for investigation. The main patterns of involvement are listed in Table 50.23 and reviewed in [1,2]. In most instances, 'internal' neutrophilic dermatoses are most common with Sweet's syndrome but several reports also include PG [3–7].

Lung lesions have been described in many reports [1,2]; they have been associated with PG, Sweet's syndrome, subcorneal pustular dermatosis and EED. Clinical features include fever, cough, dyspnoea and pleuritis. About half of the patients reported have had an associated underlying cause, most commonly haematological malignancies, and about a quarter have died despite treatment with corticosteroids as well as specific therapy for the underlying cause. Infection (including fungal infection, in the context of haematological malignancies) must be excluded; bronchial biopsies show sterile, densely neutrophilic and sometimes suppurative masses.

Table 50.23 Some examples of systemic disease associated with neutrophilic dermatoses.

Body system	Clinical features
Lung	Bronchial inflammation/pustules, infiltrates (patchy, lobar or diffuse interstitial), bronchiolitis obliterans organizing pneumonia, effusion, localized (sometimes cavitating) masses
Heart	Aortitis ± stenosis or dilatation, cardiac infiltrate, pericarditis, cardiomegaly, coronary artery occlusion
Bowel	Neutrophilic infiltrate (diffuse, ileal, pan-colitis); visceral abscesses
Liver	Hepatomegaly, elevated transaminases
Spleen	Splenomegaly, aseptic abscesses
Kidney and genitourinary tract	Mesangiocapillary glomerulonephritis, proteinuria, haematuria Prostatic PG with infarction of the urinary sphincter Sterile pyosalpinx
Muscle and tendon	Myalgia, myositis, fasciitis, tendonitis (usually symptomatic in Sweet's syndrome, may be due to exposed tendons in PG)
Bone and joint	Arthralgia, osteitis (may underlie pyoderma gangrenosum, or affect distant scattered sites), chronic recurrent multifocal osteomyelitis, SAPHO, sterile arthritis
Neurological	Neuro-Sweet's syndrome (mainly menigoencephalitis), headache, consciousness disturbance, convulsions, pareses, psychiatric symptoms, brainstem disease, Guillain–Barré disease, bilateral progressive deafness, polyneuropathy, retinal vasculitis
Ocular	Conjunctivitis, scleritis, iritis, uveitis (all non-specific); nodular episcleritis, peripheral ulcerative keratitis
Subcutaneous	Neutrophilic panniculitis, subcutaneous Sweet's disease (see p. 50.90)

SAPHO, synovitis, acne, pustulosis, hyperostosis, osteomyelitis.

Joint disease includes monoarthritis, seronegative polyarthritis and a destructive axial and peripheral polyarthritis. Bone disease is most common in children, as a chronic multifocal osteomyelitis. However, bone involvement may occur underlying ulcerative pyoderma gangrenosum. In one case, retrosternal cavitation due to pyoderma gangrenosum was successfully treated with local infusion of corticosteroids [7]. Myalgia in Sweet's syndrome is a non-specific finding, but rare cases of true myositis have been reported [1,8]; this seems to be particularly associated with use of all-*trans*-retinoic acid for acute promyelocytic leukaemia [8] (a drug also reported to cause cutaneous Sweet's syndrome [9]).

Neurological involvement is uncommon, but causes particular diagnostic problems due to the range of symptoms that can occur (Table 50.23) [1,2,10,11]. Encephalitis and meningitis are the most common patterns. One of the most difficult differential diagnoses is from neuro-Behçet's disease; the presence of HLA-Cw1 (and HLA-B54 in Japanese patients) rather than HLA-B51 is helpful, as is the absence of other features of Behçet's disease (p. 50.56). In the cerebrospinal fluid, neutrophil counts correlate well with levels of the chemoattractant IL-8 [12]. A prompt response to corticosteroids is expected [11], although recurrences may occur; indometacin, dapsone, colchicine and potassium iodide have also

been used, especially in recurrent disease. Diagnostic criteria are listed in [11].

Aseptic neutrophilic abscesses are viewed as part of the spectrum of neutrophilic disorders. They may be solitary, but are usually multifocal [1,2,13]. The most common sites of involvement are the spleen, intra-abdominal lymph nodes, around abdominal viscera, liver, lung, pancreas and others. In some cases the skin or subcutaneous tissues may also be involved [1,14,15]. Most cases are associated with inflammatory bowel disease [13,14]; associated neutrophilic dermatoses include Sweet's syndrome (most frequently), PG, relapsing polychondritis, subcorneal pustular dermatosis and intraepidermal IgA pustulosis.

References

1 Vignon-Pennamen MD. The extracutaneous involvement in the neutrophilic dermatoses. *Clin Dermatol* 2000; **18**: 339–47.
2 Rodot S, Lacour JP, van Elslande L *et al*. Manifestations extra-cutanées des dermatoses neutrophiliques. *Ann Dermatol Venereol* 1996; **123**: 129–34.
3 Brown TS, Marshall GS, Callen JP. Cavitating pulmonary infiltrate in an adolescent with pyoderma gangrenosum: a rarely recognized extracutaneous manifestation of a neutrophilic dermatosis. *J Am Acad Dermatol* 2000; **43**: 108–12.
4 Urano S, Kodama K, Nogura K. Pyoderma gangrenosum with systemic involvement. *J Dermatol* 1995; **22**: 515–9.
5 Vignon-Pennamen MD, Wallach D. Neutrophilic disease: a review of extracutaneous manifestations. *Eur J Dermatol* 1995; **5**: 449–55.
6 Vignon-Pennamen MD, Zelinsky-Gurung A, Janssen F *et al*. Pyoderma gangrenosum with pulmonary involvement. *Arch Dermatol* 1989; **125**: 1239–42.
7 Tallon B, Rademaker M, Parkinson G, *et al*. Cavitary pyoderma gangrenosum treated with local infusion of corticosteroid. *J Am Acad Dermatol* 2007; **56**: 696–9.
8 Christ E, Linka A, Jacky E *et al*. Sweet's syndrome involving the musculoskeletal system during treatment of promyelocytic leukaemia with all-trans-retinoic acid. *Leukaemia* 1996; **10**: 731–4.
9 Cox NH, O'Brien HAW. Sweet's syndrome associated with *trans*-retinoic acid treatment in acute promyelocytic leukemia. *Clin Exp Dermatol* 1994; **19**: 51–2.
10 Nobeyama Y, Kamide R. Sweet's syndrome with neurologic manifestation: case report and literature review. *Int J Dermatol* 2003; **42**: 438–43.
11 Hisanaga K, Iwasaki Y, Itoyama Y *et al*. Neuro-Sweet disease. Clinical manifestations and criteria for diagnosis. *Neurology* 2005; **64**: 1756–61.
12 Kimura A, Sakurai T, Koumura A *et al*. Longitudinal analysis of cytokines and chemokines in the cerebrospinal fluid of a patient with neuro-Sweet disease presenting with recurrent meningoencephalitis. *Intern Med* 2008; **47**: 135–41.
13 André MFC, Piette JC, Kémény JL *et al*. Aseptic abscesses: a study of 30 patients with or without inflammatory bowel disease and review of the literature. *Medicine Baltimore* 2007; **86**: 145–61.
14 André M, Aumaître O, Papo T *et al*. Disseminated aseptic abscesses associated with Crohn's disease. A new entity? *Dig Dis Sci* 1998; **43**: 420–8.
15 Carvalho P, Cordel N, Courville P *et al*. Cutaneous aseptic abscesses, manifestations of neutrophilic diseases. *Ann Dermatol Venereol* 2001; **128**: 641–3.

Erythema nodosum

Synonyms
- Erythema nodosum migrans
- Subacute nodular migratory panniculitis
- Chronic erythema nodosum

Definition. Erythema nodosum (EN) is characterized by painful erythematous, and sometimes ecchymotic, nodules on the anterior surface of the legs. The condition may be idiopathic or secondary to various internal diseases or treatments. The incidence of EN is 1–5 in 100 000 population per year, with women accounting for about 80% of cases, and mainly affecting subjects aged 15 to 40 years [1–5].

History and nomenclature.

EN was initially described by Willan in 1798 [6] and was further discussed by Wilson in 1842, who believed it to be a type of erythema multiforme. In 1860, Hebra further described the clinical manifestations of the condition, and suggested 'dermatitis contusiformis' as a name for the disorder [7]. A more chronic variant was described almost a century later, and has been termed 'erythema nodosum migrans', 'chronic erythema nodosum' or 'subacute nodular migratory panniculitis' [8–10].

References

1 MacPherson P. A survey of erythema nodosum in a rural community between 1954 and 1968. *Tubercle* 1970; **51**: 324–7.

2 Erez A, Horowitz J, Sukenik S. Erythema nodosum in the Negev area: a survey of 50 patients. *Isr J Med Sci* 1987; **23**: 1228–31.

3 Cribier B, Caille A, Heid E, Grosshans E. Erythema nodosum and associated diseases: a study of 129 cases. *Int J Dermatol* 1998; **37**: 667–72.

4 Hannuksela M. Erythema nodosum. *Ann Clin Res* 1971; **3** (Suppl. 7): 4.

5 Garcia-Porrua C, Gonzalez-Gay MA, Vazquez-Caruncho M *et al*. Erythema nodosum: aetiologic and predictive factors in a defined population. *Arthritis Rheum* 2000; **43**: 584–92.

6 Willan R. *On Cutaneous Diseases*, Vol. 1. London: J. Johnson, St Paul's Church-Yard, 1798.

7 Hebra F. *Diseases of the Skin*, Vol. 1. London: New Sydenham Society, 1860.

8 Bäfverstedt B. Erythema nodosum migrans. *Acta Derm Venereol (Stockh)* 1954; **34**: 181–93.

9 Fine RM, Meltzer HD. Chronic erythema nodosum. *Arch Dermatol* 1969; **100**: 33–8.

10 Perry HO, Winkelmann RK. Subacute nodular migratory panniculitis. *Arch Dermatol* 1964; **89**: 170–9.

Aetiology and pathogenesis.

EN is thought to be a hypersensitivity reaction that may be triggered by antigens usually associated with infections, typically group A β-haemolytic *Streptococcus*. There are several large patient series [1–9], and some smaller series in paediatric patients [10,11], as well as detailed reviews [12,13], that document presumed aetiological triggers and coexisting diseases. A list of drugs that have been implicated is provided in [14]. The most frequent underlying causes vary somewhat depending on the country, age group, and specialty of the authors. In children, infections predominate as the trigger—typically upper respiratory tract (mainly streptococcal), but *Yersinia* and tuberculosis can be found [10,11]. In adults, streptococcal infection usually accounts for about 10–30% of cases, other infections for 5–10%, sarcoidosis for 10–35%, rheumatological and autoimmune diseases for about 5%, inflammatory bowel diseases for 2–3%, medications for about 5–15% (including oral contraceptives), pregnancy for 2% and malignancies rarely [1–9,12,13]; streptococcal infections, and especially tuberculosis, are less prominent in more recent studies, in which sarcoidosis tends to be a more important trigger. EN is also common in sarcoidosis; in a series of patients with respiratory sarcoidosis who had skin lesions, 20% had EN [15]. In about a third (25–50%) of patients with EN, the cause is unknown.

Triggers of the chronic EN variant are generally unknown, although pregnancy and oral contraceptives have been implicated [9,12,13,16,17]; overall, about a third of cases of EN have no cause

identified, and nearly a third of these have lesions that continue for over 6 months [5]. In one study with long-term follow-up, over 62% of patients with idiopathic EN had annual recurrences, but such a course was only seen in one patient with a known cause (Behçet's disease) [7]. Another study reported 56 of 438 patients (12%) to have a chronic form; nearly all were women, half had no obvious trigger (pregnancy was implicated in 40% with a possible identifiable cause) and mean duration was 4.5 months [9]. In some cases of chronic EN, the prolonged course may be determined by the course of an underlying condition, a feature particularly noted with non-Hodgkin's lymphoma [5]. In one case, chronic erythema nodosum in a child resolved when she was found to have coeliac disease and was treated with a gluten-free diet [18]. In some cases the course of erythema nodosum is marked by episodic exacerbations rather than by constant lesions, as in a patient who developed EN in the first half of each of four pregnancies and whenever she used oral contraceptives [17].

The exact pathogenesis of EN is not understood, although it is thought that it may be the result of deposition of immune complexes in the venules of the septae of subcutaneous fat, causing a neutrophilic panniculitis. A study of ten patients with EN showed that they had a fourfold higher percentage of 'primed' neutrophils, assessed by production of reactive oxygen intermediates, in comparison with healthy controls [19]; there was also a correlation with disease activity, but it is not clear whether this is a cause or an effect. There may also be a genetic predisposition to EN; in a study that examined genetic polymorphisms associated with high TNF-α production in a group of patients with EN, with or without sarcoidosis, there was a strong correlation of sarcoidosis-associated EN with TNF AII allele [20]. Erythema nodosum was a frequent finding in a series of patients with fever, arthralgia, mucosal ulcers, erythema multiforme-like and Sweet's syndrome-like lesions, in whom a form of superantigen-induced id reaction was proposed as the mechanism [21]; implicated infections included streptococcus, parvovirus B19, cytomegalovirus, mycoplasma, *Klebsiella* and *Borrelia burgdorferi*. A more detailed list of causes, especially of infectious aetiologies, is provided in Table 50.24 [1–17,21–64].

Drug-induced erythema nodosum is well recorded [1–9,12–14]. In the case of antibiotics, it may be difficult to separate infection-induced from drug-induced EN, but penicillins and sulphonamides have been implicated in several series of patients with EN. Oral contraceptives are a fairly convincing cause; in one series, use of oral contraceptives was 2.5-fold the expected level compared with overall national sales figures [9]. Hepatitis B vaccine has been implicated as a cause in several reports [56,57]. Isotretinoin is of some interest as patients with EN have often had acne fulminans, and some have had immune complexes demonstrated [58,59]; this does create some uncertainty about whether antigens due to inflammatory acne, or *Propionibacterium acnes* itself [60], is actually the cause. Acne fulminans has also been documented as a cause of erythema nodosum migrans [61]. Glatiramer acetate-induced EN is also of interest in having a likely immunological explanation; this drug is a polymer that mimics major basic protein (MBP) and is used to treat multiple sclerosis, in which situation it is known to generate polyclonal antibodies that cross-react with MBP epitopes and that have been implicated in anaphylaxis,

Table 50.24 Causes of erythema nodosum [1–18,21–64].

Idiopathic [1–12]

Medical causes, excluding infections
Sarcoidosis [1–9,12,13,15] and other granulomatous disease (granulomatous mastitis [20])
Inflammatory bowel disease (see also Chapter 62) [1–9,11–13,23,24] and diverticulitis [13]
Rheumatological and autoimmune disease, including lupus erythematosus, Reiter's syndrome, Sjögren's syndrome, Behçet's disease, coeliac disease, autoimmune hepatitis [1–9,12,13,18]
Malignancy (uncommon, mainly haematological but others are recorded including lung, pancreas, renal, stomach, colon, uterus, cervix and others) [1–9,11–13,25–28]
Haematological stem cell transplantation [29]
Pregnancy [1–9,12,13]
Acne fulminans (sometimes with isotretinoin) [58–61]

Infections [1–13,21]
1 Bacterial
Group A β-haemolytic *Streptococcus* [1–13,21], uncommonly Group C streptococci
Other bacterial upper respiratory infections, e.g. *Moraxella* [30], meningococcus
Staphylococcus aureus (uncommon) [1–3]; also breast abscesses, probably staphylococcal [31]
Tuberculosis (uncommon but over 10% in some geographical areas) [1–9,11–13]
Leprosy (see Chapter 32) [32]; erythema nodosum leprosum may be chronic [33]
Atypical mycobacterial infection [12]
Yersinia (up to 15% in children) [10,34]
Gastrointestinal infections: *Salmonella* [35], *Shigella* [36], *Klebsiella* [21], *Campylobacter* [37,38]
Escherichia coli [2]
Brucellosis [39,40]
Cat scratch fever [41]
Borrelia burgdorferi [21]
Mycoplasma [1, 21]
Genitourinary: syphilis, gonorrhoea, lymphogranuloma venereum, chancroid [13]
Others: Q fever, tularaemia, *Pasteurella pseudotuberculosis*, leptospirosis, rickettsiae [12,13]
2 Other infections
Unspecified upper respiratory infections
Chlamydia (including psittacosis) [40–44]
Coccidioidomycosis [45]
Histoplasmosis [46]
Blastomycosis [47]
Dermatophytes [48]
Hepatitis B [1,49] and C [50]
Parvovirus B19 [13,21,51]
Cytomegalovirus [21]
Toxoplasmosis [8,52]
Visceral larva migrans [53]
Others: amoebiasis/giardiasis (both in the same individual), herpes simplex, varicella-zoster, HIV, infectious mononucleosis, measles, aspergillosis, trichomonas, ascariasis [12,13]

Medications
Sulphonamides, penicillins [1–9,14]
Halides [1–9,14]
Oral contraceptive pill [1–9,12,13,17]
Hepatitis B vaccine [56,57]
Isotretinoin [58,59]
Imatinib mesylate [64]
Others (see text and [12–14])

livedo-like dermatitis and lymphocytic infiltration [62]. Amongst more recently-introduced drugs causing EN, selective serotonin reuptake inhibitors should be noted as they are so widely used [63]. Imatinib mesylate, a now standard drug in treatment of chronic myeloid leukaemia, causes many skin reactions, but amongst these are several neutrophilic dermatoses including Sweet's syndrome, neutrophilic eccrine hidradenitis and EN [64]. Dermatologists also need to be aware of azathioprine as a possible cause of EN, which may cause diagnostic difficulty as it is also used to treat EN in EN leprosum or in inflammatory bowel disease [65].

References

1 Cribier B, Caille A, Heid E, Grosshans E. Erythema nodosum and associated diseases: a study of 129 cases. *Int J Dermatol* 1998; **37**: 667–72.
2 Garcia-Porrua C, Gonzalez-Gay MA, Vazquez-Caruncho M *et al.* Erythema nodosum: aetiologic and predictive factors in a defined population. *Arthritis Rheum* 2000; **43**: 584–92.
3 Psychos DN, Voulgari PV, Skopouli FN *et al.* Erythema nodosum: the underlying conditions. *Clin Rheumatol* 2000; **19**: 212–6.
4 El-Zawahry M. Erythema nodosum: a study of 60 cases. *Int J Dermatol* 1971; **10**: 145–50.
5 Bohn S, Buchner S, Itin P. Erythema nodosum: 112 cases. Epidemiology, clinical aspects and histopathology. *Schweiz Med Wochenschr* 1997; **127**: 1168–76.
6 Tantisirin O, Puavilia S. Long-term follow-up of erythema nodosum. *J Med Assoc Thai* 2003; **86**: 1095–100.
7 Mert A, Kumbasar H, Ozaras R *et al.* Erythema nodosum: an evaluation of 100 cases. *Clin Exp Rheumatol* 2007; **25**: 563–70.
8 Atanes A, Gómez N, Aspe B *et al.* Erythema nodosum: a study of 160 cases. *Med Clin Barc* 1991; **96**: 169–72.
9 Hannuksela M. Erythema nodosum migrans. *Acta Dern Venereol* 1973; **53**: 313–7.
10 Labbé L, Perel Y, Maleville J, Taïeb A. Erythema nodosum in children: a study of 27 patients. *Pediatr Dermatol* 1996; **13**: 447–50.
11 Kakourou T, Drosatou P, Psychou F *et al.* Erythema nodosum in children: a prospective study. *J Am Acad Dermatol* 2001; **44**: 17–21.
12 White JM Jr. Erythema nodosum. *Dermatol Clin* 1985; **3**: 119–27.
13 Requena L, Sánchez Yus E. Erythema nodosum. *Semin Cutan Med Surg* 2007; **26**: 114–25.
14 Litt JZ. *Drug Eruption Reference Manual*, 12th edn. London: Taylor and Francis, 2006: 619.
15 Yanardag H, Pamuk ON, Karayel T. Cutaneous involvement in sarcoidosis: analysis of the features in 170 patients. *Respir Med* 2003; **97**: 978–82.
16 Förström L, Winkelmann RK. Granulomatous panniculitis in erythema nodosum. *Arch Dermatol* 1975; **111**: 335–40.
17 Bombardieri S, Munno OD, Di Punzio C, Pasero G. Erythema nodosum associated with pregnancy and oral contraceptives. *BMJ* 1977; **i**: 1509–10.
18 Bartyik K, Várkonyi Á, Kirschner Á *et al.* Erythema nodosum in association with celiac disease. *Pediatr Dermatol* 2004; **21**: 227–30.
19 Kunz M, Beutel S, Bröcker E-B. Leukocyte activation in erythema nodosum. *Clin Exp Dermatol* 1999; **24**: 396–401.
20 Labunski S, Posern G, Ludwig S *et al.* Tumour necrosis factor-alpha promoter polymorphism in erythema nodosum. *Acta Derm Venereol* 2001; **81**: 18–21.
21 Magro CM, Crowson AN. A distinctive cutaneous reaction pattern indicative of infection by reactive arthropathy-associated microbial pathogens: the superantigen id reaction. *J Cutan Pathol* 1998; **10**: 538–44.
22 Al-Khaffaf BH, Shanks JH, Bundred N. Erythema nodosum—an extramammary manifestation of granulomatous mastitis. *Breast J* 2006; **12**: 696–70.
23 Kethu SR. Extraintestinal manifestations of inflammatory bowel diseases. *J Clin Gastroenterol* 2006; **40**: 567–75.
24 Trost LB, McDonnell JK. Important cutaneous manifestations of inflammatory bowel disease. *Postgrad Med J* 2005; **81**: 580–5.
25 La Spina M, Russo G. Presentation of childhood myeloid leukaemia with erythema nodosum. *J Clin Oncol* 2007; **25**: 4011–2.

26 Maxit MJ, Paz RA. Diffuse plane xanthoma with arthritis, serositis, erythema nodosum, vasculitis and myelomonocytic leukaemia. *Medicina B Aires* 2001; **61**: 187–90.

27 Almoznino SD, Dotan E, Sandbank J *et al*. Unusual manifestations of myelofibrosis in a patient with congenital asplenia. *Acta Haematol* 2007; **118**: 226–30.

28 Perez NB, Bernad B, Narváez J, Valverde J. Erythema nodosum and lung cancer. *Joint Bone Spine* 2006; **73**: 336–7.

29 Canninga-van-Dijk MR, Sanders CJ, Verdonck LF *et al*. Differential diagnosis of skin lesions after allogeneic haematological stem cell transplantation. *Histopathology* 2003; **42**: 313–30.

30 Periyakoil V, Krasner C. *Moraxella catarrhalis* bacteremia as a cause of erythema nodosum. *Clin Infect Dis* 1996; **23**: 650–1.

31 Ujiie H, Swamura D, Yokata K *et al*. Intractable erythema nodosum associated with breast abscesses: report of two cases. *Clin Exp Dermatol* 2005; **30**: 584–5.

32 Van Brakel WH, Khawas IB, Lucas SB. Reactions in leprosy: an epidemiological study of 386 patients in west Nepal. *Lepr Rev* 1994; **65**: 190–203.

33 Walker SL, Waters MFR, Lockwood DNJ. The role of thalidomide in the treatment of erythema nodosum leprosum. *Lepr Rev* 2007; **78**: 197–215.

34 Mygind N, Thulin H. *Yersinia enterocolitica*: a new cause of erythema nodosum. *Br J Dermatol* 1970; **82**: 351–4.

35 Scott BB. *Salmonella* gastroenteritis: another cause of erythema nodosum. *Br J Dermatol* 1980; **102**: 339–40.

36 Eastmond CJ. Gram-negative bacteria and B27 disease. *Br J Rheumatol* 1983; **22** (4 Suppl. 2): 67.

37 Lambert M, Marion E, Coche E *et al*. *Campylobacter enteritis* and erythema nodosum. *Lancet* 1982; **1**: 1409.

38 Galeazzi M, Palombi L, Mancinelli S *et al*. *Campylobacter* infections and erythema nodosum. *Eur J Epidemiol* 1986; **2**: 80–1.

39 Tanyel E, Fisgin NT, Yildiz L *et al*. Panniculitis as the initial manifestation of brucellosis: a case report. *Am J Dermatopathol* 2008; **30**: 169–71.

40 Akcali C, Savas L, Baba M *et al*. Cutaneous manifestations in brucellosis: a prospective study. *Adv Ther* 2007; **24**: 706–11.

41 Ridder GJ, Boedeker CC, Technau IK, Sander A. Cat scratch disease: otolaryngologic manifestations and management. *Otolaryngol Head Neck Surg* 2005; **132**: 353–8.

42 Sarner M, Wilson RJ. Erythema nodosum and psittacosis: report of five cases. *BMJ* 1965; **2**: 1469.

43 Sharma OP. Erythema nodosum and psittacosis pneumonia: a report of unusual clinical association. *Indian J Dermatol* 1970; **16**: 7 passim.

44 Kousa M, Saikku P, Kanerva L. Erythema nodosum in chlamydial infections. *Acta Derm Venereol* 1980; **60**: 319–22.

45 Erntell M, Ljunggren K, Gadd T *et al*. Erythema nodosum: a manifestation of chlamydial pneumoniae (strain TWAR) infection. *Scand J Infect Dis* 1989; **21**: 693–6.

46 Sundelof B, Gnarpe H, Gnarpe H. An unusual manifestation of *Chlamydia pneumoniae* infection: meningitis, hepatitis, iritis and atypical erythema nodosum. *Scand J Infect Dis* 1993; **25**: 259–61.

47 Blair JE. State-of-the-art treatment of coccidioidomycosis: skin and soft tissue infections. *Ann N Y Acad Sci* 2007; **1111**: 411–21.

48 Ozols II, Wheat LJ. Erythema nodosum in an epidemic of histoplasmosis in Indianapolis. *Arch Dermatol* 1981; **117**: 709–12.

49 Miller DD, Davies SF, Sarosi GA. Erythema nodosum and blastomycosis. *Arch Intern Med* 1982; **142**: 1839.

50 Hicks JH. Erythema nodosum in patients with tinea pedis and onychomycosis. *South Med J* 1977; **70**: 27–8.

51 Maggiore G, Grifeo S, Marzani MD. Erythema nodosum and hepatitis B virus (HBV) infection. *J Am Acad Dermatol* 1983; **9**: 602–3.

52 Calista D, Landi G. Lichen planus, erythema nodosum, and erythema multiforme in a patient with chronic hepatitis C. *Cutis* 2001; **67**: 454–6.

53 Katta R. Parvovirus B19: a review. *Dermatol Clin* 2002; **20**: 333–42.

54 Longmore HJ. Toxoplasmosis and erythema nodosum. *BMJ* 1977; **i**: 490.

55 Hartleb M, Januszewski K. Severe hepatic involvement in visceral larva migrans. *Eur J Gastroenterol Hepatol* 2001; **13**: 1245–9.

56 Rogerson SJ, Nye FJ. Hepatitis B vaccine associated with erythema nodosum and polyarthritis. *BMJ* 1990; **301**: 345.

57 Goolsby PL. Erythema nodosum after Recombivax hepatitis B vaccine. *N Engl J Med* 1989; **321**: 1198–9.

58 Kellet JK, Beck MH, Chalmers RJ. Erythema nodosum and circulating immune complexes in acne fulminans after treatment with isotretinoin. *BMJ* 1985; **290**: 820.

59 Tan BB, Lear JT, Smith AG. Acne fulminans and erythema nodosum during isotretinoin therapy responding to dapsone. *Clin Exp Dermatol* 1997; **22**: 26–7.

60 Williamson DM, Cunliffe WJ, Gatecliff M *et al*. Acute ulcerative acne (acne fulminans) with erythema nodosum. *Clin Exp Dermatol* 1977; **2**: 351–4.

61 Reizis Z, Trattner A, Hodak E *et al*. Acne fulminans with hepatosplenomegaly and erythema nodosum migrans. *J Am Acad Dermatol* 1991; **24**: 886–8.

62 Thouvenot E, Hillaire-Buys D, Bos-Thompson MA *et al*. Erythema nodosum and glatiramer acetate treatment in relapsing-remitting multiple sclerosis. *Mult Scler* 2007; **13**: 941–4.

63 Krasowska D, Szymanek M, Schwartz RA, Myslinski W. Cutaneous effects of the most commonly used antidepressant medication, the selective serotonin reuptake inhibitors. *J Am Acad Dermatol* 2007; **56**: 848–53.

64 Scheinfeld N. Imatinib mesylate and dermatology. Part 2: a review of the cutaneous side effects of imatinib mesylate. *J Drugs Dermatol* 2006; **5**: 228–31.

65 de Fonclare AL, Khosrotehrani K, Sélim A *et al*. Erythema nodosum-like eruption as a manifestation of azathioprine hypersensitivity in patients with inflammatory bowel disease. *Arch Dermatol* 2007; **143**: 744–8.

Histopathology. The histopathology of EN is quite varied and more than one biopsy may be required if there is diagnostic uncertainty. The classical picture is of a septal panniculitis without vasculitis [1–4]. Early lesions of EN demonstrate septal oedema and a lymphohistiocytic infiltrate, with an admixture of neutrophils and eosinophils. The inflammation is typically concentrated at the periphery of the septae and spreads into surrounding fat lobules between adipocytes. Miescher's radial granulomata, which are clusters of macrophages around small vessels or a slit-like space, are also seen in these lesions [1–6]; although characteristic of EN, they are also seen in other disorders that might clinically resemble EN, such as erythema induratum, nodular lesions in systemic fibrosing dermopathy, Sweet's syndrome and Behçet's disease. Finally, there may be oedema and lymphocytic infiltration of the walls of veins, although the amount of vascular involvement is variable [1–4]. Pathologists are divided on whether vasculitis within EN is consistent with the diagnosis; some would say that vasculitis does not occur [2], whereas others describe small vessel vasculitis, and even medium vessel arteritis, in at least some vessels [4]. It is probably reasonable to accept the possibility of some vasculitis at sites of severe inflammation where it may be secondary; in contrast, the erythema nodosum-like lesions of Behçet's disease may have foci of leukocytoclastic vasculitis, lymphocytic vasculitis, arteritis or venulitis scattered throughout lesions [7]. Ulceration should suggest that the diagnosis is not one of ordinary EN.

Many of the varied features of EN pathologically are explained by the chronology of lesions [8]. Older lesions of EN demonstrate widened septae with peripheral fibrosis, and inflammation extending into peripheral regions of fat lobules. There are fewer vascular changes and a shift from a primarily neutrophilic infiltrate to one of primarily lipid-rich macrophages with a 'foam-cell' appearance; in some cases, this lymphohistiocytic lobular infiltrate may predominate [4]. Macrophages without phagocytosed lipid surround multinucleated giant cells, forming granulomas. Histologically, chronic EN has similar features to the later findings in lesions of acute EN. However, vascular proliferation is accompanied by endothelial thickening and extravasation of red blood cells [9], along with more marked formation of granulomas and lipogranulomas.

Histopathologically, the differential diagnosis includes other causes of septal panniculitis [1–4], although many are distinguished by longer duration (lipodermatosclerosis, localized morphoea), a different clinical picture (eosinophilic fasciitis), or associated features (Behçet's disease). Early lesions of erythema induratum have a greater vasculitic component. Infective causes of panniculitis may be difficult to distinguish. Subcutaneous variants of neutrophilic dermatoses, such as Sweet's disease, cause particular difficulty, especially as some of the aetiologies of these disorders are the same as for EN (and, indeed, the two conditions occasionally coexist [10]); a septal neutrophilic infiltrate in some cases of Sweet's syndrome, and even the presence of Miescher's radial granulomas [11], make the histopathological differential diagnosis difficult.

References

1 Requena L, Sánchez Yus E. Panniculitis. Part II. Mostly septal panniculitis. *J Am Acad Dermatol* 2001; **45**: 163–83.
2 Ter Poorten MC, Thiers BH. Panniculitis. *Dermatol Clin* 2002; **20**: 421–33.
3 Requena L, Sánchez Yus E. Erythema nodosum. *Semin Cutan Med Surg* 2007; **26**: 114–25.
4 Thurber S, Kohler S. Histopathologic spectrum of erythema nodosum. *J Cutan Pathol* 2006; **33**: 18–26.
5 Miescher G. Zur histology des erythema nodosum. *Acta Derm Venereol (Stockh)* 1947; **27**: 447.
6 Sánchez Yus E, Sanz V, de Diego V. Miescher's radial granuloma: a characteristic marker of erythema nodosum. *Am J Dermatopathol* 1989; **11**: 434–42.
7 Kim B, LeBoit PE. Histopathologic features of erythema nodosum-like lesions in Behçet's disease: a comparison with erythema nodosum focusing on the role of vasculitis. *Am J Dermatopathol* 2000; **22**: 379–90.
8 White WL, Hitchcock MG. Diagnosis: erythema nodosum or not? *Semin Cutan Med Surg* 1999; **18**: 47–55.
9 Winkelmann RK, Förström L. New observations in the histopathology of erythema nodosum. *J Invest Dermatol* 1975; **65**: 441–6.
10 Waltz KM, Long D, Marks JG Jr, Billingsley EM. Sweet's syndrome and erythema nodosum: the simultaneous occurrence of 2 reactive dermatoses. *Arch Dermatol* 1999; **135**: 62–6.
11 Blaustein A, Moreno A, Noguera J, de Moragas JM. Septal granulomatous panniculitis in Sweet's syndrome. Report of two cases. *Arch Dermatol* 1985; **121**: 785–8.

Clinical features [1–3]. EN is typically manifest by the sudden onset of painful, erythematous, warm nodules and plaques, typically on the shins, knees and ankles. Lesions may occur at any body site, even the face, but are less common than on the lower legs. The lesions are often more easily palpated than visualized, and are typically bilateral and symmetrical, ranging between 1 and 5 cm in diameter. The nodules may coalesce to form plaques (Fig. 50.44). After several days, the erythematous nodules often flatten and become ecchymotic in colour, finally taking on a yellow-green appearance (similar to an old ecchymosis), sometimes referred to as 'erythema contusiformis'. This transformation is characteristic of EN, making retrospective diagnosis possible. Lesions of EN never ulcerate, atrophy or scar. Lesions erupt and are usually present for 3–6 weeks. In addition to cutaneous manifestations of EN, constitutional signs and symptoms may also be present. Fever, fatigue, malaise, gastrointestinal upset, headache and arthralgia may accompany the characteristic lesions of EN, as may ocular manifestations such as conjunctivitis; laboratory

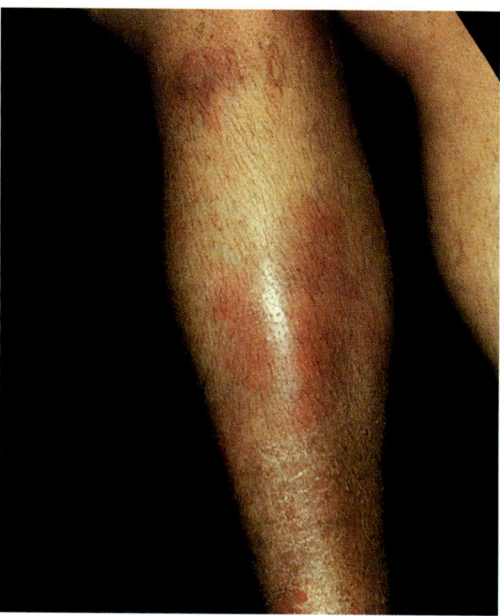

Fig. 50.44 Erythema nodosum. Note the location of the plaques on the anterior aspect of the lower leg.

markers of inflammation such as ESR and CRP may be elevated. All of these factors should raise suspicion of secondary rather than primary (idiopathic) EN [4]. A relapsing course appears to be most common in idiopathic cases or those associated with upper respiratory infections.

In the chronic EN variant, lesions may be solitary or few, usually on the lateral part of the lower leg. They are initially nodular but become broader and flatter, vaguely circular or arciform in shape, and often last several months.

Diagnosis. The diagnosis of EN is clinical, although histopathological evaluation may sometimes be necessary to support the diagnosis. Other forms of panniculitis are the main diagnostic consideration on the legs, and primary infective processes must be considered at any body site. In atypical cases of suspected EN (such as the absence of lesions on the legs, persistence or ulceration of the lesions), a deep elliptical biopsy of an active lesion should be performed. A medication history should be considered and a search should be performed for an underlying cause. A chest X-ray, tuberculin skin test and antistreptolysin (ASO) titre may be obtained in such instances to exclude causes such as sarcoidosis, tuberculosis or streptococcal infection.

Treatment. If there is a treatable, or removable (e.g. medication), cause then this should be addressed, as rapid resolution is anticipated. Even without specific therapy for a causative condition, EN typically resolves without treatment, therefore symptomatic support may be all that is necessary for the majority of patients. NSAIDs may also be used [1,2,5], as may potassium iodide 360–900 mg/day [6–9]. The concept that potassium iodide causes release of heparin from mast cells, and that this suppresses delayed hypersensitivity reactions, suggested the use of topical heparinoids [1]. Dapsone can be effective in some cases, as can colchicine. Hydroxychloroquine has been used in chronic erythema

Table 50.25 Therapeutic ladder for erythema nodosum.

Non-steroidal anti-inflammatory drugs (3)
Intralesional corticosteroid (3)
Heparinoid ointment under occlusion (3)
Potassium iodide (2)
Colchicine (3)
Hydroxychloroquine (3)
Dapsone (3)
Methotrexate (3)
Thalidomide (3)
Prednisone (3)
Anti-TNF monoclonal antibodies (3)

1, double-blind studies; 2, case series; 3, case reports.

nodosum. Systemic corticosteroids are infrequently required for the treatment of EN and may worsen underlying disease such as tuberculosis; intralesional steroids may be beneficial. Recent reports include use of anti-TNF biological agents [10,11], but these are contraindicated in the presence of infections (in particular, in the context of EN, tuberculosis must be excluded); they may have a place in cases due to inflammatory bowel disease as they could treat this and EN together [11]. A therapeutic ladder for EN is depicted in Table 50.25.

References

1 Requena L, Sánchez Yus E. Erythema nodosum. *Semin Cutan Med Surg* 2007; **26**: 114–25.
2 Mana J, Marcoval J. Erythema nodosum. *Clin Dermatol* 2007; **25**: 288–94.
3 Bohn S, Buchner S, Itin P. Erythema nodosum: 112 cases. Epidemiology, clinical aspects and histopathology. *Schweiz Med Wochenschr* 1997; **127**: 1168–76.
4 Mert A, Kumbasar H, Ozaras R *et al.* Erythema nodosum: an evaluation of 100 cases. *Clin Exp Rheumatol* 2007; **25**: 563–70.
5 Ubogy Z, Persellin RH. Suppression of erythema nodosum by indometacin. *Acta Derm Venereol* 1982; **62**: 265–6.
6 Schulz EJ, Whiting DA. Treatment of erythema nodosum and nodular vasculitis with potassium iodide. *Br J Dermatol* 1976; **94**: 75–8.
7 Marshall JK, Irvine EJ. Successful therapy of refractory erythema nodosum associated with Crohn's disease using potassium iodide. *Can J Gastroenterol* 1997; **11**: 501–2.
8 Horio T, Imamura S, Danno K *et al.* Potassium iodide in the treatment of erythema nodosum and nodular vasculitis. *Arch Dermatol* 1981; **117**: 29–31.
9 Horio T, Danno K, Okamoto H *et al.* Potassium iodide in erythema nodosum and other erythematous dermatoses. *J Am Acad Dermatol* 1983; **9**: 77–81.
10 Boyd AS. Etanercept treatment of erythema nodosum. *Skinmed* 2007; **6**: 197–9.
11 Quin A, Kane S, Ulitsky O. A case of fistulizing Crohn's disease and erythema nodosum managed with adalimumab. *Nat Clin Pract Gastroenterol Hepatol* 2008; **5**: 278–81.

Bowel-associated dermatosis–arthritis syndrome
(see also Chapter 62)

Definition. Bowel-associated dermatosis–arthritis syndrome (BADAS) is defined by the presence of pustular vasculitic lesions associated with blind loops of bowel or other causes of stasis of bowel content.

History and nomenclature. BADAS was first described in 1971 as pustular vasculitis, cutaneous lesions and serum sickness-like reactions in patients who had undergone jejunoileal bypass surgery

for morbid obesity [1–4]. The term has been extended to include the same syndrome in patients with IBD, those who have had creation of a blind loop following surgery for peptic ulcer disease [5,6], or with other causes of stasis of bowel content, such as in achalasia or related to a defunctioning colostomy.

Aetiology and pathogenesis. Blood vessel damage secondary to bowel flora antigen-associated circulating immune complexes is thought to be the pathogenesis of the cutaneous lesions. In these patients, peptidoglycans from gastrointestinal flora may be the antigenic trigger for immune complex-mediated vessel damage [4]. Therapeutic response to antimicrobials in some cases supports this concept, and immune complexes have been demonstrated [5,7]. The various underlying conditions can be divided into two main categories:

1 Related to surgery: jejunoileal bypass [1–4,8], gastric resection [5], blind loops (Bilroth II or Roux-en-Y [5,6]), defunctioning ileoanal pouch procedures [9], biliopancreatic diversion [10] and others
2 Related to bowel disease: ulcerative colitis [5,11], Crohn's disease [5,12], diverticulitis of colon [13], jejunal diverticula [14], appendicitis [15] and achalasia of the cardia [16].

In some cases there are combined causes (e.g. surgery for inflammatory bowel disease). In most instances related to surgery, the loop of bypassed bowel, or a blind loop, is in continuity with the intestine, but may be separated as a defunctioning bowel segment [9].

Histopathology. The changes noted in dermal blood vessels from early lesions of pustular vasculitis in patients with BADAS are similar to those in biopsies from patients with Sweet's syndrome [4–8] and Behçet's disease. Several cases have both clinical and pathological overlap with other neutrophilic dermatoses.

Clinical features. The cutaneous manifestations of BADAS begin as small macular lesions that progress into papules and later pustules on a purpuric base, most often on the arms and other areas of the upper body (Fig. 50.45). These pustules measure 0.5–1.5 cm in diameter and typically occur in crops, with each crop lasting up to 2 weeks, and recurring at intervals of several months [4,5,8].

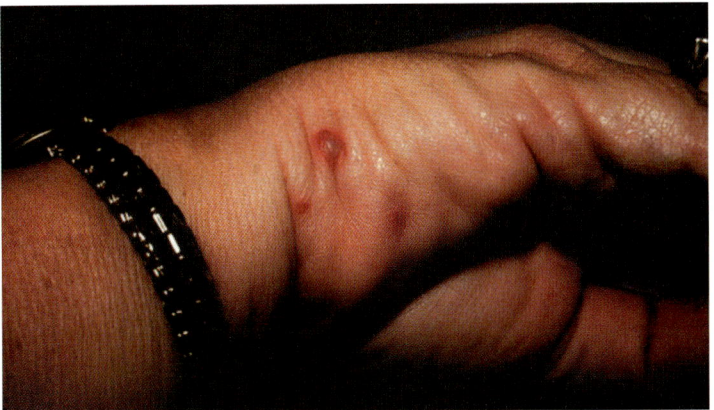

Fig. 50.45 Bowel-associated dermatosis–arthritis syndrome, showing a papule on an erythematous base.

Larger, erythema nodosum-like, lesions also occur, and sometimes larger pyoderma gangrenosum-like pustular lesions. Like Behçet's disease and pyoderma gangrenosum, pathergy seems to have a role in the distribution of the lesions. The cutaneous lesions may be preceded by constitutional signs and symptoms such as fever, flu-like symptoms or myalgia, or by gastrointestinal upset. Arthralgia or non-erosive polyarthritis affecting hands, wrists and other peripheral joints are common; ocular symptoms such as episcleritis [12], and haematuria or proteinuria [8,15] may also occur. Rarely, severe skin lesions and marked systemic manifestations may occur [17].

Diagnosis. It is important to distinguish between BADAS and Behçet's disease, as both may include oral aphthosis and lesions of pustular vasculitis. In order to distinguish between these two disease processes, an evaluation of the bowel, which may include barium studies as well as endoscopy, should follow a thorough patient history and physical examination. Clinicopathological evaluation of skin lesions is required but does not exclude lesions of Behçet's disease or early lesions of either PG or Sweet's syndrome; some patients appear to exhibit a spectrum of neutrophilic dermatoses [12], and a patient with previous pyoderma gangrenosum developed BADAS due to a defunctioning bowel segment after surgery for her ulcerative colitis [9]. Sweet's syndrome is associated with inflammatory bowel disease (p. 50.74) but has also been described with diverticular disease [18], supporting an overlap of diseases.

It is advisable to perform urinalysis in patients with BADAS as, unlike classical Sweet's syndrome, there may be haematuria or proteinuria, possibly representing an immune complex-initiated glomerulonephritis [8].

Treatment. For patients with BADAS following bowel bypass surgery, surgical correction of bowel anatomy often eliminates the signs and symptoms. In other cases, such as patients with blind loops (whether surgically created or due to bowel disease), surgical correction may be difficult and resolution of symptoms is therefore less likely. Manifestations of BADAS may be effectively controlled by the use of systemic tetracycline, metronidazole, ciprofloxacin or erythromycin [4,5,10,19]. Systemic corticosteroids are typically unnecessary for the treatment of BADAS but may be justified either depending on the degree of skin, joint or systemic symptoms, or to concurrently treat inflammatory bowel disease. Other treatments outlined for patients with cutaneous small vessel vasculitis, especially oral colchicine, dapsone or thalidomide have been used (Table 50.26); systemic drugs with an immunosuppressive action may need to be combined with an appropriate antibiotic.

References

1 Shagrin JW, Frame B, Duncan H. Polyarthritis in obese patients with intestinal bypass. *Ann Intern Med* 1971; **75**: 377–80.
2 Drenick EJ, Ament MR, Finegold SM *et al.* Bypass enteropathy: intestinal and systemic manifestations following small bowel bypass. *JAMA* 1976; **236**: 269–72.
3 Campbell JM, Hunt TK, Karam JH, Forsham PH. Jejunoileal bypass as a treatment for morbid obesity. *Arch Intern Med* 1977; **137**: 602–10.

Table 50.26 Treatment of bowel-associated dermatosis–arthritis syndrome.

Surgical correction of bowel anatomy if possible (may not eliminate symptoms if following blind loop)
Symptoms not secondary to or correctable by surgery, or temporary treatment prior to surgical correction
    Systemic tetracycline
    Systemic metronidazole
    Systemic erythromycin
Other systemic treatments that may be used depending on severity of symptoms and associated bowel condition
    Corticosteroids
    Colchicine
    Dapsone
    Mycophenolate mofetil
    Thalidomide

4 Ely PH. The bowel bypass syndrome: a response to bacterial peptidoglycans. *J Am Acad Dermatol* 1980; **2**: 473–87.
5 Jorizzo JL, Apisarnthanarax P, Subrt P *et al.* Bowel-bypass syndrome without bowel bypass: bowel-associated dermatosis–arthritis syndrome. *Arch Intern Med* 1983; **143**: 457–61.
6 Dicken CH. Bowel-associated dermatosis–arthritis syndrome: bowel bypass syndrome without bowel bypass. *Mayo Clinic Proc* 1984; **59**: 43–6.
7 Jorizzo JL, Schmalstieg FC, Dinehart SM *et al.* Bowel-associated dermatosis–arthritis syndrome: immune complex-mediated vessel damage and increased neutrophil migration. *Arch Intern Med* 1984; **144**: 738–40.
8 Gamble CN, Kinchi A, Depner TA, Christensen D. Immune complex glomerulonephritis and dermal vasculitis following intestinal bypass for morbid obesity. *Am J Clin Pathol* 1982; **77**: 347–52.
9 Cox NH, Palmer JG. Bowel-associated dermatitis-arthritis syndrome associated with ileo-anal pouch anastamosis, and treatment with mycophenolate mofetil. *Br J Dermatol* 2003; **149**: 1296–7.
10 Slater GH, Kerlin P, Beorghiou PR, Fielding GA. Bowel-associated dermatosis-arthritis syndrome after biliopancreatic diversion. *Obes Surg* 2004; **14**: 133–5.
11 Vázquez J, Almagro M, del Pozo J, Fonseca A. Neutrophilic pustulosis and ulcerative colitis. *J Eur Acad Dermatol Venereol* 2003; **17**: 77–9.
12 Mendoza JL, García-Paredes J, Peña AS *et al.* A continuous spectrum of neutrophilic dermatoses in Crohn's disease. *Rev Esp Enferm Dig* 2003; **95**: 233–6.
13 Brouard MC, Chavez P, Borradori L. Acute pustulosis of the legs in diverticulitis with sigmoid stenosis: an overlap between bowel-associated dermatosis-arthritis syndrome and pustular pyoderma gangrenosum. *J Eur Acad Dermatol Venereol* 2004; **18**: 89–92.
14 Fairris GM, Ashworth J, Cotterill JA. A dermatosis associated with bacterial overgrowth in jejunal diverticula. *Br J Dermatol* 1985; **112**: 709–13.
15 Prpic ML, Kastelan M, Brajac I *et al.* Bowel-associated dermatosis-arthritis syndrome in a patient with appendicitis. *Med Sci Monit* 2007; **13**: CS97–100.
16 Tucker SC, Chalmers RJG, Andrew SM, Odom NJ. Pustular vasculitis secondary to achalasia of the cardia. *Br J Dermatol* 2000; **142**: 373–4.
17 Kawakami A, Saga K, Hida T *et al.* Fulminant bowel-associated dermatosis-arthritis syndrome that clinically showed necrotizing fasciitis-like skin and systemic manifestations. *J Eur Acad Dermatol Venereol* 2006; **20**: 751–3.
18 Rosati E, Aracri N, Bottone A *et al.* Sweet syndrome in a female patient with multiple intestinal lipomas and diverticular disease of the colon. *Recent Prog Med* 2001; **92**: 599–601.
19 Geary RJ, Long LL, Mutasim DF. Bowel bypass syndrome without bowel bypass. *Cutis* 1999; **63**: 17–20.

Pustular neutrophilic dermatoses

This is not a specific entity, but aims to draw together some overlapping disorders and to consider their differential diagnoses. It should be accepted that some of these are probably synonymous terms (Table 50.27) although whether they are viewed as part of Sweet's syndrome, pustular PG [1,2] or simply viewed as

Table 50.27 Nomenclature of some pustular eruptions in the spectrum of neutrophilic dermatoses.

Term	Comment
Pustular PG	Discussed above
Pustular vasculitis/neutrophilic pustulosis	In Behçet's disease, bowel-associated dermatosis-arthritis syndrome; less commonly in systemic lupus erythematosus, primary biliary cirrhosis
Diffuse pustular eruption of ulcerative colitis Vesicopustular eruption of ulcerative colitis Neutrophilic pustulosis in ulcerative colitis [3–7]	Synonymous disorders, appearances vary from Sweet's syndrome to pustular PG Often associated with disease flare, pyrexia, malaise
Vesicopustular eruption associated with hepatobiliary disease [8]	Also viewed as pustular PG Lesions are often necrotizing, although some lesions resemble Sweet's syndrome Associated diseases include autoimmune hepatitis, sclerosing cholangitis, primary biliary cirrhosis and others [8]
Disseminated pustular dermatosis of polycythaemia rubra vera (PRV) [9]	Sweet's syndrome variant with response to dapsone Scattered pustules but also semiconfluent acral grouping and facial plaques, with pustular glossitis, stomatitis and nail dystrophy
Palmar, plantar or vulval pustulosis in Sweet's syndrome [10,11]	May be a presenting feature; distinct from the dorsal hand eruption
Neutrophilic spongiosis (synonym granulocytic spongiotic papulovesiculosis) [12,13]	Intermittent eruption of neutrophilic vesicles, mainly facial and mucosal (see text)
Pyostomatitis vegetans	Oral lesions, 50% with skin involvement: oral lesions may be IBD-associated variant of pustular PG, discussed earlier

unspecified neutrophilic dermatoses is less relevant than recognizing the occurrence of pustular lesions within this spectrum.

Pustular eruptions that are likely to enter the differential diagnosis of the above conditions are numerous. Localized infections such as mycobacterial or fungal infections have been discussed in the differential diagnosis of localized PG. Infections (e.g. streptococcal), folliculitis (sterile or infective), pustular psoriasis, impetigo herpetiformis and acute generalized eruptive pustulosis (AGEP) are all generalized eruptions that may be considered. Non-spongiform pustules have been described due to chronic internal infection, and related to tobacco smoking. At acral sites in infants, scabies and infantile acropustulosis are considerations, and in adults Reiter's syndrome, acropustulosis of Hallopeau or idiopathic acral pustulosis. Both generalized and palmoplantar pustular lesions have been reported in Kawasaki disease [14,15]. Other disorders that fall into the vasculitis or neutrophilic dermatosis spectrum may resemble or coexist with lesions listed in Table 50.27, including intraepidermal neutrophilic IgA dermatosis, subcorneal pustular dermatosis and CSVV.

Some disorders require special consideration as differential diagnoses, either because of close clinical similarity to neutrophilic dermatoses or because their systemic disease associations may require interpretation.

Pyoderma vegetans/blastomycosis-like pyoderma (has also been termed mycosis-like pyoderma, pyostomatitis vegetans and pyodermatitis-pyostomatitis vegetans) [16–19]. This may resemble PG, especially of vegetans type, as a verrucous plaque studded with pustules, and having pseudoepitheliomatous hyperplasia and neutrophilic microabscesses on histology. To further mimic PG, it may occur at sites of injection or tattooing (resembling a pathergic reaction), and, although not exclusively, most patients are immunosuppressed, malnourished or have diseases that have been associated with PG (including IBD (especially ulcerative colitis), leukaemias, lymphoma, diabetes, acne conglobata, hidradenitis suppurativa and dissecting cellulitis of the scalp). However, it can occur in young and fit patients. Oral lesions (which may be the only feature) may occur, especially in those with IBD (the nosology of this 'pyostomatitis vegetans' pattern, and its relationship to PG is discussed on p. 50.70); dorsal hand lesions that are morphologically very similar to neutrophilic dermatosis of the dorsal hands [19] also occur, and a rash very reminiscent of Sweet's syndrome [20]. Various bacteria (not fungi) have been reported as a cause, and the disorder may represent an abnormal response to such organisms. Antimicrobials, rather than corticosteroids or antineutrophil therapies, are indicated if the cause is uncertain, although they do not always eradicate it; the oral disease may respond to topical corticosteroids or tacrolimus, and Crohn's disease-associated cases have been treated with methotrexate and infliximab. Possible diagnostic clues include some cases with raised IgE level, and eosinophilia which is present in 50–90%.

Erosive pustular dermatitis of the leg. Although likely to be suspected when it occurs on the scalp, the commonest site, erosive pustular dermatitis of the leg is a rare condition and may resemble PG. Skin atrophy is typical and may suggest this diagnosis rather than PG; additionally, most patients are aged over 65 years, whereas most PG occurs in younger subjects, but this is not reliable. Several cases (reviewed in [21]) have had bowel problems, some with ostomies, further raising the possibility of PG (although the underlying condition in such cases has been mainly diverticular disease), and the histology shows neutrophilic spongiosis and an upper dermal neutrophilic or mixed neutrophilic and lymphocytic infiltrate. Reported responses to oral or topical corticosteroids, topical tacrolimus and colchicine, and recurrence around skin grafts as an attempted treatment, also suggest the possibility of PG. As occurs in *amicrobial pustulosis* (below), zinc deficiency, and therapeutic response to zinc, may be a feature [22].

Amicrobial pustulosis associated with autoimmune diseases

(APAD; also termed amicrobial pustulosis, follicular impetigo or pyodermatitis vegetans associated with lupus erythematosus or other autoimmune diseases). This is a condition of rapidly evolving, small, semi-confluent pustules that predominantly affects the face, scalp (causing alopecia) and flexures, reviewed in [23]. There is neutrophilic epidermal and ostial exocytosis and spongiform pustules; positive direct immunofluorescence for IgM, C3 and less often IgG is variable and may be vascular or a lupus band. Most cases are in patients with systemic lupus erythematosus, but coeliac disease and other autoimmune conditions occur; corticosteroids or dapsone may be effective, and oral zinc was effective in two cases [23].

Localized reaction to granulocyte colony-stimulating factor (GCF).

Colony-stimulating factors are a well-documented triggering factor for neutrophilic dermatoses of different types [24]. A localized form at injection sites may be less recognized. Histology may be Sweet's syndrome-like, a necrotizing vasculitis or predominantly eosinophilic [25].

Neutrophilic spongiosis

[12] (originally described as granulocytic spongiotic papulovesiculosis [13]). This was described two decades ago but never fully explained. The cases described had intermittent outbreaks of myriad, semi-confluent, small vesicopustules, predominantly on the face, neck or upper trunk but sometimes at other sites such as axillae. In one case, severe mucosal involvement occurred with significant malaise. One case had dermoepidermal IgA (distinguishing it from intraepidermal neutrophilic IgA dermatosis, which is usually flexural, with annular lesions, no mucosal disease, and intercellular IgA), the other had negative immunofluorescence but did have an admixture of eosinophils in the infiltrate. Neither case had a consistent relationship with medications, making acute, generalized, exanthematous pustulosis unlikely, and neither had any evolution suggesting early spongiotic changes of pemphigus. The illustrated morphology, epidermal neutrophilic disease and extent of mucosal disease were not typical for Sweet's disease, but this might be considered.

References

1 Powell FC, Su WPD. Pyoderma gangrenosum: classification and management. *J Am Acad Dermatol* 1996; **34**: 395–409.

2 Ahmadi S, Powell FC. Pyoderma gangrenosum: uncommon presentations. *Clin Dermatol* 2005; **23**: 612–20.

3 O'Loughlin S, Perry HO. A diffuse pustular eruption associated with ulcerative colitis. *Arch Dermatol* 1978; **114**: 1061–4.

4 Fenske NA, Gern JE, Pierce D *et al*. Vesicopustular eruption of ulcerative colitis. *Arch Dermatol* 1983; **119**: 664–9.

5 Callen JP, Woo TY. Vesicopustular eruption in a patient with ulcerative colitis. *Arch Dermatol* 1985; **121**: 399.

6 Sarkany RPE, Burrows NP, Grant JW *et al*. The pustular eruption of ulcerative colitis. A variant of Sweet's syndrome? *Br J Dermatol* 1998; **138**: 365–6.

7 Váquez J, Almaro M, del Pozo J, Fonseca E. Neutrophilic pustulosis and ulcerative colitis. *J Eur Acad Dermatol Venereol* 2003; **17**: 77–9.

8 Magro CM, Crowson NA. A distinctive vesicopustular eruption associated with hepatobiliary disease. *Int J Dermatol* 1997; **36**: 837–44.

9 Grob JJ, Mege JL, Prax AM, Bonerandi JJ. Disseminated pustular dermatosis in polycythaemia rubra vera. Relationship with neutrophilic dermatosis of myeloproliferative disorders: study of neutrophil function. *J Am Acad Dermatol* 1988; **18**: 1212–8.

10 Keefe M, Wakeel RA, Kerr REI. Sweet's syndrome, plantar pustulosis and vulval pustules. *Clin Exp Dermatol* 1988; **13**: 344–6.

11 Sommer S, Wilkinson SM, Merchant WM, Goulden V. Sweet's syndrome presenting as palmoplantar pustulosis. *J Am Acad Dermatol* 2000; **42**: 32–4.

12 Sayami S, Tagami H. Granulocytic spongiotic papulovesiculosis. A new entity? *Br J Dermatol* 1984; **110**: 504–6.

13 Batista G, Santos ANC, Sampáio SAP. Neutrophilic spongiosis. A new entity? *Br J Dermatol* 1986; **114**: 131–4.

14 Ulloa-Gutierrez R, Acón-Rojas F, Camancho-Badilla K, Soriano-Fallas A. Pustular rash in Kawasaki syndrome. *Pediatr Infect Dis J* 2007; **26**: 1163–5.

15 Mizuno Y, Suga Y, Muramatsu S *et al*. Psoriasiform and palmoplantar pustular lesions induced after Kawasaki disease. *Int J Dermatol* 2006; **45**: 1080–2.

16 Su WPD, Duncan SC, Perry HO. Blastomycosis-like pyoderma. *Arch Dermatol* 1979; **115**: 170–3.

17 Papadopoulos AJ, Schwarz RA, Kapila R *et al*. Pyoderma vegetans. *J Cutan Med Surg* 2001; **5**: 223–7.

18 Magee KH, Pollack BP, Raugi GJ. Pustule-studded plaques after abrasion injury (blastomycosis-like pyoderma). *Arch Dermatol* 2006; **142**: 1643–8.

19 Sodemoto K, Kinbara T, Kitagawa T *et al*. Multiple pustulogranulomatous plaques in the elderly (Pyoderma vegetans). *Clin Exp Dermatol* 2006; **31**: 489–90.

20 Mehravaran M, Kemény L, Husz S *et al*. Pyoderma—pyostomatitis vegetans. *Br J Dermatol* 1997; **137**: 266–9.

21 Brouard MC, Prins C, Chavaz P *et al*. Erosive pustular dermatosis of the leg: report of three cases. *Br J Dermatol* 2002; **147**: 765–9.

22 Salavert M, Franck F, Amarger S *et al*. Erosive pustular dermatosis of the leg: role of zinc deficiency? *Ann Dermatol Venereol* 2006; **133**: 975–8.

23 Bénéton N, Wolkenstein P, Bagot M *et al*. Amicrobial pustulosis associated with autoimmune diseases: healing with zinc supplementation. *Br J Dermatol* 2000; **143**: 1311–5.

24 Johnson ML, Grimwood RE. Leukocyte colony-stimulating factors. A review of associated neutrophilic dermatoses and vasculitides. *Arch Dermatol* 1994; **130**: 77–81.

25 Samlaska CP, Noyes DK. Localized reactions to granulocyte colony-stimulating factor. *Arch Dermatol* 1993; **129**: 645–6.

Other neutrophilic dermatoses and overlapping or associated variants

Subcutaneous Sweet's syndrome and neutrophilic panniculitis

These relatively rare disorders represent a further part of the spectrum of neutrophilic dermatoses that histologically resemble Sweet's syndrome. Terminology varies between authors. Sutra-Loubet and colleagues reviewed these conditions and suggested a classification of neutrophilic dermatoses, in which 'neutrophilic panniculitis' was distinguished by affecting the fat lobules, whereas 'Sweet's syndrome with subcutaneous involvement' was the term applied if there was involvement of the septae [1]. Lesions that extend more deeply from the fat, or that are non-cutaneous, were termed aseptic neutrophilic abscesses (p. 50.82). However, Cohen [2] preferred to use 'subcutaneous Sweet's syndrome' to describe any variant in which there is neutrophilic panniculitis affecting the lobules, septae or both, with or without associated dermal involvement, suggesting that neutrophilic lobular panniculitis is best viewed as a descriptive term of which subcutaneous Sweet's syndrome is one cause. Whichever term is preferred, the typical pathological pattern, as in Sweet's syndrome, is dominated by neutrophils, without vasculitis, and the involvement of fat is primary rather than simply deep extension of a dermal lesion [1–4]. Immature myeloid cells may be predominant [5]; the septal variant may be granulomatous [6].

Subcutaneous involvement can occur in patients with Sweet's syndrome or pyoderma gangrenosum, but is increasingly recognized in isolation; dermal/subcutaneous aseptic abscesses can occur in conjunction with abscesses at other sites, or combined with various neutrophilic dermatoses. Subcutaneous Sweet's syndrome is predominantly associated with myelodysplasia [1–4]; as in standard Sweet's syndrome, provocation by all-*trans*-retinoic acid [7] and by colony-stimulating factors [8] have been reported, although in one case it is likely that disease progression rather than granulocyte colony-stimulating factor (used uneventfully for the preceding year) was the cause of subcutaneous Sweet's syndrome [9]. A case related to breast carcinoma has also been reported, and some cases have had preceding viral infections.

Clinically, lesions present as subcutaneous nodules, infiltrated plaques or erythema nodosum-like lesions, at any body site, with or without more typical Sweet's syndrome lesions or occasionally pustules [10]. Fever, malaise, arthralgia, and peripheral blood eosinophilia are all common.

Important differential diagnoses, clinically and/or pathologically, include infections (especially in patients with myelodysplasia), α-1-antitrypsin deficiency, and hepatitis C infection [11]; neutrophilic lobular panniculitis also occurs in rheumatoid disease [12].

References
1 Sutra-Loubet C, Carlotti A, Guillemette J, Wallach D. Neutrophilic panniculitis. *J Am Acad Dermatol* 2004; **50**: 280–5.
2 Cohen PR. Subcutaneous Sweet's syndrome: a variant of acute febrile neutrophilic dermatosis that is included in the histopathological differential diagnosis of neutrophilic panniculitis. *J Am Acad Dermatol* 2005; **52**: 927–8.
3 Jordaan HF. Acute febrile neutrophilic dermatosis: a histopathological study of 37 patients and a review of the literature. *Am J Dermatopathol* 1989; **11**: 99–111.
4 Matsumura Y, Tanabe H, Wada Y *et al*. Neutrophilic panniculitis associated with myelodysplastic syndromes. *Br J Dermatol* 1997; **136**: 142–3.
5 Chow S, Pasternak S, Green P *et al*. Histiocytoid neutrophilic dermatoses and panniculitides: variations on a theme. *Am J Dermatopathol* 2007; **29**: 334–41.
6 Blaustein A, Moreno A, Noguera J, de Moragas JM. Septal granulomatous panniculitis in Sweet's syndrome. Report of two cases. *Arch Dermatol* 1985; **121**: 785–8.
7 Jagdea J, Campbell R, Long T *et al*. Sweet's syndrome-like neutrophilic lobular panniculitis associated with all-*trans*-retinoic acid chemotherapy in a patient with acute promyelocytic leukaemia. *J Am Acad Dermatol* 2007; **56**: 690–3.
8 Hasegawa M, Sato S, Nakada M *et al*. Sweet's syndrome associated with granulocyte colony-stimulating factor. *Eur J Dermatol* 1988; **8**: 503–5.
9 Raj K, Ho A, Creamer JD *et al*. Complete response of deep neutrophilic dermatosis associated with myelodysplastic syndrome to 5-azacytidine. *Br J Dermatol* 2007; **156**: 1039–41.
10 Chen HC, Kao WY, Chang DM *et al*. Neutrophilic panniculitis with myelodysplastic syndromes presenting as pustulosis: case report and review of the literature. *Am J Hematol* 2004; **76**: 61–5.
11 Crowson AN, Nuovo G, Ferri C, Magro CM. The dermatopathologic manifestations of hepatitis C infection: a clinical, histological, and molecular assessment of 35 cases. *Hum Pathol* 2003; **34**: 573–9.
12 Tran TA, DuPree M, Carlson JA. Neutrophilic lobular (pustular) panniculitis associated with rheumatoid arthritis: a case report and review of the literature. *Am J Dermatopathol* 1999; **21**: 247–52.

Relapsing polychondritis

Relapsing polychondritis is an inflammatory condition associated with antibodies against type II collagen, which is predominant in cartilage. The nose, ears, larynx, trachea, bronchi, joints and eyes are the most obvious sites affected, often with general malaise or fever during episodes of inflammation. Neurological (headache, nerve palsies, hemiplegia and others), cardiovascular (valvular regurgitation, aortic aneurysm, myocarditis, pericarditis, conduction defects and myocardial infarction) and renal (various forms of nephritis) features are also a consequence [1]. Issues regarding the pathogenesis and effects of the disease, and its treatment, are discussed in Chapter 51. However, features that link it with vasculitides and neutrophilic dermatoses are discussed here; in particular, it both occurs with, and has many disease associations in common with, paraneoplastic vasculitis and with neutrophilic dermatoses, and may appropriately be classified as a neutrophilic dermatosis [2], particularly given the view that neutrophilic dermatoses are a continuum of disease with vasculitides.

Some of the diseases that are associated with relapsing polychondritis as well as with vasculitis or neutrophilic dermatoses are listed in Table 50.28; vasculitides and neutrophilic dermatoses that have been reported in association with relapsing polychondritis are listed in Table 50.29. Myelodysplastic syndromes are an important association [1,3–5], possibly associated in a quarter of cases [4] although others suggest around 10% [6,7]; both Hodgkin's and non-Hodgkin's lymphomas are also reported [1,3], as well as a patient who developed paraneoplastic relapsing polychondritis associated with chemotherapy-induced erythroleukaemia after treatment for Hodgkin's disease [8]. Patients

Table 50.28 Diseases that are associated with both relapsing polychondritis and with vasculitis or neutrophilic dermatoses [1,5,7].

Disease category	Examples
Haematological malignancies	Myelodysplastic syndromes (most)
	Leukaemia
	Aplastic anaemia
	Lymphoma
	Multiple myeloma (usually IgA)
Collagen vascular disorders and autoimmune	Rheumatoid disease
	Systemic lupus erythematosus
	Dermatomyositis
	Sjögren's syndrome
	Still's disease
	Crohn's disease
	Autoimmune thyroid disease
Infections	Hepatitis C virus infection
	HIV infection
Other neoplasms [5]	Carcinomas of bladder (in a patient with Sweet's syndrome), breast, pancreas, lung/bronchus, colon/rectum, larynx; sarcomas (rarely)

Table 50.29 Vasculitides, neutrophilic dermatoses and associated clinical cutaneous findings that have been associated with relapsing polychondritis.

Disease category	Examples
Vasculitis	Wegener's granulomatosis
	Churg–Strauss syndrome
	Takayasu's arteritis
	Erythema elevatum diutinum
	Behçet's disease
	Temporal arteritis
	Leukocytoclastic vasculitis
	Lymphocytic vasculitis
	Pustular vasculitis
Neutrophilic dermatoses	Sweet's syndrome
	Erythema nodosum
	Neutrophilic panniculitis
Clinical findings	Oral and genital aphthae
	Non-follicular sterile pustules
	Thrombophlebitis
	Purpura
	Livedo reticularis
	Digital infarcts and necrosis
	Acral erythema nodosum-like nodules
	Subcutaneous nodules (representing thromboses and various panniculitides)

with an underlying myelodysplastic syndrome were statistically more likely to be male, older and to have additional skin findings in a large case series [7]. Cutaneous features other than those directly related to underlying inflammation of cartilage (e.g. auricular inflammation sparing the lobe, nasal inflammation and saddle nose) are documented in reviews and large case series [1,5,7], and are listed in Table 50.29. In one large series, over a third had dermatological findings in addition to those directly due to associated disorders (such as haematological or collagen vascular disorders); these features occurred with or separate from episodes of chondritis in approximately equal numbers (each about 10%), and 10% had cutaneous vasculitis (90% leukocytoclastic) [7].

Of the associated neutrophilic dermatoses, Sweet's syndrome has particularly been reported [9–11]; erythema nodosum, acral erythema nodosum-like nodules, neutrophilic panniculitis, non-follicular sterile pustules, and oral and genital aphthae occur and are part of the same spectrum [1,5,7]. Other neutrophilic disorders reported with relapsing polychondritis include pyoderma gangrenosum [12,13], aseptic abscesses [14], and erythema elevatum diutinum [15] (which we would classify as a vasculitis rather than a neutrophilic dermatosis, but which is viewed by some authors as a neutrophilic dermatosis [2]).

References

1 Somach SC. Relapsing polychondritis. In: Morgan MB, Smoller BR, Somach SC. *Deadly Dermatologic Diseases. Clinicopathologic Atlas And Text.* New York: Springer, 2007: 161–4.

2 de Moragos JM, Pujol RM. Neutrophilic dermatoses. *Curr Opin Dermatol* 1997; **4**: 13–20.

3 Cohen PR. Granuloma annulare, relapsing polychondritis, sarcoidosis, and systemic lupus erythematosus: conditions whose dermatologic manifestations may occur as hematologic malignancy-associated mucocutaneous paraneoplastic syndromes. *Int J Dermatol* 2006; **45**: 70–80.

4 Hall R, Hopkinson N, Hamblin T. Relapsing polychondritis, smouldering non-secretory myeloma and early myelodsplastic syndrome in the same patient: three difficult diagnoses produce a life threatening illness. *Leuk Res* 2000; **24**: 91–3.

5 Zeuner M, Straub RH, Rauh G *et al.* Relapsing polychondritis: clinical and immunogenetic analysis of 62 patients. *J Rheumatol* 1997; **24**: 96–101.

6 Provost TT, Flynn JA. Relapsing polychondritis. In: Provost TT, Flynn JA, eds. *Cutaneous Medicine: Cutaneous Manifestations of Systemic Disease.* Hamilton, Ontario: Decker, 2001: 158–64.

7 Francès C, el-Rassi R, Laporte JL *et al.* Dermatologic manifestations of relapsing polychondritis. A study of 200 cases at a single center. *Medicine (Baltimore)* 2001; **80**: 173–9.

8 Scully RE, Mark EJ, McNeely WF *et al.* Case Records of the Massachusetts General Hospital. Case 38–1997. *N Engl J Med* 1997; **337**: 1753–60.

9 Fujimoto N, Tajima S, Ishibashi A *et al.* Acute febrile neutrophilic dermatosis (Sweet's syndrome) in a patient with relapsing polychondritis. *Br J Dermatol* 1998; **139**: 930–1.

10 Astudillo L, Launay F, Lamant L *et al.* Sweet's syndrome revealing relapsing polychondritis. *Int J Dermatol* 2004; **43**: 720–2.

11 Vignon-Pennamen MD, Juillard C, Rybojad M *et al.* Chronic recurrent lymphocytic Sweet syndrome as a predictive marker of myelodysplasia: a report of 9 cases. *Arch Dermatol* 2006; **142**: 1170–6.

12 Check IJ, Ellington EP, Moreland A, McKay M. T helper-suppressor cell imbalance in pyoderma gangrenosum, with relapsing polychondritis and corneal keratolysis. *Am J Clin Pathol* 1983; **80**: 396–9.

13 Tsanadis GD, Chouliara ST, Voulgari PV *et al.* Outcome of pregnancy in a patient with relapsing polychondritis and pyoderma gangrenosum. *Clin Rheumatol* 2002; **21**: 538.

14 André MFC, Piette JC, Kémény JL *et al.* Aseptic abscesses: a study of 30 patients with or without inflammatory bowel disease and review of the literature. *Medicine (Baltimore)* 2007; **86**: 145–61.

15 Bernard P, Bedane C, Delrous JL *et al.* Erythema elevatum diutinum in a patient with relapsing polychondritis. *J Am Acad Dermatol* 1992; **26**: 312–5.

Rheumatoid neutrophilic dermatosis [1–6]

Rheumatoid neutrophilic dermatosis was described by Ackerman in 1978 [3], and a number of cases have been described subsequently, although it is an uncommon disorder. It is thought likely to be immune complex-mediated, and tends to occur in patients with severe, active rheumatoid disease. A significantly elevated rheumatoid factor may be found, but several patients with sero-negative disease have been reported [4,7], including patients with rheumatoid nodules and rheumatoid papules [8]. Lesions occur at any site, mainly the limbs and face, and may consist of papules, nodules or plaques, sometimes with an annular morphology (Fig. 50.46). Urticated, vesicular, crusted and ulcerated lesions may all occur. Rarely, lesions may be bullous [9]. Sweet's syndrome may be difficult to distinguish, and coexistence of the two entities has been reported [7,10], as well as rheumatoid neutrophilic dermatosis associated with pyoderma gangrenosum [11].

Histologically, there is a dense neutrophilic infiltrate that may extend into the epidermis or deeply into the subcutaneous fat; papillary microabscesses may be present [1]. Vasculitis is not seen but leukocytoclasis may occur. The picture is similar to that of Sweet's syndrome, but the latter usually has more prominent dermal oedema and less admixture with other cell types (some eosinophils, plasma cells and lymphocytes may be present in rheumatoid neutrophilic dermatosis) [4].

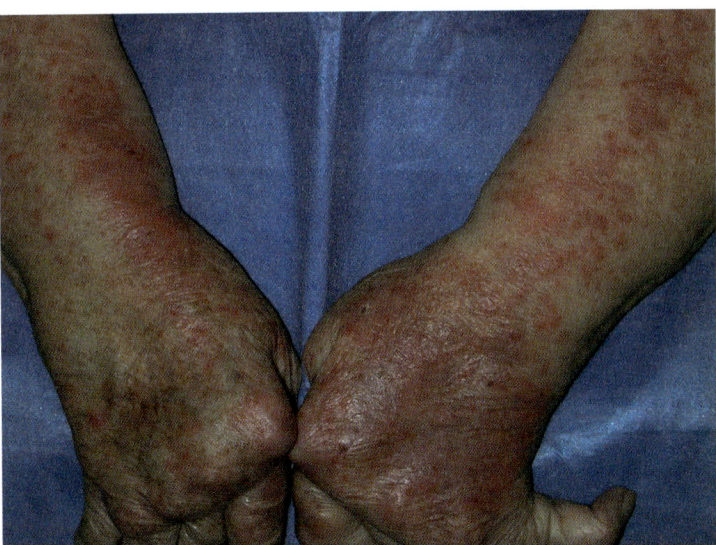

Fig. 50.46 Rheumatoid neutrophilic dermatosis affecting the hands.

Lesions may resolve spontaneously or as a result of treatment of the rheumatoid disease with immunosuppressive agents. Some plaques may be chronic over a period of months [6]. Topical or oral corticosteroids, dapsone and hydroxychloroquine have all been used with benefit.

A disorder termed 'neutrophilic lobular panniculitis associated with rheumatoid arthritis' is of uncertain aetiology, and has been classified as a lobular panniculitis with vasculitis. Histologically, it is in the differential diagnosis of subcutaneous Sweet's syndrome, discussed above. The few cases reported had a perivascular neutrophilic infiltrate and leukocytoclasis without fibrinoid change or definite vasculitis, although one had associated leukocytoclastic vasculitis in the upper dermis [12].

References

1 Huang W, McNeely MC. Neutrophilic tissue reactions. *Adv Dermatol* 1998; **13**: 33–63.

2 Mashek HA, Pham CT, Helm TN, Klaus M. Rheumatoid neutrophilic dermatitis. *Arch Dermatol* 1997; **133**: 757–60.

3 Ackerman AB. *Histologic Diagnosis of Skin Diseases: A Method by Pattern Analysis.* Philadelphia: Lea & Febiger, 1978: 449–51.

4 Sayah A, English JC 3rd. Rheumatoid arthritis: a review of the cutaneous manifestations. *J Am Acad Dermatol* 2005; **53**: 191–209.

5 Lowe L, Kornfeld B, Clayman J, Golitz LE. Rheumatoid neutrophilic dermatitis. *J Cutan Pathol* 1992; **19**: 48–53.

6 Scherbenske JM, Benson PM, Lupton GP, Samlaska CP. Rheumatoid neutrophilic dermatosis. *Arch Dermatol* 1989; **125**: 1105–8.

7 Gay-Crosier F, Dayer JM, Chavaz P, Hauser C. Rheumatoid neutrophilic dermatitis / Sweet's syndrome in a patient with seronegative rheumatoid arthritis. *Dermatology* 2000; **201**: 185–7.

8 Yamamoto T, Matsunaga T, Nishioka K. Rheumatoid neutrophilic dermatitis, rheumatoid papules, and rheumatoid nodules in a patient with seronegative rheumatoid arthritis. *J Am Acad Dermatol* 2003; **48**: 634–5.

9 Kreuter A, Rose C, Zillikens D, Altmeyer P. Bullous rheumatoid neutrophilic dermatitis. *J Am Acad Dermatol* 2005; **52**: 916–8.

10 Wilson DM, John GR, Callen JP. Peripheral ulcerative keratitis—an extracutaneous neutrophilic disorder: report of a patient with rheumatoid arthritis, pustular vasculitis, pyoderma gangrenosum, and Sweet's syndrome with an excellent response to cyclosporine therapy. *J Am Acad Dermatol* 1999; **40**: 331–4.

11 MacAya A, Servitje O, Jucglà A, Peyri J. Rheumatoid neutrophilic dermatosis associated with pyoderma gangrenosum. *Br J Dermatol* 2000; **142**: 1246–8.

12 Requena L, Sánchez Yus E. Panniculitis Part II. Mostly lobular panniculitis. *J Am Acad Dermatol* 2001; **45**: 325–61.

Neutrophilic eccrine hidradenitis

Neutrophilic eccrine hidradenitis (NEH) has been reviewed in detail in [1,2]. It is characterized by a neutrophilic infiltrate that is centred on and extends into the eccrine coils. Typically, the eccrine apparatus shows vacuolar degeneration or necrosis, and there may be mucinous degeneration around eccrine glands and squamous metaplasia of eccrine ducts. There is usually, but not always, a neutrophilic infiltrate that surrounds the eccrine coil and ducts, forms focal dermal abscesses and may surround vessels, without vasculitis. Oedema and/or haemorrhage may be present [2].

Early reports [3,4] implicated chemotherapeutic agents as the cause, and approximately 90% of cases still occur in the setting of leukaemia (usually acute myeloid type) undergoing induction chemotherapy with cytarabine and anthracyclines. However, other causes have subsequently been recorded, and in some of the patients with leukaemia the eruption precedes the diagnosis or treatment. Most cases occur in the setting of neutropenia; in neutropenia associated with acute myelogenous leukaemia (AML), 2–3% of patients may develop a neutrophilic dermatosis [5]. NEH may occur more frequently in AML subtypes FAB 4 and 5 in which leukaemia cutis and skin tropism of blast cells is more common [6]. In some cases, NEH recurs during successive cycles of chemotherapy, and it can also occur recurrently during chemotherapy for relapses of leukaemia, but not in association with consolidation chemotherapy to maintain remission; it is unclear whether this represents altered type or dose of drug therapy, or an altered drug–disease interaction. Thus, NEH represents a reaction pattern with several causes. Nevertheless, cytotoxicity of drugs on the eccrine coil remains the likely explanation for this dermatosis in most cases. The causes can be summarized into a few main groups (Table 50.30).

Clinically, lesions may resemble those of Sweet's syndrome. They may affect predominantly the head (especially the periorbital regions), neck and upper trunk; in some cases they may be generalized, but in others they are limited (for example, to the limbs, face or ears, or, in one case, around the breasts). The palms or dorsa of the hands are occasionally affected, and lesions have been reported at injection sites as a pathergic phenomenon [5]. If recurrent, they may affect similar sites to those previously affected. Lesions may be plaques, papules, nodules, erythema multiforme-like, or urticated, and may be grouped. Annular lesions have been reported on the dorsa of the hands [7]. Pustules, vesicles and occasionally purpura may be present. The lesions may be painful or tender, but can be asymptomatic, and associated fever is common. Most chemotherapy-related cases occur about 2 weeks after starting treatment, and resolve spontaneously after 2–3 weeks. Associated neutrophilic abscess formation occurred in a patient whose cultures grew 'slight' *Staphylococcus aureus* but in whom the lesions all responded to corticosteroids and not to antibiotics [8].

Treatment options, if required, include topical or systemic corticosteroids and non-steroidal anti-inflammatory agents [1]. Dapsone was used to prevent recurrent episodes in a patient receiving lomustine; it was started 2 days before the chemotherapy and

Table 50.30 Causes of neutrophilic eccrine hidradenitis [see also 1,2]*.

Type of process	Specific group	Examples
Malignant disease	Haematological malignancy	Leukaemias (especially acute myelogenous; also acute myelomonocytic, acute lymphoblastic, chronic lymphocytic, others)
		Hodgkin's lymphoma
		Non-Hodgkin's lymphoma
	Other malignant disease	Testicular carcinoma
		Osteosarcoma
		Wilm's tumour
		Breast carcinoma
		Lung carcinoma
Drugs	Chemotherapy agents	Cytosine arabinoside
		Anthracyclines (daunorubicin, doxorubicin)
		Vincristine, vinblastine
		Bleomycin
		Lomustine
		Mitoxantrone
		Cisplatin
		Dacarbazine
		Etoposide
		6-Thioguanine
		Cyclophosphamide
		Chlorambucil
		Methotrexate
		5-Fluorouracil
		Topotecan
		Imatinib mesylate
	Other drugs	Paracetamol (acetaminophen)
		Zidovudine
		Granulocyte colony-stimulating factor
		Amoxycillin
		Minocycline
Other diseases	Infections	*Serratia marcescens*
		Enterobacter cloacae
		Staphylococcus aureus
		Streptococcal endocarditis
		HIV infection (includes untreated cases)
		Hepatitis C
		Nocardiasis
	Other	Idiopathic neutropenia
		Behçet's disease
		Actinic reticuloid (methotrexate treatment)
No apparent disease association		Rare

*It should be noted that many cases have occurred in the setting of haematological malignancy and multiple-drug schedules, so interpretation of a specific cause is difficult in some instances.

continued for 14 days [9]. It was also successful in a patient with chronic NEH associated with Behçet's disease [10]. Colchicine was effective in a patient with apparently idiopathic, persistent, NEH [11].

A paediatric variant of neutrophilic hidradenitis, variously termed 'idiopathic plantar hidradenitis' or 'recurrent palmoplantar hidradenitis' [1], is discussed in Chapter 44. These disorders are not discussed further here as they are primarily neutrophilic eccrine rather than neutrophilic vascular reactions.

References

1 Huang W, McNeely MC. Neutrophilic tissue reactions. *Adv Dermatol* 1998; **13**: 33–63.

2 Bachmeyer C, Aractingi S. Neutrophilic eccrine hidradenitis. *Clin Dermatol* 2000; **18**: 319–30.

3 Flynn TC, Harrist TJ, Murphy GF *et al.* Neutrophilic eccrine hidradenitis: a distinctive rash associated with cytarabine therapy and acute leukaemia. *J Am Acad Dermatol* 1984; **11**: 584–90.

4 Scallan PJ, Kettler AH, Levy ML, Tschen JA. Neutrophilic eccrine hidradenitis. Evidence implicating bleomycin as a causative agent. *Cancer* 1988; **62**: 2532–6.

5 Aractingi S, Mallet V, Pinquier L *et al*. Neutrophilic dermatoses during granulocytopenia. *Arch Dermatol* 1995; **131**: 1141–5.

6 Cancelas-Perez JA, Perez de Oteyza J, Megido M *et al*. Chemotherapy-induced neutrophilic eccrine hidradenitis in acute myelogenous leukaemia. *Acta Haematol* 1992; **87**: 167–8.

7 Scong VY, Appell ML, Omura EF *et al*. Annular plaques on the dorsa of the hands. *Arch Dermatol* 1991; **127**: 1398–1402.

8 Horiguchi Y, Lee SG, Matsumoto I *et al*. Abscess-forming neutrophilic dermatosis: report of three cases associated with hemoglobinopathies. *Dermatology (Basel)* 1998; **197**: 174–7.

9 Shear NH, Knowles SR, Shapiro L, Poldre P. Dapsone in prevention of recurrent neutrophilic eccrine hidradenitis. *J Am Acad Dermatol* 1996; **35**: 819–22.

10 Nijsten TEC, Meuleman L, Lambert J. Chronic pruritic neutrophil eccrine hidradenitis in a patient with Behçet's disease. *Br J Dermatol* 2002; **147**: 797–800.

11 Belot V, Perrinaud A, Corven C *et al*. Adult idiopathic neutrophil eccrine hidradenitis treated with colchicines. *Presse Med* 2006; **35**: 1475–8.

Subcorneal pustular dermatosis and neutrophilic bullous disorders

Subcorneal pustular dermatosis is a rare neutrophilic dermatosis that is associated with monoclonal gammopathy, multiple myeloma, lymphomas, pyoderma gangrenosum, connective tissue disease and IBD [1,2]. Intraepidermal (neutrophilic) IgA pustulosis has some similarities, and has also been linked with monoclonal gammopathy (in 20% of cases) and with lymphomas. These disorders are bullous and are not discussed further here as they do not include a neutrophilic vascular reaction.

References

1 Reed J, Wilkinson J. Subcorneal pustular dermatosis. *Clin Dermatol* 2000; **18**: 301–13.

2 Cheng S, Edmonds E, Ben-Gashir M, Yu RC. Subcorneal pustular dermatosis: 50 years on. *Clin Exp Dermatol* 2008; **33**: 229–33.

CHAPTER 51

The 'Connective Tissue Diseases'

M.J.D. Goodfield[1], S.K. Jones[2] & D.J. Veale[3]

[1]Department of Dermatology, Leeds General Infirmary, Leeds, UK
[2]Department of Dermatology, Clatterbridge Hospital, Wirral, UK
[3]St Vincent's University Hospital, Dublin, Ireland

Introduction

Many single diseases can produce pathology in one or multiple organ systems. However, not all of the conditions that can affect multiple organ systems are related to each other, so what is it that determines the classification of diseases as 'connective tissue diseases'? We recognize that there are certain features common to all of them—the existence of autoimmunity in the form of autoantibody production or disordered cell-mediated immunity, vascular abnormalities characterized by Raynaud's phenomenon, occlusive vascular disease and vasculitis (although the pathology is not entirely a result of vascular inflammation), arthritis or arthralgia, and skin disease. However, dependence on clinical patterning is unreliable because similar patterns of disease may be seen with widely different pathologies. For instance, the primary vasculitides such as Wegener's granulomatosis or polyarteritis nodosa may share many systemic features of the connective tissue disorders, but so may sarcoidosis with a granulomatous pathology but without autoantibody production.

Despite this problem, it is still true that those disorders contained within the umbrella of the 'connective tissue diseases' share many clinical and pathological features. Indeed, it was this pathological similarity that first suggested that abnormalities of the connective tissue might be the common factor linking these conditions. In 1933, Klinge [1] was the first to propose that rheumatic fever and rheumatoid arthritis were disorders of the entire connective tissue. The changes in the intercellular components of the connective tissue, the presence of fibrinoid necrosis in collagenous tissue and the myxomatous swelling of ground substance were similar to those seen in experimental animals made hypersensitive to foreign protein, and for these reasons he concluded that the rheumatic diseases were caused by hypersensitivity. He included other conditions in which fibrinoid necrosis was a feature, such as polyarteritis nodosa, dermatomyositis and malignant hypertension. The presence of widespread fibrinoid change in the vessels led to the inclusion of systemic sclerosis by Masugi and Yä-Shu [2], and also of systemic lupus erythematosus. However, Klemperer *et al.* [3], with whose work the term 'collagen disease' is associated, struck a note of caution by pointing out that fibrinoid necrosis could be seen in the absence of hypersensitivity mechanisms, for example, in the base of peptic ulcers. It has been stated [4] that the presence of fibrinoid degeneration does not warrant the grouping of the conditions showing this change, nor does it imply an allergic mechanism. It is now recognized that there are various types of fibrinoid with somewhat similar staining properties. They have multiple origins from the degeneration of collagen, from ground substance, muscle, fibrin and other plasma proteins.

In 1950, Klemperer [5] stated: 'The term diffuse collagen disease was originally applied to acute and chronic maladies which are characterized anatomically by generalized alterations of the connective tissue, particularly by abnormalities of its extracellular components. In this case the term can include rheumatic fever, rheumatoid arthritis, polyarteritis nodosa, acute lupus erythematosus, generalized scleroderma and dermatomyositis'. Klemperer disliked the widespread indiscriminate use of the term 'collagen

Rook's Textbook of Dermatology, 8th edition. Edited by DA Burns, SM Breathnach, NH Cox and CEM Griffiths. © 2010 Blackwell Publishing Ltd.

disease' for disorders with unusual clinical or pathological features. He confirmed that his sole intention was to put forward the concept that, 'in certain diseases anatomical investigations reveal conspicuous alterations in the intermediary substances of the connective tissue in a systemic manner'. It is now realized that the connective tissue is not the only tissue involved in these disorders.

It has been customary to consider that systemic and discoid lupus erythematosus (SLE and DLE), systemic sclerosis, localized and generalized morphoea, dermatomyositis, rheumatoid arthritis and Sjögren's syndrome should be grouped together, and this has been supported by evidence of clinical, pathological and immunological overlap. The primary vasculitides, such as polyarteritis nodosa, Wegener's granulomatosis and giant cell arteritis, are sufficiently distinct to be considered separately, although there is much clinical overlap with these diseases too. However, these groupings may not be justified and may even hamper our understanding of these diseases. On the other hand, certain patients with evidence of clinical overlap can be distinguished by characteristic immunological abnormalities, associated with differences in outcome and response to therapy. With the passage of time, other conditions, sometimes newly described, such as eosinophilic fasciitis [6], may have to be added to the group.

When adequate criteria and modern investigative techniques are used, it is apparent that each disorder can usually be distinguished as a separate entity. For example, evidence has been produced that DLE is a separate disorder and not a benign variant of SLE [7–9]. Often, subsets can be distinguished clinically, pathologically or immunologically. Immunological subgroupings are becoming more numerous and complex with the identification of new antigens and the reacting autoantibodies. Specific antibodies may be strongly associated with particular disease patterns, such as the antibody to extractable nuclear antigen found in mixed connective disease or anti-Ro or anti-La antibodies in a clinically distinctive type of lupus erythematosus called subacute cutaneous lupus erythematosus (SCLE; see p. 51.22). Moreover, certain diseases that appear clinically homogeneous may be genetically heterogeneous. The separate genotypes in DLE related to age of onset [8,9], the clinical subsets in SLE and the severity of disease in systemic sclerosis related to HLA-B8 [10] are good examples.

Despite these improvements in investigational techniques, diagnosis of these disorders is sometimes far from easy. Results have to be interpreted in the context of the clinical presentation. Patients are not helped by a diagnosis of 'collagen vascular disease' or 'collagenosis' when suffering from an illness with obscure symptoms and signs, possibly associated with an elevated plasma viscosity, and a weakly positive antinuclear antibody. There is, however, often an early stage in the history of a patient's illness when the full pattern has not evolved. These patients may be said to have an 'undifferentiated connective tissue disease', but the disease usually reveals itself and it is usually ultimately possible to make a precise diagnosis. This is very important for the patient and critical for research, both epidemiological and therapeutic. It is more than an academic exercise as, in the future, specific therapy may well depend on the precision of diagnosis.

Accurate naming of diseases is important for patients, but is also relevant to this chapter. Is the term 'the connective tissue diseases' [11] the most appropriate title for this contribution? We believe that it is because there seems to be no better alternative. Some authorities prefer the older term, 'collagen disease'; others [12] apply it to all inherited or acquired disorders of the connective tissue system. 'Collagen disease' is incorrect because there is no evidence that collagen is primarily at fault. 'Collagen vascular disease' conveys a little more detail, but is still incorrect. The increasing emphasis on immunological abnormalities in these conditions has brought the terms 'autoimmune disease' [13] and 'immunological disease' [14] some popularity, but both are over-inclusive. To avoid the premature coining of a confusing new term we have preferred to continue to refer to 'connective tissue disease' wherever the use of a collective term is unavoidable.

References

1 Klinge F. Der rheumatismus pathologisch-anatomische und experimentell-pathologische tatsachen und ihre auswertung für das ärztliche rheumaproblem. *Ergebed Allg Path Path Anat* 1933; **27**: 1–336.

2 Masugi M, Yä-Shu. Die diffuse Sklerodermie und ihre Gefäss-veränderung. *Virchows Arch Path Anat Physiol* 1938; **302**: 39–62.

3 Klemperer P, Pollack AD, Bachr G. Diffuse collagen disease: acute lupus erythematosus and diffuse scleroderma. *JAMA* 1942; **119**: 331–2.

4 Baehr G, Pollack AD. Disseminated lupus erythematosus and diffuse scleroderma. *JAMA* 1947; **134**: 1169–74.

5 Klemperer P. The concept of collagen diseases. *Am J Pathol* 1950; **26**: 505–19.

6 Shulman LE. Diffuse fasciitis with hypergammaglobulinaemia and eosinophilia: a new syndrome? *J Rheumatol* 1974; **1** (Suppl. 1): 82.

7 Beck JS, Rowell NR. Discoid lupus erythematosus. *QJM* 1966; **35**: 119–36.

8 Burch PRJ, Rowell NR. Lupus erythematosus: analysis of the sex- and age-distribution of the discoid and systemic forms of the disease in different countries. *Acta Derm Venereol (Stockh)* 1966; **50**: 293–301.

9 Millard LG, Rowell NR, Rajah SM. Histocompatibility antigens in discoid and systemic lupus erythematosus. *Br J Dermatol* 1977; **96**: 139–44.

10 Hughes P, Gelsthorpe K, Doughty RW et al. The association of HLA-B8 with visceral disease in systemic sclerosis. *Clin Exp Immunol* 1978; **31**: 351–6.

11 Hughes GRV. *Connective Tissue Diseases*. Oxford: Blackwell Scientific Publications, 1978.

12 Gardner DL. *Pathology of the Connective Tissue Diseases*. London: Arnold, 1965.

13 Mackay IR, Burnet FM. *Autoimmune Diseases*. Springfield: Thomas, 1963.

14 Samter M, Alexander HL, eds. *Immunological Diseases*. London: Churchill, 1965.

Lupus erythematosus [1,2]

Lupus erythematosus (LE) is usually divided into two main types: DLE and SLE (defined on pp. 51.4 and 51.27 respectively). Although some authors [3] would prefer the term cutaneous LE to DLE, we are continuing to use the term DLE in view of the long usage and to avoid confusion with SCLE. Others [4] suggest classifying LE into three groups—cutaneous LE, intermediate LE and SLE, but this is still controversial. DLE can be subdivided into a localized form in which lesions are confined to the face above the chin, the scalp and the ears, and a disseminated form in which lesions also occur elsewhere on the body [5,6]. Although haematological and serological abnormalities occur slightly more frequently in the disseminated form, the natural history of the two subgroups is similar, and it is likely that they are subsets of the same disorder. SCLE has been described as a subset intermediate between DLE and SLE [7].

Table 51.1 Comparison of data on a series of patients with discoid and systemic lupus erythematosus seen by the authors.

	Discoid lupus erythematosus (n 120) (%)	Systemic lupus erythematosus (n 40) (%)
Rash	100	80
Joint pains	23	70
Fever	0	40
Raynaud's phenomenon	14	35
Chilblains	22	22
Poor peripheral circulation	26	32
ESR > 20 mm/h	20	85
Serum globulin >3 g (%)	29	76
LE cells	1.7	83
Antinuclear factor(s)	35	87
Homogeneous	24	74
Speckled	11	26
Nucleolar	0	5.4
Precipitating autoantibodies	4	42
WR positive	5	22
Rheumatoid factor positive	15	37
Direct Coombs' test positive	2.5	15
Leukopenia	12.5	37
Thrombocytopenia	5	21

ESR, erythrocyte sedimentation rate; LE, lupus erythematosus; WR, Wassermann reaction.

The more controversial point is whether DLE and SLE are variants of the same disease. The evidence in favour of this may be summarized as follows:

1 The cutaneous lesions of SLE and DLE may be clinically and histologically indistinguishable.
2 Certain clinical features are found in both conditions (Table 51.1).
3 Similar haematological, biochemical and immunohistochemical abnormalities can be demonstrated in both conditions (Table 51.1), although the incidence of abnormalities is lower in DLE.
4 Patients with DLE occasionally develop evidence of overt SLE.
5 Patients with SLE may develop typical lesions of DLE in the chronic phase of their disease [8].
6 Conditions such as lupus panniculitis, a recognizable clinical and pathological entity, occur in both DLE and SLE.

This seems to be formidable evidence, but the following observations require explanation.

1 The risk of a patient with DLE developing overt SLE is small. It varies from 1.3% [9] to about 6.5% [2,10]. The risk is higher in patients with disseminated DLE (22%) than in DLE confined to the head and neck (1.2%) [10]. In some series [11], such conversion was not encountered despite follow-up for nearly 30 years. A retrospective study [12] of 127 patients with SLE showed that eight patients had had discoid lesions from 2 to 29 years.
2 The presence of laboratory abnormalities in DLE does not in itself appear to predispose to the development of SLE [13],

although they are common in disseminated DLE [10,14]. The same prognosis was found in a subgroup intermediate between discoid and SLE as in patients with uncomplicated LE [11].
3 Immunoglobulins and complement are present in uninvolved skin of patients with SLE and absent in patients with DLE [15].
4 Most patients with DLE exposed to UV radiation, stress, trauma, etc., do not develop the systemic disease.
5 The age and sex distribution of SLE [16] is strikingly different from that of DLE [17]. It has been proposed [2,18] that both SLE and DLE are initiated by the occurrence of somatic mutations in lymphocytic stem cells of predisposed individuals, and that they are genetically distinct. There are at least three genotypes related to age of onset in DLE [19] and the female/male ratios found in each disease suggest that there is only one X-linked allele involved in genotype 2 and two in genotype 3. On the simplest interpretation, three 'forbidden clones' [20] of lymphocytes synthesizing cellular autoantibodies develop in SLE, whereas only one 'forbidden clone' is involved in DLE. Autosomal predisposing alleles are probably also present in all the genotypes in both SLE and DLE. The nature of these somatic mutations and the predisposing alleles remain unknown, but almost certainly include polymorphisms of genes determining the production of inflammatory cytokines [21].
6 Further evidence that DLE and SLE are genetically different disorders is now available from studies of histocompatibility antigens in the two diseases [22]. There is a significant difference in the incidence of HLA-B8 in female patients developing each disease between the ages of 15 and 39 years. It is considered that patients may have the predisposition to SLE, DLE or both. Those patients who 'convert' from DLE to SLE, and those patients with SLE who have discoid skin lesions, must be genetically predisposed to both conditions. Those patients with only a genotype for DLE will never convert, even when subjected to environmental factors, such as drugs, bacterial or viral infections, UV radiation and stress. More recent molecular genetic data give further support to this concept [23].

At present, it is not possible to determine the genetic pattern of individual patients or to predict accurately the small proportion of patients with DLE-like lesions who will develop SLE, although the link with HLA-B8 has already been discussed [22]. Humoral autoantibodies are not the primary pathogen in these diseases [24], but they probably reflect the underlying cell-bound autoimmunity that causes the disease. Nevertheless, they may enhance tissue damage [25], and specific antibodies may be responsible for certain features such as the risk of neonatal LE (anti-Ro) and for thrombosis (the lupus anticoagulant). The ability to synthesize particular antinuclear antibodies may depend on additional genetic factors, and this could account for the absence of such antibodies in certain patients with active disease. If the possession of a serological abnormality in DLE implies a predisposition to transformation into systemic disease, we would expect the sex ratio of this group to be similar to that for SLE. This is not the case. The sex ratio in patients with DLE and laboratory abnormalities is not significantly different from the sex ratio in patients without abnormalities.

From consideration of the clinical features, the natural history, the age and sex distribution, and studies of histocompatibility antigens, it is concluded that patients with DLE and haematological and serological abnormalities are not cases of SLE in disguise, but are cases of DLE, which is a separate entity from SLE, and has a different genetic background. Each of these entities, however, consists of several subsets, also genetically determined.

References

1 Rowell NR. Some historical aspects of skin disease in lupus erythematosus. *Lupus* 1997; **6**: 76–83.
2 Rowell NR. The natural history of lupus erythematosus. *Clin Exp Dermatol* 1984; **9**: 217–31.
3 Provost T. The relationship between discoid and systemic lupus erythematosus. *Arch Dermatol* 1994; **130**: 1308–9.
4 Halmi BH, Dileomondo M, Jacoby RA. Classification of lupus erythematosus. *Int J Dermatol* 1993; **32**: 643–4.
5 Dubois EL, ed. *Lupus Erythematosus*, 2nd edn. Berkeley, CA: University of Southern California Press, 1976: 446.
6 Kierland RR. Classification of cutaneous manifestations of lupus erythematosus. *Proc Staff Meet Mayo Clin* 1940; **15**: 674.
7 Sontheimer RD, Thomas JR, Gilliam JN. Subacute cutaneous lupus erythematosus. *Arch Dermatol* 1979; **115**: 1409–15.
8 Ganor S, Sagher F. Systemic lupus erythematosus changing to the chronic discoid type. *Dermatologica* 1962; **125**: 81–92.
9 Cannon EF, Curtis AC. A survey of lupus erythematosus in the University of Michigan Hospital since 1948. *Arch Dermatol* 1958; **78**: 196–9.
10 Millard LG, Rowell NR. Abnormal laboratory test results and their relationship to prognosis in discoid lupus erythematosus. *Arch Dermatol* 1979; **115**: 1055–8.
11 Shrank AB, Doniach D. Discoid lupus erythematosus. *Arch Dermatol* 1963; **87**: 677–85.
12 Rothfield N, March CH, Miescher P *et al.* Chronic discoid lupus erythematosus: study of 65 patients and 65 controls. *N Engl J Med* 1963; **269**: 1155–61.
13 Rowell NR. Laboratory abnormalities in the diagnosis and management of lupus erythematosus. *Br J Dermatol* 1971; **84**: 210–6.
14 Healy E, Kieran E, Rogers S. Cutaneous lupus erythematosus—a study of clinical and laboratory prognostic factors in 65 patients. *Ir J Med Sci* 1995; **164**: 113–5.
15 Tuffanelli DL. Cutaneous immunopathology: recent observations. *J Invest Dermatol* 1975; **65**: 143–53.
16 Burch PRJ, Rowell NR. Systemic lupus erythematosus. *Am J Med* 1965; **38**: 793–801.
17 Burch PRJ, Rowell NR. Autoimmunity: aetiological aspects of chronic discoid and systemic lupus erythematosus, systemic sclerosis and Hashimoto's thyroiditis. *Lancet* 1963; **ii**: 507–13.
18 Burch PRJ, Rowell NR. The sex and age-distribution of chronic discoid lupus erythematosus in four countries. *Acta Derm Venereol (Stockh)* 1968; **48**: 33–46.
19 Burch PRJ, Rowell NR. Lupus erythematosus. Analysis of the sex- and age-distributions of the discoid and systemic forms of the disease in different countries. *Acta Derm Venereol (Stockh)* 1970; **50**: 293–301.
20 Burnet FM. *The Clonal Selection Theory of Acquired Immunity*. Nashville, TN: Vanderbilt University Press, 1959.
21 Tsuchiya N, Ohashi J, Tokunaga K. Variations in immune response genes and their associations with multifactorial immune disorders. *Immunol Rev* 2002; **190**: 169–81.
22 Millard LG, Rowell NR, Rajah SM. Histocompatibility antigens in discoid and systemic lupus erythematosus. *Br J Dermatol* 1977; **96**: 139–44.
23 van der Linden MW, van der Slik AR, Zanelli E *et al.* Six microsatellite markers on the short arm of chromosome 6 in relation to HLA-DR3 and TNF-308A in systemic lupus erythematosus. *Genes Immun* 2001; **2**: 373–80.
24 Beck JS, Oakley CL, Rowell NR. Transplacental passage of anti-nuclear antibody. *Arch Dermatol* 1966; **93**: 656–63.
25 Hughes P, Rowell NR. Aggravation of turpentine-induced pleurisy in rats by 'homogeneous' and 'speckled' antinuclear antibodies. *J Pathol* 1970; **101**: 141–55.

Discoid lupus erythematosus

Synonyms
• Cutaneous lupus erythematosus
• Chronic discoid lupus erythematosus

Definition. DLE is a benign disorder of the skin, most frequently involving the face, and characterized by well-defined, red scaly patches of variable size, which heal with atrophy, scarring and pigmentary changes. The histology is characteristic. There are haematological and serological changes in approximately half of patients, and these changes, with other evidence, suggest an autoimmune aetiology.

Aetiology. This disorder has a characteristic age and sex pattern. The disease affects twice as many females as males, with a peak age of onset in the fourth decade in females and slightly later in males, although it can occur at any age. In a series of 1045 cases, 3% began under 15 years of age and 2.5% at over 70 years [1].

Genetic factors. Familial cases of DLE do occur. A family history was found in 4% of one series [2]. Steagall *et al.* [3] reported the condition in identical twin sisters, and listed 25 families with two or more members who had DLE or SLE. Studies also indicated a striking relationship between polymorphic light eruption and DLE, first in twins [4] and then in a large cohort of patients and their relatives, suggesting a common genetic background for these disorders [5]. Differences in the incidence of histocompatibility antigens [6–8] have supported the concept of multiple genotypes. Positive associations with HLA-B7, -B8, -Cw7, -DR2, -DR3 and -DQw1 are reported [9], but not always confirmed. The relative risk is increased with certain combinations of antigens—HLA-Cw7, -DR3 and -DQw1 and for HLA-B7, -Cw7 and -DR3. The extended haplotype—HLA*01, B*08, DRB1*0301—is associated with both SCLE and DLE, and the A*03, B*07, DRB1*15 haplotype has been associated with DLE alone [9]. Patients of both sexes developing lesions between the ages of 15 and 39 years have an increased incidence of HLA-B7, and females over the age of 40 years of HLA-B8, compared with controls [7].

Before the modern understanding of lymphocyte function [10], it was proposed that genetic factors, including somatic mutations, are implicated in the pathogenesis of the disease [11,12]. These studies suggested that there are at least three. The initiation of the disease may result from the occurrence of random events, either related to somatic mutation or to environmental factors. The model suggests that: (i) three mutations affecting autosomal genes; (ii) four mutations (one of which affects an X-linked gene); or (iii) five mutations (one involving an X-linked gene) could explain the three genotypes. The mutations interfere with control of lymphocytes; after a latent period of approximately 4 years in females and 2 years in males, clinical signs of the disease become manifest. Normally, an endogenous defence mechanism would control lymphocyte function and prevent self-harm. Environmental factors, by interfering with this defence mechanism, can precipitate or exacerbate the disease (Table 51.2). Supporting this view, DLE-like lesions have occurred after allogeneic bone marrow transplantation [13].

Table 51.2 Environmental factors associated with the onset or exacerbation of discoid lupus erythematosus [14–24].

Environmental factors	Frequency
Trauma (including X rays, diathermy, chemical burns)	11%
Stress	12%
Ultraviolet exposure (including PUVA and laser light)	5%
Infection (including herpes zoster and old smallpox vaccination)	3%
Drugs (including isoniazid, penicillamine, griseofulvin, dapsone)	Unknown
Seasonal exacerbation	Winter 10% Summer 50%
Cold exposure	2% (17% disease exacerbation)
Pregnancy	1% (onset)
Pre-menstrual	13% (disease flare)
Hormone replacement therapy	Unknown

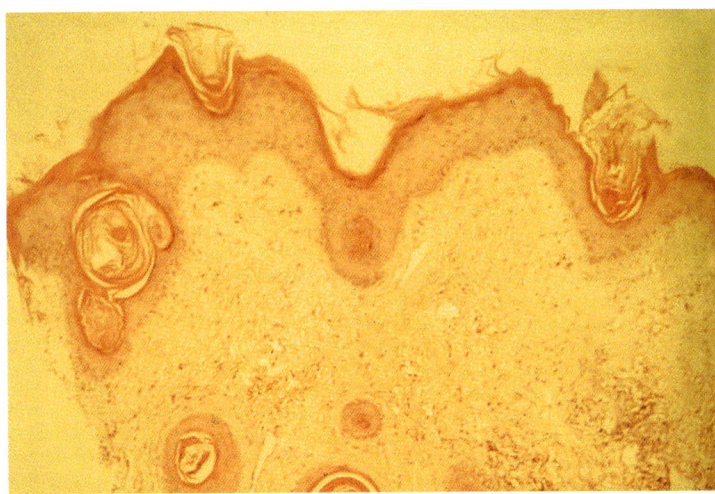

Fig. 51.1 Discoid lupus erythematosus: there is atrophy of the epidermis, keratotic plugging, liquefaction degeneration of the basal layer, oedema and hyalinization of the connective tissue below the epidermis and a marked inflammatory infiltrate.

Ultraviolet light and disease exacerbation [25]. In 120 patients at Leeds, UK a history of exacerbations with sunlight was found in 68%. In those with photo-aggravated disease, both wavelengths shorter than 329 nm and the whole range through UVB, UVA and visible light can produce lesions under experimental conditions. Skin lesions clinically and histologically compatible with lupus erythematosus (LE) were induced by UVB and UVA radiation in 42% of patients with DLE, 64% of patients with SCLE and 25% of patients with SLE.

Viruses. The finding of antibodies to reovirus RNA in 42% of patients suggests that viruses may have a role in DLE [20].

References

1 Damm J, Sonnischsen N. Clinical examinations of chronic lupus erythematosus. *Dermatol Wochenschr* 1964; **150**: 268.

2 Bielsa I, Herrero C, Ercilla G *et al.* Immunogenetic findings in cutaneous lupus erythematosus. *J Am Acad Dermatol* 1991; **25**: 251–7.

3 Steagall RW, Ash HT, Fentanco LB. Familial lupus erythematosus. *Arch Dermatol* 1962; **85**: 394–6.

4 Wojnarowska F. Simultaneous occurrence in identical twins of discoid lupus erythematosus and polymorphic light eruption. *J R Soc Med* 1983; **76**: 791–2.

5 Millard TP, Lewis CM, Khamashta MA *et al.* Familial clustering of polymorphic light eruption in relatives of patients with lupus erythematosus: evidence of a shared pathogenesis. *Br J Dermatol* 2001; **144**: 334–8.

6 Fowler JF, Callen JP, Stelzer FT *et al.* Human histocompatibility antigen associations in patients with chronic cutaneous lupus erythematosus. *J Am Acad Dermatol* 1985; **12**: 73–7.

7 Millard LG, Rowell NR, Rajah SM. Histocompatibility antigens in discoid and systemic lupus erythematosus. *Br J Dermatol* 1977; **96**: 139.

8 Tongio MM, Fersing J, Hauptmann G *et al.* HLA antigens in discoid lupus erythematosus. *Acta Derm Venereol (Stockh)* 1982; **62**: 155–7.

9 Millard TP, Kondeatis E, Vaughan RW *et al.* Polymorphic light eruption and the HLA DRB1*0301 extended haplotype are independent risk factors for cutaneous lupus erythematosus. *Lupus* 2001; **10**: 473–9.

10 Bock G, Goode J, eds. *Generation and Effector Functions of Regulatory Lymphocytes*. Chichester: John Wiley & Sons, 2004.

11 Burch PRJ, Rowell NR. The sex- and age-distributions of chronic discoid lupus erythematosus in four countries. *Acta Derm Venereol (Stockh)* 1968; **48**: 33–46.

12 Burch PRJ, Rowell NR. Lupus erythematosus: analysis of the sex- and age-distributions of the discoid and systemic forms of the disease in different countries. *Acta Derm Venereol (Stockh)* 1970; **50**: 293–301.

13 Gratwhol AA, Haralampos M, Moutsopoulos M *et al.* Sjögren-type syndrome after allogenic bone-marrow transplantation. *Ann Intern Med* 1977; **87**: 703–6.

14 Lodin A. Discoid lupus erythematosus and trauma. *Acta Derm Venereol (Stockh)* 1963; **43**: 142.

15 Lupton GP. Discoid lupus erythematosus occurring in a smallpox vaccination scar. *J Am Acad Dermatol* 1987; **89**: 688–90.

16 Eedy DJ, Corbett JR. Discoid lupus erythematosus exacerbated by X-ray irradiation. *Clin Exp Dermatol* 1988; **13**: 202–3.

17 Schmitt CL, Silverman A. Discoid lupus erythematosus in an arc welder. *Cutis* 1971; **8**: 476–7.

18 Domke HF, Ludwigsen E, Thormann J. Discoid lupus erythematosus possibly due to photochemotherapy. *Arch Dermatol* 1979; **115**: 642.

19 Wolfe JT, Weinberg JM, Elenitses R *et al.* Cutaneous lupus erythematosus following laser-induced thermal injury. *Arch Dermatol* 1997; **133**: 392–3.

20 Grundwald M, David M, Feuerman EJ. Appearance of lupus erythematosus in a patient with lichen planus treated by isoniazid. *Dermatologica* 1982; **162**: 172–7.

21 Burns DA, Sarkany I. Penicillamine-induced discoid lupus erythematosus. *Clin Exp Dermatol* 1979; **4**: 389–92.

22 Alexander S. Lupus erythematosus in two patients after griseofulvin treatment of *Trichophyton rubrum* infection. *Br J Dermatol* 1962; **74**: 72–4.

23 Shlepakov VM. Effect of gestation in the course of chronic lupus erythematosus. *Soviet Med* 1969; **32**: 111–6.

24 Yell JA, Burge SM. The effect of hormonal changes on cutaneous disease in lupus erythematosus. *Br J Dermatol* 1993; **129**: 18–22.

25 Bijl M, Kallenberg CG. Ultraviolet light and cutaneous lupus. *Lupus* 2006; **15**: 724–7.

Pathology [1]. The various clinical types of LE show an essentially similar histological picture (Figs 51.1 & 51.2), and the subsets of LE cannot be easily distinguished histologically [2]. The salient features are as follows:

1 Liquefaction degeneration of the basal cell layer of the epidermis

2 Degenerative changes in the connective tissue, consisting of hyalinization, oedema and fibrinoid change, most marked immediately below the epidermis

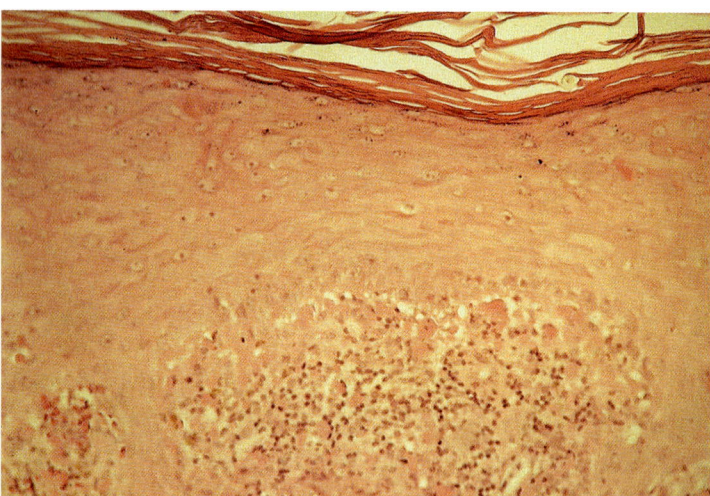

Fig. 51.2 Discoid lupus erythematosus: the degeneration of the basal layer and predominantly lymphocytic infiltration are well shown.

3 A patchy dermal lymphocytic infiltrate with a few plasma cells and histiocytes, particularly around the appendages, which may be atrophic.

The presence of at least two of these is essential to the histological diagnosis of LE. The following changes may also be found, but are less important:

1 Epidermal atrophy with relative hyperkeratosis and plugging of the follicular mouths, associated with pilosebaceous atrophy
2 Thickening of the basement membrane of the epidermis and sometimes of small vessels
3 Premature elastotic degeneration of collagen in light-exposed areas.

In more acute forms there is less hyperkeratosis and dermal infiltration, but more dermal oedema, liquefaction necrosis and atrophy. Disruption of the elastic lamina and, rarely, endothelial proliferation and thrombosis of the deeper vessels of the dermis have been reported [3]. Biopsy material from lesions on the palms stained for alkaline phosphatase activity shows irregular capillary loops with branching, 'dead end' spurs and coiling [4]. In SLE, similar changes are found in involved and uninvolved skin. In tumid lesions the dermal infiltrate can be very dense, and sometimes almost granulomatous. Dermal deposits of mucin occur [5], which may be diffuse or localized, and form nodular lesions. Deposits may be very gross [6]. Occasionally, irregular hyperplasia of the epidermis occurs, and there may be clefts, or even bullae, between the dermis and epidermis. Although keratotic plugs are usually found in the openings of the hair follicles, they may also block the sweat ducts or occur independently of either structure. Sometimes, the hair follicles contain concentric layers of keratin instead of hairs. Atrophy of the prickle cell layer occurs to a variable extent, and sometimes there may be acanthosis. Melanin may be found in the upper dermis as the result of pigmentary incontinence. Blood vessels are dilated and the upper dermis is oedematous.

Immunopathology. Immunohistology [7] shows the presence of immunoglobulins IgG, IgA, IgM and complement at the dermal–

Table 51.3 Diseases associated with the presence of immunoreactants at the dermal–epidermal junction that may be confused with lupus erythematosus.

Mixed connective tissue disease
Systemic sclerosis
Dermatomyositis
Sjögren's syndrome
Myasthenia gravis
Porphyrias
Granuloma annulare
Necrobiosis lipoidica
Amyloidosis
Graft-versus-host disease
Psoriasis
Pyoderma gangrenosum
Sarcoidosis
Leprosy
Erythema multiforme
Pityriasis lichenoides acuta
Granuloma faciale
Keratoacanthoma
Scabies
Facial telangiectases
Bullous pemphigoid

epidermal junction, in skin lesions present for 6 weeks or more, in approximately 80% of patients [8]. Homogeneous, granular or thready patterns occur, but the deposition is usually homogeneous in older lesions. They are more frequent on the face and in untreated lesions, but are rare on the trunk [9], and decrease after treatment with topical corticosteroids. They do not occur in uninvolved skin, unlike the majority of cases of SLE. For the diagnosis of DLE lesions, light microscopy is most valuable and should be carried out before direct immunofluorescence [10]. Immunoreactants are also found in oral mucosa and the conjunctiva [11]. C1q deposits are found in 29% of patients with immunofluorescent-positive DLE, compared with 90% in SLE, and the presence of such deposits implies an increased risk of eventual systemic disease [12]. Deposits at the dermal–epidermal junction are not specific to LE and have been found in many other circumstances (Table 51.3). However, in these diseases the deposits are less prominent at the dermal–epidermal junction and are more striking in the blood vessel walls. In LE, the deposits are heavy and contain several immunoglobulin classes, whereas in the other diseases only a single immunoglobulin class is usually present. In scarring alopecia caused by LE, the deposits occur around hair follicles, a feature not seen in other types of scarring alopecia [13].

Properdin, indicating complement activation, has been demonstrated at the dermal–epidermal junction in 70% of lesions, usually in association with deposition of immunoglobulin, C3 and C4 [14]. It may also be found in non-lesional skin. Serum properdin levels are raised in DLE and SLE [14].

References

1 Montgomery H. Pathology of lupus erythematosus. *J Invest Dermatol* 1939; **2**: 343–59.
2 Jerdan MS, Hood AF, Moore GW, Callen JP. Histopathologic comparison of the subsets of lupus erythematosus. *Arch Dermatol* 1990; **126**: 52–5.

3 Panja RK, Sengupta KP, Aikat BK. Vascular changes in the cutaneous lesions of lupus erythematosus and scleroderma. *Br J Dermatol* 1966; **78**: 34–42.

4 Kurban AK, Farah FS, Chaglassian HT. Capillary changes in some connective tissue diseases. *Dermatologica* 1964; **129**: 257–65.

5 Lee WS, Chung J, Ahn SK. Mucinous alopecia associated with papulonodular mucinosis as a new manifestation of lupus erythematosus. *Int J Dermatol* 1996; **35**: 72–3.

6 Weigand DA, Bungdorf HC, Gregg LJ. Dermal mucinosis in discoid lupus erythematosus. *Arch Dermatol* 1981; **117**: 735–8.

7 Rowell NR, Scott DG. Immunohistological studies with anti-connective tissue and anti-immunoglobulin antisera of the skin in lupus erythematosus and scleroderma. *Br J Dermatol* 1975; **93**: 431–41.

8 Prystowsky SD, Gilliam JN. Discoid lupus erythematosus as part of a larger disease spectrum: correlation of clinical features with laboratory findings in lupus erythematosus. *Arch Dermatol* 1975; **111**: 1448–52.

9 Weigand DA. Lupus band test: anatomic regional variations in discoid lupus erythematosus. *J Am Acad Dermatol* 1981; **14**: 426–8.

10 Williams REA, MacKie RM, O'Keefe R *et al*. The contribution of direct immunofluorescence to the diagnosis of lupus erythematosus. *J Cutan Pathol* 1989; **16**: 122–5.

11 Burge SM, Frith PA, Millard PR *et al*. The lupus band test in oral mucosa, conjunctiva and skin. *Br J Dermatol* 1989; **121**: 743–52.

12 Leibowitch M, Droz D, Noel LH *et al*. C1q deposits at the dermoepidermal junction: a marker discriminating for discoid and systemic lupus erythematosus. *J Clin Immunol* 1981; **2**: 119–24.

13 Amato L, Mei S, Massi D *et al*. Cicatricial alopecia: a dermatopathologic and immunopathologic study of 33 patients (pseudopelade of Brocq is not a specific clinicopathologic entity). *Int J Dermatol* 2002; **41**: 8–15.

14 Schrager MA, Rothfield NF. Pathways of complement activation in chronic discoid lupus. *Arthritis Rheum* 1977; **20**: 637–45.

Immunocytochemistry. The majority of infiltrating lymphocytes are T lymphocytes and express Ia-like antigens, as well as the γδ T-cell receptor. There is some evidence of clonal selection of T-cell receptors, suggesting an antigen driven response in the skin. Infiltrating cells are a mixture of CD4$^+$, CD8$^+$ and HLA-DR$^+$ cells in all types of cutaneous LE, with CD4$^+$ cells slightly predominating [1]. There are also populations of mainly CD45RO$^+$ memory cells, with few activated CD45RA$^+$ differentiated effector cells [2]. In addition, there is evidence of vascular activation with up-regulation of ICAM-1, vascular adhesion molecule-1, E-selectin and P-selectin [3].

The description of the presence of skin-homing cytotoxic lymphocytes, expressing granzyme B, in association with a Th1 pattern of cytokine expression, and targeting the epidermal adnexal structures, is an important step in our understanding of the process of inflammation and scarring in cutaneous LE [4]. Although the pattern of cytokine expression may be variable, with interleukins 2 (IL-2) and -4 absent, and IL-5 and IL-10 variably present, the expression of predominantly type 1 interferons is likely to induce auto-reactive cytotoxic lymphocytes as indicated by Wenzel *et al.* [5].

Identification of the target antigen that drives this response is urgently needed to understand the pathogenesis of the discoid pattern of cutaneous lupus. Information on the interplay of the genetic control of cytokine profiles also gives important clues to the pathogenesis of the various sub-types of cutaneous lupus, particularly the role of TNF-α and IL-10 and their balance [6].

References

1 Volcplatzer B, Alpetz B, Milota S *et al*. Accumulation of gammadelta T-cells in chronic cutaneous lupus erythematosus. *J Invest Dermatol* 1993; **100**: S84–S91.

2 Kohchiyama A, Oka D, Ueki H. T cell subsets in lesions of systemic and discoid lupus erythematosus. *J Cutan Pathol* 1985; **12**: 493–9.

3 Kuhn A, Sonntag M, Lehmann P *et al*. Characterization of the inflammatory infiltrate and expression of endothelial cell adhesion molecules in lupus erythematosus tumidus. *Arch Dermatol Res* 2002; **294**: 6–13.

4 Stein LF, Saed GM, Finerson DP. T cell cytokine network in cutaneous lupus erythematosus. *J Am Acad Dermatol* 1997; **36**: 191–6.

5 Wenzel J, Uerlich E, Worrenkamper S *et al*. Scarring skin lesions of discoid lupus erythematosus are characterised by high numbers of skin-homing cytotoxic lymphocytes associated with strong expression of the type 1 interferon-induced protein MxA. *Br J Dermatol* 2005; **153**: 1011–7.

6 Suarez A, Lopez P, Mozo L, Gutierrez C. Differential effect of IL10 and TNFα genotypes on determining susceptibility to discoid and systemic lupus erythematosus. *Ann Rheum Dis* 2005; **64**: 1605–10.

Histopathological differential diagnosis. Chronic DLE must be differentiated from other conditions in which lymphocytic infiltrations of the dermis occur.

1 In Jessner's lymphocytic infiltration [1], the dermis shows large circumscribed aggregations of lymphocytes, often concentrated round the dermal appendages and blood vessels, with a normal epidermis. Sometimes, the infiltrate may extend into the fat of the subcutaneous tissues. Immunohistochemical studies show that the cells are predominantly T lymphocytes [2], as they are in DLE and SLE [3]. Monoclonal antibody studies show an increase in natural killer (NK) cells and activated cytotoxic T lymphocytes in Jessner's lymphocytic infiltration [4].

2 In polymorphic light eruption (PLE), the infiltrate is less prominent and more likely to occur around blood vessels than cutaneous appendages. Liquefaction degeneration is infrequent but, if present, it may be difficult to distinguish from that of DLE. There may be spongiotic changes in the epidermis and parakeratosis (the histology has some features of eczema, but the dermal infiltrate is usually denser). Lever and Schaumburg-Lever [5] believe that most cases of Jessner's lymphocytic infiltration and the plaque-type of PLE represent variants of chronic DLE, but immunoglobulin does not occur at the dermal–epidermal junction in either of the first two conditions [6,7].

3 Scattered patches of lymphocytes occur in the dermis in lymphocytic lymphoma, but there are no epidermal changes.

4 The infiltrate in lymphocytoma cutis (Spiegler–Fendt sarcoid; see Chapter 57) is usually separated from the normal epidermis by a band of normal collagen, and consists of lymphocytes and a few histiocytes. Sometimes, a follicular arrangement is present, with lymphocytes surrounding islands of histiocytes resembling lymph node follicles.

5 In benign lymphocytic infiltration, polyclonal T and B cells form aggregates in the dermis.

Sometimes, patients show clinical, histopathological and immunofluorescence overlap between DLE and lichen planus. In such cases, a definite diagnosis cannot always be made, and it is likely that such patients have both diseases [8].

References

1 Jessner M, Kanof NB. Lymphocytic infiltration of the skin. *Arch Dermatol Syphilol* 1953; **68**: 447–9.

2 Willemze R, Dijkstra A, Meijer CJLM. Lymphocytic infiltration of the skin (Jessner): a T-cell lymphoproliferative disease. *Br J Dermatol* 1983; **110**: 523–8.

3 Konttinen YT, Reitamo S, Ranki A *et al*. T-lymphocytes and monoclonal phagocytes in the skin infiltrate of systemic and discoid lupus erythematosus and Jessner's lymphocytic infiltrate. *Br J Dermatol* 1981; **104**: 141–5.

4 Viljaranta S, Ranki A, Kariniemi A-L *et al.* Distribution of natural killer cells and lymphocyte subclasses in Jessner's lymphocytic infiltration of the skin and in cutaneous lesions of discoid and systemic lupus erythematosus. *Br J Dermatol* 1987; **116**: 831–8.

5 Lever WF, Schaumburg-Lever G. *Histopathology of the Skin*, 6th edn. Philadelphia: Lippincott, 1983: 457.

6 Fisher DA, Epstein JH, Kay DN *et al.* Polymorphous light eruption and lupus erythematosus. *Arch Dermatol* 1970; **101**: 458–61.

7 Ten Have-Opbroek AAW. On the differential diagnosis between chronic discoid lupus erythematosus and lymphocytic infiltration of the skin (Jessner) with emphasis on fluorescence microscopy. *Dermatologica* 1966; **132**: 109–14.

8 Potts EDA, Rowell NR. Lichen planus: a distinct entity from lupus erythematosus. *Acta Derm Venereol (Stockh)* 1981; **61**: 413–6.

Incidence. Because the condition is persistent, DLE appears to be more common than it really is. The incidence among new patients in the Department of Dermatology at Leeds is approximately 4 or 5 in 1000. It is said that it is only half as frequent in black people [1], although the distribution is worldwide.

Reference

1 Cummer CL. Aetiology of lupus erythematosus. *Arch Dermatol Syphilol* 1936; **33**: 434–45.

Clinical features

Symptoms. The patient usually presents with a rash, but on questioning a history of Raynaud's phenomenon, chilblains or poor peripheral circulation is often obtained. In 120 patients at Leeds, 14% had Raynaud's phenomenon and 22% had chilblains; a poor peripheral circulation, without a definite story of Raynaud's phenomenon, was noted in a further 26% of patients. Joint pains are complained of by approximately one-quarter of patients, but this is similar to the incidence in controls [1]. Most patients have no symptoms of systemic upset, even with widespread cutaneous disease, although fatigue is not uncommon in those with severe disease.

Most patients have disease limited to the head and neck (localized DLE), but a few have much more extensive disease, potentially affecting any area of the skin (disseminated DLE).

Localized disease. The face is most commonly affected, and the scalp, ears, nose, arms, legs and trunk to a lesser extent. The circumscribed or discoid type is the most frequent (Fig. 51.3), and occurs particularly on the cheeks, the bridge of the nose, the ears, the side of the neck and the scalp. Lesions may be bilateral, although not necessarily symmetrical, or unilateral. Alopecia occurs in the scalp lesions in approximately one-third of patients [2], and is usually permanent (Fig. 51.4). The eyebrows may be sparse, with erythema of the eyebrow skin. Usually, lesions occur as well-defined erythematous patches, varying in size from a few millimetres to 10–15 cm. There is adherent scale in many cases, and when this is removed its undersurface shows horny plugs which have occupied dilated pilosebaceous canals. This so-called 'tin-tack' sign can sometimes also be seen in localized pemphigus foliaceus [3]. When not obscured by scaling, these horny plugs can be seen on direct examination. The surface may present a dirty brownish yellow appearance that is rough to the touch, because of the follicular plugging. If hyperkeratosis is marked, a warty

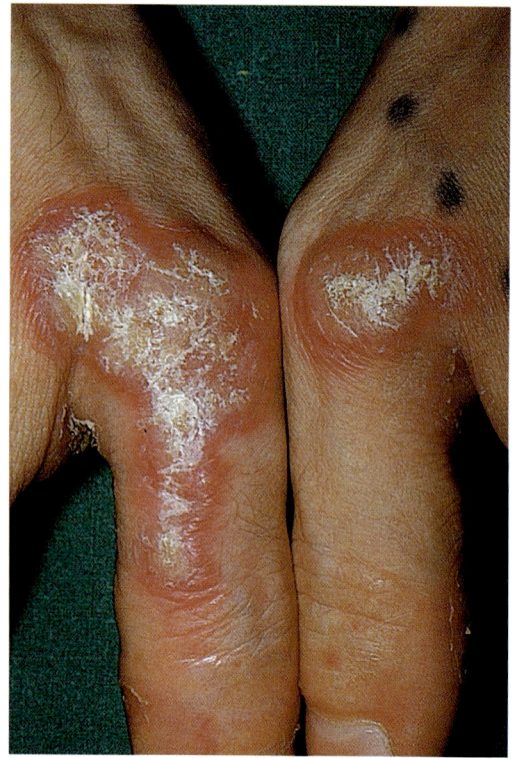

Fig. 51.3 Discoid lupus erythematosus: the typical scaling is well shown.

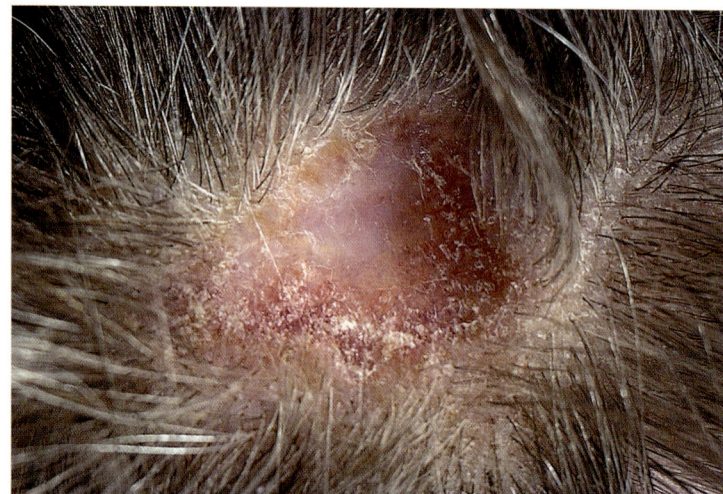

Fig. 51.4 Discoid lupus erythematosus of the scalp: note the follicular plugging.

lesion with a red, slightly raised edge results. This warty type of LE is most commonly seen on the nose, temples, ears and scalp, but may also occur on the palms and soles and causes difficulty with walking (Fig. 51.5) [4].

Non-itching hyperkeratotic papulonodular lesions on the arms and hands, resembling keratoacanthoma, hypertrophic lichen planus or nodular prurigo, also occur [5]. Sometimes, the appearance resembles psoriasis. In other cases, there may be very little hyperkeratosis. Lesions then present as reddish, well-defined, almost smooth plaques with little or no scaling. Sometimes, these plaques may show prominent flattening in the centre, giving rise to annular lesions. Over the course of some months, particularly

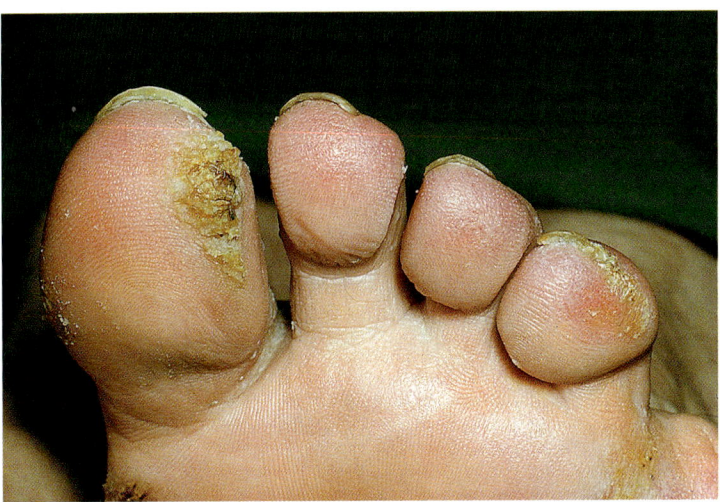

Fig. 51.5 Warty lesions of the feet in chronic lupus erythematosus.

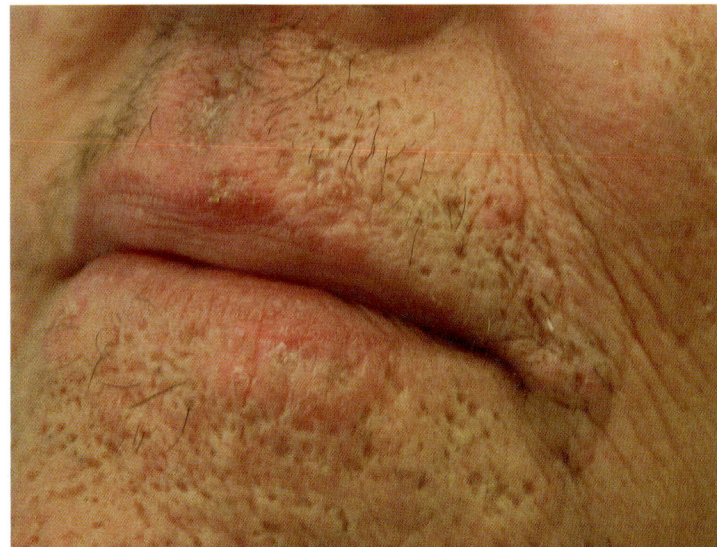

Fig. 51.7 Cribriform scarring in discoid lupus erythematosus.

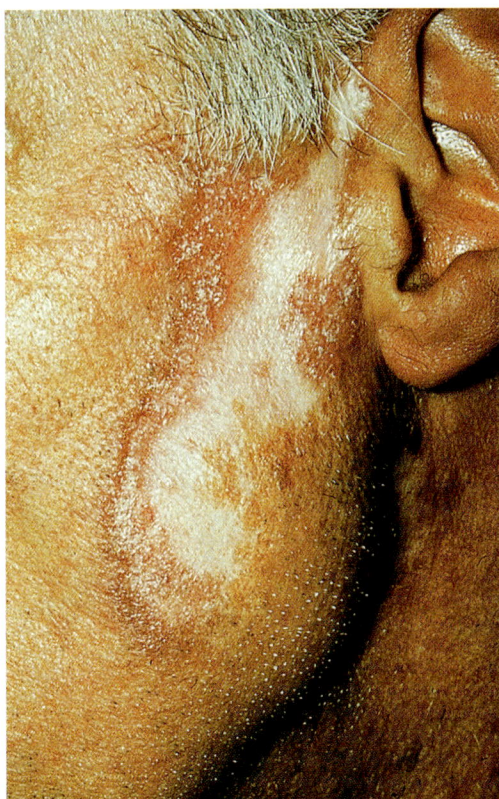

Fig. 51.6 Discoid lupus erythematosus: the pre-auricular type with pigmentation around the scarred area.

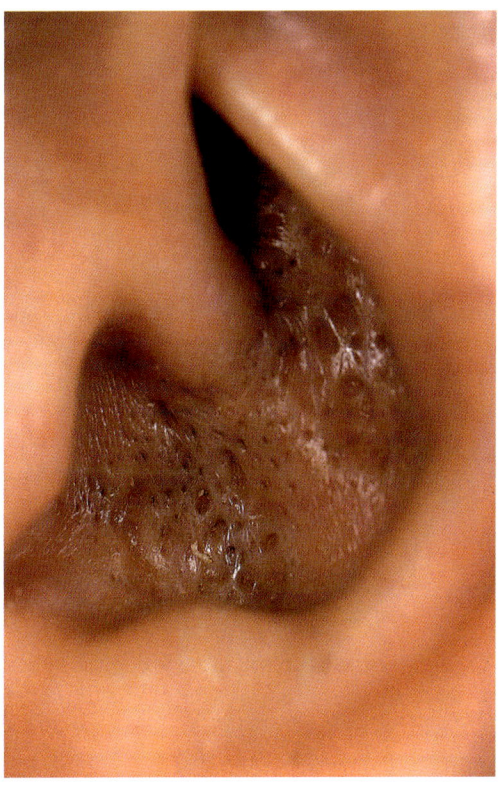

Fig. 51.8 Typical lesions in the ear.

if treated, lesions flatten and may clear completely without much scarring. More frequently, a thin white scarred area, often with a slightly raised, red border or zone of hyperpigmentation, remains (Fig. 51.6). Localized cribriform scarring occurs, particularly on the face (Fig. 51.7). Wide follicular pits, sometimes containing scale or blackheads, occur mainly in the concha or triangular fossa of the ear (Fig. 51.8). They occur in up to one-third of cases [6] of DLE but they also occur in SLE. In approximately 7.5% of patients, the lesions on the face resemble rosacea, and differentiation from true rosacea can be difficult, particularly as in approximately 15% of cases patients with true rosacea show exacerbation by sunlight. Low titre ANA also occurs in rosacea, complicating assessment, but has no clinical relevance [7]. LE of this rosaceous type presents with reddish nodular lesions on the nose, cheeks, forehead and sometimes chin, and is associated with a diffuse erythema of the face and easy flushing. Usually, unlike true rosacea, there are no pustules (Fig. 51.9) [8]. Biopsy is required to distinguish between LE and rosacea.

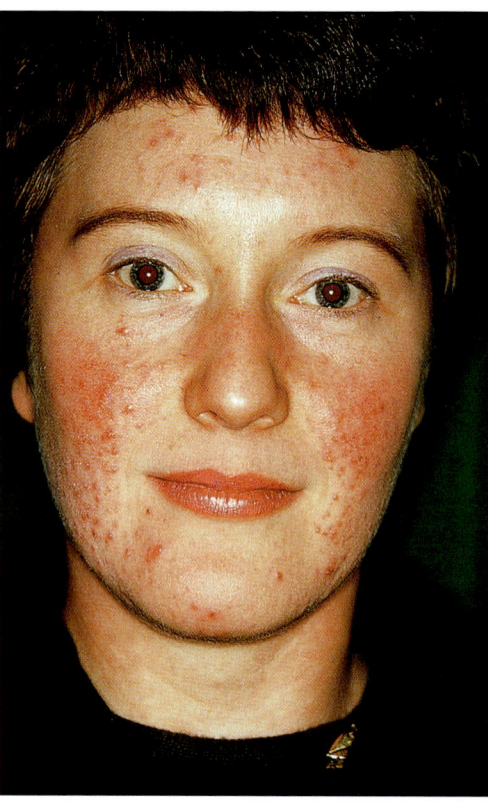

Fig. 51.9 Discoid lupus erythematosus: a rosaceous pattern seen in 7.5% of patients.

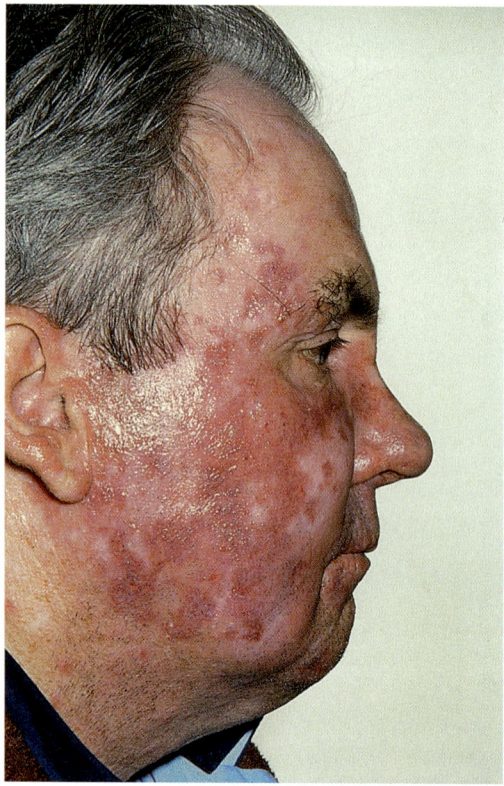

Fig. 51.10 Discoid lupus erythematosus: tumid lesions of the face.

Tumid lesions may occur, in which the tissues are swollen, brawny, warm and tense (Fig. 51.10). The surface shows a reddish, mottled appearance resulting from scarring. This type of lesion may be many centimetres in diameter and involve the whole of one cheek, or even the whole of a limb. Another clinical type of DLE results in annular atrophic plaques [8] on the face, neck and behind the ears. The centre of the plaques is depressed and sclerotic, and the lesions resemble morphoea, lichen sclerosus or 'annular atrophic plaques' [9]. Early lesions show IgG and complement at the dermal–epidermal junction [8], but repeated biopsies may be necessary to confirm the diagnosis.

Scarring. Pigmentary disturbances are common, especially in dark-skinned people, and there is some evidence that DLE is more severe in black people (Figs 51.11 & 51.12) [10]. Patches of leukoderma may be interspersed with hyperpigmented areas. If relapse occurs, it usually starts in the reddish zone surrounding the scar. Calcification may occur in the plaques [11]. Lesions on the ear lead to considerable atrophy and scarring (Fig. 51.13).

Disseminated DLE (DDLE). Characteristic lesions of DLE may occur in a widespread pattern on the trunk and limbs, or may be localized to other body sites. This occurs almost always in women, and they are usually cigarette smokers. The appearance may be indistinguishable from the papulosquamous type of SCLE (see p. 51.23), but scarring occurs in most patients. This variety tends to be persistent, resistant to therapy and associated with severe psychological upset. Lesions on the dorsa of the hands (Fig. 51.14),

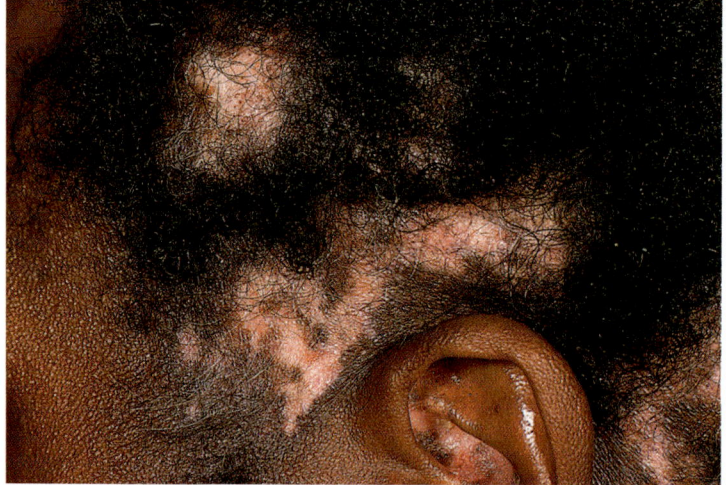

Fig. 51.11 Discoid lupus erythematosus in a black person.

palms [4] or toes (Fig. 51.15) [12] occurred in 6% of patients at Leeds. Purplish plaques may occur on the front of the knees and on the back of the heels. Another disseminated variety results in a reticulate telangiectasia, usually seen on the arms, legs and the back of the calves. This type of telangiectasia is probably similar to 'lupus erythematosus telangiectoides', first described by Crocker [13]. The appearances are characterized by a persistent, blotchy, reticulate telangiectasia, which occurs on the face, neck, ears, dorsa of the hands, breasts, heels and on the sides of the feet (Fig. 51.16). Healing occurs with punctate atrophic scarring. The histology of this type of lesion shows an atrophic epidermis, with dilata-

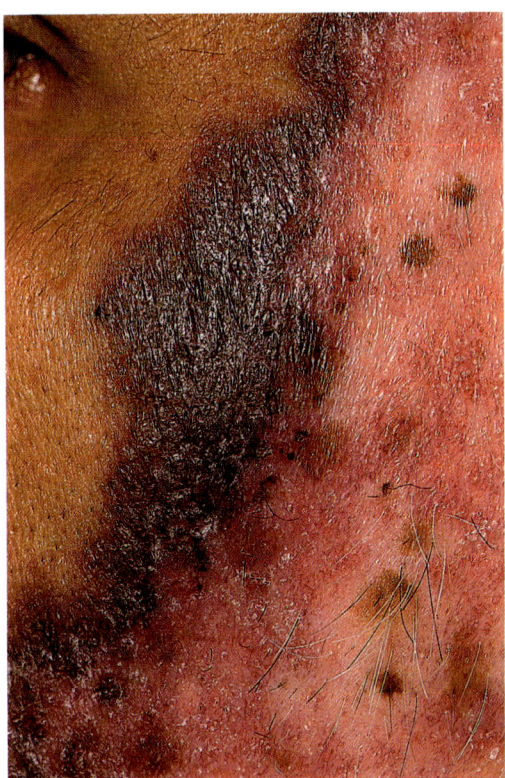

Fig. 51.12 Discoid lupus erythematosus in an Asian patient, showing marked hyperpigmentation at the border of the affected area.

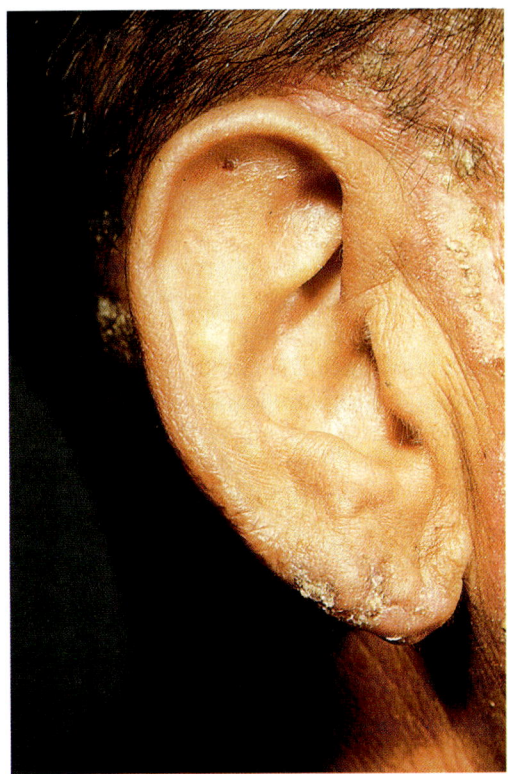

Fig. 51.13 Discoid lupus erythematosus of the ear with scarring and atrophy.

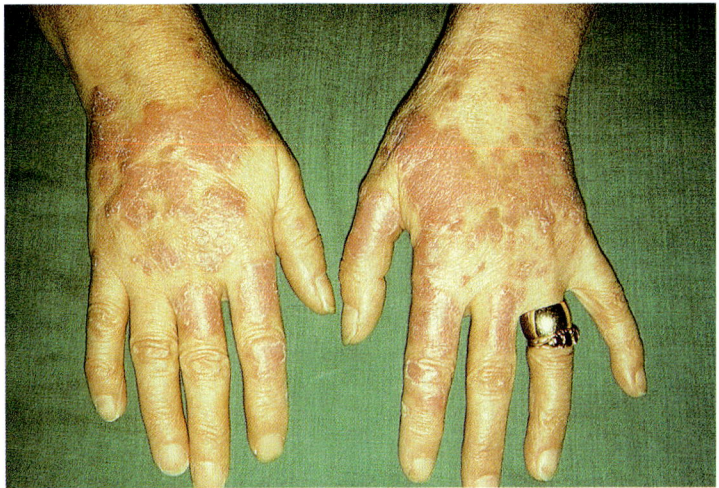

Fig. 51.14 Discoid lupus erythematosus: plaques on the back of the hands.

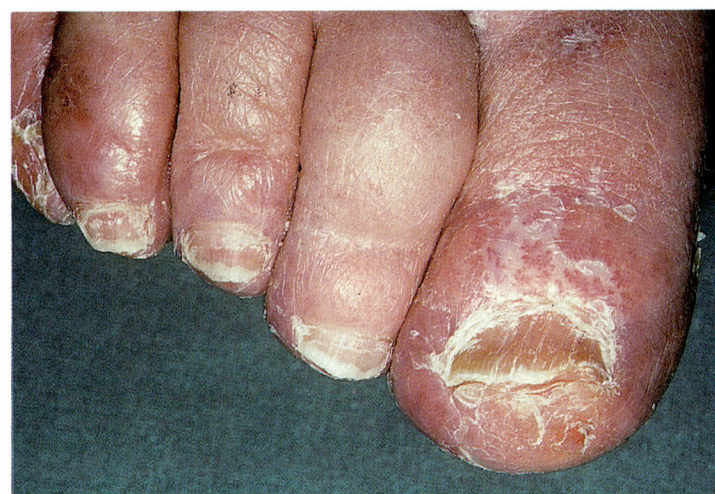

Fig. 51.15 Discoid lupus erythematosus: characteristic redness and scaling of the toes.

tion of the superficial vessels of the skin and slight infiltration of the papillary part of the corium. A further, more annular variant has been called 'lupus erythematosus gyratus repens' and consists of a migratory gyrate annular erythema with the histological features of LE (Fig. 51.17), although the lupus band test is negative [14]. There may be an underlying carcinoma. A pruritic, chronic, discrete, umbilicated papular eruption may occur on the back, and results in acneiform hypertrophic follicular scars [15].

Occasionally, one or more fingers may show a curious atrophic spindling, sometimes with hyperextension of the terminal phalanges and dystrophy of the nails (Fig. 51.18). The fingers and toes may become markedly atrophic, with patchy erythema and tuft resorption on X-ray. Rarely, bullous lesions [16] may occur. Arteritic lesions resembling those of Degos' syndrome or disseminated atrophie blanche occasionally occur, and linear lesions following Blaschko's lines have been reported [17].

'Chilblain lupus' (Fig. 51.19) [18]. Approximately 6% of patients, predominantly female, develop chilblain-like lesions chiefly on the toes and fingers, but also on the heels, calves, knees, knuckles,

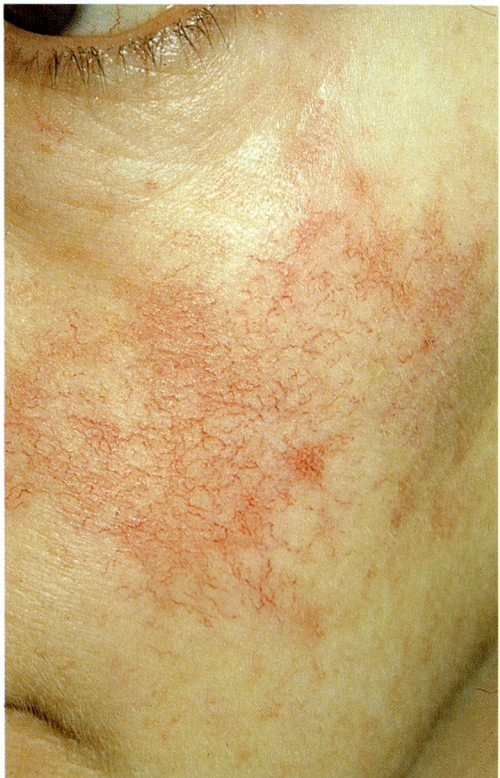

Fig. 51.16 Telangiectatic lupus erythematosus of the cheek.

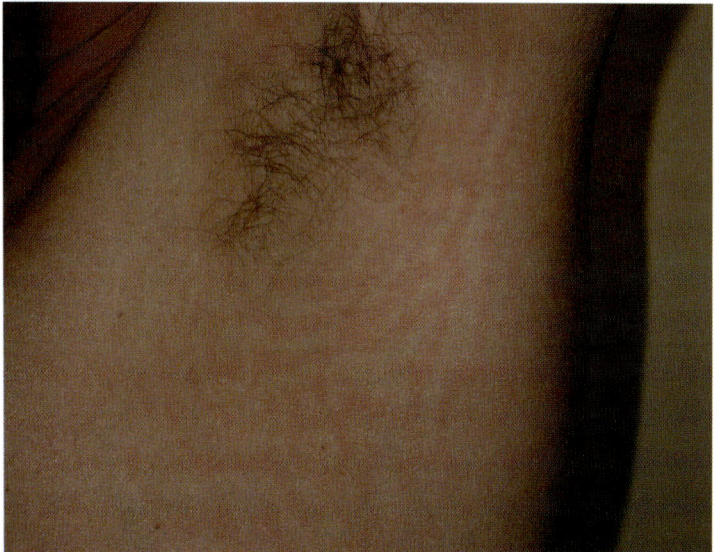

Fig. 51.17 Gyrate erythema in lupus.

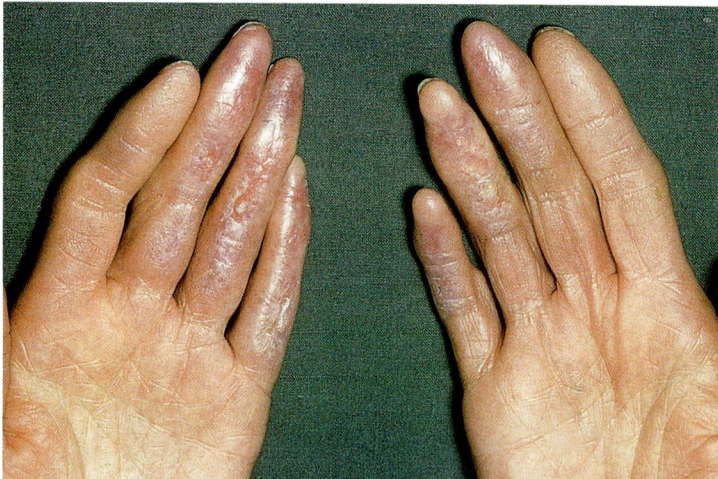

Fig. 51.18 Unusual spindling of the fingers and hyperextension of the distal phalanges in discoid lupus erythematosus.

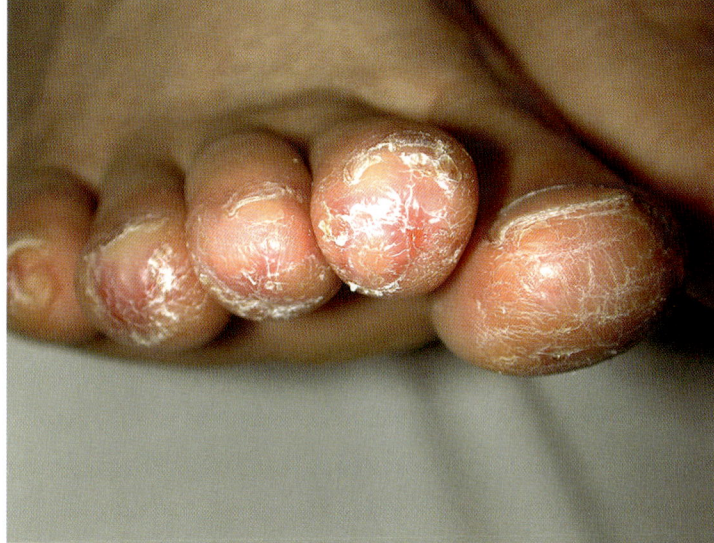

Fig. 51.19 'Chilblain' lesions in a patient with Ro-positive systemic lupus erythematosus.

elbows, nose and ears. Usually, but not always, the chilblain lesions occur some years after the development of discoid lesions on the face. It can be precipitated by pregnancy [19]. When the discoid lesions remit with treatment, the chilblains persist. Less commonly, discoid and perniotic lesions start simultaneously, and sometimes perniotic lesions occur alone. Histology and immunohistology is that of DLE, and the non-lesional skin gives a negative fluorescent band test. Some patients may have cryofibrinogenaemia or cold agglutinins. Patients are usually Ro antibody-positive [20]. They are also either smokers, or have markedly abnormal peripheral circulation with low resting blood flow. Approximately 15% of patients develop SLE, and this occurs more frequently in those who develop both forms of cutaneous LE simultaneously and in those with the erythema multiforme syndrome.

Nail changes. Subungual hyperkeratosis is more common than the red-blue colouring of the nail plate with longitudinal striae and crumbling away of the nail [21]. The changes may respond to chloroquine.

Mucous membranes [22]. These are involved in approximately 24% of patients. Nasal mucosal lesions occur in 9% and hyperkeratotic lichen planus-like plaques on the buccal mucosa and palate in a similar number. The lips show slight thickening and roughness and redness, sometimes with superficial ulceration and crusting. Healing occurs with some scarring. Erythematous patches

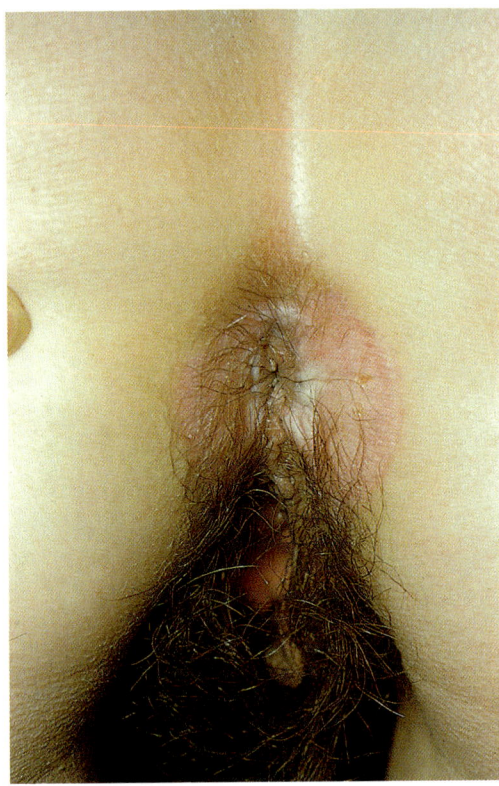

Fig. 51.20 Discoid lupus erythematosus of the perianal area.

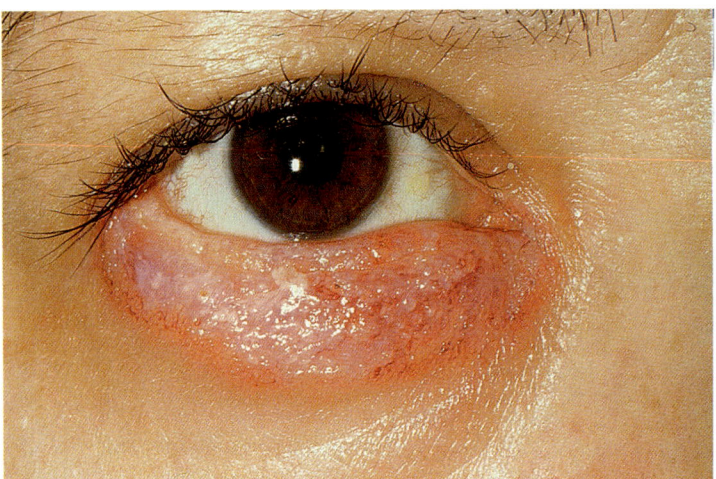

Fig. 51.21 Discoid lupus erythematosus of the lower eyelid.

with a depressed centre and superficial ulceration occur on the inner cheeks, tongue and on the palate. Oral lesions may resemble leukoplakia [23]. Erythematous lesions occur on the vulva in 5%, or around the anus (Fig. 51.20) [24].

Eye lesions. Velvety oedema and marked redness of the conjunctiva may occur. Palpebral lesions have been reported without lesions elsewhere on the face [25]. The eyelids are red, especially peripherally, and are slightly infiltrated and always scaly. Lesions are most common on the lower eyelids, especially on the outer third. The free edge is rarely completely involved. Erythematous plaques on the lower eyelids occur in 6%, and may be associated with conjunctival scarring (Fig. 51.21), and symblepharon [26]. The lesions may itch, and are exacerbated by trauma and sunlight. Corneal involvement is rare. Superficial punctate keratopathy and stromal keratitis have been reported [27]. Acute mucinosis of the eyelids and periorbital skin can occur [28].

References

1 Rothfield N, March CH, Miescher P *et al.* Chronic discoid lupus erythematosus. *N Engl J Med* 1963; **269**: 1155–61.
2 Wilson CL, Burge SM, Dean D *et al.* Scarring alopecia in discoid lupus erythematosus. *Br J Dermatol* 1992; **126**: 307–14.
3 Paramsothy Y, Lawrence CM. 'Tin-tack' sign in localized pemphigus foliaceus. *Br J Dermatol* 1987; **116**: 127–9.
4 Parish LC, Kennedy RJ, Hurley HJ. Palmar lesions in lupus erythematosus. *Arch Dermatol* 1967; **96**: 273–6.
5 Uitto J, Santa-Cruz DJ, Eisen AZ *et al.* Verrucous lesions in patients with discoid lupus erythematosus. *Br J Dermatol* 1978; **98**: 507–20.
6 Shuster S. A simple sign of discoid lupus erythematosus. *Br J Dermatol* 1981; **104**: 350–1.
7 Black AA, McCauliffe DP, Sontheimer RD. Prevalence of acne rosacea in a rheumatic skin disease subspeciality unit. *Lupus* 1992; **1**: 222–37.

8 Chorzelski TP, Jablonska S, Blaszczyk M *et al.* Annular atrophic plaques of the face. *Arch Dermatol* 1976; **112**: 1143–5.
9 Christiansen HB, Mitchell WT. Annular atrophic plaques of the face. *Arch Dermatol* 1969; **100**: 703–16.
10 Prystowsky SD, Hernadon JH, Gilliam JN. Chronic cutaneous lupus erythematosus (DLE). *Medicine* 1975; **55**: 183–91.
11 Kabin DI, Malkinson FD. Lupus erythematosus and calcinosis cutis. *Arch Dermatol* 1969; **100**: 17–22.
12 Pramatarov K. Discoid lupus erythematosus of the soles. *J Dermatol* 1989; **16**: 511.
13 Crocker HR. *Diseases of the Skin: Their Description, Pathology, Diagnosis and Treatment.* Philadelphia: Blakiston, 1888.
14 Blanc D, Kienzler JL. Lupus erythematosus gyratus repens: report of a case associated with a lung carcinoma. *Clin Exp Dermatol* 1982; **7**: 129.
15 Haroon TS, Fleming KA. An unusual presentation of discoid lupus erythematosus. *Br J Dermatol* 1972; **87**: 642–9.
16 Nagy E, Balogh E. Bullous form of chronic discoid erythematodes accompanied by LE-cell symptoms. *Dermatologica* 1961; **122**: 6–10.
17 Green JJ, Baker DJ. Linear childhood discoid lupus erythematosus following the lines of Blaschko: a case report with review of the linear manifestations of lupus erythematosus. *Pediatr Dermatol* 1999; **16**: 128–33.
18 Millard LG, Rowell NR. Chilblain lupus erythematosus (Hutchinson). *Br J Dermatol* 1978; **98**: 497–506.
19 Stainforth J, Goodfield MJD, Taylor PV. Pregnancy-induced chilblain lupus erythematosus. *Clin Exp Dermatol* 1992; **18**: 449–51.
20 Aoki T, Ishizawa T, Hozumi Y *et al.* Chilblain lupus erythematosus of Hutchinson responding to surgical treatment: a report of two patients with anti-Ro/SS-A antibodies. *Br J Dermatol* 1996; **134**: 533–7.
21 Kint A, van Herpe L. Ungual anomalies in lupus erythematosus discoides. *Dermatologica* 1976; **153**: 298–302.
22 Burge SM, Frith PA, Juniper RP *et al.* Mucosal involvement in systemic and chronic cutaneous lupus erythematosus. *Br J Dermatol* 1989; **121**: 727–41.
23 Schidt M, Anderson L, Shear M *et al.* Leukoplakia-like lesions developing in patients with oral discoid lupus erythematosus. *Acta Odontol Scand* 1981; **39**: 209–16.
24 Roundtree J, Weigand D, Burgdorf W. Lupus erythematosus with oral and perianal mucous membrane involvement. *Arch Dermatol* 1982; **118**: 55–6.
25 Tosti A, Tosti G, Giovannini A. Discoid lupus erythematosus solely involving the eyelids: report of three cases. *J Am Acad Dermatol* 1987; **16**: 1259–60.
26 Frith P, Burge SM, Millard PR, Wojnarowska F. External ocular findings in lupus erythematosus: a clinical and immunopathological study. *Br J Ophthalmol* 1990; **74**: 163–7.
27 Raizman MB, Baum J. Discoid lupus keratitis. *Arch Ophthalmol* 1989; **107**: 545–7.
28 Williams WL, Ramos-Caro FA. Acute periorbital mucinosis in discoid lupus erythematosus. *J Am Acad Dermatol* 1999; **41**: 871–3.

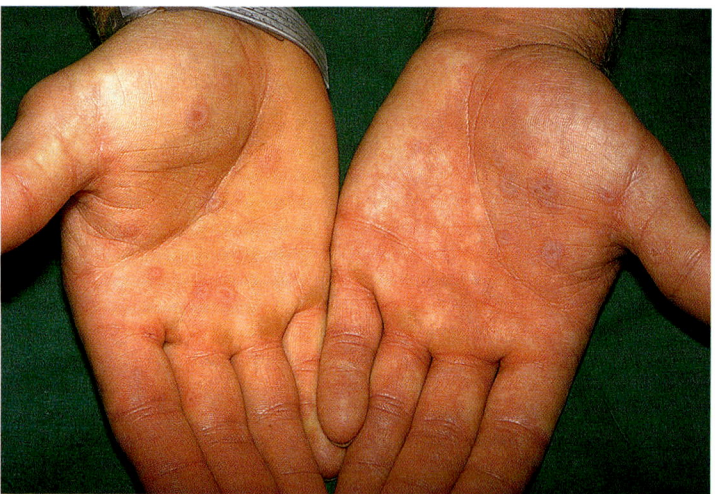

Fig. 51.22 Annular lesions of discoid lupus erythematosus resembling erythema multiforme and associated with characteristic immunological abnormalities (Rowell's syndrome).

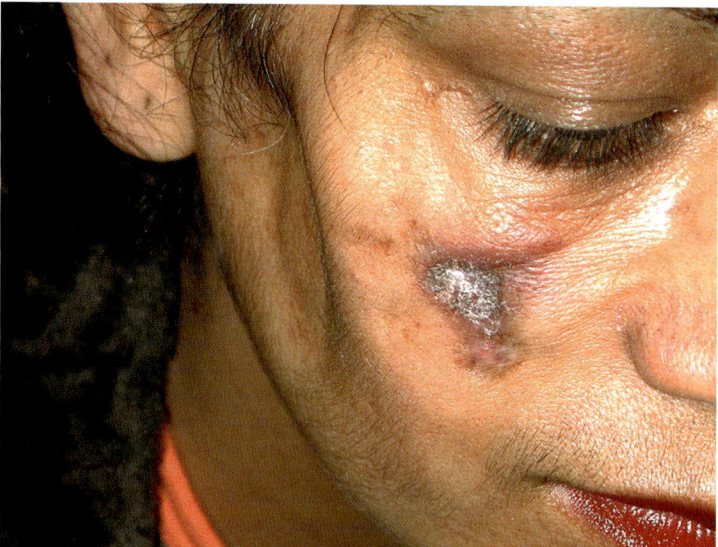

Fig. 51.23 Lupus erythematosus profundus.

Lupus erythematosus and erythema multiforme-like syndrome [1,2]

Synonym
- Rowell's syndrome

The distinctive syndrome of cutaneous LE, either discoid or systemic, occurring with lesions resembling erythema multiforme on the face, neck, hands, chest and in the mouth (Fig. 51.22) was first described by Rowell in 1963 in patients with discoid LE, but may be seen in both subacute and systemic disease. Characteristically, it lasts from a few days to over a month, but episodes may occur at intervals over a period of 20 years. No precipitating factor can be elicited. The lesions are at first papular, but later a ring forms and the edge becomes vesicular. Bullae, necrosis and ulceration may develop if the reaction is intense, although sometimes healing occurs without scarring. Patients with this syndrome also frequently have perniotic lesions [3]. They show a characteristic pattern of serological abnormality, in that the speckled type of antinuclear factor is associated with rheumatoid factor and the same precipitating antibody to saline extract of human tissues (anti-SjT). Anti-SjT is now thought to be identical to anti-La (SS-B). The syndrome has been reported in identical twin sisters, one of whom had DLE and the other SLE [4]. In patients with SLE, the homogeneous type of antinuclear antibody may also be present in the serum. When the syndrome occurs in DLE, the dermal–epidermal band test is positive in the discoid lesions and negative in the erythema multiforme lesions. If the LE is systemic, the bullous lesions show positive findings comparable with those seen in the uninvolved skin of patients with SLE [5]. The syndrome may be confused with patients showing coincidental LE and erythema multiforme [6]. In one case, anti-SS-B antibody and rheumatoid factor only developed after the erythema multiforme-like lesions appeared, suggesting that these factors are not just incidental findings but may have a role in the clinical presentation [7].

References
1 Rowell NR, Swanson-Beck J, Anderson JR. Lupus erythematosus and erythema multiforme-like lesions. *Arch Dermatol* 1963; **88**: 176–80.
2 Aydogan K, Karadogan S, Balaban AS, Tunali S. Lupus erythematosus associated with erythema multiforme: report of two cases and review of the literature. *Eur J Dermatol Venereol* 2005; **19**: 621–7.
3 Millard LG, Rowell NR. Chilblain lupus erythematosus, Hutchinson. *Br J Dermatol* 1978; **98**: 497–506.
4 Parodi A, Drago F, Varaldo G, *et al.* Rowell's syndrome. *J Am Acad Dermatol* 1989; **21**: 374–7.
5 Jablonska S, Blaszcyk M, Chorzelski T. Syndrome de Rowell: Lupus erythemateux avec les lesions coexistentes de type erytheme polymorphe bulleux. *Med Hyg* 1972; **1026**: 1390–3.
6 Lawrence CM, Marshall TL, Byrne JPH. Lupus erythematosus associated with erythema multiforme-like lesions in identical twins. *Br J Dermatol* 1982; **107**: 349–56.
7 Fiallo P, Tagliapetra A-G, Santaro G. Rowell's syndrome. *Int J Dermatol* 1995; **34**: 635–6.

Childhood DLE [1]
DLE is uncommon in childhood. There appears to be no female preponderance, there is less photosensitivity and the frequency of progression to systemic disease is higher. The other clinical features are similar to those in adults.

Reference
1 George PM, Tunnessen WW. Childhood discoid lupus erythematosus. *Arch Dermatol* 1993; **129**: 613–7.

Lupus erythematosus profundus (panniculitis) (Fig. 51.23) [1]
This is an unusual clinical variety of LE in which the cutaneous infiltrate occurs primarily (but not always exclusively) in deeper portions of the corium, with only microscopic epidermal changes, giving rise to firm, sharply defined nodules from one to several centimetres in diameter, lying beneath clinically normal skin [2]. The histopathology is sufficiently characteristic to establish the diagnosis in the absence of other cutaneous or systemic lesions of LE [1]. Clinical LE profundus occurred in 3–5% of patients with DLE [3,4], but histological disease may be found in up to 30% [5]. It can occur at any age and has been described in childhood [6].

The age and sex distribution of published cases is similar to that of DLE [7], and the disease may occur in childhood [8]. Familial cases have been reported [2,9].

Kaposi first described subcutaneous nodules in LE in 1883 [10], but Irgang [11] first used the term 'lupus erythematosus profundus' in 1940. Some authors [12] have considered the lesions to be sarcoid, but it is now usually accepted as a variant of LE [13], related more to DLE than SLE [14]. It was initially considered that it was different from 'lupus erythematosus hypertrophicus et profundus' described by Behçet [5], but the only difference is the involvement of the overlying skin in the version described by Behçet. Serological abnormalities occur when panniculitis is associated with SLE [15].

Histopathology. Microscopically [1], there may be epidermal atrophy, hydropic degeneration of the basal layer, follicular plugging and necrosis of the dermal collagen, suggesting LE. Collections of lymphocytes may occur around skin appendages and vessels in the mid-dermis. There is a striking lower dermal and subcutaneous necrobiosis, with some vasculitis and little cellular response. The collagen fibres in the lower dermis, in the septa and between the fat cells are swollen and poorly stained, and in some areas homogeneous masses and amorphous eosinophilic material replace the collagen. It is very important to exclude subcutaneous panniculitis-like T-cell lymphoma and this may require immunocytochemical investigation [16]. Immunofluorescence microscopy frequently shows linear staining at the basement-membrane zone [17]. Immune complexes can be demonstrated by direct fluorescence in small deep vessels in the dermis [18].

Clinical features. The nodular lesions are of varying size, but are usually one to several centimetres in diameter. They are usually firm, rubbery, sharply defined and persistent. The overlying skin usually appears normal, although histologically there are changes at the dermal–epidermal junction in two-thirds [1]. Typical lesions of DLE may be found elsewhere, most frequently on the cheeks. Healing usually leads to the development of depressed areas, and

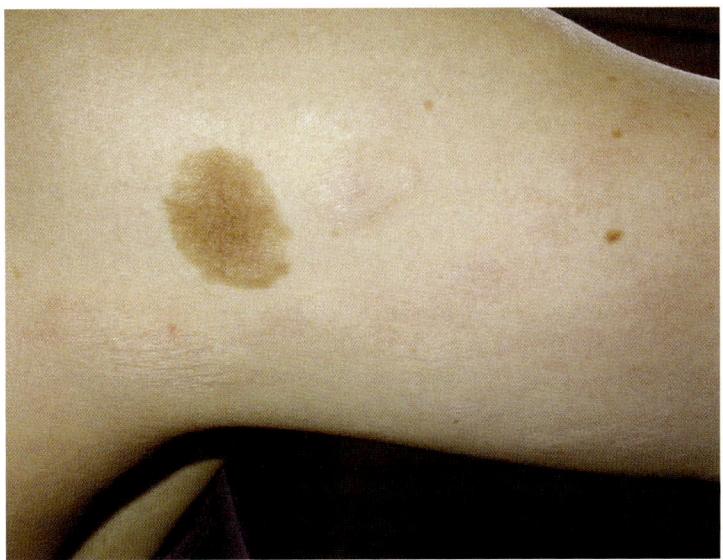

Fig. 51.24 Anetoderma secondary to lupus erythematosus profundus.

rarely to soft, slightly pink areas of anetoderma (Fig. 51.24) up to 4 cm in diameter. Cutis laxa followed one case [19]. Lupus profundus confined to the breast has been called lupus mastitis and may herald SLE. It may be confused with carcinoma [20]. LE profundus may affect the periorbital tissues and cause severe localized oedema [21]. It may occur with eyelid plaques [22]. Wherever it occurs, the nodules are persistent, and lesions in the cheeks may lead to marked disfigurement.

LE hypertrophicus et profundus starts as a violaceous, scaly, tender lesion, which rapidly enlarges, developing a warty hypertrophic surface with coarse adherent scales, which form a hard brown-black tar-like plaque [18]. Patients with LE hypertrophicus et profundus may have extensive serological abnormalities [18], and antibodies to extractable nuclear antigen (ENA) may sometimes be present [23]. On the legs, it may initially resemble thrombophlebitis [24]. Calcification can occur, and may be extensive, with the extrusion of thick, yellowish white material through ulcerated areas.

Associated diseases. LE profundus followed thrombocytopenic purpura in one case [15]. Lesions can occur after trauma or surgical biopsy [18], and have been precipitated by electromyography [25]. Monoclonal gammopathy has been reported in LE profundus [26].

Treatment. Clobetasol propionate cream (Dermovate) under a hydrocolloid occlusive dressing (Granuflex) is worth trying [27]. Antimalarial drugs are helpful [2,3,7], including in children [28]. Intralesional injections of triamcinolone (5 mg/mL) may be helpful [29]. Oral thalidomide has resolved resistant lesions, and this has been confirmed in a patient with associated partial C4 deficiency [30].

References
1 Ng PP, Tan SH, Tan T. Lupus erythematosus panniculitis: a clinicopathologic study. *Int J Dermatol* 2002; **41**: 488–90.
2 Arnold HL. Lupus erythematosus profundus. *Arch Dermatol* 1956; **73**: 15–33.
3 Tuffanelli DL. Lupus erythematosus panniculitis (profundus). *Arch Dermatol* 1971; **103**: 231–42.
4 de Berker D, Dissaneyeka M, Burge S. The sequelae of chronic cutaneous lupus erythematosus. *Lupus* 1992; **1**: 181–6.
5 Behçet PE. Lupus erythematosus hypertrophicus et profundus. *Arch Dermatol Syphilol* 1950; **61**: 495–8.
6 Marks R, Levene GM. Discoid lupus erythematosus and lupus erythematosus profundus in a child. *Clin Exp Dermatol* 1976; **1**: 187.
7 Thurston CS, Curtis AC. Lupus erythematosus profundus (Kaposi–Irgang). *Arch Dermatol* 1966; **93**: 577–82.
8 Kind P, Schreier-Rometh U, Wahn V *et al.* Lupus panniculitis: lupus erythematodesus profundus. *Gfr Klin Padiatr* 1986; **198**: 62–4.
9 Reed WB, Bergeron RF, Tuffanelli D *et al.* Hereditary inflammatory vasculitis with persistent nodules. *Br J Dermatol* 1972; **87**: 299–307.
10 Kaposi M. *Pathologie und Therapie der Hautkrankheiten*, 2nd edn. Vienna: Urban & Schwarzenberg, 1883: 642.
11 Irgang S. Lupus erythematosus profundus. *Arch Dermatol Syphilol* 1940; **42**: 97–102.
12 Pautrier LM. Apropos du pseudo-lupus erythemateux profond (Kaposi–Irgang). *Ann Dermatol Syphilol* 1953; **80**: 233–53.
13 Pascher F, Sims CF, Pensky N. Lupus erythematosus (Kaposi–Irgang). Reprint of case including comparative study of histopathology with that of chronic discoid lupus erythematosus. *J Invest Dermatol* 1955; **25**: 347–62.
14 Watanabe T, Tsuchida T. Lupus erythematosus profundus: a cutaneous marker for a distinct clinical subset? *Br J Dermatol* 1996; **134**: 123–5.

15 Zweiman B, Tomar RH, Gross PR. Lupus erythematosus profundus following thrombocytopenic purpura. *Arch Dermatol* 1975; **111**: 347–51.

16 Massone C, Kodama K, Salmhofer K *et al*. Lupus erythematosus panniculitis (lupus profundus): clinical, histopathological, and molecular analysis of nine cases. *J Cutan Pathol* 2005; **32**: 396–404.

17 Dammert K. Lupus erythematosus hypertrophicus et profundus. *Acta Derm Venereol (Stockh)* 1971; **51**: 315–20.

18 Otani A. Lupus erythematosus hypertrophicus et profundus. *Br J Dermatol* 1977; **96**: 75–8.

19 Delisee BR, Schanne R, Gilbert M. Cutis laxa généralisée post-inflammatoire associée a une panniculite lupique. *Ann Dermatol Vénéréol* 1990; **117**: 841–4.

20 de Bandt M, Meyer O, Grossin M *et al*. Lupus mastitis heralding systemic lupus erythematosus with anti-phospholipid syndrome. *J Rheumatol* 1993; **20**: 1217–20.

21 Sheehan-Dare RA, Cunliffe WJ. Severe periorbital oedema in association with lupus erythematosus profundus. *Clin Exp Dermatol* 1988; **13**: 406–7.

22 Inuzuka, M, Tomita K, Tokura K, Takigawa M. Lupus erythematosus profundus with unusual skin manifestation: subcutaneous nodules coexisting with eyelid plaques. *J Dermatol* 2001; **28**: 437–41.

23 Spann CR, Callen JP, Klein JB *et al*. Clinical, serologic and immunogenetic studies in patients with chronic cutaneous (discoid) lupus erythematosus who have verrucous and/or hypertrophic skin lesions. *J Rheumatol* 1988; **15**: 256–61.

24 Yeung M, Wood, MS, Grondin C, Chalmers A. Lupus profundus presenting as thrombophlebitis. *J Rheumatol* 1989; **16**: 625–6.

25 Fahrner L, Duvic M. Lupus panniculitis. *Arch Dematol* 1986; **122**: 625–6.

26 Fuerman EJ, Halevy S. Lupus erythematosus profundus (Kaposi–Irgang) with monoclonal gammopathy. *Br J Dermatol* 1977; **96**: 79–82.

27 Yell JA, Burge SM. Lupus erythematosus profundus treated with clobetasol propionate under a hydrocolloid dressing. *Br J Dermatol* 1993; **128**: 103.

28 Fox JN, Klapman MH, Rowe L. Lupus profundus in children: treatment with hydroxychloroquine. *J Am Acad Dermatol* 1987; **16**: 839–44.

29 Rowell NR. Treatment of chronic discoid lupus erythematosus with intralesional triamcinolone. *Br J Dermatol* 1962; **74**: 354–7.

30 Burrows NP, Walport MJ, Hammond AH *et al*. Lupus erythematosus profundus with partial C4 deficiency responding to thalidomide. *Br J Dermatol* 1991; **125**: 62–7.

Associated features. Small telangiectases on the face occur in approximately 20% of patients. These dilated vessels may sometimes resemble spider naevi, but are usually small capillaries of irregular size and distribution, particularly on the cheeks. Dilated nail fold capillaries, similar to those seen in SLE and dermatomyositis, may be visible with the naked eye in 3%, and sometimes there may be erythema of the pulps of the fingers. More than half of patients state that they have a dry skin. Very occasionally, mild diffuse alopecia may occur, similar to that found in SLE, and alopecia areata has occurred in 10% of one series of DLE and mild SLE [1].

Bilateral enlargement of the parotids has been reported [2]. Histologically, there is lymphocytic infiltration of the parotid, which is said to be like that of LE profundus [2]. The parotid swelling may increase with exposure to sunlight and decrease during treatment with antimalarials and corticosteroids [2].

Livedo reticularis on the legs has been reported in DLE, and in one case cryoglobulins were intermittently demonstrated in the serum [3]. Table 51.4 lists the other conditions associated with DLE.

References

1 Werth VP, White WL, Sanchez MR. Incidence of alopecia areata in lupus erythematosus. *Arch Dermatol* 1992; **128**: 368–71.

2 Trapl J, Sabatova M. Lupus erythematosus and parotitis. *Dermatol Wochenschr* 1960; **142**: 817–9.

Table 51.4 Diseases reported in association with lupus erythematosus [4–14].

Porphyria
Cutanea tarda
Variegate
Acute intermittent
Erythropoietic protoporphyria
Pemphigus
Myasthenia gravis
Thymoma
Chronic lymphocytic leukaemia
Macroglobulinaemia
Benign monoclonal gammopathy
Multiple myeloma
Polychondritis
Thyroiditis
Carpal tunnel syndrome
Polymorphic light eruption
Sheehan's syndrome

3 Nelson CT. Discoid lupus, reticulate livedo of legs, cryoglobulinemia. *Arch Dermatol* 1959; **80**: 497–8.

4 Callen JP, Ross L. Subacute cutaneous lupus erythematosus and porphyria cutanea tarda. *J Am Acad Dermatol* 1981; **5**: 269–73.

5 Cram DL, Epstein JH, Tuffanelli DL. Lupus erythematosus and porphyria. *Arch Dermatol* 1973; **108**: 779–84.

6 O'Reilly FM, O'Loughlin S, Murphy GM. Discoid lupus erythematosus and porphyria cutanea tarda. *J R Soc Med* 1996; **89**: 523–4.

7 Mutasim DF, Pelc NJ. Erythropoietic protoporphyria and lupus erythematosus: case report and review of the literature. *Arch Dermatol* 1994; **130**: 1330–2.

8 Cruz PD Jr, Coldiron BM, Sontheimer RD. Concurrent features of cutaneous lupus erythematosus and pemphigus erythematosus following myasthenia gravis and thymoma. *J Am Acad Dermatol* 1987; **16**: 472–80.

9 Abdou NL, Abdou NI. Discoid lupus erythematosus with macroglobulinemia. *Am J Med* 1974; **57**: 631–7.

10 Hughes RAC, Berry CL, Seifert M *et al*. Relapsing polychondritis. *QJM* 1972; **41**: 363–80.

11 Van der Meer-Roosen CH, Maes EPJ, Faber WR. Cutaneous lupus erythematosus and autoimmune thyroiditis. *Br J Dermatol* 1979; **101**: 91–2.

12 Winkelmann RK, Connolly SM, Doyle JA. Carpal tunnel syndrome in cutaneous connective tissue disease: generalized morphoea, lichen sclerosus, fasciitis, discoid lupus erythematosus and lupus panniculitis. *J Am Acad Dermatol* 1982; **7**: 94.

13 Wojnarowska F. Simultaneous occurrence in identical twins of discoid lupus erythematosus and polymorphic light eruption. *J R Soc Med* 1983; **76**: 791–2.

14 Green S, Trattner A, Weingarten MW. Discoid lupus erythematosus coexistent with Sheehan's syndrome. *Int J Dermatol* 1992; **31**: 182–3.

Chronic granulomatous disease. Two siblings showing an autosomal form of chronic granulomatous disease with DLE-like lesions have been reported [1]. An illness resembling LE, especially of the discoid type, occurs in mothers of boys with X-linked chronic granulomatous disease. In these maternal carriers, a population of defective leukocytes can be demonstrated. Photosensitivity, chilblain LE of the fingers and toes, rosaceous lesions on the face, LE profundus and Jessner's lymphocytic infiltration-like lesions and stomatitis occur [2,3].

References

1 Stalder JF, Dreno B, Bureau B *et al*. Discoid lupus erythematosus-like lesions in an autosomal form of chronic granulomatous disease. *Br J Dermatol* 1986; **114**: 251–4.

2 Garioch JJ, Sampson JR, Seywright M et al. Dermatoses in five related female carriers of X-linked chronic granulomatous disease. Br J Dermatol 1989; 121: 391–6.

3 Smitt JHS, Weening RS, Krieg SR et al. Discoid lupus erythematosus-like lesions in carriers of X-linked chronic granulomatous disease. Br J Dermatol 1990; 122: 643–50.

Complement abnormalities associated with DLE.

Hereditary C2 deficiency occurs in association with skin lesions resembling the discoid lesion of SLE [1]. Homozygous C2 deficiency in females is the most common association, but DLE has also been reported in heterozygous C2 deficiency [2]. Low levels of C4 have been demonstrated in two sisters [3]. Hereditary deficiency of the third [4] and of the fifth component of complement has also been associated with a lupus-like syndrome [5]. DLE has also occurred with C1q deficiency [6]. Identical twin boys have been reported with DLE skin lesions, immunological abnormalities of SLE and hereditary angio-oedema with low C1-esterase inhibitor and C4 [7]. DLE is associated with classical hereditary angio-oedema with reduced levels of C1-esterase inhibitor [8]. Approximately 2% of patients with hereditary angio-oedema have LE-like disease [9].

References

1 Stern R, Fu SM, Fotino M et al. Hereditary C2 deficiency: association with skin lesions resembling the discoid lesion of systemic lupus erythematosus. Arthritis Rheum 1976; 19: 517–22.

2 Belin CD, Bordwell BJ, Einarson ME et al. Familial discoid lupus erythematosus and C2 deficiency. Arthritis Rheum 1980; 23: 898–903.

3 Voigtlander V, Bahmer F, Hauptmann G. Familial discoid lupus erythematosus associated with heterozygous C4 deficiency. Acta Derm Venereol (Stockh) 1984; 64: 552–4.

4 Boom BW, Daha MR. Inherited deficiency of the third component of complement, associated with cutaneous lupus erythematosus. Br J Dermatol 1989; 121: 809–12.

5 Rosenfeld SI, Kelly ME, Leddy JP. Hereditary deficiency of the fifth component of complement in man. J Clin Invest 1976; 57: 1626–34.

6 Uenaka A, Akimoto T, Aoki T et al. A complete selective C1q deficiency in a patient with discoid lupus erythematosus (DLE). Clin Exp Immunol 1982; 48: 353–8.

7 Kohler PF, Percy J, Campion WM et al. Hereditary angioedema and 'familial' lupus erythematosus in identical twin boys. Am J Med 1974; 56: 406–11.

8 Duhra P, Holmes J, Porter DI. Discoid lupus erythematosus associated with hereditary angioneurotic oedema. Br J Dermatol 1990; 123: 241–4.

9 Donaldson VH, Hess EV, McAdams AJ. Lupus erythematosus-like disease in three unrelated women with hereditary angioneurotic oedema. Ann Intern Med 1977; 86: 312–3.

Laboratory abnormalities in DLE.

The incidence of laboratory abnormalities in 120 patients is shown in Table 51.5 [1]. Abnormalities were found in 55% of patients. T-cell counts are significantly lower than in controls, although B cells are not reduced [2]. Kidney biopsy has shown silent lupus nephritis in patients with hypocomplementaemia [3].

Autoantibodies.

Antinuclear antibodies are found in between 5 and 60% of cases depending on patient selection and laboratory techniques: the 'homogeneous' type of antinuclear factor being twice as frequent as the 'speckled' type. Antinuclear antibodies (ANA) are more common in older patients, in those who have had the disease for a long time and when there is extensive skin involvement. They are also more common in patients with chilblains, Raynaud's phenomenon and joint pains [4–7]. The incidence of anti-DNA antibodies varies from 0% [5,8] to 27% [9]. In the latter series, patients did not show any evidence of systemic involvement, and follow-up 3 years later showed no evidence of SLE [10], although progression has been reported [11]. Antibodies to single-stranded DNA (IgM in 20% [8]) occur in nearly one-fifth and may indicate widespread and progressive disease [12]. DNA antibody titres fall with chloroquine therapy. One-fifth of patients have IgM antibodies to single-stranded DNA [8]. Low-titre anti-Ro antibodies are found in 10% of patients with DLE, but are not related to photosensitivity and do not imply an increased risk of developing SCLE [13]. Antibody to extractable nuclear antigen is not found, but lymphocytotoxic antibodies have been demonstrated in 23% of patients in one series [14], but not found in another [5]. Precipitating autoantibodies are found in approximately 4% of patients. The SjT type of antibody (anti-La [SS-B]) is associated with 'speckled' antinuclear factor and rheumatoid factor in those patients with DLE and erythema multiforme [15]. Soluble IL-2 receptors may be found [16].

A high incidence of antithyroid antibodies has been found in DLE, particularly in females [17], and gastric parietal cell cytoplasmic antibodies occur in 13% of patients [17], but this incidence may not be higher than in controls.

References

1 Rowell NR. Laboratory abnormalities in the diagnosis and management of lupus erythematosus. Br J Dermatol 1971; 84: 210–6.

2 Von Vlasin Z, Kratochvil F, Rozprimova V. Spiegel der Immunoglobuline IgG, IgM, und IgA im Serum von Kranken mit einem chronischen Diskoiden erythematodes. Dermatol Monatsschr 1961; 159: 886–91.

3 Powell FC, Greipp PR, Su WP. Discoid lupus erythematosus and monoclonal gammopathy. Br J Dermatol 1983; 109: 355–60.

4 Beck JS, Rowell NR. Discoid lupus erythematosus. QJM 1966; 35: 119–36.

5 Prystowsky SD, Gilliam JN. Discoid lupus erythematosus as part of a larger disease spectrum. Arch Dermatol 1975; 111: 1448–52.

6 Doeglas HMG. Follow-up of patients with chronic discoid lupus erythematosus. Dermatologica 1963; 127: 211–5.

7 Peterson WC, Fusaro RM. Antinuclear factor in light sensitivity and lupus erythematosus. Arch Dermatol 1963; 87: 563–5.

8 Kulick KB, Provost TT, Reichlin M. Antibodies to single-stranded DNA in patients with discoid lupus erythematosus. Arthritis Rheum 1982; 25: 639–46.

9 Davis P, Atkins B, Hughes GRV. Antibodies to native DNA in discoid lupus erythematosus. Br J Dermatol 1974; 91: 175–81.

10 Bresnihan B, Hughes GRV. Anti-DNA antibodies in discoid lupus erythematosus. Ann Rheum Dis 1977; 36: 476–7.

11 Mandel MJ, Carr RI, Weston WL et al. Anti-native DNA antibodies in discoid lupus erythematosus. Arch Dermatol 1972; 106: 668–70.

12 Callen JP, Fowler JF, Kulick KB. Serologic and clinical features of patients with discoid lupus erythematosus: relationship of antibodies to single-stranded

Table 51.5 Laboratory abnormalities in discoid lupus erythematosus.

Laboratory abnormalities	Frequency (%)
Anaemia, leukopenia or thrombocytopenia	30
Raised erythrocyte sedimentation rate (ESR)	20
Raised serum globulin	29
Positive Coombs' test	2.5
Positive cryoglobulins	<1
Positive cold agglutinins	<1
False-positive syphilis serology	26
Positive anticardiolipin antibodies (mainly IgM)	15
Positive LE cell test	1.7
Positive rheumatoid factor	17

deoxyribonucleic acid and of other anti-nuclear antibody subsets to clinical manifestations. *J Am Acad Dermatol* 1985; **13**: 748–55.

13 Lee LA, Roberts CM, Frank MB *et al.* The antibody response to Ro/SSA in cutaneous lupus erythematosus. *Arch Dermatol* 1994; **130**: 1262–8.

14 Stenszky V, Nagy E, Szerze P. Examination of HLA antigens and lymphocytotoxic antibodies in discoid lupus erythematosus. *Acta Derm Venereol (Stockh)* 1975; **55**: 131–3.

15 Rowell NR, Swanson Beck J, Anderson JR. Lupus erythematosus and erythema multiforme-like lesions. *Arch Dermatol* 1963; **88**: 176–80.

16 Blum C, Zillikens D, Tony HP *et al.* Soluble interleukin-2 receptor as a parameter for disease activity in the serum of systemic and discoid lupus erythematosus. *Hautarzt* 1993; **44**: 290–5.

17 Shrank AB, Doniach D. Discoid lupus erythematosus. *Arch Dermatol* 1963; **87**: 677–85.

Differential diagnosis. The relationship of DLE to SLE has been discussed elsewhere (see p. 51.2). The cutaneous lesions may be very similar, although patients with DLE of the face usually show more scaling, pigmentary disturbances, atrophy and scarring. In those with extensive DDLE, positive antibodies and mild systemic symptoms, it can be difficult to fit the patient into a precise diagnostic category, but patients may fulfil the ARA criteria for the diagnosis of SLE (see p. 51.27), so discussion of 'progression of disease' in these patients is often unhelpful.

The annular atrophic plaque variety of DLE may resemble morphoea or lichen sclerosus [1]. Jessner's lymphocytic infiltration may be confused with the more acute localized oedematous lesions of LE, but the marked histological lymphocytic infiltration in the former should help to distinguish it from the latter, and immunoglobulin deposition does not occur at the dermal–epidermal junction in Jessner's infiltration [2]. Evidence has been produced from a study of 100 patients that Jessner's lymphocytic infiltration is a distinct entity, which does not seem to proceed to DLE, PLE or lymphoma [3], and studies of lymphoid infiltrates using the monoclonal antibody Leu-8 tend to confirm the difference between DLE and Jessner's lymphocytic infiltrate [4]; however, there is still disagreement on the relationship between DLE and Jessner's infiltrate, and others believe the latter to be a precursor of classical cutaneous lupus [5]. Benign lymphocytic infiltration of the skin may be a further form of cutaneous LE as indicated by phototesting [6]. Reticular erythematous mucinosis (REM) syndrome (see Chapter 59), which can show clinical and histological features similar to DLE, may also be induced by ultraviolet radiation, but is a discrete clinical entity.

The history and the presence of lesions elsewhere should exclude contact eczema, seborrhoeic eczema and psoriasis. Lupus vulgaris may resemble DLE, but the lesions of the former usually occur at an early age, are rarely symmetrical, may be ulcerated and usually show characteristic 'apple-jelly nodules'. Necrobiosis lipoidica can give facial lesions like DLE. The rosaceous type of LE can usually be differentiated from true rosacea by the absence of pustules and the histology.

Chronic DLE has been found in 12% of patients diagnosed as having scarring alopecia of the pseudopelade type [7]. Lesions on the lips, tongue, scalp and buccal mucosa may be confused with lichen planus, and the skin of some patients may show clinical, histological and immunological features of both diseases [8,9]. Overlap cases, in addition to LE-like lesions, have lichenoid papules, verrucous lesions, anonychia, and oral and vulval lesions resembling lichen planus. Patients with lichen planus do not have features of LE immunopathologically or by HLA typing [10]. Overlap cases either have both diseases or are variants of LE. In favour of the latter, the verrucous lesions show immunofluorescent findings of LE, and electron microscopy reveals tubuloreticular inclusions in endothelial cells of dermal blood vessels—which are found in LE but not in lichen planus [11].

LE of the legs and feet may resemble chilblains. Plaques of sarcoidosis and lesions of eosinophilic granuloma may cause diagnostic difficulties that can only be resolved histologically. Occasionally, lesions resembling DLE are caused by dermatophytes [12].

The distinction from PLE may be difficult, but the absence of antinuclear factor from the serum [13] and of dermal–epidermal immunoglobulin deposits [14] in PLE may be helpful. PLE and DLE may coexist, or PLE may precede DLE by many years [15]. PLE is more common in the relatives of patients with LE; as many as 65% of patients with cutaneous LE have symptoms indistinguishable from those of PLE [16].

Infants may show sharply marginated, erythematous, finely scaling plaques on the cheeks and bridge of the nose, sometimes exacerbated by the sun [17], or a transitory rash with telangiectases on the face, particularly around the eyes, which clinically and histologically resembles LE [18]. These rashes probably are part of so-called neonatal LE (see p. 51.49). The annular erythemas of infancy have been reviewed [15].

An LE-like rash on the face with sun sensitivity occurs in Bloom's syndrome (see Chapter 15), which is thought to be caused by an autosomal recessive gene. A congenital telangiectatic erythema occurs in well-proportioned dwarfs, who look alike because of their bird-like facial appearance. The skin changes occur in infancy and may be associated with ectodermal and mesodermal defects.

References

1 Chorzelski TP, Jablonska S, Blaszczyk M *et al.* Annular atrophic plaques of the face. *Arch Dermatol* 1976; **112**: 1143–5.

2 Ten Have-Opbroek AAW. On the differential diagnosis between chronic discoid lupus erythematodes and lymphocytic infiltration of the skin (Jessner) with emphasis on fluorescence microscopy. *Dermatologica* 1966; **132**: 109.

3 Toonstra J, Wildschut A, Boer J *et al.* Jessner's lymphocytic infiltration of the skin. *Arch Dermatol* 1989; **125**: 1525–30.

4 Ashworth J, Turbitt M, MacKie R. A comparison of the dermal lymphoid infiltrates in discoid lupus erythematosus and Jessner's lymphocytic infiltrate of the skin using the monoclonal antibody Leu 8. *J Cutan Pathol* 1987; **14**: 198–201.

5 Lipsker D, Mitschler A, Grosshans E, Cribier B. Could Jessner's lymphocytic infiltrate of the skin be a dermal variant of lupus erythematosus? An analysis of 210 cases. *Dermatology* 2006; **213**: 15–22.

6 Adamski H, Labrousse AL, Sparsa A *et al.* Positive photobiological investigation in Jessner's lymphocytic infiltration of the skin. *Ann Dermatol Vénéréol* 2002; **129**: 1370–3.

7 Braun-Falco O, Bergner T, Heilgemier GP. Pseudopelade alopecia. *Hautarzt* 1989; **40**: 77–83.

8 Davies MG, Gorkiewicz A, Knight A *et al.* Is there a relationship between lupus erythematosus and lichen planus? *Br J Dermatol* 1977; **96**: 145–54.

9 Van der Horst JC, Cirkel PKS, Nieboer C. Mixed lichen planus/lupus erythematosus disease: a distinct entity? Clinical, histopathological and immunopathological studies in six patients. *Clin Exp Dermatol* 1983; **8**: 631–40.

10 Potts EDA, Rowell NR. Lichen planus: a distinct entity from lupus erythematosus. *Arch Dermatol* 1981; **61**: 413–6.

11 Santa Cruz DJ, Uitto J, Eisen AZ *et al.* Verrucous lupus erythematosus: ultra-structural studies on a distinct variant of chronic discoid lupus erythematosus. *J Am Acad Dermatol* 1983; **9**: 82–90.

12 Shanon J, Raubitschek F. Tinea faciei simulating chronic discoid lupus erythematosus. *Arch Dermatol* 1960; **82**: 268–71.

13 Ive FA, Sanderson KV. A lupus erythematosus-like eruption in infants. *Trans St John's Hosp Dermatol Soc* 1964; **50**: 144.

14 Vonderheid EC, Koblenzer PJ, Ming PML *et al.* Neonatal lupus erythematosus. *Arch Dermatol* 1976; **112**: 698–705.

15 Cox NH, McQueen A, Evans TJ *et al.* An annular erythema of infancy. *Arch Dermatol* 1987; **123**: 510–3.

16 Peterson WC, Fusaro RM. Antinuclear factor in light sensitivity and lupus erythematosus. *Arch Dermatol* 1963; **87**: 563–5.

17 Fisher DA, Epstein JH, Kay DN *et al.* Polymorphous light eruption and lupus erythematosus. *Arch Dermatol* 1970; **101**: 458–61.

18 Nyberg F, Hasan T, Puska P *et al.* Occurrence of polymorphic light eruption in lupus erythematosus. *Br J Dermatol* 1997; **136**: 217–21.

Prognosis

Prognosis [1]. The untreated skin lesions of DLE tend to be persistent. With treatment, the more tumid lesions with little scaling may clear completely in the course of a month or two. Lesions of longer standing with much scaling and some scarring are slower to remit. Ultimately, scarring is found in 57%, with scarring alopecia in 35%; 35% also have pigmentary abnormalities [2]. Areas of activity at the edge of such scars may take years to settle. Twenty per cent of female patients notice a premenstrual flare, but there is no evidence of a deterioration of the condition on hormone replacement therapy [3]. Complete remission in the course of years can be expected in over 50% [1]. Long duration and lack of remission are related to Raynaud's phenomenon, scalp involvement and chilblain-like lesions [4]. Relapses occurring with sunlight, cold, trauma or mental stress after months or years of remission are not infrequent. In spite of the chronic and relapsing nature of the condition, the patient usually remains in good health.

Despite the fact that over half of patients have haematological and serological abnormalities, the risk of developing overt SLE is only approximately 6.5% [4,5]. The risk is higher in patients with disseminated DLE (22%) than in DLE confined to the head and neck (1.2%). Females developing DLE before the age of 40 years, with HLA-B8 in their histocompatibility type, have an increased risk of 'converting' to SLE [6]. Neither immunological nor biochemical abnormalities appear to alter the patient's progress [5,7]. Patients with active discoid skin lesions rarely have severe renal disease [8]. Patients with DLE showing signs of nephropathy, arthralgia and ANA titres of 1:320 or more should be carefully monitored [9].

References

1 Rowell NR. The natural history of lupus erythematosus. *Clin Exp Dermatol* 1984; **9**: 217–31.

2 de Berker D, Burge S, Dissaneyeka M. The sequelae of chronic cutaneous lupus erythematosus. *Lupus* 1992; **1**: 181–6.

3 Yell SA, Burge SM. The effect of hormonal changes on cutaneous disease in lupus erythematosus. *Br J Dermatol* 1993; **129**: 18–22.

4 Millard LG, Rowell NR. Abnormal laboratory test results and their relationship to prognosis in discoid lupus erythematosus. *Arch Dermatol* 1979; **115**: 1055–8.

5 Rowell NR. Laboratory abnormalities in the diagnosis and management of lupus erythematosus. *Br J Dermatol* 1971; **84**: 210–6.

6 Millard LG, Rowell NR, Rajah SM. Histocompatibility antigens in discoid and systemic lupus erythematosus. *Br J Dermatol* 1977; **96**: 139–44.

7 Beck JS, Rowell NR. Discoid lupus erythematosus. *QJM* 1966; **35**: 119–36.

8 Prystowsky SD, Gilliam JN. Discoid lupus erythematosus as part of a larger spectrum. *Arch Dermatol* 1975; **111**: 1448–52.

9 Tebbe B, Mansmann U, Wollina U *et al.* Markers in cutaneous lupus erythematosus indicating systemic involvement: a multicentre study of 296 patients. *Acta Derm Venereol (Stockh)* 1997; **77**: 305–8.

Neoplastic change in DLE

Neoplastic change in DLE. Squamous cell and, less commonly, basal cell carcinomas occasionally occur in the scars of DLE, particularly on the scalp, ears, lips and nose. An incidence of 3.3% has been noted in a series of 120 white patients with DLE [1]. They are said to be more common in middle-aged males [2], but in either sex occur only in cases of 20 years' duration or more. Black people with DLE may also develop carcinoma [3,4], especially of the lip. Death may occur from multiple metastases [1,5]. Keratoacanthoma [6], malignant fibrous histiocytoma [7] and atypical fibroxanthoma [8] in lesions have been reported.

References

1 Millard LG, Barker DJ. Development of squamous cell carcinoma in chronic DLE. *Clin Exp Dermatol* 1978; **3**: 161.

2 Epstein JH, Tuffanelli DL. In: Dubois EL, ed. *Lupus Erythematosus*. New York: McGraw-Hill, 1966: 124.

3 Caruso WR, Stewart ML, Nanda VK *et al.* Squamous cell carcinoma of the skin in black patients with discoid lupus erythematosus. *J Rheumatol* 1987; **14**: 156–9.

4 Keith WD, Kelly AP, Sumrall AJ *et al.* Squamous cell carcinoma arising in lesions of discoid lupus erythematosus in black persons. *Arch Dermatol* 1980; **116**: 315–7.

5 Martin S, Rosen T, Locker E. Metastatic squamous cell carcinoma of the lip. *Arch Dermatol* 1979; **115**: 1214.

6 Fanti PA, Tosti A, Peluso AM *et al.* Multiple keratoacanthoma in discoid lupus erythematosus. *J Am Acad Dermatol* 1989; **21**: 809–10.

7 Farber JN, Koh HK. Malignant fibrous histiocytoma arising from discoid lupus erythematosus. *Arch Dermatol* 1988; **124**: 114–6.

8 de Berker D, Burge S, Dissaneyeka M. The sequelae of chronic cutaneous lupus erythematosus. *Lupus* 1992; **1**: 181–6.

Treatment

Treatment [1]. It is important to carry out a complete medical survey of the patient at the first attendance. Such a survey should establish a diagnosis of the sub-type of DLE, a likely prognosis and a baseline by which later progress may be judged. From the outset, general measures play a large part in successful management. Overwork, mental stress and fatigue are often factors in deteriorating disease, and patients with facial scarring often suffer severe psychological upset and depression [2]. Effective forms of camouflage by covering creams are available and help morale. Patients should be warned against excessive exposure to sunlight and they should be advised to wear a broad-brimmed hat, and avoid short-sleeved shirts and shorts. A sunscreen cream or lotion should be prescribed, and a preparation with a UVB protection factor of at least 15 is required; UVA protection is at least as important. Application should be frequent—probably every 2–3 h in bright sunlight. There are many suitable preparations, and patient acceptability is an important element in the choice of agent [3]. It is important that patients understand the preventative action of these preparations.

The management of cutaneous lupus has been well reviewed [1], as has that of 'resistant' disease [4]. Topical therapy can frequently control and sometimes clear lesions without systemic treatment. In one series [5], 43 out of 59 patients could be

Table 51.6 Oral agents useful in discoid lupus erythematosus.

Drug	Daily dosage	Response rate (%) (as first-line treatment)	Response rate (%) (as second-line treatment)	Side effects
Hydroxychloroquine	200–400 mg	60–75	20	See Table 51.7
Chloroquine	200–400 mg	60–75	20	See Table 51.7
Acitretin [21,22]	25–100 mg	50–75	15–20	Dry skin, hair loss, liver or lipid abnormalities, bony ankylosis
Auranofin [23]	3–9 mg	50	15–20	GI upset, haematological, renal or liver abnormality
Dapsone [24]	50–150 mg	25–50	10–20	Rash, haemolysis, dapsone syndrome
Methotrexate [25]	5–30 mg	–	25–50	GI upset, hepatitis, hepatic fibrosis, pulmonary fibrosis
Ciclosporin [26]	2.5–5 mg/kg	–	30–50	Hypertension, renal function abnormalities
Sulfasalazine [27]	1.5 g	–	5–15	
Isotretinoin [28,29]	20–80 mg	–	15–20	
Thalidomide [30–32]	50–150 mg	80–90	40–50	Drowsiness, constipation, teratogenicity, polyneuropathy
Clofazimine [33]	50–150 mg	40–60	5–15	
Phenytoin [34]	200–300 mg	–	–	
Azathioprine [35]	75–200 mg	–	20–30	
Cyclophosphamide [36]	50–200 mg	–	–	
Interferon α2a [37]		–		

controlled by applications of 0.025% fluocinolone cream, and 0.1% betamethasone 17-valerate cream alone was effective in 68 out of 78 patients without inducing epidermal atrophy [6]. There are few data supporting the use of one topical steroid over another, although more potent agents appear generally more effective. The efficacy in resistant cases may be enhanced by applications of steroid creams under plastic occlusion, using a self-adherent plastic dressing (e.g. Tegaderm [7]), or a moulded plastic prosthesis for more difficult anatomical areas such as the ears [8]. Fludroxycortide (Haelan) tape (in which steroid is impregnated onto the tacky side of polythene tape) can be cut to size and stuck on individual lesions.

Intralesional corticosteroid injections are helpful in resistant cases [9], even on lips, mouth and ears. Multiple and repeated injections may be required. Reversible, and occasionally irreversible, atrophy may result. Intralesional therapy is sometimes surprisingly effective in lesions on the nose and ears and it may also help resistant lesions on the palms and soles [10]. Intralesional chloroquine [11] has been tried with limited success. There can be considerable local pain and inflammation. Interferon-α (IFN-α) has also been used intralesionally with success [12]. Among other local measures, cryotherapy, surgical excision [13], painting small lesions with trichloracetic acid and local laser therapy may be helpful. The carbon dioxide laser, and both the pulsed-dye and argon lasers may be valuable for telangiectatic LE [14].

Oral therapy (Table 51.6). Most patients referred to hospital will need oral therapy in addition to local and general methods. In addition, vasodilator drugs, particularly calcium-channel blockers such as nifedipine, are helpful in those with Raynaud's phenomenon and chilblain lesions, and intravenous prostacyclin may be very helpful in winter, and used before intensive oral therapy in these patients.

For patients with severe, extensive or scarring disease, particularly affecting the scalp, oral prednisolone is often the most helpful initial treatment. A dosage of 0.5 mg/kg, rapidly tapered over 6

Table 51.7 Side effects of antimalarials.

Mild
    Nausea, vomiting, abdominal pain
Severe
    Corneal deposits
    Retinopathy
    Pigmentation of palate, nails and legs
    Bleaching of hair
    Exfoliative dermatitis
    Lichenoid rashes
    Myasthenia
    Myopathy
    Extrapyramidal involuntary movements
    Neuropathy
    Psychiatric syndromes

weeks, is quickly effective, minimizes scarring, and allows the slower acting agents such as antimalarials to work. Long-term therapy with oral steroids is best avoided because of side effects, but may be necessary in a small number of patients resistant to other maintenance therapy. In such circumstances, patients should also receive bone protection with bi-phosphonates or related drugs to avoid osteoporosis. Methylprednisolone 500–1000 mg/day for 2 or 3 days, given as intravenous pulse therapy, may help resistant lesions.

There is little doubt that in most cases first-line oral treatment should be with one of the antimalarials (see Chapter 74). Most would start therapy with hydroxychloroquine, initially at 200 mg twice daily, reducing to 200 mg/day once a response is achieved. Chloroquine sulphate is equally effective, usually at a dosage of 200 mg twice daily, but hydroxychloroquine is used first by most prescribers because side effects (Table 51.7), particularly eye toxicity, are less likely provided that the dosage limitations of 6.5 mg/kg lean body weight are adhered to [15]. The comparable safe daily dosage for chloroquine is unclear, but is probably around

2.5 mg/kg/day of chloroquine base. Cumulative toxicity is rarely a problem with hydroxychloroquine, although it can occur with chloroquine [16]. For this reason, courses of treatment lasting approximately 6 months are preferred, but this may not be possible in the most severely affected patients who will require ongoing therapy. Mepacrine is also useful, and is safe from an ophthalmological point of view [16], but it is often reserved for later use (because of skin pigmentation). It may be used alone, or as part of a combination of antimalarials, which may be more effective than the equivalent amount of each drug given individually [17].

The response to therapy varies; usually, the more tumid, less scaly lesions responding more rapidly than chronic, atrophic and scarring lesions. Most patients who are going to respond to antimalarials usually do so within 6 weeks.

The occurrence of side effects with one agent does not necessarily mean that they will occur with another antimalarial, so it is always worth trying an alternative drug. Taking an ophthalmological history and arranging for an examination by an optician before treatment in any patient with symptoms not corrected by spectacles may help in avoidance of the ocular manifestations. Monitoring during therapy should include taking an ophthalmic history, and testing reading ability with appropriate charts [15]. More elaborate tests, such as the electro-oculogram and electroretinogram, are no longer believed to be helpful [15].

Approximately 60–75% of all patients are helped by antimalarials. Cigarette smoking reduces the efficacy of treatment with antimalarials, probably by modifying metabolism [18]. Of those who respond, approximately 50% relapse within 6 months of stopping treatment, and repeated courses of therapy are usually required. Nevertheless, over the course of several years, most cases treated with intermittent oral antimalarials and topical corticosteroids tend to improve, and some clear completely. There is no evidence that the continuation of antimalarials after clearance prevents relapses. Hydroxychloroquine appears to be safe in pregnancy [19]. Responses to all other agents are very limited once topical therapy and antimalarials have failed [20].

For cases not responding to topical steroids, antimalarials and sunscreens, oral thalidomide has proved remarkably effective in suppressing lesions [30], and also in the treatment of chilblain LE. The originally employed dosages of 400 mg/day [31] are unnecessary, and 100 mg/day seems to be equally effective. If used as initial therapy, response rates of 80–90% may be achieved, but when used as second-line treatment the response rate is nearer 50% [20,32]. Short courses are preferable because of the risk of polyneuropathy and the teratogenic effects. The prescription of thalidomide is tightly regulated, with prescribers, dispensers and patients all having to be registered in a pregnancy prevention programme: patients are allowed only monthly amounts of drug, and all potentially fertile women should be using double contraception and require monthly pregnancy tests.

When all of the above have failed in patients with severe and persistent disease, other forms of systemic treatment may be used. Intravenous pulses of cyclophosphamide may be used, usually at a dosage of 10 mg/kg, at 3–4 weekly intervals. It is usually given in combination with intravenous methylprednisolone [36]. Most recently, the biological agents aimed at specific cytokine

molecules have been used, with benefit following use of efalizumab [38].

Excision of oral lesions also may be practicable [39]. The carbon dioxide [40] and argon lasers [41] may produce improvement of disfiguring LE, although the latter may precipitate DLE [42]. Dermabrasion may help cribriform scarring of the face [43], as may carbon dioxide laser-brasion. Excision without grafting was successful in a case of verrucous LE following a burn [44].

References

1 Callen JP. Update on the management of cutaneous lupus erythematosus. *Br J Dermatol* 2004; **151**: 731–6.

2 Johnson P, Goodfield MJD. The psychological consequences of discoid lupus erythematosus. *Br J Dermatol* 2001; **145** (Suppl. 59): 71.

3 Hawk JLM, Challoner AVJ, Chaddock L. The efficacy of sunscreening agents: protection factors and transmission spectra. *Clin Exp Dermatol* 1982; **7**: 21–31.

4 Callen JP. Management of 'refractory' skin disease in patients with lupus erythematosus. *Baillieres Best Pract Res Clin Rheumatol* 2005; **19**: 767–84.

5 Jansen GT, Villaha CJ, Honeycutt WM. Discoid lupus erythematosus. *Arch Dermatol* 1965; **82**: 283–5.

6 Reymann E. Treatment of discoid lupus erythematosus with betametasone valerate cream 1%. *Dermatologica* 1974; **149**: 65–8.

7 Doeglas HMG. Chronic discoid lupus erythematosus treated with triamcinolone and plastic occlusion. *Dermatologica* 1964; **128**: 384.

8 Stevenson JR, Harman LE. Occlusive therapy of the ears in discoid lupus erythematosus. *Arch Dermatol* 1964; **89**: 391–2.

9 Rowell NR. Treatment of chronic discoid lupus erythematosus with intralesional triamcinolone. *Br J Dermatol* 1962; **74**: 354–7.

10 Callen JP. Intralesional triamcinolone is effective for discoid lupus erythematosus of the palms and soles. *J Rheumatol* 1985; **12**: 630–3.

11 Pelzig A, Witten VH, Sulzberger MB. Chloroquine for chronic discoid lupus erythematosus. *Arch Dermatol* 1961; **83**: 146–8.

12 Martinez J, De Misa RF, Torrelo A, Ledo A. Low dose intralesional interferon-α for discoid lupus erythematosus. *J Am Acad Dermatol* 1992; **26**: 494–6.

13 Ronchese F. Chronic discoid lupus erythematosus treated by plastic surgery. *Chron Dermatol* 1971; **2**: 105–6.

14 Zachariae H, Bjerring P, Cramers M. Argon laser treatment of cutaneous vascular lesions in connective tissue disease. *Acta Derm Venereol (Stockh)* 1988; **68**: 179–82.

15 Fielder A, Graham E, Jones SK et al. Royal College of Ophthalmologists guidelines: ocular toxicity and hydroxychloroquine. *Eye* 1998; **12**: 907–9.

16 Aylward JM. Hydroxychloroquine and chloroquine: assessing the risk of retinal toxicity. *J Am Optom Assoc* 1993; **64**: 787–97.

17 Feldmann R, Saloan D, Saurat JH. The association of the two antimalarials chloroquine and quinacrine for treatment resistant chronic and sub-acute cutaneous lupus erythematosus. *Dermatology* 1994; **189**: 425–7.

18 Jewell ML, McCauliffe DP. Patients with cutaneous lupus erythematosus who smoke are less responsive to antimalarial therapy. *J Am Acad Dermatol* 2000; **42**: 983–7.

19 Buchanan NMM, Toubi E, Khamashta MA et al. Hydroxychloroquine and lupus pregnancy: review of a series of 36 cases. *Ann Rheum Dis* 1996; **55**: 486–8.

20 Sommer S, Hoye NA, Goodfield MJD. Therapy of discoid lupus erythematosus (DLE)—a retrospective study of therapeutic benefit and risk factors. *Br J Dermatol* 2000; **142** (Suppl.): 64.

21 Ruzicka T, Meurer M, Bieber T. Efficiency of acitretin in the treatment of cutaneous lupus erythematosus. *Arch Dermatol* 1988; **124**: 897–902.

22 Ruzicka T, Sommerburg C, Goerz G et al. Treatment of cutaneous lupus erythematosus with acitretin and hydroxychloroquine. *Br J Dermatol* 1992; **127**: 513–8.

23 Dalziel K, Going S, Cartwright PH et al. Treatment of chronic discoid lupus erythematosus with an oral gold compound (auranofin). *Br J Dermatol* 1986; **115**: 211–6.

24 Coburn PR, Shuster S. Dapsone and discoid lupus erythematosus. *Br J Dermatol* 1982; **106**: 105–6.

25 Bottomley WW, Goodfield MJD. Methotrexate for the treatment of discoid lupus erythematosus. *Br J Dermatol* 1995; **133**: 655–6.

26 Yell JA, Burge SM. Cyclosporin and discoid lupus erythematosus. *Br J Dermatol* 1994; **131**: 132–3.

27 Delaporte E, Catteau B, Sabbagh N *et al.* Treatment of discoid lupus erythematosus with sulfasalazine: 11 cases. *Ann Dermatol Venereol* 1997; **124**: 151–6.

28 Shornick JK, Formica N, Parke AL. Isotretinoin for refractory lupus erythematosus. *J Am Acad Dermatol* 1991; **24**: 49–52.

29 Green SG, Piette WW. Successful treatment of hypertrophic lupus erythematosus with isotretinoin. *J Am Acad Dermatol* 1987; **17**: 364–8.

30 Knop J, Bonomann G, Happle R *et al.* Thalidomide in the treatment of 60 cases of chronic discoid lupus erythematosus. *Br J Dermatol* 1983; **108**: 461–6.

31 Stevens RJ, Andujar C, Edwards CJ *et al.* Thalidomide in the treatment of cutaneous manifestations of lupus erythematosus: experience in 16 consecutive patients. *Br J Rheumatol* 1997; **36**: 353–9.

32 Housman TS, Jorizzo JL, McCarty MA *et al.* Low-dose thalidomide therapy for refractory cutaneous lesions of lupus erythematosus. *Arch Dermatol* 2003; **139**: 50–4.

33 Mackey JP, Barnes J. Clofazimine in the treatment of discoid lupus erythematosus. *Br J Dermatol* 1974; **91**: 93–6.

34 Rodriguez-Castellanos MA, Rubio JB, Gomez JFB, Mendoza AG. Phenytoin in the treatment of discoid lupus erythematosus. *Arch Dermatol* 1995; **131**: 620–1.

35 Callen JP, Spencer LV, Burrows JB, Holtman J. Azathioprine: an effective corticosteroid-sparing therapy for patients with recalcitrant cutaneous lupus erythematosus or with recalcitrant cutaneous leukocytoclastic vasculitis. *Arch Dermatol* 1991; **127**: 515–22.

36 Schulz EJ, Menter MA. Treatment of discoid and subacute lupus erythematosus with cyclophosphamide. *Br J Dermatol* 1971; **85**: 60–5.

37 Thivolet J, Nicolas JF, Kanitakis J *et al.* Recombinant interferon-α2a is effective in the treatment of discoid and subacute cutaneous lupus erythematosus. *Br J Dermatol* 1990; **122**: 405–9.

38 Usmani N, Goodfield M. Efalizumab in the treatment of discoid lupus erythematosus. *Arch Dermatol* 2007; **143**: 873–7.

39 Schioidt M. Local excision in the treatment of oral discoid lupus erythematosus. *Acta Derm Venereol (Stockh)* 1978; **58**: 274–6.

40 Henderson DL, Odom JC. Laser treatment of discoid lupus erythematosus. *Lasers Surg Med* 1986; **6**: 12–5.

41 Zachariae H, Bjering P, Cramers M. Argon laser treatment of cutaneous vascular lesions in connective tissue disease. *Acta Derm Venereol (Stockh)* 1988; **68**: 175–82.

42 Wolfe JT, Weinberg JM, Elenitsas R, Uberti-Benz M. Cutaneous lupus erythematosus following laser-induced thermal injury. *Arch Dermatol* 1997; **133**: 392–3.

43 Ratner D, Skouge JW. Discoid lupus erythematosus scarring and dermabrasion: a case report and discussion. *J Am Acad Dermatol* 1990; **2**: 314–6.

44 Eskreis BD, Eng AM, Furey NL. Surgical excision of trauma-induced verrucous lupus erythematosus. *J Dermatol Surg Oncol* 1988; **14**: 1296–9.

Subacute cutaneous lupus erythematosus

Definition. Subacute cutaneous lupus erythematosus (SCLE) is a specific 'subset' of lupus first described by Sontheimer *et al.* in 1979 [1]. Patients exhibit mainly cutaneous disease and usually have a good prognosis. Antibodies to the Ro/SS-A antigen are closely associated with this subgroup.

Aetiology. Antibodies to the Ro/SS-A antigen are an almost universal finding in this subset of lupus. That these antibodies may be pathogenic was first suggested by LeFeber *et al.* [2], who demonstrated that sublethal doses of ultraviolet light (UVL) induced the synthesis of Ro/SS-A antigen by cultured human keratinocytes. In addition, they also showed that UVL promoted the expression of Ro/SS-A antigens on the surface of cultured human keratinocytes where they might bind antibodies. In 1988, Ro/SS-A antigen was identified in both adult and neonatal epidermis *in vivo* [3], and subsequent studies have confirmed that UVL increases Ro/SS-A antigen expression on the surface of keratinocytes [2,4,5]

and that this is increased by oestrogen [6–8]. Thus, it has been postulated that in photosensitive lupus, UVL exposure leads to increased synthesis and subsequent expression of Ro/SS-A antigen on the surface of keratinocytes where it binds antibody and initiates disease [9,10]. Further support for this hypothesis comes from a study which showed that photosensitivity and the titre of Ro/SS-A antibodies correlated with the expression of Ro/SS-A in skin specimens of patients with LE [11].

Although attractive, this hypothesis does not explain why other patients with Ro/SS-A antibodies (e.g. patients with Sjögren's syndrome) do not exhibit photosensitivity and why in the clinical setting Ro/SS-A titres rarely reflect disease activity [12], although one study has suggested that titres of Ro/SS-A are higher in SCLE patients with systemic involvement than in those without [13].

HLA antigen status may have a role in disease susceptibility. The most common haplotype in SCLE is HLA-DR3 and B8, -DR3 being most commonly associated with the annular phenotype and the expression of Ro/SS-A antibodies [14]. A more recent study has suggested an association with HLA-A1, B8, DR3, DQ2, DRw2 and C4 null haplotype [15]. DR2 has been associated with an older age of disease onset and papulosquamous lesions [16]. Complement genes are located in the HLA region and patients with SCLE have been reported to have deficiencies in the 2nd [17], 3rd [18] and 4th components [19]. A single nucleotide polymorphism leading to decreased levels of C1q antigen has been reported in patients with SCLE, the only genetic association of SCLE that lies outside the HLA region [20]. In addition, the expression of the human leukocyte antigen-DR and CD25 on circulating T cells in cutaneous lupus has been reported to correlate with disease activity [21].

Two studies [22,23] have reported an association of SCLE with the tumour necrosis factor-α (TNF-α) 308A polymorphism, which may be pathogenic or act as a marker for the HLA A1, B8, DRB1*0301 haplotype associated with other autoimmune conditions. Studies of Ro60 exons to see whether sequence alterations might be associated with SCLE have not shown differences between patients with SCLE, DLE or controls [24].

Autoantibody status. SCLE was originally labelled ANA-negative lupus, as these patients often exhibited negative autoantibody screens. This was probably because of the use of test substrates that did not contain suitable antigens for the antibodies found in this group of patients. Using human cell lines as substrates, homogeneous antinuclear antibodies are found in approximately 60% and anti-Ro/SS-A antibodies in approximately 80% of patients [1], rising to higher levels in females [25]. Anticardiolipin antibodies occur in 16% [26].

Histopathology. Histopathologically, SCLE can be differentiated from DLE by the presence of more epidermal atrophy and less hyperkeratosis, basement-membrane thickening, follicular plugging and inflammatory infiltration [27,28]. Colloid bodies and epidermal necrosis are present in more than 50%, especially in those with Ro/SS-A antibodies [29]. Dust-like particles of inter- and intracellular IgG in the basement layers of the epidermis may be a specific feature [30]. It has been suggested that pilosebaceous atrophy is the only significant predictor of DLE versus SCLE

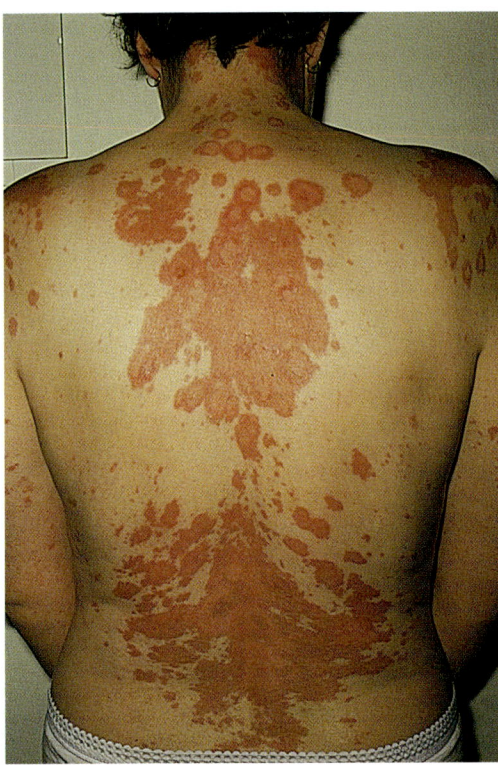

Fig. 51.25 Subacute cutaneous lupus erythematosus.

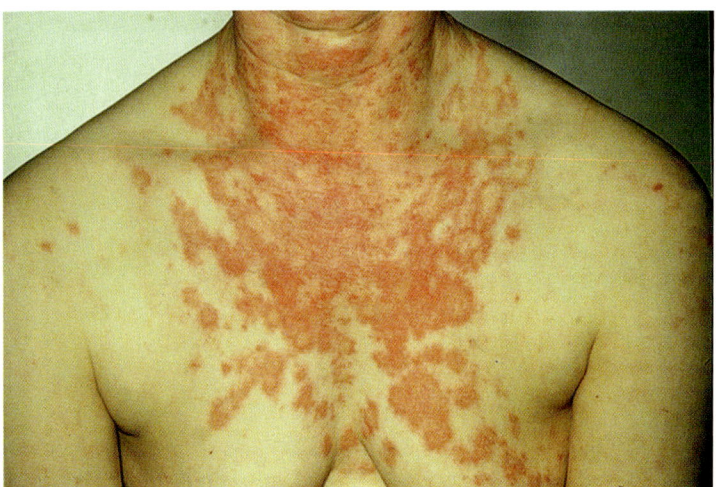

Fig. 51.26 Subacute cutaneous lupus erythematosus, showing annular polycyclic lesions.

[29,31]. Lesional subepidermal immunoglobulin is found in approximately 60%, and is more frequent in papulosquamous (88%) than annular lesions (29%) [1]. Recent studies have shown significant numbers of chemokine receptor CCR4 and cytotoxic T cells in the basal layers of the epidermis where keratinocytes showed apoptotic death [32] and strongly positive staining for TNF-α in involved skin [33].

Clinical features. This subset [1,34,35], which comprises approximately 10% of patients with LE, have either non-scarring papulosquamous (two-thirds) or annular polycyclic (one-third) lesions. The disease predominantly affects adults, although SCLE has been reported in a child [36,37]. Lesions usually occur above the waist and particularly around the neck, on the trunk and on the outer aspects of the arms (Figs. 51.25 & 51.26) and have been reported to occur along the lines of Blaschko [38]. The borders may show vesiculation and crusting and occasionally bullae [39,40] which may be associated with co-existent porphyria cutanea tarda [41]. Follicular plugging and hyperkeratosis are not prominent, and the lesions resolve leaving grey-white hypopigmentation and telangiectases. The pigmentary changes usually resolve completely. Diffuse non-scarring alopecia and photosensitivity occur in approximately half of patients, and other features include mouth ulceration (especially of the palate), reticular livedo, periungual telangiectasia and Raynaud's phenomenon. Presentation with pityriasiform lesions [2], erythroderma [42] and poikilodermatous lesions [43,44] has been described. Morphoea [45] and dystrophic calcinosis cutis [46] have followed SCLE. Some develop lesions related to mucin deposition [47].

Approximately half of patients fulfil the criteria for SLE of the American Rheumatism Association (ARA) [48], with arthritis the most frequent feature. Fever, malaise and central nervous system involvement occur, but renal disease is mild and infrequent, although a recent study suggested that the latter may occur in up to 16% of patients, a similar frequency to that seen in those with SLE in their series [49]. Urticarial vasculitis has been reported [50]. Chronic interstitial pneumonitis has been reported [51], as has hypokalaemic tetraparesis [52]. Occasionally, the annular lesions may resemble the lesions of Rowell's syndrome or the gyrate erythema secondary to occult malignancy [53]. Some patients also have Sjögren's syndrome [54], rheumatoid arthritis, Sweet's syndrome [55], Crohn's disease [56], lichen planus [57], psoriasis [58,59], hereditary angio-oedema [60,61], porphyria cutanea tarda [62], gluten-sensitive enteropathy [63], toxic epidermal necrolysis [64], inclusion body myositis [65] or calcifying lupus panniculitis [66] and Kikuchi's disease (necrotizing lymphadenitis) [67].

A number of drugs have been reported to precipitate or exacerbate SCLE and these are listed in Table 51.8.

SCLE may occur in the course of PUVA treatment of psoriasis [107], radiation therapy [108] and IFN-β1a therapy [109]. There have been occasional reports of associations with cancer, namely breast carcinoma [110], meningioma [111], hepatocellular carcinoma [112], Hodgkin's disease [113], lung cancer [114], prostate cancer [115] and squamous carcinoma of the head and neck [116]. Occasional patients develop overt SLE with severe visceral disease [117].

Treatment. The condition in most patients is controlled by sunscreens [118,119], topical or intralesional corticosteroids [120–122] or the macrolides pimecrolimus [123] and tacrolimus [124–128]. In those not responding to these agents, antimalarial drugs are often helpful [129]. These can be used as either hydroxychloroquine or chloroquine base, although the former is safer from the ophthalmological point of view and requires less ophthalmological monitoring [130]. The antimalarial mepacrine (quinacrine) does not have ocular side effects but does induce yellow discoloration of the skin. There is evidence that a combination of antimalarials may be more effective than either alone [131] and that they are less effective in smokers [132]. Patients not responding to antimalarials

Table 51.8 Drugs associated with subacute cutaneous lupus erythematosus.

Thiazide diuretics [68–72]
Griseofulvin [73]
Terbinafine [74–77]
Calcium channel blockers [78–81]
Tamoxifen [82]
Acebutalol [83]
Lansoprazole [84]
Statins [85]
ACE inhibitors [86–88]
Etanercept [89]
Efalizumab [90]
Infliximab [91]
Leflunomide [92–94]
Carbamazepine [95,96]
Cinnarizine [97]
Inhaled tiotropium bromide [98]
Bupropion [99,100]
Docetaxel (Taxotere) [101]
Ticlopidine [102]
Gold [103]
Naproxen [104]
Aldactone [105]
Fertilizer- and pesticide-containing hay [106]

may respond to oral corticosteroids or methylprednisolone [133], etretinate [134], acitretin [135], isotretinoin [136,137], dapsone [138], oral, intravenous and subcutaneous methotrexate [139–142], thalidomide [143–147], UVA [148], IFN-α [149], long-term cefuroxime axetil [150], mycophenolate mofetil [151], intravenous immunoglobulin [152,153], etanercept [154] and efalizumab [155].

References

1 Sontheimer RD, Thomas JR, Gilliam JN. Subacute cutaneous lupus erythematosus: a cutaneous marker for a distinct lupus erythematosus subset. *Arch Dermatol* 1979; **115**: 1409–15.

2 LeFeber WP, Norris DA, Ryan SR *et al*. Ultraviolet light induces binding of antibodies to selected nuclear antigens on cultured human keratinocytes. *J Clin Invest* 1984; **74**: 1545–51.

3 Jones SK, Coulter S, Harmon C *et al*. Ro/SSA antigen in human epidermis. *Br J Dermatol* 1988; **118**: 363–7.

4 Furukawa F, Kashihara-Sawami M, Lyons MB *et al*. Binding of antibodies to the extractable nuclear antigens SSA/Ro and SSB/La is induced on the surface of human keratinocytes by ultraviolet light (UVL): implications for the pathogenesis of photosensitive cutaneous lupus. *J Invest Dermatol* 1990; **94**: 77–85.

5 Jones SK. Ultraviolet radiation (UVR) induces cell-surface Ro/SSA antigen expression by human keratinocytes *in vitro*: a possible mechanism for the UVR induction of cutaneous lupus lesions. *Br J Dermatol* 1992; **126**: 546–53.

6 Furukawa F, Lyons MB, Lee LA *et al*. Estradiol enhances binding to cultured human keratinocytes of antibodies specific for SS-A/Ro and SS-B/La; another possible mechanism for estradiol influence of lupus erythematosus. *J Immunol* 1988; **141**: 1480–8.

7 Jones SK. The effects of hormonal and other stimuli on cell-surface Ro/SSA antigen expression by human keratinocytes *in vitro*: their possible role in the induction of cutaneous lupus lesions. *Br J Dermatol* 1992; **126**: 554–60.

8 Wang D, Chan EKL. 17β-Estradiol increases expression of 52-kDa and 60-kDa SS-A/Ro autoantigens in human keratinocytes and breast cancer cell line MCF-7. *J Invest Dermatol* 1996; **107**: 610–4.

9 Norris DA. Pathomechanisms of photosensitive lupus erythematosus. *J Invest Dermatol* 1993; **100**: 58S–68S.

10 Mellers S, Winterberg F, Gilliet M *et al*. Ultraviolet radiation-induced injury, chemokines and leukocyte recruitment. *Arthritis Rheum* 2005; **52**: 1504–16.

11 Ioannides D, Golden BD, Buyon JP *et al*. Expression of SS-A/Ro and SS-B/La antigens in skin biopsy specimens of patients with photosensitive forms of lupus erythematosus. *Arch Dermatol* 2000; **136**: 340–6.

12 Purcell SM, Lieu TS, Davis BM *et al*. Relationship between circulating anti-Ro/SS-A antibody levels and skin disease activity in subacute cutaneous lupus erythematosus. *Br J Dermatol* 1987; **117**: 277–87.

13 Popovic K, Brauner S, Ek M *et al*. Fine specificity of the Ro/SSA autoantibody response in relation to serological and clinical findings in 96 patients with self-reported cutaneous symptoms induced by sun. *Lupus* 2007; **16**: 10–7.

14 Sontheimer RD, Stastny P, Gilliam JN. Human histocompatibility antigen associations in subacute cutaneous lupus erythematosus. *J Clin Invest* 1981; **67**: 312–6.

15 Millard TP, McGregor JM. Molecular genetics of cutaneous lupus erythematosus. *Clin Exp Dermatol* 2001; **26**: 184–91.

16 Johansson-Stephansson E, Koskimies S, Partanen J *et al*. Subacute cutaneous lupus erythematosus: genetic markers and clinical and immunological findings in patients. *Arch Dermatol* 1989; **125**: 791–6.

17 Callen JP, Hodge SJ, Kulick KB *et al*. Subacute cutaneous lupus erythematosus in multiple members of a family with C2 deficiency. *Arch Dermatol* 1987; **123**: 66–70.

18 Van Hees CLM, Boom BW, Vermeer BJ *et al*. Subacute lupus erythematosus in a patient with inherited deficiency of the third component of complement. *Arch Dermatol* 1992; **128**: 700–1.

19 Partanen J, Koskimies S, Johansson E. C4 null phenotypes among lupus erythematosus patients are predominantly the result of deletions covering C4 and closely linked 21-hydroxylase A genes. *J Med Genet* 1988; **25**: 387–91.

20 Sontheimer RD. Subacute cutaneous lupus: a 25 year evolution of a prototypic subset (subphenotype) of lupus erythematosus defined by characteristic cutaneous, pathological, immunological and genetic findings. *Autoimmun Rev* 2005; **4**: 253–63.

21 Wenzel J, Henze S, Brahler S *et al*. The expression of human leukocyte antigen-DR and CD25 on circulating T cells in cutaneous lupus erythematosus and correlation with disease activity. *Exp Dermatol* 2005; **14**: 454–9.

22 Werth VP, Zhang W, Dortzbach K *et al*. Association of a promotor polymorphism of tumor necrosis factor-α with subacute cutaneous lupus erythematosus and distinct photoregulation of transcription. *J Invest Dermatol* 2000; **115**: 726–30.

23 Millard TP, Kondeatis E, Cox A *et al*. A candidate gene analysis of three photosensitivity disorders: cutaneous lupus erythematosus, polymorphic light eruption and actinic prurigo. *Br J Dermatol* 2001; **145**: 229–36.

24 Millard, TP, Ashton GHS, Kondeatis E *et al*. Human Ro60 (SSA2) genomic organization and sequence alterations, examined in cutaneous lupus erythematosus. *Br J Dermatol* 2002; **146**: 210–5.

25 Provost TT, Watson RM. Anti-Ro (SSA), HLA DR3-positive females: the interrelationship between some ANA negative, SS, SCLE, and NLE mothers and SS/LE overlap female patients. *J Invest Dermatol* 1993; **100**: 14S–20S.

26 Fonseca E, Alvarez R, Gonzalez MR *et al*. Prevalence of anticardiolipin antibodies in subacute cutaneous lupus erythematosus. *Lupus* 1992; **1**: 265–8.

27 Bangert JL, Freeman RG, Sontheimer RD *et al*. Subacute cutaneous lupus erythematosus and discoid lupus erythematosus. *Arch Dermatol* 1984; **120**: 332–7.

28 David-Bajar KM, Bennion SD, DeSpain JD *et al*. Clinical, histological and immunofluorescent distinctions between subacute cutaneous lupus erythematosus and discoid lupus erythematosus. *J Invest Dermatol* 1992; **99**: 251–7.

29 Bielsa I, Herrero C, Collado A *et al*. Histopathologic findings in cutaneous lupus erythematosus. *Arch Dermatol* 1994; **130**: 54–8.

30 Nieboer C, Tak-Diamand Z, Van Leeuwen-Wallau HE. Dust-like particles: a specific direct immunofluorescence pattern in subacute cutaneous lupus erythematosus. *Br J Dermatol* 1988; **118**: 725–9.

31 Jerdan MS, Hood AF, Moore GW *et al*. Histopathologic comparison of the subsets of lupus erythematosus. *Arch Dermatol* 1990; **126**: 52–5.

32 Wenzel J, Henze S, Worenkamper E *et al*. Role of the chemokine receptor CCR4 and its ligand thymus- and activation-regulated chemokine/CCL17 for lymphocyte recruitment in cutaneous lupus erythematosus. *J Invest Dermatol* 2005; **124**: 1241–8.

33 Zampieri S, Alaibac M, Iaccarino L *et al*. Tumour necrosis factor α is expressed in refractory skin lesions from patients with subacute cutaneous lupus erythematosus. *Ann Rheum Dis* 2006; **65**: 545–8.

34 Sontheimer RD. Subacute cutaneous lupus erythematosus: a decade's perspective. *Med Clin North Am* 1989; **73**: 1073–90.

35 David-Bajar KM. Subacute cutaneous lupus syndromes. *J Invest Dermatol* 1993; **100**: 2S–8S.

36 Ciconte A, Mills AE, Shipley A, Marks R. Subacute cutaneous lupus presenting in a child. *Australas J Dermatol* 2002; **43**: 62–4.

37 Amato L, Coronella G, Berti S *et al*. Subacute cutaneous lupus erythematosus in childhood. *Paediatr Dermatol* 2003; **20**: 31–4.

38 Rockmann H, Feller G, Schadenforf D *et al*. Subacute cutaneous lupus on the lines of Blaschko. *Eur J Dermatol* 2006; **16**: 302–6.

39 Perera GK, Black MM, McGibbon DH. Bullous subacute cutaneous lupus erythematosus. *Clin Exp Dermatol* 2004; **29**: 265–7.

40 Mutasim DF. Severe subacute cutaneous lupus erythematosus presenting with generalized erythroderma and bullae. *J Am Acad Dermatol* 2003; **48**: 947–9.

41 Peitsch WK, Lorentz K, Goebeler M *et al*. Subacute cutaneous lupus erythematosus with bullae associated with porphyria cutanea tarda. *J Dtsch Dermatol Ges* 2007; **5**: 220–2.

42 De Spain J, Clark DP. Subacute cutaneous lupus erythematosus presenting as erythroderma. *J Am Acad Dermatol* 1988; **19**: 388–92.

43 Pramatarov K, Vassileva S, Miteva L. Subacute cutaneous lupus erythematosus presenting with generalized poikiloderma. *J Am Acad Dermatol* 2000; **42**: 286–8.

44 Marzano AV, Facchetti M, Alessi E. Poikilodermatous subacute cutaneous lupus erythematosus. *Dermatol* 2003; **207**: 285–90.

45 Rao BK, Coldiron BM, Freeman RF *et al*. Subacute lupus erythematosus lesions progressing to morphoea. *J Am Acad Dermatol* 1990; **23**: 1019–22.

46 Marzano AV, Kolesnikova LV, Gasparini G *et al*. Dystrophic calcinosis cutis in subacute lupus. *Dermatology* 1999; **198**: 90–2.

47 Sonntag M, Lehmann P, Megahed M *et al*. Papulonodular mucinosis associated with subacute cutaneous lupus erythematosus. *Dermatology* 2003; **206**: 326–9.

48 Callen JP, Klein J. Subacute cutaneous lupus erythematosus: clinical, serologic, immunogenetic, and therapeutic considerations in 72 patients. *Arthritis Rheum* 1988; **31**: 1007–13.

49 Black DR, Hornung CA, Schneider PD *et al*. Frequency and severity of systemic disease in patients with subacute cutaneous lupus erythematosus. *Arch Dermatol* 2002; **138**: 1175–8.

50 Berti S, Moretti S, Lucin C *et al*. Urticarial vasculitis and subacute cutaneous lupus erythematosus. *Lupus* 2005; **14**: 489–92.

51 Heymann WR, Manders SM, Gottlieb GJ *et al*. Subacute cutaneous lupus erythematosus associated with chronic interstitial pneumonitis. *Int J Dermatol* 1995; **34**: 354–6.

52 De-Silva BD, Plant W, Kemmett D. Subacute cutaneous lupus erythematosus and life-threatening hypokalaemic tetraparesis: a rare complication. *Br J Dermatol* 2001; **144**: 622–4.

53 Kreft B, Marsch WC. Lupus erythematosus gyratum repens. *Eur J Dermatol* 2007; **17**: 79–82.

54 Provost TT, Talal N, Harley JB *et al*. The relationship between anti-Ro (SS-A) antibody-positive Sjögren's syndrome and anti-Ro (SS-A) antibody-positive lupus erythematosus. *Arch Dermatol* 1988; **124**: 63–71.

55 Goette DK. Sweet's syndrome in subacute cutaneous lupus erythematosus. *Arch Dermatol* 1985; **121**: 789–91.

56 Ashworth J. Subacute cutaneous lupus erythematosus in a patient with Crohn's disease. *Clin Exp Dermatol* 1992; **17**: 135–6.

57 Grabbe S, Kolde G. Coexisting lichen planus and subacute lupus erythematosus. *Clin Exp Dermatol* 1995; **20**: 249–56.

58 Kontochristopoulos GK, Giannadaki M, Doulaveri G *et al*. Psoriasis co-existing with subacute cutaneous lupus erythematosus. *Eur Acad Dermatol Venereol* 2004; **18**: 385–6.

59 Ferahbas A, Utas S, Canoz O *et al*. The co-existence of subacute cutaneous lupus erythematosus and psoriasis. *Eur Acad Dermatol Venereol* 2004; **18**: 390–1.

60 Gudat W, Bork K. Hereditary angioedema associated with subacute cutaneous lupus erythematosus. *Dermatologica* 1989; **179**: 211–3.

61 Guillet G, Sassolas B, Plantin P *et al*. Anti-Ro-positive lupus and hereditary angioneurotic oedema. *Dermatologica* 1988; **177**: 370–5.

62 Camp PB, Davis LS. Coexistence of subacute cutaneous lupus erythematosus and porphyria cutanea tarda: a case report. *Cutis* 1997; **59**: 216E.

63 Roberts DL. Subacute cutaneous lupus erythematosus and gluten sensitive enteropathy. *Br J Dermatol* 1988; **118**: 731–2.

64 Bielsa I, Herrero C, Font J *et al*. Lupus erythematosus and toxic epidermal necrolysis. *J Am Acad Dermatol* 1987; **16**: 1265–7.

65 Wenzel J, Uerlich M, Gerdsen R *et al*. Association of inclusion body myositis with subacute cutaneous lupus erythematosus. *Rheumatol Int* 2001; **21**: 75–7.

66 Morgan KW, Callen JP. Calcifying lupus panniculitis in a patient with subacute cutaneous lupus erythematosus: response to diltiazem and chloroquine. *J Rheumatol* 2001; **28**: 2129–32.

67 Toll A, Gilaberte M, Matias-Guiu X *et al*. Kikuchi's disease (necrotizing lymphadenitis) with cutaneous involvement associated with subacute cutaneous lupus erythematosus. *Clin Exp Dermatol* 2004; **29**: 240–3.

68 Brown C, Deng J. Thiazide diuretic induces cutaneous lupus-like cutaneous reaction. *J Toxicol Clin Toxicol* 1995; **33**: 729–33.

69 Reed BR, Huff JC, Jones SK *et al*. Subacute cutaneous lupus erythematosus associated with hydrochlorothiazide therapy. *Ann Intern Med* 1985; **103**: 49–51.

70 Parodi A, Romagnoli M, Rebora A. Subacute cutaneous lupus erythematosus-like eruption caused by hydrochlorothiazide. *Photodermatol* 1989; **6**: 100–2.

71 Wollenberg A, Meurer M. Thiazide diuretic induced subacute cutaneous lupus. *Hautarzt* 1991; **42**: 709–12.

72 Darken M, McBurney E. Subacute cutaneous lupus erythematosus-like drug eruption due to combination diuretic hydrochlorothiazide and triamterine. *J Am Acad Dermatol* 1988; **18**: 38–42.

73 Miyagawa S, Okuchi T, Shiomi Y *et al*. Subacute cutaneous lupus erythematosus lesions precipitated by griseofulvin. *J Am Acad Dermatol* 1989; **21**: 343–6.

74 Callen JP, Hughes AP, Kulp-Shorten C. Subacute cutaneous lupus erythematosus induced or exacerbated by terbinafine. *Arch Dermatol* 2001; **137**: 1196–8.

75 Bonsmann G, Schiller M, Luger TA *et al*. Terbinafine-induced subacute cutaneous lupus erythematosus. *J Am Acad Dermatol* 2001; **44**: 925–31.

76 McKellar G, Porter D, Burden D. Terbinafine as a cause of cutaneous lupus erythematosus. *Rheumatology (Oxford)* 2004; **43**: 249.

77 Farhi D, Viguier M, Cosnes A *et al*. Terbinafine-induced subacute cutaneous lupus erythematosus. *Dermatology* 2006; **212**: 59–65.

78 Crowson AN, Magro CM. Subacute cutaneous lupus erythematosus arising in the setting of calcium channel blocker therapy. *Hum Pathol* 1997; **28**: 67–73.

79 Gubinelli E, Cocuroccia B, Girolomoni G. Subacute cutaneous lupus erythematosus induced by nifedipine. *J Cutan Med Surg* 2003; **7**: 243–6.

80 Marzano AV, Borghi A, Mercogliano M *et al*. Nitrendipine-induced subacute cutaneous lupus erythematosus. *Eur J Dermatology* 2003; **13**: 213–6.

81 Kurtis B, Larson MJ, Hoang MP *et al*. Verapamil-induced subacute cutaneous lupus erythematosus. *J Drugs Dermatol* 2005; **4**: 506–8.

82 Fumal I, Danchin A, Cosserat F *et al*. Subacute cutaneous lupus erythematosus associated with tamoxifen therapy: two cases. *Dermatology* 2005; **210**: 251–2.

83 Fenniche S, Dhaoui A, Amma FB *et al*. Acebutalol-induced subacute cutaneous lupus erythematosus. *Skin Pharmacol Physiol* 2005; **18**: 230–3.

84 Bracke A, Nijsten T, Vandermaesen J *et al*. Lansoprazole-induced subacute cutaneous lupus erythematosus: two cases. *Acta Derm Venereol* 2005; **85**: 353–4.

85 Noel B. Lupus erythematosus and other autoimmune diseases related to statin therapy: a systematic review. *J Eur Acad Dermatol Venereol* 2007; **21**: 17–24.

86 Srivastava M, Rencic A, Diglio G *et al*. Drug induced Ro/SSA positive cutaneous lupus erythematosus. *Arch Dermatol* 2003; **139**: 45–9.

87 Patri P, Nigro A, Rebora A. Lupus erythematosus like eruption from captopril. *Acta Derm Venereol* 1985; **65**: 447–8.

88 Fernandez-Diaz M, Herranz P, Suarez-Marrero M *et al*. Subacute cutaneous lupus erythematosus associated with cilazapril. *Lancet* 1995; **345**: 398.

89 Bleumink GS, Ter-Borg EJ, Ramselaar CG *et al*. Etanercept-induced subacute cutaneous lupus. *Rheumatology* 2001; **40**: 1317–9.

90 Bentley DD, Graves JE, Smith DI *et al*. Efalizumab-induced subacute cutaneous lupus erythematosus. *J Am Acad Dermatol* 2006; **54**: S242–3.

91 High WA, Muldrow ME, Fitzpatrick JE *et al*. Cutaneous lupus erythematosus induced by infliximab. *J Am Acad Dermatol* 2005; **52**: e7–8.

92 Gensburger D, Kawashima M, Marotte H *et al*. Lupus erythematosus with leflunomide: induction or reactivation? *Ann Rheum Dis* 2005; **64**: 153–5.

93 Chan SK, Hazleman BL, Burrows NP. Subacute cutaneous lupus erythematosus precipitated by leflunomide. *Clin Exp Dermatol* 2005; **30**: 724–5.

94 Goeb V, Bertholet JM, Joly P *et al.* Leflunomide-induced subacute cutaneous lupus erythematosus. *Rheumatol* 2005; **44**: 823–4.

95 Capponi A, De Simone C, Guerriero C *et al.* Ro/SSA Positive cutaneous lupus erythematosus induced by carbamazepine. *Arch Dermatol* 2005; **141**: 103–4.

96 Ameio P, Innocente C, Feliciani C *et al.* Drug-induced cutaneous lupus erythematosus after 5 years of treatment with carbamazepine. *Eur J Dermatol* 2006; **16**: 281–3.

97 Toll A, Campo-Pisa P, Gonzalez-Castro J *et al.* Subacute cutaneous lupus erythematosus associated with cinnarizine and thiethylperazine therapy. *Lupus* 1998; **7**: 364–6.

98 Pham HC, Saurat JH. Inhalation route inducing subacute cutaneous lupus erythematosus with tiotropium. *Arch Dermatol* 2005; **141**: 911–2.

99 Cassis TB, Callen JP. Bupropion induced subacute cutaneous lupus erythematosus. *Australas J Dermatol* 2005; **46**: 266–9.

100 Jumez N, Dereure O, Bessis D *et al.* Flare of cutaneous lupus erythematosus induced by bupropion (Zyban). *Dermatology* 2004; **208**: 362.

101 Chen M, Crowson AN, Woofter M *et al.* Docetaxel (taxotere) induced subacute cutaneous lupus erythematosus: report of 4 cases. *J Rheumatol* 2004; **31**: 818–20.

102 Reich A, Bialynick-Birula R, Szepietowski JC. Drug-induced subacute cutaneous lupus erythematosus resulting from ticlopidine. *Int J Dermatol* 2006; **45**: 1112–4.

103 Balsa A, Bernad M, de Miguel E *et al.* Lupus eritematoso cutanoe subagudo por la crisoterapia en una arthritis reumatoide. *Rev Clin Esp* 1988; **182**: 505–6.

104 Parodi A, Rivara G, Guarrera M. Possible naproxen induced relapse of subacute cutaneous lupus erythematosus. *JAMA* 1992; **268**: 51–2.

105 Leroy D, Dompmartin A, Le Jean S *et al.* Dermatitis caused by aldactone of a lupic annular erythema type. *Ann Dermatol Venereol* 1987; **114**: 1237–40.

106 Shapiro M, Sosis AC, Junkins-Hopkins JM *et al.* Lupus erythematosus induced by medications, ultraviolet radiation, and other exogenous agents: a review, with special focus on the development of subacute cutaneous lupus erythematosus in a genetically predisposed individual. *Int J Dermatol* 2004; **43**: 87–94.

107 Dowdy MJ, Nigra TP, Barth WF. Subacute cutaneous lupus erythematosus during PUVA therapy for psoriasis: case report and review of the literature. *Arthritis Rheum* 1989; **32**: 343–6.

108 Balabanova MB, Botev IN, Michailova JI. Subacute cutaneous lupus induced by radiation therapy. *Br J Dermatol* 1997; **137**: 648–9.

109 Nousari HC, Kimyai-Asadi A, Tausk FA. Subacute cutaneous lupus erythematosus associated with interferon-β1a. *Lancet* 1998; **352**: 1825–6.

110 Schewach-Millet M, Shpiro D, Ziv R *et al.* Subacute cutaneous lupus erythematosus associated with breast carcinoma. *J Am Acad Dermatol* 1988; **19**: 406–8.

111 Richardson TT, Cohen PR. Subacute cutaneous lupus erythematosus: report of a patient who subsequently developed a meningioma and whose skin lesions were treated with isotretinoin. *Cutis* 2000; **66**: 183–8.

112 Ho C, Shumack SP, Morris D. Subacute cutaneous lupus erythematosus associated with hepatocellular carcinoma. *Australas J Dermatol* 2001; **42**: 110–3.

113 Castenet J, Taillan B, Lacour JP *et al.* Subacute cutaneous lupus erythematosus associated with Hodgkin's disease. *Clin Rheumatol* 1995; **14**: 692–4.

114 Brenner S, Golan H, Gat A *et al.* Paraneoplastic subacute cutaneous lupus erythematosus: report of a case associated with cancer of the lung. *Dermatology* 1997; **194**: 172–4.

115 Vogt T, Coras B, Hafner C *et al.* Antiangiogenic therapy in metastatic prostate carcinoma complicated by cutaneous lupus erythematosus. *Lancet Oncol* 2006; **7**: 695–7.

116 Chaudry SI, Murphy LA, White IR. Subacute cutaneous lupus: a paraneoplastic dermatosis. *Clin Exp Dermatol* 2005; **30**: 655–8.

117 Weinstein CL, Littlejohn GO, Thomson NM *et al.* Severe visceral disease in subacute cutaneous lupus erythematosus. *Arch Dermatol* 1987; **123**: 638–40.

118 Callen JP, Roth DE, McGrath C *et al.* Safety and efficacy of a broad-spectrum sunscreen in patients with discoid or subacute cutaneous lupus erythematosus. *Cutis* 1991; **47**: 130–6.

119 Herzinger T, Plewig G, Rocken M. Use of sunscreens to protect against ultraviolet induced lupus erythematosus. *Arthritis Rheum* 2004; **50**: 3045–8.

120 Drake LA, Dinehart SM, Farmer ER *et al.* Guidelines of care for cutaneous lupus erythematosus. *J Am Acad Dermatol* 1996; **34**: 830–6.

121 Heath M, Raugi GJ. Evidence-based evaluation of immunomodulatory therapy for the cutaneous manifestations of lupus. *Adv Dermatol* 2004; **20**: 257–91.

122 Callen JP. Cutaneous lupus erythematosus: a personal approach to management. *Australas J Dermatol* 2006; **47**: 13–27.

123 Kreuter A, Gambichler T, Breukmann F *et al.* Pimecrolimus 1% cream for cutaneous lupus erythematosus. *J Am Acad Dermatol* 2004; **51**: 407–10.

124 Bohm M, Gaubitz M, Luger TA *et al.* Topical tacrolimus as a therapeutic adjunct in patients with cutaneous lupus erythematosus. *Dermatology* 2003; **207**: 381–5.

125 Lampropoulos CE, Sangle S, Harrison P *et al.* Topical tacrolimus therapy of resistant cutaneous lesions in lupus erythematosus: a possible alternative. *Rheumatology* 2004; **43**: 1383–5.

126 Tzung TY, Liu YS, Chang HW. Tacrolimus vs clobetasol proprionate in the treatment of facial lupus erythematosus: a randomized, double blind, bilateral comparison study. *Br J Dermatol* 2007; **156**: 191–2.

127 Von Pelchrzim R, Schmook T, Friedrich M *et al.* Efficacy of topical tacrolimus in the treatment of various cutaneous manifestations of lupus erythematosus. *Int J Dermatol* 2006; **45**: 84–5.

128 Druke A, Gambichler T, Altmeyer P *et al.* 0.1% tacrolimus ointment in a patient with subacute cutaneous lupus erythematosus. *J Dermatolog Treat* 2004; **15**: 63–4.

129 Wozniacka A, Carter A, McCauliffe DP. Antimalarials in cutaneous lupus erythematosus: mechanisms of therapeutic benefit. *Lupus* 2002; **11**: 71–81.

130 Fielder A, Graham E, Jones SK *et al.* Royal College of Ophthalmologists guidelines: ocular toxicity and hydroxychloroquine. *Eye* 1998; **12**: 907–9.

131 Feldmann R, Salomon D, Saurat JH. The association of the two antimalarials chloroquine and quinacrine for treatment-resistant chronic and subacute cutaneous lupus erythematosus. *Dermatology* 1994; **189**: 425–7.

132 Jewell ML, McCauliffe DP. Patients with cutaneous lupus erythematosus who smoke are less responsive to antimalarial therapy. *J Am Acad Dermatol* 2000; **42**: 983–7.

133 Goldberg JW, Lidsky MD. Pulse methylprednisolone therapy for persistent subacute cutaneous lupus. *Arthritis Rheum* 1984; **27**: 837–8.

134 Ruzicka T, Meurer M, Braun-Falco O. Treatment of cutaneous lupus erythematosus with etretinate. *Acta Derm Venereol (Stockh)* 1985; **65**: 324–9.

135 Ruzicka T, Meurer M, Bieber T. Efficiency of acitretin in the treatment of cutaneous lupus erythematosus. *Arch Dermatol* 1988; **124**: 897–902.

136 Newton RC, Jorizzo JL, Solomon AR *et al.* Mechanism-oriented assessment of isotretinoin in chronic or subacute cutaneous lupus erythematosus. *Arch Dermatol* 1986; **122**: 170–6.

137 Richardson TT, Cohen PR. Subacute cutaneous lupus erythematosus: report of a patient who subsequently developed a meningioma and whose skin lesions were treated with isotretinoin. *Cutis* 2000; **66**: 183–8.

138 Tsutsui K, Imai T, Hatta N *et al.* Widespread pruritic plaques in a patient with subacute cutaneous lupus erythematosus and hypocomplementaemia: response to dapsone therapy. *J Am Acad Dermatol* 1996; **35**: 313–5.

139 Bohm L, Uerlich M, Bauer R. Rapid improvement of subacute cutaneous lupus erythematosus with low-dose methotrexate. *Dermatology* 1997; **194**: 307–8.

140 Kuhn A, Specker C, Ruzicka T *et al.* Methotrexate treatment for refractory subacute cutaneous lupus erythematosus. *J Am Acad Dermatol* 2002; **46**: 600–3.

141 Wenzel J, Brahler S, Bauer R *et al.* Efficacy and safety of methotrexate in recalcitrant cutaneous lupus erythematosus: results of a retrospective study in 43 patients. *Br J Dermatol* 2005; **153**: 157–62.

142 Huber A, Tuting T, Bauer R *et al.* Methotrexate treatment in cutaneous lupus erythematosus: subcutaneous application is as effective as intravenous administration. *Br J Dermatol* 2006; **155**: 861–2.

143 Stevens RJ, Andujar C, Edwards CJ *et al.* Thalidomide in the treatment of the cutaneous manifestations of lupus erythematosus: experience in 16 consecutive patients. *Br J Rheumatol* 1997; **36**: 353–9.

144 Ordi-Ros J, Cortes F, Cucurull E *et al.* Thalidomide in the treatment of cutaneous lupus refractory to conventional therapy. *Rheumatol* 2000; **27**: 1429–33.

145 Bohmeyer J, Achenbach A, Westenberger M *et al.* Thalidomide therapy of cutaneous lupus erythematosus. *Hautarzt* 2002; **53**: 744–8.

146 Housman TS, Jorizzo JL, McCarty MA *et al.* Low-dose thalidomide therapy for refractory cutaneous lesions of lupus erythematosus. *Arch Dermatol* 2003; **139**: 50–4.

147 Cuadrado MJ, Karim Y, Sanna G *et al.* Thalidomide for the treatment of resistant cutaneous lupus: efficacy and safety of different therapeutic regimes. *Am J Med* 2005; **118**: 246–50.

148 Sonnichsen N, Meffert H, Kunzelmann V *et al.* UVA-1 Therapie bei subakut-kutanem Lupus Erythematodes. *Hautarzt* 1993; **44**: 723–5.

149 Nicolas JF, Thivolet J. Interferon-α therapy in severe unresponsive subacute cutaneous lupus erythematosus. *N Engl J Med* 1989; **321**: 1550–1.

150 Rudnicka L, Szymanska E, Walecka I *et al.* Long-term cefuroxime axetil in subacute cutaneous lupus erythematosus: a report of three cases. *Dermatology* 2000; **200**: 129–31.

151 Schanz S, Ulmer A, Rassner G *et al.* Successful treatment of subacute cutaneous lupus erythematosus with mycophenolate mofetil. *Br J Dermatol* 2002; **147**: 174–8.

152 Goodfield, MJD, Davison K, Bowden K. Intravenous immunoglobulin (IVIg) for therapy-resistant cutaneous lupus erythematosus. *J Dermatolog Treat* 2004; **15**: 46–50.

153 Kreuter A, Hyun J, Altmeyer P *et al.* Intravenous immunoglobulin for recalcitrant subacute cutaneous lupus erythematosus. *Acta Derm Venereol* 2005; **85**: 545–7.

154 Fautrel B, Foltz V, Frances C *et al.* Regression of subacute cutaneous lupus erythematosus in a patient with rheumatoid arthritis treated with a biologic tumour necrosis factor α blocking agent: comment on the article by Pisetsky and the letter from Aringer. *Arthritis Rheum* 2002; **46**: 1408–9.

155 Layton TH, Ogden S, Goodfield MJG. Treatment of refractory subacute cutaneous lupus erythematosus with efalizumab. *J Am Acad Dermatol* 2005; **54**: 892–5.

Systemic lupus erythematosus [1,2]

Definition. A systemic disease characterized by multisystem organ inflammation, most commonly the skin, joints and vasculature, and associated immunological abnormalities. The main clinical features include fever, rashes and arthritis, but renal, pulmonary, cardiac and neurological involvement may occur, with increased mortality. For any individual patient, the ARA criteria may be used as an aid to diagnosis (Table 51.9).

Incidence. SLE is an uncommon disease [3–9], with incidence estimated at 1–12.5 in 100 000 per year at Leeds General Infirmary; for every case of SLE there are six cases of pernicious anaemia and 10 of leukaemia. The condition is universal, but is three times more common in black people than in white people [3]. Younger black American females are particularly predisposed to the disease [4],

Table 51.9 American Rheumatism Association criteria for diagnosis of systemic lupus erythematosus.

1 Malar rash

2 Discoid rash

3 Photosensitivity

4 Oral ulcers

5 Non-erosive arthritis

6 Serositis—pleurisy or pericarditis

7 Renal disorder—persistent proteinuria (>0.5 g/day) or cellular casts

8 Neurological disorder—seizures or psychosis

9 Haematological disorder—haemolytic anaemia or leukopenia (<4000/mm) or lymphopenia (<1500/mm) or thrombocytopenia (<100 000/mm)

10 Immunological disorder—LE cells or anti-DNA antibody or anti-Sm antibody or false-positive serology for syphilis (longer than 6 months)

11 Antinuclear antibodies

LE, lupus erythematosus.

although it is rare in native Africans. It is also common in the Chinese and in New Zealand Polynesians [5]. The pattern of disease appears to be different in such ethnic subgroups, with black Americans and Hispanics having the highest rate of internal organ damage [6]. A study in Hawaii gave similar racial variation, with the prevalence in those of Chinese origin being 24.1 in 100 000, whereas that in whites was 5.8 in 100 000 [7]. The incidence of newly diagnosed cases in New York is 10–14 per million population [8]. The prevalence varies from less than 1 in 1000 for black females in New York [9] to approximately 1 in 2000 white females in San Francisco, and figures for England and Wales suggest a prevalence of 12.5 in 100 000 women, although this is an underestimate [10]. The observed annual incidence increased from 25 per million in 1955 to 50 per million in 1959 [11]. In Hong Kong, in 1987, the incidence was 2.4 in 100 000 [11], and in Baltimore, in 1985, it was 4.6 in 100 000, a twofold increase over the preceding 15 years. Self-reported physician-diagnosed SLE occurred in 124 in 100 000 in the USA [12]. This suggests that the disorder may be more common than it used to be, but it may also represent better awareness and earlier diagnosis. An epidemiological survey in New York showed that morbidity and mortality rates were highest among black people, followed in descending order by Puerto Ricans and then other white people. Racial differences were independent of housing, overcrowding and migration, but were associated with racial variation in normal gammaglobulin levels, which were higher in black people [6]. A more recent study from England confirms the increased risk of SLE in Afro-Caribbeans and Asians, irrespective of their place of birth [13]. Familial cases occur in approximately 10% [14,15]; relatives of patients with SLE also have an increased incidence of SLE and DLE, rheumatoid arthritis, rheumatic fever, polyarteritis nodosa, dermatomyositis and poikiloderma atrophicans vasculare [16].

The condition tends to occur in early adult life, and the peak age of onset of the first symptom or sign in females is approximately 38 years (35.5 in black women, and 40.7 in white women); it is 44.2 in men [17]. The incidence of the disease is the same in all age ranges, although serositis and Sjögren's syndrome are more common disease manifestations in the elderly [18]. Most authors agree that females outnumber males by a ratio of approximately 8:1, but the features in males are the same as in females [19].

References

1 Wallace DJ, Hahn BH, eds. *Dubois' Lupus Erythematosus*, 4th edn. Philadelphia: Lee and Febiger, 1993.

2 Rowell NR. The natural history of lupus erythematosus. *Clin Exp Dermatol* 1984; **9**: 217–31.

3 Siegel M, Holley HL, Lee SL. Epidemiologic studies on systemic lupus erythematosus. *Arthritis Rheum* 1970; **13**: 802–11.

4 Ballou SP, Khan MA, Kushner I. Clinical features of systemic lupus erythematosus. *Arthritis Rheum* 1982; **25**: 55–60.

5 Hart HH, Grigor RR, Caughey DE. Ethnic difference in the prevalence of systemic lupus erythematosus. *Ann Rheum Dis* 1983; **42**: 529–32.

6 Segel M, Seelenfreund M. Racial and social factors in systemic lupus erythematosus. *JAMA* 1965; **191**: 77–80.

7 Serdula MK, Rhoads GG. The frequency of systemic lupus erythematosus in different groups in Hawaii. *Arthritis Rheum* 1979; **22**: 328–33.

8 Siegel M, Reilly EB, Lee SL *et al.* Epidemiology of systemic lupus erythematosus: time trend and racial differences. *Am J Public Health* 1964; **54**: 33–43.

9 Siegal M, Lees SL. The epidemiology of systemic lupus erythematosus. *Semin Arthritis Rheum* 1973; **3**: 1–54.

10 Hochberg MC. Prevalence of systemic lupus erythematosus in England and Wales, 1981–2. *Ann Rheum Dis* 1987; **46**: 664–6.

11 Woo J, Wong RWS, Wang SWS *et al.* Patterns of rheumatoid arthritis and systemic lupus erythematosus in Hong Kong. *Ann Rheum Dis* 1987; **46**: 644–5.

12 Hochberg MC, Perlmutter DL, Medsger TA *et al.* Prevalence of self-reported physician diagnosed systemic lupus erythematosus in the USA. *Lupus* 1995; **4**: 454–6.

13 Johnson AE, Gordon C, Palmer RG *et al.* The prevalence and incidence of systemic lupus erythematosus in Birmingham, England. *Arthritis Rheum* 1995; **38**: 551–8.

14 Arnett FC, Shulman LE. Studies in familial systemic lupus erythematosus. *Medicine* 1976; **55**: 313–22.

15 Reveille JD, Bias WB, Winkelstein JA *et al.* Familial lupus erythematosus: immunogenetic studies in eight families. *Medicine* 1983; **62**: 21–35.

16 Tuffanelli DL, Dubois EL. Cutaneous manifestations of systemic lupus erythematosus. *Arch Dermatol* 1964; **90**: 377–86.

17 Hochberg MC. The incidence of systemic lupus erythematosus in Baltimore, Maryland, 1970–77. *Arthritis Rheum* 1985; **28**: 80–6.

18 Jonsson H, Nived O, Sturfelt G. The effect of age on clinical and serological manifestations in unselected patients with systemic lupus erythematosus. *J Rheumatol* 1988; **15**: 505–9.

19 Miller MH, Urowitz MB, Gladman DD. Systemic lupus erythematosus in males. *Medicine* 1983; **62**: 327–34.

Aetiology. The aetiology of SLE remains unknown. Aetiological theories must account for the known variations in the incidence of the disease, the marked immune dysfunction, known precipitating factors and the clear familial predisposition.

Genetic factors. There is considerable evidence to suggest that genetic factors play a part in the pathogenesis [1]. The condition has been reported in identical twins [2,3], with a concordance rate of 65% [2]. Of all cases, 4% are familial [4], with marked concordance of disease expression between parents and offspring. The onset of SLE in identical twins occurred within 2 years, compared with an interval of 9 years between siblings and 20 years between parents and offspring [5]. However, the onset of disease in siblings is temporally rather than age-related, indicating a possible environmental factor [6]. Occasionally, identical twins may be discordant for SLE. In this case, the non-affected twin does not have abnormalities of helper and suppressor T-cell numbers and activity, and has different cellular immune responses [7,8]. The incidence of SLE is probably higher in XXY males with Klinefelter's syndrome [9]. Relatives of patients with SLE have a higher incidence of connective tissue disease, hyperglobulinaemia and antinuclear factor than the relatives of matched controls [10,11]. They may also show increased incidence of anti-RNA and lymphocytotoxic antibodies, specific anti-DNA antibody idiotypes [12], anticardiolipin antibodies [13] and impaired suppressor T-lymphocyte function [14], although these are not related to disease expression [15].

Studies of histocompatibility antigens further support a genetic predisposition. White people with SLE have increased frequencies of HLA-B8 [16], -DR3, -A1 and -DR2 [17]. Similar associations have been confirmed in black people [18,19], as has an association with immunoglobulin allotypes Gm 1 and 17 [20]. HLA-DQ antigens may be even more closely related to the risk of developing the disease, and different alleles may be implicated in the risk of

developing the disease from those that influence its expression [21]. There is evidence of linkage disequilibrium between B8-DR3 and alleles at the DQ locus, which is prevalent in patients who express anti-Ro antibodies [22].

Eighty per cent of patients (compared with 40% of controls) have null complement alleles [23], mainly at the C4A or B locus [24]. HLA-DR2 and the C4A null allele are independent and additive risk factors in SLE [25]. Deficiency of complement factors C5–9 is relatively common in familial cases of SLE. Genetic factors other than HLA and complement component deficiencies may also be involved [26]. The results of genome scanning of family pedigrees multiplex for SLE, including over 400 sib pairs and 175 affected relatives, suggest an epistatic interaction between chromosome 14p16–15.2 and chromosome 5p15 in European American families [27].

References

1 Criswell LA. The genetic contribution to systemic lupus erythematosus. *Bull NYU Hosp Jt Dis* 2008; **66**: 176–83.

2 Block SR, Winfield JB, Lockshin MD *et al.* Studies of twins with systemic lupus erythematosus. *Am J Med* 1975; **59**: 533–52.

3 Block SR, Lockshin MD, Winfield JB *et al.* Immunologic observations on nine sets of twins either concordant or discordant for SLE. *Arthritis Rheum* 1976; **19**: 545–54.

4 Estes D, Christian CL. The natural history of systemic lupus erythematosus by prospective analysis. *Medicine* 1971; **50**: 85–95.

5 Alvarellos A, Ahearn JM, Provost TT *et al.* Relationships of HLA-DR and MT antigens to autoantibody expression in systemic lupus erythematosus. *Arthritis Rheum* 1983; **26**: 1533–4.

6 Kaplan D. The onset of disease in twins and siblings with systemic lupus erythematosus. *J Rheumatol* 1984; **11**: 648–52.

7 Brunner CM, Horwitz DA, Shan MK *et al.* Clinical and immunologic studies in identical twins discordant for systemic lupus erythematosus. *Am J Med* 1973; **55**: 249–54.

8 Soppi E, Eskola J, Lehtonen A. Evidence against HLA and immunological dependence of disease outbreak in SLE: immunological characterization of identical twins clinically discordant for SLE. *Ann Rheum Dis* 1985; **44**: 45–9.

9 Burch PRJ, Rowell NR. Systemic lupus erythematosus and Klinefelter's syndrome. *Lancet* 1976; **i**: 1021.

10 Leonhardt T. Family studies in systemic lupus erythematosus. *Acta Med Scand* 1964; **176** (Suppl.): 416.

11 Lowenstein MB, Rothfield NF. Family study of systemic lupus erythematosus. *Arthritis Rheum* 1977; **20**: 1293–303.

12 Isenberg DA, Shoenfeld Y, Walport M *et al.* Detection of crossreactive anti-DNA antibody idiotypes in the serum of systemic lupus erythematosus patients and of their relatives. *Arthritis Rheum* 1985; **28**: 999–1007.

13 Mackworth-Young C, Chan J, Harris N *et al.* High incidence of anticardiolipin antibodies in relatives of patients with systemic lupus erythematosus. *J Rheumatol* 1987; **14**: 723–6.

14 Miller KB, Schwartz RS. Familial abnormalities of suppressor-cell function in systemic lupus erythematosus. *N Engl J Med* 1979; **301**: 803–9.

15 Dudeney C, Shoenfeld Y, Rauch J *et al.* A study of anti-poly (ADP-ribose) antibodies and an anti-DNA antibody idiotype and other immunological abnormalities in lupus family members. *Ann Rheum Dis* 1986; **45**: 502–7.

16 Millard LG, Rowell NR, Rajah SM. Histocompatibility antigens in discoid and systemic lupus erythematosus. *Br J Dermatol* 1977; **96**: 139–44.

17 Walport MJ, Black CM, Batchelor JR. The immunogenetics of SLE. *Clin Rheum Dis* 1982; **8**: 3–21.

18 Goldberg MA, Arnett FC, Bias WB *et al.* Histocompatibility antigens in systemic lupus erythematosus. *Arthritis Rheum* 1976; **19**: 129–32.

19 Kachru RAJB, Sequeira W, Mittal KK *et al.* A significant increase of HLA-DR3 and DR2 in systemic lupus erythematosus among Blacks. *J Rheumatol* 1984; **11**: 471–4.

20 Fielder AHL, Walport MJ, Batchelor JR *et al.* Family study of the major histocompatibility complex in patients with systemic lupus erythematosus: import-

ance of null alleles of C4A and C4B in determining disease susceptibility. *BMJ* 1983; **286**: 425–8.

21 Harley JB, Sestak AL, Willis LG *et al.* A model for disease heterogeneity in systemic lupus erythematosus. *Arthritis Rheum* 1989; **32**: 826–36.

22 Reveille JD, Macleod MJ, Whittington K *et al.* Specific amino acid residues in the second hypervariable region of HLA-DQA1 and DQB1 chain genes promote the Ro (SS-A)/La autoantibody responses. *J Immunol* 1991; **146**: 3871–6.

23 Foad B, Litwin A, Zimmer H *et al.* Acetylator phenotype in systemic lupus erythematosus. *Arthritis Rheum* 1977; **20**: 815–8.

24 Fedrick JA, Pardey JP, Chen Z *et al.* Gm allotypes in blacks with systemic lupus erythematosus. *Hum Immunol* 1983; **8**: 177–81.

25 Howard PF, Hochberg MC, Bias WB *et al.* Relationship between C4 null genes, HLA-D region antigens, and genetic susceptibility to systemic lupus erythematosus in caucasian and black Americans. *Am J Med* 1986; **81**: 187–93.

26 Reveille JD, Bias WB, Winkelstein JA *et al.* Familial systemic lupus erythematosus: immunogenetic studies in eight families. *Medicine* 1983; **62**: 21–35.

27 Gray-McGuire C, Moser KL, Gaffney PM *et al.* Genome scan of human systemic lupus erythematosus by regression modeling: evidence of linkage and epistasis at 4p16–15.2. *Am J Hum Genet* 2000; **67**: 1460–9.

Autoantibodies [1,2]. Non-organ-specific humoral autoantibodies are the hallmark of SLE. A range of autoantibodies may be present in the disease, although some are more disease-specific (anti-double-stranded DNA and anti-Sm antibodies), and some are much more commonly found (antinuclear and anti-Ro antibodies). The disease could be produced by the development of such antibodies against tissue antigens to which tolerance has been lost by failure of homeostatic immunological mechanisms. This could occur either because of polyclonal B-cell activation or specific antigenic drive. There is evidence for both mechanisms of production of autoantibodies [3]. There is also considerable evidence that such non-organ-specific autoantibodies are not the primary pathogens: they are not specific to any disease, they are not present in all cases, their titres are independent of the activity of the disease, they are transmitted across the placenta without apparently harming the fetus [4] and they can be transfused into human volunteers without causing any apparent disease. In animal models, however, antinuclear antibodies can intensify experimental inflammatory lesions [5]; there is also evidence for involvement of immune complexes containing antinuclear antibody (either deposited or formed *in situ*) in the renal lesion of SLE as well as in tissue damage in other sites [6]. Recent evidence suggests that these antibodies may be formed against DNA-containing debris which is packaged into a vesicle after cells have undergone apoptosis, so-called 'apoptotic bodies' [7,8]. Anti-DNA antibodies bind the DNA receptor on white blood cells and block the binding and sequestration of free DNA by mononuclear cells [9]. These antibodies also produce the release of IFN-γ from mononuclear cells, enhancing immunological and inflammatory reactions [10]. Anti-Ro or closely related antibodies are implicated in the development of the rash and heart block found in neonatal LE (see p. 51.49), and possibly in other childhood SLE. The antiphospholipid antibodies, including the so-called lupus anticoagulant, are linked to thrombosis and abortion in patients with SLE (see p. 51.48). Conversely, neurofilament autoantibodies occur in 21% of patients with SLE, but do not correlate with neurological involvement [11]. Antiribosomal P proteins are highly specific for lupus psychosis [12]. Recent evidence suggests that there is switching of antibody types between the active and quiescent stages of the disease, with low-affinity IgM antibodies present when the disease

is controlled, and high-affinity IgG, often directed against endothelial cells, being present when the disease is active [13]. Antiendothelial cell antibodies are associated with renal and vascular complications [14].

Idiotypes and anti-idiotypes [15]. Idiotypes are the antigenic determinants of immunoglobulin molecules and are found in the variable region of these molecules and the T-cell receptor. Antibodies to these antigens develop (anti-idiotype antibodies), and are themselves capable of stimulating anti-anti-idiotype antibodies. Thus, complicated networks of antibodies develop, which are involved in the mechanisms of autoimmunity and self-recognition. Anti-idiotype antibodies may have some of the capabilities of the original antigen, and may also cross-react with other self-antigens, interfering with the development of tolerance produced by the removal of self-reactive T cells. This interference would allow the development of the 'forbidden clones' originally predicted by Burch and Rowell [16]. Cross-reaction between self-antigens and those derived from extraneous sources such as infection or other environmental agents may provide the original source of anti-idiotype antibodies [17].

References

1 Alarcón-Segoviá D. The pathogenesis of immune dysregulation in systemic lupus erythematosus. A Troika. *J Rheumatol* 1984; **11**: 588–90.

2 Beck JS, Rowell NR. Discoid lupus erythematosus: a study of the clinical features and biochemical and serological abnormalities in 120 patients with observations on the relationship of this disease to systemic lupus erythematosus. *QJM* 1966; **35**: 119–36.

3 Hardin JA. The lupus autoantigens and the pathogenesis of systemic lupus erythematosus. *Arthritis Rheum* 1986; **29**: 457–60.

4 Beck JS, Oakley CL, Rowell NR. Transplacental passage of antinuclear antibody. *Arch Dermatol* 1966; **93**: 656–63.

5 Hughes P, Rowell NR. Aggravation of turpentine-induced pleurisy in rats by 'homogeneous' and 'speckled' antinuclear antibodies. *J Pathol* 1970; **101**: 141–55.

6 Brentjens J, Ossie E, Albini B *et al.* Disseminated immune deposits in lupus erythematosus. *Arthritis Rheum* 1977; **20**: 962–8.

7 Lorenz HM, Herrmann M, Winkler T *et al.* Role of apoptosis in autoimmunity. *Apoptosis* 2000; **5**: 443–9.

8 Schmidt-Acevedo S, Perez-Romano B, Ruiz-Arguelles A. 'LE cells' result from phagocytosis of apoptotic bodies induced by antinuclear antibodies. *J Autoimmun* 2000; **15**: 15–20.

9 Bennett RM, Peller JS, Merritt MM. Defective DNA-receptor function in systemic lupus erythematosus and related diseases: evidence for an autoantibody influencing cell physiology. *Lancet* 1986; **i**: 186–8.

10 Ramirez F, Williams RC, Sibbitt WL *et al.* Immunoglobulin from systemic lupus erythematosus serum induces interferon release by normal mononuclear cells. *Arthritis Rheum* 1986; **29**: 326–36.

11 Kurki P, Helve T, Dahl D *et al.* Neurofilament autoantibodies in systemic lupus erythematosus. *J Rheumatol* 1986; **13**: 69–73.

12 Teh LS, Isenberg DA. Antiribosomal P protein antibodies in systemic lupus erythematosus: a reappraisal. *Arthritis Rheum* 1994; **37**: 307–15.

13 Ehrenstein M, Longhurst C, Isenberg DA. Production and analysis of IgG monoclonal anti-DNA antibodies from systemic lupus erythematosus (SLE) patients. *Clin Exp Immunol* 1993; **92**: 39–45.

14 Cervera R, Khamashta MA, Font J *et al.* Endothelial anticellular antibodies in systemic lupus erythematosus: association with vascular and kidney lesions. *Med Clin (Barc)* 1992; **99**: 605–8.

15 Jerne NK. Towards a network theory of the immune system. *Ann Immunol (Paris)* 1974; **125c**: 373–89.

16 Burch PRJ, Rowell NR. Systemic lupus erythematosus: aetiological aspects. *Am J Med* 1965; **38**: 793–801.

17 George J, Shoenfeld Y. Infection, idiotypes and SLE. *Lupus* 1995; **4**: 333–5.

Other immune factors. Cell-mediated immunity is abnormal in SLE [1]. Lymphocyte transformation responses to common antigens [2] and decreased skin-test responses to purified protein derivative, candidin and streptokinase-dornase [3] are related to disease activity [4]. T-cell counts are diminished [5] and null cells are increased [6] in active disease. It would appear that there is an imbalance between T and B lymphocytes in the disease, with depressed cellular immunity and an overactive humoral antibody response, possibly related to a relative lack of suppressor and/or inducer T cells, although all T-cell types are reduced, and their function is impaired. IL-2 production by peripheral blood leukocytes is impaired, reducing the inhibitory effects of T cells on activated B cells [7].

There is a reduction in activated B cells, but hyperactive B cells are increased in SLE [8], and their differentiation abnormally stimulated by monocytes [9]. There is some evidence that in remission there is a return of immunological suppressor function despite a persisting impairment of T-lymphocyte reactivity [10]. Antibody-dependent cellular cytotoxicity may be another pathogenic factor, and antibodies directed against lymphocyte membranes are found in SLE. Serum-induced cytotoxicity occurs to T cells [11], and immune complexes may be implicated [12]. Circulating immune complexes occur in approximately half of patients, especially those with active and extensive disease [13]. Killer cell activity is increased [14], and complement activation occurs, and the anaphylatoxins C3a and C5a are increased during disease exacerbations, possibly contributing to the pathogenesis of the vascular lesions [15].

References

1 Rönnblom L, Pascual V. The innate immune system in SLE: type I interferons and dendritic cells. *Lupus* 2008; **17**: 394–9.
2 Hughes P, Holt S, Rowell NR *et al*. Relationship of phytohaemagglutinin-induced lymphocyte transformation to disease activity in systemic lupus erythematosus. *Ann Rheum Dis* 1976; **35**: 97–105.
3 Paty JG Jr, Sienknecht CW, Townes AS *et al*. Impaired cell-mediated immunity in systemic lupus erythematosus (SLE): a controlled study of 23 untreated patients. *Am J Med* 1975; **59**: 769–79.
4 Horwitz DA, Cousar JB. A relationship between impaired cellular immunity, humoral suppression of lymphocyte function and severity of systemic lupus erythematosus. *Am J Med* 1975; **58**: 829–35.
5 Hughes P, Holt S, Rowell NR *et al*. Thymus-dependent (T) lymphocyte deficiency in progressive systemic sclerosis. *Br J Dermatol* 1976; **95**: 469–73.
6 Scheinberg MA, Cathcart ES, Goldstein AL. Thymosin-induced reduction of 'null cells' in peripheral-blood lymphocytes of patients with systemic lupus erythematosus. *Lancet* 1975; **i**: 424–6.
7 McKenna RM, Wilkins JA, Warrington RJ. Lymphokine production in rheumatoid arthritis and systemic lupus erythematosus. *J Rheumatol* 1988; **15**: 1639–42.
8 Sakane T, Suzuki N, Takeda S *et al*. B cell hyperactivity and its relation to distinct clinical features and the degree of disease activity in patients with systemic lupus erythematosus. *Arthritis Rheum* 1988; **31**: 80–7.
9 Jandl RC, Adirein TA. Stimulation of B cell differentiation by adherent mononuclear cells in systemic lupus erythematosus. *Arthritis Rheum* 1987; **30**: 861–8.
10 Breshihan B, Jasin HE. Suppressor function of peripheral blood mononuclear cells in normal individuals and in patients with SLE. *J Clin Invest* 1977; **59**: 106–16.
11 Kumagai S, Steinberg AD, Green I. Antibodies to T cells in patients with systemic lupus erythematosus can induce antibody dependent cell-mediated cytotoxicity against human T cells. *J Clin Invest* 1981; **67**: 605–14.
12 Penning CA, Hughes P, Rowell NR. The production of antibody dependent cellular cytotoxicity by immune complexes in systemic lupus erythematosus. *J Clin Lab Immunol* 1984; **13**: 123–7.
13 Hughes P, Cunningham J, Day M *et al*. Immune complexes in systemic sclerosis; detection by C1q binding k-cell inhibition and raji cell radioimmunoassays. *J Clin Lab Immunol* 1983; **10**: 133–8.
14 Blasczyk M, Majewski S, Wasik N *et al*. Natural killer cell activity of peripheral blood mononuclear cells from patients with various forms of lupus erythematosus. *Br J Dermatol* 1987; **117**: 709–14.
15 Belmont MH, Hopkins P, Edelson HS *et al*. Complement activation during systemic lupus erythematosus. *Arthritis Rheum* 1986; **29**: 1085–9.

UV radiation. This may precipitate the onset or exacerbate the course of SLE in up to 60% of patients [1]. Phototesting to UVB and UVA [2] shows reduced minimal erythema doses and the development of skin lesions in patients with LE. The mechanism of action of UV radiation in SLE remains unknown, although antibodies to UV radiation-denatured DNA can be demonstrated. There is no defect of DNA repair in SLE [3], and the antibodies to denatured DNA have no clinical or immunological correlations [4]. The expression of Ro antibody can be induced on cultured keratinocytes by UV radiation [5], and this antibody is commonly found in photosensitive patients. However, there is no relationship between absolute levels of Ro and disease activity [6].

References

1 Werth VP. Cutaneous lupus: insights into pathogenesis and disease classification. *Bull NYU Hosp Jt Dis* 2007; **65**: 200–4.
2 Lehmann P, Holzle E, Kind P *et al*. Experimental reproduction of skin lesions in lupus erythematosus by UVA and UVB radiation. *J Am Acad Dermatol* 1990; **22**: 181–7.
3 Palmer RG, Smith-Burchnell CA, Dore CJ *et al*. Sensitivity of lymphocytes from patients with systemic lupus erythematosus to the induction of sister chromatid exchanges by alkylating agents and bromodeoxyuridine. *Ann Rheum Dis* 1987; **46**: 110–3.
4 Davis P. Antibodies to UV DNA and photosensitivity. *Br J Dermatol* 1977; **97**: 197–200.
5 Le Feber WP, Norris DA, Ryan SS *et al*. Ultraviolet light induces expression of selected nuclear antigens in cultured human keratinocytes. *Clin Invest* 1984; **74**: 1545–51.
6 Purcell SM, Lien JS, Davis BM *et al*. Relationship between circulating anti Ro/SSA antibody levels and skin disease activity in subacute cutaneous lupus erythematosus. *Br J Dermatol* 1987; **117**: 277–87.

Environmental factors. Lupus-like disorders have been reported in association with a variety of environmental factors [1]. Although early reports suggested that silicone breast implants are more frequently associated with connective tissue diseases including lupus-like syndromes, scleroderma, fibrositis, inflammatory myopathy and autoimmune thyroid disease [2], later studies show that the incidence is no higher than in control populations [3]. Haemolytic anaemia with high titres of antinuclear and anti-dsDNA antibodies has followed the ingestion of sprouts, seeds and dietary supplements of alfalfa, which contains the amino acid L-canavanine [4]. Heavy metals including cadmium, mercury and gold have also been associated with autoimmunity [5]. Other industrial factors include silica [6,7] and trichlorethylene [8].

References

1 Love LA. New environmental agents associated with lupus-like disorders. *Lupus* 1994; **3**: 467–71.
2 Sanchez-Guerrero J, Schur PH, Sergent JS *et al*. Silicone breast implants and rheumatic disease: clinical, immunological and epidemiological studies. *Arthritis Rheum* 1994; **37**: 158–68.

3 Edworthy SM, Martin L, Barr SG et al. A clinical study of the relationship between silicone breast implants and connective tissue disease. *J Rheumatol* 1998; **25**: 254–60.

4 Montanaro A, Bardana EJ. Dietary amino-acid-induced lupus erythematosus. *Rheum Dis Clin North Am* 1991; **17**: 323–32.

5 Bigazzi PE. Auto-immunity and heavy metals. *Lupus* 1994; **3**: 449–52.

6 Sanchez-Roman J, Wichmann I, Salaberri J et al. Multiple clinical and biological autoimmune manifestations in 50 workers after occupational exposure to silica. *Ann Rheum Dis* 1993; **52**: 534–8.

7 Conrad K, Mehlhoin J, Luthke K et al. Systemic lupus erythematosus after heavy exposure to quartz dust in uranium mines: clinical and serological characteristics. *Lupus* 1996; **5**: 62–9.

8 Kilburn KH, Warshaw RH. Prevalence of symptoms of systemic lupus erythematosus (SLE) and of fluorescent antinuclear antibodies associated with chronic exposure to trichlorethylene and other chemicals in well waters. *Environ Res* 1992; **57**: 1–9.

8 Lahita RG, Bucala R, Bradlow HL et al. Determination of 16α-hydroxyestrone by radioimmunoassay in systemic lupus erythematosus. *Arthritis Rheum* 1985; **28**: 1122–7.

9 Jimenez-Balderas FJ, Tapia-Serrano R, Fonseca ME et al. High frequency of association of rheumatic/autoimmune diseases and untreated male hypogonadism with severe testicular dysfunction. *Arthritis Res* 2001; **3**: 362–7.

10 Gutierrez MA, Molina JF, Jara LJ et al. Prolactin and systemic lupus erythematosus: prolactin secretion by SLE lymphocytes and proliferative (autocrine) activity. *Lupus* 1995; **4**: 348–52.

11 Denman AM. Sex hormones, auto-immune diseases, and immune responses. *BMJ* 1991; **303**: 2–3.

12 Nagata C, Fujita S, Iwata H et al. Systemic lupus erythematosus: a case–control epidemiologic study in Japan. *Int J Dermatol* 1995; **34**: 333–7.

13 Rogers MP, Dubey D, Reich P. The influence of the psyche and the brain on immunity and disease susceptibility: a critical review. *Psychosom Med* 1979; **41**: 147–64.

Infections, stress, hormonal factors. Other factors may precipitate the onset of SLE, and these include bacterial infection and mental or physical stress. A role for antigens derived from infecting organisms in the generation of anti-idiotype antigens [1] has been suggested, and microbial superantigens may stimulate abnormal T- and B-cell interactions, resulting in the state of autoimmunity found in SLE [2]. Infection is more common in SLE than in those not affected, and depressed generation of serum chemotactic factors may contribute to this increase [3]. Initial phagocytosis by polymorphonuclear neutrophils and macrophages is reduced [4].

As markedly more females than males are affected in early adult life, it has been suggested that endocrine factors may be involved [5]. In addition, 20% of female patients have premenstrual flares of skin disease, and a small number present after initiation of oestrogen-containing contraceptive therapy [6]. Levels of circulating androgens are reduced in women with SLE compared with normal controls [7], and men with SLE have reduced testosterone levels [8], indeed hypogonadism from whatever cause may be an aetiological factor in SLE [9]. Prolactin is an immunoregulator, and is secreted by immunologically active cells, suggesting an autocrine effect [10]. Normal humoral and cellular immune responses are greater in females than in males, but this may be a result of the influence of oestrogen on gene expression, rather than on immune responses [11]. A late menarche is associated with an increased risk of SLE in Japanese patients [12]. There is some evidence that neuroendocrine factors play a part in immunity, which could to some extent explain the influence of stress factors in the disease [13].

References
1 George J, Shoenfeld Y. Infection, idiotypes and SLE. *Lupus* 1995; **4**: 333–5.
2 Friedman SM, Posnett DN, Tumang JR et al. A potential role for microbial superantigens in the pathogenesis of systemic autoimmune disease. *Arthritis Rheum* 1991; **34**: 468–80.
3 Clark RA, Kimball HR, Decker JL. Neutrophil chemotaxis in systemic lupus erythematosus. *Ann Rheum Dis* 1974; **33**: 167–72.
4 Landry M. Phagocyte function and cell-mediated immunity in systemic lupus erythematosus. *Arch Dermatol* 1977; **113**: 147–54.
5 Talal N. Sex hormones and modulation of immune response in SLE. *Clin Rheum Dis* 1982; **8**: 23–8.
6 Yell JA, Burge SM. The effect of hormonal changes on cutaneous disease in lupus erythematosus. *Br J Dermatol* 1993; **129**: 18–22.
7 Lahita RG, Bradlow HL, Ginzler E et al. Low plasma androgens in women with systemic lupus erythematosus. *Arthritis Rheum* 1987; **30**: 241–8.

Viruses. An infective cause for SLE has long been postulated, and the role of acute viral infection has been reviewed recently [1]. The high incidence of antibodies to reovirus double-stranded RNA (70%) [2] and raised titres of antibody to measles and rubella antigens [3], suggest potential viral involvement, but this may be only an expression of T-cell suppression in this disease. There is no evidence of retrovirus infection in SLE [4], but endogenous retroviral DNA sequences are found [5].

References
1 Ramos-Casals M, Cuadrado MJ, Alba P et al. Acute viral infections in patients with systemic lupus erythematosus: description of 23 cases and review of the literature. *Medicine (Baltimore)* 2008; **87**: 311–8.
2 Sylvester RA, Attias M, Talal N et al. Antibodies to viral and synthetic double-stranded RNA in discoid lupus erythematosus. *Arthritis Rheum* 1973; **16**: 383–7.
3 Laitinen O, Vaheri A. Very high measles and rubella virus antibody titres associated with hepatitis, systemic lupus erythematosus and infectious mononucleosis. *Lancet* 1974; **i**: 194–8.
4 Pelton BK, North M, Palmer RG et al. A search for retrovirus infection in systemic lupus erythematosus and rheumatoid arthritis. *Ann Rheum Dis* 1988; **47**: 206–9.
5 Walchner M, Leibmosch C, Messer G, Kind P. Endogenous retroviral sequences as a pathogenic factor in systemic lupus erythematosus. *Hautarzt* 1996; **47**: 502–9.

Drugs. The precipitation of SLE by drugs [1,2], especially the antihypertensive hydralazine, is well known. However, there are features to suggest that drug-induced SLE differs from the spontaneous disease: it is uncommon in black people, it occurs in an older age group, renal and central nervous system involvement are infrequent, antihistone antibodies are frequent, anti-DNA antibodies are absent and serum complement is normal. Hydralazine is known to inhibit binding of complement component C4, and this action, with subsequent lack of control of complement activity, may explain the development of lupus-like syndromes.

Cutaneous involvement in drug-induced SLE may be vasculitic, bullous, erythema multiforme-like or resemble pyoderma gangrenosum. Cases have been reported of hydralazine-induced lupus with Sweet's syndrome [3]. It was thought that the clinical manifestations of drug-induced lupus resolved when the drug was withdrawn, but this is not necessarily so, and patients with hydralazine-induced syndromes may have hyperglobulinaemia and other abnormalities before the administration of hydralazine [4]. Patients who develop antinuclear antibodies during drug treatment need not have the drug stopped unless they have

Table 51.10 Drugs inducing systemic lupus erythematosus-like syndromes.

Acebutolol	Oral contraceptives, including:
Allopurinol	Chlormadinone
Aminoglutethimide	Ethinylestradiol
p-Aminosalicylic acid	Etynodiol diacetate
Atenolol	Medroxyprogesterone
Captopril	Mestranol
Carbamazepine	Norethindrone
Chlorpromazine	Norethisterone
Clobazam	Norethynodrel
Clofibrate	Oxyphenisatin
Co-trimoxazole	Oxprenolol
Diphenylhydantoin	Penicillamine
Ethosuximide	Penicillin
Gold salts	Phenothiazine
Griseofulvin	Phenylbutazone
Guanoxan	Phenytoin
Hydralazine	Pindolol
Hydrochlorothiazide	Piroxicam
Hydroxyurea (hydroxycarbamide)	Practolol
Ibuprofen	Primidone
Infliximab	Procainamide
Interferon	Propranolol
Isonicotinic acid hydrazide	Propylthiouracil
Isoquinazepon	Quinine
Labetalol	Recombinant interferon
Leuprolide acetate	Streptomycin
Lithium carbonate	Sulfasalazine
Methyldopa	Sulphonamides
Methylphenylethylhydantoin	Tertalol
Methylthiouracil	Tetracycline
Methysergide	Timolol eye drops
Minocycline	Trimethadione
Minoxidil	Valproate
Nitrofurantoin	Venocuran
	Vostatin/simvastatin

features of the lupus syndrome [5]. Twenty-four cases of lupus induced by minocycline [6] have been reported. It usually occurs after 2 years of therapy. Patients who require more than 1 year's therapy should have ANA and liver function tests monitored. Other drugs, particularly certain anticonvulsants, are known to precipitate SLE-like syndromes (Table 51.10). The biological agents targeting TNF-α are now well known to produce ANF, and occasionally clinical manifestations of lupus.

Drugs have been implicated in precipitating or activating SLE in 3–12% of cases [7]. There is an increased incidence of HLA-DR4 in drug-induced SLE [8] and the ratio of females to males is 4 : 1, indicating a possible genetic predisposition. It appears that individuals who are slow acetylators are more likely to develop drug-induced LE or LE-like syndromes [9]. The determination of acetylator type and DR typing may enable susceptible patients to be identified. In spontaneous SLE, however, there appears to be a preponderance of slow acetylators [10], although this is disputed [11].

Antihistone antibodies are not drug-specific, although different drugs do induce antibodies to different histone epitopes, and the antibodies are often present well before clinical manifestations occur [12]. Indeed, 50% of procainamide-treated patients develop immunological abnormalities, whereas only 20% develop clinical disease [13]. Of patients with drug-induced lupus syndromes, 82% have antihistone antibodies, compared with 32% of those with serological changes only [12].

References

1 Vedove CD, Del Giglio M, Schena D, Girolomoni G. Drug-induced lupus erythematosus. *Arch Dermatol Res* 2009; **301**: 99–105.
2 Borchers AT, Keen CL, Gershwin ME. Drug-induced lupus. *Ann N Y Acad Sci* 2007; **1108**: 166–82.
3 Ramsay-Goldman R, Franz T, Solano FX *et al.* Hydralazine induced lupus and Sweet's syndrome. *J Rheumatol* 1990; **17**: 682–4.
4 Blumenkrantz N, Christiansen AH, Ullman S, Asboe-Hansen G. Hydralazine-induced lupoid syndrome. *Acta Med Scand* 1974; **195**: 443–9.
5 Mansilla-Tinoco R, Harland SJ, Ryan PJ *et al.* Hydralazine, antinuclear antibodies and the lupus syndrome. *BMJ* 1982; **284**: 936–9.
6 Knowles SR, Shapiro L, Shear NH. Serious adverse reactions induced by minocycline. *Arch Dermatol* 1996; **132**: 934–9.
7 Lee SL, Rivero I, Siegel M. Activation of systemic lupus erythematosus by drugs. *Arch Intern Med* 1966; **117**: 620–6.
8 Batchelor JR, Welsh KI, Tinoco RM *et al.* Hydralazine-induced systemic lupus erythematosus: influence of HLA-DR and sex on susceptibility. *Lancet* 1980; **i**: 1107–9.
9 Godeau P, Aubert M, Imbert JC *et al.* Lupus erythemateux dissemine et taux d'isoniazide actif: étude de 47 observations. *Ann Intern Med* 1973; **124**: 181–6.
10 Larsson R, Karlsson E, Molin L. Spontaneous systemic lupus erythematosus and acetylator phenotype. *Acta Med Scand* 1977; **201**: 223–6.
11 Harland SJ, Facchini V, Timbrell JA. Hydralazine-induced lupus erythematosus-like syndrome in a patient of the rapid acetylator phenotype. *BMJ* 1980; **281**: 273–4.
12 Rubin RL, Nusinow SR, Johnson AD *et al.* Serological changes during induction of lupus-like disease by procainamide. *Am J Med* 1986; **80**: 999–1002.
13 Blamgren SE. Drug-induced lupus erythematosus. *Semin Hematol* 1973; **10**: 345–9.

Relationship of genetic and environmental factors and autoimmunity [1]. The relationship of genetic factors, possible virus infection and depression of cell-mediated immunity has led to the suggestion that genetic factors might allow virus replication in the thymus and in T cells, inducing damage to these cells and hence defective cellular immunity. The age pattern of the disease and its female predominance suggest that these abnormalities appear to affect only a specific susceptible genotype, involving three dominant X-linked alleles. Phenotypic expression then depends on accumulated randomly occurring changes in lymphoid stem cells, with three 'forbidden' clones of lymphocytes developing [2], and with hyperglobulinaemia and autoantibody formation from hyperactive B cells and the lack of T-cell suppression following. Normal defence mechanisms, which are more effective in females, prevent these changes persisting, but may be impaired by infections, drugs, UV radiation and stress, thus precipitating the disease. Organ involvement is determined by genetically controlled antigenic expression in target tissues. Such a concept would explain the sex differences, the occurrence of clinical and subclinical autoimmune disease and antibodies in the relatives of patients, the apparent spontaneous onset in many cases, and the precipitation and exacerbation of clinical manifestations by factors impairing the defence mechanisms.

Table 51.11 Pathological features of systemic lupus erythematosus.

Macroscopic
Pleurisy
Pericarditis
Libman–Sacks endocarditis
Lymphadenopathy
Splenomegaly
May be none

Microscopic
Immunoglobulins and complement at the dermal–epidermal junction in skin lesions
(90%) and uninvolved skin (60%)
Haematoxylin bodies in the endocardium, renal glomeruli and elsewhere
Periarterial fibrosis of the spleen
Wire loop lesions in the kidneys

References
1 Jönsen A, Bengtsson AA, Nived O *et al.* Gene–environment interactions in the aetiology of systemic lupus erythematosus. *Autoimmunity* 2007; **40**: 613–7.
2 Burch PRJ, Rowell NR. Lupus erythematosus: analysis of the sex- and age-distribution of the discoid and systemic forms of the disease in different countries. *Acta Derm Venereol (Stockh)* 1970; **50**: 293–301.

Pathology (Table 51.11). The pathological changes of SLE have been well described. The primary lesions of SLE are fibrinoid necrosis, collagen sclerosis, necrosis and basophilic body formation, and vascular endothelial thickening. The basophilic (haematoxylin) bodies are aggregates of homogeneous material staining blue with haematoxylin and staining positively for DNA by the Feulgen technique. This material is similar to that of the homogeneous nuclear material of the LE cell.

Macroscopic appearances. Despite the widespread clinical manifestations and fatal outcome, it is often disappointing to find no macroscopic changes at autopsy. Sometimes, terminal changes and infection obscure the picture. Frequent macroscopic findings include pleurisy with adhesions and effusion, and pericarditis, especially if the patient has died with uraemia. The verrucose vegetations of Libman–Sacks endocarditis are diagnostic (Fig. 51.27) [1]. These are small firm warty deposits, up to 0.5 cm in diameter, adherent to the valves of both sides of the heart and adjacent endocardium of the ventricles, chordae tendinae and on the papillary muscles. Sometimes, lesions of subacute bacterial endocarditis may be superimposed on the warty lesions.

Microscopic appearances. Usually, pathological diagnosis requires histology, but in some cases histological changes can be demonstrated only by immunohistological techniques (Fig. 51.28) [2]. Immunohistology is also useful in diagnosing SLE in patients with a rash.

Skin. There is no single diagnostic pathological feature in the skin, but a combination of features aids diagnosis [3]. Some changes, such as hyperkeratosis without parakeratosis, and keratotic plugging of the hair follicles and glandular orifices, are similar to those found in chronic DLE. There may also be some atrophy or acanthosis of the prickle cell layer. Liquefaction degeneration of the basal cell layer is common. Epidermal necrolysis has

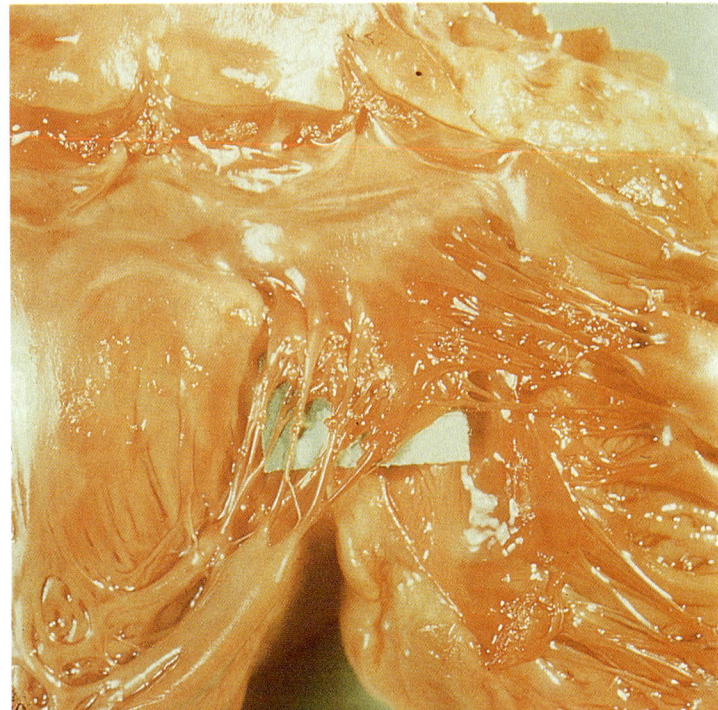

Fig. 51.27 Libman–Sacks endocarditis. Note the warty vegetations on the heart valves.

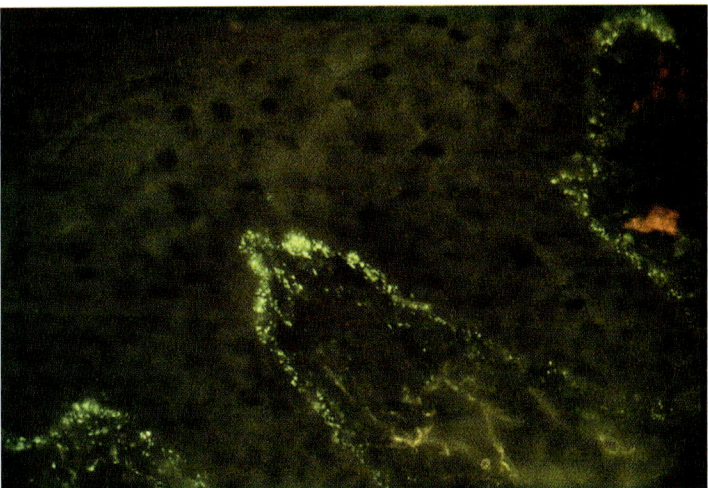

Fig. 51.28 Immunoglobulin at the dermal–epidermal junction in systemic lupus erythematosus.

been reported [4]. The dermal tissues may be oedematous, and sometimes vesicle formation occurs at the dermal–epidermal junction, with dilatation of the superficial vessels and perivascular lymphocytic infiltration. Occasionally, dermal mucinosis occurs, especially in papular lesions [5] and in areas of alopecia [6]. Pigment-containing chromatophores may occur in the infiltrate. Sometimes, the infiltrate is widely distributed in the upper portion of the dermis, being most pronounced in the more chronic type of lesions. Using monoclonal antibodies, the infiltrate is shown to consist of abundant T cells and Ia-positive cells, with rather fewer B cells and macrophages. Helper or inducer T cells and suppressor or cytotoxic T cells occur in equal numbers [7]. Fragmentation, splintering and oedema of the elastic tissue occur. Changes in the walls of blood vessels are relatively infrequent, but hyaline changes and fibrinoid degeneration occur.

Immunohistology [8,9]. Immunoglobulins, predominantly IgG, but less frequently IgM and IgA, together with complement (C1, C3) can be demonstrated at the dermal–epidermal junction by immunofluorescence techniques [10,11]. They occur in more than 80% of skin lesions of DLE and SLE, and may be preceded by basement membrane abnormalities in erythematous and purpuric lesions [12]. Deposits occur more frequently in light-exposed areas and are invariably present in acute lesions, although in early and late stages the test may be negative. If IgG, IgM and IgA are all present, the diagnosis of SLE is likely, and the more common combination of IgG and IgM is also suggestive. Single immuno-globulins favour another diagnosis (see DLE). The basement-membrane phenomenon can also be demonstrated in the uninvolved skin in three-quarters of active cases of SLE if the biopsy specimens are taken from the exposed skin, preferably from the dorsum of the wrist or forearm. Biopsy specimens from the unexposed skin are positive in only approximately 50% of cases, which may or may not have more severe renal disease and decreased long-term survival [13,14]. Variability in the presence of immunoglobulins and complement in adjacent sites of both light-exposed and light-protected areas probably accounts for differences between series. Biopsy specimens taken from oedematous areas may be negative. The presence of IgG in unexposed normal skin rarely occurs without SLE, and indicates a poorer prognosis than the presence of IgM or the absence of deposits. An IgM band may be found in other diseases, and without other evidence is not sufficient to make a diagnosis of LE [15]. IgM can be found in 80% of lesion-free sun-exposed skin in patients with actinic keratoses [16]. Deposits also occur in patients without rashes or may be present before other features of LE develop. Positive tests may come and go depending on activity, and decrease after treatment or in remission. Deposits in uninvolved skin may occasionally occur in systemic sclerosis, mixed connective tissue disease, der-matomyositis, anaphylactoid purpura, hypocomplementaemic vasculitis, rheumatoid arthritis, pemphigoid and dermatitis her-petiformis. This basement-membrane phenomenon can also be demonstrated in the uninvolved skin in patients with the so-called transitory type of DLE [17]. This is a subgroup of DLE, described by Baart De La Faille-Kuyper [18], with cutaneous lesions of DLE and immunoglobulins at the dermal–epidermal junction in unin-volved skin, as in SLE, but no definite clinical or serological evi-dence of the latter. The basement-membrane phenomenon is negative in uninvolved skin in other cases of DLE. The staining may be homogeneous or granular, or there may be larger aggre-gates under the dermal–epidermal zone [19]. Burnham and Fine describe homogeneous, thready and stippled patterns [20], which are different from the 'tubular' band of bullous pemphigoid [21]. The stippled band occurs in uninvolved skin, thready bands in new lesions and homogeneous bands in older chronic lesions. The band type depends on the type of skin lesion and does not distin-guish between DLE and SLE. The presence of complement at the dermal–epidermal junction in patients with widespread SLE without renal disease may be associated with a lowering of the serum complement [22]. Both fibrin and properdin have been demonstrated in the lesions of SLE [23]. Properdin deposition in normal skin appears to correlate with disease activity [24]. The presence of properdin suggests that the alternative pathway of complement activation is involved, but nevertheless the classical pathway is the primary complement pathway involved in SLE. In drug-induced SLE, deposits of IgG, IgM and C3 at the dermal–epidermal junction may disappear when clinical symptoms regress [25].

Epidermal nuclear deposits, usually giving a speckled IgG pattern, occur in the basal epidermal nuclei and cells of the lower epidermis in nearly one-third of patients [26]. Immunoglobulin (IgG, IgA and IgM), with or without complement, can be found in the walls of blood vessels in skin lesions and uninvolved skin. There may be homogeneous fluorescence of the subendothelial part of the vessel wall, or intramural or perivascular granular fluo-rescence, and these changes are present in discoid, transitory and systemic LE. Homogeneous staining occurs in the uninvolved skin of 20% of patients with DLE and over 80% of patients with transi-tory or systemic LE. Electron microscopy of involved and unin-volved skin has shown deposits of proteins on the dermal side of the dermal–epidermal junction and in small blood vessels, resem-bling morphologically those present in 'wire-loop' lesions in the kidney [27].

Internal organs. The characteristic microscopic features in the internal organs include haematoxylin bodies in the heart valves and elsewhere, periarterial fibrosis of the spleen, and the so-called 'wire-loop' lesions in the kidneys. In the heart, microscopic changes, including fibrinoid necrosis, may occur in normal-looking valves. The vegetations of Libman–Sacks endocarditis [1] occur in 50% of cases coming to autopsy [28], and arise from proliferation of ground substance and connective tissue cells [29], which raise the endothelium. Focal necrosis occurs in these areas, and basophilic bodies are frequently seen. Later, infiltration with inflammatory cells occurs, together with fibrosis. Focal atrophy and fibrosis occur in the myocardium, but myocarditis is unusual.

The lungs frequently show pulmonary oedema and infective changes, but specific abnormalities are uncommon. Pulmonary parenchymal lesions or pleuritis occurred in 18% of one series [30], and other findings included interstitial fibrosis, pulmonary vascu-litis, haematoxylin bodies and pneumonitis. A mucinous baso-philic oedema of the alveolar walls occurs, with a hyaline alveolar lining membrane similar to hyaline membrane disease of the newborn. Alveolar wall thickening and vascular changes similar to those of Hamman–Rich syndrome may be found.

The liver may show infiltration of the portal tracts with lym-phocytes, histiocytes and plasma cells. The so-called 'onion skin' appearance in the spleen is caused by concentric periarterial fibro-sis around central and penicilliary arteries.

The lymph-node enlargement is usually associated with reten-tion of normal architecture, but sometimes necrosis and haema-toxylin bodies may be found.

The so-called 'wire-loop' appearance in the kidneys is caused by thickening and hyalinization of the capillary basement mem-brane of the glomerular tufts. Although this change may be seen in other diseases such as systemic sclerosis, chronic glomerulonephritis and malignant nephrosclerosis, the changes in SLE are more likely to be localized to one part of the glomerulus. Thickening of the glomerular capillary basement membrane and alterations in reticular tissue in the media of arterioles are associated with deposits of IgG and C3 [31]. Lupus nephritis has been divided into three types [32]: focal proliferative (lupus glomerulitis) and membranous, which are relatively benign, and diffuse proliferative (lupus) glomerulonephritis, which has a poor prognosis. In focal proliferative nephritis, a mild proliferation is confined to parts of some of the glomeruli and electron microscopy shows no electron-dense material. In membranous lupus nephropathy, there is irregular thickening of the glomerular basement membrane with epimembranous deposition of electron-dense material. The most common renal disorder is diffuse proliferative nephritis, in which there is irregular endothelial cell proliferation, fibrinoid necrosis, hyaline thrombi and interstitial inflammatory changes. Electron-dense deposits are seen on electron microscopy in subendothelial, subepithelial and mesangial areas. Heavy proteinuria with large numbers of red and white cells and casts in the urine suggests glomerulonephritis [33]. Although most cases of the nephrotic syndrome and renal vein thrombosis show membranous glomerulonephritis, focal proliferative glomerulonephritis has also been reported [34].

Germinal centres in the thymus are frequently increased [35]. Abnormal epithelial hyperplasia in the thymus is said to occur in all cases of SLE, but the change is not specific [36].

There may be evidence of widespread vasculitis in other organs and in the central nervous system. Although the vasculitis in the nervous system is usually mild, it can be florid [37]. Gammaglobulin deposits and complement have been found in the choroid plexus when immunohistology of the cerebrum, cerebellum and brainstem has shown no abnormality [38]. This, together with the finding of low cerebrospinal fluid complement levels [39], suggests an immune-complex pathogenesis for the involvement of the central nervous system.

References

1 Libman E, Sacks B. A hitherto undescribed form of valvular and mural endocarditis. *Arch Intern Med* 1924; **33**: 701–38.
2 Rowell NR. Laboratory abnormalities in the diagnosis and management of lupus erythematosus. *Br J Dermatol* 1971; **84**: 210–6.
3 McCreight WG, Montgomery H. Cutaneous changes in lupus erythematosus. *Arch Dermatol Syphilol* 1950; **61**: 1–11.
4 Pinol-Aguadé J, Palou J, Lecha M, Castel T. Focal epidermal necrolysis: a variation of lupus erythematosus or a new disease? *Med Cutan Ibero Lat Am* 1977; **5**: 1–11.
5 Revier J, Kienzler JL, Blanc D *et al.* Mucinose papuleuse et lupus erythemateux. *Ann Dermatol Vénéréol* 1982; **109**: 331–8.
6 Lee WS, Chung J, Ahn SK. Mucinous lupus alopecia associated with papulonodular mucinosis as a new manifestation of lupus erythematosus (Letter). *Int J Dermatol* 1996; **35**: 72–3.
7 Synkowski DR, Provost TT. Characterization of the inflammatory infiltrate in lupus erythematosus lesions using monoclonal antibodies. *J Rheumatol* 1983; **10**: 920–4.
8 Dahl MV. Usefulness of direct immunofluorescence in patients with lupus erythematosus. *Arch Dermatol* 1983; **119**: 1010–7.
9 Monroe EW. Lupus band test. *Arch Dermatol* 1977; **113**: 830–4.
10 Co-operative study. Uses for immunofluorescence tests of skin and sera. *Arch Dermatol* 1975; **111**: 371–81.
11 Tuffanelli DL. Cutaneous immunopathology. *J Invest Dermatol* 1975; **65**: 143–53.
12 Rowell NR, Scott DG. Immunohistological studies, with anti-connective tissue and anti-immunoglobulin antisera, of the skin in lupus erythematosus and scleroderma. *Br J Dermatol* 1975; **93**: 431–41.
13 Davis BM, Gilliam JN. Prognostic significance of subepidermal immune deposits in uninvolved skin of patients with systemic lupus erythematosus: a 10-year longitudinal study. *J Invest Dermatol* 1984; **83**: 242–7.
14 Wertheimer D, Barland P. Clinical significance of immune deposits in the skin in SLE. *Arthritis Rheum* 1976; **19**: 1249–55.
15 Wojnarowska F, Bhogal B, Black MM. The significance of an IgM band at the dermo-epidermal junction. *J Cutan Pathol* 1986; **13**: 359–62.
16 Gruschwitz M, Keller J, Hornstein OP. Deposits of immunoglobulins at the dermo-epidermal junction in chronic light-exposed skin: what is the value of the lupus band test? *Clin Exp Dermatol* 1988; **13**: 303–8.
17 Baart De La Faille-Kuyper EH. *Grafisch Bedriff*. Utrecht: Schotanus, Jens, 1969.
18 Baart De La Faille-Kuyper EH. *In vivo* nuclear localization of immunoglobulins in clinically normal skin in systemic and procainamide-induced LE. *Neth J Med* 1974; **17**: 58.
19 Tuffanelli DL. Dermal-epidermal junction in lupus erythematosus. *Arch Dermatol* 1969; **99**: 652–62.
20 Burnham TK, Fine G. The immunofluorescent 'band' test for lupus erythematosus. I. Morphologic variations of the band of localized immunoglobulins at the dermal-epidermal junction in lupus erythematosus. *Arch Dermatol* 1969; **99**: 413–20.
21 Burnham TK, Fine G. The immunofluorescent 'band' test for lupus erythematosus. 3. Employing clinically normal skin. *Arch Dermatol* 1971; **103**: 24–32.
22 Marshall DA, Nesbitt LT, Biundo JJ. Serum complement related to skin lesions of SLE. *South Med J* 1974; **67**: 1275–9.
23 Jordon RE, Schroeter AL, Winkelmann RK. Dermal-epidermal deposition of complement components and properdin in systemic lupus erythematosus. *Br J Dermatol* 1975; **92**: 263–71.
24 Schrager MA, Rothfield NF. Clinical significance of serum properdin level and properdin deposition in the dermal–epidermal junction in systemic lupus erythematosus. *J Clin Invest* 1976; **57**: 212–21.
25 Ullman S, Wiik A, Kobayasi T *et al.* Drug-induced lupus erythematosus syndrome. *Acta Derm Venereol (Stockh)* 1974; **54**: 387–90.
26 Ze-Yi Chen, Dobson RL, Ainsworth SK *et al.* Epidermal nuclear immunofluorescence: serological correlations supporting an *in vivo* reaction. *Br J Dermatol* 1985; **112**: 15–22.
27 Grishman E, Churg J. Ultrastructure of dermal lesions in systemic lupus erythematosus. *Lab Invest* 1970; **22**: 189–97.
28 Bulkley BH, Roberts WC. The heart in systemic lupus erythematosus and the changes induced in it by corticosteroid therapy. *Am J Med* 1975; **58**: 243–64.
29 Gardner DL. *Pathology of the Connective Tissues*. London: Arnold, 1965.
30 Haupt HM, Moore GW, Hutchins GH. The lung in systemic lupus erythematosus. *Am J Med* 1981; **71**: 791–8.
31 Scott DG, Rowell NR. Immunohistological studies of the kidney in systemic lupus erythematosus and systemic sclerosis using antisera to IgG, C3 fibrin and human renal glomeruli. *Ann Rheum Dis* 1974; **33**: 473–81.
32 Baldwin DS, Lowenstein J, Rothfield NF *et al.* The clinical course of proliferative and membranous forms of lupus nephritis. *Ann Intern Med* 1970; **73**: 929–42.
33 Pollak VE, Pirani CL. Renal histologic findings in systemic lupus erythematosus. *Mayo Clin Proc* 1969; **44**: 630–44.
34 Millet VG, Usera G, Alcazardelaossa JM *et al.* Renal vein thrombosis, nephrotic syndrome and focal lupus glomerulonephritis. *BMJ* 1978; **i**: 24–5.
35 Mackay IR, Degail P. Thymic 'germinal centres' and plasma cells in systemic lupus erythematosus. *Lancet* 1963; **ii**: 667.
36 Hutchins GM, Harvey AM. The thymus in systemic lupus erythematosus. *Bull Johns Hopkins Hosp* 1964; **115**: 355–78.
37 Bunning RD, Laureno R, Barth WF. Florid central nervous system vasculitis in a fatal case of systemic lupus erythematosus. *J Rheumatol* 1982; **9**: 735–8.
38 Gershwin ME, Hyman LR, Steinberg AD. The choroid plexus in CNS involvement of systemic lupus erythematosus. *J Pediatr* 1975; **87**: 588–90.
39 Petz LW, Sharp GC, Cooper NR *et al.* Serum and cerebral spinal fluid complement and serum autoantibodies in systemic lupus erythematosus. *Medicine* 1971; **50**: 259–75.

Clinical features. See Table 51.12 for an analysis of the clinical features of several series.

Table 51.12 Clinical features of systemic lupus erythematosus.

Clinical feature	Percentage
Fever	90
Arthritis and arthralgia	90
Skin lesions	80
Renal involvement	67
Lymphadenopathy	50
Pleurisy	40
Raynaud's phenomenon	35
Pericarditis	25
Hepatomegaly	25
Central nervous system involvement	25
Abdominal symptoms	20
Splenomegaly	15

Table 51.13 Cutaneous features of systemic lupus erythematosus in 73 patients. (From Yell et al. [2].)

Cutaneous feature	Percentage
Butterfly rash	51
Facial oedema	4
Subacute cutaneous LE	7
Chronic discoid LE	25
Scarring DLE alopecia	14
Non-scarring alopecia	40
Chilblain lupus	20
Mouth ulceration	31
Bullous eruptions	8
Photosensitivity	63
Raynaud's phenomenon	60
Chronic urticaria (>36 h)	44
Cutaneous vasculitis	11
Livedo reticularis	4
Episcleritis	4
Cheilitis	4

DLE, discoid lupus erythematosus; LE, lupus erythematosus.

Presenting symptoms. The disease may affect many systems of the body, and the presentation and course are by no means uniform. Large series of cases have been reported [1–8], including one from the Far East [9]. The subject has been reviewed [8,10]. Despite the female sex predominance, clinical gender differences are not found, although men may be more liable to fits and renal failure [11].

The initial manifestations vary. In one series of 200 cases, the first changes were articular in 58% and cutaneous in 13.5% [12]. Presentation with renal abnormalities, psychiatric disturbances, pericarditis, pleurisy, abdominal pain and pyrexia of uncertain origin are less common.

In fulminating cases, there is usually marked constitutional disturbance, with fever, loss of weight, anorexia, malaise and joint pains; the skin may be involved later, if at all. On the other hand, the evolution can be gradual, starting with localized skin lesions and systemic involvement developing later. Fatigue is a prominent symptom, both at presentation and subsequently [13]. The diagnosis in many cases is made only by considering the condition in a patient with an obscure illness. As most cases are females, sex is an important diagnostic point. Although weight loss is a feature in nearly 50% of the cases, some patients may gain weight, and 18% actually did so in the Leeds series, which included several patients with long histories. Menstruation is irregular in 18% and absent in 75%. The onset in 15% of females is after the menopause. Sometimes, there is a previous history of sensitivity to drugs such as penicillin, gold or sulphonamides. Raynaud's phenomenon occurs in the course of the illness in approximately 35% of patients, and others frequently have chilblains and a poor peripheral circulation. Approximately 2% of patients with Raynaud's phenomenon eventually develop SLE. Sometimes, there may be other apparent precipitating factors, such as exposure to the sun, stress, trauma and infection. Rarely, hypothermia may occur, often precipitated by therapy [14].

References

1 Dubois EL, Tuffanelli DL. Clinical manifestations of systemic lupus erythematosus. *JAMA* 1964; **190**: 104–11.
2 Fries JF, Holman HR. Systemic lupus erythematosus: a clinical analysis. *J Invest Dermatol* 1976; **67**: 554–5.
3 Grigor R, Edmonds J, Lewkonia R *et al*. Systemic lupus erythematosus: a prospective analysis. *Ann Rheum Dis* 1978; **37**: 121–8.
4 Harvey AM, Shulman LE, Tumulty PA *et al*. Systemic lupus erythematosus: review of the literature and clinical analysis of 138 cases. *Medicine* 1954; **33**: 291–437.
5 Larson DL. *Systemic Lupus Erythematosus*. London: Churchill, 1961.
6 Lee P, Urowitz MB, Bookman AAM *et al*. Systemic lupus erythematosus: a review of 110 cases with references to nephritis, the nervous system, infections, aseptic necrosis and prognosis. *QJM* 1977; **46**: 1–32.
7 Ropes MW. *Systemic Lupus Erythematosus*. Cambridge, MA: Harvard University Press, 1976.
8 Wallace DJ, Hahn BH, Quismorio FP, Klinenberg JR, eds. *Dubois' Lupus Erythematosus*, 7th edn. Philadelphia: Lippincott Williams & Wilkins, 2007.
9 Tay CH, Khoo OT. Neurological involvement in systemic lupus erythematosus. *Singapore Med J* 1971; **12**: 18–23.
10 Klippel JH, ed. Systemic lupus erythematosus. *Rheum Dis Clin North Am* 1988; **14**: 1.
11 Ward MM, Studenski S. Systemic lupus erythematosus in men: a multivariate analysis of gender differences in clinical manifestations. *J Rheumatol* 1990; **17**: 220–4.
12 Smolen JS, Zielinski CC. *Systemic Lupus Erythematosus*. Berlin: Springer-Verlag, 1987.
13 Krupp LB, LaRocca NG, Muir J, Steinberg AD. A study of fatigue in systemic lupus erythematosus. *J Rheumatol* 1990; **17**: 1450–2.
14 Kugler SL, Costakos DT, Aron AM, Spiera H. Hypothermia and systemic lupus erythematosus. *J Rheumatol* 1990; **17**: 680–1.

Skin. Approximately 80% of cases have a rash at some stage, and in up to 25% it is the presenting sign [1]. The prevalence varies between series. Findings from a typical UK population are shown in Table 51.13 [2].

The cutaneous changes may be broadly divided between: (i) those specific for LE, and showing the characteristic histopathological appearances of LE; and (ii) those that are less specific in their origin and not showing LE histological changes. Many of these are also seen in the other connective tissue diseases.

Specific changes. Cutaneous erythema is the most common feature, particularly on light-exposed areas (Fig. 51.29). A butterfly

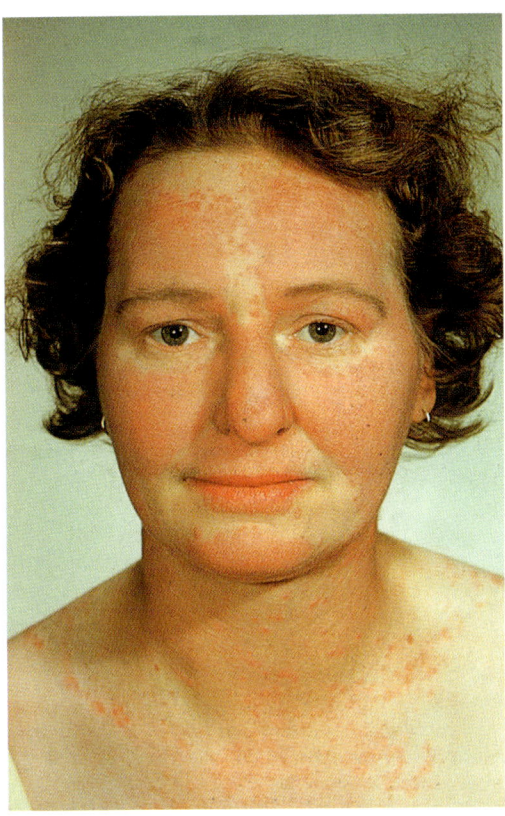

Fig. 51.29 Systemic lupus erythematosus: typical symmetrical slightly scaling erythema of the face and neck.

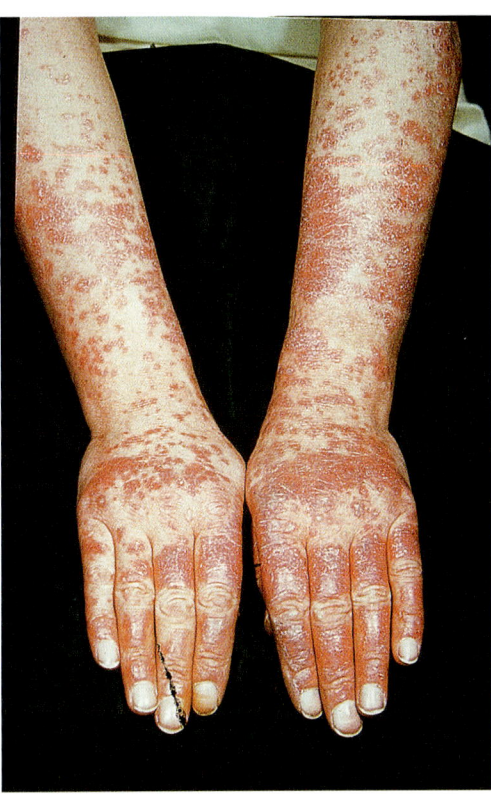

Fig. 51.30 Systemic lupus erythematosus of the dorsa of hands and forearms. Identical changes may occur in discoid lupus erythematosus. Note the chloroquine pigmentation of the distal part of the nails.

blush or discrete maculopapular eruption with fine scaling on the butterfly area of the cheeks or elsewhere is also frequently found (Fig. 51.30). Photoaggravation occurs in approximately 33% of patients at Leeds, but up to 73% has been reported from America [3]. This may relate to the amount of sunlight. UV radiation such as that found in discos [4], fluorescent lighting [5] and UVA from photocopiers [6] may also cause exacerbations. Oedema, especially of the face, may resemble contact dermatitis, seborrhoeic eczema, dermatomyositis or erysipelas, and can follow tooth extraction [7]. Occasionally, more acute lesions with bullae may follow exposure to the sun (Fig. 51.31), and bullae may be haemorrhagic [8,9].

Epidermal necrosis may give an appearance resembling toxic epidermal necrolysis [10]. In other cases, lesions are like those of erythema multiforme (Rowell's syndrome; see p. 51.14). Very rarely, the skin may show centrifugal annular erythema like that of SCLE. Lesions resembling chronic discoid lesions are initial manifestations in approximately 10% of patients and occur in the course of the disease in approximately 33%; they may be more common in men [11].

References

1 Tuffanelli DL, Dubois EL. Cutaneous manifestations of systemic lupus erythematosus. *Arch Dermatol* 1964; **90**: 377–86.
2 Yell JA, Mbuagbaw J, Burge SM. Cutaneous manifestations of systemic lupus erythematosus. *Br J Dermatol* 1996; **135**: 355–62.
3 Wysenbeek AJ, Block DA, Fries JF. Prevalence and expression of photosensitivity in systemic lupus erythematosus. *Ann Rheum Dis* 1989; **48**: 461–3.

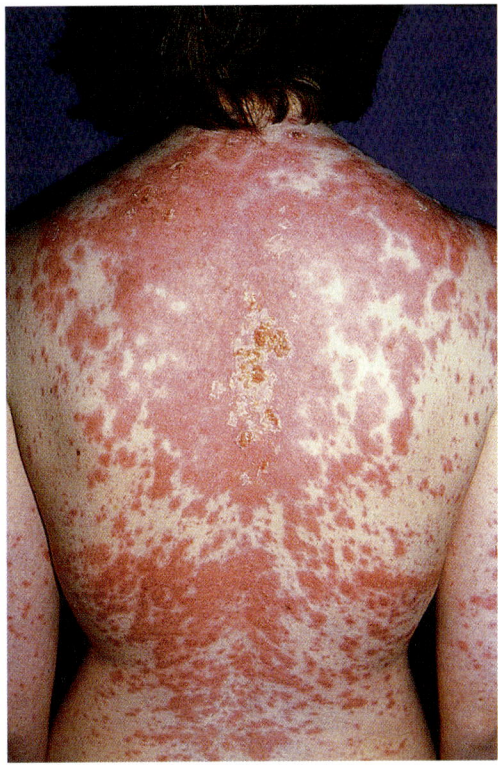

Fig. 51.31 Systemic lupus erythematosus: gross involvement of the back.

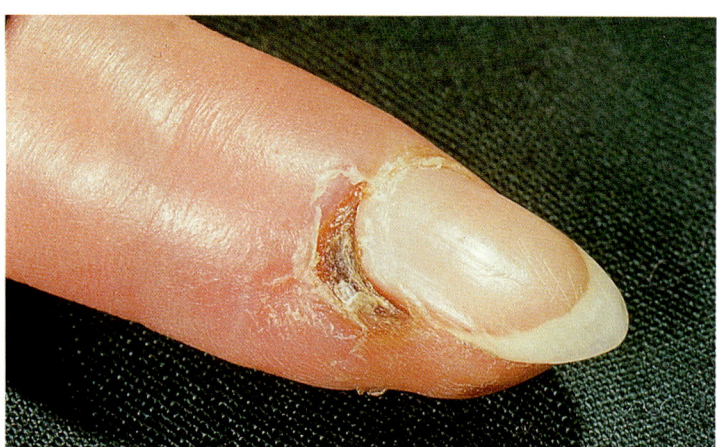

Fig. 51.32 Necrosis of the nail fold in systemic lupus erythematosus.

4 Seibold JR, Lynch CJ. Disco lupus: a new disease syndrome. *Arthritis Rheum* 1980; **23**: 962–3.

5 Martin L, Chalmers IM. Photosensitivity to fluorescent light in a patient with lupus erythematosus. *J Rheumatol* 1983; **10**: 811–2.

6 Klein LR, Elmers CA, Callen JP. Photoexacerbation of cutaneous lupus erythematosus due to ultraviolet A emissions from a photocopier. *Arthritis Rheum* 1995; **38**: 1152–6.

7 Lóescher A, Edmondson HD. Lupus erythematosus: a case of facial swelling. *Br J Oral Maxillofac Surg* 1988; **26**: 129–42.

8 Patcharee B, Sunthonpalin PB, MacGuire HC. Blister fluid in bullous systemic lupus erythematosus. *Br J Dermatol* 1970; **82**: 125–8.

9 Tromovitch TA, Hyman AB. Systemic lupus erythematosus with hemorrhagic bullae. *Arch Dermatol* 1961; **83**: 910–4.

10 Gilliam JN, Sontheimer RD. Skin manifestations of SLE. *Clin Rheum Dis* 1982; **8**: 207.

11 Font J, Pallares L, Cervera R *et al.* Systemic lupus erythematosus: clinical and immunological study of 300 patients. *Med Clinica 100* 1993; **16**: 601–5.

Non-specific changes. Sometimes, lesions may be minimal. This is particularly so in the case of the reticulate telangiectatic erythema seen on the thenar and hypothenar eminences of the palms, on the pulps and dorsum of the fingers and, to a lesser extent, on the toes and over the lateral borders of the feet and heels. The lesions on the palms may be confused with the palmar erythema of liver disease. They are bluish red and may show small whitish areas of scarring. The changes occur particularly on the dorsa of the distal phalanges and between the joints, but sometimes there may be small vascular necroses on the tips of the fingers and alongside the nails (Fig. 51.32). The nail folds may show hyperkeratotic and ragged cuticles (Fig. 51.33). Splinter haemorrhages may sometimes be seen in the nails [1], and other changes include pitting, ridging, onycholysis, striate leukonychia [2] and red lunulae [3]. Nail changes occur in approximately 25% of patients [4]. Recurrent Osler's nodes may occur in the absence of infective endocarditis [5]. Clubbing has been reported [6]. Dilatation of the nail fold capillaries also occurs, but this is seen in other conditions. Biopsies from the nails and from areas of palmar erythema show marked dilatation of superficial capillaries [7].

References

1 Mintz G, Fraga A. Arteritis in systemic lupus erythematosus. *Arch Intern Med* 1965; **116**: 55–66.

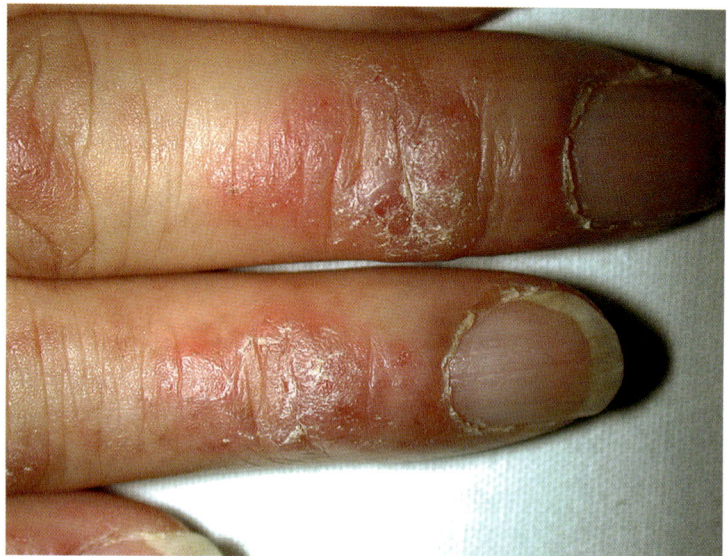

Fig. 51.33 White nail and ragged cuticle in systemic lupus erythematosus.

2 Friedman SJ. Leukonychia striata associated with systemic lupus erythematosus. *J Am Acad Dermatol* 1986; **15**: 536–8.

3 Garcia-Patos V, Bartralot R, Ordi J *et al.* Systemic lupus erythematosus presenting with red lunulae. *J Am Acad Dermatol* 1997; **36**: 834–6.

4 Urowitz MB, Gladman DD, Chalmers A *et al.* Nail lesions in systemic lupus erythematosus. *J Rheumatol* 1978; **5**: 441–7.

5 Rudusky BM. Recurrent Osler's nodes in systemic lupus erythematosus. *Angiology* 1969; **20**: 33–7.

6 MacKie RM. Lupus erythematosus in association with finger-clubbing. *Br J Dermatol* 1973; **89**: 533–5.

7 Smith EW, Kurban A. Capillary alterations in lupus erythematosus. *Bull Johns Hopkins Hosp* 1962; **110**: 202–11.

Hair changes. Alopecia occurs in over 50% of patients, especially in the active phase of the disease. This takes the form of diffuse loss of hair with a reddish scalp or, less frequently, permanent scarring alopecia, similar to that found in DLE. The hair is usually coarse, dry and fragile, especially on the frontal margin. This leads to an unruly appearance with short, broken-off hair, the so-called 'lupus hair' (Fig. 51.34) [1]. This occurs in 30% of patients, predominantly females [2]. The hair recovers as the disease becomes inactive, but 'lupus hair' usually persists longer than alopecia. The shortened hairs are unbroken and are probably brought about by slowed anagen growth.

References

1 Armas-Cruz R, Harnecker J, Ducach G *et al.* Clinical diagnosis of systemic lupus erythematosus. *Am J Med* 1958; **25**: 409–19.

2 Alarcon-Segovia D, Cetina JA. Lupus hair. *Am J Med Sci* 1974; **267**: 241–2.

Urticarial lesions and vasculitis. Persistent non-itching urticaria-like weals are common, and may respond to dapsone if associated with C1q deficiency. Urticarial lesions occurred in 7% of one series, but in 20% of patients at Leeds, and were considered to be brought about by immune-complex deposition [1]. SLE may present as hypocomplementaemic urticarial vasculitis [2]. Widespread purpura, resulting from thrombocytopenia or cutaneous vasculitis, is a common finding. Leukocytoclastic vasculitis may lead to purpuric macules, up to 1 cm in diameter, and in certain cases

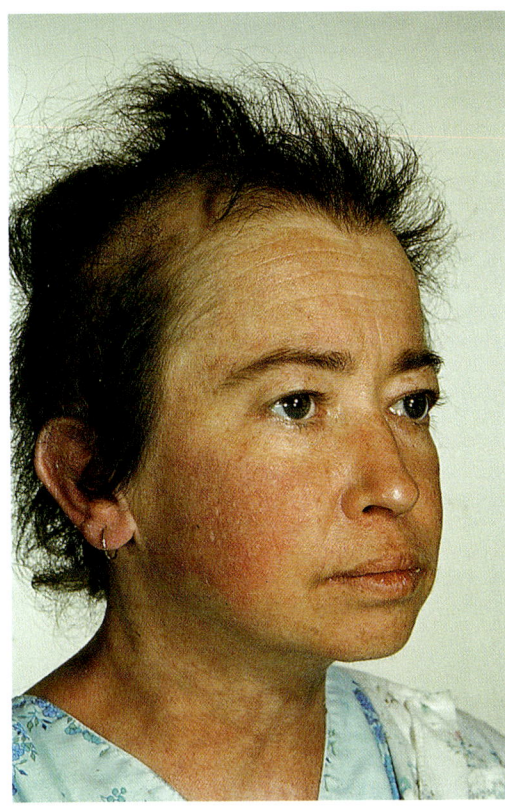

Fig. 51.34 Unruly 'lupus hair' with diffuse alopecia.

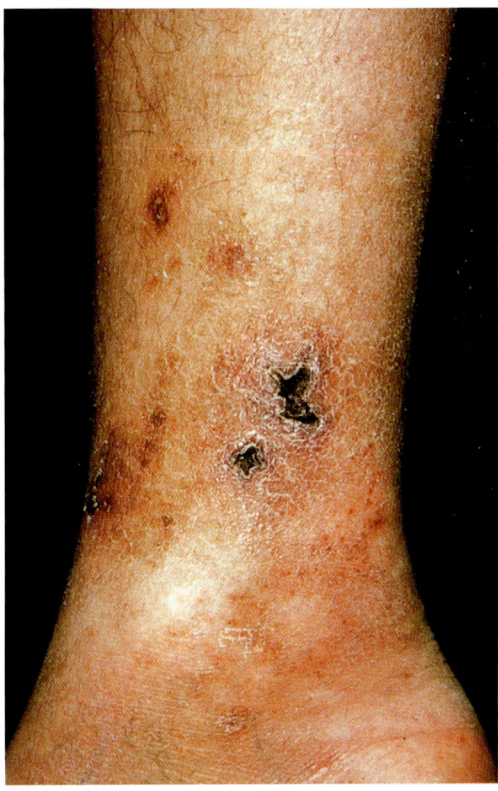

Fig. 51.35 Necrotic crusted leg ulcers in systemic lupus erythematosus.

purpuric urticarial lesions may be found. Purpura can also be a result of corticosteroid therapy. Livedo reticularis, a mottled or bluish red discoloration, which blanches on pressure and is not affected by temperature changes, may develop, especially on the outer aspects of the arms. It occurs most frequently in patients who later develop central nervous system lupus [3]. The appearance of livedo reticularis in association with flares of cerebral vasculitis has been noted [4]. Superficial ulceration can occur in areas of livedo. Atrophie blanche [5] and lesions similar to those of malignant atrophic papulosis (Degos' disease) [6] are other features of vasculitis. Patients with the perniotic lesions of 'chilblain lupus' (see p. 51.11) may go on to develop SLE. These lesions may ulcerate, as may the hyperkeratotic keratodermatous skin sometimes found. A subset has been described in which perniotic lesions on the dorsum of the knuckles and toes, fingers and the pulps and palmar and plantar surfaces is associated with anti-Ro antibody [7]. Chronic pyoderma gangrenosum occurs, and has been the presenting feature of hydralazine-induced SLE [8]. Follicular pyoderma resulting from infection has also been described [9].

References

1 Provost TT, Zone JJ, Synkowski D *et al.* Unusual cutaneous manifestations of systemic lupus erythematosus. *J Invest Dermatol* 1980; **75**: 495–9.
2 Coca A, Font J, Herrero C *et al.* Hypocomplementaemic vasculitis and systemic lupus erythematosus. *J Rheumatol* 1987; **14**: 854–5.
3 Yasue T. Livedoid vasculitis and central nervous system involvement in systemic lupus erythematosus. *Arch Dermatol* 1986; **122**: 66–70.
4 Grigor R, Edmonds J, Lewkonia R *et al.* Systemic lupus erythematosus. *Ann Rheum Dis* 1978; **37**: 121–8.
5 Stevanovicà DV. Atrophie blanche. *Arch Dermatol* 1974; **109**: 858–62.
6 Török L. Symptomatic atrophic papulosis in a patient with systemic lupus erythematosus. *Clin Exp Dermatol* 1996; **21**: 390–2.
7 Bottomley W, Goodfield M. A distinctive form of peripheral cutaneous involvement in Ro antibody positive systemic lupus erythematosus. *Lupus* 1995; **4** (Suppl. 2): 154.
8 Peterson LL. Hydralazine-induced systemic lupus erythematosus presenting as pyoderma gangrenosum-like ulcers. *J Am Acad Dermatol* 1984; **10**: 379–84.
9 Lazzari T, Parodi A, Rebora A. Follicular impetigo as a presenting sign of systemic lupus erythematosus. *Dermatologica* 1991; **182**: 233–4.

Large vessel disease. Gangrene of the tips of the fingers and toes [1] may develop insidiously. At first the digits become blue and cold and may be painful. Radiography of the fingers in cases with peripheral ischaemia shows absorption of the distal part of the terminal phalanges, as in systemic sclerosis. Later, the phalanges may become exposed, and spontaneous separation of the tips of the fingers may occur. Amputation of digits may be required. Occlusion of large- and medium-sized arteries can occur suddenly and result in gangrene requiring amputation of a limb [2,3]. This may be the result of vasculitis or thrombosis. Patients with thrombosis frequently have antiphospholipid antibodies [3]. Major vessel occlusion can occur in childhood [4]. Leg ulcers (Fig. 51.35) occur in approximately 10% of patients, usually near the malleoli but sometimes on the feet and elsewhere, from breakdown in reticular livedo and in areas of cutaneous vasculitis. Erythromelalgia (pain in the feet aggravated by heat and dependence and relieved by cooling and elevation) may be a presenting feature [5].

References

1 Dubois EL, Arterberry JD. Gangrene as a manifestation of systemic lupus erythematosus. *JAMA* 1962; **181**: 366–74.
2 Alarcón-Segoviá D, Cardiel MH, Reyes E. Antiphospholipid arterial vasculopathy. *J Rheumatol* 1989; **16**: 762–7.
3 Asherson RA, Derksen RHWM, Harris EN *et al.* Large vessel occlusion and gangrene in systemic lupus erythematosus and 'lupus-like' disease: a report of six cases. *J Rheumatol* 1986; **13**: 740–7.
4 Kaufman JL, Bancilla E, Slade J. Lupus vasculitis with tibial artery thrombosis and gangrene. *Arthritis Rheum* 1986; **29**: 1291–2.
5 Alarcón-Segoviá D, Rabb RR, Fairbairn JF. Systemic lupus erythematosus with erythromelalgia. *Arch Dermatol* 1963; **112**: 688–92.

Mucinosis. Although mucin deposition is a common and often prominent histological feature of cutaneous lupus, specific clinical patterns of mucinosis also occur. Papular or nodular lesions resulting from mucinous deposits in the dermis without microscopic features of LE have been reported [1], and form a distinct entity which may be the presenting feature of LE [2]. Multiple firm non-tender dermal papules and nodules, between 5 and 15 mm in diameter, occur on the upper part of the body and extremities [3–6]. The overlying epidermis appeared normal. Hyperpigmented acral papular mucinosis has also occurred in one patient with total alopecia [6].

References

1 Rongioletti F, Parodi A, Rebora A. Papular and nodular mucinosis as a sign of LE. *Dermatologica* 1990; **180**: 221–3.
2 Sonntag M, Lehmann P, Megahed M *et al.* Papulonodular mucinosis associated with subacute cutaneous lupus erythematosus. *Dermatology* 2003; **206**: 326–9.
3 Fowler JF Jr, Callen JP. Cutaneous mucinosis associated with lupus erythematosus. *J Rheumatol* 1984; **11**: 280–3.
4 Gammon WR, Caro I, Long JC *et al.* Secondary cutaneous mucinosis with systemic lupus erythematosus. *Arch Dermatol* 1978; **114**: 432–5.
5 Gold SC. An unusual papular eruption associated with lupus erythematosus. *Br J Dermatol* 1954; **66**: 429–33.
6 Lacour JP, Juhlin L, Blaze PE *et al.* Hyperpigmented acral papular mucinosis, systemic lupus erythematosus and universal alopecia. *Acta Derm Venereol (Stockh)* 1989; **69**: 212–6.

Connective tissue changes. Hardening, binding-down and pigmentation of the skin of the face and limbs may resemble systemic sclerosis, although the typical mat-like telangiectases of the latter are usually absent. Calcinosis is rare [1], but occasionally widespread and large palpable deposits may develop [2] or be found radiologically [3]. Subcutaneous nodules occur in approximately 5% of patients [4]. They resemble rheumatoid nodules, although there may be no evidence of arthritis. They occur mainly over the backs of the proximal phalangeal joints and wrists, but are also found on the elbows, knees, occiput and the flexor aspects of the fingers. They may respond to hydroxychloroquine [5]. Some are histologically identical with classic rheumatoid nodules [6], others are probably caused by vasculitis and thrombosis [7]. Panniculitis, similar to LE profundus, can occur in the course of the disease or can be the presenting sign [8–10]. Lesions may break down, resolve with oral corticosteroids or require surgery and grafting. Relapsing nasal and auricular chondritis have been described [11]. The nose and ears are tender, warm, swollen and red, but cartilage collapse does not occur as in polychondritis. Treatment with corticosteroids is effective.

References

1 Tay CH. Cutaneous manifestation of systemic lupus erythematosus: a clinical study from Singapore. *Australas J Dermatol* 1970; **11**: 30–41.
2 Nomura M, Okada N, Okada M, Yoshikawa K. Large subcutaneous calcification in systemic lupus erythematosus. *Arch Dermatol* 1990; **126**: 1057–9.
3 Rothe MJ, Grant-Kels JM, Rothfield NF. Extensive calcinosis cutis with systemic lupus erythematosus. *Arch Dermatol* 1990; **126**: 1060–3.
4 Hahn BH, Yardley JH, Stevens MB. 'Rheumatoid' nodules in systemic lupus erythematosus. *Arch Dermatol* 1970; **72**: 49–58.
5 Schofield JK, Cerio R, Grice K. Systemic lupus erythematosus presenting with 'rheumatoid nodules'. *Clin Exp Dermatol* 1992; **17**: 53–5.
6 Dubois EL, Friou GJ, Chandor S. Rheumatoid nodules and rheumatoid granulomas in systemic lupus erythematosus. *JAMA* 1972; **220**: 515–8.
7 Bywaters EGL, Glynn LE, Zeldis A. Subcutaneous nodules of Still's disease. *Ann Rheum Dis* 1958; **17**: 278–85.
8 Diaz-Jouanen E, DeHoratius RJ, Alarcón-Segoviá D *et al.* Systemic lupus erythematosus presenting as panniculitis. *Ann Intern Med* 1975; **82**: 376–9.
9 Tuffanelli DL. Lupus erythematosus panniculitis (profundus). *Arch Dermatol* 1971; **103**: 231–42.
10 Winkelmann RK. Panniculitis and systemic lupus erythematosus. *JAMA* 1970; **211**: 472–5.
11 Kitridou RC, Wittmann AL, Quismorio FP Jr. Chondritis in systemic lupus erythematosus: clinical and immunopathologic studies. *Clin Exp Rheumatol* 1987; **5**: 349–53.

Pigmentary changes. Pigmentary disturbances are not uncommon. Whole areas can show hypopigmentation. A bluish black pigmentation of the skin results from antimalarial therapy [1].

Other cutaneous changes. In the Chinese, hyperkeratotic follicular erythematous papules, sometimes becoming pigmented or confluent, occur on the trunk and limbs. Psoriasiform lesions and hyperkeratosis of the palms and soles are found [2,3]. Widespread ichthyosis and warty excrescences on knees and elbows may occur [4]. Eruptive dermatofibromas have been reported [5]. Acanthosis nigricans has been reported in lupoid hepatitis [6]. Herpes zoster is more frequent than expected in SLE [7], and scabies is more severe and may be of the crusted type [8].

References

1 Wallace DJ. Management and prognosis of systemic lupus erythematosus. In: Wallace DJ, Hahn B, Dubois EL, eds. *Dubois' Lupus Erythematosus*, 4th edn. Philadelphia: Lea and Febiger, 1993: 521–3.
2 Issacs P. Myasthenia with systemic lupus and palmoplantar keratosis. *BMJ* 1971; **iv**: 339–40.
3 Wong KO. Systemic lupus erythematosus: a report of 45 cases with unusual clinical and immunological features. *Br J Dermatol* 1969; **81**: 186–90.
4 Buck DC, Dodd HJ, Sarkany I. Hypertrophic lupus erythematosus. *Br J Dermatol* 1988; **119**: 72–4.
5 Kravitz P. Dermatofibromas and systemic lupus erythematosus. *Arch Dermatol* 1980; **116**: 1347.
6 Tuffanelli DL. Acanthosis nigricans with lupoid hepatitis. *JAMA* 1964; **189**: 584–5.
7 Moutsopoulos HM, Gallagher JD, Decker JL *et al.* Herpes zoster in patients with systemic lupus erythematosus. *Arthritis Rheum* 1978; **21**: 798–802.
8 Ting HC, Wang F. Scabies and systemic lupus erythematosus. *Int J Dermatol* 1983; **22**: 473–6.

Bullous SLE (Fig. 51.36) [1]. Blistering is uncommon in SLE. In the classic disease, separation of the epidermis and dermis occurs as a result of severe liquefaction degeneration of the basal layer and dermal oedema. A separate subset called bullous SLE has been defined, with distinct clinical and histopathological features, the

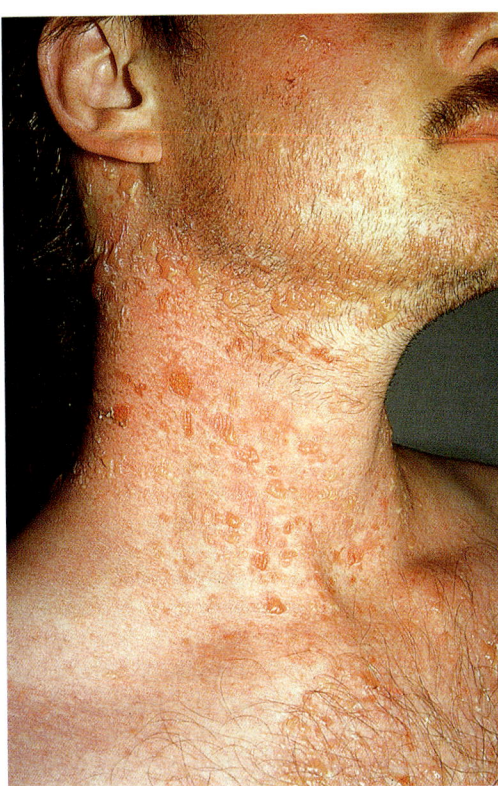

Fig. 51.36 Bullous lupus erythematosus of the face and neck.

latter resembling dermatitis herpetiformis [2]. Subepidermal vesicles contain neutrophils with microabscesses, and nuclear 'dust' and fibrin at the tips of dermal papillae. Immunohistology, however, shows linear deposition of IgA, IgG and IgM and, to a lesser extent, C3 at the basement membrane, resembling bullous pemphigoid and unlike the IgA seen in the dermal papillae in dermatitis herpetiformis. Electron microscopy shows the immunoreactants to be in the sublamina densa [3] and not in the lamina lucida as in pemphigoid, although the immunopathological changes are variable and may indicate that a number of basement-membrane antigens can act as targets [4]. This has subsequently been confirmed [5]. In particular, a form resembling epidermolysis bullosa acquisita (EBA) has been described [6]. The target antigen in some patients is type VII collagen, but other antigens may be involved in bulla formation [7].

Clinically, the bullous lesions are predominantly on the face, neck and upper trunk, but may be more widespread, and may heal with milia formation. One-third have mouth lesions. Photosensitivity may occur. The patient may initially present with lesions resembling erythema multiforme [8]. Glomerulonephritis is common, and associated with hypocomplementaemia and anti-DNA antibodies. Circulating antibasement-zone antibodies have many features of EBA antibodies. The demonstration of such antibodies may precede the development of SLE by many years [9]. It is not yet established whether patients with EBA antibodies are a unique subset of bullous LE or whether they represent the coexistence of two separate diseases, although it has been suggested that the spectrum of bullous LE should include all cases of bullous disease occurring in patients with SLE [1]. Rarely, drugs, including

hydralazine [10] and IFN-α [11], may precipitate bullous SLE. Dapsone alone or in combination with prednisone is the treatment of choice. It is not always successful and may even exacerbate the disease [7]. The authors have used thalidomide successfully in these resistant cases.

References

1 Yell JA, Allen J, Wojnarowska F, Kirtschig G, Burge SM. Bullous systemic lupus erythematosus: revised criteria for diagnosis. *Br J Dermatol* 1995; **132**: 921–8.
2 Camisa C. Vesiculobullous systemic lupus erythematosus. *J Am Acad Dermatol* 1988; **18**: 93–100.
3 Rappersberger K, Tschachler E, Tani M *et al.* Bullous disease in systemic lupus erythematosus. *J Am Acad Dermatol* 1989; **21**: 745–52.
4 Burge S, Schomberg K, Wojnarowska F. Bullous eruption of SLE: a case report and investigation of the relationship of anti-basement-membrane zone antibodies to blistering. *Clin Exp Dermatol* 1991; **16**: 133–8.
5 Chan LS, Lapiere JC, Chen M *et al.* Bullous systemic lupus erythematosus with autoantibodies recognizing multiple skin basement membrane components, bullous pemphigoid antigen 1, laminin 5, laminin 6, and type VII collagen. *Arch Dermatol* 1999; **135**: 569–73.
6 Burrows NP, Bhogal BS, Black MM *et al.* Bullous eruption of systemic lupus erythematosus: a clinicopathological study of four cases. *Br J Dermatol* 1993; **128**: 332–8.
7 Yell JA, Wojnarowska F, Allen J, Burge SM. Bullous systemic lupus erythematosus: a variable disease. *Lupus* 1993; **2**: 383–5.
8 Barton DD, Fine J-D, Gammon WR *et al.* Bullous systemic lupus erythematosus: an unusual clinical course and detectable circulating autoantibodies to the epidermolysis bullosa acquisita antigen. *J Am Acad Dermatol* 1986; **15**: 369–73.
9 Boh E, Roberts LJ, Lieu TS *et al.* Epidermolysis bullosa acquisita preceding the development of systemic lupus erythematosus. *J Am Acad Dermatol* 1990; **22**: 587–93.
10 Fleming MG, Bergfeld WF, Tomecki KJ *et al.* Bullous systemic lupus erythematosus. *Int J Dermatol* 1989; **28**: 321–6.
11 Pouthier D, Theissen F, Humbel RL. Lupus syndrome, hypothyroidism and bullous skin lesions after interferon-α for hepatitis C in a haemodialysis patient. *Nephrol Dial Transplant* 2002; **17**: 174.

Pemphigus erythematosus [1]. Erythematous, scaly, hyperkeratotic or crusted lesions, sometimes adversely affected by the sun, occur in a butterfly distribution on the cheeks and in a seborrhoeic distribution on the trunk of patients with Senear–Usher syndrome (see Chapter 40). This combines the immunological features of pemphigus and LE. Direct immunofluorescence shows immunoglobulin and complement in the intercellular substance and at the dermal–epidermal junction of perilesional and, to a lesser extent, of light-exposed and non-exposed skin. Circulating pemphigus-like antibodies and antinuclear factor occur in 80–100%, but anti-DNA and ENA antibodies are not found. Antidesmoglein antibodies have also been demonstrated [2]. The condition occurs spontaneously, but has been induced by penicillamine, propranolol, captopril, pyritinol and thiopronine. Topical steroids alone may control the condition, but systemic steroids, immunosuppressives or dapsone may be required.

References

1 Amerian ML, Ahmed RA. Pemphigus erythematosus: presentation of four cases and review of literature. *J Am Acad Dermatol* 1984; **10**: 215–22.
2 Gomi H, Kawada A, Amajai M, Matsuo I. Pemphigus erythematosus: detection of anti-desmoglein-1 antibodies by ELISA. *Dermatology* 1999; **199**: 188–99.

Mucous membrane lesions [1–3]. Mucous membrane lesions occur in 26% of cases, usually on the palate (82%) (Fig. 51.37),

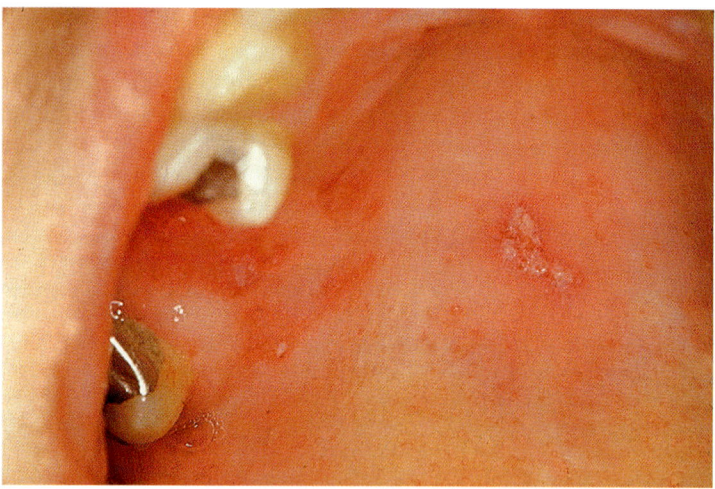

Fig. 51.37 Systemic lupus erythematosus involving the palate.

buccal mucosa or gums, in active phases of the disease [3]. Lesions start as small erythematous or purpuric areas, which break down to form shallow and sometimes painful ulcers, with a dirty yellow base and surrounding reddish halo. There may be difficulty in swallowing. Histology and immunohistology show changes similar to those in the skin. Light microscopy can usually distinguish between LE and lichen planus [4]. Immunofluorescence is usually positive [5]. Repeated sore throats and oral ulceration may be presenting features [6]. The appearances can resemble a *Candida* infection, and sometimes *Candida* is present as a secondary infection. The lips may become cracked, oedematous and crusted in acute cases. Infarction of the tongue, with anticardiolipin antibodies, was the presenting feature in one case [7]. Cheilitis occurs in approximately 6%, the lips having a silvery appearance, with erythema, scaling and blurring of the vermilion border [1]. The larynx is occasionally involved. Ulceration of the mucosa of the nasal septum occurs in approximately 5%. Perforation of the nasal septum is a complication of exacerbations and presents with epistaxis [8]. Erythema of the vulva and perianal area occurs and vulval ulceration may develop, but is less common than oral ulcers. Patients may present with vulval and vaginal ulceration. Orogenital ulceration has been reported with hydralazine-induced lupus [9].

References

1 Burge SM, Frith PA, Juniper RP *et al.* Mucosal involvement in systemic and chronic cutaneous lupus erythematosus. *Br J Dermatol* 1989; **121**: 727–41.
2 Schiodt M. Oral manifestations of lupus erythematosus. *Int J Oral Surg* 1984; **13**: 101–47.
3 Urman JD, Lowenstein MB, Abeles M *et al.* Oral mucosal ulceration in systemic lupus erythematosus. *Arthritis Rheum* 1978; **21**: 58–61.
4 Karjalainen TK, Tomich CE. A histopathologic study of oral mucosal lupus erythematosus. *Oral Surg Oral Med Oral Pathol* 1989; **67**: 547–54.
5 Jonsson R, Heyden G, Gunnar Westberg N *et al.* Oral mucosal lesions in systemic lupus erythematosus. *J Rheumatol* 1984; **11**: 38–42.
6 O'Neill SM, Thomson J, Strong AMM *et al.* Systemic lupus erythematosus presenting as a recurrent sore throat and oral ulceration: a case report. *Br J Dermatol* 1977; **96**: 211–3.
7 Korn S, Huppert A, Spitzer S *et al.* Systemic lupus erythematosus presenting with lingual infarction. *J Rheumatol* 1988; **15**: 1281–3.
8 Synder GG, McCarthy RE, Toomey JM *et al.* Nasal septal perforation in systemic lupus erythematosus. *Arch Otolaryngol* 1974; **99**: 456–7.

Table 51.14 Features distinguishing systemic lupus erythematosus (SLE) from rheumatoid arthritis (RA).

Distinguishing feature	SLE (%)	RA (%)
Deforming arthritis	25	Common
Subcutaneous nodules	5	25
Radiological erosions	Rare	Common
Involvement of kidneys	Common	Rare
Positive LE cell test	80	15
Positive ANA test	90	20
Rheumatoid factor present	40	80

ANA, antinuclear antibody; LE, lupus erythematosus.

9 Neville E, Graham PY, Brewis RAL. Orogenital ulcers, SLE and hydralazine. *Postgrad Med J* 1981; **57**: 378–9.

Arthritis [1]. Involvement of the joints occurs at some time in approximately 90% of patients, arthralgia being more common than arthritis. A rheumatoid-like deformity is present in approximately 25% of cases, with marked soft-tissue swelling, especially of the dorsa of the fingers, hands and wrists, although joint erosions on X-ray are not a feature. The deformity is usually less, but the soft-tissue swelling is more marked than in rheumatoid arthritis [2]. Jaccoud's syndrome, severe deformity of the hands with ulnar deviation and swan-neck configuration, often with little pain and good function, occurred in 13% and fixed flexion contractures of the elbows in 11% in one series [3]. Arthritis mutilans of the distal interphalangeal joints of the hands can occur [4]. The elbows, shoulders, knees and feet may also be involved and soft-tissue nodules may occur, usually indicating calcinosis. Temporomandibular joint involvement may be indicated by locking or dislocation, tenderness and pain on mastication [5]. Features distinguishing SLE from rheumatoid arthritis are shown in Table 51.14. Migratory polyarthritis with inflammation, effusion and erythema occur less frequently. Sacroiliitis occurs in male patients [6]. SLE may rarely present with polymyalgia rheumatica [7]. *Salmonella* infections occur in patients with SLE, and may be associated with septic arthritis [8,9].

References

1 Labowitz R, Schumacher HR Jr. Articular manifestations of systemic lupus erythematosus. *Ann Intern Med* 1971; **74**: 911–21.
2 Russell AS, Percy JS, Rigal MM *et al.* Deforming arthropathy in systemic lupus erythematosus. *Ann Rheum Dis* 1974; **33**: 204–9.
3 Esdaile JM, Danoff D, Rosenthall L *et al.* Deforming arthritis in systemic lupus erythematosus. *Ann Rheum Dis* 1981; **40**: 124–6.
4 Martinez-Cordero E, Lopez Zepeda J, Andrade-Ortega L *et al.* Mutilans arthropathy in systemic lupus erythematosus. *Clin Exp Rheumatol* 1989; **7**: 427–9.
5 Jonsson R, Lindvall AM, Nyberg G. Temporomandibular joint involvement in systemic lupus erythematosus. *Arthritis Rheum* 1983; **26**: 1506–10.
6 Nassonova VA, Alekberova ZS, Folomeyev MY *et al.* Sacroiliitis in male systemic lupus erythematosus. *Scand J Rheumatol* 1983; **52**: 23–9.
7 Foley J. Systemic lupus erythematosus presenting as polymyalgia rheumatica. *Ann Rheum Dis* 1987; **46**: 351.
8 Medina F, Fraga A, Lavalle C. Salmonella septic arthritis in systemic lupus erythematosus: the importance of chronic carrier state. *J Rheumatol* 1989; **16**: 203–8.
9 Van De Laar MAFJ, Meenhorst PL, Van Soesbergen RM *et al.* Polyarticular salmonella bacterial arthritis in a patient with systemic lupus erythematosus. *J Rheumatol* 1989; **16**: 231–4.

Heart. Cardiac involvement in SLE is common, and increases with the duration of the disease [1]. Pericarditis is the most frequent cardiac manifestation, but the incidence of 87% in one review [2] must have been the result of selection. Fibrinous pericarditis is frequently found, but sometimes a large effusion may occur and reabsorb on adequate corticosteroid therapy. Rarely, a large effusion can develop within hours, giving rise to cardiac tamponade [3] and requiring aspiration. The incidence of classic endocardial lesions (Libman–Sacks endocarditis) is difficult to estimate, but the diagnosis is rarely made clinically. Lesions were found at autopsy in only four out of 30 patients in one series [4] and in 50% of patients in another [5]. The valves on the left side of the heart are commonly involved. Both systolic and diastolic murmurs may be found depending upon the site of the lesion, and bacterial endocarditis can occur on the damaged heart valves. Aortic incompetence may occur without involvement of the mitral valve [6] at an early stage of the disease before steroids are used, or when the condition is well controlled. Tricuspid regurgitation has been reported [7]. Echocardiography is helpful in diagnosis [8], and valve replacement has been successful [9].

Coronary arteritis results in myocardial infarction [10]. Infarction may also result from atherosclerosis in young patients [11]. Antiphospholipid antibodies may be demonstrated in such patients [12]. The myocardium may also be affected and results in cardiac failure [13]. The diagnosis can be confirmed by endomyocardial biopsy [14]. Alterations in rhythm include atrial fibrillation and heart block of all types. This may be associated with both Ro and U$_1$-RNP antibodies [15].

Hypertension occurs in approximately 35% of patients. Alterations in the electrocardiogram (ECG) in the course of the illness may be helpful in diagnosing or in confirming the presence of cardiac involvement. There is some evidence that treatment with corticosteroids increases the incidence and degree of hypertension, coronary atherosclerosis and heart failure [5]. Reduced exercise tolerance occurs and may be caused by abnormal myocardial dynamics on exercise [16].

References
1 Giunta A, Picillo U, Maione S *et al.* Spectrum of cardiac involvement in systemic lupus erythematosus: echocardiographic, echo-Doppler observations and immunological investigation. *Acta Cardiol* 1993; **48**: 183–97.
2 Brigden W, Bywaters EGL, Lessof MH *et al.* The heart in systemic lupus erythematosus. *Br Heart J* 1960; **22**: 1–16.
3 Zashin SJ, Lipsky PE. Pericardial tamponade complicating systemic lupus erythematosus. *J Rheumatol* 1989; **16**: 374–7.
4 Kong TQ, Kellum RE, Haserick JR. Clinical diagnosis of cardiac involvement in systemic lupus erythematosus. *Circulation* 1962; **26**: 7–11.
5 Bulkley BH, Roberts WC. The heart in systemic lupus erythematosus and the changes induced in it by corticosteroid therapy. *Am J Med* 1975; **58**: 243–64.
6 El-Ghobarey A, Grennan DM, Hadidi T *et al.* Aortic incompetence in systemic lupus erythematosus. *BMJ* 1976; **ii**: 915–6.
7 Laufer J, Frand M, Milo S. Valve replacement for severe tricuspid regurgitation caused by Libman–Sacks endocarditis. *Br Heart J* 1982; **48**: 294–7.
8 Kalke S, Balakrishanan C, Mangat G *et al.* Echocardiography in systemic lupus erythematosus. *Lupus* 1998; **7**: 540–4.
9 Isaacs AJ. Aortic incompetence in systemic lupus erythematosus. *BMJ* 1976; **ii**: 1260.
10 Bonfiglio TA, Botti RE, Hagstrom JWC. Coronary arteritis and myocardial infarction due to lupus erythematosus. *Am Heart J* 1972; **83**: 153–8.
11 Spiera H, Rothenberg RR. Myocardial infarction in four young patients with SLE. *J Rheumatol* 1983; **10**: 464–6.
12 Asherson RA, Khamashta MA, Baguley E *et al.* Myocardial infarction and antiphospholipid antibodies in SLE and related disorders. *QJM* 1989; **272**: 1103–15.
13 Gur H, Keren G, Averbuch M *et al.* Severe congestive lupus cardiomyopathy complicated by an intracavitary thrombus: a clinical and echocardiographic follow-up. *J Rheumatol* 1988; **15**: 1278–83.
14 Fairfax MJ, Osborn TG, Williams GA *et al.* Endomyocardial biopsy in patients with systemic lupus erythematosus. *J Rheumatol* 1988; **15**: 593–6.
15 Fonseca E, Crespo M, Sobrino JA. Complete heart block in an adult with systemic lupus erythematosus. *Lupus* 1994; **3**: 129–31.
16 Winslow TM, Ossipov M, Redberg RF *et al.* Exercise capacity and haemodynamics in systemic lupus erythematosus: a Doppler echocardiographic exercise study. *Am Heart J* 1993; **126**: 410–4.

Lungs [1]. The incidence of involvement of the pulmonary system varies between series, and the radiological changes [2] depend on the stage of the disease. Transient pleurisy is the most common feature, and in approximately two-thirds of these cases some fluid develops, occasionally haemorrhagic. Pleural thickening can be shown radiographically. Involvement of the lungs is less frequent, and is shown mainly as transient infiltration, sometimes with mottling and reticulation (Fig. 51.38) [3]. Acute pneumonitis with severe dyspnoea and fever may be a presenting manifestation of SLE [4], and cases have been reported with disseminated intravascular coagulation [5]. There is a high incidence of anti-Ro antibodies in pneumonitis [6]. Diffuse fibrosis, like that occurring in systemic sclerosis, is not found [1]. Shrinking lung syndrome is probably caused by diaphragmatic fibrosis [7]. Pulmonary hypertension occurs [8], and pulmonary haemorrhage can be dangerous [9]. When dyspnoea, pleuritic pain and fever occur with linear shadows on radiography, recurrent pulmonary infarction may be simulated. Fibrosing alveolitis has been reported, as well as haemopneumothorax [10]. Hilar lymphadenopathy may cause confusion with other diseases [11]. Unlike those of systemic sclerosis, the pulmonary changes may resolve with steroid therapy.

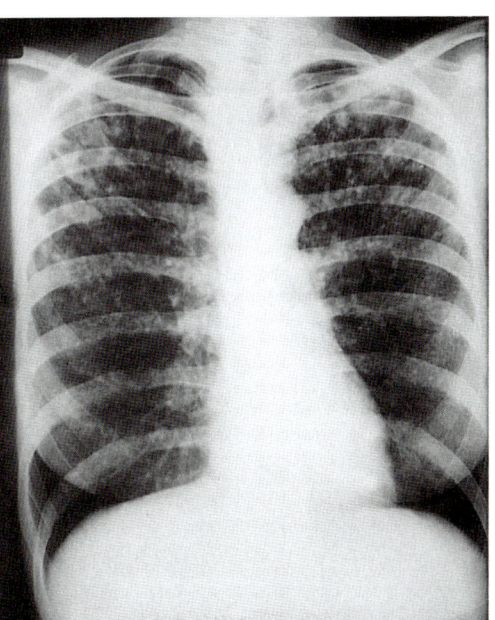

Fig. 51.38 Pulmonary infiltration in systemic lupus erythematosus. This cleared in approximately 2 years on treatment with corticosteroids.

Impairment of pulmonary diffusion (transfer factor) occurred in 42–80% [12], and is more common than reduction in lung volumes [13]. Function of the diaphragm may also be deficient [12], and bilateral elevation of the diaphragm with linear shadows over the lower zones is characteristic of SLE. *Pneumocystis carinii* infections should be considered in all steroid-treated patients who present with respiratory distress and pulmonary infiltration [14]. Nocardial infection with lung abscesses [15] and Legionnaires' disease [16] have been reported. Laryngeal involvement is rare and indicated by stridor and hoarseness, and may be life-threatening. It can occur in inactive disease, and may be complicated by nocardiosis [17].

References

1 Memet B, Ginzler EM. Pulmonary manifestations of systemic lupus erythematosus. *Semin Respir Crit Care Med* 2007; **28**: 441–50.

2 Swigris JJ, Fischer A, Gillis J *et al.* Pulmonary and thrombotic manifestations of systemic lupus erythematosus. *Chest* 2008; **133**: 271–80.

3 Eisenberg H, Dubois EL, Sherwin RP *et al.* Diffuse interstitial lung disease in systemic lupus erythematosus. *Ann Intern Med* 1973; **79**: 37–45.

4 Matthay RA, Schwarz ML, Petty TL. Pulmonary manifestations of systemic lupus erythematosus. *Medicine* 1974; **54**: 397–409.

5 Chellingsworth M, Scott DGI. Acute systemic lupus erythematosus with fatal pneumonitis and disseminated intravascular coagulation. *Ann Rheum Dis* 1985; **44**: 67–9.

6 Boulware DW, Hedgpeth MT. Lupus pneumonitis and anti-SSA (Ro) antibodies. *J Rheumatol* 1989; **16**: 479–81.

7 Rubin LA, Urowitz MB. Shrinking lung syndrome in SLE: a clinical pathologic study. *J Rheumatol* 1983; **10**: 973–6.

8 Simonson JS, Schiller NB, Petri M *et al.* Pulmonary hypertension in systemic lupus erythematosus. *J Rheumatol* 1989; **16**: 918–25.

9 Onomura K, Nakata H, Tanaka Y, Tsuda T. Pulmonary hemorrhage in patients with systemic lupus erythematosus. *J Thorac Imaging* 1991; **6**: 57–61.

10 Passero FC, Myers AR. Hemopneumothorax in systemic lupus erythematosus. *J Rheumatol* 1980; **7**: 183–6.

11 Kassan SS, Moss ML, Reddick RL. Progressive hilar and mediastinal lymphadenopathy in systemic lupus erythematosus on corticosteroid therapy. *N Engl J Med* 1976; **294**: 1382–3.

12 Gibson GJ, Edmonds JP, Hughes GRU. Diaphragm function and lung involvement in systemic lupus erythematosus. *Am J Med* 1977; **63**: 926–32.

13 Silberstein SL, Barland P, Grayzel AI *et al.* Pulmonary dysfunction in systemic lupus erythematosus: prevalence, classification and correlation with other organ involvement. *J Rheumatol* 1980; **7**: 187–95.

14 Lee P, Urowitz MB, Brookman AAM *et al.* Systemic lupus erythematosus. *QJM* 1977; **46**: 1–32.

15 Gorevic PD, Katler EI, Agus B. Pulmonary nocardiosis. *Arch Intern Med* 1980; **140**: 361–3.

16 Jacox RF, Stuard ID. Legionnaires' disease in a patient with systemic lupus erythematosus. *Arthritis Rheum* 1978; **21**: 975–7.

17 Petri M, Katzenstein P, Hellmann D. Laryngeal infection in lupus: report of nocardiosis and review of laryngeal involvement in lupus. *J Rheumatol* 1988; **15**: 1014–5.

Renal changes. The renal changes [1] in SLE are very important in assessing the prognosis (see p. 51.60). Most patients will have renal involvement, as histological evidence of nephritis may occur without proteinuria or microscopic urinary abnormality and with normal renal function [2]. Sometimes, proteinuria and casts may occur transiently with febrile exacerbations. Renal disease in lupus accounts for 3% of end-stage renal failure, and is an important cause of mortality in SLE [3]. The need for regular screening by urinalysis, blood pressure monitoring, assessment of renal function and early renal biopsy is critical. Usually, renal exacerbations are associated with high titres of antinuclear factor, elevated DNA binding and low serum complement, but occasionally these features may revert to normal in severe relapse [4]. Impaired renal tubular potassium secretion can lead to persistent hyperkalaemia [5].

The course is variable, and albuminuria and casts may persist for years without marked deterioration in renal function. Kidney damage, if this is going to develop, usually appears early (within the first 3 years) and is more frequent and severe in younger patients [1]. However, renal involvement may appear as long as 34 years after diagnosis of SLE [6]. A relatively benign course is associated with membranous lupus nephropathy. This occurs in approximately 8% of patients with SLE. Clinically, proteinuria and microscopic haematuria occur some years after other evidence of the disease. Prednisone treatment does not seem to influence proteinuria or renal function in this type [7].

Some cases develop typical signs of the nephrotic syndrome, and renal vein thrombosis has been reported. The development of pleuritic pain in a patient with SLE and the nephrotic syndrome should alert the clinician to the possibility of renal vein thrombosis and pulmonary emboli [8]. Cystitis with reduction of bladder capacity and thickening of the bladder wall may be a primary manifestation of SLE [9]. A strong correlation between lupus cystitis and gastrointestinal involvement has been noted [10].

References

1 Sauter M, Anders HJ. Lupus nephritis. *Minerva Med* 2007; **98**: 749–58.

2 Pollak VE, Pirani CL, Schwartz FD. The natural history of the renal manifestations of systemic lupus erythematosus. *J Lab Clin Med* 1964; **63**: 537–50.

3 Austin HA, Klippel JH, Balow JE *et al.* Therapy of lupus nephritis: controlled trial of prednisolone and cytotoxic drugs. *N Engl J Med* 1991; **314**: 614–9.

4 White NJ, Winearls CG, Ledingham JGG. Systemic lupus erythematosus and nephritis: severe relapse with disappearance of antinuclear antibodies. *BMJ* 1980; **ii**: 194–5.

5 Defronze RA, Cooke CR, Goldberg M *et al.* Impaired renal tubular potassium secretion in systemic lupus erythematosus. *Ann Intern Med* 1977; **86**: 268–71.

6 Adelman DC, Wallace DJ, Klinenberg JR. Thirty-four year delayed-onset lupus nephritis: a case report. *Arthritis Rheum* 1987; **30**: 479–80.

7 Marks SD, Tullus K, Sebire NJ. Current issues in pediatric lupus nephritis: role of revised histopathological classification. *Fetal Pediatr Pathol* 2006; **25**: 297–309.

8 Appel GB, Williams GS, Meltzer JI *et al.* Renal vein thrombosis, nephrotic syndrome and systemic lupus erythematosus. *Ann Intern Med* 1966; **85**: 310–7.

9 Orth RW, Weisman MH, Cohen AH *et al.* Lupus cystitis: primary bladder manifestations of systemic lupus erythematosus. *Ann Intern Med* 1983; **98**: 323–6.

10 Moriuchi J, Ichikawa Y, Takaya M *et al.* Lupus cystitis and perforation of the small bowel in a patient with systemic lupus erythematosus and overlapping syndrome. *Clin Exp Rheumatol* 1989; **7**: 533–6.

Gastrointestinal tract [1]. Anorexia, nausea and vomiting sometimes occur, and impairment of oesophageal motility has been reported [2], especially in patients with Raynaud's phenomenon. Motility studies show absent or impaired contractions in one-third of patients [3]. Abnormalities may occur in any part of the oesophagus but particularly in the upper third, and such dysfunction is not related to activity of the disease. Fewer patients complain of dysphagia or show radiological abnormalities. Pain, vomiting, diarrhoea, malabsorption [4,5], gluten-sensitive enteropathy [6] and protein-losing enteropathy [7], or evidence of obstruction or bleeding, result from intestinal involvement. Pneumatosis cystoides intestinalis and spontaneous pneumoperitoneum are rare [8], but have been reported in a patient with antinuclear-negative SLE [9]. Patients with arteritis may present as an acute surgical emergency, and this complication may be fatal [10]. Small intestinal ulceration occurs in patients with antiphospholipid antibodies [11]. Mesenteric arteriography may be helpful in showing irregularities of the small intestinal arteries [12]. Pancreatitis [13] occurs in both children and adults and is often fatal. It can be associated with subcutaneous fat necrosis and calcinosis cutis [14]. Ulcerative colitis [15] and colonic perforation [16] also occur. Mesenteric lymphadenopathy may be associated with hilar lymphadenopathy [17].

Lymphangiographical changes can resemble those seen in early malignant lymphoma [18]. Painless ascites, in the absence of the nephrotic syndrome, congestive heart failure or hepatic cirrhosis, may be the presenting feature [19]. It is presumably a result of peritoneal serositis. Infarction of the tongue can be another presentation [20].

References

1 Alarcón-Segoviá D, Cardiel MA. Connective tissue disorders and the bowel. *Baillière's Clin Rheumatol* 1989; **3**: 371–92.
2 Stevens MB, Hookman P, Siegel CI *et al.* Aperistalsis of the oesophagus in patients with connective tissue disorders and Raynaud's phenomenon. *N Engl J Med* 1964; **270**: 1218–22.
3 Ramirez-Mata M, Reyes PA, Alarcón-Segoviá D *et al.* Oesophageal motility in systemic lupus erythematosus. *Am J Dig Dis* 1974; **19**: 132–6.
4 Bazinet P, Marin GA. Malabsorption in systemic lupus erythematosus. *Am J Dig Dis* 1971; **16**: 460–6.
5 Siurala M, Julkunen H, Toivonen S *et al.* Digestive tract in collagen diseases. *Acta Med Scand* 1965; **178**: 13–25.
6 Rustgi AK, Peppercorn MA. Gluten-sensitive enteropathy and systemic lupus erythematosus. *Arch Intern Med* 1988; **148**: 1583–4.
7 Wood ML, Foulds IS, French MA. Protein losing enteropathy due to systemic lupus erythematosus. *Gut* 1984; **25**: 1013–5.
8 Laing TJ. Gastrointestinal vasculitis and pneumatosis intestinalis due to systemic lupus erythematosus: successful treatment with pulse intravenous cyclophosphamide. *Am J Med* 1988; **85**: 555–8.
9 Pruitt RE, Tumminello VV, Reveille JD. Pneumatosis cystoides intestinalis and benign pneumoperitoneum in a patient with antinuclear antibody-negative systemic lupus erythematosus. *J Rheumatol* 1988; **15**: 1575–7.
10 Zizic TM, Classen JN, Stevens MB. Acute abdominal complications of systemic lupus erythematosus and polyarteritis nodosa. *Am J Med* 1982; **73**: 525–31.
11 Sasamura H, Nakamoto H, Ryuzaki M *et al.* Repeated intestinal ulcerations in a patient with systemic lupus erythematosus and high serum anti-phospholipid antibody levels. *South Med J* 1991; **84**: 515–7.
12 Phillips JC, Howland WJ. Mesenteric arteritis in systemic lupus erythematosus. *JAMA* 1968; **206**: 1569–70.
13 Wolman R, De Gara C, Isenberg D. Acute pancreatitis in systemic lupus erythematosus: report of a case unrelated to drug therapy. *Ann Rheum Dis* 1988; **47**: 77–9.
14 Simons-Ling N, Schachner L, Penneys N *et al.* Childhood systemic lupus erythematosus. *Arch Dermatol* 1983; **119**: 491–4.
15 Alarcón-Segoviá D, Herskovic T, Dearing WH *et al.* Lupus erythematosus cell phenomenon in patients with chronic ulcerative colitis. *Gut* 1965; **6**: 39–47.
16 Zizic TM, Shulma LE, Stevens MB. Colonic perforations in systemic lupus erythematosus. *Medicine* 1975; **54**: 411–26.
17 Kassan SS, Moss ML, Reddick RL. Progressive hilar and mediastinal lymphadenopathy in systemic lupus erythematosus on corticosteroid therapy. *N Engl J Med* 1976; **294**: 1382–3.
18 Wiljasalo M, Ikkala E. Lymphography in systemic lupus erythematosus. *Ann Clin Res* 1964; **3**: 231–5.
19 Averbuch M, Levo Y. Long-standing intractable ascites as the initial and predominant manifestation of systemic lupus erythematosus. *J Rheumatol* 1986; **13**: 442–3.
20 Korn S, Huppert A, Spitzer S *et al.* Systemic lupus erythematosus presenting with lingual infarction. *J Rheumatol* 1988; **15**: 1281–3.

Hepatic lesions [1]. These may be more common than previously recognized. Liver disease is present in approximately one-third of patients, but it is usually mild and often asymptomatic. Histology usually shows steatosis or mild hepatitis. Lesions include granulomatous hepatitis, chronic active hepatitis, cirrhosis, death from liver failure and hepatic infarction. The role of hepatitis C infection has been reviewed [2]. Nodular regenerative hyperplasia occurs [3], and hepatic veno-occlusive disease has been reported [4]. Subclinical liver disease indicated by mild transaminase elevation occurs in approximately 10%. LE cells are sometimes found in hepatitis. The condition, inappropriately named 'lupoid hepatitis', involves mainly young females who have a benign cirrhosis and evidence of adrenal overactivity such as acne, hirsutism, pigmentation, amenorrhoea and abdominal striae. Other features include febrile upsets, polyarthritis, hyperglobulinaemia and other protein abnormalities. Smooth muscle and mitochondrial antibodies may be demonstrated. Patients with chronic active hepatitis may show extensive purplish telangiectasia [5].

Thyroid disease. Both hyperthyroidism and hypothyroidism occur in SLE, and there is a high frequency of abnormal thyroid function tests and thyroid autoantibodies in patients without diagnosed thyroid disease [6].

Nervous system [7,8]. Approximately 50% develop neuropsychiatric features from the disease itself [8]. There is no direct correlation between neurological and psychiatric disease and clinical or laboratory indices of disease activity. Livedoid vasculitis of the skin may be an important prodromal sign of central nervous system (CNS) lupus [9]. Anticardiolipin antibodies may or may not be present. Migraine can be a feature [10]. Epilepsy, resulting from small thromboses in cerebral vessels affected by vasculitis, can be the presenting manifestation of SLE, particularly in patients with high titres of anticardiolipin antibodies. The incidence of epilepsy is difficult to evaluate, owing to selection of cases in series from special clinics. Peripheral sensorimotor [11] and autonomic neuropathy occurs [12], brought about by vasculitis in the vasa nervorum. It is important to distinguish this from the neuropathy induced by chloroquine [13]. Trigeminal neuropathy, with numbness and pain in the face [14], deafness [15], transverse myelitis [16], optic neuritis [17], aseptic meningitis [18], Guillain–Barré syndrome, and a case presenting as disseminated encephalomyelitis, have been reported [19]. Patients may present with clinical features of multiple sclerosis, and in this variant there is a high incidence of chronic biological false-positive Wassermann reactions and mitochondrial antibodies [20]. Occasionally, a single cranial nerve may be involved. Sometimes, signs simulate an intracranial mass [21], and pseudotumour cerebri because of raised intracranial pressure occurs [22]. Subarachnoid haemorrhage [23] and massive spontaneous subdural haematoma have been reported [24]. Parkinsonism is rare [25]. The association of chorea with SLE has been reviewed [26]: two cases of chorea were reported in a series of 175 patients with SLE [27], and the authors have seen this association in two girls aged 3 and 16 years. Chorea gravidarum also occurs [28]. SLE may also cause psychiatric symptoms, including anxiety, hypomania, emotional lability, memory defects and depression. Psychiatric symptoms are found in approximately 20–30% [29]. Patients may respond to the disease with hypochondriasis, depression and hysteria, and pseudocyesis has been reported [30].

The electroencephalogram (EEG), conventional CT scanning, MRI scanning and oxygen-15 brain scanning may be helpful in the diagnosis of cerebral LE, and abnormalities are related to clinical progress [31]. Cranial computed tomography (CT) may show focal areas of infarction and cerebral atrophy or calcification [31]. The former may be caused by steroid therapy rather than the disease. Autoantibodies to neuronal antigens can be demonstrated in approximately 20% of patients with SLE, especially in those with neuropsychiatric features [32,33]. Antiribosomal P protein antibodies seem to be associated with psychosis [34]. Patients with multiple strokes followed by dementia are likely to have antiphospholipid antibodies [35]. Depressed levels of C4 in the cerebrospinal fluid (CSF) are found in patients with CNS involvement, but not in patients with active SLE without CNS manifestations [36].

Toxoplasmosis of the brain may occur as an opportunistic infection in patients with SLE and the manifestations resemble cerebral lupus [37].

References

1 Leggett BA. The liver in systemic lupus erythematosus. *J Gastroenterol Hepatol* 1993; **8**: 84–8.

2 Lormeau C, Falgarone G, Roulot D, Boissier MC. Rheumatologic manifestations of chronic hepatitis C infection. *Joint Bone Spine* 2006; **73**: 633–8.

3 Klemp P, Timme AH, Sayers GM. Systemic lupus erythematosus and nodular regenerative hyperplasia of the liver. *Ann Rheum Dis* 1986; **45**: 167–70.

4 Pappas SC, Malone DG, Rabin L et al. Hepatic veno-occlusive disease in a patient with systemic lupus erythematosus. *Arthritis Rheum* 1984; **27**: 104–8.

5 Green T, Champion RH. Extensive telangiectasia with chronic active hepatitis and systemic lupus erythematosus. *Br J Dermatol* 1989; **121**: 116.

6 Miller FW, Moore GF, Weintraub BD et al. Prevalence of thyroid disease and abnormal thyroid function test results in patients with systemic lupus erythematosus. *Arthritis Rheum* 1987; **30**: 1124–31.

7 Moskowitz N. Systemic lupus erythematosus of the central nervous system. I. Classification, epidemiology, pathology, diagnosis and therapy. *Mount Sinai J Med* 1988; **55**: 147–53.

8 Rhiannon JJ. Systemic lupus erythematosus involving the nervous system: presentation, pathogenesis, and management. *Clin Rev Allergy Immunol* 2008; **34**: 356–60.

9 Yasue T. Livedoid vasculitis and central nervous system involvement in systemic lupus erythematosus. *Arch Dermatol* 1986; **122**: 66–70.

10 Isenberg DA, Meyrick-Thomas D, Snaith ML et al. A study of migraine in systemic lupus erythematosus. *Ann Rheum Dis* 1982; **41**: 30–2.

11 McCombe PA, McLeod JG, Pollard JD et al. Peripheral sensorimotor and autonomic neuropathy associated with systemic lupus erythematosus. *Brain* 1987; **110**: 533–49.

12 Hirohata S, Iwamoto S, Miyamoto T et al. Acute autonomic neuropathy in association with systemic lupus erythematosus. *Ann Rheum Dis* 1985; **44**: 420–4.

13 Whisnant JP, Espinosa RE, Kierland RR et al. Chloroquine neuromyopathy. *Proc Staff Meetings Mayo Clin* 1963; **38**: 501–13.

14 Bailey A, Sayre GP, Clark EC. Neuritis associated with systemic lupus erythematosus. *Arch Neurol Psychiatr* 1956; **75**: 251–9.

15 Hamblin TJ, Mufti GJ, Bracewell A. Severe deafness in systemic lupus erythematosus: its immediate relief by plasma exchange. *BMJ* 1982; **284**: 1374.

16 Propper DJ, Bucknall RC. Acute transverse myelopathy complicating systemic lupus erythematosus. *Ann Rheum Dis* 1989; **48**: 512–5.

17 Kenik JG, Krohn K, Kelly RB et al. Transverse myelitis and optic neuritis in systemic lupus erythematosus: a case report with magnetic resonance imaging findings. *Arthritis Rheum* 1987; **30**: 947–50.

18 Canoso JJ, Cohen AS. Aseptic meningitis in systemic lupus erythematosus. *Arthritis Rheum* 1975; **18**: 369–74.

19 Vejjajiva A. Systemic lupus erythematosus presenting as acute disseminated encephalomyelitis. *Lancet* 1965; **i**: 352.

20 Fulford KWM, Catterall RD, Delhanty JJ et al. A collagen disorder of the nervous system presenting as multiple sclerosis. *Brain* 1972; **95**: 373–86.

21 Meagher JN, McCoy F, Rossel C. Disseminated lupus erythematosus simulating intracranial mass lesion: report of an unusual case. *Neurology* 1961; **11**: 862.

22 Li EK, Ho PCP. Pseudotumor cerebri in systemic lupus erythematosus. *J Rheumatol* 1989; **16**: 113–6.

23 Casey EB, Symon L. Systemic lupus erythematosus presenting as subarachnoid haemorrhage and space occupying lesion. *Br J Dermatol* 1971; **84**: 157–60.

24 Futran J, Shore A, Urowitz MB et al. Subdural hematoma in systemic lupus erythematosus: report and review of the literature. *J Rheumatol* 1987; **14**: 378–81.

25 Miyoshi Y, Atsumi T, Kitagawa H et al. Parkinsonism-like symptoms as a manifestation of systemic lupus erythematosus. *Lupus* 1993; **2**: 199–201.

26 Lusins JO, Szilagyi PA. Clinical features of chorea associated with systemic lupus erythematosus. *Am J Med* 1974; **58**: 857–61.

27 Lessof MH. Sydenham's chorea. *Guy's Hosp Rep* 1958; **107**: 185.

28 Wolf RE, McBeath JG. Chorea gravidarum in systemic lupus erythematosus. *J Rheumatol* 1985; **12**: 992–3.

29 Stojanovich L, Zandman-Goddard G, Pavlovich S, Sikanich N. Psychiatric manifestations in systemic lupus erythematosus. *Autoimmun Rev* 2007; **6**: 421–6.

30 Rodriguez IH, Morreno MJ, Morano LE et al. Systemic lupus erythematosus presenting as pseudocyesis. *Br J Rheumatol* 1994; **33**: 400–2.

31 Castellino G, Govoni M, Giacuzzo S, Trotta F. Optimizing clinical monitoring of central nervous system involvement in SLE. *Autoimmun Rev* 2008; **7**: 297–304.

32 Appenzeller S, Pike GB, Clarke AE. Magnetic resonance imaging in the evaluation of central nervous system manifestations in systemic lupus erythematosus. *Clin Rev Allergy Immunol* 2008; **34**: 361–6.

33 Kelly MC, Denburg JA. Cerebrospinal fluid immunoglobulins and neuronal antibodies in neuropsychiatric systemic lupus erythematosus and related conditions. *J Rheumatol* 1987; **14**: 740–4.

34 Isshi K, Hirohata S. Association of anti-ribosomal P protein antibodies with neuropsychiatric systemic lupus erythematosus. *Arthritis Rheum* 1996; **39**: 1483–90.

35 Asherson RA, Khamashta MA, Gil A et al. Cerebrovascular disease and antiphospholipid antibodies in systemic lupus erythematosus, lupus-like disease, and the primary antiphospholipid syndrome. *Am J Med* 1989; **86**: 391–9.

36 Petz LD, Sharp GC, Cooper NR et al. Serum and cerebral spinal fluid complement and serum autoantibodies in systemic lupus erythematosus. *Medicine* 1971; **50**: 259–75.

37 Deleze M, Mintz G, Del Carmen Mejia M. *Toxoplasma gondii* encephalitis in systemic lupus erythematosus: a neglected cause of treatable nervous system infection. *J Rheumatol* 1985; **12**: 994–6.

Involvement of the eyes. Eye changes in SLE are not uncommon [1]. They include lid oedema, conjunctivitis and subconjunctival haemorrhages, lacrimal hyposecretion, episcleritis, scleritis, anterior and posterior uveitis, retinal cytoid bodies, retinal haemorrhages and branch- and main-trunk arterial and venous occlusions. Optic neuritis is uncommon but may be the presenting feature, causing confusion with multiple sclerosis [2]. The retinal cytoid bodies—oval, whitish areas alongside arteries and veins—are not specific to SLE, and are thought to be brought about by damage to the endothelium of capillaries, which allows the passage of plasma and red cells into the nerve fibre layer. Depigmentation of the retina may be present. Retinal lesions rarely cause visual impairment, but blindness can occur [3]. Lupus retinopathy was found in approximately 8% in one large series and was associated with active disease and lupus cerebritis, and was a marker for poor prognosis [4]. Retinal changes can be demonstrated in nearly one-third of patients by fluorescein angiography, and are associated with active disease [5]. Visual impairment may be the presenting symptom of SLE [6]. Symptoms of corneal involvement occur in more than half of patients, and 88% have corneal staining with fluorescein [7].

References

1 Lessell S. Some ophthalmological and neurological aspects of systemic lupus erythematosus. *J Rheumatol* 1980; **7**: 398–404.
2 Smith CA, Pinals RS. Optic neuritis in systemic lupus erythematosus. *J Rheumatol* 1982; **9**: 963–6.
3 Bishko F. Retinopathy in systemic lupus erythematosus. *Arthritis Rheum* 1972; **15**: 57–63.
4 Stafford-Brady FJ, Urowitz MB, Gladman DD *et al*. Lupus retinopathy. *Arthritis Rheum* 1988; **31**: 1105–10.
5 Lanham JG, Barrie T, Kohner EM *et al*. SLE retinopathy: evaluation by fluorescein angiography. *Ann Rheum Dis* 1982; **41**: 473–8.
6 Wong K, Ai E, Jones JV *et al*. Visual loss as the initial symptom of systemic lupus erythematosus. *Am J Ophthalmol* 1981; **92**: 238–44.
7 Spaeth GL. Corneal staining in systemic lupus erythematosus. *N Engl J Med* 1967; **21**: 1168–71.

Involvement of the ears. Sudden bilateral loss of hearing, presumably because of vasculitis of the arteries of the cochlea, may be dramatic and permanent. One patient's hearing responded to plasma exchange [1].

Reference

1 Hamblin TJ, Mufti GJ, Bracewell A. Severe deafness in systemic lupus erythematosus: its immediate relief by plasma exchange. *BMJ* 1982; **284**: 1374.

Muscle changes. Muscle pain occurs in approximately 50% of patients, and this may be confused with the pain of arthritis. Muscle weakness is a less common feature. Electromyographic abnormalities correlate better with weakness than myalgia. The serum aldolase level is frequently raised but the serum creatine phosphokinase is usually normal [1]. A vacuolar myopathy is considered to be specific [2]. Calcinosis may occasionally occur [3]. Very rarely, there may be a myasthenic reaction and SLE can follow, or be associated with myasthenia gravis [4]. A thymoma may sometimes be found [5].

References

1 Tsokos GC, Moutsopoulos HM, Steinberg AD. Muscle involvement in systemic lupus erythematosus. *JAMA* 1981; **246**: 766–7.
2 Lang PA, Smith GH, Green WO. Vacuolar myopathy in lupus erythematosus. *JAMA* 1965; **191**: 49–51.
3 Quismorio FP, Dubois EL, Chandon SB. Soft tissue calcification in systemic lupus erythematosus. *Arch Dermatol* 1975; **111**: 352–6.
4 Makela TE, Ruosteenoja R, Wager O *et al*. Myasthenia gravis and systemic lupus erythematosus. *Acta Med Scand* 1964; **175**: 777–80.
5 Funkhouser JW. Thymoma associated with myocarditis and the LE-cell phenomenon. *N Engl J Med* 1961; **264**: 34–6.

Involvement of tendons [1]. Tendon rupture is rare, and involves particularly the weight-bearing tendons such as the patellar, quadriceps and Achilles tendons, but it may occur in any tendon [2,3]. Tendinous laxity may precede rupture and be partly attributable to hyperparathyroidism secondary to chronic renal failure [4], although long-term corticosteroid therapy may be relevant. Abnormalities of the feet with clawing of the toes and flexion contractures have been designated 'lupus foot' [5].

References

1 Potasman I, Bass HM. Multiple tendon rupture in systemic lupus erythematosus: case report and review of the literature. *Ann Rheum Dis* 1984; **43**: 347–8.
2 Lotem J, Maor P, Levi M. Rupture of the extensor tendons of the hand in lupus erythematosus disseminatus. *Ann Rheum Dis* 1973; **32**: 457–9.
3 Hanley JG, Urowitz MB. Tendon rupture in systemic lupus erythematosus. *Ann Rheum Dis* 1986; **45**: 349.
4 Babini SM, Maldonado Cocco JA, De La Sota M *et al*. Tendinous laxity and Jaccoud's syndrome in patients with systemic lupus erythematosus: possible role of secondary hyperparathyroidism. *J Rheumatol* 1989; **16**: 494–8.
5 Morley KD, Leung A, Rynes RI. Lupus foot. *BMJ* 1984; **284**: 557–8.

Calcification. Calcification may occasionally occur. Nine patients in one series of 130 cases had calcification [1]. This is more frequent in the legs, and may be bilateral and diffuse in the skin or deeper soft tissues, or be unilateral and localized. Sometimes, there are large deposits or nodules in the subcutaneous tissues [2]. It can occur without preceding local inflammation or ulceration, and may antedate other manifestations of SLE by as long as 7 years [3]. Periarticular calcification in the hand has been reported [1]. Calcification of the arteries of the legs may occur in early adult life. The myopathy of SLE may result in calcification [4]. A case of SLE with hypercalcaemia has been reported [5]. The serum calcium returned to normal when the patient had responded to treatment with corticosteroids and intravenous pulse cyclophosphamide.

References

1 Budin JA, Feldman F. Soft tissue calcifications in systemic lupus erythematosus. *Am J Roentgenol* 1975; **124**: 358–64.
2 Nomura M, Okada N, Okada M, Yoshikawa K. Large subcutaneous calcification in systemic lupus erythematosus. *Arch Dermatol* 1990; **126**: 1057–9.
3 Kabir DI, Malkinson FD. Lupus erythematosus and calcinosis cutis. *Arch Dermatol* 1969; **100**: 17–25.
4 Quismorio FP, Dubois EL, Chandor SB. Soft tissue calcification in systemic lupus erythematosus. *Arch Dermatol* 1975; **111**: 352–6.
5 Deftos LJ, Burton DW, Baird SM *et al*. Hypercalcaemia and systemic lupus erythematosus. *Arthritis Rheum* 1996; **39**: 2066–9.

Bone changes. Avascular bone necrosis [1] occurs in 5–7% or more of patients and is considered to be part of the disease, although it may be exacerbated by corticosteroid treatment [2], especially in high doses. It may be more frequent in patients with the lupus anticoagulant [3]. It may occur in relatively mild cases of SLE [4], but the risk is increased in patients with Raynaud's phenomenon [5]. The femoral head or condyle is most frequently involved [6], but the condition also may involve the knees, ankles, humerus, metatarsals and the carpal bones causing wrist pain [7]. It is commonly bilateral, with involvement of multiple joints. It is rarely crippling, although it may proceed to destruction of the joint. X-rays may be normal, but the diagnosis is often clear on MRI [8]. The condition is thought to be associated with increased pressure in the bone marrow because of altered venous drainage, and core decompression may be successful [9]. Total hip replacement may be required if it fails, or in the late stages. There may be patchy sclerosis and cystic changes in the bones of the hands and feet, and metacarpophalangeal and metatarsophalangeal joints may rarely show subcondylar erosions and adjacent sclerosis [10]. Osteonecrosis, possibly resulting from infarction, has been found in as many as 13 joints during corticosteroid treatment [11].

Other manifestations of systemic involvement include lymphadenopathy, which occurs in more than 50% of cases, and splenomegaly. Swelling of the parotid, submaxillary and lacrimal glands sometimes develops. Some features of Sjögren's syndrome have been found in practically all cases of SLE on detailed investigation [12].

References

1 Dubois EL, Cozen L. Avascular (aseptic) bone necrosis associated with systemic lupus erythematosus. *JAMA* 1960; **174**: 966–71.
2 Kalla AA, Learmonth ID, Klemp P. Early treatment of avascular necrosis in systemic lupus erythematosus. *Ann Rheum Dis* 1986; **45**: 649–52.
3 Migliaresi S, Picillo U, Ambrosone L. Avascular osteonecrosis in patients with SLE: relation to corticosteroid therapy and anti-cardiolipin antibodies. *Lupus* 1994; **3**: 37–41.
4 Siemsen JK, Brook J, Meister L. Lupus erythematosus and avascular bone necrosis: a clinical study of three cases and review of the literature. *Arthritis Rheum* 1962; **5**: 492–501.
5 Zizic TM, Hungerford DS, Stevens MB. Ischaemic bone necrosis in systemic lupus erythematosus. *Medicine* 1980; **59**: 134–42.
6 Klipper AR, Stevens MB, Zizic TM *et al.* Ischaemic necrosis of bone in systemic lupus erythematosus. *Medicine* 1976; **55**: 251–7.
7 Urman JD, Abeles M, Houghton AN *et al.* Aseptic necrosis presenting as wrist pain in SLE. *Arthritis Rheum* 1977; **20**: 825–8.
8 Halland AM, Klemp P, Botes D *et al.* Avascular necrosis of the hip in systemic lupus erythematosus: the role of magnetic resonance imaging. *Br J Rheumatol* 1993; **32**: 972–6.
9 Hungerford DS, Zizic TM. The treatment of ischemic necrosis of bone in systemic lupus erythematosus. *Medicine* 1980; **59**: 143–8.
10 Green N, Osmer JC. Small bone changes secondary to systemic lupus erythematosus. *Radiology* 1968; **90**: 118–23.
11 Fishel B, Caspi D, Eventov I *et al.* Multiple osteonecrotic lesions in systemic lupus erythematosus. *J Rheumatol* 1987; **14**: 601–4.
12 Alarcón-Segoviá D, Ibanez G, Velazquez-Forero F *et al.* Sjögren's syndrome in systemic lupus erythematosus: clinical and subclinical manifestations. *Ann Intern Med* 1974; **81**: 577–83.

SLE in childhood [1]. The clinical picture, course and treatment are similar to the disorder in adults, but on the whole children have more severe disease [2]. The earliest age of onset reported is 3 months [3]. Bullous SLE may resemble chronic bullous disease of childhood [4]. In one series [5], 30% had CNS involvement and 87% had renal disease (diffuse proliferative lupus nephritis, 34%). Overall survival was 85% at 10 years and 77% at 15 years after onset. Children with CNS lupus did no worse than other patients, and this has been noted by others [6]. The prognosis of patients with renal disease is now better than earlier reports suggested. Enlargement of the liver, spleen and lymph nodes is more common in childhood cases. Pancreatitis associated with cutaneous panniculitis and calcinosis has been reported [7]. Prolonged therapy with high-dose steroids may increase disease-related damage; this may be avoided by judicious use of immunosuppressives [8]. Autologous stem cell transplantation has been used successfully [9].

SLE in the elderly [10]. The onset of disease over 60 years occurs in nearly 20% of patients and is often insidious. There is an increased incidence of lung disease and Sjögren's syndrome, and a lower incidence of renal disease and mesenteric vasculitis [11], and antibodies to Ro and La are frequent. There appears to be an association with HLA-DR3.

References

1 Tucker LB. Making the diagnosis of systemic lupus erythematosus in children and adolescents. *Lupus* 2007; **16**: 546–9.
2 Tucker LB, Menon S, Schally JG *et al.* Adult and childhood onset systemic lupus erythematosus: a comparison of onset, clinical features, serology and outcome. *Br J Rheumatol* 1995; **34**: 866–72.
3 Cummings NP, Hansen J, Hollister JR. Systemic lupus erythematosus in a premature infant. *Arthritis Rheum* 1985; **28**: 573–5.
4 Kettler AH, Bean SF, Duffy JO *et al.* Systemic lupus erythematosus presenting as a bullous eruption in a child. *Arch Dermatol* 1988; **124**: 1083–7.
5 Plat JL, Burke BA, Fish AJ *et al.* Systemic lupus erythematosus in the first two decades of life. *Am J Kidney Dis* 1982; **2** (Suppl. 1): 212–22.
6 Yancey CL, Doughty RA, Athneya BH. Central nervous system involvement in childhood systemic lupus erythematosus. *JAMA* 1981; **24**: 1389–95.
7 Simons-Ling N, Schachner L, Penneys N *et al.* Childhood systemic lupus erythematosus. *Arch Dermatol* 1983; **119**: 491–4.
8 Brunner HI, Silverman ED, To T *et al.* Risk factors for damage in childhood-onset systemic lupus erythematosus: cumulative disease activity and medication use predict disease damage. *Arthritis Rheum* 2002; **46**: 436–44.
9 Wulffraat NM, Sanders EA, Kamphuis SS *et al.* Prolonged remission without treatment after autologous stem cell transplantation for refractory childhood systemic lupus erythematosus. *Arthritis Rheum* 2001; **44**: 728–31.
10 Maddison PJ. Systemic lupus erythematosus in the elderly. *J Rheumatol* 1987; **13**: 182–7.
11 Hochberg MC, Boyd RE, Ahearn JM *et al.* Systemic lupus erythematosus: a review of clinico-laboratory features and immunogenetic markers in 150 patients with emphasis on demographic subsets. *Medicine* 1985; **64**: 285–95.

SLE in pregnancy [1,2]. Fertility is normal if renal function is good. Worsening of SLE is uncommon in pregnancy, especially in those on immunosuppressive therapy [3]. Clinical remission for 6 months before conception should indicate an uncomplicated pregnancy and a live birth [4]. The outcome with renal involvement is comparable with those whose kidneys are not affected [5]. There is a higher risk of premature delivery, fetal loss and perinatal mortality in all patients. Abortion occurred in 8% and perinatal mortality was 13% in one series [6]. The increased risk of fetal death may be because of immune complex deposition on the trophoblast basement membrane [7], or the transplacental passage of antiphospholipid antibodies. Anticardiolipin antibodies, especially of the IgG isotype [8] or the lupus anticoagulant, are associated with a markedly increased fetal loss in all stages of pregnancy, but the presence of these antibodies without a previous history of fetal loss or thrombosis is not an indication for treatment [1]. With a history of recurrent fetal loss, treatment with prednisone and aspirin may be effective [9]. With good obstetric care, close follow-up, and treatment with low-dose aspirin if antiphospholipid antibody is present, a success rate of 71% has been reported [10]. The authors have seen successful pregnancies following *in vitro* fertilization in patients with SLE and the lupus anticoagulant.

Therapeutic abortion is not indicated and only causes added stress, nor is caesarean section required. It is important to avoid excessive trauma, haemorrhage or shock. The dosage of corticosteroids should be temporarily increased at the time of delivery and postpartum. Corticosteroids do not appear to cause impairment of growth or malformation in the fetus, but high-dose steroids during early pregnancy can cause cleft palate. Babies of mothers with untreated SLE are usually smaller than expected, and corticosteroids may assist growth of the fetus *in utero* [5]. If the patient is on azathioprine, this should be continued as there is no evidence of an increase in the malformation rate [11].

Oestrogen-containing contraceptives, even at low dosage, should be avoided in women with SLE. If mechanical methods of contraception or intrauterine devices are not possible, pure progestogens may be an alternative [12]. Breastfeeding is probably safe if the patient is on aspirin or low-dose steroids, but should probably be avoided if other immunosuppressives are used.

References
1 Clowse ME. Lupus activity in pregnancy. *Rheum Dis Clin North Am* 2007; **33**: 237–52.
2 Petri M. The Hopkins Lupus Pregnancy Center: ten key issues in management. *Rheum Dis Clin North Am* 2007; **33**: 227–35.
3 Meehan RT, Dorsey JK. Pregnancy among patients with systemic lupus erythematosus receiving immunosuppressive therapy. *J Rheumatol* 1987; **14**: 252–8.
4 Hayslett JP. Effect of pregnancy in patients with SLE. *Am J Kidney Dis* 1982; **2** (Suppl. 1): 223–8.
5 Oviasu E, Hicks J, Cameron JS. The outcome of pregnancy in women with lupus nephritis. *Lupus* 1991; **1**: 19–25.
6 Varner MW, Meehan RT, Syrop CH *et al.* Pregnancy in patients with systemic lupus erythematosus. *Am J Obstet Gynecol* 1983; **145**: 1025–40.
7 Grennan DM, McCormick JN, Wojtacha D *et al.* Immunological studies of the placenta in systemic lupus erythematosus. *Ann Rheum Dis* 1978; **37**: 129–34.
8 Deleze M, Alarcón-Segoviá D, Valdes-Macho E *et al.* Relationship between antiphospholipid antibodies and recurrent fetal loss in patients with systemic lupus erythematosus and apparently healthy women. *J Rheumatol* 1989; **16**: 768–72.
9 Ordi J, Barquinero J, Vilardell M *et al.* Fetal loss treatment in patients with antiphospholipid antibodies. *Ann Rheum Dis* 1989; **48**: 798–802.
10 Derksen RHWM, Bruinse HW, de Groot PG *et al.* Pregnancy in systemic lupus erythematosus: a prospective study. *Lupus* 1994; **3**: 149–55.
11 Martinez-Ruada JO, Arce-Salinas CA, Kraus A *et al.* Factors associated with foetal losses in severe systemic lupus erythematosus. *Lupus* 1996; **5**: 113–9.
12 Jungers P, Dougados M, Pélissier C *et al.* Influence of oral contraceptive therapy on the activity of systemic lupus erythematosus. *Arthritis Rheum* 1982; **25**: 618–23.

Neonatal lupus erythematosus

Definition. Neonatal lupus erythematosus (NLE) is a disorder thought to be caused by the transplacental passage of maternal antibodies. The most frequent clinical manifestations are cutaneous lesions and congenital heart block (CHB).

Aetiology. Aylward [1] was the first to report CHB in the siblings of a mother with Mikulicz's disease (Sjögren's syndrome) in 1928. McCuiston and Schoch [2], however, were the first to suggest that the association of NLE and maternal systemic lupus may be related to the transplacental transfer of 'a transmittable aetiological agent' (maternal antibodies). This suggestion subsequently gained credence from the fact that the NLE skin lesions resolve as maternal antibodies are cleared from the infant's serum [3].

The first associated antibody described [4] and the serological marker most commonly associated with NLE is the Ro/SS-A antibody. This has been reported to be present in between 82% of infants and 92% of mothers [5] and 100% of NLE patients [6–8]. Two main Ro/SS-A proteins exist (52 and 60 kDa), and studies have suggested that the former is more frequently found in CHB [9,10], whereas the latter is more frequently associated with cutaneous disease [11], although this is by no means a universal finding [12]. It has been claimed that the aa200–239 (p200) locus on the 52-kDa Ro/SS-A protein is a more specific predictor of CHB [13],

but a further study found this occurred with a similar frequency in children without CHB [14]. La/SS-B antibodies are less frequently found, one study detecting these in approximately 50% of NLE infants and 60% of mothers (usually in association with Ro/SS-A antibodies) [5]. A further study suggested that 50-kDa La/SS-B antibodies were associated with cutaneous disease [15], and another suggested that anti-idiotype antibodies to La/SS-B antibodies were protective against the development of NLE [16]. U_1-RNP antibodies are much less frequently found but have been reported as the only antibody in some patients with cutaneous NLE [17,18]. In this and subsequent reports, U_1-RNP antibodies have not been associated with CHB.

Evidence that these antibodies may be pathogenic comes from the studies of Lee *et al.* [19] who showed that purified Ro antibody bound to human skin grafted onto nude mice, in a pattern similar to that found in typical LE lesions. In addition, Ro/SS-A antigen is present in neonatal skin [20]. These antibodies have also been shown to bind to Ro/SS-A and La/SS-B antigen in human fetal cardiac conducting tissue [21–23] where they can cause conduction abnormalities [24,25]. A sequence of apoptosis, opsonization and fibrosis has been proposed [26].

It is unlikely that these antibodies represent the whole story, however, as they are non-specific for NLE, occurring in Sjögren's syndrome and SCLE. They are also found in approximately 0.5–2% of the normal population when assessed by immunodiffusion and in 5–11% when assessed by enzyme-linked immunoabsorbent assay (ELISA) [5]. Some studies have suggested that disease expression may be related to HLA status, the HLA-DR3 haplotype (especially when associated with DQA1 and DQB1) having been associated with the immune response to Ro/SS-A [27,28]. These, and a previous study [8], suggest that the HLA haplotype is important for antigen production in the mother but not necessarily relevant in the infants. Other workers argue that these antibodies are only indirectly related to disease, the disease process being caused by either: (i) the 52-kDa Ro/SS-A showing homology with the 5-HT_4 serotoninergic receptor, binding to which then mediates cardiac damage [10]; (ii) the presence of antibodies to a completely separate 57-kDa protein [29]; (iii) the prescience of the TNF-α 308A allele (associated with high TNF-α production), HLA-DRQB1*02, HLA DRB1*03 and TGF-β polymorphisms [30]; or (iv) via maternal microchimerisms [31,32]. A single case report has implicated α-interferon therapy in the aetiology of neonatal lupus [33].

Clinical features
Cutaneous. Approximately half of NLE infants manifest skin lesions [5], which may be present at birth or occur in the first few weeks of life. The most common finding is an erythematous, slightly scaly eruption on the face and periorbital skin (raccoon sign/owl-eye/eye mask) (Fig. 51.39), with the scalp, trunk, extremities, neck and intertriginous areas involved in decreasing order of frequency [34]. The eruption can be exacerbated by UV exposure and there are reports of the rash being precipitated by phototherapy for neonatal jaundice [35,36], although the rash is sometimes present at birth, which would make it difficult to implicate UV exposure in the aetiology [37]. Other manifestations include a vitiligo-like eruption in a black infant [38], morphoea-like lesions [39] and papules on the feet [40].

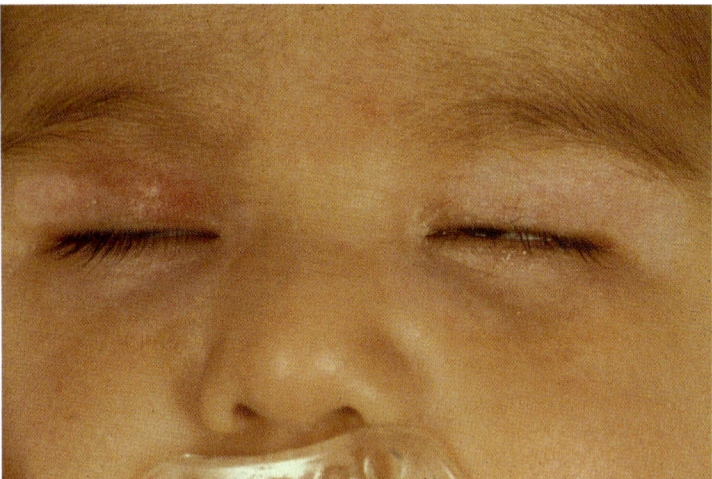

Fig. 51.39 Typical 'raccoon' eyelid lesions in neonatal lupus erythematosus.

The rash improves over the first few months of life and has usually resolved without scarring by 12 months of age. Occasional patients exhibit residual telangiectasiae [41], dyspigmentation or atrophy [34] and atrophic scarring [42].

Cardiac. Complete heart block occurs in approximately 60% of white patients [5], although it may be less common in Japanese patients [43]. Associated features may also include pericardial effusions, pleural effusions, ascites, intrauterine growth retardation and hydrops fetalis [44]. Up to 50% will require pacing in the neonatal period and others will require a pacemaker at a later date [45]. Dilated cardiomyopathy occurs in up to 20%, and has a significant mortality in the first year of life [45].

Haematological. Thrombocytopenia may occur in up to 20% of cases [41,46], is transient and does not usually require treatment, although it has been associated with petechial and purpuric lesions. Neutropenia, haemolytic anaemia and aplastic anaemia have also been reported [47,48].

Hepatic. Hepatomegaly and splenomegaly have been reported in NLE [49], with histological changes of 'neonatal hepatitis' and, on occasions, fibrosis. Cholestasis has been reported [49,50], as has cholestatic hepatitis [51,52]. A recent study showed hepatobiliary disease in 19 of 219 patients with NLE, and in three this was the only finding [53].

Miscellaneous. Case reports have associated NLE with pneumonitis [6], haemochromatosis [54], aseptic meningitis [55], myelopathy [56], transient myasthenia gravis [57], spastic paraparesis [41,58] and chondrodysplasia punctata [59]. One study demonstrated brain CT abnormalities in 10 of 11 infants with NLE although there was no clinical evidence of neurological disease, the authors emphasizing that it is important to be aware of these findings to avoid misdiagnosis of congenital viral infection in a newborn with multisystem NLE [60]. Hydrocephalus has been reported [61], affecting 8% of NLE infants in one study [62].

Treatment

Cutaneous lesions. Skin disease is often mild and requires no treatment. Sun avoidance should be advised and low-potency topical steroids may be of benefit [5,45]. Persistent telangiectasiae have been reported to respond to the tunable dye laser [63].

Cardiac. Up to 50% may require pacing in the newborn period, and others may require pacemaker insertion at a later date [44]. There is little information with regard to whether CHB and its consequences can be prevented or treated *in utero*. One study reviewed outcomes in pregnancies of mothers with Ro antibodies who had received systemic steroids during pregnancy [64]. When steroids had been given during the first 16 weeks of pregnancy, no conduction defects occurred, suggesting that they may have possibly suppressed disease initiation during this period of gestation. Corticosteroids administered after the first 16 weeks, however, were not beneficial and did not reverse established complete heart block. Another study compared outcome in fetuses whose mothers were treated with oral corticosteroids at various stages during pregnancy. Although there was no improvement in established complete heart block, the treated group showed less progression from first- to second-degree block to complete block and some improvement in pleural effusions, ascites and hydrops [43]. Anecdotally, a mother with the HLA-DR3 phenotype, high titres of Ro/SS-A and La/SS-B antibodies and an existing child with neonatal lupus, delivered a healthy infant after plasmapheresis three times weekly and systemic steroids during gestation [55].

The role of 'placenta crossing' steroids such as dexamethasone in at-risk infants is unclear at present, although a treatment algorithm has been suggested [26] and the results of a multicentre, prospective trial are awaited.

Haematological. Most resolve spontaneously without treatment, although prednisolone at a dose of 2 mg/kg/day for 14 days resulted in a dramatic improvement in thrombocytopenia in one patient [51].

Hepatic. Most resolve spontaneously without treatment.

Pregnancy. A pregnant patient who is known to have Ro/SS-A or La/SS-B antibodies should be made aware of the possible problems, and their obstetrician alerted. The risk of NLE in a Ro/SS-A positive mother without connective tissue disease or a previous history of NLE is probably low, perhaps about 2%. The risk may or may not be higher for symptomatic Ro/SS-A positive mothers, but for women who have already had a baby with NLE, the estimated risk of having another affected child ranges widely between studies, but is probably about 25% [65]. Perhaps in this latter group, the recommendation of serial fetal echocardiography by an experienced paediatric cardiologist [26] should be considered.

Although Ro/SS-A and La/SS-B antibodies have been demonstrated in human breast milk, a large study found no evidence to suggest that they had any pathological consequences. However, in the unusual circumstances of a worsening rash or developing cardiomyopathy, the authors suggested considering discontinuation of breastfeeding [66].

Prognosis

Infant. Although follow-up data are limited, some children have gone on to develop autoimmune disease, even in childhood [65], and one child developed a CNS vasculopathy at the age of 17 years [67]. Follow-up is therefore advised.

Mother. Although mothers are often asymptomatic at the time of the birth, long-term follow-up studies by several groups have shown that many develop signs and symptoms of autoimmune disease, especially Sjögren's syndrome, systemic lupus erythematosus and undifferentiated connective tissue disease [65]. Follow-up is therefore advised.

References

1 Aylward RD. Congenital heart block. *BMJ* 1928; **1**: 943.
2 McCuiston CH, Schoch EP. Possible discoid lupus erythematosus in newborn infant: report of a case with subsequent development of acute systemic lupus erythematosus in mother. *Arch Dermatol* 1954; **70**: 782–5.
3 McCauliff DP. Neonatal lupus erythematosus: a transplacentally acquired autoimmune disorder. *Semin Dermatol* 1995; **1**: 47–53.
4 Franco HL, Weston WL, Tan E *et al.* Association of antibodies to sicca syndrome antigens in newborns with lupus erythematosus and their mothers. *Clin Res* 1980; **28**: 134A.
5 Petri M, Watson R, Hochberg MC. Anti-Ro antibodies and neonatal lupus. *Rheum Dis Clin North Am* 1989; **15**: 335–60.
6 Watson RM, Lane AT, Barnett NK *et al.* Neonatal lupus erythematosus: a clinical, serological and immunogenetic study with review of the literature. *Medicine* 1984; **63**: 362–78.
7 Taylor PV, Taylor KF, Norman A *et al.* Prevalence of maternal Ro (SS-A) and La (SS-B) autoantibodies in relation to congenital heart block. *Br J Rheumatol* 1988; **27**: 128–32.
8 Lee LA, Weston WL. New findings in neonatal lupus syndrome. *Am J Dis Child* 1984; **138**: 233–6.
9 Viana VST, Garcia S, Nascimento JHM *et al.* Induction of *in vitro* heart block is not restricted to affinity purified anti-52 kDa Ro/SSA antibody from mothers of children with neonatal lupus. *Lupus* 1998; **7**: 141–7.
10 Eftekhari P, Salle L, Lezoualch F *et al.* Anti-SSA/Ro52 autoantibodies blocking the cardiac 5-HT$_4$ serotoninergic receptor could explain neonatal lupus congenital heart block. *Eur J Immunol* 2000; **30**: 2782–90.
11 Lee LA, Frank MB, McCubbin VR *et al.* Autoantibodies of neonatal lupus erythematosus. *J Invest Dermatol* 1994; **102**: 963–6.
12 Gordon P, Khamashta MA, Rosenthal E *et al.* Anti-52kDa Ro, anti-60 kDa Ro, and anti-La antibody profiles in neonatal lupus. *J Rheumatol* 2004; **31**: 2480–7.
13 Salomonsson S, Dorner T, Theander E *et al.* A serologic marker for fetal risk of congenital heart block. *Arthritis Rheum* 2002; **46**: 1233–41.
14 Clancy RM, Buyon JP, Ikeda K *et al.* Maternal antibody responses to the 52-kd SSA/Ro p200 peptide and the development of fetal conduction defects. *Arthritis Rheum* 2005; **52**: 3079–86.
15 Yukiko N. Immune responses to SS-A 52-kDa and 60-kDa proteins and to SS-B 50-kDa protein in mothers of infants with neonatal lupus erythematosus. *Br J Dermatol* 2000; **142**: 908–12.
16 Stea-Eleni A, Routsias JG, Clancy RM *et al.* Anti-La/SSB anti-idiotypic antibodies in maternal serum: a marker of low risk for neonatal lupus in an offspring. *Arthritis Rheum* 2006; **54**: 2228–34.
17 Provost TT, Watson R, Gammon WR *et al.* The neonatal lupus syndrome associated with U$_1$-RNP (nRNP) antibodies. *N Engl J Med* 1987; **316**: 1135–8.
18 Su CT, Huang CB, Chung MY. Neonatal lupus erythematosus in association with an anti-RNP antibody: a case report. *Am J Perinatol* 2001; **18**: 421–6.
19 Lee LA, Gaither KK, Coulter SN *et al.* Pattern of cutaneous immunoglobulin G deposits in subacute cutaneous lupus erythematosus reproduced by infusing purified anti-Ro (SSA) autoantibodies into human skin-grafted mice. *J Clin Invest* 1989; **83**: 1556–62.
20 Jones SK, Coulter S, Harmon C *et al.* Ro/SSA antigen in human epidermis. *Br J Dermatol* 1988; **118**: 363–7.
21 Deng JS, Blair LW, Shen-Schwartz S *et al.* Localization of Ro (SS-A) antigen in the cardiac conduction system. *Arthritis Rheum* 1987; **30**: 1232–8.
22 Horsfall AC, Venables PJW, Taylor PV *et al.* Ro and La antigens and maternal anti-La idiotype on the surface of myocardial fibres in congenital heart block. *J Autoimmun* 1991; **4**: 165–76.
23 Reichlin M, Brucato A, Frank MB *et al.* Concentration of autoantibodies to native 60-kD Ro/SS-A and denatured 52 kD Ro/SS-A in eluates from the heart of a child who died with congenital complete heart block. *Arthritis Rheum* 1994; **37**: 1698–703.
24 Alexander E, Buyon JP, Provost TT *et al.* Anti-Ro/SS-A antibodies in the pathophysiology of congenital heart block in neonatal lupus syndrome: an experimental model. *Arthritis Rheum* 1992; **35**: 176–89.
25 Garcia S, Nascimento JHM, Bonfa E *et al.* Cellular mechanism of the conduction abnormalities induced by serum from anti-Ro/SSA-positive patients in rabbit hearts. *J Clin Invest* 1994; **93**: 718–24.
26 Buyon JP, Clancy RM. Neonatal lupus: basic research and clinical perspectives. *Rheum Dis Clin N Am* 2005; **31**: 299–313.
27 Stephens HAF, McHugh NJ, Maddison PJ *et al.* HLA class II restriction of autoantibody production in patients with systemic lupus erythematosus. *Immunogenetics* 1991; **33**: 276–80.
28 Reveille JD, Macloed MJ, Whittington K *et al.* Specific amino acid residues in the second hypervariable region of HLA-DQA1 and DQB1 chain genes promote the Ro(SSA)/La(SSB) autoantibody responses. *J Immunol* 1991; **146**: 3871–6.
29 Maddison PJ, Lee L, Reichlin M *et al.* Anti-P57: a novel association with neonatal lupus. *Clin Exp Immunol* 1995; **99**: 42–8.
30 Clancy RM, Backer CB, Yin X *et al.* Genetic association of cutaneous neonatal lupus with HLA class II and tumor necrosis factor α. Implications for pathogenesis. *Arthritis Rheum* 2004; **50**: 2598–603.
31 Stevens AM, Hermes HM, Rutledge JC *et al.* Myocardial-tissue—specific phenotype of maternal microchimerism in neonatal lupus congenital heart block. *Lancet* 2003; **362**: 1617–23.
32 Stevens AM, Hermes HM, Lambert NC *et al.* Maternal and sibling microchimerism in twins and triplets discordant for neonatal lupus syndrome-congenital heart block. *Rheumatology* 2004; **44**: 187–91.
33 Fritz M, Vats K, Goyal RK. Neonatal lupus and IUGR following alpha-interferon therapy during pregnancy. *J Perinatol* 2005; **25**: 552–4.
34 Weston WL, Morelli JG, Lee LA. The clinical spectrum of anti-Ro positive neonatal lupus erythematosus. *J Am Acad Dermatol* 1999; **40**: 675–81.
35 Gawkrodger DJ, Beveridge GW. Neonatal lupus erythematosus in four successive siblings born to a mother with discoid lupus erythematosus. *Br J Dermatol* 1984; **111**: 683–7.
36 Luo SF, Huang CC, Wang JW. Neonatal lupus erythematosus: report of a case. *J Formos Med Assoc* 1989; **88**: 832–5.
37 Cimaz R, Biggioggero M, Catelli L *et al.* Ultraviolet light exposure is not a requirement for the development of cutaneous neonatal lupus. *Lupus* 2002; **11**: 257–60.
38 Jenkins RE, Kurwa AR, Atherton DJ *et al.* Neonatal lupus erythematosus. *Clin Exp Dermatol* 1994; **19**: 409–11.
39 Ohtaki N, Miyamoto C, Orita M *et al.* Concurrent multiple morphea and neonatal lupus erythematosus in an infant boy born to a mother with SLE. *Br J Dermatol* 1986; **115**: 85–90.
40 See A, Wargon O, Lim A *et al.* Neonatal lupus presenting as papules on the feet. *Australas J Dermatol* 2005; **46**: 172–6.
41 Bourke JF, Burns DA. Neonatal lupus erythematosus with persistent telangiectasia and spastic paraparesis. *Clin Exp Dermatol* 1993; **18**: 271–3.
42 High WA, Costner MI. Persistent scarring, atrophy, and dyspigmentation in a preteen girl with neonatal lupus erythematosus. *J Am Acad Dermatol* 2003; **48**: 626–8.
43 Kaneko F, Tanji O, Hasegawa T *et al.* Neonatal lupus erythematosus in Japan. *J Am Acad Dermatol* 1992; **26**: 397–403.
44 Saleeb S, Copel J, Friedman D *et al.* Comparison of treatment with fluorinated glucocorticoids to the natural history of autoantibody-associated congenital heart block: retrospective review of the research registry for neonatal lupus. *Arthitis Rheum* 1999; **42**: 2335–45.
45 Eronen M, Siren MK, Ekblad H *et al.* Short- and long-term outcome of children with congenital complete heart block diagnosed *in utero* or as a newborn. *Paediatrics* 2000; **106**: 86–91.

46 Provost TT, Watson R, Gaither KK *et al*. The neonatal lupus erythematosus syndrome. *J Rheumatol* 1987; **14** (Suppl. 13): 199–205.

47 Watson R, Kang JE, May M *et al*. Thrombocytopaenia in the neonatal lupus syndrome. *Arch Dermatol* 1988; **124**: 560–3.

48 Wolach B, Choc L, Pomeranz A *et al*. Aplastic anaemia in neonatal lupus erythematosus. *Am J Dis Child* 1993; **147**: 941–4.

49 Laxer RM, Roberts EA, Gross KR *et al*. Liver disease in neonatal lupus erythematosus. *J Paediatr* 1990; **116**: 238–42.

50 Rosh JR, Silvermann ED, Groisman G *et al*. Intrahepatic cholestasis in neonatal lupus erythematosus. *J Paediatr Gastroenterol Nutr* 1993; **17**: 310–2.

51 Lin SC, Shyur SD, Huang LH *et al*. Neonatal lupus erythematosus with cholestatic hepatitis. *J Microbiol Immunol Infect* 2004; **37**: 131–4.

52 Erbey F, Cuhaci A, Incecik F *et al*. Neonatal lupus erythematosus presenting with cholestatic hepatitis: a case report and review of the literature. *Turk J Paediatr* 2005; **47**: 63–6.

53 Lee LA, Sokol R, Buyon JP. Hepatobiliary disease in neonatal lupus: prevalence and clinical characteristics in cases enrolled in a national registry. *Pediatrics* 2002; **109**: E11.

54 Schoenlebe J, Buyon JP, Zitelli BJ *et al*. Neonatal haemochromatosis associated with maternal antibodies against Ro/SS-A and La/SS-B ribonucleoprotein. *Am J Dis Child* 1993; **147**: 1072–5.

55 Buyon JP, Roubey R, Swersky S *et al*. Complete congenital heart block: risk of occurrence and therapeutic approach to prevention. *J Rheum* 1998; **15**: 1104–8.

56 Kaye EM, Butler IJ, Conley S. Myelopathy in neonatal and infantile lupus erythematosus. *J Neurol Neurosurg Psychiatry* 1987; **50**: 923.

57 Rider LG, Sherry DD, Glass ST. Neonatal lupus erythematosus simulating transient myasthenia gravis at presentation. *J Paediatr* 1991; **118**: 417–9.

58 Besson-Leaud L, Fontan D, Billeaud C *et al*. Lupus neonatal et atteinte neurologique: une association fortuite? *Arch Pediatr* 2002; **9**: 503–5.

59 Austin-Ward E, Castillo S, Cuchacovich M *et al*. Neonatal lupus syndrome: a case with chondrodysplasia punctata and other unusual features. *J Med Genet* 1998; **35**: 695–7.

60 Prendiville JS, Cabal DA, Poskitt KJ *et al*. Central nervous system involvement in neonatal lupus erythematosus. *Paediatr Dermatol* 2003; **20**: 60–7.

61 Nakayama-Furukawa F, Takigawa M, Iwatsuki K *et al*. Hydrocephalus in two female siblings with neonatal lupus erythematosus. *Arch Dermatol* 1994; **130**: 1210–2.

62 Boros CA, Spence D, Blaser S *et al*. Hydrocephalus and macrocephaly: new manifestations of neonatal lupus erythematosus. *Arthritis Rheum* 2007; **57**: 261–6.

63 Thornton CM, Eichenfield LF, Shinall EA *et al*. Cutaneous telangiectases in neonatal lupus erythematosus. *J Am Acad Dermatol* 1995; **33**: 19–25.

64 Shinohara K, Miyagawa S, Fujita T *et al*. Neonatal lupus erythematosus: results of maternal corticosteroid therapy. *Obstet Gynaecol* 1999; **93**: 952–7.

65 Lee LA. Transient autoimmunity related to maternal autoantibodies: neonatal lupus. *Autoimmun Rev* 2005; **4**: 207–13.

66 Askanase AD, Miranda-Carus ME, Tang X *et al*. The presence of IgG antibodies reactive with components of the SSA/Ro-SSB/La complex in human breast milk: implications in neonatal lupus. *Arthritis Rheum* 2002; **46**: 269–71.

67 Inoue K, Fukushige J, Ohno T *et al*. Central nervous system vasculopathy associated with neonatal lupus. *Pediatr Neurol* 2002; **26**: 68–70.

Laboratory investigations [1]. Laboratory investigations are frequently necessary to confirm the diagnosis, although even after extensive investigations it may be impossible to be entirely dogmatic, in view of the overlap of the manifestations of connective tissue diseases. Anaemia, of some degree, is found in approximately 75% of patients and is brought about by deficiency of iron, haemolysis or renal failure. The serum iron is usually low and may rise after corticosteroid therapy [2]. A positive Coombs' test can occur in the absence of haemolytic anaemia, and was present in 15% in a series of cases seen by the authors. Pure red cell aplasia has been reported [3]. Although leukopenia, specifically a lymphopenia, is a characteristic feature of the condition, and a white cell count of below 5000/mm² occurs in more than 33% of patients,

leukocytosis may occasionally be found. The platelet count is reduced in approximately 20% of cases and is usually below 40 000/mm² in patients presenting with thrombocytopenic purpura. Thrombocytopenia may appear only during exacerbations or be a mild persisting feature [4]. Hyposplenism may occur [5]. The ESR is raised at some time in nearly 90% of patients; the C-reactive protein (CRP) is usually normal in the absence of infection, but some patients have a normal ESR throughout. The plasma viscosity may be raised, although initially thought unreliable, a more consistent assay is now being more widely used as an indicator of activity [6]. Serum globulins are frequently raised, with a rise in the gammaglobulin usually, although α_2-globulin may be elevated and the albumin decreased. IgE antibodies may be raised [7,8], particularly in patients with arthritis. False-positive serological tests for syphilis are found in approximately 25% of patients [9] and an atypical 'beaded' pattern of fluorescence of the *Treponema pallidum* antigen occurs when sera from certain patients are tested in the fluorescent treponemal antibody absorption (FTA-ABS) test [10]. Rheumatoid factor occurs in approximately 40%. Thrombosis occurs with the lupus anticoagulant (see p. 51.63), but occasionally haemorrhage results from other haematological abnormalities [11]. The lupus anticoagulant is one of a number of antiphospholipid antibodies that may be found in up to 50% of patients with SLE. As well as thrombosis, CNS disease is strongly related to the presence of these antibodies [12].

The LE cell phenomenon, first described by Hargraves *et al*. [13], is the basis for the LE cell test, which is positive in over 80% of patients. LE cells are polymorphonuclear leukocytes which have ingested nuclear material from degenerative white cells, in the presence of an antibody to deoxyribonucleoprotein (the LE cell factor) (Fig. 51.40). Sometimes, large masses of nuclear material are found extracellularly and, with surrounding leukocytes, form rosettes. LE cells, if present in large numbers, are highly suggestive of SLE, but the occasional LE cell is sometimes demonstrated in other conditions, including chronic DLE, systemic sclerosis and rheumatoid arthritis [14]. A positive LE cell test is a feature of drug-induced LE; LE cells were demonstrated in 60 out of 66

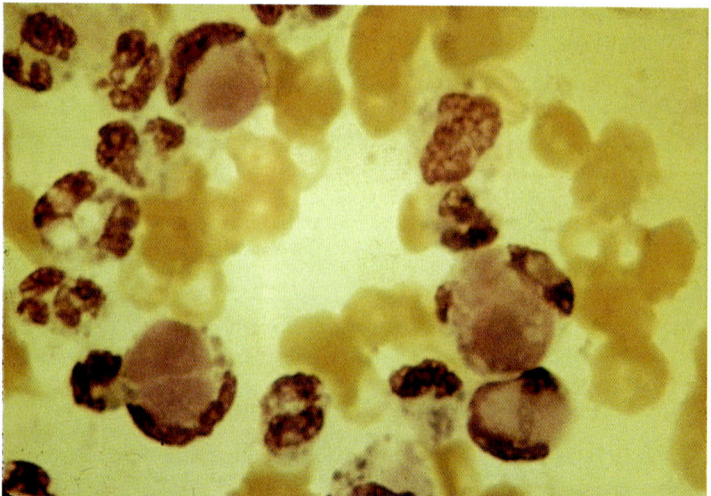

Fig. 51.40 Lupus erythematosus cells: the phagocytosed nuclear material is homogeneous and displaces the polymorph nucleus to one side.

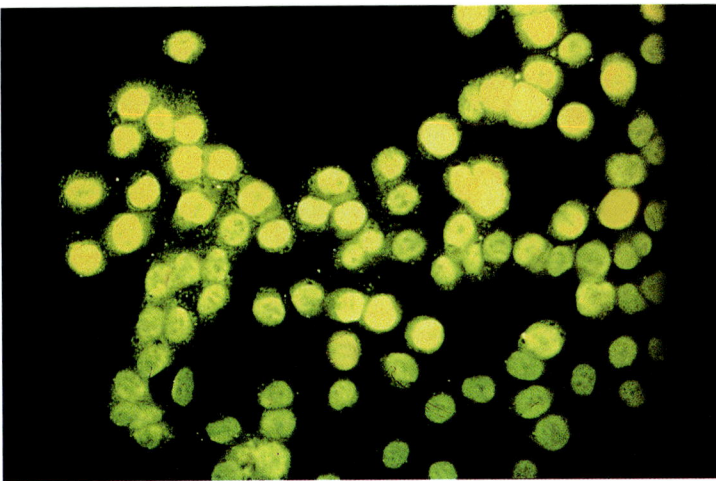

Fig. 51.41 Homogeneous type of antinuclear factor demonstrated on Hep-2 cells.

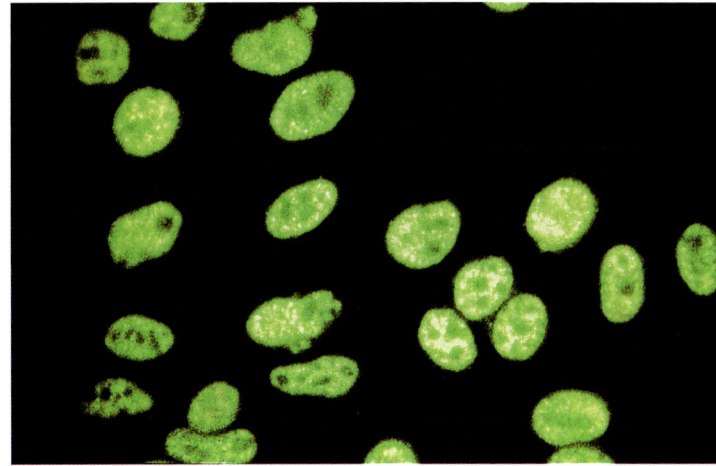

Fig. 51.43 Speckled type of antinuclear factor demonstrated on Hep-2 cells.

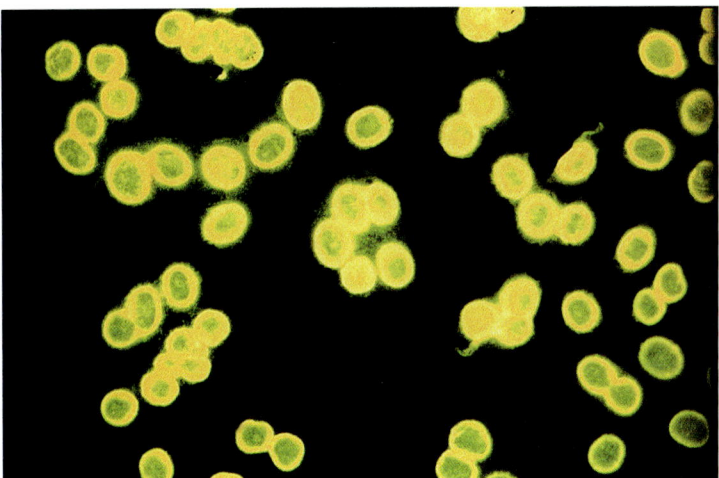

Fig. 51.42 Peripheral type of antinuclear factor demonstrated on Hep-2 cells.

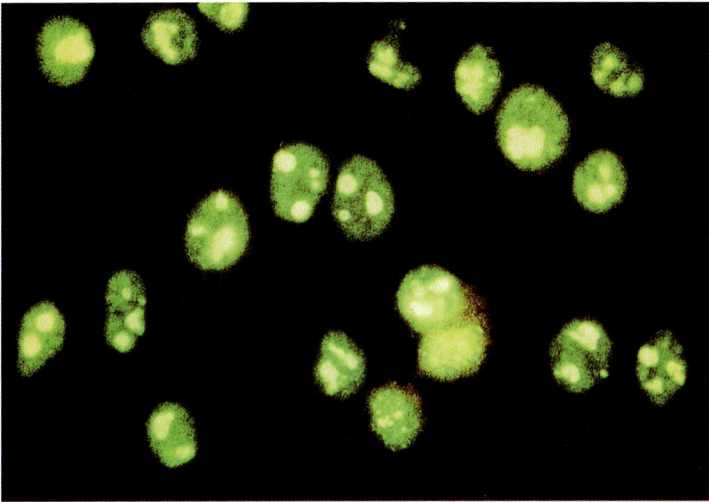

Fig. 51.44 Nucleolar type of antinuclear factor demonstrated on Hep-2 cells.

patients with procainamide-induced lupus [15]. The LE cell test has now been superseded by tests for antinuclear factors and anti-DNA antibodies.

One or more antinuclear antibodies can be detected by fluorescent antibody techniques in over 80% of cases. The incidence depends on the substrate used. Most British laboratories now use human cell lines for antibody testing, particularly Hep-2 cells derived from a human laryngeal cell line. This produces a reduction in the proportion of patients said to be antinuclear factor negative. Previously, the standard substrate was rat or mouse liver. Using rat liver, four staining patterns can be demonstrated [16], representing four systems of antinuclear antibodies (Figs 51.41–51.44).

1 In the *homogeneous pattern*, produced by antinucleohistone, the nuclei are stained all over.
2 The *speckled pattern* shows minute points of fluorescence scattered all over the nucleus, the antigens being saline-soluble proteins.
3 The *nucleolar pattern* shows uniform staining of each nucleolus.

4 Sera containing anti-DNA antibody give rise to the fourth *peripheral or membranous pattern* [16,17], in which staining occurs at the periphery of the nucleus.

These staining patterns are produced by separate antibodies, but more than one antibody may be present in a single serum, usually in different titres. No particular antibody is specific for any disease. Discrepancies in the incidence between series probably depend on differences in techniques and the substrate used.

Homogeneous antinuclear factor (which is the same factor as the LE cell factor, although the fluorescent antibody test is more sensitive than the LE cell test) is more than twice as common as the speckled factor, but antinucleolar antibody is only occasionally found. The peripheral factor is present in high titre in more than 50% in the active phase of the disease [18], and is infrequent in other diseases. The so-called shrunken peripheral pattern is thought to be associated with a poor prognosis and a high incidence of renal disease [19]. It may appear 10–15 days before an exacerbation of the disease and be associated with a fall in serum complement [20]. In a series of 63 cases of SLE seen by the authors, one or more antinuclear factors were demonstrated in 55 patients

(87%). Homogeneous staining was present in 46 cases, speckled staining in 18 and nucleolar staining in five. Titres up to 1:32000 occur, but the titre frequently bears no relation to the activity, progress or duration of the disease. A high titre (over 1:64) of antinuclear factor(s), in a patient with symptoms and signs of a multiple system disorder, suggests the possibility of SLE or systemic sclerosis, and almost certainly excludes polyarteritis nodosa or cutaneous vasculitis. Any person in apparently good health found to have a high titre of antinuclear factor should be followed-up for years, as there is a considerable likelihood of developing LE or systemic sclerosis. A low titre (less than 1:16), in the absence of clinical symptoms and signs, can be ignored [21].

When Hep-2 cells are used as substrate, as well as being more sensitive to the presence of antinuclear antibody, further patterns can be identified [22]. These include centromere staining (see p. 51.103) associated with the CREST syndrome and in 6% of patients with SLE, homogeneous, peripheral (specific to SLE), fine and coarse speckles and a ground-glass appearance produced by Scl-70 antibody (see p. 51.103) found in systemic sclerosis. There are also several patterns of nucleolar staining: homogeneous, speckled and clumpy. The full clinical association of these antibodies has not been determined.

Circulating antibodies to DNA are almost always present in active disease [23,14] and may occur in the absence of antinuclear factors [24], although this is very uncommon using Hep-2 cells. Their demonstration by the Farr technique is the most specific aid to diagnosis, and levels often correlate with disease activity, although DNA antibodies should not be the only criterion [25]. Radiolabelled DNA is incubated with the test serum and any DNA–anti-DNA complexes formed are precipitated by 50% ammonium sulphate. Comparison of the radioactivity in the supernatant and precipitate gives the so-called DNA-binding activity. Values above 30% are abnormal. The level was raised in 83% of patients with SLE and in 100% of those with active disease. A rise in the index may precede an exacerbation of the disease, and levels fall with remission [26]. Normal values are found in drug-induced LE and in other disorders in which antinuclear antibodies occur. A high binding capacity is associated with poor prognosis and renal disorder [16]. The peripheral staining pattern of antinuclear antibody does not correlate with anti-DNA antibodies or with disease activity [27].

Several other antibodies occur in patients with SLE. Patients with antihistone antibodies have a lower incidence of renal and CNS disease, alopecia, anaemia and decreased complement [28]. Antibodies to soluble cellular antigens include anti-Sm antibody, which is found in 15–25% of patients and appears to be specific for the disease, occurring particularly in patients with renal disease, CNS disease and vasculitis. Anti-RNP antibodies occur in 25% of patients [29], but are characteristic of mixed connective tissue disease (see p. 51.111). It has been reported that titres correlate with disease activity [30].

Anti-Ro [31] antibody occurs in 30% of patients who have an increased tendency to photosensitivity [32,33], renal disease, Sjögren's syndrome and rheumatoid factor, as well as being a marker for neonatal lupus (see p. 51.49). It is also found in SCLE (see p. 51.22). Anti-Ro is an antibody to an RNP derived from RNA polymerase III-transcribed hY RNAs with a protein component that appears to be the main target. Two different proteins, one of 60 kDa and another of 52 kDa, react with most positive sera. The 60-kDa protein predominates in SLE, the 52-kDa in Sjögren's syndrome [34]. Patients with anti-Ro antibodies are more likely to have HLA-B8 and -DRw3 [35]. Anti-La, an antibody to another RNP product of RNA polymerase III, is present in 10–15% of patients, often with Sjögren's syndrome and with anti-Ro antibody. Although several different antibodies occur in the same patient, they fluctuate independently, and the antibody profile may alter over the years. The only characteristic pattern of antibody appears to occur in the LE–erythema multiforme syndrome [36], in which there is speckled type of antinuclear factor, a specific precipitating antibody (originally designated SjT but now thought to be anti-La) and rheumatoid factor. This syndrome is occasionally found in cases of systemic as well as DLE, in which it was originally described (see p. 51.14). In cases associated with SLE, homogeneous antinuclear factor is also usually present.

Cryoglobulins may be found in 11% of patients. Cryoglobulinaemia may precede the manifestations of SLE by many years [37]. Cold agglutinins occur in 6%. Serum complement is frequently low [38], especially in patients with active nephritis. A decrease in levels may precede clinical evidence of an exacerbation of disease, and return to normal with remission but, in general, estimations of CH50, C3, C4 and circulating immune complexes are rarely helpful in assessing disease activity [39]. Other possible indicators of disease activity include β_2-macroglobulin [40] and serum IFN [41]. Increased levels of plasma anaphylatoxins (C3a) may predict exacerbations [42]. The intracutaneous injection of DNA solution, which has been advocated as a skin test [43], is not specific. Occasionally, circulating anticoagulants may be demonstrated [44,45]. Factor II may be absent and return with steroid therapy [46].

Inherited deficiencies of the major complement components occur with SLE [47], usually as autosomal recessive traits [48]. These include C1 [49], C2 [50] and C4 [51], as well as C5–C9. The most common is homozygous C2 deficiency in which SLE occurs in one-third of patients. Clinically, the lupus-like syndrome in C2 deficiency shows a low incidence of renal disease, low incidence and low titres of anti-DNA antibodies, infrequent occurrence of immunoglobulin and complement deposits in the skin, and frequent anti-Ro antibodies [46]. Isolated C1q deficiency has also been reported [52], and there is an association between C1-esterase inhibitor deficiency and SLE [53]. Patients may be helped by danazol [54]. Hereditary angio-oedema and SLE were found in the mother of twin boys who had DLE and angio-oedema, and this was associated with low C1 inhibitor and C4 levels [55]. Antibodies to Australia antigen can be demonstrated in 25% of cases [56]. Serum CRP levels are usually normal or only slightly elevated. A level higher than 60 mg/L suggests the presence of superimposed infection [57]. A number of soluble cytokines or their receptors may be found in serum of patients with SLE, and may correlate with disease activity: intercellular adhesion molecule-1 (ICAM-1) [58], TNF receptor [59] and IL-10 [60]. There is differential overexpression of heat-shock proteins in patients with differing patterns of systemic involvement [61]. Urinary levels of neopterin [62], or of IL-6 [63], may also be useful to monitor disease activity.

References

1 Wallace DJ, Hahn BH, eds. *Dubois' Systemic Lupus Erythematosus*, 4th edn. Philadelphia: Lea and Febiger, 1993.

2 Whittingham S, Balazs NDH, MacKay IR. The effect of corticosteroid drugs on serum iron levels in systemic lupus erythematosus and rheumatoid arthritis. *Med J Aust* 1967; **ii**: 639–41.

3 Nitsche A, Taborda GD, Bouveta HM *et al.* Pure red cell aplasia in a patient with systemic lupus erythematosus. *J Rheumatol* 1988; **15**: 1012–3.

4 Miller MH, Urowitz MB, Gladman DD. The significance of thrombocytopenia in systemic lupus erythematosus. *Arthritis Rheum* 1983; **26**: 1181–6.

5 Dillon AM, Stein HB, English RA. Splenic atrophy in systemic lupus erythematosus. *Ann Intern Med* 1982; **96**: 40–3.

6 Hazelton RA, Lowe GDO, Forbes CD *et al.* Increased blood and plasma viscosity in systemic lupus erythematosus (SLE). *J Rheumatol* 1985; **12**: 616–7.

7 Goldman JA, Klimek GA, Ali R. Allergy in systemic lupus erythematosus. *Arthritis Rheum* 1976; **19**: 669–76.

8 Gruber BL, Kaufman LD, Marchese MJ *et al.* Anti-IgE autoantibodies in systemic lupus erythematosus. *Arthritis Rheum* 1988; **31**: 1000–6.

9 Shore RN, Faricelli JA. Borderline and reactive FTA-ABS results in lupus erythematosus. *Arch Dermatol* 1977; **113**: 37–41.

10 Kraus SJ, Daniels KC. Atypical FTA-ABS test reaction. *Arch Dermatol* 1971; **104**: 260–1.

11 Quismorio FP Jr. Hemic and lymphatic abnormalities in SLE. In: *Dubois' Systemic Lupus Erythematosus*, 4th edn. Philadelphia: Lea & Febiger, 1993: 418–30.

12 Derksen RHWM, Stephens CJM. The antiphospholipid syndrome. In: Kater L, Barte de la Faille H, eds. *Multi-systemic Auto-immune Diseases: An Integrated Approach*. Amsterdam: Elsevier, 1995.

13 Hargraves MM, Richmond H, Morton R. Presentation of two bone marrow elements: the 'tart' cell and the 'LE' cell. *Proc Staff Meetings Mayo Clin* 1948; **23**: 26–8.

14 Hughes GRV. Lupus erythematosus. In: Walker G, ed. *9th Symposium of Advanced Medicine*. London: Pitman, 1973: 67.

15 Condemi JJ, Blomgren SE, Vaughan JH. Procaineamide induced LE. *Bull Rheum Dis* 1970; **20**: 604.

16 Beck JS. Auto-antibodies to cell nuclei. *Scott Med J* 1963; **8**: 373–88.

17 Casals SP, Friou GJ, O'Teague PO. Specific nuclear reaction pattern of antibody to DNA in lupus erythematosus sera. *J Lab Clin Med* 1963; **62**: 625–31.

18 Nisengard RJ, Jablonska S, Chorzelski TP *et al.* Diagnosis of systemic lupus erythematosus. *Arch Dermatol* 1975; **111**: 1298–300.

19 Burnham TK. Antinuclear antibodies. *Arch Dermatol* 1975; **111**: 203–7.

20 Mandl MAJ, Watson JI. Nuclear immunofluorescence: a guide to treatment in SLE. *Lancet* 1969; **ii**: 848.

21 Rowell NR, Swanson Beck J. The diagnostic value of an antinuclear antibody test in clinical dermatology. *Arch Dermatol* 1967; **96**: 290–5.

22 Bernstein RM, Steigenwald JC, Tan EM. Association of antinuclear and antinucleolar antibodies in progressive systemic sclerosis. *Clin Exp Immunol* 1982; **48**: 43–51.

23 Ballou SP, Kushner I. Lupus patients who lack detectable anti-DNA: clinical features and survival. *Arthritis Rheum* 1982; **25**: 1126–9.

24 Lindstedt G, Lundberg PA, Westberg G *et al.* SLE nephritis with positive tests for antibodies against native DNA but negative tests for antinuclear antibodies. *Lancet* 1977; **ii**: 135.

25 Davis P, Percy JS, Russell AS. Correlation between levels of DNA antibodies and clinical disease activity in SLE. *Ann Rheum Dis* 1977; **36**: 157–9.

26 Swaak AJG, Groenwold J, Aarden LA *et al.* Prognostic value of anti-dsDNA in SLE. *Ann Rheum Dis* 1982; **41**: 388–95.

27 Weitzman RJ, Walker SE. Relation of titred peripheral pattern ANA to anti-DNA and disease activity in systemic lupus erythematosus. *Ann Rheum Dis* 1977; **36**: 44–9.

28 Fritzler M, Ryan P, Kinsella TD. Clinical features of systemic lupus erythematosus patients with antihistone antibodies. *J Rheumatol* 1982; **9**: 46–51.

29 Aitcheson CT, Tan EM. Autoantibodies in connective tissue disease. In: Panayi GS, ed. *Scientific Basis of Rheumatology*. Edinburgh: Churchill Livingstone, 1982: 87–113.

30 Nishikai M, Okano Y, Mukohda Y *et al.* Serial estimation of anti-RNP antibody titers in systemic lupus erythematosus, mixed connective tissue disease and rheumatoid arthritis. *J Clin Lab Immunol* 1984; **13**: 15–9.

31 Provost TT, Watson R, Simmons-O'Brien E. Anti-Ro (SSA) antibody positive Sjögren's/lupus erythematosus overlap syndrome. *Lupus* 1997; **6**: 105–11.

32 Provost TT, Watson R, Simmonds-O'Brien E. Significance of the anti-Ro (SS-A) autoantibody in evaluation of patients with cutaneous manifestations of a connective tissue disease. *J Am Acad Dermatol* 1996; **35**: 147–69.

33 Mond CB, Peterson MGE, Rothfield NF. Correlation of anti-Ro antibody with photosensitivity rash in systemic lupus erythematosus patients. *Arthritis Rheum* 1989; **32**: 202–4.

34 Ben-Chetrit E, Fox RI, Tan EM. Dissociation of immune response to the SS-A (Ro) 52 kD and 60 kD polypeptides in systemic lupus erythematosus and Sjögren's syndrome. *Arthritis Rheum* 1990; **33**: 349–55.

35 Bell DA, Maddison PJ. Serologic subsets in systemic lupus erythematosus. *Arthritis Rheum* 1980; **23**: 1268–73.

36 Rowell NR, Swanson Beck J, Anderson JR. Lupus erythematosus and erythema multiforme-like lesions. *Arch Dermatol* 1963; **88**: 176–80.

37 Perek J, Mittelman M, Eisbruch A *et al.* Systemic lupus erythematosus preceded by long-term cryoglobulinaemia. *Ann Rheum Dis* 1984; **43**: 339–40.

38 Schur PH, Sanderson J. Immunologic factors and clinical activity in systemic lupus erythematosus. *N Engl J Med* 1968; **278**: 533–8.

39 Valentijn RM, van Overhagen H, Hazevoet M *et al.* The value of complement and immune complex determinations in monitoring disease activity in patients with systemic lupus erythematosus. *Arthritis Rheum* 1985; **28**: 904–13.

40 Yeung C-K, Wong K-L, Wong W-S *et al.* β_2-Microglobulin and systemic lupus erythematosus. *J Rheumatol* 1986; **13**: 1053–8.

41 Shou-Nee S, Fang FS, Yumei W *et al.* Serum interferon in systemic lupus erythematosus. *Br J Dermatol* 1987; **117**: 155–9.

42 Hopkins P, Belmont HM, Buyon J *et al.* Increased levels of plasma anaphylatoxins in systemic lupus erythematosus predict flares of the disease and may elicit vascular injury in lupus cerebritis. *Arthritis Rheum* 1988; **31**: 632–41.

43 Ores RO, Lange K. Skin test for the diagnosis of systemic lupus erythematosus. *Am J Med Sci* 1964; **248**: 562.

44 Lee SL, Miotti AB. Disorders of hemostatic function in patients with systemic lupus erythematosus. *Semin Arthritis Rheum* 1975; **4**: 241.

45 Castro O. Circulating anticoagulants against factors IX and XI in systemic lupus erythematosus. *Ann Intern Med* 1972; **77**: 543–8.

46 Natelson EA, Cyprus GS, Heltig RA. Absent factor II in systemic lupus erythematosus. *Arthritis Rheum* 1976; **19**: 79–82.

47 Walport MJ. Complement deficiency and disease. *Br J Rheumatol* 1993; **32**: 269–73.

48 Agnello V. Complement deficiency states. *Medicine* 1978; **57**: 1–23.

49 Moncada B, Day NKB, Good RA *et al.* Lupus erythematosus-like syndrome with a familial defect of complement. *N Engl J Med* 1972; **286**: 689–93.

50 Rynes RI, Urizar RE, Pickerling RJ. Genetic deficiency of the second component of complement (C2) associated with systemic lupus erythematosus. *Am J Med* 1977; **63**: 278–88.

51 Tappeiner G, Hintner H, Scholz S *et al.* Systemic lupus erythematosus in hereditary deficiency of the fourth component of complement. *J Am Acad Dermatol* 1982; **7**: 66–79.

52 Steinsson K, McLean RH, Merrow M *et al.* Selective complete C1q deficiency associated with systemic lupus erythematosus. *J Rheumatol* 1983; **10**: 590–4.

53 Bagot M, Revuz J, Intrator L *et al.* Oedème angioneurotique acquis révélant un lupus erythemateux disseminé. *Ann Dermatol Vénéréol* 1987; **114**: 1331–3.

54 Donaldson VH, Hess EV. Effect of danazol on lupus erythematosus-like disease in hereditary angioneurotic oedema. *Lancet* 1980; **ii**: 1145.

55 Kohler PF, Percy J, Campion WM *et al.* Hereditary angioedema and 'familial' lupus erythematosus in identical twin boys. *Am J Med* 1974; **56**: 406–11.

56 Alarcón-Segoviá D, Fishbein E. Australia antigen in systemic lupus. *N Engl J Med* 1971; **284**: 448.

57 Pepys MB, Lanham JG, De Beer FC. C-reactive protein in systemic lupus erythematosus. *Clin Rheum Dis* 1982; **8**: 91–103.

58 Sfikakis PP, Charalambopoulos D, Vayiopoulos G *et al.* Increased levels of intercellular adhesion molecule-1 in the serum of patients with systemic lupus erythematosus. *Clin Exp Rheumatol* 1994; **12**: 1–9.

59 Aderna D, Wysenbeek A, Engelmann H *et al.* Correlation between serum levels of soluble tumour necrosis factor receptor and disease activity in systemic lupus erythematosus. *Arthritis Rheum* 1993; **36**: 1111–20.

60 Houssiau FA, Lefebvre C, Vandenberghe M *et al.* Serum interleukin 10 titres in systemic lupus erythematosus reflect disease activity. *Lupus* 1995; **4**: 393–5.

61 Dhillon VB, McCallum S, Norton P *et al.* Differential heat shock protein overexpression and its clinical relevance in systemic lupus erythematosus. *Ann Rheum Dis* 1993; **52**: 436–42.

62 Lim KL, Jones AC, Brown NS, Powell RJ. Urine neopterin as a parameter of disease activity in patients with systemic lupus erythematosus: comparisons with serum sIL-2r and antibodies to dsDNA, erythrocyte sedimentation rate, and plasma C3, C4, and plasma C3 degradation products. *Ann Rheum Dis* 1993; **52**: 429–35.

63 Iwano M, Dohi K, Hirata E *et al.* Urinary levels of IL-6 in patients with active lupus nephritis. *Clin Nephrol* 1993; **40**: 16–21.

Antinuclear antibody-negative SLE

Antinuclear antibody-negative SLE [1,2]. Patients originally described under this title have many similarities with patients suffering from SCLE (see p. 51.22). Because the cutaneous involvement is usually the predominant feature, many patients present initially to dermatologists. Clinically, a non-scarring malar flush, oral ulceration and photosensitivity, with papulosquamous or annular lesions on the face, trunk and arms, are prominent, but arthritis, serositis, renal disease and haematological involvement are less frequent than expected in SLE. In approximately 5–10% of patients with SLE, antinuclear factor cannot be demonstrated using standard substrates such as rat or mouse liver. This is a problem in less than 1% if Hep-2 cells are used. These patients frequently have anticytoplasmic antibodies. Over 60% of patients have anti-Ro antibodies and approximately one-third have anti-La antibody (anti-La rarely occurs without anti-Ro). Twenty-five per cent have antibodies to single-stranded DNA. There is no difference in the histology of the skin between antinuclear-negative and -positive cases. Immunoglobulins and complement are found at the dermal–epidermal junction in 70% of patients, but are rare in the non-light-exposed uninvolved skin. Topical steroid therapy may be helpful, but oral antimalarials and steroids may be required. Approximately 10% of patients eventually become antinuclear factor-positive, although the pattern of anticytoplasmic antibodies does not alter.

References

1 Ahmed R, Workman S. ANA-negative systemic lupus erythematosus. *Clin Exp Dermatol* 1983; **8**: 369–77.

2 Maddison PJ, Provost TT, Reichlin M. Serological findings in patients with ANA-negative systemic lupus erythematosus. *Medicine* 1981; **60**: 87–94.

Assessment of disease activity

Assessment of disease activity. A number of attempts have been made to devise definitions of disease activity, accompanied by scoring systems using combinations of clinical and laboratory parameters to allow comparative and longitudinal studies. Global measures such as European Community Lupus Activity Measure (ECLAM) [1], Systemic Lupus Erythematosus Disease Activity Index (SLEDAI) [2] and the more detailed British Isles Lupus Activity Grading (BILAG) [3] are useful in the context of clinical trials in patients with active systemic disease. However, none is specifically designed for the assessment of patients who most concern dermatologists, and do not grade skin disease in any meaningful way. The CLASI has been described for assessment of cutaneous disease, but is not yet in routine clinical use [4].

References

1 Vitali C, Bencivelli W, Isenberg DA *et al.* Disease activity in systemic lupus erythematosus: report of the consensus study group of the European workshop for rheumatology research. II. Identification of the variables indicative of disease activity and their use in the development of an activity score. *Clin Exp Rheumatol* 1992; **10**: 541–7.

2 Bombardier C, Gladman DD, Urowitz MB *et al.* Derivation of SLEDAI: a disease activity index for lupus patients. *Arthritis Rheum* 1992; **35**: 630–40.

3 Hay EM, Bacon PA, Gordon C *et al.* The BILAG index: a reliable and valid instrument for measuring clinical disease activity in systemic lupus erythematosus. *QJM* 1993; **86**: 447–58.

4 Albrecht J, Taylor L, Berlin JA *et al.* The CLASI (Cutaneous Lupus Erythematosus Disease Area and Severity Index): an outcome instrument for cutaneous lupus erythematosus. *J Invest Dermatol* 2005; **125**: 889–94.

Association with other diseases

Association with other diseases. SLE can occur concurrently with rheumatoid arthritis [1], and may present with polymyalgia in elderly patients [2]. Systemic sclerosis and SLE may occur in the same patient [3], and the demonstration of immunoglobulins at the dermal–epidermal junction may be helpful in confirming the presence of both diseases [4]. SLE occurs with lichen sclerosus and with 'en coup de sabre' morphoea [5], and linear and plaque morphoea [6]. Sjögren's syndrome and SLE occur together [7–9] but the former is usually mild, and is unlike secondary Sjögren's syndrome occurring with rheumatoid arthritis. Patients with hyperglobulinaemic purpura may have antinuclear factor; this condition may, in certain cases, have features of SLE [10]. The finding of LE cells in young females with liver disease has already been mentioned. SLE can follow primary biliary cirrhosis [11], and may occasionally occur in association with necrotizing angiitis [12] and giant cell arteritis [13]. Patients who have LE and psoriasis often have anti-Ro antibodies [14].

Myasthenia gravis may follow SLE [15], and SLE may follow thymectomy for myasthenia gravis [16] or be associated with a thymoma [17]. Myasthenia gravis, thymoma and pemphigus may occur together in patients with SLE [18], and heterozygous C2 deficiency associated with angio-oedema, myasthenia gravis and SLE also occurs [19]. Angio-oedema resulting from C1-esterase deficiency can be associated with SLE [20], and protein S deficiency can occur in these patients [21].

SLE has been reported with Hashimoto's thyroiditis and pernicious anaemia [22]. It was associated with seminoma of the ovary in one case. Removal of the tumour led to an apparent permanent cure of the LE [23]. Lymphatic leukaemia or Hodgkin's disease has followed SLE [24], and lymphoma has been reported [25]. Amyloidosis [26] can develop in SLE, and in one case this led to adrenal insufficiency and was followed by malignant lymphoma [27]. The presentation with haemolytic anaemia [28] or thrombocytopenic purpura [29] is well documented, and overt SLE may appear after splenectomy for 'idiopathic thrombocytopenic purpura'. If this occurs, it is likely that the thrombocytopenia is an early manifestation of SLE. It may also occur in association with thrombotic thrombocytopenic purpura [30], pernicious anaemia [31], von Willebrand's disease [32], myelofibrosis [33,34], selective IgA deficiency [35], erythroleukaemia [36], red cell aplasia [37], monoclonal gammopathy and multiple myeloma [38], biclonal gammopathy [39], myelofibrosis [39], hyperviscosity syndrome [40], Whipple's disease [41] and ulcerative colitis [42]. SLE also occurs with pemphigoid [43] and cicatricial pemphigoid [44], pemphigus [45], dermatitis herpetiformis [46], linear IgA disease [47], epidermolysis bullosa dystrophica [48], porphyria cutanea tarda [49] (although the association has not been confirmed) [50], and occasionally with porphyria variegata or acute intermittent porphyria [51–53]. The disease has been reported in patients with Sweet's syndrome [54], Klinefelter's syndrome [55], hypoparathyroidism [56], partial lipodystrophy [57], relapsing polychondritis [58], pyoderma gangrenosum [59] and Kikuchi's disease [60]. In one case it has been associated with retroperitoneal fibrosis [61], and in another with eosinophilic fasciitis and retroperitoneal fibrosis [62]. It uncommonly occurs with gout [63] and sarcoidosis [64]. An unusual syndrome of breast hypertrophy, erythema annulare centrifugum, generalized melanoderma and immunodeficiency to viral warts has been associated with SLE [65]. Twelve per cent of patients with SLE have warts, which is a higher incidence than in a control population [66]. Senear–Usher syndrome (pemphigus and LE) has been associated with internal malignancy [67], but an overall increased incidence of malignancy in SLE is debatable. Malignancy occurred in 4.7% in one series [68]. Epidermodysplasia verruciformis occurs presumably as a result of immunodeficiency or prolonged treatment with corticosteroids [69]. Among other rare associations are Kaposi's sarcoma [70] and Kawasaki disease [71].

The relationship to DLE is discussed on p. 51.2. Patients with persistent false-positive serological tests for syphilis [72] may later develop SLE.

References

1 Cohen MG, Webb J. Concurrence of rheumatoid arthritis and systemic lupus erythematosus: report of 11 cases. *Ann Rheum Dis* 1987; **46**: 853–8.

2 Hutton CW, Maddison PJ. Systemic lupus erythematosus presenting as polymyalgia rheumatica in the elderly. *Ann Rheum Dis* 1986; **45**: 641–4.

3 Rowell NR. Lupus erythematosus cells in systemic sclerosis. *Ann Rheum Dis* 1962; **21**: 70–5.

4 Chorzelski J, Jablonska S. Coexistence of lupus erythematosus and scleroderma in light of immunopathological investigations. *Acta Derm Venereol (Stockh)* 1970; **50**: 81.

5 Mackel SE, Kozin F, Ryan LM *et al.* Concurrent linear scleroderma and systemic lupus erythematosus. *J Invest Dermatol* 1979; **73**: 368–72.

6 Mitchell AJ, Rusin LJ, Diaz LA. Circumscribed scleroderma with immunologic evidence of systemic lupus erythematosus. *Arch Dermatol* 1980; **116**: 69–73.

7 Alarcón-Segoviá D, Ibanez G, Velazquez-Forero F *et al.* Sjögren's syndrome in systemic lupus erythematosus. *Ann Intern Med* 1974; **81**: 577–83.

8 Andonopoulos AP, Skopouli FN, Dimou GS *et al.* Sjögren's syndrome in systemic lupus erythematosus. *J Rheumatol* 1990; **17**: 201–4.

9 Zuffery P, Meyer OC, Bourgeois P *et al.* Primary systemic Sjögren syndrome (SS) preceding systemic lupus erythematosus: a retrospective study of 4 cases in a cohort of 55 SS patients. *Lupus* 1995; **4**: 23–7.

10 Waldenstrom J. *The Harvey Lectures Series 56.* New York: Academic Press, 1961: 211.

11 Hall S, Axelsen PH, Larson DE *et al.* Systemic lupus erythematosus developing in patients with primary biliary cirrhosis. *Ann Intern Med* 1984; **100**: 388–9.

12 Winkelmann RK, Ditto WB. Cutaneous and visceral syndromes of necrotizing or 'allergic' angiitis. *Medicine* 1964; **43**: 59–89.

13 Bunker CB, Dowd PM. Giant cell arteritis and systemic lupus erythematosus. *Br J Dermatol* 1988; **33**: 71–2.

14 Kulick KB, Mogavero H, Provost TT *et al.* Serologic studies in patients with lupus erythematosus and psoriasis. *J Am Acad Dermatol* 1983; **8**: 631–4.

15 Denney D, Rose RL. Myasthenia gravis followed by systemic lupus erythematosus. *Neurology* 1961; **11**: 710–3.

16 Alarcón-Segoviá D, Galbraith RF, Maldonado JE *et al.* Systemic lupus erythematosus following thymectomy for myasthenia gravis. *Lancet* 1963; **ii**: 662–5.

17 Steven MM, Westedt ML, Eulderink F *et al.* Systemic lupus erythematosus and invasive thymoma: report of two cases. *Ann Rheum Dis* 1984; **43**: 25–8.

18 Cooper A, Wells JV. Pemphigus foliaceus, myasthenia gravis and thymoma in a patient with serological evidence of SLE. *Aust NZ J Med* 1981; **11**: 277–80.

19 Efthimiou J, D'Cruz D, Kaplan P *et al.* Heterozygous C2 deficiency associated with angioedema, myasthenia gravis, and systemic lupus erythematosus. *Ann Rheum Dis* 1986; **45**: 428–30.

20 Bagot M, Revuz J, Intrator L *et al.* Oedème angioneurotique acquis révélant un lupus erythemateux disseminé. *Ann Dermatol Vénéréol* 1987; **114**: 1331–3.

21 Perkins W, Stables GI, Lever RS. Protein S deficiency in lupus erythematosus secondary to hereditary angio-oedema. *Br J Dermatol* 1994; **130**: 381–4.

22 Hamilton DV. Systemic lupus erythematosus in a patient with Hashimoto's thyroiditis and pernicious anaemia. *J R Soc Med* 1978; **71**: 147–9.

23 Rotman M, Dorfmann H, Sèze S *et al.* Coexistence d'un lupus erythemateux disseminé et d'un seminome de l'ovarie: guerison apparente rapide du lupus aprés ablation de la tumeur. *Nouv Presse Med* 1972; **1**: 853–7.

24 Morgenfeld MC, Magnin PH. Enfermedad de Hodgkin asociada con lupus eritematoss diseminado. *Pren Med Argent* 1970; **57**: 1899–901.

25 Green JA, Dawson AA, Walker W. Systemic lupus erythematosus and lymphoma. *Lancet* 1978; **ii**: 753–6.

26 Nomura S, Kumagai N, Kanoh T *et al.* Pulmonary amyloidosis associated with systemic lupus erythematosus. *Arthritis Rheum* 1986; **29**: 680–2.

27 Schleissner LA, Sheehan WW, Orselli RC. Lupus erythematosus in a patient with amyloidosis, adrenal insufficiency and subsequent immunoblastic sarcoma. *Arthritis Rheum* 1976; **19**: 249–54.

28 Dubois EL. Acquired hemolytic anaemia as the presenting syndrome of lupus erythematosus disseminatus. *Am J Med* 1952; **12**: 197–204.

29 Rabinowitz Y, Dameshek W. Systemic lupus erythematosus after 'idiopathic' thrombocytopenic purpura. *Ann Intern Med* 1960; **52**: 1–28.

30 Fox DA, Faix JD, Coblyn J *et al.* Thrombotic thrombocytopenic purpura and systemic lupus erythematosus. *Ann Rheum Dis* 1986; **45**: 319–22.

31 Korbet SM, Corwin HL. Pernicious anaemia associated with systemic lupus erythematosus. *J Rheumatol* 1986; **13**: 193–4.

32 Poole-Wilson PA. Acquired von Willebrand's syndrome and systemic lupus erythematosus. *Proc R Soc Med* 1972; **65**: 561–2.

33 Rosen PJ, Cramer AD, Dubois EL *et al.* Systemic lupus erythematosus (SLE) and myelofibrosis. *Clin Res* 1973; **21**: 565.

34 Kaelin WG, Spivak JL. Systemic lupus erythematosus and myelofibrosis. *Am J Med* 1986; **81**: 935–8.

35 Ammann AJ, Hong R. Selective IgA deficiency: presentation of 30 cases and a review of the literature. *Medicine* 1971; **50**: 223–36.

36 Ng HS, Ng HW, Sinniah R *et al.* A case of systemic lupus erythematosus with sideroblastic anaemia terminating in erythroleukaemia. *Ann Rheum Dis* 1981; **40**: 422–6.

37 Cassileth PA, Myers AR. Erythroid aplasia in systemic lupus erythematosus. *Am J Med* 1973; **55**: 706–10.

38 Powell FC, Greipp PR, Su WPD. Discoid lupus erythematosus and monoclonal gammopathy. *Br J Dermatol* 1983; **109**: 355–60.

39 Leach IH, Jenkins JS, Murray-Leslie CF *et al.* Heavy chain and monoclonal IgG K paraproteinaemia in systemic lupus erythematosus. *Br J Rheumatol* 1987; **26**: 460–2.

40 Jara LJ, Capin NR, Lavalle C. Hyperviscosity syndrome as the initial manifestation of systemic lupus erythematosus. *J Rheumatol* 1989; **16**: 225–30.

41 Ehrenfeld M, Urowitz MB, Platts ME. Selective C4 deficiency, systemic lupus erythematosus and Whipple's disease. *Ann Rheum Dis* 1984; **43**: 91–4.

42 Stevens HP, Ostlere LS, Rustin MHA. Systemic lupus erythematosus in association with ulcerative colitis: related auto-immune diseases. *Br J Dermatol* 1994; **130**: 385–9.

43 Stoll DM, King LE. Association of bullous pemphigoid with systemic lupus erythematosus. *Arch Dermatol* 1984; **120**: 362–6.

44 Redman RS, Thorne EG. Cicatricial pemphigoid in a patient with systemic lupus erythematosus. *Arch Dermatol* 1981; **117**: 109–10.

45 Bean SF, Lynch FW. Senear–Usher syndrome (pemphigus erythematosus). *Arch Dermatol* 1970; **101**: 642–5.

46 Thomas JR, Su WPD. Concurrence of lupus erythematosus and dermatitis herpetiformis. *Arch Dermatol* 1983; **119**: 740–5.

47 Lau M, Kaufmann-Grunzinger I, Raghunath MR. A case report of a patient with features of systemic lupus erythematosus and linear IgA disease. *Br J Dermatol* 1991; **124**: 498–502.

48 Archibald GC. Epidermolysis bullosa dystrophica and systemic lupus erythematosus. *Proc R Soc Med* 1976; **69**: 881–4.

49 Clemmensen O, Thomsen K. Porphyria cutanea tarda and systemic lupus erythematosus. *Arch Dermatol* 1982; **118**: 160–2.

50 Griso D, Macri A, Biolcati G *et al.* Does an association exist between PCT and SLE? Results of a study on autoantibodies in 158 patients affected with PCT. *Arch Dermatol Res* 1989; **281**: 291–2.

51 Allard SA, Scott JT. Systemic lupus erythematosus and acute intermittent porphyria. *Br J Rheumatol* 1989; **28**: 254–6.

52 Hetherington GW, Jetton RL, Knox JM. The association of lupus erythematosus and porphyria. *Br J Dermatol* 1970; **82**: 118–24.

53 Cram DL, Epstein JH, Tuffanelli DL. Lupus erythematosus and porphyria. *Arch Dermatol* 1973; **108**: 779–84.

54 Ramsay-Goldman R, Franz T, Solano A, Medsger TA. Hydralazine induced lupus and Sweet's syndrome: report and review of the literature. *J Rheumatol* 1990; **17**: 682–4.

55 Burch PRJ, Rowell NR. Systemic lupus erythematosus and Klinefelter's syndrome. *Lancet* 1976; **i**: 1021.

56 Hajiroussou VJ. Hypoparathyroidism associated with systemic lupus erythematosus. *Postgrad Med J* 1981; **57**: 597–8.

57 Font J, Herrero C, Bosch X *et al.* Systemic lupus erythematosus in a patient with partial lipodystrophy. *J Am Acad Dermatol* 1990; **22**: 337–40.

58 Job-Deslandre C, Delrieu F, Delbarre F *et al.* Relapsing polychondritis and systemic lupus erythematosus. *J Rheumatol* 1983; **10**: 666–8.

59 Pinto GM, Cabecas MA, Riscado M, Goncalves H. Pyoderma gangrenosum associated with systemic lupus erythematosus: response to pulse steroid therapy. *J Am Acad Dermatol* 1991; **24**: 818–21.

60 Litwin MD, Kirkham B, Henderson DRF *et al.* Histiocytic necrotising lymphadenitis in systemic lupus erythematosus. *Ann Rheum Dis* 1992; **51**: 805–7.

61 Lloyd DD, Balfe JW, Barkin M *et al.* Systemic lupus erythematosus with signs of retroperitoneal fibrosis. *J Pediatr* 1974; **85**: 226–8.

62 Garcia-Morteo O, Nitsche A, Maldonado-Cocco JA *et al.* Eosinophilic fasciitis and retroperitoneal fibrosis in a patient with systemic lupus erythematosus. *Arthritis Rheum* 1987; **30**: 1314–5.

63 Decastro P, Jorizzo JL, Solomon AR *et al.* Coexistent systemic lupus erythematosus and tophaceous gout. *J Am Acad Dermatol* 1985; **13**: 650–4.

64 Fivenson DP, Crump G, Scheele P *et al.* Systemic lupus erythematosus developing in a patient with long-standing pulmonary sarcoidosis. *J Rheumatol* 1989; **16**: 1116–9.

65 Shelley WB. An unusual auto-immune syndrome. *Acta Derm Venereol (Stockh)* 1972; **52**: 33.

66 Yell JA, Burge SM. Warts and lupus erythematosus. *Lupus* 1993; **2**: 21–3.

67 Saikia NK, MacConnell LES. Senear–Usher syndrome and internal malignancy. *Br J Dermatol* 1972; **87**: 1–5.

68 Menon S, Snaith ML, Isenberg DA. The association of malignancy with SLE: an analysis of 150 patients under long-term review. *Lupus* 1993; **2**: 177–81.

69 Tanigaki T, Kanda R, Sato K. Epidermodysplasia verruciformis in a patient with systemic lupus erythematosus. *Arch Dermatol Res* 1986; **278**: 247–8.

70 Greenfield DI, Trinh P, Fulenwider A *et al.* Kaposi's sarcoma in a patient with SLE. *J Rheumatol* 1986; **13**: 637–40.

71 Laxer RM, Cameron BJ, Silverman ED. Occurrence of Kawasaki disease and systemic lupus erythematosus in a single patient. *J Rheumatol* 1988; **15**: 515–6.

72 Catterall RD. Collagen disease and the chronic biological false positive phenomenon. *QJM* 1961; **30**: 41–55.

Kikuchi's disease and SLE.

Histiocytic necrotizing lymphadenitis was first described independently by Kikuchi [1] and Fujimoto *et al.* [2] from Japan in 1972. Cases are predominantly female, but it can occur in males, and can occur at all ages. Usually, patients present with lymphadenopathy, frequently cervical, although other nodes can be involved. Fever, weight loss and night sweats are found in the more severely affected cases. There may be leukopenia and elevation of the ESR. Skin changes occur in 30% of patients [3]. They are all non-specific and include multiple, indurated, red papules on the back and arms [4], erythematous plaques resembling lymphoma, erythema and acneiform eruptions on the

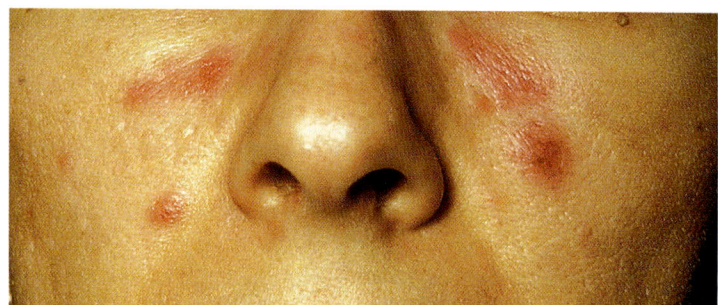

Fig. 51.45 Erythematous facial plaques in Kikuchi's disease.

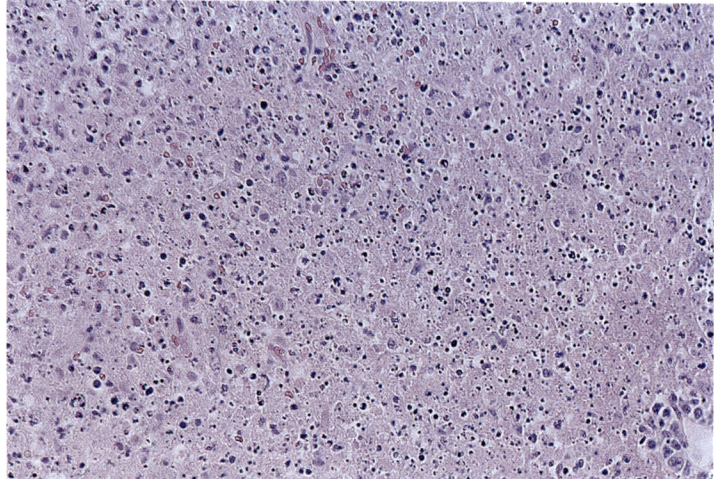

Fig. 51.46 Histiocytic necrotizing lymphadenitis (Kikuchi's disease). Lymph node. (Courtesy of Dr W. Merchant, Leeds General Infirmary, Leeds, UK.)

face (Fig. 51.45), and morbilliform, urticarial and rubella-like eruptions elsewhere. The oropharynx may be red or ulcerated.

Histology of the skin shows oedema of the papillary dermis, with a patchy perivascular infiltrate in the dermis and subcutaneous fat. The infiltrate consists of histiocytes containing nuclear debris, and small lymphocytes. The nuclei of the histiocytes may be deformed. The lymph nodes show focal or complete loss of follicular architecture, with necrosis of cortical and paracortical areas (Fig. 51.46). The extensive infiltrate consists of small lymphocytes, immunoblasts, macrophages and so-called plasmacytoid T cells [5]. Neutrophils are rarely seen, a feature that may help to distinguish this condition from SLE. The natural history is for spontaneous healing in a few months but it can be fatal as a result of heart failure brought about by microscopic myocardial necrosis [6]. There was a 3.3% recurrence rate in one series [7]. In most cases, no treatment is required, but a course of prednisolone may speed resolution. Various triggers have been incriminated, including the human herpesvirus 6 [8], parvovirus B19 [9], Epstein–Barr virus [5], dengue virus [10] and infection by *Yersinia enterocolitica*, *Toxoplasma*, cytomegalovirus and human immunodeficiency virus (HIV) [11], and rupture of a silicone breast implant [12]. The condition is occasionally associated with SLE. It may precede SLE [13], may be the presenting feature of SLE [14] and, rarely, SLE may precede it [15]. The association was found in two of 108 patients with Kikuchi's disease studied by Dorfman [16], and two of eight patients studied by El-Ramaki *et al.* [17]. It has occurred with DLE in a case encountered by the authors, and may be associated with other cutaneous manifestations of lupus [18]. Other associated conditions include Still's disease [19,20] and Sweet's syndrome [21]. In addition to SLE, the disorder can occur with lymphoma, tuberculous lymphadenitis, viral lymphadenitis, infectious mononucleosis and drug eruptions.

References

1 Kikuchi M. Lymphadenitis showing focal reticular cell hyperplasia with nuclear debris and phagocytes. *Acta Hem Jpn* 1972; **35**: 379–80.

2 Fujimoto Y, Kojima Y, Yamaguchi K. Cervical subacute necrotizing lymphadenitis. *Naika* 1972; **30**: 920–7.

3 Kuo T. Cutaneous manifestation of Kikuchi's histiocytic necrotizing lymphadenitis. *Am J Surg Pathol* 1990; **14**: 872–6.

4 Seno A, Torigoe R, Shimoe K *et al.* Kikuchi's disease (histiocytic necrotizing lymphadenitis) with cutaneous involvement. *J Am Acad Dermatol* 1994; **30**: 504–6.

5 Rivano MT, Falini B, Stein M *et al.* Histiocytic necrotizing lymphadenitis without granulocyte infiltration (Kikuchi lymphadenitis): morphological and immunohistochemical study of eight cases. *Histopathology* 1987; **11**: 1013–27.

6 Chan JK, Wong KC, Ng CS. A fatal case of multicentric Kikuchi's histiocytic necrotizing lymphadenitis. *Cancer* 1989; **63**: 1856–62.

7 Kuo TT. Kikuchi's disease (histiocytic necrotizing lymphadenitis): a clinicopathologic study of 79 cases with an analysis of histological subtypes, immunohistology, and DNA ploidy. *Am J Surg Pathol* 1995; **19**: 789–809.

8 Hoffmann A, Kirn E, Kuerteu A *et al.* Active human herpes virus-6 (HHV-6) infection associated with Kikuchi–Fujimoto disease and systemic lupus erythematosus (SLE). *In Vivo* 1991; **5**: 265–9.

9 Meyer O, Ribard P, Belmatoug N *et al.* Three cases of Kikuchi lymphadenitis in systemic lupus erythematosus: role of the parvovirus B19. *Ann Med Interne (Paris)* 1991; **142**: 259–64.

10 Harris VK, Danda D, Murali NS *et al.* Unusual association of Kikuchi's disease and dengue virus infection evolving into systemic lupus erythematosus. *J Indian Med Assoc* 2000; **98**: 391–3.

11 Bataille V, Harland CC, Behrens J *et al.* Kikuchi disease (histiocytic necrotizing lymphadenitis) in association with HTLV1. *Br J Dermatol* 1997; **136**: 610–2.

12 Sever CE, Leith CP, Appenzeller J, Foucar K. Kikuchi's histiocytic necrotizing lymphadenitis associated with ruptured silicone breast implant. *Arch Pathol Lab Med* 1996; **120**: 380–5.

13 Komocsi A, Tovari E, Pajor L, Czirjak L. Histiocytic necrotizing lymphadenitis preceding systemic lupus erythematosus. *J Eur Acad Dermatol Venereol* 2001; **15**: 476–80.

14 Dalkilic E, Karakoc Y, Tolunay S, Yurtkuran M. Systemic lupus erythematosus presenting as Kikuchi–Fujimoto disease. *Clin Exp Rheumatol* 2001; **19**: 226.

15 Tumiati B, Bellelli A, Portioli I *et al.* Kikuchi disease in systemic lupus erythematosus: an independent or dependent event? *Clin Rheumatol* 1991; **10**: 90–3.

16 Dorfman RF, Berry GJ. Kikuchi histiocytic necrotizing lymphadenitis: an analysis of 108 cases with emphasis on differential diagnosis. *Semin Diagn Pathol* 1988; **5**: 329–45.

17 El-Ramaki KM, Karran A, Ali MA. Kikuchi disease and its association with systemic lupus erythematosus. *Lupus* 1994; **3**: 409–11.

18 Kaur S, Thami GP, Kanawar AJ *et al.* Kikuchi's disease, skin and systemic lupus erythematosus. *Br J Dermatol* 2002; **146**: 167–8.

19 Ohta A, Matsumoto J, Ohta T *et al.* Still disease associated with necrotizing lymphadenitis (Kikuchi disease): report of 3 cases. *J Rheumatol* 1988; **15**: 981–3.

20 Lyberatos C. Two more cases of Still and Kikuchi. *J Rheumatol* 1990; **17**: 568–9.

21 Itoh H, Shimasaki S, Nakashima A *et al.* Sweet's syndrome associated with subacute necrotizing lymphadenitis. *Intern Med* 1992; **31**: 686–9.

Differential diagnosis. The conditions mentioned in the above section must be differentiated from LE. Many patients suspected of having a connective tissue disease may, even after investigation, present problems of categorization. The criteria for SLE of the ARA (1982) are shown in Table 51.9 [1]. The presence of four or more of the 11 manifestations, serially or simultaneously, is compatible with SLE (96% sensitive, 96% specific).

Other features, such as cutaneous LE lesions of any type, diffuse alopecia, involvement of the scalp or mucous membranes, preferably confirmed by histopathology, or direct immunofluorescence, may be helpful.

Several practical points are important. The ESR need not be elevated. In patients at Leeds, 15% followed up for at least 5 years have never had an ESR above 20 mm in the first hour. Several of these have had high titres of antinuclear factor, raised levels of anti-DNA antibodies and lowered serum complement. Diagnosis thus depends upon the association of features rather than on any specific abnormality. The demonstration of a high titre of antinuclear factor is important. In the acute phase, the membranous types of antinuclear factor may be present as well as a raised level of anti-DNA antibody, anti-Sm antibody and a reduction in the serum complement. In the authors' experience, the presence of antinuclear factor in high titre almost certainly excludes polyarteritis nodosa and other arteritic disorders. When a raised ESR, raised serum globulin, leukopenia and evidence of renal disease are added, the diagnosis becomes highly probable. It is important to remember that antinuclear factor is not always present in SLE, and in such cases alopecia, Raynaud's phenomenon and oral ulceration commonly occur [2]. The demonstration of immunoglobulins in the dermal–epidermal junction of uninvolved as well as involved skin may be very helpful (see p. 51.34). The combination of IgG and IgM at the dermal–epidermal junction of involved and uninvolved skin, raised DNA binding, antinuclear antibody in a titre of more than 1:64 and decreased C3 or C4 is highly suggestive of SLE [3]. In drug-induced LE, anti-DNA antibodies are absent, serum complement is normal and globulin is not found in the uninvolved skin. Acute febrile neutrophilic dermatosis (Sweet's syndrome) may mimic SLE when a 'butterfly rash' is associated with fever, myalgia, arthralgia, hepatosplenomegaly, renal disease and hyperglobulinaemia [4].

References

1 Tan EM, Cohen AS, Fries JF *et al.* The 1982 revised criteria for the classification of systemic lupus erythematosus. *Arthritis Rheum* 1982; **25**: 1271–7.

2 Fessel WJ. ANA-negative systemic lupus erythematosus. *Am J Med* 1970; **64**: 80–6.

3 Williams REA, O'Keefe R, MacKie RM *et al.* The contributions of direct immunofluorescence (DIF) to the diagnosis of lupus erythematosus. *Br J Dermatol* 1988; **119**: 520.

4 Frayha R, Matta M, Kurban A. Sweet's syndrome simulating systemic lupus erythematosus. *Dermatologica* 1972; **144**: 321–4.

Prognosis [1]. The course of SLE is very variable [2]. Acute fulminating cases are much less common than subacute cases, which smoulder on for many years. Mortality rates declined in both England and Wales in the 10-year period 1974–83 [3] and in the USA [4]. Although, in pre-steroid days, 52% of patients in one series [5] died within 2 years, in another series 54% of patients survived 11 years [6], compared with controls, of whom 97% survived a similar time. In 1977, an overall 5-year survival of 91% was reported [7], and 98% in another series in 1978 [8], although a 5-year survival of only 88% was reported from a rheumatological clinic in 1990 [9]. Approximately three-quarters will now survive

15 years [10]. Survival is related to organ involvement and to frequency of exacerbations [11]. Of those without renal involvement, 84% survive 15 years, compared with 57% whose kidneys are affected [10]. Spontaneous remissions, sometimes lasting 10–20 years, occurred in 35% of Dubois and Tuffanelli's [12] patients, the longest being 26 years. Serological as well as clinical remission occurred in 4% of 305 patients [13]. Exacerbations are more frequent in the first 5 years of the disease [14]. Pregnancy does not affect long-term survival. Prolonged survival is associated with an increased risk of atherosclerosis, avascular necrosis and neuropsychiatric dysfunction [15]. In elderly people the presentation is insidious and the clinical course is relatively benign. Renal disease and serological abnormalities are less frequent, and arthritis, with subcutaneous nodules, and pleuropericarditis are more prominent in elderly people [16].

The better prognosis of the more recent series is a result, not only of the administration of corticosteroids, but also of earlier diagnosis, the avoidance of stress and drugs such as sulphonamides, and the control of infections by antibiotics. The cause of death is frequently progressive renal failure, occasionally with anuria. Secondary infection, particularly bronchopneumonia, was a much more common cause of death in the pre-antibiotic era, although infection may still be more important than renal failure. The high infection rate is not caused solely by steroid [17] or antimetabolite therapy. Spontaneous peritonitis caused by Gram-positive bacteria is a complication of lupus nephritis treated with corticosteroids [18]. Unusual infections such as pneumococcal epiglottitis have been reported [19]. There is an increased risk of *Salmonella* bacteraemia [20] and rapidly fatal pneumococcal septicaemia [21]. Repeated skin infections may be a presenting feature. Cellulitis of the periorbital area caused by *Staphylococcus aureus* and group A haemolytic streptococci has been reported [22,23]. Neisserial infections may also occur [24]. Death may result from vasculitis of the CNS in patients presenting with convulsions, psychoses and paralysis. Patients with CNS lesions and psychosis have a poor prognosis. Deaths from CNS involvement become more important in the later stages of the disease [25]. Others may die from heart failure or the side effects of therapy [26].

A bimodal pattern of mortality has been described [27], but not confirmed, in black patients [28]. Patients who die early in the disease die from active LE, including renal involvement, receive large doses of steroids and have a high incidence of infection. Those who die later have relatively inactive disease, long duration of steroid therapy and a high incidence of atherosclerotic heart disease and myocardial infarction [11]. Nevertheless, it is the authors' experience that death from infection is common, even in long-standing cases. The maximum disease activity occurs early, and patients rarely develop new organ involvement after the first few years [8,14]. Late reactivation of SLE can occur [29].

Although the disease is much more common in females, the prognosis is worse in males [30–33]. Males are more likely to develop renal failure [34]. Although race and ethnic origin have been claimed not to influence prognosis [35], increased mortality has been noted in Asians [36] and black people [37], probably in part because of socioeconomic conditions. The degree of renal involvement is probably the most important factor in prognosis.

Patients with nephrotic syndrome at the onset of nephritis do badly and may die within a few months, but development later in the disease does not have an adverse effect. Patients with albuminuria may survive on small doses of steroids for many years, and the overall prognosis of patients with renal involvement is not as bad as early studies suggested. Patients with cutaneous lesions of DLE and laboratory abnormalities have the same prognosis as uncomplicated cases of DLE [38]. Patients with arteritis, antiphospholipid syndrome, thrombocytopenia, haemolytic anaemia and CNS involvement have a poorer prognosis than those whose illness mainly involves the joints. There appears to be no increased risk of malignancy [39], although earlier reports suggested this might be so [40,41].

References

1 Bresnihan B. Outcome and survival in systemic lupus erythematosus. *Ann Rheum Dis* 1989; **48**: 443–5.

2 Ropes MW. *Systemic Lupus Erythematosus.* Cambridge: Harvard University Press, 1976.

3 Hochberg MC. Mortality from systemic lupus erythematosus in England and Wales, 1974–83. *Br J Rheumatol* 1987; **26**: 437–41.

4 Ginzler E, Berg A. Mortality in systemic lupus erythematosus. *J Rheumatol* 1987; **14**: 218–22.

5 Bywaters EGL, Bauer W. (Quoted by Bywaters EGL, Scott TJ. 1939.) In: Dixon A StJ, ed. *Progress in Clinical Rheumatology.* London: Churchill, 1965: 132.

6 Kellum RE, Haserick JR. Systemic lupus erythematosus. *Arch Intern Med* 1964; **113**: 200–7.

7 Lee P, Urowitz MB, Bookman AAM *et al.* Systemic lupus erythematosus. *QJM* 1977; **46**: 1–32.

8 Grigor R, Edmonds J, Lewkonia R *et al.* Systemic lupus erythematosus. *Ann Rheum Dis* 1978; **37**: 121–8.

9 Worrall JG, Snaith ML, Batchelor JR, Isenberg DA. SLE: a rheumatological view. Analysis of the clinical features, serology, and immunogenetics of 100 SLE patients during long-term follow-up. *QJM* 1990; **74**: 319–30.

10 Wallace DJ, Podell T, Weiner J *et al.* Systemic lupus erythematosus survival patterns. *JAMA* 1981; **245**: 934–8.

11 Swaak AJG, Nossent JC, Bronsveld W *et al.* Systemic lupus erythematosus. I. Outcome and survival: Dutch experience with 110 patients studied prospectively. *Ann Rheum Dis* 1989; **48**: 447–54.

12 Dubois EL, Tuffanelli DL. Clinical manifestations of systemic lupus erythematosus. *JAMA* 1964; **190**: 104–11.

13 Heller CA, Schur PH. Serological and clinical remission in systemic lupus erythematosus. *J Rheumatol* 1985; **12**: 916–8.

14 Swaak AJG, Nossent JC, Bronsvel W *et al.* Systemic lupus erythematosus. II. Observations on the occurrence of exacerbations in the disease course: Dutch experience with 110 patients studied prospectively. *Ann Rheum Dis* 1989; **48**: 455–60.

15 Gladman DD, Urowitz MB. Morbidity in systemic lupus erythematosus. *J Rheumatol* 1987; **14**: 223–6.

16 Wilson HA, Hamilton ME, Spyker DA *et al.* Age influence on the clinical and serologic expression of systemic lupus erythematosus. *Arthritis Rheum* 1981; **24**: 1230–5.

17 Staples PJ, Gerding DN, Decker JL *et al.* Incidence of infection in systemic lupus erythematosus. *Arthritis Rheum* 1974; **17**: 1–10.

18 Lipsky PE, Hardin JA, Schour L *et al.* Spontaneous peritonitis and systemic lupus erythematosus. *JAMA* 1975; **232**: 929–31.

19 Shalit M, Gross DJ, Levo V. Pneumococcal epiglottitis in systemic lupus erythematosus on high-dosage corticosteroids. *Ann Rheum Dis* 1982; **41**: 615–6.

20 Abramson S, Kramer SB, Radin A *et al.* Salmonella bacteremia in systemic lupus erythematosus. *Arthritis Rheum* 1985; **28**: 75–9.

21 Van Der Straeten C, Wei N, Rothschild J *et al.* Rapidly fatal pneumococcal septicaemia in systemic lupus erythematosus. *J Rheumatol* 1987; **14**: 1177–80.

22 Derksen RHWM, Overbeek BP, Poeschmann PH. Serious bacterial cellulitis of the periorbital area in two patients with systemic lupus erythematosus. *J Rheumatol* 1988; **15**: 840–4.

23 Rebora A, Scala D, Paneaglio E *et al.* Repeated skin infections as a manifestation of lupus erythematosus. *Arch Dermatol* 1982; **118**: 213–4.

24 Mitchell SR, Nguyen PQ, Katz P. Increased risk of Neisserial infections in systemic lupus erythematosus. *Semin Arthritis Rheum* 1990; **20**: 174–84.

25 Cheatum DE, Hurd ER, Strunk SW *et al.* Renal histology and clinical course of systemic lupus erythematosus. *Arthritis Rheum* 1973; **16**: 670–6.

26 Feng PH, Cheah PS, Lee YK. Mortality in systemic lupus erythematosus. *BMJ* 1973; **iv**: 772–4.

27 Urowitz MB, Bookman AAM, Koehler BE *et al.* The bimodal mortality pattern of systemic lupus erythematosus. *Am J Med* 1976; **60**: 221–5.

28 Harisdangkul V, Nilganuwonge S, Rockhold L. Cause of death in systemic lupus erythematosus: a pattern based on age at onset. *South Med J* 1987; **80**: 1249–53.

29 Urowitz MB, Gladman DD. Late mortality in SLE. *J Rheumatol* 1980; **7**: 412–6.

30 Rubin LA, Urowitz MB, Gladman DD. Mortality in systemic lupus erythematosus: the bimodal pattern revisited. *QJM* 1985; **216**: 87–98.

31 Fries JF, Holman HR. Systemic lupus erythematosus. *J Invest Dermatol* 1976; **67**: 554–5.

32 Kaufman LD, Gomez-Reino JJ, Keinicke MH. Male lupus: retrospective analysis of the clinical and laboratory features of 52 patients with a review of the literature. *Semin Arthritis Rheum* 1989; **18**: 189–97.

33 Folomeer M, Alekberova Z. Survival pattern of 120 males with systemic lupus erythematosus. *J Rheumatol* 1990; **17**: 856–7.

34 Zimmerman SW. Survival patterns in systemic lupus erythematosus. *JAMA* 1981; **246**: 2323.

35 Ginzler EM, Diamond HS, Weiner M *et al.* A multicentre study of outcome in systemic lupus erythematosus. *Arthritis Rheum* 1982; **25**: 601–11.

36 Kaslow RA. High rate of death caused by systemic lupus erythematosus among US residents of Asian descent. *Arthritis Rheum* 1982; **25**: 414–8.

37 Gordon MF, Stolley PD, Schinnar R. Trends in recent systemic lupus erythematosus mortality rates. *Arthritis Rheum* 1981; **24**: 762–9.

38 Beck JS, Rowell NR. Discoid lupus erythematosus. *QJM* 1966; **35**: 119–36.

39 Rosner SM, Ginzler EM, Diamond HS *et al.* A multicenter study of outcome in systemic lupus erythematosus. *Arthritis Rheum* 1982; **25**: 612–7.

40 Canoso JJ, Cohen AS. Malignancy in a series of 70 patients with systemic lupus erythematosus. *Arthritis Rheum* 1974; **17**: 383–90.

41 Lewis RB, Castor CW, Kuisley RE *et al.* Frequency of neoplasia in systemic lupus erythematosus and rheumatoid arthritis. *Arthritis Rheum* 1976; **19**: 1256–60.

Genetic counselling. The clinical genetics of lupus has been reviewed [1]. Approximately 5% of first-degree relatives of patients may have or may develop lupus. The risk is doubled if there are two affected first-degree relatives, and this risk is even greater if further family members are affected. The risk for female relatives is greater than for males and may also be increased for those with hyperglobulinaemia or antinuclear antibodies. Mothers with anti-Ro and anti-La antibodies may have children with neonatal lupus and heart block. When a child has neonatal lupus or CHB, the risk of a subsequent child having heart block is approximately 25%.

Reference
1 Lewkonia SM. The clinical genetics of lupus. *Lupus* 1992; **1**: 55–62.

Treatment [1]. The aim is to try to maintain optimal function with the minimum of therapy. SLE is an episodic disease, and treatment must be tailored to the patient's requirements and morale must be maintained. In acute cases, and during severe exacerbations, bed rest is required. Undue exposure to the sun should be avoided and patients should be advised to wear broad-brimmed hats, to cover the 'V' of the neck and the arms, and to use a sunscreen. Mental stress, physical overexertion and secondary infection should be avoided.

Hypertension must be treated aggressively and diuretics may be required for the nephrotic syndrome or cardiac failure, and anticonvulsants for epilepsy. Chlorpromazine is a good sedative for psychosis. Symptomatic therapy for joint pain using NSAIDs is valuable. Ischaemic necrosis of bone may be best treated early by core decompression [2].

Corticosteroids are required in acute cases, and should be given in adequate regimens. Prednisolone in doses up to 60 mg/day is the steroid of choice initially. It is rare for higher dosage to be needed. Once the condition appears to be under control, the dosage may be reduced gradually, until a maintenance dosage of approximately 5–15 mg/day is reached. A single dose daily, given in the morning [3], produces fewer side effects and does not impair the therapeutic response.

Not all patients require steroids, especially if there is no internal organ involvement [1]. It is important to assess the patient's progress by their general well-being and relief of symptoms, rather than by strict attention to laboratory abnormalities [4]. The ESR and DNA antibodies are variable and a poor guide to the adequacy of therapy; the titre of antinuclear antibodies often persists unchanged despite clinical remission. Anti-DNA antibody and serum complement levels may be helpful in predicting exacerbations [5]. Low C3 often indicates severe renal disease. There is some evidence that a return of serological abnormalities to normal is followed by a prolonged remission [6], but exceptions indicate that serological data alone cannot be used as a basis of therapy.

Some fulminating cases have been treated with massive doses of steroids but the advantages of such therapy rarely outweigh the risks, and complications such as steroid-induced psychosis can occur even in patients with CNS disease [7]. Prolonged high dosage of corticosteroids (e.g. prednisolone 60 mg/day for 6 months) is said to improve renal lesions more than small suppressive doses [8], but more aggressive immunosuppressive regimens are now preferred. Steroid myopathy can occur with high doses and is easily missed.

In mild cases, the administration of chloroquine or hydroxychloroquine may allow the dosage of steroids to be reduced, but the reduction may not be clinically meaningful [9]. Antimalarials are less useful than in DLE, but may have a place in patients with photosensitivity. Their use does not preclude pregnancy, as healthy live babies have been delivered by women on antimalarial therapy throughout pregnancy [10].

Immunosuppressive drugs have been used for patients not responding to corticosteroids, or to act as steroid-sparing agents [11]. The role of azathioprine is accepted, but at least some studies show that it adds nothing to high-dose prednisolone treatment in mild or moderate renal disease [12]. Another controlled trial, comparing azathioprine plus prednisolone with prednisolone alone, did not show any significant difference in the number of deaths, renal or extrarenal manifestations, serum complement levels, DNA antibodies, LE cells, antinuclear antibody titres, or Coombs' antibodies, or any evidence of a steroid-sparing effect [13]. Sudden withdrawal may be followed by relapse [14]. Cyclophosphamide is useful in SLE [15,16], although not all support routine use. Nevertheless, pulsed therapy with cyclophosphamide may be useful for renal disease and is as effective as pulsed methylprednisolone [17].

Chlorambucil has been used [18], but methotrexate is now a more widely accepted drug in SLE. Methotrexate 7.5 mg/week has improved steroid-resistant patients [19] and patients without renal or CNS involvement [20], and 10–20 mg/week is useful for mucocutaneous lesions [21].

The long-term risk of malignancy must be considered whenever immunosuppressive drugs are used. Cyclophosphamide has been associated with bladder cancer [22], acute non-lymphocytic leukaemia and solid tumours. Mesna may reduce urotoxic side effects, but 50% of patients develop rashes which may be confused with an exacerbation of SLE [23]. Reticulum cell sarcoma [24] and non-Hodgkin's lymphoma [25] are hazards of azathioprine therapy.

Ciclosporin has been used in resistant cases in a dosage of 3–5 mg/kg [26]. Pulse therapy with methylprednisolone 1 g given intravenously in 500 ml normal saline over 4 h on 3 successive days to in-patients may be helpful in individuals who are not controlled by oral prednisolone and immunosuppressives [27]. Given monthly it may prevent deterioration in renal function in patients with nephritis [28]. Mycophenolate mofetil has been used for non-renal SLE [29], and alternatives to cyclophosphamide as a modifier of B cell function have been found to be increasingly useful. Rituximab, an antibody targeting the CD20 marker antigen of B cell precursors, has been valuable for those in whom conventional therapy has failed [30].

Plasmapheresis of 2 L/day for 3–4 days each week over a period of 2–3 weeks may be helpful in a small number of patients with a high level of immune complexes, whose condition is deteriorating despite other therapy, but controlled trials have not been convincing [31]. Any benefit lasts only approximately 2–3 weeks. Plasmapheresis may be useful in managing life-threatening complications such as fulminating vasculitis or CNS disease [32]. Intravenous gammaglobulin 1 g/kg/day for 3 days improved four out of five patients. The effect lasts 4–6 weeks [33]. Provisional studies of extracorporeal photochemotherapy have shown improvement in a few patients, and treatment was not associated with any side effects [34]. Anticoagulants may be required for patients with lupus anticoagulant or anticardiolipin antibodies who have thrombotic episodes. Danazol 400–600 mg/day may help patients with premenstrual exacerbations [35], and sometimes has a marked effect on thrombocytopenia [36]. Oral levamisole, in a dosage of 150 mg three times daily has been found helpful by some [37], but not by others [38]. Antilymphocyte and antithymocyte antisera may help patients with nephritis not responding to either corticosteroids or azathioprine [39].

A new and surprising therapeutic approach is that although UV light can exacerbate SLE, it has been found in a controlled trial that exposure to UVA-1 (340–400 mm) at a dosage of 60 kJ/m^2 three times weekly reduced disease activity, reduced the need for medication and decreased antibody levels [40]. A low-fat, high marine oil diet (eicosapentaenoic acid: Maxepa 20 g/day) modified disease activity in 27 patients in a placebo-controlled trial over 3 months [41].

Some patients with cutaneous disease as their main form of disease expression will require specific treatment as for DLE. In these patients, dapsone may be helpful for urticarial lesions [42], bullous eruptions [43] and for thrombocytopenia [44].

References

1 Vasoo S, Hughes GR. Theory, targets and therapy in systemic lupus erythematosus. *Lupus* 2005; **14**: 181–8.

2 Hungerford DS, Zizic TM. The treatment of ischemic necrosis of bone in systemic lupus erythematosus. *Medicine* 1980; **59**: 143–8.

3 Ackerman GL, Nolan CM. Adrenocortical responsiveness after alternate-day corticosteroid therapy. *N Engl J Med* 1968; **278**: 405–9.

4 Rowell NR. Laboratory abnormalities in the diagnosis and management of lupus erythematosus. *Br J Dermatol* 1971; **84**: 210–6.

5 Swaak AJG, Groenwold J, Bronsveld W. Predictive value of complement profiles and anti-dsDNA in systemic lupus erythematosus. *Ann Rheum Dis* 1986; **45**: 359–66.

6 Lightfoot RW Jr, Hughes GRV. Significance of persisting serologic abnormalities in SLE. *Arthritis Rheum* 1976; **19**: 837–43.

7 Hirohata S, Iwamoto S, Mayamoto T et al. A patient with SLE presenting with both CNS lupus and steroid-induced psychosis. *J Rheumatol* 1988; **15**: 706–10.

8 Pollak VE, Pirani CL, Schwartz FD. The natural history of the renal manifestations of systemic lupus erythematosus. *J Lab Clin Med* 1964; **63**: 537–50.

9 Rothfield N. Efficacy of antimalarials in systemic lupus erythematosus. *Am J Med* 1988; **85**: 53–6.

10 Parke L. Antimalarial drugs, systemic lupus erythematosus and pregnancy. *J Rheumatol* 1988; **15**: 607–10.

11 Sabbour MS, Osman LM. Comparison of chlorambucil, azathioprine or cyclophosphamide combined with corticosteroids in the treatment of lupus nephritis. *Br J Dermatol* 1979; **100**: 113–25.

12 Donadio JV, Holley KE, Wagoner RD et al. Further observations on the treatment of lupus nephritis with prednisone and combined prednisone and azathioprine. *Arthritis Rheum* 1974; **17**: 573–81.

13 Hahn BH, Kantor OS, Osterland CK. Azathioprine plus prednisone compared with prednisone alone in the treatment of systemic lupus erythematosus. *Ann Intern Med* 1975; **83**: 597–605.

14 Sharon E, Kaplan D, Diamond HS. Exacerbation of systemic lupus erythematosus after withdrawal of azathioprine therapy. *N Engl J Med* 1973; **288**: 122–4.

15 Ioannou Y, Isenberg DA. Current concepts for the management of systemic lupus erythematosus in adults: a therapeutic challenge. *Postgrad Med J* 2002; **78**: 599–606.

16 Karim MY, Pisoni CN, Khamashta MA. Update on immunotherapy for systemic lupus erythematosus—what's hot and what's not! *Rheumatology (Oxford)* 2009; **48**: 332–41.

17 Sesso R, Monteiro M, Sato E et al. A controlled trial of pulse cyclophosphamide versus pulse methylprednisolone in severe lupus nephritis. *Lupus* 1994; **3**: 107–12.

18 Snaith ML, Holt JM, Oliver DO et al. Treatment of patients with systemic lupus erythematosus, including nephritis, with chlorambucil. *BMJ* 1973; **ii**: 197–201.

19 Wilke WS, Krall PL, Scheetz RJ et al. Methotrexate for systemic lupus erythematosus: a retrospective analysis of 17 unselected cases. *Clin Exp Rheumatol* 1991; **9**: 581–7.

20 Gansauge S, Breitbart A, Rinaldi N et al. Methotrexate in patients with moderate systemic lupus erythematosus (exclusion of renal and central nervous system disease). *Ann Rheum Dis* 1997; **56**: 382–5.

21 Bottomley WW, Goodfield MJD. Methotrexate for the treatment of severe mucocutaneous lupus erythematosus. *Br J Dermatol* 1995; **133**: 311–4.

22 Chow SK, Looi LM, Loh CS, Yeap SS. Cyclophosphamide-induced transitional cell carcinoma of bladder in lupus nephritis. *Int Med J* 2002; **32**: 114–6.

23 Zonzito E, Aberer W, Tappeiner G. Drug reactions from Mesna. *Arch Dermatol* 1992; **128**: 80–3.

24 Hehir ME, Sewell JR, Hughes GR. Reticulum cell sarcoma in azathioprine-treated systemic lupus erythematosus. *Ann Rheum Dis* 1979; **38**: 94–5.

25 Pitt PI, Sultan AH, Malone M et al. Association between azathioprine therapy and lymphoma in rheumatoid disease. *J R Soc Med* 1987; **80**: 428–9.

26 Manger K, Kalden JR, Manger B. Cyclosporin A in the treatment of systemic lupus erythematosus: results of an open clinical study. *Br J Rheumatol* 1996; **35**: 669–75.

27 Isenberg DA, Morrow WJW, Snaith ML. Methyl prednisolone pulse therapy in the treatment of systemic lupus erythematosus. *Ann Rheum Dis* 1982; **41**: 347–51.

28 Liebling MR, McLaughlin K, Boonsue S et al. Monthly pulses of methyl prednisolone in SLE nephritis. *J Rheumatol* 1982; **9**: 543–8.

29 Mok CC. Mycophenolate mofetil for non-renal manifestations of systemic lupus erythematosus: a systematic review. *Scand J Rheumatol* 2007; **36**: 329–37.

30 Ramos-Casals M, Brito-Zerón P, Muñoz S *et al*. A systematic review of the off-label use of biological therapies in systemic autoimmune diseases. *Medicine (Baltimore)* 2008; **87**: 345–64.

31 Wei N, Huston DP, Lawley TJ *et al*. Randomized trial of plasma exchange in mild systemic lupus erythematosus. *Lancet* 1983; **i**: 17–21.

32 Wallace DJ. Plasmapheresis in lupus. *Lupus* 1993; **2**: 141–3.

33 Winder A, Molad Y, Ostfeld I *et al*. Treatment of systemic lupus erythematosus by prolonged administration of high-dose intravenous immunoglobulin: a report of two cases. *J Rheumatol* 1993; **20**: 495–8.

34 Knobler RM, Graninger W, Graninger W *et al*. Extracorporeal phototherapy for the treatment of systemic lupus erythematosus: a pilot study. *Arthritis Rheum* 1992; **35**: 319–24.

35 Morley KD, Parke A, Hughes GRV. Systemic lupus erythematosus. *BMJ* 1982; **284**: 1431–2.

36 West SG, Johnson SC. Danazol for the treatment of refractory autoimmune thrombocytopenia in systemic lupus erythematosus. *Ann Intern Med* 1988; **108**: 703–6.

37 Rovensky J, Cebecauer L, Zitnan D *et al*. Levamisole treatment of systemic lupus erythematosus. *Arthritis Rheum* 1982; **25**: 470–1.

38 Hadidi T, Decker JL, El-Nagdy L *et al*. Ineffectiveness of levamisole in systemic lupus erythematosus. *Arthritis Rheum* 1981; **24**: 60–3.

39 Pirofsky B, Bardana EJ, Bayracki C *et al*. Antilymphocyte antisera in immunological mediated renal disease. *JAMA* 1969; **210**: 1059–64.

40 McGrath H Jr, Martinez-Osuna P, Lee FA. Ultraviolet-A1 (340–400 nm) irradiation therapy in systemic lupus erythematosus. *Lupus* 1996; **5**: 269–74.

41 Walton AJE, Snaith ML, Locniskar M *et al*. Dietary fish oil and the severity of symptoms in patients with systemic lupus erythematosus. *Ann Rheum Dis* 1991; **50**: 463–6.

42 Ruzicka T, Goerz A. Dapsone in the treatment of lupus erythematosus. *Br J Dermatol* 1981; **104**: 53–6.

43 Hall RP, Lawley TJ, Smith HR *et al*. Bullous eruption of systemic lupus erythematosus. *Ann Intern Med* 1982; **97**: 165–70.

44 Moss C, Hamilton PJ. Thrombocytopenia in systemic lupus erythematosus responsive to dapsone. *BMJ* 1988; **297**: 266.

Table 51.15 Clinical features associated with the lupus anticoagulant.

Libman–Sacks endocarditis [15]
Chorea [16]
Labile hypertension
Epilepsy
Myelitis
Myocardial infarction
Valvular heart disease
Haemolytic anaemia
Retinopathy [17]
Addison's disease [18]
Avascular necrosis of bone [19]

The features associated with the lupus anticoagulant are caused by an acquired immunoglobulin (IgG or IgM), identified by prolonged activated partial thromboplastin and kaolin clotting times, which cannot be corrected by normal plasma. There may also be IgA antiphospholipid antibodies [12]. There are now a number of methods for detecting the abnormalities, and these have been reviewed [13]. The antibodies are directed against a range of phospholipids, including cardiolipin. The route by which thrombosis is induced remains unclear, but some antiphospholipid antibodies interact with a complex of phospholipid and β_2-glycoprotein-I to inhibit factor XII activation, platelet activation and prothrombinase activity [14].

Clinical features. The clinical features of the syndrome associated with the presence of the lupus anticoagulant are protean, and many are shown in Table 51.15. Rarely, patients develop vascular occlusions in multiple organs [20]. This catastrophic variety may be fatal. There is also a syndrome in which a severe reduction in clotting occurs because of a different set of antiphospholipid antibodies—the haemorrhagic lupus anticoagulant syndrome [21].

Cutaneous lesions [22] include thrombophlebitis, purpura and ecchymoses, livedo reticularis, leg ulcers, cutaneous necrosis, gangrene and subungual splinter haemorrhages. Histologically, non-inflammatory thrombosis of small dermal blood vessels can be demonstrated, but necrotizing vasculitis is not a feature [23]. Thromboses in the placenta lead to fetal death, and may recur in subsequent pregnancies. Thrombocytopenia also occurs. All women with SLE who have recurrent abortions and thrombotic episodes, or who are biological false-positive reactors, should be screened for the lupus anticoagulant, as treatment with prednisone 40–80 mg/day and aspirin 75 mg/day may result in successful pregnancy. One patient with repeated fetal loss was successfully treated with intravenous human gammaglobulin [24]. Full anticoagulation (international normalized ratio (INR) greater than 3), with or without aspirin, appears to be the most effective therapy in the non-pregnant patient [25]. The presence of the antibodies without clinical features is not an indication for either steroid therapy or anticoagulation.

The lupus anticoagulant, anticardiolipin antibodies and the antiphospholipid antibody syndrome [1]

The lupus anticoagulant was first described in SLE [2], but it also occurs in drug-induced SLE, other connective tissue diseases, polymyalgia rheumatica/giant cell arteritis (where 40–50% of patients may have antibodies [3]) and carcinoma and lymphoma [4]. It may be induced by infection, including that caused by Epstein–Barr virus [5] and varicella [6]. It also occurs as the causative abnormality of the primary antiphospholipid (Hughes') syndrome [7], although a small proportion of those classified as having the primary syndrome will progress to lupus or a lupus-like syndrome [8].

The lupus anticoagulant is only one of several antiphospholipid antibodies, which include the anticardiolipin antibody demonstrated by ELISA. IgG anticardiolipin antibody has been found in 23% of patients with SLE [9], and is associated with similar clinical features to those seen with the lupus anticoagulant [10]. The presence and titre seem to depend on disease activity and decrease with treatment, particularly when of IgM type. In a study of healthy blood donors, anticardiolipin antibodies and the lupus anticoagulant were found in 4–6% of 499 donors, mainly young females [11].

References

1 Wilson WA, Gharavi AE, Piette JC. International classification criteria for antiphospholipid syndrome: synopsis of a post-conference workshop held at the Ninth International (Tours) aPL Symposium. *Lupus* 2001; **10**: 457–60.

2 Boey ML, Colaco CB, Gharavi AE *et al.* Thrombosis in systemic lupus erythematosus. *BMJ* 1983; **287**: 1021–3.

3 Espinoza LR, Jara LJ, Silveira LH *et al.* Anticardiolipin antibodies in polymyalgia rheumatica–giant cell arteritis: association with severe vascular complications. *Am J Med* 1991; **90**: 474–8.

4 Shaw BE, Perry D, Hoffbrand AV. Progressive arterial thrombosis in a patient with non-Hodgkin's lymphoma, a lupus anticoagulant, factor V Leiden mutation and paraprotein, following chemotherapy. *Leuk Lymphoma* 2001; **42**: 221–3.

5 Shiomou K, Galanakis E, Tzoufi M *et al.* Transient lupus anticoagulant and prolonged activated partial thromboplastin time secondary to Epstein–Barr virus infection. *Scand J Infect Dis* 2002; **34**: 67–9.

6 Kurogol Z, Vardar F, Ozkinay F *et al.* Lupus anticoagulant and protein S deficiency in otherwise healthy children with acute varicella infection. *Acta Paediatr* 2000; **89**: 1186–9.

7 Ames PRJ, Khamashta MA, Hughes GRV. Clinical and therapeutic aspects of the antiphospholipid syndrome. *Lupus* 1995; **4** (Suppl. 1): S23–5.

8 Mujic F, Cuadrado MJ, Lloyd M *et al.* Primary antiphospholipid syndrome evolving into systemic lupus erythematosus. *J Rheumatol* 1995; **22**: 1589–92.

9 McHugh NJ, Maymo J, Skinner RP *et al.* Anticardiolipin antibodies, livedo reticularis, and major cerebrovascular and renal disease in systemic lupus erythematosus. *Ann Rheum Dis* 1988; **47**: 110–5.

10 Laskin CA, Clark CA, Spitzer KA. Antiphospholipid syndrome in systemic lupus erythematosus: is the whole greater than the sum of the parts? *Rheum Dis Clin North Am* 2005; **31**: 255–72.

11 Shi W, Krilis SA, Chong BH *et al.* Prevalence of lupus anticoagulant and anticardiolipin antibodies in a healthy population. *Aust NZ J Med* 1990; **20**: 231–6.

12 Bertolaccini ML, Atsumi T, Escudero-Contreras A *et al.* The value of IgA antiphospholipid testing for diagnosis of antiphospholipid (Hughes) syndrome in systemic lupus erythematosus. *J Rheumatol* 2001; **28**: 2637–43.

13 Bertolaccini ML, Hughes GR. Antiphospholipid antibody testing: which are the most useful for diagnosis? *Rheum Dis Clin North Am* 2006; **32**: 455–63.

14 Pierangeli SS, Chen PP, Gonzalez EB. Antiphospholipid antibodies and the antiphospholipid syndrome: an update on treatment and pathogenic mechanisms. *Curr Opin Hematol* 2006; **13**: 366–75.

15 Ford PM, Ford SE, Lillicrap DP. Association of lupus anticoagulant with severe valvular heart disease in systemic lupus erythematosus. *J Rheumatol* 1988; **15**: 597–600.

16 Hatron P-Y, Bouchez B, Wattel A *et al.* Chorea, systemic lupus erythematosus, circulating lupus anticoagulant. *J Rheumatol* 1986; **13**: 991–3.

17 Acheson JF, Gregson RMC, Merry P, Schulenburg WE. Vaso-occlusive retinopathy in the primary anti-phospholipid antibody syndrome. *Eye* 1991; **5**: 48–55.

18 Hughes GRV. The antiphospholipid syndrome: 10 years on. *Lancet* 1993; **342**: 341–4.

19 Mok MY, Farewell VT, Isenberg DA *et al.* Risk factors for avascular necrosis of bone in patients with systemic lupus erythematosus: is there a role for antiphospholipid antibodies? *Ann Rheum Dis* 2000; **59**: 462–7.

20 Asherson RA. The catastrophic antiphospholipid syndrome. *J Rheumatol* 1992; **19**: 508–12.

21 Schmugge M, Tolle S, Marbet GA *et al.* Gingival bleeding, epistaxis and haematoma three days after gastroenteritis: the haemorrhagic lupus anticoagulant syndrome. *Eur J Pediatr* 2001; **160**: 43–6.

22 Asherson RA, Frances C, Iaccurino L *et al.* The antiphospholipid syndrome: diagnosis, skin manifestations and current therapy. *Clin Exp Rheumatol* 2006; **24**: 846–51.

23 Alegre VA, Winkelmann RK. Histopathologic and immunofluorescence study of skin lesions associated with circulating lupus anticoagulant. *J Am Acad Dermatol* 1988; **19**: 117–24.

24 Carreras LO, Perez GN, Vega HR *et al.* Lupus anticoagulant and recurrent fetal loss: successful treatment with gammaglobulin. *Lancet* 1988; **ii**: 393–4.

25 Ruiz-Irastorza G, Khamashta MA, Hunt BJ *et al.* Bleeding and recurrent thrombosis in definite antiphospholipid syndrome: analysis of a series of 66 patients treated with oral anticoagulation to a target international normalized ratio of 3:5. *Arch Intern Med* 2002; **27**: 1164–9.

Scleroderma [1]

Sclerosis of the skin occurs in a variety of conditions, such as dermatomyositis and LE, and invariably occurs as part of the cutaneous manifestations of systemic sclerosis, which is described elsewhere. However, the term 'scleroderma' should strictly be confined to sclerosis of the skin, either localized or generalized, occurring in patients as the only or prominent feature. In such circumstances it is better to use the term 'morphoea'. There has been much discussion and confusion about the relationship of morphoea to systemic sclerosis (see below), but the two conditions, despite certain similarities, are best considered as distinct entities.

Reference

1 Jablonska S. The concept of scleroderma and its classification. In: Jablonska S, ed. *Scleroderma and Pseudoscleroderma*. Warsaw: Polish Medical Publishers, 1975: 3–10.

Localized morphoea

Synonyms
- Localized scleroderma
- Circumscribed scleroderma

Definition. A disorder of unknown cause in which there is localized sclerosis of the skin. The condition has traditionally been subdivided clinically into the following types [1]:

1 Circumscribed plaques
2 Morphoea profundus/subcutaneous (deep)
3 Bullous morphoea
4 Linear morphoea
5 Frontoparietal lesions (en coup de sabre), with or without hemiatrophy of the face.

It is apparent, however, that there is sometimes overlap between these types, this occurring in up to 15% of cases in children [2]. Recently, a new classification for childhood localized scleroderma has been proposed, to include circumscribed morphoea (superficial and deep), linear scleroderma (trunk/limbs and head), generalized morphoea, pansclerotic morphoea and mixed morphoea [3].

Although some conditions, such as atrophoderma of Pasini and Pierini, eosinophilic fasciitis and lichen sclerosus, are sometimes included in the classification of morphoea, this is not widely accepted [2].

References

1 Peterson LS, Nelson AM, Su WP. Classification of morphoea (localized scleroderma). *Mayo Clin Proc* 1995; **70**: 1068–76.

2 Laxer RM, Zulian F. Localized scleroderma. *Curr Opin Rheumatol* 2006; **18**: 606–13.

3 Zulian F, Martini G. Preliminary classification criteria for juvenile systemic sclerosis. In: Zulian F, Ruperto N, eds. *Proceedings of the II Workshop on Nomenclature and Diagnostic Criteria for Juvenile Scleroderma Syndromes*; 3–6 June 2004; Padua. Padua: Associazione II Volo, 2005: 5–16.

Aetiology. The cause of morphoea is unknown. A number of studies, however, have shown *in vitro* abnormalities in fibroblasts from patients with morphoea. These include fibroblast promotion of migration of mononuclear leukocytes across endothelial cell monolayers [1], increased platelet-derived growth factor and receptor expression [2], and increased transforming growth factor-β (TGF-β) receptor expression [3]. It is postulated that this may lead to increased connective tissue growth factor (CTGF) gene expression and ultimately fibrosis [4,5]; possibly being mediated via activation of Smad and ERX1/2 [6] or integrin alphavbeta5 pathways [7]. That morphoea is an immunologically-mediated disease also gains support from studies that have found increased levels of circulating cytokines in patients with morphoea. These include IL-2 receptor [8,9], IL-6 receptor [10], IL-13 and TNF [11], soluble CD4 and CD8 [12], CD23 [13], CD30 [14], TNF-α [15], a B-cell activating factor belonging to the tumour necrosis factor family (BAFF) [16], soluble vascular cell adhesion molecule-1 (VCAM-1) and E-selectin [17], antiendothelial cell antibodies [18], and antibodies to fibrillin 1 [19] and superoxide dismutase [20]. That they may be involved in disease activity is supported by some studies, which have found increased levels of, for instance, soluble IL-2 receptor in active but not inactive disease [8,9], although such findings are by no means universal. Additional support for an autoimmune aetiology is the occurrence of scleroderma-like lesions in chronic graft-versus-host disease, and an association with idiopathic thrombocytopenic purpura [21]. A comprehensive review of chemokines and chemokine receptors in scleroderma has been published [22].

A number of studies have reported assays which may correlate with disease activity including levels of matrix metalloproteinase-13 [23], antiagalactosyl IgG antibodies [24] and manganese superoxide dismutase [25].

Experimental exchange of Thiersch grafts between normal and affected sites resulted in rapid transformation of the normal graft to morphoea and vice versa [26]. Trauma may be a triggering factor [27,28] and may precede the onset by many months. Immobilization has also been reported as a cause [29]. Morphoea has also occurred after bacille Calmette–Guérin (BCG) vaccination [30], following varicella [31], injections of vitamin K [32] and B12 [33], after antitetanus vaccination [34], after DTP and MMR vaccinations [35] and after herpes zoster [36]. There are several reports of morphoea occurring at the site of, and extending outside the field of, previous radiotherapy [37–41], and after fluoroscopy [42]. Surgical trauma has been reported as a stimulus for the development of lesions after arteriovenous fistula formation [43], rhinoplasty [44] and laparotomy [45], and recently mechanical compression from clothing has been suggested to trigger lesions [46]. A single case of linear morphoea occurring after linear lichen aureus has been reported [47]. Hormonal factors may influence the disease; morphoea may develop during, or be exacerbated by, pregnancy, but the influence of the menopause is less clear.

Infection with borrelial organisms has been implicated in the aetiology of morphoea, some central European studies suggesting a relationship between morphoea and acrodermatitis chronica atrophicans, a disease induced by infection with *Borrelia burgdorferi* [48–50]. These studies found raised levels of antibodies against this organism in patients with morphoea compared with controls, and described the presence of viable organisms in biopsies from morphoeic lesions. In addition, using the polymerase chain reaction, *Borrelia* DNA has been found in skin biopsies from patients with morphoea [51]. However, other studies [52–56] have shown no evidence of *Borrelia* antibodies or DNA in morphoea of patients from Scandinavia, Germany, Spain or America. A recent review [57] has suggested that the reason for these contradictory findings is that either *Borrelia* infection is not the cause of morphoea or that

a subset of morphoea is caused by a special species of *Borrelia* present in some parts of Europe and Asia but not in the USA and other parts of Europe.

The genetic influence on morphoea is unclear. A familial incidence has been noticed [58], and localized and systemic scleroderma has been noted in monozygotic twins [59]. Some cases of the frontal type appear to have a genetic basis [60], but there are no significant HLA associations [61]. There is an increase in the incidence of organ-specific autoantibodies in patients and relatives [62]. Morphoea has been associated with phenylketonuria, and improvement has occurred with a low-phenylalanine diet, but excretion of phenylalanine and *o*-hydroxyphenylacetic acid in nine children with morphoea was normal [63].

Morphoea has been reported after therapy with a number of drugs. Morphoea-like plaques occurred in a patient on penicillamine therapy and remitted within a year of stopping treatment [64]. Cutaneous lesions have also been reported after therapy with bromocriptine [65], hydroxytryptophan and carbidopa [66,67], valproic acid [68], pentazocine [69,70], docetaxel [71] and the related drug paclitaxel [72], bleomycin [73,74] and after melphalan limb perfusion [75]. These localized lesions are in contrast with the systemic sclerosis-like reactions reported later in this chapter.

Although the clinical picture of morphoea is usually distinctive, and different from systemic sclerosis, the histology and histochemistry [76–78] of the skin are similar, and X-ray diffraction, historadiographical and electron microscope investigations [63,79–81] show no differences. Electron microscopy may show changes in the underlying muscle fibres in both conditions, but only in systemic sclerosis are endothelial changes found in the muscle capillaries [82]. Skin collagen may be increased in morphoeic plaques [83], possibly because of clonal overactivity of fibroblasts [84], but is decreased in the involved skin in systemic sclerosis [85]. The two disorders rarely occur together. Nail fold capillaroscopy may reveal abnormal capillaries in such patients [86].

Finally, the similarities between scleroderma and chronic graft-versus-host disease has led to studies which have shown the presence of microchimerisms in the peripheral blood mononuclear cells of patients with systemic sclerosis [87], and the presence of chimeric cells (including dendritic cells and B lymphocytes) in localized scleroderma lesions, suggesting a possible pathogenic role [88].

References

1 Denton CP, Shi-Wen X, Sutton A *et al.* Scleroderma fibroblasts promote migration of mononuclear leucocytes across endothelial cell monolayers. *Clin Exp Immunol* 1998; **114**: 293–300.

2 Zheng XY, Zhang JZ, Tu P *et al.* Expression of platelet-derived growth factor B-chain and platelet-derived growth factor β-receptor in fibroblasts of scleroderma. *J Dermatol Sci* 1998; **18**: 90–7.

3 Kubo M, Ihn H, Yamane K *et al.* Up-regulated expression of transforming growth factor β receptors in dermal fibroblasts in skin sections from patients with localized scleroderma. *Arthritis Rheum* 2001; **44**: 731–4.

4 Igarashi A, Nashiro K, Kikuchi K *et al.* Connective tissue growth factor gene expression in tissue sections from localized scleroderma, keloid and other fibrotic skin disorders. *J Invest Dermatol* 1996; **106**: 729–33.

5 Stratton R, Shiwen X, Martini G *et al.* Iloprost suppresses connective tissue growth factor production in fibroblasts and in the skin of scleroderma patients. *J Clin Invest* 2001; **108**: 241–50.

6 Pannu J, Nakerakanti S, Smith E *et al.* Transforming growth factor-β receptor type 1-dependent fibrogenic gene program is mediated via activation of Smad 1 and ERK1/2 pathways. *J Biol Chem* 2006; **282**: 1405–13.

7 Asano Y, Ihn H, Jinnin M *et al.* Involvement of alphavbeta5 integrin in the establishment of autocrine TGF—beta signaling in dermal fibroblasts derived from localized scleroderma. *J Invest Dermatol* 2006; **126**: 1761–9.

8 Ihn H, Sato S, Fujimoto M *et al.* Clinical significance of serum levels of soluble interleukin-2 receptor in patients with localized scleroderma. *Br J Dermatol* 1996; **134**: 843–7.

9 Uziel Y, Krafchik BR, Feldman B *et al.* Serum levels of soluble interleukin-2 receptor: a marker of disease activity in localized scleroderma. *Arthritis Rheum* 1994; **37**: 898–901.

10 Nagaoka T, Sato S, Hasegawa M *et al.* Serum levels of soluble interleukin 6 receptor and soluble gp130 are elevated in patients with localized scleroderma. *J Rheumatol* 2000; **27**: 1917–21.

11 Hasegawa M, Sato S, Nagaoka T *et al.* Serum levels of tumour necrosis factor and interleukin-13 are elevated in patients with localized scleroderma. *Dermatol* 2003; **207**: 141–7.

12 Sato S, Fujimoto M, Kikuchi K *et al.* Soluble CD4 and CD8 in serum from patients with localized scleroderma. *Arch Dermatol Res* 1996; **288**: 358–62.

13 Sato S, Fujimoto M, Kikuchi K *et al.* Elevated soluble CD23 levels in the sera from patients with localized scleroderma. *Arch Dermatol Res* 1996; **288**: 74–8.

14 Ihn H, Yazawa N, Kubo M *et al.* Circulating levels of soluble CD30 are increased in patients with localized scleroderma and correlated with serological and clinical features of the disease. *J Rheumatol* 2000; **27**: 698–702.

15 Majewski S, Wojas-Pelc A, Malejczyk M *et al.* Serum levels of soluble TNF-α receptor type 1 and the severity of systemic sclerosis. *Acta Derm Venereol (Stockh)* 1999; **79**: 207–10.

16 Matsushita T, Hasegawa M, Matsushita Y *et al.* Elevated serum BAFF levels in patients with localized scleroderma in contrast to other organ-specific autoimmune diseases. *Exp Dermatol* 2006; **16**: 87–93.

17 Yamane K, Ihn H, Kubo M *et al.* Increased serum levels of soluble vascular cell adhesion molecule 1 and E-selectin in patients with localized scleroderma. *J Am Acad Dermatol* 2000; **42**: 64–9.

18 Salojin KV, Le-Tonqueze M, Saraux A *et al.* Antiendothelial cell antibodies: useful markers of systemic sclerosis. *Am J Med* 1997; **102**: 178–85.

19 Arnett FC, Tan FK, Uziel Y *et al.* Autoantibodies to the extracellular matrix microfibrillar protein, fibrillin 1, in patients with localized scleroderma. *Arthritis Rheum* 1999; **42**: 2656–9.

20 Nagai M, Hasegawa M, Takehara K *et al.* Novel autoantibody to Cu/Zn super-oxide dismutase in patients with localized scleroderma. *J Invest Dermatol* 2004; **122**: 594–601.

21 Leibovici V, Zlotogorski A, Kanner A *et al.* Generalized morphoea and idiopathic thrombocytopenia. *J Am Acad Dermatol* 1988; **18**: 1194–6.

22 Yamamoto T. Chemokines and chemokine receptors in scleroderma. *Int Arch Allergol Immunol* 2006; **140**: 345–56.

23 Asano Y, Ihn H, Kubo M *et al.* Clinical significance of matrix metalloproteinase-13 levels in patients with localized scleroderma. *Clin Exp Rheumatol* 2006; **24**: 394–9.

24 Mimura Y, Ihn H, Jinnin M *et al.* Anti-agalactosyl immunoglobulin G antibodies in localized scleroderma. *Int J Dermatol* 2005; **44**: 817–20.

25 Jinnin M, Ihn H, Yazawa N *et al.* Serum levels of manganese superoxide dismutase in patients with localized scleroderma. *Exp Dermatol* 2004; **13**: 357–60.

26 Haxthausen H. Studies on the pathogenesis of morphea, vitiligo and acrodermatitis atrophicans by means of transplantation experiments. *Acta Derm Venereol (Stockh)* 1947; **27**: 352–67.

27 Komocsi A, Tovari E, Kovacs J *et al.* Physical injury as a provoking factor in three patients with scleroderma. *Clin Exp Rheumatol* 2000; **18**: 622–4.

28 Yamanaka CT, Gibbs NF. Trauma induced scleroderma. *Cutis* 1999; **63**: 29–32.

29 Varga J, Jimenez SA. Development of severe limited scleroderma in complicated Raynaud's phenomenon after limb immobilization: report of two cases and study of collagen biosynthesis. *Arthritis Rheum* 1986; **29**: 1160–5.

30 Mork NJ. Clinical and histopathologic morphoea with immunological evidence of lupus erythematosus: a case report. *Acta Derm Venereol (Stockh)* 1981; **61**: 367–8.

31 Sahl WJ. Koebner phenomenon, morphoea and viral exanthems. *Lancet* 1978; **i**: 832.

32 Alonso-Llamazares J, Ahmad I. Vitamin K1-induced localized scleroderma (morphea) with linear deposition of IgA in the basement membrane zone. *J Am Acad Dermatol* 1998; **38**: 322–4.

33 Ho J, Rothchild YH, Sengelmann R. Vitamin B12-associated localized scleroderma and its treatment. *Dermatol Surg* 2004; **30**: 1252–5.

34 Drago F, Rampini P, Lugani C *et al.* Generalized morphoea after antitetanus vaccination. *Clin Exp Dermatol* 1998; **23**: 142.

35 Torrelo A, Suarez J, Colmenero I *et al.* Deep morphoea after vaccination in two young children. *Paediatr Dermatol* 2006; **23**: 484–7.

36 Forschner A, Metzler G, Rassner G *et al.* Morphea with features of lichen sclerosus et atrophicus at the site of a herpes zoster scar: another case of an isotopic response. *Int J Dermatol* 2005; **44**: 524–5.

37 Colver GB, Rodger A, Mortimer PS *et al.* Post-irradiation morphoea. *Br J Dermatol* 1989; **120**: 831–5.

38 Schaffer JV, Carroll C, Dvoretsky I *et al.* Post-irradiation morphoea of the breast: presentation of two cases and review of the literature. *Dermatology* 2000; **200**: 67–71.

39 Ullen H, Bjorkholm E. Localized scleroderma in a woman irradiated at two sites for endometrial and breast carcinoma: a case history and a review of the literature. *Int J Gynecol Cancer* 2003; **13**: 77–82.

40 Reddy S, Pui JC, Gold LI *et al.* Postirradiation morphoea and subcutaneous polyarteritis nodosa: case report and literature review. *Semin Arthritis Rheum* 2004; **34**: 728–34.

41 McClelland M, VanLock S, Patterson JW *et al.* Radiation-induced morphoea occuring after fluoroscopy. *J Am Acad Dermatol* 2002; **47**: 962–4.

42 Ardern-Jones MR, Black MM. Widespread morphoea following radiotherapy for carcinoma of the breast. *Clin Exp Dermatol* 2003; **28**: 160–2.

43 Quan VA, Black CM, Scoble JE. Cutaneous scleroderma following bilateral arteriovenous fistula formation. *Nephrol Dial Transplant* 1997; **12**: 1719–20.

44 Ozgur F, Kayikcioglu A. Linear scleroderma after rhinoplasty. *Plast Reconstr Surg* 1998; **101**: 539–40.

45 Terao M, Murota H, Song M *et al.* Case of morphoea occuring on a scar after laparoscopy. *J Dermatol* 2006; **33**: 722–3.

46 Ehara M, Oono T, Yamasaki O *et al.* Generalized morphea-like lesions arising in mechanically-compressed areas by underclothes. *Eur J Dermatol* 2006; **16**: 307–9.

47 Bell HK, Obson CM, Jackson SP *et al.* Localized morphoea preceded by a pigmented purpuric dermatosis. *Clin Exp Dermatol* 2003; **28**: 369–71.

48 Aberer E, Neumann R, Stanek G. Is localized scleroderma a *Borrelia* infection? *Lancet* 1985; **ii**: 278.

49 Aberer E, Kollegger H, Kristoferitsch W *et al.* Neuroborreliosis in morphoea and lichen sclerosus et atrophicus. *J Am Acad Dermatol* 1988; **19**: 820–5.

50 Aberer E, Stanek G, Ertl M *et al.* Evidence for spirochetal origin of circumscribed scleroderma (morphea). *Acta Derm Venereol (Stockh)* 1987; **67**: 225–31.

51 Schempp C, Bocklage H, Lange R *et al.* Further evidence for *Borrelia burgdorferi* infection in morphoea and lichen sclerosus et atrophicus confirmed by DNA amplification. *J Invest Dermatol* 1993; **100**: 717–20.

52 Halkier-Sorensen L, Kragballe K, Hansen K. Antibodies to the *Borrelia burgdorferi* flagellum in patients with scleroderma, granuloma annulare and porphyria cutanea tarda. *Acta Derm Venereol (Stockh)* 1989; **69**: 116–9.

53 Hoesly JM, Mertz LE, Winkelmann RK. Localized scleroderma (morphea) and antibody to *Borrelia burgdorferi*. *J Am Acad Dermatol* 1987; **17**: 455–8.

54 Weinecke R, Schlupen EM, Zochling N *et al.* No evidence of *Borrelia burgdorferi*-specific DNA in lesions of localized scleroderma. *J Invest Dermatol* 1995; **104**: 23–6.

55 Alonso-Llamazares J, Persing DH, Anda P *et al.* No evidence for *Borrelia burgdorferi* infection in lesions of morphoea and lichen sclerosus in Spain: a prospective study and literature review. *Acta Derm Venereol* 1997; **77**: 299–304.

56 Dillon WI, Saed GM, Fivenson DP. *Borrelia burgdorferi* DNA is undetectable by polymerase chain reaction in skin lesions of morphea, scleroderma, or lichen sclerosus et atrophicus of patients from North America. *J Am Acad Dermatol* 1995; **33**: 617–20.

57 Weide B, Walz T, Garbe C. Is morphoea caused by *Borrelia burgdorferi*: a review. *Br J Dermatol* 2000; **142**: 636–44.

58 Wuthrich RC, Roenigk HH, Steck WD. Localized scleroderma. *Arch Dermatol* 1975; **111**: 98–100.

59 DeKeyser F, Peene I, Joos R *et al.* Occurrence of scleroderma in monozygotic twins. *J Rheumatol* 2000; **27**: 2267–9.

60 Francheschetti A, Koenig H. L'importance du facteur heredo-degeneratif dans L'hemiatrophie faciale progressive (Romberg) etude des complications oculaires dans ce syndrome. *J Genet Hum* 1952; **1**: 27–64.

61 Kuhnl P, Sibrowski W, Boehm BO *et al.* Association of HLA antigens with progressive systemic sclerosis and morphoea. *Tissue Antigens* 1989; **34**: 207–9.

62 Harrington CI, Dunsmore IR. An investigation into the incidence of autoimmune disorders in patients with localized morphoea. *Br J Dermatol* 1989; **120**: 645–8.

63 Kornreich HK, Shaw KNF, Koch R *et al.* Phenylketonuria and scleroderma. *J Pediatr* 1968; **73**: 571–5.

64 Berstein RM, Hall MA, Gostelow BE. Morphoea-like reaction to D-penicillamine therapy. *Ann Rheum Dis* 1981; **40**: 42–4.

65 Leshin B, Piette WW, Caplan RM. Morphea after bromocriptine therapy. *Int J Dermatol* 1989; **28**: 177–9.

66 Joly P, Lampert A, Thomine E *et al.* Development of pseudobullous morphoea and scleroderma-like illness during therapy with L-5-hydroxytryptophan and carbidopa. *J Am Acad Dermatol* 1991; **25**: 332–3.

67 Morgan JM, Adams SJ. Scleroderma and autoimmune thrombocytopenia associated with ingestion of L-tryptophan. *Br J Dermatol* 1993; **128**: 581–3.

68 Ferzli GT, El-Tal A, Kibbi A *et al.* Localized morphoea: a rare adverse effect of valproic acid. *Paediatr Neurol* 2003; **29**: 253–5.

69 Wanchu A, Misra R. Limited cutaneous scleroderma induced by pentazocine abuse. *J Assoc Phys Ind* 1995; **43**: 145.

70 Bellman B, Berman B. Localized indurated brown plaques on arms and right buttock: pentazocine-induced morphoea. *Arch Dermatol* 1996; **132**: 1366–9.

71 Battafarano DF, Zimmerman GC, Older SA *et al.* Docetaxel (Taxotere) associated scleroderma-like changes of the lower extremities: report of three cases. *Cancer* 1995; **76**: 110–5.

72 Kupfer I, Balguerie X, Courville P *et al.* Scleroderma-like cutaneous lesions induced by paclitaxel: a case study. *J Am Acad Dermatol* 2003; **48**: 279–81.

73 Kim KH, Yoon TJ, Oh CW *et al.* A case of bleomycin induced scleroderma. *J Korean Med Sci* 1996; **11**: 454–6.

74 Passiu G, Cauli A, Atzeni F *et al.* Bleomycin-induced scleroderma: report of a case with a chronic course rather than the typical acute/subacute self-limiting form. *Clin Rheumatol* 1999; **18**: 422–4.

75 Landau M, Brenner S, Gat A *et al.* Reticulate scleroderma after isolated limb perfusion with melphalan. *J Am Acad Dermatol* 1998; **39**: 1011–2.

76 Braun-Falco O. Über das Verhalten der interfibrillaren Grundsubstanz bei Sklerodermie. *Dermatol Wochenschr* 1957; **136**: 1085–92.

77 Szodorav L, Tuza C. On the histochemistry of scleroderma. *Hautarzt* 1960; **11**: 63–7.

78 Keech MK. The effect of collagenase on the fixed and unfixed skin lesions of morphoea: an electron-microscope study. *J Pathol Bacteriol* 1959; **77**: 351–69.

79 Macher E. Feinstrukturuntersuchungen an der Haut bei Sklerodermia diffusa und circumscriptum. *Arch Klin Exp Dermatol* 1957; **206**: 739–45.

80 Macher E, Brehler B. Röntgeninterferenz untersuchungen bei Sklerodermia diffusa und circumscriptum. *Hautarzt* 1958; **9**: 409–14.

81 Niebauer G. Zur feingeweblichen Untersuchung der Sklerodermie. *Acta Neuroreg* 1960; **21**: 271–86.

82 Michalowski R. Ultrastructural study of skeletal muscle in morphoea. *Br J Dermatol* 1970; **82**: 137–41.

83 Shuster S, Raffle EJ, Bottoms E. Quantitative changes in skin collagen in morphoea. *Br J Dermatol* 1967; **79**: 456–9.

84 Kahari VM, Sandberg M, Kalimo H *et al.* Identification of fibroblasts responsible for increased collagen production in localized scleroderma by *in situ* hybridization. *J Invest Dermatol* 1988; **90**: 664–70.

85 Black MM, Bottoms E, Shuster S. Skin collagen content and thickness in systemic sclerosis. *Br J Dermatol* 1970; **83**: 552–5.

86 Maricq HR. Capillary abnormalities, Raynaud's phenomenon and systemic sclerosis in patients with localized scleroderma. *Arch Dermatol* 1992; **128**: 630–2.

87 Lambert NC, Erickson TD, Yan Z *et al.* Quantification of maternal microchimerism by HLA-specific real-time polymerase chain reaction. Studies of healthy women and women with scleroderma. *Arthritis Rheum* 2004; **50**: 906–14.

88 McNallan KT, Aponte C, El-Azhary R *et al.* Immunophenotyping of chimeric cells in localized scleroderma. *Rheumatology* 2007; **46**: 398–402.

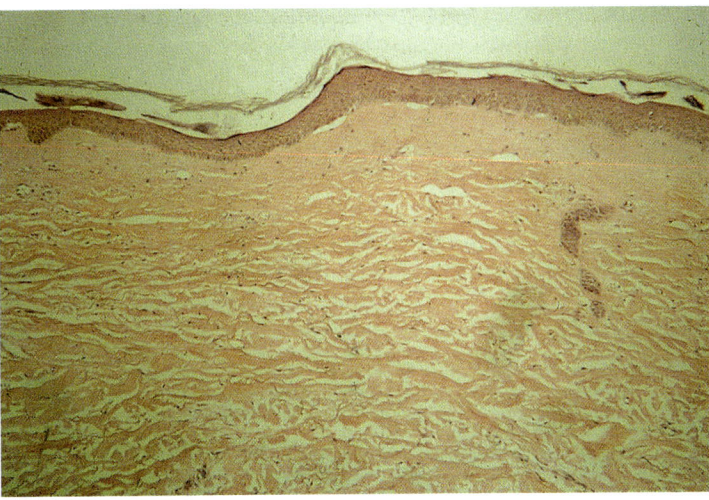

Fig. 51.47 Morphoea: slight atrophy of the epidermis with loss of dermal appendages and degeneration of dermal collagen.

be a scanty perivascular lymphocytic infiltrate. Cellular infiltrates of lymphocytes, plasma cells and macrophages, either perivascular or diffuse, occurred in 84% in one series, and there is some evidence that the infiltrate may precede fibrosis [1,2]. Later, the dermis is markedly thickened, with dense collagen and relatively few recognizable fibroblasts. The elastic tissue is reduced. The dermal appendages and dermal and subcutaneous fat are progressively lost. Some sweat glands may survive, deep in the dense sclerotic mass. Small dermal blood vessels may show intimal thickening.

Immunohistochemistry studies have shown that the main changes in morphoea consist of foci of intercollagenous staining for connective tissue antigens in the reticular layer of the dermis [3], and that there is a reduction in the size and number of dermal papillae, with increased angiogenesis in the early inflammatory stage and various numbers of enlarged vessels in inactive lesions [4]. A further study has reported an increase in dermal microvascular pericytes in the peripheral zones of active lesions, supporting the concept of a vascular pathogenesis of scleroderma [5]. IgM and C3 are found at the basement membrane and in dermal blood vessels, particularly in more extensive and deeper lesions, but there is no relation to systemic disease [6]. A study of glycosaminoglycans in normal and sclerodermatous skin has shown an increase in hyaluronic acid and altered dermatan sulphate in involved skin [7]. The histological features are similar to those seen in generalized morphoea and in the skin in systemic sclerosis.

References

1 Fleischmajer R, Perlish JS, Reeves JRT. Cellular infiltrates in scleroderma skin. *Arthritis Rheum* 1977; **20**: 975–84.

2 Winkelmann RK, Connolly SM, Doyle JA. Localized scleroderma and systemic disease. In: Kukita A, Serji M, eds. *Proceedings of the XVI International Congress of Dermatology Tokyo*. Tokyo: University of Tokyo Press, 1982: 305.

3 Rowell NR, Scott DG. Immunohistological studies with anti-connective tissue and anti-immunoglobulin antisera of the skin in lupus erythematosus and scleroderma. *Br J Dermatol* 1975; **93**: 431–41.

4 Kowalewski C, Kozlowska A, Gorska M *et al.* Alterations of basement membrane zone and cutaneous microvasculature in morphoea and extragenital lichen sclerosus. *Am J Dermatopathol* 2005; **27**: 489–96.

Pathology (Fig. 51.47). The epidermis may be normal, or flattened and atrophic with loss of the rete ridges. At first the dermis is oedematous, with swelling and degeneration of the collagen fibrils, which become homogeneous and eosinophilic. There may

5 Helmbold P, Fiedler E, Fischer M *et al.* Hyperplasia of dermal microvascular pericytes in scleroderma. *J Cutan Pathol* 2004; **31**: 431–40.

6 Vincent F, Prokopetz R, Miller RAW. Plasma cell panniculitis: a unique clinical and pathologic presentation of linear scleroderma. *J Am Acad Dermatol* 1989; **21**: 357–60.

7 Passos CO, Werneck CC, Onofre GR. Comparative biochemistry of human skin: glycosaminoglycans from different body sites in normal subjects and in patients with localized scleroderma. *J Eur Acad Dermatol Venereol* 2003; **17**: 14–9.

Incidence. All ages are affected, the peak incidence occurring between 20 and 40 years of age, although 15% begin below the age of 10 years [1,2], in which age group the linear lesions predominate. The female to male ratio is around 3:1 in most studies. Most linear lesions (75%) occur before the age of 40 years, whereas 75% of localized plaques arise between the ages of 20 and 40 years [2]. In one series, localized plaques occurred in 60 patients, with linear lesions in 33 and guttate in 13 [3], but in another series [2] there were more patients with linear lesions than with plaques. A worldwide study of 750 children with juvenile localized scleroderma showed linear lesions in 65%, plaques lesions in 26%, generalized involvement in 12% and deep lesions in 2%, with 15% exhibiting a mixed subtype [4]. Six patients (0.8%) had linear lesions present at birth and were considered as having congenital scleroderma [5]. The condition is said to be rare in black people [3]. A recent epidemiological study of morphoea in the USA has found a female to male ratio of 2.5:1, an incidence of 2.7 in 10 000 and a prevalence at 80 years of age of 1 in 500 [6].

References

1 Heite HJ. Ergebnisse häufigkeitanalytischer Untersuchungen bei der Sklerodermie. *Arch Dermatol Syphilol* 1955; **200**: 426–33.

2 Christianson HB, Dorsey CS, O'Leary PA *et al.* Localized scleroderma: a clinical study of 235 cases. *Arch Dermatol* 1956; **74**: 629–39.

3 Curtis AC, Jansen TG. The prognosis of localized scleroderma. *Arch Dermatol* 1958; **78**: 749–57.

4 Zulian F, Athreya BH, Laxer R *et al.* Juvenile localized scleroderma: clinical and epidemiological features in 750 children. An international study. *Rheumatology* 2006; **45**: 614–20.

5 Zulian F, Vallongo C, De-Oliveira SKF *et al.* Congenital localized scleroderma. *J Paediatr* 2006; **149**: 248–51.

6 Peterson LS, Nelson AM, Su WPD *et al.* The epidemiology of morphea (localized scleroderma) in Olmsted County, 1960–93. *J Rheumatol* 1997; **24**: 73–80.

Clinical features

Plaque lesions. These occur as indurated areas of skin, which at first are faintly purplish or mauve in colour. After some weeks or months they lose their colour (Fig. 51.48), especially in the centre, and appear as thickened waxy areas, which are ivory in colour, with a characteristic lilac-coloured edge (Fig. 51.49). The surface is usually smooth and shiny but may be nodular [1]. The hairs are absent, and usually the area ceases to sweat. Vesicles, bullae [2] and haemorrhages may occasionally occur, and sometimes telangiectases may be seen. The plaque is attached to the deeper tissues and, if thick, may be hypoaesthetic. The lesions are round or oval, sometimes irregular, and vary in size from approximately 2 to 15 cm or more in diameter. They are usually multiple, and often bilateral, but asymmetrical. They occur on the trunk and limbs, face and genitalia. They are less commonly found in the axillae and perineum and around the nipples. Sometimes, plaques accompany linear lesions.

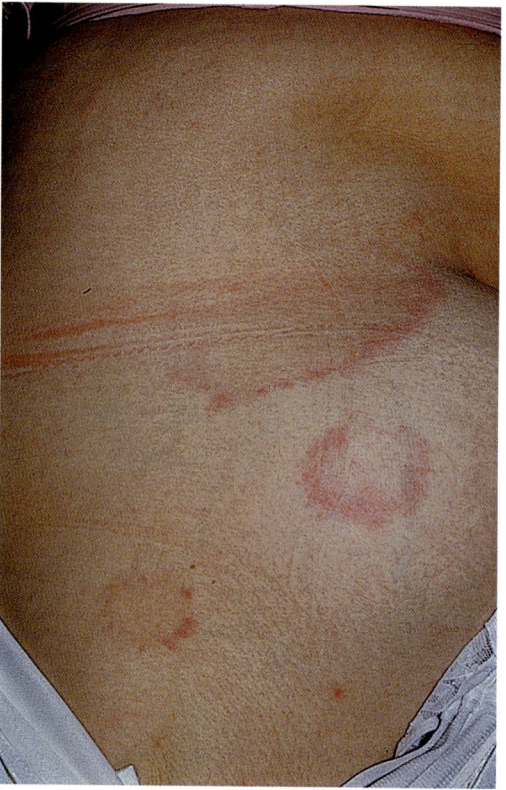

Fig. 51.48 Localized morphoea: plaque-like lesions on the abdomen.

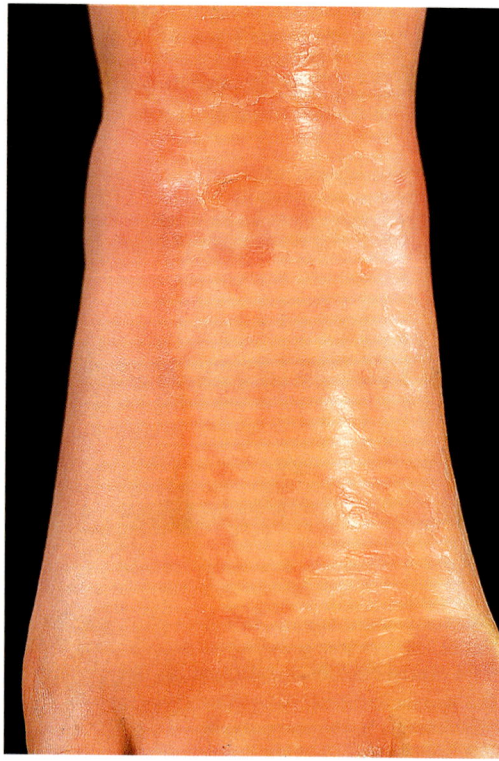

Fig. 51.49 Localized morphoea on the foot: late stage but still showing lilac border.

Although the onset of lesions is usually insidious, they can occasionally occur rapidly, with erythema and oedema. Sometimes they may be preceded by pigmentation (Fig. 51.50). In subcutaneous morphoea, induration is indistinct and the lilac ring is

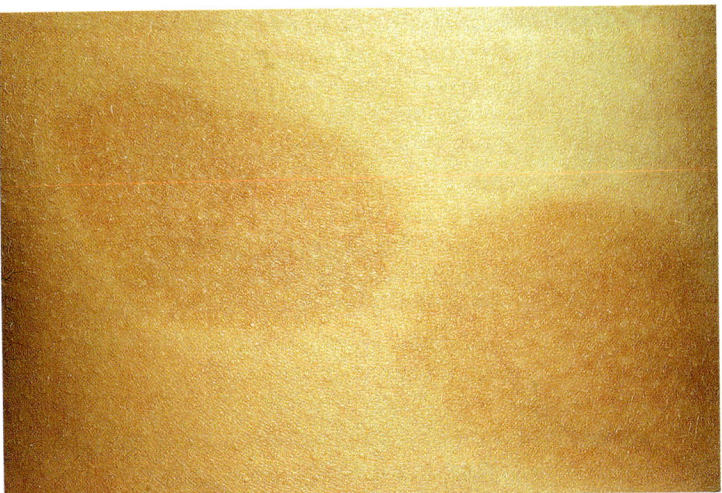

Fig. 51.50 Localized morphoea: pigmentation usually occurs as the lesion resolves but may occur at the onset.

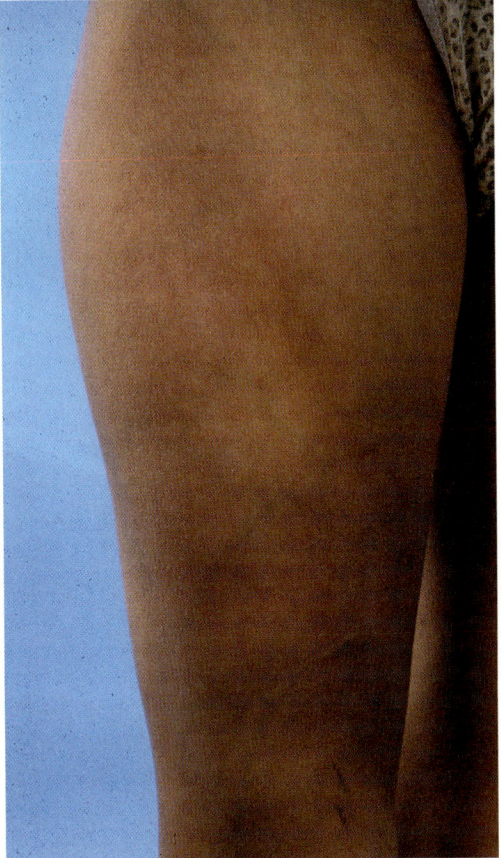

Fig. 51.51 Linear morphoea.

absent. Deep involvement of underlying structures in morphoea of the trunk is unusual, but occurs occasionally and may be followed by deep atrophy [3]. Obscure abdominal pain and migraine were features in approximately 15% of patients in one series [4], but usually any pain is limited to the skin lesions. One study detected abnormalities of the vertebral column in 47% of those X-rayed, with spina bifida occulta occurring in 20 patients. These findings were most common in those with linear lesions, occurring in 26 of these 108 patients [4]. Other studies have not, however, reported such findings.

Recently, the term 'superficial morphoea' has been proposed for lesions with minimal induration [5]. Most cases occur in females although a single case in a male has been reported [6]. It has been suggested that atrophoderma of Pasini and Pierini may also be a primary abortive form of morphoea [7] in which induration fails to occur. Some authors argue that these two conditions are one and the same [8].

Guttate lesions. In true guttate morphoea, the lesions are similar to, but smaller and more numerous than, plaque lesions. Some cases may represent lichen sclerosus et atrophicus (white spot disease) rather than true morphoea. It has been suggested that these two diseases may have a similar pathogenesis [9] or coexist [10,11].

Bullous lesions. Peterson's classification [12], describes bullous morphoea as a distinct entity. However, blisters have been described in all types of morphoea and have been thought to result from lymphatic dilatation along with the release of major basic protein from eosinophils [13]. Others have suggested that, at least in some cases, the blisters represent the development of associated lichen sclerosus [14].

Subcutaneous morphoea/deep morphoea/morphoea profundus. Nodular [1], keloidal [15,16] or subcutaneous morphoea are variants of morphoea that exhibit differing amounts and depths of inflammatory changes and sclerosis. The term morphoea profundus was first suggested by Whittaker *et al.* [17], in 1989, to describe a solitary fibrotic plaque on the shoulder, back, neck or paraspinal area, which histologically showed fibrosis, hyalinization of collagen fibres and a deep dermal and subcutaneous inflammatory infiltrate. The overlying skin may be pigmented or hypopigmented. Osteoma cutis can develop within such lesions [18,19] and contracture of the flexor muscles of the finger has been reported in subcutaneous morphoea [20]. Most lesions of morphoea profundus are said to be non-progressive [21].

Linear lesions (Fig. 51.51). The essential features are similar to the plaque lesions, but the lilac ring is inconspicuous or only present at the advancing border. They are usually single and unilateral, although occasionally bilateral lesions occur. They can follow the lines of Blaschko [22–24]. The limbs are frequently affected, the legs more than the arms. They may also occur on the anterior aspect of the thorax, and sometimes the abdomen or buttocks are affected. Lesions involving one arm and one leg are usually homolateral. Rarely, half of the body (face, arm, trunk and leg) is involved [25]. Occasionally, a linear lesion on the leg is preceded by oedema of the limb. Lesions take the form of linear areas of induration, similar to those found in the plaques, but sometimes the condition may extend to involve the underlying muscles, or even bone, with resulting disturbances in growth in approximately 20% (Fig. 51.52) [26] and possibly severe flexion deformity [27,28]. The surface may show patchy hyperkeratosis. Usually, lesions occur along the length of the limb or around the trunk, but sometimes a band surrounds a limb or a finger, resembling ainhum [29,30]. The tissues

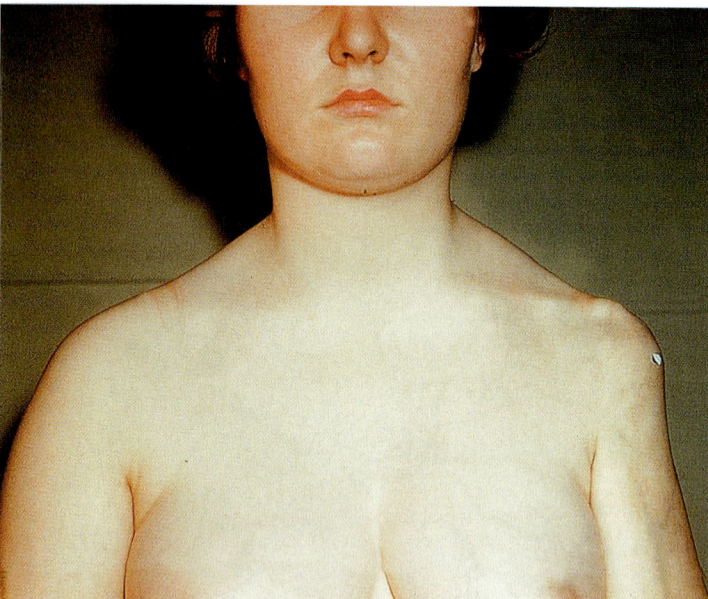

Fig. 51.52 Localized morphoea of the arm showing growth retardation.

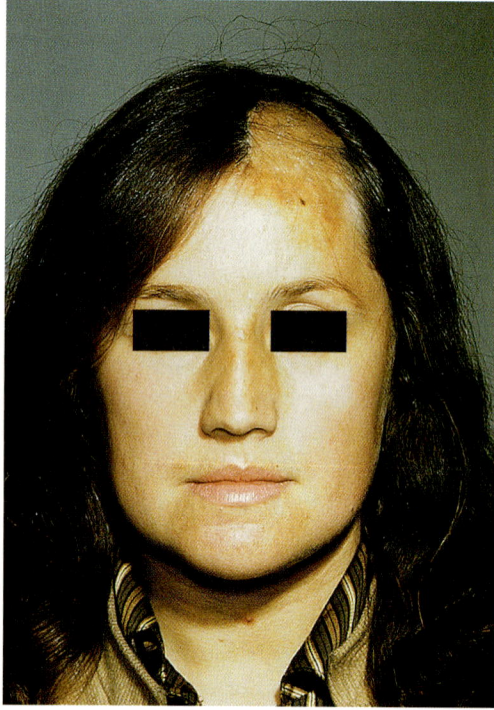

Fig. 51.53 Frontoparietal morphoea ('en coup de sabre').

distal to such a band may be oedematous and depigmented [26]. The fibrosis may spare areas within an otherwise linear lesion, producing 'skip' lesions.

Linear scleroderma has been associated with hypertrichosis [31], melorheostosis [32–34], and ulcerated dystrophic calcinosis cutis [35]. Nodular morphoea has been reported in a linear pattern [36].

Frontoparietal lesions (Fig. 51.53) 'en coup de sabre' (from its resemblance to a sabre cut), with or without hemiatrophy. These

lesions usually start with contraction and firmness of the skin over the affected area. Subsequently, an ivory irregular sclerotic plaque develops, sometimes with telangiectatic vessels coursing over it, together with hyperpigmentation at the edge. Eventually, a linear depressed groove appears on the frontoparietal region, extending into the scalp, producing a linear zone of alopecia, which may be preceded by bleaching of the hair. The groove may extend downwards into the cheek, nose and upper lip, and involve the mouth and gum. In severe cases, it extends as far as the chin and neck. The condition may affect the gingivae [37] and the jaw may also be involved, with alteration of the spacing and direction of the teeth [38]. The corresponding side of the tongue may be atrophic, although sometimes the lesion is in the midline of the tongue. Not infrequently, there is atrophy of the corresponding part of the face and cheek, with facial asymmetry, and this usually occurs within a year. The Parry–Romberg syndrome of hemifacial atrophy looks very similar, but there should be no cutaneous sclerosis at any stage [39]. Both problems may co-exist [40]. Rarely, frontoparietal lesions may be bilateral [41,42] or trilinear [43] and may follow Blaschko's lines [44]. Sometimes, there may be morphoeic plaques elsewhere on the body or evidence of linear morphoea on the extremities and trunk [45]. Facial atrophy without frontoparietal morphoea can be associated with morphoea elsewhere. Ipsilateral wasting of the upper limb occurs in less than 10% of cases [46]. Total hemiatrophy of one side of the body can occur.

Contralateral or bilateral atrophy is rare. The bones of the skull can be involved and the EEG may show evidence of dysrhythmia, maximal over the affected area. Neurological abnormalities have been reported [47–49]. A variety of ocular lesions occur [50], including enophthalmos, involvement of the lids, oculomotor muscles, iris and fundus, myopathy of the external eye muscles [51] and vasculitis [52]. Atrophy of the nasal part of the iris and loss of cilia on the upper eyelid followed exactly the line of the skin lesions in one case [53]. Heterochromia of the iris also occurs [54]. 'En coup de sabre' morphoea has presented as unilateral eyelid oedema [55]. Ossification occasionally occurs [56].

References

1 Micalizzi C, Parodi A, Rebora A. Morphoea with nodular lesions. *Br J Dermatol* 1994; **131**: 298–301.

2 Garb J, Sims CF. Scleroderma with bullous lesions: report of a case and review of the literature. *Dermatologica* 1959; **119**: 341–59.

3 Frankel H. Ein dermatologisch-neurologischer Grenzfall. *Nervenarzt* 1957; **28**: 84.

4 Christianson HB, Dorsey ES, O'Leary PA, Kierland R. Localized scleroderma: a clinical study of 235 cases. *Arch Dermatol* 1956; **74**: 629–39.

5 Jacobson L, Palazij R, Jaworsky C. Superficial morphoea. *J Am Acad Dermatol* 2003; **49**: 323–5.

6 Srinivasan SK, DiMaio D. Superficial morphoea in a man. *J Am Acad Dermatol* 2004; **51**: S156–8.

7 Kencka D, Blaszczyk M, Jablonska S. Atrophoderma Pasini–Pierini is a primary atrophic abortive morphea. *Dermatology* 1995; **190**: 203–6.

8 Jablonska S, Blaszczyk M. Is superficial morphoea synonymous with atrophoderma Pasini-Pierini? *J Am Acad Dermatol* 2003; **50**: 979–80.

9 Sawamura D, Yaguchi T, Hashimoto I *et al.* Coexistence of generalized morphea with histological changes in lichen sclerosus et atrophicus and lichen planus. *J Dermatol* 1998; **25**: 409–11.

10 Shono S, Imura M, Ota M *et al.* Lichen sclerosus et atrophicus, morphea, and coexistence of both diseases: histological studies using lectins. *Arch Dermatol* 1991; **127**: 1352–6.

11 Farrell AM, Marren PM, Wojnarowska F. Genital lichen sclerosus associated with morphoea or systemic sclerosus: clinical and HLA characteristics. *Br J Dermatol* 2000; **143**: 598–603.

12 Peterson LS, Nelson AM, Su WP. Classification of morphoea (localized scleroderma). *Mayo Clin Proc* 1995; **70**: 1068–76.

13 Daoud MS, Su WPD, Leiferman KM, Perniciaro C. Bullous morphea: clinical, pathologic, and immunopathologic evaluation of 13 cases. *J Am Acad Dermatol* 1994; **30**: 937–43.

14 Trattner A, David M, Sandbank M. Bullous morphea: a distinct entity? *Am J Dermatopathol* 1994; **16**: 414–7.

15 Perez-Wilson J, Pujol RM, Alejo M *et al.* Nodular (keloidal) scleroderma. *Int J Dermatol* 1992; **31**: 422–3.

16 Labandiera J, Leon-Mateos A, Suarez-Penaranda JM *et al.* What is nodular-keloidal scleroderma? *Dermatology* 2003; **207**: 130–2.

17 Whittaker SJ, Smith NP, Jones RR. Solitary morphoea profunda. *Br J Dermatol* 1989; **120**: 431–40.

18 Ahn SK, Won JH, Choi EH *et al.* Perforating plate-like osteoma cutis in a man with solitary morphoea profunda. *Br J Dermatol* 1996; **134**: 949–52.

19 Hulian CG, Bowers PW. Osteoma cutis in a lesion of solitary morphoea profundus. *Clin Exp Dermatol* 2003; **28**: 673–4.

20 Harris A, Burge SM, Wordsworth P *et al.* Subcutaneous morphoea with contracture of the flexor muscles of the finger. *Br J Dermatol* 1997; **136**: 476–7.

21 Azad J, Dawn G, Shaffrali FCG *et al.* Does solitary morphoea profundus progress? *Clin Exp Dermatol* 2004; **29**: 25–7.

22 Soma Y, Kawakami T, Yamasaki E *et al.* Linear scleroderma along Blaschko's lines in a patient with systematized morphoea. *Acta Derm Venereol* 2003; **83**: 362–4.

23 Mukhopadhyay A. Linear scleroderma following Blaschko's lines. *Indian J Dermatol Venereol Leprol* 2005; **71**: 421–2.

24 Hauser C, Skaria A, Harms M *et al.* Morphoea following Blaschko's lines. *Br J Dermatol* 1996; **134**: 594–5.

25 Bramley P, Forbes A. A case of progressive hemiatrophy presenting with spontaneous fractures of the lower jaw. *BMJ* 1960; **i**: 1476–8.

26 Larregue M, Ziegler JE, Lauret P *et al.* Sclerodermie en bande chez l'enfant (a propos de 27 cas). *Ann Dermatol Vénéréol* 1986; **113**: 207–24.

27 Longacre JJ, Wagner EA. The surgical management of disabling contractures due to linear scleroderma. *Plast Reconstr Surg* 1952; **9**: 367–80.

28 Weill J, Dubois M, Lewin *et al.* Sclerodermie en bandes et atrophies tissulaires multiples. *Bull Mem Soc Med Hop Paris* 1953; **69**: 490–5.

29 Tajima S, Suzuki Y, Inazumi T. A case of atypical localized scleroderma presenting with pseudoainhum: treatment with tranilast, an anti-fibrotic agent. *Acta Derm Venereol (Stockh)* 1996; **76**: 162.

30 Park BS, Hyun-Cho K, Youn JI *et al.* Pseudoainhum associated with linear scleroderma. *Arch Dermatol* 1996; **132**: 1520–1.

31 Juhn BJ, Cho YH, Lee MH. Linear scleroderma associated with hypertrichosis in the absence of melorheostosis. *Acta Derm Venereol* 2000; **80**: 62–3.

32 Alvarez MJM, Lazano MA, Espada G *et al.* Linear scleroderma and melorheostosis: case presentation and literature review. *Clin Rheumatol* 1966; **15**: 389–93.

33 Wagers LT, Young AW, Ryan SF. Linear melorheostotic scleroderma. *Br J Dermatol* 1972; **86**: 297–301.

34 Soffa DJ, Sire DJ, Dodson JH. Melorheostosis with linear sclerodermatous skin changes. *Radiology* 1975; **114**: 577–8.

35 Vereecken P, Stallenberg B, Tas S *et al.* Ulcerated dystrophic calcinosis cutis secondary to localized linear scleroderma. *Int J Clin Prac* 1998; **52**: 593–4.

36 Hsu S, Lee MWC, Carlton S *et al.* Nodular morphea in a linear pattern. *Int J Dermatol* 1999; **38**: 529–30.

37 Davis WC, Saunders TS. Scleroderma of the face involving the gingiva. *Arch Dermatol Syphilol* 1946; **54**: 133–5.

38 Looby JB, Burket LW. Scleroderma of the face with involvement of the alveolar process. *Am J Orthodontol* 1942; **28**: 493.

39 Jappe U, Holzle E, Ring J. Parry–Romberg syndrom Zussamenfassung und neue Erkenntnisse anlablich einer ungewhnlichen Kasuistik. *Hautarzt* 1996; **47**: 599–603.

40 Tollefson MM, Witman PM. En coup de sabre morphoea and Parry-Romberg syndrome: a retrospective review of 54 patients. *J Am Acad Dermatol* 2007; **56**: 257–63.

41 Dilley JJ, Perry HO. Bilateral linear scleroderma en coup de sabre. *Arch Dermatol* 1968; **97**: 688–9.

42 Rai R, Handa S, Gupta S *et al.* Bilateral en coup de sabre: a rare entity. *Pediatr Dermatol* 2000; **17**: 222–4.

43 McKenna DB, Benton EC. A tri-linear pattern of scleroderma 'en coup de sabre' following Blaschko's lines. *Clin Exp Dermatol* 1999; **24**: 467–8.

44 Soma Y, Fujimoto M. Frontoparietal scleroderma (en coup de sabre) following Blaschko's lines. *J Am Acad Dermatol* 1998; **38**: 366–8.

45 Unterberger I, Trinka E, Englhadt K *et al.* Linear scleroderma 'en coup de sabre' coexisting with plaque-morphoea: neurological manifestation and response to corticosteroids. *J Neurol Neurosurg Psych* 2003; **74**: 661–4.

46 Lakhani PK, David TJ. Progressive hemifacial atrophy with scleroderma and ipsilateral limb wasting (Parry–Romberg syndrome). *J R Soc Med* 1984; **77**: 138–9.

47 Menni S, Marzano AV, Passoni E. Neurologic abnormalities in two patients with facial hemiatrophy and sclerosis coexisting with morphoea. *Pediatr Dermatol* 1997; **14**: 113–6.

48 Appenzeller S, Montenegro MA, Dertkigil S *et al.* Neuroimaging findings in scleroderma en coup de sabre. *Neurology* 2004; **62**: 1585–9.

49 Holland KE, Steffes B, Nocton JJ *et al.* Linear scleroderma en coup de sabre with associated neurologic abnormalities. *Paediatrics* 2006; **117**: e132–6.

50 Segal P, Jablonska S, Mrzyglod S. Ocular changes in linear scleroderma. *Am J Ophthalmol* 1961; **51**: 807–13.

51 Serup J, Serup L, Sjo O. Localized scleroderma 'en coup de sabre' with external eye muscle involvement at the same time. *Clin Exp Dermatol* 1984; **9**: 196–200.

52 Holl-Wieden A, Klink T, Klink J *et al.* Linear scleroderma 'en coup de sabre' associated with cerebral and ocular vasculitis. *Scand J Rheumatol* 2006; **35**: 402–4.

53 Serup J, Alsbirk PH. Localized scleroderma 'en coup de sabre' and iridopalpebral atrophy at the same time. *Acta Derm Venereol (Stockh)* 1983; **63**: 75–7.

54 Stone RA, Scheie HG. Periorbital scleroderma associated with heterochromia iridis. *Am J Ophthalmol* 1980; **90**: 858–61.

55 Long PR, Miller OF. Linear scleroderma. *J Am Acad Dermatol* 1982; **7**: 541–4.

56 Handfield-Jones SE, Peachey RDG, Moss ALH *et al.* Ossification in linear morphoea with hemifacial atrophy: treatment by surgical excision. *Clin Exp Dermatol* 1988; **13**: 385–8.

Localized scleroderma in childhood [1–3]. Childhood onset occurs in 2–3% of all cases of scleroderma. Most present with morphoea-type lesions (particularly linear) although systemic sclerosis does occur. The clinical features are similar to adult cases but localized trauma a few months before onset of morphoeic lesions has been reported to occur in one-quarter of childhood patients. A recent large series of 750 children from 70 European centres [4] showed linear scleroderma to be the commonest subtype (65%) followed by plaque morphoea (26%), generalized morphoea (7%) and deep morphoea (2%), and 15% had a mixed subtype. Twelve per cent had a positive family history for rheumatic or autoimmune diseases and 13% reported environmental events as a possible trigger. ANA was positive in 42%, rheumatoid factor in 16%, anticardiolipin antibody in 13%, anti-double-stranded DNA in 4%, Scl-70 in 3% and anticentromere antibody in 2%.

Disabling pansclerotic morphoea of children [5]. This is a rare, severe, mutilating form of morphoea involving the dermis, fat, fascia, muscle and even bone, usually starting before the age of 14 years, although adult-onset cases have been reported [6]. It may develop from linear morphoea. Superficial and deep cutaneous sclerosis involves the trunk and extremities, scalp and face, with sparing of the fingertips and toes (Fig. 51.54). There may be a claw deformity of the hands, and patients may walk on tiptoe because of contracture of the Achilles tendons (Fig. 51.55). Arthralgia and stiffness occur at the onset, and intense pain may be a problem,

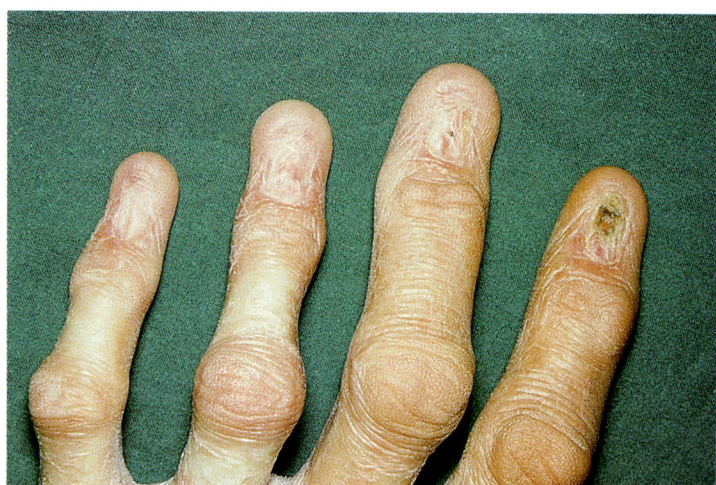

Fig. 51.54 Disabling pansclerotic morphoea of the fingers.

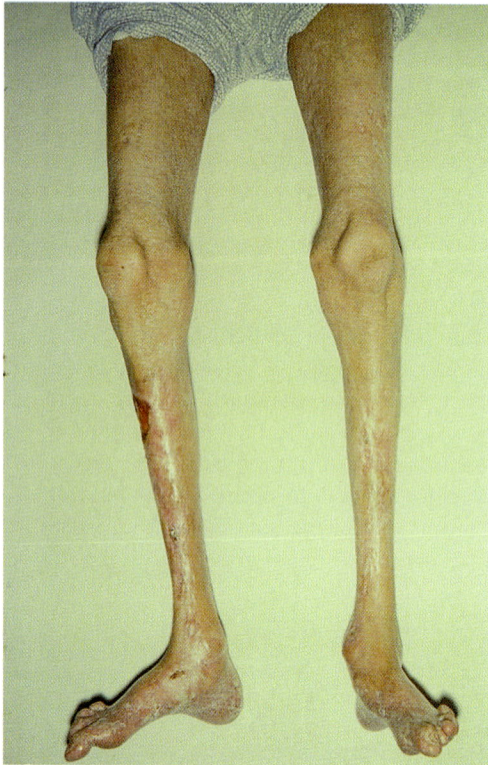

Fig. 51.55 Disabling pansclerotic morphoea of the legs.

presumably because of involvement of cutaneous nerves [7]. Raynaud's phenomenon is not found, but a few cases have had oesophageal, pulmonary and periodontal changes. Flexion contractures, osteoporosis and other bone changes are frequent. The electromyogram and histology of muscle may be abnormal, but creatine phosphokinase is normal. Elevation of ESR, hypergammaglobulinaemia and eosinophilia are frequent. Treatment with PUVA [8], low-dosage UVA-1 [9] and ciclosporin [10] has been reported. The response is often poor, however, and in most patients the condition is progressive [11] and occasionally fatal [5].

References

1 Vancheeswaran R, Black CM, David J *et al.* Childhood-onset scleroderma: is it different from adult-onset disease? *Arthritis Rheum* 1996; **39**: 1041–9.
2 Emery H. Paediatric scleroderma. *Semin Cutan Med Surg* 1998; **17**: 41–7.
3 Black CM. Scleroderma in childhood. *Adv Exp Med Biol* 1999; **45**: 35–48.
4 Zulian F, Athreya BH, Laxer R *et al.* Juvenile localized scleroderma: clinical and epidemiological features in 750 children. An international study. *Rheumatology* 2006; **45**: 614–20.
5 Diaz-Perez JL, Connolly SM, Winkelmann RK. Disabling pansclerotic morphoea of children. *Arch Dermatol* 1980; **116**: 169–73.
6 Maragh SH, Davis MDP, Bruce AJ *et al.* Disabling pansclerotic morphea: clinical presentation in two adults. *J Am Acad Dermatol* 2005; **53**: S115–9.
7 Rowell NR. Acral pansclerotic morphoea with intractable pain. In: Burgdorf WHC, Katz SI, eds. *Clinical Dermatology: the CMO Case Collection/World Congress of Dermatology*. Berlin: Scheltauer, 1987: 178–80.
8 Scharffetter-Kochanek K, Goldermann R, Lehmann P *et al.* PUVA therapy in disabling pansclerotic morphoea of children. *Br J Dermatol* 1995; **132**: 830–1.
9 Gruss C, Stucker M, Von Kobyletski G *et al.* Low dose UVA-1 phototherapy in disabling pansclerotic morphoea of childhood. *Br J Dermatol* 1997; **136**: 293–4.
10 Peter RU, Rizicka T, Eckert F. Low-dose cyclosporine A in the treatment of disabling morphoea. *Arch Dermatol* 1991; **127**: 1420–1.
11 Wollina U, Wollina K. Pansclerotic morphoea of childhood: follow-up over 6 years. *Paediatr Dermatol* 1999; **16**: 245–7.

Associated lesions. Arthralgia, sometimes localized to the sclerodermatous extremity, unilateral Raynaud's phenomenon, a history of migraine and intermittent recurrent colicky abdominal pain are sometimes found [1]. Abnormal radiological appearances of the spine occurred in 47% of patients in one series [1], particularly those with linear scleroderma. Spina bifida was found in 20 patients and was most common in patients with linear morphoea of the legs, lower abdomen and buttocks. Other abnormalities included sacralization of lumbar segments, the presence of six lumbar vertebrae, prolongation of transverse arches, scoliosis and kyphosis. Pain in the lumbar region, like that of a protruded lumbar intervertebral disc, was sometimes a feature. Rib abnormalities such as rudimentary or cervical ribs, torticollis, atrophic clavicle, absent pectoralis muscle, contracted pelvis, shortened ulna and deformities of the feet and toes have been reported [1], but other studies have not reported similar findings. Associated cutaneous abnormalities include warty, vascular or pigmented naevi, usually with linear morphoea on the same side, café-au-lait spots, alopecia areata, vitiligo [2], generalized ichthyosis or pigmentation, dystrophy of the nails, hirsutism and coarctation of the aorta [3]. Localized morphoea occurred in a pigmented area of Becker's melanosis [4]. A variant occurring later in life, in which morphoea confined to the face and anterior part of the scalp is associated with tissue calcification, hair loss and beaking of the nose, has been reported [5]. Sclerotic panatrophy, disseminated granuloma annulare and morphoea have occurred in the same patient [6].

Children may be intellectually precocious [1]. A recent review of 750 children with localized scleroderma from 70 European centres [7] showed that almost one-quarter had extracutaneous manifestations, including articular (47%), neurological (17%), vascular (9%), ocular (8%), gastrointestinal (6%), respiratory (3%), cardiac (1%) and renal (1%) abnormalities. Other autoimmune conditions were present in 7%.

Occasionally, morphoeic lesions may occur in association with lesions of lichen sclerosus et atrophicus. Localized patches of morphoea may occur in patients with systemic sclerosis [8] and occasionally patients with localized patches of morphoea may later develop systemic sclerosis [1,9]. Although no systemic abnormalities were found in 27 autopsies on patients with localized morphoea [10], changes in the oesophagus, muscles and joints may occur in as many as 27% of cases [11]. The diagnosis of systemic sclerosis was confirmed at autopsy in a 71-year-old woman with two patches of localized morphoea on the front of the chest, who subsequently developed cardiac enlargement, pulmonary fibrosis and a dilated aperistaltic oesophagus [12]. Typical morphoeic patches on the skin and gastrointestinal radiological changes typical of systemic sclerosis were found in another patient [13].

Morphoea has occurred with DLE [14], mixed connective tissue disease [15] and eosinophilic fasciitis [16], and frontoparietal morphoea has been associated with SLE [17]. Morphoea has followed SCLE [18] and may also occur with dermatomyositis [19], carpal tunnel syndrome [20], nephritis [21], vitiligo [22], pemphigus [23], primary biliary cirrhosis [24] and myasthenia gravis [25]. The coexistence of morphoea, localized bullous pemphigoid and subcorneal pustulosis has been reported [26]. Elastosis perforans serpiginosa has also occurred with morphoea [27]. Localized scleroderma can follow augmentation mammoplasty [28], and linear oedema, nodularity and scarring, with hidebound skin, has been attributed to leaking of silicone into an arm [29].

There is no relationship between localized morphoea and internal malignancy [30], although systemic sclerosis has been associated with carcinoma of the lung, skin and liver [30,31]. The morphoea-like changes found in patients with carcinoid syndrome are thought to occur as a result of serotonin release by the tumour [31]. Squamous cell carcinoma has been reported in patients with long-standing pansclerotic morphoea [32] and in localized scleroderma in a patient treated with azathioprine [33].

References

1 Christianson HB, Dorsey ES, O'Leary PA *et al*. Localized scleroderma: a clinical study of 235 cases. *Arch Dermatol* 1956; **74**: 629–39.
2 Bonifati C, Impara G, Morrone A *et al*. Simultaneous occurrence of linear scleroderma and homolateral segmental vitiligo. *J Eur Acad Dermatol Venereol* 2006; **20**: 63–5.
3 Basu S, Ganguly S. Homolateral linear morphea with coarctation of aorta. *Indian Paediatr* 2003; **40**: 1108–9.
4 Rufli T. Melanosis Becker mit lokalisierter Sklerodermie. *Dermatologica* 1972; **145**: 222–9.
5 Hazen PG, Askari A. Localized scleroderma with cutaneous calcinosis. *Arch Dermatol* 1979; **115**: 871–2.
6 Holmes RC, Meara RH. Morphoea, sclerotic panatrophy and disseminated granuloma annulare. *Clin Exp Dermatol* 1983; **8**: 201–3.
7 Zulian F, Vallongo C, Woo P *et al*. Localized scleroderma in childhood is not just a skin disease. *Arthritis Rheum* 2005; **52**: 2873–81.
8 Truelove SC, Whyte HM. Acrosclerosis. *BMJ* 1951; **ii**: 873–6.
9 Curtis AC, Jansen TG. The prognosis of localized scleroderma. *Arch Dermatol* 1958; **78**: 749–57.
10 Piper WN, Helwig EB. Progressive systemic sclerosis: visceral manifestations in generalized scleroderma. *Arch Dermatol* 1955; **72**: 535–46.
11 Luderschmidt C, Konig G, Leisner B *et al*. Zirkumskripte Sklerodermie: Interne manifestationen und signikante korrelation zu HLA-DR1 und DR-5. *Hautarzt* 1985; **36**: 516–21.
12 Rodnan GP, Fennell RH. Progressive systemic sclerosis sine scleroderma. *JAMA* 1962; **180**: 665–70.
13 Donaldson EM. Morphoea (localized scleroderma) with visceral changes. *Br J Dermatol* 1962; **74**: 105.

14 Umbert P, Winkelmann RK. Concurrent localized scleroderma and discoid lupus erythematosus. *Arch Dermatol* 1978; **114**: 1473–8.
15 Golding DN. Morphoea (localized scleroderma) in a patient with mixed connective tissue disease. *Ann Rheum Dis* 1986; **45**: 523–5.
16 Piette WW, Dorsey JK, Foucar E. Clinical and serologic expression of localized scleroderma. *J Am Acad Dermatol* 1985; **13**: 342–50.
17 Mackel SE, Kozin F, Ryan LM *et al*. Concurrent linear scleroderma and systemic lupus erythematosus. *J Invest Dermatol* 1979; **73**: 368–72.
18 Rao BK, Coldiron B, Freeman RG *et al*. Subacute lupus erythematosus lesions progressing to morphoea. *J Am Acad Dermatol* 1990; **23**: 1019–22.
19 Štáva Z. Zirkumskripte Sklerodermie (klinische analyse von 50 ausgewählten fällen). *Dermatol Wochenschr* 1959; **139**: 513–23.
20 Winkelmann RK, Connolly SM, Doyle JA. Carpal tunnel syndrome in cutaneous connective tissue disease: generalized morphea, lichen sclerosus, fasciitis, discoid lupus erythematosus and lupus panniculitis. *J Am Acad Dermatol* 1982; **7**: 94–9.
21 Bourgeois-Droin C, Touraine R. Sclerodermie en plaques, perturbations immunologiques et viscerales. *Ann Med Interne* 1978; **129**: 107–12.
22 Finkelstein E, Amichai B, Metzker A. Coexistence of vitiligo and morphoea: a case report and review of the literature. *J Dermatol* 1995; **22**: 351–3.
23 Chan LS, Cooper KD. Coexistence of pemphigus vulgaris and progressive localized scleroderma. *Arch Dermatol* 1989; **125**: 1555–7.
24 Reed JR, De Luca N, McIntyre AS *et al*. Localized morphoea, xanthomatosis and primary biliary cirrhosis. *Br J Dermatol* 2000; **143**: 652–3.
25 Kim HS, Chun YS, Hann SK *et al*. A case of linear scleroderma and myasthenia gravis. *J Dermatol* 2000; **27**: 31–4.
26 Bernstein JE, Medenica M, Soltani K. Coexistence of localized bullous pemphigoid, morphoea and subcorneal pustulosis. *Arch Dermatol* 1981; **117**: 725–7.
27 Barr RJ, Siegel JM, Graham JH. Elastosis perforans serpiginosa associated with morphoea. *J Am Acad Dermatol* 1981; **3**: 19–22.
28 Spiera H. Scleroderma after silicone augmentation mammoplasty. *JAMA* 1988; **260**: 236–8.
29 Teuber SS, Ito LK, Anderson M, Gershwin ME. Silicone breast implant-associated scarring dystrophy of the arm. *Arch Dermatol* 1995; **131**: 54–6.
30 Rosenthal AK, McLaughlin JK, Gridley G *et al*. Incidence of cancer among patients with systemic sclerosis. *Cancer* 1995; **76**: 910–4.
31 Jablonska S. Scleroderma and malignancy. In: Jablonska S, ed. *Scleroderma and Pseudoscleroderma*. Warsaw: Polish Medical Publishers, 1975; 606–9.
32 Parodi F, Stolz W, Volkenandt M *et al*. Squamous cell carcinoma in a patient with long-standing pansclerotic morphoea. *Br J Dermatol* 2001; **144**: 417–9.
33 Nachbar F, Stolz W, Volkenandt M *et al*. Squamous cell carcinoma in localized scleroderma following immunosuppression with azathioprine. *Acta Derm Venereol* 1993; **73**: 217–9.

Laboratory abnormalities. ESR and serum protein assays are usually normal, but eosinophilia may occur [1]. Anti-single-stranded DNA antibodies are more frequent in generalized morphoea (75%) and linear morphoea (53.3%) than in localized morphoea (27.3%) [2]. Antihistone antibodies have been detected in 32% of patients with linear morphoea and in 25% with localized morphoea in one study [3] and in 71% of children and 65% of adults with linear morphoea in another [4]. In the latter and one further study [5], it has been suggested that they mirror disease activity. Hereditary deficiency of complement factor C2 is reported [6]. Organ-specific autoantibodies are more commonly found than in controls [7]. Thrombocytopenia responding to corticosteroid therapy has been reported in two patients [8]. Approximately 40% of patients with linear morphoea have positive antinuclear antibodies, and the presence of these antibodies (with homogeneous and nucleolar patterns), antibodies to single-stranded DNA and the presence of eosinophilia may indicate disease activity [9] and the late development of systemic complications [10]. Serum procollagen type 1 carboxy-terminal propeptide has been reported to be raised in 30% of patients with localized morphoea, correlating with the number of lesions. Levels are lower than in generalized morphoea and may be a useful indicator of disease activity [11]. Type 3 procollagen propeptide has also been reported to be raised [12]. However, others have not found these markers as useful.

Topoisomerase 1 (Scl-70) is unusual in localized scleroderma but a recent study has found autoantibodies to topoisomerase 11α in 70% of patients with localized scleroderma and 85% of patients with generalized morphoea [13]. IgM rheumatoid factor has been suggested to be a useful marker of disease severity [14], and IgM anticardiolipin antibodies have been reported as associated with a greater number of lesions [15]. In another study, antinucleosome antibodies were found to have a higher prevalence in localized scleroderma [16]. All the serological changes associated with localized scleroderma have been recently reviewed [17].

In children, in a recent large series from 70 European centres [18], ANA was positive in 42%, rheumatoid factor in 16%, anticardiolipin antibody in 13%, anti-double-stranded DNA in 4%, Scl-70 in 3% and anticentromere antibody in 2%.

Ultrasound scanning has been reported as being helpful in diagnosing morphoea [19], in differentiating morphoea from lichen sclerosus et atrophicus [20], and in monitoring the course of localized morphoea [21]. The dermatoscope has been reported as a useful tool for assessing nail fold capillary abnormalities [22].

Prognosis. Plaque-like lesions tend to improve with time. The induration lessens and the lesions blend in with the rest of the skin, leaving a brownish stain, which may persist for a long time. The duration of activity is usually between 3 and 5 years, but some lesions last up to 25 years. It is common to find fresh lesions developing on new sites as other lesions resolve. Residual pigmentation persists for a long time in approximately one-third of patients. Linear lesions tend to persist for longer than plaque lesions, but on the whole improve with time. Calcinosis occasionally occurs in linear lesions, and sometimes requires surgical removal. Contractures may limit movement of joints and give rise to clawing of the hand. Unilateral atrophy of one or more limbs may occur. Facial hemiatrophy is usually persistent, but frontoparietal scleroderma may clear, and may be accompanied by regrowth of hair. In 63 of 88 children with morphoea, lesions resolved with minimal cosmetic disability [23]. Very rarely, patients with localized morphoea may subsequently develop classical systemic sclerosis [23,24]. It has been suggested that the presence of anti-Ku antibody may be a prognostic indicator of such progression [24].

Differential diagnosis. The diagnosis is usually not difficult, the insidious development of indurated plaques and bands in the skin, with or without hemiatrophy, being unlikely to occur in other conditions. If there is a lilac-coloured border diagnosis is easier. Reticulate lilac lesions with minimal induration can resemble cutaneous polyarteritis nodosa. Morphoeic lesions occur in sarcoidosis [25]. Lesions can start as a vascular blush, and may be mistaken for a macular vascular naevus. In the acute phase, the condition must be distinguished from scleroedema of Buschke, but in this condition the onset is much more acute, and the lesions may follow an infectious episode. Fading pigmented lesions are sometimes very difficult to diagnose, but the previous history of

some induration in the area is usually helpful. Atrophic pigmented lesions resembling lesions of the atrophy of Pierini and Pasini (see Chapter 45) [26] occurred in 47% of the patients in one series [27]. Abdominal lesions may be confused with so-called lipodystrophia centrifugalis abdominalis infantilis (see Chapter 46) [28,29]. Atrophic morphoeic plaques can result from intramuscular injections of vitamin K [30] or subcutaneous corticosteroid injections [31]. Conditions producing pseudoscleroderma (see p. 51.79) may have to be considered. Melorheostosis is a rare condition in which there are painful abnormalities of the skeleton and adjacent soft tissues, usually limited to a single limb. Linear endosteal bony densities of the long bones are seen on radiography, and resemble candle wax flowing along the affected bone. In children, the usual presentation is with asymmetrical contractures of a limb, occurring in association with thickening of the overlying skin and fascia, and distal vascular problems exacerbated by attempted surgical correction of the orthopaedic problem, including angiomas and arteriovenous malformations [32]. It is suggested that the distribution of these lesions represents the sclerotome, or the areas of the body supplied by a spinal sensory nerve, and that skin and muscle involvement occur in the relevant dermatome and myotome [33]. The cutaneous lesions are almost certainly a part of the developmental abnormality, rather than coexisting linear morphoea [34].

Treatment. As the expected natural history is towards spontaneous resolution, the condition may be allowed to take its natural course, if uncomplicated. If intervention is required, localized treatment with topical or intralesional steroids may be helpful [35]. More recently, calcipotriol has been shown to inhibit the growth of morphoea fibroblasts *in vitro* [36], and has proved beneficial when used topically *in vivo*, both alone [37,38] and in combination with UVA-1 in children [39]. Topical tacrolimus has been reported as being beneficial in seven patients [40] as has 5% imiquimod cream [41].

Numerous systemic agents have been reported to be helpful in morphoea (on the basis of case reports or small open studies), including phenytoin [42], *p*-aminobenzoate [43], griseofulvin [44], etretinate [45], vitamin E [46], chloroquine and hydroxychloroquine [47]. Tranilast was reported as helpful in a boy with linear morphoea and contractures [48], and plasmapheresis was helpful (in combination with systemic corticosteroids) in three patients with localized scleroderma and antinuclear antibodies [49]. Regression of plaques of morphoea after tamoxifen therapy has been reported in one patient [50], and a child with pansclerotic morphoea showed significant improvement after 3 months' therapy with the oral endothelin receptor antagonist bosentan [51]. Topical photodynamic therapy was reported as being helpful in five patients with localized disease [52].

Systemic corticosteroids have been found to be helpful in an open trial [53], although they are probably only beneficial in the inflammatory stage of the disease [35]. d-Penicillamine has been reported as helpful in open trials [54–56] in regimens of 2–5 mg/kg/day, with or without pyridoxine 20 mg/day. However, there is a risk of renal damage [54]. Ciclosporin was found to be helpful in open studies in localized morphoea [57,58] and in a single case of linear scleroderma in a child [59]. Oral calcitriol, in regimens of 0.5–0.75 μg/day, has been reported as helpful in a small study

[60], but a recent double-blind placebo controlled trial did not confirm this [61].

In recent years, UVA irradiation, both alone at low [62–65], medium [66] and high doses [67], as bath or oral photochemotherapy [68–71], and in combination with calcipotriol [39], has been reported as helpful. Two randomized controlled trials have both confirmed that low-dose broad-band UVA (UVA1) is as effective as medium- or high-dose UVA regimens or narrow-band UVB [72,73]. The effect is thought to result from increased production of collagenase and IFN-δ, and decreased TGF-β and collagen production [74]. A single case report has suggested that low-dose UVA was helpful in softening lesions in a case of pansclerotic morphoea in an 8-year-old girl [75]. The main therapeutic advance for morphoea, however, is the greater use of methotrexate. In low dose, this agent has proved useful in both widespread morphoea [76,77] and in localized morphoea in children when used in combination with systemic corticosteroids [78–82].

Physical therapy in the form of physiotherapy may be helpful in preventing joint deformities and contractures, and in maintaining joint movement and muscle strength. It may also help to prevent sclerosis secondary to lymphoedema in the limbs of patients with linear morphoea [35]. Surgical intervention for the relief of contractures [83], the lengthening of limbs and the correction of deformities may have to be carried out in certain cases. Various plastic surgery techniques can help patients with 'en coup de sabre' morphoea [84–95] and those with ossification [96]. Ulcers associated with bullous lesions have been treated with 'tissue-engineered' skin [97]. For those patients in whom the sclerotic processes have extended into the jaw to involve the teeth, dental treatment may be required.

References

1 Giordano M, Ara M, Valentini G et al. Presence of eosinophilia in progressive systemic sclerosis and localized scleroderma. Arch Dermatol Res 1981; 271: 411–7.

2 Ruffatti A, Peserico A, Rondinone R et al. Prevalence and characteristics of anti-single-stranded DNA antibodies in localized scleroderma. Arch Dermatol 1991; 127: 1180–3.

3 Sato S, Ihn H, Soma Y et al. Antihistone antibodies in patients with localized scleroderma. Arthritis Rheum 1993; 36: 1137–41.

4 El-Azhary RA, Aponte CC, Nelson AM et al. Antihistone antibodies in linear scleroderma variants. Int J Dermatol 2006; 45: 1296–9.

5 El-Azhary RA, Aponte CC, Nelson AM et al. Do antihistone autoantibodies reflect disease activity in linear scleroderma? Arch Dermatol 2004; 140: 759–60.

6 Hulsmans RFHJ, Asghar SS, Siddiqui AH et al. Hereditary deficiency of C2 in association with linear scleroderma 'en coup de sabre'. Arch Dermatol 1986; 122: 76–9.

7 Harrington I, Dunsmore IR. An investigation into the incidence of auto-immune disorders in patients with localized morphoea. Br J Dermatol 1989; 120: 645–8.

8 Neucks SH, Moore TL, Lichtenstein JR et al. Localized scleroderma and idiopathic thrombocytopenia. J Rheumatol 1980; 7: 741–4.

9 Falanga V, Medsger TA, Reichlin M et al. Linear scleroderma: clinical spectrum, prognosis and laboratory abnormalities. Ann Intern Med 1986; 104: 849–57.

10 Woo TY, Rasmussen JE. Juvenile linear scleroderma associated with serologic abnormalities. Arch Dermatol 1985; 121: 1403–5.

11 Kikuchi K, Sato S, Kadono T et al. Serum concentration of procollagen type 1 carboxy-terminal propeptide in localized scleroderma. Arch Dermatol 1994; 130: 1269–72.

12 Zachariae H, Halkier-Sorensen L, Heickendorff L. Serum aminoterminal propeptide of type III procollagen in progressive systemic sclerosis and localized scleroderma. Acta Derm Venereol (Stockh) 1989; 69: 66–70.

13 Hayakawa I, Hasegawa M, Takehara K et al. Anti-topoisomerase 11α autoantibodies in localized scleroderma. Arthritis Rheum 2004; 50: 227–32.

14 Mimura Y, Ihn H, Jinnin M et al. Rheumatoid factor isotypes in localized scleroderma. Clin Exp Dermatol 2005; 30: 405–8.

15 Sato S, Fujimoto M, Hasegawa M et al. Antiphospholipid antibody in localised scleroderma. Ann Rheum Dis 2003; 62: 771–4.

16 Sato S, Kodera M, Hasegawa M et al. Antinucleosome antibody is a major autoantibody in localized scleroderma. Br J Dermatol 2004; 151: 1182–8.

17 Takehara K, Sato S. Localized scleroderma is an autoimmune disorder. Rheumatology 2005; 44: 274–9.

18 Zulian F, Athreya BH, Laxer R et al. Juvenile localized scleroderma: clinical and epidemiological features in 750 children. An international study. Rheumatology 2006; 45: 614–20.

19 Cosnes A, Anglade M-C, Revuz J et al. Thirteen-megahertz ultrasound probe: its role in diagnosing localized scleroderma. Br J Dermatol 2003; 148: 724–9.

20 Chen HC, Kadono T, Mimura Y et al. High frequency ultrasound as a useful device in the preliminary differentiation of lichen sclerosus et atrophicus from morphea. J Dermatol 2004; 31: 556–9.

21 Hoffman K, Gerbaulet U, El-Gammal S et al. 20-Mhz B-mode ultrasound in monitoring the course of localized scleroderma (morphoea). Acta Derm Venereol 1991; 164: 3–16.

22 Bergman R, Sharony L, Schapira D et al. The handheld dermatoscope as a nailfold capillaroscopic instrument. Arch Dermatol 2003; 139: 1027–30.

23 Torok E, Ablonczy E. Morphoea in children. Clin Exp Dermatol 1986; 11: 607–12.

24 Birdi N, Laxer RM, Thorner P et al. Localized scleroderma progressing to systemic disease: case report and review of the literature. Arthritis Rheum 1993; 36: 410–5.

25 Hess SP, Agudelo WL, White WL et al. Ichthyosiform and morpheaform sarcoidosis. Clin Exp Rheumatol 1990; 8: 171–5.

26 Jablonska S, Szczepanski A. Atrophoderma Pasini–Pierini. In: Jablonska S, ed. Scleroderma and Pseudoscleroderma. Warsaw: Polish Medical Publishers, 1975: 521–36.

27 Serup J. Clinical appearance of skin lesions and disturbances of pigmentation in localized scleroderma. Acta Derm Venereol (Stockh) 1984; 64: 485–92.

28 Imamura S, Yamada M, Ikeda T. Lipodystrophia centrifugalis abdominalis infantilis. Arch Dermatol 1971; 104: 291–8.

29 Zachary CB, Wells RS. Centrifugal lipodystrophia. Br J Dermatol 1984; 110: 107–10.

30 Texier L, Gendre P, Gauthier O et al. Hypodermites sclerodermiformes lombo-fessieres induites par des injections medicamenteuses intramusculaires associées a la vitamine K. Ann Dermatol Syphiligr 1972; 99: 363–71.

31 Holt PJA, Marks R, Waddington E. 'Pseudomorphoea': a side effect of subcutaneous corticosteroid injection. Br J Dermatol 1975; 92: 689–91.

32 Younge D, Drummond D, Herring J et al. Melorheostosis in children. J Bone Joint Surg 1979; 61: 415–8.

33 Murray RO, McCredie J. Melorheostosis and the sclerotomes: a radiological correlation. Skeletal Radiol 1979; 4: 57–71.

34 Muller SA, Henderson ED. Melorheostosis with linear scleroderma. Arch Dermatol 1963; 88: 142–5.

35 Hunzelmann N, Kochanek KS, Hager C et al. Management of localized scleroderma. Semin Cutan Med Surg 1998; 17: 34–40.

36 Bottomley WW, Jutley J, Wood EJ et al. The action of calcipotriol on fibroblasts from patients with active morphoea. Acta Derm Venereol (Stockh) 1995; 75: 364–6.

37 Cunningham BB, Landells ID, Langman C et al. Topical calcipotriene for morphea/linear scleroderma. J Am Acad Dermatol 1998; 39: 211–5.

38 Tay YK. Topical calcipotriol ointment in the treatment of morphea. J Dermatolog Treat 2002; 14: 219–21.

39 Kreuter A, Gambichler T, Avermaete A et al. Combined treatment with calcipotriol ointment and low dose ultraviolet A1 phototherapy in childhood morphoea. Paediatr Dermatol 2001; 18: 241–5.

40 Mancuso G, Berdondini RM. Localized scleroderma: response to occlusive treatment with tacrolimus ointment. Br J Dermatol 2005; 152: 180–2.

41 Dytoc M, Ting PT, Man J et al. First case series on the use of imiquimod for morphoea. Br J Dermatol 2005; 153: 815–20.

42 Nelder K. Treatment of localized linear scleroderma with phenytoin. Cutis 1978; 22: 569–72.

43 Zarafonetis CJD. Treatment of localized form of scleroderma. Am J Med Sci 1962; 243: 147–58.

44 Giordano M, Ara M, Capelli L, Tirri G. Griseofulvin in scleroderma. In: Black CM, Myers AR, eds. *Systemic Sclerosis (Scleroderma)*. New York, NY: Gower Medical, 1985: 423–7.

45 Neuhofer J, Fritsch P. Treatment of localized scleroderma and lichen sclerosus with etretinate. *Acta Derm Venereol (Stockh)* 1984; **64**: 171–4.

46 Ayres S, Mihan R. Is vitamin E involved in the autoimmune mechanism? *Cutis* 1978; **21**: 321–5.

47 Nagy E, Ladanyi E. Behandlung de umschriebenen Sklerodermie im Kindesalter. *Z Hautkr* 1987; **62**: 547–9.

48 Taniguchi S, Yorifiji T, Hamada T. Treatment of linear localized scleroderma with the anti-allergic drug, Tranilast. *Clin Exp Dermatol* 1994; **19**: 391–3.

49 Wach F, Ullrich H, Schmitz G *et al*. Treatment of severe localized sclero-derma by plasmapheresis: report of three cases. *Br J Dermatol* 1995; **133**: 605–9.

50 Ayoub N, Bouaziz JD, Barete S *et al*. Regression of morphoea plaques after tamoxifen therapy. *J Eur Acad Dermatol Venereol* 2004; **18**: 637–8.

51 Roldan R, Morote G, Castro M *et al*. Efficacy of bosentan in treatment of unre-sponsive cutaneous ulceration in disabling pansclerotic morphea in children. *J Rheumatol* 2006; **33**: 2538–40.

52 Karrer S, Abels C, Landthaler M *et al*. Topical photodynamic therapy for local-ized scleroderma. *Acta Derm Venereol* 2000; **80**: 26–7.

53 Joly P, Bamberger N, Crickx B *et al*. Treatment of severe forms of localized sclero-derma with oral corticosteroids: follow-up study on 17 patients. *Arch Dermatol* 1994; **130**: 663–4.

54 Moynahan EJ. Morphoea (localized cutaneous scleroderma) treated with low-dosage penicillamine. *Proc R Soc Med* 1973; **66**: 1083–5.

55 Falanga V, Medsger TA. D-Penicillamine in the treatment of localized sclero-derma. *Arch Dermatol* 1990; **126**: 609–12.

56 Satta MA, Guindi RT, Sugathan TN. Penicillamine in systemic sclerosis: a reap-praisal. *Clin Rheumatol* 1990; **9**: 517–22.

57 Peter RU, Ruzicka T. Cyclosporin A in der Therapie entzündlicher Dermatosen. *Hautarzt* 1992; **43**: 687–94.

58 Peter RU, Ruzicka T, Eckert F. Low dose cyclosporine A in the treatment of dis-abling morphoea. *Arch Dermatol* 1991; **127**: 1420–1.

59 Strauss RM, Bhushan M, Goodfield MJD. Good response of linear scleroderma in a child to ciclosporin. *Br J Dermatol* 2004; **150**: 790–2.

60 Humbert PG, Dupond JL, Rochefort A *et al*. Localized scleroderma: response to 1,25-dihydroxyvitamin D$_3$. *Clin Exp Dermatol* 1990; **15**: 396–8.

61 Hulshof MM, Bavinck JNB, Bergman W *et al*. Double-blind, placebo controlled study of oral calcitriol for the treatment of localized and systemic scleroderma. *J Am Acad Dermatol* 2000; **43**: 1017–23.

62 Kerscher M, Dirschke T, Volkenandt M. Treatment of localized scleroderma by UVA-1 phototherapy. *Lancet* 1995; **348**: 1166.

63 Kerscher M, Volkenandt M, Gruss C *et al*. Low-dose UVA phototherapy for treat-ment of localized scleroderma. *J Am Acad Dermatol* 1999; **40**: 787–8.

64 El Mofty M, Zahr H, Bosseila M *et al*. Low-dose broad-band UVA in morphoea using a new method for evaluation. *Photodermatol Photoimmunol Photomed* 2000; **16**: 43–9.

65 Gruss CJ, Von Kobyletzki G, Behrens-Williams SC *et al*. Effects of low dose ultraviolet A-1 phototherapy on morphoea. *Photodermatol Photoimmunol Pho-tomed* 2001; **45**: 697–9.

66 Camacho NR, Sanchez JE, Martin RF *et al*. Medium dose phototherapy in local-ized scleroderma and its effect in CD34-positive dendritic cells. *J Am Acad Der-matol* 2001; **45**: 697–9.

67 Stege H, Berneburg M, Humke S *et al*. High-dose UVA1 radiation therapy for localized scleroderma. *J Am Acad Dermatol* 1997; **36**: 938–44.

68 Kerscher M, Meurer M, Sandu C *et al*. PUVA bath photochemotherapy for local-ized scleroderma: evaluation of 17 consecutive patients. *Arch Dermatol* 1996; **132**: 1280–2.

69 Morison WL. Psoralen UVA therapy for linear and generalized morphoea. *J Am Acad Dermatol* 1997; **37**: 657–9.

70 Kanekura T, Fukumara S, Matsushita S *et al*. Successful treatment of scleroderma with PUVA therapy. *J Dermatol* 1996; **23**: 455–9.

71 De Rie MA, Bos JD. Photochemotherapy for systemic and localized scleroderma. *J Am Acad Dermatol* 2000; **43**: 725–6.

72 El Mofty M, Mostafa W, El-Darouty M *et al*. Different low doses of broad-band UVA in the treatment of morphea and systemic sclerosis. A clinico-pathologic study. *Photodermatol Photoimmunol Photomed* 2004; **20**: 148–56.

73 Kreuter A, Hyun J, Stucker M *et al*. A randomized controlled study of low-dose UVA1, medium-dose UVA1 and narrowband UVB phototherapy in the treat-ment of localized scleroderma. *J Am Acad Dermatol* 2006; **54**: 440–7.

74 El Mofty M, Mostafa W, Esmat S *et al*. Suggested mehanisms of action of UVA phototherapy in morphea: a molecular study. *Photodermatol Photoimmunol Pho-tomed* 2004; **20**: 93–100.

75 Yildirim M, Baysal V, Aridogan BC *et al*. Pansclerotic morphea treated with UVA: a case report. *J Dermatol* 2003; **30**: 625–7.

76 Seyger MMB, Van Den Hoogen FHJ, De Boo T *et al*. Low-dose methotrexate in the treatment of widespread morphea. *J Am Acad Dermatol* 1998; **39**: 220–5.

77 Seyger MM, Van Den Hoogen FH, Van Vlijem-Willems IM *et al*. Localized and systemic scleroderma show different histological responses to methotrexate therapy. *J Pathol* 2001; **193**: 511–6.

78 Uziel Y, Feldman BM, Krafchik BR *et al*. Methotrexate and corticosteroid therapy for pediatric localized scleroderma. *J Pediatr* 2000; **136**: 91–5.

79 Kreuter A, Gambichler T, Breukmann F *et al*. Pulsed high-dose corticosteroids combined with low-dose methotrexate in severe localized scleroderma. *Arch Dermatol* 2005; **141**: 847–52.

80 Fitch PG, Rettig P, Burnham JM *et al*. Treatment of paediatric localized sclero-derma with methotrexate. *J Rheumatol* 2006; **33**: 609–14.

81 Weibel L, Sampaio MC, Visentin MT *et al*. Evaluation of methotrexate and corti-costeroids for the treatment of localized scleroderma (morphoea) in children. *Br J Dermatol* 2006; **155**: 1013–20.

82 Weibel L, Harper JI, Howell KJ. Morphea (localized scleroderma). *J Pediatr* 2007; **150**: 560.

83 Longacre JJ, Wagner GA. The surgical management of disabling contractures due to linear scleroderma. *Plast Reconstr Surg* 1952; **9**: 367–80.

84 Neumann CG. The use of large buried pedicle flaps of dermis on fat: clinical and pathological evaluation in the treatment of progressive facial hemiatrophy. *Plast Reconstr Surg* 1953; **11**: 315–32.

85 Sengezer M, Deveci M, Selmanpakoglu N. Repair of 'coup de sabre': a linear form of scleroderma. *Ann Plast Surg* 1996; **37**: 428–32.

86 Eguchi T, Harii K, Sugawara Y. Repair of a large 'coup de sabre' with soft-tissue expansion and artificial bone graft. *Ann Plast Surg* 1999; **42**: 207–10.

87 Lapiere JC, Aasi S, Cook B *et al*. Successful correction of depressed scars of the forehead secondary to trauma and en coup de sabre by en bloc autologous dermal fat graft. *Dermatol Surg* 2000; **26**: 793–7.

88 Danino AM, Ichinose M, Yoshimoto S *et al*. Repair of wide coup de sabre without cutaneous excision by means of pericranial–galeal padding flap. *Plast Reconstr Surg* 1999; **104**: 2108–11.

89 Oh CK, Lee J, Jang BS *et al*. Treatment of atrophies secondary to trilinear sclero-derma en coup de sabre by autologous tissue cocktail injection. *Dermatol Surg* 2003; **29**: 1073–5.

90 Nguyen XH, Hansen R, Valencia F. Severe ankle deformity secondary to pan-sclerotic morphea in a 9-year-old girl: correction involving arthrodesis and free flap coverage. *Pediatr Dermatol* 2002; **19**: 560–3.

91 Serel S, Uluc A, Can Z. Treatment of coup de sabre facial contour deformity with hydroxyapatite paste. *Ann Plast Surg* 2006; **57**: 241.

92 Copcu E. Treatment of coup de sabre deformity with porous polyethylene implant. *Plast Reconstr Surg* 2004; **113**: 758–9.

93 Hartwright D, Leslie IJ, Clarke S. Management of tenosynovitis in linear sclero-derma. *Rheumatology* 2006; **45**: 640–1.

94 Smucker J, Heller JG, Bohleman HH *et al*. Surgical treatment of destructive cal-cific lesions of the cervical spine in scleroderma: case series and review of the literature. *Spine* 2006; **31**: 2002–8.

95 Worret WI, Jessberger B. Effectiveness of LPG treatment in morphea. *J Eur Acad Dermatol Venereol* 2004; **18**: 527–30.

96 Handfield-Jones SE, Peachey RDG, Moss ALH, Dawson A. Ossification in linear morphoea with hemifacial atrophy: treatment by surgical excision. *Clin Exp Dermatol* 1988; **13**: 385–8.

97 Martin LK, Kirsner RS. Ulcers caused by bullous morphea treated with tissue-engineered skin. *Int J Dermatol* 2003; **42**: 402–4.

Generalized morphoea

Synonym
- Generalized scleroderma

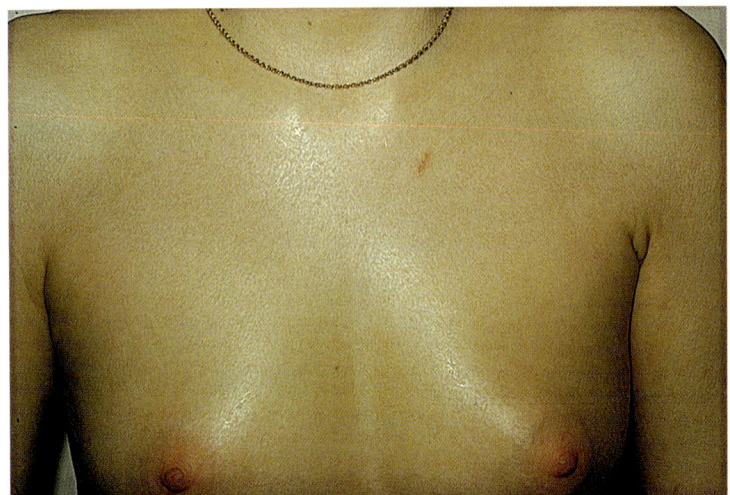

Fig. 51.56 Generalized morphoea showing diffuse tightness of the skin of the chest.

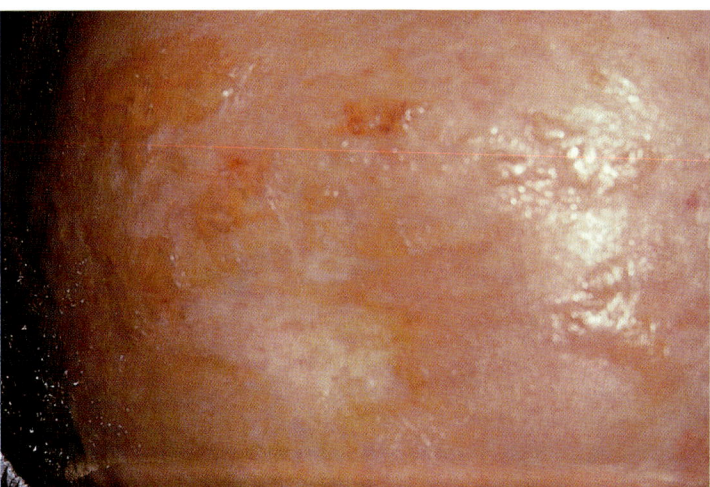

Fig. 51.57 Bullous lesions in generalized morphoea.

Definition. A rare condition in which idiopathic sclerosis of the skin occurs in a widespread manner. It usually starts on the trunk and is not associated with systemic disturbances.

Aetiology. The aetiology is unknown. The most frequent age of onset is between 30 and 40 years, and lesions start between the ages of 11 and 50 years in 80% of patients [1]. Approximately three females are affected for every male. The occurrence of generalized morphoea and localized morphoea in two sisters has been reported [2].

Pathology. This is identical to that of localized morphoea. It has been suggested that in the early stages an inflammatory infiltrate of lymphocytes, histiocytes and plasma cells is found, primarily in the subcutaneous tissue. Later, the subcutaneous tissue is replaced by hyalinized connective tissue and this is responsible for the induration of the skin. Direct immunofluorescence shows changes in approximately one-third of cases, with IgM in the basement membrane and IgM and C3 in the dermal blood vessels being the most frequent findings. Similar changes may occur less frequently in linear morphoea.

Clinical features (Fig. 51.56). The onset is usually insidious, and the patient notices the development of plaques resembling those of localized morphoea. A lilac-coloured border surrounding the indurated ivory-white shiny lesions is usually seen in the early stages. The plaques are commonly much larger than those seen in localized morphoea, being many centimetres in diameter. Usually, plaques start on the trunk and gradually increase in size, with the development of new plaques over the first year or two. The main areas involved are the upper trunk, breasts, abdomen and upper thighs. The arms may also be involved, and in some cases the hands resemble those seen in the tumid phase of systemic sclerosis, with spindling of the fingers, binding of the skin to the underlying tissues and semiflexion of the hands and fingers. The legs, face, neck and scalp may also be involved. Scarring alopecia can result from involvement of the scalp. In some cases, the whole of the body may be involved from the top of the head to the feet,

although this occurred in only one out of 44 cases in one series [1]. Mechanical compression has been suggested as an aetiological factor [3]. If the chest wall is markedly involved there may be difficulty in breathing because of constriction of the thorax. The intercostal muscles may also be involved, and death may result from respiratory failure [4]. The face is expressionless, the skin being shiny, often brown, and indurated. Telangiectasia of the face is not a feature, and although mouth opening may be restricted, the radial furrowing of systemic sclerosis is not seen. Raynaud's phenomenon occurs occasionally but is not a characteristic feature. Sometimes, especially after trauma, the hands may develop whitlows, but there is no atrophy as seen in systemic sclerosis. The tissues of the trunk and limbs sometimes show a brawny non-pitting oedema and acute widespread oedema associated with hypoproteinaemia has been observed [5]. Bullae may develop in localized areas, particularly on the abdomen (Fig. 51.57). Nodular lesions may also occur [6], and multiple keloids may be the first manifestation of the disease [7]. Acral myofibromas have been reported [8]. If the condition is generalized, it may be impossible to see any area showing a lilac border. Pigmentation is common, and in some patients may be generalized. Amyloid deposition [9] and amyloidosis cutis dyschromica [10] have been reported. Keratoses and calcinosis can occur.

Contractures occur in limbs, which become thin and hard. Some patients complain of considerable soreness in the acute phase, especially of the trunk and breasts. Joint pains occur in approximately 50% of patients, particularly in the fingers, wrists, elbows and knees. Definite rheumatoid arthritis may be found. Very occasionally, severe contractures, atrophy and infection may be associated with intractable pain in the limbs, and amputation may be required. Squamous cell carcinoma may develop in lesions of over 20 years' duration [11,12].

Sometimes generalized morphoea may develop as an extension of localized morphoea or be associated with lesions of lichen sclerosus et atrophicus [13]. Subcutaneous morphoea [14] seems to be more inflammatory than generalized morphoea of the dermis, and may respond to anti-inflammatory agents. Such cases may be more likely to develop mild systemic involvement and have eosinophilia. Generalized morphoea has been associated with polymyositis and the sick sinus syndrome [15], and necrotizing vasculitis [16], primary biliary cirrhosis [17] and fasciitis [18].

Laboratory investigations. Investigation for systemic disease is usually negative. Eosinophilia, elevated ESR and hypocomplementaemia occasionally occur. Anti-single-stranded DNA antibody occurs, but anti-double-stranded DNA antibody is rare. Serum procollagen type 1 carboxy-terminal propeptide may be a useful index of activity. Levels are higher than in localized morphoea [19]. Scl-70 antibodies are rarely found.

Differential diagnosis. The following points help to distinguish morphoea from systemic sclerosis. Raynaud's phenomenon is uncommon in generalized morphoea and is almost universal in systemic sclerosis. The distribution of the lesions also differs. In generalized morphoea, the trunk is more frequently involved, whereas the face, hands and, to a lesser extent, the feet, are most commonly involved in systemic sclerosis. Generalized morphoea usually slowly improves over the years. Scleroedema of Buschke is usually a more acute and less widespread disorder. Morphoea must also be distinguished from the various conditions described below under 'pseudoscleroderma'. Generalized morphoea may have to be distinguished from eosinophilic fasciitis (see p. 51.86).

Prognosis. Some improvement is usually seen in the course of 3–5 years, but the disease may last for many years and one patient still showed changes 33 years after diagnosis [1]. In most cases, the skin slowly softens and the pigmentation decreases. With time, the tendency to ulceration, with trauma and blistering, decreases. Although some patients may be severely disabled by the immobility associated with the sclerotic changes and contractures, others with widespread sclerosis may remain surprisingly active. Patients usually remain in good health although one patient died of bronchiolitis obliterans organizing pneumonia [20].

Treatment. The general measures outlined previously for the treatment of localized disease are just as important for patients with generalized disease.

A number of systemic agents may help generalized disease, including systemic steroids, penicillamine, antimalarials and low-dose methotrexate. In addition, individual case reports suggest a role for agents such as sulfasalazine [21], salazopyrin [22], grenz ray treatment [23] and extracorporeal photochemotherapy [24]. Initial reports suggested a role for oral calcitriol but a recent double-blind study has not confirmed this.

An increasing body of literature suggests that ciclosporin may be helpful for generalized morphoea either alone [25,26], or in combination with PUVA [27], although controlled studies are lacking. The last-mentioned case report also suggests a role for PUVA in combination with mycophenolate mofetil. Ciclosporin must be used with care, however, as side effects are common. Severe renal disease may result, although this is perhaps more likely in patients with active systemic disease [28,29]. As for localized disease, methotrexate in combination with steroids is emerg-

ing as a useful therapeutic regimen [30]. UVA phototherapy and photochemotherapy may be helpful.

References

1 Christianson HB, Dorsey ES, O'Leary PA et al. Localized scleroderma: a clinical study of 235 cases. *Arch Dermatol* 1956; **74**: 581–9.
2 Burge KM, Perry HO, Stickler GB. 'Familial' scleroderma. *Arch Dermatol* 1969; **99**: 681–7.
3 Ehara M, Oono T, Yamasaki O et al. Generalized morphoea like lesions arising in mechanically compressed areas by underclothes. *Eur J Dermatol* 2006; **16**: 307–9.
4 Russell DC, Maloney A, Muir AL. Progressive generalized scleroderma: respiratory failure from primary chest wall involvement. *Thorax* 1981; **36**: 219–20.
5 Rose RF, Goodfield MJD, Gilbey SG. Acute widespread oedema, hypoproteinaemia and generalized morphoea. *Clin Exp Dermatol* 2005; **30**: 303–4.
6 Micalizzi C, Parodi A, Rebora A. Morphoea with nodular lesions. *Br J Dermatol* 1994; **131**: 298–301.
7 Akintewe TA, Alabi GO. Scleroderma presenting with multiple keloids. *BMJ* 1985; **291**: 448–9.
8 English JC, Derdeyn AS, Smith PD et al. Adult acral cutaneous myofibromas in a patient with generalized morphoea. *J Am Acad Dermatol* 2002; **46**: 953–6.
9 Sumi K, Yamamoto T, Yokozeki H et al. Amyloid deposition associated with generalized morphea-like scleroderma. *Eur J Dermatol* 2003; **13**: 509–11.
10 Morales Callaghan AM, Vila JB, Fraile HA et al. Amyloidosis cutis dyschromica in a patient with generalized morphoea. *Br J Dermatol* 2004; **150**: 616–7.
11 Michalowski R. Diffuse morphoea with calcinosis cutis and squamous-cell carcinoma. *Br J Dermatol* 1967; **79**: 453–5.
12 Greco M, Kupfer BL, Delahaye JF et al. Multiple cutaneous squamous carcinomas arising in a patient with generalized morphea. *Eur J Dermatol* 2006; **16**: 90–1.
13 Patterson JAR, Ackerman AB. Lichen sclerosus et atrophicus is not related to morphoea: a clinical and histologic study of 24 patients in whom both conditions were reputed to be present simultaneously. *Am J Dermatopathol* 1984; **6**: 323–35.
14 Person JR, Su WPD. Subcutaneous morphoea: a clinical study of 16 cases. *Br J Dermatol* 1979; **100**: 371–80.
15 Nagai Y, Ishikawa O. A case of generalized morphea and polymyositis accompanied by sick sinus syndrome. *J Dermatol* 2001; **28**: 576–7.
16 Morita A, Tsuji T. Necrotizing vasculitis in a patient with generalized morphea. *J Am Acad Dermatol* 2001; **45**: S215–7.
17 Gonzalez-Lopez MA, Drake M, Gonzalez-vela MC et al. Generalized morphea and primary biliary cirrhosis coexisting in a male patient. *J Dermatol* 2006; **33**: 709–13.
18 Takamure M, Murata K, Kawahara M et al. Fasciitis associated with generalized morphea. *Intern Med* 2005; **44**: 679–81.
19 Kikuchi K, Sato S, Kadono T et al. Serum concentration of procollagen type 1 carboxy-terminal propeptide in localized scleroderma. *Arch Dermatol* 1994; **130**: 1269–72.
20 Cheung ST, Khair OA, Maheshwari MB et al. Fatal outcome of generalized morphea with bronchiolitis obliterans organizing pneumonia. *Clin Exp Dermatol* 2006; **31**: 722–3.
21 Taveira M, Selores M, Costa V et al. Generalized morphea and lichen sclerosus et atrophicus successfully treated with sulphasalazine. *J Eur Acad Dermatol Venereol* 1999; **12**: 283–4.
22 Micalizzi C, Parodi A, Rebora A. Generalized bullous morphea: efficacy of salazopyrin. *Clin Exp Dermatol* 1996; **21**: 246–7.
23 Molin L. Reduced skin stiffness by grenz ray treatment in generalized morphea. *Adv Exp Med Biol* 1999; **45**: 317–8.
24 Cribier B, Faradji T, Le-Coz C et al. Extracorporeal photochemotherapy in systemic sclerosis and severe morphea. *Dermatology* 1995; **191**: 25–31.
25 Stevens HP, Ostlere LS, Black CM et al. Generalized morphoea secondary to porphyria cutanea tarda. *Br J Dermatol* 1993; **129**: 455–7.
26 Worle B, Hein R, Krieg T et al. Cyclosporin in localized and systemic scleroderma: a clinical study. *Dermatologica* 1990; **181**: 215–20.
27 Rose RF, Goodfield MJD. Combining PUVA therapy with systemic immunosuppression to treat progressive diffuse morphoea. *Clin Exp Dermatol* 2005; **30**: 226–8.
28 Morton SJ, Powell RJ. Cyclosporin and tacrolimus: their use in a routine clinical setting for scleroderma. *Rheumatology* 2000; **39**: 865–9.

29 Clements PJ, Lachenbruch PA, Sterz M *et al.* Cyclosporine in systemic sclerosis: results of a 48 week open safety study in 10 patients. *Arthritis Rheum* 1994; **37**: 301–2.

30 Kawashima H, Watanabe C, Yasuyo K *et al.* Therapy of generalized morphea: case reports and reviews of the Japanese cases. *Pediatr Int* 2006; **48**: 342–5.

Pseudoscleroderma

Sclerosis of the skin may be seen in several conditions other than morphoea or systemic sclerosis [1]. It comprises a major feature of eosinophilic fasciitis and may also be seen in dermatomyositis and SLE, and this is covered elsewhere in this chapter. Pseudosclerodermatous changes may also be seen in rheumatoid arthritis [2] and acrodermatitis atrophicans, a disease found in central and eastern Europe which resembles localized morphoea (see Chapter 45). Scleroderma-like changes may also be found in a number of other conditions, and these are set out below using the classification of a review article [1].

References

1 Haustein U. Scleroderma and pseudoscleroderma: uncommon presentations. *Clin Dermatol* 2005; **23**: 480–90.

2 Bergouignan M, Arne L, Guerin A, Texier L. Sclérodermie progressive, dystrophie musculaire, syndrome endocrinien. *Rev Neurol* 1950; **83**: 126–30.

Metabolic disorders

Scleroderma-like changes are sometimes seen in porphyria cutanea tarda [1,2] and in phenylketonuria [3,4], when they usually appear in the first year of life. In the latter condition, irregular indurations appear first in the muscles and subcutis of the thighs and buttocks, and later the changes extend to the trunk and proximal parts of the limbs. Contractures, especially of the legs, are characteristic. Histology shows proliferation of histiocytes and fibroblasts in the connective tissue stroma, atrophy of the skin appendages and an inflammatory infiltrate. Improvement in the skin lesions occurs with exclusion of phenylalanine from the diet. In older children, the lesions and histology resemble morphoea. Two mentally retarded siblings with phenylketonuria had morphoea and atrophoderma of Pasini and Pierini, respectively [5], suggesting that these conditions may be related. Scleroderma-like lesions have been observed in cases of muscle glycogenosis with an undetermined enzyme defect [6], when induration and atrophy occur in the skin and muscles in the first few months of life. The proximal parts of the limbs are involved early and contractures occur, particularly in the legs, giving a characteristic bent-knee gait. Mental retardation may be a feature. Sclerosis of the legs may be found in patients with the carcinoid syndrome [7,8], and sclerosis of the skin occurs in the GEMSS syndrome (glaucoma, lens ectopia, microspherophakia, stiffness of the joints and shortness due to increased production of normal collagen) [9]. The skin may be oedematous and indurated in hypothyroidism, and atrophic changes in the skin in postpartum hypopituitarism may resemble scleroderma. Pseudosclerodermatous changes may also be seen in patients with long-standing diabetes mellitus in which limited joint mobility, termed cheiroarthropathy, is associated with thickening of the skin. The changes are most marked on the hands [10].

A recent report linked the onset of scleroderma-like changes to the diagnosis of cancer, this being postulated to be due to elevated expression of basic fibroblast growth factor [11].

References

1 Stevens HP, Ostlere LS, Black CM *et al.* Generalized morphoea secondary to porphyria cutanea tarda. *Br J Dermatol* 1993; **129**: 455–7.

2 Wilson PR. Porphyria cutanea tarda with cutaneous 'scleroderma' and calcification. *Australas J Dermatol* 1989; **30**: 93–6.

3 Jablonska S, Stachow A. Scleroderma-like lesions in phenylketonuria. In: Jablonska S, ed. *Scleroderma and Pseudoscleroderma.* Warsaw: Polish Medical Publishers, 1975: 489–98.

4 Nova MP, Kaufman M, Halpenin A. Scleroderma-like skin indurations in a child with phenylketonuria: a clinicopathologic correlation and review of the literature. *J Am Acad Dermatol* 1992; **26**: 329–33.

5 Lasser AE, Schultz BC, Beaff D *et al.* Phenylketonuria and scleroderma. *Arch Dermatol* 1978; **114**: 1215–7.

6 Jablonska S, Stachow A. Pseudoscleroderma concomitant with a muscular glycogenosis of unknown enzymatic defect. *Acta Derm Venereol (Stockh)* 1972; **52**: 379–85.

7 Fries JF, Lindgren JA, Bull JM. Scleroderma-like lesions and the carcinoid syndrome. *Arch Intern Med* 1973; **131**: 550–3.

8 Handley J, Walsh M, Armstrong K *et al.* Malignant carcinoid syndrome associated with cutaneous scleroderma. *Br J Dermatol* 1993; **129**: 222–3.

9 Kunz M, Paulins W, Sollberg S *et al.* Sclerosis of the skin in the GEMMS syndrome: an overproduction of normal collagen. *Arch Dermatol* 1995; **131**: 1170–4.

10 Seibold JR. Digital sclerosis in children with insulin-dependent diabetes mellitus. *Arthritis Rheum* 1982; **25**: 1357–61.

11 Kikuchi K, Hoashi T, Yazawa N *et al.* Pseudoscleroderma associated with cancer. *Clin Exp Dermatol* 2005; **31**: 381–3.

Deposition disorders

Scleroedema of Buschke is usually triggered by a febrile illness and comprises non-pitting induration of the face, neck, shoulders, arms and sometimes trunk. Scleromyxoedema also presents with thickening and tethering of the skin and is usually associated with a circulating paraprotein. The scleroderma-like lesions of primary systemic amyloidosis, with or without multiple myeloma, may be difficult to distinguish if not accompanied by nodular and papular lesions, particularly about the shoulders and neck, and by macroglossia. Primary localized cutaneous amyloidosis occurs in systemic sclerosis [1]. Pseudoscleroderma also occurs in multiple myeloma [2] and paraproteinaemia [3].

References

1 Black MM. Primary localized cutaneous amyloidosis in systemic sclerosis. *Trans St John's Hosp Dermatol Soc* 1971; **57**: 177–80.

2 Jablonska S, Stachow A. Scleroderma-like lesions in multiple myeloma. *Dermatologica* 1972; **144**: 257–69.

3 Oikarinen A, Ala-Kokko L, Palatsi R *et al.* Scleroderma and paraproteinemia. *Arch Dermatol* 1987; **123**: 226–9.

Genetic disorders

Atrophy of the acral parts occurs in Werner's syndrome and progeria; acrogeria and poikilodermatous epidermolysis bullosa [1] are other rare conditions in which scleroderma-like lesions occur. Sclerosis of the skin also occurs in the Moore–Federman syndrome (short stature, stiffness of joints, characteristic facies). The 'stiff skin syndrome' describes patients who from childhood develop stone-hard, subcutaneous indurations, which on MRI scan are seen to be derived from the fascia. The lesions are most pronounced on the buttocks, hips and knees, often leading to contractures. The children develop normally and no treatment other than physiotherapy is required [2,3].

References

1 Jablonska S, Blaszczyk M. Poikiloderma with scleroderma-like lesions. In: Jablonska S, ed. *Scleroderma and Pseudoscleroderma*. Warsaw: Polish Medical Publishers, 1975: 421–4.
2 Esterly NB, McKusick VA. Stiff skin syndrome. *Pediatrics* 1971; **47**: 360–9.
3 Jablonska S, Blaszczyk M. Scleroderma-like indurations involving fascias: an abortive form of congenital fascial dystrophy (stiff skin syndrome). *Pediatr Dermatol* 2000; **17**: 105–10.

Occupational causes

A number of chemicals have been reported to cause a scleroderma-like picture.

Vinyl chloride disease [1–4]

One to six per cent of polyvinyl chloride (PVC) workers, particularly reactor cleaners, develop coldness, stiffness, numbness, burning pain and discoloration of the fingers and hands, and to a lesser extent the feet, on exposure to cold. Other symptoms include loss of energy, loss of libido, impotence, dyspnoea and feeling light-headed, with irrational laughter and whistling. The skin of the hands, forearms, face and trunk may be thickened. The hands show mottled pink, purple or white areas. The terminal phalanges are shortened and bulbous, and the nails are curved. Telangiectases occur on the face, resembling those of systemic sclerosis, and there may be difficulty in opening the mouth, although radial furrowing and pigmentation are not features. Usually, it is possible to distinguish between classic systemic sclerosis and vinyl chloride disease [5]. Parotitis [6], hepatomegaly and splenomegaly occur. X-rays show erosion of the tufts of the terminal phalanges and thinning of the other phalanges of the fingers and toes. Erosions also occur in the metatarsals, pelvic bones, clavicles and bones of the arms and legs. Nail fold capillaroscopy shows changes similar to those seen in systemic sclerosis. Narrowing of digital arteries and hypervascularity of the digital tufts are seen on arteriography.

Histologically, there is thickening and separation of collagen fibres and fragmentation of elastic fibres in the dermis. Immunohistology reveals an immune-complex vasculitis with deposits of IgG, complement and fibrin in the media of small- and medium-sized arterioles [7]. Other immunological features include low levels of non-organ-specific autoantibodies, polyclonal hyperglobulinaemia, cryoglobulinaemia, cryofibrinogenaemia, *in vivo* complement activation and conversion, reduced T cells and moderate B-cell proliferation. Anticentromere or anti-Scl-70 antibodies cannot usually be demonstrated [8], although a patient who presented with 'pneumoconiosis' and systemic sclerosis features 10 years after exposure did have a positive ANA and Scl-70 antibodies [9]. Thrombocytopenia, abnormal platelet aggregation, abnormal liver function tests, raised serum creatine phosphokinase indicating muscle involvement, patchy defects of pulmonary ventilation and perfusion, hepatic fibrosis and oesophageal varices also occur.

The prognosis is unknown, and many men have not improved after removal from exposure. There is no effective treatment. Angiosarcoma of the liver is a serious complication. If the level of exposure to vinyl chloride monomer in PVC manufacturing plants is kept below five parts per million, further cases of vinyl chloride disease should not occur. A genetic susceptibility is shown by an increase in HLA-DR5 in all patients and of -B8 and -DR3 in those severely affected [8]. Acro-osteolysis has also been reported in a worker not exposed to vinyl chloride [10].

Scleroderma-like lesions resulting from perchlorethylene, trichlorethylene and organic solvents

A disorder, resembling vinyl chloride disease, has been reported after exposure to perchlorethylene, a solvent used in dry cleaning of clothes [11,12]. Acrocyanosis and acrosclerosis were associated with polymyopathy and hepatic damage. Some of the features, including the presence of speckled antinuclear factor and favourable response to prednisone, were suggestive of 'mixed connective tissue disease'. Exposure to trichlorethylene may be associated with scleroderma [13–16], possibly after even a single prolonged exposure. Of patients with systemic sclerosis in an eastern European series, 28% had suffered significant exposure to organic solvents [17]. Similarly, an Italian study has confirmed an aetiological role of exposure to solvents in scleroderma [18]. A man who used trichlorethylene for cleaning metal also had peripheral neuropathy, Raynaud's phenomenon, impotence, gynaecomastia, hepatomegaly, lymphadenopathy and pigmentation [16]. He was probably a case of Crow–Fukase (POEMS) syndrome. In a Japanese series, generalized morphoeic lesions, similar to those found in occupational scleroderma, were found in nine of 115 patients with systemic sclerosis. Seven had been exposed to organic solvents before the onset of Raynaud's phenomenon. Some had visceral changes of systemic sclerosis [19]. The same authors induced sclerotic skin changes in mice by the intraperitoneal injection of naphtha, *n*-hexane and hexachlorethane. A sclerodermatous syndrome consisting of cold sensitivity, restrictive lung defect, peripheral neuropathy, oesophageal dysfunction, labile hypertension and monoclonal paraproteinaemia has been reported in a man who had worked with many solvents. These included benzene, toluenes, toluidines, xylenes, xylidenes, aniline compounds, and ethanolamine and its derivatives [20]. Solvents recorded in other reports include isopropylalcohol, ethyl acetate, naphthalene, trimethylbenzene and terpene derivatives [21]. Systemic sclerosis occurred in two workers handling *meta*-phenylenediamine [22].

Scleroderma-like lesions resulting from pesticides

Sclerodermatous changes can occur in workers handling pesticides. Substances possibly incriminated include chlordane, heptochlor, malathion, parathion, DDT, sodium dinitro-orthocresolate and 7-chlorocyclohexane [2,23,24]. Raynaud's phenomenon occurs, but there is no evidence of involvement of internal organs. Hyperkeratosis of palms and soles with sclerodactyly of the fingers and toes has been reported in a weed sprayer with chloracne [25].

Scleroderma-like lesions resulting from epoxy resin

Six Japanese men exposed to the vapour of epoxy resins in the production of transformers for television sets developed scleroderma-like skin changes and erythema, with fatigue, loss of weight, myalgia and arthralgia [26]. The histological changes were those of scleroderma, but there was no definite evidence of systemic involvement. A hardener—1,1'-*bis*(3-methyl)-4-amino(cyclohexyl)methane—was thought to be the cause.

Improvement occurred when the men stopped work, and the disorder resolved completely within 5 years without any internal organ involvement developing [27]. One patient developed systemic sclerosis sine scleroderma after exposure to epoxy resin [28].

Silicosis and scleroderma

The association of silicosis and scleroderma has been reported in Italy [18], in South African coal mines [29] and in coal mines in other countries where silica is present [30–33]. Men in other occupations, such as sandblasters and quarrymen, may be affected. Because of the occupational risk, the condition occurs predominantly in men, particularly those suffering from silicosis. In East Germany, 93 of 120 male patients with systemic sclerosis had suffered long-term silica exposure, and 49 had coexisting silicosis [34]. The lung changes frequently precede the scleroderma. Visceral manifestations resembling those of systemic sclerosis occur in approximately half of cases, and antinuclear factor can be demonstrated in one-third. In these cases, the clinical and immunological changes are indistinguishable from those found in systemic sclerosis without any environmental exposure [35]. Systemic sclerosis-like syndromes may follow exposure to urea formaldehyde foam insulation [36].

References

1 Grainger RG, Walker AE, Ward AM. Vinyl chloride monomer-induced disease: clinical, radiological and immunological aspects. In: Preger L, ed. *Induced Disease: Drug, Irradiation, Occupation*. New York: Grune and Stratton, 1979: 191–214.

2 Lange CE, Juhe S, Stein G *et al*. Die sogenannte Vinylchlorid-Krankhe eine berufsbedingte Systemsklerose? *Intern Arch Arbeitsmed* 1974; **32**: 1–32.

3 Markowitz SS, McDonald CJ, Fethiere W *et al*. Occupational acro-osteolysis. *Arch Dermatol* 1972; **106**: 219–23.

4 Walker A. Occupational acro-osteolysis. *Proc R Soc Med* 1975; **68**: 343–4.

5 Ostlere LS, Harris D, Buckley C *et al*. Atypical systemic sclerosis following exposure to vinyl chloride monomer: a case report and review of the cutaneous aspects of vinyl chloride disease. *Clin Exp Dermatol* 1992; **17**: 208–10.

6 Watkinson J. Recurrent parotitis complicating a 'vinyl chloride-like' connective tissue disorder. *BMJ* 1985; **291**: 1094.

7 Ward AM, Udnoon S, Watkins J *et al*. Immunological mechanisms in the pathogenesis of vinyl chloride disease. *BMJ* 1976; **i**: 936–8.

8 Black CM, Welsh KI, Walker AE *et al*. Genetic susceptibility to scleroderma-like syndrome induced by vinyl chloride. *Lancet* 1983; **i**: 53–5.

9 Studnicka MJ, Menzinger G, Drlicek M *et al*. Pneumoconiosis and systemic sclerosis following 10 years of exposure to polyvinyl chloride dust. *Thorax* 1995; **50**: 583–5.

10 Meyerson LB, Meier CC. Cutaneous lesions in acro-osteolysis. *Arch Dermatol* 1972; **106**: 224–7.

11 Sparrow GP. A connective tissue disorder similar to vinyl chloride disease in a patient exposed to perchlorethylene. *Clin Exp Dermatol* 1977; **2**: 17–22.

12 Hinnen U, Schmid-Grendelmeier P, Muller E *et al*. Losungsmittelexposition bei Sklerodermie: disseminierte zirkumskripte Sklerodermie (Morphea) bei einem Perchlorethylen-exponierten Lackierer. *Schweiz Med Wochenschr* 1995; **125**: 2433–7.

13 Flindt-Hansen H, Isager H. Scleroderma after occupational exposure to trichlorethylene and trichlorethane. *Acta Derm Venereol (Stockh)* 1987; **67**: 263–4.

14 Lockey JE, Kelly CR, Cannon GW *et al*. Progressive systemic sclerosis associated with exposure to trichloroethylene. *J Occup Med* 1987; **29**: 493–5.

15 Reinl W. Sklerodermie durch Trichloräthylen-Einwirkung? *Zentralbl Arbeitsmed* 1957; **17**: 58–60.

16 Saihan EM, Burton JL, Heaton KW. A new syndrome with pigmentation, scleroderma, gynaecomastia, Raynaud's phenomenon and peripheral neuropathy. *Br J Dermatol* 1978; **99**: 437–40.

17 Czirjak L, Bokk A, Csontos G *et al*. Clinical findings in 61 patients with progressive systemic sclerosis. *Acta Derm Venereol (Stockh)* 1989; **69**: 533–6.

18 Bovenzi M, Barbone F, Betta A *et al*. Scleroderma and occupational exposure. *Scand J Work Environ Health* 1995; **21**: 289–92.

19 Yamakage A, Ishikawa H. Generalized morphea-like scleroderma occurring in people exposed to organic solvents. *Dermatologica* 1982; **165**: 186–93.

20 Bottomley WW, Sheehan-Dare RA, Hughes P *et al*. A sclerodermatous syndrome with unusual features following prolonged occupational exposure to organic solvents. *Br J Dermatol* 1993; **128**: 203–6.

21 Brasington RD, Thorpe Swenson AJ. Systemic sclerosis associated with cutaneous exposure to solvent: case report and review of the literature. *Arthritis Rheum* 1991; **34**: 631–3.

22 Owens GR, Medsger TA. Systemic sclerosis secondary to occupational exposure. *Am J Med* 1988; **85**: 114–6.

23 Couperus M. Discussion. *Arch Dermatol* 1973; **107**: 768.

24 Jablonska S. Scleroderma-like lesions produced by pesticides. In: Jablonska S, ed. *Scleroderma and Pseudoscleroderma*. Warsaw: Polish Medical Publishers, 1975: 603.

25 Poskitt LB, Duffill MB, Rademaker M. Chloracne, palmoplantar keratoderma and localized scleroderma in a weed sprayer. *Clin Exp Dermatol* 1994; **19**: 264–7.

26 Yamakage A, Ishikawa H, Saito Y *et al*. Occupational scleroderma-like disorder occurring in men engaged in the polymerization of epoxy resins. *Dermatologica* 1980; **161**: 33–44.

27 Ishikawa O, Warita S, Tamura A *et al*. Occupational scleroderma: a 17-year follow-up study. *Br J Dermatol* 1995; **133**: 786–9.

28 Inachi S, Mizutani H, Ando Y *et al*. Progressive systemic sclerosis sine scleroderma which developed after exposure to epoxy resin polymerization. *J Dermatol* 1996; **23**: 344–6.

29 Erasmus LD. Scleroderma in gold miners in the Witwatersrand, with particular reference to pulmonary manifestations. *S Afr J Lab Clin Med* 1957; **3**: 209–31.

30 Jablonska S. Scleroderma-like lesions of occupational origin. In: Jablonska S, ed. *Scleroderma and Pseudoscleroderma*. Warsaw: Polish Medical Publishers, 1975: 601–5.

31 Rodnan GP. A review of recent observations and current theories on the aetiology and pathogenesis of progressive systemic sclerosis (diffuse scleroderma). *J Chron Dis* 1963; **16**: 929–49.

32 Ebihara I, Kawami M. Mineral dust exposure and systemic diseases. *J Environ Pathol Toxicol Oncol* 2000; **19**: 109–27.

33 Ziegler V, Pampel W, Zschunke E *et al*. Kristalliner Quarz- (eine) Ursache der progressiven Sklerodermie? *Dermatol Monatsschr* 1982; **168**: 398–401.

34 Haustein U-F, Ziegler V, Herrman K *et al*. Silica-induced scleroderma. *J Am Acad Dermatol* 1990; **22**: 444–8.

35 Rustin MHA, Bull HA, Ziegler V *et al*. Silica-associated systemic sclerosis is clinically, serologically and immunologically indistinguishable from idiopathic systemic sclerosis. *Br J Dermatol* 1990; **123**: 725–34.

36 Rush PJ, Chaiton A. Scleroderma, renal failure and death associated with exposure to urea formaldehyde foam insulation. *J Rheumatol* 1986; **13**: 475–6.

Exogenous/iatrogenic scleroderma

Scleroderma-like changes resulting from bleomycin [1,2]

Cutaneous fibrosis with acrocyanosis, acrosclerosis, pigmentation, hair loss, flexion contractures and ulceration occurs in patients treated with the antitumour agent bleomycin. Pulmonary fibrosis is a prominent feature. Remission occurs some months after withdrawal of the drug. Cisplatin can cause similar changes.

Scleroderma resulting from other drugs

Carbidopa [3], pentazocine [4], cocaine [5] and appetite suppressants [6] have all been implicated in the development of sclerodermatous disease.

Scleroderma induced by silicone or paraffin implants (human adjuvant disease) [7]

Skin sclerosis, sometimes resembling morphoea, occurs at the site of injection of silicone for cosmetic breast surgery. It may act by the release of silica. Sometimes, more widespread connective tissue disease resembling systemic sclerosis [8], mixed connective tissue disease, SLE, rheumatoid arthritis, primary biliary cirrhosis, Sjögren's syndrome [9] or eosinophilic fasciitis [10] occurs. Paraffin injections may be a more important factor than silica in causing systemic sclerosis-like disease [11]. A causal link between silicone breast implants and autoimmune diseases seems to have been discounted [12].

References

1 Cohen IS, Mosher MB, O'Keefe EJ *et al.* Cutaneous toxicity of bleomycin therapy. *Arch Dermatol* 1973; **107**: 553–5.
2 Finch WR, Rodnan GP, Buckingham RB, Prince RK, Winkerstein A. Bleomycin-induced scleroderma. *J Rheumatol* 1980; **7**: 651–9.
3 Sternberg EM, Van Woert MH, Young SN *et al.* Development of scleroderma-like illness during therapy with L-5-hydroxytryptophan and carbidopa. *N Engl J Med* 1980; **303**: 782–7.
4 Palestine RF, Millns JL, Spigel GT *et al.* Skin manifestations of pentazocine abuse. *J Am Acad Dermatol* 1980; **2**: 47–55.
5 Trozac DJ, Gould WM. Cocaine abuse and connective tissue disease. *J Am Acad Dermatol* 1984; **10**: 525.
6 Tomlinson IM, Jayson MI. Systemic sclerosis after therapy with appetite suppressants. *J Rheumatol* 1984; **11**: 254–5.
7 Varga J, Jimenez SA. Augmentation mammoplasty and scleroderma: is there an association? *Arch Dermatol* 1990; **126**: 1220–1.
8 Varga J, Schumacher HR, Jimenez SA. Systemic sclerosis after augmentation mammoplasty with silicone implants. *Ann Intern Med* 1989; **111**: 377–83.
9 Okano Y, Nishikai M, Sato A. Scleroderma, primary biliary cirrhosis and Sjögren's syndrome after cosmetic breast augmentation with silicone injection. *Ann Rheum Dis* 1984; **43**: 520–2.
10 Spiera H. Scleroderma after silicone augmentation mammoplasty. *JAMA* 1988; **260**: 236–8.
11 Kumagai Y, Shiokawa Y, Medsger TA *et al.* Clinical spectrum of connective tissue disease after cosmetic surgery. *Arthritis Rheum* 1984; **27**: 1–12.
12 Cooper C, Dennison E. Do silicone breast implants cause connective tissue disease? *BMJ* 1998; **316**: 403–4.

'Toxic oil' epidemic syndrome [1,2]

In 1981, in certain areas of Spain, the ingestion of rapeseed oil denatured with aniline caused a multisystem disease affecting 18 000 people. The most prominent pathological feature was a widespread non-necrotizing intimal vasculitis in practically every organ [3]. The early phase, lasting 2–3 months, consisted of atypical pneumonia, gastrointestinal and neurological symptoms and a pruritic rash. The rash involved the limbs, abdomen and trunk, and resembled a viral exanthem lasting approximately 5–20 days. Occasionally, palpable purpura or erythema multiforme occurred. Eosinophilia was always present, antinuclear antibodies were frequently found, and elevation of IgE and abnormal liver function tests could be demonstrated in one-third of cases. Histology showed dilatation of blood vessels, and an inflammatory exudate including eosinophils in the dermis. Three to four months after the onset, 10% of patients developed a transitory eruption consisting of multiple yellowish or brownish papules of all areas except palms and soles. Five to six months after the onset, patients, mainly women, developed a neuromyopathy, and either localized or generalized morphoea or a disorder resembling systemic scle-

rosis, with dysphagia, oesophageal changes and occasionally renal involvement. Sicca syndrome and pulmonary hypertension were prominent features in some cases. Histology of the skin showed dermal infiltration and sclerosis with interfibrillar mucin deposits, but immunology was negative.

Most patients recovered to some extent, although 50% had persistent symptoms when reviewed in 1984 [4]. The cause is unknown. An immune reaction to an unknown antigen seems likely. HLA typing showed an increased incidence of HLA-DR3 and -DR4 in females with chronic disease [5].

References

1 Iglesias JL, De Moragas JM. The cutaneous lesions of the Spanish toxic oil syndrome. *J Am Acad Dermatol* 1983; **9**: 159–60.
2 Toxic Epidemic Syndrome Study Group. Toxicepidermic syndrome, Spain, 1981; *Lancet* 1982; **ii**: 697–702.
3 Martinez-Tello FJ, Navas-Palacios JJ, Ricoy JR *et al.* Pathology of a new toxic syndrome caused by ingestion of adulterated oil in Spain. *Virchows Arch (Pathol Anat)* 1982; **397**: 261–85.
4 Gilsanz V, Alvarez JL, Serrano S *et al.* Evolution of the alimentary toxic oil syndrome due to ingestion of denatured rapeseed oil. *Arch Intern Med* 1984; **44**: 254–6.
5 Vicario JL, Serrano-Rios M, Son Andres F *et al.* HLA-DR3, DR4 increase in chronic stage of Spanish oil disease. *Lancet* 1982; **i**: 276.

Nephrogenic systemic fibrosis (NSF)

> **Synonym**
> • Nephrogenic fibrosing dermopathy (NFD)

Nephrogenic systemic fibrosis is a relatively recently described scleroderma-like fibrosing disorder first reported in 2000 [1]. By 2003, over 100 US cases had been reported to the NFD registry established at Yale University. The lesions of NFD are skin coloured to erythematous papules that coalesce into erythematous/brawny plaques with a peau d'orange appearance. Nodules have been described. The involved skin becomes thickened and 'woody', resembling the skin lesions seen in eosinophilic fasciitis. Joint contractures may develop rapidly, with patients becoming wheelchair-bound within days to weeks. The lesions are typically symmetrical and develop on the limbs (often between the ankles and mid-thighs and between the wrists and mid-upper arms) and trunk. Plantar flexion of the feet may make walking impossible. Patients often experience pain and pruritis, but arthritis, fever and myalgia are uncommon [2]. Some patients, however, exhibit systemic features, with involvement of the striated muscles, pleura, pericardium and myocardium. The disease has been reported in both adults and children [3].

No single test is pathognomonic but a deep skin biopsy of involved skin will show fibrosis extending into the subcutaneous fat and sometimes fascia.

All reported patients have had renal disease and initially it was thought that the condition might be triggered by surgery, coexistent hepatic or pulmonary disease, a coexistent hypercoagulable state or following erythropoietin therapy in these patients.

Recently, however, it has become clear that the triggering factor is the use of gadolinium-based contrast agents in patients with renal disease, transmetallation of gadolinium chelates possibly leading to the precipitation of free gadolinium in the dermis or other organs [4]. Surgery and erythropoietin may be also be contributory factors [5]. Alternative imaging should be considered in these patients.

Treatment is unsatisfactory, although some success has been reported with intravenous immunoglobulin, topical and systemic steroids, calcipotriol ointment, d-penicillamine, ciclosporin, cyclophosphamide, thalidomide, interferon-α, UVA-1, extracorporeal photophoresis and photodynamic therapy [3].

References

1 Cowper SE, Robin HS, Steinberg SM *et al.* Scleromyxoedema-like cutaneous diseases in renal dialysis patients. *Lancet* 2000; **356**: 1000–1.
2 Cowper SE. Nephrogenic fibrosing dermopathy: the first 6 years. *Curr Opin Rheum* 2003; **15**: 785–90.
3 Lim YL, Lee HY, Low SCS *et al.* Possible role of gadolinium in nephrogenic systemic fibrosis: report of two cases and review of the literature. *Clin Exp Dermatol* 2007; **32**: 353–8.
4 Grobner T. Gadolinium—a specific trigger for the development of nephrogenic fibrosing dermopathy and nephrogenic systemic fibrosis? *Nephrol Dial Transplant* 2006; **21**: 1104–8.
5 Pryor JG, Poggioli G, Galaria N *et al.* Nephrogenic systemic fibrosis: a clinicopathologic study of six cases. *J Am Acad Dermatol* 2007; **57**: 105–11.

Graft-versus-host disease [1–3]

Definition. Graft-versus-host disease (GVHD) occurs when immunocompetent T cells from a donor recognize and react against 'foreign' tissue antigens in an immunocompromised host. Originally reported following bone marrow transplantation (regularly used in the management of leukaemias, lymphoma, immunodeficiency and inborn errors of metabolism), GVHD is now recognized to occur following transfusion of non-irradiated blood, after maternofetal transfer of lymphoid cells, and following peripheral blood stem cell transfer [4]. Post-transfusion-related GVHD is an uncommon but potentially fatal complication of transfusing blood between immunologically related individuals. It appears that transfused white blood cells are not recognized as foreign, and react against host tissue. The reaction seems to depend on heterozygosity of class I antigens. The two recognized forms of the disease are acute and chronic.

Incidence. Even using prophylactic therapy to prevent its occurrence, GVHD occurs in approximately 50% of patients receiving successful marrow allografts for various disorders, including immunodeficiency diseases, aplastic anaemia, acute leukaemia and radiation exposure, despite careful histocompatibility matching [3]. The frequency is the same in those receiving peripheral blood stem cell grafts [5]. It is clear that the typical acute form of the syndrome can also occur after syngeneic (identical twin) or autologous bone marrow grafting, in which genetically identical material is transplanted, and may occur in approximately 10% of such cases [7].

Aetiology [3]. Billingham described the original criteria for the development of a graft-versus-host reaction in 1966:
1 Genetically determined histocompatibility differences between donor and recipient
2 Immunocompetent cells in the grafted tissue able to recognize foreign histocompatibility antigens in the host and to react against them

3 Inability of the host to recognize and react against the grafted tissue.

It is clear from animal experiments [7], as well as the occurrence of typical GVHD in human syngeneic transplants, that criterion **1** is no longer an essential prerequisite for the development of the acute form of the syndrome. GVHD in this situation occurs because of MHC class II differences. It usually only occurs after the withdrawal of immunosuppression [8].

A similar syndrome occurs in recipients of IL-2 treatment and lymphocytes activated by this stimulating lymphokine given as treatment for widespread malignancy. Cells activated by this technique are non-specifically cytotoxic, capable of self-reactivity and may have the features of NK cells. In animal models, and in humans, HLA-DR-bearing Langerhans' cells are reduced in the acute form of the disease, and T cells directed against these cells are found. In addition, IFN production by activated T cells induces HLA-DR expression on keratinocytes, making them targets for a similar reaction [9,10]. The risk of developing GVHD may be related to cytokine gene polymorphisms [11]. T-cell depletion reduces GVHD in mouse models [12] but the effect on human GVHD is no different from conventional prophylactic regimens [13].

A possible hypothesis is suggested by Ferrara [14]; immunologically competent donor T lymphocytes are not destroyed in the host because they are not recognized as foreign. Activated T cells release IL-2, IFN and probably other lymphokines. IL-2 activates cytotoxic cells (probably NK cells), and HLA-DR-bearing epidermal cells and Langerhans' cells may be specifically attacked, giving rise to acute GVHD. The same, or similar, cells recognize any persisting malignant cells in the host, and it is suggested that graft-versus-leukaemia reactions explain the lowered incidence of recurrence of the original malignancy in patients with GVHD. However, there are some criticisms of the theory of T-cell-mediated cutaneous pathogenesis, mainly that early graft-versus-host reactions do not show T-cell infiltration of the skin [15]. There are also stimulatory antibodies to PDGF and its receptor [16], as well as high levels of B cell activating factors [12], suggesting a role for B cells in the pathogenesis. In addition, successful treatment of GVHD is accompanied by the induction of apoptosis in T cells and some epidermal cells. This suggests that a failure of programmed cell death may be a feature of pathogenesis [17]. Nevertheless, the use of T-cell-depleted marrow for grafting reduces the incidence of GVHD and prevents HLA-DR expression on keratinocytes, but unfortunately the failure rate of the transplant is markedly increased.

Pathology [18]. For acute GVHD, the cutaneous histological changes have been graded for severity.

Grade I	Basal cell vacuolation with or without mononuclear cell infiltration
Grade II	Solitary epidermal cell necrosis, surrounded by mononuclear cells
Grade III	Regional epidermal cell necrosis with bullae
Grade IV	Toxic epidermal necrolysis.

Less severe histological grades may be impossible to differentiate from drug-induced reactions. At an immunocytochemical level, the earliest (preclinical) changes are an increase in dermal macrophages expressing α_1-antichymotrypsin. In grade I disease, there is keratinocyte HLA-DR and ICAM-1 expression, and in the later stages, CD25 T cells, L1 antigen-positive keratinocytes, and VCAM-1 macrophages are increased [19].

In chronic GVHD, histological changes are lichenoid, or resemble scleroderma. IgM may occur at the dermal–epidermal junction, with granular deposits of IgM, IgA and C3 in the walls of dermal vessels. There is associated microvascular disease mediated by cytotoxic T cells [20].

References

1 Harper JI. Graft-versus-host reaction: aetiological and clinical aspects in connective tissue diseases. *Semin Dermatol* 1985; **4**: 144–51.
2 Parkman R. Graft-versus-host disease. *Ann Rev Med* 1991; **42**: 189–97.
3 Perez-Simon JA, Sanchez-Abarca I, Diez-Campelo M *et al.* Chronic graft-versus-host disease: pathogenesis and clinical management. *Drugs* 2006; **66**: 1041–57.
4 Schaffer JV. The changing face of graft-versus-host disease. *Semin Cutan Med Surg* 2006; **25**: 190–200.
5 Flowers ME, Parker PM, Johnston LJ *et al.* Comparison of chronic graft versus host disease after transplantation of peripheral blood stem cells versus bone marrow in allogeneic recipients: long-term follow-up of a randomized trial. *Blood* 2000; **15**: 415–9.
6 Hood AF, Vogelsang CB, Black LP *et al.* Acute graft-versus-host disease. *Arch Dermatol* 1987; **123**: 745–50.
7 Clazier A, Tutschka PI, Farmer ER. Graft-versus-host disease in cyclosporine A-treated rats after syngeneic and autologous bone marrow reconstitution. *J Exp Med* 1983; **158**: 1–8.
8 Hess AD, Horwitz L, Beschorner WE, Santos GW. Development of graft vs host disease-like syndrome in cyclosporine treated rats after syngeneic bone marrow transplantation. I. Development of cytotoxic T lymphocytes with apparent polyclonal anti-Ia specificity, including autoreactivity. *J Exp Med* 1985; **161**: 718–30.
9 Ferrara J, Guillen FJ, Sleckman B *et al.* Cutaneous acute graft-versus-host disease to minor histocompatibility antigens in a murine model: histologic analysis and correlation to clinical disease. *J Invest Dermatol* 1986; **86**: 371–5.
10 Paller AS, Nelson A, Steffen L *et al.* T-lymphocyte subsets in the lesional skin of allogeneic and autologous bone marrow transplant patients. *Arch Dermatol* 1988; **124**: 1795–801.
11 Dickinson AM, Cavet J, Cullup H *et al.* GvHD risk assessment in haemopoietic stem cell transplantation: role of cytokine gene polymorphisms and an *in vitro* human skin explant model. *Hum Immunol* 2001; **62**: 1266–76.
12 Chao NJ. Are there effective new strategies for the treatment of acute and chronic GvHD? *Best Pract Res Clin Haematol* 2008; **21**: 93–8.
13 Wagner JE, Thompson JS, Carter SL, Kernan NA. Effect of graft-versus-host disease prophylaxis on 3-year disease-free survival in recipients of unrelated donor bone marrow (T-cell depletion trial): a multi-centre, randomised phase II-III trial. *Lancet* 2005; **366**: 733–41.
14 Ferrara JLM. Syngeneic graft-vs-host disease. *Arch Dermatol* 1987; **123**: 741–2.
15 Sloane JP, Dilley SA. Pathogenesis of graft-versus-host disease. *Histopathology* 1988; **12**: 105–10.
16 Svegliati S, Olivieri A, Campelli N *et al.* Stimulatory autoantibodies to PDGF in patients with extensive chronic graft-versus-host disease. *Blood* 2007; **110**: 237–41.
17 Bladon J, Taylor PC. Extracorporeal photophoresis in cutaneous T cell lymphoma and graft versus host disease induces both immediate and progressive apoptotic processes. *Br J Dermatol* 2002; **146**: 59–68.
18 Pintar T, Zorc-Pleskovic R, Alessiani M *et al.* Prognostic value of skin histology in GVHD after intestinal transplantation. *Eur J Pediatr Surg* 2007; **17**: 412–5.
19 Norton J, Sloane JP. A prospective study of cellular and immunological changes in skin of allogeneic bone marrow recipients: relationship to clinical and histological features of acute graft versus host disease. *Am J Clin Pathol* 1994; **101**: 597–602.
20 Biedermann BC, Sahner S, Gregor M *et al.* Endothelial injury mediated by cytotoxic T lymphocytes and loss of microvessels in chronic graft versus host disease. *Lancet* 2002; **359**: 2078–83.

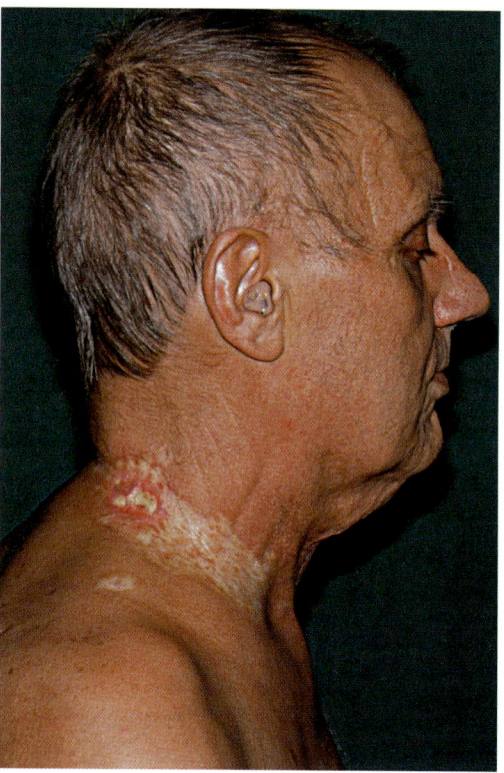

Fig. 51.58 Localized eroded sclerotic graft-versus-host disease.

Clinical features [1,2]. Acute GVHD usually occurs within 60 days of a bone marrow transplant, and most often after 7–12 days, when it is termed hyperacute. Mild fever is followed by a faint red maculopapular rash on the hands, feet, face and forehead. This spreads to the trunk and limbs, becoming deeper in colour. Desquamation or even toxic epidermal necrolysis follows. Bullous and ulcerated forms are described, and a follicular pattern may indicate more severe disease [3]. Hepatitis (indicated by raised bilirubin and alkaline phosphatase) and bloody diarrhoea resulting from enteritis are other features and, in severe cases, death occurs by the 21st day. In the original cases, it was rare to have liver and gut involvement without cutaneous pathology, and skin biopsy was the simplest reliable test for diagnosis. However, the introduction of T-cell depletion as a prophylactic measure has changed the pattern of disease so that skin disease may be mild, while liver and bowel disease may be severe. Clinical stagings for each organ system, and grading for the overall clinical picture, have been proposed [2].

Chronic GVHD may be localized (Fig. 51.58) or generalized, and principally involves the skin and the liver. The former occurs in 10% of patients as hyperpigmented nodular areas, which may be guttate, and eventually soften and atrophy. The early phase of generalized GVHD generally appears up to the 100th post-transplant day and usually, but not always, follows acute GVHD. Initially, a slowly progressive erythematous rash on the face, palms and soles becomes lichenoid, with changes resembling lichen planus in many sites. Lichenoid changes may be limited to the nails [4]. Later, scleroderma-like changes occur, which are sometimes widespread and disabling. The condition resembles systemic sclerosis, with tightening of the skin of the face, hands and feet. Autoantibody changes similar to those found in systemic sclerosis may occur [5]. Disease may be localized to the extremities and associated with a polyneuropathy [6]. There may also be eczematoid changes [7].

Oesophageal changes and subcutaneous calcification may occur. Morphoea-like changes have been reported [8]. Eruptive violaceous vascular tumours on the legs may occur [9]. Reticulate patchy hyperpigmentation and, less commonly, hypopigmentation, poikiloderma, vitiligo (which may be total [10]), erythema, atrophy, alopecia, multiple follicular papules, deep ulcerations of the buttocks and legs, and dystrophic nail changes are other features [11]. Panniculitis may occur [12]. Gastrointestinal symptoms, a Sjögren-like syndrome [13], polymyositis [14], abnormal liver function tests, primary biliary cirrhosis [15] and other organ changes occur [14].

That there may be some interaction between viral infections and minor histocompatibility differences in the pathogenesis of chronic GVHD is suggested by the development of scleroderma-like skin changes in areas affected by measles in a patient 8 months after bone marrow transplantation [16]. Similarly, pathogen-free transplanted animals do not develop GVHD until given bacteria or endotoxin, and patients nursed in laminar flow isolation remain disease-free until they are removed from this environment [17].

References

1 Goltz RW. The graft-vs-host reaction. *Arch Dermatol* 1988; **124**: 1849–50.
2 Perez-Simon JA, Sanchez-Abarca I, Diez-Campelo M *et al.* Chronic graft-versus-host disease: pathogenesis and clinical management. *Drugs* 2006; **66**: 1041–57.
3 Lycka BAS, Kaye VN. Acute follicular graft-vs-host disease. *Arch Dermatol* 1988; **124**: 1442–4.
4 Palencia SI, Rodriguez-Peralto JL, Castano E *et al.* Lichenoid nail changes as sole external manifestation of graft vs. host disease. *Int J Dermatol* 2002; **41**: 44–5.
5 Bell SA, Faust H, Mittermuller J *et al.* Specificity of antinuclear antibodies in scleroderma-like chronic graft versus host disease: clinical correlation and histocompatibility locus antigen association. *Br J Dermatol* 1996; **134**: 848–54.
6 Aractingi S, Socie G, Devergie A *et al.* Localized scleroderma-like lesions on the legs in bone marrow transplant recipients: association with polyneuropathy in the same distribution. *Br J Dermatol* 1993; **129**: 201–3.
7 Creamer D, Martyn-Simmons CL, Osborne G *et al.* Eczematoid graft-vs-host disease: a novel form of chronic cutaneous graft-vs-host disease and its response to psoralen UV-A therapy. *Arch Dermatol* 2007; **143**: 1157–62.
8 Graham-Brown RAC, Sarkany I. Scleroderma-like changes due to chronic graft-versus-host disease. *Clin Exp Dermatol* 1983; **8**: 531–8.
9 Gamis S, Billick RC, Strolovitz H. Eruptive vascular tumours associated with chronic graft-versus-host disease. *J Am Acad Dermatol* 1984; **10**: 918–21.
10 Nagler A, Goldenhersh MA, Levi-Schaffo F, Bystryn JC. Total leukoderma: a rare manifestation of chronic graft versus host disease. *Br J Dermatol* 1996; **134**: 780–3.
11 Esterly NB. Nail dystrophy in dyskeratosis congenita and chronic graft-vs-host disease. *Arch Dermatol* 1986; **122**: 506–7.
12 Naschitz JE, Boss JH. Fasciitis and fasciitis-panniculitis in chronic graft-versus-host disease. *Ann Intern Med* 1995; **122**: 155–6.
13 Gratwhol AA, Moutsopoulos HM, Chused TM *et al.* Sjögren-type syndrome after allogeneic bone-marrow transplantation. *Ann Intern Med* 1977; **87**: 703–6.
14 Anderson BA, Young PV, Kean WF *et al.* Polymyositis in chronic graft vs host disease. *Arch Neurol* 1982; **39**: 188–90.
15 Epstein O, Thomas HC, Sherlock S. Primary biliary cirrhosis is a dry gland syndrome with features of chronic graft-versus-host disease. *Lancet* 1980; **i**: 1166–8.
16 Fenvk JR Jr, Warkentin PI, Coltz RW *et al.* Sclerodermatous graft-versus-host disease limited to an area of measles exanthem. *Lancet* 1978; **i**: 472–3.
17 Parkman R. Clonal analysis of murine graft-versus-host disease. I. Phenotypic and functional analysis of T lymphocyte clones. *J Immunol* 1986; **136**: 3543–8.

Treatment [1]. Prophylactic use of ciclosporin, methotrexate and prednisolone and, in particular, combinations of these agents, has reduced the incidence of acute GVHD. None of these regimens has produced a definite reduction in the incidence of chronic GVHD, and recent studies indicate no benefit in 24-month rather than 6-month ciclosporin therapy in this situation [2]. T-cell depletion by using anti-T-cell receptor antibodies is successful in reducing the frequency of acute GVHD when used with post-transplant ciclosporin [3]. Combination therapy appears to be better at preventing GVHD than monotherapy, but overall survival is unchanged in younger patients because of higher leukaemic relapse. Older patients survive longer on combination therapy (methotrexate with ciclosporin or T-cell depletion) [4]. Granulocyte colony-stimulating factor, used to enhance engraftment, may reduce the incidence of GVHD [5].

Once the disease is established, treatment with high-dose corticosteroids or ciclosporin is of value symptomatically, and antilymphocyte globulin may be of additional benefit [6], particularly if combined with tacrolimus [7]. Treatment with prednisone and azathioprine for at least 9–12 months helps generalized chronic GVHD in one-third of patients [8], but complications are common, and survival may be reduced by the addition of azathioprine. Thalidomide, used in both low dosage (100 mg/day) and high dosage (400 mg/day), has been of value, but may result in severe cutaneous ulceration [9,10]. PUVA therapy [11], UVB [12], UVA-1 [13] and extracorporeal photophoresis may be of benefit, even in severe disease [14]. Biological therapies [15], including etanercept [16] and particularly rituximab [17], may be helpful for steroid-resistant disease.

Prognosis. Forty to fifty per cent of patients with chronic GVHD are dead within 10 years of developing the disease. Mortality is caused both by the disease itself, and by severe superinfection, related, at least in part, to the immunosuppressive effects of treatment. Recurrence of the original disease is also a problem. Patients who develop chronic GVHD after the acute form, those with the lichenoid type of eruption, and those with significant liver disease have a worse prognosis, with 80% mortality at 10 years [18].

References

1 Bacigalupo A. Management of acute graft-versus-host disease. *Brit J Haematol* 2007; **137**: 87–98.
2 Kansu E, Gooley T, Flowers ME *et al.* Administration of cyclosporine for 24 months compared with 6 months for prevention of graft versus host disease: a prospective randomized clinical trial. *Blood* 2001; **98**: 3868–70.
3 Drobyski WR, Ash RC, Casper JT *et al.* Effect of T cell depletion as graft versus host disease prophylaxis on engraftment, relapse and disease free survival in unrelated marrow transplantation for chronic myelogenous leukaemia. *Blood* 1994; **83**: 1980–7.
4 Aschan J, Ringden O. Prognostic factors for long-term survival in leukaemic marrow recipients with special emphasis on age and prophylaxis for graft versus host disease. *Clin Transplant* 1994; **8**: 258–70.
5 Dey BR, Shaffer J, Yee AJ *et al.* Comparison of outcomes after transplantation of peripheral blood stem cells versus bone marrow following an identical nonmyeloablative conditioning regimen. *Bone Marrow Transplant* 2007; **40**: 19–27.
6 Sullivan KM, Witherspoon RP, Storb R *et al.* Prednisolone and antilymphocyte globulin versus prednisolone and placebo for treatment of chronic graft-versus-host disease: prognostic influence of prolonged thrombocytopaenia after allograft marrow transplantation. *Blood* 1988; **72**: 546–54.

7 Mollee P, Morton AJ, Irving I, Durrant S. Combination therapy with tacrolimus and anti-thymocyte globulin for the treatment of steroid-resistant acute graft versus host disease developing during cyclosporine prophylaxis. *Br J Haematol* 2001; **113**: 217–23.

8 Deeg HJ, Storb R, Thomas FD. Bone marrow transplantations: a review of delayed complications. *Br J Haematol* 1984; **57**: 185–208.

9 Koe S, Leisenring W, Flowers ME *et al.* Thalidomide for treatment of patients with chronic graft versus host disease. *Blood* 2000; **96**: 3995–6.

10 Schlossberg H, Klumpp T, Sabol P *et al.* Severe cutaneous ulceration following treatment with thalidomide for GVHD. *Bone Marrow Transplant* 2001; **27**: 229–30.

11 Hymes SR, Morison WL, Farmer ER *et al.* Methoxsalen and ultraviolet A radiation in treatment of chronic cutaneous graft-versus-host reaction. *J Am Acad Dermatol* 1985; **12**: 30–7.

12 Dooren-Greebe RJ, Schattenberg A, Koopman RJ. Chronic cutaneous graft versus host disease: successful treatment with UVB. *Br J Dermatol* 1991; **125**: 498–9.

13 Stander H, Schiller M, Schwarz T. UVA-1 therapy for sclerodermic graft-versus-host disease of the skin. *J Am Acad Dermatol* 2002; **46**: 799–800.

14 Setterblad N, Garban F, Weigl R *et al.* Extracorporeal photophoresis increases sensitivity of monocytes from patients with graft-versus-host disease to HLA-DR-mediated cell death. *Transfusion* 2008; **48**: 169–77.

15 Rivkina AM, Stump LS. Infliximab in graft versus host disease. *Am J Health Syst Pharm* 2002; **59**: 1271–5.

16 Perez-Simon JA, Sanchez-Abarca I, Diez-Campelo M *et al.* Chronic graft-versus-host disease: pathogenesis and clinical management. *Drugs* 2006; **66**: 1041–57.

17 Cutler C, Miklos D, Kim HT *et al.* Rituximab for steroid-refractory chronic graft-versus-host disease. *Blood* 2006; **108**: 756–62.

18 Wingard JR, Iantadosi S, Vogelsang CB *et al.* Predictors of death from chronic graft-versus-host disease after bone marrow transplantation. *Blood* 1989; **74**: 1428–35.

Eosinophilic fasciitis [1,2]

Synonym
- Shulman's syndrome

This scleroderma-like syndrome appears to be a distinct entity, although some have suggested that it is an early variant of systemic sclerosis [3] or linear scleroderma [4], or that it may occur in conjunction with other connective tissue disease [5]. It occurs in children and adults, more commonly in males than females. In children, persistent sclerosis may occur [6]. The clinical features are the acute onset of pain, swelling and tenderness of the distal part of the limbs, which become indurated. There is limitation of movement of the feet and hands. Occasionally, the face or abdomen can be affected, and there may be superficial blistering and haemorrhage. A relationship to strenuous exertion or trauma has been suggested. Twenty-nine per cent of 52 patients showed lesions of localized morphoea at some stage [7]. Raynaud's phenomenon is rare, there is limited evidence of involvement of internal organs such as occurs in systemic sclerosis, and no history of a previous infection to suggest scleroedema. Blood eosinophilia up to 30% is a striking feature, occurring in approximately 70% of cases [7]; it is associated with elevation of the ESR and hyperglobulinaemia, but these are not present in all cases. Rarely, aplastic anaemia and thrombocytopenia occur [8].

Histologically, there is dermal sclerosis, with inflammation and fibrosis of the fat and deep fascia. The fascia is thickened and infiltrated with lymphocytes, plasma cells, histiocytes and eosinophils. IgG and C3 deposits can be demonstrated in the deep fascia. The inflammatory infiltrate consists of macrophages and predominantly CD8⁺ T cells with eosinophils [9]. MHC class 1 antigens are

Table 51.16 Factors associated with onset of eosinophilic fasciitis.

Neoplasia [18]
Atorvastatin [19]
Autoimmune thyroiditis [20]
Eosinophilic colitis [21]
Hypercalcaemia [22]
Amegakaryocytic thrombocytopenic purpura [23]

over expressed [8]. Cytokine production is enhanced with a mixed Th1/Th2 profile [10]. Antinuclear antibodies cannot be demonstrated and serum complement levels are normal.

An eosinophilic fasciitis-like syndrome occurs after recent ingestion of L-tryptophan [11]. In addition to the usual features of fasciitis, there is muscle weakness and elevated muscle enzyme levels. This may be demonstrated by nuclear magnetic resonance imaging [12]. Enhanced type I procollagen gene expression in the skin has been demonstrated [13]. Myalgia, eosinophilia, dyspnoea, oedema, arthralgia, neuropathy and rashes occur in the eosinophilia–myalgia syndrome [14] which can also be precipitated by tryptophan. Cutaneous manifestations include localized and generalized morphoeic lesions and urticarial and papular lesions [14].

Clinical improvement and disappearance of eosinophilia follow corticosteroid therapy, but spontaneous remission has been reported. Methotrexate may be useful [15]. Phototherapy [16], ciclosporin [17] and other cytotoxic agents may rarely be necessary.

Other factors associated with disease onset are shown in Table 51.16.

References

1 Shulman LE. Diffuse fasciitis with hypergammaglobulinemia and eosinophilia. *J Rheumatol* 1974; **1** (Suppl. 1): 46.

2 Antic M, Lautenschlager S, Itin PH. Eosinophilic fasciitis 30 years after—what do we really know? Report of 11 patients and review of the literature. *Dermatology* 2006; **213**: 93–101.

3 Britt WJ, Duray PH, Dahl MN *et al.* Diffuse fasciitis with eosinophilia: a steroid responsive variant of scleroderma. *J Pediatr* 1980; **97**: 432–4.

4 Williams HJ, Zifer FA, Banta CA. Childhood eosinophilic fasciitis: progression to linear scleroderma. *J Rheumatol* 1986; **13**: 961–2.

5 Mensing H, Schmidt K-U. Diffuse fasciitis with eosinophilia associated with morphoea and lichen sclerosus et atrophicus. *Acta Derm Venereol (Stockh)* 1985; **65**: 80–3.

6 Farrington ML, Haas JE, Nazar-Stewart V, Mellins ED. Eosinophilic fasciitis in children frequently progresses to scleroderma-like cutaneous fibrosis. *J Rheumatol* 1993; **20**: 128–32.

7 Lakhampal S, Ginsberg WW, Michet CJ *et al.* Eosinophilic fasciitis: clinical spectrum and therapeutic response in 52 cases. *Semin Arthritis Rheum* 1988; **17**: 221–31.

8 Shulman LE, Hoffman R, Dainiak N *et al.* Antibody-mediated aplastic anaemia and thrombocytopenic purpura in diffuse eosinophilic fasciitis. *Clin Res* 1979; **27**: 514A.

9 Toquet C, Hamidou MA, Renaudin K *et al.* In situ immunophenotype of the inflammatory infiltrate in eosinophilic fasciitis. *J Rheumatol* 2003; **30**: 1811–5.

10 Viallard JF, Taupin JL, Ranchin V *et al.* Analysis of leukemia inhibitory factor, type 1 and type 2 cytokine production in patients with eosinophilic fasciitis. *J Rheumatol* 2001; **28**: 75–80.

11 Varga J, Peltonen J, Uitto J *et al.* Development of diffuse fasciitis with eosinophilia during L-tryptophan treatment: demonstration of elevated Type 1 collagen expression in affected tissues: a clinico-pathological study of four patients. *Ann Intern Med* 1990; **112**: 344–51.

12 Kaufman LD. The eosinophilia–myalgia syndrome: current concepts and future directions. *Clin Exp Rheumatol* 1992; **10**: 87–91.

13 Douglas AS, Eagles JM, Mowat NAC. Eosinophilia myalgia syndrome associated with tryptophan. *BMJ* 1990; **301**: 387.

14 Oursler JR, Farmer ER, Roubenoff R *et al.* Cutaneous manifestations of the eosinophilia–myalgia syndrome. *Br J Dermatol* 1992; **127**: 138–46.

15 Pouplin S, Daragon A, Le Loët X. Treatment of eosinophilic fasciitis with methotrexate. *J Rheumatol* 1998; **25**: 606–7.

16 Horacek E, Sator PG, Gschnait F. 'Venous Furrowing': a clue to the diagnosis of eosinophilic fasciitis. A case of eosinophilic fasciitis ultimately treated with oral PUVA therapy. *Dermatology* 2007; **215**: 89–90.

17 Bukiej A, Dropiski J, Dyduch G, Szczeklik A. Eosinophilic fasciitis successfully treated with cyclosporine. *Clin Rheumatol* 2005; **24**: 634–6.

18 Philpott H, Hissaria P, Warren L *et al.* Eosinophilic fasciitis as a paraneoplastic phenomenon associated with metastatic colorectal carcinoma. *Australas J Dermatol* 2008; **49**: 27–9.

19 DeGiovanni C, Chard M, Woollons A. Eosinophilic fasciitis secondary to treatment with atorvastatin. *Clin Exp Dermatol* 2006; **31**: 131–2.

20 Hur JW, Lee HS, Uhm WS *et al.* Eosinophilic fasciitis associated with autoimmune thyroiditis. *Korean J Intern Med* 2005; **20**: 180–2.

21 Suresh E, Doherty V, Schofield O *et al.* Eosinophilic fasciitis and eosinophilic colitis: a rare association. *Rheumatology (Oxford)* 2005; **44**: 411–3.

22 Rutter MM, Prahalad S, Passo M, Backeljauw PF. Idiopathic hypercalcemia and eosinophilic fasciitis: a novel association. *J Pediatr Endocrinol Metab* 2004; **17**: 1251–4.

23 Chaudhary UB, Eberwine SF, Hege KM. Acquired amegakaryocytic thrombocytopenic purpura and eosinophilic fasciitis: a long relapsing and remitting course. *Am J Hematol* 2004; **75**: 146–50.

Connective tissue panniculitis (see Chapter 46)

This term has been used [1] for focal nodular or atrophic linear or plaque-like lesions on the face, upper trunk or extremities, which histologically show lymphocytic panniculitis with caseation necrosis. The lesions may respond to chloroquine.

Reference

1 Winkelmann R, Padilha-Goncalves A. Connective tissue panniculitis. *Arch Dermatol* 1980; **116**: 291–4.

Relapsing eosinophilic perimyositis [1]

This rare disorder is in the spectrum of eosinophilic myositis, and is characterized by inflammation within the perimysium (and often epimysium) without necrosis, as opposed to polymyositis and eosinophilic myositis in which necrosis and inflammation occur in the endomysium.

Clinically, patients may present with episodic swelling of the muscles, fatigue and fever. Skin lesions include blotchy erythema over the swollen muscles and erythematous papular lesions of the palms. There is peripheral blood eosinophilia and hyperglobulinaemia, but the muscle enzyme levels are normal or only slightly elevated. Histologically, there are perimysial eosinophilic infiltrates.

The aetiology is unknown. The prognosis is good, although the patient should be followed up in case of the development of lymphoproliferative disease. Most patients respond to moderate doses of steroids or indometacin.

Reference

1 Trueb RM, Becker-Wegerich P, Hafner J *et al.* Relapsing eosinophilic perimyositis. *Br J Dermatol* 1995; **133**: 109–14.

Systemic sclerosis [1,2]

Synonyms
- Progressive systemic sclerosis
- Systemic scleroderma
- Acrosclerosis

Definition. Systemic sclerosis is a multisystem disorder characterized by vascular abnormalities, connective tissue sclerosis and atrophy, and autoantibodies (see p. 51.91 for diagnostic criteria) [2].

The name progressive systemic sclerosis was coined by Goetz in 1945; however, the term 'progressive' is now omitted by most authors because of the variable course of the disease [2–5].

Incidence. Systemic sclerosis is a rare disorder, with an incidence between 2.3 and 10 per million population [6–8]. The prevalence rates in a British study were 13 per million males and 48 per million females, although these figures may represent the minimum [9]; there may be considerable regional variations, possibly as a result of environmental factors [10]. Estimates of prevalence from South Carolina are much higher (67–265 in 100 000) [11]. The ratio of females to males is between 3 and 6 : 1 depending on the source [8,9,12]. The peak onset is in the fourth decade in females and usually later in males; however, overall, 85% of patients present between the ages of 20 and 60 years [8]. In men, the condition has a number of occupational associations, especially miners and stonemasons, and it has been suggested that pneumoconiosis and silicosis are predisposing factors [13]. It occurs in all races, but appears to be less frequent in Asians [14]. There is evidence that African American women with systemic sclerosis are more likely to develop diffuse disease at a younger age and have decreased survival compared with Caucasians [15].

References

1 Varga J. Systemic sclerosis: an update. *Bull NYU Hosp Jt Dis* 2008; **66**: 198–202.

2 Rowell NR. Systemic sclerosis. *J R Coll Phys Lond* 1985; **19**: 23–30.

3 Jayson MIV. Systemic sclerosis: a microvascular disorder? *J R Soc Med* 1983; **76**: 635–42.

4 Krieg T, Meurer M. Systemic scleroderma. *J Am Acad Dermatol* 1988; **18**: 457–81.

5 LeRoy EC. Scleroderma (systemic sclerosis). In: Kelley WN, Harris ED, Ruddy S *et al.*, eds. *Textbook of Rheumatology*. London: Saunders, 1981: 1221–8.

6 Eason RJ, Tan PL, Cow PJ. Progressive systemic sclerosis in Auckland: a 10-year review with emphasis on prognostic features. *Aust NZ J Med* 1981; **11**: 657–62.

7 Kurland LT, Hauser WA, Ferguson RH *et al.* Epidemiologic features of diffuse connective tissue disorders in Rochester, Minn., 1951 through 1967, with special reference to systemic lupus erythematosus. *Mayo Clin Proc* 1969; **44**: 649–63.

8 Medsger TA, Masi AT. Epidemiology of systemic sclerosis (scleroderma). *Ann Intern Med* 1971; **74**: 714–21.

9 Silman A, Jannini S, Symmons D *et al.* An epidemiological study of scleroderma in the West Midlands. *Br J Rheumatol* 1988; **27**: 286–90.

10 Silman AJ, Howard Y, Hicklin AJ, Black C. Geographical clustering of scleroderma in south and west London. *Br J Rheumatol* 1990; **29**: 92–6.

11 Maricq HR, Weinrich MC, Keil JE *et al.* Prevalence of scleroderma spectrum disorders in the general population of South Carolina. *Arthritis Rheum* 1989; **32**: 998–1006.

12 Medsger TA. Epidemiology of progressive systemic sclerosis. In: Black CM, Myers AR, eds. *Systemic Sclerosis (Scleroderma)*. New York: Gower, 1985: 53–60.

13 Rodnan GP, Benedek TC, Medsger TA *et al.* The association of progressive systemic sclerosis (scleroderma) with coal miners pneumoconiosis and other forms of silicosis. *Ann Intern Med* 1967; **66**: 323–34.

14 Tay CH, Khoo OT. Progressive systemic sclerosis (scleroderma). *Aust Ann Med* 1970; **2**: 145–50.

15 Laing TJ, Gillespie BW, Toth MB *et al.* Racial differences in scleroderma among women in Michigan. *Arthritis Rheum* 1997; **40**: 734–52.

Aetiology [1]. The aetiology of systemic sclerosis is unknown. The presence of vascular symptoms in virtually all patients, and the fact that these may predate the development of classic fibrotic change, and the presence of markers of vascular damage (e.g. elevated circulating von Willebrand factor antigen and endothelial adhesion molecules [2,3]), suggest the endothelial cell is either an initial target or the primary dysfunctional cell in this disease. Vascular abnormalities are not limited to the clinically abnormal skin [4]. Damage to the endothelial cell may initiate the fibrotic process, either through ischaemia/reperfusion or via growth factors released from platelets and inflammatory cells. However, the pathological changes in the internal organs do not always seem to be directly related to changes in the small blood vessels of the same area.

There is now clear evidence of endothelial injury and death [5], in addition to myofibroblast dysfunction, and the primary pathology in vascular endothelium appears to be a fibromucinous change [6]. Serum from patients with the disease is cytotoxic to endothelial cells, either directly [7] or by antibody-dependent cellular cytotoxicity [8] and, although patients' serum has no effect on unstimulated release of prostacyclin [9], stimulated release may be impaired [10]. The influence of sera from affected patients on angiogenesis varies with the phase and type of disease, being stimulatory in early limited disease, but inhibitory in chronic diffuse disease [11]. Damage to endothelium is followed by vascular occlusion resulting from thrombus formation, and tissue ischaemia follows. Abnormalities in various blood components contribute to this tissue anoxia: red cell deformability is reduced [12], platelet aggregation to collagen may be specifically enhanced [13] and *in vivo* markers of platelet activation are increased [14]. Levels of fibrinogen, von Willebrand factor antigen (possibly indicating the degree of vascular damage) [15] and other plasma proteins are also raised, contributing to increased plasma viscosity, further reducing microvascular blood flow. Anticardiolipin antibodies may be present and responsible for increased endothelial cell damage and risk of thrombosis [16].

The associated fibrosis in systemic sclerosis is caused by the increased production of collagen in the subcutaneous tissue. Scleroderma fibroblasts synthesize more collagen than those from normal controls [17,18], and collagenase activity is normal [19]. The deposited collagen is similar in composition to that deposited in other fibrotic disorders, with a normal ratio of type I to type III collagen [19]. The cause of this excessive production is unknown; both intrinsic overactivity and excessive stimulation of fibroblasts may occur. Fibroblast function is modified by endothelial cell products released in a cell culture system [20]. Small collagen fibres are increased, and the response of systemic sclerosis fibroblasts to most mitogens is normal, or reduced, indicating overstimulation [21]. Raised levels of growth factors, both platelet-derived [22] and non-platelet-derived [23], support this suggestion. In addition, glycosaminoglycan synthesis is increased in fibroblasts from patients with the disease, and is stimulated by a mononuclear cell product (possibly IL-1) [24], although other mononuclear cell products can inhibit collagen overproduction [25]. Other connective tissue proteins, including tenascin, are increased [26]. However, there is evidence for an expanded clone of overactive fibroblasts in systemic sclerosis [27], possibly derived from fibroblasts from the deeper dermis [28,29]. There is also an excessive response of fibroblasts to connective-tissue growth factor (CTGF) [30], TGF-β [31], to platelet growth factors [32] and to serum from patients with the disease [33]. TGF-β may have a role both in fibroblast stimulation and in endothelial inhibition [21]. There is a failure of the inhibitory feedback of the amino-propeptide of type I collagen on the fibroblasts [34]. Soluble cytokine receptors [35] and levels of adhesion molecules [36] are often raised in the serum of patients, reflecting disease activity. Circulating anticollagen antibodies to collagen types I and IV occur in patients with systemic sclerosis [37], but these appear to be inversely related to the severity of the disease. They occur in approximately half of British patients and in at least one relative in over 80% of their families. It has been suggested that serotonin hypersensitivity may be a factor in both the vascular and fibrous changes of the disease [38]. Abnormal metabolism of, and responses to, serotonin and tryptophan may contribute to both fibrosis and vascular abnormalities [39]. Raised numbers of mast cells in affected skin may similarly contribute.

References

1 Black CM. The aetiopathogenesis of systemic sclerosis: thick skin—thin hypotheses. *J R Coll Physicians Lond* 1995; **29**: 119–30.

2 Greaves M, Malia RC, Milford Ward A *et al.* Elevated von Willebrand factor antigen in systemic sclerosis: relationship to visceral disease. *Br J Rheumatol* 1988; **27**: 281–5.

3 Kahaleh MB, Osborn I, LeRoy EC. Increased factor VIII/von Willebrand factor antigen and von Willebrand factor activity in scleroderma and in Raynaud's phenomenon. *Ann Intern Med* 1981; **94**: 482–4.

4 Fremont AJ, Hoyland J, Fielding P *et al.* Studies of the microvascular endothelium in uninvolved skin of patients with systemic sclerosis: direct evidence for a generalized microangiopathy. *Br J Dermatol* 1992; **126**: 561–8.

5 Nunzi E, Neboro A. Are endothelial cells stimulated by autoantibody in progressive systemic sclerosis? *Acta Derm Venereol (Stockh)* 1983; **63**: 458–9.

6 Winkelmann RK. Pathogenesis and staging of scleroderma. *Acta Derm Venereol (Stockh)* 1976; **56**: 83–92.

7 Kahaleh MB, Sherer GK, LeRoy EC. Endothelial injury in scleroderma. *J Exp Med* 1979; **149**: 1326–35.

8 Penning CA, Cunningham J, French MAH *et al.* Antibody dependent cellular cytotoxicity of human vascular endothelium in systemic sclerosis. *Clin Exp Immunol* 1984; **57**: 548–56.

9 Holt CM, Moult J, Lindsey N *et al.* Prostacyclin production by human umbilical vein endothelium in response to serum from patients with systemic sclerosis. *Br J Rheumatol* 1989; **28**: 216–20.

10 Rustin MHA, Bull HA, Machin SJ *et al.* Serum from patients with Raynaud's phenomenon inhibits prostacyclin production. *J Invest Dermatol* 1987; **89**: 555–9.

11 Majewski S, Skopinska-Rozewska E, Jablonska S *et al.* Modulatory effect of sera from scleroderma patients on lymphocyte-induced angiogenesis. *Arthritis Rheum* 1985; **28**: 1133–9.

12 Kovacs IB, Sowemimo-Coker SD, Kirby JDT *et al.* Altered behaviour of erythrocytes in scleroderma. *Clin Sci* 1975; **65**: 515–22.

13 Goodfield MJD, Orchard MA, Rowell NR. Increased platelet sensitivity to collagen induced aggregation in whole blood in patients with systemic sclerosis. *Clin Exp Rheumatol* 1988; **6**: 285–8.

14 Kahaleh MB, Scharstein KK, LeRoy EC. Enhanced platelet adhesion to collagen in scleroderma: effect of scleroderma plasma and scleroderma platelets. *J Rheumatol* 1985; **12**: 468–71.

15 Goodfield MJD, Orchard M, Rowell NR. Whole blood platelet aggregation and coagulation factors in patients with systemic sclerosis. *Br J Haematol* 1993; **84**: 675–80.

16 Malia RC, Greaves M, Rowlands LM *et al*. Anticardiolipin antibodies in systemic sclerosis: immunological and clinical associations. *Clin Exp Immunol* 1988; **73**: 456–60.

17 Buckingham RB, Prince RK, Rodnan GP *et al*. Increased collagen accumulation in dermal fibroblast cultures from patients with progressive systemic sclerosis (scleroderma). *J Lab Clin Med* 1978; **92**: 5–21.

18 LeRoy EC. Increased collagen synthesis by scleroderma skin fibroblasts *in vitro*. *J Clin Invest* 1974; **54**: 880–9.

19 Uitto J, Bauer EA, Eisen EZ. Scleroderma: increased biosynthesis of triple helical type I and type III procollagen with unaltered expression of collagenase by skin fibroblasts in culture. *J Clin Invest* 1979; **64**: 921–30.

20 Denton CP, Xu SW, Welsh KI *et al*. Scleroderma fibroblast phenotype is modulated by endothelial cell co-culture. *J Rheumatol* 1996; **23**: 633–8.

21 LeRoy EC, Mercurio S, Sherer CK. Replication and phenotypic expression of control and scleroderma fibroblasts: responses to growth factors. *Proc Natl Acad Sci USA* 1982; **79**: 1288–90.

22 Pandolfi A, Florita M, Altomare C *et al*. Increased plasma levels of platelet-derived growth factor activity with progressive systemic sclerosis. *Proc Soc Exp Biol Med* 1989; **19**: 1–4.

23 Potter SR, Bienenstock J, Goldstein S *et al*. Fibroblast growth factors in scleroderma. *J Rheumatol* 1989; **12**: 1129–35.

24 Whiteside TL, Inoshita T, Roumm AD *et al*. T-lymphocytes in progressive systemic sclerosis. In: Black CM, Myers AR, eds. *Systemic Sclerosis (Scleroderma)*. New York: Gower, 1985: 326–37.

25 Jimenez SA, McArthur WM, Bashey RI *et al*. Selective inhibition of excessive scleroderma fibroblast collagen production by lymphokines from normal human mononuclear cells. *Arthritis Rheum* 1985; **28**: 502–10.

26 Lacour JP, Vitetta A, Chiquet-Ehrismann R *et al*. Increased expression of tenascin in the dermis in scleroderma. *Br J Dermatol* 1992; **127**: 328–34.

27 Maxwell DB, Grotendorst CA, Grotendorst CR *et al*. Fibroblast heterogeneity in scleroderma: C1q studies. *J Rheumatol* 1987; **14**: 756–9.

28 Harper RA, Grove G. Human skin fibroblasts derived from papillary and reticular dermis: differences in growth potential *in vitro*. *Science* 1979; **204**: 525–7.

29 Krieg T, Langer I, Gerstmeier H *et al*. Type III collagen aminopropeptide levels in serum of patients with progressive systemic scleroderma. *J Invest Dermatol* 1986; **87**: 788–91.

30 Fonseca C, Lindahl GE, Ponticos M *et al*. A polymorphism in the CTGF promoter region associated with systemic sclerosis. *N Engl J Med* 2007; **357**: 1210–20.

31 Falanga V, Tiegs SL, Alstadt SP *et al*. Transforming growth factor-β: selective increase in glycosaminoglycan synthesis by cultures of fibroblasts from patients with progressive systemic sclerosis. *J Invest Dermatol* 1987; **89**: 100–4.

32 Falanga V, Hebdo PA, Eaglestein WH. Effect of platelet homogenate on *in vitro* glycosaminoglycan production by dermal fibroblasts from systemic sclerosis patients and normal controls. *Br J Dermatol* 1985; **113**: 237–43.

33 Potter SR, Bienenstock SR, Lee P *et al*. Clinical associations of fibroblast growth promotion factor in scleroderma. *J Rheumatol* 1984; **11**: 43–7.

34 Perlish JS, Lemlich C, Fleischmajer R. Identification of collagen fibrils in scleroderma skin. *J Invest Dermatol* 1988; **90**: 48–54.

35 Steen VD, Engel EE, Charley MR, Medsger TA. Soluble serum interleukin-2 receptors in patients with systemic sclerosis. *J Rheumatol* 1996; **23**: 646–9.

36 Denton CP, Bickerstaff MCM, Shiwen X *et al*. Serial circulating adhesion molecule levels reflect disease severity in systemic sclerosis. *Br J Rheumatol* 1995; **34**: 1048–54.

37 Mackel AM, DeLustro F, Harper FE *et al*. Antibodies to collagen in scleroderma. *Arthritis Rheum* 1982; **25**: 522–31.

38 Winkelmann RK, Goldyne MF, Linscheid RLL. Hypersensitivity of scleroderma cutaneous vascular smooth muscle to 5-hydroxytryptamine. *Br J Dermatol* 1976; **95**: 51–6.

39 Stachow A, Jablonska S, Skiendzielewska A. 5-Hydroxytryptamine and tryptamine pathways in scleroderma. *Br J Dermatol* 1977; **97**: 147–54.

Autoimmunity. The presence of antinuclear antibodies in over 80% of patients and specific autoantibodies—anti-isotopomerase (22%) and anticentromere (up to 30%)—suggests an autoimmune response. However, it is not clear if this is a primary abnormality or results from cellular damage. A role for immune factors in endothelial injury is also suggested by the presence of antiendothelial cell antibodies in 30% of patients [1,2], the ability of endothelial cells to act as a modulator of immune responses [3] and the finding of an IgM vasculopathy in acute-onset systemic sclerosis. Furthermore, circulating immune complexes occur in over 50% of cases [4], but their significance is unknown.

There is evidence of abnormal cellular immunity in patients with systemic sclerosis, with leukocyte migration inhibition to a variety of autologous, homologous and heterologous antigens [5]. However, the development of delayed cutaneous hypersensitivity is normal [6]. Patients have a deficiency of circulating T lymphocytes [7] and impaired lymphocyte transformation in response to phytohaemagglutinin (PHA) [8]. Both these features are related to the severity of the disease and the degree of visceral involvement, and also to an increased incidence of HLA-B8 [9]. The haplotype B8/DR3 is associated with decreased cellular immunity [10]. Helper cells [11], T cells possibly activated by raised levels of IL-2 [12] and NK cells are increased [13], whereas suppressor T cells are decreased [14]. These T-cell changes are more marked in the later stages of generalized disease. Patients with extensive disease have reduced antibody-dependent cytotoxicity, PHA-induced T-cell cytotoxicity [15] and NK-cell cytotoxicity to Chang liver cells [16], although others have found enhanced NK activity [17]. Some patients with systemic sclerosis develop a delayed cutaneous reaction to autologous leukocytes [18]. Scleroderma-like changes have been reported after allogeneic bone marrow transplantation, suggesting a graft-versus-host response (see p. 51.83).

References

1 Baguley E, Brown KA, Haskard D *et al*. Antiendothelial cell antibodies in connective tissue diseases. *Br J Rheumatol* 1989; **26**: 95–101.

2 Hashemi S, Smith CD, Izaguirre CA. Antiendothelial cell antibodies: detection and characterization using a cellular enzyme-linked immunosorbent assay. *J Lab Clin Med* 1987; **109**: 434–40.

3 Pober JS, Collins T, Cimbrone MA *et al*. Inducible expression of class II major histocompatibility complex antigens and the immunogenicity of vascular endothelium. *Transplantation* 1986; **41**: 141–6.

4 Hughes P, Cunningham J, Day M *et al*. Immune complexes in systemic sclerosis. *J Clin Lab Immunol* 1983; **10**: 133–8.

5 Hughes P, Holt S, Rowell NR. Leukocyte migration inhibition in progressive systemic sclerosis. *Br J Dermatol* 1974; **91**: 1–6.

6 Lupoli S, Amlot P, Black C. Normal immune responses in systemic sclerosis. *J Rheumatol* 1990; **17**: 323–7.

7 Hughes P, Holt S, Rowell NR *et al*. Thymus-dependent (T) lymphocyte deficiency in progressive systemic sclerosis. *Br J Dermatol* 1976; **95**: 469–73.

8 Hughes P, Holt S, Rowell NR *et al*. The relationship of defective cell-mediated immunity to visceral disease in systemic sclerosis. *Clin Exp Immunol* 1977; **28**: 233–40.

9 Hughes P, Gelsthorpe K, Doughty RW *et al*. The association of HLA-B8 with visceral disease in systemic sclerosis. *Clin Exp Immunol* 1978; **31**: 351–6.

10 Kallenberg CGM, Van der Voort-Beelen JM, D'Aman J *et al*. Increased frequency of B8/DR3 in scleroderma and association of the haplotype with impaired cellular immune response. *Clin Exp Immunol* 1981; **43**: 478–85.

11 Krakauer RS, Sundeen J, Sauder DN *et al*. Abnormalities of immunoregulation in progressive systemic sclerosis. *Arch Dermatol* 1981; **117**: 80–2.

12 Kahaleh MB, LeRoy EC. Interleukin-2 in scleroderma: correlation of serum level with extent of skin involvement and disease duration. *Ann Intern Med* 1989; **110**: 446–50.

13 Jablonska S. *Scleroderma and Pseudoscleroderma*. Warsaw: Polish Medical Publishers, 1975.

14 Whiteside TL, Kumagai Y, Roumm AD *et al.* Suppressor cell function and T-lymphocyte subpopulations in peripheral blood of patients with progressive systemic sclerosis. *Arthritis Rheum* 1983; **26**: 841–7.

15 Wright JK, Hughes P, Rowell NR *et al.* Antibody-dependent and phytohaemagglutinin-induced lymphocyte cytotoxicity in systemic sclerosis. *Clin Exp Immunol* 1979; **36**: 175–82.

16 Wright JK, Hughes P, Rowell NR. Spontaneous lymphocyte-mediated (NK cell) cytotoxicity in systemic sclerosis: a comparison with antibody-dependent lymphocyte (K-cell) cytotoxicity. *Ann Rheum Dis* 1982; **41**: 409–13.

17 Cifone MG, Giacomelli R, Famularo G *et al.* Natural killer activity and antibody-dependent cellular cytotoxicity in progressive systemic sclerosis. *Clin Exp Immunol* 1990; **80**: 360–5.

18 Tuffanelli DL. Cutaneous hypersensitivity to leukocytes in scleroderma. *J Invest Dermatol* 1964; **42**: 179–84.

Genetic factors. Despite the rarity of familial cases of systemic sclerosis [1–4], abnormalities of the serum immunoglobulins [5] and the high incidence of antinuclear factor in first-degree relatives of patients with systemic sclerosis [6], together with an increased incidence of HLA-B8 in the more severe cases [7], suggest that genetic factors play a part in the aetiology. Clinical and immunological subsets may be genetically determined, but to date there appears to be no clear relationship between HLA, autoantibodies and clinical manifestations [8]. Chromosomal abnormalities have been described in patients with the disease [9,10] and in their relatives, and a serum factor may be responsible for this abnormality. HLA-DR typing shows an increase in DR2, DR3 and DR5 [11]. There is an association between the B8-DR3-DR52-DQB2 haplotype and the development of pulmonary fibrosis [12]. Patients with mild disease have raised DR2 and DR5 and anticentromere antibodies. No relationship between HLA type and Scl-70 antibodies has yet been demonstrated. In identical twins discordant for the disease, autoantibodies [13], T-cell abnormalities and abnormal fibroblast response to mononuclear cell stimulation were found only in the affected twin [14].

An intriguing hypothesis suggests that transfer of fetal cells to the mother or vice versa during pregnancy may result in microchimerism, which has been demonstrated in higher frequency in systemic sclerosis [15]; this may then stimulate a unique immune response.

The age distribution of the disease suggests that the susceptible genotype is probably characterized by a single inherited dominant allele on the X chromosome, explaining the female predominance, together with autosomal factors. Initiation would depend on the occurrence of specific random events believed to be somatic mutations in lymphoid stem cells [16], producing 'forbidden' clones of lymphocytes. These synthesize cellular autoantibodies that are pathogenic, damaging endothelial cells. After a variable latent period, damage to tissue occurs. Antinuclear factors are the result of the disease. Normal defence mechanisms (more efficient in females) may be inhibited by precipitating factors such as silica or other environmental hazards. The pattern of organ involvement may be related to particular forbidden clones that are active, or to local tissue differences.

References

1 Dubois FL, Chandor S, Friou GJ *et al.* Progressive systemic sclerosis (PSS) and localized scleroderma (morphoea) with positive LE cell test. *Medicine* 1971; **50**: 199–222.

2 Gregor RE. Familial progressive systemic scleroderma. *Arch Dermatol* 1975; **111**: 81–5.

3 Rendall JR, McKenzie AW. Familial scleroderma. *Br J Dermatol* 1974; **91**: 517–22.

4 Sasaki S, Yoshino H. Systemic scleroderma in mother and daughter. *Arch Dermatol* 1977; **113**: 378–9.

5 Corcos JM, Robbins WC, Rogoff B *et al.* Some serum protein abnormalities in patients with progressive systemic sclerosis and their relatives. *Arthritis Rheum* 1961; **4**: 107.

6 Pereira S, Black C, Welsh K *et al.* Autoantibodies and immunogenetics in 30 patients with systemic sclerosis and their families. *J Rheumatol* 1987; **14**: 760–5.

7 Hughes P, Gelsthorpe K, Doughty RW *et al.* The association of HLA-B8 with visceral disease in systemic sclerosis. *Clin Exp Immunol* 1978; **31**: 351–6.

8 Black CM, Briggs D, Welsh K. The immunogenetic background of scleroderma: an overview. *Clin Exp Dermatol* 1992; **17**: 73–8.

9 Emerit I. Chromosomal breakage in systemic sclerosis and related disorders. *Dermatologica* 1982; **153**: 145–56.

10 Sherer CK, Jackson BB, LeRoy EC. Chromosome-breakage and sister chromatid exchange frequencies in scleroderma. *Arthritis Rheum* 1981; **24**: 1409–13.

11 Black CM, Welsh KI, Maddison PJ *et al.* HLA antigens, autoantibodies and clinical subsets in scleroderma. *Br J Rheumatol* 1984; **23**: 267–75.

12 Briggs DC, Vaughan R, Welsh KI *et al.* Immunogenetic prediction of pulmonary fibrosis in systemic sclerosis. *Lancet* 1992; **338**: 661–2.

13 McHugh NJ, Harvey GR, Whyte J, Dorsey JK. Segregation of auto-antibodies with disease in monozygotic twin pairs discordant for systemic sclerosis: three further cases. *Arthritis Rheum* 1995; **38**: 1845–50.

14 Dustoor MM, McInerney MM, Mazanec DJ *et al.* Abnormal lymphocyte function in scleroderma: a study on identical twins. *Clin Immunol Immunopathol* 1987; **44**: 20–30.

15 Johnson KL, Nelson JL, Furst DE *et al.* Fetal cell microchimerism in tissue from multiple sites in women with systemic sclerosis. *Arthritis Rheum* 2001; **44**: 1848–54.

16 Rowell NR. Systemic sclerosis. *J R Coll Phys Lond* 1985; **19**: 23–30.

Other factors. There is no evidence of a chemical cause, although cocaine has been suggested as a trigger in some cases [1]. The role of silicone gel prostheses used for breast augmentation has been much discussed, but there is now agreement that there is no relationship between this procedure and the development of systemic sclerosis [2,3] (see Chapter 70). Physical trauma appears to precipitate the disease in genetically predisposed individuals [4], who may have the allele HLA-DR52 [5]. Virus-like particles have been observed by electron microscopy in striated muscle [6], and acid-fast bacilli, closely allied to mycobacteria, have been found in skin biopsies [7] in systemic sclerosis, but their significance is not known. Glucose-tolerance curves may suggest latent diabetes [8]. A prolongation of sensory chronaxia has been found in both normal and abnormal skin [9], and it has been suggested that the condition is a primary abnormality of the central autonomic nervous system. Reciprocal skin grafting has shown that if sclerodermatous skin is placed in a normal bed, it remains sclerodermatous, and if clinically normal skin is placed in a sclerodermatous area it becomes sclerodermatous [10]. Thus, in systemic sclerosis, the skin involvement is generalized or irreversible, in contrast with morphoea, in which the disorder is localized and reversible.

References

1 Kilaru P, Kim W, Sequerina W. Cocaine and scleroderma: is there an association? *J Rheumatol* 1991; **18**: 1753–5.

2 Englert H, Morris D, March L. Scleroderma and silicone gel breast prostheses: the Sydney study revisited. *Aust NZ J Med* 1996; **26**: 349–55.

3 Hochberg MC, Perlmutter DL, Medsger TA *et al.* Lack of association between augmentation mammoplasty and systemic sclerosis (scleroderma). *Arthritis Rheum* 1996; **39**: 1125–31.

4 Lee P. Systemic sclerosis following physical trauma. *J Rheumatol* 1996; **23**: 1689–90.

5 Rahman MAA, Jayson MIV, Black CM. Five patients who developed systemic sclerosis shortly after episodes of physical trauma. *J Rheumatol* 1996; **23**: 1816–7.

6 Kudejko J. Virus-like particles observed in the striated muscles in patients with acroscleroderma. *Dermatologica* 1966; **133**: 495–502.

7 Cantwell AR Jr, Craggs E, Wilson JW *et al.* Acid-fast bacteria as a possible cause of scleroderma. *Dermatologica* 1968; **136**: 141–50.

8 Fleischmajer R, Faludi C. A study of carbohydrate metabolism in scleroderma. *J Invest Dermatol* 1969; **52**: 326–7.

9 Jablonska S. *Scleroderma and Pseudoscleroderma*. Warsaw: Polish Medical Publishers, 1975.

10 Fries JF, Hoopes JE, Shulman LE. Reciprocal skin grafts in systemic sclerosis (scleroderma). *Arthritis Rheum* 1971; **14**: 571–8.

Diagnosis. The criteria for diagnosis have been established by the Subcommittee for Scleroderma Criteria of the ARA [1] and are generally accepted. Patients should have either:

1 Scleroderma proximal to the digits, affecting limbs, face, neck or trunk—this is the single major criterion; or

2 At least two minor criteria, consisting of:
   (a) sclerodactyly
   (b) digital pitted scarring
   (c) bilateral basal pulmonary fibrosis.

These criteria have 97% sensitivity and 98% specificity, and difficulty arises principally in males who have a sclerodermatous condition brought about by occupational exposure to, for example, silica or vinyl chloride. These patients often fulfil two minor criteria, and indeed share many characteristics, both clinical and immunological, with true systemic sclerosis [2].

Classification of systemic sclerosis. There have been many attempts to classify the disease [3–6]. Most recently, a simplified classification has been proposed [7]. In this system, patients are classified as having diffuse cutaneous systemic sclerosis (dSSc), or limited cutaneous systemic sclerosis (lSSc). The distinction is made principally on the basis of the extent of cutaneous involvement, but also includes certain other clinical and immunological features (Table 51.17). This system appears satisfactory because systemic involvement, which determines the prognosis of the disease, is less frequent in patients with limited cutaneous disease.

References
1 Subcommittee for Scleroderma Criteria of the American Rheumatism Association Diagnostic and Therapeutic Criteria Committee. Preliminary criteria for the classification of systemic sclerosis. *Arthritis Rheum* 1980; **23**: 581–90.

2 Rustin MHA, Bull HA, Ziegler V *et al.* Silica exposure and silica associated systemic sclerosis. *Br J Dermatol* 1989; **121** (Suppl. 34): 29.

3 Arbeitsgruppe Sklerodermie der Arbeitsgemeinschaft Dermatologische Forschung (ADF). Klinik der progressiven systemischen Sklerodermie (PSS). *Hautarzt* 1986; **37**: 320–4.

4 Barnett AJ. *Scleroderma. Progressive Systemic Sclerosis*. Springfield: Thomas, 1974.

5 Rodnan CP, Jablonska S, Medsger TA. Classification and nomenclature of progressive systemic sclerosis (scleroderma). *Clin Rheum Dis* 1976; **5**: 5–13.

6 Winkelmann RK. Pathogenesis and staging of scleroderma. *Acta Derm Venereol (Stockh)* 1976; **56**: 83–92.

Table 51.17 Classification of systemic sclerosis.

Diffuse cutaneous systemic sclerosis
Short interval (<1 year) between the onset of Raynaud's phenomenon and the development of skin changes
Truncal and peripheral skin involvement
Tendon friction rubs
Pulmonary fibrosis, renal failure, gastrointestinal disease, myocardial involvement
Capillary drop-out visible in nail folds
Scl-70 antibody-positive
Anticentromere antibody-negative
Limited cutaneous systemic sclerosis
Long history of Raynaud's phenomenon
Limited skin involvement (peripheral only)
Calcification, telangiectasia, late onset of pulmonary hypertension
Capillary dilatation visible in nail folds
Anticentromere antibody-positive

7 LeRoy EC, Black C, Fleischmajer R *et al.* Scleroderma (systemic sclerosis): classification, subsets and pathogenesis. *J Rheumatol* 1988; **15**: 202–5.

Pathology [1]. It is important to realize that this widespread disease does not involve all organs in any patient; in certain cases it may be limited to one or two organs. Even when changes are present in an organ, the distribution of these changes is by no means uniform. Although a striking abnormality in systemic sclerosis is the sclerotic change in tissues such as the heart, lungs, submucosa and muscularis of the gastrointestinal tract, widespread vascular lesions may be a prominent feature of certain cases. The digital arteries may be severely involved, and changes of endarteritis may be seen in the lungs, heart, gastrointestinal tract, muscle and kidney. Infiltrations of inflammatory cells, particularly lymphocytes, may occur in the joints, mucosa and submucosa of the gastrointestinal tract, and in striated muscle.

In the skin, the dermis shows hyalinization of the collagen, often with associated abnormalities of elastic tissue and reticulin. The changes may be slight and difficult to detect unless the histological technique is excellent. In particular, standard fixatives must be used if hyalinization of the collagen is to be assessed. In severely involved skin, the epidermis and its appendages are usually atrophic, with loss of the rete ridges. Sometimes, there is hyperkeratosis, and the dermis shows variable degrees of homogenization of the collagen, and occasionally a light dermal lymphocytic infiltrate. In the tumid or 'inflammatory' phase in the fingers, the dermis may show a striking infiltrate, with lymphocytes predominating. Cellular infiltrates of lymphocytes, plasma cells, fibroblastic-type cells and macrophages, either perivascular or diffuse, occurred in 49% of patients of one series [2], but there was no correlation with serum serological abnormalities. Electron microscopy has shown that both T and B lymphocytes are present in the infiltrates [3], although most are activated helper T cells. Hyalinization and intimal thickening of the blood vessels may occur, but fibrinoid change is uncommon. Evidence from electron microscopy [4] and the normal distribution of cutaneous enzymes, acid mucopolysaccharides and other ground substances, together with the absence of any abnormal gammaglobulin, fibrinogen or albumin, using fluorescent antibody techniques, suggests that the

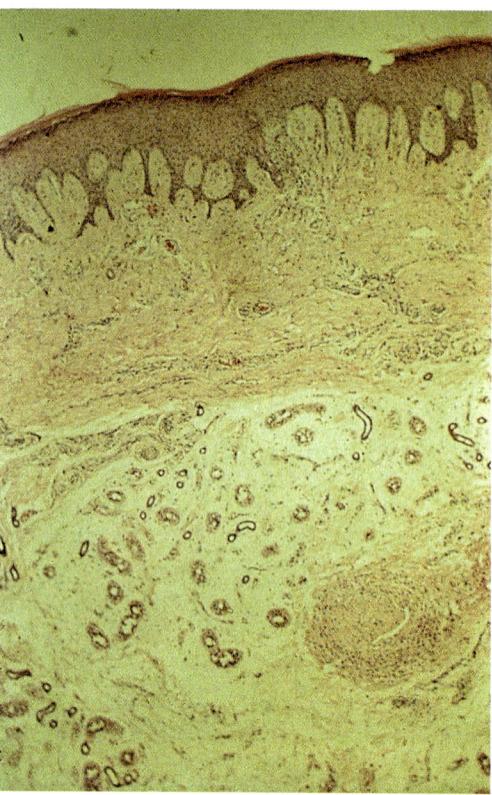

Fig. 51.59 Systemic sclerosis: section of finger showing thickened dermis with hyalinization of the collagen and almost complete occlusion of a digital vessel.

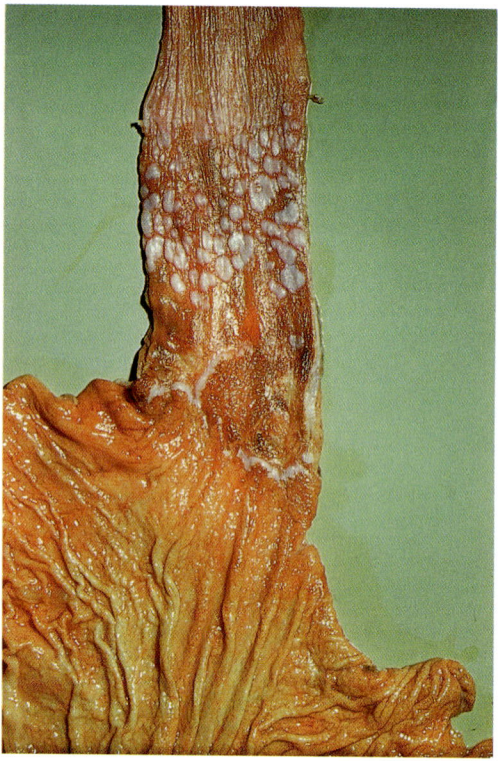

Fig. 51.60 Pearly white plaques in the oesophagus in systemic sclerosis, giving a cobblestone appearance.

alterations in dermal collagen are the result of a simple increase in the number of fibrils. Quantitatively increased fibrillogenesis, with an increased proportion of thin fibrils of type III collagen [5] in the dermis, has led some authors [6] to conclude that qualitative and quantitative disturbances in mesenchymal ground substances may play an important part in the increased formation of qualitatively normal collagen fibrils in scleroderma [7]. Further evidence that the ground substance is the tissue mainly involved has been provided by the finding of a normal concentration of water and hydroxyproline in the dermis [8]. Some authors believe that the main alterations in the skin in systemic sclerosis take place in the subcutaneous tissue and not in the dermis [9]. It is suggested that the replacement of subcutaneous tissue by connective tissue is the cause of the induration of the skin.

Histology, histochemistry, immunopathology and electron microscopy of depigmented areas of skin show changes similar to those found in vitiligo [10]. The digital vessels frequently show intimal and medial thickening, which may be so gross as to almost occlude the vessel (Fig. 51.59); this accounts in certain cases for gangrene of the fingers. Occasionally, fresh thromboses may be seen. Similar but less marked changes are found in the digital arteries of the toes, and the vessels of the leg may also show intimal thickening, which results in ischaemia and gangrene. The intimal thickening is very similar to that seen in the peripheral vascular obstruction that occurs in rheumatoid arthritis. Thromboses of major arteries can also occur [11], and reduction of local tissue fibrinolytic activity can be demonstrated in the involved vessels. Giant cell granulomatous necrosis of the intima of vessels and fat in nodular lesions of the skin has been described [12].

Immunoglobulins and complement may be demonstrated by fluorescent antibody techniques at the dermal–epidermal junction in telangiectases, but not in the indurated skin without telangiectasia [13]. Biopsies should not be taken from telangiectatic areas. The main immunohistological changes in the skin in systemic sclerosis consist of foci of intercollagenous staining for connective tissue antigens in the reticular layer of the dermis [14]. The absence of immunoglobulin and complement from the dermal–epidermal junction may be useful in distinguishing systemic sclerosis from SLE, in which the major changes are at the dermal–epidermal junction. Patients who have both systemic sclerosis and SLE have deposits of immunoglobulin and complement at the dermal–epidermal junction in involved and uninvolved skin as well as changes in the dermal collagen. Patients with scleroderma as part of 'mixed connective tissue disease' have positive immunofluorescence at the dermal–epidermal junction [15].

The gastrointestinal tract is frequently involved. The oesophagus may show areas of epithelium looking like pearly white plaques, giving a cobblestone appearance (Fig. 51.60). Microscopically, subepithelial fibrosis is the most common finding, but fibrosis may also occur in areas of muscular atrophy. The smaller arteries may show endarteritis, and some cellular infiltration also occurs. In the duodenum, jejunum, ileum and colon there is a patchy disappearance of muscle, especially of the circular layer, with replacement by fibrous tissue. The subserosal and submucosal tissues may also be thickened and fibrosed. Vessels in these areas may show sclerosis and intimal fibrosis.

Pathological changes in the lungs may be seen, even in the absence of symptoms or radiological signs of pulmonary involvement and even in the presence of normal pulmonary function.

Progressive diffuse alveolar fibrosis occurs with obliteration of capillaries and alveolar spaces, but is preceded by an inflammatory alveolitis [16,17]. In other cases, hyaline degeneration and fibrosis of alveolar walls result in the disappearance of the alveolar parenchyma and of the capillaries. Rupture of the thinned alveolar walls gives rise to cysts that are lined by cuboidal or columnar epithelium, which may be ciliated. Electron microscopy [18] may show thickening of the alveolar–capillary basement membrane. Arterial lesions in the lungs take the form of concentric thickening of the intima by loose myxomatous tissue and, later, sclerosis. In certain cases, the vessels may be almost completely occluded. Neoplastic change is a rare complication of the pulmonary abnormalities in systemic sclerosis. Various types of neoplasm have been reported [19,20], including malignant pulmonary adenomatosis, alveolar cell carcinoma, adenocarcinoma, oat cell carcinoma and squamous cell carcinoma.

The heart may show no change macroscopically, although showing widespread histological changes. The major coronary arteries are usually patent. Pericarditis, sometimes with effusion, is not uncommon, and sometimes the myocardium shows considerable streaky or focal fibrosis. Occasionally, the mitral or tricuspid valve is involved [21], and Libman–Sacks type of non-bacterial endocarditis has been reported [22]. Histologically, the myocardium may show focal or diffuse fibrosis, associated with degeneration or atrophy of some of the muscle fibres. Occasionally, smaller arteries and arterioles show thickening of the walls. Sometimes, an aneurysm of the myocardial wall develops, and the aorta may show adventitial fibrosis with a focal necrotizing panaortitis and valvulitis.

Involvement of the kidneys used to be the most common cause of serious morbidity and mortality, but this is now uncommon, probably because of the early and improved control of hypertension. In one of the first pathological studies, renal lesions were found in 74% of patients at autopsy [23], and in 90% in another series [24]. It has been suggested [25] that a triad of intimal proliferation of the small intralobular arteries and arterioles, fibrinoid necrosis of the walls of the afferent arterioles and sometimes the glomerular loops, together with cortical infarction characterizes renal lesions in systemic sclerosis. Vascular luminal occlusion may occur, particularly in patients with renal crisis [26]. These changes are not always found, and there are probably no absolutely specific features. Other changes include a mucoid appearance of the intimal thickening of the proximal part of the intralobular arteries. Hypercellularity of the glomeruli and fibrinoid necrosis of the basement membrane of the glomerular tufts may be found. The tubules may be atrophic and surrounded by increased connective tissue, or be dilated and full of hyaline eosinophilic material. A hyaline droplet nephrosis may occur. In the more chronic cases, glomerular hyalinization and interstitial fibrosis predominate. Immunohistological techniques show thickening of the glomerular capillary basement membrane and alteration in the reticular tissue of arterioles associated with deposits of fibrin and very occasionally with the presence of IgG and C3 [27].

The liver is usually normal in systemic sclerosis, although mild fibrosis of the portal tracts and around the bile ducts can occur. The gall bladder may be fibrosed. The spleen may show fibrinoid necrosis of arterioles and endarteritis obliterans, and endarteritis

is also found in the adrenals, mammary glands, pancreas, uterus and ovaries.

Histological changes in the muscles are similar to, if not identical with, those of dermatomyositis. Muscle fibres show varying degrees of degeneration, such as loss of cross-striations, hyalinization of bundles, vacuolation and splitting, with interstitial and focal infiltration of lymphocytes. Later, sclerosis develops and the vessel walls may be thickened. There may also be some thickening of the endomysium and perimysium. The thyroid [28] and parathyroid [29] glands may be involved in the fibrotic process, and the thymus may show cortical atrophy [30].

Widening of, and vascular changes in the periodontal membrane of the teeth occur.

The CNS is rarely involved, but occasionally there may be thickening of the walls of vessels in the white matter, and meningeal lymphocytic or granulomatous infiltrates. Peripheral neurological involvement is characterized by increased collagen deposition in the epi- and perineuria, and intimal thickening of the vasa nervorum [31].

References

1 D'Angelo WA, Fries JF, Masi AT *et al.* Pathologic observations in systemic sclerosis (scleroderma). *Am J Med* 1969; **46**: 428–40.

2 Fleischmajer R, Perlish JS, Reeves JRT. Cellular infiltrates in scleroderma skin. *Arthritis Rheum* 1977; **20**: 975–84.

3 Fleischmajer R, Perlish JS, West WP. Ultrastructure of cutaneous cellular infiltrates in scleroderma. *Arch Dermatol* 1977; **113**: 1661–6.

4 Fisher ER, Rodman GP. Pathologic observations concerning the cutaneous lesion of progressive systemic sclerosis. *Arthritis Rheum* 1960; **3**: 536–45.

5 Perlish JS, Lemlich G, Fleischmajer R. Identification of collagen fibrils in scleroderma skin. *J Invest Dermatol* 1988; **90**: 48–54.

6 Rupec M, Braun-Falco O. Elektronenmikroskopische Untersuchungen über das Verhalten der kollagenfibrillen der Haut bei Sklerodermie. *Arch Klin Exp Dermatol* 1964; **218**: 543–60.

7 Braun-Falco O, Rupec M. Collagen fibrils of the scleroderma in ultra-thin skin sections. *Nature* 1964; **202**: 708–9.

8 Fleischmajer R. The collagen in scleroderma. *Arch Dermatol* 1964; **89**: 437–41.

9 Fleischmajer R, Damiano V, Nedwich A. Alteration of subcutaneous tissue in systemic scleroderma. *Arch Dermatol* 1972; **105**: 59–66.

10 Sanchez JL, Vazquez M, Sanchez NP. Vitiligo-like macules in systemic scleroderma. *Arch Dermatol* 1983; **119**: 129–33.

11 Furey NL, Schmid FR, Kwaan HC *et al.* Arterial thrombosis in scleroderma. *Br J Dermatol* 1975; **93**: 683–93.

12 Sannicandro F. Nodulare, granulomatose Riesenzellen-Arteriitis der Haut, vergesellschaftet mit Akrosklerodermia. *Dermatologica* 1963; **127**: 467–75.

13 Jablonska S, Chorzelski T, Maciejowska E. The scope and limitations of the immunofluorescence method in the diagnosis of lupus erythematosus. *Br J Dermatol* 1970; **83**: 242–7.

14 Rowell NR, Scott DG. Immunohistological studies, with anti-connective tissue and anti-immunoglobulin antisera of the skin in lupus erythematosus and scleroderma. *Br J Dermatol* 1975; **93**: 431–41.

15 Winkelmann RK, Carapeto FJ, Jordon RE. Direct immunofluorescence in the diagnosis of scleroderma syndromes. *Br J Dermatol* 1977; **96**: 231–8.

16 Rossi GA, Bitterman PB, Rennard SI *et al.* Evidence for chronic inflammation as a component of the interstitial lung disease associated with progressive systemic sclerosis. *Ann Rev Respir Dis* 1985; **131**: 612–7.

17 Silver RM, Metcalf DF, Stanley JH *et al.* Interstitial lung disease in scleroderma. *Arthritis Rheum* 1984; **27**: 1254–62.

18 Wilson RJ, Rodman GP, Robin ED. An early pulmonary physiologic abnormality in progressive systemic sclerosis (diffuse scleroderma). *Am J Med* 1964; **36**: 361–9.

19 Haggani MT, Holti G. Systemic sclerosis with pulmonary fibrosis and oat cell carcinoma. *Acta Derm Venereol (Stockh)* 1973; **53**: 369–74.

20 Tomkin CH. Systemic sclerosis associated with carcinoma of the lung. *Br J Dermatol* 1969; **81**: 213–6.

21 Oram S, Stokes W. The heart in scleroderma. *Br Heart J* 1961; **23**: 243–59.

22 von Spuhler O, Morandi L. Sklerodermie und ihre Beziehungen zu Libman–Sacks-Syndrome, Dermatomyositis und rheumatischen Infektionskreis. *Helv Med Acta* 1949; **16**: 147–63.

23 Piper WN, Helwig EB. Progressive systemic sclerosis. *Arch Dermatol* 1955; **72**: 535–46.

24 Cannon PJ, Hassar M, Case DB *et al.* The relationship of hypertension and renal failure in scleroderma to structural and functional abnormalities of the renal cortical circulation. *Medicine* 1974; **53**: 1–46.

25 Levine RJ, Boshell BR. Renal involvement in progressive systemic sclerosis (scleroderma). *Ann Intern Med* 1960; **52**: 517–29.

26 Trostle DC, Bedetti CD, Steen VD *et al.* Renal vascular histology and morphometry in systemic sclerosis. *Arthritis Rheum* 1988; **31**: 393–400.

27 Scott DG, Rowell NR. Immunohistological studies of the kidney in systemic lupus erythematosus and systemic sclerosis using antisera to IgG, C3, fibrin, and human renal glomeruli. *Ann Rheum Dis* 1974; **33**: 473–81.

28 Serup J, Hagdrup H. Thyroid hormones in generalized scleroderma. *Acta Derm Venereol (Stockh)* 1986; **66**: 35–8.

29 Sentochnik DE, Hoffman GS. Hypoparathyroidism due to progressive systemic sclerosis. *J Rheumatol* 1988; **15**: 711–3.

30 Carter J, Ewen SWB, Gray E *et al.* The thymus in systemic sclerosis. *J Pathol* 1973; **110**: 97–100.

31 Di Trapani C, Tulli A, Lacarva A. Peripheral neuropathy in the course of progressive systemic sclerosis. *Acta Neuropathol* 1986; **72**: 103–10.

Natural history. In the majority of patients, the onset is with Raynaud's phenomenon, although this may have been present for many years, and the cutaneous changes occur after an interval. This is much shorter in males—in whom it is usually under a year—than in females, in whom it is usually approximately 5 years, but may be as long as 30 years [1]. Occasionally, Raynaud's phenomenon and cutaneous sclerosis are noticed at the same time, and sometimes Raynaud's phenomenon may follow the onset of cutaneous or other manifestations, or be absent. The risk of anyone with Raynaud's phenomenon developing systemic sclerosis is relatively small, although it seems to be greater in males than in females [2]. Sclerodactyly may be found in approximately 10% of patients with Raynaud's disease, but systemic sclerosis occurs in approximately 4% of patients with this combination [3]. The differentiation between severe Raynaud's disease and early systemic sclerosis is difficult, but may be aided by nail fold capillaroscopy and the presence or absence of autoantibody [2]. The main cause of mortality used to be renal disease, but recent studies show a preponderance of cardiovascular problems, with coronary and cerebrovascular events [4]. In addition to the microvascular changes described, it is now apparent that large vessel changes similar to atherosclerosis are also increased in systemic sclerosis [5].

References

1 Rowell NR. The prognosis of systemic sclerosis. *Br J Dermatol* 1976; **95**: 57–60.

2 Veale D, Belch JJF. Management of Raynaud's phenomenon. *Rheumatol Rev* 1993; **2**: 133–45.

3 Farmer RG, Gifford RW, Hines EA. Raynaud's disease with sclerodactylia. *Circulation* 1961; **23**: 13–5.

4 Bryan C, Knight C, Black CM, Silman AJ. Prediction of 5-year survival following presentation with scleroderma: development of a simple model using three disease factors at first visit. *Arthritis Rheum* 1999; **42**: 2660–5.

5 Ho M, Veale D, Eastmond C *et al.* Macrovascular disease and systemic sclerosis. *Ann Rheum Dis* 2000; **59**: 39–43.

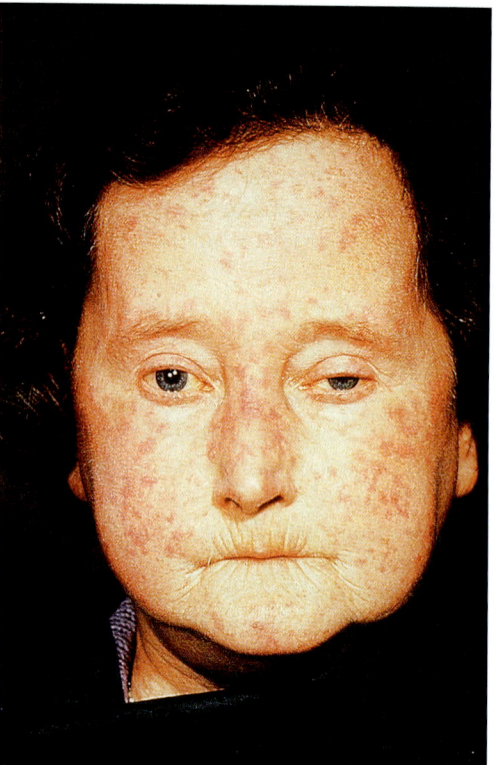

Fig. 51.61 Systemic sclerosis: typical beaked nose, telangiectasia and radial furrowing round the mouth.

Clinical features. The earliest feature is usually, but not invariably, Raynaud's phenomenon. Other early presenting symptoms and signs include swelling of the hands in approximately 15% of patients, swelling of joints, ulceration of the fingers, whitlows and even gangrene. Occasionally, the diagnosis may be made in a patient presenting with leg ulcers or calcinosis cutis. With the increased availability of laser treatments, some patients' first presentation is for treatment of telangiectasia. Less common early symptoms include gastro-oesophageal reflux and dysphagia; constipation, diarrhoea and abdominal pain are usually late features.

Cutaneous changes. The hands and face are the most frequently involved, but the changes may extend proximally to involve the forearms and upper arms, usually but not always in a continuous fashion. The fingers may be oedematous and swollen, and the skin feels tight and has a shiny appearance. With increasing severity, the skin becomes immovable or hidebound. The clinical impression of thickness and toughness of the skin is enhanced because of binding down of the skin to deeper structures. The collagen content is decreased but the density is normal [1]. Sometimes, the chest becomes tight, shiny and pigmented. The facial appearance in a well-developed case is characteristic. The forehead is smooth and shiny, the skin is bound down and hard, the lines of expression are smoothed out and the nose becomes small and pinched (Fig. 51.61). The mouth opening is constricted and radial furrows appear, giving a pursed appearance (Fig. 51.62). The lower eyelids cannot be depressed by the fingers to show the conjunctivae, because of atrophy of the tissues. Very rarely, periorbital oedema

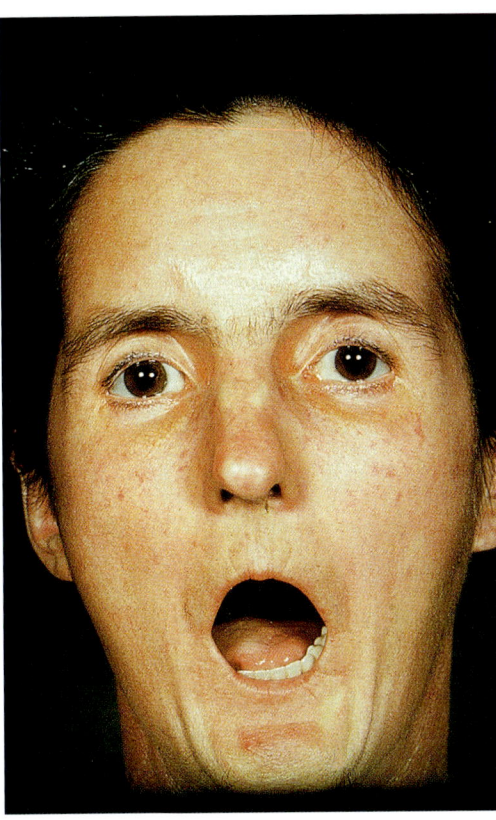

Fig. 51.62 Systemic sclerosis: restricted mouth opening.

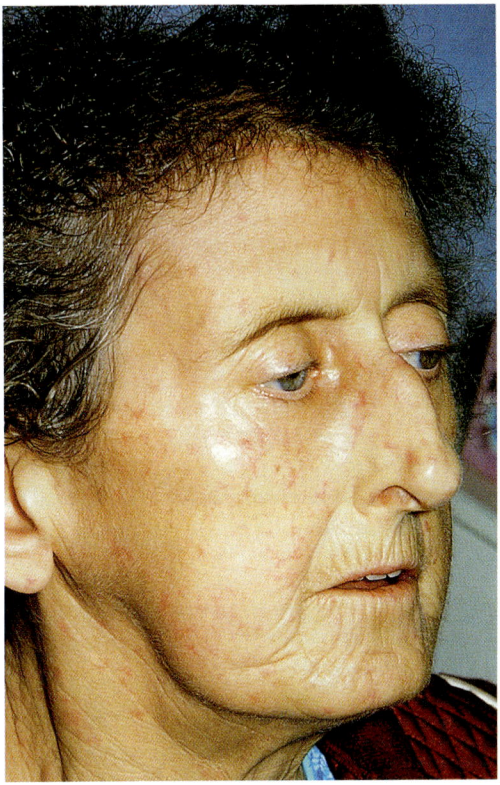

Fig. 51.63 Systemic sclerosis: mandibular atrophy. (Courtesy of Dr J. Cotterill, Leeds, UK.)

can occur [2]. Small mat-like telangiectases are frequently found on the face. Sometimes, the changes on the face are minimal and detected only by an astute observer after the diagnosis has been suspected because of other changes. Mandibular atrophy can occur (Fig. 51.63). Chondrodermatitis nodularis helicis was found in three of 21 patients with limited cutaneous disease [3].

Just as the face may be involved to a greater or lesser extent, the hands may also show great variability in their appearance (Fig. 51.64). Sometimes, in the early stages, only a little atrophy can be seen. Occasionally, the fingers and hands are swollen and rather tumid, and there is difficulty obtaining full extension. The terminal phalanges may be bulbous. Later, however, the changes are easily recognized. Atrophy occurs first in the pulps of the fingers, and small painful ulcers are formed, which heal leaving depressed scars (Fig. 51.65). Pitted scars occur in over one-third of patients, not only on the tips of the fingers but also in a linear distribution on the ulnar border of the thumb and radial borders of the index and middle fingers, as well as the dorsa of the fingers over the joints [4]. Later, sclerosis of the overlying skin of the fingers develops, giving the fingers a smooth shiny tapered appearance, with the nails curving over the atrophic phalanges. Later still, the nails become very small and the whole of the distal part of the finger atrophies. The nail folds may show ragged cuticles. Pterygium inversum unguis-like changes are sometimes found [5]. Slow-healing whitlows and paronychia are common, and ulcers may also occur over the knuckles. Later, the atrophy and sclerosis extends to involve the whole hand, which is held in semi-flexion, full extension of the fingers and metacarpal joints being impossi-

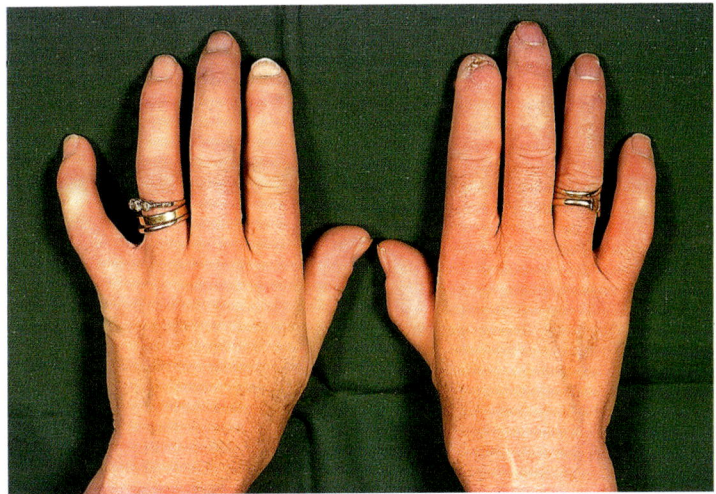

Fig. 51.64 The hands in systemic sclerosis: oedematous phase.

ble. Gangrene of the fingers is not uncommon, and may occur surprisingly early in the disease. It does not necessarily indicate a poor prognosis. Digital arteriography confirms narrowing of the digital arteries [6].

Telangiectases are often found on the palms and on the rest of the hands. Calcium deposits occur in the skin of the fingers and hands, and may break down to discharge chalky material. Calcinosis may also be found around the elbow, where the olecranon bursa may be involved. Erythema may be seen on the thenar and hypothenar eminences. Hyperkeratotic plaques over the phalan-

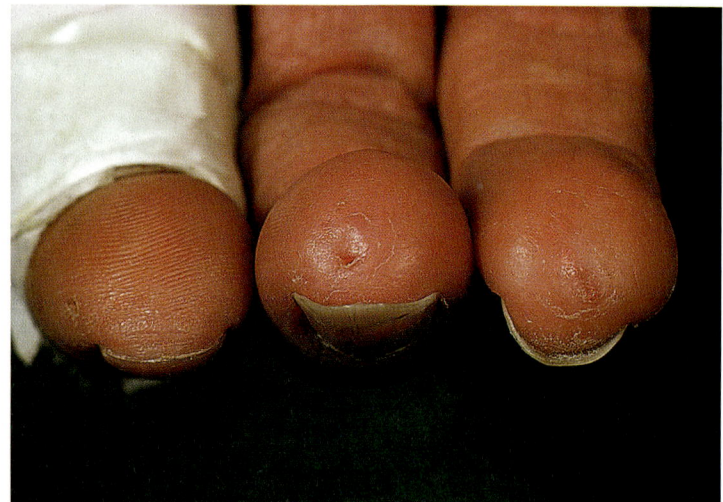

Fig. 51.65 Systemic sclerosis: healed ulceration of the fingertips.

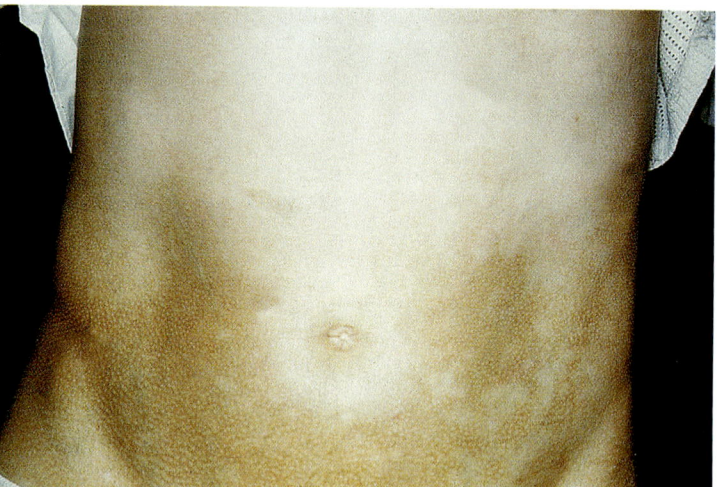

Fig. 51.67 Systemic sclerosis: pigmentation of the abdomen.

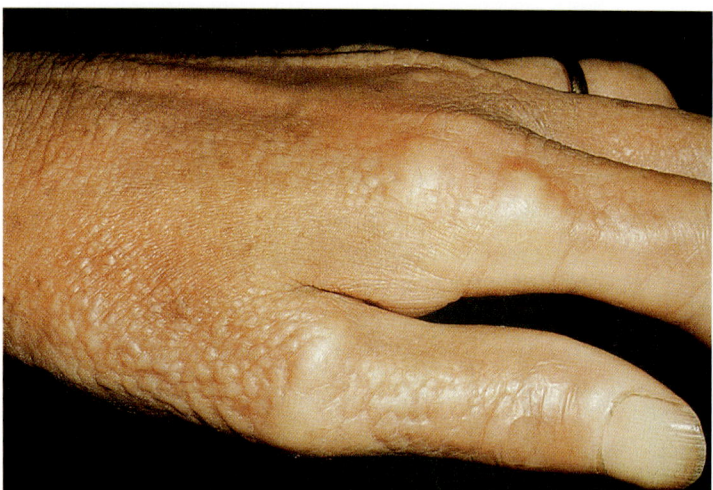

Fig. 51.66 Systemic sclerosis: 'cobblestone' appearance on the dorsum of the hand.

ges may indicate amyloid material deposited in the dermal papillae [7]. Multiple small papules of lymphangiectasia may occur in 'hidebound' skin because of obstruction of lymphatic channels by the sclerosing process (Fig. 51.66) [8]. Ivory-coloured subcutaneous nodules 3–20 mm in diameter occur rarely on the trunk and limbs. Histology shows fibromatous changes [9] or fibrinoid necrosis [10].

Similar, although less severe changes occur on the feet, and not infrequently the tips of the toes become black with incipient gangrene. The feet become encased in tight, firm skin with mottled patches of pigmentation and atrophy. These changes may extend up the legs and be present on the thighs.

In a series of patients at Leeds, changes on the hands occurred in 95% of cases, on the face in 90%, beneath the clavicles in 30% and on the feet in 15%. The changes on the face, hands and feet tend to be progressive, but changes on the trunk have been seen to regress over the years. Dilated nail fold capillaries visible without a lens occur in approximately 10% of patients and, occasionally, heliotrope cyanosis around the eye suggests a diagnosis of dermatomyositis. There is some evidence that the degree of nail

fold capillary dilatation correlates with the severity of organ involvement [11], but this has not been confirmed [12]. Nail fold capillary abnormalities have been correlated with Raynaud's phenomenon, digital pitted scars and low finger temperature [13]. Using wide-field microscopy, the capillaries are enlarged and distorted. There is loss of capillaries with disruption of the capillary bed in approximately 90% of patients. These features may indicate those patients with Raynaud's phenomenon who will go on to develop systemic sclerosis [14,15], but do not distinguish between different connective tissue diseases [16]. Transient nodules resembling erythema nodosum occasionally occur; the histology of these shows panniculitis and endarteritis.

Telangiectases varying from 2 to 20 mm in diameter, blanching on pressure and refilling from several different foci, occur in 75% of patients. They are found mainly on the face, lips, mouth, upper trunk and hands, but may extend as far as the upper thighs. These mat-like telangiectases are not absolutely diagnostic of systemic sclerosis. Pigmentation occurs in approximately 50% of the patients, most frequently on the face, and to a lesser extent on the legs, thighs, lower abdomen (Fig. 51.67), axillary folds and dorsa of the hands. Occasionally, the pigmentation is so gross as to lead to a suspicion of Addison's disease [17], and sometimes gives a mottled appearance. Dense warty pigmentation in the axillae can resemble acanthosis nigricans [18]. Leg ulcers occur in 40% of patients and are difficult to heal. Livedo reticularis [19] and small white areas of atrophie blanche develop around the ankles, even without ulceration. These features can occur in patients without hypertension. A case has been reported of large soft cystic lesions over the interphalangeal joints of both hands. Aspiration revealed mucoid material, and the histology suggested focal mucinosis [20]. Rarely, papular and nodular mucinosis may occur and may be a presenting feature [21]. Lesions resembling acrokeratoelastoidosis have been described [22].

References

1 Black MM, Bottoms E, Shuster S. Skin collagen content and thickness in systemic sclerosis. *Br J Dermatol* 1970; **83**: 552–5.

2 Dorwart BB. Periorbital edema in progressive systemic sclerosis. *Ann Intern Med* 1974; **80**: 273.

3 Bottomley WW, Goodfield MJD. Chondrodermatitis nodularis helicis occurring with systemic sclerosis: an under-reported association? *Clin Exp Dermatol* 1994; **19**: 219–20.

4 Maeda M, Matubara K, Hirano H *et al.* Pitting scars in progressive systemic sclerosis. *Dermatology* 1993; **187**: 104–8.

5 Patterson JW. Pterygium inversum unguis-like changes in scleroderma. *Arch Dermatol* 1977; **113**: 1429–30.

6 Dabich L, Bookstein JJ, Zweiffer A *et al.* Digital arteries in patients with scleroderma. *Arch Intern Med* 1972; **130**: 708–14.

7 Black MM. Primary localized cutaneous amyloidosis in systemic sclerosis. *Trans St John's Hosp Dermatol Soc* 1971; **57**: 177–80.

8 Tuffanelli DL. Lymphangiectasis due to scleroderma. *Arch Dermatol* 1975; **111**: 1216.

9 Bettley FR, Seville RH. Nodular scleroderma. *Proceedings of the 10th International Congress on Dermatology*. London: BMA, 1952: 479–81.

10 Kennedy C, Leigh IM. Systemic sclerosis with subcutaneous nodules. *Br J Dermatol* 1979; **101**: 93–6.

11 Maricq HR, Spencer-Green G, LeRoy EC. Skin capillary abnormalities as indicators of organ involvement in scleroderma, Raynaud's syndrome and dermatomyositis. *Am J Med* 1976; **61**: 862–70.

12 Statham BN, Rowell NR. Quantification of the nail fold capillary abnormalities in systemic sclerosis and Raynaud's syndrome. *Acta Derm Venereol (Stockh)* 1986; **66**: 139–43.

13 Ohtsuka T, Ishikawa H. Statistical definition of nail fold capillary pattern in patients with systemic sclerosis. *Dermatology* 1994; **188**: 286–9.

14 Lee P, Sarkozi J, Bookman AA *et al.* Digital blood flow and nail fold capillary microscopy in Raynaud's phenomenon. *J Rheumatol* 1986; **13**: 564–9.

15 Maricq HR, LeRoy EC, D'Angelo WA *et al.* Diagnostic potential of *in vivo* capillary microscopy in scleroderma and related disorders. *Arthritis Rheum* 1980; **23**: 183–90.

16 Houtman PM, Kallenberg CGM, Fidler V *et al.* Diagnostic significance of nailfold capillary patterns in patients with Raynaud's phenomenon. *J Rheumatol* 1986; **3**: 556–63.

17 Talbott JH, Gall EA, Consolazio WV *et al.* Dermatomyositis with scleroderma, calcinosis and renal endarteritis associated with focal cortical necrosis. *Arch Intern Med* 1939; **63**: 476–96.

18 Clinicopathological Conference. A case of scleroderma with pseudoacanthosis nigricans. *BMJ* 1966; **ii**: 1642–5.

19 Thomas JR, Winkelmann RH. Vascular ulcers in scleroderma. *Arch Dermatol* 1983; **119**: 803–7.

20 Marzano AV, Berti E, Gasparini G *et al.* Unique digital skin lesions associated with systemic sclerosis. *Br J Dermatol* 1997; **136**: 598–600.

21 Van Zander J, Shaw JC. Papular and nodular mucinosis as a presenting sign of progressive systemic sclerosis. *J Am Acad Dermatol* 2002; **46**: 304–6.

22 Tajima S, Tanaka N, Ishibashi A, Suzuki K. A variant of acrokeratoelastoidosis in systemic sclerosis: report of 7 cases. *J Am Acad Dermatol* 2002; **46**: 767–70.

Systemic sclerosis without skin involvement

[1–4]. Although skin lesions and Raynaud's phenomenon usually precede systemic changes, there is no doubt that occasionally the situation is reversed. In these cases, diagnosis may be difficult until the disease has progressed further to give characteristic changes in other organs.

References

1 Crown S. Visceral scleroderma without skin involvement. *BMJ* 1961; **ii**: 1541–3.

2 Herington JL Jr. Scleroderma as a cause of small bowel obstruction: successful treatment by intestinal resection. *AMA Arch Surg* 1959; **78**: 17–25.

3 McBrien DT, Mummer HEL. Steatorrhoea in progressive systemic sclerosis (scleroderma). *BMJ* 1962; **2**: 1653–4.

4 Rodnan GP, Fennell RH. Progressive systemic sclerosis sine scleroderma. *JAMA* 1962; **180**: 665–70.

Calcinosis. Weber [1] described calcinosis in scleroderma long before Thibierge and Weissenbach [2], whose names are usually associated with the syndrome. Calcification in systemic sclerosis occurs most commonly (25%) in the fingers, especially on the palmar aspects of the terminal phalanges. It is less common than absorption of the phalanges, but sometimes occurs in the absence of any radiological bone change. Digital calcification is approximately 10 times as common in females as in males. Calcification also occurs in the soft tissues around the iliac crests, alongside the spine between the vertebrae, around the knees, on the dorsa of the feet and around the elbows. Occasionally, ulceration of superficial nodules occurs, with discharge of chalky material. Deposits tend to be of considerable size and less diffuse than the calcification seen in the muscles of healed dermatomyositis. Calcification may occur in the internal organs. A suggestion that warfarin may inhibit and reverse calcification requires confirmation [3].

References

1 Weber H. Case presentation. *Korrephl Schweizer Aerzte* 1878; **8**: 623.

2 Thibierge G, Weissenbach R. Concretions calcaires sous-cutanées et sclerodermie. *Ann Dermatol Syphilol* 1911; **2**: 129.

3 Moore SE, Jump AA, Smiley JD. Effect of warfarin sodium therapy on excretion of 4-carboxy-l-glutamic acid in scleroderma, dermatomyositis, and myositis ossificans progressiva. *Arthritis Rheum* 1986; **29**: 344–51.

Bone changes. Absorption of the terminal phalanges is a feature of both systemic sclerosis and Raynaud's phenomenon, but systemic sclerosis is the only condition in which phalangeal absorption is associated with calcinosis (Fig. 51.68) [1]. Approximately 70% of patients show absorption, which may be minimal and only involve one terminal phalanx, or be gross and involve several phalanges, including the middle or even proximal phalanges. An erosive arthropathy, with 'pestle and mortar' deformity of the distal interphalangeal joints, resembles that seen in psoriatic arthropathy [2]. It must also be distinguished from gouty arthritis [3]. Pain in the temporomandibular area and a grinding sensation on chewing may be associated with bone resorption of the angle of the mandible [4] and zygomatic arches [5]. Other bone changes in systemic sclerosis include an increased intraosseous deposition

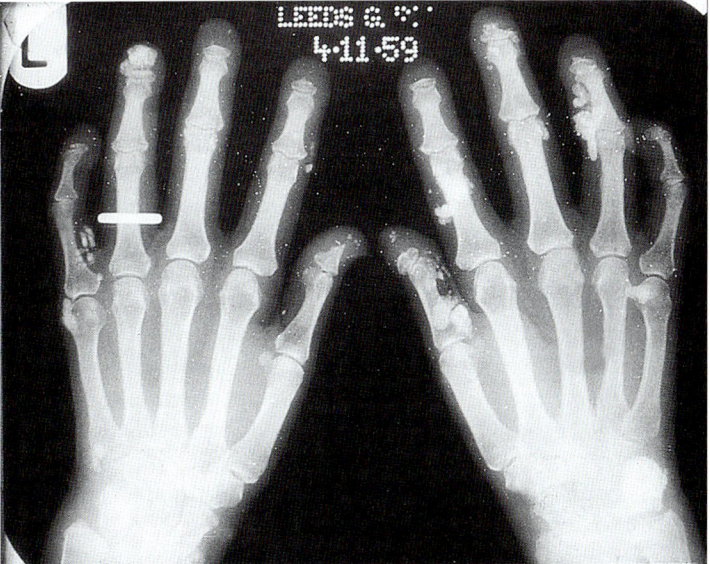

Fig. 51.68 Systemic sclerosis: terminal absorption of the phalanges and calcinosis.

of calcium [6,7] and osteopoikilosis, a rare condition in which multiple small islands of dense bone occur at the epiphyses and metaphyses [8–10]. Osteolysis also occurs in the distal end of the radius and ulna, humerus [11], acromioclavicular joint, ribs and cervical spine [12]. Avascular necrosis of the head of the femur, presumably resulting from vasculitis, has been described [13,14].

References

1 Yune HY, Vix VA, Klatte EC. Early fingertip changes in scleroderma. *JAMA* 1971; **215**: 1113–6.
2 Wild W, Beetham WP. Erosive arthropathy in systemic scleroderma. *JAMA* 1975; **232**: 511–2.
3 Durback MA, Schumacher HR Jr. Acute gouty arthritis in four patients with systemic sclerosis. *J Rheumatol* 1988; **15**: 1503–5.
4 Seifert MH, Steigerwald JC, Cliff MM. Bone resorption of the mandible in progressive systemic sclerosis. *Arthritis Rheum* 1975; **18**: 507–12.
5 Ryatt KS, Hopper FE, Cotterill JA. Mandibular resorption in systemic sclerosis. *Br J Dermatol* 1982; **107**: 711–4.
6 Edeiken L. Scleroderma with sclerodactylia. *Am J Roentgenol* 1929; **22**: 42–4.
7 Podkaminsky NA. Acrosclerosis hyperplastica intraossea. *Am J Roentgenol* 1937; **38**: 889–92.
8 von Bernuthe F. Über Sklerodermie, Osteopoikilie und Kalkgicht im Kindesalter. *Z Kinderheilk* 1932; **54**: 103–16.
9 Tuffanelli DL, Winkelmann RK. Systemic scleroderma. *Arch Dermatol* 1961; **84**: 359–71.
10 Weissman C. Scleroderma associated with osteopoikilosis. *Arch Intern Med* 1958; **101**: 108–13.
11 Khonstanteen I, Wright B, Russell ML. Localized bone resorption in systemic sclerosis. *J Rheumatol* 1988; **15**: 1435–7.
12 Haverbush TJ, Wilde AH, Hawk WA *et al.* Osteolysis of the ribs and cervical spine in progressive systemic sclerosis (scleroderma). *J Bone Joint Surg Am* 1974; **56**: 637–40.
13 Taccari E, Spadaro A, Riccieri V *et al.* Avascular necrosis of the femoral head in long-term follow-up of systemic sclerosis: report of two cases. *Clin Rheumatol* 1989; **8**: 386–92.
14 Wilde AH, Mankin HJ, Rodnan CP. Avascular necrosis of the femoral head in scleroderma. *Arthritis Rheum* 1970; **13**: 445–7.

Pulmonary involvement. Lung involvment predominantly represents diffuse pulmonary fibrosis associated with diffuse disease or pulmonary hypertension, which is more associated with limited disease or CREST syndrome [1]. Symptoms may only develop some time after the lung disease, so they are a poor predictor of lung involvement. Dyspnoea on exertion is usually the first symptom, and this may progress until the patient is distressed even at rest. Cough, usually without sputum, is also a common symptom, and may be troublesome at night, suggesting aspiration; haemoptysis is rare. Cyanosis and occasionally finger clubbing may occur in patients with severe involvement, and these signs may indicate cor pulmonale. Recurrent episodes of pneumothorax, pleurisy, pulmonary effusion and pneumonia are less common features. Considerable loss of weight may also be a prominent feature at this stage. The earliest change consists of diffuse reticular shadowing extending from the cardiac borders to the peripheral and basal parts of the lungs, usually in the lower lung fields. Sometimes, nodular changes are seen, and occasionally the apices are involved (Fig. 51.69). Cystic changes are frequent. The cysts are usually small, but if extensive the appearances are those of 'honeycomb lung'. Pneumothorax may occur [2]. Pulmonary calcification has rarely been reported [3,4], as has telangiectasia [5].

Pulmonary function is frequently abnormal when radiology shows no abnormality [6]. A sensitive test of pulmonary function

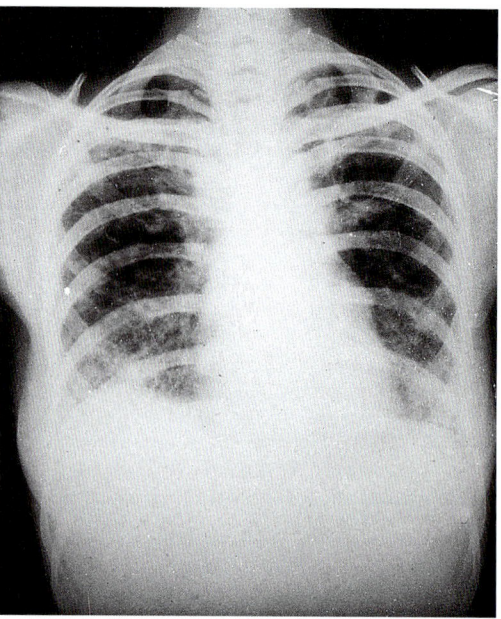

Fig. 51.69 Pulmonary involvement in systemic sclerosis: nodules are prominent, particularly in the upper zones, and there is some reticulation in the lower zones.

is the estimation of diffusing capacity (transfer factor); this test is impaired in 75% of patients. The DL_{co} may give an indication of survival; if it is less than 40% there is a 10% 5-year survival, compared with 75% if it is greater than 40%. Pulmonary involvement is more frequent in more severe and rapidly progressing disease, especially in males [7], but occurs in the CREST syndrome [8], and may precede cutaneous changes [9]. The presence of antihistone and antitopoisomerase (Scl-70) are associated with pulmonary fibrosis [10]. Small airway disease may precede measurable impairment of gas diffusion [11]. In severely affected cases, the vital capacity and maximum breathing capacity are both abnormal. Serial observations of pulmonary function may be helpful [12]. Pulmonary hypertension, sometimes severe, can occur, and does not necessarily correlate with tests of pulmonary function [1]. It is not yet possible to say whether impairment of pulmonary diffusion is caused by vascular changes or thickening of the alveolar wall and interstitial tissue. Pulmonary hypertension tends to be progressive and fatal, although new therapeutic options are available. Lung radiography may be normal in the face of symptoms and abnormal lung function, so the investigation of choice for pulmonary fibrosis is high-resolution CT scan, which is non-invasive. One series showed that high-resolution CT was 24% more accurate than radiography in demonstrating minimal evidence of fibrosing alveolitis [13]. The role of bronchoalveolar lavage is still debatable, but in expert centres it may provide additional information.

References

1 Antoniou KM, Wells AU. Scleroderma lung disease: evolving understanding in light of newer studies. *Curr Opin Rheumatol* 2008; **20**: 686–91.
2 Lang B, Ortleib H, Meske S *et al.* Progressive systemic sclerosis presenting with spontaneous pneumothorax. *J Rheumatol* 1989; **16**: 254–6.
3 Puddu V. Un caso di sclerodermia con calcificazioni operato di paratiroidectomia. *Policlinico* 1934; **41**: 1801–7.

4 Ravault PP, Moulin G, Moinex R. Apropos of a case of multiple pulmonary calcifications during scleroderma. *Lyon Med* 1960; **92**: 425–34.

5 Newman ED, Harrington TM, Amoroso A. Haemoptysis secondary to respiratory tract telangiectasia in CREST syndrome. *J Rheumatol* 1988; **15**: 1874–5.

6 Steen VD, Graham G, Conte C *et al.* Isolated diffusing capacity reduction in systemic sclerosis. *Arthritis Rheum* 1992; **35**: 765–70.

7 König G, Luderschmidt C, Hammer C *et al.* Lung involvement in scleroderma. *Chest* 1984; **85**: 318–24.

8 Steen VD, Owens CR, Fino CJ *et al.* Pulmonary involvement in systemic sclerosis (scleroderma). *Arthritis Rheum* 1985; **28**: 759–67.

9 Lomeo RM, Cornella RJ, Schabel SI *et al.* Progressive systemic sclerosis sine scleroderma presenting as pulmonary interstitial fibrosis. *Am J Med* 1989; **87**: 525–7.

10 Sato S, Ihn H, Kikuchi K *et al.* Antihistone antibodies in systemic sclerosis. *Arthritis Rheum* 1994; **37**: 391–4.

11 Guttadauria M, Ellman H, Emmanuel IG *et al.* Pulmonary function in scleroderma. *Arthritis Rheum* 1977; **20**: 1071–9.

12 Schneider PD, Wise RA, Hochberg MC *et al.* Serial pulmonary function in systemic sclerosis. *Am J Med* 1982; **73**: 385–94.

13 Strickland B, Strickland NH. The value of high definition, narrow section computed tomography in fibrosing alveolitis. *Clin Radiol* 1988; **39**: 589–94.

Involvement of the gastrointestinal tract [1].

Macroglossia may occur. The oesophagus is involved in approximately 75% of all patients and is the most frequent part of the gastrointestinal tract to be affected. Oesophageal manometry and radionuclide transit are better than radiography for showing motor abnormalities [2,3], although the changes are non-specific [4]. Although dysphagia is usually regarded as being the predominant symptom, this is not correct, as symptoms of oesophageal reflux are twice as common. The typical radiological appearance is that of an atonic dilated oesophagus, which contains air in the resting state (Fig. 51.70).

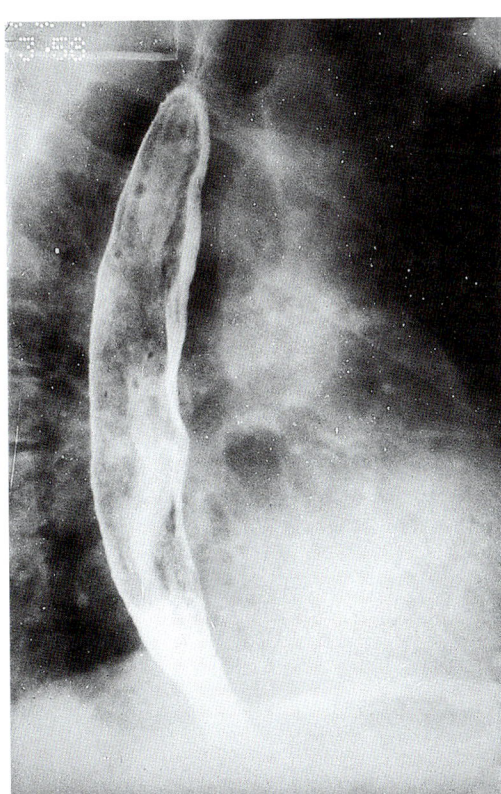

Fig. 51.70 The typical atonic, dilated, air-containing oesophagus in systemic sclerosis.

Oesophageal dilatation and abnormal peristalsis do not necessarily occur together. Stricture of the lower end of the oesophagus occurs in just over 10% of patients, is not necessarily related to gastro-oesophageal reflux or hernia, and can occur without any symptoms of dysphagia. Dysphagia is much more commonly the result of loss of propulsive activity in the oesophagus, and may occasionally be related to candidal overgrowth [5]. Hiatus hernia occurs in approximately 25% of patients. It is important to remember that approximately four out of every 10 patients with radiological changes have no symptoms. Carcinoma of the oesophagus has been reported [6,7]. Occasionally, dysphagia may be localized to the neck because of thickening of the pharyngo-oesophageal muscles [8].

Oesophageal aperistalsis has been reported in SLE and Raynaud's syndrome [9,10], but whenever aperistalsis is found systemic sclerosis must be suspected. Diffuse spasm may be detected by oesophageal manometry in approximately 5% of patients with systemic sclerosis [11].

The stomach shows dilatation and lack of peristalsis in approximately 6% of cases. Involvement of the stomach may be more common in Asians [12]. Carcinoma of the stomach has been reported [13]. Bleeding can occur from telangiectasia in all parts of the gastrointestinal tract, especially the stomach [14]. Systemic sclerosis is one cause of gastric antral vascular ectasia—the so-called 'watermelon stomach', because of the striped appearance on endoscopy. Gastric bleeding may occur at any time and may precede other signs of systemic sclerosis [15].

The duodenum shows changes of dilatation and lack of peristalsis in approximately one-third of patients. This does not appear to be a result of excess collagen deposition [16]. The changes are most pronounced in the second and third parts. Duodenal ulceration has been reported, but is probably not significant in comparison with its incidence in the normal population.

Intestinal involvement is infrequently noted in patients who have no relevant symptoms, but colicky abdominal pain and abdominal distension, with a pattern of distended loops visible through the abdominal wall, together with diarrhoea or, alternatively, constipation, may lead to a clinical diagnosis of obstruction, and death may follow from paralytic ileus. Volvulus of the small intestine may occur [17]. There may be bleeding from telangiectases. Radiological changes consist of dilated loops of bowel, with impairment of peristalsis and segments of normal or narrowed intestine. Strictures are rare. Jejunal sacculation has been reported [18,19]. Radiological changes occurred in approximately 10% of patients in the Leeds series, but others [20] found changes in 57%. Intestinal motility studies may be useful in determining changes in the small bowel [21]. If the abdomen is opened, distended loops of bowel may be seen showing a blue-grey serosal surface with numerous dilated lacteals. Small intestine involvement, determined by jejunal biopsy, small bowel radiology and tests for bacterial overgrowth and malabsorption, occurs in 55% of patients [18].

Steatorrhoea, malabsorption of glucose, calcium, vitamin B_{12} and folic acid may occasionally occur. It is important to remember that malabsorption of one or more of these substances may occur in the presence of normal fat absorption. Osteomalacia or skin changes have not been seen as the result of malabsorption.

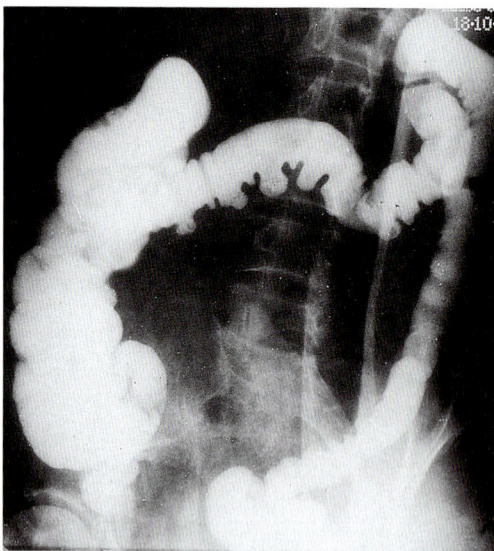

Fig. 51.71 Wide-mouthed diverticula of the colon in systemic sclerosis.

Excessive enteric loss of protein is sometimes a feature [22]. There is evidence [18] that bacterial overgrowth in the intestinal lumen as a result of stagnation because of abnormal peristalsis is a major cause of malabsorption in systemic sclerosis, and this may be corrected by therapy with tetracycline. Intestinal permeability is normal [23]. Pancreatic function is abnormal in 15% of cases [24], and death may occur from pancreatic necrosis [25].

Pneumatosis cystoides intestinalis may complicate small intestine involvement [26]. Patients present with recurrent acute or subacute intestinal obstruction [27] and rupture of cysts can cause pneumoperitoneum [28]. Treatment with respiration of high concentrations of oxygen has been successful [29].

The colon is frequently involved. In the Leeds series it occurred in 43% of cases. The patients may complain of constipation or diarrhoea. The most striking radiological change is the presence of wide-mouthed diverticula, best demonstrated on post-evacuation roentgenograms (Fig. 51.71). They usually occur on the inferior surface of the transverse colon and in the descending colon, which may be dilated and atonic; occasionally, the appearance may resemble that of ulcerative colitis [30]. Perforation of colonic diverticula may result in death from peritonitis [31]. Volvulus has been reported [32]. Colonic telangiectasia with consequent iron-deficiency anaemia may occur [33]. The mucosa of the colon has been described as being pale, dry and rather rigid on sigmoidoscopy [34], but this must be very uncommon. Anorectal pressure measurements show abnormal motility in 74% of patients [35]; symptoms are very much less common. Rectal prolapse and faecal incontinence may result. Primary exudative ascites has been reported [36].

References

1 Marie I. Gastrointestinal involvement in systemic sclerosis. *Presse Med* 2006; **35**: 1952–65.

2 Davidson A, Russell C, Littlejohn CO. Assessment of oesophageal abnormalities in progressive systemic sclerosis using radionuclide transit. *J Rheumatol* 1985; **12**: 472–7.

3 Weihrauch TR, Korting CW. Manometric assessment of oesophageal involvement in progressive systemic sclerosis, morphoea and Raynaud's disease. *Br J Dermatol* 1982; **107**: 325–32.

4 Schneider HA, Yonker RA, Longley S *et al.* Scleroderma oesophagus: a non-specific entity. *Ann Intern Med* 1984; **100**: 848–50.

5 Geirsson AJ, Akesson A, Gustafson T *et al.* Cineradiography identifies oesophageal candidiasis in progressive systemic sclerosis. *Clin Exp Rheumatol* 1989; **7**: 43–6.

6 Kilton L, Gottlieb JA. Scleroderma and carcinoma of the oesophagus. *Lancet* 1971; **ii**: 707.

7 Segel MC, Campbell WL, Medsger TAJR *et al.* Systemic sclerosis (scleroderma) and esophageal adenocarcinoma: is increased patient screening necessary? *Gastroenterology* 1985; **89**: 485–8.

8 Rajapakse CNA, Bancewicz J, Jones CJP *et al.* Pharyngo-oesophageal dysphagia in systemic sclerosis. *Ann Rheum Dis* 1981; **40**: 612–4.

9 Ramirez-Mata M, Reyes P, Alarcón-Segovia D *et al.* Oesophageal motility in systemic lupus erythematosus. *Am J Dig Dis* 1974; **19**: 132–6.

10 Stevens MB, Hookman P, Siegel CI *et al.* Aperistalsis disorders and Raynaud's phenomenon. *N Engl J Med* 1964; **270**: 1218–22.

11 Garrett JM, Winkelmann RH, Schlegel JF *et al.* Oesophageal deterioration in scleroderma. *Mayo Clin Proc* 1971; **46**: 92–6.

12 Tay CH, Khoo OT. Progressive systemic sclerosis (scleroderma). *Aust Ann Med* 1970; **2**: 145–50.

13 Rogé J, Delavierre P, Durand H *et al.* Sclérodermie et cancer d'estomac. *Semin Hôp Paris* 1971; **47**: 1211–3.

14 Rosekrans PCM, de Rooy DJ, Bosman FT *et al.* Gastrointestinal telangiectasia as a cause of severe blood loss in systemic sclerosis. *Endoscopy* 1980; **12**: 200–4.

15 Carbone LD, McKown KM, St Hilaire RJ *et al.* Scleroderma and the watermelon stomach. *Ann Rheum Dis* 1996; **55**: 560–1.

16 Hendel L, Ammitzbooll T, Dirksen K *et al.* Collagen components in the duodenal and rectal mucosa in progressive systemic sclerosis and other disease. *Acta Derm Venereol (Stockh)* 1986; **66**: 220–4.

17 Hendy MS, Torrance HB, Warnes TW. Small-bowel volvulus in association with progressive systemic sclerosis. *BMJ* 1979; **i**: 1051–2.

18 Cobden I, Axon ATR, Choneim AT *et al.* Small intestinal bacterial overgrowth in systemic sclerosis. *Clin Exp Dermatol* 1980; **5**: 37–42.

19 Queloz IM, Woloshin JH. Sacculation of the small intestine in scleroderma. *Radiology* 1972; **105**: 513–5.

20 Bluestone R, MacMahon M, Dawson JM. Systemic sclerosis and small bowel involvement. *Gut* 1969; **10**: 185–93.

21 Treacy WL, Bunting WL, Gambill EE *et al.* Scleroderma presenting as obstruction of the small bowel. *Proc Staff Meetings Mayo Clin* 1962; **37**: 607–16.

22 Greenberger NJ, Dobbins WO, Ruppert RD *et al.* Intestinal atony in progressive systemic sclerosis (scleroderma). *Am J Med* 1968; **45**: 301–8.

23 Cobden I, Rothwell J, Axon ATR *et al.* Small intestinal structure and passive permeability in systemic sclerosis. *Gut* 1980; **21**: 293–8.

24 Cobden I, Axon ATR, Rowell NR. Pancreatic exocrine function in systemic sclerosis. *Br J Dermatol* 1981; **105**: 189–93.

25 Abraham AA, Joos A. Pancreatic necrosis in progressive systemic sclerosis. *Ann Rheum Dis* 1980; **39**: 396–8.

26 Quiroz ES, Flannery MT, Martinez EJ, Warner EA. Pneumatosis cystoides intestinalis in progressive systemic sclerosis. *Am J Med Sci* 1995; **310**: 252–5.

27 Williamson DM, Bell LC. Pneumatosis cystoides intestinalis in systemic sclerosis. *Br J Dermatol* 1976; **94**: 85–8.

28 Meihoff WE, Hirschfield JS, Kem F. Small intestinal scleroderma with malabsorption and pneumatosis cystoides intestinalis. *JAMA* 1968; **204**: 854–8.

29 Watson RDS. Successful treatment of pneumatosis coli with oxygen. *BMJ* 1976; **i**: 199.

30 Wallace HJ. Ulcerative colitis, systemic sclerosis and necrobiosis. *Br J Dermatol* 1974; **91** (Suppl. 10): 45–6.

31 Robinson JC, Teitelbaum SL. Stercoral ulceration and perforation of the sclerodermatous colon: report of two cases and review of the literature. *Dis Col Rectum* 1974; **17**: 622–32.

32 Budd DC, Nirdlinger EL, Sturtz DL *et al.* Transverse colon volvulus associated with scleroderma. *Am J Surg* 1977; **113**: 370–2.

33 Baron M, Srolovitz H. Colonic telangiectasias in a patient with progressive systemic sclerosis. *Arthritis Rheum* 1986; **29**: 282–5.

34 Cullinan ER. Discussion on scleroderma. *Proc R Soc Med* 1953; **46**: 507–11.

35 Hamel-Roy J, Devroede C, Arhan P *et al.* Comparative oesophageal and anorectal motility in scleroderma. *Gastroenterology* 1985; **88**: 1–7.
36 Todd DJ, McMillan C. Primary exudative ascites in systemic sclerosis. *Int J Dermatol* 1992; **31**: 451–2.

Hepatic involvement. The liver is usually normal in systemic sclerosis, although cirrhosis and portal hypertension are occasionally found. It is by no means substantiated that such fibrosis is caused by systemic sclerosis. Bleeding from oesophageal varices may occur [1]. Systemic sclerosis has been reported in 17% of patients with primary biliary cirrhosis [2,3]. Ascites can occur without liver disease [4].

References
1 Calvert RJ, Barling B, Sopher M *et al.* Systemic scleroderma with portal hypertension. *BMJ* 1958; **i**: 22–5.
2 Clarke AK, Galbraith RM, Hamilton EBD *et al.* Rheumatic disorders in primary biliary cirrhosis. *Ann Rheum Dis* 1978; **37**: 42–7.
3 Reynolds TB, Denison EK, Frankl HD *et al.* Primary biliary cirrhosis with scleroderma, Raynaud's phenomenon and telangiectasia. *Am J Med* 1971; **50**: 302–12.
4 Quagliata F, Sebes J, Pinstein ML *et al.* Long bone erosions and ascites in progressive systemic sclerosis (scleroderma). *J Rheumatol* 1982; **9**: 641–4.

Cardiac involvement [1,2]. The resting ECG is abnormal in approximately 50% of cases, and cold-induced changes also occur [3]; however, the changes may be the result of other causes. Abnormalities of rhythm occur and these include paroxysmal atrial tachycardia, atrial fibrillation and flutter. Partial or complete heart block is not uncommon. In addition to abnormalities of rhythm, ECG may show bifid P waves and T-wave changes, indicating atrial or ventricular myocardial involvement. The conduction system seems to be relatively spared in systemic sclerosis and the high incidence of conduction disturbances may be the consequence of damage to the working myocardium [4]. Dyspnoea may be present but pain in the chest is not a prominent feature. Pericardial involvement occurs and is usually asymptomatic [5]. Mitral valve prolapse occurs more frequently in a number of connective tissue diseases, including systemic sclerosis, than in normal controls [6]. Other valvular abnormalities are rare [7]. Coronary reserve is reduced [8]. General enlargement of the heart, left-ventricular hypertrophy or a triangular outline are the most frequent radiological abnormalities. Radionuclide scanning [9], echocardiography [10], and 24-h ECG monitoring [11] are useful in the detection of abnormalities of the myocardium. More recently, studies using novel imaging technology including CT and magnetic resonance imaging (MRI) have demonstrated evidence of cardiac fibrosis [12].

References
1 Buckley BH. Progressive systemic sclerosis: cardiac involvement. *Clin Rheum Dis* 1979; **5**: 131–49.
2 Oram S, Stokes W. The heart in scleroderma. *Br Heart J* 1961; **23**: 243–59.
3 Gustafsson R, Kazzam E, Mannting F *et al.* Cold-induced reversible myocardial ischaemia in systemic sclerosis. *Lancet* 1989; **i**: 475–9.
4 Ridolfi RL, Bulkley BH, Hutchins CM. The cardiac conduction system in progressive systemic sclerosis. *Am J Med* 1976; **61**: 361–6.
5 Byers RJ, Marshall DAS, Freemont AJ. Pericardial involvement in systemic sclerosis. *Ann Rheum Dis* 1997; **56**: 393–4.
6 Comens SM, Alpert MA, Sharp GC *et al.* Frequency of mitral valve prolapse in systemic lupus erythematosus, progressive systemic sclerosis and mixed connective tissue disease. *Am J Cardiol* 1989; **63**: 369–70.
7 Yunus MB, Radford CM, Masi AT *et al.* Aortic regurgitation in scleroderma. *J Rheumatol* 1984; **11**: 384–6.
8 Kahan A, Nitenberg A, Foult JM *et al.* Decreased coronary reserve in primary scleroderma myocardial disease. *Arthritis Rheum* 1985; **28**: 637–46.
9 Ellis WW, Baer AN, Robertson RM *et al.* Left ventricular dysfunction induced by cold exposure in patients with systemic sclerosis. *Am J Med* 1986; **80**: 385–92.
10 Ferri C, Bernini L, Bongiorni MC *et al.* Non-invasive evaluation of cardiac dysrhythmias, and their relationship with multisystemic symptoms, in progressive systemic sclerosis patients. *Arthritis Rheum* 1985; **28**: 1259–66.
11 Geirsson AJ, Blom-Bulow B, Pahlm O *et al.* Cardiac involvement in systemic sclerosis. *Semin Arthritis Rheum* 1989; **19**: 110–6.
12 Hachulla AL, Launay D, Gaxotte V *et al.* Cardiac magnetic resonance imaging in systemic sclerosis: a cross-sectional observational study of 52 patients. *Ann Rheum Dis* 2009; **68**: 1878–84.

Renal involvement. Pathological changes in the kidney used to lead frequently to serious clinical problems, but the management of hypertension, and in particular the introduction of modern drugs such as inhibitors of angiotensin-converting enzyme (ACE), have revolutionized this aspect of the disease. Slight proteinuria is considered to be the most common clinical feature, often early in the disease. Proteinuria occurred in 36%, hypertension in 24%, azotaemia in 19% and malignant hypertension in 7% of one series [1]. One or more markers were found in 45% of patients. Approximately 40% of patients show disturbances of creatinine clearance. Nephrotic syndrome is increasingly rare [2]. Approximately 8% of patients with renal involvement develop malignant hypertension [3]. This may develop rapidly in the course of a few weeks, with headaches, nausea, vomiting and deterioration of vision in a patient whose renal function has previously been normal. Prior to 1971, survival beyond 1 year was unusual, the usual survival being 1–3 months. The prognosis, even with renal crisis, has improved dramatically since the introduction of ACE inhibitors (see p. 51.108). Although renal involvement has an adverse effect on survival in systemic sclerosis, patients with mild impairment of renal function may live for years.

References
1 Cannon PJ, Hassar M, Case DB *et al.* The relationship of hypertension and renal failure in scleroderma (progressive systemic sclerosis) to structural and functional abnormalities in the renal cortical circulation. *Medicine* 1974; **53**: 1–46.
2 Palma A, Sanchez-Palencia A, Armas JR *et al.* Progressive systemic sclerosis and nephrotic syndrome. *Arch Intern Med* 1981; **141**: 520–1.
3 Steen VD, Medsger TA Jr. Long-term outcomes of scleroderma renal crisis. *Ann Intern Med* 2000; **133**: 600–3.

Muscle involvement [1,2]. Muscle weakness may occur, and differentiation from dermatomyositis may be difficult, especially if there is a heliotrope appearance and oedema of the eyelids, and dilatation of the nail fold capillaries. In one series [3], the two diseases could not be distinguished in 36 of 727 patients. Muscles of the forearms and hands are affected as well as the proximal muscles. Creatine phosphokinase elevation and excessive creatinuria correlate well with muscle weakness. Electromyography is abnormal in 50% of patients early in the disease and in 93% in late stages [4], and histological changes are present in approximately 40%. MRI and spectroscopy can be useful non-invasive monitors of disease activity [5]. There does not appear to be any evidence that systemic sclerosis occurs as a cutaneous marker of internal malignancy, although carcinoma of the lung may develop in patients with pulmonary involvement [6].

Tendon involvement. Leathery, palpable and audible friction rubs occur over the limbs and tendons [7] in approximately 25% of cases. Rupture of the extensor tendons of the hand has been reported [8]. The tendon was infiltrated with amyloid.

References

1 Clements PJ, Furst DE, Campions DS *et al.* Muscle disease in progressive systemic sclerosis. *Arthritis Rheum* 1978; **21**: 62–71.
2 Medsger TA, Rodnan GP, Moossy J *et al.* Skeletal muscle involvement in progressive systemic sclerosis (scleroderma). *Arthritis Rheum* 1968; **11**: 554–68.
3 Tuffanelli DL, Winkelmann RK. Scleroderma and its relationship to the 'collagenoses': dermatomyositis, lupus erythematosus, rheumatoid arthritis and Sjögren's syndrome. *Am J Med Sci* 1962; **243**: 133–46.
4 Hausmanowa-Petrusewicz L, Jablonska S, Blaszczyk M *et al.* Electro-myographic findings in various forms of progressive systemic sclerosis. *Arthritis Rheum* 1982; **25**: 61–5.
5 King LE, Olsen NJ, Vital TL, Park JH. Quantitative evaluation of muscle weakness in scleroderma patients using magnetic resonance imaging and spectroscopy. *Arch Dermatol* 1993; **129**: 246–7.
6 Roumm AD, Medsger TA. Cancer and systemic sclerosis. *Arthritis Rheum* 1985; **28**: 1336–40.
7 Shulman LE, Kurban AK, Harvey AM. Tendon friction rubs in progressive systemic sclerosis (scleroderma). *Trans Assoc Am Physicians* 1961; **74**: 378–88.
8 Horwitz HM, DiBeneditto JD, Allegra SR *et al.* Scleroderma, amyloidosis and extensor tendon rupture. *Arthritis Rheum* 1982; **25**: 1141–3.

Joint involvement [1–3]. Arthritic pain is not uncommon in the early stages of systemic sclerosis, and sometimes rheumatoid arthritis is the initial diagnosis made. Radiological changes indistinguishable from rheumatoid arthritis occur, especially in the hands, but there are no specific changes ascribable to systemic sclerosis. They include periarticular osteoporosis, joint-space narrowing, erosions and, rarely, avascular necrosis [4], erosions of long bones [5], bone ankylosis [6] and erosive osteoarthritis.

References

1 Baron M, Lee P, Kaystone EC. The articular manifestations of progressive systemic sclerosis (scleroderma). *Ann Rheum Dis* 1982; **41**: 147–52.
2 Blocka KLN, Bassett LW, Furst DE *et al.* The arthropathy of advanced progressive systemic sclerosis. *Arthritis Rheum* 1981; **24**: 874–84.
3 Misra R, Darton K, Jeurkea RF *et al.* Arthritis in scleroderma. *Br J Rheumatol* 1995; **34**: 831–7.
4 Wilde AH, Mankin JH, Rodnan CP. Avascular necrosis of the femoral head in scleroderma. *Arthritis Rheum* 1970; **13**: 445–7.
5 Quagliata F, Sebes J, Pinstein ML *et al.* Long bone erosions and ascites in progressive systemic sclerosis (scleroderma). *J Rheumatol* 1982; **9**: 641–4.
6 Huyck CJ, Hoffman GS. Bony ankylosis of the hips in progressive systemic sclerosis. *Arthritis Rheum* 1982; **25**: 1497–500.

Dental changes (see Chapter 69) [1]. Widening of the periodontal membrane because of fibrosis, with thickening of the vessel walls, occurs in approximately 30% of cases (Fig. 51.72). Usually the whole root is involved. Anterior as well as posterior teeth are affected, and the lamina dura may or may not be abnormal. Thickening of the periodontal membrane is not related to the duration of Raynaud's phenomenon, calcinosis, involvement of internal organs, antinuclear factor or prognosis. Thickening of the periodontal membrane is not diagnostic of systemic sclerosis and is also found in periapical infection. Widening of the peri-

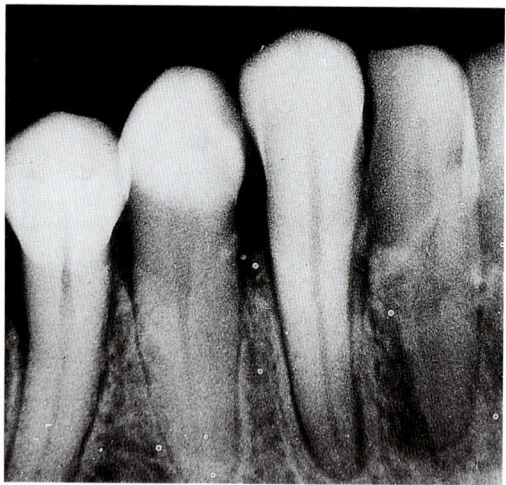

Fig. 51.72 Widening of the periodontal membrane in systemic sclerosis.

odontal membrane in only one tooth is usually a result of such infection.

Osteolysis of the mandibular angle and coronoid process occurs with equal frequency [2], and these osteolytic areas may fracture [3]. A patient who had multiple external and internal root resorptions for which all the teeth were removed was successfully treated with osseointegrated implants [4].

References

1 Rowell NR, Hopper FE. The periodontal membrane in systemic sclerosis. *Br J Dermatol* 1977; **96**: 15–20.
2 White SC, Frey NW, Blaschke DD *et al.* Oral radiographic changes in patients with progressive systemic sclerosis (scleroderma). *J Am Dent Assoc* 1977; **94**: 1178–82.
3 Weber DD, Blunt MH, Caldwell JB *et al.* Fracture of mandibular rami complicated by scleroderma: report of case. *J Oral Surg* 1970; **28**: 860–3.
4 Jensen J, Sindet-Pedersen S. Osseointegrated implants for prosthetic reconstruction in a patient with scleroderma: report of a case. *J Oral Maxillofac Surg* 1990; **48**: 739–41.

Central nervous system [1,2]. The nervous system is involved in fewer than 10% of cases [3], although asymptomatic involvement may be more common [4], and others have found involvement in 40% of patients, which can be associated with ulceration of the skin [5]. Neuropathy has been reported [6,7]: autonomic neuropathy may not be uncommon [8,9]; trigeminal neuropathy presents with numbness and pain in the face [10], and occurs in 4% of patients [11]. Of 22 cases with chronic trigeminal sensory neuropathy, nine had systemic sclerosis [12]. It is unilateral at first but later becomes bilateral. Other cranial nerves may be involved [13]. Carpal tunnel syndrome and meralgia paraesthetica may occur. Local anaesthetics may have an abnormally prolonged action [1]. Subacute combined degeneration is the result of vitamin B_{12} deficiency caused by malabsorption secondary to involvement of the small intestine by systemic sclerosis [14]. Spinal cord compression may occur because of soft-tissue calcification [15]. The EEG is not specific. Sensory chronaxia is prolonged in both abnormal and normal skin. Such prolongation in normal skin does not occur in any other condition apart from tabes dorsalis [16]. Impotence has been reported as an initial manifestation of the disease [17,18].

References

1 Berth-Jones J, Coates PAA, Graham-Brown RAC *et al.* Neurological complications of systemic sclerosis: a report of three cases and review of the literature. *Clin Exp Dermatol* 1990; **15**: 91–4.

2 Gordon RM, Silverstein A. Neurologic manifestations in progressive systemic sclerosis. *Arch Neurol* 1970; **22**: 126–34.

3 Lee P, Bruni J, Sukenik S. Neurological manifestations in systemic sclerosis (scleroderma). *J Rheumatol* 1984; **11**: 480–3.

4 Dierckx RA, Aichner F, Gerstenbrand F *et al.* Progressive systemic sclerosis and nervous system involvement. *Eur Neurol* 1987; **26**: 134–40.

5 Averbuch-Heller L, Steiner I, Abramsky O. Neurological manifestations of progressive systemic sclerosis. *Arch Neurol* 1992; **49**: 1292–5.

6 Hagberg B, Leonhardt T, Skogh M. Familial occurrence of collagen diseases. *Acta Med Scand* 1961; **169**: 727–34.

7 Rodnan CP. The natural history of progressive systemic sclerosis (diffuse scleroderma). *Bull Rheum Dis* 1963; **13**: 301–4.

8 Klimiuk PS, Taylor L, Baker RD *et al.* Autonomic neuropathy in systemic sclerosis. *Ann Rheum Dis* 1988; **47**: 542–5.

9 Sonnex C, Paice E, White AC. Autonomic neuropathy in systemic sclerosis: a case report and evaluation of six patients. *Ann Rheum Dis* 1986; **45**: 957–60.

10 Ashworth B, Tait CBW. Trigeminal neuropathy in connective tissue disease. *Neurology* 1971; **21**: 609–14.

11 Farrell DA, Medsger TA Jr. Trigeminal neuropathy in progressive systemic sclerosis. *Am J Med* 1982; **73**: 57–62.

12 Lecky BRF, Hughes RAC, Murray NMF. Trigeminal sensory neuropathy. *Brain* 1987; **110**: 1463–85.

13 Teasdall RD, Frayha RA, Shulman LE. Cranial nerve involvement in systemic sclerosis (scleroderma). *Medicine* 1980; **59**: 149–59.

14 Bjerregaard B, Hojgaard K. Neurological symptoms in scleroderma. *Arch Dermatol* 1976; **112**: 1030–1.

15 Petrocelli AR, Bassett LW, Mirra J *et al.* Scleroderma: dystrophic calcification with spinal cord compression. *J Rheumatol* 1988; **15**: 1733–5.

16 Jablonska S. Measurement of sensory chronaxie as a diagnostic procedure in scleroderma. *Br J Dermatol* 1975; **92**: 223–7.

17 Lally EV, Jimenez SA. Impotence in progressive systemic sclerosis. *Ann Intern Med* 1981; **95**: 150–3.

18 Sukenik S, Horowitz J, Busilka D *et al.* Impotence in systemic sclerosis. *Ann Intern Med* 1987; **106**: 910–1.

Eye changes. Tightness of the lids, diminished tear secretion, keratoconjunctivitis sicca and shallow fornices are specific ophthalmic changes [1]. Sjögren's syndrome occurs in 15% of cases. Retinopathy, with haemorrhages, exudates and cytoid bodies may occur with a relatively low blood pressure, and has been attributed to direct vascular involvement by systemic sclerosis [2]. Fluorescein angiography shows vascular abnormalities in the choroid in 50% and in the retina in 10% of patients [3]. Central retinal vein occlusion has been reported [4].

References

1 Horan EC. Ophthalmic manifestations of progressive systemic sclerosis. *Br J Ophthalmol* 1969; **53**: 388–92.

2 Ashton N, Coomes EN, Carner A *et al.* Retinopathy due to progressive systemic sclerosis. *J Pathol Bacteriol* 1968; **96**: 259–68.

3 Grennan DM, Forrester I. Involvement of the eye in SLE and scleroderma. *Ann Rheum Dis* 1977; **36**: 152–6.

4 Saari KM, Rudenberg HA, Laitinen O. Bilateral central retinal vein occlusion in a patient with scleroderma. *Ophthalmologica* 1981; **182**: 7–12.

Laboratory investigations. Anaemia may be found in patients with renal failure, gastrointestinal bleeding or malabsorption. The ESR is raised in approximately half of patients, as is the serum globulin level. Elevation of gammaglobulin occurs more frequently than elevation of α_2-globulin. Other acute-phase reactants are

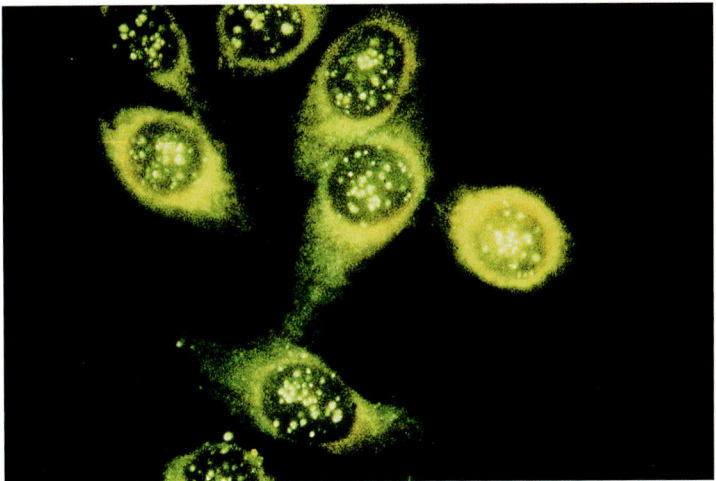

Fig. 51.73 Anticentromere antibody demonstrated on Hep-2 cells.

usually normal, although there are defects in the acute-phase response to some stimuli [1]. False-positive serology occurs in approximately 5%. Cold agglutinins may be found in 25% of cases. The Coombs' test is usually negative, although Coombs'-positive haemolytic anaemia and pancytopenia have been reported [2]. Circulating anticoagulant has been demonstrated in one case [3], but was not found in 24 patients at Leeds [4]. Anticardiolipin antibodies are found in 25% of cases overall, and occur more frequently in those severely affected [5]. Cryoglobulins are only rarely detected. Cryofibrinogenaemia has been held responsible for ulceration and gangrene of the fingers in some cases. Rheumatoid factor is present in approximately 30% of patients. Serum complement levels are usually normal. LE cells may be demonstrated in 8% of patients. Sometimes, SLE may occur in association with systemic sclerosis [6,7], but the presence of LE cells in systemic sclerosis does not necessarily imply coexistent SLE. Antinuclear antibodies have been demonstrated in 78% of patients using rat liver [8], and in 97% using Hep-2 cells [9] as substrate. Using Hep-2 cells, both speckled and homogeneous types occur, and nucleolar patterns—speckled, homogeneous and clumpy—are demonstrated more frequently than in other diseases. Centromere staining, resulting from an antibody that reacts with the kinetocore of metaphase chromosomes, occurs in 40–70% of milder (or CREST) cases [9,10] who have longer duration of disease and little renal involvement (Fig. 51.73). Anticentromere antibodies may be present in patients with Raynaud's phenomenon before the clinical features of systemic sclerosis appear. They seem to be indicative of a favourable prognosis [11]. They also occur in 6% of patients with SLE (including drug-induced lupus) [12], 6% of patients with mixed connective tissue disease, 17% of patients with primary biliary cirrhosis and systemic sclerosis [13], 11% of patients with primary biliary cirrhosis alone and 5% of patients with morphoea [14]. A diffuse 'frosted glass' staining of nuclei of Hep-2 cells is caused by Scl-70 antibody, a precipitating antibody to topoisomerase I, which is unique to systemic sclerosis and occurs in approximately 20% of patients, particularly those with lung involvement (Fig. 51.74) [10,15]. Higher frequencies are described, even in patients with acrosclerosis alone [16]. Scl-70 and anticentromere antibody occur together in 5% of cases [17], but

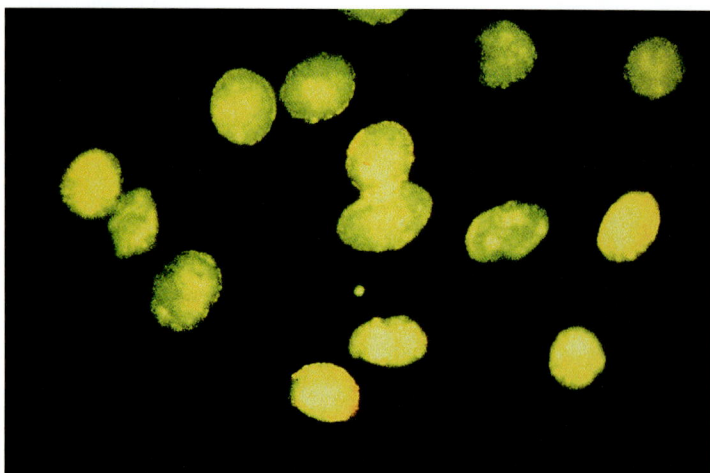

Fig. 51.74 Scl-70 antibody demonstrated on Hep-2 cells.

when occurring alone may define separate subsets of the disease. There is no relationship between Scl-70 and disease survival [18]. Scl-86 is a related antigen [19]. Other antibodies occur, presumably indicating immunological subsets, and include antibody to centriole [20,21], anti-Jo-1 [22] and anti-Ro/SS-A [23]. More intensive investigation of autoantibodies may reveal additional subsets of the disease [24]. Several patterns of nucleolar staining have been described [25]. A homogeneous pattern was associated with polymyositis/scleroderma overlap, a clumpy pattern with diffuse cutaneous systemic sclerosis and a speckled pattern with localized cutaneous systemic sclerosis. Anti-DNA antibodies are not found [26]. Anti-IgE antibodies occur [27]. Other precipitating antibodies to saline extracts of human tissue [8] may be found in 15% of patients. Anti-smooth-muscle and antiendothelial antibodies have been reported [28,29]. Antineutrophil cytoplasmic antibodies occur in 9% [30] and antihistone antibodies in 42% [31]. The latter was more frequent in patients with cardiac and renal involvement. Serum type III procollagen peptide concentrations are raised and reflect disease activity [32,33]. Urinary excretion of 5-hydroxyindole-acetic acid is normal, as is thyroid function.

References

1 Whicher JT, Bell AM, Martin MFR *et al.* Prostaglandins cause an increase in serum acute-phase proteins in man, which is diminished in systemic sclerosis. *Clin Sci* 1984; **66**: 165–71.
2 Carcassonne Y, Gastaut JA. Pancytopenia and scleroderma. *BMJ* 1976; **i**: 1446.
3 Albert J, Ekoe JM, Cunningham M *et al.* Circulating anticoagulant in CREST syndrome. *Br J Rheumatol* 1984; **23**: 20–3.
4 Rowell NR, Tate GM. Failure to demonstrate the lupus anticoagulant in systemic sclerosis. *Br J Dermatol* 1988; **119**: 549.
5 Malia RG, Greaves M, Rowlands LM *et al.* Anticardiolipin antibodies in systemic sclerosis: immunological and clinical associations. *Clin Exp Immunol* 1988; **73**: 456–60.
6 Dubois EL, Chandor S, Friou CJ *et al.* Progressive systemic sclerosis (PSS) and localized scleroderma (morphea) with positive LE cell test. *Medicine* 1971; **50**: 199–222.
7 Rowell NR. Lupus erythematosus cells in systemic sclerosis. *Ann Rheum Dis* 1962; **21**: 70–5.
8 Beck JS, Anderson JR, Gray KG *et al.* Antinuclear and precipitating autoantibodies in progressive systemic sclerosis. *Lancet* 1963; **ii**: 1188–90.
9 Bernstein RM, Steigerwald JC, Tan EM. Association of antinuclear and antinucleolar antibodies in progressive systemic sclerosis. *Clin Exp Immunol* 1982; **48**: 43–51.
10 Catoggio LJ, Bernstein RM, Black CM. Serological markers in progressive systemic sclerosis: clinical correlations. *Ann Rheum Dis* 1983; **42**: 23–7.
11 Miller MH, Littlejohn CO, Davidson A *et al.* The clinical significance of the anticentromere antibody. *Br J Rheumatol* 1987; **26**: 17–21.
12 Wade JP, Sack B, Schur PH. Anticentromere antibodies: clinical correlates. *J Rheumatol* 1988; **15**: 1759–63.
13 Bernstein RM, Callender ME, Neuberger JM *et al.* Anticentromere antibody in primary biliary cirrhosis. *Ann Rheum Dis* 1982; **41**: 612–4.
14 Powell FC, Winklemann RH, Venencie-Lemarchano F *et al.* The anticentromere antibody: disease specificity and clinical significance. *Proc Mayo Clin* 1984; **59**: 700–6.
15 Shero JH, Bordwell B, Rothfield NF *et al.* Antibodies to topoisomerase 1 in sera from patients with scleroderma. *J Rheumatol* 1987; **14**: 138–40.
16 Jarzabek-Chorzelska M, Blaszczyk M, Jablonska S *et al.* Scl 70 antibody: a specific marker of systemic sclerosis. *Br J Dermatol* 1986; **115**: 393–401.
17 Jarzabek-Chorzelska M, Blaszczyk M, Kolacinska-Strasz Z *et al.* Are AcA and Scl 70 antibodies mutually exclusive? *Br J Dermatol* 1990; **122**: 201–8.
18 Steen VD, Powell DL, Medsger JR. Clinical correlations and prognosis based on serum autoantibodies in patients with systemic sclerosis. *Arthritis Rheum* 1988; **31**: 196–203.
19 Van Venrooij WJ, Stapel SO, Houben H *et al.* Scl-86, a marker antigen for diffuse scleroderma. *J Clin Invest* 1985; **75**: 1053–60.
20 Tuffanelli DL, McKeon F, Kleinsmith DM *et al.* Anticentromere and anticentriole antibodies in the scleroderma spectrum. *Arch Dermatol* 1983; **119**: 560–6.
21 Sato S, Fujimoto M, Ihn H *et al.* Antibodies to centromere and centriole in scleroderma spectrum disorders. *Dermatology* 1994; **189**: 23–6.
22 Bernstein RM, Morgan SH, Chapman J *et al.* Anti-Jo-1 antibody: a marker for myositis with interstitial lung disease. *BMJ* 1984; **289**: 151–2.
23 Bell S, Krieg T, Meurer M. Antibodies to Ro/SSA detected by ELISA: correlation with clinical features in systemic scleroderma. *Br J Dermatol* 1989; **121**: 35–41.
24 Reimer C, Steen VD, Penning CA *et al.* Correlates between autoantibodies to nucleolar antigens and clinical features in patients with systemic sclerosis (scleroderma). *Arthritis Rheum* 1988; **31**: 525–32.
25 Blaszczyk M, Jarzabek-Cawzelka M, Jablonska S *et al.* Autoantibodies to nucleolar antigens in systemic scleroderma: clinical correlations. *Br J Dermatol* 1990; **123**: 421–30.
26 Hughes GRV. Significance of anti-DNA antibodies in systemic lupus erythematosus. *Lancet* 1971; **ii**: 861–3.
27 Kaufman LD, Gruber BL, Marchese MJ *et al.* Anti-IgE autoantibodies in systemic sclerosis (scleroderma). *Ann Rheum Dis* 1989; **48**: 201–5.
28 Kitridou RC, Fleischmajer R, Lagosky P. Antismooth muscle antibody in scleroderma. *Clin Res* 1974; **22**: 703A.
29 Rosenbaum J, Pottinger BE, Woo P. Measurement and characterisation of circulating anti-endothelial cell IgG in connective tissue diseases. *Clin Exp Immunol* 1988; **72**: 450–6.
30 Akimoto S, Ishikawa O, Tamura T *et al.* Antineutrophil cytoplasmic autoantibodies in patients with systemic sclerosis. *Br J Dermatol* 1996; **134**: 407–10.
31 Parodi A, Drosera M, Barbieri L, Rebora A. Antihistone antibodies in systemic sclerosis. *Dermatology* 1995; **191**: 16–8.
32 Black CM, McWhirter A, Harrison NK *et al.* Serum type III procollagen peptide concentrations in systemic sclerosis and Raynaud's phenomenon: relationship to disease activity and duration. *Br J Rheumatol* 1989; **28**: 98–103.
33 Krieg T, Langer I, Gerstmeier H. Type III collagen aminopropeptide levels in serum of patients with progressive systemic scleroderma. *J Invest Dermatol* 1986; **87**: 788–91.

Variations. Patients with calcinosis, Raynaud's phenomenon, sclerodactyly and telangiectasia may form a separate entity known as CRST syndrome [1], or CREST syndrome if oesophageal (esophageal) involvement is included. This is unlikely to be a separate syndrome, distinct from systemic sclerosis [2]. The variability of expression and course of the authors' series of patients with systemic sclerosis suggests that this type of case is only a subgroup of systemic sclerosis. This has been confirmed by other workers [3,4]. However, the delineation of this group of patients emphasizes that the diagnosis of systemic sclerosis does not always imply such a poor prognosis as has hitherto been considered.

The suggestion that 'systemic scleroderma' should be divided into two groups—diffuse scleroderma and acrosclerosis—remains to be confirmed [5]. The former, a relatively small group, can be distinguished from acrosclerosis in that the sex distribution is equal, the age of onset is later, Raynaud's phenomenon is absent, cutaneous sclerosis is the usual presenting feature, the sclerosis of the skin is usually generalized rather than acral, and the course is more rapid and fulminating, with death in a few years. However, both types show similar visceral involvement and laboratory abnormalities, and some patients with acrosclerosis have a short course, and Raynaud's phenomenon is not invariable. Occasionally, acute diffuse scleroderma may be much more benign than expected [6]. These two groups are probably clinical variants of systemic sclerosis. A more recent attempt at subdivision of the disease into diffuse and localized forms has met with more agreement (see p. 51.91) [7].

References

1 Winterbauer RH. Multiple telangiectasia, Raynaud's phenomenon, sclerodactyly, and subcutaneous calcinosis. *Bull Johns Hopkins Hosp* 1964; **114**: 361–83.
2 Rowell NR. The prognosis of systemic sclerosis. *Br J Dermatol* 1976; **95**: 57–60.
3 Mintz C, Fraga A, Orozco JH. The CRST syndrome: a non-entity. *J Rheumatol* 1974; **1** (Suppl. 1): 95.
4 Salerni R, Rodnan CP, Leon DF *et al.* Pulmonary hypertension in the CREST syndrome variant of progressive systemic sclerosis (scleroderma). *Ann Intern Med* 1977; **86**: 394–9.
5 Tuffanelli DL, Winkelmann RK. Diffuse systemic scleroderma. *Ann Intern Med* 1962; **57**: 198–203.
6 Nynzi E, Rebora A, Cormane RH. Acute diffuse scleroderma. *Acta Derm Venereol (Stockh)* 1981; **61**: 173–6.
7 LeRoy EC, Black C, Fleischmajer R *et al.* Scleroderma (systemic sclerosis): classification subsets and pathogenesis. *J Rheumatol* 1988; **15**: 202–5.

Systemic sclerosis in childhood. Systemic sclerosis occurs in childhood, and the clinical features resemble those seen in adult cases. Raynaud's phenomenon is less frequent and renal disease is rare [1]. The course of systemic sclerosis in childhood is said to be slower, and the disability and visceral involvement less severe than in adults [2], but fatal cases have been reported [3]. The problem has been reviewed in depth [4].

References

1 Larrègue M, Cannel C, Bazex J *et al.* Scléroderme systémique de l'enfant. *Ann Dermatol Vénéréol* 1983; **110**: 317–26.
2 Jaffe MO, Winkelmann RK. Generalized scleroderma in children. *Arch Dermatol* 1961; **83**: 402–13.
3 Kass H, Hanson V, Patrick J. Scleroderma in childhood. *J Pediatr* 1966; **68**: 243–56.
4 Singsen BH. Scleroderma in childhood. *Pediatr Clin North Am* 1986; **33**: 1119–39.

Involvement of the genital tract [1]. Vaginal dryness, ulcerations and dyspareunia are significantly more frequent in patients with systemic sclerosis when compared with controls. Frequency of sexual intercourse and sexual satisfaction is decreased, and the menopause may be early.

Reference

1 Bhadauria S, Moser DK, Clements PJ *et al.* Genital tract abnormalities and female sex function impairment in systemic sclerosis. *Am J Obstet Gynecol* 1995; **172**: 580–7.

Pregnancy [1]. Systemic sclerosis usually remains unchanged during pregnancy, but postpartum renal failure and peripheral gangrene have been described [2]. Severe renal, pulmonary or cardiac disease in the mother may be an indication for termination of the pregnancy [3], and such complications may occur late in pregnancy. ACE inhibitors may be of value for hypertension in pregnancy, although there are potential risks to the fetus [4]. There is conflicting evidence regarding the incidence of abortion and stillbirth [5,6]. Fertility may be impaired.

In some cases, pregnancy seems to precipitate the disease.

References

1 Black CM. Systemic sclerosis and pregnancy. *Baillière's Clin Rheumatol* 1990; **4**: 105–24.
2 Smith CA, Pinals RS. Progressive systemic sclerosis and postpartum renal failure complicated by peripheral gangrene. *J Rheumatol* 1982; **9**: 455–8.
3 Maymon R, Fejgin M. Scleroderma in pregnancy. *Obstet Gynecol Surv* 1989; **44**: 530–4.
4 Baethge BA, Wolf RE. Successful pregnancy with scleroderma, renal disease and pulmonary hypertension in a patient using angiotensin converting enzyme inhibitors. *Ann Rheum Dis* 1989; **48**: 776–8.
5 McHugh NJ, Reilly PA, McHugh LA. Pregnancy outcome and autoantibodies in connective tissue disease. *J Rheumatol* 1989; **16**: 42–6.
6 Steen VD. Pregnancy in women with systemic sclerosis. *Obstet Gynecol* 1999; **94**: 15–20.

Associations. Sometimes, systemic sclerosis occurs in association with other conditions, particularly those considered to have some autoimmune features. Usually, it is possible to differentiate between the diseases, but occasionally there is clinical and immunological overlap. The relationship to SLE and dermatomyositis has already been mentioned. Immunohistology of involved and uninvolved skin is of value. Sjögren's syndrome, the most common features of which are dryness and atrophy of the conjunctiva, cornea and buccal mucosa, together with arthritis, occurs with systemic sclerosis in approximately 17–20% of patients [1,2], and resembles the primary form of Sjögren's syndrome [3]. Extensive investigation reveals at least one abnormal test of the sicca syndrome in all cases [4]. Salivary flow is normal, but deficient in IgA [5]. Antibodies to Ro and La are useful markers of the presence of Sjögren's syndrome in systemic sclerosis [6], occurring in 60% of cases [7]. Other muscle disorders that have been reported in association with systemic sclerosis include polymyositis [8], myasthenia gravis [9] and muscular dystrophy [10]. Pathological features of systemic sclerosis are sometimes found in patients with polyarteritis nodosa [11–13], but there is not the same clinical or immunological overlap as seen with SLE. Temporal arteritis has been reported [14,15], and the condition has also occurred with malignant atrophic papulosis (Degos' syndrome) [16], thrombophlebitis and cryofibrinogenaemia. The association with Hashimoto's thyroiditis is rare. Unsuspected hypothyroidism may occur [17]. Systemic sclerosis is one of the disorders that are sometimes associated with congenital agammaglobulinaemia and IgA deficiency [18]. It may occur with autoimmune haemolytic anaemia [19], autoimmune neutropenia [20], thrombocytopenic purpura [21], microangiopathic haemolytic anaemia [22], urticaria pigmentosa [23], pemphigus vulgaris [24], monoclonal gammopathy [25], primary biliary cirrhosis [26,27], nodular hyperplasia of the liver [28], coeliac disease [29], pseudoxanthoma elasticum [30], elastosis perforans serpiginosa [31], lymphoma [32] and multiple sclerosis [33]. Reversible myasthenia gravis may occur on treatment with penicillamine [34].

References

1 Cipoletti JF, Buckingham RB, Barnes EL et al. Sjögren's syndrome in progressive systemic sclerosis. Ann Intern Med 1977; 87: 535–41.

2 Andonopoulos AP, Drosos AA, Skopouli FN et al. Sjögren's syndrome in rheumatoid arthritis and progressive systemic sclerosis: a comparative study. Clin Exp Rheumatol 1989; 7: 203–5.

3 Drosos AA, Andonopoulos AP, Costopoulos JS et al. Sjögren's syndrome in progressive systemic sclerosis. J Rheumatol 1988; 15: 965–8.

4 Alarcón-Segovia D, Ibáñez G, Hernández-Ortiz J et al. Sjögren's syndrome in progressive systemic sclerosis (scleroderma). Am J Med 1974; 57: 78–85.

5 Matthews RW, Bhoola KD, Rasker JJ et al. Salivary secretion and connective tissue disease in man. Ann Rheum Dis 1985; 44: 20–6.

6 Osial TA, Whiteside TL, Buckingham RB et al. Clinical and serologic study of Sjögren's syndrome in patients with progressive systemic sclerosis. Arthritis Rheum 1983; 26: 500–8.

7 Bell S, Krieg T, Meurer M. Antibodies to Ro/SSA detected by ELISA: correlation with clinical findings in systemic sclerosis. Br J Dermatol 1989; 121: 35–41.

8 Pock GF. Acute polymyositis scleroderma. Rev Assoc Med Argent 1959; 73: 266–70.

9 Weber FP, Bode OB. Sclerodermia and myasthenia gravis. Proc R Soc Med 1931–32; 25: 966.

10 Bergouignan M, Guerin A, Texier L. Sclerodermie progressive, dystrophie musculaire, syndrome endocrinien. Rev Neurol 1950; 83: 126.

11 Calvert RI, Owen TK. True scleroderma kidney. Lancet 1956; ii: 19–22.

12 Platt R, Davson J. A clinical and pathological study of renal disease. QJM 1950; 19: 33–56.

13 Swarm RL, Cermuth FC. Renal lesions in scleroderma. Am J Pathol 1953; 29: 577–8.

14 Perez-Jiminez F, Lopez-Rubio F, Canadillas F et al. Giant cell arteritis associated with progressive systemic sclerosis. Arthritis Rheum 1982; 25: 717–8.

15 Wyble M, Schirnek RA. The simultaneous occurrence of two collagen diseases in the same patient. Trans Am Acad Ophthalmol Otolaryngol 1962; 66: 632–41.

16 Durie BCM, Stroud JD, Kahn JA. Progressive systemic sclerosis with malignant atrophic papulosis. Arch Dermatol 1969; 100: 575–81.

17 Gordon MB, Klein I, Dekker A et al. Thyroid disease in progressive systemic sclerosis: increased frequency of glandular fibrosis and hypothyroidism. Ann Intern Med 1981; 95: 431–5.

18 Jay S, Helm S, Wray BB. Progressive systemic scleroderma with IgA deficiency in a child. Am J Dis Child 1981; 135: 965–6.

19 Sumithran E. Progressive systemic sclerosis and autoimmune haemolytic anaemia. Postgrad Med J 1976; 52: 173–6.

20 Waugh D, Ibels L. Malignant scleroderma associated with autoimmune neutropenia. BMJ 1980; 280: 1577–8.

21 Ivey KJ, Hwang YF, Sheets RF. Scleroderma associated with thrombocytopenia and Coombs-positive haemolytic anaemia. Am J Med 1971; 51: 815–7.

22 Sayer WR, Sayer DC, Heptinstall RH. Scleroderma and microangiopathic haemolytic anaemia. Ann Intern Med 1973; 78: 895–7.

23 Basler RSW, Harrell ER. Urticaria pigmentosa associated with scleroderma. Arch Dermatol 1974; 109: 393–4.

24 Woscoff A, Remondino C, Jaimovich L et al. Progressive systemic sclerosis and pemphigus vulgaris. J Am Acad Dermatol 1989; 21: 142–4.

25 Nishikai M, Funatsu Y, Homma M. Monoclonal gammopathy, penicillamine-induced polymyositis and systemic sclerosis. Arch Dermatol 1974; 110: 253–5.

26 Murray-Lyon IM, Thompson RPH, Ansell ID et al. Scleroderma and primary biliary cirrhosis. BMJ 1970; iii: 258–9.

27 Reynolds TB, Denison EK, Frankl HD et al. Primary biliary cirrhosis with scleroderma, Raynaud's phenomenon and telangiectasia. Am J Med 1971; 50: 302–12.

28 Russell ML, Kahn JH. Nodular regenerative hyperplasia of the liver associated with progressive systemic sclerosis. J Rheumatol 1983; 10: 748–52.

29 Cooper BT, Holmes GKT, Cooke WT. Coeliac disease and immunological disorders. BMJ 1978; i: 537–9.

30 Wilkinson JD. Pseudoxanthoma elasticum and acrosclerosis. Proc R Soc Med 1977; 70: 567–70.

31 May NC, Lester RS. Elastosis perforans serpiginosa associated with systemic sclerosis. J Am Acad Dermatol 1982; 6: 945.

32 Vignon-Pennamen MD, Janvier M, Wallach D. Sclerodermie systemique et lymphome malin ganglionnaire. Ann Dermatol Vénéréol 1983; 110: 779–80.

33 Trostle DC, Helfrich D, Medsger TA. Systemic sclerosis (scleroderma) and multiple sclerosis. Arthritis Rheum 1986; 29: 124–7.

34 Torres CF, Griggs RC, Baum J et al. Penicillamine-induced myasthenia gravis in progressive systemic sclerosis. Arthritis Rheum 1980; 23: 505–8.

Differential diagnosis. Well-developed cases of systemic sclerosis presenting with Raynaud's phenomenon and typical cutaneous changes on the face and hands are easy to recognize. Generalized morphoea may sometimes cause confusion. However, Raynaud's phenomenon is less common in the latter, and the distribution of the skin changes is different in so far as generalized morphoea involves the trunk, as well as the limbs. Systemic involvement is unusual, although not unknown, and the course is usually towards improvement over the years.

Localized morphoea should present little difficulty, although occasionally morphoeic patches may be seen in systemic sclerosis, and systemic lesions may occasionally be found in morphoea [1–3]. Sometimes, patients with localized morphoea may later develop systemic sclerosis. Morphoeic lesions were seen in 6.7% of Japanese patients with systemic sclerosis [4]. Patients with atrophoderma of Pasini and Pierini may progress to systemic sclerosis [5]. Acrosclerotic skin changes occasionally occur in SLE and dermatomyositis. Cold blue hands with inability to extend the fingers has been reported in bisalbuminaemia [6]. The pigmentation of systemic sclerosis may be confused with Addison's disease [7,8]. Cutaneous changes resembling systemic sclerosis have been reported in an unusual type of porphyria with features of erythropoietic protoporphyria and hepatic cutaneous porphyria [9]. A case of primary amyloidosis presenting as scleroderma has been described [10]. There is no Raynaud's phenomenon in familial sclerodactyly [11].

The stiff-skin syndrome [12], or congenital fascial dystrophy [13], is a rare condition presenting in childhood, in which stone-hard indurations of the fascia and dermal collagen occur. There is no systemic involvement, and the resulting disability is permanent. Patients with scleromyxoedema—a variant of lichen myxoedematosus—may resemble systemic sclerosis but there is no Raynaud's phenomenon or systemic involvement apart from the characteristic slow paraprotein in the serum. The POEMS (polyneuropathy, organomegaly, endocrinopathy, M protein, skin changes) or Crow–Fukase syndrome also shows a monoclonal paraprotein among a large number of potential features, including diffuse hyperpigmentation, scleroderma, hypertrichosis and lymphadenopathy, as well as the features indicated by its acronym. Of these patients, 50% have multiple myeloma [14]. Differentiation from systemic sclerosis relies on the presence of neuropathy and gammopathy [15,16].

Raynaud's phenomenon, firmness of the skin of the fingers, radiological absorption of the terminal phalanges and thickening of the walls of dermal arteries occur in workers engaged in the polymerization of vinyl chloride (see p. 51.80). The cutaneous changes of systemic sclerosis may resemble acrogeria (see Chapter 45), but the latter dates from birth. The condition may have to be distinguished from leprosy if a peripheral neuropathy is present

[17]. Up to 40% of insulin-dependent juvenile diabetics have contractures at the proximal interphalangeal joints, with thickening of the skin of the fingers (diabetic cheiroarthropathy) [18,19].

References

1 Donaldson EM. Morphoea (localized scleroderma) with visceral changes. *Br J Dermatol* 1962; **74**: 105.
2 Leinwand I, Duryee AW, Richter MN. Scleroderma. *Ann Intern Med* 1954; **41**: 1003–41.
3 Rodnan GP, Fennell RH. Progressive systemic sclerosis sine scleroderma. *JAMA* 1962; **180**: 665–70.
4 Soma Y, Tamaki T, Kikuchi K *et al.* Coexistence of morphoea and systemic sclerosis. *Dermatology* 1993; **186**: 103–5.
5 Bisaccia EP, Scarborourgh DA, Lowney ED. Atrophoderma of Pasini and Pierini and systemic scleroderma. *Arch Dermatol* 1982; **118**: 1–2.
6 Byrne JPH. Bisalbuminaemia. *Br J Dermatol* 1977; **95** (Suppl. 14): 54–5.
7 Banks BM. Is there a common denominator in scleroderma, dermatomyositis, disseminated lupus erythematosus, the Libman–Sacks syndrome and polyarteritis nodosa? *N Engl J Med* 1941; **255**: 433–4.
8 Talbott JH, Gall EA, Consolazio WV *et al.* Dermatomyositis with scleroderma, calcinosis and renal endarteritis associated with focal cortical necrosis. *Arch Intern Med* 1939; **63**: 476–96.
9 Simon N, Berko GY, Schneider I. Hepato erythropoietic porphyria presenting as scleroderma and acrosclerosis in a sibling pair. *Br J Dermatol* 1977; **96**: 663–8.
10 Leach WB, Vassar PS, Culling CFA. Primary systemic amyloidosis presenting as scleroderma. *Can Med Assoc J* 1960; **83**: 263–5.
11 Dijk EV. Familial sclerodactyly. *Dermatologica* 1971; **143**: 253.
12 Esterly NS, McKusick VA. Stiff skin syndrome. *Pediatrics* 1971; **47**: 360–9.
13 Jablonska S, Groniowski J, Krieg T *et al.* Congenital fascial dystrophy: a non-inflammatory disease of fascia: the stiff skin syndrome. *Pediatr Dermatol* 1984; **2**: 87–97.
14 Nakanishi T, Sobue I, Toyokura Y *et al.* The Crow–Fukase syndrome: a study of 102 cases in Japan. *Neurology* 1984; **34**: 712–20.
15 Burton JL. Peripheral neuropathy associated with dysproteinaemia, skin changes, and endocrinopathy. *BMJ* 1986; **292**: 1415.
16 Viard JP, Lesavre P, Boitard C *et al.* POEMS syndrome presenting as systemic sclerosis. *Am J Med* 1988; **84**: 524–8.
17 Lapido GOA. Progressive systemic sclerosis (scleroderma). *Dermatologica* 1976; **153**: 196–201.
18 Garza-Elizondo MA, Diaz-Jonanen E, Franco-Casique JJ *et al.* Joint contractures and scleroderma-like skin changes in the hands of insulin-dependent juvenile diabetics. *J Rheumatol* 1983; **10**: 797–800.
19 Seibold JR. Digital sclerosis in children with insulin-dependent diabetes mellitus. *Arthritis Rheum* 1982; **25**: 1357–61.

Prognosis [1–3]. The prognosis for this disorder is variable. Some patients die within a year or two and others live for many years, even those whose course may initially have been rapid with gangrene of the extremities. Males have a poorer prognosis than females [2,3], although in a recent series [4] the reverse was true. Overall, there is a fourfold increase in mortality in patients with systemic sclerosis. Patients with extensive skin and visceral involvement have a poorer prognosis [5], as do approximately 20% with rapidly progressive disease [6]. Pulmonary involvement is permanent; patients with 60% or greater reduction in pulmonary diffusing capacity have a 5-year survival of less than 10% [7]. Renal involvement is also an adverse factor, although some patients live for years. Patients with telangiectases and calcinosis have the same prognosis as other patients. Those with changes confined to the hands have a good prognosis [8]. Five-year survival varies between series from 34 to 80%, the difference probably depending on the proportion of females. Cumulative survival rate in one series [9] was 80% at 2 years, 50% at 8.5 years and 30% at

12 years. There is no relation to the presence or type of antinuclear factor. Patients with depression of T cells and decreased cell-mediated immunity [10], and with histocompatibility type HLA-B8, appear to have extensive disease and a poor prognosis [11]. The usual causes of death are from intercurrent infection, respiratory failure, cardiac failure, renal failure sometimes with malignant hypertension, and perforation of the gastrointestinal tract. Occasionally, patients with pulmonary involvement develop carcinoma of the lung [12], but the association of isolated cases of carcinoma of the thyroid, ovary, cervix, brain, oesophagus, stomach, breast [13], lymphoma and leukaemia with systemic sclerosis may be fortuitous [14]. Occasionally, the two diseases occur simultaneously, and a rare improvement of systemic sclerosis with treatment of the malignancy has been observed [15]. Localized radiotherapy for solid malignant tumours in patients with systemic sclerosis has been noted to exaggerate the cutaneous and internal fibrotic reaction in the irradiated areas [16].

References

1 Bennett R, Bluestone R, Holt PJL *et al.* Survival in scleroderma. *Ann Rheum Dis* 1971; **30**: 581–8.
2 Medsger TA, Masi AT, Rodnan GP *et al.* Survival with systemic sclerosis (scleroderma). *Ann Intern Med* 1971; **75**: 369–76.
3 Rowell NR. The prognosis of systemic sclerosis. *Br J Dermatol* 1976; **95**: 57–60.
4 Bryan C, Howard Y, Brennan P *et al.* Survival following the onset of scleroderma: results from a retrospective inception cohort study of the UK patient population. *Br J Rheumatol* 1996; **35**: 1122–6.
5 Barnett AJ, Miller MH, Littlejohn GO. A survival study of patients with scleroderma diagnosed over 30 years (1953–83): the value of a simple cutaneous classification in the early stages of the disease. *J Rheumatol* 1988; **15**: 276–83.
6 Lally EV, Jimenez SA, Kaplan SR. Progressive systemic sclerosis: mode of presentation, rapidly progressive disease course, and mortality based on an analysis of 91 patients. *Semin Arthritis Rheum* 1988; **18**: 1–13.
7 Peters-Golden M, Wise RA, Hochberg M *et al.* Carbon monoxide diffusing capacity as a predictor of outcome in systemic sclerosis. *Am J Med* 1984; **77**: 1027–34.
8 Barnett AJ, Coventry DA. Scleroderma. 1. Clinical features, course of illness and response to treatment in 61 cases. *Med J Aust* 1969; **1**: 992–1001.
9 Altman RD, Medsger TA, Bloch DA *et al.* Predictors of survival in systemic sclerosis (scleroderma). *Arthritis Rheum* 1991; **34**: 403–13.
10 Hughes P, Holt S, Rowell NR *et al.* The relationship of defective cell-mediated immunity to visceral disease in systemic sclerosis. *Clin Exp Immunol* 1977; **28**: 233–40.
11 Hughes P, Gelsthorpe K, Doughty RW *et al.* The association of HLA-B8 with visceral disease in systemic sclerosis. *Clin Exp Immunol* 1978; **31**: 351–6.
12 Haqquani MT, Holti G. Systemic sclerosis with pulmonary fibrosis and oat cell carcinoma. *Acta Derm Venereol (Stockh)* 1973; **53**: 369–74.
13 Kissinger A, Lemon HM, Foley JF. Carcinoma of the breast and scleroderma. *Nebraska Med J* 1973; **58**: 186–8.
14 Talbott JH, Barrocas M. Progressive systemic sclerosis (PSS) and malignancy, pulmonary and non-pulmonary. *Medicine* 1979; **58**: 182–207.
15 Duncan SC, Winkelmann RK. Cancer and scleroderma. *Arch Dermatol* 1979; **115**: 950–5.
16 Varga J, Haustein UF, Creech RH *et al.* Exaggerated radiation-induced fibrosis in patients with systemic sclerosis. *JAMA* 1991; **265**: 3292–5.

Treatment. Symptomatic management of the patient is very important. There is no specific treatment, and no therapy is known to alter the course of the disease. Corticosteroids in low dosage may give a feeling of increased well-being and reduction of articular symptoms, and in these cases maintenance on a low dosage of prednisolone, such as 5 mg once or twice daily, is justified. Larger dosage will be required for patients with associated LE. There is no evidence that corticosteroids retard the progress of the disease in any way, nor is there any real evidence that corticosteroids induce the onset of renal failure. Dexamethasone pulse therapy has been claimed to improve some patients [1]. It is important to advise the patient to keep as warm as possible, particularly in the winter months, and suitable work may have to be found to allow this. A light job in a warm atmosphere is ideal, and it is important to avoid even minor trauma of the hands. Electrically heated gloves are helpful [2], except in patients with incipient gangrene. Smoking should be discouraged [3]. There is no specific therapy for the skin, but applications of 0.025–0.05% tretinoin (Retin-A) have decreased perioral and facial tightening and creases [4]. Areas affected by calcium deposits may break down and heal with difficulty. Occasionally, deposits may have to be excised [5]. These techniques may be superseded by treatment with the carbon dioxide laser [6]. Treatment of digital calcinosis was successful in approximately two-thirds of cases. The average healing time was 6 weeks. Reconstructive surgery for sclerodactyly has sometimes given satisfactory results [7].

Vasodilators, such as oral reserpine [8], guanethidine [9], and particularly nifedipine 10–20 mg four times daily [10,11] and diltiazem [12], may improve the blood flow in the fingers. Ketanserin 20 mg twice daily to 40 mg three times daily may [13] or may not [14] be useful. Nifedipine may worsen oesophageal symptoms [15]. Prazosin 1 mg orally three times daily reduces the frequency and severity of vasospasm [16]. Simply warming the hands in hot water for 5–10 min produces considerable improvement in peripheral blood flow [17], and regular use of such a technique reduces the number and severity of attacks of Raynaud's phenomenon [18]. Intra-arterial reserpine is ineffective, and may have serious side effects [19]. Prostacyclin [20,21] and the synthetic prostacyclin analogue iloprost [22] are potent vasodilators and inhibitors of platelet aggregation, and have been found to be effective in decreasing the frequency, duration and severity of Raynaud's phenomenon, warming the hands, relieving pain and healing ischaemic ulcers. Earlier reports of the effect of prostaglandin E_1 have not been confirmed [23]. Infusion of prostacyclin via a central venous catheter over 72 h at a rate of 2.5–10 ng/kg/min produces improvement for approximately 8 weeks. Side effects include hypertension, headache, facial flushing, abdominal colic, nausea, vomiting and diarrhoea, and pain at the angle of the jaw at the beginning of mastication, disappearing within minutes. Similar results have been obtained by 5-h intravenous infusions given weekly for 3 weeks through a peripheral vein [24], a procedure that can be carried out on outpatients. Iloprost is useful in cases of incipient gangrene and digital ulcers [25]. Transdermal applications of these agents may be beneficial [26].

The use of intravenous low-molecular-weight dextran (Rheomacrodex) has been advocated [27], but controlled trials [28] have shown no consistent benefit, although in occasional patients there is healing of ulcerated fingertips. Renal failure and oliguria have followed this treatment [29]. Intravenous pentoxifylline may be of benefit in acute ischaemic lesions [30]. Cervical or lumbar sympathectomy may produce some improvement in the cutaneous circulation for a year or two, but there is no lasting benefit.

Penicillamine in regimens of from 500 to 1500 mg/day (mean 750 mg) given over approximately 2 years may decrease skin thickness, reduce the rate of further visceral involvement and improve the prognosis of patients if given early in their disease [31,32], particularly those with pulmonary involvement [33]. Other authors have found no benefit or no improvement in vascular or systemic complications, even if there is limited skin improvement [34]. In particular, progression of oesophageal disease continues [35]. Penicillamine therapy is associated with troublesome side effects [36]. In one study [37], the skin of 32% of patients improved, but deterioration occurred in the same percentage. In patients known to be sensitive to penicillin, the risk of an immediate allergic reaction is low [38]. Colchicine (1 mg/day or higher for 6 days per week) has also been advocated [39], but found to be ineffective [33]. Isotretinoin in a dosage of 1 mg/kg may help cutaneous sclerosis [40], as may factor XIII given intravenously [41]. Plasmapheresis [42] and plasma exchange [43], combined with prednisone and cyclophosphamide, have been used for patients with severe systemic sclerosis [42], with some clinical improvement and reduction of endothelial cell cytotoxicity. Extracorporeal photochemotherapy is encouraging but expensive. It has been shown to be more effective than penicillamine in decreasing clinical skin involvement and also safer in patients with disease of less than 4 years' duration [44]. Patients were treated for two consecutive days every 4 weeks for 6 months. It may be insufficient to control severe progressive disease with systemic involvement [45], and its use is controversial [46]. Azathioprine in a dosage of 150 mg/day has been subjectively helpful in approximately one-third of cases. Chlorambucil by mouth does not halt the progression of systemic sclerosis [47,48]. Intravenous 5-fluorouracil, given intermittently for 6 months, improved cutaneous and systemic features in an uncontrolled trial [49].

Ciclosporin may be of benefit [50,51]. It may improve skin induration but not visceral manifestations; adverse reactions, particularly nephrototoxicity, are frequent [52]. IFN-γ influences fibroblast behaviour *in vitro* [53]. It has reduced the skin score and improved blood gas analyses without any adverse effects over 12 months' therapy, but other systemic involvement was unchanged [54]. Others have noticed no alteration in skin score or improvement in visceral involvement [55]. IFN-α2a has also failed to improve visceral involvement [56]. Antithymocyte globulin is ineffective [57].

Symptomatic treatment for cardiac, renal and gastrointestinal symptoms may be required. Antihypertensive drugs, including minoxidil, reduce the blood pressure in malignant hypertension [58,59], and captopril, an oral ACE inhibitor, is a considerable advance in its treatment [60,61], as in most cases there is elevation of plasma renin activity. It controls blood pressure in most, if not all patients and relieves encephalopathy. It can improve renal function and, if given early, prevents renal failure and death. Improvement in renal function over 2 years has been reported [62], but is not uniform [63]. There is little evidence for a more general improvement in the disease resulting from these agents [64]. Benefit must be weighed against side effects. Haemodialysis and renal transplantation have helped patients with renal failure, with surprising improvement in the renal function and cutaneous manifestations [65]. Recovery of renal function can occur after months of dialysis. In one case, renal biopsy 14 months after transplant showed no evidence of the original disease [66]. Cimetidine or ranitidine are worth trying for the symptoms of oesophageal reflux. Gastrostomy may be required for short-term feeding difficulties if dysphagia is severe [67]. Stricture of the oesophagus may benefit from surgical intervention [68]. Although the diffusion defect in the lungs cannot be altered, patients benefit from breathing exercises, and chest infections must be treated energetically with antibiotics. Pulmonary hypertension is a serious complication that may be treated with endothelin inhibitors such as bosentan [69] or sitaxsentan [70].

Immunosuppressive agents such as cyclophosphamide have been reported as useful in the treatment of systemic aspects of disease including lung fibrosis in a number of small, open studies, and, more recently, in two randomized controlled clinical trials [71–74]. So far there are only two randomized controlled trials to evaluate such immunosuppressive drugs which have enrolled mainly patients with established or long-standing disease; therefore, the potential for these drugs early in the course of disease remains unclear.

Many other preparations, including relaxin, sulfasalazine, 3-hydroxy-2-phenylcinchoninic acid (HPC), antihistamines, dihydrotachysterol and nicotinic acid, potassium p-aminobenzoate [75,76], intravenous disodium edetate, topical dimethylsulfoxide [77], the combination of phenformin and ethylestrenol [78], and antiplatelet therapy [79] have not proved of benefit. Hyperbaric oxygen may occasionally produce some improvement [80]. Calcitriol 1.75 µg/day may be helpful [81]. Dietary essential fatty acids such as γ-linolenic acid do not improve the vascular or other features [82].

Migraine sometimes occurs with systemic sclerosis [83], and methysergide or drugs containing ergot should not be given to such patients.

References

1 Pai BS, Srinivas CR, Sabitha L *et al.* Efficacy of dexamethasone pulse therapy in progressive systemic sclerosis. *Int J Dermatol* 1995; **34**: 726–8.

2 Kempson GE, Coggon D, Acheson ED. Electrically heated gloves for intermittent digital ischaemia. *BMJ* 1983; **286**: 268.

3 Goodfield MJD, Hume A, Rowell NR. The acute effects of cigarette smoking on peripheral blood flow in patients with and without Raynaud's phenomenon. *Br J Rheumatol* 1990; **29**: 89–91.

4 Kremer JM. Treatment of systemic sclerosis with topical tretinoin: report of two cases. *Arthritis Rheum* 1996; **39**: 1070.

5 Schlenker JD, Clark DD, Weckesser EC. Calcinosis circumscripta of the hand in scleroderma. *J Bone Joint Surg Am* 1973; **55**: 1051–6.

6 Bottomley WW, Goodfield MJD, Sheehan-Dare RA. Digital calcification in systemic sclerosis: effective treatment with good tissue preservation using the carbon dioxide laser. *Br J Dermatol* 1996; **135**: 302–4.

7 Lipscomb PR, Simons GW, Winkelmann RK. Surgery for sclerodactylia of the hand. *J Bone Joint Surg Am* 1969; **51**: 1112–7.

8 Coffman JD, Cohen AS. Total and capillary fingertip blood flow in Raynaud's phenomenon. *N Engl J Med* 1971; **285**: 259–63.

9 LeRoy EC, Downey JA, Cannon PJ. Skin capillary blood flow in scleroderma. *J Clin Invest* 1971; **50**: 930–9.

10 Kahan A, Amor B, Menkes CJ *et al.* Nifedipine in digital ulceration in scleroderma. *Arthritis Rheum* 1983; **26**: 809.

11 Winston EL, Pariser KM, Miller KB *et al.* Nifedipine as a therapeutic modality for Raynaud's phenomenon. *Arthritis Rheum* 1983; **26**: 1177–80.

12 Kahan A, Amor B, Menkes CJ. A randomized double blind trial of diltiazem in the treatment of Raynaud's phenomenon. *Ann Rheum Dis* 1985; **44**: 30–3.

13 Roald OK, Seem E. Treatment of Raynaud's phenomenon with ketanserin in patients with connective tissue disorders. *BMJ* 1984; **289**: 577–9.

14 Ortonne JP, Torzoli C, Dujardin P *et al.* Ketanserin in the treatment of systemic sclerosis: a double blind trial. *Br J Dermatol* 1989; **120**: 261–6.

15 Kahan A, Bour B, Couturier D *et al.* Nifedipine and oesophageal dysfunction in progressive systemic sclerosis. *Arthritis Rheum* 1985; **28**: 490–5.

16 Surwitt RS, Gilgor RS, Allen LM *et al.* A double-blind study of prazosin in the treatment of Raynaud's phenomenon in scleroderma. *Arch Dermatol* 1984; **120**: 329–31.

17 Goodfield MJD, Hume A, Rowell NR. The effect of simple warming procedures on finger blood flow in systemic sclerosis. *Br J Dermatol* 1988; **118**: 661–8.

18 Goodfield MJD, Rowell NR. Simple hand warming as treatment for Raynaud's phenomenon in systemic sclerosis. *Br J Dermatol* 1988; **119**: 643–6.

19 Surwitt RS, Gilgor RS, Duric M *et al.* Intra-arterial reserpine for Raynaud's syndrome. *Arch Dermatol* 1983; **119**: 733–5.

20 Dowd PM, Martin MFR, Cooke ED *et al.* Treatment of Raynaud's phenomenon by intravenous infusion of prostacyclin (PG$_2$ 1). *Br J Dermatol* 1982; **106**: 81–9.

21 Martin MFR, Dowd PM, Ring EFJ *et al.* Prostaglandin E$_1$ infusions for vascular insufficiency in progressive systemic sclerosis. *Ann Rheum Dis* 1981; **40**: 350–4.

22 Rademaker M, Cooke ED, Almond NE *et al.* Comparison of intravenous infusions of iloprost and oral nifedipine in treatment of Raynaud's phenomenon in patients with systemic sclerosis: a double blind randomized study. *BMJ* 1989; **298**: 561–4.

23 Mohrland JS, Porter JM, Smith EA *et al.* A multiclinic, placebo-controlled, double-blind study of prostaglandin E$_1$ in Raynaud's syndrome. *Ann Rheum Dis* 1985; **44**: 754–60.

24 Belch JJF, Drury JK, Capell H *et al.* Intermittent epoprostenol (prostacyclin) infusion in patients with Raynaud's syndrome. *Lancet* 1983; **i**: 313–5.

25 Zachariae H, Halkier-Sorensen L, Bjerring P *et al.* Treatment of ischaemic digital ulcers and prevention of gangrene with intravenous iloprost in systemic sclerosis. *Acta Derm Venereol (Stockh)* 1996; **76**: 236–8.

26 Belch JJF, Madhok R, Shaw B *et al.* Double-blind trial of CL115,347, a transdermally absorbed prostaglandin E$_2$ analogue, in treatment of Raynaud's phenomenon. *Lancet* 1985; **i**: 1180–3.

27 Holti G. The effect of intermittent low molecular dextran infusions upon the digital circulation in systemic sclerosis. *Br J Dermatol* 1965; **77**: 560–8.

28 Dodman B, Rowell NR. Low molecular weight dextran in systemic sclerosis and Raynaud's phenomenon. *Acta Derm Venereol (Stockh)* 1982; **62**: 440–2.

29 Feest TG. Low molecular weight dextran. *BMJ* 1976; **ii**: 1300.

30 Goodfield MJD, Rowell NR. Treatment of peripheral gangrene due to systemic sclerosis with intravenous pentoxifylline. *Clin Exp Dermatol* 1989; **14**: 161–2.

31 Jimenez SA, Sigal H. A 15-year prospective study of treatment of rapidly progressive systemic sclerosis (PSS) with D-penicillamine (D-PEN). *J Rheumatol* 1991; **18**: 1496–503.

32 Clements PJ, Hurwitz EL, Wong WK *et al.* Skin thickness score as a predictor and correlate of outcome in systemic sclerosis: high-dose versus low-dose penicillamine trial. *Arthritis Rheum* 2000; **43**: 2445–54.

33 Medsger TA Jr. D-Penicillamine treatment of lung involvement in patients with systemic sclerosis (scleroderma). *Arthritis Rheum* 1987; **30**: 832–4.

34 Jayson MIV, Lovell C, Black CM *et al.* Penicillamine therapy in systemic sclerosis. *Proc R Soc Med* 1977; **70** (Suppl. 3): 82–8.

35 Hendel L, Stentoft P, Aggestrup S. The progress of oesophageal involvement in progressive systemic sclerosis during D-penicillamine treatment. *Scand J Rheumatol* 1989; **18**: 149–55.

36 Steen VD, Blair S, Medsger TA Jr. The toxicity of D-penicillamine in systemic sclerosis. *Ann Intern Med* 1986; **104**: 699–705.

37 Rook AH, Freundlich B, Jegasothy BV *et al.* Treatment of systemic sclerosis with extracorporeal photochemotherapy. *Arch Dermatol* 1992; **128**: 337–46.

38 Bell CL, Graziano FM. The safety of administration of penicillamine to penicillin-sensitive individuals. *Arthritis Rheum* 1983; **26**: 801–3.

39 Alarcón-Segovia D, Ibáñez G, Kershenobich D *et al.* Treatment of scleroderma. *Lancet* 1974; **i**: 1054–5.

40 Maurice PDL, Bunker CB, Dowd PM. Isotretinoin in the treatment of systemic sclerosis. *Br J Dermatol* 1989; **121**: 367–74.

41 Guilleven L, Euler-Ziegler L, Chouvet B *et al.* Treatment with factor XIII and long-term follow-up of 86 patients with progressive systemic sclerosis. *Presse Med* 1985; **14**: 2327–30.

42 Dau PC, Kahaleh MB, Sagebiel RW. Plasmapheresis and immuno-suppressive drug therapy in scleroderma. *Arthritis Rheum* 1981; **24**: 1128–36.

43 Mascaro G, Cadario G, Bordin G *et al.* Plasma exchange in the treatment of non-advanced stages of progressive systemic sclerosis. *J Clin Apheresis* 1987; **3**: 219–25.

44 di Spaltro FX, Cottrill C, Cahill C *et al.* Photochemotherapy for progressive systemic sclerosis. *Int J Dermatol* 1993; **32**: 417–21.

45 Zachariae H, Bjerring P, Heitckendorff L *et al.* Photophoresis and systemic sclerosis. *Arch Dermatol* 1992; **128**: 1651–3.

46 Cribier B, Faradji T, Le Coz C *et al.* Extracorporeal photochemotherapy in systemic sclerosis and severe morphoea. *Dermatology* 1995; **191**: 25–31.

47 Furst DE, Clements PJ, Hillis S *et al.* Immunosuppression with chlorambucil versus placebo for scleroderma. *Arthritis Rheum* 1989; **32**: 584–93.

48 Steigerwald JC. Chlorambucil therapy in progressive systemic sclerosis. *J Rheumatol* 1974; **1** (Suppl. 1): 74.

49 Casas JA, Subauste CP, Alarcon GS. A new promising treatment in systemic sclerosis: 5-fluorouracil. *Ann Rheum Dis* 1987; **46**: 763–7.

50 Vayssaiart M, Baudot N, Boitard C *et al.* Cyclosporine for severe systemic sclerosis associated with the anti-Scl-70 autoantibody. *J Am Acad Dermatol* 1990; **22**: 695–6.

51 Zachariae H, Halkier-Sorensen L, Heickendorff L *et al.* Cyclosporin A treatment of systemic sclerosis. *Br J Dermatol* 1990; **122**: 677–81.

52 Clements PJ, Lachenbruch PA, Sterz M *et al.* Cyclosporin in systemic sclerosis: results of a 48-week open safety study in 10 patients. *Arthritis Rheum* 1993; **36**: 75–83.

53 Rosenbloom J, Feldman G, Freundlich B *et al.* Inhibition of excessive scleroderma fibroblast collagen production by recombinant γ-interferon. *Arthritis Rheum* 1986; **29**: 851–6.

54 Hein R, Behr J, Hundegen M *et al.* Treatment of systemic sclerosis with γ-interferon. *Br J Dermatol* 1992; **126**: 496–501.

55 Hunzelmann N, Anders S, Fierbeck G *et al.* Systemic sclerosis: multicentre trial of 1 year treatment with recombinant interferon-γ. *Arch Dermatol* 1997; **133**: 609–13.

56 Stevens W, Vancheeswaran R, Black CM *et al.* Alpha interferon-2a (Roferon-A) in the treatment of diffuse cutaneous systemic sclerosis: a pilot study. *Br J Rheumatol* 1992; **31**: 683–9.

57 Matteson EL, Shbeeb MI, McCarthy TG *et al.* Pilot study of antithymocyte globulin in systemic sclerosis. *Arthritis Rheum* 1996; **39**: 1132–7.

58 Mitnick PD, Feig PU. Control of hypertension and reversal of renal failure in scleroderma. *N Engl J Med* 1978; **299**: 871–2.

59 Wasner C, Cooke CR, Fries JF. Successful medical treatment of scleroderma renal crisis. *N Engl J Med* 1978; **299**: 873–5.

60 Lopez-Ovejero JA, Saal SD, D'Angelo WA *et al.* Reversal of vascular and renal crises of scleroderma by oral angiotensin-converting-enzyme blockade. *N Engl J Med* 1979; **300**: 1417–9.

61 Whitman HH III, Case JB, Laragh JH *et al.* Variable response to oral angiotensin-converting enzyme blockade in hypertensive scleroderma patients. *Arthritis Rheum* 1982; **25**: 241–8.

62 Sorenson LB, Paunicka K, Harris M. Reversal of scleroderma renal crisis for more than 2 years in a patient treated with captopril. *Arthritis Rheum* 1983; **26**: 797–800.

63 Brown EA, MacGregor GA, Maini RN. Failure of captopril to reverse the renal crisis of scleroderma. *Ann Rheum Dis* 1983; **42**: 52–3.

64 Beckett VL, Donadio JV Jr, Brennan LA Jr *et al.* Use of captopril as early therapy for renal scleroderma: a prospective study. *Mayo Clin Proc* 1985; **60**: 763–71.

65 Simon NM, Graham MB, Kyser FA *et al.* Resolution of renal failure with malignant hypertension in scleroderma. *Am J Med* 1979; **67**: 533–9.

66 Keane WF, Danielson B, Raij L. Successful renal transplantation in progressive systemic sclerosis. *Ann Intern Med* 1976; **85**: 199–202.

67 Stainforth J, Goodfield MDJ. Severe oropharyngeal deglutition abnormalities in a patient with systemic sclerosis, managed with a gastrostomy. *Br J Dermatol* 1994; **130**: 682–3.

68 Mansour KA, Malone CE. Surgery for scleroderma of the oesophagus: a 12-year experience. *Ann Thorac Surg* 1988; **46**: 513–4.

69 Rubin LJ, Badesch DB, Barst RJ *et al.* Bosentan therapy for pulmonary arterial hypertension. *N Engl J Med* 2002; **346**: 896–903.

70 O'Callaghan DS, Gaine SP. Sitaxsentan: an endothelin-A receptor antagonist for the treatment of pulmonary arterial hypertension. *Int J Clin Pract* 2006; **60**: 475–81.

71 Griffiths B, Miles S, Moss H *et al.* Systemic sclerosis and interstitial lung disease: a pilot study using pulse intravenous methylprednisolone and cyclophosphamide to assess the effect on high resolution computed tomography scan and lung function. *J Rheumatol* 2002; **29**: 2371–8.

72 White B, Moore WC, Wigley FM *et al.* Cyclophosphamide is associated with pulmonary function and survival benefit in patients with scleroderma and alveolitis. *Ann Intern Med* 2000; **132**: 947–54.

73 Hoyles RK, Ellis RW, Wellsbury J *et al.* A multicenter, prospective, randomized, double-blind, placebo-controlled trial of corticosteroids and intravenous cyclophosphamide followed by oral azathioprine for the treatment of pulmonary fibrosis in scleroderma. *Arthritis Rheum* 2006; **54**: 3962–70.

74 Tashkin DP, Elashoff R, Clements PJ *et al.* Scleroderma Lung Study Research Group. Cyclophosphamide versus placebo in scleroderma lung disease. *N Engl J Med* 2006; **354**: 2655–66.

75 Silber W, Gitlin N. Progressive systemic sclerosis (diffuse scleroderma): a follow-up report of treatment with potaba. *South Afr Med J* 1973; **47**: 1001–2.

76 Zarafonetis CJD, Dabich L, Skovronski JJ *et al.* Retrospective studies in scleroderma: skin response to potassium para-aminobenzoate therapy. *Clin Exp Rheumatol* 1988; **6**: 261–8.

77 Binnick SA, Shore SS, Corman A *et al.* Failure of dimethyl sulfoxide in the treatment of scleroderma. *Arch Dermatol* 1977; **113**: 1398–402.

78 Paolino JS, Kaplan D, Lazarus R *et al.* Phenformin and ethyloestrenol in scleroderma. *Lancet* 1972; **i**: 1023.

79 Beckett VL, Conn DL, Fuster V *et al.* Trial of platelet inhibiting drug in scleroderma. *Arthritis Rheum* 1984; **27**: 1137–43.

80 Barr P-O, Enfors W, Eriksson G. Hyperbaric oxygen therapy in dermatology. *Br J Dermatol* 1972; **86**: 631–5.

81 Humbert P, Aubin F, Delaporte E. Oral calcitriol as a new therapeutic agent in localized and systemic scleroderma. *Arch Dermatol* 1995; **131**: 850–1.

82 Stainforth JM, Layton AM, Goodfield MJD. Clinical aspects of the use of gamma linolenic acid in systemic sclerosis. *Acta Derm Venereol (Stockh)* 1996; **76**: 144–6.

83 Goldberg NC, Duncan SC, Winkelmann RK. Migraine and systemic scleroderma. *Arch Dermatol* 1978; **114**: 550–1.

Mixed connective tissue disease [1]

Overlap syndromes occur in the connective tissue diseases, and have recently been reviewed [1]. A number of attempts at defining diagnostic criteria, along the lines of those used for SLE, have been made [2]. Some associations are more frequent than others; for example, systemic sclerosis combined with dermatomyositis is more frequent than systemic sclerosis combined with SLE [3]. Some of these patients may have 'mixed connective tissue disease', an entity associated with a specific antibody to U_1-RNP, an ENA first described by Sharp and colleagues in 1972 [4]. These patients, predominantly female, show features of SLE, systemic sclerosis, dermatomyositis and polymyositis. Raynaud's phenomenon, arthritis and arthralgia, sausage-shaped fingers and swelling of the dorsa of the hands, abnormal oesophageal motility, impaired pulmonary diffusing capacity and myositis are frequent. More than half have the abnormal nail fold capillaries seen in systemic sclerosis. Angiography shows obstruction of small blood vessels in almost 90% of cases, and peripheral gangrene may occur (Fig. 51.75) [5]. The incidence of clinical renal disease is approximately 5%, but renal histology is abnormal in 20% [6]. Aseptic meningitis, trigeminal neuropathy, transverse myelitis and psychosis are prominent neurological features. Neuropsychiatric manifestations were noted in 15% of one series. Other, less frequent features have been reviewed [7], and include orogenital ulceration, pneumatosis intestinalis, protein-losing enteropathy, panniculitis and autonomic neuropathy. Enlarged

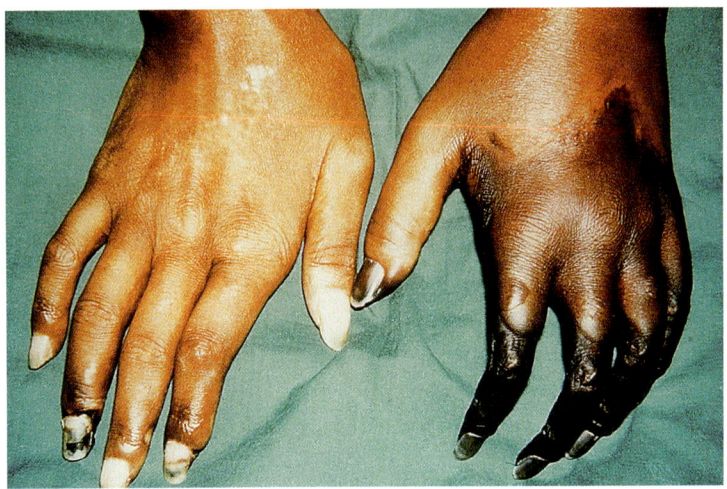

Fig. 51.75 Gangrene of the hands in mixed connective tissue disease.

nodes of Kikuchi's disease were the presenting feature in one case [8].

The response to treatment with corticosteroids is good, and other successful treatment options, including hydroxychloroquine and methotrexate, have been reviewed [9]. The characteristic antibody may be suppressed by treatment, and disappears in patients in remission [10].

Mixed connective tissue disease may be more severe in children, in whom cardiac and renal disease and arthritis are common, and thrombocytopenia may be marked, although the overall prognosis may be quite good [11]. Thrombocytopenia is also occasionally found in adult cases, and may occur with thrombotic thrombocytopenic purpura [12]. The role of silicone breast implants in the pathogenesis of the overlap syndromes is controversial, and there is probably no relationship [13]. Livedoid vasculitis [14], ankylosing spondylitis [15] and antineutrophil cytoplasmic antibody (ANCA)-related glomerulonephritis [16] are reported to occur with mixed connective tissue disease.

References

1 Venables PJ. Mixed connective tissue disease. *Lupus* 2006; **15**: 132–7.
2 Alarcón-Segoviá D, Cardiel MH. Comparison between three diagnostic criteria for mixed connective tissue disease: study of 593 patients. *J Rheumatol* 1989; **16**: 328–56.
3 Minkin W, Rabhan N. Mixed connective tissue disease. *Arch Dermatol* 1976; **112**: 1535–8.
4 Sharp GC, Irvin WS, Tan EM *et al.* Mixed connective tissue disease. *Am J Med* 1972; **52**: 148–59.
5 Kondo H. Vascular disease in mixed connective tissue disease (MCTD). *Intern Med* 2001; **40**: 1176.
6 Bennett RM, Spargo BH. Immune complex nephropathy in mixed connective tissue disease. *Am J Med* 1977; **63**: 534–41.
7 Pope JE. Other manifestations of mixed connective tissue disease. *Rheum Dis Clin North Am* 2005; **31**: 519–33.
8 Gourley I, Bell AL, Biggart D. Kikuchi's disease as a presenting feature of mixed connective tissue disease. *Clin Rheumatol* 1995; **14**: 104–7.
9 Kim P, Grossman JM. Treatment of mixed connective tissue disease. *Rheum Dis Clin North Am* 2005; **31**: 549–65.
10 Pettersson I, Wang G, Smith EI *et al.* The use of immunoblotting and immunoprecipitation of small nuclear ribonucleoproteins in the analysis of sera of patients with mixed connective tissue disease and systemic lupus erythematosus. *Arthritis Rheum* 1986; **29**: 986–96.
11 Mier RJ, Shishov M, Higginns GC *et al.* Paediatric onset mixed connective tissue disease. *Rheum Dis Clin North Am* 2005; **31**: 483–96.
12 Poullin P, Lefevre P, Durand JM. Mixed connective tissue disease with haemolytic anemia and severe thrombocytopenia due to thrombotic thrombocytopenic purpura. *Am J Hematol* 1999; **61**: 275.
13 McLaughlin JK, Lipworth L, Murphy DK, Walker PS. The safety of silicone gel-filled breast implants: a review of the epidemiologic evidence. *Ann Plast Surg* 2007; **59**: 569–80.
14 Oh YB, Jun JB, Kim CK *et al.* Mixed connective tissue disease associated with skin defects of livedoid vasculitis. *Clin Rheumatol* 2000; **19**: 381–4.
15 Lee JK, Jung SS, Kim TH *et al.* Coexistence of ankylosing spondylitis and mixed connective tissue disease in a single patient. *Clin Exp Rheumatol* 1999; **17**: 263.
16 Makita N, Katori H, Takemoto F *et al.* A case of mixed connective tissue disease (MCTD) complicated with MPO-ANCA-related necrotizing glomerulonephritis. *Clin Nephrol* 2000; **54**: 164–8.

Immunology. All patients have the speckled type of antinuclear antibody together with a high titre of antibody to ENA, which is sensitive to digestion with ribonuclease (RNase), unlike the ENA antibodies often found in patients with SLE. Different molecular forms of U_1-RNP may be associated with different clinical variants [1]. Ro and La antibodies are also frequently found, usually in association with sicca symptoms [2]. Precipitating antibodies designated PM-1 [3] and Ku [4] occur in polymyositis/systemic sclerosis overlap, and SL-Ki in patients with SLE, scleroderma and the sicca syndrome [5]. Immune complexes occur in 90% of patients, and T cells are decreased. Complement levels are normal. Sometimes, anti-DNA antibody occurs in low titre, but this usually disappears with steroid therapy. Antiendothelial antibodies occur in approximately 50% of cases, and are associated with abnormal pulmonary, neurological and cardiac function, particularly pulmonary hypertension [6]. They are also related significantly to spontaneous abortion in female patients [7]. HLA-DR4 is found more commonly in patients with arthritis than in normal controls, and is associated with a young age of onset of the condition [8]. There are also reports of familial cases [9]. Differences in HLA antigens between patients with mixed connective tissue disease and SLE indicate that they are genetically separate disorders [10].

Immunohistology of uninvolved skin, where there is basement membrane staining with IgG or M, may be helpful in distinguishing MCTD from uncomplicated systemic sclerosis where staining is absent [11].

Direct immunofluorescence study of apparently normal skin reveals particulate ('speckled') epidermal nuclear staining, and this correlates with high titres of anti-RNP. Occasionally, epidermal nucleolar staining occurs. Patients with these features [12] show a high incidence of persistent, diffuse, non-scarring and focal alopecia, hyper- and hypopigmentation with follicular retention of pigment, swollen hands with sclerodactyly, and lesions of DLE.

Although the presence of anti-RNP is usually associated with a good prognosis, death occurs in approximately 4% from pulmonary hypertension, brought about by vascular changes similar to those seen in primary pulmonary hypertension [13], nephritis, myocarditis or widespread vasculitis. Approximately one-third develop into a characteristic connective tissue disease, usually SLE or SSc [14]. A few patients with HLA-DR4 developed rheumatoid arthritis. In patients whose disease differentiated into systemic sclerosis, there was an association with HLA-DR5 [15]. The relatively good prognosis has been confirmed recently [16].

With time, more variants of the overlap syndromes are being described, both with and without U₁-RNP antibody. Hence, some authors now regard mixed connective tissue disease as one among many 'undifferentiated connective tissue diseases' or 'overlap syndromes'. Doubts about the concept of mixed connective tissue disease have been expressed, particularly in children [17]; nevertheless, it is important to recognize this group of patients because of the good prognosis and the response to steroid therapy. There may be an increased risk of malignancy, with cancer developing in 10% of cases [18].

References

1 Greidinger EL, Casciola-Rosen L, Morris SM *et al.* Autoantibody recognition of distinctly modified forms of the U1–70-kD antigen is associated with different clinical disease manifestations. *Arthritis Rheum* 2000; **43**: 881–8.
2 Setty YN, Pittman CB, Mahale AS *et al.* Sicca symptoms and anti-SSA/Ro antibodies are common in mixed connective tissue disease. *J Rheumatol* 2002; **29**: 487–9.
3 Wolf JF, Adelstein E, Sharp GC. Antinuclear antibody with distinct specificity for polymyositis. *J Clin Invest* 1977; **59**: 176–8.
4 Mimori T, Akizuki M, Yamagata H *et al.* Characterization of a high molecular weight acidic nuclear protein recognized by autoantibodies in sera from patients with polymyositis–scleroderma overlap. *J Clin Invest* 1981; **68**: 611–20.
5 Parodi A, Nigro A, Rebora A. Anti-SL-Ki antibody in a patient with fatal connective tissue overlap disease. *Br J Dermatol* 1989; **121**: 243–6.
6 Vegh J, Szodoray P, Kappelmayer J *et al.* Clinical and immunoserological characteristics of mixed connective tissue disease associated with pulmonary hypertension. *Scand J Immunol* 2006; **64**: 69–76.
7 Bodolay E, Bojan F, Szegedi G *et al.* Cytotoxic endothelial cell antibodies in mixed connective tissue disease. *Immunol Lett* 1989; **20**: 163–8.
8 Black CM, Maddison PJ, Welsh KI *et al.* HLA and immunoglobulin allotypes in mixed connective tissue disease. *Arthritis Rheum* 1988; **31**: 131–4.
9 Shiiki H, Miyagawa S, Dohi K *et al.* Anti-nuclear RNP antibodies in two sisters. *Br J Dermatol* 1985; **113**: 617–22.
10 Ruuska P, Hameenkorpi R, Forsberg S *et al.* Differences in HLA antigens between patients with mixed connective disease and systemic lupus erythematosus. *Ann Rheum Dis* 1992; **51**: 52–5.
11 Winkelmann RK, Carapeto FJ, Jordon RE. Direct immunofluorescence in the diagnosis of scleroderma syndromes. *Br J Dermatol* 1977; **96**: 231–8.
12 Gilliam JN, Prystowsky SD. Mixed connective tissue disease syndrome. *Arch Dermatol* 1977; **113**: 583–7.
13 Bull TM, Fagan KA, Badesch DB. Pulmonary vascular manifestations of mixed connective tissue disease. *Rheum Dis Clin North Am* 2005; **31**: 451–64.
14 Bodoly E, Csiki Z, Ben T *et al.* Five year follow up of 665 Hungarian patients with undifferentiated connective tissue disease (UCTD). *Clin Exp Rheumatol* 2003; **21**: 313–20.
15 Gendi NS, Welsh KI, Van-Venrooij WJ *et al.* HLA type as a predictor of mixed connective tissue disease differentiation: 10 year clinical and immunogenetic follow-up of 46 patients. *Arthritis Rheum* 1995; **38**: 259–66.
16 Lundberg IE. The prognosis of mixed connective tissue disease. *Rheum Clin North Am* 2005; **31**: 535–47.
17 Mier R, Ansell B, Hall MA *et al.* Long-term follow-up of children with mixed connective tissue disease. *Lupus* 1996; **5**: 221–6.
18 Black KA, Zilko PJ, Dawkins RL *et al.* Cancer in connective tissue disease. *Arthritis Rheum* 1982; **25**: 1130–3.

Cold, flexed fingers (Fig. 51.76)

Several female patients have been seen with cold, flexed fingers, but no evidence of systemic abnormality, despite extensive investigations including pulmonary function tests. The presenting

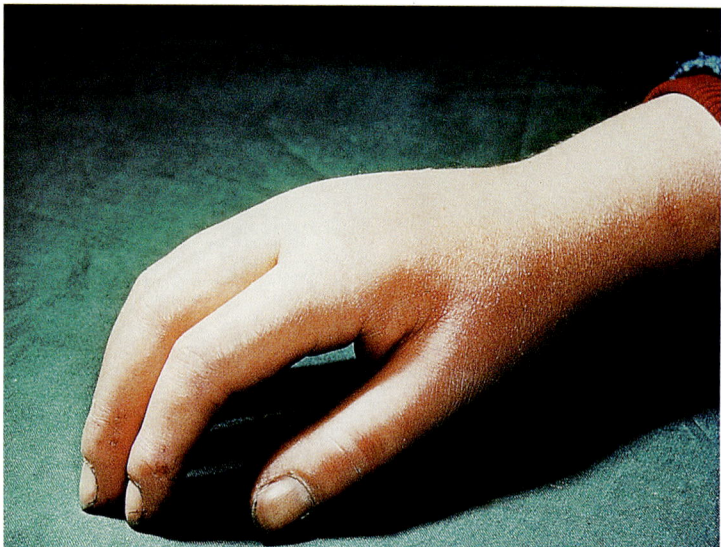

Fig. 51.76 Cold flexed fingers: note the inability to extend the fingers fully.

feature of inability to extend the fingers fully starts in the second to fourth decades. There may be difficulty in flexion of the fingers and in making a fist. All have thin, cold fingers, but there is no evidence of acrosclerosis, and Raynaud's phenomenon is not invariable. The condition remains unchanged for years and is not influenced by vasodilators or systemic corticosteroids.

Some patients may be early cases of systemic sclerosis. One patient has developed rheumatoid arthritis, with deformities of the hands.

The condition was first described in the first edition of this textbook in 1968 [1]. It appears to be similar to what has been termed 'bowed fingers' [2]. Some patients with bowed fingers had features of systemic sclerosis or mixed connective tissue disease.

References

1 Rowell NR. Cold flexed fingers. In: Rook A, Wilkinson DS, Ebling FJG, eds. *Textbook of Dermatology*. Oxford: Blackwell Scientific Publications, 1968: 564.
2 Palmer DG, Hale GM, Grennan DM. Bowed fingers: a helpful sign in the diagnosis of systemic sclerosis. *J Rheumatol* 1981; **8**: 266–72.

Lichen sclerosus [1,2]

Synonyms
- Lichen sclerosus et atrophicus
- Guttate morphoea
- Guttate scleroderma
- White-spot disease

Definition. An uncommon disease of unknown aetiology in which characteristic, easily recognized, small, white, sclerotic areas occur at any site on the skin. This frequently involves the perineal skin in the female, and the penis and foreskin in the male. It may occur in genital and non-genital skin separately or together. Hallopeau [3] first described the condition in 1887, and Darier [4] reported the histological changes in 1892. They considered the disorder to be a type of lichen planus; others thought that the condition was

Table 51.18 Associations of lichen sclerosus.

Morphoea
Vitiligo
Alopecia areata (in males)
Pernicious anaemia (in females)
Limited cutaneous systemic sclerosis
Systemic lupus erythematosus
Lichen planus

related to localized scleroderma. Most people now regard lichen sclerosus as a separate entity, because of the distinct clinical signs and pathological changes. The term 'white-spot disease' is sometimes applied to the skin lesions on the trunk and limbs, although some authors refer to these lesions as 'guttate scleroderma'. It may be closely related to morphoea, as the two conditions can occur together and, rarely, morphoea can produce similar genital lesions [5] (Table 51.18).

Incidence [6]. The condition is an uncommon one. Females predominate and patients with lichen sclerosus make up nearly 2% of general gynaecologists' practice [7]. In Wallace's [8] series of 359 patients, females outnumbered males by 10:1. Approximately 20% of patients with lichen sclerosus of the vulva had lesions on the trunk [9]. Certainly, involvement of the vulva, perineum and perianal skin in females is more common than balanitis xerotica obliterans, which is the corresponding lesion in the adult male. The condition occurs particularly around and after the menopause, but also occurs in girls between the ages of approximately 1 and 13 years. The disease is not uncommon in boys with phimosis [9], and the incidence is probably underestimated. The mean age of onset in one series of cases [10] was 50 for females and 43 for males. The condition has been seen in mother and daughter, mother and son, brother and sister, and sisters and brothers, but not in father and son. It has occurred in monozygotic female twins [11] and in non-identical female twins [12].

References

1 Tasker GL, Wojnarowska F. Lichen sclerosus. *Clin Exp Dermatol* 2003; **28**: 128–33.
2 Howard R, Tsuchiya A. Adult skin disease in the pediatric patient. *Dermatol Clin* 1998; **16**: 593–608.
3 Hallopeau H. Lichen plan, atrophique. *Ann Dermatol Syphiligr* 1887; **8**: 790–4.
4 Darier J. Lichen sclerosus. *Ann Dermatol Syphiligr* 1892; **3**: 833.
5 Bizzozero E. Scleroderma guttata, lichen sclerosus, kraurosis penis. *Arch Dermatol Syphilol* 1943; **183**: 493.
6 Pugliese JM, Morey AF, Peterson AC. Lichen sclerosus: review of the literature and current recommendations for management. *J Urol* 2007; **178**: 2268–76.
7 Goldstein AT, Marinoff SC, Christopher K, Srodon M. Prevalence of vulvar lichen sclerosus in a general gynecology practice. *J Reprod Med* 2005; **50**: 477–80.
8 Wallace HJ, Whimster I. Vulval atrophy and leukoplakia. *Br J Dermatol* 1951; **63**: 241–57.
9 Kiss A, Kiraly L, Kutasy B, Merksz M. High incidence of balanitis xerotica obliterans in boys with phimosis: prospective 10-year study. *Pediatr Dermatol* 2005; **22**: 305–8.
10 Simpkin S, Oakley A. Clinical review of 202 patients with vulval lichen sclerosus: a possible association with psoriasis. *Australas J Dermatol* 2007; **48**: 28–31.
11 Meyrick Thomas RH, Kennedy CTC. The development of lichen sclerosus et atrophicus in monozygotic twin girls. *Br J Dermatol* 1986; **114**: 377–9.
12 Cox NH, Mitchell JNS, Morley WN. Lichen sclerosus et atrophicus in non-identical female twins. *Br J Dermatol* 1986; **115**: 743–6.

Aetiology [1]. The aetiology is unknown, lesions usually appearing spontaneously without any precipitating factor. The predominance of females, the frequent onset around the menopause and the spontaneous improvement in girls after puberty suggest a hormonal factor, but no convincing causative factors have been identified.

The increased prevalence of organ-specific antibodies and of associated autoimmune diseases in both female patients and relatives suggest an autoimmune cause, but there is no difference in the natural history of those with or without antibodies [2]. The incidence of other autoimmune diseases in patients is highest when the onset is between the ages of 41 and 60 years, but is not related to the site or duration of lesions. Once the diagnosis of lichen sclerosus has been established, patients do not seem to be at continued excessive risk of developing autoimmune diseases [3]. Approximately 50% of female patients will have a personal or family history of autoimmune disease [4]. Male patients also have an increased prevalence of autoimmune disorders and autoantibodies [5]. Associations with HLA types have been inconsistent; HLA-A29 and -B44 were found to occur more frequently, both separately and together [6], but this was not confirmed [4]. The class II antigens DQ7, 8 or 9 were found to be present in 78% of patients [4], and in a large study HLA-DRB112 and its associated haplotype increased susceptibility to vulval disease, whereas DRB10301 conferred protection [7]. In men, HLA-DR11, -DR12 and -DQ7 were found to be positively associated with the development of the disease, and the association with autoimmune disease is less marked than in women [8].

A history of preceding vaginitis and, in the male, the limitation of genital involvement to the uncircumcised or very recently circumcised, who often give a history of chronic balanitis, suggests that infection may play a provocative or localizing part [9]. There may be geographical differences that explain the potential role of *Borrelia*, with evidence of infection found in Germany and Japan but not in the USA [10]. Vulval lesions are not related to parity. Trauma may act as a precipitating factor, and lichen sclerosus has been reported in a vaccination site [11], in the area of radiotherapy following mastectomy [12], after severe sunburn [13], in an old burn scar [14], as a result of welding sparks [15] and at the site of a strawberry naevus [16].

References

1 Tasker GL, Wojnarowska F. Lichen sclerosus. *Clin Exp Dermatol* 2003; **28**: 128–33.
2 Meyrick Thomas RH, Ridley CM, McGibbon DH *et al.* Lichen sclerosus et atrophicus and autoimmunity: a study of 350 women. *Br J Dermatol* 1988; **118**: 41–6.
3 Meyrick Thomas RH, Holmes RC, Rowland Payne CME *et al.* The incidence of development of autoimmune disease in women after the diagnosis of lichen sclerosus et atrophicus. *Br J Dermatol* 1982; **107** (Suppl. 22): 29.
4 Marren P, Yell J, Charnock FM *et al.* The association between lichen sclerosus and antigens of the HLA system. *Br J Dermatol* 1995; **132**: 197–203.
5 Meyrick Thomas RH, Ridley CM, Black MM. The association of lichen sclerosus et atrophicus and autoimmune-related disease in males. *Br J Dermatol* 1983; **109**: 661–4.
6 Purcell KG, Spencer LV, Simpson PM *et al.* HLA antigens in lichen sclerosus et atrophicus. *Arch Dermatol* 1990; **126**: 1043–5.

7 Gao XH, Barnardo MC, Winsey S *et al.* Agudelo JD. Zhai N. Powell JJ. Fuggle SV. Wojnarowska F. The association between HLA DR, DQ antigens, and vulval lichen sclerosus in the UK: HLA DRB112 and its associated DRB112/ DQB10301/04/09/010 haplotype confers susceptibility to vulval lichen sclerosus, and HLA DRB10301/04 and its associated DRB10301/04/DQB10201/02/03 haplotype protects from vulval lichen sclerosus. *J Invest Dermatol* 2005; **125**: 895–9.

8 Azurdia RM, Luzzi GA, Byren I *et al.* Lichen sclerosus in adult men: a study of HLA associations and susceptibility to autoimmune disease. *Br J Dermatol* 1999; **140**: 79–83.

9 Mallon E, Hawkins D, Dinneen M *et al.* Circumcision and genital dermatoses. *Arch Dermatol* 2000; **136**: 350–4.

10 Fujiwara H, Fujiwara K, Hashimoto K *et al.* Detection of *Borrelia burgdorferi* DNA (*B. garinii* or *B. afzelii*) in morphoea and lichen sclerosus et atrophicus tissues of German and Japanese but not US patients. *Arch Dermatol* 1989; **120**: 207–9.

11 Anderton RL, Abele DC. Lichen sclerosus et atrophicus in a vaccination site. *Arch Dermatol* 1976; **112**: 1787.

12 Yates VM, King CM, Dave VK. Lichen sclerosus et atrophicus following radiation therapy. *Arch Dermatol* 1985; **121**: 1044–7.

13 Milligan A, Graham-Brown RAC, Burns DA. Lichen sclerosus et atrophicus following sunburn. *Clin Exp Dermatol* 1988; **13**: 36–7.

14 Meffert JJ, Grimwood RE. Lichen sclerosus et atrophicus appearing in an old burn scar. *J Am Acad Dermatol* 1994; **31**: 671–3.

15 Tegner E, Vrana I. Lichen sclerosus et atrophicus appearing in old scars of burns from welding sparks. *Acta Derm Venereol* 2001; **81**: 211.

16 Ostlere LS, Tildsley G, Holden CA. Lichen sclerosus over a strawberry naevus: a new example of the Koebner phenomenon? *Clin Exp Dermatol* 1996; **21**: 394–5.

Pathology. The striking histological change in lichen sclerosus is a band of hyalinization of the dermal collagen below the epidermis. The hyalinized tissue appears structureless and oedematous, and contains sparse cells, but may show dilated capillaries. The epidermis shows variable thickening, hyperkeratosis and follicular plugging. Later, the epidermis becomes thinned. A band of lymphocytic infiltration may also be seen below the hyalinized area; in older lesions this may be more scanty and focal. The subepidermal elastic tissue tends to be depressed and separated from the epidermis by oedema. The infiltrate contains immunoregulatory lymphocytes [1] which may be self-recruiting [2]. T-cell-mediated inflammation and activation [3] is associated with basement membrane damage and laminin and collagen 4 and 7 over-expression [4]. There is also blood vessel proliferation [5], and over-deposition of dermal connective tissue, including hyaluronate [6], fibrillin, collagens I and III and elastin [7], with abnormal distributions of tenascin, fibronectin and fibrinogen [8]. Androgen receptors are reduced [9].

In vulval lesions, secondary infection and superficial erosion are common, and may mask the primary changes. In lesions with sclerotic change, the epidermis shows marked thickening, irregularity and hyperkeratosis. The dermal oedema tends to regress and sclerosis and dense chronic inflammation occupy the subepidermal zone. These changes are seen in over half of all biopsies of vulval lichen sclerosus, and in two-thirds when there is itching [10].

The condition must be distinguished from lichenification, in which the dermal papillae are prolonged and oedematous, with corresponding lengthening of the rete pegs. There is usually dermal oedema and epidermal spongiosis and parakeratosis. In primary atrophy of the vulva, the epidermis is thinned, the lower border is flattened and keratinization is normal or reduced. There

is also a reduction in the elastic tissue, particularly in the superficial zone, but the collagen is unaltered. Immediately beneath the epidermis there is a band of chronic inflammatory cells. In dysplastic leukoplakia, there is some degree of hyperplasia of the epidermis, with considerable irregularity in the outline of the deeper border, together with some hyperkeratosis. An inflammatory infiltrate occurs near the deeper border of the epidermis. The collagen of the superficial part of the dermis shows hyaline changes and the elastic tissue is lost.

Electron microscopy has revealed striking changes in dermal collagen fibres and increased amounts of elastin [11]. Immunoglobulins (IgG, IgM, IgA), complement and fibrin may be demonstrated in the damaged skin. IgG autoantibodies to the basement membrane zone were found and may be relevant to pathogenesis [12].

References

1 Tchorzewski H, Rotsztejn H, Banasik M *et al.* The involvement of immunoregulatory T cells in the pathogenesis of lichen sclerosus. *Med Sci Monit* 2005; **11**: CR39–43.

2 Wenzel J, Wiechert A, Merkel C *et al.* IP10/CXCL10–CXCR3 interaction: a potential self-recruiting mechanism for cytotoxic lymphocytes in lichen sclerosus et atrophicus. *Acta Derm Venereol* 2007; **87**: 112–7.

3 Hunger RE, Bronnimann M, Kappeler A *et al.* Detection of perforin and granzyme B mRNA expressing cells in lichen sclerosus. *Exp Dermatol* 2007; **16**: 416–20.

4 Cooper SM, Prenter A, Allen J *et al.* The basement membrane zone and dermal extracellular matrix in erosive lichen planus of the vulva: an immunohistochemical study demonstrating altered expression of hemidesmosome components and anchoring fibrils. *Clin Exp Dermatol* 2005; **30**: 277–81.

5 Kowalewski C, Kozlowska A, Gorska M *et al.* Alterations of basement membrane zone and cutaneous microvasculature in morphea and extragenital lichen sclerosus. *Am J Dermatopathol* 2005; **27**: 489–96.

6 Kaya G, Augsburger E, Stamenkovic I *et al.* Decrease in epidermal CD44 expression as a potential mechanism for abnormal hyaluronate accumulation in superficial dermis in lichen sclerosus et atrophicus. *J Invest Dermatol* 2000; **115**: 1054–8.

7 Farrell AM, Dean D, Millard PR *et al.* Alterations in fibrillin as well as collagens I and III and elastin occur in vulval lichen sclerosus. *J Eur Acad Dermatol Venereol* 2001; **15**: 212–7.

8 Farrell AM, Dean D, Charnock FM *et al.* Alterations in distribution of tenascin, fibronectin and fibrinogen in vulval lichen sclerosus. *Dermatology* 2000; **201**: 223–9.

9 Carlson JA, Murphy M. Androgen receptors and lichen sclerosus. *J Am Acad Dermatol* 2000; **43**: 559–60.

10 Wallace HJ. Lichen sclerosus et atrophicus. *Trans St John's Hosp Dermatol Soc* 1971; **57**: 9–30.

11 Mann PR, Cowan MA. Ultrastructural changes in four cases of lichen sclerosus et atrophicus. *Br J Dermatol* 1973; **89**: 223–31.

12 Howard A, Dean D, Cooper S *et al.* Circulating basement membrane zone antibodies are found in lichen sclerosus of the vulva. *Australas J Dermatol* 2004; **45**: 12–5.

Clinical features [1]

Non-genital lesions. The lesions on the skin are symptomless and occur on the trunk, particularly on the upper part and around the umbilicus, around the neck, in the axillae, on the flexor surfaces of the wrists (Fig. 51.77), around the eye and, very rarely, on the scalp, palms and soles [2]. They have also been described confined to the skin around the areolae [3]. Lesions can occur at sites of pressure (e.g. underneath bra straps or belts). The lesions are small, ivory or porcelain-white, shiny, round macules or papules,

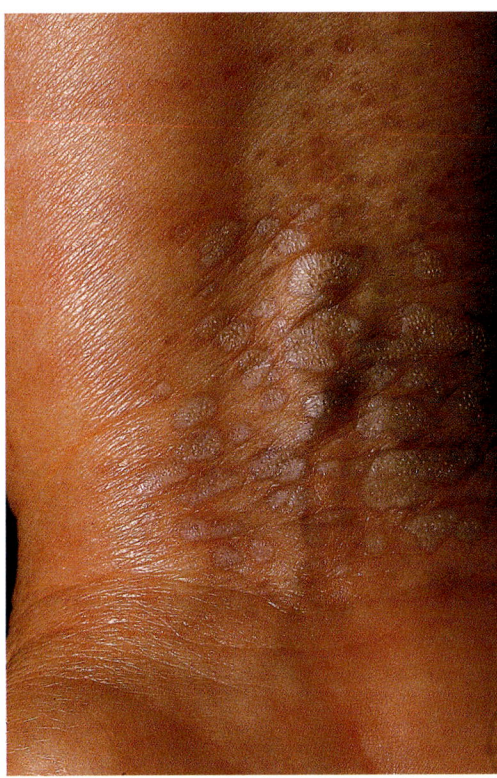

Fig. 51.77 Lichen sclerosus of the front of the wrist.

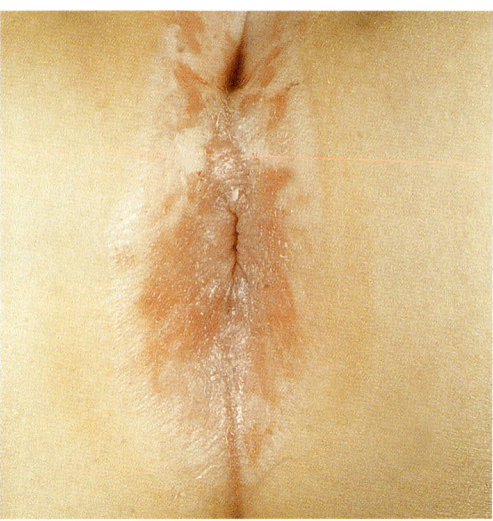

Fig. 51.78 Lichen sclerosus of the vulva and adjacent skin. (Courtesy of Professor J.L. Burton, Bristol, UK.)

7 Leppard B, Sneddon IB. Milia occurring in lichen sclerosus et atrophicus. *Arch Dermatol Syphil* 1975; **49**: 57–9.
8 Dalziel K, Reynolds AJ, Holt PJA. Lichen sclerosus et atrophicus with ocular and maxillary complications. *Br J Dermatol* 1987; **116**: 735.
9 Ramrakha-Jones VS, Paul M, McHenry B *et al*. Nail dystrophy due to lichen sclerosus? *Clin Exp Dermatol* 2001; **26**: 507–9.

a few millimetres in diameter, but occasionally, they are semitranslucent and resemble mother-of-pearl. They may be very extensive, involving most of the trunk. Lesions may follow Blaschko's lines [4] even in the face [5]. They are slightly raised, or level with the surface of the skin, and typically their surface shows prominent dilated pilosebaceous or sweat duct orifices, which often contain yellow or brown horny plugs. If the plugging is marked, the surface may be rather warty. Lichenification may occur as a result of rubbing. Occasionally, bullae, which may be very extensive [6], telangiectases and purpura may occur, and resolve leaving milia [7]. In the later stages, atrophy occurs, and the surface of the lesions becomes wrinkled, and may actually be depressed. Usually, lesions are aggregated into plaques, which resemble morphoea, but the individual lesions of lichen sclerosus can nearly always still be identified. Scarring alopecia may occur, and nail disease is reported [8]. Involvement of the tendon sheath of the superior oblique muscle of the eye can give rise to diplopia [9].

References

1 Pugliese JM. Morey AF. Peterson AC. Lichen sclerosus: review of the literature and current recommendations for management. *J Urol* 2007; **178**: 2268–76.
2 Petrozzi JW, Wood MG, Tisa V. Palmar–plantar lichen sclerosus et atrophicus. *Arch Dermatol* 1979; **115**: 884.
3 Starzycki Z. Lichen sclerosus et atrophicus confined to the areolae. *Br J Dermatol* 1993; **129**: 748–9.
4 Choi SW, Yang JE, Park HJ *et al*. A case of extragenital lichen sclerosus following Blaschko's lines. *J Am Acad Dermatol* 2000; **43**: 903–4.
5 Kim YJ, Lee ES. Case of sequentially occurring lesions of facial lichen sclerosus following the lines of Blaschko. *J Dermatol* 2007; **34**: 201–4.
6 Di Silverio A, Serri F. Generalized bullous and haemorrhagic lichen sclerosus et atrophicus. *Br J Dermatol* 1975; **93**: 215–7.

Anogenital lesions in women (see Chapter 71) [1]. The condition most commonly starts between 45 and 60 years of age but is not uncommon in childhood. Lesions occur on the vulva and around the anus, and may extend to the skin of the inner side of the thighs. The ivory-coloured atrophic papules with follicular hyperkeratosis and plugging can often be identified on the vulva but, owing to friction and moisture, the lesions frequently break down to form a red raw surface, resembling macerated intertrigo (Fig. 51.78). Vesicles and bullae, sometimes haemorrhagic, may occur. In other sites, the tops of the papules become smooth and the area becomes flat and glistening. Small telangiectases and purpuric lesions sometimes occur, probably as a result of injury to the atrophic skin. Irritation may be marked, although sometimes—particularly in children—the condition is symptomless (Fig. 51.79). Patients often complain of soreness rather than pruritus, and dyspareunia may be considerable. Atrophy is a feature, and there may be gross shrinkage of the vulva, especially of the clitoris and labia minora. Labial fusion, clitoral burial and labial resorption can all occur. The vaginal introitus may become as small as 1 cm in diameter. Despite this, pregnancy and delivery are uninfluenced [2].

Mouth lesions. Occasionally, lesions are found in the mouth. They consist of bluish-white plaques, usually on the inner surface of the cheek or on the palate. There may be superficial ulceration. Sometimes, a reticulate appearance occurs and is difficult to distinguish clinically from the lesions of lichen planus [3]. The tongue can be involved. The presence of lesions of lichen sclerosus elsewhere is helpful, as biopsies from the mouth are sometimes difficult to interpret.

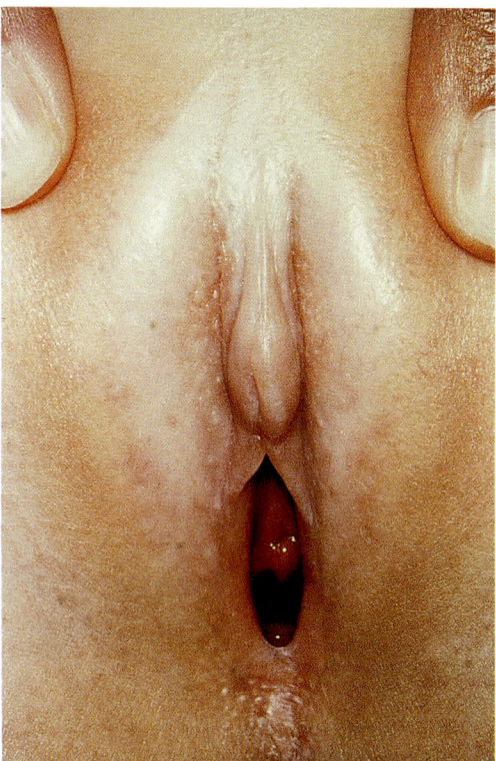

Fig. 51.79 Lichen sclerosus of the vulva in a young girl.

Malignancy in lichen sclerosus. Premalignant and frankly malignant changes can occur in patients with lichen sclerosus, with squamous carcinoma occurring in 5% [4]. It usually arises in a sclerotic area, especially on the anterior part of the vulva (Fig. 51.80). The role of the human papilloma virus in this, as in other genital malignancies, has been discussed, and HPV of the strains associated with carcinogenesis has been found in pre-pubertal females with lichen sclerosus [5].

In a review of 83 cases of squamous cell carcinoma of the vulva [6], two patients with lichen sclerosus were found. Paget's disease may rarely occur in cases of lichen sclerosus of the vulva.

Lichen sclerosus in the male (balanitis xerotica obliterans) (Fig. 51.81) (see Chapter 71). Acquired phimosis or recurrent balanitis are the presenting features [7], together with itching and soreness, and erection may be painful. The prepuce becomes sclerotic and cannot be retracted. Ulceration of the foreskin can occur. The glans and undersurface of the prepuce are shining and bluish white, and there can be considerable telangiectasia. There may be back pressure affecting the urinary tract, demonstrated by urography, as a result of meatal closure. This may require surgical correction [8]. Urethral disease may occur, and lichen sclerosus was found in 14% of 925 patients with urethral stenosis [9]. The shaft of the penis is only occasionally involved. The condition is most common between the ages of 15 and 50 years. It can be overlooked in boys unless the prepuce is examined histologically in cases of circumcision for acquired phimosis. It was found in 40% of sections from boys, with the maximum frequency in those aged 9–11 [10]. In one series, the condition only occurred in patients not circumcised early in life [11]. Carcinoma may develop, and the condition may be associated with morphoea and vitiligo.

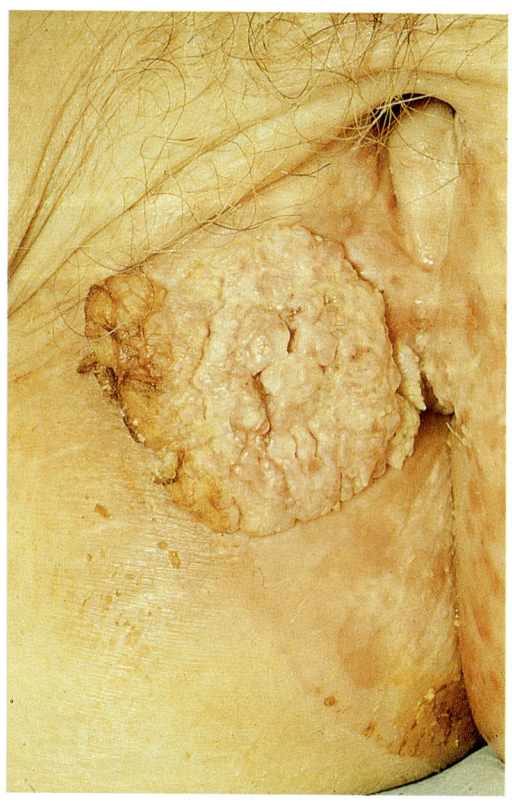

Fig. 51.80 Squamous carcinoma in an area of lichen sclerosus of the vulva.

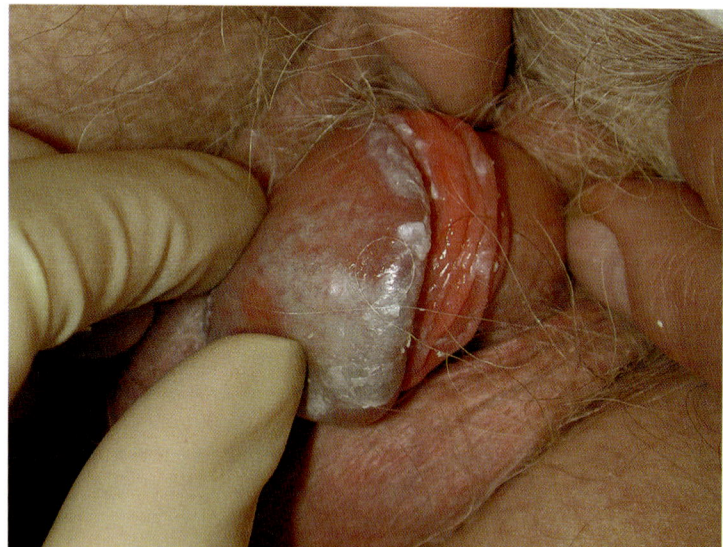

Fig. 51.81 Lichen sclerosus of the penis.

Very rarely, classical macular and papular lesions of lichen sclerosus occur on the glans and shaft of the penis and on the scrotum. The skin remains quite soft compared with the usual sclerotic skin of balanitis xerotica obliterans. Occasionally, classical lesions occur on the trunk.

References

1 Pugliese JM, Morey AF, Peterson AC. Lichen sclerosus: review of the literature and current recommendations for management. *J Urol* 2007; **178**: 2268–76.
2 Ridley CM. Lichen sclerosus et atrophicus. *Arch Dermatol* 1987; **23**: 457–60.

3 Marren P, Millard P, Chia Y *et al.* Mucosal lichen sclerosus/lichen planus overlap syndromes. *Br J Dermatol* 1994; **131**: 118–23.

4 Tasker GL. Wojnarowska. F. Lichen sclerosus. *Clin Exp Dermatol* 2003; **28**: 128–33.

5 Powell J, Strauss S, Gray J, Wojnarowska F. Genital carriage of human papilloma virus (HPV) DNA in prepubertal girls with and without vulval disease. *Pediatr Dermatol* 2003; **20**: 191–4.

6 Janovski NA, Ames S. Lichen sclerosus et atrophicus of the vulva. *Obstet Gynecol* 1963; **22**: 697–708.

7 Meyrick Thomas RH, Ridley CM, Black MM. Clinical features and therapy of lichen sclerosus et atrophicus affecting males. *Clin Exp Dermatol* 1987; **12**: 126–8.

8 Larregue M, Valayer P, Cavaroc Y *et al.* Lichen sclerosus and meatal stenosis in a child. *Ann Dermatol Vénéréol* 1989; **116**: 813–4.

9 Barbagli G, Palminteri E, Balo S *et al.* Lichen sclerosus of the male genitalia and urethral stricture diseases. *Urol Int* 2004; **73**: 1–5.

10 Kiss A, Kiraly L, Kutasy B, Merksz M. High incidence of balanitis xerotica obliterans in boys with phimosis: prospective 10-year study. *Pediatr Dermatol* 2005; **22**: 305–8.

11 Ledwig PA, Weigand DA. Late circumcision and lichen sclerosus et atrophicus of the penis. *J Am Acad Dermatol* 1989; **20**: 211–4.

Lichen sclerosus in female children [1].

The disorder is much less common in children than in adults. Published series show from 2% [2] to 15% [3] of cases begin before the age of 13 years. The earliest reported age of onset was at 6 months [4]. In Wallace's series [5], 28 of 50 started between the ages of 3 and 6 years. In this group, HLA associations are seen more frequently, although these may vary [6].

General health remains normal, and often the condition is symptomless. A vaginal discharge may precede the vulval lesions in approximately 20%, and pruritus vulvae occurs in approximately half of cases. Other presentations include pain on defecation and dysuria, resulting in constipation, nocturia and nocturnal enuresis as well as rectorrhagia [6]. Lesions have followed trauma (e.g. in operation scars and in scratch marks). The individual lesions are identical to those seen in the adult [1]. The vulva and anal region may be encircled in a figure-of-eight pattern, and shrinking of the labia and stenosis of the introitus may be marked. Follicular plugging and delling are usually absent from areas of the vulva with few or no hair follicles. Vesicles and excoriations occur. The condition may be misdiagnosed as sexual abuse [7], causing much anxiety [8], but there are suggestions that sexual abuse may precipitate the condition as a Koebner phenomenon [9]. Abnormal hirsutism may be seen on the inner side of the labia majora, disappearing with resolution of the lichen sclerosus [5]. In approximately 5% of cases, the lesions are solely outside the anogenital region, and in just over 10% lesions are found both in the anogenital region and elsewhere.

The prognosis through childhood has been studied [1]; symptoms improve, but abnormal signs persist in 75% and long-term follow-up is advised. Extragenital lesions usually clear before the menarche [5].

References

1 Poindexter G, Morrell DS. Anogenital pruritus: lichen sclerosus in children. *Pediatr Ann* 2007; **36**: 785–91.

2 Montgomery H, Hill WR. Lichen sclerosus et atrophicus. *Arch Dermatol Syphilol* 1940; **42**: 755–79.

3 Chernosky ME, Derbes VJ, Burks JW. Lichen sclerosus et atrophicus in children. *Arch Dermatol* 1957; **75**: 647–52.

4 Ridley CM. Lichen sclerosus et atrophicus. *Arch Dermatol* 1987; **123**: 457–60.

5 Wallace HJ. Lichen sclerosus et atrophicus. *Trans St John's Hosp Dermatol Soc* 1951; **57**: 9–30.

6 Powell J, Wojnarowska F, Winsey S *et al.* Lichen sclerosus premenarche: autoimmunity and immunogenetics. *Br J Dermatol* 2000; **142**: 481–4.

7 Handfield-Jones SE, Hinde FRJ, Kennedy CTC. Lichen sclerosus et atrophicus in children misdiagnosed as sexual abuse. *BMJ* 1988; **294**: 404–15.

8 Berth-Jones J, Graham-Brown RAC, Burns DA. Lichen sclerosus et atrophicus: a review of 15 cases in young girls. *Clin Exp Dermatol* 1991; **16**: 14–7.

9 Warrington SA, de San Lazaro C. Lichen sclerosus et atrophicus and sexual abuse. *Arch Dis Child* 1996; **75**: 512–6.

Laboratory investigations. Approximately three-quarters of female patients have one or more organ-specific autoantibodies [1,2], usually to thyroid microsomes, thyroglobulin, gastric parietal cells or intrinsic factor. The prevalence in males is approximately half that in females, and the antibodies are mainly to smooth muscle and gastric parietal cells [3].

References

1 Harrington CI, Dunsmore IR. An investigation into the incidence of autoimmune disorders in patients with lichen sclerosus and atrophicus. *Br J Dermatol* 1981; **104**: 563–6.

2 Meyrick Thomas RH, Holmes RC, Rowland Payne CME *et al.* The incidence of development of autoimmune diseases in women after the diagnosis of lichen sclerosus et atrophicus. *Br J Dermatol* 1982; **107** (Suppl. 22): 2.

3 Meyrick Thomas RH, Ridley CM, Black MM. The association of lichen sclerosus et atrophicus and autoimmune-related disease in males. *Br J Dermatol* 1983; **109**: 661–4.

Differential diagnosis. Lichen sclerosus of the trunk must be distinguished from plaques of morphoea, but this is rarely difficult in the presence of characteristic papules with follicular plugging. Lichen planus is distinguished by its raised, itchy, violaceous papules. The atrophic form of lichen planus may simulate lichen sclerosus quite closely [1]. Lesions of lichen sclerosus may sometimes occur in association with patches of morphoea and, in some patients, typical plaque morphoea may resolve to leave the white sclerotic features of lichen sclerosus. In patients with vulval lesions, a search should be made for lesions elsewhere on the trunk, but even if none is present, the margins of the affected area of the vulva or the perianal area usually show a few typical papules, sometimes forming a well-defined edge. The differential diagnosis of the genital lesions is discussed in Chapter 71. Vulval cicatricial pemphigoid may mimic lichen sclerosus [2]. The annular atrophic plaque type of DLE on the face may resemble lesions of lichen sclerosus [3].

References

1 Connelly MG, Winkelmann RK. Coexistence of lichen sclerosus, morphoea, and lichen planus. *J Am Acad Dermatol* 1985; **12**: 844–51.

2 Marren P, Walkden V, Mallon E, Wojnarowska F. Vulval cicatricial pemphigoid may mimic lichen sclerosus. *Br J Dermatol* 1996; **134**: 522–4.

3 Chorzelski TP, Jablonska S, Blaszczyk M *et al.* Annular atrophic plaques of the face. *Arch Dermatol* 1976; **112**: 1143–5.

Prognosis [1,2]. Lichen sclerosus is a chronic condition, but signs and symptoms may wax and wane. It is usually permanent but, occasionally, spontaneous resolution occurs. This is particularly likely in girls around the menarche. Resolution of cases appearing after puberty is uncommon, and is probably restricted to extragenital lesions arising before the age of 30 years.

References

1 Powell J, Wojnarowska F. Childhood vulvar lichen sclerosus. The course after puberty. *J Reprod Med* 2002; **47**: 706–9.
2 Simpkin S, Oakley A. Clinical review of 202 patients with vulval lichen sclerosus: a possible association with psoriasis. *Australas J Dermatol* 2007; **48**: 28–31.

Treatment. The British Association of Dermatologists provide guidelines covering the management of lichen sclerosus [1]. There is no confirmed effective treatment for extragenital lesions. Calcipotriol may be helpful [2], and phototherapy, including narrowband UVB [3] and low-dose UVA-1 [4], has been reported to be of benefit. Mycophenolate mofetil was dramatically effective in one severe case seen by the authors.

For genital lesions, there is increasing evidence that the use of potent topical steroid preparations gives both symptomatic relief and prevents scarring, and may induce complete resolution of the problem, both histologically and immunohistologically [5]. Whether this is of long-term benefit remains to be seen [6]. Oestrogen- [7] or testosterone- [8] containing creams have given symptomatic benefit, but testosterone is less effective than topical steroid [9]. No report suggests histological resolution with their use. Topical tacrolimus [10] and pimecrolimus [11] may have a role, but there are anxieties about reactivation of wart virus infection [12]. Potassium *p*-aminobenzoate, 12 g/day in divided doses, is claimed to have helped symptoms and haemorrhagic bullae, and softened the skin in some cases [13]. Etretinate may have helped both adult [14] and juvenile cases [15] and ciclosporin may be of benefit [16]. Sulfasalazine has helped a solitary case [17]. Creams containing local anaesthetic preparations should not be prescribed because of the risk of sensitization. Superficial radiation or painting with thorium X are no longer used, and are potentially dangerous.

Vulvectomy is contraindicated for uncomplicated vulval lichen sclerosus, as recurrence occurs in approximately 80% of patients. Dysplastic change should at first be treated conservatively and observed regularly. Applications of liquid nitrogen may be useful, but treatment with a nitrous oxide cryoprobe has been found to be more satisfactory [18]. The carbon dioxide laser is also effective for genital lesions in both males and females [19]. Photodynamic therapy has been used to treat vulvar disease [20]. Radical surgery is obviously required if a carcinoma develops. Surgery may also be required for severe narrowing of the introitus.

Topical corticosteroids, sometimes for short periods under a condom, or intralesional injections of triamcinolone may soften the sclerotic lesions of balanitis xerotica obliterans and reduce the phimosis. Circumcision may be helpful or even curative if the condition involves only the foreskin [21]. Meatal instillation of corticosteroid may help meatal narrowing. Attention to local hygiene and treatment of balanitis may be required.

References

1 Neill SM, Tatnall FM, Cox NH. British Association of Dermatologists. Guidelines for the management of lichen sclerosus. *Br J Dermatol* 2002; **147**: 640–9.

2 Kreuter A, Gambichler T, Sauermann K *et al.* Extragenital lichen sclerosus successfully treated with topical calcipotriol: evaluation by *in vivo* confocal laser scanning microscopy. *Br J Dermatol* 2002; **146**: 332–3.
3 Colbert RL, Chiang MP, Carlin CS, Fleming M. Progressive extragenital lichen sclerosus successfully treated with narrowband UV-B phototherapy. *Arch Dermatol* 2007; **143**: 19–20.
4 Beattie PE, Dawe RS, Ferguson J, Ibbotson SH. UVA1 phototherapy for genital lichen sclerosus. *Clin Exp Dermatol* 2006; **31**: 343–7.
5 Dalziel KL, Millard PR, Wojnarowska F. The treatment of vulval lichen sclerosus with a very potent topical steroid (clobetasol propionate 0.05%). *Br J Dermatol* 1991; **124**: 461–4.
6 Renaud-Vilmer C, Cavelier-Balloy B, Porcher R, Dubertret L. Vulvar lichen sclerosus: effect of long-term topical application of a potent steroid on the course of the disease. *Arch Dermatol* 2004; **140**: 709–12.
7 Lascano EF, Montes LF, Mazzini MA. Lichen sclerosus et atrophicus in childhood. *Obstet Gynecol* 1964; **24**: 872–7.
8 Pasieczny TAH. The treatment of balanitis xerotica obliterans with testosterone propionate ointment. *Acta Derm Venereol (Stockh)* 1977; **57**: 275–7.
9 Capobianco G, Dessole S, Cossu A *et al.* Receptor modifications in vulvar dystrophies before and after treatment with topical hormones: comparison between the dextran-charcoal technique and immunohistochemical evaluation. *Eur J Gynaecol Oncol* 2006; **27**: 411–3.
10 Hengge UR, Krause W, Hofmann H *et al.* Multicentre, phase II trial on the safety and efficacy of topical tacrolimus ointment for the treatment of lichen sclerosus. *Br J Dermatol* 2006; **155**: 1021–8.
11 Nissi R, Eriksen H, Risteli J, Niemimaa M. Pimecrolimus cream 1% in the treatment of lichen sclerosus. *Gynecol Obstet Invest* 2007; **63**: 151–4.
12 Powell J, Strauss S, Gray J, Wojnarowska F. Genital carriage of human papilloma virus (HPV) DNA in prepubertal girls with and without vulval disease. *Pediatr Dermatol* 2003; **20**: 191–4.
13 Penneys NS. Treatment of lichen sclerosus with potassium paraaminobenzoate. *J Am Acad Dermatol* 1984; **10**: 1039.
14 Mork SJ, Jensen P, Hoel PS. Lichen sclerosus et atrophicus treated with etretinate (Tigason). *Acta Derm Venereol (Stockh)* 1986; **66**: 363–5.
15 Neuhofer J, Fritsch P. Treatment of localized scleroderma and lichen sclerosus with etretinate. *Acta Derm Venereol (Stockh)* 1984; **64**: 171–4.
16 Bulbul B, Turan H, Tunali S *et al.* Open-label trial of ciclosporine for vulvar lichen sclerosus. *J Am Acad Dermatol* 2007; **57**: 276–8.
17 Taveira M, Selores M, Costa V *et al.* Generalized morphea and lichen sclerosus et atrophicus successfully treated with sulphasalazine. *J Eur Acad Dermatol Venereol* 1999; **12**: 283–4.
18 August PJ, Milward TM. Cryosurgery in the treatment of lichen sclerosus et atrophicus of the vulva. *Br J Dermatol* 1980; **103**: 667–70.
19 Kartamaa M, Reitamo S. Treatment of lichen sclerosus with carbon dioxide laser vaporization. *Br J Dermatol* 1997; **136**: 356–9.
20 Romero A, Hernandez-Nunez A, Cordoba-Guijarro S *et al.* Treatment of recalcitrant erosive vulvar lichen sclerosus with photodynamic therapy. *J Am Acad Dermatol* 2007; **57** (Suppl. 2): S46–7.
21 Meyrick Thomas RH, Ridley CM, Black MM. Clinical features and therapy of lichen sclerosus et atrophicus affecting males. *Clin Exp Dermatol* 1987; **12**: 126–8.

Scleroedema

Synonyms
- Scleroedema adultorum
- Scleroedema of Buschke

Although the name of Buschke [1] is usually associated with this condition, it was originally described by Piffard in 1876. The older term, 'scleroedema adultorum', is incorrect, as the condition can occur in childhood: 29% of cases start before the age of 10 years, and a further 22% between the ages of 10 and 20 years [2].

Definition. A rare disorder of unknown cause in which areas of induration appear in the skin, frequently after an infection but also in diabetes, and spontaneously clear in months or years. There is an excess of acid mucopolysaccharides in the dermis.

Aetiology. The aetiology is unknown. Suggestions that have been considered include obstruction to lymphatic channels by inflammation, streptococcal hypersensitivity and neurohumoral disorders. Sera from patients with paraproteinaemia stimulate collagen production in dermal fibroblast cultures [3]. Some persistent cases are associated with moderate to severe diabetes mellitus [4], and both skin and diabetes are resistant to treatment. This persistent type, with no preceding infection and a strong association with diabetes, has been called scleroedema diutinum [5].

Histology. The epidermis is normal. The dermis may be three times its normal thickness. There is swelling and splitting of the dermal collagen bundles by an increase in ground substance. Clear unstained spaces, or fenestrations, occur between the bundles in severe cases. This process extends into the subcutaneous tissues, the fat of which is replaced by coarse collagen fibres. The ground substance stains metachromatically with cresyl violet or toluidine blue. Metachromasia in scleroedema is caused by the presence of hyaluronic acid [6], and is poorly seen in formalin-fixed sections as the hyaluronic acid is removed by the fixative, and in tissues treated by hyaluronidase. There is an excess of acid mucopolysaccharides, but neutral polysaccharides are normal. Mast cells may be increased [7]. Electron microscopy [8] shows an excess of interfibrillary material, and this is associated with clumping of the collagen fibrils. The voluntary muscle and heart may be affected. Deposition of IgG, IgM and C3 at the dermal–epidermal junction has been reported.

References
1 Buschke A. Vorstellung eines Falles von Skleroderm vor der Berliner Gesellschaft fur Dermatologie. *Arch Dermatol Syphilol* 1900; **53**: 83–4.
2 von Graevenitz N. Ueber einen Fall on Skleredema adultorum Buschke. *Monatschr Kinderheilk* 1928; **39**: 257.
3 Ohta A, Uitto J, Oikarinen AI *et al.* Paraproteinemia in patients with scleroedema. *J Am Acad Dermatol* 1987; **16**: 96–107.
4 Meguerditchian C, Jacquet P, Beliard S *et al.* Scleredema adultorum of Buschke: an under-recognised skin complication of diabetes. *Diabetes Metab* 2006; **32**: 481–4.
5 Binkley GW. Scleredema adultorum of Buschke. *Arch Dermatol* 1969; **99**: 124–5.
6 Braun-Falco O. Neueres zur Histopathologie des Scleredema adultorum (Buschke). *Dermatol Wochenschr* 1952; **125**: 409–14.
7 Fleischmajer R, Lara JV. Scleredema. *Arch Dermatol* 1965; **92**: 643–52.
8 Teller H, Vester G. Elektronenmikroskopische Untersuchungsergebnisse an der Interzellularsubstanz des Coriums beim Skleroedema adultorum (Buschke). *Z Haut Geschlkrankh* 1957; **23**: 142.

Clinical features. The condition is uncommon [1]. Occasional familial cases have been reported [2]. Females are more frequently affected than males in patients without diabetes, but scleroedema associated with diabetes occurs predominantly in males [3].

Although the condition may apparently start spontaneously, there is a history of an infectious episode, from a few days to 6 weeks prior to onset, in 65–90% [4] of cases. It is usually influenza, tonsillitis, pharyngitis, measles, mumps, scarlet fever, impetigo or cellulitis; prior streptococcal infections appear to be particularly common. Sometimes, there is a history of trauma. Prodromal symptoms of slight fever, malaise, muscle and joint pains occasionally occur between the infectious episode and the onset of induration. The latter is usually symmetrical and often starts on the back and sides of the neck or on the face. This loses its expression, and the patient notices difficulty in wrinkling the forehead and in smiling. There may be difficulty in opening the mouth. The tongue and pharynx may be involved, with difficulty in swallowing. Later, the shoulders, arms, hands and upper trunk become involved, but less frequently the abdomen and legs may be affected. The condition can be limited to the thighs [5]. The induration is non-pitting and hard, and there is no sharp demarcation between normal and abnormal skin. Wrinkling occurs when the skin is compressed between the thumb and index finger, indicating that the epidermis is spared. Brownish pigmentation can be widespread in the indurated areas [6]. The onset is more insidious in diabetics, and the skin induration may be preceded by erythema or pustules [7]. Sometimes, there is stiffness and restriction of movement of joints. Pleural and pericardial effusions sometimes occur, and the skeletal and cardiac muscles can be affected. Occasionally, there are ocular manifestations. The parotid glands may be involved [8].

References
1 Parmar RC, Bavdekar SB, Bansal S *et al.* Scleredema adultorum. *J Postgrad Med* 2000; **46**: 91–3.
2 Venencie PY, Powell FC, Su WP, Perry HO. Scleroedema: a review of 33 cases. *J Am Acad Dermatol* 1984; **11**: 128–34.
3 Meguerditchian C, Jacquet P, Beliard S *et al.* Scleredema adultorum of Buschke: an under-recognised skin complication of diabetes. *Diabetes Metab* 2006; **32**: 481–4.
4 Ince A, Moore TL. Scleredema adultorum of Buschke: a case report and review of the literature. *Semin Arthritis Rheum* 2006; **35**: 355–9.
5 Farrell AM, Branfoot AC, Moso J *et al.* Scleredema diabeticorum of Buschke confined to the thighs. *Br J Dermatol* 1996; **134**: 1113–5.
6 McFadden N, Ree K, Soyland E *et al.* Scleredema adultorum associated with a monoclonal gammopathy and generalized hyperpigmentation. *Arch Dermatol* 1987; **123**: 629–32.
7 Parker SC, Fenton DA, Black MM. Scleredema. *Clin Exp Dermatol* 1989; **14**: 385–6.
8 Madison LL. Scleredema. *Am J Med* 1950; **9**: 707–13.

Laboratory investigations. The ESR may be moderately elevated, and the serum proteins usually show mild, non-specific abnormalities. IgG [1], usually IgG-kappa, and IgA paraproteinaemia [2,3], have been reported. Hyperlipoproteinaemia has been reported [4], and the antistreptolysin-O titre may be raised, especially in children.

Prognosis. The condition may completely disappear in the course of some months to a few years, but a few may persist for many years. One case [5] still had changes 38 years after the onset. A fatal case occurred following the development of IgA myeloma [4].

Differential diagnosis. The condition is usually easy to diagnose in view of the rapidity of the onset, especially if there has been a

Table 51.19 Conditions associated with scleroedema.

Malignant insulinoma [6]
Paraproteinaemia and multiple myeloma [7]
Waldenström's macroglobulinaemia [8]
Rheumatoid arthritis and Sjögren's syndrome [9]
Primary hyperparathyroidism [10]
Anaphylactoid purpura [11]

history of preceding infection. Localized and generalized morphoea are usually of much slower onset, and the ivory sclerotic areas, with a well-defined and, frequently, lilac-coloured border, are characteristic. Systemic sclerosis is usually preceded by Raynaud's phenomenon. Dermatomyositis may present more difficulty, as cutaneous oedema is a feature of both conditions. However, the presence of heliotrope cyanosis, particularly around the eyes, dilatation of nail fold capillaries and muscle weakness should distinguish the condition. Pseudoscleroderma (induration of the legs as a result of chronic oedema) and localized myxoedema should rarely cause confusion. Trichinosis may have to be considered. In the newborn, sclerema and subcutaneous fat necrosis differ in their mode of onset and course. For associated conditions see Table 51.19.

Treatment. No effective remedy is known, although multiple therapies have been tried, including systemic and intralesional corticosteroids. In a case associated with multiple myeloma, the skin softened with intravenous pulses of cyclophosphamide and oral prednisolone [12]. Improvement with ciclosporin [13] and electron beam therapy [14] have been reported, and PUVA using psoralen cream [15], UVA1 [16], extracorporeal photophoresis [17] and low-dose methotrexate are more recent suggestions [18].

References

1 Kovary PM, Vakilzadeh F, Macher E et al. Monoclonal gammopathy in scleredema. Arch Dermatol 1981; **117**: 536–9.
2 Hodak E, Tamir R, David M et al. Scleredema adultorum associated with IgG-kappa multiple myeloma: a case report and review of the literature. Clin Exp Dermatol 1988; **13**: 271–4.
3 Pajarre S. Scleredema adultorum Buschke. Acta Derm Venereol (Stockh) 1975; **55**: 158–9.
4 Sansom JE, Sheehan AL, Kennedy CTC et al. A fatal case of scleredema of Buschke. Br J Dermatol 1994; **130**: 669–70.
5 Fleischmajer R, Lara JV. Scleredema. Arch Dermatol 1965; **92**: 643–52.
6 Matsunaga J, Hara M, Tagami H. Scleredema of Buschke associated with malignant insulinoma. Br J Dermatol 1992; **126**: 527–8.
7 Korting GW, Gilfrich HJ, Meyer zum Buschenfelde KH. Scleredema adultorum associated with multiple myeloma. Arch Dermatol Forsch 1974; **248**: 379.
8 Ratip S, Akin H, Ozdemirli M et al. Scleredema of Buschke associated with Waldenstrom's macroglobulinaemia. Br J Dermatol 2000; **143**: 450–2.
9 Miyagawa S, Dohi K, Tsuruta S et al. Scleredema of Buschke associated with rheumatoid arthritis and Sjögren's syndrome. Br J Dermatol 1989; **121**: 517–20.
10 Berk MA, Lorincz AL. Scleredema adultorum of Buschke and primary hyperparathyroidism. Int J Dermatol 1988; **27**: 647–9.
11 Okuyama R, Tagami H. Scleredema adultorum associated with anaphylactoid purpura. Acta Derm Venereol (Stockh) 1997; **77**: 159–61.
12 Salisbury JA, Shallcross H, Leigh IM. Scleredema of Buschke associated with multiple myeloma. Clin Exp Dermatol 1988; **13**: 269–70.
13 Mattheon-Vakali G, Ioannides D, Thomas T et al. Cyclosporine in scleredema. J Am Acad Dermatol 1996; **35**: 990–1.
14 Angeli-Besson C, Koeppel MC, Jacquet P et al. Electron-beam therapy in scleredema adultorum with associated monoclonal hypergammaglobulinaemia. Br J Dermatol 1994; **130**: 394–7.
15 Grundmann-Kollman M, Ochsendorf F, Zollner TM et al. Cream PUVA therapy for scleredema adultorum. Br J Dermatol 2000; **142**: 1058–9.
16 Tuchinda C, Kerr HA, Taylor CR et al. UVA1 phototherapy for cutaneous diseases: and experience of 92 cases in the United States. Photodermatol Photoimmunol Photomed 2006; **22**: 247–53.
17 Stables GI, Taylor GC, Highet AS. Scleredema associated with paraproteinaemia treated by extracorporeal photopheresis. Br J Dermatol 2000; **142**: 781–3.
18 Seyger MM, van den Hoogen FH, de Mare S et al. A patient with severe scleredema diabeticorum, partially responding to low-dose methotrexate. Dermatology 1999; **198**: 177–9.

Dermatomyositis [1]

Definition. A multisystem disorder mainly affecting skin, muscle and blood vessels in which characteristic erythematous and oedematous changes in the skin are usually associated with muscle weakness and inflammation. Calcinosis is frequent, especially in childhood, and is usually associated with a more favourable prognosis for life, but functional disability may be severe. In adults, the disease is commonly associated with an underlying carcinoma or lymphoma. A wide range of systemic involvement may occur.

Incidence. Dermatomyositis is rarer than SLE, polyarteritis nodosa or systemic sclerosis. It occurs at least twice as frequently in females as in males. The incidence in children under 16 years was estimated as 1.9 per million, with the median age at onset of 6.8 years, and occurring much more frequently in girls (ratio 5:1) [2]. It may occur in infancy [3]. In adult cases, onset is predominantly between the ages of 40 and 60 years. The mean age of onset is later in men than in women [4]. Dermatomyositis affects all races and there is no obvious geographical variation, although it appears to be approximately 10 times more common in the Bantu than in the white population of the Transvaal [5].

Aetiology. The cause is not known, but there is increasing evidence of early blood vessel damage, probably humorally mediated [6]. There may be significant titres of antiendothelial cell antibodies, particularly in those patients with pulmonary involvement [7]. However, a range of factors may be relevant (Table 51.20).

Genetic factors. Familial disease is unusual [8,9], but has been found in identical twins and in first cousins. A genetic factor is suggested by the increased incidence of HLA-B8 in childhood dermatomyositis in white people but not in black people [10], and -DR3 [11] and -B14 in adult patients [12]. Other HLA haplotypes

Table 51.20 Factors important in the aetiology of dermatomyositis.

Genetics
Infections
Autoimmunity
Malignancy
Others: drugs, trauma

Table 51.21 Infections associated with dermatomyositis.

Toxoplasmosis (raised IgM antibodies) [18]
Staphylococcal osteomyelitis and arthritis [19]
Streptococcal infection (antigenic homology) [20]
Parvovirus B19 [21]
Coxsackie B virus [22]

may be associated with pulmonary disease [13]. There are associations with other type I and type II major histocompatability antigens: DRB1*0301 is a risk factor for juvenile disease, but there are also protective alleles within the DQA 1 domain [14].

Dermatomyositis has been reported in a patient with recessively inherited absence of the second component of complement (C2) [15], and antinuclear antibodies occur in a significant percentage of first-degree relatives of patients with dermatomyositis and polymyositis [16].

Infection [17]. The disorder is not consistently caused by any one infection, vaccination, immunization or drugs, but occasional cases seem to follow such events [22,23]. The infections commonly associated with the onset of dermatomyositis are indicated in Table 51.21. For *Toxoplasma* and the staphylococcal infections, treatment of the infection may produce remission of the dermatomyositis. In childhood disease, the occurrence of symptoms of respiratory or gastrointestinal infection often precedes onset of the disease [17].

Immunological abnormalities. In childhood disease, dermatomyositis appears to be a true autoimmune disorder, whereas with increasing age there is a very significant relationship with malignancy, possibly as a result of an immunological response to the neoplasm. Granular deposits of IgG, IgM and C3, alone or in combination, have been described in the walls of skeletal muscle blood vessels, especially in childhood dermatomyositis [24], and cutaneous hypersensitivity to intradermal injections of tumour extracts, but not normal tissue, has been described [25]. In some patients, myopathy seems to have been mediated by an IgGκ paraprotein with antimuscle specificity [26]. It is not clear whether paraneoplastic dermatomyositis is the same entity as the condition occurring without an associated cancer.

Autoantibodies [27]. Several precipitating autoantibodies have been demonstrated, including PM-1, Jo-1, PL-12 and, in Japanese patients, KU. There are also antibodies directed against specific myositis-related antigens, for example p155 and p155/140. Jo-1 and PL-12 antibodies are directed against tRNA synthetase enzymes and are associated with interstitial pulmonary fibrosis, and the antibody may be detected before the appearance of the lung disease [28]. It has been suggested that Jo-1 production may be linked to HLA-DR3. Patients with Jo-1 antibodies tend to have an onset of symptoms between February and July; this is not the case for the other serological subgroups of the disease [29]. In those with malignancy, there may be complement-fixing antibodies to their own tumour [30], and circulating immune complexes have been demonstrated in 70% of patients [31].

Cell-mediated immunity. There is evidence that polymyositis may be caused by lymphocyte-mediated hypersensitivity. Large numbers of T lymphocytes can be demonstrated in the infiltrates in the muscle, and there is a marked decrease of suppressor/cytotoxic cells in the blood [32]. Lymphocytes from patients with dermatomyositis and polymyositis have shown an increased response to muscle antigen in lymphocyte-stimulation tests, and the index of response showed some correlation with clinical activity. Lymphocytes from patients with dermatomyositis were cytotoxic to muscle cultures, and this cytotoxic action could be prevented by antilymphocyte serum [33].

Cytokines. Soluble CD30 levels are increased, indicating activation of T lymphocytes [34], and soluble TNF receptors are found [35]. An increased frequency of the more inflammatory polymorphisms of the TNF-α gene is found [36]. Soluble IL-2 receptor is elevated in juvenile disease [37], and expression of interferon-inducible genes in blood reflects disease activity [38].

Relationship to malignancy. Several possible mechanisms to account for the relationship with malignancy can be envisaged, but these are mainly speculative at present. Tumours are known to differ antigenically from the tissues from which they are derived, and many myositis-related antigens are expressed by tumours, possibly triggering an autoimmune response directed against muscle [39].

The primary tumour most commonly occurs in the lung, breast, female genital tract, stomach, rectum, kidney or testis. The association with a range of tumours has been reviewed [39]. In the Chinese, nasopharyngeal carcinoma accounted for 75% of malignant disease [40]. Dermatomyositis precedes the neoplasm in 40%, both conditions may occur together (26%) or the neoplasm may occur first (34%) [41]. The incidence of carcinoma in association with dermatomyositis varies from 15 to 34%. Using strict criteria, 26% of adult patients with dermatomyositis were found to have a malignancy [42]. This figure may be higher in the elderly. Patients with dermatomyositis are more likely to have a malignancy than those with polymyositis, and usually do not fare so well. Neoplasia is not associated with childhood cases. Usually, dermatomyositis worsens in parallel with the progress of the neoplasm, but it may improve when the latter is treated. Neoplasia may be missed because of failure to reinvestigate relapse of previously stable dermatomyositis [43].

Other aetiological agents. Preceding heavy muscular exertion and stress have been suggested as triggering factors [6]. Polymyositis and dermatomyositis can occur with penicillamine therapy, and may be fatal as a result of cardiac involvement [44]. A possible relationship to tamoxifen therapy for carcinoma of the breast has been reported [45]. One patient developed dermatomyositis after taking oral progesterone for dysmenorrhoea.

References

1 Lindsley CB. Juvenile dermatomyositis update. *Curr Rheumatol Rep* 2006; **8**: 174–7.
2 Symmons DPM, Sills JA, Davis SM. The incidence of juvenile dermatomyositis: results from a nationwide study. *Br J Rheumatol* 1995; **34**: 732–6.

3 Carlisle JW, Good RA. Dermatomyositis in childhood: report of studies on several cases and review of the literature. *Lancet* 1959; **79**: 266–73.

4 Degos R, Civatte J, Belaich S *et al.* The prognosis of adult dermatomyositis. *Trans St John's Hosp Dermatol Soc Lond* 1971; **57**: 98–104.

5 Findlay GH, Whiting DA, Sinson IW. Dermatomyositis in the Transvaal and its occurrence in the Bantu. *S Afr Med J* 1969; **43**: 694–7.

6 Lyon MG, Bloch DA, Hollak B *et al.* Predisposing factors in polymyositis–dermatomyositis: results of a nationwide survey. *J Rheumatol* 1989; **16**: 1218–24.

7 Cervera R, Ramirez G, Fernandez-Sola J *et al.* Antibodies to endothelial cells in dermatomyositis: association with interstitial lung disease. *BMJ* 1991; **302**: 880–1.

8 Lambie JA, Duff IF. Familial occurrence of dermatomyositis. *Ann Intern Med* 1963; **59**: 839–47.

9 Tsao CY, Mendell JR, Kissel JT. Dermatomyositis in two siblings and a brief review of familial dermatomyositis. *J Child Neurol* 2002; **17**: 540–2.

10 Friedman JM, Pachman LM, Maryjowski ML *et al.* Immunogenetic studies of juvenile dermatomyositis. *Tissue Antigens* 1983; **21**: 45–9.

11 Song MS, Farber D, Bitton A *et al.* Dermatomyositis associated with celiac disease: response to a gluten-free diet. *Can J Gastroenterol* 2006; **20**: 433–5.

12 Machulla HK, Stein J, Gautsch A *et al.* HLA-A, B, Cw, DRB1, DRB3/4/5, DQB1 in German patients suffering from rapidly progressive periodontitis (RPP) and adult periodontitis (AP). *J Clin Periodontol* 2002; **29**: 573–9.

13 Horiki T, Ichikawa Y, Moriuchi J *et al.* HLA class II haplotypes associated with pulmonary interstitial lesions of polymyositis/dermatomyositis in Japanese patients. *Tissue Antigens* 2002; **59**: 25–30.

14 Mierau R, Dick T, Bartz-Bazzanella P *et al.* Strong association of dermatomyositis-specific Mi-2 autoantibodies with a tryptophan at position 9 of the HLA-DR beta chain. *Arthritis Rheum* 1996; **39**: 868–76.

15 Leddy JP, Griggs RC, Klemperer MR *et al.* Hereditary complement (C2) deficiency with dermatomyositis. *Am J Med* 1975; **58**: 83–91.

16 Valentini G, Improta RDG, Resse M *et al.* Antinuclear antibodies in first-degree relatives of patients with polymyositis–dermatomyositis: analysis of the relationship with HLA haplotypes. *Br J Rheumatol* 1991; **30**: 429–32.

17 Pachman LM, Hayford JR, Hochberg MC *et al.* New-onset juvenile dermatomyositis: comparisons with a healthy cohort and children with juvenile rheumatoid arthritis. *Arthritis Rheum* 1997; **40**: 1526–33.

18 Harland CC, Marsden JR, Vernon SA, Allen BR. Dermatomyositis responding to treatment of associated toxoplasmosis. *Br J Dermatol* 1991; **125**: 76–8.

19 Lane S, Doherty M, Powell RJ. Dermatomyositis following chronic staphylococcal joint sepsis. *Ann Rheum Dis* 1990; **49**: 405–6.

20 Martini A, Ravelli A, Albani S *et al.* Recurrent juvenile dermatomyositis and cutaneous necrotizing arteritis with molecular mimicry between streptococcal type 5 m protein and human skeletal myosin. *J Pediatr* 1992; **121**: 739–42.

21 Crowson AN, Magro CM, Dawood MR. A causal role for parvovirus B19 infection in adult dermatomyositis and other autoimmune syndromes. *J Cutan Pathol* 2000; **27**: 505–15.

22 Christensen ML, Pachman LM, Schneiderman R *et al.* Prevalence of Coxsackie B virus antibodies in patients with juvenile dermatomyositis. *Arthritis Rheum* 1986; **11**: 1365–70.

23 Griggs RC, Karpati G. The pathogenesis of dermatomyositis. *Arch Neurol* 1991; **48**: 21–8.

24 Whitaker JN, Engel WK. Vascular deposits of immunoglobulin and complement in idiopathic inflammatory myopathy. *N Engl J Med* 1972; **286**: 333–8.

25 Curtis AC, Heckaman JH, Wheeler AH. Study of the autoimmune reaction in dermatomyositis. *JAMA* 1961; **178**: 571–3.

26 Kiprov DD, Miller RG. Polymyositis associated with monoclonal gammopathy. *Lancet* 1984; **ii**: 1183–6.

27 Benveniste O, Dubourg O, Herson S. [New classifications and pathophysiology of the inflammatory myopathies]. *Rev Med Interne* 2007; **28**: 603–12.

28 Yoshida S, Akizuki M, Mimori T *et al.* The precipitating antibody to an acidic nuclear protein antigen, the Jo-1, in connective tissue diseases. *Arthritis Rheum* 1983; **26**: 604–11.

29 Leff RL, Burgess SH, Miller FW *et al.* Distinct seasonal patterns in the onset of adult idiopathic inflammatory myopathy in patients with anti-Jo-1 and antisignal recognition particle autoantibodies. *Arthritis Rheum* 1991; **34**: 1391–6.

30 Alexander S, Forman L. Dermatomyositis and carcinoma. *Br J Dermatol* 1968; **80**: 86–9.

31 Behan WMH, Barkas T, Behan PO. Detection of immune complexes in polymyositis. *Acta Neurol Scand* 1982; **65**: 320–4.

32 Behan WMH, Micklem HS, Durward WF. Abnormalities of lymphocyte subsets in polymyositis. *BMJ* 1983; **287**: 181–2.

33 Cambridge G, Stern CM. The uptake of tritium-labelled carnitine by monolayer cultures of human fetal muscle and its potential as a label in cytotoxicity studies. *Clin Exp Immunol* 1981; **43**: 211–9.

34 Yazawa N, Ihn H, Yamane K *et al.* Elevated circulating soluble CD30 levels in patients with polymyositis/dermatomyositis. *Br J Dermatol* 2001; **145**: 676–8.

35 Shimizu T, Tomita Y, Son K *et al.* Elevation of serum soluble tumour necrosis factor receptors in patients with polymyositis and dermatomyositis. *Clin Rheumatol* 2000; **19**: 352–9.

36 Pachman LM, Fedczyna TO, Lechman TS *et al.* Juvenile dermatomyositis: the association of the TNF-α-308A allele and disease chronicity. *Curr Rheumatol Rep* 2001; **3**: 379–86.

37 Kobayashi I, Ono S, Kawamura N *et al.* Elevated serum levels of soluble interleukin-2 receptor in juvenile dermatomyositis. *Pediatr Int* 2001; **43**: 109–11.

38 Walsh RJ, Kong SW, Yao Y *et al.* Type I interferon-inducible gene expression in blood is present and reflects disease activity in dermatomyositis and polymyositis. *Arthritis Rheum* 2007; **56**: 3784–92.

39 Stockton D, Doherty VR, Brewster DH. Risk of cancer in patients with dermatomyositis or polymyositis, and follow-up implications: a Scottish population-based cohort study. *Br J Cancer* 2001; **6**: 41–5.

40 Wong KQ. Dermatomyositis: a clinical investigation of 23 cases in Hong Kong. *Br J Dermatol* 1969; **81**: 544–7.

41 Callen JP. The value of malignancy evaluation in patients with dermatomyositis. *J Am Acad Dermatol* 1982; **6**: 253–9.

42 Callen JP, Hyla JF, Bole GG *et al.* The relationship of dermatomyositis and polymyositis to internal malignancy. *Arch Dermatol* 1980; **116**: 295–8.

43 Cox NH, Lawrence CM, Langtry JAA *et al.* Dermatomyositis: disease associations and an evaluation of screening investigations for malignancy. *Arch Dermatol* 1990; **126**: 61–5.

44 Doyle DR, McCurley TL, Sergent JS. Fatal polymyositis in D-penicillamine-treated rheumatoid arthritis. *Ann Intern Med* 1983; **98**: 327–30.

45 Harris AL, Smith IE, Snaith M. Tamoxifen-induced tumour regression associated with dermatomyositis. *BMJ* 1982; **284**: 1674–5.

Pathology [1]. Dermatomyositis mainly involves the skin and muscles, although other organs, particularly the lungs, may be affected. The histological appearance of the skin depends on the stage of the disease. In acute dermatomyositis, the changes resemble those of subacute LE, although the dermal oedema may be more extensive and involve all layers of the dermis. There is usually some lymphocytic infiltrate, either perivascular or in clumps. The majority of the cells are CD4 T cells and HLA-DR-expressing macrophages. Plasmacytoid dendritic cells are present [2], but B-lymphocytes are absent [3]. The infiltrate may also include histiocytes, plasma cells and, occasionally, eosinophils. Mucin deposits commonly occur in the dermis, and mucin in an otherwise non-specific skin biopsy, although not diagnostic, is suggestive of dermatomyositis [1]. Hyperkeratosis, acanthosis and mild papillomatosis are features seen in Gottron's papules [4]. In the later stages, the collagen of the dermis may show thickening, homogenization and sclerosis, with thickening of the walls of cutaneous blood vessels. The epidermis becomes atrophic, with flattening of the rete ridges, and the basal layer may show an increase in pigment. At this stage, the appearance can be similar to that of scleroderma [5]. On direct immunofluorescence, IgM, IgG and C3 may be found at the dermal–epidermal junction in 50% of cases. Those with IgM may also have cytoid bodies [6]. The subcutaneous fat may show mucoid degeneration and lymphocytic infiltration, or sclerosis and calcification, sometimes with membranocystic changes [7].

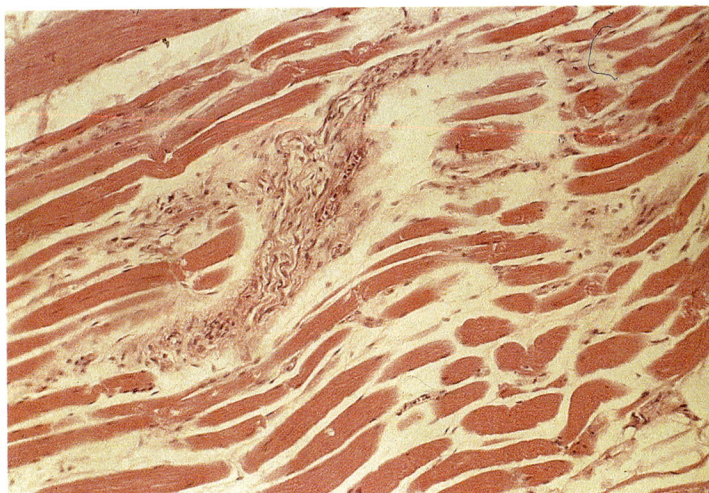

Fig. 51.82 Dermatomyositis: variable degeneration of the muscle bundles with oedema and inflammatory cells.

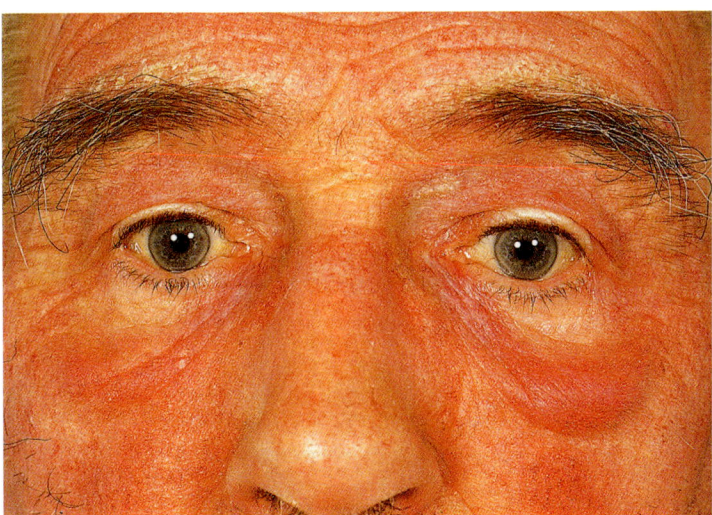

Fig. 51.83 Dermatomyositis: note the erythema and oedema of the eyelids.

The most frequently involved muscles are those of the limb girdles, the proximal parts of the limbs, the pharynx and the tongue. The muscle involvement [8] is not uniform, and histological examination of biopsy material may be negative. Biopsies should be taken from a muscle that is clinically weak, or that has been identified as abnormal on MRI scanning. The affected muscles may be pale, soft and flabby, or firm and fibrotic, depending on the stage of the disease. In patients with fibrosis, there may be calcification in the muscles and soft tissues. Histologically, in the early stages, the muscle fibres show loss of transverse striation, hyalinization of the sarcoplasm and an increase in sarcolemmal nuclei (Fig. 51.82). Later, the fibres fragment and show granular and vacuolar degeneration, and basophilic staining with histiocytic phagocytosis. There is variable cellular infiltration, mainly of lymphocytes, but also occasional plasma cells and macrophages. The blood vessels in the muscles may show eosinophilic intimal thickening, resembling the changes seen in malignant hypertension. Later still, the affected muscle fibres become atrophied and sclerosed, as in the muscles of patients with systemic sclerosis. No significant morphological differences have been found in the muscles in any of the diagnostic subgroups of polymyositis and dermatomyositis, and no consistent relationship between pathological changes in serial biopsies and clinical improvement in individual patients [9].

Intimal proliferation and thrombosis of arteries and arterioles of the skin, fat and alimentary tract [10] are sometimes seen, and the last accounts for the gastrointestinal ulceration and haemorrhage that occasionally occur. Changes resembling those seen in systemic sclerosis occur in the lungs or in the kidneys. The heart muscle may show changes similar to, but milder than, those in the voluntary muscles. Vasculitis of the cerebral and meningeal vessels has been reported, and in one case resulted in subarachnoid haemorrhage [11].

References

1 Janis JF, Winkelmann RK. Histopathology of the skin in dermatomyositis. *Arch Dermatol* 1968; **97**: 640–50.
2 Greenberg SA, Pinkus GS, Amato AA, Pinkus JL. Myeloid dendritic cells in inclusion-body myositis and polymyositis. *Muscle Nerve* 2007; **35**: 17–23.
3 Hausmann G, Herrero C, Cinta Cid M *et al.* Immunopathologic study of skin lesions in dermatomyositis. *J Am Acad Dermatol* 1991; **25**: 225–30.
4 Mendese G, Mahalingam M. Histopathology of Gottron's papules–utility in diagnosing dermatomyositis. *J Cutan Pathol* 2007; **34**: 793–6.
5 Dowling GB. Scleroderma and dermatomyositis. *Br J Dermatol* 1955; **67**: 275–90.
6 Vaughan-Jones SA, Bhogal BS, Black MM. Direct immunofluorescence findings in dermatomyositis. *Br J Dermatol* 1995; **133** (Suppl. 45): 55.
7 Ishikawa O, Tamura A, Ryuzaki K. Membranocystic changes in the panniculitis of dermatomyositis. *Br J Dermatol* 1996; **134**: 773–6.
8 Walton J. The inflammatory myopathies. *J R Soc Med* 1983; **76**: 998–1010.
9 Schwarz HA, Slavin G, Ward P *et al.* Muscle biopsy in polymyositis and dermatomyositis. *Ann Rheum Dis* 1980; **39**: 500–7.
10 Boylan RC, Sokoloff L. Vascular lesions in dermatomyositis. *Arthritis Rheum* 1960; **3**: 379–86.
11 Gotoff SP, Smith RD, Sugar O. Dermatomyositis with cerebral vasculitis in a patient with agammaglobulinaemia. *Am J Dis Child* 1972; **123**: 53–6.

Clinical features. The clinical picture is variable. Some patients with typical features of muscle involvement show little or no evidence of skin involvement, and the condition is then known as polymyositis [1]. Sometimes, the rash occurs alone [2], a condition that has been called amyopathic dermatomyositis, and this may imply a good prognosis, although the outlook is not uniformly good. Severe calcinosis may occur even in this variety [3]. The rash may precede muscle weakness in around 50% of patients [4].

The rash in well-developed cases is diagnostic. A purplish-red or heliotrope erythema occurs on the face, especially involving the eyelids, the upper cheeks, forehead and temples (Fig. 51.83). Oedema of the eyelids and periorbital tissues is not uncommon [5]. The distribution may resemble that of seborrhoeic dermatitis [6]. Oedema of the hands and arms, and sometimes of much of the body, may also be found, and this is usually associated with erythema of the backs of the forearms, the upper back and, sometimes, elsewhere. This more generalized erythema may resemble the widespread eruption of systemic lupus. In other cases, the rash is more poikilodermatous.

Small erythematous or violaceous, flat papules (Gottron's papules [7]) and small plaques occur over the knuckles, on the dorsa of the finger joints and around the nail folds (Fig. 51.84). They also occur on the dorsa of the toes, on the front of the knees

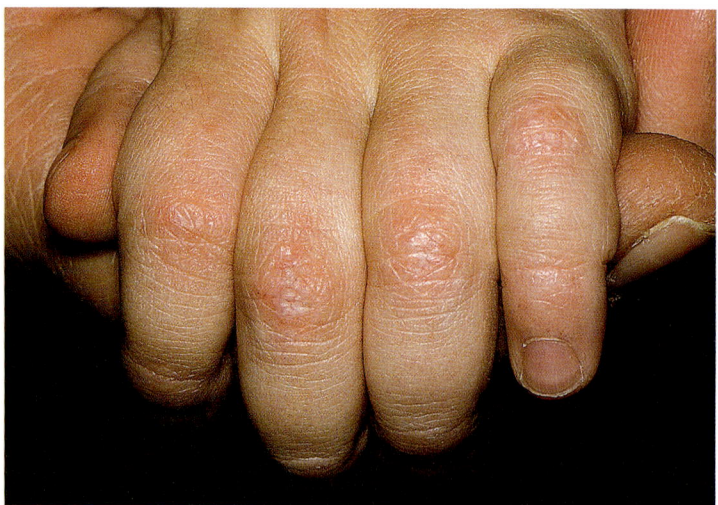

Fig. 51.84 Violaceous lesions on the dorsa of the finger joints in childhood dermatomyositis.

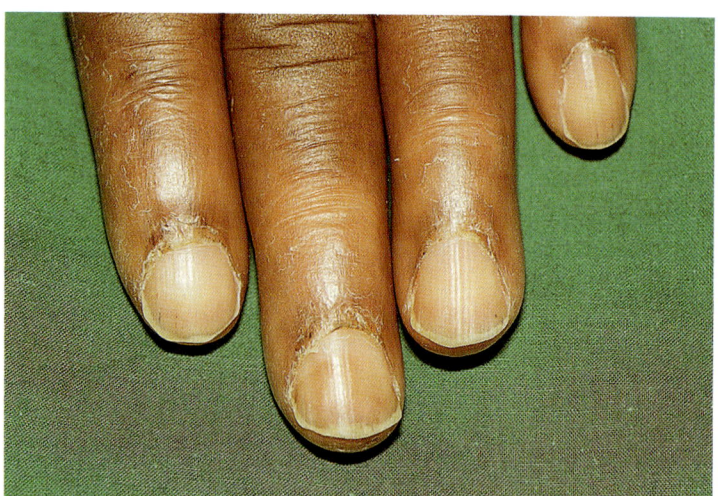

Fig. 51.86 Hyperpigmented nail fold lesions in an Afro-Caribbean patient with dermatomyositis.

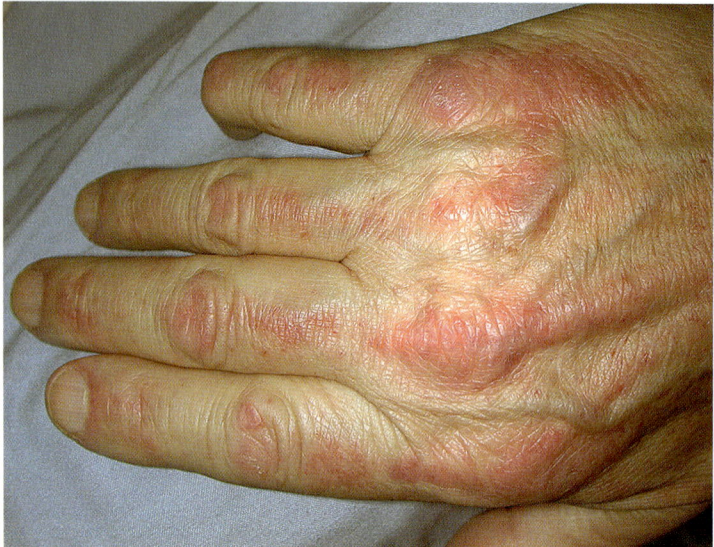

Fig. 51.85 The hands in dermatomyositis: note the linear erythema on the dorsa of the fingers.

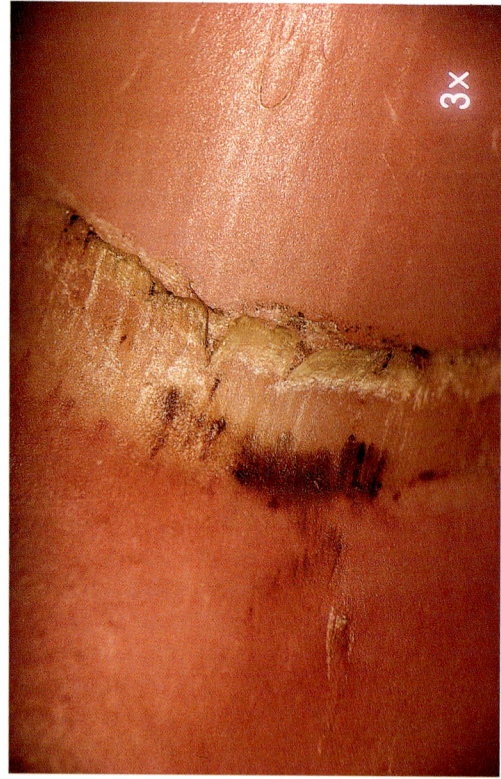

Fig. 51.87 Dermatomyositis: dilated nail fold capillaries and hypertrophic ragged cuticle.

and on the backs of the elbows. Frequently, the rash of dermatomyositis on the dorsa of the hands occurs as linear streaking over the extensor tendon sheaths (Fig. 51.85). These may be hyperpigmented as the only cutaneous sign in Afro-Caribbeans (Fig. 51.86) [8]. As well as diffuse redness and shininess of the nail folds, the capillary loops of the nail folds may be dilated, irregular and tortuous, and easily visible with or without a lens, or by capillaroscopy. The capillary changes are more marked in patients with Raynaud's phenomenon, arthritis and pulmonary involvement, but are not related to active myositis or malignancy (Fig. 51.87) [9]. Thickening, roughness, hyperkeratosis and irregularity of the cuticles, with minimal or no redness or inflammation [10], is frequent. Ragged cuticles are also found in other connective tissue diseases such as systemic sclerosis and LE.

In the Chinese, hyperkeratotic follicular erythematous papules occur on the face, back of the neck, trunk, dorsa of the hands and

feet, and palms and soles. On the dorsa of the hands and feet, the lesions occur in a linear fashion [11]. A variety of other cutaneous changes have been demonstrated (Table 51.22).

Panniculitis. In some patients, red, firm, tender areas of panniculitis develop (Fig. 51.88), and these may ulcerate or break down to form sinuses [18]. Some areas of panniculitis have their origin in vasculitis, and are often followed by severe calcification. They often occur on the buttocks and upper thighs.

Table 51.22 Less common physical signs associated with dermatomyositis [12–17].

Spreading erythema and fleeting or persistent oedema of the face and neck or of the limbs
Urticarial lesions, dermographism
Bullous lesions
Photosensitivity
Erythema nodosum, erythema multiforme
Follicular keratosis
Hypertrichosis, scalp erythema with hair loss
Hyperhidrosis
Psoriasiform eruptions and pitting of the fingernails
Gingival telangiectasia (childhood disease)
Linear, violaceous, itchy and oedematous streaks on the trunk (flagellate erythema)
Exfoliative dermatitis
Hyperpigmentation
Livedo reticularis, with ulceration

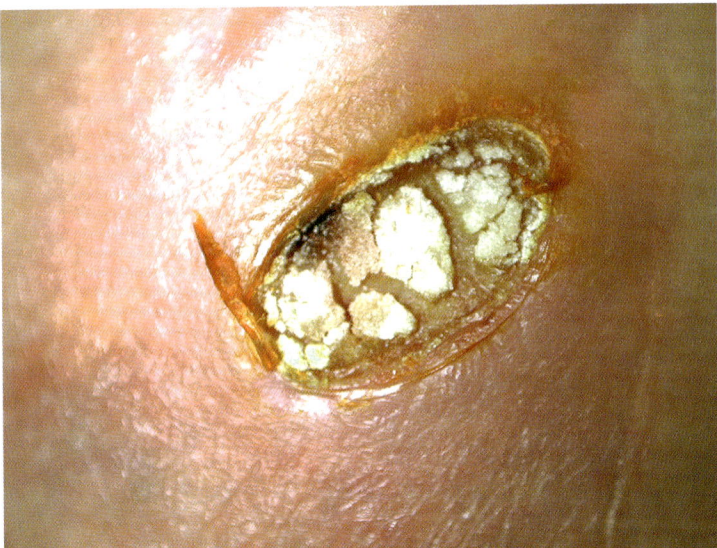

Fig. 51.88 Panniculitis with calcinosis in the thigh in dermatomyositis.

Mechanics' hands. Patients with antisynthetase antibodies may develop 'mechanics' hands'—hyperkeratosis, fissuring and linear hyperpigmentation of radial and palmar surfaces of the fingers. Histology shows hyperkeratosis, acanthosis, a mononuclear dermal infiltrate and liquefaction necrosis of the basal layer [19].

Muscle symptoms. Usually, the patient first notices aching and weakness of the muscles, which may be painful and tender, and later show some atrophy. Typical histories include difficulty in going up stairs or rising from a chair, or difficulty in raising the arms high enough to comb the hair. Usually, there is a feeling of malaise, and fever may occur. Raynaud's phenomenon occurs in approximately 10% of adults, but is very rare in children. Recurrent bursitis of shoulders and hips may precede myositis, and joint effusions occur [20].

In addition to the weakness of the limb muscles, which is mainly proximal, there may be difficulty with speech and swallowing (because of involvement of the muscles of the tongue, the pharynx and the upper third or distal part of the oesophagus [21]), diverticular out-pouching of the oesophagus [22], impaired muscular activity of the small intestine, pneumatosis intestinalis [23], sometimes with pneumoperitoneum [24], wide-mouthed diverticula of the colon, weakness of the ocular muscles and respiratory difficulty from involvement of the intercostal muscles and diaphragm which may lead to death because of respiratory infection or heart failure.

Other clinical features. Other clinical features include: interstitial pneumonitis [25], with non-productive cough, dyspnoea and hypoxaemia and radiological infiltrates or pulmonary fibrosis, may be the presenting manifestations or may occur in the course of the disease. Pulmonary hypertension, with cor pulmonale and fibrosing alveolitis, has been reported. Interstitial lung disease may be more frequent than suspected. Myocarditis, myocardial fibrosis, disorders of conduction and cardiac failure occur in approximately one-third of cases [26]. Renal lesions are uncommon [27]. Retinitis produces fluffy exudates around the papilla and along the veins; permanent visual loss occurs rarely [28]. A case of myoglobinuric acute renal failure has been reported [29].

A mild inflammatory arthritis may occur, but erosive arthritis is rare although a rheumatoid picture can occur. Patients with arthritis frequently have pulmonary involvement [30]. Trigeminal neuropathy has been reported [31].

Calcification. Calcification [32] occurs in the muscles or in areas of panniculitis in more than half of childhood cases, and approximately 15% of adults. The muscles mainly involved are those of the shoulder and pelvic girdles, and to a lesser extent those of the trunk and the limbs, especially around the elbows and hands. In adults, the distribution is less markedly around the pelvic and shoulder girdles than in childhood. Calcinosis increases over the course of months or years and, if extensive, can cause severe functional disability. Extrusion of calcium through the skin is associated with ulceration and cellulitis. Calcinosis is a good sign for survival, but functional recovery is less likely, although even severe calcinosis can resolve spontaneously. Sometimes, patients present with widespread calcification and apparently have not had a preceding myositic illness. In these cases, it is presumed—but not proved—that calcinosis is the result of old dermatomyositis. Sometimes, calcinosis developing in childhood decreases in adolescence; rarely, hypercalcaemia may occur [33].

References

1 Bohan A, Peter JB, Bowman RL *et al.* A computer-assisted analysis of 153 patients with polymyositis and dermatomyositis. *Medicine* 1977; **56**: 255–86.

2 Gerami P, Schope JM, McDonald L *et al.* A systematic review of adult-onset clinically amyopathic dermatomyositis (dermatomyositis sine myositis): a missing link within the spectrum of the idiopathic inflammatory myopathies. *J Am Acad Dermatol* 2006; **54**: 597–613.

3 Olhoffer IH, Carroll C, Watsky K. Dermatomyositis sine myositis presenting with calcinosis universalis. *Br J Dermatol* 1999; **141**: 365–6.

4 Rockerbie NR, Woo TY, Callen JP *et al.* Cutaneous changes of dermatomyositis precede muscle weakness. *J Am Acad Dermatol* 1989; **20**: 629–32.

5 Sevigny GM, Mathes BM. Periorbital oedema as the presenting sign of juvenile dermatomyositis. *Pediatr Dermatol* 1999; **16**: 43–5.

6 Katayama I, Sawada Y, Nishioka K *et al.* The seborrhoeic pattern of dermatomyositis. *Br J Dermatol* 1999; **140**: 978–9.

7 Gottron H. Hautveranuderungen bei dermatomyositis. In: Lomholt S, ed. *VIII Congres International de Dermatologie et de Syphilologie.* Copenhagen: Compts Rendus de Seances, 1930: 826.

8 Bottomley W, Goodfield MJD. A case of dermatomyositis presenting as localized hyperpigmentation of the hands and face. *Br J Dermatol* 1995; **132**: 670–1.

9 Ganczarczyk ML, Lee P, Armstrong SK. Nail fold capillary microscopy in polymyositis and dermatomyositis. *Arthritis Rheum* 1988; **31**: 116–9.

10 Samitz MH. Cuticular changes in dermatomyositis. *Arch Dermatol* 1974; **110**: 866–7.

11 Wong KO. Dermatomyositis: a clinical investigation of 23 cases in Hong Kong. *Br J Dermatol* 1969; **81**: 544–7.

12 Findley GH, Price GA, Van Rinsburg CRJ. Dermatomyositis with vesicular bullous lesions. *S Afr Med J* 1951; **25**: 60.

13 Rowland Payne CME, Meyrick Thomas RH. Dermatomyositis with urticated lesions. *J R Soc Med* 1984; **77**: 137–8.

14 Garcin R, Lapresle J, Gruner J *et al.* Les polymyosites. *Rev Neurol* 1955; **92**: 465.

15 Reich NE, Reinhart JB. Dermatomyositis associated with hypertrichosis. *Arch Dermatol Syphilol* 1948; **57**: 725–32.

16 Ghali FE, Stein LD, Fine JD *et al.* Gingival telangiectases: an underappreciated physical sign of juvenile dermatomyositis. *Arch Dermatol* 1999; **135**: 1370–4.

17 Jara M, Amerigo JA, Duce S, Borbugo J. Dermatomyositis and flagellate erythema. *Clin Exp Dermatol* 1996; **21**: 440–1.

18 Fusade T, Belanyi P, Joly P *et al.* Subcutaneous changes in dermatomyositis. *Br J Dermatol* 1993; **128**: 451–3.

19 Mitra D, Lovell CL, Macleod TIF *et al.* Clinical and histological features of 'mechanics hands' in a patient with antibodies to Jo-1: a case report. *Clin Exp Dermatol* 1994; **19**: 146–8.

20 Dorph C, Englund P, Nennesmo I, Lundberg IE. Signs of inflammation in both symptomatic and asymptomatic muscles from patients with polymyositis and dermatomyositis. *Ann Rheum Dis* 2006; **65**: 1565–71.

21 De Merieux P, Verity MA, Clements PJ *et al.* Oesophageal abnormalities and dysphagia in polymyositis and dermatomyositis. *Arthritis Rheum* 1983; **26**: 961–8.

22 O'Hara JM, Szemes G, Lowman RM. The oesophageal lesions in dermatomyositis. *Radiology* 1967; **89**: 27–31.

23 Mueller CF, Morehead R, Alter AJ *et al.* Pneumatosis intestinalis in collagen disorders. *Am J Roentgenol* 1972; **115**: 300–5.

24 Oliveros MA, Herbst JJ, Lester PD *et al.* Pneumatosis intestinalis in childhood dermatomyositis. *Pediatrics* 1973; **52**: 711–2.

25 Takizawa H, Shiga J, Moroi Y *et al.* Interstitial lung disease in dermatomyositis: clinicopathological study. *J Rheumatol* 1987; **14**: 102–7.

26 Haupt HM, Hutchins GM. The heart and cardiac conduction system in polymyositis–dermatomyositis. *Am J Cardiol* 1982; **50**: 998–1006.

27 Yen TH, Lai PC, Chen CC *et al.* Renal involvement in patients with polymyositis and dermatomyositis. *Int J Clin Pract* 2005; **59**: 188–93.

28 Kessler E, Weinberger I, Rosenfeld JB. Myoglobinuric acute renal failure in a case of dermatomyositis. *Israel J Med Sci* 1972; **8**: 978–83.

29 Yeo LMW, Swaby DSA, Sitnayake RD, Murray PI. Irreversible visual loss in dermatomyositis. *Br J Rheumatol* 1995; **34**: 1179–81.

30 Schumacher HR, Schimmer B, Gordon GV *et al.* Articular manifestations of polymyositis and dermatomyositis. *Am J Med* 1979; **67**: 287–92.

31 Ashworth B, Tait GBW. Trigeminal neuropathy in connective tissue disease. *Neurology* 1971; **21**: 609–14.

32 Muller SA, Winkelmann RK, Brunsting LA. Calcinosis in dermatomyositis. *Arch Dermatol* 1959; **79**: 669–73.

33 Ostrov BE, Goldsmith DP, Eichenfield AH, Athreya BH. Hypercalcaemia during the resolution of calcinosis universalis in juvenile dermatomyositis. *J Rheumatol* 1991; **18**: 1730–4.

Dermatomyositis in childhood.

This has been well described and reviewed [1]. It is possible that microchimerism may be an aetiological factor [2]. The condition resembles that seen in adults, but malignancy is rarely associated with it and it is usually much more severe than in adults. The prognosis is variable. Calcification occurs more frequently than in adults and contractures develop in under 5%. Widespread vasculitis affecting small arteries, capillar-

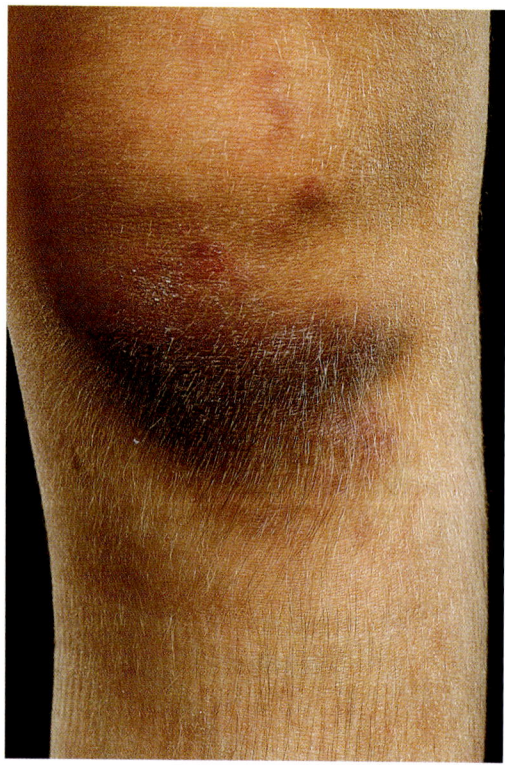

Fig. 51.89 Hypertrichosis in an area of erythema on the knee in childhood dermatomyositis.

ies and veins of the skin, muscle, subcutaneous tissue and gastrointestinal tract is a prominent feature of the so-called Banker type [3]. It may take many years for the disease to burn out but, occasionally, a child recovers without any residual disability and late recurrences are rare. Psychological difficulties occur more frequently than might be expected [4]. A rare feature is hypertrichosis (Fig. 51.89) [5]. Juvenile dermatomyositis can be associated with partial lipodystrophy [6].

References

1 Ramanan AV, Feldman BM. Clinical features and outcomes of juvenile dermatomyositis and other childhood onset myositis syndromes. *Rheum Dis Clin North Am* 2002; **28**: 833–57.

2 Artlett CM, Miller FW, Rider LG. Persistent maternally derived peripheral microchimerism is associated with the juvenile idiopathic inflammatory myopathies. *Rheumatology (Oxford)* 2001; **40**: 1279–84.

3 Banker BQ, Victor M. Dermatomyositis (systemic angiopathy) of childhood. *Medicine* 1966; **45**: 261–89.

4 Pachman LM, Cooke N. Juvenile dermatomyositis: a clinical and immunologic study. *J Pediatr* 1980; **96**: 226–34.

5 Piantanida NA, Person DA, Piantanida EW. Infrapatellar hypertrichosis: an unusual cutaneous manifestation of juvenile dermatomyositis. *Pediatr Dermatol* 2002; **19**: 132–5.

6 Kavanagh GM, Colaco B, Kennedy CTC. Juvenile dermatomyositis associated with partial lipoatrophy. *J Am Acad Dermatol* 1993; **28**: 348–51.

Sclerodermatomyositis in childhood.

This is an overlap syndrome in which cutaneous changes of systemic sclerosis and dermatomyositis are associated with myositis and the homogeneous nucleolar pattern of antinuclear antibody (anti-PM/Scl antibody). Serum muscle enzymes are normal or only slightly raised. The features of dermatomyositis are usually transient and respond to

Table 51.23 Association of dermatomyositis with other disorders.

Thymoma [1]
Hyperthyroidism [2]
Drugs:
    penicillamine [3]
    hydroxyurea [4]
Aplastic anaemia [5]
Haemolytic anaemia [6]
Agammaglobulinaemia [7]
Cystinuria [8]
Hashimoto's disease and ovarian carcinoma [9]
Generalized amyloidosis [10]
Multiple myeloma [11]
Lichen myxoedematosus [12]
Dermatitis herpetiformis [13]
Coeliac disease [14]
Bullous pemphigoid [15]
Porphyria cutanea tarda [16]
Fibrosing alveolitis [17]
Cutaneous vasculitis [18]
Sjögren's syndrome [19]
Hughes' syndrome [20]
Periorbital fasciitis [21]
Lipoatrophy [22] and lipodystrophy with phaeochromocytoma [23]

non-steroidal anti-inflammatory drugs or corticosteroids, and aggressive treatment is not usually required. The systemic sclerosis features such as Raynaud's phenomenon, calcinosis and arthritis tend to grumble on over years, but visceral involvement is not marked. One case with 'mechanics' hands'—hyperkeratosis and fissuring on the tips and sides of the fingers resembling a labourer's dirty hands—has been reported [1].

Reference

1 Garcia-Patos V, Bartralot R, Ordi J *et al.* Childhood sclerodermatomyositis: report of a case with the anti-PM/Scl antibody and mechanic's hands. *Br J Dermatol* 1996; **135**: 613–6.

Dermatomyositis in pregnancy

[1]. Dermatomyositis can start in pregnancy. The overall fetal loss is over 50%, and half of pregnancies end prematurely. Pregnancy exacerbates the disease in approximately 50% and is associated with remission in 20%. Fertility is decreased in dermatomyositis [2]. Pregnancy should be planned at a time of remission and the patient monitored at least every month. If possible, treatment should be confined to oral steroids.

References

1 Harris A, Webley M, Usherwood M *et al.* Dermatomyositis presenting in pregnancy. *Br J Dermatol* 1995; **133**: 783–5.
2 Kitridou RC. Pregnancy in mixed connective tissue disease, poly/dermatomyositis and scleroderma. *Clin Exp Rheumatol* 1988; **6**: 173–8.

Association with other disorders.

Many other diseases have been reported in conjunction with dermatomyositis (see Table 51.23).

References

1 Rundle LG, Sparks FP. Thymoma and dermatomyositis. *Arch Pathol* 1963; **75**: 276–83.

2 Shergy WJ, Caldwell DS. Polymyositis after propylthiouracil treatment for hyperthyroidism. *Ann Rheum Dis* 1988; **47**: 340–3.
3 Doyle DR, McCurley TL, Sergent JS. Fatal polymyositis in D-penicillamine-treated rheumatoid arthritis. *Ann Intern Med* 1983; **98**: 327–30.
4 Senet P, Aractingi S, Porneuf M *et al.* Hydroxyurea-induced dermatomyositis-like eruption. *Br J Dermatol* 1995; **133**: 455–9.
5 Duncan PR, Harvey PW, Seville RH. Dermatomyositis presenting as aplastic anaemia. *Br J Dermatol* 1959; **71**: 344–6.
6 Hardman CM, Garioch JJ, Leonard JN *et al.* Autoimmune haemolytic anaemia associated with dermatomyositis. *Clin Exp Dermatol* 1996; **21**: 437–9.
7 Gotoff SP, Smith RD, Sugar O. Dermatomyositis with cerebral vasculitis in a patient with agammaglobulinemia. *Am J Dis Child* 1972; **123**: 53–6.
8 Fawcett NP, Nyhan WL. Cystinuria and dermatomyositis. *Clin Pediatr* 1970; **9**: 727–32.
9 Chamberlain MJ, Whittaker SRF. Hashimoto's disease, dermatomyositis and ovarian carcinoma. *Lancet* 1963; **i**: 1398–9.
10 Gelderman AH, Levine RA, Arndt KA. Dermatomyositis complicated by generalized amyloidosis. *N Engl J Med* 1962; **267**: 858–61.
11 Zilko PJ, Dawkins RL. Amyloidosis associated with dermatomyositis and features of multiple myeloma. *Am J Med* 1975; **59**: 488–52.
12 Johnson BL, Horowitz IR, Charles CR *et al.* Dermatomyositis and lichen myxedematosus. *Dermatologica* 1973; **147**: 109–22.
13 White SW, Tesar JT. Dermatomyositis and dermatitis herpetiformis. *Arch Dermatol* 1982; **118**: 599–601.
14 Iannone F, Lapadula G. Dermatomyositis and coeliac disease association: a further case. *Clin Exp Rheumatol* 2001; **19**: 757–8.
15 Glover M, Leigh IM. Dermatomyositis pemphigoides: a case with coexistent dermatomyositis and bullous pemphigoid. *J Am Acad Dermatol* 1992; **27**: 849–52.
16 Belaich S, Crickx B, Picard C *et al.* Porphyrie cutanée tardive associée à une dermatomyosite cutanée pure. *Ann Dermatol Vénéréol* 1989; **116**: 826–7.
17 Holmes R, Black M, Farebrother MJB *et al.* Malignancy associated dermatomyositis with fibrosing alveolitis. *Clin Exp Dermatol* 1980; **5**: 415–20.
18 Feldman D, Hochberg MC, Zizic TM *et al.* Cutaneous vasculitis in adult polymyositis–dermatomyositis. *J Rheumatol* 1983; **10**: 85–9.
19 Ringel SP, Forstot JZ, Tan EM *et al.* Sjögren's syndrome and polymyositis or dermatomyositis. *Arch Neurol* 1982; **39**: 157–63.
20 Sherer Y, Livneh A, Levy Y *et al.* Dermatomyositis and polymyositis associated with the antiphospholipid syndrome: a novel overlap syndrome. *Lupus* 2000; **9**: 42–6.
21 Carruthers A, Carruthers J, Wright P. Necrotizing fasciitis with polymyositis. *BMJ* 1975; **iii**: 355–6.
22 Commens C, O'Neill P, Walker G. Dermatomyositis associated with multifocal lipoatrophy. *J Am Acad Dermatol* 1990; **22**: 966–9.
23 Huang JL. Juvenile dermatomyositis associated with partial lipodystrophy. *Br J Clin Pract* 1996; **50**: 112–3.

Differential diagnosis.

The diagnosis depends upon the association of a typical rash with muscle weakness, and is confirmed by muscle biopsy, electromyography and certain laboratory investigations. The serum creatine phosphokinase (CPK), glutamic oxalacetic transaminase (SGOT) or aldolase are frequently, but not invariably raised [1,2], and in certain cases may reflect the activity of the disease and be helpful in regulating the dosage of steroids [3]. However, some patients continue to show considerable disease activity in the presence of normal serum enzymes, so serial estimations of the 24-h urinary creatine are helpful, if available [4]. Skin and muscle biopsy are helpful, but histological changes may be absent or minimal. Radiology of the muscles in the later stages may show calcinosis, a feature that may differentiate the condition from other connective tissue diseases [5]. In dermatomyositis, the calcium deposits are widely scattered throughout the muscles and soft tissues, whereas in systemic sclerosis the calcium deposits are found mainly in the hands and around the elbows and knees.

Table 51.24 Investigation of associated malignancy in dermatomyositis.

Clinical examination (including the breasts, pelvis and rectum),
Blood count and biochemistry
Radiography of the chest
Abdominal ultrasound
Examination of the stools for occult blood
Tumour specific markers including PSA, CEA etc.

Moreover, in the latter, the tips of the terminal phalanges often show some bone resorption. MRI scanning [6] and ultrasound give useful information for longitudinal studies and are non-invasive. In patients with little or no rash, muscular dystrophies may be closely simulated [7]; electromyography [8] is helpful in distinguishing myopathy from neuropathy. Dermatomyositis is of more rapid onset and remissions are frequent.

The ESR is moderately elevated in some, but not all patients in the active phase, and there may be some elevation of the serum globulin. It has been claimed that an elevated ESR and cutaneous necrosis are potential markers of malignancy [8]. Antinuclear factor, raised DNA binding and anti-RNP may occur, especially in overlap syndromes [9]. Antibodies to aminoacyl-tRNA synthetase are antibodies to soluble nuclear antigens and are associated with myositis [10]. The association of other antibodies with particular disease profiles has already been discussed. Antibodies to cytoplasmic antigens such as anti-SRP (signal recognition particle) occur, and antibodies to the nuclear antigen Mi-2 are strongly associated with dermatomyositis [11]. Occasionally, rheumatoid factor is found. The Wassermann reaction is negative. Anticardiolipin antibodies were found in three out of 14 patients with juvenile dermatomyositis, two of whom had vascular complications [12].

In all adult cases, a determined effort to exclude internal malignancy should be carried out [13], and although most of the neoplasms can be diagnosed by physical examination and simple investigation (Table 51.24), in a minority of patients, intensive investigation may be required.

Dermatomyositis can be confused with systemic sclerosis, and the two conditions can occur together. The muscle changes may be identical in the two disorders, but visceral changes are much more common in systemic sclerosis. From the clinical point of view, differentiation between the two diseases may be difficult, particularly in those cases showing sclerosis in the healing phase. Occasionally, patients with systemic sclerosis show heliotrope cyanosis of the eyelids, and dilatation of the nail fold capillaries. Sometimes, patients with dermatomyositis resemble patients with SLE but, in the latter, antinuclear factors and anti-DNA antibodies can usually be demonstrated. Myositis is a feature of so-called mixed connective tissue disease (see p. 51.110). Neuropathy is distinguished by the electromyographic changes and the presence of a raised CPK and urinary creatine excretion. The atrophic changes of the skin in the later stages may resemble morphoea, but the history should lead to the correct diagnosis. Polymyositis [14,15] is more common than dermatomyositis. It is usually found in adults in the third to the fifth decades. Females are three times more likely to develop the disease than males. Occasionally, sclero-

edema may cause difficulty. It is important to exclude metabolic disorders in those patients with only muscle disease [16].

References

1 Bohan A, Peter JB, Bowman RL *et al*. A computer-assisted analysis of 153 patients with polymyositis and dermatomyositis. *Medicine* 1977; **56**: 255–86.
2 Carter JD, Kanik KS, Vasey FB *et al*. Dermatomyositis with normal creatine kinase and elevated aldolase levels. *J Rheumatol* 2001; **28**: 2366–7.
3 Vickers CFH. Serum transaminase estimations in the differential diagnosis of collagen diseases. *Br J Dermatol* 1961; **73**: 185–93.
4 Rowell NR, Fairris GM. Biochemical markers of myositis in dermatomyositis. *Clin Exp Dermatol* 1986; **11**: 69–72.
5 Dubois EL. Collagen disease: the overlooked diagnosis. *Med Ann DC* 1959; **28**: 681–94.
6 Park JH, Olsen NJ. Utility of magnetic resonance imaging in the evaluation of patients with inflammatory myopathies. *Curr Rheumatol Rep* 2001; **3**: 334–45.
7 Heathfield KWG, Williams JRB. Diagnosis of polymyositis. *Lancet* 1960; **i**: 1157–61.
8 Basset-Seguin N, Roujeau J-C, Gherardi R *et al*. Prognostic factors and predictive signs of malignancy in adult dermatomyositis. *Arch Dermatol* 1990; **126**: 633–7.
9 Venables PJW, Mumford PA, Maini RN. Antibodies to nuclear antigens in polymyositis. *Ann Rheum Dis* 1981; **40**: 217–23.
10 Lamedica G, Parodi A, Peris G *et al*. Polymyositis and pulmonary fibrosis associated with anti-PL-7 antibody. *J Am Acad Dermatol* 1988; **19**: 567–8.
11 Targoff IN. Humoral immunity in polymyositis/dermatomyositis. *J Invest Dermatol* 1993; **100** (Suppl.): 116S–23S.
12 Montecucco C, Ravelli A, Caporali R *et al*. Autoantibodies in juvenile dermatomyositis. *Clin Exp Rheumatol* 1990; **8**: 193–6.
13 Callen JP. The value of malignancy evaluation in patients with dermatomyositis. *J Am Acad Dermatol* 1982; **6**: 253–9.
14 Pearson CM. Patterns of polymyositis and their responses to treatment. *Ann Intern Med* 1963; **59**: 827–38.
15 Walton J, Adams RD. *Polymyositis*. Edinburgh: Livingstone, 1958.
16 Wortmann RL. Myositis or myopathy. *J Rheumatol* 1989; **16**: 1525–7.

Prognosis [1,2]. The course is variable. The prognosis is said to be better in dermatomyositis than in polymyositis; however, some have found the reverse to be true [3]. Patients without muscle involvement may have a better prognosis and may not require steroids [4]. Approximately 50% of patients seem to be responsive to therapy; the remainder appear to be relatively resistant. The overall mortality is approximately one-quarter [5], and malignancy is a significant cause of death [1]. Adverse factors include acute pulmonary infiltrations, dysphagia, cutaneous necrosis and increasing age. Fulminating cases may deteriorate rapidly despite therapy, and in the past some 20% died within the first year; other cases settle slowly and burn out in time, usually over several years. Sometimes, patients complain of vague aching in the limbs when there does not appear to be any residual activity. Some are left with minimal cutaneous change and no residual weakness. Others, particularly children, have gross disability, with contractures of the limbs and calcinosis. Of the children followed up for 5–16 years, 75% survived [6]. Removal of an underlying carcinoma in adults can lead to regression of the dermatomyositis [7].

Calcinosis is a good prognostic feature. Out of 75 adults without calcification, 26 died, usually in approximately 2 years, whereas of 12 adults with calcinosis none died [8]. Seven out of 14 children without, and only one of 17 with, calcinosis died in a mean time of approximately 16 months. Calcification can decrease without treatment. In some patients, muscle disease settles with treatment, but cutaneous disease may be persistent and resistant to therapy.

Death usually occurs from respiratory infection, cardiac failure, malnutrition, weakness or debility because of difficulty in swallowing, carcinoma, or from the side effects of steroid therapy.

References

1 Marie I, Hachulla E, Hatron PY *et al*. Polymyositis and dermatomyositis: short-term and long-term outcome, and predictive factors of prognosis. *J Rheumatol* 2001; **28**: 2230–7.

2 Medsger TA, Robinson H, Masi AT. Factors affecting survivorship in polymyositis. *Arthritis Rheum* 1971; **14**: 249–58.

3 Callen JP, Hyla JF, Bole GG *et al*. The relationship of dermatomyositis and polymyositis to internal malignancy. *Arch Dermatol* 1980; **116**: 295–8.

4 Genth E. [Inflammatory muscle diseases: dermatomyositis, polymyositis, and inclusion body myositis]. *Internist* 2005; **46**: 1218–32.

5 Airio A, Kautiainen H, Hakala M. Prognosis and mortality of polymyositis and dermatomyositis patients. *Clin Rheumatol* 2006; **25**: 234–9.

6 Henriksson KG, Sandstedt P. Polymyositis: treatment and prognosis—a study of 107 patients. *Acta Neurol Scand* 1982; **65**: 280–300.

7 Brunner MJ, Lobraico RV. Dermatomyositis as an index of malignant neoplasm. *Ann Intern Med* 1951; **34**: 1269–73.

8 Muller SA, Winkelmann RK, Brunsting LA. Calcinosis in dermatomyositis. *Arch Dermatol* 1959; **79**: 669–73.

Treatment [1]. Rest is essential in the acute phase. In adults it is important to exclude an underlying carcinoma. Treatment with corticosteroids is required in almost all cases, the dosage depending upon the degree of activity. Initial dosage of as much as 60 mg/day prednisolone may be required [1]. This dosage should be gradually reduced as the patient clinically improves and the biochemical markers improve. However, a maintenance dosage of between 5 and 15 mg/day may be required for many months, or even years, and it is important to balance the maximum therapeutic effect against the presence of side effects. If the clinical signs and serum CPK level are not improving sufficiently quickly, bolus infusions of methylprednisolone (1 g on 2–3 successive days) may be tried and are often a good alternative to a high-dose oral regimen. Alternatively, an antimetabolite should be added. Oral azathioprine (1.5–3 mg/kg/day in divided doses) as a steroid-sparing agent [2], or oral methotrexate in a small weekly dosage (7.5–15 mg) may be used to suppress disease activity [3]. Patients not responding to prednisolone and immunosuppressives may be helped by the addition of ciclosporin 5 mg/kg/day [4]. Ciclosporin is also effective in childhood in a dosage of 2.5–7.5 mg/kg [5]. A number of studies have indicated a successful role for intravenous immunoglobulin in a regimen of 1 mg/kg for 2 days each month over 4–6 months [6,7]. Cyclophosphamide 100 mg/day [8], or as pulsed intravenous therapy, is used for pulmonary interstitial fibrosis, but may also be effective for muscle and skin disease and justified in severe cases. The advent of biological agents—monoclonal antibodies directed at specific cytokines—has provided a new set of therapeutic options, and both infliximab [9] (directed against tumour necrosis factor) and more usefully rituximab [10] (directed against the CD20 molecule on B lymphocyte precursors), have been used with success.

Children with minimal myopathy may remit with indometacin without steroids [11], and antimalarials may help the rash of dermatomyositis, which may persist when muscle activity settles [12]. Topical steroid or a topical calcineurin inhibitor may be of value [13]. Less commonly, levamisole (100 mg/week) [14] or plasma exchange [15] may help patients with severe disease not responding to steroids or immunosuppressives. Improvement may occur within 48 h of plasmapheresis [16]. Extracorporeal photochemotherapy may be useful in combination with other therapies [17]. Methandienone (30 mg/day) [18], dapsone [19] and pentoxifylline [20] have all produced apparent improvement in patients unresponsive to corticosteroids. Antiplatelet agents—aspirin (650 mg/day), dipyridamole (400 mg/day) and sulfinpyrazone (400 mg/day)—helped one patient with *in vivo* platelet thrombi formation causing digital and vascular ischaemia [21].

Therapy, with either prednisolone alone or in combination with an antimetabolite, may be required for some years, and the dosage is reduced very gradually until the disease is burnt out. Any recrudescence is treated with an increase in dosage. Early treatment with low-dose steroids in children is associated with fewer relapses and lower morbidity [22]. Occasionally, weakness may arise from corticosteroid myopathy, and may be difficult to distinguish from an exacerbation of the disease. Serum enzymes are normal, but the 24-h urinary creatine excretion is raised [23]. Recovery on reduction of dosage takes up to 4 months. Weakness in dermatomyositis may occur because of hypokalaemia, the result of corticosteroid therapy. Regular electrolyte estimations are required and potassium supplements should be given.

Gastrointestinal haemorrhage may occur as a result of the disease or corticosteroid therapy. Constipation can be a feature, and octreotide may increase gastrointestinal motility. Osteoporosis is a considerable risk because of immobility and corticosteroid therapy, and prophylactic treatment should be given to both female and male patients. Treatment of calcinosis is usually ineffective, although spontaneous improvement can occur. Aluminium oxide, by producing insoluble aluminium phosphate, decreases the intestinal absorption of phosphate and has been successfully used in calcinosis in a child. Aludrox 15 mL four times daily (2.4 g/day aluminium oxide) was given by mouth [24]. Diltiazem has also been used successfully [25].

Physiotherapy plays a considerable part in preventing the development of contractures, and careful splinting may also be required. Artificial ventilation may be required in reversible transitory ventilatory failure [26], as may intravenous feeding in patients with severe oesophageal involvement. If there is definite serological evidence of recent infection with *Toxoplasma gondii*, treatment with pyrimethamine and/or sulfadiazine may be indicated [27].

References

1 Choy EH, Isenberg DA. Treatment of dermatomyositis and polymyositis. *Rheumatology* 2002; **41**: 7–13.

2 Choy EH, Hoogendijk JE, Lecky B, Winer JB. Immunosuppressant and immunomodulatory treatment for dermatomyositis and polymyositis. *Cochrane Database of Systematic Reviews* (**3**): CD003643, 2005.

3 Ramanan AV, Campbell-Webster N, Ota S *et al*. The effectiveness of treating juvenile dermatomyositis with methotrexate and aggressively tapered corticosteroids. *Arthritis Rheum* 2005; **52**: 3570–8.

4 Casato M, Bonomo L, Caccavo D *et al*. Clinical effects of cyclosporin in dermatomyositis. *Clin Exp Dermatol* 1990; **15**: 121–3.

5 Heckmat J, Saunders C, Peters AM *et al*. Cyclosporin in juvenile dermatomyositis. *Lancet* 1989; **i**: 1063–6.

6 Cherin P, Piette JC, Wechsler B *et al*. Intravenous gammaglobulin as first-line therapy in polymyositis and dermatomyositis: an open study in 11 adult patients. *J Rheumatol* 1994; **21**: 1092–7.

7 Sansome A, Dubowitz S. Intravenous immunoglobulin in juvenile dermatomyositis: 4 year review of nine cases. *Arch Dis Child* 1995; **72**: 25–8.

8 Plowman PN, Stableforth DE. Dermatomyositis with fibrosing alveolitis. *Proc R Soc Med* 1977; **70**: 738–40.

9 Dold S, Justiniano ME, Marquez J, Espinoza LR. Treatment of early and refractory dermatomyositis with infliximab: a report of two cases. *Clin Rheumatol* 2007; **26**: 1186–8.

10 Cooper MA, Willingham DL, Brown DE *et al.* Rituximab for the treatment of juvenile dermatomyositis: a report of four pediatric patients. *Arthritis Rheum* 2007; **56**: 3107–11.

11 Winkelmann RK. Dermatomyositis in childhood. *Clin Rheum Dis* 1982; **8**: 353–68.

12 Woo TY, Callen JP, Voorhees JJ *et al.* Cutaneous lesions of dermatomyositis are improved by hydroxychloroquine. *J Am Acad Dermatol* 1984; **10**: 592–600.

13 Yoshimasu T, Ohtani T, Sakamoto T *et al.* Topical FK506 (tacrolimus) therapy for facial erythematous lesions of cutaneous lupus erythematosus and dermatomyositis. *Eur J Dermatol* 2002; **12**: 50–2.

14 Rovensky J, Zitnan D, Lukac J *et al.* Effect of 'levamisole' treatment in polymyositis patients. *J Rheumatol* 1982; **9**: 158–9.

15 Dau PC. Plasmapheresis in idiopathic inflammatory myopathy. *Arch Neurol* 1981; **38**: 544–52.

16 MacPherson A, Berth-Jones J, Graham-Brown RAC. Carcinoma-associated dermatomyositis responding to plasmapheresis. *Clin Exp Dermatol* 1989; **14**: 304–5.

17 de Wilde A, DiSpaltro FX, Geller A *et al.* Extracorporeal photochemotherapy as adjunctive treatment in juvenile dermatomyositis: a case report. *Arch Dermatol* 1992; **128**: 1656–7.

18 Armstrong A, Murdoch WR. Anabolic hormone in dermatomyositis. *BMJ* 1960; **ii**: 1929–31.

19 Konohana A, Kawashima J. Successful treatment of dermatomyositis with dapsone. *Clin Exp Dermatol* 1994; **19**: 367–8.

20 Person JR. Dermatomyositis responding to pentoxifylline. *Br J Dermatol* 1996; **134**: 593–606.

21 Littlejohn GO, Deck JHN, Kelton JG *et al.* Dermatomyositis associated with platelet thrombi formation and responsive to antiplatelet therapy. *J Rheumatol* 1983; **10**: 136–9.

22 Miller G, Heckmatt JZ, Dubowitz V. Drug treatment of juvenile dermatomyositis. *Arch Dis Child* 1983; **58**: 445–50.

23 Askari A, Vignos PJ, Moskowitz RW. Steroid myopathy in connective tissue disease. *Am J Med* 1976; **61**: 485–92.

24 Nassim JR, Connolly CK. Treatment of calcinosis universalis with aluminium hydroxide. *Arch Dis Child* 1970; **45**: 118–21.

25 Palmieri GM, Sebes JI, Aelion JA *et al.* Treatment of calcinosis with diltiazem. *Arthritis Rheum* 1995; **38**: 1646–54.

26 Selva-O'Callaghan A, Sanchez-Sitjes L, Munoz-Gall X *et al.* Respiratory failure due to muscle weakness in inflammatory myopathies: maintenance therapy with home mechanical ventilation. *Rheumatology* 2000; **39**: 914–6.

27 Harland CC, Marsden JR, Vernon SA *et al.* Dermatomyositis responding to treatment of associated toxoplasmosis. *Br J Dermatol* 1991; **125**: 76–8.

Dermatological manifestations of rheumatoid disease

Although it would be unusual for patients with rheumatoid arthritis to present initially with skin problems, cutaneous disease is not uncommon, both as an intrinsic part of the condition and increasingly as a consequence of therapy (Table 51.25). Some problems, such as rheumatoid nodules and vasculitis, are well recognized, but more recently other abnormalities, such as transparent skin, linear subcutaneous bands and neutrophilic dermatoses, have been described. The array of skin problems seen in patients with rheumatoid arthritis has been well reviewed [1].

A dermatologist may also be involved in deciding between rheumatoid disease and SLE as the primary diagnosis. A skin biopsy for immunofluorescence studies may be helpful in aiding

Table 51.25 Cutaneous problems occurring in rheumatoid arthritis.

Rheumatoid nodules
Rheumatoid vasculitis (RV)
Felty's syndrome
Pyoderma gangrenosum (PG)
Interstitial granulomatous dermatitis with arthritis
Palisaded neutrophilic and granulomatous dermatitis
Rheumatoid neutrophilic dermatitis
Juvenile rheumatoid arthritis (JRA)
Adult-onset Still's disease

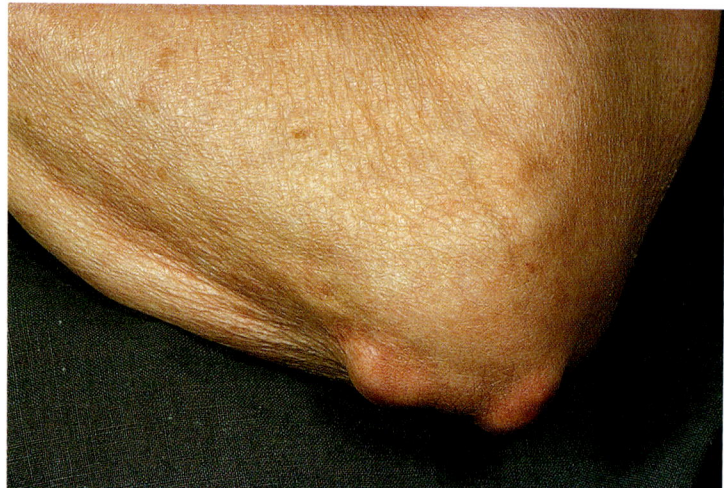

Fig. 51.90 Rheumatoid nodules on the elbow.

diagnosis because in the skin of the former, fluorescence of the dermal–epidermal junction is not found, even in cases with a high titre of antinuclear factor [2].

Pseudosclerodermatous changes, particularly of the hands, occur in rheumatoid arthritis, and there are common instances of overlap syndromes, where features of a number of more specific connective tissue diseases occur together [3].

Rheumatoid nodules [4] (Fig. 51.90)

Palpable subcutaneous nodules occur in approximately 20% of patients with rheumatoid arthritis. The most common site is on the ulnar border of the forearm. Less commonly, they occur on the dorsa of the hands, on the knees, on the ears, over the scapulae and occasionally in other areas, especially those subject to pressure, such as the sacrum, buttocks or heels. They vary in size up to several centimetres in diameter, are firm in consistency and tend to ulcerate with trauma (Fig. 51.91), particularly on the sacrum. Secondary infection with staphylococci can result in staphylococcal septicaemia and septic arthritis. Subcutaneous nodules can erode the underlying bone [5]. Sometimes, there are numerous violaceous papules with centripetal scaling. A variant of rheumatoid disease, termed 'rheumatoid nodulosis' [6], has been described, and may precede rheumatoid disease. Multiple, small nodules occur on the hands and feet with palindromic rheumatism and little evidence of synovitis. Nodules may be found in other organ systems, particularly the lungs [4].

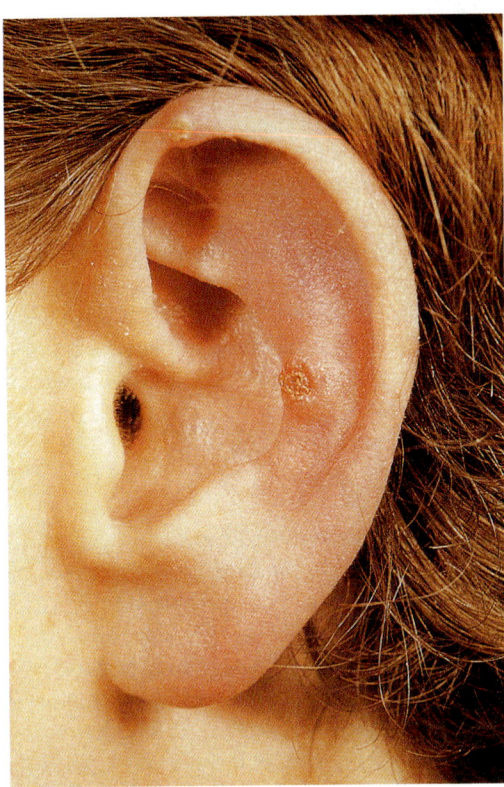

Fig. 51.91 Ulcerated rheumatoid nodule on the ear.

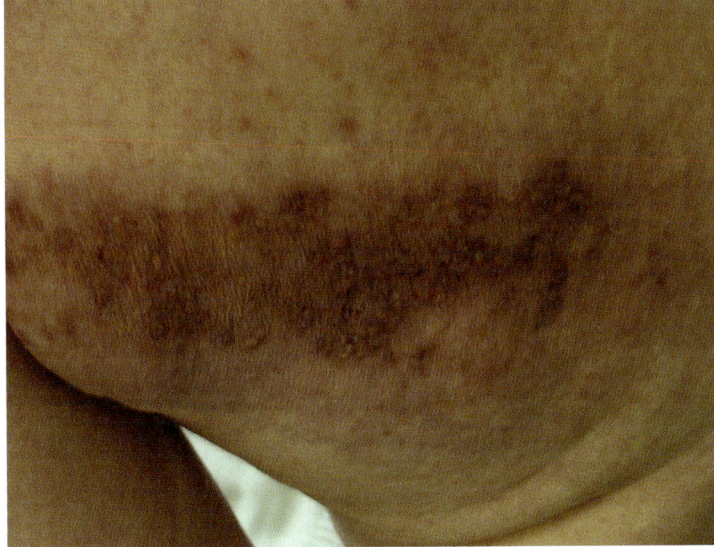

Fig. 51.92 Palisading and neutrophilic dermatosis in a patient with rheumatoid arthritis.

Nodules are almost invariably associated with more severe forms of the disease, and rheumatoid factor and antinuclear factors are frequently found in the serum. Occasionally, nodules may occur in mild rheumatoid arthritis and in anarthritic rheumatoid disease. Sometimes, they may precede rheumatoid arthritis by some years [4]. Rheumatoid nodules may rarely occur in the sclera (scleromalacia), which may perforate (scleromalacia perforans), leading to complete blindness. Severe nodulosis may be precipitated by therapies, including methotrexate and biological agents [7].

Histologically, rheumatoid nodules consist of fibrous tissue in which foci of fibrinoid necrosis are scattered, surrounded by a palisade of cells, mainly fibroblasts and histiocytes. A peripheral zone of lymphocytes and plasma cells occurs. Within the necrotic area are thin reticulum fibres, similar to those seen in young granulation tissue, amorphous material and some nuclear debris. Vasculitis can occur in rheumatoid nodules and papules. The histology has features in common with those of granuloma annulare (see Chapter 60).

The subcutaneous nodules of rheumatic fever [8] can be distinguished histologically from those of rheumatoid arthritis. There is much fibrinoid material, considerable oedema of the collagen, but relatively little infiltration with fibroblasts, histiocytes or lymphocytes. There is little attempt at zoning and fibrosis is minimal or absent. Large mononuclear cells, like those seen in Aschoff's nodes in the myocardium, may be found. Nodules from patients with Still's disease (juvenile rheumatoid arthritis) [8] resemble those seen in rheumatic fever. Another possible cause of nodulosis is the coexistence of erythema elevatum diutinum [9].

Linear subcutaneous bands and interstitial granulomatous dermatitis [10] (Fig. 51.92)

Elongated subcutaneous bands, 3–5 mm wide and 10 cm or more in length, have been described in patients with rheumatoid arthritis with nodules. Histologically, the bands show changes similar to the nodules, with interstitial granuloma formation, but no evidence of vasculitis. The bands, which are firm and non-tender, are adherent to the skin. They have so far been observed in the axilla, and extending from the axilla to the iliac crest. Similar histological appearances may be seen with a more papular clinical appearance.

Palisaded neutrophilic and granulomatous dermatitis

In addition, there are those who believe that another entity—palisaded neutrophilic and granulomatous dermatitis—may be part of a spectrum of cutaneous disease, with the degree of neutrophilic infiltration varying between patients. Others disagree, noting vasculitic histological change in those with more significant neutrophilic involvement [11]. Certainly, the two clinical patterns may occur together (Fig. 51.92).

Rheumatoid neutrophilic dermatosis. This may occur [12] in patients with severe arthritis as symmetrical erythematous nodules and 'urticaria-like' plaques on the dorsa of the hands and arms, extensor aspects of the joints, and the back of the neck and scalp and trunk. They are sometimes tender. Vertical symmetrical infiltrated linear cords on the median axillary line have been reported [11], as discussed above. Ulceration and vesiculation may occur. Histologically, there is a dense diffuse infiltrate of neutrophils in the dermis, papillary microabscesses and leukocytoclasia, but no vasculitis. The lunulae may be red [13]. Pyoderma gangrenosum may occur in association with neutrophilic dermatosis [14]. Dapsone, either alone or combined with colchicine, may help rheumatoid vasculitis and neutrophilic dermatosis [15].

Cutaneous changes due to steroid usage—purpura and paper-thin skin—are common.

References

1 Sayah A, English JC 3rd. Rheumatoid arthritis: a review of the cutaneous manifestations. *J Am Acad Dermatol* 2005; **53**: 191–209.

2 Muijs van de Moer WW, Cats A. Immunofluorescence of the skin in patients with rheumatoid arthritis. *Dermatologica* 1967; **134**: 351–5.

3 Pope JE. Musculoskeletal involvement in scleroderma. *Rheum Dis Clin North Am* 2003; **29**: 391–408.

4 Highton J, Hessian PA, Stamp L. The rheumatoid nodule: peripheral or central to rheumatoid arthritis? *Rheumatology* 2007; **46**: 1385–7.

5 Dorfman HD, Norman A, Smith RJ. Bone erosion in relation to subcutaneous rheumatoid nodules. *Arthritis Rheum* 1970; **13**: 69–73.

6 Ginsberg MH, Genant HK, Yu TF *et al.* Rheumatoid nodulosis: an unusual variant of rheumatoid disease. *Arthritis Rheum* 1963; **18**: 49–58.

7 Linksvan Ede A, den Broeder A, Wagenaar M *et al.* Etanercept-related extensive pulmonary nodulosis in a patient with rheumatoid arthritis. *J Rheumatol* 2007; **34**: 1590–2.

8 Bywaters EGL, Glynn LE, Zeldis A. Subcutaneous nodules of Still's disease. *Ann Rheum Dis* 1958; **17**: 278–83.

9 Balbir-Gurman A, Schapira D, Bergamn R, Nahir AM. Erythema elevatum diutinum: a rare cause of nodulosis in a patient with rheumatoid arthritis. *J Rheumatol* 2000; **27**: 2291–3.

10 Dykman CJ, Galens GJ, Good AE. Linear subcutaneous bands in rheumatoid arthritis. *Ann Intern Med* 1965; **63**: 134–40.

11 Al-Daraji WI, Coulson IH, Howat AJ. Palisaded neutrophilic and granulomatous dermatitis. *Clin Exp Dermatol* 2005; **30**: 578–9.

12 Mashek HA, Pham CT, Helm TN, Klaus M. Rheumatoid neutrophilic dermatitis. *Arch Dermatol* 1997; **133**: 757–60.

13 Jorizzo JL, Gonsalez EB, Daniels JC. Red lunulae in a patient with rheumatoid arthritis. *J Am Acad Dermatol* 1983; **8**: 711–4.

14 MacAya A, Servitje O, Jucqla A, Peyri J. Rheumatoid neutrophilic dermatitis associated with pyoderma gangrenosum. *Br J Dermatol* 2000; **142**: 1246–8.

15 Bernard P, Arnaud M, Treves R *et al.* Dapsone and rheumatoid vasculitis leg ulcerations. *J Am Acad Dermatol* 1988; **18**: 140–1.

Vascular lesions in rheumatoid arthritis [1,2]

The presence of vascular lesions in rheumatoid arthritis has been increasingly recognized in recent years. Raynaud's phenomenon is uncommon; it occurred in only 2.7% of one series [3]. However, there is now clear evidence of increased vascular pathology in RA, including the occurrence of large vessel atherosclerosis and cardiovascular disease [1,2].

The most characteristic lesions of arteritis in rheumatoid patients are small infarcts around the nails, sometimes at the apex of small cutaneous nodules. The lesions are usually transitory and may last only 2 or 3 days. Because they are usually painless, patients rarely complain about or even notice the lesions. Usually, a small brown spot persists a little longer, and sometimes scarring may occur. Occasionally, infarcts of the nail fold may result in grooving of the nail. Rarely, bullae may occur. The occurrence of digital necroses is closely correlated with the presence of rheumatoid factor and rheumatoid nodules [2]. Anticardiolipin antibodies can sometimes be demonstrated in patients with vasculitis, and are statistically significantly related to rheumatoid nodules but not to thrombotic events [4]. In addition to the infarcts around the nail folds, the pulps of the fingers may show small painful purpuric nodules (Bywaters' lesions). Histologically, these show leukocytoclastic vasculitis [5]. Palmar erythema is common.

In addition, the skin may show purpuric and necrotic arteritic lesions, which can be painful. The haemorrhagic areas appear without preceding trauma, and vary in size from small petechiae to areas of bruising and necrosis several centimetres in diameter. Sometimes, these areas develop black crusting, which may break down and ulcerate. The ulcers are well defined, with a surrounding bluish-red halo. Some of the ulcers are related to rheumatoid nodules. Healing occurs with scarring and may be slow. Arteritis occurs widely in rheumatoid disease, and involvement of the gastrointestinal tract [6] gives rise to abdominal pain, which may result from multiple ischaemic ulcers, gangrene of the bowel, intraperitoneal haemorrhage or splenic infarction.

Gangrene may result from changes in the digital vessels, and sometimes this may extend to involve a large part of the foot or hand, occasionally within a few days. Extensive pustular panniculitis, particularly on the legs, may occur as the result of breakdown of red, painful, nodular lesions. Treatment can be very difficult [7].

Leg ulcers. Leg ulcers are not uncommon in the rheumatoid population. Although vasculitis is an important cause, it was only considered to be a factor in 18% of rheumatoid patients in one recent series [8]. Venous insufficiency, complicated by immobility and postural factors, occurs in nearly half of cases, and trauma, pressure or arterial insufficiency are also major factors. Leg ulcers [9] may also be pyodermatous (Fig. 51.93). Arteritic ulcers are more common in males, particularly those with subcutaneous nodules and positive tests for rheumatoid factor. They are usually deep, punched out and slow healing. There is little discoloration of the legs and usually no sclerosis. Some of the ulcers may start as frankly purpuric or nodular lesions. Secondary infection is common, especially with *Staphylococcus aureus*. Response to treatment is slow and relapse frequent. Leg ulcers are more common in Felty's syndrome, in which arthritis is associated with splenomegaly and leukopenia.

Livedo reticularis [10] also occurs in rheumatoid arthritis, as does delayed pressure-induced vasculitis.

Peripheral sensory or motor neuropathy [11] is often associated with clinical evidence of arteritis elsewhere, and is caused by occlusion of the vasa nervorum by the arteritic process. These patients also have a high incidence of rheumatoid factor and nodule formation.

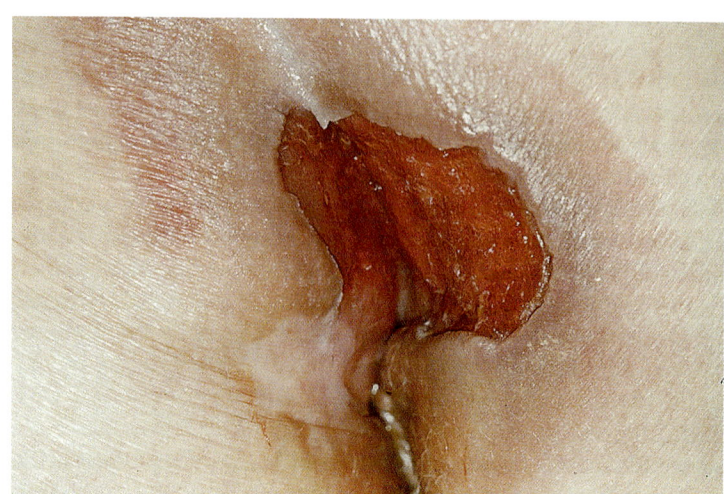

Fig. 51.93 Felty's syndrome: pyoderma gangrenosum of the perianal area.

A rash identical to that found in Still's disease (juvenile rheumatoid arthritis; see p. 51.133) occurs in adult rheumatoid arthritis, but is rare. It was found in only seven out of more than 500 patients [12].

Associations with other disorders. These have been comprehensively reviewed [13]. They include bullous pemphigoid, pemphigus vulgaris, pemphigus foliaceus, dermatitis herpetiformis, subcorneal pustular dermatosis [14], epidermolysis bullosa acquisita, yellow-nail syndrome, acquired cutis laxa [15], angioendotheliomatosis [16] and erosive pustular dermatosis of the scalp [17].

References

1 Szekanecz Z, Kerekes G, Dér H et al. Accelerated atherosclerosis in rheumatoid arthritis. Ann N Y Acad Sci 2007; **1108**: 349–58.
2 Genta MS, Genta RM, Gabay C. Systemic rheumatoid vasculitis: a review. Semin Arthritis Rheum 2006; **36**: 88–98.
3 Carroll GJ, Withers K, Bayliss CE. The prevalence of Raynaud's syndrome in rheumatoid arthritis. Ann Rheum Dis 1981; **40**: 567–70.
4 Wolf P, Gretler J, Aglas F et al. Anticardiolipin antibodies in rheumatoid arthritis: their relation to rheumatoid nodules and cutaneous vascular manifestations. Br J Dermatol 1994; **131**: 48–51.
5 Craig SD, Jorizzo JL, White WL et al. Cutaneous signs of rheumatic disease: acral purpuric papules in a patient with clinical rheumatoid arthritis. Arthritis Rheum 1994; **37**: 957–9.
6 Lindsay MK, Tavadia HB, Whyte AS et al. Acute abdomen in rheumatic arthritis due to necrotizing arteritis. BMJ 1973; **ii**: 592–3.
7 Anstey A, Wilkinson JD, Wojnarowska F et al. Pustular panniculitis in rheumatoid arthritis. J R Soc Med 1991; **84**: 307–8.
8 Pun YLW, Barraclough DRE, Muirden KD. Leg ulcers in rheumatoid arthritis. Med J Aust 1990; **153**: 585–7.
9 Wilkinson M, Kirk J. Leg ulcers complicating rheumatoid arthritis. Scott Med J 1965; **10**: 175–82.
10 Champion RH. Livedo reticularis. Br J Dermatol 1965; **77**: 167–79.
11 Said G, Lacroix C. Primary and secondary vasculitic neuropathy. J Neurol 2005; **252**: 633–41.
12 Isdale IC, Bywaters EGL. The rash of rheumatoid arthritis and Still's disease. QJM 1956; **49**: 377–87.
13 Jorizzo JL, Daniels JC. Dermatologic conditions reported in patients with rheumatoid arthritis. J Am Acad Dermatol 1983; **8**: 439–57.
14 Butt A, Burge SM. Sneddon–Wilkinson disease in association with rheumatoid arthritis. Br J Dermatol 1995; **132**: 313–5.
15 Rongioletti F, Cutolo M, Bondavalli P, Rebora A. Acral localized acquired cutis laxa associated with rheumatoid arthritis. J Am Acad Dermatol 2002; **46**: 128–30.
16 Tomasini C, Soro E, Pippione M. Angioendotheliomatosis in a woman with rheumatoid arthritis. Am J Dermatopathol 2000; **22**: 334–8.
17 Yamamoto T, Furuse Y. Erosive pustular dermatosis of the scalp in association with rheumatoid arthritis. Int J Dermatol 1995; **34**: 148.

Fibroblastic rheumatism

This entity was originally described by Chaouat et al. [1] in 1980, and since then further cases have been described, mainly in France [2]. It occurs at all ages and affects both sexes equally. Clinically, it starts suddenly with symmetrical polyarthritis and cutaneous nodules. These are between 5 and 20 cm in diameter, and can occur before the onset of arthritis. Raynaud's phenomenon, sclerodactyly with inability to join palms, joint effusions and stiffness are frequent. The nodules occur on both surfaces of the hands, usually over the joints, and on the elbows, knees, ears and neck (Fig. 51.94). They are smooth, firm and usually skin-coloured. They resolve in 6 months to a few years. Histology shows a marked proliferation of spindle cells and dermal fibrosis. The hyperplastic cells have the phenotypic features of muscle, suggesting myofibroblastic differentiation [3]. There is a reduction of collagen and

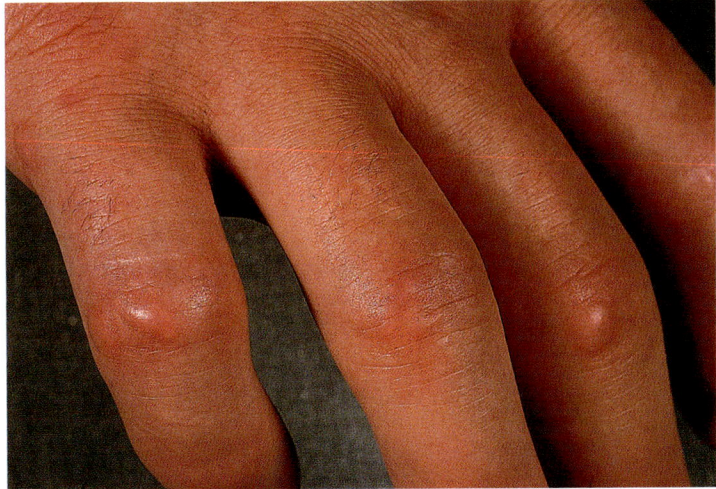

Fig. 51.94 Nodules on the dorsa of the interphalangeal joints in fibroblastic rheumatism. (Courtesy of Dr M.H.A. Rustin, The Royal Free Hospital, London, UK.)

non-collagen protein synthesis by the fibroblasts from involved skin, which contrasts markedly with the increase in collagen synthesis in scleroderma.

Systemic involvement does not usually occur—all laboratory tests are negative.

Spontaneous resolution of the nodules may be expected. Joint erosions may develop and changes tend to persist. There is little evidence indicating benefit from any treatment.

References

1 Chaouat Y, Aron-Brunetiere R, Faures B et al. Une nouvelle entite: le rheumatisme fibroblastique: a propos d'une observation. Rev Rheum Mal Osteoartic 1980; **47**: 345–51.
2 Kanzler MH, Dhillon I, Headington JT. Fibroblastic rheumatism. Arch Dermatol 1995; **131**: 710–2.
3 Lacour JP, Maquart FX, Bellow G et al. Fibroblastic rheumatism: clinical, histological, immunohistological, ultrastructural and biochemical study of a case. Br J Dermatol 1993; **128**: 194–202.

Still's disease

Synonym
• Juvenile rheumatoid arthritis

The characteristic rash [1] is seen in approximately 25% of patients with Still's disease. It occurs in boys (36%) more frequently than in girls (22%), the incidence decreasing with age. It consists of small, non-pruritic macules or papules up to 3 mm in diameter, with a slightly irregular margin. Larger lesions up to 5 cm show central pallor. The colour is bright salmon pink, often surrounded by a zone of pallor. The rash occurs most frequently on the limbs and trunk, but may occur on the face and neck, and lasts only a few hours, characteristically appearing at midday or in the evening with increased temperature of the patient or environment. It is more common in patients with fever, splenomegaly, lymphadenopathy and a raised ESR. It usually appears in the first 2 weeks of the disease but may precede other manifestations by up to 9 years. The rash may occur intermittently for many years and has no prognostic value [2].

Histologically, there is a scanty infiltrate, sometimes of neutrophils if the rash is marked, in the dermis. The rash fades as the disease settles; corticosteroids do not have a specific effect.

The rash can be distinguished from erythema marginatum by the smaller size of the lesions, their occurrence on the face and the fact that lesions are at their greatest size at the onset.

Subcutaneous nodules occur in Still's disease. The histology resembles that seen in the nodules of rheumatic fever rather than in those of rheumatoid arthritis [3]. Still's disease has been associated with Kikuchi's disease (see p. 51.58) [4,5].

References

1 Isdale IC, Bywaters EGL. The rash of rheumatoid arthritis and Still's disease. *QJM* 1956; **49**: 377–87.
2 Calabro JJ, Marchesano JM. Juvenile rheumatoid arthritis. *N Engl J Med* 1967; **277**: 696–9.
3 Bywaters EGL, Glynn LE, Zeldis A. Subcutaneous nodules of Still's disease. *Ann Rheum Dis* 1958; **17**: 278–85.
4 Lyberatos C. Two more cases of Still and Kikuchi. *J Rheumatol* 1990; **17**: 568–9.
5 Ohta A, Matsumoto J, Ohta T *et al.* Still's disease associated with necrotizing lymphadenitis (Kikuchi's disease): report of three cases. *J Rheumatol* 1988; **15**: 981–3.

Adult Still's disease [1]

In 1971, Bywaters [2] described 14 adults with arthritis and clinical features similar to those of juvenile rheumatoid arthritis. Features include a high spiking fever, sore throat, joint pain and arthritis, a transitory maculopapular rash, lymphadenopathy, hepatosplenomegaly and serositis. The white cell count is raised, and rheumatoid and antinuclear factors are usually absent. Both sexes are equally affected, and the onset is usually in the mid-twenties. The rash usually occurs in the evening, accompanied by fever in over 80% of patients, on the proximal limbs, trunk and face. Alopecia is another feature. Histologically, there is a perivascular dermal infiltrate of lymphocytes and histiocytes. Immunofluorescence is negative. The rash is an adverse prognostic indicator. Approximately one-third remit and another third become chronic; the remainder have an intermittent course. Aspirin and other nonsteroidal anti-inflammatory drugs are the first line of treatment, but systemic steroids may be required. In the more chronic cases, intramuscular or oral gold may be helpful. Methotrexate has been of benefit in refractory cases [3].

References

1 Pouchot J, Sampalis JS, Beandet F *et al.* Adult Still's disease: manifestations, disease course, and outcome in 62 patients. *Medicine* 1991; **70**: 118–36.
2 Bywaters EGL. Still's disease in the adult. *Ann Rheum Dis* 1971; **30**: 121–33.
3 Fujii T, Akizuki M, Kameda H *et al.* Methotrexate treatment in patients with adult onset Still's disease: retrospective study of 13 Japanese cases. *Ann Rheum Dis* 1997; **56**: 144–8.

Sjögren's syndrome [1]

Synonym

• Gougerot–Houwer–Sjögren syndrome

In 1933, Sjögren [2] drew attention to the syndrome that now bears his name. The first case was described in 1888, although earlier

Table 51.26 Revised classification criteria for Sjögren's syndrome (SS).

1 Ocular symptoms: at least one of:
  1 Dry eyes for more than 3 months
  2 Sensation of sand or gravel in the eyes
  3 Need for tear substitutes more than 3 times a day
2 Oral symptoms: at least one of:
  1 Dry mouth for more than 3 months
  2 Recurrently or persistently swollen salivary glands as an adult
  3 Need liquids to swallow dry food
3 Ocular signs—at least one of the following two tests positive:
  1 Schirmer's test, performed without anaesthesia (≤5 mm in 5 min)
  2 Rose Bengal score or other ocular dye score
4 Histopathology: in minor salivary glands, focal lymphocytic sialoadenitis (focus score ≥1).
5 Salivary gland involvement: a positive result for at least one of the following diagnostic tests:
  1 Unstimulated whole salivary flow (≤1.5 ml in 15 min)
  2 Parotid sialography showing the presence of diffuse sialectasias (punctate, cavitary, or destructive pattern), without evidence of obstruction in the major ducts
  3 Salivary scintigraphy showing delayed uptake, reduced concentration and/or delayed excretion of tracer
6 Autoantibodies: presence in the serum of antibodies to Ro(SSA) or La(SSB) antigens, or both

For primary SS

In patients without any potentially associated disease, primary SS may be defined as follows:

  a. The presence of any four of the six items is indicative of primary SS, as long as either item 4 (Histopathology) or 6 (Serology) is positive.
  b. The presence of any three of the four objective criteria items (that is, items 3, 4, 5, 6)

For secondary SS

In patients with a potentially associated disease, the presence of item 1 or item 2 plus any two from among items 3, 4, and 5 may be considered as indicative of secondary SS

authors, including Mikulicz, had noted several of the manifestations. The disease is caused by an immune-mediated inflammation of exocrine glands, and involves salivary, lacrimal and sweat glands. It may be primary, in which case the exocrine dysfunction occurs alone, or as secondary Sjögren's syndrome in association with a connective tissue disease. The most common features of the condition are dryness and atrophy of the conjunctiva and cornea (keratoconjunctivitis sicca), and a dry mouth (xerostomia). The diagnostic criteria, including these features and objective demonstration of exocrine dysfunction, have been reviewed, and the consensus findings are shown in Table 51.26 [3]. In addition to the commonly involved areas, other glandular structures may be affected, and there is variable internal organ involvement, but 'sicca' symptoms alone occurred in 35% of one series [4]. Malignant lymphoma is associated with the primary form of the disease [5].

Aetiology. The onset occurs most frequently in the fourth, fifth and sixth decades, and 90% of the patients with the primary form are women. A genetic predisposition is indicated by the finding of

Table 51.27 Pathological changes in Sjögren's syndrome.

Lymphocyte and plasma cell infiltration
Connective tissue proliferation
Glandular cell apoptosis, followed by atrophy of glandular structures in affected tissues (salivary glands, sebaceous glands, sweat glands etc.)
Secondary changes e.g. oedema of conjunctiva

Table 51.28 Skin manifestations in Sjögren's syndrome.

Xeroderma, pruritus and scaling
SCLE-like rashes [4], annular erythema, including Sweet's-like lesions and papular erythema [5]
Raynaud's syndrome
Hyperglobulinaemic purpura and inflammatory vasculitis, including PAN-like lesions
Vitiligo
Abnormalities of sweating
Amyloid
Alopecia—diffuse and generalized

an increased incidence of HLA-B8 and -DR3 in patients with Sjögren's syndrome, although DR4 is more closely associated with the syndrome occurring with Raynaud's phenomenon [6]. Associations with the complement allele C4AQO [7] and HLA-DRw52 [8] in Japanese patients have been reported. Antibodies to the Ro antigen occur in excess in relatives of patients with Sjögren's syndrome, especially in association with DR2 and DR3 [9]. Further evidence of an autoimmune condition is provided by the infiltration of the tissues by lymphocytes and plasma cells, and, as with the majority of autoimmune diseases, it is suggested that glandular damage, induced by a number of exogenous stimuli, leads to the expression of antigens—in this case Ro—which stimulate autoantibody production. Dendritic cells accumulate, produce interferon, which stimulates lymphocyte activation and stimulation, and glandular cell apoptosis is induced [1].

References

1 Fox RI. Sjogren's syndrome. *Lancet* 2005; **366**: 321–31.
2 Sjögren H. Zur Kenntnis der Keratoconjunctivitis sicca. *Acta Ophthalmol* 1933; **10** (Suppl. 2): 1–151.
3 Vitali C, Bombardieri S, Jonsson R *et al.* European Study Group on Classification Criteria for Sjögren's Syndrome. Classification criteria for Sjögren's syndrome: a revised version of the European criteria proposed by the American-European Consensus Group. *Ann Rheum Dis* 2002; **61**: 554–8.
4 Block KJ, Buchanan WW, Wohl MJ *et al.* Sjögren's syndrome. *Medicine* 1965; **44**: 187–231.
5 Voulgarelis M, Dafni UG, Isenberg DA *et al.* Malignant lymphoma in primary Sjögren's syndrome: a multicenter, retrospective, clinical study by the European Concerted Action of Sjögren's Syndrome. *Arthritis Rheum* 1999; **42**: 1765–72.
6 Mann DL, Moutsopoulos HM. HLA or alloantigens in different subsets of patients with Sjögren's syndrome and in family members. *Ann Rheum Dis* 1983; **42**: 533–6.
7 Mouichi J, Ichikawa Y, Takaya M *et al.* Association of the complement allele C4 AQO with primary Sjögren's syndrome in Japanese patients. *Arthritis Rheum* 1991; **34**: 224–7.
8 Miyagaura S, Dohi K, Shima H, Shirai T. HLA antigens in anti-Ro (SS-A) positive patients with recurrent annular erythema. *J Am Acad Dermatol* 1993; **28**: 185–8.
9 Arnett FC, Hamilton RG, Reveille JD *et al.* Genetic studies of Ro (SS-A) and La (SS-B) autoantibodies in familes with systemic lupus erythematosus and primary Sjögren's syndrome. *Arthritis Rheum* 1989; **32**: 413–9.

Pathology [1]. The salient pathological changes are shown in Table 51.27.

Reference

1 Morgan AD, Raven RW. Sjögren's syndrome: a general disease. *Br J Surg* 1952–53; **40**: 154–62.

Clinical features [1]. The clinical picture is extremely variable. The consequences of reduced exocrine gland activity may be a minor manifestation of a serious systemic illness, or the presenting, and for many years the only, features. In a prospective study of patients presenting with dry eyes, 43% were found to have keratoconjunctivitis sicca with xerostomia, and 23% had associated connective tissue disease, particularly rheumatoid arthritis [2]. Oral symptoms may precede ocular, or both may occur late in the disease. Some cases present with generalized or anogenital pruritus, or with diffuse alopecia. Reduction in the appreciation of taste and smell has been observed [3]. Infections, including pneumonia, oral candidosis and bacterial conjunctivitis, are frequent.

Skin involvement occurs in around 50% of patients, and may be more common but not recognized (Table 51.28). Annular erythema in Japanese patients may differ from others. In Japan, annular erythema has been subdivided into three types clinically: Sweet's disease-like annular erythema with an elevated border; SCLE-like marginally scaled erythema; and papular erythema [5]. Annular erythema of Asian patients, which is recurrent and non-scarring, may occur in patients with LE, Sjögren's syndrome or both diseases [6]. These lesions are not photosensitive in origin. Ro antibody-positive patients tend to develop annular polycyclic lesions of SCLE as well as neuropsychiatric and pulmonary disease, and have a guarded prognosis [7]. Vascular responsiveness may also be impaired [8] and nail fold capillary abnormalities are found [9].

Non-thrombocytopenic purpura may occur as recurrent crops of round pink lesions in dependent areas (Fig. 51.95), and is associated with hyperglobulinaemia. It may be confused with vasculitis, and fades to leave brown-pigmented stains, but crops occur over many years. Biopsy shows perivascular mononuclear infiltration, but no active vasculitis. However, inflammatory and often necrotizing vasculitis can occur, including an arteritis like that seen in rheumatoid arthritis, lesions indistinguishable from polyarteritis nodosa and nail fold infarcts, splinter haemorrhages and gangrene of the fingers [10].

Mouth. The saliva is at first thick and mucoid, but later salivary volume decreases. The tongue is red, smooth and dry, and in severe cases there may be difficulty in swallowing dry food. Parotid duct narrowing and web formation may develop [11]. Dental caries is often severe and progressive. The lips are red, dry and scaly. There are frequently cracks at the corners of the mouth. Chronic oral candidiasis is frequent. Recurrent episodes of swelling of one or both parotid glands or, less often, the submaxillary and sublingual glands, may be due to autoimmune inflammation or infection, which is common. Impaired glandular function may

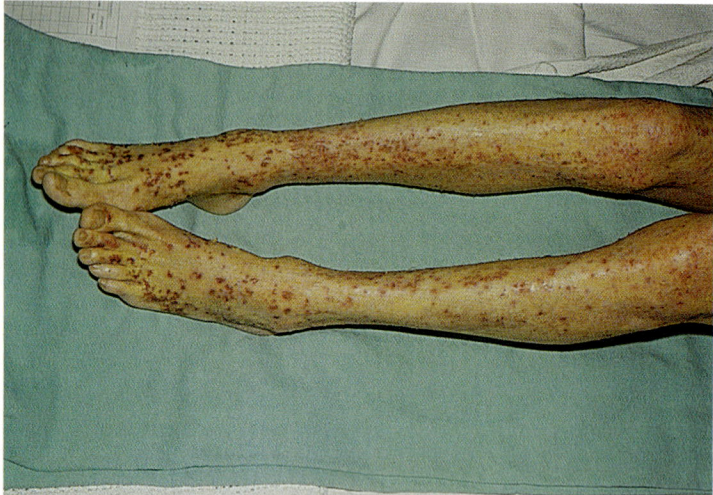

Fig. 51.95 Hyperglobulinaemic purpura in Sjögren's syndrome.

Table 51.29 Other manifestations of Sjögren's syndrome.

Joint symptoms—arthralgia and arthritis
Myalgia and myositis
ENT problems: sinusitis, hearing problems including deafness
Tracheal and oesophageal reflux
Interstitial pneumonitis, pulmonary fibrosis and pulmonary hypertension
Interstitial nephritis
Gastrointestinal conditions, including primary biliary cirrhosis
Neurological abnormalities: migraine, neuropathies, cerebral vasculitis

be due to both glandular destruction and functional changes due to altered responsiveness to neurological stimulus [12].

Other mucous membranes [11]. Atrophic changes in the mucous membranes of the upper respiratory tract lead to nasal crusting and dryness, recurrent episodes of infection, hoarseness or aphonia. Pulmonary infiltration, atelectasis or fibrosis may occur. Atrophic rhinitis can occur, and the sense of smell may be reduced. Digestive symptoms are attributable to atrophy of the gastric mucous membrane with achlorhydria. Similar changes in the vulva and vagina give rise to pruritus and vaginitis, and dryness of the anal and rectal mucous membrane leads to dyschezia and pruritus.

Other manifestations (Table 51.29) [1]. In patients without associated connective tissue disease, mild articular symptoms occur in 83%, with mild synovitis. Cervical or generalized lymphadenopathy and enlargement of the liver and spleen, which is sometimes considerable, may be found. The main renal abnormalities appear to be interstitial nephritis, renal tubular acidosis, impaired renal concentrating ability and generalized aminoaciduria [13]. Impaired renal function can occur without clinical manifestations [14]. A high prevalence of fetal loss has been recorded, but there was no correlation with anticardiolipin or anti-Ro antibodies [15].

References

1 Papiris SA, Tsonis IA, Moutsopoulos HM. Sjögren's syndrome. *Semin Respir Crit Care Med* 2007; **28**: 459–71.
2 Forstot JZ, Forstot SL, Greer RO *et al.* The incidence of Sjögren's sicca complex in a population of patients with keratoconjunctivitis sicca. *Arthritis Rheum* 1982; **25**: 156–60.
3 Henkin RI, Talal N, Larson AL *et al.* Abnormalities of taste and smell in Sjögren's syndrome. *Ann Intern Med* 1972; **76**: 375–83.
4 Ruzicka T, Faes J, Bergner T *et al.* Annular erythema associated with Sjögren's syndrome: a variant of systemic lupus erythematosus. *J Am Acad Dermatol* 1991; **25**: 557–60.
5 Teramoto N, Katayama I, Arai H *et al.* Annular erythema: a possible association with primary Sjögren's syndrome. *J Am Acad Dermatol* 1989; **20**: 596–601.
6 Watanabe T, Tsuchida T, Ito Y *et al.* Annular erythema associated with lupus erythematosus/Sjögren's syndrome. *J Am Acad Dermatol* 1997; **36**: 214–8.
7 Provost TT, Talal N, Harley JB *et al.* The relationship between anti-Ro (SS-A) antibody-positive Sjögren's syndrome and anti-Ro (SS-A) antibody-positive lupus erythematosus. *Arch Dermatol* 1988; **124**: 63–71.
8 Kovacs L, Torok T, Bari F *et al.* Impaired microvascular response to cholinergic stimuli in primary Sjögren's syndrome. *Ann Rheum Dis* 2000; **59**: 48–53.
9 Tektonidou M, Kaskani E, Skopouli FN *et al.* Microvascular abnormalities in Sjögren's syndrome: nailfold capillaroscopy. *Rheumatology (Oxford)* 1999; **38**: 826–30.
10 Claeys V, Wackens G. [Sjogren syndrome: a review of the literature and a case report]. *Revue Belge de Medecine Dentaire* 2006; **61**: 161–72.
11 Doig JA, Whaley K, Dick WC *et al.* Otolaryngological aspects of Sjögren's syndrome. *BMJ* 1971; **iv**: 460–3.
12 Soto-Rojas AE, Kraus A. The oral side of Sjogren syndrome. Diagnosis and treatment. *Arch Med Res* 2002; **33**: 95–106.
13 Tu WH, Shearn MA, Lee JC *et al.* Interstitial nephritis in Sjögren's syndrome. *Ann Intern Med* 1968; **69**: 1163–70.
14 Shiozawa S, Shiozawa K, Shimizu S *et al.* Clinical studies of renal disease in Sjögren's syndrome. *Ann Rheum Dis* 1987; **46**: 768–72.
15 Valesini G, Priori R, Borsetti A *et al.* Clinical serological correlations in the evaluation of Sjögren's syndrome. *Clin Exp Rheumatol* 1989; **7**: 197–202.

Sjögren's syndrome in childhood. Primary Sjögren's syndrome is rare in childhood. Recurrent annular erythema similar to that seen in adults has been reported on the face, trunk and limbs [1]. Episodes, with or without fever and parotid swelling, occur over years and last a few months. Anti-Ro antibodies are positive but there is no evidence of SLE. Histology of the lesions shows a dermal lymphocytic infiltration but no vasculitis, and immunohistology reveals no immunoglobulins or complement at the dermal–epidermal junction or around blood vessels. The condition responds to oral steroids.

Reference

1 Miyagawa S, Iida T, Fukumoto T *et al.* Anti-Ro/SSA-associated annular erythema in childhood. *Br J Dermatol* 1995; **133**: 779–82.

Laboratory abnormalities. Hypergammaglobulinaemia and rheumatoid factor are frequently demonstrated in the serum, even in patients without arthritis, and serum viscosity is usually raised [1]. Antinuclear antibodies are present in more than 50% of patients (homogeneous factor is more frequent than speckled, and nucleolar factor is only occasionally found). Anti-DNA antibody can occasionally be demonstrated, but anti-Sm and anti-RNP antibodies are never found in the sicca syndrome alone. Anti-Ro (also called SS-A) and anti-La (SS-B) are frequently found and are an important part of the diagnostic profile of the disease. Antibodies to Ro/La were found in 53% of patients with Sjögren's syndrome [2]. Anti-Ro antibodies are particularly associated with vasculitis, purpura, lymphadenopathy, and haematological and serological abnormalities [3]. Recurrent annular erythema is associated with anti-La antibodies in Sjögren's syndrome [4,5] but not all anti-La-positive patients have a rash, and no disease-specific epitope has been demonstrated [6]. The epitope of anti-Ro antibody is similar in the annular erythema of Sjögren's syndrome and SCLE [7]. Antibody to salivary duct epithelium can be demonstrated in approximately 50% but is also found in uncomplicated rheumatoid arthritis [8]. Thyroglobulin antibodies are present in 25% of cases [9]. Leukopenia and eosinophilia are not infrequent. Immune complexes occur in 60%, but are not related to disease activity [10].

References

1 Blaylock WM, Waller M, Normansell DE. Sjögren's syndrome: hyperviscosity and intermediate complexes. *Ann Intern Med* 1974; **80**: 27–34.
2 Pease CT, Shattles W, Charles PJ *et al.* Clinical, serological, and HLA phenotype subsets in Sjögren's syndrome. *Clin Exp Rheumatol* 1989; **7**: 185–90.
3 Alexander EL, Hirsch TJ, Arnett FC *et al.* Ro (SSA) and La (SSB) antibodies in the clinical spectrum of Sjögren's syndrome. *J Rheumatol* 1982; **9**: 239–46.
4 Teramoto N, Katayama I, Arai H *et al.* Annular erythema: a possible association with primary Sjögren's syndrome. *J Am Acad Dermatol* 1991; **20**: 596–601.
5 Ruzicka T, Faes J, Bergman T *et al.* Annular erythema associated with Sjögren's syndrome: a variant of systemic lupus erythematosus. *J Am Acad Dermatol* 1991; **25**: 557–60.
6 Yoshino Y, Hashimoto T, Mimori T *et al.* Recurrent annular erythema associated with anti-SS-B/La antibodies: analysis of the disease-specific epitope. *Br J Dermatol* 1992; **127**: 608–13.
7 McCauliffe DP, Faircloth E, Wang L *et al.* Similar Ro/SS-A autoantibody epitope and titre responses in annular erythema of Sjögren's syndrome and subacute cutaneous lupus erythematosus. *Arch Dermatol* 1996; **132**: 528–31.
8 MacSween RNM, Goudie RB, Anderson JR *et al.* Occurrence of antibody to salivary duct epithelium in Sjögren's disease, rheumatoid arthritis and other arthritides. *Ann Rheum Dis* 1967; **26**: 402–11.
9 Bloch KJ, Buchanan WW, Wohl MJ *et al.* Sjögren's syndrome. *Medicine* 1965; **44**: 187–231.
10 Fishbach M, Char D, Christensen M *et al.* Immune complexes in Sjögren's syndrome. *Arthritis Rheum* 1980; **23**: 791–5.

Associations [1]. Diseases reported in association with Sjögren's syndrome are listed in Table 51.30. Drug allergy, especially to penicillin [18], is also more common than expected.

Table 51.30 Diseases reported in association with Sjögren's syndrome.

Connective tissue disease (rheumatoid arthritis (26%), systemic sclerosis (22%)) [2]
Sweet's syndrome [3]
Lymphoproliferative disorders—B and T cell, and MALT associated [4]
Primary biliary cirrhosis, chronic hepatitis [5]
Lipodystrophy [6]
Granulomatous panniculitis [7]
Behçet's disease [8]
Coeliac disease [9]
Hypothyroidism and thyroiditis [10]
Myasthenia gravis [11]
Haemochromatosis [12]
Dermatitis herpetiformis [13]
Darier's disease [14]
Multicentric reticulohistiocytosis [15]
Sarcoidosis [16]
Waldenström's hyperglobulinaemic purpura [17]

References

1 Fox RI. Sjogren's syndrome. *Lancet* 2005; **366**: 321–31.
2 Coll J, Rives A, Grino MC *et al.* Prevalence of Sjögren's syndrome in autoimmune diseases. *Ann Rheum Dis* 1987; **46**: 286–9.
3 Levanstein MM, Fisher BK, Fisher L *et al.* Simultaneous occurrence of subacute cutaneous lupus erythematosus and Sweet syndrome: a marker of Sjögren syndrome? *Int J Dermatol* 1991; **30**: 640–3.
4 Smedby KE, Baecklund E, Askling J. Malignant lymphomas in autoimmunity and inflammation: a review of risks, risk factors, and lymphoma characteristics. *Cancer Epidemiol Biomarkers Prev* 2006; **15**: 2069–77.
5 Golding PL, Brown R, Mason AMS *et al.* 'Sicca complex' in liver disease. *BMJ* 1970; **iv**: 340–2.
6 Alarcón-Segoviá D, Ramos-Niembro F. Association of partial lipodystrophy and Sjögren's syndrome. *Ann Intern Med* 1976; **85**: 474–5.
7 Tait CP, Yu LL, Rohr J. Sjögren's syndrome and granulomatous panniculitis. *Australas J Dermatol* 2000; **41**: 187–9.
8 Ramirez-Peredo J, Cetina JA, Alarcón-Segoviá D. Sjögren's syndrome in Bechçet's disease. *Lancet* 1973; **ii**: 732.
9 Maclaurin BP, Matthews N, Kilpatrick JA. Coeliac disease associated with autoimmune thyroiditis, Sjögren's syndrome and a lymphocytotoxic serum factor. *Aust NZ J Med* 1972; **2**: 405–11.
10 Edmonds ME, Saunders A, Sturrock RD. Rheumatoid arthritis associated with hypoparathyroidism and Sjögren's syndrome. *J R Soc Med* 1979; **72**: 856–8.
11 Ito Y, Kanda N, Mitsui H *et al.* Cutaneous manifestations of Sjögren's syndrome associated with myasthenia gravis. *Br J Dermatol* 1999; **141**: 362–3.
12 Blandford RL, Dowdle JR, Stephens MR *et al.* Sicca syndrome associated with idiopathic haemochromatosis. *BMJ* 1979; **i**: 1323.
13 Fraser NG, Rennie AGR, Donald D. Dermatitis herpetiformis and Sjögren's syndrome. *Br J Dermatol* 1979; **100**: 213–5.
14 Oxholm A, da Cunha Bang F, Oxholm P. Simultaneous occurrence of Darier's disease and primary Sjögren's syndrome. *Arthritis Rheum* 1986; **29**: 1052.
15 Carey RD, Blotzer JW, Wolfe ID *et al.* Multicentric reticulohistiocytosis and Sjögren's syndrome. *J Rheumatol* 1985; **12**: 1193–5.
16 Cox NH, McCrea JD. A case of Sjögren's syndrome, sarcoidosis, previous ulcerative colitis and gastric autoantibodies. *Br J Dermatol* 1996; **134**: 1138–40.
17 Miyagaura S, Fukumoto T, Kananchi M *et al.* Hypergammaglobulinaemic purpura of Waldenstrom and Ro/SSA antibodies. *Br J Dermatol* 1996; **134**: 919–23.
18 Williams BO, St Onge RA, Young A *et al.* Penicillin allergy in rheumatoid arthritis. *Ann Rheum Dis* 1969; **28**: 607–11.

Diagnosis. So variable is the clinical picture that the diagnosis is easily overlooked, except in the more obvious cases presenting with ocular or oral symptoms.

It should also be suspected in the presence of anogenital pruritus in association with ocular and oral changes or with rheumatoid disease, and should be confirmed by specialist ophthalmological examination. Biopsy of labial salivary glands [1] or nasal mucosa [2] is useful, and the value of lip biopsy has been stressed, but a negative biopsy does not exclude the diagnosis [3]. The demonstration of anti-Ro (SS-A) and anti-La (SS-B) antibodies may be helpful in diagnosis, and anti-La may antedate clinical evidence of Sjögren's syndrome by months or even years [4]. Contrast sialography is useful [5], and sequential salivary scintigraphy [6] gives objective and sensitive estimation of salivary gland function. Once a diagnosis is made, every case requires detailed investigation to determine the extent and nature of the associated abnormalities.

Treatment. Symptomatic treatment for the dryness of the eyes is best accomplished by lubricating agents, such as 0.5% methylcellulose eye drops instilled into the eyes four or five times daily. Bromhexine 16 mg three times daily has been found to increase the lacrimal secretion, but has no effect on salivary flow [7]. However, it does change the salivary composition towards normal [8]. Artificial saliva can be prescribed, and steam inhalations or an air humidifier may help dryness of the respiratory tract. Patients with Sjögren's syndrome associated with SLE seem to improve more than those with primary Sjögren's syndrome. Systemic corticosteroids are effective in reducing parotid swelling, but rarely increase parotid or lacrimal secretion. The immunological abnormalities in the serum are not markedly altered by corticosteroids. Chloroquine or hydroxychloroquine sulphate by mouth have been found useful by some authors [9] but not by others [10]. Ciclosporin improved subjective xerostomia and may reduce histopathological progression [11]. Nifedipine may help pulmonary Raynaud's phenomenon [12]. A patient with associated polymyositis improved with monthly intravenous pulse cyclophosphamide therapy [13]. The annular erythema in Japanese patients may be controlled by prednisolone 10–20 mg/day or by dapsone. There is no single therapy that helps hyperglobulinaemic purpura, although graduated compression hosiery may be significantly valuable. The role of biological therapies, particularly rituximab, is being evaluated [14].

References

1 Daniels TE. Labial salivary gland biopsy in Sjögren's syndrome: assessment as a diagnostic criterion in 362 suspected cases. *Arthritis Rheum* 1984; **27**: 147–56.

2 Powell RD, Larson AL, Henkin RI. Nasal mucous membrane biopsy in Sjögren's syndrome. *Ann Intern Med* 1974; **81**: 25–31.

3 Valesini G, Priori R, Borsetti A *et al.* Clinical and serological correlations in the evaluation of Sjögren's syndrome. *Clin Exp Rheumatol* 1989; **7**: 197–202.

4 Isenberg DA, Hammond L, Fisher C *et al.* Predictive value of SS-B precipitating antibodies in Sjögren's syndrome. *BMJ* 1982; **284**: 1738–40.

5 Miyachi K, Naito M, Maeno Y *et al.* Sialographic study in patients with and without antibodies to Sjögren's syndrome A (Ro). *J Rheumatol* 1983; **10**: 387–94.

6 Schall GL, Anderson LG, Wolf RO *et al.* Xerostomia in Sjögren's syndrome. *JAMA* 1971; **216**: 2109–16.

7 Frost-Larsen K, Isager H, Manthorpe R. Sjögren's syndrome treated with bromhexine: a randomized clinical study. *BMJ* 1978; **i**: 1579–81.

8 Nahir AM, Aryeh HB, Szargel R *et al.* Sialochemistry in evaluating bromhexine treatment of Sjögren's syndrome. *BMJ* 1979; **ii**: 833.

9 Fox RI, Chan E, Benton L *et al.* Treatment of primary Sjögren's syndrome with hydroxychloroquine. *Am J Med* 1988; **85**: 62–7.

10 Bloch KJ, Buchanan WW, Wohl MJ *et al.* Sjögren's syndrome. *Medicine* 1965; **44**: 187–231.

11 Drosos AA, Skopouli FN, Costopoulos JS *et al.* Cyclosporin A (CyA) in primary Sjögren's syndrome: a double-blind study. *Ann Rheum Dis* 1986; **45**: 732–5.

12 Joseph BZ, Organek HW, Grant A *et al.* Effects of nifedipine therapy on pulmonary Raynaud's in primary Sjögren's syndrome. *Clin Exp Rheum* 1988; **6**: 409–10.

13 Leroy JP, Drosos AA, Yiannopoulos DI *et al.* Intravenous pulse cyclosphosphamide therapy in myositis and Sjögren's syndrome. *Arthritis Rheum* 1990; **33**: 1579–81.

14 Bryce AH, Dispenzieri A, Kyle RA *et al.* Response to rituximab in patients with type II cryoglobulinemia. *Clin Lymphoma Myeloma* 2006; **7**: 140–4.

Rheumatic fever

Erythema marginatum is the characteristic rash of rheumatic fever, and occurs in 25% of cases [1]. It appears as evanescent, asymptomatic, pinkish superficial semicircles and rings, which disappear without scaling or pigmentation in a few days. Histologically, there is a perivascular infiltration of neutrophils in the papillary dermis, and biopsy may help in the early diagnosis of rheumatic fever when the rash precedes arthritis and carditis [2]. Erythema multiforme, petechiae and urticaria may sometimes be seen in rheumatic fever. Livedo reticularis has been reported [3]. The overall clinical picture must be distinguished from post-streptococcal reactive arthritis [4].

Subcutaneous nodules occur, particularly on the occiput, wrist and the backs of the forearms, and are smaller and more transient than those seen in rheumatoid arthritis, from which they can be distinguished histologically [5]. Generalized eruptive histiocytomas [6] and erythema elevatum diutinum [7] have also occurred with rheumatic fever.

References

1 Hill AGS. Skin manifestations in rheumatic disorders. *Trans St John's Hosp Dermatol Soc* 1964; **50**: 105–12.

2 Troyer C. Erythema marginatum in rheumatic fever: early diagnosis by skin biopsy. *J Am Acad Dermatol* 1983; **8**: 724–8.

3 Haber H. Zur Ätiologie der Livedo racemosa. *Arch Dermatol Syphilol* 1931; **163**: 1–5.

4 Jansen TL, Janssen M, de Jong AJ, Jeurissen ME. Post-streptococcal reactive arthritis: a clinical and serological description, revealing its distinction from acute rheumatic fever. *J Intern Med* 1999; **245**: 261–7.

5 Bennett GA, Zeller JW, Bauer W. Subcutaneous nodules of rheumatoid arthritis and rheumatic fever. *Arch Pathol* 1940; **30**: 70–89.

6 Matsushima Y, Ohnishi K, Ishikawa O. Generalized eruptive histiocytoma of childhood associated with rheumatic fever. *Eur J Dermatol* 1999; **9**: 548–50.

7 Wahl CE, Bouldin MB, Gibson LE. Erythema elevatum diutinum: clinical, histopathologic and immunohistochemical characteristics of six patients. *Am J Dermatopathol* 2005; **27**: 397–400.

CHAPTER 52

Non-Melanoma Skin Cancer and Other Epidermal Skin Tumours

A.G. Quinn[1] & W. Perkins[2]

[1]Synageva BioPharma Corporation, Waltham, Massachusetts, USA
[2]Nottingham University Hospital, Queen's Medical Centre, Nottingham, UK

Introduction

The complexity of the cellular composition of the skin means that the range of tumours that can arise within it is very wide. This chapter deals chiefly with the benign and malignant tumours arising from epidermal keratinocytes. Non-melanoma skin cancers and related premalignant lesions are dealt with in a separate section in view of their clinical importance and the overlap in the epidemiology, pathogenesis and management of these tumours. Chapter 53 is devoted to appendage tumours, Chapter 54 to tumours arising from the melanocyte and Chapter 56 to soft-tissue tumours.

A *tumour* is an abnormal mass of tissue, the growth of which exceeds and is uncoordinated with that of normal tissues. Although most tumours retain a resemblance to the normal tissue from which they arise, they can show an extraordinary variation in their structure and it is this variation that causes difficulties in some cases in establishing a definitive pathological diagnosis. Most of the keratinocyte-derived tumours described in this chapter are *benign*, which is the term used to describe tumours where the cells remain at their site of origin, forming a single mass of tumour cells. *Hamartomas* are difficult to distinguish from true benign tumours clinically. They are not true tumours and best considered as a localized overproduction of one or more elements of a tissue but without the progressive growth characteristics of a tumour. *Malignant* tumours are composed of cells that have acquired the ability to invade through a basement membrane and this is associated with the capacity to metastasize to other organs via the lymphatics and blood vessels. In addition, malignant tumours frequently show more rapid growth and less differentiation than benign tumours, which is reflected histologically by higher mitotic

Rook's Textbook of Dermatology, 8th edition. Edited by DA Burns, SM Breathnach, NH Cox and CEM Griffiths. © 2010 Blackwell Publishing Ltd.

rates, cellular and nuclear pleomorphism and abnormal mitoses. Differentiation between benign and malignant tumours is one of the major responsibilities of a dermatopathologist. The distinction, however, can be difficult with small tissue samples and is not absolute, which means it is vital that there is good communication between the clinician and pathologist, particularly when the pathology report suggests biological behaviour not in keeping with the clinical impression [1,2].

References

1 Leigh IM, Newton-Bishop J, Kripke ML, eds. *Skin Cancer*. Cancer Surveys no. 26. New York: Cold Spring Harbor, 1996.
2 Mackie RM. *Skin Cancer*, 2nd edn. London: Dunitz, 1996.

Non-melanoma skin cancer and related premalignant lesions

Non-melanoma skin cancer (NMSC) is the most common human cancer. The term encompasses basal cell carcinoma (BCC) and squamous cell carcinoma (SCC) of the skin, which are both derived from epidermal keratinocytes. Although these tumours are clinically and pathologically distinctive, they share some characteristics and are frequently classified under the term NMSC for health care planning, cancer registry reporting and epidemiological purposes. In contrast to other common epithelial cancers, NMSCs rarely metastasize, which means that the case fatality rate for these cancers is low. This low mortality from NMSC has contributed to the widespread under-reporting of this cancer to disease registries in many countries which makes it challenging to quantify accurately the morbidity and health care costs associated with this disease. Nevertheless, given the high prevalence of NMSC and the frequent occurrence of multiple primary tumours in affected individuals, there is little disagreement amongst dermatologists that NMSC is an important and frequently underestimated public health problem.

Patients at risk for development of NMSC are also predisposed to the development of actinic keratoses (AK) and Bowen's disease, which are premalignant lesions that show some of the histological characteristics of SCC. The prevalence of AK and the multiplicity of lesions within individual subjects is considerably greater than that for NMSC. While there is some controversy about the premalignant potential of AK and Bowen's disease and their relationship to SCC, these lesions are, in themselves, an important clinical problem for three reasons. First, they need to be distinguished from SCC; secondly, they cause concern and anxiety in patients, particularly in those with a previous history of NMSC; and, thirdly, the scaling and inflammation associated with these lesions is an important contributor to the overall morbidity associated with photoageing.

Epidemiology and risk factors for non-melanoma skin cancer development

Epidemiological surveys have a key role in the generation of incidence and prevalence data for NMSC in populations, quantification of the clinical impression of increasing skin cancer incidence and identification of environmental and host factors important in NMSC development.

Incidence and mortality

Whilst the prevalence of NMSC is recognized as being high and represents a substantial economic burden to health providers, accurate figures for NMSC are unavailable in most geographical regions as these cancers are not reported in many national cancer registries. Giles *et al.* [1], in an Australian postal survey of 31 000 individuals, conducted in 1985, reported 652 BCCs and 160 SCCs and an increased incidence of SCCs from 166 to 250 per 100 000 over the 5-year period, and an 11% increase in the incidence of BCCs [2]. In the USA, a population-based study [3] quotes an incidence of 38 SCCs per 100 000 population, with a 3 : 1, male : female preponderance. Miller and Weinstock [4] have estimated that in 1994 there were 1 million new cases of NMSC in the USA. Mortality from NMSC in the USA is estimated at $0.44/10^5$ per year [5], with the main cause of death being metastases from SCC. There are a few recorded deaths from BCC, most of these being related to refusal of surgical treatment. The annual cost of treating NMSC in the USA has been estimated at over $500 million [6].

The incidence of NMSC has increased dramatically over the last 30–40 years in many populations worldwide. In addition to the study by Giles in Australia showing a 50% increase in the incidence of SCC and an 11% increase in the incidence of BCCs between 1985 and 1990 [2], Miller and Weinstock have reported a threefold increase in NMSC incidence in the USA over the past two decades with a continuing rise at a rate of 8% per year [4]. Increases in NMSC incidence have also been reported in Europe. In Wales, a population-based study has shown that the crude incidence for NMSC has increased from 173.5 to 265.4 per 100 000 population per annum between 1988 and 1998 [7]. Although differences in the methodologies between reported population-based studies make it difficult to directly compare NMSC incidence in different countries, comparison of age-specific incidence rates of BCCs in two studies from Sweden and Australia indicate that the rate in northern Europe is approximately three to four times less than that seen in the Australian population [1,7,8].

Most studies indicate that BCCs account for more than 70% of the cases of NMSC in areas with both high and low ambient sun exposure. Although a ratio of 4 : 1, BCC : SCC has been described as a relatively consistent finding in studies of NMSC incidence in non-immunosuppressed, white-skinned individuals, closer examination of the available information shows that this ratio differs between countries with low and high ambient sun exposure, which reflects a disproportionate increase in SCC relative to BCC with increasing sun exposure. In some groups such as white Maryland fisherman with very high occupational ultraviolet radiation (UVR) exposure, the ratio of BCC : SCC is almost 1 : 1 [9].

References

1 Giles GG, Marks R, Foley P. The incidence of non-melanocytic skin cancer in Australia. *BMJ* 1988; **296**: 13–7.
2 Marks R, Staples M, Giles G. Trends in non-melanocytic skin cancer treated in Australia: the second national survey. *Int J Cancer* 1993; **53**: 585–90.
3 Chuang TY, Popescu NA, Su D *et al.* Squamous cell carcinoma: a population-based incidence study in Rochester, Minnesota. *Arch Dermatol* 1990; **126**: 185–8.
4 Miller DL, Weinstock MA. Non-melanoma skin cancer in the United States: incidence. *J Am Acad Dermatol* 1994; **30**: 774–8.
5 Weinstock MA, Bogars HA, Ashley M *et al.* Non-melanoma skin cancer mortality. *Arch Dermatol* 1991; **127**: 1194–7.

6 Gloster HM Jr, Brodland DG. The epidemiology of skin cancer. *Dermatol Surg* 1996; **22**: 217–26.

7 Holme SA, Malinovszky K, Roberts DL. Changing trends in non-melanoma skin cancer in South Wales, 1988–98. *Br J Dermatol* 2000; **143**: 1224–9.

8 Dahl E, Aberg M, Rausing A, Rausing EL. Basal cell carcinoma: an epidemiologic study in a defined population. *Cancer* 1992; **70**: 104–8.

9 Vitasa BC, Taylor HR, Strickland PT *et al.* Association of non-melanoma skin cancer and actinic keratosis with cumulative solar ultraviolet exposure in Maryland watermen. *Cancer* 1990; **65**: 2811–7.

Environmental risk factors

Ultraviolet radiation

Ultraviolet radiation (UVR) is by far the most important and best understood risk factor for NMSC development. An association between sun exposure and NMSC was first suggested by Thiersch and Unna at the end of the 19th century and substantiated by the work of Hyde [1] and Dubreuilh independently at the beginning of the 20th century [2]. Since then, a large body of information from epidemiological, clinical and experimental observations has been generated to substantiate the proposed causal link between the sun and NMSC development. This evidence includes: the increased frequency of NMSC in areas of high ambient sun exposure; the latitude gradient in the annual age-adjusted incidence in the USA for cutaneous SCCs, with an increasing incidence the nearer one gets to the equator because of greater levels of the UVB component of terrestrial sunlight [3]; the increased incidence of NMSC in sun-sensitive people, which is dramatically highlighted by the differences in NMSC risk between albinos and non-albinos in countries such as Tanzania with high ambient sun exposure [4]; the association between NMSC and 'benign' sun-related conditions such as photoageing and solar telangiectasia; and the marked increase in NMSC incidence with increasing age resulting from cumulative sun exposure, which reflects both the intensity and duration of this exposure [3,5]. The strength of the evidence led the International Agency for Research on Cancer to conclude in 1992 that sun exposure is carcinogenic in humans and that it has a causal role in development of NMSC [6].

The rising incidence of NMSC over the last 30 years is largely the result of increased recreational sun exposure and there are many parallels between the changing epidemiology of NMSC with that other well-known 20th century epidemic, smoking-related lung cancer. Sunbathing, like cigarette smoking, became popular in the early half of the century with the popularization of the bronzed look by Coco Chanel in the 1930s. Although the development of sunbathing as a popular leisure pursuit has lagged behind cigarette smoking, changes in attitudes about the desirability of a tan, coupled with increased leisure time, the introduction of paid holidays and the development of cheap package holidays have seen a marked increase in the level of individual sun exposure in the latter half of the 20th century. In parallel with smoking-related lung cancer, the incidence rate for NMSC has lagged behind the changes in carcinogen exposure, which means that the current clinical impression of increasing NMSC incidence is likely to be a prelude to reporting on a more substantial scale over the next 30–40 years.

The relationship between exposure to UVR and skin cancer development is complex. Epidemiological studies have had an important role in the identification of differences between BCC and SCC with respect to age and pattern of sun exposure. Migrant studies have established that high sun exposure in childhood is especially important in determining NMSC risk and that there is a sharp change in relative risk of NMSC between arrival before and after 10 years of age [7]. Although the basis for this age effect is still unclear, an important consideration is the possibility that the skin is more susceptible to the carcinogenic effects of UVR in childhood. The concept that the response of the skin with respect to cancer susceptibility may be qualitatively different in early life is supported by the observation that susceptibility to melanocytic naevus formation is also greatest during this period [8]. Although the incidence of both BCC and SCC rises with increasing ambient sun exposure, there is a proportionately greater effect of increasing sun exposure on SCC risk [9]. Other observations suggest that the relationship between sun exposure is not the same for BCC and SCC. These observations include the greater preponderance of BCCs on intermittently sun-exposed areas, the plateauing of BCC but not SCC risk after moderate solar exposure, and the finding that for occupational sun exposure SCC but not BCC risk is related to hours of exposure, whereas BCC risk but not SCC risk is increased by sun exposure occurring during holidays [6,10].

UVR comprises a broad band of energy extending from 200 nm to visible light in the lower 400 nm range (see Chapter 29). The UV part of the solar electromagnetic spectrum is subdivided into three broad regions: UVA, UVB and UVC. Although UVB is the main wave band responsible for skin cancer induction, there is increasing interest in the carcinogenic potential of UVA. Exposure to UVA has increased considerably over the last 20 years for two reasons. First, UVB blocking sunscreens have allowed sunbathers to spend longer in the sun and, secondly, the desire to achieve a tan has led to the growth in popularity of UVA sunbeds. Experimental evidence suggests that UVA is carcinogenic [11] but it has been difficult to assess the risk of NMSC development from commercial tanning equipment, as people who tend to use sunbeds also tend to have greater levels of exposure to natural sunlight. Support for a role for UVA in NMSC induction in humans comes from recent reports of both precancerous lesions and NMSC in some individuals in areas of skin exposed almost exclusively to artificial UVA sources [12,13].

References

1 Hyde JN. On the influence of light in the production of cancer of the skin. *Am J Med Sci* 1906; **131**: 1–22.

2 Dubreuilh W. Epitheliomatose d'origine solaire. *Ann Dermatol Syphilol* 1907; **45**: 387–416.

3 Fears TR, Scotto J. Estimating increases in skin cancer morbidity due to increases in ultraviolet radiation exposure. *Cancer Invest* 1983; **1**: 119–26.

4 Luande J, Henschke CI, Mohammed N. The Tanzanian human albino skin: natural history. *Cancer* 1985; **55**: 1823–8.

5 Roberts DL. Incidence of non-melanoma skin cancer in West Glamorgan, South Wales. *Br J Dermatol* 1990; **122**: 399–403.

6 International Agency for Research on Cancer (IARC). Solar and ultra-violet radiation. *IARC Monographs on the Evaluation of Carcinogenic Risks to Humans*, Vol. 55. Lyons: IARC, 1992.

7 Armstrong BK, Kricker A. Epidemiology of sun exposure and skin cancer. *Cancer Surv* 1996; **26**: 133–53.

8 English DR, Armstrong BK. Melanocytic nevi in children. I. Anatomic sites and demographic and host factors. *Am J Epidemiol* 1994; **139**: 390–401.

9 Kricker A, Armstrong BK, English DR, Heenan PJ. A dose–response curve for sun exposure and basal cell carcinoma. *Int J Cancer* 1995; **60**: 482–8.

10 Rosso S, Zanetti R, Martinez C *et al*. The multicentre south European study 'Helios'. II. Different sun exposure patterns in the aetiology of basal cell and squamous cell carcinomas of the skin. *Br J Cancer* 1996; **73**: 1447–54.

11 de Laat JM, de Gruijl FR. The role of UVA in the aetiology of non-melanoma skin cancer. *Cancer Surv* 1996; **26**: 173–91.

12 Roest MA, Keane FM, Agnew K *et al*. Multiple squamous skin carcinomas following excess sunbed use. *J R Soc Med* 2001; **94**: 636–7.

13 Speight EL, Dahl MG, Farr PM. Actinic keratosis induced by use of sunbed. *BMJ* 1994; **308** (6925): 415.

Photochemotherapy (PUVA) and UVB phototherapy

Photochemotherapy and UVB phototherapy are widely used by dermatologists and are recognized as highly effective treatments for a variety of skin diseases. On theoretical grounds, repeated exposure of the skin to artificial UVR or PUVA would be expected to result in cumulative actinic damage and an increased risk of NMSC. Demonstration of increased skin cancer risk and the relative risk of different types of phototherapy has, however, been challenging. This is supported by mathematical modelling approaches which demonstrate that the carcinogenic potential of UVB phototherapy can only be demonstrated with confidence in large multicentre audits with lengthy follow-up [1]. A meta-analysis has estimated an excess skin cancer incidence in patients treated with UVB phototherapy of between 0.6 and 2 extra skin cancers per 100 patients treated per year [2] which in itself is insufficient evidence to definitively establish that phototherapy for psoriasis and other dermatological problems increases skin cancer risk. Given the links between sun exposure and NMSC and the methodological challenges however, it is prudent to continue to ensure monitoring and accurate record keeping of cumulative doses of UV, particularly with the newer phototherapeutic modalities such as narrow-band UVB (TL01) and high-dose UVA1 regimens while this uncertainty remains.

In marked contrast to the lack of clinical evidence of carcinogenicity of UVB phototherapy, there is strong evidence that PUVA increases the risk of developing SCC. The carcinogenic potential of PUVA in humans was first described in 1979 [3] and there is now a substantial amount of information documenting the long-term clinical effects of PUVA [4,5]. NMSC risk in PUVA-treated patients is correlated with cumulative UVA dose and, although earlier data suggested that PUVA may increase susceptibility to both BCCs and SCCs, more recent studies indicate that the increased skin cancer risk is almost exclusively a result of increased SCC risk. Although at a population level it is clear that high-dose PUVA (defined as more than 200 treatments or 2000 J/cm^2) is associated with a 14-fold (95% CI 8.3–24.1) increase in NMSC incidence rate compared to low-dose patients [5], there is evidence that the risk is not uniformly distributed in high-exposure patients, which suggests that other factors may have an important role in modifying risk. High UVB exposure in PUVA patients has been shown to be associated with a small but significant increase in SCC risk [6]. Host factors may also be important as evidenced by the observations from a clinical review of patients exposed to more than 2000 J/cm^2 which revealed that only 50% of patients had SCCs or premalignant lesions [7]. Interestingly, none of the 13% of patients in this study without PUVA lentigines had dysplastic lesions, which suggests that the absence of lentigines may be helpful in the identification of patients at low risk of PUVA malignancy.

References

1 Diffey BL, Farr PM. The challenge of follow-up in narrowband ultraviolet B phototherapy. *Br J Dermatol* 2007; **157**: 344–9.

2 Pasker-de Jong PC, Wielink G, van der Valk PG, van der Wilt GJ. Treatment with UV-B for psoriasis and non-melanoma skin cancer: a systematic review of the literature. *Arch Dermatol* 1999; **135**: 834–40.

3 Stern RS, Thibodeau LA, Kleinerman RA *et al*. Risk of cutaneous carcinoma in patients treated with oral methoxsalen photochemotherapy for psoriasis. *N Engl J Med* 1979; **300**: 809–13.

4 Henseler T, Christophers E, Honigsmann H, Wolff K. Skin tumors in the European PUVA Study. Eight-year follow-up of 1643 patients treated with PUVA for psoriasis. *J Am Acad Dermatol* 1987; **16**: 108–16.

5 Stern RS, Lunder EJ. Risk of squamous cell carcinoma and methoxsalen (psoralen) and UV-A radiation (PUVA): a meta-analysis. *Arch Dermatol* 1998; **134**: 1582–5.

6 Lim JL, Stern RS. High levels of ultraviolet B exposure increase the risk of non-melanoma skin cancer in psoralen and ultraviolet A-treated patients. *J Invest Dermatol* 2005; **124**: 505–13.

7 Lever LR, Farr PM. Skin cancers or premalignant lesions occur in half of high-dose PUVA patients. *Br J Dermatol* 1994; **131**: 215–9.

Chemical carcinogens

The importance of exogenous carcinogens in human skin carcinogenesis was first suggested by Sir Percival Potts, based on observations of an increased incidence of scrotal cancers in chimney sweeps [1]. This hypothesis was supported by observations made by Volkmann in 1874 of a high incidence of NMSC in workers exposed to tar and mineral oil. These observations, and the occurrence of NMSC in other occupational groups exposed to aromatic hydrocarbons at work, served as a stimulus for the large body of experimental studies with chemical carcinogens in animals, which have provided considerable insight into the biology of cancer. The epidemiology of skin cancers resulting from the occupational environment has been extensively reviewed [2]. Many aspects of occupational skin cancers parallel observations made in animal chemical carcinogenesis models. The prevalence of industrial skin cancer is determined by the potency of the carcinogens and by the thoroughness of the measures used to protect workers from them. The likelihood of an individual developing tumours is influenced by the duration of the exposure. An inverse relationship has been established between the age at first exposure and the length of the latent period following exposure to cutting oils and some other industrial carcinogens [3]. The long latent period between exposure and NMSC development and the observation that cancers can develop without a requirement for ongoing exposure means it is likely that many cases of occupational-induced skin cancers are not recognized. Therefore, and by implication, the published figures are likely to reflect a lowest approximation of the true incidence.

Arsenic is another important chemical carcinogen implicated in NMSC development. The association between arsenic administration and the subsequent development of both cutaneous and systemic malignancies was first recognized by Sir Jonathan Hutchinson in 1887. Unlike aromatic hydrocarbons where exposure was frequently occupationally related, arsenic exposure in the first half of the 20th century was more often caused by the ingestion of medical arsenic in the form of potassium arsenite (Fowler's solution) used to treat asthma and psoriasis [4]. Medicinal arsenic exposure remains a problem in some regions where local medicines may still contain arsenic in asthma remedies (Asiatic pills), Chinese herbal medicines and traditional Indian medicines [5]. Most arsenic exposure today, however, results from its high levels in well water from either natural sources or as a result of contamination from mining waste [6]. In some provinces in China the burning of high arsenic coal in unventilated indoor stoves has recently been identified as an important cause of endemic arsenic exposure [7].

References

1 Potter M. *Percival Potts' Contribution to Cancer Research*. National Cancer Institute. Monograph 10. Washington DC: Washington Government, 1974: 1–19.
2 Hueper WC. *Chemically Induced Skin Cancers in Man*. Monograph 10. Washington DC: National Cancer Institute, 1963: 377–91.
3 Waterhouse JAH. Cutting oils and cancer. *Ann Occup Hyg* 1971; **14**: 161–70.
4 Neubauer O. Arsenical cancer: a review. *Br J Cancer* 1947; **1**: 192–251.
5 Prasad HR, Malhotra AK, Hanna N *et al*. Arsenicosis from homeopathic medicines: a growing concern. *Clin Exp Dermatol* 2006; **31**: 497–8.
6 Tseng WP, Chu HM, How SW *et al*. Prevalence of skin cancer in an endemic area of chronic arsenicism in Taiwan. *J Natl Cancer Inst* 1968; **40**: 453–63.
7 Zhang A, Feng H, Yang G *et al*. Unventilated indoor coal-fired stoves in Guizhou province, China: cellular and genetic damage in villagers exposed to arsenic in food and air. *Environ Health Perspect* 2007; **115**: 653–8.

X-rays and thermal radiation

Physical agents other than solar radiation are less frequent causes of NMSC but are an important aetiological factor in some subject groups. The carcinogenic effects of X-rays on the skin were first recognized by Frieben in 1902. NMSCs resulting from X-rays still occur in some at-risk occupational groups such as dentists, radiographers, physicians and engineers. Other at-risk groups include patients treated with Grenz rays for other dermatological conditions such as scalp ringworm, and patients who have received radiotherapy for the treatment of ankylosing spondylitis [1], lymphomas and other malignancies. Exposure to X-rays in childhood appears to be an important risk factor for BCC development [2]. The long latent period between exposure to ionizing radiation and NMSC development means that cases of radiation-induced NMSC may be overlooked if a careful history is not taken, particularly if they occur on sun-exposed sites. Recent studies have highlighted the increased risk of NMSC in childhood cancer survivors with a 6.3 times increase in risk and a high frequency of multiple cancers in affected individuals. The high frequency of tumours (>90%) in irradiated fields supports the importance of ionizing radiation as a risk factor in this group [3]. Patients who develop large numbers of BCCs within an irradiated field should be examined for signs of the naevoid basal cell carcinoma syndrome (Gorlin's syndrome) as some patients with this syndrome show a marked increase in susceptibility to ionizing radiation-induced BCCs [4,5].

Chronic exposure to thermal radiation is also recognized as a risk factor for NMSC development. Most of the evidence comes from studies of different cultural groups where an increased incidence of NMSC has been linked to common practices within these groups. Examples include Kangri cancer in the people of the Kashmir, resulting from repeated contact of abdominal skin with an earthenware brazier containing burning charcoal [6]. Additional clinical signs implicating thermal radiation include erythema ab igne and/or thermal keratoses, which frequently co-localize with thermal-induced cutaneous SCCs [7,8].

References

1 Meara RH. Epitheliomata after radiotherapy of the spine. *Br J Dermatol* 1968; **80**: 620.
2 Shore RE, Albert RE, Reed M *et al*. Skin cancer incidence among children irradiated for ringworm of the scalp. *Radiat Res* 1984; **100**: 192–204.
3 Perkins JL, Liu Y, Mitby PA *et al*. Nonmelanoma skin cancer in survivors of childhood and adolescent cancer: a report from the childhood cancer survivor study. *J Clin Oncol* 2005; **23**: 3733–41.
4 Evans DG, Farndon PA, Burnell LD *et al*. The incidence of Gorlin syndrome in 173 consecutive cases of medulloblastoma. *Br J Cancer* 1991; **64**: 959–61.
5 Zvulunov A, Strother D, Zirbel G *et al*. Nevoid basal cell carcinoma syndrome: report of a case with associated Hodgkin's disease. *J Pediatr Hematol Oncol* 1995; **17**: 66–70.
6 Aziz SA, Hussain KS, Ahmad KN *et al*. Profile of Kangari cancer: a prospective study. *Burns* 1998; **24**: 763–6.
7 Rudolph CM, Soyer HP, Wolf P, Kerl H. Squamous epithelial carcinoma in erythema ab igne. *Hautarzt* 2000; **51**: 260.
8 Akasaka T, Kon S. Two cases of squamous cell carcinoma arising from erythema ab igne. *Nippon Hifuka Gakkai Zasshi* 1989; **99**: 735–74.

Human papillomavirus

The association between human papillomavirus (HPV) and squamous cell neoplasia is best established for cervical and anogenital cancers, which have served as a useful paradigm for unravelling the complex relationship between HPV and cancer development. HPV infection of mucosal keratinocytes is common and the prevalence is increased in women at high risk of cervical cancer. Epidemiological HPV typing studies had a key role in defining two distinct groups of genital HPV types that show marked differences in their strength of association with cancer development. 'High-risk' types (HPV16, 18, 31, 33 and 35) were found to be strongly associated with cancer development while 'low-risk' types (HPV6, 11, 42, 43 and 44) were not [1]. HPV typing studies to date have not generated convincing evidence that implicates high-risk genital HPV types with the development of most cutaneous squamous cell neoplasms. HPV16 and other high-risk genital HPV types have, however, been linked to the clinically distinctive cutaneous squamous cell neoplasms, periungual SCC and palmoplantar Bowen's disease. It is likely in these tumours that the oncogenic effects are mediated by mechanisms similar to those operating in mucosal keratinocytes [2]. The observed association between the skin lesions and aggressive vulval and/or cervical carcinomas in some patients highlights the importance of ensuring that patients with these neoplasms are screened for genital malignancies [3].

Observational studies of patients with the rare inherited condition epidermodysplasia verruciformis (EV) highlighted an association between cutaneous viral warts and NMSC many years before the epidemiological studies linking HPV infection to cervical cancer [4]. Patients with EV develop extensive cutaneous plane and common warts at an early age and in later life frequently develop SCCs on sun-exposed areas. Although the genetic basis for EV is still unclear, HPV typing suggests that there may be an aetiological link between HPV and skin cancer development as over 90% of the EV-associated skin cancers contain HPV types 5 and 8. A high burden of persistent viral warts, keratotic skin lesions and skin cancers in organ-transplant recipients which resembles the phenotype of patients with EV has led to speculation that HPV may also contribute to the increased risk of NMSC development in these patients [5]. This hypothesis is supported by the frequent detection of β-papillomaviruses, formerly called epidermodysplasia verruciformis (EV)-associated human papillomavirus types, in actinic keratoses and other keratotic skin lesions of organ-transplant recipients [6].

HPV DNA has been reported to be present in more than 80% of NMSC from immunosuppressed patients with a lower frequency (less than 40%) in NMSC from immunocompetent individuals [6]. HPV DNA can be detected in SCCs, BCCs and premalignant lesions in both immunocompetent and immunosuppressed patients and the most common HPV types are the β type. In a follow-up study using the same molecular strategy, HPV DNA was detected in 87% of normal skin samples from renal transplant recipients and 35% of samples from immune competent subjects. Although the prevalence and spectrum of HPV types in normal skin was not found to be impacted by sun exposure, multivariate analysis demonstrated that there was an association between the presence of β-HPV types in normal skin and skin cancer status (odds ratio of 6.41; 95% confidence interval 1.79–22.9) [7].

References

1 zur Hausen HH. Papillomaviruses and cancer: from basic studies to clinical application. *Nat Rev Cancer* 2002; **2**: 342–50.
2 McGrae JD Jr, Greer CE, Manos MM. Multiple Bowen's disease of the fingers associated with human papilloma virus type 16. *Int J Dermatol* 1993; **32**: 104–7.
3 Hara H, Honda A, Suzuki H *et al*. Detection of human papillomavirus type 58 in polydactylous Bowen's disease on the fingers and toes of a woman—concurrent occurrence of invasive vulval and cervical carcinomas. *Dermatology* 2004; **209**: 218–22.
4 Majewski S, Jablonska S. Epidermodysplasia verruciformis as a model of human papillomavirus-induced genetic cancer of the skin. *Arch Dermatol* 1995; **131**: 1312–8.
5 Bouwes Bavinck JN, Euvrard S, Naldi L *et al*. Keratotic skin lesions and other risk factors are associated with skin cancer in organ-transplant recipients: a case-control study in The Netherlands, United Kingdom, Germany, France, and Italy. *J Invest Dermatol* 2007; **127**: 1647–56.
6 Harwood CA, Surentheran T, McGregor JM *et al*. Human papillomavirus infection and non-melanoma skin cancer in immunosuppressed and immunocompetent individuals. *J Med Virol* 2000; **61**: 289–97.
7 Harwood CA, Surentheran T, Sasieni P *et al*. Increased risk of skin cancer associated with the presence of epidermodysplasia verruciformis human papillomavirus types in normal skin. *Br J Dermatol* 2004; **150**: 949–57.

Host susceptibility factors

Familial cancer syndromes

Interindividual differences in the susceptibility to NMSC development have been recognized for many years and epidemiological studies have identified a number of phenotypic features, such as hair and skin colour, freckling tendency and ability to tan, which show a consistent correlation with NMSC risk. Genes that determine inherited susceptibility to NMSC development can be divided broadly into two main types. The first type are genes associated with rare, highly penetrant cancer predisposition syndromes and includes conditions such as the naevoid basal cell carcinoma syndrome (NBCCS), Gorlin's syndrome (MIM 109400), Bazex's syndrome (MIM 301845) and xeroderma pigmentosum. The second type are multiple low-penetrant genetic loci that may

contribute to susceptibility in the general population. Evidence for the importance of these latter genes has come from quantitative trait loci mapping of other cancers in murine models. Although mapping of similar loci in humans is difficult, association studies provide some evidence to support a role for high-frequency, low-penetrant traits such as DNA damage repair capacity and xenobiotic metabolism in BCC susceptibility.

Naevoid basal cell carcinoma syndrome [1,2]

> **Synonyms**
> - Basal cell naevus syndrome
> - Gorlin's syndrome

Definition. An autosomal dominant familial cancer syndrome in which affected individuals are predisposed to the development of multiple BCCs at an early age and a variable combination of other phenotypic abnormalities including a highly characteristic facies (with large forehead), bifid or otherwise misshapen ribs, vertebral and other skeletal anomalies, pits of the skin of the palms and soles, dysgenesis of the corpus callosum, calcification of the falx cerebri (at an earlier age than is seen in non-affected individuals) and macrocephaly.

Aetiology and incidence. Population-based studies suggest that the prevalence of this disorder in the UK is approximately 1 in 56 000 of the population [3]. The high rate of new mutations and the variable expressivity of the condition, however, makes full ascertainment difficult, particularly in mildly affected individuals where there is no family history of the condition. Although NBCCS differs from other autosomal dominant cancer syndromes in that many of the associated features are developmental abnormalities, the presence of multiple BCCs at an early age is consistent with the 'two hit model' for inherited cancers first proposed by Knudson. The NBCCS gene was mapped to chromosome 9q22.3–3.1 and, like other tumour suppressor genes, shows frequent deletion in both sporadic and familial BCCs [4]. The NBCCS gene was identified in 1996 with the identification of mutations in the *PATCHED* (*PTCH1*) gene in the germ line of NBCCS patients and in sporadic BCC tumour samples [5]. *PTCH1* is the human homologue of PTC, which was first identified as a key regulator of the evolutionarily conserved Hedgehog (Hh) signalling pathway in elegant genetic studies of embryonic segmentation and imaginal disc specification in *Drosophila*. This finding was the first reported example of a link between genes important in development and cancer, and provided a completely new insight into the molecular pathways important in the development of this common skin cancer. The importance of Hedgehog signalling during normal development explains many of the other phenotypic abnormalities seen in patients with NBCCS and these features are consistent with findings from studies of heterozygote *PTCH1* knock-out mice [6]. The *PTCH1* mutation rate in NBCCS in published studies appears to range between 40% and 80%. A variety of mutations have been described in these studies including nonsense mutations, in-frame deletion, frame shifts due to deletions and insertions and splice-site mutations [7]. In addition to point mutations a small number of patients have been described with larger deletions detected by comparative genomic hybridization methodologies. These patients tend to present with additional clinical features which may be caused by codeletion of other genes in addition to *PTCH1* [8,9].

Clinical features [10]. The skin manifestations of the syndrome are varied and include BCCs, skin tags, palmoplantar pits, milia, epidermoid cysts and lesions that clinically resemble dermal naevi. Skin lesions including BCCs may be present at birth or develop in infancy but more frequently develop between puberty and 35 years of age. The number and type of skin lesions is very variable both within and between families and there is a marked difference between white people and African Americans in the number of BCCs [11]. It is not uncommon to find affected individuals with several hundred lesions. With the exception of the pits that are localized only on the palms and soles, skin lesions can occur in any region. The eyelids, nose, cheeks and forehead are the usual sites, but the neck, trunk and axillae are quite frequently involved. The scalp and limbs are usually spared.

The individual lesions are smooth surfaced, rounded, elevated papules, flesh-coloured or pigmented, varying in size from 1 to 15 mm in diameter. The lesions tend to increase in size and number up to late adolescence. There may be fine telangiectasia and milium-like bodies just below the surface. Tumours of the axillae, neck and eyelids tend to be pedunculated. Most lesions appear to behave in a relatively benign fashion with barely discernible growth and/or evidence of clinical progression. As is the case for patients with sporadic BCCs, some patients with NBCCS develop more aggressive tumours, which can be more difficult to treat and may cause significant morbidity or, rarely, death resulting from extensive invasion and/or recurrence following treatment. The proportion of NBCCS patients who develop very aggressive tumours and the risk factors for this have not been established. Aggressive tumours appear to occur more frequently on the eyelids or nose, and can cause gross destruction. In one study, four of five cases with aggressive BCCs in a series of 36 NBCCS patients received radiotherapy as the initial therapy, which suggests that radiotherapy may be a contributing factor to tumour aggressiveness in some NBCCS patients [12]. A variety of other skin manifestations have also been described, including multiple epidermoid cysts, milia and palmoplantar pits. The pits are a useful diagnostic feature that occur in about 65% of adults with NBCCS but are relatively rare in children. They are characterized by small, more or less circular pits, which may have an erythematous base and are usually 1–2 mm deep. In a recent study, re-examination of the skin phenotype in the context of data implicating Hh signalling in hair follicle biology led to the identification of discrete patches of unusually long, pigmented hair on the skin of three patients with NBCCS from two unrelated families with confirmed heterozygous mutations in the *PTCH* gene [13].

Other diagnostically useful phenotypic abnormalities in NBCCS patients include jaw cysts, a highly characteristic facies (broad nasal root, hypertelorism, frontal bossing), bifid or otherwise misshapen ribs, vertebral and other skeletal anomalies, dysgenesis of the corpus callosum, calcification of the falx cerebri (at an earlier age than is seen in non-NBCCS individuals) and macrocephaly [2]. The dental cysts are usually multiple, occurring in one or both jaws, and are odontogenic keratocysts [14]. Skeletal abnormalities include spina bifida occulta, bifid or splayed ribs, scoliosis or kyphosis, and occur with one-third of the frequency of the cysts or the basal cell naevi [15]. Less common associated anomalies include syndactyly, shortened metacarpals, cleft lip and palate, bicornuate uterus, hypogonadism in males, lymphatic cysts of the mesentery, ocular abnormalities including dystopia canthorum, cataracts and congenital blindness, and a variety of neurological disorders [16–21]. In addition to BCCs, the syndrome is associated with an increased susceptibility to other neoplasms including rhabdomyosarcoma, ovarian and cardiac fibromas and, in particular, medulloblastoma. Approximately 3% of NBCCS patients develop medulloblastomas, and approximately 3% of patients with medulloblastomas have NBCCS [22]. Atypical clinical features such as brachydactyly, pulmonary valve stenosis and mental retardation should prompt consideration of a contiguous gene deletion syndrome.

Pathology [23]. The histopathological appearance of BCCs from patients with NBCCS are indistinguishable from those seen in sporadic forms. The tumours induce a fibrous stroma as occurs with trichoepithelioma or nodular BCC, and the lesions may become papular or pedunculated. Deeper penetration, ulceration and invasion can occur, with lymphocytic infiltration. There may be pigmentation in and around the masses. The presence of calcification and the general architecture can resemble trichoepithelioma. Palmoplantar pits show focal absence of the stratum corneum with vacuolization of the spinous layer. At an ultrastructural level, pits show evidence of premature desquamation with a reduction in desmosomes and tonofibrils resulting from delay in maturation of the epidermal basal cells [24,25]. BCCs have developed in palmar pits [25–27].

Diagnosis. In many cases, the skin lesions resemble melanocytic naevi, von Recklinghausen's neurofibromatosis or skin tags rather than BCC, and their true nature may be suspected only because of associated features or family history. The correlation between the clinical and pathological features of the range of skin lesions seen in NBCCS patients is still poorly understood, which makes it difficult to draw firm conclusions about the natural history of the different skin lesions in these patients.

Treatment. The large number of lesions in patients with NBCCS means that primary excision of all lesions is not always practicable. Radiotherapy is contraindicated as many patients show an accelerated rate of development of new BCCs within an irradiated field, and where recurrences do occur they frequently are more aggressive and difficult to manage than the initial primary tumour. Surveillance of NBCCS patients who have developed BCCs can be useful for the early detection and treatment of new lesions. Although no controlled trials have established that reduced sun exposure can reduce the rate of BCC development in NBCCS patients, the reduced prevalence of BCCs in African Americans with this syndrome suggests that advice on reducing sun exposure is important [11].

Treatment of individual lesions should be guided by anatomical location, tumour size, clinical appearance and histology, with primary excision the treatment of choice for BCCs on the central face near critical structures. For superficial BCC on the trunk, approaches such as curettage and cautery or cryotherapy are useful. While the recurrence rate is potentially greater with these therapies, they are an effective, convenient alternative for small or superficial BCCs distant from critical sites in patients with large numbers of lesions. Where the presence of large numbers of superficial lesions limits the acceptability of conventional therapies, then photodynamic therapy with a systemic or topical photosensitizer and an appropriate laser or non-laser light source can be a useful and effective treatment option. Other non-surgical approaches that can be useful in the management of superficial lesions at non-critical sites include topical 5-fluorouracil and imiquimod formulations. These approaches have been shown to induce histological clearing of some BCCs and can reduce but not replace the need for more conventional therapies in patients with large numbers of lesions [28,29]. The value of systemic chemoprevention strategies in the management of patients with NBCCS is still unclear. A few studies suggest that systemic retinoids (isotretinoin (>4 mg/kg) and etretinate (0.7–1 mg/kg)) may reduce the rate of development of new BCCs [30,31]. The clinical benefits, however, appear small relative to those seen in patients with multiple cutaneous SCCs.

References

1 Gorlin RJ, Vickers RA, Kelln E *et al.* The multiple basal-cell naevi syndrome: analysis of a syndrome consisting of multiple naevoid basal-cell carcinoma, jaw cysts, skeletal anomalies, medulloblastoma, and hyporesponsiveness to parathormone. *Cancer* 1965; **18**: 89–104.

2 Gorlin RJ. The naevoid basal cell carcinoma syndrome. *Medicine* 1987; **66**: 98–113.

3 Evans DG, Ladusans EJ, Rimmer S *et al.* Complications of the naevoid basal cell carcinoma syndrome: results of a population-based study. *J Med Genet* 1993; **30**: 460–4.

4 Quinn AG. Molecular genetics of human non-melanoma skin cancer. *Cancer Surv* 1996; **26**: 89–114.

5 Johnson RL, Rothman AL, Xie J *et al.* Human homolog of patched, a candidate gene for the basal cell naevus syndrome. *Science* 1996; **272**: 1668–71.

6 Bale AE, Gailani MR, Leffell DJ. The Gorlin syndrome gene: a tumor suppressor active in basal cell carcinogenesis and embryonic development. *Proc Assoc Am Physicians* 1995; **107**: 253–7.

7 Soufir N, Gerard B, Portela M *et al.* PTCH mutations and deletions in patients with typical nevoid basal cell carcinoma syndrome and in patients with a suspected genetic predisposition to basal cell carcinoma: a French study. *Br J Cancer* 2006; **95**: 548–53.

8 Nowakowska B, Kutkowska-Kazmierczak A, Stankiewicz P *et al.* A girl with deletion 9q22.1-q22.32 including the PTCH and ROR2 genes identified by genome-wide array-CGH. *Am J Med Genet A* 2007; **143**: 1885–9.

9 Olivieri C, Maraschio P, Caselli D *et al.* Interstitial deletion of chromosome 9, int del(9)(9q22.31-q31.2), including the genes causing multiple basal cell nevus syndrome and Robinow/brachydactyly 1 syndrome. *Eur J Pediatr* 2003; **162**: 100–3.

10 Howell JB. Naevoid basal cell carcinoma syndrome: profile of genetic and environmental features in oncogenesis. *J Am Acad Dermatol* 1984; **11**: 98–104.

11 Kimonis VE, Goldstein AM, Pastakia B *et al.* Clinical manifestations in 105 persons with nevoid basal cell carcinoma syndrome. *Am J Med Genet* 1997; **69**: 299–308.

12 Southwick GJ, Schwartz RA. The basal cell naevus syndrome: disasters occurring among a series of 36 patients. *Cancer* 1979; **44**: 2294–305.

13 Wilson LC, Ajayi-Obe E, Bernhard B *et al.* Patched mutations and hairy skin patches: a new sign in Gorlin syndrome. *Am J Med Genet A* 2006; **140**: 2625–30.

14 Binkley GW, Johnson HH. Epithelioma adenoides cysticum: basal cell naevi, agenesis of the corpus callosum and dental cysts. *Arch Dermatol* 1951; **63**: 73–84.

15 Anderson DE, Taylor WB, Falls MF *et al.* The naevoid basal cell carcinoma syndrome. *Am J Hum Genet* 1967; **19**: 12–22.

16 Berlin NI, van Scott EJ, Clendenning WE *et al.* Basal cell naevus syndrome: combined clinical staff conference at the National Institute of Health. *Ann Intern Med* 1966; **64**: 403–21.

17 Clendenning WE, Block JB, Radde IC. Basal cell naevus syndrome. *Arch Dermatol* 1964; **90**: 38–53.

18 Gorlin RJ, Goltz RW. Multiple naevoid basal-cell epithelioma, jaw cysts and bifid rib: a syndrome. *N Engl J Med* 1960; **262**: 908–12.

19 Gorlin RJ, Yunis JJ, Tuna N. Multiple naevoid basal cell carcinoma, odontogenic keratocysts and skeletal anomalies: a syndrome. *Acta Derm Venereol (Stockh)* 1963; **43**: 39–55.

20 Howell JB, Caro MR. The basal-cell naevus: its relationship to multiple cutaneous cancers and associated anomalies of development. *AMA Arch Dermatol* 1959; **79**: 67–80.

21 Van Dijk E, Sanderink JFH. Basal cell naevus syndrome. *Dermatologica* 1967; **134**: 101–6.

22 Evans DG, Farndon PA, Burnell LD *et al.* The incidence of Gorlin syndrome in 173 consecutive cases of medulloblastoma. *Br J Cancer* 1991; **64**: 959–61.

23 Zackheim HS, Howell JB, Loud AV. Naevoid basal cell carcinoma syndrome: some histologic observations on the cutaneous lesions. *Arch Dermatol* 1966; **93**: 317–23.

24 Howell JB, Mehregan AH. Pursuit of the pits in the naevoid basal cell carcinoma syndrome. *Arch Dermatol* 1970; **102**: 586–97.

25 Holubar K, Matras H, Smalik AV. Multiple palmar basal cell epitheliomas in basal cell naevus syndrome. *Arch Dermatol* 1970; **10**: 679–82.

26 Howell JB, Freeman RG. Structure and significance of the pits and their tumours in the naevoid basal cell carcinoma syndrome. *J Am Acad Dermatol* 1980; **2**: 224–38.

27 Mason JK, Helwig EB, Graham JH. Pathology of the naevoid basal cell carcinoma syndrome. *Arch Pathol* 1965; **79**: 401–8.

28 Goette DK. Topical chemotherapy with 5-fluorouracil: a review. *J Am Acad Dermatol* 1981; **4**: 633–49.

29 Micali G, De Pasquale R, Caltabiano R *et al.* Topical imiquimod treatment of superficial and nodular basal cell carcinomas in patients affected by basal cell naevus syndrome: a preliminary report. *J Dermatolog Treat* 2002; **13**: 123–7.

30 Goldberg LH, Rubin HA. Management of basal cell carcinoma: which option is best? *Postgrad Med* 1989; **85**: 57–8, 61–3.

31 Cristofolini M, Zumiani G, Scappini P, Piscioli F. Aromatic retinoid in the chemoprevention of the progression of naevoid basal-cell carcinoma syndrome. *J Dermatol Surg Oncol* 1984; **10**: 778–81.

Follicular atrophoderma and basal cell carcinoma

Synonym
• Bazex–Dupré–Christol syndrome

This syndrome is a rare genodermatosis that also predisposes affected individuals to multiple BCCs [1,2]. Additional clinical features that allow distinction from NBCCS include follicular atrophoderma, hypotrichosis and hypohidrosis. Follicular atrophoderma is present at birth or in early childhood, and shows as 'ice-pick marks', enlarged follicular ostia on the dorsa of hands, elbows, feet and face. The follicular changes are not caused by injury or inflammation but there may be facial eczema soon after birth. There may be anhidrosis of the face and head, and hypotrichosis. The BCCs appear on the face in the second or third decade and resemble cellular naevi [3].The absence of male–male transmission is suggestive of X-linked inheritance, and this has been confirmed by linkage analysis, which has mapped the gene to Xq24–q27 [4]. The association between BCCs and clinical abnormalities of the hair follicle is of interest as BCCs have the same cytokeratin profile as a subpopulation of follicular keratinocytes

[5]. The importance of the Hedgehog signalling pathway in BCC development in patients from affected families with this disorder is not yet known.

References

1 Plosila M, Kiistala R, Niemi K-M. The Bazex syndrome: follicular atrophoderma with multiple basal cell carcinomas, hypotrichosis and hypohidrosis. *Clin Exp Dermatol* 1981; **6**: 31–41.

2 Bazex A, Dupré A, Christol B. Atrophodermie folliculaire proliférations basocellulaires et hypotrichose. *Ann Dermatol Syphiligr* 1966; **93**: 241–54.

3 Viksnin SP, Berlin A. Follicular atrophoderma and basal cell carcinomas. *Arch Dermatol* 1977; **113**: 948–51.

4 Vabres P, Lacombe D, Rabinowitz LG *et al.* The gene for Bazex–Dupré–Christol syndrome maps to chromosome Xq. *J Invest Dermatol* 1995; **105**: 87–91.

5 Markey AC, Lane EB, Macdonald DM, Leigh IM. Keratin expression in basal cell carcinomas. *Br J Dermatol* 1992; **126**: 154–60.

Rombo syndrome

Rombo syndrome is a very rare, autosomal dominant syndrome first described in 1981 (MIM 180730). Affected individuals develop vermiculate atrophoderma, milia, hypotrichosis, trichoepitheliomas and peripheral vasodilatation in addition to BCCs [1,2]. Although there are some similarities with Bazex's syndrome (follicular atrophoderma and milia), there are a number of distinctive features including cyanotic discoloration of the hands and lips in childhood, and telangiectasia. The genetic locus for Rombo syndrome has not yet been mapped.

References

1 Michaelsson G, Olsson E, Westermark P. The Rombo syndrome: a familial disorder with vermiculate atrophoderma, milia, hypotrichosis, trichoepitheliomas, basal cell carcinomas and peripheral vasodilation with cyanosis. *Acta Derm Venereol* 1981; **61**: 497–503.

2 van Steensel MA, Jaspers NG, Steijlen PM. A case of Rombo syndrome. *Br J Dermatol* 2001; **144**: 1215–81.

Self-healing epitheliomas

Synonym
• Multiple self-healing epithelioma of Ferguson-Smith (MSHE)

This condition is an autosomal dominant condition first described by Ferguson-Smith in the 1930s, characterized by the intermittent development of spontaneously regressing skin tumours histologically identical to well-differentiated SCCs.

Incidence and aetiology. The incidence is unknown but the condition is very rare. Two large Scottish kindreds are well described in the literature [1–3], and accurate genetic pedigree analysis has suggested that the condition may have arisen in these two families from a single mutation around 1790. Recent haplotype analysis for polymorphic markers segregating with MSHE in non-Scottish and Scottish families has shown differences which suggest that MSHE may not be caused by a founder mutation and that the syndrome may be more common than originally thought [4]. The gene has been mapped to chromosome 9q22 in a region of less than 4 cm between the markers D9S197 and D9S1809 but has not yet been identified [5]. Other sporadic cases have been reported. The lesions develop most frequently on light-exposed skin and it is postulated

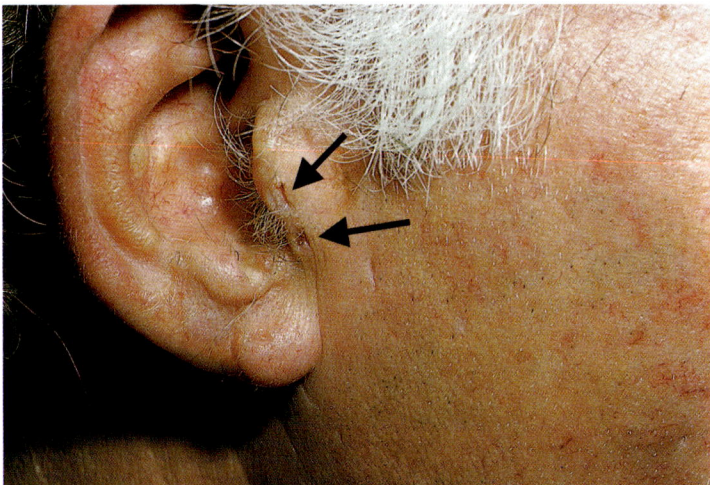

Fig. 52.1 Scarring seen in patient with multiple self-healing squamous epitheliomas of Ferguson-Smith.

that UVR is an important co-factor in the development of these tumours.

Clinical features [6]. The first lesions usually appear in the second decade of life, and each patient tends to have a fairly specific pattern of development, duration and evolution. Knowledge of the 'normal' pattern for the patient is of great value in the management of individual lesions.

The lesions develop predominantly on exposed skin and may cluster around the nose or ears. In the majority of reported cases, one or more lesions have been present in the scalp, a site rarely affected by keratoacanthoma. A small, raised, red nodule is the first sign of a new lesion. This may grow over 2–4 weeks to a diameter of 2–3 cm and may become crusted or ulcerated. The lesion then may remain unchanged for 1–2 months, and then gradually shrink, leaving behind a very characteristic and unsightly, crenellated scar (Fig. 52.1). Lesions develop singly or in crops. In one case they were strikingly confined to half of the body [7].

Pathology. The lesions have features that are indistinguishable from invasive SCCs, but are quite distinct in most cases from multiple keratoacanthoma with which they should not be confused. The epidermis may be ulcerated, and demonstrates marked cellular atypia and loss of polarity. Invasive tongues of epithelial cells will be seen at the base of the lesion and isolated invasive clumps of cells may be seen detached from the main tumour mass, which is still adherent to the epidermis. There is no marked 'shouldering' of the lesion by normal keratinocytes as is seen in keratoacanthoma, and the leukocyte abscesses characteristic of the older keratoacanthoma are absent.

Management. Although spontaneous involution does occur, the resultant scar is unsightly and the end results of shaving or curetting the lesions at an early stage in their development are more acceptable. Cryotherapy of a lesion in the early stages produces an excellent result.

References
1 Charteris AA. Self-healing epithelioma of the skin. *Am J Roentgenol* 1951; **65**: 459–64.
2 Currie AR, Smith JF. Multiple primary spontaneous-healing squamous-cell carcinomata of the skin. *J Pathol Bacteriol* 1952; **64**: 827–39.
3 Ferguson-Smith MA, Wallace D, James Z *et al.* Multiple self-healing epitheliomata. *Birth Defects* 1971; **7**: 157–63.
4 D'Alessandro M, Coats SE, Morley SM *et al.* Multiple self-healing squamous epithelioma in different ethnic groups: more than a founder mutation disorder? *J Invest Dermatol* 2007; **127**: 2336–44.
5 Bose S, Morgan LJ, Booth DR *et al.* The elusive multiple self-healing squamous epithelioma (MSSE) gene: further mapping, analysis of candidates, and loss of heterozygosity. *Oncogene* 2006; **25**: 806–12.
6 Witten VH, Zak FG. Multiple, primary, self-healing prickle-cell epithelioma of the skin. *Cancer* 1952; **5**: 539–50.
7 Rook A, Moffatt JL. Multiple self-healing epithelioma of Ferguson-Smith type: report of a case of unilateral distribution. *Arch Dermatol* 1956; **74**: 525–32.

Xeroderma pigmentosum

This is a rare autosomal recessive disorder characterized by extreme sun sensitivity, associated with a marked increase in skin cancer susceptibility. Affected individuals develop multiple precancerous lesions and skin cancers at an early age (see Chapter 15). From a historical perspective, this condition is important as it is one of the key pieces of evidence that highlighted the carcinogenic potential of UVR and was the first model in humans that supported the somatic mutation theory of the initiation of cancer. Recent evidence from studies of other genetic sun-sensitive syndromes in humans has challenged the original assumption that the increased cancer susceptibility in xeroderma pigmentosum (XP) patients is exclusively the result of persistent DNA lesions caused by defective DNA repair following exposure to UVR. The new data have come from elegant studies of patients with trichothiodystrophy (TTD) who show photosensitivity and defective nucleotide excision repair that resembles that seen in XP patients [1]. In contrast to XP patients where there is a more than 2000-fold increase in skin cancer incidence, TTD does not appear to be associated with skin cancer. The basis for these differences in cancer susceptibility between XP and TTD, however, remains an enigma [2].

References
1 Stary A, Sarasin A. The genetic basis of xeroderma pigmentosum and trichothiodystrophy syndromes. *Cancer Surv* 1996; **26**: 155–71.
2 Cleaver JE. Cancer in xeroderma pigmentosum and related disorders of DNA repair. *Nat Rev Cancer* 2005; **5**: 564–73.

Muir–Torre syndrome

Synonym
• Hereditary non-polyposis colorectal cancer

This autosomal dominant syndrome, originally described in 1967, is characterized by the presence of one or more sebaceous neoplasms in association with internal malignancies, most frequently carcinoma of the colon [1]. The clinical and pathological features overlap with hereditary non-polyposis colorectal cancer (HNPCC) syndromes. Mutations reported to cause Muir–Torre syndrome include the mismatch repair genes *MLH1* and *MSH2*, *MYH* and *MSH6* [2,3]. Tumours in patients with Muir–Torre syndrome are characterized by alterations in the length of DNA sequences called microsatellites. This microsatellite instability has been identified in sebaceous neoplasms from patients with Muir–Torre syndrome [4]. A number of other skin tumours, including SCC, BCC, keratoacanthoma and AK, have also been described in patients with this syndrome but the significance of these findings has been difficult to establish as the high frequency of undiagnosed NMSC in the population makes it hard to differentiate a real increase from an increase resulting from ascertainment bias. The identification of microsatellite instability in skin tumours other than sebaceous neoplasms indicates that the NMSC noted in previous clinical studies of Muir–Torre kindreds are also likely to reflect a true increased susceptibility and not simply a result of ascertainment bias [5,6]. Recent work suggests that immunosuppression may aggravate the Muir–Torre syndrome phenotype and it is interesting that switching from tacrolimus to a sirolimus-based regimen resulted in arrest of the disease [7,8].

References
1 Jones B, Oh C, Mangold E *et al.* Muir–Torre syndrome: diagnostic and screening guidelines. *Australas J Dermatol* 2006; **47**: 266–9.
2 Ponti G, Losi L, Pedroni M *et al.* Value of MLH1 and MSH2 mutations in the appearance of Muir-Torre syndrome phenotype in HNPCC patients presenting sebaceous gland tumors or keratoacanthomas. *J Invest Dermatol* 2006; **126**: 2302–7.
3 Arnold A, Payne S, Fisher S *et al.* An individual with Muir–Torre syndrome found to have a pathogenic MSH6 gene mutation. *Fam Cancer* 2007; **6**: 317–21.
4 Honchel R, Halling KC, Schaid DJ *et al.* Microsatellite instability in Muir–Torre syndrome. *Cancer Res* 1994; **54**: 1159–63.
5 Quinn AG, Healy E, Rehman I *et al.* Microsatellite instability in human non-melanoma and melanoma skin cancer. *J Invest Dermatol* 1995; **104**: 309–12.
6 Swale VJ, Quinn AG, Wheeler JM *et al.* Microsatellite instability in benign skin lesions in hereditary non-polyposis colorectal cancer syndrome. *J Invest Dermatol* 1999; **113**: 901–5.
7 Harwood CA, Swale VJ, Bataille VA *et al.* An association between sebaceous carcinoma and microsatellite instability in immunosuppressed organ transplant recipients. *J Invest Dermatol* 2001; **116**: 246–53.
8 Levi Z, Hazazi R, Kedar-Barnes I *et al.* Switching from tacrolimus to sirolimus halts the appearance of new sebaceous neoplasms in Muir-Torre syndrome. *Am J Transplant* 2007; **7**: 476–9.

Other cancer susceptibility modifying genes

In addition to the rare, highly penetrant skin cancer predisposition syndromes described above, there is increasing evidence that other genetic loci can contribute to sporadic NMSC risk. The importance of these so-called modifying genes has been highlighted in studies using mouse cancer models in which genes have been identified that markedly reduce the rate of cancer development in mice carrying germ-line mutations in known tumour-suppressor genes [1,2]. It is likely that similar, as yet unidentified genes in humans account for the marked variations in the susceptibility to BCC development seen both within and between families with NBCCS. At present, identification of these high-frequency low-penetrant genes in humans involves educated guesswork based on consideration of factors that might contribute to NMSC development. Epidemiological studies have already identified a number of complex phenotypic traits such as skin colour, ethnicity and freckling tendency, which are associated with an increased risk of NMSC development [3]. In addition to the well-recognized importance of differences in skin pigmentation, variations in UVR, DNA repair capacity and xenobiotic metabolism have been implicated as important modifiers of sporadic NMSC risk [4]. The published information on DNA repair enzyme polymorphisms and NMSC susceptibility is difficult to interpret at present. This is because of contradictory findings which may be due to methodological differences and/or complex gene–environment interactions in different ethnic groups exposed to a range of exposure to environmental carcinogens [5,6].

References

1 Eads CA, Nickel AE, Laird PW. Complete genetic suppression of polyp formation and reduction of CpG-island hypermethylation in Apc (Min/) Dnmt1-hypomorphic mice. *Cancer Res* 2002; **62**: 1296–9.
2 MacPhee M, Chepenik KP, Liddell RA et al. The secretory phospholipase A2 gene is a candidate for the Mom1 locus, a major modifier of ApcMin-induced intestinal neoplasia. *Cell* 1995; **81**: 957–66.
3 Armstrong BK, Kricker A. Epidemiology of sun exposure and skin cancer. *Cancer Surv* 1996; **26**: 133–53.
4 Lear JT, Smith AG, Strange RC, Fryer AA. Detoxifying enzyme genotypes and susceptibility to cutaneous malignancy. *Br J Dermatol* 2000; **142**: 8–15.
5 Kang SY, Lee KG, Lee W et al. Polymorphisms in the DNA repair gene XRCC1 associated with basal cell carcinoma and squamous cell carcinoma of the skin in a Korean population. *Cancer Sci* 2007; **98**: 716–20.
6 McCarty KM, Ryan L, Houseman EA et al. A case-control study of GST polymorphisms and arsenic related skin lesions. *Environ Health* 2007; **6**: 5.

Chronic injury and scarring

It has been recognized for many years that NMSC can arise at sites of chronic inflammation and/or scarring. Although there is a substantial literature on this subject, it is difficult to assess the risk as there are no prospective studies of patients with conditions recognized as being associated with NMSC development. Conditions linked to NMSC development include burns [1,2], discoid lupus erythematosus [3], necrobiosis lipoidica [4,5], lupus vulgaris and skin fistulae resulting from discharging sinuses. A particularly strong clinical association has been identified between patients with recessive dystrophic Epidemolysis bullosa (EB) and SCC development [6,7]. The basis for the association between deficiency in type VII collagen resulting from germ-line gene mutations and SCC risk in dystrophic EB patients is not known. In contrast to other forms of EB, fibroblast collagenase is increased in dystrophic EB and this has recently been shown to be associated with marked elevation of urinary excretion of basic fibroblast growth factor [8]. Further studies of SCC development in patients with dystrophic EBV may provide new insight into the long-recognized association between wounding and SCC development.

References

1 Edwards MJ, Hirsch RM, Broadwater JR et al. Squamous cell carcinoma arising in previously burned or irradiated skin. *Arch Surg* 1989; **124**: 115–7.
2 Ikegawa S, Saida T, Takizawa Y et al. Vimentin-positive squamous cell carcinoma arising in a burn scar: a highly malignant neoplasm composed of acantholytic round keratinocytes. *Arch Dermatol* 1989; **125**: 1672–6.
3 Sulica VI, Kao GF. Squamous-cell carcinoma of the scalp arising in lesions of discoid lupus erythematosus. *Am J Dermatopathol* 1988; **10**: 137–41.
4 Imtiaz KE, Khaleeli AA. Squamous cell carcinoma developing in necrobiosis lipoidica. *Diabet Med* 2001; **18**: 325–8.

5 Beljaards RC, Groen J, Starink TM. Bilateral squamous cell carcinomas arising in long-standing necrobiosis lipoidica. *Dermatologica* 1990; **180**: 96–8.
6 Newman C, Wagner RF Jr, Tyring SK, Spigel GT. Squamous cell carcinoma secondary to recessive dystrophic epidermolysis bullosa: a report of 4 patients with 17 primary cutaneous malignancies. *J Dermatol Surg Oncol* 1992; **18**: 301–5.
7 Bosch RJ, Gallardo MA, Ruiz DP et al. Squamous cell carcinoma secondary to recessive dystrophic epidermolysis bullosa: report of eight tumours in four patients. *J Eur Acad Dermatol Venereol* 1999; **13**: 198–204.
8 Arbiser JL, Fine JD, Murrell D et al. Basic fibroblast growth factor: a missing link between collagen VII, increased collagenase, and squamous cell carcinoma in recessive dystrophic epidermolysis bullosa. *Mol Med* 1998; **4**: 191–5.

Immunosuppression

Immunosuppressed patients show a marked increase in susceptibility to NMSC development, with an earlier age of onset and a higher incidence of multiple primary tumours relative to immunocompetent patients. This marked increase in NMSC incidence in these patients is powerful evidence of the importance of the immune system in limiting NMSC development in humans. The cumulative incidence for NMSC uncorrected for age has been shown to vary between 27 and 40% after 20–25 years of immunosuppression in different populations within Europe [1,2]. In Australia, the cumulative incidence appears to be significantly higher after only 10 years of immunosuppression, highlighting the importance of UVR as a co-factor for cancer development in these patients [3]. The risk of NMSC development in renal transplant recipients, which is the best-studied group of immunosuppressed patients, is very variable between different centres as a result of differences between populations including the age distribution of the transplanted patients, the duration of transplantation and the ambient sun exposure of the country. In the UK, a 50-fold increase in the risk of developing SCCs and a fivefold increase in BCC risk has been described in renal allograft recipients [1]. Even greater increases in risk have been described in another European study with a 250-fold increase in SCC incidence and a 10-fold increase in the incidence of BCCs [4]. Epidemiological studies have established that in immunosuppressed patients there is a close association between the development of NMSC and premalignant lesions and the presence of viral warts [5]. The viral warts and skin cancers both preferentially co-localize to areas of sun-exposed skin, although there are some interesting differences between immunocompetent and immunosuppressed patients in SCC distribution with a greater proportion on the hands and forearms in immunosuppressed patients [6].

References

1 McGregor JM, Proby CM. Skin cancer in transplant recipients. *Lancet* 1995; **346**: 964–5.
2 Hartevelt MM, Bavinck JN, Kootte AM et al. Incidence of skin cancer after renal transplantation in the Netherlands. *Transplantation* 1990; **49**: 506–9.
3 Hardie IR, Strong RW, Hartley LC et al. Skin cancer in Caucasian renal allograft recipients living in a subtropical climate. *Surgery* 1980; **87**: 177–83.
4 Bouwes Bavinck JN. Epidemiological aspects of immunosuppression: role of exposure to sunlight and human papillomavirus on the development of skin cancer. *Hum Exp Toxicol* 1995; **14**: 98.
5 Bouwes Bavinck JN, Feltkamp M, Struijk L, ter Scheggett J. Human papillomavirus infection and skin cancer risk in organ transplant recipients. *J Invest Dermatol Symp Proc* 2001; **6**: 207–11.
6 Taylor AE, Shuster S. Skin cancer after renal transplantation: the causal role of azathioprine. *Acta Derm Venereol* 1992; **72**: 115–9.

The molecular and cellular biology of non-melanoma skin cancer

NMSC is unique among human cancers in that the main aetiological factors have been identified and the accessibility of the skin has facilitated analysis of the clinical, pathological and molecular characteristics of these tumours. Advances in molecular and cell biology over the last 10 years have seen an enormous growth in the amount of descriptive data cataloguing changes at the DNA, RNA and protein level in NMSC [1]. While this information in itself has provided an insight into the basis for some of the clinicopathological differences between BCCs, SCCs and related pre-malignant lesions, a fuller understanding of the biology of NMSC will be critically dependent on approaches that integrate emerging molecular data with the clinical and epidemiological aspects of this important disease. This section outlines current concepts and summarizes some of the more important advances in the biology of NMSC, which have important clinical implications. Topics discussed include cancer genetics, multistage carcinogenesis, UV carcinogenesis and the role of HPV infection in NMSC development.

Cancer as a genetic disease

Cancers are, with few exceptions, clonal; they are derived from a single somatic cell and have accumulated a series of changes that lead to complex and persistent changes in gene expression and cell behaviour. Although it has long been thought that these phenotypic changes require the stepwise accumulation of growth-advantageous heritable changes, direct evidence of the importance of genetic alterations in tumorigenesis has only come within the last decade [2]. Genes important in cancer development can be broadly divided into three categories:

1 Proto-oncogenes that encode for proteins that regulate cellular proliferation and differentiation. These genes are inappropriately activated in cancer cells by point mutations, gene amplification or chromosome translocation.

2 Tumour suppressor genes that maintain a normal phenotype by limiting growth, invasiveness and other features of malignant cells. Mutations are recessive at the cellular level, which means that the effects of alterations in these genes are only seen when both copies are inactivated.

3 Mutator genes encode for proteins that play a critical part in maintaining genomic integrity. The importance of this class of genes in determining cancer susceptibility was first recognized in studies of patients with rare autosomal cancer susceptibility syndromes such as XP, Bloom's syndrome and ataxia telangiectasia where there are abnormalities in the recognition, response and/or repair of DNA damage [3]. Further evidence of the importance of 'mutator' genes has come with the demonstration of instability of dinucleotide repeats in a number of common cancers that are caused by either germ-line or somatic mutations in enzymes important in mismatch repair [4]. More recently, a number of groups have shown that genetic factors also influence genetic stability at a chromosome level and there is increasing evidence that the destabilizing of the genome by mutations in genes that normally maintain chromosomal stability plays an important part in the development of some cancers [5].

Molecular genetic analysis of human NMSC has to date focused on four main areas: the role of genes identified in other human cancers; the mapping of chromosome copy number changes; the mapping and positional cloning of familial NMSC susceptibility genes; and comparisons of genetic changes in SCCs with AK and Bowen's disease [1]. As has been the case for other epithelial cancers such as breast and colon cancer, most of the genes implicated to date in NMSC development are tumour-suppressor genes. DNA sequencing has identified mutations in the *p16* and *p53* tumour-suppressor genes. Comparison of the mutational spectra of these genes in NMSC and internal malignancies has confirmed the importance of UVR-induced mutagenesis in NMSC development [6]. Although the *p53* gene has been linked to genetic instability in other cancers, the mutation frequency in BCC and SCC appears broadly similar, which raises interesting questions about the functional effects of *p53* mutations in keratinocytes. Loss of heterozygosity (LOH) studies have revealed that BCCs and SCCs show marked differences in the pattern and extent of chromosome loss. BCCs differ from SCCs and other epithelial neoplasms in that chromosome losses are largely confined to the long arm of chromosome 9 where the *PATCHED1* tumour-suppressor gene that plays a key role in BCC development maps. Allelotype analysis of cutaneous SCCs has demonstrated more widespread allelic losses with frequent loss of 9p, 13q, 17p, 17q and 3p [1]. Similar findings have recently been described in BCCs and SCCs using single nucleotide polymorphism (SNP) microarray analysis [7,8]. The methods used in these studies have revealed that some LOH events in BCCs and SCCs reflect uniparental disomy (loss of one allele and gain of the remaining allele) and that non-random allelic gains occur in SCCs on 3q and 8q. Although the high frequency of copy number changes and imbalances on these chromosome arms suggests that these regions may contain one or more genes important in the development of cutaneous SCCs, with the exception of *p16* and the protein tyrosine phosphatase receptor type D (PTPRD) locus on 9p and *p53* on 17p chromosome, the identities of the candidate tumour-suppressor genes on these chromosome arms are unknown.

Multistage carcinogenesis in the murine skin model

Mouse skin has, for more than 50 years, played a critical role in the development of the concept of multistage carcinogenesis that has underpinned studies of the biology and molecular genetics of the carcinogenic process. While there are important differences between murine and human skin in the response to both chemical carcinogens and UVR, many of the basic concepts identified using this system have been shown to be generally applicable to many human cancers including NMSC. Observational studies of skin tumour induction by chemical carcinogens led to the concept of 'initiation', 'promotion' and 'progression', which represent different stages of the carcinogenic process [9]. 'Initiation' is characterized by the acquisition of an irreversible change in a cell that in the presence of appropriate growth selection pressures ('promotion') can clonally expand to form a benign tumour (papilloma). The probability of papilloma formation within a given mouse strain is dependent on the nature of the carcinogen, the dose applied and the time course over which the mouse is observed. In the murine two-stage skin carcinogenesis model, 'initiation' is accompanied by mutations in the H-*ras* proto-oncogene and the position and type of mutation within this gene is carcinogen-specific. Dimethylbenzanthracene (DMBA)-induced skin tumours predominately have a mutation at the middle adenosine of Ha-*ras* codon 61 (C**A**A → C**T**A)s, whereas methylnitrosurea (MNU)-induced tumours have a G → A transition at codon 12 [10]. This concept of a 'signature' mutation in critical target genes identified in the murine model has underpinned the studies of mutation spectra in the *p53* tumour-suppressor gene and other genes in UVR-induced human NMSC.

The latency period for tumour formation following the application of an initiator is significantly reduced by the application of 'promoters' such as 12-*O*-tetradecanoyl-phorbol-13-acetate (TPA) and other phorbol esters. In contrast to an 'initiator', a 'promoter' generally has to be applied repeatedly and the frequent visible consequences of promoter application, such as hyperkeratosis and scaling of the skin, subside if the application is discontinued. The observation of latency has parallels with the recent observations in humans that clones of *p53* mutant keratinocyte exist within the normal sun-exposed epidermis many years before clinical lesions become detectable [11].

Initiation and promotion, for example using DMBA and TPA, result in the development of multiple papillomas, which rarely progress to invasive carcinoma. The rate of progression of papilloma to carcinoma can be increased by application of the initiator to a papilloma after it has developed or by repeated application of the initiator to 'normal' skin before promotion. Progression is distinct from promotion in that it is considered to reflect accumulation of additional genetic changes and is generally regarded as irreversible. Support for this concept comes from studies of mouse skin tumours, which have established that the transition from benign papilloma to carcinoma is accompanied by an increase in the number of genetic abnormalities in the tumours. This requirement to accumulate additional genetic changes to facilitate tumour progression can occur without further application of an initiator in tumour cells that show 'genetic instability' as this increases the probability of additional genetic changes, which allow histological progression, invasion and metastasis.

Differences between mouse strains and between species in both their susceptibility to cancer induction and the types of tumours induced by identical regimens highlight the importance of other genetic factors in determining cancer susceptibility. The well-defined mouse model system has allowed mapping of these 'modifier' genes and it has now been established that these genes frequently exert their effect by acting in combination and that the same allele can exert opposite effects in different strains of mice [12]. These observations highlight the difficulties in interpreting results from cancer gene association studies in humans.

Ultraviolet radiation mutagenesis and DNA repair

The overwhelming evidence from clinical and epidemiological studies implicating UVR as the most important skin carcinogen makes it easy for us to answer the question, 'Does the sun cause skin cancer?' Answering the question, 'How does the sun cause skin cancer?' is much more challenging and from the information available at present it is still unclear which one or combination of the multitude of effects that UVR has on the skin is critical for all of its carcinogenic properties.

The UV part of the solar electromagnetic spectrum is subdivided into three broad regions:

- UVC (200–280 nm)
- UVB (280–315 nm)
- UVA (315–400 nm).

UVC is widely used in *in vitro* studies of the effects of UVR but is not relevant to human skin cancer as it is efficiently attenuated by the Earth's atmosphere. Although it accounts for less than 10% of the spectral energy of sunlight, UVB is the main waveband responsible for sunburn and skin cancer induction. UVA differs from UVB in a number of ways. It is the main (more than 90%) component of terrestrial sunlight but is less biologically active than UVB. Both UVB and UVA are complete carcinogens in that they are both capable of inducing benign papillomas and SCCs in murine skin.

The effects of UVR on the skin are complex and it is likely that a number of these effects contribute to its initiating and promoting properties. Exposure to both UVB and UVA cause genetic changes in many biological systems [13]. Dose for dose, UVB is a much more efficient mutagen than UVA and the types of mutations induced by these different wavebands are distinct. The action spectra for DNA damage and skin cancer induction are very similar for UVB and closely coincide with the absorption spectra of DNA, which suggests that direct DNA damage by UVB is an important contributor to its carcinogenic effect. Cyclobutane or pyrimidine dimers and the 6–4 photoproduct are the predominant photolesions induced by UVB and these are the preferential sites for UVB-induced mutagenesis [14]. For UVA, the spectra for DNA damage diverges from that of DNA absorption and it has been inferred that DNA damage by wavelengths above 347 nm is not caused by direct absorption by DNA but is more probably a consequence of indirect effects caused by the generation of reactive oxygen species [15]. The types of DNA damage associated with exposure to UVA are DNA strand breaks and DNA protein cross-links.

The mutagenic effects of UVR on keratinocytes within the skin are dependent on the amount and wavelength of the exposure, cellular antioxidant defences [16], the effectiveness of DNA repair mechanisms and the characteristics of the target keratinocyte. Studies in *Escherichia coli* have demonstrated that UVB induces a characteristic spectrum of mutations that is sufficiently distinctive to serve as a molecular 'signature' or 'fingerprint' of DNA damage [17]. This 'fingerprint' is characterized by the presence of C → T transitions at dipyrimidine sites, either singly (C → T) or as a tandem double bases substitution (CC → TT). The identification of mutations that show this molecular fingerprint in human NMSC [6] and in mouse skin tumours induced by UV provides important evidence at the molecular level of the importance of UVB as a mutagen in skin carcinogenesis [18]. Considerably less is known about the characteristics of mutations induced by UVA. As the DNA damage with UVA is predominately indirect, it is more difficult to extrapolate findings from *in vitro* studies using bacteria or mammalian cells. *In vivo* studies using a transgenic mouse model have shown a predominance of GC → AT transitions at non-pyrimidine dimer sites, which is consistent with the proposed involvement of oxidative DNA damage [19].

Mutations induced by UVR are a result of persistence of unrepaired photoproducts at the time of DNA replication. During DNA replication, the DNA polymerase complex misreads the photoproduct on the template strand and this leads to the insertion of a default adenine residue at this position. At subsequent cell divisions, this adenine pairs with thymine and the net result is the conversion of a cytosine base to a thymine base on the originally damaged strand. A number of studies have shown that there appears to be a close relationship between photoproduct formation and carcinogenesis in that enzymatic repair of photoproducts by endogenously activated photolyase [20] or by topical application of T_4 endonuclease in liposomes [21] reduces the incidence of tumour formation. Although these studies are consistent with the original XP paradigm, which directly links unrepaired DNA lesions, mutations and cancer, recent observations from studies of patients with TTD indicate that the marked increase in susceptibility to UV carcinogenesis seen in XP patients is a result of other effects and not simply a reflection of an increased mutation rate [22]. Detailed comparisons between XP and TTD cells have revealed a number of differences in the repair efficiency and mutational spectrum, but it is still unclear which of these underpin the differences in cancer susceptibility between these syndromes [23,24].

Immunological effects of ultraviolet radiation

The importance of the immune system in human skin carcinogenesis is dramatically illustrated by the marked increases in NMSC incidence in immunosuppressed patients. UVR, in addition to its mutagenic and other direct effects on keratinocytes, has been shown in murine models to exert an immunosuppressive effect that interferes with the ability of the immune system to eliminate UV-induced skin tumours. These observations and the importance of immunosuppressants as a risk factor for NMSC development in humans has led to speculation that UV-induced immunological injury may be an important contributor to the carcinogenic effects of UVR. In mice, skin tumours induced by UVR differ from chemical carcinogen-induced skin tumours in that they are highly immunogenic and are rejected when transplanted into genetically identical recipient mice. The importance of UV-induced immunosuppression in UV carcinogenesis was first recognized in the 1970s when Kripke [25] made the seminal observation that irradiation of recipient mice abolished the ability to reject the transplanted tumours. This work and subsequent studies established that immunosuppression could be transferred to unirradiated animals by adoptive transfer of splenic lymphocytes and that UVR exerted similar effects on the normal immunological reactions to sensitizing chemicals such as dinitrochlorobenzene in contact hypersensitivity reactions. Further investigation of the immunological effects of UVR using skin contact hypersensitivity has revealed that there are marked differences between mice strains in their susceptibility to UVR-induced immunosuppression. Genetic studies have demonstrated that the UV-susceptibility phenotype is dominantly inherited and two genetic loci have been identified that are thought to mediate this effect [26]. Recent studies using genetically modified mice suggest

that deficiencies in IL-10 decrease and in IL-12 increase susceptibility to UV-induced immune suppression and accelerate UV-induced skin carcinogenesis [27,28].

The significance of UVR-induced immunosuppression in humans is still unclear. There are some similarities with the findings in mice in that UV irradiation decreases the ability to mount a delayed-type hypersensitivity response when the immunization occurs on exposed skin and there appears to be interindividual differences in the susceptibility to this effect [29–31]. One study suggests that the UV-susceptibility phenotype is more common in patients with NMSC and that 50% of such patients develop hapten-specific tolerance using this test system [32]. While these observations raise the possibility that exposure to UVR may interfere with the ability of the immune system to eliminate UV-induced skin tumours in humans, the clinical importance of this effect is unclear. The observation that pharmacological inhibition of the immune system has a profound clinical effect on NMSC development suggests that the impact of UVR-induced immunosuppression on NMSC development may not be as great as that seen in murine models. However, further work is required to better understand the impact and clinical significance of other, more subtle aspects of the effects of UVR on cutaneous immunity and the implications of these effects in determining NMSC susceptibility in humans.

Human papillomaviruses

The subdivision of HPV types, based on clinical biology and epidemiological studies of anogenital cancers, played a critical part in the dissection of the molecular mechanisms of HPV carcinogenesis. This allowed identification of the characteristics specifically associated with the carcinogenic properties of the high-risk HPV types [33]. Cell biology and molecular studies have shown a good correlation between high- and low-risk HPVs and their ability to transform primary human keratinocytes [34]. The major transforming proteins of the high-risk genital HPVs are the E6 and E7 proteins, which target and inactivate tumour-suppressor genes including *p53* and the retinoblastoma gene.

Clinical and epidemiological studies have also provided compelling evidence of a link between cutaneous viral warts and NMSC and recent molecular studies have allowed analysis of HPV types. Although the increased prevalence of HPV infection in NMSC from high-risk organ transplant recipients is less compelling compared to the information from studies of other HPV-associated cancers, there are some other pieces of evidence that point to a possible direct role for HPV in NMSC development. Genetic analysis of squamous cell neoplasms from immunocompetent and immunosuppressed patients has revealed that there are significant differences between these two patient groups, with significantly less chromosome loss in SCCs from immunosuppressed patients [35]. Further support for a causal role for HPV in NMSC development has come from recent molecular studies that have shown that the E6 protein from some cutaneous HPVs blocks the epidermal apoptotic response to UVR by targeting the pro-apoptotic Bak protein for proteolytic degradation [36]. This finding and the demonstration of an inverse correlation between Bak protein levels and HPV positivity in cutaneous SCCs suggests that cutaneous HPV may promote SCC development by blocking the normal epidermal apoptotic response to UVR [37].

References

1 Quinn AG. Molecular genetics of human non-melanoma skin cancer. *Cancer Surv* 1996; **26**: 89–114.

2 Vogelstein B, Kinzler KW. Cancer genes and the pathways they control. *Nat Med* 2004; **10**: 789–99.

3 Hoeijmakers JH. Genome maintenance mechanisms for preventing cancer. *Nature* 2001; **411**: 366–74.

4 Jiricny J, Nystrom-Lahti M. Mismatch repair defects in cancer. *Curr Opin Genet Dev* 2000; **10**: 157–61.

5 Lengauer C, Kinzler KW, Vogelstein B. Genetic instabilities in human cancers. *Nature* 1998; **396**: 643–9.

6 Brash DE, Rudolph JA, Simon JA *et al.* A role for sunlight in skin cancer: UV-induced *p53* mutations in squamous cell carcinoma. *Proc Natl Acad Sci USA* 1991; **88**: 10124–8.

7 Teh MT, Blaydon D, Chaplin T *et al.* Genomewide single nucleotide polymorphism microarray mapping in basal cell carcinomas unveils uniparental disomy as a key somatic event. *Cancer Res* 2005; **65**: 8597–603.

8 Purdie KJ, Lambert SR, Teh MT *et al.* Allelic imbalances and microdeletions affecting the PTPRD gene in cutaneous squamous cell carcinomas detected using single nucleotide polymorphism microarray analysis. *Genes Chromosomes Cancer* 2007; **46**: 661–9.

9 Yuspa SH, Dlugosz AA, Denning MF, Glick AB. Multistage carcinogenesis in the skin. *J Invest Dermatol Symp Proc* 1996; **1**: 147–50.

10 Burns PA, Bremner R, Balmain A. Genetic changes during mouse skin tumorigenesis. *Environ Health Perspect* 1991; **93**: 41–4.

11 Jonason AS, Kunala S, Price GJ *et al.* Frequent clones of *p53*-mutated keratinocytes in normal human skin. *Proc Natl Acad Sci USA* 1996; **93**: 14025–9.

12 Nagase H, Mao JH, Balmain A. A subset of skin tumor modifier loci determines survival time of tumor-bearing mice. *Proc Natl Acad Sci USA* 1999; **96**: 15032–7.

13 Peak MJ, Peak JG. Solar-ultraviolet-induced damage to DNA. *Photodermatol* 1989; **6**: 1–15.

14 Ziegler A, Jonason AS, Leffell DJ *et al.* Sunburn and *p53* in the onset of skin cancer. *Nature* 1994; **372**: 773–6.

15 Peak MJ, Peak JG. DNA-to-protein crosslinks and backbone breaks caused by far- and near-ultraviolet, and visible light radiations in mammalian cells. *Basic Life Sci* 1986; **38**: 193–202.

16 Applegate LA, Frenk E. Oxidative defense in cultured human skin fibroblasts and keratinocytes from sun-exposed and non-exposed skin. *Photodermatol Photoimmunol Photomed* 1995; **11**: 95–101.

17 Mitchell DL, Jen J, Cleaver JE. Sequence specificity of cyclobutane pyrimidine dimers in DNA treated with solar (ultraviolet B) radiation. *Nucl Acids Res* 1992; **20**: 225–9.

18 Ananthaswamy HN, Fourtanier A, Evans RL *et al.* p53 Mutations in hairless SKH-hr1 mouse skin tumors induced by a solar simulator. *Photochem Photobiol* 1998; **67**: 227–32.

19 Gorelick NJ. Overview of mutation assays in transgenic mice for routine testing. *Environ Mol Mutagen* 1995; **25**: 218–30.

20 Ley RD, Applegate LA, Freeman SE. Photorepair of ultraviolet radiation-induced pyrimidine dimers in corneal DNA. *Mutat Res* 1988; **194**: 49–55.

21 Yarosh D, Klein J, Kibitel J *et al.* Enzyme therapy of xeroderma pigmentosum: safety and efficacy testing of T4N5 liposome lotion containing a prokaryotic DNA repair enzyme. *Photodermatol Photoimmunol Photomed* 1996; **12**: 122–30.

22 Stary A, Sarasin A. The genetic basis of xeroderma pigmentosum and trichothiodystrophy syndromes. *Cancer Surv* 1996; **26**: 155–71.

23 Eveno E, Bourre F, Quilliet X *et al.* Different removal of ultraviolet photoproducts in genetically related xeroderma pigmentosum and trichothiodystrophy diseases. *Cancer Res* 1995; **55**: 4325–32.

24 Madzak C, Armier J, Stary A *et al.* UV-induced mutations in a shuttle vector replicated in repair deficient trichothiodystrophy cells differ with those in genetically-related cancer prone xeroderma pigmentosum. *Carcinogenesis* 1993; **14**: 1255–60.

25 Kripke ML. Ultraviolet radiation and immunology: something new under the sun. Presidential address. *Cancer Res* 1994; **54**: 6102–5.

26 Streilein JW. Immunogenetics of sunlight-induced skin cancer. *Photochem Photobiol* 1996; **63**: 422–4.

27 Loser K, Apelt J, Voskort M *et al.* IL-10 controls ultraviolet-induced carcinogenesis in mice. *J Immunol* 2007; **179**: 365–71.

28 Meeran SM, Mantena SK, Meleth S *et al.* Interleukin-12-deficient mice are at greater risk of UV radiation-induced skin tumors and malignant transformation of papillomas to carcinomas. *Mol Cancer Ther* 2006; **5**: 825–32.

29 Yoshikawa T, Rae V, Bruins-Slot W *et al.* Susceptibility to effects of UVB radiation on induction of contact hypersensitivity as a risk factor for skin cancer in humans. *J Invest Dermatol* 1990; **9**: 530–6.

30 Cooper KD, Oberhelman L, Hamilton TA *et al.* UV exposure reduces immunization rates and promotes tolerance to epicutaneous antigens in humans: relationship to dose, CD1a-DR epidermal macrophage induction, and Langerhans' cell depletion. *Proc Natl Acad Sci USA* 1992; **89**: 8497–501.

31 Tie C, Golomb C, Taylor JR, Streilein JW. Suppressive and enhancing effects of ultraviolet B radiation on expression of contact hypersensitivity in man. *J Invest Dermatol* 1995; **104**: 18–22.

32 Streilein JW, Taylor JR, Vincek V *et al.* Relationship between ultraviolet radiation-induced immunosuppression and carcinogenesis. *J Invest Dermatol* 1994; **103** (Suppl. 5): 107S–11S.

33 Zur-Hausen H. Papillomaviruses and cancer: from basic studies to clinical application. *Nat Rev Cancer* 2002; **2**: 342–50.

34 Kaur P, McDougall JK. Characterization of primary human keratinocytes transformed by human papillomavirus type 18. *J Virol* 1988; **62**: 1917–24.

35 Rehman I, Quinn AG, Takata M *et al.* Low frequency of allelic loss in skin tumours from immunosuppressed individuals. *Br J Cancer* 1997; **76**: 757–9.

36 Jackson S, Harwood C, Thomas M *et al.* Role of Bak in UV-induced apoptosis in skin cancer and abrogation by HPV E6 proteins. *Genes Dev* 2000; **14**: 3065–73.

37 Storey A. Papillomaviruses: death-defying acts in skin cancer. *Trends Mol Med* 2002; **8**: 417.

General principles in the management of patients with non-melanoma skin cancer

Many aspects of the management of patients with BCC and SCC are common to both tumour types and these general principles are discussed in this section. Tumour-specific issues are discussed in the treatment section for the relevant tumour. Management of patients with NMSC requires early detection and accurate diagnosis, selection of the appropriate treatment modality based on the clinical and/or pathological findings, consideration of patient-specific risk factors and institution of preventative measures if appropriate.

Detection and diagnosis

Early detection of NMSC is critically dependent on a good awareness of risk factors and the characteristics of tumour development in at-risk groups. Although most patients with NMSC initially present with a lesion requiring a therapeutic intervention, the high prevalence of benign skin disease and the increasing use of medical screening examinations means that there are opportunities for identifying at-risk individuals sooner than they might present with an obvious clinical lesion. Superficial BCCs on the back, Bowen's disease on the leg and AK are not uncommonly either not noticed or dismissed as a normal consequence of ageing. Although early detection of such lesions may have little impact on the clinical prognosis of the identified tumour, the ability to identify at-risk individuals means that advice on preventative measures such as sun awareness and protection can be initiated much earlier than otherwise would have been the case.

Selection of appropriate therapeutic modality for tumour treatment

The aims of any treatment directed against an NMSC are the removal or destruction of the primary tumour mass and, in the case of SCC, the prevention of metastasis. A broad range of thera-peutic options are available to achieve these aims and while surgi-cal excision is frequently the treatment of choice, there are patient-related factors which may influence treatment choices. These factors include the patient's general health, concomitant medication such as anticoagulants and antiplatelet agents, home circumstance and responsibilities due to employment or carer duties and previous experience of treatment for NMSC. Treatment selection is dependent on a good understanding of the clinical and/or pathological aspects of NMSC that affect prognosis and clinical experience of the pros and cons of the various therapeutic modalities.

The different modalities we may consider include: curettage and cautery, cryosurgery, radiotherapy, photodynamic therapy, topical imiquimod, laser surgery, conventional surgical excision and Mohs micrographic surgery (described in detail in Chapters 77 and 78).

Treatments can be broadly divided into destructive or exci-sional, the latter providing histologic evaluation of the diagnosis, adequacy of removal and information on the risk associated with that tumour. Destructive treatments may be based on a firm clin-ical diagnosis of basal cell carcinoma but diagnostic doubt should lead to histological confirmation of the diagnosis before treatment. In general, destructive treatments should be used for lower-risk tumours with the exception of radiotherapy, which will be dealt with in more detail later.

Cryosurgery. The application of liquid nitrogen to skin lesions aiming to cause destruction of the tissue and a margin of sur-rounding tissue requires the achievement of lesional temperatures of −50 to −60°C. This can be achieved by a number of techniques including single or double freeze–thaw cycles [1,2]. This modality has been recommended for the treatment of AK, Bowen's disease, superficial BCC, small nodular BCC and small well-differentiated SCC. While freezing with liquid nitrogen is a quick and relatively tolerable procedure that does not require local anaesthesia, it can be associated with significant morbidity, particularly when tumours selected for treatment require prolonged freeze times to ensure adequate treatment. Although hypopigmentation is a fre-quent consequence of cryosurgery for skin tumours, wounds tend to heal without significant tissue contraction and this can give rise to excellent cosmetic results for some patients [3,4]. This form of treatment is considered in more detail in Chapter 78.

Curettage and cautery. This modality can be used for the same spectrum of lesions as cryotherapy. Curettage with traditional Volkman spoon reusable curettes is critically dependent on the friable nature of the tumours, which leads to a selective removal of abnormal tissue. This differential effect on tumour tissue is an effective way of delineating the extent of some tumours and can be useful before standard or Mohs excision of some BCCs to define more accurately lateral tumour spread within the epider-mis [5]. With the advent of disposable loop curettes, which have a much sharper edge, the technique has been modified to include a more gentle initial curettage to delineate the tumour followed by greater pressure after this point. When used therapeutically it is important that the stroma and surrounding dermis are charred

with diathermy or cautery to a depth of 1 mm following initial curettage and that this is repeated on two further occasions with curetting of the charred tumour base. As the procedure does not divide the upper dermis connective tissue network, healing is usually predictable and occurs in most cases with mild scarring. However, hypopigmentation or hypertrophic scar formation may occur, the latter particularly when the upper trunk is treated.

Radiotherapy. Most NMSCs are sensitive to ionizing radiation. Radiotherapy offers the potential to treat large tumours and a surrounding area of normal skin with minimal tissue damage. The effectiveness and cosmetic end result of this therapy is critically dependent on the treatment regimen administered. This operator dependence, which makes comparison of published studies diffi-cult, is also an important contributor to the misconceptions that some physicians have about the value of this approach. Radio-therapy can be an effective cosmetically acceptable treatment for NMSC including BCC, SCC and premalignant lesions such as Bowen's disease. Although it is often stated that radiotherapy is best suited for elderly patients, the inconvenience and practical difficulties of frequent outpatient appointments required for a full fractionated course need to be taken into account when it is con-sidered as an alternative to conventional surgical approaches. In addition to a primary therapy, radiotherapy is also an important adjuvant following excisional surgery for the treatment of residual microscopic disease and as a prophylaxis against systemic metas-tases. Situations where radiotherapy is best avoided include NMSC on the lower limbs, ear and eyelid, recurrent tumours, lesions previously treated with radiotherapy, tumours with poorly defined clinical margins and patients with multiple NMSCs and severe actinic damage. The technical details of radiotherapy are discussed elsewhere.

Photodynamic therapy. The development of topically active pho-tosensitizing agents 5-aminolevulinate (licensed as Levulan in the United States) and its methyl ester (licensed as Metvix in Europe) has led to studies on the role of photodynamic therapy (PDT) for the treatment of NMSC. These are pro-drugs which are naturally metabolized via the haem biosynthetic pathway to protoporphy-rin IX, a powerful photosensitizer. It would appear that there is a relatively selective metabolism in tumour cells allowing the therapy to target premalignant and malignant skin lesions. This therapy appears particularly effective for AK of the face and scalp. Multicentre, randomized, controlled trials have shown greater than 80% clearance of superficial AKs on the face and scalp and similar figures for the treatment of Bowen's disease and superfi-cial basal cell carcinoma. Recurrence rates of up to 20% at 5 years make this at least as effective as other destructive treatments but it may well have advantages over other therapies with respect to tolerability and cosmesis [6–8]. There are now several guidelines on the use of PDT including advice from the National Institute for Health and Clinical Excellence [6, 9–11]. So far, PDT for nodular basal cell carcinoma has been less successful than for superficial BCC but may have a place in selected patients [12]. Interestingly, PDT may have potential to delay the onset of skin tumours in at-risk groups as studies in a mouse model of BCC demonstrated an effect in terms of delayed onset of tumours [13].

Laser therapy. This therapy is rarely used to treat NMSC. Little evidence of its efficacy exists and there are no comparisons with other treatment modalities. One study utilizing the carbon dioxide ultrapulse laser in multiple, low-risk BCCs in the context of the naevoid basal cell naevus syndrome showed some efficacy [14].

Topical immune response modifiers. These are a new class of recently introduced topical therapies which stimulate innate and cell mediated immune responses by activating Toll signalling pathways and inducing cytokine production. Efficacy has been demonstrated in placebo-controlled, randomized clinical trials for imiquimod and it has been approved by regulatory authorities for the treatment of superficial BCCs and AKs in addition to its initial approval for the treatment of genital warts. Clearance of lesions is accompanied by a localized inflammation of variable severity in most subjects. Severe reactions occur in approximately 20% of subjects and may require either temporary treatment interruption or in rare cases discontinuation. Efficacy has also been observed in off-label studies of patients with Bowen's disease [15].

Conventional surgical excision. This is regarded by many as the treatment of choice for primary NMSC. Excision with primary closure, local rotational or advancement flaps or full-thickness graft to repair the defect, when carried out by a trained operator, usually produces a good cosmetic result and provides the pathologist with a specimen that allows confirmation of the completeness of excision and identification of histological factors associated with increased risk of local or systemic recurrence. Although under treatment because of lateral or deep tumour extension may be identified in conventionally processed surgical specimens, there is potential to miss cases of incomplete excision as only a small proportion of the tumour edge is examined using conventional histopathological techniques [16].

Mohs micrographic surgery. This technique combines excision with complete histological examination of the resection margins of skin tumours and has been shown to be very effective in removing NMSC [17,18] and preserves uninvolved tissues. It is only effective in tumours which extend in continuity and is particularly useful in high-risk or recurrent tumours or where tissue conservation is of importance such as the nasal tip and eyelids. Current guidance in the UK suggests that it is the treatment of choice for the highest risk BCCs and SCCs and may be particularly useful where there is evidence of perineural involvement of SCC [19,20]. The Mohs technique is described in detail in Chapter 77.

Selection of the optimal treatment modality

The selection of the most appropriate therapy for a patient is determined by three key factors: tumour size; tumour location; and the likely tumour characteristics based on clinical and, where available, pathological assessment. Low-risk NMSC and related premalignant lesions including AK, Bowen's disease and superficial BCC can usually be adequately dealt with using curettage and cautery, cryotherapy, PDT or topical imiquimod. Although the recurrence rate for these types of lesions with these modalities when used appropriately is slightly higher than that achieved with surgical excision, this needs to be balanced against the fact

that these less invasive procedures are relatively simple to carry out, often associated with less short-term morbidity and more predictably give a good cosmetic result compared to excision. Excellent cure rates for curettage and cautery and/or cryotherapy have also been reported for small (less than 1 cm) nodular BCCs and well-differentiated slow-growing SCCs on sun-exposed skin [21,22]. For intermediate-risk NMSC (tumours less than 2 cm, well-defined clinical margins), the location of the tumour is an important determinant of treatment choice. A specific advantage of surgical excision over other destructive therapies is the provision of tissue for histological examination, which provides confirmation of the diagnosis, information on the adequacy of excision and may allow recognition of histological features associated with a high risk of local recurrence and risk of metastasis. For BCC, these features include location on the central face and a morphoeic histological pattern. For SCC, depth of invasion greater than 4 mm or extension into subcutaneous fat, poor differentiation and perineural involvement have all been associated with increased risk of local recurrence and metastatic disease [20]. For high-risk NMSC, the treatment of choice is Mohs surgery.

For the management of most NMSCs a treatment plan can be defined based on a clear understanding of the pros and cons of the different treatment modalities and a careful consideration of the tumour characteristics. In some cases, such as high-risk patients with multiple NMSCs, high-risk tumours, recurrent tumours or incompletely excised NMSC, optimal selection of therapy may be best achieved in the context of a multidisciplinary tumour clinic with input from dermatologists, plastic surgeons, oncologists and radiotherapists.

Chemoprevention and management of high-risk patients

The surgical treatment of high-risk NMSC differs from that of high-risk patients with many other common cancers such as colon, breast and bladder cancer in that it is not possible to completely remove the target organ. While excision or destruction of lesions is well suited for the management of small numbers of NMSCs or related premalignant lesions, these approaches become increasingly impractical and distressing for high-risk NMSC patients with multiple lesions. Examples of patient groups where this problem arises include patients with NBCCS, immunosuppressed organ transplant recipients, high-dose PUVA patients and patients with severe actinic damage. From our current understanding of the epidemiology and biology of NMSC, the number of high-risk patients is likely to increase considerably over the next 25 years as a result of the changing age structure of the population and increased recreational sun exposure. The management of patients with multiple NMSCs is a considerable therapeutic challenge, which is not helped by the limited number of treatment options available and the lack of controlled clinical studies.

Topical 5-fluorouracil is a valuable therapy for the treatment of Bowen's disease and for patients with multiple AK. For reasons that are still not understood, 5-fluorouracil acts on both clinically detectable lesions and subclinical lesions, which means that application to a contiguous area of skin may target a greater number of lesions than would be achieved using destructive therapies of visible clinical lesions. Although there is some evidence to suggest that 5-fluorouracil may reduce the rate of development of new AK, there is no conclusive evidence at present favouring a role for 5-fluorouracil in the prevention of NMSC [23,24].

A number of systemic approaches have been investigated as chemopreventive agents for high-risk skin cancer patients (reviewed in [25,26]). Oral retinoids are used to treat patients with multiple SCCs where the rate of new SCC development makes management by surgical intervention difficult. Although oral retinoids show clinical efficacy and are the only agent proved to be chemopreventative, there are many unanswered questions on their mode of action and long-term effects as there are very few controlled trials on their use. Etretinate has been shown to be superior to placebo in the treatment of high-risk patients with AK, some of whom also had at least one NMSC [27].

References

1 Graham G. Statistical data on malignant tumours in cryosurgery: 1982. *J Dermatol Surg Oncol* 1983; **9**: 238–9.

2 Zacharian SA. Cryosurgery of cutaneous carcinomas. An 18 year study of 3022 patients with 4228 carcinomas. *J Am Acad Dermatol* 1983; **9**: 947–56.

3 Kokoszka A, Scheinfeld N. Evidence based review of the use of cryosurgery in the treatment of basal cell carcinoma. *Dermatol Surg* 2003; **29**: 566–71.

4 Jamarilo-Ayerbe F. Cryosurgery in difficult to treat basal cell carcinoma. *Int J Dermatol* 2000; **39**: 223–9.

5 Johnson TM, Tromovitch TA, Swanson NA. Combined curettage and excision: a treatment method for primary basal cell carcinoma. *J Am Acad Dermatol* 1991; **24**: 613–7.

6 Morton CA, McKenna KE, Rhodes LE. Guidelines for topical photodynamic therapy: update. *Br J Dermatol* 2008; **159**: 1245–66.

7 Kalka K, Merk H, Mukhtar H. Photodynamic therapy in dermatology. *J Am Acad Dermatol* 2000; **42**: 389–413.

8 Morton CA. The emerging role of 5-ALA-PDT in dermatology: is PDT superior to standard treatments? *J Dermatolog Treat* 2002; **13** (Suppl. 1): S25–9.

9 Haller JC, Cairnduff F, Slack G *et al*. Routine double treatments of superficial basal cell carcinomas using aminolaevulinic acid-based photodynamic therapy. *Br J Dermatol* 2000; **143**: 1270–5.

10 Braathen LR, Szeimies R-M, Basset-Sequin N *et al*. Guidelines on the use of photodynamic therapy for nonmelanoma skin cancer: an international consensus. *J Am Acad Dermatol* 2007; **56**: 125–43.

11 National Institute for Health and Clinical Excellence. *Photodynamic Therapy for Non-melanoma Skin Tumours (Including Premalignant and Primary Non-metastatic Skin Lesions)*, 2006. www.nice.org.uk/nicemedia/pdf/ip/IPG155publicinfo.pdf

12 Rhodes LE, de Rei MA, Leifsdottir R *et al*. Five year follow-up of a randomized, prospective trial of topical methyl aminolevulinate photodynamic therapy vs surgery for nodular basal cell carcinoma. *Arch Dermatol* 2007; **143**: 1131–6.

13 Caty V, Liu Y, Viau G, Bissonnette R. Multiple large surface photodynamic therapy sessions with topical methyl aminolaevulinate in PTCH heterozygous mice. *Br J Dermatol* 2006; **154**: 740–2.

14 Nouri K, Chang A, Trent JT, Jimenez GP. Ultrapulse CO_2 used for the successful treatment of basal cell carcinomas found in patients with basal cell naevus syndrome. *Dermatol Surg* 2002; **28**: 287–90.

15 Mackenzie-Wood A, Kossard S, de Launey J *et al*. Imiquimod 5% cream in the treatment of Bowen's disease. *J Am Acad Dermatol* 2001; **44**: 462–70.

16 Abide JM, Nahai F, Bennett RG. The meaning of surgical margins. *Plast Reconstr Surg* 1984; **73**: 492–7.

17 Lawrence CM. Mohs micrographic surgery for basal cell carcinoma. *Clin Exp Dermatol* 1999; **24**: 130–3.

18 Shriner DL, McCoy DK, Goldberg DJ, Wagner RF Jr. Mohs micrographic surgery. *J Am Acad Dermatol* 1998; **39**: 79–97.

19 Telfer NR, Colver GB, Morton CA. Guidelines for the management of basal cell carcinoma. *Br J Dermatol* 2008; **159**: 35–48.

20 Motley RJ, Preston PW, Lawrence CM. *Multiprofessional Guidelines for the Management of the Patient with Primary Cutaneous Squamous Cell Carcinoma*. www.bad.org.uk.

21 Tromovitch TA. Skin cancer: treatment by curettage and electrodesiccation. *Calif Med* 1965; **103**: 107–8.

22 Freeman RG, Knox JM, Heaton CL. The treatment of skin cancer: a statistical study of 1341 skin tumours comparing results obtained with irradiation, surgery and curettage followed by electrodesiccation. *Cancer* 1964; **17**: 535–8.

23 Simmonds WL. Management of actinic keratoses with topical 5-fluorouracil. *Cutis* 1976; **18**: 298–300.

24 Carter VH, Smith KW, Noojin RO. Xeroderma pigmentosum: treatment with topically applied fluorouracil. *Arch Dermatol* 1968; **98**: 526–7.

25 Wright TI, Spencer JM, Flowers FP. Chemoprevention of nonmelanoma skin cancer. *J Am Acad Dermatol* 2006; **54**: 933–46.

26 Bath-Hextall FJ, Leonardi-Bee J, Somchand N *et al*. *Interventions for Preventing Non-melanoma Skin Cancers in High-risk Groups*. www.cochrane.org/reviews.

27 Moriarty M, Dunn J, Darragh A *et al*. Etretinate in treatment of actinic keratoses: a double-blind crossover study. *Lancet* 1982; **1**: 364–5.

Basal cell carcinoma [1–3]

Synonyms
- Basalioma
- Rodent ulcer

Definition. A malignant tumour that rarely metastasizes, composed of cells similar to those in the basal area of the epidermis and its appendages. The histology of the tumour and the surrounding stroma is characteristic.

Incidence and aetiology. BCC is the most common malignant tumour of the skin and the most common cancer in some countries, including the USA and Australia. Although the prevalence of this tumour increases within a population as exposure to sunlight increases, the distribution of the lesions does not correlate well with the area of maximum exposure to UVR in that BCCs are common on the eyelids, at the inner canthus and behind the ear, but uncommon on the back of the hand and forearm. The palm, sole and vermilion of the lips are rarely, if ever, involved. The basis for the different susceptibility of skin at different sites to BCC development is not known.

BCC is more common in males than females. A population-based incidence study in Minnesota gives annual incidence figures for males and females of 175 and 124 per 100 000, respectively [4], and an Australian survey gives an incidence in that country of 849 and 605 per 100 000 for males and females, respectively, in 1990 [5], while figures from Hawaii show an incidence of 576 per 100 000 for males and 298 in 100 000 for females [6].

A Canadian case–control study has identified outdoor occupations (particularly farming), freckling, and Scottish or Irish descent as particular risk factors [7]. The Australian case–control study by Kricker *et al.* [8,9] of 226 patients with BCC suggests that the tumour is more common in those born in Australia than in immigrants, that southern European ancestry is protective, and that poor tanners are more at risk than those who tan easily. The presence of large numbers of naevi, freckles and solar elastosis all add to the BCC risk, while a past history of acne is protective [8,9]. A large European study of 1549 southern European patients with BCC reports that those with fair or red hair, those who tan poorly and those who have a history of childhood sunburn are at greater risk, and that acute episodes of intense burning sun exposure are a greater risk factor than cumulative lifetime sun exposure [10,11].

Some clues on the potential importance of exposure to hazardous air pollutants, arsenic, ionizing radiations and burns have come from a recent European multicentre study which showed that the frequency of BCCs was highest in miners and quarrymen, railway engine drivers and firemen [12].

BCC is extremely uncommon in dark-skinned races, and less common in Chinese, Japanese and other oriental populations than in white populations [13,14]. Although it may occur at any age from childhood, more than three-quarters of patients are over 40 years old. It occurs earlier and multiple tumours are more common in those with a fair freckled complexion. On the lower leg, the incidence in women is three times as great as in men [13]. BCC appears to arise more frequently and at a younger age in patients who are immunosuppressed. These lesions are frequently aggressive [15]. It is occasionally seen adjacent to leg ulcers [16].

BCC may arise in skin damaged by sunlight and ionizing radiation. It may occur in burn scars [17] or vaccination scars [18,19]. Arsenic salts are also a proven cause [20]. BCC has been reported in identical twins [21]. The increased risk of BCC development in naevus sebaceus and other adnexal hamartomas is well recognized [22–24].

The identification of mutations in the *PTCH1* gene has provided important insights into the pathogenesis of this common skin cancer and points to a key role for the Hedgehog (Hh) signalling pathway in its pathogenesis (see above and [25,26]).

Histogenesis. Theories about the nature and origin of the cells of BCC have been put forward at intervals over the last 80 years or more. The histological variability does not accord with a derivation from any individual epithelial structure, and is now generally considered to stem from the pluripotentiality of immature cells of the epidermis. It is thus capable of maturing towards any of the epithelial structures, and its behaviour is governed, as is the normal immature cell, by the connective tissue in its proximity. Thus, the stroma dependence, the range of histological patterns and the way these merge with the more organized hamartomas are explained. It has been rightly emphasized that the stroma is an essential part of the neoplastic process and it must also be removed in treatment.

Clinical features [27]. The early tumours are commonly small, translucent or pearly, raised and rounded areas covered by thin epidermis through which a few dilated, superficial vessels show (Fig. 52.2). Tiny flecks of pigment may be seen with a hand lens. Other modes of presentation are a small, pearly, erythematous, lichenoid papule or plaque, as a keratotic and slightly indurated area, or as a small and superficial ulcer resembling an excoriation by a fingernail. It may occasionally be pedunculated and telangiectatic, resembling a pyogenic granuloma.

The more advanced tumours have as wide a variety of forms as the early lesions and tend to maintain the same pattern of growth throughout their course. One common type grows slowly as a well-marginated expanding nodule or thickened plaque. The thinned epidermis closely covers the tumour and may periodically scale or erode and crust. In this variety, ulceration occurs relatively late, and may re-epithelialize and break down several times before becoming permanent. The surface contour usually

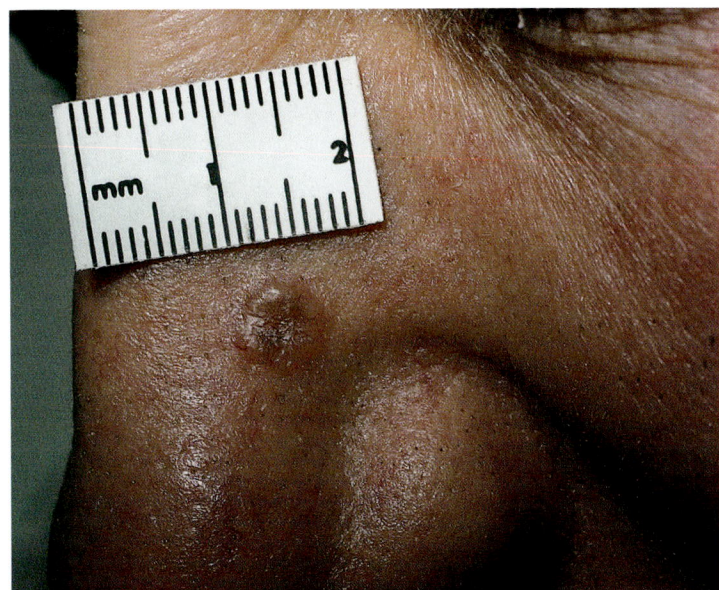

Fig. 52.2 Typical early basal cell carcinoma on the nose.

becomes more irregular as the lesion grows. The degree of vascularity varies. There may be surface telangiectasia over a flesh-coloured mass or the tumour may be pink or red in colour. Pigment, when present, is usually unevenly distributed through the tumour. Some or all of the component nodules may have cystic centres, which add to the translucent appearance; the cystic parts may be more deeply pigmented than the peripheral parts.

Less commonly, the tumour spreads only superficially. It is bounded by a slightly raised thread-like margin, which is irregular in outline and may be deficient at part of the circumference. The epidermis covering the central zone is usually atrophic and may be scaly. This, combined with an increased vascularity, gives a resemblance to Paget's disease of the nipple. There may be a series of thickened papular islands of growth within the margin, and these may be crusted or eroded. Superficial tumours are often pigmented.

The atypical rodent ulcer has an indurated edge and base, but no thread-like margin. The edge is usually raised above the normal level but in some areas, particularly in the nasolabial furrows, it may be flush with the surface. The floor of the ulcer is depressed below the skin surface, fleshy in appearance and not very vascular. However, there is more or less inflammation around the tumour. Such an ulcerated lesion may have begun as a nodule, but more frequently it is crusted or eroded from an early stage of its evolution. If left, the tumour and its following ulcer may spread deeply and cause great destruction, especially around the eye, nose or ear (Fig. 52.3). There may be wide extension in the periorbital tissues; the bones of the face, the skull and even the meninges may be invaded, and advanced cases amply justify the title 'ulcus terebrans' (penetrating ulcer).

The morphoeic or sclerodermiform BCC is uncommon, and is so named because dense fibrosis of the stroma produces a thickened plaque rather than a tumour. The exact margin of the lesion is impossible to define, but palpation reveals a firm skin texture that extends irregularly beyond the visible changes (Fig. 52.4) [28].

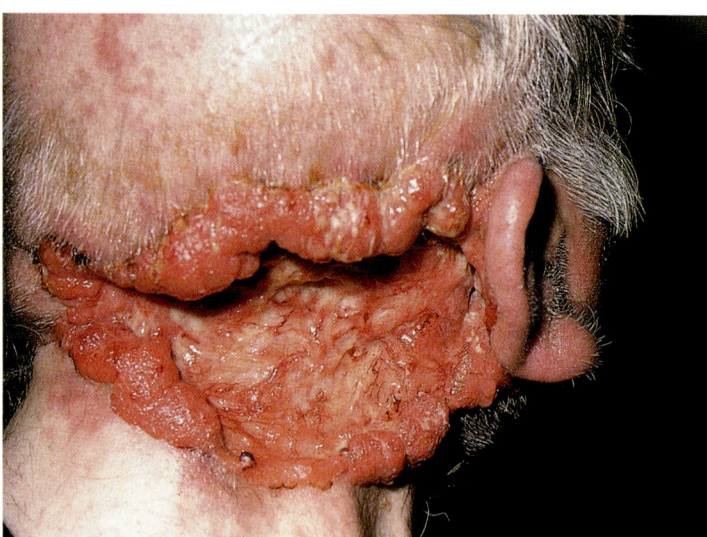

Fig. 52.3 Extensive, ignored basal cell carcinoma on the back of the neck in an elderly man presenting to a British hospital in 1988.

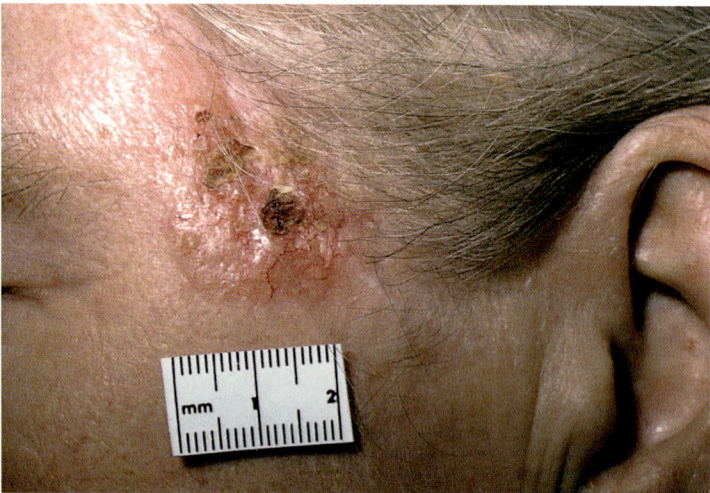

Fig. 52.4 Recurrent basal cell carcinoma that has arisen on the basis of pre-existing morphoeic basal cell carcinoma which was incompletely excised.

The surface is smooth and may be slightly raised above, or sometimes slightly depressed below, the normal level. The colour is yellowish and has been compared with old ivory. Ulceration is uncommon and only very superficial when it does occur. Many patients, and doctors, may take little notice of this type of BCC until its slow extension produces a sizeable lesion.

The majority of BCCs arise on the head and neck, with a particular predilection for the upper central part of the face. The morphoeic type occurs almost exclusively on the face. The superficial type, however, is found mainly on the trunk. The palms and soles are rarely affected. BCCs may be multiple.

Post-irradiation tumours of the scalp [29] and those that occur in sun-damaged skin of the face may be multiple and show various stages of development. A few cases of genuine BCCs have been reported to arise from the epidermis over histiocytomas, but the not uncommon basaloid buds seen in sections of histiocytoma are of doubtful significance.

The typical BCC runs a slow progressive course of peripheral extension, which produces the thread-like margin, the nodule with a central depression or the expanding rodent ulcer. Some tumours grow at so slow a rate that they are, for all practical purposes, benign. This is true for many of the superficial lesions and some of the nodular cystic lesions also. There may be spontaneous fluctuation in size, and areas of scarring can be found within many superficial tumours. A patient who has had one BCC treated should always be followed up, not only for local recurrence but also to detect fresh tumours arising elsewhere. There is no recognized premalignant stage of BCC equivalent to solar keratoses or Bowen's disease for SCC.

Rapid growth is so uncommon as to throw doubt on the accuracy of the patient's history. Invasive rodent ulcers, if neglected, may cause death. This is preceded by prolonged mutilation of the face or scalp [30], with destruction of the nose or eye and exposure of the paranasal sinuses or the skull, dura or brain. A few giant exophytic tumours have occurred on the back [31].

In rare cases, the tumour may disseminate [32–37]. When the ulceration involves the airway, fragments of tumour cells and stroma may be inhaled and become implanted in the lungs [35]. Authentic cases of bloodstream metastasis are on record in which, for example, deposits in the viscera or spinal column have caused the presenting symptoms of the terminal illness. Other cases have spread via lymphatics to the regional lymph nodes before disseminating.

Pathology [38–40]. The tumour cells resemble those of the basal layer of the epidermis and the matrix cells of the appendages, in the relatively small amount of cytoplasm they possess and in their ability to interact with the dermis adjacent to them. Their nuclei are compact, rather darkly staining and closely set. Their cytoplasm stains poorly and the cell margins are rather indistinct. Adjacent cells are connected by bridges. The sparsity of keratin fibrils gives these connections a different appearance from the 'prickles' of the Malpighian layer, but the presence of desmosomes and tonofibrils has been shown by electron microscopy. The interaction with the dermis, which is one of the principal functions of the normal epidermal basal cell, produces the characteristic marginal palisade of tumour cells and the well-organized stroma that surrounds it. The dependence of the tumour on its stroma has been shown by transplantation experiments [41]. The cells within the palisade usually show little evidence of organization or differentiation. Mitotic figures may be frequent, and it is speculated that the combination of large numbers of mitoses and a slow growth rate result from a high rate of apoptosis. Data on cell kinetics indicate that a considerable proportion of cells in the tumour die fairly rapidly [42]. Bizarre and atypical cells occur commonly in arsenic-induced tumours [20]. In some tumours, the cells may become acantholytic and amyloid may be identified [38].

In early lesions, the tumour buds can be seen arising from the epidermis. In very small lesions, multiple buds have been seen. These very soon become confluent, and the three-dimensional examination of superficial BCC shows a coherent margin of tumour with a reticular pattern of growth along the interpapillary ridges and larger, more discrete masses centrally [39]. As the tumour progresses, the masses extend into the dermis, and may separate from each other and from their point of origin. Growth in one area may be accompanied by involution of the tumour in nearby areas leaving an atrophic epidermis. A common site of origin in humans and in the experimental tumours of the rat is the junction between a pilosebaceous duct and the epidermis. From here the tumour may extend along the epidermis and down the duct. It is difficult to prove a purely adnexal origin for BCC, but some lesions behave as though this were so. In all considerations about the origin of the tumour, one must remember that the tumour can either sever its connection with epithelial structures or establish a secondary connection to structures to which it has grown close.

The variability of the natural history of BCCs is reflected in its pattern of growth. Most tumours are composed of rounded expansile islands. These throw out small buds that grow in the same way to produce multilobular masses with thin strands or septa of fibrous tissue penetrating them [39,40]. In some regions, a limited capacity to grow around and enclose adjacent connective tissue may be associated with a reticular or cystic pattern of growth. The capacity to invade in thin strands is often accompanied by an excessive and almost exclusive fibroblastic response, in contrast with the lymphocytic response around the expansile masses. Invasive strands may spread for long distances along nerve sheaths. BCC is truly invasive in only a small proportion of cases. In these, the tumours show no tendency to grow as rounded masses, have no palisade or organized stroma, and penetrate the dermis and deeper structures, destroying them as they go. Such tumours are almost always ulcerated, usually from an early stage. In the less invasive tumour, ulceration occurs when the epidermis is replaced by the tumour. An eroded, vegetating type of growth is rather uncommon.

Most BCCs provoke a round-cell inflammatory reaction of some degree. It increases in extent with ulceration and is often conspicuous in the papillary body, with superficial patterns of growth. Mast cells are often present in numbers among the fibroblasts of the stroma, and Langerhans' cells have been demonstrated within and near the tumour. This infiltrate has recently been correlated with the aggressive nature of the tumour [43].

The diversity of histological patterns of BCC is caused in part by features that have no direct bearing on the clinical course of the tumour. Not infrequently, melanocytes proliferate within the tumour. The melanin they produce causes the tumour to be pigmented, and numerous melanophages collect in the stroma, and sometimes in cystic cavities. Mucin is commonly found in the stroma, particularly at the margin of the tumour, and may be encysted within it. Cystic cavities also form when the centrally placed cells undergo necrosis. There is no evidence that such cavities represent glandular differentiation. Evidence of true sebaceous or sweat gland differentiation has been seen, but is very rare. Within some tumours there are strands of fusiform cells with more abundant eosinophilic cytoplasm, which may form whorls or keratinizing cysts, and which probably represent rudimentary differentiation towards hair roots. Citrulline can be demonstrated as a histochemical confirmation in such cases but does not help in the sometimes difficult separation from trichoepithelioma. Histochemical and electron microscopy investigations show little evidence of differentiation of the tumour cells. However, *in vitro*

culture of tumour cells from nodular tumours produces evidence of keratinization after 30 days, suggesting that the cells possess the biochemical mechanisms for keratinization but that some factor, possibly dermal in origin, inhibits them.

Diagnosis. The common nodular type of tumour has a distinctive appearance when it is more than a few millimetres in diameter. In the initial stages it may be hard to separate from a melanocytic naevus (especially when pigmented), molluscum contagiosum or senile sebaceous hyperplasia without the aid of a biopsy. Naevi can be distinguished if hairs grow from the surface, and in molluscum contagiosum and sebaceous hyperplasia there is a central keratin-filled pit. Scaling or crusting on the surface can cause confusion with warts, keratoacanthoma, SCC or molluscum contagiosum. In all cases, the debris should be removed, and this is easily done in BCC. The friable, relatively avascular tissue beneath is characteristic, and if fragments are removed and smeared on a slide the diagnosis can be confirmed by cytology. Darkly pigmented, ulcerated tumours are occasionally confused with malignant melanoma. The margin of BCC is usually rolled, telangiectatic and multinodular, and there is no pigmented halo. The colour tends to be more definitely brown, in contrast with the dusky greyish brown of malignant melanoma.

Perhaps the most difficult problems (although least crucial from the patient's viewpoint) are found with superficial BCCs. Casual inspection may suggest that these are patches of eczema, psoriasis or Bowen's disease. When the scale is removed and the edge stretched, the thread-like margin will reveal the true diagnosis [44]. Careful inspection will almost always rule out eczema or psoriasis, which the patient's history will have also made unlikely. There are some cases, however, where distinction from Bowen's disease can be made only after biopsy. The consistency of a morphoeic BCC may resemble morphoea; the outline is usually less sharp and the evolution more gradual and relentless. A recently described elastotic nodule on the anterior crus of the antihelix of the ear in sun-damaged skin may resemble a nodular BCC on cursory examination.

Clinical diagnostic accuracy in the diagnosis of BCC, widely regarded by most dermatologists as being the easiest tumour to recognize, is surprisingly poor. One study reported a diagnostic accuracy rate of 70% for academic dermatologists, 65% for dermatologists in private practice and 64% for residents [45].

Treatment. As stated previously there are many factors that influence the treatment of BCC, these include: tumour characteristics; patient characteristics; experience of the clinician; and local facilities. In the case of BCC the factors that influence prognosis are shown in Table 52.1 and should be considered when choosing treatment options.

The aim of any therapy selected for BCC is to ensure complete removal or destruction of the primary tumour to prevent local recurrence and the need for further therapeutic intervention whilst exposing the patient to the least risk of complications and producing an acceptable cosmetic result. The wide range in natural history and biology of the different subtypes of BCC and the large number of treatment modalities available for the removal and destruction of skin tumours means it is difficult to draw up rigid

Table 52.1 Factors influencing prognosis in basal cell carcinoma.

Tumour characteristics	Risk
Tumour size	Increasing size increases risk, especially over 20 mm
Site of tumour	Risk increased with central face, periocular, nasal, ears and lips
Definition of margin	Lesions that are clinically poorly defined are of higher risk
Immunosuppressed patient	Possible higher risk
Recurrent disease	Increased risk
Histological subtype	Morphoeic/infiltrative, micronodular, basosquamous all increase risk
Aggressive histological features	Perineural or vascular invasion increased risk

guidelines for the management of this common cancer. Successful management of BCC requires a clear understanding of the clinicopathological factors that affect prognosis and a good theoretical and practical knowledge of the strengths and limitations of the many different treatments available. From published series on outcomes it is clear that successful treatment can be achieved by any one of the large range of therapies, subject to appropriate matching of the treatment to the tumour characteristics [46,47]. In most cases, treatment selection is usually based on a clinical assessment which considers a number of factors that are known to influence tumour prognosis. These factors include tumour size, location, clinical subtype and defined margin. In addition to the tumour characteristics, other factors such as the patient's age, adequacy and success of previous treatments and coexisting medical conditions that influence tumour biology or treatment tolerability need to be considered. For reasons that are still unclear, BCCs recurring following radiotherapy are particularly difficult to eradicate by conventional surgical excision and this needs to be taken into account when selecting the most appropriate therapy [48].

Destructive therapies used appropriately, mainly for low-risk tumours, can offer an effective alternative to surgical excision for small primary tumours at non-critical sites. A number of studies have shown that curettage and cautery of low-risk BCCs can give cure rates of up to 97% [49]. Similar high cure rates have also been reported for cryotherapy for low-risk BCCs [50,51]. Tumour size has an important effect on prognosis for BCCs and there is good evidence that the recurrence rate following curettage and cautery or cryotherapy increases significantly with increasing size [52,53]. In addition to risk of recurrence, it is also important to bear in mind that the morbidity associated with cryotherapy also increases with increasing size.

Conventional surgical excision with predetermined margins based on the clinical characteristics of the tumour is regarded by many as the most appropriate therapy for most nodular BCCs and provides a specimen for histological examination and assessment of the lateral and deep margins yielding <2% recurrence rate at 5 years post surgery [54,55]. Studies of Mohs surgical specimens have provided useful information about the probability of achieving complete excision in tumours with predetermined margins in different sized BCCs. For BCCs less than 2 cm in diameter with

well-defined clinical margins, a 3-mm margin will clear the tumour in 85% of cases and a 4–5-mm margin in 95% of cases [56–58]. Although it has been estimated that careful inspection of the common nodular and plaque forms of the tumour with a loupe allows the margin to be determined to within 0.5 mm of the histologically proven border, inaccuracies in the clinical assessment of tumour margins are an important cause of incomplete excision of nodular BCCs. Small ulcerated nodular BCCs, which present as non-healing erosions, not infrequently extend several millimetres beyond the clinically defined margin. For these tumours and others where the margin is less clearly defined, curettage prior to excision is a useful technique for more accurately defining the true borders of the BCC [59,60]. Even in experienced hands there is a risk that nodular BCCs with apparently well-defined clinical margins may have infiltrated more extensively, leading to incomplete excision with residual tumour. In some cases, strands of cells extend along nerves for a considerable distance beyond the obvious clinical edge of the tumour [61,62]. The outlook is poor when cartilage, bone or the orbit have been invaded.

Studies of incompletely excised BCCs have demonstrated that not all incompletely excised tumours will recur but that between 21 and 41% will do so over a 2 to 5 year period [63–67]. Based on information generated over the years on residual tumour in re-excision specimens and recurrence rates of incompletely excised tumours, it may be reasonable in cases where there is incomplete excision of the lateral margin only, not to re-excise if the BCC is a primary tumour on a non-critical site with a non-aggressive histology. For all other cases and in those where the surgical defect has been repaired using a skin graft or local flaps, immediate re-excision with frozen section control or using Mohs micrographic surgery is the treatment of choice [47].

The management of morphoeic BCC, large BCCs (more than 2 cm in diameter), some smaller nodular BCCs with poorly defined clinical margins and recurrent BCCs needs to take into account the increased likelihood of subclinical extension. In the absence of either frozen section control or Mohs surgery, these tumours will require large predetermined margins; even a 5-mm margin will only give complete excision of 82% of morphoeic BCCs [56]. Management of recurrent BCCs is a difficult problem as cure rates are consistently poorer than those achieved for primary tumour. Mohs surgery is an important treatment option for the treatment of high-risk BCCs as it offers consistent high cure rates for even the most difficult BCCs. For primary BCCs and recurrent BCCs, treated with Mohs surgery, 5-year cure rates of 98.6% and 96% respectively have been reported [68]. The proportion of BCCs treated using Mohs surgery varies considerably between different countries as it is a relatively specialized technique and is more resource-intensive than simple surgical excision. Tumour characteristics that warrant consideration of Mohs surgery include BCCs at high-risk sites (nasolabial fold, periocular and nose), BCCs greater than 2 cm in diameter, morphoeic, infiltrative or micronodular BCCs and recurrent BCCs [46,47].

Basisquamous or metatypical basal cell carcinoma [69,70]

This term is used for tumours that on pathological study appear to have features of both BCC and SCC. The biological significance is that this pathological pattern is associated with a significantly higher incidence of metastatic spread [71]. The pattern in these lesions is of small aggregates of cells lacking classic palisading and embedded in dense and profuse fibrous stroma. The cells are larger with a larger paler nucleus than in the classic BCC and have a more eosinophilic cytoplasm.

References

1 Miller SJ. Biology of basal cell carcinoma. I. *J Am Acad Dermatol* 1991; **24**: 1–13.

2 Miller SJ. Biology of basal cell carcinoma. II. *J Am Acad Dermatol* 1991; **24**: 161–75.

3 Pollack SV, Goslen JB, Sherertz EF *et al.* The biology of basal cell carcinoma: a review. *J Am Acad Dermatol* 1982; **7**: 569–77.

4 Chuang TY, Popescu A, Su WPD *et al.* Basal cell carcinoma: a population-based incidence study. *J Am Acad Dermatol* 1990; **22**: 413–7.

5 Marks R, Staples M, Giles GG. Trends in non-melanocytic skin cancer treated in Australia: the second national survey. *Int J Cancer* 1993; **53**: 585–90.

6 Reizner GT, Chuang TY, Elpern DJ *et al.* Basal cell carcinoma in Kauai, Hawaii: the highest documented incidence in the United States. *J Am Acad Dermatol* 1993; **29**: 184–9.

7 Hogan DJ, To T, Gran L *et al.* Risk factors for basal carcinoma. *Int J Dermatol* 1989; **28**: 591–4.

8 Kricker A, Armstrong BK, English DR, Heenan PJ. A dose–response curve for sun exposure and basal cell carcinoma. *Int J Cancer* 1995; **60**: 482–8.

9 Kricker A, Armstrong BK, English DR, Heenan PJ. Does intermittent sun exposure cause basal cell carcinoma? A case–control study in Western Australia. *Int J Cancer* 1995; **60**: 489–94.

10 Rosso S, Zanetti R, Martinez C *et al.* The multicentre south European study 'Helios' II. Different sun exposure pattern in the aetiology of basal cell and squamous cell carcinomas of the skin. *Br J Cancer* 1996; **73**: 1447–54.

11 Zanetti R, Rosso S, Martinez C *et al.* The multicentre European Helios study I. Skin characteristics and sunburns in basal and squamous cell carcinomas of the skin. *Br J Cancer* 1996; **73**: 1440–6.

12 Suarez B, Lopez-Abente G, Martinez C *et al.* Occupation and skin cancer: the results of the HELIOS-I multicenter case-control study. *BMC Public Health* 2007; **7**: 180.

13 Miki Y. Basal cell epithelioma among Japanese. *Australas J Dermatol* 1968; **9**: 304–13.

14 Shanmugaranam K, Labrooy EB. *Skin Cancer in Singapore*. Monograph 10. Washington DC: National Cancer Institute, 1963: 127–40.

15 Weimar VW, Ceilley RI, Goeken JA. Aggressive biologic behavior of basal- and squamous-cell cancers in patients with chronic lymphocytic leukemia or chronic lymphocytic lymphoma. *J Dermatol Surg Oncol* 1979; **5**: 609–14.

16 Gaugman LJ, Bergeron JR, Mullins JF. Giant basal cell epithelioma developing in acute burn site. *Arch Dermatol* 1969; **99**: 594–5.

17 Burns DA, Calnan CD. Basal cell epithelioma in a chronic leg ulcer. *Clin Exp Dermatol* 1978; **3**: 443–5.

18 Hendricks WM. Basal cell carcinoma arising in chickenpox scar. *Arch Dermatol* 1980; **116**: 1304–5.

19 Rich JD, Shesol BF, Horne DW III. Basal cell carcinoma arising in a smallpox vaccination site. *J Clin Pathol* 1980; **33**: 134–5.

20 Yeh S, How SW, Lin CS. Arsenical cancer of skin: histologic study with special reference to Bowen's disease. *Cancer* 1968; **21**: 312–39.

21 Oettle AG. Rodent ulcers in identical twins. *AMA Arch Dermatol* 1956; **74**: 167–72.

22 Fergin PE, Chu AD, MacDonald DM. Basal cell carcinoma complicating naevus sebaceus. *Clin Exp Dermatol* 1981; **6**: 111–5.

23 Golberg HS. Basal cell epitheliomas developing in a localized linear epidermal naevus. *Cutis* 1980; **25**: 295–7, 299.

24 Lillis PJ, Ceilley RI. Multiple tumors arising in naevus sebaceus. *Cutis* 1979; **23**: 310–4.

25 Bale AE, Yu KP. The hedgehog pathway and basal cell carcinomas. *Hum Mol Genet* 2001; **10**: 757–62.

26 Epstein E Jr. Genetic determinants of basal cell carcinoma risk. *Med Oncol* 2001; **36**: 555–8.

27 Afzelius L-E, Ehnhage A, Nordgren H. Basal cell carcinoma in the head and neck. *Acta Pathol Microbiol Scand* 1980; **88A**: 5–9.

28 Litzow TJ, Perry HO, Soderstrom CW. Morpheaform basal cell carcinoma. *Am J Surg* 1968; **116**: 499–505.

29 Ridley CM, Spittle MF. Epitheliomas of the scalp after irradiation. *Lancet* 1974; **i**: 509 (Letter).

30 Gormley LJDE, Hirsch P. Aggressive basal cell carcinoma of the scalp. *Arch Dermatol* 1978; **114**: 782–3.

31 Curry MC, Montgomery H, Winkelmann RK. Giant basal cell carcinoma. *Arch Dermatol* 1977; **113**: 316–9.

32 Blewitt RW. Why does basal cell carcinoma metastasize so rarely? *Int J Dermatol* 1980; **19**: 144–6.

33 Von Domarus H, Stevens PJ. Metastatic basal cell carcinoma: report of five cases and review of 170 cases in the literature. *J Am Acad Dermatol* 1984; **10**: 1043–60.

34 Farmer ER, Helwig EB. Metastatic basal cell carcinoma: a clinico-pathologic study of 17 cases. *Cancer* 1980; **46**: 748–57.

35 Larson DL, Gillespie JJ, Parsons RW. Metastatic basal cell carcinoma of the lung. *South Med J* 1980; **73**: 647–9.

36 Snow SN, Sahl W, Lo JS *et al.* Metastatic basal cell carcinoma. *Cancer* 1994; **73**: 328–35.

37 Stell JS, Moyer DG, Dehne E. Basal cell epithelioma metastatic to bone. *Arch Dermatol* 1966; **93**: 338–40.

38 Weedon D, Shand E. Amyloid in basal cell carcinomas. *Br J Dermatol* 1979; **101**: 141–6.

39 Madsen A. Studies on basal-cell epithelioma of the skin: the architecture, manner of growth, and histogenesis of the tumours—whole tumours examined in serial sections cut parallel to the skin surface. *Acta Pathol Microbiol Scand Suppl* 1965; **117**: 3–63.

40 Sanderson KV. The architecture of basal-cell carcinoma. *Br J Dermatol* 1961; **73**: 455–74.

41 Van Scott EJ, Reinertson RP. The modulating influence of stromal environment on epithelial cells studied in human autotransplants. *J Invest Dermatol* 1961; **36**: 109–17.

42 Weinstein GD, Frost P. Cell proliferation in human basal cell carcinoma. *Cancer Res* 1970; **30**: 724–8.

43 Sherertz EF, Pollack SV, Jegasothy BV. Correlation of basal cell epithelioma aggressiveness with local inhibition of host lymphocyte response. *Clin Res* 1982; **30**: 266 (Abstract).

44 Epstein E. How accurate is visual assessment of basal carcinoma margins? *Br J Dermatol* 1973; **89**: 37–43.

45 Presser SE, Taylor JR. Clinical diagnostic accuracy of basal cell carcinoma. *J Am Acad Dermatol* 1987; **16**: 988–90.

46 Fleming ID, Amonette R, Monaghan T, Fleming MD. Principles of management of basal and squamous cell carcinoma of the skin. *Cancer* 1995; **75** (Suppl. 2): 699–704.

47 Telfer NR, Colver GB, Morton CA. Guidelines for the management of basal cell carcinoma. *Br J Dermatol* 2008; **159**: 35–48.

48 Smith SP, Grande DJ. Basal cell carcinoma recurring after radiotherapy: a unique, difficult treatment subclass of recurrent basal cell carcinoma. *J Dermatol Surg Oncol* 1991; **17**: 26–30.

49 Spiller WF, Spiller RF. Treatment of basal cell epithelioma by curettage and electrodesiccation. *J Am Acad Dermatol* 1984; **11**: 808–14.

50 Holt PJ. Cryotherapy for skin cancer: results over a 5-year period using liquid nitrogen spray cryosurgery. *Br J Dermatol* 1988; **119**: 231–40.

51 Kuflik EG, Gage AA. The five-year cure rate achieved by cryosurgery for skin cancer. *J Am Acad Dermatol* 1991; **24**: 1002.

52 Silverman MK, Kopf AW, Grin CM *et al.* Recurrence rates of treated basal cell carcinomas. II. Curettage-electrodesiccation. *J Dermatol Surg Oncol* 1991; **17**: 720–6.

53 Zacarian SA. Cryosurgery of cutaneous carcinomas: an 18-year study of 3022 patients with 4228 carcinomas. *J Am Acad Dermatol* 1983; **9**: 947–56.

54 Walker P, Hill D. Surgical treatment of basal cell carcinomas using standard post operative histological assessment. *Australas J Dermatol* 2006; **47**: 1–12.

55 Marchac D, Papadopoulos O, Duport G. Curative and aesthetic results of surgical treatment of 138 basal cell carcinomas. *J Dermatol Surg Oncol* 1982; **8**: 379–87.

56 Breuninger H, Dietz K. Prediction of subclinical tumor infiltration in basal cell carcinoma. *J Dermatol Surg Oncol* 1991; **17**: 574–8.

57 Wolf DJ, Zitelli JA. Surgical margins for basal cell carcinoma. *Arch Dermatol* 1987; **123**: 340–4.

58 Kimyai-Asadi A, Goldberg LH, Peterson SR *et al*. Efficacy of narrow-margin excision of well-demarcated primary facial basal cell carcinomas. *J Am Acad Dermatol* 2005; **53**: 464–8.

59 Johnson TM, Tromovitch TA, Swanson NA. Combined curettage and excision: a treatment method for primary basal cell carcinoma. *J Am Acad Dermatol* 1991; **24**: 613–7.

60 Chiller K, Passaro D, McCalmont T, Vin-Christian K. Efficacy of curettage before excision in clearing surgical margins in non-melanoma skin cancer. *Arch Dermatol* 2000; **136**: 1327–32.

61 Farley RL, Manolidis S, Ratner D. Aggressive basal cell carcinoma with invasion of the parotid gland, facial nerve and temporal bone. *Dermatol Surg* 2006; **32**: 307–15.

62 Williams LS, Mancuso AA, Mendenhall WM. Perineural spread of cutaneous squamous and basal cell carcinoma. CT and MR detection and its impact on patient management and prognosis. *Int J Radiat Oncol Biol Phys* 2001; **49**: 1061–9.

63 Sussman LA, Liggins DF. Incompletely excised basal cell carcinoma: a management dilemma? *Aust NZ J Surg* 1996; **66**: 276–8.

64 Richmond JD, Davie RM. The significance of incomplete excision in patients with basal cell carcinoma. *Br J Plast Surg* 1987; **40**: 63–7.

65 Park AJ, Strick M, Watson JD. Basal cell carcinomas: do they need to be followed up? *J R Coll Surg Edinb* 1994; **39**: 109–11.

66 De Silva SP, Dellon AL. Recurrence rate of positive margin basal cell carcinoma: results of a five-year prospective study. *J Surg Oncol* 1985; **28**: 72–4.

67 Wilson AW, Howsam G, Santhanam V *et al*. Surgical management of incompletely excised basal cell carcinomas of the head and neck. *Br J Oral Maxillofac Surg* 2004; **42**: 311–4.

68 Leibovitch I, Huilgol SC, Selva D *et al*. Basal cell carcinoma treated with Mohs surgery in Australia II. Outcome at 5 year follow up. *J Am Acad Dermatol* 2005; **53**: 452–7.

69 Bianchini R, Wolter M. Fatal outcome in a metatypical, giant, 'horrifying' basal cell carcinoma. *J Dermatol Surg Oncol* 1987; **13**: 556–7.

70 Farmer ER, Helwig EB. Metastatic basal cell carcinoma: a clinicopathologic study of 17 cases. *Cancer* 1980; **46**: 748–57.

71 Smith JM, Irons GB. Metastatic basal cell carcinoma: review of the literature and report of three cases. *Ann Plast Surg* 1983; **11**: 551–3.

Squamous cell carcinoma

Definition. A malignant tumour arising from the keratinocytes of the epidermis.

Incidence and aetiology. The epidemiology and risk factors important for cutaneous squamous cell carcinoma (SCC) development have been described in detail in the previous sections on NMSC. SCC of the skin is a heterogeneous disease both aetiologically and clinically, with different risk factors implicated in its development in different populations. The epidemiology of the disease has changed over the last 50 years, with a decrease in the importance of occupational exposure to chemical carcinogens and an increase in the proportion of cases caused by recreational sun exposure. In addition, new diseases, such as HIV infection, and therapeutic advances, such as the introduction of effective immunosuppressive therapies to prevent rejection of transplanted organs and PUVA therapy, have resulted in the emergence of new populations that are highly susceptible to cutaneous SCC development [1,2].

Cutaneous SCC is predominately a disease of white populations and is especially prevalent in this group in areas of high ambient sun exposure [3,4]. Although the incidence is low in non-white populations, SCC is still the most common skin cancer in these populations but shows differences in the anatomical location of

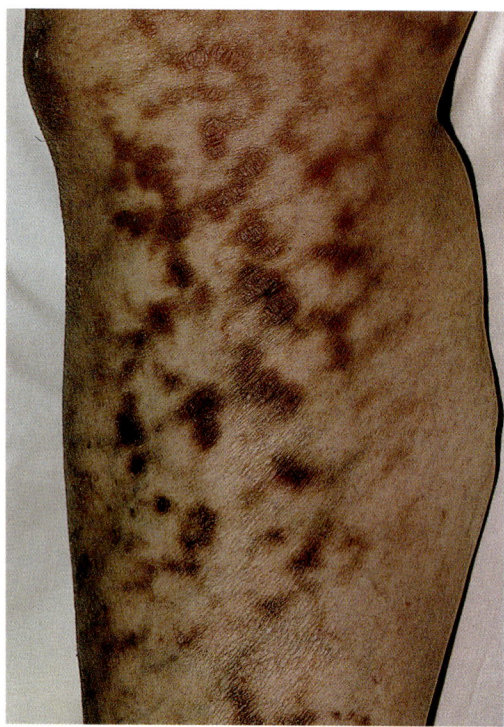

Fig. 52.5 Area of erythema ab igne on the lower leg of an elderly female.

the tumours, recognized aetiological factors and prognosis [5]. Factors implicated in the pathogenesis of cutaneous malignancy in Africans and African Americans include trauma, albinism, burn scars, ionizing radiation, chronic inflammation and chronic discoid lupus erythematosus [5,6]. There is a high incidence of SCC in albinos in Tanzania but no evidence of an increased incidence in vitiliginous skin of black people [6,7]. Additional aetiological factors implicated in development of cutaneous SCC in some populations include chronic exposure to thermal radiation and scarring. Radiant heat from coal and peat fires may cause SCC in women who habitually sit with their legs close to the fire [8,9]. The preceding lesion is called erythema ab igne (Fig. 52.5). SCC is also an occasional complication of long-standing chronic granulomas such as venereal granulomas, syphilis, lupus vulgaris and leprosy and lupus erythematosus, chronic ulcers, osteomyelitis sinuses, old burn scars and hidradenitis suppurativa. It may complicate scarring dermatoses such as poikiloderma congenitale, dystrophic epidermolysis bullosa [10] and porokeratosis of Mibelli [11].

Clinical features (Figs 52.6 & 52.7). SCC does not often arise from healthy-looking skin. Commonly, there are signs of photodamage: solar elastosis of the dermis, hyperkeratosis, irregular pigmentation and telangiectasia, or leukokeratosis and fissuring of the lip. The first clinical evidence of malignancy is induration. The area may be plaque-like, verrucous, tumid or ulcerated, but in all cases the lesion feels firm when pressed between the finger and thumb. The limits of the induration are not sharp and usually extend beyond the visible margin of the lesion. The resistance to pressure is much greater than that given by an inflammatory lesion or benign epithelial hyperplasia.

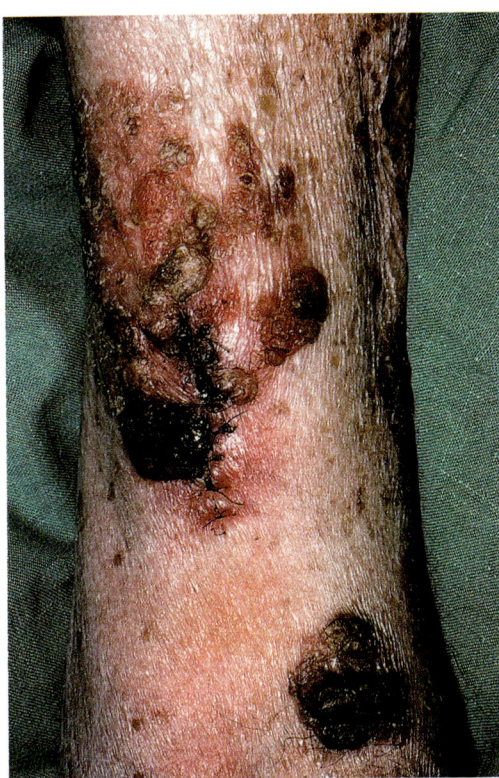

Fig. 52.6 Multiple invasive squamous cell carcinomas in a patient with a history of exposure to arsenic.

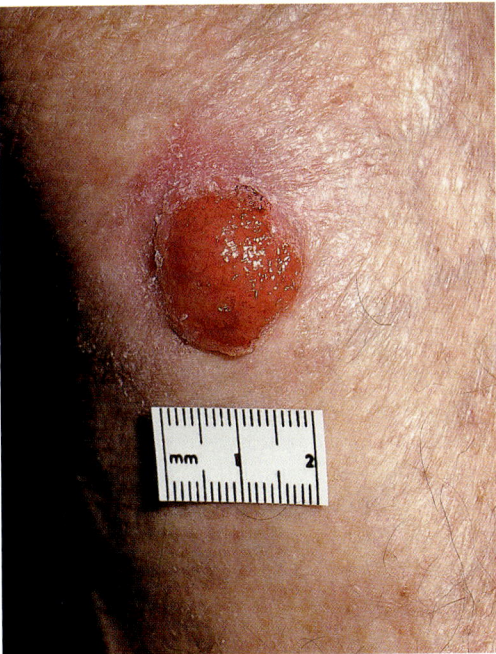

Fig. 52.7 Raised erythematous invasive squamous cell carcinoma in an elderly patient on a light-exposed site.

The tissue around the tumour is inflamed and the edge is an opaque yellowish red colour. The better-differentiated tumours are usually papillomatous and are capped by a keratotic crust in the earlier stages. This may be shed later to reveal an ulcer or eroded tumour with an indurated margin and a purulent, exuding surface that bleeds rather easily. The outline may be rounded, but is often irregular, and in premalignant lesions the induration and elevation is often asymmetrical at first. On mobile structures such as the lip or genitalia the presenting sign may be a fissure or small erosion or ulcer which fails to heal and bleeds recurrently.

The most common sites for SCC are those most exposed to the sun. They occur on the backs of the hands and forearms, the upper part of the face and, especially in males, on the lower lip and pinna.

The histological susceptibility of the scrotum in chimney sweeps, mule spinners and capstan-lathe operators was a result of the retention of the carcinogen on the skin surface. The relatively high incidence of lesions on the lower leg in the natives of tropical countries is related to the frequency of ulcers and scars. The nailbed is an uncommon site, which may be overlooked until the lesion is large enough to produce radiographical changes in the distal phalanx [12].

The evolution of SCC is usually faster than that of BCC, but is conspicuously slower than that of keratoacanthoma, which may attain the same size in as many weeks as SCC does in months or even years. Tumours arising in keratoses on the dorsum of the hand are particularly indolent and late in metastasizing. Early ulceration, and the absence of tumid outgrowth, are usually a result of an anaplastic lesion [13], and are more commonly seen on the lip and genital area than elsewhere. Regional nodes may become enlarged, either as a result of infection of the ulcer or from metastases. In the latter case, they feel harder, are more irregular and become fixed to the adjacent tissues. Spread by the bloodstream is uncommon [14].

Pathology [15–17]. SCC is a tumour that may arise in any epithelium, and its behaviour in the skin is essentially similar to its behaviour in the respiratory tract and elsewhere. Because of the accessibility of the skin, the precancerous changes that lead to the tumour are more easily observed and followed.

Potentially precancerous conditions include actinic keratoses, Bowen's disease and leukoplakia. Invasive SCC begins when atypical keratinocytes breach the dermal basement membrane and invade the dermis (Fig. 52.8). The distinction is thus architectural rather than cytological, and is based on the presence of descending strands of morphologically malignant keratinocytes, which can no longer be regarded as distorted interpapillary ridges. The distinction may be further complicated by the phenomenon of pseudo-epitheliomatous hyperplasia [15], which may occur at an ulcer margin or over certain inflammatory or neoplastic states in the dermis (see below).

The cells of SCC vary from large, well-differentiated, polygonal cells with vesicular nuclei, prominent nucleoli and an abundant cytoplasm containing numerous tonofibrils and well-developed intercellular bridges, through to completely anaplastic cells with basophilic cytoplasm, which provide no cytological evidence of their origin. Some tumours have large bizarre cells, in others the cells may have a clear, almost vacuolated cytoplasm and in yet others the cells may be spindle-shaped. Well-differentiated tumours show areas of maturation that form parakeratotic horny pearls and individually keratinized cells, and also dyskeratosis, with lacunae and lumina that contain shed rounded, degenerating

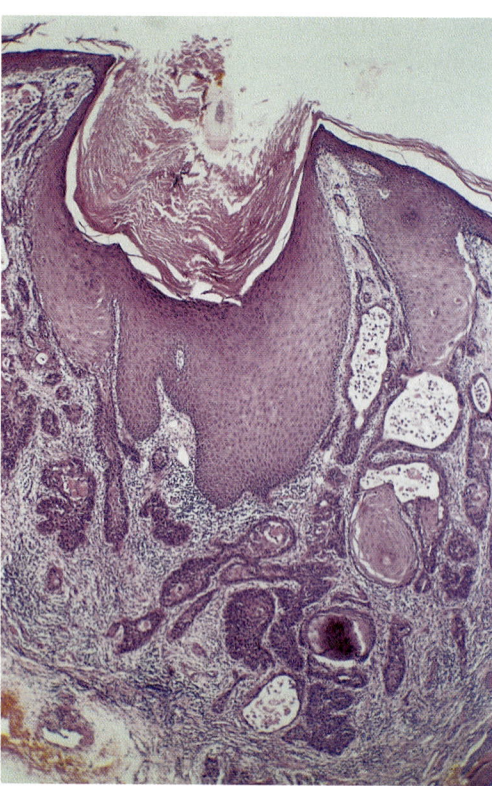

Fig. 52.8 Pathological features of well-differentiated, early invasive squamous cell carcinoma, showing differentiated keratinocytes invading the underlying dermis.

cells. The latter appearance is pseudoglandular, and is termed adenoid or acantholytic SCC [16,17].

Most tumours invade as coherent strands and columns, and reproduce the same pattern in their metastases. Many are composed of cells uniform in type and showing only moderate mitotic activity. They stimulate an inflammatory reaction in the dermis. The capillary pattern is abnormal and the number of vessels considerably increased [18]. Increasing anaplasia is associated with hyperchromatic nuclei, decreasing eosinophilia and tonofibril formation in the cytoplasm, and lessened intercellular adhesions. The cell outlines may be rounded or spindle-shaped. Mitotic figures become more frequent, and abnormal mitoses can be found. Even in extensively ulcerated tumours, the connection with the epidermis is usually maintained, and the origin can be traced to atypical epidermal cells, which may enable a distinction to be made from an anaplastic amelanotic melanoma. Its origin from an area of abnormal epidermis distinguishes it from keratoacanthoma. In rare instances, SCC may appear to arise in a keratinous cyst. Many reported instances of this occurrence, however, can now be considered as proliferating trichilemmal cysts.

Local extension of SCC may occur around nerves, sometimes for considerable distances, and may require extensive surgery [19]. Biological differences in the aggressiveness of SCCs arising in different locations and/or resulting from different aetiological factors are well recognized [20]. It is unusual for SCC originating in an AK on the hand or arm to show evidence of anaplasia or to metastasize until well advanced. In a Scandinavian series [21], fewer than 8% of tumours of the upper limb metastasized. Lesions of the vermilion of the lip, and to a lesser extent of the ear, metas-

tasize much earlier even when they are relatively well differentiated. Those elsewhere on the face appear to be less aggressive. SCC of the external genitalia is also inclined to early invasion and metastasis. Spread is almost always by the lymphatic route.

Various ways of predicting the likelihood of metastasis from the histological features have been suggested. One that has been widely used is Broders' classification based on the proportion of differentiated to atypical tumour cells. From the practical point of view, this method needs to be supplemented by the depth of invasion. For tumours of the hand, for instance, metastasis is unlikely when the penetration does not extend deeper than the sweat coils [16]. At the two extremes of differentiation this criterion does not apply. A well-differentiated lesion such as 'epithelioma cuniculatum' may invade the soft tissues of the foot extensively without metastasis [22,23], while a completely undifferentiated tumour, of the lip for instance, may disseminate at an early stage.

Epithelioma cuniculatum [24] **and verrucous carcinoma** [25]. There are several uncommon tumours that are so well differentiated that the diagnosis may be in doubt if the unrelenting course is not taken into account. One such has been reported as the 'epithelioma cuniculatum' [22]. There is a soft bulbous mass with a squashy consistency on the distal part of the sole of the foot. Multiple sinuses open on the surface and, when pressed, greasy, rancid and foul-smelling material can be expressed. It is possible that the appearance of a vegetating pyoderma may at times be caused by the same process. In such cases, the distinction from pseudoepitheliomatous hyperplasia may be very difficult. A few examples of 'giant condyloma acuminatum' have eventually become low-grade SCC [26,27].

In both the oral cavity and on the genital mucosa [28], a strikingly verrucous lesion may develop [25,29]. These lesions, because of the site involved, may become massive, moist, cauliflower-like and often malodorous because of secondary infection. The clinically apparent relentless growth contrasts with the pathologically less aggressive appearance characterized by a lack of mitotic figures and a well-demarcated lower margin with no strands of cells becoming detached from the main bulk of the lesion.

At the other extreme, anaplastic SCC rarely may arise from skin not showing a premalignant lesion and in a form very difficult to recognize. The lesion is a red papule or nodule, relatively fast growing and looking inflammatory rather than neoplastic. It tends to ulcerate early. It may resemble a keratoacanthoma, but the central keratin core is usually absent. Induration is present, but may be less marked than in well-differentiated tumours. It can infiltrate deeply and metastasize quite early. It has been designated 'squamous cell carcinoma *de novo*' [30].

Squamous cell carcinoma following immunosuppression after organ transplantation. Recipients of organ transplants receiving immunosuppressive therapy have a much higher than expected incidence of SCC [1,31,32]. The development of carcinomas is directly related to time from transplantation, and appears to be independent of the immunosuppressive regimen used. The normal ratio of BCC:SCC is reversed, and SCC is more common. The lesions are most numerous on sun-exposed sites and are frequently multiple. They may clinically be deceptively banal, and resemble either keratoacanthoma or actinic keratosis. All such lesions should be regarded with suspicion in transplant patients, and biopsied to establish their true nature. Female transplant recipients also have a much higher than expected incidence of genital premalignancy.

Careful, regular supervision of transplant patients by a dermatologist is required, and advice on sun avoidance should be part of the post-transplant care regimen.

Diagnosis. The indurated, well-differentiated SCC arising in skin damaged by sunlight presents no problems in diagnosis. The distinction from keratoacanthoma is usually easy, as the rate of growth and domed appearance of keratoacanthomas are characteristic. On occasions, however, a tumour develops like a typical keratoacanthoma, but proves by its progress to be an SCC [33]. In such cases, the histology of the early stage may not be conclusive one way or the other. The most important clinical distinction is between a poorly differentiated carcinoma arising *de novo* from normal skin, and an inflammatory ulcer or granuloma on the one hand, or an amelanotic melanoma or BCC on the other. The characteristic induration and opaque colour are the most important signs but any doubt is usually clarified by biopsy. Warty lesions such as viral warts or seborrhoeic keratoses are not indurated and are frequently multiple.

Treatment. The aims of any therapy selected for the treatment of cutaneous SCCs are to ensure complete removal and destruction of the primary tumour and to prevent metastasis. From published series on treatment outcomes it is clear that these aims can be achieved by any one of a range of therapies subject to appropriate matching of the therapy to the tumour characteristics [34]. There are a number of factors which influence the metastatic risk of cutaneous SCC, including clinical features such as size, site, rate of growth, aetiology and presence of immunosuppression. Histologic features influencing risk of metastases include tumour thickness, depth of invasion and degree of differentiation may or may not be available at the time of treatment planning but if available will aid in treatment decision making. Unfortunately, many of these factors are not routinely reported in the publications of outcomes of treatment in case series and there are few randomized trials comparing treatments to guide our decisions. Whilst published case series have provided insights into factors that impact metastases risk, the information is uncontrolled and does not take into account the impact of important factors such as differences between SCCs seen in office practice compared to secondary or tertiary care settings [20,34–42]. Treatment selection in clinical practice is based on an assessment of the clinical and, if available, pathologic tumour characteristics mentioned above that have been shown to be important in determining the level of therapy required and in identifying tumours with a poor prognosis. Identification of aggressive cutaneous SCCs is important as the overall 5-year rates of recurrence and metastasis for these tumours is 20–25% which is approximately three times greater than that for primary skin SCC (8%) [35].

Although there are considerable international differences in clinical practices, it is possible to make some generalizations. Destructive therapies used appropriately by experienced clinicians with careful tumour selection can offer an effective alternative to surgical excision for small (less than 1 cm in diameter), slow-growing, well-differentiated SCCs on sun-exposed sites [34,43]. For similar well-defined, low-risk tumours less than 2 cm in diameter, surgical excision with at least a 4-mm clinical margin is an appropriate starting point with anticipated complete excision rates of 95% [44]. Higher-risk tumours which are more than 2 cm, moderately or poorly differentiated, extending into the subcutis or on high-risk sites including the scalp, ears, nose, lip or eyelid require wider margins of more than 6 mm and may well benefit from histological examination of the margins with techniques such as Mohs surgery [44]. Tumour size has an important effect on the probability of both local recurrence and metastatic risk, with a doubling of local recurrence risk and a threefold increase in metastatic risk for SCCs greater than 2 cm in diameter. In addition to tumour size, other criteria used in the selection of appropriate therapy include the location of the tumour, the likely aetiological factor and histopathological characteristics [34,37,38]. UVR-associated SCCs on the ear, lip, scalp, eyelids and nose have a worse prognosis than UVR-associated SCCs at other sites. The basis for this difference has not been established but it is possible that some of the increased risk for cutaneous tumours may result from technical considerations at the time of surgery. SCCs on non-sun-exposed sites where aetiological factors other than UVR exposure are important are also associated with a worse prognosis. It has long been recognized that SCCs at sites of scarring, ulcers, chronic sinuses or previous thermal or ionizing radiation injury have a worse prognosis. SCCs arising in areas of Bowen's disease are also thought to have greater malignant potential. Although deaths resulting from metastatic cutaneous SCCs are more common in immunosuppressed patients, it is not clear if this increase is brought about by differences in the biology of SCCs in these patients or a reflection of the marked increase in the prevalence of SCCs in this group, which in itself could lead to more deaths from metastatic disease [45,46]. A further histopathological characteristic associated with a worse prognosis is the presence of perineural involvement [36,47,48]. SCCs extending into the subcutaneous fat or greater than 4 mm in depth are almost eight times (45.7% metastatic rate) more likely to recur than SCCs confined to the upper dermis (6.7% metastatic rate). Poorly differentiated tumours have a doubling in the incidence of local recurrence and a threefold increase in metastatic rate [34,49,50]. The worse prognosis and difficulties in managing recurrent SCCs highlight the importance of adequate initial treatment based on accurate clinical assessment and appropriate selection of therapy.

Radiotherapy is rarely the treatment of choice but may be indicated for some very large or rapidly enlarging tumours or in patients where aggressive surgical management may not be tolerated. It may also be better for certain sites where functional and cosmetic outcomes for surgery are less than ideal such as the lips, lower eyelid and occasionally the ear. Radiotherapy may also have a role as an adjuvant therapy in some high-risk SCCs where there are concerns about residual microscopic disease, for example in perineural involvement [51]. Mohs micrographic surgery offers advantages over conventional surgical excision and is widely regarded as the treatment of choice for high-risk SCCs as it reduces the risk of local recurrence and metastatic disease.

For patients with aggressive cutaneous SCCs, there are currently no recommended adjuvant chemotherapy regimes after definitive surgical or radiation treatment. A recent trial evaluating the effectiveness of adjuvant 13-*cis*-retinoic acid (13cRA) plus interferon alfa (IFN-α) failed to demonstrate benefit in the prevention of tumour recurrence or second primary tumour development [52].

The final results of any of the methods depend on the experience of the person using it rather than the technique itself. In experienced hands, all the techniques give 5-year cure rates of approximately 90% in a wide variety of SCCs at different sites. Patients with high-risk SCC and those who have evidence clinically of nodal disease are best managed with the help of a multidisciplinary team, which may comprise dermatologists, dermatopathologists, radiation oncologists, plastic surgeons, skin cancer specialist nurse and radiologist. In situations where treatment can at best be palliative, the involvement of the palliative care team may also be required [43].

Prevention. Patients presenting with SCCs or related premalignant lesions on sun-exposed skin should be advised about the importance of reducing exposure to solar radiation. In high-risk patients, regular follow-up and targeted treatment of small, low-risk tumours with cryotherapy and other destructive therapies may help reduce the frequency of tumours requiring surgical excision. Although intermittent 5-fluorouracil use may improve skin texture and reduce the rate of development of AK, there is no published evidence at present that this is associated with a decrease in the rate of development of invasive SCCs. In patients such as organ transplant recipients and patients with xeroderma pigmentosum, where the rate of new SCC development makes surgical management difficult, then it may be necessary to consider treatment with systemic retinoids to reduce the rate of development of new lesions and help target surgical excision to retinoid-unresponsive tumours. Etretinate and isotretinoin have both been shown to reduce the rate of development of new lesions in XP patients [53,54]. More recently, acitretin has been shown to reduce the rate of development of new SCCs [55,56]. In contrast to cytotoxic drugs, retinoids do not appear to eliminate neoplastic clones from the epidermis and discontinuation of therapy is associated with the rapid growth of numerous dysplastic lesions that were growth inhibited but not eliminated by retinoid therapy.

References

1 Nguyen P, Vin-Christian K, Ming ME, Berger T. Aggressive squamous cell carcinomas in persons infected with the human immunodeficiency virus. *Arch Dermatol* 2002; **138**: 758–63.

2 Ramsay HM, Fryer AA, Hawley CM *et al*. Non-melanoma skin cancer risk in the Queensland renal transplant population. *Br J Dermatol* 2002; **147**: 950–6.

3 Marks R, Staples M, Giles GG. Trends in non-melanocytic skin cancer treated in Australia: the second national survey. *Int J Cancer* 1993; **53**: 585–90.

4 Chuang TY, Popescu NA, Su WDP *et al*. Squamous cell carcinoma: a population based incidence study in Rochester Minnesota. *Arch Dermatol* 1990; **126**: 185–8.

5 Halder RM, Bridgeman-Shah S. Skin cancer in African Americans. *Cancer* 1995; **75** (Suppl. 2): 667–73.

6 Oettle AG. *Skin Cancer in Africa*. Monograph 10. Washington DC: National Cancer Institute, 1963: 197–214.

7 Okoro AN. Albinism in Nigeria. *Br J Dermatol* 1975; **92**: 485–92.

8 Cross F. On a turf (peat) fire cancer: malignant change superimposed on erythema ab igne. *Proc R Soc Med* 1967; **60**: 1307–8.

9 Peterkin GAG. Malignant change in erythema ab igne. *BMJ* 1955; **ii**: 1599–602.

10 Weschler HL, Krugh FJ, Domonkos A *et al*. Polydysplastic epidermolysis bullosa and development of epidermal neoplasms. *Arch Dermatol* 1970; **102**: 374–80.

11 Oberste-Lehn H, Moll B. Porokeratosis Mibelli und Stachelzellcarcinom. *Hautarzt* 1968; **19**: 399–403.

12 Hay DM, Cole FM. Postgranulomatous epidermoid carcinoma of the vulva. *Am J Obstet Gynecol* 1970; **108**: 479–84.

13 Johnson RE, Ackerman LV. Epidermoid carcinoma of the hand. *Cancer* 1950; **3**: 657–66.

14 Johnson WC, Helwig EB. Adenoid squamous cell carcinoma (adenoacanthoma): a clinicopathologic study of 155 patients. *Cancer* 1966; **19**: 1639–50.

15 Lund HZ. Tumors of the skin. In: *Atlas of Tumor Pathology*, Section 1, Fasc. 2. Washington DC: Armed Forces Institute of Pathology, 1957: 235.

16 Stout AP. Gross pathology of cutaneous cancer. *Arch Dermatol Syphilol* 1946; **53**: 597–8.

17 Willis RA, ed. *Pathology of Tumours*, 3rd edn. London: Butterworths, 1960.

18 Urbach F. *Anatomy and Pathophysiology of Skin Tumor Capillaries*. Monograph 10. Washington DC: National Cancer Institute, 1963: 539–59.

19 Dandy DJ, Munro DD. Squamous cell carcinoma of skin involving the median nerve. *Br J Dermatol* 1973; **89**: 527–31.

20 Kwa RE, Campana K, Moy RL. Biology of cutaneous squamous cell carcinoma. *J Am Acad Dermatol* 1992; **26**: 1–26.

21 Swanbeck G, Hillström L. Analysis of etiological factors of squamous cell skin cancer or different locations. III. The arm and the hand. *Acta Derm Venereol (Stockh)* 1970; **50**: 350–4.

22 Aird I, Johnson HD, Lennox B *et al*. Epithelioma cuniculatum: a variety of squamous carcinoma peculiar to the foot. *Br J Surg* 1954; **42**: 245–50.

23 Driban NE, Lacognata JJ. Subungal squamous cell carcinoma. *Dermatologica* 1975; **150**: 186–90.

24 Headington JT. Verrucous carcinoma. *Cutis* 1978; **21**: 207–11.

25 Ackermann LV. Verrucous carcinoma of the oral cavity. *Surgery* 1948; **23**: 670–9.

26 Davies SW. Giant condyloma acuminata: incidence among cases diagnosed as carcinoma of the penis. *J Clin Pathol* 1965; **18**: 142–9.

27 South LM, O'Sullivan JP, Gazet JC. Giant condylomata of Buschke and Loewenstein. *Clin Oncol* 1977; **3**: 107–15.

28 Foye G, Marshall MR, Minkowitz S. Verrucous carcinoma of the vulva. *Obstet Gynaecol* 1969; **34**: 384–90.

29 Kao G, Graham JH, Helwig EB. Carcinoma cuniculatum. *Cancer* 1982; **49**: 2395–403.

30 Graham JH, Helwig EB. *Cutaneous Precancerous Conditions in Man*. Monograph 10. Washington DC: National Cancer Institute, 1963: 323–3.

31 McGregor JM, Proby CM. Skin cancer in transplant recipients. *Lancet* 1995; **346**: 964–5.

32 Hartevelt MM, Bavinck JN, Kootte AM *et al*. Incidence of skin cancer after renal transplantation in the Netherlands. *Transplantation* 1990; **49**: 506–9.

33 Boyle J, MacKie RM, Briggs JD *et al*. Cancer warts and sunshine in renal transplant patients. *Lancet* 1984; **i**: 702–5.

34 Rowe DE, Carroll RJ, Day CL Jr. Prognostic factors for local recurrence, metastasis, and survival rates in squamous cell carcinoma of the skin, ear, and lip: implications for treatment modality selection. *J Am Acad Dermatol* 1992; **26**: 976–90.

35 Clayman GL, Lee JJ, Holsinger FC *et al*. Mortality risk from squamous cell skin cancer. *J Clin Oncol* 2005; **23**: 759–65.

36 Moore BA, Weber RS, Prieto V *et al*. Lymph node metastases from cutaneous squamous cell carcinoma of the head and neck. *Laryngoscope* 2005; **115**: 1561–7.

37 Veness MJ, Palme CE, Morgan GJ. High-risk cutaneous squamous cell carcinoma of the head and neck. Results from 266 treated patients with metastatic lymph node disease. *Cancer* 2006; **106**: 2389–96.

38 Mullen JT, Feng L, Xing Y *et al*. Invasive squamous cell carcinoma of the skin: defining a high-risk group. *Ann Surg Oncol* 2006; **13**: 902–9.

39 Dzubow LM, Rigel DS, Robins P. Risk factors for local recurrence of primary cutaneous squamous cell carcinomas. *Arch Dermatol* 1982; **118**: 900–2.

40 Epstein E. Malignant sun-induced squamous cell carcinoma of the skin. *J Dermatol Surg Oncol* 1983; **9**: 505–6.

41 Eroglu A, Berberoglu U, Berberoglu S. Risk factors related to locoregional recurrence in squamous cell carcinoma of the skin. *J Surg Oncol* 1996; **61**: 124–30.

42 Friedman NR. Prognostic factors for local recurrence, metastases and survival rates in squamous cell carcinoma of the skin, ear and lip. *J Am Acad Dermatol* 1993; **28**: 281–2.

43 Motley RJ, Preston PW, Lawrence CM. *Multiprofessional Guidelines for the Management of the Patient with Primary Cutaneous Squamous Cell Carcinoma.* www.bad. org.uk

44 Brodland DG, Zitelli JA. Surgical margins for excision of primary cutaneous squamous cell carcinoma. *J Am Acad Dermatol* 1992; **27**: 241–8.

45 Veness MJ, Quinn DI, Ong CS *et al.* Aggressive cutaneous malignancies following cardiothoracic transplantation: the Australian experience. *Cancer* 1999; **85**: 1758–64.

46 Barksdale SK, O'Connor N, Barnhill R. Prognostic factors for cutaneous squamous cell and basal cell carcinoma. Determinants of risk of recurrence, metastasis and development of subsequent skin cancers. *Surg Oncol Clin N Am* 1997; **6**: 625–38.

47 Mendenhall WM, Parsons JT, Mendenhall NP *et al.* Carcinoma of the skin of the head and neck with perineural invasion. *Head Neck* 1989; **11**: 301–8.

48 Cottel WI. Perineural invasion by squamous cell carcinoma. *J Dermatol Surg Oncol* 1982; **8**: 589–600.

49 Friedman HI, Cooper PH, Wanebo HJ. Prognostic and therapeutic use of microstaging in cutaneous squamous cell carcinoma of the trunk and extremities. *Cancer* 1985; **56**: 1099–105.

50 Breuninger H, Black B, Rassner G. Microstaging of squamous cell carcinomas. *Am J Clin Pathol* 1990; **94**: 624–7.

51 Han A, Ratner D. What is the role of adjuvant radiotherapy in the treatment of cutaneous squamous cell carcinoma with perineural invasion? *Cancer* 2007; **109**: 1053–9.

52 Brewster AM, Lee JJ, Clayman GL *et al.* Randomized trial of adjuvant 13-cis-retinoic acid and interferon alfa for patients with aggressive skin squamous cell carcinoma. *J Clin Oncol* 2007; **25**: 1974–8.

53 Kraemer KH, DiGiovanna JJ, Moshell AN *et al.* Prevention of skin cancer in xeroderma pigmentosum with the use of oral isotretinoin. *N Engl J Med* 1988; **318**: 1633–7.

54 Schnitzler L. [Retinoids and the prevention of cutaneous epitheliomas: 1977–87]. *Ann Dermatol Vénéréol* 1987; **114**: 1537–43.

55 George R, Weightman W, Russ GR *et al.* Acitretin for chemoprevention of non-melanoma skin cancers in renal transplant recipients. *Australas J Dermatol* 2002; **43**: 269–73.

56 Kovach BT, Sams HH, Stasko T. Systemic strategies for chemoprevention of skin cancers in transplant recipients. *Clin Transplant* 2005; **19**: 726–34.

Premalignant epithelial lesions

Premalignant epithelial lesions are conditions that can be recognized clinically or histopathologically and are associated with an increased risk of cancer development. Although premalignant lesions frequently share many of the histopathological changes seen in invasive cancers, the ability to order lesions on the basis of severity does not in itself imply that the lesions identified represent consecutive changes in a neoplastic process [1]. The histopathological changes seen in premalignant lesions include nuclear pleomorphism, increased mitotic rate, abnormal mitotic figures and abnormal differentiation. In the skin, a number of premalignant epithelial lesions have been identified and there is convincing clinical and epidemiological evidence of an association between many of these lesions and an increased risk of NMSC. Some lesions, such as AK and leukoplakia of mucosal surfaces, may show relatively little evidence of cellular atypia, whereas others, including Bowen's disease and erythroplasia of Queyrat, can show marked dysplasia of the epidermis that is histologically indistinguishable from the changes seen in well-differentiated SCC. Pre-

malignant lesions are distinguished from their invasive counterparts by the absence of histological invasion with the microscopical features of intraepidermal carcinoma confined above the dermal–epidermal junction. In addition to the epidermal changes, a common feature of many premalignant lesions is the presence of a chronic inflammatory cell infiltrate in the papillary dermis immediately beneath the abnormal epidermis [2]. The importance of premalignant lesions as indicators of increased NMSC risk is well illustrated by AK, Bowen's disease, tar keratoses, ionizing radiation keratoses and arsenical keratoses, which are frequently found in patients with NMSC or at high risk of developing this type of cancer. With the exception of arsenical keratoses, which are the result of systemic carcinogen exposure, all of the other premalignant lesions localize to areas of skin exposed to the carcinogen and these areas are the same as those at risk of NMSC development. Premalignant lesions frequently occur before the development of invasive cancers and can be useful in identifying individuals at high risk of NMSC development.

Conventional models of multistage carcinogenesis, such as the human colon cancer model and murine skin cancer models, are based on tumour systems that show an orderly progression through well-defined clinicopathological changes. In these models, cancer development is indirect, progressing through discrete clinicopathological changes and this is supported by molecular studies, which have shown that 'early' lesions have less genetic abnormalities than do 'late' lesions. Other tumours develop in the absence of any recognizable precursor lesions, that is they arise directly. Clinical observation suggests that most human cancers, including cutaneous SCCs, may not progress through intermediate stages and that progression of AK and Bowen's disease to invasive SCC may be the exception rather than the rule [1]. A full consideration of the natural history of most premalignant lesions, including AK and Bowen's disease, is difficult as therapeutic removal or destruction provides evidence of what the lesion looks like but destroys any chance of consideration of future behaviour. Notwithstanding these limitations, a number of longitudinal studies indicate that AKs frequently undergo spontaneous regression and have a low potential for developing into invasive SCCs [3,4]. Support for the hypothesis that most AKs are unlikely to progress into invasive SCCs comes from molecular studies. These studies have shown that AKs frequently show more extensive chromosome losses than do SCCs, in contrast to findings in the colon cancer model where indirect cancer development as part of a linear progression process is the norm [5,6]. These findings do not undermine the importance of regular skin examination of high-risk skin cancer patients and the treatment of lesions based on clinical need but they do not support the concept that aggressive treatment of some types of premalignant lesions such as AK will prevent cancer development in these patients.

References

1 Foulds L. *Neoplastic Development*, Vol. 1. New York: Academic Press, 1969.
2 Pinkus H, Jallad M, Mehregan AH. The inflammatory infiltrate of precancerous skin lesions. *J Invest Dermatol* 1963; **41**: 247–8.
3 Frost C, Williams G, Green A. High incidence and regression rates of solar keratoses in a Queensland community. *J Invest Dermatol* 2000; **115**: 273–7.
4 Marks R, Foley P, Goodman G *et al.* Spontaneous remission of solar keratoses: the case for conservative management. *Br J Dermatol* 1986; **115**: 649–55.

5 Rehman I, Quinn AG, Healy E, Rees JL. High frequency of loss of heterozygosity in actinic keratoses, a usually benign disease. *Lancet* 1994; **344**: 788–9.

6 Kushida Y, Miki H, Ohmori M. Loss of heterozygosity in actinic keratosis, squamous cell carcinoma and sun-exposed normal-appearing skin in Japanese: difference between Japanese and Caucasians. *Cancer Lett* 1999; **140**: 169–75.

Actinic keratosis [1–3]

Synonyms
- Solar keratosis
- Keratosis senilis

Definition. Hyperkeratotic lesions occurring on chronically light-exposed adult skin, which are focal areas of abnormal proliferation and differentiation that carry a low risk of progression to invasive SCC.

Aetiology and incidence. The great majority of actinic keratoses (AKs) occur on sun-exposed sites in fair-skinned people who have had excessive exposure to solar UVR [4]. Lesions with similar clinical and histological features may be induced by ionizing radiation or radiant heat and in workers exposed to pitch and other products of coal distillation.

The prevalence of these lesions is high in many countries and is influenced by the amount of ambient UV, the proportion of susceptible individuals in the population, the age structure of the population and the time spent in outdoor occupations and recreations. In the UK, a recent study has reported an overall prevalence of 15.4% in men and 5.9% in women over the age of 40 years and 34% and 18% in men and women, respectively, aged 70 years and over [5]. In areas with high ambient UVR levels such as Australia, a prevalence rate of 43% with 18% (of a population of 197) having more than 10 AKs is recorded [3]. Longitudinal studies in patients with AK have established, firstly, that there is a high probability of developing new lesions and, secondly, that many lesions undergo spontaneous resolution [6]. Although the rate of progression of an individual AK to invasive SCC has been estimated to be low (less than 0.1%), the presence of AK is an important biomarker of excessive UV exposure and increased NMSC risk [7].

Clinical features [8–10]. These lesions occur usually in middle-aged or elderly subjects on habitually sun-exposed areas such as the face, scalp and dorsa of the hands. The sides of the neck are involved in both sexes, but the ears predominantly in men. The vermilion of the lower lip but not often of the upper lip may also show keratosis, with a much higher incidence in men than women. Lesions are usually multiple and comprised of either macules or papules with a rough scaly surface resulting from disorganized keratinization and a variable degree of inflammation. Lesions vary in size from less than 1 mm to over 2 cm and are usually asymptomatic. In many individuals, the number of lesions can be better appreciated by skin palpation, which is a sensitive way of detecting the characteristic roughness associated with smaller lesions. Many of these small lesions may pass unnoticed by most patients, and the diagnostic changes often only appear later as a dry, rough, adherent and often yellow- or brown-coloured scale (Fig. 52.9).

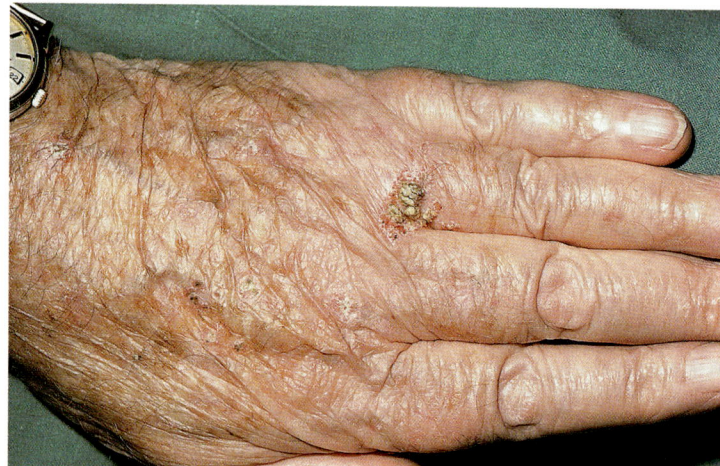

Fig. 52.9 Multiple actinic keratoses on the dorsum of the hand of an outdoor worker.

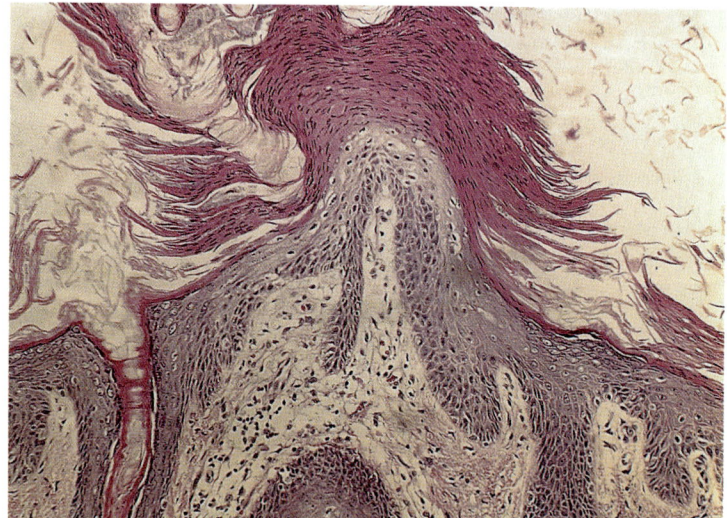

Fig. 52.10 Pathological features of actinic keratoses showing alternating parakeratosis and hyperkeratosis.

The adherent scale can only be picked off with difficulty, revealing a hyperaemic base with punctate bleeding points. In some cases, scaling may be prominent and in time may become thick and horny. The edge of the keratosis is usually sharply demarcated and the reddening is usually closely confined to the area immediately below the area of abnormal scaling. The flat, atrophic or lichenoid variety is most commonly seen on the face.

Many patients give a history of relapsing and/or remitting lesions, which can often disappear either spontaneously or after sun avoidance and use of sunscreens.

Pathology. The boundary between unaffected and affected epidermis is a sharp line that slopes upwards and inwards, and there is a similar margin where the appendage ducts perforate the epidermis as funnel-shaped columns of orthokeratosis. The epidermal cells have a paler cytoplasm and mature through an absent or diminished granular layer to form a parakeratotic scale of varying thickness. There is usually some acanthosis, and the more dysplastic lesions show epidermal hypertrophy with hyperkeratosis and parakeratosis (Fig. 52.10). The interpapillary ridges may be reduced in number and broader than normal. The affected zone tends to grow under the normal epidermis and around the ductal epithelium, and may separate from it by a cleft. The basement membrane is intact but basaloid cells may form multiple buds at the junction; the combination of clefting, budding and papillomatosis produces a Darier-like change. Within the epidermis there may be a simple dysplasia or a range of abnormalities up to a picture indistinguishable from Bowen's disease. These are the Bowenoid AK.

The papillary vessels are irregularly increased and there is a lymphoid infiltrate beneath the lesion. There is a variable degeneration of dermal collagen and deposition of material staining like elastin in the upper half of the dermis, except for a narrow band at the basement membrane; this change is more or less uniform, unlike the discontinuous keratosis.

The flat type of AK, most common on the face, may resemble discoid lupus erythematosus. The distinction is made by the altered epidermal cells, deficient granular layer and parakeratosis, the band-like rather than perivascular inflammatory reaction, and the absence of immunoglobulin in the basement membrane region. Occasionally, the appearance may appear pseudoepitheliomatous [8] or similar to lichen planus [9].

The occurrence of funnel-shaped columns of normal epidermis, derived from appendage ducts that appear to be trying to cover the diseased epidermis like an umbrella, suggests an effort at biological compensation [10]. It must be remembered, however, that in keratoses and Bowen's disease, sleeves of dysplastic cells growing down appendage ducts may survive damage by freezing or cytotoxic applications. The presence of an inflammatory response appears to be a warning sign of early malignant transformation [11].

Diagnosis. The diagnosis is usually based on clinical findings which take into account the morphology of individual lesions and the clinical setting. For lesions less than 3 mm, clinical discrimination from an early SCC may be difficult. This diagnostic uncertainty, particularly for small lesions, is one of the reasons why it is difficult to establish accurate rates of progression for AK to SCC. Clinical pointers favouring the diagnosis of an early invasive SCC include the presence of tenderness, induration or a raised shoulder that extends beyond the area of disorganized scaling. Other diagnoses that need to considered, particularly in patients with large confluent areas of erythema and scaling, include discoid lupus erythematosus. The brown colour of lichenoid AK, particularly when these lesions have only minimal scaling, can sometimes cause these to be mistaken for focal areas of lichen planus. When an AK is pigmented, it may resemble a superficial seborrhoeic keratosis, but can usually be distinguished from such lesions by the lack of organization of the hyperkeratosis. Bowen's disease on exposed areas usually has a more irregular contour and a more erythematous base.

Treatment. Management of patients with AK needs to begin with a thorough explanation of the nature, natural history and risks associated with the presence of these lesions. As AKs are a highly sensitive marker of levels of UV exposure capable of inducing premalignant and therefore malignant skin lesions, patients should be educated in the signs and symptoms of skin malignancy and given information in written and pictorial format to assist them in recognizing skin cancers when they occur. Having explained the above and discussed the treatment options, asymptomatic patients may decide that no treatment is required. Other patients may wish to simply use emollients. However, treatment decisions will be influenced by the symptoms the patient experiences, the confidence of the clinical diagnosis and patient anxiety about the potential for skin malignancy. Although AKs are frequently asymptomatic, the skin roughness may cause considerable distress and can be complicated by bleeding and pain because of low-grade skin trauma leading to detachment of the overlying scale. The presence of very large numbers of lesions can make it difficult for the patient or carers to see invasive malignancies at an early stage. The similarities between AK and SCC mean that there is always a small risk, particularly for small lesions less than 3 mm in diameter, that the lesion may not be an AK. Effective management of this risk requires a careful clinical assessment, a therapy plan and clear communication with the patient.

Once a decision that treatment aimed at clearing the AK has been made there are a number of options available [12]. Cryotherapy is effective for patients with a small number of lesions, and apart from hypopigmentation, generally gives excellent cosmetic results. This treatment does require a visit to a clinic and only deals with lesions within the treated area [13,14]. Other destructive therapies, such as curettage and cautery, can be useful for larger lesions and have the advantage of providing a specimen for histological assessment. However, a deep shave biopsy would provide better material for histological examination for evidence of invasion. Alternatively, small hyperkeratotic lesions treated by curettage and cautery with two or more cycles would have adequately treated a small, low-risk, well-differentiated SCC. Where there is significant diagnostic uncertainty, lesions are best excised for pathological examination of the base to be certain that the lesion is not an early invasive SCC.

In many patients, the number of lesions or the rate of development of new lesions makes management more difficult using approaches such as cryotherapy. For patients with extensive clinical lesions, a number of approaches are available that allow treatment of large areas of AK in severely photodamaged skin. Many of these treatments offer the added advantage that they also target early lesions, which means that a more sustained clinical effect may be achieved. These treatments can be subdivided into two broad groups based on their ease of use. The first group includes topical 5-fluorouracil, diclofenac in hyaluron gel and imiquimod which are effective therapies for AK [15–18]. Although 5-fluorouracil is an effective therapy, the marked local inflammation that commonly develops after 2–4 weeks of treatment may make it unacceptable to patients. Once-weekly application for 9 weeks with 5-fluorouracil has been shown, in a small study, to reduce the treatment-induced inflammation while maintaining efficacy [19]. A recent study has surprisingly reported greater efficacy and fewer side effects in patients treated with 0.5% fluorouracil cream compared with 5% fluorouracil cream [20]. The relative effectiveness and tolerability of 5-fluorouracil and diclofenac in hyaluron gel have not as yet been formally addressed in a clinical trial. A number of other approaches, including retinoids, are currently being investigated as topical therapies for AK [21]. The second group of therapies involves procedures that are normally carried out in the office or clinic setting and includes PDT, dermabrasion and chemical peels. PDT with topical 6-aminolaevulinic acid has been shown to be an effective, well-tolerated therapy for patients with widespread photodamage and AK [22]. A recent comparison of PDT with cryotherapy has established that PDT is as effective as cryotherapy and superior to the latter in patient satisfaction and cosmetic result [23–25]. Dermabrasion and chemical peels have been widely used in some countries for the treatment of AK and severe photodamage. There is some evidence that this approach may provide more long-term, effective prophylaxis against AK [26].

The demonstration that regular sunscreen use reduces the rate of development of new AK indicates that continuing UVR exposure plays an important role in promoting the development of clinical lesions and highlights the importance of ensuring that patients with AK are provided with practical advice on sun-avoidance strategies [27].

References

1 Marks R. Non-melanoma skin cancer and solar keratoses in Australia. *Eur J Epidemiol* 1985; **1**: 319–22.

2 Marks R, Ponsford MW, Selwood TS *et al.* Non-melanotic skin cancer and solar keratoses in Victoria. *Med J Aust* 1983; **2**: 619–22.

3 Frost CA, Green AC, Williams GM. The prevalence and determinants of solar keratoses at subtropical latitude. *Br J Dermatol* 1998; **139**: 1033–9.

4 Freeman RG. Carcinogenic effect of solar radiation and prevention measures. *Cancer* 1968; **21**: 1114–20.

5 Memon AA, Tomenson JA, Bothwell J, Friedmann PS. Prevalence of solar damage and actinic keratosis in a Merseyside population. *Br J Dermatol* 2000; **142**: 1154–9.

6 Marks R, Foley P, Goodman G *et al.* Spontaneous remission of solar keratoses: the case for conservative management. *Br J Dermatol* 1986; **115**: 649–55.

7 Salasche SJ. Epidemiology of actinic keratoses and squamous cell carcinoma. *J Am Acad Dermatol* 2000; **42**: 4–7.

8 Pinkus H. Keratosis senilis: a biologic concept of its pathogenesis and diagnosis based on the study of normal epidermis and 1730 seborrhoeic and senile keratoses. *Am J Clin Pathol* 1958; **29**: 193–207.

9 Shapiro L, Ackermann AB. Solitary lichen planus like actinic keratoses. *Dermatologica* 1966; **132**: 386–92.

10 Civatte J, Schnitzler L, Belaïch S. Hyperplasie pseudo-épithéliomateuse du dos des mains. *Ann Dermatol Syphiligr* 1973; **100**: 29–48.

11 Berhane T, Halliday GM, Cooke B, Barnetson RS. Inflammation is associated with progression of actinic keratoses to squamous cell carcinoma in humans. *Br J Dermatol* 2002; **146**: 810–5.

12 de Berker D, McGregor JM, Hughes BR, on behalf of the British Association of Dermatologists Therapy Guidelines and Audit Subcommittee. Guidelines for the management of actinic keratoses. *Br J Dermatol* 2007; **156**: 222–30.

13 Szeimies RM, Karrer S, Radakovic-Fijan S *et al.* Photodynamic therapy using topical methyl 5-aminolevulinate compared with cryotherapy for actinic keratosis: a prospective, randomized study. *J Am Acad Dermatol* 2002; **47**: 258–62.

14 Freeman M, Vinciullo C, Francis D *et al.* A comparison of photodynamic therapy using topical methyl aminolevulinate (Metvix) with single cycle cryotherapy in patients with actinic keratosis: a prospective, randomized study. *Dermatolog Treat* 2003; **14**: 99–106.

15 Goette DK. Topical chemotherapy with 5-fluorouracil: a review. *J Am Acad Dermatol* 1981; **4**: 633–49.

16 Rivers JK, Arlette J, Shear N *et al.* Topical treatment of actinic keratoses with 3.0% diclofenac in 2.5% hyaluronan gel. *Br J Dermatol* 2002; **146**: 94–100.

17 Wolf JE, Taylor JR, Tschen E, Kang S. Topical 3% diclofenac in 22.5% hyaluronan gel in the treatment of actinic keratoses. *Int J Dermatol* 2001; **40**: 709–13.

18 Hadley G, Derry S, Moore RA. Imiquimod for actinic keratosis: systematic review and meta analysis. *J Dermatol* 2006; **126**: 1251–5.

19 Pearlman DL. Weekly pulse dosing: effective and comfortable 5-fluorouracil treatment of multiple facial actinic keratoses. *J Am Acad Dermatol* 1991; **25**: 665–7.

20 Loven K, Stein L, Furst K, Levy S. Evaluation of the efficacy and tolerability of 0.5% fluouracil cream and 5% fluouracil cream applied to each side of the face in patients with actinic keratoses. *Clin Ther* 2002; **24**: 990–1000.

21 Kang S, Goldfarb MT, Weiss JB *et al.* Assessment of adapalene gel for the treatment of actinic keratoses and lentigines: a randomized trial. *J Am Acad Dermatol* 2003; **49**: 83–90.

22 Dijkstra AT, Majoie IM, van Dongen JW *et al.* Photodynamic therapy with violet light and topical 6-aminolaevulinic acid in the treatment of actinic keratosis, Bowen's disease and basal cell carcinoma. *J Eur Acad Dermatol Venereol* 2001; **15**: 550–4.

23 Szeimies RM, Karrer S, Radakovic-Fijan S *et al.* Photodynamic therapy using topical methyl 5-aminolevulinate compared with cryotherapy for actinic keratosis: a prospective, randomized study. *J Am Acad Dermatol* 2002; **47**: 258–62.

24 Morton CA, Campbell S, Gupta G *et al.* Intraindividual, right-left comparison of topical methyl aminolaevulinate-photodynamic therapy and cryotherapy in subjects with actinic keratoses: a multicentre, randomized controlled study. *Br J Dermatol* 2006; **155**: 1029–36.

25 Kaufmann R, Spelman L, Weightman W *et al.* Multicentre intra-individual randomized trial of topical methyl aminolaevulinate-photodynamic therapy vs. cryotherapy for multiple actinic keratoses on the extremities. *Br J Dermatol* 2008; **158**: 994–9.

26 Coleman WP III, Yarborough JM, Mandy SH. Dermabrasion for prophylaxis and treatment of actinic keratoses. *Dermatol Surg* 1996; **22**: 17–21.

27 Thompson SC, Jolley D, Marks R. Reduction of solar keratoses by regular sunscreen use. *N Engl J Med* 1993; **329**: 1147–51.

Bowen's disease [1,2]

Definition. A form of intraepidermal SCC characterized by a persistent, non-elevated, red, scaly or crusted plaque with a small potential for invasive malignancy. Progressive growth is usual but spontaneous partial regression occurs occasionally.

Aetiology and incidence. Most cases of typical Bowen's disease in white populations are found on the lower legs of elderly women. The distribution in the context of differences between men and women in coverage of the lower leg by clothing and molecular epidemiological evidence of UVR-specific *p53* mutations in typical Bowen's disease suggests that exposure to solar radiation is an important cause of these lesions [3]. Bowen's disease is uncommon in individuals with pigmented skin and, in these individuals, aetiological factors other than UVR exposure may be important [4].

In the past, arsenic exposure was also important [5]. Although fewer than 5% of a large series of patients with Bowen's disease gave a history of ingestion of arsenic containing medications, arsenic was found in a significantly higher proportion of the skin of patients than in that of the controls [6]. The possible sources of arsenic vary in different localities. Agricultural workers may be exposed to arsenic salts used as a fungicide, weedkiller, sheep dip or pesticide, and they frequently take inadequate precautions against accidental ingestion or inhalation. It may be a hazard in smelting and other industrial processes. In some countries, notably parts of Argentina, Bangladesh and Taiwan, the water supply has been contaminated [7].

Clinical features [8,9]. Although the lesions may occur anywhere on the skin surface or on mucosal surfaces, they are most frequently found on the lower legs of elderly women. The initial

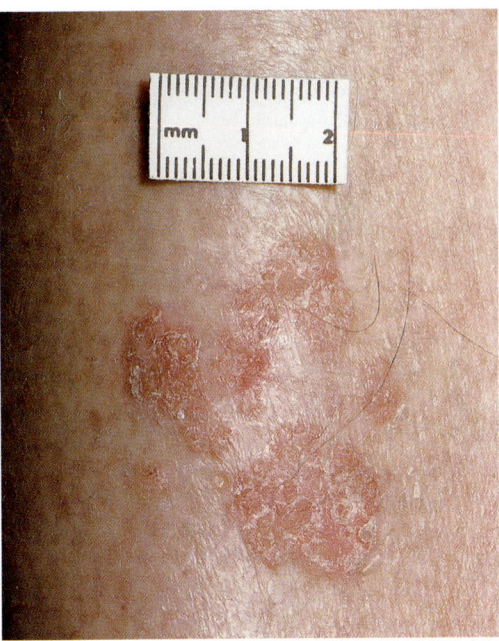

Fig. 52.11 Area of Bowen's disease on lower leg.

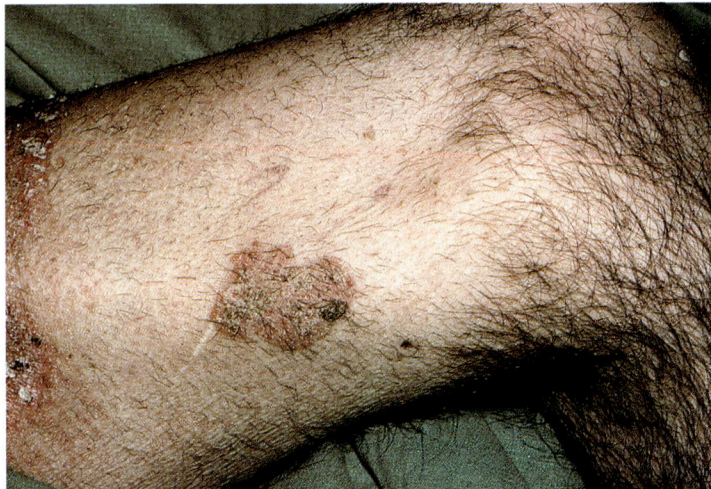

Fig. 52.12 Bowen's disease on the lower leg of a patient with a history of arsenic contact.

change is a small, red and slightly scaly area, which is symptomless and gradually enlarges in a somewhat irregular fashion. The white or yellowish scale is detached without much difficulty to give a moist, reddened and at times granular surface, but without producing bleeding (Fig. 52.11). The margin is well-demarcated and the lesion slightly raised; the surface is usually flat, but may become hyperkeratotic or crusted. Ulceration is usually a sign of development of invasive carcinoma, and may be delayed for many years after the appearance of the intraepidermal change. Persistent superficial ulceration may, however, be the early clinical evidence of Bowen's disease of palmar skin without invasion. There may be several lesions, either widely spread or sometimes close together and becoming confluent with extension.

When there is good evidence of chronic arsenicalism (Fig. 52.12), either from the history or because of associated changes such as pigmentation or punctate palmoplantar keratoses, the possible evolution of a visceral malignancy, especially of the lung, should be borne in mind. Although studies in the 1950s suggested that there was a significant link between the presence of Bowen's disease on the skin and internal malignancy [10–14], more recent studies using carefully selected control populations have failed to confirm these results [15–19].

Pathology [20]. The normal epidermis is replaced by abnormal keratinocytes, which show disordered differentiation and loss of epithelial polarity. There is variable acanthosis, with increase in the length and thickness of the interpapillary ridges but retention of a distinct dermal–epidermal junction. The atypical cells have hyperchromatic nuclei, often larger than normal, giving an irregular appearance to the epidermis. Giant forms and multinucleate cells are seen and mitotic figures can be frequent (Fig. 52.13). There is a conspicuous disturbance of epidermal organization, and cells keratinize prematurely and lose their intercellular connections. The surface is formed by a thickened, loose, parakeratotic scale.

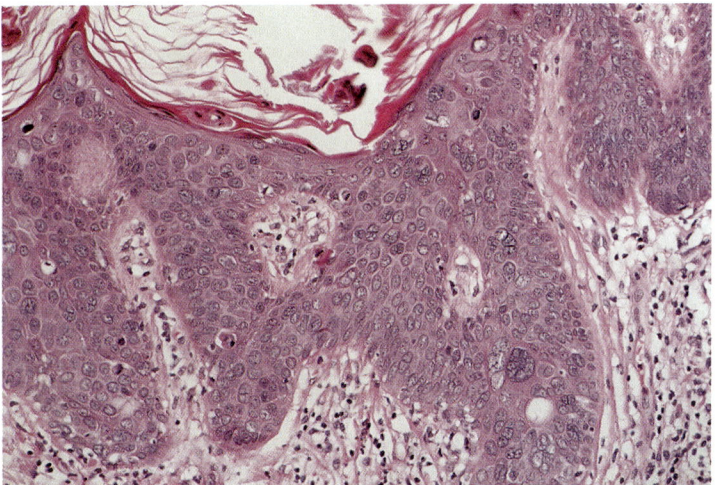

Fig. 52.13 Typical pathological features of Bowen's disease showing loss of polarity of the epidermis and the presence of atypical mitoses and giant cells.

The papillary body shows an inflammatory infiltrate that is often quite dense. In some cases, the proliferating cells may be surrounded by relatively normal epidermal cells to give a 'Borst–Jadassohn' appearance. The epidermis above the ducts of appendages may be normal, as in AK, but the cells of the lesion of Bowen's disease often grow down around the ducts like a collar. The condition can become invasive, and when it does it is always squamous cell in type. Arsenical Bowen's disease is said to be characterized by the presence of numerous vacuolated atypical cells. Electron microscope features have been described [21–24].

Diagnosis. The condition must be distinguished from lichen simplex, psoriasis and other papulosquamous dermatoses. If the diagnosis is uncertain on the first examination, the lack of improvement when steroids are applied is suggestive of Bowen's disease. The superficial ('pagetoid') type of BCC can produce a very similar appearance, but can usually be differentiated by the finely elevated, 'thread-like' margin. Bowen's disease and superficial BCC can be seen in the same patient. Differentiation from the flat type of solar keratosis may be impossible.

Treatment [24]. There is a wide range of therapeutic options available for the treatment of Bowen's disease including: cryotherapy; curettage and cautery; PDT; laser destruction; excision; 5-fluorouracil cream; imiquimod cream; and radiotherapy. The preferred treatment option is based on a number of factors including size of lesion, site, previous treatment, experience of the various treatments and the number of lesions. Destructive therapies such as curettage and cautery, or cryotherapy are widely used in clinical practice. Comparison of the relative effectiveness of different therapies and regimens is difficult as published studies do not fully control for factors such as site and size and there are inconsistencies between treatment regimens used at different centres. Cryotherapy is an effective therapy with a recurrence rate when used optimally of less than 10% at 12 months. Regimens used include single freeze–thaw cycles, single freeze–thaw cycles repeated on more than one visit and multiple freeze–thaw cycles repeated at a single visit [25–27]. Prolonged single freeze cycles for larger lesions is painful and may be better performed under local anaesthesia. Slow healing can be a problem, particularly for lesions on the lower leg. Curettage and cautery is widely used in practice but poorly studied. Reported recurrence rates are higher than those described with cryotherapy but these findings are difficult to interpret as treatment regimens and equipment are poorly described. Surgical excision is a useful approach, particularly for small lesions in poor healing sites, perineal lesions and digital lesions.

Local cytotoxic agents such as 5-fluorouracil can be applied to good effect. Treatment regimens vary and include once daily application of a 5% cream for 4–8 weeks or more prolonged treatment using a once-weekly application. There is some evidence that occlusion may increase efficacy. Recurrences are common, and may come from extensions of the carcinoma *in situ* around appendage ducts that were unaffected by treatment. Current studies suggest that PDT, using a topical photosensitizer such as aminolaevulinic acid and a laser or non-laser light source may also be an effective method of treatment [24,27–29]. Imiquimod has been used in uncontrolled trials for the treatment of Bowen's disease and in one randomized controlled trial [30] which demonstrated good efficacy but with a suboptimal dosing schedule. Further work is required.

References

1 Bowen JT. Precancerous dermatosis. *J Cutan Dis* 1912; **30**: 241–55.
2 Bowen JT. Precancerous dermatosis: the further course of two cases previously reported. *Arch Dermatol* 1920; **1**: 23–4.
3 Campbell C, Quinn AG, Ro YS *et al*. p53 mutations are common and early events that precede tumor invasion in squamous cell neoplasia of the skin. *J Invest Dermatol* 1993; **100**: 746.
4 Sau P, McMarlin SL, Sperling LC, Katz R. Bowen's disease of the nail bed and periungual area: a clinicopathologic analysis of seven cases. *Arch Dermatol* 1994; **130**: 204–9.
5 Graham JH, Helwig EB. Bowen's disease and its relationship to systemic cancer. *Arch Dermatol* 1959; **80**: 133–59.
6 Graham JH, Mazzanti GR, Helwig EB. Chemistry of Bowen's disease: relationship to arsenic. *J Invest Dermatol* 1961; **37**: 317–32.
7 Tseng WP, Chu HM, How SW *et al*. Prevalence of skin cancer in an endemic area of chronic arsenicism in Taiwan. *J Natl Cancer Inst* 1968; **40**: 453–63.
8 Callen JP, Headington J. Bowen's and non-Bowen's squamous intraepidermal neoplasia of the skin. *Arch Dermatol* 1980; **116**: 422–6.
9 Sanderson KV. Multicentric pigmented Bowen's disease. *Proc R Soc Med* 1974; **67**: 23–4.
10 Andersen SLC, Nielsen A, Reymann F. Relationship between Bowen's disease and internal malignant tumours. *Arch Dermatol* 1973; **108**: 367–70.
11 Epstein E. Association of Bowen's disease with visceral cancer. *Arch Dermatol* 1960; **82**: 349–51.
12 Kao GF. Carcinoma arising in Bowen's disease. *Arch Dermatol* 1986; **122**: 1124–6.
13 Kao GF, Graham JH. Premalignant and malignant cutaneous disorders of the head and neck. In: English GM, *Otolaryngology*, Vol 5. New York: Harper & Row, 1986.
14 Peterka ES, Lynch FW, Goltz RW. An association between Bowen's disease and internal cancer. *Arch Dermatol* 1961; **84**: 623–9.
15 Arbesmann H, Ranshoff DF. Is Bowen's disease a predictor for the development of internal malignancy? A methodological critique of the literature. *JAMA* 1987; **257**: 516–8.
16 Chuang TY, Reizner GT. Bowen's disease and internal malignancy. *J Am Acad Dermatol* 1988; **19**: 47–51.
17 Lycka BAS. Bowen's disease and internal malignancy: a meta-analysis. *Int J Dermatol* 1989; **28**: 531–3.
18 Moller R, Nielsen A, Reymann F *et al*. Squamous cell carcinoma of the skin and internal malignant neoplasms. *Arch Dermatol* 1979; **115**: 304–5.
19 Reymann F, Ravnborg L, Schon G *et al*. Bowen's disease and internal malignant disease. *Arch Dermatol* 1988; **124**: 677–9.
20 Brownstein MH, Rabinowitz AD. The precursors of squamous cell carcinoma. *Int J Dermatol* 1979; **18**: 1–16.
21 Ehlers G. Klinische und histologische Untersuchungen zur frage arzneimittel-bedingter Arsen-Tumoren. *Z Haut Geschlechts-Krankheiten* 1968; **43**: 763–74.
22 Seiji M, Mizuno F. Electron microscopic study of Bowen's disease. *Arch Dermatol* 1969; **99**: 3–16.
23 Yeh S, Chen HC, How SW *et al*. Fine structure of Bowen's disease in chronic arsenicalism. *J Natl Cancer Inst* 1975; **53**: 31–3.
24 Cox NH, Eedy DJ, Morton CA. Guidelines for management of Bowen's disease. British Association of Dermatologists. *Br J Dermatol* 2007; **156**: 11–21.
25 Holt PJ. Cryotherapy for skin cancer: results over a 5-year period using liquid nitrogen spray cryosurgery. *Br J Dermatol* 1988; **119**: 231–40.
26 Cox NH, Dyson P. Wound healing on the lower leg after radiotherapy or cryotherapy of Bowen's disease and other malignant skin lesions. *Br J Dermatol* 1995; **133**: 60–5.
27 Morton CA, Whitehurst C, Moseley H *et al*. Comparison of photodynamic therapy with cryotherapy in the treatment of Bowen's disease. *Br J Dermatol* 1996; **135**: 766–71.
28 Morton CA, Whitehurst C, McColl JH *et al*. Photodynamic therapy for large or multiple patches of Bowen disease and basal cell carcinoma. *Arch Dermatol* 2001; **137**: 319–24.
29 Morton CA, Horn M, Leman J *et al*. Comparison of topical methyl aminolevulinate photodynamic therapy with cryotherapy or fluorouracil for treatment of squamous cell carcinoma in situ: results of a multicenter randomized trial. *Arch Dermatol* 2006; **142**: 729–35.
30 Patel GK, Goodwin R, Chawla M *et al*. Imiquimod 5% cream monotherapy for cutaneous squamous cell carcinoma in situ (Bowen's disease): a randomised, double-blind, placebo-controlled trial. *J Am Acad Dermatol* 2006; **54**: 1025–32.

Arsenical keratosis

Definition. A corn-like, punctate keratosis caused by arsenic, characteristically affecting the palms and soles, which may progress to SCC.

Incidence. A considerable proportion of any population exposed to chronic arsenic intoxication develops keratoses, the frequency increasing with the degree of intoxication and its duration [1]. There is great individual variation in tolerance, and it is not possible, on present data, to construct a precise dose–response curve. The problem is greatest in parts of Bangladesh, West Bengal and Taiwan resulting from well water contamination [2].

Clinical features. The keratoses usually begin on the palms or soles as small areas of hyperkeratosis resembling corns. These enlarge, thicken and increase in number. The fingers, backs of the hands and more proximal parts of the extremities may be involved. Induration, inflammation and ulceration occur when the lesion becomes malignant. There may be areas of Bowen's disease in other sites and multiple BCCs, mainly of the trunk, may occur in association.

Pathology. A range of changes may be seen from a benign-looking hyperplasia or dysplasia, through mild or moderate atypia, to frank Bowen's disease [3–5]. There is no microscopic feature that allows a positive diagnosis of arsenic as the cause. In most lesions there is no elastotic degeneration of the upper dermis.

Diagnosis. The palmar lesions have to be differentiated from the various types of punctate keratosis, such as disseminated punctate keratoderma (see Chapter 19), which usually appears in early life, and Darier's disease and lichen planus, which usually have characteristic lesions elsewhere. Plantar warts differ in being papillomatous.

Treatment. The multiplicity of the keratoses makes treatment difficult. Where it is necessary, the use of a keratolytic ointment and trimming down of the surface is helpful. Two recent case reports suggest that oral acetretin may be beneficial [6]. All affected patients should be examined periodically for evidence of malignant change and for signs of visceral malignancy.

References
1 Montgomery H, Waisman M. Epithelioma attributable to arsenic. *J Invest Dermatol* 1941; **4**: 365–83.
2 Rahman MM, Chowdury UK, Mukherjee SC *et al.* Chronic arsenic toxicity in Bangladesh and West Bengal: a review and commentary. *J Toxicol Clin Toxicol* 2001; **39**: 683–700.
3 Hundeiker M, Petres J. Morphogenese und formenreichtum der arseninduzierten Präkanzerosen. *Arch Klin Exp Dermatol* 1968; **231**: 355–65.
4 Yeh S, How SW, Lin CS. Arsenical cancer of skin: histologic study with special reference to Bowen's disease. *Cancer* 1968; **21**: 312–39.
5 Centeno JA, Mullick FG, Martinez L *et al.* Pathology related to chronic arsenic exposure. *Environ Health Perspect* 2002; **110** (Suppl. 5): 883–6.
6 Yerebakan O, Ermis O, Yilmaz E, Basaran E. Treatment of arsenical keratoses and Bowen's disease with acetretin. *Int J Dermatol* 2002; **41**: 84–7.

Disseminated superficial 'actinic' porokeratosis

This disorder was first recognized in Texas [1,2], and is common in Australia [3]. It appears on sun-exposed areas of white-skinned individuals, becomes more prominent in summer and may improve in winter. New lesions have been provoked by exposure to a UV sun lamp [4]. The tendency to develop these lesions is inherited as an autosomal dominant [4]. The preponderance of females in reported cases has been attributed to their greater tendency to seek help for skin problems. The average age at which Texan patients first notice it is about 40 years, and its frequency in members of affected families increases with age. There are UK

patients with multiple lesions who have never lived abroad, and the true role of the sun in the aetiology of the condition has been questioned, as has its degree of premalignant potential [5,6]. Genetic studies have mapped a gene, *DSAP1*, for this condition to chromosome 12q23.2–24.1 and a Chinese family with disseminated superficial 'actinic' porokeratosis (DSAP) has recently been reported with a second affected locus, *DSAP2*, on chromosome 15q25.1–26.1 [7].

Clinical features [2]. The lesion begins as a 1–3 mm conical papule, brownish red or brown in colour, and usually around a follicle containing a keratotic plug. It expands and a sharp, slightly raised, keratotic ring, a fraction of a millimetre thick, develops and spreads out to a diameter of 10 mm or more. The skin within the ring is somewhat atrophic and mildly reddened or hyperpigmented, but a hypopigmented ring may be seen just inside the ridge. The ridge itself is sometimes darkly pigmented. The central thickening usually disappears, but it may persist with an attached scale, follicular plug or central dell. Sweating is absent within the lesions. Sun exposure may cause them to itch. In sunny areas, lesions may be present in very large numbers and may change from a circular to a polycyclic outline. In less sunny climates, such as the UK, patients have fewer lesions, which tend to remain circular (Fig. 52.14). In a few cases, the centre of the area has become considerably inflamed and covered by thick hyperkeratosis, or has even ulcerated and crusted. The disorder affects areas exposed to sunlight, appearing mainly on the distal extremities and arising more frequently on the lower legs in women than men. The malar regions and the cheeks may be affected. It has not been seen on areas habitually covered by clothes, or on the palms or soles.

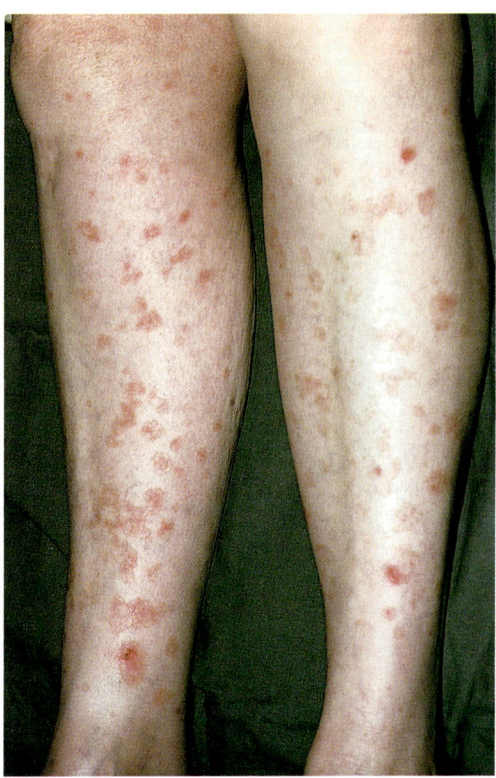

Fig. 52.14 Disseminated superficial actinic porokeratosis on the lower legs.

Pathology [8]. There is no microscopic feature that separates this disorder from porokeratosis of Mibelli (see Chapter 19), and both have been explained as the result of localized clones of abnormal epidermal cells [8], an idea supported by the successful autotransplantation of the disseminated superficial variety [4].

The distinctive pathological feature of porokeratosis is the cornoid lamella at the margin. This is a narrow column of altered or parakeratotic keratin, seated in a slight depression in the epidermis and directed obliquely inwards in some cases. It may involve the ostia of follicles and sweat ducts. The granular layer of the indented epidermis is usually missing and there may be dyskeratotic cells. The epidermis enclosed by the ridge is usually thinned, the interpapillary ridges and dermal papillae may be flattened, and the basal cells may show liquefaction degeneration. In addition to solar elastosis, decrease in collagen and telangiectasia, the upper dermis may have a non-specific inflammatory infiltrate with vascular proliferation, oedema and fibrosis. Malignant change has not been recorded.

Diagnosis. Porokeratosis is distinguished from other dermatoses by its sharp margin and history of outward expansion. The rim of DSAP is very much smaller than in Mibelli's porokeratosis and never contains a cleft. The onset of Mibelli's porokeratosis is often in childhood, and the lesions are usually solitary or few in number and do not necessarily affect exposed parts. Where the central keratosis and inflammation are prominent, the disseminated superficial variety may be mistaken for solar keratosis if the marginal ridge is not noticed.

Treatment. Lesions respond satisfactorily to cryotherapy with liquid nitrogen, but new lesions tend to develop [2,3].

References
1 Chernosky ME, Anderson DE. Disseminated superficial actinic porokeratosis: genetic aspects. *Arch Dermatol* 1969; **99**: 408–12.
2 Chernosky ME, Freeman RG. Disseminated superficial actinic porokeratosis (DSAP). *Arch Dermatol* 1967; **96**: 611–24.
3 Donald GF, Hunter GA. Disseminated superficial actinic porokeratosis: a report of eight cases. *Aust J Dermatol* 1968; **9**: 335–44.
4 Chernosky ME, Anderson DE. Disseminated superficial actinic porokeratosis. *Arch Dermatol* 1969; **99**: 401–7.
5 Goerttler EA, Jung EG. Porokeratosis Mibelli and skin carcinoma: a critical review. *Humangenetik* 1975; **26**: 291–6.
6 Shumack SP, Commens CA. Disseminated superficial actinic porokeratosis: a clinical study. *J Am Acad Dermatol* 1989; **20**: 1015–8.
7 Xia K, Deng H, Xia HJ *et al.* A novel locus for disseminated superficial actinic porokeratosis maps to chromosome 15q25.1–26.1. *Br J Dermatol* 2002; **147**: 650–4.
8 Reed RJ, Leone P. Porokeratosis: a mutant clonal keratosis of the epidermis. *Arch Dermatol* 1970; **101**: 340–3.

Cutaneous horn [1]

This is a clinical diagnosis. Horny plugs or outgrowths may be caused by various epidermal changes, such as epidermal naevus, virus wart, molluscum contagiosum, keratoacanthoma, seborrhoeic keratosis, or marsupialized trichilemmal or epidermoid cyst (Fig. 52.15). In most of these cases, the primary diagnosis is suggested by the appearance and clinical course and, in most, the horn has a friable quality.

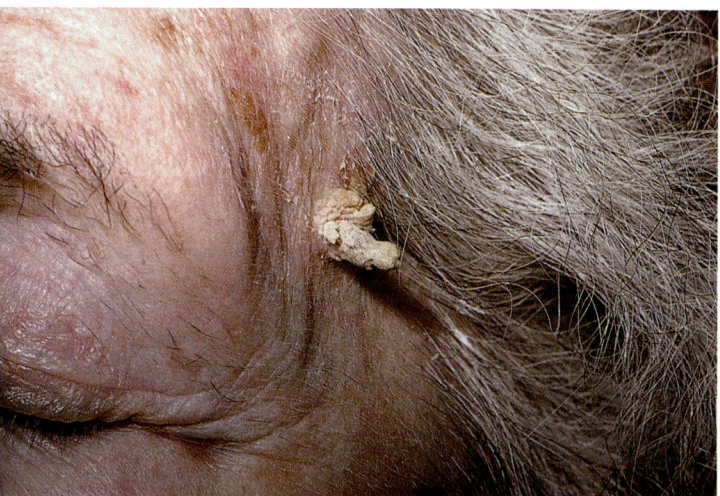

Fig. 52.15 Typical cutaneous horn. Underlying this lesion, a carcinoma *in situ* was identified after biopsy.

Clinical features. Clinical examination shows a hard, yellowish brown horn, often curved and having circumferential ridges, which is surrounded either by normal-looking epidermis or by an acanthotic collarette. Recurrent injury may cause the base to be inflamed; a combination of inflammation and induration beneath the horn is suggestive of malignant transformation. The lesions are most common on the exposed areas—particularly the upper part of the face and the ears. They are commonly single, but may be multiple; it is usual to find some more typical solar keratosis or other evidence of solar damage. Nodular AKs, which are largely confined to the dorsum of the hand and forearm and in which the histology may show an almost pseudoepitheliomatous picture, occupy a position midway between cutaneous horns and the more usual flat AKs.

Pathology. The gradual continuing development from relatively normal-looking skin to a hard keratotic protrusion resembling an animal horn in miniature is the result of dysplastic epidermal changes similar to those in a solar keratosis. Histologically, there is usually no atypicality or loss of polarity of the epidermal cells, but the granular layer is deficient or absent. In long-established lesions there may be budding from the basal layer, indicating early development of an SCC.

Reference
1 Bondeson J. Everard Home, John Hunter and cutaneous horns: a historical review. *Am J Dermatopathol* 2001; **23**: 362–9.

Erythroplasia of Queyrat [1–3]

This condition is described with the genital disorders (see Chapter 71). The histological appearance and natural history suggest that the lesion is Bowen's disease of the mucosa of the penis. However, its prevalence only in the uncircumcised indicates a different and locally acting cause.

References
1 Queyrat L. Erythroplasie du gland. *Bull Fr Soc Dermatol Syph* 1911; **22**: 378–82.
2 Goette DK. Erythroplasia of Queyrat. *Arch Dermatol* 1974; **110**: 271–3.

3 Porter WM, Hawkins D, Dineen M, Bunker CB. Penile intraepithelial neoplasis: clinical spectrum and treatment of 35 cases. *Br J Dermatol* 2002; **147**: 1159–65.

Bowenoid papulosis of the genitalia [1]

This entity is fully discussed in Chapter 71. Bowenoid papulosis (BP) is characterized clinically by lesions with a benign appearance which show histological features suggestive of squamous cell neoplasia. Most of the lesions either regress spontaneously over time or undergo resolution after local treatment. BP is now generally viewed as a localized form of *in situ* SCC which develops as a consequence of infection by high-risk human papillomavirus, especially HPV 16 and HPV 18 (reviewed in [2]). In the older literature, cases which would today be classified as BP have been reported as Bowen's disease [3–5]. Treatment of BP traditionally has included locally destructive therapies such as excisional surgery, electrocoagulation, cryotherapy and 5-fluorouracil. A number of groups have recently reported successful clearance of Bowenoid papulosis using imiquimod cream 5% [6,7].

References

1 Wade TR, Kopf AW, Ackerman AB. Bowenoid papulosis of the genitalia. *Arch Dermatol* 1979; **115**: 306–8.
2 Liu H, Urabe K, Moroi Y *et al.* Expression of p16 and hTERT protein is associated with the presence of high-risk human papillomavirus in Bowenoid papulosis. *J Cutan Pathol* 2006; **33**: 551–8.
3 Emmerson RW. Multicentric pigmented Bowen's disease of the perineum. *Proc R Soc Med* 1975; **68**: 345–6.
4 Lloyd KM. Multicentric pigmented Bowen's disease of the groin. *Arch Dermatol* 1970; **101**: 48–51.
5 Berger BW, Hori Y. Multicentric Bowen's disease of the genitalia. *Arch Dermatol* 1978; **114**: 1698–9.
6 Goorney BP, Polori R. A case of Bowenoid papulosis of the penis successfully treated with topical imiquimod cream 5%. *Int J STD AIDS* 2004; **15**: 833–5.
7 Richter ON, Petrow W, Wardelmann E *et al.* Bowenoid papulosis of the vulva—immunotherapeutical approach with topical imiquimod. *Arch Gynecol Obstet* 2003; **268**: 333–6.

Intraepidermal carcinoma of the eyelid margin

This condition (see Chapter 67), which may resemble a banal warty lesion in its early stages, represented about 6% of all eyelid malignancies in one series [1]. Occupational exposure to oils and grease may be important. The dysplastic changes seen on biopsy may not be sufficiently severe to warn of the dangers of inadequate treatment. One clue is the way the intraepidermal carcinoma invades the deepest ciliary adnexae, causing loss of eyelashes and nodularity of the margin on clinical examination. SCC may supervene and complete excision is essential.

Reference

1 McCallum DI, Kinmont PDC, Williams DW *et al.* Intra-epidermal carcinoma of the eyelid margin. *Br J Dermatol* 1975; **93**: 239–52.

Leukokeratosis of the lips

Synonym
• Actinic cheilitis [1]

Actinic cheilitis is a pathologic condition which affects predominately the lower lip and is caused by chronic and excessive exposure of the lips to solar radiation. This disorder is described in more detail in Chapter 69. Patients are frequently male outdoor workers who usually give a history of recurrent sunburn of the lips. The lower lip often shows persistent dry scaling, a tendency to fissure and atrophic changes beneath and around the keratosis. The use of lipstick by women may be protective [2], especially in preventing dehydration. Actinic cheilitis is relatively common in renal transplant recipients [3]. A number of studies suggest that progression to SCC may be more common than previously recognized. In one series, 11 of 65 cases progressed to SCC [4]. Careful follow-up is important as it is also recognized that SCC of the lip metastasize four times as frequently as cutaneous ones [5].

Treatment. A number of treatments have been described including surgical excision, cryotherapy, carbon dioxide laser ablation, electrosurgery and the topical use of 5-fluorouracil. Successful treatment has also been described with newer modalities including PDT [6].

References

1 Kaugars GE, Pillion T, Svirsky JA *et al.* Actinic cheilitis: a review of 152 cases. *Oral Med Oral Surg Oral Pathol* 1999; **88**: 181–6.
2 Wynder EL, Bross IJ. Aetiological factors in mouth cancer. *BMJ* 1957; **i**: 1137–43.
3 King GN, Healy CM, Glover MT *et al.* Increased prevalence of dysplastic and malignant lip lesions in renal-transplant recipients. *N Engl J Med* 1995; **332**: 1052–7.
4 Markopoulos A, Banidou-Farmaki E, Kayavis I. Actinic cheilitis: clinical and pathologic characteristics in 65 cases. *Oral Dis* 2004; **10**: 212–6.
5 Stender IM, Wulf HC. Photodynamic therapy with 5-aminolevulinic acid in the treatment of actinic cheilitis. *Br J Dermatol* 1996; **135**: 454–6.
6 Berking C, Herzinger T, Flaig MJ *et al.* The efficacy of photodynamic therapy in actinic cheilitis of the lower lip: a prospective study of 15 patients. *Dermatol Surg* 2007; **33**: 825–30.

Post-ionizing radiation keratoses

These may occur in an area of scarring following radiotherapy or excessive fluoroscopy where there is obvious dermal damage. They may also be seen in radiologists, surgeons, dentists and others who have exposed their skin to frequent small doses of X-rays and where the dermis is less grossly changed, although such cases are now rare. The epidermal changes are similar to solar keratosis. Histologically, the dermis shows a much more extensive replacement of collagen by scar and elastotic material, obliterative changes in the vessels and, at times, the presence of abnormally large and irregular fibroblasts (Fig. 52.16).

Tar keratoses [1–4]

These are now very rare entities. In the past, they were seen in workers with tar and pitch. There were small keratotic plaques, not unlike plane warts, or flat seborrhoeic keratoses on the face and hands, which have the microscopic features of benign acanthomas. These usually disappeared when the exposure ceased. There were also lesions resembling solar keratoses, which persisted and a few became malignant. Other lesions with the appearance of keratoacanthomas were seen. Their course was usually more prolonged and, particularly on the scrotum, a relatively high proportion became malignant.

References

1 Fisher REW. *Proceedings of the 13th International Congress on Occupational Health.* 1961: 250.

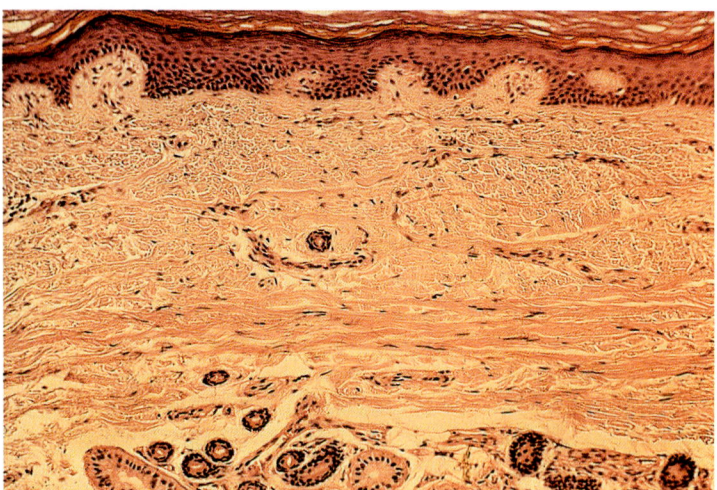

Fig. 52.16 Pathological appearance of radiodermatitis showing a scarred dermis with loss of skin appendages.

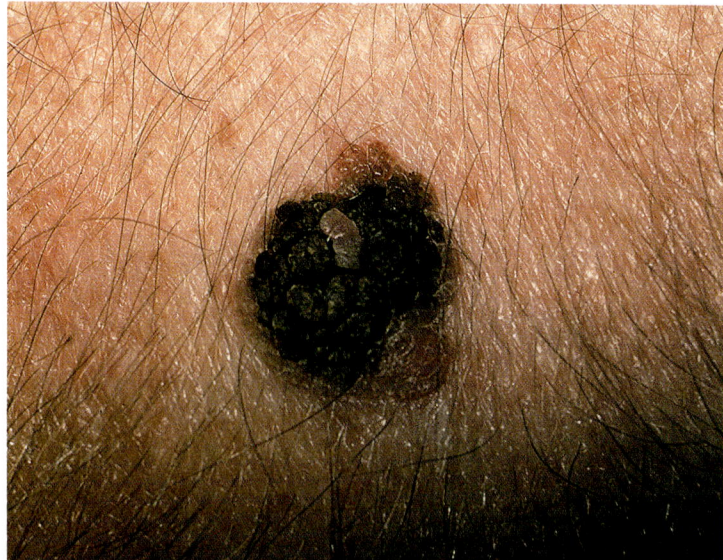

Fig. 52.17 Seborrhoeic keratosis showing dull, non-reflective, hyperkeratotic surface. This contrasts with melanocytic lesions.

2 Fisher REW. *Trans Assoc Ind Med Off* 1965; **15**: 122.
3 Colomb D, Descos L, Gauthier D. Kérato-acanthomes multiples et maladie du brai de houille. *Rev Lyonnaise Med* 1966; **15**: 449–62.
4 Letzel S, Drexler H. Occupationally related tumors in tar refinery workers. *J Am Acad Dermatol* 1998; **39**: 712–20.

Benign epidermal tumours

Seborrhoeic keratosis

Synonyms
- Seborrhoeic wart
- Senile wart
- Basal cell papilloma

Definition. A benign tumour, frequently pigmented, more common in the elderly and composed of epidermal keratinocytes.

Aetiology and incidence. Seborrhoeic keratoses (SKs) are common skin lesions that occur with increasing age; usually appear in the fifth decade in a temperate climate but may develop earlier in tropical regions. There is little tendency to spontaneous disappearance and new lesions may continue to appear for many years. Males and females are equally affected.

Although extremely common, the epidemiology is not well characterized in most populations. In studies from Australia these lesions were identified in 30% of subjects under the age of 30 years increasing to 100% of subjects older than 50 years [1]. The overall prevalence in a UK population was slightly lower with lesions identified in approximately 75% of subjects over the age of 70 years [2]. The total number and size of SKs has also been shown to increase with age. Most lesions are found on the trunk with a smaller number on the limbs, head and neck; in the Australian population no correlation was found with traditional markers of skin sensitivity to ultraviolet radiation. The rapid development of large numbers of SKs can occur in patients with an inflammatory dermatosis [3] or in association with underlying malignancies where it is known as the sign of Leser–Trélat [4]. The neoplasms most commonly associated with this skin manifestation include stomach and colon cancer and in some patients it may be associated with the development of acanthosis nigricans. It has been recognized for some time that although SK and epidermal naevi have different natural histories they share some clinical and histological characteristics, including acanthosis, papillomatosis, and variable degrees of hyperkeratosis and hyperpigmentation. These similarities and the identification of mutations in the fibroblast growth factor 3 receptor in epidermal naevi [5] triggered analysis of SKs for *FGFR3* mutations. Mutations were identified in 39% of SKs and the genetic changes identified were identical to those found in patients with a rare dwarfing chondrodysplasia and thanatophoric dysplasia, which are both also associated with acanthosis nigricans [6]. More recently, additional molecular insights into SK aetiology have emerged with the identification of activating *PIK3CA* mutations in 16% of SKs examined [7].

Clinical features. Seborrhoeic keratoses occur on any body site. They are usually asymptomatic but may be itchy. They are most frequent on the face and the upper trunk. The first evidence is slight hyperpigmentation. On the hand and face, seborrhoeic keratoses may remain superficial for a long period, and can be mistaken for melanocytic lesions. It may be difficult to distinguish superficial seborrhoeic keratoses from lentigo maligna and pigmented AK. More florid examples may be pedunculated or acanthotic, smooth-surfaced, domed and heavily pigmented, but in contrast to melanocytic naevi do not reflect light and usually have plugged follicular orifices on the surface, giving an almost cerebriform appearance. Most seborrhoeic keratoses have fewer hairs than the skin they arise from. The most common appearance is that of a very superficial verrucous plaque which appears to be stuck on the epidermis, varying from dirty yellow to black in colour and having loosely adherent, greasy keratin on the surface (Fig. 52.17). The shape is round or oval and multiple lesions may

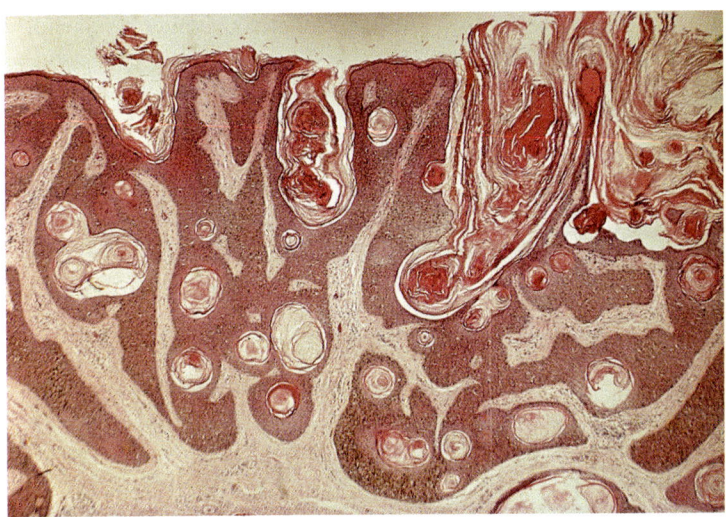

Fig. 52.18 Histology of classic seborrhoeic keratosis showing hyperkeratotic surface and numerous horn cysts.

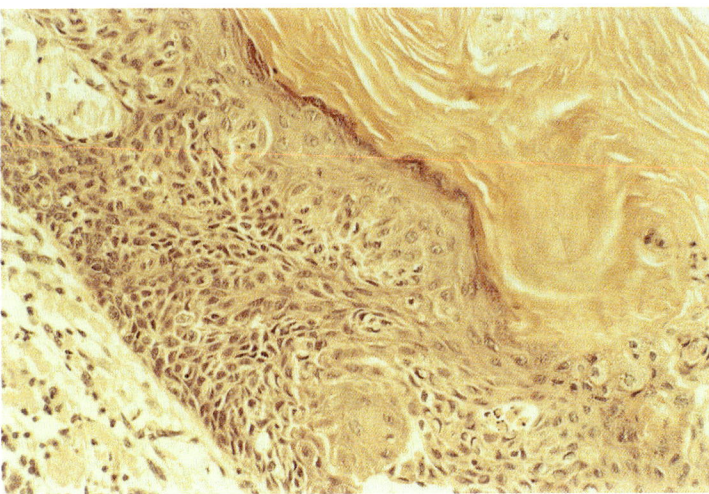

Fig. 52.19 Histology of irritated seborrhoeic keratosis. The squamous eddies are clearly seen in this illustration.

be aligned in the direction of the skin folds. The size varies from 1 mm to several centimetres. The smallest lesions occur around follicular orifices, particularly on the trunk. On the eyelids and major flexures, SKs may be pedunculated and less keratotic. Irritation or infection causes swelling, sometimes bleeding, oozing and crusting, and a deepening of the colour because of inflammation.

Pathology [8]. The essential change is an accumulation of normal keratinocytes between the basal layer and the keratinizing surface of the epidermis. Melanocytes may proliferate among these immature keratinocytes and transfer melanin to them. The dermal papillae may be elongated. Focal keratinization may occur within the mass of immature cells to produce horn cysts, which enlarge, may coalesce and can be carried to the surface by the tide of epidermal cells. If the formation and discharge of horn cysts is excessive, a verrucous surface will be formed. Marked papillomatosis will also cause an irregular 'church steeple' outer border which retains keratin. If, in contrast, the main mass of the lesion is composed of immature cells, the surface will be smooth and rounded, and the melanocyte population and degree of pigmentation will vary, so that the lesions may be deeply pigmented. The parenchymal cells are rather small and polygonal, possessing tonofibrils and intercellular bridges, and they are arranged in an orderly fashion.

The most common pathological type is the solid variant, in which a mass of immature keratinocytes is seen mainly above the level of the surrounding epidermis (Fig. 52.18). Occasional cystic areas containing fragments of stratum corneum are seen at these sites. A rarer variant is the hyperkeratotic variety, which may be clinically mistaken for an AK. The reticular form is a third variant, composed of strands of keratinocytes; this type is frequently seen as a flat lesion on the face.

If an SK becomes irritated, or develops a pattern of apparently inverted growth, frequently in association with a hair follicle opening, the pathological differential diagnosis may include an early invasive SCC. An irritated SK shows focal areas of whorls

of keratinocytes in so-called squamous eddies, but mitotic figures are rare, and the base of the lesion shows a clear separation from dermal tissue, with no single-cell invasion (Fig. 52.19).

Diagnosis. The superficial type of SK has to be distinguished from simple and malignant lentigo (see Chapter 54) and from AK, especially on the face. The patterned fine fissures on the surface may be helpful. The pigmented domed variety may closely resemble a melanocytic naevus, but the surface is less lustrous and the follicular orifices are plugged. An inflamed keratosis may be confused with a malignant melanoma. If the lesion is treated with a topical antibiotic and occluded for 3–5 days the diagnosis may become obvious, but if clinical doubt persists an excision biopsy and pathological examination is indicated. Pigmented BCCs may also have to be considered in the differential diagnosis. They are usually rather irregular with a rolled edge, a thin shiny epidermis with telangiectases and a depressed or ulcerated centre.

Treatment. Removal with a small sharp curette leaves a flat surface that becomes covered by normal epidermis in a week. Cautery or diathermy should be used as little as possible to avoid scarring. Satisfactory results can be obtained by freezing briefly, a technique especially suitable for large superficial lesions, or by carefully painting the surface with pure trichloracetic acid and repeating if the full thickness is not removed on the first occasion. Seborrhoeic keratoses tend to recur, and it is often wise to encourage patients to accept them rather than to keep returning for further treatment.

Melanoacanthoma

This term has been used for a very rare lesion, originally described by Bloch as 'non-naevoid melanoepithelioma, type 1', and has been considered to be a benign neoplasm composed of epidermal keratinocytes and large dendritic melanocytes [9]. The current general view is that this is not a discrete entity. Some deeply pigmented acanthotic seborrhoeic keratoses contain, dispersed among the parenchymal cells, numerous dendritic melanocytes, which are demonstrable by the dopa technique [10]. Normally, they transfer melanin to the surrounding immature keratinocytes. However, if irritation or inflammation caused the parenchymal cells to become more mature, the transfer of melanin would be impeded and pigment might be retained in the melanocytes, producing a microscopic appearance similar to that described as melanoacanthoma.

Stucco keratosis [11,12]

This title has been given to small, rough, whitish, keratotic plaques that are easily lifted off the skin with a fingernail and come away without causing bleeding. They are situated principally on the extremities, especially the ankle region, and occur in middle-aged or elderly persons. They have the same stuck-on appearance of SKs and a similar microscopic architecture. Basaloid cells and horn cysts are not seen and the histology is more that of a regular spiky papillomatosis, with loose lamellated hyperkeratosis capping the epidermis. If treatment is called for, curettage or cryotherapy are effective.

References

1 Yeatman JM, Kilkenny M, Marks R. The prevalence of seborrhoeic keratoses in an Australian population: does exposure to sunlight play a part in their frequency? *Br J Dermatol* 1997; **137**: 411–4.
2 Memon AA, Tomenson JA, Bothwell J *et al*. Prevalence of solar damage and actinic keratosis in a Merseyside population. *Br J Dermatol* 2000; **142**: 1154–9.
3 Williams MG. Acanthomata appearing after eczema. *Br J Dermatol* 1956; **68**: 268–71.
4 Dantzig PI. Sign of Leser-Trélat. *Arch Dermatol* 1973; **108**: 700–1.
5 Hafner C, van Oers JM, Vogt T *et al*. Mosaicism of activating FGFR3 mutations in human skin causes epidermal nevi. *J Clin Invest* 2006; **116**: 2201–7.
6 Logie A, Dunois-Larde C, Rosty C *et al*. Activating mutations of the tyrosine kinase receptor FGFR3 are associated with benign skin tumors in mice and humans. *Hum Mol Genet* 2005; **14**: 1153–60.
7 Hafner C, Lopez-Knowles E, Luis NM *et al*. Oncogenic PIK3CA mutations occur in epidermal nevi and seborrheic keratoses with a characteristic mutation pattern. *Proc Natl Acad Sci USA* 2007; **104**: 13450–4.
8 Sanderson KV. The structure of seborrhoeic keratoses. *Br J Dermatol* 1968; **80**: 588–93.
9 Mishima Y, Pinkus H. Benign mixed tumor of melanocytes and malpighian cells. *AMA Arch Dermatol* 1960; **81**: 539–50.
10 Molokhia MM, Portnoy B. A study of dendritic cells in seborrhoeic warts. *Br J Dermatol* 1971; **85**: 254–8.
11 Willoughby C, Soter NA. Stucco keratosis. *Arch Dermatol* 1972; **105**: 859–61.
12 Kocsard E, Carter JJ. The papillomatous keratoses: the nature and differential diagnosis of stucco keratosis. *Australas J Dermatol* 1971; **12**: 80–8.

Dermatosis papulosa nigra

Definition. A pigmented papular eruption of the face and neck caused by a naevoid developmental defect of the pilosebaceous follicles, with histology resembling seborrhoeic keratoses. The condition is most common in black races.

Aetiology [1]. This lesion is probably genetically determined. The incidence in black people rises from about 5% in the first decade to over 40% by the third, and is rather higher in females than males.

Clinical features [1–3]. The individual lesions are black or dark brown, flattened or cupuliform papules 1–5 mm in diameter. They are rare under the age of 7 years, after which they increase steadily in frequency, number and size. They are most numerous in the malar regions and on the forehead. They are rare on the lower parts of the face and the chin, but in a few individuals may be found on the neck, chest and back [2].

Pathology [1,4]. The lesions, which are naevoid developmental defects of the pilosebaceous follicles, show irregular acanthosis and hyperkeratosis, and somewhat resemble seborrhoeic keratoses.

Treatment. Treatment is seldom requested. Removal with the diathermy or cautery is effective.

References

1 Hairston MA Jr, Reed RJ, Derbes VJ. Dermatosis papulosa nigra. *Arch Dermatol* 1964; **89**: 655–8.
2 Castellani A. Observations on some diseases of Central America. *J Trop Med Hyg* 1925; **28**: 1–14.
3 Michael JC, Searle ER. Dermatosis papulosa nigra. *Arch Dermatol Syphilol* 1929; **20**: 629–40.
4 Diasio FA. Dermatosis papulosa nigra (Castellani) of unusual distribution (acanthosis papulosa nigra). *Arch Dermatol Syphilol* 1933; **27**: 751–5.

Skin tags

> **Synonyms**
> • Soft warts
> • Achrochordon

Definition. A common, benign lesion composed of loose fibrous tissue and occurring mainly on the neck and major flexures as a small, soft, pedunculated protrusion.

Incidence and aetiology. These lesions are very common, particularly in women at the menopause or later. They are frequently found together with seborrhoeic keratoses.

Clinical features. The lesions are pedunculated and may have a long stalk. They vary in size and are about 2 mm in diameter on average. They are round, soft and inelastic. The colour may be unchanged, but they are frequently hyperpigmented. The most common site is on the sides of the neck, where they may be mixed with typical small, sessile, seborrhoeic keratoses. When more profuse, they can extend on to the face or down to the back and chest. Similar lesions may be found in and around the axillae and groins.

Pathology. The protruding mass is connected to the skin by a narrow pedicle. The bulk of the lesion is loose fibrous tissue, similar to that of the papillary dermis. The epidermis is thin, and the basal cell layer is flat and often hyperpigmented. Melanocytic proliferation and naevus cells are not usually seen and the majority of such lesions probably come within the seborrhoeic keratosis spectrum. However, there is an overlap with melanocytic naevi and neurofibromas. Some skin tags may be the last remnants of a pre-existing melanocytic naevus.

Diagnosis. The lesions are unmistakable. They are smaller than the average pedunculated melanocytic naevus or the lesions of neurofibromatosis.

Treatment. Both cautery and cryotherapy with liquid nitrogen are effective.

Haber's syndrome

Definition. A familial condition characterized by a persistent rosacea-like eruption, associated in some cases with keratotic plaques on the trunk and limbs.

Incidence. A family in which five members were affected was originally described [1]. Another case, with 15 affected relatives, has been described from Japan [2]. The rosacea-like eruption appears in childhood, and the keratotic lesions somewhat later. The mode of inheritance seems to be a simple autosomal dominant.

Clinical features. The cheeks, nose, forehead and chin are permanently flushed. The skin surface shows a combination of erythema and telangiectasia, prominent follicles, comedones, small papules, some of which are scaly, and tiny atrophic pitted areas. There is little fluctuation in the erythema, although sunlight may aggravate it. The warty lesions occur mainly on the trunk and thighs and are static, scaly or keratotic, flat and non-indurated plaques.

Pathology. The facial eruption shows perivascular inflammation leading to fibrosis, acanthosis and parakeratosis of the epidermis, distortion of pilosebaceous complexes with dilated follicular orifices, and proliferation of immature glands and basal cell strands. The warty lesions are produced by papillomatosis, acanthosis in the interpapillary ridges and dyskeratosis with areas of pale-staining cells giving a parakeratotic stratum corneum. Mitotic figures are present, but there is no evidence of malignancy.

Treatment. The facial eruption was controlled in the young patient in the first family and in the Japanese patients by steroid creams locally. The warty lesions respond to radiotherapy. Simple destructive measures are also effective.

References
1 Sanderson KV, Wilson HTH. Haber's syndrome: familial rosacea-like eruption with intraepidermal epithelioma. *Br J Dermatol* 1965; **77**: 1–8.
2 Seiji M, Otaki N. Haber's syndrome: familial rosacea-like dermatosis with keratotic plaques and pitted scars. *Arch Dermatol* 1971; **103**: 452–5.

Clear cell acanthoma [1–3]

Synonyms
- Degos' acanthoma
- Acanthome a 'cellules claires'

Definition. A scaly plaque or nodule that has a characteristic accumulation of clear glycogen-containing cells in the epidermis.

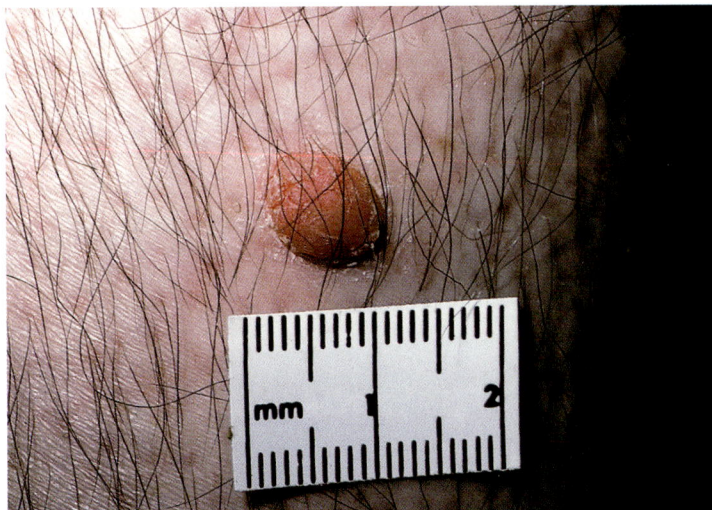

Fig. 52.20 Clear cell acanthoma.

Incidence and aetiology. Clear cell acanthoma is a relatively uncommon condition of adults. The sexes are equally affected [3]. The cause is unknown [4].

Clinical features (Fig. 52.20) [1,3,5]. The lesion is usually solitary. It is a slightly elevated to dome-shaped plaque or nodule with an abrupt margin and a wafer-like scale adherent at the periphery, which leaves a moist or bleeding surface when removed. The colour varies from pink to brown, but is most characteristically red with vascular puncta and it blanches on diascopy. It varies from 3 to 20 mm in diameter, and occurs most commonly on the lower limbs. The duration may be of many years, and there are usually no symptoms. The diagnosis can be suspected on the clinical evidence. The lesion may be mistaken for a histiocytoma, seborrhoeic keratosis or pyogenic granuloma.

Pathology [1,6,7]. The epidermis is thickened and papillomatous with sharply demarcated areas of light-coloured cells, which contrast with the normal basal cells below and Malpighian cells around them (Fig. 52.21). The cytoplasm of the clear cells contains an abundance of glycogen, which on electron microscopy is seen to displace tonofibrils [7,8]. The cells do not have the enzymes characteristic of eccrine sweat glands. There is intercellular oedema and an infiltrate often containing many polymorphonuclear leukocytes. The papillary body is oedematous and the superficial capillaries and veins are increased in number. There may be syringomatous sweat gland elements and evidence of sebaceous differentiation beneath the lesion [9].

Treatment. Excision is often needed to confirm the diagnosis [1].

References
1 Degos R, Civatte J. Clear-cell acanthoma: experience of 8 years. *Br J Dermatol* 1970; **83**: 248–54.
2 Wells GC, Wilson Jones E. Degos acanthoma (acanthoma à cellules claires): a report of five cases with particular reference to the histochemistry. *Br J Dermatol* 1967; **79**: 249–58.

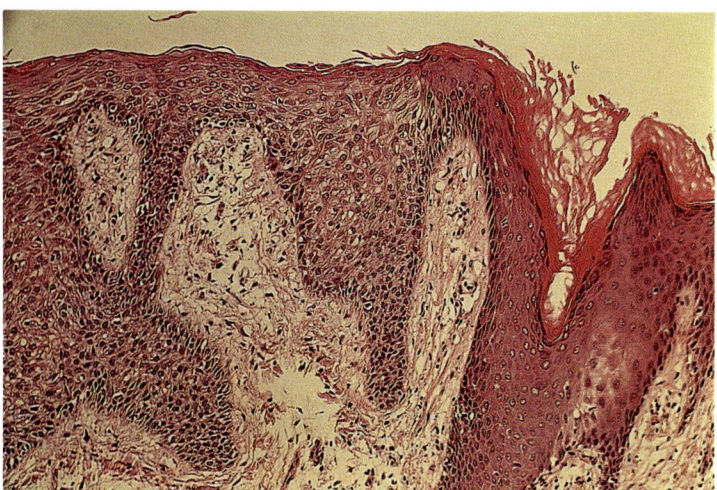

Fig. 52.21 Pathology of clear cell acanthoma of Degos, showing sharp margin between normal skin to the right and epidermis involved with the clear cells to the left.

3 Zak FG, Girerd RJ. Das blasszellige Akanthom (Degos). *Hautarzt* 1968; **19**: 559–61.

4 Duperrat B, Mascaro JM. L'acanthome a cellules unique: rapport de deux cas. *Ann Dermatol Syphiligr* 1965; **92**: 5–6.

5 Fine RM, Chernosky ME. Clinical recognition of clear-cell acanthomas (Degos'). *Arch Dermatol* 1969; **100**: 559–63.

6 Brownstein MH, Fernando S, Shapiro L. Clear cell acanthoma: clinicopathologic analysis of 37 new cases. *Am J Clin Pathol* 1973; **59**: 306–11.

7 Funan H, Sisson JK. The ultrastructure of the pale cell acanthoma. *J Invest Dermatol* 1969; **52**: 185–8.

8 Hollman KH, Civatte J. Etude au microscope électronique de l'acanthome à cellules claires. *Ann Dermatol Syphiligr* 1968; **95**: 139–46.

9 Cramer HJ. Klarzellenakanthom (Degos) mit Syringomatösen und naevus-sebaceus-artigen Anteilen. *Dermatologica* 1971; **143**: 265–70.

Keratoacanthoma

> **Synonym**
> • Molluscum sebaceum

Definition. A rapidly evolving tumour of the skin, composed of keratinizing squamous cells originating in pilosebaceous follicles and resolving spontaneously if untreated.

Incidence. Keratoacanthoma is relatively common, and in white races tends to occur with about one-third of the frequency of SCC, whatever the environmental UV levels [1]. It is uncommon in dark-skinned races and in the Japanese [2]. Males are affected about three times more often than females. The adjusted age distribution shows that it is most frequent in middle-life and does not increase in incidence in old age, unlike BCC and SCC.

Aetiology. The epidemiological data suggest that the incidence of keratocanthoma is related to sun exposure, and the localization of the tumours mainly on the head and upper limb supports this. Contact with tar and mineral oil has also been shown to cause an increased incidence [3,4] and very similar lesions have been produced in animals by painting with carcinogenic hydrocarbons. In some cases, the lesion follows injury to the skin, which suggests that infection may play a part in its origin, a view supported by the occurrence of multiple keratoacanthomas in skin grafts of patients with the tumour in the recipient site [5], the donor site [6] or both [7]. Proof of a viral cause is lacking. Cases are reported of keratoacanthoma associated with carcinoma of the larynx [8], multiple internal malignancy [9], leukaemia [10], deficient cell-mediated immunity [11] and in transplant recipients [12]. Most recently, the solid tumour multikinase inhibitor Sorafenib has been reported to lead to the development of keratoacanthomas, which resolved or stopped developing when therapy was stopped; this may give us a new insight into the aetiology of the condition [13,14].

Clinical features [1,15,16]. The first evidence of keratoacanthoma is a firm, rounded, flesh-coloured or reddish papule, which may resemble molluscum contagiosum or, if keratotic, a virus wart. The patient rarely seeks advice at this stage. There is then a rapid growth phase and in a few weeks it may become 10–20 mm across. There is no infiltration at the base. The epidermis over the nodule is smooth and shiny; the lesion is skin-coloured to red with telangiectases just beneath the surface. The centre contains a horny plug or is covered by a crust which conceals a keratin-filled crater (Fig. 52.22). As the lesion matures, the accumulating keratin expands the outermost part making the edge overhang the base somewhat, but the radial symmetry is usually well preserved. The keratin may project like a horn or it may soften and break down. Spontaneous resolution is achieved by the epidermal covering receding towards the base and the horny core being shed. The base is revealed as irregular and puckered and the edge may remain as soft but thickened epidermis, either as a continuous rim or a series of tags. The process of spontaneous healing usually takes about 3 months.

A small proportion of keratoacanthomas grow to much larger dimensions—5 cm or more in diameter being not exceptional on the forearm. One lesion on the chest was more than 15 cm in diameter [17]. In some cases, the maximum size may be reached in a month or two; others may enlarge over many months. After growth ceases, involution may not occur for some months or may occur at part of the periphery while growth continues elsewhere. There may be recurrences after curettage or excision, more frequently in lesions on the lips and fingers and when treatment is carried out in the early stages [18]. Recurrence may happen after spontaneous resolution [19].

The most frequently affected area is the central part of the face, that is the nose, cheeks, eyelids and lips. The dorsum of the hand, wrist and forearm are commonly affected; the thigh, chest, shoulder and scalp less so; and the anogenital area uncommonly except in those exposed to occupational hazards. Lesions have occurred subungually [20,21], in the vermilion of the lips [18] and on the buccal mucosa.

In most cases, the tumour presents as a solitary lesion. Multiple or recurrent tumours are more likely to be present in several circumstances. Recurrent lesions occur in patients who have been exposed to pitch or tar [3] and in rare cases as a familial disorder, although there are reasons to keep this Ferguson-Smith type as a separate entity. There are a few cases of eruptive keratoacanthoma recorded. Multiple lesions have occurred with defective cell-

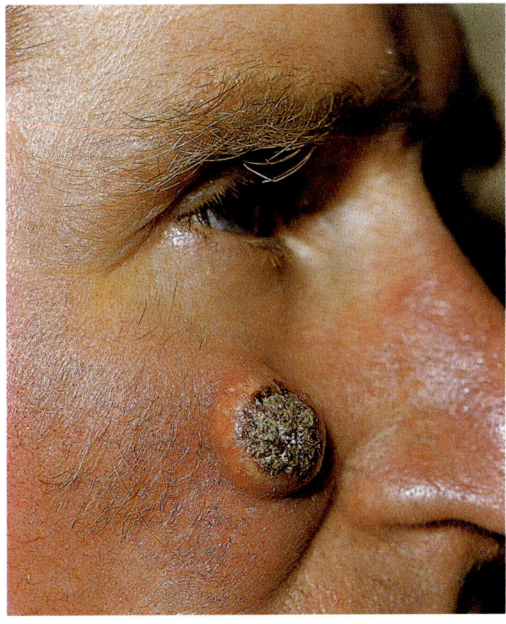
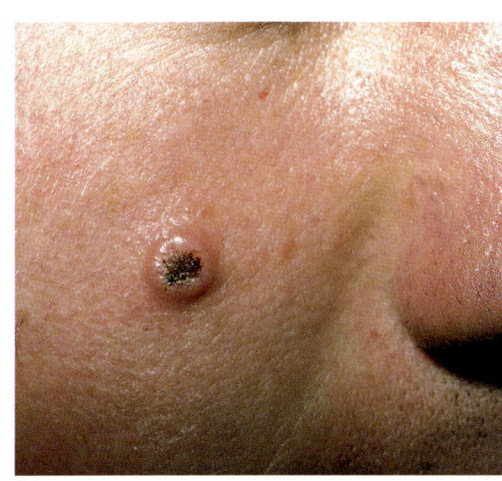

Fig. 52.22 Typical keratoacanthomas, on the face, showing raised margin and central keratin-filled crater.

(a)   (b)

mediated immunity and also as part of Torre's syndrome, with multiple internal malignancies [9] and with sebaceous adenomas (see Chapter 53).

Pathology. The distinctive features are best seen when the fixed specimen is being cut before processing or in sections under low magnification. The tumour has a symmetrical, more-or-less globular form and is situated in the dermis, usually extending down no deeper than the sweat glands, although deep penetration has occasionally been recorded. The epidermis around the tumour is normal or slightly acanthotic, but becomes thinned as it rises over the tumour. A narrow spur of connective tissue separates the epidermis from the proliferating squamous cells, except where the two connect at the mouth of the keratin-filled crypt. Serial sections of an early lesion have shown connection of the masses of squamous cells with the upper part of a hyperplastic follicle [22].

The histological features vary with the stage of evolution. The early lesion is composed of a mass of rapidly multiplying squamous cells. These are large and rather pale with vesicular nuclei, prominent nucleoli and frequent mitoses. Hyperchromatic cells, atypical mitotic figures, individual cell keratinization and other evidence of loss of polarity may be found. The marginal cells invade the surrounding dermis aggressively, while those more centrally placed keratinize to form a branched core of keratin that communicates with the surface. The stroma is vascular and infiltrated with round cells and histiocytes.

Resolution occurs through maturation of the hyperplastic masses. The accumulating keratin dilates the central pore, the epidermal lips recede from the centre and the lesion opens like a flower bud. When the horn is finally shed, the irregular epithelium beneath it replicates the scalloped outline of the active mass. The cells take on the morphology of epidermis, and a scar is formed, which is depressed and may have papillomatous tags at the margin, the remnants of the epidermal lip. Older lesions frequently show clusters of leukocyte microabscesses at the base. Thus, the

pathological features vary with the stage of evolution of the keratoacanthoma and, if an adequate specimen is not submitted, it may be impossible for the reporting pathologist to confidently rule out early invasive SCC. Keratoacanthomas may also rarely progress to SCC. In one case [23], it may have been precipitated by treatment with oral methotrexate for a recurrence. The conjunction of two independent lesions in sun-damaged skin may account for the finding of a BCC in the scar of keratoacanthoma in this and other cases.

Experimentally produced lesions differ in their form, depending on whether the hair follicles are in anagen or telogen when the proliferation begins [24,25]. Virus-like particles have been seen under electron microscopy [26].

Diagnosis. The most important differential diagnosis is to distinguish keratoacanthoma from SCC. In most cases, the more rapid evolution to a relatively large size, the regular crateriform shape and keratotic plug, the undamaged surrounding skin and the younger age of onset make a distinction relatively easy for the clinician. Spontaneous healing adds support to the diagnosis of keratoacanthoma. The problem is made more difficult in sunny areas where actinic damage and SCC are more common, and the most important single point is the history of rapid growth. The differential diagnosis includes cutaneous horn and hypertrophic AK, viral wart, molluscum contagiosum, pseudoepitheliomatous hyperplasia and granulomas of various types. Secondary deposits from non-cutaneous malignancies can also occasionally mimic keratoacanthoma.

Treatment. The end result of leaving the tumour to regress is usually a rather unsightly scar. Curettage and coagulation of the base, or excision and suture, produce a much more acceptable result. Excision is desirable if the diagnosis is in doubt, because curetted specimens yield poor sections. Radiotherapy shortens the course and improves the scar, and can be used in patients who refuse surgery. A total of 2000 cGy in two closely spaced doses of adequate penetration can be given.

The application of 5-fluorouracil ointment twice daily may reduce the time taken for natural resolution and diminish scarring [27]. If there is real doubt about the diagnosis, surgical removal or radiotherapy should be carried out as for SCC, and the patient followed up.

Generalized eruptive keratoacanthoma [9,28]

A small number of cases of widely disseminated lesions, some of them typical keratoacanthomas, have been reported. Both sexes have been affected. The primary lesions are flesh-coloured to red, dome-shaped follicular papules, 1–3 mm in size and affecting particularly the face (where they may be confluent), the trunk and the roots of the limbs. Itching is a prominent symptom, and ectropion and narrowing of the mouth may be produced by the keratotic facial change. Scattered among the papules are larger, more typical keratoacanthomas, which resolve spontaneously. The palms and soles are spared, but the oral and laryngeal epithelium can be involved.

Pathology. Histological examination shows the papules to consist of a dilated and plugged follicle duct with acanthotic follicular epidermis around it; the mucosal lesions are irregular acanthosis; and the nodules are keratoacanthomas, but with no inflammatory changes.

Management. The nodular lesions heal in a few months. The papules are not influenced by cytotoxic drugs, but one case responded to topical retinol [25].

References

1 Rook A, Champion RH. *Keratoacanthoma*. Monograph 10. Washington DC: National Cancer Institute, 1963: 257–73.
2 Miyaji T. *Skin Cancers in Japan: a Nationwide 5-Year Survey, 1956–60*. Monograph 10. Washington DC: National Cancer Institute, 1963: 55–70.
3 Colomb D, Descos L, Gauthier D. Kératoacanthomes multiples et maladie du brac de houille. *Rev Lyonaise Med* 1966; **15**: 449–62.
4 Ghadially FN, Barton BW, Kerridge DF. The etiology of keratoacanthoma. *Cancer* 1963; **16**: 603–11.
5 Pillsbury DM, Beerman H. Multiple keratoacanthoma. *Am J Med Sci* 1958; **236**: 614–24.
6 Wulsin JH. Keratoacanthoma: a benign cutaneous tumor arising in a skin graft. *Am Surg* 1958; **24**: 689–92.
7 Dibden FA, Fowler M. The multiple growth of molluscum sebaceum in donor and recipient sites of skin graft. *Aust NZ J Surg* 1955; **25**: 157–9.
8 Chapman RS, Finn OA. Carcinoma of the larynx in two patients with keratoacanthoma. *Br J Dermatol* 1974; **90**: 685–8.
9 Poleksic S. Keratoacanthoma and multiple carcinomas. *Br J Dermatol* 1974; **91**: 461–3.
10 Weber G, Stetter H, Pliess G. Assozilertes Vorkommen von eruptiven Keratoacanthomen, Tubercarcinom und Paramyeloblasten-leukamie. *Arch Klin Exp Dermatol* 1970; **238**: 107–19.
11 Claudy A, Thivolet J. Multiple keratoacanthomas: association with deficient cell mediated immunity. *Br J Dermatol* 1975; **93**: 593–5.
12 Bordea C, Wojnarowska F, Millard PR *et al*. Skin cancers in renal-transplant recipients occur more frequently than previously recognized in a temperate climate. *Transplantation* 2004; **77**: 574–9.
13 Smith KJ, Haley H, Hamza S, Skelton HG. Eruptive keratoacanthoma-type squamous cell carcinomas in patients taking sorafenib for the treatment of solid tumors. *Dermatol Surg* 2009, in press.
14 Kong HH, Cowen EW, Azad NS, Dahut W *et al*. Keratoacanthomas associated with sorafenib therapy. *J Am Acad Dermatol* 2007; **56**: 171–2.
15 Kingman J, Callen JP. Keratoacanthoma: a clinical study. *Arch Dermatol* 1984; **120**: 736–40.
16 Calnan CD, Haber H. Molluscum sebaceum. *J Pathol Bacteriol* 1955; **69**: 61–6.
17 Duany NP. Squamous cell pseudoepithelioma (keratoacanthoma): a new clinical variety, gigantic, multiple, and localized. *AMA Arch Dermatol* 1958; **78**: 703–9.
18 Stevanovic DV. Keratoacanthoma: mucous membranes as the site of its localization. *Dermatologica* 1960; **121**: 278–84.
19 Beare JM. Recurrent molluscum sebaceum. *Lancet* 1955; **i**: 182–3.
20 Lamp JC, Graham JH, Urbach F *et al*. Keratoacanthoma of the subungual region. *J Bone Joint Surg Am* 1964; **46**: 1721–31.
21 Shapiro L, Baraf CS. Subungal epidermoid carcinoma and keratoacanthoma. *Cancer* 1970; **25**: 141–52.
22 Kalkoff KW, Macher E. On the histogenesis of keratoacanthoma. *Hautarzt* 1961; **12**: 8–15.
23 Burge KM, Winkelmann RK. Keratoacanthoma: association with basal and squamous cell carcinoma. *Arch Dermatol* 1969; **100**: 306–11.
24 Ghadially FN. The role of the hair follicle in the origin and evolution of some cutaneous neoplasms of man and experimental animals. *Cancer* 1961; **14**: 801–16.
25 Whiteley HJ. The effect of the hair growth cycle on experimental skin carcinogenesis in the rabbit. *Br J Cancer* 1957; **11**: 196–205.
26 Zelickson AS. Virus-like particles demonstrated in keratoacanthomas by electron microscopy. *Acta Derm Venereol (Stockh)* 1962; **42**: 23–6.
27 Grupper C. Treatment of keratoacanthomas by local applications of 5-fluorouracil (5-FU) ointment. *Dermatologica* 1970; **140** (Suppl. 1): 127–32.
28 Winkelmann RK, Brown J. Generalized eruptive keratoacanthoma: report of cases. *Arch Dermatol* 1968; **97**: 615–23.

Pseudoepitheliomatous hyperplasia [1]

Aetiology. Epidermal hyperplasia is an early and essential feature in the healing of any breach of the skin surface. Ordinarily, this is coordinated with the repair of the dermis, and epidermal downgrowths eventually dissipate [2]. When the dermis is diseased, however, a persistent and much more extensive hyperplasia may occur. This is seen, for instance, at the margin of chronic leg ulcers, over chronic cutaneous granulomas such as lupus vulgaris, tuberculosis verrucosa cutis, insect-bite granulomas and halogen granulomas and, in a rather unusual form, over a small proportion of histiocytomas. It is also a component of some cases of lupus erythematosus and of lichen planus of the hypertrophic type. It may occur in association with tumours, particularly granular cell myoblastoma and malignant melanoma.

Clinical features. The appearance will vary with the primary disorder. Granulomas may be covered by a thickened, warty or heaped-up epidermis, perhaps best seen in chromomycosis. In chronic ulcers, the margin is heaped-up, often giving the appearance of being rolled, and has an irregular surface. The edge is not usually indurated to the extent that occurs in SCC. It is characteristic that the hyperplasia will subside as the ulcer is treated and heals. It is wise to remember that an ulcer whose margin has been affected by pseudoepitheliomatous hyperplasia in the past may eventually be the cause of metastasizing SCC.

Pathology. The nature of the primary disorder modifies the picture greatly. In simple ulcers and inflammatory lesions—by far the most common causes—there is disturbance of the upper part of the dermis, often with young fibroblasts and a rather myxomatous connective tissue stroma replacing the normal dermal collagen. Columns of prickle cells grow down into the dermis in an irregular fashion. In some areas, there is maturation of the central parts of the columns to produce horny pearls. The general appearance is that of invasive proliferation of the epithelium. The individual cells, however, do not show the atypical features suggestive of malignancy. The columns may be penetrated by inflammatory cells, a feature that is not seen in malignant proliferations. In most instances, a weighing of dermal against epidermal changes suggests that the former are the cause and not the consequence of the latter.

Diagnosis. A good-sized biopsy from a representative area of the lesion is essential.

References

1 Winer LH. Pseudoepitheliomatous hyperplasia. *Arch Dermatol Syphilol* 1940; **42**: 856–67.
2 Gillman T. The possible importance of dermal-epidermal interactions in the pathogenesis of human and experimental wound healing and skin cancers. In: Rook A, Champion RH, eds. *Progress in the Biological Sciences in Relation to Dermatology*. Cambridge: Cambridge University Press, 1964: 113.

Cysts

Nomenclature. The term *sebaceous cyst* should be used only to describe steatocystoma multiplex, which contains oily sebum. Histological examination of all other cysts reveals the lining wall to be keratinous in nature. Keratinous cysts can be divided into two types, those with a lining identical in its stratification with epidermis and pilosebaceous duct, and those with a lining resembling the external root sheath of the follicle. The latter variety is less common, and is often familial, multiple and largely confined to the scalp [1]. This type is the trichilemmal cyst [2].

The cysts found in Gardner's syndrome are epidermoid in type [3] and are characterized by their appearance in childhood. There is no genetic overlap between trichilemmal cysts, cysts of Gardner's syndrome or steatocystoma multiplex, although all have an autosomal dominant mode of inheritance.

Histogenesis. Steatocystoma multiplex is most likely to be a genetically determined failure of canalization between the sebaceous lobules and the follicular pore. The common epidermoid cyst is the result of squamous metaplasia in a damaged sebaceous gland. Milia may result from either keratinization within the sebaceous anagen ('collars') of vellus hair follicles or cystic dilatation of an interrupted sweat duct. Trichilemmal cysts may be caused by survival of fragmented segments of the hair root during catagen.

The following cysts are described in this section or elsewhere in the book:
1 Keratinous cysts, both epidermoid and trichilemmal
2 Dermoid (see Chapters 69 and 71)
3 Milium
4 Steatocystoma multiplex
5 Eccrine hidrocystoma (see Chapter 53)
6 Apocrine hidrocystoma (see Chapter 53)
7 Bartholin's cyst (see Chapter 71)
8 Myxoid cyst of the skin (see Chapter 62)
9 Branchial cyst (see Chapter 18).

Epidermoid cyst

Synonym
- Epithelial cyst (sebaceous cyst is a misnomer)

Definition. A cyst containing keratin and its breakdown products, surrounded by an epidermoid wall.

Incidence and aetiology. Epidermoid cysts are common, most frequently affecting young and middle-aged adults. They are rare in childhood. Many are the result of inflammation around a pilosebaceous follicle, and are frequently seen following the more severe lesions of acne vulgaris. Some may result from deep implantation of a fragment of epidermis by a blunt penetrating injury. Those that occur as a part of Gardner's syndrome and of the NBCCS are probably caused by a developmental defect.

Clinical features. An epidermoid cyst is situated in the dermis and raises the epidermis to produce a firm, elastic, dome-shaped protuberance that is mobile over the deeper structures. It is tethered to the epidermis, and there may be a central keratin-filled punctum. The spherical form can be felt where the skin is sufficiently lax. Cysts near the surface, as in the ear lobe or scrotum, are yellowish or white. The size varies from a few millimetres to more than 5 cm in diameter. The common sites are the face, neck, shoulders and chest, which are areas favoured by acne vulgaris. Lesions may be solitary but are commonly multiple. They enlarge slowly and may become inflamed and tender. Suppuration may occur. Cysts that follow acne and have been subject to recurrent inflammation may be difficult to remove completely. Calcification of the contents of epidermoid cysts cannot usually be detected clinically; when it occurs in multiple cysts of the upper part of the trunk it can give a confusing picture on chest X-ray.

Traumatic inclusion cysts usually occur on the palmar or plantar surfaces, buttock or knee. A history of penetrating injury is not always obtained.

Pathology. An epidermoid cyst is unilocular and spherical, unless flattened by firm tissue beneath it. There may be an obvious connection with the surface by a keratin-filled duct, but this is probably less common than surgical texts would suggest. The cyst is situated within the dermis. The lining wall reproduces the layers of the epidermis, although attenuated in large cysts. The keratin is lamellated and birefringent. Cholesterol clefts may be seen. The basal layer may be flattened and surrounded by fibrosis, or may show papillary indentations similar to the epidermis. Some cysts have a chronic inflammatory or foreign-body type of reaction around them, at times producing (or caused by) partial disruption of the wall. Occasionally, a hair shaft may be found coiled within the cyst. These cysts probably result from inflammatory destruction of the sebaceous matrix cells and connective tissue investment of the gland and subsequent re-epithelialization of the abscess cavity, or from squamous metaplasia following impaction of a hair shaft within the sebaceous gland.

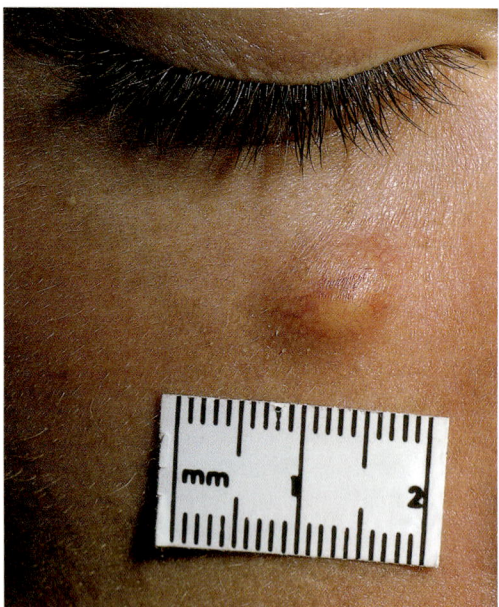

Fig. 52.23 Calcified cyst just below the eyelid margin.

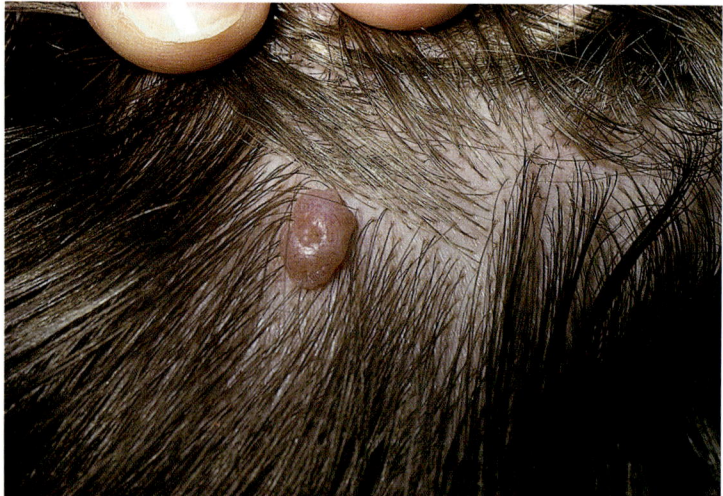

Fig. 52.25 Clinical illustration of typical pilar cyst on the scalp.

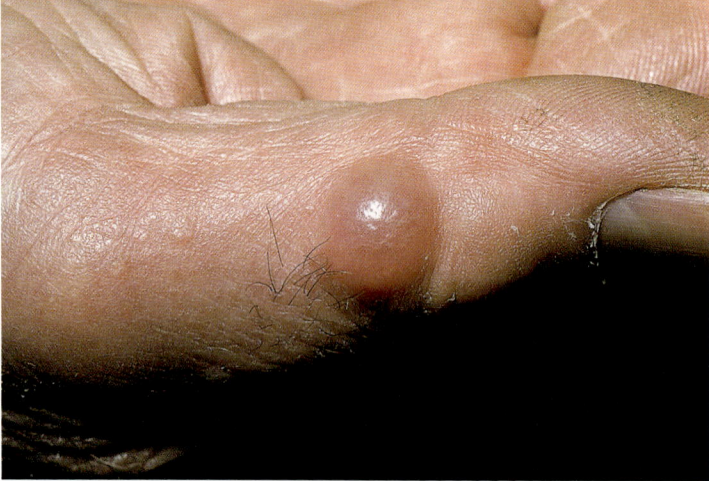

Fig. 52.24 Inclusion cyst following trauma to the thumb.

Diagnosis. The uncomplicated cyst can usually be diagnosed with confidence. Other benign and rounded dermal tumours may be mistaken for epidermoid cysts, and inflammatory granulomas such as cutaneous leishmaniasis may mimic an inflamed cyst (Figs 52.23 & 52.24).

Treatment. A cyst that has not recently been inflamed can be dissected out. An inflamed cyst is better incised, drained and phenolized.

Trichilemmal cyst

Synonym
• Pilar cyst

Definition. A cyst containing keratin and its breakdown products, usually situated on the scalp, with a wall resembling external hair root sheath [4].

Incidence and aetiology. This is a fairly common condition, and accounts for about 5–10% of keratinous cysts seen by surgical pathology services. Women are affected more frequently than men. It is seen mainly in middle age [5] and is inherited as an autosomal dominant disorder [1,6].

Clinical features. The lesion occurs mainly on the scalp, and is a smooth, mobile, firm and rounded nodule (Fig. 52.25). Larger lesions may be lobular and multiple cysts are commonly found. Tenderness occurs with inflammation, and the surface may break down with infection. The cyst wall may fuse with the epidermis to form a crypt (marsupialized cyst), which can occasionally terminate by discharging its contents and healing spontaneously [6]. In contrast, the contents may protrude above the surface to form a soft cutaneous horn.

Pathology. Trichilemmal cysts differ from epidermoid cysts in the way the lining cells mature. They do not flatten and form a granular layer, and keratinization seems to occur mainly in the region of the cell membrane. The cells appear to disintegrate at the inner margin of the lining. The contents are not brightly birefringent lamellae, but may calcify (Fig. 52.26).

The wall of a trichilemmal cyst may become ruptured and the contents invaded by granulation tissue. The reaction is much less acute than in ruptured epidermoid cysts and produces proliferation rather than destruction of the wall. The proliferation may be progressive and simulate, clinically and histologically, a well-differentiated SCC [7]. Cases of proven malignant degeneration in scalp cysts are very rare.

Treatment. Uncomplicated cysts shell out of the dermis with remarkable ease. Proliferating cysts need to be excised with a margin because they will recur if tissue is left behind.

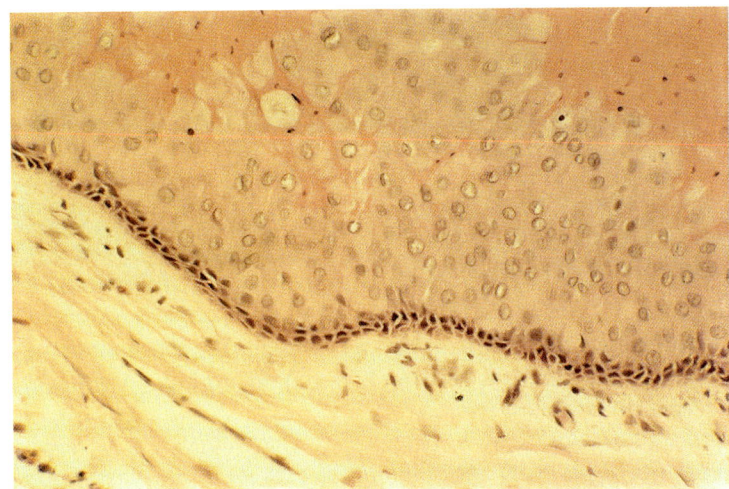

Fig. 52.26 Pilar cyst showing typical pathological features (see text).

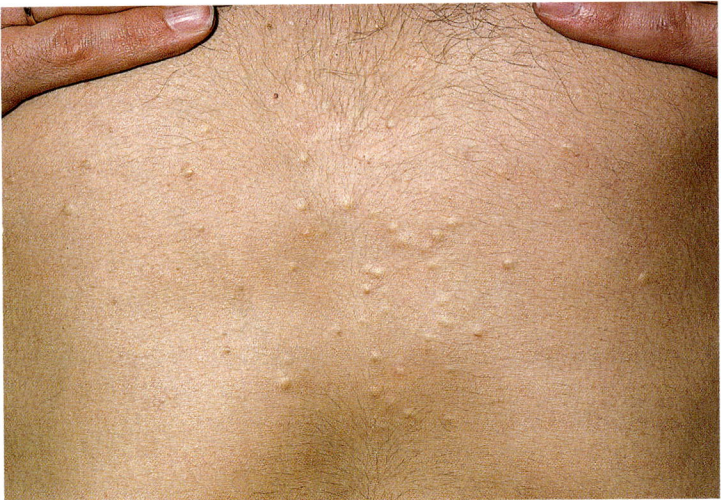

Fig. 52.27 Clinical illustration of steatocystoma multiplex on the chest.

Steatocystoma multiplex

> **Synonyms**
> - Sebocystomatosis
> - Hereditary epidermal polycystic disease

Definition. Multiple cysts in the dermis having sebaceous gland lobules in their wall and containing sebum.

Incidence and aetiology. It is a very uncommon condition, which usually begins in adolescence or early adult life [8]. It is inherited as an autosomal dominant condition in many cases [9,10]. The sexes are affected equally [11].

Clinical features. Multiple, smooth, compressible nodules are present within the dermis, varying in diameter from a few milli-metres to 20 mm or more (Fig. 52.27). They usually first appear or become larger at puberty. The trunk and proximal part of the limbs are most commonly involved, particularly the presternal

area. No punctum is usually apparent over the cyst, but there may be widespread comedones [12]. The more superficial lesions may have a yellowish colour. If pricked, an oily fluid can be expressed. Some lesions become inflamed, suppurate and heal with scarring.

Pathology. The cyst is situated in the mid-dermis. The wall is thin and composed of keratinizing epithelium. In some sections, lobules of sebaceous glands can be seen to form part of the wall or to empty by ducts into the cyst. The contents are oily, and are com-posed of the unsplit esters of sebum [13]. They may contain hairs. Hair roots and, occasionally, sweat glands may be found con-nected with the cyst, and the whole complex is joined to the epi-dermis by a short strand of undifferentiated cells [14].

Treatment. The number of cysts makes excision impractical in most cases. There is no reason, apart from cosmetic, for treating them.

Milium

Definition. A small subepidermal keratin cyst.

Incidence and aetiology. Milia are quite common at all ages from infancy onwards. Many arise in undeveloped sebaceous glands. This may occur in young women as an eruptive phenomenon, and is sometimes a sequel to sunbathing. Others may arise in the proximal part of divided sweat ducts. The cause of the duct damage is usually avulsion accompanying an acute subepidermal bulla, particularly in second-degree burns, epidermolysis bullosa, porphyria cutanea tarda and bullous lichen planus. They may also follow dermabrasion and occur in areas of chronic topical cortico-steroid-induced atrophy. Destruction of skin appendages by radiotherapy may result in a ring of milium-like lesions at the margin of an area treated with tumour doses. These, unlike other forms, can be expressed easily.

Clinical features. The lesions are firm, white or yellowish, rarely more than 1 or 2 mm in diameter and appear to be immediately beneath the epidermis. They are usually noticed only on the face, and occur in the areas of vellus hair follicles, on the cheeks and eyelids particularly. Those that follow blisters are scattered more or less at random in the affected area (Fig. 52.28).

Pathology. The lesion is so easily treated that specimens for his-tological examination are uncommon. However, the milia that follow blistering can often be traced to eccrine sweat ducts in serial sections. Those at the margin of an irradiated area are usually situ-ated in the distorted remnant of the pilosebaceous duct. The much more common milia of the face are found within the undifferenti-ated sebaceous collar that encircles many vellus hair follicles. The white milium body is composed of lamellated keratin.

Diagnosis. Milia are recognized as groups of small uniform spherical white papules with a smooth non-umbilicated top. They are usually whiter and more translucent than syringomas, which appear clinically to be more deeply situated in the skin. Milia tend

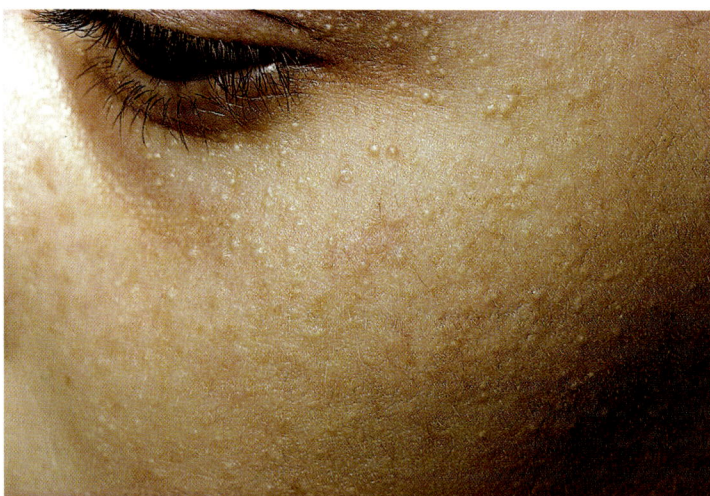

Fig. 52.28 Multiple milia on the upper cheek area.

to occur in isolation and are not associated with papules, comedones and cysts such as may be seen in closed comedones associated with acne and chloracne. Trichoepithelioma may rarely cause confusion, but tend to be larger, more multi-lobulated structures even on clinical examination.

Treatment. Incision of the epidermis over the milium with a cutting edge needle or sharp-pointed scalpel and squeezing out the contents is usually effective. Recurrence is uncommon. Spontaneous disappearance occurs in many milia in infants.

References

1 Leppard BJ, Sanderson KV, Wells RS. Hereditary trichilemmal cysts: hereditary pilar cysts. *Clin Exp Dermatol* 1977; **2**: 23–32.
2 Pinkus H. 'Sebaceous cysts' are trichilemmal cysts. *Arch Dermatol* 1969; **99**: 544–55.
3 Leppard BJ, Bussey HJR. Gardner's syndrome with epidermoid cysts showing features of pilomatrixomas. *Clin Exp Dermatol* 1976; **1**: 75–82.
4 McGauran MH, Binnington B. Keratinous cysts of the skin: identification and differentiation of pilar cysts from epidermal cysts. *Arch Dermatol* 1966; **94**: 499–508.
5 Holmes EJ. Tumors of lower hair sheath: common histogenesis of certain so-called 'sebaceous cysts', acanthomas and 'sebaceous carcinomas'. *Cancer* 1968; **21**: 234–48.
6 Leppard BJ, Sanderson KV. The natural history of trichilemmal cysts. *Br J Dermatol* 1976; **94**: 379–90.
7 Wilson Jones E. Proliferating epidermoid cysts. *Arch Dermatol* 1966; **94**: 11–9.
8 Mount LB. Steatocystome multiplex. *Arch Dermatol Syphilol* 1937; **36**: 31–9.
9 Noojin RO, Reynolds JP. Familial steatocystome multiplex: twelve cases in three generations. *Arch Dermatol Syphilol* 1948; **57**: 1013–8.
10 Sachs W. Steatocystome multiplex congenitale: ten cases in three generations. *Arch Dermatol Syphilol* 1938; **38**: 877–80.
11 Amerlinck F. Sébocystomatose héréditaire. *Arch Belges Dermatol Syphiligr* 1949; **5**: 187–91.
12 Schiff BL, Kern AB, Ronchese F. Steatocystoma multiplex. *Arch Dermatol* 1958; **77**: 516–8.
13 Nicolaides N, Wells GC. On the biogenesis of the free fatty acids in human skin surface fat. *J Invest Dermatol* 1957; **29**: 423.
14 Kligman AM, Kirschbaum JD. Steatocystoma multiplex: a dermoid tumor. *J Invest Dermatol* 1964; **42**: 383–7.

Premalignant fibroepithelial tumour (of Pinkus)

Definition. A premalignant tumour composed of cells resembling those of BCC arranged in a thin honeycomb around a prominent, overgrown papillary stroma.

Incidence. Relatively uncommon. Several examples have arisen in areas treated by radiotherapy for ankylosing spondylitis [1,2]. The author has seen one case on the chest of a patient with multiple postarsenical BCC.

Clinical features. The tumour is sessile with a domed surface and is firm and flesh-coloured. Most of the recorded lesions have been found on the abdomen or loins. There may be seborrhoeic keratoses or BCCs, or both, elsewhere [3]. Increase in size, when it occurs, is slow. The tumour is most likely to be diagnosed as a fibroma.

Pathology. The outline is domed and the surface is formed of normal epidermis. The bulk of the tumour is composed of considerably enlarged dermal papillae, more cellular and fibrotic than normal, which are surrounded by strands of small dark cells that extend down from the underside of the epidermis. Small buds of cells may arise from the strands and enlarge to form BCC, replacing part or all of the tumour [4].

Treatment. The lesions should be surgically excised.

References

1 Colomb D, Vittori F, Perraud R. Les épithéliomas baso-cellulaires et les tumeurs fibro-épithéliales de Pinkus multiples de la région lumbosacrée: discussion de role déclenchant d'un traitement radio-therapique antérieur—a propos de 4 observations. *Semin Hop Paris* 1975; **51**: 2655–64.
2 Sarkany I, Fountain RB, Evans CD *et al.* Multiple basal-cell epitheliomata following radiotherapy of the spine. *Br J Dermatol* 1968; **80**: 90–6.
3 Jaeger H, Delacrétaz J. Tumeurs fibro-épithéliales prémalignes de Pinkus: relation de deux nouveaux cas. *Dermatologica* 1956; **112**: 364–70.
4 Degos R, Hewitt J. Tumeurs fibro-épithéliales prémalignes de Pinkus et épithélioma basocellulaire: a propos de deux cas nouveaux. *Ann Dermatol Syphiligr* 1995; **82**: 124–39.

CHAPTER 53

Tumours of the Skin Appendages

E. Calonje

St John's Institute of Dermatology, St Thomas' Hospital, London, UK

Introduction

The anatomical relationships of the epidermis and dermis are fully discussed in Chapter 3. The skin appendages are of particular interest in this respect, in that they clearly show a morphological and, in some instances, functional interrelationship. The appendageal tumours discussed in this chapter either differentiate towards or arise from the pilosebaceous apparatus (including the apocrine gland) and eccrine sweat gland [1–9].

The pilosebaceous apparatus can be divided into the hair follicle, the adjacent sebaceous gland and in some body sites the apocrine glands. Small strips of smooth muscle, the arrector pili muscle, are also found in association with these structures.

The pilosebaceous apparatus is concentrated in the head and neck area, with the pilar element predominant on the scalp and the sebaceous element on the face, chest and upper back. Thus, tumours arising from these structures are found predominantly at these anatomical sites.

The eccrine sweat glands are, in contrast, found on all body sites and comprise a double-layered, deeply situated secretory structure and a more superficial excretory duct winding through the dermis and spiralling through the epidermis to reach the surface of the skin.

The excretory (ductal) portions of the eccrine and apocrine glands are identical and cannot be differentiated on morphological grounds unless the apocrine duct can be identified entering the hair follicle. To complicate matters further, the apocrine duct rarely opens directly into the epidermis, and there are no histochemical or immunohistochemical stains that allow distinction

Rook's Textbook of Dermatology, 8th edition. Edited by DA Burns, SM Breathnach, NH Cox and CEM Griffiths. © 2010 Blackwell Publishing Ltd.

between eccrine and apocrine tumours. From this, it can be inferred that adnexal tumours showing ductal differentiation may be either eccrine or apocrine, and distinction is not possible unless there is concomitant follicular differentiation. It has therefore been proposed that the classification of adnexal tumours should follow a more logical approach that takes this into consideration [6]. It has become apparent that tumours traditionally considered to be of eccrine differentiation, such as cylindroma, spiradenoma and mixed tumour (so-called chondroid syringoma) may show either line of differentiation and this is probably most often apocrine. Even a classical eccrine tumour such as poroma has been described occasionally as differentiating towards the apocrine duct [7].

A wide range of cells make up the secretory and excretory components of the appendage ducts, the hair follicles and the sebaceous glands. As each cell type capable of dividing can give rise to a tumour as a result of inappropriate transfer of genetic material and cell division, it follows that an equal number of tumours are theoretically possible. The great majority of these appendage-derived tumours are relatively benign, with behaviour and prognosis similar to that seen in basal cell carcinoma. Thus, although local recurrence is well recorded, metastases are rare, with the exception of the malignant eccrine and apocrine gland-derived tumours and ocular sebaceous carcinoma. It is important to take into account that malignant adnexal tumours with metastasis are over-reported in the literature and that this has led to overestimation of their true malignant potential.

Appendage tumours are relatively rare, and their clinical appearance is commonly non-specific. The great majority are not diagnosed as such until after excision and pathological study. Classification systems for these lesions tend to be controversial, but in general the system groups lesions according to their morphological similarity to normal appendage structures.

References

1 Brownstein MH. The genodermatology of adnexal tumors. *J Cutan Pathol* 1984; **11**: 457–65.
2 Hashimoto K, Lever WF. *Appendage Tumors of the Skin*. Springfield: Thomas, 1968.
3 Various authors. *J Cutan Pathol* 1984; **11** [whole issue].
4 Kligman AM, Pinkus H. The histogenesis of nevoid tumors of the skin. *Arch Dermatol* 1960; **81**: 922–30.
5 Lever WF. Pathogenesis of benign tumors of cutaneous appendages and of basal cell epithelioma. *Arch Dermatol Syphilol* 1948; **57**: 679–724.
6 McCalmont TH. A call for logic in the classification of adnexal neoplasms. *Am J Dermatopathol* 1996; **18**: 104–9.
7 Mehregan AH. The origin of the adnexal tumors of the skin: a viewpoint. *J Cutan Pathol* 1985; **12**: 459–67.
8 Pinkus H. Premalignant fibroepithelial tumors of the skin. *Arch Dermatol Syphilol* 1953; **67**: 598–615.
9 Wick MR, ed. *Pathology of Unusual Malignant Cutaneous Tumours*. New York: Dekker, 1985.

Hair-follicle tumours

A large number of tumours are theoretically capable of arising from the hair follicle and matrix, depending on the exact type of cell and its situation within the dermis. A representative selection of these tumours will be described here. For a comprehensive list, the reader is referred to specialized publications [1,2]. Studies on the role of the sonic hedgehog gene and related proteins in basal cell carcinoma (see Chapter 52) have been extended to hair-follicle tumours [3]. The patched gene is located on chromosome 9q22.3, and loss of heterozygosity has been identified in sporadic trichoepitheliomas [4]. Overexpression of Gli-1, which is integral to this pathway, has been observed in trichoepitheliomas in mice [5].

β-Catenin plays a key role in signal transduction and subsequent tissue modelling, and mutations in the β-catenin gene have been recorded in pilomatricomas [6,7].

References

1 Ackermann AB. *Neoplasms with Follicular Differentiation*. New York: Lea & Febiger, 1993.
2 Headington JT. Tumours of the hair follicle: a review. *Am J Clin Pathol* 1976; **85**: 480–514.
3 Callahan CA, Oro AE. Regulating hair follicle progenitors through sonic hedgehog signalling. *Curr Opinion Genet Dev* 2001; **11**: 541–6.
4 Matt D, Xin H, Vortmeyer AO *et al*. Sporadic trichoepithelioma demonstrates deletions at 9q22.3. *Arch Dermatol* 2000; **136**: 657–60.
5 Nilsson M, Unden AB, Krause D *et al*. Induction of basal cell carcinomas and trichoepitheliomas in mice overexpressing Gli 1. *Proc Natl Acad Sci USA* 2000; **97**: 3438–43.
6 Kajino Y, Yamaguchi A, Hashimoto N *et al*. Beta catenin gene mutation in human hair follicle related tumours. *Path Int* 2001; **51**: 543–8.
7 Park SW, Suh KS, Wang HY *et al*. Beta catenin expression in the transitional cell zone of pilomatricoma. *Br J Dermatol* 2001; **145**: 624–9.

Inverted follicular keratosis [1–3]

Definition. A localized area of hyperkeratosis found in association with the pilosebaceous orifice. A number of these lesions arise as a result of infection of the infundibulum of the hair follicle by human papillomavirus (HPV). It is likely that a majority of these lesions may be regarded as the most superficial tumour of the follicular infundibulum (see below), arising as the result of irritation.

Clinical features. In common with many of the lesions described in this chapter, this lesion presents as a solitary papule on the head and neck area. It may reach a considerable size, and be inflamed and pruritic.

Pathology. The pathological features show an endophytic lesion connected to the infundibulum of the hair follicle. Irritated keratinocytes form whorls of cells, so-called 'squamous eddies', and keratin cysts. All of these features may give rise to problems with the differential diagnosis of squamous cell carcinoma, especially on small biopsies. This can be relatively easily distinguished on low-power examination, as there is no individual cell invasion into the dermis. At higher power, mitotic figures may be seen, but they are not abnormal mitoses. The appearances are identical to an irritated seborrhoeic keratosis, but the latter is exophytic.

Management. Local surgical excision is generally needed, for both diagnostic and therapeutic purposes. Occasionally, the lesions recur [3].

References

1 Azzopardi JG, Laurini R. Inverted follicular keratosis. *J Clin Pathol* 1975; **28**: 465–71.

2 Mehregan AH. Inverted follicular keratosis. *Arch Dermatol* 1964; **89**: 229–35.
3 Schweitzer JG, Yanoff M. Inverted follicular keratosis: a report of two recurrent cases. *J Ophthalmol* 1987; **94**: 1465–8.

Dilated pore [1,2]

> **Synonyms**
> • Wiener's pore
> • Infundibuloma

Definition. An area of expanded follicular infundibulum with a dilated poral opening extending down to subcutaneous fat [2].

Clinical features. The pore is a comedo-like lesion found mainly on the head and neck area of the elderly.

Pathology. There is a wide, crater-like cavity, from which acanthotic areas of follicular epithelium radiate. The follicle is lined by outer root-sheath epithelium, and there is little evidence of a sebaceous gland or a well-formed emerging hair. Rare lesions may be associated with trichoblastoma [3] and exceptionally with either basal cell carcinoma [4] or squamous cell carcinoma [5].

References
1 Wiener L. The dilated pore, a trichoepithelioma. *J Invest Dermatol* 1954; **23**: 181–8.
2 Steffen C. Wiener's dilated pore: the infundibuloma. *Am J Dermatopathol* 2001; **23**: 246–53.
3 Misago N, Sada A, Narisawa Y. Thichoblastoma within a dilated pore. *J Am Acad Dermatol* 2006; **54**: 357–8.
4 Weigand DA, MacFarlane DF. Regarding trichoid basal cell carcinoma found in a dilated pore on the nose. *Dermatol Surg* 2000; **26**: 1084.
5 Zhao L, Xu J, Fang F *et al.* Squamous cell carcinoma found in a dilated pore. *J Eur Acad Dermatol Venereol* 2007; **21**: 277–8.

Tumour of the follicular infundibulum [1]

Definition. This lesion may be considered the hair-follicle equivalent of the eccrine dermal duct tumour (p. 53.24).

Clinical features. These lesions are usually found on facial skin and may be relatively large, irregular nodules. They are usually biopsied or excised to obtain a diagnosis, as the clinical appearance is not specific. It has been suggested that they can be divided into four main groups: solitary lesions; those in association with Cowden's disease; multiple eruptive tumours [2]; and follicular infundibulum-like changes in the epidermis [1].

Pathology [3–5]. The pathology is that of a large, horizontally orientated plate of small, dark cells situated in the superficial dermis, usually with multiple connections to the overlying epidermis. The cellular detail is focally similar to that seen in the trichilemmoma, with large numbers of small polygonal cells with clear cytoplasm contained within a palisaded border. Basaloid cells are often seen. The resemblance to basal cell carcinoma is striking, but the stromal element is lacking. Occasionally, sebaceous differentiation may be seen [6]. These lesions with sebaceous differentiation have been termed superficial epithelioma with sebaceous differentiation [7] and acanthomatous superficial sebaceous hamartoma [8].

References
1 Cribier B, Grosshans E. Tumours of the follicular infundibulum: a clinicopathological study. *J Am Acad Dermatol* 1995; **33**: 979–84.
2 Cheng AC, Chang YL, Wu YY *et al.* Multiple tumors of the follicular infundibulum. *Dermatol Surg* 2004; **30**: 1246–8.
3 Mehregan AH. Tumor of follicular infundibulum. *Dermatologica* 1971; **142**: 177–83.
4 Mehregan AH, Buttler JD. A tumor of follicular infundibulum. *Arch Dermatol* 1961; **83**: 924–7.
5 Mehregan AH. Infundibular tumours of the skin. *J Cutan Pathol* 1984; **11**: 387–9.
6 Mahalingam M, Bhawan J, Finn R *et al.* Tumor of the follicular infundibulum with sebaceous differentiation. *J Cutan Pathol* 2001; **28**: 314–7.
7 Rothko K, Farmer ER, Zeligman I. Superficial epithelioma with sebaceous differentiation. *Arch Dermatol* 1980; **116**: 329–31.
8 Leboeuf NR, Mahalingam M. Acanthomatous superficial sebaceous hamartoma? A study of six cases with clarification of the nomenclature. *J Cutan Pathol* 2007; **34**: 865–70.

Pilar sheath acanthoma [1]

Clinical features. These lesions are very rare and are most commonly seen on the upper lip area of the elderly [2,3].

Pathology. The pathology is that of an expanded area of the outer root-sheath epithelium within an irregularly branched cystic cavity, with large lobules of epithelial cells radiating outwards from this cavity area.

References
1 Mehregan AH, Brownstein MH. Pilar sheath acanthoma. *Arch Dermatol* 1978; **114**: 1495–7.
2 Bhawan J. Pilar sheath acanthoma. A new benign follicular tumor. *J Cutan Pathol* 1979; **6**: 438–40.
3 Vakilzadeh F. Haarscheidenakanthom. *Hautarzt* 1987; **38**: 40–2.

Trichoadenoma [1–5]

Definition. A rare benign tumour, with multiple cystic structures closely resembling the infundibular portion of the hair follicle. The keratin profile expression supports the theory that this tumour differentiates towards the follicular infundibulum and the follicular bulge region [6].

Clinical features. This lesion presents as a non-specific nodule, usually on the face, although there are some reports of lesions on the buttocks. An exceptional congenital case has been reported [7] and lesions may occur within a naevus sebaceus [8] or coexist with an intradermal naevus [9].

Pathology. The lesions are in the upper dermis, and on light-microscope scanning power give the impression of a cluster of cysts. On higher power, these cyst-like structures have an appearance similar to the infundibular portion of the hair follicle but turned through 90°; no recognizable hair shafts are seen.

References
1 Rahbari H, Mehregan AM, Pinkus H. Trichoadenoma of Nikolowski. *J Cutan Pathol* 1977; **4**: 90–8.

2 Nikolowski W. Trichoadenom. *Arch Klin Exp Dermatol* 1958; **207**: 34–45.

3 Nikolowski W. Trichoadenom. *Z Hautkrankh* 1977; **53**: 87–90.

4 Undeutsch W, Rassner G. Das Trichoadenom (Nikolowski). *Hautarzt* 1984; **35**: 650–2.

5 Rahbari H, Mehregan A, Pinkus H. Trichoadenoma of Nikolowski. *J Cutan Pathol* 1977; **4**: 90–8.

6 Kurokawa I, Mizutani H, Nishijima S *et al.* Trichoadenoma: cytokeratin expression suggesting differentiation towards the follicular infundibulum and follicular bulge regions. *Br J Dermatol* 2005; **153**: 1084–6.

7 Lee WS, Oh ST, Lee JY *et al.* Congenital trichoadenoma with an unusual clinical manifestation. *J Am Acad Dermatol* 2007; **57**: 905–6.

8 Miller CJ, Ioffreda MD, Billingsley EM. Sebaceous carcinoma, basal cell carcinoma, trichoadenoma, trichoblastoma, and syringocystadenoma papilliferum arising within a nevus sebaceous. *Dermatol Surg* 2004; **30**: 1546–9.

9 González-Vela MC, Val-Bernal JF, García-Alberdi E *et al.* Trichoadenoma associated with an intradermal melanocytic nevus: a combined malformation. *Am J Dermatopathol* 2007; **29**: 92–5.

Comedo naevus [1–3]

Definition. A rare abnormality of the follicular infundibulum presenting as a group of comedo-like lesions.

Clinical features. These lesions are rare and are seen mainly on the head and neck area. Cases may also occur at other sites including the palm and wrist [4]. The palm is not an area that contains hair follicles and the unusual presentation of nevus comedonicus in this location has led to the suggestion that these lesions may really represent variants of sweat duct naevus [5]. They may be present at birth or develop throughout adult life. They appear as a cluster of comedones or as a single giant lesion [3].

Pathology. A rudimentary pilosebaceous follicle is present, with a large overlying keratin-filled crater. The surface of the keratinous material oxidizes to give the comedone-like appearance. Rarely, lesions develop trichilemmal cysts [6].

References

1 Nabai H, Mehregan AH. Naevus comedonicus. *Acta Derm Venereol* 1973; **53**: 71–4.

2 Cestari TF, Rubim M, Valentini BC. Naevus comedonicus. *Paediatr Dermatol* 1991; **8**: 300–5.

3 Fletcher CL, Acland KM, Powles AV. Unusual giant comedo naevus. *Clin Exp Dermatol* 1999; **24**: 186–8.

4 Harper KE, Spielvogel RL. Nevus comedonicus of the palm and wrist. Case report with review of five previously unreported cases. *J Am Acad Dermatol* 1985; **12**: 185–8.

5 Marsden RA, Fleming K, Dawber RP. Comedo naevus of the palm—a sweat duct naevus? *Br J Dermatol* 1979; **101**: 717–22.

6 Leppard BJ. Trichilemmal cysts arising in an intensive comedo naevus. *Br J Dermatol* 1977; **96**: 545–8.

External root-sheath tumours

Trichilemmal cyst

Definition. A cyst apparently arising from the external root sheath, containing keratin and breakdown products [1,2].

Clinical features. These lesions are mainly seen on the scalp and are relatively common. They may be familial, inherited by autosomal-dominant transmission [3]. Females are affected more often than males. They present clinically as firm nodules, which may become infected or inflamed after minor trauma. They are commonly multiple. Unusual locations include the extremities and even the pulp of a finger [4]. A case of Merkel cell carcinoma arising from a trichilemmal cyst has been reported [5]. A further case of multiple trichilemmal cysts following Blaschko's lines and associated with filiform hyperkeratosis and referred to as trichilemmal cyst naevus has also been published [6].

Pathology. These cysts are well circumscribed in the dermis and lined by two or three layers of small, dark keratinocytes. There is then an abrupt transition, towards the centre of the lesion, to large, pale cells with features of root-sheath cells. A granular cell layer is absent. The centre of the cyst contains keratin debris. Some lesions are hybrid and show focal changes of an epidermoid cyst, with formation of a granular cell layer [7]. Occasional lesions have a verrucous lining and in one of these lesions, human papillomavirus has been identified [8].

Management. These are commonly excised to obtain a diagnosis. Lesions that are shelled out may recur [9].

References

1 McGauran MH, Binnington B. Keratinous cysts of the skin: identification and differentiation of pilar cysts from epidermal cysts. *Arch Dermatol* 1966; **94**: 499–508.

2 Pinkus H. Sebaceous cysts are trichilemmal cysts. *Arch Dermatol* 1969; **99**: 544–5.

3 Leppard BJ, Sanderson KV, Wells RS. Hereditary trichilemmal cysts. *Clin Exp Dermatol* 1977; **2**: 23–32.

4 Ikegami T, Kameyama M, Orikasa H *et al.* Trichilemmal cyst in the pulp of the index finger: a case report. *Hand Surg* 2003; **8**: 253–5.

5 Ivan D, Bengana C, Lazar AJ *et al.* Merkel cell tumor in a trichilemmal cyst: collision or association? *Am J Dermatopathol* 2007; **29**: 180–3.

6 Tantcheva-Poor I, Reinhold K, Krieg T *et al.* Trichilemmal cyst nevus: a new complex organoid epidermal nevus. *J Am Acad Dermatol* 2007; **57**: 572–7.

7 Takeda H, Miura A, Katagata Y *et al.* Hybrid cyst: case reports and review of 15 cases in Japan. *J Eur Acad Dermatol Venereol* 2003; **17**: 83–6.

8 Misago N, Narisawa Y. Verrucous trichilemmal cyst containing human papillomavirus. *Clin Exp Dermatol* 2005; **30**: 38–9.

9 Leppard BJ, Sanderson KV. The natural history of trichilemmal cysts. *Br J Dermatol* 1976; **94**: 379–90.

Proliferating trichilemmal tumour

Synonym
• Proliferating trichilemmal cyst

Clinical features. The tumour presents as a rapidly growing, large nodule, commonly on the head (scalp and less commonly the face) and neck area followed by the trunk of the elderly with predilection for females [1,2]. Some lesions are very large and may be more than 10 cm in diameter. The history of rapid expansion frequently gives rise to concern about malignancy. Malignant change has been rarely reported in these lesions (see below). Occasionally, tumours may develop within a pre-existing naevus sebaceus [3]. Multiple lesions are exceptional [4].

Pathology. These lesions may arise from pre-existing trichilemmal cysts, and remnants of a classic trichilemmal cyst may be present [1,2]. The architecture is lobular and expansile, without an infiltrative growth pattern. Tumour lobules are cystic and composed of pale squamous cells with mild atypia. However, tumour cells in the periphery of the lobules may display more prominent cytological atypia and mitotic activity. This is particularly true in early lesions that are actively growing. The surrounding stroma may be fibrotic with inflammation consisting of lymphocytes and plasma cells and a foreign body granulomatous reaction may be seen in areas where cystic structures have ruptured. Cholesterol clefts and areas of calcification may also be seen. Rarely sebaceous, apocrine and matrical differentiation may be present [5,6]. Exceptionally a malignant spindle cell component has been described [7,8]. If there is frank invasion into adjacent structures in association with tumour necrosis, cytological atypia and increased mitotic activity, the diagnosis of a malignant proliferating trichilemmal tumour should be made [9–11]. Such tumours are often characterized clinically by rapid growth and large size [11]. Metastases may occur, leading to death. The diagnosis is often very difficult in small samples of tissue, and ideally the whole tumour should be submitted for histological examination to avoid confusion with a squamous cell carcinoma. The increased expression of p53 by tumour cells similar to that seen in ordinary squamous cell carcinoma but much lower than that seen in trichilemmal cysts suggests that all these lesions may represent low-grade malignancies [12].

Management. Local recurrence takes place and complete excision is therefore necessary.

References

1 Wilson-Jones E. Proliferating epidermoid cysts. *Arch Dermatol* 1966; **94**: 11–9.
2 Sau P, Graham JH, Helwig EB. Proliferating epithelial cysts: an analysis of 96 cases. *J Cutan Pathol* 1995; **22**: 394–406.
3 Rahbari H, Pinkus H. Developmet of proliferating trichilemmal cyst in organoid nevus. Presentation of two cases. *J Am Acad Dermatol* 1986; **14**: 123–6.
4 Hendricks DL, Liang MD, Borochovitz D *et al*. A case of multiple pilar tumors and pilar cysts involving the scalp and back. *Plasr Reconstr Surg* 1991; **87**: 763–7.
5 Sakamoto F, Ito M, Nakamura A *et al*. Proliferating trichilemmal cyst with apocrine-acrosyringeal and sebaceous differentiation. *J Cutan Pathol* 1991; **18**: 137–41.
6 Noto G, Pravatà G, Aricó M. 'Shadow' cell in proliferating trichilemmal tumors. *Am J Dermatopathol* 1990; **12**: 319–20.
7 Mori O, Hachisuka H, Sasai Y. Proliferating trichilemmal cyst with spindle cell carcinoma. *Am J Dermatopathol* 1990; **12**: 479–84.
8 Plumb SJ, Stone MS. Proliferating trichilemmal tumor with a malignant spindle cell component. *J Cutan Pathol* 2002; **29**: 506–9.
9 Weis J, Heine M, Grimmel M *et al*. Malignant proliferating trichilemmal cyst. *J Am Acad Dermatol* 1995; **32**: 870–3.
10 Sethi S, Singh UR. Proliferating trichilemmal cyst: report of 2 cases—one benign, the other malignant. *J Dermatol* 2002; **29**: 214–20.
11 Folpe AL, Reisenauer AK, Mentzel T *et al*. Proliferating trichilemmal tumors: clinicopathologic evaluation is a guide to biologic behavior. *J Cutan Pathol* 2003; **30**: 492–8.
12 Fernández-Figueras MT, Casalots A, Puig L *et al*. Proliferating trichilemmal tumour: p53 immunoreactivity in association with p27Kip1 over-expression indicates low-grade carcinoma profile. *Histopathology* 2001; **38**: 454–7.

Trichilemmoma [1–3]

Definition. This lesion is classically considered to be a proliferation of the external root sheath of the hair follicle [4,5]. However, immunohistochemical studies with different molecular weight keratins normally expressed by different components of the hair follicle have not only confirmed the latter but suggest that the lesion also displays infundibular keratinization [6].

Clinical features. Clinically, these lesions are small, non-specific papules on facial skin; they present in young and middle-aged adults. Their importance lies in the fact that patients with Cowden's syndrome or multiple hamartoma and neoplasia syndrome [7–14]—which is associated with a very high incidence of breast, thyroid and gastrointestinal carcinomas—have large numbers of trichilemmomas. The diagnosis of multiple trichilemmomas should therefore stimulate a search for other evidence of Cowden's syndrome. This includes a characteristic 'cobblestone' appearance of the oral epithelium, multiple skin tags, squamous papillomas and sclerotic fibromas (storiform collagenomas). Mutations of the *PTEN* tumour suppressor gene on chromosome 10q23 are found in Cowden's syndrome [15,16]. The number of mutations identified is large and continues to increase [16]. It seems that the benign lesions in Cowden's syndrome occur without loss of the second *PTEN* allele while the malignant tumours require inactivation of both alleles and additional somatic mutations [17].

Pathology. These lesions are well-circumscribed, lobular tumours extending down from the epidermis and often connected to a hair follicle. Tumour cells display prominent clear cytoplasm secondary to the deposition of glycogen. The presence of glycogen can be confirmed with a positive periodic acid–Schiff (PAS) stain, which becomes negative after treatment with diastase. There is an irregular enclosing PAS-positive, diastase-resistant membrane. In a number of cases, there is prominent hyperplasia of the surface epithelium, with hypergranulosis, clumping of keratohyalin granules and hyperkeratosis. This suggests induction of some lesions by HPV. A viral aetiology has been confirmed by demonstration of HPV DNA by polymerase chain reaction in some [18] but not all cases of the tumour [19]. Trichilemmomas are often found within a naevus sebaceus.

A variant of trichilemmoma, described as desmoplastic trichilemmoma, has been reported [20]. The periphery of this lesion has histological features identical to those of ordinary trichilemmoma, but towards the centre there are strands of squamous cells embedded in a desmoplastic stroma. This stroma appears to contain type I collagen and tenascin but not laminin or type IV collagen [21]. This results in an infiltrative appearance that may be confused with a squamous cell carcinoma, particularly in small biopsy samples.

References

1 Brownstein MH, Shapiro L. Trichilemmoma. *Arch Dermatol* 1973; **107**: 866–9.
2 Headington JT, French AJ. Primary neoplasms of the hair follicle. *Arch Dermatol* 1962; **86**: 430–41.
3 Ingrish FM, Reed RJ. Trichilemmoma. *Dermatol Int* 1968; **7**: 182–90.
4 Brownstein MH, Shapiro EE. Trichilemmal horn: cutaneous horn overlying trichilemmoma. *Clin Exp Dermatol* 1979; **4**: 59–63.

5 Mehregan AH, Medenica M, Whitney D. A clear cell pilar sheath tumor of scalp: case report. *J Cutan Pathol* 1988; **15**: 380–4.

6 Kurokawa I, Nishijima S, Kusomoto K *et al*. Trichilemmomas: an immunohisto-chemical study of cytokeratins. *Br J Dermatol* 2003; **149**: 99–104.

7 Allen BS, Fitch MH, Smith JG Jr. Multiple hamartoma syndrome. *J Am Acad Dermatol* 1980; **2**: 303–8.

8 Brownstein MH, Mehregan AH, Bikowski B *et al*. The dermatopathology of Cowden's syndrome. *Br J Dermatol* 1979; **100**: 667–73.

9 Brownstein MH, Wolf M, Bikowski JB. Cowden's disease: a cutaneous marker of breast cancer. *Cancer* 1978; **41**: 2393–8.

10 Grattan CEH, Hamburger J. Cowden's disease in two sisters, one showing partial expression. *Clin Exp Dermatol* 1987; **12**: 360–3.

11 Starink TM, Hausman R. The cutaneous pathology of extrafacial lesions in Cowden's disease. *J Cutan Pathol* 1984; **11**: 338–44.

12 Taylor AJ, Dodds WJ, Stewart ET *et al*. Alimentary tract lesions in Cowden's disease. *Br J Radiol* 1989; **62**: 890–2.

13 Thyresson HN, Doyle JA. Cowden's disease (multiple hamartoma syndrome) (review). *Mayo Clin Proc* 1981; **56**: 179–84.

14 Weary PE, Gorlin RJ, Gentry WC Jr *et al*. Multiple hamartoma syndrome (Cowden's disease). *Arch Dermatol* 1972; **106**: 682–90.

15 Liew D, Marsh DJ, Li J *et al*. Germline mutations of the PTEN gene in Cowden's disease. *Nat Genet* 1997; **16**: 64–7.

16 Bussaglia E, Pujol RM, Gil MJ *et al*. PTEN mutations in eight Spanish families and one Brazilian family with Cowden syndrome. *J Invest Dermatol* 2002; **118**: 639–44.

17 Reifenberger J, Rauch L, Beckmann MW *et al*. Cowden's disease: clinical and molecular genetic findings in a patient with a novel PTEN germline mutations. *Br J Dermatol* 2003; **148**: 1040–6.

18 Rohwedder A, Keminer O, Hendricks C *et al*. Detection of HPV DNA in trichil-emmomas by polymerase chain reaction. *J Med Virol* 1997; **51**: 119–25.

19 Leonardi CL, Zhu WY, Kinsey WH *et al*. Trichilemmomas are not associated with human papillomavirus DNA. *J Cutan Pathol* 1991; **18**: 193–7.

20 Hunt SJ, Kilzer B, Santa Cruz DJ. Desmoplastic trichilemmoma: histologic variant resembling invasive carcinoma. *J Cutan Pathol* 1990; **17**: 45–52.

21 Massi D, Franchi A. Desmoplastic trichilemmoma: a case report with immuno-histochemical characterization of the extra cellular matrix components. *Acta Derm Venereol* 1997; **77**: 347–9.

Trichilemmal carcinoma [1–4]

Definition. A very rare tumour with metastatic capacity, usually arising in sun-exposed skin of the elderly.

Clinical features. This lesion presents as a solitary, expanding, often ulcerating lesion on the face. Clinically it may be misdiag-nosed as a basal cell carcinoma. Exceptionally, multiple tumours have been described [5]. Trichilemmal carcinoma may arise from a trichoblastoma and in the context of a naevus sebaceus [6]. It has also been described in the setting of solid organ transplantation [7,8].

Pathology. These lesions invade downwards from the epidermis or outer root-sheath areas in a multilobular and infiltrative fashion. They may have a surrounding PAS-positive membrane, and there is central trichilemmal keratinization. There is a high mitotic rate, with abnormal mitoses present. The diagnosis of trichilemmal carcinoma should only be made in the presence of clear evidence of trichilemmal differentiation. The presence of clear-cell change is not enough to make this diagnosis. Most malignant cutaneous tumours with clear-cell change are squamous cell carcinomas and often show at least focal evidence of keratinization. An exceptional case of trichilemmal carcinoma with neuroendocrine differentia-tion has been reported [9]. Immunohistochemical studies in a

single case of trichilemmal carcinoma, suggest that the tumour shows differentiation towards the follicular infundibulum rather than towards the outer root sheath as ordinary trichilemmomas usually do [10]. However, the latter also show infundibular follicular differentiation and it is possible that malignant counterparts lose the expression of markers of outer-sheath differentiation.

Management. Surgical excision with clear margins is the treat-ment of choice.

References

1 Ten Seldam REJ. Tricholemmocarcinoma. *Aust J Dermatol* 1977; **18**: 62–72.

2 Wong TY, Suster S. Trichilemmal carcinoma. *Am J Dermatopathol* 1994; **16**: 463–73.

3 Headington JT. Trichilemmal carcinoma. *J Cutan Pathol* 1992; **16**: 31–9.

4 Reis JP, Tellechea O, Unha MF *et al*. Trichilemmal carcinoma: a study of seven cases. *J Cutan Pathol* 1993; **20**: 44–9.

5 Chan KO, Lim IJ, Baladas HG, Tan WT. Multiple tumour presentation of trichi-lemmal carcinoma. *Br J Plast Surg* 1999; **52**: 665–7.

6 Misago N, Narisawa Y. Tricholemmal carcinoma in continuity with trichoblas-toma within nevus sebaceous. *Am J Dermatopathol* 2002; **24**: 149–55.

7 Kanitakis J, Euvard S, Sebbag L *et al*. Trichilemmal carcinoma of the skin mimick-ing a keloid in a heart transplant patient. *J Heart Lung Transplant* 2007; **26**: 649–51.

8 Garrett AB, Scott KA. Trichilemmal carcinoma: a case report of a rare skin cancer occurring in a renal transplant patient. *Transplantation* 2003; **76**: 1131.

9 Pozo L, Díaz-Cano SJ. Trichilemmal carcinoma with neuroendocrine differentia-tion. *Clin Exp Dermatol* 2008; **33**: 128–31.

10 Kurokawa I, Senba Y, Nishimara K *et al*. Cytokeratin expression in trichilemmal carcinoma suggests differentiation towards follicular infundibulum. *In Vivo* 2006; **20**: 583–5.

Hamartomas and hair germ tumours and cysts

Hair-follicle naevus [1,2]

Clinical features. These naevi are very rare and are recognized as plaque-like lesions with small tufts of hairs. They present in chil-dren and may be congenital. The so-called 'faun tail naevus' is a hair-follicle naevus on the sacral skin. Rare cases occur following Blaschko's lines [3]. A rare association with frontonasal dysplasia has been reported [4]. It is not clear whether some hair follicle naevi are variants of accessory tragi [5].

Pathology. The pathology of this entity consists of a group of normal vellus hair follicles clustered together.

References

1 Choi EH, Ahn SK, Lee SH, Bang D. Hair follicle naevus. *Int J Dermatol* 1992; **31**: 578–81.

2 Labandeira J, Peteiro C, Toribio J. Hair follicle naevus: case report and review. *Am J Dermatopathol* 1996; **18**: 90–3.

3 Germain M, Smith KJ. Hair follicle nevus in a distribution following Blaschko's lines. *J Am Acad Dermatol* 2002; **46**: S125–7.

4 Kuwahara H, Lao LM, Kiyohara T *et al*. Hair follicle nevus occurring in fronto-nasal dysplasia: an electron microscopic observation. *J Dermatol* 2001; **28**: 324–8.

5 Ban M, Kamiya H, Yamada T *et al*. Hair follicle nevi and accessory tragic: variable quantity of adipose tissue in connective tissue framework. *Pediatr Dermatol* 1997; **14**: 433–6.

Eruptive vellus cyst

Definition. Occlusion and cystic dilatation of vellus hair follicles.

Clinical features. These present as small red or brown papules on the chest, commonly in the second decade of life [1]. They are usually multiple, and family clusters have been reported with some lesions showing features of eruptive vellus hair cysts, other lesions showing features of steatocystoma and some displaying hybrid features [2,3]. Lesions may rarely be unilateral [4] or even generalized [5] and have been reported in chronic renal failure [6]. They are commoner than expected in patients who also have pachonychia congenita [7,8].

Pathology. Cysts are located in the mid-dermis, and are lined by squamous epithelium. They contain vellus hair and keratin debris. Biopsies from some lesions show features indistinguishable from steatocystoma, with absence of vellus hairs. This finding shows that there is an overlap with steatocystoma multiplex [9,10].

Management. If treatment is requested, the lesions may clear after application of topical retinoids [11]. Curettage and laser therapy may also be effective, but it is easy to cause scarring. Pulsed carbon dioxide laser is useful for facial lesions but this treatment may induce hypertrophic scarring if used for truncal lesions. Success has been reported at the latter site with erbium:YAG laser [12]. However, when this treatment is used on facial lesions, although initial results are good, there is tendency for local recurrence. This is due to the fact that the depth of ablation of facial lesions is superficial to avoid scarring and atrophy [13].

References
1 Esterly NB, Fretzin DF, Pinkus H. Eruptive vellus hair cysts. *Arch Dermatol* 1977; **113**: 500–3.
2 Mayron R, Grimwood RE. Familial occurrence of eruptive vellus cysts. *Paediatr Dermatol* 1992; **9**: 98–102.
3 Patrizi A, Neri I, Guerrini V *et al*. Persistent milia, steatocystoma multiplex and eruptive vellus hair cysts: variable expression of multiple pilosebaceous cysts within an affected family. *Dermatology* 1998; **196**: 392–6.
4 Lew BL, Lee MH, Haw CR. Unilateral eruptive vellus hair cysts occurring on the face. *J Eur Acad Dermatol Venereol* 2006; **20**: 1314–6.
5 Kwon KS, Lee HT, Jang HS *et al*. A case of generalized eruptive vellus hair cysts. *J Dermatol* 1997; **24**: 556–7.
6 Mieno H, Fujimoto N, Tajima S. Eruptive vellus hair cyst in patients with chronic renal failure. *Dermatology* 2004; **208**: 67–9.
7 Takeshita T, Takeshita H, Irie K. Eruptive vellus hair cyst and epidermoid cyst in a patient with pachonychia congenita. *J Dermatol* 2000; **27**: 655–7.
8 Lee HT, Chang SH, Yoon TY. Eruptive vellus hair cysts in a patient with pachonychia congenita. *J Dermatol* 1999; **26**: 402–4.
9 Patrizi A, Neri I, Guerrini V *et al*. Persistent milia, steatocystoma multiplex and eruptive vellus hair cysts: variable expression of multiple pilosebaceous cysts within an affected family. *Dermatology* 1998; **196**: 392–6.
10 Kiene P, Hauschild A, Christopher E. Eruptive vellus hair cysts and steatocystoma multiplex variants of one entity? *Dermatology* 1996; **134**: 365–7.
11 Urbina-González F, Aguilar-Martínez A, Cristóbal-Gil MC, Sánchez de Paz F. The treatment of eruptive vellus hair cysts with isotretinoin. *Br J Dermatol* 1987; **116**: 465–6.
12 Kageyama N, Tope WD. Treatment of multiple eruptive hair cysts with erbium:YAG laser. *Dermatol Surg* 1999; **25**: 819–22.

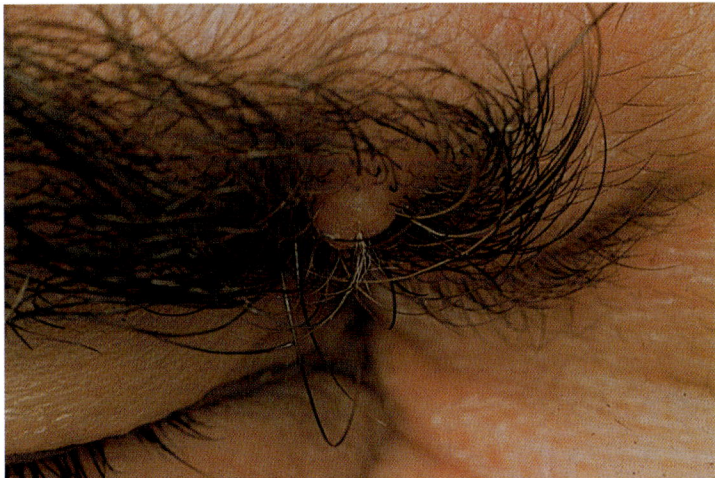

Fig. 53.1 Typical example of a trichofolliculoma, with a small tuft of hairs in the centre.

13 Coras B, Hohenleutner U, Landthaler M *et al*. Early recurrence of eruptive vellus cysts after Er:YAG laser therapy: case report and review of the literature. *Dermatol Surg* 2005; **31**: 1741–4.

Trichofolliculoma [1]

Definition. This lesion is a hamartoma of the pilosebaceous follicle, which results in several hairs being formed within the follicular opening and all protruding onto the epidermal surface from the one pilosebaceous orifice [2–6].

Clinical features. Most cases occur in young adults with predilection for the head and neck, particularly the face. Occasionally, tumours present in the vulva [7]. Clinically, lesions can be recognized as small, raised nodules with two or three hairs protruding together in a small tuft (Fig. 53.1).

Pathology. The pathological appearance is that of a dilated and abnormally large pilosebaceous canal containing numerous, poorly formed hairs, with several pilosebaceous-like structures opening into the canal (Fig. 53.2). The components of the lesion undergo evolutionary changes similar to those of the normal hair follicle [8]. Malignant change has been suggested in a single case with perineural invasion [9]. The so-called folliculosebaceous cystic hamartoma is considered by some authors to be a variant of trichofolliculoma in a late stage of development [10]. This view, however, is not agreed upon by other authors [11].

Management. Simple surgical excision is the treatment of choice.

References
1 Gray HR, Helwig EB. Trichofolliculoma. *Arch Dermatol* 1962; **86**: 619–25.
2 Hyman AB, Clayman SJ. Hair follicle nevus. *Arch Dermatol* 1957; **75**: 678–84.
3 Kligman AM, Pinkus H. The histogenesis of nevoid tumors of the skin. *Arch Dermatol* 1960; **81**: 922–30.
4 Pinkus H, Sutton RL Jr. Trichofolliculoma. *Arch Dermatol* 1965; **91**: 46–9.
5 Plewig G. Sebaceous trichofolliculoma. *J Cutan Pathol* 1980; **7**: 394–403.
6 Sanderson KV. Hair follicle naevus. *Trans St John's Hosp Dermatol Soc* 1961; **47**: 154–6.

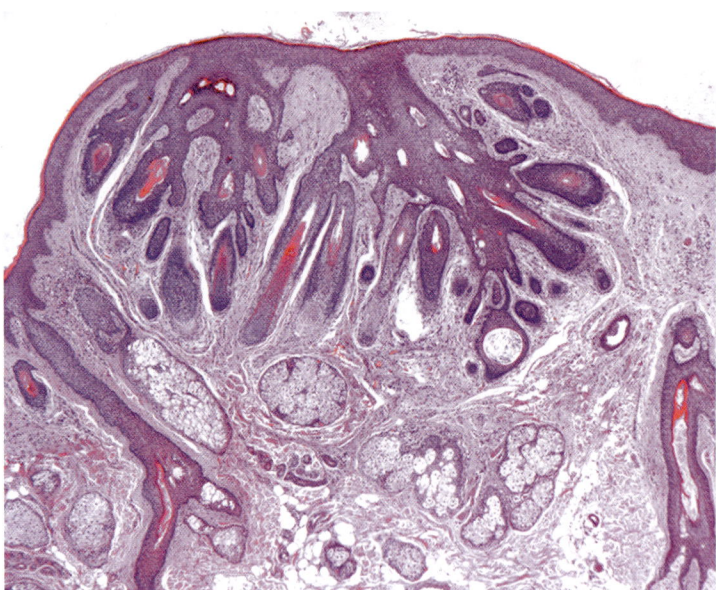

Fig. 53.2 Trichofolliculoma. A large, central follicular structure from which immature follicular structures radiate.

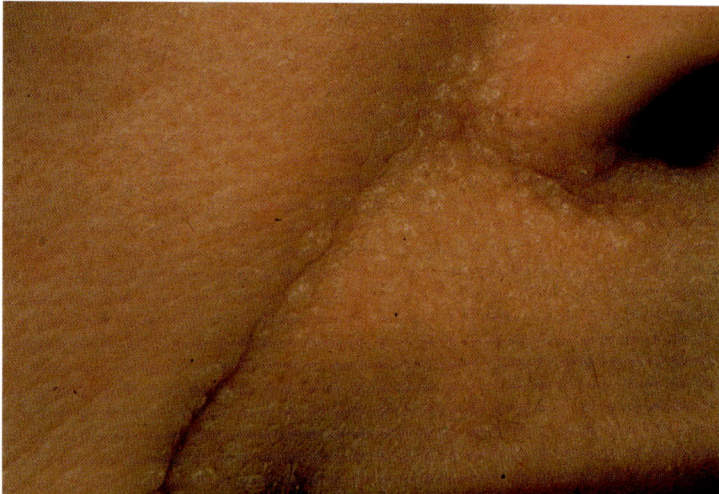

Fig. 53.3 Multiple trichoepitheliomas on the central face.

7 Peterdy GA, Huettner PC, Rajaram V *et al.* Trichofolliculoma of the vulva associated with vulvar intraepithelial neoplasia: report of three cases and review of the literature. *Int J Gynecol Pathol* 2002; **21**: 224–30.
8 Schulz T, Hartschuh W. The trichofolliculoma undergoes changes corresponding to the regressing normal hair follicle in its cycle. *J Cutan Pathol* 1998; **25**: 341–53.
9 Stern JB, Stout DA. Trichofolliculoma showing perineural invasion: trichofolliculocarcinoma? *Arch Dermatol* 1979; **115**: 1003–4.
10 Schulz T, Hartschuh W. Folliculo-sebaceous cystic hamartoma is a trichofolliculoma at its very late stage. *J Cutan Pathol* 1998; **25**: 354–64.
11 Tanimura S, Arita K, Iwao F *et al.* Two cases of folliculosebaceous cystic hamartoma. *Clin Exp Dermatol* 2006; **31**: 68–70.

Trichoepithelioma [1]

Synonyms
- Epithelioma adenoides cysticum
- Brooke's tumour

Definition. A hamartoma of the hair germ composed of immature islands of basaloid cells with focal, primitive follicular differentiation and induction of a cellular stroma. Trichoepithelioma is regarded nowadays as part of the spectrum of trichoblastoma and it is increasingly described under the same heading in some textbooks.

Clinical features. The presentation of a solitary lesion is that of a smooth nodule, usually on the face, which clinically resembles a non-ulcerated basal cell carcinoma. Most affected patients are young adults. Multiple lesions, which are inherited by autosomal-dominant transmission, are seen as multiple, small, pearly lesions, mainly on centrofacial skin (Fig. 53.3). Malignant transformation of trichoepithelioma is extremely rare [2].

Pathology [3–5]. The pathology is identical for solitary or multiple lesions and consists of lobules of small, dark basaloid cells,

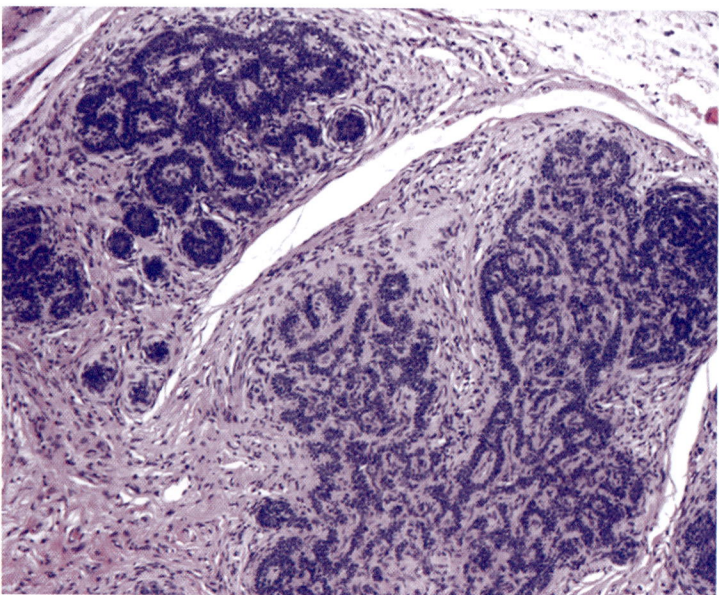

Fig. 53.4 Trichoepithelioma. A lobular basaloid tumour with induction of stroma and immature follicular differentiation.

often with a degree of peripheral palisading surrounding a central area of eosinophilic amorphous material (Fig. 53.4). Occasionally, hair shaft-like structures can be seen in these central areas. A fibrous cellular stroma is seen around the cellular lobules. There is frequently a strong resemblance to basal cell carcinoma, and at times differentiating between the two can be very difficult. However, the stroma in trichoepithelioma is distinctive in that it contains clefts, with an absence of retraction artefact between tumour cells and the surrounding stroma.

The gene for multiple trichoepitheliomas has been mapped to a locus on chromosome 9p21 [6]. The commoner sporadic cases of trichoepithelioma have, in a proportion of cases, deletions at chromosome 9q22.3, the site of the human homologue of the *Drosophila* patched gene [7]. Familial basal cell carcinomas and some cases of sporadic basal cell carcinomas also show this deletion. It has been proposed that in multiple trichoepitheliomas tumours develop from undifferentiated germinative cells of the pilosebaceous–apocrine unit [8]. This explains why in some cases tumours have features of spiradenoma and/or cylindroma, particularly in the Brooke–Spiegler syndrome. The Brooke–Spiegler syndrome inherited by autosomal dominant transmission consists of multiple trichoepitheliomas, cylindromas and spiradenomas and the gene for this syndrome has been mapped to chromosome 16q12–13 [9]. Mutations in the gene *CYLD*, a tumour suppressor gene, are responsible for the manifestations of the disease [9].

In multiple lesions, which are present in epithelioma adenoides cysticum [10–14], larger lesions may be yellow, pink, or sometimes bluish from pigmentation, and there may be dilated blood vessels over the surface. Individual tumours reach a limiting size, but the numbers may increase over the years.

Treatment. Any suspicion of malignant change calls for adequate excision and histological examination. The only other reason for treatment is cosmetic. Partial destruction is usually followed by regrowth. Many treatment modalities may be used including surgical excision, curettage, cryotherapy and dermabrasion. High energy pulsed carbon dioxide laser has also been advocated as a useful treatment [15,16].

References

1 Lever WF. Pathogenesis of benign tumors of cutaneous appendages and of basal cell epithelioma. *Arch Dermatol Syphilol* 1948; **57**: 679–724.

2 Lee KH, Kim JE, Cho BK *et al.* Malignant transformation of multiple familial trichoepithelioma: case report and literature review. *Acta Derm Venereol* 2008; **88**: 43–6.

3 Kopf AW. The distribution of alkaline phosphatase in normal and pathologic human skin. *Arch Dermatol* 1957; **75**: 1–37.

4 Müller-Hess S, Delacrétaz J. Trichoepitheliom mit Strukturen eines apokrinen Adenoms. *Dermatologica* 1973; **146**: 170–6.

5 Bettencourt MS, Prieto VG, Shea R. Trichoepithelioma: a 19-year clinicopathologic re-evaluation. *J Cutan Pathol* 1999; **26**: 398–404.

6 Harada H, Hashimoto KY, Ko MSH. The gene for multiple trichoepitheliomas maps to chromosome 9p21. *J Invest Dermatol* 1996; **107**: 41–3.

7 Matt D, Xin H, Vortmeyer AO *et al.* Sporadic trichoepithelioma demonstrates deletions at 9q22.3. *Arch Dermatol* 2000; **136**: 657–60.

8 Clarke J, Ioffreda M, Helm KE. Multiple familial trichoepitheliomas: a folliculo-sebaceous-apocrine genodermatosis. *Am J Dermatopathol* 2002; **24**: 402–5.

9 Hu G, Onder M, Gill M *et al.* A novel missense mutation in CYLD in a family with Brooke-Spiegler syndrome. *J Invest Dermatol* 2003; **121**: 732–4.

10 Gray HR, Helwig EB. Epithelioma adenoides cysticum and solitary trichoepithelioma. *Arch Dermatol* 1963; **87**: 102–14.

11 Anderson DE, Howell JB. Epithelioma adenoides cysticum: genetic update. *Br J Dermatol* 1976; **95**: 225–32.

12 Gaul LE. Heredity of multiple benign cystic epithelioma. *Arch Dermatol Syphilol* 1953; **68**: 517–24.

13 Pariser RJ. Multiple hereditary trichoepitheliomas and basal cell carcinomas. *J Cutan Pathol* 1986; **13**: 111–7.

14 Ziprkowski L, Schewach-Millet M. Multiple trichoepithelioma in a mother and two children. *Dermatologica* 1966; **132**: 248–56.

15 Rosenbach A, Alster TS. Multiple trichoepitheliomas successfully treated with a high energy, pulsed carbon dioxide laser. *Dermatol Surg* 1997; **23**: 708–10.

16 Retamar RA, Stengel F, Saadi ME *et al.* Brooke-Spiegler syndrome—report of four families: treatment with CO$_2$ laser. *Int J Dermatol* 2007; **46**: 583–6.

Desmoplastic trichoepithelioma [1–3]

Synonym
- Sclerosing epithelial hamartoma

These two terms were introduced almost simultaneously. The US group of Brownstein and Shapiro used the term 'desmoplastic trichoepithelioma' [2], while MacDonald, Wilson Jones and Marks in the UK suggested the term 'sclerosing epithelial hamartoma' [3].

Definition. A slowly expanding plaque of tissue containing hair follicle-like structures.

Clinical features. Lesions are found mainly on the face of young patients and have a depressed centre and a raised, rolled edge in many cases, causing clinical confusion with basal cell carcinoma. To date, more females than males have been reported with the condition. Exceptionally, lesions may be familial [4] and a congenital case has been described [5].

Pathology. Tumours are symmetrical on scanning magnification. The three features that characterize this lesion are large numbers of small, keratin-filled cysts, strands and ribbons of small, dark, epithelioid cells, and a dense fibrous stroma surrounding the first two structures. Perineural invasion is not a feature.

The striking palisading of the basal cell carcinoma is absent. There is, however, a considerable similarity to the sclerosing (morphoeic) variant of basal cell carcinoma, although the number of cysts is very much greater in the desmoplastic trichoepithelioma. Distinction from microcystic adnexal carcinoma may be impossible in a small and superficial biopsy. The latter, however, shows a diffuse infiltrative pattern, with prominent perineural invasion. Merkel cells are present in desmoplastic trichoepithelioma and absent in microcystic adnexal carcinoma and in most cases of morphoeic basal cell carcinoma [6]. Immunostaining with cytokeratin 20, to identify Merkel cells, is therefore useful in the differential diagnosis of these neoplasms.

An electron microscopic and immunohistochemical study with different types of keratins has suggested that this tumour derives from basal cells in the outer root sheath of the hair follicle which can differentiate into various components of the folliculosebaceous and apocrine unit [7].

Occasional desmoplastic trichoepitheliomas are combined with a benign melanocytic naevus [8].

Treatment. Local excision is effective in the majority of cases.

References

1 Dupré A, Bonafé JL, Lassere J. Hamartome épithélial sclérosant: forme clinique du trichoépithéliome. *Ann Dermatol Vénéréol* 1980; **107**: 649–54.

2 Brownstein MH, Shapiro L. Desmoplastic trichoepithelioma. *Cancer* 1977; **40**: 2979–86.

3 MacDonald DM, Wilson Jones E, Marks R. Sclerosing epithelial hamartoma. *Clin Exp Dermatol* 1977; **2**: 153–60.

4 Wang SH, Tsai RY, Chi CC. Familial desmoplastic trichoepithelioma. *Int J Dermatol* 2006; **45**: 756–8.

5 Carter JJ, Kaur MR, Hargitai B *et al.* Congenital desmoplastic trichoepithelioma. *Clin Exp Dermatol* 2007; **32**: 522–4.

6 Abesamis-Cubillan E, El-Shabrawi-Caelen L, LeBoit P. Merkel cells and sclerosing epithelial neoplasms. *Am J Dermatopathol* 2000; **22**: 311–5.

7 Yamamoto O, Hamada T, Doi Y *et al.* Immunohistochemical and ultrastructural observations of desmoplastic trichoepithelioma with a special reference to a morphological comparison with normal apocrine acrosyringium. *J Cutan Pathol* 2002; **29**: 15–26.

8 Niimi Y, Kawana S. Desmoplastic trichoepithelioma: the association with compound nevus and ossification. *Eur J Dermatol* 2002; **12**: 90–2.

Solitary giant trichoepithelioma [1,2]

Synonym

- Giant trichoblastoma

This is a rare variant of trichoblastoma with a dramatic clinical presentation that may cause concern about a rapidly growing malignancy. It has also been described under the name 'trichoblastic fibroma'. Trichoepithelioma and giant trichoepithelioma represent the more mature end of the spectrum of trichoblastoma. These tumours are described separately because they represent distinctive clinicopathological entities. However, it should be remembered that histological overlap is often seen.

Clinical features [3–5]. The clinical presentation is of a very large, polypoid lesion presenting on the lower trunk, frequently in the perianal area, with a history of recent rapid growth. The lesions may cause considerable discomfort because of their size. They affect both sexes equally.

Pathology. The pathology shows the features of the smaller, classical trichoepithelioma but the lesions are much larger, deeper and often located in the subcutaneous fat. An oedematous myxoid stroma is frequently seen and focally, various stages of follicular differentiation are identified. Mitotic figures are frequent, but abnormal mitoses are not seen.

Management. Excision is required, both to confirm the diagnosis and because of discomfort as local recurrence is exceptional [6]. Malignant change into basal cell carcinoma has been reported in a giant trichoepithelioma in a patient with multiple trichoepitheliomas [7].

References

1 Tatnall FM, Wilson-Jones E. Giant solitary trichoepitheliomas located in the perianal area: a report of three cases. *Br J Dermatol* 1986; **115**: 91–9.
2 Zeligma I. Solitary trichoepithelioma. *Arch Dermatol* 1960; **82**: 35–40.
3 Czernobilsky B. Giant solitary trichoepithelioma. *Arch Dermatol* 1972; **105**: 587–8.
4 Filho GB, Toppa NH, Miranda D *et al.* Giant solitary tricho-epithelioma. *Arch Dermatol* 1984; **120**: 797–8.
5 Jemec B, Lovgreen Nielsen P, Jemec GB *et al.* Giant solitary trichoepithelioma. *Dermatol Online J* 1999; **5**: 1.
6 Beck S, Cotton DW. Recurrent giant solitary giant trichoepithelioma located in the perianal area: a case report. *Br J Dermatol* 1988; **118**: 563–6.
7 Martínez CA, Priolli DG, Piovesan H *et al.* Nonsolitary giant perianal trichoepithelioma with malignant transformation into basal cell carcinoma: report of a case and review of the literature. *Dis Colon Rectum* 2004; **47**: 773–7.

Trichoblastoma [1–4]

Synonyms

- Trichogenic fibroma
- Trichoblastic fibroma

Definition. Tumours of the hair germ composed of follicular germinative cells.

Clinical features. These are deeply or superficially situated dermal and/or subcutaneous nodules [5], found—as is common with follicular tumours—on the head and neck. Often lesions are found within naevus sebaceus [6] and trichoblastoma is regarded as the most common neoplasm occurring in this hamartoma [7]. Tumours may be induced by low-dose X-ray depilatory treatment such as was used in the past to treat ringworm [8].

Pathology. Nests of basophilic basaloid cells with a lobular architecture and prominent induction of stroma are seen in the dermis and/or subcutaneous tissue. Focal evidence of follicular differentiation is seen, but this usually consists of less mature structures than those seen in trichoepithelioma. Characteristically, condensation of cellular stroma is seen around aggregates of basaloid cells but true follicular papillae are not formed as the stroma does not invaginate into the epithelial component. Mitotic figures vary and may be frequent. Usually, the tumour is not connected to the epidermis. According to the degree of follicular differentiation and the amount of stroma induced, lesions have been subclassified into different categories, including trichogenic and trichoblastic fibromas. However, all tumours in this category are best classified as variants of trichoblastoma. Some tumours display sebaceous and even ductal (apocrine) differentiation confirming the theory that they differentiate towards the folliculosebaceous and apocrine germ [9,10]. Melanin deposition is often seen, may be prominent and is not uncommonly associated with the presence of melanocytes [11] within the tumour as seen in normal hair follicles. In some cases, rows of tumours cells are arranged parallel to each other in a pattern that has been described as rippled trichoblastoma [12]. Occasional neoplasms consist mainly of clear cells, a change that indicates trichilemmal differentiation [13]. Histological overlap with trichoepithelioma is often seen and there is a tendency to regard all these tumours as part of the same spectrum. Distinction between nodular trichoblastoma and follicular basal cell carcinoma may be very difficult, particularly in small biopsies. Distinction is usually based on the presence of a deep infiltrative pattern in the latter [14]. The presence of Merkel cells in trichoblastoma identified by immunohistochemical markers (cytokeratin 20, chromogranin) is useful in the differentiation from basal cell carcinoma which lacks these cells [15]. Based on clinicopathological features and the presence of Merkel cells in the neoplasm it has been proposed that fibroepithelioma of Pinkus is a variant of trichoblastoma rather than a variant of basal cell carcinoma [16]. A further aid in the differential diagnosis between basal cell carcinoma and trichoblastoma is the immunohistochemical expression of androgen receptor. The latter is usually positive in basal cell carcinoma and negative in benign follicular neoplasms [17].

Management. Behaviour is usually benign but malignant transformation of the epithelial or even the mesenchymal component (trichoblastic carcinoma/sarcoma) may occasionally occur [18,19]. Complete excision is often desirable as exclusion of a basal cell carcinoma may be difficult in small biopsies.

References

1 Slater D. Trichoblastic fibroma. *Histopathology* 1987; **11**: 327–31.

2 Wong TY, Reed JA, Suster S. Benign trichogenic tumours: a report of two cases supporting a simplified nomenclature. *Histopathology* 1993; **22**: 575–80.

3 Blake Gilks C, Clement CB, Wood WS. Trichoblastic fibroma. *Am J Dermatopathol* 1989; **11**: 397–402.

4 Altman DA, Mikhail GR, Johnson TM *et al.* Trichoblastic fibroma. *Arch Dermatol* 1995; **131**: 198–201.

5 Kaddu S, Schaeppi H, Kerl H *et al.* Subcutaneous trichoblastoma. *J Cutan Pathol* 1999; **26**: 490–6.

6 Cribier B, Scrivener Y, Grosshans E. Tumors arising in nevus sebaceus: A study of 596 cases. *J Am Acad Dermatol* 2000; **42**: 263–8.

7 Jaqueti G, Requena L, Sánchez-Yus E. Trichoblastoma is the most common neoplasm developed in nevus sebaceus of Jadassohn: a clinicopathologuic study of a series of 155 cases. *Am J Dermatopathol* 2000; **22**: 108–18.

8 Fazaa B, Cribier B, Zaraa I *et al.* Low-dose X-ray depilatory treatment induces trichoblastic tumors of the scalp. *Dermatology* 2007; **215**: 301–7.

9 Chang SN, Chung YL, Kim SC *et al.* Trichoblastoma with sebaceous and sweat gland differentiation. *Br J Dermatol* 2001; **144**: 1090–2.

10 Yu DK, Joo YH, Cho KH. Trichoblastoma with apocrine and sebaceous differentiation. *Am J Dermatopathol* 2005; **27**: 6–8.

11 Kanitakis J, Brutzkus A, Butnaru AC *et al.* Melanotrichoblastoma: immunohistochemical study of a variant of pigmented trichoblastoma. *Am J Dermatopathol* 2002; **24**: 498–501.

12 Yamamoto O, Hisaoka M, Yasuda H *et al.* A rippled-pattern trichoblastoma: an immunohistochemical study. *J Cutan Pathol* 2000; **27**: 460–5.

13 Kazakov DV, Mentzel T, Erlandson RA *et al.* Clear cell trichoblastoma: a clinicopathological and ultrastructural study of two cases. *Am J Dermatopathol* 2006; **28**: 197–201.

14 Cowen EW, Helm KF, Billingsley EM. An unusually aggressive trichoblastoma. *J Am Acad Dermatol* 2000; **42**: 374–7.

15 Collina G, Eusebi V, Capella C *et al.* Merkel cell differentiation in trichoblastoma. *Virchows Arch* 1998; **433**: 291–6.

16 Bowen AR, LeBoit PE. Fibroepithelioma of Pinkus is a fenestrated trichoblastoma. *Am J Dermatopathol* 2005; **27**: 149–54.

17 Izikson L, Bhan A, Zembowicz A. Androgen receptor expression helps to differentiate basal cell carcinoma from benign trichoblastic tumors. *Am J Dermatopathol* 2005; **27**: 91–5.

18 Regauer S, Beham-Schmid C, Okcu M *et al.* Trichoblastic carcinoma ('malignant trichoblastoma') with lymphatic and hematogenous metastases. *Mod Pathol* 2000; **13**: 673–8.

19 Rosso R, Lucioni M, Savio T *et al.* Trichoblastic sarcoma: a high-grade stromal tumor arising in a trichoblastoma. *Am J Dermatopathol* 2007; **29**: 79–83.

Cutaneous lymphadenoma [1–7]

Synonym
• Adamantinoid trichoblastoma

Definition. This entity was first described in 1991 [1], and to date there are around 35 reported cases in the literature. Follicular, sebaceous and ductal differentiation has been demonstrated and therefore this tumour is regarded as a variant of trichoblastoma, a neoplasm differentiating towards the folliculosebaceous and apocrine germ [4,8].

Clinical features. The lesions are seen mainly on the head and neck area, and present as non-specific papules or nodules. Both sexes are affected equally. The preoperative clinical diagnosis is frequently either basal cell carcinoma or intradermal naevus.

Pathology. The tumour consists of nests and lobules of basaloid cells in the reticular dermis, with no connection to the epidermis.

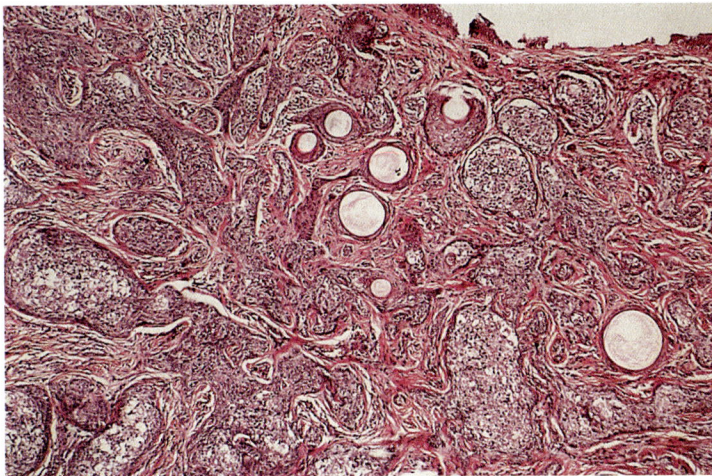

Fig. 53.5 Lymphadenoma. Nests and lobules of epithelial cells with prominent infiltration by lymphocytes.

These aggregates of cells are embedded in a fibrous stroma. Tumour cells are bland and display focal peripheral palisading. A striking feature is the presence of prominent infiltration of tumour lobules and nests by T lymphocytes and histiocytes (Fig. 53.5). These inflammatory cells are mainly located in the centre of the tumour lobules. No cellular atypia is seen, and mitotic figures are rare. Focal areas of keratinization are seen in some cases.

Treatment. Local excision is recommended. The behaviour is entirely benign.

References

1 Santa Cruz DJ, Barr RJ, Headington JT. Cutaneous lymphadenoma. *Am J Surg Pathol* 1991; **15**: 101–10.

2 Botella R, MacKie R. Cutaneous lymphadenoma: a case report and review of the literature. *Br J Dermatol* 1993; **128**: 339–41.

3 Civatte J, Moulonguet-Michau I, Marinho E *et al.* Tumeur epithelio-lymphohistiocytaire: à propos de 3 cas. *Ann Dermatol Vénéréol* 1990; **117**: 441–4.

4 Díaz-Cascajo C, Borghi S, Rey López A *et al.* Cutaneous lymphadenoma: a peculiar variant of nodular trichoblastoma. *Am J Dermatopathol* 1996; **18**: 186–92.

5 Requena L, Sánchez Yus E. Cutaneous lymphadenoma with ductal differentiation. *J Cutan Pathol* 1992; **19**: 429–33.

6 Pardal de Oliviera F, Sánchez A. Cutaneous lymphadenoma. *Histopathology* 1994; **25**: 384–7.

7 Murphy M, Brierley T, Pennoyer J *et al.* Lymphotropic adamantinoids trichoblastoma. *Pediatr Dermatol* 2007; **24**: 157–61.

8 McNiff JM, Eisen RN, Glusac EJ. Immunohistochemical comparison of cutaneous lymphadenoma, trichoblastoma, and basal cell carcinoma: support for classification of lymphadenoma as a variant of trichoblastoma. *J Cutan Pathol* 1999; **26**: 119–24.

Basaloid follicular hamartoma [1–4]

Definition. A hamartoma consisting of a proliferation of basaloid cells, with frequent involvement of hair follicles.

Clinical features. These lesions are usually small multiple papules that may become confluent to form a plaque. Involvement of the face is common but lesions may also present on the trunk. Presentation may be generalized or localized and the latter may be linear [4,5]. They may be present in isolation or inherited as an autosomal-dominant trait [6,7]. Association with autoimmune diseases and alopecia has been described particularly in the generalized variant [8]. The autoimmune diseases include lupus erythematosus [9] and myasthenia gravis [5]. Other rare associations include cystic fibrosis [10], milia and hypohidrosis [11]. In exceptional cases, basal cell carcinomas may develop within the lesions [12].

Pathology. A multifocal proliferation of cords, strands and nests of basaloid cells is seen, with frequent connections to the epidermis. Basaloid cells focally replace neighbouring hair follicles. In addition, immature follicular bulbs may also be seen.

References

1 Mehregan AH, Baker S. Basaloid follicular hamartoma: three cases with localized and systematized unilateral lesions. *J Cutan Pathol* 1985; **12**: 55–65.

2 Brownstein MH. Basaloid follicular hamartoma: solitary and multiple types. *J Am Acad Dermatol* 1992; **22**: 237–40.

3 Walsh N, Ackerman AB. Basaloid follicular hamartoma. *J Am Acad Dermatol* 1993; **29**: 125–7.

4 Lee MW, Choi JH, Moon KC *et al*. Linear basaloid follicular hamartoma on the Blaschko's lines of the face. *Clin Exp Dermatol* 2005; **30**: 30–4.

5 El-Dorouti MA, Marzouk SA, Abdel-Halim MR *et al*. Basaloid follicular hamartoma. *Int J Dermatol* 2005; **44**: 361–5.

6 Wheeler CE, Carroll MA, Groben PA *et al*. Autosomal dominantly inherited generalized basaloid follicular hamartoma syndrome: report of a new disease in a North Carolina family. *J Am Acad Dermatol* 2000; **43**: 189–206.

7 Lee PL, Lourduraj LT, Palko MJ 3rd *et al*. Hereditary basaloid follicular hamartoma syndrome. *Cutis* 2006; **78**: 42–6.

8 Smith KJ, Skelton H. Basaloid follicular hamartoma associated with autoimmune disease: a possible role for retinoids in therapy. *J Am Acad Dermatol* 2003; **49**: 1067–70.

9 Morton S, Stevens A, Powell RJ. Basaloid follicular hamartoma, total body hair loss and SLE. *Lupus* 1998; **7**: 207–9.

10 Mascaró JM Jr, Ferrando J, Bombi JA *et al*. Congenital generalized follicular hamartoma associated with alopecia and cystic fibrosis in three siblings. *Arch Dermatol* 1995; **131**: 454–8.

11 Katayama I, Hirayama M, Eishi K. Basaloid follicular hamartoma with eruptive milia and hypohidrosis: is there is a pathogenic relationship? *Eur J Dermatol* 2003; **13**: 505–8.

12 Yoshida Y, Urabe K, Mashino T *et al*. Basal cell carcinomas in association with basaloid follicular hamartoma. *Dermatology* 2003; **207**: 57–60.

Hair matrix tumours

Pilomatricoma [1–4]

Synonyms
- Benign calcifying epithelioma of Malherbe
- Trichomatricoma
- Pilomatrixoma

Definition. A benign tumour considered to be a hamartoma of the hair matrix composed of cells resembling those of the hair matrix and cortex and inner root sheath. The cells usually undergo 'mummification'.

Incidence. This lesion makes up around 20% of all hair follicle-related tumours in most series and is therefore the commonest

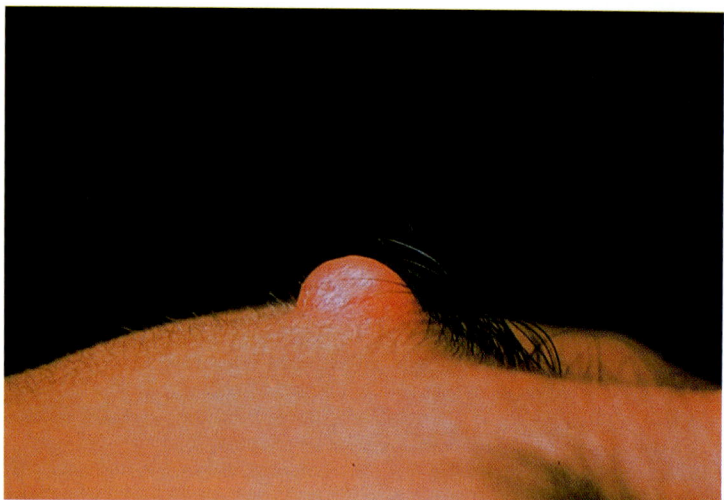

Fig. 53.6 Pilomatricoma. Small, red, firm papule.

hair-follicle tumour. It may occur at any age from infancy and is frequently seen in children [5]. The majority of patients are under 20 years of age, and females are affected more often than males. A number of familial cases are recorded [6]. Association with myotonic dystrophy [6], Turner's syndrome [7] and Rubinstein–Taybi syndrome have been described [8]. *MYH*-associated polyposis is an autosomal recessive variant of familial adenomatous polyposis with susceptibility to colorectal carcinoma and association in some affected individuals with multiple pilomatricomas [9].

Clinical features [10–16]. The lesion is usually a solitary, deep, dermal or subcutaneous tumour 3–30 mm in diameter situated on the head, neck or upper extremities (Fig. 53.6). Very large tumours occur occasionally [17]. The skin over the tumour is normal and the lesion has a firm to stone-hard consistency and a lobular shape on palpation. In adult life, there may be quite a short history [4] and there is usually no evidence of a preceding cyst. It may be subject to periodic inflammation and can present as a granulomatous swelling. Rarely, ulcerated lesions may show transepithelial elimination [18]. An unusual case associated with hypercalcaemia and high levels of parathyroid hormone has been described [19]. Malignant change is very rare (see below).

Pathology [20–27]. The tumour is situated in the dermis, and is composed of well-circumscribed, rounded islands giving a lobulated contour. The outer cells are small, and their rounded nuclei crowded together make this region deeply basophilic. Normal mitotic figures can usually be seen and are often numerous. The cytoplasm is scanty and the cell margins indistinct, but intercellular connections can be seen. Towards the centre of the mass, the cytoplasm becomes more abundant and eosinophilic. The nuclear outline persists, but the chromatin is sparse and clumped in dark granules; when all basophilic material disappears, a mummified 'ghost cell' remains (Fig. 53.7). The ultrastructural and histochemical characteristics of these cells mark them as hair-matrix cells maturing towards cortex or root sheath [3,26,27]. The central areas

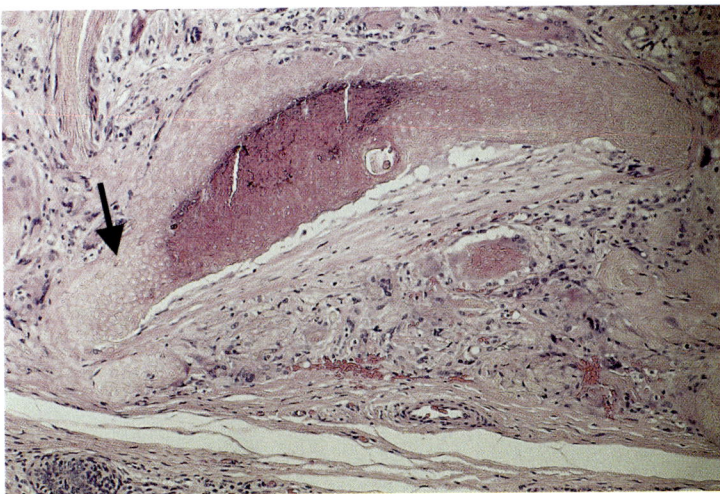

Fig. 53.7 Pilomatricoma. Lobules of basaloid cells intermixed with pale pink areas containing ghost cells.

often calcify, and calcium can be demonstrated in the basophilic areas of the tumour. In older lesions, the basophilic cells may be greatly reduced or disappear entirely. Melanin may be present, and dendritic melanocytes have been found between the tumour cells. The stroma that encapsulates the masses usually contains inflammatory and foreign-body giant cells, and occasionally ossifies. A rare variant of superficial pilomatricoma presenting clinically as a cutaneous horn and with an intraepidermal location has been reported [28]. A bullous appearance may occur consequent on lymphangiectasia [29], and anetoderma can occur in the dermis surrounding the tumour [30]. Occasional hybrid cysts may show areas of pilomatrical differentiation identical to pilomatricoma [31].

Studies have shown that 75% of pilomatricomas possess activating mutations of the β-catenin gene [32–34]. The sites of β-catenin expression within pilomatricomas suggest that this may affect cell–cell adhesion [35].

Diagnosis. The diagnosis can be suspected if a subcutaneous nodule feels hard and lobular. The presence of calcium salts may be apparent on radiographs, but these can also be deposited in other cysts and tumours of the skin. The microscopic picture is, however, diagnostic.

Malignant change is recorded in several cases, and appears to arise chiefly in large pilomatricomas that have been present for many years (see below).

Management. Local excision is required for benign lesions, as there is a tendency for local recurrence. Wider excision will be needed if malignancy is suspected.

References

1 Forbis R Jr, Helwig EB. Pilomatrixoma (calcifying epithelioma). *Arch Dermatol* 1961; **83**: 606–18.
2 Hashimoto K, Lever WF. Histogenesis of skin appendage tumors. *Arch Dermatol* 1969; **100**: 356–69.
3 McGavran MH. Ultrastructure of pilomatrixoma (calcifying epithelioma). *Cancer* 1965; **18**: 1445–56.
4 Swerlick RA, Cooper PH, Mackel SE. Rapid enlargement of pilomatricoma. *J Am Acad Dermatol* 1982; **7**: 54–6.
5 Schlechter MD, Hartsough NA, Guttman FM. Multiple pilomatricomas. *Paediatr Dermatol* 1984; **2**: 23–5.
6 Chiaramonti A, Gilgor RS. Pilomatricomas associated with myotonic dystrophy. *Arch Dermatol* 1978; **114**: 1363–5.
7 Noguchi H, Kayashima K, Nishiyama S *et al*. Two cases of pilomatrixoma in Turner's syndrome. *Dermatology* 1999; **199**: 338–40.
8 Cambiaghi S, Ermacora E, Brusasco A *et al*. Multiple pilomatricomas in Rubinstein–Taybi syndrome: a case report. *Pediatr Dermatol* 1994; **11**: 21–5.
9 Baglioni S, Melean G, Gensini F *et al*. A kindred with *MYH*-associated polyposis and pilomatricomas. *Am J Med Genet* A 2005; **134**: 212–4.
10 Lopansri S, Mihm MC Jr. Pilomatrix carcinoma or calcifying epitheliocarcinoma of Malherbe. *Cancer* 1980; **45**: 2368–73.
11 Cazers JS, Okun MR, Pearson SH. Pigmented calcifying epithelioma. *Arch Dermatol* 1974; **110**: 773–4.
12 Geiser JD. L'épithélioma calcifié de Malherbe. *Ann Dermatol Syphilol* 1959; **86**: 383–403.
13 Hadlich J, Linse R. Zur klinischen Diagnostik des Epithelioma calcificans Malherbe. *Dermatol Monatsschr* 1979; **165**: 432–9.
14 Moehlenbeck F. Pilomatrixoma (calcifying epithelioma). *Arch Dermatol* 1973; **108**: 532–4.
15 Peterson WC Jr, Hult AM. Calcifying epithelioma of Malherbe. *Arch Dermatol* 1964; **90**: 404–10.
16 Julian CG, Bowers PW. A clinical review of 209 pilomatricomas. *J Am Acad Dermatol* 1998; **39**: 191–5.
17 Lozzi GP, Soyer HP, Fruehauf J *et al*. Giant pilomatricoma. *Am J Dermatopathol* 2007; **29**: 286–9.
18 Honda Y, Ohi T, Koga M *et al*. Perforating pilomatricoma. *J Dermatol* 2002; **29**: 100–3.
19 Kambe Y, Nakano H, Kaneko T *et al*. Giant pilomatricoma associated with hypercalcaemia and elevated levels of parathyroid hormone-related protein. *Br J Dermatol* 2006; **155**: 208–10.
20 Hashimoto K, Nelson RG, Lever WF. Calcifying epithelioma of Malherbe: histochemical and electron microscopic studies. *J Invest Dermatol* 1966; **46**: 391–408.
21 Kaddu S, Soyer HP, Hodl S *et al*. Morphological stages of pilomatricoma. *Am J Dermatopathol* 1996; **18**: 333–8.
22 Lever WF, Griesemer RD. Calcifying epithelioma of Malherbe. *Arch Dermatol Syphilol* 1949; **59**: 506–18.
23 Solanki P, Ramzy I, Durr N *et al*. Pilomatrixoma. *Arch Pathol* 1987; **111**: 294–7.
24 Turhan B, Krainer L. Bemerkungen über die sogenannten verkalkenden Epitheliome der Haut und ihre Genese. *Dermatologica* 1942; **85**: 73–90.
25 Uchiyama N, Shindo Y, Saida T. Perforating pilomatricomas. *J Cutan Pathol* 1986; **13**: 312–8.
26 Wiedersberg H. Das Epithelioma calcificans Malherbe. *Dermatol Monatsschr* 1971; **157**: 867–83.
27 Lever WF, Hashimoto K. Die Histogenese einiger Hautanhangs-Tumoren im Lichte histochemischer und elektronenmikroskopischer Befunde. *Hautarzt* 1966; **17**: 161–73.
28 de la Torre JP, Saiz A, García-Arpa M *et al*. Pilomatrical horn: a new superficial variant of pilomatricoma. *Am J Dermatopathol* 2006; **28**: 426–8.
29 Yigun J, Jianfang S. Pilomatricoma with a bullous appearance. *J Cutan Pathol* 2004; **31**: 558–60.
30 Fernández-Flores A, Gonzalez-Montero JM. Anetodermic variant of pilomatricoma. *Int J Dermatol* 2005; **44**: 876–7.
31 May SA, Quirey R, Cockerell CJ. Follicular hybrid cysts with infundibular, isthmic-catagen, and pilomatrical differentiation: a report of 2 patients. *Ann Diagn Pathol* 2006; **10**: 110–3.
32 Gat U, DasGupta R, Degenstein L *et al*. De novo hair follicle morphogenesis and hair tumors in mice expressing a truncated beta catenin in skin. *Cell* 1998; **95**: 605–14.
33 Chan EF, Gat U, McNiff JM *et al*. A common skin tumour is caused by activating mutations in beta catenin. *Nat Genet* 1999; **21**: 410–3.
34 Durand M, Moles JP. Beta catenin mutations in a common skin cancer: pilomatricoma. *Bull Cancer* 1999; **86**: 725–6.
35 Park SW, Suh KS, Wang HY *et al*. Beta catenin expression in the transitional zone of pilomatricoma. *Br J Dermatol* 2001; **145**: 624–9.

Pilomatricarcinoma [1–4]

Definition. The malignant counterpart of the pilomatricoma, possessing metastatic potential.

Clinical features. A rapidly expanding firm nodule. Approximately 70 cases are reported in the literature, and the average age of the patients is 70 years. Males are more often affected than females. Most tumours develop on the head and neck followed much less frequently by the trunk [5].

Pathology. Many pilomatricarcinomas appear to arise on long-standing benign pilomatricomas. Definition of malignancy is usually very difficult on histological grounds. Malignant tumours usually have a very large predominant basaloid component, an infiltrative growth pattern and extensive necrosis. In addition, there are numerous abnormal mitotic figures, and both lymphatic and vascular invasion may be seen. There may be metastases to distant organs such as the lungs, bone and lymph nodes [6–9]. At least two cases have proved fatal.

As in pilomatricoma, mutations in β-catenin have been demonstrated in pilomatricarcinomas suggesting the activation of a common cellular pathway in both types of neoplasms despite the difference in clinical behaviour [10,11].

Management. Wide local excision is usually curative, but follow-up is required because of the possibility of metastatic spread.

References

1 Green DE, Sanusi ID, Fowler MR. Pilomatrix carcinoma. *J Am Acad Dermatol* 1987; **17**: 264–70.
2 Weedon D, Bell J, Mayze J. Matrical carcinoma of the skin. *J Cutan Pathol* 1980; **7**: 39–42.
3 Wood MG, Parhizzar B, Beerman H. Malignant pilomatricoma. *Arch Dermatol* 1984; **120**: 770–3.
4 Van Der Walt JD, Rohlova B. Carcinomatous transformation in a pilomatrixoma. *Am J Dermatopathol* 1984; **6**: 63–4.
5 Hardisson D, Linares MD, Cuevas-Santos J *et al.* Pilomatrix carcinoma: a clinicopathologic study of six cases and review of the literature. *Am J Dermatopathol* 2001; **23**: 394–401.
6 Gould E, Kurzon R, Kowalczyk P *et al.* Pilomatrix carcinoma with pulmonary metastases. *Cancer* 1984; **54**: 370–2.
7 Mir R, Cortes E, Papantoniou PA *et al.* Metastatic trichomatricial carcinoma. *Arch Pathol* 1986; **110**: 660–3.
8 Hardisson D, Linares D, Cuevas Santos J *et al.* Pilomatrix carcinoma. *Am J Dermatopathol* 2001; **23**: 394–401.
9 Sassmannhausen J, Chaffins M. Pilomatrix carcinoma. *J Am Acad Dermatol* 2001; **44**: 358–61.
10 Lazar AJ, Calonje E, Grayson W *et al.* Pilomatrix carcinoma contain mutations in CTNNB1, the gene encoding beta-catenin. *J Cutan Pathol* 2005; **32**: 148–57.
11 Hassanein AM, Glanz SM. Beta-catenin expression in benign and malignant pilomatrix neoplasms. *Br J Dermatol* 2004; **150**: 511–6.

Lesions of hair-follicle mesenchyme

Trichodiscoma [1]

Definition. This lesion is a hamartomatous proliferation of the mesodermal component of the *Haarscheibe* described by Pinkus [1]. The *Haarscheibe* is considered to be a slowly reacting mechanoreceptor associated with the hair follicle.

Clinical features. The clinical appearance of the trichodiscoma is that of multiple, discrete, flat-topped papules 2–3 mm in diameter. They occur mainly in the central area of the face. Familial cases are recorded [2,3]. Multiple trichodiscomas, trichofolliculomas and acrochordon-like lesions have been described as part of the Birt–Hogg–Dubé syndrome [4]. This syndrome is an autosomal dominant genodermatosis also associated with lung cysts, spontaneous pneumothorax and renal neoplasms (chromophobe renal carcinoma and oncocytoma) [5]. The causative gene, *FLCN*, has been mapped to chromosome 17p12q11. Interestingly, the acrochordon-like lesions display the histological features of either trichodiscomas or trichofolliculomas [6].

Pathology. A discrete but non-encapsulated area of myxoid, poorly cellular stroma with focal collagen deposition is seen in the dermis, associated with a proliferation of blood vessels, some of which are thick-walled. The proliferating cells are CD34 positive [7]. A variant with a cellular spindle-cell component has been described [8]. Pilosebaceous units are often seen on both sides of the myxoid stroma. Trichodiscomas and trichofolliculomas usually show histological overlap.

References

1 Pinkus H, Cosket R, Burgess GH. Trichodiscoma. *J Invest Dermatol* 1974; **63**: 212–8.
2 Balus L, Crovato F, Breathnach AS. Familial multiple trichodiscomas. *J Am Acad Dermatol* 1986; **15**: 603–7.
3 Camarasa JG, Calderon P, Moreno A. Familial multiple trichodiscomas. *Acta Derm Venereol* 1988; **68**: 163–5.
4 Schmidt L, Warren M, Nickerson M *et al.* Birt–Hogg–Dubé syndrome, a genodermatosis associated with spontaneous pneumothorax and kidney neoplasia, maps to chromosome 17p11.2. *Am J Hum Genet* 2002; **69**: 876–82.
5 Leter EM, Koopmans AK, Gille JJ *et al.* Birt–Hogg–Dubé síndrome: clinical and genetic studies of 20 families. *J Invest Dermatol* 2008; **128**: 45–9.
6 De la Torre C, Ocampo C, Doval IG *et al.* Acrochordons are not a component of the Birt–Hogg–Dubé syndrome: does this syndrome exist? Case reports and review of the literature. *Am J Dermatopathol* 1999; **21**: 369–74.
7 Chartier M, Reed ML, Mandavilli S *et al.* CD34-reactive trichodiscoma. *J Cutan Pathol* 2004; **31**: 398–400.
8 Kutzner H, Requena L, Rütten A *et al.* Spindle cell predominant trichodiscoma: a fibrofolliculoma/trichodiscoma variant considered formerly to be a neurofollicular hamartoma: a clinicopathological and immunohistochemical analysis of 17 cases. *Am J Dermatopathol* 2006; **28**: 1–8.

Perifollicular fibroma [1,2]

The clinical appearance of these lesions has not been well described. The pathology is that of a striking fibrous proliferation around a relatively normal pilosebaceous apparatus.

References

1 Freeman RG, Chernosky ME. Perifollicular fibroma. *Arch Dermatol* 1969; **100**: 66–9.
2 Zackheim HS, Pinkus H. Perifollicular fibromas. *Arch Dermatol* 1960; **82**: 913–7.

Fibrofolliculoma

Definition. Rare lesions of perifollicular connective tissue [1].

Clinical features. These lesions usually first appear in middle age and tend to affect the upper part of the body. Multiple lesions are seen in the Birt–Hogg–Dubé syndrome, which is an autosomal-dominant condition mapped to chromosome 17p11.2 [2–5]. In this syndrome, fibrofolliculomas are seen in association with trichodiscomas, acrochordon-like lesions, renal tumours most commonly chromophobe carcinoma and spontaneous pneumothorax [6,7]. Colonic neoplasms do not seem to be increased in this syndrome, as previously suggested [6].

Pathology. Histology shows multiple, small, poorly formed pilosebaceous follicles set in a very striking fibrous stroma. There is also an obvious proliferation of the outer root sheath similar to that seen in the perifollicular fibroma.

References

1 Scully K, Bargman H, Assaad D. Solitary fibrofolliculoma. *J Am Acad Dermatol* 1984; **11**: 361–3.

2 Birt AR, Hogg GR, Dubé J. Hereditary multiple fibrofolliculomas with trichodiscomas and acrochordons. *Arch Dermatol* 1977; **113**: 1674–7.

3 Weintraub R, Pinkus H. Multiple fibrofolliculomas (Birt–Hogg–Dubé) associated with a large connective tissue nevus. *J Cutan Pathol* 1977; **4**: 289–99.

4 Fujita WH, Barr RJ, Headley JL. Multiple fibrofolliculomas with trichodiscomas and acrochordons. *Arch Dermatol* 1981; **117**: 32–5.

5 Schmidt L, Warren MB, Nickerson ML *et al.* Birt–Hogg–Dubé syndrome, a genodermatosis associated with spontaneous pneumothorax and kidney neoplasia, maps to chromosome 17p11.2. *Am J Hum Genet* 2001; **69**: 876–82.

6 Zbar B, Alvord WG, Glenn G *et al.* Risk of renal and colonic neoplasms and spontaneous pneumothorax in the Birt–Hogg–Dubé syndrome. *Cancer Epidemiol Biomarkers Prev* 2002; **11**: 393–400.

7 Toro JR, Glenn G, Duray P *et al.* Birt–Hogg–Dubé syndrome: a novel marker of kidney neoplasia. *Arch Dermatol* 1999; **135**: 1195–202.

Sebaceous gland tumours [1]

The following tumours or tumour-like conditions of sebaceous glands are considered elsewhere in the book:
1 Naevus sebaceus (Chapter 18);
2 Senile sebaceous hyperplasia (Chapter 42);
3 'Sebaceous' cyst (Chapter 42);
4 Steatocystoma multiplex (Chapter 52).
The two main conditions discussed in this section are sebaceous adenomas and sebaceomas, and sebaceous carcinoma. The old term 'sebaceous epithelioma' is no longer used, as it causes confusion with the exceptionally rare basal cell carcinoma with sebaceous differentiation.

Sebaceous adenomas and sebaceomas [1–5]

Definition. Benign tumours composed of incompletely differentiated sebaceous cells of varying degrees of maturity. Sebaceous adenoma and sebaceoma are described together, as they do not have distinctive clinical features and, although histological separation is possible in most cases, there is also some degree of overlap.

Incidence and aetiology. These are fairly rare tumours [4]. The solitary type may occur in either sex, and most cases have occurred in the elderly. They may be associated with a cutaneous horn [6]. There is no evidence that actinic radiation or other recognized carcinogens are to blame.

Patients with multiple benign sebaceous tumours (other than sebaceous hyperplasia) should be suspected of having the Muir–Torre syndrome, associated with multiple visceral malignancies [7–18]. It is important to note, however, that a single sebaceous neoplasm and more uncommonly a sebaceous carcinoma particularly in an extraocular location may represent a marker of the syndrome [19]. It has also been demonstrated that a single sebaceous tumour outside the head and trunk is a strong indicator of the syndrome [20]. Muir–Torre syndrome is a rare subset of the hereditary non-polyposis colorectal carcinoma, representing 1–2% of cases of the latter [21,22]. It is characterized by cutaneous sebaceous tumours, gastrointestinal malignancies, especially colonic and, more rarely, renal, uterine and breast neoplasms [5]. The internal malignancies tend to be fairly low grade, and often patients develop them earlier in life than the equivalent neoplasm in the general population. Sebaceous neoplasms tend to develop later in life. Patients with Muir–Torre syndrome may also develop sebaceous keratoacanthomas [20], thus diagnosis of one of these tumours should raise the possibility of the syndrome. Microsatellite instability has been reported in the Muir–Torre syndrome [23,24], which results in the loss of a number of mismatch repair proteins particularly MLH1 and MSH2 and less commonly MSH6. Loss of expression of these proteins is a marker of patients who carry the syndrome and are therefore at risk of systemic malignancy [25,26]. The loss of expression of MLH1, MSH2 and MSH6 may be demonstrated by immunohistochemical methods [25]. In Muir–Torre syndrome, MSH2 is lost 10 times more frequently than MLH1 [21].

Clinical features. Tumours are usually rounded, raised and either sessile or somewhat pedunculated (Fig. 53.8). They are normally less than 10 mm in diameter, but older lesions may form plaques or ulcerate. Occasional tumours are more deeply located and appear cystic. The colour is fleshy or of a waxy, yellowish hue,

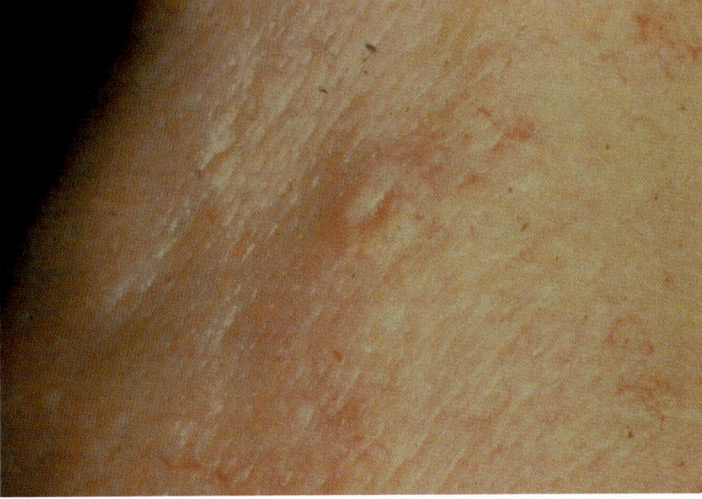

Fig. 53.8 Sebaceous adenoma. Small, yellowish papule.

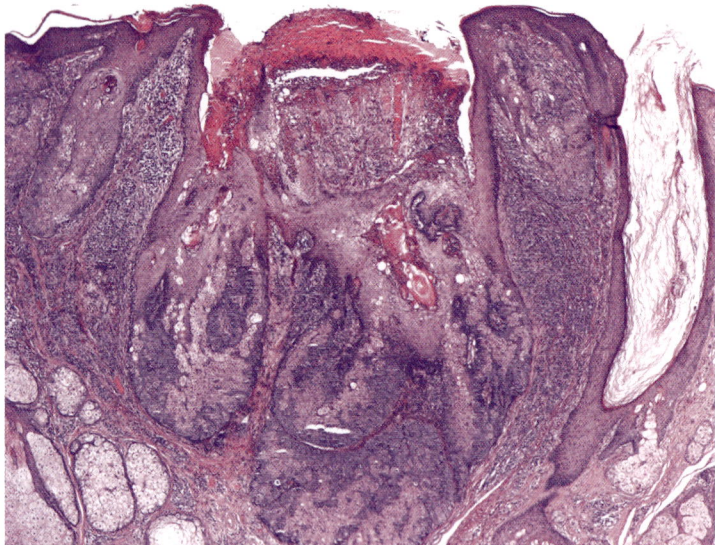

Fig. 53.9 Sebaceous adenoma. Lobular lesion with prominent maturation in the centre and immature cells in the periphery.

and the surface may be papilliferous. The common situation is the face or scalp, and it may occur on the eyelid. It usually grows slowly, but a sudden increase in growth rate can occur.

Diagnosis. A yellow-tinged facial nodule may be suggestive, but clinical differentiation from other epithelial tumours, especially basal cell carcinoma, may be impossible. The microscopic diagnosis is more certain when fat can be demonstrated, but sebaceous differentiation can usually be distinguished in ordinary sections.

Pathology [3,6,15,27]. The tumours are multilobular and usually connected to the epidermis. The lobules are well-defined, composed of variable numbers of small, basophilic, sebaceous matrix cells peripherally and larger cells—mature sebaceous cells—containing cytoplasmic fat globules. The proportion of immature, transitional and mature sebaceous cells may vary widely from one area to another. In sebaceous adenoma, mature sebaceous cells predominate in the centre of the lobules (Fig. 53.9), whilst in sebaceoma, immature basaloid sebaceous cells predominate, occupying large areas of the lobules. In both tumours, there may also be cystic spaces lined by a thin layer of eosinophilic material similar to the intraglandular sebaceous ducts. The outline of the tumour is less regular than normal sebaceous glands, and may be irregular. However, some sebaceous adenomas closely mimic the normal sebaceous gland, except for an increase in the number of immature sebaceous cells. Mitotic figures are frequent in the immature sebaceous cells, and this feature should not be regarded as evidence of malignancy. Larger and deeper tumours with cystic degeneration usually represent sebaceomas, but adenomas may also be seen. Some of these tumours have atypical histological features [28]. The cystic space contains abundant holocrine (sebaceous) material. It has been suggested that these cystic sebaceous tumours are a marker for the mismatch, repair-deficient subtype of Muir–Torre syndrome, which has a high risk of internal malignancies [28]. However, a more recent study although demonstrating that sebaceous keratoacanthomas are often associated with the syn-

drome failed to show the same correlation with cystic sebaceous neoplasms [20]. Glandular apocrine differentiation may occur rarely in some sebaceous neoplasms [29].

Treatment. The best treatment is surgical excision. Patients with tumours showing loss of expression of mismatch proteins should be screened for internal malignancy, particularly of the colon.

References

1 Prioleau PG, Santa Cruz DJ. Sebaceous gland neoplasms. *J Cutan Pathol* 1984; **11**: 396–414.

2 Lever WF. Sebaceous adenoma: review of the literature and report of a case. *Arch Dermatol Syphilol* 1948; **57**: 102–11.

3 Troy JL, Ackerman AB. Sebaceoma: a distinctive benign neoplasm of adnexal epithelium differentiating toward sebaceous cells. *Am J Dermatopathol* 1984; **6**: 7–13.

4 Dineen AM, Mehregan DR. Sebaceous epithelioma: a review of 21 cases. *J Am Acad Dermatol* 1996; **34**: 47–50.

5 Lazar AJF, Lyle S, Calonje E. Sebaceous neoplasia and Torre–Muir syndrome. *Curr Diagn Pathol* 2007; **13**: 301–19.

6 Thornton CM, Hunt SJ. Sebaceous adenoma with a cutaneous horn. *J Cutan Pathol* 1995; **22**: 185–7.

7 Muir EG, Yates-Bell AJ, Barlow KA. Multiple primary carcinomata of the colon, duodenum and larynx associated with keratoacanthoma of the face. *Br J Surg* 1967; **54**: 191–5.

8 Bakker PM, Tjon A, Joe SS. Multiple sebaceous gland tumours, with multiple tumours of internal organs: a new syndrome? *Dermatologica* 1971; **142**: 50–7.

9 Banse-Kupin L, Morales A, Barlow M. Torre's syndrome. *J Am Acad Dermatol* 1984; **10**: 803–17.

10 Burgdorf WHC, Pitha J, Fahmy A. Muir–Torre syndrome: histologic spectrum of sebaceous proliferation. *Am J Dermatopathol* 1986; **8**: 202–8.

11 Fathizadeh A, Medenica MM, Soltani K et al. Aggressive keratoacanthoma and internal malignant neoplasm. *Arch Dermatol* 1982; **118**: 112–4.

12 Finan MC, Connolly SM. Sebaceous gland tumors and systemic disease: a clinicopathologic analysis. *Medicine* 1984; **63**: 232–42.

13 Graham R, McKee P, McGibbon D et al. Torre–Muir syndrome: an association with isolated sebaceous carcinoma. *Cancer* 1985; **55**: 2868–73.

14 Lynch HT, Fusaro RM, Roberts L et al. Muir–Torre syndrome in several members of a family with a variant of the cancer family syndrome. *Br J Dermatol* 1985; **113**: 295–301.

15 Rulon DB, Helwig EB. Multiple sebaceous neoplasms of the skin: an association with multiple visceral carcinomas, especially of the colon. *Am J Clin Pathol* 1973; **60**: 745–52.

16 Schwartz RA, Torre DP. The Muir–Torré syndrome: a 25-year retrospect. *J Am Acad Dermatol* 1995; **33**: 90–104.

17 Torré D. Multiple sebaceous tumors. *Arch Dermatol* 1968; **98**: 549–51.

18 Worret WJ, Burgdorf WHC, Fahmi A et al. Torre–Muir syndrome. *Hautarzt* 1981; **32**: 519–24.

19 Donati P. Solitary sebaceoma in Muire–Torre syndrome. *Int J Dermatol* 1996; **35**: 601–2.

20 Singh RS, Grayson W, Redston M et al. Site and tumor type predicts DNA mismatch repair status in cutaneous sebaceous neoplasia. *Am J Surg Pathol* 2008; **32**: 936–42.

21 Mangold E, Pagenstecher C, Leister M et al. A genotype-phenotype correlation in HNPCC: strong predominance of msh2 mutations in 41 patients with Muir–Torre syndrome. *J Med Genet* 2004; **41**: 567–72.

22 Barana D, van der Klift H, Wijnen J et al. Spectrum of genetic alterations in Muir–Torre syndrome is the same as in HNPCC. *Am J Med Genet* 2004; **125**: 318–9.

23 Honchel R, Halling KC, Schaid DJ et al. Microsatellite instability in the Muir–Torre syndrome. *Cancer Res* 1994; **54**: 1159–63.

24 Southey MC, Young MA, Whitty J et al. Molecular pathologic analysis enhances diagnosis and management of the Muir–Torre syndrome and gives an insight into its underlying molecular pathogenesis. *Am J Surg Pathol* 2001; **25**: 936–41.

25 Mathiak M, Rutten A, Mangold E et al. Loss of DNA mismatch repair proteins from patients with Muir–Torre syndrome: establishment of immunohistochemical analysis as a screening test. *Am J Surg Pathol* 2002; **26**: 338–43.

26 Machin P, Catasus L, Pons C *et al.* Microsatellite instability and immunostaining for MSH-2 and MLH-1 in cutaneous and internal tumors from patients with the Muir–Torre syndrome. *J Cutan Pathol* 2002; **29**: 415–20.

27 Misago N, Mihara I, Ansai S *et al.* Sebaceoma and related neoplasms with sebaceous differentiation: a clinicopathologic study of 30 cases. *Am J Dermatopathol* 2002; **24**: 294–304.

28 Rutten A, Burgdorf W, Hugel H *et al.* Cystic sebaceous tumors as marker lesions for the Muir–Torre syndrome: a histopathologic and molecular genetic study. *Am J Dermatopathol* 1999; **21**: 405–13.

29 Kazakov DV, Calonje E, Rütten A *et al.* Cutaneous sebaceous neoplasms with a focal glandular pattern (seboapocrine lesions): a clinicopathological study of three cases. *Am J Dermatopathol* 2007; **29**: 359–64.

Superficial epithelioma with sebaceous differentiation [1–4]

This is a rare tumour that has no distinctive clinical features and presents as a solitary papule on the face or trunk of adults. Occasionally, lesions are multiple. Histological features consist of a multifocal, plate-like proliferation of basaloid cells with focal sebaceous differentiation and connections to the epidermis.

References
1 Rothko K, Farmer ER, Zeligman I. Superficial epithelioma with sebaceous differentiation. *Arch Dermatol* 1980; **116**: 329–31.

2 Kato N, Ueno H. Superficial epithelioma with sebaceous differentiation. *J Dermatol* 1992; **19**: 190–4.

3 Vaughan TK, Sau P. Superficial epithelioma with sebaceous differentiation. *J Am Acad Dermatol* 1990; **23**: 760–2.

4 Friedman KJ, Boudreau S, Farmer ER. Superficial epithelioma with sebaceous differentiation. *J Cutan Pathol* 1987; **14**: 193–7.

Sebaceous carcinoma [1–3]

Definition. A malignant tumour composed of cells showing differentiation toward sebaceous epithelium.

Incidence. The variable incidence reported for this tumour reflects the differing diagnostic criteria of different workers. It is, however, rare, comprising less than 1% of all skin malignancies. The tumour has been reported following radiodermatitis [4], and in a patient with multiple arsenical skin cancers. Lesions may rarely occur in naevus sebaceus [5]. It is likely that a number of sebaceomas with high mitotic activity have been reported in the past as sebaceous carcinomas.

Clinical features [6–14]. Most lesions occur in middle-aged and particularly old individuals. Exceptional cases have been reported in children [15]. The tumour is solitary, firm, sometimes translucent and covered with normal or slightly verrucose epidermis. The colour may be yellow or orange. The face and scalp [16] are the commonest sites, especially the eyelid (Fig. 53.10). The evolution may be very slow, and a size of 5 cm or more may be reached after many years without metastasis. Some tumours grow rapidly and invade early, but metastasis is uncommon [17,18]. In the absence of the yellow colour there is no feature to indicate the diagnosis clinically. Sebaceous carcinomas may occur in immunosuppressed organ-transplant patients, and these tumours are associated with microsatellite instability [19]. Sebaceous carcinoma may be associated with the Muir–Torre syndrome [20]. The latter association is

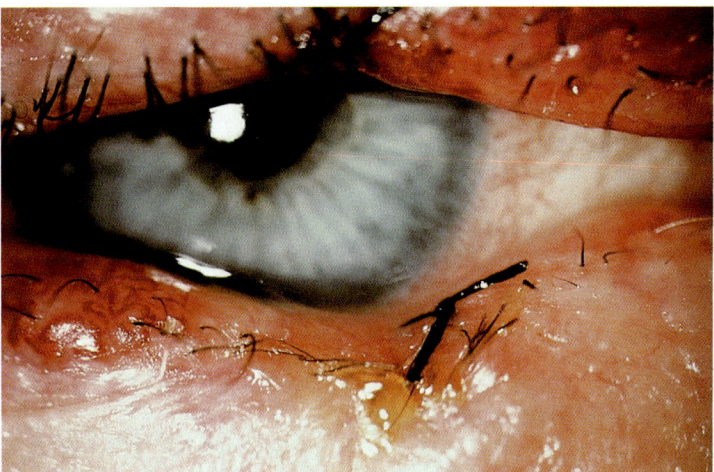

Fig. 53.10 Sebaceous carcinoma. Ulcerated, yellowish lesion of the eyelid.

mainly seen with extraocular carcinomas and those tumours occurring outside the head and neck area [21].

Pathology. The same problem of terminology exists with sebaceous carcinoma as with the adenomas. Basal cell carcinoma with sebaceous differentiation is not included in the description of sebaceous carcinoma. It is uncommon for the lesion to be aggressively invasive on the skin, although it frequently is when situated on the eyelid [6–10]. There are, however, individual case reports of aggressive lesions with occasional metastatic spread [22,23].

The essential feature is cytological evidence of sebaceous differentiation. The proportion of cells showing fat globules and the degree of cytoplasmic vacuolation are variable. The undifferentiated cells are of moderate size, with round, centrally placed nuclei and rather basophilic cytoplasm, and they tend to group themselves in masses of a multilobular configuration. The differentiating cells tend to be more central. There are, in addition, cytological features of malignancy and evidence of an infiltrative growth pattern. Mitotic figures including atypical forms are frequent. Pagetoid infiltration of the epidermis is frequent, particularly in tumours arising around the eye [6].

Treatment. Complete surgical excision is required [12,24]. Reports of excellent results with Mohs surgery suggest that this may be the treatment of choice [25].

References
1 Nelson BR, Hamlet KR, Gillard M *et al.* Sebaceous carcinoma. *J Am Acad Dermatol* 1995; **33**: 1–15.

2 Prioleau PG, Santa Cruz DJ. Sebaceous gland neoplasia. *J Cutan Pathol* 1984; **11**: 396–414.

3 Wick MR, Goellner JR, Wolfe JT III *et al.* Adnexal carcinomas of the skin, 2: extraocular sebaceous carcinomas. *Cancer* 1985; **56**: 1163–72.

4 Hood IC, Oizilbash AH, Salama SS *et al.* Sebaceous carcinoma of the face following irradiation. *Am J Dermatopathol* 1986; **8**: 505–8.

5 Kazakov DV, Calonje E, Zelger B *et al.* Sebaceous carcinoma arising in nevus sebaceous of Jadassohn: a clinicopathological study of five cases. *Am J Dermatopathol* 2007; **29**: 242–8.

6 Dixons RS, Mikhail GR, Slater HC. Sebaceous carcinoma of the eyelid. *J Am Acad Dermatol* 1980; **3**: 241–3.

7 Doxanas MT, Green WR. Sebaceous gland carcinoma: a review of 40 cases. *Arch Ophthalmol* 1984; **102**: 245–9.

8 Rulon DB, Helwig EB. Cutaneous sebaceous neoplasms. *Cancer* 1974; **33**: 83–102.

9 Urban FH, Winkelmann RK. Sebaceous malignancy. *Arch Dermatol* 1961; **84**: 63–72.

10 Russell WG, Hough AG, Rogers LW. Sebaceous carcinoma of Meibomian gland origin. *Am J Clin Pathol* 1980; **73**: 504–11.

11 Graham R, McKee P, McGibbon D. Torre–Muir syndrome: an association with isolated sebaceous carcinoma. *Cancer* 1985; **55**: 2868–73.

12 Hernández-Pérez E, Baños E. Sebaceous carcinoma: report of two cases with metastasis. *Dermatologica* 1978; **156**: 184–8.

13 Justi RA. Sebaceous carcinoma. *Arch Dermatol* 1958; **77**: 195–200.

14 Rao NA, Hidayat AA, McLeon IW. Sebaceous carcinomas of the ocular adnexa: a clinicopathologic study of 104 cases, with five-year follow-up data. *Hum Pathol* 1982; **13**: 113–22.

15 Omura NE, Collison DW, Perry AE *et al.* Sebaceous carcinoma in children. *J Am Acad Dermatol* 2002; **47**: 950–3.

16 Mellette JR, Amonette RA, Gardner JH *et al.* Carcinoma of sebaceous glands on the head and neck. *J Dermatol Surg Oncol* 1981; **7**: 404–7.

17 King DT, Hirose FM, Gurevitch AW. Sebaceous carcinoma of the skin with visceral metastases. *Arch Dermatol* 1979; **115**: 862–3.

18 Leonard DD, Deaton WR Jr. Multiple sebaceous gland tumors and visceral carcinomas. *Arch Dermatol* 1974; **110**: 917–20.

19 Harwood CA, Swale VJ, Bataille VA *et al.* An association between sebaceous carcinoma and microsatellite instability in immunosuppressed organ transplant recipients. *J Invest Dermatol* 2001; **116**: 246–53.

20 Schwartz RA, Torre DP. The Muir–Torre syndrome: a 25-year retrospect. *J Am Acad Dermatol* 1995; **33**: 90–104.

21 Singh RS, Grayson W, Redston M *et al.* Site and tumor type predicts DNA mismatch repair status in cutaneous sebaceous neoplasia. *Am J Surg Pathol* 2008; **32**: 936–42.

22 Moreno C, Jacyk WK, Judd MJ *et al.* Highly aggressive extraocular sebaceous carcinoma. *Am J Dermatopathol* 2001; **23**: 450–5.

23 Duman DG, Ceyhan BB, Celikel T *et al.* Extraorbital sebaceous carcinoma with rapidly developing visceral metastases. *Dermatol Surg* 2003; **29**: 987–9.

24 Dowd MB, Kumar RJ, Sharma R *et al.* Diagnosis and management of sebaceous carcinoma: an Australian experience. *ANZ J Surg* 2008; **78**: 158–63.

25 Spencer JM, Nossa R, Tse DT *et al.* Sebaceous carcinoma of the eyelid treated by Mohs micrographic surgery. *J Am Acad Dermatol* 2001; **44**: 1004–9.

Apocrine gland tumours [1]

Apocrine hidrocystoma [2]

Synonym
- Apocrine cystadenoma

Definition. A lesion produced by cystic dilatation of apocrine secretory glands. Although the terms apocrine hidrocystoma and cystadenoma have been used as synonyms, and the clinical features of both lesions are identical, there are a number of histological findings that set them apart (see below).

Incidence. The lesion is not uncommon, but is most often seen in ophthalmological or surgical clinics. It occurs in adult life, in no particular age group. Males and females are equally affected.

Clinical features [3–6]. The lesions are solitary or occasionally multiple, well-defined, dome-shaped, translucent nodules [7]. The surface is smooth and the colour varies from a skin colour to greyish or blue-black; pigmentation may affect only part of the cyst. The commonest site is around the eye, particularly lateral to the outer canthus (Fig. 53.11). It has also been reported on the

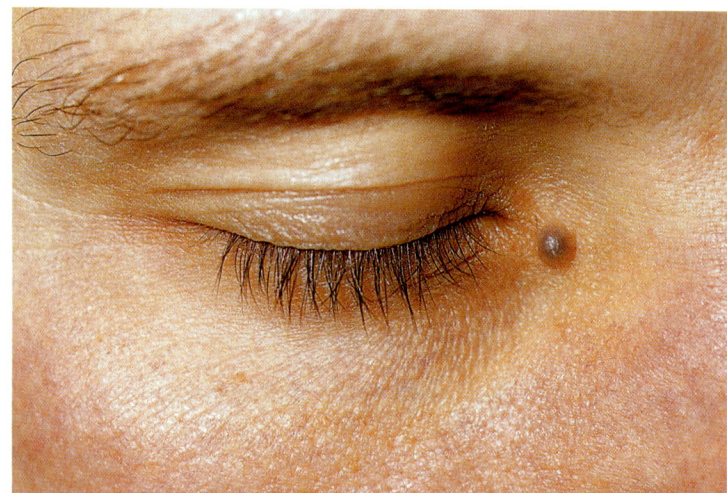

Fig. 53.11 Apocrine hidrocystoma. Cystic, translucent papule on the right inner canthus.

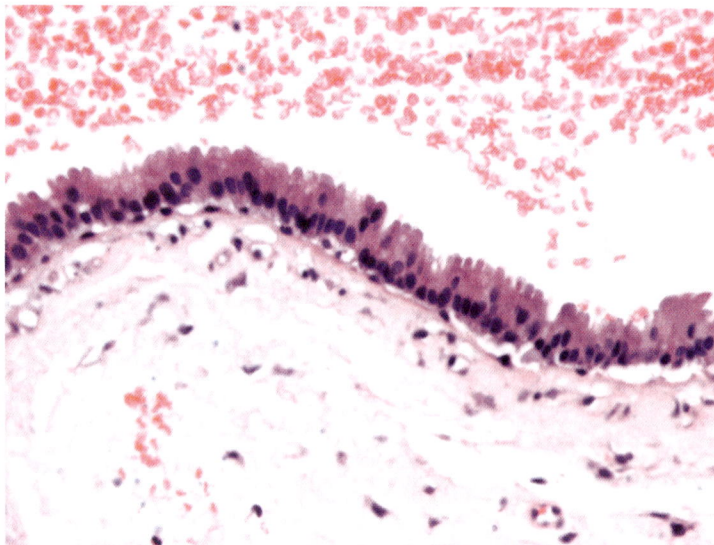

Fig. 53.12 Apocrine hidrocystoma. Cystic cavity lined by cuboidal cells with pink cytoplasm and decapitation secretion.

penis [1], fingers [8] and multiple lesions bilaterally in both axillae [9]. There are no symptoms. The cyst increases slowly in size, and may become 10 mm or more in diameter. Multiple lesions may be seen in Schöpf–Schulz–Passarge syndrome (a form of ectodermal dysplasia syndrome characterized by hypotrichosis, hypodontia, nail dystrophy, palmoplantar keratoderma and periocular apocrine hidrocystomas) [10].

Pathology [11–13]. Large cystic cavities are found in the dermis if the lesion has been carefully dissected out. Commonly, the cyst is punctured and has collapsed before fixation. The cavities are lined by cuboidal or high-columnar apocrine secretory cells with decapitation secretion and a peripheral layer of myoepithelial cells (Fig. 53.12). Papillary projections or solid buds of secretory cells may break the smooth contour of the cyst lining. The secretory cells may contain pigment [5,6], which is neither melanin nor haemosiderin. The secretions in the cysts may be coagulated and stained using the PAS technique. There is a well-organized fibrous stroma. Electron microscopy confirms the apocrine nature of the secretory epithelium [14]. Lesions designated as apocrine cystadenoma are regarded as proliferative lesions with true papillary projections (containing a fibrous core) and often display focal cytological atypia and mitotic activity. Based on these atypical features in cystadenoma, complete excision is suggested for tumours classified as such [15].

Diagnosis. Basal cell carcinoma is usually of a firmer consistency, less regular in its surface contour, and has surface telangiectases. The cystic nature of the lesion, which can often be shown by transillumination, separates it from blue naevi and malignant melanoma when pigment is present.

Treatment. The tumour is cured by surgical removal, which is commonly also needed for diagnosis. Other treatment modalities are the same as those used for eccrine hidrocystomas (see p. 53.22). Multiple lesions have been treated successfully with trichloroacetic acid [16].

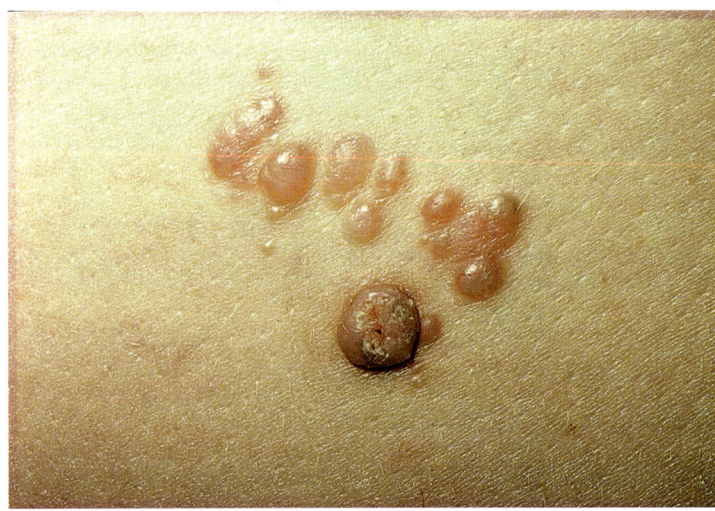

Fig. 53.13 Syringocystadenoma papilliferum. Papular lesion with superficial erosion.

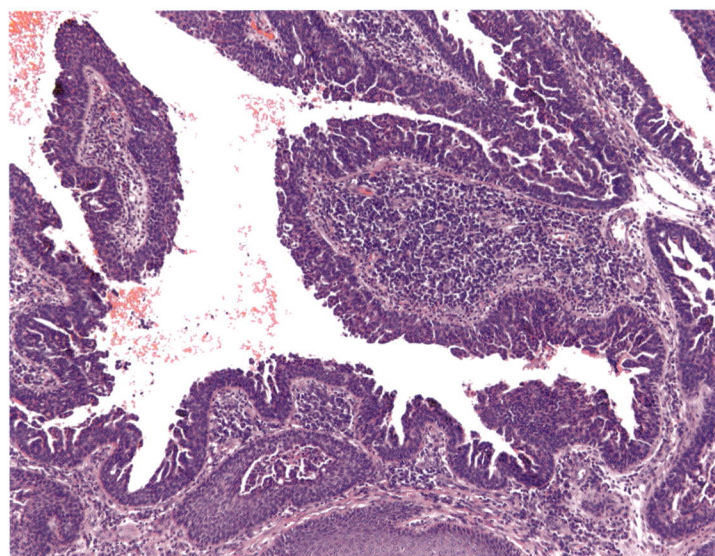

Fig. 53.14 Syringocystadenoma papilliferum. Papillary projections with a fibrovascular stroma.

References

1 Warkel RL. Selected apocrine neoplasms. *J Cutan Pathol* 1984; **11**: 437–49.
2 Hashimoto K, Lever WF. *Appendage Tumors of the Skin*. Springfield: Thomas, 1968: 52–4.
3 Benisch B, Peison B. Apocrine hidrocystoma of the shoulder. *Arch Dermatol* 1977; **113**: 71–2.
4 Hassan MO, Khan MA, Kruse TV. Apocrine cystadenoma. *Arch Dermatol* 1979; **115**: 194–200.
5 Smith JD, Chernosky ME. Apocrine hidrocystoma (cystadenoma). *Arch Dermatol* 1974; **109**: 700–2.
6 Mehregan AH. Apocrine cystadenoma. *Arch Dermatol* 1964; **90**: 274–9.
7 Schaumburg-Lever G, Lever WF. Secretion from human apocrine glands. *J Invest Dermatol* 1975; **64**: 38–41.
8 De Fontaine S, Van Geertruyden J, Vandeweyer E. Apocrine hidrocystoma of the finger. *J Hand Surg (Br)* 1998; **25**: 182–4.
9 Obaidat NA, Ghazarian DM. Bilateral multiple axillary apocrine hidrocystomas associated with benign apocrine hyperplasia. *J Cutan Pathol* 2006; **59**: 779.
10 Hampton PJ, Angus B, Carmichael AJ. A case of Schöpf–Schulz–Passarge syndrome. *Clin Exp Dermatol* 2005; **30**: 528–30.
11 Cramer HJ. Das schwarze Hidrocystom (Monfort). *Dermatol Monatsschr* 1980; **166**: 114–8.
12 Malhotra R, Bhawan J. The nature of the pigment in pigmented apocrine hidrocystoma. *J Cutan Pathol* 1985; **12**: 106–9.
13 Gross BG. The fine structure of apocrine hidrocystoma. *Arch Dermatol* 1965; **92**: 706–12.
14 Kruse TV, Khan MA, Hassan MO. Multiple apocrine cystadenomas. *Br J Dermatol* 1979; **100**: 675–81.
15 Sugiyama A, Sugiura M, Piris A *et al*. Apocrine cystadenoma and apocrine hidrocystoma: examination of 21 cases with emphasis on nomenclature according to proliferative features. *J Cutan Pathol* 2007; **34**: 912–7.
16 Dailey RA, Saulny SM, Tower RN. Treatment of multiple apocrine hidrocystomas with trichloroacetic acid. *Ophthal Plast Reconstr Surg* 2005; **21**: 148–50.

Syringocystadenoma papilliferum [1,2]

Definition. An exuberant proliferating lesion, commonly seen on the scalp in association with an organoid naevus, and showing differentiation in an apocrine pattern [3].

Clinical features [4]. These lesions may be present at birth or in childhood [5], but the majority are seen on the face and scalp of young adults. There is frequently a history of papillomatous expansion of a small pre-existing lesion at or around puberty and lesions often occur in a pre-existing organoid naevus. The lesion is composed of multiple warty papules, some of which are translucent and pigmented (Fig. 53.13). Tumours may be seen in other locations including the vulva [6], external ear [7], lower leg [8], scrotum [9] and breast [10].

Pathology [11–14]. The epidermal surface shows papillomatous expansion, and from these areas cystic invaginations are seen. The cystic structures are lined by papillae that have a lining of a double layer of columnar epithelium, which shows an apocrine pattern of secretion (Fig. 53.14) [15,16]. The underlying stroma is rich in plasma cells [17]. Sebaceous differentiation may occasionally be seen [18]. Occasionally, basal cell carcinoma, a squamous cell carcinoma (including verrucous carcinoma) [19] or a ductal carcinoma [20] develops on a pre-existing syringocystadenoma papilliferum. *In-situ* carcinoma [21] and invasive apocrine carcinoma are exceptional. Molecular biological studies have identified loss of heterozygosity at chromosome 9q22, the locus of the patched gene [22]. Superficial lesions on apocrine tubular adenoma (see below) may overlap histologically with those of syringocystadenoma papilliferum [23].

Management. Surgical excision is recommended, both to confirm the diagnosis and for cosmetic reasons.

References

1 Hashimoto K, Lever WF. *Appendage Tumors of the Skin.* Springfield: Thomas, 1968: 47.
2 Pinkus H. Life history of naevus syringadenomatosus papilliferus. *Arch Dermatol Syphilol* 1954; **69**: 305–22.
3 Krinitz K. Naevus syringocystadenomatosus papilliferus in lineärer Anordnung. *Hautarzt* 1966; **17**: 260–5.
4 Lever WF. Pathogenesis of benign tumors of cutaneous appendages and of basal cell epithelioma. *Arch Dermatol Syphilol* 1948; **57**: 679–724.
5 Townsend TC, Bowen AR, Nobuhara KK. Syringocystadenoma papilliferum: an unusual cutaneous lesion in a pediatric patient. *J Pediatr* 2004; **145**: 131–3.
6 Al-Brahim N, Daya D, Alowami S. A 64-year-old woman with vulvar papule. Vulvar syringocystadenoma papilliferum. *Arch Pathol Lab Med* 2005; **129**: e126–7.
7 Kamakura T, Horii A, Mishiro Y *et al.* Magnetic resonance imaging of syringocystadenoma papilliferum of the external auditory canal. *Auris Nasus Larynx* 2006; **33**: 53–6.
8 Yoshii N, Kanekura T, Setoyama M *et al.* Syringocystadenoma papilliferum: report of the first case on the lower leg. *J Dermatol* 2004; **31**: 939–42.
9 Goshima J, Hara H, Okada T *et al.* Syringocystadenoma papilliferum arising on the scrotum. *Eur J Dermatol* 2003; **13**: 271.
10 Singh UR. Syringocystadenoma papilliferum mimicking breast carcinoma. *Am J Dermatopathol* 2000; **22**: 91.
11 Fusaro RM, Goltz RW. Histochemically demonstrable carbohydrates of appendageal tumors of the skin, 2: benign apocrine gland tumors. *J Invest Dermatol* 1962; **38**: 137–42.
12 Hashimoto K. Syringocystadenoma papilliferum: an electron microscopic study. *Arch Dermatol Forsch* 1972; **245**: 353–69.
13 Helwig EB, Hackney VC. Syringadenoma papilliferum. *Arch Dermatol* 1955; **71**: 361–72.
14 Landry M, Winkelmann RK. An unusual tubular apocrine adenoma. *Arch Dermatol* 1972; **105**: 869–79.
15 Mazoujian G, Margolis R. Immunohistochemical study of gross cystic disease fluid protein (GCDFP-15) in 65 benign sweat gland tumors of the skin. *Am J Dermatopathol* 1988; **10**: 28–35.
16 Niizuma K. Syringocystadenoma papilliferum: light and electron microscopic studies. *Acta Derm Venereol (Stockh)* 1976; **56**: 327–36.
17 Numata M, Hosoe S, Itoh N *et al.* Syringadenocarcinoma papilliferum. *J Cutan Pathol* 1985; **12**: 3–7.
18 Vazmitel M, Michal M, Mukensnabl P *et al.* Syringocystadenoma papilliferum with sebaceous differentiation in an intradermal tubular apocrine component. *Am J Dermatopathol* 2008; **30**: 51–3.
19 Montinniolo NL, Schmidt JD, Morgan MB. Verrucous carcinoma arising within syringocystadenoma papilliferum. *Ann Clin Lab Sci* 2002; **32**: 434–7.
20 Hügel H, Requena L. Ductal carcinoma arising from a syrincystadenoma papilliferum in a nevus sebaceous of Jadassohn. *Am J Dermatopathol* 2003; **25**: 490–3.
21 Arai Y, Kusakabe H, Kiyokane K. A case of syringocystadenocarcinoma papilliferum in situ occurring partially in syringocystadenoma papilliferum. *J Dermatol* 2003; **30**: 146–50.
22 Boni R, Xin H, Hohl D *et al.* Syringocystadenoma papilliferum: a study of potential tumor suppressor genes. *Am J Dermatopathol* 2001; **23**: 87–9.
23 Kazakov DV, Bisceglia M, Calonje E *et al.* Tubular adenoma and syringocystadenoma papilliferum: a reappraisal of their relationship. An interobserver study of a series, by a panel of dermatopathologists. *Am J Dermatopathol* 2007; **29**: 256–63.

Hidradenoma papilliferum

Definition. A skin tumour of the anogenital area of adult females, composed of frond-like papillae lined by apocrine epithelium.

Incidence. This is an uncommon tumour, which occurs predominantly in women. In one large series, the subjects were exclusively white, and 75% were between the ages of 25 and 40 years. It occurs four times as commonly on the vulva as in the perianal area [1].

Clinical features [2–4]. The patients usually seek advice for a lump in the vulval or perianal area, which may be symptomless or, less frequently, may be tender or liable to bleed. The tumour is rounded, freely mobile, often elevated and may feel firm, soft or even cystic. It may range in size from 1 to 40 mm. The commonest site is the labium majus, but it may occur elsewhere on the vulva or perianal area and, exceptionally, in other sites such as the eyelid [4,5], nose [6], arm [7] and chest [8]. Coexistence with a naevus comedonicus has been described [9].

Occasionally, the epithelial surface will ulcerate and the tumour becomes everted to form a reddish-brown papillary mass, which may be suspected of being malignant [1]. Malignant transformation, however, has not been reported.

Pathology. The tumour is well-circumscribed and located just below the skin surface. It is usually spherical in shape and enclosed by compressed connective tissue stroma. Lesions are composed partly of slender fronds of connective tissue lined by one or two layers of epithelial cells, and partly of glandular structures (Fig. 53.15). The epithelial cells have histochemical characteristics in keeping with an apocrine origin [10,11]. Sebaceous differentiation is seen occasionally [5]. Mitotic figures vary and may be frequent. In the absence of other features indicative of malignancy, the mitotic count does not imply malignant behaviour [12]. Rare cases overlap with syringocystadenoma papilliferum [13].

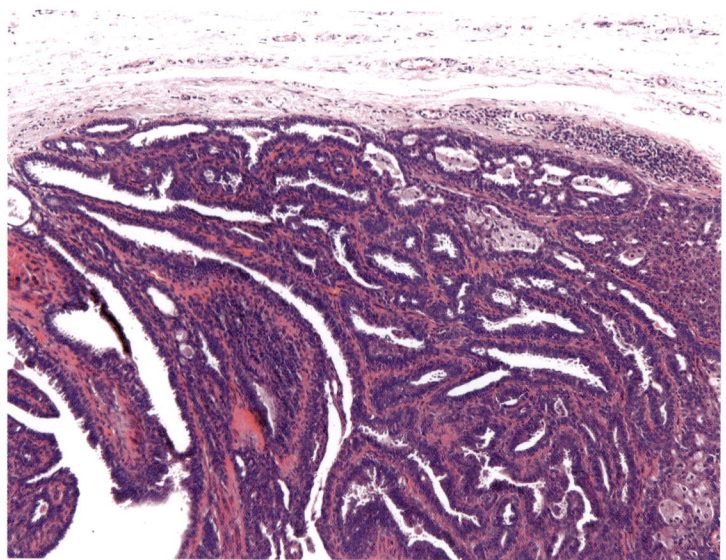

Fig. 53.15 Hidradenoma papilliferum. Well-circumscribed tumour with glands and papillary projections displaying apocrine differentiation.

Diagnosis. The tumour is usually mistaken for a cyst, polyp, angioma or haemorrhoid. A prolonged history and a firm, spherical form make the last three diagnoses unlikely.

Treatment. Simple excision is curative.

References

1 Shenoy YMV. Malignant perianal papillary hidradenoma. *Arch Dermatol* 1961; **83**: 965–7.
2 Meeker HJ, Neubecker RD, Helwig EG. Hidradenoma papilliferum. *Am J Clin Pathol* 1962; **37**: 182–95.
3 Virgili A, Marzola A, Corazza M. Vulvar hidradenoma papilliferum. A review of 10.5 years' experience. *J Reprod Med* 2000; **45**: 616–8.
4 Santa Cruz DJ, Prioleau PG, Smith ME. Hidradenoma papilliferum of the eyelid. *Arch Dermatol* 1981; **117**: 55–6.
5 Minami S, Sadanobu N, Ito T *et al*. Non-anogenital (ectopic) hidradenoma papilliferum with sebaceous differentiation: a case report and review of reported cases. *J Dermatol* 2006; **33**: 256–9.
6 Smith FB, Shemen LJ, Guerreri C *et al*. Hidradenoma papilliferum of nasal skin. *Arch Pathol Lab Med* 2003; **127**: E86–8.
7 Vang R, Cohen PR. Ectopic hidradenoma papilliferum: a case report and review of the literature. *J Am Acad Dermatol* 1999; **41**: 115–8.
8 Tanaka M, Shimizu S. Hidradenoma papilliferum occurring on the chest of a man. *J Am Acad Dermatol* 2003; **48**: S20–1.
9 Lee HJ, Chun EY, Kim YC *et al*. Nevus comedonicus with hidradenoma papilliferum and syringocystadenoma papilliferum in the female genital area. *Int J Dermatol* 2002; **41**: 933–6.
10 Hashimoto K. Hidradenoma papilliferum: an electron microscopic study. *Acta Derm Venereol (Stockh)* 1973; **53**: 22–30.
11 Tappeiner J, Wolff K. Hidradenoma papilliferum. Eine enzym-histochemische und elektronenmikroskopische Studie. *Hautarzt* 1969; **19**: 101–9.
12 Sington J, Chandrapala R, Manek S *et al*. Mitotic count is not predictive of clinical behavior in hidradenoma papilliferum of the vulva: a clinicopathologic study of 19 cases. *Am J Dermatopathol* 2006; **28**: 322–6.
13 Nishie W, Sawamura D, Mayuzumi M *et al*. Hidradenoma papilliferum with mixed histological features of syrincystadenoma papilliferum and anogenital mammary-like glands. *J Cutan Pathol* 2004; **31**: 561–4.

For erosive adenomatosis of the nipple, see Chapter 70.

Apocrine tubular adenoma [1–3]

Definition. A rare tumour usually arising on the scalp.

Clinical features. These are usually large, slowly expanding lesions on the scalp. The lesion often arises in association with a naevus sebaceus.

Pathology. Clusters of tubular structures are seen in the dermis, with a lining of cells showing decapitation secretion. There is no surrounding inflammatory response. Cytological atypia and an infiltrative margin are absent. As with many adnexal tumours, often one finds histological overlap between tubular apocrine adenoma and papillary eccrine adenoma [3,4]. Overlapping features with syringocystadenoma papilliferum are also seen, especially in superficial tumours [5].

References

1 Warkel RL, Helwig EB. Apocrine gland adenoma and adenocarcinoma of the axilla. *Arch Dermatol* 1978; **114**: 198–203.
2 Toribio J, Zulaica A, Peteiro C. Tubular apocrine adenoma. *J Cutan Pathol* 1987; **14**: 114–7.
3 Fox SB, Cotton D. Tubular apocrine adenoma and papillary eccrine adenoma: entities or unity? *Am J Dermatopathol* 1992; **14**: 149–54.
4 Ishiko A, Shimizu H, Inamoto N *et al*. Is tubular apocrine adenoma a distinct clinical entity? *Am J Dermatopathol* 1993; **15**: 482–7.
5 Kazakov DV, Bisceglia M, Calonje E *et al*. Tubular adenoma and syringcystadenoma papilliferum: a reappraisal of their relationship. An interobserver study of a series, by a panel of dermatopathologists. *Am J Dermatopathol* 2007; **29**: 256–63.

Apocrine carcinoma [1–3]

Definition. A malignant adnexal carcinoma showing clear evidence of apocrine differentiation—large cells with abundant pink cytoplasm and decapitation secretion.

Clinical features. This is a rare entity. Lesions have been reported mainly from the head and neck area, including the eyelid and external ear, anogenital skin and also the axilla [4]. It is not possible on morphological grounds or with the help of immunohistochemistry to separate a cutaneous axillary apocrine carcinoma from an apocrine breast carcinoma spreading or invading the skin by direct extension. It is therefore always important to rule out a primary breast tumour. Some tumours arise within a naevus sebaceus [5,6]. The tumour presents as a nodule, usually measuring more than 1 cm in diameter. Rare cases may be bilateral [7]. There is a slight predilection for females, and patients are middle-aged or elderly. Metastatic spread to regional lymph nodes and internal organs occurs in between 20 to 30% of the cases [6,8].

Pathology. Three histological patterns may be seen: tubular, tubulopapillary and solid (Fig. 53.16). The degree of differentiation varies, and the diagnosis is often difficult in poorly differentiated tumours. Mitotic figures, local invasion and nuclear pleomorphism all suggest a malignant lesion. The most specific pathological feature is the presence of decapitation secretion [1].

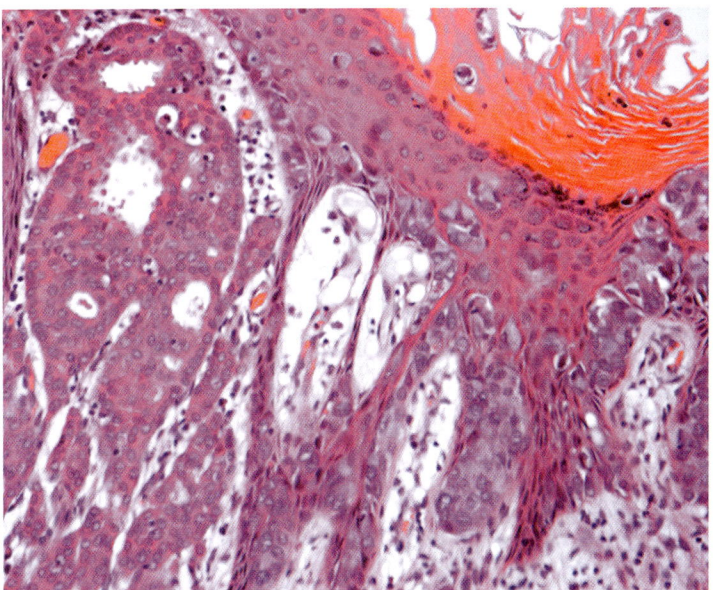

Fig. 53.16 Apocrine carcinoma. Prominent glands with decapitation secretion. Note the epidermotropism.

Some cases are associated with prominent pagetoid spread, particularly those presenting on genital skin [9]. Tumour cells are positive for gross cystic disease fluid protein-15 (GCDFP-15) [10], and they show positivity for oestrogen, progesterone and androgen receptors in up to a third of cases [6].

Treatment. It has been found that grading tumours according to the modified Bloom–Richardson method of grading breast carcinoma is very useful in establishing prognosis [6]. Patients with grade 3 tumours have a poor prognosis [6]. Wide excision and close follow-up are required. Based on the similarities between breast and apocrine carcinoma it may be of benefit to treat patients with high risk tumours and positivity for steroid receptors with medications such as tamoxifen [6].

References
1 Cooper PH. Carcinomas of the sweat glands. *Pathol Annu* 1987; **22**: 83–124.
2 Katagiri Y, Ansai S. Two cases of cutaneous apocrine ductal carcinoma of the axilla: case report and review of the literature. *Dermatology* 1999; **199**: 332–7.
3 Chamberlain RS, Huber K, White JC, Travaglino-Parda R. Apocrine gland carcinoma of the axilla: review of the literature and recommendations for treatment. *Am J Clin Oncol* 1999; **22**: 98–101.
4 Shintaku M, Tsuta K, Yoshida H *et al.* Apocrine adenocarcinoma of the eyelid with aggressive biological behavior: report of a case. *Pathol Int* 2002; **52**: 169–73.
5 Jacyk WK, Requena L, Sánchez Yus E *et al.* Tubular apocrine carcinoma arising in a nevus sebaceous of Jadassohn. *Am J Dermatopathol* 1998; **20**: 389–92.
6 Robson A, Lazar AJF, Ben Nagi J *et al.* Primary cutaneous apocrine carcinoma. A clinico-pathologic analysis of 24 cases. *Am J Surg Pathol* 2008; **32**: 682–90.
7 Nishikawa Y, Tokusashi Y, Saito Y *et al.* Apocrine adenocarcinoma associated with hamartomatous apocrine gland hyperplasia of both axillae. *Am J Pathol* 1994; **18**: 832–6.
8 Paties C, Taccagni L, Papotti M *et al.* Apocrine carcinoma of the skin. *Cancer* 1993; **71**: 375–81.
9 Castelli E, Wollina U, Anzarone A *et al.* Extramammary Paget disease of the axilla associated with comedo-like apocrine carcinoma of the skin. *Am J Dermatopathol* 2002; **24**: 351–7.
10 Ansai S, Koseki S, Hozumi Y *et al.* An immunohistochemical study of lysozyme CD-15 and gross cystic disease fluid protein 15 in various skin tumours. *Am J Dermatopathol* 1995; **17**: 249–55.

Eccrine gland tumours [1]

Eccrine gland-derived lesions make up a large and relatively common group of appendage tumours. Hidroacanthoma simplex, dermal duct tumour and eccrine poromas form a fairly homogeneous family derived from eccrine duct and pore. However, there are clear examples of apocrine poroma. Eccrine syringofibradenoma probably also belongs in this subsection. Eccrine hidradenoma, although closely related, has features suggesting both secretory and ductal differentiation, which makes the term 'acrospiroma' misleading, thus is perhaps best kept in a separate category.

Malignant tumours of sweat glands are relatively rare, but important to recognize. Their morphology and behaviour are variable.

Reference
1 Weedon D. Eccrine tumours: a selective review. *J Cutan Pathol* 1984; **11**: 421–36.

Eccrine hidrocystoma [1–7]

Definition. A tumour produced by mature, deformed eccrine sweat units, whose secretions dilate the ducts. Lesions are usually situated on the face and are often multiple.

Incidence and aetiology. This is a rare tumour that occurs mainly in middle-aged women. It was formerly reported as being more common in those who had to work exposed to heat, such as cooks. A report indicating that the lesion is usually solitary and situated close to the eyelid underlines the problem of differentiating eccrine from apocrine hidrocystomas [1].

Clinical features [1]. The lesions are largely confined to the cheeks and eyelids. They are cystic, often blue in colour and there is frequently a history of enlargement when the skin is exposed to heat and flattening of the lesion when the skin is exposed to cold. Administration of atropine also induces disappearance of the cyst [5]. The lesions may be multiple and pigmented [6]. Exceptionally, multiple eccrine hidrocystomas have been reported in Graves' disease with resolution after treatment of the condition [8].

Pathology [2–4]. The general features are those of a dermal cystic lesion uni- or multilocular lined by two layers of cells. The inner layer of cells is columnar and the outer layer consists of elongated myoepithelial cells. In cases with prominent dilatation, the epithelium appears flattened. Distinction from apocrine hidrocystoma is based on the presence of decapitation secretion in the cells of the inner layer.

Treatment. Treatment may consist of topical atropine or scopolamine but this is usually discontinued due to side effects [9]. Electrodesiccation, carbon dioxide laser and pulse dye laser have been used with good results [7,10]. Excision produces satisfactory results.

References
1 Smith JD, Chernosky ME. Hidrocystomas. *Arch Dermatol* 1973; **108**: 676–9.
2 Cordero AA, Montes LF. Eccrine hidrocystoma. *J Cutan Pathol* 1976; **3**: 292–3.
3 Ebner J, Erlach E. Ekkrine Hidrozystome. *Dermatol Monatsschr* 1975; **161**: 739–44.
4 Herzberg JJ. Ekkrines Syringocystadenom. *Arch Klin Exp Dermatol* 1962; **214**: 600–21.
5 Sperling LC, Sakas EL. Eccrine hidrocystomas. *J Am Acad Dermatol* 1982; **7**: 763–70.
6 Bourke JF, Colloby P, Graham Brown RC. Multiple pigmented eccrine hydrocystomas. *J Am Acad Dermatol* 1996; **35**: 480–1.
7 Sarabi K, Khachemoune A. Hidrocystoma—a brief review. *MedGenMed* 2006; **8**: 57.
8 Kim YD, Lee EJ, Song MH *et al.* Multiple hidrocystomas associated with Graves' disease. *Int J Dermatol* 2002; **41**: 231–6.
9 Armstrong DK, Walsh MY, Corbett JR. Multiple facial eccrine hidrocystomas: effective topical therapy with atropine. *Br J Dermatol* 1998; **139**: 558–9.
10 Tanzi E, Alster T. Pulsed dye laser treatment of multiple eccrine hydrocystomas: a novel approach. *Dermatol Surg* 2001; **27**: 898–900.

Hidroacanthoma simplex [1–4]

Definition. An intraepidermal tumour derived from the eccrine duct epithelium, which could be considered an intradermal eccrine poroma.

Clinical features. Hidroacanthoma simplex is a verrucous plaque or ring with a hyperkeratotic usually brown surface. It often mimics a flat seborrhoeic keratosis. Ulceration or elevation of the lesion suggests a dermal component. From the few reports available, it appears that the limbs are more likely to be involved than the head or trunk.

Pathology. Nests of clearly discrete, small, rounded cells are seen within the normal epidermal cells. They are smaller and more cuboidal than surrounding keratinocytes and are rich in glycogen and the glycolytic enzymes. These lesions may be confused with intraepidermal or clonal seborrhoeic keratoses, demonstrating what has in the past been called the 'Borst–Jadassohn phenomenon' [5]. The individual cells in these lesions are larger and less rich in glycogen. However, for the diagnosis to be made, ductal differentiation should be demonstrated.

Management. Excision is recommended both to confirm the diagnosis and for management. Malignant change has been reported in hidroacanthoma simplex including pigmented and clear cell variants [6–10]. If malignant change occurs, wider excision and follow-up is advisable.

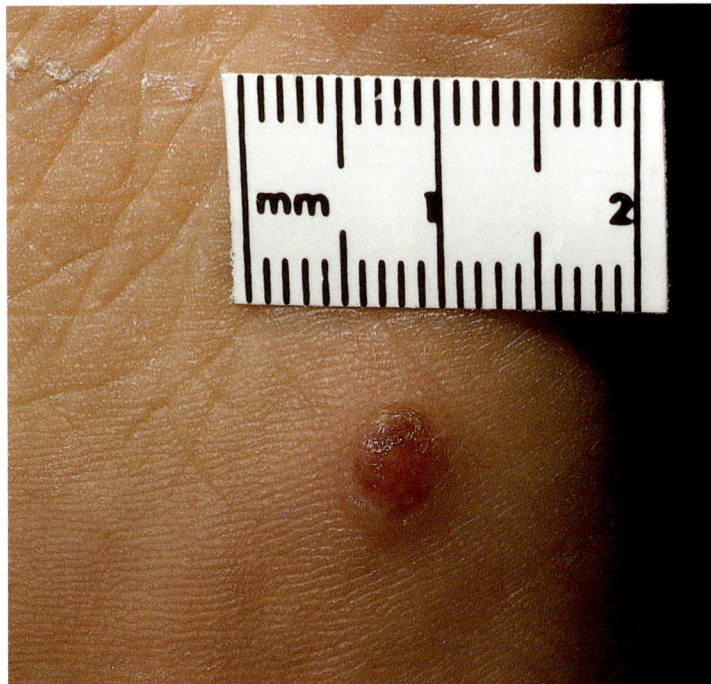

Fig. 53.17 Poroma. Note the red, shiny surface, which often leads to misdiagnosis of a pyogenic granuloma.

References
1 Smith JLS, Coburn JG. Hidroacanthoma simplex. *Br J Dermatol* 1956; **68**: 400–18.
2 Pernicario C, Muller SA, Zelickson BD, Snow JL. Hidroacanthoma simplex. *J Cutan Pathol* 1994; **21**: 274–9.
3 Rahbari H. Hidroacanthoma simplex. *Br J Dermatol* 1983; **109**: 219–25.
4 Anzai S, Arakawa S, Fujiwara S *et al.* Hidroacanthoma simplex: a case report and analysis of 70 Japanese cases. *Dermatology* 2005; **210**: 363–5.
5 Warner T, Goell W, Cripps D. Hidroacanthoma simplex: an ultrastructural study. *J Cutan Pathol* 1982; **9**: 189–95.
6 Ansai S, Koseki S, Hozumi Y *et al.* Malignant transformation of hidradenoma simplex. *Dermatology* 1994; **188**: 57–61.
7 Bardach H. Hidroacanthoma simplex with in situ porocarcinoma. *J Cutan Pathol* 1978; **5**: 236–48.
8 Piqué E, Olivares M, Espinel ML *et al.* Malignant hidroacanthoma simplex. *Dermatology* 1995; **190**: 72–6.
9 Lee JY, Lin MH. Pigmented malignant hidroacanthoma simplex mimicking irritated seborrhoeic keratosis. *J Cutan Pathol* 2006; **33**: 705–8.
10 Rütten A, Requena L, Requena C. Clear-cell porocarcinoma in situ: a cytologic variant of porocarcinoma in situ. *Am J Dermatopathol* 2002; **24**: 67–71.

Eccrine poroma [1,2]

Definition. A tumour arising from the eccrine duct epithelium in the epidermis (acrosyringium). Traditionally, all poromas have been regarded as eccrine. However, a number of lesions may show apocrine differentiation.

Clinical features [1–11]. This lesion is one of the easiest of the appendage tumours to recognize in the clinic. The great majority of these lesions are found on the palms and soles (Fig. 53.17), in contrast to other skin-appendage tumours which tend to be concentrated around the head and neck area. The anatomical distribution is, however, wide. There is no sex predilection. Most patients are adults, tumours rarely presenting in children [12]. They are moist, exophytic lesions, pink or red in colour, and may reach 1–2 cm in diameter. Occasional lesions are pigmented and look similar to pigmented basal cell carcinoma under dermatoscopy [13,14]. Exceptional examples of poroma have been reported in a naevus sebaceus [15], with rapid growth during pregnancy [16], after electron beam therapy for mycosis fungoides [10], after radiotherapy [10] and at the site of a burn [17]. Multiple poromas have been reported in a case of hidrotic ectodermal dysplasia [18].

Pathology [19–21]. These lesions are relatively easy to diagnose, with a clear margin between adjacent, normal epidermal keratinocytes and a population of smaller cuboidal cells, usually with darker nuclei protruding down into the underlying dermis (Fig. 53.18). The cells are strongly PAS-positive and are similar to those seen in the dermal duct tumour [22]. Reports, however, have stressed the fact that some poromas may show either sebaceous or apocrine differentiation [23–25]—highlighting the fact that adnexal tumours with ductal differentiation may be either eccrine or apocrine, as the ducts of both structures are identical.

Malignant change has been recorded on many occasions (see under porocarcinoma).

Management. Benign eccrine poromas are treated by surgical excision.

References
1 Hashimoto K, Lever WF. Histogenesis of skin appendage tumors. *Arch Dermatol* 1969; **100**: 356–69.
2 Hyman AB, Brownstein MH. Eccrine poroma: an analysis of 45 new cases. *Dermatologica* 1969; **138**: 29–38.
3 Goldner R. Eccrine poromatosis. *Arch Dermatol* 1970; **101**: 606–8.
4 Knox JM, Spiller WF. Eccrine poroma. *Arch Dermatol* 1958; **77**: 726–9.

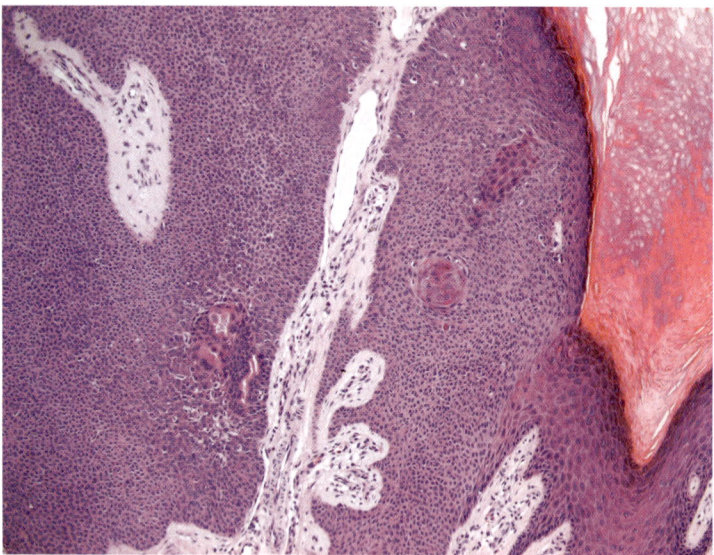

Fig. 53.18 Poroma. Note the clear demarcation between the tumour and the neighbouring epidermis.

5 Krinitz K. Ein Beitrag zur Klinik und Histologie des ekkrinen Poroms. *Hautarzt* 1967; **18**: 504–8.

6 Pinkus H, Rogin JR, Goldman P. Eccrine poroma. *Arch Dermatol* 1956; **74**: 511–21.

7 Freeman RG, Knox JM, Spiller WF. Eccrine poroma. *Am J Clin Pathol* 1961; **36**: 444–50.

8 Ogino A. Linear eccrine poroma. *Arch Dermatol* 1976; **112**: 841–4.

9 Okun MR, Anse UHB. Eccrine poroma. *Arch Dermatol* 1963; **88**: 561–6.

10 Penneys NS, Ackerman AB, Indgin SN *et al*. Eccrine poroma: two unusual variants. *Br J Dermatol* 1970; **82**: 613–5.

11 Chen CC, Chang YT, Liu HN. Clinical and histological characteristics of poroid neoplasms: a study of 25 cases in Taiwan. *Int J Dermatol* 2006; **45**: 722–7.

12 Orlandi C, Arcangeli F, Patrizi A *et al*. Eccrine poroma in child. *Pediatr Dermatol* 2005; **22**: 279–80.

13 Ohata U, Hara H, Suzuki H. Pigmented eccrine poroma occurring in the scalp: Derivation of melanocytes in the tumor. *Am J Dermatopathol* 2006; **28**: 138–41.

14 Kuo HW, Ohara K. Pigmented eccrine poroma: a report of two cases and study with dermatoscopy. *Dermatol Surg* 2033; **29**: 1076–9.

15 Jaqueti G, Requena L, Sànchez Yus E. Trichoblastoma is the most common neoplasm developed in nevus sebaceous of Jadassohn: a clinicopathologic study of a series of 155 cases. *Am J Dermatopathol* 2000; **22**: 108–18.

16 Ban M, Kitajima Y. A case of rapidly-growing eccrine poroma during pregnancy. *J Dermatol* 1997; **24**: 554–5.

17 Wakamatsu J, Yamamoto T, Minemura T *et al*. The occurrence of eccrine poroma on a burn site. *J Eur Acad Dermatol Venereol* 2007; **21**: 1128–9.

18 Wilkinson RD, Schopflocher P, Rozenfled M. Hidrotic ectodermal dysplasia with diffuse eccrine poromatosis. *Arch Dermatol* 1977; **113**: 472–6.

19 Mishima Y. Epitheliomatous differentiation of the intraepidermal eccrine sweat duct. *J Invest Dermatol* 1969; **52**: 233–46.

20 Rahbari H. Syringoacanthoma: acanthotic lesion of the acro-syringium. *Arch Dermatol* 1984; **120**: 751–6.

21 Hashimoto K, Lever WF. Eccrine poroma: histochemical and electron microscopic studies. *J Invest Dermatol* 1964; **43**: 237–47.

22 Hu CH, Marques AS, Winkelmann RK. Dermal duct tumor. *Arch Dermatol* 1978; **114**: 1659–64.

23 Moore TO, Orman HL, Orman SK *et al*. Poromas of the head and neck. *J Am Acad Dermatol* 2001; **44**: 48–52.

24 Lee NH, Lee SH, Ahn SK. Apocrine poroma with sebaceous differentiation. *Am J Dermatopathol* 2000; **22**: 261–3.

25 Kazakov DV, Kutzner H, Spagnolo DV *et al*. Sebaceous differentiation in poroid neoplasms: repoprt of 11 cases, including a case of metasplatic carcinoma associated with apocrine poroma (sarcomatoid apocrine porocarcinoma). *Am J Dermatopathol* 2008; **30**: 21–6.

Eccrine dermal duct tumour [1,2]

Definition. A benign proliferation of the eccrine dermal duct situated in the papillary dermis.

Clinical features. The clinical picture is that of a dermal nodule, occasionally with verrucous change overlying it.

Pathology. The pathology is similar to that of the hidroacanthoma simplex, but the nests of tumour cells making up the lesion are located in the dermis. The cells are small, cuboidal, regular and stain strongly with PAS. Ductal structures are often seen. An intraepidermal component may be seen in some cases, confirming that this lesion is part of the spectrum of eccrine poroma. In some cases, there is prominent clear-cell change [3].

Poroid hidradenoma is regarded as a variant of poroma with overlapping features of hidradenoma (dermal solid and cystic nests) and poroma (poroid cells and ductal differentiation) [4]. This lesion more likely represents part of the spectrum of dermal duct tumour.

Management. Excision is required for diagnostic and therapeutic purposes.

References

1 Winkelmann RK, McLeod WA. The dermal duct tumour. *Arch Dermatol* 1966; **94**: 50–5.

2 Aloi FG, Pippione M. Dermal duct tumor. *Appl Pathol* 1986; **4**: 175–8.

3 Rütten A, Hantschke M, Angulo J *et al*. Clear-cell dermal duct tumour: another distinctive, previously underrecognized cutaneous adnexal neoplasm. *Histopathology* 2007; **51**: 805–13.

4 Requena L, Sánchez M. Poroid hidradenoma: a light microscopy and immunohistochemical study. *Cutis* 1992; **50**: 43–6.

Eccrine syringofibroadenoma [1]

Clinical features. This is a rare entity, and may present as a solitary, often warty nodule on the arms or legs, especially on distal sites. The lesion may be reactive, representing hyperplasia as a result of diverse stimuli, or may be neoplastic usually presenting as a single lesion. Unusual presentations include plaques and multiple lesions [2], occasionally with a linear distribution, may be seen [3]. Coexistence with a squamous cell carcinoma and porocarcinoma has rarely been described [4,5] and lesions may rarely present within naevus sebaceus [6]. Syringofibroadenomatous hyperplasia of sweat ducts is seen in the background of other tumours, a healing ulcer, stasis, a reparative process after bullous diseases, in skin affected by leprosy, in peristomal skin, in burn scars and in association with ectodermal dysplasia [7–13]. In small biopsies, this type of hyperplasia may be confused with a syringofibroadenoma.

Pathology. A network of epithelial cells extends down from the epidermis, forming a mesh-like structure in the underlying epidermis. These cords are composed of smaller cells than in the overlying epidermis, and may contain ductal structures. This mesh is surrounded by a fibrovascular stroma. Unlike basal cell carcinoma, there is no palisading [14,15]. Clear cells may occasionally predominate [16].

Management. Simple excision is the treatment of choice.

References

1 Mascaró J. Considérations sur les tumeurs fibroepithélials. *Ann Derm Syph* 1963; **90**: 146–53.
2 Van Leeuwen RL, Lavrijsen AP, Starink TM. Eccrine syringofibroadenoma: the simultaneous occurrence of two histopathological variants (conventional and clear cell type) in one patient. *Br J Dermatol* 1999; **141**: 947–9.
3 Starink TM. Eccrine syringofibroadenoma multiple lesions representing a new cutaneous marker of the Schopf syndrome, and solitary nonhereditary tumors. *J Am Acad Dermatol* 1997; **36**: 569–76.
4 Bjarke T, Ternesten-Bratel A, Hedblad M *et al*. Carcinoma and eccrine syringofibroadenoma: a report of five cases. *J Cutan Pathol* 2003; **30**: 382–92.
5 Schadt CR, Boyd AS. Eccrine syringofibroadenoma with co-existent squamous cell carcinoma. *J Cutan Pathol* 2007; **34**: 71–4.
6 Noguchi M, Akiyama M, Kawakami M *et al*. Eccrine syringofibroadenoma arising in a sebaceous naevus. *Br J Dermatol* 2000; **142**: 1050–1.
7 Rongioletti F, Gambini C, Parodi A *et al*. Mossy leg with eccrine syringofibroadenomatous hyperplasia resembling multiple eccrine syringofibroadenoma. *Clin Exp Dermatol* 1996; **21**: 454–6.
8 Gambini C, Rongioletti F, Semino MT *et al*. Solitary eccrine syringofibroadenoma (or eccrine syringofibroadenomatous hyperplasia?) and diabetic polyneuropathy. *Dermatology* 1996; **193**: 68–9.
9 Nomura K, Kogawa T, Hashimoto I *et al*. Eccrine syringofibroadenomatous hyperplasia in a patient with bullous pemphigoid: a case report and review of the literature. *Dermatologica* 1991; **182**: 59–62.
10 Tey HL, Chong WS, Wong SN. Leprosy-associated eccrine syringofibroadenoma of Mascaro. *Clin Exp Dermatol* 2007; **32**: 533–5.
11 Clarke LE, Ioffreda M, Abt AB. Eccrine syringofibroadenoma arising in peristomal skin: a report of two cases. *Int J Surg Pathol* 2003; **11**: 61–3.
12 Ichikawa E, Fujisawa Y, Tateishi Y *et al*. Eccrine syringofibradenoma in a patient with a burn scar ulcer. *Br J Dermatol* 2000; **143**: 591–4.
13 Utani A, Hatton Y. A reactive acrosyringeal proliferation in a patient with ectodermal dysplasia: eccrine syringofibradenoma-like lesion. *J Dermatol* 1999; **26**: 36–43.
14 Mehregan AN, Marufi N, Medenica M. Eccrine syringofibroadenoma. *J Am Acad Dermatol* 1985; **13**: 433–6.
15 Ohnishi T, Suzuki T, Watanabe S. Eccrine syringofibradenoma. *Br J Dermatol* 1995; **134**: 449–54.
16 Hu S, Bakshandeh H, Kerdel FA *et al*. Eccrine syringofibroadenoma of clear cell variant: an immunohistochemical study. *Am J Dermatopathol* 2005; **27**: 228–31.

Syringoma [1–3]

Synonyms
- Hidradenomes eruptifs
- Syringocystadenoma
- Syringocystoma

Definition. A benign skin tumour that is usually multiple. The histology is characteristic.

Incidence. It is a relatively uncommon lesion, occurring more commonly in females. It is most likely to appear at adolescence, and further lesions may develop during adult life. It does not appear to be hereditary.

Clinical features [4–11]. The individual small dermal papules [12] are skin-coloured, yellowish or mauve, but sometimes appear translucent and cystic. The surface may be rounded or flat-topped

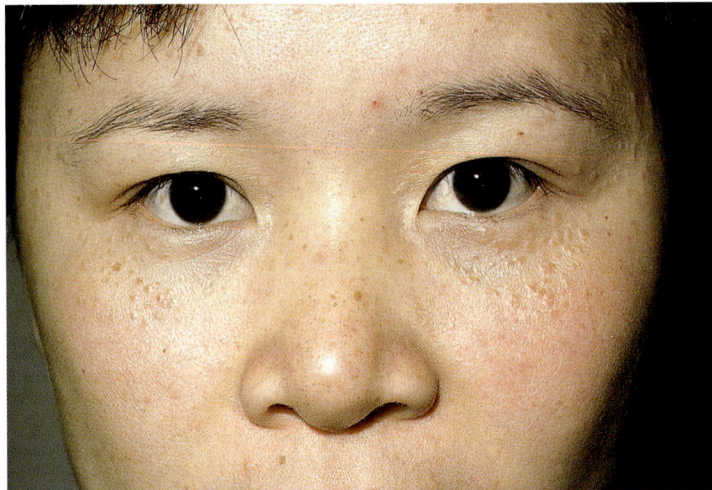

Fig. 53.19 Multiple syringomas on the upper cheek area.

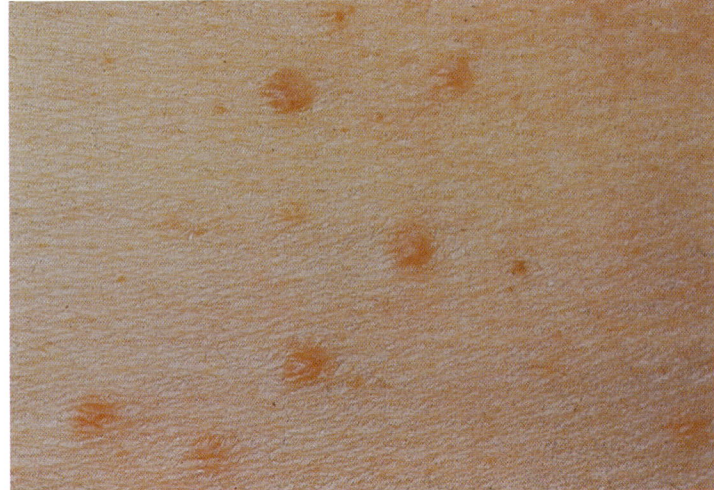

Fig. 53.20 Eruptive syringomas. Multiple, tiny, brownish or red lesions are often seen on trunk and limbs.

and the outline sometimes angular. Rarely, injury to the surface will allow a drop of clear, watery fluid to escape. They vary in size from 1 to 5 mm, but most are less than 3 mm. Some cases resemble milia and in these cases, the histology reveals a number of cystically dilated structures [13]. In most cases, there are multiple tumours, and they tend to have a bilateral symmetry in distribution. The front of the chest, face and neck are the chief areas affected. A few lesions are usually found on the eyelids when the cheeks are involved (Fig. 53.19). Eruptive syringomas have predilection for the neck, chest, abdomen, pubic area and more rarely on the buttocks [14,15]. They are more frequent in women and tend to occur in teenagers and young adults. Syringomas are seen more often than expected in patients with Down's syndrome [16,17] and may erupt dramatically (Fig. 53.20) [18]. Lesions may rarely occur on the vulva and are associated with pruritus [19,20]. Familial cases rarely occur [21]. A case of multiple syringomas probably sun-induced and in an acral location has been described [22]. Multiple syringomas have also been reported during radiotherapy for breast cancer [23]. The lesions regressed after cessation of radiotherapy.

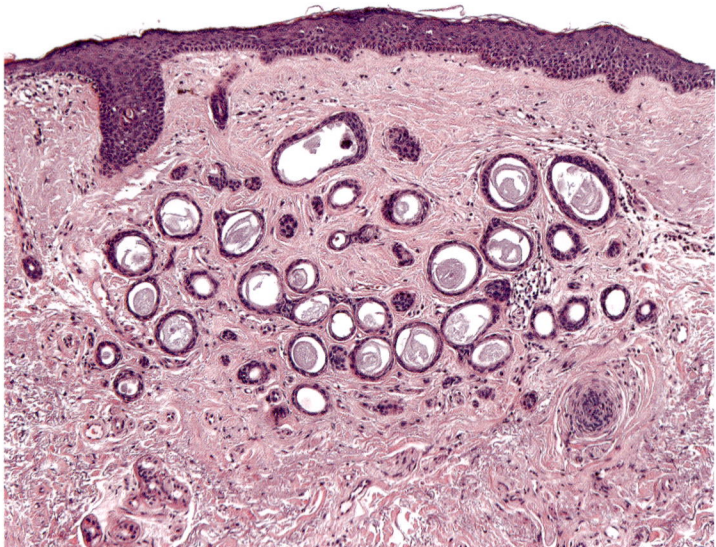

Fig. 53.21 Syringoma. Typical ductal structures with a tadpole appearance.

Pathology [24–26]. The lesion has a characteristic architectural pattern on light-microscope scanning power. Collections of convoluted and cystic ducts are seen in the upper half of the dermis. Most are lined by a double layer of cells similar to, but flatter than, those that line normal eccrine ducts. The lumina contain amorphous debris. A characteristic feature is the tail-like strand of cells projecting from one side of the duct into the stroma, giving a resemblance to a tadpole or comma (Fig. 53.21). The ducts may be enclosed in a fibrous stroma similar to the hair-follicle hamartomas, but in most cases it is narrower and less cellular. When the stroma is dense, it may be difficult to differentiate from the morphoeic basal cell carcinoma, in which, however, well-developed duct structures are not associated with cellular strands and there is a clear infiltrative margin with frequent perineurial invasion.

Diagnosis. Syringoma is most likely to be confused with trichoepithelioma on the face. The syringomas tend to be smaller, rather less superficial, more flat-topped and disposed more evenly over the cheeks and eyelids, rather than favouring the nasolabial creases. There is no family history. Lesions on the lids may be mistaken for xanthelasma, but lack the orange colour. Those erupting on the trunk may be mistaken for disseminated granuloma annulare.

Treatment. The main reason for treatment is cosmetic. Careful destruction with diathermy can produce good cosmetic results.

References
1 Hashimoto K, Lever WF. Histogenesis of skin appendage tumors. *Arch Dermatol* 1969; **100**: 356–69.
2 Lever WF. Pathogenesis of benign tumors of cutaneous appendages and of basal cell epithelioma. *Arch Dermatol Syphilol* 1948; **57**: 679–724.
3 Winkelmann RK, Muller SA. Sweat gland tumors. *Arch Dermatol* 1964; **89**: 827–31.
4 Dupre A, Bonafe JL, Christol B. Syringoma as a causative factor for cicatricial alopecia [letter]. *Arch Dermatol* 1981; **117**: 315.
5 Feibelman CE, Maize JC. Clear-cell syringoma. *Am J Dermatopathol* 1984; **6**: 139–50.

6 Friedman SJ, Butler DF. Syringoma presenting as milia. *J Am Acad Dermatol* 1987; **16**: 310–4.
7 Pujol R, Moreno A, Gonzàlez MJ *et al.* Syringoma du cuir chevelu. *Ann Dermatol Vénéréol* 1986; **113**: 693–5.
8 Shelley WB, Wood MG. Occult syringomas of scalp associated with progressive hair loss. *Arch Dermatol* 1980; **116**: 843–4.
9 Spitz DF, Stadecker MJ, Grande DJ. Subclinical syringoma coexisting with basal cell carcinoma. *J Dermatol Surg Oncol* 1987; **13**: 793–5.
10 Thomas J, Majmudar B, Gorelkin L. Syringoma localized to the vulva. *Arch Dermatol* 1979; **115**: 95–6.
11 Yung CW, Soltani K, Bernstein JE *et al.* Unilateral linear nevoidal syringoma. *J Am Acad Dermatol* 1981; **4**: 412–6.
12 Hashimoto K, Dibella RJ, Borsuk GM *et al.* Eruptive hidradenoma and syringoma. *Arch Dermatol* 1967; **96**: 500–19.
13 Wang KH, Chu JS, Lin YH *et al.* Milium-like syringoma: a case study on histogenesis. *J Cutan Pathol* 2004; **31**: 336–40.
14 Soler-Carrillo J, Estrach T, Mascaró JM. Eruptive syringoma: 27 new cases and review of the literature. *J Eur Acad Dermatol Venereol* 2001; **15**: 242–6.
15 Powell CL, Smith EP, Graham BS. Eruptive syringomas: an unusual presentation on the buttocks. *Cutis* 2005; **76**: 267–9.
16 Urban CD, Cannon JR, Cole RD. Eruptive syringomas in Down's syndrome. *Arch Dermatol* 1985; **117**: 374–9.
17 Daneshpazhooh M, Nazemi TM, Bidgeloo L *et al.* Mucocutaneous findings in 100 children with Down syndrome. *Pediatr Dermatol* 2007; **24**: 317–20.
18 Soler Carillo J, Estrach T, Mascaro JM. Eruptive syringoma: 27 new cases and a review of the literature. *J Eur Derm Venereol* 2001; **15**: 242–6.
19 Garman M, Metry D. Vulval syringomas in a 9-year-old child with review of the literature. *Pediatr Dermatol* 2006; **23**: 369–72.
20 Tay YK, Tham SN, Teo R. Localized vulvar syringomas—an unusual cause of pruritus vulvae. *Dermatology* 1996; **192**: 62–3.
21 Draznin M. Hereditary syringomas: a case report. *Dermatol Online J* 2004; **10**: 19.
22 Martin-García RF, Muñoz CM. Acral syringoma presenting as a photosensitive papular eruption. *Cutis* 2006; **77**: 33–6.
23 Yoshii N, Kanekura T, Churei H *et al.* Syringoma-like eccrine sweat duct proliferation induced by radiation. *J Dermatol* 2006; **33**: 36–9.
24 Asai Y, Ishii M, Hamada T. Acral syringoma: electron microscopic studies on its origin. *Acta Derm Venereol (Stockh)* 1982; **62**: 64–8.
25 Hashimoto K, Gross BG, Lever WF. Syringoma: histochemical and electron microscopic studies. *J Invest Dermatol* 1966; **46**: 150–66.
26 Headington JT, Koski J, Murphy PJ. Clear cell glycogenosis in multiple syringomas. *Arch Dermatol* 1972; **106**: 353–6.

Papillary eccrine adenoma

Definition. This rare lesion was first described in 1977 [1]. A solitary nodule, usually on the limbs of darker-skinned individuals it is controversial whether papillary eccrine adenoma represents the same entity as tubular apocrine adenoma [2]. The issue has not been settled but it seems that most tumours are probably apocrine and this is confirmed by examples that display follicular and sebaceous differentiation [3]. True eccrine lesions are unusual and are those arising in areas where no apocrine glands are present normally, such as the limbs [4].

Clinical features. It presents in a non-diagnostic manner as a slowly growing nodule on the limbs [5].

Pathology. The lesion is in the papillary dermis and consists of ductal structures with papillary projections. These ductal structures may display either eccrine or apocrine differentiation (decapitation secretion). Dilated ducts form a complex honeycomb-like structure.

References

1 Rulon DB, Helwig EB. Papillary eccrine adenoma. *Arch Dermatol* 1977; **113**: 596–8.

2 Tellechea O, Reis JP, Marques C *et al*. Tubular apocrine adenoma with eccrine and apocrine immunophenotypes or papillary tubular adenoma? *Am J Dermatopathol* 1995; **17**: 499–505.

3 Kazakov DV, Mukensnabl P, Michal M. Tubular adenoma of the skin with follicular and sebaceous differentiation: A report of two cases. *Am J Dermatopathol* 2006; **28**: 142–6.

4 Mizuoka H, Senzaki H, Shikata N *et al*. Papillary eccrine adenoma: immunohistochemical study and literature review. *J Cutan Pathol* 1998; **25**: 59–64.

5 Sexton M, Maize JC. Papillary eccrine adenoma: a light microscopic and immunohistochemical study. *J Am Acad Dermatol* 1988; **18**: 1114–20.

Eccrine or apocrine/follicular tumours

In recent years, it has become apparent that a number of adnexal tumours that were regarded as exclusively showing eccrine ductal differentiation often display ductal apocrine differentiation. Because of the close relationship between the apocrine and the pilosebaceous unit, these tumours may also show evidence of focal follicular and even sebaceous differentiation [1,2]. The list of tumours with potential to display apocrine ductal differentiation continues to expand and even includes rare examples of poromas showing apocrine differentiation (see p. 53.23).

References

1 McCalmont TH. A call for logic in the classification of adnexal neoplasms. *Am J Dermatopathol* 1996; **18**: 104–9.

2 Wong TY, Suster S, Cheek RF, Mihm MC Jr. Benign cutaneous adnexal tumours with combined folliculosebaceous, apocrine, and eccrine differentiation: study of eight cases. *Am J Dermatopathol* 1996; **18**: 124–36.

Hidradenoma [1]

> **Synonyms**
> - Nodulocystic hidradenoma
> - Clear-cell hidradenoma
> - Acrospiroma

Definition. A relatively rare tumour of sweat gland origin. Although traditionally regarded as displaying eccrine differentiation, it is now accepted that tumours can show either eccrine or apocrine differentiation [2].

Clinical features [3]. This is an uncommon tumour, found mainly in adults, and is excised more commonly in women than in men. Lesions in children are very rare [4]. The tumours are firm dermal nodules, 5–30 mm in size, and may be attached to the overlying epidermis, which can be either thickened or ulcerated (Fig. 53.22). Growth is slow and there may be a history of serous discharge. The lesions are usually solitary and are most likely to be found on the scalp, face, anterior trunk and proximal limbs.

Pathology [5–8]. The tumour may connect with the epidermis. It forms lobulated, circumscribed masses and is composed of two cell types—polygonal cells, whose glycogen content may give the cytoplasm a clear appearance; and elongated, darker and smaller

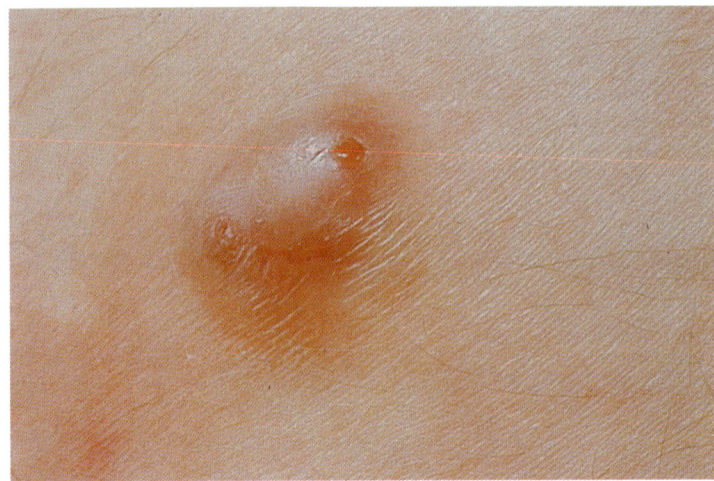

Fig. 53.22 Hidradenoma. Red–brown irregular papule.

cells, which may occur at the periphery. Often, tumours do not contain cells with clear cytoplasm, and the name 'clear-cell hidradenoma' is therefore misleading. Cuboidal or columnar cells are seen lining duct-like spaces and clefts. In cases with a connection to the epidermis, the superficial component displays poromatous features. Focal squamous differentiation may be seen [9] and occasional mucinous cells are also present. The latter is often seen in lesions with apocrine differentiation.

Malignant transformation is very rare, and the diagnosis relies on identification of the pre-existing benign component [10–13].

Diagnosis. When the tumour is attached to the epidermis, the diagnosis may be suspected on clinical grounds, especially if there is a history of discharge. Ulcerated lesions may resemble basal cell carcinoma. Dermal nodules are non-diagnostic by clinical inspection.

Treatment. Surgical excision will cure benign lesions. Local recurrences are rare [14]. Malignant eccrine hidradenoma may metastasize.

References

1 Hashimoto K, Di Bella RJ, Lever WF. Clear cell hidradenoma: histologic, histochemical, and electron microscopic study. *Arch Dermatol* 1967; **96**: 18–38.

2 Gianotti F, Alessi E. Clear cell hidradenoma associated with the folliculo-sebaceous-apocrine unit. Histologic study of five cases. *Am J Dermatopathol* 1997; **19**: 351–7.

3 Winkelmann RK, Wolff K. Solid-cystic hidradenoma of the skin. *Arch Dermatol* 1968; **97**: 651–61.

4 Faulhaber D, Wörle B, Trautner B *et al*. Clear cell hidradenoma in a young girl. *J Am Acad Dermatol* 2000; **42**: 693–5.

5 Ozawa T, Fujiwara M, Nose K *et al*. Clear cell hidradenoma of the forearm in a young boy. *Pediatr Dermatol* 2005; **22**: 450–2.

6 Hernàndez-Perez E, Cestoni-Parducci R. Nodular hidradenoma and hidradenocarcinoma. *J Am Acad Dermatol* 1985; **12**: 15–20.

7 Lever WF, Castleman B. Clear cell myoepithelioma of the skin. *Am J Pathol* 1952; **28**: 691–9.

8 O'Hara JM, Bensch K, Ioannides G *et al*. Eccrine sweat gland adenoma, clear cell type. *Cancer* 1966; **19**: 1438–50.

9 Stanley RJ, Sánchez NP, Massa MC *et al*. Epidermoid hidradenoma. *J Cutan Pathol* 1982; **9**: 293–302.

10 Hernández Pérez E, Cestoni Parducci R. Nodular hidradenoma and hidradenocarcinoma. *J Am Acad Dermatol* 1985; **12**: 15–20.

11 Yildrim S, Akoz T, Apaydin I *et al.* Malignant clear cell hidradenoma with giant metastasis to the axilla. *Ann Plast Surg* 2000; **45**: 102.

12 Vaideeswar P, Madhiwale CV, Deshpande JR. Malignant hidradenoma: a rare sweat gland tumour. *J Postgrad Med* 1999; **45**: 56–7.

13 Lim SC, Lee MJ, Lee MS *et al.* Giant hidradenocarcinoma: a report of malignant transformation from nodular hidradenoma. *Pathol Int* 1998; **48**: 818–23.

14 Will R, Coldiron B. Recurrent clear cell hidradenoma of the foot. *Dermatol Surg* 2000; **26**: 685–6.

Cylindroma [1–5]

Synonyms
- Turban tumour
- Spiegler's tumour

Definition. A skin tumour of uncertain origin with a characteristic histology (see below) that usually manifests as nodules or tumours of the scalp.

Incidence. This is an uncommon tumour, affecting females more frequently than males. It is frequently familial and an autosomal-dominant gene determines its inheritance [6,7]. It has been reported to follow radiotherapy epilation of the scalp. The onset is usually in early adult life, but may be in childhood or adolescence.

Clinical features [8,9]. The tumours are frequently multiple, smooth, firm, pink to red in colour and often somewhat pedunculated (Fig. 53.23). The lesions may be familial and a suppressor gene (cylindromatosis gene, *CYLD*) has been identified on chromosome 16q12–13, loss of which is associated with cylindroma development [10–12]. Somatic mutations have also been identified in sporadic cases. The loss of this gene causes activation of NF-B which is a transcription factor with antiapoptotic activity [13]. Based on genetic studies and the identification of mutations in the same gene in the Brooke–Spiegler syndrome, multiple familial trichoepitheliomas and familial cylindromatosis it is suggested that the three diseases have the same genetic basis and are phenotypic expressions of the same disease [14,15]. The rate of growth of cylindroma is slow and often seems to cease when a certain size has been reached. Some tumours become 5 cm or more in diameter, but most are smaller. Pain is an occasional symptom. The commonest site is the scalp and adjacent skin. Tumours on the scalp may be almost hairless when pedunculated, but the smaller lesions form dermal nodules with little loss of overlying hair. Multiple tumours have attracted much attention in the literature, but solitary lesions are not uncommonly seen by surgical pathology services. A proportion of lesions occur on the face and neck away from the scalp margin; in fewer than 10% of cases, they are situated on the trunk and limbs. Rare lesions may occur in the breast sporadically or in association with Brooke–Spiegler syndrome [16]. When the lesions are multiple, new tumours arise over the years. In some patients, there may be an admixture with trichoepithelioma, either in separate tumours or sometimes in the same tumour. This is a clear confirmation of what can be inferred from the syndromes associated with cylindromas and follicular neoplasms which is that cylindromas are more likely to be related to the apocrine gland than to the eccrine gland.

Pathology [17–23]. The tumours have a rounded outline and are composed of closely set mosaic-like masses ('jigsaw-puzzle' appearance) and columns of cells that are invested by a hyaline basal membrane of variable thickness. Thin bands of stroma (Fig. 53.24) separate tumour lobules from one another. The cells are of two types—one large, with a moderate amount of cytoplasm and a vesicular nucleus; and the other small, with little cytoplasm and

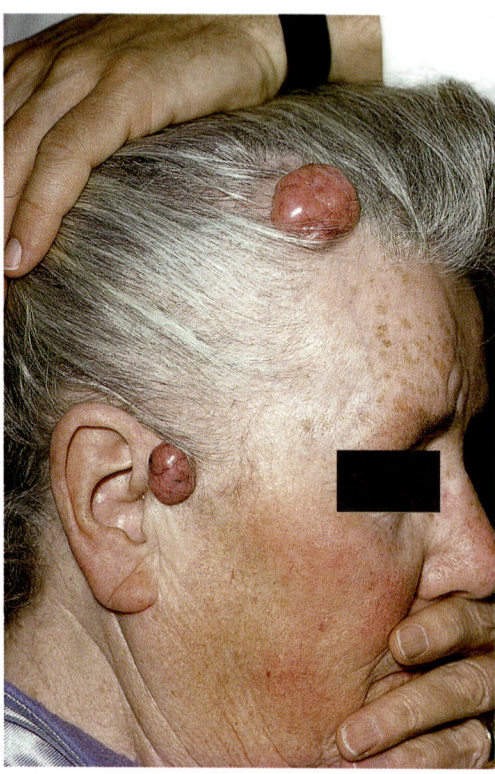

Fig. 53.23 Cylindroma. Two large tumours on the head of an elderly woman.

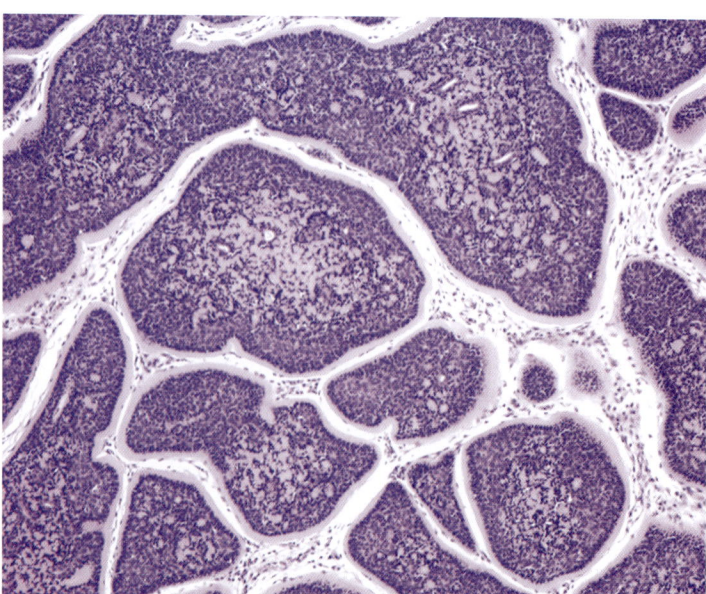

Fig. 53.24 Cylindroma. Classical jigsaw-puzzle architecture, with tumour lobules displaying a thick basal membrane.

a compact nucleus. The small cells tend to be peripheral; they also surround duct-like spaces or masses of hyaline material within the tumour lobule. There are strong immunohistochemical similarities between cylindromas and spiradenomas, and they may coexist in the same individual [24,25]. Malignant transformation is very rare and a sarcomatous component may exceptionally be seen [26–28].

Diagnosis. The multiple type on the scalp is most likely to be confused with tricholemmal cyst, which is, however, usually smoother, firmer and more mobile. Small tumours are difficult to diagnose, and must be distinguished from trichoepithelioma, steatocystoma, or basal cell carcinoma if solitary. Large, pedunculated and lobular tumours are almost unmistakable.

Treatment. Surgery is the treatment of choice. Extensive involvement of the scalp may require wide excision and replacement of the whole area by a graft. Topical salicylic acid has been used with some success in patients with multiple cylindromas [29].

References

1 Crain RC, Helwig EB. Dermal cylindroma (dermal eccrine cylindroma). *Am J Clin Pathol* 1961; **35**: 504–15.
2 Guggenheim W, Schnyder UW. Zur Nosologie der Spiegler-Brookeschen Tumoren. *Dermatologica* 1961; **122**: 274–8.
3 Hashimoto K, Lever WF. Histogenesis of skin appendage tumors. *Arch Dermatol* 1969; **100**: 356–69.
4 Holubar K, Wolff K. Zur Histogenese des Cylindromas. Eine enzymhistochemische Studie. *Arch Klin Exp Dermatol* 1967; **229**: 205–16.
5 Lever WF. Pathogenesis of benign tumors of cutaneous appendages and of basal cell epithelioma. *Arch Dermatol Syphilol* 1948; **57**: 679–724.
6 Kleine-Natrop HE. Gleichzeitige Generalisation gutartiger Basaliome der beiden Typen Spiegler und Brooke. *Arch Klin Exp Dermatol* 1959; **209**: 45–55.
7 Knoth W. Epitheliomatose Phakomatose Brooke–Spiegler (Epithelioma adenoides cysticum und Zylindrome). *Dermatol Monatschr* 1978; **164**: 63–4.
8 Guillot B, Buffiere I, Barneon G *et al*. Tricho-epitheliomas multiples, cylindromes, grain de milium. *Ann Dermatol Vénéréol* 1987; **114**: 175–82.
9 Tellechea O, Reis JP, Ilheu O, Baptista AP. Dermal cylindroma. *Am J Dermatopathol* 1995; **17**: 260–5.
10 Biggs PJ, Chapman P, Lakhani SR *et al*. The cylindromatosis gene on chromosome 16q may be the only tumour suppressor gene involved in the development of cylindromas. *Oncogene* 1996; **12**: 1375–7.
11 Takahashi M, Rapley E, Biggs PJ *et al*. Linkage and LOH studies in 19 cylindromatosis families show no evidence of genetic heterogeneity and refine the CYLD locus on chromosome 16q12-q13. *Hum Genet* 2000; **106**: 58–65.
12 Gerretson AL, Beemer FA, Deenstra W *et al*. Familial cutaneous cylindromas. *J Am Acad Dermatol* 1995; **33**: 199–206.
13 Brummelkamp TR, Nijman SM, Dirac AM *et al*. Loss of the cylindromatous tumour suppressor inhibits apoptosis by activating NF-kappaB. *Nature* 2003; **424**: 797–801.
14 Massoumi R, Paus R. Cylindromatosis and the CYLD gene: new lessons on the molecular principles of epithelial growth control. *BioEssays* 2007; **29**: 1203–14.
15 Bowen S, Gill M, Lee DA *et al*. Mutations in the CYLD gene in Brooke-Spiegler syndrome, familial cylindromatosis, and multiple familial trichoepithelioma: lack of genotype-phenotype correlation. *J Invest Dermatol* 2005; **124**: 919–20.
16 Nonaka D, Rosai J, Spagnolo D *et al*. Cylindroma of the breast of skin adnexal type: a study of 4 cases. *Am J Surg Pathol* 2004; **28**: 1070–5.
17 Ferrándiz C, Campo E, Baumann E. Dermal cylindromas (turban tumours) and eccrine spiradenomas in a patient. *J Cutan Pathol* 1985; **12**: 72–9.
18 Goette DK, McConnell MA, Fowler VR. Cylindroma and eccrine spiradenoma coexistent in the same lesion. *Arch Dermatol* 1982; **118**: 273–4.
19 Gottschalk HR, Graham JH, Aston EEIV. Dermal eccrine cylindroma, epithelioma adenoides cysticum, and eccrine spiradenoma. *Arch Dermatol* 1974; **110**: 473–4.
20 Lauseker H. Beitrag zu den Naevo-epitheliomen. *Arch Dermatol Syphilol* 1952; **194**: 639–62.
21 Gebhart W, Kokoschka WM, Wick J. The cylindroma: a model for human epithelial basement membrane [abstract]. *J Invest Dermatol* 1975; **64**: 286.
22 Mazoujian G, Margolis R. Immunohistochemistry of gross cystic disease fluid protein (GCDFP-15) in 65 benign sweat gland tumors of the skin. *Am J Dermatopathol* 1988; **10**: 28–35.
23 Munger BL, Graham JH, Helwig EB. Ultrastructure and histochemical characteristics of dermal eccrine cylindroma (turban tumor). *J Invest Dermatol* 1962; **39**: 577–94.
24 Meybehm M, Fischer HP. Spiradenoma and dermal cylindroma. *Am J Dermatopathol* 1997; **19**: 154–61.
25 Lee MW, Kelly JW. Dermal cylindroma and eccrine spiradenoma. *Australas J Dermatol* 1996; **37**: 48–9.
26 De Francesco V, Frattasio A, Pillon B *et al*. Carcinosarcoma arising in a patient with multiple cylindromas. *Am J Dermatopathol* 2005; **27**: 21–6.
27 Carlsten JR, Lewis MD, Saddler K *et al*. Spiradenocylindrocarcinoma: a malignant hybrid tumor. *J Cutan Pathol* 2005; **32**: 166–71.
28 Durani BK, Kurzen H, Jaeckel A *et al*. Malignant transformation of multiple dermal cylindromas. *Br J Dermatol* 2001; **145**: 653–6.
29 Oosterkamp HM, Neering H, Nijman SM *et al*. An evaluation of the efficacy of topical application of salicylic acid for the treatment of familial cylindromatosis. *Br J Dermatol* 2006; **155**: 182–5.

Spiradenoma [1,2]

Synonym
• Eccrine spiradenoma

Definition. A benign tumour of sweat gland origin, which is usually solitary and is distinguished by its histology (see below).

Incidence. It is relatively uncommon, appears mainly in young adults, equally in both sexes and is rarely familial (see under cylindroma).

Clinical features [3,4]. The lesion is usually solitary and painful and consists of a firm, rounded, bluish, dermal nodule 3–50 mm in diameter [3]. The usual site is on the front of the trunk and proximal limbs. Rare sites include the vulva, breast and the external ear. Congenital tumours are exceptional, and in one case lesions followed Blaschko's lines on the face [5]. Multiple neoplasms in a linear or zosteriform distribution may also be seen [6,7] and tumours may rarely be seen in a naevus sebaceus [8]. Lesions with features of spiradenoma may be part of the Brooke–Spiegler syndrome [9]. Spiradenoma often overlaps with cylindroma and this gives support to the theory that they are part of the same spectrum (see under cylindroma) [10]. Furthermore, the coexistence of spiradenoma with follicular tumours confirms an apocrine line of differentiation at least in a percentage of these tumours.

Pathology [11,12]. The tumour is lobular, with two cell types in the islands (Fig. 53.25). Larger, paler cells may be grouped around lumina, and smaller, darker cells form the periphery. Small, tubular structures or cystic spaces may occur, and large, thin-walled, dilated vascular channels are also present [13,14]. The lobules are surrounded by condensed connective tissue, which may encroach on the islands as hyaline droplets. Degenerative changes in old tumours are often prominent. Haemorrhage and

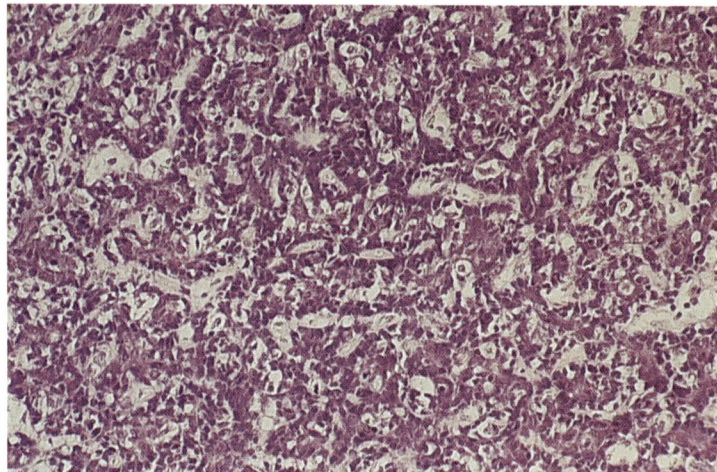

Fig. 53.25 Eccrine spiradenoma. Ductal structures and intermixed pale and dark cells.

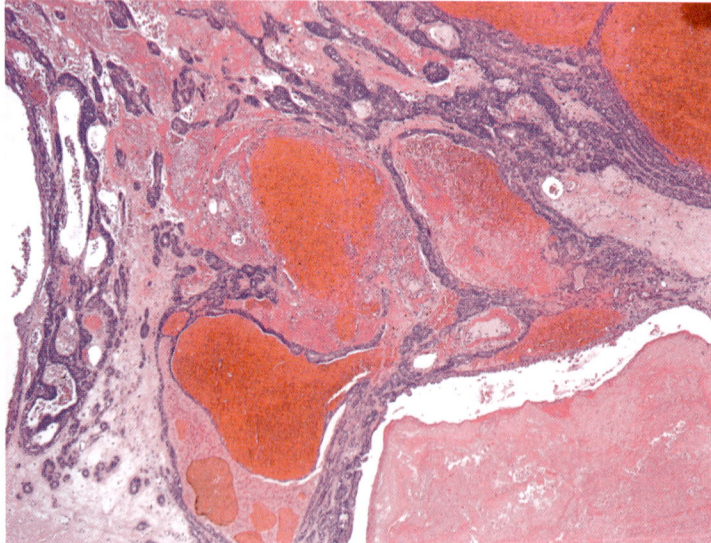

Fig. 53.26 Eccrine spiradenoma. Extensive haemorrhage with or without ischaemic necrosis may result in rapid clinical growth. Only small areas of residual spiradenoma remain.

ischaemic necrosis as a result of degeneration often obscure the histological features, and only focal areas display the typical features of a spiradenoma (Fig. 53.26). Old tumours with degenerative changes tend to be very large. Malignant transformation may occur and usually presents in long-standing tumours [15–20]; lesions may have features of cylindroma and spiradenoma [10]. The diagnosis of a malignant spiradenoma is often only made after a residual benign component is identified. Rare tumours have a sarcomatous component [21]. Malignant tumours may metastasize but it is difficult to be certain of how aggressive these neoplasms are because of their rarity and the bias to report mainly cases with aggressive behaviour.

Diagnosis. Clinical differentiation from other dermal tumours and cysts may be made if the tumour is firm, dark blue and domed.

Treatment. Surgical excision should be complete, as there may be recurrence.

References
1 Castro C, Winkelmann RK. Spiradenoma: histochemical and electron microscopic study. *Arch Dermatol* 1974; **109**: 40–8.
2 Hashimoto K, Kanzaki T. Appendage tumors of the skin: histogenesis and ultrastructure. *J Cutan Pathol* 1984; **11**: 365–81.
3 Kersting DW, Helwig EB. Eccrine spiradenoma. *Arch Dermatol* 1956; **73**: 199–227.
4 Lever WF. Myoepithelial sweat gland tumor: myoepithelioma. *Arch Dermatol Syphilol* 1948; **57**: 332–47.
5 Ekmekci TR, Koslu A, Sakiz D. Congenital blaschkoid eccrine spiradenoma on the face. *Eur J Dermatol* 2005; **15**: 73–4.
6 Yoshida A, Sato T, Sugawara Y *et al*. Two cases of multiple eccrine spiradenoma with linear or localized formation. *J Dermatol* 2004; **31**: 564–8.
7 Gupta S, Jain VK, Singh U *et al*. Multiple eccrine spiradenomas in zosteriform distribution in a child. *Pediatr Dermatol* 2000; **17**: 384–6.
8 Shapiro M, Johnson B Jr, Witmer W *et al*. Spiradenoma arising in a nevus sebaceous of Jadassohn: case report and literature review. *Am J Dermatopathol* 1999; **21**: 462–7.
9 Kim C, Kovich OI, Dosik J. Brooke-Spigler syndrome. *Dermatol Online* 2007; **13**: 10.
10 Michal M, Lamovec J, Mukensnabl P *et al*. Spiradenocylindromas of the skin: tumors with morphological features of spiradenoma and cylindroma in the same lesion: report of 12 cases. *Pathol Int* 1999; **49**: 419–25.
11 Hashimoto K, Lever WF. Histogenesis of skin appendage tumors. *Arch Dermatol* 1969; **100**: 356–69.
12 Hashimoto K, Gross BG, Nelson RG *et al*. Eccrine spiradenoma: histochemical and electron microscopic studies. *J Invest Dermatol* 1966; **46**: 347–65.
13 Munger BL, Berghorn BM, Helwig EB. A light and electron-microscopic study of a case of multiple eccrine spiradenoma. *J Invest Dermatol* 1962; **38**: 289–97.
14 van den Oord JJ, de Woolf-Peeters C. Perivascular spaces in eccrine spiradenoma. *Am J Dermatopathol* 1995; **17**: 266–70.
15 Cooper PH, Frierson HF Jr, Morrison C. Malignant transformation of eccrine spiradenoma. *Arch Dermatol* 1985; **121**: 1445–8.
16 Dabska M. Malignant transformation of eccrine spiradenoma. *Polish Med J* 1972; **11**: 388–96.
17 Evans HL, Su WPD, Smith JL *et al*. Carcinoma arising in eccrine spiradenoma. *Cancer* 1979; **43**: 1881–4.
18 Caladari C, Mehregan AH, Lee KC. Malignant transformation of eccrine tumors. *J Cutan Pathol* 1987; **14**: 15–22.
19 Mambo NC. Eccrine spiradenoma: clinical and pathologic study of 49 tumors. *J Cutan Pathol* 1983; **10**: 312–20.
20 Granter SR, Seeger K, Calonje E *et al*. Malignant eccrine spiradenoma (spiradenocarcinoma): a clinicopathologic study of 12 cases. *Am J Dermatopathol* 2000; **22**: 97–103.
21 McCluggage WG, Fon LJ, O'Rourke D *et al*. Malignant eccrine spiradenoma with carcinomatous and sarcomatous elements. *J Clin Pathol* 1997; **50**: 871–3.

Mixed tumour of the skin [1]

Synonym
• Chondroid syringoma

Definition. Although traditionally regarded as a tumour showing eccrine derivation, it has been demonstrated that a majority of lesions are folliculosebaceous-apocrine and only rare tumours are truly eccrine [2].

Clinical features [1,3–5]. This tumour is usually found on the head and neck, followed by the trunk and the extremities, as a solitary nodule. The lesions are frequently large and nodular,

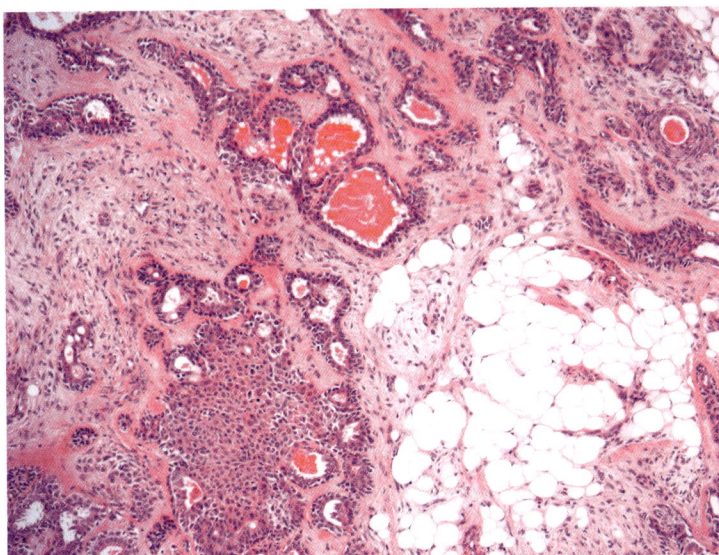

Fig. 53.27 Apocrine mixed tumour. Notice the apocrine glands with a surrounding myxoid/hyalinized stroma with fatty metaplasia.

sometimes with a diameter of 5–10 cm, and occur most commonly in middle-aged males. Lesions in children are rare [6]. Local recurrence is rarely seen.

Pathology [7–13]. This is usually a large, multilobulated tumour located in the dermis and/or subcutaneous tissue. Tumour lobules are separated by fibrous septa. A myxoid, hyalinized or chondroid stroma is variably seen in all tumours. The epithelial component consists of nests and strands of cells with pink cytoplasm and vesicular nuclei with a single, inconspicuous nucleolus. Cytological atypia is absent, and mitotic figures are sometimes seen. Tubular structures and ductal differentiation are frequently seen. Epithelial cells may show various types of metaplasia and differentiation including squamous and mucinous metaplasia and clear cell change and columnar and oxyphilic change [2]. Larger tumour cells with a plasmacytoid appearance are a frequent finding and suggest myoepithelial differentiation. Myoepithelial cells may also be spindle-shaped or display hyaline or clear cell change and collagenous spherulosis [2]. Ductal structures usually have a peripheral layer of flattened myoepithelial cells. Immunohistochemical studies reveal positivity for keratin and focal positivity for S100 and smooth muscle actin, confirming myoepithelial differentiation. Areas clearly indicative of apocrine (Fig. 53.27) and follicular differentiation are often identified [9,10,14,15]. Tumours with follicular differentiation often show numerous keratocysts indicating infundibular differentiation. Staining with cytokeratin 20 may be helpful to identify Merkel cells which, when present, confirms follicular differentiation [16]. The stroma stains positively with Alcian blue, indicating the presence of chondroitin sulphate and hyaluronic acid. Focal calcification, mature fat and bone formation may also be seen [2,17]. From this description, it is clear that all the different cellular elements in mixed tumours including the epithelial, myoepithelial and stromal components may show a wide spectrum of differentiation and metaplastic changes that may make histological interpretation difficult and a potential source of pitfalls [2]. Tumours composed exclusively of

myoepithelial cells are regarded as myoepitheliomas [18]. In some cases of mixed tumours, focal architectural and cytological atypia may be seen but this does not seem to imply a more aggressive behaviour [19].

Malignant chondroid syringomas have been reported [20–27], including rare cases with metastasis [28,29].

Management. Local excision is recommended. If there is any suspicion of malignancy, wide excision and follow-up are required.

References

1 Hirsch P, Helwig EB. Chondroid syringoma. *Arch Dermatol* 1961; **84**: 835–47.
2 Kazakov DV, Belousova IE, Bisceglia M *et al*. Apocrine mixed tumor of the skin ('mixed tumor of the folliculosebaceous-apocrine complex'). Spectrum of differentiation and metaplastic changes in the epithelial, nyoepithelial, and stromal components based on a histopathologic study of 244 cases. *J Am Acad Dermatol* 2007; **57**: 467–83.
3 Kresbach H. Ein Beitrag zum sogenannten Mischtumor der Haut. *Arch Klin Exp Dermatol* 1964; **221**: 59–74.
4 Tsoitis G, Brisou B, Destombes P. Mummified cutaneous mixed tumor. *Arch Dermatol* 1975; **111**: 194–6.
5 Welkes S, Goos M. Das chondroide Syringom. *Hautarzt* 1982; **33**: 15–7.
6 Turhan-Haktanir N, Sahin O, Bukulmez A *et al*. Chondroid syringoma in a child. *Pediatr Dermatol* 2007; **24**: 505–7.
7 Headington JT. Mixed tumors of the skin: eccrine and apocrine types. *Arch Dermatol* 1961; **84**: 989–96.
8 Gartmann H, Pullmann H. Chondroides Syringom. *Z Hautkrankh* 1979; **54**: 908–13.
9 Gartmann H, Pullmann H. Apokriner und ekkriner Mischtumor der Kopfhaut. *Z Hautkrankh* 1979; **54**: 952–8.
10 Haensch R. Apokriner Mischtumor. *Z Hautkrankh* 1983; **58**: 575–9.
11 Kanitakis J, Zambruno G, Viac J *et al*. Expression of neural-tissue markers (S-100 protein and Leu-7 antigen) by sweat gland tumors of the skin. *J Am Acad Dermatol* 1987; **17**: 187–91.
12 Mazoujian G, Margolis R. Immunohistochemistry of gross cystic disease fluid protein (GCDFP-15) in 65 benign sweat gland tumors of the skin. *Am J Dermatopathol* 1988; **10**: 28–35.
13 Hernández FJ. Mixed tumors of the skin of the salivary gland type: a light and electron microscopic study. *J Invest Dermatol* 1976; **66**: 49–52.
14 Requena L, Sánchez Yus E, Santa Cruz DJ. Apocrine type of cutaneous mixed tumor with follicular and sebaceous differentiation. *Am J Dermatopathol* 1992; **14**: 186–94.
15 Yamamoto O, Yasuda H. An immunohistochemical study of the apocrine type of cutaneous mixed tumors, with special reference to their follicular and sebaceous differentiation. *J Cutan Pathol* 1999; **26**: 232–41.
16 Salama ME, Azam M, Ma CK *et al*. Chodroid syringoma. Cytokeratin 20 immunolocalization of Merkel cells and reappraisal of apocrine folliculo-sebaceous differentiation. *Arch Pathol Lab Med* 2004; **128**: 986–90.
17 Miracco C, De Santi MM, Lalinga AV *et al*. Lipomatous mixed tumor of the skin: a histological, immunohistochemical and ultrastructural study. *Br J Dermatol* 2002; **146**: 899–903.
18 Mentzel T, Requena L, Kaddu S *et al*. Cutaneous myoepithelial neoplasms: clinicopathologic and immunohistochemical study of 20 cases suggesting a continuous spectrum ranging from benign mixed tumor of the skin to cutaneous myoepithelioma and myoepithelial carcinoma. *J Cutan Pathol* 2003; **30**: 293–302.
19 Kazakov DV, Bisceglia M, Spagnolo DV *et al*. Apocrine mixed tumors of the skin with architectural and/or cytologic atypia: a retrospective clinicopathologic study of 18 cases. *Am J Surg Pathol* 2007; **31**: 1094–102.
20 Botha JBC, Kahn LB. Aggressive chondroid syringoma. *Arch Dermatol* 1978; **114**: 954–5.
21 Devine P, Sarno RC, Ucci AA. Malignant cutaneous mixed tumor. *Arch Dermatol* 1984; **120**: 576–7.
22 Harrist TJ, Aretz TH, Mihm MC Jr *et al*. Malignant chondroid syringoma. *Arch Dermatol* 1981; **117**: 719–24.

23 Hilton JMN, Blackwell JB. Metastasizing chondroid syringoma. *J Pathol* 1973; **109**: 167–70.

24 Ishimura E, Iwamoto H, Kobashi Y *et al.* Malignant chondroid syringoma. *Cancer* 1983; **52**: 1966–73.

25 Matz LR, McCully DJ, Stokes BAR. Metastasizing chondroid syringoma: case report. *Pathology* 1969; **1**: 77–81.

26 Metzler G, Schaumburg-Lever G, Hornstein O *et al.* Malignant chondroid syringoma. *Am J Dermatopathol* 1996; **18**: 83–9.

27 Redono C, Rocamora A, Villoria F *et al.* Malignant mixed tumor of the skin: malignant chondroid syringoma. *Cancer* 1982; **49**: 1690–6.

28 Shvili D, Rothem A. Fulminant metastasizing chondroid syringoma of the skin. *Am J Dermatopathol* 1986; **8**: 321–5.

29 Kiely JL, Dunne B, McCabe M *et al.* Malignant chondroid syringoma presenting as multiple pulmonary nodules. *Thorax* 1997; **52**: 395–6.

Sweat gland carcinomas, including ductal apocrine/follicular carcinomas

These lesions can be divided into two broad groups. The first group represents the situation in which malignant change develops in a pre-existing, apparently benign lesion, such as hidradenoma, mixed tumour, spiradenoma, cylindroma and eccrine poroma. The latter is the most commonly recorded example of such malignant progression [1,2]. In most adnexal tumours, with the exception of malignant eccrine poroma, the diagnosis usually requires identification of a benign component. Even when there is unmistakable cytological evidence of malignancy, the biological behaviour of malignant tumours of skin appendages is generally relatively benign, with local recurrence being much more common than cutaneous metastases.

The second group of carcinomas consists of lesions that develop as carcinomas *ab initio*. The primary eccrine carcinomas include microcystic adnexal carcinoma, eccrine epithelioma (regarded by many as part of the spectrum of microcystic adnexal carcinoma), aggressive digital papillary adenocarcinoma, mucinous carcinoma and adenoid cystic carcinoma. Lymphoepithelioma-like carcinoma of the skin is also included in this group.

A review of 60 sweat gland carcinomas reported 41 porocarcinomas, three syringomatous carcinomas, eight ductal carcinomas, five adenoid cystic carcinomas and three mucinous carcinomas [1]. The rarity of sweat gland carcinomas makes it difficult to say whether or not this distribution is the norm, but porocarcinoma does appear to be a relatively common lesion.

References

1 Urso C, Bondi R, Paglierani M *et al.* Carcinomas of sweat glands: report of 60 cases. *Arch Pathol Lab Med* 2001; **125**: 498–505.

2 Robson A, Greene J, Ansari N *et al.* Eccrine porocarcinoma: a clinicopathologic study of 69 cases. *Am J Surg Pathol* 2001; **25**: 710–20.

Eccrine gland carcinomas

Malignant eccrine poroma [1,2]

Synonym
- Porocarcinoma

Definition. A malignant tumour with metastatic potential arising from intraepidermal eccrine duct epithelium. In up to 18% of cases, tumours arise from a pre-existing benign eccrine poroma [3].

Clinical features [4–7]. These are relatively common malignancies (0.01–0.005% of all cutaneous tumours), arising most often on the lower limbs (44% of cases) in older patients, with an average age at presentation of 73 years. Females are more commonly affected than males. The lesion presents as an endoexophytic tumour, which is often ulcerated. Tumours may attain a very large size and are frequently long standing. Local recurrence is seen in 17% of cases. Regional lymph-node metastases and systemic metastases occur in 19% and 11% of patients, respectively [3]. A small number of patients present with multiple lesions, and it is not clear whether this represents epidermotropic metastasis or true multifocality [1,3,8]. An exceptional case has been reported arising in a scar [9], and a further metastatic lesion was associated with exposure to poison gas [10]. A neoplasm developed from a poroma in a child [11].

Pathology [3,12–14]. Tumours show multiple connections to the epidermis, and a pre-existing benign eccrine poroma may be present. *In-situ* lesions are seen occasionally [3,15]. The tumour infiltrates the dermis and the subcutaneous tissue in nests and lobules composed of relatively small cells that do not have a basaloid appearance. Peripheral palisading is absent. Ductal differentiation is necessary for the diagnosis to be made. This may be demonstrated by the use of immunohistochemical stains for carcinoembryonic antigen (CEA) and epithelial membrane antigen (EMA). A PAS stain may also be used, but this only highlights the ducts in very well-differentiated tumours forming ducts with a cuticle. Comedo necrosis is often present. Clear-cell change and squamous differentiation may be seen, and the latter may be prominent in some cases making it difficult to decide whether the tumour represents a squamous cell carcinoma with ductal differentiation or a porocarcinoma with squamous differentiation [16]. Sarcomatoid change may be seen in rare cases [17].

Poor prognostic factors are a large number of mitotic figures, lymphovascular invasion, tumour depth greater than 7 mm and an infiltrating rather than a pushing border [3].

Treatment. Wide excision and follow-up are required. Two series, including a total of 93 cases, suggest that these lesions may have less metastatic capacity than thought previously [3,18]. In a smaller series of 12 cases, half displayed metastases to regional lymph nodes [19]. Mohs micrographic surgery is useful in those cases with a prominent infiltrative growth pattern [20].

References

1 Pinkus H, Mehregan AH. Epidermotropic eccrine carcinoma. *Arch Dermatol* 1963; **88**: 597–606.

2 Mishima Y, Morioka S. Oncogenic differentiation of the intraepidermal eccrine sweat duct: eccrine poroma, poroepithelioma and porocarcinoma. *Dermatologica* 1969; **138**: 238–50.

3 Robson A, Greene J, Ansari N *et al.* Eccrine porocarcinoma: a clinicopathologic study of 69 cases. *Am J Surg Pathol* 2001; **25**: 710–20.

4 Miura Y. Epidermotropic eccrine carcinoma. *Jpn J Dermatol (Series B)* 1968; **78**: 226–30.

5 Bottles K, Sagebiel RW, McNutt NS *et al*. Malignant eccrine poroma. *Cancer* 1984; **53**: 1579–83.

6 Gschnait F, Horn F, Lindlbauer R *et al*. Eccrine porocarcinoma. *J Cutan Pathol* 1980; **7**: 349–53.

7 Ishikawa K. Malignant hidroacanthoma simplex. *Arch Dermatol* 1971; **104**: 529–32.

8 Landa NG, Winkelmann RK. Epidermotropic eccrine porocarcinoma. *J Am Acad Dermatol* 1991; **24**: 27–31.

9 Nemoto I, Akiyama N, Aoyagi S *et al*. Eccrine porocarcinoma and eccrine porosa arising in a scar. *Br J Dermatol* 2004; **150**: 1232–3.

10 Helmke B, Stara H, Bachter D *et al*. Metastasising porocarcinoma following exposure to poison gas. *Lancet* 2002; **359**: 1685.

11 Valverde K, Senger C, Ngan BY *et al*. Eccrine porocarcinoma in a child that evolved rapidly from an eccrine porosa. *Med Pediatr Oncol* 2001; **23**: 402–6.

12 Krinitz K. Malignes intraepidermales ekkrines Porom. *Z Hautkrankh* 1972; **47**: 9–17.

13 Mohri S, Chika K, Saito I *et al*. A case of porocarcinoma. *J Dermatol* 1980; **7**: 431–4.

14 Shaw M, McKee PH, Lowe D, Black MM. Malignant eccrine poroma: a study of 27 cases. *Br J Dermatol* 1982; **107**: 675–80.

15 Rutten A, Requena L, Requena C. Clear cell porocarcinoma in situ. *Am J Dermatopathol* 2002; **24**: 67–71.

16 Perna C, Cuevas J, Jiménez-Hefferman JA *et al*. Eccrine porocarcinoma (malignant eccrine poroma). *Am J Surg Pathol* 2002; **26**: 272–3.

17 Mahomed F, Blok J, Grayson W. The squamous variant of eccrine porocarcinoma: a clinicopathological study of 21 cases. *J Clin Pathol* 2008; **61**: 361–5.

18 Goh SG, Dayrit JF, Calonje E. Sarcomatoid eccrine porocarcinoma: report of two cases and a review of the literature. *J Cutan Pathol* 2007; **34**: 55–60.

19 Shiohara J, Koga H, Uhara H *et al*. Eccrine porocarcinoma: clinical and pathological study of 12 cases. *J Dermatol* 2007; **34**: 516–22.

20 Wittenberg GP, Robertson DB, Solomon AR *et al*. Eccrine porocarcinoma treated with Mohs micrographic surgery: a report of five cases. *Dermatol Surg* 1999; **25**: 911–3.

Aggressive digital papillary adenocarcinoma

Definition. A rare tumour found on the hands and feet, with a high risk both of local recurrence and metastasis. Prior publications have described both a benign, aggressive digital papillary adenoma and a carcinoma [1,2], but the lack of pathologically diagnostic or prognostic differentiating features suggests that all lesions in this category should be treated as carcinomas.

Clinical features. Both sexes are affected and although most patients are young adults, the age range is wide and an exceptional case in a teenager has been reported [3]. The lesion presents as a non-diagnostic, asymptomatic nodule on the fingers, toes, palms or soles. Delayed diagnosis is frequent [1,2,4,5]. Lesions may masquerade as either a fibrokeratoma [6] or paronychia [7].

Pathology [1,2,5]. The lesions are obviously cystic on low-power microscopic examination, and have papillary projections into the cystic cavities. Ductal and tubuloalveolar structures are also present. There may be focal necrosis and both nuclear hyperchromatism and a high mitotic count. In some cases, a tubular architecture tends to predominate and papillary projections may not be so prominent. Histological features do not allow accurate prediction of behaviour, as tumours with low-grade histology may metastasize [2].

Tumours may invade surrounding soft tissues and blood vessels and can destroy bone.

Treatment. Wide local excision including amputation of the affected digit and follow-up are recommended in view of the high recurrence rate, both locally and via metastatic spread [1,2,8,9]. It has been suggested that sentinel lymph-node biopsy is appropriate for these lesions [10].

References

1 Kao GF, Helwig EB, Graham JH. Aggressive digital papillary adenoma and adenocarcinoma: a clinicopathological study of 57 cases. *J Cutan Pathol* 1987; **14**: 129–46.

2 Duke WH, Sherod TT, Lupton GP. Aggressive digital papillary adenocarcinoma (aggressive digital papillary adenoma and adenocarcinoma revisited). *Am J Surg Pathol* 2000; **24**: 775–84.

3 Bazil MK, Henshaw RM, Werner A *et al*. Aggressive digital papillary adenocarcinoma in a 15-year-old girl. *J Pediatr Hematol Oncol* 2006; **28**: 529–30.

4 Ceballos PI, Penneys NS, Acosta R. Aggressive digital papillary adenocarcinoma. *J Am Acad Dermatol* 1990; **19**: 899–900.

5 Jih DM, Elenitsas R, Vottorio CC *et al*. Aggressive digital papillary adenocarcinoma: a case report and review of the literature. *Am J Dermatopathol* 2001; **23**: 154–7.

6 Chi CC, Kuo TT, Wang SH. Aggressive digital papillary adenocarcinoma: a silent malignancy masquerading as acquired digital fibrokeratoma. *Am J Clin Dermatol* 2007; **8**: 243–5.

7 Gorva AD, Mohil R, Srinivasan MS. Aggressive digital papillary adenocarcinoma presenting as paronychia of the finger. *J Hand Surg (Br)* 2005; **30**: 534.

8 Bakotic B, Antonescu CR. Aggressive digital papillary adenocarcinoma of the foot. *J Foot Ankle Surg* 2000; **39**: 402–5.

9 Altman CE, Hamill RL, Elston DM. Metastatic aggressive digital papillary adenocarcinoma. *Cutis* 2003; **72**: 145–7.

10 Malafa M, McKesey P, Stone S *et al*. Sentinel node biopsy for staging of digital papillary adenocarcinoma. *Dermatol Surg* 2000; **26**: 580–3.

Eccrine or apocrine/follicular carcinomas

Malignant cylindroma [1–7]

Definition. A rare tumour, which develops from a pre-existing benign dermal cylindroma.

Clinical features. These unusual tumours develop as expanding nodules, usually on the scalp or very rarely in the external ear [8]. They may be suspected by expansion of a previously static dermal cylindroma or turban tumour. They have been reported in familial cases of cylindromas [1,2].

Pathology. These lesions have the characteristic architecture of a dermal cylindroma, with deeply basophilic small cells surrounded by an eosinophilic basement membrane [3–6]. In addition, however, there is marked nuclear atypia, irregularity of cell size and an infiltrative growth pattern. Mitotic figures, both normal and abnormal, are present. Exceptionally, a sarcomatous component may be seen [9].

Treatment. Wide local excision and follow-up are required.

References

1 Pizinger K, Michal M. Malignant cylindroma in Brooke–Spiegler syndrome. *Dermatology* 2000; **201**: 255–7.

2 Galadari E, Mehregan AH, Lee KC. Malignant transformation of eccrine tumors. *J Cutan Pathol* 1987; **14**: 15–22.

3 Greither A, Rehrmann A. Spiegler-Karzinome mit assoziierten Symptomen. *Dermatologica* 1980; **160**: 361–70.

4 Korting GW, Hoede N, Gebhardt R. Kurzer Bericht über einen malignen entarteten Spiegler-Tumor. *Dermatol Monatsschr* 1970; **156**: 141–7.

5 Lyon JB, Rouillard LM. Malignant degeneration of turban tumour of scalp. *Trans St John's Hosp Dermatol Soc* 1961; **46**: 74–7.

6 Urbach F, Graham JH, Goldstein J et al. Dermal eccrine cylindroma. *Arch Dermatol* 1963; **88**: 880–94.

7 Iyer PV, Leong AS. Malignant dermal cylindromas: do they exist? A morphological and immunohistochemical study and review of the literature. *Pathology* 1989; **21**: 269–74.

8 Mashkevich G, Undavia S, Iacob C et al. Malignant cylindroma of the external auditory canal. *Otol Neurotol* 2006; **27**: 21–6.

9 De Francesco V, Frattasio A, Pillon B et al. Carcinosarcoma arising in a patient with multiple cylindromas. *Am J Dermatopathol* 2005; **27**: 21–6.

Malignant hidradenoma

Synonyms
- Hidradenocarcinoma
- Malignant acrospiroma

Definition. A malignant tumour traditionally regarded as displaying eccrine differentiation and arising from a pre-existing hidradenoma.

Clinical features. These lesions are most often recorded as red, ulcerated nodules on the face, hands or feet. They are commonest in older adults, but cases have been recorded in children [1–4]. They may be very aggressive and pulmonary metastases have occurred.

Pathology. Large clusters of glycogen-rich clear cells are present in some cases, but others may resemble basal cell carcinoma [5–9]. Focal necrosis may be present, and the range of mitoses is highly variable. Squamous differentiation may be prominent [10]. Tumour cells are usually positive for EMA, CEA, S-100, gross-cystic disease fluid protein-15, the keratin cocktail AE1/AE3 and cytokeratin 5/6 [11]. Tumours may be eccrine or apocrine. Amplification of the Her-2/neu gene has been demonstrated in a single case with lymph node metastases [12]; based on this finding the patient was treated with trastuzumab.

Treatment. Wide local excision is recommended. Mohs surgery has been used successfully for lesions on the foot [13]. Follow-up is essential, as the lesions may recur locally and/or metastasize [14]. Sentinel lymph node biopsy has been used exceptionally to demonstrate early metastatic disease [15].

References

1 Headington JT, Niederhuber JE, Beals TF. Malignant clear cell acrospiroma. *Cancer* 1978; **41**: 641–7.

2 Johnson BL Jr, Helwig EB. Eccrine acrospiroma. *Cancer* 1969; **23**: 641–57.

3 Keasbey LE, Hadley GC. Clear-cell hidradenoma: report of three cases with widespread metastases. *Cancer* 1954; **7**: 934–52.

4 Kersting DW. Clear cell hidradenoma and hidradenocarcinoma. *Arch Dermatol* 1963; **87**: 323–33.

5 Mambo NC. The significance of atypical nuclear changes in benign eccrine acrospiromas: a clinical and pathological study of 18 cases. *J Cutan Pathol* 1984; **11**: 35–44.

6 Mehregan AH, Hashimoto K, Rahbari H. Eccrine adenocarcinoma: a clinico-pathologic study of 35 cases. *Arch Dermatol* 1983; **119**: 104–14.

7 Santler R, Everhartinger C. Malignes Klarzellen-Myoepitheliom. *Dermatologica* 1965; **130**: 340–7.

8 Schroeder WA Jr, Hosler MW. Malignant clear cell hidradenoma of the lip. *Mil Med* 1989; **154**: 508–11.

9 Vaideeeswar P, Madiwhale CV, Deshpande JR. Malignant hidradenoma: a rare sweat gland tumour. *J Postgrad Med* 1999; **456**: 56–7.

10 Will R, Coldiron B. Recurrent clear cell hidradenoma of the foot. *Dermatol Surg* 2000; **26**: 685–6.

11 Ko CJ, Cochran AJ, Eng W et al. Hidradenocarcinoma: a histological and immunohistochemical study. *J Cutan Pathol* 2006; **33**: 726–30.

12 Nash JW, Barrett TL, Kies M et al. Metastatic hidradenocarcinoma with demonstration of Her-2/neu gene amplification by fluorescence in-situ hybridization: potential treatment implications. *J Cutan Pathol* 2007; **34**: 49–54.

13 Park HJ, Kim YC, Cinn YW. Nodular hidradenocarcinoma with prominent squamous differentiation: case report and immunohistochemical study. *J Cutan Pathol* 2000; **27**: 423–7.

14 Jouary T, Kaiafa A, Lipinski P et al. Metastatic hidradenocarcinoma: efficacy of capecitabine. *Arch Dermatol* 2006; **142**: 1366–7.

15 Bogner PN, Fullen DR, Lowe L et al. Lymphatic mapping and sentinel lymph node biopsy in the detection of early metastasis from sweat gland carcinoma. *Cancer* 2003; **97**: 2285–9.

Malignant spiradenoma

Synonym
- Spiradenocarcinoma

Definition. A rare tumour, which usually arises in a pre-existing spiradenoma.

Clinical features. Sudden expansion of a pre-existing nodule is the most likely presentation [1]. A study of 12 cases reports the commonest site as the trunk, with limbs, head and neck less frequently involved [2]. The sex distribution appears equal, and presentation is usually in the seventh decade.

Pathology [2–4]. These lesions usually show evidence of origin from a pre-existing benign spiradenoma. Necrosis, a high mitotic count, loss of the dual cell population and an infiltrative growth pattern are features that raise the possibility of malignant transformation.

Treatment. Excision and follow-up are required. Up to 20% of these tumours have been reported to metastasize [2–5].

References

1 Biernat W, Wozniak I. Spiradenocarcinoma: a clinicopathological study of 3 cases. *Am J Dermatopathol* 1994; **16**: 377–82.

2 Granter SR, Seeger K, Calonje E, Busam K, McKee PH. Malignant eccrine spiradenoma: a study of 12 cases. *Am J Dermatopathol* 2000; **22**: 97–103.

3 Mirza I, Kloss R, Sieber SC. Malignant eccrine spiradenoma. *Arch Path Laboratory Med* 2002; **126**: 591–4.

4 Ishikawa M, Nakanishi Y, Yamazaki N, Yamamoto A. Malignant eccrine spiradenoma: a case report and review of the literature. *Dermatol Surg* 2001; **27**: 67–70.

5 Fernández-Acenero MJ, Manzerbeita F, Mestre de Juan MJ, Requena L. Malignant spiradenoma. *J Am Acad Dermatol* 2001; **44** (Suppl. 2): 395–8.

Microcystic adnexal carcinoma

Synonyms
- Sclerosing/syringomatous sweat duct carcinoma
- Malignant syringoma

Clinical features. This tumour is relatively rare, has an equal sex incidence and a predilection for the central area of the face, often as an inconspicuous, elevated or depressed sclerotic plaque or nodule in the upper lip area [1–4]. The trunk is also rarely involved. The age range is very wide, but young and middle-aged patients are more frequently affected. If the lesion is not promptly treated, or if local recurrence occurs, the lesions may present with pain or a burning sensation because of perineural spread. Cases have been reported both in patients with generalized immunosuppression and in sites of previous radiotherapy [5–7]. It has also rarely been reported arising within a naevus sebaceus [8]. Multiple tumours are exceptional [9]. The rate of local recurrence is very high (up to 40%). Bone involvement is rarely seen [10].

Pathology [11,12]. The salient histological features are the presence of cords of cytologically banal epithelial cells with focal, variable ductal differentiation set in a very sclerotic desmoplastic stroma [2–4]. Horn cysts are seen in many cases and pilar and sebaceous differentiation may also occur (Fig. 53.28) [11–14]. Superficial areas show a resemblance to syringoma, desmoplastic trichoepithelioma and, in some cases, to infiltrative basal cell carcinoma. The diagnosis can therefore be impossible if only a small, superficial biopsy is evaluated, as clues to the correct diagnosis reside in an infiltrative growth pattern and prominent perineural invasion. Immunohistochemistry is of limited value as an aid in the histological diagnosis of microcystic adnexal carcinoma. Although it has been claimed that BerEP4 is consistently negative in microcystic adnexal carcinoma [15] and this may allow distinction from infiltrative basal cell carcinoma, which is consistently

positive for this marker, this finding is contradicted by a more recent study in which 38% of microcystic adnexal carcinomas were positive for this marker [15]. Although desmoplastic trichoepithelioma and microcystic adnexal carcinoma may both show positivity for CK15 and BerEP4, it has been shown that CK15 tends to be negative in infiltrative basal cell carcinoma and this may be a useful marker in the histological differential diagnosis of both tumours [16]. Cytogenetic analysis of a case of microcystic adnexal carcinoma has shown a deletion on chromosome 6q (23–25) [17].

Management. The importance of this tumour is that perineural permeation is common, and for this reason microscopically controlled surgical excision is recommended. Mohs surgery has been recommended as the surgical approach of choice [18].

Metastatic spread is very rare [19,20], but extensive local recurrence can be a major problem. Tumours may rarely extend into the brain as a result of perineural invasion.

References
1 Cooper PH. Sclerosing carcinomas of sweat ducts (microcystic adnexal carcinoma). *Arch Dermatol* 1986; **122**: 261–4.
2 Chiller K, Passaro D, Scheuller M *et al.* Microcystic adnexal carcinoma: forty-eight cases, their treatment, and their outcome. *Arch Dermatol* 2000; **136**: 1355–9.
3 Snow S, Madjar MDD, Hardy S *et al.* Microcystic adnexal carcinoma: a report of 13 cases. *Dermatol Surg* 2001; **27**: 401–8.
4 Ohtsuka H, Nagamatsu S. Microcystic adnexal carcinoma: review of 51 Japanese patients. *Dermatology* 2002; **204**: 190–3.
5 Lei JY, Wang J, Jaffe E *et al.* Microcystic adnexal carcinoma associated with primary immunodeficiency. *Am J Dermatopathol* 2000; **22**: 524–9.
6 Carroll P, Goldstein GD, Brown CW. Metastatic microcystic adnexal carcinoma in an immunocompromised patient. *Dermatol Surg* 2000; **26**: 531–4.
7 Antley CA, Carney M, Smoller BR. Microcystic adnexal carcinoma arising in the site of previous radiation therapy. *J Cutan Pathol* 1999; **26**: 48–50.
8 Lountzis N, Junkins-Hopkins J, Uberti-Benz M *et al.* Microcystic adnexal carcinoma arising within a nevus sebaceus. *Cutis* 2007; **80**: 352–6.
9 Page RN, Hanggi MC, King R *et al.* Multiple microcystic adnexal carcinomas. *Cutis* 2007; **79**: 299–303.
10 Nagatsuka H, Riveras RS, Gunduz M *et al.* Microcystic adnexal carcinoma with mandibular bone marrow involvement: a case report with immunohistochemistry. *Am J Dermatopathol* 2006; **28**: 518–22.
11 Goldstein D, Barr R, Santa Cruz D. Microcystic adnexal carcinoma: a distinct clinicopathologic entity. *Cancer* 1982; **50**: 566–72.
12 Nickoloff BJ, Fleischmann HE, Carmel J *et al.* Microcystic adnexal carcinoma: immunohistologic observations suggesting dual (pilar and eccrine) differentiation. *Arch Dermatol* 1986; **122**: 290–4.
13 Callahan EF, Vidimos AT, Bergfeld WF. Microcystic adnexal carcinoma of the scalp with extensive pilar differentiation. *Dermatol Surg* 2002; **28**: 536–9.
14 Friedman PM, Friedman RH, Jiang SB *et al.* Microcystic adnexal carcinoma: collaborative series review and update. *J Am Acad Dermatol* 1999; **41**: 225–31.
15 Krahl D, Sellheyer K. Monoclonal antibody Ber-EP4 reliably discriminates between microcystic adnexal carcinoma and basal cell carcinoma. *J Cutan Pathol* 2007; **34**: 782–7.
16 Hoang MP, Dresser KA, Kapur P *et al.* Microcystic adnexal carcinoma: an immunohistochemical reappraisal. *Mod Pathol* 2008; **21**: 175–85.
17 Wohlfahrt C, Ternesten A, Sahlin P *et al.* Cytogenetic and fluorescence in-situ hybridization analysis of a microcystic adnexal carcinoma with del (6) (q23 q25). *Cancer Genet Cytogenet* 1997; **98**: 106–12.
18 Khachemoune A, Olbricht SM, Johnson DS. Microcystic adnexal carcinoma: report of four cases treated with Mohs' micrographic surgical technique. *Int J Dermatol* 2005; **44**: 507–12.
19 Gabillot-Carré M, Weill F, Mamelle G *et al.* Microcystic adnexal carcinoma: report of seven cases including one with lung metastasis. *Dermatology* 2006; **212**: 221–8.

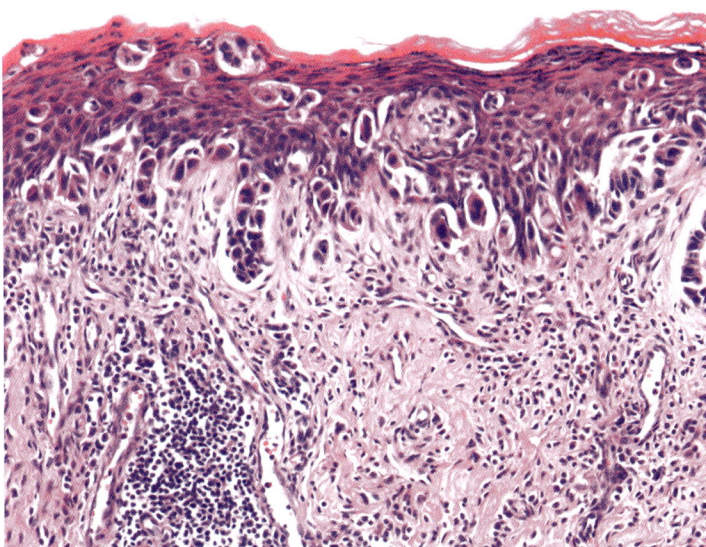

Fig. 53.28 Microcystic adnexal carcinoma. Strands and small nests of bland epithelial cells with an infiltrative growth pattern.

20 Ohta M, Hiramoto M, Ohtsuka H. Metastatic microcystic adnexal carcinoma: an autopsy case. *Dermatol Surg* 2004; **30**: 957–60.

Eccrine epithelioma [1–4]

Synonyms
- Basal cell carcinoma with eccrine differentiation
- Syringoid eccrine carcinoma

Freeman and Winkelmann, who considered it to be a basal cell tumour with eccrine differentiation [1,2], first described this rare tumour in 1969. However, the tumour does not represent a basal cell carcinoma with eccrine differentiation [3]. Some authors have proposed that it is part of the spectrum of microcystic adnexal carcinoma. At least 12 cases are currently reported in the world literature. The lesion has some resemblance to both benign syringoma and to dermal cylindroma.

Clinical features. Two-thirds of the cases so far reported have occurred on the scalp as large, non-specific, sometimes ulcerated nodules. They may be painful, due to their position in the deep dermis.

Pathology. The tumour consists of cords and clusters of small, dark-staining, cuboidal basophilic cells set in a very dense stroma. The cells are cytologically abnormal, with a high nuclear/cytoplasmic ratio, and mitotic figures are seen. These features occur in the lower part of the dermis, extending into the subcutaneous fat. The islets of cells have a surrounding PAS-positive membrane.

Management. Wide local excision is required. Follow-up is essential, as repeated local recurrences are common. In one case, metastasis to a local lymph node was recorded.

References
1 Freeman RC, Winkelmann RK. Basal cell tumor with eccrine differentiation. *Arch Dermatol* 1969; **100**: 234–42.
2 Sánchez NP, Winkelmann RK. Basal cell tumor with eccrine differentiation (eccrine epithelioma). *J Am Acad Dermatol* 1982; **6**: 514–8.
3 Urso C, Bondi R. Eccrine epithelioma: an enigma or a chimera? *Am J Dermatopathol* 1992; **14**: 179–80.
4 McKee PH, Fletcher CD, Rasbridge SA. The enigmatic eccrine epitheliomas (eccrine syringomatous carcinoma). *Am J Dermatopathol* 1990; **12**: 552–61.

Mucinous carcinoma

Definition. A rare, adnexal apocrine mucin-producing carcinoma arising on the head and neck area in more than 90% of the cases. This tumour is very similar to mucinous carcinoma of the breast [1].

Clinical features. The most frequently described clinical presentation is that of a grey nodule on the face of an elderly male, often in the periorbital area [2–6]. Occasional tumours present in younger patients [7]. Rarely tumours are bilateral [8]. An important clinical differential diagnosis is a cutaneous secondary deposit from a more common site for mucinous carcinoma such as the stomach

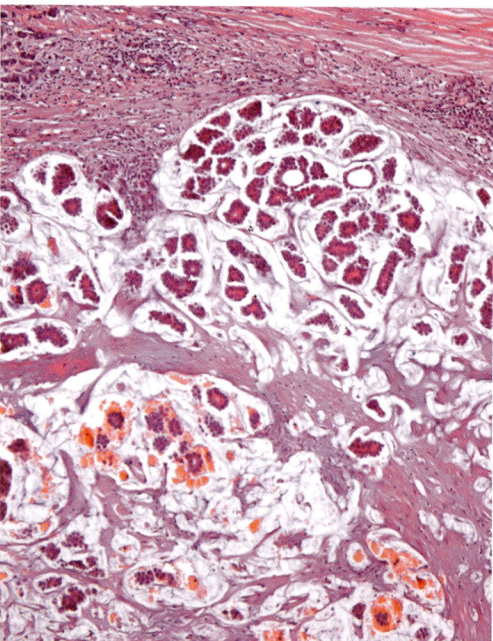

Fig. 53.29 Mucinous carcinoma. Nests of tumour cells surrounded by pools of mucin.

and breast [9]. The distinction between a primary skin tumour and a metastasis is often very difficult and has to rely on some histological features (see below), clinicopathological correlation and additional studies to rule out an internal primary. In the case of a suspected metastatic mucinous breast carcinoma, staining for oestrogen and progesterone receptors is not useful, as primary cutaneous mucinous carcinomas are often positive for these markers [10].

Pathology. These lesions are relatively deeply situated and consist of clusters of cells with pink cytoplasm and some degree of cytological atypia. The central cells are paler and surrounded by darker-staining cells arranged in a palisaded fashion. Broad, fibrous septa run between these cytologically malignant cells, and both cells and septa are separated by lakes of mucin (Fig. 53.29) [11,12]. The mucin stains with diastase-resistant PAS, and acid Alcian blue (pH 2.5). Distinction from metastatic breast of gastrointestinal mucinous carcinoma is difficult. In many cases of primary cutaneous mucinous carcinoma there is evidence of an *in situ* component in neighbouring glands and this confirms a tumour as primary arising in the skin [1,13]. Tumours presenting in the trunk often originate in the breast and those with dirty necrosis usually represent a metastasis from a gastrointestinal primary [1].

Management. Wide local excision, possibly with Mohs micrographic surgery, is recommended [14,15]. Extensive metastatic spread and invasion of bone is very rare [16,17]. Local recurrence is often seen and the risk of metastatic spread to regional lymph nodes increases after a recurrence.

References
1 Kazakov DV, Suster S, LeBoit P *et al*. Mucinous carcinoma of the skin, primary and secondary: a clinicopathologic study of 63 cases with emphasis on the

morphologic spectrum of primary cutaneous forms: homologies with mucinous lesions in the breast. *Am J Surg Pathol* 2005; **29**: 764–82.

2 Baandrup U, Sogaard H. Mucinous (adenocystic) carcinoma of the skin. *Dermatologica* 1982; **164**: 338–42.

3 Balin AK, Fine RM, Golitz LE. Mucinous carcinoma. *J Dermatol Surg Oncol* 1988; **14**: 521–4.

4 Headington JT. Primary mucinous carcinoma of the skin. *Cancer* 1977; **39**: 1055–63.

5 Breier F, Clabian M, Pokieser W *et al.* Primary mucinous carcinoma of scalp. *Dermatology* 2000; **200**: 250–3.

6 Snow SN, Reizner GT. Mucinous eccrine carcinoma of the eyelid. *Cancer* 1992; **15**: 2099–104.

7 Bindra M, Keegan DJ, Guenther T *et al.* Primary cutaneous mucinous carcinoma of the eyelid in a young male. *Orbit* 2005; **24**: 211–4.

8 Bertagnoli R, Cook DL, Goldman GD. Bilateral primary mucinous carcinoma of the eyelid treated with Mohs surgery. *Dermatol Surg* 1999; **25**: 566–8.

9 Nahass GT, Otrakji CJ, Gould E. Mucinous breast carcinoma: single cutaneous metastasis. *J Dermatol Surg Oncol* 1993; **19**: 878–80.

10 Hanby AM, McKee P, Jeffery M *et al.* Primary mucinous carcinomas of the skin express TFF1, TFF3, estrogen receptor and progesterone receptors. *Am J Surg Pathol* 1998; **22**: 1125–31.

11 Mendoza S, Helwig EB. Mucinous (adenocystic) carcinoma of the skin. *Arch Dermatol* 1971; **103**: 68–78.

12 Santa Cruz DJ, Meyers JH, Gnepp DR *et al.* Primary mucinous carcinoma of the skin. *Br J Dermatol* 1978; **98**: 645–53.

13 Qureshi HS, Salama ME, Chitale D *et al.* Primary cutaneous mucinous carcinoma: presence of myoepithelial cells as a clue to the cutaneous origin. *Am J Dermatopathol* 2004; **26**: 353–8.

14 Cecchi R, Rapicano V. Primary cutaneous mucinous carcinoma: report of two cases treated with Moh's micrographic surgery. *Australas J Dermatol* 2006; **47**: 192–4.

15 Marra DE, Schanbacher CF, Torres A. Mohs micrographic surgery of primary cutaneous mucinous carcinoma using immunohistochemistry for margin control. *Dermatol Surg* 2004; **30**: 799–802.

16 Yeung KY, Stinson JC. Mucinous (adenocystic) carcinoma of sweat glands with widespread metastases: case report with ultrastructural study. *Cancer* 1977; **39**: 2556–62.

17 Tanaka A, Hatoko M, Kuwahara M *et al.* Recurrent mucinous carcinoma of the skin invading to the frontal skull base. *Br J Dermatol* 2000; **143**: 458–9.

Adenoid cystic carcinoma [1–3]

Synonym
• Primary cutaneous adenocystic carcinoma

This is a particularly rare variant of adnexal carcinoma, which has only been recognized as an entity since 1975. Adenoid cystic carcinomas arise relatively frequently from salivary glands, and direct spread or even metastasis from this site should be ruled out before the diagnosis of primary cutaneous adenoid cystic carcinoma is made [4]. Around 50 cases are presently recorded in the literature.

Clinical features [1,2]. These lesions are non-specific, sometimes painful, nodules on the head and neck area. The pain is attributed to perineural spread. Rarely, tumours develop elsewhere in the skin including the scrotum [3].

Pathology [5–8]. The pathology is that of large masses of cells with mild or no cytological atypia, arranged in a distinct adenoid or cribriform pattern. The cystic spaces are occupied by mucin, which stains with Alcian blue (pH 2.5). The lesion occupies the middle to deep dermis and may extend to the subcutaneous

tissue. A more solid variant may be seen occasionally. Many of these tumours show at least focal evidence of myoepithelial differentiation.

Management. The management of these lesions is by wide local excision and Mohs surgery is a good treatment option [9]. Local recurrence is common and metastasis to the lung and regional lymph nodes has rarely been reported [6,10–13]. Metastatic spread to the lungs has also been reported, rarely many years after removal of the primary cutaneous tumour [14]. Erosion of bone at the primary site has also been recorded.

References

1 Boggio R. Adenoid cystic carcinoma of the scalp. *Arch Dermatol* 1975; **111**: 793–4.

2 Headington JT, Tesars R, Niederhuber JE *et al.* Primary adenoid cystic carcinoma of the skin. *Arch Dermatol* 1978; **114**: 421–4.

3 Koh BK, Choi JM, Yi JY *et al.* Recurrent primary cutaneous adenoid cystic carcinoma of the scrotum. *Int J Dermatol* 2001; **40**: 724–5.

4 Pérez DE, Magrin J, de Almeida OP *et al.* Multiple cutaneous metastases from a parotid adenoid cystic carcinoma. *Pathol Oncol Res* 2007; **13**: 167–9.

5 Cooper PH, Adelson GL, Holthaus WH. Primary cutaneous adenoid cystic carcinoma. *Arch Dermatol* 1984; **120**: 774–7.

6 Seab JA, Graham JH. Primary cutaneous adenoid cystic carcinoma. *J Am Acad Dermatol* 1987; **17**: 113–8.

7 Thomas RM, Lowe DG, Munro DD *et al.* Primary adenoid cystic carcinoma of the skin. *Clin Exp Dermatol* 1987; **12**: 378–80.

8 Wick MR, Swanson PE. Primary adenoid cystic carcinoma of the skin. *Am J Dermatopathol* 1986; **8**: 2–13.

9 Krunic AL, Kim S, Medenica M *et al.* Recurrent adenoid cystic carcinoma of the scalp treated with Mohs micrographic surgery. *Dermatol Surg* 2003; **29**: 647–9.

10 Chu SS, Chang YL, Lou PJ. Primary cutaneous adenoid cystic carcinoma with regional lymph node metastasis. *J Laryngol Otol* 2001; **115**: 673–5.

11 Weekly M, Lydiatt DD, Lydiatt WM *et al.* Primary cutaneous adenoid cystic carcinoma metastatic to cervical lymph nodes. *Head Neck* 2000; **22**: 84–6.

12 Chang SE, Ahn SJ, Choi JH *et al.* Primary adenoid cystic carcinoma of skin with lung metastasis. *J Am Acad Dermatol* 1999; **40**: 640–2.

13 Doganay L, Bilgi S, Aygit C *et al.* Primary cutaneous adenoid cystic carcinomas with lung and lymph node metastases. *J Eur Acad Dermatol Venereol* 2004; **18**: 383–5.

14 Pappo O, Gez E, Craciun I *et al.* Growth rate analysis of lung metastases appearing 18 years after resection of cutaneous adenoid cystic carcinoma: case report and review of the literature. *Arch Pathol Lab Med* 1992; **116**: 76–9.

Miscellaneous tumours

Tumours of anogenital mammary-like glands

For many years it was assumed that a number of female genital tumours with features identical to those arising in the breast were derived from ectopic mammary gland tissue along the milk lines. Van der Putte, however, has proposed that this theory is not accurate as primordia of mammary glands do not extend beyond the axillary–pectoralis area [1]. His proposal is that there is a group of distinctive, mammary-like genital glands that share features with true mammary glands and eccrine and apocrine glands and from which most genital glandular neoplasms arise [1,2]. The latter include hidrocystoma, hidradenoma papilliferum, extramammary Paget's disease and tumours identical to those arising in breast tissue including fibroadenoma, cystosarcoma phylloides and adenocarcinoma [3–7].

References

1 van der Putte SC. Mammary-like glands of the vulva and their disorders. *Int J Gynecol Pathol* 1994; **13**: 150–60.

2 van der Putte SC, van Gorp LH. Adenocarcinoma of the mammary-like glands of the vulva: a concept unifying sweat gland carcinoma of the vulva, carcinoma of supranummerary mammary glands and extramammary Paget's disease. *J Cutan Pathol* 1994; **21**: 157–63.

3 Castro CY, Deavers M. Ductal carcinoma in-situ arising in mammary-like glands of the vulva. *Int J Gynecol Pathol* 2001; **20**: 277–83.

4 Sington JD, Manek S, Hollowood K. Fibroadenoma of the mammary-like glands of the vulva. *Histopathology* 2002; **41**: 563–5.

5 Ohira S, Itoh K, Osada K *et al.* Vulval Paget's disease with underlying adenocarcinoma simulating breast carcinoma: case report and review of the literature. *Int J Gynecol Cancer* 2004; **14**: 1012–7.

6 Abbott JJ, Ahmed J. Adenocarcinoma of the mammary-like glands of the vulva: Report of a case and review of the literature. *Am J Dermatopathol* 2006; **28**: 127–33.

7 Giger OT, Lacoste E, Honegger C *et al.* Expression of the breast differentiation antigen NY-BR1 in a phyllodes tumor of the vulva. *Virchows Arch* 2007; **450**: 471–4.

Paget's disease of the nipple [1]

Definition. A progressive, marginated, scaling or crusting of the nipple and areola due to invasion of the epidermis by malignant cells, which are currently thought to originate in the intraduct carcinoma of the breast that frequently accompanies the condition.

There is a strong, current view that Paget's disease arises from apocrine duct-derived epithelial cells.

Incidence and aetiology [2]. Paget's disease of the nipple is an uncommon occurrence, considering the frequency of breast cancer [3,4]. In one series, it occurred in fewer than 3% of breast cancers. It occurs chiefly in women, although rare cases have been recorded in men [5] and is exceptionally bilateral [6]. It is rare before the fourth decade and is most frequent in the fifth and sixth. Published cases suggest that the disease is more common in Anglo-Saxon countries. The current view is that the majority of cases of Paget's disease arise from either invasive or *in-situ* ductal carcinoma in the deeper breast tissue. In a minority of cases no underlying *in-situ* or invasive carcinoma is found [7]. Although the incidence of breast cancer is increasing, the incidence of Paget's disease has decreased by 45% in the USA in the last decades [8]. Equally, the incidence of Paget's disease associated with underlying invasive cancer of ductal carcinoma *in situ* has also decreased [8].

Clinical features [9,10]. The early changes may be minimal, with a small, crusted and intermittently moist area on the nipple giving a brownish stain on clothing, or producing itching, pricking or burning sensations. Less often, there is a serous or blood-stained discharge from the nipple, or a lump may be noticed in the breast (Fig. 53.30). The surface changes persist and gradually spread to produce an eczematous appearance. The nipple, areola and, at a later stage, skin of the breast are erythematous and moist or crusted (Fig. 53.31). The change is sharply marginated and may spare a segment of the areola. The edge is slightly raised and irregular in outline. If the crusts are removed, a red, glazed, moist or vegetating surface is revealed. Itching may be a prominent

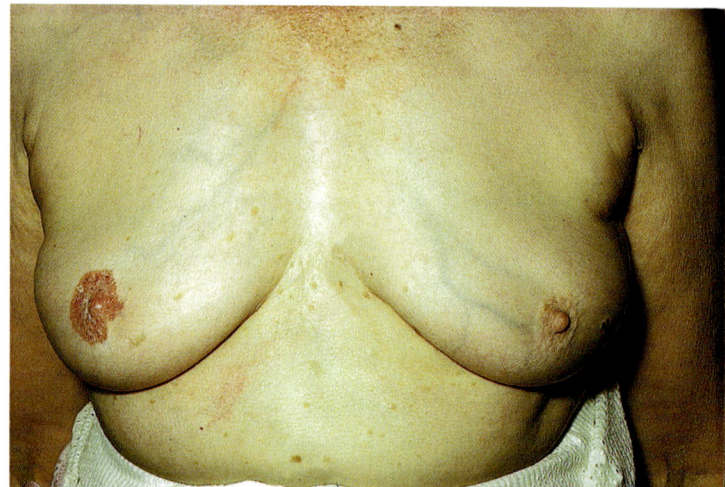

Fig. 53.30 Paget's disease of the nipple. Distant clinical view, showing unilateral lesion.

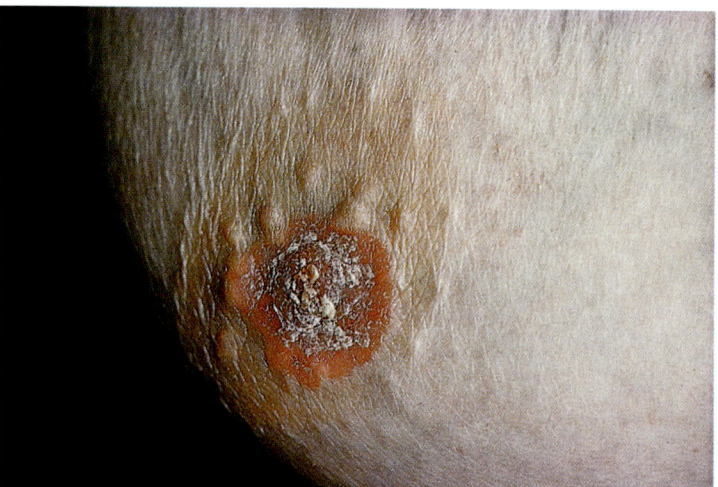

Fig. 53.31 Paget's disease of the nipple. Close-up view, showing erythema and well-marked lateral edge of the lesion.

symptom and excoriations may be found in the established lesion. Some areas may be ulcerated. The nipple itself may be retracted, and a subjacent mass or a lump deeper in the breast may be felt. The regional glands should be examined; they are rarely enlarged when a mass cannot be felt, but are enlarged in more than half the cases with a detectable tumour. The rate of spread of the skin changes is slow, and patients often wait a year or more before seeking advice. The change may occasionally involve not only the skin of the breast but also spread on to the chest wall. Poor prognosis is associated with invasive disease and the presence of a palpable mass [11]. An exceptional case has been recorded in which the patient presented with ipsilateral eruptive seborrhoeic keratoses of the nipple and areola (Leser-Trelat sign) [12].

Pathology [13–15]. The epidermis is thickened, with papillomatosis, enlargement of the interpapillary ridges and hyperkeratosis or parakeratosis on the surface (Fig. 53.32). Within the epidermis, characteristic Paget's cells are dispersed between the prickle cells. They vary in number, and when profuse the Malpighian layers

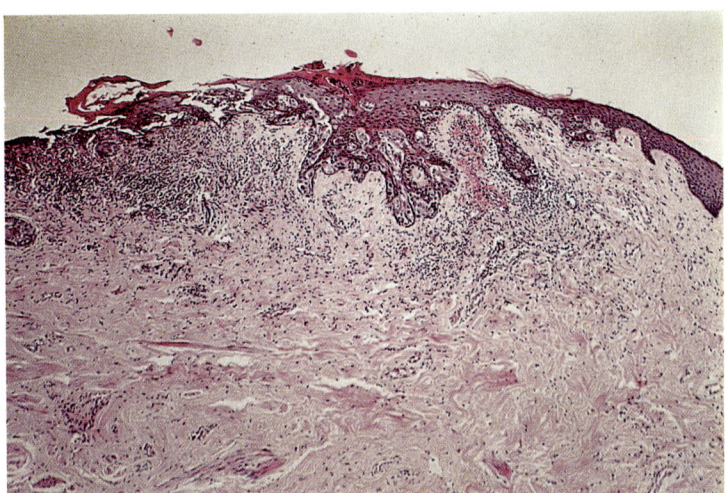

Fig. 53.32 Pathology of Paget's disease of the nipple, showing epidermal ulceration, colonization of the epidermis by large pale Paget's cells and an underlying brisk lymphocytic infiltrate.

may be disrupted and the surface covered by a crust. There is a chronic inflammatory reaction in the upper dermis. In the later stages, the epidermis may be atrophic or eroded. On scanning microscopy, the differential diagnosis may include superficial spreading malignant melanoma.

The Paget's cells have a clear, abundant cytoplasm and do not establish intercellular bridges with the adjacent normal keratinocytes. Both the cells and their nuclei are rounded; the nuclei are vesicular or hyperchromatic with a high nuclear/cytoplasmic ratio. The cytoplasm is PAS-positive and diastase-resistant [16], which indicates the presence of neutral polysaccharides and supports the glandular origin of the cells [17]. Staining with antibodies to CEA is also positive [18,19]. The cells are distributed singly among the prickle cells, or in clusters in a pattern similar to that seen in superficial spreading melanoma. The Paget's cells may also be seen in appendage ducts, so that it can be impossible to determine if these cells are migrating from these ducts to the epidermis, or invading downwards into the ducts from the epidermis.

An underlying breast carcinoma, if present, is not always seen on biopsy, as it may be deeply set. Careful examination of the amputated breast may show an intraduct carcinoma, sometimes of quite small dimensions, usually situated most distally, but sometimes in the terminal ducts, and often appearing to spread between the two layers of epithelial cells of the duct. The cells may accumulate within and distend the ducts and spread in both directions. A number of ducts are usually involved. At a later stage, the carcinoma becomes invasive and behaves like classic breast carcinoma.

Diagnosis. The principal differential diagnosis is eczema of the nipple. This is frequently bilateral and runs a more fluctuating course, improving in response to local treatment and spreading rapidly when irritated. Eczema lacks the sharp, raised and rounded margin and the superficial induration of Paget's disease. In doubtful cases, biopsy will be required. Bowen's disease and superficial basal cell carcinoma may also produce a similar clinical picture.

They are both very uncommon on the nipple and can be differentiated histologically. Psoriasis and erosive adenomatosis of the nipple may also need to be considered in the clinical differential diagnosis, and again a biopsy to obtain pathology will clarify the situation. The chief pathological challenge is to distinguish Paget's disease from malignant melanoma, the latter exceptionally presenting in the nipple [20,21]. Paget's disease cells will be CEA-positive, EMA-positive and Cam 5.2-positive, while those of melanoma will be positive for Melan A mart melanoma antigens [18,19]. Positivity to antibody to S100 protein is not useful, as although it is positive in the great majority of melanomas, this is also the case in a proportion of cases of Paget's disease. The absence of melanophages and the presence of neutral mucopolysaccharides in the cells are also helpful.

Treatment [22]. All patients should have a mammogram or ultrasound to establish whether or not there is deeper pathology in the underlying breast, as this will help determine the extent of surgery required. Surgery should be carried out as for carcinoma of the breast. In patients with no evidence of an underlying breast carcinoma, conservation may be a realistic option [23,24]. A recent study has confirmed this, recommending breast conserving therapy with or without radiotherapy according to the presence or absence of an invasive component as the treatment of choice. Sentinel lymph node biopsy is performed in cases with an invasive component [7]. Surgery should always include the whole of the nipple–areolar complex [7].

References

1 Lloyd J, Flanagan AM. Mammary and extramammary Paget's disease. *J Clin Pathol* 2000; **53**: 742–9.

2 Ordoñez NG, Awalt H, MacKay B. Mammary and extramammary Paget's disease. *Cancer* 1987; **59**: 1173–83.

3 Paget J. A disease of the mammary areola preceding cancer of the mammary gland. *St Bartholomew's Hosp Rep* 1874; **10**: 87–91.

4 Kollmorgen DR, Varanasi JS, Edge SB *et al*. Paget's disease of the breast: a 33 year experience. *J Am Coll Surg* 1998; **187**: 171–7.

5 Desai DC, Brennan EJ, Carp NZ. Paget's disease of the male breast. *Am J Surg* 1996; **62**: 1068–72.

6 Ucar AE, Korukluoglu B, Ergul E *et al*. Bilateral paget disease of the male nipple: First report. *Breast* 2008; **17**: 317–8.

7 Caliskan M, Gatti G, Sosnovskikh I *et al*. Paget's disease of the breast: the experience of the European Institute of Oncology and review of the literature. *Breast Cancer Res Treat* 2008; **112**: 513–21.

8 Chen CY, Sun LM, Anderson BO. Paget disease of the breast: changing patterns of incidence, clinical presentation, and treatment in the U.S. *Cancer* 2006; **107**: 1448–58.

9 Yim JH, Wick MR, Philpott GW *et al*. Underlying pathology in mammary Paget's disease. *Ann Surg Oncol* 1997; **4**: 287–92.

10 Kay S. Paget's disease of the nipple. *Surg Gynecol Obstet* 1966; **123**: 1010–4.

11 Dalberg K, Hellborg H, Wärnberg F. Paget's disease of the nipple in a population based cohort. *Breast Cancer Res Treat* 2008; **111**: 313–9.

12 Shamsadini S, Wadji MB, Shamsadini A. Surrounding ipsilateral eruptive seborrhoeic keratosis as a warning sign of intraductal breast carcinoma and Paget's disease (Leser Trelat sign). *Dermatol Online* 2006; **12**: 27.

13 Ashikari H, Park K, Huvós AG. Paget's disease of the breast. *Cancer* 1970; **26**: 680–5.

14 Culberson JD, Horn RC Jr. Paget's disease of the nipple: review of twenty-five cases with special reference to melanin pigmentation of 'Paget cells'. *Arch Surg* 1956; **72**: 224–31.

15 Orr JW, Parish DJ. The nature of the nipple changes in Paget's disease. *J Pathol Bacteriol* 1962; **84**: 201–8.

16 Cawley LP. Extramammary Paget's disease: report of a case. *Am J Clin Pathol* 1957; **27**: 559–66.

17 Nicolau SG, Balus L. Considérations pathogéniques sur la maladie de Paget, à l'occasion de l'étude d'un cas à localisation extra-mammaire. *Dermatologica* 1959; **119**: 93–105.

18 Kariniemi AL, Forsman L, Wahlstrohm T *et al.* Expression of differentiation antigens in mammary and extramammary Paget's disease. *Br J Dermatol* 1984; **110**: 203–10.

19 Reed W, Oppedal BR, Eeg Larsen T. Immunohistology is valuable in distinguishing between Paget's disease, Bowen's disease and superficial spreading melanoma. *Histopathology* 1990; **16**: 583–8.

20 Lin CH, Lee HS, Yu JC. Melanoma of the nipple mimicking Paget's disease. *Dermatol Online J* 2007; **13**: 18.

21 Kinoshita S, Yoshimoto K, Kyoda S *et al.* Malignant melanoma originating on the female nipple: a case report. *Breast Cancer* 2007; **14**: 105–8.

22 Paone JF, Baker RR. Pathogenesis and treatment of Paget's disease of the breast. *Cancer* 1981; **48**: 825–9.

23 Lagios MD, Westdahl PR, Rose MR. Paget's disease of the nipple: Alternative management in cases without or with minimal extent of underlying breast carcinoma. *Cancer* 1984; **54**: 545–51.

24 Fourquet A, Campana F, Vielh P *et al.* Paget's disease of the nipple without detectable breast tumour: conservative management with radiation therapy. *Int J Radiat Oncol Biol Phys* 1987; **13**: 1463–5.

Extramammary Paget's disease [1]

Definition. A marginated plaque resembling Paget's disease clinically and histologically, but occurring in sites rich in apocrine glands, such as the vulva, anogenital region and axilla.

There is currently controversy as to how often this condition arises on the background of an underlying carcinoma, and how often it arises primarily in the epidermis or apocrine ductal tissue of the affected area. This has given rise to the concept of primary and secondary extramammary Paget's disease [2].

Incidence and aetiology. This is a rare disease. It occurs more frequently in women and starts usually in the fifth decade or after. The current view is that in about 75% of cases, extramammary Paget's disease arises as a primary intraepidermal neoplasm, possibly from apocrine gland ductal cells or from keratinocyte stem cells. It has also been suggested that the disease may originate from Toker's cells [3]. In the remaining 25% of cases, an underlying primary adenocarcinoma is found. These cases are referred to as secondary Paget's disease.

Clinical features. The lesion has many features in common with Paget's disease of the nipple. The margin is sharp, rounded and slightly raised, and encloses an area that is pink or red. The surface may be scaly, and small, greyish crusts may cover erosions. Itching is a prominent feature and there may be excoriations or lichenification. Variable hyperpigmentation may be present, adding to the pathological confusion between extramammary Paget's disease and superficial spreading melanoma. In a proportion of cases, there may be leukoplakia.

The appearance varies somewhat according to the site. The commonest area involved is the vulva [4–6] (Fig. 53.33), followed by the perianal area, which is more frequently affected in men than women, the scrotum, penis and axilla [7,8]. The first symptom, especially in vulval lesions, is itching and burning, which may be persistent and spread. Quite often it is regarded as a dermatitis,

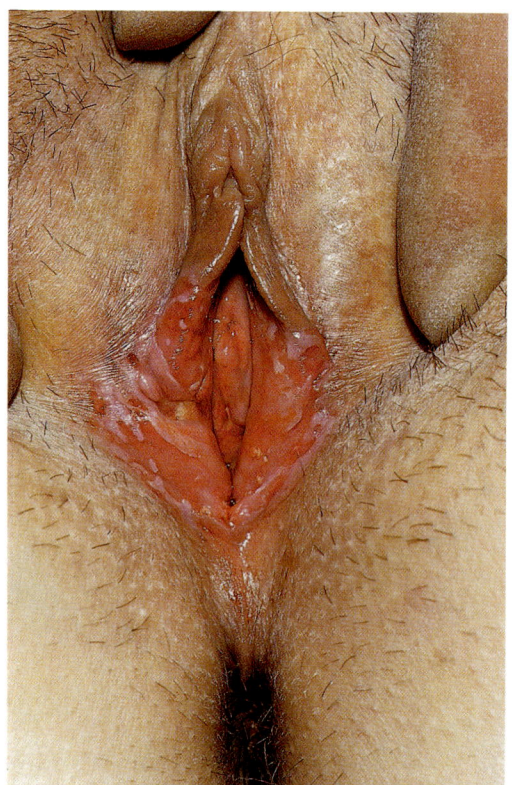

Fig. 53.33 Extramammary Paget's disease of the vulva showing inflamed eczematous presentation.

and may be irritated by topical therapy. The mucosal surfaces of the labia are frequently a rather more vivid red than the skin when both areas are involved, and the change may spread to the thighs, mons pubis and into the vaginal introitus. There may occasionally be a papillomatous surface. Perianal lesions may extend up into the anal canal. Lesions on the scrotum spread to the thigh or onto the shaft of the penis. Very occasionally, extramammary Paget's disease may be present on the eyelids or ears. Characteristic clinical features include the relentless progression, despite all local applications, and the sharp margin. Eventually, one area may become thickened and ulcerated as evidence of invasion downwards. Lymph node or distant metastases can occur.

Although most of the cases in which a primary carcinoma is found result from an underlying sweat gland adenocarcinoma, it is necessary to examine the patient for evidence of an adenocarcinoma elsewhere, particularly of the cervix and rectum.

Pathology. The changes in the epidermis are essentially similar to Paget's disease. The cells stain positively for acid as well as neutral mucopolysaccharides. They may contain melanin granules. Immunohistochemistry shows cells positive for CEA and Cam 5.2 and other low-molecular-weight keratins such as CK7 and CK8/18 [9]. GCDFP-15 is a marker of apocrine epithelium [10] and is frequently strongly expressed in primary vulval or perianal Paget's disease with no detectable underlying malignancy. Cytokeratin 20 is usually negative in primary cases and tends to be positive in lesions associated with an internal gastrointestinal tumour. Apomucin expression may be of help in establishing the origin of cases of extramammary Paget's disease [11]. Cases of intraepidermal vulval and penile and scrotal extramammary Paget's disease usually have a phenotype that is MUC1 positive, MUC2 negative and MUC5AC positive. In contrast, mammary Paget's disease is usually negative for the latter marker and perianal lesions associated with underlying rectal adenocarcinoma are positive for MUC2 and only variably positive for MUC1 and MUC5AC. Vulval lesions with underlying apocrine carcinoma tend to be negative for MUC5AC.

Comparative genomic hybridization studies in cases of extramammary Paget's disease have shown that the most common change is amplification at chromosomes Xcent-q21 and 19 and losses at chromosome 10q24-qter [12].

Diagnosis. The differential diagnosis from eczema, intertrigo and pruritus vulvae is made by the steady spread, lack of response to topical anti-inflammatory agents and the sharp and extending margin. Bowen's disease is usually more raised and verrucous, and superficial basal cell carcinoma has a thread-like margin. It may be difficult to differentiate leukoplakia or Bowen's disease of the mucosal surfaces, and biopsy may be required. As with mammary Paget's disease, superficial spreading melanoma is an important pathological differential diagnosis.

Prognosis and treatment. Local recurrence is common, even in cases with a wider excision [13]. Poor prognosis is associated with depth of invasion and with elevated serum levels of CEA [14]. Adequate tissue sampling and other investigations are essential to establish whether or not there is an associated underlying malignancy requiring surgical excision. If an underlying malignancy is present, it should be excised together with all clinically abnormal epithelium. If no underlying malignancy is detected on careful examination, the entire affected area of epithelium should be excised. Mohs surgery with careful control of excision margins may be useful, as a common cause of recurrence is inadequate excision of the lesion [15–17].

Promising results are reported with photodynamic therapy, but larger series and longer periods of follow-up are required [18,19]. In cases with limited disease, the use of topical imiquimod has been advocated with good results [20]. However, reports are mainly anecdotal. Radiotherapy has been advocated either as an adjunct to surgical therapy [21] or as an alternative therapy for elderly patients in whom surgery may be difficult [22].

References
1 Crocker HR. Paget's disease affecting the scrotum and penis. *Trans Pathol Soc London* 1888–1889; **40**: 187–91.
2 Lloyd J, Flanagan AM. Mammary and extramammary Paget's disease. *J Clin Pathol* 2000; **53**: 742–9.
3 Willman JH, Golitz LE, Fitzpatrick JE. Vulva clear cells of Toker: precursors of extramammary Paget's disease. *Am J Dermatopathol* 2005; **27**: 185–8.
4 Curtin JP, Rubin SC, Jones WB. Paget's disease of the vulva. *Gynaecol Oncol* 1990; **39**: 374–7.
5 Goldblum JR, Hart WR. Vulvar Paget's disease. *Am J Surg Pathol* 1997; **21**: 1178–87.
6 Fanning J, Lambert HC, Hale TM *et al.* Paget's disease of the vulva: prevalence of associated vulvar adenocarcinoma invasive Paget's disease, and recurrence after surgical excision. *Am J Obstet Gynaecol* 1999; **180**: 24–7.
7 Powell FC, Bjornsson J, Doyle JA *et al.* Genital Paget's disease and urinary tract malignancy. *J Am Acad Dermatol* 1985; **13**: 84–90.
8 Allen SJR, Mclaren K, Aldridge RD. Paget's disease of the scrotum: a case exhibiting positive prostate specific antigen staining and associated prostatic carcinoma. *Br J Dermatol* 1998; **138**: 689–91.
9 Liegl B, Liegl S, Gogg-Kamerer M *et al.* Mammary and extramammary Paget's disease: an immunohistochemical study of 83 cases. *Histopathology* 2007; **50**: 439–47.
10 Kohler S, Smoller BR. Gross cystic disease fluid protein-15 reactivity in extramammary Paget's disease with and without internal malignancy. *Am J Dermatopathol* 1996; **11**: 79–92.
11 Kuan SF, Montag AG, Hart J *et al.* Differential expression of mucin genes in mammary and extramammary Paget's disease. *Am J Surg Pathol* 2001; **25**: 1469–77.
12 Lee MW, Jee KJ, Gong GY *et al.* Comparative genomic hybridization in extramammary Paget's disease. *Br J Dermatol* 2005; **153**: 290–4.
13 Black D, Tornos C, Soslow RA *et al.* The outcomes of patients with positive margins after excision for intraepithelial Paget's disease of the vulva. *Gynecol Oncol* 2007; **104**: 547–50.
14 Hatta N, Yamada M, Hirano T *et al.* Extramammary Paget's disease: treatment, prognostic factors and outcome in 76 patients. *Br J Dermatol* 2008; **158**: 313–8.
15 Lloyd J, Evans DJ, Flanagan A. Extension of extramammary Paget's disease of the vulva to the cervix. *J Clin Pathol* 1999; **52**: 538–40.
16 Stacy D, Burrell MO, Franklin EW. Extramammary Paget's disease of the vulva and anus: use of intraoperative frozen sections. *Am J Obstet Gynaecol* 1986; **155**: 519–22.
17 Thomas CJ, Wood GC, Marks VJ. Mohs micrographic surgery in the treatment of rare aggressive cutaneous tumours: the Geisinger experience. *Dermatol Surg* 2007; **33**: 333–9.
18 Shieh S, Dee AS, Cheney RT *et al.* Photodynamic therapy for the treatment of extramammary Paget's disease. *Br J Dermatol* 2002; **146**: 1000–5.
19 Raspagliesi F, Fontanelli R, Rossi G *et al.* Photodynamic therapy using a methyl ester of 5 aminolevulinic acid in recurrent Paget's disease of the vulva: a pilot study. *Gynecol Oncol* 2006; **103**: 581–6.
20 Berman B, Spencer J, Villa A *et al.* Successful treatment of extramammary Paget's disease of the scrotum with Imiquimod 5% cream. *Clin Exp Dermatol* 2003; **28**: 36–8.
21 Guerrieri M, Back MF. Extramammary Paget's disease: role of radiation therapy. *Australas Radiol* 2002; **46**: 204–8.
22 Yanagi T, Kato N, Yamane N *et al.* Radiotherapy for extramammary Paget's disease: histopathological findings after radiotherapy. *Clin Exp Dermatol* 2007; **32**: 506–8.

Lymphoepithelioma-like carcinoma

Lymphoepitheliomas are well-recognized tumours of the nasopharynx, and an entity with similar histological features has also been observed in the skin [1]. However, the latter is not associated with Epstein–Barr virus (EBV) infection and its behaviour appears to be less aggressive than that of upper respiratory tract lesions [2,3]. Association with other viruses including HPV and simian virus 40 has not been found either [4].

Clinical features. The clinical appearance is of non-specific nodules on the head and neck area of older patients. Occasional cases present on the eyelid [5] and the trunk and vulva [6] are also rarely involved.

Pathology. The pathological features are those of a very dense infiltrate of inflammatory mononuclear cells, including lymphocytes and histiocytes, with small strands and nests of atypical epithelial cells. Inflammatory cells extensively infiltrate nests and strands of tumour cells, and the epithelial nature of these cells is often not immediately apparent unless more or less intact nests of epithelial cells are found. Confusion with a lymphoma is therefore a possibility, and often immunostaining for keratin and lymphoid cells is necessary to distinguish the two populations of cells. Cytological atypia is usually present, and mitotic figures are common. Focal evidence of adnexal differentiation and even neuroendocrine differentiation may be seen [7–12]. Some tumours appear to be arising from a squamous cell carcinoma. A sarcomatoid component may be seen [13]. It has therefore been suggested that this is not a distinctive entity but a morphological pattern in various cutaneous carcinomas [14].

Treatment. Surgery followed by radiotherapy is recommended. Some cases have been treated by Mohs surgery [15]. However, the lesions are aggressive, and both local recurrence and distant metastases, with one tumour-associated death, have been recorded [8,10,16].

References

1 Swanson SA, Cooper PH, Mills SE et al. Lymphoepithelioma-like carcinoma of the skin. *Mod Pathol* 1988; **1**: 359–65.
2 Ferlicot S, Plantier F, Rethers L et al. Lymphoepithelioma-like carcinoma of the skin: a report of 3 Epstein–Barr virus (EBV)-negative additional cases—immunohistochemical study of the stroma reaction. *J Cutan Pathol* 2000; **27**: 306–11.
3 Iezzoni JC, Gaffey MJ, Weiss LM. The role of Epstein–Barr virus in lymphoepithelioma-like carcinomas. *Am J Clin Pathol* 1995; **103**: 308–15.
4 Kazakov DV, Nemcova J, Mykiskova I et al. Absence of Epstein-Barr virus, human papillomavirus, and simian virus 40 in patients of central European origin with lymphoepithelioma-like carcinoma of the skin. *Am J Dermatopathol* 2007; **29**: 365–9.
5 Ho W, Taylor A, Kemp E et al. Lymphoepithelioma-like carcinoma of the eyelid: a report of two cases. *Br J Ophthalmol* 2005; **89**: 1222–3.
6 Axelsen SM, Stamp IM. Lymphoepithelioma-like carcinoma of the vulvar region. *Histopathology* 1995; **27**: 281–3.
7 Ortiz Fruitos FJ, Zarco C, Gil R et al. Lymphoepithelioma-like carcinoma of the skin. *Clin Exp Dermatol* 1993; **18**: 83–6.
8 Takayasu S, Yoshiyama M, Kutata S et al. Lymphoepithelioma-like carcinoma of the skin. *J Dermatol* 1996; **23**: 472–6.
9 Walker AN, Kent D, Mitchel AR. Lymphoepithelioma-like carcinoma of the skin. *J Am Acad Dermatol* 1990; **22**: 691–3.
10 Wick MR, Swanson PE, LeBoit PE et al. Lymphoepithelioma-like carcinoma of the skin with adnexal differentiation. *J Cutan Pathol* 1991; **18**: 93–102.
11 Otsuki T, Watanabe D, Yako K et al. Lymphoepithelioma-like carcinoma of the skin with potential for sweat gland differentiation. *J Dermatol* 2005; **32**: 393–6.
12 Ríos-Martín JJ, Solorzano-Amoreti A, Gonzalez-Cámpora R et al. Neuroendocrine carcinoma of the skin with a lymphoepithelioma-like histological pattern. *Br J Dermatol* 2000; **143**: 460–2.
13 Clarke LE, Ioffreda MD. Lymphoepithelioma-like carcinoma of the skin with spindle cell differentiation. *J Cutan Pathol* 2005; **32**: 419–23.
14 Lind AC, Breer WA, Wick MR. Lymphoepithelioma-like carcinoma of the skin with apparent origin in the epidermis—a pattern or an entity? A case report. *Cancer* 1999; **15**: 884–90.
15 Glaich AS, Behroozan DS, Cohen JL et al. Lymphoepithelioma-like carcinoma of the skin: a report of two cases treated with complete microscopic margin control and review of the literature. *Dermatol Surg* 2006; **32**: 316–9.
16 Hall G, Duncan A, Azurdia R et al. Lymphoepithelioma-like carcinoma of the skin: a case with lymph node metastasis at presentation. *Am J Dermatopathol* 2007; **29**: 365–9.

Merkel cell carcinoma [1]

Synonyms
- Trabecular cell carcinoma of skin
- Primary neuroendocrine carcinoma of the skin

Definition. An aggressive and frequently lethal tumour thought to arise from the cutaneous Merkel cell, a neuroendocrine cell [2].

Incidence and aetiology. The first definitive report of Merkel cell tumour dates from 1978 [2], although there are reports in 1972 of 'trabecular cell carcinoma of skin' [1], which is synonymous. De Wolf-Peeters *et al.* [3] were the first to suggest the use of the term 'Merkel-cell tumour'. More than 2000 cases have been recorded to date. This is a rare tumour of the elderly presenting mainly in Caucasians (0.23 annual age adjusted incidence per 100 000) [4], with a high concentration of primary tumours on sun-exposed sites. There are also a high number of cases in association with immunosuppression [5], including not only transplant patients but also those with HIV infection [6]. Incidence in patients with chronic lymphocytic leukaemia is much higher than in the general population [5]. The general incidence seems to be rising [7]. Tumours very rarely occur in patients with dark skin. An unexpectedly high proportion of Merkel cell tumours arise in association with either squamous cell or basal cell carcinomas, or in patients who have a past history of such lesions [8]. These facts suggest that excessive ultraviolet exposure may play an aetiological role in the development of Merkel cell tumours. Recently, it has been suggested that a novel type of polyomavirus (named Merkel cell polyomavirus) may play a role in the aetiology of the neoplasm as clonal integration of the virus was demonstrated in eight out of 10 cases of Merkel cell carcinoma tested [9].

Clinical features [10]. The lesions appear to have few distinctive features, and are described as raised, reddish-blue nodules, which may develop on any body site, although the head and neck area is over-represented in terms of surface area. Tumours are asymptomatic in the majority of cases and grow rapidly with most lesions measuring between 0.5 and 2 cm. Spontaneous regression of Merkel cell carcinoma has occasionally been reported [11,12]. Partial regression has been reported as a result of withdrawal of azathioprine in an immunosuppressed patient [13], although rapid growth of a tumour was described after treatment with rituximab [14].

Pathology [15,16]. The cells making up the tumour may be either a solid mass or a more diffuse collection of cells, initially situated in the mid-dermis. They are intensely basophilic, with abundant mitotic figures and also many apoptotic cells (Fig. 53.34). Lymphatic and vascular invasion is frequently present. On light microscopy, they may resemble small lymphocytes or a poorly differentiated metastatic deposit, particularly of small cell carcinoma of lung or of naevoid melanoma. The cells are argyrophilic, with sparse cytoplasm, dispersed chromatin and inconspicuous nucleoli. There may be a dense lymphoid infiltrate [17]. Exceptional cases are restricted to the epidermis (*in situ*) [18].

Electron microscopy [19] may be used for positive identification of the multiple, round, secretory granules that pack the cytoplasm of these cells. However, cytomorphology of tumour cells and immunohistochemistry is enough to establish a diagnosis.

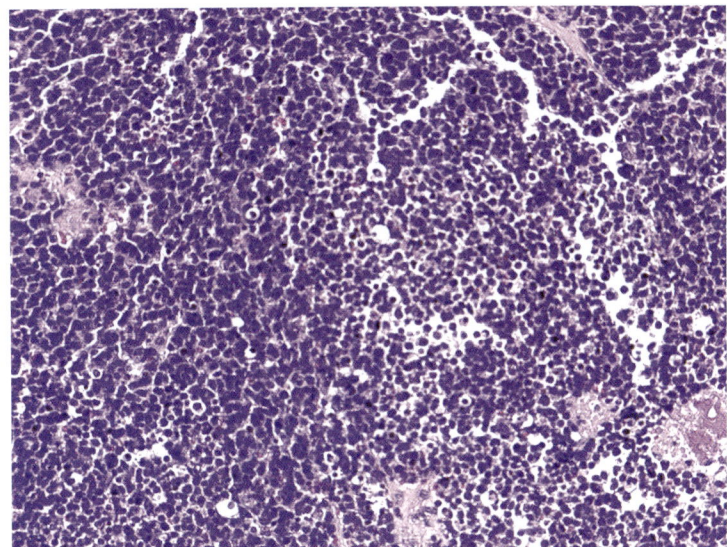

Fig. 53.34 Merkel cell carcinoma. Hyperchromatic medium-sized cells with scanty cytoplasm, prominent apoptosis and high mitotic activity.

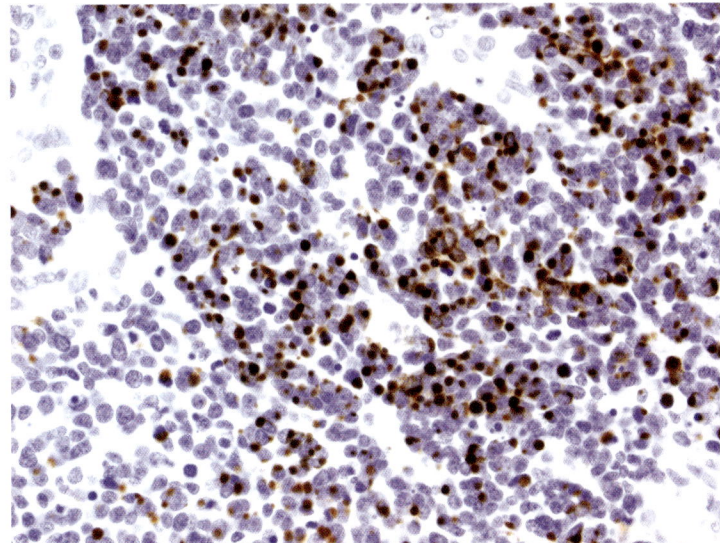

Fig. 53.35 Merkel cell carcinoma. Characteristic dot-like perinuclear positivity of cytokeratin 20.

Immunohistochemistry is useful in confirming the diagnosis. Merkel cells show a characteristic 'dot' positivity with antibodies to low-molecular-weight keratins such as cam 5.2 and CK20 (Fig. 53.35). CK20 is particularly useful in the differential diagnosis from metastatic neuroendocrine carcinomas arising in other organs. The latter except for neuroendocrine carcinoma of salivary glands tend to be negative for this marker [20]. They are also positive for neurone-specific enolase, CD56 and variably positive for chromogranin and synaptophysin. The latter is much more sensitive than chromogranin. A small subset of cases has been identified in which tumour cells are negative for cytokeratin 20 but positive for cytokeratin 7 [21]. These tumours are otherwise typical Merkel cell carcinomas.

Histological features associated with poor outcome include tumour size (≥5 mm), extension into the subcutaneous tissue, diffuse growth pattern and a heavy mononuclear inflammatory cell infiltrate [22]. A further study, however, has found that absence of lymphocytic infiltration adversely influences disease-free survival. In the same study a further important adverse variable was the presence of positivity of more than 50% of tumour cells for Ki-67 [23]. Expression of p63 by tumour cells has also been found to be an independent factor indicating poor prognosis [24]. Tumour thickness does not seem to influence prognosis [25].

Treatment. Surgical excision is required [26], but metastases occur early and 30–50% of patients may die from metastases. Arterial limb perfusion has been used for lesions on limbs and may be beneficial [27]. Merkel cell tumours are considered to be radiosensitive, and trials of postoperative radiotherapy suggest a survival advantage [28]. Sentinel lymph node biopsy is a useful procedure not only to demonstrate spread in patients that have been understaged by clinical and radiological (CT scan) examination but is also important in predicting prognosis and improving survival in patients with positive results who undergo lymph node dissection [29]. The detection of micrometastasis in sentinel lymph nodes is increased by the use of immunohistochemistry for cytokeratin 20

[30]. The preferred treatment at present is surgical excision with sentinel lymph node biopsy followed by lymph node dissection if the latter is positive. Postoperative radiotherapy is also given and this approach improves locoregional control and also improves disease-free survival [31,32]. Treatment of involved regional lymph nodes, with or without lymphadenectomy, has also been found to increase survival [33]. Chemotherapy is not routinely recommended as there is lack of evidence that it increases survival, there is important morbidity and mortality associated with this modality of treatment and resistance to chemotherapy quickly develops in many patients [34].

References
1 Toker C. Trabecular cell carcinoma of the skin. *Arch Dermatol* 1972; **105**: 107–10.
2 Tang C, Toker C. Trabecular cell carcinoma of the skin: an ultrastructural study. *Cancer* 1978; **42**: 2311–21.
3 De Wolf-Peeters C, Marien K, Mebis J *et al.* A cutaneous APUDoma or Merkel cell tumor? A morphologically recognizable tumor with a biological and histological malignant aspect in contrast with its clinical behavior. *Cancer* 1980; **46**: 1810–6.
4 Miller RW, Rabkin CS. Merkel cell carcinoma and melanoma: etiological similarities and differences. *Cancer Epidemiol Biomarkers Prev* 1999; **8**: 153–8.
5 Heath M, Jaimes N, Lemos B *et al.* Clinical characteristics of Merkel cell carcinoma at diagnosis in 195 patients: the AEIOU features. *J Am Acad Dermatol* 2008; **58**: 375–81.
6 Manganoni MA, Farisoglio C, Tucci G *et al.* Merkel cell carcinoma and HIV infection: a case report and review of the literature. *AIDS Patient Care STDS* 2007; **21**: 447–51.
7 Lemos B, Nghiem P. Merkel cell carcinoma: more deaths but still no pathway to blame. *J Invest Dermatol* 2007; **127**: 2100–3.
8 Dancey AL, Rayatt SS, Soon C *et al.* Merkel cell carcinoma: a report of 34 cases and literature review. *J Plast Reconstr Aesthet Surg* 2006; **59**: 1294–9.
9 Feng H, Shuda M, Chang Y *et al.* Clonal integration of a polyomavirus in human Merkel cell carcinoma. *Science* 2008; **319**: 1096–100.
10 Akhtar S, Oza KK, Wright J. Merkel cell carcinoma: report of 10 cases and review of the literature. *J Am Acad Dermatol* 2000; **43**: 755–67.
11 Kubo H, Matsushita S, Fukushige T *et al.* Spontaneous regression of recurrent and metastatic Merkel cell carcinoma. *J Dermatol* 2007; **34**: 773–7.
12 Vesely MJ, Murray DJ, Neligan PC *et al.* Complete spontaneous regression of Merkel cell carcinoma. *J Plast Reconstr Aesthet Surg* 2008; **61**: 165–71.

13 Muirhead R, Ritchie DM. Partial regression of Merkel cell carcinoma in response to withdrawal of azathioprine in an immunosuppression-induced case of metastatic Merkel cell carcinoma. *Clin Oncol (R Coll Radiol)* 2007; **19**: 96.

14 Wirges ML, Saporito F, Smith J. Rapid growth of Merkel cell carcinoma after treatment with rituximab. *J Drugs Dermatol* 2006; **5**: 180–1.

15 Skelton HG, Smith KJ, Hitchcock CL *et al.* Merkel cell carcinoma: analysis of clinical, histologic and immunohistochemical features of 132 cases with relation to survival. *J Am Acad Dernatol* 1997; **175**: 734–9.

16 Smith PD, Patterson JW. Merkel cell carcinoma (neuroendocrine carcinoma of the skin). *Am J Clin Pathol* 2001; **115** (Suppl.): S68–78.

17 Kasami M, Murmatsu K, Kawahata K *et al.* Large-cell neuroendocrine carcinoma of the skin, with lymphoid stroma. *Am J Dermatopathol* 2007; **29**: 578–80.

18 Ferringer T, Rogers HC, Metcalf JS. Merkel cell carcinoma in situ. *J Cutan Pathol* 2005; **32**: 162–5.

19 Haneke E. Electron microscopy of Merkel cell carcinoma from formalin fixed tissue. *J Am Acad Dermatol* 1985; **12**: 487–92.

20 Chan JK, Suster S, Wenig BM *et al.* Cytokeratin 20 immunoreactivity distinguishes Merkel cell (primary cutaneous neuroendocrine) carcinomas and salivary gland small carcinomas from small cell carcinomas of various sites. *Am J Surg Pathol* 1997; **21**: 226–34.

21 Calder KB, Coplowitz S, Schlauder S *et al.* A case series and immunophenotypic analysis of CK20-/CK7 + primary neuroendocrine carcinoma of the skin. *J Cutan Pathol* 2007; **34**: 918–23.

22 Mott RT, Smoller BR, Morgan MB. Merkel cell carcinoma: a clinicopathologic study with prognostic implications. *J Cutan Pathol* 2004; **31**: 217–23.

23 Llombart B, Monteagudo C, López-Guerrero JA *et al.* Clinicopathological and immunohistochemical analysis of 20 cases of Merkel cell carcinoma in search of prognostic markers. *Histopathology* 2005; **46**: 622–34.

24 Asioli S, Righi A, Volante M *et al.* p63 expression as a new prognostic marker in Merkel cell carcinoma. *Cancer* 2007; **110**: 640–7.

25 Goldberg SR, Neifield JP, Frable WJ. Prognostic value of tumor thickness in patients with Merkel cell carcinoma. *J Surg Oncol* 2007; **95**: 618–22.

26 Wong KC, Zuletta F, Clark SJ *et al.* Clinical management and treatment outcomes of Merkel cell carcinoma. *Aust NZ J Surg* 1998; **68**: 354–8.

27 Dawson R, Williams OM, Mansel RE. Isolated hyperthermic limb perfusion chemotherapy in Merkel cell tumour. *J R Coll Surg Edinb* 1996; **41**: 255–6.

28 Kokoska ER, Kokoska MS, Collins BT *et al.* Early aggressive treatment for Merkel cell carcinoma improves outcome. *Am J Surg* 1997; **174**: 688–93.

29 Gupta SG, Wang LC, Peñas PF *et al.* Sentinel lymph node biopsy for evaluation and treatment of patients with Merkel cell carcinoma: The Dana-Faber experience and meta-analysis of the literature. *Arch Dermatol* 2006; **142**: 685–90.

30 Su LD, Lowe L, Bradford CR *et al.* Immunostaining for cytokeratin 20 improves detection of micrometastatic Merkel cell carcinoma in sentinel lymph nodes. *J Am Acad Dermatol* 2002; **46**: 661–6.

31 Mojica P, Smith D, Ellenhom JD. Adjuvant radiation therapy is associated with improved survival in Merkel cell carcinoma of the skin. *J Clin Oncol* 2007; **25**: 1043–7.

32 Eng TY, Boersma MG, Fuller CD *et al.* A comprehensive review of the treatment of Merkel cell carcinoma. *Am J Clin Oncol* 2007; **30**: 624–36.

33 Jabbour J, Cumming R, Scolyer RA *et al.* Merkel cell carcinoma: assessing the effect of wide local excision, lymph node dissection, and radiotherapy on recurrence and survival in early-stage disease—results from a review of 82 consecutive cases diagnosed between 1992 and 2004. *Ann Surg Oncol* 2007; **14**: 1943–52.

34 Garneski KM, Nghiem P. Merkel cell carcinoma adjuvant therapy: current data support radiation but not chemotherapy. *J Am Acad Dermatol* 2007; **57**: 166–9.

CHAPTER 54

Lentigos, Melanocytic Naevi and Melanoma

J.A. Newton Bishop

Leeds Institute of Molecular Medicine, St James's University Hospital, Leeds, UK

Introduction

Factors responsible for variation in skin pigmentation are discussed in Chapter 58. Melanin pigment is synthesized and distributed to adjacent cells by cutaneous melanocytes, which are found in normal skin in the basal layer of the epidermis. Melanocytes lie in continuity with adjacent keratinocytes into which they transfer melanosomes. Melanocytes and keratinocytes are therefore biologically interdependent and cells of both lineages may be involved in many of the entities discussed below. Melanin synthesis and distribution is accelerated by exposure to UV radiation. Cutaneous pathology attributable to the melanocyte may arise as a result of overproduction of melanin by a normal quota of melanocytes as in the simple freckle, by proliferation of benign melanocytes as in a melanocytic naevus, or as a result of malignant transformation of the melanocyte as in malignant melanoma (henceforth referred to as melanoma).

The freckle or ephelis

Definition. A pale-brown, macular lesion, usually less than 3 mm in diameter with a poorly defined lateral margin, which appears and darkens on light-exposed skin sites during periods of UV exposure.

Clinical features. At any age, simple freckles are commoner in individuals who are red- or fair-haired and fair-skinned (Fig. 54.1). They fade during the winter months.

The clinical distinction between a freckle and a lentigo is that the lentigo persists in the absence of UV stimulation, and histologically a lentigo has a linear increase of melanocytes at the dermal–epidermal junction, but the two entities coexist in the same individuals and the risk factors for both are generally the same.

Pathology. The simple freckle shows no anatomical abnormality on biopsy [1,2]. It arises as a result of temporary overproduction of melanin by a normal quota of melanocytes due to stimulation

Rook's Textbook of Dermatology, 8th edition. Edited by DA Burns, SM Breathnach, NH Cox and CEM Griffiths. © 2010 Blackwell Publishing Ltd.

by UV radiation. It has been claimed that the melanocortin 1 receptor gene (MCR1) is the major freckle gene, and that *MC1R* gene variants are required for the development of freckles [3], but it is still unclear what mechanism underlies this. Elder and Murphy have even speculated that the signal for increased transfer of pigment from the melanocyte might come from the keratinocyte [4].

Diagnosis. This is usually obvious with the presence of regular macular brown lesions on light-exposed skin. The freckles and

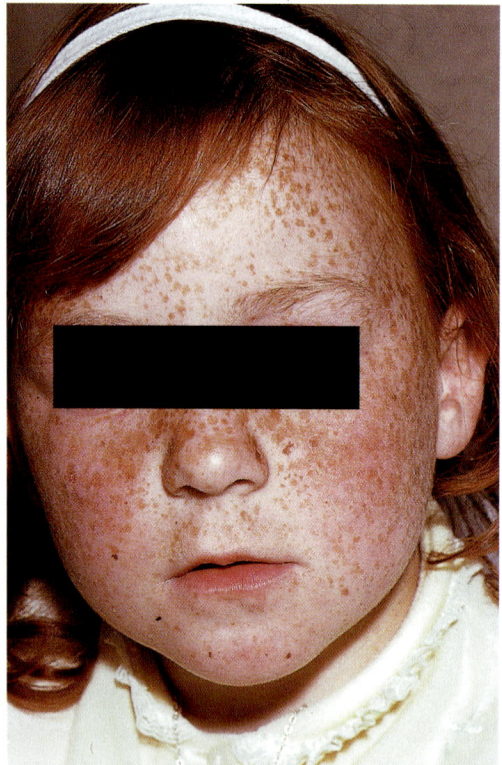

Fig. 54.1 Freckles in a child with red hair: freckles are indicative of fair skin vulnerable to sunburn.

café-au-lait spots of neurofibromatosis (Chapter 15) are distinguished as they are commonly on the trunk and axilla, and other features of neurofibromatosis may be present.

Management. No treatment is needed for these benign lesions, and their biological significance lies in the fact that they have been identified in case–control studies as an independent risk factor for skin cancer and in particular for melanoma: in a meta-analysis a high density of freckles was associated with a relative risk of melanoma of 2.10 (95% CI 1.80–2.45) [5].

Lentigines (Table 54.1)

These are also macular hyperpigmented skin lesions, but they persist throughout the year, and on microscopy have an increase in the number of melanocytes at the dermal–epidermal junction compared to that expected for the body site in question. The proliferation of melanocytes occurs usually in response to sun exposure in fair-skinned people (common lentigines). Rarely, syndromal lentigines occur when melanocyte proliferation is determined by inherited genetic anomalies.

Common lentigines are usually seen in fair-skinned people, and represent proliferative responses of melanocytes to the sun. They are commonly subclassified, but excessive exposure to natural or artificial UV radiation is the major aetiological factor for all of the following: simple lentigines, actinic (or solar) lentigines, psoralen UVA (PUVA) lentigines and the ink-spot lentigo. To some extent, the distinction between these subtypes is artificial as they represent a continuum or variations on a theme. Their features are described below, and compared in Table 54.1.

Rare forms of lentiginoses are also seen as characteristic features of a number of rare but potentially serious hereditary multisystem syndromes associated with an increased risk of tumours (Fig. 54.2; Chapter 15).

Very rarely, segmental lentiginoses may be seen; these emerge during childhood and are presumed to represent mosaicism of an unidentified gene [6]. Usually there are no other congenital anom-

Table 54.1 Comparison of freckles, lentigines and related disorders.

Lesion	Distribution	Melanocyte number	Significance
Freckle	Sun-exposed skin	Not increased	Risk factor for skin cancer and sunburn
Simple lentigo	Sun-exposed skin	Increased	Risk factor for skin cancer and sunburn
Solar lentigo	Sun-exposed skin	Increased and accompanied by pathological evidence of solar damage	Risk factor for skin cancer and sunburn
PUVA lentigo	Anywhere	Increased	Risk factor for skin cancer
Ink-spot lentigo	Anywhere but commonly shoulders	Increased and accompanied by pigment in the epidermis and dermis	Probably a risk factor for skin cancer and sunburn but no data are available
Hereditary lentiginoses	Generalized and not preferentially sun-exposed skin. Mucosal surfaces also often involved	Increased	Marker of risk of hamartomas and cancer
Genital melanosis	Genital skin	Debated: no (or extremely subtle) increase in number	None: if *in situ* melanoma excluded by biopsy
Labial melanotic macule	Lower lip generally	Debated: no (or extremely subtle) increase in number	Sun protection required

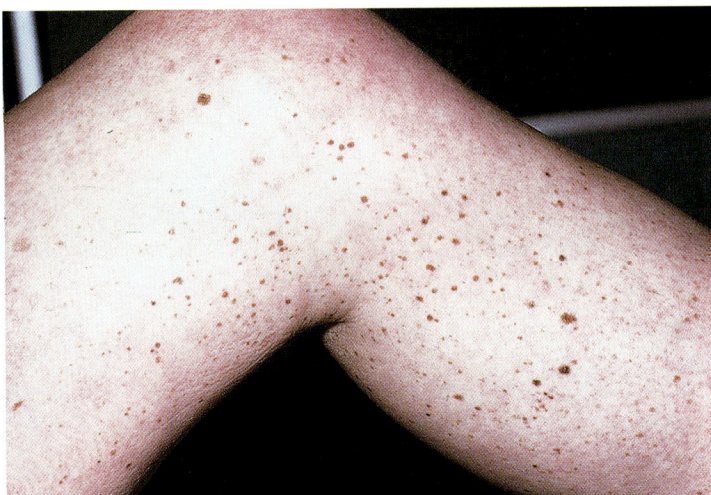

Fig. 54.2 Multiple lentigos in a patient with hereditary lentiginosis and cardiac anomalies.

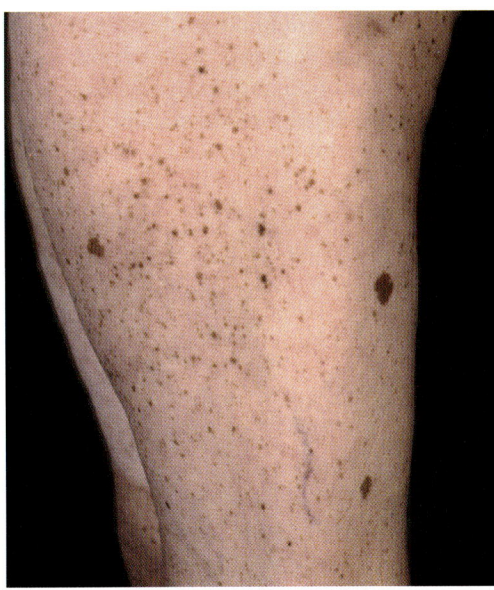

Fig. 54.4 Generalized lentiginosis in a patient who developed cutaneous melanoma in her 50s.

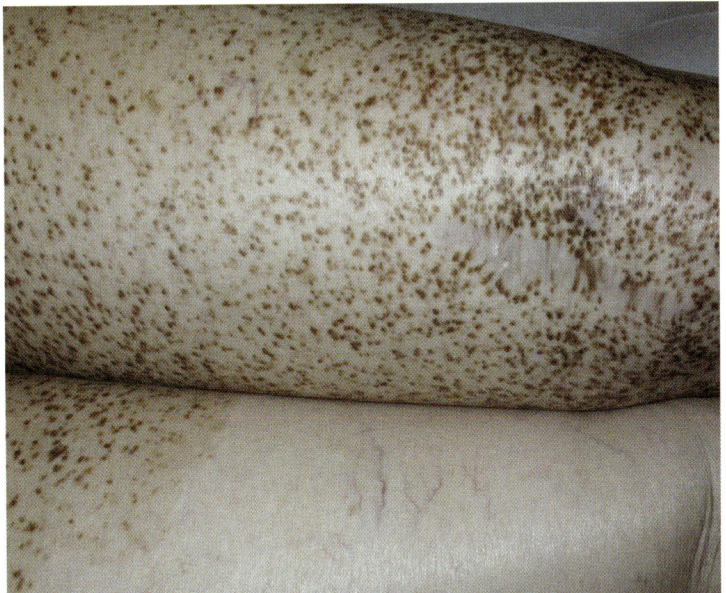

Fig. 54.3 A systematized lentiginosis in which a superficial spreading melanoma developed on the knee.

alies and the differential diagnosis includes neurofibromatosis type 1. Melanoma may occur in patients with segmental or generalized lentiginosis (Figs 54.3 & 54.4).

Simple lentigo

Definition. A brown macule, arising as a result of an increased number of melanocytes at the dermoepidermal junction, without evidence of proliferation of these melanocytes downwards into the dermis.

Aetiology and incidence. Multiple, benign lentigines occurring as an isolated phenomenon are very common, particularly in those with red hair and fair skin with melanocytes which produce a high phaeomelanin/eumelanin ratio.

Clinical features. A lentigo is a macular area of brown or brown-black pigmentation, usually circular or oval, although several individual lentigines may coalesce. There may be slight scaling of the surface, but the skin markings are unaltered. The pigmentation is usually light brown and fairly uniform. Lentigines usually start to appear in childhood and increase in number in the second and third decades. Rarely, they may erupt in large numbers [7], sometimes after inflammation, or related to use of immunosuppressive agents [8,9]. The majority of lentigines remain static in adult life. Most commonly, lentigos occur on sun exposed skin as they are part of the spectrum of lesions (ephiledes, simple lentigos, solar lentigos) which occur in fair-skinned people exposed to excessive amounts of sun exposure for their phenotype.

Whilst a lentigo, by definition, is characterized by an increased number of melanocytes, there is a clinical and even a pathological overlap with lesions in which there is an increased number of melanocytes but in which there is also a proliferation of keratinocytes; these are often referred to as 'flat seborrhoeic keratoses' or, on the back of the hands, as 'liver spots'. In practice, this overlap is of little clinical importance; all are markers of fair skin, excessive sun exposure and some risk of skin cancer. All are to be distinguished from lentigo maligna, which is usually relatively easy.

There are a number of hereditary disorders, however, in which multiple lentigines are markers of syndromes characterized by hyperplasias, hamartomas and neoplasia [10], and in these people the lentigos develop much earlier in life and are not restricted in site to sun-exposed skin. In some of these, the causal genetic mutations specifically affect tissues sharing a common origin in the neural crest [11,12] such as melanocytes and cardiac tissues. The familial lentigines include Peutz–Jeghers syndrome [13], the LEOPARD syndrome (*l*entigines, *e*lectrocardiogram anomalies, *o*cular anomalies, *p*ulmonary stenosis, *a*bnormal genitalia, *r*etardation of growth and *d*eafness), in which mutations in the *PTEN* gene have been described [14], the Carney complex and the closely related NAME and LAMB syndromes. The genetic origin of these syndromes appears to involve diverse pathways which are supposed to converge in embryogenesis and the development of systems including the neural crest [10]. Rarely, lentiginoses may develop in childhood in the absence of multisystem disease [15].

Even more rarely, multiple lentigines may be seen in patients with an evident increased susceptibility to melanoma (Fig. 54.4). A single case report of a patient with lentiginoses and gastrointestinal stromal tumours in the presence of a hereditary *c-kit* mutation suggests that this may represent a further, extremely rare, new subtype [16].

Pathology. There is a linear increase in the number of melanocytes along the dermal–epidermal junction. There is more melanin than normal in the adjacent epidermis and stratum corneum, and melanophages are abundant in the papillary body. The papillae and interpapillary ridges may be elongated—hence the overlap with pigmented seborrhoeic keratoses.

Diagnosis. Lentigines are distinguished from freckles by their darker colour, comparative sparseness and scattered distribution, and by the fact that they do not darken or increase in number on sun exposure, and do not disappear during the winter months. It is often impossible to distinguish lentigines from flat junctional or compound naevi on clinical grounds.

Treatment. As common lentigines are usually multiple, and have no pre-malignant potential, the patient should be reassured. They are however a marker of fair skin, as are freckles. For treatment, see Solar or actinic lentigo, below. Patients with lentiginoses presenting in childhood or early adult life, on non-sun-exposed sites, should be examined for multisystem disease. Extremely rare patients who present with systematized or generalized lentiginoses may be at increased risk of melanoma, and so should be educated about avoidance of sunburn and about self-examination.

Solar or actinic lentigo

Definition. A macular area of brown pigmentation appearing after either acute or chronic sun exposure.

Clinical features. In younger patients, solar lentigines are most commonly seen on sun-exposed sites, such as the face in both sexes and the shoulders in males. They are macular, tan coloured and may be very large, with a striking irregular border. There is frequently a history of acute sunburn, followed by the sudden appearance of large numbers of these irregular macular lesions [17,18]. In the UK, they are rare before the age of 12 years but in sunnier countries they may appear at a very young age.

Solar lentigines are also seen on older fair-skinned patients who have had excessive sun exposure [19]. The backs of the hands and the face are common sites. Once again the lesions are large and macular, have an irregular edge and are usually a uniform shade of brown. They are situated in an area of obviously sun-damaged epidermis and as above there is a clinical and pathological overlap with flat seborrhoeic keratoses.

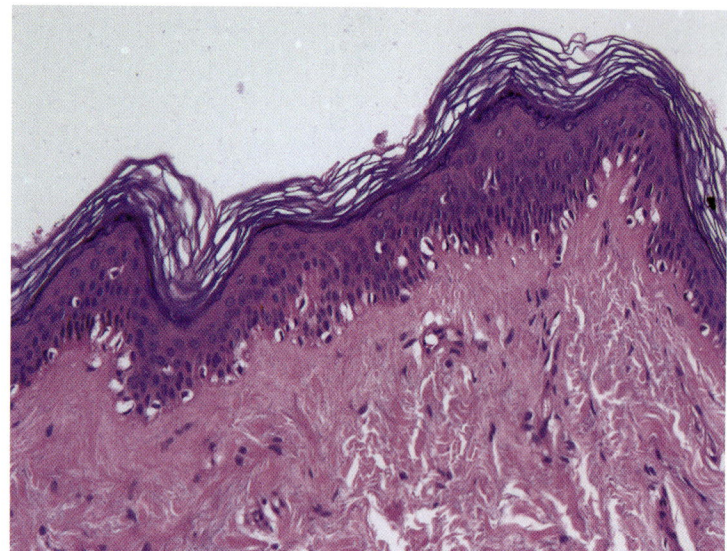

Fig. 54.5 An increased number of melanocytes is seen in this solar lentigo. The dermis also shows elastosis as evidence of sun damage. (Courtesy of Dr S. Edward, Leeds Teaching Hospitals Trust, Leeds, UK.)

Pathology. The pathological features of a solar lentigo are a continuum of those seen in the smaller simple lentigines. There is a linear increase of melanocytes at the dermal–epidermal junction, but no cytological atypia of these melanocytes, and no budding down of these cells into the underlying dermis. There is frequently associated actinic damage to the adjacent dermal collagen (Fig. 54.5).

Treatment. Because of the large size and unsightly appearance of some actinic lentigines, patients frequently request treatment. Prevention of further UV-induced damage should be encouraged by sun avoidance and the use of a high sun-protection factor, broad-spectrum sunscreen. With these measures, there is often some spontaneous resolution of existing lesions. A consensus supported the use of cryotherapy as first line therapy, where cosmesis is required [20]. There is, however, an extensive literature on the cosmetic treatment of lentigines using a variety of additional treatments including intense pulsed light [21,22], laser therapy and topical agents such as retinoids [23]. A review suggested that superficial pigmented lesions of this type respond well to the high-energy QS red and infrared lasers [24].

The majority of solar lentigos progress little over time. A small proportion, however, do slowly progress to become lentigo malignas over many years (Fig. 54.6). A well-defined, large solar lentigo on the face of a younger patient should therefore probably be treated although there are no data to support this advice.

Photochemotherapy (PUVA) lentigo

Lentigines are a well-recognized complication of long-term use of PUVA therapy [25]. They were reported in 20% of a small series of 198 patients given a mean cumulative dose of UVA of 169.5 J/cm² [26], and PUVA lentigines of any degree (slight, moderate or extensive) were noted on the buttocks of 53% of 1380 psoriatic patients an average of 5.7 years after starting PUVA [27]. They are

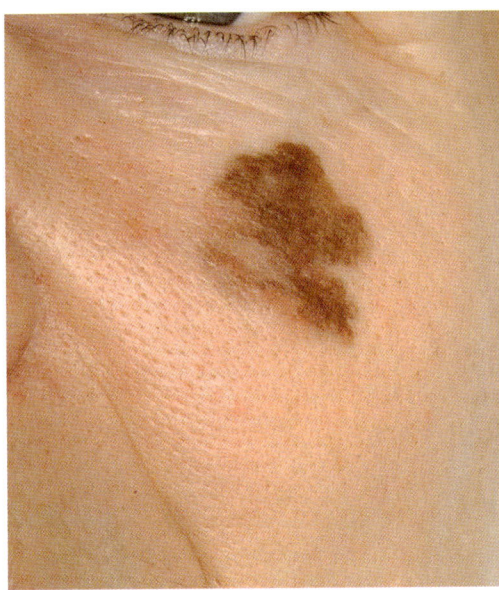

Fig. 54.6 This lentigo maligna developed from a tiny lentigo over a period of 30 years.

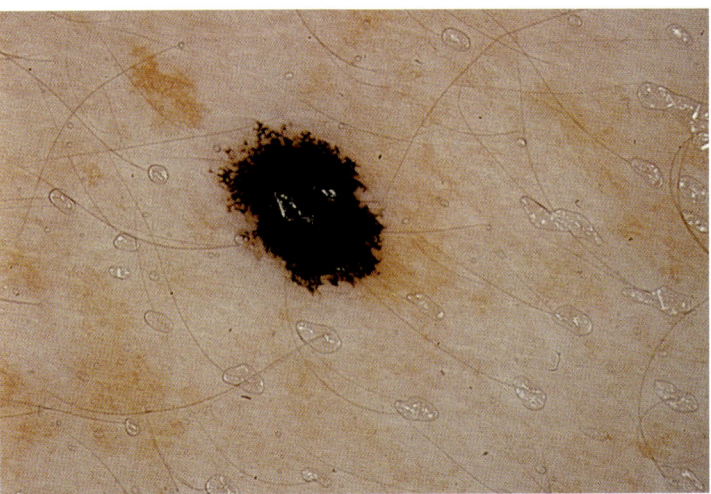

Fig. 54.7 An ink-spot lentigo.

relatively large, macular, pigmented lesions, which develop on the skin of patients receiving photochemotherapy. The number of melanocytes in the relevant body site is increased, and ultrastructural examination reveals morphological abnormalities of the melanosomes [28]. Follow-up of PUVA-treated patients in the USA has indicated that PUVA lentigines are a marker of patients at increased risk of non-melanoma skin cancer [29]. The association of risk of melanoma with PUVA treatment generally is less clear, as although an increased risk was seen in a series from the USA [30] this was not seen in a series from Scandinavia [31].

Ink-spot lentigo

Definition. A small (less than 5 mm in diameter), densely black, irregular macule, usually on sun-exposed skin (such as the upper back in a very fair-skinned person who has had a good deal of sun exposure), which resembles an ink spot (Fig. 54.7) [32].

Clinical features. These lesions commonly cause concern because they are so black and irregular in shape. The clinical diagnosis is obvious, however, when the dermoscope is used (Fig. 54.8).

Pathology. The pathology of the lesion is that of a lentigo, with a linear increase in melanocytes in the basal layer of the epidermis, and an associated increase in melanin pigmentation both in the basal cells of the epidermis and also lying free in the underlying epidermis. The melanocytes are normal, and there is no evidence of cellular atypia.

Management. These lesions do not require treatment.

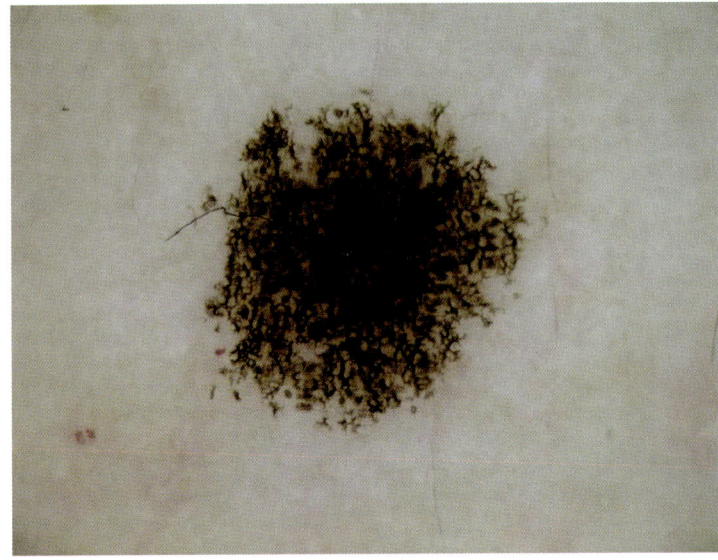

Fig. 54.8 The dermoscopic appearance of an ink-spot lentigo. (Courtesy of Dr S. Puig, Hospital Clinic Barcelona, IDIBAPS.)

References

1 Breathnach AS. Melanocyte distribution in forearm epidermis of freckled human subjects. *J Invest Dermatol* 1957; **29**: 253–61.

2 Breathnach AS, Wyllie LM. Electron microscopy of melanocytes and melanosomes in freckled human epidermis. *J Invest Dermatol* 1964; **42**: 389–94.

3 Bastiaens M, ter Huurne J, Gruis N *et al*. The melanocortin-1-receptor gene is the major freckle gene. *Hum Mol Genet* 2001; **10**: 1701–8.

4 Elder DE, Murphy GF. *Melanocytic Tumors of the Skin*. Washington, DC: American Registry of Pathology, in press.

5 Gandini S, Sera F, Cattaruzza MS *et al*. Meta-analysis of risk factors for cutaneous melanoma: III. Family history, actinic damage and phenotypic factors. *Eur J Cancer* 2005; **41**: 2040–59.

6 Toelle SP, Boltshauser E, Wirth MG, Itin P. Association of lentiginous mosaicism and congenital cataract in a girl. *Eur J Dermatol* 2006; **16**: 360–2.

7 Na JI, Park KC, Youn SW. Familial eruptive lentiginosis. *J Am Acad Dermatol* 2006; **55**: S38–40.

8 Hickey JR, Robson A, Barker JN, Smith CH. Does topical tacrolimus induce lentigines in children with atopic dermatitis? A report of three cases. *Br J Dermatol* 2005; **152**: 152–4.

9 Tosti A, Piraccini BM, Misciali C, Vincenzi C. Lentiginous eruption due to topical immunotherapy. *Arch Dermatol* 2003; **139**: 544–5.

10 Bauer AJ, Stratakis CA. The lentiginoses: cutaneous markers of systemic disease and a window to new aspects of tumourigenesis. *J Med Genet* 2005; **42**: 801–10.

11 Abdelmalek NF, Gerber TL, Menter A. Cardiocutaneous syndromes and associations. *J Am Acad Dermatol* 2002; **46**: 161–83, quiz 183.

12 Ho JC, Chan YC, Giam YC *et al*. Flexural pigmentation with multiple lentigines: a new primary pigmentary disorder? *Br J Dermatol* 2006; **154**: 382–4.

13 Stratakis CA. Genetics of Peutz–Jeghers syndrome, Carney complex and other familial lentiginoses. *Hormone Res* 2000; **54**: 334–43.

14 Digilio MC, Conti E, Sarkozy A *et al*. Grouping of multiple-lentigines/LEOPARD and Noonan syndromes on the *PTEN11* gene. *Am J Hum Genet* 2002; **71**: 389–94.

15 Chong WS, Klanwarin W, Giam YC. Generalized lentiginosis in two children lacking systemic associations: case report and review of the literature. *Pediatr Dermatol* 2004; **21**: 139–45.

16 Shibusawa Y, Tamura A, Mochiki E *et al*. c-kit Mutation in generalized lentigines associated with gastrointestinal stromal tumor. *Dermatology* 2004; **208**: 217–20.

17 Derancourt C, Bourdon-Lanoy E, Grob JJ *et al*. Multiple large solar lentigos on the upper back as clinical markers of past severe sunburn: a case–control study. *Dermatology* 2007; **214**: 25–31.

18 McLean DL, Gallagher RP. Sunburn freckles, cafe-au-lait macules, and other pigmented lesions of schoolchildren: The Vancouver Mole Study. *J Am Acad Dermatol* 1995; **32**: 565–70.

19 Monestier S, Gaudy C, Gouvernet J *et al*. Multiple senile lentigos of the face, a skin ageing pattern resulting from a life excess of intermittent sun exposure in dark-skinned caucasians: a case–control study. *Br J Dermatol* 2006; **154**: 438–44.

20 Ortonne JP, Pandya AG, Lui H, Hexsel D. Treatment of solar lentigines. *J Am Acad Dermatol* 2006; **54**: S262–71.

21 Kawana S, Ochiai H, Tachihara R. Objective evaluation of the effect of intense pulsed light on rosacea and solar lentigines by spectrophotometric analysis of skin color. *Dermatol Surg* 2007; **33**: 449–54.

22 Yamashita T, Negishi K, Hariya T *et al*. Intense pulsed light therapy for superficial pigmented lesions evaluated by reflectance-mode confocal microscopy and optical coherence tomography. *J Invest Dermatol* 2006; **126**: 2281–6.

23 Ortonne JP. Retinoid therapy of pigmentary disorders. *Dermatol Ther* 2006; **19**: 280–8.

24 Tanzi EL, Lupton JR, Alster TS. Lasers in dermatology: four decades of progress. *J Am Acad Dermatol* 2003; **49**: 1–31, quiz 31–4.

25 Basarab T, Millard TP, McGregor JM, Barker JN. Atypical pigmented lesions following extensive PUVA therapy. *Clin Exp Dermatol* 2000; **25**: 135–7.

26 Abdullah AN, Keczkes K. Cutaneous and ocular side-effects of PUVA photochemotherapy—a 10-year follow-up study. *Clin Exp Dermatol* 1989; **14**: 421–4.

27 Rhodes AR, Stern RS, Melski JW. The PUVA lentigo: an analysis of predisposing factors. *J Invest Dermatol* 1983; **81**: 459–63.

28 Nakagawa H, Rhodes AR, Momtaz TK, Fitzpatrick TB. Morphologic alterations of epidermal melanocytes and melanosomes in PUVA lentigines: a comparative ultrastructural investigation of lentigines induced by PUVA and sunlight. *J Invest Dermatol* 1984; **82**: 101–7.

29 Stern RS. Risks of cancer associated with long-term exposure to PUVA in humans: current status—1991. *Blood Cells* 1992; **18**: 91–7, discussion 98–9.

30 Stern RS. The risk of melanoma in association with long-term exposure to PUVA. *J Am Acad Dermatol* 2001; **44**: 755–61.

31 Lindelof B, Sigurgeirsson B, Tegner E *et al*. PUVA and cancer risk: the Swedish follow-up study. *Br J Dermatol* 1999; **141**: 108–12.

32 Bolognia JL. Reticulated black solar lentigo ('ink spot' lentigo). *Arch Dermatol* 1992; **128**: 934–40.

Mucosal melanotic lesions

Pigmented melanotic macules (mucosal melanosis/genital lentiginosis)

Some macular pigmentation of the mucosa in the mouth or on the genitalia is normal; the pigmentation may be increased at sites of trauma and is generally subtle. In the mouth, smoking is thought to induce melanosis and post-inflammatory pigmentation occurs. Lentines may also occur in familial lentiginoses discussed above.

More discrete, more deeply pigmented macules are also common on the vulva and sometimes on the glans penis, when they are usually referred to as genital melanotic macules, or mucosal mela-

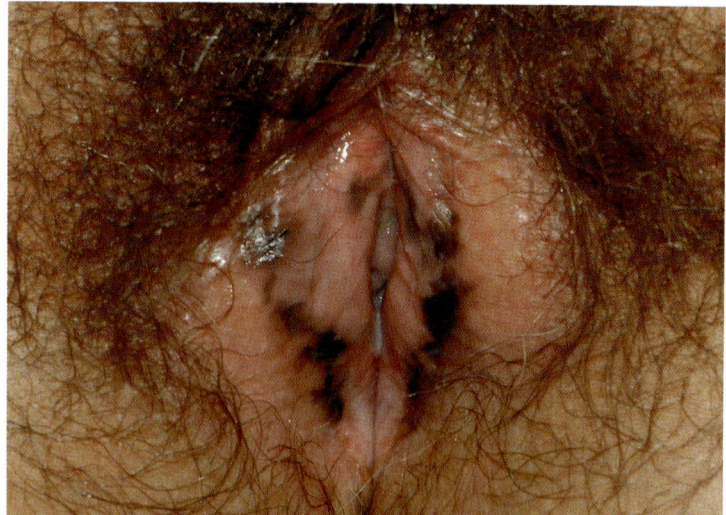

Fig. 54.9 Genital melanosis; a benign condition of unknown aetiology which none-the-less can cause considerable clinical concern.

nosis. These macules result from local excessive pigment production with normal numbers of melanocytes [1]. There is confusion around aetiology and nomenclature so that some authors refer to melanoses, others to lentiginoses, but the entities probably overlap.

Rarely, these melanotic macules may expand to several centimetres in size, they may be patchy in distribution and may develop irregular deep pigmentation, which resembles melanoma and causes concern. Melanoma must be excluded by biopsy as melanoma in the genital area may begin with a protracted *in situ* phase, but normally the histological appearance of such lesions is banal, although it has been suggested that the majority have a subtle increase in melanocyte number [2]. The aetiology of genital melanosis is unclear; the presence of pruritus has led to suggestions of a precursor inflammation but none has been clearly identified [1].

The presence of pigmented patches in the genital skin of women affected by lichen sclerosus et atrophicus has been reported [3]. Biopsy of these lesions has shown the lesions to be atypical melanocytic naevi. There is no obvious explanation for the development of these naevi in lichen sclerosus et atrophicus, but it is important to be aware of this association, as clinically the lesions may suggest melanoma.

Clinical features. These lesions are relatively large macular areas of uniform brown, black or grey pigmentation (Fig. 54.9). They may have slowly expanded to reach a large diameter over several years. The differential diagnosis in the mouth is that of oral melanoma which is a rare tumour, representing 0.5% of oral cancers [4]. Oral melanomas may be subtle in appearance (see Fig. 54.64 below) and are described as a smooth swelling which might be evenly hyperpigmented or irregularly pigmented.

Pathology. The pathology of mucosal melanosis is usually much less dramatic than their clinical appearance. There is a clear increase of melanin pigment in the basal layer keratinocytes with some overspill into the dermis, resulting in pigment-laden macrophages. The melanocyte count is relatively normal with only a slight linear increase and no junctional activity.

Treatment. No treatment is required if an incisional biopsy of appropriate area(s) has confidently excluded a significant lentiginosis or melanoma. The often dramatically intense pigmentation, however, usually leads to persistent concern and it is therefore reasonable to keep under review, although the issue is actually only one of excluding *in situ* melanoma; mucosal melanosis without the proliferation of atypical melanocytes is held not to be pre-malignant. A change in appearance would merit another biopsy, as the differential diagnosis is *in situ* melanoma.

If there is a significantly increased number of melanocytes, particularly if there is confluent proliferation resembling lentigo maligna, then treatment is required. The treatment options are limited in these circumstances. In the presence of clear *in situ* change, then surgery would be the normal treatment choice. The mutilating effect of this surgery, however, is such that a therapeutic trial of topical imiquimod might be justified with biopsy after treatment [5], although patients may find it difficult to tolerate in this site.

Labial melanotic macules [6,7]

Definition. Flat areas of benign, non-progressive melanin pigmentation on the lips, which may be best viewed as a type of freckle or a lesion akin to a simple lentigo [8].

Clinical features. Labial melanotic macules usually affect the lower lip in the central third. More females than males seek treatment for these lesions. The site suggests that excessive exposure to natural UV radiation may be an aetiological factor. The natural history is of the relatively rapid appearance of a brown to black macule on the lower lip in a young adult. The macules rarely become larger than 0.5 cm in diameter, and are usually single lesions (Fig. 54.10). The differential diagnosis includes an amalgam tattoo.

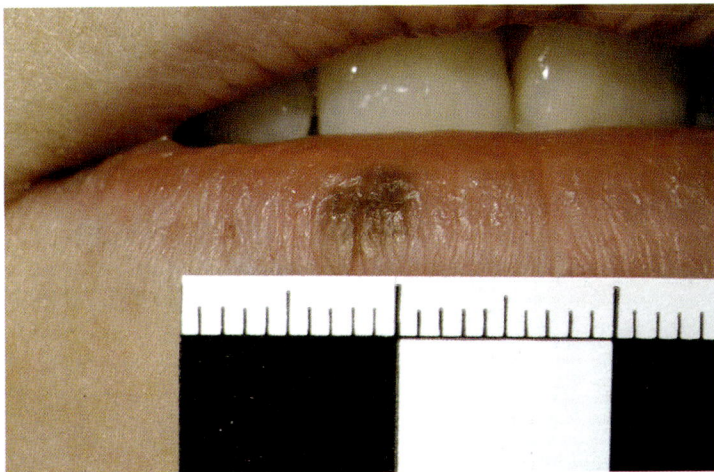

Fig. 54.10 A labial melanotic macule. This is a benign lesion seen in fair-skinned people, which is thought to be related to sun damage.

Pathology. The pathology is that of linear increase in melanin pigment in the basal cells. There may be a very modest increase in the number of melanocytes [8]. Malignant transformation has not been reported in these lesions.

Treatment. Reassurance is all that is needed on medical grounds. If removal is requested for cosmetic reasons, cryotherapy, use of the infrared coagulator or laser therapy [9] may all be effective.

References
1 Lenane P, Keane CO, Connell BO *et al.* Genital melanotic macules: clinical, histologic, immunohistochemical, and ultrastructural features. *J Am Acad Dermatol* 2000; **42**: 640–4.
2 Barnhill RL, Albert LS, Shama SK *et al.* Genital lentiginosis: a clinical and histopathologic study. *J Am Acad Dermatol* 1990; **22**: 453–60.
3 Carlson JA, Mu XC, Slominski A *et al.* Melanocytic proliferations associated with lichen sclerosus. *Arch Dermatol* 2002; **138**: 77–87.
4 Meleti M, Rene Leemans C, Mooi WJ *et al.* Oral malignant melanoma: a review of the literature. *Oral Oncol* 2007; **43**: 116–21.
5 Rajpar SF, Marsden JR. Imiquimod in the treatment of lentigo maligna. *Br J Dermatol* 2006; **155**: 653–6.
6 Gupta G, Williams RE, Mackie RM. The labial melanotic macule: a review of 79 cases. *Br J Dermatol* 1997; **136**: 772–5.
7 Weathers DR, Corio RL, Crawford BE *et al.* The labial melanotic macule. *Oral Surg Oral Med Oral Pathol* 1976; **42**: 196–205.
8 Maize JC. Mucosal melanosis. *Dermatol Clin* 1988; **6**: 283–93.
9 Gupta G, MacKay IR, MacKie RM. Q-switched ruby laser in the treatment of labial melanotic macules. *Lasers Surg Med* 1999; **25**: 219–22.

Dermal melanocytic lesions [1]

Common acquired melanocytic naevi described later in this chapter are believed, on the basis of biopsies from multiple lesions in patients at varying ages, to develop from epidermal melanocytes that completed their migration from the neural crest to the dermal–epidermal junction in fetal life, proliferated and then senesced (i.e. ceased proliferation). By contrast, the dermal lesions described here differ in that they are believed to arise from dermal melanocytes that have become arrested in the dermis during fetal life and tissue modelling and have not reached their normal site in the basal layer of the epidermis. Many mammals have a population of dermal melanocytes normally but these are not commonly observed in human dermis, with the possible exception of the Mongolian spot.

Mongolian spot

Definition. Macular blue-grey pigmentation present at birth on the sacral area in normal infants.

Incidence. The incidence of Mongolian spot varies with skin colour. They are rare in white-skinned European infants (the highest prevalence in Europe being in the Mediterranean region). By comparison, the majority of babies born to families from the Far East have a Mongolian spot. The incidence in other populations lies between these extremes. It has been found in some 26% of Turkish babies [2] and 71% of Iranian babies [3]. The relationship with skin colour raises the possibility that such lesions are

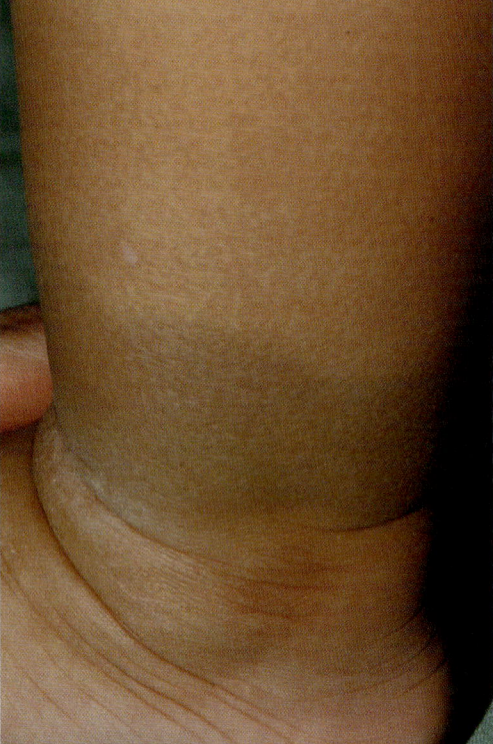

Fig. 54.11 A Mongolian spot which was evident on the limbs as well as in the lumbosacral area.

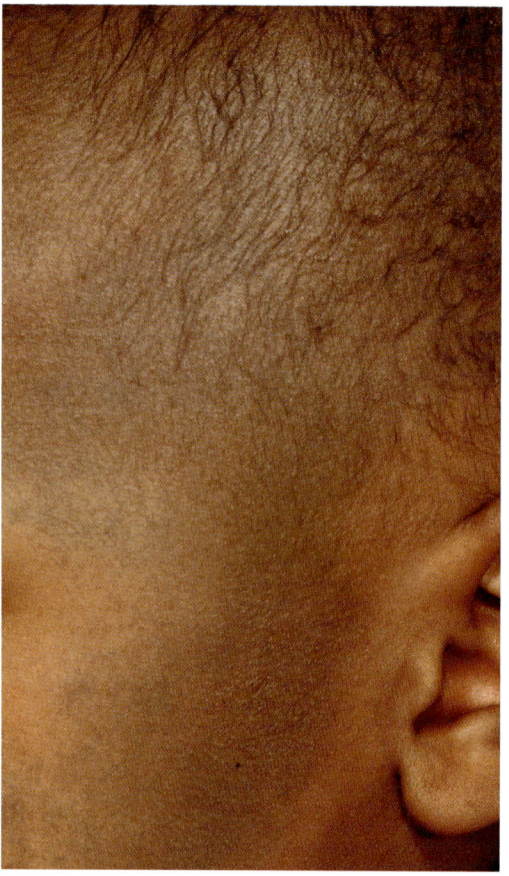

Fig. 54.12 A naevus of Ota visible in a young child.

merely more obvious in the skin where the patient has melanocytes producing a good deal of pigment.

Clinical features. The pigmentation is macular, diffuse and more or less uniform, slate blue to grey and usually relatively faint. The patches are usually rounded or oval in shape, up to 10 cm or so in diameter, and usually single but occasionally multiple. The lumbosacral region is the common site, and the buttocks, flanks or even shoulders and lower legs (Fig. 54.11) may be affected in extensive lesions. The pigmentation develops in fetal life, increases in depth for a period after birth and then diminishes. It usually disappears during the first decade, but has occasionally persisted into adult life.

Pathology. Melanocytes are dispersed in a ribbon-like pattern between the collagen fibres and around the neurovascular bundles of the dermis. They run parallel to the skin surface and contain very fine granules of melanin. There is no disturbance of the pattern of collagen and elastic fibres. Melanophages are not found. The last two characteristics enable it to be differentiated from blue naevus.

Management. No treatment is needed.

Naevus of Ota

Synonym
- Naevus fuscocaeruleus ophthalmomaxillaris

Definition. An extensive, blue, patch-like area of dermal melanocytic pigmentation of the sclera and the skin adjacent to the eye due to the presence of dermal melanocytes. The melanocytes may also extend into the uveal tract, dura and nasopharynx.

Incidence. This disorder is most common in Asian people (but still seen in less than 1%) [4] but is very rare in other groups. Unlike the Mongolian spot, it is not usually visible at birth, but becomes progressively darker in childhood (Fig. 54.12) and persists in adult life. There are published cases in which these lesions are acquired in adult life (Fig. 54.13) [5].

Clinical features. The pigmentation is often speckled and is composed of deeper bluish and more superficial brownish elements, which do not always coincide. The two colours are perhaps best seen in the eye, where the affected sclera is blue and the conjunctiva brown. The brown pigmentation is patchy and may be patterned in a reticular or geographical way; the blue pigmentation is more diffuse. The areas involved are the eyelids, the bulbar and palpebral conjunctiva and the sclera, and the cheeks, forehead, scalp, alae nasi and ears. The mucosa of the palate and cheeks may also be affected. The distribution is usually restricted to the first and second divisions of the trigeminal nerve, but rarely patches may occur on the trunk.

The pigmented spots usually appear in childhood and increase in number and extent to become confluent in some areas. There is one report of the onset following trauma, and in another the ocular

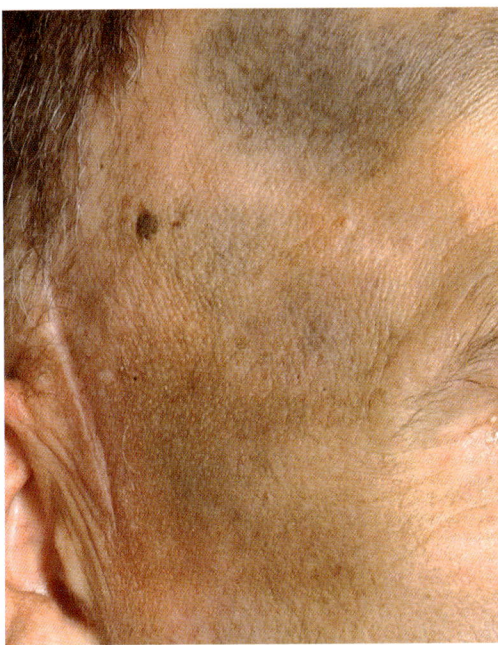

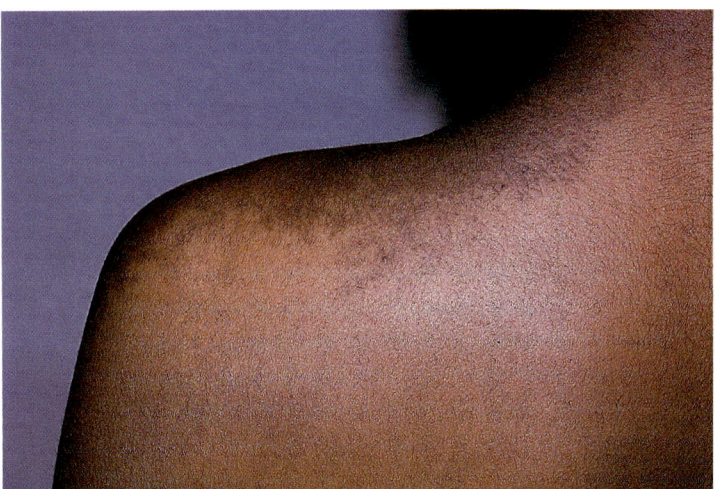

Fig. 54.14 Naevus of Ito, showing typical distribution over the shoulder area.

Fig. 54.13 This patient acquired a naevus of Ota in adult life and then developed a meningeal melanoma in relation to this blue naevus.

pigmentation became much more pronounced after an attack of conjunctivitis. The distribution is usually, but not always, unilateral.

Benign intracerebral proliferations, known as melanocytomas, are described as complications of these lesions [6]. In very rare instances malignant melanoma has developed in naevus of Ota, and this may also occur within the meninges, as in the patient seen in Fig. 54.13, or in the choroid [7,8]. Survival after excision of meningeal melanoma in these circumstances may have a surprisingly good prognosis [9].

Pathology. The features are the same as those of Mongolian spot. A variety is described called Naevus fusco-caeruleus zygomaticus [10] in which speckled naevi are seen on the upper cheek, and microscopy shows bipolar pigment-bearing cells in the upper dermis only, in contrast to the naevus of Ota in which pigment-bearing cells are seen throughout the dermis.

Treatment. Laser therapy may be of value [11], although post-treatment hypopigmentation may result [12], and cosmetic camouflage may also be useful.

Naevus of Ito

This type of dermal melanocytosis involves the acromioclavicular region and the upper chest and, like the naevus of Ota, is largely confined to the Japanese (Fig. 54.14).

References

1 Zembowicz A, Mihm MC. Dermal dendritic melanocytic proliferations: an update. *Histopathology* 2004; **45**: 433–51.
2 Egemen A, Ikizoglu T, Ergor S *et al*. Frequency and characteristics of Mongolian spots among Turkish children in Aegean region. *Turkish J Pediatr* 2006; **48**: 232–6.
3 Moosavi Z, Hosseini T. One-year survey of cutaneous lesions in 1000 consecutive Iranian newborns. *Pediatr Dermatol* 2006; **23**: 61–3.
4 Chan HH, Kono T. Nevus of Ota: clinical aspects and management. *Skinmed* 2003; **2**: 89–96, quiz 97–8.
5 Stanford DG, Georgouras KE. Dermal melanocytosis: a clinical spectrum. *Australas J Dermatol* 1996; **37**: 19–25.
6 Rahimi-Movaghar V, Karimi M. Meningeal melanocytoma of the brain and oculodermal melanocytosis (nevus of Ota): case report and literature review. *Surg Neurol* 2003; **59**: 200–10.
7 Baroody M, Holds JB. Extensive locoregional malignant melanoma transformation in a patient with oculodermal melanocytosis. *Plast Reconstr Surg* 2004; **113**: 317–22.
8 Sharan S, Grigg JR, Billson FA. Bilateral naevus of Ota with choroidal melanoma and diffuse retinal pigmentation in a dark skinned person. *Br J Ophthalmol* 2005; **89**: 1529.
9 Theunissen P, Spincemaille G, Pannebakker M, Lambers J. Meningeal melanoma associated with nevus of Ota: case report and review. *Clinical Neuropathol* 1993; **12**: 125–9.
10 Sun CC, Lu YC, Lee EF, Nakagawa H. Naevus fusco-caeruleus zygomaticus. *Br J Dermatol* 1987; **117**: 545–53.
11 Lu Z, Fang L, Jiao S *et al*. Treatment of 522 patients with Nevus of Ota with Q-switched Alexandrite laser. *Chin Med J* 2003; **116**: 226–30.
12 Kono T, Nozaki M, Chan HH, Mikashima Y. A retrospective study looking at the long-term complications of Q-switched ruby laser in the treatment of nevus of Ota. *Lasers Surg Med* 2001; **29**: 156–9.

Melanocytic naevi

Epidemiology. Melanocytic naevi are normal, benign proliferations of melanocytes. Although the risk of a naevus evolving into a melanoma is extremely small, melanocytic naevi are both risk factors for melanoma and precursors of melanoma.

The prevalence of pigmented lesions present at birth varies considerably between published series; this is principally because of the ethnic mix of the patients examined, as congenital melanocytic naevi may be more common in black or Asian children [1], but they are generally considered to be present in between 1 and 2% of newborns [2]. Most congenital naevi are deeply pigmented at birth but it may be difficult to differentiate congenital naevi from café-au-lait spots clinically. There is very limited sequential information about the eruption of acquired naevi in the period immediately after birth, but it is thought that naevi clinically and

Table 54.2 Terms commonly used in the description of melanocytic naevi.

Melanocyte	A pigment-producing cell characterized by its ability to synthesize melanosomes. Contains the enzyme 3,4-dihydroxyphenylalanine (DOPA)
Theque	A group of melanocytes (generally four or more) in contact with the basal layer of the epidermis but budding downwards into the dermis
Freckle	An area of increased melanin pigmentation
	The only histological abnormality is an excess of melanin pigment; the lesion would therefore appear to be the result of functionally overactive melanocyte/keratinocyte units
	These lesions are stimulated by UV irradiation
Lentigo	An area of increased melanin pigmentation, which shows histologically a linear replacement of keratinocytes in the basal layer of the epidermis by melanocytes
	This replacement does not reach the level of theque formation; if this were the case, the term junctional naevus would be appropriate
Junctional activity	The presence at the dermal–epidermal junction of theques of melanocytes
Junctional naevus	A pigmented melanocytic naevus in which the main histological feature is that of junctional activity
	A few naevus cells are usually observed scattered in the underlying dermis
Compound naevus	A pigmented melanocytic naevus in which the histological features include both junctional activity and the presence of naevus cells in the dermis
	Such naevi usually contain melanin
Intradermal naevus	A melanocytic naevus in which there is little or no abnormality of melanocytes in the epidermis
	The main feature is the presence of packets of naevus cells in the dermis
	Melanin pigmentation is often absent and such naevi may be clinically non-pigmented
	The deepest dermal cells tend to neural or fibroblastic differentiation

histologically similar to the congenital type may erupt within the first year of life. In adults, it has been reported that around 2% of individuals have congenital naevus-like lesions [3]. In the only sequential study reported to date of acquired naevi in the same cohort of children [4], 0.5% of 1012 babies examined at birth had melanocytic naevi compared with 35% at the age of 1 year.

Terminology commonly used in describing melanocytic naevi is included in Table 54.2.

References

1 Castilla E, Da Graca Dutra M, Orioli-Parreiras I. Epidemiology of congenital pigmented naevi: risk factors. *Br J Dermatol* 1981; **104**: 421–7.
2 Osburn K, Schosser RH, Everett MA. Congenital pigmented and vascular lesions in newborn infants. *J Am Acad Dermatol* 1987; **16**: 788–92.
3 Kopf AW, Levine LJ, Rigel DS *et al*. Prevalence of congenital-nevus-like nevi, nevi spili, and café au lait spots. *Arch Dermatol* 1985; **121**: 766–9.
4 Goss B, Forman D, Ansell P *et al*. The prevalence and characteristics of congenital pigmented lesions in newborn babies in Oxford. *Paed Perinatal Epidemiol* 1990; **4**: 448–57.

Congenital melanocytic naevi

Congenital melanocytic naevi have been arbitrarily divided into three size ranges in order to develop consistent approaches to prognosis and management. Of those melanomas that have evolved from or within congenital naevi, the majority have occurred in large naevi; because of this, great distinction has been drawn between congenital naevi less than 10 cm in diameter and larger ones. Most authors use the American National Institutes of Health (NIH) consensus definition to categorize these naevi according to size. In this document, small congenital naevi are defined as under 1.5 cm in diameter, large as having a diameter between 1.5 and 20 cm and giant naevi as having a diameter of 20 cm or more [1] (Table 54.3). The great majority of congenital

Table 54.3 Overview of congenital melanocytic naevi.

Naevus type	Subtype	Characteristic pathology	Significance	Treatment
Congenital melanocytic naevus, evident at birth	Small (<1.5 cm) May appear in the first 2 years of life	Deeper naevus cells exhibiting a tendency to extend deeply in relation to skin appendages	Very small risk of melanoma	None, other than self-examination Consider excision in sites where review is difficult such as the scalp
	Large (1.5 to 20 cm)	Deeper naevus cells exhibiting a tendency to extend deeply in relation to skin appendages	Increased risk of melanoma	Excise if technically feasible with good cosmetic result
	Giant (>20 cm)	Deeper naevus cells exhibiting a tendency to extend deeply in relation to skin appendages May be associated with benign but atypical proliferations such as hamartomas	Increased risk of melanoma especially if over the trunk and associated with many satellite naevi Lifetime risk is poorly quantified but is likely to be less than 14%	Removal of risk not possible because such lesions cannot be fully excised Surgical decisions should be based upon the cosmetic likelihood of success and should be deferred to assess spontaneous improvement in the first few years of life
Naevi thought to be variants of congenital naevi but which appear in childhood	Speckled naevus	Banal naevi arising in a macular lentigo with subtle increase in melanocyte number	Uncommon cases of melanoma described arising in such naevi	Education about self-examination
	Agminate Spitz naevus	Spitzoid proliferations arising in a macular area of pigmentation	Similar to a speckled naevus but with spitzoid elements	Review at intervals and excise changing elements within

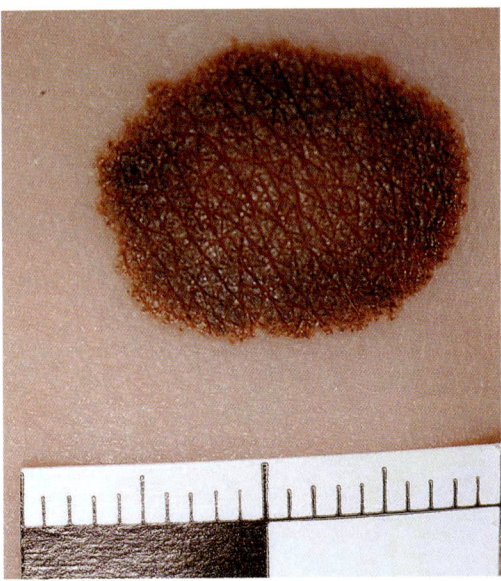

Fig. 54.15 A small congenital melanocytic naevus in a child.

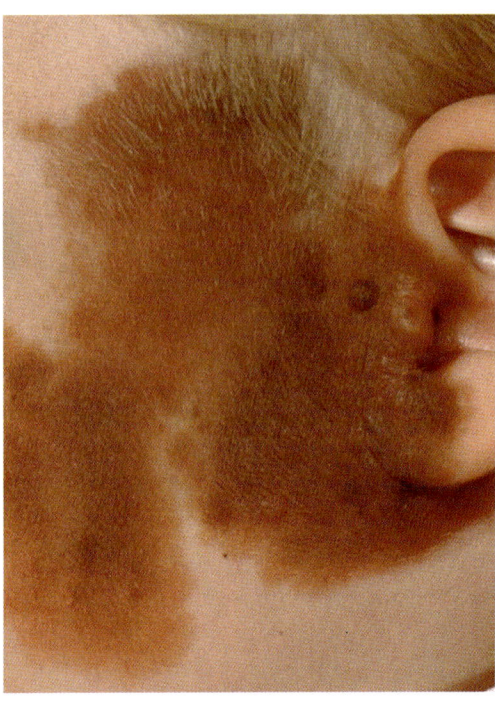

Fig. 54.16 A large congenital melanocytic naevus with junctional and compound elements.

naevi are small, although the published studies in the literature, particularly in relation to the malignant potential of congenital naevi, mainly relate to the giant, or garment, type. The giant type is rare; Castilla *et al.* described a study of 500 000 infants in South America in which one naevus at least 10 cm in diameter was identified per 20 445 subjects [2].

Clinical features. Congenital naevi are usually obvious and deeply pigmented at birth, although occasional naevi may be initially obscured by vernix and a proportion appear in the months after birth (Figs 54.15 & 54.16). The majority are macular at birth.

As the child grows the naevus usually grows in proportion. At some sites, such as the scalp, there is commonly a considerable increase in terminal hair (which is often darker than normal hair and more wiry), soon after birth, which causes alarm. In other sites, an increase in terminal hair tends to occur more subtly over time and may be accompanied by the development of rugosity. A significant proportion of naevi become paler in the first 1 to 2 years of life, and at sites such as the scalp may fade to cosmetic insignificance [3] (Fig. 54.17). There is, therefore, much to be said for deferring treatment decisions until after this period if surgery is being considered for cosmetic reasons, as, in a good proportion, the cosmetic appearance of the naevus will have considerably improved and this may influence decisions regarding the need for surgery.

The giant, garment or bathing-trunk naevus is very rare but is a considerable cosmetic problem for children and their families. The common site is the lower back and thigh area and a very large proportion of the infant's surface area may be involved (Fig. 54.18). There may also be large numbers of smaller congenital naevi present elsewhere on the infant's skin; increased numbers of these will develop over time. Such so-called satellite naevi (Fig. 54.19) were reported in 74% of one series [4]. In the same series, 31% of the patients also had naevi on mucous membranes.

As the infant grows, the surface of the naevus may become rugose or warty and nodules can develop within a large naevus (Fig. 54.20). The hairy component, which occurs in 95% of lesions, tends to become more prominent in late childhood, but at this stage the naevus itself ceases to thicken and may become paler. The hair growth pattern may have a 'vortex' distribution, often centred on the midline in giant naevi of the back. Some lesions involve both the opposed surfaces of the upper and lower eyelid so that when the eyes are shut the naevus takes its normal rounded shape. This shows that the site of the naevus was determined during the period when the lids were fused, that is between the second and sixth month of fetal life.

Neurocutaneous melanosis may produce raised intracranial pressure, hydrocephalus or space-occupying spinal lesions; this is a very rare complication. In a series of 80 Mexican patients with giant naevi only one case of hydrocephalus was reported [4]. There may be associated abnormalities such as meningeal involvement, spina bifida or meningocoele when the naevus is over the vertebral column, or club-foot and hypertrophy or atrophy of the deeper structures of a limb. Absence of subcutaneous fat is the most common associated anomaly and may be symptomatic in sites such as over the sacrum.

Congenital melanocytic naevi are said to occur in the epidermal naevus syndrome [5]. There is also a less well-substantiated association with neurofibromatosis [6].

Pathology. The majority of congenital naevi are dermal or compound melanocytic naevi with naevus cells typically extending more deeply into the dermis (within appendages and even into striated muscle and fat) than those of acquired naevi [7]. It was suggested, on the basis of histological studies, that congenital

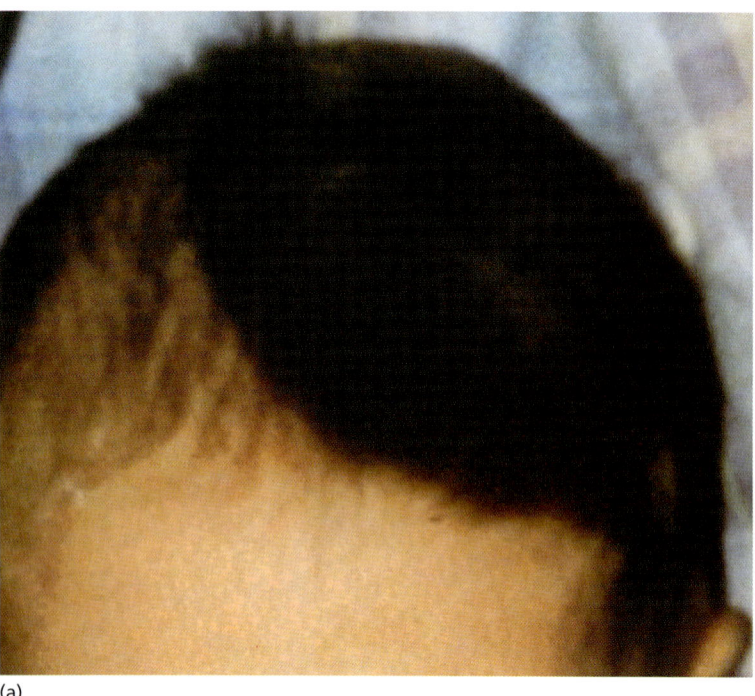

(a)

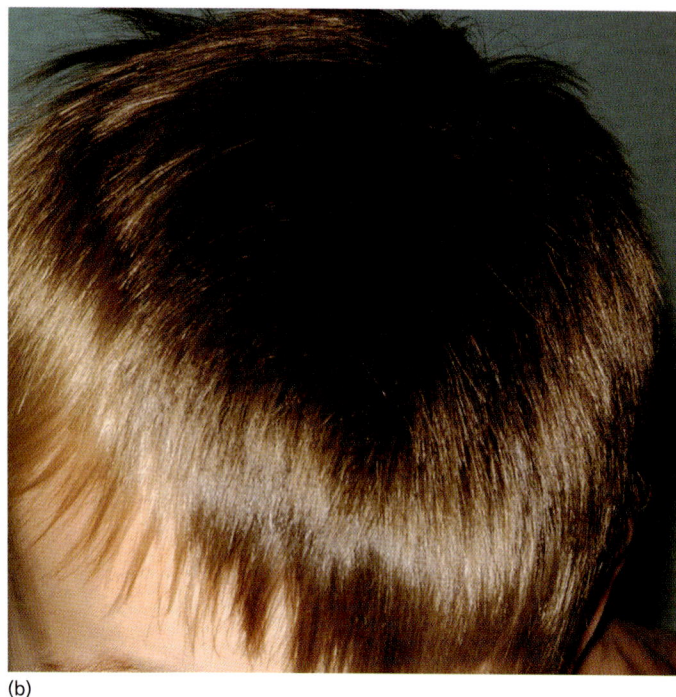

(b)

Fig. 54.17 (a) A large congenital melanocytic naevus of the scalp, which faded dramatically (b) until there was nothing visible on the skin in the first few years of life.

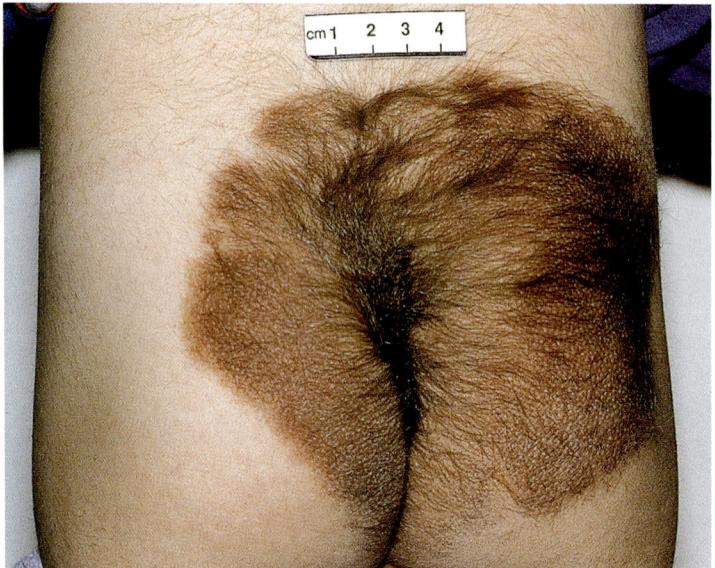

Fig. 54.18 Giant or garment congenital naevus on the lower back area of a child.

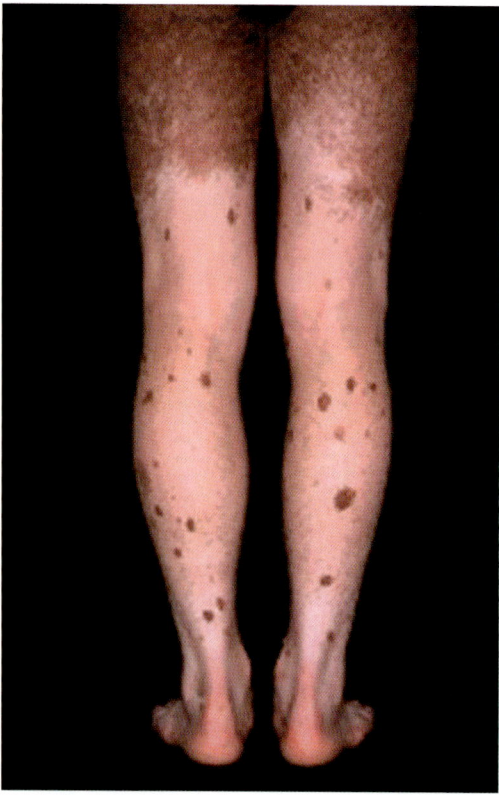

Fig. 54.19 Multiple satellite naevi in an adult with a giant congenital melanocytic naevus. These naevi usually emerge in children with giant congenital naevi, in the first 2 years of life.

naevi evolve within the first few months of life from junctional to deep lesions and it was thought that this transition offered the possibility of early treatment having an effect on long-term distribution of naevus cells, giving potential for early treatment by dermabrasion [8–10]. The current view, however, is that variation in depth of melanocytes reflects variation between individuals rather than being time-dependent.

There are a variety of proliferative neoplasms that may develop in congenital melanocytic naevi, which cause great consternation

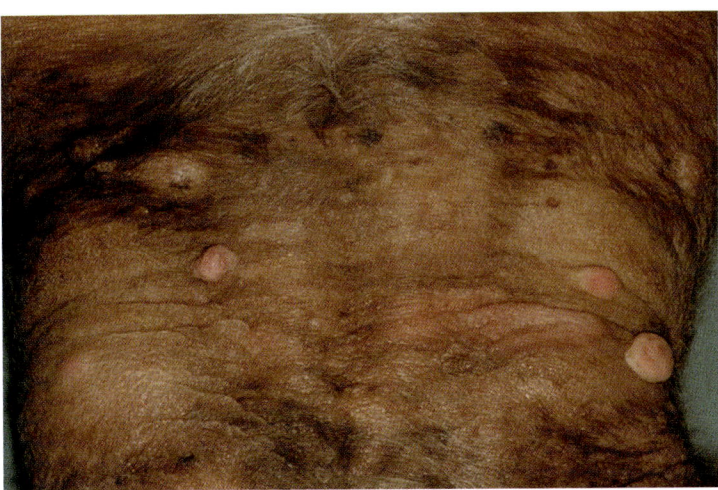

Fig. 54.20 Hypertrichosis and benign hamartomatous proliferations in a toddler with a particularly troublesome giant congenital melanocytic naevus.

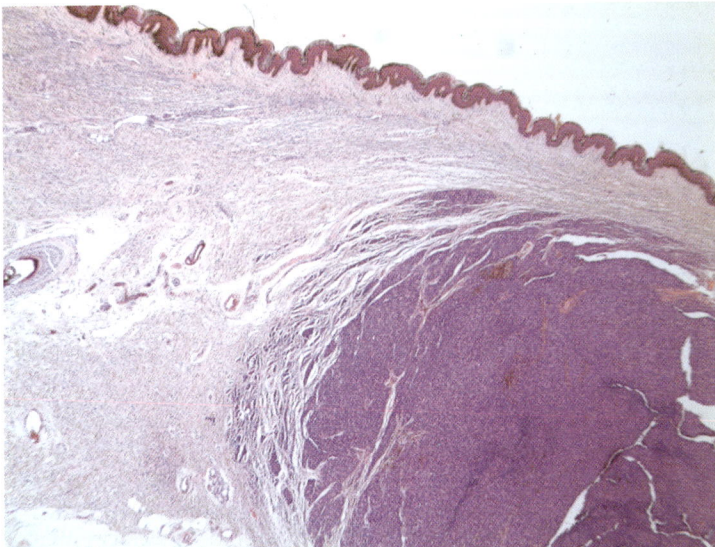

Fig. 54.21 The histological appearance of a benign proliferative nodule which arose in a giant congenital pigmented naevus in a child aged 12 years. (Courtesy of Dr S. Edward, Leeds Teaching Hospitals Trust, Leeds, UK.)

and confusion (Fig. 54.21). Certainly, malignant melanoma may arise [11]. In addition, a rapidly growing, ulcerative tumour called nodular proliferative neurocristic hamartoma has been described at birth [12]. This fetal hamartoma consists of diverse tissues of neuroectodermal and ectomesenchymal origin. The greatest diagnostic difficulty occurs when simulants of melanoma occur, characterized by the proliferation of epithelioid melanocytes.

Genetic counselling. Congenital naevi are essentially considered to be developmental abnormalities of the skin, with a very low risk of recurrence in subsequent pregnancies, which is particularly important when reassuring parents who have a child with a giant melanocytic naevus [13]. However, there are extremely rare instances of families in which more than one case has occurred, raising the possibility that, at least in these families, there may be an inherited tendency to develop giant congenital naevi. Such risks, however, are very low.

Prognosis and complications. Superficial spreading melanoma is the most significant complication of congenital naevi but the level of that risk remains the most controversial, mainly because most of the reported series come from large referral centres and may therefore suffer from ascertainment bias.

There seems to be no doubt that there is an increased risk of melanoma in patients with very large naevi. In the series reported by Swerdlow *et al.* [14], two melanomas, both fatal, occurred in 265 patients with melanoma covering at least 5% of their body area. The melanomas occurred at the ages of 18 and 20 years. In a second series of 80 patients, three melanomas occurred [4], including two in children under the age of 3 years. In giant naevi there therefore appears to be a definite risk, with the age of onset of the melanoma being very much earlier than in the general population. In contrast to the normal development pattern of melanomas, those occurring within congenital naevi may arise from below the dermoepidermal junction, which may delay diagnosis [15]. There have been several attempts to estimate lifetime risk, giving values between 4.6 and 14% [16]. Krengel *et al.* performed a useful review of a total of 6571 patients with congenital melanocytic naevi, followed up for a mean of 3.4–23.7 years, and 46 patients (0.7%) developed 49 melanomas [17]. The mean age at diagnosis of melanoma was 15.5 years (median 7 years). Primary melanomas arose inside the naevi in 33 of 49 cases (67%). In seven cases (14%), metastatic melanoma with unknown primary was encountered; in four cases (8%) the melanoma developed at an extracutaneous site. The risk of developing melanoma and the rate of fatal courses were highest by far in congenital melanocytic naevi 40 cm or greater in diameter.

There are numerous case reports of melanoma arising in smaller congenital naevi [18] but such naevi are relatively common and it is very difficult from studies reported so far to compare, for example, the relative risk of melanoma arising from a small congenital naevus with that of a melanoma arising in an acquired naevus. It seems likely, as congenital naevi tend to be bigger, that the risk might be greater at least in proportion to the melanocyte mass. Various estimates of risk have been made. Rhodes and coworkers have estimated a lifetime risk of between 2.6 and 4.9% [18,19] in naevi less than 4.5 cm in diameter. However, Swerdlow *et al.* [14] failed to demonstrate any increased risk for naevi smaller than those covering 5% of the body surface. It seems unlikely that the true risk from a small congenital naevus will ever be established accurately because of the impossibility of gathering a sufficiently large cohort of patients whose congenital naevi are left *in situ*.

Rarely, intracerebral primary melanoma may complicate leptomeningeal melanocytosis [20].

Treatment. An MRI scan should be considered in babies with naevi over the cranium or spine to exclude significant leptomeningeal melanocytosis. However, although MRI anomalies are common, occurring in around 30% [21], symptomatic neurocutaneous melanosis is rare, so the value of scanning seems questionable in the absence of neurological signs. Regular neurological examination, however, is clearly important.

The aims of treatment are to improve the cosmetic effect of naevi and to reduce the risk of malignant transformation. To date, there is no proof that any treatment regimen fulfils the second aim for giant naevi in which there is no possibility of complete excision of the naevus, because of the surface area of skin involved and the depth of the naevus within the skin and subcutis. There is perhaps a stronger argument for prophylactic excision of large naevi where complete excision of the naevus is technically possible with reasonable cosmetic result. The most common treatment is surgical, using a variety of plastic surgical techniques such as multistep surgery, the use of tissue expanders and grafting. Tissue expansion is usually used for the head and neck, but in other sites excision and grafting are more usual, with consequently poorer cosmetic results. The cosmetic results of surgery for giant naevi on the trunk are generally poor and there have been attempts to improve results, mainly by treatment within the first few weeks of life by dermabrasion or curettage [22]. The rationale for this is that there may be a natural plane of cleavage within the upper dermis very early in life which may be exploited by the curette to reduce the risk of subsequent scarring [23]. It is difficult from the literature to assess the long-term cosmetic results of the approach of curettage but those from dermabrasion seem disappointing. A review of 215 patients treated in Germany reported hypertrophic scars in 15% (particularly on the lower back) but there was good, permanent reduction in pigmentation in 34% (which was more likely when treatment was carried out early) [24]. A smaller series of 12 neonates treated by dermabrasion reported good results in 10, although six went on to have surgery later [25]. The long-term cosmetic results of surgery may therefore be disappointing, although children in one study reported a preference for a surgical scar rather than the naevus [26]. Other ablative techniques have been tried such as cryotherapy and, more recently, the Q-switched ruby laser. This laser emits light at 694 nm, which is relatively selectively taken up by melanin, but its value remains unclear.

Overall, the choice about intervention in children born with large or giant naevi is made on the basis of balancing a risk of melanoma (which is poorly quantified), and the cosmetic deficit of the naevus, against the risks of surgery. The psychological impact of giant congenital naevi is great and the risk of melanoma established, so that there is a need to establish better approaches for removal. Currently available methods leave much to be desired and it is eminently possible to operate on children to little overall benefit indeed, even do harm. The decision as to whether to proceed to surgery or not may be very difficult for families.

Parents of children with congenital naevi left *in situ* should be advised to keep the naevus under review and to seek advice if it changes in shape, size or colour. As such naevi do change through life in an entirely benign way, education about the nature of changes which would cause concern is essential. Photographs of the child's naevus and images of melanomas are useful for the family to take home. It would seem reasonable to prophylactically excise small naevi that are difficult to keep under review, such as those in the scalp or in the middle of the back, particularly if they have any atypical features such as intense or irregular pigmentation which persists beyond infancy.

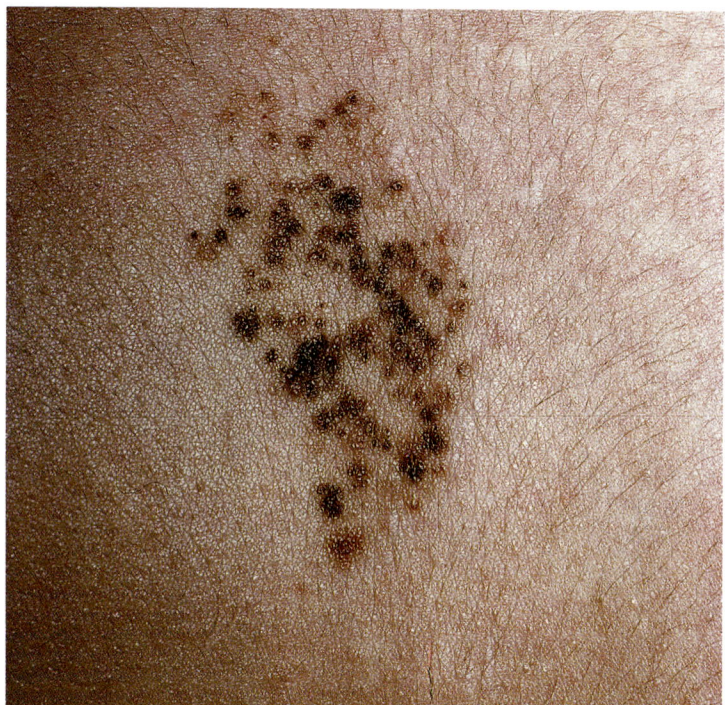

Fig. 54.22 Speckled and lentiginous naevus. Note the variation in colour of this lesion.

Speckled and lentiginous naevus

This term is recommended in preference to the term naevus spilus. Such naevi may be viewed as a type of congenital melanocytic lesion which is lentiginous in early childhood and which might develop palpable components at puberty in a 'speckled' distribution.

Clinical features. Speckled and lentiginous naevus is a relatively uncommon entity. It is comprised of a flat, macular component, subtly darker shade than the surrounding skin, resembling a café-au-lait spot. Within this pale background there are lentigo-like lesions and also elevated darker-brown naevi (Fig. 54.22). It may also coexist with other types of melanocytic naevus such as a blue [27] or Spitz naevus, indeed there is a clinical overlap with the agminate Spitz naevus described below (see also Table 54.3).

Pathology. Pathological examination shows, as the clinical appearance suggests, a background macular lesion with a very subtle increase in melanocytes, and lentigos with superimposed individual compound naevi.

Management. There have been reports of malignant change in these lesions [27,28]. There are no data however on which to estimate the risk of such a change and it is likely that the risk is very low. Patients should generally, therefore, be counselled as to self examination as is done for patients with congenital melanocytic naevi. There are very rare patients in which the naevus develops atypical melanocytic proliferations at puberty and in these patients excision should be considered if technically feasible.

References

1 Anon. Consensus conference: Precursors to malignant melanoma. *JAMA* 1984; **251**: 1864–6.

2 Castilla E, Dutra M, Orioli-Parreiras I. Epidemiology of congenital pigmented nevi. Incidence rates and relative frequencies. *Br J Dermatol* 1981; **104**: 307–15.

3 Strauss RM, Newton Bishop JA. Spontaneous involution of congenital melanocytic nevi of the scalp. *J Am Acad Dermatol* 2008; **58**: 508–11.

4 Ruiz-Maldonado R, Tamayo L, Laterza AM, Duran C. Giant pigmented nevi: clinical, histopathologic, and therapeutic considerations. *J Pediatr* 1992; **120**: 906–11.

5 Carney J, Gordon H, Carpenter P *et al*. The complex of myxomas, spotty pigmentation and endocrine overactivity. *Medicine* 1985; **64**: 270–83.

6 Marghoob AA, Orlow SJ, Kopf AW. Continuing medical education—syndromes associated with melanocytic nevi. *J Am Acad Dermatol* 1993; **29**: 373–88.

7 Rhodes AR, Silverman RA, Harrist TJ, Melski JW. A histologic comparison of congenital and acquired nevomelanocytic nevi. *Arch Dermatol* 1985; **121**: 1266–73.

8 Walton R, Jacobs A, Cox A. Pigmented lesions in newborn infants. *Br J Dermatol* 1976; **95**: 389–96.

9 Johnson H. Permanent removal of pigmentation from giant hairy nevi by dermabrasion in early age. *Br J PLast Surg* 1977; **30**: 321.

10 Mark F, Mihm M, Litelpo M *et al*. Congenital melanocytic naevi of the small and garment type. *Hum Pathol* 1973; **4**: 396–418.

11 Borges AF, Lineberger AS. Malignant melanoma without metastasis in a giant nevus. *Ann Plast Surg* 1984; **12**: 454–60.

12 Mancianti M-L, Clark WH, Hayes FA, Herlyn M. Malignant melanoma simulants arising in congenital melanocytic nevi do not show experimental evidence for a malignant phenotype. *Am J Pathol* 1990; **136**: 817–29.

13 Goodman RM, Caren J, Ziprkowski M *et al*. Genetic considerations in giant pigmented hairy naevus. *Br J Dermatol* 1971; **85**: 150–7.

14 Swerdlow AJ, English JSC, Qiao Z. The risk of melanoma in patients with congenital nevi: A cohort study. *J Am Acad Dermatol* 1995; **32**: 595–9.

15 Reed R, Martin P. Variants of melanoma. *Semin Cutan Med Surg* 1997; **16**: 137–58.

16 Illig L, Weidner F, Hundeiker M *et al*. Congenital nevi ≤10 cm as precursors to melanoma. 52 cases, a review, and a new conception. *Arch Dermatol* 1985; **121**: 1274–81.

17 Krengel S, Hauschild A, Schafer T. Melanoma risk in congenital melanocytic naevi: a systematic review. *Br J Dermatol* 2006; **155**: 1–8.

18 Rhodes A, Melski J. Small congenital nevocellular nevi and the risk of cutaneous melanoma. *J Pediatrics* 1982; **100**: 219–24.

19 Rhodes A, Sober A, Day C *et al*. The malignant potential of small congenital naevi. *J Am Acad Dermatol* 1982; **6**: 230–41.

20 Slaughter J, Hardman J, Kemple L *et al*. Neurocutaneous melanosis and leptomeningeal melanocytosis in children. *Arch Dermatol* 1969; **88**: 298–304.

21 Foster RD, Williams ML, Barkovich AJ *et al*. Giant congenital melanocytic nevi: the significance of neurocutaneous melanosis in neurologically asymptomatic children. *Plast Reconstr Surg* 2001; **107**: 933–41.

22 Miller C, Becker DJ. Removing pigmentation by dermabrading nevi in infancy. *Plast Reconstr Surg* 1979; **32**: 124–6.

23 De Raeve LE, De Coninck AL, Dierickx PR, Roseeuw DI. Neonatal curettage of giant congenital melanocytic nevi. *Arch Dermatol* 1996; **132**: 20–2.

24 Rompel R, Moser M, Petres J. Dermabrasion of congenital nevocellular nevi: experience in 215 patients. *Dermatology* 1997; **194**: 261–7.

25 Bohn J, Svensson H, Aberg M. Dermabrasion of large congenital melanocytic naevi in neonates. *Scand J Plast Reconstr Surg Hand Surg* 2000; **34**: 321–6.

26 Koot H, de Waard-van der Spek F, Peer C *et al*. Psychological sequelae in 29 children with giant congenital naevi. *Clin Dermatol* 2000; **25**: 598–3.

27 Cox NH, Malcolm A, Long ED. Cases of superficial spreading melanoma and of blue naevus within naevus spilus, with ultrastructural assessment of giant pigment granules. *Dermatology* 1997; **194**: 213–6.

28 Piana S, Gelli MC, Grenzi L *et al*. Multifocal melanoma arising on nevus spilus. *Int J Dermatol* 2006; **45**: 1380–1.

Acquired melanocytic naevi

Synonyms
- Cellular naevus
- Naevocytic naevus
- Mole

Definition. A benign cluster of melanocytic naevus cells arising as a result of proliferation of melanocytes at the dermal–epidermal junction. These may all remain in contact with the basal layer of the epidermis, giving rise to the junctional naevus. In other naevi, some of the naevus cells may migrate into the dermis over time, giving rise to the compound naevus. The end stage of this process is when there are no naevus cells attached to the epidermis and all are lying free in the dermis. This pattern is that of the mature intradermal naevus. A melanocytic naevus is therefore a benign tumour of melanocytes, in which the melanocytes (naevus cells) proliferate for some time but then cease proliferation and differentiate (or senesce) and come to resemble cells of neural or fibroblast lineage. Different types are summarized in Table 54.4.

Aetiology and incidence. Melanocytic naevi are almost universal. They develop through childhood and twin studies provide good evidence that naevus number is predominantly genetically determined [1] with a smaller effect of sun exposure [2]. There are a number of studies from Europe and Australia, which suggest that naevus number is higher in children exposed to more sun, particularly intermittent sun exposure as on sunny holidays [3–6].

Naevi continue to erupt in adult life so that the mean number bigger than 2 mm in diameter in 754 healthy women between the ages of 18 and 46 in the UK was 57 [7]. After this age naevi then involute so that the elderly usually have very few. In a UK study, 30% of 20 to 34 year olds had 50 or more moles compared with 4% of patients between 65 and 75 years old [8]. This natural history of naevi means, therefore, that new naevi developing in later life should be viewed with more suspicion than naevi of similar appearance in younger individuals.

The number of melanocytic naevi is the strongest phenotypic risk factor for melanoma [9] and the genes that control naevus number are therefore candidate melanoma susceptibility genes.

There is some, as yet unexplained, variation in naevus number. Patients with atopic dermatitis may have significantly lower naevus counts than age-matched controls [10] and individuals with Turner's syndrome have larger than average numbers of naevi, although there is no evidence that they have an increased risk of melanoma [11]. Children who have been treated for leukaemia [12] and recipients of renal transplants [13] also have increased numbers of naevi, which is postulated to be a consequence of immune suppression. There is some evidence that survivors of childhood cancer do appear to be at increased risk of melanoma [14] although, as melanoma was not increased as a second malignancy after haematological malignancies, other than possibly after Hodgkin lymphoma [15], it is not clear whether that increased risk is treatment related or genetic.

Clinical features. The new naevus is a junctional naevus and is a macular brown lesion, which may show pigment lying along the normal skin markings. It may have a slightly irregular lateral margin because of this, and may have a large diameter of up to 10 mm. The pigmentation tends to be uniform and regular (Fig. 54.23). In some body sites, such as the limbs, junctional naevi may

Table 54.4 Overview of acquired melanocytic naevi.

Naevus type	Subtype	Pathological characteristics	Significance	Treatment
Common acquired melanocytic naevus	Junctional	Benign proliferations of melanocytes in the epidermis	Normal finding but increased numbers of naevi are a risk factor for melanoma	None
	Compound	Benign proliferations of melanocytes in the epidermis, showing evidence of migration of cells into the dermis and 'maturation' of those cells within the deeper dermis	Normal finding but increased numbers of naevi are a risk factor for melanoma	None
	Dermal	Benign tumours of melanocytes in which there is no longer epidermal proliferation; the naevus cells have migrated into the dermis and matured there	Normal finding but increased numbers of naevi are a risk factor for melanoma	None
	Balloon cell naevus	Compound naevus with balloon cells (the melanocyte cytoplasm is foamy)	None	None
	Naevi of unusual sites such as the nail bed, palms and soles and genitalia	More likely to have more atypical junctional proliferation of melanocytes. However, the criteria used for the diagnosis of melanoma in these sites remain the same	None usually	Excise if there are atypical clinical features as for any naevus elsewhere
	Halo naevus	Dense lymphocytic infiltrate in the early phase and subsequent removal of naevus cells	None	None in the absence of atypical features clinically
	Meyerson's naevus	Benign naevus with overlying spongiosis of the epidermis	None	The eczematous component should be treated and the naevus re-examined
	Naevus en cockarde	None	None: unusual rosette-like variant of no significance	None
Spitz naevus	Classical type	See text	Differentiation from melanoma is the key	Excision except for very bland lesions in young children
	Pigmented spindle cell naevus of Reed	See text	Differentiation from melanoma is the key	Excision to exclude melanoma
	Atypical spitzoid tumour of unknown malignant potential (STUMP)	See text	Should be managed as for melanoma	Treat as for melanoma
Blue naevus	Common	Spindle or dendritic melanocytes within the dermis, containing pigment even deeply in the dermis (which naevus cells in acquired naevi do not do)	None save differentiation from a melanoma	None
	Cellular blue naevus	As for the common blue naevus except that the dermal naevus cells are more numerous and extend deeply even up to the fat	None save differentiation from a melanoma	
	Combined blue and acquired naevus	Histological features of both blue and acquired naevi	None	None
	Deep penetrating naevus	Larger than most naevi with extension of naevus cells deep into the dermis with a wedge shape (base abutting onto the epidermis)	None save distinction from melanoma	Excision to exclude melanoma is usual because the appearance of the naevus may be unusual
Atypical or dysplastic naevus	Junctional or compound	Characteristic architectural and cytological atypical (see text)	Precursors, and marker, of risk for melanoma although the vast majority behave in an entirely benign way	Excise only to exclude melanoma

remain unchanged through much of adult life, but the majority do 'mature' with age, becoming first a 'compound naevus' and then an 'intradermal naevus'.

The compound naevus usually slowly becomes raised above the epidermal surface and may be round or oval (Fig. 54.24). The colour varies with the natural pigmentation of the patient and may be very dark, but the majority become paler with age. There is usually little if any pigment on the flat surrounding epidermis. It is important to recognize that slow elevation and the transformation of a macular melanocytic naevus to a palpable symmetrical,

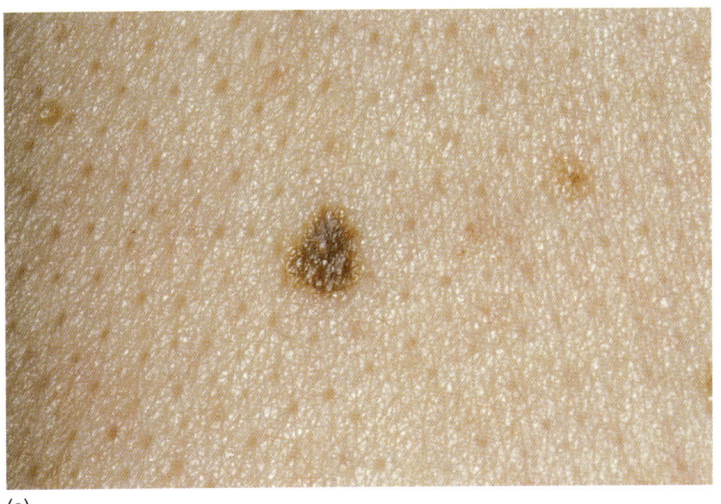

(a)

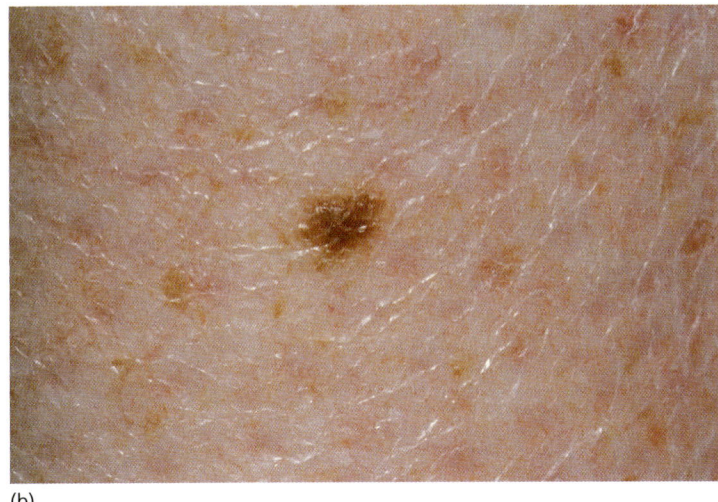

(b)

Fig. 54.23 Two junctional naevi: macular brown lesions which are composed of a proliferation of melanocytes at the dermoepidermal junction.

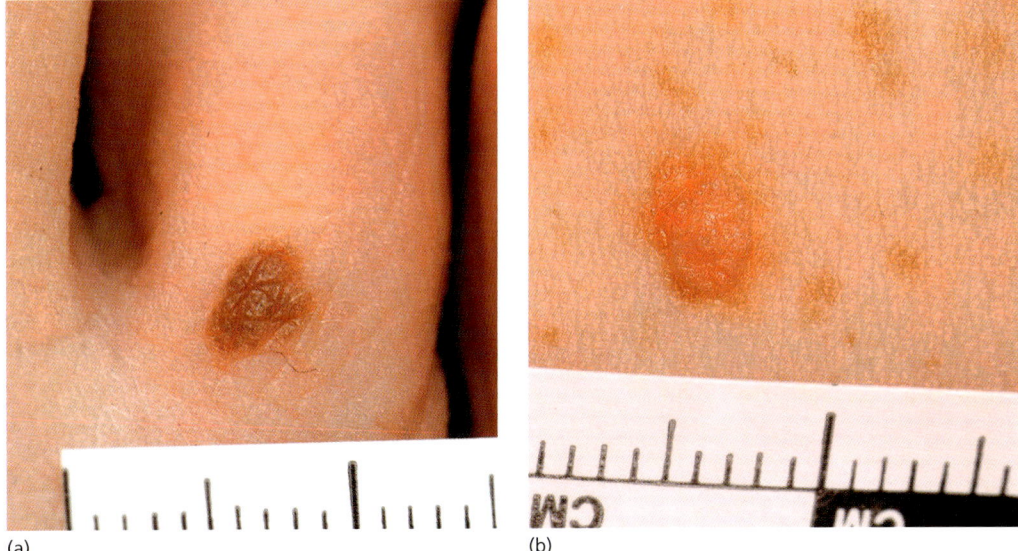

Fig. 54.24 Two compound melanocytic naevi in which junctional melanocytes persist but senescence of melanocytes has also occurred and those cells lie within the dermis.

(a)

(b)

evenly pigmented symmetrical papule over time, is not a sign of malignant change but a normal maturation pattern of these naevi.

Intradermal naevi are frequently raised, dome-shaped, non-pigmented nodules, most commonly seen on the face (Figs 54.25 & 54.26). There are often some overlying telangiectatic vessels (leading to diagnostic confusion with basal cell carcinomas) and outgrowth of one or two coarse terminal hairs is common. A proportion in some body sites, such as the flexures, may become skin tags with time.

Inflammation within intradermal naevi may occur, as a result of bacterial infection in hair follicles or granulomatous inflammation. These changes often cause alarm for patients and their family doctors, but the symptoms associated develop 'overnight' and it is useful to reassure those concerned that acute changes like this are rarely indicative of malignant change. Fragments of hair shaft can often be demonstrated histologically. The inflammation may recur and leave a fibrous nodule, or one that goes on to calcification or even ossification.

The balloon cell naevus is a subtype of compound melanocytic naevus, which has a predominant population of cells with a high volume of foamy cytoplasm [16]. These are called balloon cell naevi because of their pathological appearance. The pathological picture is striking, but there is no known biological significance. There is also a malignant counterpart of balloon cell melanoma, but the balloon cell naevus is not a precursor to balloon cell melanoma.

Naevi in unusual sites

Naevi on the palms and soles may cause concern because they are relatively infrequent and because public education has in the past suggested that they are easily confused with acral lentiginous melanoma. It is also recognized that histologically naevi in these sites show more architectural and mild cytological atypia [17]. In fact, naevi in these sites are not so rare and as they behave as do junctional naevi in other sites, they can be distinguished from melanoma. The incidence of pigmented naevi on the palms, soles

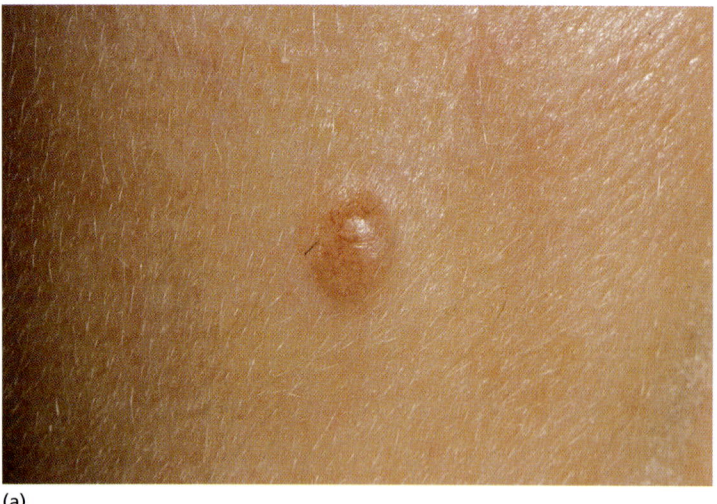

(a)

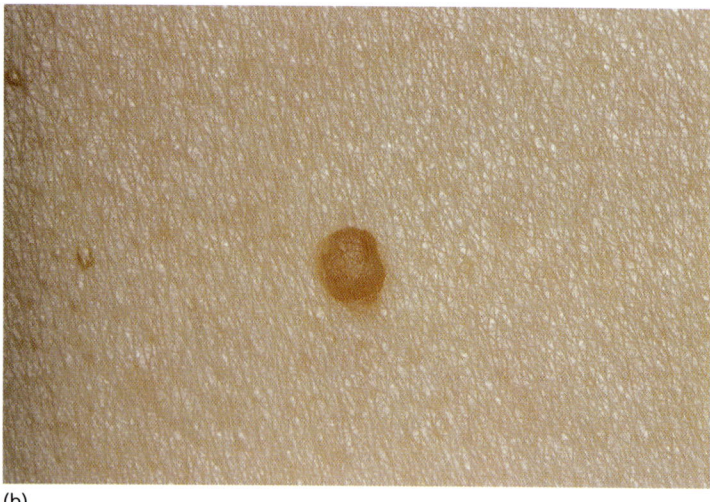

(b)

Fig. 54.25 Two mature dermal naevi, one of which has prominent vessels which can cause confusion with basal cell carcinomas. In these naevi, junctional proliferation of melanocytes has ceased and all the melanocytes are senesced and lie in the dermis.

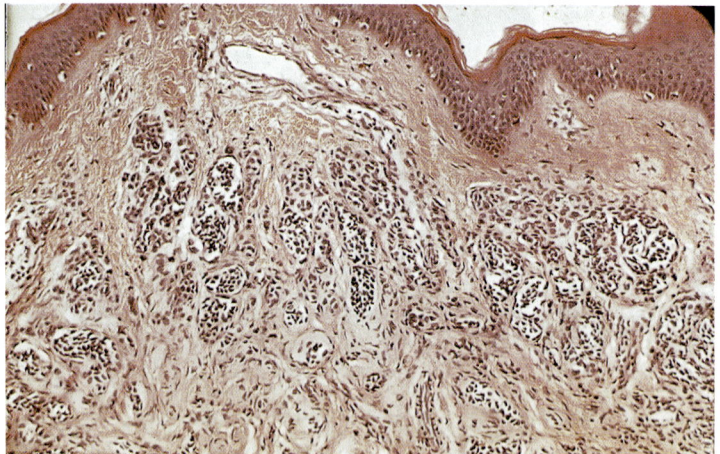

Fig. 54.26 Histology of intradermal naevus. Note the normal overlying epidermis and the maturation of dermal naevus cells, with neural appearance at lower levels.

and genitalia has been studied in a large series of normal young men [18], and more than 10% of the sample were found to have one or more. They should therefore be managed as junctional naevi elsewhere.

Conjunctival naevi are similar in their behaviour and histology to cellular naevi of the skin; and the same clinical changes would evoke the same concern.

Naevi of the nail matrix or bed may present as a longitudinal brown stripe on the underside of the nail plate (Chapter 65). There may be difficulty in distinguishing such lesions from early subungual melanoma. Benign naevi and melanoma both originate in the nail matrix and therefore typically produce a linear band of pigmentation along the length of the nail. However, as applies to melanoma at other sites, subungual melanoma has a disorganized irregular appearance, so that the pigmented band of a melanoma appears later in life than those due to naevi, tends to widen progressively and shows variable colour. Due to rapid growth, the proximal diameter is wider than the distal so the pigmented band

appears funnel-shaped (see Fig. 54.63 below). Dermoscopy can be used to improve the clinical diagnosis of such lesions, demonstrating irregular pigmentation [19,20].

Pathology. The pattern of evolution of pigmented naevi has been deduced by pathological examination of a large number of lesions removed at different ages. Elder and Murphy describe how normal melanocytes are rarely seen in contact with each other, being normally surrounded by keratinocytes even in lentigos, but in naevi proliferative groups of contiguous cells are seen [21]. In childhood, over 90% of naevi are *junctional* and show melanocyte proliferation at the dermoepidermal junction to form small clusters of cells that indent both the overlying epidermis and the underlying papillae. The cells have abundant cytoplasm containing melanin granules. The majority of naevi on the palms and soles, and also on the vulva, appear to be junctional naevi.

The next stage occurs when some of these melanocytes migrate into the dermis, where they form nests and columns of cells. In the *compound* naevus both junctional proliferation and dermal cells are present. The dermal cells accumulate in the papillary body and extend more deeply around appendages and neurovascular bundles. The more superficial cells (type A) remain recognizable as naevus cells, continuing to form melanin, which is taken up by melanophages in the stroma. The deeper cells (type B) are smaller and usually contain no melanin. The more superficial cells may throw the epidermis into a series of folds by expanding dermal papillae (so that the naevus is clinically warty in appearance). The deeper cells are arranged as a band (type B) or as arborizing columns in the deeper dermis, when the cells become spindle shaped (type C) and more closely resemble cells of neural or fibroblast lineage. Thus, as cells migrate into the dermis they are at first similar to junctional naevus cells, but over time lose the characteristics of melanocytes.

When the junctional melanocytes stop proliferating, and the overlying epidermis returns to normal, the naevus becomes *intradermal*. Many intradermal naevi have neuroid cells in their deeper parts, and some are composed of little else. These neural areas in the deeper areas of intradermal naevi are sometimes referred to as Masson's naevic corpuscles, after Pierre Masson who first evolved the theory of evolution of melanocytic naevi [22]. The stroma around the dermal naevus cells is loose and fibrillar, the nests of cells are often enclosed by flattened cells that resemble endothelium and may give an erroneous impression of naevus cells in vessels. Multinucleated naevus cells are commonly seen, but mitotic figures are rare and occur only in the type A cells. The end stage of a melanocytic naevus is a flesh-coloured, pedunculated skin tag in which very few naevus cells are observed. Pigment is sparse and fat cells may be present. The evolution of neural like cells with age has led some to suggest that melanocytic naevi are hamartomas, but they are more likely to be proliferative lesions [23] and that as the cells cease proliferation and senesce, they have a more 'neural' phenotype. Understanding why melanocytes proliferate and then senesce is crucial to understanding tumourigenesis [24].

Diagnosis. In older adults, there may be difficulty in clinical differentiation between seborrhoeic keratoses (Chapter 52) and larger papillomatous compound naevi. The seborrhoeic keratosis usually has a 'stuck-on' appearance with its bulk above the normal skin contour, and the colour is usually more grey-brown than the typical melanocytic naevus. In addition, the surface is usually dull and pitted, with a tendency to crumble, and does not reflect light in the same way as naevi.

The most important clinical differential diagnosis is from early malignant melanoma. A history of very rapid growth, over days rather than weeks, and tenderness suggests the development of an underlying infection/granuloma rather than malignant change. Features suggestive of an early malignant melanoma either developing *ab initio* or in a pre-existing naevus are progressive change in size (surface area), shape and colour. Typically, melanomas develop irregularity of outline and the presence in the lesion of several shades of brown, red, blue or black. Melanomas do sometimes itch or produce at least a changed sensation, but itch poorly differentiates between melanoma and benign naevi.

The techniques of dermoscopy and of computerized diagnosis are discussed in the section on malignant melanoma (p. 54.38). Several groups have produced useful atlases of the clinical dermatoscopic appearances of melanocytic naevi and the differences between these naevi and malignant melanoma. Dermoscopy is an essential technique used to distinguish benign from malignant, and must be learnt by all dermatologists.

Management. The management of naevi is essentially that of differentiating benign maturing naevi from those that are behaving atypically, and which therefore might either be melanomas or naevi having the potential to develop into melanomas (such as severely atypical or dysplastic naevi). The keys to the diagnosis are the history of the lesion, and its appearance to the naked eye and the dermoscopic appearance. Thus a pigmented lesion, which arises in childhood and grows progressively in size in the following months is likely to be benign, but a similar story in a 50 year old should be viewed as suspicious. Normal junctional naevi may show minor variations in shape and colour but are essentially symmetrical and the variation in colour is usually limited to shades of brown. Severely atypical naevi and melanomas tend to be asymmetrical and the colours tend to be mixtures of browns, grey/blues, reds and blacks (see Figs 54.42–54.45 below). Dermoscopy is essential in order to examine the pigment pattern for irregularity, as described below.

If a melanocytic naevus is excised for whatever reason, it should always be sent for pathological examination. Partial removal must be avoided, both because this may lead to sampling error and the wrong diagnosis, and in order to avoid failure to completely remove the deeper dermal cells. When this occurs, residual naevus cells may proliferate soon after excision and give rise to a pathological picture very like an early melanoma. This picture has been termed 'pseudomelanoma' or, more appropriately, a traumatically activated naevus. This can give rise to needless anxiety and is avoidable. Elder and Murphy suggest that the observation of pigment beyond the original scar suggests recurrent melanoma rather than the benign simulant [21].

Halo naevus

Synonym
• Sutton's naevus

Definition. A melanocytic naevus surrounded by a depigmented halo of otherwise normal skin.

Incidence and epidemiology. Halo naevi are relatively common, particularly in older children and young teenagers. They are frequently multiple. They are thought to result from immunologically mediated host responses to a naevus: there is some laboratory evidence for local and circulating immunological T-cell activation in affected patients [25].

Clinical features. These lesions have a characteristic appearance and progression. A halo of depigmentation appears around a pre-existing melanocytic naevus, and on white skin this will usually be seen during the summer months when the rest of the epidermis has acquired a tan, showing the non-tanned halo in sharp contrast to the normal skin (Fig. 54.27). The back is the commonest site and several naevi may develop haloes simultaneously, while other adjacent naevi remain unchanged. Over the next few months, the central naevus will gradually disappear leaving a macular area of non-pigmented skin. This depigmented area may persist for years and may never, or only gradually, return to a normal colour. On biopsy, all traces of the original naevus will be found to have disappeared.

Pathology. These lesions are variants of compound melanocytic naevi, and at the time of appearance of the halo they show a very striking lymphocytic infiltrate admixed with the intradermal naevus cells. The use of DOPA stains will reveal a loss of epidermal melanocytes in the halo area.

Management. Reassurance rather than excision is recommended in young people, particularly if the lesions are multiple. The patient should be warned that the depigmented areas will burn in sunlight because of the reduced numbers of melanocytes and should be advised to use a sunscreen.

In older patients, the differential diagnosis may include an early superficial spreading melanoma with surrounding depigmentation. In this case the surrounding area of depigmentation is usually irregular, and the central pigmented area may also be irregular in both shape and pigmentation. The central area has dermoscopic appearances suggestive of melanoma [26] whereas the dermoscopic appearance of a halo naevus is bland. If there is any clinical doubt, excision biopsy and pathological confirmation must be obtained.

Meyerson's naevus [27]

This name is used to describe a melanocytic naevus that has developed an associated inflammatory reaction, which looks like eczema. Meyerson's naevus is a similar lesion to the halo naevus

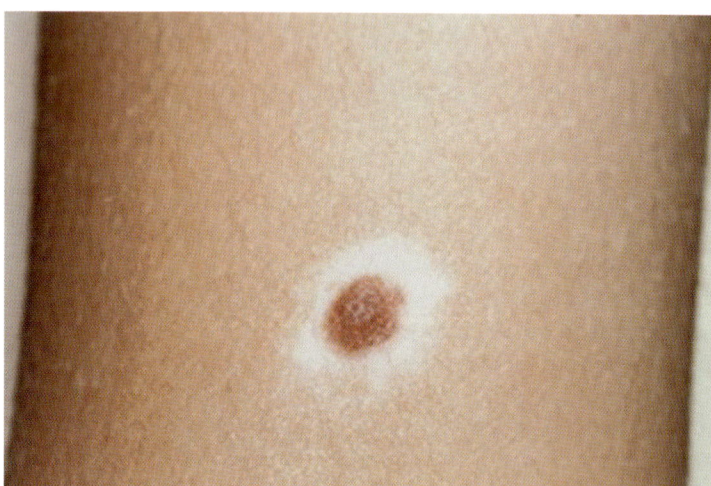

Fig. 54.27 Clinical appearance of a halo naevus.

and they may coexist although in Meyerson's naevus the central naevus does not usually subsequently disappear [28], although it may do so [29].

Clinical features. These lesions present as melanocytic naevi with associated epidermal scaling and a halo of inflammation. The original report was of multiple naevi developing this associated inflammatory reaction simultaneously. The naevus may be pruritic, and there may be overlying scaling and the appearance is of a naevus with superimposed discoid eczema.

Pathology. The pathology is usually that of a banal, usually compound, naevus with associated spongiotic dermatitis in the overlying dermis.

Treatment. These are benign naevi and it is reasonable in the first instance to treat for 1–2 weeks with a moderately potent topical steroid before re-examination. Normally, the secondary eczematous reaction will settle and examination with dermoscopy can be carried out to ensure that the underlying naevus is benign (Fig. 54.28).

Cockade naevus

Synonyms
- Kokardennaevus
- Naevus en cocarde

This rare variant of the pigmented naevus was first described by Mehregan and King in 1972 [30]. The lesion is named because of its resemblance to a rosette. All cases so far reported are in young patients with multiple, target-like naevi showing concentric circles of increased melanin pigmentation. The central lesion in all cases would appear to be a junctional naevus (Fig. 54.29).

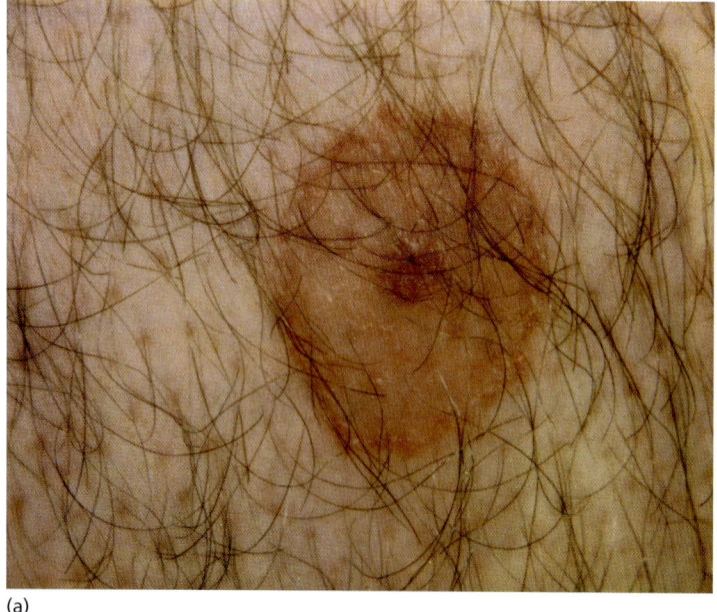

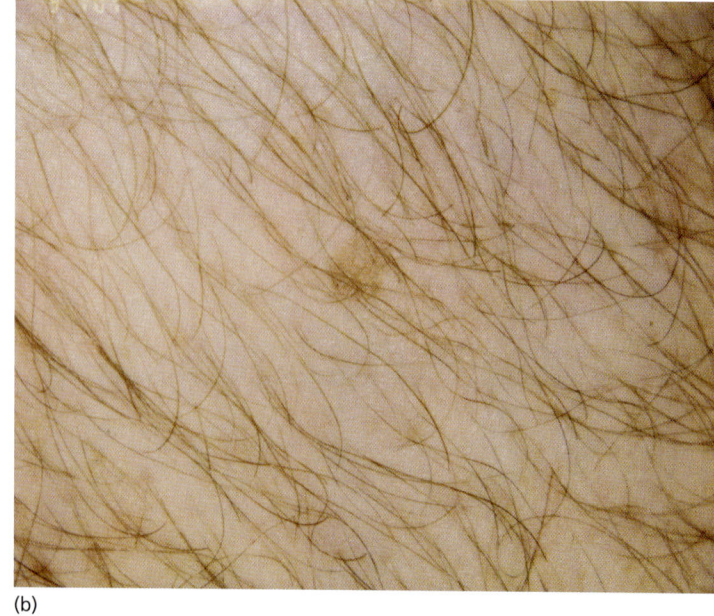

(a)   (b)

Fig. 54.28 (a) Meyerson's naevus in which an eczematous response to the naevus occurred, which cleared with 2 weeks' treatment with topical steroids (b). This allowed dermoscopic examination of the naevus, which then looked banal.

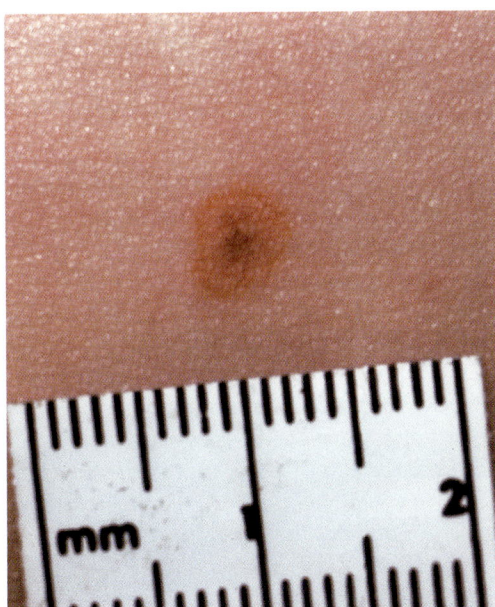

Fig. 54.29 Cockade naevus (naevus en cocarde). Note the darker outline to this lesion.

References

1 Zhu G, Duffy DL, Eldridge A *et al*. A major quantitative-trait locus for mole density is linked to the familial melanoma gene CDKN2A: a maximum-likelihood combined linkage and association analysis in twins and their sibs. *Am J Hum Genet* 1999; **65**: 483–92.

2 Wachsmuth RC, Turner F, Barrett JH *et al*. The effect of sun exposure in determining nevus density in UK adolescent twins. *J Invest Dermatol* 2005; **124**: 56–62.

3 Gefeller O, Tarantino J, Lederer P *et al*. The relation between patterns of vacation sun exposure and the development of acquired melanocytic nevi in German children 6–7 years of age. *Am J Epidemiol* 2007; **165**: 1162–9.

4 Green A, Siskind V, Hansen ME *et al*. Melanocytic nevi in schoolchildren in Queensland. *J Am Acad Dermatol* 1989; **20**: 1054–60.

5 Kelly JW, Rivers JK, MacLennan R *et al*. Sunlight: a major factor associated with the development of melanocytic nevi in Australian schoolchildren. *J Am Acad Dermatol* 1994; **30**: 40–8.

6 Rodvall Y, Wahlgren CF, Ullen H, Wiklund K. Common melanocytic nevi in 7-year-old schoolchildren residing at different latitudes in Sweden. *Cancer Epidemiol Biomarkers Prev* 2007; **16**: 122–7.

7 dos Santos Silva I, Higgins C, Abramsky T *et al*. Overseas sun exposure, nevus counts, and premature skin aging in young English women: a population-based survey. *J Invest Dermatol* 2009; **129**: 50–9.

8 Bataille V, Grulich A, Sasieni P *et al*. The association between naevi and melanoma in populations with different levels of sun exposure: a joint case-control study of melanoma in the UK and Australia. *Br J Cancer* 1998; **77**: 505–10.

9 Gandini S, Sera F, Cattaruzza MS *et al*. Meta-analysis of risk factors for cutaneous melanoma: I. Common and atypical naevi. *Eur J Cancer* 2005; **41**: 28–44.

10 Broberg A, Augustsson A. Atopic dermatitis and melanocytic naevi. *Br J Dermatol* 2000; **142**: 306–9.

11 Zvulunov A, Wyatt DT, Laud PW, Esterly NB. Influence of genetic and environmental factors on melanocytic naevi: a lesson from Turner's syndrome. *Br J Dermatol* 1998; **138**: 993–7.

12 Hughes B, Bailey CC. Excess benign melanocytic naevi. *BMJ* 1989; **299**: 854–5.

13 Szepietowski J, Wasik F, Szepietowski T. Excess benign melanocytic naevi in renal transplant recipients. *Dermatology* 1997; **194**: 17–9.

14 Inskip PD, Curtis RE. New malignancies following childhood cancer in the United States, 1973–2002. *Int J Cancer* 2007; **121**: 2233–40.

15 Maule M, Scelo G, Pastore G *et al*. Risk of second malignant neoplasms after childhood leukemia and lymphoma: an international study. *J Natl Cancer Inst* 2007; **99**: 790–800.

16 Schrader WA, Helwig EB. Balloon cell nevi. *Cancer* 1967; **20**: 1502–14.

17 Evans MJ, Gray ES, Blessing K. Histopathological features of acral melanocytic nevi in children: study of 21 cases. *Pediatr Dev Pathol* 1998; **1**: 388–92.

18 Cullen SI. Incidence of nevi. Report of survey of the palms, soles, and genitalia of 10,000 young men. *Arch Dermatol* 1962; **86**: 40–3.

19 Braun RP, Baran R, Le Gal FA *et al*. Diagnosis and management of nail pigmentations. *J Am Acad Dermatol* 2007; **56**: 835–47.

20 Thomas L, Dalle S. Dermoscopy provides useful information for the management of melanonychia striata. *Dermatol Ther* 2007; **20**: 3–10.

21 Elder DE, Murphy GF. *Melanocytic Tumors of the Skin*. Washington, DC: American Registry of Pathology, in press.

22 Masson P. My conception of cellular nevi. *Cancer* 1951; **4**: 9–38.

23 Krengel S. Nevogenesis—new thoughts regarding a classical problem. *Am J Dermatopathol* 2005; **27**: 456–65.

24 Gray-Schopfer VC, Cheong SC, Chong H *et al*. Cellular senescence in naevi and immortalisation in melanoma: a role for p16? *Br J Cancer* 2006; **95**: 496–505.

25 Baranda L, Torres-Alvarez B, Moncada B *et al*. Presence of activated lymphocytes in the peripheral blood of patients with halo nevi. *J Am Acad Dermatol* 1999; **41**: 567–72.

26 Kolm I, Di Stefani A, Hofmann-Wellenhof R *et al*. Dermoscopy patterns of halo nevi. *Arch Dermatol* 2006; **142**: 1627–32.

27 Meyerson LB. A peculiar papulosquamous eruption involving pigmented nevi. *Arch Dermatol* 1971; **103**: 510–2.

28 Brandt O, Christophers E, Folster-Holst R. Halo dermatitis followed by the development of vitiligo associated with Sutton's nevi. *J Am Acad Dermatol* 2005; **52**: S101–4.

29 Ramon R, Silvestre JF, Betlloch I *et al*. Progression of Meyerson's naevus to Sutton's naevus. *Dermatology* 2000; **200**: 337–8.

30 Mehregan AH, King JR. Multiple target-like pigmented nevi. *Arch Dermatol* 1972; **105**: 129–30.

Spitz naevus

Synonyms
- Spindle and epithelioid cell naevus
- Spitz tumour
- Juvenile melanoma

Definition. An uncommon type of melanocytic lesion, seen most commonly in children but also in adults, which has distinctive pathological features first described by Sophie Spitz as an unusual type of melanoma [1], but subsequently called benign. The entity has been controversial ever since. Whilst a characteristic clinical and histological appearance of a benign lesion usually called a Spitz naevus is recognized, there are three types of lesion that are often difficult to distinguish from each other: Spitz naevus, spitzoid melanoma and an entity that has become increasingly diagnosed an 'atypical spitzoid tumour of unknown malignant potential', reflecting the difficulties of pathological interpretation of spitzoid lesions. Much controversy still surrounds the pathology of spitzoid lesions, as reviewed [2,3], and it is clear that we have much yet to learn.

Incidence. Spitz naevi are most common under the age of 14 years; indeed 50% are thought to occur under this age, around 25% between the ages of 14 and 30 and 25% over the age of 30 years [4].

Clinical features. The classic Spitz naevus usually appears in early childhood as a firm, rounded or dome shaped, red or reddish-brown symmetrical nodule. The red colour is due to increased

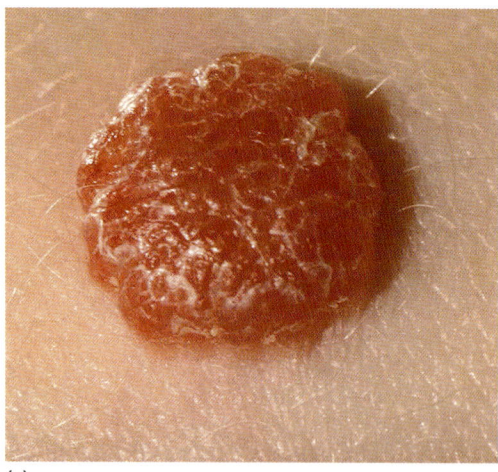

(a)

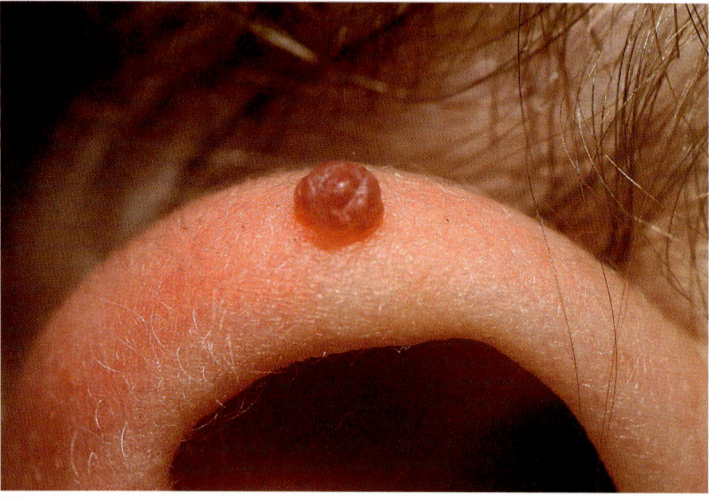

(b)

Fig. 54.30 Two classical Spitz naevi in children. The differential diagnosis is often that of a haemangioma.

vascularity and the naevus can usually be bleached by firm pressure or diascopy to show the residual degree of true melanin pigmentation (Figs 54.30 & 54.31).

The lesions usually grow rapidly over a period of 3–6 months and may reach diameters of 1–2 cm. The surface can remain smooth, with a thin, fragile, overlying epidermis. This may cause bleeding and crusting after minor injury, causing diagnostic confusion with haemangiomas or pyogenic granulomas. The commonest sites for Spitz naevi are the face, particularly the cheeks, and the legs (in young adults), but other areas may be affected. After rapid initial growth they may remain static for years. Spitz naevi may be more pigmented in some patients, particularly adults.

The spindle cell naevus of Reed is a more deeply pigmented variant, which was first described in 1975 [5]. The majority of patients reported with such lesions are young females, and they are most commonly seen on the thighs. They are densely pig-

mented, irregularly shaped dark-brown or black nodules and are usually isolated (Fig. 54.32a).

Spitz naevi may have a characteristic dermoscopic appearance, the most common being a 'starburst' pattern (Fig. 54.32b) [4]. Some have a more globular pattern however, and others a multi-component pattern.

A striking and unusual variant is that of *multiple Spitz naevi*. In these very rare cases multiple Spitz naevi erupt over a period of time [6]. The aetiology is unknown although authors have suggested that they may develop in relation to triggers [7] such as sunburn. An important differential diagnosis in these cases is epidermotropic metastatic melanoma.

Agminate Spitz naevi are lesions seen in childhood where a group of Spitz naevi develop on skin which looks normal other than for the presence of a macular pigmentary background. The individual Spitz naevi develop rapidly and thereafter remain relatively static. In some ways these lesions resemble speckled naevi and it is likely that all are subtypes of congenital pigmented naevus.

A rare subtype of the Spitz naevus is a *desmoplastic naevus* (desmoplastic Spitz naevus), seen most commonly in adults [8]. These are usually firm and may show little or no clinically visible melanocytic pigmentation, to appear as pink or red, firm, raised nodules. The lesions may be woody hard, and the clinical differential may include a keloid, although there is no history of injury (Fig. 54.33).

Some authors have developed the concept of a metastasizing Spitz as being different to melanoma. It seems unlikely, however, that there is a fundamental difference between a spitzoid lesion, which spreads to a regional node, and melanoma, although it is possible that spitzoid melanoma may have a better prognosis. This remains an area of unresolved controversy, which requires long-term investigation.

Pathology. The 'classic' Spitz naevus typically is a symmetrical and well-defined compound naevus. There is a degree of epidermal acanthosis overlying the naevus cells, in the absence of any upward epidermal invasion by naevus cells. The melanocytes at the dermal–epidermal junction are often separated from the underlying dermis by a cleft, and may be associated with amorphous pink globules. These globules are thought to be degenerating keratinocytes and are called *Kamino bodies*. They are frequently seen in Spitz naevi, but their presence is neither totally sensitive nor specific for Spitz naevi, as they may also be present in early melanoma.

The Spitz naevus cells may be either spindle-shaped, and stream into the dermis in interlacing bundles, or epithelioid, and arranged in clusters with giant and multinucleated naevus cells among them. Mitotic figures may occur but abnormal mitoses are not seen. Mitotic figures are rarer in the deeper naevus cells, and their presence should alert the observer to the possibility that the lesion is, in fact, a spitzoid melanoma. The deepest naevus cells show some degree of maturation and are usually smaller than those seen at the dermal–epidermal junction. The dermal vessels are usually dilated, and the stroma may be oedematous and infiltrated with lymphocytes. Melanin is rarely abundant, and may often be absent.

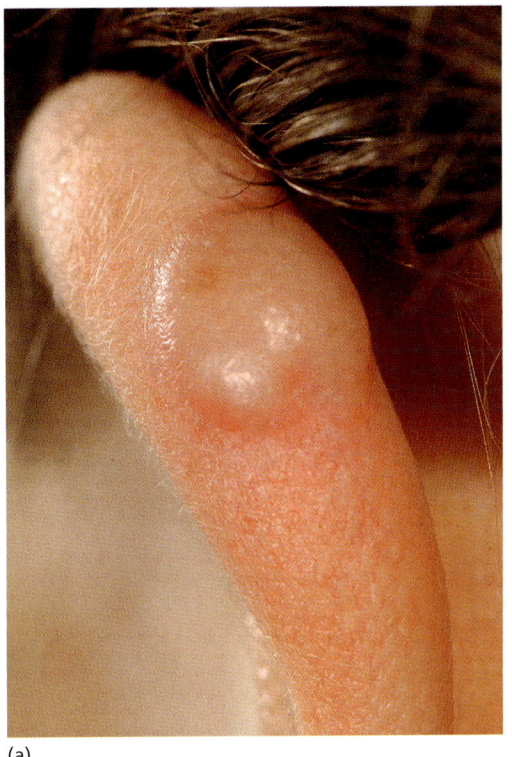
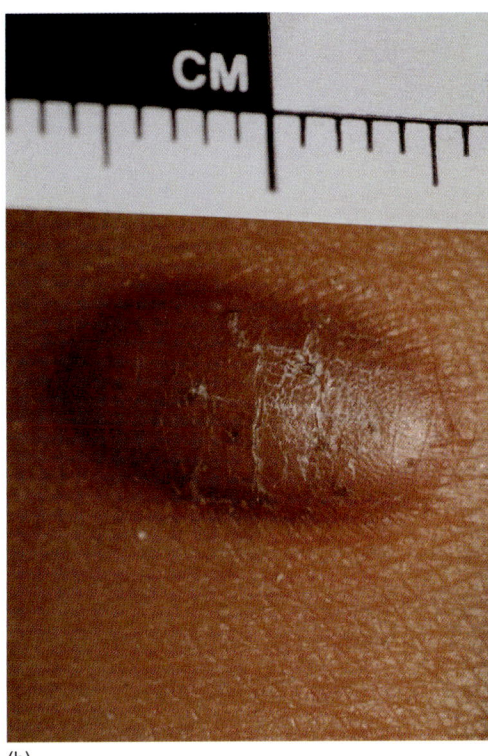

Fig. 54.31 Two Spitz naevi showing less typical appearances: both were excised.

(a)

(b)

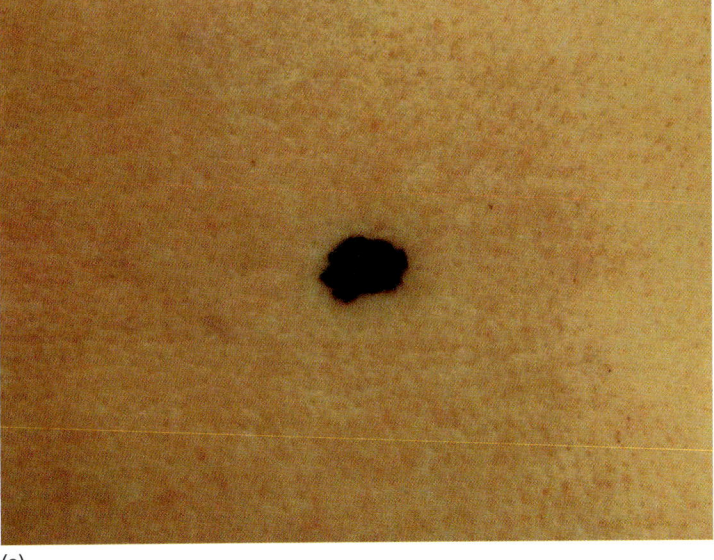

(a)

(b)

Fig. 54.32 (a) The naked-eye appearance of a typical pigmented spindle cell naevus of Reed in a child and (b) the corresponding dermoscopic appearance. (Courtesy of Dr S. Puig, Hospital Clinic Barcelona, IDIBAPS.)

In the variety known as a pigmented spindle cell naevus of Reed, there is well-demarcated junctional melanocytic activity with large quantities of melanin pigment. Spindle-shaped melanocytes proliferate downwards towards the dermis, but there is no upward movement of naevus cells through the epidermis, and usually very little, if any, intradermal component. Some naevus cells may be seen in the papillary dermis, but these naevi do not involve the reticular dermis. A sparse lymphocytic infiltrate is seen at the base of the naevus cells, but the lesion is relatively small and circumscribed. As with 'classical' Spitz naevi, symmetry is an important feature.

The problem is that many lesions with clinical and histological characteristics of Spitz naevi have some atypical features, which cause concern (Fig. 54.34), so that the most important and difficult pathological differential diagnosis is the separation of true benign Spitz naevi from spitzoid malignant melanoma. Two useful studies have tried to identify pathological factors that may help in this situation. Crotty and colleagues [9] have identified symmetry of

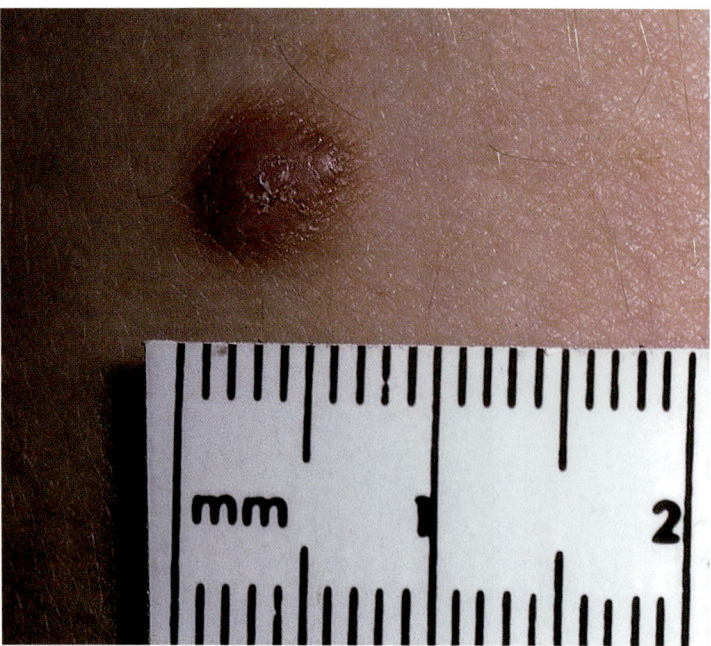

Fig. 54.33 Desmoplastic Spitz naevus.

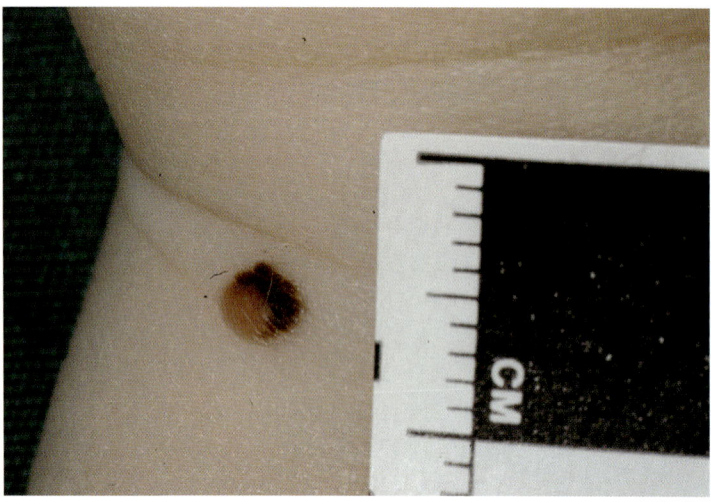

Fig. 54.34 This child developed a pigmented lesion on the wrist at the age of 1 year. At 2 and a half years the lesion was asymmetrical and showed variation in colour. Although clinically likely to be a benign Spitz nevus, prompt excision was necessary.

the lesion from side to side, the presence of Kamino bodies and the uniformity of cell nests or sheets in the dermis as features of benign Spitz naevi. In contrast, they identify abnormal mitoses, mitotic counts of over $2/\text{mm}^2$ and deep mitoses as suggestive of spitzoid melanoma. Spatz *et al*. [10] have identified age over 10 years, diameter over 10 mm, ulceration, invasion to subcutaneous fat and mitotic activity of over $6/\text{mm}^2$ as suggestive of spitzoid melanoma rather than Spitz naevi. Whilst these approaches are helpful, even between expert pathologists interobserver variation for spitzoid lesions is significant [11], and metastases have been reported from lesions categorized as 'low risk' [10]. Any atypical features should therefore be regarded with suspicion.

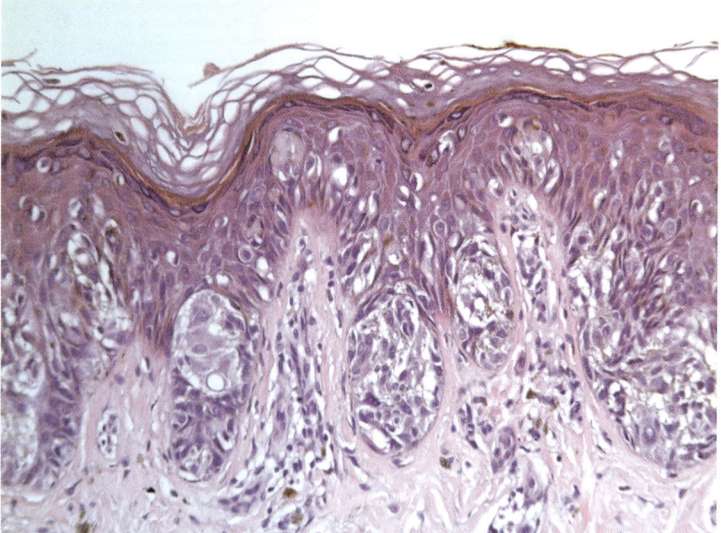

Fig. 54.35 The histological appearance of a classical Spitz naevus, with epitheliod cells and Kamino bodies. (Courtesy of Dr S. Edward, Leeds Teaching Hospitals Trust, Leeds, UK.)

In clinical practice, therefore, it is increasingly common for pathologists to report atypical Spitz naevi as 'atypical spitzoid tumours of unknown malignant potential', or STUMPs [3]. In this case, the norm is to manage the patient as if they had had a melanoma, but to reassure the patient that the lesion may, in fact, be benign although it is preferable to take a cautious view. Given the pathological difficulties around diagnosis, this seems a sensible approach to management.

Molecular biology may ultimately allow better characterization of spitzoid tumours. Comparative genomic hybridization (CGH) has been used, for example, to show differences between Spitz naevi and melanoma [12].

The pathology of the desmoplastic Spitz was well described by Barr *et al*. in 1980 [13] and it has a very striking and characteristic pathological appearance. The lesions are predominantly intradermal, and a relatively small number of naevus cells will be found embedded in thick collagen fibres. The naevus cells are usually distributed singly through the stroma rather than in clumps, and may be very large and bizarre, with copious cytoplasm, which may contain inclusions. The nuclei look unusual but not frankly malignant, and mitotic figures are rare (Fig. 54.35).

Diagnosis. Most Spitz naevi in children are red rather than brown, and may be confused clinically with vascular tumours, pyogenic granuloma, histiocytoma, juvenile xanthogranuloma or granulomas. Pigmented Spitz naevi may resemble compound melanocytic naevi or spindle cell naevi of Reed, but often cause diagnostic confusion with superficial spreading melanomas. Dermoscopy may improve the accuracy of the clinical diagnosis, especially if the lesion has the typical starburst appearance (Fig. 54.32b).

In young children, a lesion typical of a Spitz naevus, being symmetrical and red-brown in appearance, is very unlikely to be a melanoma and would normally not be excised, although review in clinic at 2 to 3 months is essential to ensure that the lesion is not developing any atypical features. In older individuals, or in

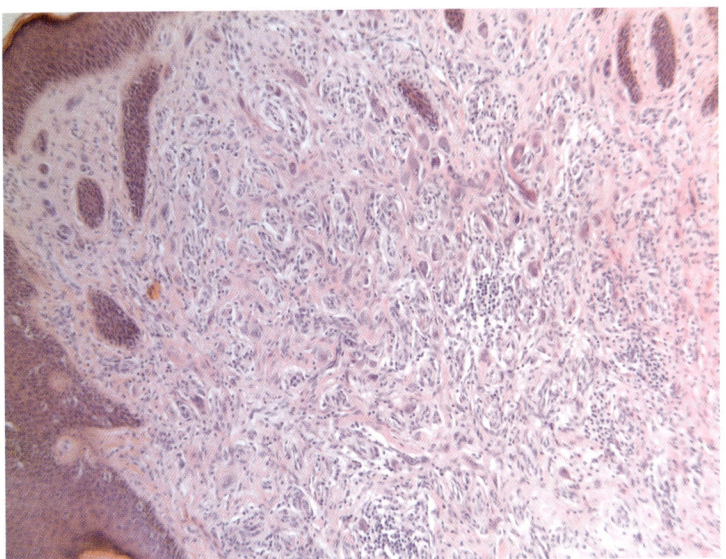

Fig. 54.36 The histological appearance of an atypical spitzoid tumour, showing relative lack of symmetry. (Courtesy of Dr S. Edward, Leeds Teaching Hospitals Trust, Leeds, UK.)

all patients (regardless of age) in which the lesion is asymmetrical or irregular in colour, excision should be carried out to exclude a 'spitzoid' melanoma (atypical spitzoid lesion) (Fig. 54.36). It is said that Spitz naevi are more common in adults on the thigh but rare on the trunk and therefore spitzoid lesions on the trunk of adults [14] would be viewed with particular suspicion. Complete excisions must be carried out, never incisional or punch biopsy. Because of the clinical and histological overlap between Spitz naevi and melanoma, some authors suggest that all spitzoid lesions should be excised [2] and Elder and Murphy suggest that a consensus is emerging towards excision of all [15]. In summary then, it seems reasonable not to remove very typical Spitz naevi in young children unable to tolerate local anaesthetic, but a 3-month review would be sensible. All other clinically spitzoid lesions should be removed in their entirety.

Treatment. Local excision with a narrow margin of 1–2 mm of normal skin is usually required to confirm the clinical diagnosis. Local recurrence has been recorded in both isolated and agminate lesions [16]. In the presence of atypical features (either clinically or histologically), or where the diagnosis of a STUMP is made, the margin of excision should be as for melanoma: 1 cm for tumours of less than 2 mm in thickness; 2 cm or more where the thickness is 2 mm or greater.

There are small reported series of sentinel node biopsies in patients with atypical spitzoid tumours that demonstrate positivity in a proportion [17], supporting the view that such lesions may be melanomas in terms of how they behave. The use of sentinel node biopsy in such patients is subject to the same limitations as for melanoma. In particular there is a no survival benefit.

References
1 Spitz S. Melanomas of childhood. *Am J Pathol* 1947; **24**: 591–609.
2 Barnhill RL. The spitzoid lesion: rethinking Spitz tumors, atypical variants, 'spitzoid melanoma' and risk assessment. *Mod Pathol* 2006; **19** (Suppl. 2): S21–33.
3 Mooi WJ, Krausz T. Spitz nevus versus spitzoid melanoma: diagnostic difficulties, conceptual controversies. *Adv Anat Pathol* 2006; **13**: 147–56.
4 Ferrara G, Argenziano G, Soyer HP *et al*. The spectrum of Spitz nevi: a clinico-pathologic study of 83 cases. *Arch Dermatol* 2005; **141**: 1381–7.
5 Reed RJ, Ichinose H, Clark WH Jr, Mihm MC Jr. Common and uncommon melanocytic nevi and borderline melanomas. *Semin Oncol* 1975; **2**: 119–47.
6 Morgan CJ, Nyak N, Cooper A *et al*. Multiple Spitz naevi: a report of both variants with clinical and histopathological correlation. *Clin Exp Dermatol* 2006; **31**: 368–71.
7 Smith SA, Day CL Jr, Vander Ploeg DE. Eruptive widespread Spitz nevi. *J Am Acad Dermatol* 1986; **15**: 1155–9.
8 Cesinaro AM, Foroni M, Sighinolfi P *et al*. Spitz nevus is relatively frequent in adults: a clinico-pathologic study of 247 cases related to patient's age. *Am J Dermatopathol* 2005; **27**: 469–75.
9 Crotty KA, Scolyer RA, Li L *et al*. Spitz naevus versus spitzoid melanoma: when and how can they be distinguished? *Pathology* 2002; **34**: 6–12.
10 Spatz A, Calonje E, Handfield-Jones S, Barnhill RL. Spitz tumors in children: a grading system for risk stratification. *Arch Dermatol* 1999; **135**: 282–5.
11 Barnhill RL, Flotte TJ, Fleischli M, Perez-Atayde A. Cutaneous melanoma and atypical Spitz tumors in childhood. *Cancer* 1995; **76**: 1833–45.
12 Bastian BC, Wesselmann U, Pinkel D, Leboit PE. Molecular cytogenetic analysis of Spitz nevi shows clear differences to melanoma. *J Invest Dermatol* 1999; **113**: 1065–9.
13 Barr RJ, Morales RV, Graham JH. Desmoplastic nevus: a distinct histologic variant of mixed spindle cell and epithelioid cell nevus. *Cancer* 1980; **46**: 557–64.
14 Schmoeckel C, Wildi G, Schafer T. Spitz nevus versus malignant melanoma: Spitz nevi predominate on the thighs in patients younger than 40 years of age, melanomas on the trunk in patients 40 years of age or older. *J Am Acad Dermatol* 2007; **56**: 753–8.
15 Elder DE, Murphy GF. *Melanocytic Tumors of the Skin*. Washington, DC: American Registry of Pathology, in press.
16 Gambini C, Rongioletti F. Recurrent Spitz nevus. Case report and review of the literature. *Am J Dermatopathol* 1994; **16**: 409–13.
17 Urso C, Borgognoni L, Saieva C *et al*. Sentinel lymph node biopsy in patients with 'atypical Spitz tumors.' A report on 12 cases. *Hum Pathol* 2006; **37**: 816–23.

Blue naevus and cellular blue naevus

Definition. A blue or blue-black melanocytic naevus comprised of aberrant collections of pigment-producing but benign melanocytes, in the dermis rather than at the dermoepidermal junction (as in common acquired naevi).

Incidence and aetiology. Blue naevi are relatively common. Their aetiology and pathogenesis is unclear. Some authors view these as equivalents of dermal melanocytic proliferations seen in animals [1]. Uncommon lesions have mixed 'blue' and 'acquired' characteristics (combined naevus, below) and this might suggest that others are variants of common acquired melanocytic naevi. Multiple epithelioid blue naevi may be associated with the Carney complex (Chapter 62).

Clinical features. There is an area of diffuse blue pigmentation, usually slightly raised and smooth surfaced. Blue naevi may be found on any site but patients with facial naevi most often request excision for cosmetic reasons. The cellular blue naevus is seen most often on the extremities, particularly the dorsa of the hands and feet (Fig. 54.37), the buttocks and the face. The onset may be before birth, but lesions frequently first appear around puberty. The blue naevus is usually very symmetrical, and has an

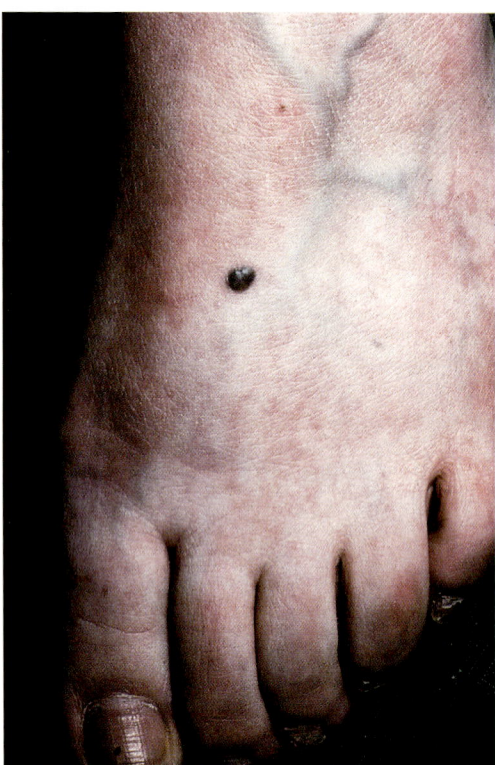

Fig. 54.37 A cellular blue naevus.

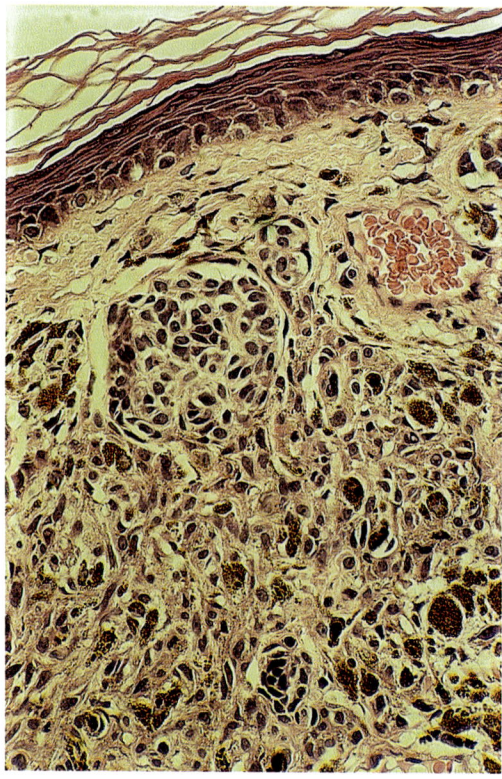

Fig. 54.38 Histology of a blue naevus. Note the normal overlying epidermis with spindle cells and dense pigmentation in underlying dermis.

amorphous, structureless pigment pattern on dermoscopy which may be blue, white or darker in colour [2].

The combined naevus is a rare variant in which there are elements of a blue naevus and a common acquired melanocytic naevus. They may cause concern clinically because of their unusual appearance and are therefore commonly removed.

The deep penetrating naevus is a further rare variant said to be more common on the head and neck [3]. Clinically, it may be a deep blue or black colour with a diffuse, irregular lateral margin. The clinical differential diagnosis is therefore frequently melanoma. The blue appearance is attributed to the 'Tyndall effect', which states that red light penetrating the skin is diffused by the dermis allowing blue light to be reflected by deep pigment.

Progressive growth in blue naevi is rare and would cause concern, although malignant transformation is very rare indeed (below). There is a view that the term malignant blue naevus is confusing and that lesions dubbed 'malignant blue naevi' are just melanomas which resemble blue naevi, or that these are very rare instances of malignant transformation in a blue naevus [4].

***

Pathology. In the common or classic variety, bipolar and dendritic melanocytes lie singly or in masses in the dermis (Fig. 54.38). The melanocytes tend to be profuse in the lower dermis and are often concentrated around appendages or in the perivascular and perineural areas. Deeper tissues may be involved. The melanocytes are relatively inconspicuous, containing fine granules of melanin dispersed through their cytoplasm. There are varying numbers of melanophages in which the melanin granules are coarse and more closely clumped.

The cellular blue naevus is composed of the same elements as the common blue naevus, but in addition possesses islands of larger cells arranged in a neuroid ('pigmented neurofibroma') or sarcomatoid fashion. The appearance may raise suspicions of malignant melanoma, but the lack of mitotic activity, vascularity or inflammatory reaction, the regularity of the cells and the absence of junctional proliferation in continuity with the cellular masses enable the distinction to be made [5,6].

The compound blue naevus is a more recently described entity [7], with additional dendritic cells in the overlying epidermis. This lesion may clinically be very similar to early malignant melanoma.

The deep penetrating naevus may be considered as a distinct entity [3] or as a variant which frequently has features of both a compound and a blue naevus or Spitz naevus, making it a variant of the so-called combined naevus but with minimal junctional activity. They are larger than most naevi, with extension of naevus cells deep into the dermis in a wedge shape, the base abutting onto the epidermis. The diagnostic feature is the presence of clusters of widely separated but deep naevus cells throughout the dermis. Frequently these clusters are around the skin appendages. The cytology is of a spindle cell population and mitotic figures are rare [8].

Malignant blue naevus is discussed below.

***

Diagnosis. The blue naevus is characterized by its colour and symmetrical shape and must be differentiated from other dermal melanoses. It is a relatively static, non-progressive lesion.

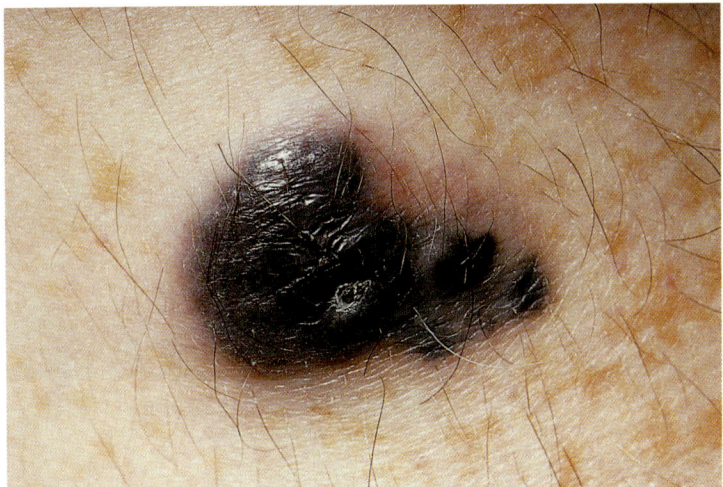

Fig. 54.39 Malignant blue naevus which has arisen in a previous cellular blue naevus. This lesion subsequently metastasized to lymph nodes.

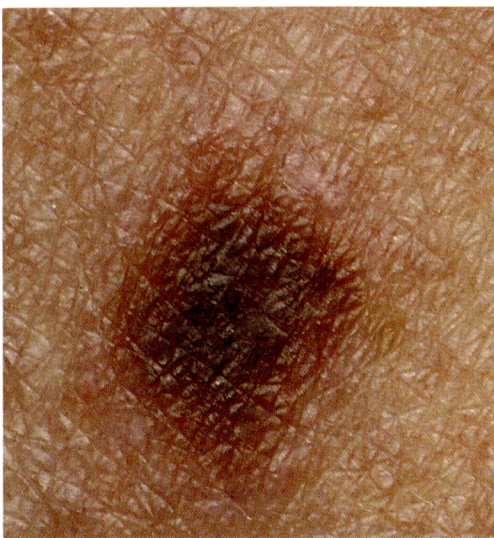

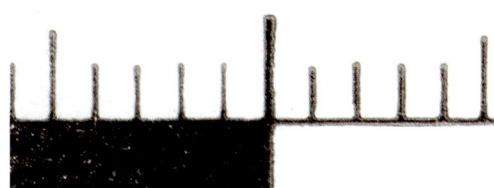

Fig. 54.40 An 'atypical' or dysplastic naevus. Such naevi are clinically defined. They are 5 mm or more in diameter, with a diffuse, or irregular edge and variable pigmentation.

Treatment. None is needed save for distinction from melanoma.

Malignant blue naevus

Definition. A very rare malignancy often confused with melanoma although it is argued that the difference is semantic [4]; in some cases it is not possible to differentiate between classic malignant melanoma and malignant change within a blue naevus.

Pathology. Malignant cells of melanocytic origin are seen in the deeper dermis with no overlying abnormality of epidermal melanocytes. Pathologically there is a sheet-like growth pattern. Necrosis and atypical mitotic figures are diagnostic features which will distinguish these lesions from benign classic or cellular blue naevi [9]. Mitotic figures are rare [10], but the presence of any at all should suggest the diagnosis of melanoma rather than a blue naevus.

Clinical features. Malignant blue naevus usually arises in a cellular blue naevus, and the scalp is the commonest site (Fig. 54.39). Expansion of a previously identified blue naevus should suggest the diagnosis. Metastases do occur [9].

Treatment. Wide surgical excision is required as for other types of melanoma.

References

1 Levene A. On the natural history and comparative pathology of the blue naevus. *Ann Roy Coll Surg* 1980; **62**: 327–34.
2 Ferrara G, Soyer HP, Malvehy J *et al*. The many faces of blue nevus: A clinicopathologic study. *J Cutan Pathol* 2007; **34**: 543–51.
3 Flauta VS, Lingamfelter DC, Dang LM, Lankachandra KM. Deep penetrating nevus: a case report and brief literature review. *Diag Pathol* 2006; **1**: 31.
4 Mones JM, Ackerman AB. 'Atypical' blue nevus, 'malignant' blue nevus, and 'metastasizing' blue nevus: a critique in historical perspective of three concepts flawed fatally. *Am J Dermatopathol* 2004; **26**: 407–30.
5 Leopold JG, Richards DB. Cellular blue naevi. *J Pathol Bacteriol* 1967; **94**: 247–55.
6 Merkow LP, Burt RC, Hayeslip DW *et al*. A cellular and malignant blue nevus: a light and electron microscopic study. *Cancer* 1969; **24**: 888–96.
7 Ferrara G, Argenziano G, Zgavec B *et al*. 'Compound blue nevus': a reappraisal of 'superficial blue nevus with prominent intraepidermal dendritic melanocytes' with emphasis on dermoscopic and histopathologic features. *J Am Acad Dermatol* 2002; **46**: 85–9.
8 Elder DE, Murphy GF. *Melanocytic Tumors of the Skin*. Washington, DC: American Registry of Pathology, in press.
9 Granter SR, McKee PH, Calonje E *et al*. Melanoma associated with blue nevus and melanoma mimicking cellular blue nevus: a clinicopathologic study of 10 cases on the spectrum of so-called 'malignant blue nevus'. *Am J Surg Pathol* 2001; **25**: 316–23.
10 Pich A, Chiusa L, Margaria E, Aloi F. Proliferative activity in the malignant cellular blue nevus. *Hum Pathol* 1993; **24**: 1323–9.

Clinically atypical naevi

Synonym
• Dysplastic naevus

Definition/pathogenesis. A melanocytic naevus, which is 5 mm or larger in diameter, with an irregular or diffuse edge and variable or mottled pigmentation (Fig. 54.40). Although there are histological correlates, the diagnosis is a clinical one.

Natural history. The natural history of acquired benign naevi is of proliferation of melanocytes until the naevus reaches up to

5 mm in diameter, and the proliferation at the dermoepidermal junction then ceases. The naevus cells migrate down into the dermis but subsequent cellular senescence occurs, resulting in the development of a compound and then a dermal cellular naevus. In an atypical naevus, the melanocyte proliferation continues so that the naevus continues to grow in size beyond the 'usual' size, and the junctional proliferative component may show some features reminiscent of an early melanoma, resulting in some irregularity of shape and colour clinically. Although in the majority of such naevi the melanocytes eventually cease proliferation, resulting in 'maturation' of the naevus as a compound and then a dermal naevus, a proportion of such naevi continue to grow and may evolve into radial growth phase melanoma. Thus, although the majority of atypical naevi behave in a benign manner, they are viewed as lesions exhibiting a more proliferative phenotype than common acquired naevi, and are therefore both markers of risk of melanoma and precursor lesions for melanoma.

Incidence and epidemiology. The term 'dysplastic naevus' was first used by Elder [1] as a pathological description of a sporadically occurring melanocytic naevus, which was clinically larger and more irregular, and showed a constellation of pathological features that also distinguished it from common or banal naevi. Earlier, Clark *et al.* [2] and Frichot *et al.* [3] had separately, but almost simultaneously, described families in which multiple primary melanomas were much more common than expected and who also had large numbers of unusual naevi—the BK mole syndrome or FAMMM syndrome (familial *a*typical *m*ultiple *m*ole *m*elanoma syndrome) [4]. The naevi seen in these syndromes have come to be recognized as 'atypical naevi'. Technically, atypical is a clinical description and dysplasia is determined histologically; although a clinically atypical naevus may not exhibit histological dysplasia, and vice versa, the terms have often been used interchangeably.

Atypical (or dysplastic) naevi are common in white-skinned peoples. In studies reported from Sweden, 18% of the population were reported to have at least one clinically diagnosed atypical naevus [5], as had 37% of young men in an Italian study [6]. In other populations the prevalence is lower, so that in a German study 5% of adults were reported to have at least one [7]. The prevalence is therefore variable and some of this variation is explained by differences in skin type, age of people studied and probably differences in clinical definitions or interobserver variability. There is no doubt, however, that they are common, although most individuals who do have some atypical naevi only have small numbers—one or two generally.

Atypical naevi are undoubtedly precursors of melanoma, although progression to melanoma is uncommon. They are also markers of risk of melanoma; in a meta-analysis the melanoma relative risk associated with the number of atypical naevi was 6.36 (95% CI 3.80–10.33) for five versus none [8]. Twin studies have provided evidence that benign naevi in general are genetically determined [9] and it is supposed that atypical naevi are also genetically determined at least in part, although with evidence that sunburn is also important [10].

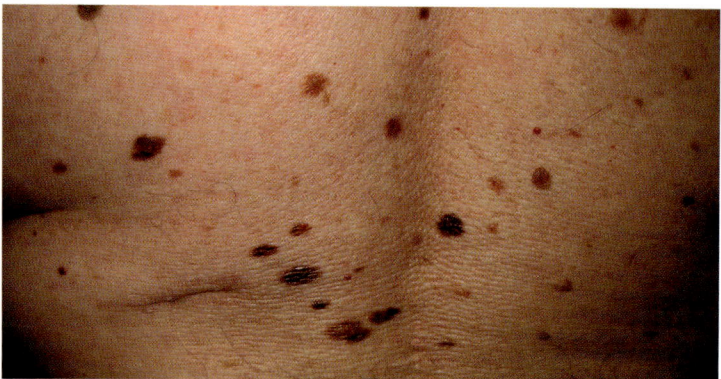

Fig. 54.41 The atypical mole syndrome is characterized by the presence of an increased number of naevi and clinically atypical naevi. This is the strongest phenotypic risk factor for melanoma.

Although small numbers of atypical naevi are common in most fair-skinned populations, as documented above, and although they are both a precursor and an associate of melanoma, the majority of people with some atypical naevi have neither a personal nor a family history of melanoma. However, many such individuals will also have increased numbers of small benign naevi (Fig. 54.41) and are recognized to be at increased risk of melanoma. The atypical mole syndrome is my preferred term to describe patients with this phenotype, but others use the 'dysplastic naevus syndrome' or the FAMMM syndrome phenotype. Their relative risk of melanoma is something around 6 to 10 times that of people with very few naevi [8,11]. The identification of this 'at risk' group, which accounts for around 2% of the UK population [12], is therefore important in terms of prevention and for education around early detection.

Clinical features. The original description of dysplastic naevi indicated that these were lesions larger than 5 mm with an irregular edge, irregular pigmentation and a degree of inflammation. Although there is a recognizable histological pattern associated with such naevi, the correlation between clinical and pathological features is poor. This, in some respects, is not a problem. The diagnosis of an atypical naevus is a clinical one. The importance of this diagnosis is only in terms of educating the patient about risk and what to look for when self-examining.

The clinical imperative is to distinguish the atypical naevus from *in situ* or early radial growth phase melanoma. In practice, the clinical features of atypical naevi are in continuum with those of *in situ* melanoma, and the clinician must have a sufficiently low threshold for excision to avoid missing the latter whilst avoiding the excision of excessive numbers of benign naevi (Figs 54.42–45).

Pathology. The great majority of atypical naevi are variants of acquired compound melanocytic naevi, although features described in atypical lesions may be seen in junctional naevi, in some congenital naevi and, occasionally, in Spitz naevi and variants.

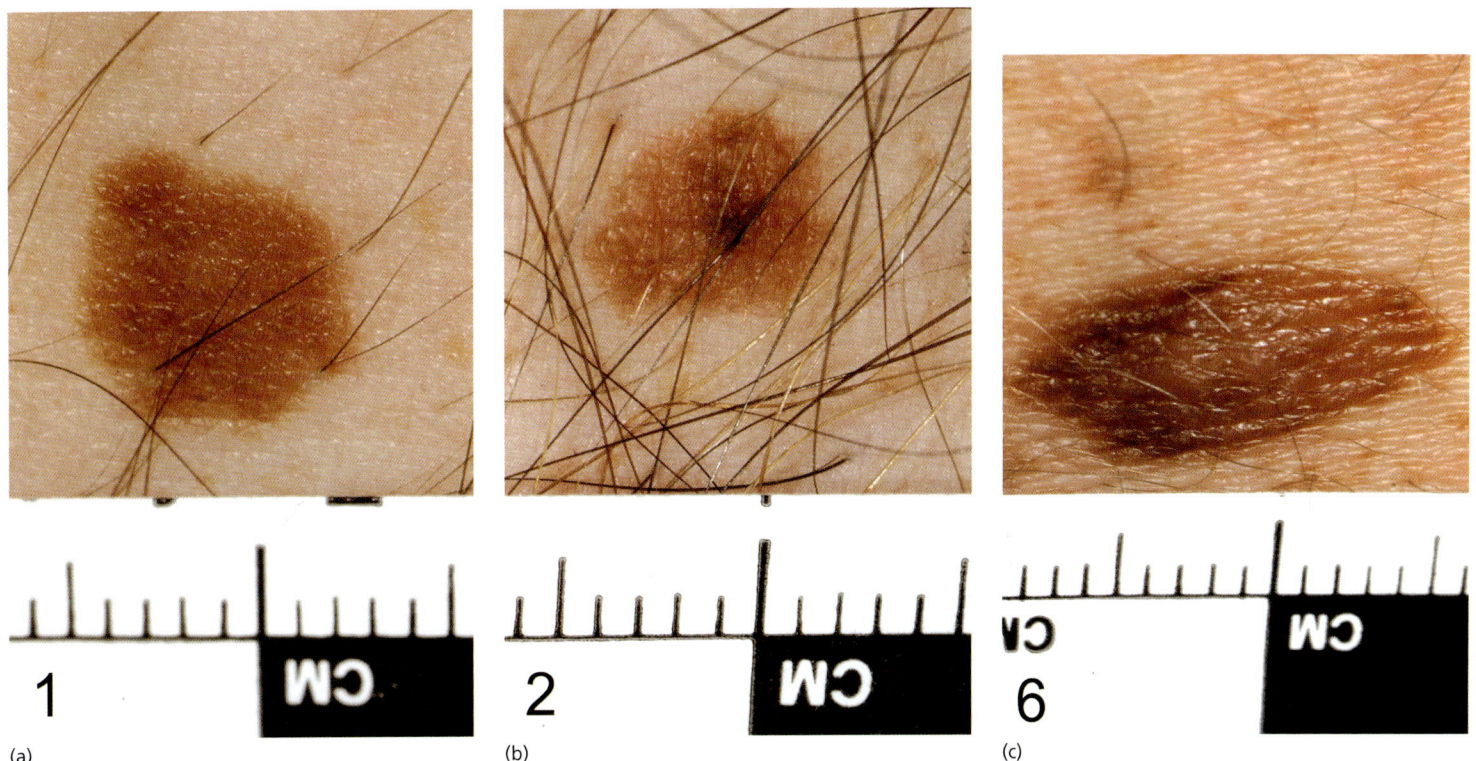

(a)   (b)   (c)

Fig. 54.42 (a, b, c) A series of bland but atypical naevi which appear to be behaving in an entirely benign fashion, showing evidence of little proliferation or stromal reaction. (c) A compound atypical naevus.

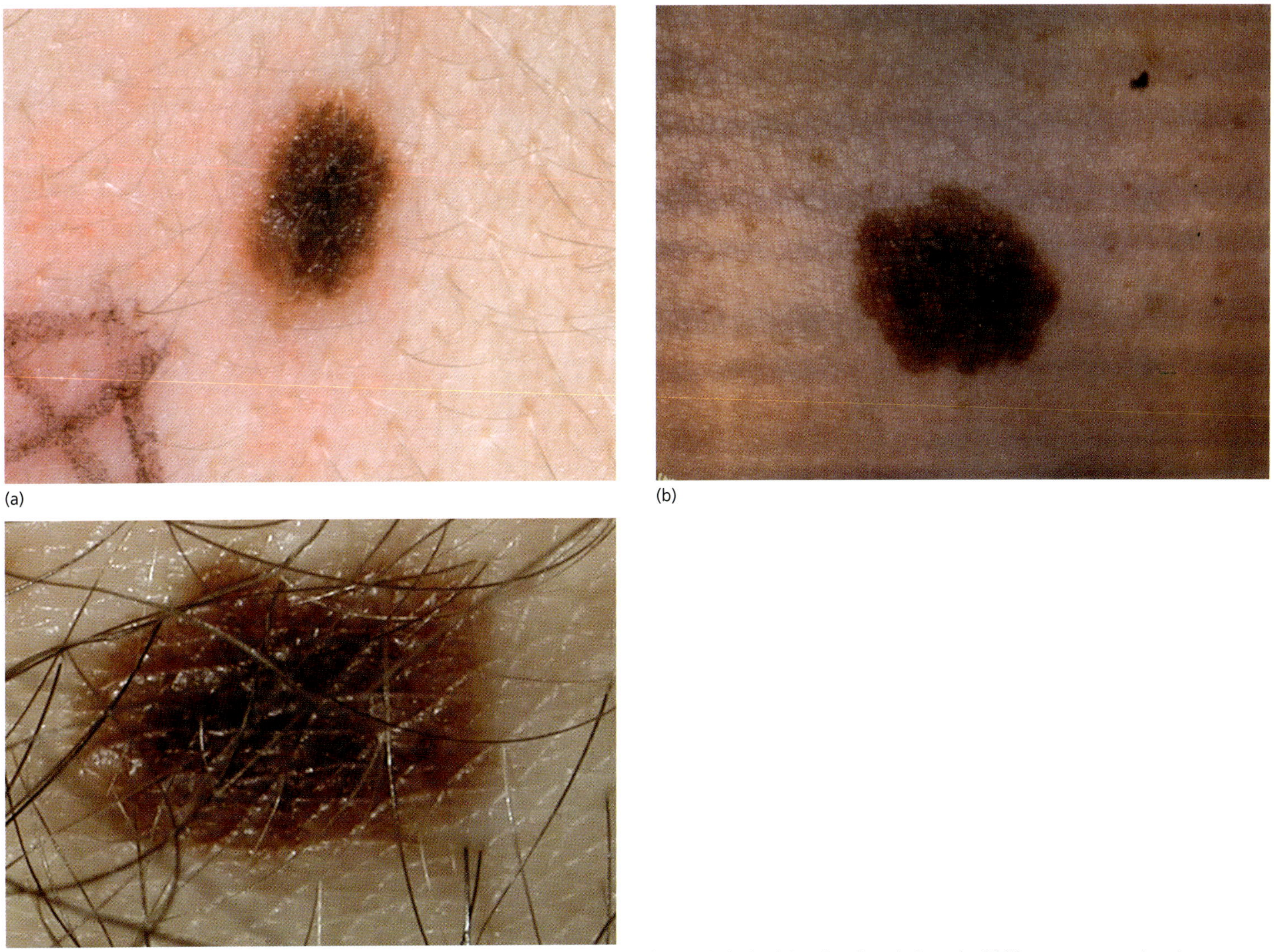

(a)   (b)

(c)   **Fig. 54.43** (a, b, c) A series of atypical naevi exhibiting a more worrying phenotype.

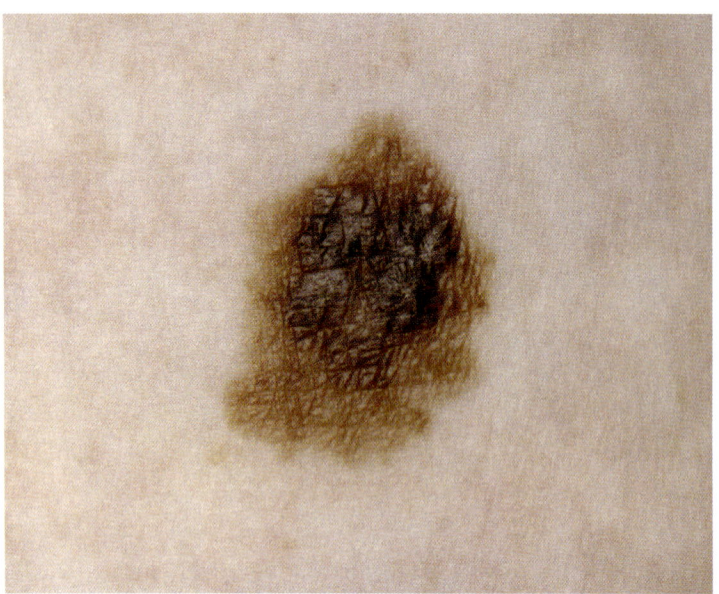

(a)

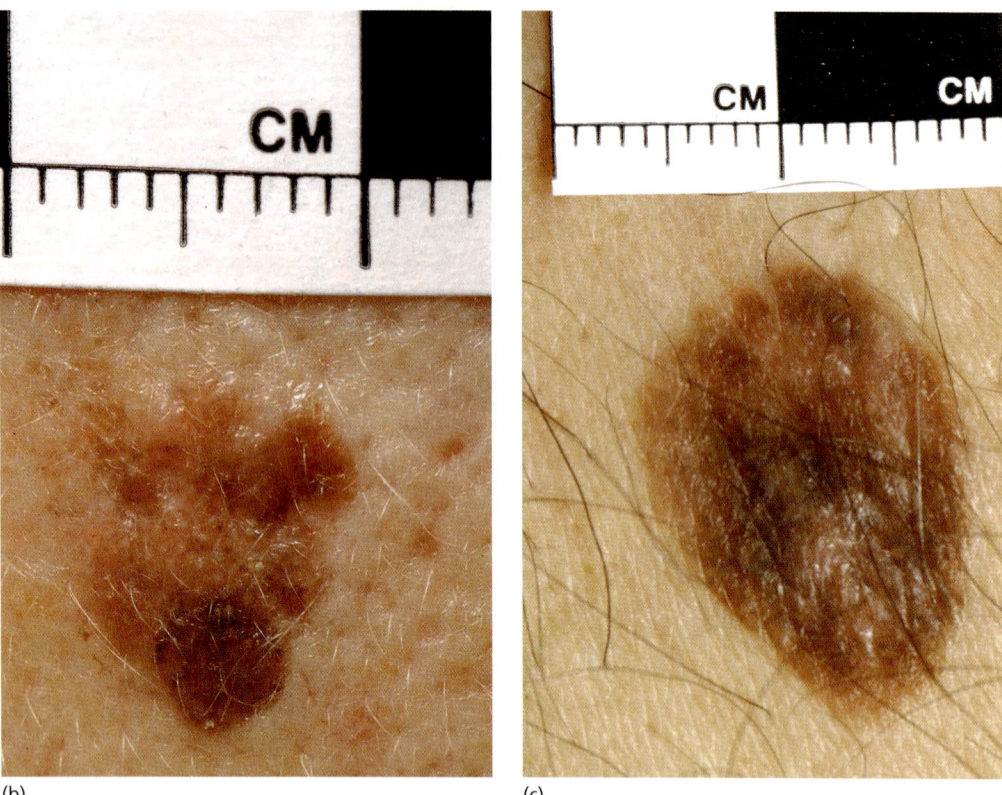

(b)   (c)

Fig. 54.44 (a, b, c) A series of *in situ* melanomas to illustrate the continuum of clinical change that is the progression from atypical naevi to melanoma.

The specific pathological features described in atypical naevi can be divided into architectural features, cytological features and features indicative of a host response to the naevus cells. The architectural features are lentiginous melanocytic hyperplasia, fusion of individual nests of naevomelanocytes and associated elongation of epidermal rete ridges (Fig. 54.46). The cytological abnormalities are the increase in the nuclear to cytoplasmic ratio of individual melanocytes, an increase in nuclear staining and occasional normal mitotic figures in melanocytes. Elder and Murphy describe random, slight to moderate atypia, occasional macronuclei, scattered epithelioid naevus cells and scattered cells with dusky pigment [13]. Most groups would not make the diagnosis on architectural features alone but consider melanocyte cytological atypia an essential feature for the diagnosis. It is preferable to report the presence of architectural and cytological atypia specifically. The three pathological features indicating a host response

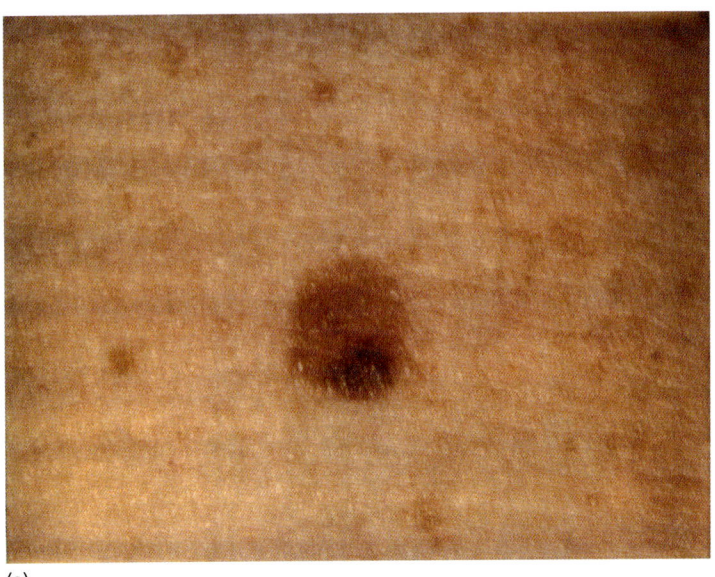

(a)

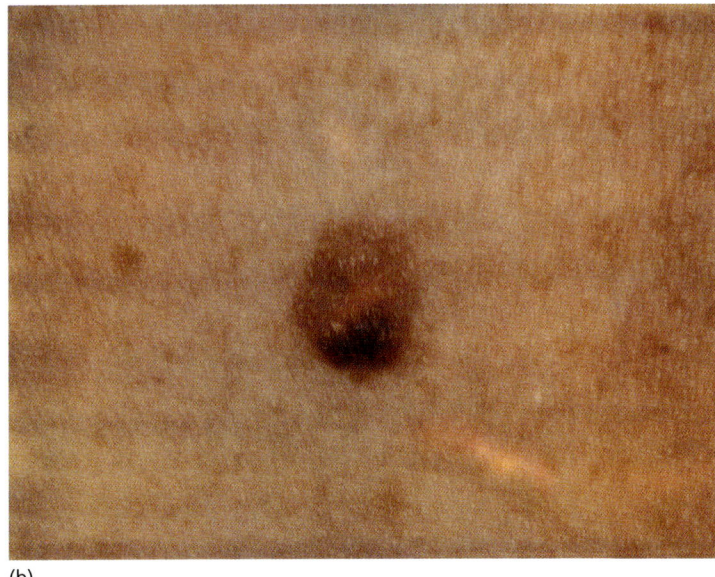

(b)

Fig. 54.45 (a, b) A change in the appearance of an atypical naevus over a 4-month period signifying evolution of an early superficial spreading melanoma in a *CDKN2A* mutation carrier.

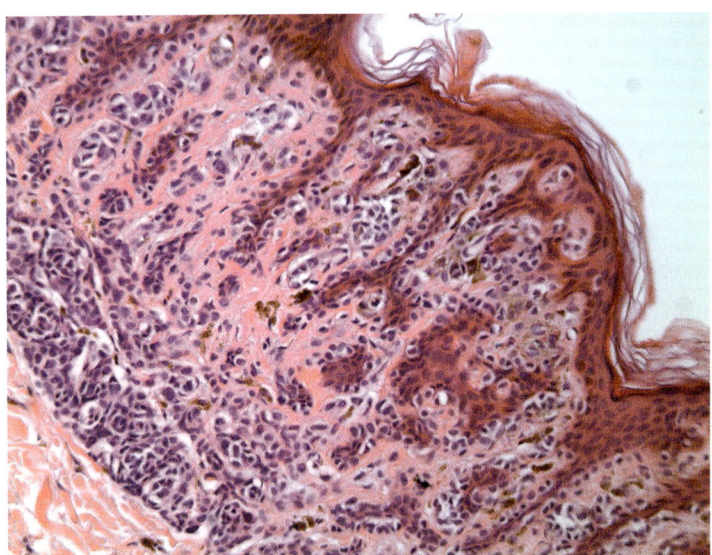

Fig. 54.46 Architectural atypia in a mildy atypical (dysplastic) compound naevus. (Courtesy of Dr S. Edward, Leeds Teaching Hospitals Trust, Leeds, UK.)

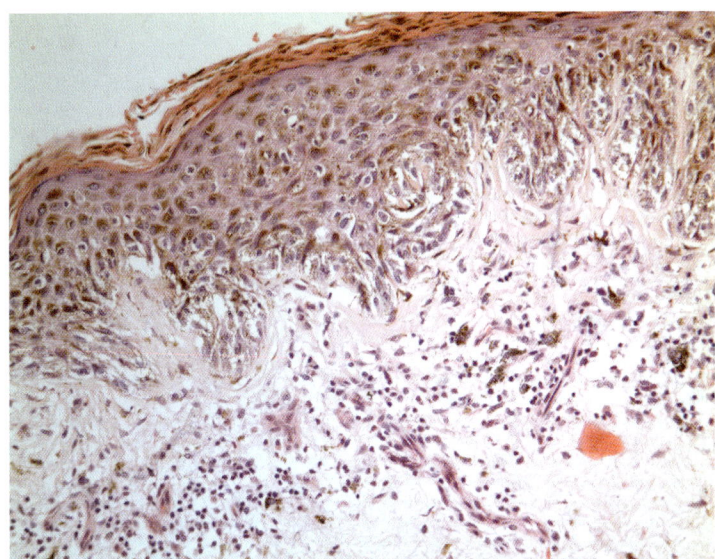

Fig. 54.47 A severely atypical (dysplastic) naevus with an inflammatory stromal reaction. (Courtesy of Dr S. Edward, Leeds Teaching Hospitals Trust, Leeds, UK.)

are the presence of a lymphocytic infiltrate, a degree of fibroplasia of the collagen of the papillary dermis and a relative increase in the vascularity of the underlying dermis (Fig. 54.47). The presence of these changes in an atypical naevus that has evolved into a melanoma may cause confusion with the possible presence of regression.

Treatment. Atypical naevi are in the majority of cases benign, stable lesions, which are bland in appearance, clinically and using dermoscopy. They can be left in place although the patient must be educated about monitoring the appearance of such naevi over time. Photographs of early melanomas are essential for this purpose, as leaflets or on line [14]. A picture of the naevus given to the patient may also be helpful.

Where the naevus is sufficiently atypical (and particularly when a single naevus is present) then it should be removed in its entirety with a 2-mm clinical margin and subjected to pathological examination, to exclude *in situ* melanoma. Such naevi should NEVER be punch biopsied or an incisional biopsy taken, as sampling error may cause an early melanoma to be missed.

Two per cent of the UK population [12] have the atypical mole syndrome in which there are multiple naevi, many of which may be clinically atypical, although this is variable. The majority have no family history of melanoma. In these patients the phenotype is a marker of risk and that risk cannot be removed by removal of the naevi. Such patients must be counselled about avoidance of sunburn for themselves and their children. They should be taught how to self examine with the aid of images [14] and a short period of follow-up is sensible, to ensure that the naevi are stable and that the patient is confident about self examination. Advice for follow-up of those with a family history of melanoma is discussed below.

References

1 Elder DE. The dysplastic nevus. *Pathology* 1985; **17**: 291–7.

2 Clark WH Jr, Reimer RR, Greene M *et al*. Origin of familial malignant melanomas from heritable melanocytic lesions. 'The B-K mole syndrome'. *Arch Dermatol* 1978; **114**: 732–8.

3 Frichot BC 3rd, Lynch HT, Guirgis HA *et al*. New cutaneous phenotype in familial malignant melanoma. *Lancet* 1977; **1**: 864–5.

4 Bergman W, Palan A, Went LN. Clinical and genetic studies in six Dutch kindreds with the dysplastic naevus syndrome. *Ann Hum Genetics* 1986; **50**: 249–58.

5 Augustsson A, Stierner U, Suurkula M, Rosdahl I. Prevalence of common and dysplastic naevi in a Swedish population. *Br J Dermatol* 1991; **124**: 152–6.

6 Ballone E, Passamonti M, Lappa G *et al*. Pigmentary traits, nevi and skin phototypes in a youth population of Central Italy. *Eur J Epidemiol* 1999; **15**: 189–95.

7 Schafer T, Merkl J, Klemm E *et al*. The epidemiology of nevi and signs of skin aging in the adult general population: Results of the KORA-survey 2000. *J Invest Dermatol* 2006; **126**: 1490–6.

8 Gandini S, Sera F, Cattaruzza MS *et al*. Meta-analysis of risk factors for cutaneous melanoma: I. Common and atypical naevi. *Eur J Cancer* 2005; **41**: 28–44.

9 Zhu G, Duffy DL, Eldridge A *et al*. A major quantitative-trait locus for mole density is linked to the familial melanoma gene CDKN2A: a maximum-likelihood combined linkage and association analysis in twins and their sibs. *Am J Hum Genet* 1999; **65**: 483–92.

10 Carli P, Biggeri A, Nardini P *et al*. Epidemiology of atypical melanocytic naevi: an analytical study in a Mediterranean population. *Eur J Cancer Prev* 1997; **6**: 506–11.

11 Bataille V, Newton Bishop JA, Sasieni P *et al*. Risk of cutaneous melanoma in relation to the numbers, types and sites of naevi: a case–control study. *Br J Cancer* 1996; **73**: 1605–11.

12 Newton JA, Bataille V, Griffiths K *et al*. How common is the atypical mole syndrome phenotype in apparently sporadic melanoma? *J Am Acad Dermatol* 1993; **29**: 989–96.

13 Elder DE, Murphy GF. *Melanocytic Tumors of the Skin*. Washington, DC: American Registry of Pathology, in press.

14 Melanoma Genetics Consortium. www.genomel.org.

Malignant melanoma of the skin (melanoma): background

Definition. A malignant tumour arising from the epidermal melanocyte.

Incidence and mortality [1]

There has been a steady rise in the incidence of melanoma of the skin in many areas of Australia, New Zealand, North America and Europe since the 1950s. The most recent incidence figures are available on line from the Globocan 2002 project at the Cancer Mondial Statistical Information website through the International Agency for Research on Cancer [2]. The highest incidence is seen in Australia and New Zealand. There has been a levelling off in incidence in many areas of Western Europe in recent years, but in Eastern and Southern Europe levels are still increasing [3]. In the

UK, there is some evidence for a levelling off in some areas [4,5] but not in all [6]. In the USA, the SEER programme reported that the incidence of melanoma continued to rise at least till 1995, with a trebling of melanoma incidence in males aged 45–64 years over the 30-year period 1969–99, from 13.5 to 40.0 per 100 000 population per annum, and a fivefold increase in older males aged over 65 years, from 18.8 to 91.9 per 100 000 population per annum. Incidence rates for females aged 45–64 years and for those aged over 65 years have also risen but less steeply than for males, while the incidence of melanoma in younger adults of both sexes aged under 45 years has only risen slightly over a 40-year period [7]. In Australia, age-standardized incidence is continuing to increase despite long-standing prevention campaigns. However, a study has provided evidence for stabilization of incidence rates in those younger than 35 years and the proportionate increase for both *in situ* and invasive lesions appears to be lower for the most recent period compared with previous periods, providing hope of a reversal in years to come [8].

Despite the increase in incidence in the north of the UK recently, mortality seems to be levelling off [6]. In Australia, melanoma mortality seems to have peaked in the 1980s [9]; statistically significant decreases in mortality rates for both men and women younger than 55 years have occurred in recent years, for 55–79 year olds, rates are now stable for both men and women whereas previously the rates were increasing. For both men and women 80 years or older, rates have continued an increase of 3–4% per year [10]. Similarly, in the USA, mortality appears to be stabilizing in women, but still rising slightly in men [7].

Overall then, melanoma is most common in white-skinned peoples living at lower latitudes such as Australia, and the incidence continues to increase in many countries but has levelled off in others. The mortality seems to have levelled off or have reduced in most areas, however, suggesting that early diagnosis may have been effective in reducing mortality. Some authors have contested this, suggesting that increased numbers of melanocytic lesions may be being removed which would not necessarily have progressed to invasive melanoma [11]. Certainly, in many areas of the world the absolute numbers of thick tumours appear to be relatively constant over time [12] suggesting persistent difficulties in early diagnosis. Thicker tumours occur particularly in older patients [6,12], and, in many series, males had a higher proportion of thicker tumours than did females [7,12]. Furthermore, in Europe generally, mortality has continued to increase in older men [13]. In terms of prevention, therefore, an important target group for early detection are older patients, particularly males.

Aetiology

Melanoma is predominantly a cancer of white-skinned peoples, which gave the first clue that sun exposure is causal. The variation in incidence amongst such populations with latitude of residence (as described above) is further evidence, the highest incidence being in Australasia where susceptible, fair-skinned peoples live in sunny climes. The aetiological factors for melanoma are therefore both genetic (related to cutaneous responses to the sun such as skin type) and environmental.

The precise type of sun exposure that is causal has been controversial but the data are now strong that the dominant cause is intermittent sun exposure. Holidays in the sun, associated with sunburn, have been identified in numerous case–control studies, and results have been subjected to meta-analysis [14]. Chronic sun exposure does not seem to be causal, at least in many areas of the world; there was even some evidence for a protective role for occupational sun exposure in the same meta-analysis [14]. In Australasia, however, solar keratoses appear to be risk factors for melanoma and it has been suggested that there are two routes to melanoma [15,16]: one associated with short sharp exposures to excessive sun exposure and sunburn and another related to chronic sun exposure which might be responsible for a greater proportion of cases in hot countries. These hypotheses are still being explored.

There is some evidence that sunbed usage is also causal for melanoma: in a meta-analysis based on 19 informative studies [17], use of sunbeds ever was positively associated with melanoma (summary relative risk 1.15; 95% CI 1.00–1.31), although there was no consistent evidence of a dose–response relationship. First exposure to sunbeds before 35 years of age significantly increased the risk of melanoma, based on seven informative studies (summary relative risk 1.75; 95% CI 1.35–2.26). It is difficult to separate the effects of sunbed use from those of sunbathing, however, and sunbed usage is likely to explain a relatively small proportion of melanoma cases.

Whether the continued increase in incidence is an artefact of the removal of increased numbers of lesions which might have progressed or not, the relationship between melanoma and intermittent sun exposure and increased mobility of fair-skinned peoples to hot countries is a cause for concern.

Phenotypic risk factors for melanoma

The strongest phenotypic risk factor for melanoma is the presence of increased numbers of melanocytic naevi. In a meta-analysis of 46 studies, 101–120 common naevi compared with less than 15 was associated with a significantly increased risk of melanoma (pooled relative risk (RR) = 6.89; 95% CI 4.63–10.25) as was the number of atypical naevi (RR = 6.36; 95% CI 3.80–10.33, for 5 versus 0) [18]. Twin studies have provided strong evidence that naevus number is predominantly genetically determined [19], with a smaller effect of environmental factors, particularly sun exposure [20]. It is theorized, therefore, that the genes that determine naevus number are also common melanoma susceptibility genes. The first evidence for inherited genes that are both naevus and melanoma susceptibility genes was published in 2009 [21].

Weaker phenotypic risk factors relate to the presence of skin that burns easily in the sun such as: skin type (I vs. IV: RR = 2.09, 95% CI 1.67–2.58), high density of freckles (RR = 2.10, 95% CI 1.80–2.45), skin colour (fair vs. dark: RR = 2.06, 95% CI 1.68–2.52), eye colour (blue vs. dark: RR = 1.47, 95% CI 1.28–1.69) and hair colour (red vs. dark: RR = 3.64, 95% CI 2.56–5.37) [22]. These phenotypes are also genetically determined; a key gene, *MC1R*, codes for the melanocortin receptor receptor, which, at least in part, determines the presence of both red hair [23] and freckles [24]. The gene mediates these effects by modulation of the ratio between the pheomelanin and eumelanin produced by the melanocyte.

Skin changes indicative of sun damage are also shown to be risk factors at meta-analysis [22], such as pre-malignant and skin cancer lesions (RR = 4.28, 95% CI 2.80–6.55) and actinic damage indicators (RR = 2.02, 95% CI 1.24–3.29).

Familial melanoma

Any family history increases the risk of melanoma. A study from the Swedish Cancer Registry estimated the standardized incidence ratio for melanoma to be 2.40 (95% CI 2.10–2.72) for offspring if one parent had a melanoma, 2.98 (95% CI 2.54–3.47) for an affected sibling and 8.92 (95% CI 4.25–15.31) if a parent and a sibling were both affected. The highest ratio was for offspring when a parent had multiple melanomas [25].

A strong family history is rare, but families with multiple cases are reported from around the world. In these families, inheritance of melanoma is consistent with inheritance of an autosomal dominant gene with incomplete penetrance (Fig. 54.48). Inheritance of mutations in the *CDKN2A* gene on chromosome 9 [26] (which codes for the cell cycle inhibitor protein, p16) explains a proportion of these families, but not all. The importance of p16 in the pathogenesis of melanoma was emphasized by the identification of germline mutations of *CDK4* as the second highest penetrance melanoma susceptibility gene [27,28], as mutations in this gene, found at chromosome 12q13, occur at the p16 binding site. Families with mutations in *CDK4* are excessively rare. Many of the reported *CDKN2A* mutations have been shown to be founder mutations, such as Gly101Trp [29], which is common in mainland Europe (France and Italy), the so-called Leiden mutation, which is an exon 2 19-bp deletion [30], and Met53Ile [31], which may be of Scottish origin. 113insArg is a Swedish founder mutation [32] and a common founder for Val126Arp has been shown by haplotype studies in North American families [33]. To date, only one mutation seems to appear repeatedly at a hotspot, a 24-bp duplication at the N-terminus [31]. An on-line database of locus specific variants, named eMelanoBase, is maintained by the Leiden Medical Center group of GenoMEL [34]. The proportion of families with identifiable mutations is higher with larger numbers of affected family members, early age of onset and if there are cases with multiple primaries, and if family members have pancreatic cancer [33], although there is variation by continent so that the association with pancreatic cancer, for example, is much less clear in Australia than it is in many parts of Europe and the USA. The majority of families appear to be predisposed to melanoma alone, if risk is assessed by pedigree examination. The gene penetrance has been estimated by GenoMEL, the Melanoma Genetics Consortium [35]. Overall, *CDKN2A* mutation penetrance was estimated to be 0.30 (95% CI 0.12–0.62), meaning that on average 30% of mutation carriers develop a melanoma by the age of 50 years and 0.67 (95% CI 0.31–0.96) by age 80 years, in 80 families pooled from the US, Australia and Europe. Not surprisingly, penetrance was higher in families living in Australia where sun exposure is more intense. A lower penetrance was reported in a population based study [36].

A significant proportion of families do not have identifiable *CDKN2A* or *CDK4* mutations and there are, therefore, other high-risk genes yet to be identified. Two possible sites are at 1p36 [37] and 1p22 [38].

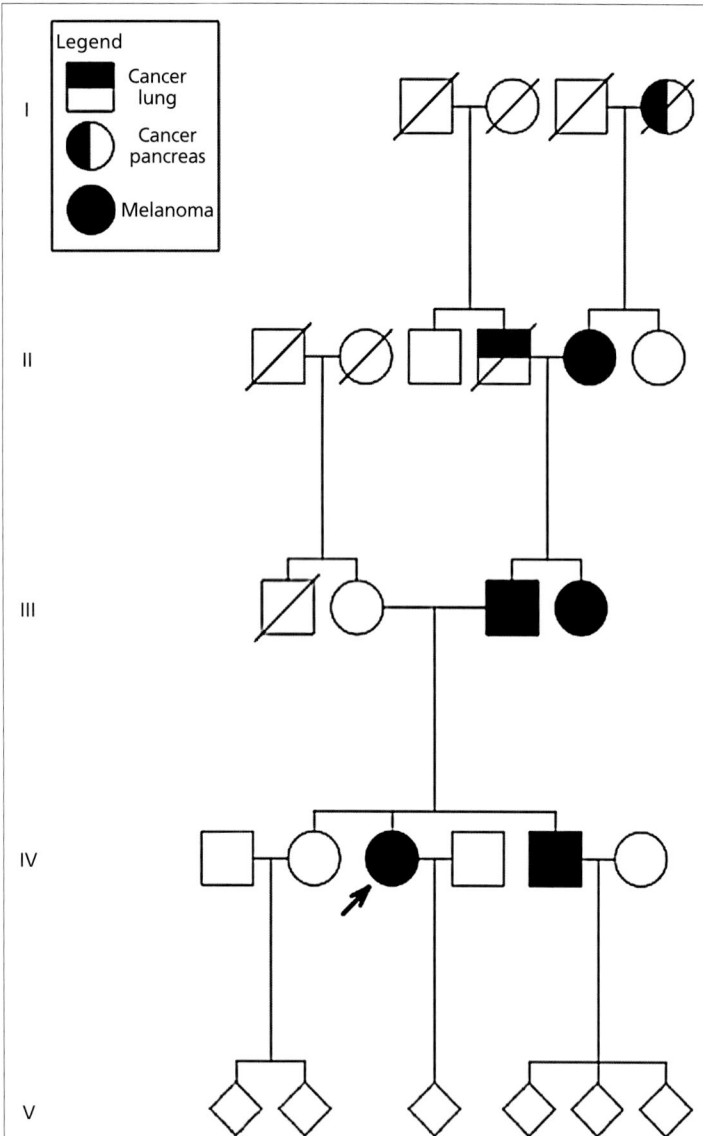

Fig. 54.48 A family tree from a family with a hereditary mutation in the *CDKN2A* gene, which is a high-risk gene for melanoma. The black circles represent melanoma cases in women, the squares, cases in men. There was a single case of pancreatic cancer.

Families with multiple cases of melanoma should be referred to specialist units for screening, education about early detection and prevention and counselling about risk. Although testing for mutations in the *CDKN2A* gene does take place in some countries, the value of the test is currently unclear and GenoMEL has taken the view that it is as yet premature [39]. GenoMEL is working to establish the information necessary to inform this counselling process in the future. The increased risk of pancreatic cancer in some countries but not in others remains confusing and may be due to variation between mutations or environmental factors. As pancreatic cancer is associated with smoking and alcohol-induced pancreatitis [40,41], it is important to advise members of melanoma families to avoid smoking and moderate alcohol intake. Screening for pancreatic cancer remains a difficult issue but there are trials currently taking place to establish the role of radiographic screening.

Identification of 'at risk' patients

The strongest risk of melanoma to an individual is that associated with familial melanoma where there are multiple cases. Within such families, all first-degree relatives are considered at risk regardless of naevus phenotype, although the presence of increased numbers of naevi increases the likelihood that the family member is a *CDKN2A* mutation carrier [42].

Patients with the atypical mole syndrome are at increased risk irrespective of family history and those with red hair and freckles are also at increased risk, although at a lower level. Algorithms have been, or are being, developed in order to estimate risk [43,44].

Prevention

The continued increase in incidence of melanoma in most white-skinned populations, and the very strong evidence that intermittent sun exposure is causal, suggests that sun exposure on holidays in sunny places is the most important behaviour to be addressed. As air fares are currently much lower than they were, there is a concern that this will prove even more difficult to modify in the next few years. It might be that directing the advice to those at increased risk will be more effective, stressing freckles, naevi and family history as risk factors for the cancer. For such people, protection using avoidance and clothing is optimal but less popular than the use of sunscreens. The wavelength of light that is causal for melanoma is still not known and therefore sunscreens should be broad-spectrum types, providing protection across both UVB and UVA ranges. Advice should be to use sunscreens that are water proof, and are applied regularly and in sufficient quantities.

Sun exposure for vitamin D synthesis is critical to human health. 1,25-dihydroxyvitamin D_3 is synthesized in the skin as a result of exposure to sunlight and is present in a few foods and dietary supplements. It has become apparent that suboptimal vitamin D levels are widespread [45], and increasing epidemiological evidence has emerged for a role for vitamin D deficiency in a number of cancers [46,47]. Most European peoples rely upon cutaneous synthesis as a result of sun exposure and the UV action spectrum for vitamin D synthesis and non-melanoma skin cancer carcinogenesis is the same [48], so that the balance between benefit and risk is close. There are, therefore, concerns that we should not give blanket advice to all to reduce their sun exposure. It seems sensible to direct advice to those at particular risk and to give the following advice:

- That people who burn in the sun, who have freckles, red hair or a larger number of melanocytic naevi, and those with a family history of skin cancer should be careful in the sun
- That these people should in particular avoid any sunburn
- That those who burn readily in the sun should probably avoid direct exposure to the sun and compensate for this avoidance by taking vitamin D supplements sufficient to maintain normal levels of vitamin D in the serum
- That dark-skinned peoples who have a low risk of skin cancer should avoid sunburn but, to avoid vitamin D depletion, which would be detrimental to their health overall, should not practise too much sun avoidance.

References

1 Parkin D, Whelan S, Ferlay J et al. Cancer Incidence in Five Continents. IARC Scientific Publications No 143, Lyon, International Agency for Research on Cancer II, 1997.

2 International Agency for Research on Cancer. CANCERMondial. http://www-dep.iarc.fr/.

3 de Vries E, Bray FI, Coebergh JW, Parkin DM. Changing epidemiology of malignant cutaneous melanoma in Europe 1953–1997: rising trends in incidence and mortality but recent stabilizations in western Europe and decreases in Scandinavia. Int J Cancer 2003; 107: 119–26.

4 MacKie RM, Bray CA, Hole DJ et al. Incidence of and survival from malignant melanoma in Scotland: an epidemiological study. Lancet 2002; 360: 587–91.

5 Newnham A, Moller H. Trends in the incidence of cutaneous malignant melanomas in the south east of England, 1960–1998. J Public Health Med 2002; 24: 268–75.

6 Downing A, Newton-Bishop JA, Forman D. Recent trends in cutaneous malignant melanoma in the Yorkshire region of England; incidence, mortality and survival in relation to stage of disease, 1993–2003. Br J Cancer 2006; 95: 91–5.

7 Jemal A, Devesa SS, Fears TR, Hartge P. Cancer surveillance series: changing patterns of cutaneous malignant melanoma mortality rates among whites in the United States. J Natl Cancer Inst 2000; 92: 811–8.

8 Coory M, Baade P, Aitken J et al. Trends for in situ and invasive melanoma in Queensland, Australia, 1982–2002. Cancer Causes Control 2006; 17: 21–7.

9 Giles GG, Armstrong BK, Burton RC et al. Has mortality from melanoma stopped rising in Australia? Analysis of trends between 1931 and 1994. BMJ 1996; 312: 1121–5.

10 Baade P, Coory M. Trends in melanoma mortality in Australia: 1950–2002 and their implications for melanoma control. Aust N Z J Public Health 2005; 29: 383–6.

11 Florez A, Cruces M. Melanoma epidemic: true or false? Int J Dermatol 2004; 43: 405–7.

12 Murray CS, Stockton DL, Doherty VR. Thick melanoma: the challenge persists. Br J Dermatol 2005; 152: 104–9.

13 de Vries E, Hontermans S, Jansses-Heijnen MLG et al. Up-to-date survival estimates and historical trends of cutaneous malignant melanoma in the south-east of the Netherlands. Ann Oncol 2007; 18: 1110–6.

14 Gandini S, Sera F, Cattaruzza MS et al. Meta-analysis of risk factors for cutaneous melanoma: II. Sun exposure. Eur J Cancer 2005; 41: 45–60.

15 Bataille V, Sasieni P, Grulich A et al. Solar keratoses: a risk factor for melanoma but negative association with melanocytic naevi. Int J Cancer 1998; 78: 8–12.

16 Whiteman DC, Watt P, Purdie DM et al. Melanocytic nevi, solar keratoses, and divergent pathways to cutaneous melanoma. J Natl Cancer Inst 2003; 95: 806–12.

17 Green A, Autier P, Boniol M et al. The association of use of sunbeds with cutaneous malignant melanoma and other skin cancers: a systematic review. Int J Cancer 2007; 120: 1116–22.

18 Gandini S, Sera F, Cattaruzza MS et al. Meta-analysis of risk factors for cutaneous melanoma: I. Common and atypical naevi. Eur J Cancer 2005; 41: 28–44.

19 Easton D, Cox G, Macdonald A, Ponder B. Genetic susceptibility to naevi—a twin study. Br J Cancer 1991; 64: 1164–7.

20 Wachsmuth RC, Turner F, Barrett JH et al. The effect of sun exposure in determining nevus density in UK adolescent twins. J Invest Dermatol 2005; 124: 56–62.

21 Falchi M, Bataille V, Hayward NK et al. Genome-wide association study identifies variants at 9p21 and 22q13 associated with development of cutaneous nevi. Nat Genet 2009.

22 Gandini S, Sera F, Cattaruzza MS et al. Meta-analysis of risk factors for cutaneous melanoma: III. Family history, actinic damage and phenotypic factors. Eur J Cancer 2005; 41: 2040–59.

23 Rees JL. Genetics of hair and skin color. Annu Rev Genet 2003; 37: 67–90.

24 Bastiaens M, ter Huurne J, Gruis N et al. The melanocortin-1-receptor gene is the major freckle gene. Hum Mol Genet 2001; 10: 1701–8.

25 Hemminki K, Zhang H, Czene K. Familial and attributable risks in cutaneous melanoma: effects of proband and age. J Invest Dermatol 2003; 120: 217–23.

26 Kamb A. Role of a cell cycle regulator in hereditary and sporadic cancer. Cold Spring Harb Symp 1994; 59: 39–47.

27 Soufir N, Avril M, Chompret A et al. Prevalence of p16 and CDK4 germline mutations in 48 melanoma-prone families in France. Hum Molec Genet 1998; 7: 209–16.

28 Zuo L, Weger J, Yang Q et al. Germline mutations in the p16^{INK4a} binding domain of CDK4 in familial melanoma. Nature Genetics 1996; 12: 97–9.

29 Ciotti P, Struewing JP, Mantelli M. A single genetic origin for the G101W CD2KN2A mutation in 20 melanoma-prone families. Am J Hum Genet 2000; 67: 311–9.

30 Gruis N, Sandkuijl L, Van der Velden P et al. CDKN2 explains part of the clinical phenotype in Dutch familial multiple-mole melanoma (FAMMM) syndrome families. Melanoma Res 1995; 5: 169–77.

31 Pollock PM, Spurr N, Bishop T et al. Haplotype analysis of two recurrent CDKN2A mutations in 10 melanoma families: evidence for common founders and independent mutations. Hum Mutat 1998; 11: 424–31.

32 Borg A, Johannsson U, Johannsson O et al. Novel germline p16 mutation in familial malignant melanoma in southern Sweden. Cancer Res 1996; 56: 2497–500.

33 Goldstein AM, Chan M, Harland M et al. Features associated with germline CDKN2A mutations: a GenoMEL study of melanoma-prone families from three continents. J Med Genet 2007; 44: 99–106.

34 Melanoma Genetics Consortium. www.genomel.org

35 Bishop DT, Demenais F, Goldstein AM et al. Geographical variation in the penetrance of CDKN2A mutations for melanoma. J Natl Cancer Inst 2002; 94: 894–903.

36 Begg CB, Orlow I, Hummer AJ et al. Lifetime risk of melanoma in CDKN2A mutation carriers in a population-based sample. J Natl Cancer Inst 2005; 97: 1507–15.

37 Bale SJ, Dracopoli NC, Tucker MA et al. Mapping the gene for hereditary cutaneous malignant melanoma-dysplastic nevus to chromosome 1p. N Engl J Med 1989; 320: 1367–72.

38 Gillanders E, Hank Juo SH, Holland EA et al. Localization of a novel melanoma susceptibility locus to 1p22. Am J Hum Genet 2003; 73: 301–13.

39 Kefford R, Bishop JN, Tucker M et al. Genetic testing for melanoma. Lancet Oncol 2002; 3: 653–4.

40 Otsuki M, Tashiro M. 4. Chronic pancreatitis and pancreatic cancer, lifestyle-related diseases. Internal Med (Tokyo, Japan) 2007; 46: 109–13.

41 Welsch T, Kleeff J, Seitz HK et al. Update on pancreatic cancer and alcohol-associated risk. J Gastroenterol Hepatol 2006; 21 (Suppl. 3): S69–75.

42 Newton Bishop JA, Bataille V, Pinney E, Bishop DT. Family studies in melanoma: identification of the atypical mole syndrome (AMS) phenotype. Melanoma Res 1994; 4: 199–206.

43 MacKie RM, Freudenberger T, Aitchison TC. Personal risk-factor chart for cutaneous melanoma. Lancet 1989; 2: 487–90.

44 Whiteman DC, Green AC. A risk prediction tool for melanoma? Cancer Epidemiol Biomarkers Prev 2005; 14: 761–3.

45 Holick MF. High prevalence of vitamin D inadequacy and implications for health. Mayo Clin Proc 2006; 81: 353–73.

46 Chen TC, Holick MF. Vitamin D and prostate cancer prevention and treatment. Trends Endocrinol Metab 2003; 14: 423–30.

47 Holick MF. Vitamin D: Its role in cancer prevention and treatment. Prog Biophys Mol Biol 2006; 92: 49–59.

48 Wolpowitz D, Gilchrest BA. The vitamin D questions: how much do you need and how should you get it? J Am Acad Dermatol 2006; 54: 301–17.

Clinicopathological variants and growth phases of primary melanoma

In 1969, Clark et al. suggested that, using a combination of clinical and pathological features, malignant melanoma could be divided into three main subsets [1]; the superficial spreading melanoma, the nodular melanoma and the lentigo maligna melanoma. In 1975, Reed et al. added a fourth group, the acral lentiginous or palmoplantar malignant melanoma [2]. There is some controversy as to whether or not these subsets are completely discrete entities, and it has been established that the clinicopathological variant is not an independent determinant of prognosis [3]. However, the four subtypes have distinct clinical features and possibly some biological distinctions, which are useful in clinical practice and each will be discussed in more detail later. The growth phases of melanoma also have clinical importance and are discussed here.

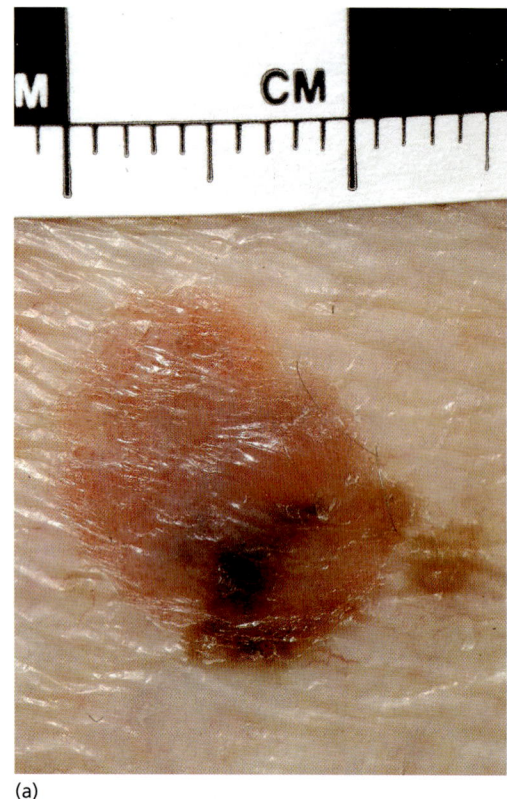

(a)

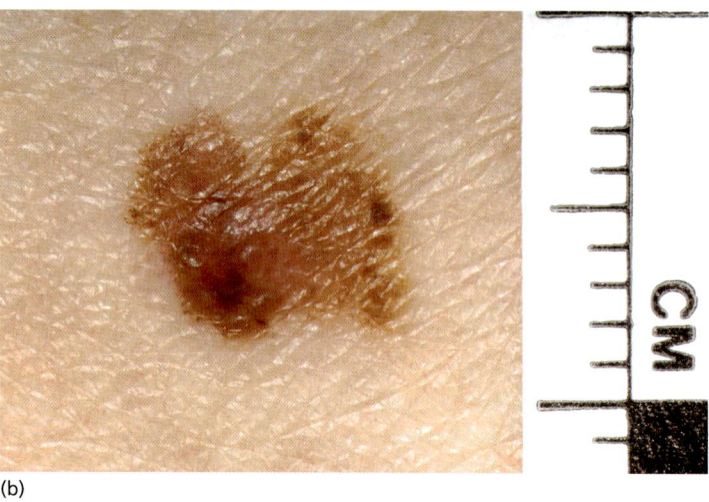

(b)

Fig. 54.49 (a, b) Two superficial spreading melanomas showing typical variation in colour and shape.

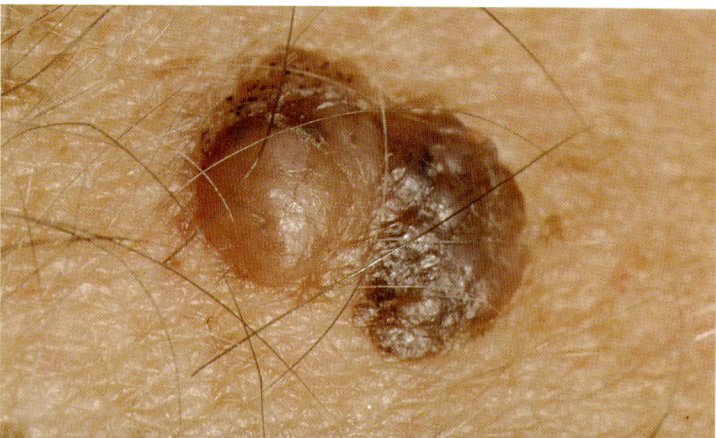

Fig. 54.50 A superficial spreading melanoma which has developed into a vertical growth phase tumour. Variable colours are seen with prominent vasculature and variable pigment. Even without a dermoscope large pigment dots can be seen.

In situ disease

Melanomas arise from melanocytes within the epidermis generally. In the majority of cases, the proliferation of melanocytes is limited to the epidermis for some time, before the cells acquire the capacity for survival and growth in the dermis. This phase is known as '*in situ*' disease, which may last for a period of years.

The commonest type of melanoma, the superficial spreading melanoma (SSM), for example, may evolve from an atypical naevus, through a borderline *in situ* lesion, to an SSM (Figs 54.49–54.51). In some subtypes of melanoma, such as lentigo maligna melanoma, acral lentiginous melanoma and genital melanoma, the *in situ* phase is particularly protracted. The *in situ* component in these rarer subtypes may, furthermore, be widespread and ill-defined and this is often known as the 'field effect'. Although ill-defined *in situ* disease typifies the subtypes of melanoma listed above, it may rarely occur on other sites, such as chronically sun-exposed skin of the arm or leg, in the skin around an SSM.

So-called nodular melanomas are the only type in which the malignant melanoma cells appear to have the capacity for invasive growth into the dermis and beyond from the beginning, without an *in situ* phase, and these tumours therefore develop much more rapidly and are much more difficult to diagnose at an early, curable stage.

Radial growth phase melanoma

The concept of evolution from *in situ* disease to invasive disease which is still unlikely to metastasize, called the 'radial growth phase', was developed by Clark and Elder [4]. Radial growth phase melanoma is strictly defined histologically. There is epidermal melanocyte proliferation and there may be some dermal cells provided that they are single or in small clusters, falling short of a dermal tumour nodule. A tumour nodule in the dermis is one which exceeds the diameter of any nest of cells along the dermo-epidermal junction [5]. The concept of radial growth phase melanoma as a lesion that should not recur means that these authors estimate a 100% expectation of survival for patients from whom such a lesion is removed.

Vertical growth phase melanoma

Melanoma in vertical growth phase is a tumour in which growth of malignant cells occurs within the dermis. These tumours have acquired the capacity for growth and, to a variable degree, the capacity for invasion of vessels and growth in other tissues. Variation in the characteristics of vertical growth phase melanoma histologically and immunohistochemically mirrors biological differences between tumours having prognostic significance, considered below.

References

1 Clark WH Jr, From L, Bernardino EA, Mihm MC. The histogenesis and biologic behavior of primary human malignant melanomas of the skin. *Cancer Res* 1969; **29**: 705–27.

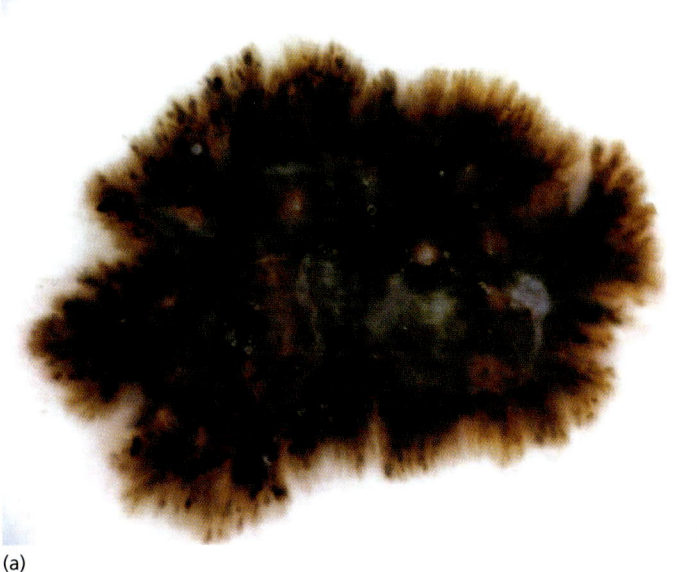
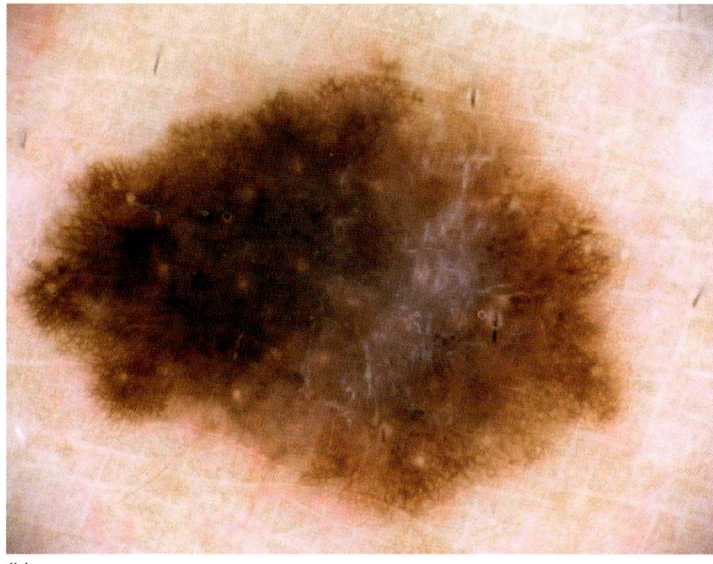

(a)

(b)

Fig. 54.51 The dermoscopic appearance of superficial spreading melanoma showing (a) an abnormal pigment network, radial streaming and large/variably sized pigment globules and (b) a melanoma with an irregular structure and pigment network and a blue/white veil.

2 Reed RJ, Ichinose H, Clark WH Jr, Mihm MC Jr. Common and uncommon melanocytic nevi and borderline melanomas. *Semin Oncol* 1975; **2**: 119–47.

3 Cox NH, Aitchison TC, Sirel JM, MacKie RM. Comparison between lentigo maligna melanoma and other histogenetic types of malignant melanoma of the head and neck. Scottish Melanoma Group. *Br J Cancer* 1996; **73**: 940–4.

4 Clark WH Jr, Elder DE, Guerry DT *et al*. Model predicting survival in stage I melanoma based on tumor progression. *J Natl Cancer Inst* 1989; **81**: 1893–904.

5 Elder DE, Murphy GF. *Melanocytic Tumors of the Skin*. Washington, DC: American Registry of Pathology, in press.

Clinical diagnostic aids

The clinical diagnosis of melanoma is based upon recognition of a progressively changing melanocytic lesion, which is growing and becoming irregular in shape and colour.

There are two diagnostic systems, which are intended to aid recognition by non-experts and the general public. Both apply mainly to the superficial spreading variant of malignant melanoma, which is the commonest subtype and generally has a relatively slow growth rate, at least in its early radial growth phase. These are the American ABCD categories and the Glasgow seven-point check-list. The American ABCD mnemonic is A = asymmetry, B = irregular border, C = irregular colour and D = diameter over 1 cm. The Glasgow seven-point check-list is divided into three major and four minor features. These are:

Major features:

1 Change in size
2 Change in shape
3 Change in colour

Minor features:

4 Diameter more than 5 mm
5 Inflammation
6 Oozing or bleeding
7 Mild itch or altered sensation.

It is suggested that any lesion with one major feature in an adult be considered for removal, and that the presence of additional minor features should add to clinical suspicion. For experts and possibly even for non-experts, however, assessment of lesions appears to be made using a 'global' assessment and it may be that widespread availability of images of melanomas may be the most effective means to promote recognition [1]. Images on the Internet may be particularly helpful here.

A number of computer-based systems are in clinical trial to aid in the diagnostic process, but these remain of unclear value.

Reference

1 Bishop JN, Bataille V, Gavin A *et al*. The prevention, diagnosis, referral and management of melanoma of the skin: concise guidelines. *Clin Med* 2007; **7**: 283–90.

Melanoma: specific histogenetic types, sites and variants

Superficial spreading melanoma

This is by far the most frequent type of melanoma. The commonest sites are the female leg and the male back, but any body site may be involved. An evolving, superficial spreading melanoma has the appearance of a flat, pigmented lesion, which becomes increasingly irregular in shape and colour over time. Shades of brown, black, red and grey or white may be present (Figs 54.49–54.51). The red colour usually indicates a degree of inflammation/vascular neogenesis and the resultant 'juicy' appearance should cause concern. White–grey areas may be indicative of a degree of regression. The lesion may still be very small, only 4–5 mm in diameter, but there may be a history of growth or change, and of subtle altered sensation, often described as a new awareness of the lesion or a tickling sensation. At this stage, the lesion will almost certainly be in the early radial growth phase, but as growth continues the lesion will become palpable, indicating that the lesion is progressing to the vertical growth phase. If the melanoma is developing in a pre-existing naevus, which occurs in approximately 50% of lesions, the irregular appearance of the growing melanoma may contrast strikingly with the more regularly pigmented and outlined residual naevus component.

Differential diagnosis. Benign naevi are usually smaller than melanoma, have a regular oval or circular outline, and are a uniform shade of brown. Seborrhoeic keratoses are dull, non-reflective lesions, which have a hyperkeratotic surface and a tendency to crumble. The main differential diagnosis in practice is between an early melanoma and a benign but atypical melanocytic naevus. A history of growth or change strongly suggests early melanoma, as does a size of 6 mm or greater, but the clinical features may be very similar in atypical naevi and early melanomas, and an excision biopsy may be needed.

Dermoscopy is an essential diagnostic aid for early melanoma. The most widely used dermoscope allows a 10-fold magnification. Fluid placed on the lesion (oil, water or even antiseptic gel) eliminates surface reflection and renders the cornified layer translucent, thus allowing a better visualization of pigmented structures within the epidermis, the dermoepidermal junction and the superficial dermis. The size and shape of vessels of the superficial vascular plexus can also be inspected. The technique of dermoscopy requires training; there are tutorials on the Internet [1–3] but it is desirable to attend a course. Benign naevi typically have an even pigment pattern on dermoscopy, which might be reticulate or globular. Melanomas typically have a disordered pigment pattern with variation in size of the pigment network, variably sized dots and often blue-grey or blue-white areas (Fig. 54.51).

There are also currently a number of computerized image analysis systems in development to aid preoperative diagnosis of malignant melanoma. These include the Mole Max system™ and spectrophotometric intracutaneous analysis using the Siascope. The absolute value of these machines in increasing both sensitivity and specificity of preoperative diagnosis of melanomas, thus reducing the number of unnecessary removals of benign naevi in routine practice, is not yet established.

Biopsy. All patients with suspected malignant melanoma should have an excision biopsy of the lesion carried out with a margin of 1–2 mm of clinically normal skin. This will enable the pathologist both to confirm the diagnosis and also to measure the thickness of the melanoma, which is an essential guide to further management. In rare situations when an excisional biopsy is not practical, such as a large possible melanoma on the face, an incisional biopsy from the area of the lesion which appears to be most invasive is acceptable, provided any necessary definitive surgery follows promptly. This procedure should probably be carried out by specialists.

Incisional or punch biopsies should not be performed in suspected melanoma because of sampling error, because an inaccurate tumour thickness may be obtained due to biopsy trauma, and also because the overall shape and symmetry of the whole lesion is important to the diagnosis of melanocytic lesions. There is a theoretical risk of displacing melanoma cells deeper into the dermis, although there is no evidence for this.

The surgeon should measure accurately the clinical excision margins, as biopsy samples shrink by 20–30% during fixation in formalin and the pathologist may report a narrower margin than was excised. It is the clinical rather than the pathologically measured excision margins that should be used in decisions concerning further surgery.

Pathology. The specimen should be examined by the pathologist in total. Features required in the biopsy report are the diagnosis, the tumour thickness, histogenetic type, growth phase, presence (and probably width) of ulceration, presence of regression, presence of tumour infiltrating lymphocytes (and whether they are brisk or non-brisk) [4], an estimate of the number of mitoses in the tumour, and whether there is evidence of vascular invasion. The presence of regression, if observed, may influence decisions on the width of definitive excision. Clark levels add little prognostic information for thicker primary melanomas, but should also be included, particularly for melanomas less than 1 mm in thickness, as Clark level 4 lesions in this thickness range appear to have a worse prognosis than level 3 lesions. In about 40% of cases [5] there will be pathological evidence of a pre-existing, benign melanocytic naevus on which the melanoma has developed. In these cases the pathologist may feel it necessary to give two tumour thicknesses, one measuring the entire thickness of the lesion and one measuring only to the deepest obvious tumour cell, ignoring any deeper apparent naevus cells. The presence of desmoplasia or neurotropism should be recorded.

The margin of excision should be recorded—both the minimum lateral margin and the deep margin in mm.

The essential pathological features of superficial spreading melanoma are the presence of a focus of malignant melanoma cells invading the dermis with areas of *in situ* malignant change in the adjacent epidermis. This consists of the presence of cytologically atypical melanocytes in the suprabasal layers of the epidermis, both singly and in clumps (Fig. 54.52). On H&E sections, the pattern may be very similar to that seen in extramammary Paget's disease, and the term pagetoid melanoma may therefore also be used to describe this lesion.

The verrucous variant. These are melanomas simulating benign warts that are easy to miss. They are characterized by gross hyperkeratosis and also epidermal hyperplasia. The significance of this lesion is the fact that it is not usually recognized clinically because of the hyperkeratosis, and it may be confused with both benign and malignant lesions derived from the keratinocyte, such as a seborrhoeic keratosis or a squamous cell carcinoma.

Pathological differential diagnosis. There are two quite distinct problems in pathological differential diagnosis of primary malignant melanoma. The first is distinguishing it from benign melanocytic naevus, the second is distinguishing non-melanocytic but malignant tumours, either primary or secondary. These are more often a problem when a clinically indeterminate, large nodule is excised.

The differentiation between benign and malignant melanocytic lesions rests on both the pattern of involvement and the cytological features of individual cells. The association of cytologically atypical melanocytic cells in the upper layers of the epidermis with apparent proliferation at the dermoepidermal junction and invasion of the underlying dermis by atypical melanocytic cells is a malignant pattern. The cells in the deeper areas of the dermis

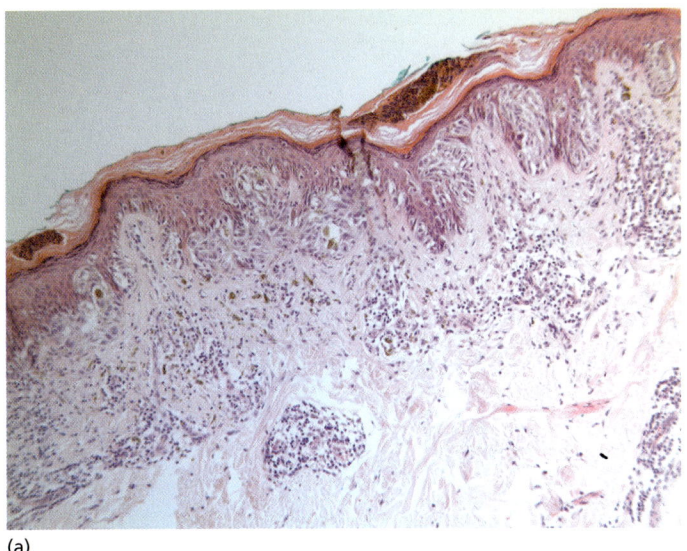
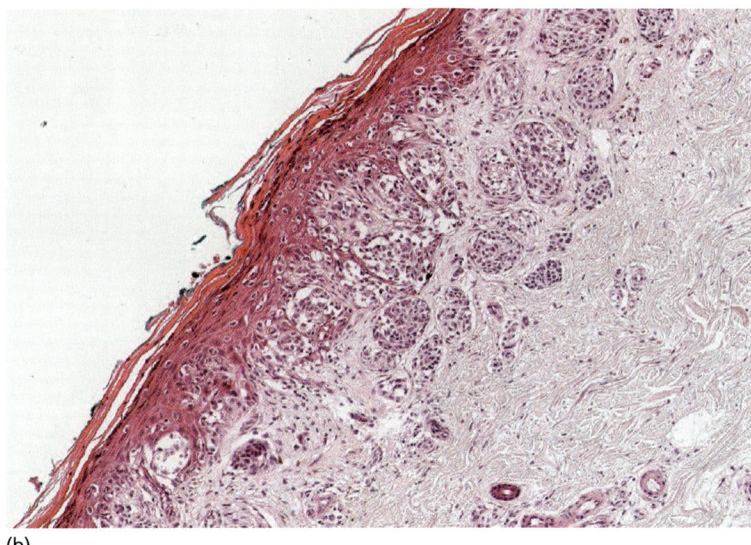

(a)   (b)

Fig. 54.52 (a) The histological appearance of an *in situ* melanoma with atypical melanocytes within the epidermis. There are dermal inflammatory cells but no tumour cells. (b) A superficial spreading melanoma showing more proliferation of tumour cells in the epidermis (known as pagetoid spread). Dermal nests of tumour cells indicate that the tumour is in vertical growth phase.

will show no maturation such as is seen in a benign naevus with dermal involvement. The cytological characteristics of malignancy are a high nuclear to cytoplasmic ratio, intense nuclear staining, size variation between adjacent cells and the presence of abnormal mitotic figures.

Two of the more difficult pathological differential diagnoses of melanoma are the halo naevus and the Spitz naevus. It is unusual for a melanoma to elicit as intense a lymphocytic response as in the halo naevus, but a careful search should be made through the lymphocytic infiltrate in a putative halo naevus for cytologically malignant cells, particularly if the clinical information suggests an unusual history, such as presence in an elderly individual.

The differentiation between malignant melanoma and Spitz naevus can be extremely difficult, as discussed above. Features suggesting that the lesion is a melanoma and not a Spitz naevus are asymmetry with a poorly defined lateral margin, the presence of abnormal (or deep) mitoses in the melanocytic cells, lack of any maturation or differentiation in the deeper naevus cells, nuclear pleomorphism, and an epithelioid cell pattern with striking lack of adhesion of one cell to the other. These features are not absolute, and there are times when it may be necessary to state that a firm diagnosis cannot be made on pathological grounds when the term STUMP is used, as discussed above. In such cases the lesion should be managed as if it was a melanoma.

A range of antibodies are currently in routine diagnostic use. They will confirm the melanocytic nature of the lesion, but cannot differentiate between benign and malignant melanocytic lesions. S100, gp100/HMB-45, typrosinase, MART-1/Melan-A and HMW_MAA are melanocyte differentiation markers. S100 is less specific than the other three, but highly sensitive and therefore is usually used in combination with at least one of the others [6].

Definitive surgical treatment to the primary site. Once the diagnosis of primary malignant melanoma is established, and the

thickness of the melanoma has been measured, the definitive excision can be planned. The extent of this excision will relate to the tumour thickness. At present, if the diagnosis is of a level 1 or *in situ* melanoma, a margin of only 2–5 mm of surrounding normal skin is considered adequate [7]. This may have been included in the diagnostic biopsy and therefore no further surgery may be necessary. There are no data, however, to support this margin, and the rare occurrence of a 'field effect' of atypical melanocytes around primary melanoma means that the patient and his doctor often elect to remove up to 1 cm of normal skin, especially if a second operation is required.

Invasive melanomas up to 2 mm thick may be safely treated with a minimal excision margin of 1 cm based upon the WHO trial [8]. Patients with thicker tumours are more likely to develop lymph node recurrence if a 1-cm margin is used [9], and therefore the recommended excision margin is 2 to 3 cm [7] where anatomically possible. Margins of this size are most difficult to achieve on the face.

In some centres, sentinel node biopsy (see p. 54.51) is offered to patients as a staging tool. Sentinel node biopsy can only be carried out at the time of wide local excision of the primary and therefore patients should be counselled about this option prior to definitive excision.

References

1 DS Medica. *Dermoscopy.* http://www.dermoscopy.org
2 New Zealand Dermatological Society. *Dermoscopy.* http://dermnetnz.org/procedures/dermoscopy.html
3 Interactive Medical Media. Dermatology lectures on line. *Dermoscopy.* http://www.dermlectures.com
4 Elder DE, Murphy GF. *Melanocytic Tumors of the Skin.* Washington, DC: American Registry of Pathology, in press.
5 Purdue MP, From L, Armstrong BK *et al.* Etiologic and other factors predicting nevus-associated cutaneous malignant melanoma. *Cancer Epidemiol Biomarkers Prev* 2005; **14**: 2015–22.
6 de Wit NJ, van Muijen GN, Ruiter DJ. Immunohistochemistry in melanocytic proliferative lesions. *Histopathology* 2004; **44**: 517–41.

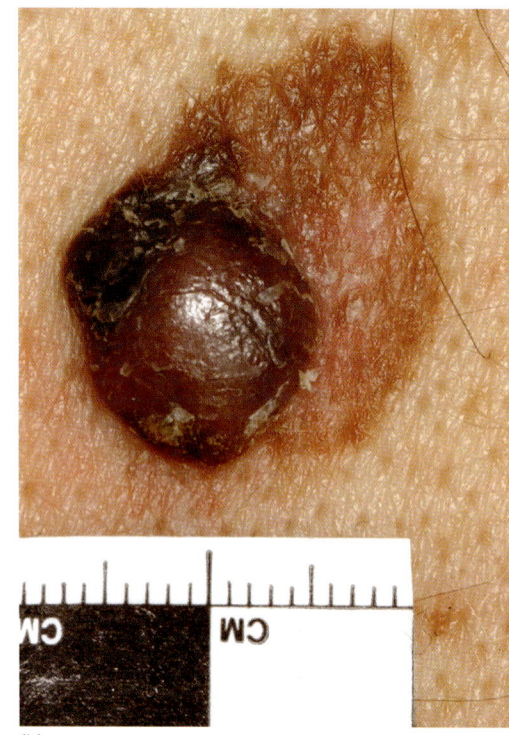

(a)   (b)

Fig. 54.53 Two nodular melanomas. (a) A melanoma that has already developed *in transit* metastases. (b) A nodular component of a melanoma that has evolved over time from an atypical naevus, which can be seen in the image.

7 Newton Bishop JA, Corrie PG, Evans J *et al*. UK guidelines for the management of cutaneous melanoma. *Br J Plast Surg* 2002; **55**: 46–54.
8 Veronesi U, Cascinelli N. Narrow excision (1-cm margin). A safe procedure for thin cutaneous melanoma. *Arch Surg* 1991; **126**: 438–41.
9 Thomas JM, Newton-Bishop J, A'Hern R *et al*. Excision margins in high-risk malignant melanoma. *N Engl J Med* 2004; **350**: 757–66.

Nodular melanoma

This variety presents most commonly in the fifth or sixth decade and occurs more frequently in males than in females. The trunk is a common site. These lesions grow rapidly and are therefore more likely to present as thicker tumours and they tend, therefore, to have a poor prognosis. Thicker tumours are more common in the elderly and diagnostic delay may be associated with living alone and lack of knowledge [1].

Nodular melanomas develop as an elevated, dome-shaped polypoid or even pedunculated structure (Fig. 54.53). Melanin pigment may be sparse in these lesions and a raised, red central area, with only a peripheral brown ring of melanin, is a common clinical pattern; in others the more typically variable pigmentation may be seen. Ulceration and bleeding from the lesion occur frequently. This variety of malignant melanoma is misdiagnosed prior to surgery more frequently than either a superficial spreading melanoma or a lentigo maligna melanoma, as they may be symmetrical and have a relative lack of melanin pigment. Thus they are not readily identified using the ABCD rule, for example.

Lesions to consider in the differential diagnosis are angioma or pigmented basal cell carcinoma. Histiocytoma or sclerosing angioma may also cause clinical confusion. Dermoscopy is very helpful in distinguishing melanoma from these benign lesions.

Pathology. The nodular melanoma has the pathological features of a focus of invasive melanoma cells in the dermis with direct contact with the immediately overlying epidermis, but no morphological abnormality apparent in the adjacent epidermis on either side of the invasive nodule (Fig. 54.54). This is, therefore, a primary melanoma with no recognizable adjacent *in situ* or radial growth phase. There is a tendency to use the term nodular melanoma inappropriately for any primary melanoma that has a visible nodule. This is incorrect usage, as superficial spreading, acral and lentigo maligna melanomas can all develop elevated nodular areas in the course of later growth.

Management. The management of nodular melanoma is the same as for superficial spreading melanoma, described above.

Reference
1 Baumert J, Plewig G, Volkenandt M, Schmid-Wendtner MH. Factors associated with a high tumour thickness in patients with melanoma. *Br J Dermatol* 2007; **156**: 938–44.

Lentigo maligna melanoma

In this histogenetic variant the preceding horizontal or *in situ* growth phase is known as a lentigo maligna (Hutchinson's melanotic freckle; melanosis circumscripta precancerosa of Dubreuilh). By comparison with the radial growth phase of the superficial spreading melanoma, lentigo maligna represents a much more prolonged period of lateral extension. Most occur on the face, commonly on the upper cheek, temple or forehead: the facial skin most exposed to the sun through life. A small proportion of lentigo malignas are observed on extrafacial exposed sites such as the arm, hand or leg.

Occasionally, periocular lentigo maligna extends into the conjunctiva. Sometimes the *in situ* component may even arise in the conjunctiva as a condition known as 'primary acquired melanosis'

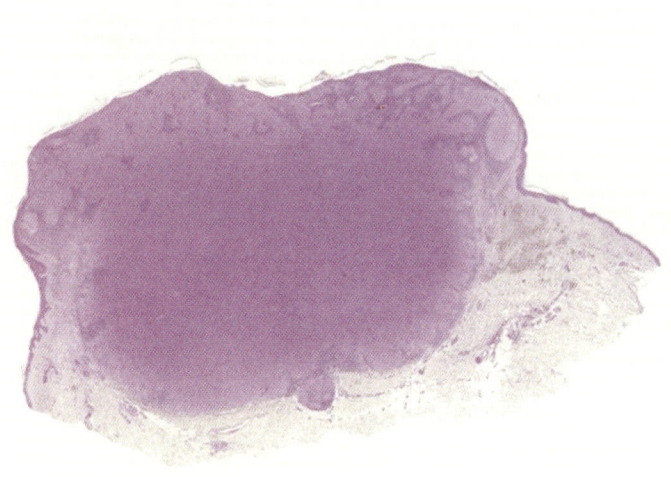

Fig. 54.54 A low power image of nodular melanoma pathology. (Courtesy of Dr S. Edward, Leeds Teaching Hospitals Trust, Leeds, UK.)

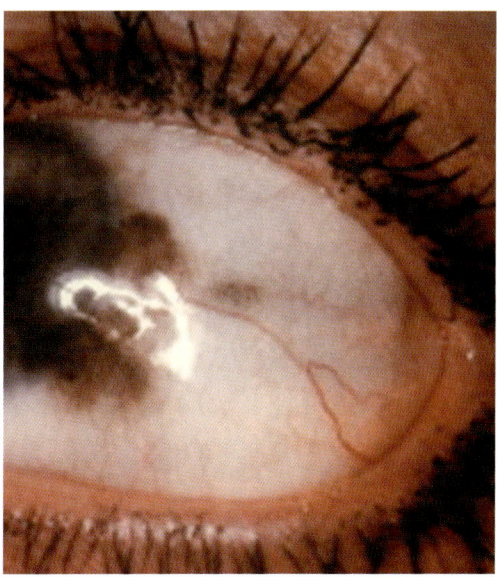

Fig. 54.55 Primary acquired melanosis of the eye, which can be likened to a continuum between an atypical naevus and *in situ* melanoma.

(PAM) [1]. PAM typically presents as irregular pigmentation at the limbus of the eye (Fig. 54.55). The pigmentation may progress very slowly over many years and then, generally, ophthalmic surgeons tend merely to observe, but a proportion do go on to invasive melanoma and melanoma may develop within the conjunctiva and in the adjacent skin. The histology of PAM has been subdivided into PAM with and without atypia, but PAM which progressed into melanoma is said to be architecturally more irregular and the melanocytes are more likely to be epithelioid in nature [1]. PAM bears some clinical and histological similarities to atypical naevi and indeed has been reported in patients with the atypical mole syndrome [2]. PAM may therefore be considered to be a continuum in the conjunctiva equivalent to the atypical naevus/*in situ* melanoma spectrum.

The *in situ* component of lentigo maligna may be extremely slow growing and probably evolves from solar lentigos (although the vast majority of solar lentigos clearly do not progress). Progression from a solar lentigo to a lentigo maligna is usually characterized by darkening, enlargement and the development of a more defined edge (Fig. 54.56). A difficulty of management is that atypical melanocytes often extend out from the edge of the lentigo for considerable distances, even involving 'skip' lesions. This is often known as the 'field effect'. Treatment may therefore initially appear to be successful, yet there may commonly be recurrence at the edge after treatment.

A proportion of lentigo malignas will evolve into invasive melanoma, developing as discrete colour change or nodules within the lentigo (Fig. 54.56). Rarely, the melanoma may be desmoplastic in type, in which case the lesion may present as a central, firm thickening, within a macular pigmented area, which may be quite subtle. These melanomas are very easy to misdiagnose; it is particularly important to write the differential diagnosis of desmoplastic melanoma on the histopathology form if there is any suspicion at all of this diagnosis, so that the pathologist will carry out an S100 stain.

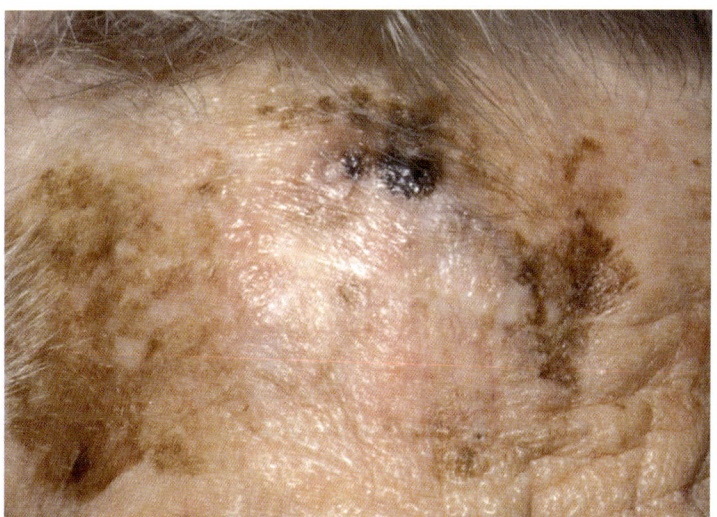

Fig. 54.56 A very extensive lentigo maligna melanoma in which a nodular element developed at the hair line.

Patients tend to be older than those presenting with the other types of melanoma. Many of the identified risk factors suggest that the aetiology of this variety of melanoma has a greater similarity to squamous cell carcinoma than to the other melanoma variants. Affected patients have evident solar damage both clinically and pathologically.

Initially the lentigo maligna is a flat, brown or black, irregularly shaped lesion. These lesions will grow very slowly, over months or years, and there may be central regression while the peripheral margin continues to extend. In time, a raised central nodule will develop, indicating transition to the vertical growth phase.

In clinic, referral of macular pigmented facial lesions is common and the differential diagnosis of very early lentigo maligna includes solar lentigo, and pigmented actinic keratoses and the flatter variant of seborrhoeic keratoses. Both of the latter tend to have more surface scaling, lack a visible melanin pigment network and have a dull, non-reflective surface. Size, depth of colour and irregularity of pigment are pointers to the diagnosis of lentigo maligna.

Pathology. This variant of melanoma is the most distinct histologically. It has a long pre-invasive or radial growth phase, during which there is striking lentiginous replacement of the basal keratinocytes by atypical melanocytes but no downward invasion into the underlying dermis, which will show actinic damage of the dermal collagen. During this phase, the names *lentigo maligna* or Hutchinson's melanotic freckle are appropriate. There is also often extensive colonization of the hair-follicle epithelium by atypical melanocytes. After a variable period of time, invasion into the underlying dermis will take place. The site of such early invasion in its earliest stages may be marked by a lymphocytic infiltrate. Once obvious dermal invasion is present, the name *lentigo maligna melanoma* is appropriate (Fig. 54.57).

Desmoplastic, neurotropic and myxoid variants. The very rare desmoplastic variant of malignant melanoma may be seen in association with chronically sun-damaged skin and overlying lentigo maligna in the epidermis. The clinical appearance may be very subtle and has few easily recognizable features. In desmoplastic melanoma arising from lentigo maligna then, the lesion may present as a subtle area of thickening associated with macular pigmentation. In other sites it may resemble a pink scar-like nodule (Fig. 54.58) and there may be an inflammatory component.

As the name suggests, this lesion represents a combination of malignant melanocytes in association with extremely dense desmoplastic change of the dermis. The stromal change in the dermis is usually much more obvious than the malignant melanocytes, which may be few in number. If an S100 stain is not carried out it may be extremely difficult to recognize the lesion as a melanoma, as the spindly dermal cells extend singly between the more obvious stromal cells.

The clinical importance of this variant is that it can be difficult to be absolutely certain that excision is complete, and local recurrence is a common problem.

In a review of published studies of desmoplastic melanoma [3], a total of 856 patients with this diagnosis were evaluated in the 17 included studies. There were 539 males (63.0%) and 317 females (37.0%). The mean age of patients varied from 55.6 to 71.3 years across the included studies, while the age range was from 4 to 99 years. The lesions were most commonly located on the head and neck (53.2%), followed by the extremities (20.6%) and the trunk (26.2%). Desmoplastic melanoma is associated with a high local recurrence rate, a lower nodal recurrence rate but systemic metastatic rates not dissimilar from melanoma as a whole [3]. Overall survival in 16 published studies ranged from 67.1 to 100%. Disease free survival in 14 studies at the end of follow-up ranged from 52 to 100%.

A pathological variant sometimes coexisting with the desmoplastic pattern is the neurotropic melanoma. In this variant, the pattern of metastatic spread is along the cutaneous nerve trunks.

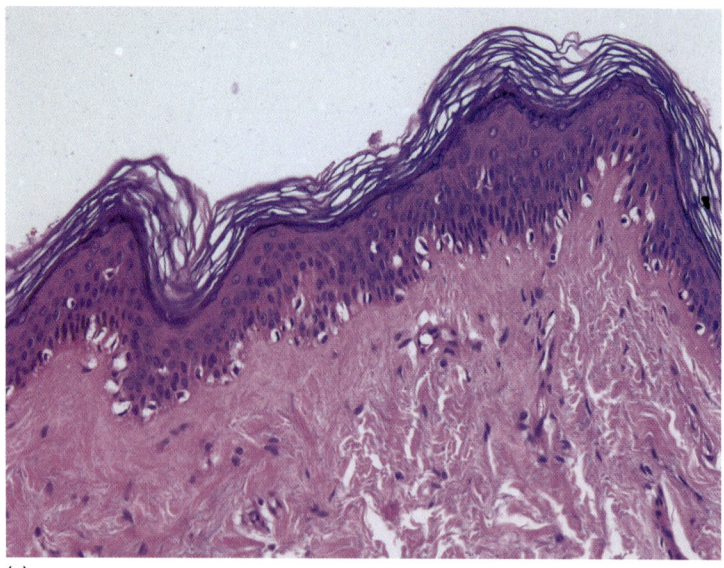

(a)

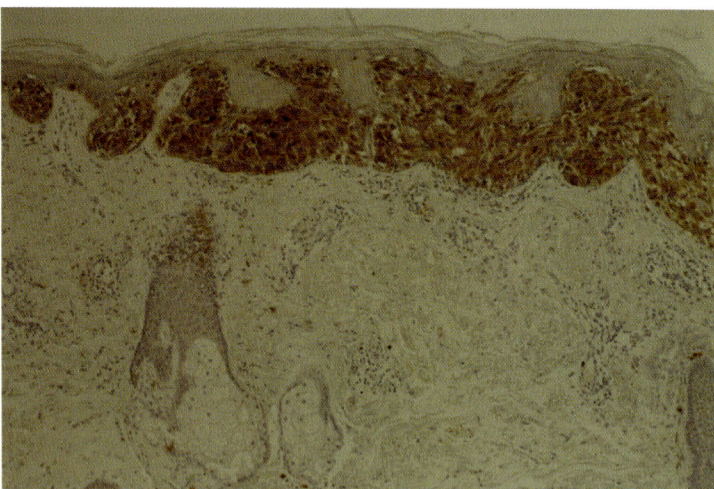

(b)

Fig. 54.57 The range of pathologies described as lentigo maligna. (a) Very early lentiginous proliferation. (b) Confluent proliferation at atypical melanocytes in a lentigo maligna melanoma; the slide has been stained with S100. (Courtesy of Dr S. Edward, Leeds Teaching Hospitals Trust, Leeds, UK.)

This is seen particularly in lesions on the head and neck area, and may cause severe, relentless pain. In a review of desmoplastic melanoma, the percentage of desmoplastic melanomas with neurotropism ranged from 16.7 to 77.8% among included studies [3]. As with the desmoplastic variant, completeness of excision can be difficult to determine. Myxoid melanoma is a rare variant in which there is a striking myxoid stroma in the dermis surrounding malignant spindle cells. The morphology has some features in common with desmoplastic melanoma.

Treatment of lentigo maligna. The diagnosis of lentigo maligna is made clinically and confirmed histologically. It is one of the very few instances where incisional biopsy of a melanocytic lesion is justifiable, where a suspicious but large macular lesion is present in a cosmetically sensitive area such as the face. The site for incisional biopsy is chosen based upon clinical examination and dermoscopy, choosing the most irregular or darkest area of pigmentation and/or any palpable or thickened areas. More than one site may be necessary. The concern is both to make the diagnosis of lentigo maligna and to determine the presence of invasion; however, exclusion of the presence of any invasive disease requires examination of the whole lesion.

If the diagnosis of lentigo maligna is confirmed, then the treatment is usually surgical excision. However, there are few clinical trial data to inform that choice. Standard excision with 5-mm margins proves to be insufficient in 50% of cases. The recurrence rate with standard excision ranges from 8 to 20%. Mohs' micrographic surgery and staged excision may offer better margin control and lower recurrence rates (0–5%) [4,5]. Estimates of recur-

rence rates following non-surgical therapies such as cryosurgery, radiotherapy, electrodesiccation and curettage, laser surgery, and topical medications range from 20 to 100% at 5 years [4]. The most pressing argument for surgical excision is the consequent ability to review the whole specimen for invasive disease, which occurs in 5 to 16% of lentigo malignas excised [6,7].

Topical imiquimod is an encouraging new therapeutic option but the data so far are few, and randomized clinical trials are needed. It may cause significant inflammation or ulceration at the site (Fig. 54.59) or, when treating the face, on the lip (Fig. 54.60). A review summarized 11 case reports and four open-label studies, with a total of 67 patients. There was significant variability in treatment schedules and regimens. Eight patients failed to respond, with lentigo maligna melanoma developing in two of these. In certain cases there were discrepancies between clinical and histological response with some patients clearing clinically but not histologically, and vice versa. Follow-up periods were short, exceeding 12 months in only five cases [8]. Some centres are using surgery as the primary treatment with imiquimod as an adjuvant but this needs to be formally evaluated. The development of lentigo maligna melanoma within lentigo maligna incompletely eradicated by imiquimod is a concern.

Treatment of lentigo maligna melanoma. The treatment of the melanoma is as for other sites in that the margin of excision for tumours thinner than 2 mm is 1 cm minimum and for thicker tumours should be 2 to 3 cm. It is recognized, however, that on the face these margins may not be attainable without unacceptable cosmetic deficit. The surgery is also subject to the same constraints as described above for lentigo maligna, in that there is a high local recurrence rate of the *in situ* component.

References

1 Sugiura M, Colby KA, Mihm MC Jr, Zembowicz A. Low-risk and high-risk histologic features in conjunctival primary acquired melanosis with atypia: Clinicopathologic analysis of 29 cases. *Am J Surg Pathol* 2007; **31**: 185–92.

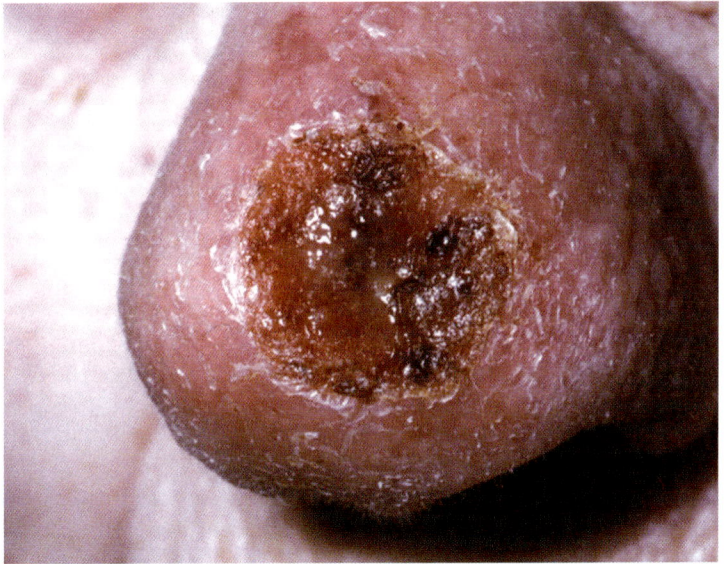

Fig. 54.58 An ill-defined, ulcerated lesion which proved to be a desmoplastic melanoma. Desmoplastic melanoma can be very difficult to diagnose clinically, being commonly sparsely pigmented but indurated to the touch.

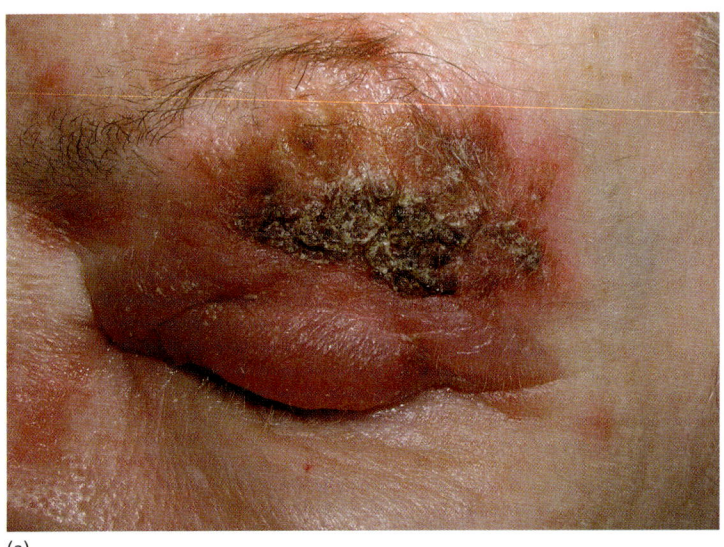

(a)

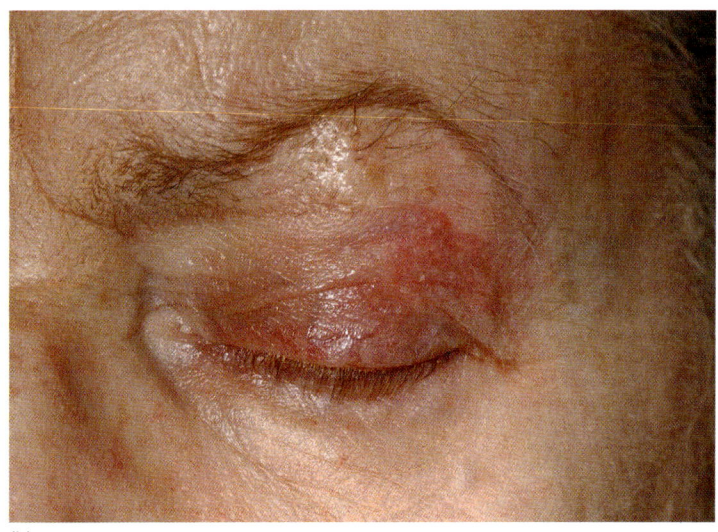

(b)

Fig. 54.59 This lady had persistent local recurrence of lentigo maligna on the eyelid. (a) She was treated with imiquimod and developed a profound inflammatory response. (b) The inflammation settled promptly and the response to treatment was clinically complete.

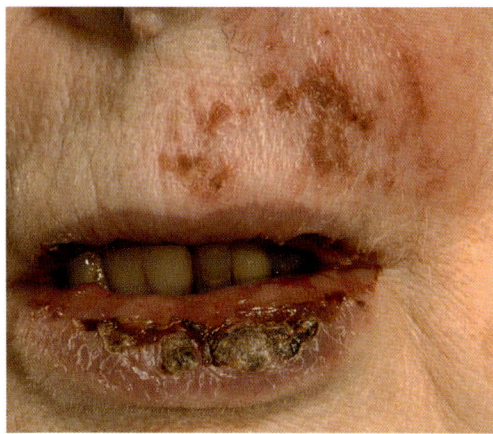

Fig. 54.60 Ulceration of the lip occurs quite commonly when imiquimod is used to treat lentigo maligna on the face. This may represent an immunological reaction to quiescent herpes.

2 Bataille V, Boyle J, Hungerford JL, Newton JA. Three cases of primary acquired melanosis of the conjunctiva as a manifestation of the atypical mole syndrome. *Br J Dermatol* 1993; **128**: 86–90.

3 Lens MB, Newton-Bishop JA, Boon AP. Desmoplastic malignant melanoma: a systematic review. *Br J Dermatol* 2005; **152**: 673–8.

4 McKenna JK, Florell SR, Goldman GD, Bowen GM. Lentigo maligna/lentigo maligna melanoma: current state of diagnosis and treatment. *Dermatol Surg* 2006; **32**: 493–504.

5 Temple CL, Arlette JP. Mohs micrographic surgery in the treatment of lentigo maligna and melanoma. *J Surg Oncol* 2006; **94**: 287–92.

6 Agarwal-Antal N, Bowen GM, Gerwels JW. Histologic evaluation of lentigo maligna with permanent sections: implications regarding current guidelines. *J Am Acad Dermatol* 2002; **47**: 743–8.

7 Bub JL, Berg D, Slee A, Odland PB. Management of lentigo maligna and lentigo maligna melanoma with staged excision: a 5-year follow-up. *Arch Dermatol* 2004; **140**: 552–8.

8 Rajpar SF, Marsden JR. Imiquimod in the treatment of lentigo maligna. *Br J Dermatol* 2006; **155**: 653–6.

Acral lentiginous melanoma (palmoplantar malignant melanoma)

This type of melanoma comprises around 10% of all melanomas on white skin but over 50% of all melanomas on darker-skinned peoples. It is the commonest type of melanoma, for example, in Japan. The recorded incidence in different ethnic groups is around 1 to 2 per million per annum [1]. The lesions are found mainly on the sole of the foot but also on the palm of the hand, and are characterized, as their name would suggest, by a large, macular, lentiginous pigmented area around an invasive, raised tumour. Approximately 50% of all melanomas on the foot are of this type (Fig. 54.61).

This precursor *in situ* component is in many ways similar to lentigo maligna in that its growth rate may be very slow, it may be very extensive, and it shows a tendency to recur because of failure to excise sufficient normal skin laterally (Fig. 54.62).

The clinical differential diagnosis may include a plantar wart, which is a common cause of delayed diagnosis, and black heel (talon noir) (Chapter 28), due to haemorrhage into the superficial layers of the epidermis. Any tender, growing nodule, or an 'ulcer' that won't heal, on the sole of the foot, should give rise to concern that the lesion is a melanoma and biopsy should be considered. The risks of missing the diagnosis are higher in circumstances where delayed healing of an ulcer is expected, such as in a diabetic ulcer.

Pathology. The essential pathological features are the presence of an extensive area of lentiginous change in the epidermis around the focus of invasive primary melanoma. In early disease, the lentiginous component may be large, but the invasive focus is small and difficult to find, requiring cutting of many sections. The basal keratinocytes are replaced by cytologically malignant melanocytes, and there is often an associated inflammatory flare of lymphoid cells in the underlying dermis. An important feature is the presence of skip areas, with foci of relatively normal epidermis in areas of gross lentiginous change, as in lentigo maligna. This feature makes it particularly important to examine the excision specimen thoroughly to determine whether or not the lesion has been completely excised.

Treatment. As for lentigo maligna, the management of acral lentiginous melanoma is one of the few occasions where incisional biopsy may be acceptable in order to plan treatment. The area chosen is that showing the most pigmentary irregularity or the most palpable nodular area.

The margins of excision are as for melanomas in other sites, 1 cm for tumours thinner than 2 mm and 2 to 3 cm for thicker tumours. As for other melanomas characterized by extensive *in situ* disease, however, there is also a need to resect adjacent precursor lentiginous hyperplasia so that the clinical margin should be measured from the most distal area of macular pigmentation. It can be easier to see this margin if emollient is applied to the sole before examination. If the patient has elected to proceed to sentinel node biopsy, this would be carried out at the time of definitive surgery. The margins used in practice are subject to the functional implications of the surgery. Acral lentiginous melanoma is commonly on the weight-bearing sole and the implications of the surgery must be discussed with the patient and in practice a compromise may be reached between margin and function.

Subungual melanoma

Subungual melanomas are rare. Like acral lentiginous (palmoplantar) melanomas they occur in people of all skin types and their aetiology is unknown. They are most common on the thumb or the great toe. It has been suggested that this indicates that trauma may play a role in their aetiology, but this localization may simply reflect the relative surface area (and therefore the number of melanocytes) of the nail matrix from which all subungual melanomas are thought to arise.

Because they arise from the nail matrix, subungual melanomas usually produce an abnormal nail and a variable degree of pigmentation of the nail itself. The classical presentation is of a new, linear, pigmented band along the length of the nail, which starts to widen progressively, especially at the base, so that the pigmented band tends to be funnel shaped. Over time, proliferation of the melanoma cells within the nail matrix then additionally

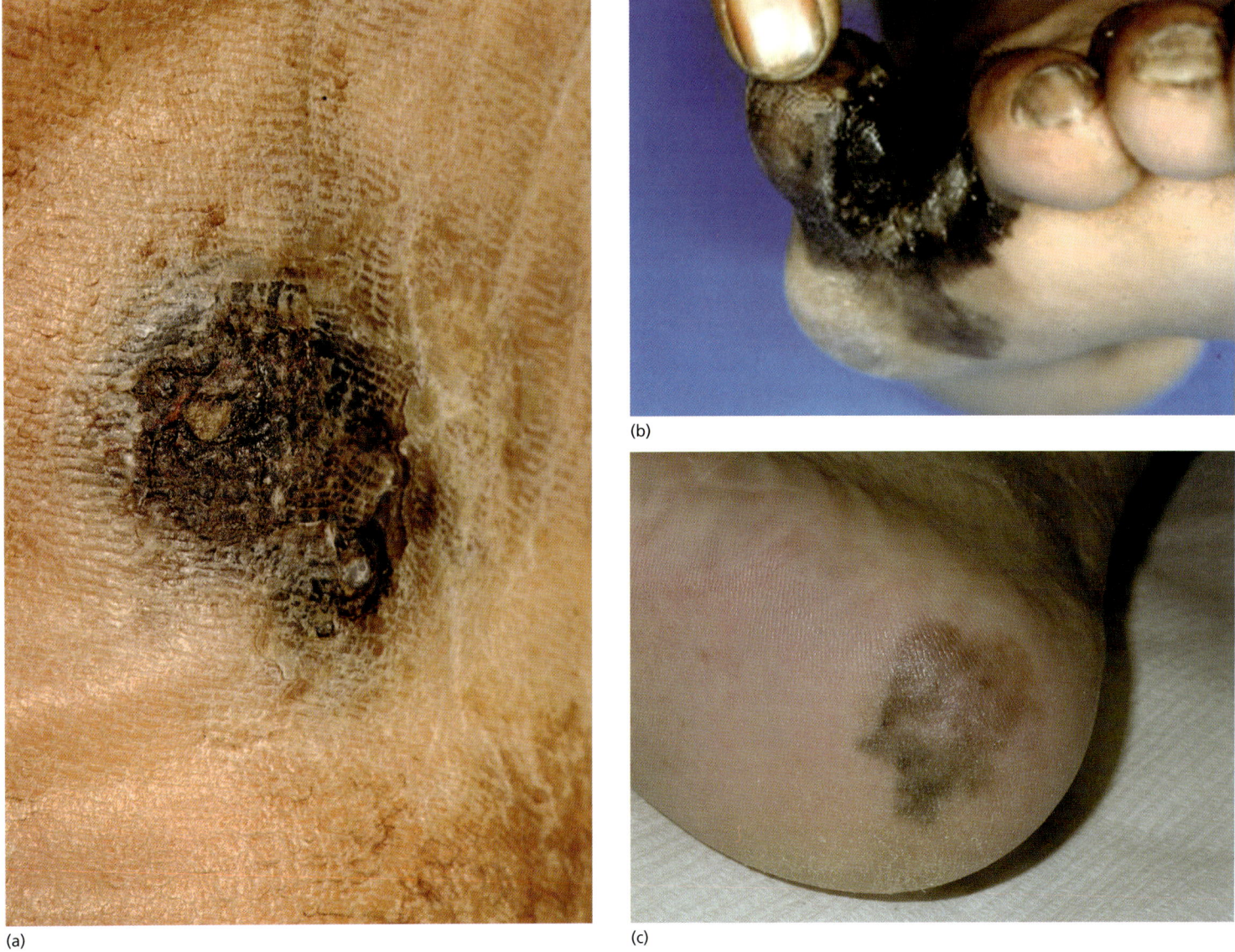

(a)

(b)

(c)

Fig. 54.61 (a, b, c) Three acral lentiginous melanomas arising on the sole of the foot in a black, asian and white-skinned person, respectively. This is the only form of melanoma to have a similar prevalence in all ethnic groups.

interferes with nail formation and a progressively dystrophic nail results (Fig. 54.63). Eventually, pigment may spread to the surrounding normal skin as 'Hutchinson's sign'.

A sizeable proportion of subungual melanomas, however, are either amelanotic or produce little pigment so that the 'classical' linear pigmented band is actually uncommon. In these tumours, therefore, the lesions present as a progressively abnormal nail, such as a fissured nail or destruction of the nail beginning proximally.

Subungual melanoma is commonly diagnosed at a late stage in development because of earlier confusion with a benign melanocytic lesion, a traumatic haemorrhage under the nail, pyogenic granuloma, persistent paronychia, a fungal infection or even a subungual wart. A high degree of suspicion is required if subungual melanoma is not to be missed. Dermoscopy may help; a band of brown to black pigment comprised of thin irregular bands which are not parallel may be seen in melanoma [2] and origin from the nail matrix may be confirmed. Subungual pigmentation due to causes other than melanoma, which must be considered as differential diagnoses, is usually distal rather than arising from the nail matrix.

Diagnosis. The diagnosis of early lesions usually requires biopsy of the nail matrix. The proximal nail plate may be reflected and the matrix biopsied. Pigment bands less than 3 mm in diameter may be biopsied using a punch biopsy, which may produce minimal damage if the lesion proves to be benign. Wider bands require elliptical biopsy, which is likely to damage the nail permanently [2]. Confirmed melanomas, or clinically obvious more advanced subungual melanomas, should be managed by expert multidisciplinary teams, as they are sufficiently rare and surgically difficult to merit pooling of experience.

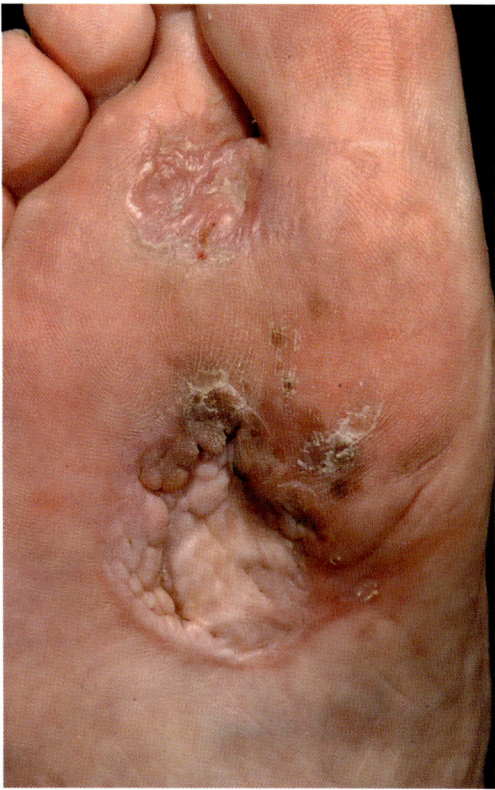

Fig. 54.62 Two skin grafts used to treat multifocal acral lentiginous melanoma. Residual *in situ* or lentiginous disease is seen between the two grafts. The whole of the area was subsequently excised. Subtle precursor lentiginous disease is common.

Treatment. The treatment of subungual melanoma is surgical. The affected digit is usually the thumb or great toe and preservation of function is therefore highly desirable. Early lesions may therefore be managed, if possible, using excision and grafting. *In situ* disease, however, is very common in the skin around the nail and therefore it is rare to achieve adequate clearance without at least partial amputation. For more advanced disease partial amputation is the norm, through either the distal interphalangeal or proximal interphalangeal joints. The choice of surgical option should be made in discussion with the patient depending on the functional implications for the patient and the thickness of the tumour. Transplantation of a toe to the thumb stump may be possible to restore function. If the patient has elected to proceed to sentinel node biopsy this must be done at the time of definitive surgery.

References

1 Stevens NG, Liff JM, Weiss NS. Plantar melanoma: is the incidence of melanoma of the sole of the foot really higher in blacks than whites? *Int J Cancer* 1990; **45**: 691–3.
2 Braun RP, Baran R, Le Gal FA *et al*. Diagnosis and management of nail pigmentations. *J Am Acad Dermatol* 2007; **56**: 835–47.

Mucosal melanoma

Mucosal melanomas are rare, but can be seen in the oral cavity, on the genital mucosa and in the perianal area. The most common presenting feature of mucosal melanoma is the presence of extensive, irregular macular pigmentation. This may be extensive but

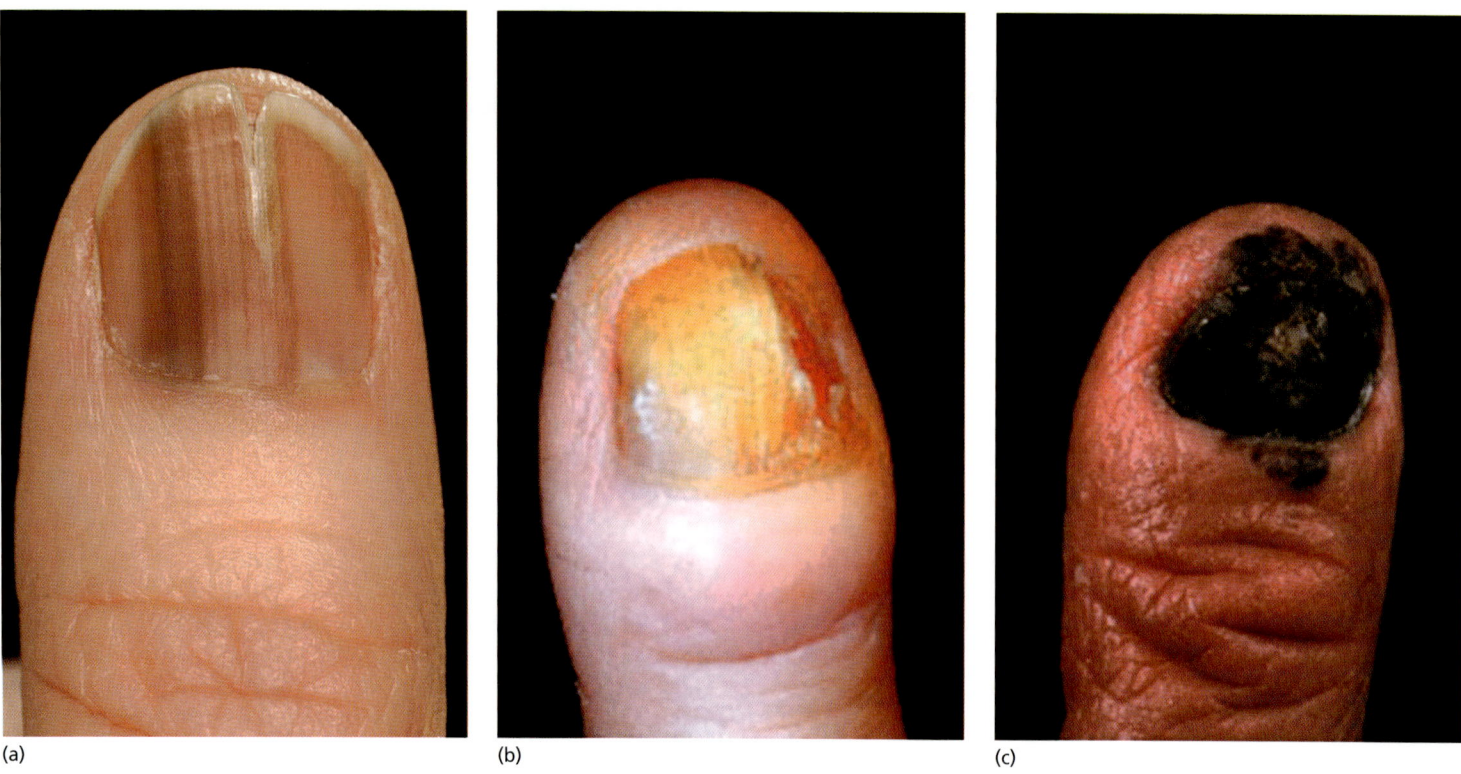

(a)   (b)   (c)

Fig. 54.63 Subungual melanoma. (a) A linear, new, pigmented band and nail dystophy. (b) An amelanotic melanoma lifting up a dystrophic nail. (c) Typical pigmentation arising proximally, irregular in shape and colour.

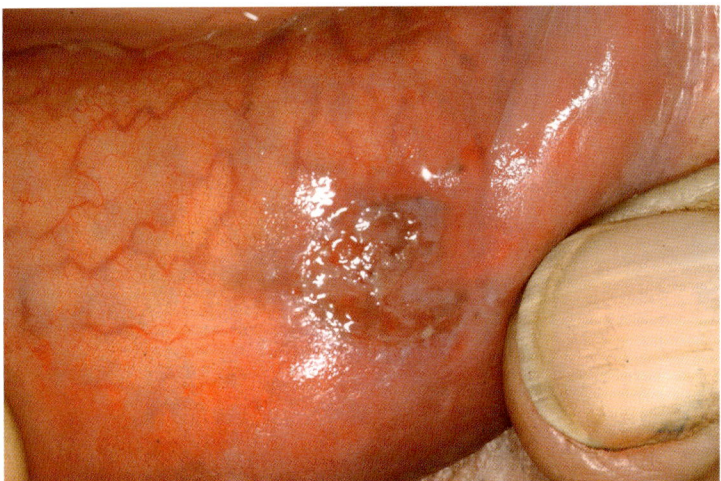

Fig. 54.64 A melanoma arising on the buccal mucosa. In this site the appearance may be subtle.

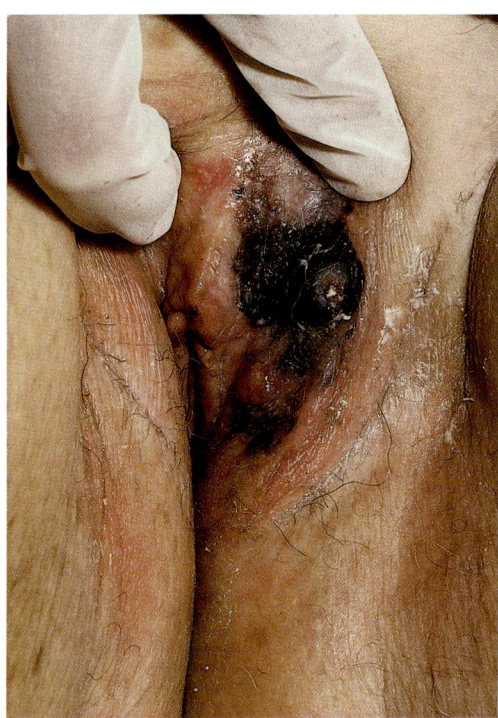

Fig. 54.65 Vulvar melanoma. This lesion is obviously deeply invasive and has a poor prognosis.

spotty and may extend laterally for years before becoming elevated. Such lesions should be biopsied without delay, although clinically they may look deceptively benign (Fig. 54.64).

Genital melanomas are also discussed on p. 54.6. They are rare variants of melanoma, which unfortunately usually still present late as a mass or with vaginal bleeding. The average age at presentation is in the seventh decade, significantly older than for cutaneous melanomas. On biopsy the majority of the tumours are in vertical growth phase and unfortunately many are thick and have a poor prognosis (Fig. 54.65).

Pathology. Primary melanomas arising on the mucosal surface of the oral cavity, the vulvovaginal and the rectal areas have some features in common with acral lentiginous melanomas, and the term palmoplantar mucosal melanoma is sometimes used to describe the entire group. Extensive lentiginous change is frequently visible, both clinically and pathologically, and the focus of invasion may be very difficult to find in early tumours, even in the presence of obvious metastases.

Treatment. Wide local excision of the melanoma is necessary. The extensive surrounding *in situ* disease makes this difficult in practice in many patients, partly because of the anatomical constraints and partly because it is very difficult clinically to distinguish involved tissue from normal. It may be necessary to do multiple biopsies prior to surgery to determine the extent of disease, and radical excision is unfortunately often necessary. Where the margins of excision are by necessity suboptimal, topical imiquimod may be used to try and remove *in situ* disease, although the treatment may be difficult to tolerate and there are insufficient data to support its use.

Secondary melanoma from an occult primary site

About 8% of melanomas present as metastatic disease from an unknown primary. The commonest site of the metastasis is regional lymph nodes but very rarely the patient may present with stage IV disease. In the majority of such patients, there is evidence of a regressed primary, presenting typically as an area of depigmentation, or a history of a lesion, which spontaneously cleared. Rare primary sites should, however, be inspected, such as the mucosae (including the anus). In a proportion, however, no origin for the metastasis can be found. As naevus cells may be seen not uncommonly in the subcapsular area of lymph glands it seems possible that melanoma may arise *de novo* in a lymph gland.

Where no origin for the melanoma can be found, the disease should be treated as usual; lymph node metastases should be treated by block dissection after imaging has been carried out.

Multiple primary malignant melanomas

At present around 5% of patients who have already had one melanoma diagnosed will develop a second and possibly a third or further primary melanoma. This is more common in patients with the atypical mole syndrome. These primaries are not infrequently in the same anatomical area, such as on one leg of a woman. This often causes concern that the second and later tumours might represent metastatic disease. It is important that the pathologist consider this as a possibility.

For patients who have had a thin melanoma diagnosed, the risk of a second primary melanoma is greater than the risk of the first melanoma metastasizing. Complete skin examination is therefore important in follow up of melanoma patients.

Treatment. Each primary should be treated by wide local excision. An important part of the management, however, is to take a family history, as the development of multiple primaries is indicative of genetic predisposition to melanoma. Patients who have a family history of melanoma comprise a proportion of those who develop multiple primary melanomas, and a small number will have mutations in the *CDKN2A* gene. In the presence of a family history of melanoma or pancreatic cancer, referral to a specialist familial melanoma clinic or clinical geneticist is appropriate.

It is supposed that the majority of those who do not have a family history have lower risk susceptibility genes and have had extensive sun exposure, although a proportion will carry high-risk genes. Patients should be advised to moderate their sun exposure and taught how to self examine. Whilst all melanoma patients should also be advised to protect the skin of their families without becoming vitamin D deficient, this is particularly appropriate in the presence of multiple primaries and a family history.

Rare histological subtypes of melanoma

Naevoid melanoma (minimal deviation melanoma, small cell melanoma). A further pathological variant is the so-called naevoid, minimal deviation or small cell melanoma. These lesions lack epidermal involvement, are fairly well defined at their lateral margins, and the small naevoid cells in the dermis, which make up the bulk of the tumour, show partial differentiation. However, careful examination will reveal the presence of abnormal mitoses in naevomelanocytes. These lesions may be confused with compound naevi.

Animal-type melanoma. This is a rare pathological variant of melanoma, which, as the name suggests, has some morphological similarities to melanoma found in grey horses. Blue-black nodules are the clinical presenting feature, and the pathology shows heavy dermal melanin pigmentation with sheets of atypical spindle cells, which may be difficult to visualize without bleaching because of the quantity of pigment present. The epidermis is usually, but not always, involved, and mitotic figures may be difficult to find. Metastases to both regional nodes and to distant organs may occur.

Melanoma of the soft parts (clear cell sarcoma). This is a further rare pathological variant of malignant melanoma. The tumours usually arise on the tendons and aponeuroses. The ankle appears to be a relatively common site, and the tumours generally appear in young people. There appears to be no epidermal component, which gives rise to diagnostic confusion with various types of sarcoma, but the malignant cells contain premelanosomes and melanosomes. Plump, pale spindle cells with clear cytoplasm are seen in the tendons (Fig. 54.66). They may be deceptively bland on microscopy as mitotic figures are difficult to find, but both local recurrence and distant metastases are relatively common.

Childhood melanomas

Incidence. Metastasizing melanoma is fortunately extremely rare in children. The true incidence of cutaneous melanoma is unknown, not least because of the difficulties of histological diagnosis of melanoma in children and, in particular, its differentiation from the Spitz naevus, but pre-pubertal melanoma is thought to be rare [1].

After puberty the incidence of melanoma starts to rise slowly [2]; melanoma is unusual amongst solid tumours in that the inci-

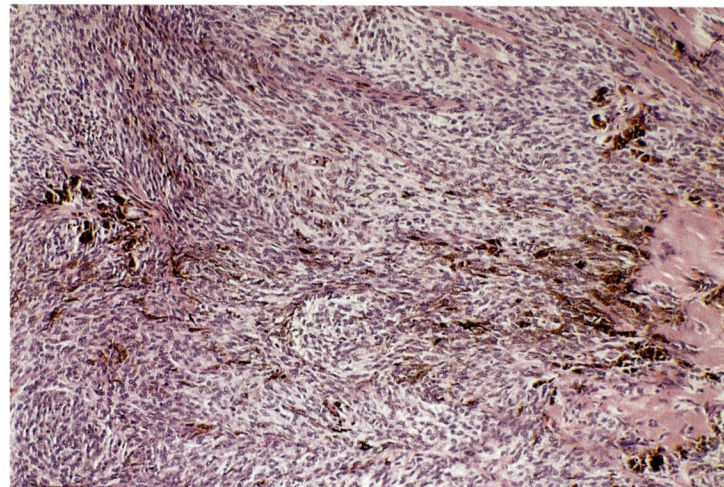

Fig. 54.66 Pathology of melanoma of the soft parts. Note the eosinophilic cytoplasm and also the pigmentation.

dence is proportionately greater in young adults. In Europe the age-standardized incidence rates for girls range from 0.2 new cases per million in Bulgaria to 3.8 in Norway [3]. Incidence is higher (as it is in adults) in Queensland, where the age-standardized incidence is 0.1/100 000 per annum in 0 to 4 year olds and 3/100 000 per annum in 10 to 14 year olds [4,5].

This section refers to melanoma in children both before and after puberty.

Aetiology. Childhood melanoma may occur in the normal host but there are three known predispositions: congenital naevi (see above), the atypical mole syndrome (AMS) (see above), familial melanoma and other cancer family syndromes such as retinoblastoma and xeroderma pigmentosum (XP) [6–8]. Melanoma accounts for 7% of second malignancies in familial retinoblastoma [8]. Many of these have developed within the field of irradiation. The role of chemotherapy in the induction of melanoma as a second malignancy is unclear. Xeroderma pigmentosum occurs as a rare autosomal recessive condition. There are a variety of subtypes with very different degrees of severity. In the severe types there is extreme photosensitivity, with freckling of the skin and the occurrence of multiple skin cancers, including melanoma. Most melanomas appear to occur in the teens [9]. In the mildest types the phenotype is similar but much less marked and there are patients described who appear to overlap clinically with Cockayne's syndrome or who do not yet fit into any well-defined entity [10].

There are several small series of childhood melanomas in the literature [1,4,11,12] and the relative importance of these predisposing conditions varies, as would be expected in such inevitably selected series. In a series of 15 cases in children under the age of 12 years from the MD Anderson Cancer Centre [2], four occurred in children with either giant congenital naevi or meningeal melanocytosis. In a review article, Williams and Pennella concluded that only 3% of reported childhood tumours occurred in giant congenital naevi [13] but 19% of the reported cases had been thought to have developed in small congenital naevi. In a series from New South Wales, none of 52 cases were associated with giant congenital naevi or xeroderma pigmentosum [4].

Although the single most common predisposition to childhood melanoma appears to be congenital naevi, the majority of childhood cases occur in patients with no obvious increased susceptibility. A case–control study from Australia of adolescent melanoma identified the same risk factors for melanoma as are seen in the adult population: family history (23/201 cases compared with 6/205 controls), red hair and an abnormal naevus phenotype; 2/147 had germline *CDKN2A* mutations [14].

Rarely, transplacental transmission of melanoma has been recorded [9,15].

References

1 Schmid-Wendtner MH, Berking C, Baumert J *et al*. Cutaneous melanoma in childhood and adolescence: an analysis of 36 patients. *J Am Acad Dermatol* 2002; **46**: 874–9.

2 Boddie A, Smith J, McBride C. Malignant melanoma in children and young adults. *Southern Med J* 1978; **71**: 1074–8.

3 Conti EM, Cercato MC, Gatta G *et al*. Childhood melanoma in Europe since 1978: a population-based survival study. *Eur J Cancer* 2001; **37**: 780–4.

4 Milton GW, Shaw HM, Thompson JF, McCarthy WH. Cutaneous melanoma in childhood: incidence and prognosis. *Australas J Dermatol* 1997; **38** (Suppl. 1): S44–8.

5 Parkin D, Whelan S, Ferlay J *et al*. *Cancer Incidence in Five Continents*. IARC Scientific Publications No 143, Lyon, International Agency for Research on Cancer II, 1997.

6 Stern JB, Peck GL, Haupt HM *et al*. Malignant melanoma in xeroderma pigmentosum: Search for a precursor lesion. *J Am Acad Dermatol* 1993; **28**: 591–4.

7 Van Der Spek PJ, Smit EME, Beverloo HB *et al*. Chromosomal localization of three repair genes: the xeroderma pigmentosum group c gene and two human homologs of yeast *RAD23*. *Genomics* 1994; **23**: 651–8.

8 Traboulsi EI, Zimmerman LE, Manz HJ. Cutaneous malignant melanoma in survivors of heritable retinoblastoma. *Arch Ophthalmology* 1988; **106**: 1059–61.

9 Roth ME, Grant-Kels JM, Kuhn MK *et al*. Melanoma in children. *J Am Acad Dermatol* 1990; **22**: 265–74.

10 Itoh T, Fujiwara Y, Ono T, Yamaizumi M. UV syndrome, a new general category of photosensitive disorder with defective DNA repair, is distinct from xeroderma pigmentosum variant and rodent complementation group 1. *Am J Hum Genet* 1995; **56**: 1267–76.

11 Ceballos P, Ruiz-Maldonado R, Mihm M. Melanoma in children. *New Eng J Med* 1995; **332**: 656–62.

12 Rao B, Hayes F, Pratt C *et al*. Malignant melanoma in children: its management and prognosis. *J Pediatric Surg* 1990; **25**: 198–203.

13 Williams M, Pennella R. Melanoma, melanocytic nevi and other risk factors in children. *J Pediatrics* 1994; **124**: 833–45.

14 Youl P, Aitken J, Hayward N *et al*. Melanoma in adolescents: a case–control study of risk factors in Queensland, Australia. *Int J Cancer* 2002; **98**: 92–8.

15 Scov-Jensen T, Hastrup J, Lambrethsen E. Malignant melanoma in children. *Cancer* 1966; **19**: 620–6.

Melanoma: prognosis and management

The estimation of prognosis for patients with melanoma

A large number of pathological features have been suggested as offering prognostic information. Tumour thickness was established by Alexander Breslow as the most valuable prognostic guide [1]. Blocks are cut from the apparently thickest area of the primary melanoma by the pathologist and the slides cut from this

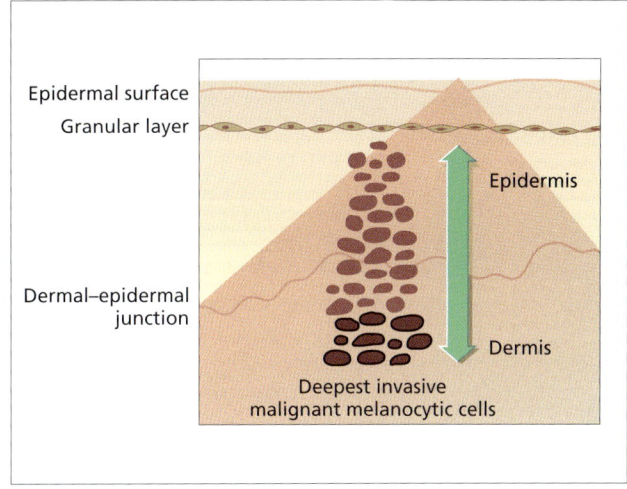

Fig. 54.67 Malignant melanoma thickness measurement (Breslow). The pathologist measures in millimetres the distance between the granular layer in the epidermis and the deepest invasive melanoma cell.

block are examined using an ocular micrometer to measure the distance between the overlying epidermal granular layer and the deepest invasive area of the primary lesion (Fig. 54.67). This figure in millimetres is the Breslow or tumour-thickness measurement and should be included in all pathology reports of primary melanoma. The thickness is indicative of the likelihood of vertical growth phase, tumour volume and correlates with biological markers of tumour progression.

Subsequently, additional histological measures predictive of survival have been established, which have been used to develop the AJCC staging system [2] (Table 54.5). In this system the key roles of thickness and ulceration of the primary in determining outcome are recognized as are the number of lymph nodes involved in metastatic disease.

With respect to primary disease, the AJCC system benefits from very large data sets and it has been validated in population-based data sets (although with a somewhat better survival in the population based SEER data set [3]). The AJCC system is still being improved and a further revision will follow soon. Attempts, however, have been made in the interim to improve the estimates by other groups, particularly the Melanoma Programme at the University of Pennsylvania. Patient sex, mitotic rate, growth phase [4] and tumour site are important determinants of survival, which are not as yet taken into account by the AJCC system; a number of algorithms have been developed that take these additional factors into consideration.

Factors associated with a higher risk of recurrence in those diagnosed with thin primaries have been identified using prognostic trees [5]. In this system the acknowledged effects of sex, site and tumour growth phase are taken into account, so that, for example, females with level II, thin, non-ulcerated tumours had 100% 10-year survival rates compared with males with level III and IV tumours and a 'mitogenic' histological subtype who had an 83.4% 10-year survival. Ultimately, additional information may come from immunohistochemistry (using dermal Ki67 expression, for example [6]), and it seems entirely preferable that this will be incorporated into web-based risk algorithm tools.

Table 54.5 The AJCC staging system [2].

Stage	Primary tumour (pT)	Lymph node (N)	Distant metastases (M)
0	*In situ* tumours	No nodes	None
IA	<1.0 mm no ulceration	No nodes	None
IB	<1.0 mm with ulceration	No nodes	None
	1.01–2.0 mm no ulceration	No nodes	None
IIA	1.01–2.0 mm with ulceration	No nodes	None
	2.01–4.0 mm no ulceration	No nodes	None
IIB	2.01–4.0 mm with ulceration	No nodes	None
	>4.0 mm no ulceration	No nodes	None
IIC	>4.0 mm with ulceration	No nodes	None
IIIA	Any Breslow no ulceration	Micrometastases in nodes	None
IIIB	Any Breslow with ulceration	Micrometastases in nodes	None
	Any Breslow no ulceration	Up to 3 palpable nodes	None
	Any Breslow ± ulceration	No nodes but *in transit*	None
		Metastases or satellite lesions	
IIIC	Any Breslow with ulceration	Up to 3 palpable nodes	None
	Any Breslow ± ulceration	4 or more palpable nodes	None
		Or matted nodes	
		Or *in transit* metastases with nodes	
IVM1			Skin, subcutaneous or distant lymph nodes
IVM2			Lung
IVM3			All other sites or any site with raised LDH

Prognostic tables published by Elder and Murphy [7] are useful aids to management of patients in the clinic, although caution must be exercised as these are not population specific and must be judged as estimates only.

The most recent TNM staging system for melanoma published by the AJCC is outlined in Table 54.5, based upon validation in 17 000 subjects. The staging system reflects the dominant effects of Breslow thickness and the presence of ulceration on outcome for primary disease but for the first time allows risk stratification by the results of sentinel node biopsy (SLNB), a positive SLNB being Stage IIIa. The staging system also reflects the poorer prognosis associated with multiple nodes, matted nodes or *in transit* disease in Stage III melanoma, and the observation that outcome for Stage IV patients is poorer with visceral metastases rather than soft tissue disease, and poorer still when lactic dehydrogenase (LDH) levels are raised. This staging system was validated in 41 417 patients in the SEER registry [3], although the survival was generally higher so that the authors suggest that population-specific figures would be preferable (although very difficult to achieve). The 10-year survival rates of the SEER registry patients are compared with the AJCC figures in Table 54.6.

References

1 Breslow A. Prognostic factors in the treatment of cutaneous melanoma. *J Cutan Pathol* 1979; **6**: 208–12.

2 Balch CM, Buzaid AC, Soong SJ *et al.* Final version of the American Joint Committee on Cancer staging system for cutaneous melanoma. *J Clin Oncol* 2001; **19**: 3635–48.

3 Gimotty PA, Botbyl J, Soong SJ, Guerry D. A population-based validation of the American Joint Committee on Cancer melanoma staging system. *J Clin Oncol* 2005; **23**: 8065–75.

4 Gimotty PA, Elder DE, Fraker DL *et al.* Identification of high-risk patients among those diagnosed with thin cutaneous melanomas. *J Clin Oncol* 2007; **25**: 1129–34.

5 Gimotty PA, Guerry D, Ming ME *et al.* Thin primary cutaneous malignant melanoma: a prognostic tree for 10-year metastasis is more accurate than American Joint Committee on Cancer staging. *J Clin Oncol* 2004; **22**: 3668–76.

6 Gimotty PA, Van Belle P, Elder DE *et al.* Biologic and prognostic significance of dermal Ki67 expression, mitoses, and tumorigenicity in thin invasive cutaneous melanoma. *J Clin Oncol* 2005; **23**: 8048–56.

7 Elder D, Murphy G. Malignant tumors (melanomas and related lesions). *Atlas of Tumor Pathology: Melanocytic Tumors of the Skin* 2 (third series). Armed Forces Institute of Pathology, 1991: 103–205.

Management of cutaneous malignant melanoma after excision of the primary

UK guidelines are available for the management of all stages of melanoma [1] and similar guidelines have been published by other national groups [2,3].

Staging

The only form of staging normally offered to the majority of patients presenting with primary melanoma is sentinel node biopsy. Some centres perform base-line chest X-ray and blood tests, including LDH, although there are no data supporting their use [4]. The likely yield of true positives on chest X-ray here is likely to be around 0%.

Staging imaging is necessary at relapse. The most typical first relapse is detected as enlarged regional lymph nodes and it would be usual to perform a CT scan prior to surgery, on the basis that the patient might choose to decline surgery if they had metastatic disease elsewhere. In practice, however, it is a very rare event to find true positive scans, and if waiting for a scan would delay surgery this may be carried out after surgery. A post-surgery scan may also be needed for trials of adjuvant therapies. For melanomas on the arm metastatic to the axilla or supraclavicular nodes,

Table 54.6 Prognosis of melanoma according to disease stage. Adapted from [2] and [3].

Substage	Characteristics of the primary such as depth and ulceration, presence of nodal or distant metastases, see Table 54.5	AJCC 10-year survival (% ± S.E.) [2]	SEER 10 year survival (% ± S.E) [3]
IA	≤1 mm	87.9 ± 1.0	97.4 ± 0.35
IB	≤1 mm with ulceration	83.1 ± 1.5	90.2 ± 1.8
	1.01–2.0 mm, no ulceration	79.2 ± 1.1	84.1 ± 1.4
IIA	1.01–2.0 mm, with ulceration	64.4 ± 2.2	65.2 ± 7.7
	2.01–4.0 mm, no ulceration	63.8 ± 1.7	67.3 ± 2.6
IIB	2.01–4.0 mm, with ulceration	50.8 ± 1.7	62.1 ± 5.9
	> 4 mm, no ulceration	53.9 ± 3.3	56.3 ± 4.4
IIC	> 4 mm, with ulceration	32.3 ± 2.1	47.5 ± 7.1
IIIA	1 micrometastases in node	62.0 ± 4.4	
	2–3 nodes	56.9 ± 6.8	
IIIB	Micrometastases and ulcerated primary	37.8 ± 4.8	
	1 palpable node	35.9 ± 7.2	49.7 ± 7.6
	2–3 nodes	47.7 ± 5.8	43.6 ± 10.6
	Satellites, no nodes	39.2 ± 5.8	59.2 ± 7.1
IIIC	1 node and ulcerated primary	24.4 ± 5.3	36.6 ± 15.7
	2–3 nodes and ulcerated primary	15.0 ± 3.9	32.9 ± 16.3
	≥4 nodes	18.4 ± 2.5	22.4 ± 6.7
IV	Overall		14.1 ± 3.2
	Skin and SC	15.7 ± 2.9	
	Lung	2.5 ± 1.5	
	Other visceral	6.0 ± 0.9	

then a scan with contrast of the chest and abdomen is the norm. For melanomas on the head and neck or upper trunk, a scan with contrast of the thorax and abdomen is usual. For melanomas on the lower leg and lower trunk including the genitalia, a scan with contrast should be performed of the thorax, abdomen and pelvis. A chest X-ray and bloods, including liver function tests and LDH, are also justified, but only as a baseline. Although LDH is commonly measured it is a poor biomarker of relapse (see below).

Patients who present with clinical signs and symptoms of Stage IV disease would normally have a CT scan with contrast of the abdomen, thorax and pelvis. As melanoma commonly metastasizes to the brain, a CT scan of the brain is also appropriate. A chest X-ray and bloods, including LDH, as a baseline are also helpful.

There is no widely used biomarker with which to monitor high-risk melanoma patients. Circulating levels of protein S100beta, melanoma-inhibitory activity (MIA), LDH, alkaline phosphatase (AP), and tyrosinase/MART-1 reverse transcription-polymerase chain reaction (RT-PCR) are biomarkers that have been evaluated. In one study of 286 patients, protein S100beta and MIA demonstrated a higher sensitivity, specificity, and diagnostic accuracy in the diagnosis of newly occurring metastasis compared with the tumour markers AP, LDH and RT-PCR diagnostics [5]. The superior value of measuring S100 compared with LDH has been reported by other groups [6,7]. When there is an effective treatment for Stage IV disease, the clinical value of markers such as S100 will be higher and it is likely that their use will increase.

Sentinel node biopsy (SLNB)

SLNB grew out of a recognition that elective lymph node dissection (ELND) does not offer a survival advantage to melanoma patients and it is worth briefly considering this history. Three randomized controlled trials that evaluated the effectiveness of ELND on survival in melanoma patients were identified with sufficient data for a meta-analysis [8–10], the Intergroup Melanoma Trial and two WHO Melanoma Trials (No.1 and No.14). The total number of participants was 1533; 768 were assigned to have ELND and 765 to delayed lymphadenectomy or no treatment. A total of 416 deaths within 5 years of the primary tumour excision were recorded in the three trials. Death occurred in 197 patients who underwent ELND compared to 219 from control groups. The pooled odds ratio was 0.86 (95% CI 0.68–1.09), showing no evidence of any therapeutic effect [11]. Whilst these trials and the subsequent meta-analysis showed no significant effect, they did not exclude a small effect and because lymphatic draining in individuals may vary, Morton developed sentinel node biopsy as a means of ensuring that the node biopsied was the one most likely to be the first draining lymph node [12]. The technique was widely adopted although the first randomized clinical trial to evaluate it was only published in 2006 [13]. In SLNB, lymphoscintigraphy is used to identify the lymphatic drainage pattern from the site of the primary melanoma, by injecting radiolabelled colloid and/or blue dye at the site of the primary melanoma. The tracer/dye are concentrated in the so-called sentinel node and are detected using a hand-held gamma probe (neoprobe) and examination by naked eye for the blue stained node. Sometimes there is more than one sentinel node and sometimes these sentinel nodes are in different lymph node basins. The node is removed, sectioned and subjected to detailed, time-consuming examination by specialist pathologists using immunohistochemistry (S100 and HMB-45). Protocols have been developed to ensure consistency between groups and the identification of small deposits in only one part of a node [14]. The Dewar classification was developed by Cook in the UK [15], to describe the anatomic metastatic deposits in the sentinel node; they were found to be subcapsular in 26.0% of patients. None of the patients with only subcapsular disease had any non-sentinel nodes involved on completion of lymphadenectomy. In the patients whose sentinel node metastases had a different microanatomic location (such as parenchymal or mixed subcapsular or parenchymal), the rate of non-sentinel node involvement was 22.2% overall. Thus it would appear that if melanoma patients have subcapsular deposits of melanoma only, they are less likely to have involvement of other glands. This finding, therefore, has prognostic importance but needs to be established in prospective trials.

The surgical technique must be learnt and false-negative results are more common in trainees, so that many centres require a training experience of around 30 cases. The pathological examination of the nodes is also a skilled procedure; naevus cells may be seen, for example, in the subcapsular area of the node and must be distinguished from melanoma cells. The technique is expensive of resources and expert time.

The likelihood of a positive SLNB result is correlated with Breslow thickness so that in a review of 4218 published cases only two were positive for patients with thickness less than 0.75 mm [16]. Patients with melanoma of Breslow thickness more than 1.0 mm and less than 1.5 mm have a low but definite risk of having micrometastases (around 8%). Use of SLNB to stage patients for trials of adjuvant therapies would appear reasonable but the patient should be aware that the risk of positivity is low. In patients with melanoma of Breslow thickness from 1.5 to 4.0 mm the risk of positive SLNBs is significantly higher at 23%. The value of SLNB in patients with tumours of Breslow thickness 4 mm or thicker is questionable (if the intent is therapeutic as well as being a staging tool) because the risk of haematogenous spread is so high. More recently, some authors have suggested that additional prognostic information does come from SLNB in these patients [17].

The first randomized clinical trial of SLNB in 1269 patients with an intermediate-thickness primary melanoma has been reported [13], and the prognostic value of SLNB was confirmed. The 5-year survival rate was 72.3 ± 4.6% among patients with tumour-positive sentinel nodes and 90.2 ± 1.3% among those with tumour-negative sentinel nodes (hazard ratio for death 2.48; 95% CI 1.54–3.98; $P < 0.001$). There was no overall survival benefit however of SLNB; the mean (±SE) estimated 5-year disease-free survival rate for the population was 78.3 ± 1.6% in the biopsy group and 73.1 ± 2.1% in the observation group (hazard ratio for death 0.74; 95% CI 0.59–0.93; $P = 0.009$). Five-year melanoma-specific survival rates were similar in the two groups (87.1 ± 1.3% and 86.6 ± 1.6%, respectively). The authors suggested that within patients with nodal metastases, there might be some benefit in that the 5-year survival rate was higher among those who underwent immediate lymphadenectomy than among those in whom lymphadenectomy was delayed (72.3 ± 4.6% vs. 52.4 ± 5.9%; hazard ratio for death 0.51; 95% CI 0.32–0.81; $P = 0.004$). This conclusion requires that an assumption is made that all patients with a positive SLNB will progress (which may not be true). The conclusion from the study may also be that SLNB could have a survival benefit for a small proportion of melanoma patients overall, but the study is as yet insufficiently powered to show this effect.

Lymphoscintigraphy for SLNB of the head and neck is technically more difficult than in other sites [18], as is the surgery [19], and is not therefore offered in all SLNB centres.

Thus, at present, SLNB is of proven staging value but of no established therapeutic value. Its use in identifying patients for adjuvant therapies means that it will continue to be used, but its role must be evaluated in the long term.

References

1 Newton Bishop JA, Corrie PG, Evans J et al. UK guidelines for the management of cutaneous melanoma. *Br J Plast Surg* 2002; **55**: 46–54.

2 Sober AJ, Chuang TY, Duvic M et al. Guidelines of care for primary cutaneous melanoma. *J Am Acad Dermatol* 2001; **45**: 579–86.

3 Kroon BB, Bergman W, Coebergh JW, Ruiter DJ. Consensus on the management of malignant melanoma of the skin in The Netherlands. Dutch Melanoma Working Party. *Melanoma Res* 1999; **9**: 207–12.

4 Wang TS, Johnson TM, Cascade PN et al. Evaluation of staging chest radiographs and serum lactate dehydrogenase for localized melanoma. *J Am Acad Dermatol* 2004; **51**: 399–405.

5 Garbe C, Leiter U, Ellwanger U et al. Diagnostic value and prognostic significance of protein S-100beta, melanoma-inhibitory activity, and tyrosinase/MART-1 reverse transcription-polymerase chain reaction in the follow-up of high-risk melanoma patients. *Cancer* 2003; **97**: 1737–45.

6 Krahn G, Kaskel P, Sander S et al. S100 beta is a more reliable tumor marker in peripheral blood for patients with newly occurred melanoma metastases compared with MIA, albumin and lactate-dehydrogenase. *Anticancer Res* 2001; **21**: 1311–6.

7 Mohammed MQ, Abraha HD, Sherwood RA et al. Serum S100beta protein as a marker of disease activity in patients with malignant melanoma. *Med Oncol (Northwood, London, England)* 2001; **18**: 109–20.

8 Balch CM, Soong SJ, Bartolucci AA et al. Efficacy of an elective regional lymph node dissection of 1 to 4 mm thick melanomas for patients 60 years of age and younger. *Ann Surg* 1996; **224**: 255–63; discussion 263–6.

9 Cascinelli N, Morabito A, Santinami M et al. Immediate or delayed dissection of regional nodes in patients with melanoma of the trunk: a randomised trial. WHO Melanoma Programme. *Lancet* 1998; **351**: 793–6.

10 Veronesi U. Delayed node dissection in stage one malignant melanoma: justification and advantages. *Cancer Invest* 1987; **5**: 47–53.

11 Lens MB, Dawes M, Goodacre T, Newton-Bishop JA. Elective lymph node dissection in patients with melanoma: systematic review and meta-analysis of randomized controlled trials. *Arch Surg* 2002; **137**: 458–61.

12 Morton DL, Wen DR, Wong JH et al. Technical details of intraoperative lymphatic mapping for early stage melanoma. *Arch Surg* 1992; **127**: 392–9.

13 Morton DL, Thompson JF, Cochran AJ et al. Sentinel-node biopsy or nodal observation in melanoma. *N Engl J Med* 2006; **355**: 1307–17.

14 Cook MG, Green MA, Anderson B et al. The development of optimal pathological assessment of sentinel lymph nodes for melanoma. *J Pathol* 2003; **200**: 314–9.

15 Dewar DJ, Newell B, Green MA et al. The microanatomic location of metastatic melanoma in sentinel lymph nodes predicts nonsentinel lymph node involvement. *J Clin Oncol* 2004; **22**: 3345–9.

16 Lens MB, Dawes M, Newton-Bishop JA, Goodacre T. Tumour thickness as a predictor of occult lymph node metastases in patients with stage I and II melanoma undergoing sentinel lymph node biopsy. *Br J Surg* 2002; **89**: 1223–7.

17 Cherpelis BS, Haddad F, Messina J et al. Sentinel lymph node micrometastasis and other histologic factors that predict outcome in patients with thicker melanomas. *J Am Acad Dermatol* 2001; **44**: 762–6.

18 Mar MV, Miller SA, Kim EE, Macapinlac HA. Evaluation and localization of lymphatic drainage and sentinel lymph nodes in patients with head and neck melanomas by hybrid SPECT/CT lymphoscintigraphic imaging. *J Nucl Med Technol* 2007; **35**: 10–6; quiz 17–20.

19 Doting EH, de Vries M, Plukker JT *et al.* Does sentinel lymph node biopsy in cutaneous head and neck melanoma alter disease outcome? *J Surg Oncol* 2006; **93**: 564–70.

Follow-up after surgery for Stage I or II melanoma

Patients who have had surgery for primary melanoma with no evidence of spread beyond the primary site have traditionally undergone a period of hospital-based follow-up at varying intervals for a varying number of years. The three main purposes of this follow-up are to detect any local recurrence around the scar of the excised melanoma, to palpate the local draining nodes for any clinically detectable evidence of nodal spread and to examine the rest of the skin surface for a second primary melanoma. Regular ultrasound examination of draining nodes is carried out in some centres and there is some evidence that this leads to earlier detection of metastatic disease, although this must be operator dependent [1].

Accepted intervals and duration of follow-up are 3-monthly intervals for 3–5 years. As, however, there is no evidence that this routine follow-up examination advances the time of diagnosing metastatic spread, and the majority of recurrences are detected between such visits, these intervals can be interpreted according to the needs of individual patients and the geographical situation. Some patients benefit emotionally from follow-up in hospital, and some find it traumatic. All patients should be taught how to look for local recurrence, how to palpate the relevant area for enlarged nodes, and be made aware of the clinical features that would suggest a second primary melanoma. They should have information about an appropriate contact in case they detect possible recurrence between regular appointments. The opportunity should also be taken to educate the family about the risk of melanoma and the avoidance of behaviours thought to be causal.

Patients with only an *in situ* melanoma do not require to be placed on a follow-up regime but can be discharged after appropriate surgery and education about self examination and sun protection.

Reference

1 Saiag P, Bernard M, Beauchet A *et al.* Ultrasonography using simple diagnostic criteria vs palpation for the detection of regional lymph node metastases of melanoma. *Arch Dermatol* 2005; **141**: 183–9.

Management of melanoma metastatic to lymph glands

Patients with a positive SLNB would normally proceed to completion lymphadenectomy, although a randomized clinical trial is currently taking place to address its value after SLNB. Axillary surgery would normally be performed to levels I, II and III. For inguinal nodes, a superficial groin dissection would normally be carried out. An additional deep ilioinguinal dissection may also be performed if a pelvic node was seen on lymphoscintigraphy which was not retrieved at SLNB, if there were multiple positive sentinel nodes superficially in the groin (often four or more is suggested), if Cloquet's node (the first of the deep pelvic nodes, lying just below the inguinal ligament) was shown to be involved with melanoma [1], or if lymphatics were seen bypassing nodes superficially and entering the pelvis directly. There are no data to support these clinical practice guidelines.

Patients who present with palpable lymph glands in the drainage area of their primary melanoma should be examined, and, in the majority of such patients, the nodes feel sufficiently firm and large (usually greater than 1 cm in diameter) for a clinical diagnosis of presumptive metastatic melanoma to be made. Patients do commonly present concerned about palpable lesions which prove to be benign such as pea sized normal lymph glands, glands which have enlarged as a result of an insult such as a recent immunization or viral illness, and lipomas.

Where there is doubt about the diagnosis, fine needle aspiration cytology should be used to aspirate a sample under vacuum for pathological examination. A slide preparation can be made in clinic and cytological examination carried out immediately in order to expedite management. An additional cytospin preparation can be examined if insufficient sample is obtained. A negative result should not be taken to exclude metastatic disease if either there was insufficient sample, or in the presence of very suggestive clinical evidence.

The examination of lymph glands is easier in some anatomical locations (inguinal and neck) than in others. The axilla may be particularly difficult, especially in larger men. In these circumstances ultrasonic examination plus fine needle aspiration cytology may be helpful.

If the diagnosis of metastatic disease is clear either clinically or cytologically, then lymphadenectomy is carried out. Again for axillary nodes, levels I, II and III should be removed. A superficial ilioinguinal dissection is usual, extended to a deep dissection if there is evidence of a pelvic node clinically or on CT scan, involvement of Cloquet's node, extensive superficial nodal involvement or a node distal to the inguinal ligament is involved [1].

Melanoma metastatic to the neck should be operated on by surgeons specialized in head and neck surgery. A functional neck dissection is usually carried out for melanoma.

Reference

1 Badgwell B, Xing Y, Gershenwald JE *et al.* Pelvic lymph node dissection is beneficial in subsets of patients with node-positive melanoma. *Ann Surg Oncol* 2007; **14**: 2867–75.

Biological therapies for melanoma

Melanoma is an immunogenic tumour; immune-mediated regression is common in primary tumours and immune-mediated vitiligo in Stage IV disease correlates with a higher chance of response to chemotherapy. Biological therapies have therefore been trialled extensively and the most widely used as an adjuvant is interferon. There have been numerous trials and much controversy but the conclusion now seems to be that interferon-alpha (IFN-α) appears to increase disease-free survival in some patients [1] but is associated with no significant overall survival benefit. Except for TNM stage, there are currently no well-recognized factors that predict outcome. There are some data however from Gogas *et al.*, which might suggest that host variation in immune response predicts outcome [2]. In a study of 200 melanoma patients treated with high-dose IFN-α 2b, the median relapse-free survival was 28.0 months, and the median overall survival was 58.7 months. Autoantibodies and clinical manifestations of autoimmunity were detected in 52 patients (26%). The median relapse-free survival was only 16.0 months among patients without autoimmunity (108 of 148 had a relapse) and more than 45 months (median not reached) in patients with autoimmunity (seven of 52 had a relapse). The median survival was 37.6 months in patients without autoimmunity (80 of 148 died) and was not reached in patients with autoimmunity (two of 52 died). The significance of this remains to be evaluated.

Of the newer biological therapies, the anti-CTLA-4 antibodies, ipilimumab and ticilumumab, intended to enhance immune response, and the antiangiogenic agent bevacizumab, are currently being investigated in clinical trials.

A series of different vaccines have been trialled, from single agents such as ganglioside vaccines to multivalent vaccines. Despite early enthusiasm however, unfortunately, as yet no adjuvant value has been established for these treatments. There is also some evidence of poorer [3] survival in patients receiving vaccine.

Interleukin 2 showed encouraging responses in conjunction with chemotherapy in Phase II clinical trials but not in Phase III trials [4]. A Cochrane review failed to show any evidence that the addition of biological therapies to chemotherapeutic regimes for melanoma increased survival [5].

Interest remains therefore in biological therapies for melanoma, but there are no established roles for these agents as yet. It is fair to say that, despite early optimism, biological therapies have proved disappointing.

Management of patients with Stage IV disease

The AJCC TNM staging revision has clearly indicated that patients with metastatic spread to certain tissues, including the lungs and soft tissue, have a better outlook than those patients with spread to the liver or central nervous system. Lung and soft tissue lesions tend to be more responsive to chemotherapy, but even for these patients such responses are rarely complete and tend to be of short duration.

Where patients have small volume disease, such as a single deposit in the liver or lung, then excision of this lesion should be considered. In these circumstances a PET scan might be used to ensure the absence of disease elsewhere.

No chemotherapeutic agent gives a high proportion of complete responses in melanoma. The current chemotherapeutic agent of choice is dacarbazine (DTIC). In large randomized trials, response rates with dacarbazine ranged from 6 to 15%. Almost all responses were partial, with a median response duration of only 7–8 months [6]. With modern antiemetics, DTIC is relatively non-toxic and can be given as an out-patient, usually at 3-week intervals. Patients should be assessed for response after four to six courses. There is no evidence that combination therapy of DTIC with other chemotherapeutic agents [2] or with biologicals [5] increases the response rate or the duration of response achieved by DTIC alone.

Temozolomide has demonstrated efficacy equal to that of dacarbazine in a randomized Phase III trial. However, unlike dacarbazine, temozolomide is a convenient oral treatment that penetrates the blood–brain barrier and that has shown activity against brain metastases. Although surgery is the preferred treatment modality for patients with solitary brain metastases from melanoma, temo-zolomide is the preferred chemotherapy for patients with brain metastases who require systemic treatment [6].

Management of recurrent disease in a limb

Recurrent disease is common in patients after resection of melanoma on a limb, particularly the leg. When recurrence occurs within 2 cm of the primary, convention is that this is called a 'local recurrence', but in fact the majority are *in transit* metastases.

More distant deposits in the skin or subcutaneous tissues are called '*in transit*' metastases. Occasionally, these may be present at diagnosis. Usually these are proximal, along the line of lymphatics, but rarely they may actually be distal to the primary tumour site. They are usually well under 1 cm in diameter at removal but larger deposits may occur. They may be pigmented or non-pigmented (Fig. 54.68). *In transit* disease is usually accompanied by regional lymph node metastases at some time or other, either simultaneously or years later. Sometimes, multiple *in transit* metastases may develop over years without spread elsewhere.

Treatment

The treatment of such lesions is essentially surgical. Tiny lesions may be removed by punch excision and if large numbers are present, these may be left to heal by secondary intention. Larger ones will require more extensive surgery, even skin grafting. The CO_2 laser may be a very useful means of removing large numbers of small lesions.

If it appears that the disease within the limb is becoming difficult to control surgically then isolated limb perfusion [7] should be considered. Isolated limb perfusion with the administration of cytotoxic drugs (primarily melphalan) has been successfully used to treat melanomas of the extremity since it was first introduced in 1958. The vessels are dissected at open surgery and cannulated. Blood transfusions, systemic drug leak, infection and damage to the blood vessels and nerves, even rare limb loss, are all potential hazards associated with this technique.

Isolated limb perfusion is used to palliate disease [8], although there is some weak evidence for an effect on survival; in a meta-analysis of four trials of 1038 patients, the analysis confirmed the reported increase in survival in two of the trials, but neither had sufficient power to detect significant benefit for perfusion [9]. There is a significant morbidity associated with the treatment and a 1% limb loss rate in most studies [10]. In order to increase the efficacy of treatment, tumour necrosis factor (TNF) may be added [11]. Perfusion with melphalan results in complete response rates of 54% (meta-analysis). The addition of TNF can improve these complete response rates (59–85%) and although no data from randomized controlled trials are available, it is said to be of value in large, bulky lesions or in patients with recurrent disease after previous isolated limb perfusion [12]. The addition of TNF adds to the toxicity. The treatment may be repeated if there is an initial good response but relapse occurs later [13]. Other cytotoxics used in isolated limb perfusion in some centres include dacarbazine and fotemustine [14].

As a result of the morbidity, an alternative, simpler technique termed isolated limb infusion (ILI), was developed by the Sydney Melanoma Unit [15]. ILI is a less invasive procedure involving the

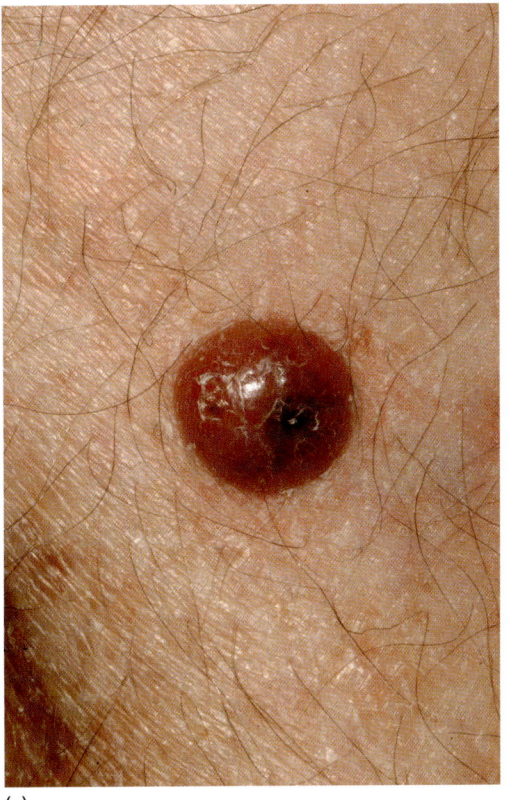

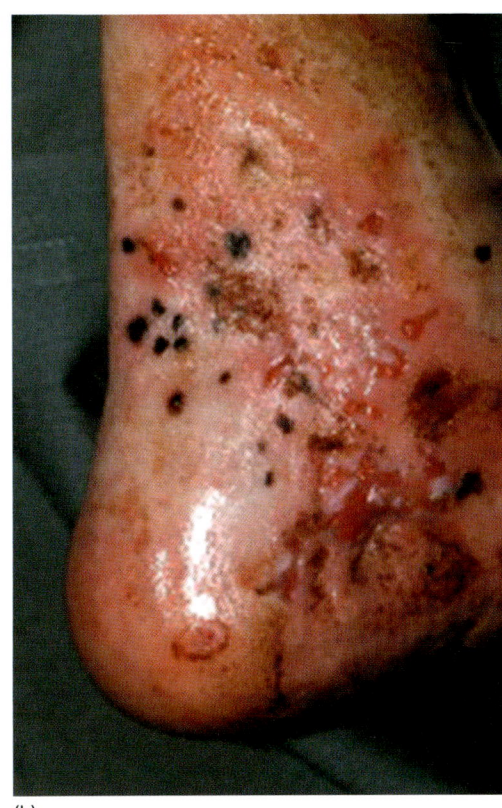

Fig. 54.68 *In transit* metastases in a limb are reasonably frequent. Some recur over long periods of time without distant relapse.

(a)   (b)

use of angiographically placed catheters inserted percutaneously through the femoral vessels, which does not require use of a heart–lung machine. It has been suggested (although based on single institution experiences) that there are fewer resultant morbidities but no compromise in patient outcomes. The overall reported response rate [16] in the treated limb of 135 patients was 85% (complete response [CR] rate 41%, partial response rate 44%). Median response duration response was 16 months (24 months for patients with CR). Median patient survival was 34 months. In those with a CR, the median survival was 42 months.

There is no value for isolated limb infusion as an adjuvant therapy [17].

The treatment of melanoma metastatic to the brain

Melanoma commonly metastasizes to the brain in Stage IV disease, presenting usually as headaches and/or fits. It can occasionally present as motor or sensory symptoms. In a series of 133 patients, 82 patients had involvement of only the cerebrum at the initial diagnosis, whereas in seven patients only the cerebellum and the brainstem were involved. Seizures (n = 29) were the single most often reported symptom. The overall median survival time was 24 weeks. Women had a significantly longer survival with 36 weeks (3–196) compared to 17 weeks (1–159) for men [18]. Although these survival figures are poor, there is a view that aggressive treatment does palliate symptoms and prolong survival [19]. The diagnosis is confirmed by CT scan, and the immediate treatment is with oral dexamethasone to control the secondary oedema.

A single (or few) brain metastasis might be amenable to surgery or stereotactic radiotherapy, and it is unclear which is most effec-

tive. Surgical resection is preferred when a pathologic diagnosis is needed, for tumours larger than 3.5 cm or when immediate tumour mass decompression is required. Stereotactic radiosurgery (SRS) is the use of highly collimated beams of radiation to deliver high-dose radiotherapy to defined areas with rapid fall off into surrounding tissues; it should be applied for single tumours less than 3.5 cm in surgically inaccessible areas and for patients who are not surgical candidates. Small tumours (i.e. <3.5 cm) that cause minimal oedema and are surgically accessible may be treated with either surgery or SRS [19]. Both surgery and SRS are normally followed by whole-brain radiotherapy, although it is not clear how much benefit this gives, and neurocognitive late effects are a side effect. There is a view that the whole-brain radiotherapy increases local control but has no effect on survival [20] and in some centres it is therefore avoided.

For unresectable lesions or multiple lesions the options are radiotherapy or chemotherapy, neither of which are very effective. Radiotherapy is usually given as whole-brain radiotherapy, but SRS may be used. In a series of 244 patients given SRS for the management of 754 metastatic tumours, the median survival was 5.3 months (mean 10 months; range, 0.2–114.3 months) [21]. Sustained local control was achieved in 86.2% of tumours. Multiple lesions and failure to provide systemic immunotherapy were predictors for the occurrence of new brain metastases, which developed in 41.7% of the patients. Symptomatic radiation changes occurred in 6.6% of the patients. Overall, 71.4% of the patients improved or remained clinically stable. Whole-brain radiotherapy is usually delivered as a short course over 1 to 2 weeks.

Temozolomide is an oral alternative to dacarbazine for the treatment of metastatic melanoma; it penetrates the blood–brain barrier and is therefore preferred treatment for brain metastases [6], although it is not yet approved in many countries. The response rates are, however, low.

References

1 Eggermont AM. Current status of interferon-alpha in the treatment of melanoma. *Cancer Chemother Biol Response Modif* 2005; **22**: 729–37.

2 Gogas H, Ioannovich J, Dafni U *et al.* Prognostic significance of autoimmunity during treatment of melanoma with interferon. *N Engl J Med* 2006; **354**: 709–18.

3 Eggermont AM. Immunotherapy: Vaccine trials in melanoma—time for reflection. *Nat Rev Clin Oncol* 2009; **6**: 256–8.

4 Buzaid AC. Biochemotherapy for advanced melanoma. *Crit Rev Oncol Hematol* 2002; **44**: 103–8.

5 Sasse AD, Sasse EC, Clark LG *et al.* Chemoimmunotherapy versus chemotherapy for metastatic malignant melanoma. *Cochrane Database Syst Rev*: CD005413, 2007.

6 Quirbt I, Verma S, Petrella T *et al.* Temozolomide for the treatment of metastatic melanoma. *Curr Oncol* 2007; **14**: 27–33.

7 McDermott P, Lawson DS, Walczak R Jr *et al.* An isolated limb infusion technique: a guide for the perfusionist. *J Extra-corp Technol* 2005; **37**: 396–9.

8 Rossi CR, Foletto M, Pilati P *et al.* Isolated limb perfusion in locally advanced cutaneous melanoma. *Semin Oncol* 2002; **29**: 400–9.

9 Lens MB, Dawes M. Isolated limb perfusion with melphalan in the treatment of malignant melanoma of the extremities: a systematic review of randomised controlled trials. *Lancet Oncol* 2003; **4**: 359–64.

10 Knorr C, Meyer T, Janssen T *et al.* Hyperthermic isolated limb perfusion (HILP) in malignant melanoma. Experience with 101 patients. *Eur J Surg Oncol* 2006; **32**: 224–7.

11 Lejeune FJ, Eggermont AM. Hyperthermic isolated limb perfusion with tumor necrosis factor is a useful therapy for advanced melanoma of the limbs. *J Clin Oncol* 2007; **25**: 1449–50; author reply 1450–1.

12 Grunhagen DJ, de Wilt JH, van Geel AN, Eggermont AM. Isolated limb perfusion for melanoma patients—a review of its indications and the role of tumour necrosis factor-alpha. *Eur J Surg Oncol* 2006; **32**: 371–80.

13 Noorda EM, Vrouenraets BC, Nieweg OE *et al.* Repeat isolated limb perfusion with TNFalpha and melphalan for recurrent limb melanoma after failure of previous perfusion. *Eur J Surg Oncol* 2006; **32**: 318–24.

14 Bonenkamp JJ, Thompson JF, de Wilt JH *et al.* Isolated limb infusion with fotemustine after dacarbazine chemosensitisation for inoperable loco-regional melanoma recurrence. *Eur J Surg Oncol* 2004; **30**: 1107–12.

15 Thompson JF, Kam PC, Waugh RC, Harman CR. Isolated limb infusion with cytotoxic agents: a simple alternative to isolated limb perfusion. *Semin Surg Oncol* 1998; **14**: 238–47.

16 Lindner P, Doubrovsky A, Kam PC, Thompson JF. Prognostic factors after isolated limb infusion with cytotoxic agents for melanoma. *Ann Surg Oncol* 2002; **9**: 127–36.

17 Koops HS, Vaglini M, Suciu S *et al.* Prophylactic isolated limb perfusion for localized, high-risk limb melanoma: results of a multicenter randomized phase III trial. European Organization for Research and Treatment of Cancer Malignant Melanoma Cooperative Group Protocol 18832, the World Health Organization Melanoma Program Trial 15, and the North American Perfusion Group Southwest Oncology Group-8593. *J Clin Oncol* 1998; **16**: 2906–12.

18 Hofmann MA, Coll SH, Kuchler I *et al.* Prognostic factors and impact of treatment in melanoma brain metastases: better prognosis for women? *Dermatology* 2007; **215**: 10–6.

19 Peacock KH, Lesser GJ. Current therapeutic approaches in patients with brain metastases. *Curr Treat Options Oncol* 2006; **7**: 479–89.

20 Bafaloukos D, Gogas H. The treatment of brain metastases in melanoma patients. *Cancer Treat Rev* 2004; **30**: 515–20.

21 Mathieu D, Kondziolka D, Cooper PB *et al.* Gamma knife radiosurgery in the management of malignant melanoma brain metastases. *Neurosurgery* 2007; **60**: 471–81; discussion 481–2.

Radiotherapy

Malignant melanoma is traditionally regarded as a radioresistant tumour but it does have a role, particularly in palliation, and there is a view that it is underused [1]. The view that melanoma is radioresistant originated from radiobiological experiments, but a modern view is that melanomas have a wide range of sensitivities and that some are radiosensitive [1]. It is usually held that melanoma responds better to hypofractionation (larger, more infrequent doses) but this remains contested.

Radiotherapy has little part to play in the management of primary tumours, although it has been recorded in the past that the lentigo maligna melanoma variant is relatively radiosensitive, and radiotherapy has been used (low-energy electron or X-ray beams with limited penetration). It may be particularly useful where extensive disease occurs in difficult sites such as at the eyelid margin. However, data are inadequate to compare treatment modalities for lentigo maligna.

Radiotherapy may have palliative value for locoregional disease, which is not amenable to surgery. Radiotherapy can also be of considerable value in the palliation of metastatic disease in relieving pain from bony metastases.

There has been a persistent interest in postoperative adjuvant radiotherapy for Stage III melanoma, particularly where there is extracapsular spread and therefore an increased risk of local recurrence. The data on efficacy are interesting but are not based upon sufficiently large randomized clinical trials [2]. Stevens and McKay, however, have compared nodal basin relapse rates after surgery alone with those after radiotherapy and local recurrence did seem to be much lower when adjuvant radiotherapy is used [1], although the morbidity in terms of lymphoedema, for example, is increased. Randomized clinical trials are needed, and one trial began in 2002 in Australia and New Zealand.

References

1 Stevens G, McKay MJ. Dispelling the myths surrounding radiotherapy for treatment of cutaneous melanoma. *Lancet Oncol* 2006; **7**: 575–83.

2 O'Brien CJ, Petersen-Schaefer K, Stevens GN *et al.* Adjuvant radiotherapy following neck dissection and parotidectomy for metastatic malignant melanoma. *Head Neck* 1997; **19**: 589–94.

Melanoma, pregnancy and female sex hormones

Concern about the effect of pregnancy on outcome from melanoma began in 1951, when Pack and Scharnagel reviewed 32 cases of melanoma diagnosed during pregnancy reporting extremely poor prognosis due to the rapid development of metastases [1]. A number of studies subsequently, however, have not shown any adverse effect on outcome [2]. A large study based on a Swedish cancer registry of 185 women diagnosed with melanoma during pregnancy and 5348 women of the same childbearing age diagnosed with melanoma while not pregnant, showed no evidence of an adverse effect of pregnancy on survival, before or after diagnosis [3]. Clinicians often advise patients with thicker primaries to defer pregnancy after diagnosis, but this is social rather than medical, based upon waiting until the period during which metastasis is most likely has passed.

Placental and fetal metastasis of melanoma is a rare but well described phenomenon. In a review of published cases the risk of fetal disease in the presence of placental metastases was estimated to be 22% [4], so that examination of the placenta at delivery in patients with poor prognosis disease is sensible.

There is no evidence that the contraceptive pill has any effect on causation of melanoma [5] and none that hormone replacement therapy should be avoided [6].

References

1 Pack GT, Scharnagel IM. The prognosis for malignant melanoma in the pregnant woman. *Cancer* 1951; **4**: 324–34.

2 O'Meara AT, Cress R, Xing G *et al.* Malignant melanoma in pregnancy. A population-based evaluation. *Cancer* 2005; **103**: 1217–26.

3 Lens MB, Rosdahl I, Ahlbom A *et al.* Effect of pregnancy on survival in women with cutaneous malignant melanoma. *J Clin Oncol* 2004; **22**: 4369–75.

4 Alexander A, Samlowski WE, Grossman D *et al.* Metastatic melanoma in pregnancy: risk of transplacental metastases in the infant. *J Clin Oncol* 2003; **21**: 2179–86.

5 Karagas MR, Stukel TA, Dykes J *et al.* A pooled analysis of 10 case-control studies of melanoma and oral contraceptive use. *Br J Cancer* 2002; **86**: 1085–92.

6 Durvasula R, Ahmed SM, Vashisht A, Studd JW. Hormone replacement therapy and malignant melanoma: to prescribe or not to prescribe? *Climacteric* 2002; **5**: 197–200.

CHAPTER 55

Histiocytoses

A.C. Chu

Hammersmith Hospital, London, UK

The histiocytoses are a heterogeneous group of diseases that are characterized by the accumulation of reactive or neoplastic histiocytes in various tissues. Many of the signs and symptoms of the histiocytoses may be the result of the functional activity of histiocytoses, and which may also be important in the pathogenesis of these diseases (Fig. 55.1).

Ontogeny of the histiocyte

Synonym
• Tissue macrophage

Histiocytes are derived from circulating monocytes and thus share a common bone marrow progenitor cell, the *neutrophil/macrophage colony-forming unit* (NM-CFU; Fig. 55.2). Promonocytes are actively dividing cells and their replication is controlled by a series of stimulatory glycoprotein hormones, colony-stimulating factor (CSF) and inhibitory prostaglandins. Colony-stimulating factor has a molecular mass of 20–50 kDa. Its main source is cells of the monocyte/macrophage lineage [1] but activated T cells [2], keratinocytes [3] and neoplastic monocytes and macrophages [4] are also capable of secreting CSF. Cell division is limited by a negative feedback mechanism involving the E prostaglandins, which are released by macrophages after stimulation by CSF.

Other factors have been shown to influence the maturation of monocyte precursors, including 1,25-dihydroxyvitamin D_3 [5], retinoic acid [6], interferon-γ (IFN-γ) [7] and phorbol esters [8]. The promonocyte matures into a monocyte, which is released into the circulation where it represents a replacement pool for tissue macrophages or histiocytes. The half-life of a circulating monocyte is about 71 h [9], after which the cells migrate into various tissues where they differentiate into histiocytes without further division. Most histiocytes do not actively divide, although in some tissues, such as the lung, they are capable of replication [10].

The Langerhans' cell is a histiocytic cell that represents a resident immigrant population in the epidermis. It is an archetypal member of a subpopulation of histiocytic cells, the dendritic cells, which play key roles in various aspects of immunity. As with all histiocytic cells, Langerhans' cells are of bone marrow origin [11] and are ultimately derived from the haemopoietic stem cell. Haemopoietic stem cells can differentiate into myeloid or lymphoid-committed precursors and Langerhans' cells can differentiate through both lineages [12]. The intermediate stages of Langerhans' cell development are unknown, but a possible intermediate cell in the bone marrow has been identified, which, in common with the Langerhans' cell, expresses the CD1 complex [13]. In the blood of healthy individuals, CD1a cells are found in very low numbers, but in cord blood [14] and blood from burns patients [15] high levels of CD1a cells are observed. It is speculated that these represent immature Langerhans' cells.

The factors that control the migration and development of Langerhans' cells in the skin are not fully understood. Langerhans' cell precursors express the cutaneous leukocyte antigen (CLA), a glycosylated form of p-selectin which acts as a homing molecule for the skin and express CCR6, the receptor for the chemokine CCL20 which is produced by epidermal keratinocytes [16]. Granulocyte/macrophage CSF (GM-CSF), interleukin (IL)-3 and tumour necrosis factor-α (TNF-α) all induce CD34 cells to

Rook's Textbook of Dermatology, 8th edition. Edited by DA Burns,
SM Breathnach, NH Cox and CEM Griffiths. © 2010 Blackwell Publishing Ltd.

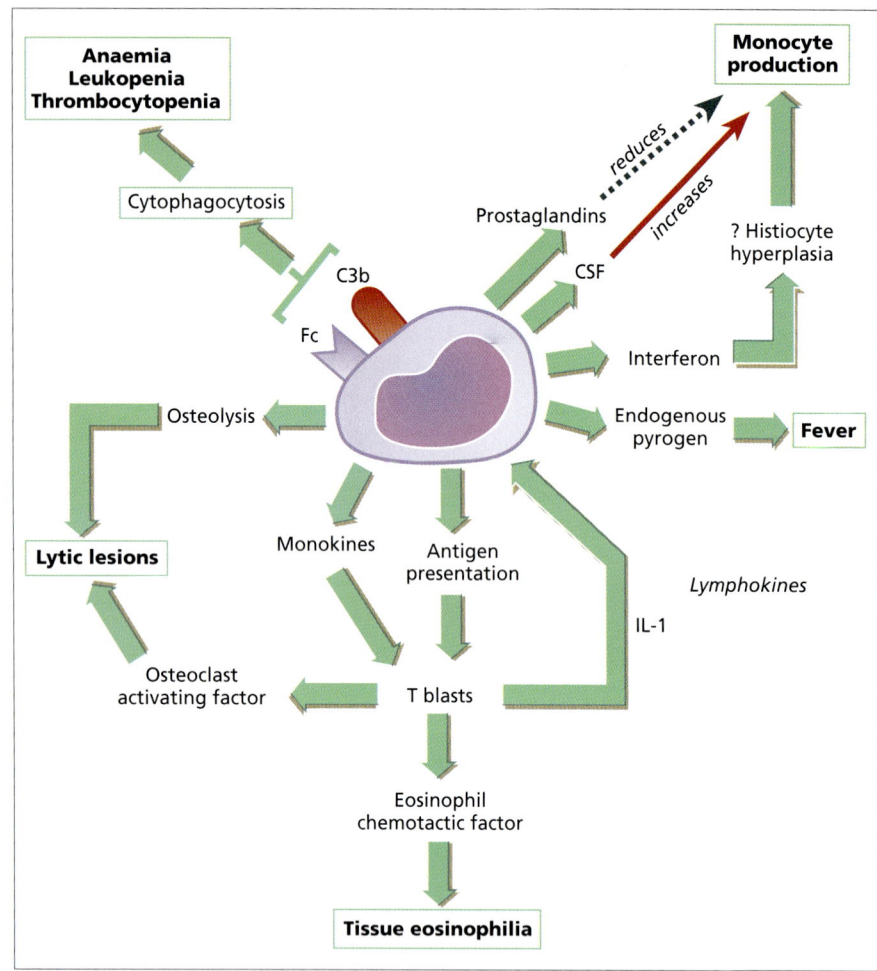

Fig. 55.1 Alteration in histiocyte function causing symptoms of the histiocytoses. CSF, colony-stimulating factor; C3b, complement 3b; Fc, heavy chain fragment of immunoglobulin; IL-1, interleukin-1; T blasts, thymus-derived lymphoblasts.

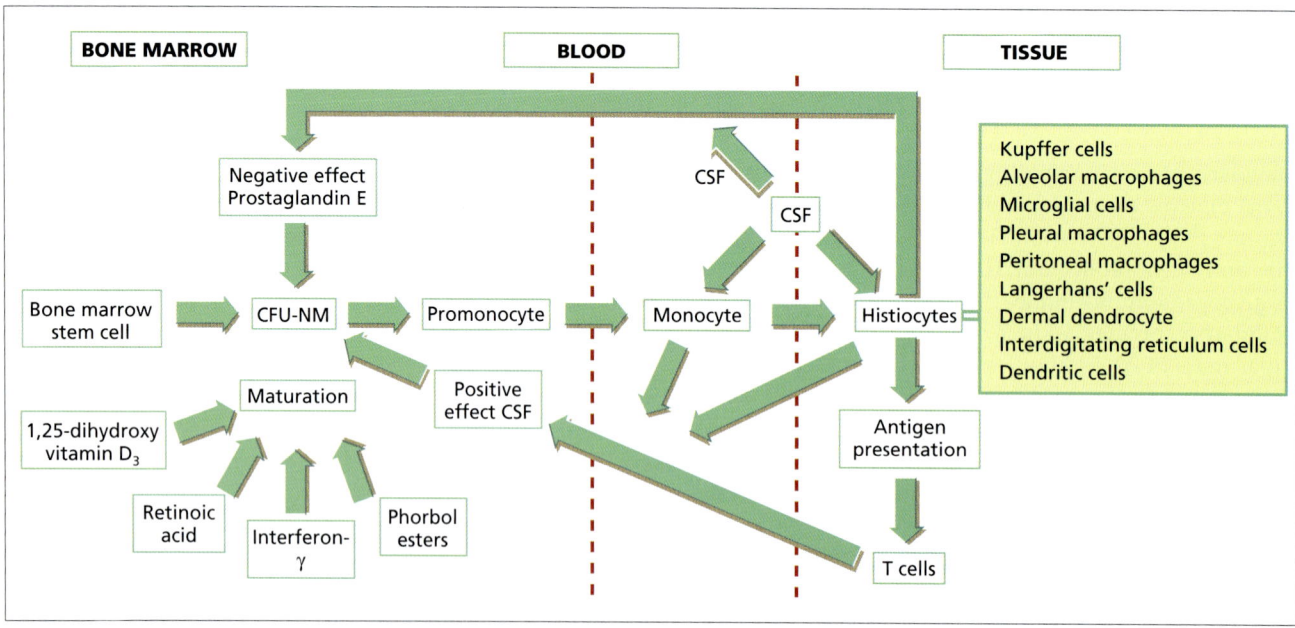

Fig. 55.2 Ontogeny of histiocytes showing factors that can influence the division and maturation of the cells. CFU-NM, neutrophil/macrophage colony-forming unit; CSF, colony-stimulating factor.

Table 55.1 Surface markers of Langerhans' cell (LC), activated LC and LC histiocytosis (LCH) cells.

Marker	LC	Activated LC	LCH cells
Surface ATPase	+	+	+
MHC II	+	+	+
MHC I	±	±	±
FcIgG receptor	+	+	+
FcIgE receptor	+	+	?
C3bi receptor	+	+	+
CD1a and CD1c	+	+	+
CD4	±	+	+
CD45	+	+	+
CD14	+	+	?
CDw29	+	+	?
IL-2 receptor	–	+	+
Langerin (CD207)	+	+	+
E-cadherin	+	–	–
Fascin	–	+	+
B7 (CD80, 86)	–	+ (cultured)	+
CD11b and CD11c	+	+	+
S100	+	+	+
Placental alkaline phosphatase	–	+ (transient)	+
Peanut agglutinin	–	–	+
IFN-γ receptor	–	–	+
Neurone-specific enolase	+	+	+
Birbeck granule	+	±	+

ATPase, adenosine triphosphatase; IFN, interferon; IL, interleukin; MHC, major histocompatibility complex.

develop the phenotypic features of Langerhans' cells. Caux *et al.* [17] generated CD1a cells from CD34 bone marrow cells using GM-CSF and TNF-α. The cells demonstrated potent antigen-presenting function. However, further research has shown that the whole field of Langerhans' cells ontogeny is more complex. Studies have now shown that GM-CSF will induce expression of CD1a, CD1b and CD1c by blood monocytes [18]. *In vitro*, human monocytes can differentiate into dendritic cells with some characteristics of Langerhans' cells on culture with GM-CSF, IL4 and TGF-β [19]. CD34+ bone marrow cells can be induced to differentiate into Langerhans' cells with GM-CSF and TNF-α [20], IL3 and TNF-α [21], or FMS-like tyrosine kinase-3 (FLT3) ligand and transforming growth factor-β (TGF-β) [22]. A possible immediate precursor of epidermal Langerhans' cell in the epidermis is the *indeterminate cell* [23], which bears a Langerhans' cell surface phenotype but lacks the characteristic Birbeck granule (see Chapter 3 and section on the phenotype of Langerhans' cells below).

Within the epidermis, Langerhans' cells are immature, able to process antigen but do not express the co-stimulatory molecules CD80 and CD86 unless activated and are poor antigen-presenting cells. Maturation and migration out of the epidermis can be stimulated by a wide variety of signals including TNF-α and IL1β, CD40 ligand, microbial products and ultraviolet radiation. Langerhans' cells down-regulate CD1a, express CD80 and CD86, lose CCR6 expression and express CCR7 which directs migration to the lymphatics and regional lymph nodes. The fate of Langerhans' cells after their development in the skin is speculative. Some authors

maintain that Langerhans' cells migrate from the skin in the efferent lymphatics as *veiled cells* and eventually develop into *interdigitating reticulum cells* in the paracortical zone of the regional lymph nodes. If Langerhans' cells are cultured *in vitro*, they lose their characteristic phenotype and adopt an interdigitating reticulum cell phenotype [24]; this phenomenon has been proposed as evidence for their extraepidermal differentiation. However, the *in vitro* culture conditions are unphysiological, and it is more probable that Langerhans' cell, veil cell and interdigitating cell are related but differentiate separately from an early common progenitor cell series.

Dermal dendrocytes, first described by Headington in 1986 [25], are highly dendritic interstitial cells of the papillary and reticular dermis. They are positive for adenosine triphosphatase (ATPase), α-napthylbutyrate esterase, β-glucuronidase and acid phosphatase, indicating they are of monocyte/macrophage lineage. They are also phagocytic *in vivo*, showing melanin and haemosiderin phagocytosis. Dermal dendrocytes are of bone marrow origin and are thought to have a possible role in phagocytosis, antigen presentation or in homeostasis of macromolecules of the dermis [26]. Elegant computer-assisted three-dimensional reconstruction of dermal dendrocytes in adult human skin has shown that in those associated with superficial blood vessels, the dendrites are thin, membrane-bound flaps that enshroud the vessel wall. In subepidermal dermal dendrocytes, the flap-like dendrites are parallel to the dermal–epidermal junction. Twenty to 40% of perivascular and some subepidermal dermal dendrocytes are closely associated with mast cells, their membrane flaps enshrouding 50–90% of the surface of the mast cell [27].

Phenotype of Langerhans' cells

For many years after the original description of Langerhans' cells [28], this epidermal clear cell was considered to be an effete melanocyte. Significant interest was generated by the finding that Langerhans' cells express a number of surface molecules, which suggested immunological importance. These molecules include major histocompatibility complex (MHC) class II molecules (which are constitutively expressed by Langerhans' cells), FcIgG receptors and C3b receptor. Langerhans' cells also express the chemokine receptors CCR5 and CCR6. A full list of the phenotypic markers of Langerhans' cells is given in Table 55.1.

A major advance was the finding that epidermal Langerhans' cells expressed the CD1 complex [29], previously considered to be restricted to cortical thymocytes. CD1 is a group of non-polymorphic membrane glycoproteins that non-covalently bind to β2-microglobulin. Five genes have been identified and cloned [30]. Four molecules have been described: CD1a, CD1b, CD1c and CD1d [31]. CD1a and CD1c are expressed by Langerhans' cells and may play a role in presenting lipid antigen to T cells [32]. Langerhans' cells have since been shown to express other molecules, identified by antibodies to CD4 and CD25, which were initially thought to be specific for lymphocytes.

The unique phenotypic feature of Langerhans' cells is the trilaminate cytoplasmic organelle, the *Birbeck granule* [33]. This organelle is only observed in Langerhans' cells, Langerhans' cell histiocytosis (LCH) cells (which are abnormal Langerhans' cells) and some hairy cell leukaemia cells. The granules are rod-shaped structures with a central lamella. They are of uniform width (33 nm) and of variable length (200–360 nm). The granules often have terminal vesicular dilations, giving rise to the characteristic 'tennis racket' appearance. The Birbeck granule was initially thought to originate from the Golgi apparatus, but studies now suggest that it arises from the cytoplasmic membrane by receptor-specific endocytosis [34]. Lag is an antigen expressed on Birbeck granules and anti-Lag antibodies can be used to identify Langerhans' cells [35].

The phenotype of the Langerhans' cell changes with activation or with culture *in vitro*. Activation involves up-regulation of human leukocyte antigen (HLA)-DR and expression of CD4 and the co-stimulatory molecules CD80 and CD86 [36]. At the same time, Birbeck granules become sparser and CD1a is down-regulated (see Table 55.1).

Phenotype of the dermal dendrocyte

In addition to showing the enzyme histochemical features of the monocyte/macrophage lineage, a characteristic feature of dermal dendrocytes is expression of factor XIIIa. The cells are always negative for CD1a, which differentiates them from Langerhans' cells, and express HLA-DR, HLA-DQ, CD36, CD68, CD34, CD11a and CD11b but neither CD15, CD54 nor CD2. Thus, they show the immunophenotype of monocyte/macrophages and antigen-presenting cells, with no features of granulocytes or T cells [37]. Following stimulation with IFN-γ, the expression of HLA-DR increases and dermal dendrocytes express CD54. In atopic dermatitis and psoriasis, cells positive for factor XIIIa, HLA-DR and CD54 are observed in the upper dermis and foci of factor XIIIa-positive cells are seen in the epidermis [37].

Dermal dendrocytes have been shown to express S100A6 [38] and type XVI collagen [39]. CD14 peripheral blood monocytes stimulated with GM-CSF and IL-4 express factor XIIIa [40] and collagen XVI [39]. It is postulated that type XVI collagen forms an intermolecular cross-link through its non-collagenous domain, contributing to the integrity of factor XIIIa.

Dermal dendrocytes also express the von Willebrand factor receptor GPIbα. Expression of this factor *in vitro* is up-regulated by mast cell degranulation [41]. Expression of GPIbα on dermal dendrocytes suggests that these cells may have a role in skin remodelling and repair.

The fate of dermal dendrocytes is unknown. The factors that influence maturation of these cells include mast cell products, although *in vitro* studies using TNF-α have failed to demonstrate up-regulation of GPIbα on factor XIIIa-positive cells [42]. When skin is maintained in organ culture, dermal dendrocytes lose their dendritic morphology and become more rounded. This change is accentuated by mast cell degranulation, regardless of stimulus. These non-dendritic cells express variable amounts of factor XIIIa, CD34 and CD68.

Function of the histiocyte

Histiocytes can be broadly divided into two functionally separate cell populations: the 'professional' phagocyte; and the antigen-presenting cell.

Phagocytes include the majority of resident tissue macrophages and immature macrophages. Immature macrophages are cells that have migrated, as monocytes, from the blood but remain responsive to chemotactic stimuli and are attracted to sites of inflammation where they become inflammatory macrophages. Phagocytes take up foreign or altered material and digest it using a number of lysosomal enzymes, they also recognize material to be taken up by a variety of different cell-surface receptors. Important in this are the carbohydrate and lectin receptors, which are involved in the phagocytosis of bacteria and possibly tumour cells. The cells also express the specific complement component receptors CR1 and CR3, which bind to C3b and C3bi respectively, and FcIgG receptors, which bind to the Fc fragment of IgG. These receptors are important in the phagocytosis of material that has bound IgG and complement, which act as opsonins and augment phagocytosis.

Phagocytosis is important in the removal of particulate matter and destruction of bacteria and parasites. The phagocytosed particles are internalized and destroyed in phagolysosomes. Partially degraded antigen may subsequently become associated with MHC class II antigens and be re-expressed on the surface of a macrophage, where it can be presented to T-helper cells.

Phagocytes also possess some antigen-presenting capacity, although this is limited—cells express class II MHC molecules and can process and re-express antigen on their surface in association with these specific molecules, but only elicit responses in specific responder T-cell populations. In general, phagocytes present antigen to sensitized T cells but not to naïve or 'memory' T cells.

Antigen-presenting cells are histiocytic cells, or in some instances other cell types, that have specialized functional activity in presenting antigen to T cells. These cells are represented in humans by the blood dendritic cell, epidermal Langerhans' cell, interdigitating reticulum cell of the lymph node paracortex and veil cell of the efferent lymph. These cells have no phagocytic activity and, unlike professional phagocytes, are unable to adhere to surfaces. They are able to internalize antigen by endocytosis, process it by lysosomal digestion and re-express the antigen on their surface in association with MHC class II molecules. In addition, these cells are potent antigen-presenting cells and are able to present antigen not only to sensitized T cells but also to memory and naïve T cells, and are also able to present self antigen to allogeneic T cells to elicit an allogeneic or mixed-cell reaction [43].

Langerhans' cells are central to the regulation of contact allergic dermatitis, responsible for cutaneous immune surveillance and the target for skin graft rejection [44]. Epidermal Langerhans' cells are immature but, following stimulation, they migrate from epidermis to lymphatics and thus to the regional lymph nodes, and during this process undergo maturation. The signals that initiate and regulate the directed movement of Langerhans' cells from skin to regional lymph nodes include chemokines and cytokines. In cutaneous sensitization, TNF-α, GM-CSF, IL-1β and IL-18 are required, while IL-4 and IL-10 antagonize this process [45,46]. Maturation of Langerhans' cells is accompanied by specific phenotypic changes, with up-regulation of HLA-DR, down-regulation of CD1a, and expression of CD4 and CD25. There is a switch in chemokine receptor expression from CCR5 and CCR6 to CCR7 and CXCR4, which enables Langerhans' cells to exit the epidermis and follow a gradient of chemokines (CCL19, CCL21 and CXCL12) to the paracortical zone of the lymph nodes [47]. Langerhans' cells also express other activation markers, including CD83 and CD40 and the T-cell co-stimulatory molecules CD80 and CD86 [48].

References

1 Golde DW, Finley TN, Cline MJ. Production of colony stimulating factor by human macrophages. *Lancet* 1972; **ii**: 1397–9.

2 Cline M, Golde DW. Production of colony-stimulating activity by human lymphocytes. *Nature* 1974; **248**: 703–4.

3 Mann A, Breuhahn K, Schirmacher P *et al.* Keratinocyte derived granulocyte-macrophage colony stimulating factor accelerates wound healing: stimulation of keratinocyte proliferation, granulation tissue formation and vascularisation. *J Invest Dermatol* 2001; **117**: 1382–90.

4 Golde DW, Rothman B, Cline MJ. Production of colony stimulating factor by malignant leukocytes. *Blood* 1974; **43**: 749–56.

5 Amento EP, Bhalla AK, Kurnick JT. 1-Alpha, 25-dihydroxyvitamin D3 induces maturation of the human monocyte cell line U937 and, in association with a factor from human T lymphocytes, augments production of the monokine, mononuclear cell factor. *J Clin Invest* 1984; **73**: 731–9.

6 Abita JP, Gauville C, Balitrand N. Binding of ^{125}I-insulin to the human histio-cytic lymphoma cell line U-937: effect of differentiation with retinoic acid. *Leuk Res* 1984; **2**: 213–21.

7 Griffin JD, Sabbath KD, Hermann F *et al.* Differential expression of HLA-DR antigen in subsets of human CFU-GM. *Blood* 1985; **66**: 788–95.

8 Nilsson K, Andersson LC, Gahmberg CG *et al.* Differentiation *in vitro* of human leukaemia and lymphoma cell lines. In: Serrou B, Rosenfeld C, eds. *International Symposium on New Trends in Human Immunology and Cancer Immunotherapy.* Paris: Doin, 1980: 271–92.

9 Van Furth R. Development of mononuclear phagocytes. In: Forster O, Landy M, eds. *Heterogeneity of Mononuclear Phagocytes.* London: Academic Press, 1981: 323–69.

10 Evans MJ, Sherman MP, Campbell LA *et al.* Proliferation of pulmonary alveolar macrophages during postnatal development of rabbit lungs. *Am Rev Respir Dis* 1987; **136**: 384–7.

11 Katz SI, Tamaki K, Sachs DH. Epidermal Langerhans cells are derived from cells originating in bone marrow. *Nature* 1979; **282**: 324–6.

12 Takeuchi S, Furue M. Dendritic cells—Ontogeny. *Allergol Internat* 2007; **56**: 215–23.

13 de Fraissinette A, Dezutter-Dambuyant C, Schmitt D *et al.* Cultured bone marrow myelomonocyte CD1 positive cells: are they Langerhans cell progenitors? *Coll Inserm* 1988; **172**: 41–53.

14 Griffiths-Chu S, Patterson J, Berger C *et al.* Characterization of immature T cell subpopulations in neonatal blood. *Blood* 1984; **64**: 296–300.

15 Gothelf Y, Hanau D, Sharon N *et al.* Precursors of Langerhans cells of the skin can be identified in the peripheral blood of burns patients. *J Invest Dermatol* 1986; **87**: 141.

16 Bartz H, Rothoeft T, Anhenn O *et al.* Large scale isolation of immature dendritic cells with features of Langerhans' cells by sorting CD34+ cord blood stem cells cultured in the presence of TGF-beta1 for cutaneous leukocyte antigen (CLA). *J Immunol Methods* 2003; **275**: 137–48.

17 Caux C, Dezutter-Dambuyant C, Schmitt D *et al.* GM-CSF and TNFα cooperate in the generation of dendritic Langerhans cells. *Nature* 1992; **360**: 258–61.

18 Kasinrerk W, Baumruker T, Majdic O *et al.* CD1 molecule expression on human monocytes induced by granulocyte-macrophage colony stimulating factor. *J Immunol* 1993; **150**: 579–84.

19 Sallusto F, Lanzavecchia A. Efficient presentation of soluble antigen by cultured human dendritic cells is maintained by granulocyte/macrophage colony-stimulating factor plus interleukin 4 and down regulated by tumour necrosis factor alpha. *J Exp Med* 1994; **179**: 1109–18.

20 Caux C, Vanbervliet B, Massacrier C *et al.* CD34+ hematopoietic progenitors from human cord blood differentiate along two independent dendritic cell pathways in response to GM-CSF + TNF alpha. *J Exp Med* 1996; **184**: 695–706.

21 Caux C, Vanbervliet B, Massacrier C *et al.* Interleukin 3 cooperates with tumour necrosis factor alpha for the development of human dendritic/Langerhans cells from cord blood CD34+ hematopoietic progenitor cells. *Blood* 1996; **87**: 2376–85.

22 Strobl H, Riedl E, Scheinecker C *et al.* TGF-beta 1 promotes in vitro development of dendritic cells from CD34+ hematopoietic progenitors. *J Immunol* 1996; **157**: 1499–507.

23 Chu A, Eisinger M, Lee JS *et al.* Immunoelectronmicroscopic identification of Langerhans cells using a new antigenic marker. *J Invest Dermatol* 1982; **28**: 177–80.

24 Romani N, Lenz A, Glossel H *et al.* Cultured human Langerhans cells resemble lymphoid dendritic cells in phenotype and function. *J Invest Dermatol* 1989; **93**: 600–9.

25 Headington JT. The dermal dendrocyte. *Adv Dermatol* 1986; **1**: 159–71.

26 Hoyo E, Kanitakis J, Schmitt D. The dermal dendrocyte. *Pathol Biol (Paris)* 1993; **41**: 613–8.

27 Sueki H, Telegan B, Murphy GF. Computer-assisted three-dimensional reconstruction of human dermal dendrocytes. *J Invest Dermatol* 1995; **105**: 704–8.

28 Langerhans P. Uber die Nerven der menschlichen Haut. *Virchows Arch (Pathol Anat Physiol)* 1868; **44**: 325–31.

29 Fithian E, Kung P, Goldstein G *et al.* Reactivity of Langerhans cells with hybridoma antibody. *Proc Natl Acad Sci USA* 1981; **78**: 2541–4.

30 Martin LH, Calabri F, Milstein C. Isolation of CD1 genes: a family of major histiocompatibility complex-related differentiation antigens. *Proc Natl Acad Sci USA* 1980; **83**: 9154–8.

31 Chu AC, Jaffe R. The normal Langerhans cell and the LCH cell. *Br J Cancer* 1994; **70**: S4–S10.

32 Zajonc DM, Crispin MD, Bowden TA *et al.* Molecular mechanism of lipopeptide presentation by CD1a. *Immunity* 2005; **22**: 209–19.

33 Birbeck MS, Breathnach AS, Everall JD. An electronmicroscopic study of basal melanocytes and high level clear cells (Langerhans cells) in vitiligo. *J Invest Dermatol* 1961; **37**: 51–64.

34 Hanau D, Gothelf Y, Fabre M *et al.* Internalisation of T6 (CD1) antigen in a subset of human cord blood mononuclear cells expressing T6 surface antigen. *J Invest Dermatol* 1986; **87**: 143.

35 Kashihara M, Ueda M, Huriguchi Y *et al.* A monoclonal antibody specifically reactive to human Langerhans cells. *J Invest Dermatol* 1986; **87**: 602–8.

36 Symington FW, Brady W, Linsley PS. Expression and function of B7 on human epidermal Langerhans cells. *J Immunol* 1993; **150**: 1286–95.

37 Cerio R, Griffiths CEM, Cooper KD *et al.* Characterization of factor XIIIa positive dermal dendritic cells in normal and inflamed skin. *Br J Dermatol* 1989; **121**: 421–31.

38 Fullen DR, Reed JA, Finnerty B, McNutt NS. S100A6 expression in fibrohistio-cytic lesions. *J Cutan Pathol* 2001; **28**: 229–34.

39 Akagi A, Tajima S, Ishibashi A *et al.* Type XVI collagen is expressed in a factor XIIIa monocyte derived dermal dendrocytes and constitutes a potential substrate for factor XIIIa. *J Invest Dermatol* 2002; **118**: 267–74.

40 Young DA, Lowe LD, Clark SC. Comparison of the effects of IL-3, granulocyte-macrophage colony-stimulating factor, and macrophage colony-stimulating factor in supporting monocyte differentiation in culture. *J Immunol* 1990; **145**: 607–15.

41 Monteiro MR, Shapiro SS, Takafuta T *et al.* Von Willebrand factor receptor GPIbα is expressed by human factor XIIIa-positive dermal dendrocytes and is upregulated by mast cell degranulation. *J Invest Dermatol* 1999; **113**: 272–6.

42 Monteiro MR, Murphy EE, Galaria NA *et al.* Cytological alterations in dermal dendrocytes *in vitro*: evidence for transformation to a non-dendritic phenotype. *Br J Dermatol* 2000; **143**: 84–90.

43 Austyn JM. Lymphoid dendritic cells. *Immunology* 1987; **62**: 161–70.

44 Wolff K, Stingl G. The Langerhans cell. *J Invest Dermatol* 1983; **80**: 17s–21s.

45 Cumberbatch M, Dearman RJ, Griffiths CEM, Kimber I. Langerhans cell migration. *Clin Exp Dermatol* 2000; **25**: 413–8.

46 Kimber I, Cumberbatch M, Dearman RJ *et al.* Cytokines and chemokines in the initiation and regulation of epidermal Langerhans cell migration. *Br J Dermatol* 2000; **142**: 401–12.

47 Sallusto F, Schaerli P, Loetscher P *et al.* A rapid and co-ordinated switch in chemokine receptor expression during dendritic cell maturation. *Eur J Immunol* 1998; **28**: 2760–9.

48 Bjorck P, Flores Romo L, Liu YJ. Human interdigitating dendritic cells directly stimulate CD40 activating naïve B cells. *Eur J Immunol* 1997; **27**: 1266–74.

Classification of the histiocytoses

Understanding of the histiocytoses has been severely hampered by the lack of a universally accepted classification of these diseases and the widespread use of eponyms to describe them. For these reasons, the Histiocyte Society published their classification of the histiocytoses for use as a standard in both diagnosis and management [1]. This classification has been generally accepted and is now widely used. In this chapter the original classification has been modified in the light of new insights into reactive histiocytoses of dermal dendrocyte phenotype. The histiocytoses are separated into four classes according to our current understanding of the biology of these diseases.

Class I: Langerhans' cell histiocytosis (LCH)

Class I histiocytoses are a diverse group of clinical diseases that are all reactive histiocytoses in which the predominant histiocyte is of Langerhans' cell phenotype. Patients with LCH can be further subdivided on the basis of the clinical organ involvement present. Bone disease and lung disease in adults appear to be significantly different in their biology from other single-system involvement and it is valid to separate them. The significance of organ involvement is discussed further in the section on LCH.

Class IIa: histiocytoses involving cells of the dermal dendrocyte lineage

Class IIa histiocytoses are reactive diseases in which cells with the phenotype of the dermal dendrocyte (positive for CD68 and factor XIIIa) accumulate in the skin and other tissues causing tissue damage. The typical histological change is a xanthogranulomatous reaction, although the histological changes reflect the cell type present. Juvenile xanthogranuloma is typical of this group of diseases, and some of the conditions described may not be specific disease entities but clinical variants of a single disease. These diseases are reactive with no clinical evidence of malignancy.

Class IIb: histiocytoses involving cells other than Langerhans' cells and dermal dendrocytes

Class IIb histiocytoses are reactive diseases in which histiocytes other than those bearing the Langerhans' cell or dermal dendrocyte phenotype accumulate in various tissues and may cause tissue damage. Within this heterogeneous group of diseases are included a number of rare and often poorly understood disorders. The major features of all these histiocytoses are that they are reactive, with no clinical or laboratory evidence of malignancy, and that Langerhans' cells and related cells are not involved.

Class III: malignant histiocytic disorders

Class III histiocytoses include all the malignant histiocytic diseases. These include monocytic leukaemias, malignant histiocytosis, which may be of the mononuclear phagocyte, dendritic cell or Langerhans' cell type, and the true histiocytic lymphoma, which once again may be of the mononuclear phagocyte, dendritic or Langerhans' cell type.

Reference

1 Chu A, D'Angio G, Favara B *et al.* Histiocytosis syndromes in children. *Lancet* 1987; **i**: 208–9.

Class I histiocytosis: Langerhans' cell histiocytosis

Synonyms
- Histiocytosis X
- Eosinophilic granuloma
- Letterer–Siwe disease
- Hand–Schüller–Christian syndrome
- Hashimoto–Pritzker syndrome
- Self-healing histiocytosis
- Pure cutaneous histiocytosis
- Langerhans' cell granulomatosis
- Type II histiocytosis
- Non-lipid reticuloendotheliosis

Definition. LCH is a reactive condition in which a clonal population of cells with the phenotype of the Langerhans' cell accumulate in various tissues and cause damage. Tissue damage appears to be due, in part, to cytokine production.

Aetiology. The aetiology of LCH is unknown but over the last century several possibilities have been considered, including tuberculosis [1] and a lipid abnormality [2,3]. The discovery of Birbeck granules in the cytoplasm of lesional cells using electron microscopy [4] led to the suggestion that these cytoplasmic bodies could be viral inclusion bodies and that LCH could be a virally mediated disease [5]. However, a large retrospective study on the fulminant form of LCH showed a random geographical distribution and little month-to-month variation in the incidence of the disease, which argued against it being due to a conventional virus [6]. A study of 56 LCH tissue samples using *in situ* hybridization and polymerase chain reaction (PCR) analysis failed to show any consistent evidence of adenovirus, cytomegalovirus, herpesvirus, parvovirus, human T-cell virus or human immunodeficiency virus infection [7].

The possibility of an immunological aetiology for LCH has been suggested by the occurrence of a number of immunological abnormalities in this disease. The fact that the lesional cell bears the phenotype of the Langerhans' cell, which is a key cell in the immune system, also suggests that the immune system is in some way involved in its pathogenesis. However, none of the immunological abnormalities have been a consistent feature, and most authors now consider them to be epiphenomena.

Serum immunoglobulins may be increased or decreased. The most common finding is that of reduced IgA and IgG levels, with normal IgE and IgM levels. In some reported cases, IgE and IgM levels were elevated [8].

In some patients, particularly those with aggressive disease, cutaneous anergy has been found on cutaneous testing, and *in vitro* studies have shown reduced T-cell responses to mitogens, recall antigens and alloantigens [9]. A reasonably consistent feature in three reported series of LCH [10–12] is a reduction of the CD8 T-cell subpopulation in the blood, with an associated normal or reduced total T-cell number. In one report [12], this reduction in the number of CD8 cells was associated with reduced suppressor T-cell activity *in vitro*.

Considering that Langerhans' cells are members of the monocyte/macrophage series of cells, very few abnormalities of this group of cells have been reported. Reduced monocyte-mediated, antibody-dependent cytotoxicity occurred in six patients with LCH, all of whom were in clinical remission [13]. This certainly warrants further study. LCH cells are unable to provide accessory cell function in a mitogen-driven T-cell response, and are inhibitory to T-cell proliferative responses [14]. Only one study has investigated the functional activity of LCH cells in depth [15]. In this report, LCH cells were shown to be functionally deficient in presenting alloantigen to T cells. It is possible that the defect in functional activity may be linked with the apparent arrest of these cells in an early stage of activation, leaving the cells immature so that they do not have the functional capacity of a normal Langerhans' cell.

Historically, LCH has been considered a malignant disease, and care of children with the disease has been in the hands of paediatric oncologists. The main reason for this is the clinical course and high mortality associated with the more fulminant forms of LCH. Flow cytometric studies have in general failed to identify aneuploidy in LCH [16,17]. In one report of an adult case with clinically and histologically confirmed LCH involving the skin, flow cytometry revealed an aneuploid peak [18]. Many features of this case were unusual and it is possible that the patient had the rare form of malignant histiocytosis of Langerhans' cell type.

Studies have demonstrated that lesional CD1a cells in LCH are clonal. Clonality studies in LCH have been difficult to perform because of the lack of cell-specific markers. Unlike the T-cell receptor in T cells and immunoglobulins in B cells, histiocytic cells have no markers that can be employed in such studies. The study of genes carried on the X chromosome have now allowed such studies in female patients with this disease. Of the gene loci examined, the human androgen receptor (HUMARA) is the most informative as there is a high degree of heterogeneity for this locus in the population. The underlying theory behind the assay is that the two alleles for HUMARA are acquired from maternal and paternal genes, each of which is a different size because of the presence of tandem repeats. Only one allele is activated, the other being inactivated by methylation, and the use of methylation-sensitive restriction enzymes in PCR allows the inactivated allele to be expanded and identified. In a normal population of cells, activation of the alleles is random so that 50% are derived from maternal and 50% from paternal genes, giving two bands on gel electrophoresis. In a clonal population of cells, all cells are derived from a single cell and therefore all these cells will have an inactivated allele, which is either maternal or paternal, giving a single band on gel electrophoresis. In a study of four female patients with LCH, purified lesional CD1a cells were shown to be clonal using this assay system [19]. Studies by Willman et al. [20] have confirmed these studies and shown that lesional cells are clonal regardless of the extent or severity of the disease. In isolated pulmonary LCH in adults, a study using X chromosome inactivation at the HUMARA locus has shown that 29% were clonal and 71% non-clonal. Discrete lung nodules from the same patient showed different allele inactivation [21]. Pulmonary LCH in adults is often an isolated disease that may remain restricted to the lungs and thus behaves in a different way biologically compared to other forms of LCH. It is possible that primary lung disease is a separate entity and only when it progresses to involve other organs does it become a clonal disease.

What clonality in LCH means is difficult to interpret. It certainly identifies the LCH cell as the primary cell in this disease but this does not mean that LCH is a malignancy. Many reactive diseases, for example lymphomatoid papulosis, have been shown to be clonal. Although of major interest, such studies have thus not altered our management of patients with this disease, nor have they identified the disease as malignant.

Pathology. The histological picture of LCH depends on the age of the lesion biopsied and the organ involved. The pathology of LCH was reviewed by the Histiocyte Society in 1987 [22], who recommended three levels of diagnostic confidence. A presumptive diagnosis is made when the histological appearance of the biopsy is consistent with the diagnosis of LCH. Diagnostic confidence increases if marker studies are performed and lesional cells are found to be positive for S100 protein, peanut agglutinin or α-D-mannosidase. If lesional cells are found to express the CD1 complex or to exhibit Birbeck granules on electron microscopy (Fig. 55.3), this constitutes a definitive diagnosis.

The characteristic histological appearance of LCH in the skin is of an upper dermal and junctional accumulation of large histiocytic cells with homogeneous pink cytoplasm. These cells have

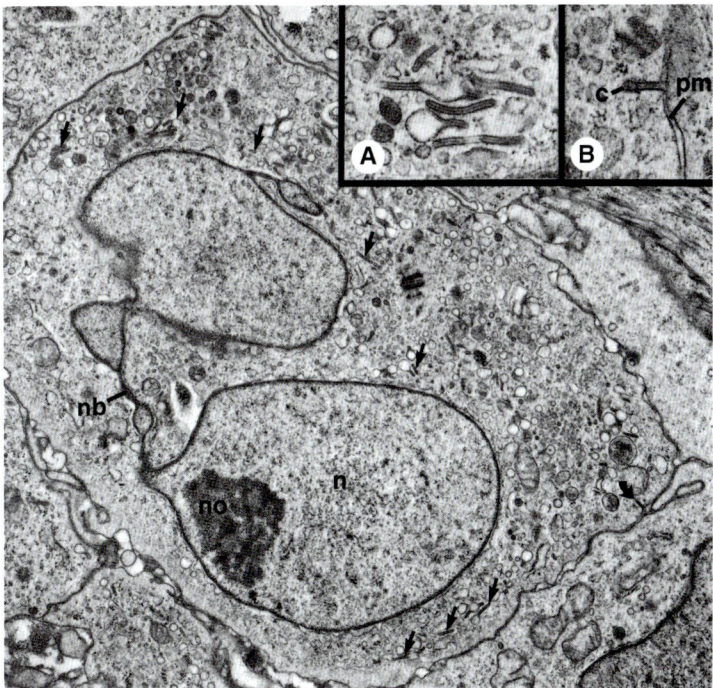

Fig. 55.3 Electron micrograph of a Langerhans' cell histiocytosis (LCH) cell in the epidermis of a patient with multisystem LCH. The cell shows a lobulated nucleus (n) with a prominent nucleolus (no) and attenuated nuclear bridge (nb). Numerous Birbeck granules (straight arrows) are evident in the cytoplasm. One granule (curved arrow) is seen projecting from the plasma membrane (× 13 000). (A) Birbeck granule in the cytoplasm. Some show characteristic vesiculation of the end, forming typical tennis-racket bodies. (B) Birbeck granules appear to be budding from the plasma membrane (pm) (× 39 000). (Courtesy of Professor R.A.J. Eady, St John's Dermatology Centre, London, UK.)

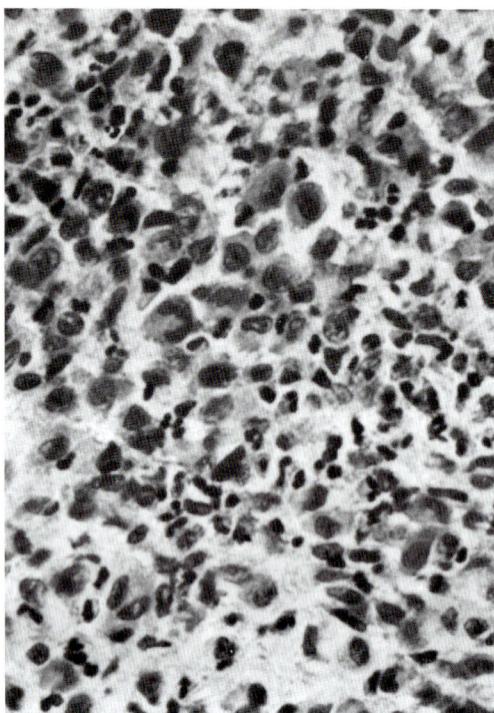

Fig. 55.4 Langerhans' cell histiocytosis cells in the dermis intermingled with polymorphs and eosinophils (H&E × 250). (Courtesy of Professor E. Wilson Jones, St John's Dermatology Centre, London, UK.)

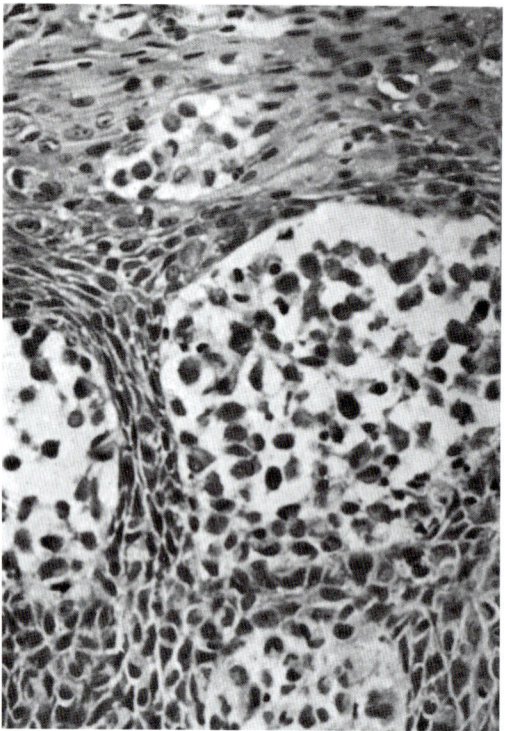

Fig. 55.5 Langerhans' cell histiocytosis (LCH). Details of a papillary tip containing LCH cells, with a small intraepidermal abscess overlying it (H&E × 250). (Courtesy of Professor E. Wilson Jones, St John's Dermatology Centre, London, UK.)

lobulated, bean-shaped or boat-shaped nuclei (Fig. 55.4). There is a variable lymphocytic infiltrate, deep to the aggregates of LCH cells. In some patients with LCH, large numbers of γ/δ T cells have been identified in the lymphocytic infiltrate [23]. Eosinophils are present in variable numbers, being rare in the more fulminant forms of LCH but present in high numbers in the less aggressive spectrum of LCH. Within the epidermis, LCH cells are often observed either singly or forming Pautrier-like microabscesses (Fig. 55.5).

With time, the histological picture changes, with fewer LCH cells present and the emergence of a more xanthomatous pattern, which is eventually followed by fibrosis. Several studies have shown no correlation between histology and extent of disease, morbidity or mortality [24–27].

In one clinical variant of LCH, described by Hashimoto and Pritzker [28], in which the disease is restricted to the skin and regresses spontaneously over a period of several months, the pathology in the skin is sufficiently different to warrant separate description. In this variant, the infiltrate is deep within the dermis, with sparing of papillary dermis and epidermis. Lesional cells are large histiocytic cells with copious glassy eosinophilic cytoplasm. Multinucleate giant cells are often observed. Up to 25% of these histiocytes contain Birbeck granules.

Immunocytochemistry. Immunohistochemical studies have demonstrated that LCH cells show many of the characteristics of the epidermal Langerhans' cell, particularly in its activated state (see Table 55.1) [29–31]. The labelling pattern with certain markers (C3b and C3bi receptors, CDW14, Ki-M1 and Ki-M6) has been shown to be variable. This does not correlate with the clinical

Table 55.2 Diagnostic markers for Langerhans' cell histiocytosis (LCH) cell.

Marker	Tissue needed
S100	Paraffin-embedded
Peanut agglutinin	Paraffin-embedded
Placental alkaline phosphatase	Paraffin-embedded
α-D-Mannosidase	Fresh
CD1a	Fresh-frozen (paraffin-embedded with 010 monoclonal antibody)
Birbeck granules	Electron microscopy prepared

course of the disease but probably reflects different phenotypic 'ages' of the Langerhans' cell [30].

Three markers have now been shown to be expressed by LCH cells but not by normal epidermal Langerhans' cells. These are peanut agglutinin, an epitope shared with IFN-γ [32,33] and placental alkaline phosphatase [34]. Placental alkaline phosphatase is negative in normal Langerhans' cells and is not observed in reactive dermatoses where Langerhans' cells are present in the dermal infiltrate. However, *in vitro* studies have shown that placental alkaline phosphatase expression is an early and transient activation marker of Langerhans' cells [35]. These observations are of particular interest, as they show that LCH cells are not merely reactive Langerhans' cells but are arrested at a particular stage of their ontogeny.

Immunohistochemistry is important in confirming the diagnosis of LCH. For retrospective studies where only formalin-fixed and paraffin-embedded tissue is available (Table 55.2), three markers are of value: S100 protein, peanut agglutinin and placental alkaline phosphatase. S100 protein staining is a consistent feature of LCH cells but is also present in normal Langerhans' cells and a variety of other skin cells and structures, including nerve tissue, melanocytes and naevus cells. In a study by Rowden *et al.* [36], the histiocytic cells and giant cells in juvenile xanthogranuloma, necrobiotic xanthogranuloma, papular xanthoma, eruptive histiocytoma and reticulohistiocytosis were all negative for S100 protein, but all LCH specimens were positive.

Peanut agglutinin shows characteristic labelling of LCH cells, with paranuclear and cell-surface deposition of reaction products. Peanut agglutinin labels other cell types in the same way, including interdigitating reticulum cells [37], but normal Langerhans' cells and other histiocytic cells show diffuse cytoplasmic labelling with this marker [32].

Placental alkaline phosphatase is normally found in placental tissue and in the female reproductive tract. It is also expressed in malignancies of the ovary and testis. In normal skin, placental alkaline phosphatase is negative and cells expressing this enzyme are absent in reactive disorders. It is perhaps the most informative marker that can be used in archival LCH material, where only the LCH cells express this enzyme [34].

Fascin is a 55-kDa actin bundling protein that is highly selective for dendritic cells of lymphoid tissue and blood. It is involved in the formation of dendritic processes in maturing epidermal Langerhans' cells and can be used to differentiate LCH from other histiocytoses. In a study of 34 samples of LCH from skin, bone, lymph node, thyroid, orbit and extradural cranial tissue, all samples stained positive for fascin, CD1a and S100. Normal epidermal Langerhans' cells were consistently negative for fascin [38].

To establish a definitive diagnosis by the criteria of the Histiocyte Society, the involved tissue must be examined for CD1a staining or for the presence of Birbeck granules (which requires fixation and processing for electron microscopy). Staining with monoclonal anti-CD1a antibodies may be carried out in paraffin-embedded tissue [39].

Incidence. The incidence of LCH is unknown because of the heterogeneity of clinical expression of the disease. In many patients, the disease is undiagnosed, with mild skin involvement being attributed to seborrhoeic dermatitis and isolated bone disease remaining undetected. Also, the diverse clinical presentation of the disease means that patients may be under the care of orthopaedic surgeons, ear, nose and throat surgeons, paediatricians, paediatric oncologists or dermatologists. In the UK, 15–20 cases are reported to the UK Children's Cancer Study Group Register each year. These represent only the more severe paediatric cases, and the real incidence in the general population is more likely to be at least four to six per million, with 50–70 new cases presenting annually.

Clinical features. LCH can affect many different organs and may cause fever, malaise and, in children, failure to thrive.

Of 58 patients with LCH seen at the Hospital for Sick Children, London, over a 7-year period, 14 had single-system disease (13 bone and one skin) and 44 had multisystem disease, of whom 50% had vital organ dysfunction [40]. At the Children's Hospital in

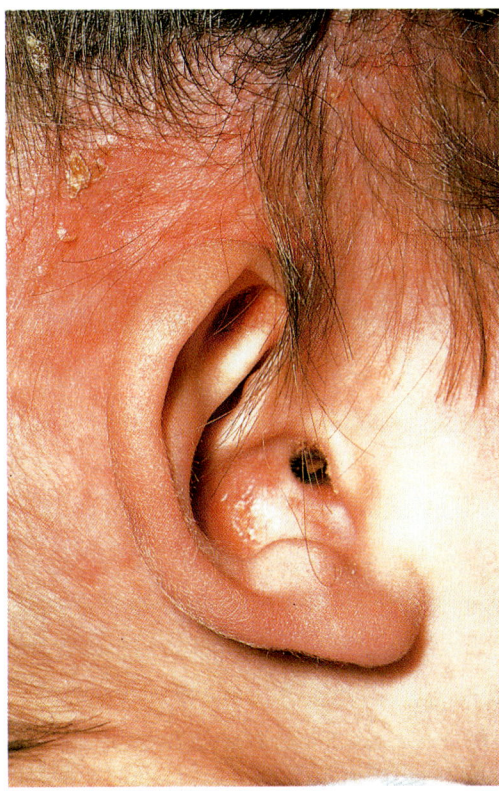

Fig. 55.6 Langerhans' cell histiocytosis of the scalp and ear of a child showing the characteristic seborrhoeic dermatitis-like eruption.

Philadelphia, 64 patients were seen over a 14-year period of whom 33 had single-organ involvement in bone (27 patients) or skin (six patients), 22 had multifocal single-organ disease affecting bone (17 patients) or soft non-osseous tissue (five patients), and nine patients had disseminated disease with dysfunction of liver or lungs [41].

In a large series of 124 patients [42], bone, lymph node and skin lesions were the most frequently seen, but 50% of patients showed liver disease and 23% lung disease with frequent haematological changes.

Skin. The most characteristic presentation is with scalp involvement. The scalp is erythematous with greasy scales, looking very like seborrhoeic dermatitis (Fig. 55.6). On the trunk, the lesions are discrete, yellow-brown, scaly papules, often showing areas of purpura (Figs 55.7 & 55.8). Lesions may become nodular and crusted or eroded. Ulceration of the flexures, groin or perianal or vulval region is a common presentation in adult patients (Fig. 55.9).

In the Hashimoto–Pritzker variant of LCH, the eruption starts in the neonatal period with nodular lesions that resemble healing chickenpox. The eruption may involve any skin surface, including palms and soles, and is self-limiting over a few weeks. In a report of four cases of Hashimoto–Pritzker LCH, follow-up showed recurrence of disease in two children, with cutaneous relapse in one at 3 months of age and bony relapse requiring systemic therapy at 6 months in the other child. Follow-up of such children is therefore necessary [43].

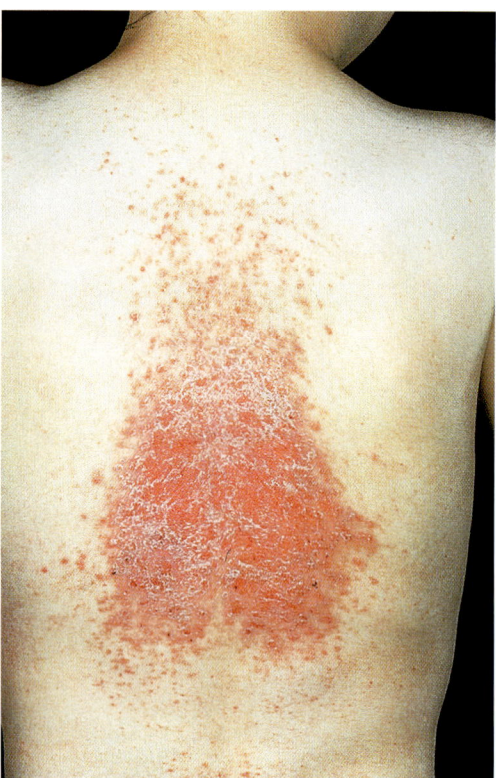

Fig. 55.7 Langerhans' cell histiocytosis in a child. Scaly maculopapular eruption on the back with mild purpura.

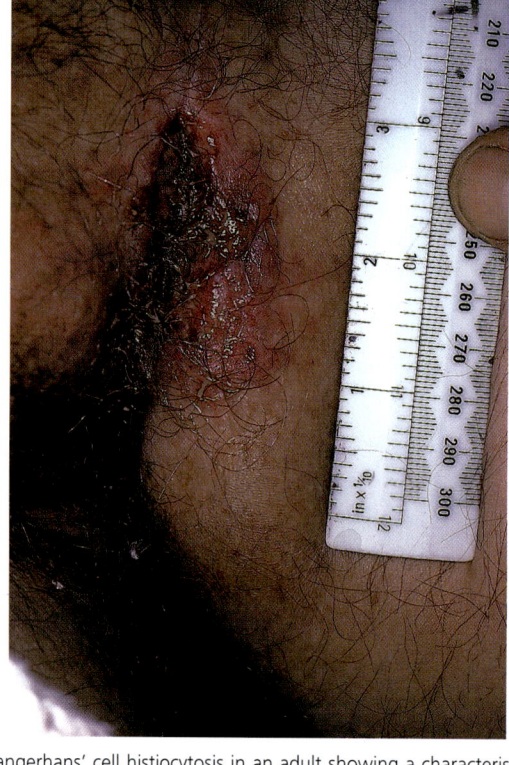

Fig. 55.9 Langerhans' cell histiocytosis in an adult showing a characteristic erosive lesion in the groin.

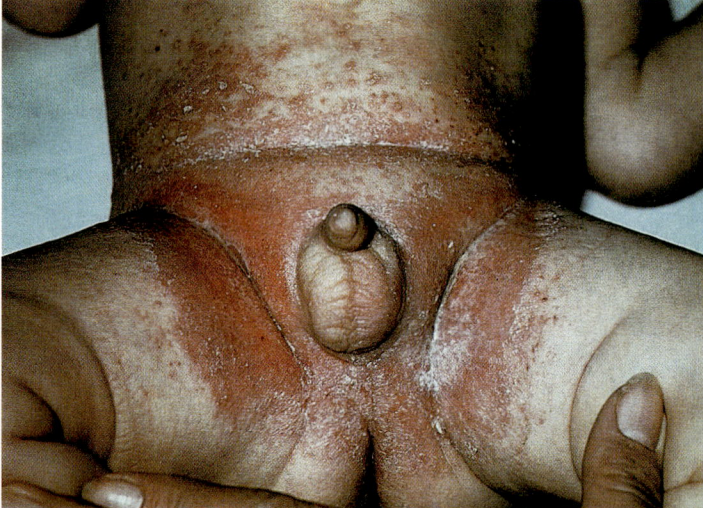

Fig. 55.8 Langerhans' cell histiocytosis in an infant showing typical eruption on the abdomen and groins mimicking seborrhoeic dermatitis and napkin eruption.

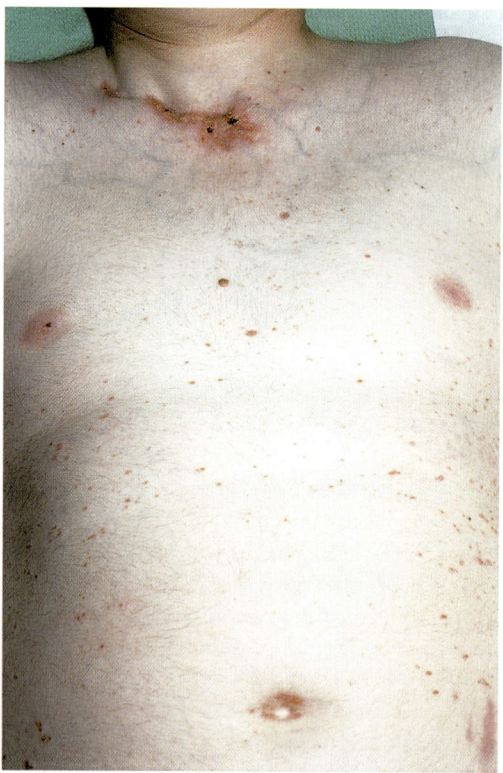

Fig. 55.10 Langerhans' cell histiocytosis in an adult with multisystem involvement. Scarring is present at sites of previous fistulae from underlying involved lymph nodes. Active skin lesions are scattered over the chest. These are scaly, erythematous, maculopapular lesions. Marked striae are the result of high-dose steroids used in therapy.

In patients with peripheral lymph node involvement, chronic draining sinuses may develop over involved sites (Fig. 55.10).

Juvenile xanthogranuloma has been associated with LCH. In a report of three children with multisystem LCH, juvenile xanthogranulomas appeared 3–6 years after the initial presentation with LCH [44]. It is possible that the juvenile xanthogranulomas developed as a reaction to the inflammatory reaction in LCH.

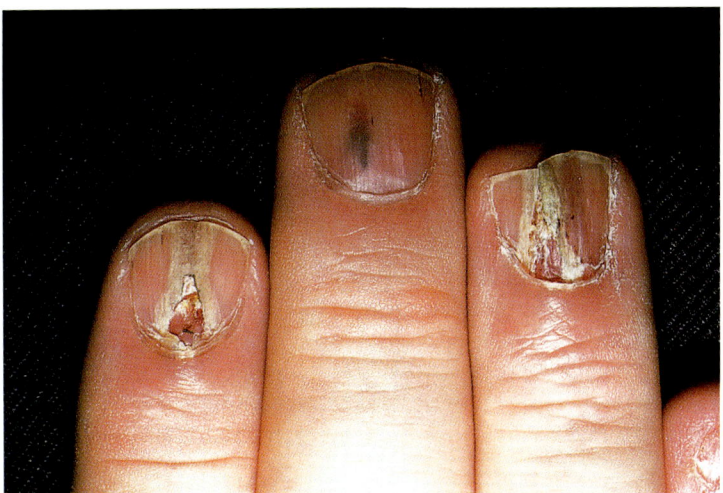

Fig. 55.11 Langerhans' cell histiocytosis: involvement of nails in an adult patient showing nail-fold destruction. (Courtesy of Dr D.A.R. de Berker, Bristol Royal Infirmary, Bristol, UK.)

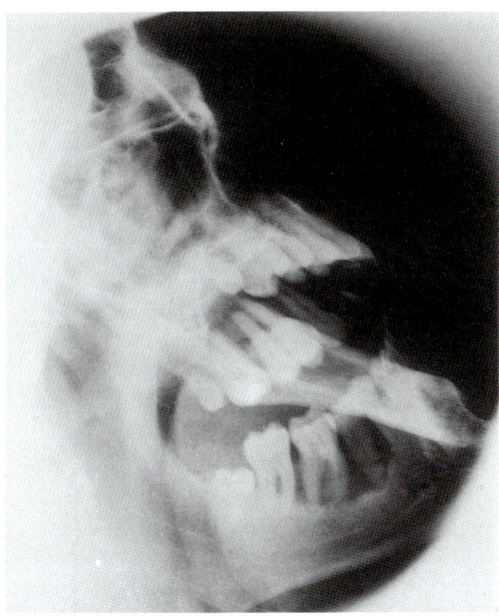

Fig. 55.12 Radiograph of the jaw of an adult with oral involvement in Langerhans' cell histiocytosis. The alveolar bone shows marked reabsorption and the teeth have become detached and appear to be floating.

Nails. Nail involvement in LCH is rare. Changes include paronychia, nail fold destruction, onycholysis and subungual expansion with nail plate loss (Fig. 55.11) [45].

Ears. Disease of the ears is common [46], with involvement of external and middle ear and mastoid. This may present with persistent aural discharge due to skin involvement or polypoid involvement of the external auditory canal. If the middle ear or mastoid is involved, deafness is common.

Oral. The commonest presentation in the mouth is with periodontal involvement, affecting particularly the lower molar areas [47]. There may be destruction of the alveolar ridge with infiltration of the gums with LCH cells resulting in the teeth floating free from their sockets (Fig. 55.12). Premature eruption of the teeth may be a presenting sign [48]. Mandible involvement is frequently observed in adults, with a palpable tender mass over the affected area. This is usually associated with oral involvement.

Bone marrow. Involvement may be occult or there may be pancytopenia. When bone marrow involvement is severe, splenomegaly is generally present. In bone marrow aspirates, LCH cells are often sparse and staining for CD1a is essential for assessment [49].

Lungs. Primary pulmonary LCH is rare and is usually seen in young or middle-aged adults. In adult patients, smoking is invariably associated with lung involvement, and in any adult smoker with LCH the lung should be examined for possible involvement. Computed tomography is usually more informative in such patients as it identifies lung disease at an earlier stage than chest X-ray. Abnormalities consist of nodular opacities representing aggregates of LCH cells which progressively show cystic central change, and cystic changes. Diagnosis is established by lung biopsy or bronchial lavage, as LCH of the lungs may be impossible to differentiate from other chronic interstitial lung diseases on clinical and radiographic findings.

Pulmonary signs and symptoms are non-specific and are rarely observed until there is frank dysfunction, with dyspnoea, tachypnoea and subcostal recession. Pain and sudden dyspnoea may indicate a pneumothorax due to rupture of a peripheral bulla. Pneumothoraces are common [50], but up to 23% may be asymptomatic.

Patients with multisystem LCH and lung involvement often have progressive lung disease and progressive dysfunction which may result in respiratory failure. Isolated pulmonary LCH may respond to cessation of smoking with regression of the nodular lesions. It is important in assessing patients with lung LCH to perform sequential lung function tests and to start treatment as soon as any fall in lung function is noted. Studies have demonstrated that lung function and gas exchange parameters correlate to cystic change but not to nodular lesions, which suggests that treatment should be directed to early nodular lesions before cystic changes lead to irreversible reduction in lung function [51].

Gastrointestinal tract. Liver involvement is very common as part of multisystem LCH, producing hepatomegaly or ascites. Cholestatic jaundice may be a late feature due to fibrotic obstruction of the biliary tree. Diarrhoea may be the result of infiltration of the lamina propria by LCH cells or may be caused by abnormal bile acid metabolism or infection within the gastrointestinal tract. Digestive tract involvement in LCH is very rare but in children even mild involvement of the gastrointestinal tract, which produces no overt symptoms of diarrhoea, may still cause failure to thrive due to mild malabsorption [52].

Central nervous system. Diabetes insipidus may be the presenting feature of LCH. Other focal lesions may occur, commonly affecting the cerebellum, temporal lobe and occipital lobe. Intracerebral disease is more frequently seen with bone involvement

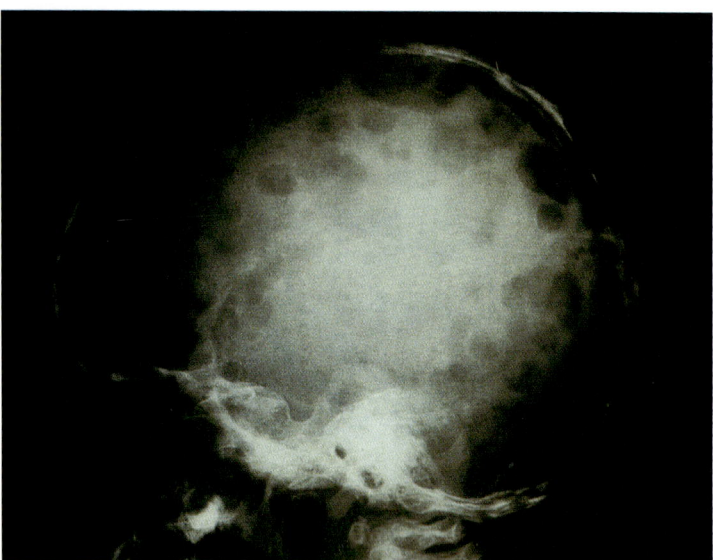

Fig. 55.13 Multiple osteolytic lesions in the skull of an infant with Langerhans' cell histiocytosis.

of the skull. A cerebellar syndrome with ataxia, dysarthria and choreoathetoid movements may be a late sequel of LCH. This is caused by progressive cerebellar atrophy. Biopsies of the cerebellum have so far failed to show infiltration with LCH cells only gliosis [53].

Bone. Solitary bone involvement with LCH is common but occasionally goes undiagnosed. The commonest sites are the bones of the calvarium, but femur, scapula, rib, mandible and vertebra are often affected [54]. Lesions may be asymptomatic or may present with swelling over the affected bone, pain or pathological fracture. Radiography is better than radionucleotide studies in detecting bone involvement in LCH [55]. Lesions appear as osteolytic areas that are sharply demarcated and may have a scalloped border (Fig. 55.13) [56]. When vertebrae are affected, the structural bone is lost and the vertebra may collapse. Spinal cord compression resulting from vertebral collapse has been reported with LCH [24]. Healing of bone lesions is usually seen as peripheral sclerosis of the lytic lesion. Radiographic changes may still be evident for long periods after the disease has been adequately treated or has undergone spontaneous remission.

Endocrine system. Diabetes insipidus is the commonest endocrine problem, the incidence in children with multisystem disease ranging from 22 to 50% [57–59]. Diabetes insipidus may result from pituitary involvement or hypothalamic involvement. Magnetic resonance imaging may show thickening of the pituitary stalk with recent-onset disease. Patients with multisystem disease and those with craniofacial bone involvement carry a significantly increased risk of developing diabetes insipidus [60]. Anterior pituitary dysfunction is always accompanied by diabetes insipidus and may develop slowly after the initial diagnosis of diabetes insipidus is made [61]. In the author's experience, men with LCH-related diabetes insipidus often develop hypoandrogenism and require testosterone replacement.

Short stature in children with LCH has been associated with growth hormone deficiency, which may be secondary to hypothalamic involvement [62]. Some of these children respond to treatment with growth hormone [58,62]. Hypogonadism with delayed puberty and thyroid involvement have also been reported [63,64].

Prognosis. Three important, independent, prognostic indices in LCH are the age of the patient, the extent of the disease and the presence of vital organ failure.

Children under the age of 2 years with multisystem disease have a much poorer prognosis than older children. In a study by Komp *et al.* [65], the mortality in children under the age of 2 years with disseminated LCH was 37% compared with 16% in the group aged over 2 years.

Lahey [66] found a positive relationship between increased mortality rate and widespread organ involvement, but Greenberger *et al.* [67] found that organ failure was a better prognostic indicator than organ involvement. Organ failure relates to lung, liver and bone marrow in children and lung and liver in adults. Studies have also suggested that survival in children is better if they respond to treatment in the first 6 weeks of therapy [68]. Both Lahey and Greenberger *et al.* [66,67] looked at prognosis in relation to mortality, but since LCH is a reactive rather than a malignant disease, prognosis should consider morbidity as well as mortality. The long-term sequelae of LCH can be related to both disease and treatment. Morbidity caused by the disease itself may be minor (e.g. skin lesions) or there may be major consequences if organs such as the liver, lungs and brain are damaged. Treatment with cytotoxic reagents may result in sterility and may cause leukaemias and other secondary malignancies. In a long-term follow-up of children with LCH over a 16-year period, only 33% of children with multisystem disease were alive and healthy without sequelae; 15% had diabetes insipidus, 10% had CNS complications and 11% had late-stage pulmonary disease [69].

Diagnosis. Pathological diagnosis is most important as many diseases can clinically mimic LCH, and S100 staining or even CD1a staining is insufficient to establish a diagnosis of LCH if the histological picture is not consistent. The differential diagnosis in cutaneous LCH includes seborrhoeic dermatitis, juvenile xanthogranuloma, xanthoma disseminatum and benign cephalic histiocytosis. In disseminated LCH there may be diagnostic problems with familial haemophagocytic lymphohistiocytosis, sinus histiocytosis with massive lymphadenopathy (SHML) and virus-associated haemophagocytic syndrome. Histological examination of tissue biopsy with specific marker studies is usually sufficient to differentiate LCH from these other conditions.

Investigation. LCH may present in various organs and it is important to investigate the patient for other sites of disease so that treatment can be properly planned. Patients may present with skin, bone, lymph node, pituitary, lung or liver disease as primary site but need to be fully investigated before a diagnosis of single-system disease can be made. Table 55.3 details investigations that should be conducted on all suspected cases and indication for more specialized investigations in some patients.

Table 55.3 Investigating the patient with LCH.

Investigations on all patients
Full blood count and ESR
Electrolytes, urea, liver function tests and CRP
Skeletal survey
Chest X-ray

Tests indicated in some patients
MRI of brain: lytic skull lesions, diabetes insipidus, symptoms suggestive of CNS involvement
Water deprivation test: polyuria, polydipsia
High resolution CT chest: adult smoker, respiratory symptoms
Lung function tests: lung involvement
Abdominal ultrasound, liver biopsy: abnormal liver function tests

In some patients with LCH, ESR and CRP are raised and these prove to be valuable markers of disease activity and response to treatment in these patients. A recent study has advocated the use of whole-body MRI to assess bony and extraosseous LCH, showing that it is superior to conventional X-rays and bone scintigraphy [70].

Treatment. Treatment depends on the extent and severity of disease. Patients with single-system bone or skin disease have a good prognosis and often require no or only limited treatment. In one study, McLelland *et al.* [40] showed that in 14 patients with single-system disease, eight required no treatment. In isolated bone disease, curettage to establish the diagnosis may be curative. In weight-bearing bones that are symptomatic, intralesional steroid injections are effective [9]. If vital structures are compromised, such as the optic nerve or spinal cord, low-dose radiotherapy (700–1000 cGy) can be given.

In single-system skin disease, topical treatment with 20% nitrogen mustard is effective [71]. Psoralen and UVA (PUVA) therapy may be useful for those patients who do not tolerate topical nitrogen mustard or fail to respond adequately. Reports have shown a good response of isolated skin disease to thalidomide [72], but poor responses in patients with multisystem disease [73].

Single-system bone disease may respond to simple curettage or intralesional steroid injections. Radiotherapy has been used in the past but is now generally restricted to use in single vertebral lesion or if there is a risk of pathological fracture in the greater trochanter [74].

In multisystem LCH where there is evidence of organ dysfunction, systemic chemotherapy is indicated. Treatment in children should initially be with prednisolone 2 mg/kg for a short course of about 2 months, with the dose adjusted to disease response [40]. Adults tend not to respond to systemic steroids and often suffer severe side effects from their use. In disease that is either unresponsive, aggressive or in adults, a number of chemotherapeutic agents have been tried, mainly the vinca alkaloids, especially vinblastine, but also methotrexate and 6-mercaptopurine in combination with prednisolone. Response rates of about 50–70% can be achieved using these agents. Evidence suggests that the epipodophyllotoxin etoposide as a single drug is better than other drugs tested [75], and ciclosporin and IFN-α have also been beneficial

[76]. 2-Chlorodeoxyadenosine, a purine analogue with antiproliferative effects on histiocytes and lymphocytes, has been used in recurrent or high-risk LCH. Treatment is with 5–7 mg/m^2 daily for 5 days every 21–28 days. In a study of six children with LCH, five patients remained in clinical remission with a follow-up of 15 months [77]. 2-Chlorodeoxyadenosine also seems to be of particular value for patients with lung involvement but should ideally be used when patients have nodular involvement rather than late-stage cystic change [78].

References
1 Hand A. Polyuria and tuberculosis. *Arch Pediatr* 1893; **10**: 673–8.
2 Rowland RS. Xanthomatosis and the reticulo-endothelial system. *Arch Intern Med* 1928; **42**: 611–8.
3 Thannhauser SJ. Serum lipids and their value in diagnosis. *N Engl J Med* 1947; **237**: 515–46.
4 Basset F, Turiaf J. Identification par la microscopie electronique de particles de nature probablement virale dans les lesions granulomateuses d'une histiocytose X pulmonaire. *C R Acad Sci Hebd Seances Acad Sci D* 1965; **261**: 3701–3.
5 Nezelof C, Basset F, Rousseau MF. Histiocytosis X. Histiogenetic arguments for a Langerhans cell origin. *Biomedicine* 1973; **18**: 365–71.
6 Glass AG, Miller RW. US mortality from Letterer–Siwe disease, 1960–1964. *Pediatrics* 1968; **42**: 364–7.
7 McClain K, Weiss R. Viruses and Langerhans cell histiocytosis: is there a link? *Br J Cancer* 1994; **70**: S34–6.
8 Leikin S, Puruganan G, Frankel A *et al.* Immunologic parameters in histiocytosis X. *Cancer* 1973; **32**: 796–802.
9 Nesbit ME Jr, O'Leary M, Dehner LP *et al.* The immune system and the histiocytosis syndromes. *Am J Pediatr Hematol Oncol* 1981; **3**: 141–9.
10 Broadbent V, Pritchard J, Davies EG *et al.* Spontaneous remission of multisystem histiocytosis X. *Lancet* 1986; **i**: 253–4.
11 Davies EG, Levinsky RJ, Butler M *et al.* Thymic hormone therapy for histiocytosis X. *N Engl J Med* 1983; **309**: 493–4.
12 Shannon BT, Newton WA, Jacobs D. Lack of suppressor cell activity in children with active histiocytosis X. *Med Pediatr Oncol* 1986; **14**: 111–4.
13 Kragballe K, Zachariae H, Herlin T *et al.* Histiocytosis X: an immune deficiency disease? Studies on antibody-dependent monocyte mediated cytotoxicity. *Br J Dermatol* 1981; **105**: 13–8.
14 Meacham R, Morris J, Chu AC. Morphological and immunological characteristics of histiocytosis X (HX) cells. *J Invest Dermatol* 1985; **84**: 440.
15 Yu RC, Morris JF, Pritchard J *et al.* Defective alloantigen presenting capacity of Langerhans cells histiocytosis cells. *Arch Dis Child* 1992; **67**: 1370–2.
16 McLelland J, Newton J, Malone M *et al.* Flow cytometric study of Langerhans cell histiocytosis. *Br J Dermatol* 1989; **120**: 485–91.
17 Rabkin MS, Wittmer CT, Kjeldsberg CR *et al.* Flow cytometric DNA content of histiocytosis X (Langerhans cell histiocytosis). *Am J Pathol* 1988; **131**: 283–9.
18 Goldberg NS, Bauer K, Rosen ST *et al.* Histiocytosis X: flow cytometric DNA-content and immunohistochemical and ultrastructural analysis. *Arch Dermatol* 1986; **122**: 446–50.
19 Yu RC, Chu C, Buluwela L *et al.* Clonal proliferation of Langerhans cells in Langerhans cell histiocytosis. *Lancet* 1994; **343**: 767–8.
20 Willman CL, Busque L, Griffith BD *et al.* Langerhans cell histiocytosis (histiocytosis X): a clonal proliferative disease. *N Engl J Med* 1994; **331**: 154–60.
21 Yousem SA, Colby TV, Chen YY. Pulmonary Langerhans cell histiocytosis: molecular analysis of clonality. *Am J Surg Pathol* 2001; **25**: 630–6.
22 Chu AC, D'Angio DJ, Favara B *et al.* Histiocytosis syndromes in children. *Lancet* 1987; **i**: 208–9.
23 Aliabac M, Chu AC. T-lymphocytes bearing the gamma delta T-cell receptor in cutaneous lesions of Langerhans cell histiocytosis. *Med Pediatr Oncol* 1993; **21**: 347–9.
24 Esterly NB, Maures HS, Gonzales-Crussi F. Histiocytosis X, a seven year experience at a Children's Hospital. *J Am Acad Dermatol* 1985; **13**: 481–96.
25 Nezelof C, Frileux-Herbet F, Cronier-Sachot J. Disseminated histiocytosis X: analysis of prognostic factors based on a retrospective study of 50 cases. *Cancer* 1979; **44**: 1824–38.
26 Risdall RJ, Dehner LP, Duray P *et al.* Histiocytosis X (Langerhans cell histiocytosis). Prognostic role of histopathology. *Arch Pathol* 1983; **107**: 59–63.

27 Simmons PS, Wold LE, Ivebach LR *et al.* Prognostic factors and management of histiocytosis X. *J Pediatr* 1981; **98**: 1023.

28 Hashimoto K, Pritzker MS. Electron microscopic study of reticulohistiocytoma: an unusual case of congenital, self-healing reticulohistiocytosis. *Arch Dermatol* 1973; **107**: 263–70.

29 Azumi N, Sheibani K, Swartz WG *et al.* Antigenic phenotype of Langerhans cell histiocytosis: an immunohistochemical study demonstrating the value of LN-2, LN-3 and vimentin. *Hum Pathol* 1988; **19**: 1376–82.

30 Groh V, Gadner H, Radaskiewicz T *et al.* The phenotypic spectrum of histiocytosis X cells. *J Invest Dermatol* 1988; **90**: 441–7.

31 Santamaria M, Lamas L, Ree HJ *et al.* Expression of sialyated Leu M1 antigen in histiocytosis X. *Am J Clin Pathol* 1988; **89**: 211–6.

32 McLelland J, Chu AC. Comparison of peanut agglutinin and S100 stain in the paraffin tissue diagnosis of Langerhans cell histiocytosis. *Br J Dermatol* 1988; **119**: 513–21.

33 Neumann C, Schamburg-Lever G, Dopfer R *et al.* Interferon gamma is a marker for histiocytosis X cells in the skin. *J Invest Dermatol* 1988; **91**: 280–2.

34 Hage C, Bullman CL, Favara BE *et al.* Langerhans cell histiocytosis (histiocytosis X). Immunophenotype and growth fraction. *Hum Pathol* 1993; **24**: 840–5.

35 Murray S, Hage C, Isaacson P *et al.* Expression of placental alkaline phosphatase in Langerhans cells and Langerhans cell histiocytosis (abstract). *J Invest Dermatol* 1993; **100**: 482.

36 Rowden G, Connelly EM, Winkelmann R. Cutaneous histiocytosis X. The presence of S100 protein and its use in diagnosis. *Arch Dermatol* 1983; **119**: 553–9.

37 Ree HJ, Kadin ME. Peanut agglutinin: a useful marker for histiocytosis X and interdigitating reticulum cells. *Cancer* 1986; **57**: 282–7.

38 Pincus GS, Lones MA, Matsumura F. Langerhans cell histiocytosis: immunohistochemical expression of fascin, a dendritic cell marker. *Am J Clin Pathol* 2002; **118**: 335–43.

39 Emile JE, Wechsler J, Brousse N *et al.* Langerhans cell histiocytoses. Definitive diagnosis with the use of monoclonal antibody 010 on routinely paraffin embedded samples. *Am J Surg Pathol* 1995; **19**: 636–41.

40 McLelland J, Broadbent V, Yeoman E *et al.* Langerhans cell histiocytosis: a conservative approach to treatment. *Arch Dis Child* 1990; **65**: 301–3.

41 Raney RB Jr, D'Angio GJ. Langerhans cell histiocytosis (histiocytosis X): experience at the Children's Hospital Philadelphia, 1970–1984. *Med Pediatr Oncol* 1989; **17**: 20–8.

42 Rivera-Luna R, Martinez-Guerra G, Altamirano-Awarez E *et al.* Langerhans cell histiocytosis: clinical experience with 124 patients. *Pediatr Dermatol* 1988; **5**: 145–50.

43 Longaker MA, Frieden IJ, Le Boit PT *et al.* Congenital self-limiting Langerhans cell histiocytosis: the need for long term follow up. *J Am Acad Dermatol* 1994; **31**: 910–6.

44 Hoeger PH, Diaz C, Malone M *et al.* Juvenile xanthogranuloma as a sequel to Langerhans cell histiocytosis: a report of three cases. *Clin Exp Dermatol* 2001; **26**: 391–4.

45 de Berker D, Lever LR, Windebank K. Nail features in Langerhans cell histiocytosis. *Br J Dermatol* 1994; **130**: 523–7.

46 Cunningham MJ, Curtin HD, Jaffe R *et al.* Otological manifestations of Langerhans cell histiocytosis. *Arch Otolaryngal Head Neck Surg* 1989; **115**: 807–13.

47 Artzi Z, Grosky M, Raviv M. Periodontal manifestations of adult onset histiocytosis. *J Periodontol* 1989; **60**: 57–66.

48 McDonald JS, Miller RL, Bernstein ML *et al.* Histiocytosis X, a clinical presentation. *J Oral Pathol* 1980; **9**: 342–9.

49 Minkov M, Potschger U, Grois N *et al.* Bone marrow assessment in Langerhans cell histiocytosis. *Pediatr Blood Cancer* 2007; **49**: 694–8.

50 Hoffman L, Cohn JE, Gaensler EA. Respiratory abnormalities in eosinophilic granuloma of the lung: long term study of 5 cases. *N Engl J Med* 1962; **267**: 577–89.

51 Canuet M, Kessler R, Jeung MY *et al.* Correlation between high-resolution computed tomography findings and lung function in pulmonary Langerhans cell histiocytosis. *Respiration* 2007; **74**: 640–6.

52 Hait E, Liang M, Degar B *et al.* Gastrointestinal tract involvement in Langerhans cell histiocytosis : case report and literature review. *Pediatrics* 2006; **118**: 1593–9.

53 Grois N, Prayer D, Prosch H *et al.* Neuropathology of CNS disease in Langerhans cell histiocytosis. *Brain* 2005; **128**: 829–38.

54 McGavran MH, Spady HA. Eosinophilic granuloma of bone. A study of 28 cases. *J Bone Joint Surg* 1960; **42**: 979–92.

55 Crone-Munzebrock W, Brassow F. Comparison of radiographic and bone scan findings in histiocytosis X. *Skeletal Radiol* 1983; **9**: 170–3.

56 Ochsner SF. Eosinophilic granuloma of bone: experience with 20 cases. *Am J Roentgenol Radium Ther Nucl Med* 1966; **97**: 719–26.

57 Braunstein GD, Kohler PO. Endocrine manifestations of histiocytosis. *Am J Pediatr Hematol Oncol* 1981; **3**: 67–75.

58 Greenberger JS, Cassady JR, Jaffe N *et al.* Radiation therapy in patients with histiocytosis: management of diabetes insipidus and bone lesions. *Int J Radiat Oncol Biol Phys* 1979; **5**: 1749–55.

59 Sims DG. Histiocytosis X: follow up of 43 cases. *Arch Dis Child* 1977; **52**: 433–40.

60 Grosi N, Potschger U, Prosch H *et al.* Risk factors for diabetes insipidus in Langerhans cell histiocytosis. *Pediatr Blood Cancer* 2006; **46**: 228–33.

61 Makras P, Alexandraki KI, Chrousos GP *et al.* Endocrine manifestations in Langerhans cell histiocytosis. *Trends Endocrinol Metab* 2007; **18**: 252–7.

62 Zinkham WH. Multifocal eosinophilic granulomas: natural history, etiology and management. *Am J Med* 1976; **60**: 457–63.

63 Braunstein GD, Raiti S, Hansen JW *et al.* Response of growth retarded patients with Hand–Schuller–Christian disease to growth hormone therapy. *N Engl J Med* 1975; **292**: 332–3.

64 Yagci B, Kandemir N, Yazici N *et al.* Thyroid involvement in Langerhans cell histiocytosis: a report of two cases and review of the literature. *Eur J Pediatr* 2007; **166**: 901–4.

65 Komp DM, Herson J, Starling KA *et al.* A staging system for histiocytosis X. A Southwest Oncology Group study. *Cancer* 1981; **47**: 798–800.

66 Lahey ME. Prognosis in reticuloendotheliosis in children. *J Pediatr* 1962; **60**: 664–71.

67 Greenberger JS, Crocker AC, Vawter G *et al.* Results of treatment of 127 patients with systemic histiocytosis (Letterer–Siwe syndrome, Schuller–Christian syndrome and multifocal eosinophilic granuloma). *Medicine (Baltimore)* 1981; **60**: 311–38.

68 Campos MK, Viana MB, de Oliveira BM *et al.* Langerhans cell histiocytosis: a 16 year experience. *J Pediatr* 2007; **83**: 79–86.

69 Bernstrand C, Sandstedt B, Ahstrom L *et al.* Long-term follow-up of Langerhans cell histiocytosis: 39 years' experience at a single centre. *Acta Paediatr* 2005; **94**: 1073–84.

70 Goo HW, Yang DH, Ra YS *et al.* Whole body MRI of Langerhans cell histiocytosis: comparison with radiography and bone scintigraphy. *Pediatr Radiol* 2006; **36**: 1019–31.

71 Wong E, Holden CA, Broadbent V *et al.* Histiocytosis X presenting as intertrigo and responding to topical nitrogen mustard. *Clin Exp Dermatol* 1986; **11**: 183–7.

72 Meunier L, Marck Y, Ribeyre C *et al.* Adult cutaneous Langerhans cell histiocytosis: remission with thalidomide treatment (letter). *Br J Dermatol* 1995; **132**: 168.

73 McClain KL, Kosinetz CA. A phase II trial using thalidomide for Langerhans cell histiocytosis. *Pediatr Blood Cancer* 2007; **48**: 44–9.

74 Allen CE, McClain KL. Langerhans cell histiocytosis: A review of past, current and future therapies. *Drugs Today* 2007; **43**: 627–43.

75 Broadbent V, Pritchard J, Yeoman E. Etoposide (VP16) in the treatment of multisystem Langerhans cell histiocytosis. *Med Pediatr Oncol* 1989; **17**: 97–100.

76 McLelland J, Pritchard J, Chu AC. Current controversies. *Hematol Oncol Clin North Am* 1987; **1**: 147–62.

77 Rodriguez-Galindo C, Kelly P, Jeng M *et al.* Treatment of children with Langerhans cell histiocytosis with 2-chlorodeoxyadenosine. *Am J Hematol* 2002; **69**: 179–84.

78 Aerni MR, Aubry CM, Myers JL *et al.* Complete remission of nodular pulmonary Langerhans cell histiocytosis lesions induced by 2-chlorodeoxyadenosine in a non-smoker. *Respir Med* 2008; **102**: 316–9.

Class IIa histiocytosis: histiocytoses involving cells of the dermal dendrocyte lineage

Class IIa histiocytoses are non-malignant diseases in which mononuclear phagocytic cells with the dermal dendrocyte phenotype accumulate in various tissues where they may or may not cause symptoms.

In many of these diseases the histological features are of a xanthogranulomatous reaction in the skin. This pattern is seen in juvenile xanthogranuloma, benign cephalic histiocytosis, generalized eruptive histiocytosis, xanthoma disseminatum and necrobiotic xanthogranuloma. In some, such as progressive nodular histiocytosis, the cells have a more spindle-shaped appearance in a storiform pattern, particularly as the lesions progress.

Histopathological studies have suggested that benign cephalic histiocytosis represents a clinical variant of a xanthogranulomatous reaction rather than being a distinct entity in its own right. In one study [1], biopsies from benign cephalic histiocytosis, generalized eruptive histiocytosis, papular xanthoma and juvenile xanthogranuloma were examined in an observer blinded fashion. In all specimens examined, three distinct patterns of histiocyte proliferation were observed—papillary dermal, lichenoid and diffuse. Benign cephalic histiocytosis, generalized eruptive histiocytosis and early non-xanthomatous juvenile xanthogranuloma could not be specifically differentiated on histopathological grounds. This study certainly suggests that benign cephalic histiocytosis may be a localized form of generalized eruptive histiocytosis or an aborted phase of juvenile xanthogranuloma. In a further study, sequential biopsies were taken from a patient with solitary giant xanthogranuloma and from a patient with benign cephalic histiocytosis. In both cases, early stages of the disease showed infiltration with histiocytes positive for Ki-M1p, HAM56 and factor XIIIa. This was followed by a polymorphic infiltrate of mononuclear and multinuclear histiocytes, which were CD68 positive. This study suggests that both entities are variants of a xanthogranulomatous reaction [2]. In one case report, a 2-year-old girl with clinical, histopathological and ultrastructural benign cephalic histiocytosis developed a varicella-zoster infection with evolution of her skin disease both clinically and histologically to juvenile xanthogranuloma [3]. In a further report of a child with generalized eruptive histiocytosis, where the diagnosis was made on clinical, histological and ultrastructural grounds, the disease progressed with the growth of yellowish confluent papules and the development of diabetes insipidus. At this stage the diagnosis was changed to xanthoma disseminatum [4].

The dermal dendrocytes involved in these diseases show a spectrum of maturation of the cells. In juvenile xanthogranuloma and benign cephalic histiocytosis, the cells are morphologically the most immature and the disease has the shortest life span. Generalized eruptive histiocytosis and xanthoma disseminatum show increasing maturation of the cells and at the other end of the spectrum, progressive nodular histiocytosis shows mature spindle shaped cells with no tendency to spontaneous remission of the disease [5].

References

1 Gianotti R, Allessi E, Caputo R. Benign cephalic histiocytosis: a distinctive entity or a part of a widespread spectrum of histiocytic proliferative disorders of children? A histopathological study. *Am J Dermatopathol* 1993; **15**: 315–9.

2 Zelger BG, Zelger B, Steiner H *et al.* Solitary giant xanthogranuloma and benign cephalic histiocytosis: variants of juvenile xanthogranuloma. *Br J Dermatol* 1995; **133**: 598–600.

3 Rodriguez-Jurado R, Duran-McKinster R, Ruis-Maldonado R. Benign cephalic histiocytosis progressing into juvenile xanthogranuloma: a non-Langerhans cell histiocytosis transforming under the influence of a virus. *Am J Dermatopathol* 2000; **22**: 70–4.

4 Repiso T, Roca-Miralles M, Kanitakis J. Generalised eruptive histiocytosis evolving into xanthoma disseminatum in a 4 year old boy. *Br J Dermatol* 1995; **132**: 978–82.

5 Chu AC. The confusing state of the histiocytoses. *Br J Dermatol* 2000; **143**: 475–6.

Dermatofibroma

This benign, nodular, dermal lesion is discussed in Chapter 56.

Juvenile xanthogranuloma

Synonyms
- Naevoxanthoendothelioma
- Xanthoma multiplex
- Juvenile xanthoma
- Multiple eruptive xanthoma in infancy
- Congenital xanthoma tuberosum
- Xanthoma naeviforme
- Juvenile giant-cell granuloma

Definition. Juvenile xanthogranulomas are benign tumours of histiocytic cells that occur predominantly in infancy and early childhood and spontaneously regress.

Aetiology. The aetiology of juvenile xanthogranuloma is unknown. The tumours represent accumulations of differentiated histiocytes. These cells express the phenotype of the dermal dendrocyte, although it has been suggested that the cell of origin could be the plasmacytoid monocyte [1]. The appearance of giant cells and foamy lipid-laden histiocytes occurs late, and they are almost certainly secondary events, possibly in response to cytokine production by the lesional histiocyte. Serum lipid levels are normal. Conflicting reports have suggested that juvenile xanthogranuloma can be associated with cytomegalovirus infection. A study by Vasconcelos *et al.* [2] has demonstrated early and late cytomegalovirus antigens in some histiocytes in a case of oral juvenile xanthogranuloma.

Pathology. An established lesion shows a mixed cellular dermal infiltrate with histiocytes, lymphocytes, eosinophils and occasional neutrophils and plasma cells. This extends from the epidermis into the subcutaneous fat but epidermal involvement is rare. A typical feature is the presence of giant cells with a wreath-like arrangement of nuclei (Touton giant cells).

In very early lesions, only spindle-shaped fibrohistiocytic cells are seen. In older lesions, foamy lipid-laden histiocytes appear, and resolution is marked by gradual replacement by fibrous tissue. A spindle cell variant of juvenile xanthogranuloma has been described [3]. In deep juvenile xanthogranuloma the lesions tend to be more cellular with fewer Touton giant cells [4].

Immunocytochemical examination in most cases shows that lesional cells are positive for lysozyme, α_1-antichymotrypsin, CD68, Ki-MIP [5], fascin, factor XIIIa and may express HLA-DR and CD4, but are negative for S100 protein [6]. However, Tahan *et al.* [7] found a small population of S100 dendritic cells in juvenile xanthogranuloma, which they felt were important in pathogenesis, and Kraus *et al.* [1] have shown reactivity to polyclonal S100 in six of eight specimens they examined. Cells are always CD1a negative.

At the ultrastructural level, the lesional histiocytes do not exhibit Birbeck granules but do show complex interdigitation of the cytoplasmic membrane [8].

Incidence. Half of the cases of juvenile xanthogranuloma have been reported in infants less than 6 months of age. Lesions may occur in children over 3 years of age and cases have been reported in adults [9]. There is no sex association and no familial tendency. Juvenile xanthogranuloma is 10 times more frequent in white than in black people.

Clinical features. The characteristic clinical features of juvenile xanthogranuloma are its onset in infancy, sudden appearance of lesions and spontaneous regression. Most patients develop single lesions, but in others several lesions may develop and occasionally hundreds of lesions may be present. In one case report, a generalized lichenoid variant of xanthogranuloma was described. The eruption consisted of small, flat, shiny papules, which resolved spontaneously [10]. The lesions most commonly occur on the upper part of the body, particularly affecting the face, neck, scalp and upper trunk (Fig. 55.14). Lesions may occur in the oral mucosa with or without skin involvement [11]. They generally start as reddish-yellow papules, which may enlarge up to 1 cm in diameter and evolve into yellow–brown plaques and macules. The lesions are firm and rubbery and can develop surface telangiectasia. Larger lesions, up to 2–3 cm in size, have been reported [12] and ulceration and satellite lesions have been described [13]. Deep dermal lesions may occur which may infiltrate skeletal muscle. Such lesions may exhibit a more aggressive biological behaviour [4]. Resolution occurs spontaneously over a period of months or years, leaving small atrophic scars. There are no subjective symptoms.

Visceral involvement may occur in lung, liver, spleen, testes [14], pericardium, gastrointestinal tract, kidney [15,16], deeper soft tissues [17] and central nervous system. Eye involvement occurs in up to 10% of cases [18] and may lead to secondary glaucoma or may be mistaken for a malignant tumour, such as melanoma or neuroblastoma. The iris is most commonly affected, producing haemorrhage into the anterior chamber, which may result in secondary glaucoma. Infiltration of the orbit, iris, ciliary body and episclera may occur, with unilateral glaucoma, recurrent hyphaema, uveitis, heterochromia, iritis or severe and sudden proptosis [19]. Eye lesions may precede the appearance of skin lesions. Central nervous system involvement is rare but several reports have been published. Lesions may present as isolated or multiple tumours of the brain involving the cortex and cerebellum [20,21], and extensive involvement of cranial nerves has been reported [22]. Central nervous system involvement may occur with or without cutaneous involvement.

Juvenile xanthogranuloma has been associated with neurofibromatosis [23], Niemann–Pick disease [24], myelogenous leukaemia [25], lymphocytic leukaemia [26], urticaria pigmentosa [27] and LCH [28].

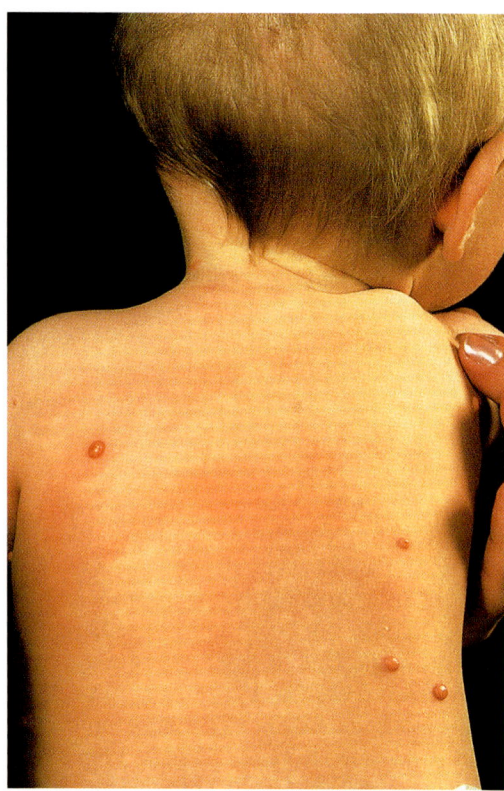

Fig. 55.14 Juvenile xanthogranuloma in an infant with typical lesions on the back.

Prognosis. Juvenile xanthogranuloma is a self-healing tumour and lesions generally resolve in 1–5 years. Disseminated neonatal juvenile xanthogranuloma may be more aggressive and fatalities in this group have been reported [29]. In addition, a recent case report describes juvenile xanthogranuloma diffusely involved the brain in an 11-year-old boy. Initial partial response was achieved with 2-cholorodeoxyadenosine but the patient then failed to respond to further chemotherapy, with dissemination of the disease to the peritoneum and bone marrow. Biopsy at this stage showed pleomorphic histiocytes with tetraploidy suggesting malignant transformation. Despite continued chemotherapy the patient died [30].

Diagnosis. Juvenile xanthogranuloma can be differentiated from xanthomas by the distribution of the lesions and the absence of lipid abnormalities. Papular urticaria can be distinguished by the symptomatic nature of the lesions and histology. The major difficulty in clinical diagnosis is with the nodular forms of LCH. Histology and immunocytochemistry will easily differentiate the two disorders.

Treatment. No treatment is necessary for the cutaneous lesions as they are self-healing. Where treatment is indicated in ocular, upper airways and central nervous system lesions, surgery or radiotherapy gives good results [31,32]. In patients with multiple cutaneous juvenile xanthogranulomas, carbon dioxide laser has been successfully used [33]. In patients with symptomatic visceral involvement, systemic steroids [16] with or without chemotherapy with vinca alkaloids have been used successfully [34]. Patients with aggressive disease with vital organ involvement, that is lungs, liver and bone marrow, are generally treated with multiagent chemotherapy, including cytarabine, methotrexate, vincristine and prednisolone [29].

References

1 Kraus MD, Haley JC, Ruiz R *et al.* 'Juvenile' xanthogranuloma: an immunophenotypic study with a reappraisal of histiogenesis. *Am J Dermatopathol* 2001; **23**: 104–11.

2 Vasconcelos FO, Oliveira LA, Naves MD *et al.* Juvenile xanthogranuloma: case report with immunohistochemical identification of early and late cytomegalovirus antigens. *J Oral Sci* 2001; **43**: 21–5.

3 DeStafeno JJ, Carlson JA, Meyer DR. Solitary spindle-cell xanthogranuloma of the eyelid. *Ophthalmology* 2002; **109**: 258–61.

4 Barroca H, Farinha NJ, Lobo A *et al.* Deep-seated congenital juvenile xanthogranuloma: report of a case with emphasis on cytologic features. *Acta Cytol* 2007; **51**: 473–6.

5 Janssen D, Harms D. Juvenile xanthogranuloma in childhood and adolescence: a clinicopathologic study of 129 patients from the kiel pediatric tumor registry. *Am J Surg Pathol* 2005; **29**: 21–8.

6 Sonda T, Hashimoto H, Enjoji M. Juvenile xanthogranuloma. Clinicopathologic analysis and immunohistochemical study of 57 patients. *Cancer* 1985; **56**: 2280–6.

7 Tahan SR, Pastel-Levy C, Bhan AK *et al.* Juvenile xanthogranuloma. Clinical and pathological characterisation. *Arch Pathol Lab Med* 1989; **113**: 1057–61.

8 Seifert HW. Membrane activity in juvenile xanthogranuloma. *J Cutan Pathol* 1981; **8**: 24–33.

9 Rodriguez J, Ackerman AB. Xanthogranuloma in adults. *Arch Dermatol* 1976; **112**: 43–4.

10 Holde G, Bonsmann G. Generalised lichenoid juvenile xanthogranuloma. *Br J Dermatol* 1992; **120**: 66–70.

11 Flaitz C, Allen C, Neville B *et al.* Juvenile xanthogranuloma of the oral cavity in children: a clinicopathological study. *Oral Surg Oral Med Oral Pathol* 2002; **94**: 345–52.

12 Fishman SJ, Brodie S, Popkin G. Juvenile xanthogranuloma. *Cutis* 1973; **11**: 499–501.

13 Gartmann H, Tritsch H. Small and large nodular nevoxanthoendothelioma: report of 13 cases. *Arch Klin Exp Dermatol Syphilol* 1963; **215**: 409–27.

14 Townell NH, Gledhill A, Robinson T *et al.* Juvenile xanthogranuloma of the testis. *J Urol* 1985; **133**: 1054–5.

15 Gilbert TJ, Parker BR. Juvenile xanthogranuloma of the kidney. *Pediatr Radiol* 1988; **18**: 169–71.

16 Unuvar E, Devecioglu O, Akay A *et al.* Successful therapy of systemic xanthogranuloma in a child. *J Pediatr Hematol Oncol* 2007; **29**: 425–7.

17 Webster SB, Reister HC, Harman LE. Juvenile xanthogranuloma with extracutaneous lesions. *Arch Dermatol* 1966; **93**: 71–6.

18 Roper SR, Spraker MK. Cutaneous histiocytosis syndromes. *Pediatr Dermatol* 1985; **3**: 19–30.

19 Labelette P, Guilbert F, Jourdel D *et al.* Bilateral multifocal uveal juvenile xanthogranuloma in a young boy with systemic disease. *Graefes Arch Clin Exp Ophthalmol* 2002; **240**: 506–9.

20 Bostrom J, Janssen G, Messing-Junger M *et al.* Multiple intracranial juvenile xanthogranulomas. Case report. *J Neurosurg* 2000; **93**: 335–41.

21 Cauro F, Houtteville JP, Mesnil JL *et al.* Cerebellar, pulmonary and cutaneous localizations of juvenile xanthogranuloma. *Ann Dermatol Vénéréol* 2002; **129**: 307–10.

22 Ernemann U, Skalej M, Hermisson M *et al.* Primary cerebral non-Langerhans cell histiocytosis: MRI and differential diagnosis. *Neuroradiology* 2002; **44**: 759–63.

23 Jensen NE. Nevoxanthoendothelioma and neurofibromatosis. *Br J Dermatol* 1971; **85**: 326–31.

24 Sibulkin D, Olichney JJ. Juvenile xanthogranuloma in a patient with Nieman–Pick disease. *Arch Dermatol* 1973; **108**: 829–34.

25 Cooper PH, Frierson HF, Kayne AL *et al.* Association of juvenile xanthogranuloma with juvenile myeloid leukaemia. *Arch Dermatol* 1984; **120**: 371–5.

26 Sarthou-Bruere S, Milpied-Homsi B, Mahe B *et al.* Eruptive xanthogranulomatosis in a trisomy 21 patient with acute lymphoblastic leukemia. *Ann Dermatol Vénéréol* 2000; **127**: 80–2.

27 DeVillez RL, Limmer BL. Juvenile xanthogranuloma and urticaria pigmentosa. *Arch Dermatol* 1975; **111**: 365–6.

28 Hoeger PH, Diaz C, Malone M *et al.* Juvenile xanthogranuloma as a sequel to Langerhans cell histiocytosis: a report of three cases. *Clin Exp Dermatol* 2001; **26**: 391–4.

29 Nakatani T, Morimoto A, Kato R *et al.* Successful treatment of congenital systemic juvenile xanthogranuloma with Langerhans cell histiocytosis-based chemotherapy. *J Pediatr Hematol Oncol* 2004; **26**: 371–4.

30 Orsey A, Paessler M, Lange BJ *et al.* Central nervous system juvenile xanthogranuloma with malignant transformation. *Pediatr Blood Cancer* 2008; **50**: 927–30.

31 MacLeod PM. Juvenile xanthogranuloma of the iris managed with superficial radiotherapy. *Clin Radiol* 1986; **37**: 295–6.

32 Somorai M, Goldstein NA, Alexis R *et al.* Managing isolated subglottic juvenile xanthogranuloma without tracheostomy: case report and review of the literature. *Pediatr Pulmonol* 2007; **42**: 181–5.

33 Klemke CD, Held B, Dippel E *et al.* Multiple juvenile xanthogranulomas successfully treated with CO_2 laser. *J Dtsch Dermatol Ges* 2007; **5**: 30–2.

34 Freyer DR, Kennedy R, Bostrom BC *et al.* Juvenile xanthogranuloma: forms of systemic disease and their clinical implications. *J Pediatr* 1996; **129**: 227–37.

Benign cephalic histiocytosis

Synonym
• Papular histiocytosis of the head

This is a rare, self-limiting histiocytosis that typically starts in early childhood [1]. As stated before, many now feel that benign cephalic histiocytosis represents a clinical variant of juvenile xanthogranuloma [2] but the clinical features of the disease are distinct enough to maintain a separate nomenclature. Erythematous papules, nodules and macules develop on the cheeks and spread to the forehead, earlobes and neck. The lesions, which are asymptomatic, gradually become reddish-brown and may spread onto the trunk, upper limbs and rarely the buttocks. Mucous membrane involvement has not been described.

No sex predisposition has been reported. In a review of the literature, the average age of onset was 15 months (range 2 to 66 months). The disease is self-limiting, and in 39 cases the mean age at resolution was 50 months in 10 patients where this detail was recorded [3]. In one case report, a 5-year-old girl developed diabetes insipidus 1 year after presenting with typical benign cephalic histiocytosis. Imaging demonstrated infiltration of the pituitary stalk [4]. Histologically, the epidermis is thinned over a well-circumscribed histiocytic infiltrate in the superficial and mid-dermis. Histiocytic cells have oval to reniform nuclei and occasionally may be pleomorphic. In older lesions, a few giant cells may be present. The cells are S100 and CD1a negative [5] but stain positively for OKM1, Leu-3 and factor XIIIa [3]. Electron microscopy shows that 5–30% of the infiltrating cells have cytoplasm rich in comma-shaped bodies and coated vesicles [3]. Dense bodies may be present and worm-like bodies have been described [6]. Since the condition is self-limiting, no therapy is indicated.

References

1 Pena Penabad C, Unamuno P, Garcia Silva J *et al.* Benign cephalic histiocytosis: case report and literature review. *Pediatr Dermatol* 1994; **11**: 164–7.

2 Sidwell RU, Francis N, Slater DN *et al.* Is disseminated juvenile xanthogranulomatosis benign cephalic histiocytosis? *Pediatr Dermatol* 2005; **22**: 40–3.

3 Jih DM, Salcedo SL, Jaworsky C. Benign cephalic histiocytosis: a case report and review. *J Am Acad Dermatol* 2002; **47**: 908–13.

4 Weston WL, Travers SH, Mierau GW *et al.* Benign cephalic histiocytosis with diabetes insipidus. *Pediatr Dermatol* 2000; **17**: 296–8.

5 de Luna ML, Glikin I, Golberg J *et al.* Benign cephalic histiocytosis: report of four cases. *Pediatr Dermatol* 1989; **6**: 198–201.

6 Eisenberg EL, Bronson DM, Barsky S. Benign cephalic histiocytosis. A case report and ultrastructural study. *J Am Acad Dermatol* 1985; **12**: 328–31.

Erdheim–Chester disease

Synonym
• Uber lipoidgranulomatose

This is a rare lipoid granulomatosis characterized by infiltration of viscera, bones, retroperitoneum and skin. It was first described by William Chester while working in the laboratory of Jakob Erdheim in 1930 [1] and the eponym was first used by Jaffe in 1972 [2].

Veyssier-Belot *et al.* [3] reviewed the literature on Erdheim–Chester disease in a comprehensive study of 59 patients. The age range was 7–84 years with a mean of 53 ± 14 years, and there was a male to female ratio of 33 : 26. The most common presentation is with chronic mild bone pain, particularly of the lower limbs. Radiography shows symmetrical sclerosis, typically affecting the long bones, with involvement of the diaphyseal and metaphyseal regions; 86% of reported cases have involvement of the long bones [4], with the distal femur, proximal tibia and fibula being most commonly affected [5]. Up to 30% of patients show lytic lesions of flat bones, which can cause problems in differentiating this disease from LCH.

Half of patients have extraosseous involvement of the retroperitoneal space, lungs, heart, kidneys, liver, pituitary, central nervous system, orbit and skin. Approximately 30% of patients have exophthalmos (Fig. 55.15), diabetes insipidus or retroperitoneal

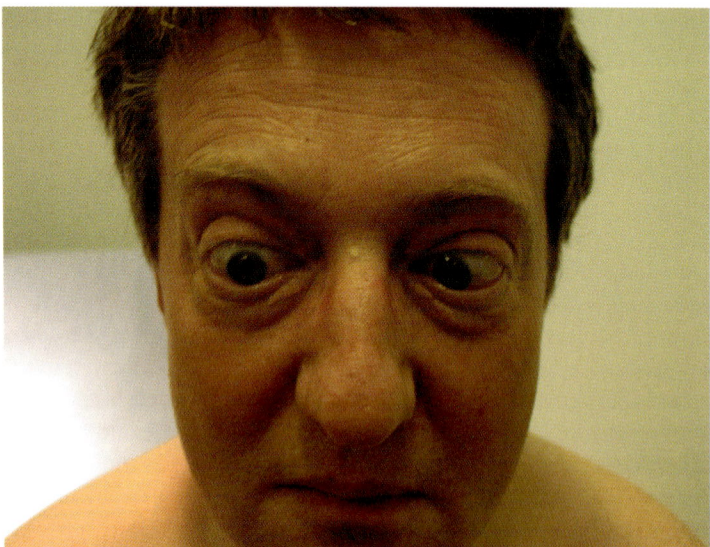

Fig. 55.15 Erdheim–Chester disease: a 47-year-old man presented with diplopia and unsteady gait. Clinically he had exophthalmos and MRI of brain showed retro-orbital masses and lesions in the mid-brain and temporal lobes. CT scan of the abdomen showed thickening of perirenal fascia and hydronephrosis demonstrating extensive disease in the retroperitoneal space.

involvement. Retroperitoneal disease is often asymptomatic and may develop over many years. It may present with dysuria, abdominal pain, obstructive renal damage or renal artery stenosis [6]. Adrenal infiltration may occur and in a study of 22 patients with Erdheim–Chester disease, 31.8% showed CT evidence of adrenal involvement and one patient developed clinical adrenal insufficiency [7].

Skin involvement is seen in about 20% of patients, usually presenting with xanthoma-like lesions, usually on the eyelids but occasionally on the trunk and submammary area. Two patients have been reported with cutaneous masses. Lung disease is seen in 35% of patients, with accumulation of histiocytes and fibrosis in a perilymphatic and subpleural pattern. It is generally asymptomatic and found on chest X-ray with diffuse interstitial fibrosis or infiltration. Advanced pulmonary involvement is associated with extensive fibrosis, which may result in cardiopulmonary failure. Prognosis tends to be poor despite treatment [8].

Cardiovascular involvement with Erdheim–Chester disease is relatively common. In a review of 72 patients with cardiovascular involvement, 55.6% had periaortic fibrosis, 44.4% had pericardial involvement and 30.6% had myocardial involvement. Six patients had a right atrial tumour and six had symptomatic valvular heart disease; 26.4% developed heart failure and 11 patients died of cardiovascular complications [9].

Central nervous system involvement is seen in 15% of patients, presenting with ataxia, paraparesis, hemiparesis or change in mental state. Imaging has shown thickening of the dura, with infiltration extending into the cerebellum. More rarely, intracerebral masses have been described. In a review of 66 patients with Erdheim–Chester disease and neurological involvement, cerebellar and pyramidal syndromes were the most common clinical manifestation, affecting 41% and 45% respectively. Seizures, headache, neuropsychiatric and cognitive problems, sensory disturbances and cranial nerve paralysis have been reported. Neurological involvement resulted in severe functional handicap in almost all of the reported patients and resulted in death in six of them. Three patterns of involvement have been demonstrated by imaging: infiltrative in 44% with widespread nodules or masses, meningeal in 37% with thickening of the dura or meningioma-like tumours, and composite in 19% with elements of both [10]. A case of slowly progressive cerebellar syndrome, similar to that seen in LCH, has been reported in a 50-year-old patient with Erdheim–Chester disease associated with unilateral exophthalmos, secondary hypogonadism and skin lesions [11].

Histological examination shows a xanthogranulomatous infiltration by lipid-laden histiocytes within a mesh and surrounded by fibrosis. Touton giant cells and eosinophils may be prominent. Cells are positive for CD68 and factor XIIIa [6] but negative for CD1a and S100 [12]. In one study of a 35-year-old woman with Erdheim–Chester disease, clonality studies based on the *HUMARA* assay in paraffin-embedded tissue showed only random distribution of allele activation and thus no evidence of clonality [13]. In a further male patient, balanced chromosomal translocation t(12; 15; 20)(q11; q24; p13.3) was identified amongst other chromosomal abnormalities, suggesting that Erdheim–Chester disease could be a clonal neoplastic disorder [14]. Further studies are needed to confirm this.

A variety of treatments have been used in Erdheim–Chester disease, including IFN-α [15,16], corticosteroids, radiotherapy, vinblastine, vincristine, cyclophosphamide [3] and 2-chlorodeoxy-adenosine [17], with variable responses. There is no clear consensus as to the best therapeutic regimen. Overall mortality is 57%, with death resulting from pulmonary, cardiac or renal failure [3].

References

1 Chester W. Uber Lipoidgranulomatose. *Virchows Arch Pathol Anat* 1930; **279**: 561–602.

2 Jaffe HL. Gaucher's disease and certain other inborn metabolic disorders: lipid (cholesterol) granulomatosis. In: Jaffe HL, ed. *Metabolic, Degenerative and Inflammatory Diseases of Bones and Joints*. Philadelphia: Lea & Febiger, 1972: 535.

3 Veyssier-Belot C, Cacoub P, Caparros-Lafebvre D *et al.* Erdheim–Chester disease: clinical and radiological characteristics of 59 cases. *Medicine (Baltimore)* 1996; **75**: 157–69.

4 Tan APA, Tan LKA, Choo IHF. Erdheim–Chester disease involving breast and muscles: imaging findings. *Am J Rheumatol* 1995; **164**: 1115–7.

5 Egan AJM, Bordman LA, Tazelaar HD *et al.* Erdheim–Chester disease: clinical, radiological and histopathological findings in five patients with interstitial lung disease. *Am J Surg Pathol* 1999; **23**: 17–26.

6 Leluc O, Andre M, Marchano S *et al.* Retroperitoneal complications of Erdheim–Chester disease. *J Radiol* 2001; **82**: 580–2.

7 Haroche J, Amoura Z, Touraine P *et al.* Bilateral adrenal infiltration with Erdheim-Chester disease. Report of seven cases and literature review. *J Clin Endocrinol Metab* 2007; **92**: 2007–12.

8 Shamburek RD, Brewer HB, Gochuico BR. Erdheim–Chester disease: a rare multisystem histiocytic disorder associated with interstitial lung disease. *Am J Med Sci* 2001; **321**: 65–75.

9 Haroche J, Amoura Z, Dion E *et al.* Cardiovascular involvement, an overlooked feature of Erdheim Chester disease. *Medicine* 2004; **83**: 371–92.

10 Lachenal F, Cotton F, Desmurs-Clavel H *et al.* Neurological manifestations and neuroradiological presentation of Erdheim-Chester disease: report of 6 cases and systematic review of the literature. *J Neurol* 2006; **253**: 1267–77.

11 Grothe C, Urbach H, Bos M *et al.* Cerebellar syndrome, exophthalmos and secondary hypogonadism in Erdheim–Chester disease. *Nervenarzt* 2001; **72**: 449–52.

12 Rush WL, Andriko JA, Galateau-Salle F *et al.* Pulmonary pathology of Erdheim–Chester disease. *Mod Pathol* 2000; **13**: 747–54.

13 Al-Quran S, Reith J, Bradley J *et al.* Erdheim–Chester disease: case report, PCR-based analysis of clonality and review of literature. *Mod Pathol* 2002; **15**: 666–72.

14 Vencio EF, Jenkins RB, Schiller JL *et al.* Clonal cytogenetic abnormalities in Erdheim-Chester disease. *Am J Surg Pathol* 2007; **31**: 319–21.

15 Esmael B, Ahmadi A, Tang R *et al.* Interferon therapy for orbital infiltration secondary to Erdheim–Chester disease. *Am J Ophthalmol* 2001; **132**: 945–7.

16 Braiteh F, Boxrud C, Esmaeli B *et al.* Successful treatment of Erdheim-Chester disease, a non-Langerhans-cell histiocytosis, with interferon-alpha. *Blood* 2005; **106**: 2992–4.

17 Myra C, Sloper L, Tighe PJ *et al.* Treatment of Erdheim-Chester disease with cladribine: a rational approach. *Br J Opthalmol* 2004; **88**: 844–7.

Fat-storing hamartoma of dermal dendrocytes

A single case report has described this entity [1]. The patient was a 30-year-old man who had a very large, circumscribed, red-brown plaque in the lumbosacral area. The plaque was composed of firm papules and nodules and was asymptomatic. The lesion had been present since birth and had slowly grown since that time.

Histology showed a slightly acanthotic epidermis and a Grenz zone, below which was a dense infiltrate of foamy histiocytes, which extended deep into the dermis. Occasional Touton giant cells were present. Lesional cells stained for factor XIIIa and vimentin and 40% of the cells labelled with Mac-387, a monoclonal antibody directed against monocyte-derived macrophages. S100 and CD1a staining were negative. Electron microscopy showed large histiocytic cells with convoluted nuclei filled with lipid droplets.

Reference

1 Bork K, Gabbert H, Knop JK. Fat-storing hamartoma of dermal dendrocytes. Clinical, histologic and ultrastructural study. *Arch Dermatol* 1990; **126**: 794–6.

Generalized eruptive histiocytoma

This is a rare cutaneous histiocytosis that mainly affects adults [1], although children with the disease have been reported [2,3]. Clinically, the disease presents as multiple, symmetrical papules that occur on the face, trunk and proximal extremities. The papules are skin coloured, brownish or blue–red and tend to come up in crops, although they are not grouped. The number of lesions is variable but may reach hundreds. Mucosal lesions are rare. The lesions are asymptomatic and resolve spontaneously to leave a macular area of hyperpigmentation.

Histology shows a proliferation of monomorphic histiocytic cells in the upper and mid dermis. No giant cells or foam cells are present. Scattered lymphocytes may be present. Ultrastructural studies have shown that the histiocytic cells lack Birbeck granules but do have cytoplasmic laminated bodies [4]. These bodies are often clustered in the cytoplasm of the cells and each measure about 1.5 μm. They are not restricted to generalized histiocytoma but have been reported in congenital self-healing histiocytosis [5].

In one case report of a 4-year-old boy with generalized eruptive histiocytoma, diagnosed using clinical, histological and ultrastructural studies, the patient subsequently developed a new eruption of yellowish confluent papules with associated diabetes insipidus. Histology of the lesions and ultrastructure confirmed the diagnosis of xanthoma disseminatum. The authors suggest that generalized eruptive histiocytoma and xanthoma disseminatum are variants of a continuous spectrum of histiocytoses [3].

The disease is generally self-limiting and often does not require treatment. PUVA has been shown to be an effective treatment in one patient with widespread disease [6].

References

1 Muller SA, Wolff K, Winkelmann RK. Generalised eruptive histiocytoma: enzyme histochemistry and electronmicroscopy. *Arch Dermatol* 1967; **96**: 11–7.

2 Winkelmann RK, Kossard S, Fraga S. Eruptive histiocytoma of childhood. *Arch Dermatol* 1980; **116**: 565–7.

3 Repiso T, Roc A, Miralles M *et al.* Generalised eruptive histiocytosis evolving into xanthoma disseminatum in a four year old boy. *Br J Dermatol* 1995; **132**: 978–82.

4 Caputo R, Alessi E, Allera F. Generalised eruptive histiocytoma: a clinical, histologic and ultrastructural study. *Arch Dermatol* 1981; **117**: 216–21.

5 Caputo R, Gianotti F. Cytoplasmic markers and ultrastructural features in histiocytic proliferations of the skin. *G Ital Dermatol Venereol* 1980; **115**: 107–20.

6 Lan M, Metze D, Luger TA *et al.* Successful treatment of generalised eruptive histiocytoma with PUVA. *J Dtsch Dermatol Ges* 2007; **5**: 131–4.

Papular xanthoma

This is a rare histiocytic disorder that was first described in adults [1] and subsequently reported in children [2]. Whether it represents a separate clinicopathological entity or a variant of other xanthogranulomatous conditions is open to debate. Clinically it can resemble juvenile xanthogranuloma but has not been associated with systemic involvement or café-au-lait spots, and may resemble xanthoma disseminatum but papules do not coalesce and there is no predilection for flexures.

Clinically, papular xanthoma is characterized by 2–15 mm yellow or reddish-yellow papules affecting both skin and mucous membranes. The back and head are most commonly affected. There are marked clinical differences between papular xanthoma occurring in adults and children. Mucous membranes are affected in adults but this has not been reported in children. In adults progressive disease has been reported [3] but in children spontaneous resolution is the norm, with involution starting after weeks or months and being complete in 1–5 years, often leaving anetoderma-like scarring [4].

Histologically, there is an upper- and mid-dermal infiltrate of foamy histiocytes and giant cells. Few inflammatory cells are present. Histiocytic cells are positive for CD68 and factor XIIIa and negative for S100 and CD1a [2,4]. More recent studies, however, have shown that the foamy cells in this disease are factor XIIIa negative [5,6]. In such a rare condition, further studies are needed to confirm the dermal dendrocyte origin of lesional cells. Electron microscopy shows similar changes to those seen in mature juvenile xanthogranuloma, with myeloid bodies filling the cytoplasm of the histiocytes with associated lysosomal inclusions, laminate bodies and lipid droplets.

No treatment is needed in children while none has been shown to be effective in adults.

References

1 Winkelmann RK. Adult histiocytic skin diseases. *G Ital Dermatol Venereol* 1980; **15**: 67–76.
2 Caputo R, Gianni E, Imondi D *et al*. Papular xanthoma in children. *J Am Acad Dermatol* 1992; **22**: 1052–6.
3 Beurey J, Lamaze B, Welere M. Xanthoma disseminatum (syndrome de Montgomery). *Ann Dermatol Vénéréol* 1979; **106**: 353–9.
4 Fonseca E, Contreras F, Cuevas J. Papular xanthoma in children: report and immunohistochemical study. *Pediatr Dermatol* 1993; **2**: 139–41.
5 Chen CG, Chen CL, Liu HN. Primary papular xanthoma of children: a clinicopathologic and ultrastructural study. *Am J Dermatopathol* 1997; **19**: 596–601.
6 Breier F, Zelger B, Reiter H *et al*. Papular xanthoma: a clinicopathological study of 10 cases. *J Cutan Pathol* 2002; **29**: 200–6.

Progressive nodular histiocytosis

Synonyms
• Progressive nodular histiocytoma
• Spindle cell xanthogranuloma

This is a rare histiocytosis first described by Taunton *et al*. [1] in 1978. The eruption consists of two different types of lesions, superficial papules and deep nodules, both of which may number into hundreds [2,3]. Papules are 2–10 mm and yellow–orange (Fig. 55.16). Nodules are 1–5 cm in diameter and may be skin coloured or reddish-orange. Distribution is random with no predilection for the flexures. Lesions may occur in the oral cavity, larynx and conjunctival mucosa.

Over the years new lesions may develop and although patients remain in good general health, the eruption may be very disfiguring causing a marked reduction in quality of life.

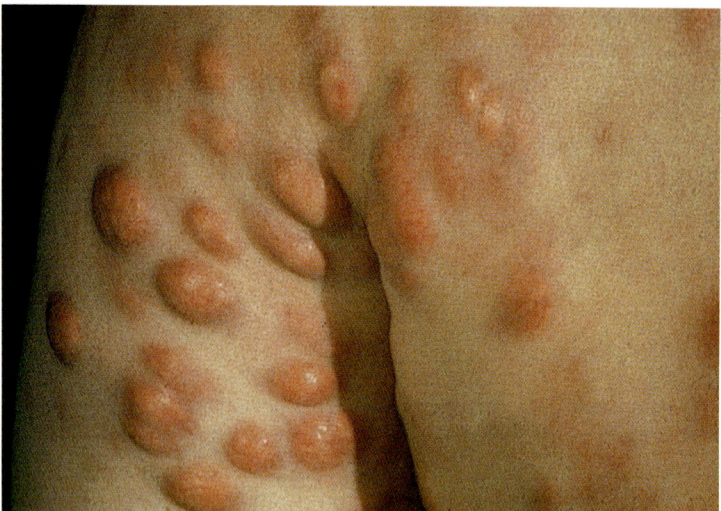

Fig. 55.16 Progressive nodular histiocytosis in a 48-year-old man with nodular lesions in the posterior axillary fold. (Courtesy of Professor J.M. Naeyaert, University Hospital, Gent, Belgium.)

Histologically, this is a dermal disease with neither epidermal involvement nor epidermotropism. Early lesions show an accumulation of xanthomatized and scalloped histiocytes with some infiltrating lymphocytes. In older lesions the histiocytes are spindle shaped and arranged in a storiform pattern. Occasional giant cells may be present. Cells are positive for CD68 and factor XIIIa and negative for S100 and CD1a [4].

Progressive nodular histiocytosis is not generally associated with systemic involvement or other disorders. In one case report, a 57-year-old man had suffered from progressive nodular histiocytosis for 26 years and during that time had developed chronic myeloid leukaemia, hepatosplenomegaly, hypothyroidism, hyperuricaemia and hypocholesterolaemia, although the relationship between progressive nodular histiocytosis and the systemic disorders remains unclear [5].

Progressive nodular histiocytosis is a benign disease and no treatment has yet been shown to be effective in reducing the size of skin lesions or in inducing remission.

References

1 Taunton OD, Yeshurun D, Jarratt M. Progressive nodular histiocytoma. *Arch Dermatol* 1978; **114**: 1505–8.
2 Gibbs NF, O'Grady TC. Progressive nodular histiocytomas. *J Am Acad Dermatol* 1996; **35**: 323–5.
3 Laftl M, Seybold H, Simon M *et al*. Progressive nodular histiocytosis—rare variant of cutaneous non-Langerhans cell histiocytosis. *J Dtsch Dermatol Ges* 2006; **4**: 236–8.
4 Zelger BWH, Standacher CH, Orchard G *et al*. Solitary and generalised variants of spindle cell xanthogranuloma (progressive nodular histiocytosis). *Histopathology* 1995; **27**: 11–9.
5 Gonzales Ruiz A, Bernal Ruiz AI, Artagoneses Fraile H *et al*. Progressive nodular histiocytosis accompanied by systemic disorders. *Br J Dermatol* 2000; **143**: 628–31.

Xanthoma disseminatum

Synonyms
• Disseminated xanthosiderohistiocytosis
• Montgomery's disease

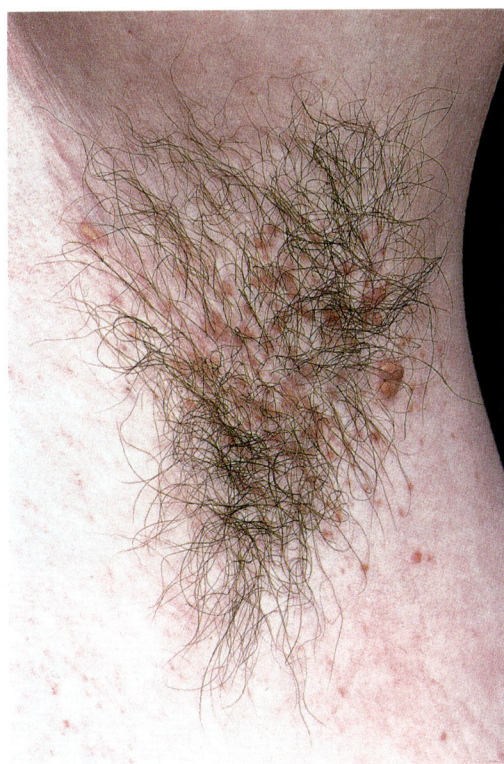

Fig. 55.17 Xanthoma disseminatum. (Courtesy of Dr R. Cerio, Royal London Hospital, London, UK.)

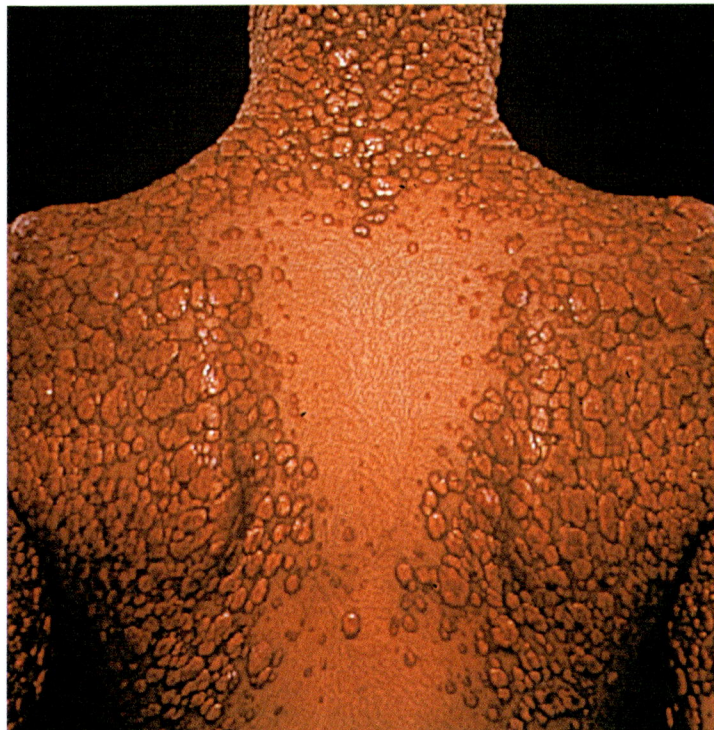

Fig. 55.18 Xanthoma disseminatum with verrucous lesions over the back of a 10-year-old boy.

This is a rare non-familial disease, characterized by proliferation of histiocytic cells in which lipid deposition is a secondary event. The disease predominantly affects male children and young adults, with involvement of the skin, mucous membranes of eyes and upper respiratory tract, the meninges and rarely other organs including liver, spleen and bone marrow [1–4].

The clinical lesions of xanthoma disseminatum are erythematous, yellow-brown papules and nodules, which are symmetrically distributed on the trunk, face and proximal extremities (Fig. 55.17). The lesions become confluent, especially in flexures, to form xanthomatous plaques, which may become verrucous (Fig. 55.18). In 30% of patients, the mucous membranes are affected, with particular involvement of the lips, pharynx, larynx, conjunctivae and bronchus. Involvement of the upper respiratory tract is not uncommon and may lead to stridor and respiratory distress requiring tracheostomy. Upper respiratory tract involvement has been fatal in one reported case of a 61-year-old woman with involvement of large and medium-sized bronchi who died of acute respiratory failure [5]. Lower respiratory tract involvement is very rare but in one 8-year-old boy, resulted in bronchiectasis [6].

Meningeal involvement is common, with infiltration at the base of the brain leading to diabetes insipidus in up to 40% of cases. Other manifestations of meningeal involvement are seizures and growth retardation. Intracranial involvement presenting as a discrete mass simulating glioma has been reported [7] and progressive intracranial disease may be fatal [8]. Progressive bone disease has been reported in xanthoma disseminatum [9,10], but this is a rare complication of the disease. Lytic bone lesions have been reported in a patient with xanthoma disseminatum, but are very rare [11,12]. Hepatic involvement is rare but a 12-year-old boy has been reported with liver dysfunction secondary to liver involvement by xanthoma disseminatum presenting as sclerosing cholangitis [13].

A clinical variant of this disease was described by Halprin and Lorincz [14] under the name xanthosiderohistiocytosis. In this variant, there is diffuse infiltration of the skin, subcutaneous tissue and muscle, giving rise to sclerodermatous changes in the skin and muscle wasting. The foamy histiocytes that are involved contain significant amounts of iron, which gives the skin a greenish-brown colour.

Histologically, xanthoma disseminatum is a dermal disease, characterized by early infiltration of the dermis with spindle-shaped mononuclear cells, foamy histiocytes, giant cells, lymphocytes, polymorphs and eosinophils. Lesional cells in xanthoma disseminatum have irregular scalloped borders with extensive cytoplasm and ovoid vesicular nuclei. Cells label strongly with factor XIIIa and KP1 [15]. Iron and lipid can be detected in the histiocytes. In older lesions, more foamy histiocytes are evident and Touton giant cells may be observed. At the ultrastructural level, histiocytic cells contain myeloid bodies and membrane-bound fat droplets.

Xanthoma disseminatum is a self-limiting disease but may persist for years. Lesions are only mildly radiosensitive. Skin lesions of xanthoma disseminatum are disfiguring and patients often request treatment. The carbon dioxide laser has been used with good results [16] and azathioprine and cyclophosphamide have been effective in some patients with cutaneous disease [17]. Conjunctival involvement can be treated with surgery. Systemic involvement with lung, liver or CNS involvement requires active treatment. Surgery has been used in CNS disease but recurrences may occur [8]. Liver involvement in one patient responded to systemic steroids and azathioprine [13]. Response to various modalities including radiotherapy, alkylating agents and antimetabolites has been variable [18].

References

1 Komatsuda A, Chubach A, Miura AB. Virus associated haemophagocytic syndrome due to measles accompanied by acute respiratory failure. *J Intern Med* 1995; **34**: 203–6.

2 Atlman J, Winklemann RK. Xanthoma disseminatum. *Arch Dermatol* 1962; **86**: 582–9.

3 Calverly DC, Wismer J, Rosonthal D *et al.* Xanthoma disseminatum in an infant with skeletal and marrow involvement. *J Pediatr Hematol Oncol* 1995; **17**: 61–5.

4 Fleishmajer R. Xanthoma disseminatum. In: Fleishmajer R, ed. *Dyslipoides.* Springfield, IL: Thomas, 1960: 176–83.

5 Davies CW, Marran P, Juniper MC *et al.* Xanthoma disseminatum with respiratory tract involvement and fatal outcome. *Thorax* 2000; **55**: 170–2.

6 Ozcelik U, Dogru D, Akcoren Z *et al.* Xanthoma disseminatum: a child with respiratory system involvement and bronchiectasis. *Pediatr Pulmonol* 2005; **39**: 84–7.

7 Chepuri NB, Challa VR. Xanthoma disseminatum: a rare intracranial mass. *Am J Neuroradiol* 2003; **24**: 105–8.

8 Zak IT, Altinok D, Neilsen SSF *et al.* Xanthoma disseminatum of the central nervous system and cranium. *Am J Neuroradiol* 2006; **27**: 919–21.

9 Blobstein SH, Caldwell D, Carter M. Bone lesions in xanthoma disseminatum. *Arch Dermatol* 1985; **121**: 1313–7.

10 Szekeres E, Tibia A, Korom I. Xanthoma disseminatum: a rare condition with non-X, non-lipid cutaneous histiocytopathy. *J Dermatol Surg Oncol* 1988; **14**: 1021–4.

11 Calverly DCV, Wismer J, Rosenthal D *et al.* Xanthoma disseminatum in an infant with skeletal and marrow involvement. *J Pediatr Hematol Oncol* 1995; **17**: 61–5.

12 Khandpur S, Manchanda Y, Sharma VK *et al.* Rare association of xanthoma disseminatum with skeletal involvement. *Australas J Dermatol* 2003; **44**: 190–3.

13 Buyukavci M, Selimoglu A, Yildrim U *et al.* Xanthoma disseminatum with hepatic involvement in a child. *Pediatr Dermatol* 2005; **22**: 550–3.

14 Halprin KM, Lorincz AL. Disseminated xanthosiderohistiocytosis (xanthoma disseminatum). Report of a case and discussion of possible relationship to other disorders showing histiocytic proliferation. *Arch Dermatol* 1960; **82**: 171–4.

15 Zelger B, Cerio R, Orchard G *et al.* Histologic and immunohistochemical study comparing xanthoma disseminatum and histiocytosis X. *Arch Dermatol* 1992; **128**: 1207–12.

16 Carpo BG, Grevelink SV, Brady S *et al.* Treatment of cutaneous lesions of xanthoma disseminatum with CO_2 laser. *Dermatol Surg* 1999; **25**: 751–4.

17 Seaton ED, Pillai GJ, Chu AC. Treatment of xanthoma disseminatum with cyclophosphamide. *Br J Dermatol* 2004; **150**: 346–9.

18 Alexander AS, Turner R, Uniate L *et al.* Xanthoma disseminatum: a case report and literature review. *Br J Radiol* 2005; **78**: 153–7.

Diffuse plane xanthomatosis

> **Synonyms**
> - Atypical xanthoma disseminatum
> - Diffuse normolipaemic plane xanthomatosis

This is a rare, non-lipaemic disease in which xanthomatous lesions develop in the skin in association with paraproteinaemia. The disease generally occurs in adults but rare paediatric cases have been reported [1]. Patients present with large, flat, plaque-like, xanthomatous skin lesions involving the eyelids, neck, upper trunk, buttocks and flexures [2,3]. Serum lipids are usually normal. About 50% of patients have a myeloproliferative disorder with multiple myeloma, granulocytic or lymphocytic leukaemia [4]. One patient with tumour stage cutaneous T-cell lymphoma

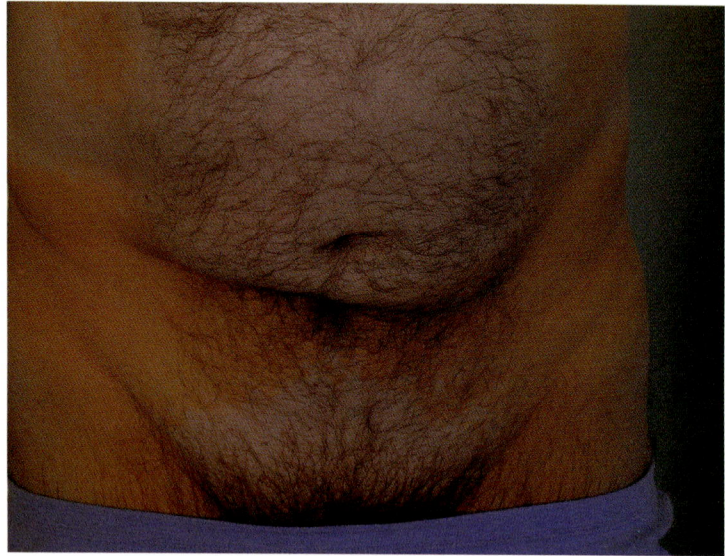

Fig. 55.19 Diffuse plane xanthomatosis in a 73-year-old man of 7 years' duration with associated IgGκ paraprotein.

developed diffuse plane xanthomatosis coincident with the appearance of new lymphoma lesions [5]. The majority of patients have a circulating paraprotein and have some abnormalities of serum complement [6,7].

The histological features include both xanthomatous and inflammatory elements. Accumulations of foamy macrophages infiltrate the dermis, with a distinct perivascular accentuation, and are associated to a variable degree with a mixed inflammatory cell reaction. There are no reported immunohistochemical studies in the world literature but a recent patient we have seen with characteristic skin changes (Fig. 55.19) and an IgGκ paraprotein, showed that the foamy macrophages were CD1a negative but strongly positive for CD68 and factor XIIIa.

The condition arises as a result of perivascular deposition of lipoprotein–immunoglobulin complexes. Antilipoprotein antibodies are formed in association with paraproteinaemia [7]. Although serum lipid levels are usually normal, they may be raised, possibly due to reduced clearance of lipoprotein–antibody complexes. Treatment of this condition is that of the underlying myeloproliferative disease or paraprotein. Theoretically, plasma exchange should be of value but its use has not yet been reported.

References

1 Hofmann M, Zappel K, Trefzer U *et al.* Diffuse normolipemic plane xanthoma in a 9 year old boy. *Pediatr Dermatol* 2005; **22**: 127–9.

2 Altman J, Winklemann RK. Diffuse normolipemic plane xanthoma. *Arch Dermatol* 1962; **85**: 115–22.

3 Lynch P, Winklemann RK. Generalized plane xanthoma and systemic disease. *Arch Dermatol* 1966; **93**: 639–46.

4 Macfarlane AW, Verbov JL. Necrobiotic xanthogranuloma with paraproteinaemia. *Br J Dermatol* 1985; **113**: 339–43.

5 Garcia-Arpa M, Rodriguez-Vazquez M, Vera E *et al.* Normolipaemic plane xanthomas and mycosis fungoides. *Actas Dermosifiliogr* 2005; **96**: 307–10.

6 Jordon RE, McDuffie FC, Good RA *et al.* Diffuse normolipemic plane xanthomatosis. An abnormal complement component profile. *Clin Exp Immunol* 1974; **18**: 407–15.

7 Russell Jones R, Baughan ASJ, Cream JJ *et al.* Complement abnormalities in plane xanthomata with paraproteinaemia. *Br J Dermatol* 1979; **101**: 711–6.

Class IIb histiocytosis: histiocytoses involving cells other than Langerhans' cells and dermal dendrocytes

Reticulohistiocytoma

Synonyms
- Solitary epithelioid histiocytoma
- Solitary histiocytoma

This is an uncommon tumour which is generally solitary and asymptomatic. Lesions less than 1 cm in diameter, presenting as papules or dome-shaped nodules, tend to occur in young adults but may appear from early childhood to old age. Lesions may occur anywhere on the body including the genitalia. Oral mucosal lesions have been reported [1].

Histology shows nodules of epithelioid histiocytes with abundant, glassy cytoplasm extending from the papillary dermis to the mid-dermis associated with lymphoid cells and occasionally neutrophils. Cells may have a lacuna space-like clearing at the periphery and scalloped cytoplasm. Cells are CD68 and CD163 positive and generally CD1a and S100 negative. In a study of five cases of solitary reticulohistiocytoma, factor XIIIa was found to be positive [2] but in a larger study of 44 cases, factor XIIIa was generally negative; however in five cases, histiocytic cells close to the dermoepidermal junction were found to be variably positive for factor XIIIa [1].

Treatment is surgical excision. Follow-up in 12 patients, with a median follow-up of 13 years, showed no recurrence following primary excision.

References
1 Miettinen M, Fetsch JF. Reticulohistiocytoma (solitary epithelioid histiocytoma): A clinicopathological and immunohistochemical study of 44 cases. *Am J Surg Pathol* 2006; **30**: 512–58.
2 Zelger B, Cerio R, Soyer HP *et al.* Reticulohistiocytoma and multicentric reticulohistiocytosis. *Am J Surg Pathol* 1994; **16**: 577–84.

Multicentric reticulohistiocytosis

Synonyms
- Reticulohistiocytic granuloma
- Lipoid dermatoarthritis
- Giant-cell histiocytoma
- Reticulohistiocytoma cutis
- Multicentric giant-cell reticulohistiocytosis

Definition. This is a rare histiocytic proliferative disease in which joints, skin and mucous membranes are affected [1]. The arthropathy usually precedes nodular skin involvement and mucosal infiltration. Other organs may be involved and 20% of patients have an associated internal malignancy. This must be differentiated from solitary or multiple reticulohistiocytomas that are restricted to skin with neither associated arthropathy nor internal malignancy.

Aetiology. Pathogenesis is unknown. The cells involved are phagocytic histiocytes, and the disease is considered to be a reac-

tive histiocytosis. No infective agent has been implicated but there is evidence of exposure to tuberculosis in some patients. In one study, 33% of patients had evidence of exposure to tuberculosis and 5% of patients had active tuberculosis on clinical examination [2]. There is no recorded genetic link. Those cases with internal malignancy have no clinical or pathological differences from those without associated malignancy.

Pathology. The characteristic pathological picture in the skin and mucous membranes is of infiltration by mononucleated and multinucleated giant cells with voluminous ground-glass cytoplasm. In early lesions, the predominant infiltrating cells are histiocytes, lymphocytes and eosinophils, with few giant cells, but the giant cell infiltrate quickly follows. The giant cells are large (100 μm) with 1–20 nuclei. The cells are periodic acid–Schiff (PAS) positive, contain diastase resistant material and variable amounts of lipid and free or esterified cholesterol. In older lesions, fibrosis usually signals regression of the lesions, with a reduction in the inflammatory cell infiltrate.

Ultrastructural studies have shown inclusions of type IV collagen inclusions in multicentric reticulohistiocytosis. These inclusions were both intracytoplasmic and extracytoplasmic. Such inclusions are usually found in lymphohistiocytic neoplasms, suggesting that multicentric reticulohistiocytosis is a proliferative rather than an inflammatory disorder [3].

Immunocytochemical studies show a histiocytic phenotype of the cells, which are positive for acid phosphatase, ATPase, lysozyme and α_1-antitrypsin [4]. The cells are also positive for vimentin, CD45 and CD68, but negative for CD1, S100 and CD34 and factor XIIIa [5]. Cells contain TNF-α, IL-1β and IL-12 [6]. Ultrastructural studies have shown that the cells contain dense bodies, coated vesicles, fat droplets in limiting membranes and myeloid bodies [7].

Clinical features. The disease typically affects women, with a female to male ratio of 3 : 1 [8]. It is a disease of middle age, and rarely affects children [9] or adolescents. Some 60% of patients present with polyarthritis, which typically affects the hands. The interphalangeal joints are affected symmetrically and are erythematous with an accompanying deforming polyarthritis, which ultimately results in shortening of the fingers and mutilation (Fig. 55.20). Other joints may be involved, including the knees, shoulders, wrists, hips, ankles, feet, elbows, spine and temporomandibular joints. Radiography of the affected joints shows destruction of the articular surfaces, with bone resorption and eventually secondary osteoarthritis [10]. Two case reports have highlighted the presence of osteolytic bone damage in this disease, in one patient affecting the bones of the upper limb [11] and in the second the skull, mimicking Langerhans' cell histiocytosis [12]. The authors suggest that the osteolytic lesions are due to the action of proinflammatory cytokines, TNF-α and IL-1, in inducing osteoclastic activity [12].

The classical skin lesions are firm brown or yellow papules and plaques, which predominantly affect extensor surfaces, particularly on the hands and forearms. The face (Fig. 55.21), scalp, hands and ears are often affected but involvement of the lower trunk and legs is rare. Coral bead-like lesions may occur around the nail

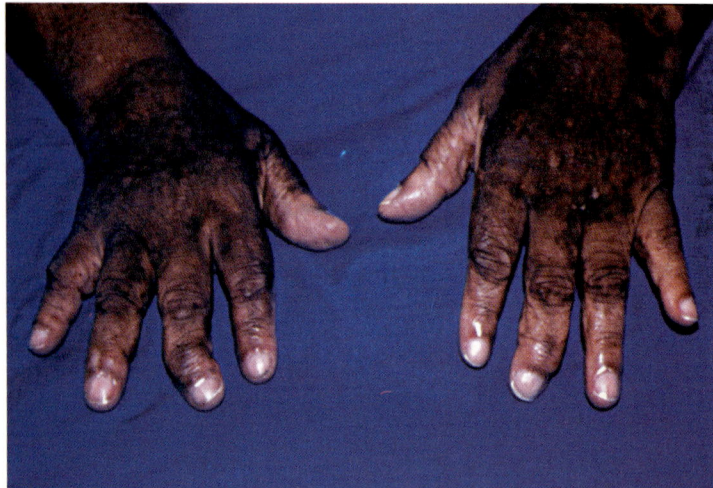

Fig. 55.20 Multicentric reticulohistiocytosis showing the characteristic skin changes, with multiple firm papular lesions on the sides of the fingers and obvious destructive arthropathy. (Courtesy of Professor N. Saxe, Groote Schuur Hospital, Cape Town, South Africa.)

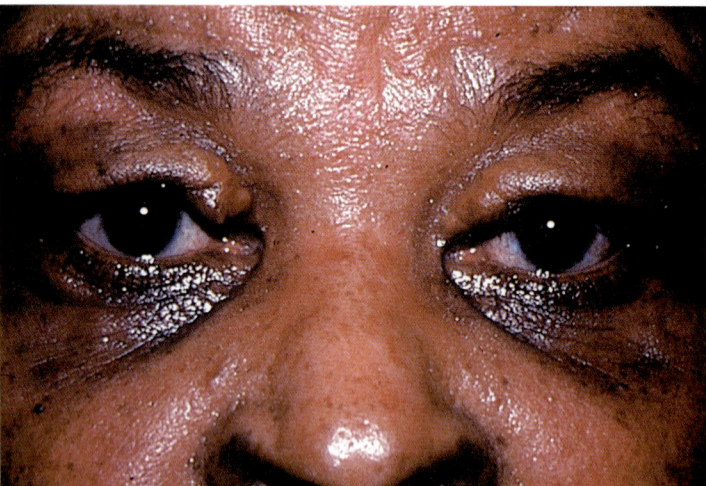

Fig. 55.21 Multicentric reticulohistiocytoma with characteristic lesions around the eyes. (Courtesy of Professor N. Saxe, Groote Schuur Hospital, Cape Town, South Africa.)

folds, which may result in nail dystrophy. Skin lesions are of variable size and rarely ulcerate. Large nodular lesions in proximity to affected joints and cystic swellings of tendon sheaths may occur. About 25% of patients complain of pruritus associated with skin lesions. Diffuse cutaneous reticulohistiocytosis without arthropathy [9] and isolated reticulohistiocytomas [13] have been described. The cutaneous lesions have the same histology as lesions in multicentric reticulohistiocytosis but are not associated with joint problems or neoplasms.

More than 50% of patients have mucosal involvement affecting the mouth, gingiva, pharynx, larynx and sclera. Characteristically, the lips and tongue are involved [14], and 30% of patients have abnormalities of serum lipids. Laboratory findings are normal with a negative rheumatoid factor. Even in the most active stages of the disease, the erythrocyte sedimentation rate is only marginally elevated.

Constitutional symptoms of pyrexia and weight loss may occur. Involvement of bone marrow, skeletal muscle, lymph nodes, heart, pericardium, lungs, pleura, bones, liver, duodenal mesentery and kidney have been reported. Deaths have occurred with cardiac involvement [15]. Multicentric reticulohistiocytosis has been reported in association with Sjögren's syndrome [16] and thyroid involvement [17].

Around 20% of patients have been found to have an associated internal malignancy. The commonest tumours are gastric, ovarian [18], breast and uterine carcinomas [19], myeloma [20], melanoma [21] and lymphomas. Rare case reports have described Ki-1 lymphoma occurring in association with multicentric reticulohistiocytosis [22]. Myelodysplastic syndrome has been reported in one patient with multicentric reticulohistiocytosis, although this patient had been treated with cytotoxic drugs for many years and the myelodysplasia may have been drug related [23]. The diagnosis of multicentric reticulohistiocytosis precedes that of the neoplasm in most cases, and the disease may relapse with recurrence of the neoplasm [24].

Prognosis. The prognosis is good if there is no systemic malignancy, the disease becoming quiescent in 7–8 years. Fatal cardiac involvement may occur with widespread systemic involvement [15]. It does, however, leave considerable morbidity, with a crippling arthropathy and scarred skin.

Diagnosis. Multicentric reticulohistiocytosis has been clinically mistaken for dermatomyositis in a patient with a macular eruption in a photodistribution [25], lupus erythematosus [26] and lepromatous leprosy [27]. Biopsy of skin nodules helps to differentiate multicentric reticulohistiocytosis from eruptive xanthomas and juvenile xanthogranulomas. The disease can usually be clinically differentiated from other disorders involving cutaneous nodules and arthritis (e.g. rheumatoid arthritis, sarcoidosis, gout and xanthomatosis).

Treatment. No treatment is of consistent value in this disease. Systemic steroids may be successful for brief periods but their long-term value is uncertain. Combination of systemic steroids with azathioprine has been used with success [28]. One case report of a patient with joint and skin involvement showed persistent improvement in all sites with the bisphosphonate, alendronate [29]. Non-steroidal anti-inflammatory agents have no effect on the arthropathy. Immunosuppressive drugs give variable results. Cyclophosphamide is reported to give high success rates [30], and ciclosporin has been reported to give good results [31]. Some case reports suggest that TNF-α antagonists may have a role in the treatment of this disease [32,33].

References

1 Luz FB, Gaspar NK, Gaspar AP *et al.* Multicentric reticulohistiocytosis: a proliferation of macrophages with tropism for skin and joints, part II. *Skinmed* 2007; **6**: 227–33.

2 Campbell DA, Edwards NL. Multicentric reticulohistiocytosis: systemic macrophage disorder. *Baillieres Clin Rheumatol* 1991; **5**: 301–19.

3 Fortier-Beaulieu M, Thomine E, Boullie MC *et al.* New electron microscopic findings in a case of multicentric reticulohistiocytosis. Long spacing collagen inclusions. *Am J Dermatopathol* 1993; **15**: 587–9.

4 Heathcote JG, Guenther LC, Wallace AC. Multicentric reticulohistiocytosis: a report of a case and review of the pathology. *Pathology* 1985; **17**: 601–8.

5 Luz FB, Gaspar AP, Ramos-e-Silva M *et al*. Immunohistochemical profile of multicentric reticulohistiocytosis. *Skinmed* 2005; **4**: 71–7.

6 Gorman JD, Danning C, Schmacher HR. Multicentric reticulohistiocytosis: case report with immunohistochemical analysis and literature review. *Arthritis Rheum* 2000; **43**: 930–8.

7 Flam M, Ryan SC, Mah-Poy GL *et al*. Multicentric reticulohistiocytosis: report of a case with atypical features and electron microscopy study of skin lesions. *Am J Med* 1972; **52**: 841–8.

8 Barrow MV, Holubar K. Multicentric reticulosis: a review of thirty-three patients. *Medicine (Baltimore)* 1969; **48**: 287–305.

9 Raphael SA, Cowery SL, Faeber EN *et al*. Multicentric reticulohistiocytosis in a child. *J Pediatr* 1989; **114**: 266–9.

10 Toporcer MB, Kantor GR, Benedetto AV. Multiple cutaneous reticulohistiocytosis. *J Am Acad Dermatol* 1991; **25**: 948–51.

11 Chen CH, Chen CH, Chen HA *et al*. Multicentric reticulohistiocytosis presenting with destructive polyarthritis, laryngopharyngeal dysfunction, and a huge reticulohistiocytoma. *J Clin Rheumatol* 2006; **12**: 252–4.

12 Ho SG, Yu RC. A case of multicentric reticulohistiocytosis with multiple lytic skull lesions. *Clin Exp Dermatol* 2005; **30**: 515–8.

13 Anaguchi S, Sinomiya S, Kinebuchi S *et al*. Solitary reticulohistiocytic granuloma: a report of three cases and a review of the literature. *Nippon Hifuka Gakkai Zasshi* 1991; **101**: 735–42.

14 Katz RW, Anderson KF. Multicentric reticulohistiocytosis. *Oral Surg Oral Med Oral Pathol* 1988; **65**: 721–5.

15 Yee KC, Bowker CM, Tam CY *et al*. Cardiac and systemic complications in multicentric reticulohistiocytosis. *Clin Exp Dermatol* 1993; **18**: 558–68.

16 Carey RN, Blotzer JW, Wolfe ID *et al*. Multicentric reticulohistiocytosis and Sjogren's syndrome. *J Rheumatol* 1985; **12**: 1193–5.

17 Finelli LG, Tenner LK, Ratz JL *et al*. A case of multicentric reticulohistiocytosis with thyroid involvement. *J Am Acad Dermatol* 1986; **15**: 1097–100.

18 Kishikawa T, Miyashita T, Fujiwara E *et al*. Multicentric reticulohistiocytosis associated with ovarian cancer. *Mod Rheumatol* 2007; **17**: 422–5.

19 Malik MK, Regan L, Robinson-Bostom L *et al*. Proliferating multicentric reticulohistiocytosis associated with papillary serous carcinoma of the endometrium. *J Am Acad Dermatol* 2005; **53**: 1075–9.

20 Fenniche S, Haoulet S, Hauman H *et al*. Multicentric histiocytosis revealing multiple myeloma. *Eur J Dermatol* 1996; **6**: 450–7.

21 Snow JC, Muller SA. Malignancy associated histiocytosis: a clinical, histiological and immunophenotypic study. *Br J Dermatol* 1995; **133**: 71–6.

22 Kuramoto Y, Lizawa O, Matsunaga J *et al*. Development of Ki-1 lymphoma in a child suffering from multicentric reticulohistiocytosis. *Acta Derm Venereol (Stockh)* 1991; **71**: 448–9.

23 Bauer A, Garbe C, Detmar M *et al*. Multicentric reticulohistiocytosis and myelodysplastic syndrome. *Hautarzt* 1994; **45**: 91–6.

24 Nunnink JC, Krusinski PA, Yates JW. Multicentric reticulohistiocytosis and cancer: a case report and review of the literature. *Med Pediatr Oncol* 1985; **13**: 273–9.

25 Muñoz-Santos C, Sàbat M, Sáez A *et al*. Multicentric reticulohistiocytosis-mimicking dermatomyositis. Case report and review of the literature. *Dermatology* 2007; **214**: 268–71.

26 Badlissi F, Setty Y, Folzenlogen D. A case of multicentric reticulohistiocytosis initially misdiagnosed as lupus. *J Clin Rheumatol* 2002; **8**: 232–3.

27 Agarwal US, Mathur DK, Jain R *et al*. Multicentric reticulohistiocytosis misdiagnosed as lepromatous leprosy. *Indian J Lepr* 2003; **75**: 259–62.

28 Fedler R, Grantzmann Y, Schwarze EW *et al*. Multicentric reticulohistiocytosis. Therapy with azathiopine and prednisolone. *Hautarzt* 1995; **46**: 118–20.

29 Goto H, Inaba M, Imanishi Y *et al*. Successful treatment of multicentric reticulohistiocytosis with alendronate: evidence for direct effect of bisphosphonate on histiocytes. *Arthritis Rheum* 2003; **48**: 3538–41.

30 Ginsberg WW, O'Duffy JD, Morris JL *et al*. Multicentric reticulohistiocytosis: response to alkylating agents in six patients. *Ann Intern Med* 1989; **111**: 384–8.

31 Saito K, Fujii K, Awazu Y *et al*. A case of systemic lupus erythematosus complicated with multicentric reticulohistiocytosis (MRH): successful treatment of MRH and lupus nephritis with cyclosporin A. *Lupus* 2001; **10**: 129–32.

32 Lovelace K, Loyd A, Adelson D *et al*. Etanercept and the treatment of multicentric reticulohistiocytosis. *Arch Dermatol* 2005; **141**: 1167–8.

33 Sellam J, Deslandre CJ, Dubreuil F *et al*. Refractory multicentric reticulohistiocytosis treated by infliximab: two cases. *Clin Exp Rheumatol* 2005; **23**: 97–9.

Familial haemophagocytic lymphohistiocytosis

Synonyms
- Familial haemophagocytic reticulosis
- Generalized lymphohistiocytic infiltration
- Familial erythrophagocytic lymphohistiocytosis
- Familial histiocytic reticulosis
- Familial lymphohistiocytosis
- Farquhar's disease

This is a rare reactive histiocytosis in which there is widespread infiltration of multiple organs by lymphocytes and mature histiocytes showing prominent cytophagocytosis. It is rapidly fatal in most patients. The incidence is 1.2 per million children [1], with a slight preponderance in boys. Three-quarters of cases are familial, and it is generally considered to be an autosomal recessive disease [2].

The genes responsible in some cases have been identified and studies have identified subsets of familial haemophagocytic lymphohistiocytosis (FHL) depending on the genetic defect. In one patient a constitutional inversion in chromosome 9 (p23;q31) was observed in cells from bone marrow, lymphocytes and fibroblasts [3]. This locus accounts for approximately 10% of cases (FHL-1) [4]. FHL-2 represents 20–30% of all cases and is characterized by mutation in genes coding for perforin, a lytic granule constituent (*PRF-1*; MIMI 70280). The mutation in the perforin gene occurs at position 374, resulting in a premature stop codon. A study of 34 families and linkage studies of a subset of consanguineous families indicates that perforin mutations account for 20–40% of cases of FHL [4]. FHL-3 represents 20–25% of all cases and is characterized by mutations in *MUNC13–14* genes [4]. Other mutations include nonsense and missense mutations and deletions of amino acids [5].

Fever is usually the first sign of the disease, with symptoms of an upper respiratory or gastrointestinal tract infection in 30%. Pallor, anorexia, vomiting and irritability are often noted. Hepatosplenomegaly is usually present at presentation and is progressive. Moderate lymphadenopathy is common. Around 50% of patients develop a transient, non-specific, maculopapular rash, which is often seen at times of high fever, but no persistent skin infiltration is seen. About 20% of patients have neurological symptoms, due to meningeal involvement, usually with convulsions but also with other signs of meningeal irritation.

Laboratory tests show anaemia, thrombocytopenia and raised liver enzymes and hyperbilirubin. Hyperlipidaemia (with elevation of triglycerides and very low-density lipoproteins) and hypofibrinogenaemia are common.

Immunological testing shows abnormalities of both the humoral and cellular limbs of the immune system. Natural antibody titres are low, antibody titres after previous immunization are low and there is an impaired response to primary immunization. All T-cell responses to mitogens, antigens and alloantigens are reduced. There is also a T-cell-suppressor factor, probably related to triglycerides, in the plasma of the patients [6]. Cytotoxic T-cell and natural killer cell activity is markedly reduced or absent in affected patients.

A number of studies have now demonstrated hypercytokinaemia in this disease, with elevated amounts of circulating IFN-γ, TNF-γ and IL-6 during active disease [7]. Serum levels of IL-6 have been shown to be of no prognostic importance [8]. Soluble CD8 has also been shown to be elevated, suggesting a role for cytotoxic T cells in the pathogenesis of this disease.

Histologically, the involved tissue shows a diffuse infiltrate with lymphocytes and mature histiocytes. The histiocytes exhibit active phagocytosis, especially of erythrocytes but also of leukocytes and occasionally platelets. The histiocytes stain positively for acid phosphatase, non-specific esterase, lysozyme and α₁-antichymotrypsin. A striking histological finding is lymphocyte depletion of lymph nodes, spleen and thymus.

Prognosis is poor, with median survival of 2–3 months [9] from diagnosis and 96% dying within 12 months. Central nervous system disease and persistently low natural killer cell activity are associated with poorer prognosis [10]. Long-term survivors have been reported after chemotherapy, but maintenance therapy is always required.

Initial treatment regimens used splenectomy, exchange transfusion [11] and chemotherapy [12], including vinblastine and intrathecal methotrexate. Henter *et al.* [13] reported a more successful regimen using etoposide and teniposide with prednisolone and intrathecal methotrexate until remission is achieved, followed by maintenance therapy with teniposide or etoposide. A recent study advocated the use of antithymocyte globulin in early stages of the disease showing low toxicity and good responses [14].

Bone marrow transplantation and haemopoietic stem cell transplantation [15] are now regarded as being the most effective treatments for this disease. Results are much better when HLA-identical siblings are used as donors. Studies have now shown that even partial engraftment is compatible with long-term remission [10,16].

References

1 Henter J-I. Familial haemophagocytic lymphohistiocytosis. A clinical, metabolic and immunological study of lymphohistiocytic inflammatory disorder. *Kongl Carolinska Medico Chirurgiska Institutet (Stockh)* 1990.

2 Genik A, Signer E, Muller H. Genetic analysis of familial erythrophagocytic lymphohistiocytosis. *Eur J Pediatr* 1984; **142**: 248–52.

3 Hasle H, Brandt C, Kerndrup G et al. Haemophagocytic lymphohistiocytosis associated with constitutional inversion of chromosome 9. *Br J Haematol* 1996; **93**: 808–9.

4 Ishii E, Ueda I, Shirakawa R et al. Genetic subtypes of familial hemophagocytic lymphohistiocytosis: correlations with clinical features and cytotoxic T lymphocyte/natural killer cell functions. *Blood* 2005; **105**: 3442–8.

5 Janka G, Schneider M, Gurgey A et al. Spectrum of perforin gene mutations in familial haemophagocytic lymphohistiocytosis. *Am J Hum Genet* 2001; **68**: 590–7.

6 Ladisch S, Poplack DG, Holiman B et al. Immunodeficiency in familial erythrophagocytic lymphohistiocytosis. *Lancet* 1978; **i**: 581–3.

7 Henter J-I, Elinder G, Soder O et al. Hypercytokinaemia in familial haemophagocytic lymphohistiocytosis. *Blood* 1991; **78**: 2918–22.

8 Imashuku S, Hibi S, Gujiwara F et al. Hyperinterleukinaemia (IL)6 in haemophagocytic lymphohistiocytosis. *Br J Haematol* 1996; **93**: 803–7.

9 Janka G. Familial haemophagocytic lymphohistiocytosis. *Eur J Pediatr* 1983; **140**: 221–30.

10 Imashuku S, Hyakuna N, Funabiki T et al. Central nervous system as a high risk prognostic indicator in young patients with familial haemophagocytic lymphohistiocytosis. *Cancer* 2002; **94**: 3023–31.

11 Ladisch S, Ho W, Matheson D et al. Immunologic and clinical effects of repeated blood exchange in familial erythrophagocytic lymphohistiocytosis. *Blood* 1982; **60**: 814–21.

12 Lillyman JS. The treatment of familial erythrophagocytic lymphohistiocytosis. *Cancer* 1980; **46**: 468–70.

13 Henter J-I, Elinder G, Finkel Y et al. Successful induction with chemotherapy including teniposide in familial erythrophagocytic lymphohistiocytosis. *Lancet* 1986; **ii**: 1402.

14 Mahlaoui N, Ouachee-Chardin M, de Saint Basile G et al. Immunotherapy of familial hemophagocytis lymphohistiocytosis with antithymocyte globulins: a single centre retrospective report of 38 patients. *Pediatrics* 2007; **120**: 622–8.

15 Ouachee-Chardin M, Elie C, de saint Basile G et al. Hematopoietic stem cell transplantation in hemophagocytic lymphohistiocytosis: a single centre report of 48 patients. *Pediatrics* 2006; **117**: 743–50.

16 Landman-Parker J, LeDeist F, Blaise A et al. Partial engraftment of donor bone marrow cells associated with long term remission of haemophagocytic lymphohistiocytosis. *Br J Haematol* 1993; **81**: 37–41.

Familial sea-blue histiocytosis

This is a rare inherited abnormality of lipid metabolism [1] in which characteristic histiocytic cells are found in the bone marrow and other tissues. The histiocytes are identified by the May–Gruenwald stain, which colours the cytoplasmic granules a deep azure blue, hence the name 'sea-blue histiocytosis'.

Familial sea-blue histiocytosis in an autosomal recessive trait [2]. It usually presents in young adulthood with hepatosplenomegaly and thrombocytopenia, although the age at presentation ranges from 1 to 83 years. The skin, lungs, gastrointestinal tract, eye and nervous system may be involved. In the skin, patchy and irregular brownish-grey pigmentation of the face, upper chest and shoulders has been reported. In one case [3], skin involvement, with eyelid swelling and facial nodules, was confirmed histologically. In the eye, white stippled deposits may be observed at the margins of the fovea or macula, with discoloration of the macular region. Neurological symptoms occur early, with ataxia, epilepsy and dementia.

Sea-blue histiocytosis is not malignant, but it may disseminate and lead to death from liver or lung involvement. The biological abnormality is poorly understood, but the condition probably represents a storage disease in which glycolipid, phospholipid or both accumulate in histiocytic cells in various organs. Sea-blue histiocytes have also been described in chronic myelogenous leukaemia [4,5], adult Niemann–Pick disease [6], following the prolonged use of intravenous fat emulsions in children [7] and in partial sphingomyelinase deficiency [8].

References

1 Wewalka F. Zur Frage der 'blauen pigment Makrophagen in sternal Punktat. *Wien Klin Wochenschr* 1950; **62**: 788–91.

2 Sawitsky A, Rodner F, Chodsky S. The sea blue histiocyte syndrome, a review: genetic and biochemical studies. *Semin Hematol* 1972; **9**: 285–97.

3 Zina AM, Bundino S, Pippione M. Sea blue histiocyte syndrome with cutaneous involvement. Case report with ultrastructural findings. *Dermatologica* 1987; **174**: 39–44.

4 Dosik H, Rosner F, Sawitsky A. Acquired lipidoses: Gaucher-like cells and blue cells in chronic myeloid leukaemia. *Semin Hematol* 1972; **9**: 309–16.

5 Hogan SF, Osborne BM, Butler JJ. Unexpected splenic nodules in leukaemic patients. *Hum Pathol* 1989; **20**: 62–8.

6 Dewhurst N, Besley GTN, Finlayson NDC *et al.* Sea blue histiocytosis in a patient with chronic non-neuropathic Niemann–Pick disease. *J Clin Pathol* 1979; **32**: 1121–7.

7 Goulet O, Girot R, Maier-Redelsperger M *et al.* Hematologic disorders following prolonged use of intravenous fat emulsions in children. *J Parenter Enteral Nutr* 1986; **10**: 284–8.

8 Konagaya M, Konishi T, Konagaya Y *et al.* Partial sphingomyelinase deficiency with sea blue histiocytosis and neurovisceral dysfunction. *Jpn J Med* 1989; **28**: 85–8.

Hereditary progressive mucinous histiocytosis

This is a rare autosomal dominant genodermatosis, which was first described in 1988. All case reports to date have been in women, thus suggesting a link to hormones [1]. Skin lesions appear in the first decade of life and gradually increase throughout life. Lesions consist of skin-coloured to red-brown papules that characteristically affect the nose, hands, forearms and thighs. Two sets of case reports have described mothers and daughters who have both presented with the disease [2,3]. Histologically, the epidermis is normal but within the dermis there are small collections of epithelioid histiocytes with telangiectatic vessels in the upper dermis in early lesions. As tumours develop, the infiltrate changes to nodular mid-dermal aggregates of tightly packed, spindle-shaped cells. In both early and established lesions, there is moderate to extensive mucin production by the epithelioid histiocytes and spindle-shaped cells. On electron microscopy, the spindle-shaped cells are shown to be dendritic histiocytes with abundant lysosomal storage organelles, myelin bodies and zebra bodies.

Immunohistochemically, these cells stain with CD68 and MS1 [3]. The condition is progressive, with gradual increase in numbers of tumours throughout life. These patients show no evidence of spontaneous resolution. No systemic involvement has been described and no treatment seems to have any impact on the disease [4,5].

References

1 Antoni-Bach N, Pfister R, Grosshans E *et al.* Hereditary progressive mucinous histiocytosis. *Ann Dermatol Venereol* 2000; **127**: 400–4.

2 Bork K. Hereditary progressive mucinous histiocytosis. Immunohistochemical and ultrastructural studies in an additional family. *Arch Dermatol* 1994; **130**: 1300–4.

3 Schroder K, Hettmannsperger U, Schmid M *et al.* Hereditary progressive mucinous histiocytosis. *J Am Acad Dermatol* 1996; **35**: 298–303.

4 Wong D, Killingsworth M, Crosland G *et al.* Hereditary progressive mucinous histiocytosis. *Br J Dermatol* 1999; **141**: 1101–5.

5 Young A, Olivere J, Yoo S *et al.* Two sporadic cases of adult onset progressive mucinous histiocytosis. *J Cutan Pathol* 2006; **32**: 166–70.

Malakoplakia

Malakoplakia is an immunodeficiency disease in which macrophages fail to phagocytose and digest bacteria adequately. The term 'malakoplakia', which means soft plaque, was adopted as a descriptive term [1].

Malakoplakia can affect many organs but most commonly affects the urinary and gastrointestinal tracts [2,3]. Cutaneous lesions are rare, non-specific and variable. Draining abscesses, sinuses, ulcers, fluctuant masses, isolated tender nodules and grouped papules have been reported. Mucous membranes may be affected, including the tongue [4] and cervix [5]. The disease generally runs a benign self-limiting course, but fatal cases have been reported [6].

Histologically, sheets of large histiocytic cells with abundant cytoplasm are present in the skin, affecting any level from epidermis to subcutaneous fat. The cells have fine eosinophilic granules in their cytoplasm and are referred to as Hansemann cells. They also contain one or more round basophilic inclusion bodies (Michaelis–Gutmann bodies). Michaelis–Gutmann bodies are 5–15 µm and stain positively with PAS, von Kossa stain (for calcium) and Perls ferrocyanide reaction (for ferric iron). They are considered pathognomonic for this disease and are thought to represent abnormal degradation of bacteria, with calcium and iron deposited on the remaining glycolipid.

The commonest bacterium found in this disease is *Escherichia coli* [7,8], although *Staphylococcus aureus* has also been cultured [9]. Mycobacteria have been identified in two cases of cutaneous malakoplakia using polyclonal anti-*Mycobacteria bovis* antibodies [10]. In some patients, the disease is related to drug-induced immunosuppression [11]. In one patient [6], intracellular cyclic guanosine monophosphate (cGMP) levels were found to be low, and *in vivo* and *in vitro* treatment of the cells with bethanechol chloride, a cholinergic agonist, increased cGMP and restored their bactericidal activity.

References

1 Michaelis L, Gutmann C. Uber Einschlusse in Blastentumoren. *Z Klin Med* 1902; **47**: 208–15.

2 Long JP Jr, Althausen AF. Malakoplakia: a 25 year experience with a review of the literature. *J Urol* 1989; **141**: 1328–31.

3 Yousef GM, Naghibi B. Malakoplakia outside the urinary tract. *Arch Pathol Lab Med* 2007; **131**: 297–300.

4 Love RB, Bernard PA, Carpenter BF. Malakoplakia of the tongue. *J Otolaryngol* 1985; **14**: 179–82.

5 Falcon-Escobedo R, Mora Tiscareno A, Pubeblitz-Peredo S *et al.* Malakoplakia of the uterine cervix: histologic, cytologic and ultrastructural study of a case. *Acta Cytol* 1986; **30**: 281–4.

6 Dervan PA, Teeling M, Dempsey J *et al.* Lymphadenopathy due to fatal histiocytic proliferative disorder containing Michaelis Gutmann bodies. *Cancer* 1986; **57**: 1337–40.

7 Abdou NI, Pombejara C, Sagawa A *et al.* Malakoplakia: evidence for monocyte lysosomal abnormality correctable by cholinergic agonist *in vitro* and *in vivo*. *N Engl J Med* 1977; **297**: 1413–9.

8 Nieland ML, Borochovitz D, Silverman AR *et al.* Cutaneous malakoplakia. *Am J Dermatopathol* 1981; **3**: 287–94.

9 Sencer O, Sencer H, Uluoglu O *et al.* Malakoplakia of the skin. *Arch Pathol* 1979; **103**: 446–50.

10 Mehregan DR, Mehregan AM, Mehregan DA. Cutaneous malakoplakia: a report of two cases with use of anti-BCG for detection of micro-organisms. *J Am Acad Dermatol* 2000; **43**: 351–4.

11 Sian CS, McCabe RE, Lattes CG. Malakoplakia of the skin and subcutaneous tissue in a renal transplant recipient. *Arch Dermatol* 1981; **117**: 654–5.

Necrobiotic xanthogranuloma

The syndrome of necrobiosis with xanthomatous granulomas and an associated paraprotein has been recognized since 1966 [1–3], but it was not until 1980 that it was recognized as a distinct dermatosis [4].

The characteristic clinical lesions are periorbital nodular and ulcerative lesions, which have the reddish-yellow colour of xanthomas (Fig. 55.22). On the trunk and limbs, subcutaneous nodules and xanthomatous plaques are present with atrophy and

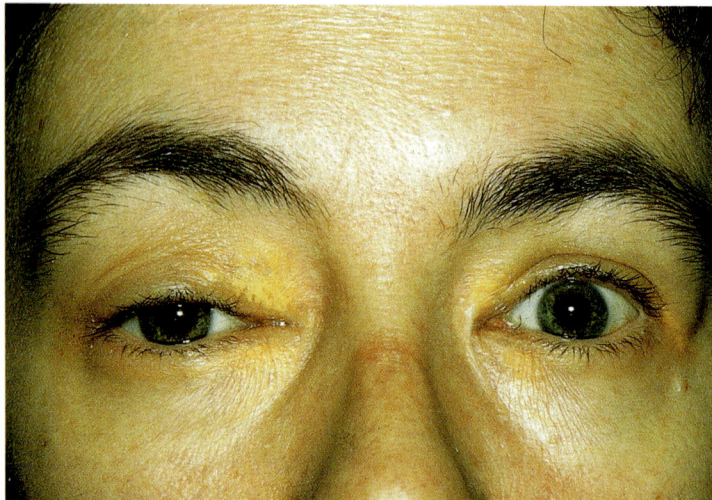

Fig. 55.22 Early lesions of necrobiotic xanthogranuloma with characteristic distribution in the periorbital area. (Courtesy of Dr A. Layton, Leeds General Infirmary, Leeds, UK.)

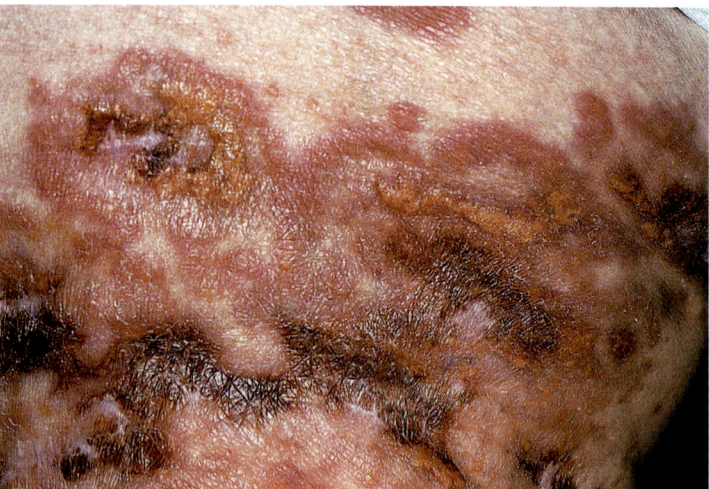

Fig. 55.23 Established lesions of necrobiotic xanthogranuloma on the abdomen showing xanthomatous plaques and atrophy. (Courtesy of Dr P. Holt, University Hospital, Cardiff, UK.)

ulceration (Fig. 55.23). The eyes are often affected with conjunctivitis, keratitis, uveitis, iritis and proptosis. Blindness has been reported in two affected patients [4]. Only one case report of a patient with typical cutaneous lesions and cerebral involvement presenting as tonic–clonic seizures has been published [5]. Systemic symptoms have been reported, including nausea, vomiting, fatigue, epistaxis, back pain and Raynaud's phenomenon. Atypical forms of necrobiotic xanthogranuloma have been reported, including solitary tumours of the skin [6].

The majority of cases have an associated paraprotein, usually an IgG κ or λ monoclonal protein. In a series of 22 patients, 16 had IgG monoclonal protein, three had multiple myeloma, three had cryoglobulinaemia and one had normal serum protein electrophoresis [7].

Decreased levels of C1 inhibitor have been reported in some patients with necrobiotic xanthogranuloma, occasionally associ-

ated with angio-oedema. Immune complex formation resulting from autoantibodies against the paraproteins have been implicated in the depletion of C1 inactivator [8].

Histologically, confluent granulomatous masses are present as either sheets or nodules, replacing much of the dermis and extending into the subcutaneous tissue [9]. Hyaline areas of necrobiosis separate individual nodules. Numerous giant cells are present, with Touton cells and bizarre angulated giant cells. Cholesterol clefts, lymphoid nodules (some of which develop germinal centres) and perivascular aggregates of plasma cells are frequent features. Less common, but characteristic when present, are palisading cholesterol cleft granulomas and xanthogranulomatous panniculitis. Granulomatous invasion of blood vessels with thrombosis has been described.

The pathogenesis of necrobiotic xanthogranuloma is unknown. Bullock *et al.* [10] suggested that the abnormal paraprotein becomes complexed with lipid and deposited in the skin, where it produces a foreign-body granulomatous reaction.

Treatment is generally directed to the associated paraproteinaemia. Alkylating agents such as melphalan, with or without prednisolone, have resulted in temporary clearing of the skin [11]. In one patient where cytotoxic drugs had failed, plasmapheresis reduced the level of the circulating monoclonal IgG and resulted in clearing of the skin [12]. Successful treatment with chlorambucil 2 mg/day for 7 months has been reported in a 51-year-old man with necrobiotic xanthogranuloma and associated paraproteinaemia [13]. Radiotherapy was successful in one case involving the eye [14]. Cutaneous disease has been successfully treated with carbon dioxide laser with no evidence of relapse after 12 months [15].

References

1 Frank SB. Xanthomatous granuloma. *Arch Dermatol* 1977; **113**: 1450–8.
2 Muller SA, Winkelmann RK. Atypical forms of necrobiosis lipoidica diabeticorum: a report of 3 cases. *Arch Pathol* 1966; **81**: 352–61.
3 Risdall RJ, Venhegan RI, Robb-Smith AH *et al.* Atypical multicentric reticulohistiocytosis with paraproteinaemia. *Arch Dermatol* 1977; **113**: 1576–82.
4 Kossard S, Winkelmann RK. Necrobiotic xanthogranuloma with paraproteinaemia. *J Am Acad Dermatol* 1980; **3**: 257–70.
5 Shah KC, Poonnoose SI, George R *et al.* Necrobiotic xanthogranuloma with cutaneous and cerebral manifestations. *J Neurosurg* 2004; **100**: 1111–4.
6 Stork J, Kodetova D, Vosmik F *et al.* Necrobiotic xanthogranuloma presenting as a solitary tumour. *Am J Dermatopathol* 2000; **22**: 453–6.
7 Finan MC, Winklemann RK. Necrobiotic xanthogranuloma with paraproteinaemia. A review of 22 cases. *Medicine (Baltimore)* 1986; **65**: 376–88.
8 Finan MC, Winkelmann RK. Histopathology of necrobiotic xanthogranuloma with paraproteinaemia. *J Cutan Pathol* 1987; **14**: 92–9.
9 Hafner O, Witte T, Schmidt RE *et al.* Nekrobiotisches xanthogranulom bei IgG-kappa plasmazytom und Quincke odem. *Hautarzt* 1994; **45**: 339–43.
10 Bullock JD, Bartley GB, Cambell RJ *et al.* Necrobiotic xanthogranuloma with paraproteinaemia. Case report and a pathogenetic theory. *Ophthalmology* 1986; **93**: 1233–6.
11 Macfarlane AW, Verbov JL. Necrobiotic xanthogranuloma with paraproteinaemia. *Br J Dermatol* 1985; **113**: 339–43.
12 Finelli LG, Ratz JL. Plasmapheresis, a treatment modality for necrobiotic xanthogranuloma. *J Am Acad Dermatol* 1987; **17**: 351–4.
13 Machado S, Alves R, Lima M *et al.* Cutaneous necrobiotic xanthogranuloma (NXG): successfully treated with low dose chlorambucil. *Eur J Dermatol* 2001; **11**: 458–62.
14 Char DH, LeBoit PE, Ljung BM *et al.* Radiation therapy for ocular necrobiotic xanthogranuloma. *Arch Ophthalmol* 1987; **105**: 174–5.

15 Vieira V, Del Pozo J, Martinez W *et al*. Necrobiotic xanthogranuloma associated with lymphoplasmacytic lymphoma. Palliative treatment with carbon dioxide laser. *Eur J Dermatol* 2005; **15**: 182–5.

Sinus histiocytosis with massive lymphadenopathy

Synonym
• Rosai–Dorfman disease

Sinus histiocytosis with massive lymphadenopathy (SHML) is a rare histiocytic proliferative disorder that is defined by its histopathological features [1,2]. A registry of this disease contains information on 423 patients [3].

SHML is currently considered to be a reactive rather than a malignant histiocytosis [4]. An infectious cause has been suggested by the occurrence of fever and pharyngitis, which often precede the onset of SHML. However, the search for a possible infectious agent has been inconclusive. Some patients show evidence of Epstein–Barr virus infection while others have demonstrable infection with *Klebsiella rhinoscleroma* and *Brucella*, but these are not consistent findings. A study failed to show evidence of human herpesvirus 6 and 8 in skin lesions [5].

The onset of SHML is usually in young adults, with a range from birth to 74 years. The sex incidence is equal. Clinical presentation is usually with painless lymph node enlargement, which may reach massive proportions. About 90% of patients present with cervical adenopathy, the rest presenting with axillary, inguinal or mediastinal node enlargement. Fever, weight loss, malaise and night sweats have been reported, usually at presentation.

Extranodal involvement is common, with 43% of patients having at least one extranodal site of involvement. Skin is the most common extranodal site and may be involved without nodal disease. Pure cutaneous SHML may remain localized to the skin with no systemic involvement even with long-term follow-up [6]. Skin lesions are usually yellow, but may be violaceous or purple. Macular erythema, papules, nodules or infiltrated plaques have been reported (Fig. 55.24). Scaling is often present and telangiectasia may be observed. Skin lesions may occur at any site [7]. Of patients with skin SHML, 50% have evidence of one or more additional extranodal sites, particularly involving the nasal cavity, with polyps and paranasal sinuses.

Other organs involved in SHML include bone with lytic bone lesions [8], salivary gland, central nervous system, genitourinary system, lower respiratory tract, liver, gastrointestinal tract, heart and thyroid gland. Isolated central nervous system involvement in SHML is well recognized. In a report of 11 cases, seven were male and four female, with an age range of 22–64 years. Presentation was with headaches, seizures, numbness or paraplegia. Eight cases involved the cranial area and three the spinal cord. Most lesions were dura based and only one case involved the brain parenchyma [9]. Treatment of these patients was surgical, with one patient dying of surgical complications and nine showing no evidence of disease progression after a mean of 15 months follow-up.

Laboratory investigations usually show a mild normochromic normocytic anaemia or hypochromic microcytic anaemia with

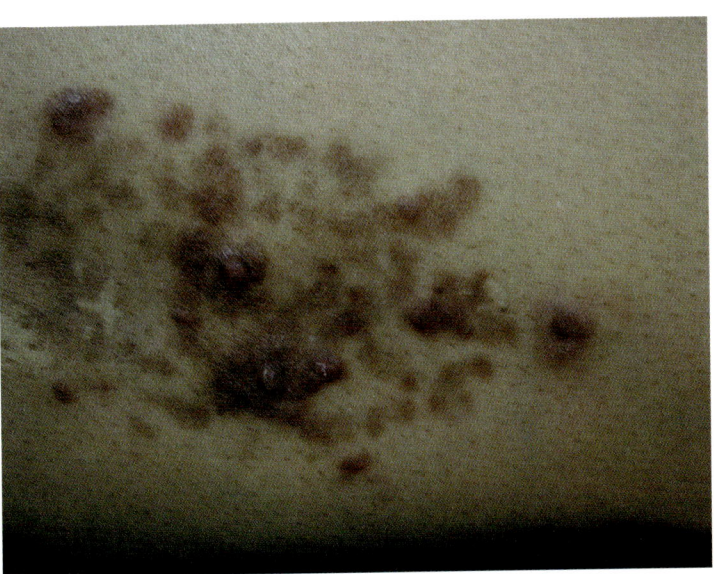

Fig. 55.24 A 41-year-old Asian woman with cutaneous SHML presenting as a pruritic papular and plaque lesion on the upper thigh.

elevation of erythrocyte sedimentation rate. Serum proteins are often abnormal, with a low serum albumin and polyclonal gammopathy. Serum lipids are normal.

Histology of involved nodes reveals the pathognomonic features of SHML. The sinuses are expanded by large pale histiocytes. The histiocytes have abundant pale-pink cytoplasm and indistinct margins or may have glassy eosinophilic cytoplasm and well-defined cytoplasmic membrane. Nuclei are round or oval, usually with a single small nucleolus. Occasionally, multinucleate cells or cells showing nuclear atypia are present but mitoses are rare. Lymphophagocytosis or emperipolesis (phagocytosis of leukocytes, particularly lymphocytes) is always present, and less frequently intracytoplasmic plasma cells, neutrophils and red blood cells may be seen. Between the expanded sinuses, lymphocytes and plasma cells are present and reactive germinal centres are occasionally seen. Rarely, neutrophils are observed scattered throughout the involved node. Electron microscopy shows numerous lipid vacuoles and moderate numbers of lysosomes in the cytoplasm of the histiocytes. The surface of the cells is often thrown into complex, convoluted, villous processes.

In extranodal SHML, the histological picture is strikingly similar to that seen with nodal disease, with what appears to be abnormal lymph node architecture, dilated sinuses and reactive germinal centres in the extranodal site. Extranodal SHML usually shows more fibrosis and lymphophagocytosis.

On immunophenotypic analysis, SHML cells show pan-macrophage markers (EBM11, HAM56 and Leu M3, FcIgG and C3 receptors), monocyte markers (OKM5 and Leu M1), activation antigens (Ki-1, transferrin receptor and CD25) and lysosomal enzymes (lysozyme and α_1-antichymotrypsin) [10]. Surprisingly, however, these cells also display factor XIIIa, a marker of dermal dendrocytes [11], and the S100 antigen that is usually present on dendritic cells; and of two frozen samples tested, both were positive for NA1/34, one for OKT6 but neither for Leu 6. These three monoclonal antibodies react with different epitopes on CD1a, which is characteristic for Langerhans' cells. The exact cell lineage is therefore still uncertain.

The prognosis in SHML is reasonably good. In 238 patients followed for more than a year [7], 49 were well and clear of the disease, 126 had persistent disease, three had progressive disease and 21 patients died, although four deaths were unrelated to SHML. Poor prognostic features in this disease are immunological abnormalities and multiple extranodal sites of disease.

Many treatments have been tried, including the vinca alkaloids, etoposide, ciclosporin and X-rays but no ideal treatment has been identified and the response is poor [12]. A review of the literature showed that 32 of 40 patients received no treatment and underwent spontaneous regression. Radiotherapy gave complete remission in three of nine patients. Surgical debulking was successful in eight of nine patients, resulting in complete remission. Chemotherapy was generally unsuccessful [13], but a case report showed complete resolution of disease with low-dose 2-chlorodeoxyadenosine in a child with nodal and extranodal disease [8].

References

1 Rosai J, Dorfman RF. Sinus histiocytosis with massive lymphadenopathy: a newly recognised benign clinicopathological entity. *Arch Dermatol* 1969; **87**: 63–70.

2 Rosai J, Dorfman RF. Sinus histiocytosis with massive lymphadenopathy: a pseudolymphomatous benign disorder. Analysis of 34 cases. *Cancer* 1972; **30**: 1174–88.

3 Foucar E, Rosai J, Dorfman R. Sinus histiocytosis with massive lymphadenopathy (Rosai–Dorfman disease): review of the entity. *Semin Diagn Pathol* 1990; **7**: 19–73.

4 Gaitonde S. Multifocal sinus histiocytosis with massive lymphadenopathy: an overview. *Arch Pathol Lab Med* 2007; **131**: 1117–21.

5 Ortonne N, Fillet AM, Kosuge H *et al.* Cutaneous Destombes–Rosai–Dorfman disease: absence of detection of HHV-6 and HHV-8 in skin. *J Cutan Pathol* 2002; **29**: 113–8.

6 Frater JL, Maddox JS, Obadiah JM *et al.* Cuttaneous Rosai-Dorfman disease: comprehensive review of cases reported in the medical literature since 1990 and presentation of an illustrative case. *J Cutan Med Surg* 2006; **10**: 281–90.

7 Perez A, Rodriguez M, Febrer I *et al.* Sinus histiocytosis confined to the skin. Case report and review of the literature. *Am J Dermatopathol* 1995; **17**: 384–8.

8 Tasso M, Esquembre C, Blanco E *et al.* Sinus histiocytosis with massive lymphadenopathy (Rosai-Dorfman disease) treated with 2-chlorodeoxyadenosine. *Pediatr Blood Cancer* 2006; **47**: 612–5.

9 Andriko JA, Morrison A, Colegial CH *et al.* Rosai–Dorfman disease isolated to the central nervous system: a report of 11 cases. *Mod Pathol* 2001; **14**: 172–8.

10 Eisen RN, Buckley PJ, Rosai J. Immunophenotypic characterisation of sinus histiocytosis with massive lymphadenopathy (Rosai–Dorfman disease). *Semin Diagn Pathol* 1990; **7**: 74–82.

11 Perrin C, Michiels JF, Lacour JP *et al.* Sinus histiocytosis (Rosai–Dorfman disease) clinically limited to the skin. An immunohistochemical and ultra structural study. *J Cutan Pathol* 1993; **20**: 368–74.

12 Komp D. The treatment of sinus histiocytosis with massive lymphadenopathy (Rosai–Dorfman disease). *Semin Diagn Pathol* 1990; **7**: 83–6.

13 Pulsoni A, Anghel G, Falcucci P *et al.* Treatment of sinus histiocytosis with massive lymphadenopathy (Rosai-Dorfman disease): report on a case and literature review. *Am J Hematol* 2002; **69**: 67–77.

Virus-associated haemophagocytic syndrome

Synonyms
• Virus-induced histiocytosis with erythrophagocytosis
• Virus-induced histiocytic medullary reticulosis

Virus-associated haemophagocytic syndrome is a rare reactive histiocytosis in patients with an active viral infection. Patients can be divided into two groups: group 1 have no evidence of underlying disease; group 2 are receiving immunosuppressive therapy for underlying disease [1–3]. The disease results from a cytokine storm derived from an inappropriate immune reaction caused by proliferating or activated T cells or natural killer cells associated with macrophage activation or inadequate apoptosis of immuno-responsive cells.

Any age group can be affected and, although children and neonates are often affected, many adult cases have been reported. The syndrome presents suddenly with fever, constitutional symptoms, hepatosplenomegaly, lymphadenopathy, pancytopenia, coagulopathies with thrombocytopenia and hypofibrinogenaemia, raised liver enzymes and bilirubin, pulmonary involvement and skin rashes. Non-specific, generalized, macular eruptions occur fairly frequently.

The viruses implicated include adenovirus, herpesvirus [4], human herpesvirus 6 [5], Epstein–Barr virus, measles virus [6], parainfluenza virus type 2, enterovirus, cytomegalovirus [7] and influenza A (H3N2) [8]. In the bone marrow, lymph nodes and other involved tissue, there is infiltration by histiocytes showing erythrophagocytosis. These cells are banal looking histiocytes with no cytological evidence of malignancy.

The differential diagnosis includes familial haemophagocytic lymphohistiocytosis, malignant histiocytosis and LCH. In the past, many patients with virus-associated haemophagocytic syndrome have been misdiagnosed as malignant histiocytosis and given inappropriate treatment with cytotoxic drugs. It is important to differentiate between these two entities, as the administration of cytotoxic drugs in a viral disease such as virus-associated haemophagocytic syndrome can precipitate a fulminant fatal infection.

The prognosis is variable. In a series of 19 patients [9], 30% died in the acute stages of the disease. The other patients recovered completely in 1–8 weeks with no recurrence in a follow-up period of 32 months. Prognosis is related to prompt introduction of immunosuppressive therapy to control the cytokine storm; ciclosporin or systemic steroids are used in low-risk groups and etoposide-containing regimens in high-risk groups [10].

References

1 Bishop JW, Marsh WL, Keonig HM. Hemophagocytic syndrome in Kawasaki disease. *Clin Res* 1980; **28**: 111A.

2 Manoharan A, Catovsky D, Lampert IA *et al.* Histiocytic medullary reticulosis complicating chronic lymphocytic leukaemia: malignant or reactive? *Scand J Haematol* 1981; **26**: 5–13.

3 Rendall RJ, McKenna RW, Nesbit ME *et al.* Virus-associated hemophagocytic syndrome. A benign histiocytic proliferation distinct from malignant histiocytosis. *Cancer* 1979; **44**: 993–1002.

4 Rosai J, Dorfman RF. Sinus histiocytosis with massive lymphadenopathy: a newly recognised benign clinicopathological entity. *Arch Dermatol* 1969; **87**: 63–70.

5 Liu DL, Teng RJ, Ho MM *et al.* Human herpes virus 6 associated haemophagocyte syndrome in beta thalassemia: report of one case. *Acta Paediatr Sin* 1995; **36**: 373–5.

6 Komatsuda A, Chubach A, Miura AB. Virus associated haemophagocytic syndrome due to measles accompanied by acute respiratory failure. *J Intern Med* 1995; **34**: 203–6.

7 Kashiwagi Y, Kawashima H, Sato S *et al.* Virological and immunological characteristics of fatal virus-associated haemophagocytic syndrome (VAHS). *Microbiol Immunol* 2007; **51**: 53–62.

8 Ando M, Miyazaki E, Hiroshige S *et al.* Virus associated hemophagocytic syndrome accompanied by acute respiratory failure caused by influenza A (H3N2). *Intern Med* 2006; **45**: 1183–6.

9 Wilson ER, Malluh A, Stagno S *et al.* Fatal Epstein–Barr virus associated hemophagocytic syndrome. *J Pediatr* 1981; **98**: 260–2.

10 Imashuku S, Teramura T, Morimoto A *et al.* Recent developments in the management of hemophagocytic lymphohistiocytosis. *Expert Opin Pharmacother* 2001; **2**: 1437–48.

Class III histiocytosis: malignant histiocytoses

Class III histiocytoses are malignancies of the monocyte/macrophage series of cells. These diseases are separated into monocytic leukaemia, malignant histiocytosis and true histiocytic lymphoma on clinical criteria, but there is an enormous overlap and it may not always be possible to differentiate them.

In monocytic leukaemia, the malignancy primarily affects the bone marrow and blood but extramedullary involvement is common. In malignant histiocytosis, the histiocytes retain their ability to migrate through the body, which results in widespread involvement of the reticuloendothelial system. In true histiocytic lymphoma, the cells are derived from fixed tissue histiocytes and the tumours are localized, although they may disseminate.

In a study by the International Lymphoma Study Group [1], tumours of histiocytes were phenotypically assessed using a panel of markers. Four groups were identified:

1 Histiocytic sarcoma: CD68 and lysozyme positive, CD1a and CD21/35 negative, with 33% showing S100 reactivity. This tumour was predominantly extranodal and associated with a high mortality.

2 Langerhans' cell sarcoma: CD68, lysozyme, CD1a and S100 positive but CD21/35 negative. This tumour was predominantly extranodal, with a 50% mortality rate.

3 Follicular dendritic cell sarcoma: CD21/35 positive. This tumour was localized to lymph nodes and associated with a low mortality.

4 Interdigitating dendritic cell sarcoma: S100 positive, 50% CD68 positive, CD1a and CD21/35 negative.

Most of these tumours were localized to lymph nodes and associated with a low mortality. This is a useful phenotypic aid for recognizing tumours of histiocytic origin. In the Histiocyte Society classification, malignant histiocytosis and true histiocytic lymphoma can be subdivided into tumours of these four phenotypes.

Reference

1 Pileri SA, Grogan TM, Harris NL *et al.* Tumours of histiocytes and accessory dendritic cells: an immunohistochemical approach to classification from the International Lymphoma Study Group based on 61 cases. *Histopathology* 2002; **41**: 1–29.

Monocytic leukaemia

Definition. Monocytic leukaemia may be acute or chronic. The acute myelogenous leukaemias have been classified in the Franco–American–British classification according to the characteristics of the cells involved. Acute myelomonocytic leukaemia is classified as M5. Acute myeloid leukaemia (AML) M(5) can be immunophenotypically subdivided into AML-M(5a) and AML-M(5b) with AML-M(5a) expressing higher levels of CD68 and CD11b. Prognosis does not seem to differ in these two subtypes [1]. The chronic myelomonocytic/monocytic leukaemias usually transform into acute forms of the leukaemia in a matter of months.

The monocytic leukaemias typically exhibit increased extramedullary disease and organomegaly, and are associated with reduced remission rates and a poorer prognosis.

Aetiology. The aetiology of monocytic leukaemias is unknown. A characteristic karyotype has been reported in M5 leukaemias, translocation t(9;11)(p22;q23).

Pathology. Leukaemic cells in monocytic leukaemia show varying degrees of monocyte differentiation. In acute forms of the disease, the cells stain positively for peroxidase, Sudan black B and non-specific esterase. The cells also contain granules that stain for α-naphthylbutyrate esterase [2]. The cells demonstrate CD13 and CD33, with 30% of cells exhibiting HLA-DR. Monocyte-associated membrane antigen (CD14) expression is variable [3].

Ultrastructurally, the cells have irregular nuclei with nuclear blebs, numerous pinocytic vesicles and perinuclear fibrillar bodies [4].

Skin infiltration favours the lower dermis and subcutaneous fat, with prominent involvement of adnexal structures, nerves and vessels of the superficial and deep plexus. Cellular atypia may be prominent and mitotic figures are common. Differentiation from other forms of leukaemia depends on examination of the blood and bone marrow and special stains in skin sections. The best marker for monocytic leukaemia is non-specific esterase.

Clinical features. Skin lesions in monocytic leukaemia may be specific, for example leukaemia cutis, or non-specific, related to anaemia, thrombocytopenia, infection or drugs. Leukaemia cutis occurs in about 20% of patients with acute monocytic leukaemia [3,5]. Specific skin lesions are light-red, brown or violaceous macules and nodules [6]. These are firm and generally asymptomatic. Skin lesions may undergo rapid cycles of development and spontaneous regression. Skin involvement is not related to the circulating white cell count. Gum involvement occurs in 25–50% of patients.

The prognosis in acute monocytic leukaemia is not related to skin involvement, and leukaemia cutis may spontaneously regress. The prognosis depends on the age of the patient, presence of renal failure and serum β_2-microglobulin levels. Aggressive chemotherapy is associated with complete remission in 60% of patients.

Diagnosis. Diagnosis is made on clinicopathological features of the disease. Differentiation from other forms of leukaemia cutis demands examination of the blood or bone marrow and the use of special stains. M4 and M5 leukaemias are associated with elevated serum lysozyme levels [2].

Treatment. Treatment of leukaemia cutis is that of the underlying leukaemia. Leukaemia cutis in monocytic leukaemia has a tendency to spontaneous regression, but large lesions or ulcerating lesions may be treated with local radiotherapy. Acute monocytic leukaemia is sensitive to the currently used chemotherapeutic regimes used in acute myeloid leukaemia with similar response rates to the other acute myeloid leukaemias [7].

References

1 Liu LB, Li L, Xiao J *et al.* Comparison of immunophenotype and clinical manifestations between patients with M5a and M5b of acute monocytic leukaemia. *Zhongguo Shi Yan Xue Ye Xue Za Zhi* 2006; **14**: 1079–82.

2 Baker AM, Falk RE, Greaves MR. Detection of monocyte specific antigen on human acute leukaemia cells. *Br J Haematol* 1976; **32**: 13–9.

3 Scott CS, Stark AN, Limbert J *et al.* Diagnostic and prognostic factors in acute monocytic leukaemia: an analysis of 51 cases. *Br J Haematol* 1988; **69**: 247–52.

4 Freeman AI, Journey LJ. Ultrastructural studies on monocytic leukaemias. *Br J Haematol* 1971; **20**: 225–31.

5 Baden TJ, Gammon WR. Leukaemia cutis in acute myelomonocytic leukaemia. *Arch Dermatol* 1987; **123**: 88–90.

6 Bernasconi C, Serri F. Skin manifestations of monocytic and myelomonocytic leukaemias. *G Ital Dermatol Venereol* 1980; **115**: 91–100.

7 Tallman MS, Kim HT, Paietta E *et al.* Acute monocytic leukaemia (French-American-British classifiaction M5) does not have a worse prognosis than other subtypes of acute myeloid leukemia: a report from the Eastern Cooperative Oncology Group. *J Clin Oncol* 2004; **22**: 1276–86.

Malignant histiocytosis

Synonyms
- Malignant reticulohistiocytosis
- Malignant reticulosis
- Histiocytic medullary reticulosis
- Sinusoidal haematolymphoid malignancy
- Malignant astrocytosis
- Aleukaemic reticulosis
- Histiocytic reticulosis

Definition. Malignant histiocytosis is a widespread neoplastic proliferation of histiocytic cells that typically involves liver, spleen, lymph nodes and bone marrow. The cells usually arise from sinusoidal histiocytes, although very rare cases of malignant histiocytosis of Langerhans' cell phenotype have been reported.

Aetiology. Malignant histiocytosis is a neoplastic proliferation of cells of the mononuclear phagocyte system. There is no evidence of a viral aetiology in this disease and no reported familial incidence. There have been reports of a characteristic chromosomal translocation t(5;6)(q35;p21) in malignant histiocytosis [1,2]. The major problem with these reports is that the large cell anaplastic lymphoma (Ki-1-positive lymphoma) is often grouped with malignant histiocytosis, but these are T-cell lymphomas. However, the 5q35 break-point does appear to be specific for malignant histiocytosis [3].

Incidence. Malignant histiocytosis is a rare disease with a male to female ratio of 3.5 : 1. It has been reported in all age groups, with a median age of 35 years [4]. Childhood disease is uncommon with few reported series [5]. The disease tends to occur earlier in women (second to third decades) than in men (third to fourth decades) [6]. Reports have suggested an increased incidence of this disease in parts of tropical Africa, with reports from Malawi [7] and Uganda [8].

Pathology. The histological picture in skin and lymph nodes is similar and the diagnosis can be established in either site. Characteristically, there is an infiltrate of histiocytic cells showing varying degrees of atypia that are typically non-cohesive. Cells are large (up to 50 μm in diameter) with abundant cytoplasm and distinct cytoplasmic membranes.

The histiocytic cells are heterogeneous. Some show more marked histiocytic differentiation, with pale cytoplasm, prominent vacuolation or even foamy cytoplasm, and exhibit phagocytosis of erythrocytes, leukocytes and cellular debris. Other cells are more 'primitive', with deeply eosinophilic or amorphous cytoplasm. Nuclei are usually lobulated, with finely granular or reticulated chromatin and prominent or bizarre nucleoli. Nuclear membranes tend to be thickened. Mitoses are common.

Cytochemical and immunohistochemical studies have shown that the cells in malignant histiocytosis are negative for chloracetate esterase, Sudan black B, alkaline phosphatase and β-glucuronidase [9]. Presence of non-specific esterase, acid phosphatase and lysozyme is variable, with the better differentiated cells showing these enzymes [10]. The more differentiated phagocytosing cells usually stain for factor XIIIa and the antimonocyte monoclonal antibody MOI [11]. In some cases, EMA, HLA-DR, CD25, CD30, CD68 and CD71 have been detected. In rare cases, CD1a or CD21/35 may be found. In lymph nodes, the architecture is disarranged but not effaced by the malignant cells.

In the skin, there is extensive perivascular and periappendageal infiltration of the dermis, with extension into subcutaneous fat. In advanced lesions, fat necrosis may occur. The epidermis and papillary dermis are characteristically spared but in the more tumid lesions epidermal ulceration may be present.

Clinical features. Malignant histiocytosis is usually of acute onset, with fever, sweats, wasting, generalized painful lymphoadenopathy and hepatosplenomegaly. As the disease progresses, jaundice, purpura, anaemia and leukopenia occur. In 50% of patients, extranodal extension of the disease is seen, most commonly affecting the skin, bone and gastrointestinal tract.

In the skin, single or multiple lesions may be present [12,13], ranging from skin coloured to violaceous. Large lesions may ulcerate. A widespread, papulonodular eruption similar to that in acute monocytic leukaemia may also be seen.

In bone, the lesions are focal, destructive, lytic and may become widespread with associated hypercalcaemia. Gastrointestinal involvement is usually observed late in the disease. Small and large bowel may be involved, with infiltration of the lamina propria and local intraluminal masses. This presents with obstruction or haemorrhage or both. A rare presentation with multiple lesions is with malabsorption.

In the past, this disease has been associated with a poor prognosis. However, with aggressive management (radiotherapy or radiotherapy and chemotherapy) complete remission has been reported in up to 50% of cases, with a mean duration of complete remission of over 12 months [4]. Microscopic evidence of vascular invasion carries a poor prognosis.

Diagnosis. The major differential diagnosis is with large cell anaplastic lymphomas, in which the clinical and histological features may be similar. Other diseases that may be confused with malignant histiocytosis are familial haemophagocytic lymphohistiocytosis, virus-associated haemophagocytic syndrome, Hodgkin's disease and SHML. Diagnosis can usually be established on clinicopathological features of the disease, although special stains may be needed to exclude large cell anaplastic lymphoma.

Treatment. Malignant histiocytosis is sensitive to both radiotherapy and chemotherapy but treatment must be started early, as many patients die before therapy can be started [5]. Chemotherapy is usually with a combination regimen, which includes doxorubicin and radiotherapy. In one series, complete remission was achieved in seven of nine patients treated [4]. In a study of 27 children with malignant histiocytosis, complete remission was achieved in 22 children using a regimen of vincristine, cyclophosphamide, doxorubicin and prednisolone, with a 5-year survival of 81% [14]. In patients who relapse after conventional chemotherapy, autologous bone marrow transplantation has successfully achieved long-term remission [15]. Large skin tumours or ulcerated tumours can be treated with local radiotherapy. A review of the treatment of malignant histiocytosis has been published [16]. Conventional chemotherapy and radiotherapy are still the mainstay of treatment.

References
1 Kamesaki H, Koya M, Miwa H *et al.* Malignant histiocytosis with rearrangement of the heavy gene and evidence of monocyte-macrophage lineage. *Cancer* 1988; **62**: 1306–9.
2 Morgan R, Smith SD, Hecht BK *et al.* Lack of involvement of the c-fos and N-myc genes by chromosomal translocation t(2;5)(p23;q35) common to malignancies with features of so-called malignant histiocytosis. *Blood* 1989; **73**: 2155–64.
3 Nezelof C, Barbey S, Gogusen J *et al.* Malignant histiocytosis in childhood: a distinct CD30 positive clinicopathological entity associated with a chromosomal translocation involving 5q35. *Semin Diagn Pathol* 1992; **9**: 75–89.
4 Rilke F, Carbone A, Musumed T *et al.* Malignant histiocytosis: a clinico-pathological study of 18 consecutive cases. *Tumori* 1978; **64**: 221–7.
5 Ornvold K, Nielsen MH, Clausen N. Malignant histiocytosis in childhood: clinicopathological study of 14 cases. *Acta Pathol Microbiol Immunol Scand* 1986; **94**: 291–6.
6 Warnke RA, Kim H, Dorfman RF. Malignant histiocytosis (histiocytic medullary reticulosis). 1. Clinicopathological study of 29 cases. *Cancer* 1975; **35**: 215–30.
7 Molyneux ME, Tozer RA, Hutt MSR. Histiocytic medullary reticulosis in Africa. *Lancet* 1978; **ii**: 259.
8 Amsel S, Bijlsma F. Histiocytic medullary reticulosis. Clinical and pathological studies in Uganda. *Trop Geogr Med* 1974; **26**: 31–8.
9 Carbone A, Micheau C, Caillard J-M *et al.* A cytochemical and immunohistochemical approach to malignant histiocytosis. *Cancer* 1981; **47**: 2862–71.
10 Van Heerde P, Feltkamp CA, Hart AAM *et al.* Malignant histiocytosis and related tumours. A clinicopathological study of 42 cases using cytological, histochemical and ultrastructural parameters. *Hematol Oncol* 1984; **2**: 13–32.
11 Nemes Z, Thomazy V. Diagnostic significance of histiocyte-related markers in malignant histiocytosis and true histiocytic lymphoma. *Cancer* 1988; **62**: 1970–80.
12 Ducatman BS, Wick MR, Morgan TW *et al.* Malignant histiocytosis: a clinical, histologic and immunohistochemical study of 20 cases. *Hum Pathol* 1984; **15**: 368–77.
13 Willemze R, Ruiter DJ, Willem A *et al.* Reticulum cell sarcomas (large cell lymphomas) presenting in the skin. High frequency of true histiocytic lymphoma. *Cancer* 1982; **50**: 1367–79.
14 Brugieres L, Caillaud JM, Patte C *et al.* Malignant histiocytosis: therapeutic results in 27 children treated with single polychemotherapy regimes. *Med Pediatr Oncol* 1989; **17**: 193–6.
15 Berry J, Russel JA. Salvage of relapsed malignant histiocytosis by autologous bone marrow transplantation. *Bone Marrow Transplant* 1989; **4**: 123–4.
16 Bucsky P, Egeler RM. Malignant histiocytic disorders in children. Clinical and therapeutic approaches with a nostalgic discussion. *Hematol Oncol Clin North Am* 1998; **12**: 465–71.

True histiocytic lymphoma

Synonyms
- Reticulum cell sarcoma
- Histiosarcoma
- Monocytic sarcoma

Definition. A malignant histiocytic neoplasm that may disseminate.

Aetiology. The aetiology is unknown. The disease represents malignant proliferation of non-Langerhans' cell histiocytes or more rarely of Langerhans' cells. Differentiation from malignant histiocytosis may be difficult.

Pathology. True histiocytic lymphoma exhibits many of the features described in malignant histiocytosis, infiltrating cells being predominantly dermal and non-cohesive. Nemes and Thomazy [1] suggest that the cells in true histiocytic lymphoma are more differentiated than those in malignant histiocytosis and that the cell population is more homogeneous, showing phagocytosis and labelling for factor XIIIa. These cells stain with macrophage markers CD11c and CD68 and are negative for T- and B-cell markers [2]. A rare spindle cell variant has been described which expressed CD163, CD68, CD45, lysozyme and NSE [3].

Clinical features. This is a localized tumour of malignant histiocytes that may be nodal or extranodal. In 40% of patients, presentation is with the painless enlargement of one or more groups of superficial lymph nodes. Constitutional symptoms of malaise, anorexia, sweating and fever may be present.

Extranodal presentation may be with bone, gastrointestinal tract or skin lesions. Bone and gastrointestinal tract lesions are as described in malignant histiocytosis. Skin lesions are localized bluish-red tumours that can attain a large size. An isolated skin tumour of true histiocytic lymphoma in a 79-year-old patient has been described that reached 20 cm in diameter at presentation [4]. In one case report from Japan, an isolated dark-red skin tumour developed on the leg of a 49-year-old woman. Histology showed a monomorphous infiltrate of large cells, with erosion of the overlying epidermis. These cells were CD1a positive and on electron microscopy contained multiple Birbeck granules. This Langerhans' cell, true histiocytic lymphoma disseminated to regional lymph nodes, liver, lungs, kidneys, bone marrow and skin and the patient died 3 years after diagnosis [5]. Hepatosplenomegaly occurs in only a minority of patients with true histiocytic lymphoma, and peripheral blood involvement is rare. In one case report, a 44-year-old man with true histiocytic lymphoma was treated with autologous bone marrow transplantation and subsequently developed histiocytic leukaemia classified as M5c monocytic leukaemia [6].

Prognosis.   True histiocytic lymphoma is treatable, and the prognosis is probably better than in malignant histiocytosis.

Treatment.   True histiocytic lymphoma is both radiosensitive and chemosensitive. Complete remission has been achieved in localized skin disease using electron-beam therapy [4]. Reports of therapeutic responses are difficult to evaluate because of doubt over the diagnosis in older series.

References

1 Nemes Z, Thomazy V. Diagnostic significance of histiocyte-related markers in malignant histiocytosis and true histiocytic lymphoma. *Cancer* 1988; **62**: 1970–80.

2 Soriac Orradre JL, Garcia Almagro D, Martinez B *et al.* True histiocytic lymphoma (monocytic sarcoma). *Am J Dermatopathol* 1992; **14**: 511–7.

3 Alexiev BA, Sailey CJ, McClure SA *et al.* Primary histiocytic sarcoma arising in the head and neck with predominant spindle cell component. *Diagn Pathol* 2007; **26**: 2–7.

4 Forestier JY, Schmitt D, Thivolet J. Malignant and isolated cutaneous tumour of pure histiocytic origin (cutaneous histiocytosarcoma). *G Ital Dermatol Venereol* 1980; **115**: 143–5.

5 Tani M, Ishii N, Kumagai M *et al.* Malignant Langerhans cell tumour. *Br J Dermatol* 1992; **126**: 398–403.

6 Esteve J, Rozman M, Campo E *et al.* Leukaemia after true histiocytic lymphoma: another type of acute monocytic leukaemia with histiocytic differentiation (AMC-M5c). *Leukaemia* 1995; **9**: 1389–91.

CHAPTER 56

Soft-Tissue Tumours and Tumour-like Conditions

E. Calonje
St John's Institute of Dermatology, St Thomas' Hospital, London, UK

Rook's Textbook of Dermatology, 8th edition. Edited by DA Burns,
SM Breathnach, NH Cox and CEM Griffiths. © 2010 Blackwell Publishing Ltd.

Introduction

For many clinical dermatologists, soft-tissue tumours arising in the dermis, subcutis or deeper soft tissues are a confusing group of lesions. This is probably partly explained by the facts that there is a very long list of soft-tissue tumours, and that a large majority of these can arise in the skin or affect it secondarily. Most of these tumours have no characteristic clinical appearance, and present as non-specific, dermal, or deep-seated nodules. However, it is necessary for all clinical dermatologists to have an understanding of the range of tumours that may arise in the dermis, and also of the likely biological behaviour of individual lesions. Although cutaneous malignant soft-tissue tumours are rare, many benign lesions may be histologically confused with a malignancy. Furthermore, there is a group of soft-tissue tumours that have low-grade malignant potential (intermediate malignancy) with frequent local recurrences but little or no potential for metastatic spread (e.g. dermatofibrosarcoma protuberans). These tumours may cause important morbidity, and their recognition is therefore essential for the planning of treatment and follow-up. Recognizing a wide range of soft-tissue tumours is also important as a number of these lesions—particularly when multiple—may be markers of genetic syndromes (for example, multiple neurofibromas and plexiform neurofibroma in neurofibromatosis type I).

A broad division can be made between tumours according to the morphological lines of differentiation. The latter include fibroblastic, myofibroblastic, neural, vascular, muscular and adipocytic types. In a number of tumours, the line of differentiation is not clear, as a normal cell of origin cannot be identified (e.g. epithelioid sarcoma). In a still larger group of tumours, their origin is descriptively ascribed to fibrohistiocytic cells, but with mounting evidence that many of these lesions have fibroblast and/or myofibroblastic differentiation and almost none display true histiocytic differentiation. The list of tumours discussed in this chapter is not all-inclusive. For a full account of the very wide range of these tumours, the reader is referred to the standard major work in this field [1]. True histiocytic tumours are discussed in Chapter 55, and keloids and hypertrophic scars in Chapter 45. Metastatic malignant tumours are covered in Chapter 62.

The most useful biological triage is into totally benign lesions; lesions that may recur locally but never or almost never metastasize; and those that are truly malignant and may metastasize. The great majority of dermal or superficial soft-tissue tumours come into the first two categories, whilst truly malignant soft-tissue tumours much more frequently arise below the deep fascia. In the case of these rare malignant tumours, there is a relationship between bulk and prognosis, smaller lesions carrying a better prognosis. More superficially situated lesions tend to carry a better prognosis than those deeply situated. Mitoses (particularly abnormal mitotic figures) and necrosis both tend to be associated with malignant rather than benign lesions.

The usual clinical presentation of many of the tumours described in this chapter is of a non-specific lump or nodule. An incisional biopsy should be arranged, and it must be adequately deep so that the nature of the lesion at its deepest margin can be determined. Once the pathologist has established the nature of the tumour, appropriate definitive surgery can be planned. Prior consultation with the pathologist is strongly recommended, as samples may be needed for cytogenetics, electron microscopy or immunohistochemistry. All of these may be helpful in arriving at an accurate diagnosis.

Reference

1 Weiss SW, Goldblum JR. *Enzinger and Weiss's Soft Tissue Tumours*, 5th edn. St Louis: Mosby, 2007.

Fibrous and myofibroblastic tumours

Fibrous papule of the face [1]

Synonym
- Fibrous papule of the nose

Definition and incidence. A small facial papule with a distinctive fibrovascular component on histological examination. The condition is relatively common, and several large series have been reported [2–4].

Clinical features [2–4]. The lesions usually occur singly on the nose. Occasionally, they may occur on the forehead, cheeks, chin or neck, and there may be several lesions [5]. The lesion usually presents in middle life, and both sexes are equally affected.

The papule develops slowly as a dome-shaped, skin-coloured or slightly red or pigmented lesion, which is usually sessile. Most are asymptomatic, but about one-third bleed on minor trauma.

Pathology [2–4]. The epidermis appears normal, although there may be an increased number of clear cells overlying the lesion. In the dermis there is increased collagen with a hyalinized appearance and scattered, somewhat dilated vascular channels (Fig. 56.1). In the background there is increased cellularity with mono- and multinucleated cells with a histiocyte-like appearance. In some lesions epithelioid or clear cells may predominate [6,7]. There are prominent dilated capillaries, but relatively few elastic fibres.

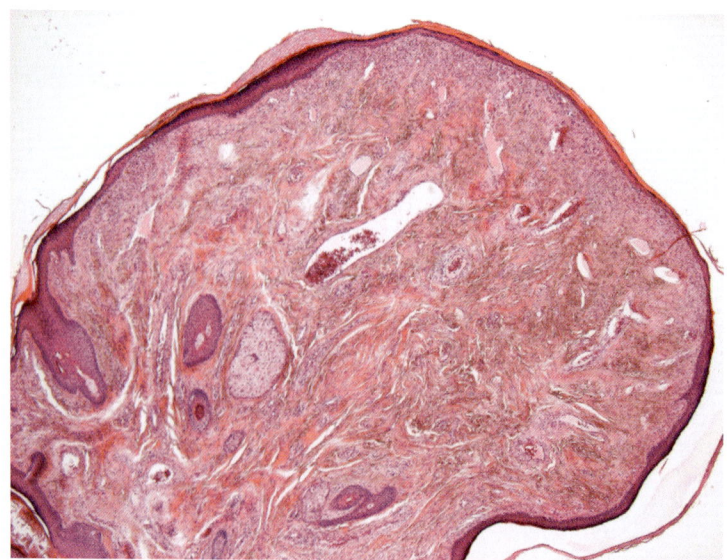

Fig. 56.1 Fibrous papule with hyalinized collagen bundles and increased dilated vascular channels.

It has been suggested that the condition may be a variant of a melanocytic naevus [2,4], but others disagree [3]. S100 protein, which is an immunohistochemical marker of neuroepithelial elements, is present neither in the stellate cells in the papillary dermis nor in the mesenchymal 'naevus' cells [8].

Treatment. The lesion is benign, but it may easily be excised or surgically pared for cosmetic reasons.

References
1 Okun M. Fibrous papules and nevocellular nevi. *J Am Acad Dermatol* 1984; **10**: 670–1.
2 Graham JH, Sanders JB, Johnson WC *et al.* Fibrous papule of the nose. *J Invest Dermatol* 1965; **45**: 194–203.
3 Meigel WN, Ackerman AB. Fibrous papule of face. *Am J Dermatopathol* 1979; **1**: 329–40.
4 Saylan T, Marks R, Wilson Jones E. Fibrous papule of the nose. *Br J Dermatol* 1971; **85**: 111–8.
5 Yamamoto T, Katayama I, Nishioka K. Fibropapule multiplex of the nose: a variant of Cowden's disease? *Dermatology* 1996; **192**: 379–81.
6 Kucher C, McNiff JM. Epithelioid fibrous papule—a new variant. *J Cutan Pathol* 2007; **34**: 571–5.
7 Lee AN, Stein SL, Cohen LM. Clear cell fibrous papule with NKI/C3 expression: clinical and histologic features in six cases. *Am J Dermatopathol* 2005; **27**: 296–300.
8 Spiegel J, Nadji M, Penneys NS. Fibrous papule: an immunohistochemical study with an antibody to S-100 protein. *J Am Acad Dermatol* 1963; **9**: 360–2.

Storiform collagenoma [1,2]

Synonym
• Sclerotic fibroma

Definition. Storiform collagenoma is a fibrous hypocellular cutaneous lesion which, when multiple, may be associated with Cowden's disease or PTEN hamartoma syndrome (multiple hamartoma and neoplasia syndrome; see Chapter 62) [3].

Clinical features. It usually presents as a small, solitary, asymptomatic papule in adults of either sex, with wide anatomical distribution.

Pathology. It typically consists of a fairly well-circumscribed dermal nodule with prominent, hypocellular, hyalinized collagen bundles in a storiform pattern (Fig. 56.2). Bland spindle-shaped cells are rare. A similar histological pattern may be seen in the late stages of lesions as diverse as pleomorphic fibroma, fibrous histiocytoma (FH) and myofibroma and it has been proposed that it does not represent a distinctive entity but a reaction pattern [4,5].

A more cellular variant containing multinucleated bizarre cells has been described as giant cell collagenoma [6]. The latter is a potential link between pleomorphic fibroma (see below) and sclerotic fibroma as it has been proposed that both entities are part of the same spectrum [7].

Treatment. Simple excision is curative.

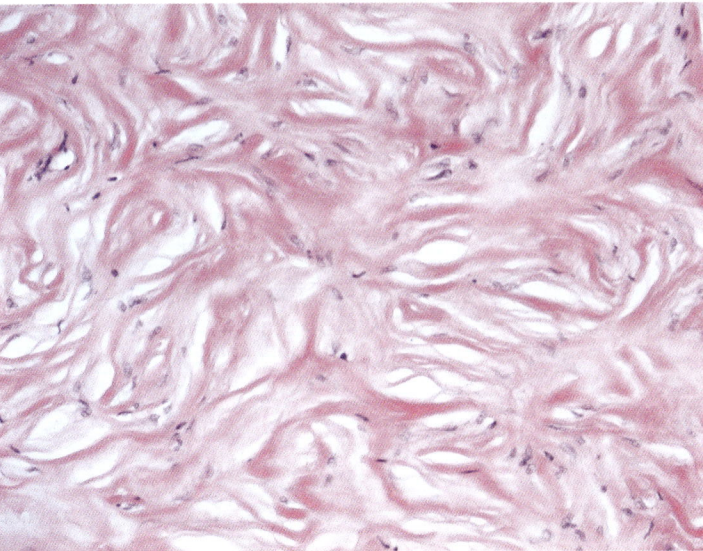

Fig. 56.2 Storiform collagenoma. Poorly cellular stroma composed of hyalinized collagen in a storiform pattern.

References
1 Rapini RP, Golitz LE. Sclerotic fibromas of the skin. *J Am Acad Dermatol* 1989; **20**: 266–71.
2 Metcalf JS, Maize JC, LeBoit PE. Circumscribed storiform collagenoma (sclerosing fibroma). *Am J Dermatopathol* 1991; **13**: 122–9.
3 Starink TM, Meijer CJLM, Brownstein MH. The cutaneous pathology of Cowden's disease: new findings. *J Cutan Pathol* 1985; **12**: 83–93.
4 Chen TM, Purohit SK, Wang AR. Pleomorphic sclerotic fibroma: a case report and literature review. *Am J Dermatopathol* 2002; **24**: 54–8.
5 High WA, Stewart D, Essary LR *et al.* Sclerotic fibroma-like change in various neoplastic and inflammatory skin lesions: is sclerotic fibroma a distinct entity? *J Cutan Pathol* 2004; **31**: 373–8.
6 Rudolph P, Schubert C, Harms D *et al.* Giant cell collagenoma: a benign dermal tumor with distinctive multinucleate cells. *Am J Surg Pathol* 1998; **22**: 57–63.
7 García Doval I, Casas L, Toribio J. Pleomorphic fibroma of the skin, a form of sclerotic fibroma: an immunohistochemical study. *Clin Exp Dermatol* 1998; **23**: 22–4.

Pleomorphic fibroma

Definition [1]. Pleomorphic fibroma is a relatively rare lesion with features very similar to those of a fibroepithelial polyp (skin tag), but characterized histologically by bizarre mono- or multinucleated stromal cells.

Clinical features. Lesions present in adults as a polyp, with no sex predilection and a wide anatomical distribution, including a subungual location [2].

Pathology. Normal or mildly acanthotic epidermis surrounds a collagenous and vascular stroma containing scattered bizarre mono- or multinucleated cells with hyperchromatic and pleomorphic nuclei. Mitotic figures are rare.

Treatment. Simple excision is curative, and there is no tendency for local recurrence.

References
1 Kamino H, Lee JY, Berke A. Pleomorphic fibroma of the skin: a benign neoplasm with cytologic atypia—a clinicopathologic study of eight cases. *Am J Surg Pathol* 1989; **13**: 107–13.

2 Hsieh YJ, Lin YC, Wu YH *et al*. Subungual pleomorphic fibroma. *J Cutan Pathol* 2003; **30**: 567–71.

Acquired digital fibrokeratoma [1]

Definition. A benign lesion, possibly a reaction to trauma, which occurs on the fingers and toes [2] (Fig. 56.3), although the palms and the soles have occasionally been involved.

Clinical features. The lesion usually occurs in adults as a solitary, dome-shaped lesion, with a collarette of slightly raised skin at its base. Occasionally, it may be elongated or pedunculated. Giant lesions may occasionally occur [3]. The surface may appear to be slightly warty.

There is a wide clinical differential diagnosis, which includes dermatofibroma, viral wart, supernumerary digit and cutaneous horn. Histologically, the lesion is extremely similar to the Koenen tumour [4], the periungual fibrous papule that arises from the nail fold in tuberous sclerosis.

Pathology. The histology shows thick collagen bundles, thin elastic fibres and increased vascularity. Occasionally, there is an obvious increase in fibroblasts, and rarely the collagen bundles may be separated by oedema [5]. The epidermis is relatively normal, but acanthosis and hyperkeratosis may occur.

Treatment. Acquired digital fibrokeratoma is cured by simple excision.

References

1 Hare PJ, Smith AJ. Acquired digital fibrokeratoma. *Br J Dermatol* 1969; **81**: 667–70.
2 Berger RS, Spielvogel RL. Dermal papule on a distal digit. *Arch Dermatol* 1988; **124**: 1559.
3 Kakurai M, Yamada T, Kiyosawa T *et al*. Giant acquired digital fibrokeratoma. *J Am Acad Dermatol* 2003; **48** (5 Suppl.): S67–8.

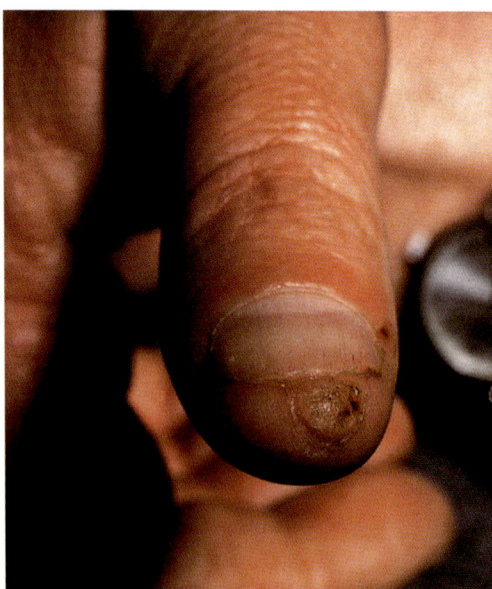

Fig. 56.3 Clinical appearance of an acquired digital fibrokeratoma.

4 Kint A, Baran R. Histopathologic study of Koenen tumors: are they different from acquired digital fibrokeratoma? *J Am Acad Dermatol* 1988; **18**: 369–72.
5 Kint A, Baran R, de Keyser H. Acquired (digital) fibrokeratoma. *J Am Acad Dermatol* 1985; **12**: 816–21.

Nodular fasciitis [1–4]

> **Synonym**
> • Subcutaneous pseudosarcomatous fibromatosis

Definition. A rapidly enlarging subcutaneous nodule, which is due to a benign proliferation of myofibroblasts and fibroblasts and has a superficial resemblance to a sarcoma.

Incidence and aetiology. A number of quite large series have been published in the last 10 years, suggesting that the condition is not uncommon. It is most frequent in young adults, but has been reported in patients from 5 months to 75 years. There is no predilection for either sex. It is not associated with other diseases. There is no evidence that trauma initiates the lesions.

Clinical features [1–4]. The majority of tumours appear as tender, rapidly growing masses beneath the skin. The average size is 1–3 cm in diameter. The commonest situation is the upper extremities, particularly the forearm, but the lesion can occur anywhere, including the orbit and the mouth [5]. Lesions on the head and neck often present in children. In nearly half the patients, the tumour has been noticed for only 2 weeks or less when they come for advice.

Pathology [1–4]. These lesions may look extremely worrying in view of the high mitotic rate and rapid growth (see below). The tumour is only focally circumscribed and it is composed of bundles of fairly uniform fibroblasts and myofibroblasts with pink cytoplasm, vesicular nuclei and a single, small nucleolus. Myxoid change and mucin deposition is often prominent, resulting in a typical tissue culture-like appearance (Fig. 56.4). In the background, there are numerous small, delicate blood vessels, extravasated red blood cells and scattered mononuclear inflammatory cells. Multinucleated giant cells may be seen, and they resemble osteoclasts. Mitoses are usually numerous, but there are no abnormal forms. Hyalinized collagen bundles are often present and may display a keloidal appearance. At the periphery, compact bundles of fibroblasts and capillaries probe the fascial planes and may infiltrate fat or skeletal muscle. It is not surprising that this histological picture is relatively often confused with that of a malignant tumour. Variants of nodular fasciitis include those with metaplastic bone (ossifying fasciitis); a variant that involves the periosteum (periosteal fasciitis); a variant that involves the scalp and tends to occur in children (cranial fasciitis); and a variant within the lumen of a blood vessel (intravascular fasciitis) [6]. A rare variant of intradermal nodular fasciitis has also been described [6,7]. Intra-articular location may also be seen [8]. Tumour cells are variably positive for smooth muscle actin and calponin [9] and usually negative for smooth-muscle markers including desmin and h-caldesmon [10]. The histological diagnosis may be very difficult, especially in small biopsies. Confusion with a sarcoma

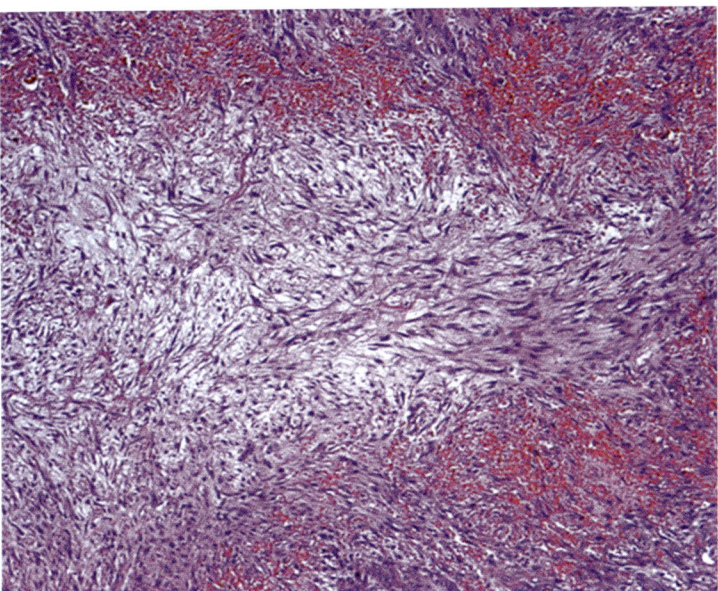

Fig. 56.4 Typical tissue culture-like appearance of nodular fasciitis with prominent myxoid background.

or with fibromatosis are major pitfalls, with obvious detrimental consequences.

Immunohistochemistry may be useful in the distinction between fibromatosis and nodular fasciitis. The former tend to display nuclear beta-catenin positivity, while the latter are usually negative or display cytoplasmic positivity only [11]. However, some fibromatoses, especially those superficially located, are negative for this marker and the diagnosis should be based on careful clinicopathological correlation.

Treatment. Resolution usually follows incomplete surgical removal. Simple excision is therefore an adequate treatment. Local recurrence is exceptional.

References
1 Bernstein KE, Lattes R. Nodular (pseudosarcomatous) fasciitis, a nonrecurrent lesion: clinicopathologic study of 134 cases. *Cancer* 1982; **49**: 1668–78.
2 Konwaler BE, Keasbey L, Kaplan L. Subcutaneous pseudosarcomatous fibromatosis (fasciitis). *J Clin Pathol* 1955; **25**: 241–52.
3 Shimizu S, Hashimoto H, Enjoji M. Nodular fasciitis: an analysis of 250 patients. *Pathology* 1984; **16**: 161–6.
4 Hutter RVP, Stewart FW, Foote FW. Fasciitis: a report of 70 cases with follow-up proving the benignity of the lesion. *Cancer* 1962; **15**: 992–1003.
5 Dayan D, Nasrallah V, Vered M. Clinicopathologic correlations of myofibroblastic tumors of the oral cavity: 1. Nodular fasciitis. *J Oral Pathol Med* 2005; **34**: 426–35.
6 Price S, Kahn L, Saxe N. Dermal and intravascular fasciitis. *Am J Dermatopathol* 1993; **15**: 539–43.
7 Nishi SP, Brey NV, Sanchez RL. Dermal nodular fasciitis: three case reports of the head and neck and literature review. *J Cutan Pathol* 2006; **33**: 378–82.
8 Hornick JL, Fletcher CD. Intrarticular nodular fasciitis—a rare lesion: clinicopathologic analysis of a series. *Am J Surg Pathol* 2006; **30**: 237–41.
9 Pérez-Montiel MD, Plaza JA, Domínguez-Malagón H *et al*. Differential expression of smooth muscle myosin, smooth muscle actin, h-caldesmon, and calponin in the diagnosis of myofibroblastic and smooth muscle lesions of skin and soft tissue. *Am J Dermatopathol* 2006; **28**: 105–11.
10 Ceballos KM, Nielsen GP, Selig MK *et al*. Is anti-h-caldesmon useful for distinguishing smooth muscle and myofibroblastic tumors? An immunohistochemical study. *Am J Clin Pathol* 2000; **114**: 746–53.
11 Bhattacharya B, Dilworth HP, Iocabuzio-Donahue C *et al*. Nuclear beta-catenin expression distinguishes deep fibromatosis from other benign and malignant fibroblastic and myofibroblastic lesions. *Am J Surg Pathol* 2005; **29**: 653–9.

Fibro-osseous pseudotumour of the digits [1,2]

Definition. This is a reactive myofibroblastic proliferation with bone formation, which occurs exclusively on the digits.

Clinical features. It presents predominantly in young adults, with a predilection for females. The fingers are more commonly affected than the toes. The lesion grows rapidly and it is not attached to bone.

Pathology. The tumour is ill-defined and similar to nodular fasciitis, except for the fact that there is formation of osteoid and mature bone. Oedematous stroma, vascular proliferation and bundles of spindle-shaped myofibroblast-like cells are seen intermixed with osteoid and mature bone. Mitotic figures are found and their number depends on the age of the lesion.

Treatment. Local recurrence is rare, and excision is the treatment of choice.

References
1 Dupree WB, Enzinger FM. Fibro-osseous pseudotumor of the digits. *Cancer* 1986; **58**: 2103–9.
2 de Silva MV, Reid R. Myositis ossificans and fibroosseous pseudotumor of digits: a clinicopathological review of 64 cases with emphasis on diagnostic pitfalls. *Int J Surg Pathol* 2003; **11**: 187–95.

Ischaemic fasciitis [1–4]

Synonym
• Atypical decubitus fibroplasia

Definition. Ischaemic fasciitis is a reactive fibroblastic/myofibroblastic proliferation that simulates malignancy and occurs as a result of alterations in local circulation and sustained pressure.

Clinical features. Most patients are elderly and immobilized, and there is a slight predilection for females. The lesion presents as an asymptomatic subcutaneous mass, predominantly over bony prominences that may extend to deeper soft tissues and to the overlying dermis.

Pathology. The lesion is poorly circumscribed and contains areas of fibrosis, vascular proliferation, necrosis and focal myxoid change. Thrombosed blood vessels with recanalization and areas of fibrinoid necrosis, focal haemorrhage and mononuclear inflammatory cells are additional features. In the background, there are variable numbers of spindle-shaped myofibroblasts/fibroblasts with vesicular or hyperchromatic nuclei and a prominent nucleolus. Mitotic figures may be seen, but are not prominent.

Treatment. Excision of the lesion is an adequate treatment.

References

1 Montgomery EA, Meis JM, Mitchell MS *et al.* Atypical decubital fibroplasia: a distinctive fibroblastic pseudotumor occurring in debilitated patients. *Am J Surg Pathol* 1992; **16**: 708–15.
2 Baldassano MF, Rosenberg AE, Flotte TJ. Atypical decubital fibroplasia: a series of three cases. *J Cutan Pathol* 1998; **25**: 149–52.
3 Perosio PM, Weiss SW. Ischemic fasciitis: a juxta-skeletal fibroblastic proliferation with a predilection for elderly patients. *Mod Pathol* 1993; **6**: 69–72.
4 Scanlon R, Kelehan P, Flannelly G *et al.* Ischemic fasciitis: an unsual vulvovaginal spindle cell lesion. *Int J Gynecol Pathol* 2004; **23**: 65–7.

Superficial acral fibromyxoma [1,2]

Definition. Superficial acral fibromyxoma is a distinctive, recently delineated, benign, dermal and/or subcutaneous, fibroblastic tumour with a strong predilection for hands and feet.

Incidence and aetiology. Lesions are relatively rare and are regarded as neoplastic.

Clinical features. Most cases present as a long-standing, solitary mass measuring between 1 and 2 cm, on the hands and feet (particularly the digits, often in a subungual location), of middle-aged adults and with some predilection for males.

Pathology. Tumours are circumscribed and consist of bland stellate and spindle-shaped cells in a variably prominent myxoid and collagenous stroma and with small blood vessels in the background. Some lesions are more cellular and have been described in the literature under the rubric of cellular fibroma of the digits [3]. In myxoid areas, mast cells are often seen. Scattered multinucleated cells may be seen in some cases. Mitotic figures are very rare. Tumour cells are diffusely positive for CD34 and may be focally positive for EMA and CD99.

In the past, it is likely that these tumours were classified as neurofibromas because of the cytomorphology of tumour cells and the myxoid background, with fairly frequent mast cells. However, neurofibroma is rare in acral sites and tumour cells are positive for S100 and only focally positive for CD34.

Prognosis and treatment. These lesions are entirely benign and local recurrence is very rare. Simple local excision is the treatment of choice.

References

1 Fetsch JF, Laskin WB, Mietinnen M. Superficial acral fibromyxoma: a clinicopathologic and immunohistochemical analysis of 37 cases of a distinctive soft tissue tumour with a predilection for the fingers and toes. *Hum Pathol* 2001; **32**: 704–14.
2 André J, Theunis A, Richert B *et al.* Superficial acral fibromyxoma: clinical and pathological features. *Am J Dermatopathol* 2004; **26**: 472–4.
3 McNiff JM, Subtil A, Cowper SE *et al.* Cellular digital fibromas: distinctive CD34-positive lesions that may mimic dermatofibrosarcoma protuberans. *J Cutan Pathol* 2005; **32**: 413–8.

Fibrous hamartoma of infancy [1–5]

Definition. This is a benign, fibroblastic/myofibroblastic, deep dermal and subcutaneous tumour presenting in children and characterized by three distinctive pathological components, as described below.

Incidence and aetiology. This is a rare tumour, often considered to be a hamartoma, but probably neoplastic in nature.

Clinical features. Most cases present in children aged under 2 years, as an asymptomatic, solitary, skin-coloured plaque/nodule only a few centimetres in diameter. Rarely, pigmentary changes and or hypertrichosis may be seen [6]. A quarter of the cases present at birth. Males are more affected than females. The tumour grows rapidly and has a predilection for the axillae, arm and shoulder girdle [1–3]. A familial association has not been reported.

Pathology. The tumour is composed of three components:
1 Bundles of interlacing, elongated, bland, wavy spindle-shaped cells in a variable collagenous background
2 Nests of more immature round cells with focal myxoid change
3 Mature adipose tissue.
A focal resemblance to a neurofibroma may be seen when the first component predominates, but tumour cells are actin-positive and S100-negative [7].

In the dermis overlying the tumour, eccrine glands may show secondary changes including hyperplasia, papillary projections and squamous syringometaplasia [8].

Treatment. Simple excision is the treatment of choice [5]; recurrences are exceptional.

References

1 Enzinger FM. Fibrous hamartoma of infancy. *Cancer* 1965; **18**: 241–8.
2 Mitchell ML, di Sant'Agnese PA, Gerber JE. Fibrous hamartoma of infancy. *Hum Pathol* 1982; **13**: 586–8.
3 Paller AS, Gonzalez-Crussi F, Sherman JO. Fibrous hamartoma of infancy: eight additional cases and a review of the literature. *Arch Dermatol* 1989; **125**: 88–91.
4 Sotelo-Avila C, Bale PM. Subdermal fibrous hamartoma of infancy: pathology of 40 cases and differential diagnosis. *Pediatr Pathol* 1994; **14**: 39–52.
5 Carretto E, Dall'Igna P, Alaggio R *et al.* Fibrous hamartoma of infancy: an Italian multi-institutional experience. *J Am Acad Dermatol* 2006; **54**: 800–3.
6 Yon TY, Kim JW. Fibrous hamartoma of infancy manifesting as multiple nodules with hypertrichosis. *J Dermatol* 2006; **33**: 427–9.
7 Groisman G, Lichtig C. Fibrous hamartoma of infancy: an immunohistochemical and ultrastructural study. *Hum Pathol* 1991; **22**: 914–8.
8 Grynspan D, Meir K, Senger C *et al.* Cutaneous changes in fibrous hamartoma of infancy. *J Cutan Pathol* 2007; **34**: 39–43.

Calcifying fibrous tumour/pseudotumour [1–3]

Definition. This is a rare, benign, hypocellular tumour characterized by dense collagen bundles, areas of calcification and a patchy mononuclear cell infiltrate. This lesion has no relation with inflammatory myofibroblastic tumour as was originally suggested [3].

Clinical features. Most lesions occur in children, and less commonly in young adults, as a fairly large, subcutaneous or deeper asymptomatic mass with a wide anatomical distribution. Cases may also occur in internal organs [3].

Pathology. The tumour typically consists of haphazardly arranged collagen bundles with scattered bland fibroblasts, focal small calcifications and focal aggregates of lymphocytes and plasma cells. Tumour cells are positive for CD34 and may be focally positive for smooth-muscle actin and more rarely for desmin [3].

Treatment. Local recurrence is rare, and the treatment of choice is simple excision.

References
1 Rosenthal NS, Abdul-Karim FW. Childhood fibrous tumor with psammoma bodies. *Arch Pathol Lab Med* 1988; **112**: 565–8.
2 Fetsch JF, Montgomery EA, Meis JM. Calcifying fibrous pseudotumour. *Am J Surg Pathol* 1993; **17**: 502–8.
3 Nascimento AF, Ruiz R, Hornick JL *et al.* Calcifying fibrous 'pseudotumor': clinicopathologic study of 15 cases and analysis of its relationship to inflammatory myofibroblastic tumor. *Int J Surg Pathol* 2002; **10**: 189–96.

Calcifying aponeurotic fibroma [1,2]

Definition. This is a rare, fibroblastic tumour characterized by a nodular proliferation of bland spindle-shaped cells surrounding nodules at different stages of calcification. Cartilage and, less commonly, bone formation may be seen.

Clinical features [1]. Most cases present in children, with a predilection for the hands and, less commonly, the feet. Occurrence at other sites is rare but tumours may present in places as diverse as the knee, the back and the thigh [2]. Tumours are small, slowly growing and usually asymptomatic. Multiple lesions are exceptional [3].

Pathology. The growth pattern is multinodular. Tumour cells are elongated, with scanty pink cytoplasm, vesicular nuclei and very rare mitotic figures. Tumour nodules frequently contain areas of calcification, which are surrounded by tumour cells in a pattern reminiscent of palisading.

Treatment. Local recurrence is observed in up to 50% of the cases, but malignant transformation is exceptional [4] and conservative treatment is therefore indicated.

References
1 Allen PW, Enzinger FM. Juvenile aponeurotic fibroma. *Cancer* 1970; **26**: 857–67.
2 Fetsch JF, Miettinen M. Calcifying aponeurotic fibroma: a clinicopathologic study of 22 cases arising in uncommon sites. *Hum Pathol* 1998; **29**: 1504–10.
3 Hassel B. Calcifying aponeurotic fibroma. A case of multiple primary tumours. Case report. *Scand J Plast Reconstr Surg Hand Surg* 1992; **26**: 115–6.
4 Lafferty KA, Nelson EL, Demuth RJ *et al.* Juvenile aponeurotic fibroma with disseminated fibrosarcoma. *J Hand Surg (Am)* 1986; **11**: 737–40.

Dermatomyofibroma

> **Synonym**
> • Dermal plaque-like fibromatosis

Definition [1–4]. A benign, dermal and superficial subcutaneous myofibroblastic proliferation microscopically mimicking a fibro-

matosis. The tumour, however, has no potential for local recurrence and lacks an infiltrative growth pattern.

Clinical features. It presents as a solitary, asymptomatic, skin-coloured or hypopigmented plaque measuring less than 4 cm in diameter. Multiple lesions are rarely seen and an exceptional case has presented with a linear pattern [5]. Most lesions occur on the trunk, and there is a predilection for young adults, particularly females. Children are only exceptionally affected [6].

Pathology. Low-power examination reveals a plaque-like proliferation of fascicles of myofibroblast-like cells with an almost parallel orientation to the epidermis. Tumour cells are bland, and mitotic figures are very rare. The tumour does not destroy adnexal structures, but may extend focally into the subcutaneous tissue. Rare cases with haemorrhage may mimic plaque-stage Kaposi's sarcoma [7]. The latter, however, is always positive for human herpes virus 8 (HHV8). Tumour cells are variably positive for smooth-muscle actin and calponin.

Treatment. Simple excision is curative.

References
1 Hugol H. Die plaqueformige dermale Fibromatose. *Hautarzt* 1991; **42**: 223–6.
2 Kamino H, Reddy VB, Gero M *et al.* Dermatomyofibroma: a benign cutaneous plaque-like proliferation of fibroblasts and myofibroblasts in young adults. *J Cutan Pathol* 1992; **19**: 85–91.
3 Mentzel T, Calonje E, Fletcher CDM. Dermatomyofibroma-additional observations of a distinctive cutaneous myofibroblastic tumour with emphasis on differential diagnosis. *Br J Dermatol* 1993; **129**: 69–73.
4 Colome MI, Sanchez RL. Dermatomyofibroma: report of two cases. *J Cutan Pathol* 1994; **21**: 371–6.
5 Trotter MJ, McGregor GI, O'Connell JX. Linear dermatomyofibroma. *Clin Exp Dermatol* 1996; **21**: 307–9.
6 Mortimore RJ, Whitehead KJ. Dermatomyofibroma: a report of two cases, one occurring in a child. *Australas J Dermatol* 2001; **42**: 22–5.
7 Mentzel T, Kutzner H. Haemorrhagic dermatomyofibroma (plaque-like dermal fibromatosis): clinicopathological and immunohistochemical analysis of three cases resembling plaque-stage Kaposi's sarcoma. *Histopathology* 2003; **29**: 426–9.

Angiomyofibroblastoma [1–4]

Definition. Angiomyofibroblastoma is a distinctive, benign neoplasia that occurs almost always in the pelvis and perineum, particularly affecting the vulva. There is some overlap with another tumour that presents in the pelvis and perineum (cellular angiofibroma, see below) and also with aggressive angiomyxoma [5].

Clinical features. Tumours are rare and present mainly in the vulva of young to middle-aged females and rarely elderly women. Cases in males are exceptional and usually affect the scrotum. Lesions are subcutaneous, asymptomatic and measure less than 5 cm in diameter.

Pathology. Lesions are well-circumscribed and consist of a mixture of round and spindle-shaped bland cells in a myxoid or oedematous stroma with numerous small, dilated blood vessels. There is a tendency for tumour cells to surround the vascular channels. Mitotic activity is not usually present. In a number of cases there are collections of mature adipocytes [4].

Cytological atypia secondary to degeneration is sometimes seen. Tumour cells are positive for desmin and for oestrogen and progesterone receptors. They are only focally positive for smooth-muscle actin and muscle-specific actin. Some tumours are variably positive for CD34.

Prognosis and treatment. Tumours are benign with no tendency for local recurrence. The treatment is simple excision. Only one malignant tumour has been reported [6].

References

1 Fletcher CD, Tsang WY, Fisher C *et al*. Angiomyofibroblastoma of the vulva. A benign neoplasm distinct from aggressive angiomyxoma. *Am J Surg Pathol* 1992; **16**: 373–82.
2 Hisaoka M, Kouho H, Aoki T *et al*. Angiomyofibroblastoma of the vulva: a clinicopathologic analysis of 7 cases. *Pathol Int* 1995; **45**: 487–92.
3 Nielsen GP, Rosenberg AE, Young RH *et al*. Angiomyofibroblastoma of the vulva and vagina. *Mod Pathol* 1996; **9**: 284–91.
4 Laskin WB, Fetsch JF, Tavasoli FA. Angiomyofibroblastoma of the female genital tract analysis of 17 cases including a lipomatous variant. *Hum Pathol* 1997; **28**: 1046–55.
5 Granter SR, Nucci MR, Fletcher CD. Aggressive angiomyxoma: reappraisal of its relationship to angiomyofibroblastoma in a series of 16 cases. *Histopathology* 1997; **30**: 3–10.
6 Nielsen GP, Young RH, Dickersin GR *et al*. Angiomyofibroblastoma of the vulva with sarcomatous transformation ('angiomyofibrosarcoma'). *Am J Surg Pathol* 1997; **21**: 1104–8.

Cellular angiofibroma [1–4]

> **Synonym**
> • Male angiomyofibroblastoma-like tumour

Definition. Cellular angiofibroma is a distinctive, benign neoplasm that occurs almost exclusively in the vulva and less commonly in the scrotum and inguinal soft tissues of men. Some cases overlap histologically with angiomyofibroblastoma and a relationship with spindle cell lipoma has been suggested [2].

Clinical features. Tumours are relatively rare, affecting mainly females and presenting as a small, well-circumscribed, asymptomatic, subcutaneous nodule. In males tumours tend to be larger and may be related to a hydrocele or a hernia [2].

Pathology. Tumours are sharply circumscribed but not encapsulated and are characterized by short, usually bland, spindle-shaped cells with scanty, ill-defined pale pink cytoplasm. These cells are arranged in bundles and the degree of cellularity varies. In the background there are thin collagen bundles and numerous small to medium-sized blood vessels. Mitotic figures are rare and cytological atypia may be occasionally seen in some cases. Scattered mononuclear inflammatory cells, mainly lymphocytes, and degenerative changes are often identified. The latter consist of haemorrhage, thrombosis, hyalinization and haemosiderin deposition. In myxoid areas, mast cells are present and many tumours contain variable numbers of mature adipocytes. The most consistent immunohistochemical finding is the presence of diffuse positivity

for CD34 in many cases. Muscular markers including actin and desmin tend to be negative but positivity has been reported in male tumours. In a few cases, there is focal positivity for oestrogen and progesterone receptors.

Prognosis and behaviour. Lesions are benign and there is no tendency for local recurrence. Simple excision is the treatment of choice.

References

1 Nucci MR, Granter SR, Fletcher CD. Cellular angiofibroma: a benign neoplasm distinct from angiomyofibroblastoma and spindle cell lipoma. *Am J Surg Pathol* 1997; **21**: 636–644
2 Laskin WB, Fetsch JF, Mostofi FK. Angiomyofibroblastoma-like tumor of the male genital tract: analysis of 11 cases with comparison to female angiomyofibroblastoma and spindle cell lipoma. *Am J Surg Pathol* 1998; **22**: 6–16.
3 Lane JE, Walker AN, Mullis EN Jr *et al*. Cellular angiofibroma of the vulva. *Gynecol Oncol* 2001; **81**: 326–9.
4 Curry JL, Olejnik JL, Wojcik EM. Cellular angiofibroma of the vulva with DNA ploidy analysis. *Int J Gynecol Pathol* 2001; **20**: 200–3.

Elastofibroma [1–3]

Definition. Elastofibroma is a reactive, probably degenerative, process of the elastic fibres of deep soft tissues that occurs almost exclusively around the shoulder. Although the lesion is regarded as degenerative, the finding of chromosomal alterations (see below), and of clonality in some cases, has led to the suggestion that it represents a neoplastic process [4].

Clinical features. It presents as an asymptomatic, slowly growing mass on the posterior upper trunk of middle-aged individuals. Lesions in other locations, including internal organs, are exceptional. Multiple lesions are usually bilateral and may be symmetrical [5].

Pathology. The mass is poorly circumscribed, and the appearances are characteristic. Abundant hypocellular hyalinized collagen containing numerous large, thick eosinophilic elastic fibres is the most distinctive feature. Sometimes the fibres are beaded and fragmented. Staining for elastic tissue nicely highlights the changes. Comparative genomic hybridization in a series of elastofibromas has found chromosomal alterations in a percentage of cases. The most common alteration consists of gains at chromosome Xq12-q22 [6].

Treatment. Simple excision is all that is necessary, as the tumours do not have a tendency to recur.

References

1 Jarvi OH, Saxen AE, Hopsu HV *et al*. Elastofibroma: a degenerative pseudotumor. *Cancer* 1969; **23**: 42–63.
2 Nagamine N, Nohara Y, Ito E. Elastofibroma in Okinawa: a clinicopathologic study of 170 cases. *Cancer* 1982; **50**: 1794–805.
3 Fukuda Y, Miyake H, Masuda Y *et al*. Histogenesis of unique elastinophilic fibers of elastofibroma: ultrastructural and immunohistochemical studies. *Hum Pathol* 1987; **18**: 424–9.
4 Hisaoka M, Hashimoto H. Elastofibroma: clonal fibrous proliferation with predominant CD34-positive cells. *Virchows Arch* 2006; **448**: 195–9.

5 Shimizu S, Yasui C, Tateno M *et al*. Multiple elastofibromas. *J Am Acad Dermatol* 2004; **50**: 126–9.
6 Nishio JN, Iwasaki H, Ohjimi Y *et al*. Gain of Xq detected by comparative genomic hybridization in elastofibroma. *Int J Mol Med* 2002; **10**: 277–80.

Infantile myofibromatosis and adult myofibroma [1–6]

> **Synonyms**
> • Congenital generalized fibromatosis
> • Infantile haemangiopericytoma

Definition. This tumour is composed of cells showing differentiation towards perivascular contractile cells, and has been described in the past as infantile haemangiopericytoma [7]. Infantile myofibromatosis and adult myofibroma/myofibromatosis are best regarded as part of the spectrum of lesions recently described as myopericytomas (see section on tumours of perivascular cells, p. 56.42) [8,9].

Clinical features [1–3]. Most cases of infantile myofibromatosis present before the age of 2 years, with slight male predominance. Congenital tumours occur in up to a third of the cases. Multiple lesions are present in 25% of patients. The preferred sites are the head and neck, followed by the trunk. Familial cases are rare. Involvement of other organs, including the gastrointestinal tract, lungs and bone, is seen in some cases. Multicentric involvement may be associated with mortality. Multiple lesions in the skin and soft tissues behave in a benign fashion and may regress spontaneously. Solitary myofibroma tends to occur in adults, with the same anatomical distribution as that of cutaneous and soft-tissue lesions presenting in infantile myofibromatosis [5,6]; multiple superficial tumours are rarely seen in adults. Intraoral lesions tend to be more common in young adults [10,11]. Exceptionally, associated thrombocytopenia has been reported [12].

Pathology [1,2,5–8]. Tumours have a distinctive biphasic growth pattern:
1 Areas composed of bundles of mature, spindle-shaped myofibroblasts with pink cytoplasm and vesicular nuclei
2 Areas composed of immature round cells, with scanty cytoplasm arranged around small blood vessels, often displaying a haemangiopericytoma-like pattern ('staghorn-like').
    Protrusion of tumour cells into vascular lumina is frequent, often mimicking vascular invasion. Old lesions often undergo hyalinization of the more mature areas. Mitotic figures and necrosis are relatively common. Tumour cells, particularly in the mature areas, are focally positive for actin.

Treatment. Lesions tend to regress spontaneously, but it is important to remember that patients with visceral tumours may die from the disease. Solitary lesions are treated by simple excision and do not tend to recur locally.

References
1 Chung EB, Enzinger FM. Infantile myofibromatosis. *Cancer* 1981; **48**: 1807–18.

2 Goldberg NS, Bauer BS, Kraus H *et al*. Infantile myofibromatosis: a review of clinicopathology with perspectives on new treatment choices. *Pediatr Dermatol* 1988; **5**: 37–46.
3 Coffin CM, Neilson KA, Ingels S *et al*. Congenital generalized myofibromatosis: a disseminated angiocentric myofibromatosis. *Pediatr Pathol Lab Med* 1995; **15**: 571–87.
4 Roggli VL, Kim HS, Hawkins E. Congenital generalized fibromatosis with visceral involvement: a case report. *Cancer* 1980; **45**: 954–60.
5 Beham A, Badve S, Suster S *et al*. Solitary myofibroma in adults: clinicopathological analysis of a series. *Histopathology* 1993; **22**: 335–41.
6 Daimaru Y, Hashimoto H, Enjoji M. Myofibromatosis in adults (adult counterpart of infantile myofibromatosis). *Am J Surg Pathol* 1989; **13**: 859–65.
7 Mentzel T, Calonje E, Nascimento AG *et al*. Infantile hemangiopericytoma versus infantile myofibromatosis: study of a series suggesting a continuous spectrum of infantile myofibroblastic lesions. *Am J Surg Pathol* 1994; **18**: 922–30.
8 Granter SR, Badizadegan K, Fletcher CDM. Myofibromatosis in adults, glomangiopericytoma and myopericytoma: a spectrum of tumors showing perivascular myoid differentiation. *Am J Surg Pathol* 1998; **22**: 513–25.
9 Mentzel T, Dei Tos AP, Sapi Z *et al*. Myopericytoma of skin and soft tissues: clinicopathologic and immunohistochemical study of 54 cases. *Am J Surg Pathol* 2006; **30**: 104–13.
10 Vered M, Allon J, Buchner A *et al*. Clinico-pathologic correlations of myofibroblastic tumors of the oral cavity. II. Myofibroma and myofibromatosis of the oral soft tissues. *J Oral Pathol Med* 2007; **36**: 304–14.
11 Foss RD, Ellis GL. Myofibromas and myofibromatosis of the oral region: A clinicopathologic analysis of 79 cases. *Oral Surg Oral Med* 2000; **89**: 57–65.
12 Leon-Villapalos J, Wolfe K, Calonje E *et al*. Involuting solitary cutaneous infantile myofibroma and thrombocytopaenia: a previously unreported clinical association. *J Plast Reconstr Aesthet Surg* 2007; **60**: 1260–2.

Inclusion body (digital) fibromatosis [1–3]

> **Synonym**
> • Infantile digital fibromatosis

Definition. Inclusion body fibromatosis is a fibro/myofibroblastic proliferation that almost only occurs on the fingers and toes. It is characterized by bright, round, intracytoplasmic, eosinophilic inclusions.

Clinical features. Most lesions present either at birth or during the first year of life as small, multiple nodules with predilection for the third, fourth and fifth digits. Involvement of the first digits (thumb and hallux) does not occur. New lesions often develop over a long period of time. Only rare cases have been described at other sites or in adults [4,5]. Spontaneous regression is sometimes seen [6]. Aggressive behaviour has not been described.

Pathology. Monomorphic bundles of bland, myofibroblast-like cells are seen in the dermis (Fig. 56.5a) and often the subcutis. Tumour cells have vesicular nuclei, an inconspicuous nucleolus and pink cytoplasm. Some mitotic figures may be seen. A distinctive feature is the presence of variable numbers of small, round, eosinophilic, intracytoplasmic inclusions in tumour cells (Fig. 56.5b). These are periodic acid–Schiff (PAS)-negative, but stain red with Masson's trichrome. They also stain for actin.

Treatment. Simple excision may be required for lesions that interfere with function, but simple observation of histologically confirmed lesions may be all that is necessary.

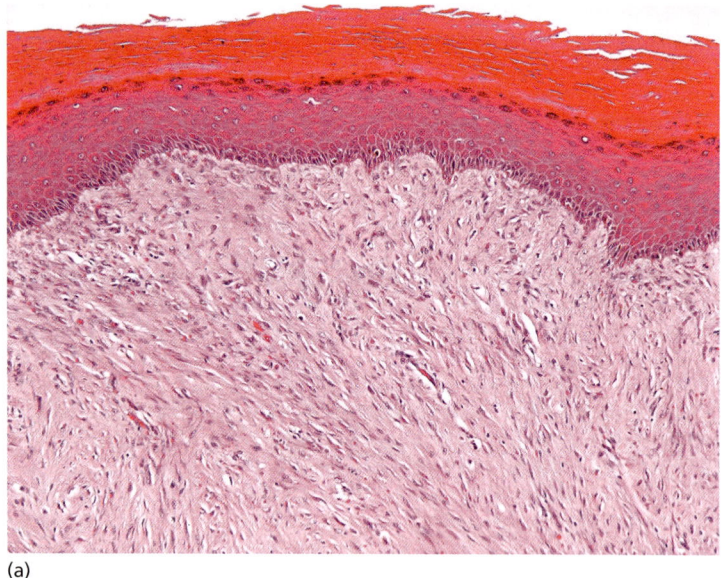

(a)

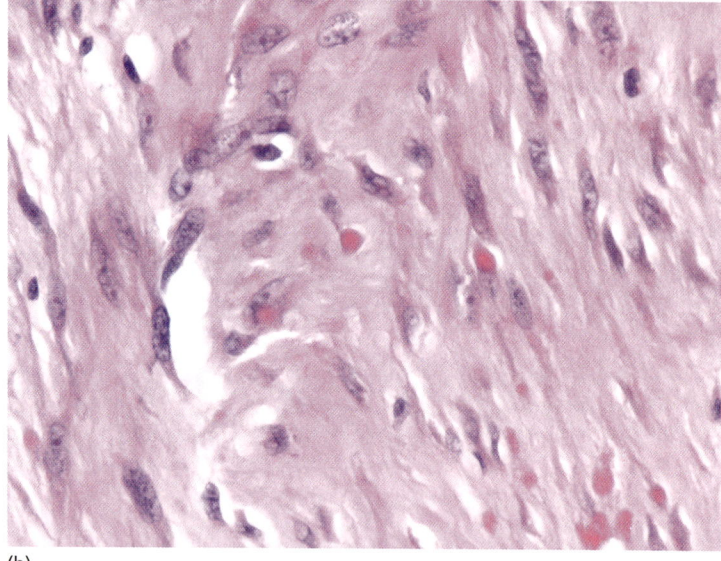

(b)

Fig. 56.5 (a) Bundles of bland myofibroblast-like cells in the dermis in a case of inclusion body fibromatosis. (b) Numerous typical eosinophilic intracytoplasmic eosinophilic inclusions.

References

1 Reye R. Recurring digital fibrous tumors of childhood. *Arch Pathol* 1965; **80**: 228–36.
2 Beckett JH, Jacobs AH. Recurring digital fibrous tumors of childhood: a review. *Pediatrics* 1977; **59**: 401–6.
3 Choi KC, Hashimoto K, Setoyama M *et al.* Infantile digital fibromatosis: immunohistochemical and immunoelectron microscopic studies. *J Cutan Pathol* 1990; **17**: 225–32.
4 Purdy LJ, Colby TV. Infantile digital fibromatosis occurring outside the digit. *Am J Surg Pathol* 1984; **8**: 787–90.
5 Viale G, Doglioni C, Iuzzolino P *et al.* Infantile digital fibromatosis-like tumor (inclusion body fibromatosis) of adulthood: report of two cases with ultrastructural and immunocytochemical findings. *Histopathology* 1988; **12**: 415–24.
6 Kawaguchi M, Mitsuhashi Y, Hozumi Y *et al.* A case of infantile digital fibromatosis with spontaneous regression. *J Dermatol* 1998; **25**: 523–6.

Fibroma of tendon sheath [1,2]

Definition. This is a distinctive, well-circumscribed fibroblastic tumour, presenting almost exclusively on the distal extremities.

Clinical features [1,2]. It is a small, slowly growing, asymptomatic tumour, presenting in young to middle-aged adults and with a marked predilection for the distal upper limb, particularly the hand and fingers. Rare lesions may present with carpal tunnel syndrome [3]. Lesions on the foot are much less common.

Pathology [1,2]. The neoplasm is multilobular and well-circumscribed and consists of cellular or poorly cellular areas on a background of variably hyalinized stroma. Stromal clefting is usually prominent. Tumour cells are spindle-shaped, with scanty cytoplasm and vesicular nuclei. Cytological atypia tends to be absent, and the mitotic count is low. A t(2;11)(q31-32;q12) has been demonstrated in a case of fibroma of tendon sheath [4].

Treatment. About 25% of cases recur locally, but the growth is not destructive. Simple excision is therefore the treatment of choice.

References

1 Chung EB, Enzinger FM. Fibroma of tendon sheath. *Cancer* 1979; **19**: 45–54.
2 Pulitzer DR, Martin PC, Reed RJ. Fibroma of tendon sheath: a clinicopathologic study of 32 cases. *Am J Surg Pathol* 1989; **13**: 472–9.
3 Tiong WH, Ismael TS, Regan PJ. Fibroma of tendon sheath: a rare cause of carpal tunnel syndrome. *J Hand Surg (Br)* 2006; **31**: 579–80.
4 Dal Cin P, Sciot R, De Smet L *et al.* Translocation 2;11 in a fibroma of tendon sheath. *Histopathology* 1998; **32**: 433–5.

Collagenous fibroma [1,2]

> **Synonym**
> • Desmoplastic fibroblastoma

Definition. Collagenous fibroma represents a distinctive, subcutaneous, fibroblastic tumour consisting of a prominent collagenous stroma.

Clinical features. It is relatively common and presents in adults as an asymptomatic nodule less than 4 cm in diameter, at any body site.

Pathology. This is a well-circumscribed tumour composed of bland elongated or stellate cells, with a background collagenous stroma and focal myxoid change. Mitotic figures are very rare. A translocation t(2;11)(q31;q12) has been found in two cases of collagenous fibroma suggesting that this is a non-random association in this type of tumour [3].

Treatment. Simple excision is the treatment of choice, as there is no tendency for local recurrence.

References

1 Evans HL. Desmoplastic fibroblastoma: a report of seven cases. *Am J Surg Pathol* 1995; **19**: 1077–81.

2 Mietinnen M, Fetsch JF. Collagenous fibroma (desmoplastic fibroblastoma): a clinicopathological analysis of 63 cases of a distinctive soft tissue lesion with stellate-shaped fibroblasts. *Hum Pathol* 1998; **29**: 676–82.
3 Bernal K, Nelson M, Neff JR *et al.* Translocation (2;11)(q31;q12) is recurrent in collagenous fibroma (desmoplastic fibroblastoma). *Cancer Genet Cytogenet* 2004; **149**: 161–3.

Nuchal fibroma [1,2]

Definition. Nuchal fibroma is a dermal or subcutaneous tumour consisting of hypocellular dense collagen.

Clinical features. Tumours are rare and occur in adult males. Patients often have diabetes. The great majority of cases present on the nape of the neck. Coexistence with scleroedema is possible, probably reflecting the association with diabetes, and lesions identical to nuchal fibroma are now recognized to occur in Gardner's syndrome (Chapter 62) and are known as Gardner-associated fibromas [3,4]. The latter may be multiple, present in various locations and may recur. These lesions may be the first clue as to the existence of Gardner's syndrome.

Pathology. Dense aggregates of collagen with very few cells and entrapment of adipose tissue.

Treatment. Simple excision is the treatment of choice but local recurrence is possible.

References
1 Balachandran K, Allen RW, McCormac LB. Nuchal fibroma: a clinicopathological analysis of nine cases. *Am J Surg Pathol* 1995; **19**: 313–7.
2 Michal M, Fetsch JF, Hes O *et al.* Nuchal-type fibroma: a clinicopathologic study of 52 cases. *Cancer* 1999; **85**: 156–63.
3 Wehrli BM, Weiss SW, Yandow S *et al.* Gardner-associated fibromas (GAF) in young patients: a distinct fibrous lesion that identifies unsuspected Gardner syndrome and risk for fibromatosis. *Am J Surg Pathol* 2001; **25**: 645–61.
4 Non-nuchal-type fibroma associated with Gardner's syndrome. A hitherto-unreported mesenchymal tumor different from fibromatosis and nuchal-type fibroma. *Pathol Res Pract* 2000; **196**: 857–60.

Palmar and plantar fibromatosis (superficial fibromatoses) [1,2]

Synonym Plantar fibromatosis
- Ledderhose's disease

Synonyms Palmar fibromatosis
- Dupuytren's disease
- Dupuytren's contracture

Definition. Palmar and plantar fibromatoses are superficial neoplastic proliferations of fibroblasts and myofibroblasts that have a tendency for local recurrence, but do not metastasize.

Incidence and aetiology. Palmar fibromatosis is more common than plantar fibromatosis. Both lesions are more common in men, but the sex difference is more marked in palmar lesions. Both conditions affect middle-aged to elderly patients and are more uncommon in younger individuals. However, children may rarely

be affected, particularly by plantar fibromatosis [3]. Affected patients are mainly of Northern European origin; non-whites are rarely affected. Coexistence between the two variants of fibromatoses and desmoid tumours, penile fibromatosis (Peyronie's disease) and knuckle pads may be seen. Genetic predisposition, as well as trauma, is thought to play an important role in the pathogenesis of these conditions. Associations with diabetes, alcoholic liver disease and epilepsy have also been described.

Clinical features. Palmar fibromatosis presents as indurated nodules or as an ill-defined area of thickening, bilateral in about 50% of cases, that may result in contracture. Plantar fibromatosis usually consists of a single nodule. Functional limitation is common.

Pathology. Early lesions are fairly cellular and consist of bundles of bland fibroblasts with some collagen deposition. The latter increases considerably in older lesions. Interestingly, although superficial fibromatoses are very similar histologically to deep fibromatosis (abdominal, extra-abdominal and mesenteric fibromatosis), the behaviour of superficial fibromatosis is not usually aggressive. This may be due to the fact that deep fibromatosis often display mutations of the *APC* gene or somatic mutations of the gene encoding beta-catenin, while these mutations are absent in superficial fibromatosis. Intriguingly however, although deep fibromatoses often display nuclear expression of beta-catenin, this is also seen in a smaller percentage of superficial fibromatoses without gene mutations [4].

Treatment. Complete excision is desirable, as there is otherwise a risk of local recurrence.

References
1 Allen PW. The fibromatoses: a clinicopathologic classification based on 140 cases. *Am J Surg Pathol* 1977; **1**: 255–70.
2 Mikkelsen OA. Dupuytren's disease: initial symptoms, age of onset and spontaneous course. *Hand* 1977; **9**: 11–5.
3 Fetsch JF, Laskin WB, Miettinen M. Palmar-plantar fibromatosis in children and pre-adolescents: a clinicopathologic study of 56 cases with newly recognized demographics and extended follow-up information. *Am J Surg Pathol* 2005; **29**: 1095–105.
4 Montgomery E, Lee JH, Abraham SC *et al.* Superficial fibromatoses are genetically distinct from deep fibromatosis. *Mod Pathol* 2001; **14**: 695–701.

Penile fibromatosis [1–3]

Synonym
- Peyronie's disease

Definition. Although usually regarded as a variant of superficial fibromatosis, it is more likely that this disease represents a reactive fibrotic disorder of unknown aetiology.

Clinical features. It presents as a solitary nodule or multiple nodules close to the corpus cavernosum on the dorsal surface of the shaft. Most patients are middle-aged, and in most the lesion is small. Pain and curvature of the penis on erection are frequent complaints. The presence of diabetes mellitus increases the severity of the disease [4].

Pathology. In early lesions, there is a patchy chronic mononuclear inflammatory cell infiltrate and focal vasculitic changes. These changes lead to dense bands of hyalinized collagen in late stages.

References

1 Smith BH. Peyronie's disease. *Am J Clin Pathol* 1966; **85**: 670–8.
2 McRoberts JW. Peyronie's disease. *Surg Gynecol Obstet* 1969; **129**: 1291–4.
3 Billig R, Baker R, Immergut Maxted W. Peyronie's disease. *Urology* 1975; **6**: 409–18.
4 Kendirci M, Trost L, Sikka SC *et al.* Diabetes mellitus is associated with severe Peyronie's disease. *BJU Int* 2007; **99**: 383–6.

Lipofibromatosis [1]

Definition. Lipofibromatosis is a locally aggressive childhood tumour composed of variable amounts of mature adipose and fibroblastic elements.

Clinical features. Tumours present in infants and children, with the majority of cases presenting in the first decade of life. Some tumours are congenital. There is a male predominance. The classical presentation is of a slowly growing, ill-defined mass. There is a predilection for the hands and feet, but other sites in the limbs, and less commonly on the trunk, may be affected. The rate of local recurrence is high.

Pathology. Tumours are infiltrative and consist of lobules of mature adipose tissue intermixed with bundles of fibroblast-like cells with no cytological atypia and low mitotic activity. By immunohistochemistry, tumour cells are focally positive for S100 protein, CD34, bcl-2, actin, EMA and CD99. The lesion closely resembles a fibrous hamartoma of infancy but has more prominent adipose tissue and lacks the third cellular component seen in the latter, which consists of round, primitive-looking cells in a myxoid background.

Prognosis and treatment. In view of the local aggressive nature of this tumour, complete excision is desirable.

Reference

1 Fetsch JF, Miettinen M, Laskin WB *et al.* A clinicopathologic study of 45 soft tissue tumors with an admixture of adipose tissue and fibroblastic elements, and a proposal for classification as lipofibromatosis. *Am J Surg Pathol* 2000; **24**: 1491–500.

Dermatofibrosarcoma protuberans [1–3]

Definition. Dermatofibrosarcoma protuberans (DFSP) is a locally invasive tumour arising in the dermis and showing fibroblastic differentiation.

Incidence and aetiology [1–3]. DFSP is uncommon, more common in black than in white patients, and slightly more common in females than males [4]. Most patients present in the third and fourth decades of life. The incidence in the USA has been estimated as 4.2 cases per million [4]. Some cases develop at the site of previous trauma, reports have included a burn scar [5] and the

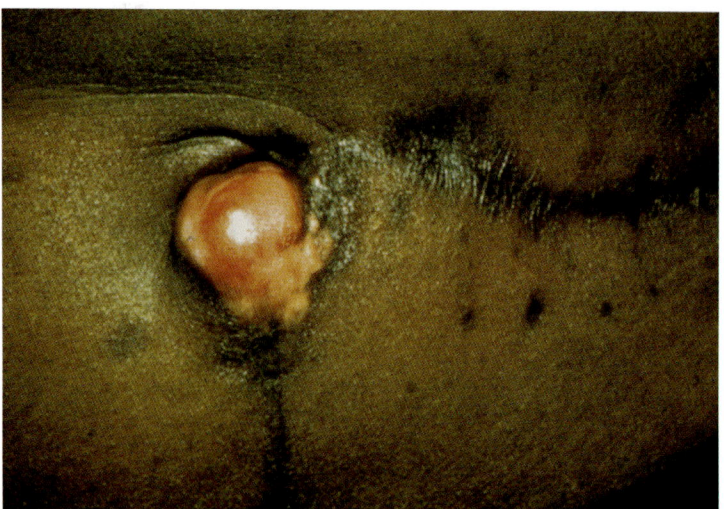

Fig. 56.6 Recurrent abdominal dermatofibrosarcoma protuberans.

site of vaccination. Exceptional cases have been associated with previous radiotherapy to the area [6].

Clinical features. The tumour is more often situated on the trunk (up to half of the cases), particularly in the flexural regions, than on the extremities or the head [1,2]. Involvement of the limbs is usually proximal. Presentation on hands and feet, particularly on the digits, is vanishingly rare. It may begin in early adult life with one or more small, firm, painless, flesh-coloured or red dermal nodules (Fig. 56.6). There are rare examples of DFSP occurring in infancy [7–9], and congenital cases have been described [9,10].

The tumour starts as a plaque, which may occasionally be atrophic [8,11]. Progression is usually very slow, and may occur over many years; a significant proportion of tumours only become protuberant after a long period of time [12]. Eventually, nodules develop, coalesce and extend, becoming redder or bluish as they enlarge to form irregular, protuberant swellings. At this stage, the base of the lesion is a hard, indurated plaque of irregular outline. In the later stages, a proportion of lesions become painful and there may be rapid growth, ulceration and discharge.

Local recurrence of ordinary DFSP is reported to vary from 15% to up to 60% [3,13,14], and that of the fibrosarcomatous variant is as high as 75% [15–18]. Metastases to lymph nodes and internal organs tend to be extremely rare in pure DFSP [15,19,20] but occur in up to 20% of cases with fibrosarcomatous transformation [16–18].

Pathology [1–3,13]. The tumour is usually a solitary, multinodular mass. The dermis and subcutaneous tissue are replaced by bundles of uniform, spindle-shaped cells with little cytoplasm and elongated hyperchromatic, but not pleomorphic, nuclei. Usually there is little mitotic activity. Deeper involvement may be seen in some cases. Laterally, the tumour cells infiltrate widely between collagen bundles of the deeper dermis and blend into the normal dermis, forming quite definite bands, which interweave or radiate like spokes of a wheel; this is described as a 'storiform' pattern (Fig. 56.7). The interstitial tissue contains collagen fibres, except in the most cellular parts of the tumour. The subcutaneous tissue is

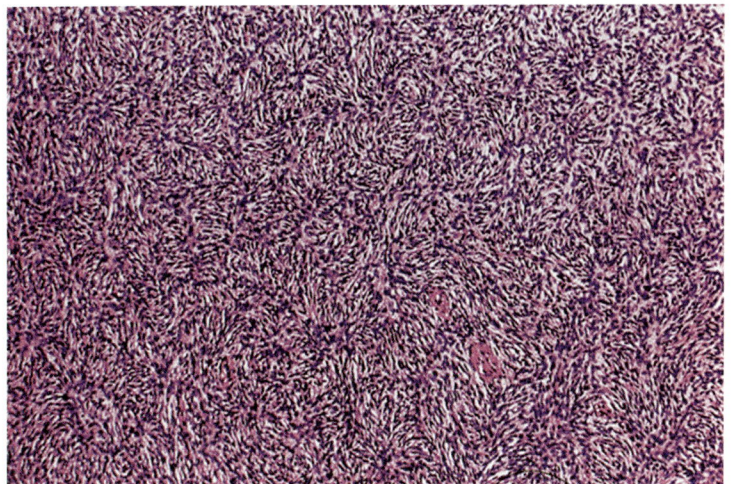

Fig. 56.7 Pathological appearance of dermatofibrosarcoma protuberans, showing the storiform or 'cartwheel' distribution of the fairly uniform, spindle-shaped tumour cells.

extensively infiltrated and replaced in a typical lace-like pattern. Myxoid change may be focal or, rarely, prominent; in the latter setting, the histological diagnosis is difficult [21,22]. Some tumours are colonized by scattered, deeply pigmented melanocytes, a variant known as pigmented DFSP (Bednar tumour) [23,24]. A further variant consists of myoid nodules and is thought to represent myofibroblastic differentiation [25]. Rare cases show focal granular cell change.

Fibrosarcomatous DFSP [16–18,26] is an important variant of this tumour, which is recognized by the focal presence of areas with long, sweeping fascicles of tumour cells intersecting at acute angles in a typical 'herring-bone' pattern, almost identical to that seen in fibrosarcoma. In these areas, mitoses are increased and there is more nuclear hyperchromatism. P53 expression is increased in fibrosarcomatous areas [26]. Identification of the presence of this pattern, and its quantity, is very important, as it is related to metastatic potential. Fibrosarcomatous areas are more common in recurrent tumours.

Very rare variants of DFSP may show areas of high-grade sarcoma either in the primary tumour or in a recurrence [27].

DFSP may show areas of giant cell fibroblastoma (see below) and either tumour may recur, displaying features of the other tumour [28].

The majority of the lesions are positive on staining with the antibody CD34, although this is not specific for DFSP [13]. Other markers are usually negative but in some cases focal positivity for epithelial membrane antigen may be seen. Fibrosarcomatous areas often show decreased staining with CD34 [18].

Cytogenetic studies are helpful, as ring chromosomes indicative of a 17;22 translocation are invariably found [28]. However, it is important to highlight that some cases demonstrate a variant ring chromosome with cryptic rearrangements of chromosomes 17 and 22 [29]. This chromosomal translocation involves the collagen type I alpha 1 (*COL1A1*) gene on chromosome 17 and the platelet-derived growth factor B (*PDGFB*) gene on chromosome 22. The abnormal fusion transcripts resulting from this translocation leads to autocrine stimulation of PDGFB and platelet-derived growth factor receptor beta (PDGFRB) and cell proliferation. The fusion

transcript is found in almost all examples of the tumour by polymerase chain reaction (PCR) and fluorescence *in situ* hybridization (FISH) [30]. The same cytogenetic abnormality is found in giant cell fibroblastoma, confirming that both tumours are part of the same spectrum (see below).

Diagnosis. In the early stages, it may be impossible to distinguish this tumour from a histiocytoma or a keloid. Some lesions may also be confused with morphoea profunda. The slow progression, deep red or bluish-red colour, and the characteristic irregular contour and extended plaque-like base, are strongly suggestive of DFSP.

Treatment. The tumour should be excised completely, with a generous margin of healthy tissue [31]. The best chance of achieving a complete cure with no recurrence is early detection of small tumours. Local recurrence invariably follows inadequate removal; the clearance necessary to cure the tumour is often underestimated [32]. A margin of between 2 and 4 cm has been recommended [14,33]. Mohs micrographic surgery has been reported as effective in reducing the rate of local recurrence [34,35]. If this type of treatment is used it should be performed using formalin-fixed paraffin-embedded sections rather than frozen sections, and evaluation should be by an experienced pathologist. Although Mohs surgery clearly reduces the rate of local recurrences, the latter still occur and sometimes this happens more than 5 years after surgery [36]. Postsurgical radiotherapy has been advocated to reduce the rate of local recurrence [37] but this type of treatment has not been assessed in large series of patients. In recent years, it has been demonstrated that imatinib mesylate, a potent inhibitor of a number of protein kinases including the platelet-derived growth factor receptor, results in good clinical response in patients with large unresectable or metastatic tumours [38–42].

References

1 Taylor HB, Helwig EB. Dermatofibrosarcoma protuberans: a study of 115 cases. *Cancer* 1962; **15**: 717–25.

2 Burkhardt BR, Soule EH, Winkelmann RK *et al.* Dermatofibrosarcoma protuberans: study of 56 cases. *Am J Surg* 1966; **111**: 638–44.

3 Gloster HM. Dermatofibrosarcoma protuberans. *J Am Acad Dermatol* 1996; **35**: 355–74.

4 Criscione VD, Weinstock MA. Descriptive epidemiology of dermatofibrosarcoma protuberans in the United States, 1973 to 2002. *J Am Acad Dermatol* 2007; **56**: 968–73.

5 Tanaka A, Hatoko M, Tada H *et al.* Dermatofibrosarcoma protuberans arising from a burn scar of the axilla. *Ann Plast Surg* 2004; **52**: 423–5.

6 Huber GF, Matthews TW, Dort JC. Radiation-induced soft tissue sarcomas of the head and neck. *J Otolaryngol* 2007; **36**: 93–7.

7 McKee PH, Fletcher CDM. Dermatofibrosarcoma presenting in infancy and childhood. *J Cutan Pathol* 1991; **18**: 241–6.

8 Martin L, Combemale P, Dupin MJ *et al.* The atrophic variant of dermatofibrosarcoma protuberans in childhood: a report of six cases. *Br J Dermatol* 1998; **139**: 719–25.

9 Checketts SR, Hamilton TK, Baughman RD. Congenital and childhood dermatofibrosarcoma protuberans: a case report and review of the literature. *J Am Acad Dermatol* 2000; **42**: 907–13.

10 Maire G, Fraitag S, Galmiche L *et al.* A clinical, histologic, and molecular analysis of 9 cases of congenital dermatofibrosarcoma protuberans. *Arch Dermatol* 2007; **143**: 203–10.

11 Zelger BW, Ofner D, Zelger BG. Atrophic variants of dermatofibroma and dermatofibrosarcoma protuberans. *Histopathology* 1995; **26**: 519–27.

12 Martin L, Piette F, Blanc P *et al.* Clinical variants of the preprotuberant stage of dermatofibrosarcoma protuberans. *Br J Dermatol* 2005; **153**: 932–6.

13 Fletcher CDM, Evans BJ, Macartney JC *et al.* Dermatofibrosarcoma protuberans: a clinicopathological and immunohistochemical study with a review of the literature. *Histopathology* 1985; **9**: 921–38.

14 Rutgers EJ, Kroon BB, Albus-Lutter CE *et al.* Dermatofibrosarcoma protuberans: treatment and prognosis. *Eur J Surg Oncol* 1992; **18**: 241–8.

15 McPeak CJ, Cruz T, Nicastri AD. Dermatofibrosarcoma protuberans: an analysis of 86 cases—five with metastasis. *Ann Surg* 1967; **166**: 803–16.

16 Ding J, Hashimoto H, Enjoji M. Dermatofibrosarcoma protuberans with fibrosarcomatous areas: a clinicopathologic study of nine cases and a comparison with allied tumors. *Cancer* 1989; **64**: 721–9.

17 Conelly JH, Evans HL. Dermatofibrosarcoma protuberans: a clinicopathologic review with emphasis on fibrosarcomatous areas. *Am J Surg Pathol* 1992; **16**: 921–5.

18 Mentzel T, Beham A, Katenkamp D *et al.* Fibrosarcomatous ('high grade') dermatofibrosarcoma protuberans. Clinicopathologic study and immunohistochemical study of a series of 41 cases with emphasis on prognostic significance. *Am J Surg Pathol* 1998; **22**: 576–87.

19 Fisher ER, Helstrom HR. Dermatofibrosarcoma with metastases simulating Hodgkin's disease and reticulum cell sarcoma. *Cancer* 1966; **19**: 1165–71.

20 Brenner W, Schaefler K, Chhabra H *et al.* Dermatofibrosarcoma protuberans metastatic to a regional lymph node: report of a case and review. *Cancer* 1975; **36**: 1897–902.

21 Reimann JD, Fletcher CD. Myxoid dermatofibrosarcomas protuberans: a rare variant analyzed in a series of 23 cases. *Am J Surg Pathol* 2007; **31**: 1371–7.

22 Mentzel T, Sharer L, Kazakov DV *et al.* Myxoid dermatofibrosarcoma protuberans: clinicopathologic, immunohistochemical, and molecular analysis of eight cases. *Am J Dermatopathol* 2007; **29**: 443–8.

23 Bednar B. Storiform neurofibromas of the skin, pigmented and nonpigmented. *Cancer* 1957; **10**: 368–75.

24 Fletcher CDM, Theaker JM, Flanagan A *et al.* Pigmented dermatofibrosarcoma protuberans (Bednar tumour): melanocytic colonization or neuroectodermal differentiation? A clinicopathological and immunohistological study. *Histopathology* 1988; **13**: 631–43.

25 Calonje E, Fletcher CDM. Myoid differentiation in dermatofibrosarcoma protuberans and its fibrosarcomatous variant: clinicopathologic analysis of 5 cases. *J Cutan Pathol* 1996; **23**: 30–6.

26 Abbott JJ, Oliveira AM, Nascimento AG. The prognostic significance of fibrosarcomatous transformation in dermatofibrosarcoma protuberans. *Am J Surg Pathol* 2006; **30**: 436–43.

27 Szollosi Z, Nemes Z. Transformed dermatofibrosarcoma protuberans: a clinicopathological study of eight cases. *J Clin Pathol* 2005; **58**: 751–6.

28 Rubin B, Fletcher J, Fletcher CD. The histologic, genetic and histological relationship between dermatofibrosarcoma protuberans and giant cell fibroblastoma: an unexpected story. *Adv Anat Pathol* 1997; **4**: 336–41.

29 Bigby SM, Oei P, Lambie NK *et al.* Dermatofibrosarcoma protuberans: report of a case with a variant ring chromosome and metastases following pregnancy. *J Cutan Pathol* 2006; **33**: 383–8.

30 Patel KU, Szabo SS, Hernandez VS *et al.* Dermatofibrosarcoma protuberans COL1A1-PDGFB fusion is identified in virtually all dermatofibrosarcoma protuberans cases when investigated by newly developed multiplex reverse transcription polymerase chain reaction and fluorescence in situ hybridization assays. *Hum Pathol* 2008; **39**: 184–93.

31 Fiore M, Miceli R, Mussi C *et al.* Dermatofibrosarcoma protuberans treated at a single institution: a surgical disease with a high cure rate. *J Clin Oncol* 2005; **23**: 7669–75.

32 Smola MG, Soyer HP, Scharnagl E. Surgical treatment of dermatofibrosarcoma protuberans: a retrospective study of 20 cases with review of literature. *Eur J Surg Oncol* 1991; **17**: 447–53.

33 Roses DF, Valensi Q, LaTrenta G *et al.* Surgical treatment of dermatofibrosarcoma protuberans. *Surg Gynecol Obstet* 1986; **162**: 449–52.

34 Robinson JK. Dermatofibrosarcoma protuberans resected by Mohs' surgery (chemosurgery): a 5-year prospective study. *J Am Acad Dermatol* 1985; **12**: 1093–8.

35 Thomas CJ, Wood GC, Marks VJ. Mohs micrographic surgery in the treatment of rare aggressive cutaneous tumors: the Geisinger experience. *Dermatol Surg* 2007; **33**: 333–9.

36 Snow SN, Gordon EM, Larson PO *et al.* Dermatofibrosarcoma protuberans: a report on 29 cases treated by Mohs micrographic surgery with long-term follow-up and review of the literature. *Cancer* 2004; **101**: 28–38.

37 Dagan R, Morris CG, Zlotecki RA *et al.* Radiotherapy in the treatment of dermatofibrosarcoma protuberans. *Am J Clin Oncol* 2005; **28**: 537–9.

38 McArthur GA. Molecular targeting of dermatofibrosarcoma protuberans: a new approach to a surgical disease. *J Natl Compr Canc Netw* 2007; **5**: 557–62.

39 Sjöblom T, Shimizu A, O'Brien KP *et al.* Growth inhibition of dermatofibrosarcoma protuberans tumors by the platelet-derived growth factor receptor antagonist ST1571 through induction of apoptosis. *Cancer Res* 2001; **61**: 5778–83.

40 Kondapalli L, Soltani K, Lacouture ME. The promise of molecular targeted therapies: protein kinases inhibitors in the treatment of cutaneous malignancies. *J Am Acad Dermatol* 2005; **53**: 291–302.

41 Price VE, Fletcher JA, Zielenska M *et al.* Imatinib mesylate: an attractive alternative in young children with large, surgically challenging dermatofibrosarcoma protuberans. *Pediatr Blood Cancer* 2005; **44**: 511–5.

42 Sirvent N, Maire G, Pedeutour F. Genetics of dermatofibrosarcoma protuberans family of tumors: from ring chromosomes to tyrosinase inhibitor treatment. *Genes Chromosomes Cancer* 2003; **37**: 1–19.

Giant cell fibroblastoma [1–4]

Definition. This is a locally recurrent, fibroblastic tumour, closely related to DFSP. It is characterized by spindle-shaped, oval or stellate, mono- or multinucleated cells in a fibromyxoid stroma with irregular pseudovascular spaces lined by tumour cells.

Clinical features [1–4]. The large majority of cases present as a subcutaneous, ill-defined mass in the first few years of life. It is rare in young adults and more exceptional in older adults. The trunk is much more commonly involved than the proximal limbs. Tumours measure a few centimetres in diameter, have a predilection for males and tend to be asymptomatic.

Pathology. Solid fibromyxoid areas with variable collagen deposition contain stellate and spindle-shaped mono- and multinucleated tumour cells with hyperchromatic nuclei. Dilated, irregularly branching pseudovascular spaces are commonly seen scattered throughout the lesion. These spaces are lined by tumour cells, which often appear multinucleated (Fig. 56.8). Mitotic figures are exceptional. Aggregates of perivascular lymphocytes in an onion-ring pattern and focal haemorrhage are often seen [4]. Focal areas identical to DFSP may be seen and can occupy a substantial part of the tumour. Excised lesions can recur as a pure giant cell fibroblastoma, as a tumour with focal DFSP, or as pure DFSP [4–7]. Tumour cells are focally positive for CD34 and only very focally positive for actin. Ring chromosomes with sequences of chromosomes 17 and 22, identical to those found in DFSP, have been described in this tumour, confirming their close histogenetic relationship [8,9].

Treatment. Recurrence may be seen in about half of the cases, but metastasis has not been reported.

References

1 Dymock RB, Allen PW, Stirling JW, Gilbert EF, Thornbery JM. Giant cell fibroblastoma: a distinctive, recurrent tumour of childhood. *Am J Surg Pathol* 1987; **11**: 263–71.

2 Shmookler BM, Enzinger FM. Giant cell fibroblastoma: a juvenile form of dermatofibrosarcoma protuberans. *Cancer* 1989; **64**: 2154–61.

3 Chou P, Gonzalez-Crussi G, Mangkornikanok M. Giant cell fibroblastoma. *Cancer* 1989; **63**: 756–62.

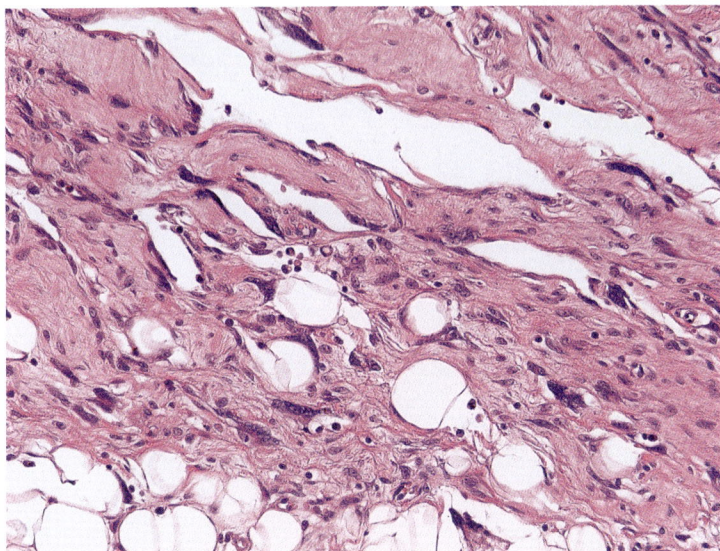

Fig. 56.8 Typical pseudovascular spaces focally lined by multinucleated cells in a case of giant cell fibroblastoma.

4 Jha P, Moosavi C, Fanburg-Smith JC. Giant cell fibroblastoma: un update and addition of 86 cases from the Armed Forces Institute of Pathology, in honor of Dr. Franz M. Enzinger. *Ann Diagn Pathol* 2007; **11**: 81–8.

5 Alguacil-García A. Giant cell fibroblastoma recurring as dermatofibrosarcoma protuberans. *Am J Surg Pathol* 1991; **21**: 184–7.

6 Harvell JD, Kilpatrick SE, White WL. Histogenetic relations between giant cell fibroblastoma and dermatofibrosarcoma protuberans. *Am J Dermatopathol* 1998; **20**: 339–45.

7 Beham A, Fletcher CD. Dermatofibrosarcoma protuberans with areas resembling giant cell fibroblastoma: report of two cases. *Histopathology* 1990; **17**: 165–7.

8 Dal Cin P, Sciot R, de Wever I *et al.* Cytogenetic and immunohistochemical evidence that giant cell fibroblastoma is related to dermatofibrosarcoma protuberans. *Genes Chrom Cancer* 1996; **15**: 73–5.

9 Terrier-Lacombe MJ, Guillou L, Maire G *et al.* Dermatofibrosarcoma protuberans, giant cell fibroblastoma and hybrid lesions in children: clinicopathologic comparative analysis of 28 cases with molecular data—a study of the French Federation of Cancer Centers Sarcoma Group. *Am J Surg Pathol* 2003; **27**: 27–9.

Myxoinflammatory fibroblastic sarcoma [1–3]

> **Synonyms**
> - Inflammatory myxohyaline tumour of the distal extremities with virocyte or Reed–Sternberg-like cells
> - Acral myxoinflammatory fibroblastic sarcoma

Definition. Myxoinflammatory fibroblastic sarcoma is a distinctive, neoplastic process with marked predilection for acral sites, and with histological features closely mimicking an inflammatory process due to the presence of prominent inflammation and virocyte-like inclusions in the nuclei of tumour cells. The latter features were initially thought to indicate an infectious aetiology. However, no firm evidence of this has yet emerged.

Clinical features. Most patients are middle-aged adults with an equal sex incidence. Characteristically, tumours are long-standing, asymptomatic and slowly growing, usually measuring no more than 4 cm. The great majority occur on acral sites, particularly the hands and wrists, followed by the feet. However, lesions may rarely present elsewhere on the limbs (arm, forearm and thigh) [4]

and exceptionally elsewhere in the body, including the neck [5]. Most cases are clinically diagnosed as a ganglion cyst or as a giant cell tumour of tendon sheath.

Pathology. Lesions are lobulated and poorly circumscribed and involve the subcutaneous fat and often extend to the dermis and deeper tissues, sparing bone. Low-power examination is misleading and the initial impression is that of an inflammatory process. Lobules of hyalinized and myxoid tissue containing variable numbers of inflammatory cells are seen. The latter include lymphocytes, histiocytes, neutrophils and less commonly eosinophils and plasma cells. Closer examination reveals variable numbers of neoplastic cells that vary from round to spindle-shaped. Some of these cells may be multinucleated. Round cells mimic ganglion cells with nucleoli resembling viral inclusions. Less commonly, vacuolated tumour cells resembling lipoblasts are seen. Mitotic activity is very low. Immunohistochemistry shows that tumour cells are variably positive for CD34 and CD68 and are rarely positive for smooth-muscle actin and exceptionally for keratin. Very few cases have been subjected to cytogenetic studies [6,7]. In two cases published, one showed a complex karyotype with a reciprocal translocation t(1;10)(p22;q24) and loss of chromosomes 3 and 13 [6] and the other a translocation t(2;6)(q31;p21.3) [7]. These findings support the theory that these lesions are neoplastic.

Prognosis and treatment. The rate of local recurrence is high, varying from 11 to 67% in different series [1,2]. Distal metastases are exceptional and are mainly to regional lymph nodes. The treatment of choice is wide local excision and this often implies amputation.

References

1 Montgomery EA, Devaney KO, Giordano TJ *et al.* Inflammatory myxohyaline tumor of distal extremities with virocyte or Reed-Sternberg-like cells: a distinctive lesion with features simulating inflammatory conditions, Hodgkin's disease, and various sarcomas. *Mod Pathol* 1998; **11**: 384–91.

2 Meis-Kindblom JM, Kindblom LG. Acral myxoinflammatory fibroblastic sarcoma: a low-grade tumor of the hands and feet. *Am J Surg Pathol* 1998; **22**: 911–24.

3 Sakaki M, Hirokawa M, Wakatsuki S *et al.* Acral myxoinflammatory fibroblastic sarcoma: a report of five cases and review of the literature. *Virchows Arch* 2003; **442**: 25–30.

4 Jurcić V, Zidar A, Montiel MD *et al.* Myxoinflammatory fibroblastic sarcoma: a tumor not restricted to acral sites. *Ann Diagn Pathol* 2002; **6**: 272–80.

5 McFarlane R, Meyers AD, Golitz L. Myxoinflammatory fibroblastic sarcoma of the neck. *J Cutan Pathol* 2005; **32**: 375–8.

6 Lambert I, Debiec-Rychter M, Guelinckx P *et al.* Acral myxoinflammatory fibroblastic sarcoma with unique clonal chromosomal changes. *Virchows Arch* 2001; **438**: 509–12.

7 Ida CM, Rolig KA, Hulshizer RL *et al.* Myxoinflammatory fibroblastic sarcoma showing t(2;6)(q31;p21.3) as a sole cytogenetic abnormality. *Cancer Genet Cytogenet* 2007; **177**: 139–42.

Fibrohistiocytic tumours

Giant cell tumour of tendon sheath [1–3]

Definition. This is a benign tumour that in its localized variant occurs mainly on the hands, and consists of a nodular proliferation of histiocyte-like cells with scattered multinucleated giant cells and variable numbers of mononuclear inflammatory cells. The diffuse variant of this tumour that involves joints is not discussed further in this chapter.

Clinical features. Tumours present mainly on the hands with predilection for the fingers. They are typically between 1 and 3 cm in diameter and asymptomatic, although they may interfere with function. There is a predilection for young females. Multiple tumours are very rare [4].

Pathology. It is a multinodular lesion composed of sheets of histiocyte-like cells with bland vesicular nuclei, intermixed with multinucleated giant cells, foamy cells, siderophages and scattered mononuclear inflammatory cells. Hyalinization, haemosiderin deposition and cholesterol clefts are often seen. No histological features predict lesions that recur locally [3].

Treatment. Excision is the treatment of choice; the rate of local recurrence is around 30%.

References

1 Myers BW, Masi AT, Feigenbaum SL. Pigmented villonodular synovitis and tenosynovitis: a clinical epidemiologic study of 166 cases and literature review. *Medicine* 1980; **59**: 223–38.
2 Ushjima M, Hashimoto H, Tsuneyoshi M *et al*. Giant cell tumor of the tendon sheath (nodular tenosynovitis): a study of 207 cases to compare the large joint group with the common digit group. *Cancer* 1986; **57**: 875–84.
3 Mohaghan H, Salter DM, Al-Nafussi A. Giant cell tumour of tendon sheath (localised nodular tenosynovitis): clinicopathological features of 71 cases. *J Clin Pathol* 2001; **54**: 404–7.
4 Park JW. Multiple separated giant cell tumors of the tendon sheath in a thumb. *J Am Acad Dermatol* 2006; **54**: 540–2.

Fibrous histiocytoma (dermatofibroma) [1–4]

Synonyms
- Histiocytoma cutis
- Subepidermal nodular fibrosis
- Sclerosing angioma

Definition. Fibrous histiocytoma (FH) is a benign dermal and often superficial subcutaneous proliferation of oval cells resembling histiocytes, and spindle-shaped cells resembling fibroblasts and myofibroblasts. Their line of differentiation remains uncertain, but these lesions are descriptively classified as fibrohistiocytic tumours because of the microscopic appearance of the tumour cells. The aetiology of FH is unknown, but recent cytogenetic studies demonstrating clonality favour these lesions being neoplastic [5,6]. The neoplastic nature of FH is also suggested by their clinical persistence and by the frequency of local recurrence of some variants (cellular, aneurysmal and atypical; see below) as well as the exceptional anecdotal metastases of some tumours (cellular and atypical types). The previous theory that they are a dermal response to injury, such as an insect bite, has been challenged [7].

Clinical features. FH is commonest on the limbs and appears as a firm papule, which is frequently yellow-brown in colour and

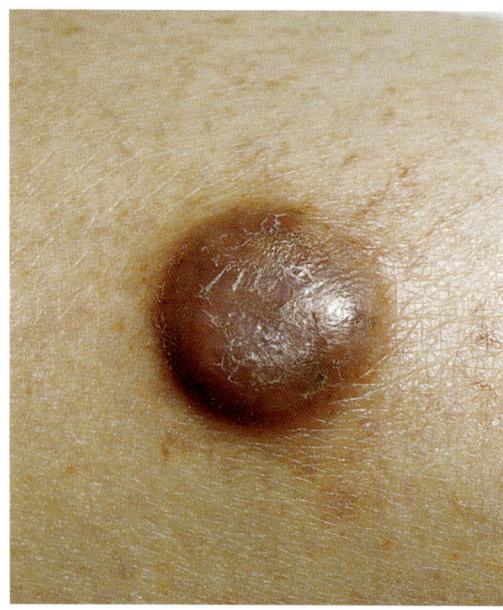

Fig. 56.9 Clinical appearance of a fibrous histiocytoma or dermatofibroma.

slightly scaly (Fig. 56.9). If the overlying epidermis is squeezed, the 'dimple sign' will be seen, indicating tethering of the overlying epidermis to the underlying lesion. Giant lesions (>5 cm in diameter) are occasionally seen [8] and large tumours are more often encountered in some of the variants (see below). Multiple lesions may develop and eruptive variants have been described. The latter may be familial [9], or may be associated with immunosuppression (HIV) [10], with systemic disease, including autoimmune diseases such as lupus erythematosus and neoplasia, particularly haematological malignancies [11–15], and even with highly active antiretroviral therapy (HAART) [16].

A number of clinicopathological variants of FH have been described, which should be recognized by clinicians and pathologists in order to avoid a misdiagnosis of malignancy. These variants include: cellular FH [17,18], aneurysmal FH [19,20], atypical FH (pseudosarcomatous FH, dermatofibroma with monster cells) [21,22] and epithelioid FH [23,24]. A further variant, described as 'atrophic' [25], may mimic a scar and does not usually pose a problem in differential diagnosis. Rare cases may be ulcerated, erosive or lichenoid [26].

Cellular FH represents less than 5% of all FHs [17]. Like ordinary FH, it has a predilection for the limbs of young adults, but it tends to occur more commonly in males. However, the distribution of age and site is wide; cellular FH is not infrequent in children, and on sites such as the head, neck, fingers and toes. The size of these lesions is also larger than that of ordinary FH. Most cellular FHs are less than 2 cm in diameter, but lesions measuring more than 5 cm may occur. Recognition of this variant is important, because it has a local recurrence rate of 25%, and metastases have been reported anecdotally in a small number of cases [18,27].

Aneurysmal FH has the same age and sex distribution as ordinary FH [19,20]. Tumours are usually rapidly growing and may attain a very large size. They clinically mimic a vascular tumour.

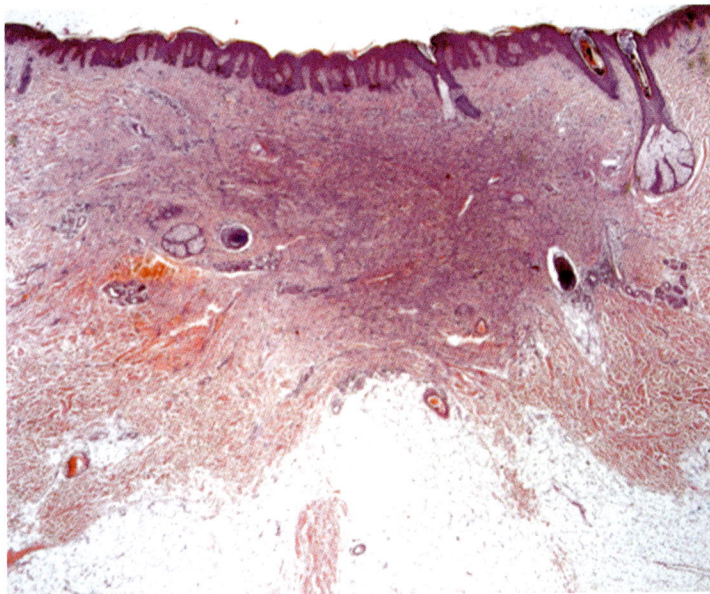

Fig. 56.10 Histological appearance of dermatofibroma, showing epidermal hyperplasia overlying the dermal sclerotic component.

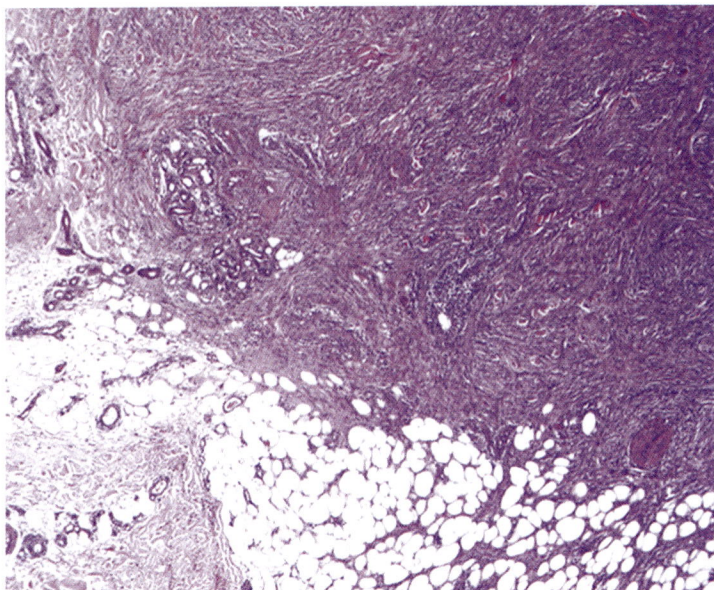

Fig. 56.11 Cellular fibrous histiocytoma. Note the increased cellularity, fascicular appearance and focal extension into the subcutis.

Exceptional tumours are multiple [28]. The rate of local recurrence is 19% [19].

Atypical FH presents mainly in young adults, with a predilection for the lower limbs [21,22]. It is commoner in males than in females. The clinical presentation is that of a papule, nodule or plaque, usually less than 1.5 cm in diameter. The rate of local recurrence is around 14%, and exceptional metastases have been reported [22].

Epithelioid FH [23,24] presents on the limbs of young patients, with a predilection for females. The typical clinical appearance is that of a polypoid, often vascular, lesion resembling a non-ulcerated pyogenic granuloma.

Pathology. The overlying epidermis frequently shows a degree of epidermal hyperplasia [29] (Fig. 56.10). The latter displays different patterns including changes mimicking a squamous papilloma, a seborrhoeic keratosis and lichen simplex chronicus. Occasionally, the epidermal proliferation is associated with immature follicular structures, which are often confused with a basal cell carcinoma. In the dermis, there is a localized proliferation of histiocyte-like cells and fibroblast-like cells, associated with variable numbers of mononuclear inflammatory cells. Foamy macrophages, siderophages and multinucleated giant cells are also variably present. A focal storiform pattern is often seen. The tumour blends with the surrounding dermis. Collagen bundles at the periphery of the lesion are surrounded by scattered tumour cells and appear somewhat hyalinized. As variable expression of factor XIIIa antigen is often seen, it has been suggested that this tumour shows differentiation towards dermal dendrocytes [30]. Focal myofibroblastic differentiation is often suggested, particularly in the cellular variant. Older lesions show focal proliferation of small blood vessels in association with haemosiderin deposition and fibrosis, hence the older name of 'sclerosing haemangioma'.

Cellular FH [17] also shows epidermal hyperplasia, but the lesions are more cellular, less polymorphic and consist of bundles of spindle-shaped cells with pink cytoplasm and a focal storiform pattern (Fig. 56.11). The mitotic rate varies, and necrosis may be found in up to 12% of cases. Extension into the subcutaneous tissue is more prominent than that seen in ordinary FH. However, the pattern of infiltration is mainly along the septae, and only focally into the subcutaneous lobule in a lace-like pattern. The cellularity and growth pattern often make distinction from DFSP difficult, particularly in small biopsies. DFSP is, however, more monomorphic, tends to infiltrate the subcutaneous tissue diffusely and is generally uniformly positive for CD34 [30]. Cellular FH may be focally positive for CD34, but this is predominantly seen at the periphery of the tumour. Staining for FXIIIa is positive in FH and negative in DFSP. Furthermore, cellular FH is often focally positive for smooth muscle actin, whereas this marker is negative in DFSP.

Aneurysmal FH [19,20] shows extensive haemorrhage, with prominent cavernous-like pseudovascular spaces (Fig. 56.12) which are not lined by endothelial cells. The mitotic rate varies, but may be prominent. The background is that of an ordinary FH.

Atypical FH [21,22] shows variable numbers of mono- or multi-nucleated, pleomorphic, spindle-shaped or histiocyte-like cells on a background of an ordinary FH. These cells may be very prominent, making the histological diagnosis difficult. Mitotic figures, including atypical forms, may be seen. These lesions used to be classified as 'atypical fibroxanthoma occurring in non-sun-exposed skin of young patients'.

Epithelioid FH [23,24] contains a predominant population of cells with abundant pink cytoplasm and vesicular nuclei, and there is often myxoid change and a prominent vascular component. Distinction from a Spitz naevus may be difficult, but in epithelioid

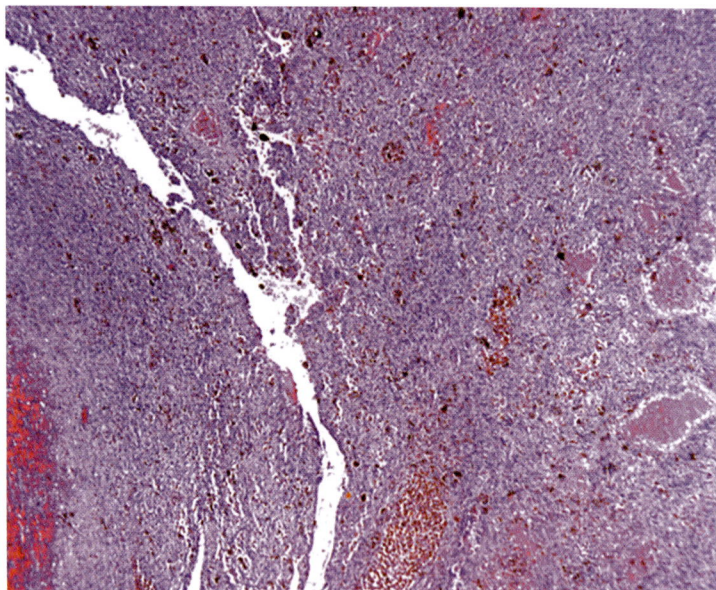

Fig. 56.12 Aneurysmal fibrous histiocytoma. Prominent haemorrhage and cavernous-like spaces obscure the typical background of a fibrous histiocytoma.

FH there is no junctional component, tumour cells are not nested and they are negative for S100.

Many histological variants of FH have been described; recognizing these variants is important to avoid misdiagnosis. They include lesions with palisading, granular cell change [31], abundant lipid (ankle-type) [32], clear cell change [33], balloon cell change [34] and keloidal change [35]. The presence of lipid within lesions of FH is not usually associated with systemic lipid abnormalities [36].

Treatment. Most FHs are no more than a cosmetic nuisance, and no treatment is necessary. However, cellular, atypical and aneurysmal variants should be completely removed, because of the risk of local recurrence and the occurrence of occasional distant metastases in the first two variants.

References

1 Niemi KM. The benign fibrohistiocytic tumours of the skin. *Acta Dermatol Venereol (Stockh)* 1970; **50** (Suppl. 63): 7–42.
2 Vilanova JR, Flint A. The morphologic variants of histiocytomas. *J Cutan Pathol* 1974; **1**: 155–64.
3 Gonzáles S, Duarte I. Benign fibrous histiocytoma of the skin: a morphologic study of 290 cases. *Pathol Res Pract* 1982; **174**: 379–91.
4 Calonje E, Fletcher CDM. Cutaneous fibrohistiocytic tumors: an update. *Adv Anat Pathol* 1994; **1**: 2–15.
5 Vanni R, Marras S, Faa G *et al.* Cellular fibrous histiocytoma of the skin: evidence of a clonal process with different karyotype from dermatofibrosarcoma. *Genes Chromosomes Cancer* 1997; **18**: 314–7.
6 Calonje E. Dermatofibroma (fibrous histiocytoma): an inflammatory or neoplastic disorder? *Histopathology* 2001; **39**: 213.
7 Evans J, Clarke T, Mattacks CA *et al.* Dermatofibromas and arthropod bites: is there any evidence to link the two? *Lancet* 1989; **ii**: 36–7.
8 Requena L, Farina MC, Fuente C *et al.* Giant dermatofibroma. *J Am Acad Dermatol* 1994; **30**: 714–8.
9 Yazici AC, Baz K, Ikizoglu G *et al.* Familial eruptive dermatofibromas in atopic dermatitis. *J Eur Acad Dermatol Venereol* 2006; **20**: 90–2.
10 Kanitakis J, Carbonnel E, Delmonte S *et al.* Multiple eruptive dermatofibromas in a patient with HIV infection: case report and literature review. *J Cutan Pathol* 2000; **27**: 54–6.

11 Niiyama S, Katsuoka K, Happle R *et al.* Multiple eruptive dermatofibromas: a review of the literature. *Acta Derm Venereol* 2002; **82**: 241–4.
12 Yamamoto T, Sumi K, Yokozeki H *et al.* Multiple cutaneous fibrous histiocytomas in association with systemic lupus erythematosus. *J Dermatol* 2005; **32**: 645–9.
13 Lee HW, Lee DK, Oh SH *et al.* Multiple eruptive dermatofibromas in a patient with primary pulmonary hypertension. *Br J Dermatol* 2005; **153**: 845–7.
14 Alexandrescu DT, Wiernik PH. Multiple eruptive dermatofibromas occurring in a patient with chronic myelogenous leukaemia. *Arch Dermatol* 2005; **141**: 397–8.
15 Chang SE, Choi JH, Sung KJ *et al.* Multiple eruptive dermatofibromas occurring in a patient with acute myeloid leukaemia. *Br J Dermatol* 2000; **142**: 1062–3.
16 Bachmeyer C, Cordier F, Blum L *et al.* Multiple eruptive dermatofibromas after highly active antiretroviral therapy. *Br J Dermatol* 2000; **143**: 1336–7.
17 Calonje E, Mentzel T, Fletcher CDM. Cellular benign fibrous histiocytoma: clinicopathologic analysis of 74 cases of a distinctive variant of cutaneous fibrous histiocytoma with frequent recurrence. *Am J Surg Pathol* 1994; **18**: 668–76.
18 Colome-Grimmer MI, Evans HL. Metastasizing cellular dermatofibroma: a report of two cases. *Am J Surg Pathol* 1996; **20**: 1361–7.
19 Santa Cruz DJ, Kyriakos M. Aneurysmal ('angiomatoid') fibrous histiocytoma of the skin. *Cancer* 1981; **47**: 2053–61.
20 Calonje E, Fletcher CDM. Aneurysmal benign cutaneous fibrous histiocytoma: clinicopathologic analysis of a tumor frequently misdiagnosed as a vascular lesion. *Histopathology* 1995; **26**: 323–31.
21 Leyva WH, Santa Cruz DJ. Atypical cutaneous fibrous histiocytoma. *Am J Dermatopathol* 1986; **8**: 467–71.
22 Kaddu S, McMenamin M, Fletcher CD. Atypical fibrous histiocytoma of the skin: clinicopathologic analysis of 59 cases with evidence of infrequent metastasis. *Am J Surg Pathol* 2002; **26**: 35–46.
23 Wilson Jones E, Cerio R, Smith NP. Epithelioid cell histiocytoma: a new entity. *Br J Dermatol* 1989; **120**: 185–95.
24 Glusac EJ, Barr RJ, Everett MA *et al.* Epithelioid cell histiocytoma: a report of 10 cases including a new cellular variant. *Am J Surg Pathol* 1994; **18**: 583–90.
25 Hendi A, Jukic DM, Kress DW *et al.* Atrophic dermatofibroma: a case report and review of the literature. *Dermatol Surg* 2002; **28**: 1085–7.
26 Sánchez Yus E, Soria L, de Eusebio E *et al.* Lichenoid, erosive and ulcerated dermatofibromas. Three additional clinico-pathologic variants. *J Cutan Pathol* 2000; **27**: 112–7.
27 Gu M, Sohn K, Kim D *et al.* Metastasizing dermatofibroma in lung. *Ann Diagn Pathol* 2007; **11**: 64–7.
28 Ichikawa N, Kobayashi M, Kimoto M *et al.* A case of multiple aneurysmal fibrous histiocytomas. *Br J Dermatol* 2005; **153**: 664–5.
29 Schoenfeld RJ. Epidermal proliferations overlying histiocytomas. *Arch Dermatol* 1964; **90**: 266–70.
30 Abenoza P, Lillemoe T. CD 34 and factor 13a in the differential diagnosis of dermatofibroma and dermatofibrosarcoma protuberans. *Am J Dermatopathol* 1993; **15**: 429–34.
31 Soyer HP, Metze D, Kerl H. Granular cell dermatofibroma. *Am J Dermatopathol* 1997; **19**: 168–73.
32 Iwata J, Fletcher CDM. Lipidized fibrous histiocytoma: clinicopathologic analysis of 22 cases. *Am J Dermatopathol* 2000; **22**: 126–34.
33 Zelger BW, Steiner H, Kutzner H. Clear cell dermatofibroma: case report of an unusual fibrohistiocytic lesion. *Am J Surg Pathol* 1996; **20**: 483–91.
34 Tran TA, Hayner-Buchan A, Jones DM *et al.* Cutaneous balloon cell dermatofibroma (fibrous histiocytoma). *Am J Dermatopathol* 2007; **29**: 197–200.
35 Kuo TT, Hu S, Chan HL. Keloidal dermatofibroma: report of 10 cases of a new variant. *Am J Surg Pathol* 1998; **22**: 564–8.
36 Wagamon K, Somach SC, Bass J *et al.* Lipidized dermatofibromas and their relationship to serum lipids. *J Am Acad Dermatol* 2006; **54**: 494–8.

Medallion-like dermal dendrocytic hamartoma [1,2]

Definition. This is a very rare lesion that appears to derive from dermal dendrocytes and is usually congenital.

Clinical features. The handful of cases described have occurred in females with predilection for the trunk. Lesions are round or oval and have an atrophic appearance and a yellow–red colour.

Pathology. The epidermis appears atrophic and in the dermis there is a fairly monotonous proliferation of spindle-shaped bland cells. These cells are positive for CD34, factor XIIIa and fascin. The appearance may resemble DFSP, which may occasionally be congenital, and distinction between the two conditions is very important. However, medallion-like dermal dendrocytic hamartoma does not replace the subcutaneous tissue in a lace-like pattern and the proliferating cells are positive not only for CD34 but also for FXIIIa, a marker that is usually negative in dermatofibrosarcoma protuberans.

Treatment. Simple excision is the treatment of choice.

References
1 Rodríguez-Jurado R, Palacio C, Durán-McKinster C *et al*. Medallion-like dermal dendrocyte hamartoma: a new clinically and histopathologically distinct lesion. *J Am Acad Dermatol* 2004; **51**: 359–63.
2 Shah KN, Anderson E, Junkins-Hopkins J *et al*. Medallion-like dermal dendrocyte hamartoma. *Pediatr Dermatol* 2007; **24**: 632–6.

Hemosiderotic fibrohistiocytic lipomatous lesion [1,2]

> **Synonym**
> • Haemosiderotic fibrolipomatous tumour

Definition. This is a distinctive, benign, rare lesion that occurs almost exclusively on the foot, particularly the ankle, and that was initially thought to represent a reactive process [1]. A relationship with impaired circulation, particularly stasis, has been suggested [3]. However, other authors suggest that it is more likely to be neoplastic and related to a lesion described as pleomorphic angiectatic hyalinizing tumour [4]. The latter is regarded as a tumour of intermediate malignancy that occurs in most cases in deeper soft tissues and will not be described further in this chapter.

Clinical features. Lesions present as a slowly growing, fairly well-defined subcutaneous tumour, which tends to be asymptomatic and has some predilection for middle-aged to elderly females. Size is variable and may be several centimetres in diameter.

Pathology. The tumour is fairly circumscribed and it is composed of lobules of mature adipose tissue with scattered areas containing variable numbers of spindle-shaped cells which may be slightly hyperchromatic and often contain abundant intracytoplasmic haemosiderin. Histiocyte-like cells may also be seen. These cells are bland and only rarely slightly atypical. In the background there may be a few mononuclear inflammatory cells, mainly lymphocytes. Mitotic figures are exceptional. Spindle cells are positive for calponin and CD34 and may be positive for CD68 but negative for other markers, including desmin and h-caldesmon.

Prognosis and management. Tumours are benign and local recurrences occur rarely. The treatment of choice is simple excision.

References
1 Marshall-Taylor C, Farnburg-Smith JC. Hemosiderotic fibrohistiocytic lipomatous lesion: ten cases of a previously undescribed fatty lesion of the foot/ankle. *Mod Pathol* 2000; **13**: 1192–9.
2 Browne TJ, Fletcher CD. Haemosiderotic fibrolipomatous tumour (so-called haemosiderotic fibrohistiocytic lipomatous tumour): analysis of 13 new cases in support of a distinct entity. *Histopathology* 2006; **48**: 453–61.
3 Kazakov DV, Sima R, Michal M. Hemosiderotic fibrohistiocytic lipomatous lesion: clinical correlation with venous stasis. *Virchows Arch* 2005; **447**: 103–6.
4 Folpe AL, Weiss SW. Pleomorphic hyalinizing angiectatic tumor: analysis of 41 cases supporting evolution from a distinctive precursor lesion. *Am J Surg Pathol* 2004; **28**: 1417–25.

Angiomatoid fibrous histiocytoma [1–5]

> **Synonym**
> • Previously known as angiomatoid malignant fibrous histiocytoma

Definition. Angiomatoid FH was initially described as a variant of malignant FH [1]. It has recently been reclassified as a neoplasm with low-grade malignant behaviour, unrelated to malignant FH. Although it is considered to be 'fibrohistiocytic' due to the cytological resemblance of tumour cells to histiocytes, focal positivity of these cells to desmin raises the possibility of muscular differentiation. However, the lesion is now regarded as of uncertain histiogenesis.

Clinical features. It presents in children and young adults, with no sex predilection, as an asymptomatic blue or skin-coloured, subcutaneous or deeper mass. Primary dermal tumours are exceptional. Most cases occur on the limbs and patients may present with systemic symptoms including fever, anaemia and weight loss. Generalized lymphadenopathy may also be seen.

Pathology [1–4]. Low-power examination reveals haemorrhagic, pseudovascular, cavernous-like, cystic spaces filled with red blood cells. Mononuclear inflammatory cells are prominent and germinal centres are present in some cases. Tumour cells are arranged in sheets and consist of short spindle-shaped and round cells with pink cytoplasm and vesicular nuclei. Cytological atypia is sometimes present, and the mitotic count tends to be low. Tumour cells are focally positive in some cases to desmin [3,4], muscle-specific actin, calponin, CD99 and CD68, but not for smooth muscle actin.

Initial cytogenetic studies demonstrated a translocation between chromosomes 16p11 involving the *FUS* (*TLS*) gene and chromosome 12q13 involving the *ATF1* gene. The resultant protein (FUS/ATF1) is similar to the protein present in clear cell sarcoma (EWS/ATF1) involving t(12;22)(q13;q12) [6]. However, other cases show a different fusion gene, *EWSR1-CREB1*, which seems to be, in fact, the most common fusion gene in these tumours [7].

Prognosis and management. Most cases are cured after adequate excision, but local recurrence is observed in about 15% of patients and, exceptionally, metastasis to neighbouring soft tissues or regional lymph nodes may occur. Complete excision and follow-up are therefore indicated. Local recurrence is more likely with deep tumours, those with an infiltrative growth pattern and those that are incompletely removed [2].

References

1 Enzinger FM. Angiomatoid malignant fibrous histiocytoma: a distinct fibrohistiocytic tumor of children and young adults simulating a vascular neoplasm. *Cancer* 1979; **44**: 2147–57.

2 Costa MJ, Weiss SW. Angiomatoid malignant fibrous histiocytoma: a follow-up study of 108 cases with evaluation of possible predictors of outcome. *Am J Surg Pathol* 1990; **14**: 1126–32.

3 Fletcher CD. Angiomatoid 'malignant fibrous histiocytoma': an immunohistochemical study indicative of myoid differentiation. *Hum Pathol* 1991; **22**: 563–8.

4 Fanburgh-Smith JC, Miettinen M. Angiomatoid 'malignant' fibrous histiocytoma: a clinicopathologic study of 158 cases and further exploration of the myoid phenotype. *Hum Pathol* 1999; **30**: 1336–43.

5 Billings SD, Folpe AL. Cutaneous and subcutaneous fibrohistiocytic tumors of intermediate malignancy: an update. *Am J Dermatopathol* 2004; **26**: 141–55.

6 Waters BL, Panagopoulos I, Allen EF. Genetic characterization of angiomatoid fibrous histiocytoma identifies fusion of the FUS and ATF-1 genes induced by a chromosomal translocation involving bands 12q13 and 16p11. *Cancer Genet Cytogenet* 2000; **121**: 109–16.

7 Antonescu CR, Dal Cin P, Nafa K *et al*. EWSR1-CREB1 is the predominant gene fusion in angiomatoid fibrous histiocytoma. *Genes Chromosomes Cancer* 2007; **46**: 1051–60.

Plexiform fibrous histiocytoma [1–4]

> **Synonym**
> • Plexiform fibrohistiocytic tumour

Definition. Plexiform FH is a distinctive, predominantly subcutaneous tumour with two distinctive components:
1 A fibro/myofibroblastic fascicular component
2 A nodular histiocytic-like component, which also includes giant cells.

Despite its new name, it does not represent a plexiform variant of an ordinary FH (dermatofibroma).

Clinical features [1–4]. It mainly occurs in children and young adults, most commonly in females, and has a predilection for the upper limbs. An exceptional case has been congenital [5]. The tumour is solitary, measures no more than a few centimetres in diameter and is asymptomatic.

Pathology [1–4]. Low-power examination reveals a predominantly subcutaneous tumour, with focal involvement of the dermis and a distinctive plexiform growth pattern. Purely dermal lesions are occasionally seen [6]. Two components are usually identified and consist of fascicles of bland spindle-shaped fibro/myofibroblast-like cells and nodules of histiocyte-like cells with scattered giant cells, focal haemorrhage and haemosiderin deposition. In some tumours, one of the components may predominate. The spindle-shaped cells stain focally for smooth muscle actin, and the cells in the nodules are focally positive for CD68.

Prognosis and treatment. Local recurrences are observed in up to 30% of cases. Metastases to regional lymph nodes or to the lungs

have been reported [1,3,7]. Complete surgical excision and follow-up are therefore indicated. The histological features do not predict cases with more aggressive behaviour.

References

1 Enzinger FM, Zhang R. Plexiform fibrohistiocytic tumor presenting in children and young adults: an analysis of 65 cases. *Am J Surg Pathol* 1988; **12**: 816–26.

2 Hollowood K, Holley MP, Fletcher CD. Plexiform fibrohistiocytic tumour: clinicopathological, immunohistochemical and ultrastructural analysis in favour of a myofibroblastic lesion. *Histopathology* 1991; **19**: 503–13.

3 Remstein ED, Arndt CA, Nascimento AG. Plexiform fibrohistiocytic tumor. Clinicopathologic analysis of 22 cases. *Am J Surg Pathol* 1999; **23**: 662–70.

4 Taher A, Pushpanathan C. Plexiform fibrohistiocytic tumor: a brief review. *Arch Pathol Lab Med* 2007; **131**: 1135–8.

5 Leclerc S, Hamel-Teillac D, Oner P *et al*. Plexiform fibrohistiocytic tumor: three unusual cases occurring in infancy. *J Cutan Pathol* 2005; **32**: 572–6.

6 Zelger B, Weinlich G, Steiner H *et al*. Dermal and subcutaneous variants of plexiform fibrohistiocytic tumor. *Am J Surg Pathol* 1997; **21**: 235–41.

7 Salomao D, Nascimento A. Plexiform fibrohistiocytic tumor with systemic metastases: a case report. *Am J Surg Pathol* 1997; **21**: 469–76.

Atypical fibroxanthoma [1–4]

Definition. Atypical fibroxanthoma (AFX), by definition, arises in sun-damaged skin of elderly people. Ultraviolet radiation-induced *p53* mutations have been observed in these lesions, confirming the association with sun-damaged skin [5]. Tumours described in younger patients in non-sun-damaged skin represent examples of atypical FH.

Clinical features. The lesions occur most frequently on the ears, bald scalp and cheeks of elderly males (Fig. 56.13). Females are

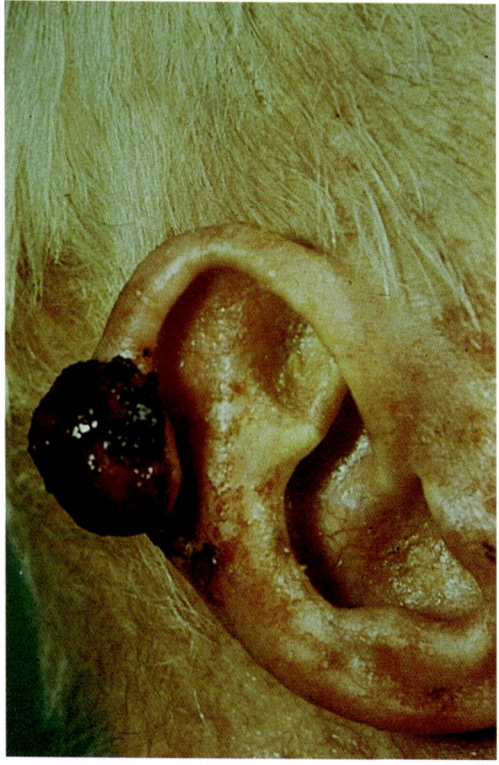

Fig. 56.13 Typical clinical appearance of an atypical fibroxanthoma with a polypoid architecture.

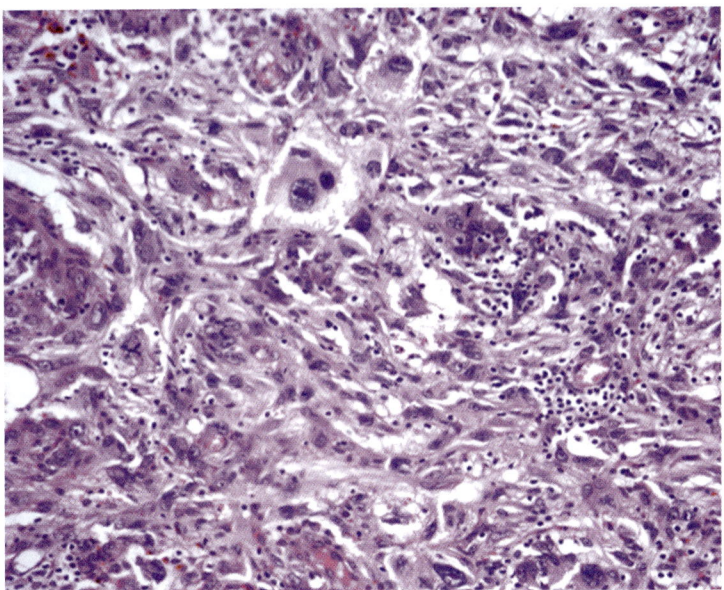

Fig. 56.14 Prominent cellular pleomorphism in a case of atypical fibroxanthoma.

much less frequently affected. The lesions are often ulcerated and have a red, fleshy appearance; they rarely exceed 30 mm in diameter, and are usually of less than 6 months' duration. Exceptional cases occur in association with xeroderma pigmentosum [6] or as a result of immunosuppression in cardiac transplant [7]. Multiple lesions have been reported [8]. Local recurrence may be seen in about 10% of cases and metastases to lymph nodes and internal organs are occasionally reported [9,10]. However, since the advent of immunohistochemistry, reports of metastatic tumours have been very rare. This suggests that many lesions reported in the past as metastatic AFX, which were diagnosed by examination of haematoxylin and eosin stained slides alone, probably represented other tumours, such as spindle cell melanomas or sarcomatoid squamous cell carcinoma.

Pathology. The tumours are exophytic, fairly well circumscribed and surrounded by an epidermal collarette. The remarkable and paradoxical feature of AFX is its histological resemblance to a highly malignant soft tissue sarcoma (Fig. 56.14) [11–13]. It arises in the dermis and may extend into the fat, but the edge is pushing rather than infiltrative. It is composed of large, spindle-shaped and histiocyte-like pleomorphic cells, many of which appear multinucleated. The cells are arranged in a haphazard fashion and mitotic figures, including atypical forms, are frequent. The histiocytic cells may contain lipid or haemosiderin [14,15]. A series of a less pleomorphic spindle cell variant, which may cause considerable problems in differential diagnosis, has been described [16]. Rare cases display prominent sclerosis [17] which may indicate regression. In some tumours there is focal or prominent clear or granular cell change [18–20]. The diagnosis of AFX is a diagnosis of exclusion. An immunohistochemical panel to rule out melanoma (S100), sarcomatoid squamous cell carcinoma (pan-keratin, mainly MNF 116 and AE1/AE3, as the low molecular weight keratin Cam 5.2 is usually negative in sarcomatoid squamous cell carcinoma of the skin) and even leiomyosarcoma (desmin, h-caldesmon) should be performed in all cases. The basic panel

should be enough to accurately diagnose most cases of AFX. Other markers have been described that are often positive in AFX, and tend to be negative in other tumours that enter the differential diagnosis. These include CD99, CD10 and pro-collagen 1 [21–23].

Treatment. The benign behaviour of the tumour enables it to be treated by limited local removal. Although rare cases are treated by Mohs micrographic surgery [24], tumours are usually relatively well-circumscribed and the former treatment is rarely needed to achieve good clearance. Radiotherapy is not recommended.

References

1 Bourne RG. Paradoxical fibrosarcoma of skin: a review of 13 cases. *Med J Aust* 1963; **50**: 504–10.
2 Fretzin DF, Helwig EB. Atypical fibroxanthoma of the skin: a clinicopathological study of 140 cases. *Cancer* 1973; **31**: 1541–52.
3 Kempson RL, McGavran MH. Atypical fibroxanthomas of the skin. *Cancer* 1964; **17**: 1463–71.
4 Mirza B, Weedon D. Atypical fibroxanthoma: a clinicopathological study of 89 cases. *Australas J Dermatol* 2005; **46**: 235–8.
5 dei Tos AP, Maestro R, Doglione C *et al*. UV-induced p53 mutations in atypical fibroxanthoma. *Am J Pathol* 1994; **145**: 11–7.
6 Berk DR, Lind AC, Tapia B *et al*. Atypical fibroxanthoma in a child with xeroderma pigmentosum. *Pediatr Dermatol* 2007; **24**: 450–2.
7 Kovach BT, Sams HH, Stasko T. Multiple atypical fibroxanthomas in a cardiac transplant patient. *Dermatol Surg* 2005; **31**: 467–70.
8 Jensen KJ, Peterson SR. Multiple recurrent atypical fibroxanthomas/superficial malignant fibrous histiocytomas of the forehead excised with Mohs micrographic surgery. *Dermatol Surg* 2006; **32**: 588–91.
9 Cooper JZ, Newman SR, Scott GA *et al*. Metastasizing atypical fibroxanthoma (cutaneous malignant histiocytoma): report of five cases. *Dermatol Surg* 2005; **31**: 221–5.
10 Lum DJ, King AR. Peritoneal metastases from an atypical fibroxanthoma. *Am J Surg Pathol* 2006; **30**: 1041–6.
11 Dahl I. Atypical fibroxanthoma of the skin: a clinico-pathological study of 57 cases. *Acta Pathol Microbiol Scand* 1976; **84**: 183–97.
12 Kroe OJ, Pitcock JA. Atypical fibroxanthoma of the skin. *Am J Clin Pathol* 1969; **51**: 487–92.
13 Kuwano H, Hashimoto H, Enjoji M. Atypical fibroxanthoma distinguishable from spindle cell carcinoma in sarcoma-like skin lesions. *Cancer* 1985; **55**: 172–80.
14 Leong ASY, Milios J. Atypical fibroxanthoma of the skin: a clinicopathological and immunohistochemical study and a discussion of its histogenesis. *Histopathology* 1987; **11**: 463–75.
15 Reed RJ. Atypical fibroxanthomas and spindle cell carcinomas of the skin. *Bull Tulane Univ Med Fac* 1967; **26**: 75–89.
16 Calonje E, Wadden C, Wilson Jones E *et al*. Spindle cell nonpleomorphic atypical fibroxanthoma. *Histopathology* 1993; **22**: 247–54.
17 Bruecks AK, Medlicott SA, Trotter MJ. Atypical fibroxanthoma with prominent sclerosis. *J Cutan Pathol* 2003; **30**: 336–9.
18 Rudisaile SN, Hurt MA, Santa Cruz DJ. Granular cell atypical fibroxanthoma. *J Cutan Pathol* 2005; **32**: 314–7.
19 Rios-Martín JJ, Delgado MD, Moreno-Ramírez D *et al*. Granular cell atypical fibroxanthoma: report of two cases. *Am J Dermatopathol* 2007; **29**: 84–7.
20 Lázaro-Santander R, Andrés-Gozalbo C, Rodríguez-Pereira C *et al*. Clear cell atypical fibroxanthoma. *Histopathology* 1999; **35**: 484–5.
21 Hultgren TL, DiMaio DJ. Immunohistochemical staining of CD10 in atypical fibroxanthomas. *J Cutan Pathol* 2007; **34**: 415–9.
22 Hartel PH, Jackson J, Ducatman BS *et al*. CD99 immunoreactivity in atypical fibroxanthoma and pleomorphic malignant fibrous histiocytoma: a useful diagnostic marker. *J Cutan Pathol* 2006; **33** (Suppl. 2): 24–8.
23 Jensen K, Wilkinson B, Wines N *et al*. Procollagen 1 expression in atypical fibroxanthoma and other tumors. *J Cutan Pathol* 2004; **31**: 57–61.

24 Seavolt M, McCall M. Atypical fibroxanthoma: review of the literature and summary of 13 patients treated with Mohs micrographic surgery. *Dermatol Surg* 2006; **32**: 435–41.

Malignant fibrous histiocytoma [1–4]

Definition. 'Malignant FH' is an umbrella term encompassing a heterogeneous group of neoplasms that initially included five different clinicopathologic subtypes: pleomorphic, myxoid, giant cell, inflammatory and angiomatoid. There is little relation between the different subtypes; the angiomatoid variant has recently been reclassified in the group of fibrohistiocytic tumours and the name changed to 'angiomatoid FH'. The concept of pleomorphic malignant FH has been challenged as not representing a distinct group of neoplasms but a heterogeneous category, including pleomorphic poorly differentiated sarcomas. If cases classified as such are extensively studied with ancillary studies including immunohistochemistry, electron microscopy and more recently cytogenetics [5,6], a large percentage may be reclassified as pleomorphic variants of other soft-tissue tumours, including liposarcoma, rhabdomyosarcoma and leiomyosarcoma. The myxoid variant of malignant FH is now known as 'myxofibrosarcoma', and it is likely to show fibroblastic differentiation; this tumour often involves the skin because of its frequent origin in the subcutis, and it will therefore be discussed in more detail below. Angiomatoid FH has been described under fibrohistiocytic tumours. The inflammatory and giant cell variants of malignant FH hardly ever involve the skin and will not be discussed further.

References

1 Fletcher CDM, McKee PH. Sarcomas: a clinicopathological guide with particular reference to cutaneous manifestation, 1. *Clin Exp Dermatol* 1984; **9**: 451–65.
2 Lawson CW, Fisher C, Gatter KC. An immunohistochemical study of differentiation in malignant fibrous histiocytoma. *Histopathology* 1987; **11**: 375–83.
3 Weiss SW, Enzinger FM. Malignant fibrous histiocytoma: an analysis of 200 cases. *Cancer* 1978; **41**: 2250–66.
4 Enzinger FM. Malignant fibrous histiocytoma 20 years after Stout. *Am J Surg Pathol* 1986; **10**: 43–53.
5 Fletcher CD. Pleomorphic malignant fibrous histiocytoma: fact or fiction? A critical reappraisal based on 159 tumors diagnosed as pleomorphic sarcoma. *Am J Surg Pathol* 1992; **16**: 213–28.
6 Nakayama R, Nemoto T, Takahashi H *et al*. Gene expression analysis of soft tissue sarcomas: characterization and reclassification of malignant fibrous histiocytoma. *Mod Pathol* 2007; **20**: 749–59.

Myxofibrosarcoma [1–4]

Synonym
• Myxoid malignant fibrous histiocytoma

Definition. Myxofibrosarcoma is a neoplasm of the subcutis and deeper soft tissues with variable cellularity, myxoid change and cells with pleomorphic nuclei. The cellular end of the spectrum is identical to a pleomorphic malignant FH, and the diagnosis is made based on the presence of myxoid areas with less cellularity and a lobular pattern. The myxoid change should be seen in 10% or more of the tumour before a lesion is classified as myxofibrosarcoma.

Clinical features. This tumour mainly presents in middle-aged to old adults, with a slight predilection for females and for involvement of the extremities, particularly the lower limbs and followed by the trunk [4]. Typically, an asymptomatic mass, measuring several centimetres in diameter, is found in the subcutis or deeper soft tissues. This is one of the sarcomas that more often involves the dermis as a result of extension from the subcutis or deeper soft tissues, rather than having a dermal origin.

Pathology [4]. These tumours have a lobular growth pattern. They are classified according to the degree of cellularity and pleomorphism into low, medium and high grade. Low-grade tumours are paucicellular and consist of round or elongated bland and pleomorphic cells in a prominent myxoid stroma. The atypical cells have irregular hyperchromatic nuclei, and mitotic figures are relatively frequent. In the background, a fairly prominent number of thin-walled vascular channels with a typical curvilinear pattern are seen. Vacuolated, Alcian blue-positive cells, focally mimicking lipoblasts, are relatively frequent. In some tumours, hypocellular areas blend with more cellular areas containing cells with increased pleomorphism; such tumours are classified as intermediate-grade. Tumours with high cellularity (high-grade) are indistinguishable from the so-called pleomorphic malignant FH and may have necrosis. Grading of lesions is important, because the rate of local recurrence and metastasis varies (see below). Some tumours, particularly high-grade lesions, may have epithelioid morphology [5]. Tumour cells are positive for vimentin and only rarely display very focal positivity for actin.

Prognosis and treatment [4]. Excision with clear margins is essential. High-grade lesions have a higher tendency for local recurrence and for metastatic spread to regional lymph nodes. The overall 5-year survival is around 60%. Tumours with epithelioid morphology appear to have a more aggressive behaviour [5].

References

1 Angervall L, Kindblom LG, Merck C. Myxofibrosarcoma: a study of 30 cases. *Acta Pathol Microbiol Scand* 1977; **85**: 127–40.
2 Weiss SW, Enzinger FM. Myxoid variant of malignant fibrous histiocytoma. *Cancer* 1977; **39**: 1672–85.
3 Merck C, Angervall L, Kindblom LG *et al*. Myxofibrosarcoma, a malignant soft tissue tumor of fibroblastic-histiocytic origin: a clinicopathologic and prognostic study of 110 cases using multivariate analysis. *Acta Pathol Microbiol Immunol Scand* 1983; **91**: 3–40.
4 Mentzel T, Calonje E, Wadden C *et al*. Myxofibrosarcoma: clinicopathologic analysis of 75 cases with emphasis on the low-grade variant. *Am J Surg Pathol* 1996; **20**: 391–405.
5 Nascimento AF, Bertoni F, Fletcher CD. Epithelioid variant of myxofibrosarcoma: expanding the clinicomorphologic spectrum of myxofibrosarcoma in a series of 17 cases. *Am J Surg Pathol* 2007; **31**: 99–105.

Low-grade fibromyxoid sarcoma [1–3]

Synonym
• Hyalinizing spindle cell tumour with giant rosettes

Definition. This distinctive neoplasm is regarded as a low-grade variant of fibrosarcoma and it is characterized by deceptive, bland spindle-shaped cells in a stroma with curvilinear blood vessels and either collagenous or myxoid background.

Clinical features. The tumour usually presents as a slowly growing lesion in young to middle-aged adults, with an equal sex incidence; it has a predilection for the proximal extremities, followed by the trunk. Tumours tend to be long-standing and asymptomatic and present as a mass, measuring several centimetres in diameter, and located in the subcutis or deeper soft tissues. Subcutaneous lesions are often clinically diagnosed as a lipoma.

Pathology [1–3]. The tumour consists of a proliferation of wavy, bland, spindle-shaped cells arranged in short fascicles and surrounded by a collagenous or myxoid stroma. Cellularity varies and tumour cells are usually bland with very rare mitotic figures. Frequent, elongated, thin-walled blood vessels are seen throughout the tumour. Only a small number of cases display some degree of cytological atypia. As a result of the deceiving histological appearances, the tumour is often diagnosed as benign. In a proportion of cases there are focal areas with hyalinized collagen surrounded by epithelioid tumour cells forming rosettes. This variant of the tumour was originally described as hyalinizing spindle cell tumour with giant rosettes [4]. The presence of rosettes does not influence the behaviour of the neoplasm. Immunohistochemistry is of limited value as tumour cells are negative for most markers. They may be, however, positive for epithelial membrane antigen (EMA) and this may lead to a misdiagnosis of perineurioma.

Tumours show a distinctive translocation, t(7;16)(q33;p11), leading to fusion of the *FUS* and *CREB3L2* genes [5]. This finding is very useful for confirmation of the diagnosis by fluorescent in situ hybridization (FISH).

Prognosis and treatment. Excision with clear margins is essential. In the largest series of cases reported so far it has been shown that local recurrence occurs in 9% of cases, metastases in 9% and mortality in 2% [6]. It seems that areas with higher grade morphology do not confer a more aggressive behaviour. However, this needs to be confirmed in further studies. Metastatic spread may occur many years after the original diagnosis and therefore long-term follow-up is indicated.

References
1 Evans HL. Low-grade fibromyxoid sarcoma: A report of 12 cases. *Am J Surg Pathol* 1993; **17**: 595–600.
2 Goodlad JR, Mentzel T, Fletcher CD. Low-grade fibromyxoid sarcoma: clinicopathological analysis of eleven new cases in support of a distinct entity. *Histopathology* 1995; **26**: 229–37.
3 Zamecnik M, Michal M. Low-grade fibromyxoid sarcoma: a report of 8 cases with histologic, immunohistochemical, and ultrastructural study. *Ann Diagn Pathol* 2000; **4**: 207–17.
4 Lane KL, Shannon RJ, Weiss SW. Hyalinizing spindle cell tumor with giant rosettes: a distinctive tumor closely resembling low-grade fibromyxoid sarcoma. *Am J Surg Pathol* 1997; **21**: 1481–8.
5 Folpe AL, Lane KL, Paull G *et al.* Low-grade fibromyxoid sarcoma and hyalinizing spindle cell tumor with giant rosettes: a clinicopathologic study of 73 cases supporting their identity and assessing the impact of high-grade areas. *Am J Surg Pathol* 2000; **24**: 1353–60.
6 Panagopoulos I, Storlazzi CT, Fletcher CD *et al.* The chimeric FUS/CREB3l2 gene is specific for low-grade fibromyxoid sarcoma. *Genes Chromosomes Cancer* 2004; **40**: 218–28.

Vascular tumours

Reviews of vascular tumours may be found in [1,2]. The vascular ectasias, verrucous haemangioma, tufted angioma, cavernous and capillary haemangiomas and congenital haemangiomas are described in Chapter 18.

References
1 Calonje E, Fletcher CDM. Tumors of blood vessels/lymphatics. In: Fletcher CDM, ed. *Diagnostic Histopathology of Tumors*, 3rd edition. London: Churchill Livingstone, 2007: 45–86.
2 Weiss SW, Goldblum JR. *Enzinger and Weiss's Soft Tissue Tumours*, 5th edn. St Louis: Mosby, 2007: 837–1036.

Reactive vascular lesions

Intravascular papillary endothelial hyperplasia [1–4]

Synonyms
- Masson's pseudoangiosarcoma
- Masson's vegetant intravascular haemangioendothelioma

Definition. Intravascular papillary endothelial hyperplasia is regarded as a form of organizing thrombus in which endothelial cells line hyalinized papillae.

Incidence and aetiology. This is a relatively common lesion, which usually presents as a primary phenomenon within a thrombosed blood vessel, usually a vein [2–4]. The secondary variant is commonly seen as an incidental finding within other vascular tumours, or in lesions such as haemorrhoids. Exceptionally, the same phenomenon is seen within a haematoma [4]. The primary form presents in young adults, with a slight predilection for females.

Clinical features. The primary form presents as a slowly growing solitary asymptomatic or slightly painful bluish nodule less than 20 mm in diameter. The site of predilection is the head and neck, followed by the hand (particularly the fingers). Multiple lesions are exceptional [5].

Pathology. The pathology is that of a widely dilated vascular channel in the dermis or subcutis, containing an organizing thrombus and prominent papillary projections with a hyalinized collagenous core. The papillae are lined by a single layer of usually bland endothelial cells with few mitotic figures. The presence of hyalinized collagen lined by endothelial cells produces an appearance similar to the 'dissection of collagen bundles' described in angiosarcoma. Distinction from angiosarcoma, however, is easy, as the latter is only exceptionally purely intravascular; it also displays cytological atypia, multilayering and mitotic figures. In secondary forms of Masson's tumour, the changes are seen within one or several vascular channels of a vascular tumour, usually a cavernous haemangioma or a vascular malformation.

Diagnosis. The clinical diagnosis suggested is usually that of a vascular tumour.

Treatment. Simple excision is usually curative and there is no tendency for local recurrence.

References

1 Masson P. Hémangioendothéliome végétant intra-vasculaire. *Bull Soc Anat* 1923; **93**: 517–23.
2 Kuo T, Sayers CP, Rosai J. Masson's 'vegetant intravascular hemangioendo-thelioma', a lesion often mistaken for angiosarcoma: study of seventeen cases located in the skin and soft tissues. *Cancer* 1976; **38**: 1227–36.
3 Hashimoto H, Daimaru Y, Enjoji M. Intravascular papillary endothelial hyperpla-sia: a clinicopathologic study of 91 cases. *Am J Dermatopathol* 1983; **5**: 539–45.
4 Pins MR, Rosenthal DI, Springfield DS *et al.* Florid extravascular papillary endo-thelial hyperplasia (Masson's pseudoangiosarcoma) presenting as a soft tissue sarcoma. *Arch Pathol Lab Med* 1993; **117**: 259–63.
5 Reed CN, Cooper PH, Swerlick RA. Intravascular papillary endothelial hyperpla-sia: multiple lesions simulating Kaposi's sarcoma. *J Am Acad Dermatol* 1984; **10**: 110–3.

Reactive angioendotheliomatosis [1–3]

Definition. A reactive vascular proliferation, which is usually multifocal and which is associated with a number of systemic diseases. In the past, it was divided into a reactive and a malignant form. With the advent of immunohistochemistry, it became appar-ent that the malignant form is a variant of aggressive intravascular lymphoma (see Chapter 57).

Incidence and aetiology. This condition is rare and involves adults, with a wide age range and no sex predilection. Most cases present with cutaneous involvement only and are idiopathic. It has been described in association with systemic diseases, including bacterial endocarditis, peripheral vascular athero-sclerotic disease, cryoglobulinaemia [2], liver and renal disease, antiphospholipid syndrome [4], amyloidosis [5] and sarcoidosis [6]. It is not clear how systemic diseases induce this vascular proliferation.

Clinical features. Most patients present with multiple erythema-tous and/or haemorrhagic macules, papules and plaques on the trunk and limbs. Patients with fewer, more localized, lesions may also be seen. In the latter cases, the association with systemic disease is not usually present. In patients with antiphospholipid syndrome or cryoglobulinaemia, ulcerated lesions may be present.

Pathology [7]. The dermis and, in some cases, the subcutis show a multifocal proliferation of clusters of capillaries lined by plump endothelial cells with little or no cytological atypia. A layer of pericytes surrounds each capillary. In some areas, dilated capil-laries appear to contain smaller vascular channels within their lumina. Patients with cryoglobulinaemia show thrombosis of capillaries by hyaline eosinophilic globules.

Treatment. There is no treatment available, but the condition is usually self-limited and resolves spontaneously within a few weeks.

References

1 Wick MR, Rocamora A. Reactive and malignant 'angioendotheliomatosis': a discriminant clinicopathologic study. *J Cutan Pathol* 1988; **15**: 260–71.
2 Le Boit PE, Solomon AR, Santa Cruz DJ *et al.* Angiomatosis with luminal cryoprotein deposition. *J Am Acad Dermatol* 1992; **27**: 969–73.
3 Krell JM, Sanchez RL, Solomon AR. Diffuse dermal angiomatosis: a variant of reactive cutaneous angioendotheliomatosis. *J Cutan Pathol* 1994; **21**: 363–70.
4 Creamer D, Black MM, Calonje E. Reactive angioendotheliomatosis in association with the antiphospholipid syndrome. *J Am Acad Dermatol* 2000; **42**: 903–6.
5 Ortonne N, Vignon-Pennamen MD, Majdalani G *et al.* Reactive angioendothelio-matosis secondary to dermal amyloid angiopathy. *Am J Dermatopathol* 2001; **23**: 315–9.
6 Shyong EQ, Gorevic P, Lebwohl M *et al.* Reactive angioendotheliomatosis and sarcoidosis. *Int J Dermatol* 2002; **41**: 894–7.
7 McMenamin ME, Fletcher CD. Reactive angioendotheliomatosis: a study of 15 cases demonstrating a wide clinicopathologic spectrum. *Am J Surg Pathol* 2002; **26**: 685–97.

Glomeruloid haemangioma [1,2]

Definition. This is a distinctive multifocal vascular proliferation that occurs in association with POEMS syndrome (*p*olyneuropa-thy, *o*rganomegaly, *e*ndocrinopathy, *M* protein and *s*kin changes; Chapter 62) or with multicentric Castleman's disease. This condi-tion is best considered as a form of reactive angioendotheliomar-tosis in the setting of POEMS syndrome.

Incidence and aetiology. This is a rare disease that presents almost exclusively in the context of POEMS syndrome and multi-centric Castleman's disease. It presents in adults, with no sex pre-dilection. Exceptional cases with no clinical features of POEMS syndrome have been reported [3,4].

Clinical features. Patients present with multiple vascular papules on the trunk and limbs. Only a minority of these vascular lesions have the histological appearance of glomeruloid haemangioma; most have the histological appearance of cherry angiomas, or overlap with other vascular lesions, including cirsoid aneurysm (p. 56.26).

Pathology. The histological appearances in a typical case are striking, consisting of a multifocal dermal proliferation of clusters of closely packed dilated capillaries with a striking similarity to renal glomeruli. A layer of pericytes surrounds each capillary. Vacuolated cells are focally present and, in some cases, there are eosinophilic hyaline globules within the lumina of capillaries. These globules represent deposits of protein.

Treatment. The lesions do not tend to regress spontaneously. Individual lesions can be removed surgically, but because of their numbers this is not generally a practical option.

References

1 Chan JKC, Fletcher CDM, Hicklin GA *et al.* Glomeruloid hemangioma: a distinc-tive cutaneous lesion of multicentric Castleman's disease associated with POEMS syndrome. *Am J Surg Pathol* 1990; **14**: 1036–46.
2 Rongioletti F, Gambini C, Lerza R. Glomeruloid hemangioma: a cutaneous marker of POEMS syndrome. *Am J Dermatopathol* 1994; **16**: 175–8.
3 Piña-Oviedo S, López-Patiño S, Ortiz-Hidalgo C. Glomeruloid hemangioma local-ized to the skin of the trunk with no clinical features of POEMS syndrome. *Int J Dermatol* 2006; **45**: 1449–50.

4 Vélez D, Delgado-Jiménez Y, Fraga J. Solitary glomeruloid hemangioma without POEMS syndrome. *J Cutan Pathol* 2005; **32**: 449–52.

Benign vascular tumours

Lobular capillary haemangioma (pyogenic granuloma) [1,2]

Synonym
• Granuloma telangiectaticum

Definition. A vascular nodule that develops rapidly, often at the site of a recent injury, and which is composed of a lobular proliferation of capillaries in a loose stroma.

Incidence and aetiology. This is a common lesion affecting both sexes with a predilection for males [3] except for lesions that occur in the oral cavity which are more common in females [4]. It may occur at any age with a peak in the second decade of life [3], and is seen quite often in children and young adults but is unusual in the elderly [5]. In a minority of cases, a minor injury, usually of a penetrating kind, has occurred a few weeks before the nodule appears. Lesions may also occur at the sites of burns [6]. In other cases, no injury can be recollected, but this is likely on the basis of the patient's occupation or the body site affected. The balance of evidence indicates a reactive lesion.

Granuloma gravidarum is a variant of pyogenic granuloma that presents in the oral cavity during pregnancy.

Clinical features. The tumour is vascular, bright red to brownish-red or blue-black in colour. It is partially compressible, but cannot be completely blanched and does not show pulsation. The surface of early, bright-red lesions is usually thin, intact epidermis. Older and darker lesions are frequently eroded and crusted, and may bleed very easily. Occasionally, the surface is raspberry-like or even verrucous. The size is commonly between 5 and 10 mm, but may reach 50 mm. The outline is rounded. The base is often pedunculated and surrounded by a collar of acanthotic epidermis; the lesion may be sessile. The common sites are the hands, especially the fingers (Fig. 56.15), the feet, lips, head and upper trunk, and the mucosal surfaces of the mouth and perianal area. The initial evolution is rapid, but growth ceases after a few weeks. Spontaneous disappearance is rare. Lesions are not painful; patients mainly complain of the appearance or of recurrent bleeding. Rarely, pyogenic granulomas may occur within a port wine stain [7]. There are reported cases of multiple pyogenic granulomas developing after exfoliative dermatitis [8] and, in a periungual location, after HAART [9]. Lesions mimicking pyogenic granuloma may occur during therapy with gefitinib [10], systemic 5-fluorouracil [11] and capecitabine [12]. Eruptive forms of this tumour have rarely been reported [13]. In this setting, distinction from bacillary angiomatosis is crucial, as the latter often presents with multiple lesions that can be clinically and histologically difficult to distinguish from pyogenic granuloma. Multiple lesions closely resembling pyogenic granulomas have been reported after systemic [14] and topical [15] treatment with retinoids.

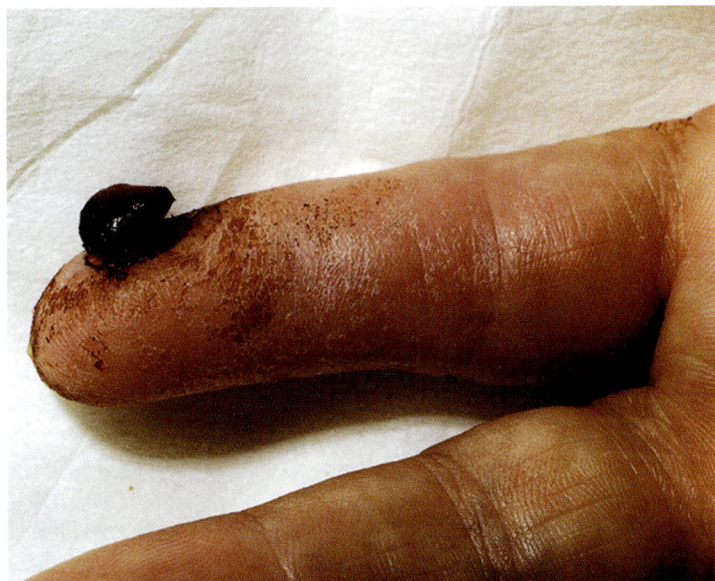

Fig. 56.15 Clinical appearance of a pyogenic granuloma on a typical site at the tip of the finger.

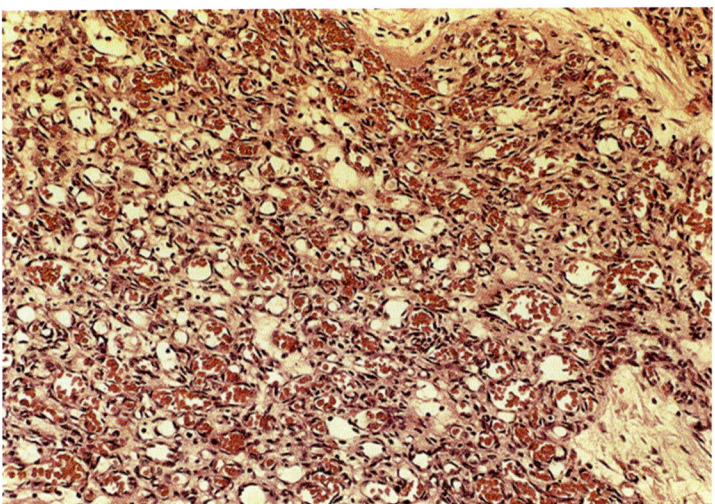

Fig. 56.16 Typical lobules of capillaries in a myxoid background, in a case of pyogenic granuloma.

Subcutaneous [16,17] and intravascular [18] variants are rarely seen and do not have distinctive clinical features. Interestingly, two cases of subcutaneous lesions have been described in patients with antiphospholipid antibodies [19].

Pathology. There is a lobular proliferation of small blood vessels, which erupt through a breach in the epidermis to produce a globular pedunculated tumour. The epidermis forms a collarette at the base of the lesion and covers part, or all, of the tumour in a thin layer. The proliferating vessels are set in a myxoid stroma, lacking in collagen in the earlier stages and relatively rich in mucin. The endothelial cells are plump, as in new granulation tissue, lining the vessels in a single layer. They are surrounded by a mixed cell population of fibroblasts, mast cells, lymphocytes, plasma cells and, where the surface is eroded, polymorphonuclear leukocytes (Fig. 56.16). Mitotic figures may be prominent. Older lesions tend to organize and partly fibrose and may show focal bone formation. Late lesions can display focal degenerative atypia, raising the possibility of malignancy. In rare instances, particularly in children, and sometimes following treatment, satellite lesions which have a similar pathology to the primary lesion may develop around a pyogenic granuloma. These respond to simple destructive measures, thus ruling out malignancy [20]. In exceptional cases extramedullary haemopoiesis may be seen [21]. Bacillary angiomatosis shows an almost identical histology to that of pyogenic granuloma [22]. However, in bacillary angiomatosis, pale epithelioid endothelial cells are prominent, neutrophils and nuclear dust are seen throughout the lesion and violaceous amorphous aggregates of bacilli which are positive with either Giemsa or Warthin–Starry stains are easily identified. The causative organism may also be identified by PCR.

Diagnosis. In most cases, the history and clinical appearance leave little doubt about the diagnosis, and microscopic confirmation is straightforward. In 38% of one case series, the clinical diagnosis of pyogenic granuloma proved to be wrong [23]. The errors included keratoacanthoma and other epithelial neoplasms, inflamed seborrhoeic keratoses, melanocytic naevi, 'juvenile' and malignant melanoma, virus warts, molluscum contagiosum, angioma, glomus tumour, eccrine poroma, Kaposi's sarcoma and metastatic carcinoma.

Treatment. The pedunculated lesions are easy to treat by curettage with cauterization or diathermy coagulation of the base. A considerable proportion of pyogenic granulomas recur after such treatment, because the proliferating vessels in the base extend in a conical manner into the deeper dermis. In some areas—for instance in the nail fold or on the palmar aspect of a finger—it may be reasonable to carry out curettage and hope for the best. Wherever possible, it is desirable to excise a narrow, but deep, ellipse of skin beneath the lesion and close the wound with sutures. A small number of lesions have been treated with topical imiquimod 5% cream both in children and adults with complete resolution [24,25]. Other treatment modalities that have been used include Nd:YAG laser [26], cryosurgery [27], intralesional steroids, flash lamp pulsed dye laser and even injection of absolute ethanol [28].

References

1 Lee FD. A comparative study of Kaposi's sarcoma and granuloma pyogenicum in Uganda. *J Clin Pathol* 1968; **21**: 119–28.
2 McGeoch AH. Pyogenic granuloma. *Aust J Dermatol* 1961; **6**: 33–40.
3 Harris MN, Desai R, Chuang TY *et al*. Lobular capillary hemangioma: An epidemiologic report, with emphasis on cutaneous lesions. *J Am Acad Dermatol* 2000; **42**: 1012–6.
4 Jafarzadeh H, Sanatkhani M, Mohtasham N. Oral pyogenic granuloma: a review. *J Oral Sci* 2006; **48**: 167–75.
5 Knoth W, Ehlers G. On the problem of the existence of telangiectatic pyogenic granuloma with special reference to its relations to hemangioma and hemangio-endothelioma. *Arch Klin Exp Dermatol* 1962; **214**: 394–414.
6 Bozkurt M, Kulahci Y, Zor F *et al*. Multiple giant disseminated pyogenic granuloma in a burn lesion. *J Burn Care Res* 2006; **27**: 247–9.
7 Sheehan DJ, Lesher JL Jr. Pyogenic granuloma arising within a port-wine stain. *Cutis* 2004; **73**: 175–80.
8 Torres JE, Sánchez JL. Disseminated pyogenic granuloma developing after an exfoliative dermatitis. *J Am Acad Dermatol* 1995; **32**: 280–2.
9 Williams LH, Fleckman P. Painless periungual pyogenic granulomata associated with reverse transcriptase inhibitor therapy in a patient with human immunodeficiency virus infection. *Br J Dermatol* 2007; **156**: 163–4.
10 High WA. Gefitinib: a cause of pyogenic granulomalike lesions of the nail. *Arch Dermatol* 2006; **142**: 939.
11 Curr N, Saunders H, Murugasu A *et al*. Multiple periungual pyogenic granulomas following systemic 5-fluorouracil. *Australas J Dermatol* 2006; **47**: 130–3.
12 Piquet V, Borradori L. Pyogenic granuloma-like lesions during capecitabine therapy. *Br J Dermatol* 2002; **147**: 1270–2.
13 Nappi O, Wick MR. Disseminated lobular capillary hemangioma (pyogenic granuloma): a clinicopathologic study of two cases. *Am J Dermatopathol* 1986; **8**: 379–85.
14 Exner JH, Dahod S, Pochi PE. Pyogenic granuloma-like acne lesions during isotretinoin therapy. *Arch Dermatol* 1983; **119**: 808–11.
15 MacKenzie-Wood AR, Wood G. Pyogenic granuloma-like lesions in a patient using topical tretinoin. *Australas J Dermatol* 1998; **39**: 248–50.
16 Cooper PH, Mills SE. Subcutaneous granuloma pyogenicum: lobular capillary hemangioma. *Arch Dermatol* 1982; **118**: 30–3.
17 Fortna RR, Junkins-Hopkins JM. A case of lobular capillary hemangioma (pyogenic granuloma). Localized to the subcutaneous tissue, and a review of the literature. *Am J Dermatopathol* 2007; **29**: 408–11.
18 Cooper PH, McAllister HA, Helwig EB. Intravenous pyogenic granuloma: a study of 18 cases. *Am J Surg Pathol* 1979; **3**: 221–8.
19 Kuroda K, Mizoguchi M. Subcutaneous granuloma pyogenicum in patients with antiphospholipid antibodies. *Dermatology* 2004; **208**: 331–4.
20 Warner J, Wilson Jones E. Pyogenic granuloma recurring with multiple satellites: a report of 11 cases. *Br J Dermatol* 1968; **80**: 218–27.
21 Vega Harring SM, Niyaz M, Okada S *et al*. Extramedullary hematopoiesis in a pyogenic granuloma: a case report and review. *J Cutan Pathol* 2004; **31**: 555–7.
22 LeBoit PE, Berger TG, Egbert BM *et al*. Bacillary angiomatosis: the histopathology and differential diagnosis of a pseudoneoplastic infection in patients with human immunodeficiency virus disease. *Am J Surg Pathol* 1989; **13**: 909–20.
23 Rowe L. Granuloma pyogenicum. *AMA Arch Dermatol* 1958; **78**: 341–7.
24 Fallah H, Fischer G, Zagarella S. Pyogenic granuloma in children: treatment with topical imiquimod. *Australas J Dermatol* 2007; **48**: 217–20.
25 Goldenberg G, Krowchuk DP, Jorizzo JL. Successful treatment of a therapy-resistant pyogenic granuloma with topical imiquimod 5% cream. *J Dermatol Treat* 2006; **17**: 121–3.
26 Bourguignon R, Paquet P, Pierard-Franchimont C *et al*. Treatment of pyogenic granulomas with Nd-YAG laser. *J Dermatol Treat* 2006; **17**: 247–9.
27 Mirshams M, Daneshpazhooh M, Mirshekari A *et al*. Cryotherapy in the treatment of pyogenic granuloma. *J Eur Acad Dermatol Venereol* 2006; **20**: 788–90.
28 Ichimiya M, Yohikawa Y, Hamamoto Y *et al*. Successful treatment of pyogenic granuloma with injection of absolute ethanol. *J Dermatol* 2004; **31**: 342–4.

Cirsoid aneurysm [1–4]

Synonyms
- Cutaneous arteriovenous haemangioma
- Acral arteriovenous tumour

Definition. Cirsoid aneurysm is a small vascular proliferation characterized by small to medium-sized channels with features of arteries and veins. As opposed to deeper tumours showing similar features, shunting is absent.

Clinical features. Most lesions present on the head and neck region of young adults, with no sex predilection, as a small, blue/red, asymptomatic papule.

Pathology. The dermis contains a mixture of scattered blood vessels with thick walls and features of veins and arteries (Fig. 56.17).

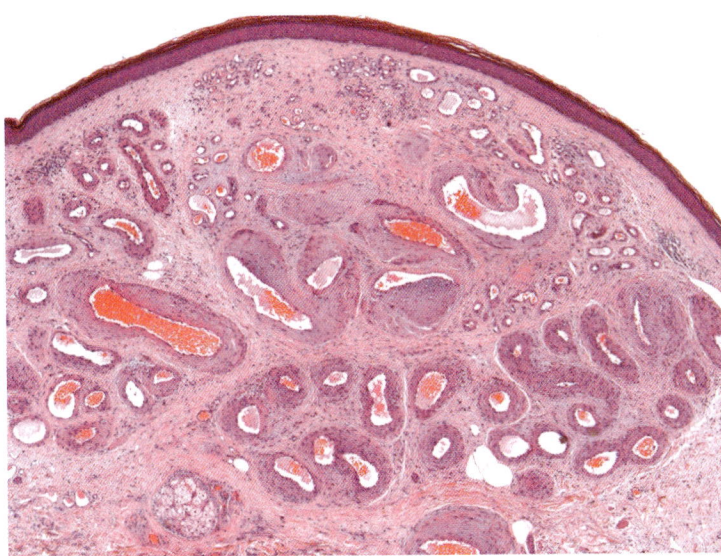

Fig. 56.17 A dermal collection of thick and thin walled blood vessels in a typical case of cirsoid aneurysm.

Treatment. As there is no associated shunting or deep component, simple excision is the treatment of choice.

References

1 Girard C, Graham JH, Johnson WC. Arteriovenous hemangioma (arteriovenous shunt): a clinicopathological and histochemical study. *J Cutan Pathol* 1974; **1**: 73–87.
2 Connelly MG, Winkelmann RK. Acral arteriovenous tumor: a clinicopathologic review. *Am J Surg Pathol* 1985; **9**: 15–21.
3 Koutlas IG, Jessurun J. Arteriovenous hemangioma: a clinicopathological and immunohistochemical study. *J Cutan Pathol* 1994; **21**: 343–9.
4 Gurbuz Y, Muezzinoglu B, Apaydin R *et al.* Acral arteriovenous tumor (cirsoid aneurysm): clinical and histopathological analysis of 6 cases. *Adv Clin Path* 2002; **6**: 25–9.

Epithelioid haemangioma [1,2]

> **Synonyms**
> * Angiolymphoid hyperplasia with eosinophilia
> * Pseudopyogenic granuloma
> * Histiocytoid haemangioma

Definition. A benign, locally proliferating lesion composed of vascular channels lined by endothelial cells with abundant pink cytoplasm and vesicular nuclei. There has, on occasion, been a difficulty with nomenclature such that the term Kimura's disease has been applied but this condition is now viewed as distinct from angiolymphoid hyperplasia with eosinophils. In Kimura's disease, the lesions occur in younger patients, are deeper-seated, are associated with lymphadenopathy, have no initial overlying skin lesions and do not contain epithelioid endothelial cells [3,4]. Furthermore, peripheral blood eosinophilia is much more common in Kimura's disease. Exceptionally, angiolymphoid hyperplasia with eosinophilia may co-exist with Kimura's disease [5].

Incidence and aetiology. These lesions have now been reported from many parts of the world. The cause is unknown, but most studies suggest a reactive process [6].

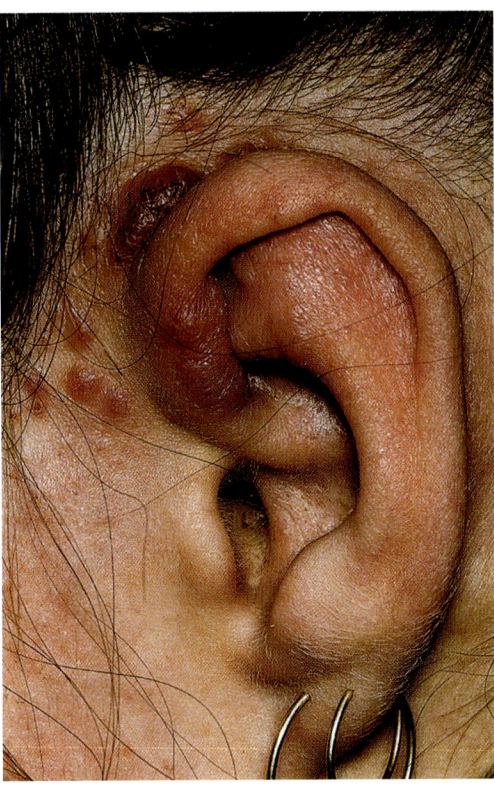

Fig. 56.18 Epithelioid haemangioma, or angiolymphoid hyperplasia with eosinophilia. (Courtesy of Dr R.H. Champion, Addenbrooke's Hospital, Cambridge, UK.)

Clinical features [7–11] (Fig. 56.18). Affected individuals are commonly young adults who present with a cluster of small, translucent nodules on the head and neck, particularly around the ear or the hairline. The lesions may also involve the oral mucosa [12]. Less frequently, lesions can involve the trunk and extremities. Involvement of deeper soft tissues and internal organs, including bone, can be seen. Both sexes are equally affected. Individual nodules rarely exceed 2–3 cm in diameter, but occasionally deeper extension and larger subcutaneous lesions occur. Spontaneous regression is seen in the majority of cases after a variable period of time. Peripheral blood eosinophilia may be present but only in less than 10% of patients.

Pathology [2,13]. A poorly circumscribed lobular lesion is seen. It is composed of clusters of proliferating capillaries and, often, thicker blood vessels lined by plump, epithelioid endothelial cells (Fig 56.19) with little cytological atypia and rare mitotic figures. Around the blood vessels there is a cellular inflammatory infiltrate composed mainly of lymphocytes and large numbers of eosinophils. However, only less than half of cases contain a prominent infiltrate. Older lesions show sclerosis of the stroma and the endothelial cells become more prominent. A frequent finding, particularly in larger lesions, is the involvement of larger blood vessels. Rare cases are entirely intravascular [14,15]. The endothelial cells stain for vascular markers including CD34, von Willebrand factor and CD31. In cutaneous cases, endothelial cells are negative for pan-keratin.

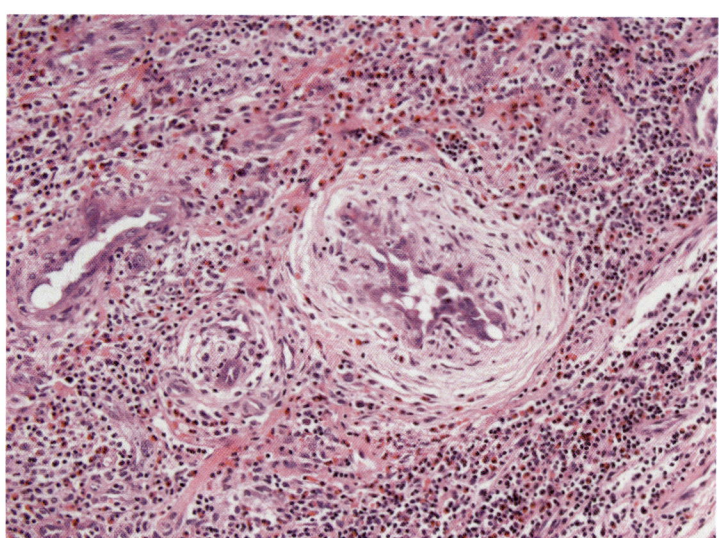

Fig. 56.19 Vascular channels lined by epithelioid endothelial cells with abundant pink cytoplasm in a case of epithelioid haemangioma.

Treatment. The natural history of the lesion is such that if a confident diagnosis is made on a small lesion, it is reasonable to observe the lesion for 3–6 months and await spontaneous regression. Both surgery and radiotherapy are effective, but local recurrences are common. Treatment with Nd-YAG laser has been effective [16] and there is an anecdotal report of response to imiquimod cream [17].

References

1 Olsen TG, Helwig EB. Angiolymphoid hyperplasia with eosinophilia. *J Am Acad Dermatol* 1985; **12**: 781–96.
2 Wells GC, Whimster IW. Subcutaneous angiolymphoid hyperplasia with eosinophilia. *Br J Dermatol* 1969; **81**: 1–15.
3 Chan JKC, Hui PK, Ng CS *et al*. Epithelioid haemangioma (angiolymphoid hyperplasia with eosinophilia) and Kimura's disease in Chinese. *Histopathology* 1989; **15**: 557–74.
4 Fetsch JF, Weiss SW. Observations concerning the pathogenesis of epithelioid haemangioma/angiolymphoid hyperplasia. *Mod Pathol* 1991; **4**: 449–55.
5 Chong WS, Thomas A, Goh CL. Kimura's disease and angiolymphoid hyperplasia with eosinophilia: two entities in the same patient: case report and review of the literature. *Int J Dermatol* 2006; **45**: 139–45.
6 Kuo TT, Shih LY, Chan HL. Kimura's disease: involvement of regional lymph nodes and distinction from angiolymphoid hyperplasia with eosinophilia. *Am J Surg Pathol* 1988; **12**: 843–54.
7 Baler GR. Angiolymphoid hyperplasia with eosinophilia: a report of two cases. *J Dermatol Surg Oncol* 1981; **7**: 229–34.
8 Grimwood R, Swinehart JM, Aeling JL. Angiolymphoid hyperplasia with eosinophilia. *Arch Dermatol* 1979; **115**: 205–7.
9 Reed RJ, Terazekis N. Subcutaneous angioblastic lymphoid hyperplasia with eosinophilia (Kimura's disease). *Cancer* 1972; **29**: 489–97.
10 Vazquez-Botet M, Sanchez JL. Angiolymphoid hyperplasia with eosinophilia: report of a case and a review of the literature. *J Dermatol Surg Oncol* 1978; **4**: 931–6.
11 Wilson Jones E. Inflammatory angiomatous nodules with abnormal blood vessels occurring about the ears and scalp (pseudo or atypical pyogenic granuloma). *Br J Dermatol* 1969; **81**: 804–16.
12 Bartralot R, Garcia Patos V, Hueto J *et al*. Angiolymphoid hyperplasia with eosinophils affecting the oral mucosa. *Br J Dermatol* 1996; **134**: 744–8.
13 Kung ITM, Gibson JB, Bannatyne PM. Kimura's disease: a clinicopathological study of 21 cases and its distinction from angiolymphoid hyperplasia with eosinophilia. *Pathology* 1984; **16**: 39–44.
14 Rosai J, Ackerman LR. Intravenous atypical vascular proliferation: a cutaneous lesion simulating a malignant blood vessel tumor. *Arch Dermatol* 1974; **109**: 714–7.
15 Koubaa W, Verdier M, Perez M *et al*. Intra-arterial angiolymphoid hyperplasia with eosinophilia. *J Cutan Pathol* 2008; **35**: 495–8.
16 Kadurina MI, Dimitrov BG, Bojinova ST *et al*. Angiolymphoid hyperplasia with eosinophilia: successful treatment with Nd:YAG laser. *J Cosmet Laser Ther* 2007; **9**: 107–11.
17 Gencoglan G, Karaca S, Ertekin B. Angiolymphoid hyperplasia with eosinophilia successfully treated with imiquimod. A case report. *Dermatology* 2007; **215**: 233–5.

Cutaneous epithelioid angiomatous nodule

Definition. This is a recently described tumour within the spectrum of vascular lesions characterized by epithelioid endothelial cells [1–3]. It is regarded by some as part of the spectrum of epithelioid haemangioma.

Clinical features. It is rare, with only a handful of cases reported. Lesions consist of a papule or nodule presenting in an adult, with a predilection for the trunk and limbs and, less commonly, involving the face. Multiple lesions are rare and there is no tendency for local recurrence.

Pathology. The majority of lesions are superficial, well-circumscribed and surrounded by an epithelial collarette. Occasional, deeper tumours may be observed. It is composed of sheets of epithelioid endothelial cells with abundant pink cytoplasm, vesicular nuclei and a single, small nucleolus. Cytological atypia is mild or absent and mitotic figures are variable. There is little tendency for formation of vascular channels but individual endothelial cells often contain intracytoplasmic vacuoles. In the background, scattered mononuclear inflammatory cells and eosinophils may be seen.

References

1 Brenn T, Fletcher CDM. Cutaneous epithelioid angiomatous nodule: a distinct lesion in the morphologic spectrum of epithelioid vascular tumors. *Am J Dermatopathol* 2004; **26**: 14–21.
2 Fernández-Flores A, Montero MG, Renedo G. Cutaneous epithelioid angiomatous nodule of the external ear. *Am J Dermatopathol* 2005; **27**: 175–6.
3 Kantrow S, Martin JD, Vnencak-Jones CL, Boyd AS. Cutaneous epithelioid angiomatous nodule: report of a case and absence of microsatellite instability. *J Cutan Pathol* 2007; **34**: 515–6.

Acquired elastotic haemangioma [1]

Definition. This is a distinctive vascular lesion that develops in sun-exposed skin in association with solar elastosis.

Incidence and aetiology. Acquired elastotic haemangioma is rare and seems to be aetiologically related to chronic sun-exposure.

Clinical features. Lesions present mainly on the forearms or neck of middle-aged to elderly patients, with a predilection for females. The clinical presentation consists of a small, red or blue, circumscribed and asymptomatic plaque.

Pathology. Lesions are well circumscribed and consist of a superficial, band-like proliferation of capillaries in the background of solar elastosis. Each capillary is surrounded by a layer of pericytes.

Treatment. Simple excision is the treatment of choice and there is no tendency to local recurrence.

Reference
1 Requena L, Kutzner H, Mentzel T. Acquired elastotic hemangioma: a clinicopathologic variant of hemangioma. *J Am Acad Dermatol* 2002; **47**: 371–6.

Hobnail haemangioma [1–4]

Synonym
- Targetoid haemosiderotic haemangioma

Definition. This is a benign vascular dermal proliferation characterized by small channels lined by endothelial cells with little cytoplasm and a prominent dark nucleus (hobnail cells). Formation of small papillae is also often seen. The original name proposed for this condition was based on a distinctive targetoid clinical appearance produced by bleeding and haemosiderin deposition. However, only a minority of lesions present with this typical appearance and, therefore, the alternative name of hobnail haemangioma has been proposed.

Incidence and aetiology. It is relatively uncommon and occurs mainly in young to middle-aged adults with a slight predilection for males. Trauma may play a part in its pathogenesis [4]. Occasionally, lesions vary according to the timing within the menstrual cycle [5].

Clinical features. This entity presents as a rapidly developing, asymptomatic, solitary red or brown lesion, which in some cases has a central, raised, violaceous papule and is surrounded by a paler brown halo (targetoid appearance) [1]. Any body site may be affected, but it has predilection for the lower limbs and trunk. The oral mucosa may also be affected [3].

Pathology. Pathological examination shows dilated vascular channels in the papillary and high reticular dermis, with a single layer of endothelial cells lining intraluminal papillary projections. These cells have a hobnail ('matchstick') appearance. They may occasionally be more numerous and appear to fill the lumen of the vessel. The vascular channels tend to disappear in the mid and lower reticular dermis, and the endothelial cells become less prominent and lose the hobnail appearance. Haemosiderin deposition is prominent and can be highlighted with a Perl's stain. The endothelial cells stain for the lymphatic marker podoplanin (D2-40), suggesting that these lesions represent lymphangiomas rather than haemangiomas [6]. The pathological appearance may resemble Kaposi's sarcoma, but this differential diagnosis can usually be resolved by clinicopathological correlation, as hobnail haemangioma is a solitary entity whereas Kaposi's sarcoma is usually composed of multiple lesions. Histological distinction can be made if attention is paid to the symmetry of the lesion, the presence of hobnail endothelial cells with papillary projections and the absence of inflammation in hobnail haemangioma. Furthermore, hobnail haemangioma is not associated with HHV8 while all cases of Kaposi's sarcoma are associated with this virus.

Diagnosis. It is usually suspected clinically if lesions have a targetoid appearance. The diagnosis is otherwise made histologically.

Treatment. Simple surgical excision is the treatment of choice; there is no tendency for recurrence.

References
1 Santa Cruz DJ, Aronberg J. Targetoid hemosiderotic hemangioma. *J Am Acad Dermatol* 1988; **19**: 550–8.
2 Torrelo A. Hobnail hemangioma. *Dermatology* 1995; **191**: 154–6.
3 Guillou L, Calonje E, Speight P *et al.* Hobnail hemangioma: a pseudomalignant vascular lesion with a reappraisal of targetoid hemosiderotic hemangioma. *Am J Surg Pathol* 1999; **23**: 97–105.
4 Mentzel T, Partanen TA, Kutzner H. Hobnail hemangioma ('targetoid hemosiderotic hemangioma'): clinicopathologic and immunohistochemical analysis of 62 cases. *J Cutan Pathol* 1999; **26**: 279–86.
5 Ortiz-Rey JA, González-Ruiz A, San Miguel P *et al.* Hobnail hemangioma associated with the menstrual cycle. *J Eur Acad Dermatol Venereol* 2005; **19**: 367–9.
6 Franke FE, Steger K, Marks A *et al.* Hobnail hemangiomas (targetoid hemosiderotic hemangiomas) are true lymphangiomas. *J Cutan Pathol* 2004; **31**: 362–7.

Microvenular haemangioma [1–3]

Definition. This is a benign dermal vascular lesion characterized by proliferation of small vascular channels with features suggestive of venules.

Incidence and aetiology. It is relatively rare and presents mainly in young adults, with no sex predilection. Presentation in children is very rare [4]. Although the histological appearances suggest venular differentiation, this has not been proven.

Clinical features. It presents as a solitary, red–brown or bluish papule, nodule or plaque with predilection for the limbs. Most lesions are less than 10 mm in diameter.

Pathology. There is a superficial and deep dermal proliferation of angulated, thin-walled, vascular channels, all of which are surrounded by a single layer of pericytes. These channels are lined by flat, bland, endothelial cells and are surrounded by somewhat hyalinized collagen. A frequent finding is the infiltration of arrector pili muscles by vascular channels. Inflammation is not usually a feature. These lesions are negative for HHV8.

Treatment. Simple surgical excision is the treatment of choice; there is no tendency for local recurrence.

References
1 Hunt SJ, Santa Cruz DJ, Barr RJ. Microvenular hemangioma. *J Cutan Pathol* 1991; **18**: 235–40.
2 Aloi F, Tomasini C, Pippione M. Microvenular hemangioma. *Am J Dermatopathol* 1993; **15**: 534–8.
3 Fukunaga M, Ushigome S. Microvenular hemangioma. *Pathol Int* 1998; **48**: 237–9.

4 Sànz-Trelles A, Ojeda-Martos A, Jiménez-Fernandéz A *et al*. Microvenular haemangioma: a new case in a child. *Histopathology* 1998; **32**: 89–90.

Sinusoidal haemangioma [1]

Definition. This is a benign dermal and/or subcutaneous variant
of cavernous haemangioma composed of thin-walled, dilated vascular spaces in a typical sieve-like distribution.

Incidence and aetiology. Lesions are rare and present in adults,
with a slight predilection for females.

Clinical features. Sinusoidal haemangioma presents as a solitary,
blue, asymptomatic nodule, particularly on the trunk or upper
limbs. The dermis and subcutaneous tissue overlying the breast
is not uncommonly involved and may suggest a diagnosis of
angiosarcoma (differentiating features are discussed below; see
also p. 56.37).

Pathology. The lesion is usually well circumscribed, but several
lobules of subcutaneous tissue may be focally affected by the
tumour. A striking feature is the presence of back-to-back, dilated
and congested thin-walled vascular channels. These channels are
interconnected, and transverse sectioning is, in part, responsible
for the distinctive sinusoidal appearance. Pseudopapillary projections are focally present and thrombosis with dystrophic calcification may also be seen. Focal cytological atypia secondary to
degenerative changes may be seen. Distinction from angiosarcoma, particularly in tumours presenting in the breast, is based
on the fact that the latter occurs in the breast parenchyma and
only invades the dermis and subcutis secondarily. Tumour cells in
angiosarcoma also display cytological atypia, multilayering and
mitotic figures.

Treatment. Simple surgical excision is the treatment of choice,
and there is no tendency for local recurrence.

Reference
1 Calonje E, Fletcher CDM. Sinusoidal hemangioma. *Am J Surg Pathol* 1991; **15**:
1130–5.

Spindle cell haemangioma [1–5]

> **Synonym**
> • Spindle cell haemangioendothelioma

Definition. This is a benign vascular tumour. Although initially
described as a low-grade malignant lesion with a high tendency
for local recurrence and minimal potential for metastasis, further
studies demonstrated that it is a benign multifocal process, often
associated with a vascular malformation [3–5]. Confirmation of its
benign nature has led to change of the name 'haemangioendothelioma' for 'haemangioma', as the former implies low-grade (intermediate-grade) malignant potential [6].

Incidence and aetiology. Spindle cell haemangioma is relatively
rare. Males and females are affected equally, and the age range is

wide. Often, lesions present in childhood or early adulthood and
tend to be long-standing. The process appears to be reactive or
may be a form of malformation, and it is often associated with
lymphoedema, Maffucci's syndrome (multiple enchondromas)
[7], early-onset varicose veins or Klippel–Trenaunay syndrome.

Clinical features. The majority of cases present in the distal limbs,
particularly the hands and feet, as multiple cutaneous or subcutaneous, red or bluish nodules. Deeper tumours are rare. Presentation at other sites including the neck and oral cavity is very rare
[8,9]. Lesions continue to appear over many years, indicating
multifocality rather than true recurrences. Most nodules are less
than a few centimetres in diameter; they may occasionally be
painful.

Pathology. Low-power magnification reveals single or multiple,
fairly well-circumscribed, haemorrhagic nodules. Origin from
a pre-existing blood vessel is often seen, and individual lesions
may be entirely intravascular. Dilated, thin-walled, congested,
cavernous-like vascular spaces are intermixed with more cellular
areas composed of bland, short, spindle-shaped cells, with formation of slit-like spaces. Scattered, more epithelioid cells, with pink
cytoplasm and prominent vacuolation, are also seen. The spindle-
shaped cells are a mixture of endothelial cells, pericytes and
fibroblasts. Focal degenerative cytological atypia may be present.
Immunohistochemistry reveals staining for CD31 and CD34 and
focal staining for smooth muscle actin.

Diagnosis. The clinical appearances usually suggest a vascular
process, but the final diagnosis usually requires histological
confirmation.

Treatment. Single lesions are easily treated with simple excision.
Treatment is more difficult in the presence of multiple lesions, as
new lesions are more likely to appear over time.

References
1 Weiss SW, Enzinger FM. Spindle cell hemangioendothelioma: a low grade angiosarcoma resembling a cavernous hemangioma and Kaposi's sarcoma. *Am J Surg
Pathol* 1986; **10**: 521–30.
2 Scott GA, Rosai J. Spindle cell hemangioendothelioma: report of seven additional
cases of a recently described vascular neoplasm. *Am J Dermatopathol* 1988; **10**:
281–8.
3 Fletcher CDM, Beham A, Schmid C. Spindle cell haemangioendothelioma: a clinicopathological and immunohistochemical study indicative of a nonneoplastic
lesion. *Histopathology* 1991; **18**: 291–301.
4 Ding J, Hashimoto H, Imayama S *et al*. Spindle cell hemangioendothelioma, probably a benign vascular lesion not a low-grade angiosarcoma: a clinicopathological,
ultrastructural and immunohistochemical study. *Virchows Arch (A)* 1992; **420**:
77–85.
5 Imayama S, Murakamai Y, Hashimoto H *et al*. Spindle cell hemangioendothelioma
exhibits the ultrastructural features of reactive vascular proliferation rather than
of angiosarcoma. *Am J Clin Pathol* 1992; **97**: 279–87.
6 Perkins P, Weiss SW. Spindle cell hemangioendothelioma: an analysis of 78 cases
with reassessment of its pathogenesis and biologic behavior. *Am J Surg Pathol*
1996; **20**: 1196–204.
7 Fanburg JC, Meis Kindblom JM, Rosenberg AE. Multiple enchondromas
associated with spindle cell hemangioendotheliomas: an overlooked variant of
Maffucci's syndrome. *Am J Surg Pathol* 1995; **19**: 1029–38.
8 Sheehan M, Roumpf SO, Summerlin DJ *et al*. Spindle cell hemangioma: report of
a case presenting in the oral cavity. *J Cutan Pathol* 2007; **34**: 797–800.

9 Tosios KI, Gouveris I, Sklavounou A *et al*. Spindle cell hemangioma (hemangioendothelioma) of the head and neck: report of an unusual (or underdiagnosed) tumor. *Oral Surg Oral Med* 2008; **105**: 216–21.

Symplastic haemangioma

Definition. This is not a distinctive variant of haemangioma but represents extensive degenerative changes in a pre-existing haemangioma, closely mimicking malignancy [1–3]. Only a handful of cases have been reported. From personal experience with a small number of cases, the pre-existing vascular lesion is often either not identifiable or it represents a cirsoid aneurysm.

Clinical features. These are not distinctive. However, the patient is usually an adult, and the description is usually of a long-standing lesion that has rapidly increased in size.

Pathology. These tumours are often polypoid and well-circumscribed and do not tend to be ulcerated. The typical histological picture consists of dilated and congested, thin to thick-walled vascular spaces surrounded by a variable cellular stroma with frequent myxoid change and haemorrhage. Stromal cells and smooth muscle cells within the vessel walls show variable cytological atypia, consisting of nuclear enlargement and hyperchromatism. The endothelial cells lining the vascular spaces may be plump but do not display cytological atypia, multilayering or mitotic activity, allowing distinction from an angiosarcoma. Often cells have a bizarre appearance and multinucleated cells are common. Mitotic figures may be found but tend to be rare. Very occasional, atypical mitotic figures may also be seen.

References

1 Tsang WYW, Chan JKC, Fletcher CDM *et al*. Symplastic hemangioma: a distinctive vascular neoplasm featuring bizarre stromal cells. *Int J Surg Pathol* 1994; **1**: 202.
2 Kutzner H, Winzer M, Mentzel T. [Symplastic hemangioma]. *Hautarzt* 2000; **51**: 327–31.
3 Goh N, Dayrit J, Calonje E. Symplastic hemangioma. Report of two cases. *J Cutan Pathol* 2006; **33**: 735–40.

Vascular tumours of intermediate malignancy

Kaposiform haemangioendothelioma [1–5]

Synonym
- Kaposi-like infantile haemangioendothelioma

Definition. Kaposiform haemangioendothelioma is a locally aggressive, vascular neoplasm, which occurs mainly in the abdominal cavity [1] but can affect primarily the skin or deeper soft tissues.

Incidence and aetiology. This tumour is rare and presents mainly in young children under the age of 2 years, with no sex predilection. Some lesions are congenital [6]. Rare cases occur in older children and adults. In 20% of cases, there is an association with lymphangiomatosis [3]. It appears clear that this lesion is truly neoplastic. Although it is not malignant, it causes morbidity and mortality due to its location and the frequent occurrence of consumption coagulopathy (Kasabach–Merritt syndrome).

Clinical features. The most common presentation by far is that of a large, retroperitoneal, infiltrative mass. Involvement of neighbouring organs and the very common association with Kasabach–Merritt syndrome may lead to death. This complication is less common in more superficial tumours, particularly those located in the dermis and subcutaneous tissue [5,7,8]. Multifocal lesions are exceptional [9].

Pathology. The growth pattern is lobular and infiltrative. Multiple nodules with haemorrhage and surrounding fibrosis are seen. Tumour lobules are composed of bland, spindle-shaped cells with poorly defined, pink cytoplasm. Cleft-like spaces are often seen between spindle-shaped cells, and the resemblance to Kaposi's sarcoma can be striking. However, numerous capillaries, often associated with microthrombi, are also present in tumour lobules. Epithelioid endothelial cells with focal vacuolation are also present. These features, along with the striking lobular architecture of the tumour and negative staining for HHV8, allow distinction from Kaposi's sarcoma. Podoplanin (D2-40), a marker of lymphatic endothelium, is positive in the spindle cells and lymphatic channels around tumour lobules [10]. This finding not only suggests a lymphatic line of differentiation for this tumour, but it is also useful in making the histological diagnosis and in differential diagnosis from other tumours such as tufted angioma in which the tumour lobules are negative for D2-40 [11]. However, it has been suggested that Kaposiform hemangioioendothelioma and tufted angioma are part of the same spectrum [12].

Treatment. Complete excision is desirable as local recurrence is frequent, but this may be difficult to achieve when involvement is extensive. Spontaneous regression does not occur. Treatment of Kasabach–-Merritt syndrome is difficult and good response has been reported with vincristine [13]. Anecdotal cases responding to interferon-α have been described [14].

References

1 Tsang WY, Chan JK. Kaposi-like infantile hemangioendothelioma: a distinctive vascular neoplasm of the retroperitoneum. *Am J Surg Pathol* 1991; **15**: 982–9.
2 Niedt GW, Alba Greco M, Wieczorek R *et al*. Hemangioma with Kaposi's sarcoma-like features: report of two cases. *Pediatr Pathol* 1989; **9**: 567–75.
3 Zukerberg LR, Nickoloff BJ, Weiss SW. Kaposiform hemangioendothelioma of infancy and childhood: an aggressive neoplasm associated with Kasabach–Merritt syndrome and lymphangiomatosis. *Am J Surg Pathol* 1993; **17**: 321–8.
4 Fukunaga M, Ushigome S, Ishikawa E. Kaposiform haemangioendothelioma associated with Kasabach–Merritt syndrome. *Histopathology* 1996; **28**: 281–4.
5 Vin-Christian K, McCalmont TH, Frieden IJ. Kaposiform hemangioendothelioma: an aggressive, locally invasive vascular tumor that can mimic hemangioma of infancy. *Arch Dermatol* 1997; **133**: 1573–8.
6 Gianotti R, Gelmetti C, Alessi E. Congenital cutaneous multifocal kaposiform hemangioendothelioma. *Am J Dermatopathol* 1999; **21**: 557–61.
7 Mentzel T, Mazzoleni G, Dei Tos AP *et al*. Kaposiform hemangioendothelioma in adults: clinicopathologic and immunohistochemical analysis of three cases. *Am J Clin Pathol* 1997; **108**: 450–5.

8 Mac-Moune Lai F, To KF, Choi PC *et al.* Kaposiform hemangioendothelioma: five patients with cutaneous lesions and long follow-up. *Mod Pathol* 2001; **14**: 1087–92.

9 Deraedt K, Vander Poorten V, Van Geet C *et al.* Multifocal kaposiform haemangioendothelioma. *Virchows Arch* 2006; **448**: 843–6.

10 Debelenko LV, Perez-Atayde AR, Mulliken JB *et al.* D2-40 immunohistochemical analysis of pediatric vascular tumors reveals positivity in kaposiform hemangioendothelioma. *Mod Pathol* 2005; **18**: 1454–60.

11 Arai E, Kuramochi A, Tsuchida T *et al.* Usefulness of D2-40 immunohistochemistry for differentiation between kaposiform hemangioendothelioma and tufted angioma. *J Cutan Pathol* 2006; **33**: 492–7.

12 Chu CY, Hsiao CH, Chiu HC. Transformation between Kaposiform hemangioendothelioma and tufted angioma. *Dermatology* 2003; **206**: 334–7.

13 Haisley-Royster C, Enjolras O, Frieden IJ *et al.* Kasabach-Merritt phenomenon: a retrospective study of treatment with vincristine. *J Pediatr Hematol Oncol* 2002; **24**: 459–62.

14 Harper L, Michel JL, Emjolras O *et al.* Successful management of a retroperitoneal kaposiform hemangioendothelioma with Kasabach-Merritt phenomenon using alpha-interferon. *Eur J Pediatr Surg* 2006; **16**: 369–372.

Giant cell angioblastoma [1,2]

Definition. This is a very rare entity of which only a handful of cases have been reported. It is not clear whether it represents a true vascular tumour and, until it is more clearly delineated and defined, it has not been included in the latest WHO classification of vascular tumours.

Clinical features. Tumours are congenital and have been described on the hand, the palate and the scalp. The tumour is diffusely infiltrative and slowly growing. Two of the reported cases showed no progression after incomplete excision.

Pathology. The tumour is composed of infiltrative vascular channels lined by a single layer of bland endothelial cells and intermixed with solid nodules composed of spindle-shaped cells, histiocyte-like cells and osteoclasts. A plexiform growth pattern is often seen.

Treatment. Two cases have been successfully treated with interferon-α-2b [3].

References

1 Gonzalez-Crussi F, Choud P, Crawford SE. Congenital infiltrating giant cell angioblastoma, a new entity? *Am J Surg Pathol* 1991; **15**: 175–83.

2 Vargas SO, Perez-Atayde AR, Gonzalez-Crussi F *et al.* Giant cell angioblastoma: three additional occurrences of a distinct pathologic entity. *Am J Surg Pathol* 2001; **25**: 185–96.

3 Marler JJ, Rubin JB, Trede NS *et al.* Successful antiangiogenic therapy of giant cell angioblastoma with interferon alfa 2b: report of two cases. *Pediatrics* 2002; **109**: E37.

Retiform haemangioendothelioma [1–3]

Synonym
• Hobnail haemangioendothelioma

Definition. Retiform haemangioendothelioma is a rare variant of low-grade angiosarcoma with a tendency for local aggressive behaviour. It is characterized by arborizing vascular channels lined by endothelial cells with hobnail morphology.

Clinical features [1–4]. Retiform haemangioendothelioma presents mainly in young adults, with no sex predilection, as a slowly growing, asymptomatic, dermal and subcutaneous plaque or nodule. Rarely lesions present as a bruise [5]. Exceptional cases present with multiple lesions [6]. Rarely there is an association with lymphoedema or radiotherapy. Local recurrence occurs in up to 60% of cases. So far, there has only been one report of a tumour metastasizing to a regional lymph node, and a further lesion has spread locally to soft tissues [7]. No tumour-related deaths have been reported.

Pathology. Scanning magnification is distinctive and reveals arborizing, thin-walled, narrow, vascular channels with a striking resemblance to the rete testis. The growth pattern is infiltrative, and the vascular spaces are lined by bland hobnail endothelial cells with prominent nuclei and scanty cytoplasm. Intravascular papillae with collagenous cores, similar to those seen in papillary endolymphatic angioendothelioma, are sometimes seen. The surrounding stroma often appears hyalinized; a prominent mononuclear inflammatory cell infiltrate is common. The endothelial cells stain for vascular markers. There is no relationship to HHV8.

Treatment. Wide local excision is the treatment of choice.

References

1 Calonje E, Fletcher CD, Wilson Jones E *et al.* Retiform hemangioendothelioma: a distinctive form of low-grade angiosarcoma delineated in a series of 15 cases. *Am J Surg Pathol* 1994; **18**: 115–25.

2 Dufau JP, Pierre C, De SaintMaur PP *et al.* Hemangioendothelioma retiforme. *Ann Pathol* 1997; **17**: 47–51.

3 Fukunaga M, Endo Y, Masui F *et al.* Retiform haemangioendothelioma. *Virchows Arch* 1996; **428**: 301–4.

4 Tan D, Kraybill W, Cheney RT *et al.* Retiform hemangioendothelioma: a case report and review of the literature. *J Cutan Pathol* 2005; **23**: 634–7.

5 Ioannidou D, Panayiotides J, Krasagakis K *et al.* Retiform hemangioendothelioma presenting as bruise-like plaque in an adult woman. *Int J Dermatol* 2006; **45**: 53–5.

6 Duke D, Dvorak AM, Harrist TJ *et al.* Multiple retiform hemangioendotheliomas: a low grade angiosarcoma. *Am J Dermatopathol* 1996; **18**: 606–10.

7 Mentzel T, Stengel B, Katenkamp D. Retiform hemangioendothelioma: clinicopathologic case report and discussion of the group of low grade malignancy vascular tumors. *Pathologe* 1997; **18**: 390–4.

Papillary intralymphatic angioendothelioma [1]

Synonyms
• Endovascular lymphatic angioendothelioma
• Dabska's tumour

Definition. Defining this entity is difficult because, since its original description in 1969, few further convincing cases have been described [1–4]. Furthermore, the original series included some examples of what is now known as retiform haemangioendothelioma. Recently, the tumour has been better characterized under the preferred name of 'papillary endolymphatic angioendothelioma' [5]. It belongs to the family of tumours with hobnail endothelial cells, and it is characterized by dilated, cavernous-like lymphatic spaces with frequent papillary projections.

Clinical features. It presents mainly in infants and children, with 25% of the cases occurring in adults. There is no sex predilection. Presentation is as a slowly growing, asymptomatic plaque or nodule with a predilection for the limbs. In the original series of six cases, a tendency for local recurrence and metastasis to regional lymph nodes was reported [1], but in a recent series of 12 cases, none of the eight cases with follow-up recurred locally or metastasized [5]. It therefore seems likely that the behaviour of this tumour is benign. Further studies are needed to confirm whether it deserves to be kept in the group of tumours of intermediate behaviour.

Pathology. This tumour is composed of dilated, thin-walled channels simulating a cavernous lymphangioma. These channels are lined by bland hobnail endothelial cells with very rare mitotic figures. A striking feature is the formation of intraluminal papillary tufts with hyaline cores. Aggregates of mononuclear inflammatory cells may be seen around the vascular channels.

Treatment. Until the issue regarding the biological behaviour of this tumour is resolved, complete excision is recommended.

References

1 Dabska M. Malignant endovascular angioendothelioma of childhood. *Cancer* 1969; **24**: 503–9.
2 Manivel JC, Wick MR, Swanson PE *et al.* Endovascular papillary angioendothelioma of childhood. *Hum Pathol* 1986; **17**: 1240–4.
3 Morgan J, Robinson NJ, Rosen LB *et al.* Malignant endovascular papillary angioendothelioma. *Am J Dermatopathol* 1989; **11**: 64–8.
4 Patterson K, Chandra RS. Malignant endovascular papillary angioendothelioma. *Arch Pathol Lab Med* 1985; **109**: 671–3.
5 Fanburgh-Smith JC, Michal M *et al.* Papillary intralymphatic angioendothelioma (PILA): a report of twelve cases of a distinctive vascular tumor with phenotypic features of lymphatic vessels. *Am J Surg Pathol* 1999; **23**: 1004–10.

Kaposi's sarcoma [1–3]

> **Synonyms**
> - Kaposi's disease
> - Granuloma multiplex haemorrhagicum
> - Idiopathic multiple pigmented sarcoma

Definition. A multifocal, endothelial proliferation predominantly involving the skin and other organs and associated with formation of vascular channels and proliferation of spindle-shaped cells. It is not clear whether Kaposi's sarcoma is a reactive vascular proliferation or a neoplastic process (see below).

Aetiology and pathogenesis. In the mid 1990's, Chang *et al.* described a new human gammaherpesvirus associated with Kaposi's sarcoma [4]. This virus is closely associated to Epstein–Barr virus, was named human herpesvirus type 8 (HHV8), and it is associated with all clinical variants of Kaposi's sarcoma (HIV/AIDS-related Kaposi's sarcoma, the African endemic type, Kaposi's sarcoma induced by iatrogenic immunosuppresion and Mediterranean endemic Kaposi's sarcoma) [5,6]. The virus can be found in the blood of patients before lesions of Kaposi's sarcoma develop [7]. This gives further support to the belief that this virus,

along with genetic, immunological and environmental factors, is closely involved in the pathogenesis of Kaposi's sarcoma [8].

The multifocal development, symmetry of lesions, slow evolution of the classic form of the disease, regression when immunosuppression is reduced or stopped, and histology both of inflammation and of cells lacking cytological atypia, has led many to suggest that Kaposi's sarcoma is a reactive condition and not a neoplastic process. A few reports demonstrating the presence of clonality tend to support the hypothesis that this disorder is neoplastic [9]. Recent studies have suggested that the disease, in fact, starts as a reactive angioproliferative and inflammatory process, but progresses to become a monoclonal neoplastic process [10,11]. This is probably the result of close complex interactions between inflammatory cytokines, angiogenic factors, HHV8 and, in HIV-positive patients, the HIV virus itself [12]. In the latter setting it has been demonstrated that the HIV-1 trans-activating protein Tat-1 promotes the development of lesions by increasing the activity of different cytokines and angiogenic factors [13].

For many years, the line of differentiation of the proliferating cell in Kaposi's sarcoma remained difficult to elucidate. The suspicion has always been that the main proliferating cells are endothelial cells with lymphatic differentiation. This has recently been substantiated by the development of lymphatic endothelium-specific antibodies, including Lyve-1, podoplanin (D2-40) and Prox-1, which are positive in the proliferating cells in Kaposi's sarcoma [14,15].

At present, there are four recognized clinical subsets of Kaposi's sarcoma. These are:

1 Classic
2 Endemic
3 Iatrogenic
4 Human immunodeficiency virus (HIV)-related (Chapter 35).

Classic Kaposi's sarcoma [16–18] is as described originally by Kaposi. It is found mainly in elderly males, particularly from Southern Europe (mainly Italian and Greek) or Jews of Eastern European origin. The lesions begin slowly and insidiously around the ankle and slowly spread up the leg (Fig. 56.20). Lymphoedema

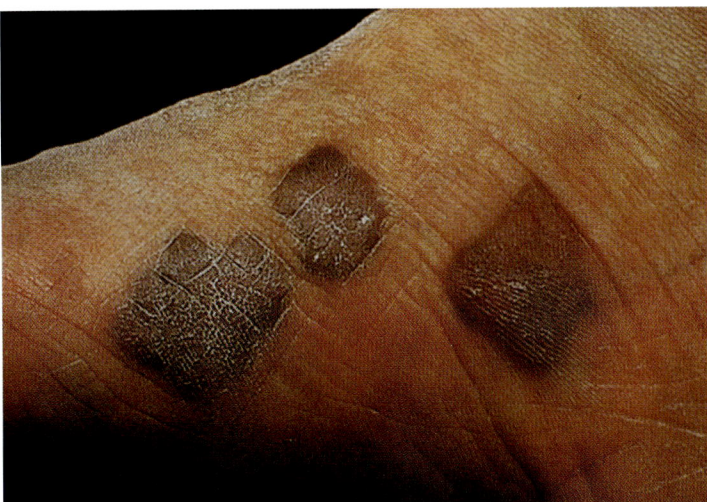

Fig. 56.20 Classic Kaposi's sarcoma arising on the feet of a male patient of Mediterranean origin.

can occur as a complication. Lesions in other locations, including the oral mucosa, are very rare. Involvement of internal organs is not usually seen. The disease is very rarely responsible for the death of the patient. An association with haemopoietic malignancies may be seen.

Endemic Kaposi's sarcoma [19,20] is found in equatorial Africa, mainly in the Democratic Republic of Congo, Uganda [21,22] and Rwanda. In adults, males predominate, but this form is also seen in children. Crops of cutaneous, vascular lesions develop, and may be associated with gross oedema. Visceral lesions may also occur; the prognosis is poor if there is extracutaneous involvement.

Iatrogenic Kaposi's sarcoma [16,23,24]. This is seen in transplant patients and after cytotoxic chemotherapy for lymphomas. Drug-induced immunosuppression to prevent rejection of transplanted organs markedly increases the risk of developing lymphomas and other tumours, including Kaposi's sarcoma. In transplant patients, Kaposi's sarcoma is 150 times more common than expected and affected patients may be younger than those with other types of Kaposi's sarcoma (excepting those with HIV infection). In a large, retrospective study over 23 years, Kaposi's sarcoma developed in 3.9% of cases of kidney transplant patients [23]. Both systemic and cutaneous involvement may occur, and the progress of the disease may be aggressive, causing the death of the patient. If it is possible to remove the immunosuppression, the lesions will regress.

Kaposi's sarcoma associated with HIV infection [25–28]. This variant was first recognized in 1979 [29,30] when an epidemic of Kaposi's sarcoma was identified in the homosexual community in New York. Since that time, it became firmly associated with the later stages of HIV infection. It is much commoner in homosexual and bisexual men than in others at risk, such as drug abusers or haemophiliacs. Kaposi's sarcoma usually develops in the later stages of the disease and it may be a presenting feature of HIV infection. With the advent of highly active antiretroviral therapy (HAART) the incidence of Kaposi's sarcoma in HIV/AIDS has decreased dramatically in the Western world [31]. As a result of HAART it is rare to see patients presenting with widespread lesions of Kaposi's sarcoma and the latter may regress as a result of this therapy, making the clinical and histological diagnosis even more difficult. This is not true, however, in third world countries, particularly in Africa [32,33] where the availability of HAART is still very limited. In patients on HAART and according to the degree of restoration of the immune system, lesions may regress; also, if they develop during treatment they are usually limited in number and extent. It is more common now to see patients with early lesions consisting of only one or two flat, macular lesions (Fig. 56.21) than with extensive nodular or plaque lesions. However, in patients with prominent immunosuppression, as still seen in many sub-Saharan African countries, the lesions may occur anywhere on the body, develop with explosive rapidity and become large nodules. The face and mucous membranes, such as the soft palate, are relatively frequently involved (Fig. 56.22). Involvement of lymph nodes, lungs and gastrointestinal tract is common.

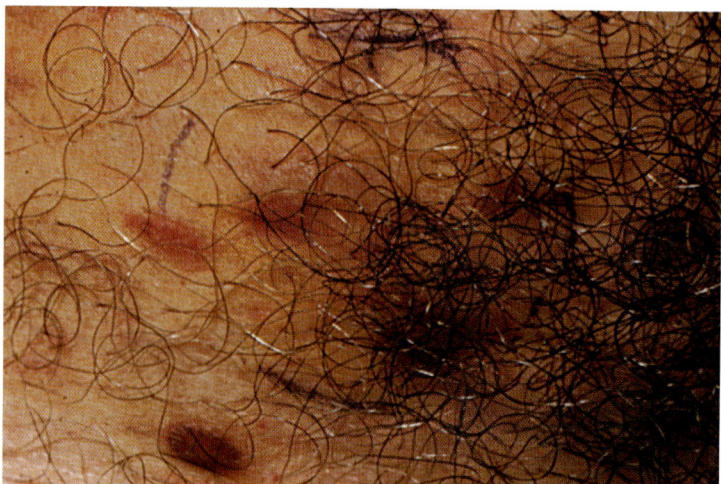

Fig. 56.21 Patch-stage Kaposi's sarcoma in an HIV-positive patient.

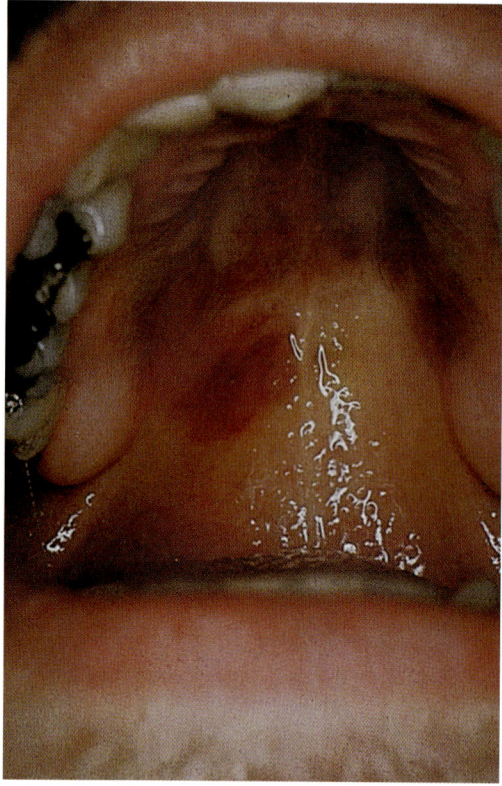

Fig. 56.22 Early lesion of Kaposi's sarcoma in an HIV-positive patient.

Clinical features [2,34–36]. Kaposi's sarcoma tends to occur in males. The lesions have a dark-blue or purplish colour. Initially, they may be almost macular and when they become tumid, pressure may produce partial blanching to reveal a brown tinge. The process usually begins on the extremities, most commonly on the feet and occasionally on the hands, ears or nose. Individual tumours enlarge to a diameter of 10–30 mm and stop growing. The process is multifocal, and adjacent areas may fuse to form a plaque or tumour. Oedema of the limb may follow, or at times precede, the appearance of the tumour. There are few subjective symptoms;

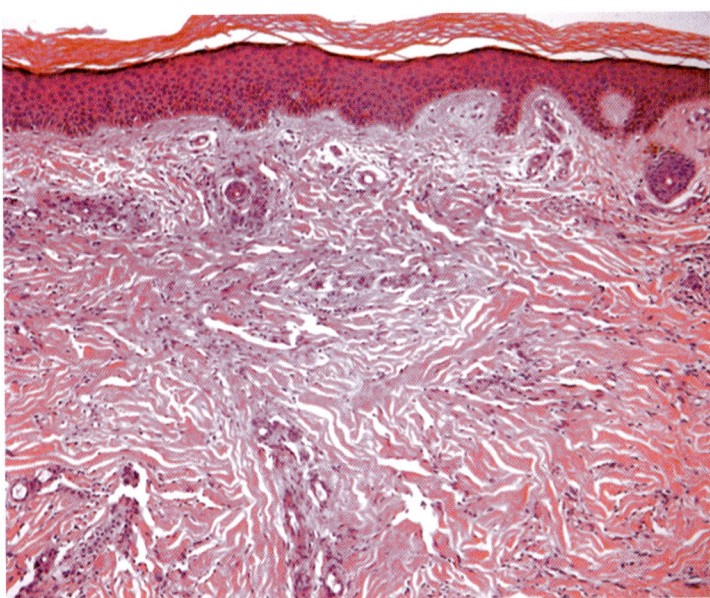

Fig. 56.23 Patch-stage Kaposi's sarcoma. Note the dermal proliferation of small, thin-walled, irregular lymphatic-like channels around pre-existing, normal blood vessels and adnexal structures.

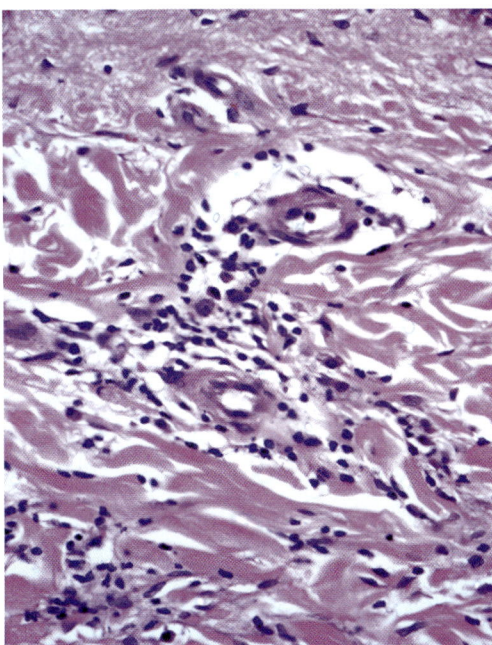

Fig. 56.24 Patch-stage Kaposi's sarcoma. Small, irregular vascular channels lined by bland endothelial cells. Note the promontory sign, in which a normal pre-existing capillary seems to be floating in a newly formed channel.

pain may be felt in nodules on pressure areas. The lesions may involute to leave pigmented scars, or may become eroded, ulcerated or fungating. New lesions may appear along the course of superficial veins, and in time most patients have more or less symmetrical lesions. The rate of spread is remarkably variable. It tends to be slow in Europeans and more rapid in Africans, where oedema is often the first sign. Lymph nodes, mucosal surfaces and internal organs, particularly the small intestine, may all be involved as the disease progresses. Kaposi's sarcoma may at times start in other organs and run its course without skin manifestation. Visceral involvement is the common pattern in African children, with lymph nodes as the main tissue involved.

Patients presenting with Kaposi's sarcoma associated with severe immunosuppression have subtle lesions, which may well be missed by the unwary [2]. They may have only one or two lesions scattered over the body, and these may resemble slight areas of trauma or a simple bruise. The lesions are therefore quite dissimilar from the classic, florid lesions developing on the lower limbs of the older patients from central Europe.

Pathology

[37–39]. The cutaneous lesions of Kaposi's sarcoma can generally be divided into patch, plaque and nodular stages. These stages often overlap clinically and histologically. In the patch stage of the disease, there is a proliferation of jagged, irregular, lymphatic-like vascular channels lined by a single layer of bland endothelial cells; these channels particularly surround pre-existing blood vessels and adnexal structures (Fig. 56.23). Normal, pre-existing capillaries and even adnexal structures seem to be floating within the newly formed channels, the so-called 'promontory sign' (Fig. 56.24). From the early stages a patchy, variably prominent, mononuclear inflammatory cell infiltrate containing plasma cells is seen. This is associated with extravasation of red blood cells and haemosiderin deposition. In some cases, numerous, irregular, widely dilated, lymphatic-like channels impart a

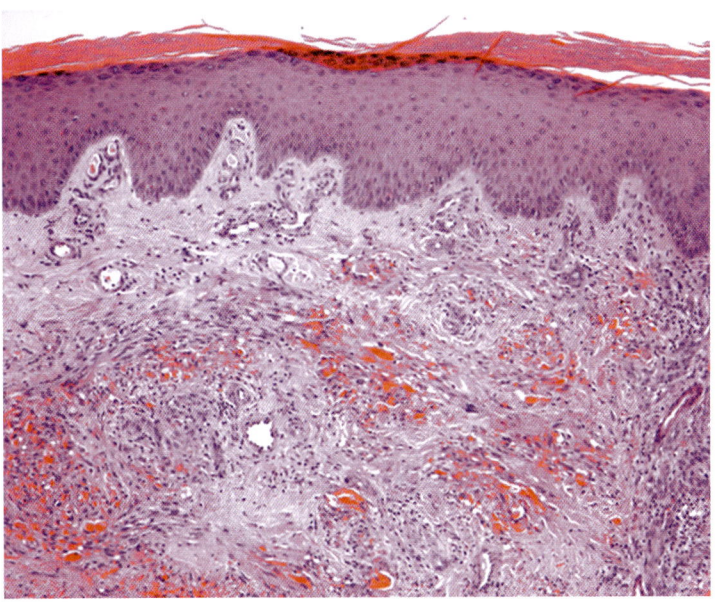

Fig. 56.25 Plaque-stage Kaposi's sarcoma. More diffuse proliferation of vascular channels with prominent haemorrhage.

prominent lymphangiomatous appearance (lymphangiomatous Kaposi's sarcoma) [40].

The plaque stage is an exaggeration of the patch stage (Fig. 56.25). The vascular channels increase in number, and a network of bland spindle-shaped cells with pink cytoplasm develops. Dilated vascular channels in a back-to-back pattern may also be seen. Intra- or extracellular, hyaline, PAS-positive, eosinophilic globules are common, and probably represent degenerate red blood cells [41]. Involvement of the whole dermis and superficial subcutis is frequent.

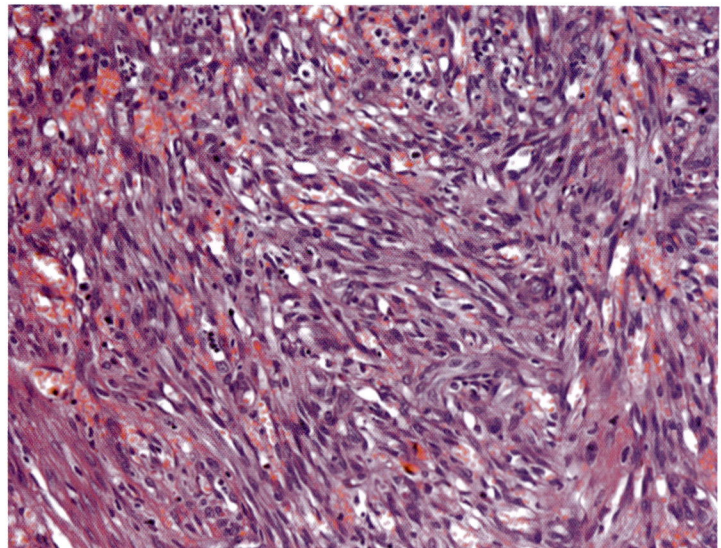

Fig. 56.26 Nodular Kaposi's sarcoma. Note the typical, sieve-like appearance, with blood cells between the cleft-like spaces.

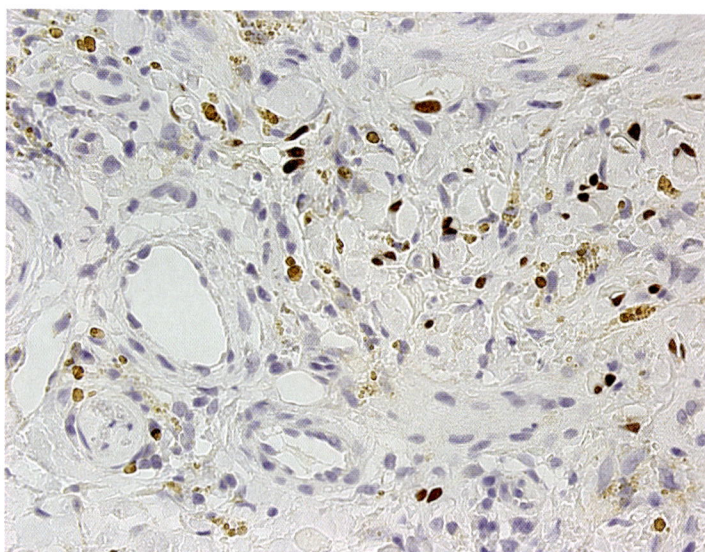

Fig. 56.27 Immunohistochemistry for the LNA of HHV8 in a case of Kaposi's sarcoma highlighting the presence of nuclear staining in the proliferating endothelial cells.

In the nodular stage, there are fairly well-circumscribed nodules of generally bland, spindle-shaped cells forming frequent cleft-like spaces that impart a typical sieve-like appearance (Fig. 56.26). Extravasated red blood cells are plentiful, as are hyaline globules. Mitotic figures are common. The periphery of the nodules may display a more angiomatous appearance.

Rarely, lesions of Kaposi's sarcoma may be partially or totally in an intravascular location, particularly within a vein [42].

Very rare examples of Kaposi's sarcoma display a high degree of cytological atypia and behave in an aggressive fashion.

The histology of lesions of Kaposi's sarcoma that have regressed after chemotherapy or with angiogenesis inhibitors, including Col-3 or HAART, may be very difficult to interpret [43]. Regression may be partial or complete. In completely regressed lesions there is absence of irregular lymphatic-like channels and spindle-shaped cells, increase in the number of capillaries in the superficial dermis and a superficial, perivascular lymphohistiocytic inflammatory cell infiltrate with variable numbers of siderophages. Partially regressed lesions show prominent decrease in the number of lymphatic-like vascular channels and spindle-shaped cells and focal inflammation with siderophages. The residual spindle-shaped cells tend to be arranged around superficial and mid-dermal capillaries. These changes are correlated with prominent decrease in the expression of LAN-1.

A useful aid in the histological diagnosis of Kaposi's sarcoma is a monoclonal antibody against the latent nuclear antigen 1 (LNA-1) of HHV8, which stains tumour cells in all cases of the disease [44]. Positive cases demonstrate granular nuclear staining (Fig. 56.27). *In situ* hybridization was the only technique initially used to demonstrate the virus, but this is a more expensive and time consuming technique and it is not widely available.

The pathological differential diagnosis includes many benign vascular tumours or reactive proliferations, including spindle cell haemangioma, tufted angioma, microvenular haemangioma,

hobnail haemangioma, progressive lymphangioma and, on the lower legs, a 'venous' dermatitis (acroangiodermatitis). Angiosarcoma is also often considered in the differential diagnosis, but in the latter there is clear evidence of cytological atypia, mitotic activity and multilayering.

Differential diagnosis. The early lesion is most likely to be confused with a wide variety of benign vascular proliferations. It must also be distinguished from fibrous histiocytoma or from other types of soft-tissue tumours. Its evolution from a macular lesion and its characteristic colour, slow development and multifocal distribution make the diagnosis likely in most instances. Cases in which the tumour is preceded by oedema may cause difficulty, as angiosarcoma may arise in chronic lymphoedema. In prolonged venous hypertension of the lower legs, or in association with underlying vascular malformations, nodules with a close resemblance to Kaposi's sarcoma may develop (acroangiodermatitis, pseudo-Kaposi's sarcoma); they differ, however, in lack of progression, and a spindle-cell proliferation is not seen in the histological sections.

Treatment. Where a small area is involved, excision or radiotherapy can be used. Superficial radiotherapy is rapid and effective, and is the treatment of choice for the majority of patients with nodular disease of the extremities. For more extensive disease a number of treatment options have been used including antiviral, cytotoxic and immunomodulator drugs. In HIV/AIDS regression of lesions may be seen with HAART [45]. Liposomal doxorubicin may also be a useful treatment and interleukin-12, either alone or in combination with the latter, may also induce remission in AIDS patients with Kaposi's sarcoma who are on HAART [46]. Pegylated liposomal doxorubicin has been used with success on its own, as second line treatment of AIDS-related Kaposi's sarcoma and in advanced, classic Kaposi's sarcoma [47,48].

References

1 Cox FH, Helwig EG. Kaposi's sarcoma: a review. *Cancer* 1959; **12**: 289–98.

2 Gottlieb G, Ackermann AB, eds. *Kaposi's Sarcoma: a Text Atlas.* Philadelphia: Lea & Febiger 1989.

3 Schwartz R. Kaposi's sarcoma: advances and perspectives. *J Am Acad Dermatol* 1996; **34**: 804–14.

4 Beral V, Peterman TA, Berkelman R *et al.* Kaposi's sarcoma among persons with AIDS: a sexually transmitted infection. *Lancet* 1990; **i**: 123–8.

5 Moore PS, Chang Y. Detection of herpes virus-like sequences in Kaposi's sarcoma in patients with and without HIV infection. *N Engl J Med* 1995; **332**: 1181–5.

6 Nickoloff BJ, Foreman KE. Charting a new course through the chaos of KS (Kaposi's sarcoma). *Am J Pathol* 1996; **148**: 1323–9.

7 Gao SJ, Kingsley L, Hoover SR *et al.* Seroconversion to antibodies against Kaposi's sarcoma-associated herpes virus-related nuclear antigens before the development of Kaposi's sarcoma. *N Engl J Med* 1996; **335**: 233–41.

8 Ensoli B, Sgadari C, Barillari G *et al.* Biology of Kaposi's sarcoma. *Eur J Cancer* 2001; **37**: 1251–69.

9 Rabkin CS, Janz S, Lash A *et al.* Monoclonal origin of multicentric Kaposi's sarcoma lesions. *N Engl J Med* 1997; **336**: 988–93.

10 Judde JG, Lacoste V, Brière J *et al.* Monoclonality or oligoclonality of human herpesvirus-8 terminal repeat sequences in Kaposi's sarcoma and other diseases. *J Nat Cancer Inst* 2000; **92**: 677.

11 Duprez R, Lacoste V, Brière J *et al.* Evidence for a multicloral origin of multicentric advanced lesions of Kaposi sarcoma. *J Natl Cancer Inst* 2007; **99**: 1086.

12 Gessain A, Duprez R. Spindle cells and their role in Kaposi's sarcoma. *Int J Biochem Cell Biol* 2005; **37**: 2457.

13 Aoki Y, Tosato G. Interactions between HIV-1 Tat and KSHV. *Curr Top Microbiol Immunol* 2007; **312**: 309.

14 Carroll PA, Brazeau E, Lagunoff M. Kaposi's sarcoma-associated herpesvirus infection of blood endothelial cells induces lymphatic differentiation. *Virology* 2004; **328**: 7.

15 Xu H, Edwards JR, Espinosa O *et al.* Expression of a lymphatic endothelial cell marker in benign and malignant vascular tumors. *Hum Pathol* 2004; **35**: 857.

16 Bluefarb SM, ed. *Kaposi's Sarcoma: Multiple Idiopathic Haemorrhagic Sarcoma.* Springfield: Thomas, 1957.

17 Losspalluti M, Mastrolonardo M, Lonosole F *et al.* Classical Kaposi's sarcoma: a survey of 163 cases observed in Bari, Italy. *Dermatology* 1995; **191**: 104–8.

18 Tedeschi CG. Some considerations concerning the nature of the so-called sarcoma of Kaposi. *AMA Arch Pathol* 1958; **66**: 656–84.

19 Oettle AG. Geographical and racial differences in the frequency of Kaposi's sarcoma as evidence of environmental or genetic causes. *Acta UICC Cancer* 1962; **18**: 330–63.

20 Olowasanmi JO, Williams AO, Alli AF. Superficial cancer in Nigeria. *Br J Cancer* 1969; **23**: 714–28.

21 Taylor JF, Templeton AC, Vogel CL *et al.* Kaposi's sarcoma in Uganda: a clinico-pathological study. *Int J Cancer* 1971; **8**: 122–35.

22 Templeton AC, Viegas OAC. Racial variations in tumour incidence in Uganda. *Trop Geogr Med* 1970; **22**: 431–8.

23 Serraino D, Angeletti C, Carrieri MP *et al.* Kaposi's sarcoma in transplant and HIV infected patients: an epidemiologic study in Italy and France. *Transplantation* 2005; **80**: 1699.

24 Moosa MR. Kaposi's sarcoma in kidney transplant recipients: a 23-year experience. *QJM* 2005; **98**: 205.

25 Lemlich G, Schwam L, Lebwohl M. Kaposi's sarcoma and acquired immunodeficiency syndrome. *J Am Acad Dermatol* 1987; **16**: 319–25.

26 Jessop S. HIV-associated Kaposi's sarcoma. *Dermatol Clin* 2006; **24**: 509.

27 Lemlich G, Schwam L, Lebwohl M. Kaposi's sarcoma and acquired immunodeficiency syndrome: postmortem findings in twenty-four cases. *J Am Acad Dermatol* 1987; **16**: 319–25.

28 Friedmann-Kien AE, Laubenstein LJ, Rubinstein P *et al.* Disseminated Kaposi's sarcoma in homosexual men. *Ann Intern Med* 1982; **96**: 693–700.

29 Gottlieb GJ, Ragaz A, Vogel JV *et al.* A preliminary communication on extensively disseminated Kaposi's sarcoma in young homosexual men. *Am J Dermatopathol* 1981; **3**: 111–4.

30 Groopman JE. Causation of AIDS revealed. *Nature* 1984; **308**: 769.

31 Biggar RJ. AIDS-related cancers in the era of highly active antiretroviral therapy. *Oncology (Williston Park)* 2001; **15**: 439–48.

32 Onunu AN, Okoduwa C, Eze EU *et al.* Kaposi's sarcoma in Nigeria. *Int J Dermatol* 2007; **46**: 204.

33 Mwanda OW, Fu P, Collea R, Whalen C *et al.* Kaposi's sarcoma in patients with and without human immunodeficiency virus infection, in a tertiary referral centre in Kenya. *Ann Trop Med Parasitol* 2005; **99**: 81.

34 Viera J, Frank E, Spira TJ *et al.* Acquired immune deficiency in Haitians: opportunistic infections in previously healthy Haitian immigrants. *N Engl J Med* 1983; **308**: 125–9.

35 Templeton AC. Kaposi's sarcoma. *Pathol Ann* 1981; **16**: 315–36.

36 Tappero JW, Connant MA, Wolfe SF *et al.* Kaposi's sarcoma: epidemiology, pathogenesis, histology, clinical spectrum, staging criteria and therapy. *J Am Acad Dermatol* 1993; **28**: 371–95.

37 Dorfman RF. Kaposi's sarcoma revisited. *Hum Pathol* 1984; **15**: 1013–7.

38 Murray JF, Lothe F. The histopathology of Kaposi's sarcoma. *Acta Unio Int Contra Cancrum* 1962; **18**: 413–28.

39 Chor PJ, Santa Cruz DJ. Kaposi's sarcoma: a clinicopathologic review and differential diagnosis. *J Cutan Pathol* 1992; **19**: 6–20.

40 Gange RW, Wilson Jones E. Lymphangioma-like Kaposi's sarcoma: a report of three cases. *Br J Dermatol* 1979; **100**: 327–34.

41 Kao GF, Johnson FB, Sulica VI. The nature of hyaline (eosinophilic) globules and vascular slits of Kaposi's sarcoma. *Am J Dermatopathol* 1990; **12**: 256–67.

42 Luzar B, Antony F, Ramdial PK *et al.* Intravascular Kaposi's sarcoma – A hitherto unrecognized phenomenon. *J Cutan Pathol* 2007; **34**: 861–4.

43 Pantanowitz L, Dezube BJ, Pinkus GS *et al.* Histological characterization of regression in acquired immunodeficiency syndrome-related Kaposi's sarcoma. *J Cutan Pathol* 2004; **31**: 26.

44 Cheuk W, Wong KO, Wong CS *et al.* Immunostaining for human herpesvirus 8 latent nuclear antigen-1 helps distinguish Kaposi's sarcoma from its mimics. *Am J Clin Pathol* 2004; **121**: 335.

45 Leder HA, Galor A, Peters GB *et al.* Resolution of conjunctival Kaposi sarcoma after institution of highly active antiretorviral therapy alone. *Br J Ophthalmol* 2008; **92**: 151.

46 Yarchoan R, Pluda JM, Wyvill KM *et al.* Treatment of AIDS-related Kaposi's sarcoma with interleukin-12: rationale and preliminary evidence of clinical activity. *Crit Rev Immunol* 2007; **27**: 401–14.

47 Udhrain A, Skubitz KM, Northflet DW. Pegylated liposomal doxorubicin in the treatment of AIDS-related Kaposi's sarcoma. *Int J Nanomedicine* 2007; **2**: 345–52.

48 Di Lorenzo G, Di Trolio R, Montesarchio V *et al.* Pegylated liposomal doxorubicin as second-like therapy in the treatment of patients with advanced classic Kaposi sarcoma. A retrospective study. *Cancer* 2008; **112**: 1147–52.

Malignant vascular tumours

Angiosarcoma [1–4]

> **Synonyms**
> - Malignant haemangioendothelioma
> - Haemangiosarcoma
> - Lymphangiosarcoma

Definition. A malignant vascular tumour, arising from both vascular and lymphatic endothelium. Except for the pure epithelioid variant of angiosarcoma (see below), cutaneous angiosarcoma almost exclusively occurs in three settings: idiopathic angiosarcoma of the face, scalp and neck [2–4], angiosarcoma associated with chronic lymphoedema (Stewart–Treves syndrome) [5–9] and post-irradiation angiosarcoma [10–12]. In this chapter, the terms 'angiosarcoma' and 'lymphangiosarcoma' are used interchangeably.

Incidence. This is a rare tumour in any form. Angiosarcoma of the scalp and face of the elderly is very rare, affects mainly males and it is almost invariably fatal.

Stewart–Treves syndrome occurs in 0.5% of patients who survive mastectomy for more than 5 years. The mean age at appearance of the angiosarcoma is 62 years, and the mean interval between mastectomy and the appearance of the tumour is 10.5 years [9]. Two cases have been reported in men following mastectomy [13]. Not all patients have received radiotherapy in association with the mastectomy, and not all have had axillary nodes removed.

Lymphoedema is not invariably present, or it may be late in appearing and antedate the tumour by only a short time. The incidence and cause of postmastectomy lymphoedema have been reviewed [14]. In the majority of cases, the clinical course and autopsy findings have shown that the treatment of the breast carcinoma was successful and that patients have had less frequent involvement of the axillary nodes than usual [9]. A small number of cases have arisen in lymphoedema of the lower limb, or in the upper limb without breast cancer and mastectomy [15]. Most of these patients were women.

Multiple primary malignancies have occurred in 8% of cases of Stewart–Treves syndrome [6] and a systemically acting carcinogen has been suggested [8,9]. There is no evidence to support this.

Post-irradiation angiosarcoma is rare and most cases arise in the skin after radiotherapy for breast or, less commonly, internal cancer [10–12].

Angiosarcoma occurring in other settings is very rare. Presentation in children is extremely rare [16]. Angiosarcoma may also exceptionally occur in benign vascular tumours including vascular malformations [17], in a large blood vessel [18], in association with a plexiform neurofibroma in neurofibromatosis [19], in a schwannoma [20], in a malignant peripheral nerve sheath tumour [21,22], in xeroderma pigmentosum [23], in a gouty tophus [24], in association with vinyl chloride exposure [25], in association with immunosuppression in organ transplantation [26] and as the mesenchymal component in a metaplastic carcinoma [27]. An exceptional case of an angiosarcoma producing granulocyte colony-stimulating factor and inducing a leukaemoid reaction has been described [28].

Clinical features [3,4,29,30].

In all types of angiosarcoma, the first sign may be an area of bruising, often thought by the patient to be traumatic (Fig. 56.28). Dusky blue or red nodules develop and grow rapidly, and fresh, discrete nodules appear nearby. In some cases, haemorrhagic blisters are a prominent feature. As the tumours grow, the oedema may increase and older lesions may ulcerate. Multifocality is a very frequent finding; this makes surgical excision very difficult, particularly in those cases occurring on the face and scalp. Dissemination occurs early, with the first visceral deposits usually being in the lung and pleural cavity.

Most studies reporting outcome have confined their attention to idiopathic angiosarcoma of the face, neck and scalp, in which the reported 5-year survival is low, at between 12% and 33% [3,31]. Angiosarcomas arising in the setting of chronic lymphoedema and after radiotherapy appear to be equally aggressive. Combined series of idiopathic angiosarcoma of the face and scalp, other cutaneous angiosarcomas and angiosarcomas occurring in internal organs report 5-year survival rates varying between 24 and 34% [1,32–34]. Features found to affect prognosis vary between different studies. Tumour size and completeness of excision appear

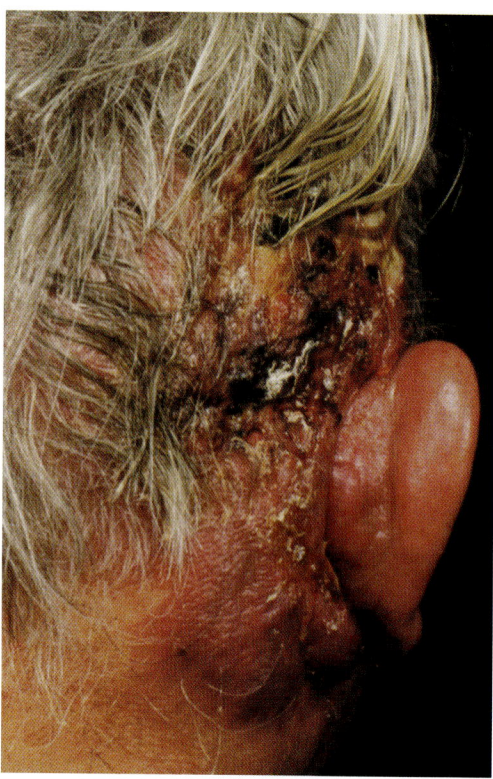

Fig. 56.28 Typical haemorrhagic appearance of an angiosarcoma.

to be more reliable factors to predict outcome [28]. It has been suggested that a high mitotic count correlates with poor prognosis and that a heavy mononuclear inflammatory cell infiltrate correlates with good prognosis [3,5,28]. A recent study of cutaneous sporadic angiosarcomas, excluding those associated with radiotherapy or with chronic lymphoedema, has found by univariate analysis that factors associated with higher mortality include older age, lesions on trunk and limbs compared to those on the head and neck, necrosis and an epithelioid cell morphology [35]. Tumours with necrosis and epithelioid morphology were classified as high risk and confirmed by multivariate analysis to be associated with higher mortality. The depth of invasion correlated with higher risk of local recurrence. The caveat with this study is that it combines traditional head and neck angiosarcomas with those showing a more pure epithelioid cell morphology that usually occur elsewhere and are usually classified under a different category.

Pathology [4,36–38].

In the well-differentiated tumour, vascular channels infiltrate the normal structures in a disorganized fashion, as if trying to line every available tissue space with a layer of endothelial cells. The collagen is characteristically lined by tumour cells in a pattern that has been described as 'dissection of collagen' (Fig. 56.29). Tumour cells may be plumper than normal, double-layered in places and form solid, intravascular buds. The pattern of growth is more suggestive of lymphatic vessels than blood vessels, but both are probably involved. Haemorrhage is often prominent. Less well-differentiated tumours show more atypical, pleomorphic, endothelial cells, often with a spindle-cell morphology, which may be heaped into several layers or become syncytial.

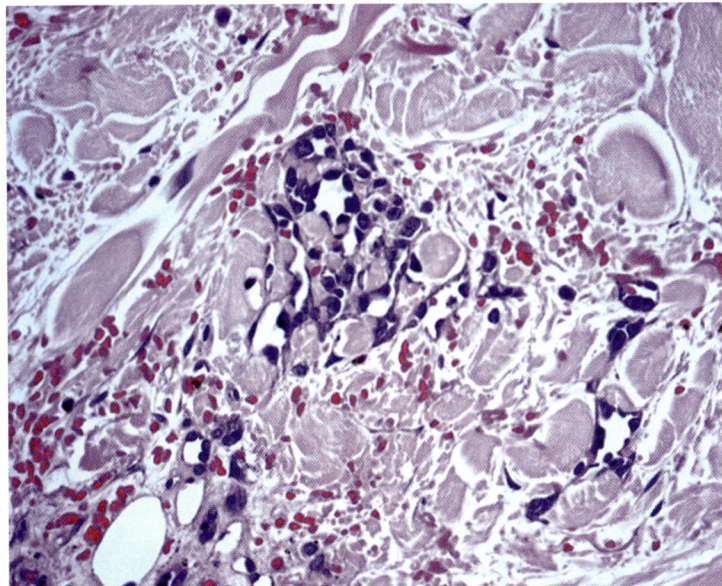

Fig. 56.29 Well-differentiated angiosarcoma, with thin-walled irregular vascular channels lined by atypical endothelial cells. Note the dissection of collagen pattern.

Advancing malignancy may be associated with loss of vascular pattern and proliferation of cell masses. Rare cases are composed of granular cells [39]. In exceptional cases, tumours may be extensively infiltrated by lymphocytes or macrophages. In these cases, distinction from a lymphoma may be difficult [40,41].

Immunohistochemical studies have indicated that antibodies to CD31 are the most reliable markers for routine use, compared with antibodies against von Willebrand factor and CD34 [7]. However, a panel of antibodies including the three markers is recommended in difficult cases as positivity to the various markers varies. Recently, an antibody against the carboxy terminal of the Fli-1 protein, a nuclear transcription factor member of the ETS family of DNA-binding transcription factors, has been shown to be a fairly specific marker of endothelial cells [42].

Cytogenetics studies of soft tissue and cutaneous angiosarcoma are limited to a few case reports. Most analyzed cases have shown complex cytogenetic aberrations [43,44].

Treatment [3]. All angiosarcomas, regardless of the setting in which they occur, have a bad prognosis. In the less malignant types, wide excision and grafting has controlled some cases. The response to radiotherapy is disappointing and is usually only palliative. In the early stages of angiosarcoma of a limb, radical amputation may offer a hope of cure. In idiopathic angiosarcoma of the head and neck, a very small percentage of patients with smaller lesions (usually less than between 5 and 10 cm in diameter at presentation) can be successfully treated with radical wide-field radiotherapy and surgery [1,32–34]. The best chance of survival in these patients resides in wide surgical excision followed by radiotherapy [45].

References

1 Mark RJ, Poen JC, Tran LM *et al*. Angiosarcoma: a review of 67 patients and review of the literature. *Cancer* 1996; **77**: 2400–6.
2 Bardwill JM, Mocega EE, Butler JJ *et al*. Angiosarcomas of the head and neck region. *Am J Surg* 1968; **11**: 548–53.
3 Holden CA, Spittle MF, Wilson Jones E. Angiosarcoma of the face and scalp: prognosis and treatment. *Cancer* 1987; **48**: 1907–21.
4 Maddox JC, Evans HL. Angiosarcoma of skin and soft tissue: a study of 44 cases. *Cancer* 1981; **48**: 1907–21.
5 Chen KTK, Gilbert EF. Angiosarcoma complicating generalized lymphangiectasia. *Arch Pathol Lab Med* 1979; **103**: 86–8.
6 Eby CS, Brennan MF, Fine G. Lymphangiosarcoma: lethal complication of chronic lymphedema—report of two cases and review of the literature. *Arch Surg* 1967; **94**: 223–30.
7 MacKenzie DH. Lymphangiosarcoma arising in chronic congenital and idiopathic lymphoedema. *J Clin Pathol* 1971; **24**: 524–9.
8 Stewart FW, Treves N. Lymphangiosarcoma in postmastectomy lymphedema: a report of six cases in elephantiasis chirurgica. *Cancer* 1948; **1**: 64–81.
9 Herrman JB. Lymphangiosarcoma of the chronically edematous extremity. *Surg Gynecol Obstet* 1965; **121**: 1107–15.
10 Goette DK, Detlefs RL. Postirradiation angiosarcoma. *J Am Acad Dermatol* 1985; **12**: 922–6.
11 Fineberg S, Rosen PP. Cutaneous angiosarcoma and atypical vascular lesions of the skin of the breast after radiation therapy for breast carcinoma. *Am J Clin Pathol* 1994; **102**: 757–63.
12 Karlsson P, Holmberg E, Johansson KA *et al*. Soft tissue sarcoma after treatment for breast cancer. *Radiother Oncol* 1996; **38**: 25–31.
13 Oettle AG, van Blerk PJP. Postmastectomy lymphostatic endothelioma of Stewart and Treves in a male. *Br J Surg* 1963; **50**: 736–43.
14 Treves N. An evaluation of the etiological factors of lymphedema following radical mastectomy: an analysis of 1007 cases. *Cancer* 1957; **10**: 444–59.
15 Scott RB, Nydick I, Conway H. Lymphangiosarcoma arising in lymphedema. *Am J Med* 1960; **28**: 1008–12.
16 Lezana-del Valle P, Gerald WL, Tsai J *et al*. Malignant vascular tumors in young patients. *Cancer* 1998; **83**: 1634–9.
17 Rossi S, Fletcher CD. Angiosarcoma arising in hemangioma/vascular malformation: report of four cases and review of the literature. *Am J Surg Pathol* 2002; **26**: 1319–29.
18 Abratt RP, Williams M, Raff M *et al*. Angiosarcoma of the superior vena cava. *Cancer* 1983; **52**: 740–3.
19 Chadhuri B, Ronan SG, Manahgod JR. Angiosarcoma arising in a plexiform neurofibroma. *Cancer* 1980; **46**: 605–10.
20 Trassard M, Le Doussal V, Bui BN *et al*. Angiosarcoma arising in a solitary schwannoma (neurilemoma) of the sciatic nerve. *Am J Surg Pathol* 1996; **20**: 1412–7.
21 Mentzel T, Katencamp D. Intraneural angiosarcoma and angiosarcoma arising in benign and malignant peripheral nerve sheath tumours: clinicopathological and immunohistochemical analysis of four cases. *Histopathology* 1999; **35**: 114–20.
22 Morphopoulos GD, Banerjee SS, Ali HH *et al*. Malignant peripheral nerve sheath tumour with vascular differentiation: a report of four cases. *Histopathology* 1996; **28**: 401–10.
23 Marcon I, Collini P, Casanova M *et al*. Cutaneous angiosarcoma in a patient with xeroderma pigmentosum. *Pediatr Hematol Oncol* 2004; **21**: 23–6.
24 Folpe AL, Johnston CA, Weiss SW. Cutaneous angiosarcoma arising in a gouty tophus: report of a unique case and a review of foreign material-associated angiosarcoma. *Am J Dermatopathol* 2000; **22**: 418–21.
25 Ghandur-Mnaymneh L, Gonzales MS. Angiosarcoma of the penis with hepatic angiomas in a patient with low vinyl chloride exposure. *Cancer* 1981; **47**: 1318.
26 Ahmed I, Hamacher KL. Angiosarcoma in a chronically immunosuppressed renal transplant recipient: report of a case and review of the literature. *Am J Dermatopathol* 2002; **24**: 330–5.
27 Kantrow SM, Boyd AS. Primary cutaneous metaplastic carcinoma: report of a case involving angiosarcoma. *Am J Dermatopathol* 2007; **29**: 270–3.
28 Nake N, Ohsawa M, Tomita Y *et al*. Prognostic factors in angiosarcoma: a multivariate analysis of 55 cases. *J Surg Oncol* 1996; **61**: 170–6.
29 Wilson Jones E. Malignant vascular tumours. *Clin Exp Dermatol* 1976; **1**: 287–312.
30 Orchard GE, Zelger B, Wilson Jones E, Russell Jones R. An immunohistochemical assessment of 19 cases of angiosarcoma. *Histopathology* 1996; **28**: 235–40.
31 Hori Y. Malignant hemangioendothelioma of the skin. *J Dermatol Surg Oncol* 1981; **7**: 130–6.

32 Morgan MB, Swann M, Somach S *et al.* Cutaneous angiosarcoma: a case series with prognostic correlations. *J Am Acad Dermatol* 2004; **50**: 867–74.

33 Abraham JA, Hamicek FJ, Kaufman AM *et al.* Treatment and outcome of 82 patients with angiosarcoma. *Ann Surg Oncol* 2007; **14**: 1953–67.

34 Mendenhall WM, Mendenhall CM, Werning JW *et al.* Cutaneous angiosarcoma. *Am J Clin Oncol* 2006; **29**: 524–8.

35 Deyrup AT, McKenney JK, Tighiouart M *et al.* Sporadic cutaneous angiosarcomas: a proposal for risk stratification based on 69 cases. *Am J Surg Pathol* 2008; **32**: 72–7.

36 Wilson Jones E. Malignant angioendothelioma of the skin. *Br J Dermatol* 1964; **76**: 21–39.

37 Girard C, Johnson WC, Graham JH. Cutaneous angiosarcoma. *Cancer* 1970; **26**: 868–83.

38 Lydiatt WM, Shaha AR, Sha JP. Angiosarcoma of the head and neck. *Am J Surg* 1994; **168**: 451–4.

39 Hitchcock MG, Hurt MA, Santa Cruz DJ. Cutaneous granular cell angiosarcoma. *J Cutan Pathol* 1994; **21**: 256–62.

40 Brightman LA, Demierre MF, Byers HR. Macrophage-rich epithelioid angiosarcoma mimicking malignant melanoma. *J Cutan Pathol* 2006; **33**: 38–42.

41 Requena L, Santonja C, Stutz N *et al.* Pseudolymphomatous cutaneous angiosarcoma: a rare variant of cutaneous angiosarcoma readily mistaken for cutaneous lymphoma. *Am J Dermatopathol* 2007; **29**: 342–50.

42 Folpe AL, Chand EM, Goldblum JR *et al.* Expression of Fli-1, a nuclear transcription factor distinguishes vascular neoplasms from potential mimics. *Am J Surg Pathol* 2001; **25**: 1061–6.

43 Schuborg C, Mertens F, Rydholm A *et al.* Cytogenetic analysis of four angiosarcomas from deep and superficial soft tissue. *Cancer Genet Cytogenet* 1998; **100**: 52–6.

44 Kindblom LG, Stenman G, Angervall L. Morphological and cytogenetic studies of angiosarcoma in Stewart-Treves syndrome. *Virchows Arch A Pathol Anat Histopathol* 1991; **419**: 439–45.

45 Pawlik TM, Paulino AF, McGinn C *et al.* Cutaneous angiosarcoma of the scalp: a multidisciplinary approach. *Cancer* 2003; **98**: 1716–26.

Epithelioid haemangioendothelioma [1–3]

Definition. Epithelioid haemangioendothelioma is a distinctive tumour characterized by epithelioid endothelial cells arranged in strands or as individual units, in a myxoid or hyalinized stroma. It was initially described as a low-grade malignant tumour, but it has recently been proposed that it should be classified as a fully malignant neoplasm, in view of the associated morbidity and mortality [3]. However, small, primary cutaneous lesions appear to have an indolent behaviour.

Clinical features [1–3]. This tumour may occur in many internal organs, and it is more commonly seen in deeper soft tissues. Involvement of the skin may occur primarily or as a result of direct extension from a deep-seated primary. Less than 10% of cases occur primarily in the skin. Tumours present in middle-aged adults, with an equal sex incidence. Cutaneous tumours are usually small, but deeper lesions are often several centimetres in diameter. Pain is a frequent complaint, probably due to angiocentricity. Involvement of other organs, including the lung, liver and bone, may be seen in some cases, and it is not clear whether this represents multicentricity or metastatic spread.

Pathology [1–3]. The neoplasm is infiltrative and is composed of strands, cords and nests of endothelial cells in a hyaline or myxoid stroma. Dermal lesions often consist of a fairly well-defined nodule. The tumour cells have epithelioid morphology and consist of pink cytoplasm, vesicular nuclei and inconspicuous nucleoli.

Angiocentricity is commonly seen. Formation of vascular channels is not readily apparent but a common finding is the presence of intracytoplasmic vacuoles with or without red blood cells. A small number of cases display cytological atypia, which may be prominent, and a high mitotic count. There is no clear correlation between cytological grade and behaviour. Occasional tumours overlap with epithelioid angiosarcoma. Staining for endothelial cell markers, especially factor VIII-related antigen and CD31, is usually positive, and 20% of cases are focally positive for keratin [3,4].

Prognosis and treatment. Purely cutaneous tumours appear to have a benign behaviour, but there is some tendency for local recurrence. Deeper tumours have a recurrence rate of up to 15% and a mortality rate of 20%. Complete excision with clear margins is therefore necessary.

References

1 Weiss SW, Enzinger FM. Epithelioid hemangioendothelioma: a vascular tumor often mistaken for a carcinoma. *Cancer* 1982; **50**: 970–81.

2 Weiss SW, Ishak KG, Dail DH *et al.* Epithelioid hemangioendothelioma and related lesions. *Semin Diagn Pathol* 1986; **3**: 259–87.

3 Mentzel T, Beham A, Calonje E *et al.* Epithelioid hemangioendothelioma of skin and soft tissues: clinicopathologic and immunohistochemical study of 30 cases. *Am J Surg Pathol* 1997; **21**: 363–74.

4 Grey MH, Rosenberg AE, Dickersin GR *et al.* Cytokeratin expression in epithelioid vascular neoplasms. *Hum Pathol* 1990; **21**: 212–7.

Epithelioid angiosarcoma [1–3]

Definition. A distinctive variant of angiosarcoma composed almost exclusively of endothelial cells with an epithelioid morphology, often mimicking a carcinoma. This tumour represents the malignant end of the spectrum of tumours with epithelioid cell morphology.

Incidence. This is a rare tumour that mainly occurs in deep soft tissue, but that may present primarily in the skin or other organs.

Clinical features [1–3]. Cutaneous tumours present in young to middle-aged adults, mainly in males, with a predilection for the extremities. The typical presentation is that of solitary, or more rarely multiple, asymptomatic papules or nodules which are often haemorrhagic. It is not clear whether multiple lesions represent multifocality or metastatic disease. Occasional cases have been reported in association with a foreign body [4], radiotherapy [1] or an arteriovenous fistula [5]. Epithelioid angiosarcoma arising in another organ may present with cutaneous metastases [6].

Pathology [1–3]. Sheets of atypical epithelioid cells with abundant pink cytoplasm, vesicular nuclei and a single eosinophilic nucleolus occupy the dermis and/or subcutis. Haemorrhage and haemosiderin deposition is often seen. Formation of vascular channels is not readily apparent, and the main feature is the presence of intracytoplasmic vacuoles with or without red blood cells in variable numbers of tumour cells. Mitotic figures are common. Tumour cells are variably positive for vascular markers including

CD31, CD34, Fli-1 and von Willebrand factor. In 50% of cases, there is positivity for cytokeratin. Focal positivity for epithelial membrane antigen is also seen in some cases. Ordinary angiosarcomas such as those occurring on the head of elderly patients, those associated with radiotherapy and those associated with chronic lymphoedema may display focal areas with epithelioid endothelial cells. This is no reason to classify these tumours as epithelioid angiosarcomas.

Prognosis and treatment. Although it was initially suggested that cutaneous epithelioid angiosarcoma has a relatively good prognosis, this was based on only very few cases with limited follow-up [2]. Overall, the behaviour of these tumours appears to be aggressive, and complete excision and close follow-up are therefore indicated.

References
1 Fletcher CDM, Beham A, Bekir S *et al.* Epithelioid angiosarcoma of deep soft tissue: a distinctive tumor readily mistaken for an epithelial neoplasm. *Am J Surg Pathol* 1991; **15**: 915–24.
2 Marrogi AJ, Hunt SJ, Santa Cruz DJ. Cutaneous epithelioid angiosarcoma. *Am J Dermatopathol* 1990; **12**: 350–6.
3 Prescott RJ, Banerjee SS, Eyden BP *et al.* Cutaneous epithelioid angiosarcoma: a clinicopathological study of four cases. *Histopathology* 1994; **25**: 421–9.
4 Jennings TA, Peterson L, Axiotis CA *et al.* Angiosarcoma associated with foreign body material. *Cancer* 1988; **62**: 2436–44.
5 Byers RJ, McMahon RFT, Freemont AJ *et al.* Epithelioid angiosarcoma arising in an arteriovenous fistula. *Histopathology* 1992; **21**: 87–9.
6 Val-Bernal JF, Figols J, Arce FP *et al.* Cardiac epithelioid angiosarcoma presenting as cutaneous metastases. *J Cutan Pathol* 2001; **28**: 265–70.

Lymphatic tumours

Cavernous lymphangioma, cystic hygroma and lymphangioma circumscriptum are described in Chapter 48.

Progressive lymphangioma

Synonym
• Benign lymphangioendothelioma

Definition This is a benign dermal tumour composed of irregular, lymphatic channels dissecting between collagen bundles.

Clinical features [1–4]. Most cases present in middle-aged adults, but the age range is wide and children may be affected. The tumour presents as a slowly enlarging red macule, usually several centimetres in diameter with predilection for the limbs. Males are slightly more affected than females. Multiple lesions are exceptional [3].

Pathology [1–4]. Low-power examination reveals an ill-defined, often pan-dermal, proliferation of irregular, thin-walled lymphatic channels dissecting between collagen bundles. These channels tend to be orientated parallel to the epidermis and are lined by a single layer of bland endothelial cells. Involvement of the subcutaneous tissue is rare. Distinction from the lymphangiomatous variant of Kaposi's sarcoma is often very difficult, but in the former there are aggregates of inflammatory cells including plasma cells, and the cells lining the vascular channels are usually positive for HHV8. Distinction from a well-differentiated angiosarcoma is based on the absence of cytological atypia and mitotic figures.

Treatment. Excision is all that is required; there is no tendency for local recurrence.

References
1 Jones EW, Winkelmann RK, Zachary CB *et al.* Benign lymphangioendothelioma. *J Am Acad Dermatol* 1990; **23**: 229–35.
2 Mehregan DR, Mehregan AH, Mehregan DA. Benign lymphangioendothelioma: report of 2 cases. *J Cutan Pathol* 1992; **19**: 502–5.
3 Watanabe M, Kishiyama K, Ohkawara A. Acquired progressive lymphangioma. *J Am Acad Dermatol* 1983; **8**: 663–7.
4 Guillou L, Flecher CDM. Benign lymphangioendothelioma (acquired progressive lymphangioma), a lesion not to be confused with well-differentiated angiosarcoma and patch stage Kaposi's sarcoma: clinicopathologic analysis of a series. *Am J Surg Pathol* 2000; **24**: 1047–57.

Atypical vascular proliferation after radiotherapy [1–7]

Definition. Atypical vascular proliferation after radiotherapy (AVPR) defines a group of vascular lesions that occur months or years after radiotherapy—mainly, but not exclusively, after breast cancer. Lesions may also present after radiotherapy for ovarian and endometrial carcinoma.

Incidence and aetiology. These lesions are rare and there is a clear aetiological link with radiotherapy [1–7]. The demonstration of staining of the endothelial cells for lymphatic markers suggests a lymphatic line of differentiation. Although it has been suggested that AVPR represents part of a spectrum of lesions with post-radiation angiosarcomas [4], this view has recently been challenged in a study that stated that all lesions in this group are benign [7]. The problem with the latter study is that follow-up was limited.

Clinical features. AVPR presents a few years or months after radiotherapy for breast cancer (by comparison, post-irradiation angiosarcomas usually but not always tend to present many years after radiotherapy) [1–3]. The clinical lesions are not distinctive and vary from macules to papules. Occasional cases may mimic lymphangioma circumscriptum. As mentioned before, it is controversial whether these lesions are uniformly benign or whether they overlap with radiation-induced angiosarcoma.

Pathology. Irregular lymphatic-like vascular channels, lined by a single layer of endothelial cells, are seen in the dermis and may be multifocal. The endothelial cells are flat or have a hobnail appearance, and papillary projections can also be found. Careful examination of multiple sections is recommended to make sure that there are no mitotic figures or cytological atypia, as distinction from a well-differentiated angiosarcoma can be very difficult.

Treatment. Complete conservative excision of these lesions with close follow-up is recommended.

References

1 Fineberg S, Rosen PP. Cutaneous angiosarcoma and atypical vascular lesion of the skin and breast after radiation therapy for breast carcinoma. *Am J Clin Pathol* 1994; **102**: 757–63.

2 Díaz-Cascajo C, Borghi S, Weyers W *et al*. Benign lymphangiomatous papules of the skin after radiotherapy: a report of five new cases and review of the literature. *Histopathology* 1999; **35**: 319–27.

3 Requena L, Kutzner H, Mentzel T *et al*. Benign vascular proliferations in irradiated skin. *Am J Surg Pathol* 2002; **26**: 328–37.

4 Brenn T, Fletcher CD. Radiation-induced cutaneous atypical vascular lesions and angiosarcoma: clinicopathologic analysis of 42 cases. *Am J Surg Pathol* 2005; **29**: 983–96.

5 Brenn T, Fletcher CD. Post-radiation vascular proliferation: an increasing problem. *Histopathology* 2006; **48**: 106.

6 Mattoch IW, Robbins JB, Kempson RL *et al*. Post-radiotherapy vascular proliferations in mammary skin: a clinicopathologic study of 11 cases. *J Am Acad Dermatol* 2007; **57**: 126–33.

7 Gengler C, Coindre JM, Leroux A *et al*. Vascular proliferations of the skin after radiation therapy for breast cancer: clinicopathologic analysis of a series in favour of a benign process: a study from the French Sarcoma Group. *Cancer* 2007; **109**: 1584–98.

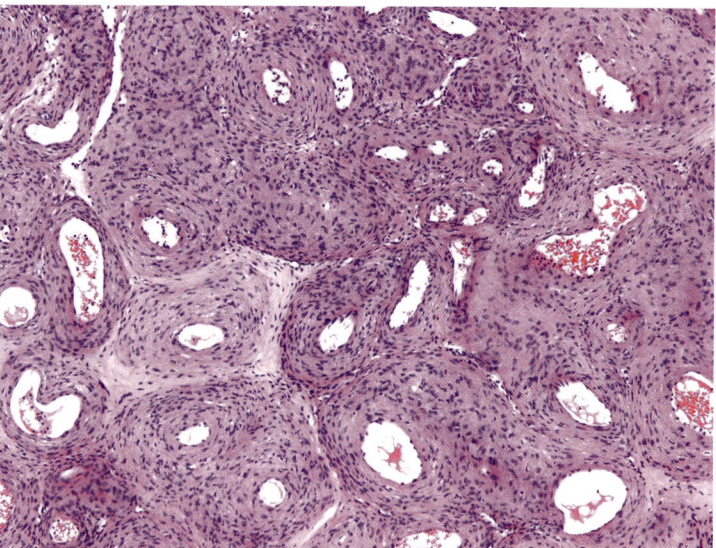

Fig. 56.30 Numerous vascular channels surrounded by layers of pericytes in an onion ring distribution in a case of myopericytoma.

Tumours of perivascular cells

Myopericytoma

Definition. For many years, tumours thought to differentiate towards pericytes (perivascular myoid cells) were divided into two main categories: infantile hemangiopericytoma and adult hemangiopericytoma. Both variants, however, appear to have very little in common except for the histological presence of a pericytomatous pattern characterized by elongated, branching thin-walled vascular spaces with a stag-horn pattern. With the combination of immunohistochemistry and electron microscopy, most tumours previously classified as adult hemangiopericytoma on light microscopy represent other tumours, including synovial sarcoma, mesenchymal chondrosarcoma and solitary fibrous tumour [1]. In very few cases the line of differentiation remains obscure, and these represent the 'true' adult hemangiopericytomas. They are more likely to arise from an undifferentiated mesenchymal cell than from a pericyte. 'True' adult hemangiopericytomas do not usually occur in the skin and will not be discussed further here.

The concept of myopericytoma was introduced to describe a group of lesions characterized by short, oval to spindle-shaped myofibroblasts and a characteristic concentric perivascular growth [2]. Tumours tend to be mainly deep dermal and subcutaneous and include lesions classified in the past as glomangiopericytoma, myopericytoma, myofibroma and myofibromatosis in adults. Infantile hemangiopericytoma and infantile myofibromatosis represent identical conditions and the former term has been abandoned.

Infantile myofibroma/myofibromatosis has already been described in the section on myofibroblastic tumours (p. 56.9).

Clinical features. Myopericytoma is relatively rare and presents mainly in middle-aged adults with a predilection for the limbs, especially the distal lower limb. Lesions are small (no more than 2 cm in diameter), long-standing, usually asymptomatic and may be solitary or, rarely, multiple [2–4]. Exceptionally they are painful. In the setting of multiple myopericytomas, these often develop simultaneously with a predilection for a single anatomic site. Very rarely, malignant examples of myopericytoma have been reported [5].

Pathology. The histological spectrum of myopericytoma is wide and varies from lesions that are very similar to myofibromatosis (p. 56.9), to tumours that closely resemble glomus tumours and even to angioleiomyoma. Lesions are well circumscribed and composed of a mixture of solid cellular areas intermixed with variable numbers of vascular channels. The later are often elongated and display prominent branching resulting in a stag-horn appearance (hemangiopericytoma-like). The cells in the solid areas are bland, round or short and spindle-shaped with eosinophilic or amphophilic cytoplasm and vesicular nuclei. Mitotic figures are exceptional. A common feature is the presence of concentric layers of tumour cells around vascular channels resulting in a typical onion ring appearance (Fig. 56.30). Myxoid change may be focally prominent. Occasional findings include hyalinization, cystic degeneration and bone formation. Nodules of tumour cells may protrude into the lumina of vascular channels. Rare examples are entirely intravascular [6]. In some cases, tumour cells closely resemble glomus cells and are characterized by round punched-out central nuclei and pale eosinophilic cytoplasm. These cases are referred to as glomangiopericytomas. Tumour cells are positive for smooth-muscle actin and in most cases negative for desmin.

References

1 Fletcher CDM. Haemangiopericytoma: a dying breed? Reappraisal of an entity and its variants. *Curr Diagn Pathol* 1994; **1**: 19–25.

2 Granter SR, Badizadegan K, Fletcher CD. Myofibromatosis in adults, glomangiopericytoma, and myopericytoma: a spectrum of tumors showing perivascular myoid differentiation. *Am J Surg Pathol* 1998; **22**: 513–25.

3 Dray MS, McCarthy SW, Palmer AA *et al*. Myopericytoma: a unifying term for a spectrum of tumors that show overlapping features with myofibroma. A review of 14 cases. *J Clin Pathol* 2006; **59**: 67–73.

4 Mentzel T, Dei Tos AP, Sapi Z *et al.* Myopericytoma of skin and soft tissues: clinicopathologic and immunohistochemical study of 54 cases. *Am J Surg Pathol* 2006; **30**: 104–13.

5 McMenamin ME, Fletcher CDM. Malignant myopericytoma: expanding the spectrum of tumors with myopericytic differentiation. *Histopathology* 2002; **41**: 450–60.

6 McMenamin ME, Calonje E. Intravascular myopericytoma. *J Cutan Pathol* 2002; **29**: 557–61.

Glomus tumour [1–3]

Synonyms
- Glomangioma
- Glomangiomyoma

Definition. A tumour of the myoarterial glomus, composed of vascular channels surrounded by proliferating glomus cells. The tumours have variable quantities of glomus cells, blood vessels and smooth muscle. According to this finding, they are classified as either solid glomus tumour, glomangioma or glomangiomyoma.

Incidence and aetiology. Glomus tumours are comparatively uncommon. Some are present at birth; they rarely appear during infancy, but from the age of 7 years onwards the incidence increases gradually. There may be a history of trauma preceding the tumour. Multiple tumours are 10 times more frequent in children than in adults [3,4]. The occurrence of familial cases with autosomal dominant inheritance [1,5,6], and the association of multiple tumours with malformation of the same limb, suggests involvement of genetic factors. This theory has been confirmed by the identification of the *glomulin* gene for multiple inherited glomangiomas (also known as glomuvenous malformations [7]) at chromosome 1p21-22 [8–10].

Clinical features. A solitary glomus tumour is a pink or purple nodule varying in size from 1 to 20 mm; it is conspicuously painful (Fig. 56.31). Pain may be provoked by direct pressure or a change in skin temperature, or may be spontaneous. There is an equal sex incidence; adults present mainly during the third or fourth decades of life. The commonest site is the hands, particularly the fingers, followed by other sites on the extremities including the head, neck and penis [11]. Tumours beneath the nail are particularly painful, and patients present for treatment while the lesions are still very small. The affected nail has a bluish-red flush. An association between subungual glomus tumour and neurofibromatosis type 1 has been reported [12]. Glomus tumours may also involve internal organs.

Multiple glomus tumours are larger and usually dark blue in colour, and are situated deep in the dermis. They are less restricted to the extremities, may be widely scattered and are not usually painful [13–16]. In some cases, grouped multiple tumours may be painful, and pain, intermittent discoloration and sweating of a limb may precede the development of a palpable tumour.

Pathology. The tumour is lobulated, well-circumscribed and situated in the dermis. The proportion of glomus cells to vascular spaces varies. The smaller, painful lesions tend to be mainly

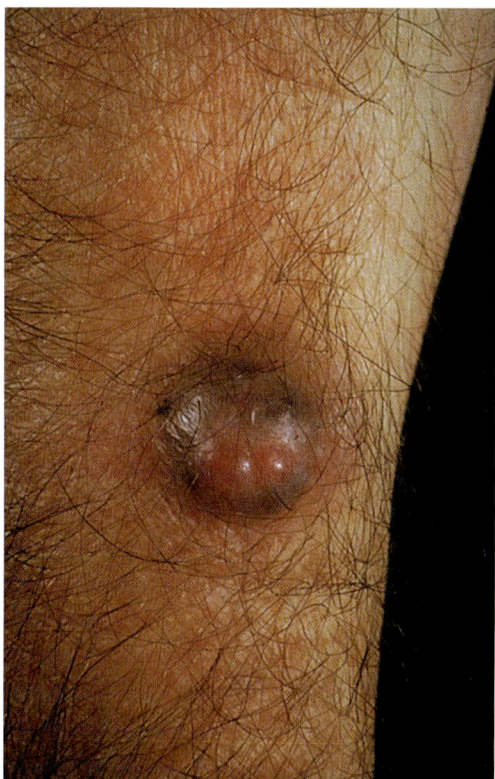

Fig. 56.31 Clinical appearance of a glomus tumour.

cellular. The larger, multiple and often painless lesions are angiomatous, with only a band of cells around the dilated vascular channels. The glomus cell is cuboidal, with a well-marked cell membrane and a round central nucleus. The cells align themselves in rows around the single layer of endothelial cells of the vascular spaces and in a somewhat less orderly fashion further out. Numerous, non-myelinated nerve fibres course through the cellular masses. More than 50% of tumours can be classified as glomangiomas, and a minority (less than 15%) are classified as glomangiomyomas (Fig. 56.32). Electron microscopy [17–19] suggests that glomus cells are transversely cut smooth muscle cells and that there are many mast cells around the tumour, but that nerve fibres are not associated with the glomus cells. Tumour cells are universally positive for smooth muscle actin and are usually negative for desmin. Positivity for CD34 may be seen [20]. An oncocytic variant has been described [21], and also variants developing within a cutaneous nerve [22] and within a vein [23]. Malignant glomus tumour (glomangiosarcoma) is exceedingly rare. Even tumours that are histologically malignant rarely metastasize, but they have a potential for local recurrence [24,25].

Diagnosis. The solitary tumour is to be distinguished from other painful tumours such as leiomyoma and eccrine spiradenoma. Distinction is usually only possible on histological examination. The multiple glomangioma may be indistinguishable clinically from a cavernous haemangioma, and is possibly identical to 'blue rubber bleb' naevus [5].

Treatment. Surgical excision is usually curative. Local recurrence is very rare and occurs mainly after incomplete excision. Most

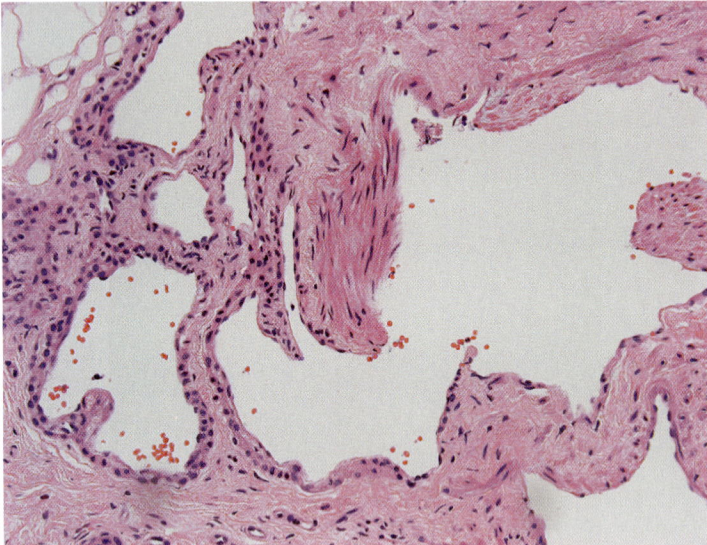

Fig. 56.32 A typical case of glomangiomyoma displaying vascular channels, smooth muscle and thin layers of glomus cells.

recurrences are seen in deeper lesions with an infiltrative growth pattern. These lesions have been described as infiltrating glomus tumours [24].

References

1 Carroll RE, Berman AT. Glomus tumors of the hand: review of the literature and report on twenty-eight cases. *J Bone Joint Surg* 1972; **54A**: 691–703.
2 Anagnostou GD, Papademetriou DG, Toumazani MN. Subcutaneous glomus tumors. *Surg Gynecol Obstet* 1973; **136**: 945–50.
3 Kohout E, Stout AP. The glomus tumor in children. *Cancer* 1961; **14**: 555–66.
4 Sluiter JT, Postma C. Multiple glomus tumours of the skin. *Acta Derm Venereol (Stockh)* 1959; **39**: 98–107.
5 De Sablet M, Mascaro JM. Tumeurs glomiques multiples et blue rubber bleb naevus. *Ann Dermatol Syphiligr* 1967; **94**: 35–46.
6 Touraine A, Renault P. Tumeurs glomiques multiples du tronc et des membres. *Bull Soc Franc Dermatol Syphiligr* 1936; **43**: 736–40.
7 Henning JS, Kovich OI, Schaffer JV. Glomuvenous malformations. *Dermatol Online J* 2007; **13**: 17.
8 Boon LM, Brouillard P, Irrthum A *et al*. A gene for inherited cutaneous venous anomalies ('glomangiomas') localizes to chromosome 1p21-22. *Am J Hum Genet* 1999; **65**: 125–33.
9 Calvert JT, Burns S, Riney TJ *et al*. Additional glomangioma family link to chromosome 1p: no evidence for genetic heterogeneity. *Hum Hered* 2001; **51**: 180.
10 Brouillard P, Boon LM, Mulliken JB *et al*. Mutations in a novel factor, glomulin, are responsible for glomuvenous malformations ('glomangiomas'). *Am J Hum Genet* 2002; **70**: 866–74.
11 Schiefer TK, Parker WL, Anakwenze OA *et al*. Extradigital glomus tumors: a 20-year experience. *Mayo Clin Proc* 2006; **81**: 1337–44.
12 Sawada S, Honda M, Kamide R *et al*. Three cases of subungual glomus tumors with von Recklinghausen neurofibromatosis. *J Am Acad Dermatol* 1995; **32**: 277–8.
13 Chevrant-Breton J, Dunn JE, Laudren A. Multiple glomus tumors associated with multiple neoplasias. *Dermatologica* 1984; **168**: 290–2.
14 Goodman TF, Abele DC. Multiple glomus tumours. *Arch Dermatol* 1971; **103**: 11–23.
15 Gorlin RJ, Fusaro RM, Benton JW. Multiple glomus tumour of the pseudocavernous hemangioma type. *Arch Dermatol* 1960; **8**: 776–8.
16 Rycroft RJG, Menter MA, Sharvill DE *et al*. Hereditary multiple glomus tumours. *Trans St John's Hosp Dermatol Soc Lond* 1975; **61**: 70–81.
17 Tarnowski WM, Hashimoto K. Multiple glomus tumors: an ultrastructural study. *J Invest Dermatol* 1969; **52**: 474–8.
18 Tsuneyoshi M, Enjoji M. Glomus tumour. *Cancer* 1982; **50**: 1601–7.
19 Venkatachalam MA, Greally JG. Fine structure of glomus tumor: similarity of glomus cells to smooth muscle. *Cancer* 1969; **23**: 1176–84.
20 Mentzel T, Hugel H, Kutzner H. CD34-positive glomus tumor: clinicopathologic and immunohistochemical analysis of six cases with myxoid stromal changes. *J Cutan Pathol* 2002; **29**: 421–5.
21 Slater DN, Cotton DWK, Azzopardi JG. Oncocytic glomus tumour: a new variant? *Histopathology* 1987; **11**: 523–31.
22 Calonje E, Fletcher CDM. Cutaneous intraneural glomus tumour. *Am J Dermatopathol* 1995; **17**: 395–8.
23 Beham A, Fletcher CDM. Intravascular glomus tumour: a previously undescribed phenomenon. *Virchows Arch (A) Pathol Anat Histol* 1991; **418**: 175–7.
24 Gould EW, Manivel JC, Albores-Saavedra J *et al*. Locally infiltrative glomus tumors and glomangiosarcoma: a clinical, ultrastructural and immunohistochemical study. *Cancer* 1990; **65**: 310–8.
25 Folpe AL, Fanburgh-Smith JC, Miettinen M *et al*. Atypical glomus tumors: analysis of 52 cases, with a proposal for the reclassification of glomus tumors. *Am J Surg Pathol* 2001; **25**: 1–12.

Peripheral neuroectodermal tumours

Reviews of neural tumours may be found in [1–4].

References

1 Argenyi ZB. Cutaneous neural heterotopias and related tumours relevant for the dermatopathologist. *Semin Diagn Pathol* 1996; **13**: 60–71.
2 Weiss SW, Goldblum JR. *Enziger and Weiss's Soft Tissue Tumors*, 5th edn. St Louis: Mosby, 2007: 1111–264.
3 Reed RJ. Cutaneous manifestation of neural crest disorders. *Int J Dermatol* 1977; **16**: 807–26.
4 Requena L, Sangueza OP. Benign neoplasms with neural differentiation. *Am J Dermatopathol* 1995; **17**: 75–96.

Neuromuscular hamartoma [1,2]

Synonym
- Triton tumour

Definition. These lesions appear to be combined hamartomas of both muscular and neural tissue.

Clinical features. The clinical appearance is of a subcutaneous mass.

Pathology. Multinodular masses of skeletal muscle are mixed with both myelinated and unmyelinated nerve fibres. Malignant triton tumours, composed of a mixture of schwannoma-like material and rhabdomyosarcoma, are very much commoner than the benign variety of triton tumour.

Management. Surgical excision is required.

References

1 Louhimo I, Rapola J. Intraneural muscular hamartoma: report of two cases in small children. *J Pediatr Surg* 1972; **7**: 696–9.
2 Markel SF, Enzinger FM. Neuromuscular hamartoma: a benign 'triton tumor' composed of mature neural and striated muscle elements. *Cancer* 1982; **49**: 140–4.

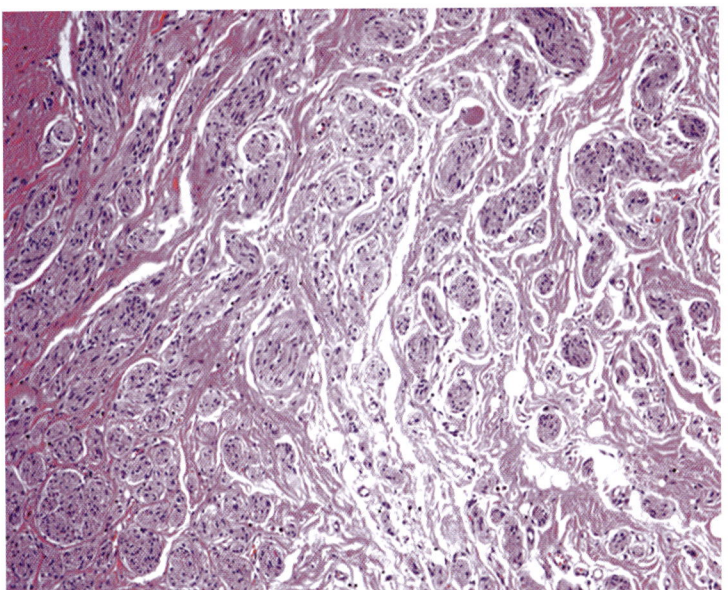

Fig. 56.33 Histological appearance of an amputation neuroma. Small nerves proliferate in the dermis in a background of fibrosis.

Multiple mucosal neuromas [1]

Synonym
- Sipple's syndrome

In Sipple's syndrome, multiple neuromas of the oral mucosa may be associated with phaeochromocytoma, parafollicular thyroid cysts secreting calcitonin, medullary thyroid carcinoma and opaque nerve fibres on the cornea (Chapters 15 and 62).

Reference
1 Gorlin RJ, Sedano HO, Vickers RA *et al.* Multiple mucosal neuromas, pheochromocytoma and medullary carcinoma of the thyroid: a syndrome. *Cancer* 1968; **22**: 293–9.

Amputation stump neuroma [1]

Synonym
- Traumatic neuroma

Definition. This is a benign response of nerve tissue to injury.

Clinical features. A small, tender nodule is found in a scar site.

Pathology. Foci of proliferating nerve tissue surrounded by scar tissue are typically seen (Fig. 56.33). Accessory digits may show a very similar pattern of tissue involvement.

Management. Surgical excision is usually required. The problem can be prevented by apposing ends of nerves at sites of injury.

Reference
1 Cieslak AK, Stout AP. Traumatic and amputation neuromas. *Arch Surg* 1946; **53**: 646–51.

Morton's neuroma [1,2]

Synonym
- Morton's metatarsalgia

Definition. This is the result of damage to the plantar digital nerve, followed by fibrosis. The condition has been associated with the use of high-heeled footwear.

Clinical features. It is most common in women, who complain of severe pain, usually between the third and fourth metatarsals, especially when walking.

Pathology. On pathological examination, there is very prominent perineurial, endoneurial and epineurial fibrosis. Perivascular fibrosis and intimal thickening are also seen.

Management. Excision is the recommended therapy and is curative.

References
1 Lassmann G, Lassmann H, Stockinger L. Morton's metatarsalgia: light and electron microscopic observations and their relation to entrapment neuropathies. *Virchows Arch (A)* 1976; **370**: 307–21.
2 Meachim G, Abberton MJ. Histological findings in Morton's metatarsalgia. *J Pathol* 1971; **103**: 209–17.

Solitary circumscribed neuroma

Synonym
- Palisaded encapsulated neuroma

Definition. This is a distinctive variant of cutaneous neuroma composed of variable proportions of the normal components of nerve tissue.

Clinical features [1–3]. It is fairly common and presents mainly on the face of adults as a small, asymptomatic papule, which may resemble a naevus. There is an equal sex incidence.

Pathology [1–3]. Examination reveals a well-circumscribed, partially encapsulated dermal nodule (Fig. 56.34), often associated with a nerve in the deep dermis. It is composed of uniform cells with pink cytoplasm in a collagenous background and with artefactual clefting between bundles. The capsule displays epithelial membrane antigen-positive perineurial cells. Most of the cells within the nodule are S100-positive, and special stains may demonstrate axons.

Treatment. Simple excision is curative.

References
1 Reed RJ, Fine RM, Meltzer HD. Palisaded, encapsulated neuromas of the skin. *Arch Dermatol* 1972; **106**: 865–70.
2 Fletcher CDM. Solitary circumscribed neuroma of the skin (so-called palisaded, encapsulated neuroma): a clinicopathologic and immunohistochemical study. *Am J Surg Pathol* 1989; **13**: 574–80.

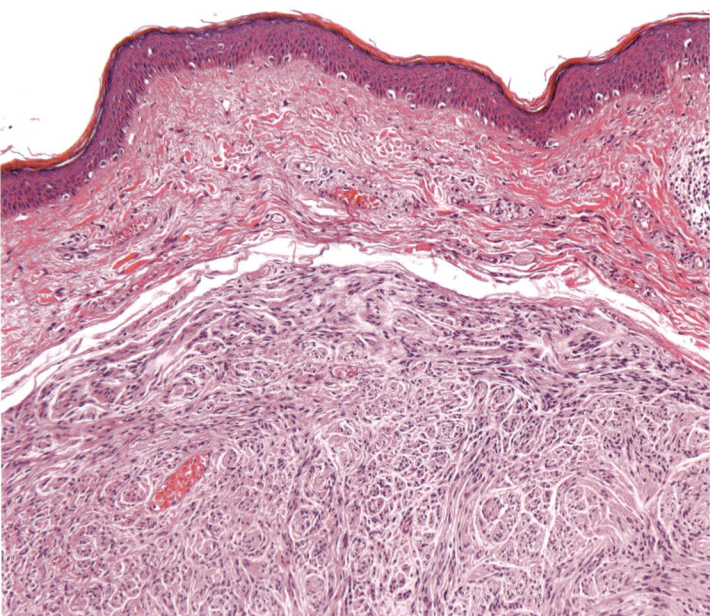

Fig. 56.34 Sharply demarcated dermal nodule in a case of solitary circumscribed neuroma.

3 Dover JS, From L, Lewis A. Palisaded encapsulated neuromas: a clinicopathologic study. *Arch Dermatol* 1989; **125**: 386–9.

Schwannoma

Synonym
- Neurilemmoma

Definition. A tumour of nerve sheaths composed of Schwann cells.

Incidence. The tumour is relatively rare in the skin and relatively uncommon in other sites including soft tissues. It arises most frequently from the acoustic nerve. Bilateral acoustic schwannomas are characteristic of neurofibromatosis type 2. A further manifestation of the latter is the occurrence of multiple cutaneous plexiform schwannomas [1]. There is no association with neurofibromatosis type 1. In the peripheral nervous system, it is usually found in association with one of the main nerves of the limbs, usually on the flexor aspect near the elbow, wrist or knee, the hands or the head and neck [2]. It may be seen on the tongue. Other sites include the wall of the gastrointestinal tract and the posterior mediastinum. It may occur at any age, but is most common in the fourth and fifth decades. Females are affected more often than males [3].

Clinical features [4]. They are rounded or ovoid, circumscribed nodules varying in size up to 5 cm, usually firm (but sometimes soft and cystic) in consistency, and sometimes painful. The colour is pink-grey or yellowish. Small lesions may be intradermal, but larger ones are subcutaneous. They usually grow slowly. Malignant transformation of a schwannoma is exceedingly rare and may contain areas of epithelioid angiosarcoma [5–7].

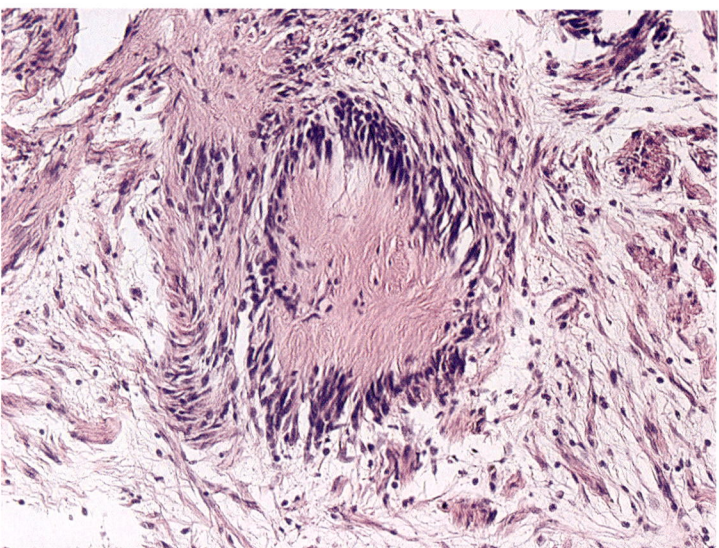

Fig. 56.35 Typical Verocay body in a case of schwannoma.

Pathology [2,8]. The tumour is rounded, circumscribed and encapsulated. It is situated in the course of a nerve, usually in the subcutaneous fat. The cells are spindle shaped with poorly defined cytoplasm and elongated, wavy, basophilic nuclei. Variable amounts of collagen are seen in the background. Cells are arranged in bands, which stream and interweave. The nuclei display palisading and are arranged in parallel rows with intervening eosinophilic cytoplasm in a typical appearance known as Verocay bodies (Fig. 56.35). Cellular areas known as Antoni A areas are intermixed with areas showing prominent myxoid change known as Antoni B areas [9]. The latter areas are likely to be the result of degeneration. In some tumours, there is mucous secretion, producing a vacuolated stroma. Scattered mononuclear inflammatory cells are often seen. In some cases, the nerve of origin may be found associated with the capsule. Electron microscopy shows that tumour cells have typical features of Schwann cells [10]. S100 protein staining is strong and uniform [11]. For many years it was thought that schwannomas lack axons and this was regarded as a useful way in distinguishing these tumours from neurofibromas which contain variable numbers of axons. The presence of the latter is demonstrated by immunostaining for neurofilaments. This view, however, has been challenged recently as both hereditary and sporadic schwannomas may contain axons, suggesting that both entities may in fact be more closely related than previously thought [12]. This explains the rare occurrence of hybrid lesions combining features of neurofibroma and schwannoma [13].

There are several variants of schwannoma, which may be confused histologically with other benign or malignant tumours.

Ancient schwannoma [14] often occurs in a deep location and is characterized by prominent degenerative changes, which often result in cytological atypia. Ectatic blood vessels, haemorrhage, haemosiderin deposition and focal inflammation consisting of lymphocytes are often seen. There is loss of Antoni A areas, which makes histological diagnosis difficult.

Cellular schwannoma [15] also tends to have a predilection for deep soft tissues. It is characterized by high cellularity, with almost complete absence of Antoni B areas. This, coupled with the presence of mitotic figures, often leads to a misdiagnosis of malignancy [16]. A multinodular plexiform variant may occur in children and some examples are congenital.

Plexiform schwannoma [17,18] tends to occur in younger patients, may be painful and has a predilection for the dermis. Multiple cellular nodules composed of bland Schwann cells are seen in the dermis. Distinction from plexiform neurofibroma is important, as these tumours are not usually associated with neurofibromatosis type 1. Multiple cutaneous plexiform schwannomas, however, are associated with neurofibromatosis type 2 [1,19].

Melanotic schwannoma [20] only exceptionally occurs in the skin; it has a predilection for spinal nerve roots. Tumour cells are epithelioid and melanin pigment is prominent. The importance of this variant is that they are capable of malignant behaviour and may be a marker of Carney complex (Chapter 62).

Pacinian schwannoma is a rare variant composed of structures closely resembling the Pacinian corpuscles.

Neuroblastoma-like schwannoma is very rare and characterized histologically by areas composed of round, blue, small Schwann cells which may form perivascular rosettes or rosettes with collagenous cores [21]. The tumour in other areas has the typical appearance of a schwannoma and the immunohistochemical profile is typical of the latter.

Epithelioid schwannoma is an infrequent type of schwannoma composed predominantly of cells with epithelioid morphology [22]. However, although these tumours are positive for S-100 protein, they lack palisading, are composed of uniform tumour cells and contain a population of CD34-positive cells. It has therefore been proposed that these lesions do not represent classical examples of schwannomas [23].

Glandular schwannoma [24,25] represents in most cases an ordinary schwannoma with entrapment of normal sweat glands.

Diagnosis. Of the various nodular dermal and hypodermal tumours, schwannoma is most likely to be mistaken for a glomus tumour when painful, and for a lipoma, epidermoid cyst, synovial ganglion, juxta-articular node or neurofibroma when asymptomatic. The diagnosis can be suspected when it is in the course of a nerve; otherwise, histological examination is necessary.

Treatment. Simple excision is curative.

References
1 Miyakawa T, Kamada N, Kobayashi T *et al*. Neurofibromatosis type 2 in an infant with multiple plexiform schwannomas as first symptom. *J Dermatol* 2007; **34**: 60–4.
2 Stout AP. The peripheral manifestations of the specific nerve sheath tumour (neurilemmoma). *Am J Cancer* 1935; **24**: 751–96.
3 Das Gupta TK, Brasfield RD, Strong EW *et al*. Benign solitary schwannomas (neurilemmomas). *Cancer* 1969; **24**: 355–66.
4 Mercantini ES, Mopper C. Neurilemmoma of the tongue. *AMA Arch Dermatol* 1959; **79**: 542–4.
5 Woodruff JM, Selig AM, Crowley K *et al*. Schwannoma (neurilemmoma) with malignant transformation: a rare, distinctive peripheral nerve tumor. *Am J Surg Pathol* 1994; **18**: 882–95.
6 Trassard M, Le Doussal V, Bui BN *et al*. Angiosarcoma arising in a solitary schwannoma (neurilemoma) of the sciatic nerve. *Am J Surg Pathol* 1996; **20**: 1412–7.
7 McMenamin ME, Fletcher CD. Expanding the spectrum of malignant change in schwannomas: epithelioid malignant change, epithelioid malignant peripheral nerve sheath tumor, and epithelioid angiosarcoma: a study of 17 cases. *Am J Surg Pathol* 2001; **25**: 13–25.
8 Geschikler CF. Tumours of the peripheral nerves. *Am J Cancer* 1935; **25**: 377–89.
9 Sian CS, Ryan SF. The ultrastructure of neurilemmoma with emphasis on Antoni B tissue. *Hum Pathol* 1981; **12**: 145–52.
10 Waggener JD. Ultrastructure of benign peripheral nerve sheath tumors. *Cancer* 1966; **19**: 699–709.
11 Weiss SW, Langloss JM, Enzinger F. The role of the S100 protein in the diagnosis of soft tissue tumours with particular reference to benign and malignant Schwann cell tumours. *Lab Invest* 1983; **49**: 299–304.
12 Nascimento AF, Fletcher CD. The controversial nosology of benign nerve sheath tumors: neurofilament protein demonstrates intratumoral axons in many sporadic schwannomas. *Am J Surg Pathol* 2007; **31**: 1363–70.
13 Feany MB, Anthony DC, Fletcher CD. Nerve sheath tumours with hybrid features of neurofibroma and schwannoma: a conceptual challenge. *Histopathology* 1998; **32**: 405–10.
14 Dahl I. Ancient neurilemmoma (schwannoma). *Acta Pathol Microbiol Scand A* 1977; **85**: 812–8.
15 White WM, Shiu MH, Rosenblum MK *et al*. Cellular schwannoma: a clinicopathologic study of 57 patients and 58 tumors. *Cancer* 1990; **66**: 1266–75.
16 Woodruff JM, Scheithauer BW, Kurtkaya-Yapicier O *et al*. Congenital and childhood plexiform (multinodular) cellular schwannoma: a troublesome mimic of malignant peripheral nerve sheath tumor. *Am J Surg Pathol* 2003; **27**: 1321–9.
17 Fletcher CDM, Davies SE. Benign plexiform (multinodular) schwannoma: a rare tumour unassociated with neurofibromatosis. *Histopathology* 1986; **10**: 971–80.
18 Kao GF, Laskin WB, Olson TG. Solitary cutaneous plexiform neurilemmoma (schwannoma): a clinicopathologic, immunohistochemical and ultrastructural study of 11 cases. *Mod Pathol* 1989; **2**: 20–6.
19 Lim HS, Jung J, Chung KY. Neurofibromatosis type 2 with multiple plexiform schwannomas. *Int J Dermatol* 2004; **43**: 336–40.
20 Carney JA. Psammomatous melanotic schwannoma: a distinctive heritable tumor with special associations including cardiac myxoma and the Cushing syndrome. *Am J Surg Pathol* 1990; **14**: 206–22.
21 Goldblum JR, Beals TF, Weiss SW. Neuroblastoma-like neurilemmoma. *Am J Surg Pathol* 1994; **18**: 266–73.
22 Smith K, Mezebish D, Williams JP *et al*. Cutaneous epithelioid schwannomas: a rare variant of a benign peripheral nerve sheath tumor. *J Cutan Pathol* 1998; **25**: 50–5.
23 Laskin WB, Fetsch JF, Lasota J *et al*. Benign epithelioid peripheral nerve sheath tumors of the soft tissues: clinicopathologic spectrum of 33 cases. *Am J Surg Pathol* 2005; **29**: 39–51.
24 Brooks JJ, Draffen RM. Benign glandular schwannoma. *Arch Pathol Lab Med* 1992; **116**: 192–5.
25 Deng A, Petrali J, Jaffe D *et al*. Benign cutaneous pseudoglandular schwannoma: a case report. *Am J Dermatopathol* 2005; **27**: 432–5.

Solitary neurofibroma [1–4]

Definition. An isolated lesion probably arising from the endoneurium and composed of a mixture of Schwann cells, fibroblasts and perineurial fibroblasts. It is not related to neurofibromatosis type 1. Although it appears to be hamartomatous in nature, the demonstration of clonality suggests a neoplastic origin [5].

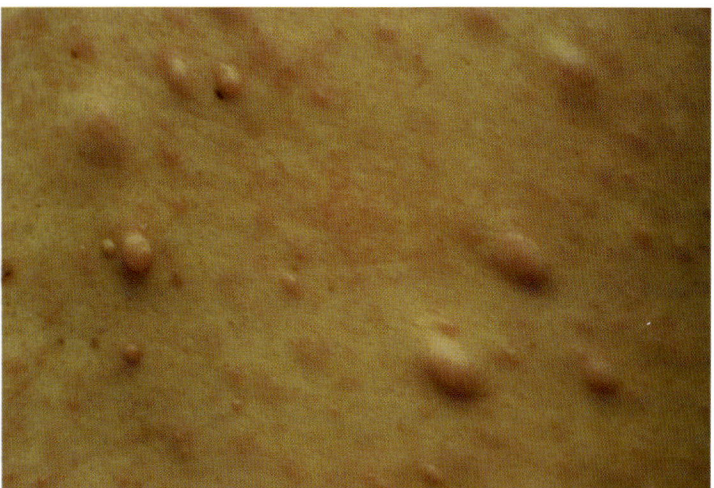

Fig. 56.36 Multiple soft papules, typical of neurofibroma in a patient with neurofibromatosis type 1.

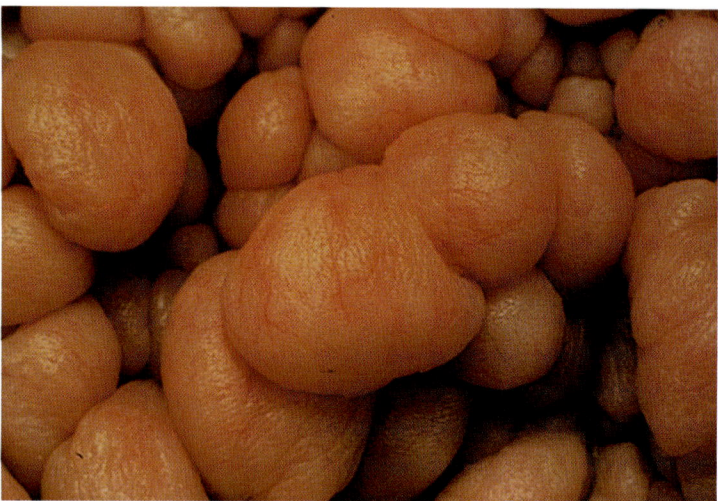

Fig. 56.37 Clinical appearance of a plexiform neurofibroma.

Clinical features. Both sexes and any body site may be affected. It usually appears during the third decade as a slow-growing, small, polypoid lesion. Multiple neurofibromas are rare outside the setting of neurofibromatosis type 1 (Fig. 56.36).

Simple excision is curative. Malignant change is said not to occur outside the setting of neurofibromatosis type 1.

Pathology. These lesions differ from neurilemmomas in that they do not have a capsule, they are only focally positive for S100 protein, and they do not usually have well-defined Antoni A and Antoni B areas. Instead, they are composed of bland, spindle-shaped cells with wavy nuclei in a myxoid or collagenous stroma. Mast cells are usually prominent. Degenerative changes are sometimes seen but mitotic activity is absent. Less than 50% of the cells in these lesions are S100-positive. There is also focal positivity for CD34 and epithelial membrane antigen (EMA).

Several histological variants of neurofibroma have been described, including epithelioid neurofibroma, granular cell neurofibroma, pigmented neurofibroma [6] and a variant with dendritic cells and pseudorosettes [3,7].

Cytogenetic analysis in a single case of solitary neurofibroma has found a reciprocal translocation t(4;9)(q31;p22) [8].

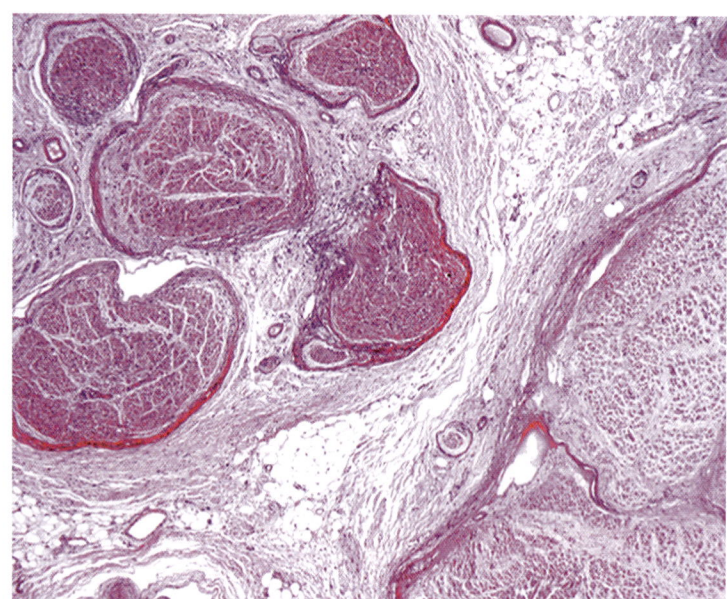

Fig. 56.38 Irregular, poorly formed nerves in a plexiform neurofibroma.

References

1 Geschikler CF. Tumours of the peripheral nerves. *Am J Cancer* 1935; **25**: 377–89.
2 Reed RJ. Cutaneous manifestations of neural crest disorders (neurocristopathies). *Int J Dermatol* 1977; **16**: 807–26.
3 Megahed M. Histopathological variants of neurofibroma: a study of 114 lesions. *Am J Dermatopathol* 1994; **16**: 486–95.
4 Erlandson RA. Peripheral nerve sheath tumors. *Ultrastruct Pathol* 1985; **9**: 113–22.
5 Colman DS, Williams CA, Wallace MR. Benign neurofibromas in type 1 neurofibromatosis (NF1) show somatic deletions of the NF1 gene. *Nature Genet* 1995; **11**: 90–2.
6 Fetsch JF, Michal M, Mietinnen M. Pigmented (melanotic) neurofibroma: a clinicopathologic and immunohistochemical analysis of 19 lesions from 17 patients. *Am J Surg Pathol* 2000; **24**: 331–43.
7 Michal M, Fanburg-Smith JC, Mentzel T *et al*. Dendritic cell neurofibroma with pseudorosettes: a report of 18 cases of a distinct and hitherto unrecognized neurofibroma variant. *Am J Surg Pathol* 2001; **25**: 587–94.
8 Sawyer JR, Parr LG, Gokden N *et al*. A reciprocal t(4;9)(q31;p22) in a solitary neurofibroma. *Cancer Genet Cytogenet* 2005; **156**: 172–4.

Plexiform neurofibroma

This tumour is considered to be pathognomonic of neurofibromatosis type I (see Chapter 15). However, it has been contested whether the presence of a single plexiform neurofibroma in the absence of other signs of neurofibroma can be regarded as pathognomonic of neurofibromatosis type I [1,2]. It presents in children and young adults of either sex, with predilection for the lower limbs and the head and neck. Tumours are large and located in the dermis, subcutis and even deeper soft tissues. The overlying skin is folded and hyperpigmented and the lesion is described as having an appearance like a 'bag of worms' (Fig. 56.37). This reflects the typical histological appearance of nerve trunks of different sizes randomly distributed throughout the involved tissues (Fig. 56.38). Careful histological examination of these lesions is necessary because the presence of any mitotic activity usually indicates malignant transformation.

Surgical removal of these lesions is usually very difficult because of the extensive involvement. When planning the surgical removal of these tumours, surgeons should remember that there is a tendency for haemorrhage within the tumour that may lead to morbidity or mortality.

References

1 Lin V, Daniel S, Forte V. Is a plexiform neurofibroma pathognomonic of neurofibromatosis type I? *Laryngoscope* 2004; **114**: 1410–4.
2 Fisher DA, Chu P, McCalmont T. Solitary plexiform neurofibroma is not pathognomonic of von Recklinghausen's neurofibromatosis: report of a case. *Int J Dermatol* 1997; **36**: 439–42.

Diffuse neurofibroma

This lesion presents as a diffuse, poorly-defined induration or plaque-like lesion of the skin and subcutaneous tissue in children or young adults, with a predilection for the trunk and head and neck area. Only a minority of cases are associated with neurofibromatosis type 1. The histological features are identical to those of a solitary neurofibroma except for the fact that there is diffuse replacement of involved tissue by the tumour. Local recurrence is frequent unless the lesion is widely excised.

Perineurioma [1–4]

Synonym
• Storiform perineural fibroma

Definition. Perineurioma is a tumour originally described in soft tissues. It is relatively common in the skin and it is composed of cells showing differentiation towards perineural fibroblasts.

Clinical features. The lesion has predilection for the lower limbs of young females. Tumours are small and asymptomatic. A distinctive, sclerosing variant has been described, affecting most commonly, but not always, the hands [4,5].

Pathology. Tumours are well-circumscribed and composed of bipolar and slender bland, thin, spindle-shaped cells with scanty cytoplasm and wavy nuclei. They are often arranged in concentric whorls (Fig. 56.39) or in a storiform pattern. Cellularity varies and is low in the sclerosing variant where hyalinized collagen predominates. The architecture may be plexiform in some cases [6]. Tumour cells are distinctively positive for EMA. They are also positive for a tight junction associated protein, claudin-1 [7]. Focal positivity for factor XIIIa and CD34 may also be seen.

Treatment. Lesions are entirely benign, and simple excision is the treatment of choice.

References

1 Robson AM, Calonje E. Cutaneous perineurioma: a poorly recognized tumour often misdiagnosed as epithelioid histiocytoma. *Histopathology* 2000; **37**: 332–9.
2 Smith K, Skelton H. Cutaneous fibrous perineuroma. *J Cutan Pathol* 1998; **25**: 333–7.

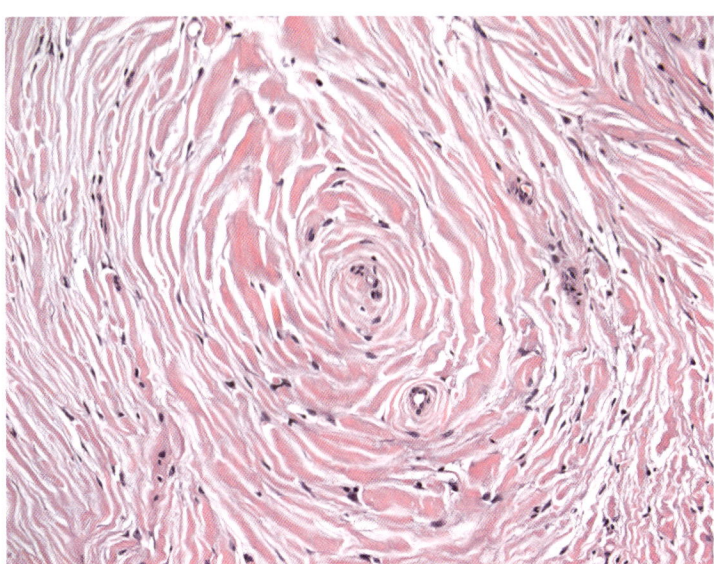

Fig. 56.39 Typical whirling appearance and some degree of sclerosis in a case of perineurioma.

3 Fetsch JF, Miettinen M. Sclerosing perineurioma: a clinicopathological study of 15 cases of a distinctive soft tissue lesion with a predilection for the fingers and palms of young adults. *Am J Surg Pathol* 1997; **21**: 1433–42.
4 Rankine AJ, Filion PR, Platten MA *et al.* Perineurioma: a clinicopathologic study of eight cases. *Pathology* 2004; **36**: 309–15.
5 Skelton HG, Williams J, Smith KJ. The clinical and histologic spectrum of cutaneous fibrous perineuriomas. *Am J Dermatopathol* 2001; **23**: 190–6.
6 Zelger B, Weinlich G, Zelger B. Perineuroma. A frequently unrecognized entity with emphasis on a plexiform variant. *Adv Clin Pathol* 2000; **4**: 25–33.
7 Folpe AL, Billings SD, McKenney JK *et al.* Expression of claudin-1, a recently described tight junction-associated protein, distinguishes soft tissue perineurioma from potential mimics. *Am J Surg Pathol* 2002; **26**: 1620–6.

Dermal nerve sheath myxoma [1–3]

Synonym
• Neurothekeoma

Definition. This is a myxoid tumour that is thought to display nerve sheath differentiation.

Clinical features [1,2,4]. It presents most commonly on the upper limbs (particularly the fingers and hands) and lower limbs (mainly the knees, shins or feet) of young adults, with a predilection for males. The trunk and head and neck are rarely affected. Lesions are long-standing, small, usually less than 1 cm, skin-coloured and asymptomatic.

Pathology [1–3]. The dermis shows a well-defined tumour composed of lobules that vary in size and shape and are separated by fibrocollagenous stroma. Each lobule is composed of slender stellate or spindle-shaped Schwann cells with bland nuclei and indistinct cytoplasm margins in the background of prominent myxoid change. Mitotic figures are very rare. Tumour cells are uniformly positive for S100. They are also positive for glial fibrillary acid protein and CD57 [4]. EMA-positive cells are seen in the periphery of tumour lobules. These tumours have no relationship with the so-called cellular neurothekeoma [5].

Treatment. Simple excision is curative. There is high tendency for local recurrence [4].

References

1 Gallager RL, Helwig EB. Neurothekeoma: a benign tumor of neural crest origin. *Am J Clin Pathol* 1980; **74**: 759–64.
2 Pulitzer DR, Reed RJ. Nerve-sheath myxoma (perineurial myxoma). *Am J Dermatopathol* 1985; **7**: 409–21.
3 Fletcher CDM, Chen JKC, McKee PH. Dermal nerve sheath myxoma: a study of three cases. *Histopathology* 1986; **10**: 135–45.
4 Fetsch JF, Laskin WB, Mietinen M. Nerve sheath myxoma: a clinicopathologic and immunohistochemical analysis of 57 morphologically distinctive, S-100 protein and GFAP positive myxoid peripheral nerve sheath tumors with a predilection for the extremities and a high local recurrence rate. *Am J Surg Pathol* 2005; **29**: 1615–24.
5 Rosati LA, Fratamico CM, Eusebi V. Cellular neurothekeoma. *Appl Pathol* 1986; **4**: 186–91.

Cellular neurothekeoma [1–4]

Definition. Despite its name, this tumour is not related to dermal nerve sheath myxoma, and its line of differentiation has not been established. It should not be confused with ordinary nerve sheath myxomas showing focal cellular areas [1–3].

Clinical features. The tumour presents as a small, asymptomatic papule in children and young adults, more common in females than males and with a predilection for the upper limbs and face and neck [4,5]. Multiple lesions are exceptional [6].

Pathology. In the dermis and frequently extending into the subcutis [5], there is an ill-defined tumour composed of nests and fascicles of epithelioid or spindle-shaped cells (Fig. 56.40) with vesicular nuclei and a single small eosinophilic nucleolus. Lesions presenting in the face may extend into the underlying skeletal muscle. Mitotic figures are relatively common and scattered multi-

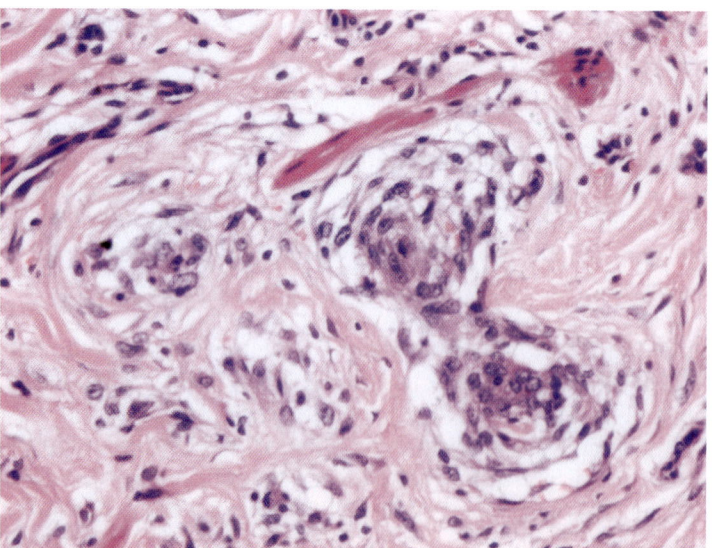

Fig. 56.40 Cellular neurothekeoma. Nests of epithelioid cells in the background of a hyalinized stroma. In cases with cytological atypia and mitotic activity, confusion with a melanoma is more likely.

nucleated cells (osteoclast-like) may be seen. Tumour cells resemble melanocytes, and this often leads to the lesion being confused with a melanoma. However, there is no junctional activity, and cells are invariably negative for S100. Some tumours have larger size, more cytological atypia and increased mitotic count, and these tumours have been classified as atypical cellular neurothekeoma [4,5]. However, this does not seem to be related to a more aggressive behaviour. Tumour cells are often positive for smooth muscle actin (in about 57% of cases), NKI-C3, neuron-specific enolase and PGP 9.5 [5].

Treatment. Simple excision is curative, and there is very little tendency for local recurrence [5].

References

1 Barnhill RL, Mihm MC. Cellular neurothekeoma: a distinctive variant of neurothekeoma mimicking nevomelanocytic tumors. *Am J Surg Pathol* 1990; **14**: 113–20.
2 Calonje E, Wilson-Jones E, Smith NP *et al.* Cellular 'neurothekeoma': an epithelioid variant of pilar leiomyoma? Morphological and immunohistochemical analysis of a series. *Histopathology* 1992; **20**: 397–404.
3 Barnhill RL, Dickersin GR, Nickeleit V *et al.* Studies on the cellular origin of neurothekeoma: clinical, light microscopic, immunohistochemical and ultrastructural observations. *J Am Acad Dermatol* 1991; **25**: 80–8.
4 Busam KJ, Mentzel T, Colpaert C *et al.* Atypical or worrisome features in cellular neurothekeoma: a study of 10 cases. *Am J Surg Pathol* 1998; **22**: 1067–72.
5 Hornick JL, Fletcher CD. Cellular neurothekeoma: detailed characterization in a series of 133 cases. *Am J Surg Pathol* 2007; **31**: 329–40.
6 Mahalingam M, Alter JN, Bhawan J. Multiple cellular neurothekeomas—a case report and review on the role of immunohistochemistry as a histologic adjunct. *J Cutan Pathol* 2006; **33**: 51–6.

Granular cell tumour [1–4]

Synonyms
- Abrikossoff's tumour
- Granular cell myoblastoma

Definition. A tumour composed of cells with characteristic granular cytoplasm. The histogenesis of the classic granular cell tumour seems to be neuroectodermal. However, it is worth remembering that many tumours of different histogenesis may show granular cell change, due to the cytoplasmic accumulation of secondary lysosomes.

Incidence. This is a rare tumour, occurring in the tongue as well as in the skin, and also in a variety of deeper locations including internal organs. Females are slightly more affected than males, and it is common in the third to fifth decade of life. It can occur in childhood [5,6].

Clinical features. The tumour is usually solitary, situated in the skin, the gingiva [7], or beneath the epithelium of the tongue. It is firm and rounded but with rather indefinite margins, sessile or pedunculated, and between 5 and 20 mm in diameter, although larger tumours may be seen. The colour may vary from flesh colour to pink or greyish-brown. It is most common in the tongue, where the epithelium over it may be thickened. On the skin surface, the epithelium covering the tumour is usually normal,

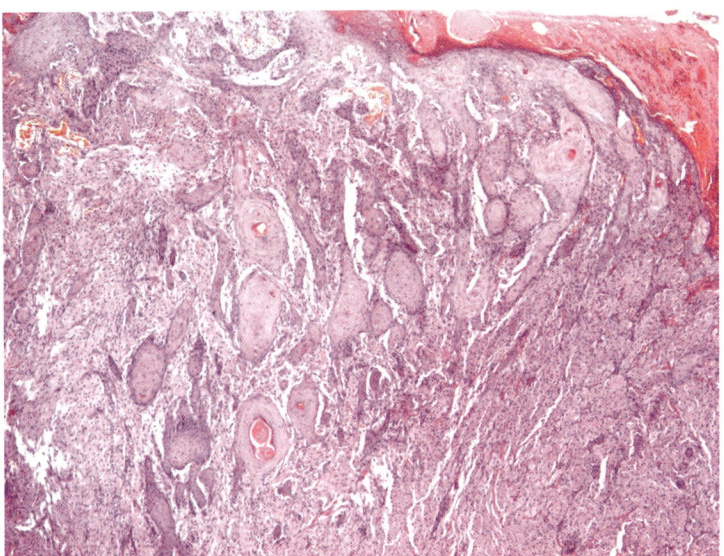

Fig. 56.41 Prominent pseudoepitheliomatous hyperplasia mimicking a squamous cell carcinoma in a case of granular cell tumour.

although it may thicken or at times ulcerate. There is no particular site of predilection. Multiple tumours may occur [8], and several have been reported in children, one of whom also had axillary freckling [5]. The tumour grows slowly.

A malignant type of granular cell tumour that metastasizes has been reported [9,10]. Among the internal sites reported are muscle, lip, jaws, parotid gland, pharynx, larynx, trachea, bronchus, lung, chest wall, breast, lacrimal sac, orbit, heart, oesophagus, common bile duct, urinary bladder, spermatic cord, male urethra, perineum, anal region, vulva and ovary [6,11].

Pathology [12,13]. Large polyhedral cells arranged in sheets, which infiltrate the dermal connective tissue and subcutaneous fat, form the tumour. The cytoplasm is pale and contains brightly acidophilic granules. The nuclei are relatively small and round, and tend to be vesicular. Clear cell change may occasionally be prominent [14]. The epithelium over the area may show pseudoepitheliomatous hyperplasia and in small biopsies this may be confused with a squamous cell carcinoma (Fig. 56.41). Perineural extension is often seen. Occasionally, tumour cells involve the epidermis and distinction from melanoma may be difficult [15]. However, although S-100 positivity is seen in both tumours, other melanocytic markers, including HMB45 and melan-A, are negative in granular cell tumour. The original suggestion that the cells are myoblasts probably arose from examination of tumours of the tongue in which infiltration between the striated muscle bundles gave the impression of origin from the muscle. The general belief now is that the cells are of neural or nerve sheath origin [16–21].

Diagnosis. Histological examination is usually necessary to separate this tumour from other tumours of the deeper dermis.

Treatment. Local recurrence, mainly due to incomplete excision, is uncommon, and simple excision is therefore the treatment of choice.

References

1 Garancis JC, Komorowski RA, Kuzma FJ. Granular cell myoblastoma. *Cancer* 1970; **25**: 542–50.
2 Pugh JI, Rigg BM, Murley RS. Granular cell myoblastoma of the breast. *Br J Surg* 1967; **54**: 590–4.
3 Stefansson K, Wollmann RL. S-100 protein in granular cell tumors (granular cell myoblastoma). *Cancer* 1982; **49**: 1834–7.
4 White SW, Gallager RL, Rodman OG. Multiple granular cell tumors. *J Dermatol Surg Oncol* 1980; **6**: 57–62.
5 Apted JH. Multiple granular cell myoblastoma (Schwannoma) in a child. *Br J Dermatol* 1968; **80**: 257–60.
6 Cave VG, Koff AW, Vegas FK. Multiple myoblastomas in children. *Arch Dermatol* 1955; **71**: 579–86.
7 Anderson PJ, Kirkland P, Schafer K *et al.* Congenital gingival granular cell tumour. *J R Soc Med* 1996; **89**: 53–4.
8 Hazan C, Fangman W. Multiple cutaneous granular-cell tumors. *Dermatol Online J* 2007; **13**: 4
9 Gamboa LG. Malignant granular cell myoblastoma. *AMA Arch Pathol* 1995; **60**: 663–8.
10 Svejd J, Horn V. A disseminated granular cell pseudotumour, so-called metastasising granular cell myoblastoma. *J Pathol Bacteriol* 1958; **76**: 343–8.
11 Seo IS, Azarelli B, Warner TF *et al.* Multiple visceral and cutaneous granular cell tumors: ultrastructural and immunocytochemical evidence of Schwann cell origin. *Cancer* 1984; **53**: 2104–10.
12 Lack EE, Worsham GF, Calliham MD *et al.* Granular cell tumor: a clinicopathologic study of 100 patients. *J Surg Oncol* 1980; **13**: 301–9.
13 Bangle R Jr. A morphological and histochemical study of the granular cell myoblastoma. *Cancer* 1952; **5**: 950–65.
14 Zedek DC, Murphy BA, Shea CR *et al.* Cutaneous clear-cell granular cell tumors: the histologic description of an unusual variant. *J Cutan Pathol* 2007; **34**: 397–404.
15 Ray S, Jukic DM. Cutaneous granular cell tumor with epidermal involvement: a potential mimic of melanocytic neoplasia. *J Cutan Pathol* 2007; **34**: 188–94.
16 Bedetti CD, Martinez AJ, Beckford NS *et al.* Granular cell tumours arising in myelinated peripheral nerves: light and electron microscopy and immunoperoxidase study. *Virchows Arch (Pathol Anat)* 1983; **402**: 175–84.
17 Chimelli L, Symon L, Scaravilli F. Granular cell tumor of the fifth cranial nerve: further evidence for Schwann cell origin. *J Neuropathol Exp Neurol* 1984; **43**: 634–40.
18 Dhillon AP, Rode J. Immunohistochemical studies of S100 protein and other neural characteristics expressed by granular cell tumour. *Diagn Histopathol* 1983; **6**: 23–8.
19 Fust JA, Custer RP. On the neurogenesis of so-called granular cell myoblastoma. *Am J Clin Pathol* 1949; **19**: 522–35.
20 Miettinen M, Lehtonen E, Lehtola H *et al.* Histogenesis of granular cell tumour: an immunological and ultrastructural study. *J Pathol* 1984; **142**: 221–31.
21 Nakazato Y, Ishizeki J, Takahashi K *et al.* Immunohistochemical localization of S-100 protein in granular cell myoblastoma. *Cancer* 1982; **49**: 1624–9.

Meningothelial heterotopias [1–8]

Synonym
• Cutaneous meningioma

Lesions with meningothelial elements presenting in the skin and soft tissue were divided into three groups by Lopez *et al.* [4]. The first two groups of lesions represent meningothelial heterotopias or hamartomas. The main difference between both groups is that affected patients are children in the first group and adults in the second group. The third group consists of intracranial meningiomas that extend secondarily into the skin or soft tissues. This group will not be discussed in more detail here.

A small number of cases of meningothelial heterotopias have been associated with von Recklinghausen's disease [1]. The tumour occurs over the scalp or in the paraspinous region of the trunk of children and young adults. Occasionally it appears to be familial [6]. The lesions resemble 'soft naevi'. On the scalp, the area may be bald. The skin is adherent to the mass, which is dermal or subcutaneous, and there may be a central depression with epidermal atrophy or ulceration. A connection with the cranial cavity is not usually demonstrated. The size ranges from 2 to 10 cm.

Pathology [6–8]. Low-power examination often reveals a lesion with a striking resemblance to a lymphangioma. Irregular dilated spaces are seen dissecting between collagen bundles. The spaces are partially lined by plump epithelioid cells, which are also seen in clusters in the surrounding stroma. Focal formation of psammoma bodies may be present. The dermal collagen and blood vessels also appear to be increased. Some lesions contain more solid areas. The presence of meningothelial cells can be demonstrated by positive staining for EMA.

References
1 Argenyi ZB, Thieberg MD, Hayes CM, Whitaker DC. Primary cutaneous meningioma associated with von Recklinghausen's disease. *J Cutan Pathol* 1994; **21**: 549–56.
2 Argenyi ZB. Cutaneous neural heterotopias and related tumours relevant for the dermatopathologist. *Semin Diagn Pathol* 1996; **13**: 60–71.
3 Bain GO, Shnitka TK. Cutaneous meningioma (psammoma). *AMA Arch Dermatol* 1956; **74**: 590–4.
4 Lopez DA, Silvers DN, Helwig EB. Cutaneous meningiomas: a clinico-pathologic study. *Cancer* 1974; **34**: 728–44.
5 Miyamoto T, Mihara M, Hagari Y *et al*. Primary cutaneous meningioma of the scalp: report of 2 siblings. *J Dermatol* 1995; **22**: 611–9.
6 Suster S, Rosai J. Hamartoma of the scalp with ectopic meningothelial elements: a distinctive soft tissue lesion that may simulate angiosarcoma. *Am J Surg Pathol* 1990; **14**: 1–11.
7 Bale PM, Hughes L, De Silva M. Sequestrated meningoceles of the scalp: extracranial meningeal hamartoma. *Hum Pathol* 1990; **21**: 1156–63.
8 Theaker JM, Fletcher CDM, Tudway AJ. Cutaneous heterotopic meningeal nodules. *Histopathology* 1990; **16**: 475–9.

Glial heterotopic nodules [1,2]

Synonym
- Nasal glioma

Definition. This represents the presence of heterotopic mature glial tissue in the dermis or subcutis, predominantly on the central face. It may be considered to be a developmental defect in the closure of the neural tube. However, rare cases occur away from the midline, suggesting a different unexplained mechanism for its occurrence [3].

Clinical features. Most lesions present in infants or children as a subcutaneous mass on the bridge of the nose. Presentation in adults is exceptional. Communication with the cranial cavity is present in up to 20% of cases.

Pathology. Nodules of astrocytes in a neurofibrillar background are characteristic. Less commonly, oligodendrocytes are seen; neuronal elements are exceptional.

Treatment. Excision is curative, but it is very important to make sure that an underlying communication with the cranial cavity is ruled out, as failure to do so may result in complications such as meningitis or cerebrospinal fluid leakage.

References
1 Fletcher CDM, Carpenter G, McKee PH. Nasal glioma: a rarity. *Am J Dermatopathol* 1986; **8**: 341–6.
2 Theaker JM, Fletcher CDM. Heterotopic glial nodules: a light microscopic and immunohistochemical study. *Histopathology* 1991; **18**: 255–60.
3 McDermott MB, Glasner SD, Nielsen PL, Dehner LP. Soft tissue gliomatosis: morphologic unity and histogenetic diversity. *Am J Surg Pathol* 1996; **20**: 148–55.

Epithelial sheath neuroma [1]

Definition. This is a novel, rare and intriguing dermal lesion that combines a neural and an epithelial component. Although some features suggest that this may be a hamartoma, the fact that it has only been described in adults makes this possibility unlikely.

Clinical features. In view of the fact that so few cases have been described, very little can be said about the clinical features. The clinical presentation is not distinctive and lesions appear to have a predilection for the back.

Pathology. Histologically there are scattered, prominent nerves in the superficial dermis, encased by mature, non-dysplastic squamous epithelium with focal keratinization and dyskeratotic cells. Immunohistochemistry displays the normal staining of nerves and epidermis respectively.

Prognosis and treatment. Lesions appear to be benign and no recurrences have been reported so far.

Reference
1 Requena L, Grosshans E, Kutzner H *et al*. Epithelial sheath neuroma: a new entity. *Am J Surg Pathol* 2000; **24**: 190–6.

Pigmented neuroectodermal tumour of infancy [1,2]

Synonyms
- Melanotic progonoma
- Retinal anlage tumour

For many years, there has been a debate as to whether this tumour is of neural or melanocytic origin [3–5]. Recent evidence seems to indicate that this tumour recapitulates the early stages of development of the retinal epithelium [6].

Clinical features. This tumour occurs most frequently in the anterior part of the maxilla, usually in infants less than 6 months old, and often presents as a pigmented oral mass [7]. It has been reported also in the anterior fontanelle, the shoulder, epididymis, femur and mediastinum. There is a slight predilection for males. It may cause a high urinary excretion of vanillylmandelic acid [3]. This tumour has been mistaken in the past for malignant melanoma, and could also be confused with a cellular blue naevus.

The clinical appearance is that of a rapidly expanding nodule in the jaw, which may affect dentition. Although classified as benign, the lesions may cause considerable local destruction, and around 5% of cases may metastasize and prove fatal [8].

Pathology [9,10]. A mass of irregular alveolar spaces surrounded by fibrous stroma is seen. Two types of cells are easily recognized: small round blue cells with scanty cytoplasm in a fibrillary matrix, and large epithelioid cells with pink cytoplasm and vesicular nuclei. These cells often contain melanin. Both types of tumour cells stain for synaptophysin and neurone-specific enolase, and are negative for S100. The large cells are positive for cytokeratin and HMB45.

Treatment. Complete surgical excision is the treatment of choice.

References
1 Koudstaal J, Oldhoff J, Panders AK *et al.* Melanotic neuroectodermal tumor of infancy. *Cancer* 1968; **22**: 151–61.
2 Krused-Lösler B, Gaertner C, Bürger H *et al.* Melanotic neuroectodermal tumor of infancy: systematic review of the literature and presentation of a case. *Oral Surg Oral Pathol* 2006; **102**: 204–16.
3 Borello ED, Gorlin RJ. Melanotic neuroectodermal tumour of infancy: a neoplasm of neural crest origin. *Cancer* 1966; **19**: 196–203.
4 Cutler LS, Chaudhury AP, Topiazian R. Melanotic neuroectodermal tumour of infancy: an ultrastructural literature review and reevaluation. *Cancer* 1981; **48**: 257–68.
5 Johnson RE, Scheithauer BW, Dahlin DC. Melanotic neuroectodermal tumour of infancy. *Cancer* 1983; **52**: 661–6.
6 Pettinato G, Manivel JC, d'Amore ESG *et al.* Melanotic neuroectodermal tumor of infancy: a reexamination of a histogenetic problem based on immunohistochemical, flow cytometric and ultrastructural study of 10 cases. *Am J Surg Pathol* 1991; **15**: 233–45.
7 Takeda Y, Kuroda M, Suzuki A. Melanocytes in odontoameloblastoma: a case report. *Acta Pathol Jpn* 1989; **39**: 465–8.
8 Dehner LP, Sibley RK, Sauk JJ *et al.* Malignant melanotic neuroectodermal tumor of infancy: a clinical, pathologic, ultrastructural and tissue culture study. *Cancer* 1979; **43**: 1389–410.
9 Johnson RE, Scheithauer BW, Dahlin DC. Melanotic neuroectodermal tumor of infancy: a review of seven cases. *Cancer* 1983; **52**: 661–6.
10 Stirling RW, Powell G, Fletcher CDM. Pigmented neuroectodermal tumour of infancy: an immunohistochemical study. *Histopathology* 1988; **12**: 425–35.

Malignant peripheral nerve sheath tumour [1,2]

Synonyms
- Neurofibrosarcoma
- Malignant schwannoma

Definition. A malignant tumour arising from the nerve sheath.

Aetiology. Cutaneous tumours usually arise from a plexiform neurofibroma in patients with neurofibromatosis type 1 [3]. Rare cutaneous lesions may arise within ordinary neurofibromas or *de novo* [4]. Deep-seated lesions arise *de novo* or in association with neurofibromatosis type 1. Patients with this disease develop malignancy in 30–50% of cases.

Incidence. It is an uncommon tumour. It occurs in young adults, or even children, when it complicates multiple neurofibromatosis. Sporadic cases occur in older individuals.

Clinical features [5]. The diagnosis should be suspected when a previously static tumour in a patient with neurofibromatosis begins to enlarge or becomes painful. The pain may become radicular as the lesion progresses but the tumours are not always associated with nerve trunks. The commoner sites are the flexor aspects of the limbs. A minority of cases occur as a complication of radiotherapy.

Pathology. The basic pattern is that of fascicles of tumour cells, often with a herringbone pattern and resembling a fibrosarcoma. Tumour cells tend to concentrate around blood vessels and myxoid change is common. The degree of pleomorphism and the number of mitotic figures varies. Immunohistochemical markers are not usually of help in the diagnosis as S-100 is only focally positive and often entirely negative.

Treatment. Wide local excision or amputation is necessary because of the aggressive behaviour of the tumour, and even then the prognosis is not good. Systemic metastases, particularly to the lungs, are common. The prognosis is worse in cases occurring after previous radiotherapy.

References
1 D'Agostino AN, Soule EH, Miller RH. Sarcomas of the peripheral nerves and somatic soft tissues associated with multiple neurofibromatosis (von Recklinghausen's disease). *Cancer* 1963; **16**: 1015–27.
2 George E, Swanson PE, Wick MR. Malignant peripheral nerve sheath tumours of the skin. *Am J Dermatopathol* 1989; **11**: 213–21.
3 Demitsu T, Murata S, Kiyosawa T *et al.* Malignant Schwannoma arising in patients with von Recklinghausen's disease. *J Dermatol* 1995; **22**: 747–54.
4 Allison KH, Patel RM, Goldblum JR *et al.* Superficial malignant peripheral nerve sheath tumor: a rare and challenging diagnosis. *Am J Clin Pathol* 2005; **124**: 685–92.
5 Giodillo PP, Helson L, Hajdu SI *et al.* Malignant schwannoma: clinical characteristics and response to therapy. *Cancer* 1981; **47**: 2503–9.

Clear cell sarcoma [1–5]

Definition. Clear cell sarcoma is a distinctive, malignant soft-tissue tumour that displays melanocytic differentiation.

Clinical features. Most cases occur on the lower limbs, with a predilection for the foot. The upper limb is affected in about 25% of cases. There is a predilection for females. Tumours tend to grow around tendons, are usually less than 3 cm in diameter and are often painful. Primary dermal tumours are exceptional.

Pathology. The lesion has a lobular growth pattern. Tumour cells are fairly homogeneous and contain clear or pale pink cytoplasm and a prominent eosinophilic nucleolus. Mitotic figures are not prominent, but multinucleated giant cells with a wreath-like arrangement of the nuclei are often identified. Loose, thin bands of collagen surround tumour cells. Secondary involvement of the dermis is relatively common. Necrosis is sometimes seen. Melanin is sometimes identified, and S100, HMB45 and melan A are usually positive. Electron-microscopic examination of tumour cells reveals the presence of melanosomes.

Cytogenetic analysis often reveals a translocation t(12; 22) (q13;q12); this translocation is not found in melanoma, which often has mutations in the *BRAF* gene (a feature not seen in clear cell sarcoma) [6,7]. The clear cell sarcoma translocation results in an *EWSR1—ATF1* fusion gene [8].

Prognosis and treatment [1–4]. About 50% of patients develop metastatic disease, often many years after the initial diagnosis. Prognosis is associated with mitotic index, size of the tumour and presence of necrosis [9,10]. The 5- and 10-year survival rates are 52% and 25% respectively [9]. Wide excision is the treatment of choice. Chemotherapy does not seem to be effective in the treatment of disseminated disease.

References

1 Enzinger FM. Clear cell sarcoma of tendons and aponeuroses: an analysis of 21 cases. *Cancer* 1965; **18**: 1163–76.
2 Eckardt JJ, Pritchard DJ, Soule EH. Clear cell sarcoma: a clinicopathologic study of 27 cases. *Cancer* 1983; **52**: 1482–8.
3 Lucas DR, Nascimento AG, Sim FH. Clear cell sarcoma of soft tissues: Mayo Clinic experience with 35 cases. *Am J Surg Pathol* 1992; **16**: 1197–204.
4 Montgomery EA, Meis JM, Ramos AG et al. Clear cell sarcoma of tendons and aponeurosis: a clinicopathologic study of 58 cases with analysis of prognostic factors. *Int J Surg Pathol* 1993; **1**: 59–62.
5 Meis-Kindblom JM. Clear cell sarcoma of tendon and aponeuroses: a historical perspective and tribute to the man behind the entity. *Adv Anat Pathol* 2006; **13**: 286–92.
6 Reeves BR, Fletcher CD, Gusterson BA. Translocation t(12;22)(q13;q13) is a nonrandom rearrangement in clear cell sarcoma. *Cancer Genet Cytogenet* 1992; **64**: 101–3.
7 Panagopoulos I, Mertens F, Isaksson M et al. Absence of mutations of the BRAF gene in malignant melanoma of soft parts (clear cell sarcoma of tendons and aponeuroses). *Cancer Genet Cytogenet* 2005; **156**: 74–6.
8 Panagopoulos I, Mertens F, Débiec-Rychter M et al. Molecular genetic characterization of the EWS/ATF1 fusion gene in clear cell sarcoma of tendons and aponeuroses. *Int J Cancer* 2002; **99**: 560–7.
9 Clark MA, Johnson MB, Thway K et al. Clear cell sarcoma (melanoma of soft parts): The Royal Marsden Hospital experience. *Eur J Surg Oncol* 2008; **34**: 800–4.
10 Coindre JM, Hostein I, Terrier P et al. Diagnosis of clear cell sarcoma by real-time reverse transcriptase-polymerase chain reaction analysis of paraffin embedded tissues: clinicopathological and molecular analysis of 44 patients from the French sarcoma group. *Cancer* 2005; **107**: 1055–64.

Peripheral primitive neuroectodermal tumour [1,2]

Synonyms
- Peripheral neuroepithelioma
- Extraosseous Ewing's sarcoma

Primary cutaneous or subcutaneous peripheral primitive neuroectodermal tumour is extremely rare, and only a handful of cases have been reported in the literature. The tumour presents in children and has no distinctive clinical features, although it is often confused with a vascular tumour. It has been suggested that superficial tumours have a better prognosis than those presenting in deeper soft tissues, but the number of cases reported and their follow-up is too limited for this to be certain. The histological diagnosis includes tumours composed of small, blue, round cells, for which immunohistochemistry plays an important role in diagnosis. Tumour cells are diffusely positive for CD99. This

tumour usually presents a reciprocal chromosome translocation t(11;22)(q24;q12) that is an important aid in diagnosis.

References

1 Banerjee SS, Agbamu DA, Eyden BP et al. Clinicopathological characteristics of peripheral neuroectodermal tumour of skin and subcutaneous tissue. *Histopathology* 1997; **31**: 355–66.
2 Hasegawa S, Davidson JM, Rutten A et al. Primary cutaneous Ewing's sarcoma: immunophenotypic and molecular cytogenetic evaluation of five cases. *Am J Surg Pathol* 1998; **22**: 310–8.

Tumours of muscle

Congenital smooth muscle hamartoma

This lesion is described in Chapter 18.

Leiomyoma [1–3]

Definition. A benign tumour of smooth muscle derived from the arrector pili muscle, from the media of blood vessels, or from smooth muscle of the scrotum, labia majora or nipples (genital leiomyoma) [4,5].

Incidence. The tumour occurs in three main types, all of which are relatively uncommon.

Pilar leiomyoma (leiomyoma cutis) originates in the pilomotor muscle and is the most frequent. It can occur at any age from birth onwards, but appears usually in early adult life. It has been reported in identical twins, in siblings and in several generations of a family [6–8]. The cases with a familial background have all had multiple tumours. The sexes are affected equally.

Genital leiomyoma (dartoic myoma) arises in the smooth muscle of the genitalia and areola of the nipple [9,10]. It can occur at any age. The cutaneous variety is about six times more frequent than the genital type [11].

Angioleiomyoma arises from the muscular coat of veins, and is seen mainly in middle age or later as a solitary nodule on a limb. It is rather more prevalent than glomus tumour in published series [6,12,13]. Females are more commonly affected than males.

Clinical features [6,14]. Pilar leiomyoma generally presents as a collection of pink, red or dusky brown, firm dermal nodules of varying size but usually less than 15 mm diameter (Fig. 56.42). The nodules are often subject to episodes of pain and may be tender. The pain can be provoked by touching or chilling the skin, or by emotional disturbance, and is often worse in winter. Some lesions contract and become paler when painful [12,15]. The condition usually begins with the appearance of one small nodule, which gradually increases in size, and further similar lesions appear nearby or at some other area. Adjacent tumours may coalesce to form a plaque. The areas most commonly affected are the extremities, with the proximal and extensor aspects somewhat favoured. The trunk is involved more often than the head and neck. Multiple lesions may be regional and unilateral, or more than one region

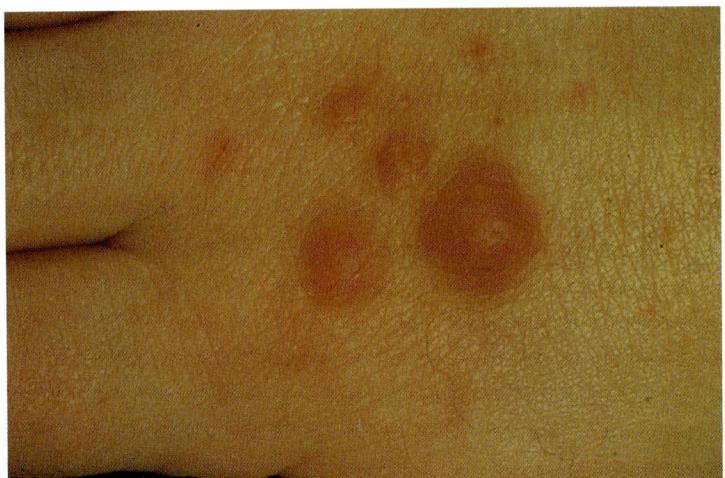

Fig. 56.42 Clinical appearance of multiple leiomyomas.

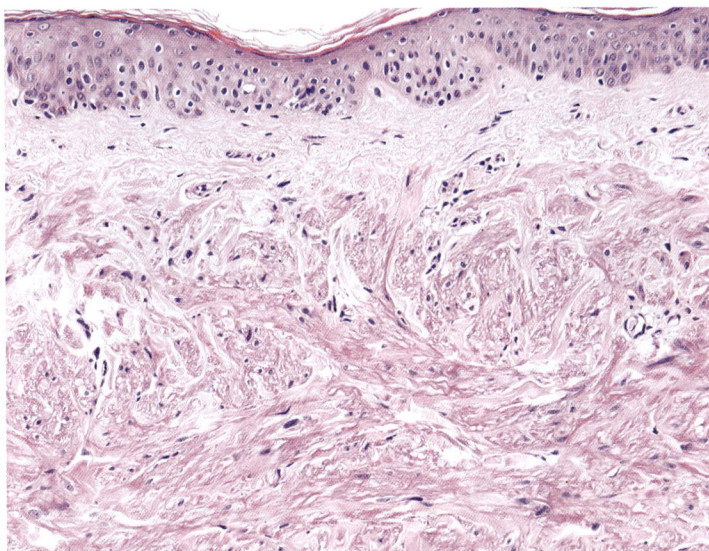

Fig. 56.43 Pathology of leiomyoma, showing spindle-shaped cells with eosinophilic cytoplasm arranged in bundles closely resembling the arrector pili muscle.

can be affected. Solitary lesions may occur, apart from the dartoic type. The gene that predisposes to multiple pilar leiomyomas has been mapped to chromosome 1q 42.3-q43 [16]. It also predisposes to uterine leiomyomas (multiple cutaneous and uterine leiomyomatosis, MCUL) and to renal cancer [17]. This is as a result of mutations in the gene encoding the enzyme fumarate hydratase [18]. In patients with associated renal cancer the syndrome is known as hereditary leiomyomatosis and renal cancer.

Genital leiomyoma is a solitary dermal nodule occurring most commonly in the scrotum, but also appearing on the penis, labia majora and nipple area. Scrotal tumours are often large. Pain is less frequent than with leiomyoma cutis. Contraction in response to stimulation by touch or cold can occur.

Angioleiomyoma is usually a solitary, flesh-coloured, rounded, subcutaneous or deep dermal tumour up to 40 mm in diameter. It is more frequent on the lower limb than the upper and may appear on the trunk or face. About half the reported cases have been painful [6,12]. Lesions are long-standing and present between the fourth and sixth decades of life. Pain may be triggered by changes in temperature, pregnancy or menses.

Pathology [12,14,19,20]. The smooth muscle cells proliferate to produce interweaving bundles of spindle-shaped cells, which are strongly eosinophilic (Fig. 56.43). The nuclei are long and thin, and the general appearance of the mass in ordinary sections may suggest a hypertrophic fibrous reaction. The smooth muscle cells can be distinguished from collagen by their different reaction with trichrome stains, and by the presence of myofibrils, which stain with phosphotungstic acid haematoxylin, and by their blunt-ended nuclei. Tumour cells are positive for actin and desmin.

The tumour of pilomotor origin (leiomyoma cutis, multiple cutaneous leiomyomas) is usually composed of numerous dermal nodules with vague margins where the cells penetrate the surrounding collagen bundles, and an upper border that approaches the papillary body. Associated epidermal hyperplasia is common. Focal nuclear atypia likely to be degenerative in origin and very low mitotic activity (up to one per 10 high-power fields) may be seen without this being indicative of malignant degeneration [21]. Genital leiomyomas are nodular tumours with a similar

appearance. Scrotal tumours are less circumscribed and more cellular than those developing in the vulva. The angiomyomas are related to veins in the subcutaneous tissue, and are rounded and well circumscribed [22]. Vessels of variable thickness are intermixed with bundles of mature smooth muscle. Focal degenerative cytological atypia may be seen, but mitotic figures are absent. Calcification, hyalinization and thrombosis of vessels are often seen.

Diagnosis. The multiple type should cause little difficulty, and even without pain it is fairly distinctive. The solitary painful lesion may be mistaken for a glomus tumour or an eccrine spiradenoma, and a history of contraction is helpful. In practice the diagnosis can be elusive.

Treatment. Surgical excision cures the solitary tumour. The severity of the pain may make the patient demand treatment, and extensive lesions require plastic surgery. Excision of an area containing multiple tumours is often followed by their appearance in the neighbourhood of the treated area. Medical treatments that may relieve pain include calcium-channel blockers and gabapentin.

References

1 Eldor A, Even-Paz Z, Polliak A. Erythrocytosis associated with multiple cutaneous leiomyomata: report of a case with demonstration of erythropoietic activity in the tumour. *Scand J Haematol* 1976; **16**: 245.

2 Merrill RG, Downs JR. Oral leiomyomas: report of two cases. *Oral Surg* 1967; **23**: 438–40.

3 Venencie PY, Puissant A, Boffa GA *et al.* Multiple cutaneous leiomyomata and erythrocytosis. *Br J Dermatol* 1982; **107**: 483–6.

4 Nascimento AG, Karas M, Rosen PP *et al.* Leiomyoma of the nipple. *Am J Surg Pathol* 1979; **3**: 151–6.

5 Prabhakar BR, Davessar K, Chitkara NL *et al.* Leiomyoma of the areolar region of the breast. *Int J Cancer* 1969; **6**: 260–1.

6 Hachisuga T, Hashimoto H, Enjoji M. Angioleiomyoma: a clinical reappraisal of 562 cases. *Cancer* 1984; **54**: 126–30.

7 Kloepfer HW, Krafchuk J, Derbes V *et al.* Hereditary multiple leiomyoma of the skin. *Am J Hum Genet* 1958; **10**: 48–52.

8 Verma KC, Chawdhry SD, Rathi KS. Cutaneous leiomyomata in two brothers. *Br J Dermatol* 1973; **90**: 351–3.

9 Matsubara J, Miura K. Leiomyoma of the scrotum: a case report and review of the literature. *Jpn J Cancer Clin* 1971; **17**: 151–4.

10 Newman PL, Fletcher CDM. Smooth muscle tumours of the external genitalia: clinicopathological analysis of a series. *Histopathology* 1991; **18**: 523–9.

11 Fisher WC, Helwig EB. Leiomyomas of the skin. *Arch Dermatol* 1963; **88**: 510–20.

12 Duhig JT, Ayer JP. Vascular leiomyoma: a study of sixty-one cases. *AMA Arch Pathol* 1959; **68**: 424–30.

13 MacDonald DM, Sanderson KV. Angioleiomyoma of the skin. *Br J Dermatol* 1974; **91**: 161–8.

14 Bardach H, Ebner H. Das Angioleiomyom der Haut. *Hautarzt* 1975; **26**: 638–44.

15 Engelke H, Christophers E. Leiomyomatosis cutis et uteri. *Acta Derm Venereol (Stockh)* 1979; **59** (Suppl. 85): 51.

16 Alam NA, Bevan S, Churchman M *et al.* Localization of a gene (MCUL1) for multiple cutaneous leiomyomata and uterine fibroids to chromosome 1q,42.3–q43. *Am J Hum Genet* 2001; **68**: 1264–9.

17 Alam NA, Barclay E, Rowan AJ, Tyrer JP *et al.* Clinical features of multiple cutaneous and uterine leiomyomatosis: an underdiagnosed tumor syndrome. *Arch Dermatol* 2005; **141**: 199–206.

18 Alam NA, Olpin S, Leigh IM. Fumarate hydratase mutations and predisposition to cutaneous leiomyomas, uterine leiomyomas and renal cancer. *Br J Dermatol* 2005; **153**: 11–7.

19 Mann PR. Leiomyoma cutis: an electron microscopy study. *Br J Dermatol* 1970; **82**: 463–9.

20 Seifert HW. Ultrastructural investigation on cutaneous angioleiomyoma. *Arch Dermatol Res* 1981; **271**: 91–9.

21 Raj S, Calonje E, Kraus M *et al.* Cutaneous pilar leiomyoma: clinicopathologic analysis of 53 lesions in 45 patients. *Am J Dermatopathol* 1997; **19**: 2–9.

22 Magner D, Hill D. Encapsulated angiomyoma of the skin and subcutaneous tissue. *Am J Clin Pathol* 1961; **35**: 137–41.

Leiomyosarcoma [1–4]

Definition. A malignant tumour displaying smooth muscle differentiation. Tumours are divided into those occurring in the subcutaneous tissue and those arising in the dermis. Pure dermal lesions have a very different behaviour from those arising in the subcutis and it is therefore important to separate them (see below).

Incidence. This is a rare tumour. Dermal leiomyosarcoma presents predominantly on the lower limbs of young adults, with a predilection for males. Subcutaneous leiomyosarcoma affects middle-aged to elderly patients with slight predilection for males.

Clinical features [5,6]. The tumour may be situated in the dermis, when it is reddish in colour and may bleed on trauma. It is usually larger than a leiomyoma and dermal lesions may be painful. The majority of tumours have, however, arisen in the subcutaneous or deeper tissues as nodular tumours, ulcerated plaques [7] or diffuse swellings [8]. It may invade underlying muscle fascia. It is most common on the thigh, followed by the head and neck, arm and trunk, and may arise from the penis [9] or vulva. It is unlikely to be diagnosed clinically. An exceptional tumour has been reported arising in a naevus sebaceous [10]. Dermal leiomyosarcomas have a 40% recurrence rate, but they almost never metastasize [11]. Subcutaneous tumours metastasize in up to 50% of cases and they are associated with a mortality of about 30%.

Pathology [3,11–15]. The lesion is distinguished from other dermal malignant tumours composed of spindle-shaped cells by the presence of fascicles of eosinophilic spindle-shaped cells with vesicular cigar-shaped nuclei. The degree of differentiation varies and necrosis tends to be present in deeper tumours, but not in those arising primarily in the dermis. Most tumours are actin- and desmin-positive, but staining for the latter may be lost in poorly differentiated variants. Dermal variants tend to be consistently positive for both markers. Rare cases have a desmoplastic stroma making histological diagnosis difficult [16,17]. About 30% of leiomyosarcomas are immunohistochemically positive for keratin, but this is less commonly seen in cutaneous examples.

Treatment. Wide surgical excision is necessary, as local recurrence follows inadequate excision.

References

1 Headington JT, Beals TF, Niederhuber JE. Primary leiomyosarcoma of skin. *J Cutan Pathol* 1977; **4**: 308–17.

2 Wang P, Hornstein OP, Schricker KTH. Kutanes Leiomyosarkom und osteomedullaeres Plasmozytom mit Nachweis von IgA kappa-Paraprotein in Serum und Hauttummor. *Hautarzt* 1976; **27**: 441–8.

3 Oliver GF, Reiman HM, Gonchoroff NT *et al.* Cutaneous and subcutaneous leiomyosarcoma: a clinicopathological review of 14 cases with reference to antidesmin staining and nuclear DNA patterns studied by flow cytometry. *Br J Dermatol* 1991; **124**: 252–7.

4 Bellezza G, Sidoni A, Cavaliere A *et al.* Primary cutaneous leiomyosarcoma: a clinicopathological and immunohistochemical study of 7 cases. *Int J Surg Pathol* 2004; **12**: 39–44.

5 Haim S, Gellei B. Leiomyosarcoma of the skin: report of two cases. *Dermatologica* 1970; **140**: 30–5.

6 Orellana-Díaz O, Hernández-Pérez E. Leiomyoma cutis and leiomyosarcoma: a 10-year study and a short review. *J Dermatol Surg Oncol* 1983; **9**: 283–7.

7 Karroum KE, Zappi EG, Cockerell CJ. Sclerotic primary cutaneous leiomyosarcoma. *Am J Dermatopathol* 1995; **17**: 292–6.

8 Phelan JT, Sherer W, Mesa P. Malignant smooth-muscle tumors (leiomyosarcomas) of soft tissue origin. *N Engl J Med* 1962; **266**: 1027–30.

9 Greenwood N, Fox H, Edwards EC. Leiomyosarcoma of the penis. *Cancer* 1972; **29**: 481–3.

10 Premalata CS, Kumar RV, Malathi M *et al.* Cutaneous leiomyosarcoma, trichoblastoma, and syringocystadenoma papilliferum arising from nevus sebaceous. *Int J Dermatol* 2007; **46**: 306–8.

11 Kaddu S, Beham A, Cerroni L *et al.* Cutaneous leiomyosarcoma. *Am J Surg Pathol* 1997; **21**: 979–87.

12 Akers WA, Prazak G. Leiomyosarcoma metastatic to scalp from primary in retroperitoneal area: report of a case. *Arch Dermatol* 1960; **81**: 953–7.

13 Cháves E, Sa HH, Gadelha N *et al.* Leiomyosarcoma in the skin. *Acta Dermatol Vénéréol* 1972; **52**: 288.

14 Dahl I, Angervall L. Cutaneous and subcutaneous leiomyosarcoma: a clinico-pathologic study of 47 patients. *Pathol Eur* 1974; **9**: 307–15.

15 Fields JP, Helwig EB. Leiomyosarcoma of the skin and subcutaneous tissue. *Cancer* 1981; **47**: 156–69.

16 Choy C, Cooper A, Kossard S. Primary cutaneous diffuse leiomyosarcoma with desmoplasia. *Australas J Dermatol* 2006; **47**: 291–5.

17 Berzal-Cantalejo F, Sabater-Marco V, Pérez-Vallés A *et al.* Desmoplastic cutaneous leiomyosarcoma: case report and review of the literature. *J Cutan Pathol* 2006; **33** (Suppl. 2): 29–31.

Skeletal muscle tumours

Rhabdomyosarcomatous congenital hamartoma

This lesion is described in Chapter 18.

Rhabdomyoma

Rhabdomyomas are divided into adult, fetal and genital types. They mainly occur in soft tissues, vulva or vagina, upper respiratory tract and internal organs. Presentation in the skin is almost never seen, and they will not be discussed further in this chapter.

Cutaneous rhabdomyosarcoma

Malignant tumours with skeletal-muscle differentiation are classified into two large groups, namely embryonal and alveolar types. Although rhabdomyosarcomas represent up to 8% of tumours in children, primary involvement of the skin by this tumour is very rare [1]. Much more common is involvement of the skin by direct extension from deeper soft tissues. Only 16 cases of primary cutaneous rhabdomyosarcoma have been reported in the literature so far, and only five of these have occurred in adults [2,3]. The most common subtype occurring in the skin is the alveolar variant. The majority of cases have presented on the face. The prognosis is difficult to estimate because of the rarity of these cases and the limited follow-up available.

References

1 Brecher AR, Reyes-Mugica M, Kamino H *et al*. Congenital primary cutaneous rhabdomyosarcoma in a neonate. *Pediatr Dermatol* 2003; **20**: 335–8.
2 Schmidt D, Fletcher CD, Harms D. Rhabdomyosarcoma with primary presentation in skin. *Pathol Res Pract* 1993; **189**: 422–7.
3 Setterfield J, Sciot R, Debiec-Rychter M *et al*. Primary cutaneous epidermotropic alveolar rhabdomyosarcoma with t(2;13) in an elderly woman: case report and review of the literature. *Am J Surg Pathol* 2002; **26**: 938–44.

Tumours of fat cells

Lipoma, angiolipoma and hibernoma

These lesions are described in Chapter 46.

Lipoblastoma and lipoblastomatosis

Definition. Lipoblastoma is a tumour that occurs almost exclusively in infants and children. It is characterized by a proliferation of immature fat cells in a myxoid stroma (that may mimic myxoid liposarcoma) and intermixed with mature adipocytes [1]. Lipoblastoma is a well-circumscribed, subcutaneous tumour; lipoblastomatosis refers to a deeper lesion or those that have an infiltrative growth pattern.

Clinical features [1–3]. Most cases present during the first few years of life, with a predilection for males. The majority of tumours occur on the limbs as an asymptomatic mass no more than a few centimetres in diameter. Lipoblastoma is much more common than lipoblastomatosis.

Pathology [1–3]. Tumours have a characteristic lobular appearance. Each tumour lobule is separated by fibrous septae and consists of a mixture of small, univacuolated, signet-ring cells, spindle-shaped or stellate cells and scattered mature adipocytes. In the background, there are prominent myxoid changes and numerous small vessels in a typical 'crow's-feet' distribution, mimicking a myxoid liposarcoma. Distinction from the latter may be very difficult, especially in small biopsies. The clinical information is therefore crucial, as myxoid liposarcoma is vanishingly rare in children and almost never occurs before the age of 10 years [4]. Furthermore, lipoblastoma tends to be less cellular than myxoid liposarcoma and has a lobular architecture. Over time, maturation occurs, and in some cases most of the tumour is composed of mature fat cells.

Cytogenetic studies in lipoblastoma have shown rearrangements on chromosome 8q [5,6].

Treatment. The tumour is benign, and simple excision is the treatment of choice. Deeper lesions have some tendency for local recurrence.

References

1 Chung EB, Enzinger FM. Benign lipoblastomatosis. *Cancer* 1973; **32**: 482–92.
2 Mentzel T, Calonje E, Fletcher CDM. Lipoblastoma and lipoblastomatosis: a clinicopathological study of 14 cases. *Histopathology* 1993; **23**: 527–33.
3 Collins MH, Chatten J. Lipoblastoma/lipoblastomatosis: a clinicopathologic study of 25 tumors. *Am J Surg Pathol* 1997; **21**: 1131–7.
4 Shmookler BM, Enzinger FM. Liposarcoma occurring in children: an analysis of 17 cases and review of the literature. *Cancer* 1983; **52**: 567–74.
5 Fletcher JA, Kozakewich HP, Schoenberg ML *et al*. Cytogenetic findings in pediatric adipose tumors: consistent rearrangement of chromosome 8 in lipoblastoma. *Genes Chromosomes Cancer* 1993; **6**: 24–9.
6 Hicks J, Dilley A, Patel D *et al*. Lipoblastoma and lipoblastomatosis in infancy and childhood: histopathologic, ultrastructural, and cytogenetic features. *Ultrastruct Pathol* 2001; **25**: 321–33.

Spindle cell and pleomorphic lipoma [1–5]

Definition. Spindle cell lipoma is composed of mature adipocytes and variable numbers of short, bland, spindle-shaped cells with indistinct cytoplasm. Pleomorphic lipoma is composed of mature adipocytes, cells with hyperchromatic nuclei and frequent multinucleation, and collagen bundles. Both types of tumour may overlap, and they are therefore considered to be part of the same spectrum.

Clinical features [1,2,4,5]. Spindle cell lipoma usually presents as a small subcutaneous nodule on the upper back or nape of the neck of middle-aged to old patients, with marked predilection for males. Occasional, purely dermal examples may be seen [6]. Multiple lesions, and familial cases, occur rarely [3]. Pleomorphic lipoma has a similar clinical presentation.

Pathology [1,2,4]. Spindle cell lipoma presents as a well-circumscribed tumour composed of mature adipocytes intermixed with short, spindle-shaped cells with wavy nuclei. Hyalinized collagen bundles and focal myxoid change are prominent. Pseudovascular spaces are prominent in some cases. The spindle-shaped cells stain for CD34 and the adipocytes are positive for S100. Pleomorphic lipoma is also well-circumscribed and composed of mature adipocytes intermixed with uninucleated or multinucleated cells with hyperchromatic nuclei. The nuclei in the multinucleated cells are often arranged in a circle (floret cell). The histological diagnosis may be quite difficult in cases with few or no mature fat cells [7]. Rare variants contain real prominent vascular spaces [8].

Cytogenetic studies of both tumours have shown variable abnormalities, most commonly in chromosome 16q and rarely in chromosomes 13q and 6p [9,10].

Treatment. There is little tendency for local recurrence, and simple excision is therefore the treatment of choice.

References

1 Enzinger FM, Harvey DA. Spindle cell lipoma. *Cancer* 1975; **36**: 1852–9.
2 Fletcher CDM, Martin-Bates E. Spindle cell lipoma: a clinicopathological study with some original observations. *Histopathology* 1987; **11**: 803–17.
3 Fanburgh-Smith JC, Devaney KO, Miettinen M, Weiss SW. Multiple spindle cell lipomas: a report of 7 familial and 11 nonfamilial cases. *Am J Surg Pathol* 1998; **22**: 40–8.
4 Schmookler BM, Enzinger FM. Pleomorphic lipoma: a benign tumor simulating liposarcoma: a clinicopathologic analysis of 48 cases. *Cancer* 1981; **47**: 126–33.
5 Griffin TD, Goldstein J, Johnson WC. Pleomorphic lipoma: case report and discussion of 'atypical' lipomatous tumors. *J Cutan Pathol* 1992; **19**: 330–3.
6 Mentzel T. Cutaneous lipomatous neoplasms. *Semin Diagn Pathol* 2001; **18**: 250–7.
7 Billings SD, Folpe AL. Diagnostically challenging spindle cell lipomas: a report of 34 'low-fat' and 'fat-free' variants. *Am J Dermatopathol* 2007; **29**: 437–42.
8 Zamecnik M, Michal M. Angiomatous spindle cell lipoma: report of three cases with immunohistochemical and ultrastructural study and reappraisal of former 'pseudoangiomatous' variant. *Pathol Int* 2007; **57**: 26–31.
9 Fletcher CD, Akerman M, Dal Cin P *et al.* Correlation between clinicopathologic features and karyotype in lipomatous tumors. *Am J Pathol* 1996; **148**: 623–30.
10 Rubin BP, Fletcher CD. The cytogenetics of lipomatous tumours. *Histopathology* 1997; **30**: 507–11.

Atypical lipomatous tumour [1–4]

> **Synonym**
> • Well-differentiated liposarcoma

Definition. This is a lesion composed of lobules of mature adipose cells, with scattered larger cells with variation in nuclear size and hyperchromatism. The term 'atypical lipomatous tumour' is usually used for neoplasms occurring in the subcutis or within skeletal muscle. Similar tumours occurring in the abdominal cavity are regarded as well-differentiated liposarcomas, in view of the fact that they have a potential to cause death as a result of extensive growth. Only subcutaneous lesions will be discussed here.

Clinical features [1–3]. Subcutaneous atypical lipomatous tumours occur in middle-aged to old adults with predilection for the lower limbs. Tumours may be large, are asymptomatic and have the same clinical appearance as a lipoma.

Pathology. Typically, lobules of mature adipose tissue, with or without fibrous tissue and myxoid change, are seen. Focal variation in the size and shape of adipocytes is seen and this is associated with nuclear enlargement and hyperchromatism. Vacuolated cells may also be found. Atypical cells are often present in the fibrous tissue. Some tumours are classified as cellular based on the presence of non-lipogenic areas of increased cellularity with low-mitotic activity [5]. Dedifferentiated tumours are lesions that develop a high-grade sarcomatous component that is associated with poor prognosis [6]. This change does not usually develop in tumours that are superficially located.

Cytogenetic studies of these neoplasms have found chromosomal abnormalities in most cases. About a third of cases show supernumerary ring chromosomes affecting chromosome 12q.13–15 [4]. This results in amplification of *MDM2* and *CDK4* genes [7]. Expression of these genes can be detected by FISH, real-time PCR or immunohistochemistry, making it a useful diagnostic aid. Of these methods, FISH and real-time PCR, but particularly the former, are more sensitive than immunohistochemistry for detection of these amplifications [8].

Prognosis and treatment. There is a tendency for local recurrence, but metastases are not seen unless the tumour undergoes dedifferentiation which does not tend to happen in superficially located tumours, particularly those in the subcutaneous tissue [6]. Complete surgical excision is indicated.

References

1 Azumi N, Curtis J, Kempson RL, Hendrickson MR. Atypical and malignant neoplasms showing lipomatous differentiation: a study of 111 cases. *Am J Surg Pathol* 1987; **11**: 161–83.
2 Evans HL, Soule EH, Winkelmann RK. Atypical lipoma, atypical intramuscular lipoma, and well-differentiated retroperitoneal liposarcoma: a reappraisal of 30 cases formerly classified as well-differentiated liposarcoma. *Cancer* 1979; **43**: 574–84.
3 Evans HL. Liposarcoma and atypical lipomatous tumors: a study of 66 cases followed for a minimum of 10 years. *Surg Pathol* 1988; **1**: 41–54.
4 Rosai J, Akerman M, Dal Cin P *et al.* Combined morphologic and karyotypic study of 59 atypical lipomatous tumors: evaluation of their relationship and differential diagnosis with other adipose tissue tumors (a report of the CHAMP Study Group). *Am J Surg Pathol* 1996; **20**: 1182–9.
5 Evans HL. Atypical lipomatous tumour, its variants, and its combined forms: a study of 61 cases, with a minimum follow-up of 10 years. *Am J Surg Pathol* 2007; **31**: 1–14.
6 Weiss SW, Rao VK. Well-differentiated liposarcoma (atypical lipoma) of deep soft tissue of the extremities, retroperitoneum, and miscellaneous sites: a follow-up study of 92 cases with analysis of the incidence of dedifferentiation. *Am J Surg Pathol* 1992; **16**: 1051–8.
7 Binh MB, Sastre-Garau X, Guillou L *et al.* MDM2 and CDK4 immunostainings are useful adjuncts in diagnosing well-differentiated and dedifferentiated liposarcoma subtypes: a comparative analysis of 559 soft tissue neoplasms with genetic data. *Am J Surg Pathol* 2005; **29**: 1340–7.
8 Sirvent N, Coindre JM, Maire G *et al.* Detection of MDM2-CDK4 amplification by fluorescence in situ hybridization in 200 paraffin-embedded tumor samples: utility in diagnosing adipocytic lesions and comparison with immunohistochemistry and real-time PCR. *Am J Surg Pathol* 2007; **31**: 1476–89.

Liposarcoma [1]

Myxoid and round cell liposarcoma and pleomorphic liposarcoma are vanishingly rare in the skin. Only a few cases of primary cutaneous liposarcoma have been described. Follow-up is limited, but the behaviour seems to be better than that of their deeper counterparts, probably reflecting early detection and treatment and the easy accessibility to the skin. Liposarcoma will not be discussed further in this chapter.

Reference

1 Dei Tos AP, Mentzel T, Fletcher CD. Primary liposarcoma of the skin: a rare neoplasm with unusual high grade features. *Am J Dermatopathol* 1998; **20**: 332–8.

Tumours of uncertain histogenesis

Superficial angiomyxoma [1,2]

Definition. Superficial angiomyxoma is a dermal or subcutaneous tumour composed of a mixture of small blood vessels and sparse spindle-shaped cells in a prominent myxoid stroma.

Clinical features [1,2]. Most cases occur in adults as an asymptomatic solitary papule or nodule with equal sex incidence. Lesions are usually less than 3 cm and have a wide anatomical distribution with a predilection for the trunk, head and neck and genital skin. In patients with multiple lesions, the possibility of Carney complex should be considered (see Chapter 62) [3].

Pathology. Tumours are multilobulated, with copious myxoid stroma, numerous delicate small blood vessels and spindle-shaped or stellate bland cells, probably representing fibroblasts. Aggregates of inflammatory cells, mainly neutrophils, are frequent. In up to 30% of cases epithelial structures, probably representing hyperplastic trapped adnexal structures (particularly hair follicles), are identified.

Treatment. Local recurrence is seen in up to 30% of cases [3], but the behaviour is benign and therefore excision is the treatment of choice.

References

1 Allen PW, Dymock RB, MacCormac WB. Superficial angiomyxoma with or without epithelial components: report of 30 tumors in 28 patients. *Am J Surg Pathol* 1988; **12**: 519–30.
2 Calonje E, Guerin D, McCormick D *et al.* Superficial angiomyxoma: clinicopathologic analysis of a series of distinctive but poorly recognized cutaneous tumors with a tendency for recurrence. *Am J Surg Pathol* 1999; **23**: 910–7.
3 Carney JA, Headington JT, Wu SP. Cutaneous myxomas: a major component of the complex of myxomas, spotty pigmentation and endocrine overactivity. *Arch Dermatol* 1986; **122**: 790–8.

Digital myxoma [1]

> **Synonym**
> • Cutaneous myxoid cyst

Digital myxoma is relatively rare and presents mainly on the fingers as a small, solitary painful nodule. Females are much more commonly affected than males and there is a tendency for local recurrence. Lesions are poorly circumscribed and consist of abundant myxoid stroma with only scattered, bland, spindle-shaped cells.

Reference

1 Johnson WC, Graham JH, Helwig EB. Cutaneous myxoid cyst: a clinicopathologic and histochemical study. *JAMA* 1965; **191**: 15–20.

Dermal non-neural granular cell tumour

> **Synonyms**
> • Primitive polypoid granular cell tumour
> • Primitive non-neural granular cell tumour

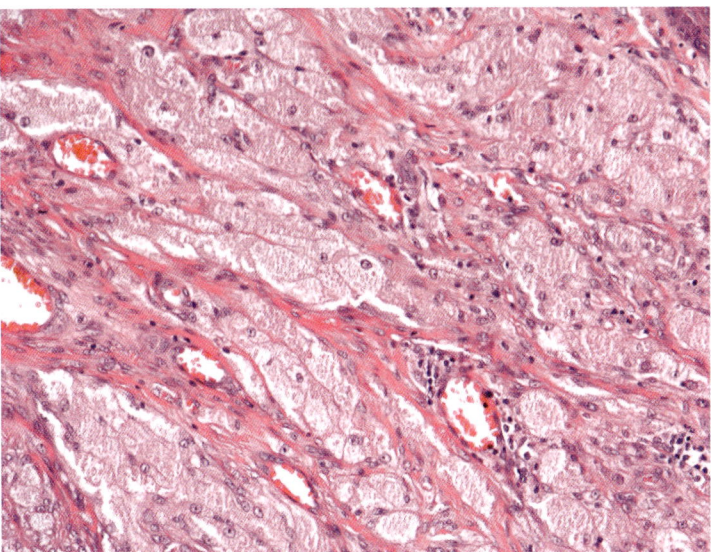

Fig. 56.44 Large cells with prominent granular cell change in a case of dermal non-neural granular cell tumour.

Definition. This is a distinctive dermal tumour with no specific line of differentiation, initially described as primitive polypoid granular cell tumour in 1991 [1]. Tumours are not related to neural granular cell tumours, which are uniformly S-100 positive. They occur both in the dermis and in subcutaneous tissue.

Clinical features. This tumour usually presents as an exophytic, small, cutaneous lesion with a wide anatomical distribution, wide age range and no sex predilection. Not all tumours are polypoid. Clinical behaviour is usually benign with only rare local recurrences [2–4]. However, a single case of metastasis to a regional lymph node has been reported [3].

Pathology. Histologically, lesions show rounded or spindle-shaped cells with prominent granular cell change (Fig. 56.44). Polypoid tumours have an epithelial collarette. Nuclear pleomorphism varies but does not tend to be prominent. Mitotic figures may be prominent. Multinucleated cells are sometimes seen. There is diffuse positivity for NKI-C3, which is a non-specific marker for lysosomes, and focal positivity for CD68 and NSE. Tumour cells do not stain for keratin, EMA, actin, desmin, H-caldesmon or S-100 [3,4].

Treatment. Complete conservative excision is the treatment of choice.

References

1 LeBoit PE, Barr RJ, Burall S *et al.* Primitive polypoid granular cell tumor and other cutaneous granular cell neoplasms of apparent non-neural origin. *Am J Surg Pathol* 1991; **15**: 48–58.
2 Lacroix-Triki M, Rochaix P, Marques B *et al.* Granular cell tumors of the skin of nonneural origin: report of 8 cases. *Ann Pathol* 1999; **19**: 94–8.
3 Lazar AJ, Fletcher CD. Primitive nonneural granular cell tumors of the skin: clinicopathologic analysis of 13 cases. *Am J Surg Pathol* 2005; **29**: 927–34.
4 Chaudhry IH, Calonje E. Dermal non-neural granular cell tumour (so-called polypoid granular cell tumour): a distinctive entity further delineated in a clinicopathological study of 11 cases. *Histopathology* 2005; **47**: 179–85.

Perivascular epithelioid cell tumour ('PEComa')

Definition. Perivascular epithelioid cell tumour is part of a spectrum of neoplasms that includes clear cell 'sugar' tumour of the lung, angiomyolipoma, lymphangioleiomyomatosis and clear cell myomelanocytic tumour of the falciform ligament [1–3]. Occurrence in the skin and soft tissue is rare but it is likely that the lesion is under-recognized. Although tumour cells are usually positive for melanocytic markers such as HMB45 and melan-A, the cell of origin has not been identified.

Clinical features. Cutaneous lesions are rare [4] and mainly occur in the lower extremities with a strong predilection for females.

Pathology [3,4]. Histology is distinctive and consists of bland epithelioid cells, typically arranged radially around thin-walled vascular channels. A smaller population of spindle cells is often seen. Tumour cells have pale pink cytoplasm and vesicular nuclei. Malignant examples may be seen but have not been reported in the skin. The immunophenotype is distinctive, as the tumour cells stain for melanocytic markers including HMB45, MITF-1, Melan-A and tyrosinase and for muscular markers including SMA and calponin. They are usually negative for S-100 and keratin.

Treatment. Simple excision is the treatment of choice.

References
1 Folpe AL, Goodman ZD, Ishak KG et al. Clear cell myomelanocytic tumor of the falciform ligament/ligamentum teres: a novel member of the perivascular epithelioid clear cell family of tumors with predilection for children and young adults. *Am J Surg Pathol* 2000; **24**: 1239–46.
2 Folpe AL, McKenney JK, Li Z et al. Clear cell myomelanocytic tumor of the thigh: report of a unique case. *Am J Surg Pathol* 2002; **26**: 809–12.
3 Hornick JL, Fletcher CD. PEComa: what do we know so far? *Histopathology* 2006; **48**: 75–82.
4 Mentzel T, Reisshauer S, Rütten A et al. Cutaneous clear cell myomelanocytic tumour: a new member of the growing family of perivascular epithelioid cell tumours (PEComas). Clinicopathological and immunohistochemical analysis of seven cases. *Histopathology* 2005; **46**: 498–504.

'Aggressive' angiomyxoma [1,2]

Definition. 'Aggressive' angiomyxoma is a distinctive tumour occurring in the genital region and pelvis, predominantly of females. It is characterized by bland, spindle-shaped cells in the background of a prominent myxoid stroma and frequent, thick-walled blood vessels.

Clinical features. This tumour occurs almost exclusively in females of reproductive age, but rare lesions have been described in males [3]. Cases in children are exceptional and may involve the spermatic cord [4]. Tumours are slowly growing and by the time of presentation they are large and ill-defined, often measuring 10 cm or more. The most commonly affected sites are the vulva and perineum. Extension into deeper soft tissues is often found.

Pathology. The lesion is infiltrative and is composed of spindle or stellate-shaped, bland cells with scanty cytoplasm, surrounded by prominent myxoid stroma. Small to medium-sized, thick-walled blood vessels are seen throughout the tumour. Mitotic figures are very rare. Rare cases contain multinucleated giant cells [5]. Interestingly, tumour cells are positive for actin and desmin. Tumour cells are often positive for oestrogen and/or progesterone receptors [6].

Cytogenetics in one case demonstrated a translocation t(8;12)(p12;p15) involving a rearrangement of *HMGIC* (a DNA architectural factor gene) [7], and analysis in a further case found a translocation t(5;8)(p15;q22) [8].

Prognosis and treatment. Local recurrence is observed in up to a third of cases, and complete surgical excision is usually difficult because of the infiltration of surrounding tissue. However, recurrences are not usually destructive, and radical surgical procedures are therefore not indicated.

References
1 Steeper TA, Rosai J. Aggressive angiomyxoma of the female pelvis and peritoneum: report of nine cases of a distinctive type of gynecologic soft tissue neoplasm. *Am J Surg Pathol* 1983; **7**: 463–75.
2 Fetsch JF, Laskin WB, Lefkowitz M et al. Aggressive angiomyxoma: a clinicopathologic study of 29 female patients. *Cancer* 1996; **78**: 79–90.
3 Tsang WY, Chang JK, Lee KC et al. Aggressive angiomyxoma: a report of four cases occurring in men. *Am J Surg Pathol* 1992; **16**: 1059–65.
4 Carlinfante G, De Marco L, Mori M et al. Aggressive angiomyxoma of the spermatic cord. Two unusual cases occurring in childhood. *Pathol Res Pract* 2001; **197**: 139–44.
5 Zamecnik M, Skalova A, Michal M et al. Aggressive angiomyxoma with multinucleated giant cells: a lesion mimicking liposarcoma. *Am J Dermatopathol* 2000; **22**: 368–71.
6 McCluggage WG, Patterson A, Maxwell P. Aggressive angiomyxoma of pelvic parts exhibits oestrogen and progesterone receptor positivity. *J Clin Pathol* 2000; **53**: 603–5.
7 Nucci MR, Weremowicz S, Neskey DM et al. Chromosomal translocation t(8;12) induces aberrant HMGIC expression in aggressive angiomyxoma of the vulva. *Gene Chromosome Canc* 2001; **32**: 172–6.
8 Tsuji T, Yoshinaga M, Inomoto Y et al. Aggressive angiomyxoma of the vulva with a sole t(5;8)(p15;q22). *Int J Gynecol Pathol* 2007; **26**: 494–6.

Epithelioid sarcoma [1–3]

Definition. A distinctive, malignant soft-tissue tumour composed of cells with epithelial differentiation. It is not clear whether this tumour represents a primary soft-tissue carcinoma or a sarcoma with epithelial differentiation.

Incidence. It is an uncommon tumour, affecting males more often than females and tending to begin in early adult life.

Clinical features [4,5]. The presenting sign can be a dermal nodule that grows outwards and may ulcerate early, a nodule or lobular subcutaneous tumour that is painless and grows slowly, or a tumour attached to deeper structures that is rather poorly defined and causes pain, paraesthesiae or muscular wasting when growing along a large trunk nerve. As a result of prominent perineurial and perivascular extension of tumour cells, multiple nodules in a sporotrichoid distribution may be seen. The distal extremities are the usual situation for the tumour, particularly the flexor aspect of the finger and the palm. It may grow at a deceptively slow rate.

A distinctive variant of epithelioid sarcoma previously described as 'extrarenal rhabdoid tumour' has been reported in older patients who present with a large mass on the proximal limbs, genitalia, buttocks, trunk or head and neck [6,7]. This variant is known as 'proximal-type epithelioid sarcoma'.

Pathology [8,9]. The tumour is composed of firm nodules, 5–50 mm or larger in diameter surrounded by fibrous tissue and fat. It is often closely associated with fascia, periosteum, tendon or nerve sheaths. The cut surface is greyish-white and flecked or mottled with yellow or brown, reflecting the presence of areas of necrosis. Microscopically, there are masses of large, round, polygonal or spindle cells with acidophilic cytoplasm. Spindle cells are often present and may predominate. The larger nodules have necrotic centres and show so-called 'geographical necrosis', which may be mistaken on scanning power microscopy for a granuloma. Mitotic figures are common, and binucleate cells occur. Variable cytological atypia is always present and may be prominent. Intercellular hyalinized collagen increases the acidophilia, while calcification, with osteoid or bone formation, may take place in the necrotic areas. The tumour spreads along dense fibrous structures and may ulcerate in areas with little subcutaneous fat. Local recurrence after excision is common, and metastasis, principally to lymph nodes, lung and pleura, may occur. Tumour cells show clear histological, ultrastructural and immunohistochemical evidence of epithelial differentiation.

The proximal type of epithelioid sarcoma shows a similar multinodular growth pattern but tumour cells are larger and with a more rhabdoid appearance consisting of abundant cytoplasm and large nuclei with or without a prominent eosinophilic nucleolus. Immunohistochemically, tumour cells in both variants of epithelioid sarcoma have the same profile. They are positive for vimentin, keratin and EMA, and 50% of cases are positive for CD34 [10].

No distinctive and consistent cytogenetic abnormality has been identified in this tumour. However, lesions often display chromosomal gains and the most frequent of these is on chromosome 22q [11,12].

Diagnosis. Superficial lesions can easily be mistaken for an ulcerating squamous cell carcinoma, deeper ones are usually regarded as inflammatory in nature. Histological diagnoses have varied, with granulomatous inflammation and synovial sarcoma being the commonest benign and malignant diagnoses, respectively.

Prognosis and treatment. Complete removal by surgical excision is essential if local recurrence and eventual metastasis are to be avoided, and the earlier this is done the less likely is the process to spread along fascial planes. Surgical excision followed by radiotherapy is often recommended. Involvement of regional lymph nodes is associated with distant metastasis and death [13]. Local recurrence and metastasis may occur years after the original diagnosis. The survival rate has been estimated at between 65% and 70% [8,13]. Features associated with poorer prognosis include male sex, older age at diagnosis, proximal location, rhabdoid phenotype, tumour size, mitotic rate, necrosis, vascular invasion, local recurrence and lymph node metastasis [3,8,9,13].

References

1 Enzinger F. Epithelioid sarcoma: a sarcoma simulating granuloma or carcinoma. *Cancer* 1970; **26**: 1029–41.
2 Fletcher CDM, McKee PH. Sarcomas: a clinicopathological guide with particular reference to cutaneous manifestation, 1. *Clin Exp Dermatol* 1984; **9**: 451–65.
3 Fisher C. Epithelioid sarcoma of Enzinger. *Adv Anat Pathol* 2006; **13**: 114–21.
4 Santiago H, Feinerman LK, Lattes R. Epithelioid sarcoma: a clinical and pathologic study of 9 cases. *Hum Pathol* 1972; **3**: 1706–10.
5 Evans HL, Baer SC. Epithelioid sarcoma: a clinicopathologic and prognostic study of 26 cases. *Semin Diagn Pathol* 1993; **10**: 286–91.
6 Guillou L, Wadden C, Coindre JM *et al*. Proximal-type epithelioid sarcoma, a distinctive aggressive neoplasm showing rhabdoid features: clinicopathologic, immunohistochemical, and ultrastructural study of a series. *Am J Surg Pathol* 1997; **21**: 130–46.
7 Hasegawa T, Matsuno Y, Shimoda T *et al*. Proximal-type epithelioid sarcoma: a clinicopathologic study of 20 cases. *Mod Pathol* 2001; **14**: 655–63.
8 Halling AC, Wollan PC, Pritchard DJ *et al*. Epithelioid sarcoma: a clinicopathologic review of 55 cases. *Mayo Clin Proc* 1996; **71**: 636–42.
9 Prat J, Woodruff JM, Marcove RC. Epithelioid sarcoma: an analysis of 22 cases indicating the prognostic significance of vascular invasion and regional lymph node metastasis. *Cancer* 1978; **41**: 1472–87.
10 Arber DA, Kandalaft PL, Mehta P *et al*. Vimentin-negative epithelioid sarcoma: the value of an immunohistochemical panel that includes CD34. *Am J Surg Pathol* 1993; **17**: 302–7.
11 Lualdi E, Modena P, Debiec-Rychter M *et al*. Molecular cytogenetic characterization of proximal-type epithelioid sarcoma. *Genes Chromosomes Cancer* 2004; **41**: 283–90.
12 Lee MW, Jee KJ, Han SS *et al*. Comparative genomic hybridization in epithelioid sarcoma. *Br J Dermatol* 2004; **151**: 1054–9.
13 Chase DR, Enzinger FM. Epithelioid sarcoma: diagnosis, prognostic indicators and treatment. *Am J Surg Pathol* 1985; **9**: 241–63.

Ossifying lesions in the dermis [1]

A wide range of subcutaneous lesions may occasionally show partial ossification. The most common are pilomatricomas and melanocytic naevi. Other soft-tissue lesions, such as soft-tissue chondromas and fibromyxoid tumours, may show metaplastic bone formation.

Reference

1 Fletcher CDM. Calcifying and ossifying soft tissue lesions presenting in the skin. *J Cutan Pathol* 1996; **23**: 297.

Osteoma cutis [1]

Definition. A true bony new growth arising within the skin from bone-forming tissue and showing no tendency to invade.

Incidence and aetiology. Osteoma cutis is a rare tumour. Most osseous nodules in the skin are not true neoplasms, but result from metaplastic ossification, which usually occurs in a focus of calcification; the initiating lesion is frequently an inflammatory granuloma or scar. The majority of these lesions are best classified as dystrophic ossification rather than as osteomas. Dystrophic ossification has been reported in scleroderma, in old acne cysts and at sites of puncture of the skin or of haematomas. They may be found in melanocytic naevus, pilomatricoma, histiocytoma and chondroid syringoma, and may be secondary to basal cell carcinoma [2,3]. Another cause is Albright's hereditary osteodystrophy, in which cutaneous ossification has recently been recognized with increasing frequency [4–6]. Rarely, multiple miliary osteomas of the skin can occur after acne [7,8], sometimes with neurotic excoriations or after dermabrasion [9]. There remain a minority of reported cases that appear to be primary osteomas, the majority of which are multiple and on the face or scalp [9–11].

There is no point in trying to estimate the age and sex incidence for a group as heterogeneous as individuals with dystrophic calcification of the skin. It seems likely that primary osteomas will become even more rare if hereditary osteodystrophy and other causes are sought.

Clinical features. Metaplastic osteomas are frequently small and clinically undetectable in the primary lesion. They are usually situated deep in the dermis or subcutaneous tissue. They may be seen when radiographs of the area are taken, but are most commonly first noticed by the histology technician as a hard body that damages the knife edge. The distinguishing feature, if the tumour is found clinically, is the stone-hard texture on palpation, similar to pilomatricoma. A case of osteoma cutis associated with diaphyseal aclasis has been reported [12].

Pathology [3]. Whether metaplastic or primary, the microscopic picture is of a small circumscribed nodule of osseous tissue with trabeculae enclosing fat and, occasionally, marrow cells.

Treatment. If required, simple excision is curative.

References
1 Reichenberger M, Löhnert J. Osteosis cutis multiplex. *Hautarzt* 1971; **22**: 73–7.
2 Duperrat B. Cutaneous osteomas: study based on 24 personal cases. *Ann Dermatol Syphiligr* 1961; **88**: 11–31.
3 Roth SL, Stowell RE, Helwig EB. Cutaneous ossification: report of 120 cases and review of the literature. *Arch Pathol* 1963; **76**: 44–54.
4 Brook CGD, Valman HB. Osteoma cutis and Albright's hereditary osteodystrophy. *Br J Dermatol* 1971; **85**: 471–5.
5 Eyre WG, Reed WB. Albright's hereditary osteodystrophy with cutaneous bone formation. *Arch Dermatol* 1971; **104**: 636–42.
6 Peterson WC, Mandel SL. Primary osteomas of skin. *Arch Dermatol* 1963; **87**: 626–32.
7 Basler RSW, Taylor WB, Peacor DR. Postacne osteoma cutis: X-ray diffraction analysis. *Arch Dermatol* 1974; **110**: 113–4.
8 Delaney TJ, Gold SC, Leppard B. Disseminated perforating granuloma annulare. *Br J Dermatol* 1974; **89**: 523–6.
9 Rossman RE, Freeman RG. Osteoma cutis, a stage of preosseous calcification. *Arch Dermatol* 1964; **89**: 68–73.
10 Helm F, De La Pava S, Klein E. Multiple miliary osteomas of the skin. *Arch Dermatol* 1967; **96**: 681–2.
11 Zabel R. Osteosis cutis multiplex faciei. *Dermatol Monatsschr* 1970; **156**: 798–801.
12 Donaldson EM, Summerly R. Primary osteoma cutis and diaphyseal aclasis. *Arch Dermatol* 1962; **85**: 261–5.

Cutaneous calculus [1,2]

Synonym
- Subepidermal calcified nodule

This small tumour, which is relatively common, has a characteristic yellowish white colour and is situated in the subepidermal tissue. It is seen most commonly on the face in children; it varies in size up to 10 mm or so, but may occasionally be larger and plaque-like, and it has a hard consistency. The epidermis over it may be verrucose. Episodes of inflammation and shedding of a portion of the lesion may occur. Microscopic examination shows calcareous bodies in the superficial part of the dermis. A histiocytic or foreign-body reaction often surrounds some of the calcified bodies. The exact histogenesis is uncertain. Calcification of naevus cells has been suggested. The lesion can be removed easily by curettage.

References
1 Hunter GA, Donald GF. Cutaneous calculus: a report of three cases. *Aust J Dermatol* 1963; **7**: 23–5.
2 Woods B, Kellaway TD. Cutaneous calculi: subepidermal calcified nodules. *Br J Dermatol* 1963; **75**: 1–11.

Progressive osseous heteroplasia

This is discussed in Chapter 45.

CHAPTER 57

Cutaneous Lymphomas and Lymphocytic Infiltrates

S.J. Whittaker

St John's Institute of Dermatology, Guy's and St Thomas' Hospital, London, UK

Introduction

Over the past 20 years, advances in understanding the biology of lymphoid cells have greatly improved our knowledge of primary cutaneous lymphomas. Various node-based classifications of lymphomas, including the Kiel classification first introduced in 1980 and updated in 1988 [1], were of relatively little value for primary cutaneous lymphoma as they were based purely on detailed pathological assessment of nodes with no clinical correlation. In contrast, the current World Health Organization/European Organization of Research and Treatment of Cancer (WHO–EORTC) classification is based on clinical, pathological, immuno-pathological, molecular and cytogenetic findings [2], and implicitly recognizes that the site of origin of extranodal lymphomas rather than just tumour morphology determines clinical behaviour, which in turn has a critical influence on prognosis and therapeutic approach.

In 1975, it was demonstrated that the great majority of lymphoid infiltrates associated with the skin were of T-cell type and Edelson introduced the term cutaneous T-cell lymphoma (CTCL) [3]. In Europe, the work of the Dutch Cutaneous Lymphoma Working Party (DCLWP) and the Graz group delineated different subsets of primary cutaneous T- and B-cell lymphomas, which led directly to the EORTC proposal for classification of primary cutaneous lymphomas and the recent WHO–EORTC classification (Table 57.1) [2,4]. This consensus is now reflected in the 2008 WHO classification of haematologic malignancies as all the primary cutaneous lymphoma variants have been recognized as distinct entities [5].

Mycosis fungoides (MF) is the most common primary CTCL subset, but other subsets with clearly identifiable clinicopathological features and varying prognoses have also been described. A critical observation has been the realization that lymphomas with a similar pathology arising in different organs have different prognoses and a distinct molecular pathogenesis; nodal CD30⁺ anaplastic large cell lymphomas are usually ALK⁺ and can be associated with a poor prognosis, especially for ALK⁻ variants, whereas primary cutaneous CD30⁺ anaplastic large cell lymphomas are invariably ALK⁻ and generally associated with a good prognosis [2]. Primary cutaneous B-cell lymphomas represent [2] about one-third of all primary cutaneous lymphomas, and primary cutaneous follicle centre lymphomas are now recognized as pathogentically distinct from nodal follicular lymphomas. The majority of these primary cutaneous B-cell lymphomas have an excellent prognosis [2].

The concept of a subset of circulating lymphocytes with a special avidity or affinity for the skin has been supported by the identification of T cells expressing the cutaneous lymphocyte antigen

Rook's Textbook of Dermatology, 8th edition. Edited by DA Burns, SM Breathnach, NH Cox and CEM Griffiths. © 2010 Blackwell Publishing Ltd.

Table 57.1 WHO–EORTC classification of primary cutaneous lymphomas (frequency and prognosis based on Dutch and Austrian clinical data).

WHO–EORTC classification	No.	Frequency (%)	Disease-specific 5-year survival (%)
Primary cutaneous T-cell lymphoma			
Indolent clinical behaviour			
Mycosis fungoides	800	44	88
Folliculotropic MF	86	4	80
Pagetoid reticulosis	14	<1	100
Granulomatous slack skin	4	<1	100
Primary cutaneous anaplastic large cell lymphoma	146	8	96
Lymphomatoid papulosis	236	12	100
Subcutaneous panniculitis-like T-cell lymphoma	18	1	82
Primary cutaneous CD4+ small/medium pleomorphic T-cell lymphoma	39	2	75
Aggressive clinical behaviour			
Sézary syndrome	52	3	24
Primary cutaneous NK/T-cell lymphoma, nasal type	7	<1	NR
Primary cutaneous aggressive CD8+ T-cell lymphoma	14	<1	18
Primary cutaneous γδ T-cell lymphoma	13	<1	NR
Primary cutaneous peripheral T-cell lymphoma, unspecified	47	2	16
Cutaneous B-cell lymphoma			
Indolent clinical behaviour			
Primary cutaneous marginal zone B-cell lymphoma	127	7	99
Primary cutaneous follicle centre lymphoma	207	11	95
Intermediate clinical behaviour			
Primary cutaneous diffuse large B-cell lymphoma, leg type	85	4	55
Primary cutaneous diffuse large B-cell lymphoma, other	4	<1	50
Primary cutaneous intravascular large B-cell lymphoma	6	<1	65

NR – not reached.

(CLA; HECA 452), which binds to its ligand, E-selectin, on dermal endothelial cells [6]. These subsets of skin trafficking T cells comprise the skin-associated lymphoid tissue (SALT), and contribute to the skin immune system (SIS), in a similar manner to other mucosal sites such as the gut mucosa-associated lymphoid tissue (MALT). The expression of the chemokine receptors CCR4 and CCR10 by tumour cells may also contribute to epidermotropism in cutaneous T-cell lymphoma (CTCL) while the expression of the lymph node chemokine receptor CCR7 may contribute to tumour dissemination in Sézary syndrome (SS) [7].

The identification of T-cell clones in skin using T-cell receptor (TCR) gene analysis has established both the neoplastic nature and lineage of a wide variety of cutaneous lymphoproliferative entities, and both TCR and immunoglobulin gene analysis are now part of the standard diagnostic assessment of cutaneous lymphoid infiltrates [8]. The presence of a lymphoid clone is not synonymous with malignancy and its significance in benign cutaneous lymphoid infiltrates is at present unknown. It is unclear whether these techniques will also provide prognostic information but they complement existing staging approaches, particularly for analysis of lymph node and peripheral blood in MF and SS.

It has been apparent for some time that the original American Joint Committee on Cancer (AJCC) staging system for MF/SS was not ideal, with markedly variable outcomes for patients with stage IIB and slightly better outcomes for stage III than stage IIB. Also there has been a lack of consensus regarding the measurement of tumour burden in peripheral blood. This has led to new staging proposals for MF/SS and non-MF/SS primary cutaneous lymphomas, which now require prospective validation [9,10].

The underlying molecular pathogenesis of CTCL is unknown but various abnormalities have been identified, including inactivation of genes controlling the cell cycle and apoptosis [11]. These abnormalities appear to be associated with disease progression and may contribute to treatment resistance. In addition, molecular cytogenetic techniques have detected a consistent pattern of chromosomal abnormalities, indicating the location of putative genes that may have a fundamental role in the pathogenesis of CTCL [11].

Several novel therapies have been licensed for CTCL, including a retinoid, bexarotene, that binds to the retinoid X receptor (RXR), a diphtheria interleukin-2 (IL-2) fusion toxin, denileukin diftitox (Onzar; Ontak), and a histone deacetylase inhibitor, suberoylanilide hydroxamic acid (SAHA/vorinostat) [12–15]. A number of other novel therapies have been proven to have efficacy in CTCL and offer promising alternatives to existing therapies [16]. These studies have also facilitated the current development of more robust response criteria for MF and SS.

References

1 Stansfield AG, Diebold J, Kapanci Y *et al*. Updated Kiel classification for lymphomas. *Lancet* 1988; **1**: 292–3.

2 Willemze R, Jaffe E, Burg G *et al*. WHO-EORTC classification for cutaneous lymphomas. *Blood* 2005; **105**: 3768–85.

3 Edelson RL. Cutaneous T-cell lymphoma: the Sézary syndrome, mycosis fungoides and other variants. *J Am Acad Dermatol* 1980; **2**: 89–106.

4 Willemze R, Kerl H, Sterry W *et al*. EORTC classification for primary cutaneous lymphomas: a proposal from the Cutaneous Lymphoma Study Group of the European Organization for Research on Treatment of Cancer. *Blood* 1997; **90**: 354–71.

5 Jaffe E, Ralfkiaer E. Mycosis fungoides and Sézary syndrome. In: *World Health Organization Classification of Tumours: Pathology and Genetics of Tumours of Haematopoietic and Lymphoid Tissues*. IARC, 2008.

6 Picker LJ, Michie SA, Rott LS, Butcher EC. A unique type of skin-associated lymphocytes in humans: preferential expression of the HECA452 epitope by benign and malignant T cells at cutaneous sites. *Am J Pathol* 1990; **136**: 1053–68.

7 Pals S, Gorter D, Spaargaren M. Lymphoma dissemination: the other face of lymphocyte homing. *Blood* 2007; **110**: 3102–11.

8 Whittaker S. T-cell receptor gene analysis in cutaneous T-cell lymphomas. *Clin Exp Dermatol* 1996; **21**: 81–7.

9 Olsen E, Vonderheid E, Pimpinelli N *et al*. Revisions to the staging and classification of mycosis fungoides and Sezary syndrome: a proposal of the International Society for Cutaneous Lymphomas (ISCL) and the cutaneous lymphoma task force of the European Organisation of Research and Treatment of Cancer (EORTC). *Blood* 2007; **110**: 1713–22.

10 Kim Y, Willemze R, Pimpinelli N *et al*. TNM classification system for primary cutaneous lymphomas other than mycosis fungoides and Sezary syndrome: a proposal of the International Society for Cutaneous Lymphoma (ISCL) and the Cutaneous Lymphoma Task Force of the European Organisation for Research and Treatment of Cancer (EORTC). *Blood* 2007; **110**: 479–84.

11 Whittaker S. Biological insights into the pathogenesis of cutaneous T-cell lymphomas (CTCL). *Semin Oncol* 2006; **33**: S3–6.

12 Duvic M, Martin A, Kim Y *et al*. Phase 2 and 3 clinical trial of oral bexarotene (Targretin capsules) for the treatment of refractory or persistent early stage cutaneous T-cell lymphoma. *Arch Dermatol* 2001; **137**: 581–93.

13 Duvic M, Hymes K, Heald P *et al*. Bexarotene is effective and safe for treatment of refractory advanced-stage cutaneous T-cell lymphoma: multinational phase II–III trial results. *J Clin Oncol* 2001; **19**: 2456–71.

14 Olsen E, Duvic M, Frankel A *et al*. Pivotal phase III trial of two dose levels of Denileukin Diftitox for the treatment of cutaneous T-cell lymphoma. *J Clin Oncol* 2001; **19**: 376–88.

15 Olsen E, Kim Y, Kuzel T *et al*. Phase IIB multicenter trial of vorinostat in patients with persistent, progressive or treatment refractory cutaneous T-cell lymphoma. *J Clin Oncol* 2007; **25**: 1–9.

16 Whittaker S, Foss F. Efficacy and tolerability of currently available therapies for the mycosis fungoides and Sezary syndrome variants of cutaneous T-cell lymphoma variants. *Cancer Treat Rev* 2007; **33**: 146–60.

Primary cutaneous T-cell lymphomas

Mycosis fungoides

Definition. The most common variant of primary CTCL, generally associated with an indolent clinical course and characterized by well-defined clinicopathological features.

Aetiology. The aetiology of MF is not yet established. The HTLV-1 retrovirus was first isolated from a patient with CTCL and subsequently it was appreciated that this patient had adult T-cell leukaemia–lymphoma (ATLL). Because of clinical and pathological similarities to cutaneous involvement in ATLL, there has been an intensive search for HTLV-1 and related viruses in MF. However, although an association with HTLV-1 has been suggested, subsequent extensive investigations have failed to identify conclusively any of the currently recognized HTLV-associated viruses in MF [1–5]. For over 20 years, one of the theories associated with the development of MF has been that this is a disease of antigen persistence associated with chronic lymphocyte stimu-

lation and eventual transformation of benign lymphocytes to a low-grade malignant T-cell lymphoma [6]. This is a plausible and attractive theory, but as yet the antigen or antigens responsible for this transformation have not been identified.

A number of case–control studies have investigated the possibility of environmental agents precipitating or aggravating early CTCL. One study from the east coast of North America [7] recorded a significantly higher incidence of allergies and of fungal and viral infections in patients who developed CTCL compared with healthy controls, and also reported that a higher proportion of CTCL patients had worked in the petrochemical, textile, machine and metal industries. Other case–control studies have suggested possible links with occupational exposure to glass, pottery and ceramics [8], as well as workers exposed to solar radiation [9]. Other studies have not confirmed these observations but did record a significantly higher incidence of atopic disease in MF patients [10] and there have been subsequent reports of CTCL developing in patients with severe atopic dermatitis [11]. An association with atopic disease has not been confirmed in another case–control study [12]. A more recent study from North America has also failed to confirm any clear occupational or environmental exposure [13] but other studies have observed a higher than expected prevalence of other malignancies, including non-lymphoma cutaneous malignancies in patients with MF [14]. Further reports have also suggested that there is a possible increased incidence of non-melanoma skin cancer, melanoma and also lung cancer in MF but whether or not this is related to prior therapy remains to be clarified [15–17].

The incidence of MF (0.64/100 000 for CTCL) is increasing but the explanation for this is unclear. The rise could represent a combination of improved diagnosis and previous coding problems as well as a genuine increasing disease incidence, as seen for non-Hodgkin's lymphoma [18].

Clinical features. Mycosis fungoides is characterized by typical cutaneous stages of disease, consisting of patches and plaques involving less than 10% of the body surface area (stage T1/IA), more than 10% of the body surface area (stage T2/IB), tumours (stage T3/IIB) and erythrodermic disease (stage T3/III). Patients may progress from having limited patches and plaques to extensive plaques or tumours and even erythroderma [19]. However, many patients do not show any evidence of progression. Stage IA MF is characterized by subtle, fine scaly and often slightly atrophic erythematous patches on the trunk, usually involving the limb girdle areas, breast and particularly the buttocks (Fig. 57.1). There may be mild pruritus but patients are often asymptomatic. At this stage, the clinical differential diagnosis includes pityriasis rosea, fungal infection, mild dermatitis or even a rather atypical form of psoriasis. Plaques are more obvious, persistent, polymorphic, erythematous lesions with a similar distribution but, with the development of stage T2/IB, there is usually involvement of the head, neck and limbs as well as the trunk (Figs 57.2 & 57.3). Individual plaques may become very large, and there may be some degree of regression, giving rise to unusual arcuate and horseshoe-shaped lesions that can show considerable variation in colour, degree of scaling and border definition. Striking psoriasiform scaling can sometimes be a feature. There is some evidence that the overall

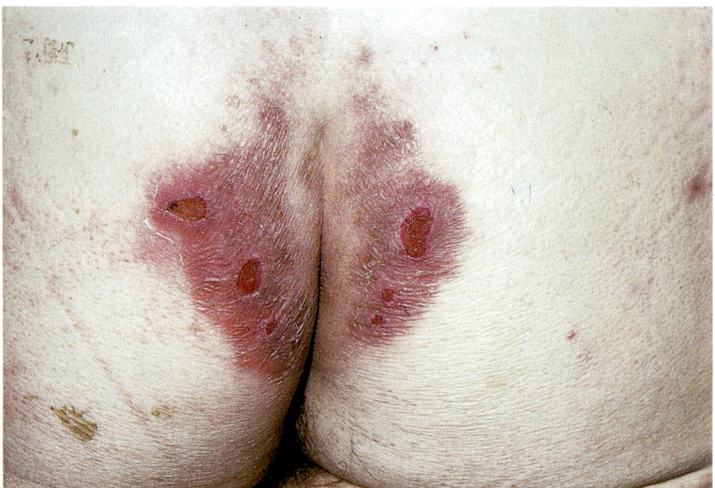

Fig. 57.1 Early mycosis fungoides showing plaques in the buttock area.

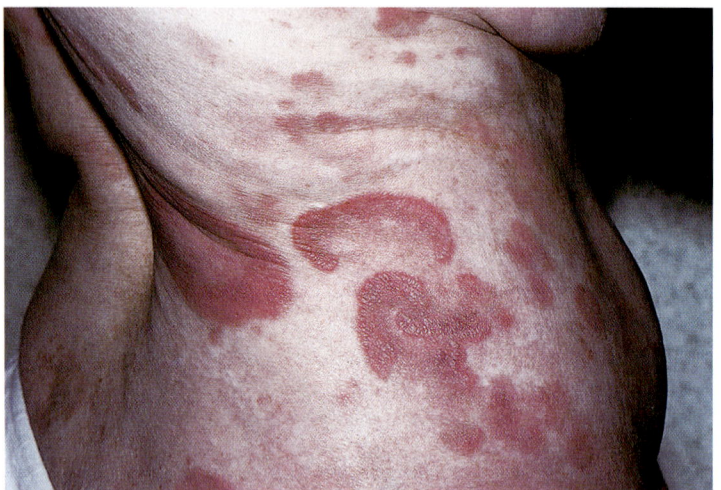

Fig. 57.2 More advanced mycosis fungoides showing typical polycyclic plaques.

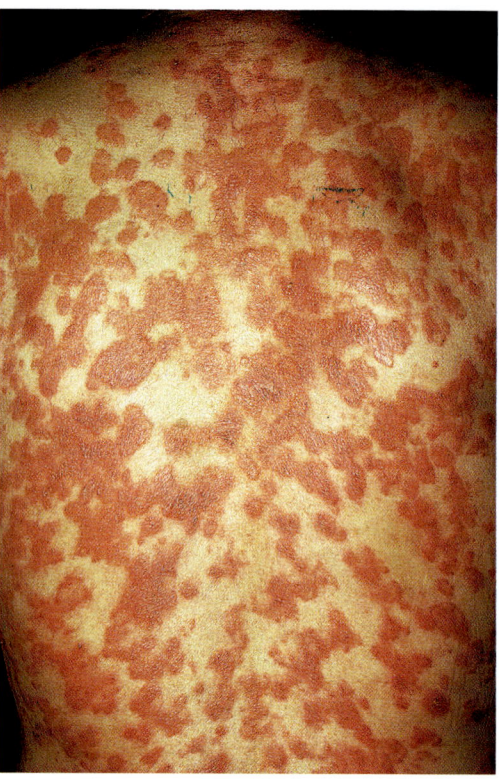

Fig. 57.3 Further stage of mycosis fungoides showing plaques involving more than 10% of the body surface.

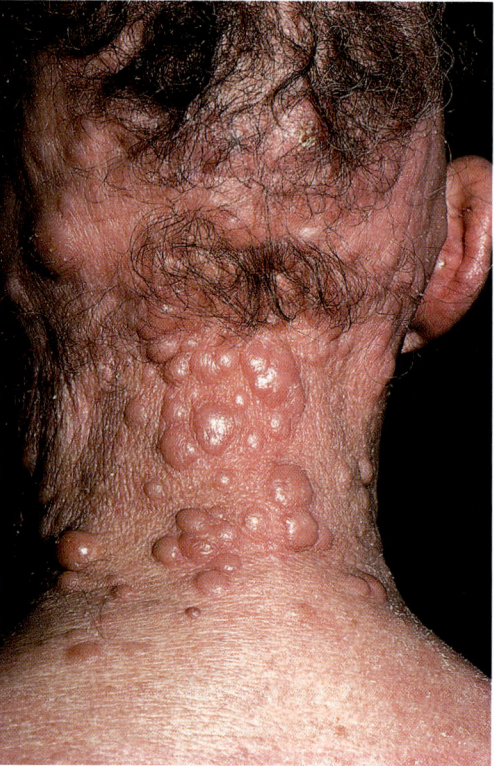

Fig. 57.4 Nodular mycosis fungoides showing striking nodules on the back of the neck. Similar lesions were present on all four limbs.

thickness of plaques in stage T2/IB may have prognostic significance [20]. Once again, patients may complain of pruritus or be asymptomatic. Rarely, individual plaques may become eroded or ulcerated and painful, which is often associated with secondary bacterial infection and such patients may have a very poor quality of life and high morbidity despite having an early stage of disease. Tumours can show considerable variation in size (Fig. 57.4), and if there are only a few small tumours it may be difficult to categorize as truly stage T3/IIB disease. Many patients with early stages (T1/IA–T2/IB) of disease do not progress but rarely patients may gradually develop an erythroderma (stage T3/III), which is usually associated with severe pruritus. A *tumeur d'emblée* form of MF, in which patients rapidly develop large nodules and tumours without the prior presence of patches and plaques, has been described in the past [21], but it is now appreciated that many of these patients have other CTCL variants, which should be excluded on the basis of a critical assessment of the histological and immunophenotypical features. Patients may also rarely present with erythrodermic stages of disease and the differential diagnosis for these patients includes inflammatory dermatoses and Sézary syndrome.

The development of peripheral lymphadenopathy in MF alters the staging regardless of the cutaneous stage of disease [22]. Although the great majority of patients with early stage disease do not develop overt clinical involvement of lymph nodes or other organs (see prognosis), a small proportion do eventually show generalized, systemic spread and may exhibit typical 'B' symptoms with fever and weight loss. Histological involvement of central lymph nodes and other organs is a very poor prognostic sign. Any systemic organ can be involved but apart from liver, spleen and bone marrow, other sites commonly involved include the pulmonary, skeletal, nasopharyngeal and central nervous systems (CNS).

There are a large number of clinical variants of MF. Some plaques have a rather verrucous [23] or hyperkeratotic appearance, and bullae may rarely develop in the course of progression of individual plaques [24]. Rare ichthyosiform variants have been described [25]. An important subset of patients have MF that appears to be associated with pilosebaceous follicles, giving rise to a follicular clinical pattern often with alopecia (pilotropic or folliculotropic MF; see below) and there is evidence that these patients may be resistant to treatment and have a poorer prognosis independent of their stage of disease [26]. Rarely, younger patients present with a purpuric eruption not unlike the pigmented purpuric dermatosis associated with capillaritis but with histological features of MF [27]. Non-white younger adult patients may also present with a hypopigmented variant of MF [28,29], characterized by striking hypopigmented scaly patches often involving the trunk and especially the pelvic girdle area rather than the limbs. Histologically, these lesions tend to show marked epidermotropism, in contrast to the subtle clinical features. In poikilodermatous MF, patients develop clinical lesions characterized by either widespread or isolated poikiloderma, which may or may not be associated with typical patches and plaques of MF. The trunk is usually involved and the breasts and pelvic girdle area may also be affected (Fig. 57.5). The poikiloderma is typically characterized by atrophy, pigmentation and telangiectasia and must be distinguished from poikiloderma resulting from other disorders by appropriate histology. Rarely, patients may have extensive poikiloderma as a feature of erythrodermic disease. These clinical variants do not have any prognostic significance with the exception of folliculotropic/pilotropic MF [26].

Clinical differential diagnosis. In the early stages of MF, the clinical differential diagnosis may include such diverse conditions as allergic contact dermatitis, atopic dermatitis, psoriasis and fungal infection. Any patient with persistent polymorphic plaques, particularly involving the pelvic girdle area, should have a skin biopsy and histological confirmation of the disease. Multiple biopsies may be required to confirm a clinical suspicion of MF in early stages of disease and criteria for the early diagnosis of MF have been published by the International Society for Cutaneous Lymphoma (ISCL) [30].

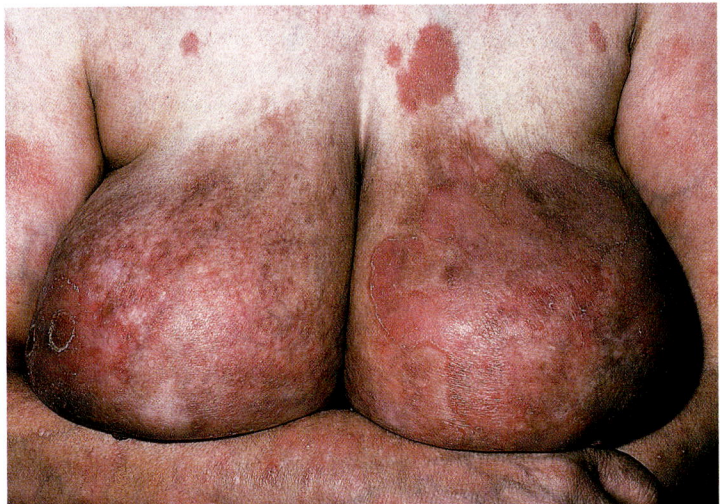

Fig. 57.5 Poikilodermatous mycosis fungoides showing involvement of both breasts.

References

1 Pancake B, Zucker-Franklin D, Coutavas E. The cutaneous T-cell lymphoma, mycosis fungoides, is a human T cell lymphotropic virus-associated disease. *J Clin Invest* 1995; **95**: 547.

2 Whittaker S, Luzatto L. HTLV-1 and mycosis fungoides. *Science* 1993; **259**: 1470–1.

3 Lisby G, Reitz MR, Vejlsgaard GL. No detection of HTLV-1 DNA in punch biopsies from patients with cutaneous T-cell lymphoma by the polymerase chain reaction. *J Invest Dermatol* 1992; **98**: 417–20.

4 Boni R, Daneschfar A, Burg G *et al.* No detection of HTLV-1 proviral DNA in lesional skin biopsies from Swiss and German patients with cutaneous T-cell lymphoma. *Br J Dermatol* 1996; **134**: 282.

5 Li G, Vowels B, Benoit B *et al.* Failure to detect human T-lymphotropic virus type 1 (HTLV-1) proviral DNA in cell lines and tissues from patients with cutaneous T-cell lymphoma. *J Invest Dermatol* 1996; **107**: 308–13.

6 Tan RSH, Butterworth CM, McLaughlin H *et al.* Mycosis fungoides: a disease of antigen persistence. *Br J Dermatol* 1974; **91**: 607–16.

7 Cohen SR, Stenn KS, Bravermann IS *et al.* Mycosis fungoides: clinicopathological relationships, survival and therapy in 59 patients with observations on occupation as a new prognostic factor. *Cancer* 1980; **46**: 2654–6.

8 Morales M, Varela R, Olsen J *et al.* Occupational risk factors for mycosis fungoides: a European multicentre case-control study. *J Occup Environ Med* 2004; **46**: 205–11.

9 Morales M, Varela R, Olsen J *et al.* Occupational sun exposure and mycosis fungoides: a European mulitcentre case-control study. *J Occup Environ Med* 2006; **48**: 390–3.

10 Tuyp E, Burgoyne A, Mackie RM. A case–control study of possible causative factors in mycosis fungoides. *Arch Dermatol* 1987; **123**: 196–200.

11 Fletcher C, Orchard G, Hubbard V *et al.* CD30+ cutaneous lymphoma in association with atopic eczema. *Arch Dermatol* 2004; **140**: 449–54.

12 Morales M, Olsen J, Johansen P *et al.* Viral infection, atopy and mycosis fungoides: a European multicentre case-control study. *Eur J Cancer* 2003; **39**: 511–6.

13 Whitmore AS, Holly EA, Lee IM *et al.* Mycosis fungoides in relation to environmental exposure and immune response. *J Natl Cancer Inst* 1989; **81**: 1560–7.

14 Huang K, Weinstock M, Clarke C *et al.* Second lymphomas and other malignant neoplasms in patients with mycosis fungoides and Sezary syndrome. *Arch Dermatol* 2007; **143**: 45–50.

15 Scarisbrick J, Child F, Evans A *et al.* Secondary malignant neoplasms in 71 patients with Sézary syndrome. *Arch Dermatol* 1999; **135**: 1381–5.

16 Vakeva L, Pukkala E, Ranki A. Increased risk of secondary cancers in patients with primary cutaneous T-cell lymphoma. *J Invest Dermatol* 2000; **115**: 62–5.

17 Evans A, Scarisbrick J, Child F *et al.* Cutaneous malignant melanoma in association with mycosis fungoides. *J Am Acad Dermatol* 2004; **50**: 701–5.

18 Criscione V, Weinstock M. Incidence of cutaneous T-cell lymphoma in the United States, 1973–2002. *Arch Dermatol* 2007; **143**: 854–9.

19 Willemze R, Jaffe E, Burg G *et al.* WHO-EORTC classification for cutaneous lymphomas. *Blood* 2005; **105**: 3768–85.

20 Kashani-Sabet M, McMillan A, Zackheim H. A modified staging classification for cutaneous T-cell lymphoma. *J Am Acad Dermatol* 2001; **45**: 700–6.

Table 57.2 TNM classification of mycosis fungoides (MF).

Cutaneous involvement (T)

T_0	Lesions clinically and/or histologically suspicious but not diagnostic
T_1	Plaques involving less than 10% of skin
T_2	Plaques involving more than 10% of skin
T_3	Tumours present
T_4	Erythroderma

Lymph nodes (N)

N_0	Clinically and pathologically normal
N_1	Palpable; pathologically not involved
N_2	Clinically non-palpable; pathologically MF
N_3	Clinically enlarged; pathologically MF

Viscera (M)

M_0	No visceral spread
M_1	Visceral spread present

Peripheral blood (B)

B_0	No atypical circulating cells
B_1	Atypical circulating cells present

Table 57.3 A staging system for mycosis fungoides related to TNM classification.

Stage	T	N	M
IA	T_1	N_0	M_0
IB	T_2	N_0	M_0
IIA	T_{1-2}	N_1	M_0
IIB	T_3	N_{0-1}	M_0
III	T_4	N_{0-1}	M_0
IVA	T_{1-4}	N_{2-3}	M_0
IVB	T_{1-4}	N_{0-3}	M_1

21 Willemze R, Beljaards RC, Meijer CJLM. Classification of primary cutaneous T cell lymphomas. *Histopathology* 1994; **24**: 405–15.

22 Sausville E, Worsham G, Matthews M *et al*. Histologic assessment of lymph nodes in mycosis fungoides/Sézary syndrome (cutaneous T-cell lymphoma): clinical correlation and prognostic import of a new classification system. *Hum Pathol* 1985; **16**: 1098–109.

23 Price NM, Fuks ZY, Hoffman TE. Hyperkeratotic and verrucous features of mycosis fungoides. *Arch Dermatol* 1977; **113**: 57–60.

24 Roenigk HH, Castrovina AJ. Mycosis fungoides bullosa. *Arch Dermatol* 1971; **104**: 402–6.

25 Eisman S, O'Toole E, Jones A, Whittaker S. Granulomatous mycosis funogides presenting as an acquired icthyosis. *Clin Exp Dermatol* 2003; **28**: 174–6.

26 Van Doorn R, Scheffer E, Willemze R. Follicular mycosis fungoides, a distinct disease entity with or without associated follicular mucinosis. *Arch Dermatol* 2002; **138**: 191–8.

27 Magro C, Schaefer J, Crowson A *et al*. Pigmented purpuric dermatosis. Classification by phenotypic and molecular profiles. *Am J Clin Pathol* 2007; **128**: 218–29.

28 Smith NP, Samman PD. Mycosis fungoides presenting with areas of cutaneous hypopigmentation. *Clin Exp Dermatol* 1978; **3**: 213–6.

29 Lambroza E, Cohen SR, Phelps R *et al*. Hypopigmented variant of mycosis fungoides: demography, histopathology and treatment of seven cases. *J Am Acad Dermatol* 1995; **32**: 987–93.

30 Pimipinelli N, Olsen E, Santucci M *et al*. Defining early mycosis fungoides. *J Am Acad Dermatol* 2005; **53**: 1053–63.

Staging. There are two staging systems in current use that have prognostic significance [1–3]. The Tumour, Nodes, Metastases classification and the staging system suggested by the North American MF Cooperative Group are given in Tables 57.2 and 57.3. All patients should have a defined stage so that appropriate advice can be given regarding prognosis and treatment.

All patients with MF should have a full clinical examination and adequate diagnostic biopsies for histology and immunophenotypic and preferably molecular studies as, even for stage IA disease, studies suggest that patients with a detectable T-cell clone have a shorter duration of response and a higher rate of treatment failure [4]. Occasionally, multiple skin biopsies and the opinion of experienced dermatopathologists are required to make a diagno-

sis. Peripheral blood samples should be taken for routine haematology, biochemistry, serum lactate dehydrogenase (LDH), Sézary cells, lymphocyte subsets, CD4 : CD8 ratio, HTLV-1 serology and, ideally, TCR gene analysis of peripheral blood mononuclear cells. These tests are necessary to distinguish patients with ATLL and those patients with peripheral blood T-cell clones identical to skin who may have a poor prognosis. Any palpable and bulky peripheral nodes should be biopsied but the practice of 'blind' lymph node biopsy of non-palpable nodes is not essential, although histological evidence of lymphoma can very rarely be detected in the absence of palpable lymphadenopathy. Chest X-ray should be performed in those with advanced stages of disease. Staging CT scans of the chest, abdomen and pelvis are indicated in all those patients with stage IIA, IIB, III and IV MF, but not in those with stage IA or IB MF [5]. Peripheral nodes with a diameter greater than 1.5 cm are considered to be abnormal in patients with cutaneous lymphomas whereas for central nodes a diameter greater than 1.0 cm is considered to be the limit. The value of PET-CT in MF has yet to be established but this may increase the detection rate of systemic disease with PET activity correlating with histologic lymph node grade [6]. Bone marrow aspirate and trephine biopsies may be indicated in patients with stage IIB, III and IV MF and those patients with peripheral blood involvement, as indicated by the presence of Sézary cell counts representing more than 5% of the total leukocyte count, although the overall positive yield will be low [7,8]. The ISCL and EORTC have published a revised staging system for MF/SS which is currently being validated in prospective studies [9]. This staging system attempts to distinguish patients with early stage IA/IB who only have patches and to stratify more accurately lymph node disease incorporating molecular analysis for T-cell clones as well as assessing the degree of peripheral blood involvement more specifically (Table 57.4). Prospective validation of this staging system will also clarify the prognostic relevance of features such as folliculotropism and large cell transformation.

References

1 Green S, Byar D, Lamberg S. Prognostic variables in mycosis fungoides. *Cancer* 1981; **47**: 2671–7.

2 Lamberg S, Green S, Byar D *et al*. Clinical staging for cutaneous T-cell lymphomas. *Ann Intern Med* 1984; **100**: 187–92.

3 Bunn P, Lamberg S. Report of the committeee on staging and classification of cutaneous T-cell lymphomas. *Cancer Treat Rep* 1979; **63**: 725–8.

4 Delfau-Larue M, Dalac S, Lepage E *et al*. Prognostic significance of a polymerase chain reaction-detectable dominant T-lymphocyte clone in cutaneous lesions of patients with mycosis fungoides. *Blood* 1998; **92**: 3376–80.

Table 57.4 Proposed revised staging classification for mycosis fungoides/Sézary syndrome.

TNMB stages	
Skin	
T_1	Limited patches, papules and plaques covering <10% of the skin surface; may further stratify into T_{1a} (patch only) vs T_{1b} (plaque ± patch)
T_2	Patches, papules and plaques covering ≥10% of the skin surface; may further stratify into T_{2a} (patch only) vs T_{2b} (plaque ± patch)
T_3	One or more tumours (≥1 cm diameter)
T_4	Confluence of erythema covering ≥80% body surface area
Node	
N_0	No clinically abnormal peripheral lymph nodes; biopsy not required
N_1	Clinically abnormal peripheral lymph nodes; histopathology Dutch grade 1 or NCI LN_{0-2}
N_{1a}	Clone negative
N_{1b}	Clone positive
N_2	Clinically abnormal peripheral lymph nodes; histopathology Dutch grade 2 or NCI LN_3
N_{2a}	Clone negative
N_{2b}	Clone positive
N_3	Clinically abnormal peripheral lymph nodes; histopathology Dutch grades 3–4 or NCI LN_4; clone positive or negative
N_X	Clinically abnormal peripheral lymph nodes; no histologic conformation
Visceral	
M_0	No visceral organ involvement
M_1	Visceral involvement (must have pathology confirmation and organ involved should be specified)
Blood	
B_0	Albescence of significant blood involvement; ≤5% of peripheral blood lymphocytes are atypical (Sézary cells)
B_{0a}	Clone negative
B_{0b}	Clone positive
B_1	Low blood tumour burden; >5% of peripheral blood lymphocytes are atypical (Sézary cells) but does not meet the criteria of B_2
B_{1a}	Clone negative
B_{1b}	Clone positive
B_2	High blood tumour burden; ≥1000/μL Sézary cells with positive clones

5 Bunn PA, Huberman MS, Whang-Peng J et al. Prospective staging evaluation of patients with cutaneous T-cell lymphomas: demonstration of a high frequency of extracutaneous dissemination. *Ann Intern Med* 1980; **93**: 223–30.

6 Tsai E, Taur A, Espinosa L et al. Staging accuracy in mycosis fungoides and Sezary syndrome using positron emission tomography and computed tomography. *Arch Dermatol* 2006; **142**: 577–84.

7 Epstein EH Jr, Levin DL, Schein P et al. Mycosis fungoides: survival, prognostic features, response to therapy, and autopsy findings. *Medicine* 1972; **51**: 61–72.

8 Sibaud V, Beylot-Barry M, Thiebaut R et al. Bone marrow histopathologic and molecular staging in epidermotropic T-cell lymphomas. *Am J Clin Pathol* 2003; **119**: 444–53.

9 Olsen E, Vonderheid E, Pimpinelli N et al. Revisions to the staging and classification of mycosis fungoides and Sezary syndrome: a proposal of the International Society for Cutaneous Lymphomas (ISCL) and the cutaneous lymphoma task force of the European Organisation of Research and Treatment of Cancer (EORTC). *Blood* 2007; **110**: 1713–22.

Prognosis (Table 57.5). Multivariate analysis has established that age at onset (over 60 years), skin stage and the presence of nodal (IVA) or visceral (IVB) disease are independent prognostic factors in MF [1–6]. Studies have confirmed that a patient's life expectancy is not adversely affected in stage IA disease [6]. Patients with stage IB–IIA disease at diagnosis have a 72–86%/49% overall 5-year survival, while patients with stage IIB disease have a 40–65% 5-year survival [6–8]. The 5-year survival of patients with erythrodermic stage III disease is 41–57%, for those with stage IVA 27–40% and for stage IVB disease 0–27% [6–8]. The presence of a peripheral blood T-cell clone may indicate which patients with early stage disease are likely to develop disease progression but this requires confirmation in large studies [9]. The development of lymph node disease has a significant impact on prognosis [10]. Sézary syndrome patients by definition are staged as T4 N1–3 M0 B1 and have a poor prognosis, with an overall median survival of 32 months from diagnosis [11]. Recent studies of erythrodermic CTCL have shown that the presence of peripheral nodal disease is the most important prognostic factor in a multivariate analysis, although the peripheral blood tumour burden is also very close to significance [12]. In addition, prognostic data on a large series of patients have suggested that patients with thick plaques may have a worse prognosis than those with thin or patch stage disease and this has formed the basis for a suggested modification of the staging system, although the reproducibility of this histological assessment has not been confirmed [13].

A high incidence of second malignancies in MF patients, notably non-melanoma skin cancer and pulmonary small cell lung cancer (including small incidence of melanoma), and also of malignancies in relatives of patients, mainly lymphomas and leukaemias, have been reported [14–16]. Other types of lymphoma–leukaemia and Hodgkin's lymphoma have also been described in association with MF and Sézary syndrome [17–20].

References

1 Fuks ZY, Bagshaw MA, Farber EM. Prognostic signs and the management of mycosis fungoides. *Cancer* 1973; **32**: 1385–95.

2 Hamminga L, Hermans J, Noordijk EM et al. Cutaneous T-cell lymphoma: clinicopathological relationship, therapy and survival in 92 patients. *Br J Dermatol* 1982; **107**: 145–56.

3 Sausville E, Eddy J, Makuch R et al. Histopathologic staging at initial diagnosis of mycosis fungoides and the Sézary syndrome: definition of three distinctive prognostic groups. *Ann Intern Med* 1988; **109**: 372–82.

4 Weinstock MA, Horne JW. Population-based estimate of survival and determinants of prognosis in patients with mycosis fungoides. *Cancer* 1988; **62**: 1658–61.

5 Marti L, Estrach T, Reverter J, Mascaro J. Prognostic clinicopathologic factors in cutaneous T-cell lymphoma. *Arch Dermatol* 1991; **127**: 1511–6.

6 Kim Y, Liu H, Mraz-Gernhard S et al. Long term outcome of 525 patients with mycosis fungoides and Sezary syndrome. *Arch Dermatol* 2003; **139**: 857–66.

7 Doorn R, Van Haselan C, Voorst Vader P et al. Mycosis fungoides: disease evolution and prognosis of 309 Dutch patients. *Arch Dermatol* 2000; **136**: 504–10.

8 Zackheim H, Amin S, Kashani-Sabet M, McMillan A. Prognosis in cutaneous T-cell lymphoma by skin stage: long term survival in 489 patients. *J Am Acad Dermatol* 1999; **40**: 418–25.

9 Fraser-Andrews E, Woolford A, Russell Jones R et al. Detection of a peripheral blood clone is an independent prognostic marker in mycosis fungoides. *J Invest Dermatol* 2000; **114**: 117–21.

10 Sausville E, Worsham G, Matthews M et al. Histologic assessment of lymph nodes in mycosis fungoides/Sézary syndrome (cutaneous T-cell lymphoma):

Table 57.5 Published prognostic data in mycosis fungoides.

	IA (%)	IB (%)	IIA (%)	IIB (%)	III (%)	IVA (%)	IVB (%)	Overall (%)	Reference	No.	Median follow up (years)
OS at 5 years	99	86	49	65		40	0	80	Doorn et al. [7]	309	5.2
	100	84		52	57				Zackheim et al. [8]	489	4.7
	97	72		40	41	27	27	68	Kim et al. [6]	525	5.5
OS at 10 years	84	61	49	27		20	0	57	Doorn et al. [7]	309	5.2
	100	67		39	41				Zackheim et al. [8]	489	4.7
	88	55		26	24			53	Kim et al. [6]	525	5.5
DSS at 5 years	100	96 (81)	68	80		40	0	89	Doorn et al. [7]	309	5.2
	100	95	84	56	65	30	30	81	Kim et al. [6]	525	5.5
DSS at 10 years	97	83 (36)	68	42		20	0	75	Doorn et al. [7]	309	5.2
DSS at 15 years	98	85	71	32	49	14	14	74	Kim et al. [6]	525	5.5
Median survival	NR	12.1 years		3.3 years	4.0 years	1.2	0.7		Kim et al. [6]	556	9.8
Disease progression (5 years)	4	21	65	32		70	100		Doorn et al. [7]	309	5.2
	10	22		56	48				Kim et al. [6]	525	5.5
Disease progression (10 years)	10	39	65	60		70	100		Doorn et al. [7]	309	5.2
	13	32		72	57				Kim et al. [6]	525	5.5
Disease progression (20 years)	16	40		81	78				Kim et al. [6]	525	5.5

DSS, disease-specific survival; NR, not reached; OS, overall survival.

Comments:

1. All actuarial survival curves calculated according to method of Kaplan–Meier and based on stage at diagnosis.

2. In the study by Doorn et al. [7] (and in a subsequent publication: van Doorn et al. Arch Dermatol 2002; **138**: 191–8), the presence of follicular mucinosis was an independent poor prognostic feature, possibly related to depth of infiltrate in patients with stage IB disease (DSS of 81% and 36% and OS of 75% and 21% at 5 and 10 years respectively). A lack of a complete response to initial therapy was also associated with a poor outcome ($P < 0.001$) in a multivariate analysis as well as increasing clinical stage and the presence of extracutaneous disease. A different staging system was used in this study (based on Hamminga et al. [2]) but for the purposes of this table the staging has been altered to be consistent. Only three patients had stage IVB disease and only 18 patients each had stage IIA and IVA disease. Therefore the results for these stages must be interpreted cautiously.

3. In the study by Zackheim et al. [8], black patients had a relatively more advanced stage of disease than white patients. The TNM classification was used in this study. Lymph node stage had an unfavourable impact on survival but this trend did not reach significance for each individual T stage because of a lack of sufficient power (an estimated 1700 subjects required) and IIA/IVA patients were not designated separately. Similar considerations apply to peripheral blood involvement. Similar outcomes for patients with stage IIB (T_3) and III (T_4) disease is consistent with other studies but this might reflect a lack of lymph node staging data included in this study.

4. The study by Kim et al. [6] included data on 525 patients and showed that the majority presented with early stage disease and that independent multivariate prognostic factors were age, skin stage and presence of extracutaneous disease at presentation. With the exception of stage IA, the relative risk for death is greater in MF than in a control population; 2.2 for stage IB/IIA; 3.9 for stage IIB/III; 12.8 for stage IV disease.

clinical correlation and prognostic import of a new classification system. *Hum Pathol* 1985; **16**: 1098–109.

11 Toro JR, Stoll HL, Stomper PC et al. Prognostic factors and evaluation of mycosis fungoides and Sézary syndrome. *J Am Acad Dermatol* 1997; **37**: 58–67.

12 Scarisbrick J, Whittaker S, Evans A et al. Prognostic significance of tumour burden in the blood of patients with erythrodermic primary cutaneous T-cell lymphoma. *Blood* 2001; **97**: 624–30.

13 Kashani-Sabet M, McMillan A, Zackheim H. A modified staging classification for cutaneous T-cell lymphoma. *J Am Acad Dermatol* 2001; **45**: 700–6.

14 Greene MH, Pinto HA, Kant JA et al. Lymphomas and leukemias in the relatives of patients with mycosis fungoides. *Cancer* 1982; **49**: 737–41.

15 Epstein EH Jr, Levin DL, Craft JD Jr et al. Mycosis fungoides: survival, prognostic features, response to therapy, and autopsy findings. *Medicine* 1972; **51**: 61–72.

16 Evans A, Scarisbrick J, Child F et al. Cutaneous malignant melanoma in association with mycosis fungoides. *J Am Acad Dermatol* 2004; **50**: 701–5.

17 Harland C, Whittaker S, Ng Y et al. Coexistent cutaneous T-cell lymphoma and B-cell chronic lymphocytic leukaemia. *Br J Dermatol* 1992; **127**: 519–23.

18 Brousset P, Lamant L, Viraben R et al. Hodgkin's disease following mycosis fungoides: phenotypic and molecular evidence for different tumour cell clones. *J Clin Pathol* 1996; **49**: 504–7.

19 Scarisbrick J, Child F, Spittle M et al. Systemic Hodgkin's lymphoma in a patient with Sézary syndrome. *Br J Dermatol* 2000; **142**: 771–5.

20 Hallerman C, Kaune M, Tiemann M et al. High frequency of primary cutaneous lymphomas associated with lymphoproliferative disorders of different lineage. *Ann Haematol* 2007; **86**: 509–15.

Pathology [1–3]. The features of MF vary according to the clinical stage. The earliest pathological features of MF are the presence of a moderate, predominantly lymphocytic infiltrate in the papillary dermis. Many of the small lymphoid cells may be hyperchromatic and show a tendency to 'line up' just below the dermal–epidermal junction. Even at this early stage, the affinity of these T lymphocytes for the epidermis and papillary dermis is apparent, as there is rarely significant involvement in the underlying reticular dermis.

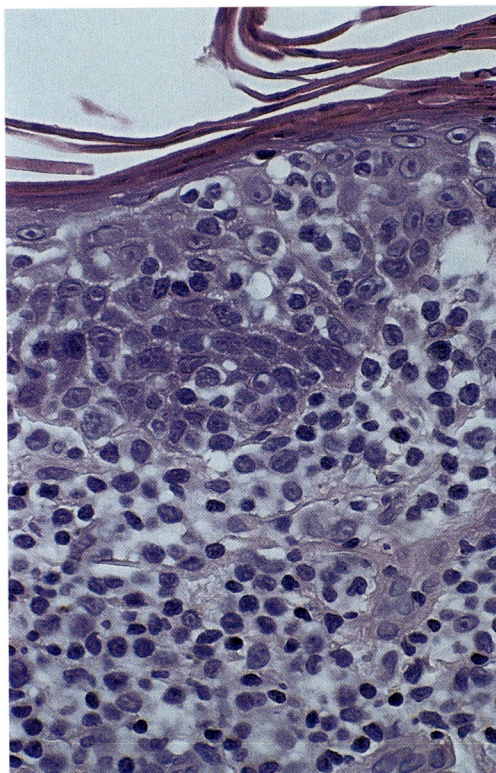

Fig. 57.6 Histology of mycosis fungoides showing striking epidermotropism with the presence in the epidermis of cytologically atypical small dark cells proven on marker studies to be CD4+ helper T lymphocytes.

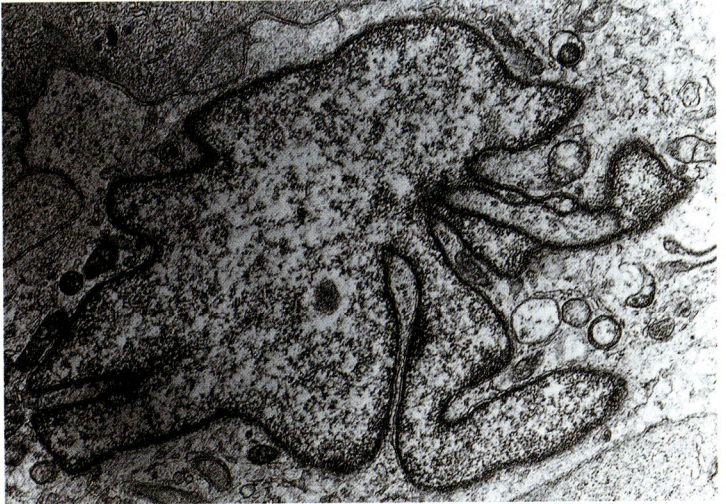

Fig. 57.7 Electron micrograph of T cell infiltrating the epidermis in mycosis fungoides, showing the striking cellular contours of the typical cell of Lutzner with a typical high nuclear contour index.

As the disease progresses with the development of thicker plaques, prominent epidermotropism (Fig. 57.6) is seen. This describes the selective colonization of the epidermis by these atypical T cells and is characterized by single-cell colonization, often along the basal layer, or by clusters of atypical lymphocytes in the epidermis—so-called Pautrier microabscesses. The lymphocytes in the epidermis are often strikingly cerebriform (Fig. 57.7), with a very

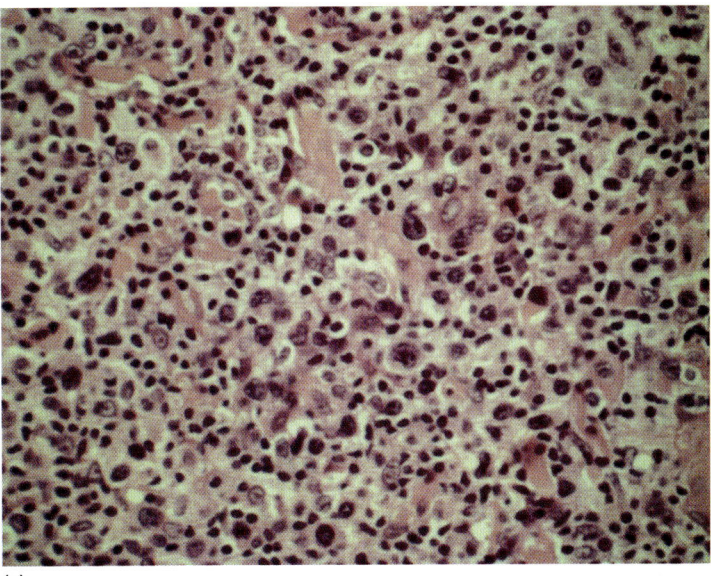

(a)

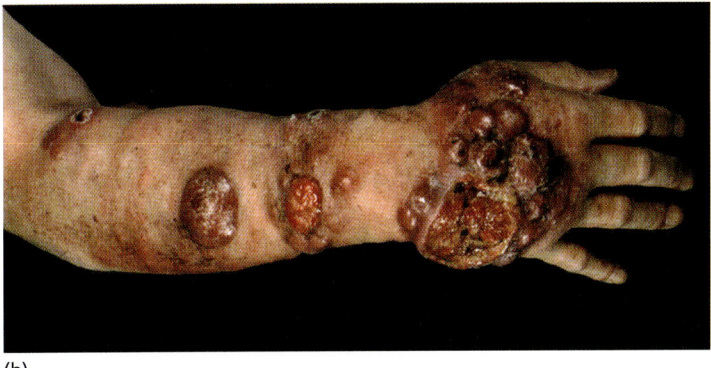

(b)

Fig. 57.8 High-power view (a) of large cell transformation in mycosis fungoides (b).

irregular nuclear outline and heavy nuclear staining as well as a characteristic halo appearance to the cells. If these cells are examined either under high power or with thin sections, the cerebriform and irregular nature of the nuclei can be better appreciated in three dimensions. In early MF, the T-cell lymphocytic infiltrate may be associated with a number of other cell types including small numbers of plasma cells or eosinophils, but as the infiltrate becomes more intense and more epidermotropic, the infiltrate becomes monotonous and monomorphic. Granulomatous features may be rarely present and a prominent histiocytic infiltrate can be seen, so called interstitial MF [4].

In more advanced stages of disease (IIB–III), the striking epidermotropic quality of the lymphocytic infiltrate may be lost, with scattered larger tumour cells showing marked cellular atypia. Large cell transformation may also occur and is a poor prognostic feature on univariate analysis, although this does not appear to be independent of age and stage of disease on multivariate analysis [5]. An earlier study showed no difference in survival for stage IIB patients showing histological features of large cell transformation compared to those without, but there was a significant difference in survival from diagnosis [6]. Large cell transformation (Fig. 57.8) is defined as the presence of more than 25–50% of large cells

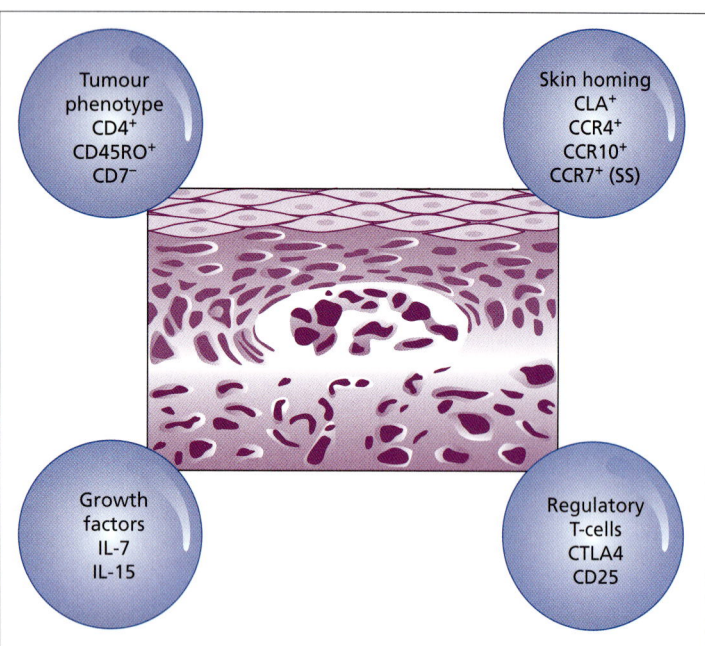

Fig. 57.9 Immunopathology of mycosis fungoides/Sézary syndrome.

(either CD30 positive or negative) within the dermal infiltrate or the development of microscopic dermal nodules consisting of larger cells with pleomorphic and occasionally anaplastic morphology [5]. It is important to distinguish large histiocytic cells from large tumour cells with an anaplastic morphology and occasionally the presence of reactive germinal centres in MF can also cause histological confusion.

The differentiation between large cell transformation in MF and the association with a primary cutaneous CD30[+] lymphoproliferative disorder such as lymphomatoid papulosis or anaplastic large cell lymphoma, which have a good prognosis, is crucial and based on a careful clinical assessment of the patient. The development of large tumours in patients with typical patches or plaques of MF would suggest large cell transformation of MF if the histological criteria were fulfilled. In contrast, the presence of very large numbers (more than 75%) of CD30[+] large cells in only one or a few isolated tumours developing in patients with no concurrent or previous clinical evidence of MF, as indicated by patches and plaques, suggests that the patient has a primary cutaneous CD30[+] lymphoproliferative disorder.

Immunopathology (Fig. 57.9). The tumour cells in MF are CD3[+], CD4[+], CD45RO[+] and usually CD7[−] T cells. This is the phenotype of a mature helper T cell of memory subtype [7]. The tumour cells are CLA[+], CCR4[+], CCR10[+] consistent with a skin homing T cell [8,9]. In rare cases, the tumour cells are CD8[+] rather than CD4[+] but this does not appear to have any prognostic significance [10]. Interestingly, CD8[+] cases of MF are more common in childhood and in hypopigmented variants [11]. CD8[+] MF must be distinguished from an epidermotropic cytotoxic variant of CTCL with a poor prognosis (see below). Occasionally, there is a very prominent infiltrate of reactive tumour infiltrating CD8[+] T cells expressing cytotoxic proteins, which may indicate a good prognosis

[12–14]. The dermal infiltrate often consists of a prominent population of CD1a[+] dendritic cells and CD68[+] histiocytic cells. In advanced disease, tumour cells may express an aberrant phenotype with either loss of T-cell surface antigens 'null-cell phenotype' or expression of the CD30 antigen either by scattered larger tumour cells or by prominent dermal nodules consisting of large pleomorphic or anaplastic tumour cells [5,7]. The latter feature may be associated with large cell transformation but CD30 expression per se does not appear to have any prognostic significance [5]. The tumour cells usually express the αβ T-cell receptor and only rarely express cytotoxic proteins with disease progression [14].

A subset of CD4[+] CD25[+] T-cells has been defined with suppressive function. These regulatory T cells (T-regs) are cytotoxic T-lymphocyte antigen 4+ (CTLA4+) and express the transcription factor FoxP3. Studies in MF/SS have analysed the expression of FoxP3, as well as T-reg function, and have established that a proportion of the intraepidermal and dermal T cells in early stages of MF are FoxP3[+] T-cells but this decreases significantly with more advanced disease [15,16]. This suggests that in MF the presence of T-regs may be a good prognostic factor and that T-regs may actually suppress the expansion of tumour cells. Whether tumour cells also function as T-regs remains to be established; CTLA4 is expressed by a proportion of Sézary cells, and Sézary cells which have immunosuppressive T-reg function have only been described in a minority of SS patients [17–19].

Pathological differential diagnosis. In early MF, the main differential diagnosis includes a dermatitis reaction. The epidermotropic quality of the T-cell infiltrate in MF may be helpful, as may the cytology of the individual T cells, as in MF these intraepidermal lymphocytes tend to be larger than surrounding keratinocytes and have intensely stained nuclei with a very irregular outline. Spongiosis, if present in association with epidermotropic T cells or Pautrier microabscesses, is minimal, whereas this tends to be more striking in dermatitis reactions. A useful clue may be the characteristic basal layer colonization and the larger size of the intraepidermal T cells compared to the dermal mononuclear cells [20].

The pathological diagnosis of early MF can still, however, be extremely subjective and is best made in full collaboration with the clinician and only after careful correlation with the clinical features. It is often wise to take several biopsies from separate lesions, and if necessary to arrange for repeat biopsies to be carried out as the clinical picture evolves over a period of months or even years. An algorithm for establishing an early clinical and histological diagnosis of MF has been proposed by the ISCL (Table 57.6) [21].

Immunophenotypic studies are usually of minimal value in differentiating early MF from other cutaneous lymphocytic infiltrates, as the majority of these cells will also be CD3[+], CD4[+] although a predominance of larger CD4[+] cells within the epidermis compared to the mixed population of smaller cells within the dermis can sometimes be helpful [7,20].

The differential diagnosis of early MF from conditions such as arthropod bites and lymphomatous drug eruptions can also be difficult, and good clinicopathological correlation is essential. In

Table 57.6 ISCL diagnostic criteria for early mycosis fungoides (4 points).

Criteria	Major (2 points)	Minor (1 point)
Clinical Persistent and/or progressive patches and plaques plus 1. Non-sun exposed location 2. Size/shape variation 3. Poikiloderma	Any 2	Any 1
Histopathological Superficial lymphoid infiltrate plus 1. Epidermotropism 2. Atypia	Both	Either
Molecular/biological Clonal TCR rearrangement		Present
Immunopathological 1. CD2, 3, 5 <50% 2. CD7 <10% 3. Epidermal discordance		Any 1

general, reactions to arthropod bites tend to show a higher proportion of eosinophils, and the disposition of the infiltrate in lymphomatous drug reactions will be perivascular rather than epidermotropic. In a proportion of cases, however, the diagnosis is suspected on clinical grounds but cannot confidently be made with certainty on histological examination. In these cases, sequential biopsies at 3–6-month intervals may be needed.

Pathology of extracutaneous disease. The usual pattern of extracutaneous spread is from the skin to the draining peripheral lymph nodes and thereafter to other organs such as the liver and spleen, but pulmonary, skeletal and CNS involvement have been documented.

An NCI classification system was proposed in 1985 (Table 57.4) [22]. In this system, lymph node architecture is preserved in LN1–3 in which dermatopathic changes may predominate. LN1 is characterized by single infrequent atypical cells, LN2 shows small clusters of atypical lymphocytes and LN3 shows larger aggregates of atypical cells in paracortical areas. LN4 is characterized by partial or complete effacement by atypical cells [22].

A further histological assessment of peripheral nodes is utilized and based on the study by Scheffer *et al.* [23]. Those biopsies with no abnormalities are recorded as LN0 while those with dermatopathic changes are designated LN1 (dermatopathic lymphadenopathy), which is characterized by enlargement of the paracortical area of the lymph node because of the presence of large numbers of macrophages and pale dendritic (interdigitating reticulum) cells (grade 1 = LN1–2). The macrophages contain aggregates both of melanin and lipid material, giving rise to the older term 'lipomelanic reticulosis'. Histological evidence of possible involvement (grade 2 = LN3) is characterized by the additional presence of small clusters of larger atypical mononuclear cells within the expanded paracortical areas (Fig. 57.10). In contrast, partial (grade 3 = LN4) or complete effacement (grade 4 = LN4) of the lymph node architecture is consistent with definite lymphomatous involvement (Fig. 57.10).

A comparison of these systems has shown that both have a poor prognosis for partial or totally effaced nodes with non-effaced nodes showing no difference in survival [24]. In the WHO classification system, a modification of these classifications has been proposed whereby LN1 and LN2 have been grouped together as grade I (no histological involvement), with LN3 as grade II and LN4 as grade III, both representing definite histological involvement, although this system has not yet been validated [25]. However, there is a subtle difference in this system because in the WHO proposal grade I can be characterized by scattered but not clusters of atypical cerebriform cells, whereas nodes showing clusters of atypical cerebriform cells are graded as II (LN3).

The ISCL EORTC revised staging classification suggests grouping lymph node biopsies N1– with no definite histologic involvement (grade 1/LN1–2), N2– possible involvement (grade 2/LN3) and N3– definite involvement (grade 3–4/LN4) with each group reflecting the results of TCR gene analysis as clone present or absent, but this has not yet been validated prospectively [26].

References

1 Nickoloff B. Light microscopic assessment of 100 patients with patch/plaque stage mycosis fungoides. *Am J Dermatopathol* 1988; **10**: 469–77.
2 Shapiro PE, Pinto FJ. The histologic spectrum of mycosis fungoides/Sézary syndrome. *Am J Surg Pathol* 1994; **18**: 645–67.
3 Smoller B, Bishop K, Glusac E, Warnke R. Reassessment of histologic parameters in the diagnosis of mycosis fungoides. *Am J Surg Pathol* 1995; **19**: 1423.
4 Scarabello A, Leinweber B, Ardigo M *et al.* Cutaneous lymphomas with prominent granulomatous reaction. *Am J Surg Pathol* 2002; **26**: 1259–68.
5 Vergier B, Muret A, Beylot-Barry M *et al.* Transformation of mycosis fungoides: clinicopathological and prognostic features. *Blood* 2000; **95**: 2212–8.
6 Cerroni l, Rieger E, Hodl S, Kerl H. Clinicopathologic and immunologic features associated with transformation of mycosis fungoides to large-cell lymphoma. *Am J Surg Pathol* 1992; **16**: 543–52.
7 Ralfkiaer E. Immunohistological markers for the diagnosis of cutaneous lymphomas. *Semin Diagn Pathol* 1991; **8**: 62–72.
8 Kallinch T, Muche M, Qin S *et al.* Chemokine receptor expression in neoplastic and reactive T cells in the skin at different stages of of mycosis fungoides. *J Invest Dermatol* 2003; **121**: 1045–52.
9 Capriotti E, Vonderheid E, Thoburn C *et al.* Chemokine receptor expression by leukemic T-cells of cutaneous T-cell lymphoma: clinical and histopathological correlations. *J Invest Dermatol* 2007; **127**: 2882–92.
10 Dummer R, Kamarashev J, Kempf W *et al.* Junctional CD8 cutaneous lymphomas with non-aggressive clinical behaviour. *Arch Dermatol* 2002; **138**: 199–203.
11 Wain M, Orchard G, Whittaker S *et al.* Outcome in 34 patients with juvenile-onset mycosis fungoides. *Cancer* 2003; **98**: 2282–90.
12 Hoppe R, Medeiros L, Warnke R *et al.* CD8-positive tumour infiltrating lymphocytes influence the long-term survival of patients with mycosis fungoides. *J Am Acad Dermatol* 1995; **32**: 448–53.
13 Vermeer M, Van Doorn R, Dukers D *et al.* CD8 T cells in cutaneous T-cell lymphoma: expression of cytotoxic proteins, Fas ligand and killing inhibitory receptors and their relationship with clinical behaviour. *J Clin Oncol* 2001; **19**: 4322–9.
14 Vermeer M, Geelen F, Kummer J *et al.* Expression of cytotoxic proteins by neoplastic T cells in mycosis fungoides increases with progression from plaque to tumor stage disease. *Am J Pathol* 1999; **154**: 1203–10.
15 Klemke C, Fritzsching B, Franz B *et al.* Paucity of FOXP3+ cells in skin and peripheral blood distinguishes Sezary syndrome from other cutaneous T-cell lymphomas. *Leukemia* 2006; **20**: 1123–9.
16 Gjerdrum L, Woetmann A, Odum N *et al.* FOXP3+ regulatory T cells in cutaneous T-cell lymphomas: association with disease stage and survival. *Leukemia* 2007; **21**: 2512–8.

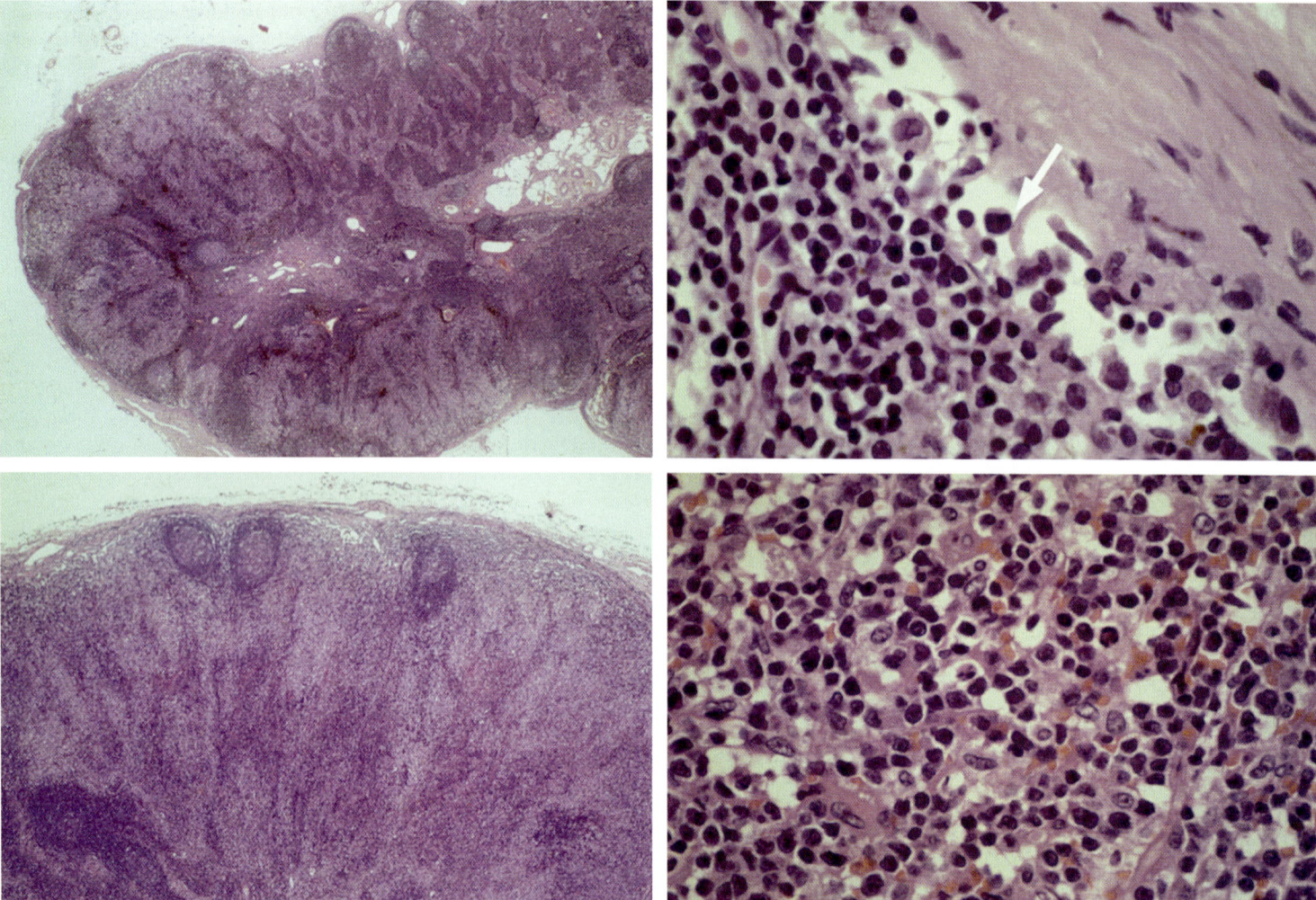

Fig. 57.10 Composite photomicrograph showing features of dermatopathic lymphadenopathy. LN1 is characterized by dermatopathic changes with melanin deposition and occasional atypical lymphocytes. LN2 with paracortical expansion of T-cell areas. LN4 showing a high-power view of lymph node effacement by small and medium sized atypical convoluted cells.

17 Wong H, Wilson A, Gibson H *et al*. Increased expression of CTLA-4 in malignant T cells from patients with mycosis fungoides—cutaneous T-cell lymphoma. *J Invest Dermatol* 2006; **126**: 212–9.

18 Berger C, Tigelaar R, Cohen J *et al*. Cutaneous T-cell lymphoma: malignant proliferation of T-regulatory cells. *Blood* 2005; **105**: 1640–7.

19 Tiemessen M, Mitchell T, Hendry L *et al*. Lack of suppressive CD4⁺ CD25⁺ FOXP3⁺ T cells in advanced stages of primary cutaneous T-cell lymphoma. *J Invest Dermatol* 2006; **126**: 2217–23.

20 Bagot M, Wechsler J, Lescs M *et al*. Intra-epidermal localization of the clone in cutaneous T-cell lymphoma. *J Am Acad Dermatol* 1992; **27**: 235–7.

21 Pimipinelli N, Olsen E, Santucci M *et al*. Defining early mycosis fungoides. *J Am Acad Dermatol* 2005; **53**: 1053–63.

22 Sausville E, Worsham G, Matthews M *et al*. Histologic assessment of lymph nodes in mycosis fungoides/Sézary syndrome (cutaneous T-cell lymphoma). *Hum Pathol* 1985; **16**: 1098–109.

23 Scheffer E, Meijer C, Van Vloten W. Dermatopathic lymphadenopathy and lymph node involvement in mycosis fungoides. *Cancer* 1980; **45**: 137–48.

24 Vonderheid E, Diamond L, Van Vloten W *et al*. Lymph node classification systems in cutaneous T-cell lymphoma. *Cancer* 1994; **73**: 207–18.

25 Jaffe E, Ralfkiaer E. Mycosis fungoides and Sézary syndrome. In: *World Health Organization Classification of Tumours: Pathology and Genetics of Tumours of Haematopoietic and Lymphoid Tissues*. IARC, 2001: 216–20.

26 Olsen E, Vonderheid E, Pimpinelli N *et al*. Revisions to the staging and classification of mycosis fungoides and Sezary syndrome: a proposal of the International Society for Cutaneous Lymphomas (ISCL) and the cutaneous lymphoma task force of the European Organisation of Research and Treatment of Cancer (EORTC). *Blood* 2007; **110**: 1713–22.

T-cell receptor gene analysis. TCR gene analysis consists of analysis of DNA from tissue samples for the detection of clonal rearrangements of the TCR genes as a marker of a monoclonal T-cell population. A similar approach can be used to identify a B-cell clone using analysis of immunoglobulin genes. A clonal lymphoid population is usually synonymous with a neoplastic proliferation but this does not signify malignancy. In contrast, the malignant potential of a lymphoid clone is related to the underlying molecular abnormalities. Analysis of TCR genes in MF is now a standard approach that has diagnostic, prognostic and therapeutic implications. Originally, Southern blot analysis of the β TCR gene was employed but this approach is time-consuming, requires large amounts of high-quality DNA and is relatively insensitive [1,2]. Consequently, most studies are now based on more sensitive PCR techniques and several different methods are employed including denaturing gradient gel electrophoresis (DGGE), temperature gradient gel electrophoresis (TGGE), single-strand conformational gel electrophoresis (SSCP) and gene scan methods for analysis of the γ TCR gene [3–8]. Although MF tumour cells usually express an αβ TCR, the γ TCR gene is rearranged in lymphocytes expressing both a γδ and an αβ TCR and this gene is much easier to analyse comprehensively than the β TCR gene. These different electrophoretic approaches have not been compared adequately but most results are broadly consistent and the standardization of this technique has been partly achieved by the use of Biomed 2 primers for the γ and βTCR genes [9].

T-cell clones can be detected in a proportion (approximately 70% overall) of patients with early stage disease and are almost invariable in patients with later stages of disease [5,6]. The lack of T-cell clones in all patients with early stages of disease almost certainly reflects a lack of sensitivity of the technique, although studies have shown that those early stage patients without a T-cell clone achieve a higher complete remission rate with skin-directed therapy than those with a T-cell clone [10]. This suggests that the proportion of non-tumour cells in the infiltrate, possibly reflecting the host immune response, may also be critical. Identical T-cell clones can be detected in peripheral blood of a proportion of patients with all stages of disease and this may have independent prognostic significance [7,11]. In contrast, non-identical peripheral blood T-cell clones can also be detected and may not be pathological, emphasizing that results from all samples must be carefully compared [12]. In patients with both MF and lymphomatoid papulosis or CD30⁺ large cell anaplastic lymphoma, identical T-cell clones can be found, suggesting a common pathogenesis [1,2,13]. T-cell clones identical to those in the skin can also be detected in dermatopathic lymph nodes (LN1–LN2) and this might provide independent prognostic information, although larger studies are required to prove this conclusively [14–16]. Assessment of enlarged lymph nodes with fine needle aspirate in CTCL has shown that T-cell clones cannot be detected with the same frequency compared to TCR gene analysis of excised nodes, suggesting sampling error [17]. Because of the sensitivity of these PCR-based techniques, T-cell clones have rarely been detected in non-neoplastic inflammatory disorders and therefore it is critical that the presence or absence of a clonal TCR gene rearrangement must always be interpreted in conjunction with the clinical and pathological features. Recent PCR-based studies have also detected clonal T-cell proliferations in some cases of pityriasis lichenoides acuta, small and large plaque parapsoriasis and pityriasis lichenoides chronica [18–23]. The clinical significance of these findings is unclear at present. Although these results would appear to support clinical impressions that large plaque parapsoriasis probably represents early stage MF, small plaque parapsoriasis has been thought to be a separate inflammatory condition that is not related to MF. The findings in pityriasis lichenoides acuta support previous suggestions that this represents part of a spectrum with lymphomatoid papulosis and, intriguingly, lesions resembling pityriasis lichenoides chronica can be associated with MF [23].

References

1 Whittaker S, Smith N, Russell Jones R, Luzatto L. Analysis of β, γ and δ T-cell receptor genes in mycosis fungoides and Sézary syndrome. *Cancer* 1991; **68**: 1572–82.

2 Zelickson B, Peters M, Muller S *et al.* T-cell receptor gene rearrangement analysis: cutaneous T-cell lymphoma, peripheral T-cell lymphoma and premalignant and benign cutaneous lymphoproliferative disorders. *J Am Acad Dermatol* 1991; **25**: 787–96.

3 Whittaker S. T-cell receptor gene analysis in cutaneous T-cell lymphomas. *Clin Exp Dermatol* 1996; **21**: 81–7.

4 Wood G, Tung R, Haeffner A *et al.* Detection of clonal T-cell receptor γ gene rearrangements in early mycosis fungoides/Sézary syndrome by polymerase chain reaction and denaturing gradient gel electrophoresis (PCR/DGGE). *J Invest Dermatol* 1994; **103**: 34–41.

5 Theodorou I, Delfau-Larue M, Bigorgne C *et al.* Cutaneous T-cell infiltrates: analysis of T-cell receptor γ gene rearrangement by polymerase chain reaction and denaturing gradient gel elctrophoresis. *Blood* 1995; **86**: 305–10.

6 Bottaro M, Berti E, Biondi A *et al.* Heteroduplex analysis of T-cell receptor γ gene rearrangements for diagnosis and monitoring of cutaneous T-cell lymphomas. *Blood* 1994; **83**: 3271–8.

7 Fraser Andrews E, Woolford A, Russell Jones R *et al.* Detection of a peripheral blood T-cell clone is an independent prognostic marker in mycosis fungoides. *J Invest Dermatol* 2000; **114**: 117–21.

8 Klemke C, Dippel E, Dembinski A *et al.* Clonal T cell receptor γ-chain gene rearrangement by PCR-based genescan analysis in the skin and blood of patients with parapsoriasis and early stage mycosis fungoides. *J Pathol* 2002; **197**: 348–54.

9 Sandberg Y, Heule F, Lam K *et al.* Molecular immunoglobulin/T-cell receptor clonality analysis in cutaneous lymphoproliferations. Experience with the Biomed-2 standardized polymerase chain reaction protocol. *Haematologica* 2003; **88**: 659–70.

10 Delfau-Larue M, Dalac S, Lepage E *et al.* Prognostic significance of a polymerase chain reaction-detectable dominant T-lymphocyte clone in cutaneous lesions of patients with mycosis fungoides. *Blood* 1998; **92**: 3376–80.

11 Muche M, Lukowsky A, Asadullah K *et al.* Demonstration of frequent occurrence of clonal T cells in the peripheral blood of patients with primary cutaneous T-cell lymphoma. *Blood* 1997; **4**: 1636–42.

12 Delfau-Larue M, Laroche L, Wechsler J *et al.* Diagnostic value of dominant T-cell clones in the peripheral blood in 363 patients presenting consecutively with a clinical suspicion of cutaneous lymphoma. *Blood* 2000; **96**: 2987–92.

13 Whittaker S, Smith N, Russell Jones R, Luzzatto L. Analysis of β, γ and δ TCR genes in lymphomatoid papulosis: cellular basis of two distinct histologic subsets. *J Invest Dermatol* 1991; **96**: 786–91.

14 Assaf C, Hummel M, Steinhoff M *et al.* Early TCR-β and TCR-γ PCR detection of T-cell clonality indicates mimimal tumour disease in lymph nodes of cutaneous T-cell lymphoma: diagnostic and prognostic implications. *Blood* 2005; **105**: 503–10.

15 Juarez T, Isenhath S, Polissar N *et al.* Analysis of T-cell receptor gene rearrangement for predicting clinical outcome in patients with cutaneous T-cell lymphoma. *Arch Dermatol* 2005; **141**: 1107–13.

16 Fraser-Andrews E, Mitchell T, Ferreira S *et al.* Molecular staging of lymph nodes from 60 patients with mycosis fungoides and Sezary syndrome: correlation with histopathology and outcome suggests prognostic relevance in mycosis fungoides. *Br J Dermatol* 2006; **155**: 756–62.

17 Galindo L, Garcia F, Hanau C *et al.* Fine needle aspiration biopsy in the evaluation of lymphadenopathy associated with cutaneous T-cell lymphoma (mycosis fungoides/Sézary syndrome). *Am J Clin Pathol* 2000; **113**: 865–71.

18 Dereure O, Levi E, Kadin M. T-cell clonality in pityriasis lichenoides et varioliformis acuta. *Arch Dermatol* 2000; **136**: 1483–6.

19 Haeffner A, Smoller B, Zepter K, Wood G. Differentiation and clonality of lesional lymphocytes in small plaque parapsoriasis. *Arch Dermatol* 1995; **131**: 321–4.

20 Simon M, Flaig M, Kind P *et al.* Large plaque parapsoriasis: clinical and genotypic correlations. *J Cutan Pathol* 2000; **27**: 57–60.

21 Shieh S, Mikkola D, Wood G. Differentiation and clonality of lesional lymphocytes in pityriasis lichenoides chronica. *Arch Dermatol* 2001; **137**: 305–8.

22 Weinberg J, Kristal L, Chooback L *et al.* The clonal nature of pityriasis lichenoides. *Arch Dermatol* 2002; **138**: 1063–7.

23 Magro C, Crowson A, Morrison C, Jingwei L. Pityriasis lichenoides chronica: stratification by molecular and phenotypic profile. *Human Pathol* 2007; **38**: 479–90.

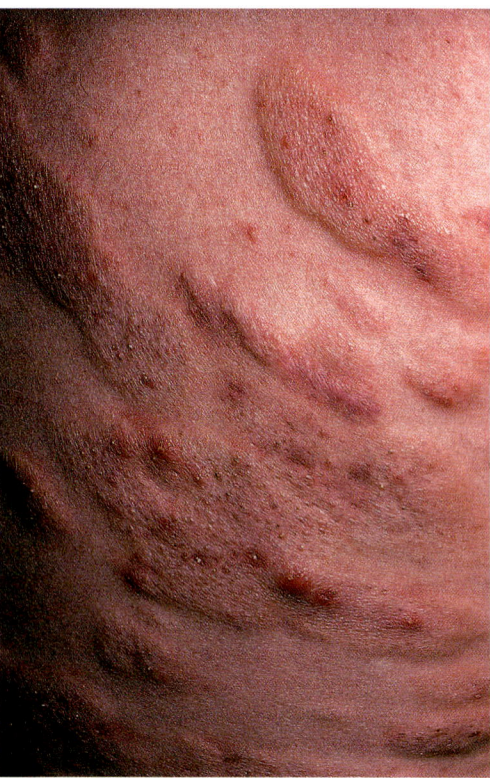

Fig. 57.11 Clinical appearance of follicular mucinosis showing boggy mucin-secreting plaques on the trunk.

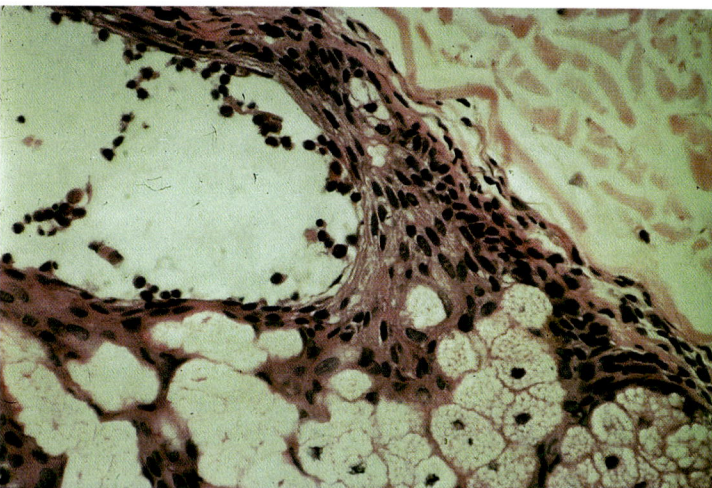

Fig. 57.12 Histology of lesion illustrated in Fig. 57.11 showing degeneration of the hair follicle.

Follicular mucinosis [1–4]

Synonym
- Alopecia mucinosa

Definition. Boggy cutaneous plaques showing follicular prominence and histological evidence of mucinous degeneration of hair follicles that is often associated with an atypical pilotropic T-cell infiltrate and clinical features of MF (pilotropic or folliculotropic MF).

Clinical features. There appear to be two distinct forms of follicular mucinosis, one associated with MF and an entirely separate, benign, inflammatory form of follicular mucinosis, which is not associated with the development of MF. The clinical features of these two types of follicular mucinosis are identical; follicular papules and plaques often associated with severe pruritus and with a predilection for the face and scalp but the trunk and limbs can be affected and the classic patches and plaques of MF may also be present. A younger age group is affected by inflammatory forms but there are no satisfactory criteria for distinguishing this from MF-associated follicular mucinosis, suggesting that both may represent forms of MF. Prominent giant comedones are often a feature with acneiform lesions (Fig. 57.11), and significant alopecia may be present, rarely with mucinorrhoea [5].

Pathology. There is degeneration of involved hair follicles, associated in MF with a prominent pilotropic atypical T-cell infiltrate. In MF there may also be associated interfollicular epidermotro-

pism. Although these histological features distinguish follicular mucinosis from pilotropic MF, both conditions may simply represent points on a spectrum [5]. Mucin stains such as alcian blue show the presence of large quantities of mucin (Fig. 57.12). In MF, a pilotropic or folliculotropic infiltrate may also occur without mucinosis. In contrast, the inflammatory form of follicular mucinosis does not show a prominent atypical pilotropic T-cell infiltrate, although repeated biopsies may be required to fully exclude MF. It may be impossible to distinguish these two forms with confidence and there is an emerging consensus that most, if not all, patients with follicular mucinosis have a form of CTCL (pilotropic mycosis fungoides) [6]. However, histologic features of follicular mucinosis, without atypia, can also occur as an incidental histological feature in the context of a variety of inflammatory dermatoses [7].

Immunophenotype. The tumour cells in both follicular mucinosis and folliculotropic/pilotropic MF are usually CD3$^+$, CD4$^+$ and CD8$^-$. Prominent CD30$^{+/-}$ blast cells may be associated with a poor prognosis [5,6]. T-cell receptor clonal gene rearrangements can be detected in both MF-associated follicular mucinosis and so-called benign forms of inflammatory follicular mucinosis, consistent with suggestions that both may represent MF variants [6,8].

Pathogenesis. It is accepted that follicular mucinosis represents a follicular (pilotropic) variant of MF with mucinous degeneration of the hair follicle, although the reason for mucin deposition is not currently known. This is supported by the presence of this clinical and histological pattern in patients with typical features of MF. The poor prognosis of folliculotropic variants may relate to the poorer efficacy of skin-directed therapies because of the depth of the associated T-cell infiltrate or a currently unknown pathogenetic difference.

Treatment. There is emerging evidence that follicular variants of MF have a worse prognosis, with disease-specific survival rates of 81% at 5 years and 36% at 10 years [5,9]. Mycosis fungoides associated with follicular mucinosis is treated with skin-directed therapy as for early stages of MF, but patients may also require systemic treatment with IFN-α or retinoids (bexarotene). Radiotherapy is ideal for isolated plaques of folliculotropic MF. Total skin electron beam therapy may be appropriate for resistant cases. Dapsone can be effective for inflammatory forms of follicular mucinosis. However, if the hair follicles have been destroyed, scarring alopecia will be present and the hair loss permanent.

References
1 Binnick AN, Wax FD, Clendenning WE. Alopecia mucinosa of the face associated with mycosis fungoides. *Arch Dermatol* 1978; **114**: 791–8.
2 Coskey RJ, Mehregan AH. Alopecia mucinosa: a follow-up study. *Arch Dermatol* 1970; **102**: 193–4.
3 Emmerson RW. Follicular mucinosis: a study of 47 patients. *Br J Dermatol* 1969; **81**: 395–413.
4 Pinkus H. Alopecia mucinosa. *Arch Dermatol* 1957; **76**: 419–26.
5 Van Doorn R, Scheffer E, Willemze R. Follicular mycosis fungoides, a distinct disease entity with or without associated follicular mucinosis. *Arch Dermatol* 2002; **138**: 191–8.
6 Cerroni L, Fink-Puches R, Back B, Kerl H. Follicular mucinosis. *Arch Dermatol* 2002; **138**: 182–9.
7 Hempstead R, Ackerman B. Follicular mucinosis: a reaction pattern in follicular epithelium. *Am J Dermatopathol* 1985; **7**: 245–57.
8 Meehan S, Jensen K, Kim Y *et al.* Use of polymerase chain reaction heteroduplex analysis in the evaluation of follicular mucinosis. *J Cutan Pathol* 1999; **26**: 458.
9 Gerami P, Rosen S, Kuzel T *et al.* Follicolotropic mycosis fungoides. An aggressive variant of cutaneous T-cell lymphoma. *Arch Dermatol* 2008; **144**: 738–46.

Pagetoid reticulosis

Synonym
• Woringer–Kolopp disease

Definition. A localized, solitary variant of CTCL, which histologically shows intense epidermotropism.

Clinical features. This entity was first described in 1939 [1] and is rare but appears to affect younger adults [2]. It is characterized by an isolated, persistent, scaly plaque, commonly involving an acral site (Fig. 57.13). The lesion may be asymptomatic and slowly

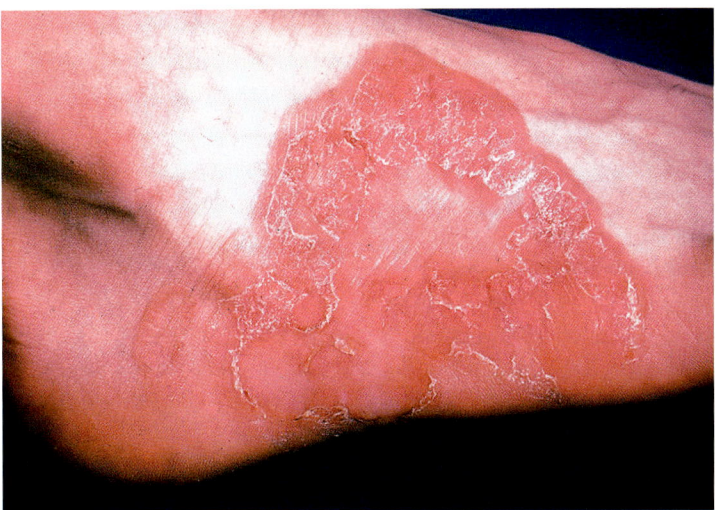

Fig. 57.13 Pagetoid reticulosis. Striking solitary scaling lesion on the side of the foot of a young male.

expands, but no further plaques develop on other body sites. A more generalized variant with multiple plaques at other sites has also been described (Ketron–Goodman), but it is likely that this represents an epidermotropic variant of MF or the more recently described CD8+ epidermotropic CTCL variant [3] (see below).

Pathology. Biopsies show very striking colonization of an acanthotic epidermis [4,5] by atypical, large, pale, mononuclear cells, which usually either fail to express lymphoid markers or express an aberrant T-cell phenotype. Originally there was controversy over whether these cells were derived from histiocytes, Langerhans' cells or Merkel cells. However, the detection of an aberrant T-cell phenotype (CD4– and CD8–) in some cases and clonal TCR gene rearrangements has clearly established that this entity represents a CTCL variant [6–8].

Pathogenesis. This entity may either represent a localized epidermotropic variant of either MF [9] or the more recently described CD8+ epidermotropic CTCL [3]. However, the underlying pathogenesis will not be understood fully until the fundamental biology of MF has been clarified.

Treatment. The natural history of this lesion is of very slow local extension with an excellent prognosis. Successful remission and probable cure has been reported with both surgical excision and low-dose superficial radiotherapy.

References
1 Woringer F, Kolopp P. Lesion erythematosquameuse polycyclique de l'avant bras evoluant depuis 6 ans chez un garcon de 13 ans: histologiquement infiltrat intraepidermique d'apparence tumorale. *Ann Dermatol Vénéréol* 1939; **10**: 945–58.
2 Mandojana RM, Helwig EB. Localized epidermotropic reticulosis (Woringer–Kolopp disease). *J Am Acad Dermatol* 1983; **8**: 813–29.
3 Berti E, Tomasini D, Vermeer M *et al.* Primary cutaneous CD8-positive epidermotropic cytotoxic T-cell lymphomas: a distinct clinicopathological entity with an aggressive clinical behaviour. *Am J Pathol* 1999; **155**: 483–92.
4 Haneke E, Tulusan AH, Weidner F. Histological features of 'pagetoid reticulosis' (Woringer–Kolopp) in premycosis fungoides. *Arch Dermatol Res* 1977; **258**: 265–73.
5 Degreef H, Holvoet C, van Vloten WA *et al.* Woringer–Kolopp disease: an epidermotropic variant of mycosis fungoides. *Cancer* 1976; **38**: 2154–65.
6 Deneau D, Wood G, Beckstead J *et al.* Worringer–Kollopp disease (pagetoid reticulosis): four cases with histopathologic, ultrastructural and immunohistologic observations. *Arch Dermatol* 1984; **120**: 1045–51.
7 MacKie RM, Turbitt ML. A case of pagetoid reticulosis bearing the T cytotoxic suppressor surface marker on the lymphoid infiltrate: further evidence that pagetoid reticulosis is not a variant of mycosis fungoides. *Br J Dermatol* 1984; **110**: 89–94.
8 Wood G, Weiss L, Hu C *et al.* T-cell antigen deficiences and clonal rearrangements of T-cell receptor genes in pagetoid reticulosis (Woringer–Kolopp disease). *N Engl J Med* 1988; **318**: 164–7.
9 Burns MK, Chan LS, Cooper KD. Woringer–Kolopp disease or unilesional mycosis fungoides? *Arch Dermatol* 1995; **131**: 325–9.

Granulomatous slack-skin disease

Definition. A rare disease characterized clinically by the slow development of pendulous folds of lax erythematous skin and histologically by dermal granulomas and elastolysis.

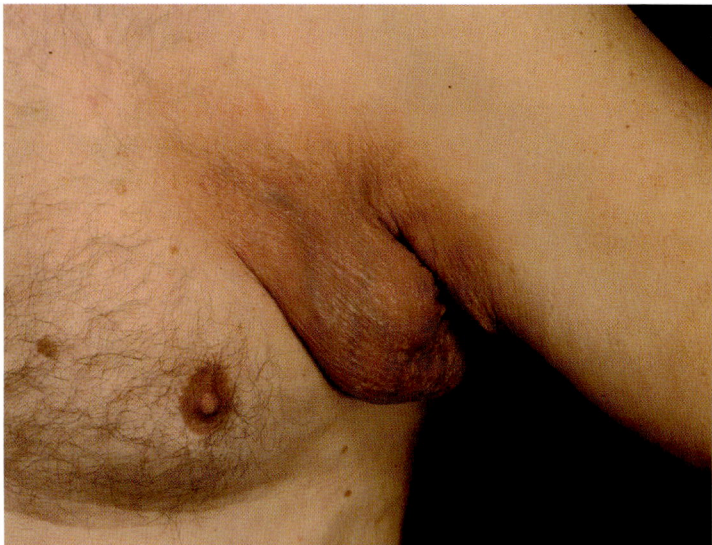

Fig. 57.14 Granulomatous slack skin showing prominent, lax folds of markedly indurated axillary skin with superficial scaling and wrinkling.

Clinical features. The lesions develop slowly, usually in middle-aged adults, and then progress over several years [1]. They are typically flexural in distribution and consist of thickened, pendulous folds (Fig. 57.14). This condition appears to be caused by cutaneous elastolysis associated with an underlying lymphoma. Several patients have died of Hodgkin's disease or non-Hodgkin's lymphoma [2–4] and the otherwise unaltered epidermis may show epidermotropism, similar to that seen in MF. The condition must be distinguished from other forms of cutis laxa.

Pathology. Histology reveals a dense granulomatous dermal infiltrate (Fig. 57.15) with destruction of dermal elastic tissue (elastolysis) [5–7]. The destruction appears to be mediated by histiocytic giant cells [8]. Similar granulomas may occasionally be found in the spleen and lymph nodes [4]. The lymphocytic infiltrate in the dermis shows some cytologic atypia and has an aberrant T-cell phenotype suggestive of lymphoma. TCR gene analysis has also confirmed that T-cell clones are present, suggesting a CTCL variant in most cases [9], but whether this condition represents a granulomatous variant of MF or a different type of CTCL is currently unclear [10], especially as a novel balanced translocation has recently been detected in granulomatous slack skin [11].

Treatment. No definitive therapy has yet been identified but radiotherapy, retinoids and surgery have been reported to be effective [12–14].

References

1 Schot JDL. Granulomatous slack skin. *Br J Dermatol* 1989; **120**: 807.
2 Degregorio R, Fenske NA, Glass LF. Granulomatous slack skin: a possible precursor of Hodgkin's disease. *J Am Acad Dermatol* 1995; **33**: 1044–7.
3 Noto G, Pravata G, Arico M. Granulomatous slack skin: report of a case associated with Hodgkin's disease and review of the literature. *Br J Dermatol* 1994; **131**: 275–9.
4 Le T, Pierard G. Granulomatous slack skin syndrome and Hodgkin's disease. *Ital Gen Rev Dermatol* 1986; **23**: 48–9.

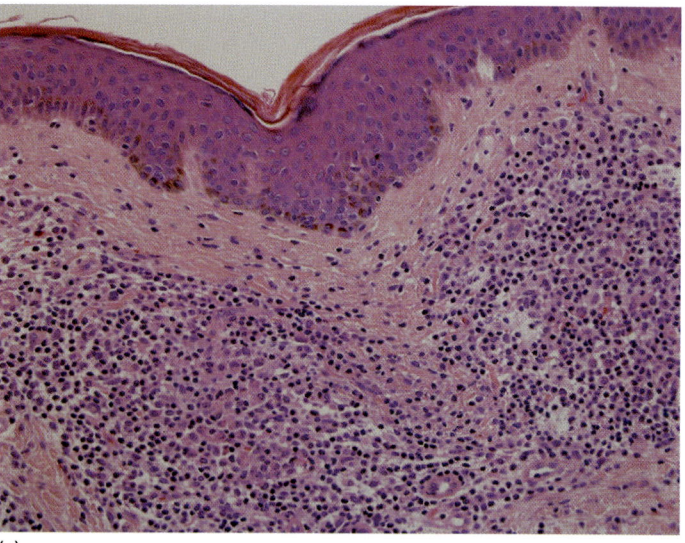

(a)

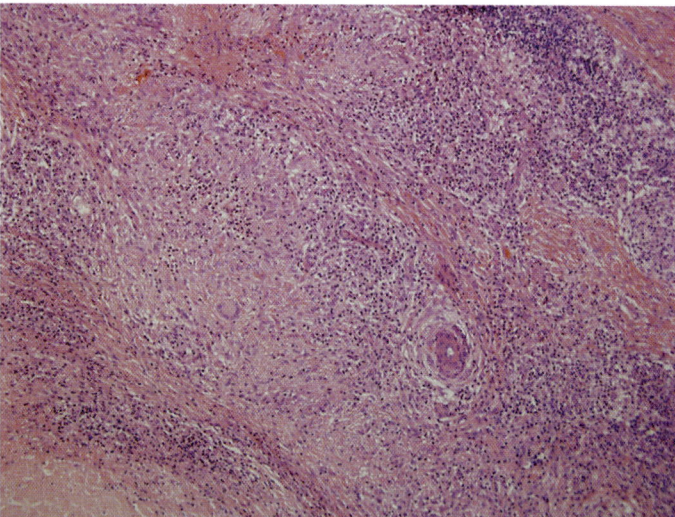

(b)

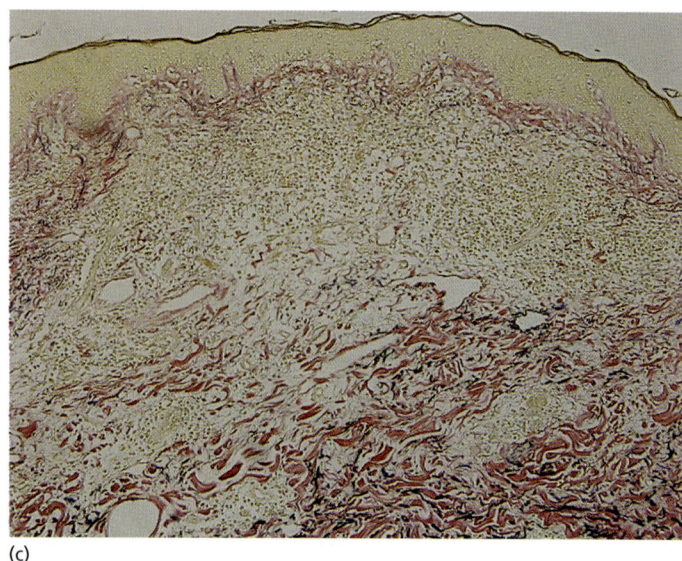

(c)

Fig. 57.15 (a) Histology showing a prominent infiltrate of histiocytic cells and lymphoid cells showing mild cytologic atypia. (b) Giant cells are present and marked loss of elastic tissue (elastolysis) shown with an elastic van Gieson stain (EVG) in the upper dermis (c).

5 Balus L, Bassetti F, Gentili G. Granulomatous slack skin. *Arch Dermatol* 1985; **121**: 250–2.

6 Convit J, Kerdel F, Goihman M *et al*. Progressive atrophying chronic granulomatous dermohypodermatitis. *Arch Dermatol* 1973; **107**: 371–4.

7 White CR, Holbrook KA, Atkin E *et al*. Granulomatous slack skin. *Arch Dermatol* 1984; **120**: 1085.

8 Helm KF, Cerio R, Winkelmann RK. Granulomatous slack skin: a clinico-pathological and immunohistochemical study of three cases. *Br J Dermatol* 1992; **126**: 142–7.

9 Le Boit PE, Beckstead K, Atkin E *et al*. Granulomatous slack skin: clonal rearrangement of the T-cell receptor β gene is evidence for the lymphoproliferative nature of the cutaneous elastolytic disorder. *J Invest Dermatol* 1987; **89**: 183–6.

10 Kempf W, Ostheeren-Michaelis S, Paulli M *et al*. Granulomatous mycosis fungoides and granulomatous slack skin. *Arch Dermatol* 2008; **144**: 1069–617.

11 Ikonomou I, Aamot V, Heim S *et al*. Granulomatous slack skin with a translocation t(3;9)(q12;24). *Am J Surg Pathol* 2007; **31**: 803–6.

12 Wollina U, Greafe T, Fuller J. Granulomatous slack skin or granulomatous mycosis fungoides: a case report. Complete response to percutaneous radiation and interferon alpha. *J Cancer Res Clin Oncol* 2002; **128**: 50–4.

13 Balus L, Manente L, Remotti D. Granulomatous slack skin: report of a case and review of the literature. *Am J Dermatopathol* 1996; **18**: 199–206.

14 Benton E, Morris S, Robson A, Whittaker S. An unusual case of granulomatous slack skin with necrobiosis. *Am J Dermatopathol* 2008; **30**: 462–5.

Sézary syndrome [1–4]

Definition. The presence of a clinical triad consisting of erythroderma, peripheral lymphadenopathy and atypical mononuclear cells (Sézary cells) comprising 5% or more of peripheral blood lymphocytes on a buffy coat smear (B1), or more than 20% of total lymphocyte count or a total Sézary count of more than 1000×10^9/L (B2). The presence of a peripheral blood T-cell clone as indicated either by a CD4:CD8 ratio greater than 10, aberrant expression of pan T-cell antigens, cytogenetics or TCR gene analysis is now also required to confirm that the patient has a malignant disease, Sézary T-cell lymphoma–leukaemia [5].

Clinical features. The majority of patients are elderly males and may develop the syndrome either *ab initio* or as progression from classical MF. Many patients describe a prolonged history of 'dermatitis'. Patients present with a generalized exfoliative erythroderma, and may have systemic problems because of shunting of blood through grossly dilated cutaneous vasculature, and resulting high-output cardiac failure. There may be associated ectropion, scalp alopecia, palmoplantar hyperkeratoses and fissuring and the nails often show gross subungual hyperkeratoses (Fig. 57.16). Peripheral lymphadenopathy is often present. The distinction from erythrodermic MF (T4 N0–3 M0/stage III–IVA) is based on the degree of peripheral blood involvement (more than 5% Sézary cells per 100 lymphocytes (T4 N0–3 M0B1/stage III–IVA) as suggested in the original National Cancer Institute (NCI) staging system) [6]. However, there has been a debate about the diagnostic and prognostic relevance of the proportion of peripheral blood Sézary cells as low numbers of Sézary cells can be detected in the peripheral blood of healthy individuals and patients with inflammatory dermatoses. In 1988, the NCI published a revised staging system, with over 20% Sézary cell count (per 100 lymphocytes) as the B1 rating [7], based on previous studies showing that this figure had prognostic significance in Sézary syndrome [8,9]. However, this has been shown to include some patients with

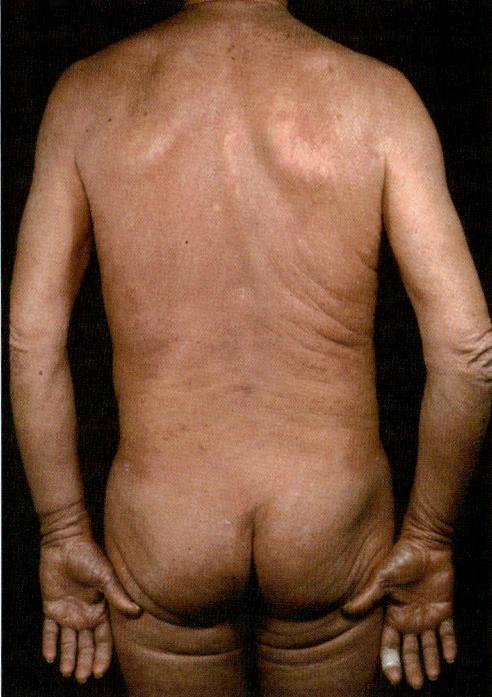

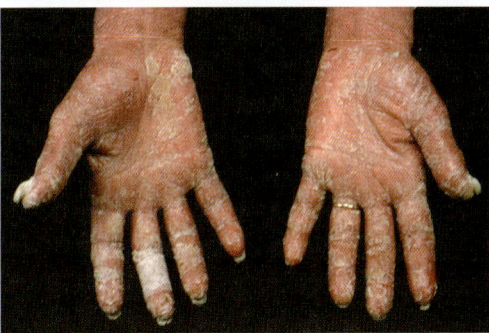

Fig. 57.16 Sézary syndrome showing erythroderma with palmoplantar hyperkeratoses and prominent nail dystrophy.

benign disorders and may actually represent a larger tumour burden (B2). An absolute Sézary cell count of over 1000/mm³ has recently been proposed as a criterion for the diagnosis of Sézary syndrome, which most closely represents the B2 rating for peripheral blood involvement, but this figure may exclude those patients with a lower tumour burden (more than 5% per 100 lymphocytes; B1), who nevertheless have a neoplastic form of SS [5,10]. The recent ISCL EORTC proposal for a revision of the staging system provides a well-defined staging of peripheral blood in SS and should clarify these issues [11]. A recent study suggests that the presence of lymph node disease in Sézary syndrome is an independent prognostic factor while the degree of peripheral blood involvement also has some prognostic significance [12]. The prognosis for patients with SS is poor, with a median survival of 35 months from diagnosis. Most die of opportunistic infection. However, with improved earlier diagnosis the prognosis may now be better.

Immunopathology. Skin biopsies can show large numbers of atypical mononuclear cells in the dermis with epidermotropism, but it has been shown that non-diagnostic and lymphomatoid

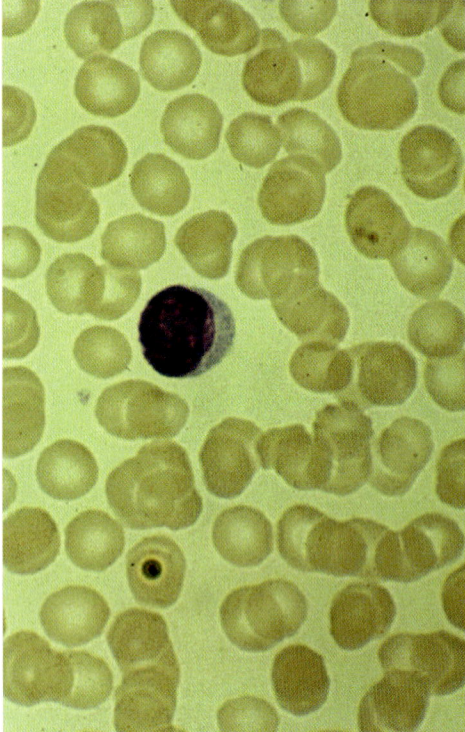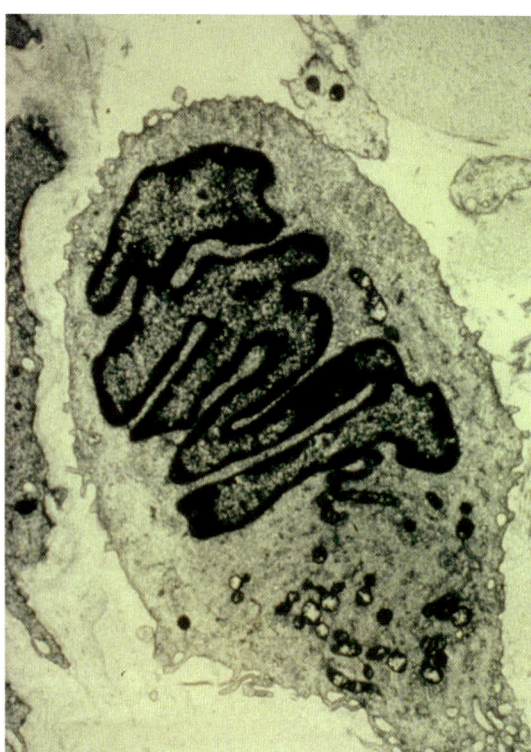

Fig. 57.17 High-power view of Sézary cells in peripheral blood showing large cell with very large nucleus and minimal cytoplasm and ultrastructural features of a typical cerebriform nucleus.

histology is frequently seen in proven cases of SS [13]. The presence of atypical (Sézary-like) peripheral blood cerebriform mononuclear cells has also been reported in a variety of inflammatory conditions including actinic reticuloid, erythroderma associated with dermatitis and psoriasis, and severe drug reactions, but in general the percentage of atypical cells in such conditions is lower than in SS (Fig. 57.17) [14,15]. In addition, T cells with the morphological and ultrastructural features of Sézary cells can be identified in the peripheral blood of normal healthy individuals [16,17]. However, it is important to realize that the total lymphocyte count does not have to be raised for the diagnosis to be made, and the presence of a normal total white cell count without careful morphological examination of the 'tail' of a blood smear or of a buffy coat preparation may mask this diagnosis. Consequently, it can be difficult to conclusively distinguish cases of T-cell leukaemia–lymphoma from inflammatory dermatoses. Large Sézary cell variants (over 16 μm diameter) are easier to recognize but small Sézary cell variants (12–14 μm) are more common and are more difficult to distinguish from activated lymphocytes [4]. Sézary cells are usually CD3+, CD4+, CD7−, CD26− T cells but CD26+, CD7+ and CD8+ variants have been reported and CD26 loss can occur in control populations albeit at low levels [18–23]. Absolute CD4 counts and CD4:CD8 ratios are elevated. A CD4:CD8 ratio greater than 10 distinguishes most cases of T-cell leukaemia–lymphoma from inflammatory dermatosis associated with Sézary cells but is not pathognomonic as it usually represents a large peripheral blood tumour burden. A consensus has now been agreed that diagnostic criteria should include the clinical triad of features plus the presence of a peripheral blood T-cell clone detected either by expression of aberrant pan T-cell antigens, cytogenetics or TCR gene analysis [5]. Those patients without evidence of a T-cell

clone may have a benign inflammatory dermatosis with an excellent prognosis [24]. Sézary syndrome should also be distinguished from other T-cell malignancies such as T-prolymphocytic leukaemia, which can present with cutaneous involvement including rarely erythroderma, although this diagnosis is usually apparent on the basis of clinicopathological and immunophenotypic features [25].

References

1 Sézary A, Bouvrain Y. Erythrodermie avec presence de cellules monstreuses dans derme et sang circulant. *Bull Soc Fr Dermatol Syphilol* 1938; **45**: 254–60.
2 Main R, Goodall H, Swanson W. Sézary's syndrome. *Br J Dermatol* 1959; **71**: 254–60.
3 Lutzner M, Jordan H. The ultrastructure of an abnormal cell in Sézary's syndrome. *Blood* 1968; **31**: 719–26.
4 Lutzner M, Emerit I, Durepaire R *et al.* Cytogenetic, cytophotometric and ultrastructural study of large cerebriform cells of the Sézary syndrome and description of the small-cell variant. *J Natl Cancer Inst* 1973; **50**: 1145–62.
5 Vonderheid E, Bernengo M, Burg G *et al.* Update on erythrodermic cutaneous T-cell lymphoma: report of the International Society for Cutaneous Lymphomas. *J Am Acad Dermatol* 2002; **46**: 95–106.
6 Lamberg SI, Bunn PA Jr. Cutaneous T-cell lymphomas: summary of the Mycosis Fungoides Cooperative Group—National Cancer Institute Workshop. *Arch Dermatol* 1979; **115**: 1103–5.
7 Sausville E, Eddy J, Makuch R *et al.* Histopathologic staging at initial diagnosis of mycosis fungoides and the Sézary syndrome: definition of three distinctive prognostic groups. *Ann Intern Med* 1988; **109**: 372–82.
8 Schechter G, Sausville E, Fischmann A *et al.* Evaluation of circulating malignant cells provides prognostic information in cutaneous T-cell lymphoma. *Blood* 1987; **69**: 841–9.
9 Vonderheid E, Sobel E, Nowell P *et al.* Diagnostic and prognostic significance of Sézary cells in peripheral blood smears from patients with cutaneous T cell lymphoma. *Blood* 1985; **66**: 358–66.
10 Russell Jones R, Whittaker S. T-cell receptor gene analysis in the diagnosis of Sézary syndrome. *J Am Acad Dermatol* 1999; **41**: 254–7.

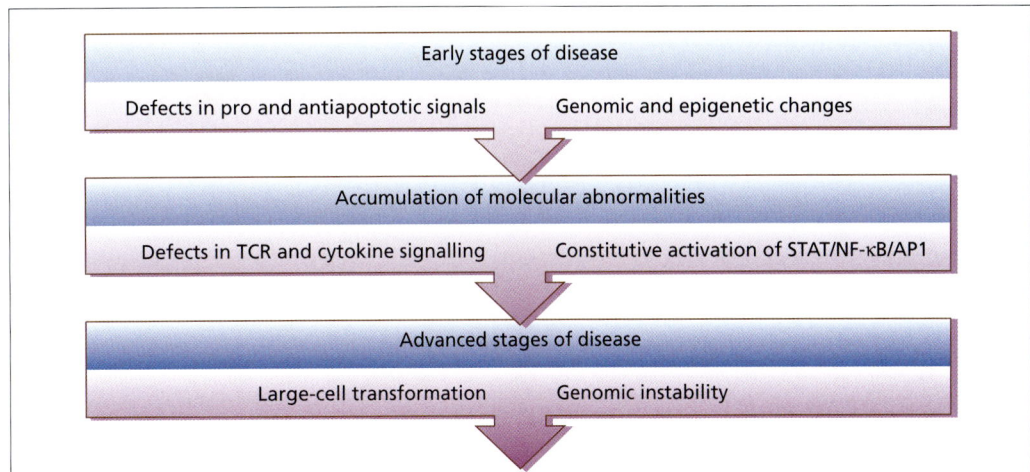

Fig. 57.18 Molecular pathogenesis of mycosis fungoides/Sézary syndrome.

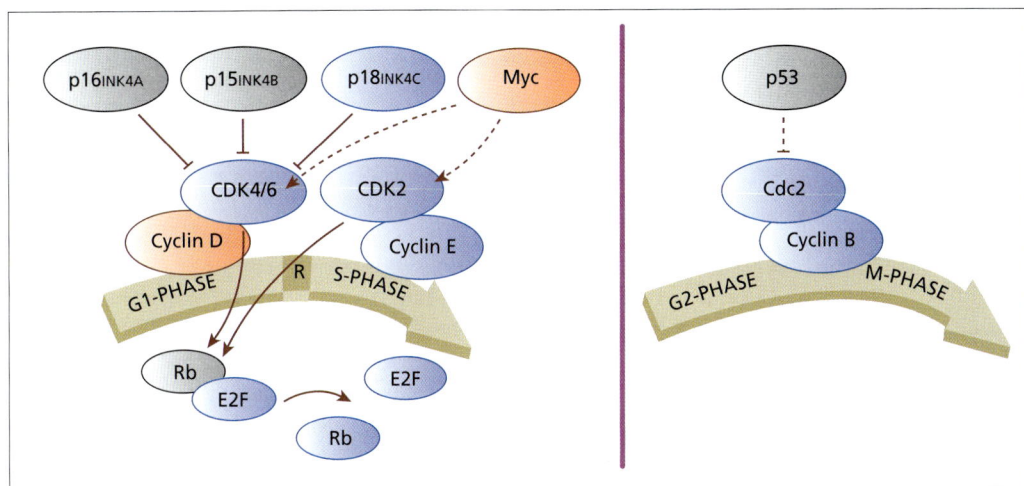

Fig. 57.19 Abnormalities of genes controlling cell-cycle checkpoints in mycosis fungoides/Sézary syndrome (grey, loss of function; red, gain of function).

11 Olsen E, Vonderheid E, Pimpinelli N *et al*. Revisions to the staging and classification of mycosis fungoides and Sezary syndrome: a proposal of the International Society for Cutaneous Lymphomas (ISCL) and the cutaneous lymphoma task force of the European Organisation of Research and Treatment of Cancer (EORTC). *Blood* 2007; **110**: 1713–22.

12 Scarisbrick J, Whittaker S, Evans A *et al*. Prognostic significance of tumour burden in the blood of patients with erythrodermic primary cutaneous T-cell lymphoma. *Blood* 2001; **97**: 624–30.

13 Trotter M, Whittaker S, Orchard G, Smith N. Cutaneous histopathology of Sézary syndrome: a study of 41 cases with a proven circulating T-cell clone. *J Cutan Pathol* 1997; **24**: 286–91.

14 Chu A, Robinson D, Hawk J *et al*. Immunologic differentiation of the Sézary syndrome due to cutaneous T-cell lymphoma and chronic actinic dermatitis. *J Invest Dermatol* 1986; **86**: 134–7.

15 D'Incan M, Souteyrand P, Bignon Y *et al*. Hydantoin-induced cutaneous pseudolymphoma with clinical, pathologic and immunologic aspects of Sézary syndrome. *Arch Dermatol* 1992; **128**: 1371–4.

16 Meijer C, Van Leeuwen A, Van der Loo E *et al*. Cerebriform (Sézary-like) mononuclear cells in healthy individuals: a morphologically distinct population of T-cells. *Arch B Cell Pathol* 1977; **25**: 95–104.

17 Matutes E, Robinson D, O'Brien M *et al*. Candiate counterparts of Sézary cells and adult T-cell lymphoma–leukaemia cells in normal peripheral blood: an ultrastructural study with immunogold method and monoclonal antibodies. *Leuk Res* 1983; **7**: 787–801.

18 Lutzner M, Edelson R, Schein P *et al*. Cutaneous T-cell lymphomas: the Sézary syndrome, mycosis fungoides, and related disorders. *Ann Intern Med* 1975; **83**: 534–52.

19 Miller RA, Coleman CN, Fawcett HD *et al*. Sézary syndrome: a model for migration of T lymphocytes to skin. *N Engl J Med* 1980; **303**: 89–92.

20 Willemze R, Van Vloten W, Hermans J *et al*. Diagnostic criteria in Sézary's syndrome: a multiparameter study of peripheral blood lymphocytes in 32 patients with erythroderma. *J Invest Dermatol* 1983; **81**: 392–7.

21 Bernengo M, Novelli M, Quaglino P *et al*. Prognostic factors in Sézary syndrome: a multivariate analysis of clinical, haematological, and immunological features. *Ann Oncol* 1998; **9**: 857–63.

22 Bernengo M, Novelli M, Quaglino P *et al*. The relevance of the CD4 CD26⁻ subset in the identication of circulating Sézary cells. *Br J Dermatol* 2001; **144**: 25–135.

23 Kelemen K, Guitart J, Kuzel T *et al*. The usefulness of CD26 in flow cytometric analysis of peripheral blood in Sezary syndrome. *Am J Clin Pathol* 2008; **129**: 146–56.

24 Fraser-Andrews E, Russell-Jones R, Woolford A *et al*. Diagnostic and prognostic importance of T-cell receptor gene analysis in patients with Sézary syndrome. *Cancer* 2001; **92**: 1745–52.

25 Matutes E, Brito-Babapulle V, Swansbury J *et al*. Clinical and laboratory features of 78 cases of T-prolymphocytic leukaemia. *Blood* 1991; **78**: 3269–74.

Molecular features (MF/SS) (Fig. 57.18). The underlying molecular pathogenesis of MF and SS has not yet been fully characterized. No disease-specific translocations have yet been identified [1], but studies have shown consistent abnormalities of cell cycle (Fig. 57.19), DNA repair and apoptotic pathways which contributes to both genomic instability and a failure of activation-induced cell

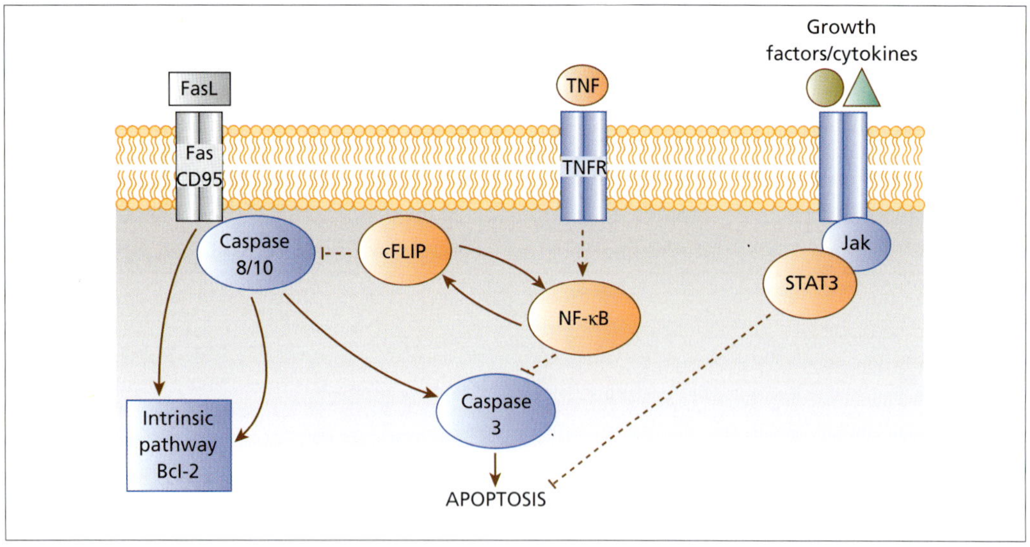

Fig. 57.20 Abnormalities of T-cell activation induced cell death in mycosis fungoides/Sézary syndrome causing defective T-cell homeostasis (grey, loss of function; red, gain of function).

death, which is primarily responsible for T-cell homeostasis (Fig. 57.20).

Extensive studies have shown complex but consistent and recurrent numerical and structural chromosomal abnormalities in all stages of disease [1–9]. In SS an abnormal karyotype is a poor prognostic factor [10]. These studies, using conventional cytogenetics, allelotyping, metaphase and array comparative genomic hybridization (CGH) techniques, have shown similar patterns of chromosomal losses (1p, 13, 19, 17p and 10q) and gains (4, 8q and 17q), and patterns of loss of heterozygosity (9p, 10q and 17p) in both MF and SS suggesting a shared pathogenesis. Minimal regions of deletion have been detected on 10q, suggesting a number of potential candidate genes [11,12]. High resolution array CGH studies have confirmed these 10q findings in SS and suggest a high frequency (40–75% of cases) of candidate gene abnormalities, including gains of cMYC and STAT3/5 and loss of cMYC antagonists including MXI1 and MNT and p53 [13]. Gains of Her 2/neu gene copy number at 17q have also been detected using fluorescent in situ hybridization (FISH) in a small series of SS patients [14]. High resolution array CGH studies in early stages of MF have also shown recurrent losses (7p, 7q, 9q, 12q, 16q and 19) with gains (8q and 21q) and specific deletions of tumour suppressor genes BCL7a, SMAC/DIABLO and RHOF [15].

Although as yet no disease-specific balanced translocation has been defined, a balanced t(12;18)(q21;21.2) translocation was recently described in a patient with SS and led to the identification of a NAV3 gene deletion on chromosome 12q21-22 using interphase FISH in a majority of MF and SS patients [16]. However, subsequent studies have not detected specific NAV3 deletions in a separate series of MF and SS patients; 12q losses were detected in a few cases but in only two cases did the 12q deletions include NAV3 [17].

Specific chromosomal abnormalities have been detected in early stages of disease, suggesting that chromosomal instability occurs early [18]. Microsatellite instability (MSI) has also been detected in some studies, and has been attributed to hypermethylation of the mismatch repair enzyme gene promoter, MLH1 [19]. Undoubtedly MSI also contributes to genomic instability in MF/SS. Telom-

erase activity is increased in MF/SS [20], which is essential to prevent tumour cell senescence but also will potentially contribute to genomic instability.

Specific gene abnormalities in MF/SS include overexpression and mutation of p53 in advanced stages of disease [21–24]. In one study, UVB-type p53 mutations were found [23]. Additional 17p copy number losses also contribute to loss of p53 function in MF/SS [6]. p53 abnormalities are not found in early stages of disease, suggesting that inactivation of p53 is related to disease progression, similar to findings in other nodal and extranodal lymphomas. At present, it is unclear if p53 abnormalities are associated with treatment resistance and a poor prognosis, as seen in other non-Hodgkin's lymphomas, but loss of p53 would contribute to both apoptotic defects and genomic instability. Inactivation of both p14, p15 and p16 genes has also been detected in MF [25–27]. This is a consequence of 9p deletions involving the CDKN2A locus and epigenetic abnormalities due to hypermethylation of gene promoter sequences rather than mutation (Fig. 57.19). It is still unclear whether this is restricted to late-stage disease and transformation. Other genes shown to be inactivated through epigenetic mechanisms involving promoter hypermethylation include tumour suppressor genes, BCL7a, PTPRG and p73 [28]. Deletions of BCL7a have also been demonstrated in early stages of MF [15]. The tumour suppressor gene on 10q, PTEN, has been shown to be homozygously deleted in a proportion of patients, suggesting that the pro-apoptotic AKT signalling pathway is dysregulated [11]. Recent studies have identified infrequent mutations of the Fas gene on 10q in early stages of MF and loss of Fas expression in advanced disease, providing a further mechanism by which tumour cells may escape apoptosis [29,30]. Fas-mediated apoptosis may also be inhibited in tumour cells by over-expression of cFLIP which inhibits the extrinsic apoptotic pathway [31] (Fig. 57.20). Dysregulation of the intrinsic apoptotic pathway has also been detected in MF/SS [32]. Gains of oncogenes, including RAF1 and CTSB, have been detected in a small series of MF/SS cases [33]. In addition, gains of JUNB on chromosome 19p have been detected in a large series of MF/SS patients and this appears to be due to chromosomal amplification in some cases with overexpression in tumour cells identified in tumour samples as well [34]. JunB is a member of the AP1 transcription factor family involved in controlling cell proliferation and differentiation. JunB is also essential for expression of a Th2 cytokine profile and so over-expression in MF/SS may explain the characteristic Th2 cytokine expression by MF/SS [35].

Gene expression studies in MF have shown abnormalities of TNF signalling pathways and gene expression signatures which reportedly distinguish inflammatory dermatoses from MF [36]. A further array cDNA study of MF has identified three signature profiles using consensus clustering which distinguishes those patients with: (i) early stage disease (IA–IIA) who respond to therapy; (ii) an intermediate group (stage IB–III) who show a degree of resistance to therapy; and (iii) a poor prognostic group (predominantly stage IIB) [37]. Both these findings have yet to be validated and may explain more about the host immune response than the actual tumour gene expression profile.

In SS, cDNA array studies have identified a gene signature that is reported to be associated with poor prognosis and a diagnostic gene signature that can be used to distinguish it from inflammatory dermatoses has also been described [38,39]. A further study using a different array platform showed expression of a tyrosine kinase receptor, *EphA4* and a transcription factor, *Twist* [40]. The functional relevance and validation of these findings requires further study. Several studies have now confirmed over-expression of T-plastin in SS. This is an actin bundling protein and the T-plastin isoform is normally only expressed in epithelial tissues and could prove to be an important biomarker [38,41].

Fundamental questions remaining include the cause(s) of the genomic instability which defines MF/SS even at early stages as well as a need to define the specific genomic abnormalities that distinguish SS from MF. However, it is apparent that critical abnormalities of apoptosis are prevalent in both MF and SS and almost certainly this affects T-cell homeostasis. Such defects are probably essential acquired abnormalities allowing tumour cells in MF/SS to adopt a malignant phenotype. Defective activation-induced cell death in MF/SS is further exemplified by other key findings (Fig. 57.21); constitutive expression of STAT3 protein

which is integral to cytokine mediated T-cell activation and inhibition of IL-2 mediated expression of STAT5 have been clearly defined in advanced stages of disease such as SS [42–44]. In addition, constitutive expression of NFkB has also been shown in both MF and SS [45,46]. The consequent dysregulation of multiple signalling pathways controlled by STAT and NFkB will contribute to prevention of tumour cell apoptosis in MF/SS and these pathways may also be potential therapeutic targets.

References

1 Thangavelu M, Finn W, Yelavarthi K *et al.* Recurring structural chromosomal abnormalities in peripheral blood lymphocytes of patients with mycosis fungoides/Sézary syndrome. *Blood* 1997; **89**: 3371.

2 Karenko L, Kahkonen M, Hyytinen E *et al.* Notable losses at specific regions of chromosome 10q and 13q in the Sézary syndrome detected by comparative genomic hybridization. *J Invest Dermatol* 1999; **112**: 392.

3 Mao X, Lillington D, Scarisbrick J *et al.* Molecular cytogenetic analysis of cutaneous T-cell lymphomas: identification of common genetic alterations in Sézary syndrome and mycosis fungoides. *Br J Dermatol* 2002; **147**: 464–75.

4 Karenko L, Sarna S, Kahkonen M, Ranki A. Chromosomal abnormalities in relation to clinical disease in patients with cutaneous T-cell lymphoma: a 5 year follow-up study. *Br J Dermatol* 2003; **148**: 55–64.

5 Scarisbrick JJ, Woolford AJ, Russell-Jones R, Whittaker SJ. Allelotyping in mycosis fungoides and Sézary syndrome: common regions of allelic loss identified on 9p, 10q, and 17p. *J Invest Dermatol* 2001; **117**: 663–70.

6 Mao X, Lillington D, Czepulkowski B *et al.* Molecular cytogenetic characterization of Sézary syndrome. *Genes Chromosomes Cancer* 2003; **36**: 250–60.

7 Batista D, Vonderheid E, Hawkins A *et al.* Multicolor fluorescence in situ hybridization (SKY) in mycosis fungoides and Sezary syndrome: search for recurrent chromosome abnormalities. *Genes Chrom Cancer* 2006; **45**: 383–91.

8 Padilla-Nash H, Wu K, Just H *et al.* Spectral karyotyping demonstrates genetically unstable skin homing T lymphocytes in cutaneous T-cell lymphoma. *Exp Dermatol* 2006; **16**: 98–103.

9 Prochazkova M, Chevret E, Mainhaguiet G *et al.* Common chromosomal abnormalities in mycosis fungoides transformation. *Genes Chrom Cancer* 2007; **46**: 828–38.

10 Whang-Peng J, Bunn P, Knutsen T *et al.* Clinical implications of cytogenetic studies in cutaneous T-cell lymphoma (CTCL). *Cancer* 1982; **50**: 1539–53.

11 Scarisbrick J, Woolford A, Russell-Jones R *et al.* Loss of heterozygosity on 10q and microsatellite instability in advanced stages of primary cutaneous T-cell lymphoma and possible association with homozygous deletion of *PTEN*. *Blood* 2000; **95**: 2937–42.

12 Wain M, Mitchell T, Russell Jones R, Whittaker S. Fine mapping of chromosome 10q deletions in mycosis fungoides and Sezary syndrome: identification of two discrete regions of deletion at 10q23.33-24.1 and 10q24.33-25.1. *Genes Chrom Cancer* 2005; **42**: 184–92.

13 Vermeer M, van Doorn R, Dijkman R *et al.* Novel and highly recurrent chromosomal alterations in Sezary syndrome. *Cancer Res* 2008; **68**: 2689–98.

14 Utikal J, Poenitz N, Gratchev A *et al.* Additional Her 2/*neu* gene copies in patients with Sezary Syndrome. *Leuk Res* 2006; **30**: 755–60.

15 Carbone A, Bernardini L, Valenzano F *et al.* Array-based comparative genomic hybridization in early-stage mycosis fungoides: recurrent deletion of tumour suppressor genes *BCL7A*, *SMAC/DIABLO* and *RHOF*. *Genes Chrom Cancer* 2008; **47**: 1067–75.

16 Karenko L, Hahtola S, Paivinen S *et al.* Primary cutaneous T-cell lymphomas show a deletion or translocation affecting *NAV3*, the human *UNC-53* homologue. *Cancer Res* 2005; **65**: 8101–10.

17 Marty M, Prochazkova M, Lahranne E *et al.* Primary cutaneous T-cell lymphomas do not show specific *NAV3* gene deletion or translocation. *J Invest Dermatol* 2008; **128**: 2458–66.

18 Barab G, Matteucci C, Girolomoni G *et al.* Comparative genomic hybridization identifies 17q11.2-q12 duplication as an early event in cutaneous T-cell lymphomas. *Cancer Gen Cytogen* 2008; **184**: 48–51.

19 Scarisbrick J, Mitchell T, Calonje E *et al.* Microsatellite instability is associated with hypermethylation of the hMLH1 gene and reduced expression in mycosis fungoides. *J Invest Dermatol* 2003; **121**: 894–901.

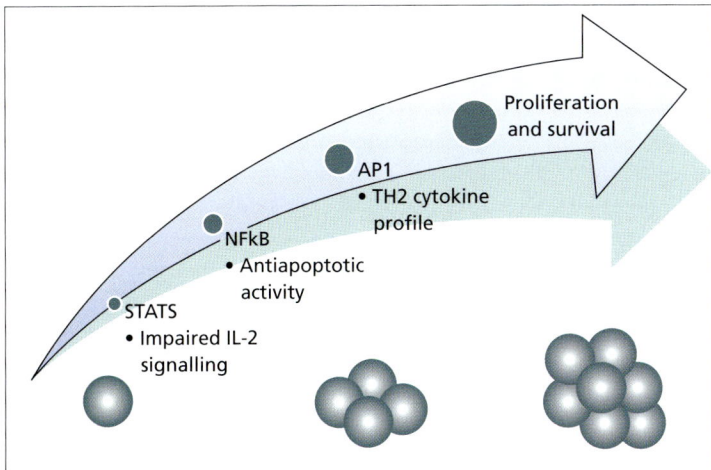

Fig. 57.21 Dysregulated T-cell signalling pathways in mycosis fungoides/Sézary syndrome.

20 Wu K, Lund M, Bang K, Thestrup-Pedersen K. Telomerase activity and telomere length in lymphocytes from patients with cutaneous T-cell lymphoma. *Cancer* 1999; **86**: 1056–63.

21 Lauritzen A, Vejlsgaard G, Hou-Jensen K *et al*. P53 protein expression in cutaneous T-cell lymphomas. *Br J Dermatol* 1995; **133**: 32–6.

22 MacGregor J, Dublin E, Levison D *et al*. P53 immunoreactivity is uncommon in primary cutaneous lymphoma. *Br J Dermatol* 1995; **132**: 353.

23 MacGregor J, Crook T, Fraser-Andrews E *et al*. Spectrum of *p53* gene mutations suggests a possible role for ultraviolet radiation in the pathogenesis of advanced cutaneous lymphomas. *J Invest Dermatol* 1999; **112**: 317–21.

24 Marrogi A, Khan M, Vonderheid E *et al*. P53 tumour suppressor gene mutations in transformed cutaneous T-cell lymphoma: a study of 12 cases. *J Cutan Pathol* 1999; **26**: 369–78.

25 Peris K, Stanta G, Fargnoli C *et al*. Reduced expression of CDKN2a/p16 in mycosis fungoides. *Arch Dermatol Res* 1999; **291**: 207–11.

26 Navas I, Oritz-Romero P, Villuendas R *et al*. P16 gene alterations are frequent in lesions of mycosis fungoides. *Am J Pathol* 2000; **156**: 1565–72.

27 Scarisbrick JJ, Woolford AJ, Calonje E *et al*. Frequent abnormalities of the *p15* and *p16* genes in mycosis fungoides and Sézary syndrome. *J Invest Dermatol* 2002; **118**: 493–9.

28 van Doorn R, Zoutman W, Dijkman R *et al*. Epigenetic profiling of cutaneous T-cell lymphoma: promoter hypermethylation of multiple tumour suppressor genes including *BCL7a, PTPRG* and *p73*. *J Clin Oncol* 2005; **23**: 3886–96.

29 Dereure O, Levi E, Vonderhied E, Kadin M. Infrequent Fas mutations but no BAX or p53 mutations in early mycosis fungoides: a possible mechanism for the accumulation of malignant T lymphocytes in the skin. *J Invest Dermatol* 2002; **118**: 949–56.

30 Zoi-Toli O, Vermmer M, De Vries E *et al*. Expression of Fas and Fas-ligand in primary cutaneous T-cell lymphoma (CTCL): association between lack of Fas expression and aggressive types of CTCL. *Br J Dermatol* 2000; **143**: 313–9.

31 Contassot E, Kerl K, Roques S *et al*. Resistance to FasL and tumour necrosis factor-related apoptosis-inducing ligand-mediated apoptosis in Sezary syndrome T-cells associated with impaired death receptor and FLICE-inhibitory protein expression. *Blood* 2006; **111**: 4780–7.

32 Zhang C-L, Kamarashev J, Qin J-Z *et al*. Expression of apoptosis regulators in cutaneous T-cell lymphoma (CTCL) cells. *J Pathol* 2003; **200**: 249–54.

33 Mao X, Orchard G, Lillington D *et al*. Amplification and overexpression of *JUNB* is associated with primary cutaneous T-cell lymphomas. *Blood* 2003; **101**: 1513–9.

34 Mao X, Orchard G, Mitchell T *et al*. A genomic and expression study of AP-1 in primary cutaneous T-cell lymphoma: evidence for dysregulated expression of JUNB and JUND in MF and SS. *J Cutan Pathol* 2008; **35**: 899–910.

35 Hahtola S, Tuomela S, Elo L *et al*. Th1 response and cytotoxicity genes are down-regulated in cutaneous T-cell lymphoma. *Clin Cancer Res* 2006; **12**: 4812–21.

36 Tracey L, Villuendas R, Dotor A *et al*. Mycosis fungoides shows concurrent deregulation of multiple genes involved in the TNF signaling pathway: an expression profile study. *Blood* 2003; **102**: 1042–50.

37 Shin J, Monti S, Aires D *et al*. Lesional gene expression profiling in cutaneous T cell lymphoma reveals natural clusters associated with disease outcome. *Blood* 2007; **110**: 3015–27.

38 Kari L, Loboda A, Nebozhyn M *et al*. Classification and prediction of survival in patients with the leukemic phase of cutaneous T cell lymphoma. *J Exp Med* 2003; **197**: 1477–88.

39 Nebozhyn M, Loboda A, Kari L *et al*. Quantitative PCR on 5 genes reliably identifies CTCL patients with 5% to 99% circulating tumour cells with 90% accuracy. *Blood* 2006; **107**: 3189–96.

40 van Doorn R, Dijkman R, Vermeer M *et al*. Aberrant expression of the tyrosine kinase receptor EphA4 and the transcription factor Twist in Sezary syndrome identified by gene expression analysis. *Cancer Res* 2004; **64**: 5578–86.

41 Su M, Dorocicz I, Dragowska W *et al*. Aberrant expression of T-plastin in Sezary cells. *Cancer Res* 2003; **63**: 7122–7.

42 Zhang Q, Nowak I, Vonderheid E *et al*. Activation of Jak/STAT proteins involved in signal transduction pathway mediated by receptor for interleukin 2 in malignant T lymphocytes derived from cutaneous anaplastic large T-cell lymphoma and Sezary syndrome. *PNAS* 1996; **93**: 9148–53.

43 Qin J-Z, Kamarashev J, Zhang C-L *et al*. Constitutive and interleukin-7 and interleukin-15 stimulated DNA binding of STAT and novel factors in cutaneous T cell lymphoma cells. *J Invest Dermatol* 2001; **117**: 583–9.

44 Mitchell T, Whittaker S, John S. Dysregulated expression of COOH-terminally truncated Stat5 and loss of IL2-inducible Stat5-dependent gene expression in Sezary syndrome. *Cancer Res* 2003; **63**: 9048–54.

45 Izban K, Ergin M, Qin J-Z *et al*. Constitutive expression of NF-kB is a characteristic feature of mycosis fungoides: implications for apoptosis resistance and pathogenesis. *Hum Pathol* 2000; **31**: 1482–90.

46 Sors A, Jean-Loius F, Pellet C *et al*. Down-regulating constitutive activation of the NFkB canonical pathway overcomes the resistance of cutaneous T-cell lymphoma to apoptosis. *Blood* 2006; **107**: 2354–63.

Treatment of mycosis fungoides and Sézary syndrome

Current therapy of MF and Sézary syndrome includes:
1 Topical steroids
2 Topical chemotherapy—mechlorethamine (nitrogen mustard) and carmustine (BCNU)
3 Phototherapy—both UVB and psoralen with UVA (PUVA) and UVA-1
4 Radiotherapy, including total skin electron beam therapy (TSEB)
5 Immunotherapy (IFN-α, IFN-γ and IL-12)
6 Retinoids
7 Combination therapies
8 Systemic single and multiagent chemotherapy
9 Photopheresis
10 Toxin therapies
11 Monoclonal antibodies
12 Histone deacetylase inhibitors
13 Other novel therapies.

The choice of initial treatment for the MF patient will depend on the stage of the disease as well as the general condition and age of the patient (performance status). At present, there are very few published studies that could form the basis for evidence-based therapy, mainly because of the rarity of the condition and also because of the variation between individual patients in disease pattern and progress. A large proportion of patients with MF are frail, elderly and likely to succumb either to other general medical problems or to the side effects of overenthusiastic therapy. In addition, the patient's quality of life should always be considered when selecting a treatment regimen. One of the few randomized trials of treatment of MF reported on 103 patients who received either TSEB (3000 cGy total skin electron beam) together with cyclophosphamide, daunorubicin, etoposide and vincristine (a rigorous 'treat to cure' regimen) or sequential topical therapy consisting of nitrogen mustard, superficial radiotherapy and TSEB, progressing to PUVA if required (a 'gentle palliative' regimen). After a median follow-up time of 75 months, there was no difference in disease-free or overall survival between the 52 patients who received TSEB plus chemotherapy and the 51 who received sequential palliative topical therapy [1]. This study established a consensus that therapy in MF should be based on stage of disease and aimed at disease palliation rather than an aggressive intent to cure. Therefore the current consensus is that patients with early

Table 57.7 Treatment algorithm for cutaneous T-cell lymphoma.

Stage Prognostic group	1st line	2nd line	3rd line
Stage IA-IIA Good prognosis	SDT	SDT + α-interferon/ bexarotene	TSEB Trials
Stage III Intermediate prognosis	PUVA ECP/bexarotene/ α-interferon	TSEB Single-agent chemotherapy Antibody therapies	Trials RISCT
Stage IIB/IV* Poor prognosis	Radiotherapy (TSEB) Chemotherapy (single/multiagent)	Trials Toxin therapy RISCT	Palliation

SDT, skin directed therapy; RISCT, reduced intensity stem cell transplant; TSEB, total skin electron beam therapy; ECP, extracorporeal photopheresis.

* Maintenance therapy with SDT ± α interferon/bexarotene for residual skin disease (patches/plaques).

stage disease should receive skin directed therapies. Systemic therapies are reserved for those with either early stage disease resistant to skin directed therapy or advanced disease (Table 57.7) [2]. The precise role of a wide variety of novel therapeutic approaches remains to be established but these studies have helped to develop an emerging consensus about the optimal methods for assessment of disease response assessment [3–4].

References
1 Kaye FJ, Bunn PA Jr, Steinberg SM *et al.* A randomized trial comparing combination electron-beam radiation and chemotherapy with topical therapy in the initial treatment of mycosis fungoides. *N Engl J Med* 1989; **321**: 1784–90.
2 Trautinger F, Knobler R, Willemze R *et al.* EORTC consensus recommendations for the treatment of mycosis fungoides/Sezary syndrome. *Eur J Cancer* 2006; **42**: 1014–30.
3 Schmid M, Bird P, Dummer R *et al.* Tumour burden index as a prognostic tool for cutaneous T-cell lymphoma. *Arch Dermatol* 1999; **135**: 1204–8.
4 Stevens S, Ke M, Parry E *et al.* Quantifying skin disease burden in mycosis fungoides-type cutaneous T-cell lymphomas. *Arch Dermatol* 2002; **138**: 42–8.

Skin directed therapy

Topical steroids

For patients with limited early stage MF, life expectancy may not be adversely affected and it is acceptable to simply use emollients with or without moderate-potency topical steroids. Potent topical corticosteroids can produce a clinical response, although this is usually short-lived [1].

Reference
1 Zackheim H, Kashani-Sabet M, Amin S. Topical corticosteroids for mycosis fungoides. *Arch Dermatol* 1998; **134**: 949–54.

Topical chemotherapy—nitrogen mustard (mechlorethamine) and carmustine (BCNU)

Topical mechlorethamine (nitrogen mustard) 0.01% or 0.02%, either as an aqueous solution (normal saline) or ointment base (emulsifying ointment), is effective for superficial disease with response rates of 51–80% for IA, 26–68% for IB and 61% for IIA disease [1–5]. The aqueous solution is relatively unstable, and the ointment base—more commonly than the aqueous solution—can

cause irritancy or an allergic dermatitis in sensitized individuals (35–58%), but efficacy is similar. This product must not be used in pregnancy and there are rare reports of non-melanoma skin cancer in patients treated with topical mechlorethamine. There is no consensus as to whether mechlorethamine should be applied to individual lesions or to the whole skin, daily or twice weekly, or about the duration of topical therapy after a clinical remission has been produced; responses can be sustained for prolonged periods.

Topical BCNU is an alternative topical chemotherapeutic agent in MF, with similar efficacy to mechlorethamine as indicated by response rates of 86% in stage IA, 47% in stage IB and 55% in stage IIA patients [6]. Alternate day or daily treatment with 10 mg BCNU in 60 mL dilute alcohol (95%) or 20–40% BCNU ointment can be used. Hypersensitivity reactions occur less often (5–10%) than with mechlorethamine. All patients treated topically with carmustine should have regular monitoring of their full blood counts and treatment is normally given for only 2–4 weeks to avoid myelosuppression; maintenance therapy is contraindicated.

References
1 Van Scott EJ, Kalmanson JD. Complete remissions of mycosis fungoides lymphoma induced by topical nitrogen mustard (HN2): control of delayed hypersensitivity to HN2 by desensitization and by induction of specific immunologic tolerance. *Cancer* 1973; **32**: 18–30.
2 Hoppe R, Abel E, Deneau D, Price N. Mycosis fungoides: management with topical nitrogen mustard. *J Clin Oncol* 1987; **5**: 1796–803.
3 Ramsay DL, Halperin PS, Zeleniuch-Jacquotte A. Topical mechlorethamine therapy for early stage mycosis fungoides. *J Am Acad Dermatol* 1988; **19**: 684–91.
4 Vonderheid E, Tan E, Kantor AF *et al.* Long-term efficacy, curative potential and carcinogenicity of mechlorethamine chemotherapy in cutaneous T-cell lymphoma. *J Am Acad Dermatol* 1989; **20**: 416–28.
5 Kim Y, Martinez G, Varghese A *et al.* Topical nitrogen mustard in the management of mycosis fungoides: update of the Stanford experience. *Arch Dermatol* 2003; **139**: 165–73.
6 Zackheim HS, Epstein EH Jr, Crain WR. Topical carmustine (BCNU) for cutaneous T cell lymphoma: a 15 year experience in 143 patients. *J Am Acad Dermatol* 1990; **22**: 802–10.

Topical retinoids

Recently, a novel retinoid, 1% Targretin (bexarotene) gel, has been approved by the Food and Drug Administration (FDA) for topical therapy in stage I MF in patients who are resistant to, or intolerant of, other topical therapies [1]. In open uncontrolled studies, response rates of 63% with 21% complete response rates have been reported in 67 patients with early stage (IA–IIA) disease. Median time to and duration of response were 20 and 99 weeks, respectively.

Other topical therapies

There has only been one randomized placebo-controlled trial of topical therapy in MF. Topical peldesine cream (BCX-34, an inhibitor of the purine nucleoside phosphorylase enzyme) showed no benefit, compared to vehicle, with complete responses of 28% and 24%, respectively, emphasizing the difficulties in interpretation of uncontrolled studies of topical therapy in early stages of MF [2].

References

1 Breneman D, Duvic M, Kuzel T *et al.* Phase I and II trial of bexarotene gel for skin-directed treatment of patients with cutaneous T-cell lymphoma. *Arch Dermatol* 2002; **138**: 325–32.

2 Duvic M, Olsen E, Omura G *et al.* A phase III, randomized, double-blind, placebo-controlled study of peldesine (BCX-34) cream as topical therapy for cutaneous T-cell lymphoma. *J Am Acad Dermatol* 2001; **44**: 940–7.

Phototherapy and photochemotherapy

The clinical benefit of PUVA (photochemotherapy) was noted over 25 years ago and complete response rates of 79–88% in stage IA and 52–59% in stage IB disease have been reported [1–5]. Flexural sites ('sanctuary sites') often fail to respond completely and the duration of response varies. There is no significant response in tumour (IIB) stage disease. One study has shown that 56% of stage IA and 39% of stage IB complete PUVA responders had no recurrence of disease after 44 months follow-up without maintenance therapy [6]. A recent retrospective study on long-term outcome for MF patients treated with PUVA reported that 50% of patients with a higher cumulative UVA dose achieved a longer duration of response but these patients also received maintenance therapy while those who relapsed early did not [7]. Furthermore, there was no difference in clinical outcome in terms of disease progression or survival in the two groups. Maintenance therapy is rarely effective at preventing relapse and therefore should be avoided if possible so as to limit the total cumulative dose, as patients will often require repeated courses over many years.

PUVA is an ideal therapy for patients with stage IB–IIA disease who are intolerant of, or fail to respond to, topical therapies such as mechlorethamine, although both therapies can be complementary for some patients. Treatment regimens have varied in reported studies of PUVA in CTCL with two to four times weekly and different protocols for incremental dosage, but usually two to three times weekly treatment is acceptable until disease clearance or best partial response. Many patients will inevitably have a high total cumulative UVA dosage and the risks of non-melanoma and melanoma skin cancer are consequently increased for these patients. Efforts should be made to restrict the total PUVA dosage to less than 200 treatment sessions or a total cumulative dose of 1200 J/cm². In some circumstances patients may receive a greater total dosage if clinically justified and with the consent of the patient. PUVA remains one of the most effective therapies for patients with early stage disease but there are surprisingly no data to establish if PUVA can improve overall survival or reduce rates of disease progression in stage IB. PUVA therapy is rarely tolerated in erythrodermic (stage III) disease but occasional patients will respond repeatedly.

Broad- and narrow-band UVB and high-dose UVA-1 phototherapy have also been used in MF with success [8–10]. There have been no adequate comparative studies of different phototherapy regimens in CTCL but narrow-band UVB therapy may be an effective option in patients with patches as opposed to plaques.

References

1 Vella Briffa D, Warin AP. Photochemotherapy in mycosis fungoides: a study of 73 patients. *Lancet* 1980; **ii**: 49–53.

2 Molin L, Thomsen K, Volden G *et al.* Photochemotherapy (PUVA) in the pre-tumour stage of mycosis fungoides. *Acta Derm Venereol (Stockh)* 1980; **61**: 47–51.

3 Gilchrest BA, Parrish JA, Tannenbaum L *et al.* Oral methoxsalen photochemotherapy of mycosis fungoides. *Cancer* 1976; **38**: 683–9.

4 Abel EA, Sendagorta E, Hoppe RT *et al.* PUVA treatment of erythrodermic and plaque-type mycosis fungoides. *Arch Dermatol* 1987; **123**: 897–901.

5 Honigsmann Brenner W, Rauschmeier W, Konrad K, Wolff K. Photochemotherapy for cutaneous T cell lymphoma. *J Am Acad Dermatol* 1984; **10**: 238–45.

6 Hermann J, Roenigk H, Hurria A *et al.* Treatment of mycosis fungoides with photochemotherapy (PUVA): long-term follow-up. *J Am Acad Dermatol* 1995; **33**: 234–42.

7 Querfeld C, Rosen S, Kuzel T *et al.* Long term follow-up of patients with early stage cutaneous T-cell lymphoma who achieved complete remission with psoralen plus UV-A monotherapy. *Arch Dermatol* 2005; **141**: 305–11.

8 Ramsey D, Lish K, Yalowitz C, Soter N. Ultraviolet-B phototherapy for early stage cutaneous T-cell lymphoma. *Arch Dermatol* 1992; **128**: 931–3.

9 Clark C, Dawe R, Evans A *et al.* Narrow-band TL-01 phototherapy for patch stage mycosis fungoides. *Arch Dermatol* 2000; **136**: 748–52.

10 Zane C, Leali C, Airo P *et al.* 'High dose' UVA-1 therapy of widespread plaque-type, nodular and erythrodermic mycosis fungoides. *J Am Acad Dermatol* 2001; **44**: 629–33.

Radiotherapy and electron beam therapy

MF and other CTCL variants are very radiosensitive malignancies and individual thick plaques, or tumours can be treated successfully with low-dose superficial radiotherapy (orthovoltage or electrons) often administered in several fractions (e.g. two or three fractions of 400 cGy at 80–120 kV). Large tumours may require a different energy source. Radiotherapy is often used with other therapeutic modalities such as PUVA, and closely adjacent and overlapping fields can often be retreated because of the low doses used [1].

Whole body TSEB therapy has been evaluated extensively in CTCL [2,3]. Different field arrangements have been used in an attempt to treat the whole skin uniformly to a depth of 1 cm with various total dosage administered and additional radiotherapy to shielded areas. A meta-analysis of open uncontrolled and mostly retrospective studies of TSEB as monotherapy in 952 patients with CTCL has established that responses are stage dependent, with complete responses of 96% in stage IA, IB and IIA disease but disease relapse rates are very high, indicating that this approach is not curative even in early stage disease [4]. In stage IIB disease, complete responses are less common (36%), but erythrodermic (stage III) disease shows complete responses of 60%. Greater skin surface dose (32–36 Gy) and higher energy (4–6 MeV electrons) are associated with a higher rate of complete response and 5-year relapse-free survivals of 10–23% were noted [4]. A retrospective study of erythrodermic disease has also shown 60% complete responses with 26% progression-free at 5 years [5]. In this study, the overall median survival was 3.4 years with a median dose of 32 Gy given as five weekly fractions over 6–9 weeks. Patients with stage III disease did best compared to those with significant nodal or haematological (IVA–B) disease. The duration of response was also longer for those who received more than 20 Gy using 4–9 MeV [5].

Comparative studies of TSEB versus topical mechlorethamine in early stage MF show similar response rates and duration of response, suggesting that TSEB therapy should be reserved for those who fail first- and second-line therapies [6,7]. Adverse effects of TSEB include temporary alopecia, telangiectasia and skin malignancies, and the treatment is only available in a limited number of centres [8]. Although TSEB is usually only given once in a lifetime, several reports have documented patients who have received two or three courses, although the total dosage tolerated and duration of response have been lower with subsequent courses [9,10]. EORTC consensus guidelines have been produced for TSEB [11].

References

1 Cotter G, Baglan R, Wasserman T, Mill W. Palliative radiation treatment of cutaneous mycosis fungoides: a dose–response. *Int J Radiat Oncol Biol Phys* 1983; **9**: 1477–80.
2 Hoppe RT, Cox RS, Fuks ZY *et al.* Electron-beam therapy for mycosis fungoides: the Stanford University experience. *Cancer Treat Rep* 1979; **63**: 691–700.
3 Spittle MF. Electron beam therapy in England. *Cancer Treat Rep* 1979; **63**: 639–41.
4 Jones G, Hoppe R, Glatstein E. Electron beam treatment for cutaneous T-cell lymphoma. *Haematol Oncol Clin North Am* 1995; **9**: 1057–76.
5 Jones G, Rosenthal D, Wilson L. Total skin electron beam radiation for patients with erythrodermic cutaneous T-cell lymphoma (mycosis fungoides and the Sézary syndrome). *Cancer* 1999; **85**: 1985–95.
6 Hamminga B, Noordijk EM, van Vloten WA. Treatment of mycosis fungoides: total-skin electron-beam irradiation versus topical mechlorethamine therapy. *Arch Dermatol* 1982; **118**: 150–3.
7 Chinn D, Chow S, Kim Y, Hoppe R. Total skin electron beam therapy with or without adjuvant topical nitrogen mustard or nitrogen mustard alone as initial treatment of T2 and T3 mycosis fungoides. *Int J Rad Onc Biol Phys* 1999; **43**: 951–8.
8 Price NM. Radiation dermatitis following electron beam therapy: an evaluation of patients 10 years after total skin irradiation for mycosis fungoides. *Arch Dermatol* 1978; **114**: 63–6.
9 Becker M, Hoppe R, Knox S. Multiple courses of high dose total skin electron beam therapy in the management of mycosis fungoides. *Int J Radiat Oncol Biol Phys* 1995; **30**: 1445–9.
10 Wilson L, Quiros P, Kolenik S *et al.* Additional courses of total skin electron beam therapy in the treatment of patients with recurrent cutaneous T-cell lymphoma. *J Am Acad Dermatol* 1996; **35**: 69–73.
11 Jones G, Kacinski B, Wilson L *et al.* Total skin electron beam radiation in the management of mycosis fungoides: consensus of the European Organisation for Research and Treatment of Cancer (EORTC) Cutaneous Lymphoma Project Group. *J Am Acad Dermatol* 2002; **47**: 364–70.

Systemic therapy
Immunotherapy

Different forms of immunotherapy have been evaluated in CTCL, with the intention of enhancing antitumour host immune responses by promoting the generation of cytotoxic T cells and Th1 cytokine responses. Studies of IFN-α have shown overall response rates of 45–74%, with complete responses of 10–27% [1–3]. Various regimens have been employed (from 3 MU three times weekly to 36 MU/day) and it appears that response rates are higher for larger-dosage regimens (overall responses of 78% compared to 37% for the lower-dosage regimen) [2]. Overall response rates are also higher in early (IB–IIA 88%) compared to late (III–IV 63%) stages of disease [2].

Other small pilot studies have shown that both IL-12 and IFN-γ can produce clinical responses in CTCL but their therapeutic value remains to be established [4,5]. Ciclosporin has been used in CTCL, particularly in erythrodermic variants, to relieve severe pruritus but there is some evidence that treatment may actually cause rapid disease progression and its use in CTCL is not recommended [6].

References

1 Bunn P, Ihde D, Foon K. The role of recombinant interferon-α2a in the therapy of cutaneous T-cell lymphomas. *Cancer* 1986; **57**: 1689–95.
2 Olsen E, Rosen S, Vollmer R *et al.* Interferon-α2a in the treatment of cutaneous T-cell lymphoma. *J Am Acad Dermatol* 1989; **20**: 395–407.
3 Papa G, Tura S, Mandelli F *et al.* Is interferon-α in cutaneous T-cell lymphoma a treatment of choice? *Br J Haematol* 1991; **79**: 48–51.
4 Rook A, Wood G, Yoo E *et al.* Interleukin-12 therapy of cutaneous T-cell lymphoma induces lesion regression and cytotoxic T-cell responses. *Blood* 1999; **94**: 902–8.
5 Kaplan E, Rosen S, Norris D *et al.* Phase II study of recombinant interferon-γ for treatment of cutaneous T-cell lymphoma. *J Natl Cancer Inst* 1990; **82**: 208–12.
6 Cooper D, Braverman I, Sarris A *et al.* Cyclosporine treatment of refractory T-cell lymphomas. *Cancer* 1993; **71**: 2335–41.

Retinoids

Oral retinoid therapy has been used both as a single agent and in combination with interferons and PUVA in the management of MF (see below). A non-randomized, small study comparing acitretin and isotretinoin in MF and SS has shown no obvious differences, with complete responses of 21% in both groups [1].

Phase II and III studies of a novel synthetic retinoid in CTCL prompted licensing of this retinoid for MF/SS [2,3]. Bexarotene (Targretin) is the only retinoid that selectively binds and activates the RXR receptor. Bexarotene has been shown to promote apoptosis and inhibit cell proliferation. It is relatively selective and therefore should have little effect on the RAR receptor involved in cell differentiation. In phase II and III studies of 152 patients with CTCL, response rates from 20% to 67% have been reported [2,3]. The most effective tolerated oral dosage is 300 mg/m^2/day, although responses improve with higher dosage. Side effects are transient and generally mild but most patients while on therapy require treatment for hyperlipidaemia and central (hypothalamic) hypothyroidism according to an algorithm [4,5]. At a dosage of 300 mg/m^2/day in early stage disease (IA, IB, IIA), overall response rates of 54% have been noted [2], while advanced MF patients (stage IIB–IVB) have shown overall response rates of 45% with a notable reduction in pruritus in stage III disease [3].

References

1 Molin L, Thomsen K, Volden G *et al.* Oral retinoids in mycosis fungoides and Sézary syndrome: a comparison of isotretinoin and etretinate. *Acta Derm Venereol (Stockh)* 1987; **67**: 232–6.
2 Duvic M, Martin A, Kim Y *et al.* Phase 2 and 3 clinical trial of oral bexarotene (Targretin capsules) for the treatment of refractory or persistent early stage cutaneous T-cell lymphoma. *Arch Dermatol* 2001; **137**: 581–93.
3 Duvic M, Hymes K, Heald P *et al.* Bexarotene is effective and safe for treatment of refractory advanced-stage cutaneous T-cell lymphoma: multinational phase II–III trial results. *J Clin Oncol* 2001; **19**: 2456–71.
4 Gniadecki R, Assaf C, Bagot M *et al.* The optimal use of Bexarotene in cutaneous T-cell lymphoma. *Br J Dermatol* 2007; **157**: 433–40.
5 Assaf C, Bagot M, Dummer R *et al.* Minimizing adverse side-effects of oral bexarotene in cutaneous T-cell lymphoma: an expert opinion. *Br J Dermatol* 2006; **155**: 261–6.

Combination therapy

Combined IFN-α and retinoids produces similar response rates to IFN alone and is not recommended [1]. Studies comparing PUVA and IFN-α with IFN-α and acitretin in early stage disease have shown complete response rates of 70% and 38%, respectively, but there are no data on duration of response [2]. Uncontrolled studies of combined PUVA and IFN-α (maximum tolerated dosage 12 MU/m² three times weekly) in MF and SS have shown overall response rates of 100%, with 62% complete response rates [3]. This combination may also be useful in patients with resistant early stage disease, such as those with thick plaques and folliculotropic disease. Open studies comparing PUVA with combined PUVA and acitretin have shown a similar complete response rate (73 and 72%, respectively), although the cumulative dose to best response was lower in patients receiving the combination therapy [4]. Current randomized controlled studies are comparing: (i) PUVA versus PUVA and IFN-α in early stage MF; (ii) the role of maintenance IFN-α after induction of a complete response with PUVA and IFN; and (iii) PUVA alone compared to PUVA combined with bexarotene. At present there are few data on the impact on disease-free and overall survival.

References

1 Dreno B, Claudy A, Meynadier J *et al*. The treatment of 45 patients with cutaneous T-cell lymphoma with low doses of interferon-α2a and etretinate. *Br J Dermatol* 1991; **125**: 456–9.

2 Stadler R, Otte H, Luger T *et al*. Prospective randomized multicentre clinical trial on the use of interferon-α2a plus acitretin versus interferon-α2a plus PUVA in patients with cutaneous T-cell lymphoma stages I and II. *Blood* 1998; **10**: 3578–81.

3 Kuzel T, Roenigk H, Samuelson E *et al*. Effectiveness of interferon-α2a combined with phototherapy for mycosis fungoides and the Sézary syndrome. *J Clin Oncol* 1995; **13**: 257–63.

4 Thomson K, Hammar H, Holin L *et al*. Retinoids plus PUVA (RePUVA) and PUVA in mycosis fungoides, plaque stage: a report from the Scandinavian mycosis fungoides group. *Acta Derm Venereol (Stockh)* 1989; **69**: 536–8.

Systemic chemotherapy

MF and SS are relatively chemoresistant and responses are usually short lived [1]. This may partly reflect the low proliferative rate of tumour cells and a high prevalence of inactivating *p53* mutations, which produce a relative resistance to tumour cell apoptosis. A systematic review of published data on different regimens has shown complete response rates of 33% in 526 patients treated with single-agent chemotherapy with a median duration of 3–22 months [2]. Combination chemotherapy regimes (including cyclophosphamide, doxorubicin, vincristine, prednisolone (CHOP)) in 331 patients produced complete response rates of 38%, with a median duration of 5–41 months [2]. CTCL patients are prone to infection and septicaemia is a common preterminal event.

Chemotherapy should not be used in patients with early stage IA, IB or IIA disease. However, treatment of stage IIB and IVA disease remains problematic. Individual tumours and effaced peripheral lymph nodes will respond to superficial radiotherapy and additional chemotherapy should be considered in patients with a good performance status (WHO 0–2). However, responses are likely to be short-lived and patients should be entered into ongoing clinical trials. Single-agent chemotherapy that has been shown to produce a clinical response in stage IIB–IVB disease, and especially erythrodermic patients, includes oral chlorambucil (four to six cycles of 0.15–0.2 mg/kg/day for 2 weeks every 28 days), methotrexate and etoposide, and the intravenous use of the purine analogues 2-deoxycoformycin, 2-chlorodeoxyadenosine and fludarabine [2]. Open studies of 2-deoxycoformycin in MF and SS have reported response rates of 35–71%, with complete

response rates of 10–33% [3,4]. Methotrexate has been reported to produce a complete response rate of 41% in 29 patients with erythrodermic (stage III/T4) disease, with a median survival of 8.4 years with single weekly doses of 5–125 mg. However, this study was uncontrolled and it is unclear if the patients included represented an usually good prognostic group [5]. In contrast, liposomal doxorubicin [6,7] and gemcitabine [8,9] have shown excellent responses in stage IIB and IVA non-erythrodermic MF with overall responses of 88% (44% complete remission (CR)) and 70–85% (10–22% CR), respectively, but once again the duration of response is often short-lived with a median duration of response of 10 months for CR patients treated with gemcitabine [9]. In a further study, liposomal doxorubicin showed similar responses (56% overall response rate (ORR) with 20% CR) in both transformed MF and erythrodermic SS patients [10].

Recent pilot studies assessing the use of TSEB and/or total body irradiation (TBI) combined with high-dose conditioning chemotherapy prior to autologous stem cell transplantation in patients with stage IIB–IVA disease have shown good clinical responses [11,12] but high relapse rates and there are no data available at present to indicate if this approach affects disease-free or overall survival. Allogeneic stem cell or bone marrow transplantation has only been used in a few patients with encouraging results [13–15], but the associated mortality suggests that this approach is difficult to justify. However, reduced intensity allogeneic stem cell transplantation has shown promising results in small studies [16] with clear evidence of a graft-versus-lymphoma effect indicating that this may potentially have a durable effect for selected CTCL patients [17].

References

1 Kaye FJ, Bunn PA Jr, Steinberg SM *et al*. A randomized trial comparing combination electron-beam radiation and chemotherapy with topical therapy in the initial treatment of mycosis fungoides. *N Engl J Med* 1989; **321**: 1784–90.

2 Bunn P, Hoffman S, Norris D, Golitz L, Aeling J. Systemic therapy of cutaneous T-cell lymphomas (mycosis fungoides and the Sézary syndrome). *Ann Intern Med* 1994; **121**: 592–602.

3 Kurzrock R, Pilat S, Duvic M. Pentostatin therapy of T-cell lymphomas with cutaneous manifestations. *J Clin Oncol* 1999; **17**: 3117–21.

4 Deardon C, Matutes E, Catovsky D. Pentostatin treatment of cutaneous T-cell lymphoma. *Oncology* 2000; **14**: 37–40.

5 Zackheim H, Kashani Sabet M, Hwang ST. Low dose methotrexate to treat erythrodermic cutaneous T cell lymphoma. *J Am Acad Dermatol* 1996; **34**: 626–31.

6 Wollina U, Graefe T, Kaatz M. Pegylated doxorubicin for primary cutaneous T-cell lymphoma: a report on 10 patients with follow-up. *J Cancer Res Clin Oncol* 2001; **127**: 128–34.

7 Wollina U, Dummer R, Brockmayer N *et al*. Multicentre study of pegylated liposomal doxorubicin in patients with cutaneous T-cell lymphoma. *Cancer* 2003; **98**: 993–1001.

8 Zinzani P, Baliva G, Magagnoli M *et al*. Gemcitabine treatment in pretreated cutaneous T-cell lymphoma: experience in 44 patients. *J Clin Oncol* 2000; **18**: 2603–6.

9 Marchi E, Alinari L, Tani M *et al*. Gemcitabine as frontline treatment for cutaneous T-cell lymphoma. *Cancer* 2005; **104**: 2437–41.

10 Quereux G, Marques S, Nguyen J-M *et al*. Prospective multicenter study of pegylated liposomal doxorubicin treatment in patients with advanced or refractory mycosis fungoides or Sezary syndrome. *Arch Dermatol* 2008; **144**: 727–33.

11 Olavarria E, Child F, Woolford A *et al*. T-cell depletion and autologous stem cell transplantation in the management of tumour stage mycosis fungoides with peripheral blood involvement. *Br J Haematol* 2001; **114**: 624–31.

12 Bigler R, Crilley P, Micaily B *et al.* Autologous bone marrow transplantation for advanced stage mycosis fungoides. *Bone Marrow Tranplant* 1991; **7**: 133–7.

13 Burt R, Guitart J, Traynor A *et al.* Allogeneic haematopoietic stem cell transplantation for advanced mycosis fungoides: evidence of a graft-versus-tumour effect. *Bone Marrow Transplant* 2000; **25**: 111–3.

14 Molina A, Nademanee A, Arber D, Forman S. Remission of refractory Sézary syndrome after bone marrow transplantation from a matched unrelated donor. *Biol Blood Marrow Transplant* 1999; **5**: 400–4.

15 Guitart J, Wickless S, Oyama Y *et al.* Long term remission after allogeneic hematopoietic stem cell transplantation for refractory cutaneous T-cell lymphoma. *Arch Dermatol* 2002; **138**: 1359–65.

16 Molina A, Zain J, Arber D *et al.* Durable clinical, cytogenetic and molecular remissions after allogeneic hematopoietic cell transplantation for refractory Sezary syndrome and mycosis fungoides. *J Clin Oncol* 2005; **23**: 6163–71.

17 Duarte R, Schmitz N, Servitje O, Sureda A. Haematopoietic stem cell transplantation for patients with primary cutaneous T-cell lymphoma. *Bone Marrow Transplant* 2008; **41**: 597–604.

Photopheresis

Extracorporeal photopheresis (ECP) involves administration of oral psoralen, followed by *ex vivo* collection of an enriched buffy coat preparation using a cell separator. These leukocytes are then passed through thin polythene tubing with exposure to UVA and the cells thereafter returned to the patient. This regimen is repeated on 2 successive days and the 2-day cycle repeated monthly or fortnightly in an accelerated regimen. A specially designed photopheresis apparatus is required for this technique. The underlying theory is that a proportion of the UVA-exposed leukocytes, including some tumour lymphocytes, undergo apoptosis and that dendritic cells are activated during the *ex vivo* circulation with induction of a host antitumour immune response after the treated cells are returned to the patient. Different models of autoimmune disease support this suggestion [1,2] and recent evidence has also shown activation of dendritic cells during an expanded period of *ex vivo* incubation overnight (transimmunization) [3].

ECP is licensed by the FDA for the treatment of CTCL but there are no randomized studies to clarify whether ECP has an impact on overall survival. The original open study of ECP in 29 patients with erythrodermic CTCL reported a response rate of 73% but response rates in patients with earlier stages of MF were much lower (38%) [4]. Subsequently, a median survival of 62 months was reported in the original cohort of 29 erythrodermic patients, which compares favourably with historical controls (30 months) [5]. A study of 33 patients with SS treated with ECP reported a median survival of 39 months, which was similar to historical controls from the same institution [6]. Other studies have shown more prolonged median survival data [7]. An accelerated regimen consisting of nine collections rather than six for each cycle and an increase to treatment every 2 weeks has shown overall response rates of 50%, with 18% complete responses in erythrodermic disease [8]. A systematic review of response rates in erythrodermic disease (stage III–IVA) with ECP has shown overall responses of 35–71%, with complete responses of 14–26% [9]. Other studies are more difficult to interpret because they have either involved small numbers, patients with earlier stages of disease and in most studies many of the patients have been on other concurrent therapies [10,11]. Preliminary pilot studies suggest that the combination of IFN-α and ECP is more effective than ECP alone but this has yet to be confirmed in randomized studies [12,13]. There are isolated case reports of combined ECP and IFN-α and/or bexarotene that have induced complete clinical and molecular responses [14–16].

Randomized, controlled trials of ECP are required to establish an effect on disease-free and overall survival. There have been claims that the CD8 count is critical in predicting whether patients will respond to ECP [5], although others have provided evidence that the total baseline Sézary count is the only predictor of response [17].

References

1 Perez M, Edelson R, Laroche L, Berger C. Inhibition of anti-skin allograft immunity by infusion with syngeneic photoinactivated effector lymphocytes. *J Invest Dermatol* 1989; **92**: 669–76.

2 Berger C, Perez M, Laroche L, Edelson R. Inhibition of autoimmune disease in a murine model of systemic lupus erythematosus induced by exposure to syngeneic photoinactivated lymphocytes. *J Invest Dermatol* 1990; **94**: 52–7.

3 Berger C, Xu A, Hanlon D *et al.* Induction of tumour loaded dendritic cells. *Int J Cancer* 2001; **91**: 438–47.

4 Edelson R, Berger C, Gasparro F *et al.* Treatment of cutaneous T cell lymphoma by extracorporeal photochemotherapy. *N Engl J Med* 1987; **316**: 297–303.

5 Heald P, Rook A, Perez M *et al.* Treatment of erythrodermic cutaneous T cell lymphoma with extracorporeal photochemotherapy. *J Am Acad Dermatol* 1992; **27**: 427–33.

6 Fraser-Andrews E, Seed P, Whittaker S, Russell-Jones R. Extracorporeal photophoresis in Sézary syndrome: no significant effect in the survival of 44 patients with a peripheral blood T-cell clone. *Arch Dermatol* 1998; **134**: 1001–5.

7 Zic J, Stricklin G, Greer J *et al.* Long-term follow-up of patients with cutaneous T-cell lymphoma treated with extracorporeal photochemotherapy. *J Am Acad Dermatol* 1996; **35**: 935–45.

8 Duvic M, Hester J, Lemak N. Photophoresis therapy for cutaneous T-cell lymphoma. *J Am Acad Dermatol* 1996; **35**: 573–9.

9 Russell-Jones R. Extracorporeal photophoresis in cutaneous T-cell lymphoma: inconsistent data underline the need for randomized studies. *Br J Dermatol* 2000; **142**: 16–21.

10 Gottleib S, Wolfe J, Fox F *et al.* Treatment of cutaneous T-cell lymphoma with extracorporeal photophoresis monotherapy and in combination with recombinant interferon-α: a 10-year experience at a single institution. *J Am Acad Dermatol* 1996; **35**: 946–57.

11 Vonderheid E, Bigler R, Greenberg A, Neukum S, Micaily B. Extracorporeal photophoresis and recombinant interferon-α2b in Sézary syndrome. *Am J Clin Oncol* 1994; **17**: 255–63.

12 Wollina U, Looks A, Meyer J *et al.* Treatment of stage II cutaneous T-cell lymphoma with interferon-α2a and extracorporeal photochemotherapy: a prospective controlled trial. *J Am Acad Dermatol* 2001; **44**: 253–60.

13 Dippel E, Schrag H, Goerdt S, Orfanos C. Extracorporeal photophoresis and interferon-α in advanced cutaneous T-cell lymphoma. *Lancet* 1997; **350**: 32–3.

14 Haley H, Davis D, Sams M. Durable loss of a malignant T-cell clone in a stage IV cutaneous T-cell lymphoma patient treated with high-dose interferon and photophoresis. *J Am Acad Dermatol* 1999; **41**: 880–3.

15 Yoo E, Cassin M, Lessin S, Rook A. Complete molecular remission during biologic response modifier therapy for Sézary syndrome is associated with enhanced helper T type I cytokine production and natural killer cell activity. *J Am Acad Dermatol* 2001; **45**: 208–16.

16 Suchin K, Cucchiara A, Gottlieb S *et al.* Treatment of cutaneous T-cell lymphoma with combined immunomodulatory therapy. *Arch Dermatol* 2002; **138**: 1054–60.

17 Evans A, Wood B, Scarisbrick J *et al.* Extracorporeal photophoresis in Sézary syndrome: haematologic parameters as predictors of response. *Blood* 2001; **98**: 1298–301.

Toxin therapies

Denileukin diftitox, a DAB_{389}–IL-2 fusion toxin (Ontak USA/Onzar Europe), received provisional FDA approval for the treatment of resistant or recurrent CTCL after completion of open-label, phase I/II studies. Onzar is a recombinant fusion protein consisting of peptide sequences for the enzymatically active domain (389) of diphtheria toxin and the membrane translocation domain of IL-2 that is capable of inhibiting protein synthesis in tumour cells expressing high levels of the IL-2 receptor, resulting in cell death. Phase III studies of 71 heavily pre-treated patients with stage IB–IVA, and more than 20% CD25$^+$ T cells, showed an overall response rate of 30%, including 10% with complete responses [1]. Patients were assessed with a rigorous skin scoring system and documented responses were defined as lasting at least 6 weeks. The median duration of response was 6.9 months (range 2.7–46.1 months). The optimally tolerated intravenous regimen is 18 μg/kg/day for 5 days, repeated every 21 days for four to eight cycles. Adverse effects include fever, chills, myalgia, nausea and vomiting, and a mild increase in transaminase levels. Acute hypersensitivity reactions occurred in 60%, invariably within 24 h and during the initial infusion but this can be prevented with steroid pre-treatment [2]. A vascular leak syndrome characterized by hypotension, hypoalbuminaemia and oedema was defined retrospectively within the first 14 days of a given dose in 25% of patients. Myelosuppression is rare. Five per cent of adverse effects are severe or life-threatening. The clinical relevance of antibody responses to denileukin diftitox is unclear. The duration of clinical response has not yet been established and current studies are comparing different regimens of Onzar and are also assessing the use of this therapy in CD25$^-$ tumours. This therapy is not likely to be appropriate for early stage disease but may be useful in advanced disease.

References
1 Olsen E, Duvic M, Frankel A *et al.* Pivotal phase III trial of two dose levels of denileukin diftitox for the treatment of cutaneous T-cell lymphoma. *J Clin Oncol* 2001; **19**: 376–88.
2 Foss F, Bacha P, Osann K *et al.* Biological correlates of acute hypersensitivity events with DAB(389)IL-2 (denileukin diftitox, ONTAK) in cutaneous T-cell lymphoma: decreased frequency and severity with steroid premedication. *Clin Lymphoma* 2001; **1**: 298–302.

Monoclonal antibody therapy
The first antibody approach was a humanized chimeric anti-CD4 monoclonal antibody used to treat eight patients with CTCL, of whom seven showed a clinical response but this was of short duration [1]. A radiolabelled anti-CD5 antibody has also been used in MF with some objective results [2] and CAMPATH (anti-CD52/alemtuzumab) has also been studied in patients (stage III) with overall responses in 55–85% and a median response duration/time to treatment failure of 12 months [3,4]. Studies of a fully humanized anti-CD4 antibody (Zanolimumab) in bexarotene-refractory MF/SS have shown overall responses of 56% and median response duration of 81 weeks [5].

References
1 Knox S, Hoppe R, Maloney D *et al.* Treatment of cutaneous T-cell lymphoma with chimeric anti-CD4 monoclonal antibody. *Blood* 1996; **87**: 893–9.
2 Foss F, Raubitscheck A, Mulshine J *et al.* Phase I study of the pharmacokinetics of a radioimmunoconjugate, 90Y–T101, in patients with CD5-expressing leukaemia and lymphoma. *Clin Cancer Res* 1998; **4**: 2691–700.
3 Lundin J, Hagberg H, Repp R *et al.* Phase 2 study of alemtuzumab (anti-CD52 monoclonal antibody) in patients with advanced mycosis fungoides/Sezary syndrome. *Blood* 2003; **101**: 4267–72.
4 Bernengo M, Quaglino P, Comessantti A *et al.* Low-dose intermittent alemtuzumab in the treatment of Sezary syndrome: clinical and immunologic findings in 14 patients. *Haematologica* 2007; **92**: 784–94
5 Kim Y, Duvic M, Obitz E *et al.* Clinical efficacy of zanolimimab (HuMax-CD4): two phase 2 studies in refractory cutaneous T-cell lymphoma. *Blood* 2007; **109**: 4655–62.

Histone deacetylase inhibitors
A novel class of drugs has been assessed in both MF and SS in a series of open label studies. These histone deacetylase (HDAC) inhibitors affect gene expression by inhibiting deacetylation of histone proteins which causes the chromatin structure to adopt an open configuration therefore allowing binding of transcription factors to promoter regions and gene transcription. While the effect of these drugs on histone proteins within chromatin is best understood there are almost certainly widespread effects on non-histone proteins as well, which may be therapeutically important. There are four classes of HDAC inhibitors and several including SAHA and depsipeptide have been studied in both MF and SS [1–3]. Phase I/II studies of SAHA (vorinostat) have shown overall response rates of 30% with a median time to progression of 5 months [1,2]. This has prompted the US Food and Drug Administration to license vorinostat for second line-therapy of MF/SS. Side-effects include lethargy, thrombocytopenia. gastrointestinal symptoms and prolongation of the QT interval. Whether HDAC inhibitors are best used as maintenance therapy or in combination for advanced disease remains unclear but constitutive expression of STAT3 may indicate resistance to histone deacetylase inhibition in MF/SS [4].

References
1 Duvic M, Talpur R, Ni X *et al.* Phase 2 trial of oral vorinostat (suberoylanilide hydroxamic acid, SAHA) for refractory cutaneous T-cell lymphoma (CTCL). *Blood* 2007; **109**: 31–9.
2 Olsen E, Kim Y, Kuzel T *et al.* Phase IIB multicenter trial of vorinostat in patients with persistent, progressive or treatment refractory cutaneous T-cell lymphoma. *J Clin Oncol* 2007; **25**: 1–9.
3 Piekarz R, Fryer A, Wright J *et al.* Cardiac studies in patients treated with depsipeptide, FK228, in a phase II trial for T-cell lymphoma. *Clin Cancer Res* 2006; **12**: 3762–73.
4 Fantin V, Lobock A, Poweletz L *et al.* Constitutive activation of signal transducers of activation and transcription predicts vorinostat resistance in cutaneous T-cell lymphoma. *Cancer Res* 2008; **68**: 3785–94.

Other novel therapies
Several novel therapies currently being assessed in open phase II studies show promise of significant efficacy in both MF and SS [1] including the proteasome inhibitor, bortezomib (Velcade) [2] but whether additional studies will confirm this promise is currently unclear.

References
1 Whittaker S and Foss F. Efficacy and tolerability of currently available therapies for the mycosis fungoides and Sezary syndrome variants of cutaneous T-cell lymphoma variants. *Cancer Treat Rev* 2007; **33**: 146–60.
2 Zinzani P, Musuraca G, Tani M *et al.* Phase II trial of proteasome inhibitor bortezomib in patients with relapsed or refractory cutaneous T-cell lymphoma. *J Clin Oncol* 2007; **25**: 4293–7.

Primary cutaneous CD30⁺ lymphoproliferative disorders

Primary cutaneous CD30⁺ lymphoproliferative disorders consist of a spectrum of conditions; lymphomatoid papulosis and CD30⁺ anaplastic large cell lymphomas which are defined on the basis of clinical and pathologic features. Where a distinction cannot be made, patients are designated as 'borderline cases'. This group represents approximately 30% of all primary cutaneous lymphomas.

In the skin, CD30⁺ lymphoproliferative disorders are invariably of T-cell origin although nodal CD30⁺ lymphomas can be derived from B, T or null cells. By definition, primary cutaneous CD30⁺ disorders do not have any systemic or nodal involvement [1–3]. CD30 positivity was originally identified on Reed–Sternberg cells in Hodgkin's disease, but is expressed on a proportion of activated T and B lymphocytes. In general, cutaneous lymphomas that are CD30⁺ *ab initio* are associated with a good prognosis, in contrast to CD30⁺ lymphomas in other anatomical sites such as the lymph nodes where CD30 positivity is more commonly associated with a poor prognosis and is invariably associated with a disease-specific t(2;5)(p23;q35) translocation not found in primary cutaneous CD30⁺ lymphoproliferative disorders [4]. In MF, the situation in which tumour cells acquire CD30 expression, during the course of disease, is also generally associated with a poor prognosis [5].

Molecular studies show the presence of the Epstein–Barr genome in a proportion of CD30⁺ infiltrates in Hodgkin's disease, but this has not been found in patients with lymphomatoid papulosis [6]. CD30 is a cell-surface receptor for tumour necrosis factor-α like cytokines [7], and it has been demonstrated that CD30 expression can be up-regulated by EBV. The pathogenesis of primary cutaneous CD30⁺ lymphoproliferative disorders remains unknown but studies have suggested that there may be restriction of the normal T-cell repertoire in peripheral blood [8] and abnormalities of Notch signalling [9].

References

1 Leboit PE. Lymphomatoid papulosis and CD30⁺ lymphoma. *Am J Dermatopathol* 1996; **18**: 221–35.
2 Kadin ME. Primary Ki positive anaplastic large cell lymphoma. *Ann Oncol* 1994; **5** (Suppl. 1): 25–30.
3 Bekkenk MW, Geelen FAMJ, van Voorst Vader PC *et al*. Primary and secondary cutaneous CD30 positive lymphoproliferative disorders: a report from the Dutch Cutaneous Lymphoma Group. *Blood* 2000; **95**: 3653–61.
4 DeCoteau J, Butmarc J, Kinney M, Kadin M. The t(2;5) chromosomal translocation is not a common feature of primary cutaneous CD30⁺ lymphoproliferative disorders: comparison with anaplastic large cell lymphoma of nodal origin. *Blood* 1996; **87**: 3437–41.
5 Willemze R, Beljaards RC. The spectrum of primary cutaneous CD30⁺ lymphoproliferative disorders: a proposed classification, and guidelines for management and treatment. *J Am Acad Dermatol* 1993; **28**: 973–80.
6 Kadin ME, Vonderheid EC, Weiss LM. Absence of Epstein–Barr viral RNA in lymphomatoid papulosis. *J Pathol* 1993; **170**: 145–8.
7 Smith CA, Gruss HJ, Davis T. CD30 antigen a marker for Hodgkin's lymphoma is a receptor whose ligand defines an emerging family of cytokines with homology to TNF. *Cell* 1993; **73**: 1349–60.
8 Humme D, Lukowsky A, Steinhoff M *et al*. Dominance of nonmalignant T-cell clones and distortion of the TCR repertoire in the peripheral blood of patients with cutaneous CD30⁺ lymphoproliferative disorders. *J Invest Dermatol* 2009; **129**: 89–98.

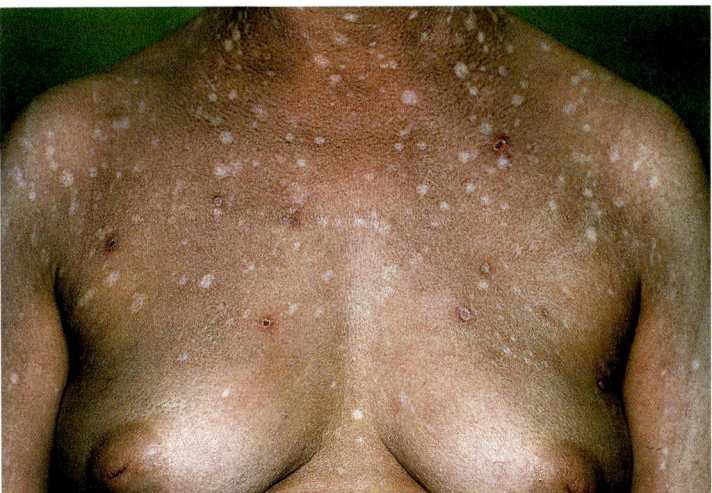

Fig. 57.22 Lymphomatoid papulosis. Note multiple scars on the upper chest area of this patient, with a small number of fresh papular lesions.

9 Kamstrup M, Ralfikiaer E, Skovgaard G, Gniadecki R. Potential involvement of Notch signalling in the pathogenesis of primary cutaneous CD30-positive lymphoproliferative disorders. *Br J Dermatol* 2008; **158**: 747–53.

Lymphomatoid papulosis

Definition. This term was first used in 1968 by Macaulay to describe a 'self-healing rhythmical paradoxical papular eruption, histologically malignant but clinically benign' [1–6]. It is a chronic recurrent self-healing papulonecrotic or papulonodular eruption with histological features of a CD30⁺ cutaneous lymphoma.

Clinical features. Affected patients have recurrent crops of papular or papulonecrotic or nodular lesions predominantly affecting the trunk, although any body site can be involved and regional localized patterns may occur (Fig. 57.22) [7]. These lesions grow rapidly over a few days and develop ulcerated necrotic centres. Healing occurs slowly over 3–12 weeks, with fine atrophic circular or varioliform scars, but the cycle recurs every few months, with no obvious initiating factor. The lesions generally occur first in adult life and may recur in crops for up to 40 years. Over time, every individual skin lesion will resolve and there may eventually be a persistent remission. A small number of cases have been reported in children [8,9].

The original description of lymphomatoid papulosis suggested a benign and non-progressive chronic pattern of the disease, but there are well-documented rare cases both of patients with lymphomatoid papulosis developing primary cutaneous or nodal CD30⁺ large cell anaplastic T-cell lymphoma or more commonly MF, and of patients with pre-existing MF developing lesions indistinguishable from those of lymphomatoid papulosis [10,11]. A follicular variant of the condition has also been described [12]. A proportion of patients have developed Hodgkin's disease, or develop lymphomatoid papulosis-like lesions with a preceding history of Hodgkin's disease [13–15].

Pathology. The histological features are a relative lack of epidermotropism and Pautrier abscesses, but the presence in the dermis

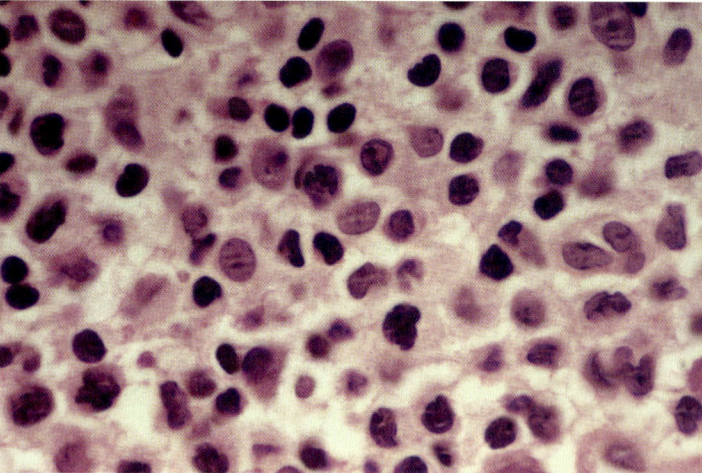

(a)

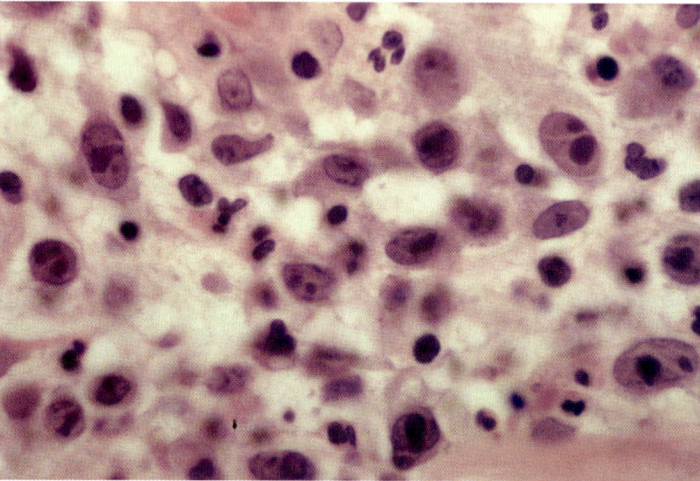

(b)

Fig. 57.23 Composite high-power view of atypical cerebriform cells in type B lymphomatoid papulosis (a) and large 'Reed–Sternberg-like' (CD30⁺) cells in type A histology (b).

of a mixed infiltrate composed of atypical lymphocytes with large nuclei and frequent abnormal mitoses, eosinophils, neutrophils, extravasated red cells and large histiocytic cells [16]. Some of these cells may show gross cytological atypia (Fig. 57.23). The epidermis may be ulcerated and the infiltrate may extend deeply into the reticular dermis. True vasculitis is rarely seen.

Lymphomatoid papulosis can be divided on histological grounds into types A, B and C subgroups [17]. In the A subgroup there appears to be a predominance of scattered large, strikingly atypical CD30⁺ cells similar to those seen in Hodgkin's disease [18]. In the B subgroup, smaller atypical T lymphocytes with convoluted nuclei similar to those seen in MF predominate and are CD3⁺ and CD4⁺ but CD30⁻. Rare cases of lymphomatoid papulosis are CD8⁺ [19]. Group C lesions have large clusters of CD30⁺ cells and an overall pattern suggestive of an anaplastic CD30⁺ large cell lymphoma. Many cases, however, have all types of lesions coexisting simultaneously or a mixed pattern of A and B. Some patients with clinical lesions resembling pityriasis lichenoides et variol's acuta (PLEVA) show a lymphomatoid histology and this probably represents a form of lymphomatoid papulosis (type B) [20,21].

Recent studies have shown that *MUM1*, a transcription factor expressed in myeloma and lymphomas with plasmacytoid differentiation as well as activated T-cells and Hodgkin's lymphoma, is expressed by the CD30⁺ cells in a majority of cases of lymphomatoid papulosis but only rarely in primary cutaneous CD30⁺ ALCL [22]. Furthermore *TRAF1*, expressed by activated T-cells and in Hodgkin's lymphoma, is also differentially expressed in PCCD30⁺ lymphoproliferative disorders, with expression restricted mostly to lymphomatoid papulosis as opposed to PCALCL [23]. The functional significance of differential *MUM1* and *TRAF1* expression in lymphomatoid papulosis remains to be confirmed.

Clonal TCR gene rearrangements can be identified and are identical in different lesions from the same patient, but some biopsies may not show a clonal pattern either because of an inability to detect a small clonal T-cell population as a result of a lack of sensitivity, or because of a non-T-cell lineage in type A lesions [4,24]. Identical T-cell clones can be detected in skin biopsies from patients with both MF and lymphomatoid papulosis [24]. Studies using laser captured CD30⁺ cells and sequencing of TCR genes have shown contradictory findings with one study suggesting that the large CD30⁺ cells show clonal TCR gene rearrangements while other studies have shown that these large CD30⁺ are polyclonal and that the monoclonal population resides in the smaller population of CD30⁻ cells [25,26]. The t(2;5) characteristic of nodal CD30⁺ lymphomas is not detected in lymphomatoid papulosis [27].

Treatment. There is no current treatment that alters the natural history of the disease but some therapies appear to accelerate healing and may reduce or prevent the frequency and severity of new crops of lesions for a short time. There is no evidence that intensive combination chemotherapy alters beneficially the course of lymphomatoid papulosis, and indeed there are individual case reports suggesting that high-dose intensive chemotherapy may cause transition to a more aggressive CD30⁺ lymphoproliferative disorder. Topical or intralesional steroids and topical nitrogen mustard applied to developing lesions may accelerate clearance, but have little effect on well-developed lesions. Narrow-band UVB therapy and PUVA both appear to benefit individual patients for short periods of time. Low-dose oral methotrexate appears to be the most useful systemic therapy, and there are reports of a beneficial effect with oral dapsone [28,29].

Long-term follow-up is necessary in all cases because of the risk of progression to a more aggressive lymphoma such as a primary cutaneous CD30⁺ anaplastic lymphoma, MF or Hodgkin's disease in less than 5% of cases. The prognosis in patients with both MF and lymphomatoid papulosis appears to be excellent [10]. There appear to be no currently available clinical or pathological prognostic markers to indicate whether such progression is likely.

An excellent recent review of 118 patients with lymphomatoid papulosis followed for many years suggests that approximately 4% will develop extracutaneous disease within 10 years [30].

References

1 Leboit P. Lymphomatoid papulosis and cutaneous CD30⁺ lymphoma. *Am J Dermatopathol* 1996; **18**: 221–35.
2 Thomsen K, Wantzin GL. Lymphomatoid papulosis: a follow-up study of 30 patients. *J Am Acad Dermatol* 1987; **17**: 632–6.

3 Weinman VF, Ackerman AB. Lymphomatoid papulosis: a critical review and new findings. *Am J Dermatopathol* 1981; **3**: 129–63.

4 Weiss LM, Wood GS, Trela M *et al.* Clonal T cell populations in lymphomatoid papulosis: evidence of a lymphoproliferative origin for a clinically benign disease. *N Engl J Med* 1986; **315**: 475–9.

5 Macaulay WL. Lymphomatoid papulosis. *Arch Dermatol* 1986; **97**: 23–30.

6 Macaulay WL. Lymphomatoid papulosis update: a historical perspective. *Arch Dermatol* 1989; **125**: 1387–9.

7 Scarisbrick J, Evans A, Woolford A *et al.* Regional lymphomatoid papulosis: a report of four cases. *Br J Dermatol* 1999; **141**: 1125–8.

8 Ashworth J, Paterson WD, MacKie RM. Lymphomatoid papulosis in two children. *Paediatr Dermatol* 1987; **4**: 238–41.

9 Zirbel GM, Gellis SE, Kadin ME, Esterly NB. Lymphomatoid papulosis in children. *J Am Acad Dermatol* 1995; **33**: 741–8.

10 Basarab T, Fraser-Andrews EA, Orchard G *et al.* Lymphomatoid papulosis in association with mycosis fungoides: a study of 15 cases. *Br J Dermatol* 1998; **139**: 630–8.

11 Kadin M. Lymphomatoid papulosis and associated lymphomas: how are they related? *Arch Dermatol* 1993; **129**: 351–2.

12 Pierard GE, Ackerman AB, Lapiere CM. Follicular lymphomatoid papulosis. *Am J Dermatopathol* 1980; **2**: 173–80.

13 Lederman JS, Sober AJ, Harrist TJ *et al.* Lymphomatoid papulosis following Hodgkin's disease. *J Am Acad Dermatol* 1987; **16**: 331–5.

14 Zackheim HS, Leboit P, Gordon BI, Glassberg A. Lymphomatoid papulosis followed by Hodgkin's lymphoma. *Arch Dermatol* 1993; **129**: 86–8.

15 Demierre MF, Goldberg LJ, Kadin ME *et al.* Is it lymphoma or lymphomatoid papulosis? *J Am Acad Dermatol* 1997; **36**: 765–72.

16 Kadin ME. Characteristic immunologic profile of large atypical cells in lymphomatoid papulosis. *Arch Dermatol* 1986; **122**: 1388–90.

17 Willemze R, Meijer CJLM, van Vloten WA, Scheffer E. The clinical and histological spectrum of lymphomatoid papulosis. *Br J Dermatol* 1982; **107**: 131–44.

18 Shabrawi-Caelen L, Kerl H, Cerroni L. Lymphomatoid papulosis. Reaapraisal of clinicopathologic presentation and classification into subtypes A, B and C. *Arch Dermatol* 2004; **140**; 441–7.

19 Magro C, Crowson A, Morrison C *et al.* CD8⁺ lymphomatoid papulosis and its differential diagnosis. *Am J Clin Pathol* 2006; **125**: 490–501.

20 Verallo VM, Haserick JR. Mucha–Habermann disease simulating lymphoma cutis: report of two cases. *Arch Dermatol* 1966; **94**: 295–9.

21 Black MM, Wilson-Jones E. 'Lymphomatoid' pityriasis lichenoides: a variant with histological features simulating a lymphoma—a clinical and histopathological study of 15 cases with details of long-term follow-up. *Br J Dermatol* 1972; **86**: 329–47.

22 Kempf W, Kutzner H, Cozzio A *et al.* MUM1 expression in cutaneous CD30⁺ lymphoproliferative disorders: a valuable tool for the distinction between lymphomatoid papulosis and primary cutaneous anaplastic large-cell lymphoma. *Br J Dermatol* 2008; **158**: 1280–7.

23 Assaf C, Hirsch B, Wagner F *et al.* Differential expression of TRAF1 aids in the distinction of cutaneous CD30-positive lymphoproliferations. *J Invest Dermatol* 2007; **127**: 1898–904.

24 Whittaker S, Smith N, Jones RR, Luzzatto L. Analysis of β, γ, and δ T-cell receptor genes in lymphomatoid papulosis: cellular basis of two distinct histologic subsets. *J Invest Dermatol* 1991; **96**: 786–91.

25 Steinhof M, Hummel M, Anagnostopoulos I *et al.* Single cell analysis of CD30⁺ cells in lymphomatoid papulosis demonstrates a common clonal T-cell origin. *Blood* 2002; **100**: 578–84.

26 Gellrich S, Wernicke M, Wilks A *et al.* The cell infiltrate in lymphomatoid papulosis comprises a mixture of polyclonal large atypical cells (CD30-positive) and smaller monoclonal T cells (CD30-negative). *J Invest Dermatol* 2004; **12**: 859–61.

27 DeCoteau J, Butmarc J, Kinney M, Kadin M. The t(2;5) chromosomal translocation is not a common feature of primary cutaneous CD30⁺ lymphoproliferative disorders: comparison with anaplastic large cell lymphoma of nodal origin. *Blood* 1996; **87**: 3437–41.

28 Vonderheid EC, Sajjadian A, Kadin M. Methotrexate is effective therapy for lymphomatoid papulosis and other primary cutaneous CD30-positive lymphoproliferative disorders. *J Am Acad Dermatol* 1996; **34**: 470–81.

29 Wantzin GL, Thomsen K. Methotrexate in lymphomatoid papulosis. *Br J Dermatol* 1984; **111**: 93–5.

30 Bekkenk MW, Geelen FAMJ, van Voorst Vader PC *et al.* Primary and secondary cutaneous CD30-positive lymphoproliferative disorders. *Blood* 2000; **95**: 3653–61.

Primary cutaneous (anaplastic) CD30⁺ large cell lymphoma

Definition. A primary cutaneous CD30⁺ anaplastic (or rarely pleomorphic or blastic) large cell lymphoma in which the CD30⁺ tumour cells comprise the majority of the infiltrate. Clinical features of mycosis fungoides are absent.

Clinical features. These lymphomas are usually seen in adults and present as large solitary or multiple and often ulcerated nodules, most often on the trunk (Fig. 57.24) [1]. There are no patches or plaques of MF elsewhere, and some individual lesions may regress spontaneously. Some individuals develop disease localized to a limb. Progression to extracutaneous sites is rare but has been recorded in approximately 10% [1,2] and recent evidence suggests that patients with extensive regional disease may be at risk of disease progression [3,4]. Careful staging consisting of bone marrow and CT scans are required to exclude systemic CD30⁺ anaplastic large T-cell proliferation in which there is secondary cutaneous involvement. Disease-related 5-year survival rates of 90% have been reported but as low as 50% for generalized tumours [1,3–5].

Flynn *et al.* described patients with large ulcerative nodules, often on the thighs and buttocks, which show variable rates of spontaneous resolution and were labelled as 'regressing atypical histiocytosis' [6]. These 'borderline cases' are now considered to be closely related to both lymphomatoid papulosis and primary cutaneous CD30⁺ large cell lymphoma with the detection of a T-cell phenotype and clonal rearrangements of the TCR gene confirming a T-cell origin [2,7,8].

A rare variant has been described in which there are palpable and pathologically involved regional lymph nodes at presenta-

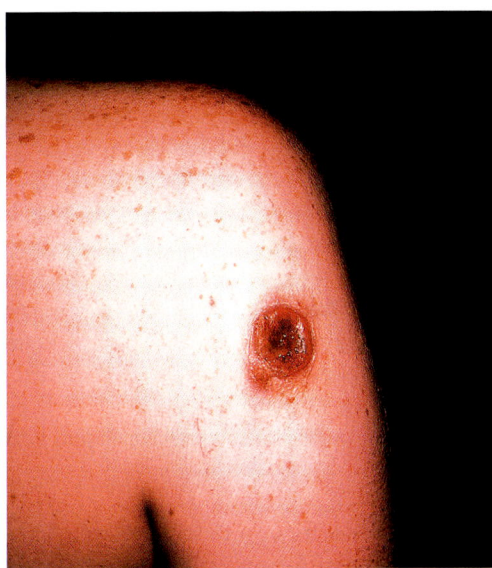

Fig. 57.24 CD30⁺ cutaneous lymphoma showing typical ulcerated lesion on shoulder.

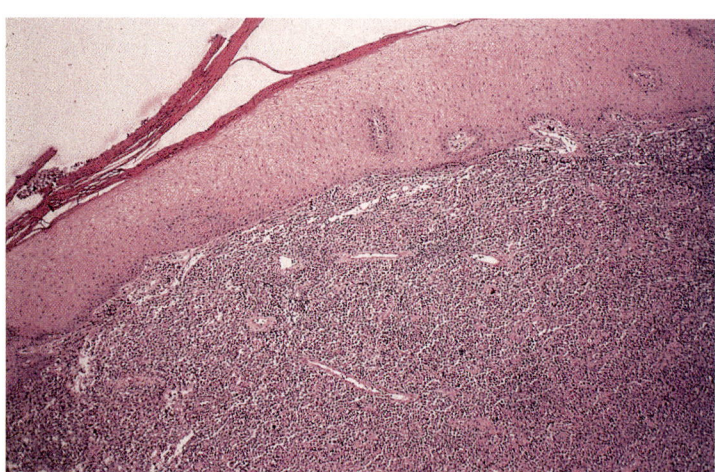

Fig. 57.25 Low-power view of CD30⁺ infiltrate showing lack of epidermotropism but dense infiltrate in the underlying dermis.

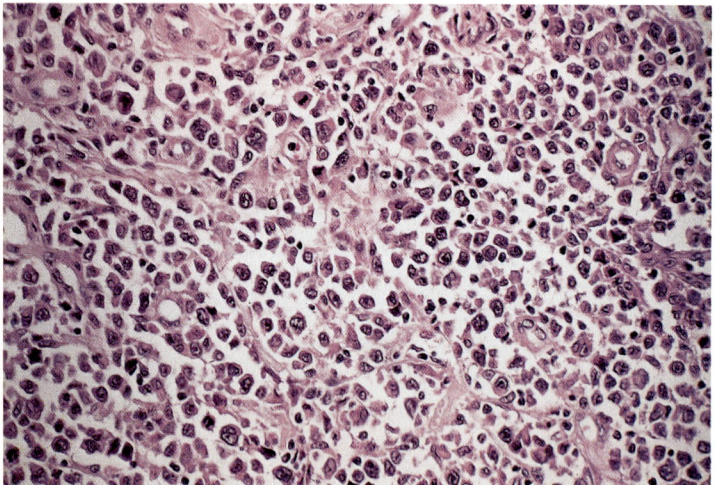

Fig. 57.26 CD30⁺ lymphocytic infiltrate showing striking large atypical cells.

tion, but no evidence of lymphoma beyond the regional nodal basin [1]. The limited evidence to date on treatment and prognosis suggests that this lymphoma is similar, if not identical, to primary cutaneous CD30⁺ anaplastic large cell lymphomas.

Pathology. Biopsy shows a dense lymphocytic infiltrate consisting of sheets of large atypical cells with an anaplastic morphology and mitoses, but usually there is no epidermotropism as seen in MF (Figs 57.25 & 57.26). The tumour cells variably express T-cell antigens and the vast majority will be CD30⁺. Some tumour cells show a pleomorphic or blast-like morphology [1,2,9,10]. Pseudo-epitheliomatous hyperplasia may occur. Clonal TCR gene rearrangements are detected in almost all cases consistent with a T-cell origin [11].

Immunophenotype. The tumour cells are generally CD4⁺ and by definition CD30⁺ with expression of cytotoxic proteins [9,10]. There is variable loss of other T-cell antigens such as CD2, CD5 and CD3. Some cases are CD8⁺. Tumour cells are EMA and CD15.

ALK is not expressed, in contrast to those systemic CD30⁺ lymphomas with secondary cutaneous involvement, but CD56 may be rarely expressed. The t(2;5) is absent [12]. While the morphology and phenotype are similar in lymphomatoid papulosis [13], the key distinguishing feature is the presence of cohesive nodules and sheets of anaplastic cells in PCALCL. Recent studies also suggest that in PCALCL the tumour cells generally do not express *MUM1* and *TRAF1* in contrast to lymphomatoid papulosis [14,15].

Pathogenesis. Primary cutaneous CD30⁺ ALCL express CCR3 and Th2 cytokines [16] as well as CCR4 as in MF/SS. There is no evidence for the t(2;5) chromosomal translocation seen in a high proportion of nodal CD30⁺ anaplastic lymphomas (NPM-ALK) [12], but molecular studies in PCCD30⁺ALCL have shown allelic loss at 9p21-22, although the frequency of p16 loss/inactivation has yet to be determined [17]. Array CGH studies have also shown chromosomal imbalances with gains of chromosomes 1p and 5 and amplification of several different oncogenes as well as *JUNB*, a member of the AP1 transcription family [18]. Recent studies have also shown over-expression of AP1 proteins in Pc CD30⁺ ALCL which might explain the characteristic Th2 cytokine profile [19].

Treatment. Both excision and localized radiotherapy are acceptable methods of treating isolated lesions [20]. The recurrence rate on the treated site is very low, but over time new lesions may develop elsewhere on the skin. Spontaneous clearance of even quite large lesions is recorded, and therefore a short period of observation after the diagnosis is made is also acceptable. Systemic chemotherapy, including CHOP, may be effective but cutaneous recurrence is likely, and chemotherapy is therefore not the treatment of choice for disease confined to the skin. Low-dose methotrexate may also be effective. Rare variants with regional nodal disease have been successfully treated with radiotherapy and do not always require systemic chemotherapy.

References

1 Bekkenk MW, Geelen FAMJ, van Voorst Vader PC *et al.* Primary and secondary cutaneous CD30-positive lymphoproliferative disorders. *Blood* 2000; **95**: 3653–61.

2 Beljaards RC, Kaudewitz P, Berti E *et al.* Primary cutaneous CD30-positive large cell lymphoma: definition of a new type of cutaneous lymphoma with a favourable prognosis. *Cancer* 1993; **71**: 2097–3002.

3 Liu H, Hoppe R, Kohler S *et al.* CD30⁺ cutaneous lymphoproliferative disorders: The Stanford experience in lymphomatoid papulosis and primary cutaneous anaplastic large cell lymphoma. *J Am Acad Dermatol* 2003; **49**: 1049–58.

4 Shehan J, Kalaaji A, Markovic S, Ahmed I. Management of multifocal primary cutaneous CD30⁺ anaplastic large cell lymphoma. *J Am Acad Dermatol* 2004; **51**: 103–10.

5 Yu J, Blitzblau R, Decker R *et al.* Analysis of primary CD30⁺ cutaneous lymphoproliferative disease and survival from the surveillance, epidemiology and end results database. *J Clin Oncol* 2008; **26**: 1438–88.

6 Flynn KJ, Dehner LP, Gajl-Peczalka K *et al.* Regressing atypical histiocytosis. *Cancer* 1982; **49**: 959–70.

7 Bernier M, Bagot M, Broyer M *et al.* Distinctive clinicopathological features associated with regressive primary CD30-positive cutaneous lymphomas: analysis of six cases. *J Cutan Pathol* 1997; **24**: 157–63.

8 Headington JT, Roth MS, Ginsburg D *et al.* T-cell receptor gene rearrangement in regressing atypical histiocytosis. *Arch Dermatol* 1987; **123**: 1183–7.

9 Beljaards RC, Meier CJ, Scheffer E *et al.* Prognostic significance of CD30 expression in primary cutaneous large cell lymphomas of T cell origin. *Am J Pathol* 1989; **44**: 119–24.

10 Krishnan J, Tomaszewski MM, Kao GF. Primary cutaneous anaplastic large cell lymphoma: report of 27 cases. *J Cutan Pathol* 1993; **20**: 193–6.

11 Greisser J, Palmedo G, Sander C *et al.* Detection of clonal rearrangement of T-cell receptor genes in the diagnosis of primary cutaneous CD30⁺ lymphoproliferative disorders. *J Cutan Pathol* 2006; **33**: 711–5.

12 DeCoteau J, Butmarc J, Kinney M, Kadin M. The t(2;5) chromosomal translocation is not a common feature of primary cutaneous CD30⁺ lymphoproliferative disorders: comparison with anaplastic large cell lymphoma of nodal origin. *Blood* 1996; **87**: 3437–41.

13 Tomaszewski MM, Lupton G, Krishnan J, May DI. A comparison of clinical morphological and immunohistochemical features of lymphomatoid papulosis and primary cutaneous CD30-positive anaplastic large cell lymphoma. *J Cutan Pathol* 1995; **22**: 310–5.

14 Kempf W, Kutzner H, Cozzio A *et al.* MUM1 expression in cutaneous CD30⁺ lymphoproliferative disorders: a valuable tool for the distinction between lymphomatoid papulosis and primary cutaneous anaplastic large-cell lymphoma. *Br J Dermatol* 2008; **158**: 1280–7.

15 Assaf C, Hirsch B, Wagner F *et al.* Differential expression of TRAF1 aids in the distinction of cutaneous CD30-positive lymphoproliferations. *J Invest Dermatol* 2007; **127**: 1898–904.

16 Kleinhans M, Tun-kyi A, Gilliet M *et al.* Functional expression of the eotaxin receptor CCR3 in CD30⁺ cutaneous T-cell lymphoma. *Blood* 2003; **101**: 1487–93.

17 Boni R, Xin H, Kamarashev J *et al.* Allelic deletion at 9p21-22 in primary cutaneous CD30⁺ large cell lymphoma. *J Invest Dermatol* 2000; **115**; 1104–7.

18 Mao X, Orchard G, Lillington D *et al.* Genetic alterations in primary cutaneous CD30⁺ anaplastic large cell lymphoma. *Genes Chrom Cancer* 2003; **37**: 176–85.

19 Mao X, Orchard G, Russell-Jones R, Whittaker S. Abnormal activator 1 protein expression in primary cutaneous CD30 positive large cell lymphomas. *Br J Dermatol* 2007; **157**: 914–21.

20 Yu J, McNiff J, Lund M, Wilson L. Treatment of primary cutaneous CD30⁺ anaplastic large cell lymphoma with radiation therapy. *Int J Radiat Oncol Biol Phys* 2008; **70**: 1542–5.

Subcutaneous panniculitis-like T-cell lymphoma (SPTL)

Definition. This is a rare cytotoxic T-cell lymphoma, representing less than 1% of all non-Hodgkin's lymphomas, which usually affects younger adults with an equal sex incidence [1,2]. Two subsets have been defined consisting of those cases derived from an αβ T cell which have an indolent course and those derived from a γδ T cell [3]. The term SPTL is now restricted to those lymphomas derived from an αβ T cell [1].

Clinical features. Patients present with indolent, slowly expanding, subcutaneous nodules usually involving the limbs, which may initially be misdiagnosed as panniculitis (Fig. 57.27) [4–6]. Occasionally, patients present with more diffuse erythematous induration mimicking a cellulitis. Ulceration is rare. Lymphadenopathy is usually absent at presentation. There is often a prolonged indolent phase before the diagnosis is established [7]. Cases must be carefully distinguished from lupus panniculitis as both conditions share similar clinical and pathological features [8,9]. Systemic symptoms may occur, particularly in those patients who develop a haemophagocytic syndrome consisting of fever, pancytopenia and hepatosplenomegaly although this is more common in those with a γδ T-cell lymphoma [10,11]. The prognosis is reasonable with a 5-year survival of 80%, and dissemination

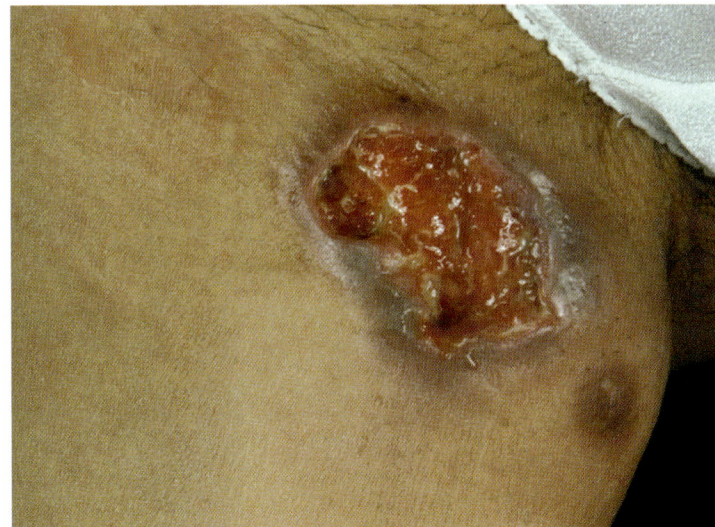

Fig. 57.27 Subcutaneous panniculitis-like T-cell lymphoma: indurated and eroded deep plaque on the thigh.

to extracutaneous sites is rare in contrast to primary cutaneous γδ T-cell lymphomas which has a poor prognosis [1].

Pathology. There is a diffuse infiltrate restricted to and extending throughout the subcutis without epidermotropism [1,3,5,11]. In contrast, primary cutaneous γδ T-cell lymphomas may show prominent involvement of the subcutis which is indistinguishable but there is invariably associated dermal and/or epidermal involvement [1]. The degree of cellular atypia can be minimal but medium-sized and occasionally large pleomorphic cells are usually present (Fig. 57.28). Rimming of the tumour cells around fat cells is a characteristic feature, although not restricted to SPTL [12]. A prominent reactive inflammatory infiltrate is common and the tumour cells may show vascular invasion with angiocentricity. Necrosis and erythrolymphophagocytosis may be present. Indolent cases were previously diagnosed as benign cytophagic histiocytosis (Weber–Christian disease) [13,14].

Immunophenotype. Tumour cells have a mature T-cell phenotype and are usually βF1⁺ CD3⁺ CD8⁺ CD4⁻ [1,3,9]. CD30 and CD56 are generally negative. They express cytotoxic molecules including granzyme B, perforin and TIA-I [15]. Clonal rearrangements of the TCR genes are present [3,16].

Pathogenesis. There is no evidence for an association with EBV, and the underlying molecular pathogenesis remains to be established but recent studies have characterized a specific pattern of chromosomal abnormalities using CGH, LOH and FISH techniques, which have shown losses of 10q, 17p and 19 similar to MF/SS, with additional 5q and 13q gains, which appear to be distinct from findings in MF/SS [17].

Treatment. Patients with αβ subcutaneous panniculitis–like T-cell lymphoma can be treated successfully with systemic steroids and there are reports of responses to ciclosporin [1,18]. Superficial radiotherapy can be used for individual lesions. Denileukin

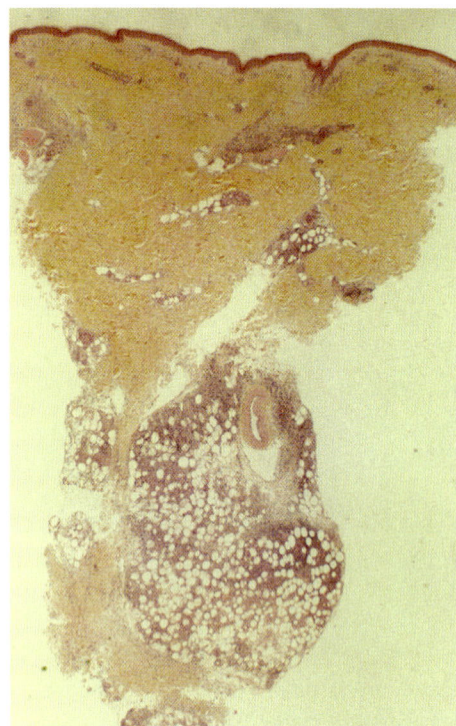

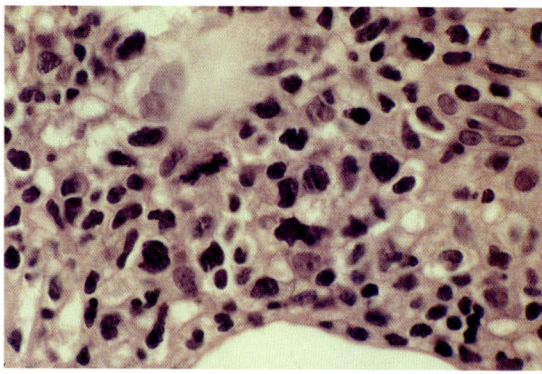

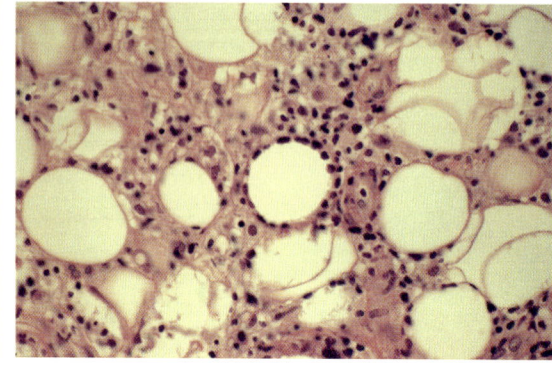

Fig. 57.28 Low-power view of subcutaneous infiltrate with high-power view showing rimming of fat cells by atypical mononuclear cells and medium/large pleomorphic tumour cells seen in subcutaneous panniculitis-like T-cell lymphoma.

diftitox has been used successfully in SPTL [19]. Combination chemotherapy can be associated with successful clinical responses and resolution of haemophagocytic syndrome, although this is usually restricted to those with extracutaneous disease [1]. High-dose therapy and autologous/allogeneic stem cell transplantation has been successful in patients with refractory disease [20,21].

References

1 Willemze R, Jansen P, Cerroni L *et al*. Subcutaneous panniculitis-like T-cell lymphoma: definition, classification and prognostic factors: an EORTC cutanoeus lymphoma group study of 83 cases. *Blood* 2008; **111**; 838–45.

2 Shabrawi-Caelen L, Cerrono L, Kerl H. The clinicopathologic spectrum of cytotoxic lymphomas of the skin. *Semin Cutan Med Surg* 2000; **19**: 118–23.

3 Salhany K, Macon W, Choi J *et al*. Subcutaneous panniculitis-like T-cell lymphoma: clinicopathologic, immunophenotypic and genotypic analysis of α/β and γ/δ subtypes. *Am J Surg Pathol* 1998; **22**: 881–93.

4 Aronson IK, West DP, Variakojis D. Panniculitis associated with cutaneous T-cell lymphoma and cytophagic histiocytosis. *Br J Dermatol* 1985; **112**: 87–96.

5 Mehregan D, Su WDP, Kurtin P. Subcutaneous T-cell lymphoma. *J Cutan Pathol* 1994; **21**: 110–7.

6 Monterrosso V, Bujan W, Jaramillo O, Medeiros J. Subcutaneous tissue involvement by T-cell lymphoma. *Arch Dermatol* 1996; **132**: 1345–50.

7 Perniciaro C, Zalla MJ, White JW. Subcutaneous T-cell lymphoma. *Arch Dermatol* 1993; **129**: 1171–6.

8 Gonzalez E, Selvi E, Lorenzini S *et al*. Subcutaneous panniculitis-like T-cell lymphoma misdiagnosed as lupus erythematosus panniculitis. *Clin Rheumatol* 2007; **26**: 244–6.

9 Massone C, Kodama K, Salmhofer W *et al*. Lupus erythematosus panniculitis (lupus profundus): clinical, histopathological and molecular analysis of nine cases. *J Cutan Pathol* 2005; **32**: 396–404.

10 Romero LS, Goltz RW, Bagi C *et al*. Subcutaneous T-cell lymphoma with associated haemophagocytic syndrome and terminal leukemic transformation. *J Am Acad Dermatol* 1996; **34**: 904–10.

11 Gonzalez C, Medeiros L, Brazieln R, Jaffe E. T-cell lymphoma involving subcutaneous tissue: a clinicopathologic entity commonly associated with haemophagocytic syndrome. *Am J Surg Pathol* 1991; **15**: 17–27.

12 Lozzi G, Massone C, Citarella L *et al*. Rimming of adipocytes by neoplastic lymphocytes: a histopathologic feature not restricted to subcutaneous T-cell lymphoma. *Am J Dermatopathol* 2006; **28**: 9–12.

13 Winkelmann R, Bowie E. Haemophagic diathesis associated with benign histiocytic, cytophagic panniculitis and systemic histiocytosis. *Arch Dermatol* 1980; **140**: 1460–3.

14 Perniciaro C, Winkelmann R, Herhardt D. Fatal systemic cytophagic histiocytic panniculitis: a histopathologic and immunohistochemical study of multiple organ sites. *J Am Acad Dermatol* 1994; **31**: 901–5.

15 Kumar S, Krenacs L, Medeiros J *et al*. Subcutaneous panniculitic T-cell lymphoma is a tumour of cytotoxic T-lymphocytes. *Hum Pathol* 1998; **29**: 397–403.

16 Hoque S, Child F, Whittaker S *et al*. Subcutaneous panniculitis-like T-cell lymphoma: a clinicopathological, immunophenotypic and molecular analysis of six patients. *Br J Dermatol* 2003; **148**: 516–25.

17 Hahtola S, Burghart E, Jeskanen L *et al*. Clinicopathological characterisation and genomic aberrations in subcutaneous panniculitis-like T-cell lymphoma. *J Invest Dermatol* 2008; **128**: 2304–9.

18 Rojnuckarin P, Nakoprn T, Assanasen T *et al*. Cyclosporin in subcutaneous panniculitis-like T-cell lymphoma. *Leuk Lymphoma* 2007; **48**: 560–3.

19 Hathaway T, Subtil A, Kuo P, Foss F. Efficacy of denileukin diftitox in subcutaneous panniculitis-like T-cell lymphoma. *Clin Lymphoma Myeloma* 2007; **7**: 541–5.

20 Alaibac M, Berti E, Pigozzi B *et al*. High-dose chemotherapy with autologous blood stem cell transplantation for aggressive subcutaneous panniculitis-like T-cell lymphoma. *J Am Acad Dermatol* 2005; **52**: S121–3.

21 Ichii M, Hatanaka K, Imakita M *et al*. Successful treatment of refractory subcutaneous panniculitis-like T-cell lymphoma with allogeneic peripheral blood stem cell transplantation from HLA-mismatched sibling donor. *Leuk Lymphoma* 2006; **47**: 2250–2.

Primary cutaneous peripheral T-cell lymphoma (unspecified)

Definition. These lymphomas represent a heterogeneous group of T-cell malignancies which are not defined by any of the recognized clinicopathologic subsets. In all cases mycosis funogides must be carefully excluded especially on the basis of the clinical features. Several subtypes (listed below) are currently considered as provisional entities based on characteristic clinical, pathologic and immunophenotypic features [1]. For patients who do not fulfil the characteristic features of these provisional entities, the designation of peripheral T-cell lymphoma (not otherwise specified (NOS)) should be used and the prognosis is generally poor with a high probability of systemic involvement. Full staging investigations are required for all patients to exclude a systemic nodal/extranodal peripheral T-cell lymphoma.

Primary cutaneous aggressive epidermotropic CD8⁺ T-cell lymphoma (provisional)

Definition. A primary cutaneous CD8⁺ T-cell lymphoma that expresses cytotoxic proteins and shows a prominent epidermotropic infiltrate [1,2]. Although there are currently few reports of this entity, the distinctive pathological and immunophenotypic features and poor prognosis suggest that it represents a distinct subtype of CTCL [1–3].

Clinical features. These patients rapidly develop generalized papules, plaques, nodules and/or tumours (Fig. 57.29a) which may show ulceration and necrosis [1,2]. Mucosal involvement may occur. The characteristic clinical features and distribution of MF, namely polymorphic patches and plaques and involvement of the limb girdle areas, are absent. Primary cutaneous CD30⁺ lymphoproliferative disorders with a CD8⁺ phenotype should also be distinguished. The prognosis is very poor, with a 5-year survival of 18% [1].

Pathology. These lymphomas show a prominent epidermotropic band-like infiltrate (pagetoid) with nodular infiltrates of large or small- to medium-sized pleomorphic or blastic T cells often accompanied by haemorrhage in the upper dermis (Fig. 57.29b). Angiocentricity and invasion can be a feature. These cutaneous lymphomas must be distinguished from MF and primary cutaneous γδ T-cell lymphomas [1,4]. An indolent CD8⁺ cutaneous lymphoma characterized by solitary nodular lesions, often around the ear, has been suggested to be a distinct entity but appears to be very rare [5], and its relationship to epidermotropic CD8⁺ T-cell lymphoma is unclear.

Immunophenotype. The tumour cells are CD8⁺ and usually βF1⁺ CD45RA⁺ and CD3⁺ [1–3]. The tumour cells also express cytotoxic proteins such as T-cell intracellular antigen-I (TIA-I), granzyme B and perforin. CD4, CD45RO, CD56 and CD30 are negative. Epstein–Barr virus (EBV) is not detected, in contrast to nasal-type natural killer (NK)/T-cell lymphomas [1,4].

Pathogenesis. This CTCL subset may previously have represented disseminated pagetoid reticuloses (Ketron–Goodman). Clonal TCR gene rearrangements are detected but the pathogenesis has not been established. Although the number of cases reported is small, these cases can be distinguished from peripheral

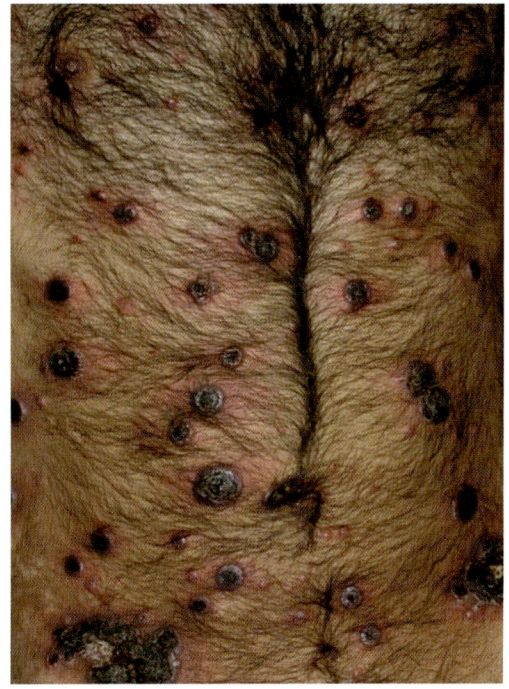

(a)

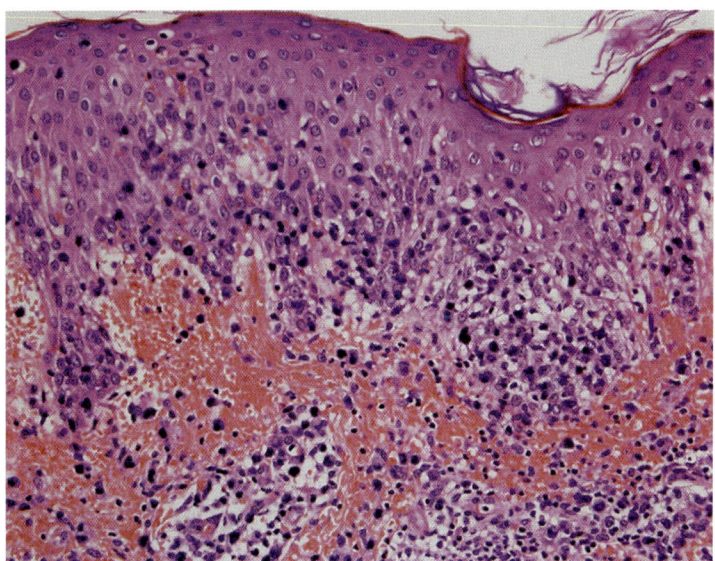

(b)

Fig. 57.29 (a) Primary cutaneous aggressive epidermotropic CD8⁺ cutaneous T-cell lymphoma showing necrotic haemorraghic plaques and (b) an epidermotropic infiltrate of large pleomorphic lymphoid cells and marked papillary dermal haemorrhage.

T-cell lymphomas derived from γδ T-cells (βF1 negative) which show clonal rearrangements of the γ TCR gene with the β TCR gene in a germline configuration [1,6].

Treatment. These patients have a very poor prognosis and dissemination to visceral sites such as CNS, testis and lung is more common than to nodal sites. Responses to radiotherapy and chemotherapy are limited and the treatment of choice may be a reduced intensity allograft procedure.

References

1 Willemze R, Jaffe E, Burg G *et al.* WHO-EORTC classification for cutaneous lymphomas. *Blood* 2005; **105**: 3768–85.

2 Berti E, Tomasini D, Vermeer M *et al.* Primary cutaneous CD8-positive epidermotropic cytotoxic T-cell lymphomas: a distinct clinicopathological entity with an aggressive clinical behaviour. *Am J Pathol* 1999; **155**: 483–92.

3 Agnarsson B, Vonderheid E, Kadin M. Cutaneous T-cell lymphoma with suppressor/cytotoxic (CD8) phenotype: identification of rapidly progressive and chronic subtypes. *J Am Acad Dermatol* 1990; **22**: 569–77.

4 Santucci M, Pimpinelli N, Massi D *et al.* Cytotoxic/natural killer cell cutaneous lymphomas. *Cancer* 2003; **97**: 610–27.

5 Petrella T, Maubec E, Cornillet-Lefebvre P *et al.* Indolent CD8-positive lymphoid proliferation of the ear: a distinct primary cutaneous T-cell lymphoma? *Am J Surg Pathol* 2007; **31**: 1887–92.

6 Munn SE, McGregor JM, Jones A *et al.* Clinical and pathological heterogeneity in cutaneous γδ T-cell lymphoma: a report of three cases and a review of the literature. *Br J Dermatol* 1996; **135**: 976–81.

Primary cutaneous γδ T-cell lymphomas (provisional entity)

Definition. A T-cell lymphoma consisting of γδ T-cells with a cytotoxic phenotype which may present primarily with skin involvement. A subgroup of patients with subcutaneous panniculitis-like T-cell lymphoma derived from γδ T-cells are included in this category [1–3].

Clinical features. The characteristic presentation is the sudden appearance of multiple cutaneous plaques, nodules or tumours which may be ulcerated and with no preceding polymorphic plaques or patches of typical MF. The clinical presentation may be similar to primary cutaneous CD8$^+$ aggressive epidermotropic lymphomas but some patients present with only subcutaneous involvement. Mucosal involvement and extranodal involvement is common. Some cases of disseminated pagetoid reticulosis (Ketron–Goodman) may have represented cutaneous γδ T-cell lymphomas [4]. A haemophagocytic syndrome may complicate some cases. The prognosis is very poor [1–3].

Pathology. Prominent nodular or diffuse infiltrates are characteristic with medium to large pleomorphic or blast like T cells. Epidermotropism may occur but the infiltrate is often extensive with dermal and subcutaneous patterns. Angiocentricity and rimming of fat cells may occur [1].

Immunophenotype. The tumour cells are usually CD2$^+$ CD3$^+$ CD5$^-$CD7$^{+/-}$ and CD56$^+$ but are CD4$^-$CD8$^-$ and βF1$^-$. EBV is negative and clonal TCR gene rearrangements are usually present.

Pathogenesis. This variant must be distinguished from transformed MF, ATLL, primary cutaneous aggressive epidermotropic cytotoxic CD8$^+$ CTCL and blastic NK-cell or extranodal NK/T-cell lymphomas (nasal type).

Treatment. Superficial radiotherapy and multiagent chemotherapy are usually required but the overall prognosis is very poor and reduced intensity allografts may be appropriate.

References

1 Willemze R, Beljaards RC, Meier CJLM. Classification of primary cutaneous T-cell lymphomas. *Histopathology* 1994; **24**: 405–15.

2 Willemze R, Jaffe E, Burg G *et al.* WHO-EORTC classification for cutaneous lymphomas. *Blood* 2005; **105**: 3768–85.

3 Toro J, Liewehr D, Pabby N *et al.* Gamma-delta T-cell phenotype is associated with significantly decreased survival in cutaneous T-cell lymphoma. *Blood* 2003; **101**: 3407–12.

4 Berti E, Cerri A, Cavicchini S *et al.* Primary cutaneous gamma/delta lymphoma presenting as disseminated pagetoid reticulosis. *J Invest Dermatol* 1991; **96**: 718–23.

Primary cutaneous CD4$^+$ small/medium sized pleomorphic T-cell lymphoma

Definition. This subtype of CTCL must be distinguished clinically from MF and is characterized by small to medium sized pleomorphic tumour cells which are CD4$^+$ [1].

Clinical features. Patients present with solitary or a few small plaques, nodules or tumours, often on the upper trunk or head and neck, without typical patches or plaques of MF. Patients are HTLV-1 negative. The estimated 5-year survival is 62–80%, but this is only based on small series [1–4]. Systemic involvement is very unusual.

Pathology. There are dense nodular or diffuse infiltrates of small to medium-sized pleomorphic T cells within the dermis, often extending into the subcutis [1–3]. Occasional larger pleomorphic cells may be present but are a minority. Epidermotropism may be present.

Immunophenotype. The tumour cells are usually CD4$^+$ and CD3$^+$ but loss of some T-cell antigens is common [1–3]. CD30 and CD8 are negative and cytotoxic proteins are not expressed. Clonal TCR gene rearrangements are present [5].

Pathogenesis. Currently, little is known about the underlying aetiology and pathogenesis of this rare group of primary cutaneous lymphomas. Cases must be distinguished from MF and pseudo T-cell lymphomas and also peripheral T-cell lymphoma (NOS) in order to avoid inappropriately aggressive therapy.

Treatment. In view of the excellent prognosis, superficial radiotherapy is appropriate for solitary lesions. Single-agent chemotherapy and IFN-α have been reported to be effective [3,4].

References

1 Willemze R, Jaffe E, Burg G *et al.* WHO-EORTC classification for cutaneous lymphomas. *Blood* 2005; **105**: 3768–85.

2 Friedmann D, Wechsler J, Delfau MH *et al.* Primary cutaneous pleomorphic small T-cell lymphoma. *Arch Dermatol* 1995; **131**: 1009–15.

3 Sterry W, Siebel A, Mielke V. HTLV-1 negative pleomorphic T-cell lymphoma of the skin. *Br J Dermatol* 1992; **126**: 456–62.

4 Garcia-Nerrera A, Colmo L, Camos M *et al.* Primary cutaneous small/medium CD4$^+$ T-cell lymphomas: a heterogenous group of tumours with different clinico-pathologic features and outcome. *J Clin Oncol* 2008; **26**: 3364–71.

5 Grogg K, Jung S, Erickson L *et al.* Primary cutaneous CD4-positive small/medium-sized pleomorphic T-cell lymphoma: a clonal T-cell lymphoproliferative disorder with indolent behaviour. *Mod Pathol* 2008; **21**: 708–15.

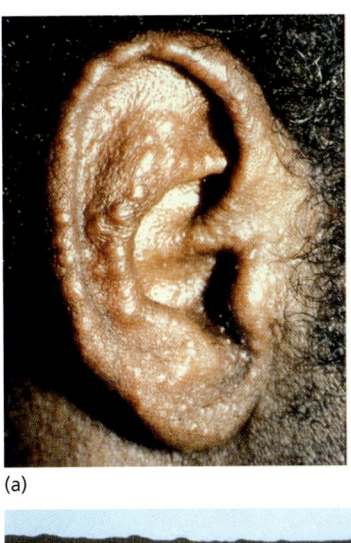

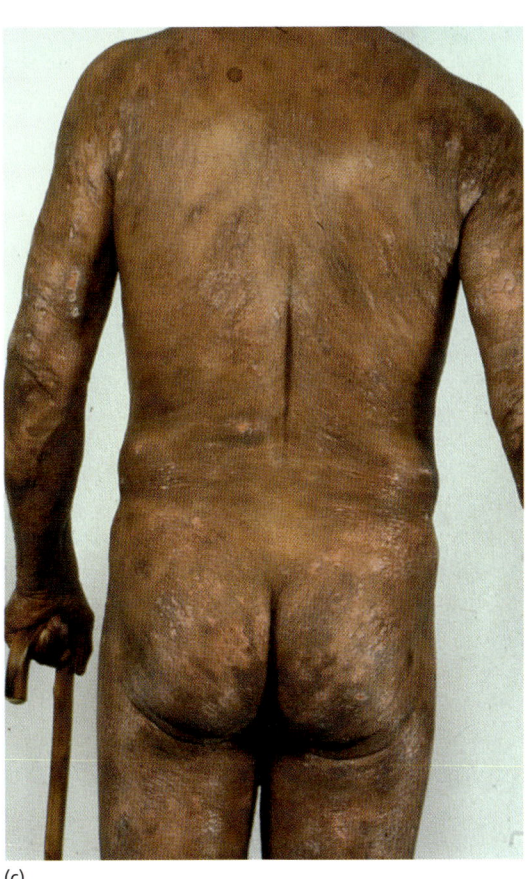

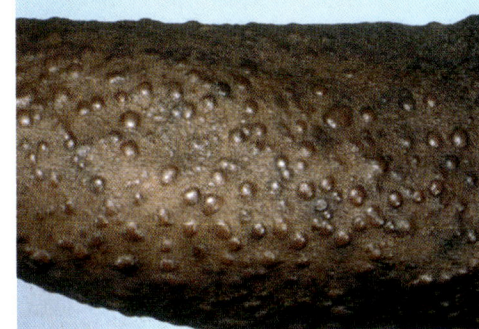

Fig. 57.30 Three clinical presentations of cutaneous adult T-cell leukaemia–lymphoma: (a) a pruritic papular eruption confined to the auricle, (b) an extensive nodular eruption on the forearm, and (c) superficial patches and plaques involving the limb girdle area similar to mycosis fungoides.

Adult T-cell leukaemia–lymphoma (HTLV-1-associated)

Definition. Adult T-cell leukaemia–lymphoma (ATLL) is a peripheral T-cell leukaemia–lymphoma caused by the human retrovirus HTLV-1. HTLV-1 infection is prevalent in certain parts of the world, including Japan, central Africa, the Caribbean and southeastern states of the USA, and consequently ATLL is endemic in these regions. Sporadic cases are found throughout the world. The disease has a long latency and the incidence of ATLL among HTLV-1 carriers has been estimated to be 2.5% [1]. The virus can be transmitted in breast milk and in blood products. There is a slight male predominance and the median age of onset is 55 years [1].

Clinical features. Patients with ATLL often have extensive lymph node and peripheral blood involvement but the skin is the most common extranodal site of disease (50% of patients) and primary cutaneous disease can occur [2,3]. Other extranodal sites of disease include bone, lung, liver, gastrointestinal tract and CNS. Cutaneous involvement is characterized by widespread or solitary papules, nodules, tumours or erythroderma, often associated with intense pruritus (Fig. 57.30) [4,5]. Patients may present with patches and plaques that are clinically indistinguishable from MF [6]. Several clinical variants have been defined [7]: an acute variant is characterized by a leukaemic phase with generalized lymphadenopathy and hepatosplenomegaly often associated with cutane-

ous involvement and hypercalcaemia with lytic bone lesions. Opportunistic infections are common because of a relative T-cell immunodeficiency. A lymphomatous variant is similar but with the absence of peripheral blood involvement. A chronic variant is typically characterized by cutaneous disease and a peripheral blood lymphocytosis without hypercalcaemia. The smouldering variant is also characterized by prominent cutaneous disease without overt peripheral blood involvement. Pulmonary lesions may occur. Progression from the chronic and smouldering variants to acute disease occurs in at least 25% of cases but often only after a long duration [6]. HTLV-1 serology is invariably positive [7]. Patients with cutaneous ATLL have shown marked photosensitivity mimicking actinic reticuloid [8,9].

Pathology. In the skin, a prominent epidermotropic infiltrate consisting of medium to large cells with a pleomorphic nuclear morphology is usually found, particularly in the acute and lymphomatous variants (Fig. 57.31) [3–7]. Blast-like cells may be present. Pautrier-like microabscesses and a cerebriform nuclear morphology can be seen, simulating MF. However, the degree of cellular atypia may also be mild, causing diagnostic difficulties. Eosinophilia is often present. Granulomatous features have been rarely described [6]. In the peripheral blood, the tumour cells have polylobulated nuclei ('flower cells'). Lymph nodes usually show a leukaemic pattern of infiltration, with preservation and dilatation of lymph node sinuses containing tumour cells. Rarely, Hodgkin-like features are present within an expanded lymph

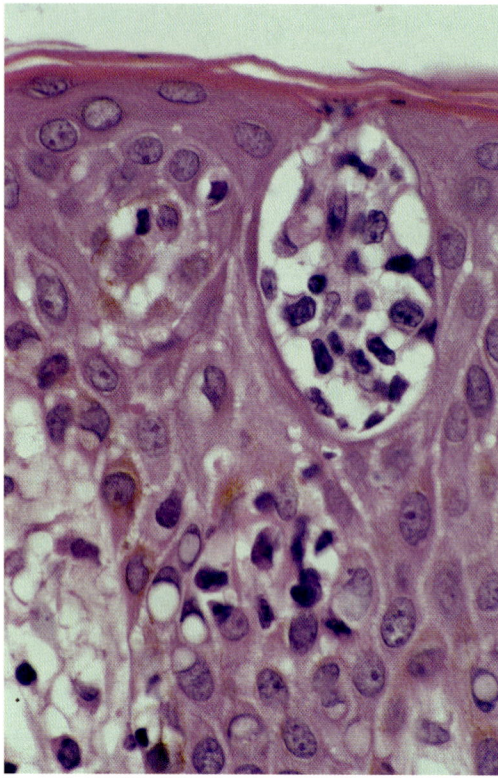
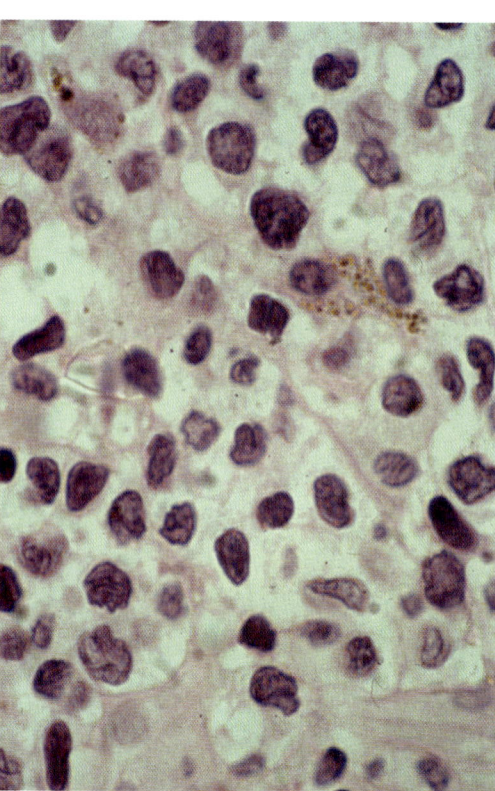

Fig. 57.31 Adult T-cell leukaemia–lymphoma: prominent atypical cells forming a Pautrier microabscess and large pleomorphic cells within the dermis.

node paracortex containing a diffuse infiltrate of small, mildly atypical lymphocytes and scattered CD30+, CD15+ Reed–Sternberg-like EBV-positive cells resulting from expansion of EBV-positive cells as a consequence of a relative T-cell immunodeficiency [10].

Immunophenotype. Tumour cells are CD2+, CD3+, CD5+ and CD7−. Most cells are CD4+, although CD8+ and CD4−, CD8− variants also occur [11]. CD25 expression is almost universal. Large blast-like cells can be CD30+ but are ALK−. Cytotoxic proteins are not expressed. Analysis of TCR genes shows clonal TCR gene rearrangements.

Pathogenesis. HTLV-1 is the underlying cause of ATLL. The virus is randomly integrated into the host genome following expression of viral reverse transcriptase, and the viral tax protein is a potent transactivation factor that induces expression of numerous host genes with additional molecular abnormalities producing a malignant phenotype [12]. The HTLV-1 proviral DNA is clonally integrated, confirming a pathogenetic role for the virus in individual cases [11]. Tumour burden can be assessed by monitoring viral RNA expression levels [13].

Treatment. Cutaneous disease can respond to skin-directed therapy but patients with the acute and lymphomatous variants have a poor prognosis (less than 10% 5-year survival) and require combination chemotherapy. In contrast, patients with the chronic (30% 5-year survival) and smouldering (65% 5-year survival) variants can have a prolonged course, although disease transformation eventually occurs for most patients [7]. Combination azathioprine and IFN therapy is a standard of care for those with chronic and smouldering variants of ATLL [14,15], and trials of antibody therapies have suggested promise for daclizumab (anti-CD25) [16]. Younger patients may be candidates for stem cell transplantation and reduced intensity allograft procedures have been shown to induce a graft-versus-lymphoma effect [17].

References

1 Yamaguchi K. Human T-lymphotropic virus type 1 in Japan. *Lancet* 1994; **343**: 213–6.

2 Bunn P, Schechter G, Jaffe E *et al*. Clinical course of retrovirus-associated adult T-cell lymphoma in the United States. *N Engl J Med* 1983; **309**: 257–64.

3 Yamaguchi T, Ohshima K, Karube K *et al*. Clinicopathological features of cutaneous lesions of adult T-cell leukaemia/lymphoma. *Br J Dermatol* 2005; **152**: 76–81.

4 Lessin SR, Vowels BR, Rook AH. Retroviruses and cutaneous lymphoma. *Dermatol Clin* 1994; **12**: 243–53.

5 Dicaudo DJ, Perniciaro C, Worrell JT *et al*. Clinical and histologic spectrum of human T-cell lymphotropic virus type 1-associated lymphoma involving the skin. *J Am Acad Dermatol* 1996; **34**: 69–76.

6 Whittaker S, Ng Y, Rustin M *et al*. HTLV-1 associated cutaneous disease: a clinicopathological and molecular study of patients from the UK. *Br J Dermatol* 1993; **128**: 483–92.

7 Shimoyama M. Diagnostic criteria and classification of clinical subtypes of adult T-cell leukaemia–lymphoma: a report from the Lymphoma Study Group (1984–87). *Br J Haematol* 1991; **79**: 428–37.

8 Ohshima K, Suzumiya J, Kato A *et al*. Clonal HTLV-1 infected CD4+ T-lymphocytes and non-clonal non-HTLV-1-infected giant cells in incipient ATLL with Hodgkin-like histologic features. *Int J Cancer* 1997; **72**: 592–8.

9 Adachi Y, Horio T. Chronic actinic dermatitis in a patient with adult T-cell leukemia. *Photodermatol Photoimmunol Photomed* 2008; **24**: 147–9.

10 Agar N, Morris S, Russell Jones R *et al*. Case report of four patients with erythrodermic cutaneous T-cell lymphoma and severe photosensitivity mimicking chronic actinic dermatitis. *Br J Dermatol* 2009; **160**: 698–703.

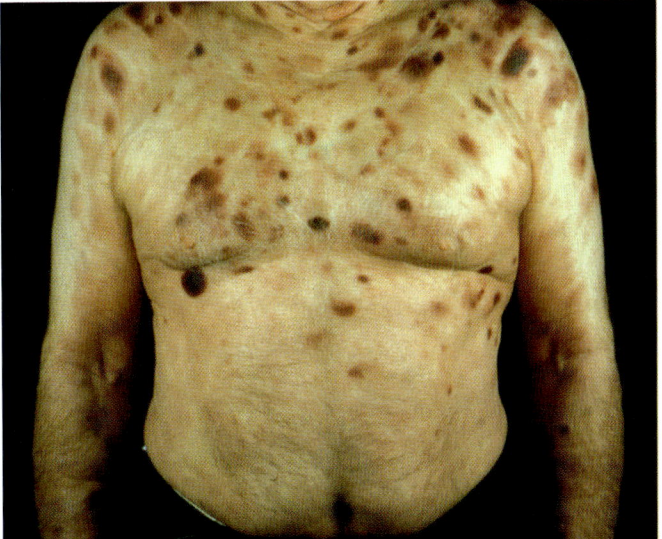 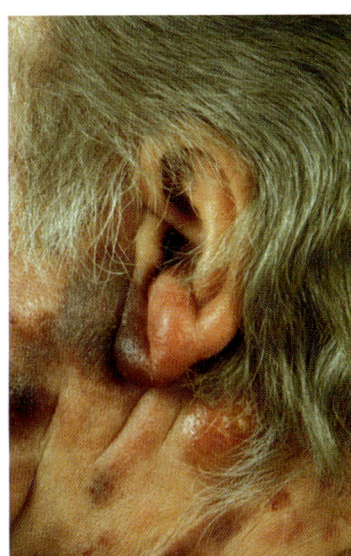

Fig. 57.32 Typical clinical presentations of blastic lymphoma in the skin with large mauvish and pigmented dermal plaques involving the head/neck and trunk.

11 Ohshima K, Suzumiya J, Sato K *et al*. Nodal T-cell lymphoma in an HTLV-1 endemic area: proviral HTLV-1 DNA, histological classification and clinical evaluation. *Br J Haematol* 1998; **101**: 444–50.

12 Taylor G. Molecular aspects of HTLV-1 infection and adult T-cell leukaemia/lymphoma. *J Clin Pathol* 2007; **60**: 1392–6.

13 Amano M, Kurokawa M, Ogata K, Itoh H *et al*. New entity, definition and diagnostic criteria of cutaneous adult T-cell leukaemia/lymphoma: human T-lymphotropic virus type 1 proviral DNA load can distinguish between cutaneous and smouldering types. *J Dermatol* 2008; **35**: 270–5.

14 Ishitsuka K, Tamura K. Treatment of adult T-cell leukemia/lymphoma: past, present and future. *Eur J Haematol* 2008; **80**: 185–96.

15 Bazarbachi A, Lepelletier Y, Nasr R *et al*. New therapeutic approaches for adult T-cell leukaemia. *Lancet Oncol* 2004; **5**: 664–72.

16 Waldmann T. Daclizumab (anti-Tac, zenapax) in the treatment of leukemia/lymphoma. *Oncogene* 2007; **28**: 3699–703.

17 Shiratori S, Yasumoto A, Tanaka J *et al*. A retrospective anyalsis of allogeneic hematopoietic stem cell transplantation for adult T cell leukemia/lymphoma (ATL): clinical impact of graft-versus-leukemia/lymphoma effect. *Biol Blood Marrow Transplant* 2008; **14**: 817–23.

CD4+/CD56+ haematodermic neoplasm (blastic NK-cell lymphoma)

Definition. This is a rare haematologic neoplasm, which is now thought to be derived from plasmacytoid dendritic cells and shows a predilection for extranodal sites, particularly the skin, and a tendency to leukaemic dissemination [1]. Previously, this tumour was erroneously thought to be derived from NK-cells because of CD56 expression. There is no racial predisposition. Elderly male patients are mostly affected and the prognosis is poor.

Clinical features. Patients usually present with multiple and rarely solitary, large, dusky mauve dermal tumours, which can become ulcerated (Fig. 57.32). There is no specific site predilection but the upper trunk is often affected. Primary cutaneous disease is common but lymphadenopathy and peripheral blood/bone marrow involvement is likely during the course of disease [2–5]. This neoplasm must be differentiated from myelomonocytic leukaemia and is closely related to 'aleukaemia' leukaemia cutis.

Pathology. A dense monomorphic infiltrate of medium-sized tumour cells with a fine chromatin resembling lymphoblasts is seen throughout the dermis with a well-defined grenz zone (Fig. 57.33) [4,5]. Occasionally, tumour cells show a rosette pattern. Necrosis and angiocentricity are usually absent.

Immunophenotype. Tumour cells are CD56+ with variable expression of CD4, CD45RA and CD43 but do not express surface CD3. CD2, CD7 and cytoplasmic CD3ε are usually negative [3–5]. Cytotoxic proteins may be rarely expressed. Rare cases are CD34+CD68+ and TdT+. Because of a morphological resemblance to myeloblastic and precursor T-lymphoblastic leukaemia which also express CD56, it is important to confirm that the tumour cells are negative for surface CD3, CD33 and myeloperoxidase/lysozyme. TCR gene analysis reveals a germline pattern for all TCR genes consistent with a non-lymphoid origin [4–6]. The tumours are CD123+ TCL1a+, confirming a derivation from rare peripheral blood plasmacytoid dendritic cells [7,8].

Pathogenesis. EBV has not been detected in tumour cells and no disease-specific cytogenetic abnormality has been detected [5,6]. Comparative genomic hybridization techniques and gene expression studies have shown a distinct pattern of chromosomal abnormalities and over-expression of the oncogene, *FLT3*, and loss of expression of the *Rb1* gene [9–12]. These studies have also shown that CD4+ CD56+ haematodermic neoplasms and cutaneous infiltrates of myeloid leukaemia have different chromosomal and gene expression profiles.

Treatment. Combination chemotherapy and radiotherapy can produce a partial remission, which is invariably short-lived, and the prognosis is very poor with a median survival of 14 months reported. Survival may be better in patients less than 40 years old and high TdT expression. Myeloid leukaemia protocols may be appropriate [12].

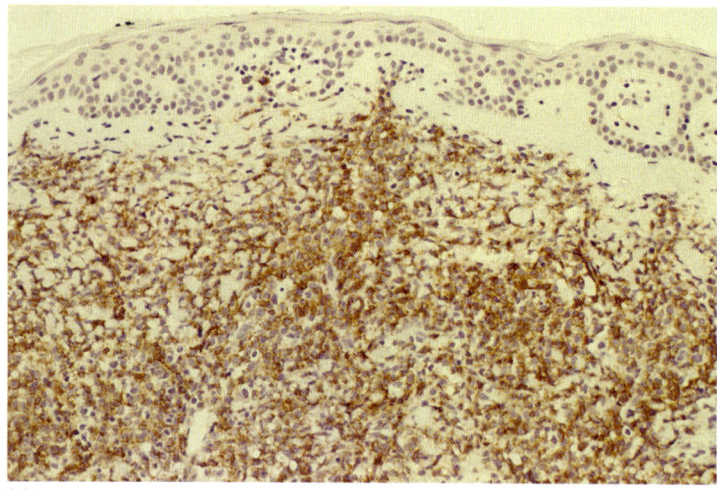

(a)

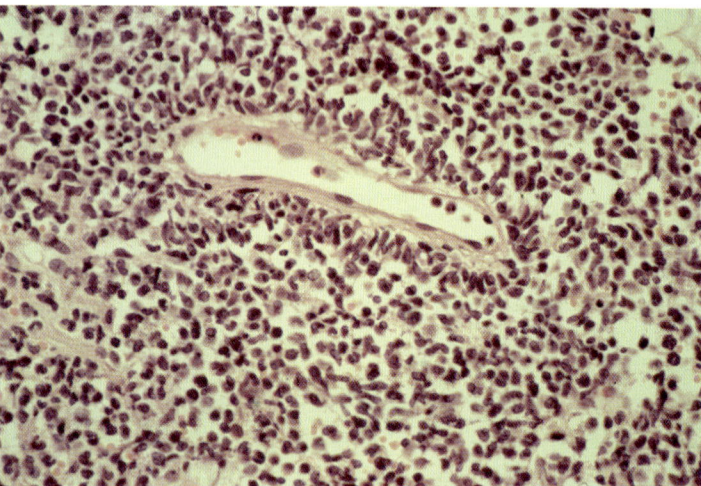

(b)

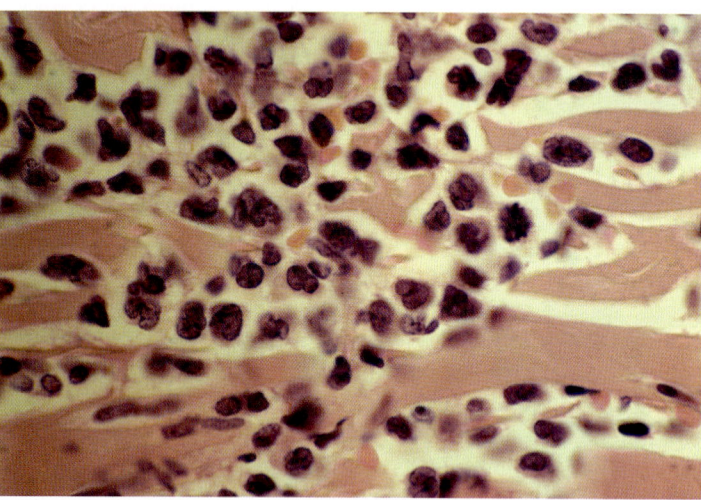

(c)

Fig. 57.33 Extranodal NK/T-cell lymphoma in the skin: (a) CD56 positivity; (b) rosetting of blood vessels; (c) large atypical mononuclear cells.

References

1 Harris N, Jaffe E, Diebold J *et al.* The World Health Organization classification of neoplastic disease of the haematopoietic and lymphoid tissues: report of the clinical advisory committee. *Histopathology* 2000; **36**: 69–87.

2 Petrella T, Dalac S, Maynadie M *et al.* CD4⁺ CD56⁺ cutaneous neoplasms: a distinct haematological entity? *Am J Surg Pathol* 1999; **23**: 137–46.

3 Shabrawi-Caelen L, Cerrono L, Kerl H. The clinicopathologic spectrum of cytotoxic lymphomas of the skin. *Semin Cutan Med Surg* 2000; **19**: 118–23.

4 Nakamura S, Suchi T, Koshikawa T *et al.* Clinicopathologic study of CD56 (NCAM)–positive angiocentric lymphoma occuring in sites other than the upper and lower respiratory tract. *Am J Surg Pathol* 1995; **19**: 284–96.

5 Chan J, Sin V, Wong K *et al.* Non-nasal lymphoma expressing the natural killer cell marker CD56: a clinicopathologic study of 49 cases of an uncommon aggressive neoplasm. *Blood* 1997; **89**: 4501–13.

6 Child F, Mitchell T, Whittaker S *et al.* Blastic natural killer cell and extranodal natural killer cell-like T-cell lymphoma presenting in the skin: report of six cases in the UK. *Br J Dermatol* 2003; **148**: 507–15.

7 Petrella T, Comeau M, Maynadie M *et al.* 'Agranular CD4⁺ CD56⁺ haematodermic neoplasm' (blastic NK-cell lymphoma) originates from a population of CD56⁺ precursor cells related to plasmacytoid monocytes. *Am J Surg Pathol* 2002; **26**: 852–62.

8 Petrella T, Meijer C, Dalac S *et al.* TCL1 and CLA expression in agranular CD4/CD56 hematodermic neoplasms (Blastic NK-cell lymphomas) and leukaemia cutis. *Am J Clin Pathol* 2004; **122**: 307–13.

9 Hallerman C, Middel P, Griesenger F *et al.* CD4⁺ CD56⁺ blastic tumour of the skin: cytogenetic observations and further evidence of an origin from plasmacytoid dendritic cells. *Eur J Dermatol* 2004; **14**: 317–22.

10 Mao X, Onadim Z, Price E *et al.* Genomic alterations in blastic natural killer/extranodal natural killer like T-cell lymphoma with cutaneous involvement. *J Invest Dermatol* 2003; **121**: 618–27.

11 Dijkman R, Van Doorn R, Szuhai K *et al.* Gene expression profiling and array based CGH classify CD4⁺ CD56⁺ haematodermic neoplasm and cutaneous myelomonocytic leukaemia as distinct disease entities. *Blood* 2007; **109**: 1720–7.

12 Bekkenk M, Jansen P, Meijer C, Willemze R. CD56⁺ hematological neoplasms presenting in the skin: a retrospective analysis of 23 new cases and 130 cases from the literature. *Ann Oncol* 2004; **15**: 1097–108.

Extranodal NK/T-cell lymphoma (nasal type)

Definition. This rare type of extranodal EBV-positive angiocentric lymphoma preferentially involves the nasal cavity and nasopharynx but also shows a predilection for the skin and used to be referred to as polymorphic reticuloses or angiocentric immunoproliferative lesion [1–4]. The disease is more prevalent in Asia and Central and South America. Most cases are derived from NK cells but rare cases have a cytotoxic T-cell phenotype.

Clinical features. Involvement of the nasal cavity, nasopharynx, paranasal sinuses, orbit and oropharynx is associated with tissue destruction ('lethal midline granuloma'). Secondary involvement of other extranodal sites including the skin and gastrointestinal tract occurs but primary cutaneous disease is rare. Cutaneous plaques, nodules and tumours may ulcerate and become necrotic. Purpura, bullous lesions, cellulitis and diffuse maculopapular rashes have been described [5–9]. A haemophagocytic syndrome can develop rarely and systemic symptoms are common. Bone marrow and peripheral blood involvement is rare but such cases can be indistinguishable from aggressive NK-cell leukaemia.

Pathology. There is a diffuse infiltrate in the dermis and often the subcutis with prominent angiocentricity and angiodestruction [1–4,6]. Extensive necrosis is common. Tumour cells can show a variable morphology with small/medium and large pleomorphic/anaplastic cells. An associated heavy mixed inflammatory infiltrate is common and pseudoepitheliomatous hyperplasia may be found, which can lead to diagnostic confusion.

Immunophenotype. Tumour cells are CD56$^+$, CD2$^+$, surface CD3$^-$ and cytoplasmic CD3ϵ^+. Most cases express cytotoxic proteins, namely granzyme B, perforin and TIA-I [1–4,6]. Rare cases are CD30$^+$ and this may confer a more favourable prognosis [6]. TCR genes are in a germline configuration consistent with an NK-cell origin. However, rare cases of extranodal NK/T-cell lymphomas have a CD56$^-$, CD3ϵ^+ cytotoxic phenotype and show a clonal TCR gene rearrangement consistent with derivation from a cytotoxic T cell [4,7,10,11].

Pathogenesis. EBV is present in almost all cases of extranodal NK/T-cell lymphoma, whether CD56$^+$ or CD56$^-$ [3]. EBV is present in a clonal episomal form, suggesting that the virus has a critical pathogenetic role. No disease-specific cytogenetic abnormality has been identified but deletions of 6q and isochromosome 6q are common and genomic abnormalities are distinct to those found in NK-cell leukaemias [12,13].

Reports have implicated EBV-infected cytotoxic T cells in the pathogenesis of both the photosensitive disorder hydroa vacciniforme and hypersensitivity to mosquito bites in patients from Asia and South America [14]. Furthermore, there is now substantial evidence that such patients are at risk of developing extranodal NK/T-cell lymphomas with a fatal outcome [15–18]. This suggests that in genetically susceptible individuals an EBV-driven NK/T-cell lymphoproliferative inflammatory disorder has the potential to transform into an aggressive EBV-associated NK/T-cell lymphoproliferative disorder [14].

Treatment. The prognosis is poor despite aggressive chemotherapy, particularly for those patients with disease outside the nasal cavity [4]. The multidrug resistance phenotype is often expressed in cutaneous cases and the median survival for patients presenting with cutaneous disease is 12–15 months although the prognosis may be better for those patients with only cutaneous involvement (27 months) [6–9].

References

1 Kern W, Spier C, Hanneman E et al. Neural cell adhesion molecule-positive peripheral T-cell lymphoma: a rare variant with a propensity for unusual sites of involvement. *Blood* 1992; **79**: 2432–7.

2 Wong K, Chan J, Ng C et al. CD56 (NCAM)–positive hematolymphoid malignancies: an aggressive neoplasm featuring frequent cutaneous/mucosal involvement, cytoplasmic azurophilic granules and angiocentricity. *Hum Pathol* 1992; **23**: 798–804.

3 Kanavaros P, Lescs M, Briere J et al. Nasal T-cell lymphoma: a clinicopathologic entity associated with peculiar phenotype and with Epstein–Barr virus. *Blood* 1993; **81**: 2688–95.

4 Chan J, Sin V, Wong K et al. Non-nasal lymphoma expressing the natural killer cell marker CD56: a clinicopathologic study of 49 cases of an uncommon aggressive neoplasm. *Blood* 1997; **89**: 4501–13.

5 Shabrawi-Caelen L, Cerrono L, Kerl H. The clinicopathologic spectrum of cytotoxic lymphomas of the skin. *Semin Cutan Med Surg* 2000; **19**: 118–23.

6 Gernhard S, Natkunam Y, Hoppe R et al. Natural killer/natural killer-like T-cell lymphoma, CD56$^+$, presenting in the skin: an increasingly recognized entity with an aggressive course. *J Clin Oncol* 2001; **19**: 2179–88.

7 Nakamura S, Suchi T, Koshikawa T et al. Clinicopathologic study of CD56 (NCAM)–positive angiocentric lymphoma occuring in sites other than the upper and lower respiratory tract. *Am J Surg Pathol* 1995; **19**: 284–96.

8 Wong K, Chan J, Ng C. CD56 (NCAM)–positive malignant lymphoma. *Leuk Lymphoma* 1994; **14**: 29–36

9 Jia H, Sun T. Extranodal NK/T-cell lymphoma mimicking cellulitis. *Leuk Lymphoma* 2004; **45**: 1467–70.

10 Massone C, Chott A, Metze D et al. Subcutaneous, blastic natural killer (NK), NK/T-cell and other cytotoxic lymphomas of the skin: a morphologic, immunophenotypic and molecular study of 50 patients. *Am J Surg Pathol* 2004; **28**: 719–35.

11 Child F, Mitchell T, Whittaker S et al. Blastic natural killer cell and extranodal natural killer cell-like T-cell lymphoma presenting in the skin: report of six cases from the UK. *Br J Dermatol* 2003; **148**: 507–15.

12 Siu L, Wong K, Chan J, Kwong Y. Comparative genomic hybridization analysis of natural killer cell lymphoma–leukaemia: recognition of consistent patterns of genetic alterations. *Am J Pathol* 1999; **155**: 1419–25.

13 Nakashima Y, Tagawa H, Suzuki R et al. Genome-wide array-based comparative genomic hybridization of natural killer cell lymphoma/leukemia: different genomic patterns of aggressive NK-cell leukemia and extranodal NK/T-cell lymphoma, nasal type. *Genes Chrom Cancer* 2005; **44**: 247–55.

14 Iwatsuki K, Satoh M, Yamamoto T et al. Pathogenic link between hydroa vacciniforme and Epstein-Barr virus-associated hematologic disorders. *Arch Dermatol* 2006; **142**: 587–95.

15 Chen H, Hsiao C, Chiu H. Hydroa vacciniforme-like primary cutaneous CD8-positive lymphoma. *Br J Dermatol* 2002; **147**: 587–91.

16 Iwatsuki K, Ohtsuka M, Akiba H, Kaneko F. Atypical hydroa vacciniforme in childhood: from a smoldering stage to Epsein-Barr virus-associated lymphoid malignancy. *J Am Acad Dermatol* 1999; **40**: 283–4.

17 Barrionuevo C, Anderson V, Zevallos-Giamietri E et al. Hydroa-like cutaneous T-cell lymphoma: a clinicopathologic and molecular genetic study of 16 pediatric cases from Peru. *Appl Immunohistochem Mol Morphol* 2002; **10**: 7–14.

18 Tomita N, Kanamori H, Fujimaki K et al. Epstein-Barr virus-associated extranodal NK/T-cell lymphoma following mosquito bites in an elderly patient without prior hypersensitivity. *Leuk Lymphoma* 2004; **45**: 2153–5.

Primary cutaneous B-cell lymphomas

Primary cutaneous B-cell lymphomas constitute approximately one-quarter of all primary cutaneous lymphomas [1]. Increasing recognition of this group of primary cutaneous lymphomas led to controversy following the first publication of the EORTC classification of primary cutaneous lymphomas which included a subgroup of diffuse large B-cell lymphomas situated almost exclusively on the leg [2]. In addition, the description of a low-grade primary cutaneous lymphoma derived from follicle centre cells, which was distinct from both nodal follicular lymphoma and primary cutaneous diffuse large B-cell lymphoma, also caused controversy although this entity was recognized in the early WHO classification [3]. However, there is now a consensus classification of cutaneous B-cell lymphomas, illustrated by the recent WHO–EORTC classification which defines three specific subtypes of primary cutaneous B-cell lymphoma: marginal zone (MZL), follicle centre cell (FCL) and diffuse large B-cell (LBCL) lymphomas [4]. Full staging investigations are essential for patients with a cutaneous B-cell lymphoma to exclude secondary cutaneous involvement with a nodal lymphoma. Most primary cutaneous B-cell lymphomas are indolent with an excellent long-term prognosis, with the exception of PCLBCL [4,5]. An ISCL–EORTC TNM classification has been proposed for staging primary cutaneous lymphomas other than MF and SS (Table 57.8) [6]. This staging classification has shown prognostic relevance for PCLBCL as multifocal disease appears to be a poor prognostic feature but the value of staging the skin tumour burden in PCMZL and PCFCL has not yet been shown to have an impact on prognosis [7,8]. Recent ISCL–EORTC

Table 57.8 Proposed staging classification of non-mycosis fungoides/Sézary syndrome primary cutaneous lymphomas.

T		
	T_1	Solitary skin involvement
	T_{1a}	a solitary lesion <5 cm diameter
	T_{1b}	a solitary lesion >5 cm diameter
	T_2	Regional skin involvement; multiple lesions limited to 1 body region or 2 contiguous body regions
	T_{2a}	all-disease-encompassing in a <15-cm diameter circular area
	T_{2b}	all-disease-encompassing in a >15- and <30-cm diameter circular area
	T_{2c}	all-disease-encompassing in a >30-cm diameter circular area
	T_3	Generalized skin involvement
	T_{3a}	multiple lesions involving 2 non-contiguous body regions
	T_{3b}	multiple lesions involving ≥3 body regions
N		
	N_0	No clinical or pathological lymph node involvement
	N_1	Involvement of 1 peripheral lymph node region that drains an area of current or prior skin involvement
	N_2	Involvement of 2 or more peripheral lymph node regions or involvement of any lymph node region that does not drain an area of current or prior skin involvement
	N_3	Involvement of central lymph nodes
M		
	M_0	No evidence of extracutaneous non-lymph node disease
	M_1	Extracutaneous non-lymph node disease present

Table 57.9 Summary of cytogenetic findings in primary cutaneous B-cell lymphomas.

Cytogenetic abnormality	PCMZL	PCFCL	PCLBCL
t(14;18) IgH:MALT1	22% (21/95)	0% (0/6)	0% (0/14)
t(14;18) IgH:BCL2	11% (9/80)	17% (24/143)	7% (4/54)
t(11;18) AP12:MALT1	4% (4/96)	0% (0/1)	0% (0/6)
t(1;14) BCL10:IgH	0% (0/63)	ND	ND
t(8;14) MYC:IgH	0% (0/9)	0% (0/6)	36% (5/14)
t(3;14) BCL6:IgH	0% (0/9)	6% (2/33)	14% (2/14)
Trisomy 3	17% (11/63)	ND	ND
Trisomy 18	6% (4/63)	ND	ND
BCL2/MALT1 amplification	0% (0/11)	8% (2/25)	60% (12/20)
BCL10 mutation	3% (1/33)	50% (2/4)	ND
BCL6 mutation	0% (0/9)	37% (7/19)	47% (15/32)
cMYC amplification	0% (0/9)	0% (0/6)	17% (3/18)
cREL amplification	ND	25% (3/12)	63% (12/19)
9p21.3 (p16/p14ARF) deletion	ND	0% (0/19)	62% (43/64)

PCMZL, primary cutaneous marginal zone lymphoma; PCFCL, primary cutaneous follicle centre cell lymphoma; PCLBCL, primary cutaneous diffuse large B-cell lymphoma; ND, not determined.

consensus recommendations for the management of primary cutaneous B-cell lymphomas have been published and conservative management is appropriate for PCMZL and PCFCL, although more aggressive therapy may be required for PCLBCL [9]. Distinction between cutaneous B-cell pseudolymphomas and marginal zone lymphomas can be particularly difficult. Systemic B-cell non-Hodgkin's lymphomas such as small cell lymphocytic lymphoma and mantle cell lymphomas are only found within skin as secondary cutaneous involvement associated with underlying nodal disease [10–11], although very rarely mantle cell lymphomas can be restricted to skin [12].

The pathogenetic relationship between these primary cutaneous B-cell lymphomas and their nodal counterparts remains unclear (Table 57.9). Specific translocations characteristic of marginal mucosa associated lymphoid tissue (MALT) lymphomas of nodal and extranodal origin have been detected in a minority of primary cutaneous marginal zone lymphomas. Genomic abnormalities detected in nodal diffuse large B-cell lymphomas have been identified in a primary cutaneous large B-cell lymphoma, suggesting a similar pathogenesis [4]. However, primary cutaneous follicle centre cell lymphomas appear to be distinct pathogenetically from nodal follicular lymphomas [4].

In 1982, Burgdorf *et al.* suggested that Lyme disease was caused by the tick *Ixodes ricinus*, and subsequently the spirochete *Borrelia burgdorferi* was recognized as being the vehicle responsible for carrying infection from the tick to human [13]. Prior to the publication by Burgdorf *et al.*, it had been recognized that patients with acrodermatitis chronica atrophicans, now known to be part of the cutaneous spectrum of Lyme disease, could develop low-grade cutaneous B-cell lymphomas [14–16]. These patients developed

multiple plaques and nodules superimposed on lesions of acrodermatitis chronica atrophicans. In a small number of reported cases, the lesions of acrodermatitis chronica atrophicans cleared with antibiotic therapy, but the B-cell lymphoma nodules often persisted [17]. Nevertheless, this suggested the possibility that *Borrelia* might have a role in the pathogenesis of PCMZL [18]. For those patients without clinical evidence of acrodermatitis the causal relationship has been more controversial, with some studies detecting positive *Borrelia* serology and the presence of *Borrelia* in tumour DNA using PCR [19,20] and others consistently reporting negative results [21–23]. Nevertheless this suggests that chronic antigenic stimulation in skin, such as the presence of *Borrelia burgdorferi* infection, may rarely encourage emergence of a neoplastic B-cell clone from a previously benign reactive proliferation of B lymphocytes.

References

1 Kerl H. The morphologic spectrum of B cell lymphomas. *Arch Dermatol* 1996; **132**: 1376–7.

2 Willemze R, Kerl H, Sterry W et al. EORTC classification for primary cutaneous lymphomas: a proposal from the Cutaneous Lymphoma Study Group of the European Organization for Research on Treatment of Cancer. *Blood* 1997; **90**: 354–71.

3 Harris N, Jaffe E, Diebold J et al. The World Health Organization classification of neoplastic disease of the haematopoietic and lymphoid tissues: report of the clinical advisory committee. *Histopathology* 2000; **36**: 69–87.

4 Willemze R, Jaffe E, Burg G et al. WHO-EORTC classification for cutaneous lymphomas. *Blood* 2005; **105**: 3768–85.

5 Pandolfino T, Siegel R, Kuzel T et al. Primary cutaneous B-cell lymphoma: review and current concepts. *J Clin Oncol* 2000; **18**: 2152–68.

6 Kim Y, Willemze R, Pimpinelli N et al. TNM classification system for primary cutaneous lymphomas other than mycosis fungoides and Sezary syndrome: a proposal of the International Society for Cutaneous Lymphoma (ISCL) and the Cutaneous Lymphoma Task Force of the European Organisation for Research and Treatment of Cancer (EORTC). *Blood* 2007; **110**: 479–84.

7 Senff N and Willemze R. The applicability and prognostic value of the new TNM classification system for primary cutaneous lymphomas other than mycosis fungoides and Sezary syndrome: results on a large cohort of primary cutaneous

B-cell lymphomas and comparison with the system used by the Dutch Cutaneous Lymphoma Group. *Br J Dermatol* 2007; **157**: 1205–11.

8 Golling P, Cozzio A, Dummer R *et al.* Primary cutaneous B-cell lymphomas—clinicopathological, prognostic and therapeutic characterisation of 54 cases according to the new WHO-EORTC classification and the ISCL/EORTC TNM classification system for primary cutaneous lymphomas other than mycosis fungoides and Sezary syndrome. *Leukaemia Lymphoma* 2008; **49**: 1094–103.

9 Senff N, Noordijk E, Kim Y *et al.* European Organization for Research and Treatment of Cancer and International Society for Cutaneous Lymphoma consensus recommendations for the management of cutaneous B-cell lymphomas. *Blood* 2008; **112**: 1600–9.

10 Bertero M, Novelli M, Fierro MT, Bernengo MG. Mantle zone lymphoma: an immunohistologic study of skin lesions. *J Am Acad Dermatol* 1994; **30**: 23–30.

11 Burg G, Kempf W, Haeffner A *et al.* Cutaneous lymphomas. *Curr Probl Dermatol* 1997; **9**: 137–204.

12 Sen F, Medeiros L, Lu D *et al.* Mantle cell lymphoma. *Skin Am J Surg Pathol* 2002; **26**: 1312–8.

13 Steere AC. Lyme disease. *N Engl J Med* 1989; **321**: 386–96.

14 Braun-Falco O, Guggenberger K, Burg G. Immunozytom unter dem Bild einer Acrodermatitis chronica atrophicans. *Hautarzt* 1978; **29**: 644–7.

15 Geiger HG, Hagedorn M, Petres J. Retikulumzellsarcom bei acrodermatitis chronica atrophicans Herxheimer. *Z Hautkr* 1974; **49**: 359–65.

16 Orfanos CE, Steigleder GK. Die tumorbilende kutane Form des morbus Waldenstrom. *Deutsch Med Wochenschr* 1967; **33**: 1449–77.

17 Garbe C, Stein H, Dienemann D, Orfanos CE. *Borrelia burgdorferi*-associated cutaneous B-cell lymphoma: clinical and immunohistologic characterization of four cases. *J Am Acad Dermatol* 1991; **24**: 584–90.

18 Weber K, Schierz G, Wilkse B. Das Lymphozytom: eine Borreliose? *Z Hautkr* 1985; **60**: 1585–98.

19 Cerroni L, Zochling N, Putz B *et al.* Infection by *Borrelia burgdorferi* and cutaneous B-cell lymphoma. *J Cutan Pathol* 1997; **24**: 457–61.

20 Goodlad J, Davidson M, Hollowood K *et al.* Primary cutaneous B-cell lymphoma and *Borrelia burgdorferi* infection in patients from the highlands of Scotland. *Am J Surg Pathol* 2000; **245**: 1279–85.

21 LeBoit P, McNutt N, Reed J *et al.* Primary cutaneous immunocytoma: a B-cell lymphoma that can easily be mistaken for cutaneous lymphoid hyperplasia. *Am J Surg Pathol* 1994; **18**: 969–78.

22 Dillon W, Saed G, Fivenson D. *Borrelia burgdorferi* DNA is undetectable by polymerase chain reaction in skin lesions of morphoea, scleroderma or lichen sclerosis et atrophicus of patients from North America. *J Am Acad Dermatol* 1995; **33**: 617–20.

23 Wood G, Kamath N, Guitart J *et al.* Absence of *Borrelia burgdorferi* DNA in cutaneous B-cell lymphomas from the United States. *J Cutan Pathol* 2001; **28**: 502–7.

Marginal zone lymphoma

Definition. An indolent cutaneous B-cell lymphoma derived from post-germinal centre cells and characterized by a proliferation of small lymphocytes, marginal zone B-cells (small centrocyte-like), lymphoplasmacytoid cells and plasma cells with monotypic cytoplasmic immunoglobulin [1–3]. Primary cutaneous marginal zone lymphoma (PCMZL) is considered part of the spectrum of extranodal marginal zone B-cell lymphomas which often involve mucosal sites (MALT lymphomas).

This category also includes primary cutaneous immunocytoma [4] and rare primary cutaneous plasmacytoma without overt evidence of underlying myeloma or localized bony or other extramedullary involvement [5,6]. Extraosseous lesions in multiple myeloma are common, and the skin is infiltrated in approximately 10% of cases [7] but primary involvement of the skin without evidence of bone involvement is extremely rare.

Clinical features. These lymphomas present as asymptomatic solitary or multiple dermal papules, plaques or nodules on any

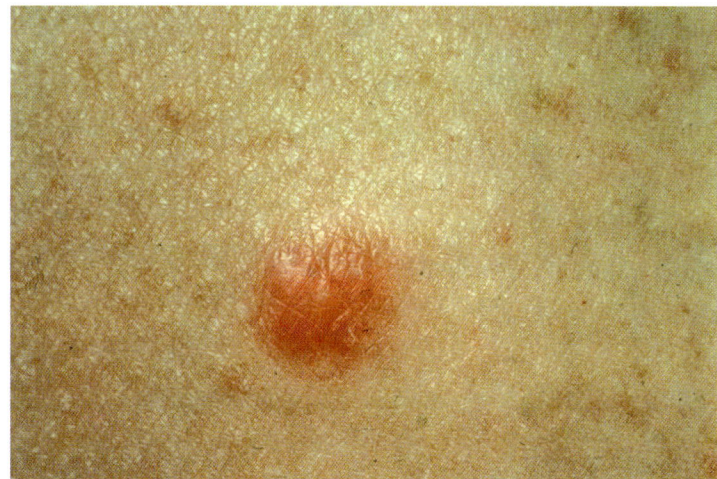

Fig. 57.34 Marginal zone primary cutaneous B-cell lymphoma: typical urticated dermal erythematous papules and plaques predominantly situated on the trunk.

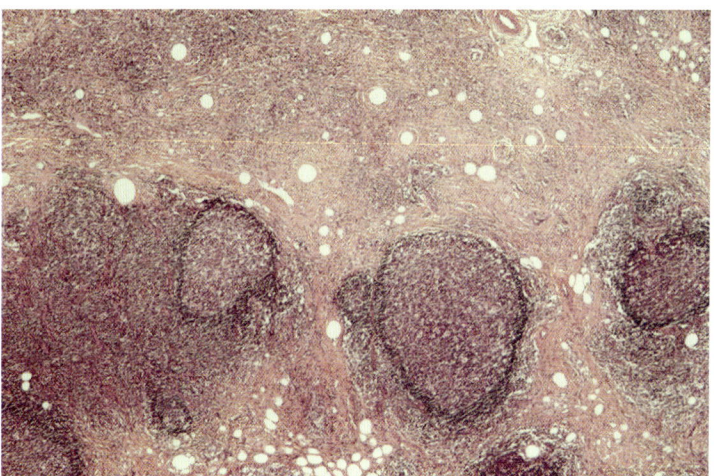

Fig. 57.35 Marginal zone primary cutaneous B-cell lymphoma: reactive germinal centres with a non-epidermotropic monomorphic infiltrate of lymphoplasmacytoid cells and mature plasma cells.

body site, although the trunk is most often involved (Fig. 57.34) [1–4]. Spontaneous resolution can occur. Full staging investigations are indicated and a benign monoclonal paraproteinaemia may be present. In cases of plasmacytoma skeletal surveys are required to exclude underlying myeloma. There is a slight male predominance. Anetoderma associated with individual lesions has been described [8]. The estimated 5-year survival is 98–100% [3,4,9].

Pathology. Histology is characterized by nodular or diffuse dermal infiltrates of small- to medium-sized lymphocytes, marginal B-cells (centrocyte-like), lymphoplasmacytoid cells and plasma cells, often with a reactive T-cell infiltrate [1–4]. There is no epidermotropism. Reactive follicular structures are often present and tumour cells present within expanded marginal zones and interfollicular areas may colonize these follicular structures (Fig. 57.35). This pattern has to be distinguished immunophenotypically from rare follicular patterns of PCFCL [10,11]. Occasional scattered centrocytes, centroblasts and immunoblasts may be present. Tumour cells, characterized by monotypic κ or λ positive larger paler lymphoplasmacytoid cells, are concentrated at the periphery of the cellular aggregates or residual follicular structures. PAS-positive intranuclear or intracytoplasmic inclusions may be present [1–3]. Cases with a monomorphic infiltrate of plasma cells (immunocytoma-like) are included [4]. Rare cases of cutaneous plasmacytoma have to be distinguished from benign reactive plasma cell infiltrates (plasmacytosis) by identifying monotypic light chain expression.

Immunophenotype.
Tumour cells express CD20, CD79a and Bcl-2, but are Bcl-6, CD5 and CD10 negative [3,12]. PCMZL of the skin should be distinguished from cutaneous infiltrates chronic B-lymphocytic leukaemia, which are CD5+. Plasma cells are CD138+ and CD79a+ (but CD19− and CD20−) and the infiltrate usually shows either κ or λ light chain restriction (although this can often be difficult to detect in cutaneous sections because of non-specific staining of collagen). Reactive follicles are Bcl-6+ and CD10+ positive but Bcl-2−.

Clonal immunoglobulin gene rearrangements are detected in most cases [13]. False-negative results may occur because of somatic hypermutation, which interferes with primer annealing in the analysis of immunoglobulin genes as for follicle centre cell lymphomas although this is less common with the current standardized Biomed primers [14]. The demonstration of light chain restriction and/or a clonal immunoglobulin gene rearrangement represents a critical technique for distinguishing these low-grade cutaneous lymphomas from reactive cutaneous B-cell infiltrates (pseudolymphomas).

Pathogenesis.
PCMZL is considered to be part of the spectrum of extranodal marginal zone B-cell lymphomas which were first described in the stomach, the so-called MALT lymphoma, and have since been described in the thyroid, salivary gland, orbit and lung as well as the skin.

As would be expected, PCMZL shows a plasma cell signature in a subset of cases [15]. No disease-specific cytogenetic abnormalities have been identified in PCMZL, although CGH techniques have shown amplification of the *BCL2* locus on chromosome 18 [16]. Fas mutations have rarely been described [17]. Studies (Table 57.9) have also clearly demonstrated that approximately 50% of PCMZL have identical translocations to those found in other extranodal MALT lymphomas, including the t(14;18) involving the *IgH* gene locus and the *MALT-1* gene, which is mostly found in monocytoid variants [18–20]. Trisomy 3 and 18 have also been detected in up to 40% of cases [20,21]. The t(11;18) which produces a fusion protein involving the *AP12* gene and the *MALT-1* gene has also been detected in PCMZL [21,22], although other studies have failed to detect this translocation [17,20,23]. Other translocations found in extranodal marginal zone B-cell lymphomas, such as the t(1;14) involving the *Bcl-10* gene on 1q, have not yet been identified in PCMZL [17,20,21,23]. The t(14;18) involving *Bcl2* has also not been consistently detected in PCMZL [20,24] except in isolated reports [18,25].

Development of immunocytomas has been reported in patients with acrodermatitis chronica atrophicans and has led to speculation about the role of *Borrelia burgdorferi* producing chronic antigen stimulation, leading to neoplastic transformation. The detection of *Borrelia* DNA in some cutaneous lesions of PCMZL, using polymerase chain reaction (PCR), has provided support for this role, but the frequency of positivity varies considerably in different geographical regions, with positive results in central Europe and Scotland [26,27] but no evidence of an association in the USA [28,29]. To date, most cases of PCMZL associated with *Borrelia* have been κ-chain positive.

Treatment.
Radiotherapy (low dose) is appropriate and some patients may be managed simply by observation in view of the excellent long-term prognosis [30–32]. Surgical excision may be used for isolated small lesions. The role of IFN-α has not been established but it may be effective either systemically or intralesionally [32]. In cases associated with *Borrelia burgdorferi* relevant antibiotic therapy is appropriate [33]. In patients with multifocal disease chlorambucil may be appropriate [31,32]. Cutaneous recurrences are common and can be treated in a similar manner.

References

1 Sander C, Kaudewitz P, Schirren C et al. Immunocytoma and marginal zone B-cell lymphoma (MALT lymphoma), presenting in skin: different entities or a spectrum of disease? *J Cutan Pathol* 1996; **23**: 59.

2 Cerroni L, Signoretti S, Hofler G et al. Primary cutaneous marginal zone B-cell lymphoma: a recently described entity of low-grade malignant cutaneous B-cell lymphoma. *Am J Surg Pathol* 1997; **21**: 1307–15.

3 Willemze R, Jaffe E, Burg G et al. WHO-EORTC classification for cutaneous lymphomas. *Blood* 2005; **105**: 3768–85.

4 Rijlaarsdam JU, Van Der Putte SCJ, Berti E et al. Cutaneous immunocytomas: a clinicopathologic study of 26 cases. *Histopathology* 1993; **23**: 117–25.

5 Johnson WH Jr, Taylor BG. Solitary extramedullary plasmacytoma of the skin: a review of the world literature and the report of an additional case. *Cancer* 1970; **26**: 65–8.

6 Wong KF, Chan JKC, Li LPK et al. Primary cutaneous plasmacytoma: report of two cases and review of the literature. *Am J Dermatopathol* 1994; **16**: 392–7.

7 Bluefarb SM. Cutaneous manifestations of multiple myeloma. *Arch Dermatol* 1955; **72**: 506–22.

8 Child F, Woolons A, Price M et al. Multiple cutaneous immunocytoma with secondary anetoderma: a report of two cases. *Br J Dermatol* 2000; **143**: 165–70.

9 Senff N, Hoefnagel J, Jansen P et al. Reclassification of 300 primary cutaneous B-cell lymphomas according to the new WHO-EORTC classification for cutaneous lymphomas: comparison with previous classifications and identification of prognostic markers. *J Clin Oncol* 2007; **25**: 1581–7.

10 de Laval Harris N, Longtime J, Ferry J, Duncan L. Cutaneous B-cell lymphomas of follicular and marginal zone types. *Am J Surg Pathol* 2001; **25**: 732–41.

11 Pimpinelli N, Santucci M, Moria M et al. Primary cutaneous B-cell lymphoma: a clinically homogeneous entity? *J Am Acad Dermatol* 1997; **37**: 1012–6.

12 Gronbaek K, Moller P, Nedergaard T et al. Primary cutaneous B-cell lymphoma: a clinical, histological, phenotypic and genotypic study of 21 cases. *Br J Dermatol* 2000; **142**: 913–23.

13 Child F, Woolford A, Calonje E et al. Molecular analysis of the immunoglobulin heavy chain gene in the diagnosis of primary cutaneous B-cell lymphoma. *J Invest Dermatol* 2001; **117**: 984–9.

14 Sandberg Y, Heule F, Lam K et al. Molecular immunoglobulin/T-cell receptor clonality in cutaneous lymphoproliferations. Experience with the BIOMED-2 standardised polymerase chain reaction protocol. *Haematologica* 2003; **88**: 659–70.

15 Storz M, van de Rijn M, Kim Y et al. Gene expression profiles of cutaneous B-cell lymphoma. *J Invest Dermatol* 2003; **120**: 865–70.

16 Mao X, Lillington D, Child F et al. Comparative genomic hybridization analysis of primary cutaneous B-cell lymphoma: identification of common genetic alterations in disease pathogenesis. *Genes Chromosomes Cancer* 2002; **35**: 144–55.

17 Gronbaek K, Ralfkiaer E, Kalla J *et al.* Infrequent somatic FAS mutations but no evidence of Bcl10 mutations or t(11;18) in primary cutaneous MALT-type lymphoma. *J Pathol* 2003 **201**: 134–40.

18 Palmedo G, Hautschke M, Rutten A *et al.* Primary cutaneous marginal zone B-cell lymphoma may exhibit both the t(14;18)(q32;21) IGH/BCL2 and the t(14;18)(q32;21) IGH/MALT1 translocation: an indicator for clonal transformation towards higher grade B-cell lymphoma. *Am J Dermatopathol* 2007; **29**: 231–6.

19 Streubel B, Lamprecht A, Dierlamm J *et al.* T(14;18)(q32;q21) involving IGH and MALT-1 is a frequent chromosomal aberration in MALT lymphoma. *Blood* 2003; **101**: 2335–9.

20 Schreuder M, Hoefnagel J, Jansen P *et al.* FISH analysis of MALT lymphoma-specific translocations and aneuploidy in primary cutaneous marginal zone lymphoma. *J Pathol* 2005; **205**: 302–10.

21 Streubel B, Simonitsch-Klupp I, Mullauer L *et al.* Variable frequency of MALT lymphoma-associated genetic aberrations in MALT lymphomas of different sites. *Leukemia* 2004; **18**: 1722–6.

22 Remstein E, James C, Kurtin P. Incidence and subtype specificity of AP12 MALT-1 fusion translocations in extranodal, nodal and splenic marginal zone lymphomas. *Am J Pathol* 2000; **156**: 1183–8.

23 Li C, Inagaki H, Kuo T *et al.* Primary cutaneous marginal zone B-cell lymphoma: a molecular and clinicopathologic study of 24 asian cases. *Am J Surg Pathol* 2003; **27**: 1061–9.

24 Child F, Russell Jones R, Woolford A *et al.* Absence of the t(14;18) translocation in primary cutaneous B-cell lymphomas. *Br J Dermatol* 2001; **144**: 735–44.

25 Servitje O, Gallardo F, Estrach T *et al.* Primary cutaneous marginal zone B-cell lymphoma: a clinical, histopathological, immunophenotypic and molecular genetic study of 22 cases. *Br J Dermatol* 2002; **147**: 1147–58.

26 Cerroni L, Zochling N, Putz B *et al.* Infection by *Borrelia burgdorferi* and cutaneous B-cell lymphoma. *J Cutan Pathol* 1997; **24**: 457–61.

27 Goodlad J, Davidson M, Hollowood K *et al.* Primary cutaneous B-cell lymphoma and *Borrelia burgdorferi* infection in patients from the highlands of Scotland. *Am J Surg Pathol* 2000; **245**: 1279–85.

28 Wood G, Kamath N, Guitart J *et al.* Absence of *Borrelia burgdorferi* DNA in cutaneous B-cell lymphomas from the United States. *J Cutan Pathol* 2001; **28**: 502–7.

29 Dillon W, Saed G, Fivenson D. *Borrelia burgdorferi* DNA is undetectable by polymerase chain reaction in skin lesions of morphoea, scleroderma or lichen sclerosis et atrophicus of patients from North America. *J Am Acad Dermatol* 1995; **33**: 617–20.

30 Santucci M, Pimpinelli N, Arganini L. Primary cutaneous B-cell lymphoma: a unique type of low grade lymphoma—clinicopathologic and immunologic study of 83 cases. *Cancer* 1991; **67**: 2311–26.

31 Hoefnagel J, Vermeer M, Jansen P *et al.* Primary cutaneous marginal zone B-cell lymphoma. *Arch Dermatol* 2005; **141**: 1139–45.

32 Senff N, Noordijk E, Kim Y *et al.* European Organization for Research and Treatment of Cancer and International Society for Cutaneous Lymphoma consensus recommendations for the management of cutaneous B-cell lymphomas. *Blood* 2008; **112**: 1600–9.

33 Kutting B, Bonsmann G, Metz D *et al. Borrelia burgdorferi*-associated primary cutaneous B-cell lymphoma: complete clearing of skin lesions after antibiotic pulse therapy or intralesional injection of interferon-α2a. *J Am Acad Dermatol* 1997; **36**: 31–4.

Follicle centre cell lymphoma

Synonym
• Crosti's lymphoma

Definition. An indolent primary cutaneous B-cell lymphoma derived from follicle centre cells (PCFCL) and consisting of a mixture of centrocytes (small/large cleaved cells) and centroblasts (larger non-cleaved cells).

Clinical features. Patients present with clinically non-specific solitary or grouped papules, nodules or tumours, most commonly on the head and neck or trunk [1–3], although any body site may

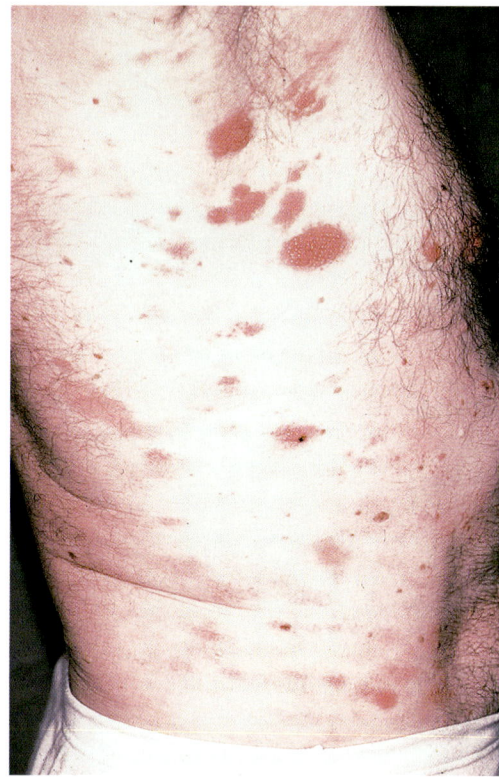

Fig. 57.36 Primary cutaneous follicle centre cell lymphoma. Extensive erythematous plaque and nodular lesions on the lower back.

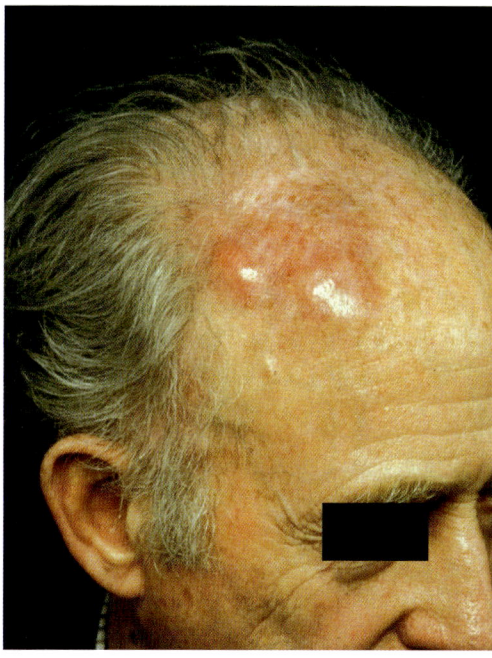

Fig. 57.37 Typical clinical presentation of primary cutaneous follicle centre cell lymphoma on the scalp.

be involved (Figs 57.36–57.38). A gradual increase in size of preexisting lesions and the appearance of new nodules over a period of years is likely without treatment [1–3]. Rarely, multifocal lesions may occur. Staging investigations including CT scans of the chest, abdomen and pelvis, and bone marrow aspirate and trephine

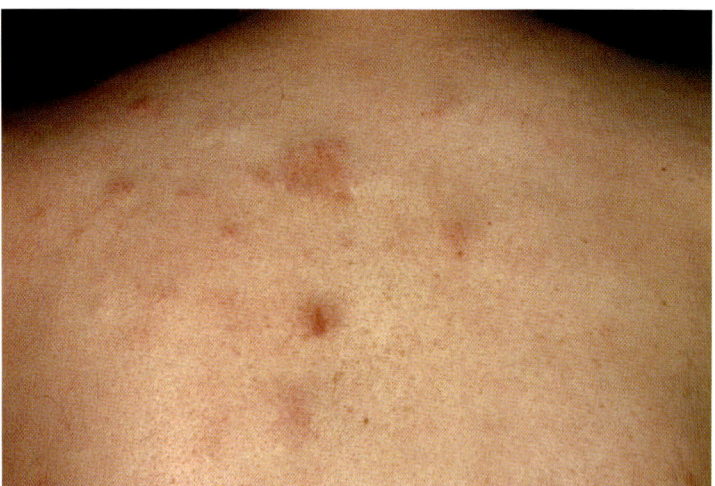

Fig. 57.38 Primary cutaneous follicle centre cell lymphoma. Cutaneous presentation of a systemic follicular t(14;18) lymphoma on the trunk with subtle dermal papules and plaques.

biopsies are negative at the time of diagnosis. The estimated 5-year survival of PCFCL is 94–97% [3,4].

Pathology. The histology of PCFCL is variable but the infiltrate shows no epidermotropism and there is a clear grenz zone in the papillary dermis. In the reticular dermis and subcutaneous fat, there is a 'bottom-heavy' nodular or diffuse infiltrate composed of a mixture of centrocytes (small/large cleaved cells), centroblasts (large non-cleaved cells with prominent nucleoli) and a prominent infiltrate of reactive T cells with the remnants of poorly formed germinal centres [1–3]. Some tumour cells show a 'strap-like' or 'fibroblast-like' morphology. The growth pattern may be follicular, follicular and diffuse, or diffuse. Individual patients may show different histological patterns in biopsies from the same group of lesions. PCFCL has to be distinguished from marginal zone lymphomas with follicular colonization of reactive germinal centres. Prominent larger tumours tend to show a more diffuse infiltrate of larger centrocytes, centroblasts and occasional immunoblasts with fewer reactive T cells and no evidence of follicular structures. Such lymphomas should be distinguished from PCLBCL although the presence of a monotonous infiltrate of centroblasts and immunoblasts should be classified as a PCLBCL [3]. A subset of PCFCL shows neoplastic follicular structures with an expansile growth pattern, a thin poorly formed mantle zone and an absence of tingible body (starry sky) macrophages similar to nodal follicular lymphoma although the phenotypic and molecular features are distinct [5].

Immunophenotype. The tumour cells express B-cell associated markers such as CD19, CD20, CD22 and CD79a but are CD5⁻ [3,6]. CD10 and monotypic cytoplasmic and/or surface immunoglobulin are variably expressed by the neoplastic cells [7]. Follicular structures can be more clearly defined by identifying networks of CD21⁺ and CD23⁺ follicular dendritic cells. The tumour cells are mostly Bcl-2 negative, in contrast to systemic nodal follicular lymphoma and diffuse large B-cell lymphoma (DLBCL) in which a significant proportion of the tumour cells are CD10⁺ and Bcl-2

positive [8]. In those cases with a follicular growth pattern CD10 may be expressed and Bcl-2 may be weakly positive. In contrast, Bcl-6 is usually expressed by PCFCL tumour cells indicative of somatic mutation, as also seen in nodal follicular lymphoma and DLBCL [4]. *MUM-1* and *FOXP1* are usually negative but may be rarely expressed [9,10]. Clonal immunoglobulin gene rearrangements are present in most cases. However false-negative cases are common, caused by somatic hypermutation affecting the primer binding for PCR immunoglobulin gene analysis [11]. Extensive somatic mutation of variable region genes has been identified, which is also consistent with an origin from germinal centre cells [12,13].

Pathogenesis. The relationship between PCFCL and nodal systemic follicular and diffuse large B-cell lymphomas remains unclear. While there are morphological similarities, PCFCL follows an indolent clinical course and the immunophenotypic features (CD10 expression is mostly confined to PCFCL with an exclusively follicular growth pattern and Bcl-2 is usually negative or rarely only weakly positive) are distinct. Microdissection of tumour cells has also confirmed the germinal centre cell origin of PCFCL Bcl-2⁻ tumour cells, with no evidence of the t(14;18) translocation, also suggesting a different pathogenesis to nodal follicular lymphoma [13]. Gene expression studies have detected a germinal centre B-cell signature in PCFCL [14] distinct from the activated B-cell signature detected in primary cutaneous DLBCL [15]. While the t(14;18), characteristic of nodal systemic follicular lymphoma and a significant proportion of DLBCLs, has not been consistently detected in most studies of PCFCL [8,16–18], other studies especially from the USA have detected the t(14;18) in a proportion of CD10⁺ and Bcl-2 positive PCFCL with a follicular growth pattern [19,20], suggesting that there might be some unexplained geographical or histological subset distinction although there are no obvious prognostic differences. A study using a FISH based technique has detected the t(14;18) translocation involving *Bcl-2* in 41% of 27 cases in which a PCR based technique had failed to identify any *Bcl-2* rearrangement [21]. However, this study restricted the cases of PCFCL to those with a follicular growth pattern only.

CGH studies have also identified patterns of chromosomal gains and losses associated with specific oncogene abnormalities in PCFCL including *c-REL* amplification but a consistent pattern has not yet emerged [22,23]. FISH studies (Table 57.9) have not identified chromosomal breakpoints involving the IgH, *myc* or *bcl-6* loci [24] although one study did show a t(3;14) in two of 27 cases involving *Bcl6* and IgH in PCFCL (21). Inactivation of both the cyclin-dependent kinase inhibitors, namely the *p15* and *p16* genes, by promoter hypermethylation has been detected in a proportion of cases but the clinical significance is unclear [25]. A recent study has identified aberrant somatic hypermutation affecting certain oncogenes in PCFCL including *BCL6*, *PAX5*, *MYC* and *RhoH/TTF* similar to findings in nodal and primary cutaneous LBCL [26].

At present, a detailed characterization of the molecular abnormalities in PCFCL is required to clarify the pathogenetic relationship between PCFCL and systemic nodal follicular and diffuse large B-cell lymphomas.

Treatment. Superficial radiotherapy is the treatment of choice for solitary, recurrent and multifocal cutaneous disease, except in rare cases with very extensive cutaneous disease or systemic involvement when single-agent treatment with chlorambucil or combination chemotherapy may be indicated [27–31]. Solitary lesions may be excised, although subsequent radiotherapy is probably advisable to reduce the risk of local recurrence [28]. Recurrences occur in approximately 30% of cases, are usually confined to the skin and do not signify a worse prognosis [30]. Therefore treatment options remain similar.

References

1 Willemze R, Meijer CJLM, Scheffer E. Diffuse large cell lymphomas of follicular centre origin presenting in the skin. *Am J Pathol* 1987; **126**: 325–33.

2 Garcia C, Weiss L, Warnke R, Wood G. Cutaneous follicular lymphoma. *Am J Surg Pathol* 1986; **10**: 454–63.

3 Willemze R, Meijer CJLM, Sentis HJ *et al.* Primary cutaneous large cell lymphomas of follicular center cell origin. *J Am Acad Dermatol* 1987; **16**: 518–26.

4 Willemze R, Jaffe E, Burg G *et al.* WHO-EORTC classification for cutaneous lymphomas. *Blood* 2005; **105**: 3768–85.

5 Cerroni L, Arzberger E, Putz B *et al.* Primary cutaneous follicle center cell lymphoma with follicular growth pattern. *Blood* 2000; **95**: 3922–8.

6 Franco R, Fernandez-Vazquez A, Rodriguez-Peralto J *et al.* Cutaneous follicular B-cell lymphoma. *Am J Surg Pathol* 2001; **25**: 875–83.

7 Gronboek Moller P, Nedergaard T *et al.* Primary cutaneous B-cell lymphoma: a clinical, histological, phenotypic and genotypic study of 21 cases. *Br J Dermatol* 2000; **142**: 913–23.

8 Cerroni L, Volkenandt M, Rieger E *et al.* Bcl-2 protein expression and correlation with the interchromosomal 14;18 translocation in cutaneous lymphomas and pseudolymphomas. *J Invest Dermatol* 1994; **102**: 231–5.

9 Kodama K, Massone C, Chott A *et al.* Primary cutaneous large B-cell lymphomas: clinicopathologic features, classification, and prognostic factors in a large series of patients. *Blood* 2005; **106**: 2491–7.

10 Senff N, Hoefnagel J, Jansen P *et al.* Reclassification of 300 primary cutaneous B-cell lymphomas according to the new WHO-EORTC classification for cutaneous lymphomas: comparison with previous classifications and identification of prognostic markers. *J Clin Oncol* 2007; **25**: 1581–7.

11 Child F, Woolford A, Calonje E *et al.* Molecular analysis of the immunoglobulin heavy chain gene in the diagnosis of primary cutaneous B-cell lymphoma. *J Invest Dermatol* 2001; **117**: 984–9.

12 Aarts W, Willemze R, Bende R *et al.* VH gene analysis of primary cutaneous B-cell lymphomas: evidence for ongoing somatic hypermutation and isotype switching. *Blood* 1998; **92**: 3857–64.

13 Gellrich S, Rutz S, Golembowski S *et al.* Primary cutaneous follicle center cell lymphomas and large B-cell lymphomas of the leg descend from germinal center cells: a single cell polymerase chain reaction analysis. *J Invest Dermatol* 2001; **117**: 1512–20.

14 Storz M, van de Rijn M, Kim Y *et al.* Gene expression profiles of cutaneous B-cell lymphoma. *J Invest Dermatol* 2003; **120**: 865–70.

15 Hoefnagel J, Dijkman R, Basso K *et al.* Distinct types of primary cutaneous large B-cell lymphoma identified by gene expression profiling. *Blood* 2005; **105**: 3671–8.

16 Child F, Russell Jones R, Woolford A, Whittaker S. Absence of the t(14;18) chromosomal translocation in primary cutaneous B-cell lymphoma. *Br J Dermatol* 2001; **144**: 735–44.

17 Goodlad J, Krajewski A, Batstone P *et al.* Primary cutaneous follicular lymphoma; a clinicopathologic and molecular study of 16 cases in support of a distinct entity. *Am J Surg Pathol* 2002; **26**: 733–41.

18 Mirza I, Macpherson N, Paproski R *et al.* Primary cutaneous follicular lymphoma: an assessment of clinical, histopathologic, immunophenotypic, and molecular features. *J Clin Oncol* 2002; **20**: 647–55.

19 Bergman R, Kurtin P, Gibson L *et al.* Clinicopathologic, immunophenotypic and molecular characterization of primary cutaneous B-cell lymphoma. *Arch Dermatol* 2001; **137**: 432–9.

20 Yang B, Tubbs R, Finn W *et al.* Clinicopathologic reassessment of primary cutaneous B-cell lymphomas with immunophenotypic and molecular genetic characterization. *Am J Surg Pathol* 2000; **24**: 694–702.

21 Streubel B, Scheucher B, Valencak J *et al.* Molecular cytogenetic evidence of t(14;18)(IGH;BCL2) in a substantial proportion of primary cutaneous follicle center lymphomas. *Am J Surg Pathol* 2006; **30**: 529–36.

22 Mao X, Lillington D, Child F *et al.* Comparative genomic hybridization analysis of primary cutaneous B-cell lymphoma: identification of common genetic alterations in disease pathogenesis. *Genes Chrom Cancer* 2002; **35**: 144–55.

23 Dijkman R, Tensen C, Jordanova E *et al.* Array based comparative hybridization analysis reveals recurrent chromosomal alterations and prognostic parameters in primary cutaneous large B-cell lymphomas. *J Clin Oncol* 2006; **24**: 296–305.

24 Hallerman C, Kaune K, Gesk S *et al.* Molecular cytogenetic analysis of chromosomal breakpoints in the IGH, MYC, BCL6 and MALT1 gene loci in primary cutaneous B-cell lymphomas. *J Invest Dermatol* 2004; **123**: 213–9.

25 Child F, Scarisbrick J, Calonje E *et al.* Inactivation of tumour suppressor genes *p15* (INK4b) and *p16* (INK4a) in primary cutaneous B cell lymphoma. *J Invest Dermatol* 2002; **118**: 941–8.

26 Dijkman R, Tensen C, Buettner M *et al.* Primary cutaneous follicle center lymphoma and primary cutaneous large B-cell lymphoma, leg type, are both targeted by aberrant somatic hypermutation but demonstrate differential expression of AID. *Blood* 2006; **107**: 4926–9.

27 Rijlaarsdam J, Toonstra J, Meijer C *et al.* Treatment of primary cutaneous B-cell lymphomas of follicle centre cell origin: a clinical follow-up study of 55 patients treated with radiotherapy or chemotherapy. *J Clin Oncol* 1996; **14**: 549–55.

28 Santucci M, Pimpinelli N, Arganini L. Primary cutaneous B-cell lymphoma: a unique type of low grade lymphoma—clinicopathologic and immunologic study of 83 cases. *Cancer* 1991; **67**: 2311–26.

29 Bekkenk M, Vermeer M, Geerts M *et al.* Treatment of multifocal primary cutaneous B-cell lymphoma: a clinical follow-up study of 29 patients. *J Clin Oncol* 1999; **17**: 2471–8.

30 Senff N, Hoefnagel J, Nelis K *et al.* Results of radiotherapy in 153 primary cutaneous B-cell lymphomas classified according to the WHO-EORTC classification. *Arch Dermatol* 2007; **143**: 1520–6.

31 Senff N, Noordijk E, Kim Y *et al.* European Organization for Research and Treatment of Cancer and International Society for Cutaneous Lymphoma consensus recommendations for the management of cutaneous B-cell lymphomas. *Blood* 2008; **112**: 1600–9.

Diffuse large B-cell lymphoma

Definition. Primary cutaneous diffuse large B-cell lymphoma (PCLBCL) is a rare primary cutaneous lymphoma characterized by a diffuse proliferation of large B cells consisting of centroblasts and immunoblasts occurring most commonly on the leg [1]. PCLBCL is closely related to systemic nodal diffuse large B-cell lymphomas, which is the most common form of non-Hodgkin's lymphoma.

Clinical features. PCLBCL affects an elderly population with a female predominance. These lymphomas tend to develop on the lower limbs, predominantly as large dermal nodules or tumours, which are either solitary or multifocal and rapidly enlarging (Fig. 57.39) [1]. PCLBCL can also rarely occur at other cutaneous sites (PCLBCL/other) [2]. Full staging investigations are critical to exclude systemic involvement. The prognosis of PCLBCL is poor, with a 5-year survival of 41–58% [1–4].

Pathology. There is a diffuse non-epidermotropic infiltrate of large cells with morphological similarity to centroblasts and immunoblasts which may extend to involve the subcutis (Fig. 57.40). The infiltrate is monotonous with relatively few associated inflammatory cells or reactive T-cells present. Germinal centres

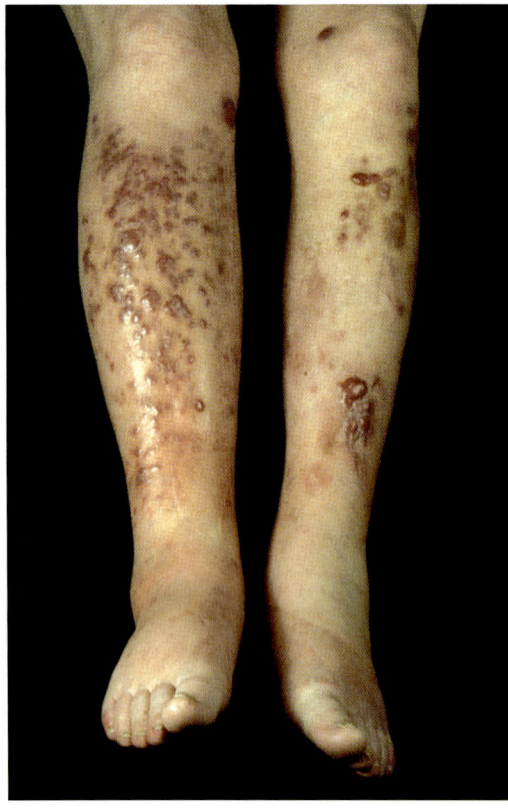
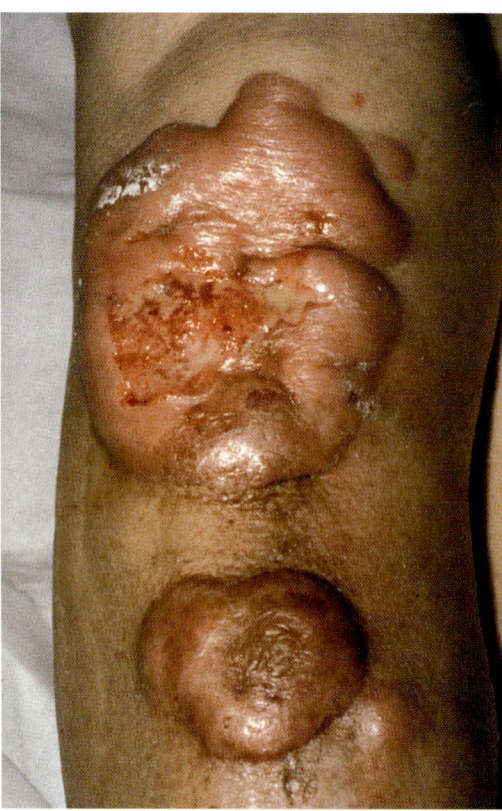

Fig. 57.39 Clinical presentation of primary cutaneous large B-cell lymphoma on the legs.

are not apparent and mitoses are prominent. Morphological variants recognized in cutaneous disease include cleaved and round cell types but the reproducibility of this distinction is poor [3]. Initially it was reported that the presence of round cell morphology was an adverse prognostic feature. However, this may be explained by subsequent recognition that the cleaved cell type, showing a predominance of large centrocytes and multilobated cells, with few exceptions represents diffuse PCFCL (Crosti's lymphoma) [2].

Immunophenotype. The tumour cells are CD19+, CD20+, CD22+ and CD79a+ with monotypic expression of surface and/or cytoplasmic immunoglobulin in some cases [2,5]. Tumour cells are usually strongly Bcl-2 positive [5,6] and Bcl-6 is also expressed by most cases with evidence of *Bcl-6* gene mutations [5,7]. CD10 expression is only rarely detected in PCLBCL [5]. *MUM-1* and *FOX-P1* are invariably expressed by tumour cells in PCLBCL in contrast to PCFCL [8].

Pathogenesis. Although PCLBCL by definition arises *de novo* in the skin, some tumours might result from high-grade transformation of a low-grade primary cutaneous B-cell lymphoma such as PCFCL [9]. At present, it is unclear whether PCLBCL has the same pathogenesis as primary nodal DLBCL. When PCLBCL presents at sites other than the leg, it is important to distinguish this from diffuse forms of PCFCL, because PCFCL has an excellent prognosis [9].

Clonal rearrangements of immunoglobulin genes are present in most cases with false-negative results resulting from somatic

hypermutation [10]. No disease-specific cytogenetic abnormalities have been identified. The t(14;18) translocation has not been identified in Bcl-2 positive cutaneous cases [11–14], except in rare cases from one series [15], The t(14;18) is a common feature of nodal DLBCL reflecting a likely transformation from nodal follicular lymphoma and is found in nodal DLBCL with secondary cutaneous involvement [12]. Unlike PCFCL and PCMZL, 6q losses and 2p, 12 and 18q gains are characteristic findings in PCLBCL and chromosomal amplification of the *bcl2* gene may account for bcl-2 overexpression in PCLBCL [15–17]. In addition, inactivation of *p15* and *p16* genes by promotor hypermethylation and deletion of the 9p21.3 locus containing the *p14/16* genes has been detected [17,18] and CGH studies have identified specific oncogene abnormalities including *c-REL* and *MALT1* gene amplification [16,17]. Recent studies suggest that *p16* loss may have prognostic significance [19]. Studies (Table 57.9) have also shown rare translocations involving *myc* and IgH in PCLBCL in contrast to PCFCL [14,15]. *BCL6* rearrangements have not been detected in PCLBCL [15] but mutations of the *BCL6* gene have been detected [7] and this provides an alternative explanation for over-expression of Bcl-6.

Recent studies in nodal DLBCL using microarray technology have confirmed that these tumours are heterogeneous in origin with the detection of three distinct gene expression profiles which also have prognostic significance: one characteristic of germinal centre cells; one with an expression profile consistent with activated peripheral blood B cells; and one with an indeterminate profile [20,21]. Studies have shown that PCLBCL has an origin from activated B-cells compared to PCFCL which show a germinal centre B-cell gene expression profile [22].

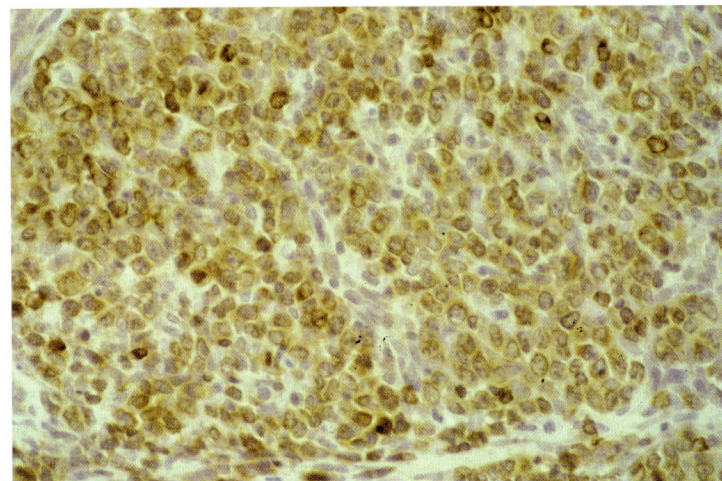

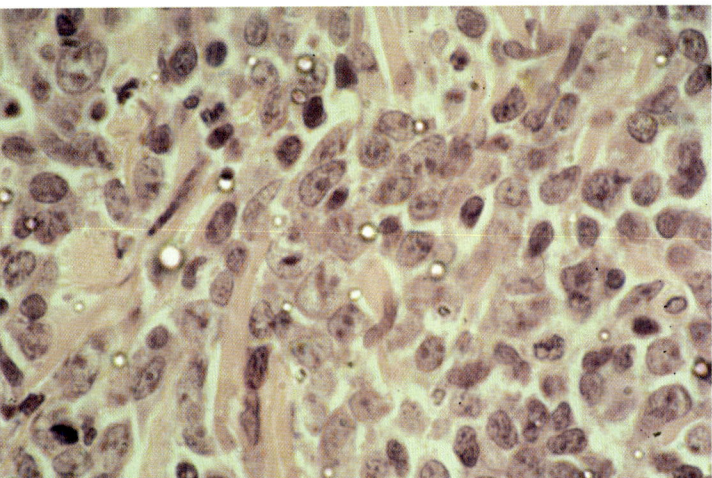

Fig. 57.40 Primary cutaneous large B-cell lymphoma showing a diffuse pattern of large mononuclear cells and strong Bcl-2 positivity.

Prognosis. The prognosis for PCLBCL is poor, with a 41–58% 5-year survival, but this is generally better than for nodal DLBCL [1–4]. Although studies initially suggested that *Bcl-2* expression was site-related (lower limbs and multifocal lesions are more frequently Bcl-2 positive) and associated with a worse prognosis [3], the prognostic significance of *Bcl-2* expression has since been disputed [23]. Recent studies have shown that multifocal disease and location on the leg, are associated with a worse prognosis in multivariate analysis [2,4,8].

Treatment. In elderly patients with solitary tumours, radiotherapy may be appropriate but multiagent chemotherapy is usually required, especially for multifocal disease [24,25,26]. The role of rituximab (a chimeric mouse/human anti-CD20 antibody which induces antibody-dependent cytotoxicity) as a single agent in cutaneous disease has yet to be determined [27,28], but CHOP chemotherapy (R-CHOP) is now the standard of care in nodal DLBCL and an appropriate consideration for patients with PCLBCL. Intralesional rituximab may prove to be effective for selected patients in whom radiotherapy or R-CHOP is not possible [29].

References

1 Vermeer MH, Geelen FAMJ, van Haselen CW *et al.* Primary cutaneous large B-cell lymphomas of the legs. *Arch Dermatol* 1996; **132**: 1304–8.

2 Willemze R, Jaffe E, Burg G *et al.* WHO-EORTC classification for cutaneous lymphomas. *Blood* 2005; **105**: 3768–85.

3 Grange F, Bekkenk M, Wechsler J *et al.* Prognostic factors in primary cutaneous large B-cell lymphomas: a European multicenter study. *J Clin Oncol* 2001; **19**: 3602–10.

4 Grange F, Beylot-Barry M, Courville P *et al.* Primary cutaneous diffuse large B-cell lymphoma, leg type. *Arch Dermatol* 2007; **143**: 1144–50.

5 Yang B, Tubbs R, Finn W *et al.* Clinicopathologic reassessment of primary cutaneous B-cell lymphomas with immunophenotypic and molecular genetic characterization. *Am J Surg Pathol* 2000; **24**: 694–702.

6 Geelen F, Vermeer M, Meijer C *et al.* Bcl-2 protein expression in primary cutaneous large B-cell lymphoma is site related. *J Clin Oncol* 1998; **16**: 2080–5.

7 Paulli M, Viglio A, Vivenza D *et al.* Primary cutaneous large B-cell lymphoma of the leg: histogenetic analysis of a controversial clinicopathologic entity. *Hum Pathol* 2002; **33**: 937–43.

8 Kodama K, Massone C, Chott A *et al.* Primary cutaneous large B-cell lymphomas: clinicopathologic features, classification, and prognostic factors in a large series of patients. *Blood* 2005; **106**: 2491–7.

9 Willemze R, Meijer CJLM, Sentis HJ *et al.* Primary cutaneous large cell lymphomas of follicular center cell origin. *J Am Acad Dermatol* 1997; **16**: 518–26.

10 Child F, Woolford A, Calonje E *et al.* Molecular analysis of the immunoglobulin heavy chain gene in the diagnosis of primary cutaneous B-cell lymphoma. *J Invest Dermatol* 2001; **117**: 984–9.

11 Child F, Russell Jones R, Woolford A, Whittaker S. Absence of the t(14;18) chromosomal translocation in primary cutaneous B-cell lymphoma. *Br J Dermatol* 2001; **144**: 735–44.

12 Kim B, Surti U, Pandya A, Swerdlow S. Primary and secondary cutaneous diffuse large B-cell lymphomas. *Am J Surg Pathol* 2003; **27**: 356–64.

13 Hallerman C, Kaune K, Siebert R *et al.* Chromosomal aberration patterns differ in subtypes of primary cutaneous B-cell lymphomas. *J Invest Dermatol* 2004; **122**: 1495–502.

14 Hallerman C, Kaune K, Gesk S *et al.* Molecular cytogenetic analysis of chromosomal breakpoints in the IGH, MYC, BCL6 and MALT1 gene loci in primary cutaneous B-cell lymphomas. *J Invest Dermatol* 2004; **123**: 213–9.

15 Wiesner T, Streubel B, Huber D, Kerl H, Chott A, Cerroni L. Genetic aberrations in primary cutaneous large B-cell lymphoma. *Am J Surg Pathol* 2005; **29**: 666–73.

16 Mao X, Lillington D, Child F *et al.* Comparative genomic hybridization analysis of primary cutaneous B-cell lymphoma: identification of common genetic alterations in disease pathogenesis. *Genes Chromosomes Cancer* 2002; **35**: 144–55.

17 Dijkman R, Tensen C, Jordanova E *et al.* Array based comparative genomic hybridisation analysis reveals recurrent chromosomal alterations and prognostic parameters in primary cutaneous large B-cell lymphoma. *J Clin Oncol* 2006; **24**: 296–305.

18 Child F, Scarisbrick J, Calonje E *et al.* Inactivation of tumour suppressor genes *p15* and *p16* in primary cutaneous B-cell lymphoma. *J Invest Dermatol* 2002; **118**: 941–8.

19 Senff NJ, Zoutman WH, Vermeer MH *et al.* Fine-mapping chromosomal loss at 9p21: correlation with prognosis in primary cutaneous diffuse large B-cell lymphoma, leg type. *J Invest Dermatol* 2009; **129**: 1149–55.

20 Rosenwald A, Wright G, Chan W *et al.* The use of molecular profiling to predict survival after chemotherapy for diffuse large B-cell lymphoma. *N Engl J Med* 2002; **346**: 1937–47.

21 Alizadeh A, Eisen M, Davis R *et al.* Distinct types of diffuse large B-cell lymphoma identified by gene expression profiling. *Nature* 2000; **403**: 503–11.

22 Hoefnagel J, Dijkman R, Basso K *et al.* Distinct types of primary cutaneous large B-cell lymphoma identified by gene expression profiling. *Blood* 2005; **105**: 3671–8.

23 Fernadez-Vazquez A, Rodriguez-Peralto J, Martinez M *et al.* Primary cutaneous large B-cell lymphoma: the relation between morphology, clinical presentation, immunohistochemical markers and survival. *Am J Surg Pathol* 2001; **25**: 307–15.

24 Brice P, Cazals D, Mounier N *et al.* Primary cutaneous large-cell lymphoma: analysis of 49 patients included in the LNH87 prospective trial of polychemotherapy for high-grade lymphomas. *Leukaemia* 1998; **12**: 213–9.

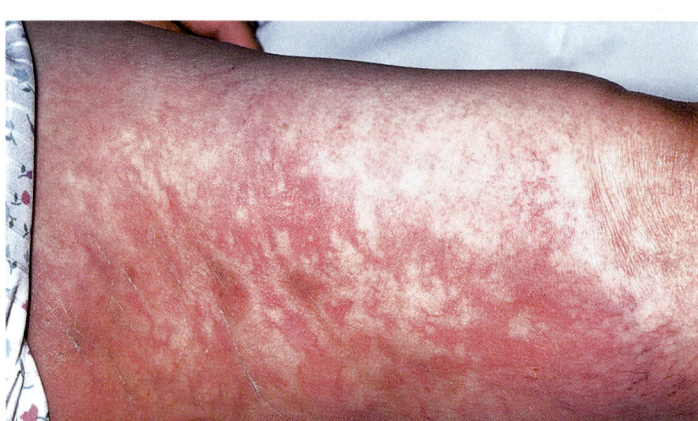

Fig. 57.41 Clinical illustration of histology illustrated in Fig. 57.42. Note marbled appearance of inner thigh which was woody hard on palpation. B-cell lymphoma showing lack of epidermotropism and clear grenz zone in the papillary dermis. (Courtesy of R.S. Lever, Western Infirmary, Glasgow, UK.)

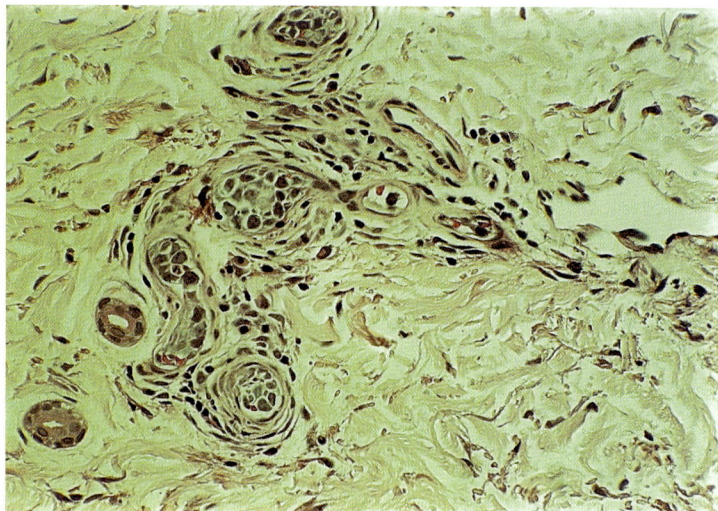

Fig. 57.42 Histology of angiocentric B-cell lymphoma showing B cells within small vascular channels in the dermis. These are stained with membrane markers for B cells, not with membrane markers for endothelial cells.

25 Bekkenk M, Vermeer M, Geerts M *et al.* Treatment of multifocal primary cutaneous B-cell lymphoma: a clinical follow-up study of 29 patients. *J Clin Oncol* 1999; **17**: 2471–8.

26 Senff N, Noordijk E, Kim Y *et al.* European Organization for Research and Treatment of Cancer and International Society for Cutaneous Lymphoma consensus recommendations for the management of cutaneous B-cell lymphomas. *Blood* 2008; **112**: 1600–9.

27 Sabroe R, Child F, Woolford A *et al.* Rituximab in cutaneous B-cell lymphoma: a report of two cases. *Br J Dermatol* 2000; **143**: 157–61.

28 Heinzerling L, Urbanek M, Funk J *et al.* Reduction of tumour burden and stabilization of disease by systemic therapy with anti-CD20 antibody (rituximab) in patients with primary cutaneous B-cell lymphoma. *Cancer* 2000; **89**: 1835–44.

29 Heinzerling L, Dummer R, Kempf W *et al.* Intralesional therapy with anti-CD20 monoclonal antibody rituximab in primary cutaneous B-cell lymphoma. *Arch Dermatol* 2000; **136**: 374–8.

Secondary cutaneous B-cell lymphomas

Intravascular large B-cell lymphoma [1–11]

Synonyms
- Malignant angioendotheliomatosis
- Angiotrophic lymphoma

Definition. A rare extranodal B-cell lymphoma characterized by accumulation of large B cells within small blood vessels. This tumour usually involves multiple extranodal sites including the CNS, lung and skin, and symptoms and/or signs at these sites may be the presenting feature.

Clinical features. Patients present with diffuse, tender, hard, infiltrated plaques, commonly on the thigh (Fig. 57.41); the clinical appearance may suggest a sclerotic connective tissue disorder or panniculitis. A variety of clinical features may occur as a consequence of occlusion of small vessels including telangiectatic skin lesions. Colonization of benign haemangiomas by tumour cells has been reported. The prognosis is poor, although rare cases with

disease confined to the skin may have a better outlook with a 3-year survival of 56% versus 22% if spread beyond the skin.

Pathology. The tumour cells are large and show striking atypia with an occasional anaplastic morphology. These cells are situated entirely within dilated vessel lumina in the dermis and subcutis (Fig. 57.42). Occlusion of vessels by tumour cells and fibrin thrombi may be present.

Immunophenotype. The tumour cells are positive for B-cell-associated antigens consistent with origin from a peripheral post-germinal centre B cell. Clonal immunoglobulin gene rearrangements are present. Rare cases are derived from T cells and show a clonal TCR gene rearrangement. Rarely, factor VIII, an endothelial cell-related antigen, may be positive but this is thought to be caused by absorption of antigen by tumour cells rather than indicating an endothelial cell origin.

Treatment. There are some reports of partial response to combination chemotherapy, but the disease has a poor prognosis and is usually fatal.

References

1 Berger TG, Dawson NA. Angioendotheliomatosis. *J Am Acad Dermatol* 1988; **18**: 407–12.

2 Dominguez FE, Rosen LB, Kramer HC. Malignant angioendotheliomatosis proliferans. *Am J Dermatopathol* 1986; **8**: 419–25.

3 Perniciaro C, Winkelmann RK, Daoud MS, Su WPD. Malignant angioendotheliomatosis is an angiotropic intravascular lymphoma. *Am J Dermatol* 1995; **17**: 242–8.

4 Petroff N, Koger OW, Fleming MG *et al.* Malignant angioendotheliomatosis: an angiotropic lymphoma. *J Am Acad Dermatol* 1989; **21**: 727–33.

5 Wick MR, Rocamora A. Reactive and malignant 'angioendotheliomatosis': a discriminant clinicopathological study. *J Cutan Pathol* 1988; **15**: 260–1.

6 Willemze R, Kruyswijk MRJ, De Bruin CD *et al.* Angiotropic (intravascular) large cell lymphoma of the skin previously classified as malignant angioendotheliomatosis. *Br J Dermatol* 1987; **116**: 393–9.

7 Braverman IM, Lerner AB. Diffuse malignant proliferation of vascular endothelium. *Arch Dermatol* 1961; **84**: 72–80.

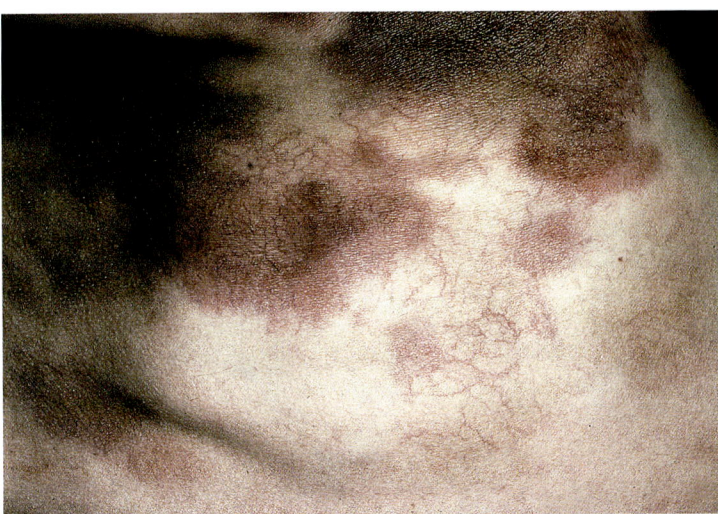

Fig. 57.43 Clinical features of lymphomatoid granulomatosis showing extensive purpuric, bruise-like lesions on the trunk.

8 Eros N, Karolyi Z, Kovacs A *et al.* Intravascular B-cell lymphoma. *J Am Acad Dermatol* 2002; **47**: S260–2.
9 Ferreri A, Campo E, Seymour J *et al.* Intravascular lymphoma: clinical presentation, natural history and prognostic factors in a series of 38 cases with special emphasis on the 'cutaneous variant'. *Br J Haematol* 2004; **127**: 173–83.
10 Rubin M, Cossman J, Freter C, Azumi N. Intravascular large cell lymphoma coexisting within hemangiomas of the skin. *Am J Surg Pathol* 1997; **21**: 860–4.
11 Kobayashi T, Munakata S, Sugiura H *et al.* Angiotropic lymphoma: proliferation of B-cells in the capillaries of cutaneous angiomas. *Br J Dermatol* 2000; **143**: 162–4.

Lymphomatoid granulomatosis

Definition. An angiocentric and angiodestructive extranodal EBV-positive B-cell lymphoma, which invariably involves the lungs and may involve the skin and CNS [1–3].

Clinical features. Patients most frequently present with pulmonary symptoms associated with systemic malaise, arthralgias, weight loss and fever. The skin (50% of cases), CNS and kidneys are also often directly involved. The cutaneous lesions described are diverse but include subcutaneous nodules and plaques, more superficial plaques and a diffuse erythematous maculopapular eruption (Fig. 57.43) with epidermal atrophy and purpura [4–10]. Necrosis and ulceration may also occur [4]. Some patients have a fluctuating course with spontaneous remissions but eventually progressive disease develops.

Pathology. The striking feature is the angiocentricity of the infiltrate and gross vessel destruction sometimes accompanied by fibrinoid necrosis (angiodestruction) [7]. The infiltrate is polymorphous and contains both lymphocytes and histiocytes with pleomorphic or large (immunoblast-like) tumour cells and often a prominent reactive T-cell infiltrate. Multinucleated cells may be present although well-formed granulomas are rare. The presence of large transformed cells is associated with a worse prognosis.

Immunophenotype. The tumour cells are EBV$^+$, express CD20 and are variably CD79a$^+$. CD30 may be expressed but the cells are CD15$^-$. The reactive T cells are CD3$^+$ and CD4$^+$. Clonal immunoglobulin gene rearrangements can be detected in most cases and Southern blot analysis usually confirms the presence of clonal episomal EBV [8].

Pathogenesis. Lymphomatoid granulomatosis is an EBV-driven lymphoproliferative disorder that can be associated with immunodeficiency states including post-transplantation and long-term therapies such as methotrexate for rheumatoid arthritis [9,10]. This lymphoma should be distinguished from extranodal NK/T-cell lymphoma (nasal type), which is also EBV$^+$ and characterized by an angiodestructive histology [8].

Treatment. Although some patients have spontaneous remissions, the development of high-grade disease is associated with a median survival of less than 2 years. Short-lived remissions with high-dose chemotherapy have been described. There are reports of responses to cyclophosphamide and IFN-α, particularly for patients with low-grade disease [11].

References
1 Liebow AA, Carrington CRB, Friedman PJ. Lymphomatoid granulomatosis. *Hum Pathol* 1972; **3**: 457–558.
2 Katzenstein A-LA, Carrington CB, Liebow AA. Lymphomatoid granulomatosis: a clinicopathologic study of 152 cases. *Cancer* 1979; **43**: 360–73.
3 Lee SC, Roth LM, Brashear RE. Lymphomatoid granulomatosis. *Cancer* 1976; **38**: 846–53.
4 Minars N, Kay S, Escobar MR. Lymphomatoid granulomatosis: a new clinicopathologic entity. *Arch Dermatol* 1975; **111**: 493–6.
5 Macdonald DM, Sarkany I. Lymphomatoid granulomatosis. *Clin Exp Dermatol* 1976; **1**: 163–73.
6 Jambrosic J, From L, Assaad DA *et al.* Lymphomatoid granulomatosis. *J Am Acad Dermatol* 1987; **17**: 621–31.
7 Madison Mcniff J, Cooper D, Howe G *et al.* Lymphomatoid granulomatosis of the skin and lung. *Arch Dermatol* 1996; **132**: 1464–70.
8 Harris N, Jaffe E, Diebold J *et al.* The World Health Organization classification of neoplastic disease of the haematopoietic and lymphoid tissues: report of the clinical advisory committee. *Histopathology* 2000; **36**: 69–87.
9 Kwon E, Katz K, Draft K *et al.* Posttransplantation lymphoproliferative disease with features of lymphomatoid granulomatosis in a lung transplant patient. *J Am Acad Dermatol* 2006; **54**: 657–63.
10 Beaty M, Toro J, Sorbara L *et al.* Cutaneous lymphomatoid granulomatosis: correlation of clinical and biologic features. *Am J Surg Pathol* 2001; **25**: 111–20.
11 Fauci AS, Haynes B, Costa J *et al.* Lymphomatoid granulomatosis; prospective clinical trial and therapeutic experience over 10 years. *N Engl J Med* 1982; **306**: 68–74.

Secondary cutaneous T-cell lymphomas

Angioimmunoblastic T-cell lymphoma

Synonym
• Angioimmunoblastic lymphadenopathy (AILD)

Definition. AILD is a nodal T-cell lymphoma derived from follicular helper T-cells and associated with a complex dysregulation of B-cells [1]. Extranodal involvement of sites, including skin, is well recognized [2].

Clinical features. Patients may present with systemic and/or peripheral lymphadenopathy often accompanied by 'B' symptoms [2]. Splenomegaly occurs in over 50% of cases and many patients will have advanced disease and bone marrow involvement at diagnosis [2]. Autoimmune phenomena are common, including neurological abnormalities, arthritis, hypergammaglobulinaemia, haemolytic anaemia and thrombocytopenic purpura [2]. Cutaneous extranodal involvement is common (45% of cases) and rarely can be a presenting feature [2]. Skin changes are highly variable and can be subtle, including maculopapular and papulonodular eruptions. Erythroderma, haemorrhagic and urticarial eruptions have been described as well as dermal plaques [3]. Occasionally, cutaneous involvement in AILD can mimic drug eruptions and infections [4,5].

Pathology. The nodal pathologic features in AILD are characterized by hyperplastic follicles and a prominent arborizing vascular proliferation with expanded follicular dendritic cells. There is an associated polymorphous infiltrate with clusters of large clear cells [1]. The infiltrate consists of CD10$^+$ T-cells and an expansion of EBV infected B-cells (EBER positive). Cutaneous involvement is characterized by variable features; a non-specific perivascular lymphocytic infiltrate with minimal atypia and capillary hyperplasia can be found in some biopsies or more prominent dermal perivascular infiltrates showing cytologically atypical pleomorphic cells and occasionally more obvious dense infiltrates of atypical lymphocytes are present [6]. Granulomatous infiltrates and vasculitis have been reported [6]. There is no epidermotropism. The atypical cells express T-cell antigens and are also CD10$^+$ [3].

Pathogenesis. Clonal rearrangements of TCR genes are detected in a majority of cases but additional monoclonal or oligoclonal IgH rearrangements are often found consistent with the characteristic EBV$^+$ B-cell proliferation seen in lymph nodes from AILD patients [1]. The recent finding of *CXCL13* expression by tumour cells in AILD has confirmed a derivation from follicular helper T cells [1]. Specific patterns of chromosomal abnormalities, including deletions of chromosome 7, have been reported but no disease-specific translocations [1].

Treatment. The disease can be indolent but transformation is associated with a poor prognosis. Immunomodulatory therapies have been used successfully including ciclosporin, steroids, thalidomide and angiogenesis inhibitors such as bevacizumab [1].

References

1 Dunleavy K, Wilson W, Jaffe E. Angioimmunoblastic T-cell lymphoma: pathobiological insights and clinical implications. *Curr Opin Haematol* 2007; **14**: 348–53.
2 Lachenal F, Berger F, Ghesquieres H *et al*. Angioimmunoblastic T-cell lymphoma. Clinical and laboratory features at diagnosis in 77 patients. *Medicine* 2007; **86**: 282–92.
3 Huang C, Chuang S. Angioimmunoblastic T-cell lymphoma with cutaneous involvement. *Arch Pathol Lab Med* 2004; **128**: 122–4.
4 Yoon G, Chang S, Kim H *et al*. Cutaneous relapse of angioimmunoblastic lymphadenopathy-type peripheral T-cell lymphoma mimicking an exanthematous drug eruption. *Int J Dermatol* 2003; **42**: 816–8.
5 Jayaraman A, Cassarino D, Advani R *et al*. Cutaneous involvement by angioimmunoblastic T-cell lymphoma: a unique histologic presentation mimicking an infectious etiology. *J Cutan Pathol* 2006; **33** (Suppl): 6–11.
6 Martel P, Laroche L, Courville P *et al*. Cutaneous involvement in patients with angioimmunoblastic lymphadenopathy with dysproteinemia: a clinical, immunohistological and molecular analysis. *Arch Dermatol* 2000; **136**: 881–6.

Post-transplant lymphoproliferative disorder (PTLD)

Definition. Lymphomas occurring in solid organ transplant recipients on immunosuppressive therapy. The incidence varies according to the organ transplanted (heart–lung : renal transplant rates of 10–1% respectively) and although extranodal lymphomas are overrepresented in PTLD, primary cutaneous involvement is very rare. Less than 20 cases have been reported of primary cutaneous B-cell PTLD and primary cutaneous T-cell PTLD is even less frequent [1–2].

Clinical features. The clinical features described are diverse; solitary or multiple plaques, nodules or tumours, with or without ulceration, have been described affecting any site. Systemic involvement and in particular involvement of the transplanted organ must be excluded in patients with primary cutaneous PTLD. Spontaneous resolution has been reported. For primary cutaneous T-cell PTLD, erythroderma is the most common clinical presentation but all types of CTCL have been described [3].

Pathology. Diffuse dermal infiltrates extending to the subcutis and consisting of large pleomorphic lymphocytes or centroblasts. Plasmacytoid differentiation and plasmablasts may be a feature. Necrosis may be present. For PC B-cell PTLD the tumour cells express B-cell antigens while PC T-cell PTLD may be CD30$^+$ but histological features mimicking all types of CTCL have been described [2,3].

Pathogenesis. B-cell PTLD is associated with EBV infection and progression from an early reactive phase can be identified. Three distinct types of PTLD are recognized: (i) plasmacytic hyperplasia is a polyclonal proliferation associated with multiple copies of EBV and occurring early after transplantation; (ii) polymorphic lymphoproliferative disorder usually occurring several years after transplantation is a monoclonal EBV proliferation with a single copy of EBV but without secondary genomic abnormalities; and (iii) malignant lymphoma is a monoclonal EBV infection with a single copy of EBV and associated secondary genomic abnormalities and widespread disease. Rare cases of PC B-cell PTLD have been associated with HHV-8 infection [4]. No viral association has been described for systemic or cutaneous T-cell PTLD although rare EBV$^+$ T-cell lymphomas have been reported. Primary cutaneous presentations can also occur in non-organ transplant recipients such as HIV$^+$ patients or those with other forms of profound immunodeficiency. Similarly EBV$^+$ lymphoproliferative disorders can develop in patients who have undergone high-dose chemotherapy for primary lymphomas although cutaneous involvement has not been reported as yet in this context.

Treatment. While surgery and radiotherapy can be used, reduction in immunosuppression is often effective [5]. Both chemotherapy and rituximab have been reported to be effective. While the prognosis for B-cell PTLD is generally good [6], both primary cutaneous and systemic T-cell PTLD have a very poor prognosis.

References

1 Blokx W, Andriessen M, Hamersvelt H, van Krieken J. Initial spontaneous regression of posttransplantation Epstein Barr virus-related B-cell lymphoproliferative disorder of the skin in a renal transplant recipient. *Am J Dermatopathol* 2002; **24**: 414–22.

2 Lok C, Viseux V, Denoeux J, Bagot M. Post-transplant cutaneous T-cell lymphomas. *Crit Rev Oncol/Haematol* 2005; **56**: 137–45.

3 Ravat F, Spittle M, Russell Jones R. Primary cutaneous T-cell lymphoma occuring after organ transplantation. *J Am Acad Dermatol* 2006; **54**: 668–75.

4 Verma S, Nuovo J, Porcu P *et al*. Epstein-Barr virus and human herpesvirus 8-associated primary cutaneous plasmablastic lymphoma in the setting of renal transplantation. *J Cutan Pathol* 2005; **32**: 35–9.

5 Mohsin N, Budruddin M, Kamble P *et al*. Complete regression of cutaneous B-cell lymphoma in a renal transplant patient after conversion from cyclosporin to sirolimus. *Transplant Proc* 2007; **39**: 1267–71.

6 McGregor J, Carmen C, Lu Q *et al*. Post-transplant cutaneous lymphoma. *J Am Acad Dermatol* 1993; **29**: 549–54.

Pseudolymphomas

Definition. Benign but persistent lymphoid proliferations in the dermis, which may be difficult to distinguish from a low-grade malignant lymphoma and possibly may rarely transform to a lymphoma in some cases [1–3]. The term cutaneous lymphoid hyperplasia has been suggested and both terms are more commonly used to describe a pathological rather than a clinical appearance. Confusion between pseudolymphoma and lymphoma can easily arise if a biopsy is submitted to the pathologist without an adequate history of recent events such as drug ingestion or scabies infestation.

Aetiology. T-cell pseudolymphomas may arise as a form of adverse drug reaction. The range of drugs causing T-cell pseudolymphomas is wide but includes anticonvulsants, angiotensin-converting enzyme inhibitors, β-blockers, cytotoxics, antirheumatics, antibiotics, antidepressants and many others [4–8]. Persistent contact dermatitis may produce a T-cell pseudolymphoma [9]. Persistent nodular scabies and arthropod bites may also cause a T-cell pseudolymphomatous histology [10], possibly caused by retained foreign material stimulating a persistent antigenic reaction [11,12]. There are three reports in the literature of putative CTCL arising in association with silicone breast implants, which may be examples of this phenomenon [13]. Actinic reticuloid (see below) may resemble a cutaneous T-cell lymphoma histologically. Jessner's lymphocytic infiltrate (see below) can also be classified as a T-cell pseudolymphoma, although there is a view that it is a variant of cutaneous lupus erythematosus.

B-cell pseudolymphomas may arise in the course of Lyme disease with *Borrelia burgdorferi* infection [14], in tattoos as a reaction to certain pigments [15,16], after vaccination and trauma [17], acupuncture [18] and within scars after herpes zoster infection

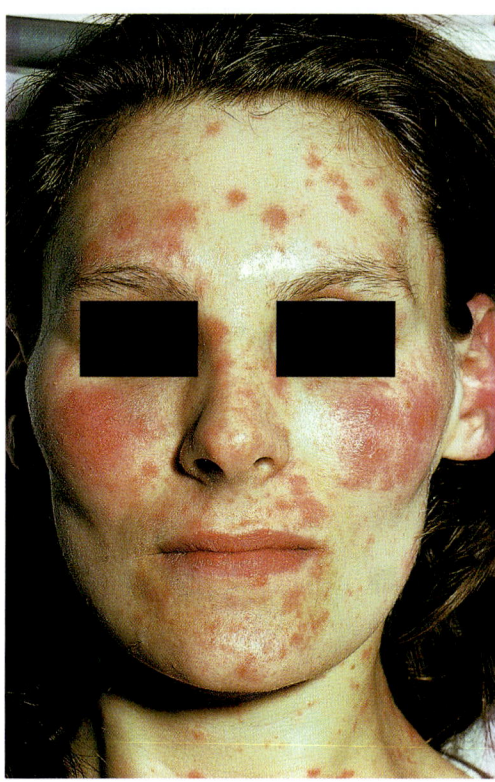

Fig. 57.44 Clinical appearance of a persistent photosensitive drug eruption induced by co-trimoxazole (Septrin).

[19]. The classic entity of lymphocytoma cutis histologically resembles a B-cell pseudolymphoma, and is at present of unknown aetiology.

It is generally wise to be guarded in the diagnosis and prognosis of pseudolymphoma, as in a number of cases clear progression from apparent pseudolymphoma to malignant lymphoma has been recorded. This appears to confirm the concept that chronic, initially benign, reactive inflammatory conditions may very rarely progress to frank lymphoma or that indeed these conditions may be low grade lymphomas initially which then transform and adopt a more obvious malignant cellular cytology/morphology.

Clinical features. Both T- and B-cell pseudolymphomas may present as multiple cutaneous nodules (Fig. 57.44) as in persistent nodular scabies or lymphocytoma cutis. T-cell pseudolymphomas may also present as persistent erythema sometimes developing into an exfoliative erythroderma [20]. This is characteristic of T-cell pseudolymphomas caused by drug reactions or contact dermatitis. B-cell pseudolymphomas may also be associated with palpable lymphadenopathy, adding to diagnostic confusion.

Pathology [21–26]. If the distinction between lymphoma and pseudolymphoma is to be made, it is vital to give the pathologist a good clinical history as the pathological, phenotypic and molecular differentiation is not absolute. The salient feature of a pseudolymphoma is the presence of T- or B-cell lymphoid proliferations. A few mitotic figures may be present, but the degree of cytologic atypia is minimal. T-cell pseudolymphomas may be band-like or nodular in distribution, whereas B-cell pseudolymphomas are usually nodular. Germinal centre formation may or may not be present in B-cell pseudolymphomas but typically reactive germinal centres have tingible body macrophages. Rarely, the lymphoid cells may be very bizarre and resemble mitogen-stimulated lymphocytes seen *in vitro* during the lymphocyte-transformation test [27]. In general, T-cell pseudolymphomas do not show significant epidermotropism such as Pautrier's microabscesses.

Immunophenotypic studies show a normal T-cell phenotype and a mixed κ/λ expression. When germinal centres are present, Bcl-2 is not expressed in B-cell pseudolymphomas [28]. TCR and immunoglobulin gene analysis usually show evidence of a polyclonal proliferation, but rarely a monoclonal pattern has been detected, suggesting a neoplastic proliferation, but the significance of this finding is unclear at present [29–33].

Management. If the diagnosis of pseudolymphoma is considered likely, the presumed cause should be removed if possible. This is probably easiest in the case of an adverse drug reaction, but it may take weeks or even months for the cutaneous reaction to subside. In the cases of persistent nodular scabies or other pseudolymphomas that cause symptomatic itch, application of topical steroids will accelerate clearance.

References

1 Ploysangam T, Breneman DL, Mutasim DF. Cutaneous pseudolymphomas. *J Am Acad Dermatol* 1998; **38**: 877–905.
2 Halevy S, Sandbank M. Transformation of lymphocytoma cutis into malignant lymphoma. *Acta Derm Venereol (Stockh)* 1987; **67**: 172–5.
3 Nakayama H, Mihara M, Shimao S. Malignant transformation of lymphadenosis benigna cutis. *J Dermatol* 1987; **14**: 266–9.
4 Furness PN, Goodfield MJ, Maclennan KA *et al.* Severe cutaneous reactions to captopril and enalapril. *J Clin Pathol* 1986; **39**: 902–7.
5 Henderson CA, Shamy HK. Atenolol induced pseudolymphoma. *Clin Exp Dermatol* 1990; **115**: 119–20.
6 Kaurdan SH, Scheffer E, Vermeer BJ. Drug-induced pseudolymphomatous reactions. *Br J Dermatol* 1988; **188**: 545–52.
7 Souteyrand P, Duncan M. Drug-induced mycosis fungoides-like lesions. *Curr Prob Dermatol* 1990; **19**: 176–82.
8 Nathan DL, Belsito DV. Carbamazepine induced pseudolymphoma with CD30 positive cells. *J Am Acad Dermatol* 1998; **38**: 806–9.
9 Ecker RI, Winkelmann RD. Lymphomatoid contact dermatitis. *Contact Dermatitis* 1981; **7**: 84–93.
10 Walton S, Bottomley WW, Wyatt EH, Bury HPR. Pseudo T-cell lymphoma due to scabies in a patient with Hodgkin's disease. *Br J Dermatol* 1991; **124**: 277–8.
11 Burg G, Dummer R, Kadin M. From inflammation to neoplasia. *Arch Dermatol* 2001; **137**: 949–52.
12 Hermes B, Haas N, Grabbe J, Cznarnetzki B. Foreign body granuloma and IgE-pseudolymphoma after multiple bee stings. *Br J Dermatol* 1994; **130**: 780–4.
13 Duvic M, Moore D, Menter A, Vonderheid EC. Cutaneous T-cell lymphoma in association with silicone breast implants. *J Am Acad Dermatol* 1995; **32**: 939–42.
14 Garbe C, Stein H, Dienemann D, Orfanos C. *Borrelia burdorferi*-associated cutaneous B-cell lymphoma. *J Am Acad Dermatol* 1991; **24**: 584–90.
15 Blumental G, Okun MR, Ponitch A. Pseudolymphomatous reactions to tattoos. *J Am Acad Dermatol* 1982; **6**: 485–8.
16 Rijlaarsdam J, Bruynzeel D, Vos W *et al.* Immunohistochemical studies of lymphadenosis benigna cutis occurring in a tattoo. *Am J Dermatopathol* 1998; **10**: 518–23.
17 Lanzafame S, Micali G. Cutaneous lymphoid hyperplasia (pseudolymphoma) secondary to vaccination. *Pathologica* 1993; **85**: 555–6.
18 Kim K, Lee M, Choi J *et al.* CD30-positive T-cell rich pseudolymphoma induced by gold acupuncture. *Br J Dermatol* 2002; **146**: 882–4.
19 Roo E, Villegas C, Lopez-Bran E *et al.* Postzoster cutaneous pseudolymphoma. *Arch Dermatol* 1994; **130**: 661–3.
20 Rijlaarsdam JU, Scheffer E, Meier CJLM, Willemze R. Cutaneous pseudo T-cell lymphomas. *Cancer* 1992; **69**: 717–24.
21 Kawada A, Mori S, Hayashi T. Lymphadenosis benigna cutis: pseudomalignant form and its imprint smear cytology. *Dermatologica* 1970; **141**: 339–47.
22 Geerts ML, Kaiserling E. A morphologic study of lymphadenosis benigna cutis. *Dermatologica* 1985; **170**: 121–7.
23 Shelley WB, Wood MG, Wilson JF *et al.* Premalignant lymphoid hyperplasia. *Arch Dermatol* 1981; **117**: 500–3.
24 Evans HL, Winkelmann RK, Banks PM. Differential diagnosis of malignant and benign cutaneous infiltrates. *Cancer* 1979; **44**: 699–717.
25 Burg G, Braun-Falco O, Schmoeckel C. Differentiation between pseudolymphomas and malignant B-cell lymphomas of the skin. In: Goos M, Christophers E, eds. *Lymphoproliferative Diseases of the Skin.* Berlin: Springer-Verlag, 1982: 101–34.
26 van der Putte SCJ, Toonstra J, Felten PC, van Vloten WA. Solitary nonepidermotropic T-cell pseudolymphoma of the skin. *J Am Acad Dermatol* 1986; **14**: 444–53.
27 Bernstein H, Shupack J, Ackerman AB. Cutaneous pseudolymphoma resulting from antigen injections. *Arch Dermatol* 1974; **110**: 756–7.
28 Chimenti S, Cerroni L, Zenahlik P *et al.* The role of MT2 and anti bcl-2 protein antibodies in the differentiation of benign from malignant cutaneous infiltrates of B lymphocytes with germinal centre formation. *J Cutan Pathol* 1996; **23**: 319–22.
29 Wood G, Ngan B, Tung R *et al.* Clonal arrangements of immunoglobulin genes and progression to B-cell lymphoma in cutaneous lymphoid hyperplasia. *Am J Pathol* 1989; **35**: 969–78.
30 Bignon YJ, Souteyrand P. Genotyping of cutaneous T-cell lymphomas and pseudolymphomas. *Curr Probl Dermatol* 1990; **19**: 114–23.
31 Zelickson BD, Peters MS, Muller SA *et al.* T-cell receptor gene rearrangement analysis. *J Am Acad Dermatol* 1991; **25**: 787–96.
32 Weinberg J, Rook A, Lessin S. Molecular diagnosis of lymphocytic infiltrates of the skin. *Arch Dermatol* 1993; **129**: 1491–500.
33 Wood GS. Analysis of clonality in cutaneous T-cell lymphoma and associated diseases. *Ann NY Acad Sci* 2001; **941**: 26–30.

Pityriasis lichenoides [1–8]

Synonym
• Mucha–Habermann disease

Definition. This disorder or group of disorders is difficult to classify. Clinically, pityriasis lichenoides is divided into two main conditions: pityriasis lichenoides chronica (PLC) and pityriasis lichenoides et varioliformis acuta (PLEVA; Mucha–Habermann disease). A third, much rarer and aggressive form, febrile ulceronecrotic Mucha–Habermann disease (FUMHD) also occurs [2,5–7]. Despite their names, the distinction between PLC and PLEVA is based on clinical morphology and histology (see below) rather than the course of the disease [6], as both conditions last for an average of about 18 months with an episodic course.

PLC is the most common type, occurring largely in children and young adults, with a male predominance [9], although a recent large study suggested that PLEVA is the most common pattern in younger children (57% compared with 37% PLC and 6% mixed pattern) [8]. In contrast, in adults there is an approximately equal sex incidence [6,9]. All types are rare in infancy and old age, but PLEVA has been reported at birth [10]. Some patients may have simultaneous lesions of both PLC and PLEVA types, or may have transitional lesions; FUMHD usually occurs in isolation but can evolve from PLC or PLEVA [7]. There is a strong male predominance in FUMHD (about 75%), and most cases occur in the second or third decade of life [6].

References

1 Patel DG, Kihiczak G, Schwartz RA *et al*. Pityriasis lichenoides. *Cutis* 2000; **65**: 17–23.

2 Tsuji T, Kasamatsu M, Yokota M *et al*. Mucha–Habermann disease and its febrile ulceronecrotic variant. *Cutis* 1996; **58**: 123–31.

3 Romani J, Puig L, Fernandez-Figueras MT, de Moragas JM. Pityriasis lichenoides in children: clinicopathologic review of 22 patients. *Pediatr Dermatol* 1998; **15**: 1–6.

4 Gelmetti C, Rigioni C, Alessi E *et al*. Pityriasis lichenoides in children: a long-term follow-up of 89 cases. *J Am Acad Dermatol* 1990; **23**: 473–8.

5 Degos R, Duperrat B, Daniel F. Le parapsoriasis ulcero-necrotique hyperthermique. *Ann Dermatol Syphiligr* 1966; **93**: 481–96.

6 Bowers S, Warshaw EM. Pityriasis lichenoides and its subtypes. *J Am Acad Dermatol* 2006; **55**: 557–72.

7 Khachemoune A, Blyumin ML. Pityriasis lichenoides. Pathophysiology, classification, and treatment. *Am J Clin Dermatol* 2007; **8**: 29–36.

8 Ersoy-Evans S, Greco F, Mancini AJ *et al*. Pityriasis lichenoides in childhood. A retrospective review of 124 patients. *J Am Acad Dermatol* 2007; **56**: 205–10.

9 Wahie S, Hiscutt E, Natarajan S, Taylor A. Pityriasis lichenoides: the differences between children and adults. *Br J Dermatol* 2007; **157**: 941–5.

10 Longley J, Demar L, Feinstein RP *et al*. Clinical and histological features of pityriasis lichenoides et varioliformis acuta in children. *Arch Dermatol* 1987; **123**: 1335–9.

Clinical features [1–10]. The skin eruption is usually the first manifestation of the disease, and generally the only manifestation in PLC, but constitutional symptoms such as fever, headache, malaise and arthralgia may precede and/or accompany the onset of PLEVA.

PLEVA. The eruption develops in crops, and consequently appears polymorphic. The initial lesion is an oedematous pink papule that undergoes central vesiculation and haemorrhagic necrosis, which may be intense. In the vesicular forms [4], the vesicles may be small or so large that the eruption appears frankly bullous. The rate of progression of individual lesions varies greatly, as does the frequency and extent. New lesions may cause irritation or a burning sensation as they appear, but often they are asymptomatic. The trunk, thighs and upper arms, especially the flexor aspects, are chiefly affected, but the eruption may be generalized. Lesions of the palms and soles are less common, and the face and scalp are often spared; erythematous or necrotic lesions of mucous membranes may be present. Lesions heal with scarring, which may be varioliform. PLEVA in pregnancy carries a potential risk of premature labour if there are mucosal lesions in the region of the cervical os [7].

FUMHD. In the acute ulceronecrotic form there is high fever and large necrotic lesions; new crops may continue to develop over many months. About 50–75% of cases occur in adults, with a fulminating course that may even be fatal [2,8–10]. General malaise, weakness, myalgia, neuropsychiatric symptoms and lymphadenopathy occur, with non-specific serological markers of inflammation such as raised ESR and C-reactive protein; there may be serological evidence of associated viral infection.

PLC. The characteristic lesion is a small, firm lichenoid papule 3–10 mm in diameter, and reddish brown in colour. An adherent 'mica-like' scale can be detached by gentle scraping to reveal a shining brown surface—a distinctive diagnostic feature. Over the course of 3 or 4 weeks the papule flattens and the scale separates spontaneously to leave a pigmented macule which gradually fades. Post-inflammatory hypopigmentation may occur, and is occasionally persistent, but scarring is unusual in PLC. The body site distribution is the same as for PLEVA but an isolated acral form may occur [11,12]; segmental forms have been reported.

The course of pityriasis lichenoides varies. If the onset is acute, new crops may cease to develop after a few weeks, and many cases are clear within 6 months. However, acute recurrences may occur over a period of years, or chronicity may supervene. In some cases, all lesions are of the chronic scaling type from the onset, and new crops of similar lesions may develop from time to time over the years. Uncommonly, acute attacks occur after chronic lesions have been present for months or years. In general, the immediate prognosis is said to be better when the onset is acute and the lesions in successive crops are also of the acute type, but one large study of 124 children showed only a small difference in clearance times between PLEVA (mean 18 months) and PLC (mean 20 months) [13]. A smaller study comparing adults and children found that the disease tended to run a longer course in children, with greater extent of lesions, more pigmentation, and poor response to conventional treatments [14].

Differential diagnosis. The acute vesicular form must be distinguished from varicella; acute necrotic lesions may suggest other necrotic skin infections, vasculitis or pyoderma gangrenosum. Lymphomatoid papulosis is a particularly difficult differential diagnosis in patients with necrotic lesions in view of its histological similarity, discussed above, although lymphomatoid papulosis is usually characterized by less vesicular and more necrotic papulonodular lesions than those of PLEVA.

PLC must be differentiated from guttate psoriasis and lichen planus. The acral form of PLC in particular may mimic psoriasis, and secondary syphilis needs to be excluded especially if the palms and soles are involved or if there are mucosal lesions. The single, detachable 'mica-like' scale on the red-brown papule is a characteristic sign of PLC. Gianotti–Crosti syndrome is less likely to be confused with pityriasis lichenoides, but insect bites and drug eruptions should be included in the differential diagnosis.

References

1 Patel DG, Kihiczak G, Schwartz RA, Janniger CK, Lambert WC. Pityriasis lichenoides. *Cutis* 2000; **65**: 17–23.

2 Tsuji T, Kasamatsu M, Yokota M *et al*. A. Mucha–Habermann disease and its febrile ulceronecrotic variant. *Cutis* 1996; **58**: 123–31.

3 Romani J, Puig L, Fernandez-Figueras MT, de Moragas JM. Pityriasis lichenoides in children: clinicopathologic review of 22 patients. *Pediatr Dermatol* 1998; **15**: 1–6.

4 Gelmetti C, Rigioni C, Alessi E *et al*. Pityriasis lichenoides in children: a long-term follow-up of 89 cases. *J Am Acad Dermatol* 1990; **23**: 473–8.

5 Bowers S, Warshaw EM. Pityriasis lichenoides and its subtypes. *J Am Acad Dermatol* 2006; **55**: 557–72.

6 Khachemoune A, Blyumin ML. Pityriasis lichenoides. Pathophysiology, classification, and treatment. *Am J Clin Dermatol* 2007; **8**: 29–36.

7 Brazzini B, Ghersetich I, Urso C *et al*. Pityriasis lichenoides et varioliformis acuta during pregnancy. *J Eur Acad Dermatol Venereol* 2001; **15**: 458–60.

8 Degos R, Duperrat B, Daniel F. Le parapsoriasis ulcero-necrotique hyperthermique. *Ann Dermatol Syphiligr* 1966; **93**: 481–96.

9 Puddu P, Cianchini G, Colonna L *et al*. Febrile ulceronecrotic Mucha–Habermann's disease with fatal outcome. *Int J Dermatol* 1997; **36**: 691–4.

10 De Cuyper C, Hindryckx P, Deroo N. Febrile ulceronecrotic pityriasis lichenoides et varioliformis acuta. *Dermatology* 1994; **189** (Suppl. 2): 50–3.

11 Kossard S. Acral pityriasis lichenoides. *Australas J Dermatol* 2002; **43**: 68–71.

12 Chung HG, Kim SC. Pityriasis lichenoides chronica with acral distribution mimicking palmoplantar syphilid. *Acta Derm Venereol* 1999; **79**: 239.

13 Ersoy-Evans S, Greco F, Mancini AJ *et al*. Pityriasis lichenoides in childhood. A retrospective review of 124 patients. *J Am Acad Dermatol* 2007; **56**: 205–10.

14 Wahie S, Hiscutt E, Natarajan S, Taylor A. Pityriasis lichenoides: the differences between children and adults. *Br J Dermatol* 2007; **157**: 941–5.

Aetiology and pathogenesis. Pityriasis lichenoides has been reported mainly from Europe and America, but there is no specific geographical variation in incidence. The aetiology is unknown. Nosologically, pityriasis lichenoides has been considered to be a variant of parapsoriasis and to show overlap with lymphomatoid papulosis [1,2]. Evidence of T-cell clonality has also been detected in most cases of PLEVA and some cases of isolated PLC without MF [4–6], and in FUMHD [7]. PLEVA has also been reported with an associated lymphoma [8]. PLC-like lesions have also been described in patients with typical features of mycosis fungoides and identical T-cell clones have been identified in both types of cutaneous lesions from the same patients which may explain the overlap with 'parapsoriasis' [9]. Therefore these findings suggest that at least some cases represent a cytotoxic CD8+ T-cell lymphoproliferative disease which may coexist with other primary cutaneous T-cell lymphomas.

Histological features of an underlying vasculitis in PLEVA suggest an immune complex-mediated pathogenesis. In support of this hypothesis there are many documented cases of infective or drug triggers (see below). Seasonal peaks of onset in autumn and winter [10], and rare familial outbreaks [11], suggest the possibility of an infectious trigger. Numerous potential infectious triggers have been summarized in reviews [1,2], and include toxoplasmosis [12,13], cytomegalovirus [14], parvovirus B19 [15], adenovirus, EBV [16], varicella-zoster virus, HIV [17], measles vaccine, streptococci [18], staphylococci and *Mycoplasma* infections. In many such reports, there is evidence of seroconversion at the time of onset or of resolution of pityriasis lichenoides when the infective trigger was treated thus supporting a casual relationship. Parvovirus B19 genomic DNA was identified in lesional skin in 30% of patients with PLEVA [19]. A therapeutic response of PLC to tonsillectomy in the setting of chronic tonsillitis has been reported [20], as well as responses to antibiotics such as erythromycin [21,22] or tetracycline [23]. Resolution has also followed pegylated interferon and ribavirin in a patient with hepatitis C infection. Other reported triggers include medications, such as chemotherapeutic agents, oral contraceptives, astemizole, and possibly herbs. Therefore the combination of several well-documented infective triggers (mainly viral) and the nature of the cellular infiltrate suggest that pityriasis lichenoides may be caused by an antiviral immune response leading to aberrant skin recruitment of CLA+ CCR4+ CD8+ T-cells [24].

These findings collectively suggest that pityriasis lichenoides is a diverse group of entities which share a similar morphologic pattern due to a variety of underlying aetiologies including a reactive immune complex mediated hypersensitivity vasculitis to different triggers, an immune response to a T-cell dyscrasia or a primary cutaneous T-cell lymphoma.

Pathology [1,2]. The histology varies with the stage, intensity and extent of the reaction; changes are more severe in PLEVA than in PLC. In early lesions, an infiltrate of predominantly small lymphocytes surrounds and involves the walls of dilated dermal capillaries, which show endothelial proliferation. In PLEVA, the infiltrate may be deep, dense and wedge-shaped rather than predominantly perivascular. The epidermis is oedematous, with an interface dermatitis comprised mainly of CD8+ lymphocytes; some necrotic keratinocytes are generally present, especially in PLEVA. Intraepidermal and perivascular extravasation of erythrocytes is typical. Later, over the centre of the lesion, a parakeratotic scale forms, containing lymphocytic pseudo-Munro abscesses and prominent exocytosis of lymphocytes and a little cytologic atypia can be present. If the reaction is still more intense, as occurs in FUMHD, frank necrosis occurs and the lesion may be difficult to distinguish from other forms of acute necrosis of the skin on histology. In FUMHD there may be marked fibrinoid necrosis of deep vessels with luminal thrombi, partial necrosis of follicles and complete necrosis of eccrine glands.

Immunofluorescent studies variably demonstrate IgM, C3 and fibrin in vessel walls of fresh lesions [2]. Macrophages are increased in number and Langerhans' cells decreased. HLA-DR is expressed by the lymphocytic infiltrate and the overlying epidermis.

There is a histological resemblance to many other conditions, including common inflammatory conditions such as psoriasis and resolving eczema. The most important is the distinction from parapsoriasis and particularly (as they may also be clinically similar) differentiation between PLEVA and lymphomatoid papulosis. The most useful distinction from lymphomatoid papulosis is that the latter shows a more pronounced collection of papulonodular lesions with a predominant population of large atypical CD30+ cells (usually CD4+ but occasionally CD8+) whereas atypical CD30+ cells in pityriasis lichenoides are usually few and invariably CD8+ [9]. *CLA* and *TIA-1* are expressed in both conditions and indicate a proliferation of cytotoxic T-cells [25].

References

1 Benmaman O, Sanchez JL. Comparative clinicopathological study on pityriasis lichenoides chronica and small plaque parapsoriasis. *Am J Dermatopathol* 1988; **10**: 189–96.

2 Bowers S, Warshaw EM. Pityriasis lichenoides and its subtypes. *J Am Acad Dermatol* 2006; **55**: 557–72.

3 Khachemoune A, Blyumin ML. Pityriasis lichenoides. Pathophysiology, classification, and treatment. *Am J Clin Dermatol* 2007; **8**: 29–36.

4 Shieh S, Mikkola DL, Wood GS. Differentiation and clonality of lesional lymphocytes in pityriasis lichenoides chronica. *Arch Dermatol* 2001; **137**: 305–8.

5 Dereure O, Levi E, Kadin ME. T-cell clonality in pityriasis lichenoides et varioliformis acuta: a heteroduplex analysis of 20 cases. *Arch Dermatol* 2000; **136**: 1483–6.

6 Weinberg JM, Kristal L, Chooback L *et al*. The clonal nature of pityriasis lichenoides. *Arch Dermatol* 2002; **138**: 1063–7.

7 Helmbold P, Gaisbauer G, Fielder E *et al*. Self-limited variant of febrile ulceronecrotic Mucha–Habermann disease with polyclonal T-cell receptor rearrangement. *J Am Acad Dermatol* 2006; **54**: 1113–4.

8 Kempf W, Kutzner H, Kettelhack N *et al*. Paraneoplastic pityriasis lichenoides in cutaneous lymphoma: case report and review of the literature on paraneoplastic reactions of the skin in lymphoma and leukaemia. *Br J Dermatol* 2005; **152**: 1327–31.

9 Magro C, Crowson A, Morrison C *et al*. Pityriasis lichenoides chronica: stratification by molecular and phenotypic profile. *Hum Pathol* 2007; **38**: 479–90.

10 Ersoy-Evans S, Greco F, Mancini AJ *et al*. Pityriasis lichenoides in childhood. A retrospective review of 124 patients. *J Am Acad Dermatol* 2007; **56**: 205–10.

11 Dupont C. Pityriasis lichenoides in a family. *Br J Dermatol* 1995; **133**: 388–9.

12 Rongioletti F, Delmonte S, Rebora A. Pityriasis lichenoides and acquired toxoplasmosis. *Int J Dermatol* 1999; **38**: 372–4.

13 Nassef NE, Hammam MA. The relation between toxoplasmosis and pityriasis lichenoides chronica. *J Egypt Soc Parasitol* 1997; **27**: 93–9.

14 Tsai KS, Hsieh HJ, Chow KC *et al*. Detection of cytomegalovirus infection in a patient with febrile ulceronecrotic Mucha–Habermann's disease. *Int J Dermatol* 2001; **40**: 694–8.

15 Labarthe MP, Salomon D, Saurat JH. Ulcers of the tongue, pityriasis lichenoides and primary parvovirus B19 infection. *Ann Dermatol Venereol* 1996; **123**: 735–8.

16 Edwards BL, Bonagura VR, Valacer DJ *et al*. Mucha–Habermann's disease and arthritis: possible association with reactivated Epstein–Barr virus infection. *J Rheumatol* 1989; **16**: 387–9.

17 Smith KJ, Nelson A, Skelton H *et al*. Pityriasis lichenoides et varioliformis acuta in HIV-1+ patients: a marker of early stage disease. *Int J Dermatol* 1997; **36**: 104–9.

18 English JC, Collins M, Bryant-Bruce C. Pityriasis lichenoides et varioliformis acuta and group A β-hemolytic streptococcal infection. *Int J Dermatol* 1995; **34**: 642–4.

19 Tomasini D, Tomasini CF, Cerri A *et al*. Pityriasis lichenoides: a cytotoxic T-cell-mediated skin disorder. Evidence of human parvovirus B19 DNA in nine cases. *J Cutan Pathol* 2004; **31**: 531–8.

20 Takahashi K, Atsumi M. Pityriasis lichenoides chronica resolving after tonsillectomy. *Br J Dermatol* 1993; **129**: 353–4.

21 Tsuji T, Kasamatsu M, Yokota M *et al*. Mucha–Habermann disease and its febrile ulceronecrotic variant. *Cutis* 1996; **58**: 123–31.

22 Romani J, Puig L, Fernandez-Figueras MT, de Moragas JM. Pityriasis lichenoides in children: clinicopathologic review of 22 patients. *Pediatr Dermatol* 1998; **15**: 1–6.

23 Piamphongsant T. Tetracycline for the treatment of pityriasis lichenoides. *Br J Dermatol* 1974; **911**: 319–22.

24 Wenzel J, Gütgemann I, Distelmaier U *et al*. The role of cytotoxic skin-homing CD8+ lymphocytes in cutaneous cytotoxic T-cell lymphoma and pityriasis lichenoides. *J Am Acad Dermatol* 2005; **53**: 422–7.

25 Jang KA, Choi JC, Choi JH. Expression of cutaneous lymphocyte-associated antigen and TIA-1 by lymphocytes in pityriasis lichenoides et varioliformis acuta and lymphomatoid papulosis: immunohistochemical study. *J Cutan Pathol* 2001; **28**: 453–9.

Treatment [1–5]. Treatment options include antibiotics such as tetracyclines or erythromycin (preferred in young children because of dental pigmentation side effects of tetracycline) [1], and phototherapy of different types, including natural sunlight, UVB [2], narrow-band UVB, UVA1 and PUVA [3]. Results of phototherapy for pityriasis lichenoides are summarized in [4]. Topical corticosteroids may improve symptoms and healing of lesions but are not felt to alter the course of the disease [1]. A report of topical tacrolimus suggested success in a refractory case of PLC [5]. In more aggressive disease of PLEVA or FUMHD pattern, and less commonly in PLC, various immunosuppressive agents and intravenous immunoglobulin have been used.

References

1 Piamphongsant T. Tetracycline for the treatment of pityriasis lichenoides. *Br J Dermatol* 1974; **911**: 319–22.

2 Le Vine MJ. Phototherapy for pityriasis lichenoides. *Arch Dermatol* 1983; **119**: 378–80.

3 Powell FC, Muller SA. Psoralens and ultraviolet A therapy of pityriasis lichenoides. *J Am Acad Dermatol* 1984; **10**: 59–64.

4 Bowers S, Warshaw EM. Pityriasis lichenoides and its subtypes. *J Am Acad Dermatol* 2006; **55**: 557–72.

5 Mallipeddi R, Evans AV. Refractory pityriasis lichenoides chronica successfully treated with topical tacrolimus. *Clin Exp Dermatol* 2003; **28**: 456–8.

Parapsoriasis

This term has caused confusion since its introduction in 1902 because of a lack of a universally agreed definition of the clinical entities to be included. For this reason, many dermatologists prefer not to use the term at all, and to substitute one of the many synonyms for clinical conditions that might be included in one of the parapsoriasis groups. There is unresolved controversy as to whether two of the parapsoriasis variants are either precursors to cutaneous lymphoma in the form of MF (so-called premycotic eruptions) or established, but early, MF from the outset. There is a broad division of parapsoriasis into small and large plaque variants, each with a number of synonyms. The evidence that the majority of cases of small-plaque parapsoriasis are a chronic, benign condition is reasonable. In contrast, large series of patients with large-plaque parapsoriasis have recorded the development of definite MF in 11% of cases but whether these cases were MF from the outset remains unclear at present [1]. Unfortunately, TCR gene rearrangement studies have been in conclusive, although the proportion of cases with evidence of monoclonality is lower in small-plaque parapsoriasis. Long-term follow-up of these cases is now required.

Small-plaque parapsoriasis [1,2]

Synonyms
- Chronic superficial scaly dermatitis
- Persistent superficial dermatitis
- Digitate dermatosis
- Xanthoerythroderma perstans

Definition. A chronic asymptomatic condition, characterized by the presence of persistent, small, scaly plaques, mainly on the trunk.

Clinical features. The lesions usually appear insidiously and asymptomatically on the trunk and, to a lesser extent, on the limbs of young adults. Individual lesions are monomorphic round or oval erythematous patches, 2.5–5 cm in diameter, with slight scaling (Fig. 57.45). Some have a slightly yellow, waxy tinge. The lesions persist for years or even decades, and may be more obvious in the winter months. There is sparing of the pelvic girdle area and the striking polymorphic appearance of individual patches in MF is lacking.

Pathology. This is non-specific. There are small focal areas of hyperkeratosis and parakeratosis, and in the underlying dermis there are small aggregates of morphologically normal CD4+ T cells, mainly around the vasculature. There is no epidermotropism, and no Pautrier's microabscesses.

Immunophenotypic studies reveal a normal mature T-cell phenotype. One report has identified a 'dominant T-cell clone' in two out of five cases of small-plaque parapsoriasis, using PCR analysis [3]. The significance of this observation in terms of relationship to MF and disease progression is not yet clear. There is also a report of a higher frequency of clonal T cells in the peripheral blood of patients with small-plaque parapsoriasis [4] with no evidence of clonality in the skin, although the significance of this finding is

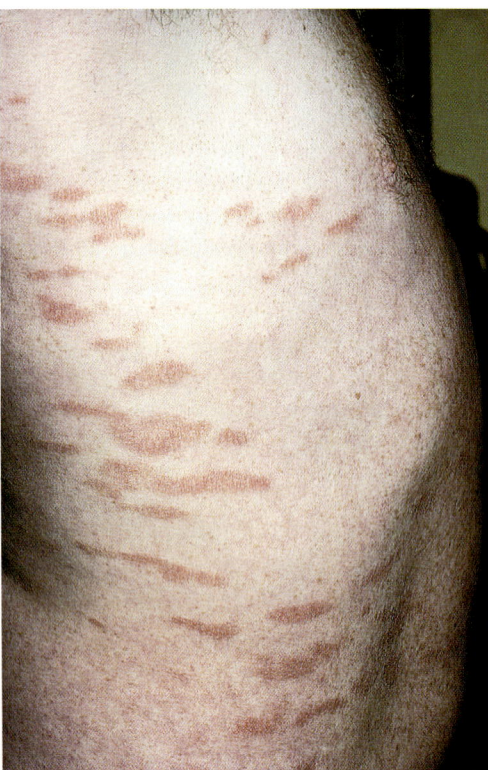

Fig. 57.45 Typical chronic superficial scaly dermatitis showing linear plaques on the trunk that change little over time.

now questionable because non-pathological T-cell clones can occasionally be found in the peripheral blood of normal, healthy volunteers.

Treatment. Often little treatment is needed. Emollients may help control the scaling, and a course of UVB phototherapy may result in temporary clearance of the lesions, but recurrence is invariable [5].

References
1 Ackerman AB, Schiff TA. If small plaque parapsoriasis is a cutaneous T-cell lymphoma, even an abortive one, it must be mycosis fungoides. *Arch Dermatol* 1996; **132**: 562–6.
2 Burg G, Dummer R. Small plaque parapsoriasis is an abortive cutaneous T-cell lymphoma, and is not mycosis fungoides. *Arch Dermatol* 1995; **131**: 336–8.
3 Haeffner AC, Smoller BR, Zepter K, Wood GS. Differentiation and clonality of lesional lymphocytes in small plaque parapsoriasis. *Arch Dermatol* 1995; **131**: 321–8.
4 Muche JM, Lukowsky A, Heim J *et al.* Demonstration of frequent occurrence of clonal T cells in the blood but not the skin of patients with small plaque parapsoriasis. *Blood* 1999; **94**: 1409–17.
5 Hofer A, Cerroni L, Kerl H, Wolf P. Narrow-band UVB therapy for small plaques parapsoriasis and early stage mycosis fungoides. *Arch Dermatol* 1999; **135**: 1377–80.

Large-plaque parapsoriasis

Synonyms
- Parakeratosis variegata
- Retiform parapsoriasis
- Atrophic parapsoriasis
- Poikilodermatous parapsoriasis

Definition. A chronic condition characterized by the presence of fixed, large, atrophic, erythematous plaques, usually on the trunk and occasionally on the limbs.

Clinical features. Patients present with persistent, large, yellow–orange atrophic patches and thin plaques on the trunk and limbs. Involvement of covered skin on the breast and buttock areas should suggest MF and in these cases patches and plaques may show striking polymorphism and poikiloderma with slow progression [1].

Pathology [2,3]. There is frequently epidermal atrophy, and a lichenoid or interface reaction may also be seen at the dermal–epidermal junction. There is a band-like lymphocytic infiltrate in the papillary dermis, and there may also be free red cells present. The histology is not diagnostic for MF and most biopsies only show a mild dermatitis.

Immunophenotypic studies reveal a normal T-cell phenotype. TCR gene rearrangement studies have shown a clonal T-cell population in the skin in six of 12 patients, but progression to overt CTCL was only noted in one of the 12 patients [4].

Treatment. Topical emollients, UVB and PUVA are all helpful in offering symptomatic relief. Topical steroids should be used with caution because of the atrophic nature of the condition.

References
1 Lambert WC, Everett MA. The nosology of parapsoriasis. *J Am Acad Dermatol* 1981; **5**: 373–95.
2 Kempf W, Dummer R, Burg G. Approach to lymphoproliferative conditions of the skin. *Am J Clin Pathol* 1999; **111** (Suppl. 1): S84–S93.
3 Liu V, McKee PH. Cutaneous lymphoproliferative disorders. *Adv Anat Pathol* 2002; **9**: 79–100.
4 Simon M, Flaig MJ, Kind P *et al.* Large plaque parapsoriasis: clinical and genotypic considerations. *J Cutan Pathol* 2000; **27**: 57–60.

Actinic reticuloid [1,2]

Definition. This condition was first described by Ive *et al.* in 1969 [3]. The original description was of a group of elderly, exclusively male patients who developed a severe and very disabling photosensitivity involving reaction to light throughout the UVB, UVA and visible part of the spectrum. A number of these patients had a past history of contact dermatitis and a milder form of photosensitivity ('persistent light reactors'), but the true relationship between contact dermatitis, particularly to plants of the Compositae family [4], persistent light reactors (chronic actinic dermatitis) and actinic reticuloid is not yet established. The photosensitivity is very severe.

Clinical features. The clinical features are the symptoms of severe and persistent photosensitivity with erythema, oedema and striking 'leonine' thickening of the light-exposed skin of the face, neck and hands which can mimic closely the features of erythrodermic MF/SS (Fig. 57.46) [5].

Patients with atopic dermatitis may be more likely to develop actinic reticuloid, and this should be considered in those with chronic atopic dermatitis who develop photosensitivity [6].

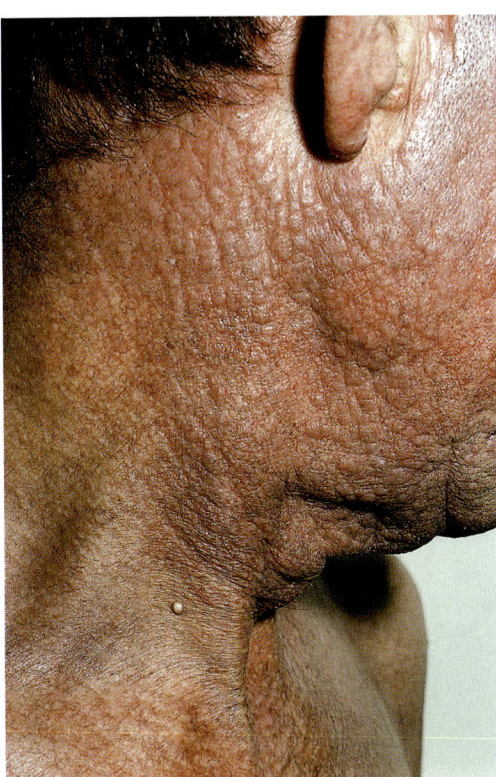

Fig. 57.46 Actinic reticuloid showing marked infiltration of light-exposed skin of the face, with a striking change in skin texture at the collar area and normal skin on the area usually covered by clothing.

Pathology. The histological picture is that of an intense, superficial and deep lymphocytic infiltrate extending from the papillary dermis deep into the reticular dermis. Signs of actinic damage to collagen are present and some of the lymphocytic cells are large and atypical mimicking a cutaneous lymphoma, hence the term 'reticuloid'. The majority of the lymphoid infiltrate consists of CD8+ T cells.

TCR gene analysis does not show a clonal T-cell population [7], but the development of a T-cell clone has been reported in a single patient with mild photosensitivity who developed MF [8]. A recent case series of patients with MF/SS and a report of a patient with cutaneous ATLL suggests that patients with cutaneous lymphomas can show marked photosensitivity with clinical features mimicking chronic actinic dermatitis/actinic reticuloid, emphasizing the importance of considering carefully a diagnosis of a cutaneous T-cell lymphoma in patients with actinic reticuloid [9,10].

Treatment. Treatment is based on light avoidance and the use of both the titanium dioxide-containing physical barrier creams and the newer, more effective chemical UVA and UVB blockers. Low-dose systemic steroid therapy, ciclosporin, hydroxyurea [11] and azathioprine [12] may be effective in some patients.

The prognosis for recovery is poor and the majority of patients tend to have severe photosensitivity for the remainder of their lives.

References

1 Dawe RS, Crombie IK, Ferguson J. The natural history of chronic actinic dermatitis. *Arch Dermatol* 2000; **136**: 1215–20.
2 Zak Prelich M, Schwartz RA. Actinic reticuloid. *Int J Dermatol* 1999; **38**: 335–42.
3 Ive FA, Magnus IA, Warin RP *et al.* 'Actinic reticuloid': a chronic dermatosis associated with severe photosensitivity and the histological resemblance to lymphoma. *Br J Dermatol* 1969; **81**: 469–85.
4 Johnson SC, Cripps DJ, Norbach DH. Actinic reticuloid: a clinical, pathologic, and action spectrum study. *Arch Dermatol* 1979; **115**: 1078–83.
5 Dawe RS, Green CM, MacLeod TM, Ferguson J. Daisy, dandelion and thistle contact allergy in the photosensitivity dermatitis and actinic reticuloid spectrum. *Contact Dermatitis* 1996; **35**: 109–10.
6 Russell S, Dawe RS, Collins P *et al.* The photosensitivity and actinic reticuloid syndrome occurring in seven young atopic dermatitis patients. *Br J Dermatol* 1998; **138**: 496–501.
7 Bakels V, Oostveen JW, Pressman AH *et al.* Differentiation between actinic reticuloid and cutaneous lymphoma by T-cell receptor gamma gene rearrangement and immunophenotyping. *J Clin Pathol* 1998; **51**: 154–8.
8 De Silva BD, McLaren K, Kavanagh GM. Photosensitive dermatitis or actinic reticuloid? *Br J Dermatol* 2000; **142**: 1221–7.
9 Agar N, Morris S, Russell Jones R *et al.* Case report of four patients with erythrodermic cutaneous T-cell lymphoma and severe photosensitivity mimicking chronic actinic dermatitis. *Br J Dermatol* 2009; **160**: 698–703.
10 Adachi Y, Horio T. Chromic actinic dermatitis in a patient with adult T-cell leukemia. *Photodermatol Photoimmunol Photomed* 2008; **24**: 147–9.
11 Gramvussakis S, George SA. Chronic actinic dermatitis: beneficial effect from hydroxyurea. *Br J Dermatol* 2000; **143**: 1340.
12 Kingston TP, Lowe NJ, Sofen HL *et al.* Actinic reticuloid in a black man: successful therapy with azathioprine. *J Am Acad Dermatol* 1987; **16**: 1079–83.

Lymphocytoma cutis

Synonyms
- Spiegler–Fendt sarcoid
- Lymphadenosis benigna cutis of Bafverstedt

Definition. Lymphocytoma cutis is a benign, cutaneous B-cell lymphoproliferative condition. It presents as papules, nodules or plaques usually on the head and neck and pursues a chronic course [1–3].

Aetiology. This is at present unknown.

Clinical features. More cases are reported in females than males. Most patients show solitary or grouped, asymptomatic, erythematous or violaceous papules, nodules or plaques, on the head, especially the ear lobes, and rarely the trunk or limbs (Fig. 57.47). Occasionally, they may have a translucent appearance. They are asymptomatic and not tender, painful or itchy. Lesions are often multiple and may be in all stages of development. They enlarge slowly and may reach a diameter of 3–5 cm. Associated sunlight sensitivity has been reported in some patients. Bafverstedt [4] has described an unusual form of lymphocytoma that presented as a solitary tumour of scrotal skin. Disseminated or miliary lymphocytoma cutis is also rare [5], and occurs in older patients on any body site.

Pathology [6,7]. The epidermis is usually unaffected and is often separated by a relatively acellular grenz zone from the dermis, which is replaced by a nodular dense infiltrate extending through the full thickness of the dermis but without cellular atypia. In

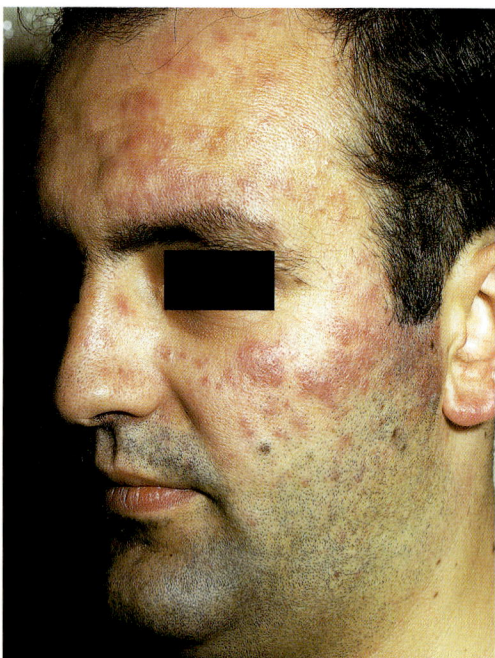

Fig. 57.47 Clinical presentation of a patient with lymphocytoma cutis.

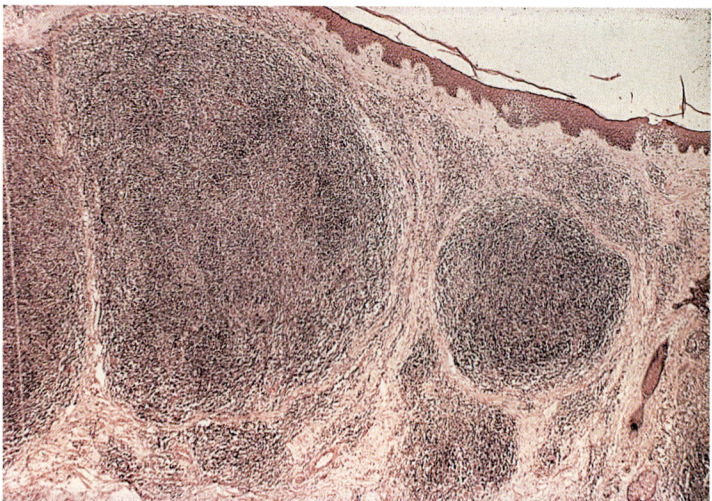

Fig. 57.48 Histology of Spiegler–Fendt sarcoid showing striking lymphoid follicles.

classic cases, lymphocytes and histiocytes form a follicular arrangement resembling the appearance of a lymph node (Fig. 57.48). Mitotic figures may be visible in the cells of the follicles and occasional eosinophils may also be present. Appendages and blood vessels are spared. In some instances, there is no tendency for lymphoid follicle formation, although the histological appearance with normal lymphocytes and histiocytes is otherwise similar. The histological differential diagnosis includes primary cutaneous lymphoma, particularly of marginal zone origin.

Immunopathology. The majority of lymphocytes in the dermis are B cells. Germinal centres are frequently seen in lymphocytoma cutis, and appropriate markers will confirm the morphological similarity of these structures to the germinal centres of lymph nodes. A cuff of reactive T cells may be seen around the periphery of the main B-cell aggregate.

Differential diagnosis. Histological examination should distinguish lymphocytoma cutis from granulomatous disorders including sarcoidosis, granuloma faciale and rosacea. Distinction from primary cutaneous B-cell marginal zone lymphoma (MZL) is difficult, although the presence of atypical lymphoid cells would suggest a primary cutaneous MZL. Insect bite reactions may also be impossible to distinguish with any confidence from lymphocytoma cutis.

Jessner's benign lymphocytic infiltration, tumid discoid lupus erythematosus (LE) and polymorphic light eruption can also cause difficulties. However, in Jessner's lymphocytic infiltrate, which characteristically waxes and wanes in severity, the dermal lymphocytic infiltrate is dominated by T cells. The presence of basal cell liquefaction degeneration and positive direct immunofluorescence helps distinguish LE.

Treatment. There is no treatment of proven value for lymphocytoma cutis. Penicillin and radiotherapy have been advocated in the past without adequate clinical trials. Intralesional steroids have also been advocated. Miliary lesions may partially respond to topical steroids. Hydroxychloroquine has also been effective.

Prognosis. Lymphocytoma cutis is a benign disorder in both localized and disseminated forms, although often running a very protracted course. Long-term follow-up of these patients suggests that a small proportion progress to or begin as a primary cutaneous B-cell lymphoma (MZL) and therefore the prognosis must be guarded [8–11].

References

1 Lange Wantzin G, Hou Jensen K, Nielsen M *et al.* Cutaneous lymphocytomas: clinical and histological aspects. *Acta Derm Venereol* 1982; **62**: 119–24.
2 Van Hale HM, Winkelmann RK. Nodular lymphoid disease of the head and neck. *J Am Acad Dermatol* 1985; **12**: 455–61.
3 Clark WH, Mihm MC, Reed RJ *et al.* The lymphoytic infiltrates of the skin. *Hum Pathol* 1974; **5**: 25–43.
4 Bafverstedt B. Unusual forms of lymphadenosis benigna cutis (LABC). *Acta Derm Venereol (Stockh)* 1962; **42**: 3–10.
5 Bafverstedt B. Lymphadenosis benigna cutis (LABC): its nature, course and prognosis. *Acta Derm Venereol (Stockh)* 1960; **40**: 10–8.
6 Mach KW, Wilgram GF. Charactersitic histopathology of cutaneous lymphoplasia. *Arch Dermatol* 1966; **94**: 26–32.
7 Kawada A, Mori S, Hayashi T. Lymphadenosis benigna cutis: pseudomalignant form and its imprint smear technology. *Dermatologica* 1970; **141**: 339–47.
8 Shelley WB, Wood MG, Wilson JF. Premalignant lymphoid hyperplasia. *Arch Dermatol* 1981; **117**: 500–3.
9 Halevy S, Sandbank M. Transformation of lymphocytoma cutis into malignant lymphoma. *Acta Derm Venereol* 1987; **67**: 172–5.
10 Evans HL, Winkelman RK, Banks PM. Differential diagnosis of malignant and benign cutaneous infiltrates. *Cancer* 1970; **44**: 699–717.
11 Burg G, Braun-Falco O, Schmoeckel C. Differentiation between pseudolymphomas and malignant B-cell lymphomas of the skin. In: Goos M, Christophers E, eds. *Lymphoproliferative Diseases of the Skin.* Berlin: Springer Verlag, 1982: 10–4.

Jessner's lymphocytic infiltrate [1]

Definition. A chronic benign T-cell lymphoproliferative disorder, usually of exposed skin.

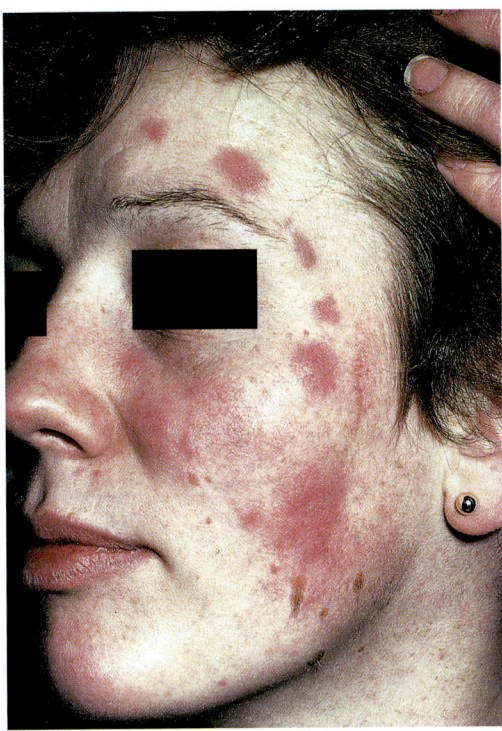

Fig. 57.49 Clinical appearance of a young woman with Jessner's lymphocytic infiltrate.

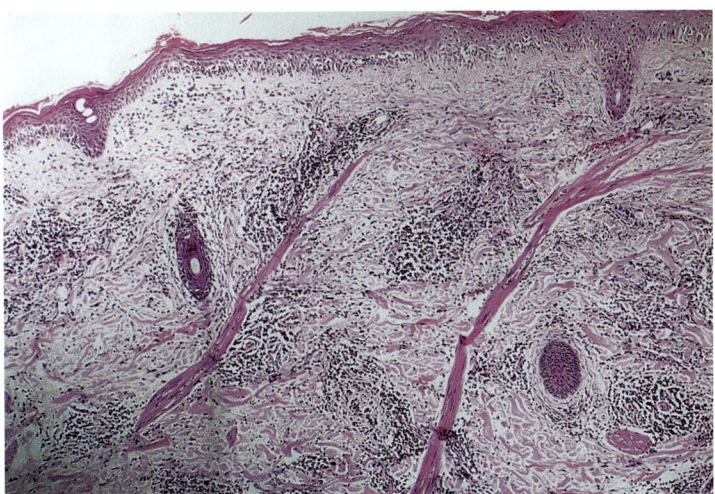

Fig. 57.50 Pathological pattern of Jessner's lymphocytic infiltrate. Note perivascular distribution and absence of epidermotropism.

Clinical features. Females are more often affected than males [2]. Both children [3,4] and familial cases [5,6] have been recorded. Benign lymphocytic infiltration of Jessner is characterized by the presence of red tumid nodules, usually on facial skin (Fig. 57.49). The lesions may involute spontaneously, but more commonly are persistent, and new lesions develop over time. There is variation in seasonal activity of the lesions, with winter exacerbations. The individual lesions are smooth raised non-scaling erythematous nodules or plaques and are commonly asymptomatic, although some patients complain of burning or pruritus.

Pathology [7–11]. Biopsies reveal a lymphocytic infiltrate predominantly in the lower dermis and concentrated tightly around blood vessels (Fig. 57.50). The epidermis and papillary dermis are relatively normal, and within the lymphocytic infiltrate there is no evidence of cellular atypia, germinal centre or follicle formation. The great majority of these cells are CD4+ T cells.

Differential diagnosis. The clinical differential diagnosis includes a fixed drug eruption and cutaneous discoid LE. The lesions are usually more numerous than would be associated with a fixed drug eruption, although the histology is very similar. The individual lesions of Jessner's lymphocytic infiltrate are smooth and non-scarring, in contrast to the scaling atrophic scarring associated with chronic discoid LE. In addition, Jessner's lymphocytic infiltrate does not demonstrate a lupus band as seen at the dermal–epidermal junction in chronic discoid LE. However, there is a view that Jessner's lymphocytic infiltrate is a variant of LE.

Treatment. This is unsatisfactory, and lesions tend both to persist and to increase in numbers. There are individual case reports of successful therapy with topical steroids, systemic steroids, PUVA, radiotherapy, dapsone, hydroxychloroquine and gold [12].

References

1 Jessner M, Kanof NB. Lymphocytic infiltration of the skin. *Arch Dermatol* 1953; **68**: 447–9.

2 Toonstra J, Wildschut A, Boer J *et al.* Jessner's lymphocytic infiltrate of the skin: a clinical study of 100 patients. *Arch Dermatol* 1989; **125**: 1525–30.

3 Mullen RH, Jacobs AH. Jessner's lymphocytic infiltrate in two girls. *Arch Dermatol* 1988; **124**: 1091–3.

4 Higgins CR, Wakeel RAP, Cerio R. Childhood Jessner's lymphocytic infiltrate of the skin. *Br J Dermatol* 1994; **131**: 99–101.

5 Toonstra J, Van der Putte SCJ, Baart de la Faille H, van Vloten W. Familial Jessner's lymphocytic infiltrate of the skin occurring in a father and daughter. *Clin Exp Dermatol* 1993; **18**: 142–5.

6 O'Toole EA, Powell F, Barnes L. Jessner's lymphocytic infiltrate and probable discoid lupus erythematosus occurring separately in two sisters. *Clin Exp Dermatol* 1999; **24**: 90–3.

7 Willemze R, Dijkstra A, Meijer CJ. Lymphocytic infiltration of the skin (Jessner): a T-cell lymphoproliferative disease. *Br J Dermatol* 1984; **110**: 523–9.

8 Calnan CD. Lymphocytic infiltration of the skin (Jessner): cutaneous Hodgkin's disease. *Br J Dermatol* 1957; **69**: 169–73.

9 Rijlaarsdam JU, Nieboer C, de Vries E *et al.* Characterization of the dermal infiltrates in Jessner's lymphocytic infiltrate of the skin. *J Cutan Pathol* 1990; **17**: 2–8.

10 Hellier FF. Lymphocytoma of the face. *Br J Dermatol* 1939; **51**: 260–5.

11 Postma C, Sluiter JTF. The relationship between Bafverstedt's benign lymphadenosis of the skin and Jessner's lymphocytic infiltration of the skin. *Acta Derm Venereol (Stockh)* 1958; **38**: 180–8.

12 Farrell AM, McGregor JM, Staughton RC, Bunker CB. Jessner's lymphocytic infiltrate treated with auranofin. *Clin Exp Dermatol* 1999; **24**: 500.

Leukaemia cutis [1–3]

Diagnosis. The diagnosis of the specific type of leukaemia depends on detailed examination of the blood and bone marrow. The cutaneous infiltrate rarely indicates the type of leukaemia involved.

Specific cutaneous lesions occur most often in myelomonocytic leukaemia and T-cell malignancies such as T-cell prolymphocytic leukaemia and T-ALL [4]. Cutaneous involvement in

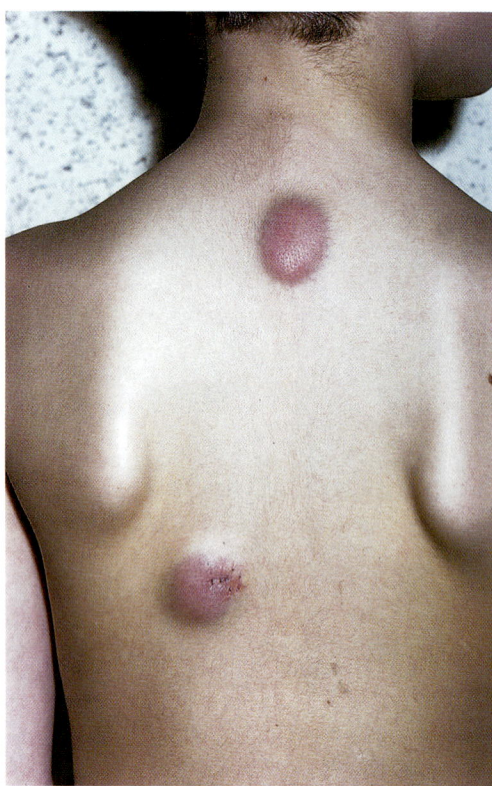

Fig. 57.51 Specific deposits in a child with leukaemia. Note two large nodular lesions on the back.

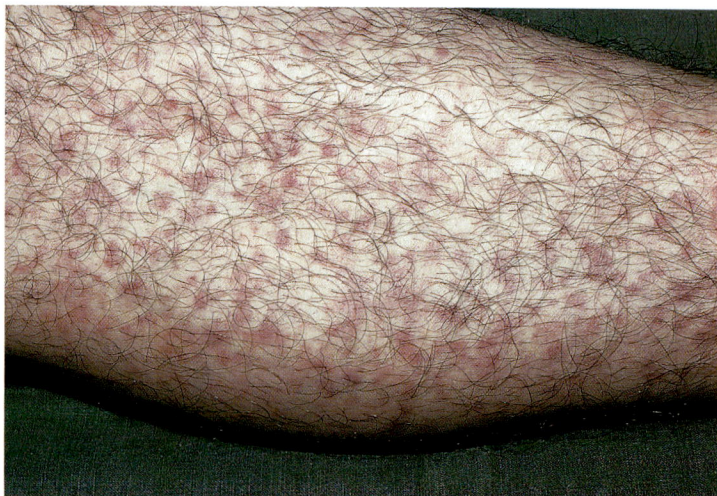

Fig. 57.52 Purpuric lesions in an adult patient with myelocytic leukaemia.

the other forms of leukaemia is unusual as a presenting feature, and usually appear after the diagnosis has been established. There are a few cases where the diagnosis of leukaemia has been established first by analysis of the skin lesions [5]. These lesions usually consist of small, reddish papules or nodules which may be fleeting or persistent. Clinically, they may resemble lesions of Sweet's syndrome, sarcoidosis, panniculitis, other granulomas or cutaneous lymphoma (Fig. 57.51). Ulceration, especially around the ankles, simulating gravitational ulceration, has been described in chronic lymphatic leukaemia and may represent the development of a leukaemic deposit in an area of low vascular resistance.

Although 'non-specific' lesions are said to be common, they are rarely reported by dermatologists. Generalized pruritus may be a presenting symptom and prurigo-like papules develop in some cases. Erythroderma has been recorded in association with an underlying T-cell leukaemia such as T-cell prolymphocytic leukaemia which must be distinguished from Sézary syndrome. There is usually marked exfoliation and the skin may be markedly thickened, especially over the face. The histological features in the skin may or may not be diagnostic.

Disseminated or unusually severe herpes zoster is common in association with all types of malignant disease. Specific leukaemic infiltrations into herpetic scars may occur and bullous lesions have been recorded [6]. In multiple myeloma, both generalized and local amyloidosis is common. Anhidrosis has been recorded. Patients with myelomatosis may subsequently develop variants of acute myelogenous leukaemia [7,8] and it has been suggested

that this complication is the result of treating the underlying disease with irradiation or alkylating agents [9].

Three cases of a perniotic syndrome associated with monocytosis and neutropenia have been described as a possible association with a preleukaemic state [10]. Sweet's disease and bullous pyoderma have also been associated with leukaemia (see Chapter 52).

Thrombocytopenic purpura is a characteristic symptom of the acute leukaemias and may occur on skin or mucous membranes, often as the presenting symptom (Fig. 57.52).

Beek [9] recorded 289 cases of lymphatic leukaemia with skin lesions and, in these, tumours were present in 50%, the head being the most common site. Erythroderma was present in 25%, herpes zoster in 26%, prurigo-like papules in 21%, bullae in 10%, variceliform eruptions and urticaria in 3%. Haemorrhagic gangrene of the skin has also been recorded. The usual age at presentation of patients with lymphatic leukaemia is 45–54 years, but those with cutaneous lesions tend to be older. Skin lesions in myelogenous leukaemia are much less frequent, with only 72 recorded cases. When the skin is involved the prognosis is poor.

A relatively specific picture is observed in a number of patients with chronic T-cell lymphatic leukaemia [6]. These patients are frequently elderly males and may present with diffuse generalized erythroderma, splenomegaly and lymphadenopathy. This may be caused by lymphokine release by the malignant T cells during their passage through the dermal vasculature, as skin biopsy of these lesions does not reveal a specific cutaneous infiltrate, or epidermotropism characteristic of MF.

Diagnosis. Diagnosis of all these conditions is based on pathological examination of material from blood, bone marrow, lymph nodes and skin [8,11–13].

Treatment. The treatment for leukaemia cutis is management of the underlying disease, with symptomatic measures for the skin lesions when required. Superficial radiotherapy may be useful, giving rapid symptomatic relief, and regression of specific cutaneous deposits.

References

1 Bonvalet D, Foldes C, Civatte J. Cutaneous manifestations in chronic lymphocytic leukaemia. *J Dermatol Surg Oncol* 1984; **10**: 278–82.

2 Buechner SA, Li CY, Su WPD. Leukaemia cutis: a histopathologic study of 42 cases. *Am J Dermatopathol* 1985; **7**: 109–19.

3 Su WPD, Buechner SA, Li CY. Clinicopathologic correlations in leukaemia cutis. *J Am Acad Dermatol* 1984; **11**: 121–8.

4 Hubler WR, Netherton EW. Cutaneous manifestations of monocytic leukaemia. *Arch Dermatol* 1947; **56**: 70–89.

5 Blaustein JC, Narany S, Palutke M *et al.* Extra-medullary (skin) presentation of acute monocytic leukaemia resembling cutaneous lymphoma. *J Cutan Pathol* 1987; **14**: 232–7.

6 Cote J, Trudel M, Gratton D. T-cell chronic lymphocytic leukaemia with bullous manifestations. *J Am Acad Dermatol* 1983; **8**: 874–8.

7 Costello MJ, Canizares O, Montague M *et al.* Cutaneous manifestations of myelogenous leukaemia. *Arch Dermatol* 1955; **71**: 605–14.

8 Eubanks SW, Patterson JW. Subacute myelomonocytic leukaemia, an unusual skin manifestation. *J Am Acad Dermatol* 1983; **9**: 581–4.

9 Beek CH. Skin manifestations associated with lymphomas and leukaemias. *Dermatologica* 1948; **96**: 350–6.

10 Marks R, Lim CC, Borrie PF. A perniotic syndrome with monocytosis and neutropenia: a possible association with a preleukaemic state. *Br J Dermatol* 1969; **81**: 327–32.

11 Arai E, Ideda S, Itoh S *et al.* Specific skin lesions as the presenting symptom of hairy cell leukaemia. *Am J Clin Pathol* 1988; **90**: 459–64.

12 Finan MC, Su WPD, Li CY. Cutaneous findings in hairy cell leukaemia. *J Am Acad Dermatol* 1984; **11**: 788–97.

13 Lawrence DM, Sun NCJ, Mena R *et al.* Cutaneous lesions in hairy cell leukaemia. *Arch Dermatol* 1983; **119**: 322–5.

Cutaneous Hodgkin's disease

The existence of a variant of Hodgkin's disease that begins in the skin is still debated, and it can be difficult if not impossible to differentiate from Hodgkin's disease beginning in the nodes, which spreads in a contiguous manner at an early stage to the skin [1–5]. Invariably, cutaneous Hodgkin's disease only occurs as direct extension from an underlying involved regional lymph node. Thus, careful clinical examination, followed if appropriate by node biopsy and CT scans, should be performed before a diagnosis of primary cutaneous Hodgkin's disease is made. In view of the cytological similarity between the cells of lymphomatoid papulosis and those of Hodgkin's disease, this differential diagnosis must be carefully considered and positively excluded.

Clinical features. One review of 1810 cases of Hodgkin's disease reports only nine (0.5%) with specific cutaneous lesions [6] but a more recent study records involvement in 16 of 465 cases (3.4%) [7]. They usually consist of small nodules, but ulcerative lesions have been recorded and rarely are the presenting symptom.

Pathology [1,2,8]. To consider the diagnosis of Hodgkin's disease either involving the skin as a secondary process, or originating in the skin, the cutaneous infiltrate should consist of nodules of atypical lymphoid and histiocytic cells, including the presence of Reed–Sternberg cells that are CD30$^+$ and lymphoid cells that are CD15$^+$ [9–11]. CD15 positivity is not seen in lymphomatoid papulosis.

Non-specific cutaneous signs associated with Hodgkin's disease [5,12] are very common and occur in 3–50% of cases. These include pigmentation, pruritus, prurigo, atrophy, alopecia, exfoliative dermatitis and herpes zoster.

Pigmentation. This is melanin pigmentation and is very common. It resembles the pigmentation of Addison's disease, being most marked in areas that normally show some darkening such as the axillae, groins and around the nipples. Less often it is more widespread, and occasionally a bizarre pigmentation occurs. The mucous membranes are usually spared.

Pruritus. This often occurs together with pigmentation. Pruritus is not infrequently the presenting feature of the disease, and may precede the presence of palpable nodes by months or years. It tends to start on the legs. It is especially severe in patients who show other general symptoms such as fever and weight loss. Both pigmentation and pruritus occur in association with enlarged mediastinal or retroperitoneal glands, the presence of which should always be suspected when itching is severe.

Prurigo. This is a development from pruritus. In addition to the widespread irritation, there are excessively itchy papules, which are scratched until the skin surface is removed and is replaced by a blood crust. The papules and crusts are usually found on the trunk. When present in association with enlarged superficial glands, this forms a very characteristic picture, often called Hodgkin's prurigo.

Ichthyosiform atrophy. An acquired ichthyosis occurring in the course of a chronic wasting disease is fairly common. Hodgkin's disease is probably the most common condition to be associated with this change. It usually starts on the legs and may remain restricted, but in severe cases progresses until it becomes universal. It resembles ichthyosis vulgaris, with thin, dry and rather firmly attached scales. It is not static and may regress for a time, only to return later. Red streaks are often visible between the scales. The patient is usually wasted and severely ill. Malabsorption from the gut may occur in some cases and contribute to this problem.

Alopecia. Hair loss is common in Hodgkin's disease. It can be caused by rubbing or scratching to relieve itching. It may also be part of the ichthyosiform atrophy or be caused by endocrine dysfunction, when specific infiltration occurs in organs such as the pituitary or adrenal. Rarely, it may be brought about by specific infiltration in the scalp.

Exfoliative dermatitis. Erythroderma and exfoliative dermatitis have been recorded as occurring in Hodgkin's disease on many occasions [4]. Most recorded cases would probably be more correctly included under ichthyosiform atrophy.

Herpes zoster. Herpes zoster is common in the course of Hodgkin's disease, but disseminated zoster is much less likely to occur in Hodgkin's disease than in chronic lymphatic leukaemia.

Miscellaneous conditions. Many other non-specific skin lesions have been described in association with Hodgkin's disease, but they are probably incidental. Erythema nodosum is seen occasionally and is apparently caused by the disease itself; in these cases, differentiation from sarcoidosis may be difficult, but the Kveim test or node biopsy should establish the diagnosis.

References

1 Carbone PP, Kaplan HS, Musshoff K *et al.* Report of the committee on Hodgkin's disease staging classification. *Cancer Res* 1971; **31**: 1860–1.
2 Franssila KO, Kalma TV, Voutilainen A. Histologic classification of Hodgkin's disease. *Cancer* 1967; **20**: 1594–601.
3 O'Bryan-Tear CG, Burke M, Coulson IH *et al.* Hodgkin's disease presenting in the skin. *Clin Exp Dermatol* 1987; **12**: 69–71.
4 Rubins J. Cutaneous Hodgkin's disease. *Cancer* 1978; **42**: 1219–21.
5 Silverman CL, Strayer DS, Wasserman TH. Cutaneous Hodgkin's disease. *Arch Dermatol* 1982; **118**: 918–21.
6 Gordon RA, Lookingbill DP, Abt AB. Skin infiltration in Hodgkin's disease. *Arch Dermatol* 1980; **116**: 1038–40.
7 White RM, Patterson JW. Cutaneous involvement in Hodgkin's disease. *Cancer* 1985; **55**: 1136–45.
8 Jaffe ES. The elusive Reed–Sternberg cell. *N Engl J Med* 1989; **320**: 529–31.
9 Kadin ME. Histogenesis of Hodgkin's disease. *Hum Pathol* 1987; **18**: 1085–8.
10 Kaplan HS. Hodgkin's disease: unfolding concepts concerning its nature, management and prognosis. *Cancer* 1980; **45**: 2439–74.
11 Schwab V, Stein H, Gerdes J *et al.* Production of a monoclonal antibody specific for Hodgkin and Sternberg–Reed cells of Hodgkin's disease and a subset of normal lymphoid cells. *Nature* 1982; **299**: 65–7.
12 Smith JL, Butler JJ. Skin involvement in Hodgkin's disease. *Cancer* 1980; **45**: 354–61.

Lennert's lymphoma

Definition. A rare variant of systemic lymphoma with a characteristic histology, first described in 1968 as a variant of Hodgkin's disease [1].

Clinical features. Most patients have lymphadenopathy, fever, fatigue and weight loss. The skin is involved very rarely as a secondary event and this usually consists of clinically non-specific papules or nodules [2]. One patient presented with chronic cutaneous infection and pyoderma [3], and another simulating atypical granuloma annulare [4].

Pathology. The characteristic pattern is an infiltrate with a high content of epithelioid histiocytes, admixed with CD4$^+$ cells. If the skin is involved, there may be a subcutaneous infiltrate consisting of epithelioid histiocytes and T cells. Reed–Sternberg cells are rare [2,3].

References

1 Lennert K, Mestdagh J. Lymphogranulomatosen mit kinstant hohem epitheloidzellgehalt. *Virchows Arch Pathol Anat* 1968; **344**: 1–20.
2 Kiesewetter F, Haneke E, Lennert K *et al.* Cutaneous lymphoepithelioid lymphoma. *Am J Dermatopathol* 1989; **11**: 549–54.
3 Zamora A, Nunez C, Hu CH. Lennert's lymphoma presenting with clusters of cutaneous infection. *J Am Acad Dermatol* 1981; **5**: 450–4.
4 Bhushan M, Craven NM, Armstrong GR, Chalmers RJG. Lymphoepitheloid cell lymphoma (Lennert's lymphoma) presenting as atypical granuloma annulare. *Br J Dermatol* 2000; **142**: 776–80.

CHAPTER 58

Disorders of Skin Colour

A.V. Anstey

Royal Gwent Hospital, Newport, Gwent, UK

The colour of the skin [1–7]

Normal skin colour is determined by a number of chromophores, the most important of which is melanin. Besides melanin, other chromophores that contribute significantly to skin colour include haemoglobin (in both the oxygenated and reduced state) and carotenoids. Racial and ethnic differences in skin colour are related to the number, size, shape, distribution and degradation of melanin-laden organelles called melanosomes. These are produced by melanocytes (Fig. 58.1) and are transferred to the surrounding epidermal keratinocytes. Two types of melanin pigmentation occur in humans [1]. The first is *constitutive* skin colour, which is the amount of melanin pigmentation that is genetically determined in the absence of sun exposure and other influences. The other is *facultative* (inducible) skin colour or 'tan', which results from sun exposure. Increased pigmentation can also be due to endocrine, paracrine and autocrine factors [1,2].

The least pigmented human subjects are almost white and have a skin colour similar to that of an albino. In contrast, the darkest pigmented human subjects are deep brown or black-brown in colour. Most peoples of the world fall between these two extremes and are moderate brown or yellow-brown in colour. The Caucasian peoples of Europe exhibit a light brown colour that can be enhanced by exposure to sunlight. The ability to tan is marked in the Mediterranean and Middle Eastern peoples. In contrast, some of those from the western parts of Northern Europe have fair skin, red hair, and a tendency to develop red-brown freckles after exposure to sunlight. The definitive method for objective measurement of skin colour uses the recording spectrophotometer adapted for reflectance readings [3]. Application of reflectance chromameters in clinical practice includes the measurement of skin colour, the measurement of ultraviolet (UV)-induced pigmentation, and the quantification of the bleaching effect of depigmenting agents [3].

In some ethnic groups, a sharply demarcated linear border is seen between more and less pigmented skin [4]. This has been studied most extensively in the Japanese and in black Americans, and is most frequently observed in darkly pigmented individuals. Six major forms (designated A–F) of natural pigmentary demarcation boundaries in the skin have been described [4]. These are summarized in Table 58.1.

A blue colour is seen in the congenital pigmentation termed 'Mongolian spot', a form of dermal pigmentation that can occur on any part of the body, although it is most commonly found in the sacral region [5,6]. These spots fade after birth, but can persist in certain sites as in the naevus of Ota (see p. 58.36). Blue naevus is an example of acquired blue pigmentation of skin. The blue coloration of the skin in both of these lesions is due to an optical effect that alters the perceived colour of brown pigment in the dermis. The melanin dispersed in the dermis absorbs incident visible light such that the diffuse reflectance in the longer (red) wavelengths is reduced, giving the pigmented sites a blue appearance.

Rook's Textbook of Dermatology, 8th edition. Edited by DA Burns,
SM Breathnach, NH Cox and CEM Griffiths. © 2010 Blackwell Publishing Ltd.

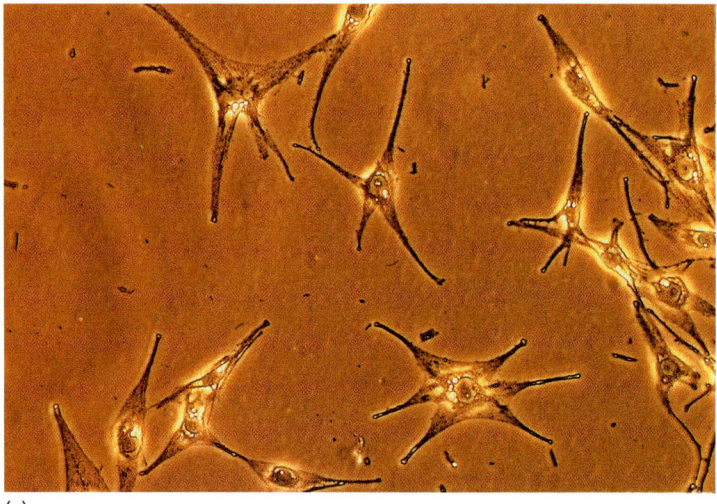
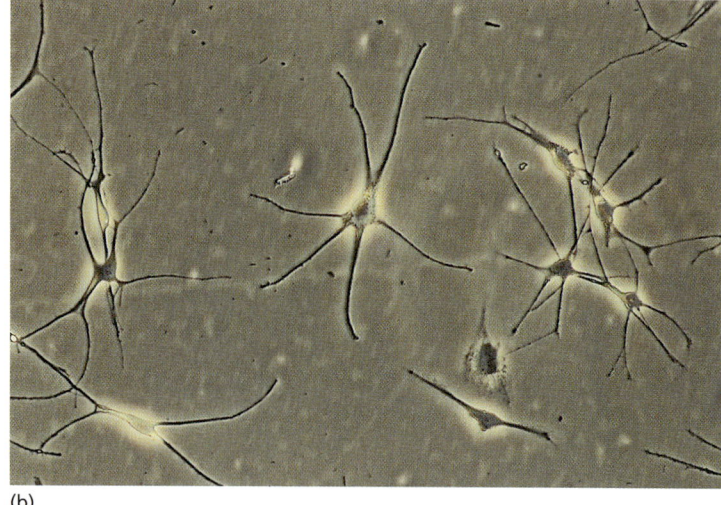

(a)   (b)

Fig. 58.1 (a,b) Melanocytes in culture. (Courtesy of Professor P. Friedmann, Royal Liverpool University Hospital, Liverpool, UK.)

Table 58.1 Pigmentary demarcation lines [4].

A: Located on the anterolateral portion of the upper arm (Futcher's line)

B: Posteromedial portion of the leg

C: Hypopigmented lines band on the mid chest in the pre- or parasternal region

D: A vertical line in the posteromedial area of the spine

E: Hypopigmented macules located on the chest extending from the clavicle to the periareolar skin

F: Lines on face

Carotenoids are lipid-soluble yellow to orange-red pigments that are exogenously produced and can be obtained only from plants in the diet. Carotenoids serve a photoprotective role in green plants, but their photoprotective effect in humans is small, even when taken in excess [7]. Carotenoids are found in the epidermis as well as the subcutaneous fat. When present in excess, carotenoids impart a yellowish hue to the skin which may sometimes be prominent [7].

The evolution of pigmentary systems and their variety throughout the animal kingdom are reviewed in Chapter 2.

References

1 Abdel-Malek Z, Kadekaro AL. Human pigmentation: its regulation by ultraviolet light and by endocrine, paracrine, and autocrine factors. In Nordlund JJ, Boissy RE, Hearing VJ *et al.*, eds. *The Pigmentary System,* 2nd edn. Oxford: Blackwell Publishing, 2006: 410–20.

2 Imokawa G. Paracrine interactions of melanocytes in pigmentary disorders. In Nordlund JJ, Boissy RE, Hearing VJ *et al.*, eds. *The Pigmentary System,* 2nd edn. Oxford: Blackwell Publishing, 2006: 421–44.

3 Westerhof W. Colourimetry. In: Serup J, Jemec GBE, Grove GL, eds. *Handbook of Non-Invasive Methods and the Skin,* 2nd edn. Florida: CRC Press, Taylor & Francis, 2006: 634–47.

4 James WD, Carter JM, Rodman OG. Pigmentary demarcation lines: a population survey. *J Am Acad Dermatol* 1987; **16**: 584–90.

5 Kikuchi I. What is a Mongolian spot? *Int J Dermatol* 1982; **21**: 131–3.

6 Kim JH, Herr H. A statistical study of Mongolian spot. *Korean J Dermatol* 1986; **24**: 373–9.

7 Anstey AV. Systemic photoprotection with alpha-tocopherol (vitamin E) and beta-carotene. *Clin Exp Dermatol* 2002; **27**: 170–6.

The melanocyte [1–3]

Epidermal melanin unit

The estimated mass of all pigment cells within the body is about 1.5 g. Most of these are melanocytes within the epidermis [1]. The process of melanin production within these melanocytes is a three-stage process, which involves not only the production of melanosomes within the melanocyte, termed melanogenesis, but also the trafficking and transfer of these pigment granules via long arborizing dendrites to surrounding epidermal keratinocytes. Each epidermal melanocyte together with the epidermal cells that it serves, comprises an 'epidermal melanin unit' as first described by Fitzpatrick and Breathnach in 1963 [2,3]. Although the number of active epidermal melanin units varies considerably in the different regions of the body (Fig. 58.2), the number of keratinocytes served by each melanocyte remains constant. It is estimated that a single melanocyte supplies melanosomes to a group of about 36 viable keratinocytes. This intricate interface between melanocytes and their keratinocytes is essential for skin pigmentation. Adequate pigmentation of the skin is as dependent upon successful transport and transfer of melanosomes to keratinocytes as it is on the formation of the organelle itself.

References

1 Rosdahl I, Rorsman H. An estimate of melanocyte mass in humans. *J Invest Dermatol* 1983; **81**: 278–81.

2 Fitzpatrick TB, Breathnach AS. Das epidermale melamim-einheit System. *Dermatol Wochenschr* 1963; **147**: 481–9.

3 Hadley MacE, Quevedo WC. Vertebrate epidermal melanin unit. *Nature* 1966; **209**: 1334–5.

Distribution of melanocytes [1–3]

Melanocytes are situated in the basal epidermis (Fig. 58.3). The number of melanocytes within the skin shows little variation between different races or between the sexes. However, the capacity of melanocytes to synthesize melanin, both in the basal state (constitutive colour) and after stimulation (facultative colour) by sunlight, shows great variation. Melanocytes in those with dark

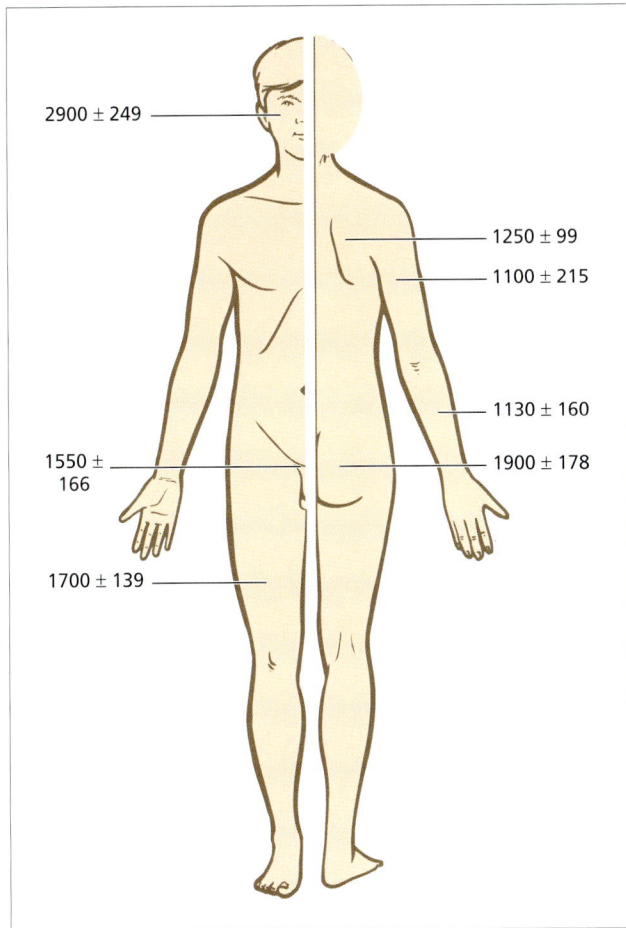

Fig. 58.2 Regional variation in the distribution of epidermal melanocytes. The figures are mean values per mm² ± standard error of the mean. (From Rosdahl & Rorsman [1].)

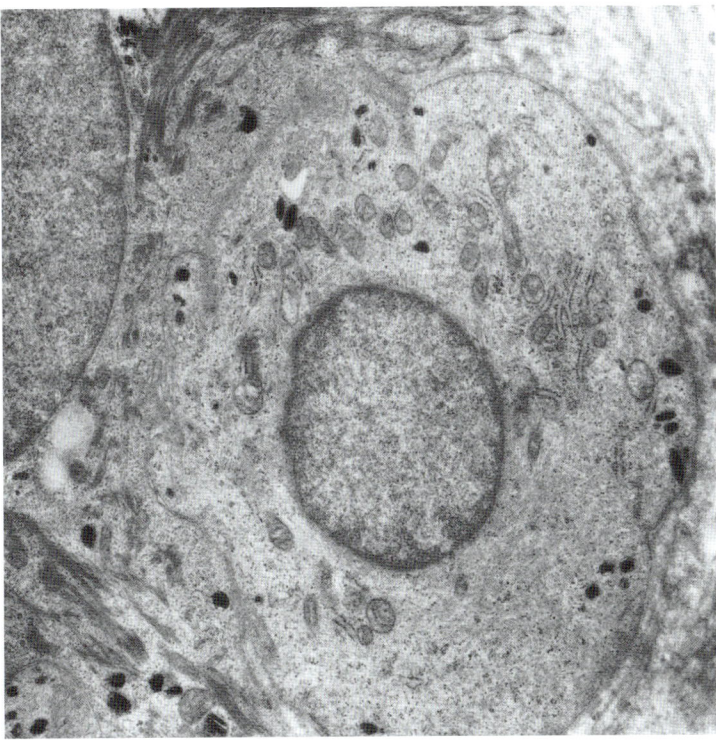

Fig. 58.3 Melanocyte in the basal layer of the epidermis, × 12 000.

skin or with the facility to tan darkly have a great capacity to synthesize melanin and to transfer it to surrounding keratinocytes. In contrast, those with fair skin and lack of tanning facility have very limited capacity. Melanocytes are found in nearly every tissue but are most numerous in the epidermis, hair follicles and the eye [1,2]. A reduction in the number of melanocytes occurs with ageing, with a decrease in melanocyte density of about 6–8% per decade [3]. The density of melanocytes is about two-fold higher in exposed than in non-exposed skin [2].

References
1 Rosdahl I, Rorsman H. An estimate of the melanocyte mass in humans. *J Invest Dermatol* 1983; **81**: 278–81.
2 Szabo G. Regional anatomy of the human integument with special reference to the distribution of hair follicles, sweat glands, and melanocytes. *Philos Trans R Soc Lond B* 1967; **252**: 447–85.
3 Gilchrest BA, Blog FB, Szabo G. Effects of aging and chronic sun exposure on melanocytes in human skin. *J Invest Dermatol* 1979; **73**: 141–3.

Melanoblast migration and differentiation

Pigment cells arise from the neural crest [1], a region of the embryonic ectoderm that originates from the margins of the neural plate at the time when it sinks in to form the tubular central nervous system. The developmental potential of neural crest cells has been studied by a variety of means including clonal analysis, cell grafting experiments and lineage-specific marker studies. Collectively, these studies indicate that most early neural crest cells are multipotent, and become fate-restricted over time [2–4]. Melanoblasts originate in the neural crest and migrate laterally, first to the dermis and then to the basal lamina of the epidermis. Immunocytochemical marker studies with the melanocyte-specific HMB-45 antibody have revealed that melanoblasts appear in the epidermis by 7 weeks' gestation, with a cell density of about 50% of that observed at birth [4]. Ultrastructural studies on early human embryos have demonstrated the presence of melanocytes containing melanosomes showing early melanization [5]. HMB-45 staining has revealed an approximately two-fold increase in melanocyte numbers between gestation weeks 10 and 14, possibly due to mitosis of cells already *in situ* rather than due to addition cell migration. Melanocytes associated with hair follicles arrive at their final location by following the downgrowth of epidermal cells in developing hair follicles [6].

Studies in mice have demonstrated that melanocyte lineage segregation starts early in neural crest development, with melanoblasts specified prior to or coincident with their emigration from the neural tube [7]. Initial segregation of melanocyte lineage involves the Wnt/β-catenin pathway [8]. The transcription factor *mi* is relatively specific for melanocytes differentiation, as was first identified in the *microthalmia (mi)* mutant. *Mi* encodes the transcription factor Mitf, which regulates several melanocyte-specific genes [9,10]. In humans, mutations in *mi* are associated with Waardenburg's syndrome type 2A, an autosomal dominant condition characterized by deafness and patchy abnormal pigmentation [11]. *Sox10* and *Pax3* are two other genes associated with Waardenburg's syndrome, probably through regulation of expression of Mitf protein [12]. *Pax3* appears to prime cells for differentiation, whereas *Wnt* signalling allows cells to proceed along this route [13].

Much of our knowledge about melanocytes development in humans has been derived from studies on mouse pigment mutants [11]. To summarize this body of work in broad terms, mouse coat colour mutants arise from three main groups: those that affect the subcellular structure of melanocytes, those that disrupt the normal synthesis of melanin and those that alter development and differentiation of normal melanocytes. Where possible in the following chapter, molecular and biochemical mechanisms for pigmentary abnormalities in humans with genetic disorders will be highlighted.

References

1 Bagnara JT, Matsumoto J, Ferris W *et al*. On the common origin of pigment cells. *Science* 1979; **203**: 410–5.

2 Le Douarin NM, Creuzet S, Couly G, Dupin E. Neural crest cell plasticity and its limits. *Development* 2004; **131**: 4637–50.

3 Weston JA. Sequential segregation and fate of developmentally restricted intermediate cell populations in the neural crest. *Curr Top Dev Biol* 1991; **25**: 133–53.

4 Holbrook KA, Vogel AM, Underwood RA, Foster CA. Melanocytes in human embryonic and fetal skin: a review and new findings. *Pig Cell Res* 1988; **1** (Suppl.): 6–17.

5 Sagebiel RW, Odland GF. In: Riley V, ed. *Pigmentation: its Genesis and Biologic Control*. New York: Appleton-Century-Crofts, 1972: 43.

6 Mishima Y, Widlan S. Embryonic development of melanocytes in human hair and epidermis. *J Invest Dermatol* 1966; **46**: 263–77.

7 Wilson YM, Richards KL, Ford-Perriss ML *et al*. Neural crest cell lineage segregation in the mouse neural tube. *Development* 2004; **131**: 6153–62.

8 Dunn JD, Brady M, Ochsebauer-Jambor C *et al*. WNT1 and WNT3a promote expansion of melanocytes through distinct modes of action. *Pigment Cell Res* 2005; **18**: 167–80.

9 Baxter LL, Pavan WJ. Pmel17 expression is Mitf-dependent and reveals cranial melanoblasts migration during murine development. *Gene Expr Patterns* 2003; **3**: 703–7.

10 Bentley NJ, Eisen T, Goding CR. Melanocyte-specific expression of the human tyrosinase promoter: activation by the microphthalmia gene product and role of the initiator. *Mol Cell Biol* 1994; **14**: 7996–8006.

11 Baxter LL, Hou L, Loftus SK, Pavan WJ. Spotlight on spotted mice: a review of white spotting mutants and associated human pigmentation disorders. *Pigment Cell Res* 2004; **17**: 215–24.

12 Potterf SB, Furumura M, Dunn KJ *et al*. Transcription factor hierarchy in Waardenburg syndrome: regulation of MITF expression by SOX10 and PAX3. *Hum Gen* 2000; **107**: 1–6.

13 Lang D, Lu MM, Huang L *et al*. Pax3 functions at a nodal point in melanocytes stem cell differentiation. *Nature* 2005; **433**: 884–7.

Melanosome transport [1–10]

Melanosome transport depends upon effective dendrite formation by melanocytes. Ultraviolet radiation and melanocyte-stimulating hormone are both known to stimulate this process [1]. Melanocyte dendrite formation requires actin polymerization, which in turn is controlled by the activity of the small guanosine triphosphate (GTP)-binding proteins Rac and Rho [2–4]. These are themselves controlled by regulatory associated proteins. Direct visualization of melanosome trafficking by video microscopy has revealed evidence to suggest that transfer of melanosomes along dendrites occurs on microtubules [5,6], a process driven by dynein (a minus end microtubule motor) and kinesin (a plus end microtubule motor) [7,8]. Dynein binds microtubules and adenosine triphosphate and produces forces which move the dynein and melanosome complex along the microtubule. Both dynein and kinesin remain bound to the melanosomes and their regulation modifies the direction of melanosome movement along the microtubules [9]. Three individual proteins work together in the final stages of melanosome trafficking. One of these, myosin Va, functions to facilitate the 'capture' of melanosomes at the actin-rich tip of the dendrite [7]. Another, Rab protein, Rab27A, associates with the membrane of melanocytes and then forms a complex with myosin Va and a third protein, melanophylin. The ability of melanophylin to bind actin, in addition to its ability to link with Rab27A and myosin Va, has led to the postulate that transfer of melanosomes from microtubules to actin filaments at the tip of melanocyte dendrites is the final part of the transport process prior to melanosome transfer [10].

References

1 Scott GA, Cassidy L. Rac1 mediates dendrite formation in response to melanocyte stimulating hormone and ultraviolet light in a murine melanoma model. *J Invest Dermatol* 1998; **111**: 243–50.

2 Busca R, Bertolotto C, Abbe P *et al*. Inhibition of Rho is required for cAMP-induced melanoma cell differentiation. *Mol Biol Cell* 1998; **9**: 1367–78.

3 Scott G, Leopardi S. The cAMP signalling pathway has opposing effects on Rac and Rho in B16F10 cells: implications for dendrite formation in melanocytic cells. *Pig Cell Res* 2003; **16**: 139–48.

4 Scott G. Rac and Rho: the story behind melanocyte dendrite formation. *Pig Cell Res* 2002; **15**: 322–30.

5 Scott G, Leopardi S, Printup S, Madden BC. Filopedia are conduits for melanosome transfer to keratinocytes. *J Cell Sci* 2002; **115**: 1441–51.

6 Wu X, Bowers B, Wei Q *et al*. Myosin V associates with melanosomes in mouse melanocytes: evidence that myosin V is an organelle motor. *J Cell Sci* 1997; **110**: 847–59.

7 Byers HR, Yaar M, Eller MS *et al*. Role of cytoplasmic dynein in melanosome transport in human melanocytes. *J Invest Dermatol* 2000; **114**: 990–7.

8 Hara M, Yaar M, Byers HR *et al*. Kinesin participates in melanosomal movement along melanocyte dendrites. *J Invest Dermatol* 2000; **114**: 438–43.

9 Gross SP, Tuma MC, Deacon SW *et al*. Interactions and regulation of molecular motors in *Xenopus* melanophores. *J Cell Biol* 2002; **156**: 855–65.

10 Strom M, Hume AN, Tarafder AK *et al*. A family of Rab27-binding proteins. Melanophilin links Rab27a and myosin Va function in melanosome transport. *J Biol Chem* 2002; **277**: 25423–30.

Melanosome transfer to keratinocytes [1–7]

The successful synthesis of a melanosome, and its transport to the tip of a dendrite, is followed by transfer of the melanosome to the keratinocyte. Both ultraviolet radiation and the hormone MSH stimulate this transfer, while niacinamide has been shown to suppress it [1]. However, the exact mechanism by which the melanosome is transferred to the keratinocyte remains unclear. One possibility is exocytosis of melanosomes from the tips of dendrites with subsequent keratinocyte uptake by endocytosis. In support of this, exocytosis-associated proteins soluble *N*-ethylmaleimide-sensitive factor attachment protein receptor (SNARE) and Rab3a have both been identified on melanosomes [2–4]. Furthermore, *in vivo* high-resolution time-lapse digital images of this process have identified long, dynamic filopedia arising from the melanocyte dendrite tips packed with melanosomes [4]. The filopedia have been observed to attach and detach from the keratinocyte membrane; melanocytes have been observed travelling in both directions within the filopedia [4]. Work from several groups has revealed that lectins and their glycosolated ligands may function as receptor-ligand pairs in these melanocyte-keratinocyte interactions [5–7].

References

1 Hakozaki T, Minwalla L, Zhuang J *et al.* The effect of niacinamide on reducing cutaneous pigmentation and suppression of melanosome transfer. *Br J Dermatol* 2002; **147**: 200–31.

2 Takai Y, Sasaki T, Shirataki H, Nakanishi H. Rab3A small GTP-binding protein in Ca(2+)-dependent exocytosis. *Genes Cells* 1996; **1**: 615–32.

3 Jahn R, Sudhof TC. Membrane fusion and exocytosis. *Ann Rev Biochem* 1999; **68**: 863–911.

4 Scott G, Zhao Q. Rab3a and SNARE proteins: potential regulators of melanosome movement. *J Invest Dermatol* 2001; **116**: 296–304.

5 Cerdan D, Grillon C, Monsigny M, Redziniak G, Keida C. Human keratinocyte membrane lectins: characterization and modulation of their expression by cytokines. *Biol Cell* 1991; **73**: 35–42.

6 Condaminet B, Redziniak G, Monsigny M, Keida C. Ultraviolet rays induced expression of lectins on the surface of a squamous carcinoma keratinocyte cell line. *Exp Cell Res* 1997; **232**: 216–24.

7 Minwalla I, Zhao Y, Cornelius J *et al.* Inhibition of melanosome transfer from melanocytes to keratinocytes by lectins and neoglycoproteins in an *in vitro* model system. *Pigment Cell Res* 2001; **14**: 185–94.

Melanocyte culture [1–8]

Melanocytes fail to grow, and usually die, in culture media used for skin fibroblasts or keratinocytes. In contrast to many other cell types, melanocytes do not produce any of the growth factors that are known to stimulate them [1]. Following an intensive search, the first highly effective natural melanocyte mitogen was identified as basic fibroblast growth factor (now termed FGF2) [2]. As more mitogens for melanocytes emerged, it was apparent that a combination of synergistic growth factors was required to stimulate quiescent or moribund melanocytes in culture [1,3]. Additional stimulatory peptides include mast cell growth factor/stem cell factor (M/SCF, also known as Kit ligand and Steel factor), hepatocyte growth factor/scatter factor (HGF/SF), endothelins and, to a lesser degree, melanocyte-stimulating hormone (MSH). In the presence of FGF2, phorbol ester and cyclic adenosine monophosphate these peptides act synergistically on melanocytes in culture [1,4]. A more recent addition to the list of melanocyte mitogens is leukaemia inhibitory factor (LIF) [5]. With the exception of FGF2, most of these factors also promote melanocyte differentiation [6,7]. Endothelin 1 (ET1) can also sustain the viability of human melanocytes in the absence of other growth factors and can also stimulate the formation and elongation of dendrites [4,8].

References

1 Halaban R. The regulation of normal melanocytes proliferation. *Pigment Cell Res* 2000; **13**: 4–14.

2 Halaban R, Ghosh S, Baird A. bFGF is the putative natural growth factor for human melanocytes. *In Vitro Cell Dev Biol* 1987; **23**: 47–52.

3 Halaban R. Growth factors and tyrosine protein kinases in normal and malignant melanocytes. *Cancer Metast Rev* 1991; **10**: 129–40.

4 Böhm M, Moellmann GE, Cheng M *et al.* Identification of p90RSK as the probable CREB-Ser 133 kinase in human melanocytes. *Cell Growth Differ* 1995; **6**: 291–302.

5 Hirobe T. Role of leukaemia inhibitory factor in the regulation of differentiation of neonatal mouse epidermal melanocytes in culture. *J Cell Physiol* 2002; **192**: 315–26.

6 Halaban R, Tyrrell L, Longley J, Yarden Y, Rubin J. Pigmentation and proliferation in human melanocytes and the effects of melanocyte-stimulating hormone and ultraviolet B light. *Ann N Y Acad Sci* 1993; **680**: 290–301.

7 Odecamp K, Kos L, Arnheiter H, Pavan WJ. Endothelin signaling in the development of neural crest-derived melanocytes. *Biochem Cell Biol* 1998; **76**: 1093–9.

8 Hara M, Yaar M, Gilchrest BA. Endothelin-1 of keratinocytes origin is a mediator of melanocytes dendricity. *J Invest Dermatol* 1995; **105**: 744–8.

Table 58.2 Main types of epidermal melanin pigments. (Courtesy of Prota [2].)

Eumelanins	Brown or black nitrogenous pigments, insoluble in all solvents, which arise by oxidative polymerization of 5,6-dihydroxyindoles derived biogenetically from tyrosine
Phaeomelanins	Alkali-soluble pigments, ranging from yellow to reddish-brown; most of them contain sulphur in addition to nitrogen and arise by oxidative polymerization of cysteinyl-dopa via 1,4-benzothiazine intermediates
Trichochromes	A variety of sulphur-containing phaeomelanic pigments with a well-defined structure, characterized by a $\Delta^{2,2'}$-bi(1,4-benzothiazine) chromophore

Biochemistry of melanogenesis [1–5]

Melanins are usually classified into two main groups: the brown to black insoluble eumelanins, and the yellow to reddish-brown alkali-soluble phaeomelanins (Table 58.2). Both pigments are derived from dopaquinone, which is formed by the oxidation of the common amino acid L-tyrosine by tyrosinase.

Eumelanin formation

Dopaquinone is a highly reactive intermediate and in the absence of sulfhydryl compounds it forms cyclodopa. The redox exchange between cyclodopa and dopaquinone then gives rise to the red intermediate dopachrome and dopa. Dopachrome then rearranges to 5,6-dihydroxyindole (DHI) and to a lesser extent to 5,6-dihydroxyindole carboxylic acid (DHICA). Finally, these two compounds are oxidized and polymerized to produce eumelanins. In addition to tyrosinase, dopachrome tautomerase and Tryp1 (DHICA oxidase) are now both recognized as having a role in the regulation and promotion of eumelanogenesis [1].

Pheomelanin formation

In contrast to eumelanins, pheomelanins contain sulphur in addition to nitrogen and are formed from cysteinyldopa (Fig. 58.4). Further oxidation of the thiol adducts leads to the formation of pheomelanin via benzothiazine intermediates. Most melanin pigments in skin are mixtures or copolymers of eumelanins and pheomelanins. However, the situation is complicated by the fact that some pheomelanin-like pigments may be structural variants of eumelanins [2]. Thus, in the presence of metal ions, black insoluble eumelanin may be oxidized chemically or photochemically to a soluble form (melanin-free acid), which is light in colour [3,4].

Trichochromes

A further complication is that red human hair contains, in addition to pheomelanins, small amounts of intensely coloured pigments known as trichochromes [2,5], originally isolated from the red feathers of New Hampshire hens. Trichochromes are sulphur-containing pigments of a well-defined structure, of which six variants have so far been identified (Fig. 58.5).

References

1 Hearing VJ. Invited editorial: unraveling the melanocytes. *Am J Hum Genet* 1993; **52**: 1–7.

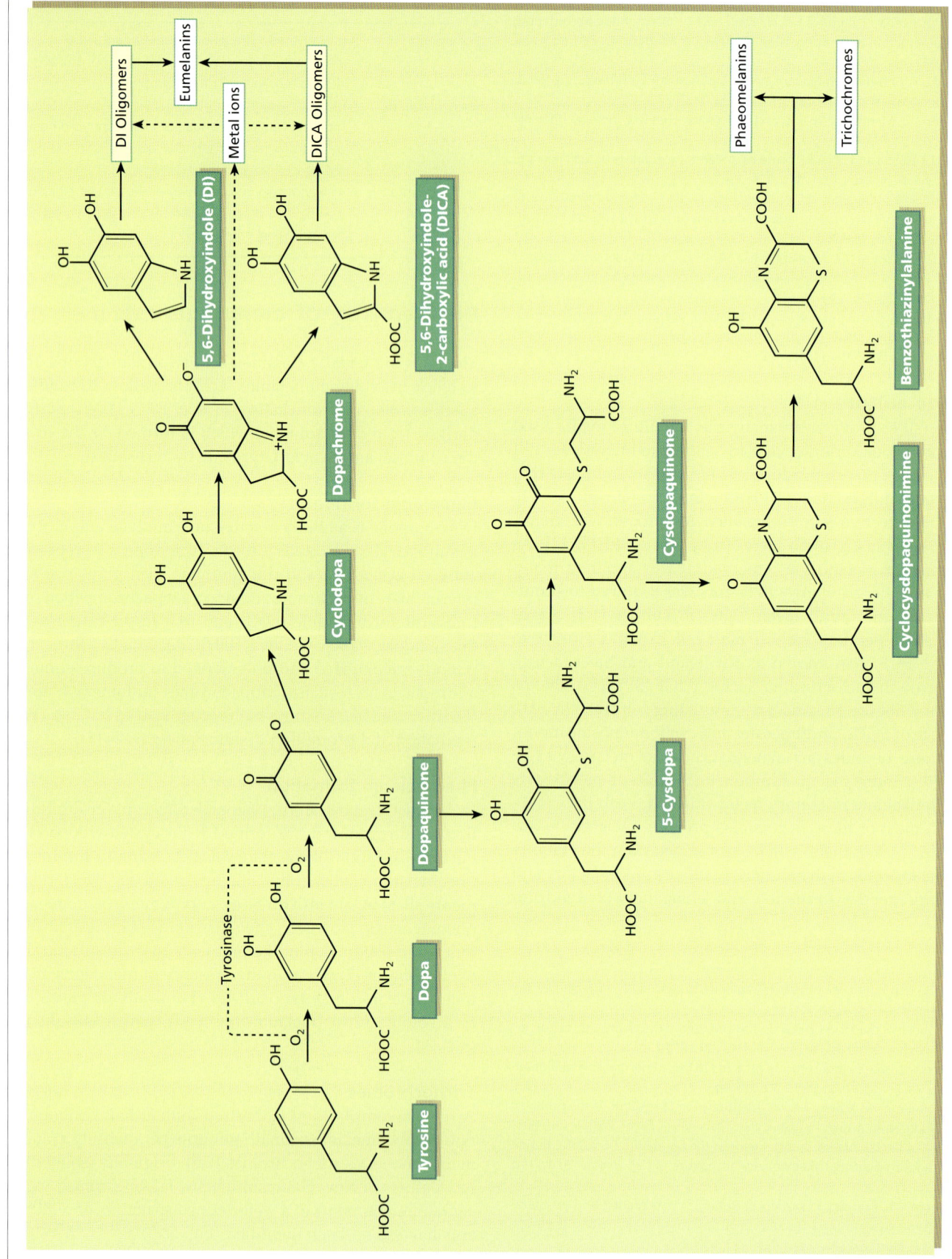

Fig. 58.4 A simplified overview of the major metabolic pathways in the synthesis of melanins and trichochromes. (From Prota [2].)

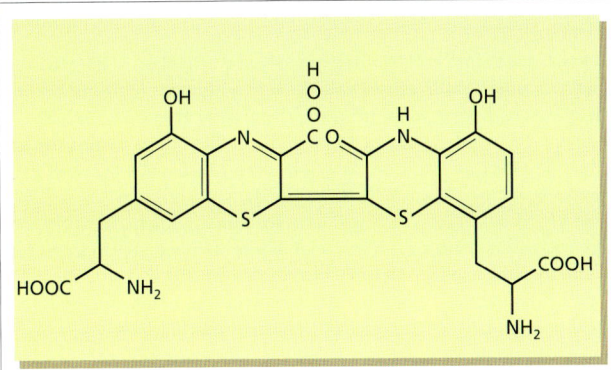

Fig. 58.5 Structure of trichochrome B, one of six trichochromes so far identified.

2 Prota G. Progress in the chemistry of melanins and related metabolites. *Med Res Rev* 1988; **8**: 525–56.
3 Albrecht L, Patil D, Wolfram LJ. Photochemical properties of pheo and eumelanins. *J Invest Dermatol* 1986; **87**: 396.
4 Chedekel MR, Bahn P, Patil D *et al*. Melanin free acid: a chemical standard for eumelanin research. *J Invest Dermatol* 1986; **87**: 397.
5 Prota G. Recent advances in the chemistry of melanogenesis in mammals. *J Invest Dermatol* 1980; **75**: 122–7.

Regulation of human pigmentation by ultraviolet light and by endocrine, paracrine and autocrine factors

Regulation of human melanocytes is complex; in addition to a direct stimulatory effect of ultraviolet radiation, there are also effects mediated by endocrine, paracrine and autocrine factors. Constitutive melanin content is determined by the rate of synthesis by melanocytes and by the rate and mode of melanosome delivery to keratinocytes. The response of cultured melanocytes to ultraviolet radiation involves growth arrest in conjunction with increased melanogenesis. A differential response is observed between melanocytes derived from individuals of skin types I or II and those from skin types V or IV, with the former showing more prolonged growth arrest, more cyclobutane pyrimidine dimers and less melanogenesis. Exposure of human skin to ultraviolet radiation induces a number of epidermal cytokines and growth factors which in turn induce proliferation of melanocytes and/or melanogenesis. Many devoted sun-worshippers know that by deliberately overdosing on sun exposure, the inflammatory sunburn that ensues is more effective at inducing tanning than a more patient, non-burning approach.

Melanocyte response to UV radiation

Sun exposure is associated with an increased number of active melanocytes in sun-protected skin in the same individual. Friedmann and Gilchrest [1] were the first to demonstrate this direct responsiveness in cultured melanocytes, by showing that irradiation with solar-simulated ultraviolet light resulted in a dose-dependent decrease in proliferation and an increase in pigmentation. More recently, research using sub-lethal doses of UVB showed inhibition of melanocyte proliferation as a result of arrest in G_2 phase of the cell cycle, and an increased tyrosinase activity and

melanin content [2]. Melanocytes derived from different skin types all showed a similar pattern of response [2]. Subsequent research has confirmed that this UV-induced growth arrest of melanocytes is related to increased levels of the tumour suppressor gene product p53, with lightly pigmented melanocytes experiencing a more prolonged growth arrest, and a more sustained increase in the p53 protein, than occurs in darkly pigmented melanocytes [3]. Furthermore, lightly pigmented melanocytes show more cyclobutane pyrimidine dimers (a reliable marker for UV-induced DNA damage) after UV irradiation than occurs in heavily pigmented melanocytes [3]. In addition to increased activity of melanocyte tyrosinase, sun exposure leads to elongation and branching of melanocyte dendrites, and an increase in the number and size of melanosomes.

Melanocyte regulation by endocrine factors

The effects of oestrogens on cutaneous pigmentation have been recognized for more than 60 years [4,5]. High levels of oestrogens during pregnancy are implicated in the increased pigmentation that occurs on the face, areola, lower central abdomen and genitalia. Oestrogens have been shown to stimulate melanogenesis in cultured melanocytes by increased tyrosinase activity [6]; these include α-oestradiol, β-oestradiol and oestriol [7]. However, no specific receptors for oestrogens have yet been identified in melanocytes.

In Addison disease the diffuse brown hyperpigmentation results from the melanogenic action of melanocortins derived from the pituitary. The melanocortins are all derived from a precursor molecule, pro-opiomelanocortin. Other melanocortins released from the pituitary in increased quantities in Addison disease include β-lipotrophin, γ-melanotrophin (γ-MSH), β-melanotropin (β-MSH) and α-melanotropin (α-MSH). These peptides all have a stimulatory effect on melanocytes [8], and, in the absence of negative feedback to inhibit their secretion, the hyperpigmentation produced is insidious and progressive (Fig. 58.6). Human melanocytes express the melanocortin 1 receptor (MC1R) that binds α-MSH and ACTH with the same affinity [9]. α-MSH causes a small rise in cAMP but has no effect on basal or ultraviolet-stimulated melanogenesis in human melanocytes [10].

Melanocyte regulation by paracrine and autocrine factors

Post-inflammatory hyperpigmentation is believed to be mediated by immune inflammatory mediators including IL-1α, IL-1β, IL-6 and TNF-α [11]. Human melanocytes have also been demonstrated to respond to, and synthesise, IL-1α and IL-1β, which suggests an autocrine as well as a paracrine regulatory role [12]. Other inflammatory mediators that act on human melanocytes include ecosanoids, metabolites of arachidonic acid. Melanocytes respond to PGE_2 with increased melanogenesis and dendrite formation [13]. Scott *et al.* demonstrated an increase in dendricity of human melanocytes in response to PGE_2 and $PGF_{2\alpha}$ [14]. Basic fibroblast growth factor was the first paracrine factor for human melanocytes to be identified. It exerts its effect by binding to a tyrosine kinase receptor that is expressed on human melanocytes [15]. In contrast to IL-1α, IL-1β, IL-6 and TNF-α and the ecosanoids, basic fibroblast growth factor is not secreted by keratinocytes; direct contact between melanocytes and keratinocytes is required for its

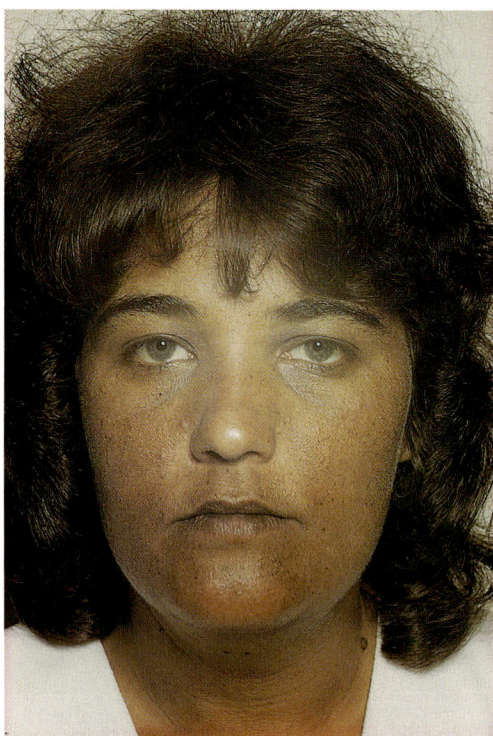

Fig. 58.6 Diffuse hyperpigmentation with darkening of hair and mucous membranes in a woman with Nelson's syndrome following bilateral adrenalectomy.

biological effects [16]. Additionally, leukotrienes C_4 and D_4 have been shown to act as potent mitogens on cultured human neonatal melanocytes [17].

Endothelins are a further important group of peptides that act upon melanocytes in a paracrine manner [18]. Endothelin-1 (ET-1) is both mitogenic and melanogenic for human melanocytes that express ET-1 receptors [19]. ET-1 acts synergistically with α-MSH and basic fibroblast growth factor to stimulate human melanocytes proliferation [20]. Endothelin-3 (ET-3) has similar effects to ET-1; both peptides bind the endothelin receptor on melanocytes with equal affinity [21]. Furthermore, endothelins appear to have a role in protecting melanocytes: Kadekaro *et al.* demonstrated that treatment of human melanocytes with ET-1 reduced UVR-induced apoptosis and prolonged melanocyte survival [22].

References

1 Friedmann PS, Gilchrest BA. Ultraviolet radiation directly induces pigment production by cultured human melanocytes. *J Cell Physiol* 1987; **133**: 88–94.
2 Abdel-Malek Z, Swope V, Smalara D *et al.* Analysis of the UV-induced melanogenesis and growth arrest in human melanocytes. *Pig Cell Res* 1994; **7**: 326–32.
3 Barker D, Dixon K, Medrano EE *et al.* Comparison of the responses of human melanocytes with different melanin contents to ultraviolet B irradiation. *Cancer Res* 1995; **55**: 4041–6.
4 Hamilton JB, Hubert G. Photographic nature of tanning of human skin as shown by studies of male hormone therapy. *Science* 1938; **88**: 481.
5 Hamilton JB. Significance of sex hormones in tanning of the skin in women. *Proc Soc Exp Biol Med* 1941; **40**: 502–3.
6 Ransom M, Posen S, Mason RS. Human melanocytes as a target tissue for hormones: in vitro studies with 1α-25, dihydroxy-vitamin D3, α-melanocyte stimulating hormone, and β-estradiol. *J Invest Dermatol* 1988; **91**: 593–8.
7 McLeod SD, Ranson M, Mason RS. Effects of estrogens on human melanocytes in vitro. *J Steroid Biochem* 1994; **49**: 9–14.
8 Shizume K. Thirty five years of progress in the study of MSH. *Yale J Biol Med* 1985; **58**: 561–70.
9 Suzuki I, Cone R, Im S *et al.* Binding capacity and activation of the MC1 receptors by melanotropic hormones correlate directly with their mitogenic and melanogenic effects on human melanocytes. *Endocrinology* 1996; **137**: 1627–33.
10 Friedmann PS, Wren F, Buffey J, MacNeil S. α-MSH causes a small rise in cAMP but has no effect on basal or ultraviolet-stimulated melanogenesis in human melanocytes. *Br J Dermatol* 1990; **123**: 145–51.
11 Swope VB, Abdel-Malek ZA, Kassem L, Nordlund JJ. Interleukins 1-α and 6 and tumor necrosis factor-α are paracrine inhibitors of human melanocytes proliferation and melanogenesis. *J Invest Dermatol* 1991; **96**: 180–5.
12 Swope VB, Sauder DN, McKenzie RC *et al.* Synthesis of interleukin-1α and β by normal human melanocytes. *J Invest Dermatol* 1994; **102**: 749–53.
13 Tomita Y, Iwamoto M, Masuda T, Tagami H. Stimulatory effect of prostaglandin E_2 on the configuration of normal human melanocytes. *J Invest Dermatol* 1987; **89**: 299–301.
14 Scott G, Leopardi S, Printup S *et al.* Proteinase-activated receptor-2 stimulates prostaglandin production in keratinocytes: analysis of prostaglandin receptors on human melanocytes and effects of PGE_2 and $PGF_{2\alpha}$ on melanocytes dendricity. *J Invest Dermatol* 2004; **122**: 1214–24.
15 Pittelkow MR, Shipley GD. Serum-free culture of normal human melanocytes: growth kinetics and growth factor requirements. *J Cell Physiol* 1989; **140**: 565–76.
16 Gordon PR, Mansur CP, Gilchrest BA. Regulation of human melanocyte growth, dendricity, and melanization by keratinocyte derived factors. *J Invest Dermatol* 1989; **92**: 565–72.
17 Morelli JG, Yohn JJ, Lyons MM *et al.* Leukotrienes C_4 and D_4 as potent mitogens for cultured human neonatal melanocytes. *J Invest Dermatol* 1989; **93**: 719–22.
18 Rubanyi GM, Polokoff MA. Endothelins: molecular biology, biochemistry, pharmacology, physiology and pathophysiology. *Pharmacol Rev* 1994; **46**: 325–415.
19 Yada Y, Higuchi K, Imokawa G. Effects of endothelins on signal transduction and proliferation in human melanocytes. *J Biol Chem* 1991; **166**: 18352–7.
20 Swope VB, Medrano EE, Smalara D, Abdel-Malek Z. Long-term proliferation of human melanocytes is supported by the physiologic mitogens α-melanotropin, endothelin-1, and basic fibroblast growth factor. *Exp Cell Res* 1995; **217**: 453–9.
21 Tada A, Suzuki I, Im S *et al.* Endothelin-1 is a paracrine growth factor that modulates melanogenesis of human melanocytes and participates in their responses to ultraviolet radiation. *Cell Growth Differ* 1998; **9**: 575–84.
22 Kadekaro AL, Kanto H, Kavanagh R *et al.* α-Melanocortin and endothelin-1 promote the survival of human melanocytes by activating anti-apoptotic pathways and enhancing the repair of DNA photoproduct. *Cancer Res* 2005; **65**: 4292–9.

Biological significance of melanin

The major biological function of melanin is generally assumed to be protection of the lower layers of the skin against UV light. If human pigment has such adaptive significance, we might expect to find that, among the races of the world, pigment is geographically distributed in relation to solar intensity. It appears to be generally true that pigmentation is greatest in the tropics and reduced in temperate zones, reappearing to some extent in northern races subjected to prolonged snow glare [1]. However, there are exceptions, for example native Americans are not notably different in skin colour throughout the whole continent, and Tasmanians are dark even though they live in a temperate climate.

The damaging role of UV light is well illustrated by the high incidence of epidermal carcinoma in Europeans exposed to excess sun. The evolutionary usefulness of pigmentation may be twofold. On the one hand, it protects against damage by sunburn. On the other, since it efficiently absorbs UV radiation and is readily activated to a free radical by incident light, it may serve to eliminate genetically damaged cells by a phototoxic mechanism.

Not all the effects of pigmentation are advantageous. There is no doubt that pigmentation increases the heat load in hot climates, so that black people absorb 30% more heat from sunlight than do white people, although this factor may be offset by more profuse sweating [2,3]. In addition, in cold climates pale skin has the advantage that heat loss by radiation is reduced.

A further disadvantage of pigmentation is that it hinders synthesis of vitamin D, so that in areas of poor nutrition black children are more liable to rickets than white children. Thus, loss of pigmentation may facilitate vitamin D synthesis in temperate climates. It might be presumed that the retention of pigment in Arctic latitudes, while providing a protection against snow glare, is only permitted by natural selection because of the high-fat diet in these areas.

Since pigmentation appears to be not entirely advantageous to life in the tropics, other hypotheses about its biological significance have been advanced. For example, Wassermann [4,5] suggested that the major adaptation of black people to tropical Africa is in the ability to survive malaria, multiple parasites and tropical diseases under the hazards of intense solar radiation and, more often than not, poor nutrition. He suggests that diseases, not climatic conditions, are the primary selective factors, and lists evidence that black Africans, in comparison with white people, show increased reticuloendothelial activity and increased serum γ-globulin fractions. These features are inversely related to the size and activity of the adrenal cortex. Because of their primary decrease in adrenocortical function, black people show increased MSH and adrenocorticotrophic hormone (ACTH) activity, which enhances melanogenesis. Pigmentation might thus be a secondary phenomenon.

References

1 Fleure HJ. The distribution of types of skin colour. *Geogr Rev* 1945; **35**: 580–95.
2 Blum HF. The physiological effects of sunlight on man. *Physiol Rev* 1945; **25**: 483–530.
3 Blum HF. Does the melanin pigment of human skin have adaptive value? An essay in human ecology and the evolution of race. *Q Rev Biol* 1961; **36**: 50–63.
4 Wassermann HP. Melanokinetics and the biological significance of melanin. *Br J Dermatol* 1970; **82**: 530–4.
5 Wassermann HP. *Ethnic Pigmentation*. Amsterdam: Excerpta Medica, 1974.

Classification of disorders of melanin pigmentation

Disorders of melanin pigmentation can be divided on morphological grounds into two types. The first is hypermelanosis, where there is an increased amount of melanin in the skin. This excess may be confined to the epidermis, when the skin appears browner than normal, or it may be present in the dermis, producing a slaty-grey or blue appearance. The second type is hypomelanosis, where there is a lack of pigment in the skin, which therefore appears white or lighter than the normal colour. Amelanosis is the term applied when there is a total lack of melanin in the skin. Hypermelanosis and hypomelanosis can be generalized and diffuse, or may be localized and circumscribed. Sometimes, localized areas may have a segmental or dermatomal pattern. The term 'depigmentation' is used to describe a loss of pre-existing pigment from

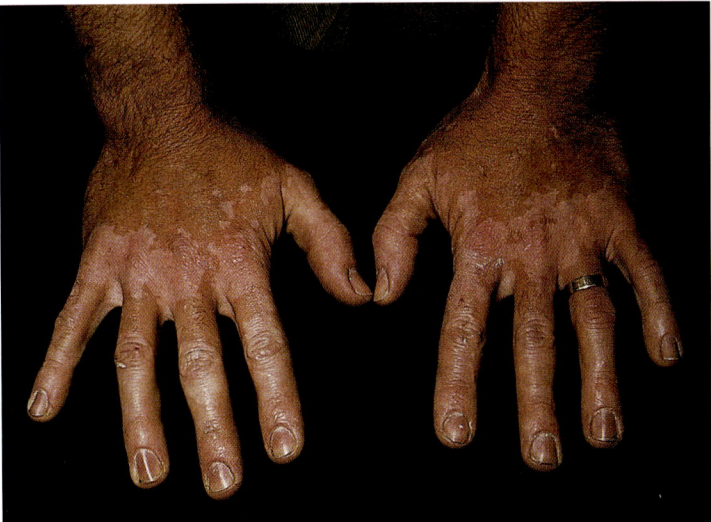

Fig. 58.7 Occupational vitiligo due to tertiary-butylphenol.

the skin. Leukoderma is a white skin that may be congenital or acquired and can be due to a variety of aetiological factors. Examination of the skin with a source of long-wave UV light, for example Wood's lamp, is often helpful in localizing abnormal variations in melanin pigmentation in the skin and as an aid to the diagnosis of various disorders [1].

Changes in pigmentation can arise in a number of ways and can be due to a variety of genetic and environmental factors. It is also pertinent to consider non-melanin pigmentation as a cause of cutaneous colour changes, as discussed at the end of this chapter.

Hypermelanosis similarly can be due to many factors, both genetic and acquired (Fig. 58.7). It can be due to an increased number of melanocytes in the skin such as occurs in the dermal melanocytoses: the naevus of Ota, the naevus of Ito and the Mongolian spot. Many of the hypermelanotic disorders are due to an increase in melanogenesis due to genetic factors. Some may be induced by UV light, hormones and chemical compounds. Finally, the degradation of melanosomes may vary in different disorders of pigmentation.

Reference

1 Gilchrest BA, Fitzpatrick TB, Anderson RR, Parrish JA. Localization of melanin pigmentation in the skin with Wood's lamp. *Br J Dermatol* 1977; **96**: 245–8.

Constitutive pigmentation, human pigmentation and the response to sun exposure

Genetic factors play the primary role in determining the degree of pigmentation that is normal for the individual. Variation in skin pigmentation is not due to differences in the number of melanocytes but is explained by differences in melanocyte structure and function; melanogenic activity, the size and number of melanosomes, the type of melanin deposited onto melanosomes, and the donation of mature melanosomes to adjacent keratinocytes all contribute to the resulting colour of the skin and are genetically determined. Thus, constitutive skin colour, as well as how the colour changes in response to exposure to sunlight, are both genetically determined, and show relatively little variation within different racial groups. There is, however, marked variation in human skin colour between the main racial groupings ranging from white (Caucasoid), through lightly pigmented (Asian and Oriental), to black (Negroid and Australoid and some Asian races). Racial differences in melanocyte morphology and function are apparent, but there is little inter-racial variation in the density of melanocytes at a particular skin site. Ultrastructural studies have shown that melanosomes in white skin are small and tend to be in membrane-bound complexes containing three or more within the keratinocytes [1]. The ellipsoidal melanosomes of aboriginals and black people are larger, about 1 μm in length, and tend to be distributed as singlets rather than being aggregated. These larger melanosomes can be found intact in the stratum corneum. The melanosomes in the complexes in white people show degradative changes even in the basal layer of the epidermis and are presumably broken up by lysosomal enzymes [2]. Whether melanosomes are individually dispersed or aggregated in melanosomal complexes appears to depend on the size of the melanosome [1].

Melanin in the skin exerts its photoprotective effect by reducing the penetration of ultraviolet light through the epidermis and by quenching reactive oxygen radicals that contribute to the sun-induced DNA damage [3]. The superior photoprotection of the black epidermis is due not only to its increased melanin content but also to melanogenic activity, the size and number of melanosomes, the type of melanin deposited onto melanosomes, and the donation of mature melanosomes to adjacent keratinocytes. A classification of sun-reactive skin types based on sunburn and tanning history has been in widespread use since its introduction (Table 58.3) [4]. Two types of pigmentation of the skin in humans occur in response to sun exposure. The first is immediate pigment darkening, sometimes referred to as the Meirowsky phenomenon or 'IPD'. This is best observed in those with hyperpigmented skins and is most effectively induced by long-wave UV light (UVA). It is transient and, although rapidly induced, soon fades. The second is the increased pigmentation that follows the erythemal response. This is the delayed tanning reaction and can be seen 48–72 h after skin exposure to UV light.

References

1 Olson RL, Gaylon J, Everett MA. Skin color, melanin and erythema. *Arch Dermatol* 1973; **108**: 541–4.
2 Hori Y, Toda K, Pathak MA *et al.* A fine-structure study of the human epidermal melanosome complex and its acid phosphatase activity. *J Ultrastruct Res* 1968; **25**: 109–20.

Table 58.3 Classification of sun-reactive skin types.

Skin type	Sun sensitivity	Pigmentary response
I	Very sensitive, always burn easily	Little or no tan
II	Very sensitive, always burn	Minimal tan
III	Sensitive, burn moderately	Tan gradually (light brown)
IV	Moderately sensitive, burn minimally	Tan easily (brown)
V	Minimally sensitive, rarely burn	Tan darkly (dark brown)
VI	Insensitive, never burn	Deeply pigmented (black)

3 Kaidbey KH, Poh Agin P, Sayre RM, Kligman AM. Photoprotection by melanin: a comparison of black and caucasian skin. *J Am Acad Dermatol* 1979; **1**: 249–60.
4 Fitzpatrick TB. The validity and practicality of sun-reaction skin types I through VI. *Arch Dermatol* 1988; **124**: 869–71.

Hypermelanosis

Ephelides

Synonym
• Freckles

Freckling is probably determined by an autosomal dominant gene [1]. It is most frequent in individuals with red or blonde hair and blue eyes, particularly in those of Celtic (Scottish, Irish, Welsh) extraction. Red-haired individuals with fair skin (and freckles) have a significantly higher incidence of the gene encoding melanocortin receptors [2,3].

Pathology [4]. There is no increase in the number of melanocytes in the pigmented macules but their melanosomes are long and rod-shaped, like those found generally in dark-skinned people. They form melanin more rapidly after exposure to sunlight than do those in the surrounding pale skin, which are spherical and often granular, and are of the type usually found in fair- and red-haired individuals. With the light microscope, the only abnormality detectable is an increase in the quantity of melanin in the epidermis.

Clinical features (Fig. 58.8). Freckles are small macules of hyperpigmentation, usually measuring 2–4 mm in size. They first appear at about the age of 5 years as light-brown pigmented macules on

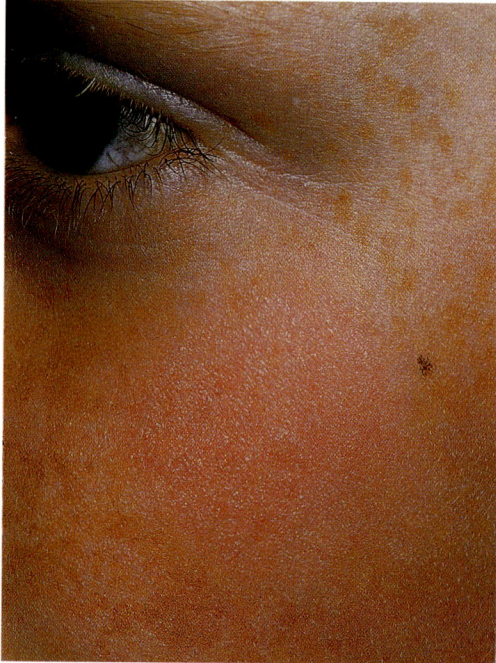

Fig. 58.8 Freckles, one area of which has been bleached by a superimposed patch of pityriasis alba.

light-exposed skin. They are most numerous on the face, upper back, and dorsal forearms and hands. They increase in number, size and depth of pigmentation during the summer months and are smaller, lighter and fewer in number in the winter. They may be cosmetically disfiguring or may enhance appearance, but are not otherwise of significance.

The incidence of melanocytic naevi is increased in freckled individuals.

Treatment. Freckles seldom require treatment and may sometimes be regarded as a desirable cutaneous feature. Application of 2–4% hydroquinone with a UVA-blocking sunscreen in the morning and retinoic acid in the evening produces significant lightening in most freckles. Alternatively, they are amenable to removal by laser [5,6]. Solar lentigines may be improved in appearance by topical treatment which includes retinoic acid [7].

Freckles in various syndromes. Freckles are a feature of a number of inherited and acquired disorders described in this chapter. These include xeroderma pigmentosum [8], neurofibromatosis, Moynahan's syndrome and progeria. The lesions in the various forms of lentiginosis (see below) must also be differentiated. Their distribution and the lack of relationship to light exposure should be noted.

References
1 Brues AM. Linkage of body build with sex, eye colour and freckling. *Am J Hum Genet* 1950; **2**: 215–39.
2 Valverde P, Healy E, Jackson I *et al*. Variants of the melanocyte-stimulating hormone-receptor gene are associated with red hair and fair skin in humans. *Nat Genet* 1995; **11**: 328–30.
3 Box NF, Wyeth JR, O'Gorman LE *et al*. Chacterization of melanocyte stimulating hormone receptor variant alleles in twins with red hair. *Hum Mol Genet* 1997; **6**: 1891–7.
4 Breathnach AS. Electron microscopy of melanocytes and melanosomes in freckled human epidermis. *J Invest Dermatol* 1964; **42**: 389–94.
5 Brazzini B, Hautmann G, Ghersitich I *et al*. Laser tissue interaction with epidermal pigmented lesions. *J Eur Acad Dermatol* 2001; **15**: 468–9.
6 Rosenbach A, Lee S-J. Treatment of medium-brown solar lentigines using an alexandrite laser designed for hair reduction. *Arch Dermatol* 2002; **138**: 547–8.
7 Fleisher AB, Schwartzel EH, Colby SI, Altman DJ. The combination of 2% 4-hydroxyanisole (Mequinol) and 0.01% tretinoin is effective in improving the appearance of solar lentigines and related hyperpigmented lesions in two double-blind multicenter clinical studies. *J Am Acad Dermatol* 2000; **42**: 459–67.
8 Ito M. Genetical studies on skin diseases: ephelides, dyschromatosis symmetrica hereditaria and xeroderma pigmentosum. *Tohoku J Exp Med* 1950; **3**: 69–72.

Lentiginosis

The histological and clinical features of lentigo, together with other lesions in which the number of melanocytes is increased, are fully described in Chapter 54. A lentigo is a benign, pigmented macule in which there is an increased number of melanocytes. The term 'lentiginosis' is applied either when lentigines are present in exceptionally large numbers, or when they occur in a distinctive distribution. The following clinical syndromes are recognized.

Generalized lentiginosis

Lentigines are commonly multiple but appear singly or in small crops at irregular intervals from infancy onwards. Their pathogenesis is unknown and in the great majority of cases no genetic factor is demonstrable.

Unilateral lentiginosis (zosteriform lentiginosis)

Lentigines may occur on one side of the body [1]. Cases have been reported with and without associated neurological abnormalities [2–4]. The lentigines can be zosteriform and occur in a dermatomal-like distribution [5–7]. These cases are usually without central nervous system abnormalities and are naevoid. Lentigines have also been reported within naevoid hypopigmentation [8]. A case of unilateral lentiginosis with contralateral naevus depigmentosus has been reported [9].

References
1 Davis DG, Shaw MW. An unusual human mosaic for skin pigmentation. *N Engl J Med* 1964; **270**: 1384–9.
2 Pickering JG. Partial unilateral lentiginosis with associated developmental abnormalities. *Guys Hosp Rep* 1973; **122**: 361–70.
3 Thompson GW, Diehl AK. Partial unilateral lentiginosis. *Arch Dermatol* 1980; **116**: 356.
4 Trattner H, Metzker A. Partial unilateral lentiginosis. *J Am Acad Dermatol* 1993; **29**: 693–5.
5 Matsudo H, Reed WB, Homme D *et al*. Zosterform lentiginous nevus. *Arch Dermatol* 1973; **107**: 902–5.
6 Port M, Courniotes J, Podwal M. Zosteriform lentiginous naevus with ipsilateral rigid left cavus foot. *Br J Dermatol* 1978; **98**: 693–8.
7 Schaffer JV, Lazova R, Bolognia JL. Partial unilateral lentiginosis with occular involvement. *J Am Acad Dermatol* 2001; **44**: 387–90.
8 Khumalo NP, Huson S, Burge S. Development of lentigines within naevoid hypopigmentation. *Br J Dermatol* 2001; **144**: 188–9.
9 Alkemade H, Juhlin L. Unilateral lentiginosis with nevus depigmentosus on the other side. *J Am Acad Dermatol* 2000; **43**: 361–3.

Inherited patterned lentiginosis in black people [1]

O'Neill reported generalized lentiginosis in 10 adult black patients, with onset in childhood; seven showed familial clustering, suggesting autosomal dominant inheritance [1]. Distribution of the lentigines included the face, lips, extremities, buttocks, palms and soles, but not mucosal surfaces.

Reference
1 O'Neill JF, James WD. Inherited patterned lentiginosis in blacks. *Arch Dermatol* 1989; **125**: 1231–5.

Eruptive lentiginosis [1,2]

Widespread occurrence of very large numbers of lentigines that develop rapidly over the course of a few months to years is typical of eruptive lentiginosis. The condition usually occurs in adolescents and young adults who show no evidence of systemic abnormalities. In 1956, Degos and Carteaud described telangiectatic papules that darkened and evolved into depressed, scaly lentigines [1]. In spite of the misleading title of their report, Eady *et al*. reported two patients in whom very large numbers of lentigines developed over 2 years; histology and electron microscopy confirmed the diagnosis of eruptive lentiginosis [2].

References
1 Degos R, Carteaud A. Lentiginose profuse kératosique. *Ann Dermatol Syphiligr* 1956; **83**: 125–9.
2 Eady RA, Gilkes JJ, Jones EW. Eruptive naevi: report of 2 cases, with enzyme histochemical, light and electron microscopical findings. *Br J Dermatol* 1977; **97**: 267–78.

Multiple lentigines syndrome (LEOPARD syndrome, MIM #151100) [1–4]

In 1969, Gorlin *et al.* postulated that multiple lentigines represented one aspect of a syndrome and proposed the acronym LEOPARD (Lentigines, Electrocardiographic abnormalities, Ocular hypertelorism, Pulmonary stenosis, Abnormalities of genitalia, Retardation of growth and Deafness of sensorineural type) [1]. It is determined by an autosomal dominant gene with high penetrance and variable expression [2]. Lentigines are present at birth or first appear early in life and increase in number until puberty. They are most numerous on the neck and upper trunk, but occur all over the body, including the scalp, genitalia, palms and soles. Cardiac abnormalities are frequent—sometimes pulmonary or subaortic stenosis but more commonly conduction defects [3]. Several patients with this syndrome have died at an early age from obstructive cardiomyopathy [4]. Growth tends to be retarded. Ocular hypertelorism and mild mandibular prognathism are the most usual of a variety of skeletal abnormalities. Inconstant features are deafness and genital abnormalities. The deafness, which may be profound, is of sensorineural type. The genital abnormalities include gonadal hypoplasia, hypospadias and delayed puberty.

References

1 Gorlin RJ, Anderson RC, Blaw M. Multiple lentigines syndrome. *Am J Dis Child* 1969; **117**: 652–62.
2 Gorlin RJ, Sedano H. Leopard syndrome. *Modern Med* 1969; **37**: 178.
3 Smith RF, Pulicicchio LV, Holmes AV. Generalized lentigo: electrocardiographic abnormalities, conduction disorders and arrhythmias in three cases. *Am J Cardiol* 1970; **25**: 501–6.
4 Polani PE, Moynahan EJ. Progressive cardiomyopathic lentiginosis. *QJM* 1972: **41**: 205–25.

Centrofacial lentiginosis (MIM 151000) [1]

This poorly defined syndrome remains an enigma more than 30 years after the last English language report of the disorder. It is characterized by a triad of clinical features: lentigines limited to the medial face, neuropsychiatric problems and dysraphic anomalies. It is apparently determined by an autosomal dominant gene. Small brown or black macules appear during the first year and increase in number up to the age of 8 or 10 years. Their distribution is restricted to a horizontal band across the centre of the face. The mucous membranes are not involved. Associated defects include coalescence of the eyebrows, a high-arched palate, absent upper median incisors, sacral hypertrichosis, spina bifida and scoliosis. Mental retardation is frequent and many affected individuals are epileptic.

Reference

1 Dociu I, Galactin-Nitelea O, Sirgită N, Murgu V. Centrofacial lentiginosis. *Br J Dermatol* 1976; **94**: 39–43.

Peutz–Jeghers syndrome (MIM 175200)

Synonym
- Periorificial lentiginosis

Definition. Peutz–Jeghers syndrome is an autosomal dominant disorder with a high degree of penetrance. It is characterized by hamartomatous polyps in the gastrointestinal tract in association with mucocutaneous melanin pigmentation and an increased rate of soft tissue malignancy. All races are affected.

History. The first reported cases of what is now known as 'Peutz–Jeghers syndrome' were twin sisters reported by a British physician, Dr Connor, in 1895 [1]. Interestingly, one of the sisters died from intestinal obstruction at the age of 20, while the other died of breast cancer aged 59 years [2,3]. They were illustrated by the British surgeon Jonathan Hutchinson in 1896 [4]. The first description of intestinal polyposis in this condition was by the Dutch physician, Dr Johannes Peutz in 1921 [5]. In 1949, Jeghers confirmed the association of intestinal polyposis with hyperpigmentation of the skin and mucous membranes and described its familial characteristics [3]. It was the American, Dr A Bruwer, who was the first to coin the term 'Peutz–Jeghers syndrome' in the title of his paper on the disorder [6].

Genetics. Variable penetrance and clinical heterogeneity make it difficult to determine the exact frequency of Peutz–Jeghers syndrome. In about 40% of cases there is no family history and these represent new mutations. The disorder is due to inactivating germline mutations in the serine–threonine kinase gene *LKB1* (*STK11/LKB1* gene), mapping to 19q13.3 [7]. This gene is now the focus of additional research interest due to its central role as a signalling pathway for tumour suppression [8].

Clinical features. A recent review of Peutz–Jeghers syndrome confirmed the variability of the manifestations [9]. The syndrome is characterized by mucocutaneous pigmentation, multiple gastrointestinal hamartomatous polyps and by an increased risk of developing malignant tumours involving several different organs [9]. Both sexes and all races may be affected. The pigmented macules usually appear in infancy and early childhood, but may be present at birth or may develop later in life. The oral mucous membrane is consistently involved; round, oval or irregular patches of brown or almost black pigmentation 1–5 mm in diameter are irregularly distributed over the buccal mucosa, gums, hard palate and lips, especially the lower lip. The pigmented macules on the face are smaller, often under 1 mm, and darker, and are concentrated around the nose and mouth. Larger macules may be present on both aspects of the hands and feet and may be conspicuous on palms and soles. The oral pigmentation is usually permanent, but the macules on the lips and skin may become less prominent after puberty. Rarely, the nails may be pigmented, diffusely or in longitudinal bands. Mucosal and facial pigmentation without evidence of intestinal polyposis may be found in relatives. Indistinguishable pigmentary changes beginning in adult life also occur sporadically in individuals without intestinal involvement.

Symptoms attributable to the polyps usually occur between the ages of 10 and 30 years, but may occur in early childhood or be delayed until later adult life. The most common symptoms are repeated attacks of abdominal pain caused by intestinal obstruction. Rectal bleeding is common and haematemesis may occur with gastric or duodenal polyps. Many patients are anaemic.

Pathology. The pigmented macules show an increase in the amount of melanin in the basal layer of the epidermis. Polyps are found throughout the gastrointestinal tract. They are most numerous in the jejunum and ileum and less frequent in the colon, rectum, stomach and duodenum. In general, the polyps are benign hamartomas. The malignant potential of the polyps is not as great as in some other genetically determined syndromes with colonic polyps, but is not negligible. There is also increased incidence of malignancy in other organs, including the pancreas, breast, uterus and ovary.

Diagnosis. The mucosal pigmentation is the most constant feature of the syndrome. Freckling occurs in those of fair complexion, but the macules in freckling are light-influenced, are not focused on the skin around the nose and mouth and do not involve the mucous membranes. Examination of relatives may assist the diagnosis. At a stage when the polyps are already giving rise to symptoms they may not always be radiologically detectable.

Management. Cancer genetic counselling is now a key component to the successful management of patients with Peutz–Jeghers syndrome [10]. This also provides an opportunity for predictive testing of at-risk family members [10]. Age-related cancer risks for *STKL/LKB1* mutation carriers may be used to inform the cancer surveillance strategy [11]. Additionally, patients with mutations on exon 6 of *LKB1* appear to be at higher risk of developing cancer, which may justify a more vigilant protocol [11]. Guidelines for Peutz–Jeghers syndrome management recommend colonoscopic polypectomies every 1–3 years [12]. In many cases, it may be appropriate to undertake regular endoscopic examinations of the upper gastrointestinal tract and of the whole colon, together with barium follow-through studies of the small intestine every 2 years or so. In females, increased risk of breast cancer and gynaecological malignancy confirm that breast and pelvic examination should be included in the cancer surveillance programme [13]. In view of the generally benign nature of the polyps, routine radical surgery is not required. Individual polyps may require endoscopic or surgical removal. Prophylactic colectomy is recommended for cases with numerous colonic polyps, dysplastic polyps and uncontrolled bleeding [12]. Screening for at-risk individuals (first degree relatives of Peutz–Jeghers syndrome patients) should be annually from birth for history and physical examination for melanotic spots, precocious puberty and testicular tumours [9]. At-risk individuals who are asymptomatic and free from stigmata at age 8 years should be offered genetic testing for mutation analysis in the *STK11/LKB1* gene [14].

References

1 Connor JT. Aesculapian society of London. *Lancet* 1895; **2**: 1169.
2 Weber FP. Patches of deep pigmentation of oral mucus membranes not connected with Addison's disease. *QJM* 1949; **12**: 404–8.
3 Jeghers H, McKusick VA, Katz KH. Generalized intestinal polyposis and melanin spots of the oral mucosa, lips and digits. *N Engl J Med* 1949; **241**: 993–1005.
4 Hutchinson J. Pigmented spots on the lips in twin sisters. *Arch Surg* 1896; **7**: 290.
5 Peutz JLA. Very remarkable case of familial polyposis of mucous membrane of intestinal tract and nasopharynx accompanied by peculiar pigmentations of skin and mucous membrane. *Ned Maandschr Geneeskd* 1921; **10**: 134–6.
6 Bruwer A, Bargen JA, Kieland RR. Surface pigmentation and generalized intestinal polyposis (Puetz–Jeghers syndrome). *Proc Mayo Clin* 1954; **29**: 168–71.
7 Jenne DE, Reimann H, Nezu J *et al*. Peutz–Jeghers syndrome is caused by mutations in a novel serine threonine kinase. *Nat Genet* 1998; **18**: 38–43.
8 Alessi DR, Dario R, Sakamoto K, Bayascas JR. LKB1-dependent signaling pathways. *Ann Rev Biochem* 2006; **75**: 137–63.
9 Giardiello FM, Trimbath JD. Peutz–Jeghers syndrome and management recommendations. *Clin Gastroenterol Hepatol* 2006; **4**: 408–15.
10 Zbuk KM, Eng C. Hamartomatous polyposis syndromes. *Nat Clin Prac Gastroenterol Hepatol* 2007; **4**: 492–502.
11 Mehenni H, Resta N, Park JG *et al*. Cancer risks in LKB1 germline mutation carriers. *Gut* 2006; **55**: 984–90.
12 Bonner MP. Gastrointestinal polyposis syndromes. *Am J Med Genet* 2003; **122A**: 335–41.
13 Hearle N, Schumacher V, Menko FH *et al*. Frequency and spectrum of cancers in Peutz-Jeghers syndrome. *Clin Cancer Res* 2006; **12**: 3209–15.
14 McGrath DR, Spigelman AD. Preventative measures in Peutz-Jeghers syndrome. *Fam Cancer* 2001; **1**: 121–5.

Polyposis, skin pigmentation, alopecia, and fingernail changes (MIM: 175500)

Synonym
• Cronkhite–Canada syndrome

Definition. Cronkhite and Canada first described the syndrome that now bears their names in 1955 [1]. The syndrome is rare, non-inherited and is characterized by generalized gastrointestinal polyposis, cutaneous hyperpigmentation, hair loss and nail atrophy.

Aetiology. Nutritional, infectious and immunological associations have been considered, but the cause of Cronkhite–Canada syndrome remains elusive. All cases have been sporadic. The skin changes are assumed to be the result of malabsorption associated with the protein-losing enteropathy.

Clinical features. Sixty per cent of reported cases occur in men. It has a worldwide distribution, with mean age of symptom onset at 59 years (range 31–86 years). No familial cases have been reported. Hyperpigmentation is present in most patients [2–4]. It consists of light to dark brown, lentigo-like macules ranging in size up to 10 cm in diameter. These hyperpigmented macules are scattered but are most numerous on upper and lower extremities, and the face. The hands tend to show diffuse pigmentation of the palms and fingers, with macular pigmentation of the dorsae. The mucosal surfaces are usually spared, although the buccal mucosa is occasionally affected. In some patients hyperpigmentation is generalized.

Diarrhoea, abdominal pain and weight loss, beginning in adult life, are the presenting manifestations. Alopecia, patchy at first but becoming total, begins a few months later, and dystrophic changes in the nails develop at the same stage. The nail dystrophy is distinctive but not pathognomonic and could be explained by the formation of ventral nail in the absence of normal nail production by the matrix [5]. Exceptionally, the nail changes may precede gastrointestinal symptoms by months or years [6].

Management. Treatment of the malabsorption leads to reversal of hyperpigmentation in most cases. However, the overall prognosis is generally poor.

References
1 Cronkhite LW, Canada WJ. Generalized gastrointestinal polyposis. *N Engl J Med* 1955; **252**: 1011–5.
2 Daniel ES, Ludwig S, Lewin KJ. The Cronkhite–Canada syndrome. *Medicine (Baltimore)* 1982; **61**: 293–309.
3 Ortonne J-P, Bazex J, Berbis P. Les troubles pigmentaire de la maladie de Cronkhite–Canada. *Ann Dermatol Vénéréol* 1985; **112**: 951–8.
4 Nishiyama S, Mori S, Harada S. Gastrointestinale Polyposis mit universelle Alopecie, Onychodystrophie und Pigmentation der Haut. *Arch Klin Exp Dermatol* 1965; **221**: 144–61.
5 Cunliffe WJ, Anderson J. Case of Cronkhite–Canada syndrome with associated jejunal diverticulosis. *BMJ* 1967; **4**: 601–2.
6 Manousos O, Webster CV. Diffuse gastrointestinal polyposis with ectodermal changes. *Gut* 1966; **7**: 375–9.

Cutaneous lentiginosis with atrial myxomas (Type I: OMIM 160980; Type II: OMIM *160980) [1–4]

Synonyms
- Carney complex
- CNC
- Carney syndrome
- NAME syndrome
- LAMB syndrome

Definition. In 1986, Carney described the complex that is now associated with this name [1]. Carney syndrome is a complex with three associated features: (i) primary pigmented nodular adrenocortical disease, a pituitary-independent, primary adrenal form of Cushing's syndrome; (ii) lentigines and blue naevi of the skin and mucosae; and (iii) a variety of non-endocrine and endocrine tumours, including atrial myxomas.

Aetiology. This inherited disorder shows an autosomal dominant pattern of inheritance. In more than 50% of patients with Carney syndrome disease-associated mutations are present in the gene encoding the R1-α regulatory subunit of cyclic monophosphate-dependent protein kinase on chromosome 2p16 [2]. Cytogenetic studies of tumours from patients with Carney syndrome suggest that the responsible gene may not have a tumour suppression function [3].

Clinical features. NAME syndrome and LAMB syndrome are simply variations of Carney syndrome and are terms that could usefully be dropped. NAME syndrome comprises *n*aevi, *a*trial myxomas, *m*yxomas of the skin and *e*phelides [4]. LAMB syndrome comprises *l*entigines, *a*trial myxomas, *m*ucocutaneous myxomas and *b*lue naevi [5]. Cardiac myxomas are the most important internal myxomas, due to the causation of cardiac symptoms and potentially life-threatening effects [6]. Carney syndrome often affects the adrenal cortex, thyroid and pituitary glands and gonads [7]. Life-long echocardigraphic screening and surveillance in all family members of affected cases is important [8].

References
1 Carney JA, Hruska LS, Beauchamp GD, Gordon H. Dominant inheritance of the complex of myxomas, spotty pigmentation, and endocrine overactivity. *Mayo Clin Proc* 1986; **61**: 165–72.
2 Aspres N, Bleasel NR, Stapleton KM. Genetic testing of the family with a Carney-complex member leads to successful early removal of an asymptomatic atrial myxoma in the mother of the patient. *Australas J Dermatol* 2003; **44**: 121–2.
3 Chrousos GP, Stratakis CA. Carney complex and the familial lentiginosis syndromes: link to inherited neoplasias and developmental disorders, and genetic loci. *J Int Med* 1998; **243**: 573–9.
4 Atherton DJ, Pitcher DW, Wells RS, MacDonald DM. A syndrome of various cutaneous pigmented lesions, myxoid neurofibromata and atrial myxoma: the NAME syndrome. *Br J Dermatol* 1980; **103**: 421–9.
5 Rhodes AR, Silverman RA, Harrist TJ *et al*. Mucocutaneous lentigines, cardiomucocutaneous myxomas and multiple blue naevi: the LAMB syndrome. *J Am Acad Dermatol* 1984; **10**: 72–82.
6 Reed OM, Mellette JR, Fitzpatrick JE. Cutaneous lentiginosis with atrial myxomas. *J Am Acad Dermatol* 1986; **15**: 398–402.
7 Handley J, Carson D, Sloan J *et al*. Multiple lentigines, myxoid tumours and endocrine overactivity; four cases of Carney's complex. *Br J Dermatol* 1992; **126**: 367–71.
8 Zahedi RG, Wald DS, Ohri S. Carney complex. *Ann Thorac Surg* 2006; **82**: 320–2.

Arterial dissections and lentiginosis (MIM: 600459)

Arterial dissections and lentiginosis is a familial syndrome that was first described in 1995 in two sets of siblings from a series of 240 patients with arterial dissections seen at the Mayo Clinic (Rochester, MN, USA) [1]. Six additional sporadic cases were also reported.

Genetics. The gene for this disorder has yet to be identified. However, disease expression in offspring from a consanguineous marriage suggests that it is autosomal recessive.

Clinical features. The lentigines are located on the trunk and the extremities, particularly the lower legs. The arteries prone to dissection include the aorta, renal artery and extra-cranial internal carotid artery. These vessels are the same that are prone to dissection in Marfan syndrome and other connective tissue diseases.

Reference
1 Schievink WI, Michels VV, Mokri B *et al*. A familial syndrome of arterial dissections with lentiginosis. *New Eng J Med* 1995; **332**: 576–9.

Laugier–Hunziker syndrome [1–5]

This rare syndrome of unknown aetiology was first recognized and described by Laugier and Hunziker in 1970 [1]. It has no known genetic basis. It is characterized by macular pigmentation of the lips and buccal mucosa together with linear black streaks of the nails [2]. Onset is usually in adult life. There have been no systemic changes reported, and the condition is therefore regarded as having a benign prognosis. Histological examination of affected skin shows accumulation of melanin in the basal layer keratinocytes and an increased number of melanophages in the papillary dermis [3]. Ultrastructural examination revealed numerous mature melanosomes in the cytoplasm of basal layer keratinocytes and melanophages in the papillary dermis [3]. Conjunctival and genital hyperpigmentation have also been reported [4]. The differential diagnosis of striate melanonychia is considered in Chapter 65. The term 'essential mucocutaneous hyperpigmentation' has been proposed to replace the eponym for this condition [5].

References
1 Laugier P, Hunziker N. Pigmentation melaniques lenticulaire essentielle de la muquese jugale et des lèvres. *Arch Belge Derm Syph* 1970; **26**: 391–9.
2 Kemmett D, Ellis J, Spencer MJ, Hunter JA. The Laugier-Hunziker syndrome. A clinical review of six cases. *Clin Exp Dermatol* 1990; **15**: 111–4.
3 Veraldi S, Cavicchini S, Benelli C, Gasparini G. Laugier-Hunziker syndrome: a clinical, histopathologic and ultrastructural study of four cases and review of the literature. *J Am Acad Dermatol* 1991; **25**: 632–6.
4 Ayoub N, Barete S, Bouaziz JD *et al.* Additional conjunctival and penile pigmentation in Laugier-Hunziker syndrome: a report of two cases. *Int J Dermatol* 2004; **43**: 571–4.
5 Seoane Leston JM, Vazwqez Garcia J, Cazenave Jiminez AM *et al.* Laugier-Hunziker syndrome. A clinical and pathological study. Presentation of 13 cases. *Revue de Stomatologie et de Chirurgie Maxillo-Faciale* 1998; **99**: 44–8.

Penile melanosis/vulvovaginal melanosis [1–4]

Acquired, irregular, brownish or slaty-brown discoloration of the glans or shaft of the penis or of the vulva and vagina may give rise to fears of malignant potential. Histologically, there is only an increase of pigment without any increase or atypia of the melanocytes.

References
1 Barnhill RL, Albert LS, Sharma SK *et al.* Genital lentiginosis: a clinical and histopathologic study. *J Am Acad Dermatol* 1990; **22**: 453–60.
2 Revuz J, Clerici T. Penile melanosis. *J Am Acad Dermatol* 1989; **20**: 567–70.
3 Hwang L, Wilson H, Orengo I. Off-center fold: irregular, pigmented genital macules. *Arch Dermatol* 2000; **136**: 1559–64.
4 Rudolph RI. Vulvar melanosis. *J Am Acad Dermatol* 1990; **23**: 982–4.

Incontinentia pigmenti (MIM #308300)

Synonyms
- Bloch–Sulzberger syndrome
- Bloch–Siemens syndrome

Historical background. A number of cases of probable incontinentia pigmenti (IP) were presented in Europe in the early 20th century. However, it was Bloch who first used the term 'incontinentia pigmenti' for this condition [1], and Sulzberger who provided a more detailed account of Bloch's patient [2].

Definition. Incontinentia pigmenti is a rare and complex hereditary syndrome in which vesicular, verrucous and pigmented cutaneous lesions are associated with developmental defects of the eye, teeth and central nervous system [3,4].

Aetiology. Most pedigrees are small, but accumulated genetic data point to an X-linked dominant trait that is lethal for hemizygous affected males [5]. The IP gene has been mapped to Xq28 [6,7]. The 23-kb gene encodes nuclear factor B essential modulator (NEMO), and consists of 10 exons. More than 80% of cases of IP are caused by a deletion of exons 4–10 [8]. Mutations involving other alleles of the NEMO gene result in phenotypes different from IP, including anhidrotic ectodermal dysplasia with immunodeficiency [9,10].

Pathology. The bullae are situated beneath the horny layer or within a spongiotic epidermis. The dermis shows non-specific inflammatory changes with a cellular infiltrate, including numer-

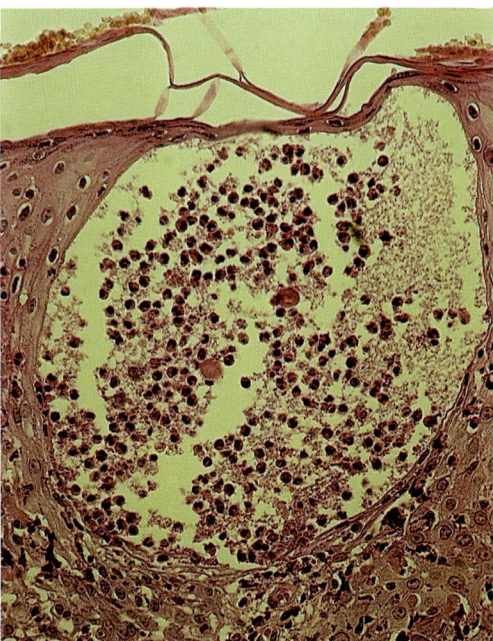

Fig. 58.9 Incontinentia pigmenti. Intraepidermal vesicle containing eosinophils. The spongiotic epidermis has been invaded by an inflammatory infiltrate that includes many eosinophils. Dyskeratotic cells are present.

ous eosinophils. The infiltrate extends into the epidermis, and the contents of the bullae may consist predominantly of eosinophils [11] (Fig. 58.9). The lichenoid papules show hyperkeratosis, acanthosis and oedema of the basal layer, many cells of which are degenerate. Macrophages laden with melanin are present in the upper dermis. In the warty lesions, the hyperkeratosis is further increased, and within the irregularly acanthotic epidermis are hyaline bodies representing individual cell keratinization. The epidermal changes at this stage may suggest pseudoepitheliomatous hyperplasia. The pigmented patches show diminution or absence of pigment in the basal cells and large quantities of melanin in melanophages in the upper dermis. The epidermis may be normal or slightly acanthotic.

Ultrastructural studies [12] show that, particularly in the early stages, there are many dyskeratotic cells in the epidermis. In addition to eosinophils, there are activated lymphocytes, basophils and mast cells, especially in the upper dermis. In all three stages, melanophages are present.

Clinical features. Two large studies have defined the clinical features of IP; Carney reviewed 653 cases from the world's literature [4], and more recently Landy and Donnai reported their experience of over 100 cases [5]. The skin changes are often present at birth, have usually developed before the end of the first week and rarely appear after the first 2 months. Four distinct clinical stages are recognized:

Stage 1: inflammatory macules, papules, vesicles and pustules
Stage 2: hyperkeratotic and verrucous lesions
Stage 3: grey-brown pigmentation
Stage 4: atrophic, hypopigmented and depigmented bands or streaks that are hairless and anhidrotic and fail to tan on sun exposure [13].

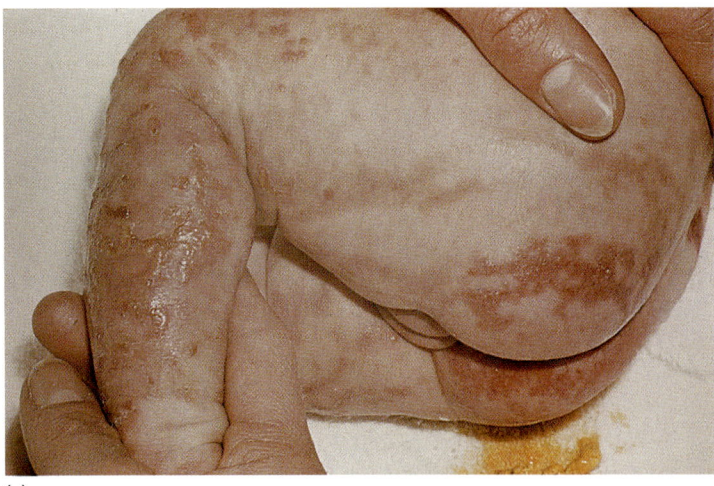

(a)

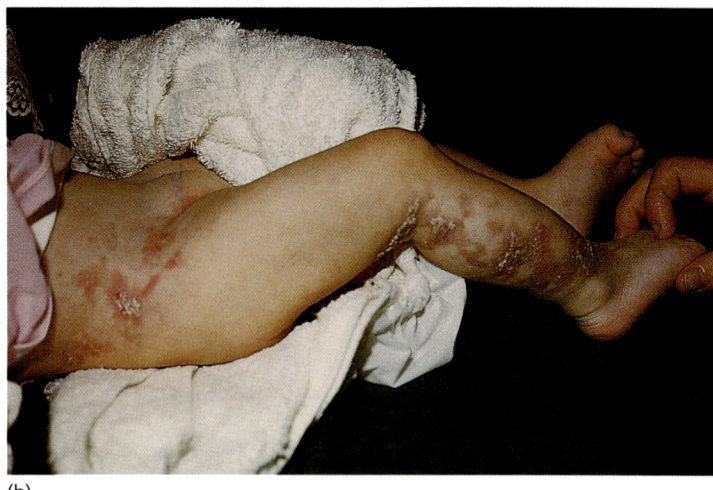

(b)

Fig. 58.10 Incontinentia pigmenti: (a) linear groups of blisters in a child aged 3 weeks; (b) linear warty lesions on the lower leg of the same child aged 3 months.

The sequence of these stages is irregular, their duration variable and they may overlap. It is possible that the earlier inflammatory stages can occur *in utero* and do not progress after birth. The most striking feature of IP is the clear, tense bullae in linear array that tend to develop along lines of Blaschko on the trunk and limbs (Fig. 58.10). These lesions are usually in recurrent crops; less often they are generalized. The crops persist for a few days or for a month or two. They are accompanied or followed by smooth red nodules or plaques, often irregularly linear, on the limbs and trunk. The plaques may be extensive and may precede the bullae. They may be bluish-purple in colour and may ulcerate. Linear warty lesions may be present on the dorsa of hands and feet at birth, but more typically develop in early infancy, tending to wane by 6 months of age. The pigmentation, which may be the only abnormality, may be present from the outset or may appear as the inflammatory lesions are subsiding. Inflammatory lesions can develop in areas that are already pigmented. Activity may rarely persist into adult life [14]. The pigmentation, ranging in colour from blue-grey or slate to brown (Fig. 58.11), is characteristic of the syndrome, and the bizarre 'Chinese letter pattern' is diagnostic. The hair is usually normal, but in about 25% of cases patches of cicatricial alopecia, resembling pseudopelade, are present from birth or develop in infancy at or near the vertex. The nails are usually normal but may be small and dystrophic.

A number of extra-cutaneous features are also reported (Table 58.4).

Diagnosis. The combination of bullae with linear nodular or warty lesions in a female infant is pathognomonic. During a purely bullous phase the following differential diagnosis should be considered and excluded: infantile pemphigoid, herpes simplex infection, mastocytosis, Langerhans' cell histiocytosis, epidermolysis bullosa. Biopsy of the skin in the blistering phase is often of help in establishing the diagnosis (see Fig. 58.10) with the presence of many eosinophils in the epidermis and dermis.

Treatment. Usually no treatment is necessary other than the control of secondary infection. Systemic therapy with corticoster-

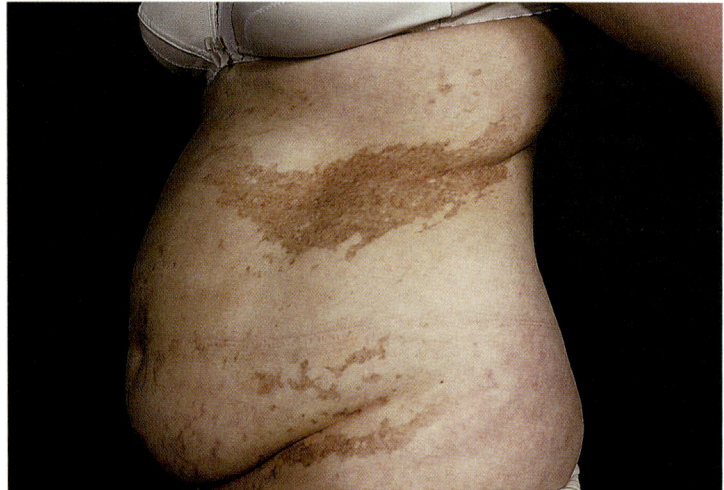

Fig. 58.11 Slate-grey pigmentation on the abdomen of a woman who had blistering lesions in childhood and who gave birth to a child with typical incontinentia pigmenti.

oids or sulfapyridine (sulphapyridine) is usually unsuccessful. Skilled dental supervision will minimize the cosmetic disability. As with other serious genetically determined disorders, family counselling should be offered. Ophthalmic examination in infancy is mandatory. Dental examination should also be carried out in the early infantile period after the age of one. If neurological features are present, the child should be seen by a neurologist.

Prognosis. The prognosis is determined by the spectrum of clinical features [5]. Thus, those with neurological features tend to do less well than those with more minor manifestations of the syndrome. The pigmentary changes typically fade during childhood years.

References

1 Bloch B. Eigentumliche, bisher nicht beschriebene pigmentaffektion (incontinentia pigmenti). *Sch Med Wochenschr* 1926; **56**: 404–5.

Table 58.4 Extra-cutaneous features of incontinentia pigmenti.

Central nervous system	Microcephaly
	Hydrocephaly
	Mental retardation
	Motor delay
	Spastic paralysis
	Ataxia
	Seizures
Ocular [15]	Blindness
	Strabismus
	Microphthalmos
	Cataracts
	Retinal detachment
	Proliferative retinopathy
	Fibrovascular retinal membrane
	Optic atrophy
Dental	Delayed eruption of teeth
	Hypodontia
	Partial anodontia
	Cone- or peg-shaped teeth
	Absence of teeth in apparently unaffected first degree relatives
Haematological	Blood eosinophilia when acute inflammatory skin changes are present
	Neutrophil and lymphocyte dysfunction
Immunological	Altered immunological reactivity is observed in some patients [16]
Skeletal abnormalities	Skull defects
	Palatal defects

2 Sulzberger MB. Uber eine bisher nicht beschriebene congenitale pigmentanomalie (incontinentia pigmenti). *Arch Dermatol Syphilol* 1927; **154**: 19–32.

3 Berlin AL, Paller AS, Chan LS. Incontinentia pigmenti: a review and update on the molecular basis of pathophysiology. *J Am Acad Dermatol* 2002; **47**: 169–87.

4 Carney RG Jr. Incontinentia pigmenti: a world statistical analysis. *Arch Dermatol* 1976; **112**: 535–42.

5 Landy SJ, Donnai D. Incontinentia pigmenti (Bloch–Sulzberger syndrome). *J Med Genet* 1993; **30**: 53–9.

6 Hyden-Granskog C, Salonen R, Von Koskull H. Three Finnish incontinentia pigmenti (IP) families with recombinations with the IP loci at Xq28 and Xp11. *Hum Genet* 1993; **91**: 185–9.

7 Smahi A, Hyden-Granskog C, Peterlin B *et al.* The gene for the familial form of incontinentia pigmenti (IP2) maps to the distal part of Xq28. *Hum Mol Genet* 1994; **3**: 273–8.

8 Aradhya S, Woffendin H, Jakins T *et al.* A recurrent deletion in the ubiquitously expressed NEMO (IKK-gamma) gene accounts for the vast majority of incontinentia mutations. *Hum Mol Genet* 2001; **I**: 2171–9.

9 Berlin AL, Paller AS, Chan LS. Incontinentia pigmenti: a review and update on the molecular basis of pathphysiology. *J Am Acad Dermatol* 2002; **124**: 169–87.

10 Smahi A, Courtois G, Rabia SH *et al.* The NF-kappaß signaling pathway in human diseases: from incontinentia pigmenti to ectodermal dysplasias and immunodeficiency syndromes. *Hum Mol Genet* 2002; **11**: 2371–5.

11 Mihm MC Jr, Murphy GF, Kwan TH *et al.* Characterisation of the nature of the inflammatory cell infiltrate of the vesicular stage of incontinentia pigmenti. In: Fitzpatrick TB, ed. *Biology and Diseases of Dermal Pigmentation.* Tokyo: University of Tokyo Press, 1981: 163–74.

12 Schaumburg-Lever G, Lever WF. Electron microscopy of incontinentia pigmenti. *J Invest Dermatol* 1973; **61**: 151–8.

13 Moss C, Ince P. Anhidrotic and achromians lesions in incontinentia pigmenti. *Br J Dermatol* 1987; **116**: 839–49.

14 Barnes CM. Incontinentia pigmenti: a report of a case with persistent activity into adult life. *Cutis* 1978; **22**: 621–4.

15 Jain RB, Willetts GS. Fundus changes in incontinentia pigmenti (Bloch–Sulzberger syndrome): a case report. *Br J Ophthalmol* 1978; **62**: 622–6.

16 Menni S, Piccinno R, Biolchini A, Plebani A. Immunologic investigations in eight patients with incontinentia pigmenti. *Pediatr Dermatol* 1990; **7**: 275–7.

Fanconi's anaemia (OMIM 227650) [1–8]

Definition. Fanconi's syndrome is a rare, autosomal recessive condition characterized by widespread, mottled skin pigmentation, bone marrow failure and a tendency to develop malignancy. The syndrome was first described in three brothers with aplastic anaemia, skeletal malformations, genital hypoplasia, retarded growth and pigmented macules on the trunk [1]. The full syndrome occurs more frequently in boys than in girls.

Pathogenesis. Most of the Fanconi genes have been cloned yet the exact function of their gene products remains uncertain [2]. Possibilities include a role in DNA repair, cell cycle control, regulation of oxidative stress or even the maintenance of apoptosis and telomeres [3].

Clinical features. The age of onset is usually between 4 and 10 years, and either cutaneous or haematological abnormalities may be the presenting manifestation [4]. In most cases there is generalized, dusky or olive-brown pigmentation, often most intense on the lower trunk, flexures and neck. Typically, scattered over the dusky areas are depigmented macules of 'raindrop' type and macules of darker pigmentation. Rarely, only café-au-lait macules are present. The oral mucosa is not involved [5].

A constant feature is progressive hypoplastic anaemia with neutropenia and thrombocytopenia, usually presenting as an increased bleeding tendency. The haematological manifestations appear earlier in males. The pancytopenia usually causes death in 2–5 years. Treatment of anaemia with anabolic steroids improves survival. Haematological defects may also be present in otherwise normal siblings. There is an increased incidence of acute leukaemia and other neoplasms.

Diagnosis. The diagnosis of Fanconi's anaemia is usually suspected in a child with hypogonadism, pigmentary changes and aplastic anaemia. The association of pigmentation of very similar type with pancytopenia is seen only in dyskeratosis congenita. Prenatal diagnosis is now possible by demonstrating increased spontaneous and induced chromosomal breakage in cultured fetal amniocytes or chorionic villous cells [6]. Complementation groups can be determined using retroviruses expressing FANCA, FANCC or FANCG cDNA [3].

Prognosis. The prognosis is poor due to aplastic anaemia. Bone marrow or cord blood transplant can be curative [7]. Average life expectancy for Fanconi's anaemia is 20 years [8].

References

1 Fanconi G. Familiarere infantile perniziosaartage anaemie (pernizioeses Blutbild und Konstitution). *Jahrbuch Kinderheild* 1927; **117**: 257–80.

2 Strathdee CA, Gavish H, Shannon WR *et al.* Cloning of cDNAs for Fanconi's anaemia by functional complentation. *Nature* 1992; **356**: 763–7.

3 Tischkowtiz MD, Hodgson SV. Fanconi anaemia. *J Med Genet* 2003; **40**: 1–10.

4 Butturini A, Gale RP, Verlander PC *et al*. Hematologic abnormalities in Fanconi anemia: an international Fanconi Anemia Registry study. *Blood* 1994; **84**: 1650–5.

5 Auerbach AD. Fanconi anemia. *Dermatol Clin* 1995; **13**: 41–9.

6 Auerbach AD, Sagi M, Adler B. Fanconi anaemia: prenatal diagnosis in 30 fetuses at risk. *Pediatrics* 1985; **76**: 794–800.

7 Alter BP. Fanconi anaemia. Current concept. *Am J Pediatr Hematol Oncol* 1992; **14**: 170–6.

8 Joenje H, Patel KJ. The emerging genetic and molecular basis of Fanconi anaemia. *Nat Rev Genet* 2001; **2**: 446–59.

McCune–Albright syndrome (OMIM 174800, 139320) [1–8]

Albright *et al*. [1] described a syndrome, in 1937, characterized by polyostotic fibrous dysplasia, skin pigmentation and (in females) precocious puberty. In McCune–Albright syndrome, fibrous dysplasia of bone occurs in association with hyperpigmented skin lesions (café-au-lait macules), gonadotropin-independent sexual precocity, and/or endocrine and non-endocrine manifestations [2].

Aetiology. McCune–Albright syndrome results from somatic mutations during early development, resulting in a widespread mosaic of normal and mutant-bearing cells. Thus, the clinical presentation of each patient is determined by the extent and distribution of abnormal cells. These mutations encode constitutively active forms of G(s)α, the ubiquitously expressed G protein α-subunit that links hormone receptors to intracellular cAMP generation. These mutations result in the loss of amino acid residues required to deactivate the G protein, leading to prolonged activation of G(s)α and its downstream effectors. This explains why McCune–Albright syndrome patients suffer from the effects of excess stimulation of multiple peripheral endocrine glands, without having appropriately raised stimulatory hormones. The skin hyperpigmentation is one such example of this phenomenon; increase in skin pigmentation is mediated through G(s)α/cAMP. Parental origin of the mutated allele influences the clinical presentation, as G(s)α is imprinted and expressed only from the maternal allele in some tissues [3].

Simple monostotic and polyostotic fibrous dysplasia affects the sexes equally and is relatively common. Fibrous dysplasia with associated pigmentation is unusual and is more frequent in females than in males. The full McCune–Albright syndrome with precocious puberty is seen mainly in girls [2–4], although males may develop isolated testicular enlargement [5].

Pathology. In the majority of patients, the number of melanocytes is not increased either in the lesions or in normal skin, and in split-skin preparations the giant pigment granules characteristically seen in Malpighian cells and melanocytes in neurofibromatosis are rarely to be found [6].

Clinical features [7]. Cutaneous pigmentation usually develops between the ages of 4 months and 2 years, but may be present at birth. Extensive light-brown patches, often with an irregular or serrated margin, occur mainly on the trunk, buttocks and thighs, but may rarely involve the face and neck. They tend to be asymmetrical and to be most extensive on the side showing the most severe bone involvement (Fig. 58.12).

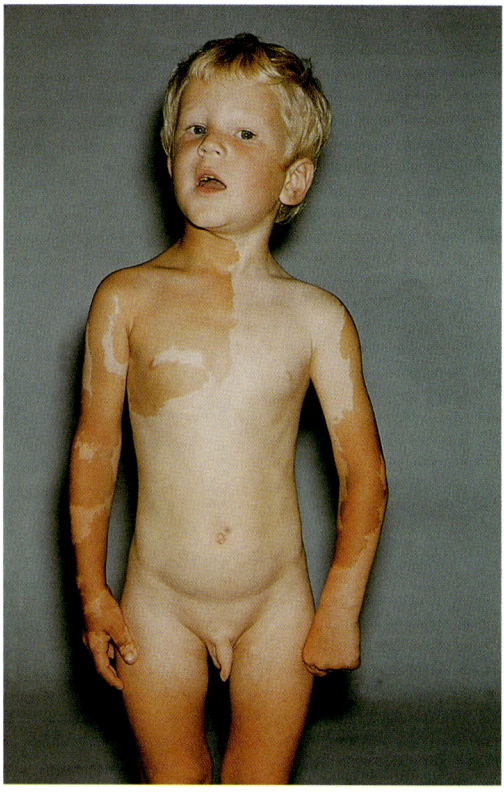

Fig. 58.12 Large pigmented macules in a child with Albright's syndrome. (Courtesy of Professor N.R. Rowell, Leeds General Infirmary, Leeds, UK.)

The bone lesions usually reveal themselves during the first decade by aching pain, pathological fractures and secondary deformities [3]. Bony overgrowth at the base of the skull may produce defective vision or proptosis. Serum calcium and phosphorus are normal but alkaline phosphatase may be elevated if the bone lesions are numerous. In females, precocious puberty, manifested by breast enlargement or by vaginal bleeding and growth of pubic hair, occurs below the age of 5 years in about 50% of cases and between 5 and 10 years in 30%. Growth in childhood is accelerated but the epiphyses unite prematurely. Other developmental abnormalities may be associated. The prognosis for life is good and the pathological fractures unite normally.

Diagnosis. There is no single clinical feature of the pigmented lesions that reliably differentiates McCune–Albright syndrome from neurofibromatosis, in which bone lesions and endocrine disturbances may also occur. The presence of many café-au-lait macules, freckles in the axillae and Lisch nodules on the iris are diagnostic for neurofibromatosis. Giant pigment granules may also rarely be found in McCune–Albright syndrome. Peptidic nucleic acid clamping is a rapid, reliable and economical method to diagnose McCune–Albright syndrome [8]. Negative results by peptidic nucleic acid clamping should be confirmed by nested polymerase chain reaction [8].

References

1 Albright F, Butler AM, Hampton AO *et al*. Syndrome characterized by osteitis fibrosa disseminata, area of pigmentation and endocrine dysfunction, with precocious puberty in females: report of five cases. *N Engl J Med* 1937; **21**: 727–46.

2 Feuillan P, Calis K, Hill S et al. Leterozole treatment of precocious puberty in girls with McCune-Albright syndrome: a pilot study. *J Clin Endocrinol Metabol* 2007; **92**: 2100–6.
3 Weinstein LS. G(s)alpha mutations in fibrous dysplasia and McCune-Albright syndrome. *J Bone Mineral Res* 2006; **21** (Suppl. 2): P120–4.
4 Sung SH, Yoon HD, Shon HS et al. A case of McCune-Albright syndrome with associated multiple endocrinopathies. *Korean J Internal Med* 2007; **22**: 45–50.
5 Rey RA, Venara M, Coutant R et al. Unexpected mosaicism of R201H-GNAS1 mutant-bearing cells in the testes underlie macro-orchidism without sexual precocity in McCune-Albright syndrome. *Hum Mol Genetics* 2006; **15**: 3538–43.
6 Benedict PH, Szabó G, Fitzpatrick TB, Sinesi SJ. Melanotic macules in Albright's syndrome and in neurofibromatosis. *JAMA* 1968; **205**: 618–26.
7 Gelfand IM, Eugster EA, DiMeglio LA. Presentation and clinical progression of pseudohypoparathyroidism with multi-hormone resistance and Albright hereditary osteodystrophy: a case series. *J Pediatrics* 2006; **149**: 877–80.
8 Kalfa N, Philibert P, Audran F et al. Searching for somatic mutations in McCune-Albright syndrome: a comparative study of the peptidic nucleic acid versus the nested PCR method based on 148 DNA samples. *Eur J Endocrinol* 2006; **155**: 839–43.

Other hereditary disorders with hypermelanosis

Increased pigmentation is an incidental or inconstant feature of many other genetically determined syndromes characterized predominantly by ectodermal dysplasia or diffuse connective-tissue defects. Such conditions are described in other chapters but are briefly mentioned below in differential diagnosis. There are also a number of unusual syndromes of which pigmentation is the most conspicuous or the only manifestation. The inter-relationships, classification and nomenclature of some of these syndromes, of which few examples have been reported, are not reliably established [1,2].

References
1 Fulk CS. Primary disorders of pigmentation. *J Am Acad Dermatol* 1984; **10**: 1–16.
2 Griffiths WAD. Reticulate pigmentary disorders: a review. *Clin Exp Dermatol* 1984; **9**: 439–50.

Familial progressive hyperpigmentation
(MIM *145250) [1–4]

Familial progressive hyperpigmentation was first reported using this diagnostic term by Chernosky et al. in 1971 [1]. They described a black family with diffuse macular areas of hyperpigmentation that were present at birth and increased in size and number with age. Pigmented macules also involved mucosal surfaces. Four individuals in two generations were affected. More recent reports in both large and small kindreds suggest autosomal dominant inheritance [2–4]. The diagnosis is made on the basis of the extent and depth of the hyperpigmentation in the absence of an alternative explanation. Histological features include markedly increased amounts of melanin throughout the epidermis, with great density in the basal layer and no pigmentation in the dermis. There is no known effective treatment, but the prognosis is good with no adverse associations.

References
1 Chernosky ME, Anderson DE, Chang JP et al. Familial progressive hyperpigmentation. *Arch Dermatol* 1971; **103**: 581–91.
2 Debao L, Ting L. Familial progressive hyperpigmentation: a family study in China. *Br J Dermatol* 1991; **125**: 607.
3 Rebora A, Parodi A. Universal inherited melanodyschromatosis: a case of melanosis universalis hereditaria. *Arch Dermatol* 1989; **125**: 1442–3.
4 Betts CM, Bardazzi F, Fanti PA et al. Progressive hyperpigmentation: case report with a clinical, histological, and ultrastructural investigation. *Dermatology* 1994; **189**: 384–91.

Periorbital hyperpigmentation

Some darkening of the skin around the eyes is not uncommon. Familial periorbital hyperpigmentation is characterized by dark circular areas around the eyes. Peters [1] reported a kindred of 20 individuals in five generations and first speculated that this might be an autosomal dominant disorder. Additional large pedigrees have confirmed the heritable nature of this condition [2–4]. The sexes are equally affected. Increased pigmentation is first noted below the lower eyelids at the approach of puberty. There is wide variation in its ultimate extent and intensity, but it is seen more frequently in individuals with dark complexions [5]. There is no known treatment for this disorder.

References
1 Peters R. Auffallende dunkelfarbung der unteren lider als erbliche anomalie. *Zbl Prakt Augenheilk* 1918; **42**: 8–11.
2 Goodman RM, Belcher RW. Periorbital hyperpigmentation. *Arch Dermatol* 1969; **100**: 169–74.
3 Franceschetti A, Jadassohn W, Paillard R. Démonstration d'un syndrome de Sjögren associé a una hyperpigmentation familiale des paupières. *Dermatologica* 1953; **106**: 277.
4 Fulk CS. Primary disorders of hyperpigmentation. *J Am Acad Dermatol* 1984; **10**: 1–16.
5 Gellin GA. Dark circles around the eyes. *J Am Med Assoc* 1981; **245**: 1165.

Naegeli–Franceschetti–Jadassohn syndrome (MIM *161000) [1–11]

Synonym
• Naegeli's syndrome

This rare syndrome, inherited as an autosomal dominant condition, is known in one large Swiss family [3]. A very similar condition with associated onychodystrophy is described in an English family [4].

Reticulate pigmentation develops during the second or third year in a previously normal child. It may become very extensive and is not preceded by any inflammation. Often the neck and axillae are particularly affected. The fine network of hyperpigmentation differs from the irregular splashes and whirls seen in incontinentia pigmenti. Keratoderma of the palms and soles is usual. Hypohidrosis with intolerance to heat is common. The hair and nails are normal, except in the English family where the fingernails and toenails are of almond shape. The teeth may be normal or defective, with yellow discoloration of the enamel. Mental and physical development is normal. In addition to pigmentary incontinence, varying amounts of colloid–amyloid bodies have been found in the superficial dermis [5].

A number of cases have been described that show a combination of some of the features of Naegeli–Franceschetti–Jadassohn syndrome and of incontinentia pigmenti [6–8].

Reticulate hyperpigmentation may be associated with alopecia, nail changes and growth retardation [7] and there may be a history of blisters [9]. There may or may not be sweating defects [10].

Reticular pigmentation with milia has also been described as a variant of Naegeli–Franceschetti–Jadassohn syndrome [11].

References

1 Fulk CS. Primary disorders of pigmentation. *J Am Acad Dermatol* 1984; **10**: 1–16.
2 Griffiths WAD. Reticulate pigmentary disorders: a review. *Clin Exp Dermatol* 1984; **9**: 439–50.
3 Franceschetti A, Jadassohn W. A propos de l'incontinentia pigmenti: délineation de deux syndromes différents figurant sous le même terme. *Dermatologica* 1954; **108**: 1–28.
4 Sparrow GP, Samman PD, Wells RS. Hyperpigmentation and hypohidrosis (the Naegeli–Franceschetti–Jadassohn syndrome). *Clin Exp Dermatol* 1976; **1**: 127–40.
5 Frenk E, Mevorah B, Hohl D. The Nägeli–Franceschetti–Jadassohn syndrome: a hereditary ectodermal defect leading to colloid–amyloid formation in the dermis. *Dermatology* 1993; **187**: 169–73.
6 Curth HO, Warburton D. The genetics of incontinentia pigmenti. *Arch Dermatol* 1965; **92**: 229–35.
7 Jäckli W. Ein Fall von infantiler Poikilodermie combiniert mit Alopeci, Mikrodontie und frühzeitiger Cataracta complicata. *Monatsschr Kinderheilkd* 1939; **78**: 773–81.
8 Kitamura K, Hirako T. Uber zwei japanische Fälle einer eigenartigen retulären Pigmentierung. *Dermatologica* 1955; **110**: 97–107.
9 Greither A, Haensch R. Syndrome d'Albright et troubles associés. *Schweiz Med Wochenschr* 1970; **100**: 228–33.
10 Vilanova X, Aguade JP. Incontinentia pigmenti. Troubles sudoripares fonctionnels dysplasiques et pigmentaires chez les ascendants. *Ann Dermatol Syphiligr* 1959; **86**: 247–58.
11 Tzermias C, Zioga A, Hatzis I. Reticular pigmented genodermatosis with milia: a special form of Naegeli–Franceschetti–Jadassohn syndrome or a new entity? *Clin Exp Dermatol* 1995; **20**: 331–5.

Dermatopathia pigmentosa reticularis (OMIM *125595)

Definition. Dermatopathia pigmentosa reticularis was first described by Hauss and Oberste-Lehn in 1958 [1]. It is characterized by widespread reticulate pigmentation in combination with alopecia, nail changes, palmoplantar hyperkeratosis and loss of dermatoglyphics.

Aetiology. It is a rare form of autosomal dominant ectodermal dysplasia, closely related to Naegeli–Franceschetti–Jadassohn syndrome. Loss of protection against proapoptotic signals by a defect in the N-terminal part of keratin molecules may partly explain the unusual features of this syndrome.

Genetics. Both Naegeli–Franceschetti–Jadassohn syndrome and dermatopathia pigmentosa reticularis have been mapped to a common 6-cM interval on 17q11.2-q21 [2,3] which supports the idea that they are allelic disorders [4].

Clinical features. Onset is usually in early childhood or from birth. There is reticulate hyperpigmentation which is most prominent on the trunk. An isolated case from the Netherlands also presented ainhum-like constrictions of the digits [5].

References

1 Hauss H, Oberste-Lehn H. Dermatopathia pigmentosa reticularis. *Dermatol Wochenschr* 1958; **138**: 1337.
2 Whittock NV, Coleman CM, McLean WH *et al*. The gene for Naegeli-Franceschetti-Jadassohn syndrome maps to 17q21. *J Invest Dermatol* 2000; **115**: 694–8.

3 Sprecher E, Itin P, Whittock MW *et al*. Refined mapping of Naegeli-Franceschetti-Jadassohn syndrome to a 6 cM interval on chromosome 17q11.2-q21 and investigation of candidate genes. *J Invest Dermatol* 2002; **119**: 692–8.
4 Itin PH, Lautenschlager S. Genodermatoses with reticulate, patchy and mottled pigmentation of the neck—a clue to rare dermatological disorders. *Dermatology* 1998; **197**: 281–90.
5 Van Der Lugt L. Dermatopathia pigmentosa reticularis hyperkeratotica et mutilans. *Dermatologica* 1970; **140**: 294–302.

Mendes da Costa–van der Valk syndrome

Synonyms
- Dystrophia bullosa hereditaria
- Typus maculatus

Patients with this rare syndrome, determined by a sex-linked recessive gene, present at birth or in early infancy with universal alopecia associated with red-brown pigmentation on the face and extremities [1]. Affected individuals, all boys, develop non-traumatic intraepidermal bullae, irregularly scattered on trunk and limbs. Conspicuous, coarsely reticulate pigmentation develops on the face and limbs in association with macular atrophy. Some patients are physically and mentally retarded and life expectancy is short [1].

Reference

1 Hassing JH, Doeglas HMG. Dystrophia bullosa hereditaria, typus maculates (Mendes da Costa-van der Valk): a rare genodermatosis. *Br J Dermatol* 1980; **102**: 474–6.

Cantú's syndrome (MIM 114620)

This is an autosomal dominant disorder characterized by hyperkeratosis and hyperpigmentation [1]. Multiple small (1 mm diameter) macules develop on the face, forearms, hands and feet during childhood and adolescence. Some of these coalesce to produce larger lesions. The palms and soles show punctate hyperkeratoderma [1].

Reference

1 Cantú JM, Sánchez-Corona J, Fragoso R *et al*. A 'new' autosomal dominant genodermatosis characterized by hyperpigmented spots and palmoplantar hyperkeratosis. *Clin Genet* 1978; **14**: 165–8.

Dyskeratosis congenita (MIM #305000, 224230, 127550)

Synonym
- Zinsser–Engman–Cole syndrome

History. The first description of dyskeratosis congenita is credited to Zinsser [1]. The condition was further defined by Engman [2] and Cole [3].

Genetics and pathogenesis. Three different patterns of inheritance have been reported for dyskeratosis congenita: X-linked recessive (MIM 305000), autosomal recessive (MIM 224230) and autosomal dominant (MIM 127550). Of these, the X-linked recessive variant is the commonest, the autosomal dominant variant the mildest with the best prognosis [4]. The gene for the X-linked variant, *DKC1*, was mapped to Xq28 [5,6] and then identified by Heiss *et al.* in 1998 [7]. The protein encoded by this gene, dyskerin, has been shown to be associated with human telomerase RNA [8]. This in turn led to the identification of *TERC*, which codes for telomerase component 3, as a candidate gene for autosomal dominant dyskeratosis congenita. Subsequent gene studies confirmed the presence of short telomeres and mutations in *TERC* in autosomal dominant dyskeratosis congenita [9,10].

Clinical features. Dyskeratosis congenita is a progressive, degenerative disorder characterized by reticulate hyperpigmentation with poikiloderma of the neck, chest and thighs. Cutaneous and mucosal changes occur in childhood, followed in the second and third decade by marrow failure and malignancy. Other features include nail dystrophy and leukoplakia of the oral, ocular and anal mucous membranes [11–13].

Management. Leukoplakia should be closely monitored for early signs of malignant transformation. Oral retinoids may help to cause regression of skin or mucous membrane dysplasia. Marrow aplasia requires treatment from a haematologist. About half of patients with dyskeratosis congenita die from bone marrow failure.

References
1 Zinsser F. Atrophia cutis reticularis cum pigmentatione, dystrophia et leukoplakia oris. *Ikonogr Dermatol* 1910; **5**: 219–23.
2 Engman FM. A unique case of reticular pigmentation of the skin with atrophy. *Arch Dermatol* 1926; **13**: 685–7.
3 Cole HN, Rauschkolb JE, Toomey J. Dyskeratosis congenita with pigmentation, dystrophia unguis, and leukokeratosis oris. *Arch Dermatol* 1929; **21**: 71–95.
4 Drachtman RA, Alter BP. Dyskeratosis congenita. *Dermatol Clin* 1995; **13**: 33–9.
5 Connor JM, Gathere D, Gray FC *et al.* Assignment of the gene for dyskeratosis congenita to Xq28. *Hum Genet* 1986; **72**: 348–51.
6 Arngrimsson R, Dokal I, Luzzatto L *et al.* Dyskeratosis congenita: three additional families show linkage to a locus in Xq28. *J Med Genet* 1993; **30**: 618–9.
7 Heiss NS, Knight SW, Vulliamy TJ *et al.* X-linked dyskeratosis is caused by mutations in a highly conserved gene with putative nucleolar functions. *Natr Genet* 1998; **19**: 32–8.
8 Mitchell JR, Wood E, Collins K. A telomerase component is defective in the human disease dyskeratosis congenita. *Nature* 1999; **402**: 551–5.
9 Vulliamy TJ, Knight SW, Mason PJ *et al.* Very short telomeres in the peripheral blood of patients with X-linked and autosomal recessive dyskeratosis congenita. *Blood Cells Mol Dis* 2001; **27**: 353–7.
10 Vuliamy TJ, Marrone A, Goldman F *et al.* The RNA component of telomerase is mutated in autosomal dominant dyskeratosis congenita. *Nature* 2001; **413**: 432–5.
11 Connor JM, Teague RH. Dyskeratosis congenita. Report of a large kindred. *Br J Dermatol* 1981; **105**: 321–5.
12 Davidson HR, Connor JM. Dyskeratosis congenita. *J Med Genet* 1988; **25**: 843–6.
13 Limmer RL, Zurowski SM, Swinfard RW. Abnormal nails in a patient with severe anaemia. Dyskeratosis congenita. *Arch Dermatol* 1997; **133**: 97–8.

Becker's syndrome [1–4]

This is different from Becker's naevus. Becker reported three sisters in 1939 with discrete or confluent brown macules on the neck and forearms, present from early infancy [1]. There was no atrophy or telangiectasia. In another case, somewhat similar mottled pigmentation of neck and elbows appeared at the age of 10 years [2].

Two other syndromes defy classification: diffuse pigmentation of the trunk and neck, beginning in the first year, with later development of small white macules in the pigmented areas [3]; and diffuse pigmentation with conspicuous macular depigmentation on the trunk, associated with macular and reticulate pigmentation of the neck [4].

References
1 Becker SW, Reuter MJ. A familial pigmentary anomaly. *Arch Dermatol Syphilol* 1939; **40**: 987–98.
2 Wodniansky P. Zur kemtris poikilodermatischer und poikilodermie: ahnlicher Pigmentverschebungen. *Z Haut-U Geschl Krankh* 1962; **32**: 33–44.
3 Pegum JS. Diffuse pigmentation in brothers. *Proc R Soc Med* 1955; **48**: 179–80.
4 Jost K. Hereditäre connatale, Pigmentanomalie. *Hautarzt* 1955; **6**: 458–60.

Acromelanosis [1–21]

Diffuse hyperpigmentation of the dorsal aspects of fingers and toes is not uncommon in individuals of dark complexion [1]. It has been reported in individuals of mixed race, white-skinned, black-skinned and oriental people. There may be more than one genotype. The pigmentation begins in infancy or childhood and increases in depth and extent [2,3]. There may be increased pigmentation in the flexures of the finger joints and in the larger joint flexures. A single case report of acromelanosis with hyperpigmentation of genital mucosa in a baby girl has been reported from Spain [4]. The condition must be differentiated from hyperpigmentation induced by repeated trauma. The term 'acromelanosis' has also been used to describe acquired hyperpigmentation of the hands or feet as a manifestation of a drug reaction [5].

Reticulate acropigmentation [6–21]

Reticulate acropigmentation generally has an autosomal dominant pattern of inheritance. Two main variants have been reported: reticulate acropigmentation of Kitamura and reticulate hyperpigmentation of Dohi.

Reticulate acropigmentation of Kitamura

Reticulate acropigmentation of Kitamura is characterized by a network of freckle-like areas of pigmentation which develop on the dorsa of the hands in the first two decades [6–9]. The reticulate pigmentation may subsequently involve most parts of the body (Fig. 58.13). Palmar pits and breakages of epidermal ridge pattern are found. Several individual cases and families have been reported with features of both Kitamura's disease and reticulate pigmented anomaly of the flexures (Dowling–Degos disease) [10–12]. Histologically, the pigment macules show epidermal atrophy and an increased number of melanocytes. It is unclear if bony abnormalities reported in a Saudi female with Kitamura's syndrome were coincidental or linked [13]. Differing patterns of inheritance suggest that this is not always an autosomal dominant disorder [14].

*Symmetrical dyschromatosis of the extremities (MIM *127400)* [15–21]

Synonyms
- Dyschromatosis symmetrica hereditaria
- Reticulate acropigmentation of Dohi

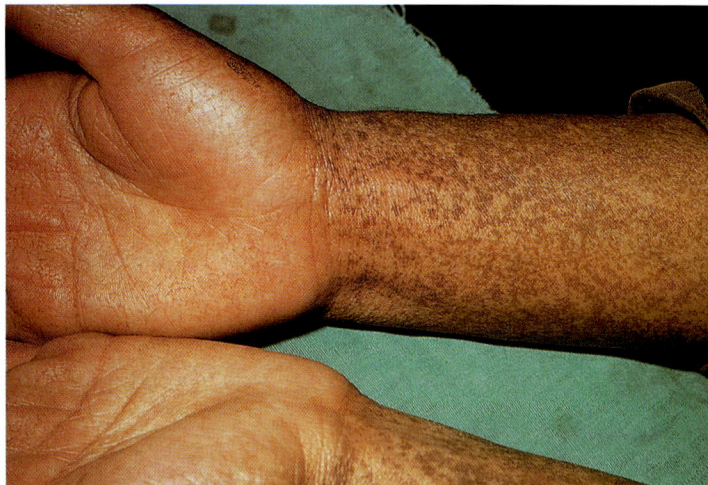

Fig. 58.13 Reticulate acropigmentation of Kitamura. (Courtesy of Dr W.A.D. Griffiths, St John's Institute of Dermatology, London, UK.)

Symmetrical dyschromatosis of the extremities is an autosomal dominant disorder caused by mutations in the double-stranded RNA-specific adenosine deaminase gene (*ADAR1* or *DSRAD*) [15,16]. The syndrome has been reported from Japan, where it is not uncommon, and also in European [17], Afro-Caribbean and Indian patients [18]. During infancy or early childhood, mottled pigmentation with areas of depigmentation develop on the dorsa of the hands and feet and sometimes on the arms and legs [19]. The face is spared, apart from a few scattered, small, discrete, pigmented macules. A single case of neurofibromatosis occurring in association with reticulate acropigmentation of Dohi has been reported from Singapore [20]. A comprehensive review of the literature on acropigmentation of Dohi that included cases reported in Japanese, identified 185 cases worldwide [21].

References

1 Weidman AI. Acropigmentation (acromelanosis). *Cutis* 1969; **5**: 1119–20.
2 Furuya T, Mishima Y. Progressive pigmentary disorder in Japanese child. *Arch Dermatol* 1962; **86**: 412–8.
3 Gonzalez JR, Botet MV. Acromelanosis. *J Am Acad Dermatol* 1980; **2**: 128–31.
4 Sopena Barona J, Gamo Villegas R, Guerra Tapia A, Iglesias Diez L. Acromelanosis. *Anales de Pediatria* 2003; **58**: 277–80.
5 Kanwar AJ, Jaswal R, Thami GP, Bedi GK. Acquired acromelanosis due to phenytoin. *Dermatology* 1997; **194**: 373–4.
6 Kitamura K, Akamatsu S, Hirokawa K. Eine besondere form der akropigmentation: Acropigmentatio reticularis. *Hautarzt* 1953; **4**: 152–6.
7 Kitamura K. Acropigmentatio reticularis, eine Allgemein in der Welt vorkommende Krankheit. *Hautarzt* 1976; **27**: 352–4.
8 Griffiths WAD. Reticulate acropigmentation of Kitamura. *Br J Dermatol* 1976; **95**: 437–43.
9 Woodley DT, Caro I, Wheeler CE. Reticulate acropigmentation of Kitamura. *Arch Dermatol* 1979; **115**: 760–1.
10 Crovato F, Rebora A. Reticulate pigmentary anomaly of the flexures associating reticulate acropigmentation: one single entity. *J Am Acad Dermatol* 1986; **14**: 359–61.
11 Berth-Jones J, Graham-Brown RA. A family with Dowling Degos disease showing features of Kitamura's reticulate acropigmentation. *Br J Dermatol* 1989; **120**: 463–6.
12 Cox NH, Long E. Dowling–Degos disease and Kitamura's reticulate acropigmentation: support for the concept of a single disease. *Br J Dermatol* 1991; **125**: 169–71.
13 el-Hoshy K, Hashimoto K. Bony anomalies in a patient with reticulate acropigmentation of Kitamura. *J Dermatol* 1996; **23**: 713–5.
14 Singal A, Bhattacharya SN, Baruah MC *et al*. Is the hereditary of reticulate acropigmentation of Kitamura always autosomal dominant? *J Dermatol* 1998; **25**: 57–9.
15 Liu Q, Liu W, Jiang L *et al*. Novel mutations of the RNA-specific adenosine deaminase gene (DSRAD) in Chinese families with dyschromatosis symmetrica hereditaria. *J Invest Dermatol* 2004; **122**: 896–9.
16 Suzuki N, Suzuki T, Inagaki K *et al*. Mutation analysis of the ADAR1 gene in dyschromatosis symmetrica hereditaria and genetic differentiation from both dyschromatosis universalis hereditaria and acropigmentation reticularis. *J Invest Dermatol* 2005; **124**: 1186–92.
17 Danese P, Zanca A, Bertazzoni MG. Familial reticulate acropigmentation of Dohi. *J Am Acad Dermatol* 1997; **37**: 884–6.
18 Ostlere LS, Ratnavel RC, Lawlor F *et al*. Reticulate acropigmentation of Dohi. *Clin Exp Dermatol* 1995; **20**: 477–9.
19 Sugai T, Saito T, Hamata T. Symmetric acroleukopathy in mother and daughter. *Arch Dermatol* 1965; **92**: 172–3.
20 Tan HH, Tay YK. Neurofibromatosis and reticulate acropigmentation of Dohi: a case report. *Pediatric Dermatology* 1997; **14**: 296–8.
21 Oyama M, Shimizu H, Ohata Y *et al*. Dyschromatosis symmetrica hereditaria (reticulate acropigmentation of Dohi): report of a Japanese family with the condition and a literature review of 185 cases. *Br J Dermatol* 1999; **140**: 491–6.

Universal acquired melanosis [1–2]

Pigmentation is usually present from early infancy but it may be progressive. It is often diffuse and generalized but may later become rather mottled.

References

1 Maldonado-Ruiz R, Tamayo L, Fernandez-Diez J. Universal acquired melanosis. *Arch Dermatol* 1978; **114**: 775–8.
2 Betts CM, Bardazzi F, Fanti PA *et al*. Progressive hyperpigmentation: case report with a clinical, histological and ultrastructural investigation. *Dermatology* 1994; **189**: 384–91.

Reticulate pigmented anomaly of the flexures (OMIM 179850) [1]

Synonym
• Dowling–Degos disease

Reticulate pigmentation of the flexures arises during childhood. The characteristic histological finding is filiform downgrowths in the epidermis with hyperpigmentation of the deepest areas [1–3].

References

1 Wilson Jones E, Grice K. Reticulate pigmented anomaly of the flexures. Dowling-Degos disease, a new genodermatosis. *Arch Dermatol* 1978; **114**: 1150–7.
2 Rebora A, Crovato F. The clinical spectrum of Dowling-Degos disease. *Br J Dermatol* 1984; **110**: 627–30.
3 Crovato F, Rebora A. Reticulate pigmented anomaly of the flexures associating reticulate acropigmentation: one single entity. *J Am Acad Dermatol* 1986; **14**: 359–61.

Zosteriform reticulate hyperpigmentation [1–3]

The description of this disorder is encapsulated by its name. There may be an associated change in the texture of the skin within the lesions. This condition arises in children. All four cases reported from Japan showed eosinophilia [1,2].

References

1 Iijima S, Naito Y, Naito S, Uyeno K. Reticulate hyperpigmentation distributed in a zosteriform fashion: a new clinical type of hyperpigmentation. *Br J Dermatol* 1987; **117**: 503–10.
2 Iijima S, Naito Y, Naito S, Uyeno K. Reticulate hyperpigmentation distributed in a zosteriform fashion: a new clinical type of hyperpigmentation. *Br J Dermatol* 1989; **121**: 280.
3 Rower JM, Carr RD, Lowney ED. Progressive cribriform and zosteriform hyper-pigmentation. *Arch Dermatol* 1978; **114**: 98–9.

Human chimera with pigment anomalies

True human chimeras, formed from more than one zygote, with pigment anomalies are described [1].

Reference

1 Findlay GH, Moores PP. Pigment anomalies of the skin in the human chimaera. *Br J Dermatol* 1980; **103**: 489–98.

Schimke immuno-osseous dysplasia (OMIM #242900) [1]

Schimke immuno-osseous dysplasia is a rare autosomal recessive spondyloepiphyseal dysplasia characterized by short stature, unusual facies, hyperpigmented macules, proteinuria with progressive renal failure, lymphopenia with recurrent infections and cerebral ischaemia. There is no effective treatment for patients suffering from this syndrome other than supportive measures.

Reference

1 Boerkoel CF, O'Neill S, Andre JL *et al.* Manifestations and treatment of Schimke immuno-osseous dysplasia: 14 new cases and a review of the literature. *Eur J Pediatr* 2000; **159**: 1–7.

Neurofibromatosis (OMIM *162200) (see Chapter 15)

Café-au-lait marks are present in 90% of patients with neurofibromatosis, particularly in those with NF-1, and may appear early. They are round or oval patches of light-brown pigmentation. They are also found in 10% of normal subjects. The presence of one or two is not diagnostic in the absence of other signs of the disease but if six or more are present, with a diameter of 5 mm or more, the probability of neurofibromatosis is high.

Extensive melanotic macules can also occur and resemble those seen in Albright's syndrome; however, these tend to be confined to a particular site and are on either side of the midline. Axillary freckling is common in neurofibromatosis and is an aid to the diagnosis. Lisch nodules and iris hamartomas are present in most patients over the age of 6 years (Fig. 58.14). Giant pigment granules (macromelanosomes) are found in the café-au-lait macules (Fig. 58.15).

NF-1 accounts for 85% of all neurofibromatosis. The NF-1 gene has been identified on the proximal long arm of chromosome 17 [1,2]. It is inherited as an autosomal dominant trait with variable penetrance and expression, and a spontaneous mutation rate of around 50%. NF-2 has the same mode of inheritance, high spontaneous mutation rate, high penetrance and variable expression as NF-1. The NF-2 gene is located near the centre of the long arm of chromosome 22 [3].

References

1 Barker D, Wright T, Neuyen K *et al.* Gene for von Recklinghausen neurofibromatosis in the pericentromeric region of chromosome 17. *Science* 1987; **236**: 1100–2.

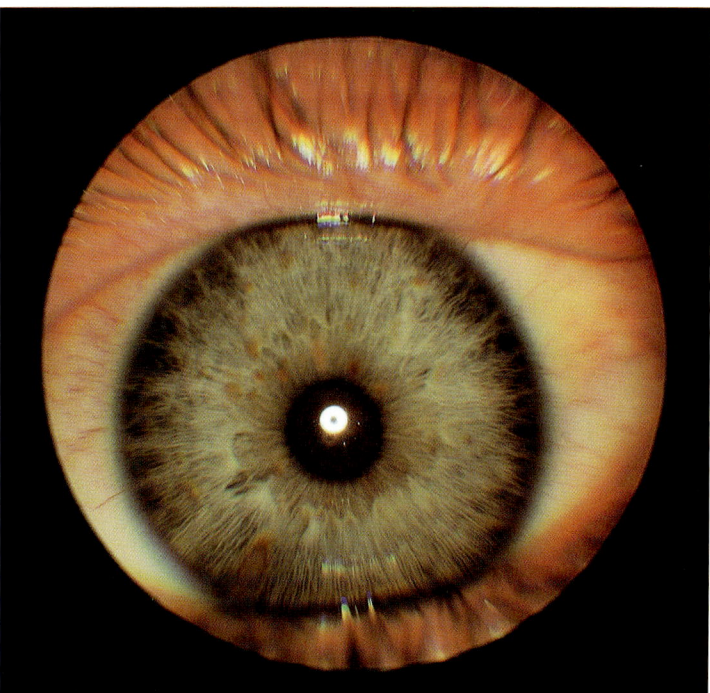

Fig. 58.14 Lisch nodules in the iris.

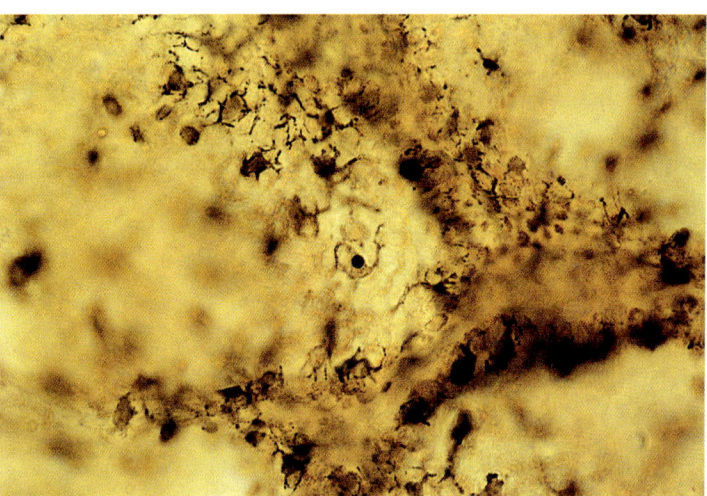

Fig. 58.15 Giant pigment granules in epidermal melanocyte in neurofibromatosis.

2 Seizinger BR, Rouleau GA, Ozelius LJ *et al.* Genetic linkage of von Recklinghausen neurofibromatosis to the nerve growth factor receptor gene. *Cell* 1987; **49**: 589–94.
3 Werteleck W, Rouleau GA, Superneau DW *et al.* Neurofibromatosis 2: clinical and DNA linkage studies of a large kindred. *N Engl J Med* 1988; **319**: 278–83.

Werner's syndrome (MIM #277700) [1–5]

Werner's syndrome is a rare, autosomal recessive disorder characterized by primary growth retardation, premature ageing, an increased prevalence of malignancy, high levels of atherosclerosis and type 2 diabetes [1]. Localized or diffuse hyperpigmentation is commonly seen [2]. Less commonly, depigmented spots with greying of the hair are present [2–3]. Most cases are caused by mutations in the gene encoding the RecQ helicase WRN [4].

Marked genomic instability explains the increased cancer risk in Werner's syndrome [5].

References

1 Davis T, Wyllie FS, Rokicki MJ *et al*. The role of cellular senescence in Werner syndrome: toward therapeutic intervention in human premature aging. *Ann N Y Acad Sci* 2007; **1100**: 455–69.
2 Hatamochi A. Dermatological features and collagen metabolism in Werner syndrome. *Gann Monogr Cancer Res* 2001; **49**: 51–9.
3 Nakayama T, Ochiai T, Takahashi Y *et al*. A novel mutation in a patient with Werner's syndrome. *Gerontology* 2002; **48**: 215–9.
4 Ramirez CL, Cadinanos J, Varela I *et al*. Human progeroid syndromes, aging and cancer: new genetic and epigenetic insights into old questions. *Cell Mol Life Sci* 2007; **64**: 155–70.
5 Crabbe L, Jauch A, Naeger CM *et al*. Telomere dysfunction as a cause of genetic instability in Werner syndrome. *Proc Natl Acad Sci USA* 2007; **104**: 2205–10.

Gaucher's disease and Niemann–Pick disease

(see Chapter 59)

Pigmentation of two types occurs in adults with Gaucher's disease: brown patches of chloasma type on the face, neck and hands; and symmetrical pigmentation of the lower legs with a sharp lower margin and an irregular upper margin. There may also be a brown, wedge-shaped thickening of the bulbar conjunctiva.

In the acute infantile form of Gaucher's disease, the skin is not pigmented, but in Niemann–Pick disease there is diffuse brown pigmentation, most marked on the face.

Xeroderma pigmentosum (see Chapter 15) [1]

Freckle-like pigmentation of the face and other exposed skin begins in infancy or early childhood. The light- or dark-brown macules are associated with telangiectases, small white atrophic spots and later with keratoses and tumours. The freckled sun-exposed skin with associated severe photosensitivity in a young child is a striking clinical phenotype not easily overlooked.

Reference

1 Kraemer KH, Lee MM, Scotto J. Xeroderma pigmentosum: cutaneous, ocular, and neurologic abnormalities in 830 published cases. *Arch Dermatol* 1987; **123**: 241–50.

Hypermelanosis in endocrine disorders

Some of the mechanisms by which endocrine glands influence melanogenesis are discussed on pp. 58.5–58.7. Here are considered clinical syndromes showing endocrine-induced pigmentary changes (see also Chapter 62).

Addison's disease [1–4]

Increased pigmentation is such a well-known feature of Addison's disease that its absence may significantly delay diagnosis and endanger life [1,2]. When present, the hyperpigmentation of Addison's disease is typically diffuse, and is most intense on areas exposed to light [3]. It is also accentuated in the flexures, at sites of pressure and friction, and in the creases of palms and soles [3]. Normally pigmented areas, such as the nipples and genital skin, darken. Pigmentation of the buccal mucous membrane is often present, and the conjunctival and vaginal mucous membranes may also be involved [3]. However, less distinctive patterns of pigmentation are not exceptional, and in any unexplained cases

of hypermelanosis adrenal function should be carefully evaluated. Similarly, patients without hyperpigmentation, but with other features suggesting Addison's disease should have adrenal function assessed. Vitiligo-like lesions may also occur in Addison's disease [3].

The hypermelanosis is the result of increased secretion of melanotrophic hormones by the pituitary. Affected patients have elevated plasma levels of β-MSH-like immunoreactivity [4]. Absence of hypermelanosis in Addison's disease was explained in a single case by a high degree of melanosome degradation in secondary lysosomes [1].

References

1 Kendereski A, Mici D, Sumarac M *et al*. White Addison's disease: what is the possible cause? *J Endocrinolog Invest* 1999; **22**: 395–400.
2 Runcie CJ, Semple CG, Slater SD. Addison's disease without pigmentation. *Scott Med J* 1986; **31**: 111–2.
3 Dunlop D. Eighty-six cases of Addison's disease. *BMJ* 1963; **ii**: 887–91.
4 Deutsch S, Mescon H. Melanin pigmentation and its endocrine control. *N Engl J Med* 1957; **257**: 222–6, 268–72.

Acromegaly

Pigmentation of Addisonian pattern is present in some cases of acromegaly, and may be a striking feature.

Cushing's syndrome [1–4]

Pigmentation of Addisonian pattern has been noted in about 10% of reported patients with Cushing's syndrome. It is an indication of secretion of ACTH and β-MSH by the pituitary and suggests the presence of a pituitary tumour. After adrenalectomy, progressive hypermelanosis develops in a proportion of patients, about 10%, in spite of adequate hormone replacement therapy. Only in half of these patients is the sella turcica enlarged [1,2]. These patients with Nelson's syndrome [3] show marked hypermelanosis, with the mucous membranes also being involved (see Fig. 58.6). The hair is often darker and there are sometimes multiple lentigines and longitudinal pigmented bands in the nails. High levels of both β-MSH and ACTH are found in the plasma, with degree of clinical hyperpigmentation correlating well with the quantity of β-MSH in the plasma [4].

References

1 McKenzie AD, McIntosh HW. Hyperpigmentation and pituitary tumor as sequelae of the surgical treatment of Cushing's syndrome. *Am J Surg* 1965; **110**: 135–41.
2 Sawin CT, Abe K, Orth DN. Hyperpigmentation due solely to increased plasma β-melanotropin. *Arch Intern Med* 1970; **125**: 708–10.
3 Nelson DH, Meakin JW, Thorn GW. ACTH-producing pituitary tumors following adrenalectomy for Cushing's syndrome. *Ann Intern Med* 1960; **52**: 560–9.
4 Abe K, Nicholson WE, Liddle GW *et al*. Normal and abnormal regulation of β-MSH in man. *J Clin Invest* 1969; **48**: 1580–5.

Hyperthyroidism

Pigmentation occurs in about 10% of patients with primary thyrotoxicosis [1]. It is usually diffuse and is broadly of Addisonian pattern, although involvement of the mucous membranes is uncommon and pigmentation of nipples and genital skin is less striking. The eyelids are occasionally conspicuously pigmented (Jellinek's sign). Some patients show chloasmal rather than diffuse pigmentation. The incidence of vitiligo is increased. Diffuse pigmentation was present at birth in the infant of a thyrotoxic mother [2].

References

1 Readett MD. Constitutional eczema and thyroid disease. *Br J Dermatol* 1964; **76**: 126–39.

2 Arakawa T. Hyperpigmentation of the skin with DOPA-uria of a newborn. *Tohoku J Exp Med* 1963; **80**: 329–37.

Pregnancy and menstruation

Increased pigmentation is almost invariable in pregnancy and is most marked in brunettes. A blotchy hypermelanosis of the face involving the cheeks, forehead and chin is frequently seen. This was called chloasma, but the term 'melasma' is now preferred (see p. 58.34). The pigmentation may involve the neck and is associated with darkening of the nipples, the linea alba to form the linea nigra, and the anogenital skin. The pigmentation usually fades after parturition, but may persist for months and years. The same pigmentation can be idiopathic and familial and is particularly seen in those who tan readily when exposed to bright sunlight [1,2]. It is noted by some women to be more apparent just prior to menstruation [3].

Oral contraceptives

Melasma (chloasma) (see p. 58.34) is frequently seen in women on oral contraceptives. No one oral contraceptive appears to be more liable than any other to cause pigmentation in predisposed subjects. The hypermelanosis is made more apparent with sun exposure. These patients also develop the same pigmentation when pregnant [4]. The pigmentation takes a long time to fade after discontinuing oral contraception and, as after pregnancy, it may never fade completely.

The mechanism is not fully elucidated and although MSH may be involved it plays a minor part. Oestrogens and progesterone are involved in the increased pigmentation but other factors are also implicated [2]. In a study of idiopathic melasma it was suggested that some of the patients had mild ovarian dysfunction [5]. Plasma concentrations of MSH are normal in patients with idiopathic melasma [5] and in those on oral contraceptives [6].

References

1 Carruthers R. Chloasma and oral contraceptives. *Med J Aust* 1966; **2**: 17–20.

2 Sanchez NP, Pathak MA, Sato S *et al*. Melasma: a clinical, light microscopic, ultrastructural and immunofluorescence study. *J Am Acad Dermatol* 1981; **4**: 698–710.

3 Snell RS, Turner R. Skin pigmentation in relation to the menstrual cycle. *J Invest Dermatol* 1966; **47**: 147–55.

4 Resnik S. Melasma induced by oral contraceptive drugs. *JAMA* 1967; **199**: 95–9.

5 Pérez M, Sánchez JL, Aguiló F. Endocrinologic profile of patients with idiopathic melasma. *J Invest Dermatol* 1981; **81**: 543–5.

6 Smith AG, Shuster S, Thody AJ, Peberdy M. Chloasma, oral contraceptives, and plasma immunoreactive β-melanocyte-stimulating hormone. *J Invest Dermatol* 1977; **68**: 169–70.

Phaeochromocytoma

Pigmentation of Addisonian pattern occurs in some cases of malignant phaeochromocytoma. Hypertension, headaches, profuse sweating, palpitation and apprehension will suggest the diagnosis, which is established by the abnormal plasma catecholamines.

Carcinoid syndrome

Hyperpigmentation of the skin has been noted in a number of patients with this syndrome.

ACTH administration [1,2]

A small proportion of patients treated with ACTH in high dosage (120 units/day) develop pigmentation of Addisonian pattern. The pigmentation, which is accompanied by a combination of Addisonian and cushingoid manifestations, fades when the dose is reduced. The incidence of melanosis appears to be rather higher in patients treated with tetracosactrin [2].

References

1 Cass LJ, Alexander L, Frederik WS *et al*. ACTH-induced Addisonian-like melanoderma in man. *Curr Ther Res* 1964; **6**: 601–7.

2 Khan SA, Smith AF. Intermittent tetracosactrin-depot therapy in dermatology. *Br J Dermatol* 1970; **82**: 389–96.

Hypermelanosis in other systemic disorders

Increased pigmentation is an inconstant feature of a wide variety of systemic disorders and may be associated with malignant disease. In most instances, the mechanism is obscure although, in some, elevated levels of β-MSH-like immunoreactivity are found. A genetic predisposition may be present in those affected. The hypermelanosis may be diffuse or localized. It may be confined to the epidermis, when the skin appears brown in colour, or it may be in the dermis, when often the skin is a slate-grey or blue colour. Pigments other than melanins may also be present.

Neoplastic disease [1–5]

In cachectic states there may be diffuse hyperpigmentation of the skin as in Addison's disease. The mechanism is uncertain. In the ectopic ACTH syndrome, which may occur in patients with oat cell carcinoma of the bronchus, pigmentation is usual. The tumour has been shown to produce a distinct MSH-like compound [1].

In adults, acquired acanthosis nigricans may rarely be associated with internal malignancy, almost invariably an adenocarcinoma. The hypermelanosis affects the axillae, nipples and umbilicus, which also show a warty papillomatosis. These skin changes may later become generalized. The mucous membranes are frequently involved.

A diffuse dermal melanosis, having a slaty-blue colour, can occur secondary to melanoma and melanogenuria [2,3]. Ultrastructural studies on this rare condition have shown in one patient [4] single-cell metastases disseminated widely through the skin; in another [5] the dermal histiocytes contained many lysosomal bodies containing electron-dense granular material, presumably melanin.

References

1 Liddle GW, Givens JR, Nicholson WE *et al*. The ectopic ACTH syndrome. *Cancer Res* 1965; **25**: 1057–61.

2 Fitzpatrick TB, Montgomery H, Lerner AB. Pathogenesis of generalised dermal pigmentation secondary to malignant melanoma and melanuria. *J Invest Dermatol* 1954; **22**: 163–72.

3 Sexton M, Snyder CR. Generalized melanosis in occult primary melanoma. *J Am Acad Dermatol* 1989; **20**: 261–6.
4 Konrad K, Wolff K. Pathogenesis of diffuse melanosis secondary to malignant melanoma. *Br J Dermatol* 1974; **91**: 635–55.
5 Adrian RM, Murphy GF, Sato S *et al.* Diffuse melanosis secondary to metastatic malignant melanoma. *J Am Acad Dermatol* 1981; **5**: 308–18.

Lymphomas [1–3]

Pigmentation is an uncommon manifestation of lymphomas, occurring in 10% of cases of Hodgkin's disease and in 1 or 2% of cases of lymphosarcoma and lymphatic leukaemia. The pigmentation is of Addisonian type, but allegedly without involvement of the mucous membranes. Malnutrition may be a factor and post-inflammatory pigmentation after scratching may modify the clinical pattern. Diffuse progressive hyperpigmentation can also be a manifestation of mycosis fungoides [1,2]. A number of different clinical patterns of early mycosis fungoides have been described, including pigmented purpura-like lesions [3]. Several of the cytostatic drugs used for the treatment of these disorders can also produce increased pigmentation of the skin.

References
1 David M, Shanon A, Hazay B, Sandbank M. Diffuse, progressive, hyperpigmentation: an unusual skin manifestation of mycosis fungoides. *J Am Acad Dermatol* 1987; **16**: 257–60.
2 Kikuchi A, Shimizu H, Nishikawa T. Mycosis fungoides with marked hyperpigmentation. *Dermatology* 1996; **192**: 360–3.
3 Barnhill RL, Braverman IM. Progression of pigmented purpura-like eruptions to mycosis fungoides: report of three cases. *J Am Acad Dermatol* 1988; **19**: 25–31.

Diseases of the nervous system [1–3]

Pigmentation, usually conforming to the Addisonian pattern, occurs in some diseases of the nervous system, particularly those involving the diencephalon and the substantia nigra. Intense pigmentation is a feature of Schilder's disease [1] but some increase in pigmentation is not uncommon in hepatolenticular degeneration [2] and in ependymomas. It is occasionally noted in chronic schizophrenia. In post-encephalitic Parkinsonism, it may be diffuse but may be melasmal. Pigmentation may sometimes develop after intense and prolonged emotional stress [3].

References
1 Derbes VJ, Fleming G, Becker SW. Generalized cutaneous pigmentation of diencephalic origin. *Arch Dermatol* 1955; **72**: 13–22.
2 Leu ML, Strickland GT, Wang CC *et al.* Skin pigmentation in Wilson's disease. *JAMA* 1970; **211**: 1542–3.
3 Meerloo JAM. Human camouflage and identification with the environment. *Psychosom Med* 1957; **19**: 89–98.

Rheumatoid arthritis and Still's disease [1,2]

Pigmentation, usually generalized, is occasionally observed in rheumatoid arthritis and is a more frequent feature of Still's disease. It may sometimes be caused by medication taken to treat the rheumatoid arthritis, such as minocycline [1] or methotrexate [2].

References
1 Langevitz P, Livneh A, Bank I, Pras M. Benefits and risks of minocycline in rheumatoid arthritis. *Drug Saf* 2000; **22**: 405–14.
2 Toussirot E, Wendling D. Methotrexate-induced hyperpigmentation in a rheumatoid arthritis patient. *Clin Exp Rheumatol* 1999; **17**: 751.

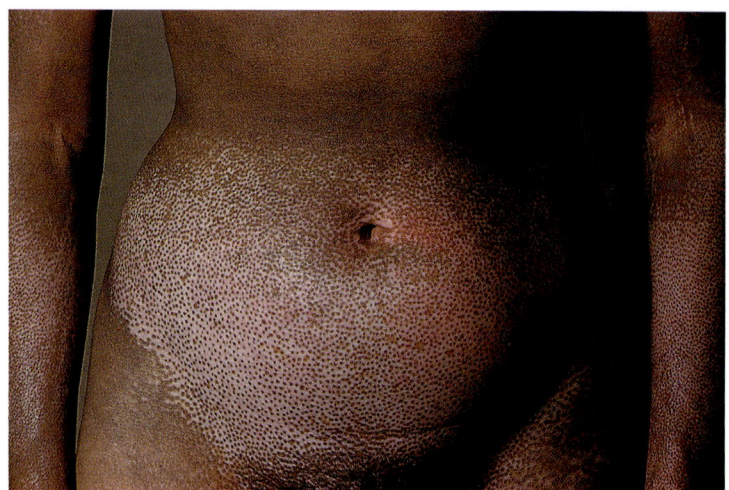

Fig. 58.16 Generalized pigmentation in a woman aged 33 years with systemic sclerosis.

Systemic sclerosis, scleroderma and morphoea [1–9]

Generalized pigmentation in systemic sclerosis and scleroderma may be intense and diffuse or of Addisonian type, but without mucous membrane involvement [1]. It may involve predominantly the face and limbs but is often far more extensive than the scleroderma (Fig. 58.16). Hyperpigmentation in systemic sclerosis is seen most commonly in patients with pigmented skin, and is less common in whites [2]. Keratinocyte endothelin-1 production has been implicated as playing a central role in the pathogenesis of cutaneous hyperpigmentation in systemic sclerosis [3], as has local expression and systemic release of a stem cell factor [4]. Levels of soluble cell surface L-selectin are elevated in systemic sclerosis with diffuse hyperpigmentation [5].

Pigmentation may also be a conspicuous feature of morphoea [6] and is occasionally the presenting symptom (Fig. 58.17). Hyperpigmentation is sometimes a feature of atrophoderma of Pasini and Pierini [7], and has also been reported in the linear atrophoderma of Moulin [8]. Prominent post-inflammatory hyperpigmentation has been reported in a case of porphyria cutanea tarda with idiopathic myelofibrosis and CREST syndrome [9]. A colorimetry device has helped to define the pigmentation changes of extensive scleroderma [10].

References
1 McFadden N, Ree K, Søyland E, Larson TE. Scleredema adultorum associated with a monoclonal gammopathy and generalised hyperpigmentation. *Arch Dermatol* 1987; **123**: 629–32.
2 Reveille JD, Fischbach M, McNearney T *et al.* Systemic sclerosis in three US ethnic groups: a comparison of clinical, sociodemographic, serologic, and immunogenetic determinants. *Semin Arthritis Rheum* 2001; **30**: 332–46.
3 Tabata H, Hara N, Otsuka S *et al.* Correlation between diffuse pigmentation and keratinocyte-derived endothelin-1 in systemic sclerosis. *Int J Dermatol* 2000; **39**: 899–902.
4 Yamamoto T, Sawada Y, Katayama I, Nishioka K. Local expression and systemic release of stem cell factor in systemic sclerosis with diffuse hyperpigmentation. *Br J Dermatol* 2001; **144**: 199–200.
5 Shimada Y, Hasegawa M, Takehara K, Sato S. Systemic sclerosis with elevated cell surface L-selectin levels. *Clin Exp Immunol* 2001; **124**: 474–9.
6 Weinberg JM, Russo M, Hirsch RJ, Don PC. Morphoea of the breast in a young girl. *Clin Exp Dermatol* 2001; **26**: 497–8.

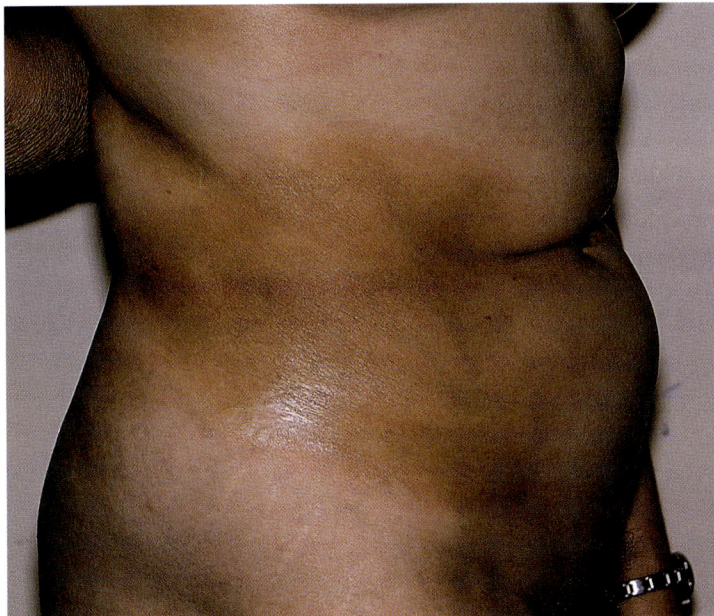

Fig. 58.17 Morphoea. Hyperpigmentation was the presenting symptom.

7 Iranzo P, Lopez I, Palou J et al. Morphoea in three siblings. *J Eur Acad Dermatol Venereol* 2001; **15**: 46–7.
8 Rompel R, Mischke AL, Langner C, Happle R. Linear atrophoderma of Moulin. *Eur J Dermatol* 2000; **10**: 611–3.
9 Lee SC, Yun SJ, Lee JB et al. A case of porphyria cutanea tarda in association with idiopathic myelofibrosis and CREST syndrome. *Br J Dermatol* 2001; **144**: 182–5.
10 Maeda M, Kachin H, Matubara K et al. Pigmentation abnormalities in systemic scleroderma examined by using a colorimeter. *J Dermatological Sci* 1996; **11**: 228–33.

Dermatomyositis and lupus erythematosus [1,3]

Diffuse pigmentation may accompany or follow the cutaneous lesions of dermatomyositis [1]. Acanthosis nigricans has also been reported in association with dermatomyositis [2]. In systemic lupus erythematosus, diffuse pigmentation of light-exposed skin occurs in about 10% of cases. It may gradually darken, although the disease is controlled by treatment. Longitudinal melanonychia may occasionally be a feature of systemic lupus erythematosus [3].

References
1 Bottomley WW, Goodfield MD. A case of dermatomyositis presenting as localized hyperpigmentation of the hands and face. *Br J Dermatol* 1995; **132**: 670–1.
2 Castro MA, Kutzbach A. Acanthosis nigricans associated with long-standing dermatomyositis. *J Rheum* 1996; **23**: 1487–8.
3 Skowron F, Combemale P, Faisant M et al. Functional melanonychia due to involvement of the nail matrix in systemic lupus erythematosus. *J Am Acad Dermatol* 2002; **47** (2 Suppl.): S187–S188.

Multiple organ failure [1]

Patients with multiple organ failure who survive for long periods are susceptible to hyperpigmentation. Renal failure, hepatic failure and polypharmacy may all contribute to this. An unusual case of intense green colour in a patient with multiple organ failure was attributed to dyes in the liquid tube feeds [1].

Reference
1 Czop M, Herr DL. Green skin discoloration associated with multiple organ failure. *Crit Care Med* 2002; **30**: 598–61.

Renal failure [1–4]

Chronic renal disease with nitrogen retention is frequently accompanied by increased pigmentation of the skin. This hypermelanosis is diffuse and brown in colour. It is most intense on the hands and face. Hyperpigmented macules are common on the palms and soles [3]. Elevated levels of β-MSH are found in the plasma of these patients [1,2] and cause the excess production of melanin in the skin. The increased levels of β-MSH-like immunoreactivity are due to slow clearance by the kidney rather than increased production by the pituitary. Lipochromes and carotenoids deposited in the skin may also play a part. Paradoxically, hypopigmentation with acquired lightening of hair is sometimes a feature of chronic renal failure [4].

References
1 Gilkes JJH, Eady RAJ, Rees LH et al. Plasma immunoreactive melanotrophic hormones in patients on maintenance haemodialysis. *BMJ* 1975; **1**: 656–7.
2 Smith AG, Shuster S, Comaish JS et al. Plasma immunoreactive β-melanocyte-stimulating hormone and skin pigmentation in chronic renal failure. *BMJ* 1975; **1**: 658–9.
3 Pico MR, Lugo-Somolinos A, Sanchez JL, Burgos-Calderon R. Cutaneous alterations in patients with chronic renal failure. *Int J Dermatol* 1992; **31**: 860–3.
4 Hmida MB, Turki H, Hachicha J et al. Hypopigmentation in haemodialysis. Acquired hair and skin fairness in a uraemic patient undergoing maintenance haemodialysis: case report and review of the literature. *Dermatology* 1996; **192**: 148–52.

Anaemia [1–8]

Hyperpigmentation of the skin occurs in vitamin B_{12} deficiency and is more common in dark-skinned races [1]. A diffuse brown pigmentation is also seen occasionally in patients with folic acid deficiency [2,4]. Pigmentation of the fingertips and nails of a patient with B_{12} deficiency has been reported [5]. The pigmentation seen in association with B_{12} deficiency often has a rather dappled and mottled appearance, and particularly affects the face, hands and feet [3,5,7]. Sometimes, only the fingers are affected. Treatment with vitamin B_{12} reverses the pigmentation of the skin to normal [7,8]. Pigmentation also occurs in megaloblastic anaemia associated with pregnancy [2]. In the haemolytic anaemias, hypermelanosis and haemosiderosis may develop on the lower legs.

References
1 Baker SJ, Ignatius M, Johnson S, Vaish SK. Hyperpigmentation of skin: a sign of vitamin B_{12} deficiency. *BMJ* 1963; **i**: 1713–5.
2 Baumslag N, Metz J. Pigmentation in megaloblastic anaemia associated with pregnancy and lactation. *BMJ* 1969; **ii**: 737–9.
3 Gilliam JN, Cox AJ. Epidermal changes in vitamin B_{12} deficiency. *Arch Dermatol* 1973; **107**: 231–61.
4 Downham TF, Rehbein HM, Taylor KE. Hyperpigmentation and folate deficiency. *Arch Dermatol* 1976; **112**: 562.
5 Ridley CM. Pigmentation of fingertips and nails in vitamin B_{12} deficiency. *Br J Dermatol* 1977; **97**: 105–6.
6 Marks VJ, Briggaman RA, Wheeler CE Jr. Hyperpigmentation in megaloblastic anaemia. *J Am Acad Dermatol* 1985; **12**: 914–7.
7 Mori K, Ando I, Kukita A. Generalized hyperpigmentation of the skin due to vitamin B12 deficiency. *J Dermatol* 2001; **28**: 282–5.

8 Sabatino D, Kosuri S, Remollino A, Shotter B. Cobalamin deficiency presenting with cutaneous hyperpigmentation: a report of two siblings. *Pediatr Hematol Oncol* 1998; **15**: 447–50.

Primary biliary cirrhosis

A diffuse hypermelanosis is seen in patients with cirrhosis due to many aetiological factors, and is particularly striking in patients with primary biliary cirrhosis. The hyperpigmentation is particularly striking on sun-exposed sites. The excess melanin is dispersed widely in the epidermis [1]. No significant difference from normal controls is observed in the levels of MSH-like peptides [1].

Reference

1 Mills PR, Skerrow CJ, MacKie RM. Melanin pigmentation of the skin in primary biliary cirrhosis. *J Cutan Pathol* 1981; **8**: 404–10.

Haemochromatosis

The disease haemochromatosis was first described by Troisier, Hanot and Chauffard in 1865 [1]. The term 'haemochromatosis' was subsequently coined by von Recklinghausen in 1899 in recognition that the skin pigmentation originated from the blood [1]. Pigmentation, bronzed or greyish in colour, initially involves exposed sites but later becomes generalized [2,3]. It is present in most cases [3], but may be subtle. The diagnosis should be suspected when pigmentation of this pattern occurs in middle-aged men in association with an enlarged liver and diabetes [4]. The diagnosis is confirmed by the high level of serum iron. Hyperpigmentation is reversible with phlebotomy [5]. Haemochromatosis is a common disease whose diagnosis is often overlooked [6]. However, only 50% of homozygous patients show clinical features of the disease [7].

References

1 Pietrangelo A. Haemochromatosis. *Gut* 2003; **52** (Suppl. 2): ii23–ii30.
2 Finch SC, Finch CA. Idiopathic hemochromatosis, an iron storage disease. *Medicine (Baltimore)* 1955; **34**: 381–430.
3 Chevrant-Breton J, Simon M, Bourel M, Ferrand B. Cutaneous manifestations of idiopathic hemochromatosis. Study of 100 cases. *Arch Dermatol* 1977; **113**: 161–5.
4 Adams PC, Deugnier Y, Moirand R, Rissot P. The relationship between iron overload, clinical symptoms and age in 410 patients with genetic hemochromatosis. *Hepatology* 1997; **25**: 162–6.
5 Barton JC, McDonnell SM, Adams PC *et al.* Management of hemochromatosis. Hemochromatosis Management Working Group. *Ann Intern Med* 1998; **129**: 932–9.
6 Bomford A. Genetics of haemochromatosis. *Lancet* 2002; **360**: 1673–81.
7 Olynyk JK, Cullen DJ, Aquilia S *et al.* A population-based study of the clinical expression of the hemochromatosis gene. *Gastroenterology* 1999; **341**: 718–24.

Amyloidosis

Localized pigmentation, often symmetrical, is seen in both lichen and macular amyloidosis [1,2]. The macular type of amyloidosis may be mistaken for post-inflammatory hyperpigmentation, but the lesions usually have a distinctive 'ripple' pattern, and microscopic studies reveal the presence of amyloid. Melanophages are found in the papillary dermis. The melanin contained in these dermal cells is derived from degenerating basal keratinocytes and melanocytes [1,3]. Macular amyloidosis is seen most commonly on the upper back (interscapular areas), chest, buttocks, forearms and shins.

References

1 Black MM, Wilson Jones E. Macular amyloidosis. *Br J Dermatol* 1971; **84**: 199–209.
2 Brownstein MH, Hashimoto K. Macular amyloidosis. *Arch Dermatol* 1972; **106**: 50–7.
3 Hori Y, Koboni T. Macular amyloidosis: clinical and pathological studies. In: Fitzpatrick TB, ed. *Biology and Diseases of Dermal Pigmentation.* Tokyo: University of Tokyo Press, 1981: 299–309.

Vitamin A deficiency

Severely malnourished patients with the ocular lesions of vitamin A deficiency tend also to show cutaneous changes. In children, dry skin is the main manifestation of vitamin A deficiency and may be associated with hyperpigmentation of the face and limbs. In adults there is dryness and scaling of the skin with desquamation and generalized hyperpigmentation. Conjunctival pigmentation has been noted particularly in oriental races and may be striking, especially in the lower fornix and bulbar conjunctiva.

Pellagra

Pellagra, the classic clinical manifestation of niacin deficiency, is characterized by erythema and hyperpigmentation of sun-exposed sites. It was first described by Gaspar Casal in the Asturias region of Spain in 1735 [1]. The nutritional basis for the disorder was established by Joseph Goldberger of the United States Public Health Service in the 1910s [2]. However, it was Conrad Elvehjem of the University of Wisconsin who finally proved that pellagra was caused by a deficiency in niacin [3]. Affected skin becomes hard, dry and cracked and in extreme cases is black in colour [4]. The sites of involvement are the sun-exposed skin of the face, neck, dorsa of hands and feet, and sometimes the forearms. Mucosal sites are also affected. Treatment of pellagra consists of 300 mg of oral niacin per day.

References

1 Sebrell WH Jr. History of pellagra. *Fed Proc* 1981; **40**: 1520–2.
2 Goldberger J, Tanner WF. Amino acid deficiency is probably the primary etiologic factor in pellagra. *Public Health Rep* 1922; **37**: 462–86.
3 Elvehjem CA, Madden RJ, Strong FM, Wooley DW. Isolation and identification of anti-black tongue factor. *J Biol Chem* 1938; **123**: 137–49.
4 Karthikeyan K, Mohan TD. Pellagra and skin. *Rev Int J Dermatol* 2002; **41**: 476–81.

Malabsorption syndromes

In sprue and other malabsorption syndromes, pigmentation is of common occurrence and may sometimes be prominent [1,2]. It may be of Addisonian type but without involvement of the mucous membranes, or may occur in well-defined patches on the face and neck and occasionally on the trunk. The scaly inflammatory plaques (see Chapter 59) that may develop in these syndromes are usually followed by intense pigmentation.

References

1 Dutly F, Altwegg M. Whipple's disease and 'trephoryma whippelii'. *Clin Microbiol Rev* 2001; **14**: 561–83.
2 Panicker JN, Vijayaraghavan L, Madhusudanan S. Whipple's disease. *J Assoc Physicians India* 2001; **49**: 853–5.

Vagabond's disease

This classically occurs in those in whom lack of food is combined with lack of cleanliness, and heavy infestation with pediculi. The pigmentation is basically of Addisonian pattern and the mucous membranes may be involved. The pathogenesis is uncertain, but the hypermelanosis is probably post-inflammatory and related to the scratching from the pediculosis infestation. Areas of hypomelanosis occur and there is a decrease in the number of melanocytes that show degenerative changes [1]. Adrenal function is in most cases normal [2].

References
1 Grosshans E, Stoebner P, Basset A. La leucomélanodermie des vagabonds. *Ann Dermatol Syphiligr* 1972; **99**: 141–59.
2 Thiers H, Colomb D, Durand B. Deux cas de mélanodermie des vagabonds. *Bull Soc Fr Dermatol Syphiligr* 1965; **72**: 82–4.

Peripheral neuropathy with dysproteinaemia, skin changes and endocrinopathy

Synonyms
- Crow–Fukase syndrome
- Shimpo's syndrome
- PEP syndrome
- POEMS syndrome

This multisystem disorder, characterized by polyneuropathy, dysglobulinaemia, anasarca, pigmentation, scleroderma, hypertrichosis, endocrinopathy, hepatosplenomegaly and lymphadenopathy, is discussed in Chapter 62.

Hypermelanosis of drug origin [1–4]

Skin pigmentation may be induced by a wide variety of drugs [1]. Several mechanisms are involved in drug-induced changes of pigmentation of the skin. These include increased melanin synthesis, increased lipofuscin synthesis, deposition of drug-related material and post-inflammatory hyperpigmentation. For example, the phenothiazines, particularly chlorpromazine, react with melanin to form drug–pigment complexes. In contrast to melanin, the chlorpromazine–melanin complexes are not metabolized by the body. On discontinuing chloropromazine and related phenthiazines, the pigmentation sometimes fades slowly, but more often is permanent. Many drugs induce hypermelanosis as a non-specific post-inflammatory change in predisposed subjects. The pigmentation following fixed drug eruptions is of this type. Other drugs induce pigmentation more directly; in the case of arsenic it is believed that it combines avidly with sulphydryl groups in the epidermal cells and promotes the action of tyrosinase. A post-inflammatory hyperpigmentation of the skin is seen following the resolution of drug-induced lichenoid reactions. Oestrogens stimulate melanin production, and drug-induced hyperpigmentation may be seen with the combined oral contraceptive. Hyperpigmentation in AIDS patients may occur as a complication of drug therapy, most notably with zidovudine which causes pigmentation of nail, skin and oral mucosa.

References
1 Dereure O. Drug-induced skin pigmentation. Epidemiology, diagnosis and treatment. *Am J Clin Dermatol* 2001; **2**: 253–62.
2 Lerner EA, Sober AJ. Chemical and pharmacologic agents that cause hyperpigmentation or hypopigmentation of the skin. *Dermatol Clin* 1988; **6**: 327–37.

3 Ferguson J, Frain-Bell W. Pigmentary disorders and systemic drug therapy. *Clin Dermatol* 1989; **7**: 44–54.
4 Ming ME, Bhawan J, Stefanato CM *et al.* Imipramine-induced hyperpigmentation: four cases and a review of the literature. *J Am Acad Dermatol* 1999; **40**: 159–66.

Chlorpromazine and related phenothiazines [1–10]

Blue-grey pigmentation of the sun-exposed areas of the skin is seen in a small percentage of patients receiving high doses of chlorpromazine for long periods [1,2]. The pigmentation is cumulative and some develop a purplish tint. Related phenothiazines may cause a similar effect, but chlorpromazine is usually implicated [3]. Some of those affected also develop cataracts, corneal opacities and pigmentation of the conjunctivae [4]. The nail beds are also affected in severe cases [2]. The mechanism is uncertain, as discussed above, but probably involves drug–melanin complexes. There is extensive deposition of melanin-like material throughout the reticuloendothelial system and involving the parenchymal cells of internal organs. The pigment found in the cells of the dermis stains as for melanin [1,2]. Electron microscopy studies [5] show increased melanin in the epidermis and perivascular macrophages in the dermis that contain electron-dense particles. Radioactively labelled chlorpromazine is found to localize in tissues containing melanin [6]. It is believed that this drug or some metabolite is bound to melanin in the tissues [8]. The level of immunoreactive β-MSH in the plasma of these patients is within the normal range [7]. A blue-grey pigmentation of the sun-exposed areas of skin has also been reported with trifluoperazine and imipramine [9,10].

References
1 Hays GB, Lyle CB, Wheeler CE. Slate-gray color in patients receiving chlorpromazine. *Arch Dermatol* 1964; **90**: 471–6.
2 Satanove A. Pigmentation due to phenothiazines in high and prolonged dosage. *JAMA* 1965; **191**: 263–8.
3 Hägermark Ö, Wennersten G, Almeyda J. Cutaneous side effects of phenothiazines. *Br J Dermatol* 1971; **84**: 605–7.
4 Greiner AC, Berry K. Skin pigmentation and corneal and lens opacities with prolonged chlorpromazine therapy. *Can Med Assoc J* 1964; **90**: 663–5.
5 Hashimoto K, Wiener W, Albert J *et al.* An electron microscopic study of chlorpromazine pigmentation. *J Invest Dermatol* 1966; **47**: 296–306.
6 Blois MS. On chlorpromazine binding *in vivo*. *J Invest Dermatol* 1965; **45**: 475–81.
7 Smith AG, Goolamali SIK, Thody AJ *et al.* Phenothiazine therapy and plasma immunoreactive β-MSH in schizophrenia and pruritic dermatoses. *Br J Dermatol* 1977; **96**: 537–9.
8 Benning TL, McCormack KM, Ingram P *et al.* Microprobe analysis of chlorpromazine pigmentation. *Arch Dermatol* 1988; **124**: 1541–4.
9 Buckley C, Thomas V, Lewin J *et al.* Stelazine-induced pigmentation. *Clin Exp Dermatol* 1994; **19**: 149–51.
10 Hashimoto K *et al.* Imipramine hyperpigmentation: a slate grey discolouration caused by long-term imipramine administration. *J Am Acad Dermatol* 1991; **25**: 357–61.

Hydantoin [1,2]

Phenytoin (diphenylhydantoin) is the prototype of the hydantoin derivatives. Some 10% of patients receiving hydantoin preparations develop pigmentation of the face and neck, resembling chloasma, which fades in a few months when the drug is stopped. It has been suggested that hydantoin exerts a direct action on the melanocytes inducing dispersion of melanin granules in the cutis, in addition to increased pigmentation of the basal epidermis.

A patient on this drug developed pigmentation of Addisonian type and other evidence of hypoadrenalism [2].

References
1 Kuske H, Krebs A. Hyperpigmentierungen vom Typus des Chloasmas nach Behandlung mit Hydantoin-Präparaten. *Dermatologica* 1964; **129**: 121–39.
2 Gottwald W, Aksoy F. Mesantoin-Begleiteffekte mit Addisonpigmentierung und cerebrale Anfalls-Rhythmik. *Hautarzt* 1965; **16**: 445–9.

Arsenic (see Chapter 75)

Prolonged ingestion of inorganic arsenic may result in diffuse pigmentation, most intense on the trunk, where macular areas of depigmentation within areas of hyperpigmentation produce the distinctive 'raindrop' appearance [1]. Many cases also show arsenical keratoses, but the severity of the two manifestations of arsenic poisoning is not necessarily proportionate and either may be present alone.

Reference
1 Meyhofer W, Knoth W. Uber die Auswirkung einer langjahrigen antipsoriatischen Arsentherapie auf mehrere Organe unter besonderer Berucksichtigung andrologischer Befunde. *Hautarzt* 1966; **17**: 309–13.

Antimalarial drugs [1–5]

About 25% of patients receiving chloroquine or hydroxychloroquine for several years develop bluish-grey pigmentation on the face and neck and sometimes the lower legs and forearms. With continued therapy, the areas darken, particularly oval patches on the shins, which increase in size. A blue-black colour may develop. Also, these patches are more pigmented in the light-exposed areas. The nail beds may be affected diffusely or in transverse bands and the hard palate may be bluish-grey. Bleaching of the colour of the hair occurs and when associated with pigmentation of the skin should suggest the diagnosis [4]. Corneal and retinal changes may develop following pigmentation of the skin due to antimalarials [3]. Chloroquine has been shown to have an affinity for dermal melanin [4]. A yellowish pigmentation of the skin is common with mepacrine [5]. Pigmentation appears to result from complexes of melanin, haemosiderin and mepacrine, in combination with sulphur [5]. Quinine and quinidine may also produce a generalized pigmentation [3,6].

References
1 Sams WM, Epstein WM. The affinity of melanin for chloroquine. *J Invest Dermatol* 1965; **45**: 482–8.
2 Shee JC, Bernard PJ. Pigmentation from amodiaquine simulating cyanosis. *Trans R Soc Trop Med Hyg* 1963; **57**: 379–81.
3 Tuffanelli D, Abraham RK, Dubois E. Pigmentation from antimalarial therapy. *Arch Dermatol* 1963; **88**: 419–26.
4 Marriott P, Borrie PF. Pigmentary changes following chloroquine. *Proc R Soc Med* 1975; **68**: 535–6.
5 Leigh IM, Kennedy CT, Ramsey JD, Henderson WJ. Mepacrine pigmentation in systemic lupus erythematosus. New data from an ultrastructural, biochemical and analytical electron microscope investigation. *Br J Dermatol* 1979; **101**: 147–53.
6 Mahler R, Sissons W, Watters K. Pigmentation induced by quinidine therapy. *Arch Dermatol* 1986; **122**: 1062–4.

Antitumour agents [1–7]

Long-term administration of busulfan (busulphan) produces a diffuse brown pigmentation, particularly in non-white people with a dark complexion. Less commonly, Addison's disease is simulated [2,3]. Light and electron microscopy studies suggest that busulfan has both a stimulatory and a toxic effect on melanocytes [4]. Both busulfan and doxorubicin cause mucous membrane pigmentation. Other cytostatic drugs that may produce hyperpigmentation include cyclophosphamide, bleomycin, fluorouracil, hydroxyurea, daunorubicin, methotrexate, mithramycin, mitomycin, thiotepa and adriamycin [6,7]. Topical cytostatic drugs that produce localized hyperpigmentation include carmustine, mechlorethamine and fluorouracil. Patients on cyclophosphamide [5], bleomycin, daunorubicin, doxorubicin and fluorouracil can develop banded or diffuse pigmentation of the nails. Hair pigmentation may be induced by methotrexate, and pigmentation of the teeth may be seen with cyclophosphamide.

References
1 Bronner AK, Hood AF. Cutaneous complications of chemotherapeutic agents. *J Am Acad Dermatol* 1983; **9**: 645–63.
2 Feingold ML, Koss LG. Effects of long-term administration of busulfan. *Arch Intern Med* 1969; **124**: 66–71.
3 Kyle RA, Schwartz RS, Oliver HL *et al.* A syndrome resembling adrenal cortical insufficiency associated with long term busulfan (myleran) therapy. *Blood* 1961; **18**: 497–510.
4 Adam BA, Ismail R, Sivanesan S. Busulfan hyperpigmentation. *J Dermatol* 1980; **7**: 405–11.
5 Shah PC, Rao KRP, Patel AR. Cyclophosphamide induced nail pigmentation. *Br J Dermatol* 1978; **98**: 675–80.
6 Kerker BJ, Hood AF. Chemotherapy-induced cutaneous reactions. *Semin Dermatol* 1989; **8**: 173–81.
7 Vassallo C, Passamonti F, Merante S *et al.* Muco-cutaneous changes during long-term therapy with hydroxyurea in chronic myeloid leukaemia. *Clin Exp Dermatol* 2001; **26**: 141–8.

Fixed eruptions [1–6]

Circumscribed areas of slate-brown pigmentation commonly follow the erythematous and bullous stages of fixed eruptions (see Chapter 75) but almost universal brown pigmentation has followed the long-continued ingestion of phenolphthalein [3]. Fixed eruptions are particularly frequent in black people. More or less symmetrical, discrete patches are usually seen but the melanosis may be diffuse or melasmal, and the mucous membranes may be involved [4,5]. The slate-brown colour in fixed drug eruption is due to pigmentary incontinence with melanophages in the upper dermis [6].

References
1 Browne SG. Fixed eruption in deeply pigmented subjects. *BMJ* 1964; **ii**: 1041–4.
2 Gelfand M. 'Melanotic' lesions in the Africans. *Cent Afr J Med* 1964; **10**: 443–7.
3 Weiss RS, Kile RL. Unusual phenolphthalein eruptions. *Arch Dermatol Syphilol* 1935; **32**: 915–21.
4 Tagami H. Pigmented macules of the tongue following fixed drug eruption. *Dermatologica* 1973; **147**: 157–60.
5 Westerhof W, Wolters EC, Brookbakker JT *et al.* Pigmented lesions of the tongue in heroin addicts: fixed drug eruption. *Br J Dermatol* 1983; **109**: 605–10.
6 Masu S, Seiji M. Pigmentary incontinence in fixed drug eruptions. *J Am Acad Dermatol* 1983; **8**: 525–32.

Post-inflammatory hypermelanosis

Hypermelanosis commonly follows acute or chronic inflammatory processes in the skin. The intensity and persistence of the hypermelanosis are greater in dark-skinned subjects. The degree of inflammation appears to be of less significance in determining the pigmentary response than the nature of the dermatosis, for it may be frequent and severe after some conditions and slight after others. Disorders where there is disruption of the basal layer of the epidermis, such as lichen planus or lupus erythematosus, frequently develop areas of slate-brown hypermelanosis. Similarly, in fixed drug eruptions, hyperpigmentation occurs owing to damage of cells in the basal layer. There is pigmentary incontinence with melanophages in the upper dermis [1]. In the late phase of chronic graft-versus-host reaction, there is a poikilodermatous appearance with hyperpigmentation [2].

Hypermelanosis of the epidermis may also occur in inflammatory disorders, but more frequently there is hypomelanosis of the skin. This results from an increased mitotic rate of keratinocytes and diminished transfer of melanosomes from the melanocyte to these cells, which also exhibit a reduced transit time from the basal layer to being shed on the skin surface. Very frequently in inflammatory disease in the skin, hypermelanosis and hypomelanosis occur together, often with a slaty-blue colour due to the presence of melanophages in the upper dermis. There may be an associated loss of functional melanocytes in the skin [3].

The cause of the pigmentation is usually obvious, although the preceding lesions have sometimes not been noticed by the patient or have been transitory or clinically imperceptible. The pattern and distribution of the pigmentation will sometimes allow a retrospective diagnosis, as in lichen planus, herpes zoster, dermatitis herpetiformis and papular urticaria. Pigmentation is often conspicuous after lichenoid drug eruptions, and is a feature of lipomelanic reticulosis.

An unexplained, but not excessively rare, clinical syndrome has been reported in some dark-skinned white people [4]. A small, irregular patch of hypermelanosis of the interscapular skin is often intensely pruritic. It seems likely that this condition is in fact notalgia paraesthetica [5,6] (see Chapter 63).

Reticulate pigmentation following the vascular network is characteristic of erythema ab igne (see Chapter 28), which may occur at any site regularly exposed to the heat of a fire or a hot-water bottle. A reticulate pigmentation is also seen in prurigo pigmentosa, a dermatosis mostly occurring in Japan [7].

Post-inflammatory hyperpigmentation may occur following trauma to the skin. It can occur following dermabrasion and particularly in those who are racially pigmented. Unusual patterns may declare their origin, for example the tooth-mark pattern on an ill-treated child [8] or the symmetrical pigmentation of the sides of the chin in a patient who, as a nervous tic, chews the buccal mucosa [9].

In late secondary syphilis, especially in women, so-called syphilitic leukoderma is occasionally seen. Diffuse hypermelanosis of the sides and back of the neck and the shoulders is mottled with depigmented macules 1–2 cm in diameter. The Wassermann reaction is always positive. A deep-blue or slate-grey hyperpigmentation is seen in late pinta (see Chapter 30).

References

1 Masu S, Seiji M. Pigmentary incontinence in fixed drug eruptions. *J Am Acad Dermatol* 1983; **8**: 525–32.
2 Touraine R, Revuz J, Dreyfus B *et al*. Graft-versus-host reaction and lichen planus. *Br J Dermatol* 1975; **92**: 589.
3 Papa CM, Kligman AM. The behaviour of melanocytes in inflammation. *J Invest Dermatol* 1965; **45**: 465–74.
4 Gibbs RC, Frank SB. A peculiar spotty pigmentation: report of five cases. *Dermatol Int* 1969; **8**: 14–6.
5 Leibson I, Honecke H, Mas P. Puzzling posterior pigmented pruritic patches. *Cutis* 1973; **23**: 471–3.
6 Weber PJ, Poullos EG. Notalgia paresthetica. *J Am Acad Dermatol* 1988; **18**: 25–30.
7 Joyce AP, Horn TD, Anhalt GJ. Prurigo pigmentosa. Report of a case and review of the literature. *Arch Dermatol* 1989; **125**: 1551–4.
8 Palomeque FE, Hairston MA. 'Battered child' syndrome. *Arch Dermatol* 1964; **90**: 326–7.
9 Penev SG. Peribuccal pigmentation as an artefact. *Br J Dermatol* 1970; **82**: 40–1.

Tanning with UV light

Tanning is the term used to describe the pigmentary response of the skin following exposure to ultraviolet radiation. Tanning occurs in three distinct phases: immediate pigment darkening, persistent pigment darkening and delayed tanning. Immediate pigment darkening (IPD) occurs in response to low doses of UVA. It appears within minutes of UV exposure and typically fades within 10–20 min. Clinically, immediate pigment darkening manifests as grey-brown pigmentation. IPD is believed to result from oxidation and redistribution of pre-existing melanin. Higher doses of UVA induce persistent pigment darkening (PPD) which persists for 2–24 h. This pigmentation is brown and is also caused by oxidation and redistribution of pre-existing melanin. Delayed tanning involves the formation of new melanin due to increased numbers of melanocytes and increased melanocyte activity. Both UVA and UVB are able to induce delayed tanning, but UVB is more effective. Delayed tanning becomes visible about 72 h after UV exposure and persists for 1–2 weeks before gradually fading as keratinocytes are shed from the skin surface.

Tanning and DNA damage are closely associated. Repeated suberythemal doses of UV light induce tanning but have also been shown to induce DNA damage [1]. Tanning salon exposure has also been demonstrated to induce cyclobutane pyrimidine dimers and p53 protein expression in epidermal keratinocytes, changes linked with the early stages of cutaneous carcinogenesis [2]. It is widely believed by lay people that a tan provides good protection against sunburn [3]. However, tanned skin has been shown to be less effective against formation of DNA photoproducts than constitutive pigmentation [3] and has a sun protection factor of 3–5 at best. Population-based surveys reveal that tanning remains popular, particularly with the young, and that episodes of sunburn remain common [4,5]. However, newer sunbeds with a greater proportion of UVB are significantly more carcinogenic than the older lamps that emitted primarily UVA, with little UVB [6,7].

References

1 Sheehan JM, Cragg N, Chadwick CA *et al*. Repeated ultraviolet exposure affords the same protection against DNA photodamage and erythema in human skin types II and IV but is associated with faster DNA repair in skin type IV. *J Invest Dermatol* 2002; **118**: 825–9.
2 Whitmore SE, Morison WL, Potten CS, Chadwick C. Tanning salon exposure and molecular alterations. *J Am Acad Dermatol* 2001; **44**: 775–80.
3 Bykov VJ, Marcusson JA, Hemminki K. Protective effects of tanning on cutaneous DNA damage in situ. *Dermatology* 2001; **202**: 22–6.
4 Boldeman C, Branstrom R, Dal H *et al*. Tanning habits and sunburn in a Swedish population age 13–50 years. *Eur J Cancer* 2001; **37**: 2441–8.

5 Pratt K, Borland R. Predictors of sun protection among adolescents at the beach. *Aust Psychol* 1994; **29**: 135–9.
6 Diffey B. Sunbeds, beauty and melanoma. *Br J Dermatol* 2007; **157**: 215–6.
7 Oliver H, Ferguson J, Moseley H. Quantitative risk assessment of sunbeds: impact of new high power lamps. *Br J Dermatol* 2007; **157**: 350–6.

Photodynamic and phototoxic reactions [1–5]

Drugs and other chemicals with photodynamic and phototoxic activity have the potential to induce skin hyperpigmentation. Tanning follows the sunburn-like reactions to drugs such as demethylchlortetracycline and imipramine, but does not usually occur after photoallergic reactions [3].

If the photodynamic agent is applied directly to the skin, the intensity of the pigmentary response is greatly enhanced. Transient hyperpigmentation has been reported due to photodynamic therapy in acne [4] and localized scleroderma [5]. Hypermelanosis may sometimes be heavy and persistent following photodynamic and phototoxic reactions. The more or less diffuse patterns of pigmentation so induced are considered below, together with other facial melanoses. Two distinctive clinical syndromes are Berloque dermatitis and phytophotodermatitis.

References
1 Epstein JH. Photoallergy. *Arch Dermatol* 1972; **106**: 741–8.
2 Epstein JH. Phototoxicity and photoallergy: clinical syndromes. In: Fitzpatrick TB, ed. *Sunlight and Man*. Tokyo: University of Tokyo Press, 1974: 459–77.
3 Hashimoto K, Joselow SA, Tye MJ. Imipramine hyperpigmentation: a slate-gray discoloration caused by long-term imipramine administration. *J Am Acad Dermatol* 1991; **25**: 357–61.
4 Hongcharu W, Taylor CR, Chang Y *et al*. Topical ALA-photodynamic therapy for the treatment of acne vulgaris. *J Invest Dermatol* 2000; **115**: 183–92.
5 Karrer S, Abels C, Landthaler M, Szeimies RM. Topical photodynamic therapy for localized scleroderma. *Acta Derm Venereol (Stockh)* 2000; **80**: 26–7.

Phytophotodermatitis

> **Synonyms**
> - Meadow dermatitis
> - Strimmer dermatitis
> - Weed-wacker dermatitis

This is an inflammatory and pigmentary reaction of the skin to light, potentiated by furocoumarins in plants (Fig. 58.18). All the plants reliably recorded as inducing this reaction in humans have been shown to contain furocoumarins, including cow parsley (*Anthrisus sylvestris*) and giant hogweed (*Heracleum sphondylium*) [1,2]. The reaction occurs in those exposed to sunlight after these plants have been crushed on the skin. There is some individual variation in susceptibility but with adequate exposure most will react. If the inflammatory phase is severe, bullae are formed. Milder cases show pigmentary changes without inflammation. Serial dilutions of psoralens may, in exceptional cases, be needed to distinguish photoallergy from phototoxicity [3].

Common clinical patterns for phytophotodermatitis include a bizarre network of pigmented streaks on the legs or arms (meadow dermatitis), and much finer spots and small streaks on forearms and legs from contact with plant material during strimming (strimmer dermatitis). Squeezing limes outside when preparing cold drinks can cause blistering of the hands if carried out on sunny days. Handling celery either at harvest or when it is sold

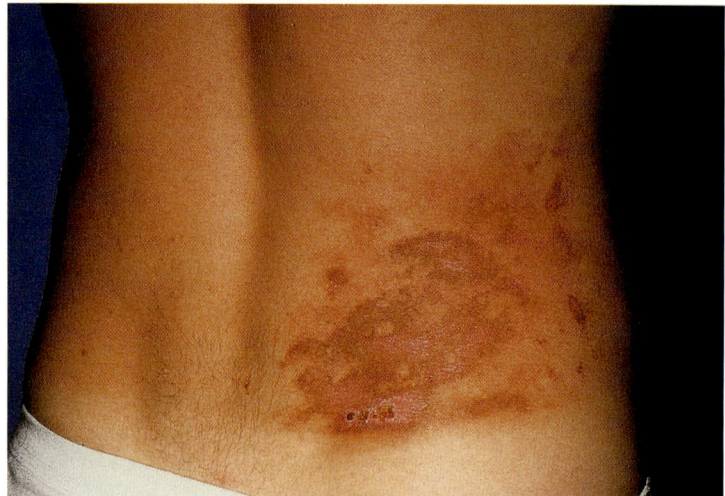

Fig. 58.18 Phytophotodermatitis. Linear, streaky pigmentation following an acute blistering reaction caused by giant hogweed and sunlight.

can cause phytophotodermatitis of the fingertips if it takes place in direct sunlight [4].

References
1 Gawkrodger DJ, Savin JA. Phytophotodermatitis due to common rue (*Ruta graveolens*). *Contact Dermatitis* 1983; **9**: 224.
2 Tunget CL, Turchen SG, Manoguerra AS *et al*. Sunlight and the plant: a toxic combination: severe phytophotodermatitis from *Cneoridium dumosum*. *Cutis* 1994; **54**: 400–2.
3 Ljunggren B. Psoralen photoallergy caused by plant contact. *Contact Dermatitis* 1977; **3**: 85–90.
4 Birmingham DJ, Key MM, Tubich GE, Perone VB. Phototoxic bullae among celery harvesters. *Arch Dermatol* 1961; **83**: 73–87.

Berloque dermatitis (Fig. 58.19) [1–4]

Berloque dermatitis results from the potentiation of UV-stimulated melanogenesis by 5-methoxypsoralen (bergapten) in perfumes containing bergamot oil. There is wide variation in susceptibility, with the reaction occurring in only a small proportion of those exposed [1]. This variation depends on the readiness with which the bergapten is absorbed, the quantity applied, and the intensity and duration of exposure to UV light. Susceptibility is increased by stripping the horny layer. Hot humid conditions favour absorption. The pigmentation occurs in susceptible subjects who have been exposed to light after the application of perfume [2,3]. The distribution of the lesions is therefore variable but their configuration is usually distinctive. Deep-brown pigmentation follows the pattern formed by the trickle of the droplets of perfume over the skin from their points of application. The pigmentation fades after weeks or months. The condition is now much less frequent, although it is a continuing cosmetic problem [4].

References
1 Marzulli FN, Maibach HT. Perfume phototoxicity. *J Soc Cosmet Chem* 1970; **21**: 695–715.
2 Harber LC, Harris H, Leider M *et al*. Berloque dermatitis. *Arch Dermatol* 1964; **90**: 572–6.
3 Burdick KH. Phototoxicity of Shalimar perfume. *Arch Dermatol* 1966; **93**: 424–5.
4 Zaynoun ST, Aftimos BA, Tenekjian KK *et al*. Berloque dermatitis: a continuing cosmetic problem. *Contact Dermatitis* 1981; **7**: 111–6.

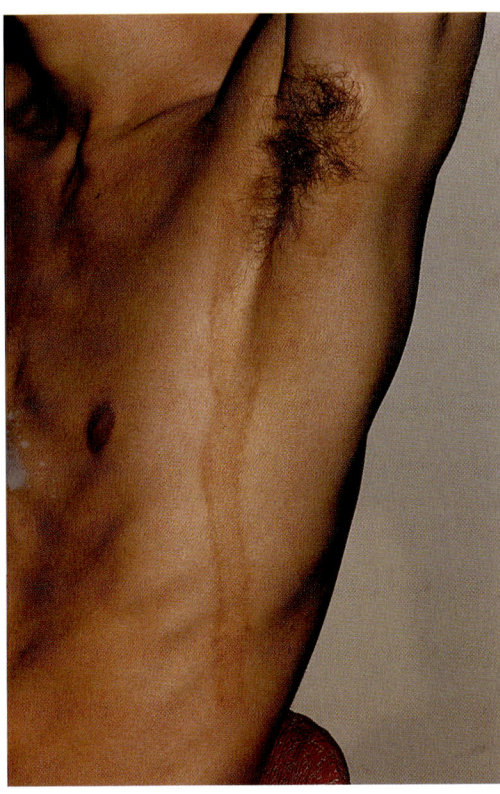

Fig. 58.19 Berloque dermatitis.

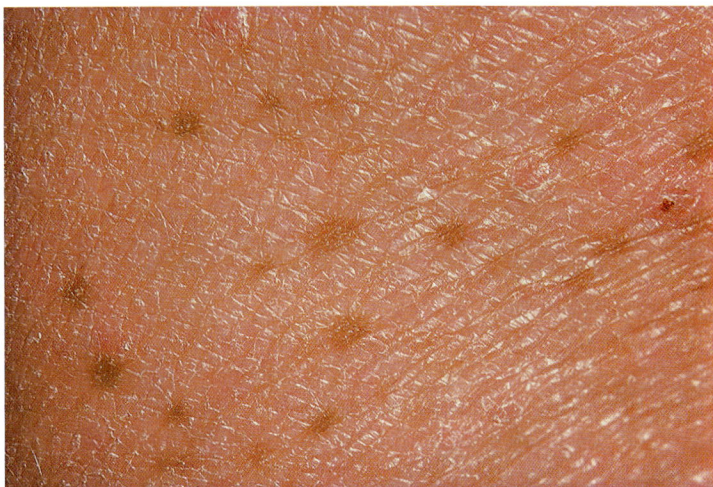

Fig. 58.20 Psoralen and UVA (PUVA)-induced freckles in a patient on long-term treatment.

PUVA lentigines [1–5]

These pigmented macules are a common complication of PUVA therapy occurring on treatment-exposed areas [1–3]. There is a dose effect with a tendency to greater numbers of lentigines in those who have had more therapy [3]. They vary in appearance and may be numerous in number and small in size. Occasionally, larger irregular lentigines are seen, some with a stellate configuration [3] (Fig. 58.20). PUVA lentigines are usually permanent and show little tendency to remit. A less common clinical pattern is localization of lentigines to sites previously affected by psoriasis, creating an appearance not unlike a naevus spilus [2]. The histology is that of a lentigo. The melanocytes are hypertrophic and some may be cytologically atypical [3]. Similar melanocytic macules have been reported following use of a sunbed [4]. PUVA has also been reported to cause hyperpigmentation of the nails [5].

References

1 Miller RA. Psoralens and UV-A-induced stellate hyperpigmented freckling. *Arch Dermatol* 1982; **118**: 619–20.
2 Helland S, Bang G. Nevus spilus-like hyperpigmentation in psoriatic lesions during PUVA therapy. *Acta Derm Venereol (Stockh)* 1980; **60**: 81–3.
3 Rhodes AR, Stern RS, Melski JW. The PUVA lentigo: an analysis of predisposing factors. *J Invest Dermatol* 1983; **81**: 459–63.
4 Kadunce DP, Piepkorn MW, Zone JJ. Persistent melanocytic lesions associated with cosmetic tanning bed use: 'sunbed lentigines'. *J Am Acad Dermatol* 1990; **23**: 1029–31.
5 Naik RP, Parameswara YR. 8-Methoxypsoralen-induced nail pigmentation. *Int J Dermatol* 1982; **21**: 275–6.

Erythema dyschromicum perstans

Synonym
• Ashy dermatosis of Ramirez

This clinical syndrome of unknown origin was first reported by Ramirez of El Salvador in 1957 [1]. He initially used the term 'los cenicientos' (the ashen ones) for the ashy discoloration of the skin, but subsequently called this condition 'erythema dyschromicum perstans' [2]. It occurs in both sexes from childhood to old age, and is not uncommon in individuals of intermediate skin colour. Most published cases have been from Central America [3]. Histologically, the active border shows vacuolar degeneration of the basal cells. The epidermis contains much pigment and there is pigmentary incontinence; the dermal vessels are sleeved with an infiltrate of lymphocytes and histiocytes, and there are many melanophages [4]. Ultrastructural studies show vacuoles within the cytoplasm of basal and suprabasal keratinocytes that contain many melanosomal complexes. One study found IgM cytoid bodies on direct immunofluorescence [5].

Clinically, the condition is characterized by numerous macules of varying shades of grey with a red, slightly raised and palpably infiltrated margin. They vary in size and tend to coalesce over extensive areas of the trunk, limbs and face. Against the general greyish background are macules of hypomelanosis or hypermelanosis. The condition is persistent and slowly extends, but causes no symptoms. The pigmented macules resemble very closely the lesions of late pinta, but the negative dark-field examinations, negative serological tests for syphilis and lack of response to penicillin are important features that allow the dermatologist to exclude this treponematosis. There is no established therapy for this condition [6].

References

1 Ramirez CO. Los cenicientos, problemo clinico. In: *Memoria del Primer Congresso Centroamericano de Dermatologica.* San Salvador, 1957: 122–30.
2 Convit J, Kerdel-Vegas F, Rodriguez G. Erythema dyschromicum perstans: a hitherto undescribed skin disease. *J Invest Dermatol* 1961; **6**: 457–62.

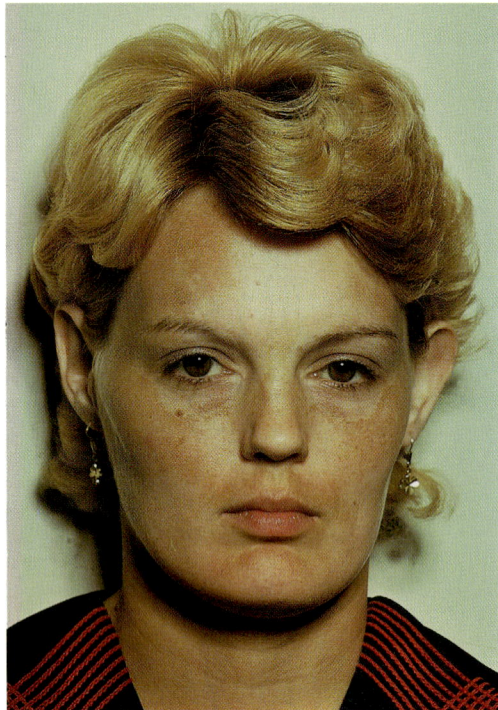

Fig. 58.21 Melasma.

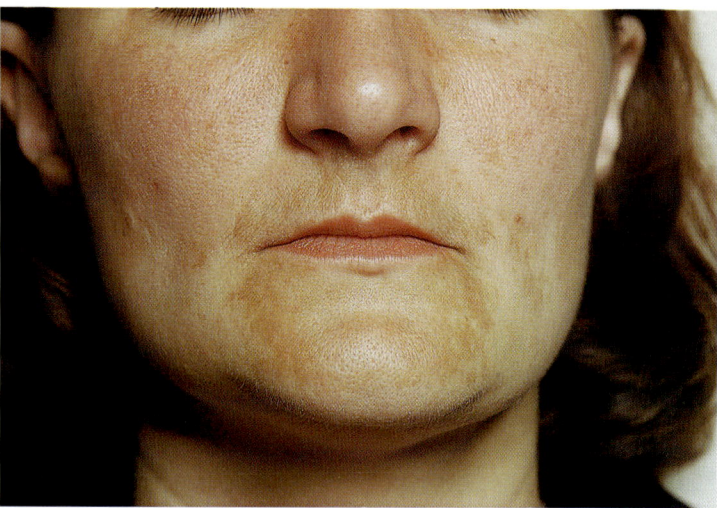

Fig. 58.22 Melasma.

3 Ramirez CO. The ashy dermatoses (erythema dyschromicum perstans). *Cutis* 1967; **3**: 244–7.

4 Migagawa S, Komatsu M, Okuchi T *et al*. Erythema dyschromicum perstans: immunopathologic studies. *J Am Acad Dermatol* 1989; **20**: 882–6.

5 Person JR, Rogers RS. Ashy dermatosis. *Arch Dermatol* 1981; **117**: 701–4.

6 Novick NL, Phelps R. Erythema dyschromicum perstans. *Int J Dermatol* 1985; **24**: 630–3.

Facial melanoses

Hypermelanosis involving predominantly the face and the neck is relatively common and often presents a complex diagnostic problem. Several more or less well-defined clinical syndromes can be recognized, but many transitional forms defy classification. The causes of the pigmentation are often obscure.

Genetic and racial factors are important, the increased pigmentation occurring more frequently in those with dark skins, especially Oriental people. Endocrine factors play a major role in melasma and are implicated to some degree in other melanoses. External agents (light and photodynamic chemicals) are essential factors in the occupational melanoses but are also concerned in Riehl's melanosis, erythrosis and poikiloderma of Civatte. Other unknown factors are certainly implicated, and wide individual variation in susceptibility must be postulated.

Cosmetics may occasionally cause facial melanosis. Facial melanosis is, of course, also a conspicuous feature of Addisonian pigmentation.

Melasma (Figs 58.21 & 58.22)

Synonyms
- Mask of pregnancy
- Chloasma

This common acquired hypermelanosis is seen mainly in women, and occurs mainly on sun-exposed skin on the face, only occasionally affecting the forearms. Many cases are attributed to pregnancy or the combined oral contraceptive pill. In the context of pregnancy melasma is regarded as a normal physiological change, along with darkening of the nipples and linea nigra. It is not uncommon at any time during the years of reproductive activity and has been attributed, without acceptable proof, to a variety of ovarian disorders. The rarity of melasma in post-menopausal women on oestrogen-containing hormone replacement therapy and the fact that men are occasionally affected suggests that oestrogen alone is not the causative agent. Despite light microscopic, ultrastructural and immunofluorescence studies, the condition remains an enigma [1]. An endocrine mechanism is postulated but the cause of melasma is unknown.

Clinical features. Hypermelanosis affects the upper lip, cheeks, forehead and chin and is more apparent following sun exposure. Affected skin is brown in colour. The pigmentary changes are usually bilateral and are frequently symmetrical. After pregnancy or after stopping oral contraceptives the condition may fade but is often persistent. Melasma-like hyperpigmentation has been reported from use of phenytoin or mephenytoin (hydantoins). Up to 10% of cases of melasma are seen in men, particularly Latin Americans and those from the Middle East or Asia.

Treatment. A variety of topical treatments are effective at lightening melasma [2–5], but these treatments should be combined with assiduous sun-protection measures if the reduced pigmentation is to be maintained.

References

1 Sanchez NP, Pathak MA, Sato S *et al*. Melasma: a clinical, light microscopic, ultrastructural and immunofluorescence study. *J Am Acad Dermatol* 1981; **4**: 698–710.

2 Pathak MA, Fitzpatrick TB, Kraus EW. Usefulness of retinoic acid in the treatment of melasma. *J Am Acad Dermatol* 1986; **15**: 894–9.

3 Grimes PE. Melasma: etiologic and therapeutic considerations. *Arch Dermatol* 1995; **131**: 1453–7.

4 Jimbow K. N-Acetyl-4-S-cysteaminylphenol as a new type of depigmenting agent for the melanoderma of patients with melasma. *Arch Dermatol* 1991; **127**: 1928–34.
5 Breathnach AS. Melanin hyperpigmentation of skin: melasma, topical treatment with azelaic acid and other therapies. *Cutis* 1996; **57**: 36–45.

Riehl's melanosis

Synonyms
- Melanodermatitis toxica
- Pigmented cosmetic dermatitis

Background. A distinctive pattern of grey-brown facial pigmentation was first described by Riehl in Vienna between 1916 and 1920 [1]. Riehl attributed this pigmentation to contact with noxious substances or to wartime living conditions. It was subsequently seen in Europe and Asia during and after the Second World War and has also occurred in Argentina [2] and in the South African Bantu [3]. The condition is more frequent in women, and tar derivatives and fragrances are suspected to be the cause [4]. An outbreak of Riehl's melanosis in Japan was attributed to contact dermatitis to cosmetic ingredients and prompted the phrase 'pigmented cosmetic dermatitis' for this condition [5].

Histopathology. In the early stages there is liquefaction degeneration of the basal layer of the epidermis and a perivascular or band-like dermal infiltrate with pigmentary incontinence. Later, the epidermis appears normal but many melanophages are present in the upper dermis [6]. Ultrastructural studies show intercellular and intracellular oedema of keratinocytes and a multilayered basal lamina, as well as many melanophages in the dermis [6].

Course, prognosis and treatment. Brownish-grey pigmentation develops quite rapidly over the greater part of the face but is more intense on the forehead and temples. Smaller pigmented macules, often perifollicular, lie beyond the indefinite margin. The pigmentation may extend to the chest, neck and scalp, and occasionally involves hands and forearms. Horny plugs fill the follicles and there may be some scaling. Where a contact cause can be identified and avoided, there follows a slow improvement over many months.

References
1 Riehl G. Über eine eigenartige Melanose. *Wien Klin Wochenschr* 1917; **30**: 780–1.
2 Peirini LE. Melanosis de Riehl. *Arch Argent Dermatol* 1952; **2**: 315.
3 Findlay GH. Some observations on melanosis of Riehl. *S Afr Med J* 1952; **26**: 373–5.
4 Serrano G, Pujol C, Cuadra J, Aliaga A. Riehl's melanosis: pigmented contact dermatitis caused by fragrances. *J Am Acad Dermatol* 1989; **21**: 1057–60.
5 Nakayama H, Harada R, Toda M. Pigmented cosmetic dermatitis. *Int J Dermatol* 1976; **15**: 673–5.
6 Nagao S, Iijima S. Light and electron microscopic study of Riehl's melanosis. *J Cutan Pathol* 1974; **1**: 165–75.

Poikiloderma of Civatte (Fig. 58.23) [1]

Background. This characteristic pattern of reticulate hyperpigmentation of the face and neck was first reported in 1923 by Civatte [1].

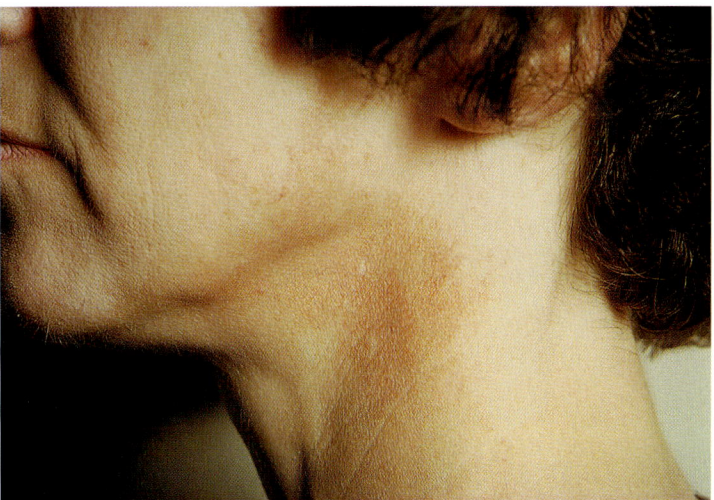

Fig. 58.23 Poikiloderma of Civatte on side of neck.

Clinical features. It tends to occur in women aged 30–50. Poikilodermatous changes develop on the sides of the neck with hyperpigmentation, telangiectasia and dermal atrophy. The submandibular and submental areas are spared thus implicating sunlight in the pathogenesis of this condition. Milder forms are common and few patients seek medical advice.

Treatment. Laser therapy with the tuneable dye laser may be effective but care is needed as it may also cause scarring and may even worsen the appearance [2]. Photoprotection with a high SPF sunscreen may help prevent disease progression.

References
1 Civatte A. Poikilodermie reticule pigmentaire du visage et du col. *Ann Dermatol Syphilol (Paris)* 1923; **6**: 605–20.
2 Wheeland RG, Applebaum J. Flashlamp-pumped pulsed dye laser therapy for poikiloderma of Civatte. *J Dermatol Surg Oncol* 1990; **16**: 12–6.

Pigmented peribuccal pigmentation of Brocq

Background. It was Brocq in 1923 who first reported a case of perioral hyperpigmentation in a clinical pattern that now bears his name [1].

Clinical features. This syndrome occurs predominantly in middle-aged women and has rarely been reported in men. A photodynamic substance in cosmetics is probably responsible. Diffuse brownish-red pigmentation develops symmetrically around the mouth but spares a narrow perioral ring. It may extend up the centre of the face to the forehead and in some cases there are well-defined patches of pigmentation over the angles of the jaw and the temples. The erythematous component, and hence the intensity of the pigmentation, may fluctuate over short periods. The pigmentation is usually persistent but tends gradually to fade if the cause is eliminated. A similar post-inflammatory hyperpigmentation is seen in some patients with perioral dermatitis and may be the result of topical steroid therapy [2].

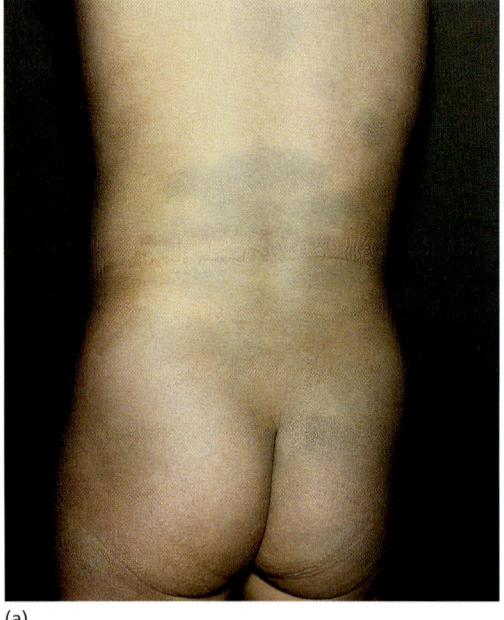
(a)

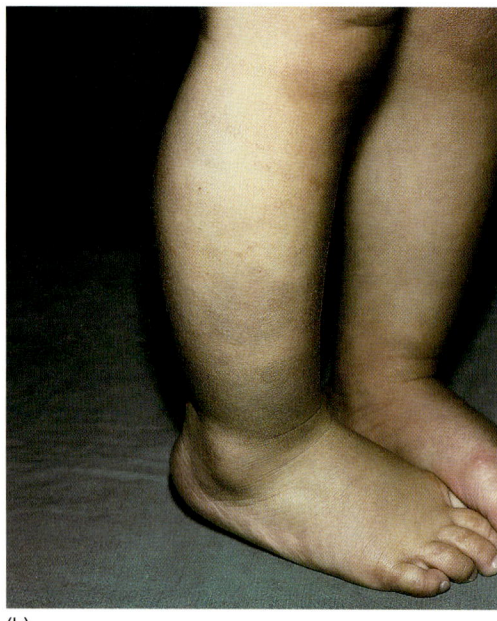
(b)

Fig. 58.24 Mongolian spot: (a) extensive blue coloration on the back of an oriental child; (b) involvement of the legs in the same child.

References
1 Brocq JL. L'eryththrose pigmentée péri-buccale. *Presse Med* 1923; **31**: 720–8.
2 Allen BR, Hunter JAA. Abnormal facial pigmentation associated with the prolonged use of topical corticosteroids. *Scott Med J* 1975; **20**: 277.

Erythromelanosis follicularis of the face and neck

This syndrome, of unknown origin, was originally described in Japan by Kitamura [1]. Affected individuals are usually young or middle-aged males [2,3] although it has also been reported in adult females [4]. Histologically, there is slight hyperkeratosis. The hair follicles are enlarged and contain lamellar horny masses. The sebaceous glands are also enlarged. The epidermis overlying the affected follicle is flattened and contains excess melanin. In the dermis, an inconspicuous lymphocytic infiltrate surrounds dilated vessels.

The clinical picture is distinctive. A background of reddish-brown pigmentation with telangiectasia is studded with pale follicular papules. The hairs are lost from the majority of affected follicles in the vellus region, but less conspicuously from the terminal hair of scalp or beard. The pigmentation involves the skin in front of, beneath and behind the ear, extending to the side of the neck. It spreads slowly, is persistent and is not influenced by treatment. The distribution and lack of clinical follicular keratosis or scarring readily distinguish erythromelanosis from the various forms of keratosis pilaris and from other facial melanoses.

References
1 Kitamura K, Kato H, Mishima Y *et al.* Erythromelanosis follicularis faciei. *Hautarzt* 1960; **11**: 391–3.
2 Watt TL, Kaiser JS. Erythromelanosis follicularis faciei et colli. *J Am Acad Dermatol* 1981; **5**: 533–4.
3 Anderson BL. Erythromelanosis follicularis faciei et colli. *Br J Dermatol* 1980; **102**: 323–5.
4 Warren FM, Davis LS. Erythromelanosis follicularis faciei in women. *J Am Acad Dermatol* 1995; **32**: 863–6.

Dermal melanocytosis

Synonym
• Ceruloderma

Hyperpigmentation of the skin may be due to the presence of functional fusiform and dendritic melanocytes that lie in the dermis [1]. Although dermal melanocytes are common in other mammals, they are not often seen in humans. These cells have failed to reach their proper location in the basal layer of the epidermis in their migration from the neural crest of the developing embryo. Several conditions are grouped under the term 'dermal melanocytosis'. In all of them, the affected areas have a slate-brown or blue colour (ceruloderma) due to an optical effect from the pigment lying in the dermis.

Mongolian spot (Fig. 58.24) [1–4]

Mongolian blue spots are seen in 90% of Oriental babies and less frequently in black babies. The usual site of involvement is the lumbosacral region. The spots are poorly circumscribed areas of slate-brown or blue-black pigmentation that are sometimes extensive and may be mistaken for bruises. A case of generalized dermal melanocytosis of the newborn has been described [2]. Mongolian blue spots usually fade in early childhood, although the aberrant extrasacral spots can persist [3]. Very extensive Mongolian blue spots may regress more slowly, and some areas may persist indefinitely. The dermal melanocytes in persistent Mongolian spots have an extracellular sheath [4], as also seen in the naevus of Ito. The aetiology of this birthmark is unknown.

Naevus of Ota

Synonyms
• Nevus fuscocaeruleus ophthalmomaxillaris
• Oculodermal melanocytosis

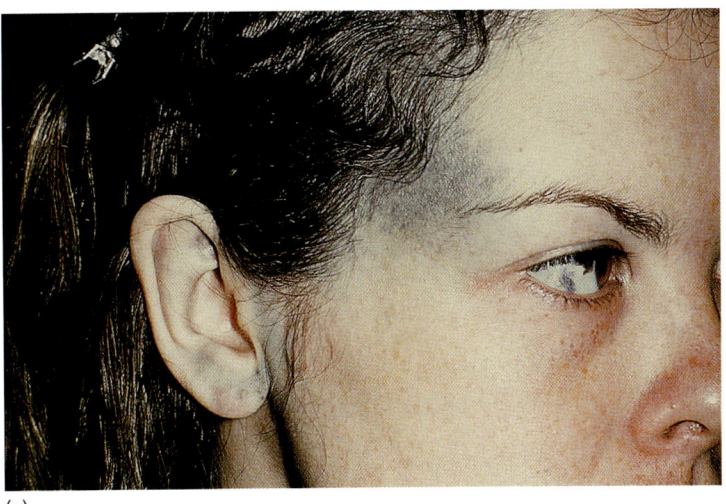
(a)

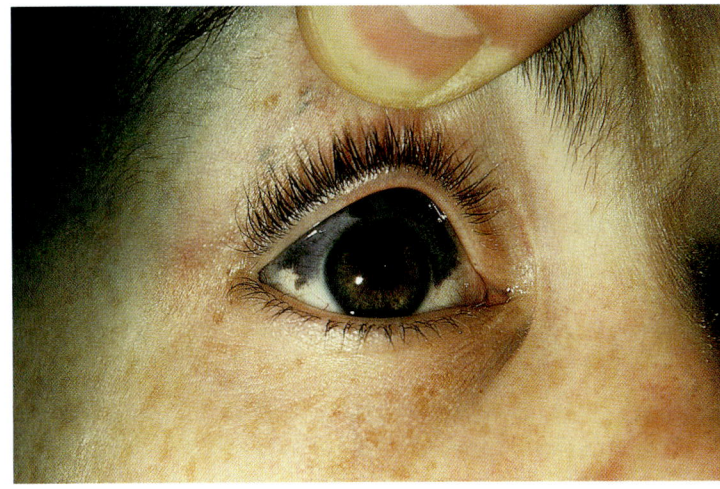
(b)

Fig. 58.25 (a) Naevus of Ota in a white subject. (b) Marked blue coloration of the sclera in the same patient.

Naevus of Ota was first described by the Japanese dermatologist Ota in 1939 [5]. The hyperpigmentation affects one side of the face in the area supplied by the ophthalmic and maxillary divisions of the trigeminal nerve [6,7]. Occasionally, it is bilateral. It is usually congenital but may appear later in life. It is more prevalent in the Japanese but is observed in other races. The colour is variable, but is usually either slate-brown or blue. The sclera is involved and there may be hyperpigmentation of the cornea, iris, retina, ocular muscles and orbit [8] (Fig. 58.25). Sometimes, there is pigmentation of the hard palate. An ipsilateral sensorineural deafness occurring in a patient with naevus of Ota has been reported [9].

Naevus of Ota does not improve with time. Malignant change in the cutaneous lesions of naevus of Ota is extremely rare. However, melanomas are more common in the choroid, iris, orbit and brain of these patients [10]. A bilateral, acquired dermal melanosis of the face resembling naevus of Ota has been described [11]. Promising results with the Q-switch ruby laser have been reported in the treatment of naevus of Ota, with multiple treatments increasing the response rate [12].

Naevus of Ito (Fig. 58.26) [4,12,13]

In this condition, the increased pigmentation affects the area supplied by the posterior supraclavicular and lateral brachial cutaneous nerves. It is relatively common in the Japanese.

Blue naevus

These commonly occur on or near the dorsa of hands and feet, usually early in life. Malignant transformation does not occur in the common blue naevus. However, the cellular blue naevus may rarely undergo malignant change.

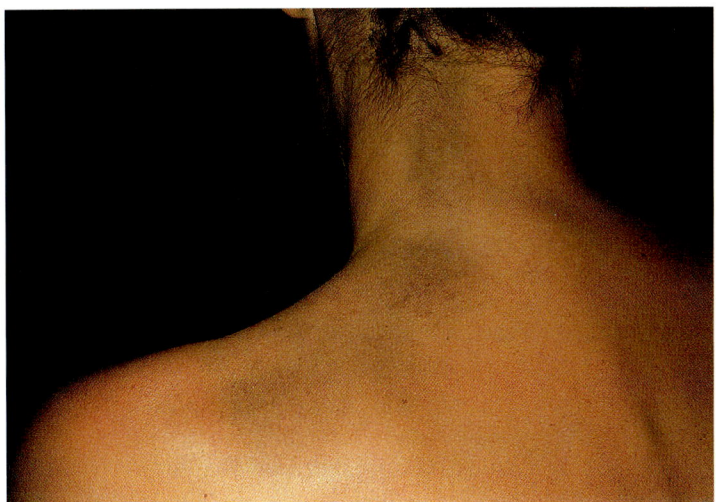

Fig. 58.26 Naevus of Ito.

References

1 Dorsey CS, Montgomery H. Blue nevus and its distinction from Mongolian spot and the nevus of Ota. *J Invest Dermatol* 1954; **22**: 225–36.

2 Bashiti HM, Blair JD, Triska RA, Keller L. Generalized dermal melanocytosis. *Arch Dermatol* 1981; **117**: 791–3.

3 Hidano A. Persistent Mongolian spot in the adult. *Arch Dermatol* 1971; **103**: 680–1.

4 Okawa Y, Yokota R, Yamauchi A. On the extracellular sheath of dermal melanocyte in nevus fuscoceruleus acromiodeltoideus (Ito) and mongolian spot. *J Invest Dermatol* 1979; **73**: 224–30.

5 Ota M, Tanino H. The naevus fusco-caeruleus opthalmomaxillaris and its relationship to pigmentary changes in the eye. *Jikeikai Med J* 1939; **63**: 1243–4.

6 Hidano A, Kajima H, Ikeda S *et al.* Natural history of nevus of Ota. *Arch Dermatol* 1967; **95**: 187–95.

7 Mishima Y, Mevorah B. Nevus Ota and nevus Ito in American Negroes. *J Invest Dermatol* 1961; **36**: 133–54.

8 Cowan TH, Balistocky M. The nevus of Ota or oculodermal melanocytosis. *Arch Ophthalmol* 1961; **65**: 483–92.

9 Reed WB, Sugarman Gi. Unilateral nevus of Ota with sensorineural deafness. *Arch Dermatol* 1974; **109**: 881–3.

10 Enriquez R, Egbert B, Bullock J. Primary malignant melanoma of the central nervous system. *Arch Pathol* 1973; **95**: 392–5.

11 Hori Y, Kawashima M, Oohara K, Kukita A. Acquired bilateral nevus of Ota-like macules. *J Am Acad Dermatol* 1984; **10**: 961–4.

12 Waatanabe S, Takahashi H. Treatment of nevus of Ota with the Q-switch ruby laser. *N Engl J Med* 1994; **331**: 1745–50.

13 Ito M. Studies on melanin XXII. Nevus fusco-ceruleus acromiodeltoideus. *Tohoku J Exp Med* 1954; **60**: 10.

Table 58.5 Hypermelanosis due to genetic and naevoid factors.

Brown colour	Grey, slate or blue colour
Ephelides (freckles)	Mongolian spot
Lentigines	Naevus of Ota
Multiple lentigines syndrome	Naevus of Ito
Peutz–Jeghers syndrome	Blue naevus
Café-au-lait and freckle-like macules in neurofibromatosis	Diffuse melanocytosis
Melanotic macules in Albright's syndrome	Incontinentia pigmenti (Bloch–Sulzberger syndrome)
Acanthosis nigricans, juvenile type	Naegeli–Franceschetti–Jadassohn syndrome
Xeroderma pigmentosum	
Fanconi's syndrome	
Dyskeratosis congenita	
Familial progressive hyperpigmentation	

Disseminated dermal melanocytosis [1]

Progressive dermal melanocytosis has been described in a patient who developed profuse, bluish, bruise-like spots in childhood. The woman died in the fifth decade from melanoma.

Reference

1 Levene A. Disseminated dermal melanocytosis terminating in melanoma. *Br J Dermatol* 1979; **101**: 197–205.

Hypermelanosis associated with other cutaneous lesions

Hypermelanosis is a characteristic feature of urticaria pigmentosa but the mechanism of its production is unknown. Tyrosinase-positive cells have been found in the upper dermis in some cases. In the childhood type, the light-brown macules often exceed 2 cm in diameter and the lesions are frequently nodular. In the adult types, the smaller and more numerous macules are purplish-brown in colour and not palpably infiltrated, and often fail to urticate on friction. They are usually widely distributed over the trunk and limbs.

The differential diagnosis of hypermelanosis

The very large number of conditions associated with widespread or localized hypermelanosis cannot readily be classified. The present classification is based on the colour of the skin and on various causative factors. The hypermelanosis may be due to genetic and naevoid factors (Table 58.5) or it is acquired and due to a variety of factors (Table 58.6).

The areas of hypermelanosis may be circumscribed or may be diffuse with intensification of the normal pattern of pigmentation. Hypermelanosis confined to the face and neck is considered on pp. 58.34–58.35. In acquired, circumscribed patches of hypermelanosis, a post-inflammatory origin should be considered (see p. 58.30).

Treatment of hypermelanosis

Hypermelanosis, particularly affecting areas on the face, can be the cause of marked cosmetic disability and give rise to much mental distress. Treatment depends essentially on establishing the

Table 58.6 Acquired hypermelanosis.

Causative factor	Brown	Grey, slate or blue
Metabolic	Liver disease	Haemochromatosis
	Haemochromatosis, hepatolenticular degeneration, biliary cirrhosis	
	Porphyria	
	Porphyria cutanea tarda and variegata, erythropoietic (congenital) porphyria	
Endocrine	ACTH and MSH-producing pituitary and other tumours	
	Addison's disease	
	ACTH therapy	
	Pregnancy	
	Contraceptive pill and oestrogens	
	Melasma (chloasma)	
Chemical	Arsenic	Minocycline
	Busulfan, bleomycin, cyclophosphamide	Fixed drug eruptions, barbiturates, phenolphthalein
	Adriamycin	
	Psoralens	Phenothiazines
	Berloque dermatitis	Chlorpromazine
	Phytophotodermatitis	
Physical	UV light, ionizing radiation, trauma	
Nutritional	Kwashiorkor	Chronic nutritional deficiency
	Pellagra	
	Sprue	
	Vitamin B_{12} deficiency	
Post-inflammatory	Eczema	Pinta
	Lichen planus, lupus erythematosus	Erythema dyschromicum perstans
	Lichen and macular amyloidosis	
	Systemic sclerosis, morphoea	
Tumours	Malignant melanoma	Metastatic melanoma with melanogenuria
	Acanthosis nigricans with adenocarcinoma	
	Malignant tumours	

ACTH, adrenocorticotrophic hormone; MSH, melanocyte-stimulating hormone.

cause and if possible reversing the conditions that have given rise to the hypermelanosis. In the majority of cases, topical therapy has no place, although some who are perturbed about their cosmetic disability will demand treatment with a skin-bleaching preparation. Because in many cases exposure to sunlight intensifies the pigmentation, a photoprotective preparation should be prescribed and applied during sunny weather. Cosmetic camouflage may also be indicated.

A number of compounds have been used in skin-bleaching preparations and of these hydroquinone is the most safe. Preparations containing 2% hydroquinone, although not very effective, are of help in producing cutaneous depigmentation [1]. Although higher concentrations of hydroquinone are more potent, these preparations frequently irritate the skin and may produce, if used for long periods of time, an exogenous ochronosis and pigmented colloid milium [2,3]. A formulation of hydroquinone and retinoic acid has some effect in depigmenting human skin and is of use in the treatment of hypermelanotic conditions such as melasma [4–6]. It is not very effective for post-inflammatory hyperpigmentation. Topical tretinoin has been found to be effective in the treatment of actinic lentigines ('liver spots') in photodamaged skin [7] and also improves melasma [8]. The monobenzylether of hydroquinone is responsible for many therapeutic and cosmetic disasters and the compound should be used only to bleach away the remaining pigmented areas in patients with extensive vitiligo [9]. Several other substituted phenols, such as 4-isopropylcatechol, can produce cutaneous depigmentation; however, this compound and others are irritant and may produce sensitization [10].

References

1 Fitzpatrick TB, Arndt KA, El Mofty AM *et al*. Hydroquinone and psoralens in the therapy of hypermelanosis and vitiligo. *Arch Dermatol* 1966; **93**: 589–600.
2 Findlay GH, Morrison JGL, Simson IW. Exogenous ochronosis and pigmented colloid milium from hydroquinone bleaching creams. *Br J Dermatol* 1975; **93**: 613–22.
3 Hoshaw RA, Zimmerman KG, Menter A. Ochronosis-like pigmentation from hydroquinone bleaching cream in American Blacks. *Arch Dermatol* 1985; **121**: 105–8.
4 Bleehen SS. Skin bleaching preparations. *J Soc Cosmet Chem* 1977; **28**: 407–12.
5 Engasser PG, Maibach HI. Cosmetics and dermatology: bleaching creams. *J Am Acad Dermatol* 1981; **5**: 143–7.
6 Kligman AM, Willis I. A new formula for depigmenting human skin. *Arch Dermatol* 1975; **111**: 40–8.
7 Rafal ES, Griffiths CEM, Ditre CM. Topical tretinoin (retinoic acid) treatment for liver spots associated with photodamage. *N Engl J Med* 1992; **326**: 368–74.
8 Griffiths CE, Finkel LT, Ditre CM *et al*. Topical tretinoin (retinoic acid) improves melasma: a vehicle controlled clinical trial. *Br J Dermatol* 1993; **129**: 415–21.
9 Mosher DB, Parrish JA, Fitzpatrick TB. Monobenzylether of hydroquinone. *Br J Dermatol* 1977; **97**: 669–79.
10 Bleehen SS. The treatment of hypermelanosis with 4-isopropyl-catechol. *Br J Dermatol* 1976; **94**: 687–94.

Hypomelanosis

Genetic and naevoid disorders

A number of genetically determined or naevoid conditions are characterized by localized and/or generalized hypomelanosis of the skin. These are listed in Table 58.7.

Albinism [1–9]

There are many distinct types of oculocutaneous albinism (OCA), each of which is characterized by partial or complete failure to produce melanin in the skin and the eyes. The classification is rapidly changing with the advent of advances in molecular genetics (e.g. rufous OCA is now *TRP-1* gene-related OCA or type III OCA). Melanocytes are present in normal distribution but fail to synthesize melanin adequately. These conditions are inherited as autosomal recessive disorders; one rare type with apparent autosomal dominant inheritance is now felt to be due to quasi-dominant pedigree patterns or to partial expression of OCA II in

Table 58.7 Hypomelanosis due to genetic and naevoid factors (MIM numbers in parentheses).

Oculocutaneous albinism (OCA)	
Tyrosinase negative (type IA, #203100)	Recessive
Yellow mutant (type IB, #606952)	Recessive
Temperature sensitive (type 1TS; included in IB #606952)	Recessive
Tyrosinase positive (type II, *203200)	Recessive
Brown	Recessive*
Minimal pigment (203280)	Recessive
Platinum	Recessive†
TRP-1 gene-related (type III) (was rufous OCA, #278400)	Recessive
Hermansky–Pudlak syndrome (203300)	Recessive
Chédiak–Higashi syndrome (#214500)	Recessive
Autosomal dominant	Dominant‡
Ocular albinism	X-linked
With deafness	X-linked, recessive, dominant
Albinoidism (*126070)	Dominant§
Cross syndrome (*257800)	Recessive
Piebaldism (#172800)	Dominant
Waardenburg syndrome (#193150, #193510)	Dominant
Phenylketonuria (*261200)	Recessive
Vitiligo	Polygenic
Tuberous sclerosis (#191100)	Dominant
Achromic naevus	
Incontinentia pigmenti achromians	

* Brown OCA is currently included as a type of OCA II.
† Platinum OCA may be an allelic variant of minimal pigment OCA.
‡ Dominant OCA probably does not exist: instances appear to be due to quasidominant pedigree patterns or to partial expression of albinism II in OCA I heterozygotes.
§ The term 'albinoidism' is applied to both pigmentary dilution (MIM *126070) and OCA II.

OCA I heterozygotes (Table 58.7). The gene encoding tyrosinase has been localized to chromosome 11 [2] and many different mutations are now recognized for OCA [3]. The gene for type II OCA has been mapped to chromosome 15q11.13 [4]. Tyrosinase-negative albinism is characterized by hair bulbs that, after plucking and incubation with tyrosine, fail to produce darkening. In tyrosinase-positive albinism, the hair bulbs do darken in this test and the precise metabolic defects have yet to be ascertained. The tyrosinase-positive types are the most common. Ultrastructural studies of skin and hair show that in tyrosinase-negative albinos most of the melanosomes are stage 1 and stage 2 without any melanization. Other types may show melanosomes up to stage 3 of their development.

In ocular albinism, only the eyes are clinically involved, although careful investigation of the melanocytes in the skin does show some changes. There are four different types, two X-linked, one dominant and one recessive. Carrier females of the X-linked types may show irregular retinal pigmentation. In two types there is an associated deafness, the melanocytes apparently failing to play a protective role in the ear. In most albinos this defect leads to little or no change in ear function.

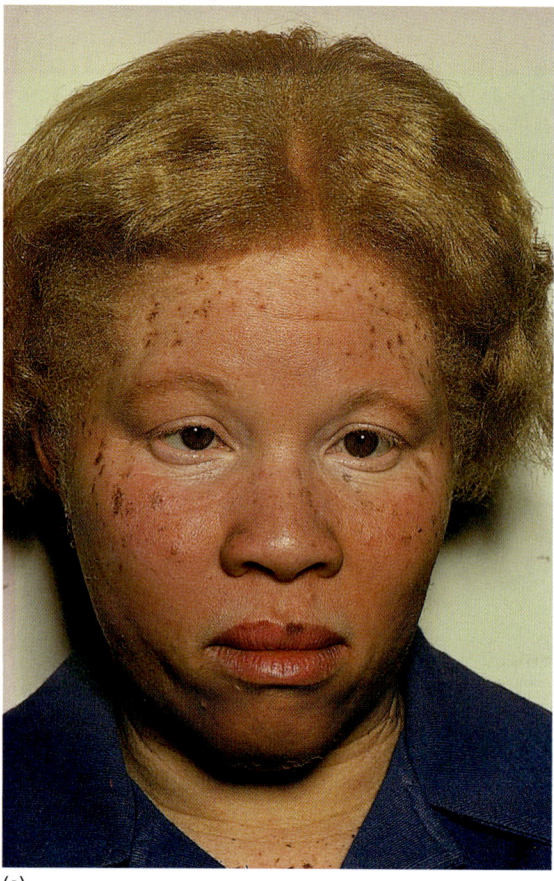

(a)

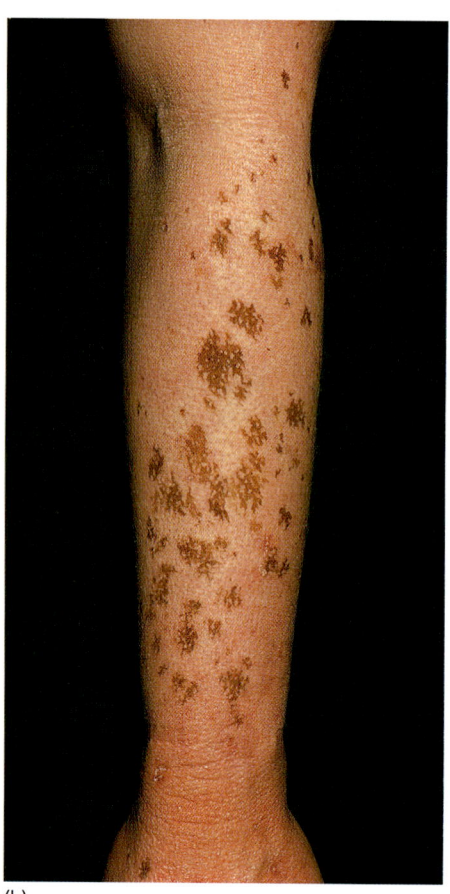

(b)

Fig. 58.27 (a) Tyrosinase-positive oculocutaneous albinism in a black woman aged 40 years. (b) Dark-brown freckles on light-exposed areas.

Incidence. Albinism is found in all races and the prevalence varies considerably. In the UK, the incidence is estimated at 1 in 20 000. In the USA, the incidence of albinism is estimated at 1 in 39 000 in Caucasians and 1 in 28 000 in Afro-Caribbeans. In some countries it is more common, particularly where there is a tendency towards inbreeding and especially in isolated communities. The Cuna tribe on the San Blas islands off the coast of Panama have the highest incidence of albinism in the world (63 per 10 000). In Nigeria, the incidence of albinism is much higher in the south [5]. There are no adequate studies of the incidence of the different genotypes of OCA in the different races.

Clinical features. In all races there is marked dilution of the pigmentation of the skin, hair and eyes. In tyrosinase-negative OCA the skin is pink in colour, the hair is white and the patients show a prominent red reflex. This is the most severe variant of OCA.

In tyrosinase-positive OCA, some pigment is formed and with increasing age is to be found in the iris, skin and hair, the latter often developing a flaxen-yellow colour. These patients may also tan and in black people the skin has a yellowish-brown colour that with age develops dark-brown freckles, particularly in sun-exposed areas (Fig. 58.27). Also in this type, the iris is less translucent and in black people may be brown in colour.

In both types, patients have photophobia; often they have a characteristic facial expression due to apparent squinting. Errors of refraction are common, especially in the tyrosinase-negative

type (OCA IA), and almost all patients have horizontal or rotatory nystagmus, sometimes with head nodding. In the tyrosinase-positive type, visual acuity may improve as patients get older and they may have less severe nystagmus [6]. There are abnormalities of the optic pathway. Foveal hypoplasia occurs in the tyrosinase-negative type [6].

In the yellow mutant type of albinism, the newborn resembles the tyrosinase-negative type, but by the age of 1 year the hair is yellow-red in colour. Hair bulbs incubated in tyrosine plus cysteine produce an intensification of the yellow-red pheomelanin. This type of albinism is prevalent in the Amish communities in the USA [7].

The other types of albinism listed in Table 58.7 have pigment changes described by their names. Each has a rather distinctive racial predisposition.

In temperate climates, the prognosis for the albino is good, the visual defects constituting the greatest disability. In the tropics the fate of albinos is grim. At an early age [8] most of them develop in solar-exposed skin many actinic keratoses, squamous cell carcinomas and, occasionally, melanomas. Some die young from these tumours [5].

Treatment. No treatment is possible other than prescribing photoprotective preparations and limiting sun exposure, vigorous enforcement of which from early childhood can be very helpful. The regular examination of all albinos for the early detection and treatment of premalignant and malignant conditions of the skin is advisable, especially in the tropics. Prenatal diagnosis of albinism has been reported [9].

References

1 Bolognia JL, Pawelek JM. Biology of hypopigmentation. *J Am Acad Dermatol* 1988; **19**: 217–55.
2 Barton DE, Kwon BS, Francke U. Human tyrosinase gene, mapped to chromosome 11 (q14–q21), defines second region of homology with mouse chromosome 7. *Genomics* 1988; **3**: 17–24.
3 Tomita Y. Tyrosinase gene mutations causing oculocutaneous albinisms. *J Invest Dermatol* 1993; **100**: 1865–905.
4 Ramsay M, Colman M-A, Stevens G *et al.* The tyrosinase-positive oculocutaneous albinism locus maps to chromosome 15q11.2–q12. *Am J Hum Genet* 1992; **51**: 879–84.
5 Okoro AN. Albinism in Nigeria. *Br J Dermatol* 1975; **92**: 485–92.
6 Mietz H, Green WR, Wolf SM, Abundo GP. Foveal hypoplasia in complete oculocutaneous albinism: a histopathologic study. *Retina* 1992; **12**: 254–60.
7 King RA, Witkop CJ. Hair-bulb tyrosinase activity in oculocutaneous albinism. *Nature* 1976; **263**: 69–71.
8 Lookingbill DP, Lookingbill GL, Leppard B. Actinic damage and skin cancer in albinos in northern Tanzania: findings in 164 patients enrolled in an outreach skin care program. *J Am Acad Dermatol* 1995; **32**: 653–8.
9 Eady RAJ, Gunner DB, Garner A, Rodeck CH. Prenatal diagnosis of oculocutaneous albinism by electron microscopy of fetal skin. *J Invest Dermatol* 1983; **80**: 210–2.

Albinoidism (MIM *126070)

Albinoidism is the name applied to families where there is some partial defect in melanin production in the skin but only minimal changes in the eyes. The biochemical basis of this is uncertain. Several families are described with this type of albinism [1,2]. Although there is hypopigmentation of the skin and hair, it is not as marked as in OCA. Slight tanning is reported and the hair-bulb test is positive. A diffuse punctate pattern of iris transillumination is seen. The eyes are usually normal, but there may be photophobia. In one large Swiss pedigree there was high-grade myopia [2]. The condition appears to have autosomal dominant inheritance, but in some families it is recessive.

References

1 Bergsma DR, Kaiser-Kupfer M. A new form of albinism. *Am J Ophthalmol* 1974; **77**: 837–44.
2 Busti-Rosner L. Deux cas d'albinisme universel incomplet (albinoidisme) d'un biotype particulier dans une souche valaisanne. *J Génét Hum* 1956; **5**: 197–215.

Hermansky–Pudlak syndrome (MIM #203300)

Hermansky–Pudlak syndrome is a rare type of OCA associated with a haemorrhagic diathesis [1]. About 250 cases have been reported, most of whom are from Puerto Rico or the south of the Netherlands [1]. Two different mutations in the gene for Hermansky–Pudlak syndrome have been identified. Tyrosinase-positive OCA occurs in association with a bleeding tendency and deposits of a ceroid-like pigment in the cells of the reticuloendothelial system [2]. The bleeding tendency is attributed to a storage-pool platelet defect. The platelets have decreased numbers of dense granules and reduced levels of serotonin and ADP [3]. Pulmonary fibrosis, granulomatous colitis and lupus nephritis have been associated [4]. There is no defect in circulating lymphocytes or neutrophils [5]. Two cases of Hermansky–Pudlak syndrome have been complicated by systemic lupus erythematosus [6].

References

1 Hermansky F, Pudlak P. Albinism associated with a haemorrhagic diathesis and unusual pigmented reticular cells in the bone marrow. *Blood* 1959; **14**: 162–9.
2 Shanahan F, Randolph L, King R *et al.* Hermansky–Pudlak syndrome: an immunologic assessment of 15 cases. *Am J Med* 1988; **85**: 823–8.
3 Garay SM, Gardella JE, Fazzini EP, Goldring RM. Hermansky–Pudlak syndrome. Pulmonary manifestations of a ceroid storage disease. *Am J Med* 1979; **66**: 737–47.
4 Schinella RA, Greco MA, Colbert BL *et al.* Hermansky–Pudlak syndrome with granulomatous colitis. *Ann Intern Med* 1980; **92**: 20–3.
5 Schachne JP, Glaser N, Lee S *et al.* Hermansky–Pudlak syndrome: case report and clinicopathologic review. *J Am Acad Dermatol* 1990; **22**: 926–32.
6 Mitsui H, Komine M, Watanabe T *et al.* Does Hermansky–Pudlak syndrome predispose to systemic lupus erythematosus? *Br J Dermatol* 2002; **146**: 908–11.

Chédiak–Higashi syndrome (MIM #214500)

Chédiak–Higashi syndrome is a rare, autosomal recessive disorder characterized by hypopigmentation of the skin and eye [1]. The skin is fair, the retinae are pale and the irides translucent. The hair is light blonde or silvery grey. These children are very susceptible to bacterial and viral infections, and intractable respiratory and cutaneous infections usually prove fatal before the age of 10 years. Longer survival is possible but later the lymph nodes, spleen and liver are enlarged and a malignant lymphoma develops. A similar condition is seen in Aleutian mink [2], Hereford cattle [3] and the beige mouse [4].

The hereditary defect concerns membrane-bound organelles of various cell types and is due to mutations in a gene encoding a protein known as lysosomal trafficking regulator. The melanocytes contain giant pigment granules (Fig. 58.28), which arise by autophagocytosis and fusion of large melanosomes that show degradative changes within the cells [5]. Similar defects of granules and other organelles occur in white cells and platelets. Cytoplasmic inclusions are present in a variety of cells of neuroectodermal origin. The white cells are defective in combating infection and if children with this condition survive infancy, they usually die later from a malignant lymphoma.

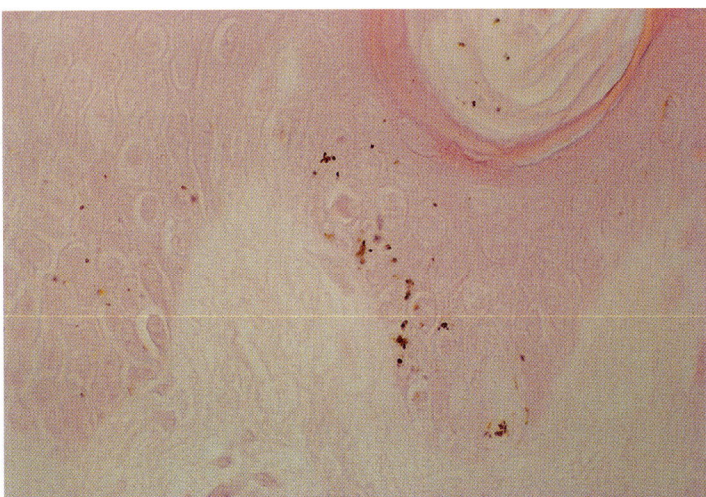

Fig. 58.28 Chédiak–Higashi syndrome. Large pigment granules in the epidermis as seen by light microscopy. Fontana stain, × 40.

References

1 Blume RS, Wolff SM. The Chediak–Higashi syndrome: studies in four patients and a review of the literature. *Medicine (Baltimore)* 1972; **51**: 247–80.
2 Windhorst DB, Zelickson AS, Good RA. A human pigmentary dilution based on a heritable subcellular structural defect. *J Invest Dermatol* 1968; **50**: 9–18.
3 Padgett GA, Reiquam CW, Gorham JR *et al*. Comparative studies of the Chediak–Higashi syndrome. *Am J Pathol* 1967; **51**: 553–71.
4 Lutzner MA, Lowrie CT, Jordan HW. Giant granules in leukocytes of the beige mouse. *J Hered* 1967; **58**: 299–300.
5 Zelickson AS, Windhorst DB, White JG, Good RA. The Chediak–Higashi syndrome: formation of giant melanosomes and the basis for hypopigmentation. *J Invest Dermatol* 1967; **49**: 575–81.

Griscelli syndromes type I (MIM #214450) and type II (MIM #607624)

Griscelli syndrome type I comprises partial albinism with neurological deficiency due to mutations in the myosin type V gene.

Griscelli syndrome type II, due to mutations in the *RAB27A* gene, combines partial albinism and immunodeficiency [1], but is distinct from Chédiak–Higashi syndrome. It is inherited as an autosomal recessive condition. In addition to pigmentary dilution, there is immune deficiency and the affected children are prone to recurrent pyogenic infection. There is hypogammaglobulinaemia and defective cell-mediated immunity with lymphohistiocytosis and haematophagocytosis.

Reference

1 Griscelli C, Durandy A, Guy-Grand D *et al*. A syndrome associating partial albinism and immunodeficiency. *Am J Med* 1978; **65**: 691–702.

Prader–Willi syndrome (MIM #176270) and Angelman syndrome (MIM #105830) [1]

Both syndromes are associated with mental retardation, abnormal behaviour and hypopigmentation. In both there are deletions of the same region of chromosome 15, with deletion on the paternal chromosome in Prader–Willi syndrome and the maternal in Angelman syndrome.

Reference

1 Kirkilionis AJ, Chudley AE, Gregory CA, Hamerton JL. Molecular and clinical overlap of Angelman and Prader–Willi syndrome phenotypes. *Am J Med Genet* 1991; **40**: 454–9.

Cross' syndrome (MIM *257800)

Synonym
• Oculocerebral syndrome with hypopigmentation

Cross' syndrome is one of the 'silvery hair' syndromes and is characterized by generalized hypopigmentation associated with ocular anomalies, mental and physical retardation, ataxia and spasticity [1]. It is probably determined by an autosomal recessive gene [2,3]. The pigmentary and ocular defects are manifest from birth. The hypopigmentation resembles albinism; blood tyrosine levels are normal and the light-coloured hair pigments poorly in tyrosine solution. The ocular defects include microphthalmos, a small opaque cornea and coarse nystagmus. Spasticity soon becomes evident, and physical and mental development is retarded [3].

References

1 Cross HE, McKusick VA, Breen W. A new oculocerebral syndrome with hypopigmentation. *J Pediatr* 1967; **70**: 398–406.
2 Lerone M, Pessagno A, Taccone A *et al*. Oculocerebral syndrome with hypopigmentation (Cross syndrome): report of a new case. *Clin Genet* 1992; **41**: 87–9.
3 Tezcan I, Demir E, Asan E *et al*. A new case of oculocerebral hypopigmentation syndrome (Cross syndrome) with additional findings. *Clin Genet* 1997; **51**: 118–21.

Piebaldism (MIM #172800) [1–11]

Piebaldism is a rare autosomal dominant condition characterized by stable areas of vitiligo-like amelanotic skin associated with a white forelock [2,3]. The incidence of piebaldism is estimated at less than 1 in 20 000. Both sexes are affected equally, and no race is spared. A similar condition of 'white spotting' is seen in mice and results from deletion or mutation of the c-*kit* proto-oncogene that codes for an embryonic growth factor called Steel factor [4]. Missense and frameshift mutations of the *kit* proto-oncogene, which encodes the cellular receptor tyrosine kinase for the mast cell/stem cell growth factor, are responsible for a range of phenotypes with piebaldism [5,6].

The plurality of defects revealed by electron microscopy suggests that a number of different gene loci are concerned. Ultrastructural studies have shown either an absence of melanocytes and melanosomes in the hypomelanotic areas or sometimes reduced numbers of abnormal large melanocytes. In the hypermelanotic islands in the areas of hypomelanosis, melanocytes are present that produce normal melanosomes but also abnormal spherical and granular melanosomes [9]. When transferred to the keratinocytes, these show abnormal degradation and fusion.

Clinical features. Patches of skin totally devoid of pigment are present at birth and usually remain unchanged throughout life. Most common is a frontal median or paramedian patch, associated with a mesh of white hair (white forelock); rarely, this may be the only lesion. Often, white patches occur on the upper chest, abdomen and limbs, bilaterally but not necessarily symmetrically (Fig. 58.29). Occasionally, they are found on the face, particularly the chin. The hands and feet, as well as the back, remain normally pigmented. Islands of normal or hypermelanotic skin occur in the white areas, or less often on normal skin.

Piebaldism can easily be distinguished from vitiligo where the lesions are acquired later in life and their configuration and distribution are quite different. In piebaldism, there is almost invariably a white forelock and the pattern of arrangement of the lesions is quite characteristic. Also the presence of islands of normal pigmented skin in the hypomelanotic areas is typical. If the interpupillary distance is increased or the patient is deaf, the diagnosis of Waardenburg's syndrome (see below) must be considered. The patterns of hypomelanosis as seen in the localized and systematized types of naevus depigmentosus differ from piebaldism. Microscopy of the skin in naevus depigmentosus reveals normal numbers of melanocytes with sometimes rather stubby dendrites [9]. A progressive variant of piebaldism has been described in association with a novel mutation in the *kit* gene [11].

Treatment. Photoprotective preparations should be prescribed to protect the amelanotic areas from burning with sun exposure.

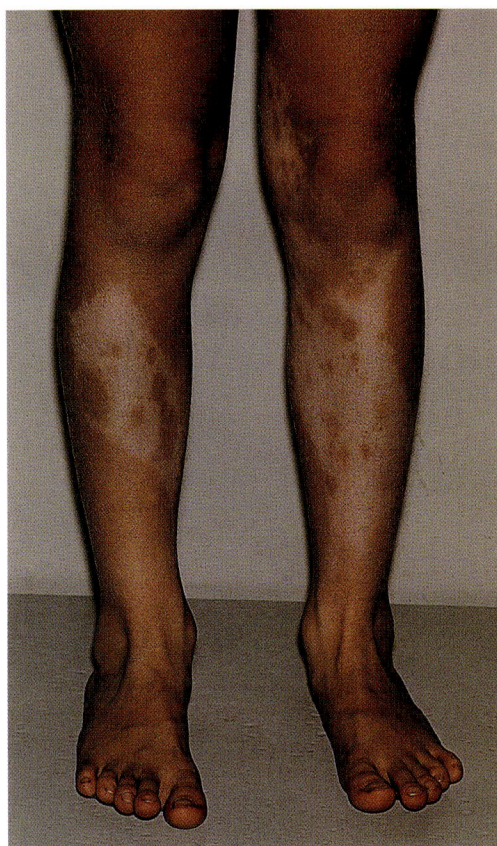

Fig. 58.29 Piebaldism. The lesions had been present from birth.

Cosmetic camouflage or skin dyes may be helpful for some patients. Skin grafts, minigrafts and grafts of autologous cultured melanocytes have some promise [12,13]. PUVA therapy is generally disappointing, as are topical corticosteroids.

References

1 Bolognia JL, Pawelek JM. Biology of hypopigmentation. *J Am Acad Dermatol* 1988; **19**: 217–55.
2 Comings DE, Odland GF. Partial albinism. *JAMA* 1966; **195**: 519–23.
3 Mosher DB, Fitzpatrick TB. Piebaldism. *Arch Dermatol* 1988; **124**: 364–5.
4 Morrison-Graham K, Takahashi Y. Steel factor and c-kit receptor. From mutants to a growth factor system. *Bioessays* 1993; **15**: 77–83.
5 Sprite RA, Holmes SA, Ramesar R *et al*. Mutations of the *kit* (mast/stem cell growth-factor receptor) proto-oncogene accounts for a continuous range of phenotypes in piebaldism. *Am J Hum Genet* 1992; **51**: 1058–65.
6 Ward KA, Moss C, Sanders DSA. Human piebaldism: relationship between phenotype and site of *kit* gene mutation. *Br J Dermatol* 1995; **132**: 929–35.
7 Breathnach AS, Fitzpatrick TB, Wyllie LM. Electron microscopy of melanocytes in human piebaldism. *J Invest Dermatol* 1965; **45**: 28–37.
8 Hayashibe K, Mishima Y. Tyrosinase-positive melanocyte distribution and induction of pigmentation in human piebald skin. *Arch Dermatol* 1988; **124**: 381–6.
9 Jimbow K, Fitzpatrick TB, Szabo G *et al*. Congenital circumscribed hypomelanosis. *J Invest Dermatol* 1975; **64**: 50–6.
10 Cooke JV. Familial white skin spotting (piebaldness) ('partial albinism') with white forelock. *J Pediatr* 1952; **41**: 1–12.
11 Richards KA, Fukai K, Oiso N, Paller AS. A novel KIT mutation results in piebaldism with progressive depigmentation. *J Am Acad Dermatol* 2001; **44**: 288–92.
12 Falabella R. Grafting and transplantation of melanocytes for repigmenting vitiligo and other types of leukoderma. *Int J Dermatol* 1989; **28**: 363–72.
13 Njoo MD, Nieuweboer-Krobotova L, Westerhof W. Repigmentation of leucodermic defects in piebaldism by dermabrasion and thin split-thickness skin grafting in combination with minigrafting. *Br J Dermatol* 1998; **139**: 829–33.

Tietz's syndrome (MIM #103500)

Tietz reported a six-generation pedigree with the constant association of total absence of pigment in the skin and hair, normal eyes, complete deaf-mutism and hypoplasia of the eyebrows [1]. An autosomal dominant gene appeared to be implicated. There is some doubt that this syndrome is a distinct entity.

The analogy with a syndrome in cats, in which severe deafness is associated with total absence of skin pigment but normal eye colour, suggests that Tietz's syndrome probably represents a 'generalized white spot' rather than albinism.

Reference

1 Tietz W. A syndrome of deaf-mutism associated with albinism showing dominant autosomal inheritance. *Am J Hum Genet* 1963; **15**: 259–64.

Waardenburg syndrome (MIM #193150) [1–8]

Historical background. Waardenburg syndrome (WS) was first described by a Dutch ophthalmologist in 1951 [1].

Aetiology. All of the abnormalities of Waardenburg syndrome involve the neural crest. Waardenburg syndrome is therefore considered to represent a global disorder of neural crest development.

Clinical features. Waardenburg syndrome is characterized by lateral displacement of the inner canthi and the lacrimal puncta, prominent nasal root and medial eyebrows, congenital deafness and heterochromic irides [2,3]. Other pigmentary changes are a 'dappled' appearance of the skin, a white forelock, and premature greying of hair, eyebrows and cilia. A few patients show piebaldism; pigment-free patches may be large and multiple or small and inconspicuous. WS has been reported in both black and white people.

Classification. Four classical clinical variants of WS have been described. Type I is the classic form [4], while type II lacks dystopia canthorum but has a high incidence of congenital sensorineural deafness and heterochromia. Type III resembles type I but is associated with limb abnormalities in addition to dystopia canthorum. Type IV, like type III, is autosomal recessive and is characterized by associated Hirschsprung's disease and, in some cases, by more extensive hypopigmentation [5]. Recent molecular genetic findings have demonstrated at least nine distinct genetic subtypes of Waardenburg syndrome, several of which correspond to distinct clinical subtypes not included in these four classical subtypes. Thus, a new and more comprehensive classification can be anticipated soon.

Incidence and genetics. It is a relatively rare autosomal dominant condition with an estimated incidence of 1 in 20–40 000 [6]. Autosomal recessive forms of Waardenburg syndrome are rare. Variable expression and penetrance explain milder or incomplete phenotypes. A number of different mutations of the *PAX*-3 gene on chromosome 2q35 have now been reported in different forms of type I and type III. None of the cases of type II have been linked to 2q markers but type IIA is now known to be due to mutations in the *MITF* gene. Mutations in the endothelin-3 gene [7] and in endothelin-B genes have been reported in type IV, and mutations in the *SOX10* gene [8] have also been implicated as causing WS. Types IIB and IIC are further subdivisions linked to genes mapping to chromosomes 1p and 8p, respectively.

References

1 Waardenburg PJ. A new syndrome combining developmental anomalies of the eyelids, eyebrows, and nose root with pigmentary defects of the iris and head hair with congenital deafness. *Am J Hum Genet* 1951; **3**: 195–253.

2 DiGeorge AM, Olmstead RW, Harley RD. Waardenburg's syndrome. *J Pediatr* 1960; **57**: 649–69.

3 Ortonne J-P. Piebaldism, Waardenburg's syndrome and related disorders. *Dermatol Clin* 1988; **6**: 205–16.

4 Farrer LA, Grundfast KM, Amos J et al. Waardenburg syndrome (WS) type I is caused by defects at multiple loci one of which is near ALPP on chromosome 2: first report of the WS consortium. *Am J Hum Genet* 1992; **50**: 902–13.

5 Shah KN. White forelock, pigmentary disorder of irides and long segment Hirschsprung disease: a possible variant of Waardenburg's syndrome. *J Pediatr* 1981; **99**: 432–5.

6 Liu XZ, Newton VE, Read AP. Waardenburg syndrome type II: phenotypic findings and diagnostic criteria. *Am J Med Genet* 1995; **55**: 95–100.

7 Edery P, Attie T, Amiel J et al. Mutation of the endothelin-3 gene in the Waardenburg–Hirschsprung disease (Shah–Waardenburg syndrome). *Nat Genet* 1996; **12**: 442–4.

8 Pingault V, Bondurand N, Kuhlbrodt K et al. SOX10 mutations in patients with Waardenburg–Hirschsprung disease. *Nat Genet* 1998; **18**: 171–3.

Albinism–deafness syndrome (MIM #300700) [1–4]

> **Synonyms**
> • Ziprkowski–Margolis syndrome
> • Woolf syndrome

Albinism–deafness syndrome (ADFN) is a rare X-linked recessive syndrome that was first described (separately) by Ziprkowski [1] and Margolis [2] in 1962. Ziprkowski reported 14 members of an Egyptian–Jewish family with males showing deaf-mutism, heterochromic irides and piebald-like hypomelanosis of skin and hair [1]. The skin appears completely amelanotic at birth, but pigmented macules develop on the extremities, trunk and scalp. The hair usually remains white. Genetic linkage studies and somatic cell hybrid mapping studies localize the *ADFN* gene to Xq26.3-q27.1 [3]. However, the gene has not yet been identified. Piebaldism in association with congenital nerve deafness [4] has been reported in two brothers with no other manifestation of ADFN. It is unclear whether this is the same or a genetically distinct condition.

References

1 Ziprkowski L, Krakowski A, Adam A et al. Partial albinism and deaf-mutism due to a recessive sex-linked gene. *Arch Dermatol* 1962; **86**: 530–9.

2 Margolis E. A new hereditary syndrome: sex-linked deaf-mutism associated with total albinism. *Acta Genet Stat Med (Basel)* 1962; **12**: 12–9.

3 Shiloh Y, Litvak G, Ziv Y et al. Genetic mapping of X-linked albinism deafness syndrome (ADFN) to xq26.3-27.1. *Am J Hum Genet* 1990; **47**: 20–7.

4 Woolf CM, Dolowitz Aldous HE. Congenital deafness associated with piebaldness. *Arch Otolaryngol* 1965; **82**: 244–50.

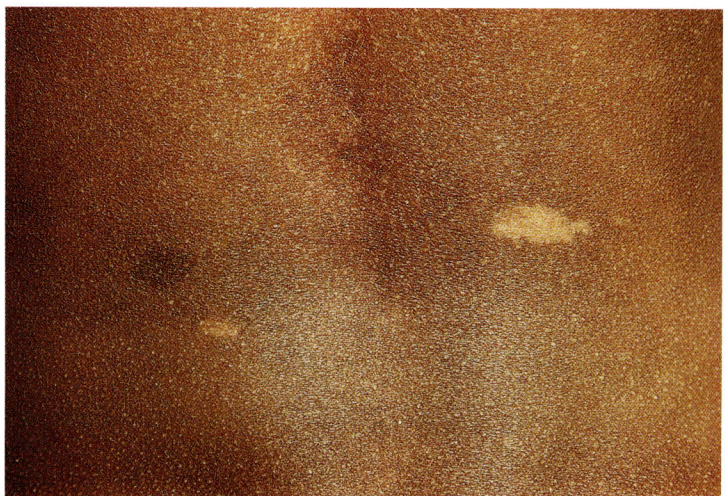

Fig. 58.30 Ash-leaf-shaped hypopigmented macules in tuberous sclerosis.

Hypomelanotic macules of tuberous sclerosis

In this neurocutaneous disorder (see Chapter 15), transmitted as an autosomal dominant trait, hypomelanotic macules are found in about 50–100% of affected babies [1–3]. It is a significant feature as it is often the earliest feature of tuberous sclerosis [1]. These macules are usually multiple, irregularly scattered and frequently have a lance–ovate shape, likened by Thomas Fitzpatrick in 1968 to the leaflet of the mountain ash [1] (Fig. 58.30). The macules are of diagnostic significance in a baby with fits, especially infantile spasms [1]. They are best identified in the fair-skinned with the aid of a Wood's lamp. Electron microscopy of the macules shows the presence of normal or reduced numbers of melanocytes that have poorly developed dendrites containing fewer and smaller melanosomes than normal [2]. The gene responsible for tuberous sclerosis has been localized to 9q34 (*TSC1*) and 16p13.3 (*TSC2*) [4,5].

References

1 Fitzpatrick TB, Szabó G, Hori Y et al. White leaf-shaped macules: earliest visible sign of tuberous sclerosis. *Arch Dermatol* 1968; **98**: 1–6.

2 Jimbow K, Fitzpatrick TB, Szabó G, Hori Y. Congenital circumscribed hypomelanosis. *J Invest Dermatol* 1975; **64**: 50–62.

3 Zulanov A, Esterly NB. Neurocutaneous syndromes associated with pigmentary skin lesions. *J Am Acad Dermatol* 1995; **32**: 915–35.

4 European Chromosome 16 Tuberous Sclerosis Consortium. Identification and characterization of the tuberous sclerosis gene on chromosome 16. *Cell* 1993; **75**: 1305–15.

5 Nellist M, Brook-Carter PT, Connor JM et al. Identification of markers flanking the tuberous sclerosis locus on chromosome 9 (TSC1). *J Med Genet* 1993; **30**: 224–7.

Naevus depigmentosus

> **Synonym**
> • Achromic naevus

Definition. This is a rare, localized area of depigmented skin, first described by Lesser in 1884 [1]. It remains stable in size and colour over time and typically has no associated findings.

Clinical features. This circumscribed area of depigmentation is congenital, but may not be apparent at birth. There are three clinical variants; the commonest is the single, circumscribed, rounded lesion. Segmental and systematized forms are very rare, and may resemble hypomelanosis of Ito. Lesions occur most commonly on the trunk. Hairs within the depigmented macules are usually depigmented. Histology may show either normal or reduced numbers of melanocytes [2]. A functional defect in melanocytes, with morphological abnormalities of melanosomes, has been identified [3].

References
1 Lesser E. In: Ziemssen HV, ed. *Hanbuchder Hautkrankheiten*, 2nd edn. Leipzig: Vogel, 1884: 183.
2 Jimbow K, Fitzpatrick TB, Szabó G, Hori Y. Congenital circumscribed hypomelanosis. *J Invest Dermatol* 1975; **64**: 50–62.
3 Lee HS, Chun YS, Hann SK. Nevus depigmentosus: clinical features and histopathologic characteristics in 67 patients. *J Am Acad Dermatol* 1999; **40**: 21–6.

Hypomelanosis of Ito (MIM *300337) [1–8]

> **Synonym**
> • Incontinentia pigmenti achromians of Ito

In 1952 the Japanese dermatologist Minor Ito described a 21-year-old woman with widespread, symmetrical, depigmented whorls and streaks that had started at the age of 5 years [1]. This neurocutaneous disorder is variable in extent and may be unilateral or bilateral. The areas of hypomelanosis occur along Blaschko's lines, a requirement for the diagnosis of this condition (Fig. 58.31). There

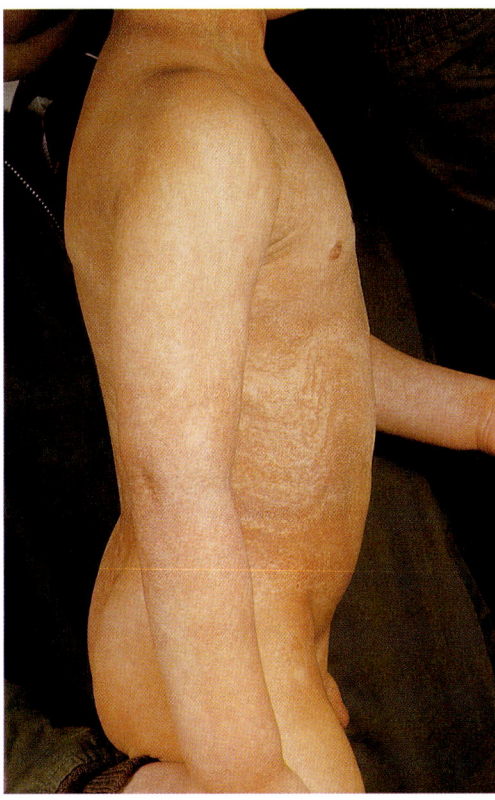

Fig. 58.31 Incontinentia pigmenti achromians of Ito.

may be associated disorders in the musculoskeletal system, teeth, eyes and central nervous system [2]. Convulsions and mental deficiency occur commonly in the reported cases [3]. The appearances resemble the late stages of incontinentia pigmenti, but this is clearly a quite separate disease without the preceding inflammatory stages and without the sex-linked inheritance of incontinentia pigmenti. There is no basal layer damage and no pigmentary incontinence. Nearly all cases are sporadic suggesting a postzygotic mutation. The mutation can only survive in a mosaic and is usually lethal when transmitted to offspring due to the lack of admixture with normal cell lines. However, one case of inheritance of hypomelanosis of Ito has been reported, consistent with X-linked dominant inheritance with lethality to male embryos [4]. The white streaks are usually present at birth and tend to progress thereafter. Eventually, they may repigment. The skin lesions have to be distinguished from the more bizarre-shaped depigmented naevi and from focal dermal hypoplasia where the skin also shows atrophic changes.

References
1 Ito M. Studies on melanin XI: Incontinentia pigmenti achromians. A singular case of nevus depigmentosus systematicus bilateralis. *Tohoku J Exp Med* 1952; **55**: 57–9.
2 Pascual-Castroviejo I, Lopez-Rodriguez L, de la Cruz Medina M *et al*. Hypomelanosis of Ito. Neurologic complications. *Can J Neurol Sci* 1988; **15**: 124–9.
3 Glover MT, Brett EM, Atherton DJ. Hypomelanosis of Ito: spectrum of the disease. *J Pediatr* 1989; **115**: 75–80.
4 Grosshans EM, Stoebner P, Bergoend H, Stoll C. Incontinentia pigmenti achromians (Ito). Etude clinique at histopathologique. *Dermatologica* 1971; **142**: 65–78.
5 Ritter CL, Steele MW, Wenger SL, Cohen BA. Chromosome mosaicism in hypomelanosis of Ito. *Am J Med Genet* 1990; **35**: 14–7.
6 Ruiz-Maldonado R, Toussaint S, Tamayo L *et al*. Hypomelanosis of Ito: diagnostic criteria and report of 41 cases. *Pediatr Dermatol* 1992; **9**: 1–10.
7 Moss C, Larkins S, Stacey M *et al*. Epidermal mosaicism and Blaschko's lines. *J Med Genet* 1993; **30**: 752–5.
8 Koiffmann CP, de Souza DH, Diament A *et al*. Incontinentia pigmenti achromians (hypomelanosis of Ito, MIM 146150): further evidence of localization at Xp11. *Am J Med Genet* 1993; **46**: 529–33.

Vogt–Koyanagi–Harada syndrome

Historical background. In 1906 Vogt reported a patient with atraumatic, idiopathic uveitis, poliosis and alopecia, a syndrome that in time would be associated with his name [1]. In 1926, Harada reported five cases of bilateral posterior uveitis and retinal detachment [2]. In 1929, Koyanagi reported 16 patients with headache, fever, dysacousia, vitiligo, poliosis, alopecia, bilateral anterior uveitis with occasional exudative retinal detachment [3]. Various combinations of synonym have been used for this disorder, which is now generally referred to with the above three names, and abbreviated to VKHS.

Aetiology. The aetiology of VKHS has yet to be established. An abnormal response to a virus, and immunological mechanisms, have been postulated.

Pathology. Electron microscopy of depigmented skin shows an absence of melanocytes as in vitiligo [4]. Colloid–amyloid bodies are also found at the dermal–epidermal junction [5]. Inflammatory skin lesions are characterized by a chronic, mixed inflammatory cell infiltrate [6].

Clinical features [7,8]. VKHS mainly affects dark-skinned people or white people with dark pigmentation. It is rare but widely distributed. Most cases occur in the third and fourth decades but children may be affected. It affects the skin, eyes, inner ears and meninges. Criteria for diagnosis are as follows:

- No history of ocular trauma or surgery preceding the initial onset of uveitis
- No clinical or laboratory evidence suggestive of ocular disease entities
- Bilateral ocular involvement: an early sign is diffuse choroiditis; a late sign is ocular depigmentation
- Neurological and auditory findings: meningismus, tinnitus, cerebrospinal fluid pleocytosis
- Skin and hair changes: alopecia, vitiligo, poliosis.

Typically, this condition is first diagnosed by ophthalmologists as the uveitis starts the march of symptoms and signs.

Diagnosis. The association of vitiligo with loss of pigment in brows and lashes and with the residual ocular defects should clearly differentiate this syndrome from any other.

References

1 Vogt A. Frühseitiges Ergrauen der Zilen und Bemerkungen über den sogenannten plötzlichen Eintritt dieser Veränderung. *Klin Monatsbl Augenheilkd* 1906; **44**: 228–42.
2 Harada Y. Beitrag zur klinischen Kenntnis von viechteitriger Choroiditis (Choroiditis diffusa acuta). *Nippon Gankai Zasshi* 1926; **30**: 356–78.
3 Koyanagi Y. Dysakusis, alopecia and poliosis bei schwerer uveitis nicht traumatischen ursprunges. *Klin Monatsbl Augenheilkd* 1929; **82**: 194–211.
4 Morohashi M, Hashimoto K, Goodman TF. Ultrastructural studies of vitiligo, Vogt–Koyanagi syndrome, and incontinentia pigmenti achromians. *Arch Dermatol* 1977; **113**: 755–66.
5 Okada T, Sakamoto T, Ishibashi T, Inomata H. Vitiligo in Vogt–Koyanagi–Harada disease: immunohistological analysis of inflammatory site. *Graefes Arch Clin Exp Ophthalmol* 1996; **234**: 359–63.
6 Tsuruta D, Hamada T, Teramae H *et al.* Inflammatory vitiligo in Vogt–Koyanagi–Harada disease. *J Am Acad Dermatol* 2001; **44**: 129–31.
7 Nordlund JJ, Albert D, Forget B, Lerner AB. Halo nevi and the Vogt–Koyanagi–Harada syndrome. *Arch Dermatol* 1980; **116**: 690–2.
8 Rabsmen PE, Gass DM. Vogt–Koyanagi–Harada syndrome: clinical course, therapy and long-term visual outcome. *Arch Ophthalmol* 1991; **10**: 682–7.

Alezzandrini's syndrome [1–4]

Historical background. Alezzandrini was involved in three papers describing the syndrome that now bears his name in the late 1950s and early 1960s [1–3].

Aetiology. The aetiology of this syndrome is unknown.

Clinical features. Alezzandrini's syndrome has only been reported in a small number of cases [1–4]. It is characterized by unilateral, facial vitiligo associated with unilateral retinal degeneration, white hair, poliosis and deafness. There are similarities with the Vogt–Koyanagi–Harada syndrome in which skin, eye and auditory changes are also observed.

References

1 Casala AM, Alezzandrini AA. Vitiligo y poliosis unilateral con retinitis pigmentaria y hypoacusia. *Arch Argent Dermatol* 1959; **9**: 449–56.
2 Cremona AC, Alezzandrini AA, Casala AM. Vitiligo, poliosis and unilateral macular degeneration. *Arch Oftalmol B Aires* 1961; **36**: 102–6.
3 Alezzandrini AA. Manifestations unilaterales degenerescence tapetoretinienne, de vitiligo, de poliose, de cheveux blancs et d'hypoacousie. *Ophthalmologica* 1964; **147**: 409–19.
4 Hoffmann MD, Dudley C. Suspected Alezandrini's syndrome in a diabetic patient with unilateral retinal detachment and ipsilateral vitiligo and poliosis. *J Am Acad Dermatol* 1992; **26**: 496–7.

Vitiligo [1–3]

Aetiology. Vitiligo affects all races and has a long history [4]. It is stated that it occurs in 1% of the world's population [2]. An epidemiological survey on the island of Bornholm in Denmark [5] found the prevalence to be 0.38%. It is likely that this figure applies also to other countries in north-west Europe. The incidence of vitiligo in those with racially pigmented skins is higher (and the social impact greater), although reliable figures are not available. There is a preponderance of females in most series based on outpatient attendances, but the frequency in the population is probably the same in both sexes [5]. Between 30 and 40% of patients have a positive family history [2], and a genetic factor is undoubtedly involved. Inheritance may be polygenic or may be determined by an autosomal dominant gene of variable penetrance. Vitiligo has been reported in monozygotic twins [6].

Various theories have been suggested for the aetiology of vitiligo; the same mechanism may not apply to all cases.

- *Autoimmune hypothesis*: this is based on the clinical association of vitiligo with a number of disorders also considered to be autoimmune (Table 58.8). Organ-specific autoantibodies to thyroid, gastric parietal cells and adrenal tissue are found in the serum more frequently in patients with vitiligo than in the general population [11,12]. A complement-fixing antibody to melanocytes has been found in the serum of several patients who in addition to vitiligo had alopecia areata, mucocutaneous candidiasis and multiple endocrine insufficiencies [11]. Antibodies to normal human melanocytes have been detected using a specific immunoprecipitation assay [13,14], and have a cytolytic effect [15]. T-cell profiles are abnormal in vitiligo, with a decrease in T-helper cells [16–18].

Table 58.8 Disorders associated with vitiligo.

Thyroid disease* (hyperthyroidism and hypothyroidism [7])
Pernicious anaemia*
Addison's disease* [8]
Diabetes mellitus* [9]
Hypoparathyroidism*
Myasthenia gravis*
Alopecia areata
Morphoea and lichen sclerosus
Halo naevus*
Malignant melanoma* [10]

* Autoantibodies demonstrable.

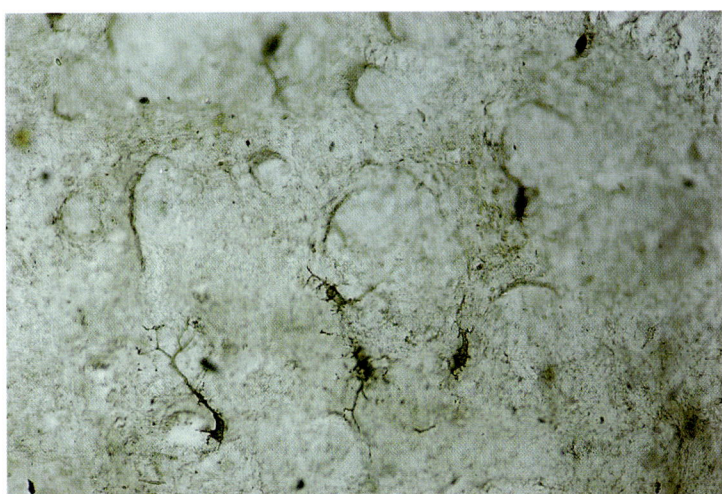

Fig. 58.32 Vitiligo. Epidermal sheet of marginal depigmented area showing marked reduction in number of melanocytes.

- *Neurogenic hypothesis* [19]: this suggests that a compound is released at peripheral nerve endings in the skin that may inhibit melanogenesis and could have a toxic effect on melanocytes. Although vitiligo may sometimes occur in a dermatomal distribution and electron microscopy shows abnormalities of terminal portions of peripheral nerves, there is little support for this hypothesis. However, recent studies on neuropeptide and neuronal markers in vitiligo suggest that neuropeptide Y may have a role [20].
- *Self-destruct theory of Lerner* [2]: this suggests that melanocytes destroy themselves due to a defect in a natural protective mechanism that removes toxic melanin precursors. This hypothesis is based on the clinical features of vitiligo and on experimental studies of cutaneous depigmentation by chemical compounds that have a selective lethal effect on functional melanocytes [21]. These compounds can produce a leukoderma indistinguishable from idiopathic vitiligo.

It has been suggested that defective keratinocyte metabolism plays a major role, with low catalase levels in the epidermis of vitiligo [22]. A new hypothesis involving defective tetrahydrobiopterin and catecholamine biosynthesis has been put forward to explain the pathogenesis of this disorder [23].

Pathology. There is a marked absence of melanocytes and melanin in the epidermis. Histochemical studies [24] show a lack of dopa-positive melanocytes in the basal layer of the epidermis (Fig. 58.32). Recent immunohistochemical studies with a large panel of antibodies show only an occasional melanocyte in lesional skin [25]. Electron microscopy studies [9,26,27] confirm the loss of melanocytes, which appear to be replaced by Langerhans' cells. In the epidermis of areas around the margins of vitiligo are abnormalities of keratinocytes [9] as well as degenerating melanocytes. There is increased cellularity of the dermis and occasional colloid amyloid bodies are found. In inflammatory vitiligo, where there is a raised erythematous border, there is an infiltrate of lymphocytes and histiocytes. This infiltrate is also found in the marginal areas of some biopsies [27].

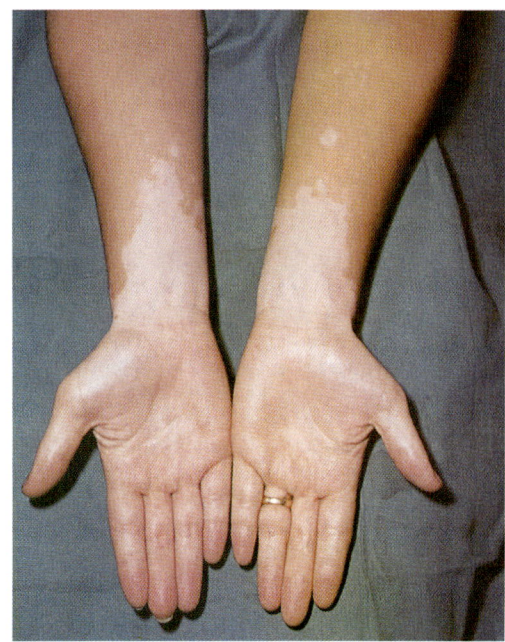

Fig. 58.33 Vitiligo.

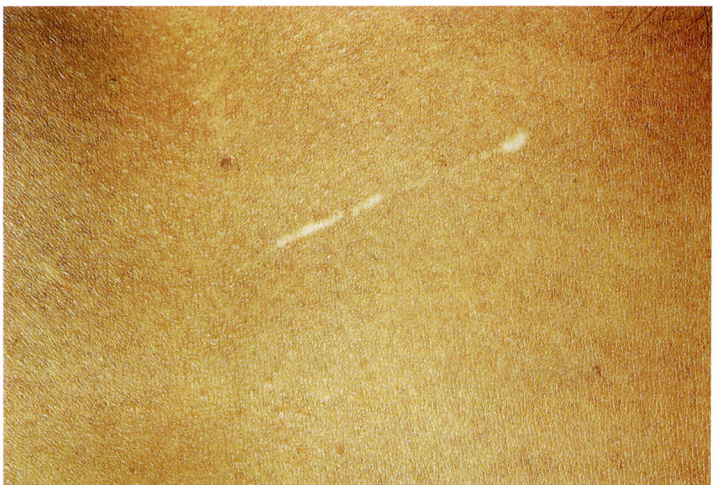

Fig. 58.34 Isomorphic or Koebner phenomenon at site of a scratch in a patient with vitiligo.

Clinical features [2,3]. Vitiligo can begin at any age, but in 50% of cases it develops before the age of 20 years. The condition is gradually progressive, sometimes extending rapidly over a period of several months and then remaining quiescent for many years.

Hypomelanotic macules are usually first noted on the sun-exposed areas of skin, on the face or on the dorsa of hands (Fig. 58.33). These areas are prone to sunburn. Rarely, itching in the absence of sunburn may occur. Damage to the 'normal' skin frequently results in an area of depigmentation—an isomorphic or Koebner phenomenon (Fig. 58.34).

The amelanotic macules in vitiligo are found particularly in areas that are normally hyperpigmented, for example the face, axillae, groins, areolae and genitalia. Areas subjected to repeated friction and trauma are also likely to be affected, for example the

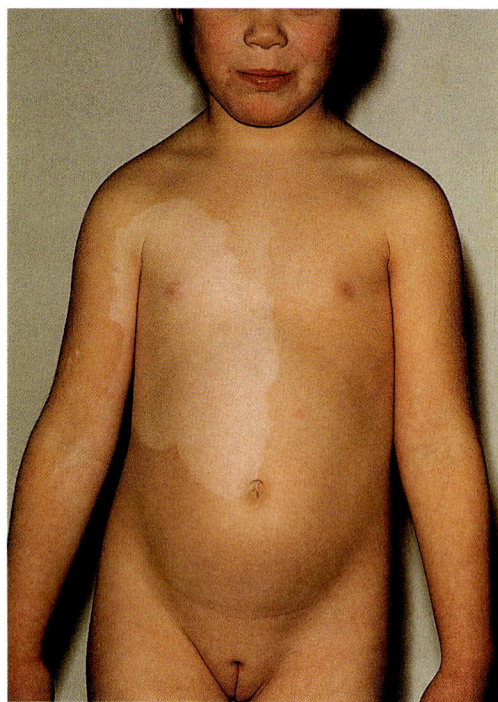

Fig. 58.35 Segmental vitiligo.

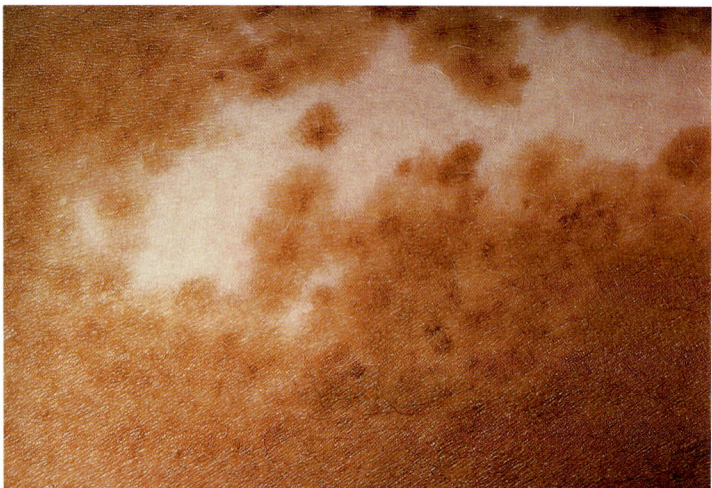

Fig. 58.36 'Trichrome' vitiligo.

dorsa of hands, feet, elbows, knees and ankles. The distribution of the lesions is usually symmetrical, although sometimes it is unilateral and may have a dermatomal arrangement (Fig. 58.35). Rarely, there is complete vitiligo, although a few pigmented areas always remain.

The pigment loss may be partial or complete, or both may occur in the same areas (trichrome vitiligo) (Fig. 58.36).

The macules have a convex outline, increase irregularly in size and fuse with neighbouring lesions to form complex patterns. The hairs in the patches frequently remain normally pigmented, but in older lesions the hairs too are often amelanotic. The margins of the lesions may become hyperpigmented. The main symptom is the cosmetic disability, although some patients present because of sunburn in the amelanotic areas. Vitiligo commonly starts in children, who are more likely to show segmental vitiligo, autoimmune diseases or to have a family history of canities [28].

Spontaneous repigmentation is noted in about 10–20% of patients, most frequently in sun-exposed areas. It is usually seen in younger patients, the repigmentation being quite trivial and mainly perifollicular.

In addition to premature greyness of the hair, uveitis also rarely occurs [29]. Careful examination of the ocular fundus may show abnormalities [30]. There have also been suggestions of an increased incidence of deafness [31].

Associated disorders. A number of conditions occur in association with vitiligo and are listed in Table 58.8. Halo naevi [2,3] occur not infrequently and often antedate the onset of vitiligo. Areas of depigmentation sometimes develop in patients with malignant melanoma [10]. Vitiligo with uveitis, central nervous system involvement and premature greying of the hair occurs in the Vogt–Koyanagi syndrome (see p. 58.45).

Diagnosis. The distribution, age of onset and hyperpigmented border will suggest the diagnosis. In piebaldism, the lesions are present at birth, are usually confined to the head and trunk, and rarely show a hyperpigmented border. Careful examination of the texture of the unpigmented skin should exclude lichen sclerosus and scleroderma. Post-inflammatory leukoderma, which is frequent in the darker races, shows an irregular mottling of hyperpigmented and hypopigmented blotches. Hypomelanosis of the affected skin is commonly seen in pityriasis alba, producing slightly scaly areas with rather ill-defined edges on children's faces. Hypopigmented slightly scaly macules are seen in pityriasis versicolor. These areas often fluoresce a golden yellow when examined under a Wood's lamp. The hypomelanotic macules in leprosy are anaesthetic.

Treatment. The treatment of vitiligo is unsatisfactory and in most cases the patient is best advised to seek effective cosmetic camouflage for the lesions on exposed skin. In sunny climates, the prescription of sunscreens is often necessary.

Treatment with systemic psoralens, 4,5′,8-trimethylpsoralen, 8-methoxypsoralen or 5-methoxypsoralen, combined with exposure to sunlight or to light sources providing high-intensity long-wave UV light, is effective in a proportion of cases [3,32,33]. The patient is instructed to take the psoralens in a dose of 0.6 mg/kg 2 h before carefully controlled, graduated exposure to sunlight, preferably around midday. Therapy is continued for at least 6 months and in some for several years. In the majority of patients, the areas retain the pigment long after psoralen therapy has been discontinued. The use of topical applications of psoralens is hazardous and may result in untoward blistering of the skin. Khellin has also been used with UVA [34].

Narrow-band UVB phototherapy has been found to be effective and safe for vitiligo [35].

In some patients, the more potent topical corticosteroid preparations, 0.1% betamethasone valerate and 0.05% clobetasol propionate, are effective in producing repigmentation of areas of vitiligo, but often at the price of some atrophy [36].

In those patients with extensive vitiligo and only a few residual areas of hyperpigmentation, skin-bleaching creams, such as 20% monobenzylether of hydroquinone, are of use [37].

The use of grafting techniques, minigrafts and autologous cultured melanocytes is interesting but may be limited by the Koebner phenomenon [38–40]. Minigrafting has been carried out with success in some patients with more widespread vitiligo [41]. A systematic review of autologous transplantation methods in vitiligo has recently been performed [42].

References

1 Bologna J, Pawelek JM. Biology of hypopigmentation. *J Am Acad Dermatol* 1988; **19**: 217–55.
2 Lerner AB. On the etiology of vitiligo and gray hair. *Am J Med* 1971; **51**: 141–7.
3 Gawkrodger DJ, Ormerod AD, Shaw L *et al.* Guideline for the diagnosis and management of vitiligo. *Br J Dermatol* 2008; **159**: 1051–76.
4 Koranue RV, Sachdeva KG. Vitiligo. *Int J Dermatol* 1988; **27**: 676–81.
5 Howitz J, Brodthagen H, Schwartz M *et al.* Prevalence of vitiligo. *Arch Dermatol* 1977; **113**: 47–52.
6 Mohr J. Vitiligo in a pair of monovular twins. *Acta Genet* 1951; **2**: 252–5.
7 Cunliffe WJ, Hall R, Newell DJ *et al.* Vitiligo, thyroid disease and autoimmunity. *Br J Dermatol* 1968; **80**: 135–9.
8 Dunlop D. Eighty-six cases of Addison's disease. *BMJ* 1963; **ii**: 887–91.
9 Dawber RPR. Clinical associations of vitiligo. *Postgrad Med J* 1970; **46**: 276–7.
10 Frenk E. Dépigmentations vitiligineuses chez des patients atteints de mélanomes malins. *Dermatologica* 1969; **139**: 84–91.
11 Betterle C, Peserico A, Bersani G. Vitiligo and autoimmune polyendocrine deficiencies with autoantibodies to melanin-producing cells. *Arch Dermatol* 1979; **115**: 364.
12 Woolfson H, Finn OA, Mackie RM *et al.* Serum anti-tumour antibodies and autoantibodies in vitiligo. *Br J Dermatol* 1975; **92**: 395–400.
13 Naughton GK, Eisinger M, Bystryn J-C. Detection of antibodies to melanocytes in vitiligo by specific immunoprecipitation. *J Invest Dermatol* 1983; **81**: 540–2.
14 Naughton GK, Reggiardo D, Bystryn J-C. Correlation between vitiligo antibodies and extent of depigmentation in vitiligo. *J Am Acad Dermatol* 1986; **15**: 978–81.
15 Cui J, Arita Y, Bystryn JC. Cytolytic antibodies to melanocytes in vitiligo. *J Invest Dermatol* 1993; **100**: 812–5.
16 Ghoneum M, Grimes E, Gill G *et al.* Natural cell-mediated cytotoxicity in vitiligo. *J Am Acad Dermatol* 1987; **17**: 600–5.
17 Grimes PE, Ghoneum M, Stockton T *et al.* T-cell profiles in vitiligo. *J Am Acad Dermatol* 1986; **14**: 196–201.
18 Mozzanica N, Frigerio U, Finzi AF *et al.* T cell subpopulations in vitiligo: a chronobiologic study. *J Am Acad Dermatol* 1990; **22**: 223–30.
19 Lerner AB. Vitiligo. *J Invest Dermatol* 1959; **32**: 285–310.
20 Al-Abadie MSK, Senior HJ, Bleehen SS, Gawkrodger DJ. Neuropeptide and neuronal marker studies in vitiligo. *Br J Dermatol* 1994; **131**: 160–5.
21 Bleehen SS, Pathak MA, Hori Y, Fitzpatrick TB. Depigmentation of skin with 4-isopropylcatechol, mercaptoamines, and other compounds. *J Invest Dermatol* 1968; **50**: 103–17.
22 Schallreuter KU, Wood JM, Berger J. Low catalase levels in epidermis of patients with vitiligo. *J Invest Dermatol* 1991; **97**: 1081–5.
23 Schallreuter KU, Wood JM, Ziegler I *et al.* Defective tetrahydrobiopterin and catecholamine biosynthesis in the depigmentation disorder vitiligo. *Biochim Biophys Acta* 1994; **122**: 181–92.
24 Jarrett A, Szabo G. The pathological varieties of vitiligo and their response to treatment with meladinine. *Br J Dermatol* 1956; **68**: 313–26.
25 Le Poole IC, van den Wijngaard RMJGF, Westerhof W *et al.* Presence or absence of melanocytes in vitiligo lesions: an immunohistochemical investigation. *J Invest Dermatol* 1993; **100**: 816–22.
26 Birbeck M. An electron microscope study of basal melanocytes and high level clear cells (Langerhans cells) in vitiligo. *J Invest Dermatol* 1961; **37**: 51–64.
27 Bleehen SS. Histology of vitiligo. In: Klaus SN, ed. *Pigment Cell*, Vol. 5. Basel: Karger, 1979: 54–61.

28 Halder RM, Grimes PE, Cowan CA *et al.* Childhood vitiligo. *J Am Acad Dermatol* 1987; **16**: 948–54.
29 Nordlund JJ, Todes Taylor N, Albert DM *et al.* The presence of vitiligo and poliosis in patients with uveitis. *J Am Acad Dermatol* 1981; **4**: 528–36.
30 Cowan CL, Halder RM, Grimes PE *et al.* Ocular disturbances in vitiligo. *J Am Acad Dermatol* 1986; **15**: 17–24.
31 Tosti A, Bardazzi F, Tosti G *et al.* Audiologic abnormalities in cases of vitiligo. *J Am Acad Dermatol* 1987; **17**: 230–3.
32 Parrish JA, Fitzpatrick TB, Shea C *et al.* Photochemotherapy of vitiligo. *Arch Dermatol* 1976; **112**: 1531–4.
33 Bleehen SS. Treatment of vitiligo with oral 4,5′,8-trimethylpsoralen (tripsoralen). *Br J Dermatol* 1972; **86**: 54–60.
34 Ortel B, Tanew A, Hönigsmann H. Treatment of vitiligo with khellin and ultraviolet A. *J Am Acad Dermatol* 1988; **18**: 693–701.
35 Scherschum L, Kim JJ, Lim HW. Narrow-band ultraviolet B is a useful and well-tolerated treatment for vitiligo. *J Am Acad Dermatol* 2001; **44**: 999–1003.
36 Kandil E. Treatment of vitiligo with 0.1% betamethasone 17-valerate in isopropyl alcohol: a double-blind trial. *Br J Dermatol* 1974; **91**: 457–60.
37 Mosher DB, Parrish JA, Fitzpatrick TB. Monobenzylether of hydroquinone. *Br J Dermatol* 1977; **97**: 669–79.
38 Lerner AB, Halaban R, Klaus SN *et al.* Transplantation of human melanocytes. *J Invest Dermatol* 1987; **89**: 219–24.
39 Falabella R. Treatment of localized vitiligo by autologous minigrafting. *Arch Dermatol* 1988; **124**: 1649–55.
40 Hatchome N, Kato T, Tagami H. Therapeutic success of epidermal grafting in generalized vitiligo is limited by the Koebner phenomenon. *Int J Dermatol* 1988; **27**: 676–81.
41 Boersma BR, Westerhof W, Bos JD. Repigmentation in vitiligo vulgaris by autologous minigrafting: results in nineteen patients. *J Am Acad Dermatol* 1995; **33**: 990–5.
42 Njoo MD, Westerhof W, Bos JD *et al.* A systematic review of autologous transplantation methods in vitiligo. *Arch Dermatol* 1998; **34**: 1543–9.

Halo naevus [1,2]

Synonyms
- Sutton's naevus
- Leukoderma acquisitum centrifugum

Definition and aetiology. Leukoderma acquisitum centrifugum designates the development of a halo of hypomelanosis around a central cutaneous tumour. This tumour is usually a benign melanocytic naevus but may be a neuroid naevus, a blue naevus, a neurofibroma, or a primary or secondary malignant melanoma [1]. The phenomenon, which is not uncommon, is usually seen in children or young adults of either sex.

Halo naevi occur with increased frequency in patients with certain organ-specific autoimmune disorders, as does vitiligo (see above), with which it is often associated. An immunological association of halo naevus with cutaneous malignant melanoma exists. Antibodies against the cytoplasm of malignant melanoma cells are found in the serum of patients with halo naevi [3]. Multiple halo naevi may occur in patients with melanoma.

Pathology [1,4]. Most halo naevi are compound naevi. There is frequently a lymphocytic infiltration of the naevus and the constituent cells may show damage. Ultrastructural studies show the apposition of mononuclear cells with naevus cells that show cytotoxic changes [5]. In the depigmented halo, there is an absence of melanocytes, but Langerhans' cells are present [6]. Melanophages are often present in the dermis.

Clinical features [1,7]. Circular areas of hypomelanosis occur around pigmented naevi, particularly on the trunk, less commonly on the head and rarely on the limbs. Multiple lesions are common, the halos being about 0.5–1.0 cm wide and developing simultaneously or at intervals around several, but not all, naevi (Fig. 58.37). The condition is usually seen in young people. The naevus tends to flatten and may disappear completely. The depigmented areas often persist, but may pigment after many years. Eczema around naevi (Meyerson's naevi) is discussed in Chapter 54.

Treatment. Normally none is required. The usual diagnostic criteria must be applied if there is any possibility that the central tumour is a melanoma. It should be remembered that a halo around a benign naevus is relatively common, whereas malignant melanoma is rare, and a melanoma surrounded by a halo is extremely rare. Mutilating surgery must never be undertaken without preliminary histological examination by an experienced pathologist.

References
1 Kopf AW, Morrill SD, Silberberg I. Broad spectrum of leukoderma acquisitum centrifugum. *Arch Dermatol* 1965; **92**: 14–35.
2 Ortonne J-P. In: Ortonne J-P, Mosher DB, Fitzpatrick TB, eds. *Vitiligo and other Hypomelanoses of Hair and Skin*. New York: Plenum, 1983: 567–82.
3 Copeman PWM, Lewis MG, Phillips TM, Elliott PG. Immunological associations of the halo naevus with cutaneous malignant melanoma. *Br J Dermatol* 1973; **88**: 127–37.
4 Wayte DM, Helwig EB. Halo nevi. *Cancer* 1968; **22**: 69–90.
5 Gauthier Y, Surleve-Bazeille JE, Gauthier O. Ultrastructure of halo nevi. *J Cutan Pathol* 1975; **2**: 71–81.
6 Swanson JL, Wayte DM, Helwig EB. Ultrastructure of halo nevi. *J Invest Dermatol* 1968; **50**: 434–7.
7 Stegmaier OC, Becker SW, Medenica M. Multiple halo nevi. *Arch Dermatol* 1965; **99**: 180–9.

Acquired hypomelanosis

The disorders in which there is frequently an acquired loss of melanin pigment not due to genetic factors are shown in Table 58.9.

Chemical depigmentation

A number of chemicals can produce cutaneous depigmentation when applied to the skin [1,2]. Several substituted phenols produce an occupational leukoderma in workers coming in contact with them (see also Chapter 27). Of these, *p*-tertiary-butylphenol is the most important [2–4]. Occupational leukoderma occurs in workers in contact with the monobenzylether of hydroquinone [5]; this compound is used in the treatment of hypermelanosis and can produce confetti-like areas of depigmentation in the treated areas [6] (Fig. 58.38). The monomethylether of hydroquinone can induce a similar leukoderma [7]. Several phenolic germicidal preparations can produce depigmentation of the skin [4]. 4-Tertiary-butylcatechol is also a cause of occupational leukoderma [8], and this may follow contact sensitization [9]. The areas most likely to be affected in occupational leukoderma are the dorsa of the hands (see Fig. 58.7), but other areas are involved, not necessarily in contact with the chemicals. The depigmented areas frequently enlarge, and new ones appear even after the patient is no longer

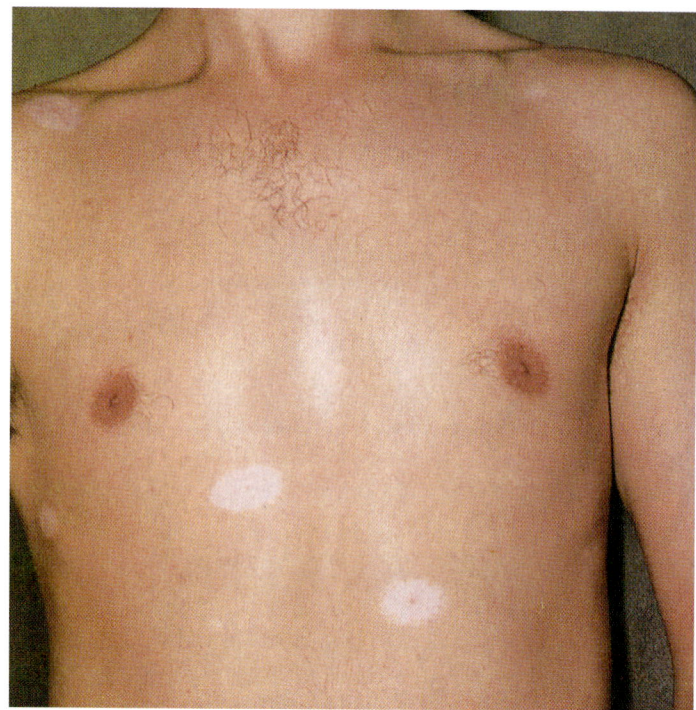

(a)

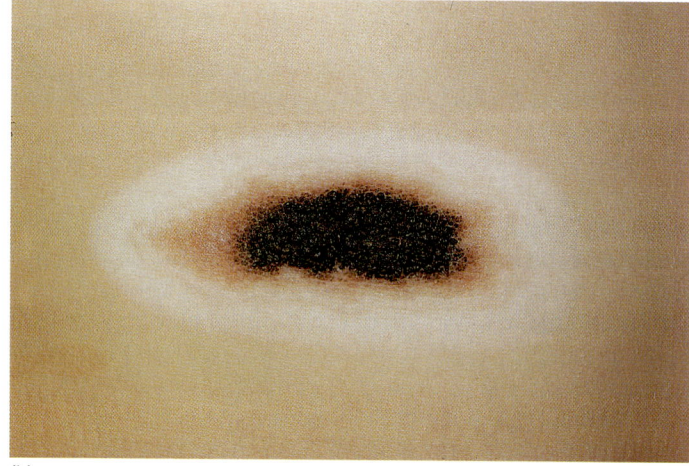

(b)

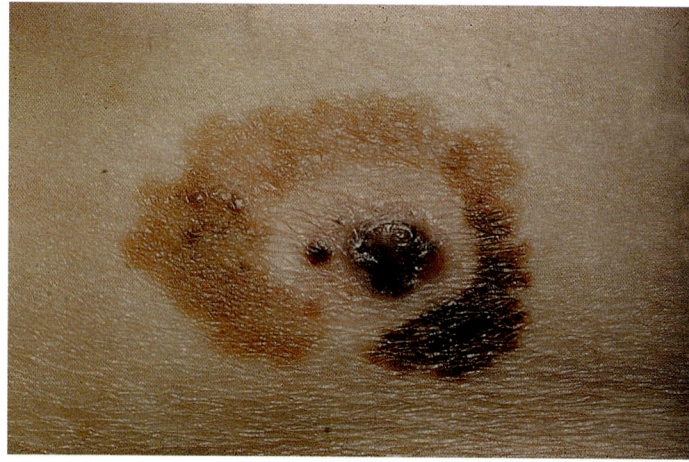

(c)

Fig. 58.37 (a) Multiple halo naevi in a young man who also had vitiligo. (b) Unusually large halo naevus. (c) Halo phenomenon developing within a malignant melanoma that later proved fatal.

Table 58.9 Acquired hypomelanosis.

Endocrine factors
Hypopituitarism*
Addison's disease[†]
Thyroid disease[†]

Chemical factors (occupational and therapeutic)
Monobenzylether of hydroquinone[†]
Monomethylether of hydroquinone
   p-tertiary-butylphenol[†]
   p-tertiary amylphenol[†]
Chloroquine and hydroxychloroquine
Arsenic[‡]

Nutritional factors
Chronic protein deficiency[§]
Pernicious anaemia[§]

Post-inflammatory and infections
Eczema (pityriasis alba)[‡]
Psoriasis[‡]
Pityriasis versicolor[‡]
Pinta[‡], syphilis[‡], yaws[‡]
Leprosy[‡]
Sarcoidosis[‡]
Lupus erythematosus[‡]
Lichen planus[‡]

Neoplasms
Halo naevus[†]
Malignant melanoma[†]

Miscellaneous
Idiopathic guttate hypomelanosis[‡]
Vogt–Koyanagi–Harada syndrome[†]

* Diffuse loss of pigment: lack of melanocyte-stimulating hormone.
[†] Circumscribed areas: vitiligo-like lesions.
[‡] Partial loss of pigment in circumscribed areas.
[§] Loss of pigment in hair.

in contact. The areas may or may not repigment. Treatment with psoralens is usually ineffective. In the hypomelanotic and amelanotic areas, there is often an almost complete absence of melanocytes [3,4]. Experimental studies [1,10] indicate that these substituted phenols have a selective lethal effect on functional melanocytes.

References

1 Bleehen SS, Pathak MA, Hori Y, Fitzpatrick TB. Depigmentation of skin with 4-isopropylcatechol, mercaptoamines and other compounds. *J Invest Dermatol* 1968; **50**: 103–17.
2 Lerner EA, Sober AJ. Chemical and pharmacologic agents that cause hyperpigmentation or hypopigmentation of the skin. *Dermatol Clin* 1988; **6**: 327–37.
3 Bleehen SS. Vitiligo-like leukoderma produced by substituted phenols. In: Seijii M, ed. *Pigment Cell 1981. Phenotypic Expression in Pigment Cells*. Tokyo: University of Tokyo Press, 1981: 461–6.
4 Kahn G. Depigmentation caused by phenolic detergent germicides. *Arch Dermatol* 1970; **102**: 177–87.
5 Oliver EA, Schwartz L, Warren LH. Occupational leukoderma. *Arch Dermatol Syphilol* 1940; **42**: 993–1014.
6 Bleehen SS. Skin bleaching preparations. *J Soc Cosmet Chem* 1977; **28**: 407–12.
7 Boyle J, Kennedy CTC. Leucoderma induced by monomethyl ether of hydroquinone. *Clin Exp Dermatol* 1985; **10**: 154–8.
8 Gellin GA, Maibach H. *Dermatopharmacology and Toxicology: Chemically Induced Depigmentation. Models in Dermatology*, Vol. 2. Basel: Karger, 1985: 282–6.
9 Gawkrodger DJ, Cork MJ, Bleehen SS. Occupational vitiligo and contact sensitisation. *Contact Dermatitis* 1991; **25**: 200–1.
10 Riley PA. Mechanism of pigment-cell toxicity produced by hydroxyanisole. *J Pathol* 1970; **101**: 163–9.

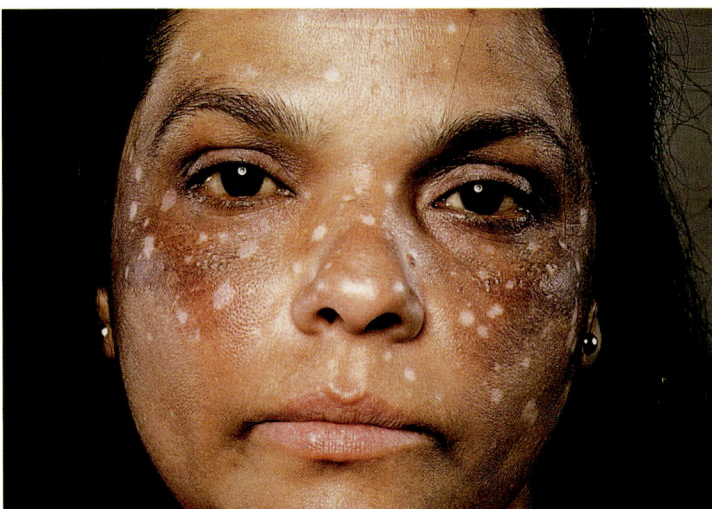

Fig. 58.38 Depigmentation on the face following treatment of melasma with monobenzylether of hydroquinone. (Courtesy of St John's Dermatology Centre, London, UK.)

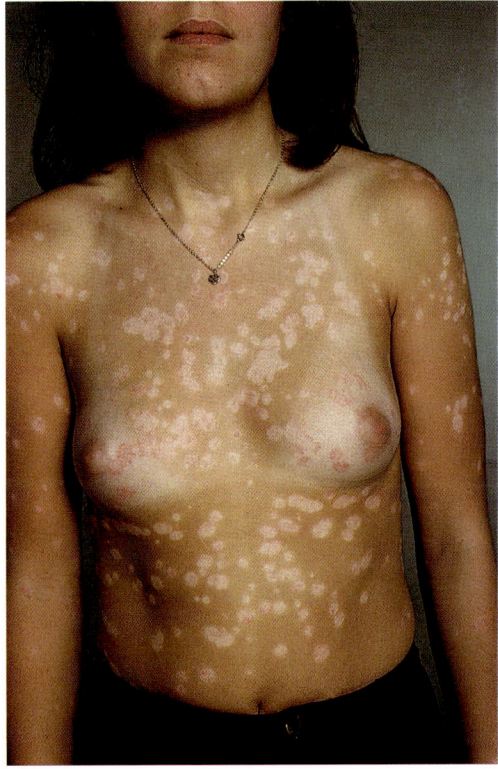

Fig. 58.39 Hypopigmentation in a girl with resolving psoriasis.

Post-inflammatory and infections

Hypomelanotic areas occur following the resolution of areas of eczema and psoriasis (Fig. 58.39). These are also seen in pityriasis lichenoides and cutaneous T-cell lymphoma [1].

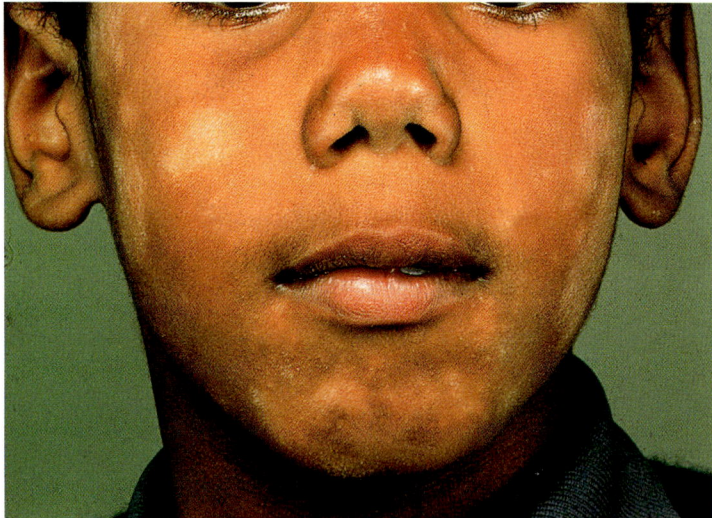

Fig. 58.40 Pityriasis alba. (Courtesy of St John's Institute of Dermatology, London, UK.)

The superficial eczema known as pityriasis alba (see Chapter 23) commonly presents with white, somewhat scaly, and not so well-defined areas of skin, which are most noticeable on the cheeks of racially pigmented children (Fig. 58.40).

Hypopigmented macules occur in the superficial fungal infection pityriasis versicolor, a condition frequently mistaken for vitiligo. Hyperpigmented areas are also present. It is suggested that the fungus forms oxidation products of unsaturated fatty acids of skin surface lipids that inhibit the tyrosinase activity of melanocytes [2]. Other mechanisms are suggested, including the fungus acting as a sun barrier in a thickened stratum corneum. Light and electron microscopy studies of hypopigmented macules [3,4] and of hyperpigmented areas [5] have been unhelpful in determining the mechanisms involved and are confusing. The lack of sunburn in the pale areas may be explained by the fact that the causative yeast produces pityriacitrin, an indole compound that has a broad spectrum of ultraviolet absorption [6].

In a number of inflammatory disorders of the skin, there are areas of hypomelanosis and in these there may be a loss of functional melanocytes. This loss is seen in lupus erythematosus and lichen planus. Hypopigmentation is seen in sarcoidosis [7,8] and leprosy [9]. A leukomelanoderma occurs in syphilis.

References
1 Whitmore SE, Simmons-O'Brein E, Rotter FS. Hypopigmented mycosis fungoides. *Arch Dermatol* 1994; **130**: 476–80.
2 Nazzaro Porro M, Passi S, Balus L. The monoene fatty acids of human surface lipids and their relation to skin melanogenesis. *Br J Dermatol* 1977; **97** (Suppl. 15): 16.
3 Galadari I, El Komy M, Mousa A *et al*. Tinea versicolor: histologic and ultrastructural investigation of pigmentary changes. *Int J Dermatol* 1992; **31**: 253–6.
4 Charles CR, Sire DJ, Johnson BL *et al*. Hypopigmentation in tinea versicolor. *Int J Dermatol* 1973; **12**: 48–58.
5 Allen HB, Charles R, Johnson BL. Hyperpigmented tinea versicolor. *Arch Dermatol* 1976; **112**: 1110–2.
6 Mayser P, Schäfer U, Krämer H-J *et al*. Pityriacitrin: an ultraviolet-absorbing indole alkaloid from the yeast *Malassezia furfur. Arch Dermatol Res* 2002; **294**: 131–4.

7 Clayton R, Breathnach A, Martin B, Feiwel M. Hypopigmented sarcoidosis in the negro. *Br J Dermatol* 1977; **96**: 119–25.
8 Cornelius CE, Stein KM, Hanshaw WJ, Sprott DA. Hypopigmentation and sarcoidosis. *Arch Dermatol* 1973; **108**: 249–51.
9 Job CK, Nayar A, Narayanan JS. Electronmicroscopic study of hypopigmented lesions in leprosy. *Br J Dermatol* 1972; **87**: 200–12.

Idiopathic guttate hypomelanosis [1–3]

This clinical entity, also known as disseminate lenticular leukoderma [4], can be mistaken for vitiligo. It is common. The lesions in white people most frequently occur in sun-exposed areas of the limbs. Solar damage is a factor in these cases. Non-actinic lesions occur in black people and may be on the trunk in unexposed areas [1].

Clinically, the lesions are porcelain-white macules, usually 2–6 mm in size but sometimes much larger. The borders are sharply defined, often angular and irregular. The skin markings are normal. Histologically, there is a decrease in pigment granules. Histochemical and ultrastructural studies [5,6] show a reduction in the number of melanocytes, many of which lack mature melanosomes. It has been suggested that this disorder results from an age-related somatic mutation of melanocytes.

References
1 Cummings KI, Cottel WI. Idiopathic guttate hypomelanosis. *Arch Dermatol* 1966; **93**: 184–6.
2 Falabella R, Escobar C, Giraldo N *et al*. On the pathogenesis of idiopathic guttate hypomelanosis. *J Am Acad Dermatol* 1987; **16**: 35–44.
3 Whitehead WJ, Moyer DG, Vander Ploeg DE. Idiopathic guttate hypomelanosis. *Arch Dermatol* 1966; **94**: 279–81.
4 Argnelles-Casals D, Gonzalez D. La leucoderme lenticulaire disséminée. *Ann Dermatol Syphiligr* 1969; **96**: 283–6.
5 Ortonne J-P, Perrot H. Idiopathic guttate hypomelanosis. *Arch Dermatol* 1980; **116**: 664–8.
6 Wilson PD, Lavker RM, Kligman AM. On the nature of idiopathic guttate hypomelanosis. *Acta Derm Venereol (Stockh)* 1982; **62**: 301–6.

Symmetrical progressive leukopathy [1]

This has been reported from Japan and Brazil, where it is relatively common. Punctate leukoderma develops in young adults, symmetrically on the front of the shins and on the extensor aspects of the arms, and less often on the abdomen and interscapular region. It is persistent.

Reference
1 Costa OG. Leucopathie symétrique progressiva des extrémités. *Ann Dermatol Syphiligr* 1951; **78**: 452–4.

Cutanous lymphoma [1,2]

Cutaneous T-cell lymphoma may sometimes show prominent hypopigmentation. In poikilodermatous mycosis fungoides, clinical lesions are characterized by widespread poikiloderma rather than plaques or nodules. On clinical examination there is alternating increase and decrease in pigmentation associated with epidermal atrophy. In hypopigmented mycosis fungoides, the areas of hypopigmentation are more prominent than in poikilodermatous mycosis fungoides [1,2].

References
1 Smith NP, Samman PD. Mycosis fungoides presenting with areas of cutaneous hypopigmentation. *Clin Exp Dermatol* 1978; **3**: 213–6.

2 Lambroza E, Cohen SR, Phelps R *et al*. Hypopigmented variant of mycosis fungoides: demography, histopathology and treatment of seven cases. *J Am Acad Dermatol* 1995; **32**: 987–93.

Endogenous non-melanin pigmentation [1]

A variety of substances that are normal constituents of the body may, if present in excess or in an abnormal form or site, give rise to alterations in skin colour. Other substances formed only by patients with certain metabolic defects may also produce pigmentary changes. Special stains of histological specimens, or techniques such as spectroscopy, may help to identify the nature of exogenous and other non-melanin pigments.

Haemosiderosis

The deposition in the tissue of the iron-containing pigment haemosiderin is commonly the result of the local destruction of red blood cells, but also occurs in haemochromatosis. The presence of haemosiderin stimulates melanogenesis, and hypermelanosis may dominate the clinical and histological picture. Such is the case in haemochromatosis (see Chapters 59 & 62). Much more frequently, haemosiderin in the skin is derived locally from red blood cells (Chapter 49); in such conditions, the pigmentation is orange–red at first, later fading through ochre and tawny shades.

Hypostatic haemosiderosis

Haemosiderosis of the lower legs is extremely common in the presence of venous insufficiency. Recently involved areas show grouped points of reddish pigment, but recurrent extravasation of red cells combined with increasing hypermelanosis soon produce a more or less uniform deep brown or coppery colour. The pigmentation usually persists even if the venous insufficiency is relieved.

Sickle-cell anaemia and congenital haemolytic anaemia

Haemosiderosis and melanosis may give rise to conspicuous pigmentation of the lower leg in the third decade or earlier.

Schamberg's disease and related disorders [2]

(see Chapter 49)

Haemosiderosis without clinically evident hypermelanosis is seen in Schamberg's disease and other types of capillaritis. Reddish-brown plaques with cayenne-pepper points beyond their margins are present on the legs and thighs and sometimes on the arms.

Small patches of haemosiderosis, most numerous on the lower legs but progressively involving thighs and buttocks, are characteristic of drug reactions to ureides. Haemosiderosis of the trunk is a feature of some reactions to clothing.

Jaundice

Jaundice results from the staining of the skin with bilirubin, which has a great affinity for elastic tissue, hence the early involvement of the sclerae. The range of yellow shades produced by bilirubin may be modified by the presence of biliverdin, which adds a greenish hue. Bronzing is the effect of added melanin pigmentation and is often seen in jaundice of long duration. The sclerae are not involved in carotenaemia and only rarely in mepacrine pigmentation (p. 58.55).

References
1 Jeghers H. Pigmentation of the skin. *N Engl J Med* 1944; **231**: 88–100.
2 Satoh T, Yokozeki H, Nishioka K. Chronic pigmented purpura associated with odontogenic infection. *J Am Acad Dermatol* 2002; **46**: 942–4.

Bronze baby syndrome [1–3]

This striking grey-brown discoloration of the skin of neonates follows phototherapy for hyperbilirubinaemia and is often associated with evidence of liver dysfunction. The serum is also brownish. The nature and origin of the pigment are uncertain. The changes are reversible unless there is some underlying liver disease.

References
1 Ashley JR, Littler CM, Burgdorf WHC. Bronze baby syndrome: report of a case. *J Am Acad Dermatol* 1985; **12**: 325–8.
2 Kopelman AE, Brown R, Odell G. The bronze baby syndrome: a complication of phototherapy. *J Pediatr* 1972; **81**: 466–72.
3 Purcell SM, Wians FH, Ackerman AB *et al*. Hyperbilirubinemia in bronze baby syndrome. *J Am Acad Dermatol* 1987; **16**: 172–7.

Riboflavinaemia [1]

Yellow skin and hair have been described in a patient with myeloma, due to riboflavin being avidly bound by a monoclonal antiflavin antibody.

Reference
1 Farhangi M, Osserman EF. Myeloma with xanthoderma due to an IgG monoclonal anti-flavin antibody. *N Engl J Med* 1976; **294**: 177–83.

Carotenaemia [1]

Carotene, a lipochrome, contributes a yellow component to the colour of normal skin. In the presence of excessive blood carotene levels, this yellow component is increased, and is most conspicuously accentuated where the horny layer is thick on the palms and soles. The sclerae are not discoloured. The most striking coloration is seen in food faddists who overindulge in oranges or carrots. Some increased yellowness is seen in conditions with hyperlipaemia, diabetes, nephritis and hypothyroidism, and where conversion of carotene to vitamin A is impaired by an inborn metabolic error [2] or by hepatic disease. However, it is now more commonly seen in young women drastically reducing their weight and eating foodstuffs with high carotene content [3,4].

Carotenaemia is seen in patients on oral supplements of β-carotene as a photoprotective agent in erythropoietic protoporphyria [5,6] and in those taking carotenoids that contain canthaxanthin.

References
1 Cohen H, Lord. Observations on carotenemia. *Ann Intern Med* 1958; **48**: 219–27.
2 Monk BE. Metabolic carotenemia. *Br J Dermatol* 1982; **106**: 485–7.
3 Bilimoria S, Keczkes K, Williamson D. Hypercarotenaemia in weight watchers. *Clin Exp Dermatol* 1979; **4**: 331–5.
4 Pops MA, Schwabe AD. Hypercarotenemia in anorexia nervosa. *JAMA* 1968; **205**: 533–4.
5 Mathews-Roth MM, Pathak MA, Fitzpatrick TB *et al*. Beta-carotene as a photoprotective agent in erythropoietic protoporphyria. *N Engl J Med* 1970; **282**: 1231–4.

6 Anstey AV. Systemic photoprotection with alpha-tocopherol (vitamin E) and beta-carotene. *Clin Exp Dermatol* 2002; **27**: 170–6.

Ochronosis (see Chapter 59)

In alkaptonuria, a deficiency in homogentisic acid oxidase causes accumulation of homogentisic acid throughout the body. Ochronosis is the term used to describe the pigmentary changes that occur in connective tissue in patients with alkaptonuria [1]. The term was coined by Virchow in 1866 for the ochre-like (pale yellow) colour of the connective tissue when viewed down a microscope. Ochronosis is present in about 75% of patients with alkaptonuria, and the majority show some pigmentation. Most frequent is darkening of the ear cartilages and of the sclerae and conjunctiva. Less often the axillary skin is pigmented and there is brown mottled pigmentation of the face, sometimes in a butterfly distribution, and of the neck and trunk. Rarely, pigmentation of the palmar and plantar skin is seen [2]. Examination of the urine establishes the diagnosis.

References

1 Lubics A, Schneider I, Sebok B, Havass Z. Extensive bluish gray skin pigmentation and severe arthropathy. Endogenous ochronosis (alkaptonuria). *Arch Dermatol* 2000; **136**: 548–52.
2 Vijaikumar M, Thappa DM, Srikanth S *et al*. Alkaptonuric ochronosis presenting as palmoplantar pigmentation. *Clin Exp Dermatol* 2000; **25**: 305–7.

Exogenous pigments

A wide variety of chemicals, either from industrial or medicinal exposure, can produce discoloration of the skin. Some of these may not only produce an alteration of pigmentation by being deposited in the dermis but may also result in an increase in the amount of melanin in the skin. Of importance are the metals silver, gold, mercury and bismuth, which are cumulatively deposited in the dermis and can produce permanent disfiguring pigmentation. A number of drugs can cause discoloration of the skin. These include the antimalarials, the phenothiazines, clofazimine and minocycline. Of less importance is the transient staining of the skin produced by picric acid, dinitrophenol and chemical dyes.

Metals

Argyria [1–8]

Silver may be deposited in the skin either from industrial exposure or as a result of medication with silver salts [2–4]. Blue macules have appeared at sites of acupuncture needles [6]. Cases have followed the use of silver salts for the irrigation of nasal, oral and urethral mucous membranes and the excessive use of an oral smoking remedy containing silver acetate [2,7]. 'Food supplements' may also contain colloidal silver [8]. The pigmentation is usually a slate-grey colour and may be clinically apparent after a few months, but usually takes many years to develop and depends on the degree of exposure. The hyperpigmentation is most apparent in sun-exposed areas of skin, especially the forehead, nose and hands (Fig. 58.41). In some patients, the entire skin has a slate blue-grey colour. The sclerae, nails and mucous membranes may become hyperpigmented. Light and electron microscopy studies

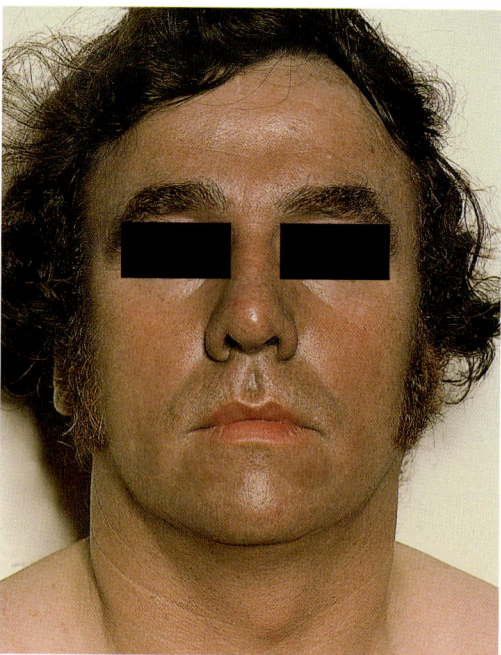

Fig. 58.41 Occupational argyria.

[1,5,6,8,9] show silver granules in the dermis that are most numerous in relation to the basal lamina of the eccrine sweat glands, and in the dermal elastic fibres. Furthermore, silver particles may be seen lying free within the cell cytoplasm of epithelial cells of the secretory segment of eccrine sweat glands and in mast cells [8,9]. Silver granules are readily visible with dark-field illumination. X-ray-dispersive microanalysis confirms that the granules contain silver [1,6]. Silver is widely deposited in the tissues as well as in the skin. The diagnosis of argyria is established by skin biopsy. The pigmentation is permanent; treatment with depigmentary preparations is not effective.

References

1 Bleehen SS, Gould DJ, Harrington CI *et al*. Occupational argyria: light and electron microscopic studies and X-ray microanalysis. *Br J Dermatol* 1981; **104**: 19–26.
2 Buckley WR, Terhaar CJ. The skin as an excretory organ in argyria. *Trans St John's Hosp Dermatol Soc Lond* 1973; **59**: 39–44.
3 Marshall JP II, Schneider RP. Systemic argyria secondary to topical silver nitrate. *Arch Dermatol* 1977; **113**: 1077–9.
4 East BW, Boddy K, Williams ED *et al*. Silver retention, total body silver and tissue silver concentrations in argyria associated with exposure to an anti-smoking remedy containing silver acetate. *Clin Exp Dermatol* 1980; **5**: 305–11.
5 Pariser RJ. Generalized argyria. *Arch Dermatol* 1978; **114**: 373–7.
6 Tanita Y, Kato T, Hanada K *et al*. Blue macules of localized argyria caused by implanted acupuncture needles. *Arch Dermatol* 1985; **121**: 1550–2.
7 Farina MC, Escalonilla P, Griilli R *et al*. Generalized argyria secondary to topical administration of silver nitrate. *Actas Dermo-Sifiliograficas* 1998; **89**: 547–52.
8 White JML, Powell AM, Brady K *et al*. Severe generalised argyria secondary to ingestion of colloidal silver protein. *Clin Exp Dermatol* 2002; **28**: 254–6.
9 Massi D, Santucci M. Human generalized argyria. A submicroscopic and X-ray spectroscopic study. *Ultrastruct Pathol* 1998; **22**: 47–53.

Chrysiasis [1–5]

Chrysiasis and chrysoderma are terms used to describe permanent pigmentation of the skin due to parenteral administration of gold salts. Excessive administration of gold leads to its deposition in connective tissue. Chrysiasis has not been observed in any patient who has received less than 50 mg/kg of gold thiosulphate, and it has not failed to develop in any patient receiving more than 150 mg/kg. It may first develop after a few months or after a long latent period. The pigmentation is blue-grey or may show a purplish hue, and is limited to light-exposed skin and to the sclerae [3]. The oral mucous membrane is not affected. The diagnosis is confirmed histologically on microscopy with dark-field illumination and on electron microscopy with electron probe microanalysis [4]. The granules of gold are larger and more irregular than those of silver. The pigmentation is permanent [5].

References
1 Altmeyer R, Hufnagl D. Chrysiasis: Nebenwirkung einer intra-muskulären Gold-therapie. *Hautarzt* 1975; **26**: 330–3.
2 Jeffery DA, Biggs DF, Percy JS, Russell AS. Quantitation of gold in skin in chrysiasis. *J Rheumatol* 1975; **2**: 28–35.
3 Leonard PA, Moatamed F, Ward JR *et al*. Chrysiasis: the role of sun exposure in dermal hyperpigmentation secondary to gold therapy. *J Rheumatol* 1986; **13**: 58–64.
4 Smith RW, Leppard B, Barnett NL *et al*. Chrysiasis revisited: a clinical and pathological study. *Br J Dermatol* 1995; **133**: 671–8.
5 Miller ML, Harford RR, Yeager JK, Johnson F. A case of chrysiasis. *Cutis* 1997; **59**: 256–8.

Mercury [1–4]

Repeated applications of mercury-containing compounds can produce localized hyperpigmentation of the treated areas [1–3]. Systemic administration of mercury results in gingival hyperpigmentation. The pigment is observed in the upper dermis around capillaries and associated with collagen and elastic fibres. Electron microscopy shows an increase in melanin pigmentation and the metal is present as granules in dermal macrophages [1,3]. A case report of homicidal subcutaneous injection of metallic mercury resulted in widespread skin lesions, remote from the radiologically visible mercury; these appeared at 40 days and began to clear at 6 months [4].

References
1 Burge KM, Winkelmann RK. Mercury pigmentation. *Arch Dermatol* 1970; **102**: 51–61.
2 Jeghers H. Pigmentation of the skin. *N Engl J Med* 1944; **231**: 181–9.
3 Kennedy C, Molland EA, Henderson WJ, Whiteley AM. Mercury pigmentation from industrial exposure. *Br J Dermatol* 1977; **96**: 367–74.
4 Souza EM, Cintra ML, Vieira RJ *et al*. Subcutaneous injection of elemental mercury with distant skin lesions. *J Toxicol* 2000; **38**: 441–3.

Bismuthia

The administration of bismuth at regular intervals over a period of years has often been practised, yet generalized pigmentation is extremely rare. The diffuse grey pigmentation resembles that of argyria and involves also the sclera and the oral and sometimes the vaginal mucous membrane [1].

A distinctive blue-black line occurs at the gingival margin. This is due to deposition of bismuth that reacts with hydrogen sulphide formed by bacteria in the mouth [2].

References
1 Dummett CO. Oral mucosal discolorations related to pharmacotherapeutics. *J Oral Ther* 1964; **1**: 106–10.

2 Lueth HC, Sutton DC, McMullen CJ *et al*. Generalized discoloration of skin resembling argyria following prolonged oral use of bismuth. *Arch Intern Med* 1936; **57**: 1115–24.

Drugs

Mepacrine [1,2]

Pigmentation of the skin is first noticed a few days after the administration of mepacrine commences and may persist for several weeks after it ceases. The dye is deposited in the skin. A bright-yellow or greenish-yellow colour develops first and remains most prominent on the face, hands and feet, but occurs diffusely with accentuation in the skin flexures. The sclerae are sometimes affected, which may mimic jaundice [2]. The melanin-containing pigment induced by antimalarials is discussed in Chapter 75.

References
1 Schachter AJ, Taylor HM. Atabrine pigmentation. *Am J Med Sci* 1936; **192**: 645–50.
2 Leigh IM, Kennedy CT, Ramsey JD, Henderson WJ. Mepacrine pigmentation in systemic lupus erythematosus. New data from an ultrastructural, biochemical and analytical electron microscopic investigation. *Br J Dermatol* 1979; **101**: 147–53.

Clofazimine (Lamprene) [1–4]

This synthetic riminohenazine dye used in the treatment of leprosy produces an initial redness of the skin due to an accumulation of the drug. Later, with prolonged treatment, a violaceous brown colour develops that is most noticeable in lesional areas [1]. Histochemical studies indicate a ceroid-lipofuscin pigment as well as clofazimine inside macrophage phagolysosomes [2,3]. Reddish-blue pigmentation has been reported within scarred areas of lupus erythematosus in one patient [4].

References
1 Pettit JHS. B 663 (Lampren) in mycobacterial infections. *Br J Dermatol* 1969; **81**: 794–5.
2 Sakurai I, Skinsnes OK. Histochemistry of B 663 pigmentation: ceroid-like pigmentation in macrophages. *Int J Lepr* 1977; **45**: 343–54.
3 Job CK, Yoder L, Jacobson RR, Hastings RC. Skin pigmentation from clofazimine therapy in leprosy patients: a reappraisal. *J Am Acad Dermatol* 1990; **23**: 236–41.
4 Kossard S, Doherty E, Mccoll I, Ryman W. Autofluorescence of clofazimine in discoid lupus erythematosus. *J Am Acad Dermatol* 1987; **17**: 867–71.

Hydroxyurea [1]

Nail pigmentation has been reported in association with use of hydroxyurea and most commonly consists of longitudinal melanonychia. Occasionally all 20 nails are affected and there is associated hyperpigmentation of the skin.

Reference
1 Aste N, Fumo G, Contu F *et al*. Nail pigmentation caused by hydroxyurea: report of nine cases. *J Am Acad Dermatol* 2002; **47**: 146–7.

Minocycline [1–8]

Long-term therapy with minocycline may result in pigmentation, but this is generally agreed to be rare. Three types of cutaneous pigmentation are seen in patients treated with minocycline [6] (Fig. 58.42):

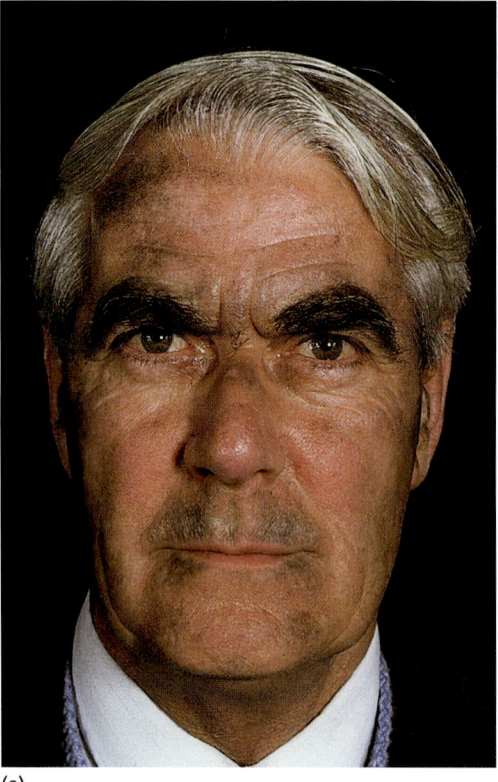
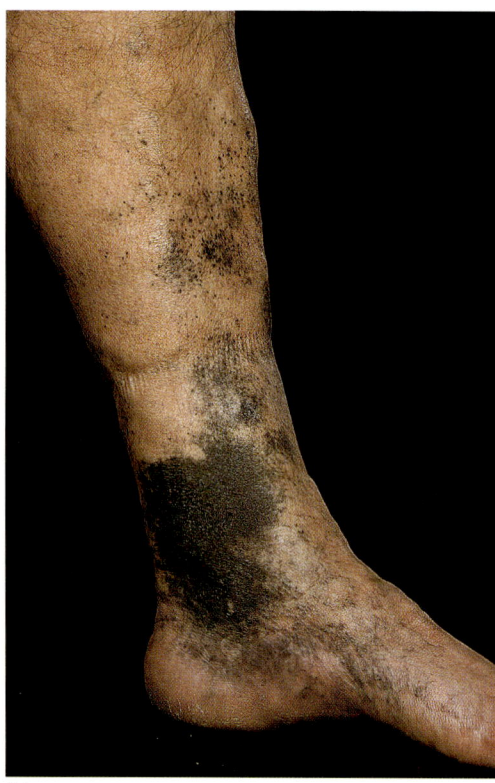

(a)   (b)

Fig. 58.42 (a) Hyperpigmentation of the skin in sun-exposed areas of the face due to long-term therapy with minocycline. (b) Blue-black pigmentation on the lower legs in the same patient.

1 A focal type with well-demarcated blue-black pigmentation at sites of previous inflammation as first described in acne scars [1]

2 A more diffuse and generalized pigmentation that is most apparent in sun-exposed areas of skin and nails [2], but may also involve the sclera [5]

3 A more persistent brown-grey change most prominent on sun-exposed sites.

The pigmentation usually occurs following prolonged courses and high doses of this drug. Histological studies show the presence of brown-black granules in the upper dermis that stain for iron [1,3]. Electron microscopy reveals electron-dense material in dermal macrophages and X-ray microanalysis confirms the presence of iron [4]. Partial resolution of the pigmentation occurs after the drug is stopped [6]. Similar blue-black pigmentation of the legs has resulted from treatment with the 4-quinolone antibiotic pefloxacin [7] and the tetracycline antibiotic methacycline [8].

References

1 Basler RSW. Minocycline-related hyperpigmentation. *Arch Dermatol* 1985; **121**: 606–8.

2 Simons JJ, Morales A. Minocycline and generalized cutaneous pigmentation. *J Am Acad Dermatol* 1980; **3**: 244–7.

3 Gordon G, Sparano BM, Iatropoulos MJ. Hyperpigmentation of the skin associated with minocycline therapy. *Arch Dermatol* 1985; **121**: 618–23.

4 Argenyi ZB, Finelli L, Bergfeld WF *et al*. Minocycline-related cutaneous hyperpigmentation as demonstrated by light microscopy, electron microscopy and X-ray energy spectroscopy. *J Cutan Pathol* 1987; **14**: 176–80.

5 Angeloni VL, Salasche SJ, Ortiz R. Nail, skin, and scleral pigmentation induced by minocin. *Cutis* 1987; **40**: 229–33.

6 Layton AM, Cunliffe WJ. Minocycline induced pigmentation in the treatment of acne: a review and personal observations. *J Dermatol Treat* 1989; **1**: 9–12.

7 Le Cleach L, Chosidow O, Peytavin G *et al*. Blue–black pigmentation of the legs associated with pefloxacin therapy. *Arch Dermatol* 1995; **131**: 856–7.

8 Moller H, Rausing A. Methacycline pigmentation: a five-year follow-up. *Acta Derm Venereol (Stockh)* 1980; **60**: 495–501.

Amiodarone [1–5]

Amiodarone is a drug used for prolonged periods in the treatment of ventricular tachycardia. It induces photosensitivity in more than 50% of patients; however, fewer than 5% develop cutaneous hyperpigmentation [1–5]. A grey-blue pigmentation of the face and other sun-exposed areas is a rare late effect of this drug, and may also involve non-exposed sites (Fig. 58.43) [1]. Yellow-brown granules are present in dermal histiocytes. Ultrastructural studies show membrane-bound dense lysosomal bodies in macrophages that probably contain degradation products of the drug bound to lipofuscin [1,2]. Dose reduction or withdrawal of amiodarone can lead to complete disappearance of the pigmentation [5].

References

1 Delage C, Legacé R, Huard J. Pseudocyanotic pigmentation of the skin induced by amiodarone. *Can Med Assoc J* 1975; **112**: 1205–8.

2 Zachary CB, Slater DN, Holt DW *et al*. The pathogenesis of amiodarone-induced pigmentation and photosensitivity. *Br J Dermatol* 1984; **110**: 451–6.

3 Ferguson J, Addo HA, Jones S *et al*. A study of cutaneous photosensitivity induced by amiodarone. *Br J Dermatol* 1985; **113**: 537–49.

4 Sivaram CA, Beckman KJ. Images in clinical medicine. Amiodarone-induced skin discoloration. *N Engl J Med* 1997; **337**: 1813.

5 Scholz S, Rompel R. Amiodarone-induced pigmentation. *Z Hautkr* 1997; **72**: 901–4.

Picric acid, dinitrophenol and other chemicals

Picric acid, self-administered by malingerers to simulate jaundice, stains the skin yellow. Dinitrophenol, formerly used in industry

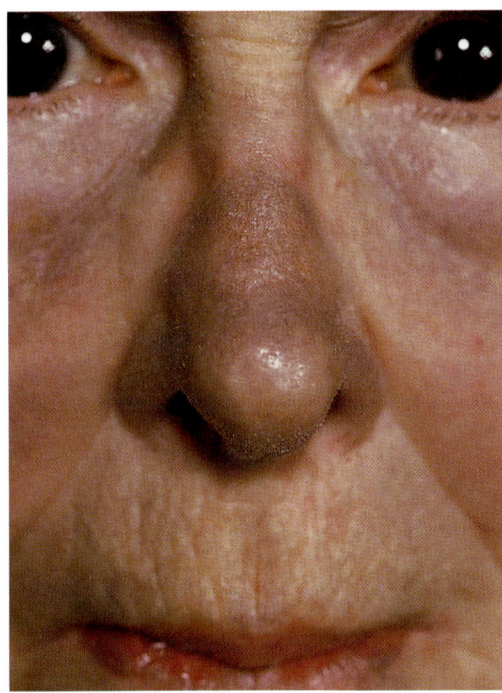

Fig. 58.43 Bluish pigmentation on the nose caused by amiodarone therapy.

and as a metabolic stimulant, also produces yellow staining of the skin and of the sclerae. Trinitrotoluene, santonin and acriflavine also stain the skin yellow.

Tattoos

Accidental tattoos
Pigmented particles may be accidentally introduced as contaminants of wounds or may, at high velocity, penetrate previously intact skin.

Superficial abrasions contaminated with chemically inert particles may be followed by disfiguring tattoos. Such irregularly spattered pigmentation is quite commonly seen after road accidents and blast injuries. Some particles may eventually be extruded, but the disfigurement is often permanent. Small lesions may be excised and larger areas treated by dermabrasion, the results of which depend on the depth to which the particles have penetrated.

Collier's stripes [1]
These are a very distinctive occupational mark in coalminers. The bluish grey, linear or angular stripes develop at the sites of abrasions. The commonest sites are the forehead, bridge of the nose, wrists and elbows. Histologically, particles of coal dust up to 100 µm in diameter are seen at all levels in the dermis. They tend to be grouped around blood vessels.

Therapeutic agents
Iron salts. The use of solutions of ferric sulphate and ferric chloride in the treatment of dermatitis has been followed by a reddish-brown tattoo [2,3]. The pigmentation may disappear after a few months or may persist indefinitely [4].

Occupational contact with iron salts [5] produced red-brown punctate perifollicular pigmentation of the forearms in a man employed in pickling metal in hydrochloric acid.

Gentian violet (pararosaniline chloride). This has, exceptionally, given rise to a tattoo when applied to a wound of the face [6].

References
1 Bettley FR. Colliers' stripes: the coal miners' dermatosis. *Br J Dermatol Syphilol* 1940; **52**: 129–30.
2 Reyner CE. Pigmentation following the use of iron salts. *Arch Dermatol Syphilol* 1939; **40**: 380–1.
3 Traub EF, Tennen JS. Permanent pigmentation following application of iron salts. *JAMA* 1936; **106**: 1711–2.
4 Sutton RL. Pigmentation of the skin due to iron (copperas) applied locally. *JAMA* 1937; **108**: 112–3.
5 Hare PJ. A case of occupational iron pigmentation of the skin. *Br J Dermatol* 1951; **63**: 63–6.
6 Sutton RL. Gentian violet as a therapeutic agent. *JAMA* 1938; **110**: 1733–8.

Decorative tattoos (see also Chapter 28) [1–5]

History and prevalence. From ancient origins the practice of tattooing has developed along more or less parallel lines in most countries. Tattoos have been used to accentuate beauty, as a permanent adornment or to make a statement. Occasionally, tattoos serve to accentuate aggression or ugliness in order to make the wearer more intimidating. Tattoos with words or a name as a symbol of dedication or devotion have always been popular. Tattoos have also been used for more sinister motives. Tattoos were used as a means of identification by the Nazis in the Second World War for members of concentration and labour camps as well as for members of the SS. Formerly associated with religious ceremonies, fertility and marriage rites, tattooing in contemporary westernized civilizations thus fulfils a number of diverse functions and in so doing it survives and flourishes.

Contemporary life finds tattooing more popular than ever [1], even among the elite [2]. Tattoos are no longer the exclusive preserve of street gangs, prisoners and members of the armed forces [1,2]. Not all who submit to tattooing are emotionally unstable, immature individuals. Indeed, tattooing is viewed by many as an acceptable fashion accessory like any other, and is increasingly popular in Western societies with the young and with women, as well as the more traditional male stereotypes [1,2]. Tattooing and body piercing are now so common that health-care workers are advised to maintain a non-judgemental attitude to tattoos [1], even in the face of the unexpected [4]. The decision to have a tattoo may be taken when an individual is in no position to make such a life-long commitment, for example when intoxicated, under peer pressure or when mentally unwell [5]. Tattoos may also be a manifestation of deliberate self-harm [6].

Another contemporary trend is the use of temporary black henna 'tattoos' [3,7]. These are not true tattoos but represent application of a black dye to produce a tattoo-like appearance that lasts for a few days. Unfortunately, a high concentration of the well-known contact sensitizer paraphenylenediamine is usually present in these 'tattoos', which results in a risk of contact allergy [3,7].

Techniques and materials. The professional tattooist uses an electric needle to introduce particles of pigment into the dermis; the amateur, often a child, pricks particles of soot or Indian ink into skin with any pointed object. The individual's choice of design may be motivated by subconscious psychological factors. The pigments commonly employed include:

- Blue-black (carbon)
- Red (cinnabar and vegetable dyes)
- Light blue (cobaltous aluminate)
- Green (chromic oxide or chromium sesquioxide)
- Yellow (cadmium sulphide)
- Brown (ochre, iron oxides).

Complications of tattoos

Unhappiness with the tattoo

Many regret having a tattoo, which may cause a significant psychological, social and financial burden [8].

Introduction of infection

Significant infection of tattoos is now unusual, and pyogenic infection, although the most frequent, is seldom serious. Erysipelas and gangrene, necessitating amputation, are mentioned in the older literature. Syphilis and tuberculosis have been inoculated by the tattoo needle, and small outbreaks have been traced to an infected operator. The tattooing of many people in rapid succession has been suspected of transmitting infective hepatitis. Also there is the risk of transmitting retrovirus infection. The transmission of leprosy is suspected [9]. Both vaccinia and warts have developed in recently inflicted tattoos.

Allergic reactions to pigment

Once the initial inflammatory changes have subsided, by far the most frequent reaction observed in tattoos is the development of allergic sensitivity to one of the pigments.

In most cases, the tattoo pigment itself, or a derived compound formed locally in the tissues, provokes the development of hypersensitivity, which is manifest clinically by the sudden onset of irritation, swelling and redness in a part of the tattoo a few weeks or many years after its infliction. In recent years, lichenoid tattoo reactions have been reported; these appear to be confined entirely to the red areas (Fig. 58.44) [10]. These resemble the reactions to cinnabar (mercuric sulphide); although this pigment has now been replaced by vegetable dyes, cases do still occur [11].

The allergic reaction can remain localized but may become generalized as a patchy eczematous eruption or an exfoliative dermatitis. In some cases, the primary sensitization is induced by some other contact with the metal, and the reaction in the tattoo accompanies or follows an attack of contact dermatitis.

Mercury [12]. The red areas of the tattoo are affected. The reaction may eventually subside spontaneously, but the risk of a generalized eruption is high. The tattoo reaction may be accompanied by erosions of the oral mucosa in contact with amalgam dental fillings [13]. Patch tests are positive to mercuric chloride and ammoniated mercury but not necessarily to cinnabar.

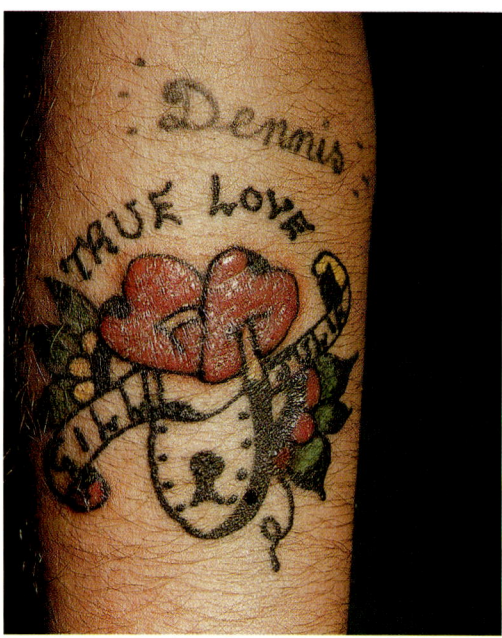

Fig. 58.44 Lichenoid reaction in red areas of a tattoo.

Chrome [14]. The green areas are affected. The patient is often primarily sensitized by exposure to cement. Patch tests with 0.5% potassium dichromate are positive.

Cobalt [15]. The light-blue areas are affected. In three patients, the tattoo reaction was accompanied by the simultaneous development of uveitis [16]. Patch tests are positive with 2% cobalt chloride.

Manganese [17]. A reaction in the purple areas of a tattoo was due to manganese.

Carbon [18]. A case is reported of a reaction in the black areas of a tattoo, presumably to carbon particles.

Light-induced reactions [19]. A high proportion of yellow tattoos develop redness and swelling only on exposure to sunlight, and the same phenomenon is occasionally observed in red tattoos. The mechanism is uncertain, although the yellow pigment, cadmium sulphide, has photoconducting properties.

Localization of skin disease in tattoos

Some skin disorders show a predilection for tattooed skin, in which they may appear first or be accentuated. Syphilis in the secondary or tertiary stage has often been observed in tattoos but tends to spare the red areas, apparently deterred by the mercury. Lichen planus and psoriasis may be localized in tattoos but show no colour predilection. Lupus erythematosus is more rarely seen. A sarcoidal granuloma in a tattoo may be the presenting manifestation of generalized sarcoidosis [20]. Melanoma has been reported in a tattoo [21], although the association may be fortuitous. Foreign-body granulomas of sarcoid type are extremely unusual after decorative tattoos, but have been reported in ochre tattoos [22]; ochre has a high silica content.

References

1 Millner VS, Eichold BH. Body piercing and tattooing perspectives. *Clin Nurs Res* 2001; **10**: 424–41.

2 Mayers LB, Judelson DA, Moriarty BW, Rundell KW. Prevalence of body art (body piercing and tattooing) in university undergraduates and incidence of medical complications. *Mayo Clin Proc* 2002; **77**: 29–34.

3 Onder M, Atahan CA, Oztas P, Oztas MO. Temporary henna tattoo reactions in children. *Int J Dermatol* 2001; **40**: 577–9.

4 Bowling JC, Groves R. An unexpected tattoo. *Lancet* 2002; **359**: 649.

5 Gittleson NL, Wallen GOP, Dowson-Butterworth K. The tattooed psychiatric patient. *Br J Psychiatry* 1969; **115**: 1249–53.

6 Joe EK, Li VW, Magro CM *et al*. Diagnostic clues to dermatitis artefacta. *Cutis* 1999; **63**: 209–14.

7 Brancaccio RR, Brown LH, Chang YT *et al*. Identification and quantification of para-phenylenediamine in a temporary henna tattoo. *Am J Contact Dermatitis* 2002; **13**: 15–8.

8 Varma S, Lanigan SW. Reasons for requesting laser removal of unwanted tattoos. *Br J Dermatol* 1999; **140**: 483–5.

9 Sehgal VN. Inoculation leprosy appearing after several years of tattooing. *Dermatologica* 1971; **142**: 58–61.

10 Taaffe A, Knight A, Marks R. Lichenoid tattoo hypersensitivity. *BMJ* 1978; **i**: 616–8.

11 Sowden JM, Byme JPH, Smith AH *et al*. Red tattoo reactions: X-ray microanalysis and patch test studies. *Br J Dermatol* 1991; **124**: 576–80.

12 Biro L, Klein WP. Unusual complication of mercurial (cinnabar) tattoo. *Arch Dermatol* 1967; **96**: 165–7.

13 Juhlin L, Oleman S. Allergic reactions to mercury in red tattoos and in mucosa adjacent to amalgam fillings. *Acta Derm Venereol (Stockh)* 1968; **48**: 103–5.

14 Björnberg A. Allergic reactions to chrome in green tattoo markings. *Acta Derm Venereol (Stockh)* 1959; **39**: 23–9.

15 Björnberg A. Allergic reactions to cobalt in light blue tattoo markings. *Acta Derm Venereol (Stockh)* 1961; **41**: 259–63.

16 Rorsman H, Dahlquist I, Jacobsson S *et al*. Tattoo granuloma and uveitis. *Lancet* 1969; **ii**: 27–8.

17 Scwartz RA, Mathias CA, Muller CH *et al*. Granulomatous reaction to purple tattoo pigment. *Contact Dermatitis* 1987; **16**: 198–202.

18 Tope WD, Arbiser JL, Duncan LM. Black tattoo reaction: the peacock's tale. *J Am Acad Dermatol* 1996; **35**: 477–9.

19 Björnberg A. Reactions to light in yellow tattoos from cadmium sulfide. *Arch Dermatol* 1963; **88**: 267–71.

20 Dickinson JA. Sarcoidal reactions in tattoos. *Arch Dermatol* 1969; **100**: 315–9.

21 Kirsch N. Malignant melanoma developing in a tattoo. *Arch Dermatol* 1969; **99**: 596–8.

22 Hoffman-Martinot R, Gratadour P. Divers modes de comportement des tatouages. A propos d'un cas clinique particulier du type granulome silicotique. *Presse Med* 1963; **71**: 2095–7.

Treatment of tattoos [1–9]. The removal of a tattoo may become essential on account of the development of one of the complications considered above, most commonly an allergic reaction within the tattoo. Some cases will settle with intralesional or even topical steroids, but more often excision of the offending area of tattoo, followed if necessary by grafting, is the only satisfactory treatment to secure elimination of all particles of pigment.

Far more frequently, removal of a tattoo is sought on aesthetic or cosmetic grounds, often only a few weeks after its infliction. If the area involved is small and simple or serial excision without grafting is practicable, this is undoubtedly the treatment of choice. If grafting is essential, the inevitable cosmetic imperfections of grafts are such that alternative procedures may be considered. Salabrasion using table salt is of use [6]. Some good results have been achieved with lasers, but scarring, at times quite troublesome, is likely to remain. The best results are with Q-switched red or near-infrared laser systems [7]. Infrared coagulation has also been used [8]. The keratotome [9] gives moderately good results and at least partially obliterates the design. For very extensive tattoos, dermabrasion or chemosurgery [4] have been advocated. The choice of technique should be influenced by personal predilections, and the experience of the plastic surgeon consulted. The patient should be warned that there is usually some residual pigment following superficial abrasion and there may be scarring.

References

1 Apfelberg DB, Maser MR, Lash H. Argon laser treatment of decorative tattoos. *Br J Plast Surg* 1979; **32**: 141–4.

2 Buncke HJ, Conway H. Surgery of decorative and traumatic tattoos. *Plast Reconstr Surg* 1957; **20**: 67–77.

3 Clabaugh W. Removal of tattoos by superficial dermabrasion. *Arch Dermatol* 1968; **98**: 515–21.

4 Lerner C. Removal of tattoo marks. *NY State J Med* 1948; **48**: 1937–9.

5 Scutt RWB. The chemical removal of tattoos. *Br J Plast Surg* 1972; **25**: 189–94.

6 Crittenden FM Jr. Salabrasion: removal of tattoos by superficial abrasion with table salt. *Cutis* 1971; **7**: 295–300.

7 Alster TS. Q-switched alexandrite laser treatment (755 nm) of professional and amateur tattoos. *J Am Acad Dermatol* 1995; **33**: 69–73.

8 Venning VA, Colver GB, Millard PR *et al*. Tattoo removal using infrared coagulation: a dose comparison. *Br J Dermatol* 1987; **117**: 99–105.

9 Grice KA. The removal of tattoos with a keratotome. *Br J Dermatol* 1964; **76**: 318–21.

CHAPTER 59

Metabolic and Nutritional Disorders

R.P.E. Sarkany[1], S.M. Breathnach[1], A.A.M. Morris[2], K. Weismann[3] & P.D. Flynn[4]

[1]St John's Institute of Dermatology, St Thomas' Hospital, London, UK
[2]Willink Biochemical Genetics Unit, Royal Manchester Children's Hospital, Manchester, UK
[3]The Skin Clinic, Privatehospital Hamlet, Søborg, Denmark
[4]Addenbrooke's Hospital, Cambridge, UK

The cutaneous porphyrias

R.P.E. Sarkany, pp. 59.1–59.21

Introduction

The porphyrias are a group of disorders caused by defects in the biosynthesis of haem. Their relevance to the skin arises from the phototoxic properties of the porphyrins, which accumulate in most porphyrias and cause photosensitivity.

Rook's Textbook of Dermatology, 8th edition. Edited by DA Burns, SM Breathnach, NH Cox and CEM Griffiths. © 2010 Blackwell Publishing Ltd.

The majority of the porphyrias are inherited. Many of them affect other organs as well as the skin. The recognition and management of both the genetic and internal consequences of porphyrias presenting in the skin are a key challenge for the dermatologist.

Clinical management in these disorders is made easier when the clinician understands their theoretical basis. Thus, this section is divided into two halves. The first provides a theoretical basis for understanding the porphyrias, the general principles of clinical management and a clinician's guide to laboratory testing. The second half covers individual porphyries in detail.

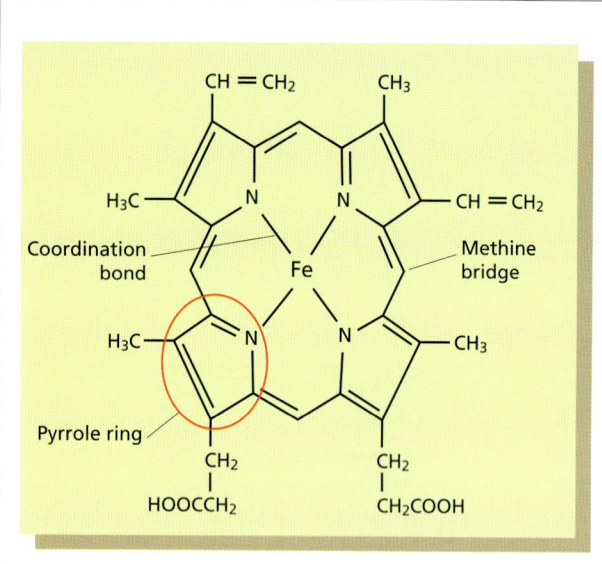

Fig. 59.1 The haem molecule and its key structural features. The alternation of single and double bonds around the tetrapyrrole ring indicates the aromaticity of the molecule, central to its chemical characteristics. The four coordination bonds between iron and nitrogen atoms are shown. The two remaining bonds between the iron and either molecular oxygen or amino acid residues lie perpendicular to the page.

General considerations: theoretical basis, clinical features and laboratory testing in porphyria

A theoretical basis for understanding the porphyrias

The phototoxicity of porphyrins

The phototoxic properties of porphyrins are responsible for the cutaneous features of the porphyrias. Porphyrins are intermediates in the biosynthesis of haem, and consideration of the chemical features of the haem and porphyrin molecules is necessary to understand the cause of porphyrin phototoxicity.

The chemistry of porphyrins and haem [1]. A pyrrole is a ring composed of four carbon atoms and one nitrogen atom. Four pyrroles linked into a ring create a tetrapyrrole, a remarkable and biologically critical molecular structure found in chlorophyll, haem and vitamin B_{12}. A porphyrin is a special type of tetrapyrrole in which four pyrrole rings are linked by methine bridges into a large ring structure.

Haem is the molecule created by the insertion of ferrous iron into the centre of the porphyrin molecule, protoporphyrin IX (Fig. 59.1). Essentially, incorporation of iron into the porphyrin molecule enables it to become biologically useful. Iron's capacity to bind to molecular oxygen, and to transfer electrons (by moving between the 2+ and 3+ oxidation states) makes it potentially useful in biological systems, but free iron precipitates in the presence of water. For iron to be useful, it has to be kept soluble by protecting its binding sites against water. In addition, subtle modification of the electronic structure of the iron atom can optimize its ability to

transfer electrons and reversibly bind molecular oxygen. Binding of iron to the porphyrin molecule solubilizes iron and also optimizes its electronic structure. The porphyrin's central cavity is the right size to fit an iron atom, and its four central nitrogen atoms occupy four of the iron's coordination binding sites, leaving only two free. A key feature of the porphyrin structure is that each double bond is adjacent to a single bond, so it is 'aromatic' with 18 of its electrons being delocalized and free to move around the molecule (Fig. 59.1). This electron current results in the central nitrogen atoms tending to donate electrons to the iron atom, as well as other subtler electronic interactions involving transient changes in the porphyrin's electronic state [2]. Haem can bind to a variety of proteins, and the nature of this interaction reflects the protein's function. In proteins with electron transport functions, such as respiratory cytochromes, amino acids bind to both remaining coordination binding sites on the iron so that haem can transfer electrons through alterations in the iron's oxidation state. In proteins with oxygen-binding functions, such as haemoglobin, an amino acid binds to one of the iron's remaining coordination binding sites, leaving the sixth site free to bind to oxygen. In summary, the aromatic porphyrin structure is well suited to complexing with iron to form haem, rendering the iron useful for electron transfer (respiratory cytochromes), reversible oxygen binding (haemoglobin and myoglobin), and oxidation and reduction reactions (cytochrome P450, catalase), with fine tuning of the iron's functionality being determined by the apoprotein which binds to the haem.

Photochemistry of the porphyrins [3,4]. The complex electronic structure of the large aromatic porphyrin molecule results in its 18 delocalized electrons having unusual excitation characteristics. These electrons are excited by relatively long wavelength light. The main absorption peak is at 408 nm ('Soret band') [3], and this long wavelength of exciting light predisposes to phototoxic behaviour by the porphyrin; these photons have insufficient energy to chemically alter the porphyrin structure, so that alternative fates for the energy, particularly fluorescence and phosphorescence, become more likely [4]. Thus, following excitation by light around the 408 nm peak, electrons either return to the non-excited ground state by releasing the energy as the characteristic red fluorescence, or the porphyrin's excited singlet state transforms (by intersystem crossing) to the longer-lived excited triplet state. Transfer of energy from this excited triplet state to neighbouring molecules leads to the phototoxicity responsible for the clinical features of the cutaneous porphyrias. Thus cutaneous disease in the porphyrias can be thought of as a by-product of the unusual porphyrin structure which enables haem-proteins to fulfil their biological functions.

References

1 Wilkins PC, Wilkins RG. *Inorganic Chemistry in Biology*. Oxford: Oxford University Press, 1997.
2 Constable EC. *Coordination Chemistry of Macrocyclic Compounds*. Oxford: Oxford University Press, 1999.
3 Drabkin DL. Selected landmarks in the history of porphyrins and their biologically functional derivatives. In: Dolphin D, ed. *The Porphyrins*. New York: Academic Press, 1979: 31–71.
4 Wayne CE, Wayne RP, eds. Photophysics. In: *Photochemistry*. Oxford: Oxford University Press, 1996: 39–58.

Enzyme deficiencies and the porphyrias

The porphyrias all result from a partial deficiency of one of the enzymes required for the biosynthesis of haem, thus causing accumulation of the enzyme's substrate. The toxicity profile of the accumulated molecule determines the clinical features of the resulting porphyria. A basic understanding of the biosynthetic pathway enables the clinician to interpret laboratory results and to predict the clinical features of each porphyria on the basis of each porphyrin's properties.

The biosynthesis of haem [1,2] (Fig. 59.2). Haem is synthesized from simple biochemicals (glycine and succinyl CoA) via an eight-step pathway, each step being catalysed by an enzyme. Synthesis of the pyrrole ring (porphobilinogen (PBG)) is followed by assembly of the tetrapyrrole structure (hydroxymethylbilane). One of the pyrrole rings (the 'D' ring) is 'flipped' around to create the III isomer (the alternative I isomer forms in the absence of the cosynthase enzyme). Next, the carboxylic acid side-chains of uroporphyrinogen III are progressively decarboxylated via coproporphyrinogen III to protoporphyrinogen, which is then oxidized to protoporphyrin IX. It is likely that the progressive decarboxylation to remove six of the eight electron-withdrawing carboxylate groups increases the flux of electrons onto the molecule's central nitrogens to facilitate coordination with iron. Finally, ferrous iron is chelated into the protoporphyrin's central cavity to form haem. Around 80% of haem is synthesized in erythroid cell precursors in the bone marrow (for haemoglobin production). The decarboxylation of uroporphyrinogen to coproporphyrinogen, and thence to protoporphyrinogen, decreases water solubility, so that uroporphyrinogen is only excreted via the kidneys whereas hydrophobic protoporphyrinogen and protoporphyrin are exclusively excreted into the bile. Coproporphyrinogen is excreted by both routes. Physiological concentrations of porphyrins stay low because of the high efficiency of haem synthesis.

References
1 Elder GH. The cutaneous porphyrias. In: Hawk JLM, ed. *Photodermatology*. London: Arnold, 1999: 171–99.
2 del C, Battle AM. Tetrapyrrole biosynthesis. *Semin Dermatol* 1986; **5**: 70–87.

Clinical features of the porphyrias: general considerations

Porphyrias present with either skin disease or acute attacks or both.

The classification of the porphyrias [1,2]

In any porphyria, a partial enzyme deficiency causes the accumulation of porphyrins. The enzyme deficiency associated with each disorder is shown in Fig. 59.3. The porphyrias have previously been classified, according to the predominant site of porphyrin accumulation, into the erythropoietic group (congenital erythropoietic porphyria and erythropoietic protoporphyria) and the hepatic group (all the others). This division is not of value clinically. For the clinician, the key division is between porphyrias that cause acute attacks and those that cause skin disease. In this chapter the following classification is used for the six common porphyrias:

1 Cutaneous disease only:
   Porphyria cutanea tarda (PCT)
   Congenital erythropoietic porphyria (CEP)
   Erythropoietic protoporphyria (EPP).
2 Cutaneous disease and acute attacks:
   Hereditary coproporphyria (HC)
   Variegate porphyria (VP).
3 Acute attacks only:
   Acute intermittent porphyria (AIP)

References
1 Elder GH. The cutaneous porphyrias. In: Hawk JLM, ed. *Photodermatology*. London: Arnold, 1999: 171–99.
2 Dean G. Historical background. In: Dean G, ed. *The Porphyrias. A Story of Inheritance and Environment*, 2nd edn. London: Pitman Medical, 1971: 14–9.

Porphyria and the skin

The cutaneous porphyrias share many features. Consideration of these underlying similarities is necessary for a logical approach to clinical management of patients.

All the cutaneous porphyrias, except EPP, present with fragility and blistering of light-exposed skin; the term 'bullous porphyrias' is often used for this group of diseases. Not only can they appear very similar clinically, but the mechanism underlying the skin disease in all cutaneous porphyrias is a local porphyrin phototoxicity reaction. This shared pathogenetic mechanism means that the histopathological appearances in each of these conditions are also similar. As a result, these disorders can only be reliably differentiated by biochemical analysis. The other important similarity between them is that they are all caused by Soret wavelength light (408 nm), so the same strategy for photoprotection applies to them all, as detailed below.

The pathogenesis of skin disease in porphyria (Fig. 59.4) [1–3]. Photons of violet light, with a wavelength peak at 408 nm, transform the porphyrin molecule into an excited singlet state. This may revert to the unexcited ground state by emission of the characteristic red porphyrin fluorescence, but intersystem crossing can convert it to the excited triplet state, long-lived enough to interact with other molecules, particularly molecular oxygen, converting it to excited singlet oxygen in the process. The singlet oxygen stimulates production of hydroxyl radicals which damage tissue directly, and also indirectly by stimulating complement activation [4], mast cell degranulation [5] and matrix metalloproteinase activity [6]. The site of this phototoxic reaction in the skin determines the clinical characteristics of the porphyria. In EPP, lipophilic protoporphyrin tends to localize to membranes including endothelial cell membranes, and to remain within erythrocytes, and the phototoxic reaction involves upper dermal blood vessels causing pain. In PCT, the water-soluble uroporphyrin diffuses easily into surrounding tissues and the phototoxic reaction occurs in the upper dermis, causing lysis of cells in the superficial dermis with the formation of membrane-limited vacuoles which merge to produce a blister under the basal lamina, producing the characteristic clinical presentation [7]. In VP, copro- and protoporphyrin accumulate (Fig. 59.3), but patients suffer from PCT-like upper dermal blisters rather than EPP-like acute pain. This is likely to be

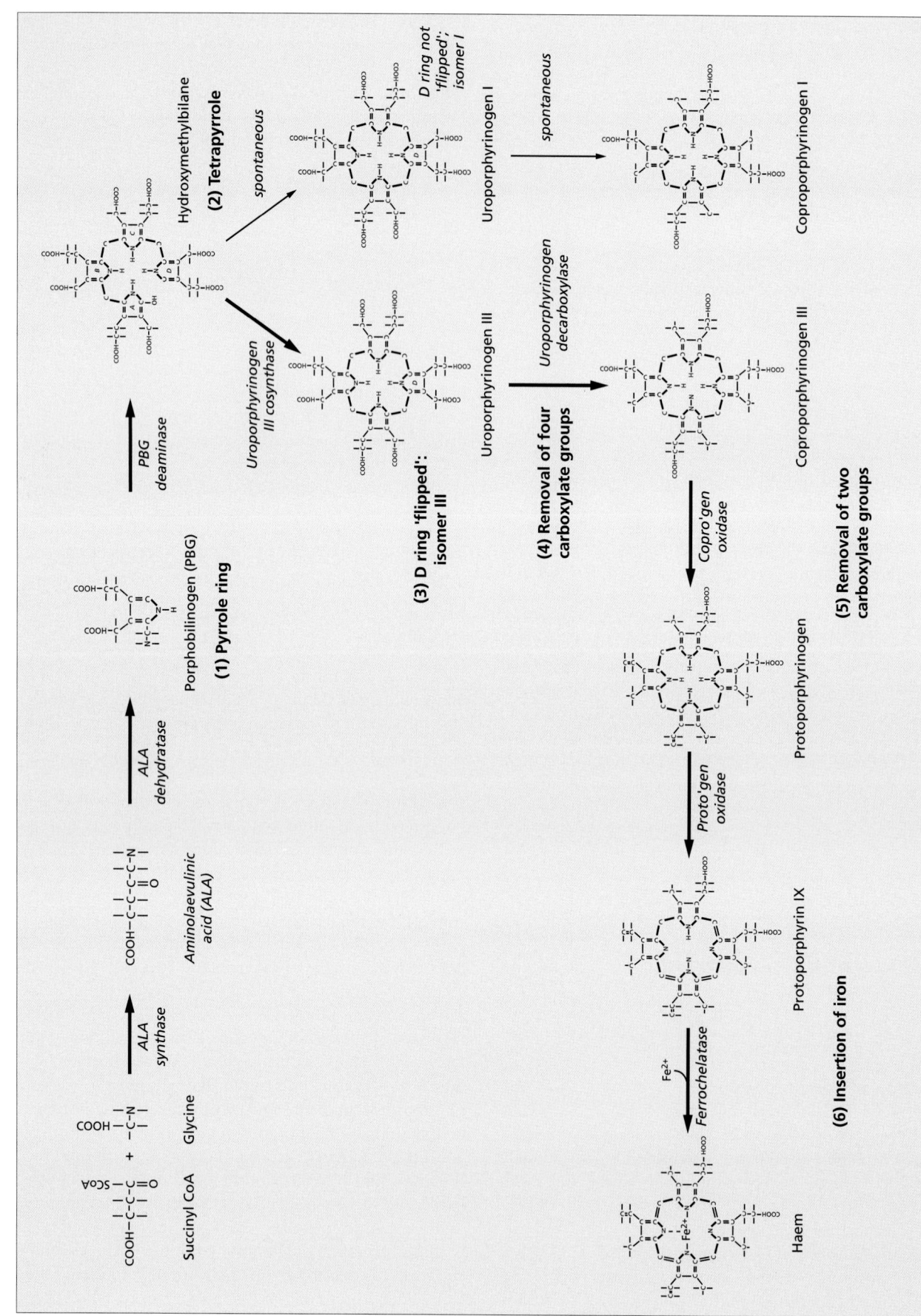

Fig. 59.2 The pathway of haem biosynthesis showing the six key structural changes.

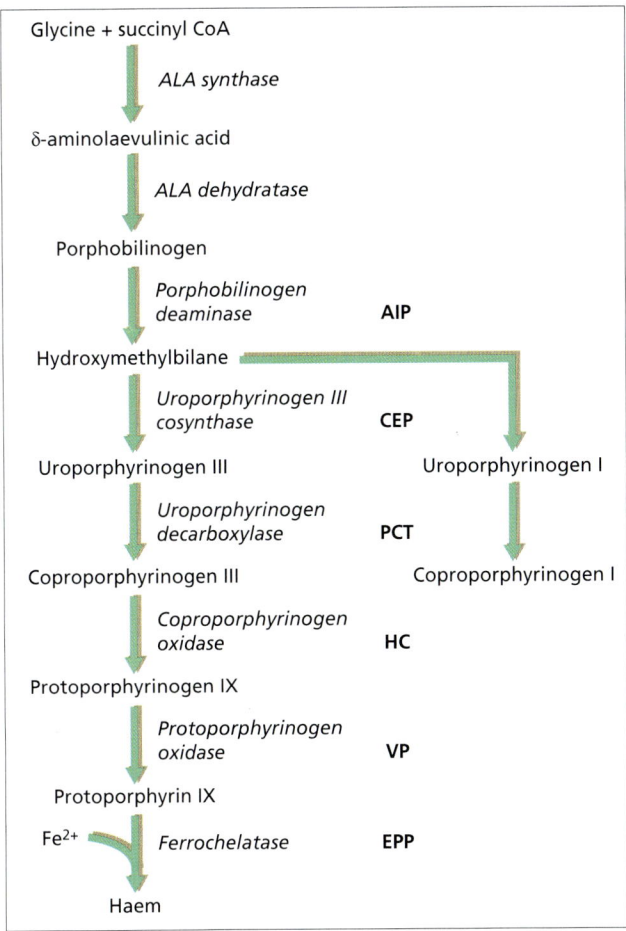

Fig. 59.3 The pathway of haem biosynthesis showing the enzyme deficiency associated with each porphyria. (The abbreviations of disease names are defined in the text relating to classification of the porphyrias.)

because, although hydrophobic porphyrins predominate in plasma in VP, hydrophilic porphyrins, particularly uroporphyrin, predominate in the skin, probably due to secondary local photoinactivation of uroporphyrinogen decarboxylase (UROD) in the skin by coproporphyrin [2]. In addition, the protoporphyrin in VP is conjugated to a peptide which may reduce its phototoxicity.

There is no simple correlation between the plasma porphyrin concentration and the severity of cutaneous disease in porphyria because of the large number of local variables which can alter the extent of the phototoxic reaction in the skin, and an increased plasma porphyrin concentration is not always associated with cutaneous disease [8].

Histopathology of the skin in porphyria [9,10]. In all the cutaneous porphyrias, homogeneous material is seen within vessel walls of the upper dermal and papillary vascular plexus. It is periodic acid–Schiff (PAS)-positive and diastase resistant, and contains a protein polysaccharide complex, lipids and tryptophan. Immunofluorescence reveals immunoglobulins (mainly IgG) in a similar vascular distribution, and IgG at the dermal–epidermal basement membrane zone, in involved skin. Electron microscopy shows reduplication of the vascular basal lamina and the presence of masses of fine fibrillar material, mainly around these blood vessels and often also at the dermal–epidermal junction. In EPP the vessel wall changes are more pronounced, whereas the basement membrane zone changes predominate in affected skin in PCT and VP. In the bullous porphyrias, bullae are subepidermal with the split occurring in the lamina lucida [11] (Fig. 59.5) leaving the dermal papilla protruding into the blister cavity, an appearance called 'festooning' [10]. The findings in bullous porphyrias are indistinguishable from those of pseudoporphyria. In EPP in the acute

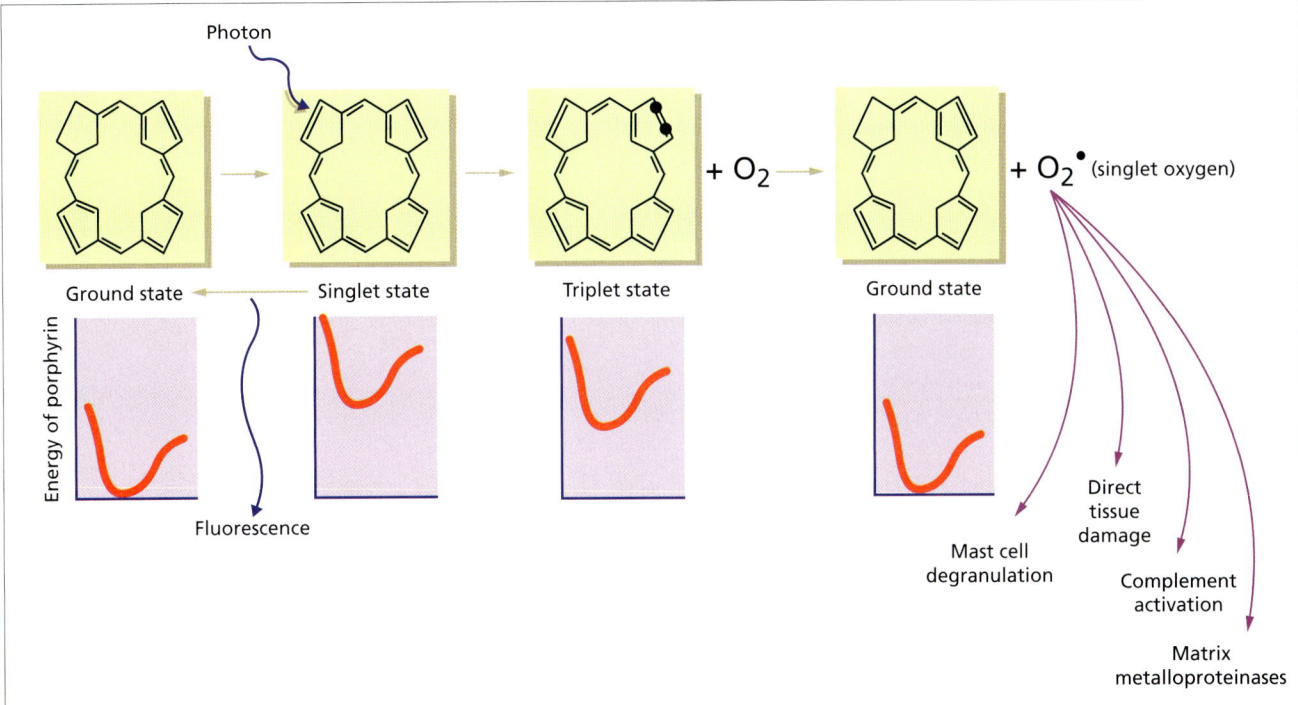

Fig. 59.4 The pathogenesis of skin disease in porphyria.

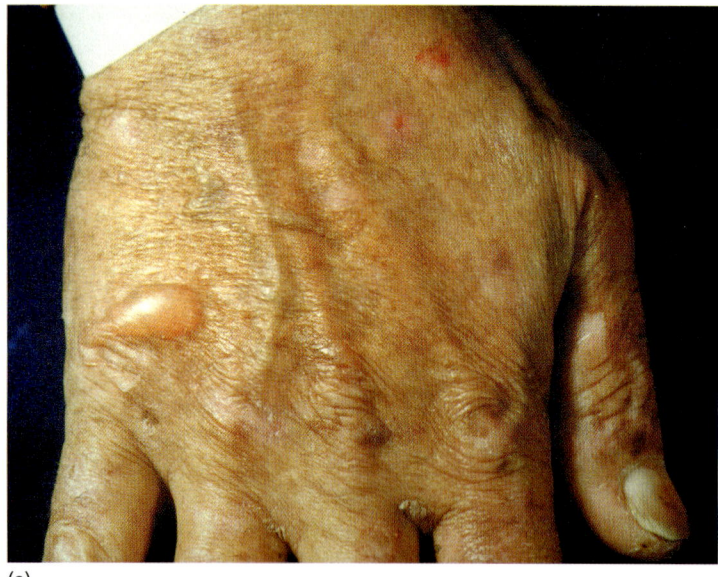

(a)

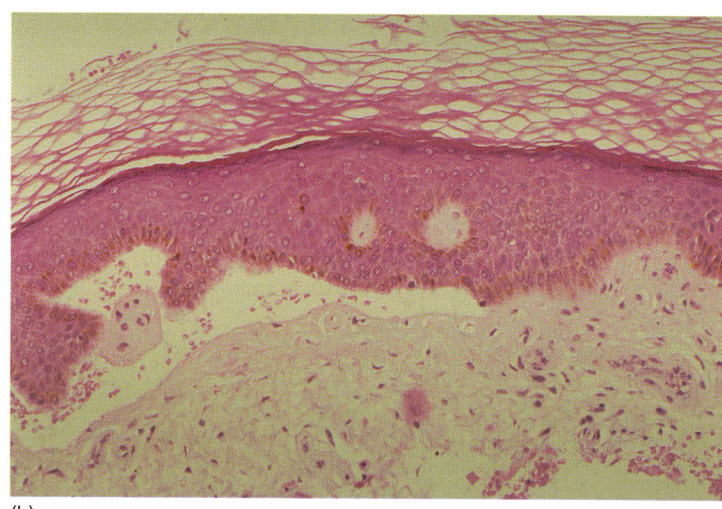

(b)

Fig. 59.5 Typical subepidermal bulla in a bullous porphyria: (a) clinical appearance, (b) histological appearance.

phase there is visible endothelial damage in superficial dermal vessels [12]. Electron microscopy shows the 'amorphous' material seen in vessel walls on light microscopy in light-exposed skin to be a replicated, layered and fragmented basement membrane, with fine fibrillar material permeating the capillary connective tissue sheath and extending beyond the vessel walls, caused by the repeated episodes of damage [13,14].

General considerations in the management of skin disease in porphyria.

Apart from PCT, and to some extent CEP, where effective specific treatments exist, the management of the skin in the other cutaneous porphyrias is based on preventing violet (Soret wavelength) light penetrating the epidermis. The connection between sun exposure and symptoms is obvious in EPP, but is not obvious to patients with the bullous porphyrias where fragility and blistering are not related to individual episodes of sun exposure. It can therefore be difficult to convince these patients of the importance of photoprotection. Basic measures include sun avoidance behaviour, sun-protective clothing and hats. Most sunscreens, including UV-absorbent chemical 'total sunblocks', do not protect against the visible violet Soret wavelength [15]; any sunscreen providing significant visible light protection will be opaque rather than transparent. Sunscreens containing reflectant particles, particularly large particle size titanium dioxide (pigmentary grade), zinc oxide and iron oxide, can effectively protect against violet light [16], and cosmetically acceptable sunscreens with reasonable protection up to 430 nm are available commercially, for example Dundee sunscreen (Tayside Pharmaceuticals, Dundee, UK) [15,16]. Dihydroxyacetone paint induces formation of a light-absorbing brown pigment in the stratum corneum, and has been used in some patients with EPP [17]. Some reasonably clear window films can absorb some violet light, and are useful on car or home windows, particularly in EPP and CEP [18]. This author generally uses two films which are clear and provide reasonable, though not complete, protection against Soret wavelength light (Dermagard

film, Bonwyke, Hants, UK; and CLS200XSR film, Madico, USA). The Madico TA81XSR film is yellower but does provide better protection. Clearly, films applied to car windows must comply with local legislation, which varies considerably in different parts of the world.

References

1 Brun A, Sandberg S. Mechanisms of photosensitivity in porphyric patients with special emphasis on erythropoietic protoporphyria. *J Photochem Photobiol B* 1991; **10**: 285–302.

2 Day RS. Variegate porphyria. *Semin Dermatol* 1986; **5**: 138–54.

3 Takeshita K, Takajo T, Hirata H *et al.* In vivo oxygen radical generation in the skin of the protoporphyria model mouse with visible light exposure: an L-band ESR study. *J Invest Dermatol* 2004; **122**: 1463–70.

4 Lim HW, Poh-Fitzpatrick M, Gigli I. Activation of the complement system in patients with porphyrias after irradiation *in vivo*. *J Clin Invest* 1984; **74**: 1961–5.

5 Glover RA, Bailey CS, Barrett KE *et al.* Histamine release from rodent and human mast cells induced by protoporphyrin and ultraviolet light: studies of the mechanism of mast-cell activation in erythropoietic protoporphyria. *Br J Dermatol* 1990; **122**: 501–12.

6 Herrmann G, Wlaschek M, Bolsen K *et al.* Photosensitization of uroporphyrin augments the ultraviolet A-induced synthesis of matrix metalloproteinases in human dermal fibroblasts. *J Invest Dermatol* 1996; **107**: 398–403.

7 Caputo R, Berti E, Gasparini G, Monti M. The morphologic events of blister formation in porphyria cutanea tarda. *Int J Dermatol* 1983; **22**: 467–72.

8 Poh-Fitzpatrick MB, Sosin AE, Bemis J. Porphyrin levels in plasma and erythrocytes of chronic hemodialysis patients. *J Am Acad Dermatol* 1982; **7**: 100–4.

9 Epstein JH, Tuffanelli DL, Epstein WL. Cutaneous changes in the porphyrias. A microscopic study. *Arch Dermatol* 1973; **107**: 689–98.

10 Wolff K, Hönigsmann H, Rauschmeier W *et al.* Microscopic and fine structural aspects of porphyrias. *Acta Derm Venereol Suppl (Stockh)* 1982; **100**: 17–28.

11 Dabski C, Beutner EH. Studies of laminin and type IV collagen in blisters of porphyria cutanea tarda and drug-induced pseudoporphyria. *J Am Acad Dermatol* 1991; **25**: 28–32.

12 Gschnait FG, Wolff K, Konrad K. Erythropoietic protoprophyria—submicroscopic events during the acute photosensitivity flare. *Br J Dermatol* 1975; **92**: 545–57.

13 Wick G, Honigsmann H, Timpl R. Immunofluorescence demonstration of type IV collagen and a noncollagenous glycoprotein in thickened vascular basal membranes in protoporphyria. *J Invest Dermatol* 1979; **73**: 335–8.

14 Ryan EA, Madill GT. Electron microscopy of the skin in erythropoietic protoporphyria. *Br J Dermatol* 1968; **80**: 561–70.

15 Moseley H, Cameron H, MacLeod T *et al.* New sunscreens confer improved protection for photosensitive patients in the blue light region. *Br J Dermatol* 2001; **145**: 789–94.

16 Kaye ET, Levin JA, Blank IH *et al.* Efficiency of opaque photoprotective agents in the visible light range. *Arch Dermatol* 1991; **127**: 351–5.

17 Johnson JA. Durable protection against long-wavelength UV-A radiation and blue light. *Arch Dermatol* 1992; **128**: 409.

18 Huang JL, Zaider E, Roth P *et al.* Congenital erythropoietic porphyria: clinical, biochemical, and enzymatic profile of a severely affected infant. *J Am Acad Dermatol* 1996; **34**: 924–7.

Acute attacks of porphyria [1,2]

AIP, HC and VP can all cause acute attacks, and HC and VP may also cause cutaneous disease. (A rare autosomal recessive acute porphyria, aminolaevulinic acid (ALA) dehydratase porphyria, has also been reported but does not cause skin disease, and will not be discussed further.)

Definition. An acute and potentially fatal illness, frequently triggered by drugs and hormones which are metabolized by cytochrome P450. It is characterized by an acute neurotoxic reaction in many tissues.

Prevalence. The commonest acute porphyria is AIP, followed by VP. HC is rare. The prevalence of clinically overt acute porphyria in Europe is 1–2/100 000 inhabitants, but over 90% of individuals possessing AIP or VP gene defects are asymptomatic, so the enzyme deficiencies are common; PBG deaminase deficiency, which causes AIP, is present in 0.2% of all blood donors [3].

Aetiology [4]. Impaired activity of PBG deaminase is associated with acute attacks. The deficiency can be primary (as in AIP) or secondary, the latter being due to inhibition of the enzyme by accumulated coproporphyrinogen and protoporphyrinogen (as in HC and VP) [5]. In the liver, haem is mostly incorporated into cytochrome P450 proteins, whose production is induced by many of the drugs and hormones metabolized by the P450 system. When a drug or hormone induces cytochrome P450, and hence acutely increases the hepatic requirement for haem, the inability of the pathway to respond adequately because of the PBG deaminase deficiency is exposed. This acute hepatic haem deficiency in turn causes secondary accumulation of ALA and increased ALA synthase activity due to loss of end-product negative feedback. The symptoms of the acute attack result from neuronal dysfunction, the pathogenesis of which is not fully understood though postulated mechanisms include disturbed metabolism of neurotransmitters (due to reduced activity of haem-containing hepatic tryptophan dioxygenase), direct neurotoxicity of accumulated ALA (which structurally resembles the neurotransmitter γ-aminobutyric acid (GABA)) and acute haem deficiency within neurones.

Factors that may precipitate an acute attack [1]. The most common precipitants are drugs and the menstrual cycle, with recurrent attacks often occurring in the late luteal phase. Alcohol, cannabis, fasting, stress and infection may also trigger attacks. It is not possible to predict whether a specific drug will provoke an attack in an individual. Drugs should be prescribed only after reference to an up-to-date drug list. The author recommends using the lists available on the Internet from the Welsh Medicines Information Centre [6] or the European Porphyria Initiative [7]. These lists are regularly reviewed and updated by experts, and are lists of drugs, by type, that are known to be safe in acute porphyria, that is the lists are designed to answer questions such as 'which antihypertensive can be safely used in a patient with acute porphyria?'. The recommendations on such lists are not absolute and do not substitute for clinical judgement. The risk of a drug provoking an attack is obviously highest where that drug has previously caused an attack in that patient, and in any patients who have previously had symptoms suggestive of an acute attack.

Clinical presentation [1,2]. Acute attacks are five times more common in females, and most frequently occur between the ages of 10 and 40 years. They are rare before puberty. The severity of acute attacks varies from mild abdominal pain, sometimes accompanied by vomiting and constipation, through to very severe attacks with bulbar palsy and respiratory paralysis. Severe, constant abdominal pain occurs in almost all acute attacks. It can be in any quadrant or even in the back, buttocks and thighs, and may require large amounts of opiate analgesia. There may be guarding but no true peritonism. Vomiting and constipation (due to partial ileus) occur in at least half of attacks. The pulse rate and blood pressure are often moderately raised, dehydration is common and hyponatraemia (probably caused by inappropriate secretion of vasopressin) may be severe enough to cause convulsions. The pain, tachycardia, hypertension and partial ileus are all caused by an acute autonomic neuropathy. Sensory or sympathetic involvement, manifest as severe dysaesthesia or causalgia, is rarer. A motor neuropathy occurs in 5–10% of cases, usually heralded by aching pains in the limbs and sometimes by disappearance of the abdominal pain. It may cause a severe acute Guillain–Barré-type syndrome. The motor neuropathy usually occurs when porphyrinogenic drugs have been administered inadvertently during the developing acute attack. Respiratory paralysis is the commonest cause of death. Confusion, abnormal behaviour, agitation and hallucinations occur in up to 50% of attacks. Porphyria is not related to any chronic psychiatric disease, except generalized anxiety.

Biochemical diagnosis of an acute attack [8,9]. The diagnostic finding is of increased urinary PBG excretion. Although qualitative screening tests may be useful in an emergency, their low sensitivity makes it essential to also carry out a quantitative assay. Commercially available kits can provide a rapid and reasonably sensitive semi-quantitative assay, after which a specific quantitative assay should be carried out (reliable quantitative assay kits are commercially available). A normal urinary PBG concentration excludes an acute porphyric attack (except in ALA dehydratase porphyria). An increased PBG concentration does not necessarily mean that an acute attack is occurring since urinary PBG falls between attacks but does not always return to normal, particularly in AIP. The higher the PBG concentration, the more likely an acute attack, but, in the presence of an increased urinary PBG, an acute attack can only be diagnosed on clinical grounds. Urinary ALA is also increased during an acute attack but to a lesser extent than PBG and is not as useful diagnostically (the only exception being ALA dehydratase porphyria in which only ALA is increased and urinary PBG is normal).

Long-term management of patients with acute porphyria [1,2].

The dermatologist may diagnose VP (or less commonly HC) on the basis of cutaneous disease before any acute attack has occurred. Once an acute porphyria has been diagnosed, the patient should be given a list of drugs with information about their safety in acute porphyria. Many lists exist both of 'safe' drugs and 'unsafe' drugs [6,7]. It is obviously vital for clinicians and patients to be clear about whether they are dealing with a list of 'safe' or of 'unsafe' drugs, and there are advantages to using a 'safe' list, as discussed above. It is important to recognize that a list of safe drugs is a guide, and that no drug can be guaranteed to be safe in an individual patient. Conversely, drugs which do not appear on a 'safe' list should not be withheld in patients who need them to treat a serious or life-threatening illness; in that situation expert advice should be sought from a specialist centre.

The patient should also be advised to abstain from alcohol, cannabis and from prolonged calorie-restricted diets, and to wear an emergency identification bracelet (e.g. MedicAlert) so that medical staff are aware of the diagnosis if the patient is ever found in an unconscious or confused state. Screening of relatives is essential to identify those with clinically latent disease, who are also at risk of acute attacks. The choice of test and interpretation of results can be complex and details are covered in the 'laboratory testing' section and under each individual disorder in this chapter. Such testing is ideally carried out in a specialist centre. Relatives diagnosed with an acute porphyria need the same advice as the index case. Conversely, patients with PCT, EPP and CEP can be reassured that acute attacks are not part of their disease.

Treatment of the acute attack [1,2].

The key to managing an acute attack is early diagnosis. Once the diagnosis has been made, avoidance of acute attack-inducing drugs is essential to prevent exacerbation. Supportive treatment includes analgesia, sedatives and antiemetics (in each case using drugs known to be safe in acute porphyria) and careful management of fluid balance with rehydration and correction of hyponatraemia. The specific treatments are intravenous haematin or haem arginate (Normosang, Orphan Pharmaceuticals), which have now replaced carbohydrate as the treatment of choice. These drugs suppress hepatic ALA synthase activity and so reduce ALA and PBG accumulation. Haem arginate is more effective when given earlier during an attack, increasing the importance of early diagnosis. Advice from a specialist centre should be sought when treating an acute attack.

References

1 Elder GH, Hift RJ, Meissner PN. The acute porphyrias. *Lancet* 1997; **349**: 1613–7.
2 Day RS. Variegate porphyria. *Semin Dermatol* 1986; **5**: 138–54.
3 Mustajoki P, Kauppinen R, Lannfelt L, Lilius L, Koistinen J. Frequency of low erythrocyte porphobilinogen deaminase activity in Finland. *J Intern Med* 1992; **231**: 389–95.
4 Meyer UA, Schuurmans MM, Lindberg RL. Acute porphyrias: pathogenesis of neurological manifestations. *Semin Liver Dis* 1998; **18**: 43–52.
5 Meissner P, Adams P, Kirsch R. Allosteric inhibition of human lymphoblast and purified porphobilinogen deaminase by protoporphyrinogen and coproporphyrinogen. A possible mechanism for the acute attack of variegate porphyria. *J Clin Invest* 1993; **91**: 1436–44.
6 Welsh Medicines Information Centre. http://www.wmic.wales.nhs.uk.
7 European Porphyria Initiative/ The European Porphyria NETwork. http://www.porphyria-europe.com
8 Deacon AC, Elder GH. ACP Best Practice No 165: front line tests for the investigation of suspected porphyria. *J Clin Pathol* 2001; **54**: 500–7.
9 Deacon A. The porphyrias and their investigation. *CPD Bull Clin Biochem* 1999; **1**: 122–6.

A clinician's guide to laboratory testing in porphyria [1–3]

Although clinical features may raise the possibility of a porphyria, the cutaneous presentations of several porphyrias are very similar. Precise diagnosis is essential in porphyria because of the great differences in clinical management between porphyrias which can be clinically indistinguishable. An accurate diagnosis can only be made on the basis of porphyrin analyses carried out in an experienced laboratory. The clinician's role is to suspect the diagnosis of cutaneous porphyria, and then to use laboratory testing to confirm whether this is the diagnosis, and if so to precisely identify the porphyria. For any porphyria characterized by acute attacks, testing for latent porphyria in relatives will then be necessary.

What samples to send.

In an adult with suspected bullous porphyria, it is generally sufficient to analyse urine and either plasma (where fluorimetry is available) or faeces (where it is not). However, urine, plasma and faeces need to be analysed in children, because of the increased complexity of the differential diagnosis. Faecal analysis is also necessary in instances when urine and plasma results do not differentiate HC from CEP, and in renal failure, where urine may be unavailable and plasma analysis unhelpful because renal failure increases plasma porphyrins. In suspected EPP, red cells and either plasma or faeces should be analysed.

Handling of samples.

Laboratory testing of body fluids measures porphyrins, since porphyrinogens are spontaneously oxidized to their respective porphyrins outside the body. PBG has a tendency to polymerize to other molecules but porphyrins are reasonably stable when protected from light and oxidants. Thus, all specimens should be kept at room temperature or at 4°C in the dark and ideally should be analysed within 48 h of collection.

For urine and faecal analysis, fresh random specimens (10–20 mL urine or 5–10 g dry weight faeces) are preferable to 24 h collections. Random specimens yield equally useful results, and 24 h collections delay samples reaching the laboratory. Very dilute urine (creatinine <4 mmol/L) is unsuitable.

Laboratory analysis of porphyrins.

Old-fashioned qualitative screening methods for detecting porphyrins in specimens (often involving a Wood's light) are insensitive, and negative results from such tests are not of value. Whether testing urine, faeces, red cells or whole blood, quantitative screening using spectrophotometric or fluorimetric techniques is necessary and yields results as a total porphyrin concentration. Whole blood or red cell porphyrin testing measures both the total and free protoporphyrin concentrations. Plasma is analysed by fluorimetric scanning, a diagnostically powerful and simple qualitative technique. In urine and faeces, the finding of an increased porphyrin concentration will lead on to high-performance liquid chromatography (HPLC) which can be used to rapidly identify the accumulated porphyrins (Fig. 59.6). For PBG measurement in urine, qualitative tests are insensitive, and quantitative measurement, usually using a kit, is required, with semi-quantitative test kits being useful in emergencies where a result is needed quickly.

Interpretation of results [4] (Table 59.1). In cutaneous porphyrias, the accumulated porphyrin can usually be detected in plasma as an emission peak on spectrofluorimetry. Uro- and copropor-

phyrin are excreted into the urine and copro- and protoporphyrin into the faeces. Protoporphyrin accumulates in red cells in EPP.

1 **Plasma spectrofluorimetry.** In plasma spectrofluorimetry, the sample is excited by 410 nm light, and fluorescent emissions detected. An emission peak at 615–620 nm indicates the presence of uro- or coproporphyrin and suggests a diagnosis of PCT, HC, CEP or HEP (urine analysis will differentiate PCT and HEP from the other two conditions). A peak at 624–626 nm indicates the presence of a porphyrin–peptide conjugate diagnostic of VP. This 624–626 nm peak is a sensitive indicator of VP and may even persist during periods of clinical remission when faecal excretion becomes normal. It is also positive in most cases of latent VP (in relatives) [5,6]. A peak around 633 nm (it can lie between 626 and 634 nm) is caused by protoporphyrin and suggests EPP, and EPP is an unlikely diagnosis in the absence of this peak. Plasma porphyrin concentrations, particularly uroporphyrin, increase in renal failure and can be as high as those found in patients with PCT.

2 **Whole blood/red cell.** An increased free protoporphyrin concentration is the diagnostic finding in EPP. The total protoporphyrin concentration includes both free and zinc-protoporphyrin. Zinc-protoporphyrin is also increased in iron deficiency, lead poisoning and certain anaemias. In a child with plasma, urine and faecal results typical of PCT, red cell UROD activity needs to be measured to exclude hepatoerythropoietic porphyria (HEP).

3 **Urinary and faecal analysis.** An increased total porphyrin concentration suggests a diagnosis of cutaneous porphyria. The total urinary porphyrin concentration is used to monitor disease activity in PCT. HPLC analysis is used to identify the porphyrins once an increased concentration has been found.

(a) **In urine.** An increase in uroporphyrin (and other highly carboxylated porphyrins especially heptacarboxy-porphyrin) is typical of PCT though this does not exclude VP. Plasma spectrofluorimetry differentiates these two conditions and faecal analysis is required where this is unavailable. When PCT goes into remission and the total urinary porphyrin concentration returns to normal, it may still be possible to diagnose PCT from the characteristic urinary HPLC pattern. Coproporphyrinuria, in the presence of normal faecal porphyrin levels, does not indicate porphyria

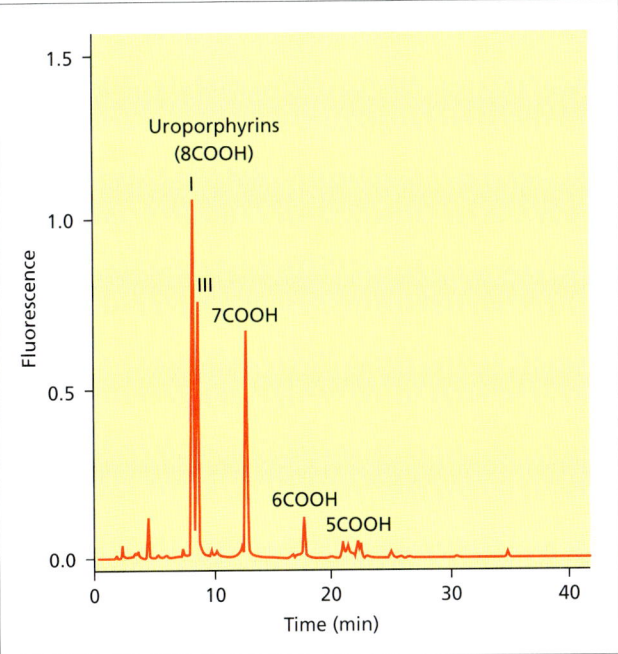

Fig. 59.6 High-performance liquid chromatography (HPLC) analysis: the more carboxylate groups it possesses, the faster a porphyrin molecule passes through the column. After passing through the column, porphyrins are detected by fluorimetry. This HPLC trace of urine shows the porphyrin profile typical of porphyria cutanea tarda (PCT). (Courtesy of Dr A. Deacon, King's College Hospital, London, UK.)

Table 59.1 The major biochemical findings in the cutaneous porphyrias. (Adapted from Deacon and Elder [4].)

	Urine	Faeces	Red cell	Plasma fluorimetry
Congenital erythropoietic porphyria	Uroporphyrin I; coproporphyrin I	Coproporphyrin I	Zinc- and free protoporphyrin; uroporphyrin I; coproporphyrin I	Peak at 615–620 nm
Porphyria cutanea tarda	Uroporphyrin III; heptacarboxy-porphyrin	Isocoproporphyrin; heptacarboxy-porphyrin	Normal	Peak at 615–620 nm
Hereditary coproporphyria	Coproporphyrin III	Coproporphyrin III	Normal	Peak at 615–620 nm
Variegate porphyria	Coproporphyrin III	Protoporphyrin; coproporphyrin III; X-porphyrin	Normal	Peak at 624–627 nm
Erythropoietic protoporphyria	Normal	Protoporphyrin (not diagnostically helpful)	Free protoporphyrin	Peak at 626–634 nm

and can be caused by certain drugs, lead toxicity and hepatobiliary disease.

(b) **In urine and faeces.** Increased coproporphyrin suggests VP, but does not exclude HC. Isomer III to isomer I ratios are increased in every porphyria except CEP (where they are decreased). In CEP, excess type I isomers of uro- and coproporphyrin are present in urine and type I coproporphyrin in faeces.

(c) **In faeces.** In the presence of a plasma spectrofluorimetry peak at 615–620 nm, if urine HPLC does not show the PCT pattern, faecal analysis is required to differentiate HC (increased coproporphyrin III concentration) from CEP (increased coproporphyrin I concentration). Increased faecal isocoproporphyrin is characteristic of PCT. In renal failure, faecal analysis is vital, since urine may be unavailable and plasma porphyrins are increased in renal failure (PCT is the porphyria most commonly associated with renal failure). Increased faecal protoporphyrin is suggestive but not diagnostic of EPP, since it can also derive from bacterial degradation of haem in the gut and may indicate gastrointestinal haemorrhage when porphyrin concentrations are normal elsewhere.

Biochemical diagnosis of an acute attack of porphyria [3,4]. This is discussed above (Acute attacks of porphyria, p. 59.7). A definitive diagnosis of VP or HC can usually be made on the basis of detailed porphyrin analysis. A definitive diagnosis of AIP requires enzyme or genetic tests.

Screening of relatives. In VP and HC, porphyrin levels are normal before puberty. Over the age of 15 years, a plasma fluorimetry scan is a reasonably sensitive biochemical test for latent VP in asymptomatic relatives of patients, picking up most cases. A positive scan is diagnostic of latent VP but a negative result is uninformative [5,6]. Faecal analysis, to measure the ratio of coproporphyrin isomers, will pick up some cases of latent HC after puberty [7]. In VP and HC, a negative porphyrin screening test in a relative needs to be followed by DNA analysis before latent disease can be excluded. The lack of any common mutations in porphyria (apart from South African VP) means that the causative mutation usually has to be identified for each family.

References
1 Kappas A, Sassa S, Galbraith RA, Nordmann Y. The porphyrias. In: Scriver CR, Beaudet AL, Sly WS, Valle D, eds. *The Metabolic and Molecular Bases of Inherited Disease*, 7th edn. New York: McGraw-Hill, 1995: 2103–59.
2 Elder GH. Testing for the cutaneous porphyrias (Appendix D). In: Hawk JLM, ed. *Photodermatology*. London: Arnold, 1999: 281–91.
3 Deacon A. The porphyrias and their investigation. *CPD Bull Clin Biochem* 1999; **1**: 122–6.
4 Deacon AC, Elder GH. ACP Best Practice No 165: front line tests for the investigation of suspected porphyria. *J Clin Pathol* 2001; **54**: 500–7.
5 Long C, Smyth SJ, Woolf J *et al.* Detection of latent variegate porphyria by fluorescence emission spectroscopy of plasma. *Br J Dermatol* 1993; **129**: 9–13.
6 Da Silva V, Simonin S, Deybach JC *et al.* Variegate porphyria: diagnostic value of fluorometric scanning of plasma porphyrins. *Clin Chim Acta* 1995; **238**: 163–8.
7 Kuhnel A, Gross U, Doss MO. Hereditary coproporphyria in Germany: clinical-biochemical studies in 53 patients. *Clin Biochem* 2000; **33**: 465–73.

The individual porphyrias

Porphyrias that cause cutaneous disease but do not cause acute attacks

Congenital erythropoietic porphyria (Günther's disease)

Definition. A severe and rare childhood porphyria causing lifelong mutilating photosensitivity and haematological disease.

Aetiology. Congenital erythropoietic porphyria (CEP) is caused by an autosomal recessive inherited deficiency of the uroporphyrinogen III cosynthase enzyme. Since this enzyme is required to form the biologically useful type III porphyrin isomers, its absence results in non-enzymatic reactions producing large amounts of type I isomer porphyrins which cannot participate in haem formation, and which massively accumulate in erythroid cells and then gradually leak into the plasma. The incidence in the UK is 2 per 3 million live births and less than 100 cases have ever been reported worldwide. Rare adult onset cases of acquired CEP have been reported secondary to myelodysplasia [1].

Clinical features [2–4]. CEP has a wide spectrum of presentation, from hydrops fetalis through to severe disease starting in infancy and also mild forms presenting later in life. The first sign of CEP is often the child's mother noting brown discoloration of amniotic fluid at the onset of labour, or observing pink or brown porphyrin staining of nappies (which fluoresce red-orange under Wood's light).

The skin in CEP [2,4]. Severe photosensitivity begins in infancy, often in the neonatal period, with blisters developing in light-exposed skin on minimal light exposure. Phototherapy for neonatal jaundice may trigger lesions. Most children are so sensitive to the light that they have problems throughout the year. Exposed (and sometimes non-exposed) skin is fragile. The repeated bouts of inflammation with vesicles and bullae, often complicated by secondary infection, cause mutilating scarring, particularly of the face and hands (Fig. 59.7). This photomutilation is associated with erosion of the terminal phalanges, onycholysis and destructive changes affecting the pinnae and nose. A diffuse pseudosclerodermatous thickening of exposed skin often gradually develops, with microstomia and sclerodactyly-like changes [4]. Hypertrichosis is found in most patients, particularly on the upper arms, temples and malar region. Patchy hypo- and hyperpigmentation occur even in minimally exposed areas.

A milder late onset form, presenting at any age from the third decade onward, has been described; this presents in a manner similar to PCT, and occurs either as a result of mild inherited gene mutations [5] or as an acquired disease secondary to bone marrow myelodysplasia [1].

Involvement of eyes and internal organs [4]:
- Eyes. Keratoconjunctivitis, blepharitis, cataracts, corneal ulcers, scars, cicatricial ectropion and scarring alopecia of eyelashes and eyebrows may all occur. Scleromalacia, pterygium formation, optic atrophy and retinal haemorrhage are less common.

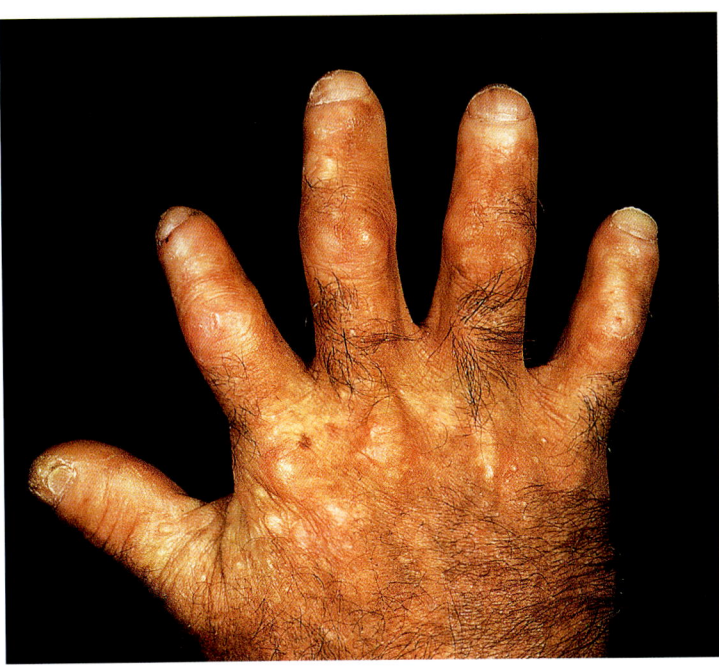

Fig. 59.7 Congenital erythropoietic porphyria (CEP): scarring of skin with resorption of terminal phalanges. (Courtesy of Dr A. du Vivier, King's College Hospital, London, UK.)

- Bones and teeth. When teeth emerge, they are almost always stained brown (and fluoresce under Wood's light). Decreased bone density, osteopenia and osteolytic lesions secondary to erosion by hyperplastic bone marrow are seen on X-ray and are associated with vertebral compression and collapse, and with pathological fractures. In the hands there is resorption of terminal phalanges with acroosteolysis and cortical bone rarefaction. Occasionally, strict avoidance of the sun may impair vitamin D metabolism.

- Haematology [2,4]. The high concentrations of porphyrins in red cells cause haemolytic anaemia, severe enough to induce marrow hyperplasia often with visible expansion of the maxillary bones in the face. Hypersplenism is common. The haemolysis can be fully compensated or may cause a severe anaemia, and is occasionally so severe that some patients become transfusion dependent. The severity of the anaemia often fluctuates strikingly over time. Very severe haemolytic anaemia may even cause hydrops fetalis. Bone marrow examination reveals normoblastic hyperplasia, and under violet illumination most normoblasts have persistent red fluorescence localized to their nuclei, with haem-containing inclusion bodies being seen in the nuclei of these fluorescent cells.

Differential diagnosis. The photosensitivity differentiates CEP from other scarring blistering disorders of childhood, including epidermolysis bullosa dystrophica. The cutaneous changes may resemble HEP (the homozygous form of familial PCT) or homozygous VP. The cutaneous disease in late-onset CEP is clinically indistinguishable from PCT or VP.

Biochemical findings [2]. The uroporphyrinogen III cosynthase enzyme deficiency results in the massive accumulation in all tissues of type I isomers of porphyrins, mainly uroporphyrin, along with coproporphyrin and smaller amounts of 7-, 6- and 5-carboxylic acid porphyrins. Red cells and urine contain large amounts of uro- and coproporphyrin (mainly type I) and faeces contains increased concentrations of coproporphyrin (mainly type I). A plasma spectrofluorimetry peak is seen at 615–620 nm. The absence of isocoproporphyrins and the normal level of 5-carboxylic porphyrin excretion in faeces distinguish CEP from HEP.

Prognosis. In the past, most patients died by the age of 40 years but improvements in supportive care (particularly use of antibiotics) have improved the prognosis, though the haematological complications may be fatal. Long-term hypertransfusion causes significant problems with iron overload as patients reach adulthood, even when iron chelation has been used. Bone marrow transplantation now holds out the promise of cure for these patients (see below).

Treatment [6]. The photosensitivity is so severe that photoprotection is crucial. Sun avoidance and use of sun protective clothing and hats are essential. Opaque sunscreens containing pigmentary grade titanium dioxide or zinc oxide, possibly with added iron oxide, may be of limited value [7,8], and amber window films on home or car windows can reduce exposure to Soret wavelength light (TA81XSR, Madico, USA) [9], though more opaque films may be necessary (which are obviously not allowed on car windows). Prompt treatment of secondary infection is important.

β-Carotene may help cutaneous disease in some patients [2].

Many therapies reduce the porphyrin concentrations by suppressing erythropoiesis. Hypertransfusion with regular blood transfusions to maintain a polycythaemia inhibits endogenous haemoglobin production and decreases porphyrin formation, and may reduce haemolysis and cutaneous symptoms in moderately affected patients. However, splenomegaly may increase transfusion requirements and the value of hypertransfusion often decreases at puberty [6]. Hypertransfusion is frequently complicated by iron overload, even when desferrioxamine has been used, and blood-borne infections can be a complication. Hydroxyurea has been used with hypertransfusion and may be useful in transfusion-dependent CEP [10]. Intravenous haematin has been tried in late-onset disease [11]. Haemolysis worsens the porphyria by causing anaemia and usually necessitates blood transfusion. Splenectomy may reduce haemolysis though the improvement may be temporary [6]. Lights during surgical procedures may cause phototoxic reactions and filters should be used over the operation lights during any unavoidable surgery, preferably a yellow filter (e.g. Madico TA81XSR).

Since 1991, allogeneic bone marrow transplantation (bone marrow or umbilical cord blood stem cells) from a human leukocyte antigen (HLA)-compatible donor has emerged as the treatment of choice in severe CEP. It provides a long-term cure [12,13] though the difficulties of finding a tissue-matched donor, and the dangers of marrow transplantation, mean that it should be reserved for the most severely affected patients [14]. Gene therapy has been successfully used *in vitro*, but no *in vivo* studies have been carried out yet [15].

Genetic counselling. Since CEP is autosomal recessive, parents will be unaware of the risk until an affected child has been born, and the risk of disease is in further offspring rather than subsequent generations. For parents of an affected child, the chance of each future offspring suffering from the disease is 25%. The diagnosis may be made before birth by measuring the uroporphyrin I concentration in amniotic fluid, which is increased as early as 16 weeks *in utero*. If the mutations in the index case have been identified, or the fetus is homozygous for the common C73R mutation, prenatal diagnosis from chorionic villous biopsy is possible [16].

References

1 Kontos AP, Ozog D, Bichakjian C, Lim HW. Congenital erythropoietic porphyria associated with myelodysplasia presenting in a 72-year-old man: report of a case and review of the literature. *Br J Dermatol* 2003; **148**: 160–4.

2 Nordmann Y, Deybach JC. Congenital erythropoietic porphyria. *Semin Dermatol* 1986; **5**: 106–14.

3 Elder GH. The cutaneous porphyrias. In: Hawk JLM, ed. *Photodermatology*. London: Arnold, 1999: 171–99.

4 Fritsch C, Bolsen K, Ruzicka T, Goerz G. Congenital erythropoietic porphyria. *J Am Acad Dermatol* 1997; **36**: 594–610.

5 Berry AA, Desnick RJ, Astrin KH *et al.* Two brothers with mild congenital erythropoietic porphyria due to a novel genotype. *Arch Dermatol* 2005; **141**: 1575–9.

6 Harada FA, Shwayder TA, Desnick RJ, Lim HW. Treatment of severe congenital erythropoietic porphyria by bone marrow transplantation. *J Am Acad Dermatol* 2001; **45**: 279–82.

7 Moseley H, Cameron H, MacLeod T *et al.* New sunscreens confer improved protection for photosensitive patients in the blue light region. *Br J Dermatol* 2001; **145**: 789–94.

8 Kaye ET, Levin JA, Blank IH, Arndt KA, Anderson RR. Efficiency of opaque photoprotective agents in the visible light range. *Arch Dermatol* 1991; **127**: 351–5.

9 Huang JL, Zaider E, Roth P *et al.* Congenital erythropoietic porphyria: clinical, biochemical, and enzymatic profile of a severely affected infant. *J Am Acad Dermatol* 1996; **34**: 924–7.

10 Guarini L, Piomelli S, Poh-Fitzpatrick MB. Hydroxyurea in congenital erythropoietic porphyria. *N Engl J Med* 1994; **330**: 1091–2.

11 Rank JM, Straka JG, Weimer MK *et al.* Hematin therapy in late onset congenital erythropoietic porphyria. *Br J Haematol* 1990; **75**: 617–8.

12 Shaw PH, Mancini AJ, McConnell JP *et al.* Treatment of congenital erythropoietic porphyria in children by allogeneic stem cell transplantation: a case report and review of the literature. *Bone Marrow Transplant* 2001; **27**: 101–5.

13 Dupuis-Girod S, Akkari V, Ged C *et al.* Successful match-unrelated donor bone marrow transplantation for congenital erythropoietic porphyria (Gunther disease). *Eur J Pediatr* 2005; **164**: 104–7.

14 Dawe SA, Peters TJ, Du Vivier A, Creamer JD. Congenital erythropoietic porphyria: dilemmas in present day management. *Clin Exp Dermatol* 2002; **27**: 680–3.

15 Geronimi F, Richard E, Lamrissi-Garcia I *et al.* Lentivirus-mediated gene transfer of uroporphyrinogen III synthase fully corrects the porphyric phenotype in human cells. *J Mol Med* 2003; **81**: 310–20.

16 Lazebnik N, Lazebnik RS. The prenatal presentation of congenital erythropoietic porphyria: report of two siblings with elevated maternal serum alpha-fetoprotein. *Prenat Diagn* 2004; **24**: 282–6.

Porphyria cutanea tarda [1,2]

Definition. Porphyria cutanea tarda (PCT) is the commonest of all the porphyrias. It is characterized by fragility and blistering of exposed skin. It is usually acquired and is often associated with liver disease. It does not cause acute attacks.

Aetiology and classification. PCT results from deficiency of UROD [3]. This causes accumulation of uroporphyrin and other highly carboxylated porphyrins. Seventy-five per cent of patients have the *type I* (*sporadic*) form in which the enzyme deficiency is acquired and restricted to hepatocytes, due to inhibition of a normal UROD enzyme [3]. Twenty-five per cent have *type II* (*familial*) disease where the enzyme deficiency is hereditary, present in all tissues and associated with a UROD gene mutation. The penetrance of this autosomal dominant inherited form is so low that a family history is present in under 7% of cases, and since at least a 75% reduction in enzyme activity is required for clinical expression, some enzyme inhibition in the liver also occurs in familial PCT. Thus, UROD mutations are increasingly thought of as a risk factor for the development of PCT, rather than as representing a completely separate familial form of the disease. *Type III* disease is rare and characterized by an hereditary enzyme deficiency localized to the liver. *Toxic porphyria*, in which halogenated aromatic hydrocarbons inhibit the enzyme, is rare and mainly affects workers making herbicides [4]. A major epidemic of toxic porphyria in the 1950s in Turkey was caused by hexachlorobenzene added as a fungicide to seed wheat [5].

In PCT, the UROD enzyme is inactivated by an inhibitor which binds to its catalytic site. The inhibitor is generated in the liver by reactive oxygen species in the presence of iron (Fig. 59.8) [6]. The

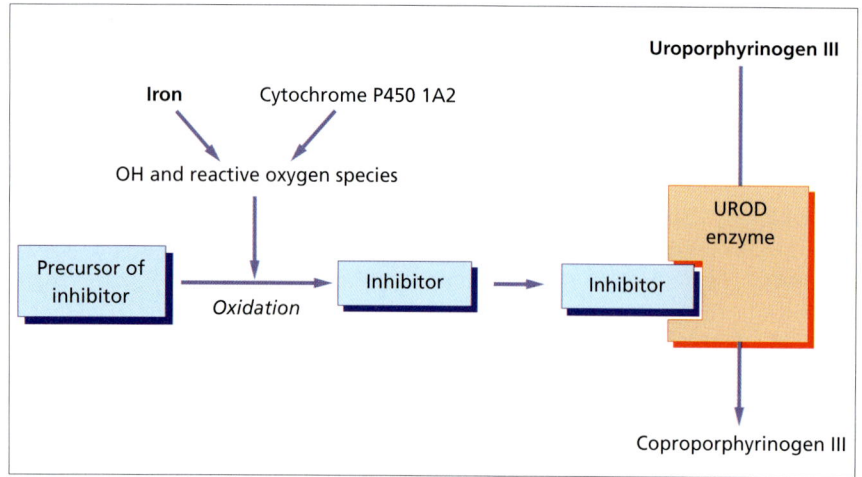

Fig. 59.8 Porphyria cutanea tarda (PCT) is caused by production of an inhibitor of uroporphyrinogen decarboxylase (UROD) in the liver, in the presence of iron. (Adapted from Elder [2].)

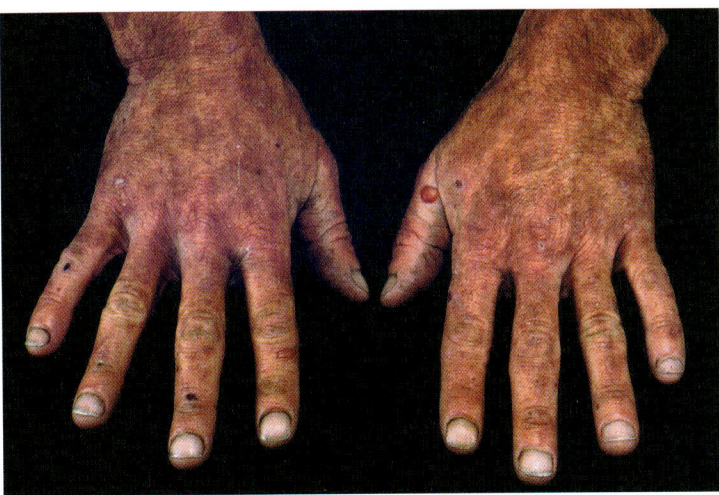

Fig. 59.9 Porphyria cutanea tarda (PCT): erosions, blisters, pigmentary changes and scarring.

accumulated uroporphyrin diffuses from the plasma into surrounding tissues, causing a phototoxic reaction in the upper dermis in sun-exposed skin. This leads to lysis of cells in the superficial dermis with the formation of membrane-limited vacuoles which merge to produce a blister cavity under the basal lamina [7].

Histopathology

Histopathology [8]. The bullae in PCT are subepidermal with a sparse inflammatory infiltrate and 'festooning' of dermal papillae into the bullae. There is deposition of PAS-positive diastase-resistant fibrillar glycoprotein material in and around upper dermal blood vessel walls, and reduplication of the basement membrane. Immunofluorescence reveals IgG, a little IgM, fibrinogen and complement at the epidermal–dermal junction. Morphoea-like lesions in PCT are histologically indistinguishable from other forms of morphoea.

Clinical features

Clinical features (Fig. 59.9) [9]. Sporadic PCT usually presents in middle age whilst the familial form can occur at a younger age. Almost all patients notice increased fragility on light-exposed skin, particularly the backs of the hands and forearms, with minor trauma shearing the skin away to leave sharply marginated erosions. Most patients suffer from bullae, which can be over 1 cm in diameter and may be painful. They crust and resolve over a few weeks, leaving atrophic scars, milia and often mottled hyper- or hypopigmentation. Patients rarely associate development of new lesions with sun exposure, but symptoms are generally worse in the summer. Other common features are: patches of scarring alopecia following resolution of bullae on the scalp; hypertrichosis, usually on the upper face and forehead, sometimes on the ears or arms [10] and occasionally affecting the whole body; hyperpigmentation in a melasma-like pattern on the cheeks and around the eyes, or in a diffuse pattern on light-exposed skin, or occasionally in a reticulate distribution [9,10]. Photo-induced onycholysis [11] and accelerated solar elastosis [10] may also occur. Morphoea-like plaques may develop, particularly on the head and upper trunk. They are histologically indistinguishable from true scleroderma and mainly occur in longstanding untreated disease. It has been

postulated that they arise as a result of the induction of collagen synthesis by uroporphyrin I [12]. These plaques may calcify, and may require excision and grafting if they ulcerate [13].

On the scalp, the morphoea-like change may cause a slowly expanding scarring alopecia starting in the frontoparietal and occipital areas [9,10,14], and even sclerodactyly or the facial changes of systemic sclerosis have been reported. Rare presentations of PCT include cicatricial conjunctivitis [15] and hair darkening [16].

Hepatoerythropoietic porphyria

Hepatoerythropoietic porphyria [10,17]. The homozygous form of familial PCT, hepatoerythropoietic porphyria (HEP), is associated with over 90% reduction in UROD activity. It usually causes a severe disease clinically similar to CEP, with photosensitivity during infancy causing immediate pain on sun exposure, blisters on sun-exposed skin, and mutilating scarring of face and fingers. Prominent hypertrichosis, fluorescent teeth, eye involvement and shortened distal phalanges also occur. Haemolysis is milder than in CEP, and life expectancy is normal. HEP can occasionally present with a milder disease similar to PCT. Since the mutated alleles in HEP have to be associated with some residual enzyme activity to be compatible with life, the UROD gene mutations in HEP patients are different to those found in type II PCT [18].

Differential diagnosis

Differential diagnosis. PCT can be clinically indistinguishable from VP, drug-induced pseudoporphyria, renal pseudoporphyria, HC, late-onset Günther's disease or mild HEP. Biochemical analysis is necessary to diagnose PCT and it is particularly important to exclude VP and HC among the differential diagnoses, since they can cause acute attacks.

Biochemical findings

Biochemical findings [2]. In PCT, the urinary porphyrin concentration is increased, consisting mainly of uroporphyrin, some heptacarboxylic acid porphyrin, and sometimes also hexa- and pentacarboxylic acid porphyrins. A plasma spectrofluorimetry peak is seen at 615–620 nm. Isocoproporphyrin accumulates in the faeces. Urine analysis alone is insufficient to diagnose PCT, since a few patients with VP have the PCT urine pattern ('dual porphyria') [19]. In patients with renal failure, faecal analysis is essential, since plasma porphyrins are increased by haemodialysis and urine collection may not be possible. The biochemical marker of disease activity and response to treatment is quantitative urinary porphyrin excretion measured in a random urine sample.

In HEP, the findings are as in PCT, but with the additional finding of a raised red cell zinc-protoporphyrin, and lower red cell UROD activity than occurs in type II PCT.

The investigation of the patient with PCT

The investigation of the patient with PCT. PCT is essentially a liver disorder with secondary effects in the skin. It is crucial to investigate patients thoroughly both regarding other systemic diseases predisposing to the development of PCT, and in order to assess the severity of any liver disease.

1 Risk factors for the development of PCT [20]. The major risk factors for developing PCT are subclinical genetic haemochromatosis, hepatitis C infection, alcohol and oestrogens. They all predispose to the inhibition of the UROD enzyme in the liver. Since some inhibition of the hepatic enzyme is also required for

clinical expression of familial PCT, the same risk factors apply to sporadic and familial PCT. Since most of the risk factors have significant implications both for treatment and for the patient's general health, it is essential to investigate for risk factors in all patients diagnosed with PCT.

(i) Haemochromatosis. As expected in a disorder where hepatic iron plays a key role, almost all patients have increased stainable iron in the liver, and total body iron stores are increased in at least 60% of patients [2,20,21]. In the USA and Northern Europe, around 20% of PCT patients have true hereditary haemochromatosis [20,22] with homozygosity for the Cys282Tyr haemochromatosis mutation. Homozygosity for this mutation increases the risk of developing PCT 60-fold [20]. The clinical relevance of heterozygosity for the mutation is unclear. In Southern Europe, haemochromatosis is a less important risk factor. The iron overload found in PCT patients who do not have haemochromatosis is milder, and its cause obscure.

(ii) Hepatitis C infection. In Southern Europe, 70–90% of all PCT patients are infected with the hepatitis C virus [23,24], compared with around 60% of patients in the USA [20] and 7–36% in Northern Europe [25,26].

(iii) Alcohol. Between 30% and 90% of PCT patients consume over 40 g of alcohol daily, and 2% of all alcoholics with cirrhosis develop PCT [6].

(iv) Oestrogens. Ingested oestrogens, in the oral contraceptive pill or in hormone replacement therapy, are the sole risk factor in over a quarter of female patients [20]. Stopping the hormone may be sufficient to induce remission if the duration of therapy has been short [27]. If it is not possible to stop the hormone therapy, transdermal drug delivery is a safer alternative than the oral route [28].

There are other less common risk factors for developing PCT: haemodialysis predisposes to PCT [10], though PCT is less common in renal failure than pseudoporphyria—faecal porphyrin analysis differentiates these disorders. Human immune deficiency virus (HIV) infection predisposes to PCT [29], an association which may be due to coinfection with the hepatitis C virus [30]. Non-insulin dependent diabetes mellitus, systemic lupus erythematosus, dermatomyositis, hepatitis A and B infection, haematological malignancy, sideroblastic anaemia, thalassaemia and the drug tamoxifen have all been reported to be associated with PCT [2,9,31,32].

Most patients possess more than one risk factor for developing PCT, with hepatitis C infection and alcohol being strongly linked in men.

2 Liver disease in PCT [21]. Since PCT is primarily a liver disorder with secondary effects in the skin, liver disease is a major concern. In almost all cases, liver biopsy reveals increased stainable iron, fatty change and intracellular porphyrin crystals. Fifty per cent of patients have more severe changes (lobular necrosis or inflamed fibrotic portal tracts), and cirrhosis occurs in 15% [21]. As one would expect, the most severe liver disease tends to occur in patients who have alcoholism, hepatitis C infection and iron overload [20]. The accumulated porphyrins are carcinogenic to the liver, and so PCT confers an additional risk for developing hepatocellular carcinoma on top of the risk con-

ferred by the hepatitis C infection present in many patients [33]. In Southern Europe around 3% of PCT patients develop hepatocellular carcinoma during the decade after presentation [34], and the incidence of hepatic malignancy is probably lower than this in countries with lower hepatitis C infection rates. Risk factors for developing hepatocellular carcinoma are thought to be a symptomatic period longer than 10 years prior to treatment, severe changes on hepatic histology at presentation, hepatitis C infection, male sex and age over 50 years at presentation [35,36]. The converse situation, where a primary hepatic tumour secretes porphyrins to cause a PCT-like skin disease, is rare [37]. Hepatic function must be assessed at presentation in all PCT patients, and patients at high risk of hepatic malignancy require regular ultrasounds and serum α-fetoprotein measurement to detect carcinoma at a treatable stage [35]. PCT should be managed as a liver disorder, and the threshold for referral to a hepatologist should be low.

Treatment

Photoprotection. Visible light sunscreens containing pigmentary grade titanium dioxide or zinc oxide, sometimes with added iron oxide [38,39], filter films for car and home windows, gloves, hats and clothes play an important role in controlling symptoms during the period of several months before specific therapies take effect.

Elimination of risk factors. Stopping oestrogen therapy [27], if it has not been used for more than 2 years, can induce remission. However, elimination of the underlying cause by abstaining from alcohol, or by treating hepatitis C with interferon-α [40], does not always induce remission. All patients should be advised to abstain from alcohol or oestrogen therapy to prevent exacerbation of the disease.

Specific treatments. Definitive treatment with venesection or low-dose antimalarials is required in almost all cases. Venesection depletes iron stores and eliminates hepatic iron overload, thus restoring normal enzyme activity. Around 500 mL of blood is removed every week or every 2 weeks, aiming to decrease transferrin saturation to 15%, haemoglobin to 11–12 g/dL and plasma ferritin to below 25 μg/L [41,42]. Blistering usually resolves within 2–3 months, skin fragility within 6–9 months [43], and porphyrin concentrations generally normalize within 13 months or so [9], at which point treatment should be stopped. Hypertrichosis [9] and sclerodermoid lesions [14] respond more slowly during the years after treatment has stopped. Excision and grafting may be needed for ulcerated sclerodermoid lesions [9]. Desferrioxamine leads to earlier remission than venesection because it rapidly chelates hepatic iron, and it may be of value in PCT with renal failure but it is expensive and requires use of a subcutaneous pump at night [44,45]. Erythropoietin mobilizes hepatic iron into haemoglobin and is the treatment of choice for PCT in renal failure where patients are too anaemic for venesection and cannot excrete chloroquine [46]. Low-dose antimalarials are a very effective treatment for PCT. They work by complexing with uroporphyrin and promoting its excretion into the bile [47]. Daily doses of chloroquine cause a potentially dangerous acute hepatitis but chloroquine at the low dose of 125 mg [48,49] or 250 mg [50,51] taken twice a week is safe and effective. It leads to clinical remission within 6 months or so and biochemical remission after 6–15 months, at which point treatment is stopped [48–51]. Retinopathy does not seem to occur with such low doses of chloroquine [50]. Hydroxychloroquine (200 mg twice weekly) can be used but duration of remission is shorter than with chloroquine [52,53].

Low-dose chloroquine is the treatment of choice except in the following situations, in which venesection is preferable: (i) patients who do not respond to chloroquine; (ii) patients with a pathologically high serum ferritin concentration or homozygous for the Cys282Tyr mutation (if genetic analysis is available), who require iron depletion to protect internal organs; and (iii) patients with significant hepatitis C liver disease, who require iron depletion since hepatic siderosis increases their virally induced liver damage [54] and reduces the effectiveness of interferon [55]. Anyway, chloroquine is usually less effective in the patients with haemochromatosis [56]. However, chloroquine is not contraindicated in these situations, and may be needed when venesection is not possible, particularly in patients with hepatitis C liver disease where venous access is impaired by previous intravenous drug abuse.

Remission with low-dose chloroquine generally lasts 17–24 months [49,50]. With venesection, relapse generally occurs around 2.5 years after the end of treatment [9,48]. Long-term follow-up is necessary for all patients to monitor for relapse (by measuring urinary porphyrin excretion), and for the management of coexisting liver disease.

Genetic counselling [57]. Familial and sporadic PCT can be differentiated by measuring red cell UROD activity. Since additional inhibition of the hepatic enzyme is required for clinical expression of disease in familial PCT, UROD mutations can be considered as a risk factor for developing the disease rather than as a different form of PCT. In view of the identical management of sporadic and familial PCT, the lack of evidence that identifying latent PCT in relatives alters outcomes, and the very low penetrance of familial PCT, it is difficult to justify family screening in familial PCT. It is therefore of little value to measure red cell UROD activity unless one is trying to differentiate HEP from PCT.

References

1 Sarkany RPE. The management of porphyria cutanea tarda. *Clin Exp Dermatol* 2001; **26**: 225–32.

2 Elder GH. Porphyria cutanea tarda. *Semin Liver Dis* 1998; **18**: 67–75.

3 Elder GH, Urquhart AJ, De Salamanca RE *et al.* Immunoreactive uroporphyrinogen decarboxylase in the liver in porphyria cutanea tarda. *Lancet* 1985; **2**: 229–33.

4 Bleiberg J, Wallew M, Brodkin K *et al.* Industrially acquired porphyria. *Arch Dermatol* 1964; **89**: 793–7.

5 Dean G. The Turkish epidemic of porphyria. In: Dean G, ed. *The Porphyrias: a Story of Inheritance and Environment*, 2nd edn. London: Pitman Medical, 1971: 67–72.

6 Elder GH. Alcohol intake and porphyria cutanea tarda. *Clin Dermatol* 1999; **17**: 431–6.

7 Caputo R, Berti E, Gasparini G, Monti M. The morphologic events of blister formation in porphyria cutanea tarda. *Int J Dermatol* 1983; **22**: 467–72.

8 Wolff K, Hönigsmann H, Rauschmeier W *et al.* Microscopic and fine structural aspects of porphyrias. *Acta Derm Venereol Suppl (Stockh)* 1982; **100**: 17–28.

9 Grossman ME, Bickers DR, Poh-Fitzpatrick MB *et al.* Porphyria cutanea tarda: clinical features and laboratory findings in 40 patients. *Am J Med* 1979; **67**: 277–86.

10 Mascaro JM, Herrero C, Lecha M *et al.* Uroporphyrinogen-decarboxylase deficiencies: porphyria cutanea tarda and related conditions. *Semin Dermatol* 1986; **5**: 115–24.

11 Byrne JP, Boss JM, Dawber RP. Contraceptive pill-induced porphyria cutanea tarda presenting with onycholysis of the finger nails. *Postgrad Med J* 1976; **52**: 535–8.

12 Varigos G, Schiltz JR, Bickers DR. Uroporphyrin I stimulation of collagen biosynthesis in human skin fibroblasts. A unique dark effect of porphyrin. *J Clin Invest* 1982; **69**: 129–35.

13 Inglese MJ, Bergamo BM. Large, nonhealing scalp ulcer associated with scarring alopecia and sclerodermatous change in a patient with porphyria cutanea tarda. *Cutis* 2005; **76**: 329–33.

14 Doyle JA, Friedman SJ. Porphyria and scleroderma. A clinical and laboratory review of 12 patients. *Australas J Dermatol* 1983; **24**: 109–14.

15 Park AJ, Webster GF, Penne RB, Raber IM. Porphyria cutanea tarda presenting as cicatricial conjunctivitis. *Am J Ophthalmol* 2002; **134**: 619–21.

16 Shaffrali FC, McDonagh AJ, Messenger AG. Hair darkening in porphyria cutanea tarda. *Br J Dermatol* 2002; **146**: 325–9.

17 Smith SG. Hepatoerythropoietic porphyria. *Semin Dermatol* 1986; **5**: 125–37.

18 Castano Suarez E, Zamarro Sanz O, Guerra Tapia A *et al.* Hepatoerythropoietic porphyria: relationship with familial porphyria cutanea tarda. *Dermatology* 1996; **193**: 332–5.

19 Sturrock ED, Meissner PN, Maeder DL, Kirsch RE. Uroporphyrinogen decarboxylase and protoporphyrinogen oxidase in dual porphyria. *S Afr Med J* 1989; **76**: 405–8.

20 Bulaj ZJ, Phillips JD, Ajioka RS *et al.* Hemochromatosis genes and other factors contributing to the pathogenesis of porphyria cutanea tarda. *Blood* 2000; **95**: 1565–71.

21 Bruguera M. Liver involvement in porphyria. *Semin Dermatol* 1986; **5**: 178–85.

22 Roberts AG, Whatley SD, Morgan RR *et al.* Increased frequency of the haemochromatosis Cys282Tyr mutation in sporadic porphyria cutanea tarda. *Lancet* 1997; **349**: 321–3.

23 Quecedo L, Costa J, Enriquez de Salamanca R. Role of hepatitis C virus in porphyria cutanea tarda hepatopathy. *Med Clin (Barc)* 1996; **106**: 321–4.

24 Fargion S, Piperno A, Cappellini MD *et al.* Hepatitis C virus and porphyria cutanea tarda: evidence of a strong association. *Hepatology* 1992; **16**: 1322–6.

25 Linde Y, Harper P, Floderus Y, Ros AM. The prevalence of hepatitis C in patients with porphyria cutanea tarda in Stockholm, Sweden. *Acta Derm Venereol* 2005; **85**: 164–6.

26 Murphy A, Dooley S, Hillary IB, Murphy GM. HCV infection in porphyria cutanea tarda. *Lancet* 1993; **341**: 1534–5.

27 Haberman HF, Rosenberg F, Menon IA. Porphyria cutanea tarda. Comparison of cases precipitated by alcohol and estrogens. *Can Med Assoc J* 1975; **113**: 653–5.

28 Bulaj ZJ, Franklin MR, Phillips JD *et al.* Transdermal estrogen replacement therapy in postmenopausal women previously treated for porphyria cutanea tarda. *J Lab Clin Med* 2000; **136**: 482–8.

29 Blauvelt A, Ross Harris H, Hogan DJ *et al.* Porphyria cutanea tarda and human immunodeficiency virus infection. *Int J Dermatol* 1992; **31**: 474–9.

30 Castanet J, Lacour JP, Bodokh J *et al.* Porphyria cutanea tarda in association with human immunodeficiency virus infection: is it related to hepatitis C virus infection? *Arch Dermatol* 1994; **130**: 664–5.

31 Cram DL, Epstein JK, Tuffanelli DL. Lupus erythematosus and porphyria. *Arch Dermatol* 1973; **108**: 779–84.

32 Agarwal R, Peters TJ, Coombes RC, Vigushin DM. Tamoxifen-related porphyria cutanea tarda. *Med Oncol* 2002; **19**: 121–3.

33 Smith AG, Francis JE, Dinsdale D *et al.* Hepatocarcinogenicity of hexachlorobenzene in rats and the sex difference in hepatic iron status and development of porphyria. *Carcinogenesis* 1985; **6**: 631–6.

34 Gisbert JP, Garcia-Buey L, Alonso A *et al.* Hepatocellular carcinoma risk in patients with porphyria cutanea tarda. *Eur J Gastroenterol Hepatol* 2004; **16**: 689–92.

35 Siersema PD, ten Kate FJW, Mulder PGH, Wilson JHP. Hepatocellular carcinoma in porphyria cutanea tarda: frequency and factors related to its occurrence. *Liver* 1992; **12**: 56–61.

36 Salata H, Cortes JM, Enriquez de Salamanca R *et al.* Porphyria cutanea tarda and hepatocellular carcinoma. Frequency of occurrence and related factors. *J Hepatol* 1985; **1**: 477–87.

37 Tio TH, Leijnse B, Jarrett A. Acquired porphyria from a liver tumor. *Clin Sci* 1957; **16**: 517–27.

38 Moseley H, Cameron H, MacLeod T *et al.* New sunscreens confer improved protection for photosensitive patients in the blue light region. *Br J Dermatol* 2001; **145**: 789–94.

39 Kaye ET, Levin JA, Blank IH, Arndt KA, Anderson RR. Efficiency of opaque photoprotective agents in the visible light range. *Arch Dermatol* 1991; **127**: 351–5.

40 Sheikh MY, Wright RA, Burruss JB. Dramatic resolution of skin lesions associated with porphyria cutanea tarda after interferon-alpha therapy in a case of chronic hepatitis C. *Dig Dis Sci* 1998; **43**: 529–33.

41 Rocchi E, Gibertini P, Cassanelli M *et al.* Serum ferritin in the assessment of liver iron overload and iron removal therapy in porphyria cutanea tarda. *J Lab Clin Med* 1986; **107**: 36–42.

42 Ratnaike S, Blake D, Campbell D *et al.* Plasma ferritin levels as a guide to the treatment of porphyria cutanea tarda by venesection. *Australas J Dermatol* 1988; **29**: 3–7.

43 Wennersten G, Ros A-M. Chloroquine in treatment of porphyria cutanea tarda. Long-term efficacy of combined phlebotomy and high-dose chloroquine therapy. *Acta Derm Venereol Suppl (Stockh)* 1982; **100**: 119–23.

44 Pitche P, Corrin E, Wolkenstein P *et al.* Successful treatment of haemodialysis-related porphyria cutanea tarda with deferoxamine. *Ann Dermatol Venereol* 2003; **130**: 37–9.

45 Rocchi E, Gibertini P, Cassanelli M *et al.* Iron removal therapy in porphyria cutanea tarda: phlebotomy versus slow subcutaneous desferrioxamine infusion. *Br J Dermatol* 1986; **114**: 621–9.

46 Sarkell B, Patterson JW. Treatment of porphyria cutanea tarda of end-stage renal disease with erythropoietin. *J Am Acad Dermatol* 1993; **29**: 499–500.

47 Scholnick PL, Epstein J, Marver HS. The molecular basis of the action of chloroquine in porphyria cutanea tarda. *J Invest Dermatol* 1973; **61**: 226–32.

48 Malina L, Chlumsky J. A comparative study of the results of phlebotomy therapy and low-dose chloroquine treatment in porphyria cutanea tarda. *Acta Derm Venereol Suppl (Stockh)* 1981; **61**: 346–50.

49 Ashton RE, Hawk JLM, Magnus IA. Low-dose oral chloroquine in the treatment of porphyria cutanea tarda. *Br J Dermatol* 1984; **111**: 609–13.

50 Valls V, Ena J, Enriquez-de-Salamanca R. Low-dose oral chloroquine in patients with porphyria cutanea tarda and low-moderate iron overload. *J Dermatol Sci* 1994; **7**: 164–75.

51 Kordac V, Kotal JP, Kalab M. Agents affecting porphyrin formation and secretion: implications for porphyria cutanea tarda treatment. *Semin Hematol* 1989; **26**: 16–23.

52 Cainelli T, Di Padova C, Marchesi L *et al.* Hydroxychloroquine versus phlebotomy in the treatment of porphyria cutanea tarda. *Br J Dermatol* 1983; **108**: 593–600.

53 Malkinson FD, Levitt L. Hydroxychloroquine treament of porphyria cutanea tarda. *Arch Dermatol* 1980; **116**: 1147–50.

54 Farinati F, Cardin R, DeMaria N *et al.* Iron storage, lipid peroxidation and glutathione turnover in chronic HCV-positive hepatitis. *J Hepatol* 1995; **22**: 449–56.

55 Roeckel IE. Commentary: iron metabolism in hepatitis C infection. *Ann Clin Lab Sci* 2000; **30**: 163–5.

56 Stolzel U, Kostler E, Schuppan D *et al.* Hemochromatosis (HFE) gene mutations and response to chloroquine in porphyria cutanea tarda. *Arch Dermatol* 2003; **139**: 309–13.

57 Elder GH. The cutaneous porphyrias. In: Hawk JLM, ed. *Photodermatology*. London: Arnold, 1999: 171–99.

Erythropoietic protoporphyria

Definition. EPP is an hereditary porphyria characterized by painful, lifelong photosensitivity and occasionally liver disease.

Incidence and aetiology. The prevalence of EPP is around 1/100 000 [1]. EPP results from deficient activity of ferrochelatase, the final enzyme of haem biosynthesis. This causes the accumulation of protoporphyrin predominantly in cells of the erythroid series, which causes a phototoxic reaction as the porphyrin-laden cells pass through small upper dermal blood vessels and are exposed to the Soret wavelength in sunlight. The photoactivated porphyrin from red cells and plasma causes an acute injury to the endothelium mediated by singlet oxygen and the hydroxyl radical [2,3]. Many ferrochelatase gene mutations have been identified in EPP patients and none are particularly common [4]. A few adult-onset cases have been reported which are associated with haematological malignancy and may be associated with chromosomal deletions involving the ferrochelatase gene [5].

Histopathology [6,7]. In the acute phase there is visible endothelial damage in superficial dermal vessels [8]. In the chronic phase, in exposed areas of skin, the repeated episodes of damage to small vessels in the upper dermis cause deposition of PAS-positive diastase-resistant hyaline material in the walls of blood vessels of the upper dermal and papillary vascular plexuses. Immunofluorescence shows immunoglobulins (mainly IgG) in a similar distribution. On electron microscopy the hyaline material can be seen to be a greatly replicated, layered and fragmented basement membrane, with fine fibrillar material permeating the capillary connective tissue sheath and extending beyond the vessel walls [6,9].

Clinical features [1,10]. Unlike the other cutaneous porphyrias, EPP causes immediate pain on exposure to bright sunlight. It presents most commonly in the first year, quite often in babies who usually present with crying in their prams in sunny weather, or crying for no obvious reason at night in the summer. Onset later in childhood does occur but onset in adulthood is rare. In spring and summer, after anything from a few minutes to an hour or two of sun exposure, patients describe discomfort, tingling or itching in exposed skin, particularly the dorsae of the hands and the face. If exposure continues, severe burning pain follows which can last anything between an hour and several days. Children often find partial relief with cold water and wet cloths, and this feature may be diagnostically useful. Usually the only physical sign during an attack is oedema, which may be subtle (Fig. 59.10). Erythema is less common. The lack of physical signs often leads to delay in diagnosis, with some patients initially being labelled as malingerers. Many patients experience a 'priming phenomenon' in which sunlight tolerance is reduced on the day after significant sun exposure [11]. In severe attacks, purpuric lesions and crusted erosions or vesicles may occur; these take a week or two to resolve after the attack settles down, and the pain may be severe enough to require hospital admission. Rare cases of EPP with prominent purpura and histological changes resembling a leukocytoclastic vasculitis [12], acute photo-onycholysis [13] or erythematous plaques [14] have been described. Physical signs may develop during childhood, with slight thickening of skin over the metacarpophalangeal and interphalangeal joints, superficial vermicular waxy scarring on the nose, shallow linear, punctate or small circular scars on cheeks and forehead and radial scars around the lips (Fig. 59.11). The skin over the nose, cheeks and forehead can become roughened and 'pebbly' in texture. Fifteen per cent of patients have no physical signs at all [1]. Children with EPP suffer from social isolation due to difficulty joining friends to play outside, and sensitivity to psychosocial issues is important for clinicians. Although EPP is lifelong, childhood and adolescence

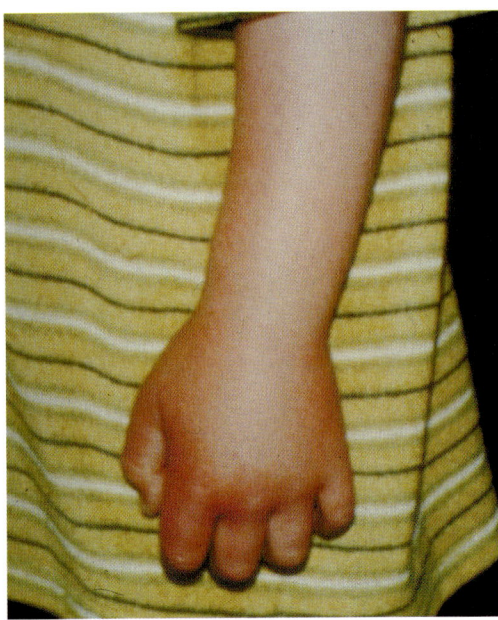

Fig. 59.10 Oedema during an acute painful attack in a child with erythropoietic protoporphyria (EPP).

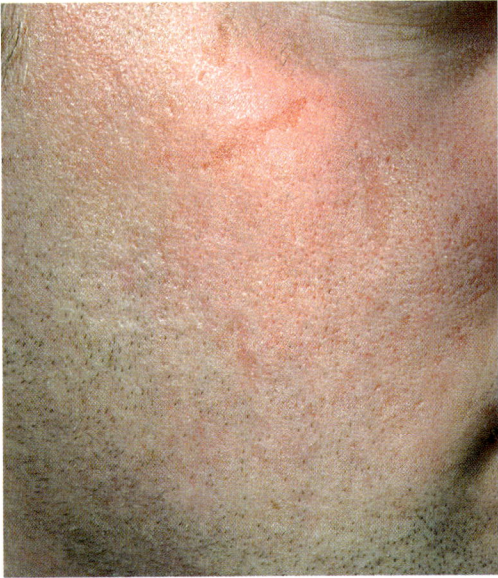

Fig. 59.11 Typical scars on the cheeks in erythropoietic protoporphyria (EPP).

are frequently the most difficult times because it is easier for adults to organize their lives to reduce sun exposure, but it is not surprising that the disease has such a profound impact on quality of life [1]. Symptoms often improve and porphyrin levels fall during pregnancy [1,15]. Patients may develop a mild hypochromic microcytic or normocytic anaemia, which can be associated with decreased serum iron levels and increased serum iron binding capacity [10]. With the exception of patients with EPP liver failure, operating theatre lights do not cause any problems during or after surgery in EPP patients [16]. Anaesthetists can also be reassured that acute attacks do not occur in EPP. In contrast, operating theatre lights can cause a devastating and potentially fatal phototoxic reaction in patients undergoing liver transplantation for protoporphyric liver failure.

Biochemical investigation [17]. The diagnostic finding is of an increased red cell free protoporphyrin concentration. Protoporphyrin is seen as a peak at 633 nm on plasma fluorimetric scanning. Sixty per cent of EPP patients have an increased faecal protoporphyrin concentration though this is not very useful diagnostically because of its lack of specificity. Urinary porphyrins are normal except in biliary impairment, when coproporphyrinuria develops.

Treatment [1]. No therapy has ever been proven to be effective in EPP mainly because of the lack of an objective test for disease activity in EPP, and high placebo rates make useful clinical trials difficult. This author's experience is that results with the specific therapies are generally fairly disappointing, and that attention to sunlight protection is the key to management.

Photoprotection. Basic measures include sun avoidance behaviour, sun-protective clothing and hats. It is important to use correct sunscreens [18,19]. Dihydroxyacetone paint has been used in some patients with EPP [20], and window films, which absorb violet light, can be useful for car or home windows, particularly in severely affected patients; all of these are discussed in detail on p. 59.6.

The acute reaction. For the acute reaction, complete sun avoidance (even through windows) leads to earlier resolution, and fans and cold water provide some pain relief. Antihistamines and most analgesics are of little value. For severe attacks, hospital admission may be necessary, for light avoidance and analgesia (usually opiate).

Specific therapies. Oral β-carotene is the most widely used treatment, usually at a dose around 180 mg daily in adults (90 mg daily in children) taken throughout the spring and summer. It is postulated to scavenge free radicals involved in the acute phototoxic reaction. Although some patients report that it reduces symptoms, others do not, and proof of efficacy from controlled trials is lacking. Patients may need to take it for several months before any effect is observed. The most common adverse effect of β-carotene is reversible skin discoloration. A controlled trial of N-acetyl cysteine has shown no benefit [21]. Short courses of a few weeks of psoralen and long-wave UV radiation (PUVA) [22] and narrow-band UVB [23] used in the early spring may be valuable, particularly in milder cases, and probably increase photoprotection by inducing epidermal thickening and pigmentation. Unlike PUVA, narrow-band UVB does not overlap with the EPP action spectrum and so cannot trigger attacks of pain. Many other systemic treatments with antioxidant or free radical scavenging properties have been used in EPP in an uncontrolled way on small numbers of patients, with conflicting and generally unconvincing results.

Genetic counselling. Although rare cases of autosomal recessive inheritance have been reported [24,25], EPP is generally an autosomal dominant disorder with incomplete penetrance, the disease resulting from co-inheritance of a gene mutation on one ferrochelatase allele with a low expression variant on the other allele. This low expression variant is present in around 10% of the Caucasian population and is associated with reduced ferrochelatase mRNA levels resulting from the presence of the polymorphic variant IVS3-48C [26]. This low expression variant is common in Japan and South-East Asia and rare in Africa, which may explain the observed variations between continents [27]. Overall, the probability of each offspring of an EPP patient suffering from the disease is under 10%, but testing for the IVS3-48C polymorphism in a patient's partner is now available and can indicate more precisely whether there is a significant probability of future offspring being affected. This is useful for patients who would not consider having children if there were a significant likelihood of them having the disease. For a disorder which is rarely life-threatening, termination of pregnancy and thus antenatal diagnosis are not relevant.

Liver disease in EPP [24]. Protoporphyrin is excreted exclusively into the bile. It precipitates to form gallstones in around 12% of patients. It is also hepatotoxic, particularly to bile canaliculi, and severe liver damage occurs in around 1% of patients. EPP liver failure is most common in the teens and twenties. Usually a patient develops jaundice, worsening photosensitivity and often upper abdominal pain over a period of weeks or months. Investigation shows severe or total cholestasis, and a dramatically high red cell protoporphyrin concentration (due to its impaired excretion), which causes the worsening photosensitivity. Liver histology reveals deposition of protoporphyrin in vacuoles within bile canaliculi and hepatocytes, which may be accompanied by cirrhosis (Fig. 59.12). Although such acute episodes may resolve spontaneously, the porphyrin-induced cholestasis may become increasingly severe and itself further increase the protoporphyrin concentration in a vicious cycle, in which case the patient will die unless a liver transplant can be performed. Under operating theatre lights during the transplant surgery, the very high protoporphyrin concentration may cause a severe phototoxic reaction with postoperative burns, massive haemolysis and a severe neuropathy. Yellow filters blocking out light below 460 nm (e.g. Madico TA81XSR) must be used over the operating theatre lights, and do not impair the surgeon's view [16]. Even if these immediate postoperative complications are avoided, protoporphyric liver disease recurs in

the graft in most patients over several years, severe enough to require retransplantation in a minority [28]. Recently, two patients with severe liver disease have been treated by bone marrow transplantation (in one of them with a liver transplant). Although the marrow transplantation does cure the EPP, the dangers of the procedure mean that it is reserved for these rare, life-threatening situations [29,30].

It is vital to recognize impending protoporphyric liver failure early enough that arrangements can be made for a liver transplant if it should become necessary. Thus, all EPP patients should have liver function tests and red cell protoporphyrin concentration checked at least once a year. The appearance of coproporphyrin in the urine has been proposed as an indicator of significant liver disease in EPP [31]. Worsening photosensitivity may be the only clinical indication of the development of severe liver disease. Although protoporphyric liver failure is rare, mild abnormalities of liver function tests are common in EPP [31]. Since the significance of these abnormalities is unclear, it is advisable to monitor closely in these patients, and to refer the patient to a hepatologist if the abnormality is persistent or deteriorating. In such patients, an ion exchange resin such as cholestyramine may protect the liver against further porphyrin toxicity. The major difficulty for the dermatologist is the lack of any means of identifying those EPP patients at risk of liver failure. Since several cases have been described in siblings, patients with a relative who has suffered protoporphyric liver failure should be treated as being at increased risk of developing it themselves. Recessive inheritance of EPP may increase the risk of severe hepatic disease, though it is not clear how significant an association this is [24].

Iron deficiency anaemia may trigger or exacerbate hepatic disease by increasing porphyrin accumulation [24], and subsequent iron replacement may make the situation temporarily worse by acutely stimulating haem biosynthesis.

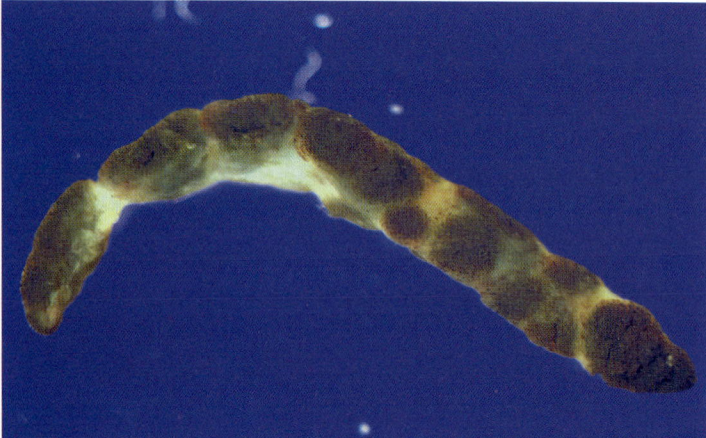

Fig. 59.12 Liver biopsy in protoporphyric liver disease, showing nodules of cirrhosis and black staining by deposits of protoporphyrin.

References
1 Holme SA, Anstey AV, Finlay AY *et al.* Erythropoietic protoporphyria in the U.K.: clinical features and effect on quality of life. *Br J Dermatol* 2006; **155**: 574–81.
2 Brun A, Sandberg S. Mechanisms of photosensitivity in porphyric patients with special emphasis on erythropoietic protoporphyria. *J Photochem Photobiol B* 1991; **10**: 285–302.
3 Takeshita K, Takajo T, Hirata H *et al.* In vivo oxygen radical generation in the skin of the protoporphyria model mouse with visible light exposure: an L-band ESR study. *J Invest Dermatol* 2004; **122**: 1463–70.
4 Minder EI, Gouya L, Schneider-Yin X, Deybach JC. A genotype–phenotype correlation between null-allele mutations in the ferrochelatase gene and liver complication in patients with erythropoietic protoporphyria. *Cell Mol Biol (Noisy-le-grand)* 2002; **48**: 91–6.
5 Sarkany RP, Ross G, Willis F. Acquired erythropoietic protoporphyria as a result of myelodysplasia causing loss of chromosome 18. *Br J Dermatol* 2006; **155**: 464–6.
6 Ryan EA, Madill GT. Electron microscopy of the skin in erythropoietic protoporphyria. *Br J Dermatol* 1968; **80**: 561–70.
7 Epstein JH, Tuffanelli DL, Epstein WL. Cutaneous changes in the porphyrias. A microscopic study. *Arch Dermatol* 1973; **107**: 689–98.
8 Gschnait FG, Wolff K, Konrad K. Erythropoietic protoporphyria—submicroscopic events during the acute photosensitivity flare. *Br J Dermatol* 1975; **92**: 545–57.
9 Wick G, Honigsmann H, Timpl R. Immunofluorescence demonstration of type IV collagen and a noncollagenous glycoprotein in thickened vascular basal membranes in protoporphyria. *J Invest Dermatol* 1979; **73**: 335–8.

10 Deleo VA, Poh-Fitzpatrick M, Mathews-Roth M, Harber LC. Erythropoietic protoporphyria. Ten years experience. *Am J Med* 1976; **60**: 8–22.

11 Poh-Fitzpatrick MB. The 'priming phenomenon' in the acute phototoxicity of erythropoietic protoporphyria. *J Am Acad Dermatol* 1989; **21**: 311.

12 Patel GK, Weston J, Derrick EK, Hawk JL. An unusual case of purpuric erythropoietic protoporphyria. *Clin Exp Dermatol* 2000; **25**: 406–8.

13 Marsden RA, Dawber RP. Erythropoietic protoporphyria with onycholysis. *Proc R Soc Med* 1977; **70**: 572–4.

14 Murphy GM, Hawk JL, Magnus IA. Late-onset erythropoietic protoporphyria with unusual cutaneous features. *Arch Dermatol* 1985; **121**: 1309–12.

15 Poh-Fitzpatrick MB. Human protoporphyria: reduced cutaneous photosensitivity and lower erythrocyte porphyrin levels during pregnancy. *J Am Acad Dermatol* 1997; **36**: 40–3.

16 Wahlin S, Harper P, Brun A. Protection from phototoxic injury in erythropoietic protoporphyria. Presented at: *Porphyrins and Porphyrias International Conference*, Rotterdam, May 2007.

17 Deacon A. The porphyrias and their investigation. *CPD Bull Clin Biochem* 1999; **1**: 122–6.

18 Moseley H, Cameron H, MacLeod T *et al.* New sunscreens confer improved protection for photosensitive patients in the blue light region. *Br J Dermatol* 2001; **145**: 789–94.

19 Kaye ET, Levin JA, Blank IH *et al.* Efficiency of opaque photoprotective agents in the visible light range. *Arch Dermatol* 1991; **127**: 351–5.

20 Johnson JA. Durable protection against long-wavelength UV-A radiation and blue light. *Arch Dermatol* 1992; **128**: 409.

21 Norris PG, Baker CS, Roberts JE, Hawk JL. Treatment of erythropoietic protoporphyria with N-acetylcysteine. *Arch Dermatol* 1995; **131**: 354–5.

22 Roelandts R. Photo (chemo) therapy and general management of erythropoietic protoporphyria. *Dermatology* 1995; **190**: 330–1.

23 Collins P, Ferguson J. Narrow-band UVB (TL-01) phototherapy. An effective preventative treatment for the photodermatoses. *Br J Dermatol* 1995; **132**: 956–63.

24 Sarkany RPE, Cox TM. Autosomal recessive erythropoietic protoporphyria: a syndrome of severe photosensitivity and hepatic failure. *QJM* 1995; **88**: 541–9.

25 Whatley SD, Mason NG, Khan M *et al.* Autosomal recessive erythropoietic protoporphyria in the United Kingdom: prevalence and relationship to liver disease. *J Med Genet* 2004; **41**: e105.

26 Gouya L, Puy H, Robreau AM *et al.* The penetrance of dominant erythropoietic protoporphyria is modulated by expression of wildtype FECH. *Nat Genet* 2002; **30**: 27–8.

27 Gouya L, Martin-Schmitt C, Robreau AM *et al.* Contribution of a common single-nucleotide polymorphism to the genetic predisposition for erythropoietic protoporphyria. *Am J Hum Genet* 2006; **78**: 2–14.

28 McGuire BM, Bonkovsky HL, Carithers RL Jr *et al.* Liver transplantation for erythropoietic protoporphyria liver disease. *Liver Transpl* 2005; **11**: 1590–6.

29 Wahlin S, Aschan J, Bjornstedt M *et al.* Curative bone marrow transplantation in erythropoietic protoporphyria after reversal of severe cholestasis. *J Hepatol* 2007; **46**: 174–9.

30 Rand EB, Bunin N, Cochran W, Ruchelli E *et al.* Sequential liver and bone marrow transplantation for treatment of erythropoietic protoporphyria. *Pediatrics* 2006; **118**: e1896–9.

31 Doss MO, Frank M. Hepatobiliary implications and complications in protoporphyria, a 20-year study. *Clin Biochem* 1989; **22**: 223–9.

Porphyrias that cause cutaneous disease and acute attacks

Hereditary coproporphyria

Like VP, this porphyria presents from puberty onwards. The skin is not affected in most patients suffering from this rare acute porphyria but around 10–20% [1] of patients have cutaneous involvement with fragility and blistering in sun-exposed areas, indistinguishable from that seen in PCT or VP. The skin disease may be triggered or exacerbated by intercurrent liver disease [2]. HC is caused by an autosomal dominant inherited deficiency of coproporphyrinogen oxidase. The biochemical findings are of a 615–620 nm peak on plasma spectrofluorimetry, increased uro- and coproporphyrin concentrations in urine, and increased coproporphyrin in faeces. Predominance of the type III isomer in faeces is a sensitive indicator of HC [1]. Rare variants include a homozygous form characterized by short stature, acute attacks and skin changes with prominent hypertrichosis and pigmentation [3], and harderoporphyria which causes haemolysis in the neonate or bullae.

References

1 Kuhnel A, Gross U, Doss MO. Hereditary coproporphyria in Germany: clinical-biochemical studies in 53 patients. *Clin Biochem* 2000; **33**: 465–73.

2 Hawk JL, Magnus IA, Parkes A *et al.* Deficiency of hepatic coproporphyrinogen oxidase in hereditary coproporphyria. *J R Soc Med* 1978; **71**: 775–7.

3 Grandchamp B, Phung N, Nordmann Y. Homozygous case of hereditary coproporphyria. *Lancet* 1977; **2**: 1348–9.

Variegate porphyria

Definition. A rare inherited disease usually characterized by photo-induced skin fragility and blistering, which may cause acute attacks.

Aetiology and incidence. VP is caused by an autosomal dominant inherited deficiency of protoporphyrinogen oxidase. In addition to causing photosensitization, accumulated coproporphyrinogen and protoporphyrinogen also inhibit PBG deaminase, the probable mechanism for acute attacks in VP [1]. In South Africa, VP is common (due to a founder effect) with a prevalence in whites and Afrikaner-descended non-whites of 1/200. Elsewhere the prevalence is around 0.5–1/100000 [2]. At least 80% of South African carriers of a pathogenic VP mutation are completely asymptomatic [3].

Pathogenesis of skin lesions in VP. It is perhaps unexpected that the accumulated copro- and protoporphyrin should cause PCT-like upper dermal blistering rather than EPP-like acute pain. This is likely to be because, although hydrophobic porphyrins predominate in plasma, hydrophilic porphyrins, especially uroporphyrin, predominate in the skin. This local accumulation is thought to result from secondary local photo-inactivation of UROD in the skin by coproporphyrin [3]. In addition, the protoporphyrin in VP is conjugated to a peptide which may reduce its phototoxicity.

Clinical features [2–4]

Skin. Of those patients with symptomatic VP, around 70% of patients have cutaneous involvement, and only around 17% of these patients will ever suffer an acute attack [5]. VP only very rarely presents before puberty, and usually the skin disease begins in adolescence or young adulthood. Patients describe skin fragility, usually fairly mild, affecting sun-exposed skin particularly on the backs of the hands [2,3]. The skin disease is generally indistinguishable from PCT, with painful tense bullae occurring in sun-exposed skin, as well as scarring, pigmentary abnormalities, sometimes pseudosclerodermatous changes of the hands and fingers, and occasionally photo-onycholysis. However, a significant number of patients do not describe worsening in the summer, and the patients who do describe seasonal variation often have their worst problems in late summer and autumn. In addition, around half of patients with VP describe mild, transient, light-related eruptions in the early summer. The examination findings of scarring, patches of hypo- and hyperpigmentation at sites of blisters, milia and mild hypertrichosis particularly around the eyes, are indistinguishable from PCT. Intercurrent biliary obstruction exacerbates the cutaneous disease since the accumulated porphyrins are excreted into the bile. Acute photosensitivity can occur in patients with disturbed liver function. Hormonally induced hepatic dysfunction may explain the exacerbations of skin disease seen in females taking oral contraceptives and during pregnancy. VP sometimes goes into clinical and biochemical remission in old age.

Acute attacks [2,3,5,6]. As in other acute porphyrias, women are three times as frequently affected as men, and 70% of acute attacks occur between the ages of 20 and 40 years. Around 17% of patients with cutaneous VP ever suffer an acute attack; the number has declined recently due to improved use of prophylactic measures. The severity of acute attacks varies from mild abdominal pain, sometimes accompanied by vomiting and constipation, through to very severe attacks with bulbar palsy and respiratory paralysis. The presentation, diagnosis and management of acute attacks is covered in the section on acute attacks of porphyria, p. 59.7.

Homozygous VP [7]. In this disease, a mutation on both proto-porphyrinogen oxidase alleles results in an enzyme activity less than 20% of normal, compared to the 50% in other VP patients. In homozygous VP, fragility, bullae and often hypertrichosis develop in exposed (and sometimes non-exposed) skin in neonates or infants and the skin disease may be severe. Delayed development, epilepsy, sensory neuropathy, nystagmus, various hand deformities and growth retardation also commonly occur. Acute attacks do not occur in these patients. The biochemical findings are the same as in VP, except for the lower enzyme activity.

Differential diagnosis. VP cutaneous disease is easily distinguished from non-photosensitive blistering disorders. It can be clinically very similar to PCT, late-onset CEP, HC and pseudoporphyria. Biochemical analysis is required to diagnose VP.

Biochemical findings. A plasma spectrofluorimetry peak around 626 nm (caused by a porphyrin–protein complex) is diagnostic of VP in the absence of a raised free red cell protoporphyrin level, and is present in virtually all symptomatic cases of VP. It may persist during periods of clinical remission when faecal excretion becomes normal and is a more sensitive test than measurement of faecal porphyrins [8]. A persistently normal faecal protoporphyrin concentration in adulthood in patients with the VP genetic defect has been proposed as a prognostic marker indicating a greater likelihood of the VP never causing any clinical problems and staying clinically latent [6]. The urine contains increased levels of coproporphyrin, and increased concentrations of copro- and protoporphyrin are found in faeces. In a few patients, the urine shows the typical PCT pattern of uroporphyrin accompanied by hepta- and sometimes hexa- and pentacarboxylic acid porphyrins, a situation known as 'dual porphyria' [9]. Thus, urinary analysis alone can result in the misdiagnosis of VP as PCT, with potentially disastrous consequences. During acute attacks, urinary PBG (and ALA) are raised. The urinary PBG usually falls to normal within weeks of the attack resolving, but may stay a little increased outside the context of an acute attack [10].

Treatment. The key to successful management of the skin disease is photoprotection with sun avoidance using clothes, hats and gloves. Opaque sunscreens, containing pigmentary grade titanium dioxide or zinc oxide sometimes with the addition of iron oxide, are protective against Soret wavelength light [11,12]. The skin disease is rarely severe enough to require filter films for car and home windows. Since the relationship between sun exposure and skin lesions is not obvious, the role of light in producing the skin lesions should be explained to the patient. β-Carotene and canthaxanthin have also been claimed to provide limited protection in some patients, and UVB phototherapy may also be of value [3]. If liver function tests indicate biliary obstruction, relief of this will reduce cutaneous symptoms. The risk of acute attacks is the key issue for safe management of patients and their families. Patients should be directed to a list of drugs to avoid [13,14], including those which can induce attacks, and also those known to induce cholestasis, and cannabis; they should also be advised to wear an emergency identification bracelet, to avoid low calorie diets, and to become teetotal. Liver transplantation has been successfully used to cure variegate porphyria (and acute intermittent porphyria) in cases where acute attacks are frequent, severe and uncontrollable by medical means [15].

Genetic counselling. It is important to identify relatives who have latent VP because of the risk of acute attacks. The plasma 624–626 nm peak is found in the majority of cases of latent VP but only from teenage onwards. A positive plasma fluorimetry result is diagnostic of latent VP but a negative result is uninformative [16,17]. The only completely reliable way to identify those carrying the VP gene defect if the plasma scan is negative is to identify the protoporphyrinogen oxidase gene mutation in the index case and then assess its presence or absence in relatives. This is labour intensive because, outside South Africa, most families have their own private mutation. Relatives found to have the gene defect are at a low risk (roughly 5–10%) of acute attacks and should take all the precautions taken by any patient diagnosed with an acute porphyria. The risk of a patient passing the mutated gene on to each offspring is 50%, and around 20% of those carrying the mutation will eventually develop symptoms of some sort.

References

1 Meissner P, Adams P, Kirsch R. Allosteric inhibition of human lymphoblast and purified porphobilinogen deaminase by protoporphyrinogen and coproporphyrinogen. A possible mechanism for the acute attack of variegate porphyria. *J Clin Invest* 1993; **91**: 1436–44.

2 Mustajoki P. Variegate porphyria. Twelve years' experience in Finland. *QJM* 1980; **49**: 191–203.

3 Day RS. Variegate porphyria. *Semin Dermatol* 1986; **5**: 138–54.

4 Timonen K, Niemi KM, Mustajoki P, Tenhunen R. Skin changes in variegate porphyria. Clinical, histopathological, and ultrastructural study. *Arch Dermatol Res* 1990; **282**: 108–14.

5 Elder GH, Hift RJ, Meissner PN. The acute porphyrias. *Lancet* 1997; **349**: 1613–7.

6 von und zu Fraunberg M, Timonen K *et al.* Clinical and biochemical characteristics and genotype-phenotype correlation in Finnish variegate porphyria patients. *Eur J Hum Genet* 2002; **10**: 649–57.

7 Hift RJ, Meissner PN, Todd G *et al.* Homozygous variegate porphyria: an evolving clinical syndrome. *Postgrad Med J* 1993; **69**: 781–6.

8 Hift RJ, Davidson BP, van der Hooft C *et al.* Plasma fluorescence scanning and fecal porphyrin analysis for the diagnosis of variegate porphyria: precise determination of sensitivity and specificity with detection of protoporphyrinogen oxidase mutations as a reference standard. *Clin Chem* 2004; **50**: 915–23.

9 Sturrock ED, Meissner PN, Maeder DL, Kirsch RE. Uroporphyrinogen decarboxylase and protoporphyrinogen oxidase in dual porphyria. *S Afr Med J* 1989; **76**: 405–8.

10 Deacon A. The porphyrias and their investigation. *CPD Bull Clin Biochem* 1999; **1**: 122–6.

11 Moseley H, Cameron H, MacLeod T *et al.* New sunscreens confer improved protection for photosensitive patients in the blue light region. *Br J Dermatol* 2001; **145**: 789–94.

12 Kaye ET, Levin JA, Blank IH *et al.* Efficiency of opaque photoprotective agents in the visible light range. *Arch Dermatol* 1991; **127**: 351–5.

13 Welsh Medicines Information Centre. http://www.wmic.wales.nhs.uk.

14 European Porphyria Initiative/The European Porphyria NETwork. http://www.porphyria-europe.com.

15 Stojeba N, Meyer C, Jeanpierre C *et al.* Recovery from a variegate porphyria by a liver transplantation. *Liver Transpl* 2004; **10**: 935–8.

16 Long C, Smyth SJ, Woolf J *et al.* Detection of latent variegate porphyria by fluorescence emission spectroscopy of plasma. *Br J Dermatol* 1993; **129**: 9–13.

17 Da Silva V, Simonin S, Deybach JC *et al.* Variegate porphyria: diagnostic value of fluorometric scanning of plasma porphyrins. *Clin Chim Acta* 1995; **238**: 163–8.

Mucinoses [1–5]

S.M. Breathnach, pp. 59.21–59.30

Mucins are jelly-like acid glycosaminoglycans (formerly known as mucopolysaccharides) of the ground substances and probably play a part in the extravascular exchange of metabolites. Mucin is normally produced in small quantities by fibroblasts. Acid glycosaminoglycans, such as hyaluronic acid and heparin, stain with toluidine blue, colloidal iron, or with Alcian blue at pH 2.5, the coloration depending on the number and nature of the acid groups [6]. Periodic acid Schiff (PAS) stains heparin, but not hyaluronic acid. In general, acid glycosaminoglycans stain much brighter in frozen fixed tissue, or in specimens preserved in 1% cetylpyridinium chloride solution [7], rather than in formalin-fixed biopsies [8].

Neutral glycosaminoglycans are glycoproteins in which the hexosamine sugar polymer is incorporated in a protein chain. Hale and Alcian blue stains are negative but PAS stain is positive. The mucins in the skin and their histochemistry have been well reviewed [9]. Histopathological examination of many cutaneous mucinoses reveals that collagen fibres are fragmented [10].

Classification of the cutaneous mucinoses [1–5]

Mucinous infiltration of the skin is found in many widely differing disorders, some affecting the skin only, others related to systemic disease [1–5,11]. The association of HIV infection with lichen myxoedematosus seems to be more than coincidental [12]. They can be classified as shown in Table 59.2.

Table 59.2 Classification of the cutaneous mucinoses.

Primary

Diffuse (degenerative-inflammatory mucinoses):
Generalized myxoedema (Chapter 62)
Pretibial myxoedema (Chapter 62)
Lichen myxoedematosus (papular mucinosis, scleromyxoedema)
   Acral persistent papular mucinosis
   Cutaneous papular mucinosis of infancy
   Self-healing papular cutaneous mucinosis; juvenile and adult
Hereditary progressive mucinous histiocytosis
Reticular erythematous mucinosis (plaque-like mucinosis)
Scleredema (Chapter 51)

Follicular forms:
Follicular mucinosis (alopecia mucinosa)
Urticaria-like follicular mucinosis

Focal (neoplastic-hamartomatous mucinoses):
Cutaneous focal mucinosis
Mucous (myxoid) cyst
Mucinous naevus
Secondary
Papular and nodular mucinosis associated with lupus erythematosus
Collagen vascular diseases (especially dermatomyositis, lupus erythematosus)
Malignant atrophic papulosis (Degos' syndrome) [13]
Papular mucinosis in L-tryptophan-induced eosinophilia–myalgia syndrome
Papular mucinosis of the toxic oil syndrome
Mucinosis accompanying mesenchymal and neural tumours

References

1 Rongioletti F, Rebora A. The new cutaneous mucinoses: a review with an up-to-date classification of cutaneous mucinoses. *J Am Acad Dermatol* 1991; **24**: 265–70.

2 Stephens CJM, McKee PH, Black MM. The dermal mucinoses. *Adv Dermatol* 1993; **8**: 201–27.

3 Truhan AP, Roenigk HH. The cutaneous mucinoses. *J Am Acad Dermatol* 1986; **14**: 1–18.

4 Rongioletti F, Rebora A. Updated classification of papular mucinosis, lichen myxedematosus, and scleromyxedema. *J Am Acad Dermatol* 2001; **44**: 273–81.

5 Rongioletti F, Rebora A. Cutaneous mucinoses: microscopic criteria for diagnosis. *Am J Dermatopathol* 2001; **23**: 257–67.

6 Scott JE, Dorling J. Differential staining of acid glycosaminoglycans (mucopolysaccharides) by alcian blue in salt solutions. *Histochemie* 1965; **5**: 221–3.

7 Matsuoka LY, Wortsmann J, Dietrich JG. Glycosaminoglycans in histologic sections. *Arch Dermatol* 1987; **123**: 862–3.

8 Cole HG, Winkelmann RK. Acid mucopolysaccharide staining in scleredema. *J Cutan Pathol* 1990; **17**: 211–3.

9 Wells GC. Mucins in the skin and their histochemistry. *Trans Rep St John's Hosp Derm Soc Lond* 1962; **48**: 35–9.

10 Alves MF, Filgueira AL, Lorena DE, Porto LC. Type I and type III collagens in cutaneous mucinosis. *Am J Dermatopathol* 1998; **20**: 41–7.

11 Reed RJ, Clark WH, Mihm MC. The cutaneous mucinoses. *Hum Pathol* 1973; **4**: 201–5.

12 Rongioletti F, Ghigliotti G, De Marchi R, Rebora A. Cutaneous mucinoses and HIV infection. *Br J Dermatol* 1998; **139**: 1077–80.

13 Black MM. Malignant atrophic papulosis (Degos' syndrome). *Br J Dermatol* 1971; **85**: 290–2.

Lichen myxoedematosus

Synonyms
- Papular mucinosis
- Lichen fibromucinodosis
- Scleromyxoedema

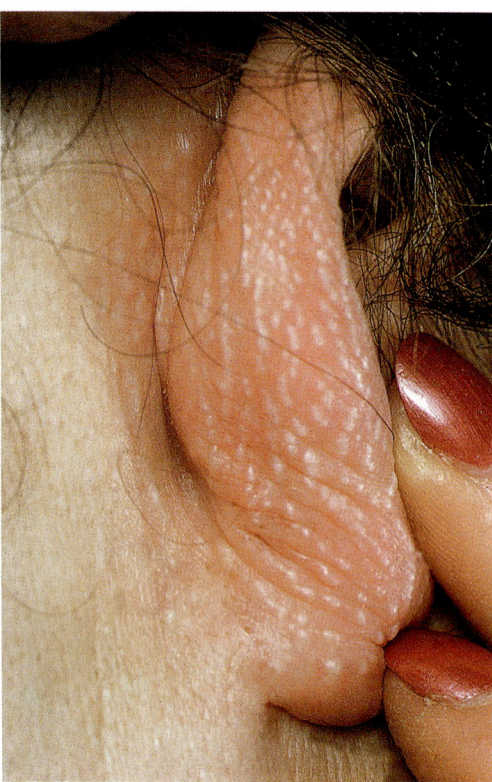

Fig. 59.13 Lichen myxoedematosus. Close-up of micropapules behind earlobe. (Courtesy of St Thomas' Hospital, London, UK.)

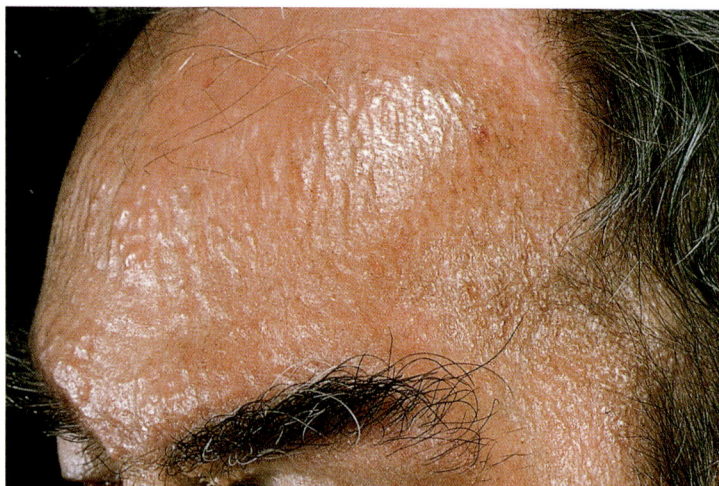

Fig. 59.14 Scleromyxoedema. View of forehead showing sclerodermoid appearance and linear papulation. (Courtesy of St Thomas' Hospital, London, UK.)

Lichen myxoedematosus is a cutaneous myxoedematous condition characterized by formation of numerous lichenoid papules which coalesce to form generalized plaques, causing extensive thickening and hardening of the skin [1–3] (Fig. 59.13). It is a rare disorder characterized by proliferation of fibroblasts with fibrosis and excessive deposition of acid glycosaminoglycans in the skin, and is distinct from scleroderma [4].

It has been proposed [2,3] that there are really only two main divisions of lichen myxoedematosus: (i) a generalized papular and sclerodermoid form (scleromyxoedema) with systemic, even lethal, manifestations; and (ii) a localized form, without a demonstrable paraprotein, which runs a more benign course. The localized form in turn is subdivided into five subtypes: (i) a discrete papular form involving any site [5]; (ii) acral persistent papular mucinosis involving only the extensor surface of the hands and wrists [6]; (iii) papular mucinosis of infancy, a paediatric variant of the discrete form or the acral form of persistent papular mucinosis; (iv) self-healing papular mucinosis, of juvenile and adult types; and (v) a nodular form.

A third group of atypical or intermediate forms, not meeting the criteria for either scleromyxoedema or the localized form, includes cases of (i) scleromyxoedema without monoclonal gammopathy; (ii) localized forms with monoclonal gammopathy and/or systemic symptoms; (iii) localized forms with mixed features of the subtypes; and (iv) poorly-specified cases and a localized papular form.

Scleromyxoedema is usually associated with a monoclonal gammopathy. Serum from patients with lichen myxoedematosus, even after elution of the IgG paraprotein, can stimulate synthesis of DNA and cell proliferation in cultured fibroblasts [7].

Histopathology [2,8,9]. Mucinous deposits occur in the middle and deeper layers of the dermis, where they displace collagen fibres, but do not involve the dermal papillae or accumulate around blood vessels. Histochemically, the mucinous deposits are heterogeneous mixtures of acid glycosaminoglycans, which stain positively with Alcian blue and toluidine blue. Large, stellate, elongated fibroblasts are present within the mucinous stroma [10]. Mucin deposition in the media and adventitia of vessels and in many organs including the myocardium is reported, and the skeletal muscles may be infiltrated with lymphocytes [11].

Clinical features [1,12–14]. In scleromyxoedema (the Arndt–Gottron syndrome) the pattern of lichen myxoedematosus is confluent, papular and sclerotic. Diffuse thickening of the skin underlies the papules. The facial features may be distorted by exaggeration of the facial ridges (Fig. 59.14), and flexion of the fingers may be limited. Multiple periorbital myxomas may progress to scleromyxoedema [15]. The involvement of the hands may simulate the sclerodactyly of scleroderma (Fig. 59.15), but the clinical appearance of numerous small papules of more or less uniform size, often in linear patterns on an erythematous and palpably thickened background, is very distinctive.

No endocrine abnormalities have been demonstrated, but cardiovascular abnormalities may occur in 10% of cases [8], whereas others may complain of extreme muscular weakness and lassitude due to myopathic or neurological involvement [16]. Occasionally, systemic involvement may occur in other internal organs [17].

An IgG class paraproteinaemia is almost always found on serum electrophoresis, although total serum protein values are usually normal [1,18]. Bone marrow studies may show a mild plasmacytic infiltration. Radiological survey of the skeletal system is normal. In one case, acid glycosaminoglycan levels in the serum were elevated [19].

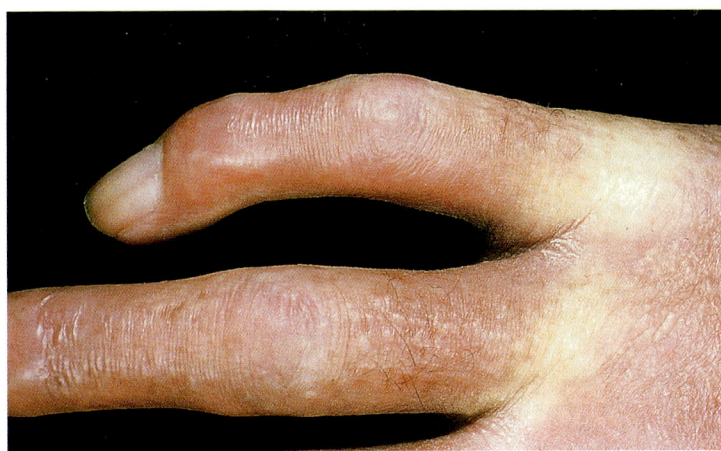

Fig. 59.15 Scleromyxoedema. Sclerodermoid appearance of finger. Same patient as shown in Fig. 59.14. (Courtesy of St Thomas' Hospital, London, UK.)

Localized lichen myxoedematosus is characterized by small, firm, waxy papules of limited distribution [1], although a rare nodular form has larger lesions.

Diagnosis. Infiltrates appearing in and around old scars may simulate 'scar sarcoidosis'. Papules on the dorsa of the hands and ears may cause confusion with granuloma annulare. Systemic scleroderma may show many features simulating scleromyxoedema. However, in scleroderma the skin is thickened and bound-down, whereas in scleromyxoedema it is also thickened but moveable over the subcutis. Papules are absent in scleroedema and scleroderma, but common in scleromyxoedema. Nephrogenic systemic fibrosis, previously known as nephrogenic fibrosing dermopathy, a fibromucinous scleromyxoedema-like disorder associated with renal dysfunction, has been linked to administration of gadolinium-based contrast medium (see Chapter 75).

Prognosis. The prognosis of scleromyxoedema is poor despite a multiplicity of potential treatments. Death may result from non-specific complications such as bronchopneumonia, coronary occlusion or from haematological malignancies.

Treatment. The potential for spontaneous long-term regression renders treatment of scleromyxoedema difficult to assess [20]. Localized lichen myxoedematosus of the discrete type has been treated with tacrolimus ointment [21]. Topical betamethasone and dimethylsulphoxide (DMSO) has produced regression in one case [22]. Systemic steroids alone may be ineffective [23,24]. Oral aromatic retinoids produce inconsistent but occasionally successful results [25,26]. Thalidomide has been advocated [27–29], as has interferon-α [30]. Plasmapheresis can be beneficial if combined with pulsed corticosteroid and/or immunosuppressive therapy [31,32]. Other therapies reported to be successful in isolated cases include extracorporeal photochemotherapy [33,34], intravenous immunoglobulin [35–37] and electron-beam therapy [38]. High-dose melphalan chemotherapy with autologous stem cell transplantation offers durable remission in most patients [39–41]. Aggressive surgical intervention for palliation of severe aesthetic and functional disability may be indicated [42].

References

1 Montgomery H, Underwood LJ. Lichen myxedematosus (differentiation from cutaneous myxedemas or mucoid states). *J Invest Dermatol* 1953; **20**: 213–36.

2 Rongioletti F, Rebora A. Updated classification of papular mucinosis, lichen myxedematosus, and scleromyxedema. *J Am Acad Dermatol* 2001; **44**: 273–81.

3 Rongioletti F. Lichen myxedematosus (papular mucinosis): new concepts and perspectives for an old disease. *Semin Cutan Med Surg* 2006; **25**: 100–4.

4 Jablonska S, Blaszczyk M. Scleromyxedema is a scleroderma-like disorder and not a coexistence of scleroderma with papular mucinosis. *Eur J Dermatol* 1999; **9**: 551–4.

5 Poswig A, Hinrichs R, Megahed M *et al.* Discrete papular mucinosis—a rare subtype of lichen myxoedematosus. *Clin Exp Dermatol* 2000; **25**: 289–92.

6 Rebora A, Rongioletti F. Acral persistent papular mucinosis and lichen myxoedematosus. *Dermatology* 1992; **185**: 81.

7 Harper RA, Rispler J. Lichen myxedematosus serum stimulating human skin fibroblast proliferation. *Science* 1978; **199**: 545–7.

8 McCuiston CH, Schoch EP. Autopsy findings in lichen myxedematosus. *Arch Dermatol* 1956; **74**: 259–62.

9 Rongioletti F, Rebora A. Cutaneous mucinoses: microscopic criteria for diagnosis. *Am J Dermatopathol* 2001; **23**: 257–67.

10 Matsuoka LY, Wortsman J, Carlisle KS *et al.* The acquired cutaneous mucinoses. *Arch Intern Med* 1984; **144**: 1974–80.

11 Dirneen AM, Dicken CH. Scleromyxedema. *J Am Acad Dermatol* 1995; **33**: 37–43.

12 Cokonis Georgakis CD, Falasca G, Georgakis A, Heymann WR. Scleromyxedema. *Clin Dermatol* 2006; **24**: 493–7.

13 Heymann WR. Scleromyxedema. *J Am Acad Dermatol* 2007; **57**: 890–1.

14 Perry HO, Montgomery H, Stickney JM. Further observations on lichen myxedematosus. *Ann Intern Med* 1960; **53**: 955–69.

15 Craig NM, Putterman AM, Roenigk RK *et al.* Multiple periorbital cutaneous myxomas progressing to scleromyxedema. *J Am Acad Dermatol* 1996; **34**: 928–30.

16 Rothe MJ, Rivas R, Gauld E *et al.* Scleromyxedema and severe myositis. *Int J Dermatol* 1989; **28**: 657–60.

17 Truhan AP, Roenigk HH. Lichen myxedematosus: an unusual case with rapid progression and possible internal involvement. *Int J Dermatol* 1987; **26**: 91–5.

18 Ayala F, Balato N, Ceparano S *et al.* Immunochemical characterization of the abnormal paraprotein in a case of scleromyxoedema. *Clin Exp Dermatol* 1984; **9**: 351–7.

19 Rudner EJ, Mehregan A, Pinkus H. Scleromyxedema. *Arch Dermatol* 1966; **93**: 3–12.

20 Boffa MJ, Ead RD. Spontaneous improvement of scleromyxoedema. *Clin Exp Dermatol* 1995; **20**: 157–60.

21 Rongioletti F, Zaccaria E, Cozzani E, Parodi A. Treatment of localized lichen myxedematosus of discrete type with tacrolimus ointment. *J Am Acad Dermatol* 2008; **58**: 530–2.

22 Bonnetblanc JM, Bedane C. Regression of scleromyxoedema with topical betamethasone and dimethyl sulfoxide: a 30-month follow-up. *Arch Dermatol* 1991; **127**: 1733–4.

23 Kreuter A, Altmeyer P. High-dose dexamethasone in scleromyxedema: report of 2 additional cases. *J Am Acad Dermatol* 2005; **53**: 739–40.

24 Lin YC, Wang HC, Shen JL. Scleromyxedema: an experience using treatment with systemic corticosteroid and review of the published work. *J Dermatol* 2006; **33**: 207–10.

25 Milam CP, Cohen LE, Fenske NA *et al.* Scleromyxoedema: therapeutic response to isotretinoin in three patients. *J Am Acad Dermatol* 1988; **19**: 469–77.

26 Hisler BM, Savoy LB, Hashimoto K. Improvement of scleromyxoedema associated with isotretinoin therapy. *J Am Acad Dermatol* 1991; **24**: 854–7.

27 Sansbury JC, Cocuroccia B, Jorizzo JL *et al.* Treatment of recalcitrant scleromyxedema with thalidomide in 3 patients. *J Am Acad Dermatol* 2004; **51**: 126–31.

28 Amini-Adle M, Thieulent N, Dalle S *et al.* Scleromyxedema: successful treatment with thalidomide in two patients. *Dermatology* 2007; **214**: 58–60.

29 Martins A, Paiva Lopes MJ, Tavares Belo R, Rodrigues JC. Scleromyxedema—thalidomide therapy. *J Eur Acad Dermatol Venereol* 2008; **22**: 622–4.

30 Tschen JA, Chang JR. Scleromyxedema: treatment with interferon alfa. *J Am Acad Dermatol* 1999; **40**: 303–7.

31 Keong CH, Asaka Y, Fukuro S *et al*. Successful treatment of scleromyxoedema with plasmapheresis and immunosuppression. *J Am Acad Dermatol* 1990; **22**: 842–4.

32 Nieves DS, Bondi EE, Wallmark J *et al*. Scleromyxedema: successful treatment of cutaneous and neurologic symptoms. *Cutis* 2000; **65**: 89–92.

33 Berkson M, Lazarus GS, Uberti-Benz M, Rook AH. Extracorporeal photo-chemotherapy: a potentially useful treatment for scleromyxoedema. *J Am Acad Dermatol* 1991; **25**: 724.

34 D'Incan M, Franck F, Kanold J *et al*. Cutaneo-systemic papulosclerotic mucinosis (scleromyxedema): remission after extracorporeal photochemotherapy and corticoid bolus. *Ann Dermatol Vénéréol* 2001; **128**: 38–41.

35 Gholam P, Hartmann M, Enk A. Arndt-Gottron scleromyxedema: successful therapy with intravenous immunoglobulins. *Br J Dermatol* 2007; **157**: 1058–60.

36 Körber A, Franckson T, Grabbe S, Dissemond J. Successful therapy of scleromyxoedema Arndt-Gottron with low-dose intravenous immunoglobulin. *J Eur Acad Dermatol Venereol* 2007; **21**: 553–4.

37 Blum M, Wigley FM, Hummers LK. Scleromyxedema: a case series highlighting long-term outcomes of treatment with intravenous immunoglobulin (IVIG). *Medicine (Baltimore)* 2008; **87**: 10–20.

38 Koeppel Rampino M, Garibaldi E, Ragona R, Ricardi U. Scleromyxedema: treatment of widespread cutaneous involvement by total skin electron-beam therapy. *Int J Dermatol* 2007; **46**: 864–7.

39 Lacy MQ, Hogan WJ, Gertz MA *et al*. Successful treatment of scleromyxedema with autologous peripheral blood stem cell transplantation. *Arch Dermatol* 2005; **141**: 1277–82.

40 Donato ML, Feasel AM, Weber DM *et al*. Scleromyxedema: role of high-dose melphalan with autologous stem cell transplantation. *Blood* 2006; **107**: 463–6.

41 Iranzo P, López-Lerma I, Bladé J *et al*. Scleromyxoedema treated with autologous stem cell transplantation. *J Eur Acad Dermatol Venereol* 2007; **21**: 129–30.

42 Elliott MP, Dooley P. Scleromyxedema (papular mucinosis): a surgical perspective. *Ann Plast Surg* 1998; **41**: 436–9.

Acral persistent papular mucinosis

Acral persistent papular mucinosis has been proposed as a distinct form of cutaneous mucinosis [1–4]. The characteristic findings include discrete papules or annular lesions on the extensor surfaces of the hands, wrists and forearms, mucinous deposits within the dermis, persisting for several years, and usually an absence of systemic abnormalities. However, a monoclonal IgA of kappa light chain isotype was detected in one case [5]. Familial occurrence has been reported in two sisters [6]. The accumulation of lysosomal structures in acral persistent papular mucinosis may be a distinctive feature of the disorder [7]. However, it is still debatable whether acral persistent papular mucinosis is a distinct entity [8] or whether it is a variant of the discrete papular form of lichen myxoedematosus [1]. A case resembling acral persistent papular mucinosis has been described in which transient carpal tunnel syndrome appeared, suggesting that extracutaneous involvement might occur [9]. 'Aypical' soft minuscule mucinous papules occurred localized to the axillae of a mother and her (identical) twin daughters; again, it is difficult to classify this entity [10].

References

1 Flowers SL, Cooper PH, Landes HB. Acral persistent papular mucinosis. *J Am Acad Dermatol* 1989; **21**: 293–7.

2 Rongioletti F, Rebora A. Acral persistent papular mucinosis: a new entity. *Arch Dermatol* 1986; **122**: 1237–9.

3 Barba A, Maruccia A, D'Onghia FS. Persistent acral papulous mucinosis. *Ann Dermatol Vénéréol* 1996; **123**: 256–8.

4 Harris JE, Purcell SM, Griffin TD. Acral persistent papular mucinosis. *J Am Acad Dermatol* 2004; **51**: 982–8.

5 Borradori L, Aractingi S, Blanc F *et al*. Acral persistent papular mucinosis and IgA monoclonal gammapathy: report of a case. *Dermatology* 1992; **185**: 134–6.

6 Menni S, Cavicchim S, Brezzi A *et al*. Acral persistent papular mucinosis in two sisters. *Clin Exp Dermatol* 1995; **20**: 431–3.

7 Heikki JA, Forsten Y, Hopsu-Havo VK. Ultrastructural signs of altered intracellular metabolism in acral persistent papular mucinosis. *J Cutan Pathol* 1991; **18**: 347–52.

8 Fosko SW, Perez MI, Longley BJ. Acral persistent papular mucinosis. *J Am Acad Dermatol* 1992; **27**: 1026–9.

9 Stephens CJM, Ross JS, Charles-Holmes R *et al*. An unusual case of transient papular mucinosis associated with carpal tunnel syndrome. *Br J Dermatol* 1993; **129**: 89–91.

10 Scheidegger EP, Itin P, Kempf W. Familial occurrence of axillary papular mucinosis. *Eur J Dermatol* 2005; **15**: 70–2.

Papular mucinosis of infancy [1–4]

In this rare condition, opalescent papules may be noted at birth [2] or develop a few months later [1,3]. The papules are scattered on the dorsa of the hands or around the elbows, and may have a linear distribution [2]. Focal mucinous material is deposited in the papillary dermis without overt fibroblast proliferation. It is not clear what the long-term outlook of cutaneous mucinosis of infancy is, but some cases appear to progress [3]. Thus, certain cases of cutaneous mucinosis of infancy are in fact the infantile presentation of lichen myxoedematosus [5].

References

1 Lum D. Cutaneous mucinosis of infancy. *Arch Dermatol* 1980; **116**: 198–200.

2 McGrae JD. Cutaneous mucinosis of infancy: a congenital and linear variant. *Arch Dermatol* 1983; **119**: 272–3.

3 Carapeto FJ, Charlez L, Marron J *et al*. Infantile and progressive papular mucinosis. *Pediatr Dermatol* 1987; **4**: 62.

4 Velho GC, Oliveira M, Alves R *et al*. Childhood cutaneous mucinosis. *J Eur Acad Dermatol Venereol* 1998; **10**: 164–6.

5 Podda M, Rongioletti F, Greiner D *et al*. Cutaneous mucinosis of infancy: is it a real entity or the paediatric form of lichen myxoedematosus (papular mucinosis)? *Br J Dermatol* 2001; **144**: 590–3.

Self-healing papular mucinosis; juvenile and adult

Self-healing juvenile cutaneous mucinosis [1–5] is a rare disorder characterized by an early age of onset accompanied by inflammatory phenomena and spontaneous resolution over a few months. The condition has also been reported in a child undergoing chemotherapy for nephroblastoma [6], and in two brothers [7]. Clinically, there are papules, nodules or plaques with a predilection for the head and trunk rather than the extremities. Histologically, there is dermal mucinosis and a mild increase in fibroblasts and mast cells. It is postulated that a temporary alteration of fibroblast synthetic function occurs, possibly as a result of a viral infection. Rare cases of self-healing cutaneous mucinosis have been reported in adults [8–10].

References

1 Pucevich MV, Latour DL, Bale GF *et al*. Self-healing juvenile cutaneous mucinosis. *J Am Acad Dermatol* 1984; **11**: 327–32.

2 Kim YJ, Kim YT, Kim JH. Self-healing juvenile cutaneous mucinosis. *J Am Acad Dermatol* 1994; **31**: 815–6.

3 Aydingoz IE, Candan I, Dervent B. Self-healing juvenile cutaneous mucinosis. *Dermatology* 1999; **199**: 57–9.

4 Cowen EW, Scott GA, Mercurio MG. Self-healing juvenile cutaneous mucinosis. *J Am Acad Dermatol* 2004; **50** (5 Suppl.): S97–100.

5 Nagaraj LV, Fangman W, White WL *et al*. Self-healing juvenile cutaneous mucinosis: cases highlighting subcutaneous/fascial involvement. *J Am Acad Dermatol* 2006; **55**: 1036–43.

6 Wadee S, Roode H, Schulz EJ. Self-healing juvenile cutaneous mucinosis in a patient with nephroblastoma. *Clin Exp Dermatol* 1994; **19**: 90–3.

7 Gonzalez-Ensenat MA, Vicente MA, Castella N *et al.* Self-healing infantile familial cutaneous mucinosis. *Pediatr Dermatol* 1997; **14**: 460–2.

8 Jang KA, Han MH, Choi JH *et al.* Recurrent self-healing cutaneous mucinosis in an adult. *Br J Dermatol* 2000; **143**: 650–1.

9 Sperber BR, Allee J, James WD. Self-healing papular mucinosis in an adult. *J Am Acad Dermatol* 2004; **50**: 121–3.

10 Yokoyama E, Muto M. Adult variant of self-healing papular mucinosis in a patient with rheumatoid arthritis: predominant proliferation of dermal dendritic cells expressing CD34 or factor XIIIa in association with dermal deposition of mucin. *J Dermatol* 2006; **33**: 30–5.

Hereditary progressive mucinous histiocytosis [1]

Hereditary progressive mucinous histiocytosis (MIM 142630) is a rare, probably autosomal dominant, disease in which small skin-coloured papules or nodules begin to appear anywhere in the first decade of life. In contrast to other benign histiocytic skin diseases there is no spontaneous resolution, so that a steadily increasing number of papules is noted. To date the disease has been confined to females. Histologically, the disease is associated with a progressive proliferation of histiocytes (non-X type) and dermal mucinosis but there is no evidence of any known lysosomal storage disease.

Reference

1 Bark K. Hereditary progressive mucinous histiocytosis: immunohistochemical and ultrastructural studies in an additional family. *Arch Dermatol* 1994; **130**: 1300–4.

Cutaneous focal mucinosis [1–3]

Cutaneous focal mucinosis has been accepted as a distinct entity, although recently it has been classified as a superficial angiomyxoma [4,5]. Clinically, it is characterized by a solitary, asymptomatic, flesh-coloured papule or nodule that can occur on the face, trunk or extremities. Histologically, there is localized accumulation of mucin in the dermis with an increased number of fibroblasts. The fibroblasts appear to function as mucoblasts with many large condensing vacuoles or secretory granules in their cytoplasm [2]. It is suggested that cutaneous focal mucinosis arises as a result of a dysfunction of the fibroblasts in a localized area only. If treatment is required, local excision is satisfactory, since recurrence is unusual. The condition may show some overlap with other mucinoses, for example REM syndrome and scleromyxoedema [6].

Focal cutaneous mucinosis forms part of the Birt–Hogg–Dubé syndrome, where it is associated with multiple fibrofolliculomas and a predisposition to renal cancer [7].

Oral focal mucinosis of the tongue, causing a clinically elevated mass, is an uncommon clinicopathological entity which is considered to be the oral counterpart of cutaneous focal mucinosis [8].

References

1 Johnson WC, Helwig EB. Cutaneous focal mucinosis: a clinico-pathological and histochemical study. *Arch Dermatol* 1966; **93**: 13–20.

2 Nishiura S, Mihara M, Shimao S *et al.* Cutaneous focal mucinosis. *Br J Dermatol* 1989; **121**: 511–5.

3 Nebrida ML, Tay YK. Cutaneous focal mucinosis: a case report. *Pediatr Dermatol* 2002; **19**: 33–5.

4 Allen PW, Dymock RB, MacCormac LB. Superficial angiomyxomas with and without epithelial components. *Am J Surg Pathol* 1988; **12**: 519–30.

5 Nakayama H, Hirol M, Kiyoku H *et al.* Superficial angiomyxoma of the right inguinal region: report of a case. *Jpn J Clin Oncol* 1997; **27**: 200–3.

6 Rongioletti F, Amantea A, Balus L *et al.* Cutaneous focal mucinosis associated with reticular erythematous mucinosis and scleromyxoedema. *J Am Acad Dermatol* 1991; **24**: 656–7.

7 Lindor NM, Hand J, Burch PA, Gibson LE. Birt–Hogg–Dubé syndrome: an autosomal dominant disorder with predisposition to cancers of the kidney, fibrofolliculomas, and focal cutaneous mucinosis. *Int J Dermatol* 2001; **40**: 653–6.

8 Soda G, Baiocchini A, Bosco D *et al.* Oral focal mucinosis of the tongue. *Pathol Oncol Res* 1998; **4**: 304–7.

Mucinous naevus

The association of dermal mucinosis in association with a congenital plaque-like lesion in the interscapular area was first reported in a 16-year-old female [1]. In the absence of an overt connective tissue naevus and associated systemic disease, it was felt the lesion represented a congenital cutaneous mucinosis (mucinous naevus). Analysis of further cases suggests that these lesions may be a connective tissue naevus of proteoglycan type, and the only type to contain hyaluronic acid [2].

References

1 Redondo Bellòn PR, Vázquez-Doval J, Idoate M, Quintanilla E. Mucinous nevus. *J Am Acad Dermatol* 1993; **28**: 797–8.

2 Rongioletti F, Rebora A. Mucinous nevus. *Arch Dermatol* 1996; **132**: 1522–3.

Reticular erythematous mucinosis [1]

Synonyms

- REM syndrome
- Plaque-like cutaneous mucinosis [2]

This syndrome comprises areas of reticular erythema on the trunk with a mucinous and round cell infiltrate in the dermis, and is frequently called the REM syndrome. Plaque-like cutaneous mucinosis is essentially the same disease process [3].

Aetiology. The aetiology is unknown, but there is some clinical and also experimental evidence that light is a factor in the pathogenesis of this disorder [4,5]. REM syndrome can be associated with the production of a monoclonal paraprotein, suggesting that the disease may involve disturbance of immune mechanisms [6]. Immunophenotypic studies have suggested a potential overlap between REM syndrome and Jessner's lymphocytic infiltration [7]. An hormonal influence may be operative [8]. Interleukin (IL)-1β may be involved in the abnormal hyaluronic acid metabolism in REM syndrome, as patient fibroblasts exhibit an abnormal response to stimulation by exogenous IL-1β [9]. Rare familial cases have been reported [10].

Pathology. The epidermis appears normal. In the papillary and upper reticular dermis there is a perivascular, and occasionally perifollicular, infiltrate largely composed of small mononuclear cells and populations of FXIIIa+/hyaluronan synthase 2+ dermal dendrocytes, which have been postulated to be responsible for accumulation of hyaluronan, rather than this being derived from fibroblasts [11]. There is separation of collagen bundles and fragmentation of elastic fibres. Histochemical stains show an increase in dermal mucin with a profile consistent with hyaluronic acid [4].

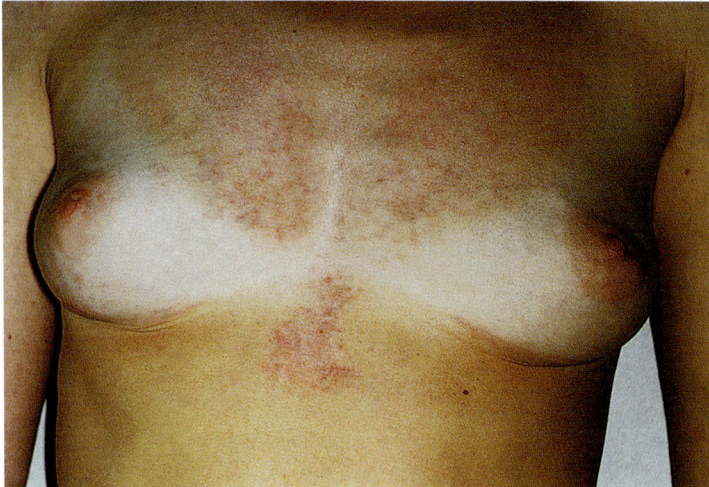

Fig. 59.16 Reticular erythematous mucinosis syndrome. View of anterior chest to show erythematous rash in photodistributed location.

Direct immunofluorescence is usually negative for immunoglobulins, fibrin and complement [4], although granular basement-membrane deposits of IgM, IgA and C3 have been described in isolated cases [5,12].

Clinical features. Most affected patients are female [1,3,4,13] and usually middle aged, but the condition has been reported in children [14]. Areas of pink, reticulate or sheet-like erythema are present on the central part of the chest and back, particularly over the sternum and on the upper back (Fig. 59.16). There is usually no pruritus, although sometimes the areas become itchy following sun exposure, and the erythema may be then more apparent. The areas become infiltrated and then slowly increase in size. Coexisting disorders reported in association with occasional cases of REM syndrome include hyperthyroidism, hypothyroidism, discoid lupus erythematosus, carcinoma and thrombocytopenic purpura [15]. Evolution of REM syndrome to systemic lupus erythematosus has been reported [16]. Mycosis fungoides presenting as reticular erythematous mucinosis has been documented [17].

Treatment. Topical steroids are ineffective, but fortunately antimalarials are almost invariably effective in controlling the eruption [1,4,13]. Ciclosporin appears to be of no value in treating REM syndrome [18]. UVB radiation combined with steroid impregnated tape [19], and use of the pulsed dye laser [20], have been beneficial.

References

1 Steigleder GK, Gartmann H, Linker V. REM syndrome: reticular erythematous mucinosis (round-cell erythematosis): a new entity? *Br J Dermatol* 1974; **91**: 191–9.
2 Perry HO, Kierland RR, Montgomery H. Plaque-like form of cutaneous mucinosis. *Arch Dermatol* 1960; **82**: 980–5.
3 Quimby SR, Perry HO. Plaque-like cutaneous mucinosis: its relationship to reticular erythematous mucinosis. *J Am Acad Dermatol* 1982; **6**: 856–61.
4 Bleehen SS, Slater DN, Mahood J et al. Reticular erythematous mucinosis: light and electron microscopy, immunofluorescence and histochemical findings. *Br J Dermatol* 1982; **106**: 9–18.
5 Dodd HJ, Sarkany I, Sadrudin A. Reticular erythematous mucinosis syndrome. *Clin Exp Dermatol* 1987; **12**: 36–9.

6 Zaki I, Shall L, Millard LG. Reticular erythematous mucinosis syndrome and a monoclonal IgG kappa paraprotein—is there an association? *Br J Dermatol* 1993; **129**: 347–56.
7 Braddock SW, Kay HD, Maemle D et al. Clinical and immunologic studies in reticular erythematous mucinosis and Jessner's lymphocytic infiltrate of skin. *J Am Acad Dermatol* 1993; **28**: 691–5.
8 Sidwell RU, Francis N, Bunker CB. Hormonal influence on reticular erythematous mucinosis. *Br J Dermatol* 2001; **144**: 633–4.
9 Izumi T, Tajima S, Harada R, Nishikawa T. Reticular erythematous mucinosis syndrome: glycosaminoglycan synthesis by fibroblasts and abnormal response to interleukin-1 beta. *Dermatology* 1996; **192**: 41–5.
10 Caputo R, Marzano AV, Tourlaki A, Marchini M. Reticular erythematous mucinosis occurring in a brother and sister. *Dermatology* 2006; **212**: 385–7.
11 Tominaga A, Tajima S, Ishibashi A, Kimata K. Reticular erythematous mucinosis syndrome with an infiltration of factor XIIIa and hyaluronan synthase 2 dermal dendrocytes. *Br J Dermatol* 2001; **145**: 141–5.
12 Del Pozo J, Martinez W, Almagro M et al. Reticular erythematous mucinosis syndrome. Report of a case with positive immunofluorescence. *Clin Exp Dermatol* 1997; **22**: 234–6.
13 Steigleder GK, Kanzow G. Muzinablagerungen in der Dermis und REM syndrom. *Hautarzt* 1980; **31**: 575–83.
14 Cohen PR, Rabinowitz AD, Ruszkowski AM et al. Reticular erythematous mucinosis syndrome: a review of the world literature and report of the syndrome in a pre-pubertal child. *Pediatr Dermatol* 1990; **7**: 1–10.
15 Braddock SW, Davis CS, Davis RB. Reticular erythematosus mucinosis and thrombocytopenic purpura. Report of a case and review of the world literature, including plaque-like cutaneous mucinosis. *J Am Acad Dermatol* 1988; **19**: 859–68.
16 Del Pozo J, Pena C, Almagro M et al. Systemic lupus erythematosus presenting with a reticular erythematous mucinosis-like condition. *Lupus* 2000; **9**: 144–6.
17 Twersky JM, Mutasim DF. Mycosis fungoides presenting as reticular erythematous mucinosis. *Int J Dermatol* 2006; **45**: 230–3.
18 Bulengo-Ramsby SM, Ellis CN, Griffiths CEM et al. Failure of reticular erythematous mucinosis to respond to cyclosporine. *J Am Acad Dermatol* 1992; **27**: 825–8.
19 Yamazaki S, Katayama I, Kurumaji Y et al. Treatment of reticular erythematous mucinosis with a large dose of ultraviolet B radiation and steroid impregnated tape. *J Dermatol* 1999; **26**: 115–8.
20 Greve B, Raulin C. Treating REM syndrome with the pulsed dye laser. *Lasers Surg Med* 2001; **29**: 248–51.

Follicular mucinosis

Synonym
• Alopecia mucinosa

Definition and nomenclature. Follicular mucinosis is an inflammatory disorder characterized clinically by infiltrated plaques with scaling and loss of hair, and histologically by the accumulation of acid glycosaminoglycans in the sebaceous gland and the outer root sheath of the hair follicles. The condition was first described by Pinkus in 1957 [1] under the name alopecia mucinosa, but alopecia is not always evident, especially when only vellus follicles are involved.

Aetiology [2–6]. The cause of follicular mucinosis is unknown, but cell-mediated immune mechanisms may play a role in its pathogenesis [7]. Follicular mucinosis may be subclassified into three groups. The first and largest group consists of patients with solitary or only a few lesions, clearing spontaneously in 2 months to 2 years. In a second group are patients in whom the lesions persist, or new lesions continue to develop over many years. In the third group (about 15% of cases [2]) the mucinosis is associated with a lymphoma [4–6]; in such cases, histological evidence of the

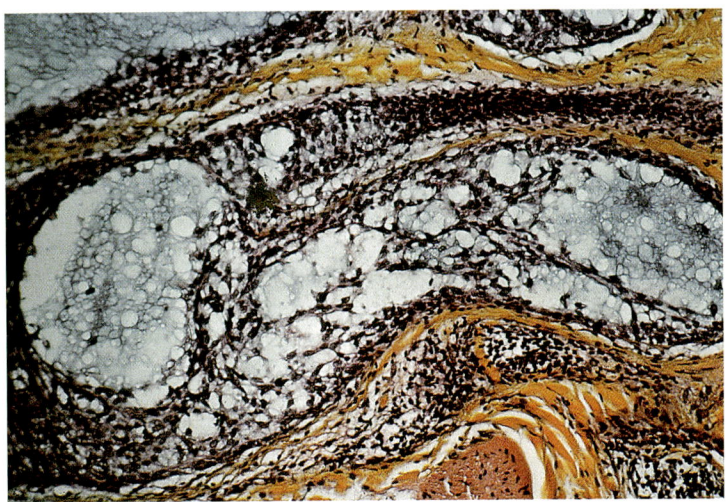

Fig. 59.17 Follicular mucinosis. Marked spongiosis and mucinous degeneration of outer root sheath of a follicle. Alcian blue, H&E, × 50. (Courtesy of St John's Institute of Dermatology, London, UK.)

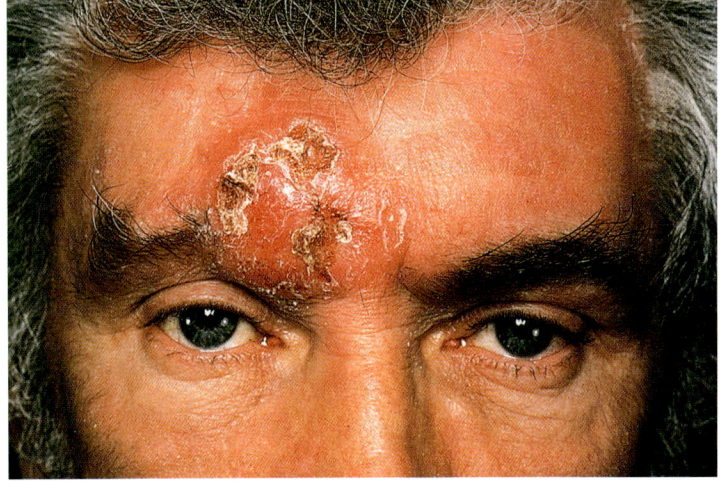

Fig. 59.18 Follicular mucinosis. 'Boggy' erythematous plaque on forehead. (Courtesy of St John's Institute of Dermatology, London, UK.)

lymphoma is present from the onset, but it may be overlooked until the sections are later re-examined with hindsight.

Patients with lymphoma-associated follicular mucinosis tend to be older (age 20–70 years; average 45 years) than those with benign disease (age 2–75 years; peak between 20 and 40 years), but there is no absolute distinction in age incidence [2,8,9].

Some authorities regard follicular mucinosis as a non-specific follicular reaction [3], as similar changes have been observed in association with lupus erythematosus, angiolymphoid hyperplasia [10], Hodgkin's disease [11], cutaneous B-cell lymphoma [12], secondary extramedullary cutaneous plasmacytoma [13] and alopecia areata [14].

Pathology

Pathology [2,3]. The earliest change appears to be oedema of the outer root sheath and sebaceous gland, with formation of cystic spaces in which mucin accumulates. The entire depth of the follicle may be involved, but the degree of damage to the hair matrix is variable. Later, the sebaceous glands may appear to be absent, or the whole follicle may be converted into a cystic cavity containing mucin and degenerate root-sheath cells (Fig. 59.17). Dermal inflammatory changes are variable, and may become granulomatous. Electron-microscopic studies [15] have shown changes in the keratinocytes of the follicular epithelium. Autoradiographic studies [16] have failed to show increased synthesis of glycosaminoglycans in affected follicles.

Histopathological findings may not allow clear-cut differentiation between idiopathic and lymphoma-associated follicular mucinosis [4]. In general, the presence of large numbers of eosinophils in the inflammatory infiltrate and marked mucinous changes in the follicular epithelium favour a benign form, whereas lymphocytic epidermotropism and a dense perifollicular infiltrate with atypical cells suggests an associated lymphoma. Similarly, monoclonal rearrangement of the T-cell receptor (TCR) gamma gene on polymerase chain reaction analysis does not reliably differentiate the benign and lymphoma-associated forms. In one study, TCR gene rearrangements were found in about 50% of tested cases from both idiopathic primary and lymphoma-associated groups of patients [5], whilst a study of patients with primary follicular mucinosis found no evidence of progression to cutaneous T-cell lymphoma despite the presence of a clonal TCR gene rearrangement [17]. When a lymphoma is demonstrated, this is usually of T-cell type [18–21], although B-cell lymphoma has been reported [12]. A follicular variant of mycosis fungoides is being increasingly recognized, although overt mucinous spongiosis is not necessarily present [21]. Syringolymphoid hyperplasia with alopecia and anhidrosis is a syringotropic variant of follicular mucinosis and should be viewed as a facultative precursor lesion of mycosis fungoides [22].

Clinical features

Clinical features [2,23]. In the acute benign form, the earliest changes are grouped, skin-coloured papules or erythematous plaques, with some scale, and with prominent follicles. Each plaque, commonly 2–5 cm in diameter but sometimes larger, changes little in appearance. Multiple lesions may be present from the onset or may develop within a period of a few weeks. The face, scalp, neck and shoulders are commonly affected. The hairs are shed from the affected follicles, so that alopecia may therefore be the presenting symptom when the scalp or eyebrow region is involved. Spontaneous recovery usually takes place within a few months, but may be delayed for a year or more.

In the chronic form, the lesions are often more numerous and more widely distributed and their morphology tends to be more variable. There may be elevated, flat or domed plaques or nodules, some of which may ulcerate. The plaques and nodules are often of soft, gelatinous consistency; sometimes mucin can be squeezed out of affected follicles (Fig. 59.18). Non-infiltrated, red, scaly plaques, patchy scaling, alopecia (Fig. 59.19) and indurated plaques may all be present. In some cases, leprosy may be simulated [24]. Presentation with an unusual acneiform eruption has been recorded [25].

Rarely, follicular papules may be generalized without obvious grouping. Irritation may be troublesome and persistent. Destruction of follicles may give rise to patches of permanent alopecia, which may be studded with horny plugs. This chronic form may

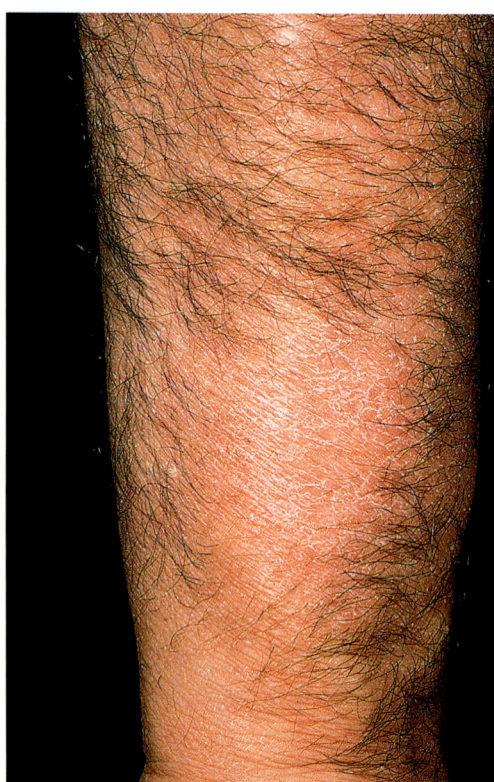

Fig. 59.19 Follicular mucinosis. Circumscribed patch of hair loss associated with erythematous plaque on forearm. (Courtesy of St John's Institute of Dermatology, UK.)

persist for many years without any evidence of associated disease. An unusual case associated with erythroderma and boggy plaques on the scalp and face, associated with alopecia and purulent paronychia and nail loss, has been described [26].

Unfortunately, no single clinical feature distinguishes lymphoma-associated cases from the chronic benign form. Extensive cystic changes have been recorded in the lymphoma-associated type [27]. Contrary to earlier opinion [2,7] lymphoma-associated follicular mucinosis has been reported where the lesions occurred on the head and neck [19,28]. The temporal relationship between lymphoma and follicular mucinosis is very variable. Gross manifestations of the lymphoma may have been present for some time before the mucinosis develops; in other cases, the first indication of the lymphoma is uncovered by histology.

Diagnosis. The loss of hair in plaques with prominent follicles but minimal inflammatory changes should suggest the diagnosis. Sometimes, mucin can be expressed from the follicle. Eczema, seborrhoeic dermatitis, lichen simplex, pityriasis rosea, traumatic alopecia and tinea capitis can all be closely simulated. Biopsy and serial sectioning of the tissue should confirm the diagnosis.

Treatment. There are no clear guidelines for treating follicular mucinosis. Some improve spontaneously, while treatment with topical and intralesional steroids has been claimed to be of benefit. Superficial radiotherapy may be beneficial in some of the lymphoma-associated cases [28], but some cases fail to respond [29]. Response to dapsone [30], isotretinoin [31] or photodynamic therapy [32] has been reported. Low-dose systemic steroids may benefit widespread pruritic follicular mucinosis, and interferon therapy, with or without acitretin, has also proved successful [33,34].

Urticaria-like follicular mucinosis

Urticaria-like follicular mucinosis appears to be a variant of follicular mucinosis, largely confined to middle-aged men, in which urticarial pruritic papules or plaques appear on the head and neck on an erythematous 'seborrhoeic' background [35]. The lesions tend to fade but recur for months to years leaving neither follicular plugging nor alopecia. Sun exposure may temporarily clear the eruption. The histopathological features are identical to follicular mucinosis but the prognosis is good, with a long, benign course.

References

1 Pinkus H. Alopecia mucinosa: inflammatory plaques with alopecia characterized by root-sheath mucinosis. *Arch Dermatol* 1957; **76**: 419–26.
2 Emmerson RW. Follicular mucinosis. A study of 47 patients. *Br J Dermatol* 1969; **81**: 395–413.
3 Hempstead RW, Ackerman AB. Follicular mucinosis: a reaction pattern in follicular epithelium. *Am J Dermatopathol* 1985; **7**: 245–57.
4 Cerroni L, Fink-Puches R, Back B, Kerl H. Follicular mucinosis. A critical reappraisal of clinicopathologic features and association with mycosis fungoides and Sézary syndrome. *Arch Dermatol* 2002; **138**: 182–9.
5 van Doorn R, Scheffer E, Willemze R. Follicular mycosis fungoides, a distinct disease entity with or without associated follicular mucinosis: a clinicopathologic and follow-up study of 51 patients. *Arch Dermatol* 2002; **138**: 191–8.
6 Cerroni L, Kerl H. Primary follicular mucinosis and association with mycosis fungoides and other cutaneous T-cell lymphomas. *J Am Acad Dermatol* 2004; **51**: 146–7.
7 Lancer HA, Bronstein BR, Nakagawa H *et al*. Follicular mucinosis: a detailed morphologic and immunopathologic study. *J Am Acad Dermatol* 1984; **10**: 760–8.
8 Plotnick H, Abrecht M. Alopecia mucinosa and lymphoma. *Arch Dermatol* 1965; **92**: 137–41.
9 Hess Schmid M, Dummer R, Kempf W *et al*. Mycosis fungoides with mucinosis follicularis in childhood. *Dermatology* 1999; **198**: 284–7.
10 Wolff HH, Kinney J, Ackermann AB. Angiolymphoid hyperplasia with follicular mucinosis. *Arch Dermatol* 1978; **114**: 229–32.
11 Stewart M, Smoller BR. Follicular mucinosis in Hodgkin's disease: a poor prognostic sign? *J Am Acad Dermatol* 1991; **24**: 784–5.
12 Benchikhi H, Wechsler J, Rethers L *et al*. Cutaneous B-cell lymphoma associated with follicular mucinosis. *J Am Acad Dermatol* 1995; **33**: 673–5.
13 Rodríguez-Lozano J, Del Pozo J, Almagro M *et al*. Localized cutaneous mucinosis as a presentation of secondary extramedullary cutaneous plasmacytoma. *Br J Dermatol* 2004; **150**: 367–9.
14 Fanti PA, Tosti A, Morelli R *et al*. Follicular mucinosis in alopecia areata. *Am J Dermatopathol* 1992; **14**: 542–5.
15 Ishibashi A, Chujo T. Ultrastructure of follicular mucinosis. *J Cutan Pathol* 1974; **1**: 126–31.
16 Langner A, Jablonska S, Darzynkiewicz Z. Studies on the origin of the mucin in mucinosis follicularis. *Acta Derm Venereol (Stockh)* 1960; **49**: 76–81.
17 Brown HA, Gibson LE, Pujol RM *et al*. Primary follicular mucinosis: long-term follow-up of patients younger than 40 years with and without clonal T-cell receptor gene rearrangement. *J Am Acad Dermatol* 2002; **47**: 856–62.
18 Wilkinson JD, Black MM, Chu A. Follicular mucinosis associated with mycosis fungoides presenting with gross cystic changes on the face. *Clin Exp Dermatol* 1982; **7**: 333–40.
19 Gibson LE, Muller SA, Leiferman KM *et al*. Follicular mucinosis: clinical and histopathologic study. *J Am Acad Dermatol* 1989; **20**: 441–6.
20 Mehregan AD, Gibson EL, Muller SA. Follicular mucinosis. A histopathologic review of 33 cases. *Mayo Clin Proc* 1991; **66**: 387–90.

21 Lacour JP, Castanet J, Perrin C *et al.* Follicular mycosis fungoides: a clinical and histologic variant of cutaneous T-cell lymphoma. *J Am Acad Dermatol* 1993; **29**: 330–4.

22 Haller A, Elzubi E, Petzelbauer P. Localized syringolymphoid hyperplasia with alopecia and anhidrosis. *J Am Acad Dermatol* 2001; **45**: 127–30.

23 Kim R, Winkelmann RK. Follicular mucinosis (alopecia mucinosa). *Arch Dermatol* 1962; **85**: 490–8.

24 Fan J, Chang HS, Ma B. Alopecia mucinosa simulating leprosy. *Arch Dermatol* 1967; **95**: 354–6.

25 Passaro EM, Silveira MT, Valente NY. Acneiform follicular mucinosis. *Clin Exp Dermatol* 2004; **29**: 396–8.

26 Fairris GM, Kirkham N, Goodwin PG *et al.* Erythrodermic follicular mucinosis. *Clin Exp Dermatol* 1987; **12**: 50–2.

27 Wilkinson JD, Ryan TJ, Dawber RPR *et al.* Follicular mucinosis (lymphoma) occurring on the head and neck. *J R Soc Med* 1979; **72**: 281–2.

28 Lacour JP, Castanet J, Lagrange JL *et al.* Follicular mycosis fungoides: a response to radiation therapy. *Br J Dermatol* 1994; **130**: 256–63.

29 Oliwiecki S, Ashworth J. Mycosis fungoides with a widespread follicular eruption, comedones and cysts. *Br J Dermatol* 1992; **127**: 54–6.

30 Kubba RK, Stewart TW. Follicular mucinosis responding to dapsone. *Br J Dermatol* 1974; **91**: 217–20.

31 Arca E, Köse O, Ta tan HB, Gür AR, Safali M. Follicular mucinosis responding to isotretinoin treatment. *J Dermatolog Treat* 2004; **15**: 391–5.

32 Fernández-Guarino M, Harto Castaño A, Carrillo R, Jaén P. Primary follicular mucinosis: excellent response to treatment with photodynamic therapy. *J Eur Acad Dermatol Venereol* 2008; **22**: 393–4.

33 Meissner K, Weyer U, Kowalzick L *et al.* Successful treatment of primary progressive follicular mucinosis with interferons. *J Am Acad Dermatol* 1991; **24**: 848–50.

34 Kontochristopoulos GJ, Exadaktylou D, Hatziolou E *et al.* Follicular mucinosis associated with early stage cutaneous T-cell lymphoma: successful treatment with interferon alpha-2b and acitretin. *J Dermatolog Treat* 2001; **12**: 117–21.

35 Govato F, Nazzari G, Nunzi E *et al.* Urticaria-like follicular mucinosis. *Dermatologica* 1985; **170**: 133–5.

Secondary mucinoses [1]

Dermal mucinosis may be associated to a greater or lesser extent with histopathological features otherwise typical of the disease in question [1]. In some, the mucinous deposition may be so striking as to suggest the diagnosis, for example Degos' disease [2]. Cutaneous mucinosis and polymyositis have been reported as presenting features of hypothyroidism [3].

Papulonodular mucinosis associated with systemic lupus erythematosus [1–6]

Papulonodular mucinosis is a distinct but rare cutaneous manifestation occurring in patients with discoid, subacute cutaneous or systemic lupus erythematosus. It presents as indolent, flesh-coloured papulonodules or plaques [7] on the neck, trunk and upper limbs due to diffuse mucinosis in the dermis. It differs from the diffuse mucinosis that may be found in lesional skin of lupus erythematosus in that it occurs in areas free of specific lupus erythematosus lesions. Clinical recognition is important because in one-third of cases it precedes both clinical and serological evidence of systemic lupus erythematosus, sometimes by several years. Cutaneous mucin deposition in papulonodular lupus erythematosus is associated with increased glycosaminoglycan production by dermal fibroblasts, which appears to be due to an unidentified serum factor [8].

References

1 Rongioletti F, Rebora A. Papular and nodular mucinosis associated with systemic lupus erythematosus. *Br J Dermatol* 1986; **115**: 631–6.

2 Lowe L, Rapini RP, Golitz LE *et al.* Papulonodular dermal mucinosis in lupus erythematosus. *J Am Acad Dermatol* 1992; **27**: 312–5.

3 Kano Y, Sagawa Y, Yagita A, Nagashima M. Nodular cutaneous lupus mucinosis: report of a case and review of previously reported cases. *Cutis* 1996; **57**: 441–4.

4 Kanda N, Tsuchida T, Watanabe T, Tamaki K. Cutaneous lupus mucinosis: a review of our cases and the possible pathogenesis. *J Cutan Pathol* 1997; **24**: 553–8.

5 Sonntag M, Lehmann P, Megahed M *et al.* Papulonodular mucinosis associated with subacute cutaneous lupus erythematosus. *Dermatology* 2003; **206**: 326–9.

6 Ortiz VG, Krishnan RS, Chen LL, Hsu S. Papulonodular mucinosis in systemic lupus erythematosus. *Dermatol Online J* 2004; **10**: 16.

7 Kobayashi T, Shimizu H, Shimizu S *et al.* Plaque-like cutaneous lupus mucinosis. *Arch Dermatol* 1993; **129**: 383–4.

8 Pandya AG, Santheimen RD, Cockerell CJ *et al.* Papulonodular mucinosis associated with systemic lupus erythematosus: possible mechanisms of increased glycosaminoglycan accumulation. *J Am Acad Dermatol* 1995; **32**: 199–205.

Collagen vascular diseases

Dermal mucinosis occurs in lupus erythematosus [1] and dermatomyositis, and has been linked in some patients to parvovirus B19 infection [2]. Marked periorbital oedema from massive mucinosis has been reported in a patient with discoid lupus erythematosus [3]. Infiltrated erythematous plaques on the back progressing to erythematous and elastic, soft, tumorous masses over 20 cm in diameter were recorded in a patient with systemic lupus erythematosus [4]. Dermatomyositis may present as plaque-like mucinosis [5,6]. Papular and nodular mucinosis has been recorded as a presenting sign of progressive systemic sclerosis [7], and development of multiple, large, soft skin lesions over the interphalangeal joints of both hands, resembling cutaneous focal mucinosis, has also been reported [8]. Lesions typical of papular mucinosis without evidence of paraproteinaemia occurred in a patient with generalized morphoea [9]. Dermal mucinosis has been associated with severe chronic cutaneous graft-versus-host disease of the sclerodermoid variety [10].

Papular mucinosis in L-tryptophan-induced eosinophilia–myalgia syndrome [11]

The L-tryptophan-induced eosinophilia–myalgia syndrome, due to ingestion of contaminants of L-tryptophan, was first recognized in 1989. The skin lesions include a diffuse morbilliform eruption, urticaria and angio-oedema, dermographism, alopecia and cutaneous induration. Papular mucinosis may coexist for a while, although the lesions slowly regress after cessation of L-tryptophan ingestion. There is associated weakness, fatigue, arthralgia and pneumonitis.

Cutaneous mucinosis in the toxic oil syndrome [12]

Toxic oil syndrome occurred in Spain in 1981 related to the ingestion of adulterated oil. During the late recovery stages, an asymptomatic papular eruption developed on the arms, thighs and legs due to dermal mucin deposition. The papular eruption gradually resolved but sometimes led to sclerodermoid changes.

References

1 Knisley RR, Kobayashi TT. Lupus mucinosis: a case report and review of cutaneous lupus. *Cutis* 2003; **72**: 366–71.

2 Magro CM, Dawood MR, Crowson AN. The cutaneous manifestations of human parvovirus B19 infection. *Hum Pathol* 2000; **31**: 488–97.

3 Williams WL, Ramos-Caro FA. Acute periorbital mucinosis in discoid lupus erythematosus. *J Am Acad Dermatol* 1999; **41**: 871–3.

4 Maruyama M, Miyauchi S, Hashimoto K. Massive cutaneous mucinosis associated with systemic lupus erythematosus. *Br J Dermatol* 1997; **137**: 450–3.

5 Kaufmann R, Greiner D, Schmidt P, Wolter M. Dermatomyositis presenting as plaque-like mucinosis. *Br J Dermatol* 1998; **138**: 889–92.

6 del Pozo J, Almagro M, Martinez W *et al.* Dermatomyositis and mucinosis. *Int J Dermatol* 2001; **40**: 120–4.

7 Van Zander J, Shaw JC. Papular and nodular mucinosis as a presenting sign of progressive systemic sclerosis. *J Am Acad Dermatol* 2002; **46**: 304–6.

8 Marzano AV, Berti E, Gasparini G *et al.* Unique digital skin lesions associated with systemic sclerosis. *Br J Dermatol* 1997; **136**: 598–600.

9 Rongioletti F, Rampini P, Parodi A, Rebora A. Papular mucinosis associated with generalized morphoea. *Br J Dermatol* 1999; **141**: 905–8.

10 Ameen M, Russell-Jones R. Macroscopic and microscopic mucinosis in chronic sclerodermoid graft-versus-host disease. *Br J Dermatol* 2000; **142**: 529–32.

11 Valicenti JMK, Fleming MG, Pearson RW *et al.* Papular mucinosis in ʟ tryptophan-induced eosinophilia–myalgia syndrome. *J Am Acad Dermatol* 1991; **25**: 54–8.

12 Fonseca E, Contreras F. Cutaneous mucinosis in the toxic oil syndrome. *J Am Acad Dermatol* 1987; **16**: 139–40.

Lysosomal storage disorders

A.A.M. Morris, pp. 59.30–59.36

Lysosomes are a major site for the degradation of macromolecules and contain more than 50 acid hydrolases. Lysosomal storage disorders are inherited conditions in which deficiency of one or more hydrolases leads to the accumulation of various molecules in lysosomes. Typically, these are progressive multisystem diseases but the clinical features vary depending on the precise disorder and the severity of the enzyme deficiency. The presence of some residual enzyme activity reduces the severity of problems, delays their onset and may completely prevent the involvement of some organs (such as the brain in some disorders). Dermatological abnormalities are seen in lysosomal disorders affecting the degradation of glycosaminoglycans, glycoproteins and sphingolipids. Two characteristic dermatological findings are angiokeratomas (discussed later) and a combination of thickened skin and hypertrichosis. This combination, together with abnormalities of the facial skeleton, gives rise to a 'coarse' facial appearance. These facial features are seen in most mucopolysaccharidoses and glycoprotein breakdown disorders and in a few sphingolipidoses. Though it is widely used among professionals, the term 'coarse' should be avoided when talking to families, as many find it offensive. Lysosomal disorders are often associated with characteristic histological abnormalities, especially on electron microscopy. If a mucopolysaccharidosis or glycoprotein breakdown disorder is suspected, the next step is analysis of urinary glycosaminoglycans and oligosaccharides. Definitive diagnosis requires demonstration of the enzyme deficiency, usually in leukocytes.

Mucopolysaccharidoses [1,2]

The mucopolysaccharidoses (MPS) result from deficiencies of the enzymes required for the normal degradation of glycosaminoglycans (GAGs, formerly known as mucopolysaccharides). GAGs are long sugar chains composed of alternating sulphated hexuronic acid and hexosamine residues; in connective tissue, they are bound to core proteins to form proteoglycans. Dermatan sulphate, heparan sulphate and keratan sulphate are the main GAGs that accumulate in the MPS disorders; one or more GAGs are found in

each disorder. Characteristic clinical features include coarse facial features, hepatosplenomegaly, bone dysplasia (known as dysostosis multiplex) and developmental regression. Some of these features, however, are absent in some disorders. Moreover, there is a considerable range of severity for each disorder; for MPS I, the spectrum is divided into Hurler syndrome (severe), Hurler–Scheie (intermediate) and Scheie syndrome (relatively mild). MPS III (Sanfilippo syndrome) can result from deficiencies of four different enzymes. The biochemical and clinical features of the different disorders are summarized in Table 59.3. The clinical features of MPS IX are not yet clear as only one case has been reported in detail [3].

Genetics. All the mucopolysaccharidoses are inherited as autosomal recessive traits except for MPS II (Hunter syndrome), which is X-linked.

Dysmorphism. MPS patients seldom show abnormalities at birth, except that some have umbilical or inguinal hernias. Patients presenting with an MPS-like phenotype at birth are likely to have mucolipidosis type II or GM_1 gangliosidosis (see below) [4]. The dysmorphism of MPS becomes more apparent with time (Fig. 59.20). Hypoplasia of the mid-facial bones leads to a flat nasal bridge. The skin is thickened, as are the lips, and the tongue is enlarged. The mouth is often slightly open due to adenoidal hypertrophy and the need for mouth breathing. Many patients have generalized hypertrichosis and some have synophrys. Corneal clouding is seen in MPS I, VI and VII. The hands appear podgy with short, broad digits. The facial dysmorphism is relatively subtle in MPS III (Sanfilippo syndrome), which presents with developmental delay. Facial abnormalities are not seen in MPS IV (Morquio disease), which presents with skeletal problems.

Dermatological features. In addition to the hypertrichosis and thickened skin mentioned above, ivory-white papules or nodules are often seen on the back of patients with severe MPS II (Hunter syndrome) [5–7]; similar pebbly skin may also occur in MPS I (Hurler and Hurler–Scheie syndromes) [8]. Individual nodules range from 1 to 10 mm in size and they may coalesce to form ridges or a reticular pattern. Typically, they are found laterally, between the angles of the scapulae and posterior axillary lines (Fig. 59.21). Papules may also be found on the upper arms and outer thighs. Typically, the papules appear at 1–4 years of age and progress for a few years; they may clear spontaneously in older patients. Mongolian blue spots are common in Hurler and Hunter syndromes and, in addition to the sacrococcygeal region, they may be found on the upper back, the anterior trunk or the limbs [9–11]. The spots fade more slowly than in the general population; in Japanese patients they persist until teenage years [11].

Other clinical features. Developmental regression is the dominant feature in MPS III. After presenting with developmental delay, patients have a period of hyperactivity, behaviour problems and sleep disturbance at 3–10 years of age; following this, they gradually deteriorate into a vegetative state. Learning difficulties are also present in Hurler syndrome and severe cases of MPS II and VII. Other neurological problems may include sei-

Table 59.3 Classification of the mucopolysaccharidoses.

Number	MIM no.	Eponym	Clinical features	Enzyme deficiency	GAGs stored and excreted
MPS IH	252800	Hurler	Dysmorphism, corneal clouding, DM, HSM, PR, heart disease, death in childhood	α-L-iduronidase	DS, HS
MPS IS	252800	Scheie	Dysmorphism, corneal clouding, DM, normal IQ and life span	α-L-iduronidase	DS, HS
MPS IH/S	252800	Hurler–Scheie	Phenotype intermediate between I H and I S	α-L-iduronidase	DS, HS
MPS II	309900	Hunter (severe)	Dysmorphism, DM, HSM, heart disease, PR, death before 15 years	Iduronate sulphatase	DS, HS
		Hunter (mild)	Normal IQ, short stature, survive to adulthood	Iduronate sulphatase	DS, HS
MPS IIIA	252900	Sanfilippo A	PR, regression, hyperactivity, mild somatic features	Heparan-N-sulphatase	HS
MPS IIIB	252920	Sanfilippo B	Similar to III A	α-N-acetyl-glucosaminidase	HS
MPS IIIC	252930	Sanfilippo C	Similar to III A	Acetyl-CoA glucosamine N-acetyl-transferase	HS
MPS IIID	252940	Sanfilippo D	Similar to III A	N-acetyl-glucosamine 6-sulphatase	HS
MPS IVA	253000	Morquio A	DM, odontoid hypoplasia, corneal clouding	Galactose-6-sulphatase	KS
MPS IVB	253010	Morquio B	Milder DM, slow neurodegeneration	β-galactosidase	KS
MPS VI	253200	Maroteaux–Lamy	Dysmorphism, DM, corneal clouding, normal IQ	N-acetyl-galactosamine 4-sulphatase	DS
MPS VII	253220	Sly	Hydrops fetalis, dysmorphism, DM, HSM, PR	β-glucoronidase	DS, HS
MPS IX	601492	Natowicz	Soft tissue masses in the one reported patient	Hyaluronidase	Hyaluronan

The terms MPS V and MPS VIII are no longer used.

IQ, intelligence quotient; DM, dysostosis multiplex; HSM, hepatosplenomegaly; PR, psychomotor retardation; DS, dermatan sulphate; HS, heparan sulphate; KS, keratan sulphate.

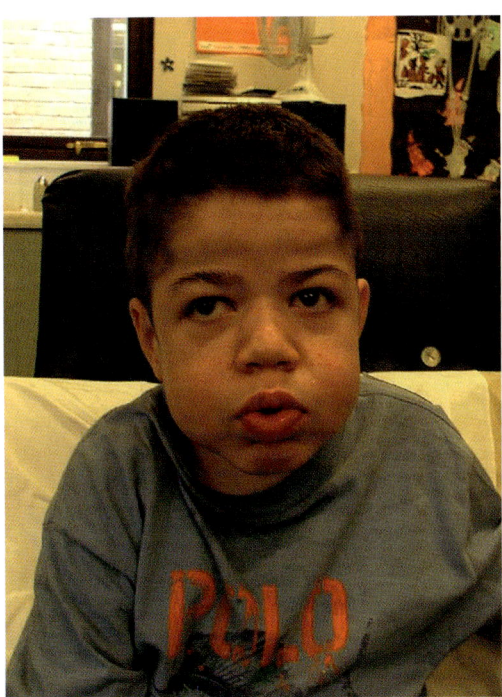

Fig. 59.20 Facial features of an 8-year-old boy with Hunter syndrome (MPS II).

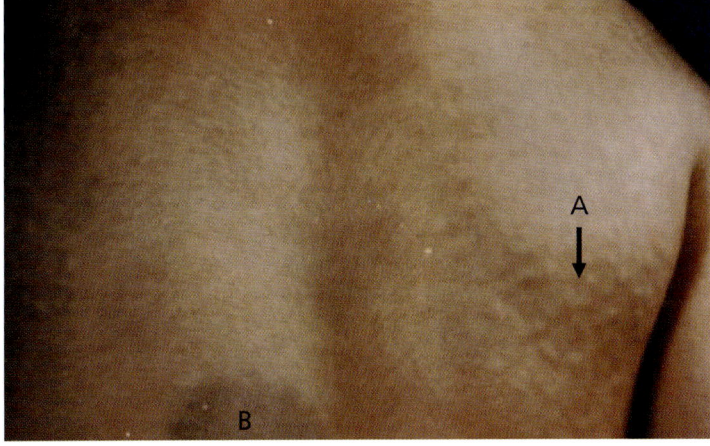

Fig. 59.21 'Pebbling' of the skin (A) and extensive Mongolian blue spot (B) on the back of a boy with Hunter syndrome (MPS II). (Reproduced from J.E. Wraith [2] with permission of author and publisher.)

zures, hydrocephalus, spinal cord compression and carpal tunnel syndrome.

Dysostosis multiplex is a particular problem in patients with MPS IV, who have very short stature and a high risk of atlanto-axial dislocation. Dysplasia of the hip and knee leads to arthritis and sometimes to dislocation. Joint problems, short stature and kyphosis are also seen in the other mucopolysaccharidoses. Ear, nose and throat infections, upper airway obstruction and deafness are common. Valvular heart disease is another frequent problem and is often the cause of death. MPS VII is rare but may present with hydrops fetalis.

Histology. The skin may show distinctive changes even in the absence of clinical skin abnormalities. A few Malpighian cells in the epidermis are distended with pale cytoplasm. Fibroblasts, Schwann cells and some smooth muscle and sweat gland cells show cytoplasmic metachromasia when stained with toluidine blue (due to the presence of GAGs) [12,13]. Fragmentation of collagen and increased tissue mucin may be seen. In Hunter syndrome, examination of the nodules shows pooling of metachromatic material between the collagen bundles of the lower reticular dermis [14].

Ultrastructurally, in all forms of MPS, dermal fibroblasts and Schwann cells contain membrane-bound cytoplasmic vacuoles; these may appear empty or contain fibrillogranular material [12–14].

Diagnosis. If MPS is suspected, it may be worth undertaking a skeletal survey to look for dysostosis multiplex. 'Spot tests' for urine GAGs are unreliable, especially for MPS III and IV. Quantitation usually shows increased amounts of GAGs in the urine but even this can miss patients at the mild end of the spectrum. Two-dimensional electrophoresis allows the clearest discrimination between different GAGs. The diagnosis can be confirmed by enzyme assay in leukocytes, plasma or fibroblasts. The main differential diagnoses are other lysosomal disorders, such as the glycoprotein breakdown disorders, mucolipidoses and the severe forms of galactosialidosis and GM_1 gangliosidosis (see below).

Treatment. Symptomatic treatment is important and requires a multidisciplinary approach. Ear, nose and throat, orthopaedic and neurosurgery may all be needed. Medication can be useful for sleep and behaviour problems, especially in MPS III. Haematopoietic stem cell transplantation (HSCT) is an established treatment for Hurler and Maroteaux–Lamy syndromes, using bone marrow or umbilical cord blood [15]. Transplantation in infancy leads to improvement in most systems and can preserve normal developmental progress in Hurler syndrome but the skeletal problems progress [16] and ophthalmological problems persist. Moreover, HSCT is associated with a high morbidity and mortality. Enzyme replacement therapy is now available for MPS I, II and VI [17–19]. Its major limitation is the inability of the enzyme to cross the blood–brain barrier. Bone and heart valve disease are also resistant to enzyme replacement therapy, though outcomes can be improved by starting treatment early.

References

1 Neufeld EF, Muenzer J. The mucopolysaccharidoses. In: Scriver CR, Beaudet AL, Sly WS *et al.*, eds. *The Metabolic and Molecular Bases of Inherited Disease*, 8th edn. New York: McGraw-Hill, 2001: 3421–52.

2 Wraith JE. Mucopolysaccharidoses and oligosaccharidoses. In: Fernandes J, Saudubray J-M, van den Berghe G, Walter JH, eds. *Inborn Metabolic Diseases*, 4th edn. Heidelberg: Springer, 2006: 495–507.

3 Natowicz MR, Short MP, Wang Y *et al.* Clinical and biochemical manifestations of hyaluronidase deficiency. *N Engl J Med* 1996; **335**: 1029–33.

4 Wraith JE. Lysosomal disorders. *Semin Neonatol* 2002; **7**: 75–83.

5 Hunter C. A rare disease in two brothers. *Proc R Soc Med* 1917; **10**: 104–16.

6 Prystowsky SD, Maumenee IH, Freeman RG *et al.* A cutaneous marker in the Hunter syndrome: a report of four cases. *Arch Dermatol* 1977; **113**: 602–5.

7 Demitsu T, Kakurai M, Okubo Y *et al.* Skin eruption as the presenting sign of Hunter syndrome IIB. *Clin Exp Dermatol* 1999; **24**: 179–82.

8 Schiro JA, Mallory SB, Demmer L *et al.* Grouped papules in Hurler–Scheie syndrome. *J Am Acad Dermatol* 1996; **5**: 68–70.

9 Grant BP, Beard JS, de Castro F *et al.* Extensive mongolian spots in an infant with Hurler syndrome. *Arch Dermatol* 1998; **134**: 108–9.

10 Sapadin AN, Friedman IS. Extensive Mongolian spots associated with Hunter syndrome. *J Am Acad Dermatol* 1998; **39**: 1013–5.

11 Ochiai T, Suzuki Y, Kato T *et al.* Natural history of extensive Mongolian spots in mucopolysaccharidosis type II (Hunter syndrome): a survey among 52 Japanese patients. *J Eur Acad Dermatol Venereol* 2007; **21**: 1082–5.

12 Belcher RW. Ultrastructure of the skin in the genetic mucopolysaccharidoses. *Arch Pathol* 1972; **94**: 511–8.

13 Alroy J, Jones MZ, Rutledge JC *et al.* The ultrastructure of skin from a patient with mucopolysaccharidosis IIID. *Acta Neuropathol (Berl)* 1997; **93**: 210–3.

14 Freeman RG. A pathological basis for the cutaneous papules of mucopolysaccharidosis II (the Hunter syndrome). *J Cutan Pathol* 1977; **4**: 318–28.

15 Staba SL, Escolar ML, Poe M *et al.* Cord-blood transplants from unrelated donors in patients with Hurler's syndrome. *N Engl J Med* 2004; **350**: 1960–9.

16 Weisstein JS, Delgado E, Steinbach LS *et al.* Musculoskeletal manifestations of Hurler syndrome: long-term follow-up after bone marrow transplantation. *J Pediatr Orthop* 2004; **24**: 97–101.

17 Kakkis ED, Muenzer J, Tiller GE *et al.* Enzyme-replacement therapy in mucopolysaccharidosis I. *N Engl J Med* 2001; **344**: 182–8.

18 Muenzer J, Wraith JE, Beck M *et al.* A phase II/III clinical study of enzyme replacement therapy with idursulfase in mucopolysaccharidosis II (Hunter syndrome). *Genet Med* 2006; **8**: 465–73.

19 Harmatz P, Giugliani R, Schwartz I *et al.* Enzyme replacement therapy for mucopolysaccharidosis VI. *J Pediatr* 2006; **148**: 533–9.

Mucolipidoses [1]

The term 'mucolipidosis' (ML) was originally used to describe lysosomal disorders with clinical features of MPS and the sphingolipidoses. ML I is now called sialidosis; it is considered with the other disorders of glycoprotein degradation. ML IV presents in infancy with psychomotor retardation and corneal clouding; though there are no dermatological problems, electron microscopy reveals a variety of inclusions in skin, as in other tissues [2].

ML II and III refer to different severities of an autosomal recessive disorder (MIM 252600), in which multiple lysosomal enzymes fail to enter their organelle. The underlying problem is a deficiency of UDP-N-acetylglucosamine-1-phosphotransferase, which is needed for lysosomal enzymes to acquire a mannose-6-phosphate residue. The transport of lysosomal enzymes into the lysosome depends on the binding of this residue to a mannose-6-phosphate receptor. ML II (I cell disease) refers to the severe end of the spectrum; patients often present at birth with coarse facial features. They also have gum hypertrophy, severe neurological involvement, dysostosis multiplex and cardiomyopathy, which is frequently the cause of death. In patients with ML III, the main problem is arthritis caused by the skeletal dysplasia. Other features may include mild learning difficulties and dysmorphism. MPS excretion is normal in ML II and III but there are abnormal urinary oligosaccharides. The diagnosis is established by demonstrating raised levels of the mistargetted lysosomal enzymes in plasma. Cultured fibroblasts from patients with ML II and III contain dense cytoplasmic inclusions, which gave rise to the name, I cell disease [3]. Histology reveals vacuoles in fibroblasts and other mesenchymal cells in skin and elsewhere; ultrastructurally, the vacuoles are membrane-bound and contain electron-lucent or fibrillogranular material [4].

References

1 Kornfeld S, Sly WS. I-cell disease and pseudo-Hurler polydystrophy: disorders of lysosomal enzyme phosphorylation. In: Scriver CR, Beaudet AL, Sly WS *et al.*, eds. *The Metabolic and Molecular Bases of Inherited Disease*, 8th edn. New York: McGraw-Hill, 2001: 3469–82.

2 Bargal R, Goebel HH, Latta E, Bach G. Mucolipidosis IV: novel mutation and diverse ultrastructural spectrum in the skin. *Neuropediatrics* 2002; **33**: 199–202.

3 Leroy JG, De Mars RI. Mutant enzymatic and cytological phenotypes in cultured human fibroblasts. *Science* 1967; **157**: 804–7.

4 Tondeur M, Vamos-Hurwitz E, Mockel-Pohl S *et al.* Clinical, biochemical and ultrastructural studies in a case of chondrodystrophy presenting the I-cell phenotype in tissue culture. *J Pediatr* 1971; **79**: 366–78.

Table 59.4 Glycoprotein storage disorders, sphingolipidoses and mucolipidoses with cutaneous features

Name	Enzyme deficiency	Cutaneous features*	Other clinical features*	Abnormal urine oligosaccharides	Sample for enzymology
Fucosidosis	α-L-fucosidase	MLF (mild), AK	PR	(+)	leukocytes
α-Mannosidosis	α-Mannosidase	MLF	PR, deafness, DM, HSM, frequent infections	+	leukocytes
β-Mannosidosis	β-Mannosidase	AK	PR, deafness, frequent infections	(+)	leukocytes
Sialidosis type I	neuraminidase		(Late onset) myoclonus, CRS	(+)	cultured cells
Sialidosis type II	neuraminidase	MLF	(Early onset) PR, DM, HSM	(+)	cultured cells
Aspartylglucosaminuria	aspartylglucosaminidase	MLF, AK	PR, regression, seizures	(+)	leukocytes
GM1 gangliosidosis	β-galactosidase	MLF, AK, T	Early onset form: hydrops, HSM, DM, PR, regression, spasticity, CRS	+	leukocytes
			Late onset: Dysarthria, dystonia, DM, PR	+	leukocytes
Galactosialidosis	PPCA	MLF, T	Early onset form: hydrops, HSM, Heart disease, DM, PR, CRS	+	leukocytes
		AK, MLF (mild)	Later onset: myoclonus, ataxia, PR, CRS	+	leukocytes
Fabry	α-galactosidase A	AK, hypohydrosis	Acroparaesthesia, renal failure, heart disease, strokes		leukocytes
Schindler	α-N-acetylgalactosaminidase		(Early onset) PR, regression, spasticity		
Kanzaki	α-N-acetylgalactosaminidase	AK, MLF (mild)	(Late onset) PR		
Niemann–Pick A	sphingomyelinase	Papules, pigmentation	HSM, lymphadenopathy, PR, regression, spasticity, CRS		leukocytes
Niemann–Pick B	sphingomyelinase	Papules, pigmentation	HSM, lung disease		leukocytes
Gaucher type I	β-glucosidase	Pigmentation, T	Bone pain, DM, HSM		leukocytes
Gaucher type II	β-glucosidase	Collodion baby	HSM, squint, stridor, dysphagia, spasticity		leukocytes
Gaucher type III	β-glucosidase		HSM, abnormal eye movements, regression		leukocytes
Farber	ceramidase	Nodules	Hoarse voice, arthritis, PR, regression, CRS		leukocytes
Mucolipidosis type II	multiple	MLF	Gum hypertrophy, DM, PR, cardiomyopathy	+	plasma
Mucolipidosis type III	multiple	MLF (mild)	Arthritis, DM, PR	+	plasma
Multiple sulphatase def.	multiple	MLF ± ichthiosis	PR, regression, HSM, DM (references A & B)	+	leukocytes
ISSD	sialic acid transporter	MLF, hypopigmentation	PR, HSM, DM, hydrops/ascites (references C & D see Table footnote)	+	cultured cells

* Features that are characteristic or have been reported in a number of patients.

MLF = Mucopolysaccharidosis-like facies; AK = angiokeratomas; T = telangiectasia; PR = psychomotor retardation; DM = dysostosis multiplex; HSM = hepatosplenomegaly; CRS cherry red spot; PPCA = protective protein/cathepsin A; ISSD = infantile free sialic acid storage disease

Mucolipidosis type I is now called sialidosis.

References:

A Díaz-Font A, Santamaría R, Cozar M, Blanco M, Chamoles N, Josep Coll M, Chabás A, Vilageliu L, Grinberg D. Clinical and mutational characterization of three patients with multiple sulfatase deficiency. *Mol Genet Metab* 2005; **86**: 205–11.

B Loffeld A, Gray RG, Green SH, Roper HP, Moss C. Mild ichthyosis in a 4-year-old boy with multiple sulphatase deficiency. *Br J Dermatol* 2002; **147**: 353–5.

C Aulla P, Gahl WA. Disorders of free sialic acid storage. In: Scriver CR, Beaudet AL, Sly WS *et al.*, eds. *The Metabolic and Molecular Bases of Inherited Disease*, 8th edn. New York: McGraw-Hill, 2001: 5109–120.

D Lemyre E, Russo P, Melancon SB, Gagne R, Potier M, Lambert M. Clinical spectrum of infantile free sialic acid storage disease. *Am J Med Genet* 1999; **82**: 385–91.

Disorders of glycoprotein degradation

Most secreted and cell surface proteins are glycosylated, with oligosaccharides attached to asparagine (N-linked glycoproteins) or to serine or threonine (O-linked glycoproteins). The oligosaccharide components of glycoproteins are degraded by lysosomal hydrolases which sequentially remove the terminal monosaccharides. Deficiency of an enzyme prevents subsequent degradation steps and leads to the storage of various oligosaccharides and/or glycopeptides, depending on the precise defect [1,2]. The disorders of glycoprotein degradation are all very rare and are sometimes called glycoproteinoses or oligosaccharidoses. They resemble the mucopolysaccharidoses in several respects, including the facial appearance in many cases. Angiokeratomas are found in some disorders. Mucopolysaccharides are not present in the urine but abnormal oligosaccharides may be detected by thin-layer chromatography and staining with orcinol (α-mannosidosis), resorcinol (sialidosis) or ninhydrin (aspartylglucosaminuria). In other disorders, abnormal oligosaccharides are not consistently detected (β-mannosidosis, fucosidosis). Enzyme assays are, therefore, important for diagnosis. Most of the assays can be performed on leukocytes but neuraminidase can only be measured reliably in cultured cells. Because it can be difficult to distinguish these disorders from the sphingolipidoses on clinical grounds, many laboratories offer a set of lysosomal enzyme assays on leukocytes for screening patients with relevant clinical features. The clinical and biochemical features of these disorders are summarized in Table 59.4 (along with relevant mucolipidoses and sphingolipidoses).

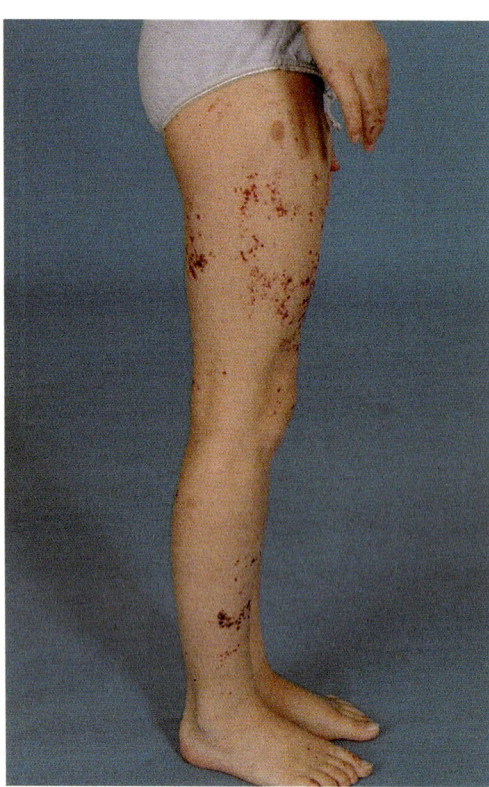

Fig. 59.22 Angiokeratoma corporis diffusum on the limbs of a 7-year-old girl with fucosidosis.

Genetics. All the disorders of glycoprotein degradation are inherited as autosomal recessive traits.

Fucosidosis (MIM 230000) [1]

Patients with α-L-fucosidase deficiency usually present by the age of 3 years with developmental delay, followed by neurological deterioration. Approximately 50% patients lose the ability to sit and talk by 10 years of age [3]. Most patients have a mild MPS-like facial appearance and short stature, with dysostosis multiplex that principally affects the spine. Angiokeratomas usually appear in mid- to late childhood and they are present in 85% of patients aged over 20 years [3]. The angiokeratomas usually have the same appearance and distribution as in Fabry's disease but they may be confined to the limbs (Fig. 59.22). Similar lesions may occur on the lips, gums or tongue [4]. Other clinical features include hypohydrosis [5], recurrent infections, hepatosplenomegaly and epilepsy. Bone marrow transplantation may improve the neurological outcome [6].

Ultrastructure of endothelial cells and fibroblasts reveals numerous cytoplasmic vacuoles that appear empty or contain fine granular material [5]; by contrast, concentric lamellar inclusions are seen in Fabry's disease. Lamellar inclusions are, however, seen in Schwann cells and in the myoepithelial cells of sweat glands in fucosidosis [5]. Fucose-containing oligosaccharides can be detected in the urine of some patients but not others. The diagnosis is confirmed by measuring enzyme activity in leukocytes or cultured fibroblasts.

The mannosidoses [1]

α-Mannosidase deficiency (MIM 248500) is associated with MPS-like facial features, learning difficulties, deafness, corneal clouding and cataracts, dysostosis multiplex, hepatosplenomegaly and frequent infections.

β-Mannosidase deficiency (MIM 248510) is associated with learning difficulties, deafness and frequent infections; the face is not coarse but angiokeratomas appear in some patients during late childhood or adulthood. Ultrastructural examination shows lysosomal vacuoles containing granular material in basal keratinocytes, endothelial cells, fibroblasts and eccrine sweat glands [7,8].

Abnormal urinary oligosaccharides can readily be detected in α-mannosidosis but the mannose-containing disaccharides excreted in β-mannosidosis can easily be missed, especially during infancy. Both diagnoses can be confirmed by enzyme measurement in leukocytes.

Sialidosis (MIM 256550) [1]

This disorder results from a deficiency of α-neuraminidase (also called sialidase). Mildly affected patients are said to have sialidosis type I: they present as adolescents or adults with myoclonus and visual impairment associated with a macular 'cherry red spot' on fundoscopy. Sialidosis type II refers to more severely affected patients, who present in infancy or childhood with an MPS-like phenotype, developmental delay, dysostosis multiplex and hepatosplenomegaly [9]. Histology shows vacuolation of many cell types, particularly reticuloendothelial cells and fibroblasts. Abnormal urinary oligosaccharides can be seen when stained with resorcinol. Cultured fibroblasts are needed to demonstrate the enzyme deficiency because normal activity is low in leukocytes.

Aspartylglucosaminuria (MIM 208400) [10]

This disease is caused by deficiency of aspartylglucosaminidase, which catalyses the final step in the lysosomal breakdown of glycoproteins. Patients usually present with developmental delay at 2–4 years of age. They make some developmental progress until puberty following which they regress and may develop epilepsy. Subtle facial dysmorphism is present in children; from adolescence onwards, there is coarsening of the facial features, with sagging skin, thick lips, a broad low nasal bridge and coarse hair [11]. Facial angiofibromas are common in adults, as are gingival overgrowths and oedema of the buccal mucosa [12]. Angiokeratomas are less common and may be confined to the limbs [13,14]. Ultrastructurally, dermal fibrocytes have enlarged lysosomes containing scanty fibrillogranular material. The diagnosis can be established by demonstrating aspartylglucosamine in the urine or by measuring the enzyme activity in leukocytes or cultured fibroblasts. The disorder is extremely rare in most countries but a common mutation in the Finnish population has led to a higher incidence there [13].

α-N-acetyl-galactosaminidase deficiency (MIM 104170) [15–17]

This extremely rare disorder leads to the accumulation of oligosaccharides, glycopeptides and glycosphingolipids with terminal α-N-acetyl-galactosamine residues. The few reported patients have presented either as infants with neurodegeneration and histologi-

Table 59.5 Lysosomal diseases associated with angiokeratomas.

Name/eponym	Enzyme deficiency	Usual age of onset	Ultrastructure of lysosomal storage in mesenchymal cells
Fabry	α-galactosidase A	>10 years (males), adulthood (females)	Dense concentric lamellar inclusions
Fucosidosis	α-L-fucosidase	Mid- to late childhood	Vacuoles with granular material
Kanzaki	α-N-acetylgalactosaminidase	Adulthood	Vacuoles with fibrillary material
Galactosialidosis	β-galactosidase and neuraminidase	Adulthood	Vacuoles with granular material
GM$_1$ gangliosidosis	β-galactosidase	Infancy	Vacuoles with fibrillogranular material
Aspartylglycosaminuria	aspartylglucosaminidase	Late childhood or adulthood	Vacuoles with fibrillogranular material
β-Mannosidosis	β-mannosidase	Late childhood or adulthood	Vacuoles with granular material

cal features of neuroaxonal dystrophy (Schindler disease) or as adults with angiokeratomas and mild learning difficulties (Kanzaki disease) [15–17]. The angiokeratomas appeared first between the knees and the umbilicus but later spread to the breasts, limbs, face, mouth and gastric mucosa. Ultrastructural examination showed clear vacuoles with scanty fibrillary contents, especially in endothelial and eccrine sweat gland cells [16]. Adult patients have slightly coarse facial features, lymphoedema in the legs and peripheral neuroaxonal degeneration [16,17].

References

1 Thomas GH. Disorders of glycoprotein degradation: α-mannosidosis, β-mannosidosis, fucosidosis and sialidosis. In: Scriver CR, Beaudet AL, Sly WS *et al.*, eds. *The Metabolic and Molecular Bases of Inherited Disease*, 8th edn. New York: McGraw-Hill, 2001: 3507–34.

2 Wraith JE. Mucopolysaccharidoses and oligosaccharidoses. In: Fernandes J, Saudubray J-M, van den Berghe G, Walter JH, eds. *Inborn Metabolic Diseases*, 4th edn. Heidelberg: Springer, 2006: 495–507.

3 Williams PJ, Gatti R, Darby JK *et al.* Fucosidosis revisited: a review of 77 patients. *Am J Med Genet* 1991; **38**: 111–31.

4 Kanitakis J, Allombert C, Doebelin B *et al.* Fucosidosis with angiokeratoma. Immunohistochemical & electronmicroscopic study of a new case and literature review. *J Cutan Pathol* 2005; **32**: 506–11.

5 Kornfeld M, Snyder RD, Wenger DA. Fucosidosis with angiokeratoma. Electron microscopic changes in the skin. *Arch Pathol Lab Med* 1977; **101**: 478–85.

6 Miano M, Lanino E, Gatti R *et al.* Four year follow-up of a case of fucosidosis treated with unrelated donor bone marrow transplantation. *Bone Marrow Transplant* 2001; **27**: 747–51.

7 Rodriguez-Serna M, Botella-Estrada R, Chabas A *et al.* Angiokeratoma corporis diffusum associated with beta-mannosidase deficiency. *Arch Dermatol* 1996; **132**: 1219–22.

8 Uchino Y, Fukushige T, Yotsumoto S *et al.* Morphological and biochemical studies of human beta-mannosidosis: identification of a novel beta-mannosidase gene mutation. *Br J Dermatol* 2003; **149**: 23–9.

9 Aylsworth AS, Thomas GH, Hood JL *et al.* A severe infantile sialidosis: clinical, biochemical and microscopic features. *J Pediatr* 1980; **96**: 662–8.

10 Aula P, Jalanko A, Peltonen L. Aspartylglucosaminuria. In: Scriver CR, Beaudet AL, Sly WS *et al.*, eds. *The Metabolic and Molecular Bases of Inherited Disease*, 8th edn. New York: McGraw-Hill, 2001: 3535–50.

11 Arvio MA, Peippo MM, Arvio PJ, Kaariainen HA. Dysmorphic facial features in aspartylglucosaminuria patients and carriers. *Clin Dysmorphol* 2004; **13**: 11–5.

12 Arvio P, Arvio M, Kero M *et al.* Overgrowth of oral mucosa and facial skin, a novel feature of aspartylglucosaminuria. *J Med Genet* 1999; **36**: 398–404.

13 Arvio M, Autio S, Louhiala P. Early clinical symptoms and incidence of aspartylglucosaminuria in Finland. *Acta Paediatr* 1993; **82**: 587–9.

14 Vargas-Diez E, Chabas A, Coll MJ *et al.* Angiokeratoma corporis diffusum in a Spanish patient with aspartylglucosaminuria. *Br J Dermatol* 2002; **147**: 760–4.

15 Deanick RJ, Schindler D. α-N-Acetylgalactosaminidase deficiency: Schindler disease. In: Scriver CR, Beaudet AL, Sly WS *et al.*, eds. *The Metabolic and Molecular Bases of Inherited Disease*, 8th edn. New York: McGraw-Hill, 2001: 3483–506.

16 Kanzaki T, Yokota M, Irie F *et al.* Angiokeratoma coporis diffusum with glycopeptiduria due to deficient lysosomal α-N-acetylgalactosaminidase activity.

17 Chabas A, Coll MJ, Aparicio M, Rodriguez DE. Mild phenotypic expression of alpha-N-acetylgalactosaminidase deficiency in two adult siblings. *J Inherit Metab Dis* 1994; **17**: 724–31.

Clinical, morphologic and biochemical studies. *Arch Dermatol* 1993; **129**: 460–5.

Angiokeratoma corporis diffusum

Angiokeratoma corporis diffusum is the dermatological hallmark of several rare inherited lysosomal disorders, summarized in Table 59.5. Fabry's disease is much the commonest of these disorders. Angiokeratomas are mainly found in the milder (late-onset) forms of galactosialidosis and α-N-acetylgalactosaminidase deficiency and they are only an occasional finding in GM$_1$ gangliosidosis, aspartylglycosaminuria and β-mannosidosis. The angiokeratomas are accompanied by various problems affecting other parts of the body, depending on the underlying diagnosis. Fucosidosis, β-mannosidosis, aspartylglycosaminuria and Kanzaki disease have been described above; the other disorders primarily affect sphingolipid degradation and are described below. There have been a few reports of patients with angiokeratoma corporis diffusum in whom no specific enzyme deficiency has been identified [1–4]. In some cases, the presence of cytoplasmic vacuolation and associated clinical features suggests an unrecognized lysosomal disorder [2]; in cases without these features, a different aetiology seems more likely [3,4].

In each of the disorders, the skin lesions develop slowly as clusters of individual telangiectases or small angiomas. The colour ranges from dark red to blue-black. They are flat or slightly raised and do not blanch with pressure. The larger and older lesions may become hyperkeratotic. Bleeding can occur from the larger angiokeratomas. In patients with sparse angiokeratomas, the differential diagnoses include purpura, angioma serpiginosum and other types of angiokeratoma: solitary, circumscriptum, Fordyce type (scrotal) and Mibelli type [5]. Angiokeratomas can be removed by argon laser treatment if bleeding is a recurrent problem or for cosmetic reasons.

References

1 Holmes RC, Fenson AH, McKee P *et al.* Angiokeratoma corporis diffusum in a patient with normal enzyme activities. *J Am Acad Dermatol* 1984; **10**: 384–7.

2 McCallum DI, Macadam RF, Johnston AW. Angiokeratoma corporis diffusum with features of a mucopolysaccharidosis. *J Med Genet* 1980; **17**: 21–6.

3 Marsden J, Allen R. Widespread angiokeratomas without evidence of metabolic disease. *Arch Dermatol* 1987; **123**: 1125–7.

4 Gasparini G, Sarchi G, Cavicchini S *et al.* Angiokeratoma corporis diffusum in a patient with normal enzyme activities and Turner's syndrome. *Clin Exp Dermatol* 1992; **17**: 56–9.

5 Schiller PI, Itin PH. Angiokeratomas: an update. *Dermatology* 1996; **193**: 275–82.

Sphingolipidoses

Sphingolipids are amphiphilic molecules found in cell membranes. In all sphingolipids, the lipophilic component is ceramide. The hydrophilic portion is phosphorylcholine in sphingomyelin and usually an oligosaccharide in the glycosphingolipids. Glycosphingolipids containing neuraminic acid are called gangliosides. Sphingolipids are degraded in a stepwise fashion by lysosomal hydrolases and deficiencies of these enzymes (or their protector/activator proteins) cause the sphingolipidoses [1]. In some sphingolipidoses (e.g. Tay–Sachs disease), problems are confined to the nervous system; these are not considered further here. Other sphingolipidoses may be associated with an MPS-like facial appearance, angiokeratomas or other dermatological abnormalities. In many of these disorders, histology reveals vacuolated cells, whose ultrastructural appearance provides clues to the diagnosis. Thin layer chromatography reveals abnormal urinary oligosaccharides in a few disorders but the diagnosis is generally established by enzyme assays on leukocytes (or cultured cells). The clinical and biochemical features of the sphingolipidoses with dermatological features are included in Table 59.4.

Genetics. All the disorders are rare and show an autosomal recessive pattern of inheritance, except Fabry's disease, which is X-linked.

GM$_1$ gangliosidosis (MIM 230500) [1,2]

Deficiency of acid β-galactosidase leads to the accumulation of GM$_1$ ganglioside, other glycosphingolipids, galactose-containing oligosaccharides and keratan sulphate. GM$_1$ gangliosidosis is very rare and has a wide range of severity. Some patients present with hydrops fetalis or as neonates with hypotonia, hepatosplenomegaly and dysmorphism. The face is often puffy, with macroglossia, gum hypertrophy and a depressed nasal bridge; radiological investigation reveals dysostosis multiplex. These patients develop spasticity, seizures, dysphagia, loss of vision and macular cherry red spots; most die by 2 years of age. Other patients present with regression in early childhood and develop a spastic quadriplegia. The most mildly affected patients present later in childhood or as adults with dysarthria, dystonia and an abnormal gait; they may have mild learning difficulties and skeletal dysplasia, affecting the spine and hip. Widespread angiokeratomas have been reported in a few infants with GM$_1$ gangliosidosis [3]; the age of onset contrasts with other disorders, in which angiokeratomas seldom appear before mid-childhood. Telangiectasia and extensive Mongolian blue spots have also been reported in some infants [3,4]. Electron microscopy shows vacuolated histiocytes, fibroblasts and endothelial cells with fibrillogranular material in the vacuoles. The diagnosis is made by demonstrating β-galactosidase deficiency in leukocytes, with normal neuraminidase activity (which excludes galactosialidosis). There is no treatment for early-onset forms but substrate reduction therapy with miglustat may help late-onset patients.

Galactosialidosis (MIM 256540) [1,5]

In this extremely rare disorder, there is a combined deficiency of neuraminidase and β-galactosidase. The primary defect is in a protein (PPCA) that normally protects the two enzymes from rapid proteolysis. The protective protein is also called cathepsin A (hence PPCA) and has peptidase activity towards certain neuropeptides. The most severely affected patients present with hydrops fetalis or with MPS-like facial dysmorphism and organomegaly in the neonatal period and die within the first year from renal or cardiac failure. Many of these patients have telangiectases [6] and a few have angiokeratomas. Other patients present in early childhood with coarse facies, organomegaly, dysostosis multiplex and neurodevelopmental problems. Mildly affected patients are mostly Japanese. They present in late childhood or adulthood with myoclonus, ataxia, mental retardation and loss of vision with cherry red spots. They have no organomegaly but do have mild MPS-like facial features and spinal abnormalities. Half of these patients have angiokeratomas, similar to those seen in Fabry's disease [7]. Electron microscopy shows vacuoles, some containing granular material, in endothelial cells and fibroblasts. The diagnosis is made by finding deficiencies of β-galactosidase, neuraminidase and cathepsin A in leukocytes or cultured fibroblasts.

References

1 Vanier M-T. Disorders of sphingolipid metabolism. In: Fernandes J, Saudubray J-M, van den Berghe G, Walter JH, eds. *Inborn Metabolic Diseases*, 4th edn. Heidelberg: Springer, 2006: 479–94.

2 Suzuki Y, Oshima A, Nanba E. β-Galactosidase deficiency: GM$_1$ gangliosidosis and Morquio B disease. In: Scriver CR, Beaudet AL, Sly WS *et al.*, eds. *The Metabolic and Molecular Bases of Inherited Disease*, 8th edn. New York: McGraw-Hill, 2001: 3775–810.

3 Beratis NG, Varvarigou-Frimas A, Beratis S, Sklower SL. Angiokeratoma corporis diffusum in GM1 gangliosidosis, type 1. *Clin Genet* 1989; **36**: 59–64.

4 Weissbluth M, Esterly NB, Caro WA. Report of an infant with GM1 gangliosidosis type I and extensive and unusual mongolian spots. *Br J Dermatol* 1981; **104**: 195–200.

5 d'Azzo A, Andria G, Strisciuglio P, Galjaard H. Galactosialidosis. In: Scriver CR, Beaudet AL, Sly WS *et al.*, eds. *The Metabolic and Molecular Bases of Inherited Disease*, 8th edn. New York: McGraw-Hill, 2001: 3811–26.

6 Patel MS, Callahan JW, Zhang S *et al.* Early infantile galactosialidosis. *Am J Med Genet* 1999; **85**: 38–47.

7 Nobeyama Y, Honda M, Niimura M. A case of galactosialidosis. *Br J Dermatol* 2003; **149**: 405–9.

Fabry's disease (MIM 301500) [1]

A.A.M. Morris & S.M. Breathnach, pp. 59.36–59.39

Synonym
- Anderson–Fabry disease

This is a rare X-linked sphingolipidosis, with an estimated incidence of 1 in 40000–60000 male births [1,2]. Affected males usually present in childhood with episodes of pain in the extremities, followed by the appearance of angiokeratomas. Most adult males develop renal failure, cardiac and cerebrovascular disease. Many heterozygous females also develop symptoms, though the onset is usually later.

Aetiology. Deficiency of the lysosomal enzyme, α-galactosidase A, leads to the accumulation of glycosphingolipids with terminal galactose residues, predominantly globotriaosylceramide (galactose–galactose–glucose–ceramide) but also galabiosylceramide (galactose–galactose–ceramide) and blood group B substances [1]. These are found in the lysosomes of endothelial, perithelial and vascular smooth muscle cells; the swollen endothelial cells encroach on the lumen of blood vessels, leading to focal increases in pressure and aneurysmal dilatation of the weakened vascular wall. Glycosphingolipids also accumulate in renal glomeruli and tubules, cardiac muscle, autonomic ganglion cells and the corneal epithelium. More than 300 mutations have been identified in the GLA gene; none are highly prevalent. Some mutations seem to be associated with mild variants (e.g. N215S with the 'cardiac' variant) [3] but others are found in both mild variants and in classical disease [3,4].

Clinical features. The first symptoms are usually episodes of severe burning pain in the palms and soles (acroparesthesiae). These occur in 70–85% of male patients, usually starting between 5 and 15 years, though it may take many years for the diagnosis to be established [4]. Acroparesthesiae occur in 50–70% of females, with a mean age of onset of 15 years [5,6]. Painful crises are often triggered by fever or exertion and may last hours or days. Pain may diminish spontaneously in older men.

Angiokeratomas are found in 65–70% of male and 35–40% of female patients [4,5,7]. In males, they often start to appear shortly before puberty (age of onset 19 ± 14 years, mean ± SD) whereas in females they usually appear later (28 ± 17 years). The initial lesion is a dark-red or black telangiectatic macule or papule up to 4 mm across, that does not blanch with pressure; there is usually mild hyperkeratosis over larger lesions. Angiokeratomas are clustered and numerous in some patients but they are sparse in most women and in many men [7]. In men, the commonest sites are around the umbilicus (Fig. 59.23) and in the bathing-trunk area, affecting the inner thighs, lower back, buttocks, penis and scrotum. Lesions may also be found on the upper arms, around the border of the lips, around the nail folds and on the palms and soles; these are usually macular angiomas with minimal hyperkeratosis [7]. In women, lesions are most frequent on the trunk and proximal limbs; genital lesions are rare. Telangiectases are present in 23% of males and 9% of females, usually on the lips, buccal mucosa, ears or conjunctivae [7,8]. The other common dermatological problem is anhidrosis or hypohidrosis (in 53% of males and 28%

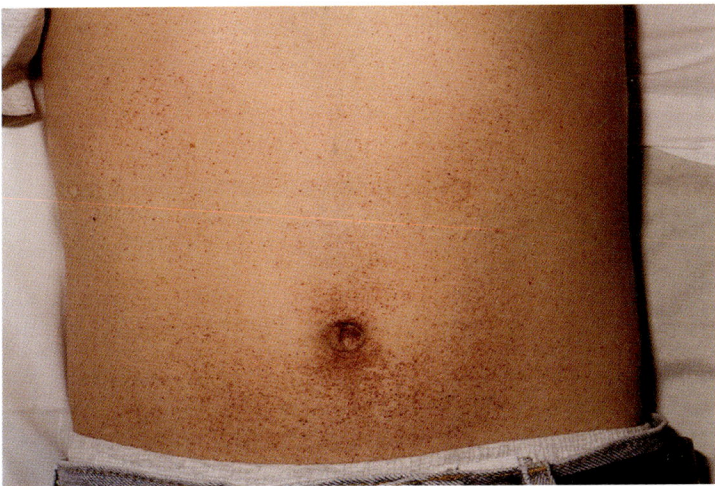

Fig. 59.23 Angiokeratoma corporis diffusum around the umbilicus in a man with Fabry's disease.

of females) [7,9]. This probably results from an autonomic neuropathy. It is associated with heat and exercise intolerance, and sometimes with unexplained bouts of fever. Onset is most often in the third decade. Hyperhidrosis occurs in about 10% of patients, predominantly females, often starting in adolescence [10]. Later, vasomotor disturbances may cause the hands to be blue or blanched, or there may be flushing of the extremities. Lymphoedema is much commoner than in the general population [7] and may be due to lymphatic microangiopathy [11].

Cardiac involvement occurs in almost all adult males [1,2,4]. It includes left ventricular dilatation and hypertrophy, mitral valve regurgitation, arrhythmias and ischaemic heart disease. Most adult males have proteinuria, hypertension and gradually deteriorating renal function. Without enzyme replacement therapy, endstage renal failure is usually reached between 40 and 50 years of age, though it can occur much earlier [1,4]. Cerebrovascular disease is also common and may lead to early strokes or transient ischaemic attacks. Other patients develop severe neurological problems without any obvious thrombotic episodes, presumably due to the involvement of multiple small vessels [1]. Vertigo, dizziness and high frequency hearing loss are common.

Most male patients have the full syndrome but atypical, milder variants have been reported. Men with the 'cardiac variant' usually present after the age of 40 years with cardiomyopathy and proteinuria [2]. Cardiac and cerebrovascular disease are commoner in heterozygous women than previously thought [5]. In a survey of 248 female patients, 26% had left ventricular hypertrophy (mean age of onset 50 years) and 7% had suffered strokes (mean age 50 years) [6].

Slit-lamp examination reveals an asymptomatic corneal dystrophy in most adult male and female patients [12]. Glycosphingolipid deposits under the epithelium initially cause superficial haziness, which progresses to characteristic whorled streaks radiating to the periphery (cornea verticillata). Identical appearances have been reported after long-term chloroquine or amiodarone [13]. Other ophthalmological findings include lens opacities and tortuosity of the conjunctival and retinal vessels.

Episodes of abdominal pain and diarrhoea are common and there may be achalasia of the oesophagus. Some patients suffer arthritis in the distal interphalangeal joint of the hand.

Prognosis. Men and women with Fabry's disease have a reduced life expectancy due to renal, cerebrovascular and cardiac disease. In a cohort of male patients, the median survival was 50 years, approximately 20 years less than the normal population [4]. School attendance, sport and social activities were all affected and only 57% of patients were in employment [4]. In a cohort of heterozygous women, the median survival was 70 years, approximately 15 years less than the normal population [5].

Histopathology. Light microscopy of the angiokeratomas shows dilated vessels in the upper dermis beneath a thinned epidermis, with or without hyperkeratosis (Fig. 59.24). Vacuolated cells are present in the media and intima of small blood vessels. The accumulated glycosphingolipids are birefringent and, in frozen sections, they appear as 'Maltese crosses' in polarized light [1]. Electron microscopy shows cytoplasmic inclusion bodies in the

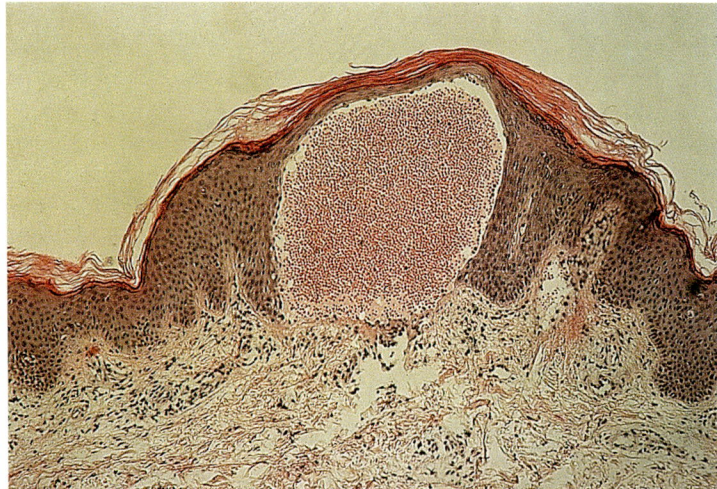

Fig. 59.24 Angiokeratoma corporis diffusum: H&E, × 4. Dilated blood-filled vessels in papillary dermis.

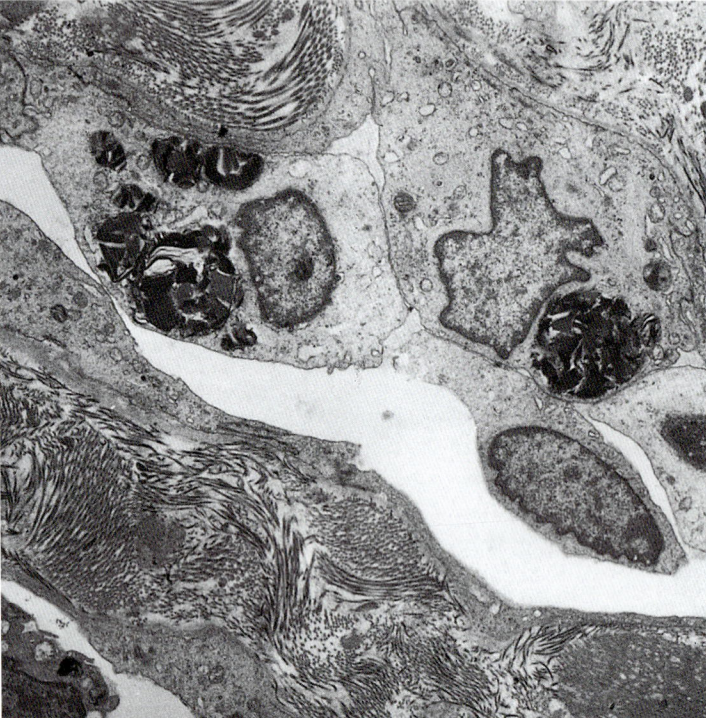

Fig. 59.25 Angiokeratoma corporis diffusum. Electron-dense cytoplasmic inclusion bodies are present within endothelial cells. (Courtesy of Dr P.H. McKee, King's College, London, UK.)

endothelial (Fig. 59.25) and perithelial cells of blood vessels, smooth muscle, perineural cells and dermal macrophages. The inclusions are electron-dense and lamellar, with a periodicity of 4–6 nm [1,14]. In contrast, other lysosomal disorders associated with angiokeratomas have electron-lucent vacuoles containing scanty fibrillary or granular material. The inclusions in Fabry's disease represent lipid deposits within lysosomes [14]. They are present in clinically unaffected skin, even in infancy [15], and in other tissues (e.g. myocardial and glomerular epithelial cells).

Diagnosis. If the angiokeratomas are sparse, it may be difficult to distinguish them from angiokeratomas without systemic disease.

The diagnosis of Fabry's disease can be established by skin histology or slit-lamp examination of the cornea. In males, it should be confirmed by demonstrating α-galactosidase A deficiency in plasma or leukocytes (or cultured skin fibroblasts). This technique is unsuitable for heterozygous females, who often have normal enzyme activity. Urinary globotriacylceramide concentrations are raised in most heterozygous females [16] but the assay is not widely available. Molecular analysis is, therefore, the preferred technique for confirming the diagnosis in women, though occasionally it is difficult to distinguish pathogenic mutations from benign polymorphisms.

Treatment. The acroparesthesiae may respond to carbamazepine, gabapentin or phenytoin [17,18] or they may require opiates. Angiokeratomas can be removed by laser therapy for cosmetic or other reasons but this is seldom requested [19]. Cardiac complications should be managed conventionally. Aspirin may reduce the risk of stroke. Smoking should be avoided; statins should be prescribed if there is hyperlipidaemia and hypertension should be controlled. ACE inhibitors should be started if there is proteinuria. Patients developing renal failure warrant dialysis or transplantation; glycolipids do not reaccumulate in the graft [20].

Enzyme replacement therapy (ERT) with recombinant human α-galactosidase A has been shown to clear microvascular deposits of globotriaosylceramide from the kidneys, heart and skin [21]. It reduces neurogenic pain [22], reduces left ventricular hypertrophy [23] and prevents the development of renal impairment in patients with normal baseline renal function [24]. In the UK, ERT is now started following diagnosis in symptomatic male patients; in female patients, it is started if there is cardiac, neurological or renal disease, troublesome gastrointestinal symptoms or pain that cannot be controlled by other means.

References

1 Desnick RJ, Ioannou YA, Eng CM. α-Galactosidase deficiency: Fabry disease. In: Scriver CR, Beaudet AL, Sly WS *et al.*, eds. *The Metabolic and Molecular Bases of Inherited Disease*, 8th edn. New York: McGraw-Hill, 2001: 3733–74.

2 Nakao S, Takenaka T, Maeda M *et al.* An atypical variant of Fabry's disease in men with left ventricular hypertrophy. *N Engl J Med* 1995; **333**: 288–93.

3 Eng CM, Resnick-Silverman LA, Niehaus DJ *et al.* Nature and frequency of mutations in the alpha-galactosidase A gene that cause Fabry disease. *Am J Hum Genet* 1993; **53**: 1186–97.

4 MacDermot KD, Holmes A, Miners AH. Anderson–Fabry disease. Clinical manifestations and impact of disease in a cohort of 98 hemizygous males. *J Med Genet* 2001; **38**: 750–60.

5 MacDermot KD, Holmes A, Miners AH. Anderson–Fabry disease. Clinical manifestations and impact of disease in a cohort of 60 obligate carrier females. *J Med Genet* 2001; **38**: 769–75.

6 Deegan PB, Baehner AF, Barba Romero MA *et al.* Natural history of Fabry disease in females in the Fabry Outcome Survey. *J Med Genet* 2006; **43**: 347–52.

7 Orteu CH, Jansen T, Lidove O *et al.* Fabry disease and the skin: data from FOS, the Fabry outcome survey. *Br J Dermatol* 2007; **157**: 331–7.

8 Chesser RS, Gentry RH, Fitzpatrick JE *et al.* Perioral telangiectases: a new cutaneous finding in Fabry's disease. *Arch Dermatol* 1990; **126**: 1655–6.

9 Lao LM, Kumakiri M, Mima H *et al.* The ultrastructural characteristics of eccrine sweat glands in a Fabry disease patient with hypohidrosis. *J Dermatol Sci* 1998; **18**: 109–17.

10 Lidove O, Ramaswami U, Jaussaud R *et al.* Hyperhidrosis: a new and often early symptom in Fabry disease. International experience and data from the Fabry Outcome Survey. *Int J Clin Pract* 2006; **60**: 1053–9.

11 Amann-Vesti BR, Gitzelmann G, Widmer U *et al.* Severe lymphatic microangiopathy in Fabry disease. *Lymphat Res Biol* 2003; **1**: 185–9.

12 Sodi A, Ioannidis AS, Mehta A *et al*. Ocular manifestations of Fabry's disease: data from the Fabry Outcome Survey. *Br J Ophthalmol* 2007; **91**: 210–4.

13 Chew E, Ghosh M, McCulloch C. Amiodarone-induced cornea verticillata. *Can J Ophthalmol* 1982; **17**: 96–9.

14 Hashimoto K, Lieberman P, Lamkin N. Angiokeratoma corporis diffusum (Fabry's disease): a lysosomal disease. *Arch Dermatol* 1976; **112**: 1416–23.

15 Breathnach SM, Black MM, Wallace HJ. Anderson–Fabry disease: characteristic ultrastructure features in cutaneous blood vessels in a 1-year-old boy. *Br J Dermatol* 1980; **103**: 81–4.

16 Young E, Mills K, Morris P *et al*. Is globotriaosylceramide a useful biomarker in Fabry disease? *Acta Paediatr Suppl* 2005; **94**: 51–4.

17 Lockman LA, Hunninglake DB, Krivit W *et al*. Relief of pain of Fabry's disease by diphenylhydantoin. *Neurology* 1973; **23**: 871–5.

18 Ries M, Mengel E, Kutschke G *et al*. Use of gabapentin to reduce chronic neuropathic pain in Fabry disease. *J Inherit Metab Dis* 2003; **26**: 413–4.

19 Mohrenschlager M, Braun-Falco M, Ring J, Abeck D. Fabry disease: recognition and management of cutaneous manifestations. *Am J Clin Dermatol* 2003; **4**: 189–96.

20 Ojo A, Meier-Kriesche HU, Friedman G *et al*. Excellent outcome of renal transplantation in patients with Fabry's disease. *Transplantation* 2000; **69**: 2337–9.

21 Eng CM, Guffon N, Wilcox WR *et al*. Safety and efficacy of recombinant human α-galactosidase A replacement therapy in Fabry's disease. *N Engl J Med* 2001; **345**: 9–16.

22 Schiffmann R, Kopp JB, Austin HA 3rd *et al*. Enzyme replacement therapy in Fabry disease: a randomized controlled trial. *JAMA* 2001; **285**: 2743–9.

23 Hughes DA, Elliott PM, Shah J *et al*. Effects of enzyme replacement therapy on the cardiomyopathy of Anderson-Fabry disease: a randomized, double-blind, placebo-controlled clinical trial of agalsidase-alfa. *Heart* 2008; **94**: 15–8.

24 Germain DP, Waldek S, Banikazemi M *et al*. Sustained, long-term renal stabilization after 54 months of agalsidase beta therapy in patients with Fabry disease. *J Am Soc Nephrol* 2007; **18**: 1547–57.

Gaucher's disease (MIM 606463) [1]

A.A.M. Morris, pp. 59.39–59.42

This autosomal recessive disorder results from deficiency of acid β-glucosidase (glucocerebrosidase). Glycosphingolipids (principally glucosylceramide, also known as glucocerebroside) accumulate in macrophages in the liver, spleen and bones. Though Gaucher's disease is rare, it is the most prevalent lysosomal disorder (1:57000 in Australia [2]).

Clinical features. Gaucher's disease is classified clinically into type 1 (non-neuronopathic), type 2 (acute neuronopathic) and type 3 (subacute neuronopathic). Type 1 is much the commonest, particularly in Ashkenazi Jews, in whom the incidence is over 1:1000, mainly due to a high prevalence of the N370S mutation. It presents in childhood or adulthood, with hepatosplenomegaly, features of hypersplenism (usually thrombocytopenia) or bone problems. Some children and adolescents suffer painful 'bone crises' due to ischaemia, typically in the femoral head or shaft. Later, loss of bone mass can lead to pathological fractures [3]. Lung infiltration is a rare but serious complication. The prognosis for type 1 Gaucher's disease depends on the severity of the mutations [4]; some patients can die by the age of 20 years without treatment, whereas some N370S homozygotes never develop symptoms.

Cutaneous features are common but not troublesome in type 1 Gaucher's disease [5]. In a series of 50 South African patients, 50% had diffuse yellow-brown pigmentation, 40% reported easy tanning, 30% had brown macules and 20% had telangiectasia [6]. Thrombocytopenia may lead to petechiae or ecchymoses.

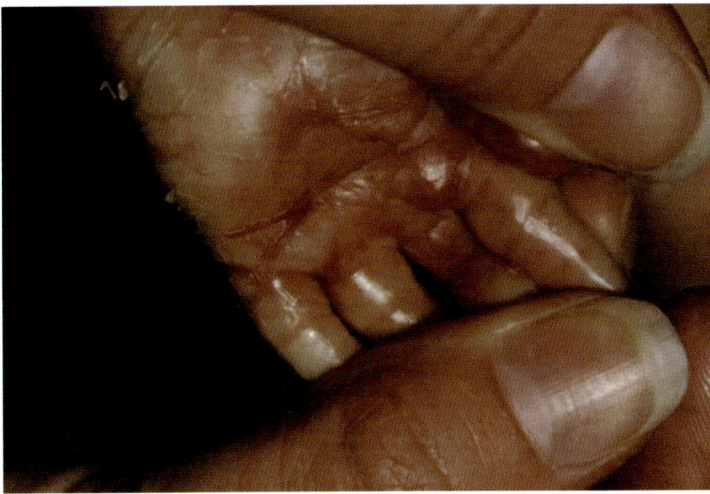

Fig. 59.26 The hand of a 'collodion baby' with Gaucher's disease type 2.

Type 2 Gaucher's disease presents during the first 6 months of life with brainstem problems, such as squint, dysphagia and hyperextension of the neck, followed by episodes of apnoea. Other features include stridor, spasticity, epilepsy, lung disease and hepatosplenomegaly. Most type 2 patients die by the age of 2 years [7]. There is also a perinatal-lethal form that usually presents with hydrops fetalis. Some of these patients have severe ichthyosis, leading to the collodion baby phenotype (Fig. 59.26) [8]. The baby is encased in thick, tight, shiny skin that cracks and desquamates to leave erythroderma. The thickened skin causes ectropia of the eyes. The skin may return to normal if the baby survives for more than a month.

Type 3 disease is particularly common in the Norrbottnian population of northern Sweden, where it is associated with homozygosity for the L444P mutation. These patients usually present with hepatosplenomegaly in infancy, followed a few years later by an eye movement disorder, impaired hearing and other neurological problems [9]. Some type 3 patients have progressive myoclonic epilepsy and dementia with less severe organomegaly.

Pathology. Numerous characteristic histiocytes (Gaucher cells) are found in the spleen, liver, bone marrow and lymph nodes, with smaller numbers in other organs. Gaucher cells are large cells with pale-staining cytoplasm that has a delicate, striated, 'wrinkled tissue paper' appearance, best seen in thicker sections (10 μm). They differ markedly from the foam cells seen in other lipidoses. Ultrastructurally, Gaucher cells have membrane bound twisted tubular inclusions that represent aggregated glucocerebroside molecules within lysosomes [1,10].

Diagnosis. The diagnosis should be confirmed by enzyme assay in lymphocytes, leukocytes or cultured fibroblasts or by mutation analysis.

Treatment. Enzyme replacement therapy (ERT) is safe and effective for the treatment of type 1 Gaucher's disease but it is expensive and requires slow intravenous infusion at least every 2 weeks [11–13]. In the UK, all paediatric patients receive ERT, as do adults with significant symptoms but not those who only have mild splenomegaly or mild skeletal abnormalities. Miglustat is an oral drug that decreases the accumulation of glucocerebroside by reducing the synthesis of glycosphingolipids (substrate reduction therapy) [14]. In the UK, it is used in mildly affected patients who are unable or unwilling to receive ERT. Diarrhoea and weight loss are common side effects. Splenectomy reduces abdominal distension and can relieve thrombocytopenia but it is seldom indicated in countries that can afford ERT. Other supportive measures include transfusion of blood products, bisphosphonates and analgesia.

There is no effective treatment for type 2 Gaucher's disease. ERT relieves the systemic complications in type 3 Gaucher's disease but it does not cross the blood–brain barrier; addition of miglustat or haematopoietic stem cell transplantation should be considered if there is neurological deterioration [15].

References

1 Beutler E, Grabowski GA. Gaucher's disease. In: Scriver CR, Beaudet AL, Sly WS *et al.*, eds. *The Metabolic and Molecular Bases of Inherited Disease*, 8th edn. New York: McGraw-Hill, 2001: 3635–68.

2 Meikle PJ, Hopwood JJ, Clague AE, Carey WF. Prevalence of lysosomal storage disorders. *JAMA* 1999; **281**: 249–54.

3 Wenstrup RJ, Roca-Espiau M, Weinreb NJ, Bembi B. Skeletal aspects of Gaucher disease: a review. *Br J Radiol* 2002; **75** (Suppl. 1): A2–12.

4 Charrow J, Andersson HC, Kaplan P *et al.* The Gaucher registry: demographics and disease characteristics of 1698 patients with Gaucher disease. *Arch Intern Med* 2000; **160**: 2835–43.

5 Reich C, Seife M, Kessler BJ. Gaucher's disease. A review and discussion of 20 cases. *Medicine (Baltimore)* 1951; **30**: 1–20.

6 Goldblatt J, Beighton P. Cutaneous manifestations of Gaucher disease. *Br J Dermatol* 1984; **111**: 331–4.

7 Mignot C, Doummar D, Maire I, De Villemeur TB. Type 2 Gaucher disease: 15 new cases and review of the literature. *Brain Dev* 2006; **28**: 39–48.

8 Stone DL, Carey WF, Christodoulou J *et al.* Type 2 Gaucher disease: the collodion baby phenotype revisited. *Arch Dis Child (Fetal Neonatal Edn)* 2000; **82**: F163–6.

9 Dreborg S, Erikson A, Hagberg B. Gaucher disease–Norrbottnian type. I. General clinical description. *Eur J Pediatr* 1980; **133**: 107–18.

10 Lee RE. The fine structure of the cerebroside occurring in Gaucher's disease. *Proc Natl Acad Sci USA* 1968; **61**: 484–9.

11 Weinreb NJ, Charrow J, Andersson HC *et al.* Effectiveness of enzyme replacement therapy in 1028 patients with type 1 Gaucher disease after 2–5 years of treatment: a report from the Gaucher Registry. *Am J Med* 2002; **113**: 112–9.

12 Baldellou A, Andria G, Campbell PE *et al.* Paediatric non-neuronopathic Gaucher disease: recommendations for treatment and monitoring. *Eur J Pediatr* 2004; **163**: 67–75.

13 Andersson HC, Charrow J, Kaplan P *et al.* Individualization of long-term enzyme replacement therapy for Gaucher disease. *Genet Med* 2005; **7**: 105–10.

14 Weinreb NJ, Barranger JA, Charrow J *et al.* Guidance on the use of miglustat for treating patients with type 1 Gaucher disease. *Am J Hematol* 2005; **80**: 223–9.

15 Capablo JL, Franco R, de Cabezon AS *et al.* Neurologic improvement in a type 3 Gaucher disease patient treated with imiglucerase/miglustat combination. *Epilepsia* 2007; **48**: 1406–8.

Niemann–Pick disease types A and B (MIM 257200) [1]

Aetiology. Niemann–Pick disease (NPD) types A and B are autosomal recessive sphingolipidoses, caused by sphingomyelinase deficiency. Sphingomyelin accumulates in histiocytes and leads to hepatosplenomegaly. In NPD type A, sphingomyelin also accumulates in the brain, leading to progressive neurodegeneration during early childhood. NPD type B is non-neuronopathic. Both types are very rare but type A is more common in Ashkenazi Jews. (NPD type C is an unrelated disorder characterized by defective intracellular lipid trafficking.)

Clinical features. Classical NPD type A patients present with diarrhoea, vomiting and failure to thrive in the first 2 months. By 6 months of age, there is hepatosplenomegaly, lymphadenopathy, trunkal hypotonia and spasticity in the limbs. Deafness and blindness are common and half the patients have retinal cherry red spots. Most patients die by 3 years of age. Other NPD type A patients have milder systemic features and juvenile or adult-onset neurological disease [2]. Type B patients usually present with splenomegaly or hepatosplenomegaly, sometimes not until adulthood. Interstitial lung disease, poor growth, hyperlipidaemia and thrombocytopenia are common. Nevertheless, some patients have a normal lifespan [3].

The skin may show patches of waxy induration and brownish-yellow pigmentation [4]. Papular, papulonodular or suppurative lesions may be found on the face or trunk [5,6], occasionally becoming confluent [6]. These may be commoner in patients with NPD of intermediate severity. Xanthomas and xanthogranulomas [7], café-au-lait macules and Mongolian blue spots have also been reported. Thrombocytopenia may lead to purpura or bruising.

Pathology. Niemann–Pick cells are the hallmark of NPD; some are present in virtually all tissues, including the skin [4,5]. They are large, usually mononucleate histiocytes, whose cytoplasm is filled with lipid droplets, giving rise to a foamy appearance. In cryostat sections, they stain readily with Sudan stains and contain doubly refractile material. Ultrastructurally, the cytoplasm contains concentric lamellar inclusions [5]. Similar cells are found in Wolman disease, cholesterol ester storage disease and lipoprotein lipase deficiency; Niemann–Pick cells stain poorly with PAS, in contrast to Gaucher cells. The diagnosis can be confirmed by measuring sphingomyelinase activity in leukocytes or cultured fibroblasts.

Treatment. There is no effective treatment for NPD type A. Trials of enzyme replacement therapy are planned for NPD type B.

References

1 Schuchman EH, Desnick RJ. Niemann–Pick disease types A and B. Acid sphingomyelinase deficiencies. In: Scriver CR, Beaudet AL, Sly WS *et al.*, eds. *The Metabolic and Molecular Bases of Inherited Disease*, 8th edn. New York: McGraw-Hill, 2001: 3589–610.

2 Wasserstein MP, Aron A, Brodie SE *et al.* Acid sphingomyelinase deficiency: prevalence and characterization of an intermediate phenotype of Niemann-Pick disease. *J Pediatr* 2006; **149**: 554–9.

3 Wasserstein MP, Desnick RJ, Schuchman EH *et al.* The natural history of type B Niemann–Pick disease: results from a 10-year longitudinal study. *Pediatrics* 2004; **114**: e672–e677.

4 Mardini MK, Gergan P, Akltar M *et al.* Niemann–Pick disease: report of a case with skin involvement. *Am J Dis Child* 1982; **136**: 650–1.

5 Toussaint M, Worret WI, Drosner M *et al.* Specific skin lesions in a patient with Niemann–Pick disease. *Br J Dermatol* 1994; **131**: 895–7.

6 Raddadi AA, Al Twaim AA. Type A Niemann-Pick disease. *J Eur Acad Dermatol Venereol* 2000; **14**: 301–3.

7 Crocker AC, Farber S. Niemann–Pick disease. A review of 18 patients. *Medicine (Baltimore)* 1958; **37**: 1–95.

Farber's disease (MIM 228000) [1]

Synonym
• Disseminated lipogranulomatosis

Farber's disease is an extremely rare autosomal recessive lipid-storage disease of infants, in which deficiency of lysosomal acid ceramidase leads to the accumulation of ceramide [1,2].

Clinical features. Patients usually present in early infancy with a hoarse cry, painful swollen joints and subcutaneous nodules. The most commonly affected joints are those of the hand and wrist, elbows, knees and ankles. The subcutaneous nodules may be associated with erythematous papules and are generally close to affected joints or over pressure points, such as the occiput and lower spine. Laryngeal involvement can lead to stridor as well as hoarseness. Most patients have psychomotor retardation, poor weight gain and die in early childhood from respiratory infections. A few patients present with hydrops fetalis or neonatal hepatosplenomegaly [2]. In other patients, neurodegeneration is the main feature [3]; these patients usually have cherry-red spots at the macula.

Histopathology. In the skin and subcutaneous tissue, dense areas of mixed granulomatous infiltration are found among a fibrovascular stroma. Groups of large, foamy histiocytes are found towards the centre of the granulomas. Ultrastructurally, the histiocytes have cytoplasmic vacuoles containing curvilinear inclusions (Farber bodies) [2,4]. Histochemical studies indicate that the storage material consists of ceramide and glycolipids [1,2]. The diagnosis can be confirmed by enzyme assay in leukocytes or fibroblasts.

Treatment. Symptomatic treatment includes analgesia and corticosteroids. Haematopoietic stem cell transplantation does not prevent neurological deterioration but may be appropriate for atypical patients without neurological involvement [5].

References
1 Moser HW, Linke T, Fensom AH, Levade T, Sandhoff K. Acid ceramidase deficiency: Farber lipogranulomatosis. In: Scriver CR, Beaudet AL, Sly WS *et al.*, eds. *The Metabolic and Molecular Basis of Inherited Disease*, 8th edn. New York: McGraw-Hill, 2001: 3573–88.
2 Qualman SJ, Moser HW, Valle D *et al.* Farber disease: pathologic diagnosis in sibs with phenotypic variability. *Am J Med Genet Suppl* 1987; **3**: 233–41.
3 Eviatar L, Sklower SL, Wisniewski K *et al.* Farber lipogranulomatosis: an unusual presentation in a black child. *Pediatr Neurol* 1986; **2**: 371–4.
4 Schmoeckel C, Hohlfell M. A specific ultrastructural marker for disseminated lipogranulomatosis (Farber). *Arch Dermatol Res* 1979; **266**: 187–96.
5 Vormoor J, Ehlert K, Groll AH *et al.* Successful hematopoietic stem cell transplantation in Farber disease. *J Pediatr* 2004; **144**: 132–4.

Lipoid proteinosis (MIM 247100) [1,2]

Synonyms
• Urbach–Wiethe disease
• Hyalinosis cutis et mucosae
• Lipoglycoproteinosis

Aetiology. Lipoid proteinosis is a very rare, autosomal recessive disorder, characterized by infiltration of hyaline material into the skin, oral cavity, larynx and internal organs. The exact nature of the hyaline material is still uncertain. The disorder is caused by mutations in the extracellular matrix protein 1 (ECM1) gene [3]. ECM1 binds to various proteins (perlecan, fibulins and matrix metalloproteinase-9) but its function is unknown [1]. Interestingly, antibodies to ECM1 are present in 75% of patients with lichen sclerosis [4]. Lipoid proteinosis is common in the Namaqualand region of South Africa, where cases can be traced back to a German immigrant [2].

Clinical features. Lipoid proteinosis usually presents in infancy with hoarseness, which can progress to complete aphonia. The vocal cords are thickened, with nodules here and on the epiglottis. Occasionally, stridor necessitates a tracheostomy [5]. The lips, pharynx, soft palate, uvula and tonsils develop yellow-white submucous infiltrates. The tongue is enlarged and firm with infiltrates on its under-surface. The frenulum becomes short and thick, restricting tongue movement, such that it cannot be protruded. There may be recurrent inflammation of the salivary glands [2].

The first skin lesions are often blisters in early childhood, which become eroded and crusted after minor trauma [2]. Acneiform, pock-like scars appear on the face and elsewhere, either following trauma or spontaneously. Infiltration of the skin can cause waxy papules, hyperkeratosis or warty plaques, which may become darker with time. These lesions may affect the palms or backs of the hands, the forehead or the elbows, where they can be prominent and resemble xanthomas. Characteristic 'beaded' papules are present along the margins of the eyelids but they may be subtle (moniliform blepharosis) (Fig. 59.27). There may be loss of eyelashes or patchy alopecia due to scalp involvement [6]. Some patients complain of itching or increased sensitivity to sunlight [2].

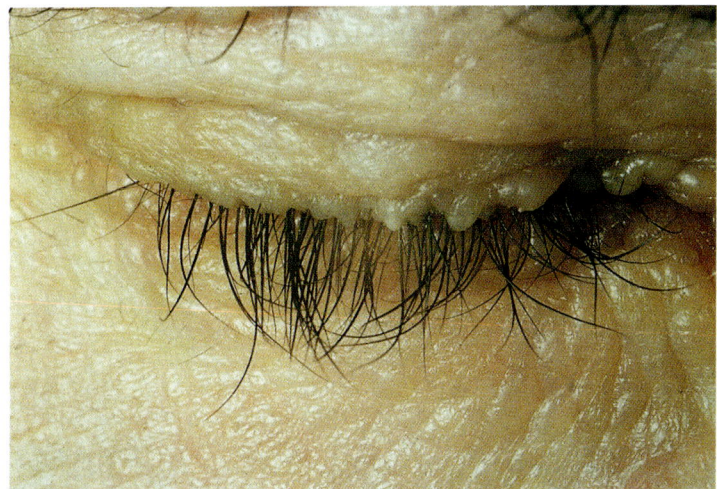

Fig. 59.27 Lipoid proteinosis. Typical 'beaded' papules present along the margins of the upper eyelids. (Courtesy of Dr R.C.D. Staughton, Chelsea and Westminster Hospital, London, UK.)

Epilepsy and psychiatric problems occur in a number of patients and may be associated with intracranial calcification (e.g. in the temporal lobes or amygdala) [7]. Visceral involvement has also been reported [8]. Problems progress until early adult life but subsequently stabilize.

Histopathology. The epidermis shows hyperkeratosis and irregular acanthosis. The dermis is thickened and the upper dermis contains large deposits of extracellular hyaline material that stains strongly with PAS. There is also thickening of the (PAS-positive) basement membranes at the dermal–epidermal junction and around blood vessels and sweat glands. Immunofluorescence labelling for type IV collagen confirms the basement membrane thickening. Staining for type I and type III collagen is decreased in the upper dermis; the deposits of hyaline material do not stain with anticollagen antibodies [6]. Ultrastructurally, there are multiple concentric rings of basement membrane around blood vessels and irregular reduplication of the lamina densa at the dermal–epidermal junction. The hyaline deposits are featureless. Lysosomes containing curved tubular inclusions have been reported in histiocytes and eccrine sweat glands [9] but this is not thought to be a primary lysosomal disorder. Histochemical diagnosis is now possible using an antibody to ECM1 [10].

Diagnosis. The combination of hoarseness from early childhood, thickening of the tongue and frenulum and cutaneous nodules suggests the diagnosis. Erythropoietic protoporphyria also causes waxy papules and depressed scars but the scars are confined to sun-exposed skin; on histology, the hyaline material is less extensive and there are fine lipid droplets. Xanthomatosis and amyloidosis are also excluded by the histological appearances. In adults, other differential diagnoses include lichen myxoedematosus and myxoedema with hoarseness.

Treatment. Microlaryngoscopy and dissection of the vocal cords can be successful. Dermabrasion [11], chemical skin peeling, blepharoplasty and carbon dioxide laser therapy [12] may be helpful. Oral dimethylsulphoxide was reported to help one patient [13] but not others [14]. Beneficial effects of etretinate [15] and of penicillamine [16] have also been reported.

References

1 Chan I, Liu L, Hamada T, Sethuraman G, McGrath JA. The molecular basis of lipoid proteinosis: mutations in extracellular matrix protein 1. *Exp Dermatol* 2007; **16**: 881–90.

2 Hougenhouck-Tulleken W, Chan I, Hamada T *et al.* Clinical and molecular characterization of lipoid proteinosis in Namaqualand, South Africa. *Br J Dermatol* 2004; **151**: 413–23.

3 Hamada T, McLean WH, Ramsay M *et al.* Lipoid proteinosis maps to 1q21 and is caused by mutations in the extracellular matrix protein 1 gene (ECM1). *Hum Mol Genet* 2002; **11**: 833–40.

4 Oyama N, Chan I, Neill SM *et al.* Autoantibodies to extracellular matrix protein 1 in lichen sclerosus. *Lancet* 2003; **362**: 118–23.

5 Konstantinov K, Kabakchiev P, Karchev T *et al.* Lipoid proteinosis. *J Am Acad Dermatol* 1992; **27**: 293–7.

6 Newton JA, Rasbridge S, Temple A *et al.* Lipoid proteinosis: new immunopathological observations. *Clin Exp Dermatol* 1991; **16**: 350–4.

7 Siebert M, Markowitsch HJ, Bartel P. Amygdala, affect and cognition: evidence from 10 patients with Urbach-Wiethe disease. *Brain* 2003; **126**: 2627–37.

8 Caplan RM. Visceral involvement in lipoid proteinosis. *Arch Dermatol* 1967; **95**: 149–55.

9 Navarro C, Fachal C, Rodriguez C *et al.* Lipoid proteinosis. A biochemical and ultrastructural investigation of two new cases. *Br J Dermatol* 1999; **141**: 326–31.

10 Chan I, South AP, McGrath JA *et al.* Rapid diagnosis of lipoid proteinosis using an anti-extracellular matrix protein 1 (ECM1) antibody. *J Dermatol Sci* 2004; **35**: 151–3.

11 Bannerot H, Aubin F, Tropet Y *et al.* Lipoid proteinosis: importance of dermabrasion. Apropos of a case. *Ann Chir Plast Esthet* 1998; **43**: 78–81.

12 Rosenthal G, Lifshitz T, Monos T *et al.* Carbon dioxide laser treatment for lipoid proteinosis (Urbach–Wiethe syndrome) involving the eyelids. *Br J Ophthalmol* 1997; **81**: 253.

13 Wong CK, Lin CS. Remarkable response of lipoid proteinosis to oral dimethyl sulphoxide. *Br J Dermatol* 1988; **119**: 541–4.

14 Ozkaya-Bayazit E, Ozarmagan G, Baykal C, Ulug T. Oral DMSO therapy in three patients with lipoidproteinosis. Results of long-term therapy. *Hautarzt* 1997; **48**: 477–81.

15 Gruber F, Manestar D, Stasic A, Grgurevic Z. Treatment of lipoid proteinosis with etretinate. *Acta Derm Venereol (Stockh)* 1996; **76**: 154–5.

16 Kaya TI, Kokturk A, Tursen U *et al.* D-penicillamine treatment for lipoid proteinosis. *J Eur Acad Dermatol Venereol* 2002; **16**: 286–8.

Amyloid and the amyloidoses of the skin
S.M. Breathnach, pp. 59.42–59.58

Amyloidosis is a generic term, originally coined by Rudolf Virchow in 1854, which denotes extracellular deposition of a proteinaceous substance composed of one of a family of biochemically unrelated proteins, depending on the underlying condition, and which is usually associated with considerable tissue dysfunction [1–7]. A classification based on the biochemical nature of amyloid fibril proteins is shown in Tables 59.6 and 59.7. Amyloidosis now tends to be classified on the basis of characterization of the fibril proteins (of which over 20 have now been identified) rather than according to clinicopathological features. Fibrils in primary and myeloma-associated systemic amyloidosis, as well as in nodular primary localized cutaneous amyloidosis, are composed of immunoglobulin protein AL, whereas in secondary systemic amyloidosis they are composed of a non-immunoglobulin protein termed protein AA. Fibrils in other forms of primary localized cutaneous amyloidosis, and in secondary localized cutaneous amyloidosis, contain material related to cytokeratin [8].

Amyloid proteins, regardless of biochemical constitution, share certain characteristic physicochemical properties, tinctorial properties (Congophilia and green birefringence under polarized light) and a fibrillar ultrastructure. Paired, 7.5–10.0 nm, rigid, linear, non-branching, aggregated, hollow fibrils of indefinite length constitute the bulk of amyloid deposits, regardless of clinicopathological type or the tissue involved, and are arranged in a loose meshwork. Amyloid fibrils have been shown by X-ray diffraction crystallography and infrared spectroscopy to have, at least in part, a beta-pleated sheet configuration; this probably accounts for their ability to bind Congo red and for the low solubility and resistance to proteolytic digestion of amyloid.

Non-fibrillar amyloid proteins
All types of amyloid contain small amounts of a protein termed amyloid P component (AP) derived from, and identical to, serum amyloid P component (SAP), present in the blood of all normal

Table 59.6 Biochemical nature of fibril proteins in systemic amyloidosis.

Clinical type of amyloidosis	Amyloid fibril protein	Precursor substance
Primary (immunocyte dyscrasia)	AL	Monoclonal immunoglobulin light chains
Myeloma-associated	AL	Monoclonal immunoglobulin light chains
Secondary (chronic active disease)	AA	Serum amyloid A protein (SAA)
Haemodialysis-associated (periarticular, bony and renal)	β2-microglobulin	
Heredofamilial		
Predominantly nephropathic		
Familial Mediterranean fever	AA	SAA
Muckle–Wells syndrome	AA	SAA
Predominantly neuropathic		
Familial amyloid polyneuropathy	Transthyretin variant or apoliprotein A1 or gelsolin	
Non-neuropathic forms (Ostertag)	Apoliprotein A1 or lysozyme variant or fibrinogen α chain	
Predominantly cardiomyopathic	Transthyretin variant	
Cardiomyopathy with persistent atrial standstill	Unknown	
Senile systemic	Transthyretin from plasma	

Table 59.7 Biochemical nature of fibril proteins in organ-limited (localized) amyloidosis.

Nodular (skin, lung, genitourinary)	AL
Primary localized cutaneous	
Nodular	AL
Macular amyloid and lichen amyloidosus	?Altered cytokeratin
Secondary localized cutaneous amyloidosis	?Altered cytokeratin
Hereditary syndromes	
Hereditary cerebral haemorrhage with amyloidosis	
Icelandic type	Cystatin C
Dutch type	β-protein
Cerebral amyloid angiopathy and cortical plaques (Alzheimer's disease, senile dementia, Down's syndrome)	Amyloid β-protein (Abeta)
Sporadic Creutzfeldt–Jakob disease, kuru	Prion protein
Focal senile amyloidosis	
Heart atria	Atrial natriuretic peptide
Joints	Unknown
Seminal vesicles	Seminal vesicle exocrine protein
Prostate	β2-microglobulin
Ocular deposits (corneal, conjunctival)	Unknown
Endocrine amyloidosis (APUD organs, APUDomas)	
Elderly non-insulin-dependent diabetics, benign insulinomas of the pancreas, normal aged pancreas	Islet amyloid polypeptide (homology with calcitonin gene-related peptide)
Medullary carcinoma of the thyroid	Precalcitonin-related

8 Chang YT, Liu HN, Wang W *et al.* A study of cytokeratin profiles in localized cutaneous amyloids. *Arch Dermatol Res* 2004; **296**: 83–8.
9 Tennent GA, Lovat LB, Pepys MB. Serum amyloid P component prevents proteolysis of the amyloid fibrils of Alzheimer disease and systemic amyloidosis. *Proc Natl Acad Sci USA* 1995; **92**: 4299–303.
10 Breathnach SM, Melrose SM, Bhogal B *et al.* Amyloid P component is located on elastic fibre microfibrils in normal human tissue. *Nature* 1981; **293**: 652–4.
11 Sepp N, Pichler E, Breathnach SM *et al.* Amyloid elastosis: analysis of the role of amyloid P component. *J Am Acad Dermatol* 1990; **22**: 27–34.
12 Husby G, Stenstad T, Magnus JH *et al.* Interaction between circulating amyloid fibril protein precursors and extracellular tissue matrix components in the pathogenesis of systemic amyloidosis. *Clin Immunol Immunopathol* 1994; **70**: 2–9.

individuals [1–3]. SAP prevents proteolysis of the amyloid fibrils of Alzheimer's disease, of AA amyloidosis and of AL amyloidosis, and may contribute to persistence of amyloid *in vivo* [9]. AP is constantly associated with the microfibrillar sheath of elastic fibres throughout the body in normal adults [10]. AP binds to isolated amyloid fibrils *in vitro* in a calcium-dependent manner, which may account for the frequent observation of amyloid deposition in the vicinity of elastic fibres [11]. Amyloid deposits also contain extracellular matrix components, including glycosaminoglycans and proteoglycans, which may be involved in the pathogenesis [12].

References
1 Lachmann HJ, Hawkins PN. Systemic amyloidosis. *Curr Opin Pharmacol* 2006; **6**: 214–20.
2 Pepys MB. Amyloidosis. *Annu Rev Med* 2006; **57**: 223–41.
3 Pepys MB. Science and serendipity. *Clin Med* 2007; **7**: 562–78.
4 Sipe JD, Cohen AS. Review: history of the amyloid fibril. *J Struct Biol* 2000; **130**: 88–98.
5 Buxbaum Bellotti V, Nuvolone M, Giorgetti S *et al.* The workings of the amyloid diseases. *Ann Med* 2007; **39**: 200–7.
6 Skinner M. AL amyloidosis: the last 30 years. *Amyloid* 2000; **7**: 13–4.
7 Westermark P, Araki S, Benson MD *et al.* Nomenclature of amyloid fibril proteins. Report from the meeting of the International Nomenclature Committee on Amyloidosis, August 8–9, 1998, Part 1. *Amyloid* 1999; **6**: 63–6.

Staining reactions [1–3]

Special stains for amyloid include the triphenyl-methane dyes methyl and cresyl violet for the demonstration of metachromasia, the PAS method, the substantive cotton dyes Congo red and Sirius red with or without fluorescence [4] or polarized light microscopy (Fig. 59.28), and fluorescence with thiazole dyes such as thioflavine T (Fig. 59.29). Immunohistochemical staining with anti-SAP has also been advocated [5].

The staining properties depend to some extent upon the duration of fixation in formalin and tend to be far brighter on frozen fixed material. Congophilia is the most specific [6]. Unfortunately, methyl violet and Congo red staining may be equivocal and inadequate for detecting small deposits of amyloid; false-positive results occur in colloid milium (which may mimic nodular amyloidosis histopathologically [7]) and in lipoid proteinosis. False-positive staining with thioflavine T is seen with stromal hyaline deposits, collagen fibres and colloid bodies in lichen planus; anti-

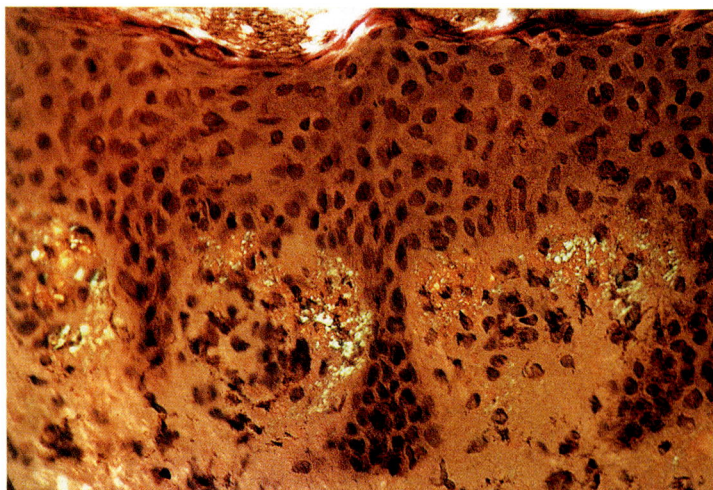

Fig. 59.28 Lichen amyloidosus. Alkaline Congo red, × 100. View under polarized light to show specific green fluorescence in amyloid deposits in papillary dermis.

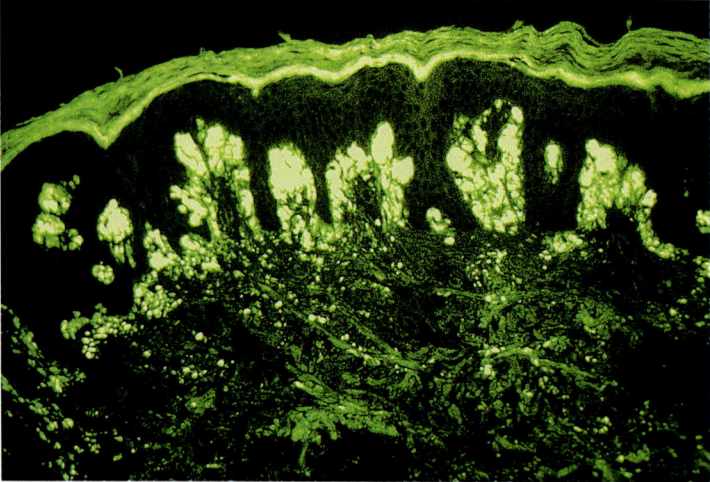

Fig. 59.29 Cutaneous amyloidosis. Thioflavine T, × 50. Viewed under fluorescence microscopy to show bright-yellow staining of amyloid deposits.

SAP also stains colloid bodies and elastotic elastic fibres. Use of a battery of stains is therefore recommended. In some cases it may be necessary to resort to electron microscopy to look for the characteristic ultrastructure of the fibrils. *In vivo* scintigraphy techniques using ^{123}I-labelled human SAP component can be used to delineate amyloid deposits in systemic amyloidosis and to monitor the effects of therapy [8].

AL type amyloid, unlike AA type amyloid, retains its affinity for Congo red and its typical polarization characteristics after exposure to potassium permanganate [9]. Immunohistochemical staining with specific antisera [10,11], or either amino acid sequencing or mass spectroscopy of material extracted from fibrillar deposits (using sections of formalin-fixed, paraffin-embedded biopsy specimens) [12], are used to differentiate between the various types of fibril protein in amyloid deposits. Immunohistochemical staining with antikeratin antibody EAB-903 using formalin-fixed tissue appears to be a useful method in the differential diagnosis of primary localized cutaneous amyloidosis [13].

References

1 Black MM. Primary localized amyloidosis of the skin: clinical variants, histochemistry and ultrastructure. In: Wegelius O, Pasternack A, eds. *Amyloidosis*. London: Academic Press, 1976: 479–513.
2 Wong CK, Breathnach SM, eds. Cutaneous amyloidosis. *Clin Dermatol* 1990; **8** (2).
3 Elghetany MT, Saleem A. Methods for staining amyloid in tissues: a review. *Stain Technol* 1988; **63**: 201–12.
4 Linke RP. Highly sensitive diagnosis of amyloid and various amyloid syndromes using Congo red fluorescence. *Virchows Arch* 2000; **436**: 439–48.
5 Breathnach SM, Bhogal B, Dyck RF *et al.* Immunohistochemical demonstration of amyloid P component in skin of normal subjects and patients with cutaneous amyloidosis. *Br J Dermatol* 1981; **105**: 115–24.
6 Cheung ST, Maheshwari MB, Tan CY. A comparative study of two Congo red stains for the detection of primary cutaneous amyloidosis. *J Am Acad Dermatol* 2006; **55**: 363–4.
7 Desai AM, Pielop JA, Smith-Zagone MJ, Hsu S. Colloid milium: a histopathologic mimicker of nodular amyloidosis. *Arch Dermatol* 2006; **142**: 784–5.
8 Hawkins PN, Richardson S, MacSweeney JE *et al.* Scintigraphic quantification and serial monitoring of human visceral amyloid deposits provide evidence for turnover and regression. *QJM* 1993; **86**: 365–74.
9 Wright JR, Calkins E, Humphrey RL. Potassium permanganate reaction in amyloidosis: a histologic method to assist in differentiating forms of this disease. *Lab Invest* 1977; **36**: 274–81.
10 Fujihara S, Balow JE, Costa JC, Glenner GG. Identification and classification of amyloid in formalin-fixed, paraffin-embedded tissue sections by the unlabelled immunoperoxidase method. *Lab Invest* 1980; **43**: 358–65.
11 Linke RP, Gartner HV, Michels H. High-sensitivity diagnosis of AA amyloidosis using Congo red and immunohistochemistry detects missed amyloid deposits. *J Histochem Cytochem* 1995; **43**: 863–9.
12 Murphy CL, Eulitz M, Hrncic R *et al.* Chemical typing of amyloid protein contained in formalin-fixed paraffin-embedded biopsy specimens. *Am J Clin Pathol* 2001; **116**: 135–42.
13 Yoneda K, Watnabe H, Yanagihara M *et al.* Immunohistochemical staining properties of amyloids with anti-keratin antibodies using formalin-fixed, paraffin-embedded sections. *J Cutan Pathol* 1989; **16**: 133–6.

Primary localized cutaneous amyloidosis

In primary localized cutaneous amyloidosis (PLCA) there is deposition of amyloid in previously apparently normal skin, with no evidence of deposits occurring in internal organs. Various subtypes of PLCA are recognized, including the more common macular and papular (lichen amyloidosus) types and the rare nodular (tumefactive) form. Both macular and papular lesions can occur in the same patient.

Aetiology. Nodular PLCA may be regarded as a form of extramedullary plasmacytoma, since the fibrils are of immunoglobulin AL type, and are thought to arise as a result of local aberrant light chain material production by clonally expanded plasma cells [1,2]. Modified β_2-microglobulin has also been reported to be a component of amyloid fibrils of primary localized cutaneous nodular amyloidosis [3].

The aetiology of other forms of PLCA remains unknown. Lichen amyloidosus is commoner among the Chinese [4]. Macular amyloidosis is rare in Europe and North America, but is much more common in Central and South America, the Middle East and Asia, suggesting the importance of genetic factors [4–9]. The occurrence of rare familial cases reinforces this view [9–16]. Familial primary localized cutaneous amyloidosis is an autosomal-dominant disorder mapped to 5p13.1-q11.2. Mutations in the OSMR gene, encoding oncostatin M-specific receptor beta (OSMRβ), have been reported [17]. OSMRβ is a component of the oncostatin M (OSM) type II receptor and the IL-31 receptor; OSM and IL-31 signalling have been implicated in keratinocyte proliferation, differentiation, apoptosis and inflammation. Primary cutaneous amyloidosis has been described in identical twins, who also had numerous congenital abnormalities [18]. A review of the current literature has revealed no instance of systemic deposition of amyloid.

Fibrils in lichen amyloidosus and macular amyloidosis do not bind antibodies to protein AA or prealbumin [19], and although immunoglobulins, κ and λ light chains, and complement are frequently observed in deposits of macular and papular PLCA [20], they are not thought to be integral constituents of the fibrils, since they are readily eluted. The close proximity of the amyloid deposits to the lower epidermis in macular amyloidosis and in lichen amyloidosus suggests that the epidermis plays a role in its pathogenesis [21,22]. It has been proposed that focal epidermal damage and filamentous degeneration of keratinocytes is followed by apoptosis and conversion of filamentous masses (colloid bodies) into amyloid material in the papillary dermis [23,24]. There may be a contribution from the dermal–epidermal junction [25]. In support of this theory is the fact that dermal amyloid deposits in these forms of PLCA react immunohistochemically with antihuman cytokeratin antibody [26–28]. It is not clear why colloid (keratin) bodies produced in other dermatoses such as lichen planus are not transformed into amyloid. It has been proposed that in lichen amyloidosus specific immunological tolerance to the presence of colloid bodies in the papillary dermis favours their transformation into amyloid by macrophages or fibroblasts, whereas in lichen planus a brisk inflammatory response ensures their removal [29].

PLCA is associated with chronic friction, perhaps causing epidermal damage, as in the so-called friction amyloidosis seen especially in the Japanese as a result of rubbing the skin vigorously with a nylon towel or brush, bath sponge, towel, plant sticks or leaves [30–33], and in nodular prurigo and lichen simplex chronicus [34]. The association of macular amyloidosis with notalgia paraesthetica supports the role of chronic pruritus in development of macular amyloidosis [35,36]. In the dyschromic forms of primary cutaneous amyloidosis, hypersensitivity to UVB with a possible DNA-repair defect may be significant [37]. An association of maculopapular amyloidosis with chronic active Epstein–Barr viral infection was reported [38].

References

1 Grunewald K, Sepp N, Weyrar K *et al.* Gene rearrangement studies in the diagnosis of primary systemic and nodular primary localized cutaneous amyloidosis. *J Invest Dermatol* 1991; **97**: 693–6.

2 Hagari Y, Mihara M, Konohana I *et al.* Nodular localized cutaneous amyloidosis: further demonstration of monoclonality of infiltrating plasma cells in four additional Japanese patients. *Br J Dermatol* 1998; **138**: 652–4.

3 Fujimoto N, Yajima M, Ohnishi Y *et al.* Advanced glycation end product-modified beta2-microglobulin is a component of amyloid fibrils of primary localized cutaneous nodular amyloidosis. *J Invest Dermatol* 2002; **118**: 479–84.

4 Wong CK. Cutaneous amyloidoses. *Int J Dermatol* 1987; **26**: 273–7.

5 Black MM. Primary localized amyloidosis of the skin: clinical variants, histochemistry and ultrastructure. In: Wegelius O, Pasternack A, eds. *Amyloidosis*. London: Academic Press, 1976: 479–513.

6 Breathnach SM. Amyloid and amyloidosis. *J Am Acad Dermatol* 1988; **18**: 1–16.

7 Wong CK, Breathnach SM, eds. Cutaneous amyloidosis. *Clin Dermatol* 1990; **8** (2).

8 Kurban AK, Malak JA, Afifi AK *et al.* Primary localized macular cutaneous amyloidosis: histochemistry and electron microscopy. *Br J Dermatol* 1971; **85**: 52–60.

9 Shanon J, Sagher F. Interscapular cutaneous amyloidosis. *Arch Dermatol* 1970; **102**: 195–8.

10 Rajagopalan K, Tay CH. Familial lichen amyloidosis. Report of 19 cases in four generations of a Chinese family in Malaysia. *Br J Dermatol* 1972; **87**: 123–9.

11 De Pietro WP. Primary familial cutaneous amyloidosis. A study of HLA antigens in a Puerto Rican family. *Arch Dermatol* 1981; **117**: 639–43.

12 Vasily DB, Bhatia SG, Uhlin SR. Familial primary cutaneous amyloidosis: clinical, genetic and immunofluorescent studies. *Arch Dermatol* 1978; **114**: 1173–6.

13 Newton JA, Jagjivan A, Bhogal B *et al.* Familial primary cutaneous amyloidosis. *Br J Dermatol* 1985; **112**: 201–8.

14 Partington MW, Marriott PJ, Prentice RSA *et al.* Familial cutaneous amyloidosis with systemic manifestations in males. *Am J Med Genet* 1991; **10**: 65–75.

15 Gallardo F, Juan A, Condom E *et al.* Familial primary localized amyloidosis L. *Br J Dermatol* 1999; **140**: 544–6.

16 Hartshorne ST. Familial primary cutaneous amyloidosis in a South African family. *Clin Exp Dermatol* 1999; **24**: 438–42.

17 Arita K, South AP, Hans-Filho G *et al.* Oncostatin M receptor-beta mutations underlie familial primary localized cutaneous amyloidosis. *Am J Hum Genet* 2008; **82**: 73–80.

18 Le Boit PH, Greene I. Primary cutaneous amyloidosis: identically distributed lesions in identical twins. *Pediatr Dermatol* 1986; **3**: 244–6.

19 Breathnach SM, Bhogal B, de Beer FC *et al.* Primary localised cutaneous amyloidosis: dermal amyloid deposits do not bind antibodies to amyloid A protein, prealbumin or fibronectin. *Br J Dermatol* 1982; **107**: 453–9.

20 Habermann MC, Montenegro MR. Primary cutaneous amyloidosis; clinical, laboratorial and histopathological study of 25 cases: identification of gamma-globulins and C3 and in the lesions by immunofluorescence. *Dermatologica* 1980; **160**: 240–8.

21 Black MM. The role of the epidermis in the histopathogenesis of lichen amyloidosis: histochemical correlations. *Br J Dermatol* 1971; **85**: 524–30.

22 Black MM, Wilson Jones E. Macular amyloidosis. *Br J Dermatol* 1971; **84**: 199–209.

23 Kumakiri M, Hashimoto K. Histogenesis of primary localized cutaneous amyloidosis: sequential change of epidermal keratinocytes to amyloid via filamentous degeneration. *J Invest Dermatol* 1979; **73**: 150–62.

24 Chang YT, Wong CK, Chow KC *et al.* Apoptosis in primary cutaneous amyloidosis. *Br J Dermatol* 1999; **140**: 210–5.

25 Horiguchi Y, Fine JD, Leigh IM *et al.* Lamina densa malformation involved in histogenesis of primary localized cutaneous amyloidosis. *J Invest Dermatol* 1992; **99**: 12–8.

26 Kobayashi H, Hashimoto K. Amyloidogenesis in organ-limited cutaneous amyloidosis: an antigenic identity between epidermal keratin and skin amyloid. *J Invest Dermatol* 1983; **80**: 66–72.

27 Huilgol SC, Ramnarain N, Carrington P *et al.* Cytokeratins in primary cutaneous amyloidosis. *Australas J Dermatol* 1998; **39**: 81–5.

28 Chang YT, Liu HN, Wang W *et al.* A study of cytokeratin profiles in localized cutaneous amyloids. *Arch Dermatol Res* 2004; **296**: 83–8.

29 Black MM. The role of the epidermis in the histopathogenesis of lichen amyloidosis: histochemical correlations. *Br J Dermatol* 1971; **85**: 524–30.

30 Wong CK, Lin CS. Friction amyloidosis. *Int J Dermatol* 1988; **27**: 302–7.

31 Sumitra S, Yesudian D. Friction amyloidosis—a variant or an etiologic factor in amyloidosis cutis? *Int J Dermatol* 1993; **32**: 422–3.

32 Hashimoto K, Ito K, Kumakiri M *et al.* Nylon brush macular amyloidosis. *Arch Dermatol* 1987; **123**: 633–7.

33 Venkataram MN, Bhushnurmath SR, Muirhead DE *et al.* Frictional amyloidosis: a study of 10 cases. *Australas J Dermatol* 2001; **42**: 176–9.

34 Weyers W. Lichen amyloidosus—Krankheitsentität oder Kratzeffekt. *Hautarzt* 1995; **46**: 165–72.

35 Goulden V, Highet AS, Sharry HK. Notalgia paraesthetica—report of an association with macular amyloidosis. *Clin Exp Dermatol* 1994; **19**: 346–9.

36 Pena-Penabad MC, Garcia-Silva J, Armijo M. Notalgia paraesthetica and macular amyloidosis: cause-effect relationship? *Clin Exp Dermatol* 1995; **20**: 279.

37 Moriwaki S, Nishigori C, Horiguchi Y *et al.* Amyloidosis cutis dyschromica: DNA repair reduction in the cellular response to UV light. *Arch Dermatol* 1992; **128**: 966–70.

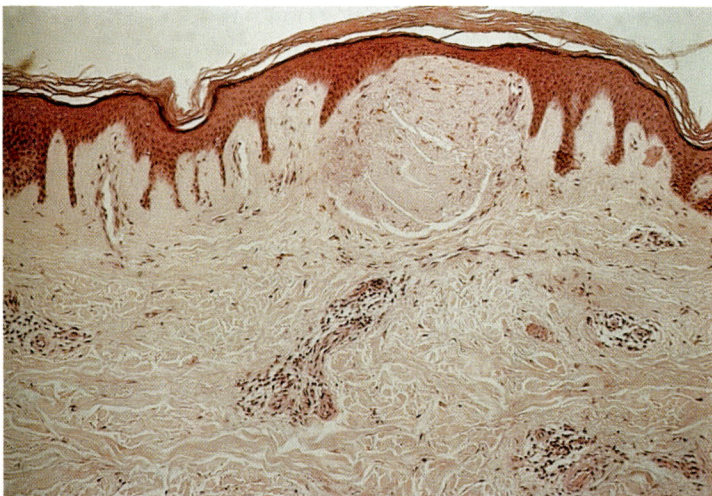

Fig. 59.30 Lichen amyloidosis. H&E, × 4. Amorphous globular hyaline amyloid deposition widening the rete ridges.

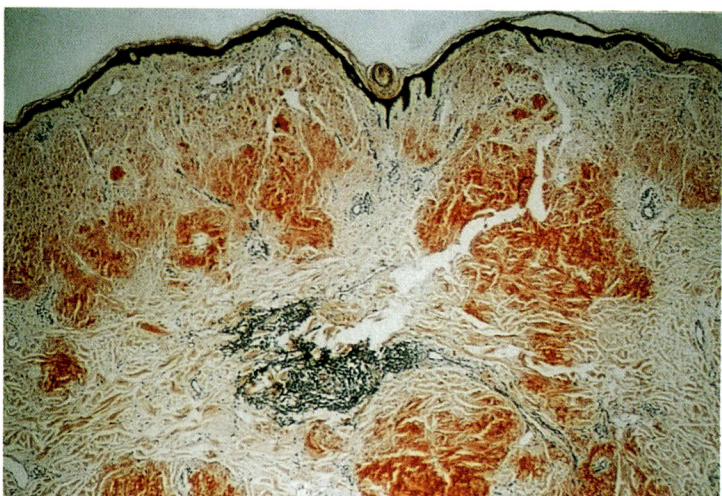

Fig. 59.31 Nodular or tumefactive cutaneous amyloidosis. Congo red, × 4. Amorphous masses of amyloid are present in the entire dermis with focal collections of plasma cells.

38 Drago F, Ranieri E, Pastorino A *et al.* Epstein–Barr virus related primary cutaneous amyloidosis and successful treatment with acyclovir and interferon-α. *Br J Dermatol* 1996; **134**: 170–4.

Pathology. In papular and macular forms of PLCA, the amyloid deposits are confined to the papillary dermis, and do not involve blood vessels or adnexal structures [1,2]. In macular amyloidosis, the deposits of amyloid are composed of small, multifaceted, amorphous globules, similar in size to the hyaline bodies found in lichen planus. They may be so sparse that more than one biopsy is necessary to confirm the diagnosis, and are easily missed without the use of special stains. The epidermis is usually of normal thickness but pigmentary incontinence with melanophages is a notable feature. In papular lichen amyloidosus, focal deposits of amyloid are often large enough to expand the dermal papillae and displace the elongated rete ridges laterally (Fig. 59.30). The overlying epidermis shows considerable irregular acanthosis and hyperkeratosis. The amyloid deposits are in close apposition to the basal layer of the epidermis and contain a few melanophages. Near the amyloid deposits, there is usually a sparse lymphohistiocytic perivascular infiltrate.

By contrast, in the nodular or tumefactive forms of PLCA the dermis, subcutis and blood vessel walls are diffusely infiltrated with amyloid as seen in primary systemic amyloidosis (Fig. 59.31). However, there is usually a perivascular infiltrate of plasma cells [3–5].

References

1 Brownstein MH, Helwig EB. The cutaneous amyloidoses. I. Localized forms. *Arch Dermatol* 1970; **102**: 8–19.
2 Black MM. Primary localized amyloidosis of the skin: clinical variants, histochemistry and ultrastructure. In: Wegelius O, Pasternack A, eds. *Amyloidosis*. London: Academic Press, 1976: 479–513.
3 Westermark P. Amyloidosis of the skin: a comparison between localized and systemic amyloidosis. *Acta Derm Venereol (Stockh)* 1979; **59**: 341–5.
4 Masuda C, Moturi S, Nakajima H. Histopathological and immunohistochemical study of amyloidosis cutis nodularis atrophicus: comparison with systemic amyloidosis. *Br J Dermatol* 1988; **119**: 33–43.
5 Nguyen TU, Oghalai JS, McGregor DK *et al.* Subcutaneous nodular amyloidosis: a case report and review of the literature. *Hum Pathol* 2001; **32**: 346–8.

Table 59.8 Clinical classification of primary localized amyloidosis.

Papular or lichen amyloidosus
Macular amyloidosus
Maculopapular amyloidosis
Nodular or tumefactive
Familial (dyschromic)

Clinical features [1–7]. Several distinctive clinical forms of PLCA have been described (Table 59.8). Because macular amyloid and lichen amyloidosus may coexist in an affected individual (biphasic amyloidosis), they are regarded as variants of a single pathological process [6].

The papular form (lichen amyloidosus) is perhaps the best known. It usually presents as a pruritic eruption of multiple, discrete, hyperkeratotic papules, scaly and often hyperpigmented, distributed principally on the shins (Figs 59.32 & 59.33). The calves, ankles, dorsa of the feet and thighs, and the extensor aspects of the arms and abdominal or chest wall, may also be involved. A rare bullous variant of lichen amyloidosus has been documented [8]. A 'thermosensitive' form sparing skin overlying the superficial limb veins has been described [9]. Papules may coalesce to form thickened plaques, closely simulating hypertrophic lichen planus or lichen simplex chronicus. The condition usually persists for many years with localized pruritus as the prominent symptom.

The predominant sign in macular amyloidosis is clusters of small, pigmented macules, about 2 or 3 mm in diameter, which may coalesce to produce macular hyperpigmented areas. A reticulate or 'rippled' pattern of pigmentation is a characteristic diagnostic feature in many cases (Figs 59.34 & 59.35). The lesions tend to be associated with mild to moderate pruritus, but pruritus may be absent in 18% of cases. The lesions may be confined to the interscapular area (Fig. 59.34), but more commonly are extensively distributed over the back or chest [10,11]. Macular amyloidosis on the back has been reported to follow prolonged chronic friction

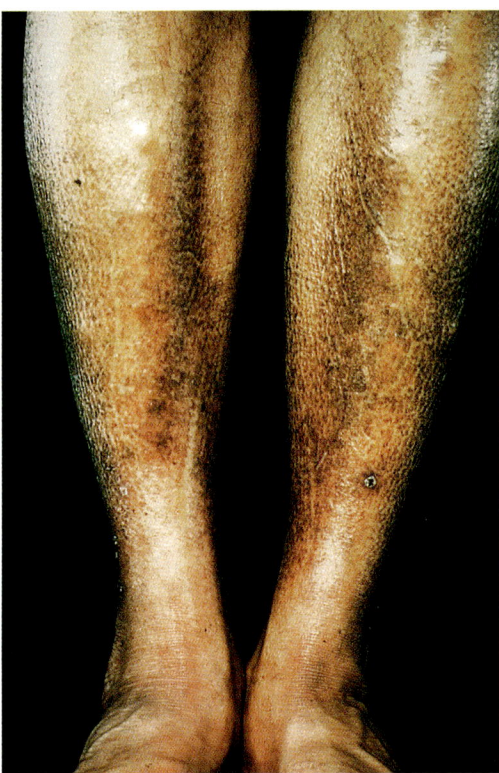

Fig. 59.32 Lichen amyloidosus (papular form). Typical appearance of pigmented pruritic papular eruption on shin in an Asian male. (Courtesy of St John's Institute of Dermatology, UK.)

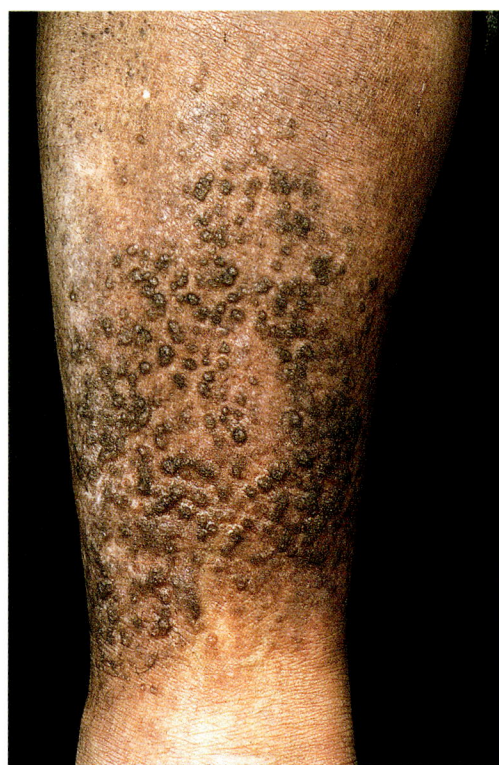

Fig. 59.33 Lichen amyloidosus (papular form). Close-up of small hyperkeratotic papules on shin. (Courtesy of St John's Institute of Dermatology, London, UK.)

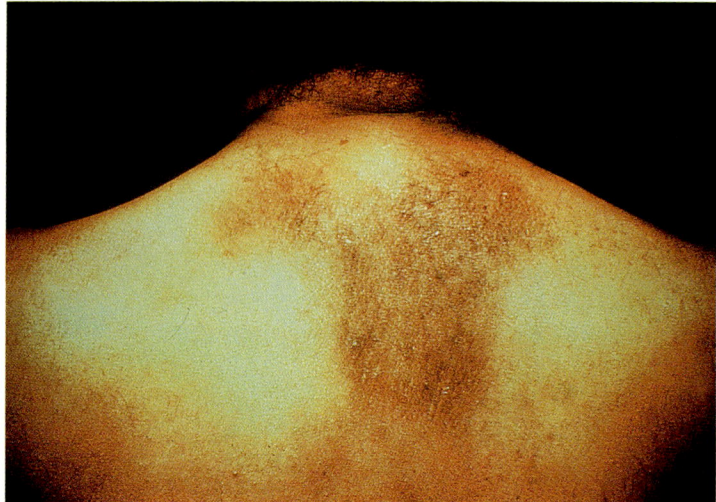

Fig. 59.34 Macular amyloidosis. Confluent pigmentation in an interscapular area in an Asian male. (Courtesy of St John's Institute of Dermatology, London, UK.)

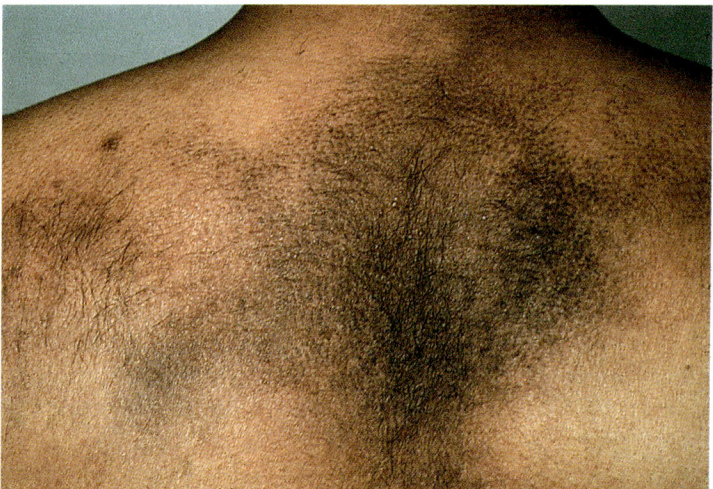

Fig. 59.35 Macular amyloidosis. Close-up to show characteristic reticular or 'rippled' pigmentation over deltoid region. (Courtesy of St John's Institute of Dermatology, London, UK.)

(see above). Lesions may also occur on the extensor aspect of extremities, and occasionally on the chest and buttocks. Hypopigmented areas may produce a 'poikilodermatous' appearance. The condition usually presents in early adult life and persists for many years; both sexes are equally affected. Macular amyloidosis can be misdiagnosed as post-inflammatory pigmentation, resolving lichen planus or neurodermatitis, or as the reticulate hyperpigmentation of the neck ('dirty neck') that has been described in association with atopic eczema [12,13]. Amyloid-like material has been demonstrated by electron microscopy, but not at light microscope level, in the atopic dirty neck [14].

Unusual variants of PLCA include: macular forms with widespread diffuse hyperpigmentation without papules but with poikiloderma-like facial involvement [15]; causing periocular hyperpigmentation [16]; simulating naevoid hyperpigmentation [17]; following Blaschko's lines [18]; resembling incontinentia pigmenti [19,20]; and a poikiloderma-like form [21–23]. Amyloidosis cutis dyschromica is assumed to be a congenital disorder with hypersensitivity to UVB radiation, with possible DNA repair defects; hyperpigmented and hypopigmented xerotic lesions with deposits of amyloid in the papillary dermis occur in sun-exposed skin [24,25]. Primary cutaneous amyloidosis of the auricular concha, in which small papules are grouped on the concha of the ear, is also believed to be a variant of PLCA, and may coexist with lichen amyloidosus [26,27].

Associations of PLCA in a few kindreds with pachyonychia congenita [28], dyskeratosis congenita [29], familial palmar–plantar keratoderma [30] and multiple endocrine neoplasia type 2a (caused by germline mutations in the RET proto-oncogene) with multiple cutaneous neuromas and medullary thyroid carcinoma, have been described; in the latter, macular lichen amyloidosus is confined to the interscapular region [31–33]. Cases of PLCA have also been described in association with a variety of connective tissue disorders: systemic lupus erythematosus [34], systemic sclerosis [35], dermatomyositis [36], primary biliary cirrhosis and scleroderma [3,37], and Raynaud's phenomenon with livedo reticularis [38]. An association with angiolymphoid hyperplasia and Kimura's disease has been reported [39,40].

Anosacral cutaneous amyloidosis is a rare syndrome described in Japanese and Chinese males, in which pigmented macules and glossy hyperkeratotic lesions radiate out from the anus [41]. Fifty per cent of patients present below the age of 60 years, and the disease may be misdiagnosed as lichen simplex chronicus, postinflammatory hyperpigmentation or tinea cruris.

The nodular or tumefactive form is a rare variant of PLCA (Fig. 59.36). Most reported patients have been females. Single or more commonly multiple nodules or plaques, indistinguishable from those associated with plasma cell dyscrasia-related systemic amyloidosis, may occur on the face, trunk, limbs, genitalia or palate [1,3,5,42–55]. They vary in size from a few millimetres to several centimetres. The overlying skin is often atrophic, and there may be petechial haemorrhages within the nodules. Some cases are associated with diabetes mellitus and Sjögren's syndrome [45,46].

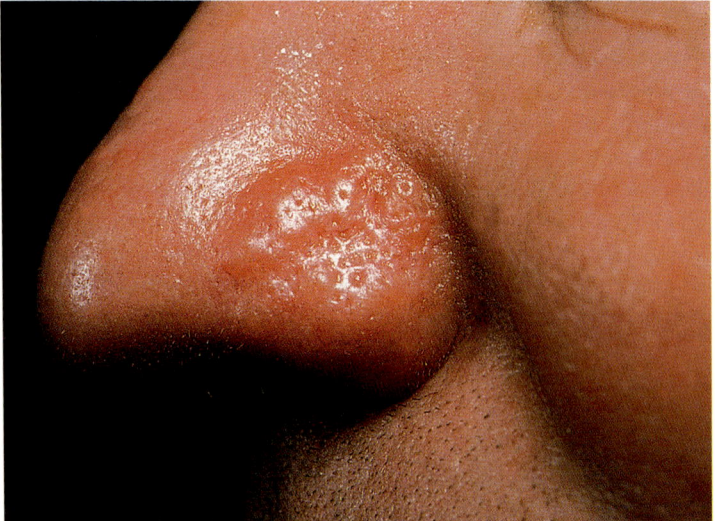

Fig. 59.36 Nodular or tumefactive cutaneous amyloidosis. Close-up of tumour on side of nose. (Courtesy of St John's Institute of Dermatology, London, UK.)

The condition, as with localized nodular amyloidosis in other organs [56], may follow a prolonged benign course over many years [47,48]; however, some patients later develop paraproteinaemia and overt systemic amyloidosis [1,3]. In a series of 16 patients, only one progressed to systemic amyloidosis over a follow-up period ranging from 8 months to 24 years (mean 10 years), and this patient had a serum monoclonal lambda protein initially [57]. Rare familial cases of nodular cutaneous amyloidosis have been reported [58].

References

1 Brownstein MH, Helwig EB. The cutaneous amyloidoses. I. Localized forms. *Arch Dermatol* 1970; **102**: 8–19.

2 Black MM, Wilson Jones E. Macular amyloidosis. *Br J Dermatol* 1971; **84**: 199–209.

3 Black MM. Primary localized amyloidosis of the skin: clinical variants, histochemistry and ultrastructure. In: Wegelius O, Pasternack A, eds. *Amyloidosis*. London: Academic Press, 1976: 479–513.

4 Wong C-K. Lichen amyloidosus: a relatively common skin disorder in Taiwan. *Arch Dermatol* 1974; **110**: 438–40.

5 Breathnach SM. Amyloid and amyloidosis. *J Am Acad Dermatol* 1988; **18**: 1–16.

6 Brownstein MH, Hashimoto K, Greenwald G. Biphasic amyloidosis: link between macular and lichenoid forms. *Br J Dermatol* 1973; **88**: 25–9.

7 Garg A, Mahalingam M, Alavian C. Pruritic patches on the back and papules on the legs. Primary localized cutaneous amyloidosis (PLCA) (cutaneous lichen amyloidosis and macular amyloidosis). *Arch Dermatol* 2007; **143**: 255–60.

8 Kuroda K, Mizoguchi M. Lichen amyloidosus with subepidermal blister formation. *Eur J Dermatol* 2004; **14**: 262–3.

9 Parsi K, Kossard S. Thermosensitive lichen amyloidosis. *Int J Dermatol* 2004; **43**: 925–8.

10 Kurban AK, Malak JA, Afifi AK *et al.* Primary localized macular cutaneous amyloidosis: histochemistry and electron microscopy. *Br J Dermatol* 1971; **85**: 52–60.

11 Shanon J, Sagher F. Interscapular cutaneous amyloidosis. *Arch Dermatol* 1970; **102**: 195–8.

12 Colver GB, Mortimer PS, Millard PR *et al.* The 'dirty neck'—reticulate pigmentation in atopics. *Clin Exp Dermatol* 1987; **12**: 1–4.

13 Hughes BR, Cunliffe WJ. Rippled hyperpigmentation resembling macular amyloidosis—a feature of atopic eczema. *Clin Exp Dermatol* 1990; **15**: 380–1.

14 Humphreys F, Spencer J, McLaren K, Tidman M. An histological and ultrastructural study of the 'dirty neck' appearance in atopic eczema. *Clin Exp Dermatol* 1996; **21**: 17–9.

15 Wang CK, Lee JY. Macular amyloidosis with widespread diffuse pigmentation. *Br J Dermatol* 1996; **135**: 135–8.

16 Van den Berg WH, Starink TM. Macular amyloidosis presenting as periocular hyperpigmentation. *Clin Exp Dermatol* 1983; **8**: 195–7.

17 Black MM, Maibach HI. Macular amyloidosis simulating naevoid hyperpigmentation. *Br J Dermatol* 1974; **90**: 461–4.

18 Bourke JF, Berth-Jones J, Burns DA. Diffuse primary cutaneous amyloidosis. *Br J Dermatol* 1992; **127**: 641–4.

19 An HT, Han KH, Cho KH. Macular amyloidosis with an incontinentia pigmenti-like pattern. *Br J Dermatol* 2000; **142**: 371–3.

20 Wu JJ, Su YN, Hsiao CH *et al.* Macular amyloidosis presenting in an incontinentia pigmenti-like pattern with subepidermal blister formation. *J Eur Acad Dermatol Venereol* 2008; **22**: 635–7.

21 Ho MH, Chong LY. Poikiloderma-like cutaneous amyloidosis in an ethnic Chinese girl. *J Dermatol* 1998; **25**: 730–4.

22 Serna-Perez MJ, Vazquez-Doval FJ, Idoate M *et al.* Extensive macular amyloidosis associated with poikiloderma. *Int J Dermatol* 1992; **31**: 277–8.

23 Pardo Arranz L, Escalonilla García-Patos P, Román Curto C *et al.* Familial poikylodermic cutaneous amyloidosis. *Eur J Dermatol* 2008; **18**: 289–91.

24 Moriwaki S, Nishigori C, Horiguchi Y *et al.* Amyloidosis cutis dyschromica: DNA repair reduction in the cellular response to UV light. *Arch Dermatol* 1992; **128**: 966–70.

25 Ozcan A, Senol M, Aydin NE, Karaca S. Amyloidosis cutis dyschromica: a case treated with acitretin. *J Dermatol* 2005; **32**: 474–7.

26 Errol C. Lichen amyloidosis of the auricular concha: report of two cases and review of the literature. *Dermatol Online J* 2006; **12**: 1.

27 Shimauchi T, Shin JH, Tokura Y. Primary cutaneous amyloidosis of the auricular concha: case report and review of published work. *J Dermatol* 2006; **33**: 128–31.

28 Tidman MJ, Wells RS, MacDonald DM. Pachyonychia congenita with cutaneous amyloidosis and hyperpigmentation—a distinct variant. *J Am Acad Dermatol* 1987; **16**: 935–40.

29 Llistosella E, Moreno A, de Moragas JM. Dyskeratosis congenita with macular amyloid deposits. *Arch Dermatol* 1984; **120**: 1381–2.

30 Graells J, Marcoval J, Moreno A *et al*. Cutaneous amyloid deposits in familial palmo-plantar keratoderma. *J Eur Acad Dermatol Venereol* 1996; **6**: 32–4.

31 Hofstra RM, Sijmons RH, Stelwagen T *et al*. RET mutation screening in familial cutaneous lichen amyloidosis and in skin amyloidosis associated with multiple endocrine neoplasia. *J Invest Dermatol* 1996; **107**: 215–8.

32 Seri M, Celli I, Betsos N *et al*. A Cys634Gly substitution of the RET proto-onco-gene in a family with recurrence of multiple endocrine neoplasia type 2A and cutaneous lichen amyloidosis. *Clin Genet* 1997; **51**: 86–90.

33 Baykal C, Buyukbabani N, Boztepe H *et al*. Multiple cutaneous neuromas and macular amyloidosis associated with medullary thyroid carcinoma. *J Am Acad Dermatol* 2007; **56** (2 Suppl.): S33–7.

34 Danielsen L, Christensen HE, Wanstrup J *et al*. Amyloidosis of the skin. In: Wegelius O, Pasternack A, eds. *Amyloidosis*. London: Academic Press, 1976: 471–7.

35 Ogiyama Y, Hayashi Y, Kou C *et al*. Cutaneous amyloidosis in patients with progressive systemic sclerosis. *Cutis* 1996; **57**: 28–32.

36 Orihara T, Yanase S, Furuya T. A case of sclerodermatomyositis with cutaneous amyloidosis. *Br J Dermatol* 1985; **112**: 213–9.

37 Fujiwara K, Kono T, Ishii M *et al*. Primary localized cutaneous amyloidosis associated with autoimmune cholangitis. *Int J Dermatol* 2000; **39**: 768–71.

38 Naldi L, Marchesi L, Locati F *et al*. Unusual manifestations of primary cutaneous amyloidosis in association with Raynaud's phenomenon and livedo reticularis. *Clin Exp Dermatol* 1992; **17**: 117–20.

39 Shankar S, Russell-Jones R. Co-existence of lichen amyloidosus and angiolym-phoid hyperplasia with eosinophilia. *Clin Exp Dermatol* 2004; **29**: 363–5.

40 Teraki Y, Katsuta M, Shiohara T. Lichen amyloidosus associated with Kimura's disease: successful treatment with cyclosporine. *Dermatology* 2002; **204**: 133–5.

41 Wang WJ, Huang CY, Chang YT *et al*. Anosacral cutaneous amyloidosis: a study of 10 Chinese cases. *Br J Dermatol* 2000; **143**: 1266–9.

42 Northcutt AD, Vanover MJ. Nodular cutaneous amyloidosis involving the vulva. *Arch Dermatol* 1985; **121**: 518–21.

43 Kitajima Y, Seno J, Aoki S *et al*. Nodular primary cutaneous amyloidosis. *Arch Dermatol* 1986; **122**: 1425–30.

44 Truhan AP, Garden JM, Roenigk HH. Nodular primary localized cutaneous amyloidosis: immunohistochemical evaluation and treatment with the carbon dioxide laser. *J Am Acad Dermatol* 1986; **14**: 1058–62.

45 Cheng-Chung A, Lin CS, Wong CK. Nodular amyloidosis. *Clin Exp Dermatol* 1988; **13**: 20–3.

46 Srivastava M. Primary cutaneous nodular amyloidosis in a patient with Sjögren's syndrome. *J Drugs Dermatol* 2006; **5**: 279–80.

47 Woollons A, Black MM. Nodular localized primary cutaneous amyloidosis: a long-term follow-up study. *Br J Dermatol* 2001; **145**: 105–9.

48 Kalajian AH, Waldman M, Knable AL. Nodular primary localized cutaneous amyloidosis after trauma: a case report and discussion of the rate of progression to systemic amyloidosis. *J Am Acad Dermatol* 2007; **57** (2 Suppl.): S26–9.

49 Kakani RS, Goldstein AE, Meisher I *et al*. Nodular amyloidosis: case report and literature review. *J Cutan Med Surg* 2001; **5**: 101–4.

50 Nguyen TU, Oghalai JS, McGregor DK *et al*. Subcutaneous nodular amyloidosis: a case report and review of the literature. *Hum Pathol* 2001; **32**: 346–8.

51 Yu LL, Heenan PJ, Randell P. Nodular amyloidosis of the lip mimicking an infiltrating neoplasm. *Australas J Dermatol* 1997; **38**: 91–2.

52 Evers M, Baron E, Zaim MT, Han A. Papules and plaques on the nose. Nodular localized primary cutaneous amyloidosis. *Arch Dermatol* 2007; **143**: 535–40.

53 Love WE, Miedler JD, Smith MK *et al*. The spectrum of primary cutaneous nodular amyloidosis: two illustrative cases. *J Am Acad Dermatol* 2008; **58** (2 Suppl.): S33–5.

54 Borrowman TA, Lutz ME, Walsh JS. Cutaneous nodular amyloidosis masquer-ading as a foot callus. *J Am Acad Dermatol* 2003; **49**: 307–10.

55 Henley E, Houghton N, Bucknall R *et al*. Localized amyloidosis of the palate. *Clin Exp Dermatol* 2008; **33**: 100–1.

56 Biewend ML, Menke DM, Calamia KT. The spectrum of localized amyloidosis: a case series of 20 patients and review of the literature. *Amyloid* 2006; **13**: 135–42.

57 Moon AO, Calamia KT, Walsh JS. Nodular amyloidosis: review and long-term follow-up of 16 cases. *Arch Dermatol* 2003; **139**: 1157–9.

58 Hashimoto H, Itami S, Kurata S *et al*. Primary localized amyloidosis in one family. *Int J Dermatol* 1991; **30**: 632–4.

Treatment. In general, the treatment of PLCA is disappointing. Milder cases can be helped by hydrocolloid dressings [1] or by using potent topical corticosteroids with or without occlusive dressings, but usually in the short term only. Calcipotriol or pho-totherapy are similarly of limited use [2,3]. There have been reports of response to topical DMSO therapy in some [4–7] but not all [8] cases. Acitretin therapy has been beneficial in some but not all patients, either alone [9–11] or in combination with bath-PUVA photochemotherapy [12]; the condition relapses after therapy is stopped. A trial of long-term cyclophosphamide 50 mg daily in lichen amyloidosus found that itching was markedly decreased within 4 months [13]. Dexamethasone cyclophosphamide pulse therapy stopped itching after five sessions and lesions cleared after nine sessions with no relapse during 30 months of follow-up [14]. Ciclosporin given to treat atopic eczema coincidentally improved lichen amyloidosus [15]. Dermabrasion may have a long-term beneficial effect on papular lichen amyloidosus of the shins [16]. Pulsed dye laser therapy has been used [17].

Nodular PLCA shows a good response to excision and grafting [18], shave removal [19], curettage and cautery [20], cryotherapy, dermabrasion [21] or the carbon dioxide or pulsed dye laser [22–24], but subsequent recurrence is likely.

References

1 Hallel-Halevy D, Finkelstein E, Grunwald MH, Halevy S. Lichen amyloidosus treated by hydrocolloid dressings. *J Eur Acad Dermatol Venereol* 2004; **18**: 691–2.

2 Khoo BP, Tay YK, Goh CL. Calcipotriol ointment vs. betamethasone 17-valerate ointment in the treatment of lichen amyloidosis. *Int J Dermatol* 1999; **38**: 539–41.

3 Jin AG, Por A, Wee LK *et al*. Comparative study of phototherapy (UVB) vs. photochemotherapy (PUVA) vs. topical steroids in the treatment of primary cutaneous lichen amyloidosis. *Photodermatol Photoimmunol Photomed* 2001; **17**: 42–3.

4 Ollague W. Primary cutaneous amyloidosis. *Int J Dermatol* 1987; **26**: 135.

5 Monfrecola G, Iandoli R, Bruno G, Martellotta D. Lichen amyloidosus: a new therapeutic approach. *Acta Derm Venereol (Stockh)* 1985; **65**: 453–5.

6 Pravata G, Pinto G, Bosco M *et al*. Unusual localization of lichen amyloidosus. Topical treatment with dimethylsulfoxide. *Acta Derm Venereol (Stockh)* 1989; **69**: 259–60.

7 Ozkaya-Bayazit E, Kavak A, Gungor H *et al*. Intermittent use of topical dimethyl sulfoxide in macular and papular amyloidosis. *Int J Dermatol* 1998; **37**: 949–54.

8 Lim KB, Tan SH, Tan KT. Lack of effect of dimethyl sulphoxide (DMSO) on amyloid deposits in lichen amyloidosus. *Br J Dermatol* 1988; **119**: 409–10.

9 Reider N, Sepp N, Fritsch P. Remission of lichen amyloidosus after treatment with acitretin. *Dermatology* 1997; **194**: 309–11.

10 Hernandez-Nunez A, Dauden E, Moreno de Vega MJ *et al*. Widespread biphasic amyloidosis: response to acitretin. *Clin Exp Dermatol* 2001; **26**: 256–9.

11 Choi JY, Sippe J, Lee S. Acitretin for lichen amyloidosus. *Australas J Dermatol* 2008; **49**: 109–13.

12 Grimmer J, Weiss T, Weber L *et al*. Successful treatment of lichen amyloidosis with combined bath PUVA photochemotherapy and oral acitretin. *Clin Exp Dermatol* 2007; **32**: 39–42.

13 Pasricha JS, Seetharam KA. Low dose cyclophosphamide therapy in lichen amyloidosis. *Indian J Dermatol Venereol Leprol* 1987; **53**: 273–4.

14 Gupta R, Gupta S. Dexamethasone cyclophosphamide pulse therapy in lichen amyloidosus: a case report. *J Dermatolog Treat* 2007; **18**: 249–51.

15 Behr FD, Levine N, Bangert J. Lichen amyloidosis associated with atopic dermatitis: clinical resolution with cyclosporine. *Arch Dermatol* 2001; **137**: 553–5.

16 Wong CK, Li WM. Dermabrasion for lichen amyloidosus. *Arch Dermatol* 1982; **118**: 302–4.

17 Sawamura D, Sato-Matsumura KC, Shibaki A *et al.* A case of lichen amyloidosis treated with pulsed dye laser. *J Eur Acad Dermatol Venereol* 2005; **19**: 262–3.

18 Bozikov K, Janezic T. Excision and split thickness skin grafting in the treatment of nodular primary localized cutaneous amyloidosis. *Eur J Dermatol* 2006; **16**: 315–6.

19 Grattan CEH, Burton JL, Dahl MGC. Two cases of nodular cutaneous amyloid with positive organ-specific antibodies, treated by shave excision. *Clin Exp Dermatol* 1988; **13**: 187–9.

20 Vestey JP, Tidman MJ, McLaren KM. Primary nodular cutaneous amyloidosis—long-term follow-up and treatment. *Clin Exp Dermatol* 1994; **19**: 159–62.

21 Lien MH, Railan D, Nelson BR. The efficacy of dermabrasion in the treatment of nodular amyloidosis. *J Am Acad Dermatol* 1997; **36**: 315–6.

22 Kakani RS, Goldstein AE, Meisher I *et al.* Nodular amyloidosis: case report and literature review. *J Cutan Med Surg* 2001; **5**: 101–4.

23 Truhan AP, Garden JM, Roenigk HH. Nodular primary localized cutaneous amyloidosis: immunohistochemical evaluation and treatment with the carbon dioxide laser. *J Am Acad Dermatol* 1986; **14**: 1058–62.

24 Alster TS, Manaloto RM. Nodular amyloidosis treated with a pulsed dye laser. *Dermatol Surg* 1999; **25**: 133–5.

Secondary localized cutaneous amyloidosis [1–3]

Microscopic deposits of amyloid material have been described in association with a variety of cutaneous tumours, including intradermal melanocytic naevus [4], sweat gland tumours, pilomatrixoma, dermatofibroma, seborrhoeic wart, photosensitive annular elastolytic giant cell granuloma [5], solar keratosis, porokeratosis of Mibelli [6,7], disseminated superficial actinic porokeratosis [8], Bowen's disease [9,10], basal cell carcinoma [11,12] and trichoepithelioma [13,14]. The amount of amyloid material in tumours is usually clinically insignificant but massive deposits may occur and cause diagnostic difficulty [15]. A similar phenomenon has been noted following PUVA therapy [16,17].

References

1 Brownstein MH, Helwig EB. The cutaneous amyloidoses. I. Localized forms. *Arch Dermatol* 1970; **102**: 8–19.

2 Malak JA, Smith EW. Secondary localised cutaneous amyloidosis. *Arch Dermatol* 1962; **86**: 465–77.

3 Runne U, Orfanos CE. Amyloid production by dermal fibroblasts. Electron microscopic studies on the origin of amyloid in various dermatoses and skin tumours. *Br J Dermatol* 1977; **97**: 155–66.

4 MacDonald DM, Black MM. Secondary localized cutaneous amyloidosis in melanocytic naevi. *Br J Dermatol* 1980; **103**: 553–6.

5 Lee Y-S, Vijayasingam S, Chan HL. Photosensitive annular elastolytic giant cell granuloma with cutaneous amyloidosis. *Am J Dermatopathol* 1989; **11**: 443–50.

6 Amantea A, Giuliano MC, Balus L. Disseminated superficial porokeratosis with dermal amyloid deposits: case report and immunohistochemical study of amyloid. *Am J Dermatopathol* 1998; **20**: 86–8.

7 Demitsu T, Okada O. Disseminated superficial porokeratosis with dermal amyloid deposition. *J Dermatol* 1999; **26**: 405–6.

8 Ginarte M, León A, Toribio J. Disseminated superficial porokeratosis with amyloid deposits. *Eur J Dermatol* 2005; **15**: 298–300.

9 Speight EL, Milne DS, Lawrence CM. Secondary localized cutaneous amyloid in Bowen's disease. *Clin Exp Dermatol* 1993; **18**: 286–8.

10 Vazquez-Doval J, Mosquera O, Iglesias ME *et al.* Bowen's disease with amyloid deposit on the palmar surface of a finger. *Eur J Dermatol* 1995; **5**: 145–7.

11 Satti MB, Azzopardi JG. Amyloid deposits in basal cell carcinoma of the skin. A pathologic study of 199 cases. *J Am Acad Dermatol* 1990; **22**: 1082–7.

12 Nojiri K, Ono T, Johno M *et al.* BCC-associated amyloidosis with a peculiar pattern of deposition. *J Dermatol* 1992; **19**: 618–21.

13 Lee YS, Fong PH. Secondary localized amyloidosis in trichoepithelioma: light microscopic and ultrastructural study. *Am J Dermatopathol* 1990; **12**: 469–78.

14 Yang JE, Kim KM, Kang H *et al.* Multiple trichoepithelioma with secondary localized amyloidosis. *Br J Dermatol* 2000; **143**: 1343–4.

15 Cox NH, Nicoll JJ, Popple AW. Amyloid deposition in basal cell carcinoma: a cause of apparent lack of sensitivity to radiotherapy. *Clin Exp Dermatol* 2001; **26**: 499–500.

16 Green I, Cox AJ. Amyloid deposition after psoriasis therapy with psoralen and long-wave ultraviolet light. *Arch Dermatol* 1979; **115**: 1200–2.

17 Hashimoto K, Kumakiri M. Colloid-amyloid bodies in PUVA-treated human psoriatic patients. *J Invest Dermatol* 1979; **72**: 70–80.

Systemic amyloidosis

Systemic types of amyloidosis include those associated with plasma cell dyscrasia, either overt as in multiple myeloma, or occult as in 'primary' systemic amyloidosis, amyloidosis secondary to a variety of chronic diseases, and in the heredofamilial amyloidoses. Clinically evident involvement of the skin is frequent in 'primary' systemic and myeloma-associated systemic amyloidosis, but occurs only rarely in secondary systemic amyloidosis. Although there is a degree of overlap, primary and myeloma-associated systemic amyloidosis typically involve the tongue, heart, gastrointestinal tract, skeletal and smooth muscle, carpal ligaments, nerves and skin, whereas secondary systemic amyloidosis affects the liver, spleen, kidneys and adrenals [1]. Skin manifestations are associated with a number of systemic heredofamilial syndromes of amyloid deposition including familial Mediterranean fever [2], the Muckle–Wells syndrome [3] and heredofamilial amyloid polyneuropathy [4].

References

1 Isobe T, Osserman EF. Patterns of amyloidosis and their association with plasma cell dyscrasia, monoclonal immunoglobulins and Bence Jones proteins. *N Engl J Med* 1974; **290**: 473–7.

2 Sohar E, Gafni J, Pras M, Heller H. Familial Mediterranean fever. A survey of 470 cases and a review of the literature. *Am J Med* 1967; **43**: 227–53.

3 Lieberman A, Grossman ME, Silvers DN. Muckle–Wells syndrome: case report and review of cutaneous pathology. *J Am Acad Dermatol* 1998; **39**: 290–1.

4 Rubinow A, Cohen AS. Skin involvement in familial amyloidotic polyneuropathy. *Neurology* 1981; **31**: 1341–5.

Primary and myeloma-associated cutaneous amyloidosis

Aetiology. In primary and myeloma-associated amyloidosis, the fibrils are composed of 'protein AL' (amyloid L-chain protein) and appear to be a consequence of plasma cell dyscrasia, although bone marrow aspiration may not reveal any abnormality. Amino acid sequence analysis has demonstrated that protein AL consists of fragments of immunoglobulin polypeptide light chain, particularly the variable (amino-terminal) region, or of an intact immunoglobulin light chain, or of both [1–4], and is usually associated with a similar abnormal immunoglobulin light chain in the serum, commonly of λ class. Abnormal light chain material is almost always present in the serum or urine, even in so-called primary systemic amyloidosis, and can be demonstrated on tissue culture of bone marrow cells from affected patients. Only a proportion of

Bence Jones proteins produce amyloid fibrils on digestion [5], which may account for the fact that amyloidosis develops in only about 15% of patients with myelomatosis. Amyloidogenic immunoglobulin AL monoclonal proteins appear to be preferentially of λ type, of lower molecular weight, and of lower isoelectric point [6]. Domains may be destabilized by specific amino acid residue changes due to point mutation, rendering them susceptible to the formation of ordered, fibril-like aggregates *in vitro* [7]. The organ tropism (i.e. whether there is predominant renal, cardiac or hepatic involvement) in AL amyloidosis may reflect germ-line gene use and plasma cell burden [8]. Rare cases of AH amyloidosis associated with monoclonal gammopathy and renal amyloid deposition, in which the amyloid fibrils are composed of immunoglobulin heavy chain variable region (VH) fragments, are recorded [9].

References

1 Glenner GG, Terry W, Horada M. Amyloid fibril proteins: proof of homology with immunoglobulin light chains by sequence analyses. *Science* 1971; **172**: 1150–1.
2 Stevens FJ, Kisilevsky R. Immunoglobulin light chains, glycosaminoglycans, and amyloid. *Cell Mol Life Sci* 2000; **57**: 441–9.
3 Skinner M. AL amyloidosis: the last 30 years. *Amyloid* 2000; **7**: 13–4.
4 Sipe JD, Cohen AS. Review: history of the amyloid fibril. *J Struct Biol* 2000; **130**: 88–98.
5 Glenner GG, Ein D, Eanes ED *et al.* Creation of 'amyloid' fibrils from Bence-Jones proteins *in vitro. Science* 1971; **174**: 712–4.
6 Bellotti V, Merlini G, Bucciarelli E *et al.* Relevance of class, molecular weight and isoelectric point in predicting human light chain amyloidogenicity. *Br J Haematol* 1990; **74**: 65–9.
7 Helms LR, Wetzel R. Specificity of abnormal assembly in immunoglobulin light chain deposition disease and amyloidosis. *J Mol Biol* 1996; **257**: 77–86.
8 Comenzo RL, Zhang Y, Martinez C *et al.* The tropism of organ involvement in primary systemic amyloidosis. Contributions of Ig V (L) germ line gene use and clonal plasma cell burden. *Blood* 2001; **98**: 714–20.
9 Miyazaki D, Yazaki M, Gono T *et al.* AH amyloidosis associated with an immunoglobulin heavy chain variable region (VH1) fragment: a case report. *Amyloid* 2008; **15**: 125–8.

Histopathology [1–5].

In primary and myeloma-associated amyloidosis, deposits of amyloid are usually superficially placed in the papillary dermis as amorphous, faintly eosinophilic, often fissured masses, with associated thinning or obliteration of the rete ridges, accounting for the papules seen clinically. Amyloid deposits in the deep reticular dermis and subcutis give rise to the clinical appearance of nodules and tumefactions, and infiltration of blood vessel walls correlates with the clinical finding of purpura. Marked thickening of blood vessel walls due to amyloid infiltration has been described [6]. Usually, there is little in the way of any inflammatory infiltrate, unlike nodular PLCA in which infiltration of plasma cells is a significant feature [3,4]. In areas of alopecia, amyloid deposits may surround and compress pilosebaceous units with resultant atrophy and loss of hair from the shafts. Amyloid may also be deposited in arrector pili muscles, in the lamina propria of sweat glands and ducts, and around individual fat cells in the subcutis as characteristic 'amyloid rings'. Amyloid deposition in the nail fold and bed of dystrophic nails has been reported [7]. An affinity for amyloid to coat elastic fibres has been noted [8].

References

1 Brownstein MH, Helwig EB. The cutaneous amyloidoses. II. Systemic forms. *Arch Dermatol* 1970; **102**: 20–8.
2 Wong CK, Breathnach SM, eds. Cutaneous amyloidosis. *Clin Dermatol* 1990; **8** (2).
3 Westermark P. Amyloidosis of the skin: a comparison between localized and systemic amyloidosis. *Acta Derm Venereol Suppl (Stockh)* 1979; **59**: 341–5.
4 Masuda C, Moturi S, Nakajima H. Histopathological and immuno-histochemical study of amyloidosis cutis nodularis atrophicus: comparison with systemic amyloidosis. *Br J Dermatol* 1988; **119**: 33–43.
5 Lee DD, Huang CY, Wong CK. Dermatopathologic findings in 20 cases of systemic amyloidosis. *Am J Dermatopathol* 1998; **20**: 438–42.
6 Henry RB, Fisher GB, Cooper PH. Vascular amyloid in a patient with multiple myeloma. *J Am Acad Dermatol* 1986; **15**: 379–82.
7 Breathnach SM, Wilkinson JD, Black MM. Systemic amyloidosis with an underlying lymphoproliferative disorder: report of a case in which nail involvement was a presenting feature. *Clin Exp Dermatol* 1979; **4**: 495–9.
8 Winkelmann RK, Peters MS, Venencie PY. Amyloid elastosis. A new cutaneous and systemic pattern of amyloidosis. *Arch Dermatol* 1985; **121**: 498–502.

Clinical features [1–10].

The mean age of onset of primary amyloidosis is about 65 years, and there is a slight male preponderance. Presenting symptoms may be rather non-specific, and include fatigue, weight loss, paresthesiae, hoarseness, oedema, dyspnoea, and syncope secondary to orthostatic hypotension. These features may predate the histological diagnosis by up to 2 years. The classical presentation with symptoms of carpal tunnel syndrome, macroglossia, specific mucocutaneous lesions which occur in up to 40% of cases, hepatomegaly and oedema should always alert the clinician to the presence of an underlying plasma cell dyscrasia.

Amyloidosis is the commonest cause of macroglossia in adults [11], and occurs in about 10% of cases. The tongue is usually diffusely enlarged and firm (Fig. 59.37), but it may also be fissured,

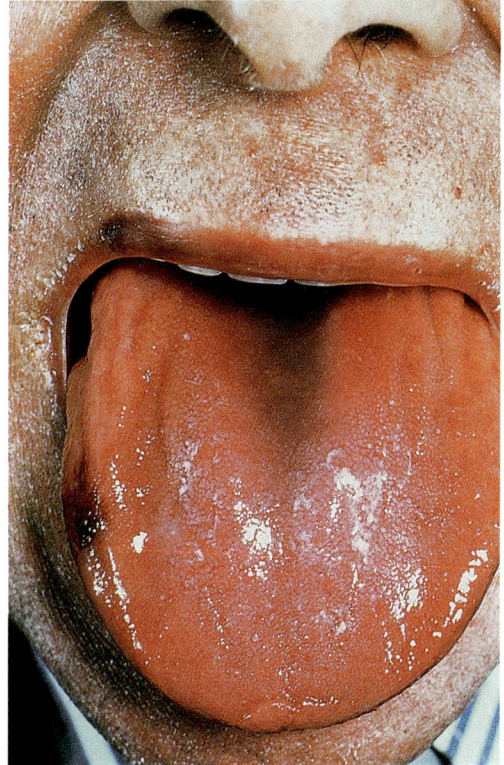

Fig. 59.37 Primary systemic amyloidosis. Macroglossia. (Courtesy of St John's Institute of Dermatology, London, UK.)

Table 59.9 Cutaneous lesions in primary and myeloma-associated systemic amyloidosis.

Common	Less common
Petechiae, purpura, ecchymoses	Pigmentary changes
Waxy, translucent or purpuric papules	Scleroderma-like infiltration
Nodules	Bullous lesions
Plaques	Alopecia
Tumefactive lesions	Cord-like blood vessel thickening
	Nail dystrophy
	Cutis laxa; localized redundant skin folds and depressions

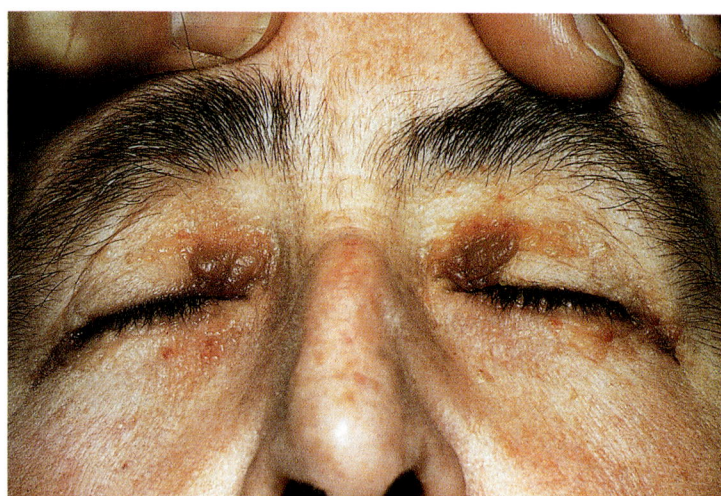

Fig. 59.39 Primary systemic amyloidosis. Purpuric plaques situated on upper eyelids. (Courtesy of St John's Institute of Dermatology, London, UK.)

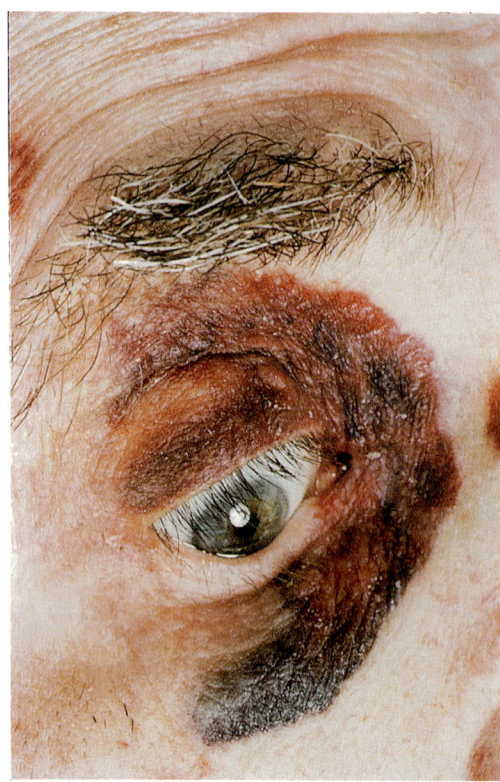

Fig. 59.38 Primary systemic amyloidosis. Prominent eyelid purpura following coughing. (Courtesy of St John's Institute of Dermatology, London, UK.)

with haemorrhagic papules, nodules, plaques or even bullae on its surface. There may be permanent tooth indentations along its lateral borders. Macroglossia may be so extensive as to cause dysphagia.

The commonest skin lesions are those related to intracutaneous haemorrhage due to infiltration of blood vessel walls by amyloid deposits (Table 59.9). Petechiae, purpura and ecchymoses may occur spontaneously or after minor trauma on normal or clinically involved skin, especially in the body folds, for example eyelids, sides of neck, axillae, umbilicus, oral and anogenital regions. Purpuric haloes may occur around long-standing Campbell de Morgan spots [12]. Eyelid purpura after pinching, and periorbital purpura after proctoscopy ('post-proctoscopic palpebral purpura'), coughing (Fig. 59.38), vomiting or the Valsalva manoeuvre, are charac-

teristic. Pigmentary changes include jaundice due to hepatic disease, cardiac failure or severe haemorrhage, pallor due to anaemia and hyperpigmentation due to haemorrhage.

Smooth, shiny, waxy papules or plaques, often with a haemorrhagic component, may also be found (Fig. 59.39). Translucent areas may resemble vesicles. Flexural areas are sites of predilection, including the eyelids, retroauricular region, neck, axillae, umbilicus, inguinal and anogenital regions. Lesions may also be found on the central face, lips, tongue and buccal mucosa. Widespread nodules may occur, coalescing to form large tumefactions. They may resemble condylomata lata on perianal and vulval skin [13,14], and when widespread may appear like xanthomas [15]. Diffuse infiltration of large areas, especially on the face, hands and feet, may simulate scleroderma [16,17], or on the face produce a myxoedema-like appearance. Alopecia may be patchy or widespread [18], and the scalp skin may be thrown into longitudinal folds resembling cutis verticis gyrata. Nail involvement due to infiltration of the nail matrix by amyloid may produce longitudinal striation (Fig. 59.40), crumbling, brittleness and partial anonychia, and may be a presenting sign [19–21]. Chronic paronychia with palmodigital erythema has also been described [22]. Signs which occur rarely include bullae of the skin or mucous membranes as a result of shearing within dermal amyloid deposits [23–27], which may result in changes resembling porphyria cutanea tarda or epidermolysis bullosa acquisita (Fig. 59.41). Extensive amyloid infiltration may lead to cord-like thickening of superficial blood vessels [28]. Extensive cutaneous ulceration has been recorded [29]. Amyloid elastosis is an unusual syndrome in which papulonodular cutaneous lesions are associated with widespread amyloid infiltration of visceral and cutaneous blood vessels, particularly in relation to elastic fibres [30,31]. Acquired cutis laxa has also been reported [32,33]. Localized elastolytic cutaneous lesions may present as soft, loose folds or indentations on the fingertips [34]. Other cases of cutis laxa may reveal fibrillar extracellular deposits, which are different from amyloid fibrils [35].

Hepatomegaly occurs in about 50%, and splenomegaly in about 10% of patients. The nephrotic syndrome or congestive cardiac failure (each of which occur in about 30% of cases), and rarely

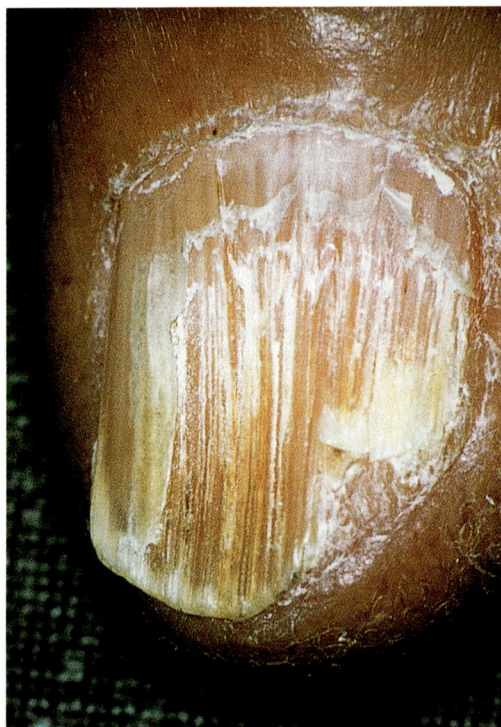

Fig. 59.40 Primary systemic amyloidosis. Close-up of thumbnail showing longitudinal ridging and splitting. A nail biopsy in this case confirmed amyloid deposition. (Courtesy of St John's Institute of Dermatology, London, UK.)

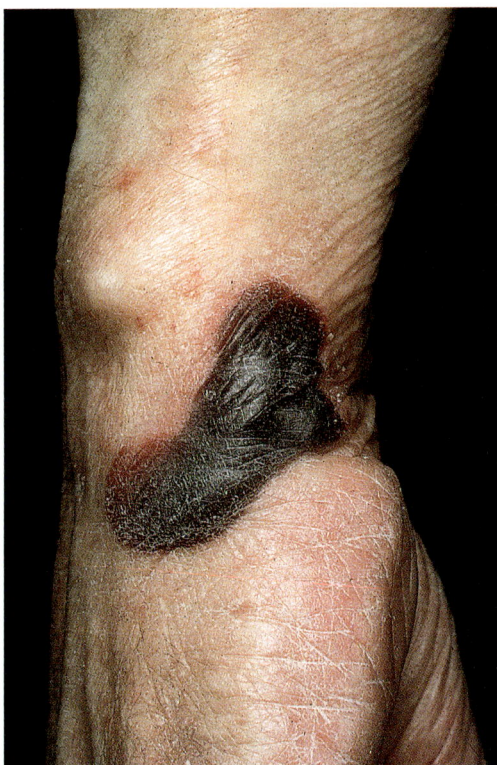

Fig. 59.41 Primary systemic amyloidosis. Haemorrhagic bulla on side of wrist. (Courtesy of St John's Institute of Dermatology, London, UK.)

protein-losing enteropathy from amyloid involvement of the small bowel, may cause pitting oedema. Ascites may develop. Cardiac infiltration results in angina, infarction, congestive cardiac failure, orthostatic hypotension or arrhythmias [36]; it accounts for death in about 40% of cases of AL type systemic amyloidosis. Pulmonary involvement is common but usually asymptomatic. Amyloid infiltration of blood vessels may lead to claudication of the legs or jaw. Gastrointestinal tract involvement [37,38] may simulate inflammatory bowel disease with haemorrhage; malabsorption is found in 5% of cases. The carpal tunnel syndrome [39] has been reported in up to 25% of patients with 'primary' systemic amyloidosis. Neurological complications [40] include peripheral neuropathy [41], initially of the lower extremities, which tends to pursue a chronic course; there may be superimposed autonomic neuropathy leading to orthostatic hypotension, diarrhoea, loss of bladder control or impotence. Muscle weakness may be caused by neuropathy, or by amyloid infiltration of muscle or its vascular supply; infiltration between muscle fibres leading to pseudohypertrophy is reported [42]. Lymphadenopathy occurs in about 10% of patients [43]. Sjögren's syndrome or sicca syndrome due to amyloid infiltration of lacrimal and parotid glands [44] are occasional presenting features. Amyloid deposition in joints may mimic rheumatoid arthritis [45], and deposition around the shoulders may cause extensive soft-tissue enlargement (the shoulder-pad sign) [46]. Giant cell arteritis and polymalgia rheumatica are recorded [47], as are isolated factor X deficiency [48], disseminated intravascular coagulation and fibrinolysis with severe bleeding.

References

1 Brownstein MH, Helwig EB. The cutaneous amyloidoses. II. Systemic forms. *Arch Dermatol* 1970; **102**: 20–8.
2 Breathnach SM. Amyloid and amyloidosis. *J Am Acad Dermatol* 1988; **18**: 1–16.
3 Wong CK, Breathnach SM, eds. Cutaneous amyloidosis. *Clin Dermatol* 1990; **8** (2).
4 Wong Wang WJ. Systemic amyloidosis. A report of 19 cases. *Dermatology* 1994; **189**: 47–51.
5 Kyle RA, Gertz MA. Primary systemic amyloidosis: clinical and laboratory features in 474 cases. *Semin Hematol* 1995; **32**: 45–59.
6 Gertz MA, Lacy MQ, Dispenzieri A. Amyloidosis: recognition, confirmation, prognosis, therapy. *Mayo Clin Proc* 1999; **74**: 490–4.
7 Kyle RA. Clinical aspects of multiple myeloma and related disorders including amyloidosis. *Pathol Biol (Paris)* 1999; **47**: 148–57.
8 Daoud MS, Lust JA, Kyle RA *et al.* Monoclonal gammopathies and associated skin disorders. *J Am Acad Dermatol* 1999; **40**: 507–35.
9 Terrier B, Jaccard A, Harousseau JL *et al.* The clinical spectrum of IgM-related amyloidosis: a French nationwide retrospective study of 72 patients. *Medicine (Baltimore)* 2008; **87**: 99–109.
10 Mason AR, Rackoff EM, Pollack RB. Primary systemic amyloidosis associated with multiple myeloma: a case report and review of the literature. *Cutis* 2007; **80**: 193–200.
11 Murthy P, Laing MR. Macroglossia. *BMJ* 1994; **309**: 1386–7.
12 Brear SG, Rademaker M, Hasleton P *et al.* Target-like skin lesions in primary amyloidosis. *Br J Dermatol* 1985; **112**: 209–11.
13 Buezo GF, Penas PF, Firaga J *et al.* Condyloma-like lesions as the presenting sign of multiple myeloma associated amyloidosis. *Br J Dermatol* 1996; **135**: 665–6.
14 Konig A, Wennemuth G, Soyer HP *et al.* Vulvar amyloidosis mimicking giant condylomata acuminata in a patient with multiple myeloma. *Eur J Dermatol* 1999; **9**: 29–31.
15 Chapman RS, Neville EA, Lawson JW. Xanthoma-like skin lesions as a presenting feature in primary systemic amyloidosis. *Br J Clin Pract* 1973; **27**: 271–3.
16 Gerster JC, Landry M, Dudler J. Scleroderma-like changes of the hands in primary amyloidosis. *J Rheumatol* 2000; **27**: 2275–7.

17 Reyes CM, Rudinskaya A, Kloss R *et al.* Scleroderma-like illness as a presenting feature of multiple myeloma and amyloidosis. *J Clin Rheumatol* 2008; **14**: 161–5.

18 Hunt SJ, Caserio RJ, Abell E. Primary systemic amyloidosis causing diffuse alopecia by telogen arrest. *Arch Dermatol* 1991; **127**: 1067–8.

19 Breathnach SM, Wilkinson JD, Black MM. Systemic amyloidosis with an underlying lymphoproliferative disorder. Report of a case in which nail involvement was a presenting feature. *Clin Exp Dermatol* 1979; **4**: 495–9.

20 Fujita Y, Tsuji-Abe Y, Sato-Matsumura KC *et al.* Nail dystrophy and blisters as sole manifestations in myeloma-associated amyloidosis. *J Am Acad Dermatol* 2006; **54**: 712–4.

21 Prat C, Moreno A, Viñas M, Jucglà A. Nail dystrophy in primary systemic amyloidosis. *J Eur Acad Dermatol Venereol* 2008; **22**: 107–9.

22 Ahmed I, Cronk JS, Crutchfield CE 3rd *et al.* Myeloma-associated systemic amyloidosis presenting as chronic paronychia and palmodigital erythematous swelling and induration of the hands. *J Am Acad Dermatol* 2000; **42**: 339–42.

23 Hunter JAA. Primary systemic amyloidosis imitating porphyria cutanea tarda. *Proc R Soc Med* 1976; **69**: 235–6.

24 Bieber T, Ruzicka T, Linke RD. Hemorrhagic bullous amyloidosis. *Arch Dermatol* 1988; **124**: 1683–6.

25 Robert C, Aractingi S, Prost C, Verola O *et al.* Bullous amyloidosis. Report of three cases and review of the literature. *Medicine (Baltimore)* 1993; **72**: 38–44.

26 Pramatarov Wang XD, Shen H, Liu ZH. Diffuse haemorrhagic bullous amyloidosis with multiple myeloma. *Clin Exp Dermatol* 2008; **33**: 94–6.

27 Rekhtman N, Hash KS, Moresi JM. Mucocutaneous bullous amyloidosis with an unusual mixed protein composition of amyloid deposits. *Br J Dermatol* 2006; **154**: 751–4.

28 Breathnach SM, Wells GC. Amyloid vascular disease: cord-like thickening of mucocutaneous arteries, intermittent claudication and angina in a case with underlying myelomatosis. *Br J Dermatol* 1980; **102**: 591–5.

29 Alhaddab M, Srolovitz H, Rosen N. Primary systemic amyloidosis presenting as extensive cutaneous ulceration. *J Cutan Med Surg* 2006; **10**: 253–6.

30 Winkelmann RK, Peters MS, Venencie PY. Amyloid elastosis. A new cutaneous and systemic pattern of amyloidosis. *Arch Dermatol* 1985; **121**: 498–502.

31 Sepp N, Pichler E, Breathnach SM *et al.* Amyloid elastosis: analysis of the role of amyloid P component. *J Am Acad Dermatol* 1990; **22**: 27–34.

32 Newton JA, McKee PH, Black MM. Cutis laxa associated with amyloidosis. *Clin Exp Dermatol* 1986; **11**: 87–91.

33 Appiah YE, Onumah N, Wu H *et al.* Multiple myeloma-associated amyloidosis and acral localized acquired cutis laxa. *J Am Acad Dermatol* 2008; **58** (2 Suppl.): S32–3.

34 Yoneda K, Kanoh T, Nomura S *et al.* Elastolytic cutaneous lesions in myeloma-associated amyloidosis. *Arch Dermatol* 1990; **126**: 657–60.

35 Niemi KM, Anton-Lamprecht A, Virtanen I *et al.* Fibrillar protein deposits with tubular substructure in a systemic disease beginning as cutis laxa. *Arch Dermatol* 1993; **129**: 757–62.

36 Dubrey SW, Cha K, Anderson J *et al.* The clinical features of immunoglobulin light-chain (AL) amyloidosis with heart involvement. *QJM* 1998; **91**: 141–57.

37 Ebert EC, Nagar M. Gastrointestinal manifestations of amyloidosis. *Am J Gastroenterol* 2008; **103**: 776–87.

38 Petre S, Shah IA, Gilani N. Review article: gastrointestinal amyloidosis—clinical features, diagnosis and therapy. *Aliment Pharmacol Ther* 2008; **27**: 1006–16.

39 Nestle FO, Burg G. Bilateral carpal tunnel syndrome as a clue for the diagnosis of systemic amyloidosis. *Dermatology* 2001; **202**: 353–5.

40 Kelly JJ. Neurologic complications of primary systemic amyloidosis. *Rev Neurol Dis* 2006; **3**: 173–81.

41 Duston MA, Skinner M, Anderson J, Cohen AS. Peripheral neuropathy as an early marker of AL amyloidosis. *Arch Intern Med* 1989; **149**: 358–60.

42 Sibelt LA, Lokhorst HM, van de Kerkhof PC, van Dooren-Greebe RJ. A 'muscle' man without exercise: muscle pseudohypertrophy in myeloma-associated generalized amyloidosis. *J Eur Acad Dermatol Venereol* 2007; **21**: 986–8.

43 Matsuda M, Gono T, Shimojima Y *et al.* AL amyloidosis manifesting as systemic lymphadenopathy. *Amyloid* 2008; **15**: 117–24.

44 Jardinet D, Westhovens R, Peeters J. Sicca syndrome as an initial symptom of amyloidosis. *Clin Rheumatol* 1998; **17**: 546–8.

45 Katoh N, Tazawa K, Ishii W, Matsuda M, Ikeda S. Systemic AL amyloidosis mimicking rheumatoid arthritis. *Intern Med* 2008; **47**: 1133–8.

46 Liepnieks JJ, Burt C, Benson MD. Shoulder-pad sign of amyloidosis: structure of an Ig κ III protein. *Scand J Immunol* 2001; **54**: 404–8.

47 Salvarani C, Gabriel SE, Gertz MA *et al.* Primary systemic amyloidosis presenting as giant cell arteritis and polymyalgia rheumatica. *Arthritis Rheum* 1994; **37**: 1621–6.

48 Marcatti M, Mauri S, Tresoldi M *et al.* Unusual bleeding manifestations in a case of primary amyloidosis with factor X deficiency but elevations of *in vivo* markers of thrombin formation and activity. *Thromb Res* 1995; **80**: 333–7.

Diagnosis. The diagnosis should always be considered when a patient presents with the triad of carpal tunnel syndrome, macroglossia and mucocutaneous skin lesions [1,2]. Biopsy of classical mucocutaneous lesions should be the procedure of first choice. Biopsy of even clinically normal forearm skin has been reported positive in up to 50% of cases of primary and myeloma-associated disease. Fine-needle biopsies of the subcutaneous fat from clinically normal abdominal skin have a high positive yield in AL- and AA-type amyloidosis as well as in heredofamilial amyloidoses [3–5]. Rectal biopsy is positive in up to 80% of cases of AL or AA amyloidosis, jejunal biopsy in about two-thirds, but gingival biopsy in only 19%. Gastric biopsy may produce a higher yield than rectal biopsy. Ninety-six per cent of hepatic, and 90% of renal and of splenic percutaneous needle biopsies, as well as carpal tunnel tissue biopsies at the time of decompression, are positive. Bone marrow aspiration may be positive in up to 45% of cases. Electrocardiography, echocardiography, angiocardiography, technetium scanning and endomyocardial biopsy are useful in the diagnosis of amyloid heart disease [6–8]. Computed tomography, ultrasound examination, and Doppler analysis of blood flow may be useful in renal amyloidosis. Sural nerve biopsy in patients with peripheral neuropathy [9], and synovial fluid analysis in patients with arthropathy, may be helpful. Scanning with ^{123}I-labelled SAP component enables specific localization and imaging of amyloid deposits *in vivo* [10,11].

Immunoelectrophoresis of both serum and concentrated urine is essential if the clinical presentation suggests the presence of a plasma cell dyscrasia, as conventional urine heat tests and simple electrophoresis of serum and urine may not detect small amounts of paraprotein or Bence Jones protein. Protein electrophoresis of serum shows a spike pattern in just under half of patients with primary AL, and in about two-thirds of those with myeloma. Immunoelectrophoresis of serum reveals a monoclonal protein in two-thirds of patients with AL amyloidosis; only 45% have a monoclonal heavy chain, while 20% have free monoclonal light chains (Bence Jones proteinaemia). Immunoelectrophoresis of concentrated urine reveals a monoclonal light chain in about two-thirds of cases (λ to κ ratio 2 : 1). When screening of both serum and urine is performed, the frequency of patients with an identifiable monoclonal protein rises to about 86%. A combination of immuno-fixation on agarose gel electrophoresis and bone marrow plasma cell light chain λ to κ ratio analysis improves diagnostic sensitivity [12]. Nevertheless, in some cases with the clinical features of AL amyloidosis it is not possible to demonstrate a paraprotein, even after prolonged follow-up for as long as 24 years [13].

Skeletal survey may be useful, as 50% of patients with myeloma-associated amyloidosis have radiological abnormalities, compared with only 6% of those with primary amyloidosis. Most myeloma cases, but no primary systemic amyloidosis cases, have more than 15% plasma cells in the marrow. In general, myeloma is not present if a patient has no lytic bone lesions, hypercalcaemia or anaemia, has only a small serum or urine monoclonal component, and has less than 25% bone marrow plasma cells.

References

1 Gertz MA, Lacy MQ, Dispenzieri A. Amyloidosis: recognition, confirmation prognosis, therapy. *Mayo Clin Proc* 1999; **74**: 490–4.

2 Kyle RA. Clinical aspects of multiple myeloma and related disorders including amyloidosis. *Pathol Biol (Paris)* 1999; **47**: 148–57.

3 Westermark P. Diagnosing amyloidosis. *Scand J Rheumatol* 1995; **24**: 327–9.

4 Guy CD, Jones CK. Abdominal fat pad aspiration biopsy for tissue confirmation of systemic amyloidosis: specificity, positive predictive value, and diagnostic pitfalls. *Diagn Cytopathol* 2001; **24**: 181–5.

5 Dhingra S, Krishnani N, Kumari N, Pandey R. Evaluation of abdominal fat pad aspiration cytology and grading for detection in systemic amyloidosis. *Acta Cytol* 2007; **51**: 860–4.

6 Bellavia D, Pellikka PA, Abraham TP *et al.* Evidence of impaired left ventricular systolic function by Doppler myocardial imaging in patients with systemic amyloidosis and no evidence of cardiac involvement by standard two-dimensional and Doppler echocardiography. *Am J Cardiol* 2008; **101**: 1039–45.

7 Vogelsberg H, Mahrholdt H, Deluigi CC *et al.* Cardiovascular magnetic resonance in clinically suspected cardiac amyloidosis: noninvasive imaging compared to endomyocardial biopsy. *J Am Coll Cardiol* 2008; **51**: 1022–30.

8 Rapezzi C, Guidalotti P, Salvi F *et al.* Usefulness of 99mTc-DPD scintigraphy in cardiac amyloidosis. *J Am Coll Cardiol* 2008; **51**: 1509–10.

9 Rajani B, Rajani V, Prayson RA. Peripheral nerve amyloidosis in sural nerve biopsies. A clinicopathologic analysis of 13 cases. *Arch Pathol Lab Med* 2000; **124**: 114–8.

10 Hawkins PN, Richardson S, MacSweeney JE *et al.* Scintigraphic quantification and serial monitoring of human visceral amyloid deposits provide evidence for turnover and regression. *QJM* 1993; **86**: 365–74.

11 Hachulla E, Maulin L, Deveaux M *et al.* Prospective and serial study of primary amyloidosis with serum amyloid P component scintigraphy: from diagnosis to prognosis. *Am J Med* 1996; **101**: 77–87.

12 Perfetti V, Garini P, Vignarelli MC *et al.* Diagnostic approach to and follow-up of difficult cases of AL amyloidosis. *Haematologica* 1995; **80**: 409–15.

13 Crow KD. Primary amyloidosis. *Br J Dermatol* 1977; **97** (Suppl. 15): 58–60.

Prognosis. Prognosis in primary systemic and myeloma-associated amyloidosis is poor, the major causes of death being cardiac and renal failure, and is linked to degree of plasma cell clonality and marrow infiltration [1]. The prognosis of AL amyloidosis has improved, with a currently reported median survival of about 40 months compared to 13 months in the early 1990s. Autologous stem cell transplantation (ASCT) achieves the highest rates of complete clonal response but is associated with substantial treatment-related mortality unless restricted to highly selected patients. Newer chemotherapy regimens which can be used more widely may achieve better safety and respectable efficacy [2]. Median survival on high-dose melphalan and autologous stem-cell transplantation was 4.6 years [3] and 4.75 years respectively [4] in other series; 21% of patients died within the first year of treatment-related complications or progressive disease, but median survival exceeded 10 years for patients achieving a complete haematological response [4]. Median survival was only 26 months in patients undergoing dialysis [5]; a good renal response after high-dose melphalan and stem cell transplantation is a favourable marker [6]. Occasional patients surviving longer than 10 years have been recorded [3,7–10]. Patients presenting with amyloid neuropathy without associated cardiac, renal or hepatic involvement may have a better prognosis (median survival 40–50 months; 5 years survival 31.6%) [11]. Survival for more than 10 years has been

recorded in a patient with primary systemic amyloidosis with sensorimotor polyneuropathy only [12].

Treatment. Most patients receive a trial of chemotherapy, usually melphalan and prednisone, with or without autologous bone marrow stem-cell transplantation [2,3,13–17]. There is a risk of development of leukaemia or a dysmyelopoietic syndrome [14]. Other chemotherapeutic regimens have been used [18–20]. Cardiac [21,22] or renal transplantation can prolong survival; renal amyloidosis is not an absolute contraindication to transplantation, although amyloid may re-accumulate in the transplanted kidney.

References

1 Perfetti V, Colli Vignarelli M, Anesi E *et al.* The degrees of plasma cell clonality and marrow infiltration adversely influence the prognosis of AL amyloidosis patients. *Haematologica* 1999; **84**: 218–21.

2 Gertz Wechalekar AD, Hawkins PN, Gillmore JD. Perspectives in treatment of AL amyloidosis. *Br J Haematol* 2008; **140**: 365–77.

3 Skinner M, Sanchorawala V, Seldin DC *et al.* High-dose melphalan and autologous stem-cell transplantation in patients with AL amyloidosis: an 8-year study. *Ann Intern Med* 2004; **140**: 85–93.

4 Sanchorawala V, Skinner M, Quillen K *et al.* Long-term outcome of patients with AL amyloidosis treated with high-dose melphalan and stem-cell transplantation. *Blood* 2007; **110**: 3561–3.

5 Bollée G, Guery B, Joly D *et al.* Presentation and outcome of patients with systemic amyloidosis undergoing dialysis. *Clin J Am Soc Nephrol* 2008; **3**: 375–81.

6 Leung N, Dispenzieri A, Fervenza FC *et al.* Renal response after high-dose melphalan and stem cell transplantation is a favorable marker in patients with primary systemic amyloidosis. *Am J Kidney Dis* 2005; **46**: 270–7.

7 Kyle RA, Gertz MA, Greipp PR *et al.* Long-term survival (10 years or more) in 30 patients with primary amyloidosis. *Blood* 1999; **93**: 1062–6.

8 Crow KD. Primary amyloidosis. *Br J Dermatol* 1977; **97** (Suppl. 15): 58–60.

9 Fritz DA, Luggen ME, Hess EV. Unusual longevity in primary systemic amyloidosis: a 19-year survivor. *Am J Med* 1989; **86**: 245–8.

10 Goldsmith DJ, Sandooran D, Short CD *et al.* Twenty-one years survival with systemic AL-amyloidosis. *Am J Kidney Dis* 1996; **28**: 278–82.

11 Duston MA, Skinner M, Anderson J, Cohen AS. Peripheral neuropathy as an early marker of AL amyloidosis. *Arch Intern Med* 1989; **149**: 358–60.

12 Rinaldi R, Azzimondi G, Preda P *et al.* Primary systemic amyloidosis presenting with polyneuropathy characterized by very long survival. *Acta Neurol Scand* 1995; **91**: 511–3.

13 Palladini G, Perfetti V, Obici L *et al.* Association of melphalan and high-dose dexamethasone is effective and well tolerated in patients with AL (primary) amyloidosis who are ineligible for stem cell transplantation. *Blood* 2004; **103**: 2936–8.

14 Jaccard A, Moreau P, Leblond V *et al.* High-dose melphalan versus melphalan plus dexamethasone for AL amyloidosis. *N Engl J Med* 2007; **357**: 1083–93.

15 Sanchorawala V, Seldin DC. An overview of high-dose melphalan and stem cell transplantation in the treatment of AL amyloidosis. *Amyloid* 2007; **14**: 261–9.

16 Akay OM, Sahin G, Kabukcuoglu S *et al.* Successful treatment of nephrotic syndrome due to systemic AL amyloidosis after autologous stem cell transplantation: renal response is an important therapeutic end point. *Clin Nephrol* 2008; **69**: 294–7.

17 Gertz MA, Kyle RA. Acute leukemia and cytogenetic abnormalities complicating melphalan treatment of primary systemic amyloidosis. *Arch Intern Med* 1990; **150**: 629–33.

18 Imagawa S, Ohmine K *et al.* Successful treatment of multiple myeloma-associated amyloidosis by interferon-α, dimethyl sulfoxide, and VAD (vincristine, adriamycin, and dexamethasone). *Int J Hematol* 2000; **72**: 491–3.

19 Kastritis E, Anagnostopoulos A, Roussou M *et al.* Treatment of light chain (AL) amyloidosis with the combination of bortezomib and dexamethasone. *Haematologica* 2007; **92**: 1351–8.

20 Matsuda M, Gono T, Katoh N *et al.* Nephrotic syndrome due to primary systemic AL amyloidosis, successfully treated with VAD (vincristine, doxorubicin and dexamethasone) alone. *Intern Med* 2008; **47**: 543–9.

21 Sack FU, Kristen A, Goldschmidt H *et al.* Treatment options for severe cardiac amyloidosis: heart transplantation combined with chemotherapy and stem cell transplantation for patients with AL-amyloidosis and heart and liver transplantation for patients with ATTR-amyloidosis. *Eur J Cardiothorac Surg* 2008; **33**: 257–62.

22 Mignot A, Bridoux F, Thierry A *et al.* Successful heart transplantation following melphalan plus dexamethasone therapy in systemic AL amyloidosis. *Haematologica* 2008; **93**: e32–5.

Secondary systemic amyloidosis

In secondary systemic amyloidosis, the fibrils are composed of a non-immunoglobulin protein designated protein AA [1]. A precursor of protein AA, known as serum amyloid A protein (protein SAA), is present in the serum of normal individuals as an apolipoprotein of high-density lipoprotein, and behaves as an acute phase reactant.

Secondary amyloidosis occurs as a complication of many chronic inflammatory diseases in which the immune system is stimulated [2,3]. These include acute recurrent and chronic infections, rheumatoid arthritis [4], juvenile chronic arthritis [5], ankylosing spondylitis [6], Reiter's syndrome, Behçet's syndrome [7], Sjögren's syndrome, dermatomyositis, scleroderma, systemic lupus erythematosus [8], inflammatory bowel disease [9], Hodgkin's disease, non-Hodgkin's lymphoma [10], histiocytosis X [11], Schnitzler's syndrome [12] and some solid non-lymphoid tumours, as well as Castleman's disease [13] and Rosai–Dorfman disease [14]. Secondary systemic amyloidosis may also arise as a complication of a number of dermatoses [15], such as venous ulceration [16], generalized psoriasis and psoriatic arthritis [17,18], pustular psoriasis [19], lepromatous leprosy [20], hidradenitis suppurativa, chronically infected burns, chronic skin infection in drug addicts [21], nodular non-suppurative panniculitis [22], giant, ulcerated or metastatic basal cell carcinoma [23], acne conglobata [24], epidermolysis bullosa of dystrophic [25,26] and aquisita types, and X-linked anhidrotic ectodermal dysplasia.

Secondary systemic amyloidosis rarely produces specific skin lesions. An elbow skin nodule due to deposition of AA amyloid was reported in a patient with primary Sjögren syndrome, myopathy, severe osteoporosis, and vertebral fractures attributed to coeliac disease [27]. By contrast, secondary systemic amyloidosis commonly involves the kidneys (causing the nephrotic syndrome), spleen, alimentary tract and adrenals; the diagnosis should be confirmed by rectal or renal biopsy. Needle aspirates of abdominal wall subcutis may yield positive histological identification of amyloid [28]. Small or minute amyloid deposits are most often found around the adnexae, sometimes in small blood vessels and in the subcutis around fat cells: 'amyloid rings'.

There is no specific treatment, and many die from progressive renal failure. Treatment of the primary disease may arrest progression of the amyloidosis. Estimated survival at 10 years was 90% in patients whose median protein SAA level was under 10 mg/L, and only 40% among those whose median SAA level exceeded this in one study [29]. Median survival after diagnosis was 133 months, with renal dysfunction being the predominant disease manifestation in another recent study, which reiterated the prognostic value of the SAA level [30]. Renal disease has responded to colchicine therapy, cyclophosphamide, or high dose melphalan and autologous stem cell transplantation [4,31,32]. Etanercept therapy is reportedly of benefit in inflammatory arthritis-related AA amyloidosis [33–35]. Renal transplantation is certainly worthy of consideration.

References

1 Cunnane G. Amyloid precursors and amyloidosis in inflammatory arthritis. *Curr Opin Rheumatol* 2001; **13**: 67–73.

2 Brownstein MH, Helwig EB. Secondary systemic amyloidosis: analysis of underlying disorders. *South Med J* 1971; **64**: 491–6.

3 Gertz MA. Secondary amyloidosis (AA). *J Intern Med* 1992; **232**: 517–8.

4 Chevrel G, Jenvrin C, McGregor B *et al.* Renal type AA amyloidosis associated with rheumatoid arthritis: a cohort study showing improved survival on treatment with pulse cyclophosphamide. *Rheumatology (Oxford)* 2001; **40**: 821–5.

5 Immonen K, Savolainen A, Kautiainen H, Hakala M. Longterm outcome of amyloidosis associated with juvenile idiopathic arthritis. *J Rheumatol* 2008; **35**: 907–12.

6 Kobak S, Oksel F, Kabasakal Y, Doganavsargil E. Ankylosing spondylitis-related secondary amyloidosis responded well to etanercept: a report of three patients. *Clin Rheumatol* 2007; **26**: 2191–4.

7 Skhiri H, Mahjoub S, Harzallah O *et al.* Secondary amyloidosis, a fatal complication of Behcet's disease: three case reports. *Saudi J Kidney Dis Transpl* 2004; **15**: 57–60.

8 Aktas Yilmaz B, Düzgün N, Mete T *et al.* AA amyloidosis associated with systemic lupus erythematosus: impact on clinical course and outcome. *Rheumatol Int* 2008; **28**: 367–70.

9 Leiper K, Howse ML, Bell GM. Resolution of nephrotic syndrome caused by amyloidosis following surgery for Crohn's disease. *Hosp Med* 2000; **61**: 802–3.

10 Piskin O, Alacacioglu I, Ozkal S *et al.* A patient with diffuse large B-cell non-Hodgkin's lymphoma and AA type amyloidosis. *J Bulkan Union Oncol* 2008; **13**: 113–6.

11 Pérez-Martínez J, Marques M, Kilmurray L *et al.* Secondary amyloidosis associated with histiocytosis X. *Amyloid* 2008; **15**: 69–71.

12 Claes K, Bammens B, Delforge M *et al.* Another devastating complication of the Schnitzler syndrome: AA amyloidosis. *Br J Dermatol* 2008; **158**: 182–4.

13 Morita-Hoshi Y, Tohda S, Miura O, Nara N. An autopsy case of multicentric Castleman's disease associated with interstitial nephritis and secondary AA amyloidosis. *Int J Hematol* 2008; **87**: 69–74.

14 Rocken C, Wieker K, Grote HJ *et al.* Rosai–Dorfman disease and generalized AA amyloidosis: a case report. *Hum Pathol* 2000; **31**: 621–4.

15 Brownstein MH, Helwig EB. Systemic amyloidosis complicating dermatoses. *Arch Dermatol* 1970; **102**: 1–7.

16 Landau M, Ophir J, Gal R *et al.* Systemic amyloidosis secondary to chronic leg ulcers. *Cutis* 1992; **50**: 47–9.

17 Wittenberg GP, Ousler JR, Peters MS. Secondary amyloidosis complicating psoriasis. *J Am Acad Dermatol* 1995; **32**: 465–8.

18 Ryan JG, Dorman AM, O'Connell PG. AA amyloidosis in psoriatic arthritis. *Ir J Med Sci* 2006; **175**: 81–2.

19 MacKie RM, Burton J. Pustular psoriasis in association with renal amyloidosis. *Br J Dermatol* 1974; **90**: 567–71.

20 McAdam KPWJ, Anders RF, Smith SR *et al.* Association of amyloidosis with erythema nodosum leprosum reactions and recurrent neutrophil leucocytosis in leprosy. *Lancet* 1975; **ii**: 572–5.

21 Neugarten J, Gallo GR, Buxbaum J *et al.* Amyloidosis in subcutaneous heroin abusers ('skin popper's amyloidosis'). *Am J Med* 1986; **81**: 635–40.

22 Pallares R, Sancho S, Nogues R *et al.* Amyloidosis (AA type) associated with nodular nonsuppurative panniculitis. *Ann Intern Med* 1983; **99**: 488–9.

23 Yamamoto S, Johno O, Kayashima K *et al.* Giant basal cell carcinoma associated with systemic amyloidosis. *J Dermatol* 1996; **23**: 329–34.

24 Pérez-Villa F, Campistol JM, Montoliu J, Trilla A. Renal amyloidosis secondary to acne conglobata. *Int J Dermatol* 1989; **28**: 132–3.

25 Bourke JF, Browne G, Gaffney EF, Young M. Fatal systemic amyloidosis (AA type) in two sisters with dystrophic epidermolysis bullosa. *J Am Acad Dermatol* 1995; **33**: 370–2.

26 Gunduz K, Vatansever S, Turel A *et al.* Recessive dystrophic epidermolysis bullosa complicated with nephrotic syndrome due to secondary amyloidosis. *Int J Dermatol* 2000; **39**: 151–3.

27 Katsikas GA, Maragou M, Rontogianni D et al. Secondary cutaneous nodular AA amyloidosis in a patient with primary Sjögren syndrome and celiac disease. *J Clin Rheumatol* 2008; **14**: 27–9.

28 Westermark P. Occurrence of amyloid deposits in the skin in secondary systemic amyloidosis. *Acta Pathol Microbiol Scand* 1972; **80**: 718–20.

29 Gillmore JD, Lovat LB, Persey MR et al. Amyloid load and clinical outcome in AA amyloidosis in relation to circulating concentration of serum amyloid A protein. *Lancet* 2001; **358**: 24–9.

30 Lachmann HJ, Goodman HJ, Gilbertson JA et al. Natural history and outcome in systemic AA amyloidosis. *N Engl J Med* 2007; **356**: 2361–71.

31 Kagan A, Husza'r M, Frumkin A et al. Reversal of nephrotic syndrome due to AA amyloidosis in psoriatic patients on long-term colchicine treatment. Case report and review of the literature. *Nephron* 1999; **82**: 348–53.

32 Ogita M, Hoshino J, Sogawa Y et al. Multicentric Castleman disease with secondary AA renal amyloidosis, nephrotic syndrome and chronic renal failure, remission after high-dose melphalan and autologous stem cell transplantation. *Clin Nephrol* 2007; **68**: 171–6.

33 Kobak S, Oksel F, Kabasakal Y, Doganavsargil E. Ankylosing spondylitis-related secondary amyloidosis responded well to etanercept: a report of three patients. *Clin Rheumatol* 2007; **26**: 2191–4.

34 Nakamura T, Higashi S, Tomoda K et al. Efficacy of etanercept in patients with AA amyloidosis secondary to rheumatoid arthritis. *Clin Exp Rheumatol* 2007; **25**: 518–22.

35 Perry ME, Stirling A, Hunter JA. Effect of etanercept on serum amyloid A protein (SAA) levels in patients with AA amyloidosis complicating inflammatory arthritis. *Clin Rheumatol* 2008; **27**: 923–5.

Dialysis-related amyloidosis

In systemic amyloidosis related to haemodialysis, the major constituent protein of amyloid fibrils is β_2-microglobulin. Most of the clinical findings are related to amyloid deposition in osseo-articular tissues [1,2]. Extensive tissue deposition of β_2-microglobulin may rarely present as masses in the buttocks [3,4], or as lichenoid lesions [5,6].

References

1 Danesh F, Ho LT. Dialysis-related amyloidosis: history and clinical manifestations. *Semin Dial* 2001; **14**: 80–5.

2 Kiss E, Keusch G, Zanetti M et al. Dialysis-related amyloidosis revisited. *Am J Roentgenol* 2005; **185**: 1460–7.

3 Lipner HI, Minkowitz S, Neiderman G et al. Dialysis-related amyloidosis manifested as masses in the buttocks. *South Med J* 1995; **88**: 876–8.

4 Takayama K, Satoh T, Maruyama R, Yokozeki H. Dialysis-related amyloidosis on the buttocks. *Acta Derm Venereol* 2008; **88**: 72–3.

5 Sato KC, Kumakiu M, Koizumi H et al. Lichenoid lesions as a sign of β_2-microglobulin-induced amyloidosis in a long-term haemodialysis patient. *Br J Dermatol* 1993; **128**: 686–9.

6 Uenotsuchi T, Imafuku S, Nagata M et al. Cutaneous and lingual papules as a sign of beta 2 microglobulin-derived amyloidosis in a long-term hemodialysis patient. *Eur J Dermatol* 2003; **13**: 393–5.

Inherited systemic amyloidosis

Several distinct genetic types of amyloidosis are recognized, which may be associated with mutations in a number of plasma proteins including transthyretin (MIM *176300), apolipoprotein AI (MIM *107680), fibrinogen A α chain (MIM *134820), lysozyme (MIM *153450), gelsolin (MIM *137350) and the 55-kDa tumour necrosis factor (TNF) receptor [1–4]. The kidney, peripheral nerves and spinal ganglia, or the heart are predominantly affected. Skin manifestations are associated with a number of systemic heredofamilial syndromes of amyloid deposition, including familial Mediterranean fever [5], the Muckle–Wells syndrome [6] and heredofamilial amyloid polyneuropathy [7–10]. The most prevalent forms of the autosomal dominantly inherited hereditary sensory neuropathies are HSN I, associated with mutations in the *SPTLC1* gene, and CMT 2b, associated with mutations in the *RAB7* gene.

Familial Mediterranean fever is inherited as an autosomal recessive disorder, and is caused by mutations in the *MEFV* gene, leading to defects in the pyrin protein which normally blunts neutrophil-mediated inflammation, probably via IL-1 down-regulation [11–13]. It may involve erysipelas-like lesions on the lower legs, urticaria, Henoch–Schönlein purpura and vasculitic nodules [5]. Associated features are intermittent fevers with abdominal pain and joint effusions, and a tendency to peritonitis, pleurisy, synovitis and renal amyloidosis. Colchicine at a dose of 1 to 2 mg daily reduces the frequency of attacks and prevents development of secondary amyloidosis. There have been case reports of benefits with catecholamine blockade (prazosin), tumour necrosis factor antagonists (etanercept, thalidomide), and IL-1 receptor blockade (anakinra) [12,13].

The Muckle–Wells syndrome, which has autosomal dominant inheritance, is characterized by periodic attacks of fever, urticaria, conjunctivitis and arthropathy with limb pains, associated with progressive perceptive nerve deafness and renal amyloidosis [6,14–16]; cold urticaria [14,15] and hyperpigmented sclerodermoid skin lesions [17] have been described. Levels of C-reactive protein, serum amyloid A, and IL-1β are elevated. Patients with Muckle–Wells syndrome have a mutation in *NALP3/CIAS1/PYPAF1*, the gene encoding cryopyrin, a component of the inflammasome that regulates the processing of IL-1β. Treatment with the recombinant human IL-1 receptor antagonist anakinra has resulted in resolution of clinical symptoms including deafness, and normalizes laboratory abnormalities [14,16].

Trophic skin changes with skin ulceration and sweating abnormalities may develop in heredofamilial amyloid polyneuropathy [7–10]. The Finnish type of heredofamilial neuropathic amyloidosis, a gelsolin-related systemic amyloidosis characterized by cranial neuropathy and corneal lattice dystrophy, may be associated with cutis laxa, blepharochalasis and lichen amyloidosus [18]. Cutis laxa is a principal clinical manifestation of hereditary gelsolin amyloidosis (AGel amyloidosis), an age-associated systemic disease with global distribution, caused by a G654A or G654T gelsolin gene mutation [19]. Heart and liver transplantation may be successful in familial amyloidotic neuropathy [20,21].

References

1 Buxbaum JN, Tagoe CE. The genetics of the amyloidoses. *Annu Rev Med* 2000; **51**: 543–69.

2 Benson MD, Liepnieks JJ, Yazaki M et al. A new human hereditary amyloidosis: the result of a stop-codon mutation in the apolipoprotein AII gene. *Genomics* 2001; **72**: 272–7.

3 Aksentijevich I, Galon J, Soares M et al. The tumor-necrosis-factor receptor-associated periodic syndrome: new mutations in TNFRSF1A, ancestral origins, genotype–phenotype studies, and evidence for further genetic heterogeneity of periodic fevers. *Am J Hum Genet* 2001; **69**: 301–14.

4 Ando Y, Ueda M. Novel methods for detecting amyloidogenic proteins in trans-thyretin related amyloidosis. *Front Biosc* 2008; **13**: 5548–58.

5 Sohar E, Gafni J, Pras M, Heller H. Familial Mediterranean fever. A survey of 470 cases and a review of the literature. *Am J Med* 1967; **43**: 227–53.

6 Lieberman A, Grossman ME, Silvers DN. Muckle–Wells syndrome: case report and review of cutaneous pathology. *J Am Acad Dermatol* 1998; **39**: 290–1.

7 Rubinow A, Cohen AS. Skin involvement in familial amyloidotic polyneuropathy. *Neurology* 1981; **31**: 1341–5.

8 Auer-Grumbach M. Hereditary sensory neuropathies. *Drugs Today (Barc)* 2004; **40**: 385–94.

9 Rocha N, Velho G, Horta M *et al*. Cutaneous manifestations of familial amyloidotic polyneuropathy. *J Eur Acad Dermatol Venereol* 2005; **19**: 605–7.

10 Auer-Grumbach M. Hereditary sensory neuropathy type I. *Orphanet J Rare Dis* 2008; **3**: 7.

11 Chae JJ, Wood G, Masters SL *et al*. The B30.2 domain of pyrin, the familial Mediterranean fever protein, interacts directly with caspase-1 to modulate IL-1beta production. *Proc Natl Acad Sci U S A* 2006; **103**: 9982–7.

12 Bhat A, Naguwa SM, Gershwin ME. Genetics and new treatment modalities for familial Mediterranean fever. *Ann N Y Acad Sci* 2007; **1110**: 201–8.

13 Sugiura T, Kawaguchi Y, Fujikawa S *et al*. Familial Mediterranean fever in three Japanese patients, and a comparison of the frequency of MEFV gene mutations in Japanese and Mediterranean populations. *Mod Rheumatol* 2008; **18**: 57–9.

14 Hawkins PN, Lachmann HJ, Aganna E, McDermott MF. Spectrum of clinical features in Muckle-Wells syndrome and response to anakinra. *Arthritis Rheum* 2004; **50**: 607–12.

15 Haas N, Küster W, Zuberbier T, Henz BM. Muckle-Wells syndrome: clinical and histological skin findings compatible with cold air urticaria in a large kindred. *Br J Dermatol* 2004; **151**: 99–104.

16 Yamazaki T, Masumoto J, Agematsu K *et al*. Anakinra improves sensory deafness in a Japanese patient with Muckle-Wells syndrome, possibly by inhibiting the cryopyrin inflammasome. *Arthritis Rheum* 2008; **58**: 864–8.

17 El-Darouti MA, Marzouk SA, Abdel-Halim MR. Muckle-Wells syndrome: report of six cases with hyperpigmented sclerodermoid skin lesions. *Int J Dermatol* 2006; **45**: 239–44.

18 Boysen G, Galassi G, Kamieniecka Z *et al*. Familial amyloidosis with cranial neuropathy and corneal lattice dystrophy. *J Neurol Neurosurg Psychiatry* 1979; **42**: 1020–30.

19 Kiuru-Enari S, Keski-Oja J, Haltia M. Cutis laxa in hereditary gelsolin amyloidosis. *Br J Dermatol* 2005; **152**: 250–7.

20 Yamamoto S, Wilczek HE, Nowak G *et al*. Liver transplantation for familial amyloidotic polyneuropathy (FAP): a single-center experience over 16 years. *Am J Transplant* 2007; **7**: 2597–604.

21 Pilato E, Dell'Amore A, Botta L, Arpesella G. Combined heart and liver transplantation for familial amyloidotic neuropathy. *Eur J Cardiothorac Surg* 2007; **32**: 180–2.

Nutrition and the skin

K. Weismann, pp. 59.58–59.81

Lack of essential nutrients is most commonly due to a reduced or insufficient intake of food, malabsorption (see below), vomiting or decreased passage time of food due to diarrhoea or fistulae. Some medications may interfere with utilization of nutrients. An increased metabolic requirement of nutrients occurs during periods of sudden weight gain, such as growth and convalescence. This may lead to relative deficiencies, as seen in patients receiving long-term parenteral nutrition who may become severely deficient in zinc (p. 59.73).

Often, the cutaneous changes of inadequate nutrition are varied, reflecting combined deficiencies. When there is an apparently isolated deficiency, an underlying genetic or enzymatic defect should be suspected.

Malabsorption

Malabsorption is a condition characterized by a decreased intestinal uptake of nutrients associated with an increased faecal excretion of fat (steatorrhoea). This leads to various degrees of lack of proteins, minerals, trace elements, fat-soluble vitamins, carbohydrates and water. Some causes of malabsorption are listed in Table 59.10.

Table 59.10 Various causes of malabsorption.

Chelating substances in the gut
  Phytates
Insufficient digestive enzyme activity
  Pancreatic diseases (pancreatitis, mucoviscidosis)
Defective micelle formation
  Obstructive jaundice, liver cirrhosis
Contaminated small bowel syndrome (i.e. presence of an abnormal bacterial flora in the small bowel)
Gastric resection (lack of hydrochloric acid production)
Stagnant loop syndrome (strictures, surgical blind loops, scleroderma, diabetic enteropathy)
Colonic reflux (intestinal fistula, extensive small bowel resection)
Agammaglobulinaemia
Defective enzyme activity or carrier function in the intestinal mucosa
  Disaccharidase deficiency
  Coeliac disease
  Acrodermatitis enteropathica (zinc deficiency)
  Hartnup disease (pellagra)
Loss of absorption capacity
  Intestinal resection and bypass operation
  Crohn's disease
  Pernicious anaemia
Interference with intestinal lymphatics
  Lymphangiectasis
  Tuberculous mesenteric adenitis
  Hodgkin's disease
Inadequate transport mechanisms in the blood
  Abetalipoproteinaemia
Miscellaneous
  Polyarteritis nodosa
  Lupus erythematosus
  Amyloidosis
  Mastocytosis
  Diabetes mellitus
  Zollinger–Ellison syndrome
  Protein-losing enteropathy
  Hyperthyroidism
  Hypothyroidism
  Cronkhite–Canada syndrome
  Dermatogenic enteropathy

Clinical features

Non-specific cutaneous symptoms [1,2]. Non-specific symptoms may be observed in patients who have lost weight due to malabsorption or malignant disease. The skin changes reflect general illness rather than specific disease.

Itching and acquired ichthyosis. Itch is mostly caused by dry skin. Elderly patients are especially prone to developing dry skin, which becomes eczematized. Patients with cancer, chronic liver or kidney diseases, or with lymphoma, may develop an itchy atrophic ichthyosis [3]. Hypoferraemia may cause itch, which disappears after initiation of iron therapy. Serum ferritin is a sensitive indicator of the state [4]. Polycythaemia rubra vera may cause generalized itch (see Chapters 21 and 62).

Melanosis. Malnutrition due to malabsorption may cause symmetrical melanin hyperpigmentation of the skin, although melanocyte-stimulating hormone (MSH) levels are seldom increased. Other skin colour changes associated with malnutrition are those due to wasting and atrophy, and pallor due to anaemia.

Arsenic pollution of drinking water in a primitive rural area caused blackening of hands and feet [5].

Skin appendages. Brittle nails and hair loss are frequent findings in poorly nourished patients. In some cases, lack of zinc, iron and vitamins is the main cause. In the majority of patients the aetiology is probably multifactorial.

Specific cutaneous effects [1]. Vitamin deficiencies occur due to malabsorption. Lack of fat-soluble vitamins, in particular, may cause skin changes including follicular hyperkeratosis (lack of vitamin A), ecchymoses and haematuria (lack of vitamin K), and cheilitis, glossitis, neuritis and dermatitis (lack of vitamin B complex). Zinc deficiency-related skin changes may be seen.

Investigations. Patients presenting with skin changes suggestive of malabsorption should have a thorough medical examination and laboratory tests to determine both the causes and the consequences of malabsorption. Relevant tests include serum calcium, zinc, folate and albumin levels, faecal fat excretion and X-ray examination of the small intestine.

Treatment. The cause of malabsorption should be treated where possible, and dietary measures instituted to ensure adequate supply of all essential nutrients from a wide variety of foods [2].

References
1 Wells GC. Skin disorders in relation to malabsorption. *BMJ* 1962; **ii**: 937–43.
2 Bender AE. Nutritional requirements. *J R Soc Health* 1985; **105**: 1–4.
3 Flint GL, Flam M, Soter NA. Acquired ichthyosis: a sign of nonlymphoproliferative malignant disorders. *Arch Dermatol* 1975; **111**: 1446–7.
4 Adams SJ. Iron deficiency, serum ferritin, generalized pruritus and systemic disease: a case-controlled study. *Br J Dermatol* 1989; **121** (Suppl. 34): 15.
5 Loewenberg S. Scientists tackle water contamination in Bangladesh. *Lancet* 2007; **370**: 471–2.

Specific syndromes with malabsorption

Cronkhite–Canada syndrome [1]
See Chapter 62.

Whipple's disease
This is a rare disease of uncertain aetiology involving the gastrointestinal tract, skin, joints, heart and lymph nodes (Chapter 62). There is diffuse hyperpigmentation of the skin, and leg nodules or erythema nodosum may occur. The involvement of the heart includes inflammatory changes of the pericardium, myocardium and endocardium and may lead to valvular insufficiency [2].

Dermatitis herpetiformis (see Chapter 40)
Enteropathy is present in at least two-thirds of all patients and may respond to a gluten-free diet. Patients may be managed on a gluten-free diet alone, and it at least enables most patients to reduce their requirement for dapsone [3].

References
1 Cronkhite LW, Canada WJ. Generalized gastrointestinal polyposis. *N Engl J Med* 1955; **252**: 1011–5.
2 McAllister HA, Fenoglio JJ. Cardiac involvement in Whipple's disease. *Circulation* 1975; **52**: 152–6.
3 Garioch JJ, Lewis HM, Sargent SA *et al.* Twenty-five years experience of a gluten-free diet in the treatment of dermatitis herpetiformis. *Br J Dermatol* 1994; **131**: 541–5.

Mucoviscidosis

Synonyms
- Fibrocystic disease
- Cystic fibrosis of the pancreas (MIM #219700)

Mucoviscidosis is an inherited disorder characterized by three major components: chronic lung disease, exocrine pancreatic insufficiency and an abnormally high sodium concentration of the sweat.

Aetiology. The mode of genetic transmission is autosomal recessive. The basic metabolic defect is unknown. The mucous secretion has an increased viscosity resulting in obstruction of the small bronchial branches, the excretory ducts of the pancreas and the bile ducts of the liver. This eventually leads to respiratory disease, pancreatic insufficiency and hepatic failure. The high sodium concentration in sweat is due to a lowered reabsorption of sodium in the sweat glands [1] (Chapter 44).

Histopathology. The exocrine sweat glands and pancreas show electron-dense bodies, and there are fewer than normal secretory vacuoles in the 'dark cells' of the sweat coils [2].

Clinical features. The main presenting features are chronic pulmonary disease, exocrine pancreatic insufficiency with malabsorption, retarded growth and hepatic disease. Skin changes in the form of acrodermatitis enteropathica-like lesions due to essential fatty acid and zinc deficiency have been seen [3,4]. Several studies have indicated that atopy is more common in patients with cystic fibrosis than in the general population [5], although the prevalence of urticaria is not increased [6]. A purpuric rash may occur in patients with cystic fibrosis.

Diagnosis. The diagnosis is established by the finding of high sodium concentration in the sweat, absence of pancreatic enzymes in the duodenum, chronic respiratory disease, retarded growth and a family history of the disease.

Aquagenic wrinkling of the palms and fingers is characterized by formation of oedematous whitish plaques on the palms on exposure to water. Cystic fibrosis should be considered in patients with this type of reaction [7].

Treatment. Respiratory infection is controlled by prolonged antibiotic therapy according to bacterial cultures. Pancreatic insufficiency is treated by pancreatic enzyme preparations orally and a diet low in fat. The liver disease and the sweat abnormality are not amenable to treatment at present.

References

1 Report of the Committee for a Study for the Evaluation of Testing for Cystic Fibrosis. *J Pediatr* 1976; **88**: 711–34.
2 Munger BL, Brunsilow SW, Cooke RE. An electron microscopic study of eccrine sweat glands in patients with cystic fibrosis of the pancreas. *J Pediatr* 1961; **59**: 497–511.
3 Hansen RC, Leme R, Revsin B. Cystic fibrosis manifesting with acrodermatitis enteropathica-like eruption. *Arch Dermatol* 1983; **119**: 51–5.
4 Schmidt CP, Tunessen W. Cystic fibrosis with periorificial dermatitis. *J Am Acad Dermatol* 1991; **25**: 896–7.
5 Tacier-Eugster H, Wuthrich B, Meyer H. Atopic allergy, serum IgE and RAST specific IgE antibodies in patients with cystic fibrosis. *Helv Paediatr Acta* 1980; **35**: 31–7.
6 Laufer P. Urticaria in cystic fibrosis. *Cutis* 1985; **36**: 245–6.
7 Katz K, Yan AC, Turner ML. Aquagenic wrinkling of the palms in patients with cystic fibrosis homozygous for the F508 CFTR mutation. *Arch Dermatol* 2005; **141**: 621–4.

Vitamins [1]

Vitamins are biologically active organic compounds, which are indispensable for the normal functions of the body. They have no direct function as an energy source or as structural tissue components, but in most cases act as coenzymes in various enzyme systems.

Reference

1 Miller S. Nutritional deficiency and the skin. *J Am Acad Dermatol* 1989; **21**: 1–30.

Vitamin A

Vitamin A (retinol) is a cyclic polyene alcohol present in yellow and green vegetables, egg yolk, butter, liver and fish oils [1]. β-Carotene occurs in fruits, carrots and green vegetables, and is absorbed and converted to vitamin A in the body. The recommended daily allowance is 5000 i.u. (equivalent to 6000–12 000 i.u. β-carotene). The plasma level in normal adults is about 600 ng/mL [2]. Vitamin A is mobilized from liver stores and transported in plasma, in which it is bound to retinol-binding protein [3].

Vitamin A is essential for the reproductive system, bone formation, vision and epithelial tissues [4]. *In vitro* studies on human keratinocytes have shown that vitamin A affects their growth and differentiation [5]. In human volunteers, 150 000 i.u. daily of vitamin A produced demonstrable retardation of keratinocyte maturation [6]. Skin disorders with abnormal keratinization, such as ichthyosis, pityriasis rubra pilaris and Darier's disease, have been treated with high doses of oral vitamin A. There is a risk of intoxication by such treatment and stereoisomers of retinoic acid are now used instead [1,7].

Vitamin A deficiency

Vitamin A deficiency is seldom seen in the Western world today. It is observed mainly in diseases causing malabsorption and is often associated with deficiency of other fat-soluble vitamins.

Clinical features. Classical manifestations of vitamin A deficiency include xerophthalmia, follicular hyperkeratosis and generalized xerosis [8]. Follicular papules are seen especially on the dorsal and lateral areas of the extremities, so-called phrynoderma. Histologically, there is lamellated hyperkeratosis around the hair follicles with keratinous plugs and atrophy of the sebaceous glands [9].

Diagnosis is confirmed by the finding of a low vitamin A level in blood and a positive response to vitamin A supplementation.

Zinc deficiency may lead to vitamin A deficiency as zinc acts on the retinol-binding protein, which is the transport protein for vitamin A and which is indispensable for mobilization of the vitamin from the liver. Furthermore, zinc acts on the oxidation–reduction interconversion of vitamin A (alcohol dehydrogenase is a zinc metalloenzyme). Lack of zinc may provoke symptoms of vitamin A deficiency [10], and night blindness in alcoholics may be due to a combined lack of vitamin A and zinc [11].

Vitamin A intoxication

Aetiology. Chronic hypervitaminosis A is observed in young children if they are persistently overdosed with strong vitamin preparations. Most reported adult cases have ingested more than 100 000 i.u. daily for several months. There is probably a risk of toxic effects if more than 50 000 i.u. daily is ingested for longer periods [1].

Clinical features. There is lethargy, anorexia, weight loss and diffuse alopecia. The skin becomes pruritic, rough and dry with desquamation. The lips are dry and cracked. Follicular keratosis, patchy erythema and purpura may occur in hypervitaminosis A or due to administration of synthetic retinoids [2]. In young children, painful swellings of the limbs due to bone changes are conspicuous.

Diagnosis. Vitamin A intoxication is diagnosed by consistent clinical findings associated with an increased vitamin A level in the blood. Radiology may demonstrate bone changes in young children and in some adults.

Treatment. No treatment is needed except immediate discontinuation of the vitamin A.

Carotenoderma

β-Carotene is the natural provitamin of vitamin A (retinol). A high intake of food containing carotene, especially carrots, causes carotenaemia (increased carotene in plasma) and may induce carotenoderma due to excess carotenes in the sweat. The condition is characterized by orange discoloration of the stratum corneum, especially on palms, soles and in areas where sebaceous glands predominate. The condition is quite harmless and subsides gradually when the dietary habits are regulated. It may occur in pregnancy as a 'pica'.

Carotenaemia is also seen in patients with hyperlipidaemia (diabetes mellitus, myxoedema) and occurs in subjects unable to convert ingested β-carotene into vitamin A [12].

β-Carotene traps free radicals and has been studied together with vitamin E and selenium as a possible dietary factor that may inhibit cancers [13], although this hypothesis remains unproven [14].

Carotenoderma provides no photoprotection [15].

References

1 Keller KL, Fenske NA. Uses of vitamins A, C, and E and related compounds in dermatology: a review. *J Am Acad Dermatol* 1998; **39**: 611–25.

2 Larsen FG, Vahlquist C, Andersson E *et al*. Oral acitretin in psoriasis: drug and vitamin A concentration in plasma, skin and adipose tissue. *Acta Derm Venereol Suppl (Stockh)* 1992; **72**: 84–8.

3 Siegenthaler G, Saurat J-H. Plasma and skin carriers for natural and synthetic retinoids. *Arch Dermatol* 1987; **123**: 1690a–2a.

4 Bollag W. Vitamin A and retinoids: from nutrition to pharmacotherapy in dermatology and oncology. *Lancet* 1983; **i**: 860–3.

5 Chopra PP, Flaxman BA. The effect of vitamin A on growth and differentiation of human keratinocytes *in vivo*. *J Invest Dermatol* 1975; **64**: 19–22.

6 Pinkus H, Hunter R. Biometric analysis of the effect of oral vitamin A on human epidermis. *J Invest Dermatol* 1964; **42**: 131–6.

7 Thomas JR, Cooke JP, Winkelmann RK. High-dose vitamin A therapy for Darier's disease. *Arch Dermatol* 1982; **118**: 891–4.

8 Frazier CN, Hu CK. Cutaneous lesions associated with a deficiency in vitamin A. *Arch Intern Med* 1931; **48**: 507–9.

9 Miller S. Nutritional deficiency of the skin. *J Am Acad Dermatol* 1989; **21**: 1–30.

10 Weismann K, Christensen E, Dreyer V. Zinc supplementation in alcoholic cirrhosis: a double-blind clinical trial. *Acta Med Scand* 1979; **205**: 361–6.

11 Solomons NW, Russel RM. The interaction of vitamin A and zinc: implications for human nutrition. *Am J Clin Nutr* 1980; **33**: 2031–40.

12 Monk BE. Metabolic carotenaemia. *Br J Dermatol* 1982; **106**: 485–8.

13 Menkes MS, Comstock GW, Vuilleumier JP *et al*. Serum beta-carotene, vitamins A and E, selenium, and the risk of lung cancer. *N Engl J Med* 1986; **315**: 1250–4.

14 Rowe PM. Beta-carotene takes a collective beating. *Lancet* 1996; **347**: 249.

15 Pathak MA. Sunscreens: topical and systemic approaches for protection of human skin against harmful effects of solar radiation. *J Am Acad Dermatol* 1982; **7**: 285–312.

Vitamin D [1,2]

Vitamin D is a group of antirachitic steroid derivatives with similar biochemical activity. It is synthesized in the body as vitamin D_3 (cholecalciferol), and is present in the diet from some animal sources (as vitamin D_3) or from plant sources as vitamin D_2 (ergocalciferol). There is little vitamin D_3 in the diet although it is present in cod-liver oil, butter, eggs and liver. Vitamin D is synthesized in the skin from 7-dehydrocholesterol, which is present in abundance, by the action of 290–320-nm UV irradiation (to previtamin D) followed by a temperature-dependent conversion stage. Vitamin D_2 is synthesized from its inactive provitamin, ergosterol, in plants, also by the action of UV irradiation. With adequate exposure to sunlight, dietary vitamin D is unnecessary [1]. Cholecalciferol is hydroxylated in the liver to form 25-hydroxyvitamin D, and further hydroxylation takes place in the kidney to form the biologically active 1,25-dihydroxyvitamin D [1,2]. Vitamin D_2 follows the same hydroxylation pathway, and is equipotent to vitamin D_3. 1α-Hydroxyvitamin D_3 is a synthetic, highly potent vitamin D analogue used in the management of hypoparathyroidism, vitamin-D-resistant rickets and osteomalacia.

Circulating vitamin D is usually measured as 25-hydroxyvitamin D, low status being defined as a level below 30–60 ng/L. Low levels do not reflect the degree of exposure to solar ultraviolet light [3]. Sunbeds (tanning parlour) have been proposed as a means to increase vitamin D status. This claim is controversial since UVA does not participate in the production of vitamin D of the skin, and UVA exposure increases the risk of skin cancer and malignant melanoma [4].

Vitamin D regulates calcium and phosphorus absorption and deposition, and influences the level of serum alkaline phosphatase. The skin is of unique importance in the synthesis, storage and release of vitamin D into the circulation [2]. Lack of vitamin D in children results in tetany and rickets (rachitis), and causes osteomalacia in adults. Elderly people produce less vitamin D_3. In children, limited exposure to sunshine may play an aetiological role; the same applies to some Asian women in the UK in whom there may be a combination of dietary deficiency and little sunlight exposure. Regular use of sunscreens may also lead to reduced synthesis of vitamin D_3 [3]. It is remarkable how exposure to sunlight a few times a week can reduce the risk of osteoporosis, osteomalacia, muscle weakness and fractures [1]. The daily need for calciferol is 400–800 i.u.

Vitamin D intoxication (long-continued administration of more than 100 000 i.u. daily) causes anorexia, vomiting, headache, diarrhoea, hypercalcaemia and hypercalciuria with osteoporosis, resembling the action of parathyroid hormone. Treatment consists of withdrawal of vitamin D, a low-calcium diet and systemic corticosteroids.

Combined calcium and vitamin D supplementation has been shown to reduce the risk of osteoporosis in people aged 50 years or older. A minimum dose of 1200 mg calcium and 800 i.u. vitamin D daily is recommended [5].

References

1 Holick MF. Sunlight 'D'ilemma. Risk of skin cancer or bone disease and muscle weakness. *Lancet* 2001; **357**: 4–6.

2 Holick MF, Smith E, Pincus S. Skin as the site of vitamin D synthesis and target tissue for 1,25-dihydroxyvitamin D_3. *Arch Dermatol* 1987; **123**: 1677–83.

3 Binkley N, Novotny R, Krueger D *et al*. Low vitamin D status despite abundant sun exposure. *J Clin Endocrinol Metab* 2007; **92**: 2130–5.

4 Levine JA, Soarce M, Spencer J *et al*. The indoor UV-tanning industry: a review of skin cancer risk, health benefit claims, and regulation. *J Am Acad Dermatol* 2005; **53**: 1038–44.

5 Reginster J-Y. Calcium and vitamin D for osteoporotic fracture risk. *Lancet* 2007; **370**: 632–3.

Vitamin E [1,2]

Synonym
- α-Tocopherol

Tocopherols are present in oils of vegetables, seeds, corn, whole wheat flour, nuts and some meats; D-α-tocopherol is the most biologically active form. The main physiological activity of tocopherol is antioxidation. Whether the vitamin is essential to humans is still a matter of debate. In rats, guinea pigs and rabbits, a true vitamin effect has been demonstrated. Various dermatological diseases and conditions have been claimed to respond to vitamin E [1–3]. So far, no true benefit has been definitely documented. Fat-soluble vitamin E is located in the stratum corneum and seems to play a role in protecting this layer from damage [2]. An inhibitory effect on hyaluronidase and a protective effect on cellular membranes and on vitamin A oxidation have been suggested, but the clinical relevance is doubtful. Neurological function in children with chronic cholestasis was improved following large doses of vitamin E [4]. Large doses of vitamin E in a controlled trial have been shown to reduce the risk of myocardial infarction [5]. Vitamin E has also been used in dermatology to reduce dapsone-induced haemolysis [6] and headache [7].

References

1 Keller KL, Fenske NA. Uses of vitamins A, C, and E and related compounds in dermatology: a review. *J Am Acad Dermatol* 1998; **39**: 611–25.

2 Edwards H. Vitamin E: an important antioxidant in the skin? *Retinoids* 2001; **17**: 43.

3 Pollack SV. Wound healing: a review. IV. Systemic medications affecting wound healing. *J Dermatol Surg Oncol* 1983; **8**: 667–72.

4 Sokol RJ, Guggenheim MA, Jannacone ST *et al.* Improved neurologic function after long-term correction of vitamin E deficiency in children with chronic cholestasis. *N Engl J Med* 1985; **313**: 1580–6.

5 Stephens NG, Parsons A, Schofield PM *et al.* Randomized controlled trial of vitamin E in patients with coronary disease: Cambridge Heart Antioxidant Study (CHAOS). *Lancet* 1996; **347**: 781–6.

6 Prussick R, Ali MA, Rosenthal D, Guyatt G. The protective effect of vitamin E on the hemolysis associated with dapsone treatment in patients with dermatitis herpetiformis. *Arch Dermatol* 1992; **128**: 210–3.

7 Cox NH. Vitamin E for dapsone-induced headache. *Br J Dermatol* 2002; **156**: 174.

Vitamin B complex

The vitamins of the B complex are of great clinical significance. Isolated deficiencies of certain B vitamins are uncommon. Mostly combined deficiencies of the vitamins belonging to the group are involved, often occurring as a result of insufficient supply of protein and other essential nutrients (zinc, essential fatty acids).

The vitamin B group includes:

1 Aneurin (thiamine) (vitamin B_1)
2 Riboflavine (vitamin B_2)
3 Niacin (nicotinic acid) (B_3)
4 Pyridoxine (vitamin B_6)
5 Cyanocobalamin (vitamin B_{12})
6 Folic acid
7 Pantothenic acid
8 Biotin (vitamin H).

Aneurin

Synonyms
- Vitamin B_1
- Thiamine

Aneurin is present in yeast, cereals, liver, meat, eggs and vegetables. It functions as cocarboxylase in carbohydrate metabolism and in numerous other enzyme systems. It is involved in growth processes and in the function of the nervous system. Deficiency results in accumulation of pyruvic and lactic acids. Dietary deficiency may be a consequence of consuming polished rice as the staple food or, more commonly, of insufficient nutrition associated with chronic alcoholism. Beer drinkers have a reduced risk of developing B vitamin deficiency due to the presence of the vitamins in beer. Hypovitaminosis B_1 may be associated with pregnancy, lactation, diabetes mellitus, ulcerative colitis, coeliac disease, achlorhydria or myxoedema [1].

Clinical features [1]. The classical form of vitamin B_1 deficiency is beriberi, characterized by anorexia, weakness, constipation, symmetrical progressive polyneuritis, cardiac insufficiency with oedema and wasting of musculature. The diagnosis is based on the history and a low urinary aneurin excretion following an injection of 1.0 mg of aneurin. Excretion of less than 50 μg indicates a deficiency state.

Treatment. Aneurin 2–3 mg is given three times daily in mild cases. With severe cardiac and gastrointestinal involvement, polyneuritis and muscular paresis, 20 mg aneurin twice a day given parenterally is indicated.

Riboflavine

Synonyms
- Vitamin B_2
- Lactoflavine

Riboflavine is a D-ribitol isoalloxazine derivative that is widely distributed in plant and animal tissues. It plays a part in intracellular redox reactions. Nutritional sources are milk and the same sources as those of vitamin B_1 [1]. The human requirement is 1–2 mg daily.

Clinical features. Deficiency becomes clinically manifest after several months of deprivation due to chronic illness and malnutrition, especially in elderly women who suffer from achlorhydria, or in malnourished children with malabsorption.

Ariboflavinosis may occur in alcoholic liver cirrhosis, and an association with other deficiencies, such as pellagra, is frequent. Clinically, there is photophobia due to conjunctivitis, sometimes with corneal vascularization, angular stomatitis (perlèche) and sore lips, tongue and mouth [1]. The tongue is purplish red and smooth. A scaly seborrhoeic dermatitis-like eruption may be seen around the nose, eyes, ears and genital area (oro-oculo-genital syndrome). There is an association with zinc deficiency as the content of the two nutrients in foodstuffs is correlated [2].

Treatment. Treatment consists of 5–15 mg riboflavine two to three times daily for 2 weeks and correction of dietary errors.

Pyridoxine

Synonyms
- Vitamin B_6
- Pyridoxal

Pyridoxine is a pyridine derivative, participating as a coenzyme in transaminase and decarboxylase reactions and in the metabolism of cystein, tryptophan and essential fatty acids. It is present in many foods including yeast, eggs and various grains. The recommended daily allowance is about 2 mg.

Although much is known about experimental deficiency in many species, the manifestations in humans are not well defined. Convulsions, anaemia and acrodynia may develop in infants [3]. Dermatitis has occurred and is attributed to disturbed metabolism of unsaturated fatty acids. Pyridoxine deficiency may follow therapy with isoniazid, hydralazine and penicillamine [4].

Vitamin B_{12}

Synonyms
- Cyanocobalamin
- Cycobemine

Vitamin B$_{12}$ is involved in nucleic acid synthesis and erythrocyte production. Deficiency may occur in vegetarians, as plants do not contain the vitamin. Most frequently it is due to lack of the 'intrinsic factor' in pernicious anaemia. Hyperpigmentation, especially in dark-skinned races, may occur. It is most pronounced in skin flexures, such as finger and palm creases, and on the knuckles. Pigmented streaks of the nails may be seen. An enlarged, red tongue is a characteristic finding [5].

Folic acid

Folic acid is a compound consisting of pteridine, *p*-aminobenzoic acid and glutamic acid. It is present in liver, meat, green leaves and milk. In the organism, folic acid is converted to folinic acid, which is the biologically active form. The conversion requires the presence of vitamin C. Folinic acid is needed for the transport of one-carbon units and plays a role in growth and erythrocyte production. The daily requirement is estimated to be about 0.4 mg.

Although no consistent or specific cutaneous changes are related to folate deficiency, greyish brown pigmentation on light-exposed parts has been described in megaloblastic anaemia [5,6]. Cheilitis, glossitis and mucosal erosions are common. Pigmentation similar to that of vitamin B$_{12}$ deficiency has been associated with folate deficiency in pregnancy and during lactation. Spotty pigmentation of palms and soles and pigmented palmar creases have been described. Folate deficiency is estimated by serum and erythrocyte folate levels. Subclinical deficiency may be present in patients with extensive skin disease.

Deficiency causing macrocytic anaemia may result in retinal haemorrhages [7].

Synthetic folic acid may cause anaphylactic reactions [8]. The requirement for folate supplementation during methotrexate therapy is discussed in Chapters 20 and 74.

Niacin

Synonyms
- Nicotinic acid
- Vitamin B$_3$

Niacin is an essential component of two coenzymes, coenzyme I (nicotinamide adenine dinucleotide, NAD) and coenzyme II (NAD phosphate, NADP), which either donate or accept hydrogen in a wide range of biochemical reactions. Tryptophan, an essential amino acid, can be transformed to niacin, which is converted to the amide in the body. Niacin is involved in the biosynthesis of ceramides as well as of other stratum corneum lipids which improve the epidermal permeability layer [9].

Pellagra [10]

Cellular deficiency of niacin, resulting from an inadequate dietary supply of niacin and tryptophan, is termed pellagra. In Western Europe and North America pellagra is only rarely encountered now, mostly in subjects living on an unbalanced diet, such as chronic alcoholics, and in patients with gastrointestinal diseases or severe psychiatric disturbances. Rare causes are functioning carcinoid tumours (Chapter 43) and Hartnup disease (p. 59.100). Therapy with isoniazid (which competes biochemically with

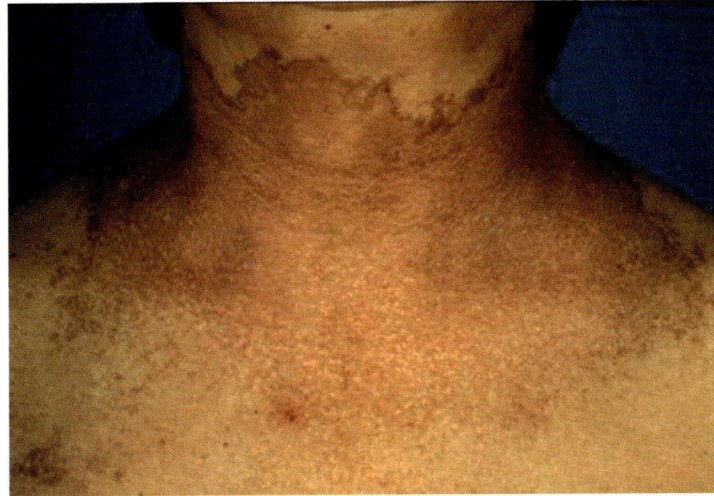

Fig. 59.42 Pellagra with erythematous, brownish scaling on the neck (Casal's necklace).

niacin owing to a close structural resemblance), 6-mercaptopurine or 5-fluorouracil may provoke pellagra.

The classical triad of clinical features is *dermatitis*, *diarrhoea* and *dementia*, not invariably appearing in this order. Redness and superficial scaling appear on areas exposed to sunlight, heat, friction or pressure. The changes resemble sunburn and subside leaving a dusky, brown-red coloration, but this occurs more slowly than typical in sunburn and exacerbation follows re-exposure to sunlight. On the face, a symmetrical 'butterfly' eruption is frequently observed and there is often a characteristic well-margin-ated eruption on the front of the neck ('Casal's necklace'). Asymmetrical lesions may appear at sites of sun exposure, eczema, injury or stasis [11–12] (Figs 59.42–59.45).

Gastrointestinal symptoms include pain, diarrhoea and achlorhydria in 50% of cases. In mild instances, the mental disturbance may pass unnoticed, patients perhaps being slightly depressed or apathetic. Sometimes, there may be frank disorientation, restlessness or other severe central nervous system symptoms [13]. Peripheral neuritis and myelitis are occasionally encountered.

Histology. Histological examination shows hyper- and parakeratosis, acanthosis and multiple melanin granules throughout the epidermis. Such changes are suggestive, but not diagnostic, of pellagra.

Drug eruptions, various forms of porphyria, photodermatitis, lupus erythematosus and actinic reticuloid may cause diagnostic difficulty. The so-called pellagrous vulvitis, vaginitis and scrotal dermatitis may be attributed to accompanying ariboflavinosis and other deficiencies of the vitamin B group and of zinc.

Therapy. In severe cases, intravenous niacin is required in doses of 50–100 mg once or twice a day. Otherwise, oral niacin amide in a total dose of 0.5 g/day should be given. The amide is to be preferred, as it does not precipitate flushing, itching and burning as is seen following ingestion of niacin in large doses. Improvement can be expected within a day or two.

Kava dermopathy. Kava, a psychoactive intoxicating beverage used ceremonially and socially by Pacific Islanders, may produce a pellagra-like ichthyosiform dermopathy with widespread acquired ichthyosis [14,15]. Kava is produced by infusing dried roots of *Piper methysticum* with water or coconut milk. The cause

of the skin disease has not been established; interference with tryptophan or niacin as previously suggested is not likely [15]. Interference with cholesterol metabolism akin to changes associated with lipid-lowering agents is a possibility. Kava dermopathy is curable with abstinence.

Biotin

Biotin is a water-soluble, sulphur-containing, heterocyclic carboxylic acid involved in bacterial metabolism and possibly functioning as a coenzyme in decarboxylation and other enzymatic processes. Deficiency can be induced by feeding raw egg-white containing avidin which binds biotin and makes it poorly absorbable [16]. Short bowel syndrome in association with parenteral nutrition may cause biotin deficiency [17,18]. Symptoms include alopecia, conjunctivitis, eczema around the nose and mouth, nail dystrophy, hyperaesthesia, paraesthesia, depression and muscle pain. A multivitamin preparation supplying 60 μg of biotin daily cured an adult patient within 3 weeks [16]. Biotin seems to possess some antiseborrhoeic actions and has been used in high doses for therapy of Leiner's disease in infants (Chapter 17) [19].

Inborn errors of biotin metabolism [20]. The genetically determined disorders of biotin metabolism consist of two separate diseases: holocarboxylase synthetase deficiency and biotinidase deficiency. Both are transmitted as an autosomal recessive trait.

Holocarboxylase deficiency (MIM #253270) presents in the neonatal period, affected subjects having severe symptoms of organic acidaemia. The patients may have shown recurrent episodes of

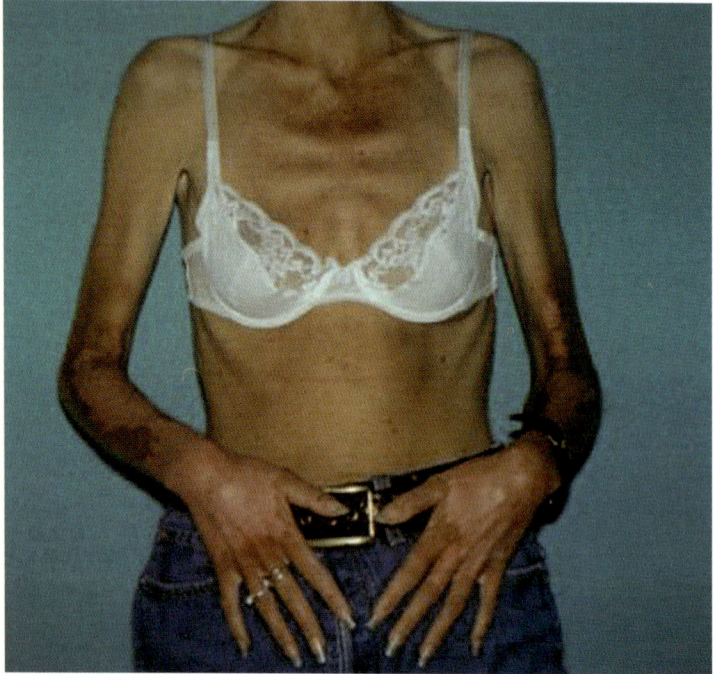

Fig. 59.43 Pellagra on the face provoked by sun exposure.

(a)

(b)

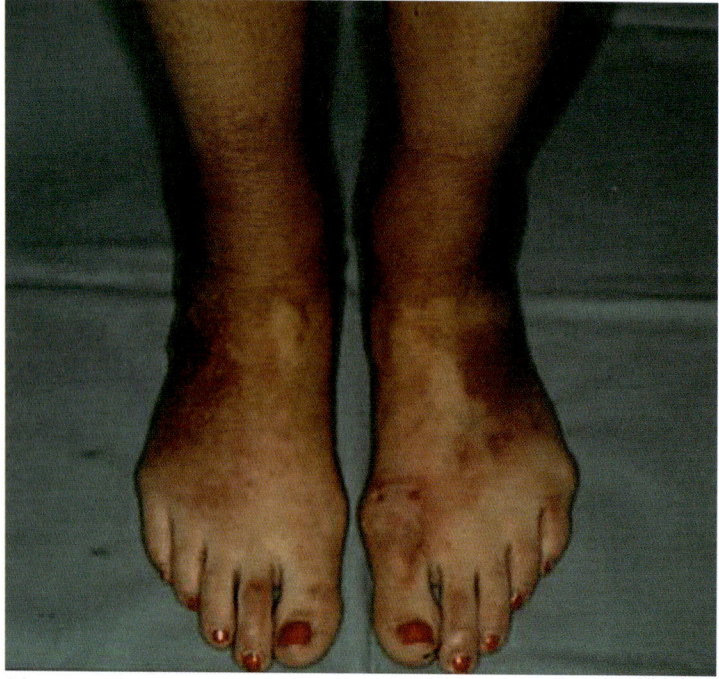

Fig. 59.44 Pellagra (a) in a patient with anorexia nervosa. (b) Note marked reaction in sun exposed areas on the feet.

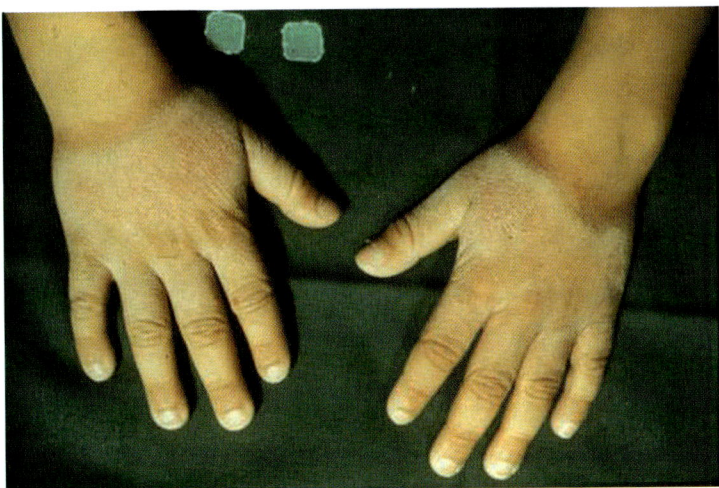

Fig. 59.45 Pellagra on sun exposed dorsal hands.

vomiting from birth and rapid respiration as a sign of severe metabolic acidosis. There are seizures, hypo- as well as hypertonia, electroencephalogram abnormalities, and the disease progresses to death unless diagnosis and effective therapy supervene. An erythematous, scaly rash is prominent over most of the body in the patients who survive the first days of life. The skin lesions may resemble ichthyosis and seborrhoeic dermatitis. The pattern of excretion of organic acids is characteristic, especially 3-hydroxy-isovaleric acid and 3-methylcrotonylglycine in urine being increased. Lactic acidaemia is striking. The molecular defect is in the enzyme holocarboxylase synthetase.

Biotinidase deficiency (multiple decarboxylase deficiency, MIM #253260) usually presents after 3 months of age. The cutaneous lesions may resemble those of acrodermatitis enteropathica, that is severe zinc deficiency, with periorificial eczematous rash on the face, nail dystrophy (onychoschizia) and skin infection. The hair is sparse, and there may be total alopecia. Neurological symptoms are prominent with myoclonic seizures, ataxia, lethargy and developmental delay [21]. There are low levels of biotin in blood and urine. The fundamental defect is in biotinidase, which normally acts on biocytin, a biotin–lysine complex, thereby separating biotin from lysine [19].

Biotin treatment. Both of the biotin-related disorders discussed above are treated with an oral dose of biotin, usually 10 mg/day but some patients need less and some have required as much as 40 mg/day.

Uncombable hair syndrome (Chapter 66) may respond to a low oral dose of biotin [22].

References

1 Miller SJ. Nutritional deficiency of the skin. *J Am Acad Dermatol* 1989; **21**: 1–30.
2 Weismann K. *Zinc Deficiency and Effects of Systemic Zinc Therapy*. Copenhagen: FADL's Forlag, 1980: 46.
3 Vilter RW, Mueller JF, Glazer HF. The effect of vitamin B_6 deficiency induced by desoxypyridoxine in human beings. *J Lab Clin Med* 1953; **42**: 335–7.
4 Capps JC, Meddler EM, Jacobs LW *et al.* Effects of orally administered *N*-acetyl-1-cysteine and *N*-acetyl-DL-penicillamine on vitamin B_6 availability and copper excretion in the rat. *Am J Clin Nutr* 1968; **21**: 715–22.
5 Noppakun N, Swasdikul D. Reversible hyperpigmentation of skin and nails with white hair due to vitamin B_{12} deficiency. *Arch Dermatol* 1986; **122**: 896–9.
6 Marks VJ, Briggaman RA, Wheeler CE. Hyperpigmentation in megaloblastic anemia. *J Am Acad Dermatol* 1985; **12**: 914–7.
7 Hughes M, Learch M. Dietary folate deficiency and bilateral retinal haemorrhages. *Lancet* 2006; **368**: 2155.
8 Stratigos JD, Katsambas A. Pellagra: a still existing disease. *Br J Dermatol* 1977; **96**: 99–106.
9 Smith J, Empson M, Wall C. Recurrent anaphylaxis to synthetic folic acid. *Lancet* 2007; **370**: 652.
10 Tanno O, Ota Y, Kitamura N, Katsube T, Inoue S. Nicotinamide increases biosynthesis of ceramides as well as other stratum corneum lipids to improve the epidermal permeability barrier. *Br J Dermatol* 2000; **143**: 524–31.
11 Findlay GH. Pellagra, kwashiorkor and sun exposure. *Br J Dermatol* 1965; **77**: 666–7.
12 Bean WR, Spies TD, Vilter RW. Asymmetric cutaneous lesions in pellagra. *Arch Dermatol Syphilol* 1944; **49**: 335–45.
13 Risum G. Pellagra et tilfælde med alvorlige symptomer central nerve systemet. *Ugeskr Læger* 1977; **113**: 935–8.
14 Ruze P. Kava-induced dermopathy: a niacin deficiency? *Lancet* 1990; **335**: 1142–5.
15 Norton SA, Ruze P. Kava dermopathy. *J Am Acad Dermatol* 1994; **31**: 89–97.
16 Roth KS. Biotin in clinical medicine—a review. *Am J Clin Nutr* 1981; **34**: 1967–74.
17 Mock DM, Delorimer AA, Liebman WM *et al.* Biotin deficiency: an unusual complication of parenteral alimentation. *N Engl J Med* 1981; **304**: 820–3.
18 McClain CI, Baker H, Onstad GR. Biotin deficiency in an adult during parenteral nutrition. *JAMA* 1982; **247**: 3116–7.
19 Nisenson A. Seborrhoeic dermatitis of infants with Leiner's disease: a biotin deficiency. *J Pediatr* 1957; **51**: 537–48.
20 Nyhan WI. Inborn errors of biotin metabolism. *Arch Dermatol* 1982; **123**: 1696–8.
21 Redondo-Maleo J, Urbon-Artero A. Facial erythema and onychoschizia. *Arch Dermatol* 2005; **141**: 1457–62.
22 Shelley WB, Shelley ED. Uncombable hair syndrome: observations on response to biotin and occurrence in siblings with ectodermal dysplasia. *J Am Acad Dermatol* 1985; **13**: 97–102.

Vitamin C [1–3]

Synonym
• Ascorbic acid

Vitamin C is a relatively strong organic acid, chemically related to the carbohydrates. Only the laevo form is biologically active. Ascorbic acid is a strong reducing agent, easily oxidized to dehydroascorbic acid, with which it constitutes a reversible redox system. Vitamin C plays a central role in collagen and ground-substance formation, metabolism of aromatic amino acids (phenylalanine, tyrosine), reduction of folic acid to folinic acid and a broad range of biochemical redox reactions, including the preservation of sulphur-containing enzymes in a reduced form. It occurs naturally in cabbage, potatoes, green vegetables and fruits. The recommended daily dose is 30–80 mg; a daily intake of 10 mg prevents scurvy.

Vitamin C deficiency

Synonyms
• Scurvy
• Scorbutus
• Hypovitaminosis C

Unlike most other animals, humans and guinea pigs are unable to synthesize ascorbic acid due to lack of the enzymatic pathways

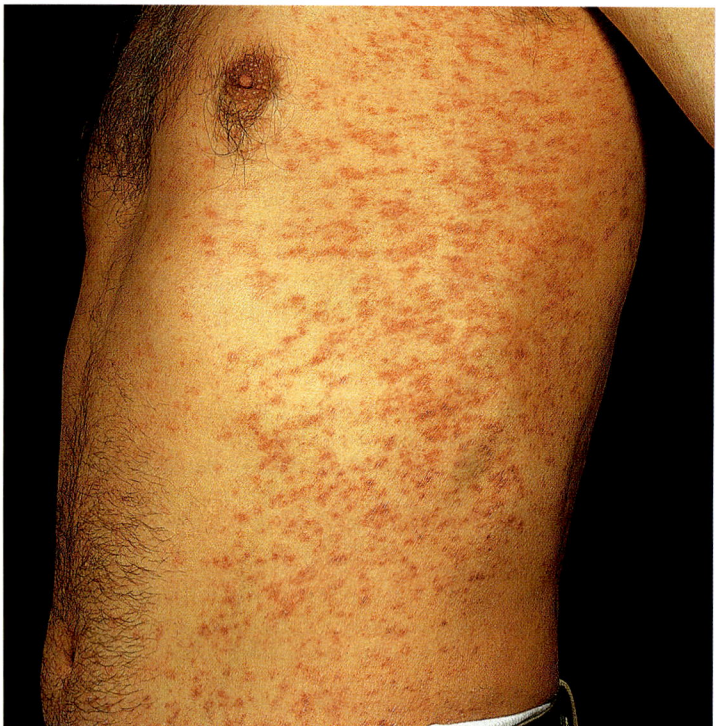

Fig. 59.46 Scurvy. Purpuric rash on the trunk. The lower extremities were also affected.

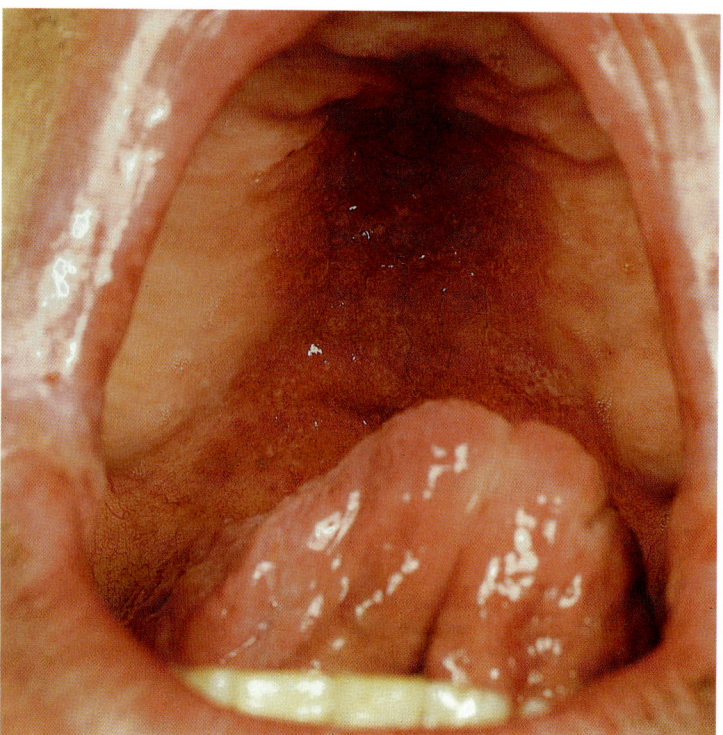

Fig. 59.47 Scurvy, showing purpura on the hard palate.

for synthesis of L-ascorbic acid from D-glucuronic acid. In the deficiency state, collagen and ground-substance synthesis are depressed, which leads to a multiplicity of symptoms involving bones, mucous membranes and skin.

Aetiology. Lack of vitamin C is still a serious problem in many parts of the world where access to fruit and vegetables is limited and where general malnutrition prevails. By contrast, most cases in developed countries are a consequence of food faddism, ignorance or alcoholism [4,5]. Danish beer no longer contains vitamin C as an antioxidant, and can therefore no longer prevent scurvy in alcoholics [6]. Malnourished children with scurvy (Barlow's disease) [7] may still be a paediatric problem [8] and vitamin C deficiency has been observed in teenagers living on processed food devoid of fresh fruit and vegetables [9]. In patients with chronic gastrointestinal disturbances, subclinical scurvy may be present. Elderly men living alone, who rarely get fresh fruit or vegetables and who may abuse alcohol, are particularly at risk.

Scurvy may be a presenting sign of undiagnosed psychiatric illness [10], and may appear with ecchymosis, perifollicular petechiae and haemorrhagic pustules on a previously injured extremity [11].

The cause of scurvy observed in liver transplant patients is not clear [12].

Clinical features [4]. (Figs 59.46 and 59.47). The initial skin change is follicular keratosis with coiled hairs on the upper arms, back, buttocks and lower extremities. Later, perifollicular haemorrhage with blood pigment discoloration especially on the legs, swollen bleeding gums, stomatitis and epistaxis occur. Large skin haemorrhages may be seen. Anaemia is usually present, and the patient

appears resentful and mentally depressed. In the infant, dental development is impaired and oral changes may be severe. Tender subperiostal haematomas may develop and dominate the picture. Chronic hypovitaminosis C with 'woody' oedema and discoloration of the legs as the presenting feature has been described. Subnormal serum levels of vitamin C are present (normal range about 17–94 μmol/L). The significance of low values without clinical symptoms is doubtful.

Treatment. The scorbutic patient should be treated with oral vitamin C 100 mg three times daily in addition to protein-rich food [4]. The response is dramatic. It is advisable to continue the therapy for several weeks to ensure repletion of the emptied body stores.

References
1 Dickman SR. The search for the specific factor in scurvy. *Perspect Biol Med* 1981; **24**: 382–6.
2 Levine M. New concepts in the biology and biochemistry of ascorbic acid. *N Engl J Med* 1986; **314**: 892–902.
3 Kutsky RJ. *Handbook of Vitamins and Hormones.* New York: Reinhold, 1973.
4 Hirschmann JV, Raugi GJ. Adult scurvy. *J Am Acad Dermatol* 1999; **41**: 895–906.
5 Leung FW, Guze PA. Adult scurvy. *Ann Emerg Med* 1981; **10**: 652–6.
6 Jørgensen J, Paulson PA, Klemp P. Skørbug. *Ugeskr Læger* 1983; **145**: 1525–7.
7 Weismann K. Infantile scurvy's true father: Vilhelm Ingerslev. *Bibl Laeger* 1996; **188**: 345–52 (Summary in English).
8 Heymann WR. Scurvy in children. *J Am Acad Dermatol* 2007; **57**: 358–9.
9 McKenna KE, Dawson JF. Scurvy occurring in a teenager. *Clin Exp Dermatol* 1993; **18**: 75–7.
10 Arron ST, Lizo W, Maurer T. Scurvy: a presenting sign of phychosis. *J Am Acad Dermatol* 2007; **57**: S8–10.
11 Walters RW. Scurvy with manifestations limited to a previously injured extremity. *J Am Acad Dermatol* 2007; **57**: S 48–9.
12 Hatuel H, Buffet M, Mateus C, Calmos Y *et al.* Scurvy in liver transplant patients. *J Am Acad Dermatol* 2006; **55**: 154–6.

Kwashiorkor and marasmus [1,2]

Kwashiorkor is a nutritional syndrome with characteristic cutaneous changes due to severe protein malnutrition with relative carbohydrate excess. In children, there is retardation of skeletal and mental development, muscular wasting, fatty infiltration of the liver and oedema. Marasmus is the result of prolonged starvation, a wasting syndrome, resulting in 40–50% reduction in body weight but with no peripheral oedema.

Kwashiorkor

Aetiology [2]. Protein–energy deficiency is one of the commonest and most widespread nutritional disorders in developing countries. The majority of kwashiorkor cases are found in countries where the diet consists of corn, rice or beans. Kwashiorkor is more common in children than in adults and is a major paediatric problem in certain parts of the world. The onset in infancy is during the weaning and postweaning period. In Europe and North America, occasional cases are seen in patients suffering from malabsorption or eating a diet that includes an inadequate amount of protein. Milder forms are probably not uncommon, particularly in the elderly.

Kwashiorkor refers to the 'deposed child' who is no longer suckled. It is a multiple deficiency syndrome. The cause is related to lack of essential amino acids, vitamins and trace elements, particularly zinc. The skin manifestations, hair changes and failure to thrive may mimic those seen in acrodermatitis enteropathica. Serum zinc is low, but this may be attributable partly to hypoalbuminaemia. Hospitalized children may show persistent hypozincaemia after clinical cure has occurred, indicating a need for zinc supplementation together with vitamins and protein-rich nutrition [3,4].

Clinical features [1,2,5]. The symptoms of kwashiorkor usually first develop between the age of 6 months and 5 years. The most important feature in the child is a failure to thrive, with inhibition of growth and mental development; oedema and muscle wasting are also found.

The skin lesions are initially erythematous and later purple or reddish brown in colour with marked exfoliation. In milder cases a lacquered 'flaky paint' ('enamel paint') or 'cracked skin' appearance is present. The hair is dry and lustreless and may become light red-brown in colour. In more severe cases it may be prematurely grey or show a 'pepper and salt' appearance, and become sparse, fine and brittle.

The skin often shows dyschromia with hypopigmentation, perhaps the result of phenylalanine deficiency, and patchy postinflammatory hyperpigmentation. In severe cases pigmentary changes are particularly striking. There is convincing evidence that the skin changes of kwashiorkor are primarily due to zinc deficiency [6]. Mucosal lesions, such as cheilosis, xerophthalmia and vulvovaginitis may be found, which are related to other deficiencies.

Mental disturbances are variable and may appear either as apathy or irritability. The child does not smile; when it does, it is a sign of recovery.

Table 59.11 Clinical features distinguishing kwashiorkor from pellagra.

Kwashiorkor	Pellagra
Children more than adults	Adults more than children
Dermatitis with systemic signs of apathy and oedema	Dermatitis precedes gastrointestinal and neuropsychiatric symptoms in most cases
Eruption generalized; pale, ill-defined; 'crackled skin'	Exposed areas; red, thickened, well-defined lesions; later, dry, branny scales
Hair light, 'pepper and salt' appearance, thin	Normal
Nails sometimes soft and thin	Normal
High mortality	Low mortality

Oedema is the result of hypoalbuminaemia (less than 2.5 g/100 mL). The α- and β-globulins are low, while an increase in gammaglobulin is usual.

Hypoglycaemia with hypothermia, coma and severe bacterial or parasitic disease are rare, often fatal, complications [7].

Mild cases of kwashiorkor appearing in the elderly show as a 'cracked skin' appearance on the front of the legs and lower abdomen. They have been reported under the title of geriatric nutritional eczema.

Prognosis. The short-term prognosis of mild cases which are given full dietary treatment is good, but mortality is high in severe and relapsing cases.

Diagnosis. Diagnostic difficulties occur in mild cases. The dietary history, 'cracked skin' and oedema, particularly when associated with pigmentary changes, should lead to the suspicion of protein deficiency. Acrodermatitis enteropathica may be mistaken for kwashiorkor. The features distinguishing kwashiorkor from pellagra are shown in Table 59.11.

Prevention and treatment. Prevention of kwashiorkor depends on increasing the supply of animal proteins, and on education and social welfare in poor areas.

In an established case, a complete and balanced diet should be given as soon as possible. Skimmed milk is the most useful treatment, presumably through its amino-acid content. Appropriate measures should be taken to correct any electrolyte disturbance.

Marasmus [1]

Aetiology. Marasmus is derived from the Greek *marasmos*, which means wasting. It is a result of severe protein and calorie deprivation for a prolonged period. Worldwide, marasmus is more frequent than kwashiorkor and is especially seen in developing countries where food is absent or scarce. Severely ill, hospitalized patients may show signs of marasmus. Low zinc levels are a predominant feature.

Clinical features. Patients have a wrinkled, loose, dry skin. There is a substantial loss of subcutaneous fat tissue, and the facial expression is described as 'monkey facies' due to loss of the buccal adipose tissue. Follicular hyperkeratosis may be prominent in adults. The hair is thin and sparse and readily lost and the nails are fissured. Skin ulceration occurs.

Diagnosis. The combined finding of a severely reduced body weight, loss of subcutaneous fat, poor hair and nail growth and a loose, wrinkled, dry skin that appears too large is diagnostic. There is no peripheral oedema.

Prevention and treatment. This is as for kwashiorkor. Skin ulceration may respond to topical zinc paste or oral zinc supplementation in addition to a protein-rich nutritional supply.

References
1 Miller SJ. Nutritional deficiency and the skin. *J Am Acad Dermatol* 1989; **21**: 1–30.
2 McLaren DS. Skin in protein energy malnutrition. *Arch Dermatol* 1987; **123**: 1674–6.
3 Golden BE, Golden MHN. Plasma zinc, rate of weight gain, and the energy cost of tissue deposition in children recovering from severe malnutrition on a cow's milk or soya protein-based diet. *Am J Clin Nutr* 1981; **34**: 892–9.
4 Hambidge KM, Walravens PA. Zinc deficiency in infants and preadolescent children. In: Prasad AS, Oberlaeas D, eds. *Trace Elements in Human Health and Disease*, Vol. 1. New York: Academic Press, 1976: 21–32.
5 Editorial. Classification of infantile nutrition. *Lancet* 1970; **2**: 302–3.
6 McLaren. Skin in protein energy malnutrition. *Arch Dermatol* 1987; **123**: 1674–6.
7 Wharton B. Hypoglycaemia in children with kwashiorkor. *Lancet* 1970; **i**: 170–20.

Calcification and ossification of the skin [1–5]

Calcification or calcinosis cutis is the result of deposition of calcium and phosphate in organic matrices of the tissues. The process occurs in a wide range of different conditions. The mineral phase may be arranged in the manner seen in normal bone formation, *ossification*. If the deposition is not organized, the condition is termed *calcification*. The organic matrix consists largely of collagen or elastic tissue. All organic matrices of calcified or ossified tissues contain protein-bound phosphorus. In pathological ectopic calcification, the matrix is altered and contains acid proteins. In pseudoxanthoma elasticum, γ-carboxyglutamic acid, an amino acid present in calcium-binding proteins, has been found in high concentrations in the dermis. The solid phase of calcified tissue is made up of hydroxyapatite and amorphous calcium phosphate. Once formed, the focus increases in size by growth and may result in disorganized masses of pasta-like material.

Aberrant calcium deposition in the skin may be divided into three main groups:
1 Associated with localized or widespread tissue changes or damage (dystrophic calcification)
2 Unassociated with tissue damage or demonstrable metabolic disorder (idiopathic calcification)
3 Associated with an abnormal calcium and phosphorus metabolism (metastatic calcification) (Table 59.12).

Dystrophic calcification [6]

The calcinosis is confined to the dermis or subcutaneous tissue and related to local connective tissue or fatty tissue damage, in the absence of any detectable abnormality of calcium metabolism. The calcification appears a variable time after the injury; for example, in dermatomyositis it occurs after a few years and in generalized

Table 59.12 Various forms of calcinosis cutis.

Dystrophic calcification
Calcification usually associated with localized injury
Congenital
Fibrodysplasia ossificans
Traumatic
Subcutaneous injection with calcium-containing heparin
Radiotherapy
Foreign-body, haematoma, fat cell necrosis
Inflammatory
Acne, varicose veins, tuberculous granuloma, postoperative inflammation in scars
Degenerative infarcts (arterial, venous), venous stasis, parasitic cysts (e.g. echinococcal cysts)
Neoplastic
Benign: sebaceous cysts, lipomas, angiomas, calcifying epithelioma of Malherbe
Malignant: some liposarcomas
Calcification associated with widespread tissue injury
Dermatomyositis
Generalized scleroderma (Thibierge–Weissenbach or CREST syndrome)
Systemic lupus erythematosus
Acrodermatitis atrophicans
Pseudoxanthoma elasticum
Ehlers–Danlos syndrome
Idiopathic calcification
Calcinosis universalis; calcinosis circumscripta
Solitary nodular calcification of the skin ('cutaneous calculus')
Pinnal calcification
Tumoral calcinosis
Metastatic calcification
Hypercalcaemic
Hyperparathyroidism
Sarcoidosis
Vitamin D excess
Milk–alkali syndrome
Destructive bone disease
Metastatic carcinoma, lymphoma, multiple myeloma, leukaemia
Paget's disease
Normocalcaemic
Chronic renal failure
Pseudohypoparathyroidism

scleroderma usually after 10 or more years. Dystrophic calcification may also occur in systemic lupus erythematosus [1,7,8].

Electrical injuries may be particularly likely to result in dystrophic calcification. An accumulation of calcium salts on dermal collagen fibres of pig skin was observed in scars following electrical injury [9]. Deposition of calcium salts in high concentration on a damaged skin surface may induce dermal calcification, as observed following electroencephalography in children [10]. In these cases, the skin was abraded prior to application of an electrode paste containing calcium chloride; lesions developed shortly after electroencephalography and disappeared in 2–6 months without therapy. An intact stratum corneum is protective.

Idiopathic calcification
Calcinosis universalis

The deposition of calcium in the dermis, subcutis and muscles is unrelated to any recognizable tissue injury or metabolic disorder.

Many cases reported in the literature under the diagnosis were probably suffering from undetected dermatomyositis, systemic lupus erythematosus or scleroderma, but there remain a number of instances in which no underlying disease is demonstrable [2].

Histopathology. Initially, calcium particles gather around fat cells. Electron microscopy of early lesions has shown apatite crystals lying in parallel to the collagen fibres [11].

Clinical features. Nodules or plaques 0.5–5.0 cm in size are symmetrically distributed over the extremities and, less commonly, the trunk. The lesions may become tender and ulcerate, discharging chalk-like creamy material consisting mainly of calcium phosphate with a small amount of calcium carbonate. After ulceration, a slowly healing sinus remains. Fingertip lesions are often painful, while in other sites there may be limitation of movement due to stiffening of the skin. The disease is eventually fatal.

X-ray examination is valuable for localizing the deeper deposits. Biochemical investigations are normal.

Treatment. Surgical removal of painful deposits may give temporary relief. In some instances, corticosteroids may be considered, although the response is variable. Cellulose phosphate combined with a low-calcium diet should be considered [12].

Calcinosis circumscripta
There may be only a few calcium deposits in the skin. Most cases of calcinosis circumscripta are found in generalized scleroderma or dermatomyositis but rarely it may occur as an idiopathic disorder [3]. Keloid formation with calcification has been described [13].

Idiopathic calcinosis of the scrotum [13,14]
Calcinosis scrotalis (Fig. 59.48) is a rare, benign disorder consisting of multiple asymtomatic firm nodules 0.2–1.0 cm in diameter. It is often misdiagnosed as scrotal cysts. Dystrophic calcification in the penis has been reported following trauma, Peyronie's disease and cytostatic therapy.

Calcifying epithelioma of Malberbe
See Chapter 53.

Tumoral calcinosis [2,15,16]
Tumoral calcinosis occurs most commonly in the native population of Africa, particularly among younger age groups. Clinically, the lesions present as swellings around the large joints (hip, elbow, ankle and scapula), but there is no actual involvement of the joint. Extrusion of calcified material, which has been likened to a suspension of procaine-penicillin, may take place. Histologically, there is initially collagen necrobiosis, which results in cyst formation and a foreign-body response. The calcification is first granular; later, dense deposits are seen [15]. The aetiology is unknown, but it is probably a form of dystrophic calcification caused by mechanical injury.

Pinnal calcification [2]
Calcified ear cartilage has been observed in several conditions such as Addison's disease, ochronosis, acromegaly, diabetes mel-

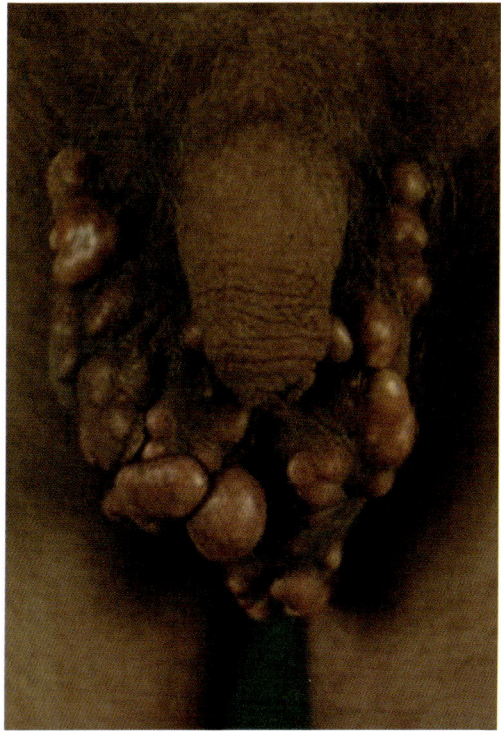

(a)

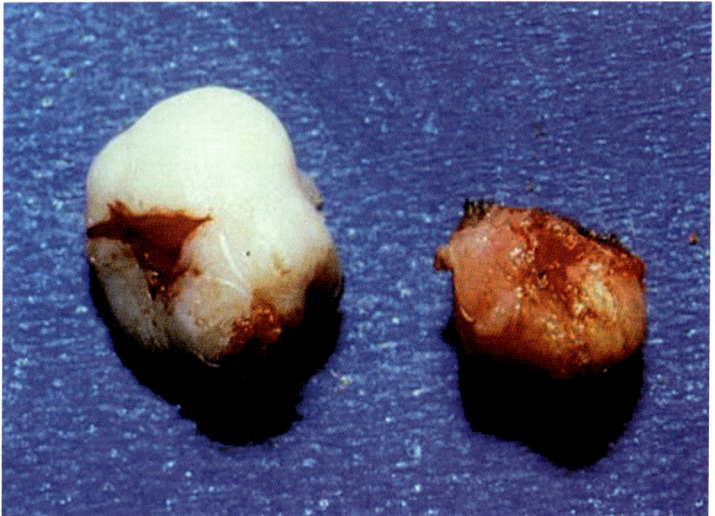

(b)

Fig. 59.48   (a) Calcinosis scrotalis; (b) solitary nodules after removal.

litus, hyperthyroidism, systemic chondromalacia (von Meyenburg's disease), familial cold hypersensitivity and frostbite.

Metastatic calcification [3,17]
In metastatic calcification, calcinosis occurs as a precipitation of calcium salts in normal skin, subcutaneous tissue, muscles and internal organs.

Aetiology. In all cases, there is an increase in the serum levels of calcium or phosphate. Hypercalcaemia may be due to hyperparathyroidism, vitamin D intoxication, milk–alkali syndrome or destructive bone disease with excessive osteoclastic activity. Metastatic carcinoma, multiple myeloma, leukaemia and Paget's disease of bone may all be associated with metastatic calcification. Calciphylaxis, now termed calcific uraemic arteriolopathy (Chapters 49 and 62), is a potentially fatal syndrome, in which there is usually a raised serum calcium phosphate product. Most cases occur in the context of chronic renal insufficiency in patients undergoing long-term renal dialysis, in whom there has been development of secondary or tertiary hyperparathyroidism [18].

Clinical features. The cutaneous manifestations are similar to those of calcinosis universalis. Additional clinical features reflect the primary disease.

Treatment. Only in hypervitaminosis D and the milk–alkali syndrome can improvement be expected by regulation of dietary habits and withdrawal of vitamin D and milk intake. In cases of renal insufficiency, restriction of dietary phosphate and oral administration of an aluminium hydroxide gel may be useful.

Ossification of the skin

Synonyms
- Osteomatosis
- Osteoma cutis

Osteomatosis represents cutaneous calcification with *de novo* bone formation in the skin [19]. It has been noted in suprapubic prostatectomy scars and in otherwise normal postoperative scars [20]. It may also occur in collagen vascular disease (lupus erythematosus, scleroderma and dermatomyositis) [21]. Cutaneous ossification without any known causative factor (also known as osteomatosis cutis, primary osteoma cutis or osteosis cutis) has been reported [17].

Post-acne osteoma cutis

This is a rare complication of long-standing acne vulgaris. It has been reported to occur as pigmented osteomas during tetracycline or minocycline therapy. The osteomas that represent metaplastic bone formation are located in the mid- or reticular dermis, and consist of concentric lamellae with lacunae, Haversian canals and marrow cavities. With the use of tetracycline, more patients develop bluish, 1–2-mm, moveable papules on the face. Treatment consists of surgery or local 0.5% tretinoin cream with resultant transepidermal elimination of the lesions [22].

References

1 Rothe MJ, Grant-Kels JM, Rothfield NF. Extensive calcinosis cutis with systemic lupus erythematosus. *Arch Dermatol* 1990; **126**: 1060–3.
2 Mehregan AH. Calcinosis cutis. A review of the clinical forms and report of 75 cases. *Semin Dermatol* 1984; **3**: 53–61.
3 Walsh JS, Fairley JA. Calcifying disorders of the skin. *J Am Acad Dermatol* 1995; **33**: 693–706.
4 Lewis VJ, Holt PJ. Subcutaneous calcification following high-dose radiotherapy. *Br J Dermatol* 2004; **150**: 1049–50.
5 Eich D, Scharffetter-Kochanek K, Weilrauch J *et al.* Calcinosis cutis and subcutis: an unusual non-immunologic adverse reaction to subcutaneous infections of low-molecular-weight calcium containing heparins. *J Am Acad Dermatol* 2004; **50**: 210–4.
6 Touart DM, Sau P. Cutaneous deposition diseases. Part II. *J Am Acad Dermatol* 1998; **39**: 527–44.
7 Bhatia S, Silverberg NB, Don PC, Weinberg JM. Extensive calcinosis cutis in association with systemic lupus erythematosus. *Acta Derm Venereol* 2001; **81**: 446–7.
8 Quismorio FP, Dubois EL, Chandor SB. Soft-tissue calcification in systemic lupus erythematosus. *Arch Dermatol* 1975; **111**: 352–6.
9 Karlsmark T, Danielsen L, Thomsen HK *et al.* Tracing the use of torture: electrically induced calcification of collagen in pig skin. *Nature* 1983; **301**: 75–8.
10 Wiley HE, Eaglstein WE. Calcinosis cutis in children following electro-encephalography. *JAMA* 1979; **242**: 455–6.
11 Cornelius CE, Tenenhouse A, Weber JC. Calcinosis cutis: metabolic, sweat, histochemical, X-ray diffraction and electron microscopic study. *Arch Dermatol* 1968; **98**: 219–29.
12 Marks J. Studies with ⁴⁷Ca in patients with calcinosis cutis. *Br J Dermatol* 1970; **82**: 1–9.
13 Song DH, Lee KH, Kang WH. Idiopathic calcinosis of the scrotum. Histopathologic observations of fifty-one nodules. *J Am Acad Dermatol* 1988; **19**: 1095–101.
14 Ito A, Sakamoto F, Ito M. Dystrophic scrotal calcinosis originating from benign eccrine epithelial cysts. *Br J Dermatol* 2001; **144**: 146–50.
15 McKee PH, Liomba NG, Hutt MSR. Tumoral calcinosis. A pathological study of 56 cases. *Br J Dermatol* 1982; **107**: 669–74.
16 Whiting DA, Simson IW, Kallmeyer JC, Dannheimer IP. Unusual cutaneous lesions in tumoral calcinosis. *Arch Dermatol* 1970; **102**: 465–73.
17 Raimer SS, Archer ME, Jorizzo JL. Metastatic calcinosis cutis. *Cutis* 1983; **32**: 463–5.
18 Kolton B, Pedersen J. Calcinosis cutis and renal failure. *Arch Dermatol* 1974; **110**: 256–7.
19 Goldminz D, Greenberg RD. Multiple miliary osteoma cutis. *J Am Acad Dermatol* 1991; **24**: 878–81.
20 Lim MO, Mukherjee AB, Hansen JW. Dysplastic cutaneous osteomatosis: a unique case of true osteoma. *Arch Dermatol* 1981; **117**: 797–801.
21 Maclean GD, Main RA, Andersen TE *et al.* Connective tissue ossification presenting in the skin. *Arch Dermatol* 1966; **94**: 168–74.
22 Moritz DL, Elewski B. Pigmented postacne osteoma cutis in a patient treated with minocycline: report and review of the literature. *J Am Acad Dermatol* 1991; **24**: 851–3.

Iron metabolism [1]

The total iron content of an adult man is 4–5 g, 60–70% of which is blood haemoglobin iron. Small amounts of ferritin iron are present in erythrocytes, plasma and leukocytes [1]. Iron is stored in the liver, spleen and bone marrow as ferritin and haemosiderin. It is released readily from these sites according to the body's needs. Serum ferritin levels vary with the iron status of the individual and with certain diseases. The body has a limited ability to excrete iron, and homeostasis is therefore regulated mainly by adjusting iron absorption. Iron compounds need to be reduced to the ferrous form (Fe^2) to be absorbed. Ascorbic acid, which can reduce and chelate iron, enhances iron absorption.

The mechanism of iron absorption is not completely understood. Recent evidence points to an iron-transport system involving the binding of iron to the plasma membrane of mucosal cells and the interaction of transferrin in plasma with these sites.

Total iron in faeces varies between 6 and 16 mg/day depending on the amount ingested. Most of it is unabsorbed food iron.

Iron deficiency

Iron deficiency is a major risk factor for disability and disease worldwide, affecting about two billion people. Targeted iron supplementation, fortification of foods and selective plant breeding are means to improve iron nutritional status in the developing world [2].

General symptoms include fatigue, palpitations on exertion, sore tongue with atrophic filiform papillae, angular cheilitis (perlèche), dysphagia and koilonychia (Chapter 65). Generalized itch may occur [3], and hair loss with or without morphological changes of the hair shaft may be seen [4,5]. In infants and children, anorexia, retarded growth and decreased resistance to infections are the outstanding features. The recommended daily allowance is 10 mg in infants, 10–15 mg in children, 18 mg in young males and females, and 10 mg in both sexes above 20 years of age [6]. Pregnant women should receive supplemental iron, as the increased need for iron can barely be met by ordinary diets [7].

The diagnosis of iron deficiency is based on low serum iron levels, clinical symptoms and improvement following iron therapy. Serum ferritin is significantly correlated to bone marrow haemosiderin iron and provides a convenient method for assessing iron stores in normal subjects [8].

Iron intoxication

Daily ingestion of 50–75 mg iron is reported as safe [1,2], and even higher intakes in some individuals turn out to be harmless. Chronic iron intoxication has been reported among Bantus consuming beer that is brewed in iron utensils. The iron is in a soluble form and may supply a substantial net supply of iron. Iron-contaminated cereals do not induce siderosis because iron is present in a less available form.

Haemochromatosis (MIM +253200 and others) [1,9]

Haemochromatosis is a syndrome characterized by the triad of hyperpigmentation, diabetes mellitus and cirrhosis of the liver, associated with increased iron deposition in the internal organs. Hypogonadism is frequently present. The female/male ratio is 1:10. Onset of symptoms is gradual, usually between 40 and 60 years.

Aetiology. Haemochromatosis can be found in the following conditions: idiopathic or primary haemochromatosis; chronic iron intoxication (e.g. Bantu haemochromatosis); chronic liver disease and iron overload (alcoholic haemochromatosis); hepatic haemosiderosis in anaemic patients with an ineffective erythropoiesis; and congenital transferrin deficiency. The cause of primary haemochromatosis is basically unknown, but a defective control of iron absorption is involved. The abnormality is inherited as an autosomal recessive trait (see Chapter 62). Erythrocyte ferritin is increased 60-fold in idiopathic haemochromatosis, which allows a distinction between this disorder and alcoholic liver disease with iron overload [10]. In alcoholic haemochromatosis, alcohol consumption, particularly red wine and iron-containing beverages, play an aetiological role. Whether the acquired form is seen in patients heterozygous for the trait is not known.

Histopathology. Liver biopsy in primary haemochromatosis shows marked iron deposits in the parenchymal cells and to a lesser degree in the Kupffer cells. The hyperpigmentation of the skin is due to increased epidermal melanin and upper dermal melanophages, but iron deposits can be identified in the deeper dermis.

Clinical features. The skin shows a distinctive grey-brown pigmentation, especially on the face, flexural creases and exposed parts. This may precede other signs by many years but can appear late in the course. Sometimes, the buccal mucosa is involved as in Addison's disease but adrenal insufficiency is not present. The various skin changes were studied in 100 patients [11]. There was almost 100% frequency of hyperpigmentation, 75% had hair loss (including axillary and pubic hair), about 50% had koilonychia and 45% had ichthyosis-like, atrophic dry skin. Less frequent signs included palmar erythema, striate onychia, leukonychia and spider angiomas (findings that may be seen in cirrhosis of any cause). Hepatomegaly, diabetes, testicular atrophy, heart disease and weight loss are additional findings. Arthropathy, present in 25–50% of the patients, resembles rheumatoid arthritis, but serology is negative.

Diagnosis. The diagnosis should be suspected in a patient with diabetes mellitus, liver cirrhosis and hyperpigmentation. Liver biopsy is usually diagnostic.

Routine laboratory tests may reveal evidence of chronic hepatic disease or of diabetes mellitus. Total serum iron is increased to the range 180–300 mg/100 mL [1], serum transferrin saturation is above 80%, and the transferrin level and the total iron binding capacity (TIBC) may be reduced [9,11]. Serum and erythrocyte ferritin is high, reflecting the increased iron stores [10]. HLA-typing has revealed an increased frequency of HLA-A3 and -B14 [12] but has largely been superseded by genotyping for the commoner haemochromatosis genes (Chapter 62).

Treatment. A liver concentration above 100 µmol/g iron weight is an indication for therapy [1,7]. Organ damage may be reversed by reducing the excessive iron stores by repeated venesection for 1–2 years. Serum iron and serum transferrin and transferrin saturation remain unchanged until excess iron has been removed. Serum or erythrocyte ferritin should be monitored as a guide to the efficacy of treatment. Family members should have their serum iron estimated and, if found to have iron overload, should be treated with prophylactic venesection.

References

1 Underwood EJ. *Trace Elements in Human and Animal Nutrition.* New York: Academic Press 1977: 13–55.

2 Zimmermann M, Hurrell R. Nutritional iron deficiency. *Lancet* 2007; **370**: 511–20.

3 Adams SJ. Iron deficiency and other haematological causes of generalized pruritus. In: Bernhard JD, ed. *Itch: Mechanisms and Management of Pruritus.* New York: McGraw-Hill, 1994: 243–50.

4 Blankship ML. Dysplastic hairs in iron deficiency anaemia. *Cutis* 1971; **7**: 467.

5 Hard S. Non-anaemic iron deficiency as an aetiological factor in diffuse loss of hair of the scalp in women. *Acta Derm Venereol Suppl (Stockh)* 1963; **43**: 652–9.

6 Food and Nutrition Board. *Recommended Dietary Allowances.* Washington, DC: National Academy of Sciences, 1974.

7 Finch CA, Monsen ER. Iron nutrition and the fortification of food with iron. *JAMA* 1972; **219**: 1462–5.

8 Millman N, Pedersen NS, Visfeldt J. Serum ferritin in healthy Danes: relation to marrow haemosiderin iron stores. *Dan Med Bull* 1983; **30**: 115–20.

9 Anhalt GJ, Dubin HV. Hemochromatosis and cirrhosis. In: Callen JP, ed. *Cutaneous Aspects of Internal Disease.* London: Year Book, 1981: 525–30.

10 Weyden MB, Vander BM, Fong H *et al.* Erythrocyte ferritin content in idiopathic haemochromatosis and alcoholic liver disease with iron overload. *BMJ* 1983; **286**: 752–4.

11 Chevrant-Breton J, Simon M, Bourel M *et al.* Cutaneous manifestations of idiopathic hemochromatosis: study of 100 cases. *Arch Dermatol* 1977; **113**: 161–5.

12 Shewan WG, Mouat SA, Allan TM. HLA antigens in haemochromatosis (Letter). *BMJ* 1976; **i**: 280–2.

Sulphur metabolism [1]

Sulphur is a vital element for the normal function of the human body. It is an essential component of the amino acids methionine and cysteine and of chondroitin sulphate, which are involved in keratinization and formation of dermal collagen, respectively. Dietary thionine and cysteine are the main precursors for the synthesis of sulphur-containing components in the body. In homocystinuria there is a metabolic block in the pathway; clinical features include tissue-paper scars on the hands and sparse, fair hair due to impaired keratin formation. When the supply of sulphur-containing amino acids is inadequate, less sulphur is available to maintain nail and hair growth, but the keratin produced seems to be normal [2]. The liver plays a central role in degradation of sulphur-containing amino acids. In chronic liver disease, low urinary levels of inorganic sulphate are present [1].

In exfoliative psoriasis with increased epidermopoiesis, relative sulphur depletion is found and the urinary excretion of inorganic sulphate is decreased. Hair loss in chronic exfoliative dermatoses may be related to diversion of sulphur-containing amino acids to synthesis of skin protein instead of hair keratin formation [2]. Mucopolysaccharide synthesis in the dermis is influenced by certain hormonal factors. Thyrotrophin (thyroid-stimulating hormone, TSH) has a stimulant action on connective tissue and the pituitary somatrophic hormone (growth hormone, GH) stimulates chondroitin sulphate formation.

Trichothiodystrophy

Trichothiodystrophy is a sulphur-deficient brittle hair syndrome associated with ectodermal dysplasias [3,4]. The hair is short and brittle with a characteristic microscopy in polarized light showing alternating light and dark bands (Chapter 66). There is a 50% decrease or more in the cysteine and sulphur content of the hair. The disease is inherited as an autosomal recessive trait; there are photosensitive (MIM #601675) and non-photosensitive (MIM #234050) variants. Collodion baby syndrome may herald trichothiodystrophy [5].

References

1 Mårtensson J. *Studies on Human Sulphur Metabolism*. Linköping: Linköping University Medical Dissertations, 1981: no. 119.
2 Roe DA. Sulphur metabolism in relation to cutaneous disease. *Br J Dermatol* 1969; **81** (Suppl. 2): 49–69.
3 Itin PH, Sarasin A, Pittelkow MR. Trichothiodystrophy: update on the sulfur-deficient brittle hair syndromes. *J Am Acad Dermatol* 2001; **44**: 891–920.
4 Richetta Giustini S, Rossi A, Calvieri S. What's new in trichothiodystrophy. *J Eur Acad Dermatol Venereol* 2001; **15**: 1–4.
5 Larrégue M, Guillet G. Collodion baby syndrome with neonatal signs of trichothiodystrophy misdiagnosed as Netherton syndrome: reassessment of a previous diagnostic error. *Ann Dermatol Venereol* 2007; **134**: 245–8.

Zinc metabolism [1–3]

Zinc belongs to the group of essential trace elements that comprises zinc, iron, copper, manganese, nickel, cobalt, molybdenum, selenium, chromium, iodine, fluorine, tin, silicon, vanadium and arsenic. High concentrations of zinc are present in shellfish, legumes, nuts, whole grain and green leafy vegetables, whereas fruits usually contain insignificant levels. Wine, beer and spirits contain very low concentrations of zinc. The zinc supply depends largely on the protein content of the food, and protein undernourishment will lead to an insufficient zinc supply.

Recommended dietary allowance of zinc [4]. The daily oral intake of zinc should average 3 mg in infants less than 6 months, 5 mg in infants 0.5–1.0 years old, 10 mg in children 1–7 years old and 16 mg from 11 years old onwards. Pregnant and lactating women should receive 20–25 mg zinc daily.

Biological functions. More than 300 catalytically active zinc metalloproteins and more than 2000 zinc-dependent transcription factors involved in gene expression of various proteins have been recognized [5]. Zinc is indispensable to the normal function of all cells, cellular systems, tissues and organs in the human body. The essentiality is related mainly to its function as the metal moiety of important enzymes, such as alkaline phosphatase, alcohol dehydrogenase and several different dehydrogenases, and digestive enzymes. Zinc regulates DNA and RNA polymerases, thymidine kinase and ribonuclease, and plays an important role in immunological functions.

Zinc deficiency

Dietary zinc deficiency, like iron deficiency, is a worldwide risk factor, most prevalent in the developing world. It is involved in severe deficiency syndromes such as kwashiorkor, marasmus and growth retardation. It affects about 2 billion people mainly living on phytate- and fibre- rich cereals, and soy products [6].

Zinc deficiency may be caused by a specific absorptive defect, acrodermatitis enteropathica, or may be due to diseases of the gastrointestinal tract causing diarrhoea and malabsorption (conditioned, or acquired, zinc deficiency).

Acrodermatitis enteropathica (MIM #201100 and others)

Acrodermatitis enteropathica was first recognized in 1936 by the Swedish dermatologist Thore Brandt [7] and further described by Danbolt and Closs [8] (Fig. 59.49). It is a rare disease believed to be transmitted as an autosomal recessive trait. In Denmark, the prevalence is about 1/500 000 inhabitants. Adema disease in black-pied cattle of Dutch descent, an autosomal recessive disease due to reduced zinc absorption, represents an animal parallel to acrodermatitis enteropathica in man [9] (Fig. 59.50).

Aetiology. Zinc absorption in acrodermatitis enteropathica is abnormally low, in young patients about 2–3% compared to 27–65% in normal adults [10]. The cause of the specific zinc malabsorption is not known. It can be overcome by an oral zinc load. Without zinc therapy, serum zinc levels are consistently low.

Clinical features. The disease typically starts after weaning or earlier if the infant is not given breast milk. The child turns peevish, withdrawn and photophobic, and develops a vesicobullous dermatitis on hands, feet and periorificial areas. The scalp hair is lost. Diarrhoea is often present. Growth is retarded and there is a decreased resistance to infections. Wound healing is poor and skin lesions tend not to heal [3,11].

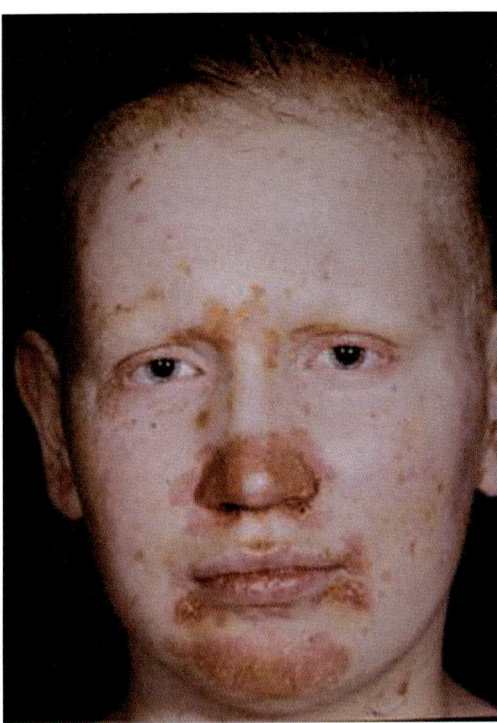

Fig. 59.49 Acrodermatitis enteropathica with typical eczematous skin lesions. The vermilion area is free, the hair growth poor and sparse.

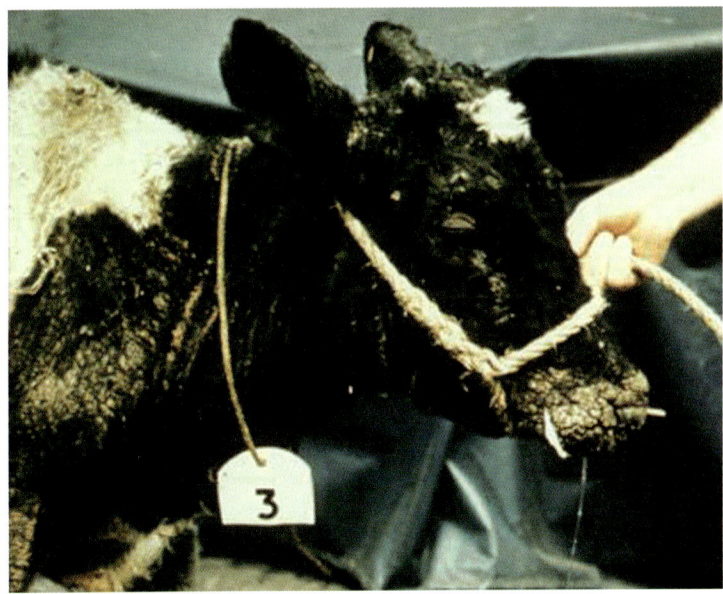

Fig. 59.50 Adema disease. The black-pied calf shows stunted growth, a poor scaly fur and characteristic keratotic muzzle eczema.

Prognosis. Without proper management, the prognosis is poor and in the past a lethal outcome within 4–5 years was the rule.

Treatment. Halogenated 8-hydroxyquinolines (e.g. diodoquin) were formerly used successfully for therapy on an empirical basis. Experimental animal studies using rats have shown that 8-hydroxyquinolines, which were used as antibacterial agents, increase ^{65}Zn absorption significantly [3]. Zinc sulphate for acrodermatitis enteropathica was introduced in the 1970s [3,11]. An oral zinc dose of 2–3 mg/kg/day cures all clinical manifestations, apart from hair and nail growth, within a few days. Prolonged high-dose therapy up to adult age is necessary, then a continuous zinc supplementation is indicated, often with oral doses of 1–2 mg zinc/kg/day.

Endemic nutritional zinc deficiency [6]
Endemic zinc deficiency presenting with dwarfism and hypogonadism as the main symptoms has been reported from rural districts in Iran, Egypt and Turkey. The chronic zinc deficiency is attributed to the diet, which consists mainly of unleavened whole grain bread with a high fibre and phytate content. Zinc deficiency has been described in severely malnourished children in Jamaica, Egypt and various parts of Africa [12]. In the Western world anorexia nervosa has been reported with symptoms of acquired zinc deficiency, often described as 'acrodermatitis enteropathica' [13] although it is acquired deficiency.

Acquired zinc deficiency
Zinc depletion syndrome. Where there is disturbed bowel function, zinc loss is increased; if combined with decreased absorption and low dietary zinc intake, severe zinc depletion will develop within 1–3 months. Zinc depletion syndrome was originally identified in patients who received prolonged total parenteral nutrition without zinc [14,15]. Most patients had undergone extensive intestinal resections. The serum zinc level was decreased, often below 20 µg/100 mL (3 µmol/L) (normal range 70–125 µg/100 ml or 10–19 µmol/L).

Zinc deficiency in breastfed infants. Premature infants receiving mother's milk are at risk of developing zinc deficiency due to rapid growth and insufficient zinc supply via the breast milk. Premature infants have an extra need for zinc, and zinc absorption is lower than in mature infants (Fig. 59.51a). Zinc deficiency may also be seen in normal infants due to low zinc levels in their mother's milk (Fig. 59.51b) [16].

Diseases of liver and pancreas. Chronic zinc deficiency has been reported in patients suffering from malabsorption–malnutrition associated with alcoholic liver cirrhosis and alcoholic pancreatitis [17]. A defective exocrine pancreatic function causing malabsorption and increased urinary zinc excretion in liver cirrhosis add to a negative zinc balance.

Cancer chemotherapy. Cancer chemotherapy for leukaemia in children may provoke zinc deficiency [18].

Zinc deficiency and the skin [19]
Acute zinc deficiency. General symptoms include septicaemia, photophobia and mental depression. Skin changes consist of eczematous eruptions on face, hands, feet, in the anogenital regions and around the body orifices. Finger and palm skin creases show characteristic flat bullous lesions surrounded by brownish erythema (Fig. 59.52). Oozing lesions may be seen on the sacral area and heels in bedridden patients. Some lesions are necrotic and burn-like. There is angular stomatitis with perioral lesions sparing the vermilion border.

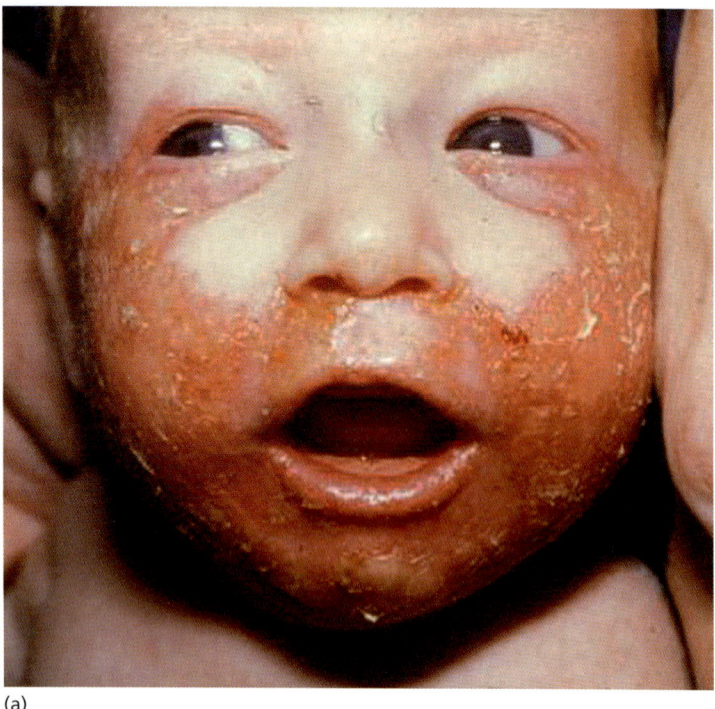

(a)

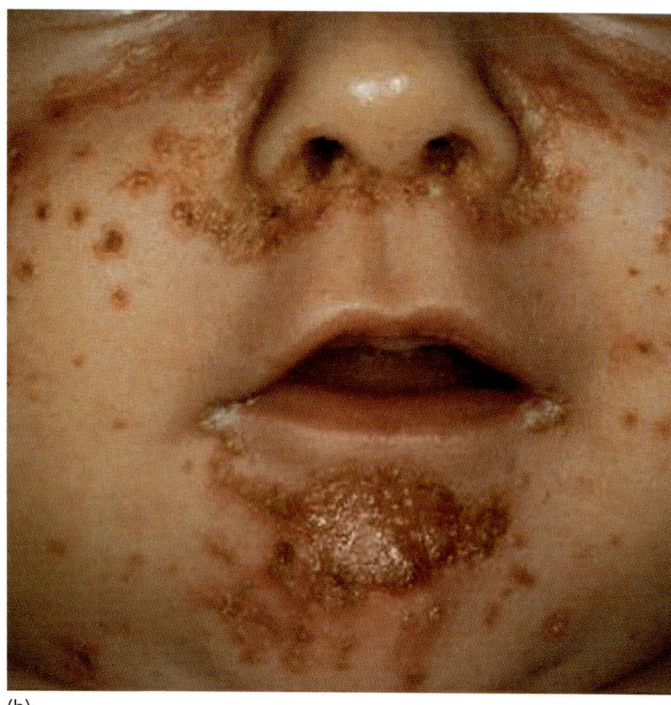

(b)

Fig. 59.51 (a) Zinc deficiency in a premature breastfed infant and (b) in a normal breastfed infant.

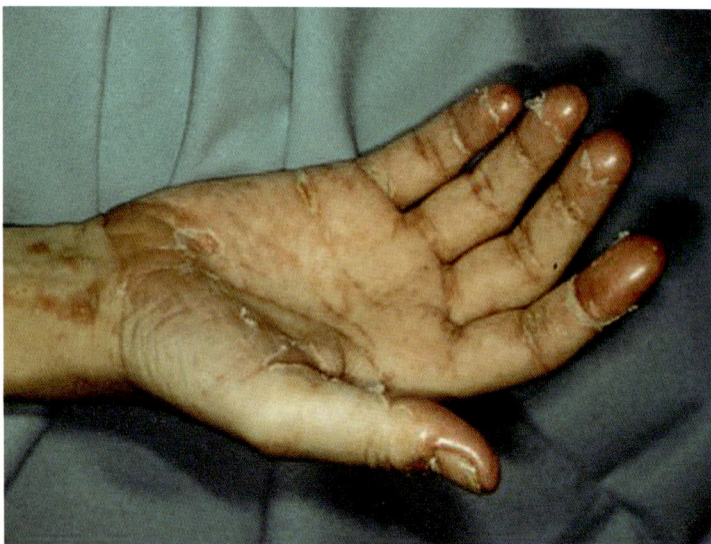

Fig. 59.52 Acute zinc depletion syndrome with denuded finger tips and bullae on finger flexural creases.

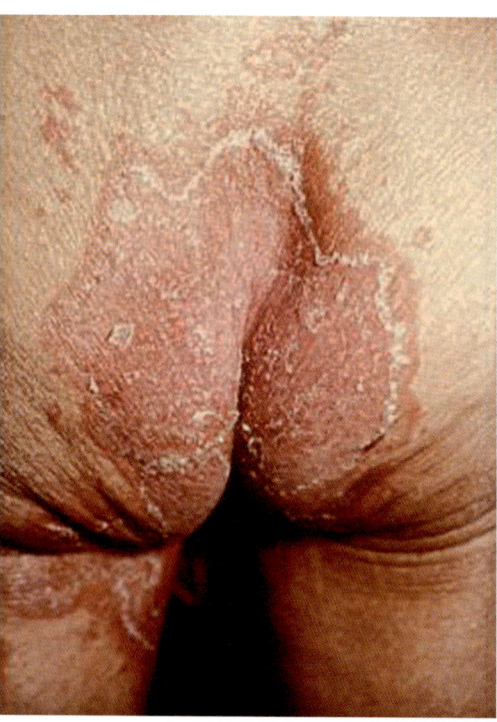

Fig. 59.53 Chronic zinc deficiency with scaly eczema on the perianal area. Note peripheral collarette scaling.

Chronic zinc deficiency. The patient is listless and mentally depressed. Skin lesions are typically seen on areas subject to repeated pressure and trauma, such as elbows, knees, knuckles, malleolar regions of the ankles and the sacral area. The lesions are brownish and scaly, sometimes psoriasis-like (Fig. 59.53). Seborrhoeic dermatitis-like changes may be seen on the face, and acne may flare.

A non-itchy, scaly dermatitis on the trunk has been described in zinc-deficient alcoholics.

Hair and nail changes. In zinc deficiency, hair and nail growth ceases or stops. Diffuse thinning of the scalp hair progresses, eventually leading to total alopecia. Structural changes of the hair may be observed, such as broken spearhead-like endings, transverse striation of the shaft, pseudomonilethrix, longitudinal splits and

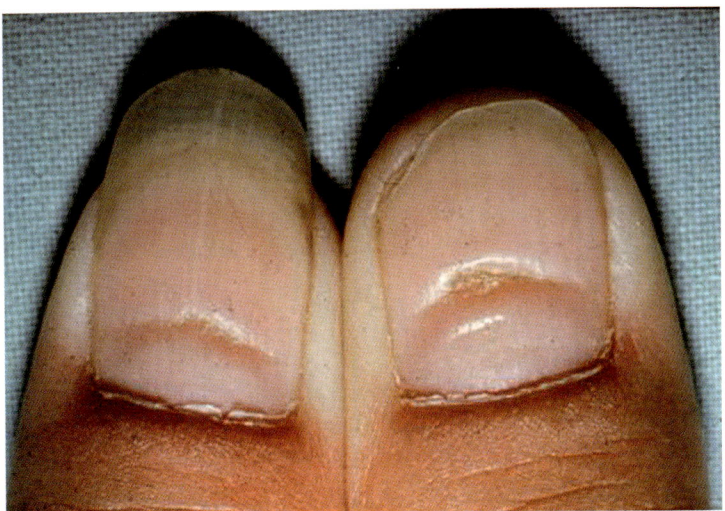

Fig. 59.54 Beau's line on thumbnail in a case of zinc depletion syndrome, appearing one month after start of zinc therapy. Note faster growth of left thumb nail, typically seen in right-handed patients.

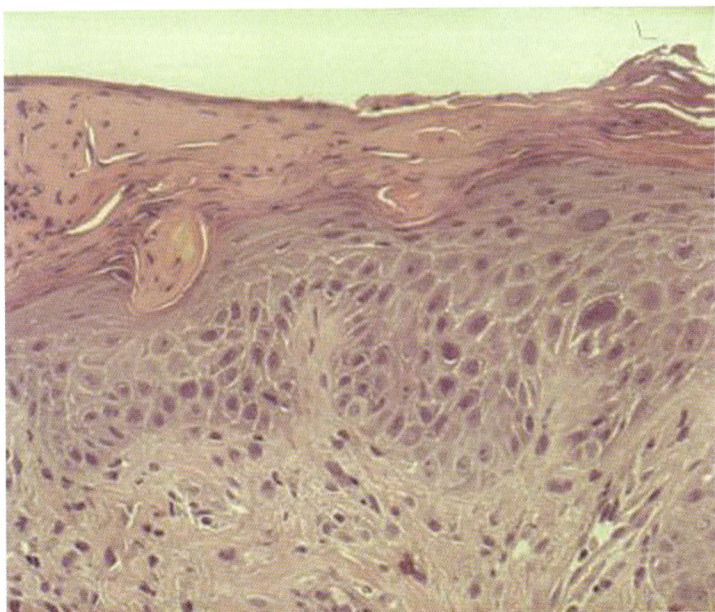

Fig. 59.56 Chronic zinc deficiency with parakeratosis, acanthosis and slight spongiosis.

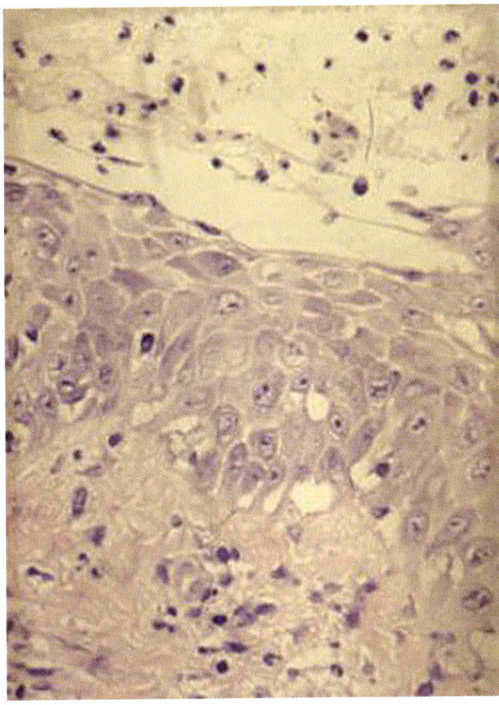

Fig. 59.55 Acute zinc deficiency with spongiotic dermatitis and degenerate basal cells.

bayonet hairs. Severe zinc deficiency causes total arrest of nail growth. Transverse depressions (Beau's lines) on the fingernails become visible about 4 weeks after zinc therapy is started and normal nail growth is re-established (Fig. 59.54) [20].

Pathology. In the acute stage, light microscopy reveals spongiosis, sometimes with suprabasal cysts and clefts (Fig. 59.55). The horny layer is often separated or lost, and necrosis of the epidermal cells may be seen. In chronic zinc deficiency, there are chronic eczema or psoriasis-like changes of the epidermis (Fig. 59.56). Electron microscopy of acute lesions shows degenerate basal cells

with slender cytoplasmic protrusions and an intact basal lamina with multiple invaginations.

Diagnosis. Severe zinc deficiency is usually suspected from the clinical findings. The serum zinc and alkaline phosphatase levels are low and will rise during zinc therapy [19]. It is important to consider the level of plasma albumin as albumin binds 60–70% of circulating zinc. As a result, hypoalbuminaemia is associated with lowered serum zinc values, which may not necessarily reflect a state of zinc deficiency.

In suspect cases, a therapeutic trial with oral or parenteral zinc should be undertaken. If no clinical improvement occurs within a few days and the serum alkaline phosphatase remains stable as the serum zinc level goes up, the patient is not deficient in zinc.

Treatment with zinc. In adult patients, oral zinc sulphate ($Zn_2SO_4 \cdot 7H_2O$) tablets of 0.2 g (45 mg elemental zinc) are given two to three times a day (about 2 mg zinc/kg/day). Similar doses on a body weight basis are given to children. Parenterally, 0.2–0.3 mg zinc/kg/day (about 10–20 mg/day in adult patients) is sufficient and safe. For prophylactic purposes, total parenteral nutrition should supply no less than 70–80 µg zinc/kg/day. Infants and premature babies on parenteral nutrition should receive a prophylactic dose of 0.1–0.3 mg/kg/day [21].

There is no evidence of benefit from the use of zinc sulphate for patients with chronic leg ulcers [22], common cold [23] or acne vulgaris [24].

A variety of cutaneous disorders not related to zinc deficiency have been reported to respond to zinc supplementation. Zinc has no known pharmacological effect, so the significance of such observations seems dubious.

References

1 Kirchgessner M, Roth HP, Weigand E. Biochemical changes in zinc deficiency. In: Prasad AS, Oberleas D, eds. *Trace Elements in Human Health and Disease.* London: Academic Press, 1976: 189–225.

2 Underwood EJ. *Trace Elements in Human and Animal Nutrition*, 4th edn. New York: Academic Press, 1977.

3 Weismann K. *Zinc Deficiency and Effects of Systemic Zinc Therapy*. Copenhagen: FADL's Forlag, 1980: 26–8.

4 Food and Nutrition Board. *Recommended Dietary Allowances*, 8th edn. Washington, DC: National Academy of Sciences, 1980.

5 Prasad AS. Zinc and enzymes. In: Prasad AS. *Biochemistry of Zinc*. New York: Plenum Press 1993: 17–33.

6 Prasad AS. Zinc deficiency. *Br J Dermatol* 2003; **326**: 409–10.

7 Brandt T. Dermatitis in children with disturbances of general condition and absorption of food. *Acta Derm Venereol Suppl (Stockh)* 1936; **17**: 513–46.

8 Danbolt N, Closs K. Acrodermatitis enteropathica. *Acta Derm Venereol Suppl (Stockh)* 1942; **23**: 127.

9 Weismann K, Flagstad T. Hereditary zinc deficiency (Adema disease) in black-pied cattle, an animal parallel to acrodermatitis enteropathica. *Acta Derm Venereol* 1976; **56**: 151–4.

10 Weismann K, Hoe S, Knuden L *et al.* [65]Zinc absorption in patients suffering from acrodermatitis enteropathica and in normal adults assessed by whole-body counting techniques. *Br J Dermatol* 1979; **101**: 573–9.

11 Michaelsson G. Zinc therapy in acrodermatitis enteropathica. *Acta Derm Venereol Suppl (Stockh)* 1974; **54**: 377–81.

12 Golden PE, Golden MHN. Plasma zinc, rate of weight gain, and the energy cost of tissue deposition in children recovering from severe malnutrition on a cow's milk or soya-protein based diet. *Am J Clin Nutr* 1981; **34**: 892–9.

13 Quirk CM, Seykora J, Wingate BJ *et al.* Acrodermatitis enteropathica associated with anorexia nervosa. *JAMA* 2002; **288**: 2655–6.

14 Weismann K, Hjorth N, Fischer A. Zinc depletion syndrome during long term intravenous feeding. *Clin Exp Dermatol* 1976; **1**: 237–42.

15 Kay RG, Tasman-Jones C, Whiting R *et al.* A syndrome of acute zinc deficiency during total parenteral alimentation in man. *Ann Surg* 1976; **183**: 331–40.

16 Ottevanger V, Hansen ER, Petersen CS, Weismann K. Severe conditioned zinc deficiency in breastfed premature infants. *Eur J Pediatr Dermatol* 1994; **4**: 13–6.

17 Vallee BL, Wacker EWC, Bartholomay F *et al.* Zinc metabolism in hepatic dysfunction. I. Serum zinc concentrations in Laënnec's cirrhosis and their validation by sequential analysis. *N Engl J Med* 1986; **255**: 403–8.

18 Cutler EA, Palmer J, Kontras SB. Chemotherapy and possible zinc deficiency. *N Engl J Med* 1977; **297**: 168–72.

19 Weismann K. Zinc metabolism and the skin. In: Rook A, Savin J, eds. *Recent Advances in Dermatology*, Vol. 5. London: Churchill Livingstone, 1980: 109–29.

20 Weismann K. Lines of Beau: possible markers of zinc deficiency. *Acta Derm Venereol Suppl (Stockh)* 1971; **57**: 88–90.

21 Shils ME, Burke AW, Greene HI *et al.* Guidelines for essential trace element preparations for parenteral use. A statement by an expert panel. *J Am Acad Dermatol* 1979; **241**: 2051–4.

22 Wilkinson EAJ, Hawke CI. Does oral zinc aid the healing of chronic leg ulcers? *Arch Dermatol* 1998; **134**: 1556–60.

23 Weismann K, Jakobsen JP, Weismann JE *et al.* Zinc gluconate for common cold. *Dan Med Bull* 1990; **37**: 279–81.

24 Weismann K, Wadskov S, Søndergaard J. Oral zinc sulphate therapy for acne vulgaris. *Acta Derm Venereol* 1977; **57**: 357–60.

Copper metabolism

The normal adult body contains about 80 mg of elemental copper. Copper in plasma occurs in two forms: about 90% is firmly bound as the blue copper protein coeruloplasmin, the remainder is loosely bound to plasma proteins, primarily albumin. Copper competes with the albumin-binding sites for zinc, so fluctuations in concentration of one of these metals are reflected by a change in concentration of the other. Coeruloplasmin is an oxidase involved in iron utilization. It does not play a role in copper transport to the tissue; this is done by albumin, which is the true transport protein. Copper is part of superoxide dismutase, catalysing superoxide anion radicals into hydrogen peroxide and oxygen.

Copper-induced green hair

Green hair is usually caused by deposition of copper from exogenous sources. Usually, the patient has blond or reddish hair that has been exposed to physical or chemical damage (sun damage or bleaching) whereby high-sulphur matrix proteins (mainly cysteine) are exposed, and are therefore available to bind copper ions. A high copper concentration may occur in swimming-pool water due to copper-containing algicides, and in household tapwater due to copper piping [1,2]. Hair shampoo with an added copper-chelating agent such as dimethylcystein (penicillamine) can remove the green discoloration.

Copper deficiency

Copper deficiency has been reported to occur in infants receiving milk low in copper, and in malnourished children given high-calorie nutrition with an insufficient copper supply. The symptoms include anaemia, neutropenia and failure to thrive.

Menkes' kinky hair syndrome (MIM #309400). This is an X-linked defect in copper absorption, resulting in low copper levels in blood, liver and hair. There is progressive mental deterioration, metaphyseal lesions, degenerative aortic elastin and defective keratinization of hair (Chapter 66). There is no effective treatment [3].

Wilson's disease (hepatolenticular degeneration syndrome) (MIM #277900). This is a rare, inborn error of copper metabolism, inherited as an autosomal recessive trait [4]. It is characterized by cirrhosis of the liver and degenerative changes in the brain, particularly the basal ganglia. Deposition of copper takes place primarily in the liver, brain, kidneys and cornea (Kayser–Fleischer ring). The patients have low coeruloplasmin and plasma copper levels.

Treatment consists of cupriuretic chelating agents such as penicillamine or by competing intestinal copper absorption with oral zinc [4].

References

1 Mascaró JM, Ferrando J, Fontarneau R *et al.* Green hair. *Cutis* 1995; **56**: 37–40.

2 Munkvad S, Weismann K. Copper-induced green hair. *Ugeskr Læger* 1996; **158**: 3791–2.

3 Danks DM. Steely hair, mottled mice and copper metabolism. *N Engl J Med* 1975; **293**: 1147–8.

4 Hoogenraad TU, van der Hamer CJA, Hattum JV. Effective treatment of Wilson's disease with oral zinc sulphate: two case reports. *BMJ* 1984; **289**: 273–6.

Selenium metabolism [1]

Selenium is an essential element of the enzyme glutathione peroxidase. It plays a role against oxidative damage by endogenous peroxides. Selenium deficiency has long been known in several animal species. Selenium-deficient rats grow slowly, develop cataracts, lose their hair and show aspermogenesis. In humans, selenium deficiency has been reported in children, causing hypopigmented skin lesions and various other symptoms. Treatment consists of supplementation of selenium in low doses of

2 mg/kg/day [2]. Patients with psoriasis, atopic dermatitis, dermatitis herpetiformis and acne vulgaris have a lower glutathione peroxidase activity than normal controls [3], although the significance of this is unclear. In a study on malignant melanoma, significantly lower serum selenium levels were demonstrated as compared with controls [4]. Serum selenium levels have been shown to be of a prognostic value in the follow-up of malignant melanoma and cutaneous T-cell lymphoma [5]. There is no apparent protective effect of selenium supplementation against the development of non-melanoma skin cancer [6–8].

Selenium is incorporated as the sulphide into shampoos for the treatment of seborrhoeic dermatitis. Selenium sulphide is water-insoluble and possesses a very low toxicity. A possible protective role of selenium on cancer, cardiovascular diseases and rheumatic diseases has attracted much attention but there is no proven reason to recommend selenium supplementation.

References

1 Underwood EJ. *Trace Elements in Human and Animal Nutrition.* New York: Academic Press, 1977: 302–46.
2 Vinton NE, Dahlstrom KA, Strobel CT *et al.* Macrocytosis and pseudoalbinism: manifestations of selenium deficiency. *J Pediatr* 1987; **111**: 711–7.
3 Juhlin L, Edqvist L-E, Ekman LG *et al.* Blood glutathione–peroxidase levels in skin disease: effect of selenium and vitamin E treatment. *Acta Derm Venereol Suppl (Stockh)* 1982; **62**: 211–4.
4 Reinhold U, Biltz H, Bayer W *et al.* Serum selenium levels in patients with malignant melanoma. *Acta Derm Venereol Suppl (Stockh)* 1989; **69**: 132–6.
5 Deffuant C, Celerier P, Boiteau HL *et al.* Serum selenium in melanoma and epidermotropic cutaneous T-cell lymphoma. *Acta Derm Venereol Suppl (Stockh)* 1994; **74**: 90–2.
6 Clark LC, Combs JF Jr, Turnbull BW *et al.* Effects of selenium supplementation for cancer prevention in patients with carcinoma of the skin. A randomized controlled trial. Nutritional Prevention of Cancer Study Group. *JAMA* 1996; **276**: 1957–63.
7 Bialy TL, Rothe MJ, Grant-Kels JM. Dietary factors in the prevention and treatment of nonmelanoma skin cancer and melanoma. *Dermatol Surg* 2002; **28**: 1143–52.
8 Fleshner N, Zlotta AR. Prostate cancer prevention: past, present and future. *Cancer* 2007; **110**: 1889–99.

Skin disorders in diabetes mellitus

Diabetes mellitus [1,2]. Diabetes mellitus is a metabolic disorder characterized by elevated fasting and postprandial blood glucose levels and a variety of multisystem complications, mainly in the blood vessels, eye, kidney, nervous system and integument. Three main types can be distinguished. Type 1, also known as insulin-dependent diabetes mellitus or juvenile-onset diabetes, is characterized by abrupt onset of symptoms, insulinopenia, dependence on insulin injections, proneness to ketoacidosis and lack of ability to produce C peptide. Type 2, non-insulin-dependent diabetes mellitus or adult-onset diabetes, is characterized by lack of keto-acidosis except under stressful circumstances, ability to produce C peptide, a tendency to obesity and improvement following loss of weight. Type 3, secondary diabetes, is an additional type of diabetes, which occurs as a complication of pancreatic, hormonal or genetic disease or following ingestion of certain drugs or chemical compounds.

There are several reviews of skin disorders associated with diabetes mellitus [2–8].

Skin symptoms due to diabetic vascular abnormalities [3–5]

Diabetic microangiopathy. Both small and large blood vessels are affected in diabetes mellitus. In diabetic microangiopathy, there is proliferation of endothelial cells and deposits of PAS-positive material in the basement membrane of arterioles, capillaries and venules with resulting decreased luminal area [9]. Basement-membrane thickening is a characteristic finding in diabetic and prediabetic patients, but it is neither absolute nor pathognomonic for the disease [10]. The diabetic microangiopathy precedes manifest abnormalities of the disease, and it is possible that vascular changes are the primary expression of the disease. Microangiopathy is responsible for the retinopathy, nephropathy and possibly also neuropathy and dermopathy associated with diabetes.

Erysipelas-like erythema [10]. This condition is seen mostly in elderly diabetic patients with an average duration of diabetes mellitus of 5 years. Well-demarcated, red areas occur on the legs or feet, and there may be underlying destructive bone disease caused by a small vessel insufficiency. Cardiac decompensation may be involved.

Wet gangrene of the foot. This is a late manifestation of diabetic microangiopathy. Non-diabetic atherosclerotic subjects tend to develop a dry form as a result of large vessel insufficiency.

Diabetic rubeosis [11]. A peculiar rosy reddening of the face, and sometimes of the hands and feet, may be seen in long-standing diabetes. The changes have been attributed to decreased vascular tone or diabetic microangiopathy. Rubeosis may have some practical diagnostic significance, especially in fair-skinned patients.

Diabetic dermopathy (diabetic shin spots). This is the most common dermatosis associated with diabetes mellitus. Microangiopathy and neuropathy are involved [12]. Lesions are predominantly situated on the shins, forearms, thighs and over bony prominences. About half of patients show such lesions, more frequently men than women. The initial lesion is an oval, dull-red papule 0.5–1 cm in diameter. It evolves slowly, producing a superficial scale, leaving an atrophic brownish scar. The colour is due to haemosiderin in histiocytes near the vessels [13] (Fig. 59.57). Microscopically, a combination of vascular disease with PAS-positive thickening of the vessel wall and minor collagen changes is found. Although not confirmed in all studies, recent research suggests that there is a significant correlation between the presence of these lesions and other complications of diabetes, such as retinopathy, nephropathy and neuropathy [14].

Large vessel disease [4]. Atherosclerosis is the second form of vascular disease frequently associated with diabetes mellitus. The patient shows intermittent claudication with pallid and cool skin distally on the extremities. The postural test discloses delayed filling of the veins. Common clinical sequelae are myocardial infarction, cerebral thrombosis, nephrosclerosis and ischaemic gangrenous lesions of the legs and feet. Microangiopathy is usually present together with large vessel involvement.

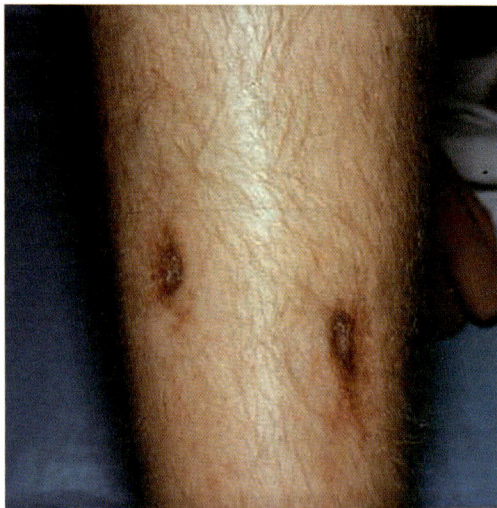

Fig. 59.57 Diabetic dermopathy on both shins.

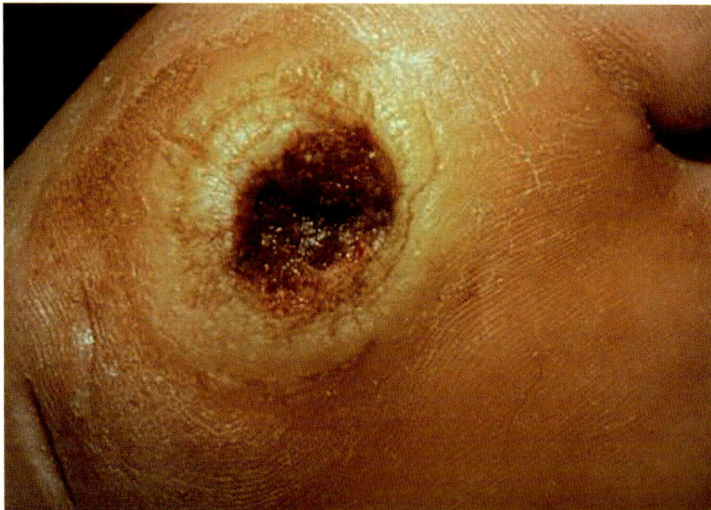

Fig. 59.58 Diabetic foot with neurotrophic ulceration and necrosis ('mal perforans').

Diabetic neuropathy

Elderly patients with an insidious onset of the disease are especially at risk. Commonly, there is a distal symmetrical polyneuropathy with mixed motor and sensory nerve involvement. The motor neuropathy of the foot is characterized by dorsally subluxed digits, distally displaced plantar fat pads, depressed metatarsal heads, hammer toes and pes cavus [3]. Proper foot care is essential to prevent formation of indolent perforating ulcers ('mal perforans'). A painless and slowly penetrating ulcer of the sole and of other pressure sites is suggestive of diabetic neuropathy. The ulcer is circular and punched out in shape, occurring in the middle of a callosity (Fig. 59.58). An initial subepidermal haemorrhagic bulla may give rise to discoloration of the surrounding skin [4]. Loss of temperature and pain sensation and absence of the ankle reflex (an early sign of diabetic neuropathy) indicate a neuropathic origin. Sensory abnormalities of the lower extremities include numbness, tingling, aching and burning. Burning feet and restless legs are common complaints, which intensify at night while lying down. Autonomic neuropathy may cause decreased

or absent sweating of the lower extremities with compensatory sweating in other skin areas. Damage to autonomic nerves of the skin in chronic advanced cases is manifested by oedema, erythema and atrophy [3].

The complex nature of the diabetic foot requires special attention. There is a multifactorial aetiology [6,8]. Predisposing factors include abnormal plantar pressure points, foot deformities and minor trauma. Peripheral neuropathy causes ulcers, loss of ankle jerks and vibration sensation. The foot has accentuated plantar arches and hammer toes, there is interdigital maceration leading to bacterial and fungal infection. Diabetic angiopathy leads to ulceration, necrosis, gangrene and osteomyelitis [15].

Local treatment of the ulcer consists of repeated debridement, treatment of infection, dressings and pressure-relieving footwear [8,16]. Simple surgery such as split skin grafting or minor toe amputations may be necessary [16], and some patients require more complex orthopaedic procedures to correct abnormal foot shape.

Cutaneous infections in diabetes mellitus

Skin infections due to *Staphylococcus aureus* and group A *Streptococcus haemolyticus* are common in diabetic patients [17]. Before insulin and antibiotics were available, infections causing severe furuncles, carbuncles and styes were frequent among diabetic individuals. Invasive *Pseudomonas* infection of the ear can progress through cellulitis and osteitis to cranial nerve damage and meningitis with a high mortality rate, so-called malignant otitis externa (Chapter 68) [18].

Non-clostridial gas gangrene. This complication develops in the soft tissues near a gangrenous focus. It was diagnosed in 17% of diabetics who were admitted to hospital because of gangrene or ulceration [19]. The commonest pathogens are *Escherichia coli*, *Klebsiella*, *Pseudomonas* and *Bacteroides* spp. in various combinations. The outcome is generally good.

Candida albicans. *Candida albicans* infections of mouth, nail folds, genitals and intertriginous skin areas are frequent in diabetics. Candidiasis may be the presenting feature of diabetes, and is frequently seen in diabetic patients whose disease is not well controlled [3]. A high glucose level of the saliva seems to account for the oral infection [20]. Phimosis is a common complaint of diabetic men, and recurring candidal infection is usually the cause. Dermatophyte infections are not more frequent in diabetic than in non-diabetic individuals [21].

Insulin resistance and acanthosis nigricans [22–24]

Tissue resistance to insulin is a major feature underlying the development of acanthosis nigricans in many diseases (e.g. Cushing's syndrome, acromegaly, Laurence–Moon–Bardet–Biedel syndrome, Prader–Willi syndrome and congenital lipodystrophy). There are two syndromes of insulin resistance. The type A syndrome has been reported in hyperandrogenetic women with clinical signs of virilization or accelerated growth (the acronym HAIR-AN has been proposed: HA, hyperandrogenism; IR, insulin resistance; AN, acanthosis nigricans). A genetic defect at the insulin receptor or in a post-receptor pathway has been postu-

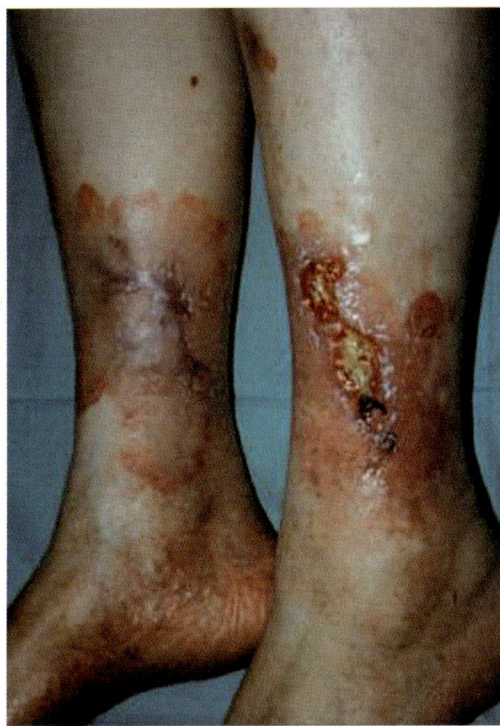

Fig. 59.59 Necrobiosis lipoidica with ulcerations on the shins.

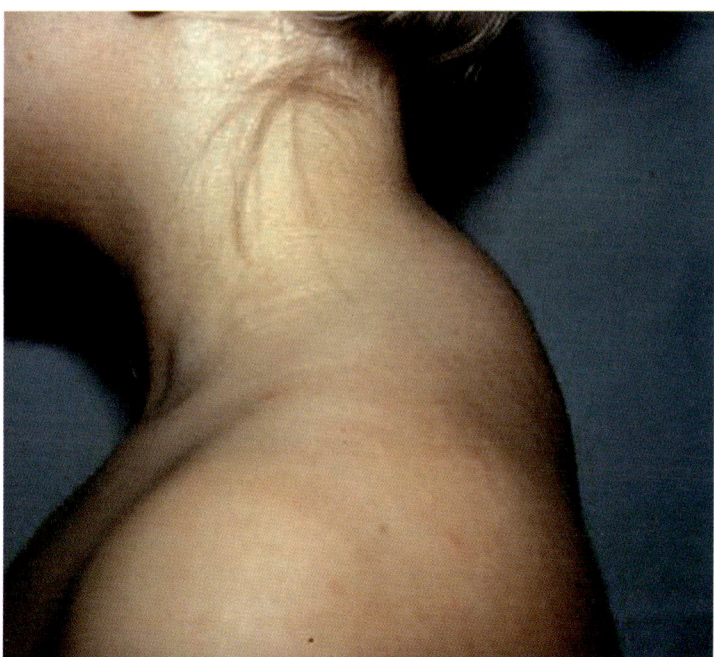

Fig. 59.60 Scleredema diabeticorum with a 'buffalo hump' in a young woman with diabetes mellitus.

lated. The type B syndrome has been reported in older women with signs of immunological dysfunction. High plasma levels of insulin are thought to contribute to the development of acanthosis nigricans.

Various skin disorders associated with diabetes mellitus

Necrobiosis lipoidica [2–8]. Necrobiosis lipoidica is associated with diabetes mellitus (Fig. 59.59). Frequencies of diabetes between 42% and 62% have been reported in patients with necrobiosis lipoidica, whereas necrobiosis lipoidica is uncommon (0.3%) among diabetic patients [3]. See also Chapter 60.

Disseminated granuloma annulare (Chapter 60). This is rarely seen in diabetic patients; the evidence that granuloma annulare is associated with diabetes mellitus is inconclusive [8,25].

Pruritus. Pruritus was once considered a typical symptom of diabetes mellitus. The frequency of generalized pruritus in diabetic patients is unknown. Anogenital pruritus may be due to secondary infection with candidiasis or haemolytic streptococci.

Stiff joints and waxy skin. Waxy tight skin on the backs of the hands and limited joint mobility may be seen in patients with insulin-dependent diabetes [8,26].

Scleredema diabeticorum. Whether post-infectious scleredema and diabetic scleredema are identical diseases, with a more severe course in the diabetes-associated form due to altered host response, is still a matter of debate [27]. The most common sites of involvement are the neck and upper back (Fig. 59.60). The condition is mainly seen in overweight adults with non-insulin-dependent diabetes, is essentially permanent, painless and causes no morbid-

ity. There is no specific treatment although penicillin, methotrexate, ciclosporin and PUVA have been used with various degrees of benefit.

Vitiligo (Chapter 58). Vitiligo occurs more frequently in diabetic individuals. In late-onset diabetes, a 4.5% frequency has been reported [28].

Lichen planus (Chapter 41). An increased incidence of abnormal glucose tolerance tests in patients with lichen planus, especially oral lichen planus, has been reported [29]. The overall support for a true association seems limited [6].

Haemochromatosis (Chapter 62). The main symptoms are liver disease, hyperpigmentation, joint disease, hypogonadism and, eventually, diabetes.

Eruptive xanthomas of the skin. Eruptive xanthomas may develop in diabetic patients with hyperlipidaemia. The lesions slowly resolve when the diabetes is properly managed (Fig. 59.61).

Finger pebbles. Among 60 patients with diabetes mellitus, 45 (75%) had a pebbly appearance of the knuckle and distal finger skin. Similar changes were observed in 21% of control subjects [30]. The changes may be of external origin (trauma) or internal (acanthosis nigricans).

Skin tags. Skin tags are small, soft, pedunculated lesions occurring on eyelids, neck and axillae, often associated with obesity. Among 216 patients with skin tags, 57 (26%) had diabetes of the non-insulin-dependent type, of whom only about one-quarter were classified as obese [31].

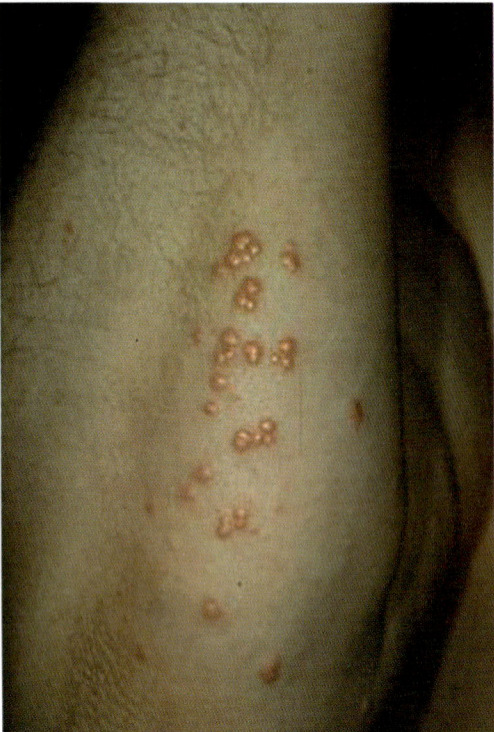

Fig. 59.61 Eruptive xanthomas in a diabetic patient with hyperlipidaemia.

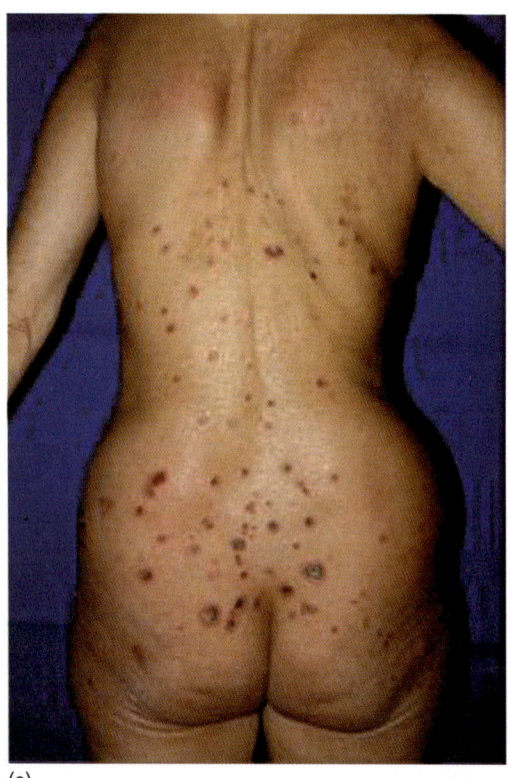

(a)

Local insulin reactions [6,32]. Insulin may cause immediate local reactions, starting as erythema, which turn urticarial within 30 min and subside within an hour; these are probably IgE mediated. Serious generalized immediate reactions are rare.

The most common reactions are delayed, starting about 2 weeks after onset of insulin therapy. An itchy nodule develops at the site of injection. It lasts for days and heals with hyperpigmentation and perhaps a scar. Delayed hypersensitivity is involved.

Insulin lipodystrophy. Insulin lipodystrophy is rare. Patients present with atrophic plaques at the sites of insulin injection. There is atrophy of the subcutaneous fat. The lesions seldom show complete spontaneous resolution. The mechanism is not known.

Reactive perforating collagenosis (folliculitis) (Fig. 59.62). There have been reports of perforating collagenosis in patients with diabetes with and without renal insufficiency. The cause is attributed to diabetic microangiopathy and lesions are due to minor injury such as pressure or scratching [8,33].

Diabetic bullae. Diabetic bullae are uncommon, but believed to be a distinct marker for diabetes [34,35]. The location is the lower legs and feet, occasionally hands and fingers. They range in size from less than one centimetre to several centimetres (Fig. 59.63). A typical blister arises on a non-inflamed base, and heals without scarring in 2–5 weeks. Histological examination shows intra- or subepidermal separation without acantholysis.

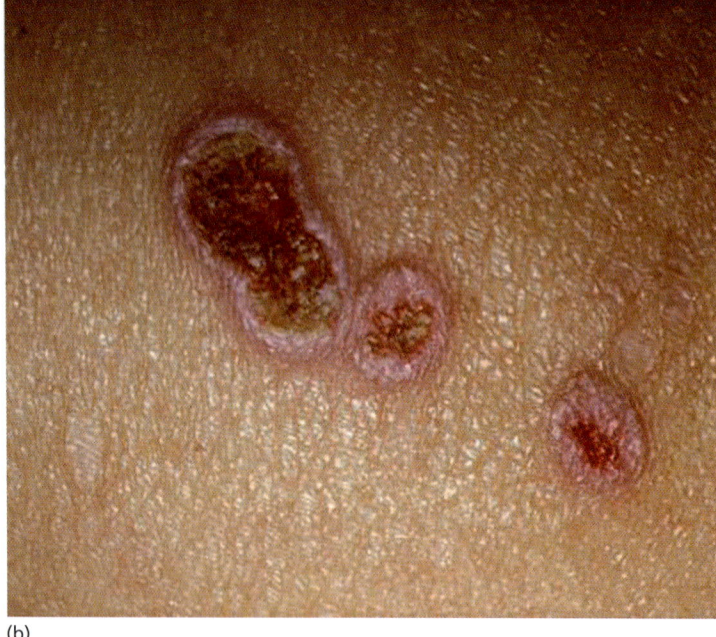

(b)

Fig. 59.62 (a) Perforating collagenosis on the back of a 64-year-old woman with diabetic retinopathy. (b) Close-up view.

References

1 National Diabetes Data Group. Classification and diagnosis of diabetes mellitus and other categories of glucose intolerance. *Diabetes* 1979; **28**: 1039–57.

2 Perez MI, Kohn SR. Cutaneous manifestations of diabetes mellitus. *J Am Acad Dermatol* 1994; **30**: 519–31.

3 Huntley AC. The cutaneous manifestations of diabetes. *J Am Acad Dermatol* 1982; **7**: 427–55.

4 Kalkoff KW. Diabetes and the skin. *Hexagon* 1982; **9**: 1–10.

5 Braverman IA. *Skin Signs of Systemic Disease*, 3rd edn. Philadelphia: Saunders, 1998: 457–64.

6 Ferringer T, Miller OF III. Cutaneous manifestations of diabetes mellitus. *Dermatol Clin* 2002; **20**: 483–92.

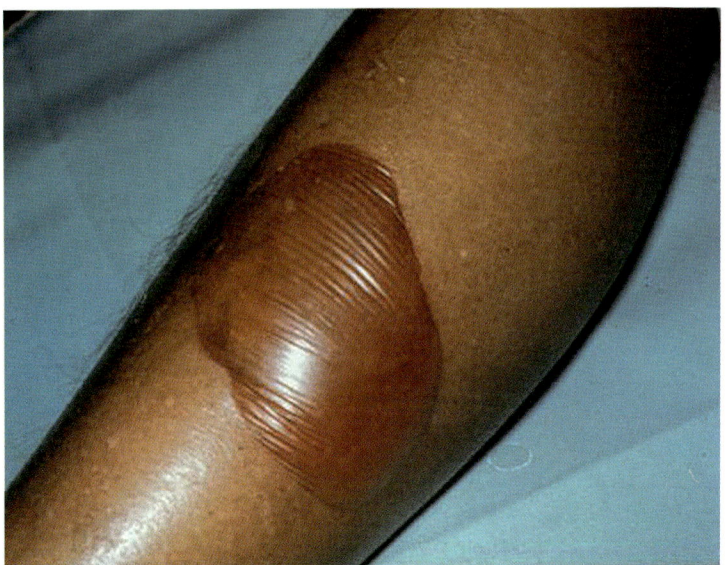

Fig. 59.63 A large diabetic bulla on the shin of a patient with diabetes mellitus.

7 Boyne M, Dobs AS, Krasner AS, Provost TT. Evaluation and treatment of endocrine disorders. In: Provost TT, Flynn JA, eds. *Cutaneous Medicine. Cutaneous Manifestations of Systemic Disease*. Hamilton, Ontario: B.C. Decker, 2001: 413–51.

8 Cox NH. Diabetes and the skin: an update for dermatologists. *Expert Rev Dermatol* 207; **2**: 305–16.

9 Ajam Z, Barton SP, Marks R. Characterization of abnormalities in the cutaneous microvasculature of diabetic subjects. *Br J Dermatol* 1982; **107** (Suppl. 22): 22–3.

10 Lithner F. Cutaneous erythema, with or without necrosis. Localized to the legs and feet—a lesion in elderly diabetics. *Acta Med Scand* 1974; **196**: 333–42.

11 Gitelson S, Wertheimer-Kaplinski N. Color of the face in diabetes mellitus: observations on a group of patients in Jerusalem. *Diabetes* 1965; **14**: 201–8.

12 Binkley GW, Giraldo B, Stoughton RB. Diabetic dermopathy—a clinical study. *Cutis* 1967; **3**: 955–8.

13 Baur FM, Levan NE. Diabetic dermangiopathy: a spectrum including pigmented pretibial patches and necrobiosis lipoidica diabeticorum. *Br J Dermatol* 1970; **83**: 528–35.

14 Shemer A, Bergman R, Linn S *et al.* Diabetic dermopathy and internal complications in diabetes mellitus. *Int J Dermatol* 1998; **37**: 113–5.

15 Lipsky BA. Diabetic foot infections. Pathophysiology, diagnosis and treatment. *Int J Dermatol* 1991; **30**: 560–2.

16 Leung PC. Diabetic foot ulcers—a comprehensive review. *Surgeon* 2007; **5**: 219–93.

17 Breen JD, Karchmer AW. *Staphylococcus aureus* infection in diabetic patients. *Infect Dis Clin N Am* 1995; **9**: 11–5.

18 Zaky DA, Bentley DW, Lowy K *et al.* Malignant external otitis: a severe form of otitis in diabetics. *Am J Med* 1976; **61**: 298–301.

19 Bessman AN, Wagner W. Nonclostridial gas gangrene. A report of 48 cases and review of the literature. *JAMA* 1975; **233**: 958–63.

20 Knight L, Fletcher J. Growth of *Candida albicans* in saliva: stimulation by glucose associated with antibiotics, corticosteroids and diabetes mellitus. *J Infect Dis* 1971; **123**: 371–7.

21 Alteras J, Saryt E. Prevalence of pathogenic fungi in the toe-webs and toenails of diabetic patients. *Mycopathologia* 1979; **67**: 157–9.

22 Barth JH, Wojnarowska F, Dawber RPR. Acanthosis nigricans, insulin resistance and cutaneous virilism. *Br J Dermatol* 1988; **118**: 613–9.

23 Rendon MI, Ponciano PD, Sontheimer RD *et al.* Acanthosis nigricans: a cutaneous marker of tissue resistance to insulin. *J Am Acad Dermatol* 1989; **21**: 461–9.

24 Schwartz RA. Acanthosis nigricans. *J Am Acad Dermatol* 1994; **31**: 1–19.

25 Andersen BL, Verdich J. Granuloma annulare and diabetes mellitus. *Clin Exp Dermatol* 1979; **4**: 31–7.

26 Rosenbloom AL, Silverstein JM, Lezotte DC *et al.* Limited joint mobility in childhood diabetes mellitus indicates increased risk of microvascular disease. *N Engl J Med* 1981; **305**: 191–4.

27 Krakowski A, Covo J, Berlin C. Diabetic scleredema. *Dermatologica* 1973; **146**: 193–8.

28 Dawber RPR. Vitiligo and diabetes mellitus (Letter). *Br J Dermatol* 1971; **84**: 600.

29 Halevy S, Feuerman EJ. Abnormal glucose tolerance associated with lichen planus. *Acta Derm Venereol Suppl (Stockh)* 1979; **59**: 167–70.

30 Huntley AC. Finger pebbles in diabetes mellitus. *J Am Acad Dermatol* 1986; **14**: 612–7.

31 Kahana M, Grossman E, Feinstein A *et al.* Skin tags: a cutaneous marker for diabetes mellitus. *Acta Derm Venereol Suppl (Stockh)* 1986; **67**: 175–7.

32 Sibbald RG, Schachter RK. Skin and diabetes mellitus. *Int J Dermatol* 1984; **23**: 567–83.

33 Cochran RJ, Tucker SB, Wilkin JK. Reactive perforating collagenosis of diabetes mellitus and renal failure. *Cutis* 1983; **31**: 55–8.

34 Bernstein JE, Medenica M, Soltani K. Bullous eruption of diabetes mellitus. *Arch Dermatol* 1979; **115**: 324–5.

35 Basarab T, Munn SE, McGrath J, Jones RR. Bullosis diabeticum. A case report and literature review. *Clin Exp Dermatol* 1995; **20**: 218–20.

Xanthomas and abnormalities of lipid metabolism and storage
P.D. Flynn, pp. 59.81–59.103

Introduction [1,2]

Disorders of lipid metabolism are heterogeneous. They include the very rare and the very common. They range from monogenic diseases with high penetrance through polygenic disorders to those that are paradigms of gene–environment interaction. Some are entirely or partially secondary to other diseases such as diabetes mellitus, hypothyroidism, renal failure or hepatic disorders. Dyslipidaemias are of relevance to all medical and surgical disciplines, and to all involved in delivering health care in the 21st century, as most are associated with an increased risk of atherosclerosis and its complications. They are of particular relevance to dermatologists because they may present with subcutaneous lipid deposits, collectively known as xanthomata. These may require treatment in their own right for the relief of the symptoms they cause; they may also allow the identification and treatment of a dyslipidaemia before the onset of premature cardiovascular disease.

This account will include a brief description of the principal lipid metabolic pathways and an overview of the classification of the dyslipidaemias, followed by a more detailed discussion of some of the individual primary lipid disorders, focusing on those most likely to be seen by dermatologists. The section will conclude with summaries of the secondary dyslipidaemias and of the overall management of dyslipidaemia.

References

1 Durrington PN. *Hyperlipidaemia: Diagnosis and Management*, 3rd edn. London: Hodder Arnold, 2007.

2 Scriver VR, Beaudet AL, Sly WS *et al. The Metabolic and Molecular Bases of Inherited Disease*, 8th edn. New York: McGraw Hill, 2001.

Lipid metabolism [1]

Most metabolic pathways initially appear daunting; those describing lipid metabolism are no exception. Circulating lipids (cholesterol, cholesterol esters, triglycerides and phospholipids) are insoluble and therefore have to be solubilized by combination

Table 59.13 Classification of lipoproteins (adapted from [1]).

Class	Density (g/ml)	Electrophoretic mobility	Lipids*	Apolipoproteins
Chylomicrons	0.93	Remains at origin	Triglycerides 86% Cholesterol 5%	Apo B-48, Apo C, Apo E
VLDL	0.93–1.006	Pre-β-lipoproteins	Triglycerides 55% Cholesterol 19%	Apo B-100, Apo C, Apo E
IDL	1.006–1.019	Slow pre-β-lipoproteins	Cholesterol 38% Triglycerides 23%	Apo B-100, Apo E
LDL	1.019–1.063	β-lipoproteins	Cholesterol 50% Triglycerides 6%	Apo B-100
HDL	1.063–1.210	α-lipoproteins	Cholesterol 19% Triglycerides 4%	Apo A-I, A-II, A-IV
Lipoprotein (a)	1.040–1.090	Slow pre-β-lipoproteins		Apo (a), Apo B-100

* Expressed as % of dry mass.

with proteins; the resulting particles are called lipoproteins and the proteins they contain are generally called apolipoproteins. Understanding of the production, clearance and interrelationships of lipoproteins is growing rapidly and the following account aims merely to provide an overview of current understanding and a framework into which future advances can (hopefully) be incorporated. It is worth remembering that the current classification of lipoproteins is a pragmatic one based on their densities, a physical property we can measure, rather than their biological functions, which we would like to measure; there is fortunately some correlation between the two but it is not always absolute. The classification is shown in Table 59.13.

To discuss the metabolic pathways linking these differing lipoprotein classes it is helpful to consider those involved in the absorption of dietary fats and their transport to places of storage (the exogenous lipid pathway), those involved in the transport of lipids from the liver to peripheral tissues where they are required (the endogenous pathway), and those involved in the return of excess cholesterol to the liver from peripheral tissues (reverse cholesterol transport). In reality all three are closely interrelated.

Reference

1 Havel RJ, Kane JP. Structure and metabolism of plasma lipoproteins. In: Scriver CR, Beaudet AL, Sly WS *et al.*, eds. *The Metabolic and Molecular Bases of Inherited Diseases*, 8th edn. New York: McGraw Hill, 1995: 2705–16.

The exogenous lipid pathway [1,2]

The majority of fat absorbed from the diet derives from triglycerides. These are hydrolysed by pancreatic lipase and the resulting free fatty acids and monoglycerides pass across the brush border of the small intestine into the enterocytes. Here they are reassembled into triglycerides which are packaged with apo B-48 and apo A-I, A-II and A-IV, and the relatively small amount of dietary cholesterol that is absorbed, to form nascent chylomicrons that are released and enter the lacteals. Chylomicron formation is completed by the transfer of apo C and apo E from high density lipoproteins (HDL) before release from the thoracic duct into the systemic circulation. Here chylomicron apo C-II is recognized by endothelial-bound lipoprotein lipase which acts to hydrolyse tri-

glycerides, releasing fatty acids that can be taken up by adipose tissue for storage, or by other cells (e.g. muscle) for oxidation to provide a source of energy, or that are released into the circulation where they are largely bound by albumin. This loss of triglyceride is accompanied by a loss of apolipoproteins (A-I, A-II, A-IV and C) producing a chylomicron remnant that is itself bound by receptors expressed on hepatocytes (principally the low-density lipoprotein (LDL) receptor and the LDL receptor related protein (LRP)) and then endocytosed. The triglycerides and cholesterol thus delivered to the hepatocyte can be stored in intracellular lipid droplets, excreted in the bile or be re-packaged into nascent lipoproteins to participate in the endogenous lipid pathway.

The endogenous lipid pathway

This lipid pathway starts in the hepatocyte where triglycerides, and to a lesser extent cholesterol and cholesterol esters, are assembled with apo B-100 to produce nascent very-low-density lipoproteins (VLDL) in a manner similar to the production of chylomicrons in enterocytes. (Indeed apo B-48 and apo B-100 are produced from the same gene, the former representing simply the amino terminal 48% of the latter.) Following secretion, VLDL accept further apo C and apo E from HDL and can thus be bound, like chylomicrons, by endothelial lipoprotein lipase with subsequent hydrolysis of their triglycerides and uptake of the released fatty acids by peripheral cells. The resulting VLDL remnants comprise a population of lipoproteins heterogeneous both in density and in affinity for the hepatic LDL receptors that mediate their removal from the circulation; the smaller remnants include intermediate density lipoproteins (IDL) which remain relatively longer in the circulation and so can be further processed, probably by hepatic lipase, to produce LDL. LDL are cleared from the circulation by LDL receptors, 90% of which are hepatic.

Reverse cholesterol transport [3–5]

The process of reverse cholesterol transport begins in peripheral tissues with the transfer of cholesterol, cholesterol esters and phospholipids to two pools of HDL precursor particles—discoidal apo A-I and A-IV, produced by the liver, and nascent pre-β HDL, produced from chylomicrons. Lipid transfer to these particles depends on the lipid transporter ATP binding cassette A-1 (ABCA1); stabilization of the newly formed HDL depends additionally on the esterification and internalization of these transferred lipids by lecithin cholesterol acyl transferase (LCAT) and phospholipid transfer protein (PLTP). The cholesterol taken up by HDL returns to the liver by two principal routes. One involves the transfer of cholesterol esters from HDL to apo B containing lipoproteins (principally VLDL) mediated by cholesterol ester transfer protein (CETP) and subsequent uptake by hepatic LDL receptors; the other is mediated by direct uptake of HDL by hepatic scavenger receptors, mainly SR-B1. Cholesterol returned to the liver by reverse cholesterol transport can be stored in hepatocytes or converted into bile acids and then excreted.

References

1 Havel RJ, Goldstein JL, Brown MS. Lipoproteins and lipid transport. In: Bondy PK, Rosenberg LE, eds. *Metabolic Control and Disease*, 8th edn. Philadelphia: Saunders, 1980: 393–494.
2 Myant NB. *The Biology of Cholesterol and Related Steroids*. London: Heinemann Medical, 1981.
3 Reichl D, Miller NE. The anatomy and physiology of reverse cholesterol transport. *Clin Sci* 1986; **70**: 221–31.
4 Barter P. High-density lipoproteins and reverse cholesterol transport. *Curr Opin Lipidol* 1993; **4**: 210–7.
5 Schmidt G, Kaminski WE, Orso E. ABC transporters in cellular lipid trafficking. *Curr Opin Lipidol* 2000; **11**: 493–501.

Lipids, lipoproteins and atherosclerosis [1–4]

There is now near universal acceptance that there is a causal relationship between circulating lipid concentrations and the development of atherosclerosis and its clinical sequelae (angina, myocardial infarctions, strokes and peripheral vascular disease). That it has taken so long to reach this point reflects both the influence of other risk factors for cardiovascular disease (and their often complicated interaction with lipid metabolism) and the complexity of the metabolism and variable atherogenicity of the different lipoproteins. It is very clear that high LDL cholesterol levels confer an increased risk of cardiovascular disease (CVD) and that this risk is decreased if LDL cholesterol levels are reduced, evidence for the latter coming most clearly from trials of the 3-hydroxy-3-methylglutaryl coenzyme A reductase (HMG CoA reductase) inhibitors, or 'statin' group of drugs. There is also evidence that some LDL are more atherogenic than others; a preponderance of small, dense LDL or increased levels of oxidized LDL are both associated with increased CVD risk. Elevated concentrations of lipoprotein(a), which differs from LDL only by the additional presence of apolipoprotein(a), are also correlated with increased risk of atherosclerosis.

Epidemiological studies have also shown a strong and consistent inverse relationship between HDL and risk of atherosclerosis, that is high HDL levels are associated with a lower risk of CVD. There are some exceptions, for example apo AI Milano, where low levels of HDL are, apparently paradoxically, linked to low levels of CVD. In fact apo AI Milano is extremely efficient both at accepting lipid species from peripheral cells and at transporting them back to the liver; at any one time there is high flux through the reverse cholesterol transport pathway but concentrations of HDL cholesterol are low. There is also growing evidence that HDL

have additional antiatherogenic properties; under appropriate conditions they can be anti-inflammatory and antioxidant. Taken together, these factors may explain the conflicting results of trials that have attempted to reduce CVD risk by increasing HDL concentration; some have yielded positive results (e.g. the Helsinki Heart Study, VA-HIT and HATS) but others have not (e.g. the WHO Clofibrate trial, FIELD and ILLUMINATE). Interpretation of such trials is further compounded by the fact that the agents used also altered other lipid risk factors including LDL cholesterol and triglycerides. A number of epidemiological studies have shown an association between high fasting triglyceride concentrations and CVD risk, albeit a rather weaker one than for LDL or HDL cholesterol and one which often loses significance in multivariate analysis, especially when correcting for HDL cholesterol concentrations with which fasting triglyceride levels are often negatively correlated. High fasting triglycerides are certainly linked to acute pancreatitis, often as a consequence but sometimes as a cause, with the risk rising significantly once levels exceed 10 mmol/L.

References

1 Ross R. The pathogenesis of atherosclerosis. An update. *N Engl J Med* 1984; **314**: 488–500.
2 Libby P, Theroux P. Pathophysiology of coronary artery disease. *Circulation* 2005; **111**: 3481–8.
3 Cholesterol Treatment Triallists' (CTT) Collaborators. Efficacy and safety of cholesterol-lowering treatment: prospective meta-analysis of data from 90,056 participants in 14 randomised trials of statins. *Lancet* 2005; **366**: 1267–78.
4 Studer M, Briel M, Leimenstall B *et al*. Effect of different antilipidemic agents and diets on mortality: a systematic review. *Arch Intern Med* 2005; **165**: 725–30.

Dyslipidaemias: classification

There are a number of classifications of disordered lipid and lipoprotein metabolism, none of them entirely satisfactory. Perhaps the most straightforward is the WHO classification, usually referred to as the Fredrickson classification, based on the class of lipoprotein present in excess (Table 59.14) [1]. However, this requires plasma ultracentrifugation, does not include disorders characterized by low levels of HDL cholesterol or secondary dyslipidaemias and is not a diagnostic classification.

Pragmatically, given that for most patients all that is likely to be available is a lipid profile comprising total cholesterol, triglycerides and HDL cholesterol with a calculated LDL cholesterol, it may be most convenient to group patients rather broadly as having hypercholesterolaemia, hypertriglyceridaemia, combined (or mixed) dyslipidaemia, or other dyslipidaemia; wherever possible, further characterization and diagnosis may be based on

Table 59.14 WHO classification of hyperlipoproteinaemias [1].

Type	Lipoprotein abnormality
I	Hyperchylomicronaemia
IIa	Elevated LDL
IIb	Elevated LDL and VLDL
III	Broad β-VLDL
IV	Elevated VLDL
V	Elevated chylomicrons and VLDL

Table 59.15 Working classification of dyslipidaemias.

	Lipid abnormalities	WHO type	Primary dyslipidaemias	Secondary causes
Hypercholesterolaemia	↑ TC ↑ LDL-C Normal Tgs	IIa	Familial hypercholesterolaemia Familial defective Apo B-100 Polygenic hypercholesterolaemia	Hypothyroidism Anorexia Cholestatic liver disease Nephrotic syndrome Acute intermittent porphyria Drugs: thiazide diuretics, corticosteroids
Combined dyslipidaemia	↑ TC ↑ LDL-C ↑ Tgs ± ↓ HDL-C	III IIb IV	Familial dysbetalipoproteinaemia Familial combined hyperlipidaemia	Diabetes mellitus Metabolic syndrome Lipodystrophies Hypothyroidism Hepatocellular liver disease Nephrotic syndrome Chronic renal failure Paraproteinaemias Pregnancy Drugs: β blockers, antiretrovirals, retinoic acid derivatives
Hypertriglyceridaemia	↑↑ Tgs ↑ TC ↓ HDL-C	I IV, V	Lipoprotein lipase deficiency Apo CII deficiency	Diabetes mellitus Alcohol excess Chronic renal failure Paraproteinaemias Pregnancy (esp. 3rd trimester) Drugs: retinoic acid derivatives, oral contraceptives
Other dyslipidaemias	↓ HDL-C only ↑ HDL-C ↓↓ LDL-C ↓ LDL-C		Tangier disease Apo AI Milano Hyperalphalipoproteinaemia Abetalipoproteinaemia Hypobetalipoproteinaemia	 Alcohol, anabolic steroids

additional tests. (The LDL cholesterol in a standard lipid profile is calculated from the Friedewald formula:

$$LDL\text{-}C = \text{total cholesterol} - HDL \text{ cholesterol} - 0.42 \times \text{triglycerides}$$

To provide a valid estimate of the LDL cholesterol the sample should be taken from a fasting subject and the triglyceride level should be below 4.5 mmol/L.) Such a working classification is shown in Table 59.15; it might at first sight seem confusing that total cholesterol is raised in conditions characterized by predominant hypertriglyceridaemia but this reflects the much increased contribution of triglyceride-rich lipoprotein cholesterol to the total cholesterol in these disorders.

Reference

1 Fredrickson DS, Levy RI, Lees RS. Fat transport in lipoproteins—an integrated approach to mechanisms and disorders. *N Engl J Med* 1967; **276**: 34–42, 94–103, 148–56, 215–25, 273–81.

Xanthomata

The term xanthoma derives from the Greek 'xanthos' meaning yellow and is used to describe a variety of subcutaneous lipid deposits, even those that do not appear particularly yellow. All xanthomata contain macrophages loaded with cholesterol and cholesterol esters ('foam cells') [1]; any distinctive features of the different types of xanthoma are discussed below.

Tendon xanthomata

These occur most commonly attached to the extensor tendons over the knuckles and in the Achilles tendon, though other tendons can sometimes be affected. In these sites they can usually be moved from side to side. Occasionally, they can involve the periosteum at the site of insertion of the patellar tendon where they cannot be moved. As the accumulation of cholesterol is deep within the tendons the overlying skin does not appear yellow. The xanthomata contain collagen in addition to foamy macrophages and so feel quite hard. They are most frequently seen in familial hypercholesterolaemia [2,3], but are also a feature of the secondary hypercholesterolaemia seen in prolonged cholestasis and the rare lipid disorders cerebrotendinous xanthomatosis [4] and sitosterolaemia [5]. In all cases other than sitosterolaemia they are indicative of raised levels of LDL cholesterol, though they do not completely resolve with LDL-lowering treatment. However, in the occasional patients where the tendon xanthomata are painful this symptom does improve with LDL cholesterol reduction.

Xanthelasmata (Fig. 59.64)

Xanthelasmata are the xanthomata that develop around the eyes, and were among the earliest recognized historically. They most

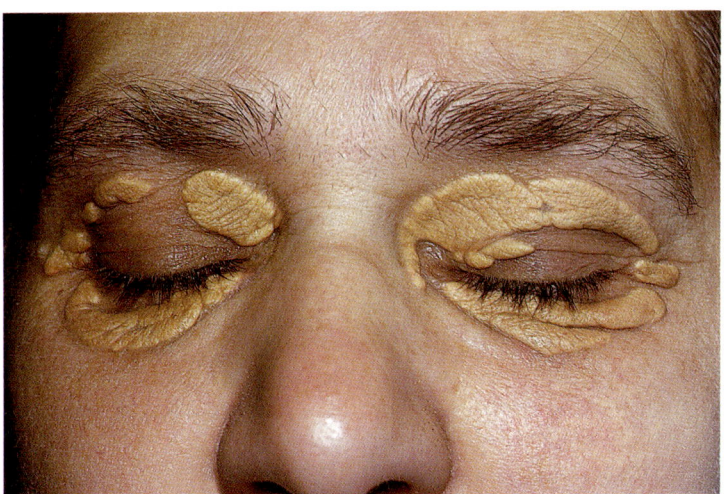

Fig. 59.64 Extensive xanthelasmas palpebrarum. (Courtesy of Addenbrooke's Hospital, Cambridge, UK.)

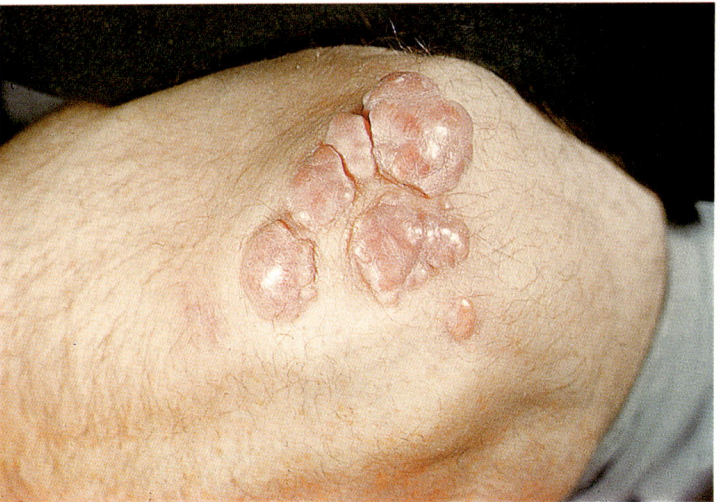

Fig. 59.65 Tuberous xanthomas. (Courtesy of Addenbrooke's Hospital, Cambridge, UK.)

commonly affect the upper eyelids and the area around the medical canthus. They are relatively soft to the touch and range from pale yellow to yellow-orange in colour. They are seen in familial hypercholesterolaemia, type III hyperlipoproteinaemia and in chronic cholestasis (especially primary biliary cirrhosis) [6], but are also often seen in people with circulating lipid levels considered normal in Western populations. Given their rather prominent site they are often noticed by patients, to whom they may be a source of considerable cosmetic distress. They can be removed surgically, or by cauterization or by application of silver nitrate but often recur, particularly if LDL cholesterol levels are high. In these circumstances subsequent treatment to lower LDL cholesterol, for example with a 'statin', seems sensible even if not yet confirmed by clinical trial. Such treatment is often associated with regression of xanthelasmata in hypercholesterolaemic patients without the need for other intervention.

Tuberous xanthomata (Fig. 59.65)
Although starting as small xanthomata, usually over the extensor aspects of the elbows and knees, these can develop into quite

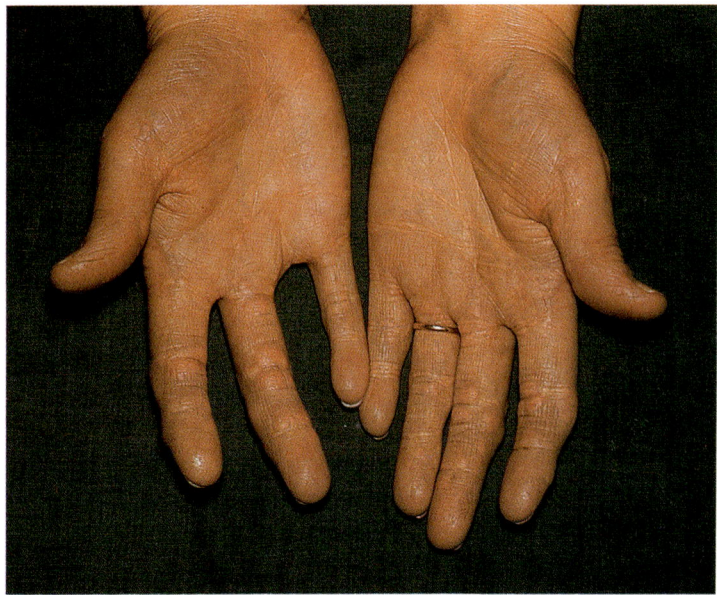

Fig. 59.66 Xanthomatosis and yellow palmar creases. (Courtesy of Addenbrooke's Hospital, Cambridge, UK.)

exuberant exophytic lesions several centimetres in diameter and height. They can develop over other pressure areas such as the heels and plantar surfaces of the feet, and very occasionally can occur in the bone marrow. They can be itchy and are susceptible to trauma given their position. They usually indicate the presence of type III hyperlipoproteinaemia [7]. They respond well to effective treatment of the combined dyslipidaemia characteristic of this disorder.

Palmar xanthomata (Fig. 59.66)
Linear palmar xanthomata consisting of an orange-yellow lipid deposition running along the palmar creases, and occasionally the flexor creases of the wrists, are pathognomonic of type III hyperlipoproteinaemia [7]. Like tuberous xanthomata they respond well to treatment of the dyslipidaemia. They were formerly known as xanthoma striata palmaris.

Eruptive xanthomata (Fig. 59.67)
These small xanthomata consist of small yellow papules 2–5 mm in diameter, arising out of a slightly wider red base and usually appear in large numbers over extensor surfaces, particularly of the buttocks, back, legs and arms. In extreme cases they can be itchy and have an even more widespread distribution, potentially leading to diagnostic confusion. Their foamy macrophages contain triglycerides as well as cholesterol [8]. They only occur with severe hypertriglyceridaemia of any cause (serum triglycerides at least greater than 20 mmol/L), and are therefore almost always accompanied by lipaemia retinalis, a creamy yellow discoloration of the retinal blood vessels, and a lipaemic appearance of blood or serum samples. Eruptive xanthomata resolve well within a couple of weeks of treatment of the hypertriglyceridaemia.

Planar xanthomata (Fig. 59.68)
These xanthomata are wide based and rather flat and can cover the areas usually affected by xanthelasmata, but are usually

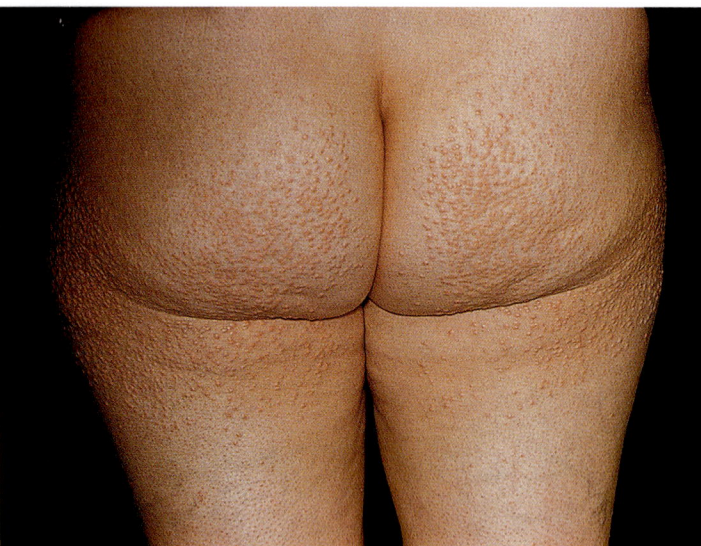

Fig. 59.67 Eruptive xanthomas. (Courtesy of Addenbrooke's Hospital, Cambridge, UK.)

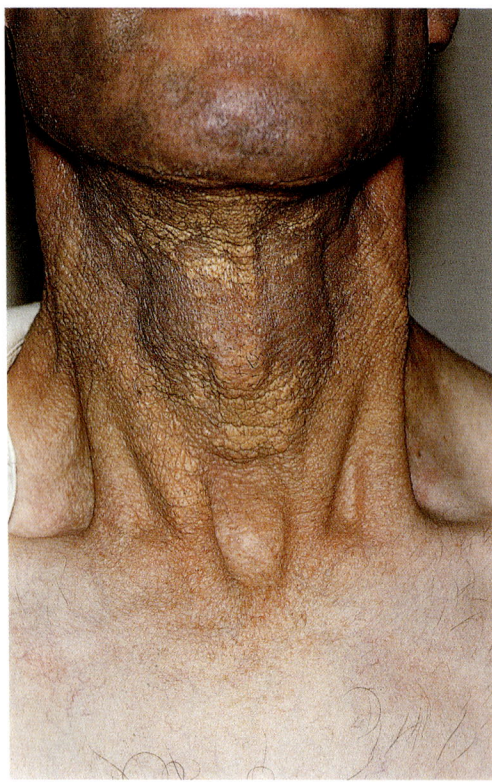

Fig. 59.68 Plane xanthomatosis. (Courtesy of Addenbrooke's Hospital, Cambridge, UK.)

broader and more widespread. They most frequently occur with paraproteinaemias (multiple myeloma or monoclonal gammopathy of uncertain significance (MGUS)) [9,10], when they often develop in areas subject to pressure from clothing or jewellery. Serum lipid levels are infrequently raised, indeed they may be below average, and the precise aetiology is unclear though complexes between immunoglobulins and lipoproteins are often

found. When hyperlipidaemia is present a type III hyperlipoproteinaemic pattern is quite common. Occasionally planar xanthomata can be seen in lymphoma and systemic lupus erythematosus; they are also a feature of homozygous familial hypercholesterolaemia. Rarely, patients with paraproteinaemia develop necrobiotic xanthogranuloma with widespread, severe xanthelasmata that can cause complete closure of the eyelids accompanied by subcutaneous xanthogranulomata of the face and body [11].

Corneal arcus

Corneal arcus is not strictly a xanthoma, but does represent the deposition of cholesterol esters in the peripheral cornea. It is commoner in young people with familial hypercholesterolaemia (it is present in 50% of heterozygotes by the age of 30), but can occur with other causes of longstanding hypercholesterolaemia and in subjects with normal circulating lipid levels. In its early stages it is not a complete ring, but comprises superior and inferior crescents that may only be evident with eyelid retraction. With increasing age its specificity for familial hypercholesterolaemia falls even further. Corneal arcus does not regress with lipid-modulating drug treatment, but neither does it ever impair vision.

References

1 Takahashi W, Naito M. Lipid storage disease: part I. Ultrastructure of xanthoma cells in various xanthomatous diseases. *Acta Pathol Jpn* 1983; **33**: 959–77.
2 Burns FS. A contribution to the study of the aetiology of xanthoma. *Arch Derm Syph* 1920; **2**: 415–29.
3 Thannhauser SJ, Magendanta H. The different clinical groups of xanthomatous diseases: a clinical physiological study of 22 cases. *Ann Intern Med* 1938; **11**: 1662–746.
4 Björkhem I, Boberg KM, Leitersdorf E. Inborn errors in bile acid biosynthesis and storage of sterols other than cholesterol. In: Scriver CR, Beaudet AL, Sly WS, Valle D, eds. *The Metabolic and Molecular Bases of Inherited Disease*, 8th edn. New York: McGraw-Hill, 2001: 2961–88.
5 Bhattacharyya AK, Conner WE. Beta-sitosterolaemia and xanthomatosis. *J Clin Invest* 1974; **53**: 1033–43.
6 Ahrens EH, Kunkel HG. The relationship between serum lipids and skin xanthomata in eighteen patients with primary biliary cirrhosis. *J Clin Invest* 1949; **28**: 1565–74.
7 Polano MK. Xanthomatosis and hyperlipoproteinaemia. *Dermatologica* 1974; **149**: 1–9.
8 Parker F, Bagdade JD, Odland GF, Bierman EL. Evidence for the chylomicron origin of lipids accumulating in diabetic eruptive xanthomas. A correlative lipid biochemical, histological and electron microscopic study. *J Clin Invest* 1970; **49**: 2172–87.
9 Groszek E, Abrams JJ, Grundy SM. Normolipidaemic planar xanthomatosis associated with benign monoclonal gammopathy. *Metabolism* 1981; **30**: 927–35.
10 Lynch PJ, Winkelmann RK. Generalised plane xanthoma and systemic disease. *Arch Dermatol* 1960; **93**: 639–46.
11 Jeziorska M, Hassan A, Mackness MI et al. Clinical, biochemical and immunohistochemical features of necrobiotic xanthogranulomatosis. *J Clin Pathol* 2003; **56**: 64–8.

Primary dyslipidaemias

Hypercholesterolaemia
Familial hypercholesterolaemia

Clinical features. Familial hypercholesterolaemia (FH) is an autosomal co-dominant condition characterized by:
- High total and LDL cholesterol, slightly low HDL cholesterol and normal triglyceride concentrations

Table 59.16 Lipid concentrations in familial hypercholesterolaemia [6].

	Total Cholesterol (mM)	LDL-Cholesterol (mM)	HDL-Cholesterol (mM)	Triglycerides (mM)
Normal	4.52 ± 0.72	2.84 ± 0.64	1.37 ± 0.33	0.68 ± 0.28
Heterozygotes	7.73 ± 1.63	6.23 ± 1.55	1.11 ± 0.31	0.93 ± 0.58
Homozygotes	17.5 ± 4.39	16.1 ± 4.13	0.88 ± 0.26	1.14 ± 0.58

- Frequent tendon xanthomata (especially of the Achilles tendons)
- Premature onset of cardiovascular disease.

The familial clustering of these three features has been recognized since at least the late 19th century and was the subject of detailed studies in the 1930s [1,2]. In the 1950s, the development of ultracentrifugation for quantifying lipoproteins revealed that the biochemical hallmark of FH is an accumulation of LDL [3], and in 1973 Goldstein and Brown discovered the LDL receptor and showed that its defective functioning was the underlying cause of the condition [4]. Homozygotes number about 1 per million in Caucasian populations and can have total cholesterol levels of 15 mmol/L or higher, may be born with tendon xanthomas and can suffer from the clinical effects of coronary heart disease as early as their teens. They can also develop a supravalvular aortic stenosis. Heterozygotes occur at a frequency of about 1 in 500 in most Caucasian populations, though with notably higher frequency in certain groups, for example Afrikaners and the Lebanese, where there are marked founder gene effects. They have less marked elevations in their cholesterol than homozygotes (Table 59.16), but of untreated males 50% will have suffered a myocardial infarction (MI) and 24% will have died by age 50 years. Heterozygous females have a slightly delayed onset of CVD compared with males but 58% will have had an MI and 15% have died by the age of 60 if not treated [5]. FH thus accounts for a significant proportion of premature cardiovascular disease and of premature sudden cardiac death. There is a striking preponderance in FH of coronary arterial disease, as opposed to cerebrovascular or peripheral vascular disease.

The presence of tendon xanthomata is the principal cutaneous manifestation of FH [1], and may often be helpful in establishing the diagnosis. They are usually present in childhood in homozygotes and become more prevalent with age in untreated heterozygotes. They occur most frequently in extensor tendons, especially the Achilles tendons and those over the knuckles. They feel rather hard as they contain fibrous tissue as well as cholesterol, and they can become inflamed. They are not invariably present, especially if treatments to reduce the LDL cholesterol are begun at a sufficiently early age. They can also occur in two other disorders of sterol metabolism, cerebrotendinous xanthomatosis [6] and sitosterolaemia [7], both of which are extremely rare. Subcutaneous planar and tuberous xanthomata may occasionally be seen in FH homozygotes, but not heterozygotes. Corneal arcus is seen in many but not all cases and lacks both sensitivity and specificity for establishing the diagnosis though it does feature in some sets of criteria. Specifically, its presence and severity does not correlate with the risk of CVD in FH. Xanthelasmata are not commonly seen in FH; where they do occur they can respond to treatment that reduces LDL cholesterol concentrations. They can also be removed surgically but can recur more markedly thereafter; the efficacy of LDL reduction in this setting awaits confirmation but is quite common clinical practice.

Genetics and diagnosis. The majority of patients with FH have mutations in their LDL receptor associated with a variable degree of loss of function. As a result there is both defective clearance of VLDL from the circulation with consequent increased conversion to LDL and impaired clearance of LDL resulting in the significant elevation of LDL cholesterol concentration which accounts for the raised plasma total cholesterol. Over 1000 disease-associated mutations have so far been described in the LDL receptor gene (which is one of the largest human genes) [8]. They have been classified on the basis of the effect they have on the synthesis, expression and processing of the LDL receptor [9]:

Type 1 prevent receptor synthesis

Type 2 impair transport of the receptor from the endoplasmic reticulum to the Golgi

Type 3 affect receptor binding of circulating LDL

Type 4 prevent clathrin-mediated receptor clustering and internalization

Type 5 interfere with receptor recycling from the endosome.

Type 1 mutations tend to result in a complete absence of LDL receptor activity ('receptor negative') while the other classes of mutations usually cause markedly reduced but not completely absent activity ('receptor defective').

In a small proportion of patients with FH (around 2%) the mutation affects not the LDL receptor but the receptor binding domain in the LDL apo B-100 (familial defective apo B-100) [10]. This is almost always due to a mutation in codon 3500 (R3500Q) resulting in a substitution of arginine for glutamine; rarely it is due to a different mutation in codon 3500 (R3500W, in which tryptophan replaces arginine) or in codon 3531. Such patients are phenotypically indistinguishable from those with LDL receptor mutations though there is some evidence that their cardiovascular risk is not as dramatically raised. Recently, a new genetic locus has been found to account for some of the previously mutation-negative cases of FH; the gene codes for proprotein convertase subtilisin kexin 9 (PCSK9) [11], a serine protease whose activity appears to decrease LDL receptor expression and LDL clearance and thus increases LDL cholesterol concentration. It has emerged that statins upregulate PCSK9, so it represents an interesting target for agents to augment the LDL-lowering effect of these drugs. Finally, a small group of patients, all from Sardinia, have a phenotype similar to homozygous FH but inherited in a recessive pattern— autosomal recessive hypercholesterolaemia (ARH) [12].

Given the genetic heterogeneity underlying FH, diagnosis has largely rested on clinical and biochemical criteria. In the United Kingdom, the criteria used by the Simon Broome Register of patients with FH have been widely adopted (Table 59.17). Other sets of diagnostic criteria have also been developed, for example the Dutch Lipid Clinic Network Criteria [13] and the Make Early Diagnosis to Prevent Early Disease on Medical Pedigree (MEDPED) system [14]. Increasingly, advances in molecular biological

Table 59.17 Simon Broome Register criteria for diagnosing familial hypercholesterolaemia. (From Scientific Steering Committee of the Simon Broome Register Group. Risk of fatal coronary heart disease in familial hypercholesterolaemia. *BMJ* 1991; **303**: 893–6.)

Definite FH

- total cholesterol above 6.7 mM or LDL cholesterol above 4.0 mM in children under 16 or total cholesterol above 7.5 mM or LDL cholesterol above 4.9 mM in adults

plus

- tendon xanthomata in patient or 1st or 2nd degree relative

or

- FH mutation detected

Possible FH

- total cholesterol above 6.7 mM or LDL cholesterol above 4.0 mM in children under 16 or total cholesterol above 7.5 mM or LDL cholesterol above 4.9 mM in adults

plus

- family history of MI <50 in 2nd degree relative or <60 in 1st degree relative

or

- family history of total cholesterol >7.5 mM in 1st or 2nd degree relative.

techniques are proving helpful in diagnosing FH; this is particularly true where a disease-causing mutation has been identified in one family member.

Treatment. The hypercholesterolaemia of FH will only respond marginally to lifestyle measures such as reducing saturated fat intake. However, encouraging patients with measures that reduce cardiovascular risk, such as avoiding smoking and exercising regularly, clearly make sense, and may help account for the reduced risk of cancer, particularly lung and colon cancer, seen in the Simon Broome Register [15]. In recent years, statins have become the mainstay of treatment and they are likely to have played a large part in the reduction of cardiovascular mortality seen in recent years in FH. In comparison with the general population, statins usually have to be started at a much earlier age in patients with FH, and to achieve the desired reduction in LDL cholesterol (recently the National Institute for Health and Clinical Excellence (NICE) in the UK has advised a greater than 50% reduction) [16], higher doses of the more potent statins may well have to be used. Referral to a specialist lipid clinic is advised to allow counselling of young patients starting lifelong therapy, especially young women where the specific issue of the potential teratogenicity of the statins and family planning needs to be fully explored. Such clinics will have experience of other therapies that can prove helpful, including the bile acid sequestrants and LDL apheresis. Ezetimibe is a relatively new agent that works to reduce intestinal cholesterol absorption mediated by the recently described transporter Niemann Pick C-1 Like Protein 1 (NPC1L1); it is well tolerated and can augment the LDL reduction achieved by statins by a further 20% [17], but evidence that it is clinically effective in reducing CVD risk is still awaited. Tendon xanthomata and xanthelasmata may respond to the reduction in LDL cholesterol; corneal arcus does not. FH homozygotes must be referred for specialist assessment and treatment; their cholesterol does not respond well to statins or other drug therapies that work by up-regulating LDL receptor expression. These patients often require LDL apheresis and occasionally liver transplantation as well as coronary revascularization and aortic valve surgery [18].

References

1 Thannhauser SJ, Magendanta H. The different clinical groups of xanthomatous diseases: a clinical physiological study of 22 cases. *Ann Intern Med* 1938; **11**: 1662–746.

2 Müller C. Angina pectoris in hereditary xanthomatosis. *Arch Intern Med* 1939; **64**: 675–700.

3 Gofman JW, De Lalla O, Glazier F *et al*. The serum lipoprotein transport system in health, metabolic diseases, atherosclerosis and coronary artery disease. *Plasma* 1954; **2**: 413–84.

4 Goldstein JL, Brown MS. Familial hypercholesterolaemia: identification of a defect in the regulation of 3-hydroxy-3-methylglutaryl coenzyme A reductase activity associated with overproduction of cholesterol. *Proc Natn Acad Sci USA* 1973; **70**: 2804–8.

5 Slack J. Risks of ischaemic heart disease in familial hyperlipoproteinaemia states. *Lancet* 1969; **ii**: 1380–2.

6 Björkhem I, Boberg KM, Leitersdorf E. Inborn errors in bile acid biosynthesis and storage of sterols other than cholesterol. In: Scriver CR, Beaudet AL, Sly WS, Valle D, eds. *The Metabolic and Molecular Bases of Inherited Disease*, 8th edn. New York: McGraw-Hill, 2001: 2961–88.

7 Bhattacharyya AK, Conner WE. Beta-sitosterolaemia and xanthomatosis. *J Clin Invest* 1974; **53**: 1033–43.

8 Villeger L, Abifadel M, Allard D *et al*. The UMD-LDLR data-base: additions to the software and 490 new entries to the data-base. *Hum Mutat* 2002; **20**: 81–7.

9 Hobbs HH, Brown MS, Goldstein JL. Molecular genetics of the LDL receptor gene in familial hypercholesterolaemia. *Hum Mutat* 1992; **1**: 445–66.

10 Myant NB. Familial defective apolipoprotein B-100: a review, including some comparisons with familial hypercholesterolaemia. *Atherosclerosis* 1993; **104**: 1–19.

11 Timms KM, Wagner S, Samuels ME *et al*. A mutation in PCSK9 causing autosomal dominant hypercholesterolaemia in a Utah pedigree. *Hum Genet* 2004; **114**: 349–53.

12 Soutar AK, Nauomova RP, Traub LM. Genetics, clinical phenotype, and molecular cell biology of autosomal recessive hypercholesterolaemia. *Arterioscler Thromb Vasc Biol* 2003; **23**: 1963–70.

13 World Health Organization. *Familial Hypercholesterolaemia*. Report of a Second WHO Consultation. WHO publication no. WHO/HGN/FH/CONS/99.2, 1999.

14 Williams RR, Hunt SC, Schumacher MC *et al*. Diagnosing heterozygous familial hypercholesterolaemia using new practical criteria validated by molecular genetics. *Am J Cardiol* 1993; **72**: 171–6.

15 Neil HAW, Hawkins MM, Durrington PN *et al*. Non-coronary heart disease mortality and risk of fatal cancer in patients with treated heterozygous familial hypercholesterolaemia: a prospective study. *Atherosclerosis* 2005; **179**: 293–7.

16 NICE guideline CG71. Identification and management of familial hypercholesterolaemia. August 2008.

17 Davidson MH, McGarry T, Bettis R *et al*. Ezetimibe coadministered with Simvastatin in patients with primary hypercholesterolaemia. *J Am Coll Cardiol* 2002; **40**: 2125–34.

18 Naoumova RP, Thompson GR, Soutar AK. Current management of severe homozygous hypercholesterolaemias. *Curr Opin Lipidol* 2004; **15**: 413–22.

Combined dyslipidaemia

Type III hyperlipoproteinaemia

Clinical features. Type III hyperlipoproteinaemia merits discussion for several reasons. It may have been the first recognized disorder of lipoprotein metabolism; Addison and Gull reported a patient with its typical cutaneous hallmarks in 1851. It has a plethora of aliases (including broad-beta disease, dysbetalipoproteinaemia and remnant removal disease) reflecting the gradual emergence of our understanding of the biochemical basis of the condition. It is an excellent example of a disease resulting from a gene–environment interaction.

There are several skin manifestations of type III hyperlipoproteinaemia. The most characteristic are linear yellow-orange lipid deposits within the palmar creases and sometimes the flexor creases of the fingers and wrists. They are called striate palmar xanthomata (Fig. 59.66). Tuberous xanthomata are also common over the tuberosities of the elbows and knees (Fig. 59.65). They start as yellowish papules that gradually coalesce to form larger, sometimes exuberant, exophytic lesions. Where a central tuberous xanthoma is surrounded by several smaller lesions they are sometimes called tuberoeruptive xanthomata. They can also occur over the heel; being subcutaneous and yellow in colour they are not difficult to distinguish from Achilles tendon xanthomata. Patients with type III hyperlipoproteinaemia with particularly high triglyceride concentrations may also develop lipaemia retinalis and eruptive xanthomata over their buttocks (Fig. 59.67). Striate palmar and tuberous xanthomata can occasionally be seen in the paraproteinaemias and systemic lupus erythmatosus.

Estimates of the frequency of type III hyperlipoproteinaemia vary, reflecting the lack of clear diagnostic criteria, but range between about 1 and 10 in 10 000. There is evidence of an increased risk of both coronary artery and peripheral arterial disease, especially in those with all the clinical and biochemical features of the disorder in whom up to 50% have premature CVD [1]. Gout also appears common in this group of patients [2]. Type III hyperlipoproteinaemia has been associated with lipoprotein glomerulopathy, manifesting as proteinuria or the nephrotic syndrome [3]. Renal biopsy shows glomerular foam cells; the condition usually resolves with successful treatment of the abnormal lipid profile.

Biochemistry and genetics. Patients with type III hyperlipoproteinaemia have a characteristic lipoprotein electrophoretic pattern; indeed this remains the gold standard diagnostic test. There is an increase in small VLDL and IDL and a decrease in LDL. VLDL isolated from type III patients is uncharacteristically enriched with cholesterol esters and gives rise to a broad-β migrating band, rather than the usual pre-β band [4,5]. This results from an accumulation of VLDL remnants and chylomicron remnants and produces a marked increase in plasma total cholesterol and triglycerides. The underlying defect is an abnormal apoE [6], the apolipoprotein in remnant lipoproteins that mediates their binding to the LDL receptor and the LRP. There are three common isoforms of apo E: apo E2, E3 and E4, each differing by one amino acid (Table 59.18).

Apo E2 homozygosity represents by far the commonest abnormality associated with type III hyperlipoproteinaemia; its cysteine at residue 112 is within the receptor binding domain of the protein and its cysteine at residue 158 affects salt bridges within the protein and thereby the conformation of the receptor binding domain. Very occasionally, other apo E mutations are associated with type III hyperlipoproteinaemia, many of which severely reduce apo E mediated receptor binding and can cause the disorder in heterozygotes [7].

However, less than 10% of subjects homozygous for apo E2 develop type III hyperlipoproteinaemia, and most of the rest have lower than average lipid levels. It is clear that a second factor is required for the development of type III hyperlipoproteinaemia, either environmental or genetic. Increased production of chylomicrons or VLDL can be one such factor and may result from excessive caloric intake, increased alcohol consumption, obesity, type 2 diabetes mellitus, the metabolic syndrome or from an interplay of multiple genetic influences on lipoprotein metabolism (as presumed to underlie familial combined hyperlipidaemia (FCH)). Equally, increasing age, hypothyroidism or post-menopausal oestrogen deficiency can further impair apo E mediated receptor catabolism of lipoproteins and result in the development of the disorder.

Treatment. Identification and treatment of any contributing lifestyle factors or diseases is clearly central to the management of patients with type III hyperlipoproteinaemia. Patients should be screened for obesity, diabetes and hypothyroidism and treated accordingly. Dietary advice should be given and exercise, which increases the activity of lipoprotein lipase and thereby reduces chylomicron and VLDL remnant production, encouraged. Such measures are often successful in improving the lipid profile on their own; in their absence drug therapy is usually less effective. Normally both statins [8] and fibrates [9] work well, both in improving the lipid profile and also in causing regression of the palmar and tuberous xanthomata. Occasionally combined statin and fibrate therapy may be required.

References

1 Morganroth J, Levy RI, Fredrickson DS: The biochemical, clinical and genetic features of type III hyperlipoproteinaemia. *Ann Intern Med* 1975; **82**: 158–74.
2 Brewer HB, Zech LA, Gregg RE *et al.* Type III hyperlipoproteinaemia. Diagnosis, molecular defects, pathology and treatment. *Ann Intern Med* 1983; **98**: 623–40.
3 Yang AH, Ng YY, Tarng DC *et al.* Association of apolipoprotein E polymorphism with lipoprotein glomerulopathy. *Nephron* 1998; **78**: 266–70.
4 Gofman IW, Rubin L, McGinley JP, Jones HB. Hyperlipoproteinaemia. *Am J Med* 1954; **17**: 514–20.
5 Gofman IW, Rubin L, Lees RS. Fat transport in lipoproteins. An integrated approach to mechanisms and disorders. *N Engl J Med* 1967; **276**: 32–44, 94–103, 148–56, 215–26, 273–81.
6 Utermann G. Apolipoprotein E polymorphisms in health and disease. *Am Heart J* 1987; **113**: 433–40.
7 Mahley RW, Rall SC. Type III hyperlipoproteinaemia (dysbetalipoproteinaemia): the role of apolipoprotein E in normal and abnormal lipoprotein metabolism. In: Scriver CR, Beaudet AL, Sly WS, Valle D, eds. *The Metabolic and Molecular Bases of Inherited Disease*, 8th edn. New York: McGraw-Hill, 2001: 2835–62.
8 Vega GL, East C, Grundy SM. Lovastatin therapy in familial dysbetalipoproteinaemia: effects on kinetics of apolipoprotein B. *Atherosclerosis* 1988; **70**: 131–43.
9 Kuo PT, Wilson AC, Kostis JB *et al.* Treatment of type III hyperlipoproteinaemia with gemfibrozil to retard progression of coronary artery disease. *Am Heart J* 1988; **116**: 85–90.

Table 59.18 The amino acid differences between the isoforms of apo E.

	E2	E3	E4
Residue 112	Cysteine	Cysteine	Arginine
Residue 158	Cysteine	Arginine	Arginine

Hypertriglyceridaemias
Type I hyperlipoproteinaemia

Clinical, biochemical and genetic features. In type I hyperlipoproteinaemia there is an accumulation of chylomicrons alone. It results from a deficiency of lipoprotein lipase (LPL), and as such shows an autosomal recessive pattern of inheritance (though there is accumulating evidence that some heterozygotes for LPL deficiency may show a milder degree of hypertriglyceridaemia). The condition is extremely rare with a frequency of perhaps 1 per million in most populations, but with higher frequency in some populations such as French Canadians due to founder gene effects. An increasing number of mutations in the LPL gene have been described. Some cases result from apo CII deficiency, an essential factor for LPL activation; this discovery followed from the observation that the hyperchylomicronaemia was alleviated in some patients following plasma infusions [1].

Familial LPL deficiency causes extremely elevated levels of serum triglycerides, often greater than 20 mM. Total cholesterol levels are often substantially elevated as well, reflecting the extreme concentrations of chylomicrons which do contain some cholesterol and cholesterol esters as well as their predominant triglycerides. Blood, serum or plasma from such patients will appear milky and a creamy layer will separate on top of the sample if centrifuged or allowed to stand for some hours. Hyperchylomicronaemia will be present from childhood onwards in homozygous LPL deficiency. It remains unclear why LPL deficiency can cause an isolated accumulation of chylomicrons, given the role of the enzyme in VLDL catabolism. However, with increasing age there is a progressive shift towards a type V hyperlipoproteinaemic pattern (see below).

The principal concern in type I hyperlipoproteinaemia is the increased risk of acute pancreatitis with its attendant morbidity and mortality [2]. Whilst hypertriglyceridaemia may be a consequence of acute pancreatitis there is clear evidence it may also be a cause, perhaps accounting for up to 10% of cases. The risk increases with increasing fasting triglyceride levels, with a threshold around 10 mmol/L, rising markedly beyond 20 mmol/L, although other factors must play a part as some patients seem remarkably immune from attacks despite grossly elevated triglyceride concentrations. The mortality is further increased because the serum amylase, so often used as a sole diagnostic test for acute pancreatitis, may well not be elevated [3]. (It is possible that the very elevated triglyceride levels interfere with the amylase assay; dilution of the serum sample can sometimes reveal the raised amylase concentration.) As a result, many such patients have undergone laparotomy to establish the cause of their severe abdominal pain and the examination findings of generalized tenderness and guarding, with the consequent physical stress further exacerbating their hypertriglyceridaemia.

The characteristic skin finding in patients with type I hyperlipoproteinaemia is eruptive xanthomata (Fig. 59.67), yellowish papules several millimetres in diameter occurring over extensor surfaces, particularly the buttocks and the backs of the legs [4]. The rash may be itchy. It usually indicates triglyceride levels in excess of 20 mmol/L, and is seen with all causes of such severe hypertriglyceridaemia. It responds to lowering of the triglycerides, though it tends to last a few days longer than the lipid abnormality. Clearance of chylomicrons from the circulation by cells of the reticuloendothelial system can result in hepatomegaly and splenomegaly, with splenic infarcts in some cases. Lipaemia retinalis, with creamy yellow discoloration of the retinal arterioles and veins, can be seen on fundoscopy and in very severe hypertriglyceridaemia can appear almost fluorescent [5].

Treatment. The principal treatment of severe hypertriglyceridaemia involves strict restriction of all dietary fats (not just saturated fats) to reduce chylomicron production as much as possible [6]. Attention must be paid to any other factors that may increase the production of, or decrease the clearance of, the triglyceride rich lipoproteins (TRLs); good control of diabetes, weight reduction where appropriate, alcohol restriction and a review of all other medications are particularly important. Intake of refined carbohydrates should also be limited. Fibrates usually have little effect in genetic LPL deficiency. Nicotinic acid derivatives can be helpful. Bile acid sequestrants are contraindicated as they may increase the triglyceride level. Infusions of fresh frozen plasma are beneficial in those with apo CII deficiency who present with acute pancreatitis. Antioxidant therapy has proved very effective in reducing the frequency of attacks of acute pancreatitis in a number of patients with severe hypertriglyceridaemia [7]. All patients with severe hypertriglyceridaemia should have access to specialist lipid clinics.

References

1 Brunzell JD, Deeb SS. Familial lipoprotein lipase deficiency, apo CII deficiency and hepatic lipase deficiency. In: Scriver CR, Beaudet AL, Sly WS, Valle D, eds. *The Metabolic and Molecular Bases of Inherited Disease*, 8th edn. New York: McGraw-Hill, 2001: 2789–816.
2 Durrington PN, Twentyman OP, Braganza JM, Miller JP. Hypertriglyceridaemia and abnormalities of triglyceride metabolism persisting after pancreatitis. *Int J Pancreatol* 1996; **1**: 195–203.
3 Fallat RW, Vestor JW, Glueck CJ. Suppression of amylase activity by hypertriglyceridaemia. *JAMA* 1973; **225**: 1331–4.
4 Parker F, Bagdade JD, Odland GF, Bierman EL. Evidence for the chylomicron origin of lipids accumulating in diabetic eruptive xanthomas. A correlative lipid biochemical, histological and electron microscopic study. *J Clin Invest* 1970; **49**: 2172–87.
5 Holt LE, Aylward FX, Timbres HG. Idiopathic familial lipaemia. *Johns Hopkins Hosp Bull* 1939; **64**: 279–314.
6 Durrington PN. Hypertriglyceridaemia. In: *Hyperlipidaemia: Diagnosis and Management*, 3rd edn. London: Hodder Arnold, 2007: 169–202.
7 Heaney AP, Sharer N, Rameh B *et al*. Prevention of recurrent pancreatitis in patients with familial lipoprotein lipase deficiency with high dose antioxidant therapy. *J Clin Endocrinol Metab* 1999; **84**: 1203–5.

Type V hyperlipoproteinaemia

Clinical and biochemical features. Type V differs from type I hyperlipoproteinaemia in that there is an accumulation of VLDL as well as chylomicrons. It is also far commoner, perhaps affecting 1 in every 5–10000, and although it can result from LPL deficiency this only accounts for a very small proportion of cases. Patient samples will demonstrate some milkiness with the separation of a creamy layer after standing or centrifugation (made up of chylomicrons) but the serum or plasma will be opaque, representing the presence of VLDL. Patients with type V hyperlipoproteinaemia may have relatives with hypertriglyceridaemia as well, though many of these will have a type IV lipoprotein pattern (see below). This has led to the hypothesis that most type V patients have a reasonably marked defect in the catabolism of TRLs combined with some additional factor that either further decreases catabolism or additionally increases the production of TRLs. Such factors include obesity, poor diabetic control, alcohol consumption, pregnancy, drugs (oral contraceptives, highly-active antiretroviral therapy, β-blockers and thiazide diuretics being the main offenders), hypothyroidism, lipodystrophy and renal failure.

Lipid levels in type V hyperlipoproteinaemia may be as markedly elevated as in type I. Acute pancreatitis, eruptive xanthomata, hepatosplenomegaly, lipaemia retinalis and all the other clinical features of type I hyperlipoproteinaemia may be present. Additionally, hyperuricaemia, glucose intolerance and hepatic steatosis are often seen.

Treatment. The treatment of type V hyperlipoproteinaemia is exactly as for type I, though fibrates are generally far more effective.

Type IV hyperlipoproteinaemia

Clinical and biochemical features. In type IV hyperlipoproteinaemia VLDL accumulate but without any increase in chylomicrons. The degree of hypertriglyceridaemia is usually much less marked than in type I or type V hyperlipoproteinaemia, with many patients having fasting triglycerides less than 6 mmol/L and most less than 10 mmol/L. Patients with type IV hyperlipoproteinaemia are heterogeneous, the common abnormality being an increased production of VLDL by the liver [1], often accompanied by a partial defect in their catabolism [2]. As with other forms of hypertriglyceridaemia, LDL tend to be smaller and denser, a pattern of abnormalities associated with increased cardiovascular risk. Apart from those rare type IV patients with marked hypertriglyceridaemia, the clinical features of type I and type V hyperlipoproteinaemia are not present.

Treatment. Lifestyle modification along the lines of that advocated for severe hypertriglyceridaemia (see above) is appropriate for type IV hyperlipoproteinaemia. However, dietary fat restriction does not have to be so marked, and can be mainly restricted to saturated fats. Indeed intake of omega-3 unsaturated fatty acids may be beneficial. The need for drug therapy will largely be guided by estimations of the 10-year CVD risk; many type IV patients will require such treatment and the first line will often be the statins because of their proven efficacy in reducing that risk, even though they do not usually much affect hypertriglyceridaemia.

References

1 Brunzell JD, Albers JJ, Chait AI *et al*. Plasma lipoproteins in familial combined hyperlipidaemia and monogenic familial hypertriglyceridaemia. *J Lipid Res* 1983; **24**: 147–55.

2 Krauss RH, Levy RI, Fredrickson RS. Selective measurement of two lipase activities in postheparin plasma from normal subjects and patients with hyperlipoproteinaemia. *J Clin Invest* 1974; **54**: 1107–24.

Other primary dyslipidaemias [1,2]

Cerebrotendinous xanthomatosis

This autosomal recessive condition is a rare cause of tendon xanthomata and xanthelasmata. It results from a defect in sterol 27-hydroxylase with consequent increased production of cholestanol and 7-hydroxycholesterol which accumulate in plasma and throughout the body. Accumulation in the central nervous system causes myelin destruction leading to mental retardation, seizures, spasticity and ataxia; peripheral neuropathy results from similar pathology in the peripheral nervous system. Presentation occurs during childhood or early adult life. Early-onset cataracts, diarrhoea and premature osteoporosis are additional features. Patients are at risk of cardiovascular disease, although plasma cholesterol levels are normal. Treatment with chenodeoxycholate reduces plasma cholestanol concentrations and improves the neurological manifestations of the disease.

Sitosterolaemia

This is another rare, autosomal recessive cause of tendon and tuberous xanthomata. It results from mutations in the genes *ABCG5* or *ABCG8* which encode the proteins sterolin-1 and sterolin-2 in enterocytes and hepatocytes. Sterolin-1 and sterolin-2 act together to form a lipid transporter that is thought to facilitate immediate excretion of any plant sterols absorbed across the small intestinal brush border. Defective function thereby allows much increased absorption of plant sterols into the body, principally β-sitosterol but also sitostanol, campesterol and stigmasterol. Patients suffer from impaired growth, anaemia, thrombocytopenia and arthritis and are at risk of premature CVD. Diagnosis is made by measuring serum plant sterol concentrations. It has recently been shown that ezetimibe reduces plant sterol levels effectively in this condition, suggesting a role for the Niemann–Pick C1-like protein in plant sterol transport in the intestine.

Tangier disease

In Tangier disease cholesterol esters accumulate in foam cells throughout the reticuloendothelial system. Clinically, this manifests most consistently as enlarged, yellow-orange tonsils, but similar deposits can also be seen in the rectal mucosa and generalized lymphadenopathy and hepatosplenomegaly can be found. Thrombocytopenia is a frequent finding, resulting usually from a combination of hypersplenism and foam cell infiltration of the bone marrow. Peripheral neuropathy and corneal opacities have also been described; the latter only evident on slit-lamp examination. The biochemical hallmark of Tangier disease is a low level of HDL-cholesterol with near complete absence of apo AI. Total cholesterol levels are also lower than average, partly because of the low HDL cholesterol but LDL cholesterol is also usually reduced. The disease results from mutations in the gene coding for ABCA1; this discovery led to the elucidation of the role of this lipid transporter in cellular cholesterol efflux, the first step in reverse cholesterol transport. It has been shown that the majority of HDL cholesterol arises from expression of ABCA1 in the liver, and that if liver ABCA1 is defective the newly secreted discoidal apo AI/AIV particles cannot be stabilized by incorporating cholesterol, are rapidly cleared by the kidney and cannot participate in peripheral cellular cholesterol efflux. (It is striking how much of our understanding of human lipoprotein metabolism has come from studies of rare dyslipidaemias.) Although there are reports of premature CVD in Tangier disease, this does not seem as common as might be expected from the low levels of HDL cholesterol.

References

1 Björkhem I, Boberg KM, Leitersdorf E. Inborn errors in bile acid biosynthesis and storage of sterols other than cholesterol. In: Scriver CR, Beaudet AL, Sly WS, Valle D, eds. *The Metabolic and Molecular Bases of Inherited Disease,* 8th edn. New York: McGraw-Hill, 2001: 2961–88.
2 Assmann G, von Eckardstein A, Brewer HB. Familial analphalipoproteinaemia: Tangier Disease. In: Scriver CR, Beaudet AL, Sly WS, Valle D, eds. *The Metabolic and Molecular Bases of Inherited Disease,* 8th edn. New York: McGraw-Hill, 2001: 2937–60.

Secondary dyslipidaemias [1]

Dyslipidaemias are frequently secondary to, or exacerbated by, a range of other diseases or medications. The following account is far from exhaustive but will concentrate on those that may produce xanthomata or follow from the use of drugs used by dermatologists.

Perhaps the commonest cause of secondary dyslipidaemia at present is diabetes mellitus. Type 1 diabetics frequently have quite high HDL cholesterol levels, but they also have a number of abnormalities of their LDL and VLDL and they are at high CVD risk. Type 2 diabetics have insulin resistance; their typical lipid profile includes relatively normal total and LDL cholesterol levels, but often somewhat increased triglyceride and reduced HDL cholesterol concentrations. These quantitative abnormalities are usually accompanied by qualitative changes in the LDL with a preponderance of highly atherogenic small dense LDL. As a result, type 2 diabetics are also at high risk of developing premature CVD. It is now recommended that statins should be considered for all diabetics over the age of 40 years, and in younger diabetic patients with other CVD risk factors including microalbuminuria. In some patients the development of type 2 diabetes, or worsening of its glycaemic control, can cause marked hypertriglyceridaemia (with a type IV or V hyperlipoproteinaemia) with all its clinical features including eruptive xanthomata, lipaemia retinalis and acute pancreatitis. This is most likely to occur on the background of some mild defect of triglyceride-rich lipoprotein clearance, and may be further exacerbated by the concomitant presence of obesity and excess alcohol intake. Diabetes can also precipitate the development of type III hyperlipoproteinaemia in those with the appropriate genetic background (usually homozygosity for apo E2); such patients may present to a dermatologist with the typical xanthomata of this condition. It follows that in any patient presenting with eruptive, tuberous or planar xanthomata a fasting glucose and/or HbA1c should be requested along with the lipid profile and other appropriate tests.

Patients with insulin resistance, but without type 2 diabetes mellitus, have a similar combined dyslipidaemia. In some a marked hypertriglyceridaemia can develop, sufficient to cause eruptive xanthomata. This is seen quite commonly in the lipodystrophies, a group of disorders with either partial or generalized loss of subcutaneous fat. They can be inherited (e.g. Dunnigan–Köbberling syndrome) or acquired. The latter is now most commonly seen in patients with human immunodeficiency virus/acquired immunedeficiency syndrome (HIV/AIDS) who are having treatment with protease inhibitors, especially saquinavir and ritonavir. Management of lipodystrophy-associated dyslipidaemia is likely to require specialist input; the principles are lifestyle change, especially strict dietary fat restriction in hypertriglyceridaemia, optimization of the drug regimen in HIV, and judicious, monitored use of lipid-modulating drug therapy, given the potential for significant interactions between statins, fibrates and the antiretroviral agents.

It has already been noted that xanthelasmata can be a feature of chronic cholestasis. This can occur, for example, in primary biliary cirrhosis and the presence of xanthelasmata should prompt a request for blood tests including a bilirubin and an alkaline phosphatase at least. Long-standing cholestasis is associated with hypercholesterolaemia due to the accumulation of an abnormal lipoprotein, lipoprotein X. It remains unclear whether this dyslipidaemia increases CVD risk, but it can cause a wide range of xanthomata as well as xanthelasmata. Both the dyslipidaemia and the xanthomata improve with relief of biliary obstruction; where this is not possible bile acid sequestrants can be helpful (and may also relieve the pruritus associated with cholestasis). Where necessary statins can be used, but cautiously to avoid accumulation and toxicity. Hepatocellular liver disease leads to specific lipoprotein abnormalities, principally abnormal HDL secondary to progressive deficiency of lecithin-cholesterol acyl transferase with mild hypertriglyceridaemia, but these are not usually severe enough to cause xanthomata.

Nephrotic syndrome is complicated by hypercholesterolaemia or a combined dyslipidaemia that can prove difficult to treat. Hypertriglyceridaemia is not usually marked though occasionally a type IV hyperlipoproteinaemia may occur. Xanthomata are not a frequent feature and the dyslipidaemia resolves if the nephrotic syndrome responds to therapy. Chronic renal failure leads to hypertriglyceridaemia, often exacerbated by haemodialysis or peritoneal dialysis, and this can sometimes lead to eruptive xanthomata especially if other risk factors are present. Lipoprotein(a) levels are elevated and may contribute to the increased CVD risk in this population but do not produce any dermatological signs.

The characteristic xanthomata associated with the paraproteinaemias (planar xanthomata and necrobiotic xanthogranuloma) have been discussed earlier. Their presence does not necessarily reflect a measurable dyslipidaemia, though a hyperlipoproteinaemia similar to type III may be present. The pathophysiology underlying paraproteinaemia-associated xanthomata and dyslipidaemia remains unclear although lipoprotein–immunoglobulin complexes are a common finding, usually involving VLDL. These abnormalities have occasionally also been reported in lymphoma and systemic lupus erythematosus. Very rarely, immunoglobulins directed against the LDL receptor can produce a hypercholesterolaemia with total and LDL cholesterol levels similar to those seen in FH homozygotes but without any tendon xanthomata. This has been referred to as 'pseudo familial hypercholesterolaemia'.

Many drugs can produce dyslipidaemia, alcohol perhaps being the commonest example and a frequent contributor to marked hypertriglyceridaemia. Of the prescription drugs used by dermatologists it is worth considering corticosteroids, ciclosporin and retinoic acid derivatives. Systemic corticosteroids increase total, LDL and HDL cholesterol levels. Unless they precipitate diabetes mellitus in a susceptible individual, they do not cause hypertriglyceridaemia. Ciclosporin increases LDL cholesterol levels, sometimes quite significantly. It also inhibits cytochrome P450 3A4, the isoform responsible for the metabolism of fluvastatin, simvastatin and atorvastatin, so patients taking these statins should be advised of the possible interaction and the risk of myalgia. In some patients (e.g. those with hepatic or renal impairment, or taking other drugs that affect CYP450 3A4), it may be appropriate to reduce the statin dose or to change to an alternative (pravastatin or rosuvastatin are less dependent on CYP450 3A4). Retinoic acid derivatives often induce hypertriglyceridaemia; this is usually mild and does not necessarily require anything other than dietary modification. Occasionally, however, marked hypertriglyceridaemia with a type IV or V hyperlipoproteinaemic pattern can be provoked—usually in a susceptible individual who may well have evidence of dyslipidaemia prior to treatment. It is therefore sensible to include a full lipid profile on any pre-treatment blood tests and to repeat this several weeks after starting any retinoids.

Reference

1 Durrington PN. Secondary hyperlipidaemia. In: Durrington PN, *Hyperlipidaemia: Diagnosis and Management,* 3rd edn. London: Hodder Arnold, 2007: 310–59.

Treatment [1]. Treatment of dyslipidaemia requires the identification and treatment of any secondary cause, dietary modification and drug therapy in appropriate cases. The mainstay of dietary therapy is a reduction in the total intake of fat, especially saturated fat. Associated dietary interventions that are worthwhile include increasing the intake of monounsaturated and omega-3 unsaturated fatty acids and of antioxidant vitamins (found in fresh fruit and vegetables); these may not alter the standard lipid profile but some do cause qualitative differences in various lipoproteins and they are of benefit in reducing cardiovascular risk. The only exception to this is in cases of severe hypertriglyceridaemia where all fat intake must be severely restricted (to 20–25 g per day) to reduce intestinal chylomicron production. Given that one of the principal aims of treating dyslipidaemia is to reduce CVD risk, dietary therapy should be accompanied by discussion of exercise, smoking cessation and weight optimization.

Statins are the most effective and best tolerated of the drugs available that reduce cholesterol levels. They act by inhibiting 3-hydroxy, 3-methyl-glutaryl CoA reductase, the rate-limiting step in intracellular cholesterol biosynthesis, with a consequent up-regulation of hepatic LDL receptor expression and increased clearance of LDL from the circulation. Throughout the various statin trials there has been a highly consistent relationship between the absolute reduction achieved in the LDL cholesterol level and the relative reduction in cardiovascular risk; other means of lowering LDL cholesterol levels (e.g. bile acid sequestrants and ileal resection) produce a strikingly similar relationship though based on a much smaller body of evidence. The role of statins in treating FH has already been discussed; they should also be offered to all patients with clinical cardiovascular disease, to all diabetics aged over 40 years (and to diabetics under age 40 years with other CVD risk factors including microalbuminuria), to patients with other diseases that predispose to CVD (e.g. renal failure, metabolic syndrome, rheumatoid arthritis, etc.), or to anyone whose 10-year CVD risk exceeds 20% after lifestyle modification. Some patients

do develop muscle problems with statin therapy; it is wise to inform patients of this possibility when starting or changing statins, with the advice that if they develop widespread muscle ache or pain they should stop the drug and seek medical review. Risk factors for developing myalgia include high statin dose, hepatic or renal impairment and co-administration of drugs that inhibit cytochrome enzymes. Females of child-bearing age should be counselled about the potential teratogenicity of the statins; current advice is that they should stop the statins 1 month before starting to try to conceive and that if they do become pregnant while taking a statin they should be seen urgently in a specialist lipid clinic. Liver enzymes should be monitored periodically after introducing statins.

Bile acid sequestrants lower total and LDL cholesterol but rather less effectively than statins. Nonetheless they have been shown to reduce CVD risk. They have the advantage that they are not absorbed from the intestine, where they work by binding the bile acids resulting from hepatic cholesterol catabolism and preventing their reabsorption in the terminal ileum. They therefore do not cause myalgia or abnormal liver function tests and are safe during pregnancy and breastfeeding. However, they have the disadvantage of being unpleasant to take and do cause gastrointestinal side effects. Ezetimibe is the latest agent that reduces total and LDL cholesterol. It works by blocking the newly described intestinal lipid transporter Niemann–Pick C1 like protein. It is well tolerated. Evidence that it reduces CVD risk is still awaited, so it remains a second- or third-line agent for those unable to tolerate statins or bile acid sequestrants or who fail to achieve satisfactory lipid profiles with them. It is the drug of choice for sitosterolaemia.

Fibrates are also well tolerated. They are now known to exert their multiple effects as agonists of peroxisome proliferators-activated receptor α (PPAR-α). Their main lipid effect is to reduce triglyceride levels by decreasing VLDL, and they also reduce β-VLDL in type III hyperlipoproteinaemia. They can increase HDL cholesterol. Trial evidence of their overall clinical effect is mixed; some trials have certainly shown reduced CVD risk with fibrates but others have not and there are as yet no clear data that they reduce overall mortality. Their main clinical role is in the treatment of severe hypertriglyceridaemia and of type III hyperlipoproteinaemia. They can also improve the lipid profile of those type 2 diabetic patients whose CVD risk remains high and largely driven by high triglycerides and low HDL cholesterol despite optimal statin therapy. Such combination therapy seems to run a lower risk of myalgia, myositis and rhabdomyolysis than once thought, but should be instituted in a clinic with experience of its monitoring. Clinical trials of statin–fibrate co-administration are under way. Fibrates can increase the serum creatinine and potentiate oral anticoagulants so renal function and INR need to be checked after initiation.

For some time, high-dose nicotinic acid has been known to have very favourable effects on the lipid profile. It lowers total and LDL cholesterol and triglycerides, increases HDL cholesterol more than any of the other drugs so far discussed and is the only drug that significantly reduces lipoprotein(a) levels. The mechanisms by which it achieves these changes are largely unknown. However, its clinical use has been much limited by its side effects: severe flushing especially at higher doses, hyperglycaemia (a particular issue for the diabetics whose lipid profile might best be helped by it), and worsening of peptic ulcer disease. A couple of trials have found a reduction in CVD or atherosclerosis progression, either in combination with diet or statins. A new preparation of nicotinic acid (Niaspan®) does seem to have a reduced tendency to cause flushing or hyperglycaemia; this is also shortly to be combined with a prostaglandin D2 receptor-1 antagonist, which promises further improvements in tolerability. At present, use of nicotinic acid derivatives remains largely confined to specialist lipid clinics.

Reference

1 Durrington PN. Lipid-modifying therapy. In: Durrington PN, *Hyperlipidaemia: Diagnosis and Management*, 3rd edn. London: Hodder Arnold, 2007: 258–91.

Conclusion

Dyslipidaemias may present to dermatologists because they may cause subcutaneous and other lipid deposits collectively known as xanthomata. Not all such xanthomata are associated with abnormal circulating lipids, but where they are the underlying dyslipidaemia is likely to be severe and to require therapy that can reduce the risks of acute pancreatitis (in severe hypertriglyceridaemia) and of premature cardiovascular disease. Appropriate recognition of xanthomata and identification and management of any underlying dyslipidaemia can therefore be as effective a life saver as DC cardioversion during an acute MI in the Emergency Department—and more timely!

Disorders of amino-acid metabolism

There is a very wide array of disorders of the metabolism of the amino acids. This section will concentrate on those with significant cutaneous components in their presentation.

Hyperphenylalaninaemia syndromes

These syndromes result from defective hydroxylation of phenylalanine to tyrosine, with the consequent accumulation of phenylalanine in plasma, since this is the principal pathway for the breakdown of phenylalanine. This reaction is catalysed by phenylalanine hydroxylase (PAH) and requires the presence of the cofactor tetrahydrobiopterin (BH_4), which is itself converted to 4α-hydroxytetrahydropterin (also called 4α-carbinolamine) in the process. BH_4 is restored by the sequential action of 4α-carbinolamine dehydratase and dihydropterin reductase (DHPR). Synthesis of BH_4 from guanosine triphosphate (GTP) is catalysed by GTP-cyclohydrolase and 6-pyruvoyl tetrahydopterin synthase (6-PTS). The commonest clinical hyperphenylalaninaemia syndrome is phenylketonuria.

Phenylketonuria (MIM *261600)

Synonyms
- Hyperphenylalaninaemia type I
- Folling's disease
- Phenylpyruvic oligophrenia

Phenylketonuria (PKU) is a rare inherited disease defined by plasma phenylalanine levels exceeding $1000\,\mu mol/L$ (normal range less than $120\,\mu mol/L$). (Patients with phenylalanine levels above the normal range but less than the defining concentration are described as having non-PKU hyperphenylalaninaemia.) PKU can be caused by primary deficiency of PAH, reduced BH_4 recycling secondary to DHPR deficiency (PKU2, MIM *261630), or impaired BH_4 synthesis secondary to GTP-cyclohydrolase or 6-PTS deficiency (MIM *261640). PAH deficiency is the commonest of these and causes 'classical' PKU; impaired BH_4 metabolism can cause plasma phenylalanine levels in excess of $1000\,\mu mol/L$, thus satisfying the biochemical diagnostic criterion for PKU, but the clinical course and treatment show some significant deviations from 'classical' PKU.

Aetiology [1,2]. Inheritance of PKU is autosomal recessive with an overall incidence of one in 8–12 000 live births. One in 50 individuals carry one of the mutant alleles. The genotype is markedly heterogeneous, PAH deficiency itself being caused by over 400 mutations at the PAH locus on chromosome 12q22–q24.1 [1]. The *DHPR* gene has been localized to chromosome 4 band 15.1p16.1 [1,3]. BH_4 deficiency is linked to three other loci: one on chromosome 4 and the others unmapped to date [3,4]. In PAH deficiency, hyperphenylalaninaemia requires exposure to phenylalanine, but in deficiencies of BH_4 recycling or synthesis PKU arises in the presence of the mutation alone. The usual gene dose effects are seen in heterozygotes.

In PKU, the accumulation of phenylalanine is accompanied by high levels of other derivatives of phenylalanine (such as phenylethylamine and phenylpyruvate, formed by decarboxylation and transamination, respectively) but there is ample evidence that it is the hyperphenylalaninaemia that is directly pathogenic. Tyrosine deficiency will reduce the availability of its metabolites, including acetoacetate and fumarate which contribute to the pool of two-carbon metabolites and glucose, so could contribute to impaired brain development. The oxidation rate in the brain is probably diminished but, although degenerative changes have been described in the cortex and basal ganglia and in the liver, they are inconstant [5–7]. In fact, there is little evidence of tyrosine deficiency in PKU, and tyrosine supplementation makes no impact on cognitive function. However, the reduction of melanin formation in the hair may be due to the inhibition of tyrosine–tyrosinase reaction by phenylalanine, and the hair will darken if large amounts of tyrosine are ingested. Disorders of BH_4 synthesis and recycling have additional pathological effects secondary to impaired tryptophan and tyrosine hydroxylation, as well as those secondary to hyperphenylalaninaemia.

Clinical features [1,5–7]. The clinical phenotype of PKU should now be a thing of the past because the damaging features of the disease can be reduced or prevented with early diagnosis and treatment. Affected infants are of average height and weight at birth, but thereafter show variable developmental delay. Unless diagnosis is made early, they present with psychomotor delay in early childhood leading on to mental retardation and often the need for long-term institutional care. Brain phenylalanine levels may better predict intellectual impairment than plasma concentrations. About 50% have epilepsy, and extrapyramidal manifestations, such as athetosis and exaggerated tendon reflexes, may be found. The electroencephalogram is abnormal in 80% of patients and correlates with the metabolic phenotype. Magnetic resonance imaging has demonstrated changes consistent with disturbance in the water content of the white matter. It is not clear whether these are of clinical significance [8].

Recent studies have suggested that other clinical features previously associated with PKU may not be linked. However, patients almost invariably have fair skin and hair (due to impaired melanin synthesis). The fair and sensitive skin readily develops eczema. This may be of the atopic variety. Although clinical light sensitivity has been reported, the ability to tan and the erythemal response to UV radiation are normal [9]. The incidence of pyogenic infections is increased. Scleroderma-like lesions with involvement of the muscles have been described [10]. Eye abnormalities associated with hypopigmentation may occur [1,11]. Impaired physical growth affects the head circumference and height (abnormal long bone metaphyseal endplates) in the untreated condition [7,11].

There is clear evidence that in mothers with PKU, phenylalanine crosses the placental barrier (along a concentration gradient) causing impaired growth, congenital malformations, microcephaly, epilepsy or mental deficiency in the fetus [6]. Treatment is therefore recommended before conception and during pregnancy.

Diagnosis. Newborn screening is the established way to determine hyperphenylalaninaemia (HPA); plasma phenylalanine determination is far more sensitive than urine testing for phenylpyruvate and it is recommended that screening is performed on blood samples during the first week of life [12]. The most widely used method is based on the Guthrie test [13]. The test is performed on a dried capillary blood sample collected on filter paper and analysed by microbiological inhibition assay (Guthrie) or by chromatography, fluorimetry or tandem mass spectrometry. The latter test has few false negatives. Where hyperphenylalaninaemia is detected it is appropriate also to establish whether this is secondary to PAH deficiency or to abnormal BH$_4$ metabolism as the latter will require specific therapy to limit disease expression.

Prenatal diagnosis. Indications for this are uncertain, as treatment is experimental. Families at risk can have prenatal diagnosis by a combination of DNA analysis, enzyme activity, or amniocyte or chorion villus sample metabolite levels [1,3,12]. There are advantages to gene testing by DNA analysis, if alleles have been identified in an affected family member.

Treatment [5–19]. The aim of treatment is to normalize phenylalanine levels as soon and for as long as possible, and particularly during pregnancy. It is vital that the diagnosis is made early so that a low phenylalanine diet can be instituted immediately to avoid cerebral damage produced by high blood phenylalanine levels. Blood phenylalanine levels are routinely measured to monitor treatment. The diet is selectively restricted in phenylalanine to about 250–550 mg/day to keep the plasma phenylalanine level below the toxic range [20], and may need supplementation with tyrosine/tryptophan. The aim is to keep the plasma phenyl-

alanine as low as possible and certainly less than 480 µmol/L. Phenylalanine is monitored twice weekly in the neonate, weekly in infants, 2–3 weekly in toddlers and ideally monthly thereafter even during adult life. This can now be achieved using dried blood spot samples. Particularly careful dietary treatment is necessary before conception and during pregnancy to reduce the risk of congenital heart disease [21–23] and abnormal brain development. Twice-weekly sampling blood tests are ideal to maintain levels of 100–250 µmol/L. There is evidence that reduction in maternal phenylalanine levels during pregnancy results in neonates with a higher birth weight [24].

The diet is based on a synthetic substitute for most of the dietary protein and should be continued throughout adult life as it has now been established that neurological sequelae can develop in the untreated affected adult [1,21,22,24,25]. Unfortunately, the response to dietary treatment is variable despite early and careful control. The amount of phenylalanine supplied in the diet should be low enough to prevent its accumulation in the blood, but high enough to allow protein synthesis and growth. Foods are given on an exchange basis using tables to indicate food with 1 g protein (equivalent 50 mg phenylalanine). Close collaboration with a metabolic dietician is an integral part of a successful treatment regimen and food diaries can also be helpful.

References

1 Scriver CR, Kaufman S. The hyperphenylalaninemias. In: Scriver CR, Beaudet AL, Sly WS, Valle D, eds. *The Metabolic and Molecular Bases of Inherited Disease,* 8th edn. New York: McGraw-Hill, 2001: 1677–725.
2 Scriver CR, Eisensmith RC, Woo SLC, Kaufman S. The hyperphenylalaninemias of man and mouse. *Annu Rev Genet* 1994; **28**: 141–65.
3 Guttler F, Guldberg P. Mutations in the phenylalanine hydroxylase gene. Genetic determinants for the phenotypic variability of hyperphenylalaninemia. *Acta Paediatr Suppl* 1994; **407**: 49–56.
4 Lidsky AS, Law ML, Morse HG *et al.* Regional mapping of the phenylalanine hydroxylase gene and the phenylketonuria locus in the human genome. *Proc Natl Acad Sci USA* 1985; **82**: 6221–5.
5 Smith I. Phenylketonuria due to phenylalanine hydroxylase deficiency, an unfolding story. Report of MRC Working Party on PKU. *BMJ* 1993; **306**: 115–9.
6 Tourian A, Sidbury JB. Phenylketonuria and hyperphenylalaninemia. In: Stanbury JB, Wyngaarden JB, Friedrickson DS, eds. *The Metabolic Basis of Inherited Disease,* 5th edn. New York: McGraw-Hill, 1983: 270–86.
7 Pitt DB, Danks DM. The natural history of untreated phenylketonuria. *J Paediatr Child Health* 1991; **27**: 189–90.
8 Cleary MA, Walter JH, Wraith JE *et al.* Magnetic resonance imaging of the brain in phenylketonuria. *Lancet* 1994; **344**: 87–90.
9 Hassell CW, Brunsting LA. Phenylpyruvic oligophrenia: an evaluation of the light-sensitive and pigmentary characteristics of seventeen patients. *Arch Dermatol* 1959; **79**: 458–65.
10 Jablonska S, Stachow A, Suffczynska M. Skin and muscle indurations in phenylketonuria. *Arch Dermatol* 1967; **95**: 443–50.
11 Walter JH. Late effects of phenylketonuria. *Arch Dis Child* 1995; **73**: 485–6.
12 MRC Working Party on Phenylketonuria. Present status of different mass screening procedures for phenylketonuria. *BMJ* 1968; **3**: 7–13.
13 Guthrie R, Susi A. A simple phenylalanine method for detecting phenylketonuria in large populations of newborn infants. *Pediatrics* 1963; **32**: 338–43.
14 Blaskovics ME, Schaeffler GE, Hack S. Phenylalaninaemia: differential diagnosis. *Arch Dis Child* 1974; **49**: 835–43.
15 Smith I. Treatment of phenylalanine hydroxylase deficiency. *Acta Paediatr* (Suppl.) 1994; **407**: 60–5.
16 Beasley MG, Costello PM, Smith I. Outcome of treatment in young adults with phenylketonuria detected by routine neonatal screening between 1964 and 1971. *QJM* 1994; **87**: 155–60.

17 Giovannini M, Biasucci G, Agostoni C et al. Lipid status and fatty acid metabolism in phenylketonuria. *J Inherit Metab Dis* 1995; **18**: 265–72.

18 Eisensmith RC, Woo SL. Gene therapy for phenylketonuria. *Acta Paediatr Suppl* 1994; **407**: 124–9.

19 Sutherland BS, Umbarger B, Berry HK. The treatment of phenylketonuria: a decade of results. *Am J Dis Child* 1966; **111**: 505–23.

20 Smith I. Recommendations on dietary management of phenylalanine. Report of MRC Working Party on phenylketonuria. *Arch Dis Child* 1993; **68**: 426–7.

21 Brenton DP, Hasler ME. Maternal phenylketonuria. In: Fernandes J, Saudubray JM, Tada K, eds. *Inborn Metabolic Diseases, Diagnosis and Management*. Berlin: Springer-Verlag, 1990: 175.

22 Dobblelaere D, Michaud L, Debrabander A et al. Evaluation of nutritional status and pathophysiology of growth retardation in patients with phenylketonuria. *J Inherit Metab Dis* 2003; **26**: 1–11.

23 Platt LD, Koch R, Azen C et al. Maternal phenylketonuria collaborative study, obstetric aspects and outcome: the first six years. *Am Obstet Gynecol* 1992; **166**: 1150–60.

24 Lenke R, Levy HL. Maternal phenylketonuria and hyperphenylalaninaemia. *New Engl J Med* 1980; **303**: 1202–8.

25 Burgard P, Link R, Schweitzer-Krantz S. Phenylketonuria: evidence-based clinical practice. Summary of the roundtable discussion. *Eur J Pediatr* 2000; **159** (Suppl. 2): S163–8.

Non-PKU hyperphenylalaninaemia (types II and III)

Where phenylalanine levels are raised but do not exceed 1000 μmol/L the patient is described as having non-PKU hyperphenylalaninaemia [1]. The clinical spectrum of this condition ranges from the apparently normal infant to those indistinguishable from classical PKU. There is a general correlation between PAH activity and blood levels of phenylalanine [2]. Accurate classification usually requires testing with phenylalanine loading and measurement of metabolites [3,4]. Treatment needs to be modified according to the severity of the enzyme deficiency, but essentially is as for PKU.

References

1 Scriver CR, Kaufman S. The hyperphenylalaninaemias. In: Scriver CR, Beaudet AL, Sly WS, Valle D, eds. *The Metabolic and Molecular Bases of Inherited Disease*, 8th edn. New York: McGraw-Hill, 2001: 1667–725.

2 Kang ES, Kaufman S, Gerald PS. Clinical and biochemical observations of patients with atypical phenylketonuria. *Pediatrics* 1970; **45**: 83–92.

3 Güttler F. Hyperphenylalaninaemia: diagnosis and classification of the various types of phenylalanine hydroxylase deficiency in childhood. *Acta Paediatr Suppl* 1980; **280**: 1–80.

4 Williamson M, Dobson JC, Koch R. Collaborative study of children treated for phenylketonuria: study design. *Pediatrics* 1977; **60**: 815–21.

Hyperphenylalaninaemia (types IV and V)

Hyperphenylalaninaemia types IV and V are due to deficiencies of tetrahydrobiopterin (BH$_4$) recycling or synthesis [1]. Together they account for 1–2% of all hyperphenylalaninaemias; failure of BH$_4$ recycling results from deficiency of dihydopteridine reductase (DHPR) and failure of synthesis from deficiency of either GTP cyclohydrase or 6-pyruvoyl tetrahydropterin synthase (6-PTS), the latter being about 20 times as common as the former.

Patients lacking DHPR have hyperphenylalaninaemia and other metabolic abnormalities reflecting the wide range of effects of DHPR [2]. They have defects of folate metabolism and are deficient in those neurotransmitters whose synthesis is dependent on tyrosine and tryptophan hydroxylation. They therefore have low urinary and cerebrospinal fluid levels of vanillyl mandelic acid (derived from norepinephrine), homovanillic acid (from dopamine) and 5-hydroxyindoleacetic acid (from 5-hydroxytryptamine). Treatment should aim to reduce plasma phenylalanine and to correct deficiencies of monoamines and folate metabolism. Thus the standard PKU diet should be instituted, together with supplementation of L-dopa (10–12 mg/kg/day) and 5-hydroxytryptophan (8–10 mg/kg/day) administered with a peripheral dopa decarboxylase inhibitor (e.g. carbidopa) to prevent nausea. Folinic acid (12.5 mg/day) is the recommended method of restoring normal folate balance. Early diagnosis is essential as in the absence of specific treatment there will be rapid neurological deterioration despite a low phenylalanine diet, and the earlier specific treatment starts the better the outcome. As the clinical picture is initially indistinguishable from PKU, biochemical diagnosis is required; urine screening for monoamine derivatives may help increase the suspicion of DHPR deficiency but direct assay of DHPR activity is now available and is the only reliable way to confirm or refute the diagnosis [3].

Patients with GTP cyclohydrolase deficiency have defective BH$_4$ synthesis [1]. They present with a progressive neurological disease with extrapyramidal features, mental retardation, seizures and occasional hyperthermia. Biochemically they have low levels of neopterin and biopterin as expected from a defect early in the biopterin synthetic pathway. Diagnosis can be confirmed by assaying GTP cyclohydrolase activity. Treatment with BH$_4$ as soon as possible is recommended, though the disorder is sufficiently rare that secure outcome data are not yet available. A commoner cause of reduced BH$_4$ synthesis is 6-PTS deficiency [4], which accounts for the commonest form of hyperphenylalaninaemia not resulting from PAH deficiency. These patients have high neopterin but low biopterin levels (and thus a high neopterin : biopterin ratio), and reduced synthesis of monoamine neurotransmitters (as in DHPR deficiency). They also present with the clinical features of PKU, with an additional progressive extrapyramidal syndrome. They typically have a low birth weight. Diagnosis rests on detection of hyperphenylalaninaemia, measurement of pterins, and correction of phenylalanine levels with test doses of BH$_4$. Treatment requires administration of BH$_4$, which is effective at reducing phenylalanine levels, but also administration of L-dopa and 5-hydroxytryptophan supplements (with a dopa decarboxylase inhibitor exactly as for DHPR deficiency) as BH$_4$ does not readily cross the blood–brain barrier.

Prenatal diagnosis. DHPR deficiency can now be detected prenatally by direct measurement of enzyme activity in amniocytes and by genetic screening in families with known mutations. GTP cyclohydrolase deficiency is more difficult to diagnose before birth as the enzyme is not expressed in amniocytes; but 6-PTS deficiency can be looked for by measurement of pterins in amniotic fluid and DNA analysis in families with previously defined mutations.

References

1 Blau N, Thony B, Cotton RGH, Hyland K. Disorders of tetrabiopterin and related biogenic amines. In: Scriver CR, Beaudet AL, Sly WS, Valle D, eds. *The Metabolic and Molecular Bases of Inherited Disease*, 8th edn. New York: McGraw-Hill, 2001: 1735–47.

2 Kaufman S, Holtzman NA, Milstien S et al. Phenylketonuria due to a deficiency of dihydrobiopterine reductase. *N Engl J Med* 1975; **293**: 785–90.

3 Dhondt JL. Strategy for the screening of tetrahydrobiopterin deficiency among hyperphenylalaninaemic patients: 15 years experience. *J Inherit Metab Dis* 1991; **14**: 117–27.
4 Naylor EW, Ennis D, Davidson AGF, Wong LT. Guanosine triphosphate cyclohydrolase I deficiency. Early diagnosis by routine urine pteridine screening. *Pediatrics* 1987; **79**: 374–8.

Tyrosinaemia

There are a number of inherited conditions that cause hypertyrosinaemia. These include inborn errors of metabolism (e.g. oculocutaneous and hepatorenal tyrosinaemia) and secondary causes (e.g. severe hepatocellular dysfunction and transient tyrosinaemia of the newborn). Tyrosine comes either from dietary intake or from hydroxylation of phenylalanine, and is the starting point of the synthetic pathways for catecholamines, thyroid hormone and melanin. Catabolism occurs mainly in hepatocytes and results in the formation of the gluconeogenic fumaric acid and the ketogenic acetoacetic acid. The inborn errors that lead to hypertyrosinaemia result from deficiency of one of the enzymes involved in this catabolic pathway.

Tyrosinaemia I (hepatorenal) (MIM *276700) [1–3]

This is a rare but well-documented, autosomal recessive disorder due to a deficiency in fumarylacetoacetic hydroxylase (FAH) which catalyses the last step in tyrosine catabolism. This enzyme has been located to chromosome 15. It can present as an acute or chronic form, and principally affects the liver, kidney and peripheral nerves.

The acute form presents in the first few weeks of life with failure to thrive, vomiting, jaundice, ascites and often gastrointestinal bleeding, and is often precipitated by infection or metabolic stress. An unusual odour said to resemble boiled cabbage may be detectable. Hepatomegaly may be present. Some acute crises proceed to liver failure and encephalopathy, while others resolve though may then recur. During acute attacks plasma tyrosine and methionine levels are high, as are transaminases (sometimes to a marked degree in severe attacks) and often α-fetoprotein.

The chronic form is characterized by chronic liver and renal disease (Fanconi-like syndrome) with death within the first decade. Some patients may develop porphyria-like neurological crises with painful paraesthesiae, autonomic dysfunction (with tachycardia and hypertension) and occasionally a progressive paralysis. These crises are due to the accumulation of succinylacetone, the most powerful known inhibitor of delta aminolaevulinic acid (δ-ALA) dehydratase [3]. Plasma tyrosine and methionine are elevated diagnostically and there is a global increase in urine amino acids, with particular increase in δ-ALA [3].

Secondary deficiency of hepatic 4-hydroxyphenylpyruvic acid dioxygenase (pHPPD) occurs in FAH deficiency, accounts for the increased tyrosine levels and was indeed originally thought to be the primary cause of hepatorenal tyrosinaemia. Some patients develop hypermethioninaemia, due to a secondary inhibition of methionine adenosyltransferase.

Cirrhosis is probably invariable in patients with hepatorenal tyrosinaemia and there is a very high incidence of hepatocellular carcinoma, though it is now thought that some of the initial estimates of this particular complication may have been overestimated [2]. Nonetheless, regular screening is recommended, despite some of the recognized pitfalls of liver ultrasound or CT in distinguishing benign and malignant nodules.

Diagnosis. Prenatal diagnosis is either by direct determination of the FAH enzyme activity or detection of succinylacetone directly or from its inhibitory activity in amniocytes or chorionic villus samples [2,4]. Neonatal screening is aimed at detecting increased levels of tyrosine, methionine or succinylacetone from blood spots on filter paper; more recently these have also been used for screening δ-ALA dehydratase. Several different mutations have been reported, and where the mutation is known, molecular analysis should be carried out.

Treatment. This is with a low tyrosine and phenylalanine diet which can reduce plasma tyrosine levels and does improve renal function, though with less certain benefit for liver disease. Treatment with NTBC (2-(nitro-4-trifluoromethylbenzoyl)-1,3-cyclohexanedione), which inhibits pHPPD, has been tried in a number of patients with hepatorenal tyrosinaemia with some benefit [5–7]. However liver transplantation, which cures the underlying metabolic defect, has revolutionized the prognosis for this condition and remains the treatment of choice [5–7].

References

1 Goldsmith LA, Laberge C. Tyrosinemia and related disorder. In: Scriver CR, Beaudet AL, Sly WS *et al.*, eds. *The Metabolic Basis of Inherited Disease*, 6th edn. New York: McGraw-Hill, 1989: 547–62.
2 Mitchell GA, Lambert M, Tanguay RM. Hypertyrosinemia. In: Scriver CR, Beaudet AL, Sly WS *et al.*, eds. *The Metabolic and Molecular Basis of Disease*, 7th edn. New York: McGraw-Hill, 1995: 1077–106.
3 Berger R. Biochemical aspects of type I hereditary tyrosinaemia. In: Bickel H, Wachtel H, eds. *Inherited Diseases of Amino Acid Metabolism*. New York: Thieme Verlag, 1985: 192.
4 Goulden KJ, Moss MA, Cole DE *et al.* Pitfalls in the initial diagnosis of the tyrosinaemia: three case reports and a review of the literature. *Clin Biochem* 1987; **20**: 207–12.
5 Kvittingen EA. Tyrosinaemia—treatment and outcome. *J Inherit Metab Dis* 1995; **18**: 375–9.
6 Mitchell GA, Grompe M, Lambert M, Tanguay RM. Hypertyrosinosinemia. In: Scriver CR, Beaudet AL, Sly WS, Valle D, eds. *The Metabolic and Molecular Bases of Inherited Disease*, 8th edn. New York: McGraw-Hill, 2001: 1777–805.
7 Gissen P, Preece MA, Willshaw HA, McKiernan PJ. Ophthalmic follow-up of patients with tyrosinaemia type 1 on NTBC. *J Inherit Metab Dis* 2003; **26**: 13–6.

Tyrosinaemia II (MIM *276710)

Synonym
- Richner–Hanhart oculocutaneous syndrome

This is a very rare disorder, inherited as an autosomal recessive trait, due to a deficiency of cytoplasmic tyrosine aminotransferase (TAT), which catalyses the first and rate-limiting step in tyrosine catabolism [1,2]. Males and females are equally affected. The skin, eyes and nervous system are the only organs affected.

The skin manifestations of oculocutaneous tyrosinaemia do not usually appear until after the first year of life. They consist of painful hyperkeratotic plaques on the soles and palms with a particular predilection for the fingertips and thenar and hypothenar eminences [3]. They do not itch but can be sufficiently painful that they prevent walking. Hyperhidrosis of the affected area may also occur, as may leukokeratosis of the tongue [4]. Skin biopsy reveals hyperkeratosis, acanthosis and parakeratosis with homogeneous refractile eosinophilic inclusions in the stratum corneum and upper Malpighian layer; none of these are pathognomonic [1]. On electron microscopy lipid-like granules, myelin-like fragments, keratinocytes with increased tonofibrils and tightly packed microtubular and tonofibrillar masses have all been described. There is minimal, if any, evidence of inflammation and tyrosine crystals are not seen, unlike the conjunctival biopsies of these patients [5].

By contrast with the skin manifestations, eye symptoms are usually present in the first year, though they can develop later. They consist of episodes of pain, photophobia, redness and lacrimation. On examination, central corneal dendritic erosions are seen with prominent neovascularization also occurring quite frequently. There can be progression to corneal opacities with consequent reduced visual acuity [6,7]. A variable degree of mental retardation is present in less than 50% of patients with oculocutaneous tyrosinaemia [3].

Biochemically, this disease produces a highly characteristic pattern with plasma tyrosine as the only elevated plasma amino acid and the only amino acid excreted in the urine. Metabolites of tyrosine are also detectable in urine [1].

Diagnosis. This is made by detection of increased blood tyrosine levels, normal phenylalanine and increased urinary metabolites of 4-hydroxyphenylacetic acid, *N*-acetyltyrosine and 4-tyramine.

Treatment. Most patients respond to dietary restriction of tyrosine and phenylalanine [1,8] with the aim of reducing blood levels to less than 600 μmol/L. Skin and eye symptoms and signs usually respond fairly rapidly, though can recur if the diet is discontinued. Oral retinoids have proved beneficial but steroids make skin symptoms worse.

References

1 Mitchell GA, Marcus G, Lambert M, Tanguay RM. Hypertyrosinemia. In: Scriver CR, Beaudet AL, Sly WS, Valle D, eds. *The Metabolic and Molecular Bases of Inherited Disease*, 8th edn. New York: McGraw-Hill, 2001: 1777–805.
2 Goldsmith LA, Thorpe J, Roe CR. Hepatic enzymes of tyrosine metabolism in tyrosinemia II. *J Invest Dermatol* 1979; **73**: 530–2.
3 Hanhart E. Neue Sonderformen von Keratosis palmoplantaris. *Dermatologica* 1947; **94**: 286–308.
4 Larrègue M, de Giacomoni P, Bressieux JM, Odievre M. Syndrome de Richner-Hanhart ou tyrosinose oculo-cutanée. A propos d'un cas. *Ann Dermatol Vénéréol* 1979; **106**: 53–62.
5 Bohnert A, Anton-Lamprecht I. Richner-Hanhart's syndrome: ultrastructural abnormalities of epidermal keratinization indicating a causal relationship to high intracellular tyrosine levels. *J Invest Dermatol* 1982; **79**: 68.
6 Bienfang DC, Kuwabara T, Pueschel SM. The Richner–Hanhart syndrome: report of a case with associated tyrosinemia. *Arch Ophthalmol* 1976; **94**: 1133–7.
7 Bardelli AM, Borgogni P, Farnetani MA *et al*. Familial tyrosinaemia with eye and skin lesions. *Ophthalmologica* 1977; **175**: 5–9.
8 Hill A, Nordin PM, Zaleski WA. Dietary treatment of tyrosinosis. *J Am Diet Assoc* 1970; **56**: 308–12.

Alkaptonuria (MIM #203500) [1,2]

This is a rare metabolic disorder first described by Garrod in 1902 [1], which results from a single gene defect. It is characterized by a discrete biochemical lesion, with deposition of oxidized homo-gentisic acid pigment throughout the body, particularly in fibrous and cartilaginous tissues. Dark urine (homogentisic aciduria), distinctive cutaneous pigmentation (ochronosis) and arthritis are characteristic. Generally, it is considered a benign degenerative disorder with normal life expectancy [2].

Aetiology [1–3]. Alkaptonuria is characterized by a constitutional deficiency of homogentisic oxidase (homogentisic 1,2-dioxygenase activity), an enzyme usually found in liver and kidney. This leads to an accumulation of homogentisic acid, an intermediate metabolite of phenylalanine and tyrosine catabolism.

Ochronosis [4,5] describes the deposition of a melanin-like brownish-black pigment, derived from the oxidized product of homogentisic acid (benzoquinone acetic acid), in connective tissues and cartilage. The enzyme homogentisic acid oxidase contains an essential sulphhydryl group, which is inhibited by certain chemicals. These include various drugs such as phenol, resorcin, mepacrine and perhaps other antimalarials that may cause acquired ochronosis. An exogenous ochronosis can also occur from hydroquinone-containing skin-bleaching creams [4].

Genetics. Alkaptonuria is an autosomal recessive condition. The gene locus (*AKU*) has been assigned to chromosome 3q by consanguinity and by comparative mapping. The gene has been cloned to 3q21–q23 with demonstration that the human 1890 gene harbours missense mutations and co-segregates with the disease [3]. The incidence is one in 200 000 but in areas of consanguinity it is higher [6].

Histopathology. There is deposition of black pigment in the cartilage, fibrous tissue, tendons and atheromatous areas. The intervertebral discs, larynx, tracheal rings and articular cartilages are jet-black as if 'dipped in Indian ink'. Differentiation of the ochronotic pigment from melanin is difficult, and stains do not consistently differentiate between the two pigments.

Clinical features [2,7]. Cardinal features are due to homogentisic acid in urine, and pigmentation of cartilage, connective tissue and joints. The patient with the hereditary type is symptom-free until adult life. The only manifestations in childhood are discoloration of the urine and 'spotting or staining' of the napkins or clothing due to alkaline pH. The clinical sequence of events is alkaptonuria, then ochronosis and lastly ochronotic arthropathy (fifth decade). The cutaneous manifestations appear in the fourth decade. One of the earliest signs is thickening of the ear cartilage, associated with blue-black or grey-blue discoloration. The pinna feels noticeably thickened and inflexible, and in later stages there may be gross calcification. Cerumen is often brown or jet black. Scleral pigmentation is noted as early as the third decade; it appears as brown or grey deposits midway between the corneal margin and the medial canthus. The skin of the eyelids and forehead is also pigmented and the tarsal plates often appear blue on transillumination. All the tendons are similarly discoloured; the dark discoloration over the extensor tendons on the knuckles is best seen when the patient makes a fist. Widespread, dusky cutaneous pigmentation may be noted, but this feature is particularly marked over the cheeks, forehead, axillae and genital regions. The buccal mucosa and larynx are also affected and the nails are sometimes distinctly coloured brown. Ochronotic changes affecting the ear drum and ossicles may produce deafness; prostatic concretions and black renal calculi, as well as calcific aortic disease, have been recorded. The urine is of normal colour but darkens on exposure to air or within seconds of adding an alkaline solution. Patients sometimes observe that both their sweat and urine discolour clothing.

Ochronotic arthropathy follows a fairly consistent clinical pattern. There is low back pain with stiffness early in the fourth decade; during the next 10 years the knees become involved and, later, the shoulders and hips. The friable articular cartilages lead to prolapsed intervertebral discs or a ruptured nucleus pulposus with accompanying acute pain. Spondylosis spreads to the thoracic spine; patients then assume a stooping posture and can lose up to 15 cm in height. Limitation of expansion of the chest provokes dyspnoea. The spinal X-ray appearances are diagnostic, consisting of narrowing of the lumbar disc spaces with intense calcification of the narrowed discs.

Marked atherosclerosis is common in the older age groups as well as valvulitis and calcification of aortic and mitral valves. In spite of their marked disability, many patients reach old age.

Diagnosis. The diagnosis is by demonstration on gas–liquid chromatography of homogentisic acid in the urine (by its reducing ability), or with specific enzyme tests [8].

Differential diagnosis. An incorrect diagnosis of glycosuria or diabetes can be made if the urine is tested with Fehling's solution (but this is rarely used now). The pigmentation of acquired ochronosis from exogenous foreign chemicals or drugs is identical to the genetic disorder, but is unaccompanied by homogentisic acid in the urine or by arthropathy.

The overall clinical picture and the localization of pigment thus distinguish the genetic disease from other pigmentation disorders such as Addison's disease, haemochromatosis, argyria, chronic photosensitivity pigmentation, cutaneous porphyria and pellagra. The ferric chloride urine test gives variable results; other phenolic compounds give similar colour reactions and thus, when the test is positive, the urine should be examined by chromatography.

Treatment [2]. Since the major damage induced by the metabolic defect is pigmentation and joint changes, treatment is directed towards reducing connective tissue damage by ascorbic acid (acting as an antioxidant), and by analgesics and physiotherapy for the arthropathy. A low protein diet limiting the amount of phenylalanine and tyrosine is not practicable as a long-term measure, although it could be used intermittently. Use of vitamins (B_{12}, C) may be helpful (for example ascorbic acid in reducing homogentisic acid oxidation).

References

1 Garrod AE. The incidence of alkaptonuria: a study in clinical individuality. *Lancet* 1908; **ii**: 73–9.

2 La Du BN. Alkaptonuria. In: Scriver CR, Beaudet AL, Sly WS, Valle D, eds. *The Metabolic and Molecular Bases of Inherited Disease*, 8th edn. New York: McGraw-Hill, 2001: 2109–23.

3 Fernandez-Canon JM, Granadino B, Beltron-Valero de Bernabe D *et al.* The molecular basis of alkaptonuria. *Nat Genet* 1996; **14**: 19–24.

4 Findlay GH, Morrison JGL, Simson IW. Exogenous onchronosis and pigmented colloid milium from hydroquinone bleaching creams. *Br J Dermatol* 1975; **93**: 613–22.

5 Woolley PB. Exogenous onchronosis. *BMJ* 1952; **2**: 760–1.

6 Lee PJ, Brenton DP. Inborn errors of amino acid and organic acid metabolism. In: Warrell DA, Cox TM, Firth JD, Benz EJ, eds. *Oxford Textbook of Medicine*, 4th edn. Oxford: Oxford University Press, 2003: 9–31.

7 O'Brien WM, La Du BN, Bunim JJ. Biochemical, pathologic and clinical aspects of alkaptonuria, ochronosis and ochronotic arthropathy. Review of world literature. *Am J Med* 1963; **34**: 813–38.

8 Seegmiller JE, Zannoni VG, Laster L, Brent N. An enzymatic spectrophotometric method for the determination of homogentisic acid in plasma and urine. *J Biol Chem* 1961; **236**: 774–7.

Homocysteinurias [1–5]

Synonym
• Homocystinurias

Homocysteinurias are a group of rare, inborn errors of amino-acid metabolism first reported in 1962 [4]. They also encompass hypermethioninaemia and cystathioninuria. The defects arise when there is abnormality in transfer of the sulphur from methionine to homocysteine in the biochemical pathway responsible for the disposal of methionine and the formation of cysteine, resulting in the accumulation of homocysteine, methionine and other sulphurated metabolites in a wide range of tissues and in the urine.

Aetiology. Initially homocysteinuria was thought to be due solely to deficiency of cystathionine-β synthase (CBS; MIM *236200), but it is now apparent that homocysteine accumulation may also result from inherited defects in the 5-methyltetrahydrofolate–homocysteine methyltransferase reaction (MIM # 236250) [1,3,6]. These can be distinguished because there is an increase in urine methionine in the CBS deficiency whereas it is low in hyperhomocystinaemia secondary to defects of the folate pathway. Secondary forms of homocysteinuria can occur in vegetarians with vitamin B_{12} deficiency, or with treatment with isonicotinic acid. The accumulated homocysteine is believed to interfere with collagen cross-linking accounting for the wide range of clinical features.

Clinical features. CBS deficiency is inherited as an autosomal recessive trait, with a world prevalence of 1 : 344 000 though with wide variation between different countries [1]. Four major systems are affected: the eye, skeletal system, central nervous system and the vascular system. The newborn infant appears clinically normal, but lens dislocation, mental deficiency, growth disorder and cutaneous signs may develop slowly over the next few years. The skin features of homocysteinuria include fine, brittle hair and thin skin. Livedo reticularis of the legs and tissue-paper scars on the hands may be present. In some cases, hair examination shows no fluorescence with acridine orange, indicating abnormality of disulphide bonds. The cysteine content is normal. Abnormal glucose tolerance and increased growth hormone levels are often present.

Osteoporosis of the spine is common and predisposes to scoliosis. Lengthening and thinning of the long bones may lead to a variety of skeletal abnormalities and their presence together with the arachnodactyly that also occurs may lead to a Marfanoid appearance. Other features include hepatomegaly (secondary to fatty change) and myopathy. Many patients with CBS deficiency exhibit some degree of mental impairment; developmental delay may be the presenting feature of the disease and about 20% also suffer seizures. Psychiatric abnormalities occur in about 50% of patients, including episodic depression (10%), chronic behavioural disorders (17%) [7], chronic obsessive–compulsive disorders (5%) and personality disorders (19%). Some children develop spontaneous venous and arterial thrombosis, probably secondary to increased platelet adhesiveness, and venous thromboembolic disease is a frequent cause of mortality [6,8]. There has been much interest in recent years in establishing whether milder forms of hyperhomocystinaemia, seen quite frequently in folate deficiency, may be associated with increased risk of cardiovascular disease [9,10]. Although the initial epidemiology seemed convincing, trials of folic acid supplementation have not generally reduced the clinical endpoints of atherosclerosis such as myocardial infarcts and strokes.

Differential diagnosis. Marfan's syndrome, an hereditary mesodermal dysplasia, exhibits visceral manifestations without mental deficiency. The hair is normal and homocysteine is absent from the urine.

Diagnosis. This is by detection of urinary homocysteine by a positive urinary cyanide–nitroprusside reaction. Recently, plasma homocysteine measurement (with increases of 50–200 µmol/L), confirmed by changes after methionine loading, is regarded as a more accurate assessment. Heterozygotes can be detected by assaying for the enzyme in the liver, phytohaemagglutinin-stimulated lymphocytes and in cultured fibroblasts. In addition, the presence of abnormal sulphur-containing metabolites can be detected in the urine after an oral load of L-methionine. CBS deficiency can be diagnosed by hypermethioninaemia or by detection of increased homocysteine in urine or blood. Methods for detecting heterozygotes rest on enzyme assays, metabolite measurements or a combination using liver tissue, cultured fibroblasts or phytohaemagglutinin-stimulated lymphocytes. Newer techniques include tandem mass spectrometry [11].

Treatment [1,12]. There are two aims of treatment: (i) control/elimination of the biochemical abnormality; and (ii) treatment of complications. Patients are usually divided into pyridoxine-responsive or non-responsive individuals, detected after the newborn period. For the newborn, diets restricting methionine and supplemented with cysteine have been used with encouraging results when started early in life. Large doses of vitamin B_6 (pyridoxine) in the form of pyridoxine hydrochloride 150–300 mg/day produce complete reversal of the biochemical abnormality in some cases. Some may become folate deficient; administration of vitamin B_{12} and folic acid improves clinical symptoms. For the non-pyridoxine responsive patients, a low protein diet with methionine-free amino acid supplements and exchanges, and minerals and vitamins may be helpful. In non-responsive patients diagnosed after birth (non-responsive after a trial of 500–1000 mg/day for several weeks), the use of betaine as a methyl donor agent to lower homocysteine levels can prove effective in lowering

plasma homocysteine levels in combination with a low-methionine diet. Aspirin can help reduce the thrombotic risk and other cardiovascular risk factors, such as hypertension, diabetes and dyslipidaemia should be sought and treated appropriately.

Prognosis. Prognosis is more favourable than might be thought, with recent surveys showing that fewer than 5% of affected individuals die by the age of 20 years [1–3].

References
1 Mudd H, Levy HL, Kraus JP. Disorders of transsulfuration. In: Scriver CR, Beaudet AL, Sly WS, Valle D, eds. *The Metabolic and Molecular Bases of Inherited Disease*, 8th edn. New York: McGraw-Hill, 2001: 2007–56.
2 Brenton DP, Cusworth DC, Dent CE, Jones EE. Homocystinuria. Clinical and dietary studies. *QJM* 1966; **35**: 325–46.
3 Carson NAJ, Cusworth DC, Dent CE *et al*. Homocystinuria. *Arch Dis Child* 1963; **38**: 425–36.
4 Field CMB *et al*. *Abstracts of the Xth International Congress of Paediatrics*. Lisbon, 1962: 274.
5 Fourth International Conference on Homocysteine Metabolism (Abstracts). *J Inherit Metab Dis* 2003; **26**: 1–129.
6 McDonald L, Bray C, Field C *et al*. Homocystinuria, thrombosis, and the blood platelets. *Lancet* 1964; **1**: 745–6.
7 Abbott MH, Folstein SE, Abbey H, Pyeritz RE. Psychiatric manifestations of homocystinuria due to cystathione-synthase deficiency. *Am J Med Genet* 1987; **26**: 959–69.
8 McKusick VA. *Heritable Disorders of Connective Tissue*, 4th edn. St Louis: Mosby, 1972: 224.
9 Scott J, Weir D. Homocyst(e)ine and cardiovascular disease (Editorial). *QJM* 1996; **89**: 571–7.
10 Wilcken DEL, Wilcken B. The natural history of vascular disease in homocystinuria and the effects of treatment. *J Inherit Metab Dis* 1997; **20**: 295–300.
11 Chace DH, Hillman SL, Millington DS *et al*. Rapid diagnosis of homocystinuria and other hypermethioninemias from newborns' blood spots by tandem mass spectrometry. *Clin Chem* 1996; **42**: 349–55.
12 Barber GW, Spaeth GL. Pyridoxine therapy in homocystinuria (Letter). *Lancet* 1967; **1**: 337.

Hartnup disease (MIM *2345000) [1–3]

This is a very rare hereditary recessive disorder of neutral amino acid transport, which is characterized by a pellagrous eruption, a temporary and intermittent cerebellar ataxia, and a characteristic renal aminoaciduria with excessive indicanuria [1].

Aetiology [1,4]. Hartnup disease is believed to be caused by a genetic defect in the specific system for transport of neutral amino acids in the kidney and across the brush border epithelium of the intestine, leading to hyperaminoaciduria and urinary excretion of indolic compounds formed by bacterial action on the unabsorbed tryptophan [5–7]. It is likely that Hartnup disorder is a monogenic defect which interacts with polygenic and environmental factors giving a wide clinical spectrum [8]. The failure of absorption of tryptophan results in a deficiency in the synthesis of nicotinamide causing a pellagra-like syndrome.

Clinical features. The onset is usually in childhood between 3 and 9 years, but the first signs are occasionally encountered as early as 10 days after birth. The cutaneous signs precede the neurological manifestations. The rash is dry, scaly and well marginated, affecting the light-exposed areas, notably the forehead, cheeks, periorbital regions, the uncovered areas of the arms and the dorsal surface of the hands. After exposure to sunlight, the skin reddens and blistering may occur. With recovery there is often desquamation and depigmentation.

Cerebellar ataxia is the most commonly encountered neurological feature. It usually develops later than the skin lesions. Other signs of cerebellar origin include nystagmus and diplopia, and occasionally tremor of the hands and tongue. Early reports suggested mental retardation, but this has not been the case with most patients. Minor cognitive defects have been reported. Less commonly, there are associated psychiatric disturbances such as depression, delusions and hallucinations. Exacerbations are most frequently seen in the spring or early summer [2], cutaneous manifestations being accompanied by transient ataxia. Rarely, the attacks are provoked by febrile illness. Other somatic abnormalities include oedema and hypoproteinaemia with fatty change in the liver [2], fever, diarrhoea and atrophic glossitis.

Intravenous tryptophan is metabolized normally and the serum amino acid profile is normal. The urine contains increased amounts of amino acids of the monoamine monocarboxylic groups [5], and it is the pattern of the amino acid excretion that confirms the diagnosis.

Differential diagnosis. The eruption in mild cases closely simulates infantile atopic eczema, seborrhoeic eczema or pityriasis alba; in Hartnup disease the covered areas are usually spared. Florid cases closely mimic nutritional pellagra. The congenital poikilodermas, particularly the light-sensitive hereditary disorders such as Cockayne's syndrome, may present diagnostic difficulties.

Treatment [2,3]. The rationale for the treatment is to replace the defect by giving nicotinamide (50–300 mg/day) orally. Treatment usually results in amelioration of the rash and may improve ataxia and psychotic behaviour. A high-protein diet may be a useful adjunct. Intravenous nutrition may be necessary in severely affected patients.

Prognosis. Symptoms become milder with increasing age.

References

1 Baron DN, Dent CE, Harris H et al. Hereditary pellagra-like skin rash with temporary cerebellar ataxia. Constant renal amino-aciduria, and other bizarre biochemical features. Lancet 1956; **2**: 421–8.
2 Halvorsen K, Halvorsen S. Hartnup disease. Pediatrics 1963; **31**: 29–38.
3 Levy HL. Hartnup disorder. In: Scriver CR, Beaudet AL, Sly WS, Valle D, eds. The Metabolic and Molecular Bases of Inherited Disease, 8th edn. New York: McGraw-Hill, 2001: 4957–81.
4 Scriver CR, Mahon B, Levy HL et al. The Hartnup phenotype: Mendelian transport disorder, multifactorial disease. Am J Hum Genet 1987; **40**: 401–12.
5 Milne MD. Disorders of amino acid transport. BMJ 1964; **1**: 327–36.
6 Milne MD, Crawford MA, Girdo CB et al. The metabolic disorder in Hartnup disease. QJM 1960; **29**: 407–21.
7 Scriver CR. Hartnup disease: a genetic modification of intestinal and renal transport of certain neutral alpha amino acids. N Engl J Med 1965; **273**: 530–2.
8 Matthews DM. Experimental approach in chemical pathology. BMJ 1971; **3**: 659–64.

Gout

This heterogeneous group of abnormalities of purine metabolism is characterized by hyperuricaemia, and recurrent attacks of acute

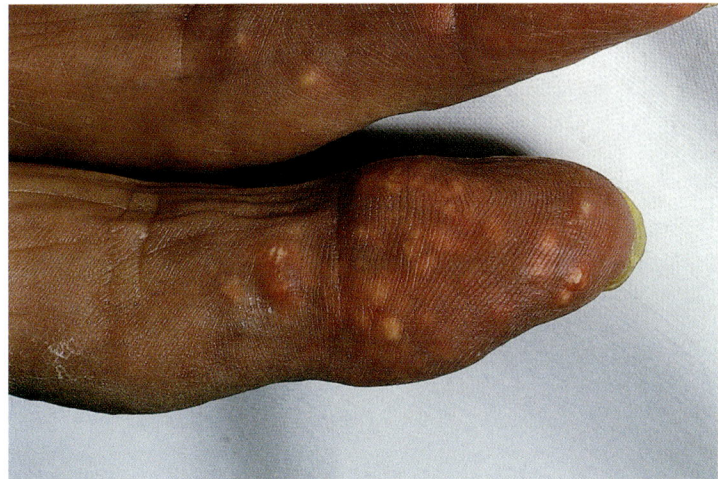

Fig. 59.69 Gouty tophi. (Courtesy of Dr R.H. Champion, West Suffolk Hospital, Bury St Edmunds, UK.)

arthritis in some cases, with the deposition of monosodium urates in the articular cartilage and urate deposits in the skin (tophi) (Fig. 59.69). Arthritis may be progressive and nephropathy is common. Nephrolithiasis due to uric acid may precede arthritis.

Aetiology [1–4]. Uric acid is the degradative product of purine metabolism in humans. Increased circulating levels of uric acid arise because of overproduction or underexcretion of uric acid. Primary gout has long been recognized as a heterogeneous disorder; in up to 40% of patients the family history suggests a genetic component [4]. Population studies suggest that the disorder is multifactorial and attributable to a combination of genetic and non-genetic factors [1]. There are two very rare specific enzyme deficiencies associated with gout, which have X-linked inheritance. These are partial deficiency of hypoxanthine–guanine phosphoribosyl transferase (HGPRT; HPRT-related gout, MIM #300323) and increased activity of phosphoribosyl-pyrophosphate (PRPP) synthetase [5]. Most patients with primary gout appear to have reduced excretion of uric acid [6,7] but the molecular mechanisms underlying this remain poorly understood. Fewer than 10% of patients with primary gout have an increase in the rate of purine biosynthesis [8].

Secondary gout may result from decreased excretion of uric acid. The most important cause of this is diuretic therapy but it may also occur in a number of disease states, especially renal tubular disease. Increased uric acid production is commonly secondary to increased turnover of nucleic acids in conditions such as polycythaemia rubra vera, lymphoma, myeloma and leukaemia especially when patients are receiving active chemotherapy. A number of other disorders may be associated with hyperuricaemia and gout. 82% of patients with pure or combined hypertriglyceridaemia have increased uric acid levels, and conversely 74% of patients with gout have raised lipoproteins (TG, VLDL [5,9] and Lp(a) [10]); the link between the two is likely to be insulin resistance. There has been a suggestion that hyperuricaemia may be a risk factor for cardiovascular disease [9,11]. Hypertension, obesity, diabetes mellitus and ethanol consumption in susceptible persons may also be associated with gout [12].

Histopathology. Sodium urate crystals may be found in joint fluid. The crystals can be identified by microscopic examination and by their ability to polarize light strongly. In the dermis and medulla of the kidney, the urate crystals provoke a giant cell reaction [12,13].

Clinical features [1,3,4,7]. Hyperuricaemia develops at around puberty in males but usually later in females, often after the menopause. Patients normally remain asymptomatic until the fourth to sixth decades when the first attack of acute gouty arthritis occurs. Recurrent, self-limiting attacks usually follow after a period of about 6 months to 2 years. Initially single joints, classically the great toe, are involved, but later the condition may become polyarticular and then usually involves the joints of the lower extremities. Later in the disease, a chronic tophus state develops with deposits in cartilage, synovial membranes, tendons and soft tissues. The classical locations for tophi are the helix and antihelix of the ear, and the index fingers (Fig. 59.69). Criteria for clinical diagnosis of acute gout have been reported [3,14].

Acute uric acid nephropathy results from precipitation of uric acid crystals in the collecting ducts of the kidney and is most commonly seen in patients with leukaemia undergoing aggressive chemotherapy. Renal stones develop in up to one-quarter of patients [12] and renal colic may be a presenting manifestation of gout. Chronic urate nephropathy is common [6,15] and contributes significantly to the morbidity and mortality of gout [15].

Differential diagnosis. Pseudogout [2,16] (calcium pyrophosphate deposition disease) shows close similarities to gout (particularly the acute attacks), and is characterized by familial incidence and later chronic arthropathy, pseudotophi and precipitation by surgical operations and diuretic therapy. The serum uric acid level is normal, calcium pyrophosphate is found in synovial fluid and X-rays show articular calcification [2]. Multicentric reticulohistiocytosis is frequently accompanied by papules and nodules on the ears and fingers with an associated arthropathy. Rheumatoid arthritis with necrobiotic nodules is usually sufficiently characteristic to avoid confusion with gout. Psoriatic arthropathy may cause diagnostic difficulties.

Treatment [1,3,15,17,18]. All patients with gout or a raised uric acid level should be investigated for its cause. Acute attacks are treated by rest of the affected joint and with regular anti-inflammatory treatment, such as indomethacin. Where non-steroidal anti-inflammatory drugs are contraindicated, corticosteroids can sometimes be helpful. Colchicine (0.5 mg 6-hourly until symptoms subside, or a maximum oral dose of 6 mg has been reached) may also be useful in acute episodes. Side effects of diarrhoea, renal and hepatic damage need to be carefully monitored during treatment with colchicine. It is a matter of clinical judgement whether to treat asymptomatic hyperuricaemia.

Antiuricaemic therapy using allopurinol, a xanthine oxidase inhibitor, is effective after the acute event and in prophylaxis. Allopurinol should be avoided in an acute attack, and its introduction sometimes precipitates an acute attack. If this happens, reintroduction of allopurinol after a suitable interval should be covered by concomitant administration of colchicine or non-steroidal anti-inflammatory drugs for the first couple of weeks. Drugs such as probenecid and sulfinpyrazone may be used to increase uric acid excretion, but are usually less effective prophylaxis. Treatment must be tailored to the needs of individual patients [8,19].

References

1 Becker MA. Hyperuricemia and gout. In: Scriver CR, Beaudet AL, Sly WS, Valle D, eds. *The Metabolic and Molecular Bases of Inherited Disease*, 8th edn. New York: McGraw-Hill, 2001: 2513–55.
2 Howell DS. Diseases due to the deposition of calcium pyrophosphate and hydroxyapatite. In: Kelley WN *et al.*, eds. *Textbook of Rheumatology*, 2nd edn. Philadelphia: Saunders, 1985.
3 Watts RWE. Disorders of purine and pyrimidine metabolism. In: Warrell DA, Cox TM, Firth JD, Benz EJ, eds. *Oxford Textbook of Medicine*, 4th edn. Oxford: Oxford University Press, 2003: 49–60.
4 Grahame R, Scott JT. Clinical survey of 354 patients with gout. *Ann Rheum Dis* 1970; **29**: 461–8.
5 Stout JT, Caskey CG. Hypoxanthine. The Lesch–Nyhan syndrome and gouty arthritis. In: Scriver CR, Beaudet AL, Sly WS, Valle D, eds. *The Metabolic Basis of Inherited Disease*, 6th edn. New York: McGraw-Hill, 1989: 1007–28.
6 Snaith ML, Scott JT. Uric acid clearance in patients with gout and normal subjects. *Ann Rheum Dis* 1971; **30**: 285–9.
7 Barlow KA, Beilin LJ. Renal disease in primary gout. *QJM* 1968; **37**: 79–96.
8 Kelley KN. Approach to the patient with hyperuricemia. In: Kelley WN *et al.*, eds. *Textbook of Rheumatology*, 2nd edn. Philadelphia: Saunders, 1985.
9 Laskarzewski PM, Khoury P, Morrison JA *et al.* Familial hyper- and hypouricaemias in random and hyperlipidaemic recall cohorts: The Princeton School District Family Study. *Metabolism* 1983; **32**: 230–43.
10 Takahashi S, Yamamoto T, Moriwaki Y *et al.* Increased concentrations of serum Lp(a) lipoprotein in patients with primary gout. *Ann Rheum Dis* 1995; **54**: 90–3.
11 Waring WS, Webb DJ, Maxwell SRJ. Uric acid as risk factors for cardiovascular disease. *QJM* 2000; **93**: 707–13.
12 Landis RC, Haskard DO. Pathogenesis of crystal-induced inflamation. *Curr Rheumatol Rep* 2001; **3**: 36–41.
13 Gutman AB, Yu TF. Uric acid nephrolithiasis. *Am J Med* 1968; **45**: 756–79.
14 Hochberg MC. Gout. In: Silman AJ, Hochberg MC, eds. *Epidemiology of the Rheumatic Diseases*, 2nd edn. Oxford: Oxford University Press, 2001: 230–42.
15 Talbott JH, Terplan KL. The kidney in gout. *Medicine* 1960; **39**: 405–67.
16 McCarty DJ, Kohn NN, Faires JS. The significance of calcium phosphate crystals in the synovial fluid of arthritic patients: the 'pseudogout' syndrome. Clinical aspects. *Ann Intern Med* 1962; **56**: 711–37.
17 Emerson BT. The management of gout. *N Engl J Med* 1996; **334**: 445–51.
18 Fam AG. Difficult gout and new approaches for control of hyperuricaemia in the allopurinol-allergic patient. *Curr Rheumatol Rep* 2001; **3**: 29–35.
19 Yu T. Milestones in the treatment of gout. *Am J Med* 1974; **56**: 676–85.

Lesch–Nyhan syndrome (MIM #300322) [1–6]

Lesch–Nyhan syndrome results from a complete lack of the purine salvage enzyme hypoxanthine-guanine phosphoribosyltransferase (HGPRT). HGPRT is coded for by a single gene on the X chromosome (Xq26-q27), and is expressed in all tissues, and at high level in the basal ganglia. This enzyme catalyses the salvage of hypoxanthine and guanine to inosine monophosphate (IMP) and guanosine monophosphate (GMP). The principal clinical features are choreoathetosis, spasticity, mental retardation and self-mutilation, particularly biting of the lower lip in childhood. There may also be a macrocytic/megaloblastic anaemia. Patients are normal at birth, but by 6 months developmental abnormalities are apparent with choreiform movements usually being the first to appear. The origin of the neurological abnormality in humans is still unknown; HGPRT-deficient mice do not show any of the neurological features of Lesch–Nyhan syndrome. It is, however, thought that it is the accumulation of purine metabolites rather than deficiency of purine nucleotides that is pathogenic with secondary effects on neurotransmitter function. Changes in terminal arborization of dopaminergic neurones have been found, probably occurring secondary to reduced concentrations of dopamine homovanillic acid, dopa and tyrosine decarboxylase in dopaminergic neurones in the putamen. Blood uric acid levels are high and, although there are no reports of gouty arthritis, renal function is impaired by deposit of urates. However, patients with partial deficiency of HGPRT may develop gouty arthritis and/or uric acid calculi though without any of the neurological and behavioural features of the full-blown syndrome.

Prenatal diagnosis. HGPRT analysis can be carried out on amniocyte or chorionic villus samples in the ninth week of pregnancy. Affected male heterozygotes can be identified by HGPRT assay on red cell lysates. Carrier females can be identified by HGPRT and HGPRT⁻ mosaicism in hair roots; mosaicism can also be identified in cultured fibroblasts [7].

Treatment. Allopurinol, in appropriate dosage, can reduce plasma urate and urinary uric acid to reduce occurrence of gouty arthritis, urate nephropathy and renal calculi. There is no effective treatment of the neurological features. However, padded wheelchairs and physical restraints may reduce spinal injury and self-mutilation. Dental extraction may also assist in preventing the latter [5,7].

References

1 Hoefnagel D, Andrew ED, Mireault NG, Berndt WO. Hereditary choreoathetosis, self-mutilation and hyperuricemia in young males. *N Engl J Med* 1965; **273**: 130–5.

2 Lesch M, Nyhan WL. A familial disorder of uric acid metabolism and central nervous system function. *Am J Med* 1964; **36**: 561–70.

3 Kelley WN, Greene ML, Rosenbloom FM, Helderson JF. Hypoxanthineguanine phosphoribosyltransferase deficiency in gout. *Ann Intern Med* 1969; **70**: 155–206.

4 Nyhan WL, Oliver WJ, Lesch M. A familial disorder of uric acid metabolism and central nervous system function. II. *J Pediatr* 1965; **67**: 257–63.

5 Jinnah HA, Friedmann T. Lesch–Nyhan disease and its variants. In: Scriver CR, Beaudet AL, Sly WS, Valle D, eds. *The Metabolic and Molecular Bases of Inherited Disease*, 8th edn. New York: McGraw-Hill, 2001: 2537–70.

6 Reed WB, Fish CH. Hyperuricemia with self-mutilation and choreoathetosis. Lesch–Nyhan syndrome. *Arch Dermatol* 1966; **94**: 194–5.

7 Watts RWE. Disorders of purine and pyrimidine metabolism. In: Warrell DA, Cox TM, Firth JD, Benz EJ, eds. *Oxford Textbook of Medicine*, 4th edn. Oxford: Oxford University Press, 2003: 49–60.

CHAPTER 60

Necrobiotic Disorders

D.A. Burns

Leicester Royal Infirmary, Leicester, UK

Granuloma annulare

Introduction. Granuloma annulare was first described by Colcott Fox in 1895 [1], and established as a specific entity by Radcliffe Crocker in 1902 [2]. It is a disease in which, in typical cases, the skin and/or subcutis is involved in a process characterized by foci of alteration of collagen (necrobiosis) surrounded by histiocytes and lymphocytes. Clinical variants include localized, generalized, perforating and subcutaneous patterns [3,4].

References

1 Fox TC. Ringed eruption of the fingers. *Br J Dermatol* 1895; **7**: 91–2.
2 Radcliffe Crocker H. Granuloma annulare. *Br J Dermatol* 1902; **14**: 1–9.
3 Muhlbauer JE. Granuloma annulare. *J Am Acad Dermatol* 1980; **3**: 217–30.
4 Smith MD, Downie JB, DiCostanzo D. Granuloma annulare. *Int J Dermatol* 1997; **36**: 326–33.

Aetiology [1–3]. Although the aetiology and pathogenesis of granuloma annulare are unclear, it appears likely that it represents a reaction pattern to a variety of triggering factors. Reported triggering factors have included insect bites [4], scabies [5], a cat bite [6], waxing-induced pseudofolliculitis [7], tuberculin tests [8], BCG vaccination [9,10], hepatitis B vaccination [11,12] and chronic hepatitis B virus infection, with resolution soon after treatment with interferon-α [13], a possible relationship to antitetanus and diphtheria toxoid vaccination [14,15], and various forms of trauma such as occupational pressure on the fingers in a milkman [16] and saphenectomy [17]. In the past, its occurrence with tuberculosis was noted in a number of reports, and cases may still be encountered in which there appears to be an association between these two disorders [18,19]. Other infectious agents that have been implicated in the causation of lesions of granuloma annulare include human papilloma virus [20], varicella/zoster virus [21–29] (although persistence of viral DNA does not appear to be related to granuloma formation [26,30]), Epstein–Barr virus (EBV) [31,32] (although EBV could not be demonstrated in lesions occurring in HIV-positive patients [33]), parvovirus B19 [34], hepatitis C virus [35] and during pegylated interferon-α treatment for hepatitis C

virus infection [36], and human immunodeficiency virus [33,37–46]. Although there has been evidence implicating *Borrelia burgdorferi* in some cases [47,48], it was absent in others [49]. Examination of several biopsy specimens using polymerase chain reaction amplification did not reveal any evidence of *Bartonella* infection [50]. Granuloma annulare at the site of an infection such as herpes zoster has been termed an 'isotopic' response.

Seasonally recurrent granuloma annulare has been described [51,52], and sun exposure may have acted as a precipitating factor in one of these cases [52]. Sun exposure is thought to have provoked or contributed to localization of lesions in a number of cases [53–56]. Disseminated granuloma annulare has occurred in a patient undergoing PUVA therapy [57]. Whether actinic granuloma is a distinct entity, or represents granuloma annulare on sun-exposed skin, has been the subject of debate [58–66].

A report of granuloma annulare occurring in the red areas of tattoos [67] prompted description of a similar case and the suggestion that both were examples of a perforating collagenosis [68].

There is a report of disseminated granuloma annulare occurring in the same sites as lesions of erythema multiforme minor [69].

Some cases of granuloma annulare-like lesions attributed to drugs may have been examples of drug-induced interstitial granulomatous reactions [70].

It has been suggested that an immunoglobulin-mediated vasculitis is the cause of the necrobiotic granulomas [2,71], but evidence from immunofluorescence studies is conflicting—some authors have demonstrated immunoreactants in vessel walls [71], whereas others have not [72,73]. An alternative view is that the pathogenetic mechanism is a delayed-type hypersensitivity response [2,73–77].

An increased prevalence of HLA-Bw35, compared with controls and those with localized lesions, has been demonstrated in individuals with generalized granuloma annulare [78].

The relationship between diabetes mellitus and granuloma annulare is discussed below, as are apparent associations with several other disorders.

References

1 Muhlbauer JE. Granuloma annulare. *J Am Acad Dermatol* 1980; **3**: 217–30.
2 Dahl MV. Speculations on the pathogenesis of granuloma annulare. *Australas J Dermatol* 1985; **26**: 49–57.

Rook's Textbook of Dermatology, 8th edition. Edited by DA Burns,
SM Breathnach, NH Cox and CEM Griffiths. © 2010 Blackwell Publishing Ltd.

3 Smith MD, Downie JB, DiCostanzo D. Granuloma annulare. *Int J Dermatol* 1997; **36**: 326–33.

4 Moyer DG. Papular granuloma annulare. *Arch Dermatol* 1964; **89**: 41–5.

5 Wilsmann TD, Wenzel J, Gerdsen R *et al.* Granuloma annulare induced by scabies. *Acta Derm Venereol* 2003; **83**: 318.

6 Trujillo-Santos AJ, Aguiar-Garcia F, González-Hermoso C. Subcutaneous nodules after a cat bite. *Arch Intern Med* 2001; **161**: 2043–4.

7 Young HS, Coulson IH. Granuloma annulare following waxing-induced folliculitis. *Clin Exp Dermatol* 2000; **25**: 274–6.

8 Beer WE, Wilson Jones E. Granuloma annulare following tuberculin Heaf tests. *Trans St. John's Hosp Dermatol Soc* 1966; **52**: 68–70.

9 Houcke-Bruge C, Delaporte E, Catteau B *et al.* Granuloma annulaire après vaccination par le BCG. *Ann Dermatol Vénéréol* 2001; **128**: 541–4.

10 Kakurai M, Kiyosawa T, Ohtsuki M, Nakagawa H. Multiple lesions of granuloma annulare following BCG vaccination: case report and review of the literature. *Int J Dermatol* 2001; **40**: 579–81.

11 Wolf F, Grezard P, Berard F *et al.* Generalized granuloma annulare and hepatitis B vaccination. *Eur J Dermatol* 1998; **8**: 435–6.

12 Criado PR, de Oliveira RR, Vasconcellos C *et al.* Two case reports of cutaneous adverse reactions following hepatitis B vaccine: lichen planus and granuloma annulare. *J Eur Acad Dermatol Venereol* 2004; **18**: 603–6.

13 Ma HJ, Zhu WY, Yue XZ. Generalized granuloma annulare associated with chronic hepatitis B virus infection. *J Eur Acad Dermatol Venereol* 2006; **20**: 186–9.

14 Baykal C, Ozkaya-Bayazit E, Kaymaz R. Granuloma annulare possibly triggered by antitetanus vaccination. *J Eur Acad Dermatol Venereol* 2002; **16**: 516–8.

15 Baskan EB, Tunali S, Kacar SD *et al.* A case of granuloma annulare in a child following tetanus and diphtheria toxoid vaccination. *J Eur Acad Dermatol Venereol* 2005; **19**: 639–40.

16 Beer WE, Wayte DM, Morgan GW. Knobbly granuloma annulare (GA) of the fingers of a milkman—a possible relationship to his work. *Clin Exp Dermatol* 1992; **17**: 63–4.

17 Borgia F, Cannavò SP, Guaneri F *et al.* Isomorphic response after saphenectomy in a patient with granuloma annulare. *J Am Acad Dermatol* 2004; **50** (Suppl. 2): S31–3.

18 Winkelmann RK. The granuloma annulare phenotype and tuberculosis. *J Am Acad Dermatol* 2002; **46**: 948–52.

19 Herron MD, Florell SR. Disseminated granuloma annulare accompanying *Mycobacterium tuberculosis* lymphadenitis. *Int J Dermatol* 2004; **43**: 961–3.

20 Ward WH. Warts and granuloma annulare. *BMJ* 1956; **2**: 1484.

21 Guill MA, Goette DK. Granuloma annulare at sites of healing herpes zoster. *Arch Dermatol* 1978; **114**: 1383.

22 Kleber R, Landthaler M, Burg G. Post-zoster granuloma annulare. *Hautarzt* 1989; **40**: 110–1.

23 Zanolli MD, Powell BL, McCalmont T *et al.* Granuloma annulare and disseminated herpes zoster. *Int J Dermatol* 1992; **31**: 55–7.

24 Hayakawa K, Mizukawa Y, Shiohara T, Nagashima M. Granuloma annulare arising after herpes zoster. *Int J Dermatol* 1992; **31**: 745–6.

25 Krahl D, Hartschuh W, Tilgen W. Granuloma annulare perforans in herpes zoster scars. *J Am Acad Dermatol* 1993; **29**: 859–62.

26 Requena L, Kutzner H, Escalonilla P *et al.* Cutaneous reactions at sites of herpes zoster scars: an expanded spectrum. *Br J Dermatol* 1998; **138**: 161–8.

27 Bygum A. Granuloma annulare after herpes zoster: isotopic response. *Ugeskr Laeger* 1998; **20**: 4429–30.

28 Ohata C, Shirabe H, Takagi K, Kawatsu T. Granuloma annulare in herpes zoster scars. *J Dermatol* 2000; **27**: 166–9.

29 Chang SE, Bae GY, Moon KC *et al.* Subcutaneous granuloma annulare following herpes zoster. *Int J Dermatol* 2004; **43**: 298–9.

30 Serfling U, Penneys NS, Zhu WY *et al.* Varicella-zoster virus DNA in granulomatous skin lesions following herpes zoster: a study by the polymerase chain reaction. *J Cutan Pathol* 1993; **20**: 28–33.

31 Spencer SA, Fenske NA, Espinoza CG *et al.* Granuloma annulare-like eruption due to chronic Epstein–Barr virus infection. *Arch Dermatol* 1988; **124**: 250–5.

32 Person JR. Generalized granuloma annulare, mononucleosis and positive rheumatoid factor. *Int J Dermatol* 1995; **34**: 40–1.

33 Toro JR, Chu P, Ben Yen T-S, LeBoit PE. Granuloma annulare and human immunodeficiency virus infection. *Arch Dermatol* 1999; **135**: 1341–6.

34 Magro CM, Dawood MR, Crowson AN. The cutaneous manifestations of human parvovirus B19 infection. *Hum Pathol* 2000; **31**: 488–97.

35 Granel B, Serratrice J, Rey J *et al.* Chronic hepatitis C virus infection associated with a generalized granuloma annulare. *J Am Acad Dermatol* 2000; **43**: 918–9.

36 Kluger N, Moguelet P, Chaslin-Ferbus D *et al.* Generalized interstitial granuloma annulare induced by pegylated interferon-alpha. *Dermatology* 2006; **213**: 248–9.

37 Huerter CJ, Bass J, Bergfeld WF, Tubbs RR. Perforating granuloma annulare in a patient with acquired immunodeficiency syndrome. *Arch Dermatol* 1987; **123**: 1217–20.

38 Bakos L, Hampe S, da Rocha JL *et al.* Generalized granuloma annulare in a patient with acquired immunodeficiency syndrome. *J Am Acad Dermatol* 1987; **17**: 844–5.

39 Jones SK, Harman RRM. Atypical granuloma annulare in patients with the acquired immunodeficiency syndrome. *J Am Acad Dermatol* 1989; **20**: 299–300.

40 Cohen PR, Grossman ME, Silvers DN, DeLeo VA. Generalized granuloma annulare located on sun-exposed areas in a human immunodeficiency virus–seropositive man with ultraviolet B photosensitivity. *Arch Dermatol* 1990; **126**: 830–1.

41 McGregor JM, McGibbon DH. Disseminated granuloma annulare as a presentation of acquired immunodeficiency syndrome (AIDS). *Clin Exp Dermatol* 1992; **17**: 60–2.

42 Muñoz-Pérez MA, García-Bravo B, Rodriguez-Pichardo A, Camacho F. Coexistence of allergic contact dermatitis and granuloma annulare in an HIV-I-infected patient: a casual association? *Am J Contact Dermatitis* 1999; **10**: 100–1.

43 Cohen PR. Granuloma annulare. A mucocutaneous condition in human immunodeficiency virus-infected patients. *Arch Dermatol* 1999; **135**: 1404–7.

44 O'Moore EJ, Nandawni R, Uthayakumar S *et al.* HIV-associated granuloma annulare (HAGA): a report of six cases. *Br J Dermatol* 2000; **142**: 1054–6.

45 Morris SD, Cerio R, Paige DG. An unusual presentation of diffuse granuloma annulare in an HIV-positive patient—immunohistochemical evidence of predominant CD8 lymphocytes. *Clin Exp Dermatol* 2002; **27**: 205–8.

46 Calista D, Landi G. Disseminated granuloma annulare in acquired immunodeficiency syndrome: case report and review of the literature. *Cutis* 1995; **55**: 158–60.

47 Strle F, Preac-Mursic V, Ruzic E *et al.* Isolation of *Borrelia burgdorferi* from a skin lesion in a patient with granuloma annulare. *Infection* 1991; **19**: 351–2.

48 Aberer E, Schmidt BL, Breier F *et al.* Amplification of DNA of *Borrelia burgdorferi* in urine samples of patients with granuloma annulare and lichen sclerosus et atrophicus. *Arch Dermatol* 1999; **135**: 210–2.

49 Halkier-Sorensen L, Kragballe K, Hansen K. Antibodies to the *Borrelia burgdorferi* flagellum in patients with scleroderma, granuloma annulare and porphyria cutanea tarda. *Acta Derm Venereol* 1989; **69**: 116–9.

50 Smoller BR, Madhusudhan KT, Scott MA, Horn TD. Granuloma annulare: another manifestation of *Bartonella* infection? *Am J Dermatopathol* 2001; **23**: 510–3.

51 McLelland J, Young S, Marks JM, Lawrence CM. Seasonally recurrent granuloma annulare of the elbows. *Clin Exp Dermatol* 1991; **16**: 129–30.

52 Uenotsuchi T, Imayama S, Furue M. Seasonally recurrent granuloma annulare on sun-exposed areas. *Br J Dermatol* 1999; **141**: 367.

53 Leppard B, Black MM. Disseminated granuloma annulare. A variant in which the lesions involve the sun-exposed areas. *Trans St John's Hosp Dermatol Soc* 1972; **58**: 186–90.

54 Duncan WC, Smith JD, Knox JM. Generalized perforating granuloma annulare. *Arch Dermatol* 1973; **108**: 570–2.

55 Izumi AK. Generalized perforating granuloma annulare. *Arch Dermatol* 1973; **108**: 708–9.

56 Derancourt C, Sensor M, Atallah L *et al.* Granuloma annulaire des zones photo-exposées chez deux malades ayant en une greff hépatique. *Ann Dermatol Vénéréol* 2000; **127**: 723–7.

57 Dorval J-C, Leroy J-P, Masse R. Granulomes annulaires disséminés après PUVA thérapie. *Ann Dermatol Vénéréol* 1979; **106**: 79–80.

58 Al-Hoqail IA, Al-Ghamdi AM, Martinka M, Crawford RI. Actinic granuloma is a unique and distinct entity. A comparative study with granuloma annulare. *Am J Dermatopathol* 2002; **24**: 209–12.

59 Ackerman AB. Vasculitis: the true and near-true. *Am J Dermatopathol* 2002; **24**: 521–2.

60 Al-Hoqail IA, Martinka M, Crawford RI. Vasculitis: the true and near-true: authors' reply. *Am J Dermatopathol* 2002; **24**: 522–3.

61 Hanke CW, Bailin PL, Roenigk HH Jr. Annular elastolytic giant cell granuloma. A clinicopathologic study of five cases and a review of similar entities. *J Am Acad Dermatol* 1979; **1**: 413–21.

62 Ragaz A, Ackerman AB. Is actinic granuloma a specific condition? *Am J Dermatopathol* 1979; **1**: 43–50.

63 Wilson Jones E. Actinic granuloma. *Am J Dermatopathol* 1980; **2**: 89–90.

64 Weedon D. Actinic granuloma: the controversy continues. *Am J Dermatopathol* 1980; **2**: 90–1.

65 Revenga F, Rovira I, Pimentel J, Alejo M. Annular elastolytic giant cell granuloma—actinic granuloma. *Clin Exp Dermatol* 1996; **21**: 51–3.

66 O'Brien JP, Regan W. Actinically degenerate elastic tissue is the likely antigenic basis of actinic granuloma of the skin and of temporal arteritis. *J Am Acad Dermatol* 1999; **40**: 214–22.

67 Gradwell E, Evans S. Perforating granuloma annulare complicating tattoos. *Br J Dermatol* 1998; **138**: 360–1.

68 Bedlow AJ, Wong E, Cook MG, Marsden RA. Perforating collagenosis due to red dye in a tattoo. *Br J Dermatol* 1998; **139**: 926–7.

69 Abraham Z, Feuerman Ej, Schafer I, Feinmesser M. Disseminated granuloma annulare following erythema multiforme minor. *Australas J Dermatol* 2000; **41**: 238–41.

70 Lim AC, Hart K, Murrell D. A granuloma annulare-like eruption associated with the use of amlodipine. *Australas J Dermatol* 2002; **43**: 24–7.

71 Dahl MV, Ullman S, Goltz RW. Vasculitis in granuloma annulare: histopathology and direct immunofluorescence. *Arch Dermatol* 1977; **113**: 463–7.

72 Umbert P, Winkelmann RK. Granuloma annulare: direct immunofluorescence study. *Br J Dermatol* 1976; **95**: 487–92.

73 Bergman R, Pam Z, Lichtig C *et al*. Localized granuloma annulare. Histopathological and direct immunofluorescence study of early lesions, and the adjacent normal-looking skin of actively spreading lesions. *Am J Dermatopathol* 1993; **15**: 544–8.

74 Cherney KJ, Lindroos WE, Goltz RW *et al*. Leukocyte function in granuloma annulare. *Br J Dermatol* 1979; **101**: 23–31.

75 Buechner SA, Winkelmann RK, Banks PM. Identification of T-cell sub-populations in granuloma annulare. *Arch Dermatol* 1983; **119**: 125–8.

76 Modlin RL, Vaccaro SA, Gottlieb B *et al*. Granuloma annulare. Identification of cells in the cutaneous infiltrate by immunoperoxidase techniques. *Arch Pathol Lab Med* 1984; **108**: 379–82.

77 Fayyazi A, Schweyer S, Eichmeyer B *et al*. Expression of IFN gamma, coexpression of TNF alpha and matrix metalloproteinases and apoptosis of T lymphocytes and macrophages in granuloma annulare. *Arch Dermatol Res* 2000; **292**: 384–90.

78 Friedman-Birnbaum R, Haim S, Gideone O, Barzilai A. Histocompatibility antigens in granuloma annulare. Comparative study of the generalized and localized types. *Br J Dermatol* 1978; **98**: 425–8.

Histopathology [1–5] (Figs 60.1 & 60.2). The most characteristic histological lesion in granuloma annulare is the necrobiotic granuloma, but there are three histological patterns that may occur: necrobiotic palisading granulomas, an interstitial form, and granulomas of sarcoidal or tuberculoid type [1]. Umbert and Winkelmann [3] found that the commonest histological pattern was the interstitial type, as did Friedmann-Birnbaum *et al*. [4]. The latter authors compared the histopathological features of localized and generalized granuloma annulare, and noted that the interstitial pattern was more frequent in localized than in generalized disease; the prevalence of the palisading granuloma pattern was almost equal in both clinical types. Dabski and Winkelmann [5] also found that the interstitial pattern was common in both these types of granuloma annulare, and in many cases it occurred alone, without palisading granulomas. However, they noted a prominent palisading pattern more frequently in localized disease than in the generalized variety. Observer variation and the existence of more than one pattern in the same section may have contributed to differences in the findings in these series.

Necrobiotic granulomas are characterized by foci of necrobiosis surrounded by histiocytes and lymphocytes, with the histiocytes

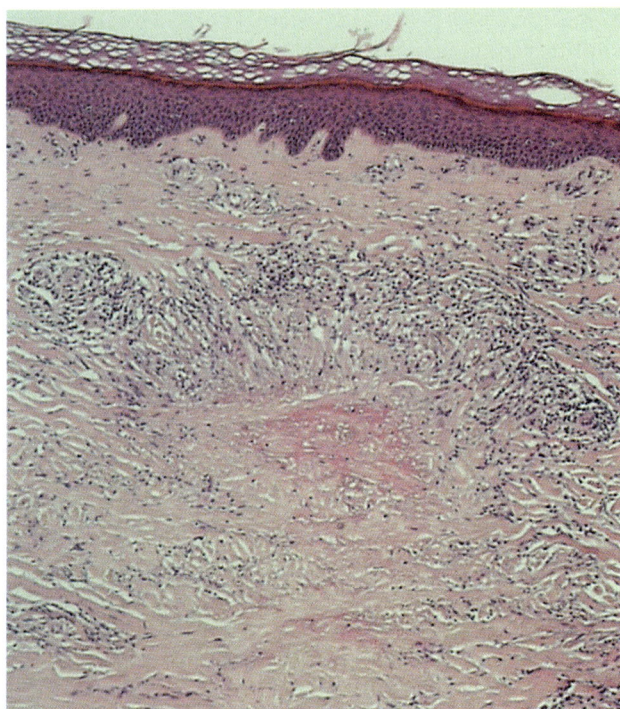

Fig. 60.1 Granuloma annulare. Nodule in upper dermis. H&E stain. (Courtesy of Dr M. Bamford, Dept. of Pathology, Leicester Royal Infirmary, Leicester, UK.)

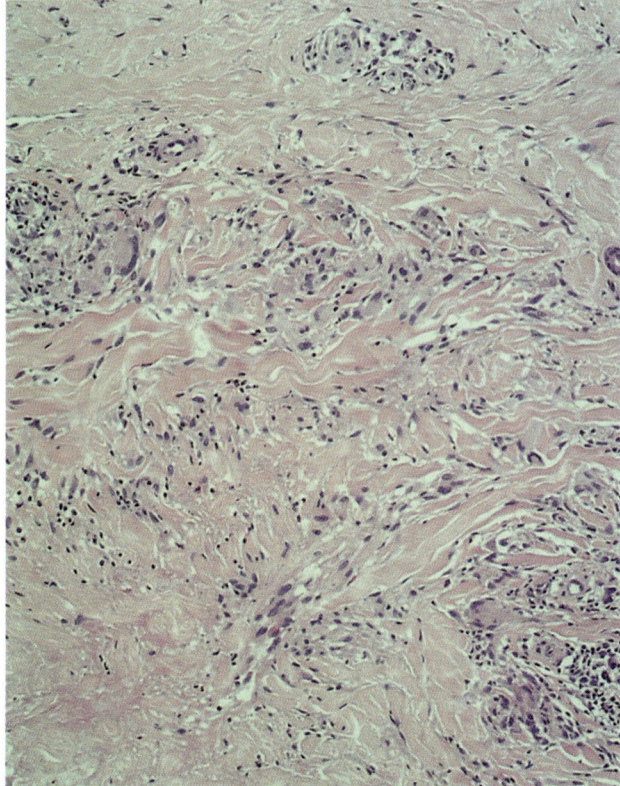

Fig. 60.2 Granuloma annulare. Nodule—well circumscribed with good palisade of histiocytes and central necrobiosis. H&E stain. (Courtesy of Dr M. Bamford, Dept. of Pathology, Leicester Royal Infirmary, Leicester, UK.)

commonly forming a palisaded pattern. There are varying numbers of multinucleate giant cells in this peripheral zone. T cells in the lymphocytic infiltrate are of the helper/inducer phenotype (CD4+) [6–8], but in two cases associated with HIV infection a predominantly T-suppressor (CD8+) infiltrate was demonstrated [9,10]. Analysis of the T-cell repertoire and cytokine pattern has shown a T-cell response characterized by a combination of a few skin-specific clones together with many non-specific T cells, and abundant production of interleukin-2 [8]. The high local production of interleukin-2 could be responsible for the non-specific attraction of T cells to the granulomas.

Mucin is present within the foci of necrobiosis, and it can be seen more readily by staining with Alcian blue or colloidal iron. Small deposits of lipid material may also be present in these areas. Some form of collagen alteration, most commonly fragmentation of collagen bundles, was observed in 79% of cases of localized and 53% of cases of generalized granuloma annulare by Dabski and Winkelmann [5]. There is a marked reduction in, or absence of, elastic fibres [11,12]. Metalloproteinases are probably involved in the damage to collagen and elastic fibres [13,14]. The granulomas are situated in the superficial and mid-dermis and, in contrast with necrobiosis lipoidica, areas between them are relatively normal.

In the interstitial pattern there are no formed areas of necrobiosis, histiocytes and lymphocytes are present around blood vessels and between collagen bundles, and collagen fibres are separated by mucin.

The sarcoidal or tuberculoid pattern is uncommon, and may cause problems in diagnosis. The presence of mucin and eosinophils can help to distinguish granuloma annulare from sarcoidosis. Blau syndrome is rare but causes histological differential diagnostic difficulties as it comprises an interstitial infiltrate as well as a sarcoidal pattern.

There is a perivascular infiltrate of lymphocytes and histiocytes. Eosinophils are variably present [15]. In one study [16], the presence of eosinophils was strongly associated with a palisaded architectural pattern and the presence of necrobiosis. Plasma cells are rare. A vasculitis has been described in or near foci of necrobiosis [17].

Histiocytes express the marker PG-M1 [18]. They may show an increased mitotic rate, and recognition of this is important, in particular in differentiating granuloma annulare from epithelioid sarcoma [19–22].

Epidermal changes are inconspicuous except in perforating granuloma annulare. In this variant there is a superficial area of necrobiosis surrounded by palisading histiocytes, situated beneath a perforation in the epidermis [1,2,23]. The necrobiotic material is extruded via the perforation. At the margins of the perforation there are varying degrees of epidermal hyperplasia.

The lesions of subcutaneous granuloma annulare often contain large areas of necrobiosis, and they are similar to rheumatoid nodules both clinically and histologically. Patterson [24] found that Alcian blue staining of mucin in lesions of granuloma annulare was the most helpful distinguishing feature.

Other disorders with similar histological features include mycosis fungoides variants [25–28], interstitial granulomatous dermatitis (interstitial granulomatous dermatitis with arthritis; interstitial granulomatous dermatitis with plaques; palisaded neutrophilic granulomatous dermatitis) [29–35], and the interstitial granulomatous drug reaction [36,37].

References

1 Weedon D. *Skin Pathology*, 2nd edn. London: Churchill Livingstone, 2002: 200–2.

2 Elder D, Elenitsas R, Jaworsky C, Johson B Jr, eds. *Lever's Histopathology of the Skin* 8th edn. Philadelphia: Lippincott-Raven, 1999: 328–30.

3 Umbert P, Winkelmann RK. Histologic, ultrastructural and histochemical studies of granuloma annulare. *Arch Dermatol* 1977; **113**: 1681–6.

4 Friedman-Birnbaum R, Weltfriend S, Munichor M, Lichtig C. A comparative histopathologic study of generalized and localized granuloma annulare. *Am J Dermatopathol* 1989; **11**: 144–8.

5 Dabski K, Winkelmann RK. Generalized granuloma annulare: histopathology and immunopathology. Systematic review of 100 cases and comparison with localized granuloma annulare. *J Am Acad Dermatol* 1989; **20**: 28–39.

6 Buechner SA, Winkelmann RK, Banks PM. Identification of T-cell subpopulations in granuloma annulare. *Arch Dermatol* 1983; **119**: 125–8.

7 Kallioinen M, Sandberg M, Kinnunen T, Oikarinen A. Collagen synthesis in granuloma annulare. *J Invest Dermatol* 1992; **98**: 463–8.

8 Mempel M, Musette P, Flageul B *et al*. T-cell receptor repertoire and cytokine pattern in granuloma annulare: defining a particular type of cutaneous granulomatous inflammation. *J Invest Dermatol* 2002; **118**: 957–66.

9 Huerter CJ, Bass J, Bergfeld WF, Tubbs RR. Perforating granuloma annulare in a patient with acquired immunodeficiency syndrome. Immunohistologic evaluation of the cellular infiltrate. *Arch Dermatol* 1987; **123**: 1217–20.

10 Morris SD, Cerio R, Paige DG. An unusual presentation of diffuse granuloma annulare in an HIV-positive patient—immunohistochemical evidence of predominant CD8 lymphocytes. *Clin Exp Dermatol* 2002; **27**: 205–8.

11 Friedman-Birnbaum R, Weltfriend S, Kerner H, Lichtig C. Elastic tissue changes in generalized granuloma annulare. *Am J Dermatopathol* 1989; **11**: 429–33.

12 Hanna WM, Moreno-Merlo F, Andrighetti L. Granuloma annulare: an elastic tissue disease? Case report and literature review. *Ultrastruct Pathol* 1999; **23**: 33–8.

13 Vaalamo M, Kariniemi A-L, Shapiro SD, Saarialho-Kere U. Enhanced expression of human metalloelastase (MMP-12) in cutaneous granulomas and macrophage migration. *J Invest Dermatol* 1999; **112**: 499–505.

14 Fayyazi A, Schweyer S, Eichmeyer B *et al*. Expression of IFNγ, coexpression of TNFα and matrix metalloproteinases and apoptosis of T lymphocytes and macrophages in granuloma annulare. *Arch Dermatol Res* 2000; **292**: 384–90.

15 Silverman RA, Rabinowitz AD. Eosinophils in the cellular infiltrate of granuloma annulare. *J Cutan Pathol* 1985; **12**: 13–17.

16 Romero LS, Kantor GR. Eosinophils are not a clue to the pathogenesis of granuloma annulare. *Am J Dermatopathol* 1998; **20**: 29–34.

17 Dahl MV, Ullman S, Goltz RW. Vasculitis in granuloma annulare: histopathology and direct immunofluorescence. *Arch Dermatol* 1977; **113**: 463–7.

18 Groisman GM, Schafer I, Amar M, Sabo E. Expression of the histiocytic marker PG-M1 in granuloma annulare and rheumatoid nodules of the skin. *J Cutan Pathol* 2002; **29**: 590–5.

19 Heenan PJ, Quirk CJ, Papadimitriou JM. Epithelioid sarcoma. A diagnostic problem. *Am J Dermatopathol* 1986; **8**: 95–104.

20 Trotter MJ, Crawford RI, O'Connell JX, Tron VA. Mitotic granuloma annulare: a clinicopathologic study of 20 cases. *J Cutan Pathol* 1996; **23**: 537–45.

21 Lopez-Rios F, Rodriguez-Peralto JL, Castano E, Gil R. Epithelioid sarcoma masquerading as perforating granuloma annulare. *Histopathology* 1997; **31**: 102–3.

22 Shmookler BM, Gunther SF. Superficial epithelioid sarcoma: a clinical and histologic simulant of benign cutaneous disease. *J Am Acad Dermatol* 1986; **14**: 893–8.

23 Peñas PF, Jones-Caballero M, Frage J *et al*. Perforating granuloma annulare. *Int J Dermatol* 1997; **36**: 340–8.

24 Patterson JW. Rheumatoid nodule and subcutaneous granuloma annulare. A comparative histologic study. *Am J Dermatopathol* 1988; **10**: 1–8.

25 Chen K-R, Tanaka M, Miyakawa S. Granulomatous mycosis fungoides with small intestinal involvement and a fatal outcome. *Br J Dermatol* 1998; **138**: 522–5.

26 Fischer M, Wohlrab J, Audring TH *et al.* Granulomatous mycosis fungoides. Report of two cases and review of the literature. *J Eur Acad Dermatol Venereol* 2000; **14:** 196–202.

27 Su LD, Kim YH, LeBoit PE *et al.* Interstitial mycosis fungoides, a variant of mycosis fungoides resembling granuloma annulare and inflammatory morphoea. *J Cutan Pathol* 2002; **29:** 135–41.

28 Eisman S, O'Toole EA, Jones A, Whittaker SJ. Granulomatous mycosis fungoides presenting as an acquired ichthyosis. *Clin Exp Dermatol* 2003; **28:** 174–6.

29 Chu P, Connolly MK, LeBoit PE. The histopathologic spectrum of palisaded neutrophilic and granulomatous dermatitis in patients with collagen vascular disease. *Arch Dermatol* 1994; **130:** 1278–83.

30 Long D, Thiboutot DM, Majeski JT *et al.* Interstitial granulomatous dermatitis with arthritis. *J Am Acad Dermatol* 1996; **34:** 957–61.

31 Ackerman AB, Chongchitnant N, Sanchez J *et al.* Interstitial granulomatous dermatitis with arthritis. In: Ackerman AB, ed. *Histologic Diagnosis of Inflammatory Skin Diseases. An Algorithmic Method Based on Pattern Analysis.* Baltimore: Williams & Wilkins, 1997: 459–62.

32 Aloi P, Tomasini C, Pippione M. Interstitial granulomatous dermatitis with plaques. *Am J Dermatopathol* 1999; **21:** 320–3.

33 Verneuil L, Dompmartin A, Comoz F *et al.* Interstitial granulomatous dermatitis with cutaneous cords and arthritis: a disorder associated with autoantibodies. *J Am Acad Dermatol* 2001; **45:** 286–91.

34 Sangueza OP, Caudell MD, Mengesha YM *et al.* Palisaded neutrophilic granulomatous dermatitis in rheumatoid arthritis. *J Am Acad Dermatol* 2002; **47:** 251–7.

35 Kroesen S, Itin PH, Hasler P. Arthritis and interstitial granulomatous dermatitis (Ackerman syndrome) with pulmonary silicosis. *Semin Arthritis Rheum* 2003; **32:** 334–40.

36 Magro CM, Crowson AN, Schapiro BL. The interstitial granulomatous drug reaction: a distinctive clinical and pathological entity. *J Cutan Pathol* 1998; **25:** 72–8.

37 Perrin C, Lacour J-P, Castanet J, Michiels J-F. Interstitial granulomatous drug reaction with a histological pattern of interstitial granulomatous dermatitis. *Am J Dermatopathol* 2001; **23:** 295–8.

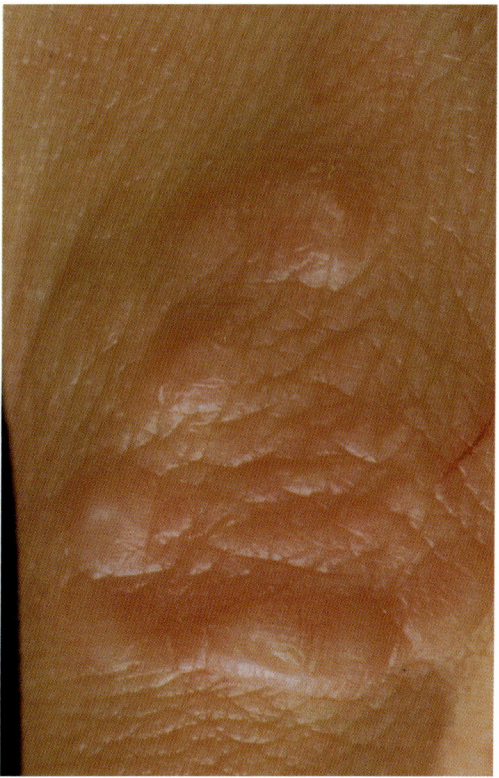

Fig. 60.3 Typical papules of granuloma annulare.

Clinical features [1,2]. Granuloma annulare can occur at almost any age—in one series the youngest patient was 1 year old and the oldest 76 [3]—but the majority of affected individuals are under 30 years of age [3]. It is twice as common in women as in men. There are a few reports of familial cases [3–9]. Clinical variants include localized, generalized, perforating and subcutaneous.

Localized granuloma annulare is the commonest form, and typically presents as a ring of small, smooth, flesh-coloured or erythematous papules (Fig. 60.3). Stretching the skin enables the papules to be seen more readily. The surface of the skin over the papules is intact and there is usually no scaling. Annular lesions tend to enlarge centrifugally. They may be solitary or multiple, and may occur anywhere on the skin, although the dorsa of the hands (Figs 60.4 & 60.5) and feet (Fig. 60.6), and the fingers (Fig. 60.7) are the commonest sites. Lesions are usually symptomless, although some may be tender to touch, and acute-onset, painful acral lesions have been described [10]. Some, often acral, lesions enlarge as nodules rather than having an annular morphology.

The other patterns of granuloma annulare may occur alone or in association with the annular lesions. In the generalized or disseminated pattern, there are numerous skin-coloured or erythematous papules, which may have an annular configuration or consist of myriad, symmetrically distributed, often coalescing lesions, on the trunk and limbs [11–14] (Fig. 60.8). The area enclosed by annular papules is often violaceous in colour. Pruritus may be a prominent complaint in generalized lesions [13]. Although generalized granuloma annulare may occur in children, the mean age

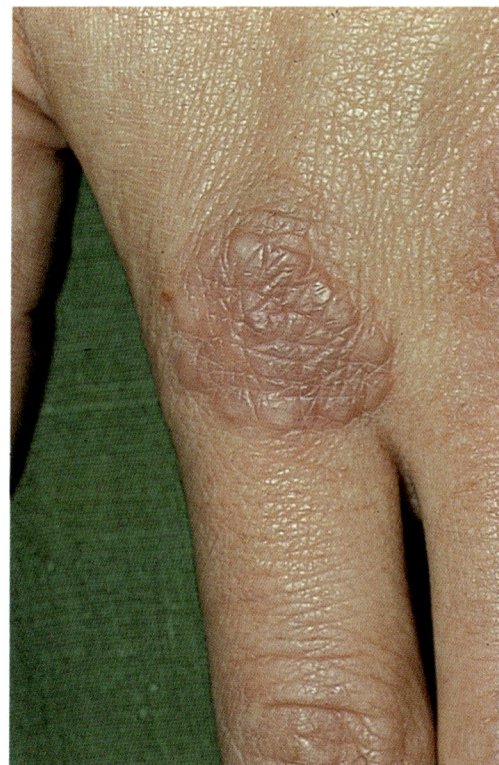

Fig. 60.4 Granuloma annulare on the dorsum of the hand—a typical site.

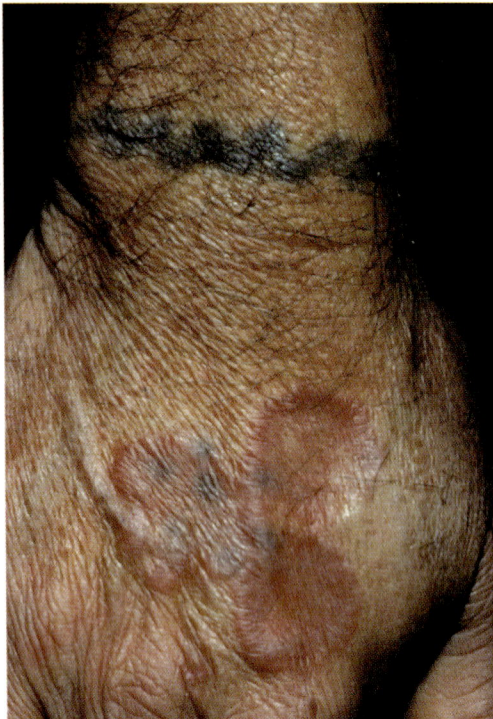

Fig. 60.5 Granuloma annulare on the dorsum of the hand. Altered pigmentation and atrophy in the centre of the lesions.

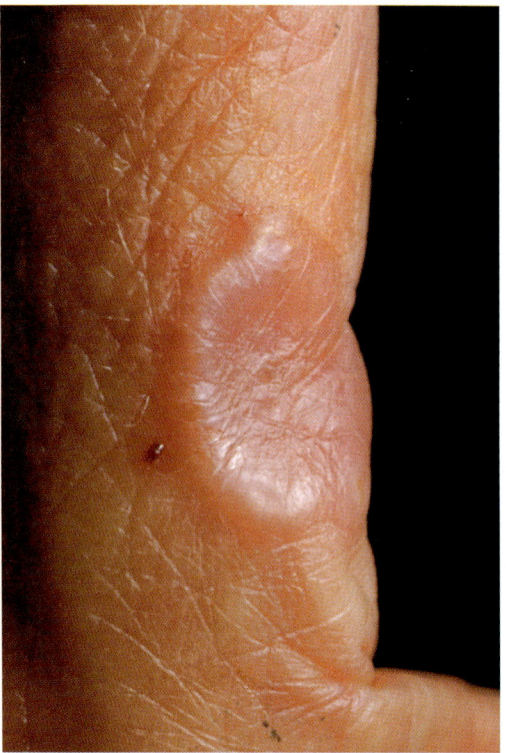

Fig. 60.7 Granuloma annulare on the side of a finger.

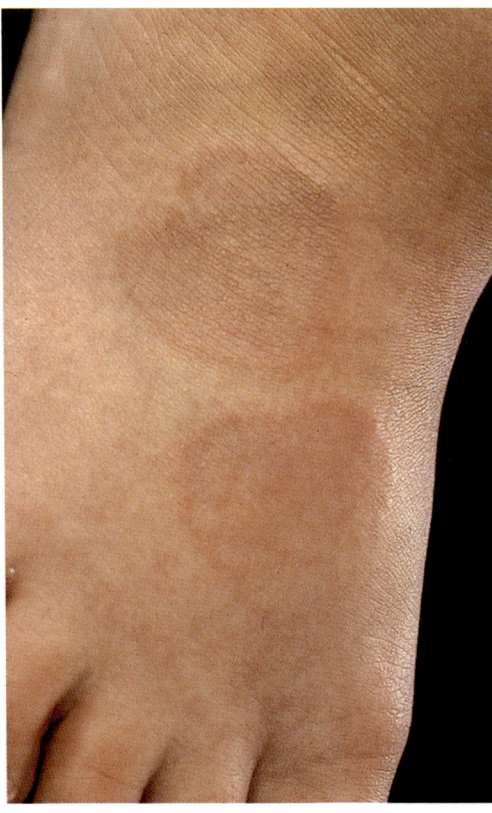

Fig. 60.6 Granuloma annulare on the dorsum of a child's foot. Often mistaken for tinea—but there is no scale and tinea in this site would be unlikely in a child.

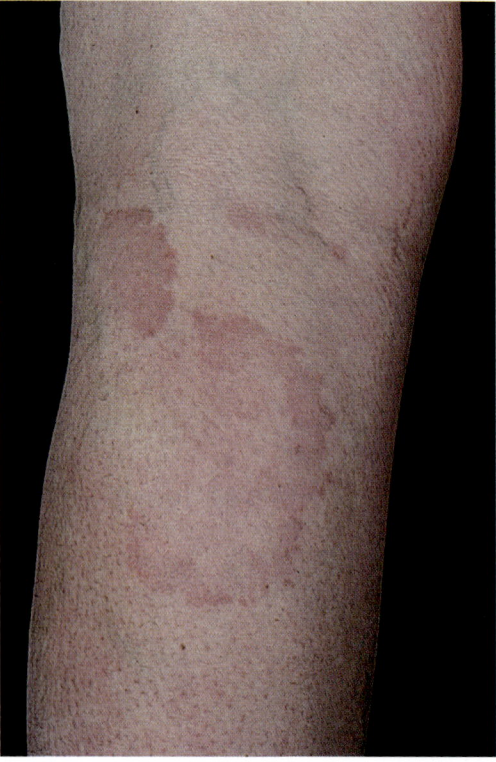

Fig. 60.8 These annular lesions were part of an extensive eruption on the limbs in a patient with generalized granuloma annulare.

at onset is later than in the localized variety, and in the series of Dabski and Winkelmann [13] it was 51.7 years. The exact incidence of the generalized pattern is unknown, but 8.9% of all patients with granuloma annulare seen at the Mayo Clinic had a generalized or disseminated pattern [13]. As in the localized form, twice as many females are affected as males. Although in immunocompetent individuals localized disease is more common than generalized granuloma annulare, in HIV-infected patients the generalized pattern predominates [14–18]. The sparing of vaccination sites in a case of generalized granuloma annulare is an interesting phenomenon [19].

Perforating granuloma annulare was named by Owens and Freeman in 1971 [20]. In this uncommon variety, some of the papules develop yellowish centres and discharge a little clear, viscous fluid. This dries to form a crust, which eventually separates, and may leave a hypo- or hyperpigmented scar. Lesions may be localized or generalized [21–24]. A high incidence of perforating granuloma annulare has been reported in the Hawaiian Islands [22,23]. Perforating lesions have been present in some of the reported HIV-positive individuals with granuloma annulare. Generalized perforating granuloma annulare has been described in an infant [25].

Subcutaneous granuloma annulare is also uncommon. It occurs predominantly in children, and has been given a variety of names, including benign rheumatoid nodules [26], pseudorheumatoid nodules [27,28], deep granuloma annulare [29,30], subcutaneous palisading granuloma [31], isolated subcutaneous granuloma and subcutaneous necrobiotic granuloma [32]. Lesions are nodular and occur predominantly on the scalp and legs, particularly in the pretibial region [4,32–34], but unusual locations include periorbital subperiosteal [35], palm [36,37] and penis [38]. A congenital case has been recorded [39]. Magnetic resonance imaging features are diagnostically helpful [40–42].

Other reported variants of granuloma annulare include a papular umbilicated form on the dorsa of the hands in children [43], a case of 'follicular pustulous' granuloma annulare, in which palisading necrobiotic granulomas occurred in a perifollicular distribution [44], pustular generalized perforating granuloma annulare, in which a dense infiltrate of neutrophils was present in areas of necrobiosis [45], linear granuloma annulare [46,47], and 'patch' granuloma annulare, in which erythematous patches occur on the trunk and limbs [48]. It has been suggested that cases with 'linear' lesions may be examples of interstitial granulomatous dermatitis, and those with 'patch' lesions may represent examples of the interstitial granulomatous form of drug reaction [49].

Uncommon sites for lesions of granuloma annulare are the ears (Fig. 60.9), where the perforating variety is particularly unusual [50], penis [51–56], palms [57] and periocular regions [58–63]. Mucous membranes are spared, although there is a report of involvement of the oral mucosa in a patient with HIV infection [64].

A destructive form has been described [65,66].

The postal questionnaire survey carried out by Wells and Smith [3] revealed that in about 50% of patients the lesions resolved within 2 years. However, about 40% of those whose lesions cleared had a recurrence, in the majority of cases at the same sites as the original lesions. In this study, there did not appear to be any dif-

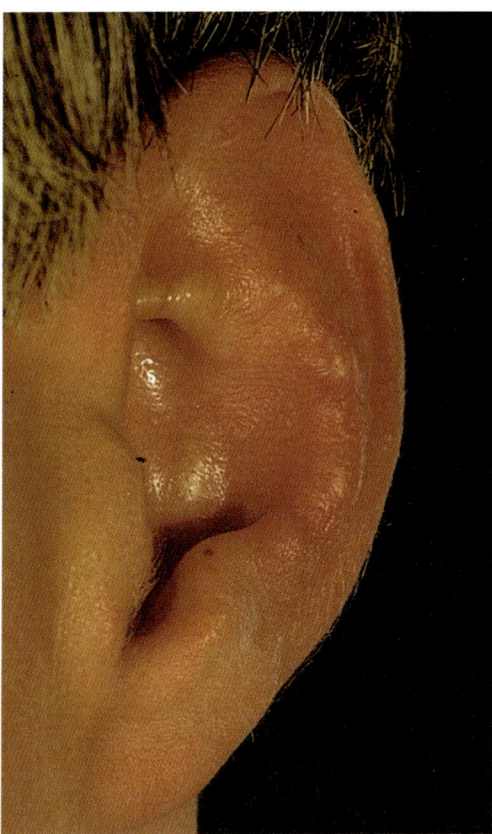

Fig. 60.9 Granuloma annulare on the ear.

ference in prognosis between individuals with single lesions and those with multiple lesions, and although there is an impression that spontaneous resolution is less likely to occur with generalized granuloma annulare there does not appear to be any documented confirmation of this.

There are reports of anetoderma secondary to generalized lesions [67], and mid-dermal elastolysis occurring with granuloma annulare [68] and subsequent to lesions resembling granuloma annulare [69]. In another case, loss of elastic fibres was presumed to be responsible for development of open comedones on the rim of granuloma annulare lesions occurring on light-exposed areas [70].

Levin *et al.* [71] have discussed the matter of resolution of lesions following biopsy, and have noted the paucity of information relating to this phenomenon in the literature. There appears to be anecdotal evidence of its occurrence, but little documentation. However, it is of interest, in this context, that scarification is one form of physical treatment that has been advocated in the past [72–74].

References

1 Muhlbauer JE. Granuloma annulare. *J Am Acad Dermatol* 1980; **3**: 217–30.
2 Smith MD, Downie JB, DiCostanzo D. Granuloma annulare. *Int J Dermatol* 1997; **36**: 326–33.
3 Wells RS, Smith MA. The natural history of granuloma annulare. *Br J Dermatol* 1963; **75**: 199–205.
4 Rubin M, Lynch FW. Subcutaneous granuloma annulare. Comment on familial granuloma annulare. *Arch Dermatol* 1966; **93**: 416–20.
5 Arner S, Aspergren N. Familial granuloma annulare. *Acta Derm Venereol (Stockh)* 1968; **48**: 253–4.

6 Goolamali SK, Stevenson CJ. Granuloma annulare in identical twins. *Br J Dermatol* 1972; **86**: 636–7.

7 Friedman SJ, Winkelmann RK. Familial granuloma annulare. Report of two cases and review of the literature. *J Am Acad Dermatol* 1987; **16**: 600–5.

8 Abrusci V, Weiss E, Planus G. Familial generalized perforating granuloma annulare. *Int J Dermatol* 1988; **27**: 126–7.

9 Suite M, Jankey N. Familial granuloma annulare. *Int J Dermatol* 1992; **31**: 818.

10 Brey NV, Malone J, Callen JP. Acute-onset, painful acral granuloma annulare. *Arch Dermatol* 2006; **142**: 49–54.

11 Stankler L, Leslie G. Generalized granuloma annulare: a report of a case and review of the literature. *Arch Dermatol* 1967; **95**: 509–13.

12 Dicken CH, Carrington SG, Winkelmann RK. Generalized granuloma annulare. *Arch Dermatol* 1969; **99**: 556–63.

13 Dabski K, Winkelmann RK. Generalized granuloma annulare: clinical and laboratory findings in 100 patients. *J Am Acad Dermatol* 1989; **20**: 39–47.

14 Bakos L, Hampe S, daRocha JL *et al.* Generalized granuloma annulare in a patient with acquired immunodeficiency syndrome. *J Am Acad Dermatol* 1987; **17**: 844–5.

15 Toro JR, Chu P, Ben Yen T-S, LeBoit PE. Granuloma annulare and human immunodeficiency virus infection. *Arch Dermatol* 1999; **135**: 1341–6.

16 Cohen PR. Granuloma annulare. A mucocutaneous condition in human immunodeficiency virus-infected patients. *Arch Dermatol* 1999; **135**: 1404–7.

17 O'Moore EJ, Nandawni R, Uthayakumar S *et al.* HIV-associated granuloma annulare (HAGA): a report of six cases. *Br J Dermatol* 2000; **142**: 1054–6.

18 Morris SD, Cerio R, Paige DG. An unusual presentation of diffuse granuloma annulare in an HIV-positive patient—immunohistochemical evidence of predominant CD8 lymphocytes. *Clin Exp Dermatol* 2002; **27**: 205–8.

19 Huilgol SC, Liddell K, Black MM. Generalized granuloma annulare sparing vaccination sites. *Clin Exp Dermatol* 1995; **20**: 51–3.

20 Owens DW, Freeman RG. Perforating granuloma annulare. *Arch Dermatol* 1971; **103**: 64–7.

21 Delaney TJ, Gold SC, Leppard B. Disseminated perforating granuloma annulare. *Br J Dermatol* 1973; **89**: 523–6.

22 Izumi AK. Generalized perforating granuloma annulare. *Arch Dermatol* 1973; **108**: 708–9.

23 Samlaska CP, Sandberg GD, Maggio KL, Sakas EL. Generalized perforating granuloma annulare. *J Am Acad Dermatol* 1992; **27**: 319–22.

24 Peñas PF, Jones-Caballero M, Fraga J *et al.* Perforating granuloma annulare. *Int J Dermatol* 1997; **36**: 340–8.

25 Choi JC, Bae JY, Cho S *et al.* Generalized perforating granuloma annulare in an infant. *Pediatr Dermatol* 2003; **20**: 131–3.

26 Simons FER, Schaller JG. Benign rheumatoid nodules. *Pediatrics* 1975; **56**: 29–33.

27 Burrington JD. 'Pseudorheumatoid' nodules in children: report of 10 cases. *Pediatrics* 1970; **45**: 473–8.

28 Barzilai A, Huszar M, Shpiro D *et al.* Pseudorheumatoid nodules in adults: a juxta-articular form of nodular granuloma annulare. *Am J Dermatopathol* 2005; **27**: 1–5.

29 McDermott MB, Lind AC, Marley EF, Dehner LP. Deep granuloma annulare (pseudorheumatoid nodule) in children: clinicopathologic study of 35 cases. *Pediatr Dev Pathol* 1998; **1**: 300–8.

30 Salomon RJ, Gardepe SF, Woodley DT. Deep granuloma annulare in adults. *Int J Dermatol* 1986; **25**: 109–12.

31 Minifee PK, Buchino JJ. Subcutaneous palisading granulomas (benign rheumatoid nodules) in children. *J Pediatr Surg* 1986; **21**: 1078–80.

32 Hutchinson ACS, Hurray DH, Smith MT, Shannon AB. Subcutaneous granuloma annulare of the scalp: a case report and case review. *Cutis* 2005; **76**: 377–82.

33 Felner EI, Steinberg JB, Weinberg AG. Subcutaneous granuloma annulare: a review of 47 cases. *Pediatrics* 1997; **100**: 965–7.

34 Grogg KL, Nascimento AG. Subcutaneous granuloma annulare in childhood: clinicopathologic features in 34 cases. *Pediatrics* 2001; **107**: E42 p.580 (Abstr.).

35 Dutton JJ, Escaravage GK Jr. Periocular subperiosteal deep granuloma annulare in a child. *Ophthalmol Plast Reconstr Surg* 2006; **22**: 141–3.

36 Takeyama J, Sanada T, Watanabe M *et al.* Subcutaneous granuloma annulare in a child's palm: a case report. *J Hand Surg Am* 2006; **31**: 103–6.

37 Mur EC, Fernández CM, Hermosa JMH. Bilateral and subcutaneous palmar nodules in a 2-year-old child suggesting deep granuloma annulare. *J Eur Acad Dermatol Venereol* 2005; **19**: 100–3.

38 Sidwell RU, Green JSA, Agnew K *et al.* Subcutaneous granuloma annulare of the penis in 2 adolescents. *J Pediatr Surg* 2005; **40**: 1329–31.

39 De Aloe G, Risulo M, Sbano P *et al.* Congenital subcutaneous granuloma annulare. *Pediatr Dermatol* 2005; **22**: 234–6.

40 Kransdorf MJ, Murphey MD, Temple HT. Subcutaneous granuloma annulare: radiologic appearance. *Skeletal Radiol* 1998; **27**: 266–70.

41 Chung S, Frush DP, Prose NS *et al.* Subcutaneous granuloma annulare: MR imaging features in six children and literature review. *Radiology* 1999; **210**: 845–9.

42 Shehan JM, El-Azhary RA. Magnetic resonance imaging features of subcutaneous granuloma annulare. *Pediatr Dermatol* 2005; **22**: 377–8.

43 Lucky AW, Prose NS, Bove K *et al.* Papular umbilicated granuloma annulare. A report of four pediatric cases. *Arch Dermatol* 1992; **128**: 1375–8.

44 Vargas-Díez E, Feal-Cortizas C, Fraga J *et al.* Follicular pustulous granuloma annulare. *Br J Dermatol* 1998; **138**: 1075–8.

45 Gamo Villegas R, Sopena Barona J, Guerra Tapia A *et al.* Pustular generalized perforating granuloma annulare. *Br J Dermatol* 2003; **149**: 866–8.

46 McDow RA, Fields JP. Linear granuloma annulare of the finger. *Cutis* 1987; **39**: 43–4.

47 Harpster EF, Mauro T, Barr RJ. Linear granuloma annulare. *J Am Acad Dermatol* 1989; **21**: 1138–41.

48 Mutasim DF, Bridges AG. Patch granuloma annulare: clinicopathologic study of 6 patients. *J Am Acad Dermatol* 2000; **42**: 417–21.

49 Weedon D. *Skin Pathology*, 2nd edn. London: Churchill Livingstone, 2002: 200.

50 Farrar CW, Bell HK, Dobson CM, Sharpe GR. Perforating granuloma annulare presenting on the ears. *Br J Dermatol* 2002; **147**: 1026–8.

51 Trap R, Wiebe B. Granuloma annulare localized to the shaft of the penis. *Scand J Urol Nephrol* 1993; **27**: 549–51.

52 Narouz N, Allan PS, Wade AH. Penile granuloma annulare. *Sex Transm Infect* 1999; **75**: 186–7.

53 Kossard S, Collins AG, Wegman A, Hughes MR. Necrobiotic granulomas localized to the penis: a possible variant of subcutaneous granuloma annulare. *J Cutan Pathol* 1990; **17**: 101–4.

54 Hillman RJ, Waldron S, Walker MM, Harris JR. Granuloma annulare of the penis. *Genitourin Med* 1992; **68**: 47–9.

55 Laird SM. Granuloma annulare of the penis. *Genitourin Med* 1992; **68**: 277.

56 Lucas F, Viraebn R. Granulome palissadique du pénis: une variante de granulome annulaire profond. *Ann Dermatol Vénéréol* 2002; **129**: 1046–8.

57 Hsu S, Lehner AC, Chang JR. Granuloma annulare localized to the palms. *J Am Acad Dermatol* 1999; **41**: 287–8.

58 Mc Farland JP, Kauh YC, Luscombe HA. Periorbital granuloma annulare. *Arch Dermatol* 1982; **118**: 190–1.

59 Bucji ER, Daicker B, Huber P, Bucker SA. Granuloma annulare des Augenlides. *Klin Montabl Augenheikd* 1995; **207**: 91–4.

60 Moegelin A, Thalmann U, Haas N. Subcutaneous granuloma annulare of the eyelid. A case report. *Int J Oral Maxillofac Surg* 1995; **24**: 236–8.

61 Sandwich JT, David LS. Granuloma annulare of the eyelid: a case report and review of the literature. *Pediatr Dermatol* 1999; **16**: 373–6.

62 Cronquist SD, Stashower ME, Benson PM. Deep dermal granuloma annulare presenting as an eyelid tumor in a child, with review of pediatric eyelid lesions. *Pediatr Dermatol* 1999; **16**: 377–80.

63 Ramaesh K, Bhagat S, Wharton SB, Singh J. Orbital nodular granuloma annulare in a juvenile diabetic. *Eye* 2002; **16**: 670–3.

64 Toro JR, Chu P, Ben Yen T-S, LeBoit PE. Granuloma annulare and human immunodeficiency virus infection. *Arch Dermatol* 1999; **135**: 1341–6.

65 Dabski K, Winkelmann RK. Destructive granuloma annulare of the skin and underlying tissues—report of two cases. *Clin Exp Dermatol* 1991; **16**: 218–21.

66 Bancroft LW, Perniciaro C, Berquist TH. Granuloma annulare: radiographic demonstration of progressive mutilating arthropathy with vanishing bones. *Skeletal Radiol* 1998; **27**: 211–4.

67 Ozkan S, Fetil E, Izler F *et al.* Anetoderma secondary to generalized granuloma annulare. *J Am Acad Dermatol* 2000; **42**: 335–8.

68 Adams BB, Mutasim DF. Colocalization of granuloma annulare and mid-dermal elastolysis. *J Am Acad Dermatol* 2003; **48**: S25–7.

69 Yen A, Tschen J, Raimer SS. Mid-dermal elastolysis in an adolescent subsequent to lesions resembling granuloma annulare. *J Am Acad Dermatol* 1997; **37**: 870–2.

70 Sudy E, Urbina F, Espinosa X. Open comedones overlying granuloma annulare in a photoexposed area. *Photodermatol Photoimmunol Photomed* 2006; **22**: 273–4.

71 Levin NA, Patterson JW, Yao LL, Wilson BB. Resolution of patch-type granuloma annulare lesions after biopsy. *J Am Acad Dermatol* 2002; **46**: 426–9.

72 Shakhnes IE. Lechenic kol'tsevidnoi granulemy methodom skarifikatsii. *Vestn Dermatol Venerol* 1977; **4**: 78–9.

73 Robinson HM Sr. Treatment for granuloma annulare. *Arch Dermatol* 1953; **67**: 320.

74 Wilkin JK, DuComb D, Castrow FF. Scarification treatment of granuloma annulare. *Arch Dermatol* 1982; **118**: 68–9.

Differential diagnosis. When the typical annular arrangement of papules is present, the diagnosis is usually straightforward. However, granuloma annulare may be mistaken for tinea, although the latter is more inflammatory, and the annular margin is scaly. Other annular lesions and granulomatous conditions may cause diagnostic confusion, including annular lichen planus, erythema annulare centrifugum, erythema multiforme, erythema migrans of Lyme disease, tuberculides [1] and tertiary syphilis [2]. The morphology and distribution of lesions may simulate mycosis fungoides [3].

With regard to subcutaneous granuloma annulare, the differential diagnosis of subcutaneous nodules of the scalp and legs in children is extensive, and includes trauma, infection and tumours, and a diagnostic biopsy will usually be necessary. In adults, nodular lesions have to be distinguished from sarcoidosis and rheumatoid nodules.

The differential diagnosis of perforating granuloma annulare includes molluscum contagiosum [4], transepithelial elimination disorders such as perforating collagenosis and acquired perforating dermatosis, sarcoidosis and papulonecrotic tuberculide [5,6]. As mentioned above, epithelioid sarcoma may masquerade as perforating granuloma annulare.

Mycobacterium marinum infection has histologically simulated interstitial granuloma annulare [7], and other histological differential diagnoses include granulomatous mycosis fungoides [8], interstitial granulomatous dermatitis and interstitial granulomatous drug reaction, as mentioned above.

References

1 Tsai J, Chen GS, Lan LH, Lan CCE. Cutaneous tuberculid clinically resembling generalized granuloma annulare. *Clin Exp Dermatol* 2007; **32**: 450–1.

2 Jones Wu S, Nguyen EQ, Nielsen TA, Pellegrini EA. Nodular tertiary syphilis mimicking granuloma annulare. *J Am Acad Dermatol* 2000; **42**: 378–80.

3 Wu H, Barusevicius A, Lessin SR. Granuloma annulare with a mycosis fungoides-like distribution and palisaded granuloma of CD68-positive histiocytes. *J Am Acad Dermatol* 2004; **51**: 39–44.

4 Kapembwa MS, Goolamali SK, Price A, Boyle S. Granuloma annulare masquerading as molluscum contagiosum-like eruption in an HIV-positive African woman. *J Am Acad Dermatol* 2003; **49** (Suppl. 2): S184–6.

5 Samlaska CP, Sandberg GD, Maggio KL, Sakas EL. Generalized perforating granuloma annulare. *J Am Acad Dermatol* 1992; **27**: 319–22.

6 Peñas PF, Jones-Caballero M, Fraga J *et al.* Perforating granuloma annulare. *Int J Dermatol* 1997; **36**: 340–8.

7 Barr KL, Lowe L, Su LD. *Mycobacterium marinum* infection simulating interstitial granuloma annulare: a report of two cases. *Am J Dermatopathol* 2003; **25**: 148–51.

8 Jouary T, Beylot-Barry M, Vergier B *et al.* Mycosis fungoides mimicking granuloma annulare. *Br J Dermatol* 2002; **146**: 1102–4.

Associations. There has been much discussion of whether there is an association between granuloma annulare and diabetes mellitus [1–13]. A number of studies have not demonstrated any relationship, whereas others suggest an association [1–12]. In the latter, some have favoured an association with generalized granuloma annulare [4–6] and others an association with localized disease [3,7], and possibly localized nodular granuloma annulare [8]. It is of interest to note that in three reports [3,7,8] the majority of diabetics were insulin-dependent (type 1). One study, employing a case–control design, did not show any association between granuloma annulare and type 2 diabetes [9]. The patient population studied did not include anyone with type 1 diabetes. In order to clarify the situation, further, large-scale studies are required, in which the pattern of granuloma annulare and type of diabetes are recorded.

Thomas *et al.* [14] reported a man with granuloma annulare of the skin, and intra-abdominal lesions, insulin-dependent diabetes and polyendocrine disease, in whom there appeared to be a relationship between diabetic control and the granuloma annulare. Granuloma annulare has been described in a child with Mauriac's syndrome (juvenile diabetes, stunted growth and hepatomegaly) [15].

There are a number of reports of the coexistence of both localized and generalized granuloma annulare and autoimmune thyroiditis in women [16–22], and results of a case–control study indicated an association between localized granuloma annulare and autoimmune thyroiditis [22]. In one case with generalized granuloma annulare the skin lesions improved in concert with disappearance of antithyroid antibodies and restoration of the euthyroid state [17]. Generalized granuloma annulare has also been reported in a patient with a toxic adenoma of the thyroid (Plummer's disease) [23].

Recent reports suggest the possibility of an association between uveitis and granuloma annulare [24,25].

Li *et al.* [26] have summarized and analyzed reports addressing a possible relationship between granuloma annulare and malignant neoplasms. In the cases reviewed, skin lesions that had histological features of granuloma annulare, but were often atypical clinically (for example, painful lesions on the palms and soles), occurred in patients with a neoplasm (in 56% of cases this was a lymphoma). They concluded that there was no definite relationship between granuloma annulare and malignant neoplasms.

There are isolated reports of the occurrence of temporal arteritis in a patient with generalized granuloma annulare [27], and of the coexistence of granuloma annulare and morphoea [28].

There are a number of reports of the occurrence of granuloma annulare and necrobiosis lipoidica in the same patient [29–32], and of the association of granuloma annulare and sarcoidosis [33–36].

References

1 Muhlbauer JE. Granuloma annulare. *J Am Acad Dermatol* 1980; **3**: 217–30.

2 Smith MD, Downie JB, DiCostanzo D. Granuloma annulare. *Int J Dermatol* 1997; **36**: 326–33.

3 Veraldi S, Bencini PL, Drudi E, Caputo R. Laboratory abnormalities in granuloma annulare: a case–control study. *Br J Dermatol* 1997; **136**: 652–3.

4 Romaine R, Rudner EJ, Altman J. Papular granuloma annulare and diabetes mellitus. Report of cases. *Arch Dermatol* 1968; **98**: 152–4.

5 Haim S, Friedman-Birnbaum R, Shafrir A. Generalized granuloma annulare: relationship to diabetes mellitus as revealed in 8 cases. *Br J Dermatol* 1970; **83**: 302–5.

6 Haim S, Friedman-Birnbaum R, Haim N *et al*. Carbohydrate intolerance in patients with granuloma annulare. Study of fifty-two cases. *Br J Dermatol* 1973; **88**: 447–51.

7 Muhlemann MF, Williams DRR. Localized granuloma annulare is associated with insulin-dependent diabetes mellitus. *Br J Dermatol* 1984; **111**: 325–9.

8 Choudry K, Charles-Holmes R. Are patients with localized nodular granuloma annulare more likely to have diabetes mellitus? *Clin Exp Dermatol* 2000; **25**: 451–3.

9 Nebesio CL, Lewis C, Chuang T-Y. Lack of an association between granuloma annulare and type 2 diabetes mellitus. *Br J Dermatol* 2002; **146**: 122–4.

10 Gannon TF, Lynch PJ. Absence of carbohydrate intolerance in granuloma annulare. *J Am Acad Dermatol* 1994; **30**: 662–3.

11 Studer EM, Calza A-M, Saurat J-H. Precipitating factors and associated diseases in 84 patients with granuloma annulare: a retrospective study. *Dermatology* 1996; **193**: 364–8.

12 Kakourou T, Psychou F, Voutetakis A *et al*. Low serum insulin values in children with multiple lesions of granuloma annulare: a prospective study. *J Eur Acad Dermatol Venereol* 2005; **19**: 30–4.

13 Cox NH. Diabetes and the skin: an update for dermatologists. *Expert Rev Dermatol* 2007; **2**: 305–16.

14 Thomas DJB, Rademaker M, Munro DD *et al*. Visceral and skin granuloma annulare, diabetes, and polyendocrine disease. *BMJ* 1986; **293**: 977–8.

15 Goldin D, Rook A, Gairdner D. Granuloma annulare in Mauriac's syndrome. *Br J Dermatol* 1975; **93** (Suppl. 11): 31.

16 Gross PR, Shelley WB. The association of generalized granuloma annulare with antithyroid antibodies. *Acta Derm Venereol (Stockh)* 1971; **51**: 59–62.

17 Willemsen MJ, de Coninck AL, Jonckheer MH, Roseeuw DI. Autoimmune thyroiditis and generalized granuloma annulare: remission of the skin lesions after thyroxine therapy. *Dermatologica* 1987; **175**: 239–43.

18 Dabski K, Winkelmann RK. Generalized granuloma annulare: clinical and laboratory findings in 100 patients. *J Am Acad Dermatol* 1989; **20**: 39–47.

19 Magro CM, Crowson AN, Regauer S. Granuloma annulare and necrobiosis lipoidica tissue reactions as a manifestation of systemic disease. *Hum Pathol* 1996; **27**: 50–6.

20 Vázquez-López F, González-López MA, Raya-Aguado C, Pérez-Oliva N. Localized granuloma annulare and autoimmune thyroiditis: a new case report. *J Am Acad Dermatol* 2000; **43**: 943–5.

21 Kappeler D, Troendle A, Mueller B. Localized granuloma annulare associated with autoimmune thyroid disease in a patient with a positive family history for autoimmune polyglandular syndrome type II. *Eur J Endocrinol* 2001; **145**: 101–2.

22 Vásquez-López F, Pereiro M Jr, Manjón Haces JA *et al*. Localized granuloma annulare and autoimmune thyroiditis in adult women: a case–control study. *J Am Acad Dermatol* 2003; **48**: 517–20.

23 Tursen U, Pata C, Kaya TI *et al*. Generalized granuloma annulare associated with Plummer's disease. *J Eur Acad Dermatol Venereol* 2002; **16**: 419–20.

24 Oz O, Tursen U, Yildirim O *et al*. Uveitis associated with granuloma annulare. *Eur J Ophthalmol* 2003; **13**: 93–5.

25 van Kooij B, Canninga van Dijk M, de Boer J *et al*. Is granuloma annulare related to intermediate uveitis with retinal vasculitis? *Br J Ophthalmol* 2003; **87**: 763–6.

26 Li A, Hogan DJ, Sanusi DI, Smoller BR. Granuloma annulare and malignant neoplasms. *Am J Dermatopathol* 2003; **25**: 113–6.

27 Fukai K, Ishii M, Kobayashi H *et al*. Generalized granuloma annulare in a patient with temporal arteritis—are these conditions associated? *Clin Exp Dermatol* 1990; **15**: 70–2.

28 Ben-Amitai D, Hodak E, Lapidoth M, David M. Coexisting morphoea and granuloma annulare—are the conditions related? *Clin Exp Dermatol* 1999; **24**: 86–9.

29 Feldman FF. Granuloma annulare and necrobiosis lipoidica in the same patient. *Arch Dermatol* 1968; **98**: 677–8.

30 Schwartz ME. Necrobiosis lipoidica and granuloma annulare. Simultaneous occurrence in a patient. *Arch Dermatol* 1982; **118**: 192–3.

31 Burton JL. Granuloma annulare, rheumatoid nodules and necrobiosis lipoidica. *Br J Dermatol* 1977; **77** (Suppl. 15): 52–4.

32 Berkson MH, Bondi EE, Margolis DJ. Ulcerated necrobiosis lipoidica diabeticorum in a patient with a history of generalized granuloma annulare. *Cutis* 1994; **53**: 85–6.

33 Umbert P, Winkelmann RK. Granuloma annulare and sarcoidosis. *Br J Dermatol* 1977; **97**: 481–6.

34 Harrison P, Shuster S. Granuloma annulare and sarcoidosis. *Br J Dermatol* 1979; **100**: 231.

35 Kato H, Yoshihiko F, Kitajima Y *et al*. A case of granuloma annulare and sarcoidosis. *J Dermatol* 1985; **12**: 63–9.

36 Ehrich EW, McGuire JL, Kim YH. Association of granuloma annulare with sarcoidosis. *Arch Dermatol* 1992; **128**: 855–6.

Treatment. The tendency of granuloma annulare to remit spontaneously complicates accurate assessment of the efficacy of any treatment, but in some patients explanation that this is the natural course of the disease is all that is required, and certainly in children it is preferable to await spontaneous resolution rather than subjecting them to the discomfort of some of the treatment methods. Potent topical steroids, with or without occlusion, are used by many dermatologists, but often with little benefit. Intralesional steroids, given by either needle injection or jet injector [1], appear to be more effective in the management of localized lesions. Cryosurgery also appears to be an effective treatment for localized disease. In a study of 31 patients, in which nitrous oxide and liquid nitrogen were employed, resolution was achieved in all, following a single freeze–thaw cycle in the majority [2]. The cosmetic result obtained by cryosurgery with nitrous oxide was independent of the size of the lesion, whereas in individuals treated with liquid nitrogen a better cosmetic result was obtained with smaller lesions. Because of this, the authors of the report proposed that use of nitrous oxide as refrigerant was preferable to liquid nitrogen.

Localized granuloma annulare has also been treated with local injections of low-dose recombinant interferon gamma [3]. Complete resolution of lesions occurred in the three treated patients, with no recurrence during 12 months of follow-up. More recently, photodynamic therapy was used successfully for localized disease [4], as was the pulsed dye laser [5].

Although some reports have indicated a beneficial effect of oral potassium iodide in the treatment of disseminated granuloma annulare [6,7], a double-blind, placebo-controlled, crossover study showed that it had no advantage over placebo [8]. PUVA therapy appears to be an effective treatment for generalized granuloma annulare, and good results have been reported using both oral and topical psoralens [9–17]. In many cases, however, maintenance therapy is required to sustain the benefit. Narrowband UVB [18] and UVA-1 phototherapy [19,20] have also been reported as effective in the treatment of generalized granuloma annulare. Etretinate [21–23] and isotretinoin [24–29] have both been of benefit in disseminated disease. Isotretinoin has also improved localized [30] and perforating granuloma annulare [31]. There are a few reports of the use of ciclosporin in generalized granuloma annulare [32–35], with good results in most cases. Other treatments which have been used with apparent benefit in isolated cases or small numbers of patients with disseminated granuloma annulare include low-dose chlorambucil [36–40], dapsone [41], antimalarials [42–44], niacinamide [45], pentoxifylline [46], tranilast [47], fumaric acid esters [48–50], clofazimine [51], topical vitamin E [52], a combination of vitamin E and a 5-lipoxygenase inhibitor [53], and defibrotide [54].

Recent reports suggest that topical imiquimod [55,56], tacrolimus [57,58] and pimecrolimus [59] may be helpful, and rapid resolution of recalcitrant disseminated lesions on treatment with infliximab [60] and efalizumab [61] has been reported. Shupack and Siu [62] noted clearing of disseminated lesions in a patient treated with etanercept, but in a series of four patients reported by Kreuter *et al.* [63] there was either no change or deterioration during therapy with this agent.

Most of the treatments mentioned above have been employed in patients with perforating lesions, with varying degrees of success [64].

Lesions of subcutaneous granuloma annulare should be left to resolve spontaneously once the diagnosis has been confirmed [65].

References

1 Sparrow G, Abell E. Granuloma annulare and necrobiosis lipoidica treated by jet injector. *Br J Dermatol* 1975; **93:** 85–9.
2 Blume-Peytavi U, Zouboulis Ch C, Jacobi H *et al.* Successful outcome of cryosurgery in patients with granuloma annulare. *Br J Dermatol* 1994; **130:** 494–7.
3 Weiss JM, Muchenberger S, Schöpf E, Simon JC. Treatment of granuloma annulare by local injections with low-dose recombinant human interferon gamma. *J Am Acad Dermatol* 1998; **39:** 117–9.
4 Kim YJ, Kang HY, Lee ES, Kim YC. Successful treatment of granuloma annulare with topical 5-aminolaevulinic acid photodynamic therapy. *J Dermatol* 2006; **33:** 642–3.
5 Sniezek PJ, De Bloom JR 2nd, Arpey CJ. Treatment of granuloma annulare with the 585 nm pulsed dye laser. *Dermatol Surg* 2005; **31:** 1370–3.
6 Giessel M, Graves K, Kalivas J. Treatment of disseminated granuloma annulare with potassium iodide. *Arch Dermatol* 1979; **115:** 639–40.
7 Caserio RJ, Eaglstein WH, Allen CM. Treatment of granuloma annulare with potassium iodide. *J Am Acad Dermatol* 1984; **10:** 294–5.
8 Smith JB, Hansen CD, Zone JJ. Potassium iodide in the treatment of disseminated granuloma annulare. *J Am Acad Dermatol* 1994; **30:** 791–2.
9 Hindson TC, Spiro JG, Cochrane H. PUVA therapy of diffuse granuloma annulare. *Clin Exp Dermatol* 1988; **13:** 26–7.
10 Kerker BJ, Huang CP, Morison WL. Photochemotherapy of generalized granuloma annulare. *Arch Dermatol* 1990; **126:** 359–61.
11 Langrock A, Weyers W, Schill WB. Balneophotochemotherapie bei disseminiertem Granuloma anulare. *Hautarzt* 1998; **49:** 303–6.
12 Setterfield J, Huilgol SC, Black MM. Generalized granuloma annulare successfully treated with PUVA. *Clin Exp Dermatol* 1999; **24:** 458–60.
13 Szegedi A, Bégány A, Hunyadi J. Successful treatment of generalized granuloma annulare with polythene sheet bath PUVA. *Acta Derm Venereol (Stockh)* 1999; **79:** 84–5.
14 Salomon N, Walchner M, Messer G *et al.* Bade-PUVA-Therapie bei Granuloma anulare. *Hautarzt* 1999; **50:** 275–9.
15 Schmutz JL. PUVA therapy of granuloma annulare. *Clin Exp Dermatol* 2000; **25:** 451–3.
16 Grundmann-Kollmann M, Ochsendorf FR, Zollner TM *et al.* Cream psoralen plus ultraviolet A therapy for granuloma annulare. *Br J Dermatol* 2001; **144:** 996–9.
17 Batchelor R, Clark S. Clearance of generalized papular umbilicated granuloma annulare in a child with bath PUVA therapy. *Pediatr Dermatol* 2006; **23:** 72–4.
18 Inui S, Nishida Y, Itami S, Katayama I. Disseminated granuloma annulare responsive to narrowband ultraviolet B therapy. *J Am Acad Dermatol* 2005; **53:** 533–4.
19 Muchenberger S, Schöpf E, Simon JC. Phototherapy with UV-A-1 for generalized granuloma annulare. *Arch Dermatol* 1997; **133:** 1605.
20 Schnopp C, Tsaneva S, Mempel M *et al.* UVA1 phototherapy for disseminated granuloma annulare. *Photodermatol Photoimmunol Photomed* 2005; **21:** 68–71.
21 Botella-Estrada R, Guillen C, Sanmartin O, Aliaga A. Disseminated granuloma annulare: resolution with etretinate therapy. *Arch Dermatol* 1992; **26:** 777–8.
22 Harth W, Richard G. Retinoide in der Therapie des Granuloma anulare disseminatum. *Hautarzt* 1993; **44:** 693–8.
23 Asano Y, Saito A, Idezuki T, Igarashi A. Generalized granuloma annulare treated with short-term administration of etretinate. *J Am Acad Dermatol* 2006; **54:** S245–7.
24 Schleicher SM, Milstein HJ. Resolution of disseminated granuloma annulare following isotretinoin therapy. *Cutis* 1985; **36:** 147–8.
25 Schleicher SM, Milstein HJ, Lim SJM, Stanton CD. Resolution of disseminated granuloma annulare with isotretinoin. *Int J Dermatol* 1992; **31:** 371–2.
26 Tang WY, Chong LY, Lo KK. Resolution of generalized granuloma annulare with isotretinoin therapy. *Int J Dermatol* 1996; **35:** 455–6.
27 Adams DC, Hogan DJ. Improvement of chronic generalized granuloma annulare with isotretinoin. *Arch Dermatol* 2002; **138:** 1518–9.
28 Looney M, Smith KM. Isotretinoin in the treatment of granuloma annulare. *Ann Pharmacother* 2004; **38:** 494–7.
29 Pasmatzi E, Georgiou S, Monastirli A, Tsambaos D. Temporary remission of disseminated granuloma annulare under oral isotretinoin therapy. *Int J Dermatol* 2005; **44:** 169–71.
30 Young HS, Coulson IH. Granuloma annulare following waxing induced folliculitis. *Clin Exp Dermatol* 2000; **25:** 274–6.
31 Ratnavel RC, Norris PG. Perforating granuloma annulare: response to treatment with isotretinoin. *J Am Acad Dermatol* 1995; **32:** 126–7.
32 Filotico R, Vena GA, Coviello C, Angelini G. Cyclosporine in the treatment of generalized granuloma annulare. *J Am Acad Dermatol* 1994; **30:** 487–8.
33 Ho VC. Cyclosporine in the treatment of generalized granuloma annulare. *J Am Acad Dermatol* 1995; **32:** 298.
34 Fiallo P. Cyclosporin for the treatment of granuloma annulare. *Br J Dermatol* 1998; **138:** 369–70.
35 Spadino S, Altomare A, Cainelli C *et al.* Disseminated granuloma annulare: efficacy of cyclosporine therapy. *Int J Immunopathol Pharmacol* 2006; **19:** 433–8.
36 Kossard S, Winkelmann RK. Response of generalized granuloma annulare to alkylating agents. *Arch Dermatol* 1978; **114:** 216–20.
37 Kossard S, Winkelmann RK. Low-dose chlorambucil in the treatment of generalized granuloma annulare. *Dermatologica* 1979; **158:** 443–50.
38 Rudolph RI. Disseminated granuloma annulare treated with low-dose chlorambucil. *Arch Dermatol* 1979; **115:** 1212–3.
39 Dabski K, Winkelmann RK. Generalized granuloma annulare: clinical and laboratory findings in 100 patients. *J Am Acad Dermatol* 1989; **20:** 39–47.
40 Winkelmann RK, Stevens JC. Successful treatment response of granuloma annulare and carpal tunnel syndrome to chlorambucil. *Mayo Clin Proc* 1994; **69:** 1163–5.
41 Saied N, Schwartz RA, Estes SA. Treatment of generalized granuloma annulare with dapsone. *Arch Dermatol* 1980; **116:** 1345–6.
42 Mandel EH. Disseminated granuloma annulare. Report of a case treated with chloroquine phosphate (Aralen). *Arch Dermatol* 1959; **79:** 352–3.
43 Stritzler C. Generalized granuloma annulare (apparently responding well to chloroquine therapy). *Arch Dermatol* 1961; **83:** 1033–4.
44 Carlin MC, Ratz JL. A case of generalized granuloma annulare responding to hydroxychloroquine. *Cleve Clin J Med* 1987; **54:** 229–32.
45 Ma A, Medenica M. Response of generalized granuloma annulare to high-dose niacinamide. *Arch Dermatol* 1983; **119:** 836–9.
46 Rubel DM, Wood G, Rosen R, Jopp-McKay A. Generalized granuloma annulare successfully treated with pentoxifylline. *Australas J Dermatol* 1993; **34:** 103–8.
47 Yamada H, Ide A, Sugiura M *et al.* Treatment of granuloma annulare with tranilast. *J Dermatol* 1995; **22:** 354–6.
48 Schulze DA, Petzoldt D. Granuloma anulare disseminatum—erfolgreiche Therapie mit Fumarsäureester. *Hautarzt* 2001; **52:** 228–30.
49 Eberlein-König B, Mempel M, Stahlecker J *et al.* Disseminated granuloma annulare—treatment with fumaric acid esters. *Dermatology* 2005; **210:** 223–6.
50 Breuer K, Gutzmer R, Völker B *et al.* Therapy of noninfectious granulomatous skin diseases with fumaric acid esters. *Br J Dermatol* 2005; **152:** 1290–5.
51 Mensing H. Clofazimine—therapeutische Alternative bei Necrobiosis lipoidica und Granuloma anulare. *Hautarzt* 1989; **40:** 99–103.
52 Burg G. Disseminated granuloma annulare: therapy with vitamin E topically. *Dermatology* 1992; **184:** 308–9.
53 Smith KJ, Norwood C, Skelton H. Treatment of disseminated granuloma annulare with a 5-lipoxygenase inhibitor and vitamin E. *Br J Dermatol* 2002; **146:** 667–70.
54 Rubegni P, Sbano P, Fimiani M. A case of disseminated granuloma annulare treated with defibrotide: complete clinical remission and progressive hair darkening. *Br J Dermatol* 2003; **149:** 437–9.
55 Kuwahara RT, Skinner RB Jr. Granuloma annulare resolved with topical application of imiquimod. *Pediatr Dermatol* 2002; **19:** 368–9.

56 Badavanis G, Monastirli A, Pasmatzi E, Tsambaos D. Successful treatment of granuloma annulare with imiquimod cream 5%: a report of four cases. *Acta Derm Venereol (Stockh)* 2005; **85**: 547–8.

57 Jain S, Stephens CJM. Successful treatment of disseminated granuloma annulare with topical tacrolimus. *Br J Dermatol* 2004; **150**: 1042–3.

58 Harth W, Linse R. Topical tacrolimus in granuloma annulare and necrobiosis lipoidica. *Br J Dermatol* 2004; **150**: 792–4.

59 Rigopoulos D, Prantsidis A, Christofidou E *et al*. Pimecrolimus 1% cream in the treatment of disseminated granuloma annulare. *Br J Dermatol* 2005; **152**: 1364–5.

60 Hertl MS, Haendle I, Schuler G, Hertl M. Rapid improvement of recalcitrant disseminated granuloma annulare upon treatment with the tumour necrosis factor-alpha inhibitor, infliximab. *Br J Dermatol* 2005; **152**: 552–5.

61 Goffe BS. Disseminated granuloma annulare resolved with the T-cell modulator efalizumab. *Arch Dermatol* 2004; **140**: 1287–8.

62 Shupack J, Siu K. Resolving granuloma annulare with etanercept. *Arch Dermatol* 2006; **142**: 394–5.

63 Kreuter A, Altmeyer P, Gambichler T. Failure of etanercept therapy in granuloma annulare. *Arch Dermatol* 2006; **142**: 1236–7.

64 Peñas PF, Jones-Caballero M, Fraga J *et al*. Perforating granuloma annulare. *Int J Dermatol* 1997; **36**: 340–8.

65 Felner EI, Steinberg JB, Weinberg AG. Subcutaneous granuloma annulare: a review of 47 cases. *Pediatrics* 1997; **100**: 965–7.

Necrobiosis lipoidica

Introduction. Necrobiosis lipoidica was first described by Oppenheim, in 1930 [1], and subsequently named *necrobiosis lipoidica diabeticorum* by Urbach, in 1932 [2]. Because it is not peculiar to diabetes, it is now usually called necrobiosis lipoidica. It is similar in histological appearance to granuloma annulare, but has a distinctive clinical appearance characterized by sharply demarcated plaques of atrophic yellowish skin, which may ulcerate.

Aetiology [3]. This condition was originally regarded as a complication of diabetes mellitus, but it was soon realized that some patients with necrobiosis lipoidica did not have overt diabetes. The precise relationship of the diabetic state to necrobiosis lipoidica is still not clear, although they are undoubtedly associated as discussed below.

Some authors have considered vascular changes to be important in the pathogenesis of necrobiosis lipoidica, but in Muller and Winkelmann's histopathological study vascular involvement was very mild in about a third of the cases [4]. An altered plasma protein profile [5], elevated factor VIII-related antigen [6] and fibronectin [7] may contribute to the vascular changes.

The possible role of an antibody-mediated vasculitis as an initiating event in necrobiosis lipoidica has provoked debate, as results of immunofluorescence studies differ. Laukkanen *et al*. [8] did not demonstrate immunoreactants in lesional skin, but others have shown immunoreactants, principally IgM, C3 and fibrin, in vessel walls in the involved skin, and IgM, C3 and fibrinogen at the dermoepidermal junction [9,10]. Dahl [11] has discussed immunofluorescence findings in necrobiosis lipoidica.

Whatever the mechanism, there is evidence of impaired microcirculation in non-diabetic individuals with necrobiosis lipoidica compared with controls, as measured by laser-Doppler flowmetry [12].

Although vascular factors may play a role, the precise pathogenesis of necrobiosis lipoidica remains unknown.

References

1 Oppenheim M. Eigentümliche disseminierte Degeneration des Bindegewebes der Haut bei einem Diabetiker. *Zentralbl Haut Geschlechtskr* 1930; **32**: 179.

2 Urbach E. Beiträge zu einer physiologischen und pathologischen Chemie der Haut; eine neue diabetische Stoffwechselsdermatose: Nekrobiosis lipoidica diabeticum. *Arch Dermatol Syph* 1932; **166**: 273–85.

3 Lowitt MH, Dover JS. Necrobiosis lipoidica. *J Am Acad Dermatol* 1991; **25**: 735–48.

4 Muller SA, Winkelmann RK. Necrobiosis lipoidica diabeticorum. Histopathologic study of 98 cases. *Arch Dermatol* 1966; **94**: 1–10.

5 Majewski BBJ, Barter S, Rhodes EL. Serum α_2 globulin levels in granuloma annulare and necrobiosis lipoidica. *Br J Dermatol* 1981; **105**: 557–62.

6 Majewski BBJ, Koh MS, Barter S, Rhodes EL. Increased factor VIII-related antigen in necrobiosis lipoidica and widespread granuloma annulare without associated diabetes. *Br J Dermatol* 1982; **107**: 641–5.

7 Koh MS, Majewski BBJ, Barter S, Rhodes EL. Increased plasma fibronectin in diabetes mellitus, necrobiosis lipoidica and widespread granuloma annulare. *Clin Exp Dermatol* 1984; **9**: 293–7.

8 Laukkanen A, Fräki JE, Väätäinen N *et al*. Necrobiosis lipoidica: clinical and immunofluorescent study. *Dermatologica* 1986; **172**: 89–92.

9 Ullman S, Dahl MV. Necrobiosis lipoidica. An immunofluorescence study. *Arch Dermatol* 1977; **113**: 1671–3.

10 Quimby SR, Muller SA, Schroeter AL. The cutaneous immunopathology of necrobiosis lipoidica diabeticorum. *Arch Dermatol* 1988; **124**: 1364–71.

11 Dahl MV. Immunofluorescence, necrobiosis lipoidica, and blood vessels. *Arch Dermatol* 1988; **124**: 1417–9.

12 Boateng B, Hiller D, Albrecht HP, Hornstein OP. Kutane Mikrozirkulation bei prätibialer Nekrobiosis lipoidica. Vergleichende Laser-Doppler Fluxmetrie und Sauerstoffpartialdruckmessungen bei Patienten und Hautgesunden. *Hautarzt* 1993; **44**: 581–6.

Histopathology [1–3] (Fig. 60.10). The histological appearances are similar to those of granuloma annulare, but some features differ. The epidermis is normal or atrophic, and absent if there is ulceration. The dermal changes involve its full thickness, and often extend into the subcutaneous fat. Early lesions show a perivascular and interstitial mixed inflammatory cell infiltrate. Areas of necrobiosis are usually more extensive and less well-defined than in granuloma annulare. There is degeneration of collagen and elastin within lesions [4]. Histiocytes border the areas of necrobiosis. There are variable numbers of Langhans' or foreign-body giant cells. A perivascular inflammatory infiltrate includes occasional eosinophils and, in contrast with granuloma annulare, plasma cells. Lymphoid nodules, containing germinal centres, may be present in the deep dermis or subcutaneous fat [5]. Lipid can be demonstrated in the necrobiotic areas, and cholesterol clefts may be present [6]. Mucin may be present in the dermis, but it is not as prominent as in granuloma annulare.

Small, superficial blood vessels are increased in number and telangiectatic. Deeper dermal blood vessels often show thickening of their walls and proliferation of endothelial cells. The walls are often infiltrated with periodic acid–Schiff-positive, diastase-negative material. Histologically, comedo-like plugs at the periphery of lesions represent elimination of necrotic material through hair follicles [7,8]. Anaesthesia in the lesions appears to be related to a decreased number of nerves within them [9]. In old, atrophic lesions there is considerable fibrosis in the dermis and subcutis.

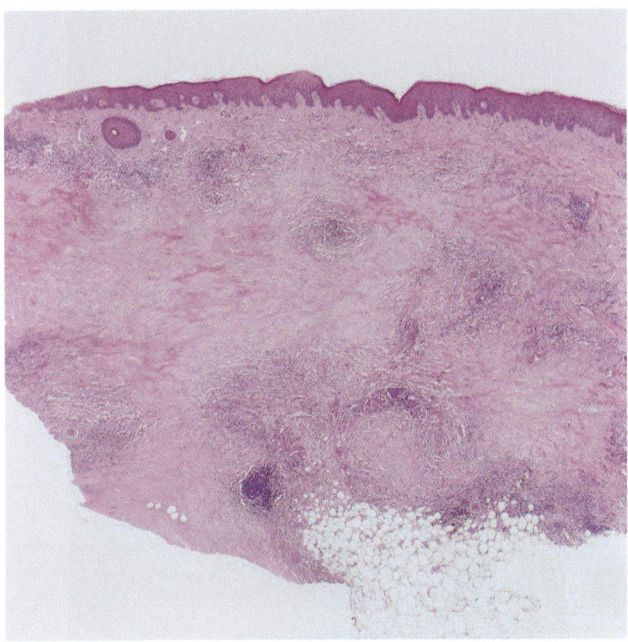

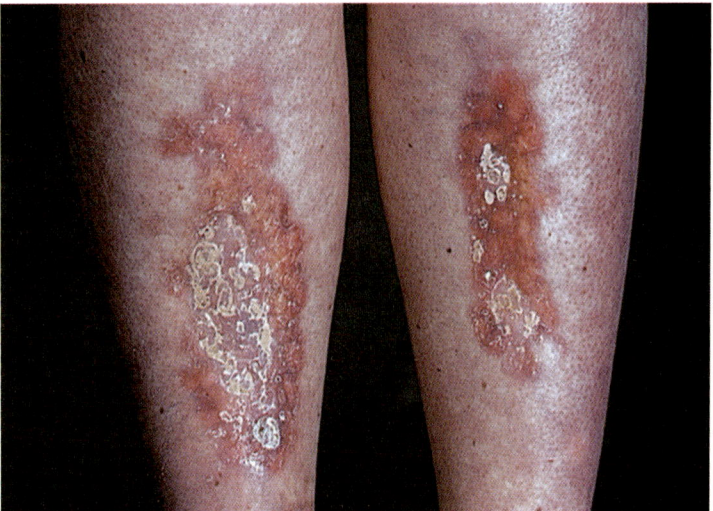

Fig. 60.11 Necrobiosis lipoidica. Lesions on both shins.

Fig. 60.10 Necrobiosis lipoidica. Extensive necrobiosis in the dermis. H&E stain. (Courtesy of Dr M. Bamford, Dept. of Pathology, Leicester Royal Infirmary, Leicester, UK.)

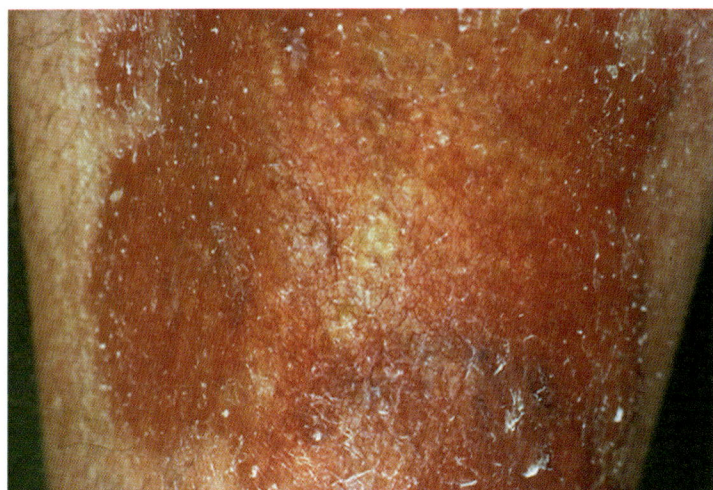

Fig. 60.12 Area of necrobiosis showing yellowish colour, atrophy and prominent vessels.

References

1 Weedon D. *Skin Pathology*, 2nd edn. London: Churchill Livingstone, 2002: 202–4.
2 Elder D, Elenitsas R, Jaworsky C, Johnson B Jr, eds. *Lever's Histopathology of the Skin*, 8th edn. Philadelphia: Lippincott-Raven, 1999: 330–3.
3 Muller SA, Winkelmann RK. Necrobiosis lipoidica diabeticorum. Histopathologic study of 98 cases. *Arch Dermatol* 1966; **94**: 1–10.
4 Oikarinen A, Mörtenhumer M, Kallionen M, Savolainen ER. Necrobiosis lipoidica: ultrastructural and biochemical demonstration of a collagen defect. *J Invest Dermatol* 1987; **88**: 227–32.
5 Alegre VA, Winkelmann RK. A new histopathologic feature of necrobiosis lipoidica diabeticorum: lymphoid nodules. *J Cutan Pathol* 1988; **15**: 75–7.
6 De la Torre C, Losada A, Cruces MJ. Necrobiosis lipoidica: a case with prominent cholesterol clefting and transepithelial elimination. *Am J Dermatopathol* 1999; **21**: 575–7.
7 Parra CA. Transepithelial elimination in necrobiosis lipoidica. *Br J Dermatol* 1977; **96**: 83–6.
8 Pestoni C, Ferreirós MMP, de la Torre C, Toribio J. Two girls with necrobiosis lipoidica and type 1 diabetes mellitus with transfollicular elimination in one girl. *Pediatr Dermatol* 2003; **20**: 211–4.
9 Boulton AJM, Cutfield RG, Abouganem D *et al*. Necrobiosis lipoidica diabeticorum: a clinicopathologic study. *J Am Acad Dermatol* 1988; **18**: 530–7.

Clinical features [1–3]. Necrobiosis lipoidica may occur at any age, but usually develops in young adults and in early middle-age. In insulin-dependent diabetics the age of onset is earlier than in non-insulin-dependent and non-diabetic individuals [4]. It is rare in childhood [5,6]. The female:male ratio is 3:1. Familial occurrence is rare [7,8].

Typical lesions occur on the pretibial skin, and begin as a firm, dull-red papule or plaque which enlarges radially to become a yellowish, atrophic plaque with an erythematous edge (Figs 60.11 & 60.12). The surface is often glazed in appearance, and telangiectatic vessels may be prominent (Fig. 60.13). Lesions are usually symptomless. Hypoaesthesia or anaesthesia, and hypohidrosis, are features of the affected skin [2,9,10]. Comedo-like plugs may occur at the periphery of lesions [11]. In most cases, lesions are bilateral, and they are similar in appearance whether occurring in diabetic or non-diabetic individuals [1]. They tend to be persistent, and some may ulcerate [12] (Fig. 60.14). In one study [4], ulceration correlated with sensory impairment. Squamous cell carcinoma may develop in long-standing lesions [13–20].

Lesions can also occur on other parts of the body, including the trunk [21] and penis [22,23], and rarely may be diffuse [24]. They may also occur at sites of trauma [25–28]. The number of lesions, and their rate of progress, are very variable. Slow extension over many years is usual, but long periods of quiescence, or resolution with variable atrophy and scarring (Fig. 60.15), may occur.

Wilson Jones [29] described an 'atypical annular form' of necrobiosis lipoidica affecting the upper face and scalp margins. The majority of affected individuals were female, and some developed lesions of necrobiosis lipoidica elsewhere. Since then, other authors have described similar annular lesions occurring predominantly on the exposed skin of the head, neck and arms, and these have been named Miescher's granuloma [30] and actinic granuloma [31]. Hanke *et al*. [32] proposed the term 'annular elastolytic giant

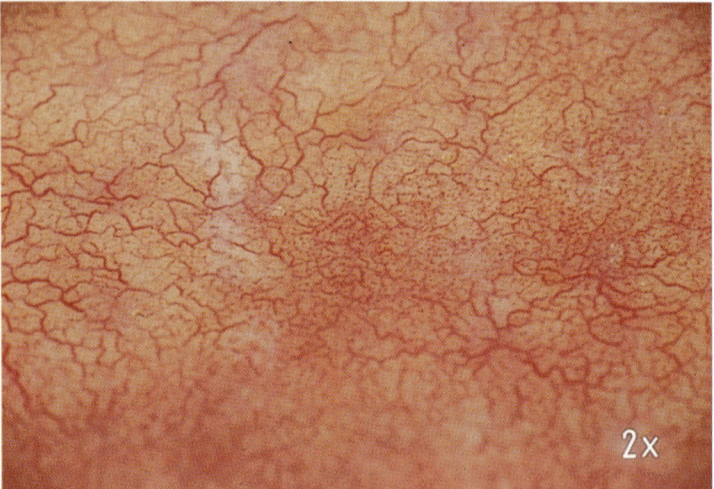

Fig. 60.13 Prominent telangiectasia in an area of necrobiosis.

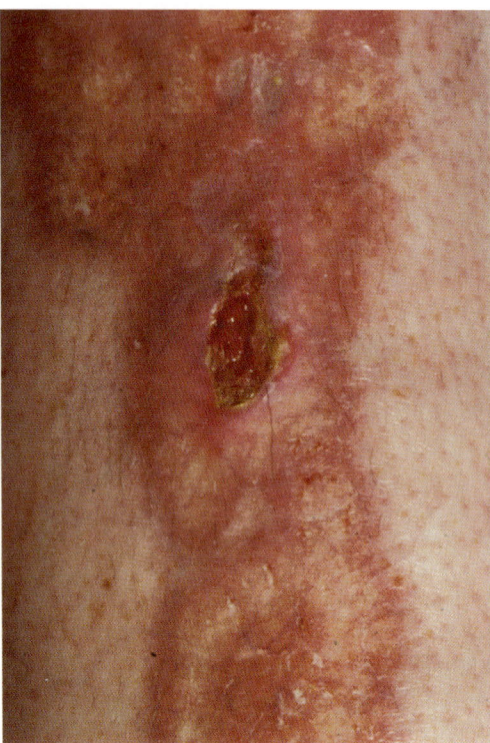

Fig. 60.14 Ulcerated necrobiosis lipoidica.

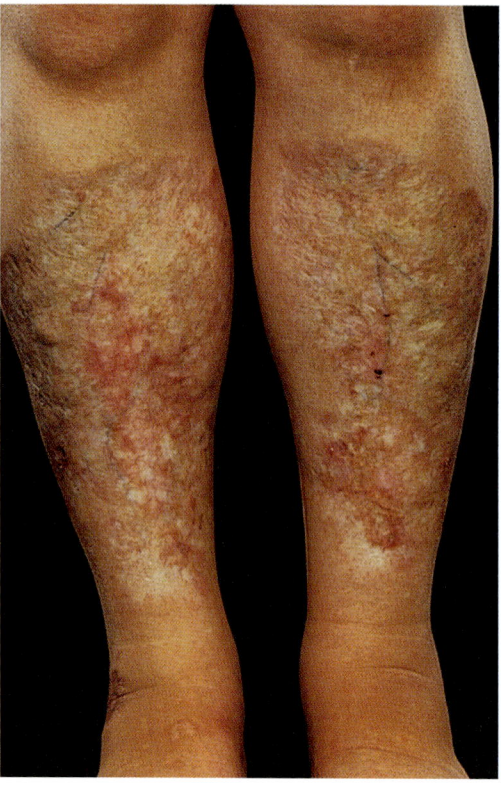

Fig. 60.15 'Burnt out' necrobiosis lipoidica—marked atrophy is evident.

cell granuloma' for these lesions. A similarity to granuloma multiforme (p. 60.17) is also apparent. The relationship of these disorders to each other, and to the necrobiotic granulomas, has provoked debate [3,33].

Differential diagnosis. Lesions with marked fatty infiltration, particularly when not on the legs, may be mistaken for xanthomas. Necrobiotic xanthogranuloma is a rare destructive xanthogranuloma, in which red-orange or yellowish indurated plaques most frequently involve the periorbital regions and trunk [34,35]. It is associated with systemic lesions and a monoclonal gammopathy (Chapter 62).

References

1 Muller SA, Winkelmann RK. Necrobiosis lipoidica diabeticorum. A clinical and pathological investigation of 171 cases. *Arch Dermatol* 1966; **93**: 272–81.

2 Boulton AJM, Cutfield RG, Abouganem D *et al*. Necrobiosis lipoidica diabeticorum. A clinicopathologic study. *J Am Acad Dermatol* 1988; **18**: 530–7.

3 Lowitt MH, Dover JS. Necrobiosis lipoidica. *J Am Acad Dermatol* 1991; **25**: 735–48.

4 Shall L, Millard LG, Stevens A *et al*. Necrobiosis lipoidica: 'the footprint not the footstep'. *Br J Dermatol* 1990; **123** (Suppl. 37): 47.

5 Chernosky ME, Guin JD. Necrobiosis lipoidica in a three-year-old girl. *Arch Dermatol* 1961; **84**: 135–6.

6 Verrotti A, Chiarelli F, Amerio P, Morgese G. Necrobiosis lipoidica diabeticorum in children and adolescents: a clue for underlying renal and retinal disease. *Pediatr Dermatol* 1995; **12**: 220–3.

7 Ho KK, O'Loughlin S, Powell FC. Familial non-diabetic necrobiosis lipoidica. *Australas J Dermatol* 1992; **33**: 31–4.

8 Findlay GH, Morrison JGL, De Beer HA. Non-diabetic necrobiosis lipoidica. *S Afr Med J* 1981; **59**: 323–6.

9 Mann RJ, Harman RRM. Cutaneous anaesthesia in necrobiosis lipoidica. *Br J Dermatol* 1984; **110**: 323–5.

10 Hatzis J, Varelzidis A, Tosca A, Stratigos J. Sweat gland disturbances in granuloma annulare and necrobiosis lipoidica. *Br J Dermatol* 1983; **108**: 705–9.

11 Parra CA. Transepithelial elimination in necrobiosis lipoidica. *Br J Dermatol* 1977; **96**: 83–6.

12 Dwyer CM, Dick D. Ulceration in necrobiosis lipoidica—a case report and study. *Clin Exp Dermatol* 1993; **18**: 366–9.

13 Clement M, Guy R, Pembroke AC. Squamous cell carcinoma arising in long standing necrobiosis lipoidica. *Arch Dermatol* 1985; **121**: 24–5.

14 Kossard S, Collins E, Wargon O, Downie D. Squamous carcinomas developing in bilateral lesions of necrobiosis lipoidica. *Australas J Dermatol* 1987; **28**: 14–7.

15 Beljaards RC, Groen J, Starink TM. Bilateral squamous cell carcinomas arising in long-standing necrobiosis lipoidica. *Dermatologica* 1990; **180**: 96–8.

16 Gudi VS, Campbell S, Gould DJ, Marshall R. Squamous cell carcinoma in an area of necrobiosis lipoidica diabeticorum: a case report. *Clin Exp Dermatol* 2000; **25**: 597–9.

17 Imtiaz KE, Kaleeli AA. Squamous cell carcinoma developing in necrobiosis lipoidica. *Diabet Med* 2001; **18**: 325–8.

18 Santos-Juanes J, Galache C, Curto JR *et al*. Squamous cell carcinoma arising in long-standing necrobiosis lipoidica. *J Eur Acad Dermatol Venereol* 2004; **18**: 199–200.

19 Vanhooteghem O, André J, de la Brassinne M. Epidermoid carcinoma and perforating necrobiosis lipoidica: a rare association. *J Eur Acad Dermatol Venereol* 2005; **19**: 756–8.

20 Lim C, Tschuchnigg M, Lim J. Squamous cell carcinoma arising in an area of long-standing necrobiosis lipoidica. *J Cutan Pathol* 2006; **33**: 581–3.

21 Kavanagh GM, Novelli M, Hartog M, Kennedy CTC. Necrobiosis lipoidica—involvement of atypical sites. *Clin Exp Dermatol* 1993; **18**: 543–4.

22 España A, Sánchez-Yus E, Serna MJ *et al*. Chronic balanitis with palisading granuloma: an atypical genital localisation of necrobiosis lipoidica responsive to pentoxifylline. *Dermatology* 1994; **188**: 222–5.

23 Velasco-Pastor AM, del Pino Gil-Mateo M, Martinéz-Aparicio A, Aliaga-Boniche A. Necrobiosis lipoidica of the glans penis. *Br J Dermatol* 1996; **135**: 154–5.

24 Imakado S, Satomi H, Ishikawa M *et al*. Diffuse necrobiosis lipoidica diabeticorum associated with non-insulin dependent diabetes mellitus. *Clin Exp Dermatol* 1998; **23**: 271–3.

25 Gebauer K, Armstrong M. Koebner phenomenon with necrobiosis lipoidica diabeticorum. *Int J Dermatol* 1993; **32**: 895–6.

26 Sahl WJ Jr. Necrobiosis lipoidica diabeticorum. Localization in surgical scars. *J Cutan Pathol* 1978; **5**: 249–53.

27 Miller RA. Koebner phenomenon in a diabetic with necrobiosis lipoidica diabeticorum. *Int J Dermatol* 1990; **29**: 52–3.

28 Ghate JV, Williford PM, Sane DC, Hitchcock MG. Necrobiosis lipoidica associated with Köbner's phenomenon in a patient with diabetes. *Cutis* 2001; **67**: 158–60.

29 Wilson Jones E. Necrobiosis lipoidica presenting on the scalp and face: an account of 29 patients and a detailed consideration of recent histochemical findings. *Trans St John's Hosp Dermatol Soc* 1971; **57**: 202–20.

30 Mehregan AH, Altman J. Miescher's granuloma of the face. *Arch Dermatol* 1973; **107**: 62–4.

31 O'Brien J. Actinic granuloma. An annular connective tissue disorder affecting sun- and heat-damaged (elastotic) skin. *Arch Dermatol* 1975; **111**: 460–6.

32 Hanke CW, Bailin PL, Roenigk HH Jr. Annular elastolytic giant cell granuloma. A clinicopathologic study of five cases and a review of similar entities. *J Am Acad Dermatol* 1979; **1**: 413–21.

33 Weedon D. *Skin Pathology*, 2nd edn. London: Churchill Livingstone, 2002: 208–10.

34 Finan MC, Winkelmann RK. Necrobiotic xanthogranuloma with paraproteinemia. A review of 22 cases. *Medicine (Baltimore)* 1986; **65**: 376–88.

35 Finan MC, Winkelmann RK. Histopathology of necrobiotic xanthogranuloma with paraproteinemia. *J Cutan Pathol* 1987; **14**: 92–9.

Associations. Although it is accepted that there is a relationship between necrobiosis lipoidica and diabetes mellitus, there is some disagreement about the closeness of this association. In Muller and Winkelmann's large series of cases, 111 of 171 patients with necrobiosis lipoidica (65%) had diabetes, and several of the non-diabetic patients subsequently had abnormal glucose tolerance tests, whereas in a study from Ireland [2], of 65 individuals with necrobiosis lipoidica only seven (11%) were known to have diabetes at the time of presentation. Necrobiosis lipoidica is relatively uncommon in diabetic patients, with reported prevalences of 0.3% [1] and 1.2% [3], and appears to be rare (0.06%) in childhood diabetes [4].

It is most commonly seen in patients with type 1 diabetes [3,5], but also occurs in type 2 diabetes, and in recent years has been reported in children and adolescents with type 2 diabetes [6–9], including diabetes associated with Prader–Willi syndrome [10]. A survey of the records of 178 patients fitting the clinical criteria for maturity-onset diabetes of the young (MODY), which is a sub-

type of non-insulin-dependent diabetes, showed a prevalence of necrobiosis lipoidica of 2.8% [8].

There is some evidence that diabetic patients who have necrobiosis lipoidica are at higher risk of retinopathy and nephropathy than diabetics who do not [5,11,12]. In the past, it was noted that good control of diabetes did not appear to have a significant effect on the course of necrobiosis lipoidica [1], but it would be of interest to reassess this aspect of the disease in the context of advances in diabetes care in recent years.

Necrobiosis lipoidica has also been reported as occurring in association with ulcerative colitis [13] and Crohn's disease [14], ataxia–telangiectasia [15], and after jejunal bypass surgery [16]. Reports of its occurrence with granuloma annulare have been mentioned previously (p. 60.9). It has also been reported in association with sarcoidosis [17,18].

Magro *et al.* [19] have demonstrated histopathological evidence of an 'active vasculopathy' in the majority of a series of cases of necrobiosis lipoidica associated with systemic disease.

References

1 Muller SA, Winkelmann RK. Necrobiosis lipoidica diabeticorum. A clinical and pathological investigation of 171 cases. *Arch Dermatol* 1966; **93**: 272–81.

2 O'Toole EA, Kennedy U, Nolan JJ *et al*. Necrobiosis lipoidica: only a minority of patients have diabetes mellitus. *Br J Dermatol* 1999; **140**: 283–6.

3 Shall L, Millard LG, Stevens A *et al*. Necrobiosis lipoidica: 'the footprint not the footstep'. *Br J Dermatol* 1990; **123** (Suppl. 37): 47.

4 de Silva BD, Schofield OMV, Walker JD. The prevalence of necrobiosis lipoidica diabeticorum in children with type 1 diabetes. *Br J Dermatol* 1999; **140**: 283–6.

5 Boulton AJM, Cutfield RG, Abouganem D *et al*. Necrobiosis lipoidica diabeticorum: a clinicopathologic study. *J Am Acad Dermatol* 1988; **18**: 530–7.

6 Szabo RM, Harris GD, Burke WA. Necrobiosis lipoidica in a 9-year-old girl with new-onset type II diabetes mellitus. *Pediatr Dermatol* 2001; **18**: 316–9.

7 Yigit S, Estrada E. Recurrent necrobiosis lipoidica diabeticorum associated with venous insufficiency in an adolescent with poorly controlled type 2 diabetes mellitus. *J Pediatr* 2002; **141**: 280–2.

8 Stride A, Lambert P, Burden ACF *et al*. Necrobiosis lipoidica is a clinical feature of maturity-onset diabetes of the young. *Diabetes Care* 2002; **25**: 1249–50.

9 Marchetti F, Gerarduzzi T, Longo F *et al*. Maturity-onset diabetes of the young with necrobiosis lipoidica and granuloma annulare. *Pediatr Dermatol* 2006; **23**: 247–50.

10 Walker JD, Warren RE. Necrobiosis lipoidica in Prader–Willi-associated diabetes mellitus. *Diabet Med* 2002; **19**: 884–5.

11 Kelly WF, Nicholas J, Adams J, Mahmood R. Necrobiosis lipoidica diabeticorum: association with background retinopathy, smoking, and proteinuria. A case controlled study. *Diabet Med* 1993; **10**: 725–8.

12 Verrotti A, Chiarelli F, Amerio P, Morgese G. Necrobiosis lipoidica diabeticorum in children and adolescents: a clue for underlying renal and retinal disease. *Pediatr Dermatol* 1995; **12**: 220–3.

13 Whorwell PJ, Haboubi NY, Du Boulay C. Nodular necrobiosis in association with ulcerative colitis. *Gut* 1986; **27**: 1517.

14 Du Boulay C, Whorwell PJ. 'Nodular necrobiosis': a new cutaneous manifestation of Crohn's disease? *Gut* 1982; **23**: 712–5.

15 Götz A, Eckert F, Landthaler M. Ataxia-telangiectasia (Louis–Bar syndrome) associated with ulcerating necrobiosis lipoidica. *J Am Acad Dermatol* 1994; **31**: 124–6.

16 Clegg DO, Zone JJ, Piepkorn MW. Necrobiosis lipoidica ssociated with jejuno-ileal bypass surgery. *Arch Dermatol* 1982; **118**: 135–6.

17 Graham-Brown RAC, Shuttleworth D, Sarkany I. Coexistence of sarcoidosis and necrobiosis lipoidica of the legs—a report of two cases. *Clin Exp Dermatol* 1985; **10**: 274–8.

18 Monk BE, Du Vivier AWP. Necrobiosis lipoidica and sarcoidosis. *Clin Exp Dermatol* 1987; **12**: 294–5.

19 Magro CM, Crowson AN, Regauer S. Granuloma annulare and necrobiosis lipoidica tissue reactions as a manifestation of systemic disease. *Hum Pathol* 1996; **27**: 50–6.

Treatment. Potent topical corticosteroids, particularly if applied beneath an occlusive dressing, and changed weekly, may help [1]. Locally injected triamcinolone, delivered by needle or jet injector [2], can improve the appearance, but atrophy usually remains. As there is evidence of extension of the inflammatory infiltrate into apparently normal skin surrounding active lesions, injection of steroids into perilesional areas might help to limit progression [3]. The use of oral steroids may be of benefit [4,5]. Petzelbauer *et al.* [5] employed short-course steroid therapy that resulted in cessation of disease activity in six patients, and no recurrence in a mean follow-up period of 7 months.

There are reports of benefit from PUVA therapy [6–12], UVA1 phototherapy—some patients improved but there was a poor response in others [13], topical tacrolimus [14], fumaric acid esters [15], thalidomide [16], chloroquine [17], photodynamic therapy [18], a combination of split-thickness autografting and immuno-modulatory therapy [19], and etanercept [20].

Other treatments that have been employed in the past, with varying degrees of success, include fibrinolytic agents [21], high-dose nicotinamide [22], clofazimine [23], pentoxifylline [24–27], tretinoin (0.05%) [28], prostaglandin E1 [29,30], and aspirin or an aspirin/dipyridamole combination [31–33]. Aspirin alone was subsequently shown to be ineffective [34,35], and in a randomized, double-blind comparison with placebo, patients treated with an aspirin/dipyridamole combination did not show any significant improvement [36].

Pulsed dye laser has been employed, and may improve the telangiectatic and erythematous components [37], but skin breakdown can occur [38]. Ulcerated necrobiosis has been treated by excision and grafting [39–41], although recurrence tends to occur unless the excision is deep [41]. Other treatments employed include oral steroid [42], ciclosporin [43–45], mycophenolate mofetil [46], topical granulocyte-macrophage colony stimulating factor [47,48], infliximab [49], intravenous immunoglobulin [50], hyperbaric oxygen [51,52], topically applied bovine collagen [53], and grafting with bioengineered dermal tissue [54,55].

References

1 Volden G. Successful treatment of chronic skin diseases with clobetasol propionate and hydrocolloid occlusive dressing. *Acta Derm Venereol (Stockh)* 1992; **72**: 69–71.

2 Sparrow G, Abell E. Granuloma annulare and necrobiosis lipoidica treated by jet injector. *Br J Dermatol* 1975; **93**: 85–9.

3 Boulton AJM, Cutfield RG, Abouganem D *et al.* Necrobiosis lipoidica diabeticorum: a clinicopathologic study. *J Am Acad Dermatol* 1988; **18**: 530–7.

4 Taniguchi Y, Sakamoto T, Shimizu M. A case of necrobiosis lipoidica treated with systemic corticosteroid. *J Dermatol* 1993; **20**: 304–7.

5 Petzelbauer P, Wolff K, Tappeiner G. Necrobiosis lipoidica: treatment with systemic corticosteroids. *Br J Dermatol* 1992; **126**: 542–5.

6 Patel GK, Rashid A, Mills CM. Topical photochemotherapy: a ray of hope for the treatment of necrobiosis lipoidica. *Br J Dermatol* 1999; **141**(Suppl. 55): 118 (Abstr).

7 McKenna DB, Cooper EJ, Tidman MJ. Topical psoralen plus ultraviolet A treatment for necrobiosis lipoidica. *Br J Dermatol* 2000; **143**: 1333–5.

8 Patel GK, Harding KG, Mills CM. Severe disabling koebnerizing ulcerated necrobiosis lipoidica successfully treated with topical PUVA. *Br J Dermatol* 2000; **143**: 668–9.

9 Patel GK, Mills CM. A prospective open study of topical psoralen-UV-A therapy for necrobiosis lipoidica. *Arch Dermatol* 2001; **137**: 1658–60.

10 de Rie MA, Sommer A, Hoekzema R, Neumann HAM. Treatment of necrobiosis lipoidica with topical psoralen plus ultraviolet A. *Br J Dermatol* 2002; **147**: 743–7.

11 Ling TC, Thomson KF, Goulden V, Goodfield MJD. PUVA therapy in necrobiosis lipoidica diabeticorum. *J Am Acad Dermatol* 2002; **46**: 3129–20.

12 Narbutt J, Torzecka JD, Sysa-Jedrzejowska A, Zalewska A. Long-term results of topical PUVA in necrobiosis lipoidica. *Clin Exp Dermatol* 2006; **31**: 65–7.

13 Beattie PE, Dawe RS, Ibbotson SH, Ferguson J. UVA1 phototherapy for treatment of necrobiosis lipoidica. *Clin Exp Dermatol* 2006; **31**: 235–8.

14 Harth W, Linse R. Topical tacrolimus in granuloma annulare and necrobiosis lipoidica. *Br J Dermatol* 2004; **150**: 792–4.

15 Kreuter A, Knierim C, Stücker M *et al.* Fumaric acid esters in necrobiosis lipoidica: results of a prospective noncontrolled study. *Br J Dermatol* 2005; **153**: 802–7.

16 Kukreja T, Petersen J. Thalidomide for the treatment of refractory necrobiosis lipoidica. *Arch Dermatol* 2006; **142**: 20–2.

17 Nguyen K, Washenik K, Shupack J. Necrobiosis lipoidica diabeticorum treated with chloroquine. *J Am Acad Dermatol* 2002; **46** (Suppl. 2): S34–6.

18 Heidenheim M, Jemec GBE. Successful treatment of necrobiosis lipoidica diabeticorum with photodynamic therapy. *Arch Dermatol* 2006; **142**: 1548–50.

19 Cummins DL, Hiatt KM, Mimouni D *et al.* Generalized necrobiosis lipoidica treated with a combination of split-thickness autografting and immunomodulatory therapy. *Int J Dermatol* 2004; **43**: 852–4.

20 Zeichner JA, Stern DWK, Lebwohl M. Treatment of necrobiosis lipoidica with the tumor necrosis factor antagonist etanercept. *J Am Acad Dermatol* 2006; **54** (Suppl. 2): S120–1.

21 Rhodes EL. Fibrinolytic agents in the treatment of necrobiosis lipoidica. *Angiology* 1978; **29**: 60–4.

22 Handfield-Jones S, Jones S, Peachey R. High dose nicotinamide in the treatment of necrobiosis lipoidica. *Br J Dermatol* 1988; **118**: 693–6.

23 Mensing H. Clofazimine—therapeutische Alternative bei Necrobiosis lipoidica und Granuloma anulare. *Hautarzt* 1989; **40**: 99–103.

24 Littler CM, Tschen EH. Pentoxifylline for necrobiosis lipoidica diabeticorum. *J Am Acad Dermatol* 1987; **17**: 314–6.

25 España A, Sánchez-Yus E, Serna MJ *et al.* Chronic balanitis with palisading granuloma: an atypical genital localisation of necrobiosis lipoidica responsive to pentoxifylline. *Dermatology* 1994; **188**: 222–5.

26 Noz KC, Korstanje MJ, Vermeer BJ. Ulcerating necrobiosis lipoidica effectively treated with pentoxifylline. *Clin Exp Dermatol* 1993; **18**: 78–9.

27 Basaria S, Braga-Basaria M. Necrobiosis lipoidica diabeticorum: response to pentoxiphylline. *J Endocrinol Invest* 2003; **26**: 1037–40.

28 Boyd AS. Tretinoin treatment of necrobiosis lipoidica diabeticorum. *Diabetes Care* 1999; **22**: 1753–4.

29 Sawada Y. Successful treatment of ulcerated necrobiosis lipoidica diabeticorum with prostaglandin E1 and skin flap transfer—a case report. *J Dermatol* 1985; **12**: 449–54.

30 Kuwert C, Abeck D, Steinkraus V *et al.* Prostaglandin E1 improves necrobiosis lipoidica. *Acta Derm Venereol (Stockh)* 1995; **75**: 319–20.

31 Heng MC, Song MK, Heng MK. Healing of necrobiotic ulcers with antiplatelet therapy. Correlation with plasma thromboxane levels. *Int J Dermatol* 1989; **28**: 195–7.

32 Quimby SR, Muller SA, Shroeter AL *et al.* Necrobiosis lipoidica diabeticorum: platelet survival and response to platelet inhibitors. *Cutis* 1989; **43**: 213–6.

33 Eldor A, Diaz EG, Naparstek E. Treatment of diabetic necrobiosis with aspirin and dipyridamole. *N Engl J Med* 1978; **298**: 1033.

34 Beck HI, Bjerring P, Rasmussen I *et al.* Treatment of necrobiosis lipoidica with low-dose acetylsalicylic acid. A randomized double-blind trial. *Acta Derm Venereol* 1985; **65**: 230–4.

35 Beck HI, Bjerring P. Skin blood flow in necrobiosis lipoidica during treatment with low-dose acetylsalicylic acid. *Acta Derm Venereol (Stockh)* 1988; **68**: 364–5.

36 Statham B, Finlay AY, Marks R. A randomised double blind comparison of an aspirin dipyridamole combination versus a placebo in the treatment of necrobiosis lipoidica. *Acta Derm Venereol (Stockh)* 1981; **61**: 270–1.

37 Moreno-Arias GA, Camps-Fresneda A. Necrobiosis lipoidica diabeticorum treated with the pulsed dye laser. *J Cosmet Laser Ther* 2001; **3**: 143–6.
38 Currie CL, Monk BE. Pulsed dye laser treatment of necrobiosis lipoidica: report of a case. *J Cutan Laser Ther* 1999; **1**: 239–41.
39 Cawley EP, Dingman RO. Necrobiosis lipoidica diabeticorum: its surgical treatment. *Arch Dermatol Syphilol* 1951; **63**: 764–7.
40 Nylen BO, Skoog T. Surgical treatment of necrobiosis lipoidica. *Acta Derm Venereol (Stockh)* 1958; **38**: 366–71.
41 Dubin BJ, Kaplan EN. The surgical treatment of necrobiosis lipoidica diabeticorum. *Plast Reconstr Surg* 1977; **60**: 421–8.
42 Dwyer CM, Dick D. Ulceration in necrobiosis lipoidica—a case report and study. *Clin Exp Dermatol* 1993; **18**: 366–9.
43 Darvay A, Acland KM, Russell-Jones R. Persistent ulcerated necrobiosis lipoidica responding to treatment with cyclosporin. *Br J Dermatol* 1999; **141**: 725–7.
44 Stinco G, Parlangeli ME, De Francesco V *et al*. Ulcerated necrobiosis lipoidica treated with cyclosporin A. *Acta Derm Venereol (Stockh)* 2003; **83**: 151–3.
45 Stanway A, Rademaker M, Newman P. Healing of severe ulcerative necrobiosis lipoidica with cyclosporin. *Australas J Dermatol* 2004; **45**: 119–22.
46 Reinhard G, Lohmann F, Uerlich M *et al*. Successful treatment of ulcerated necrobiosis lipoidica with mycophenolate mofetil. *Acta Derm Venereol (Stockh)* 2000; **80**: 312–3.
47 Remes K, Rönnemaa T. Healing of chronic leg ulcers in diabetic necrobiosis lipoidica with local granulocyte-macrophage colony stimulating factor. *J Diabetes Complications* 1999; **13**: 115–8.
48 Evans AV, Atherton DJ. Recalcitrant ulcers in necrobiosis lipoidica diabeticorum healed by topical granulocyte-macrophage colony-stimulating factor treatment. *Br J Dermatol* 2002; **147**: 1023–5.
49 Kolde G, Muche JM, Schulze P *et al*. Infliximab: a promising new treatment option for ulcerated necrobiosis lipoidica. *Dermatology* 2003; **206**: 180–1.
50 Batchelor J, Todd PM. Improvement of ulcerated necrobiosis lipoidica with intravenous immunoglobulin. *Br J Dermatol* 2007; **157** (Suppl. 1): 66.
51 Weisz G, Ramon Y, Waisman D, Melamed Y. Treatment of necrobiosis lipoidica diabeticorum by hyperbaric oxygen. *Acta Derm Venereol (Stockh)* 1993; **73**: 447–8.
52 Bouhanick B, Vervet JL, Guello JP *et al*. Necrobiosis lipoidica: treatment by hyperbaric oxygen and local corticosteroids. *Diabetes Metab* 1998; **24**: 156–9.
53 Spenceri EA, Nahass GT. Topically applied bovine collagen in the treatment of ulcerative necrobiosis lipoidica diabeticorum. *Arch Dermatol* 1997; **133**: 817–8.
54 Owen CM, Murphy H, Yates VM. Tissue-engineered dermal skin grafting in the treatment of ulcerated necrobiosis lipoidica. *Clin Exp Dermatol* 2001; **26**: 176–8.
55 Stuart L, Wiles PG. Management of ulcerated necrobiosis lipoidica: an innovative approach. *Br J Dermatol* 2001; **144**: 907–8.

Granuloma multiforme

Definition. A chronic granulomatous skin condition, characterized clinically by firm papules aggregated into plaques or forming the edges of annular lesions, and histologically by focal necrobiosis and histiocytic granulomas. It has been reported from Africa, Indonesia and India [1–8]. Leiker *et al*. [1–3] first described granuloma multiforme and distinguished it from tuberculoid leprosy. Leiker called it Mkar disease, after the town where it was first studied. The condition is endemic in certain villages in eastern Nigeria, where the local inhabitants refer to it in the Ibo tongue as 'Ununo Enyi' (elephant ringworm) [4,7].

The disease appears to occur predominantly in females over the age of 40 years [4,7,9].

Aetiology. The morphology and histological features of lesions, and their distribution predominantly on exposed parts of the body, indicate that this disorder may be granuloma annulare on light-exposed areas. It has been suggested that the primary event may be sun-induced damage to dermal connective tissue [9].

Pathology [4,10]. There are focal areas of necrobiosis, with loss of elastic tissue, surrounded by histiocytes. Multinucleated giant cells are usually a prominent feature. There is a perivascular lymphocytic infiltrate with variable numbers of plasma cells and eosinophils.

Clinical features. The upper, uncovered parts of the body are predominantly affected. The initial lesions are small, flesh-coloured papules which become aggregated into plaques or form the elevated rims of annular lesions. In larger annular lesions the central area is often hypopigmented. Pruritus may be prominent. The condition lasts for many months or years, and may persist indefinitely.

Differential diagnosis. Leprosy is endemic in the same regions where granuloma multiforme is found, and can look very similar. However, there is no loss of sensation or sweating, or other evidence of neural involvement in granuloma multiforme. In addition, the histological changes are different.

Treatment. None is known to be effective.

References
1 Leiker DL, Kok SH, Spaas JAJ. Granuloma multiforme: a new skin disease resembling leprosy. *Int J Lepr* 1964; **32**: 368–76.
2 Marshall J, Weber HW, Kok SH. Granuloma multiforme (Leiker). *Dermatologica* 1967; **134**: 193–207.
3 Leiker DL, Ziedses des Plantes M. Granuloma multiforme in Kenya. *East Afr Med J* 1967; **44**: 429–36.
4 Allenby CF, Wilson Jones E. Granuloma multiforme. *Trans St John's Hosp Dermatol Soc* 1969; **55**: 88–98.
5 Cherian S. Granuloma multiforme in India. *Int J Lepr* 1990; **58**: 719–21.
6 Verhagen ARHB, Koten JW, Chaddah VK, Patel RI. Skin diseases in Kenya: a clinical and histopathological study of 3168 patients. *Arch Dermatol* 1968; **98**: 577–86.
7 Garrett AS. Granuloma multiforme (called Nkanu disease in the 1940s and Mkar disease in 1964). *Int J Lepr* 1999; **67**: 172–4.
8 Sandhu K, Saraswat A, Gupta S *et al*. Granuloma multiforme. *Int J Dermatol* 2004; **43**: 441–3.
9 Cherian S. Is granuloma multiforme a photodermatosis? *Int J Dermatol* 1994; **33**: 21–2.
10 Meyers WM, Connor DH, Shannon R. Histologic characteristics of granuloma multiforme (Mkar disease). Including a comparison with leprosy and granuloma annulare. Report of first case from Congo (Kinshasa). *Int J Lepr* 1970; **38**: 241–9.

CHAPTER 61

Sarcoidosis

D.J. Gawkrodger
Royal Hallamshire Hospital, Sheffield, UK

Definition

There is no universally accepted definition of sarcoidosis. Many attempts have been made, but as long as its cause is unknown, definitions must be empirical and may also be inaccurate. Current definitions still have to avoid aetiological implications and the illogicalities that may result from them.

Scadding and Mitchell [1], after a full discussion of the difficulties, suggested the following: 'Sarcoidosis is a disease characterized by the formation in all or several affected organs or tissues of epithelioid cell tubercles, without caseation, although fibrinoid necrosis may be present at the centre of a few, proceeding either to resolution or to conversion of the epithelioid cell tubercles into hyaline fibrous tissue.'

The characteristic histology should be present in all affected tissue and similar in all parts of it. This excludes the sarcoid-like histology found in tuberculosis, brucellosis or leprosy. It is characterized by non-caseating epithelioid granulomas.

Main features

The most important features of sarcoidosis are as follows.
1 The disease process is usually generalized. The term is seldom applicable to a localized granulomatous reaction even though it may have similar histological findings.
2 The clinical manifestations are protean; the disease process is usually widespread; the course is protracted and usually benign, though sometimes with dangerous and disabling sequelae and complications.
3 The disease may affect any organ of the body (the adrenal gland possibly excluded). The lymph nodes, lungs, liver, spleen, skin, eyes, small bones of hands and feet, and salivary glands are most frequently affected.
4 All affected organs conform to a similar histological pattern.
5 Other changes present to a varying and inconstant degree include suppression or weakening of tuberculin and other intradermal responses, an increase in the serum gamma-globulins and a raised serum calcium level.
6 The Kveim reaction is positive in most active cases. This test is no longer available.

History [2–4]

The earliest description of a case which would now be categorized as sarcoidosis was probably Besnier's report in 1889 [5] of an association between reddish-blue lesions of the face and nose with swellings of the fingers [4]; the name 'lupus pernio' reflected his view that this might be a variant of lupus vulgaris. Tenneson in 1892 added the histological description [6]. In 1898 Hutchinson described two more cases of a skin eruption, probably sarcoidosis, to which he gave the name of 'Mortimer's malady' after one of his patients [7]. Boeck in 1899 [8] recorded his 'multiple benign sarkoid of the skin', and the current term 'sarcoidosis' stems from his misinterpretation of the histological changes. However, it was Boeck who first developed the concept of a disease involving both the skin and internal organs—a concept taken further by Schaumann [9], who again emphasized the generalized nature of the disease and showed that skin changes were not a necessary feature of it. The disease was further expanded by the inclusion of 'osteitis tuberculosa multiplex cystica' [10], uveoparotid fever [11], and pulmonary and other manifestations [12,13]. The introduction of mass radiography led to the recognition of hilar lymphadenopathy, with or without erythema nodosum, as an early benign form [14,15] and this has altered the whole concept

Rook's Textbook of Dermatology, 8th edition. Edited by DA Burns, SM Breathnach, NH Cox and CEM Griffiths. © 2010 Blackwell Publishing Ltd.

of the disease, which is now seen more often by chest and general physicians than by dermatologists.

References

1 Scadding JG, Mitchell DN, eds. *Sarcoidosis*, 2nd edn. London: Chapman & Hall, 1985: 1–12.
2 Epstein WL. What begot Boeck. *Arch Dermatol* 1982; **118**: 721–2.
3 Hutchinson J, ed. *Illustrations of Clinical Surgery*, Vol. 1. London: Churchill, 1878: 42–3.
4 Scadding JG. The eponymy of sarcoidosis. *J R Soc Med* 1981; **74**: 147–57.
5 Besnier E. Lupus pernio de la face: synovites fongueuses symétriques des extrémités supérieures. *Ann Dermatol Syphil* 1889; **10**: 333–6.
6 Tenneson M. Lupus pernio. *Bull Soc Fr Dermatol Syphil* 1892; **3**: 417–9.
7 Hutchinson J. Mortimer's malady (a form of lupus). *Arch Surg* 1898; **9**: 307–21.
8 Boeck C. Multiple benign sarkoid of the skin. *J Cutan Genitourin Dis* 1899; **17**: 543–50.
9 Schaumann J. Etude sur le lupus pernio et ses rapports avec les sarcoïdes et la tuberculose. *Ann Dermatol Syphil* 1917; **6**: 357–73.
10 Jungling O. Osteitis tuberculosa multiplex cystica. *Fortschr Röntgenstr* 1920–21; **27**: 375–83.
11 Heerfordt CF. Über eine Febrid Uveo-Parotidea Subchronica und der Glandula Parotis und der Uvea des Auges lokalisiert und häufig mit paresen cerebrospinaler Nerven kompliziert. *Arch Ophthalmol* 1909; **70**: 254–73.
12 Kusnitsky E, Bittord A. Boecksches Sarkoid mit Beteiligung innerer Organe. *Münch Med Wochenschr* 1915; **62**: 1349–53.
13 Leitner SJ, ed. *Der Morbus Besnier–Boeck–Schaumann*. Basle: Schwabe, 1949: 6.
14 James DG. Dermatological aspects of sarcoidosis. *Q J Med* 1959; **28**: 109–24.
15 Kerley P. The significance of the radiological manifestations of erythema nodosum. *Br J Radiol* 1942; **15**: 155–65.

Epidemiology [1]

The apparent increase in sarcoidosis over the last 40 years has been due partly to better detection, especially by mass radiography. However, even in countries with compulsory notification of the disease, there are bound to be many cases in an early, asymptomatic stage that remain undetected. For this reason, prevalence and incidence figures have to be interpreted with caution, though it is now clear that the disease has a worldwide distribution.

Sarcoidosis seems to be most prevalent (more than 10 per 100 000 population) in developed countries, but 'each succeeding world congress brings to the fore yet another country which has achieved manhood by joining in the world recognition of sarcoidosis' [2].

The danger of drawing inferences from unrepresentative collections of patients is well known [3], but certain groups do seem to be especially prone to sarcoidosis. It is, for example, more common in Afro-Caribbeans than in white inhabitants of the same area [4,5]. Other especially vulnerable groups include Puerto Ricans in New York and Irish immigrants to England. A useful study of 401 consecutive patients presenting to a district general hospital in the UK [6] gives a view of ethnic representation: Irish and Afro-Caribbean patients were disproportionately common in the material, but no attempt was made to assess incidence or prevalence in the population covered. Erythema nodosum was particularly common in the British and Irish; other skin manifestations occurred in 30 patients, 80% of whom were under 45 years of age.

Overall, sarcoidosis may be slightly more common in women than in men, and usually presents between the ages of 20 and 40 years. It is rare in young children [7]. The fact remains, however, that despite the voluminous data available, the factors influencing the prevalence and incidence of sarcoidosis remain obscure. Occupational, socioeconomic and climatic factors may be more important than have been recognized so far.

References

1 Sharma OP. Epidemiology of sarcoidosis: a report of the papers and posters presented at the Tenth International Conference on Sarcoidosis, Baltimore, USA, 1984. *Sarcoidosis* 1985; **2**: 9–11.
2 James DG. Sarcoidosis around the world. *Postgrad Med J* 1988; **64**: 177–9.
3 Scharkoff T. Apropos of the present level of epidemiologic knowledge on sarcoidosis. *Sarcoidosis* 1987; **4**: 152–4.
4 Benatar SR. A comparative study of sarcoidosis in white, black and coloured South Africans. In: Jones Williams W, Davies BH, eds. *Proceedings of the VIIIth International Conference on Sarcoidosis*. Cardiff: Alpha Omega, 1980: 508–13.
5 Sartwell PE. Racial differences in sarcoidosis. *Ann NY Acad Sci* 1976; **278**: 368–70.
6 Mikhail JR. Ethnicity and sarcoidosis. In: Jones Williams W, Davies BH, eds. *Proceedings of the VIIIth International Conference on Sarcoidosis*. Cardiff: Alpha Omega, 1980: 532–5.
7 O'Driscoll JB, Beck MH, Lendon M *et al*. Cutaneous presentation of sarcoid in an infant. *Clin Exp Dermatol* 1990; **15**: 60–2.

Aetiology

Despite intensive investigation, the cause of sarcoidosis remains unknown; it is not even clear whether the condition has only one or many causes. Most of the earlier theories have been discarded; others remain unproven. Evidence from genetic and environmental sources has been inconclusive, and immunological studies have, perhaps, raised more questions than they have solved. Speculations now lie in two main areas: infectious causes and genetic factors. Both may be interlinked.

Infectious agents

Many infectious agents have been put forward as the cause of sarcoidosis, but cultures are always negative and responses to treatment have not supported these beliefs. However, it remains possible that the disease represents an unusual host reaction to one or more infective agents—as yet unknown. Diagnostic confusion with tuberculosis led to speculation that *Mycobacterium tuberculosis*, perhaps in some transmuted form, might be responsible for the symptom complex of sarcoidosis. Recent evidence has lent some support for this. Serological studies have shown that patients with sarcoidosis have raised levels of antibodies to *M. paratuberculosis*, similar to those seen with Crohn's disease [1]. A polymerase chain reaction study revealed the presence of various subtypes of mycobacterial DNA (including *M. avium–intracellulare*) in 16 of 20 cases of cutaneous sarcoidosis [2]. In addition, it was reported that acid-fast cell-wall-deficient forms of *M. tuberculosis* have been grown from the blood of patients with active sarcoidosis [3]. However, a recent study failed to detect *M. tuberculosis* ribosomal RNA in fresh tissue specimens [4]. The significance of these findings is unclear at present, and the contribution of any mycobacteria to the pathogenesis of sarcoidosis is unknown. The onset of cutaneous sarcoidosis has been described following *M. marinum* infection [5]. It has been questioned as to whether *Propionibacterium acnes* may be involved in the aetiology of sarcoidosis, as *P. acnes* has been isolated from bronchial lavage in subjects with pulmonary sarcoidosis. However, it is known that *P. acnes* is a commensal in peripheral lung tissues and the findings do not appear to be specific for sarcoidosis [6].

Histoplasmosis and other fungi, which can produce granulomas exactly mimicking sarcoidosis, also have been suspected as possible causes, but their geographical limitations rule them out. Finally, it is always tempting to consider a viral cause for an obscure disease, but there is still no evidence to take this beyond mere speculation.

Genetic and familial factors

Familial sarcoidosis is well recognized and occurs more commonly than chance would predict. In ethnic groups known to have a high prevalence of sarcoidosis, the probability that an index case will have a sibling with sarcoidosis is about 10% [7]. In one study of 645 cases of sarcoidosis, 26 came from 12 families [8]. A literature search [9] found 182 affected sibling pairs; the excess of like-sex pairs was thought to reflect the effects of environmental exposure, which they are more likely to share than unlike-sex pairs. Far fewer examples of husband/wife sarcoidosis have been recorded [10] and this suggests that family aggregates occur either on a mainly genetic basis, or require a common environmental exposure during childhood. No consistent mode of inheritance has been found, although a recessive pattern may be more common [11].

Studies of human leukocyte antigens (HLAs) have not clarified the matter [12]. Differences between black and white subjects exist. Among black patients in the USA, sarcoidosis occurred significantly more frequently in individuals with BW15—but so did tuberculosis [13]. In London, white people with HLA-B8 were especially likely to have arthritis or erythema nodosum [14]. A recent Japanese study of 63 patients with sarcoidosis suggested that susceptibility for the disease may reside in the HLA-DRB1 locus, with resistance being conferred by the HLA-DRB1*1302 locus [15].

It seems likely that the HLA type can influence the pattern of the disease, rather than determine its occurrence. Recent studies suggest that the genes influencing clinical presentation of sarcoidosis in African Americans are different from those that underlie disease susceptibility [16].

Interferon-alpha (IFN-α) therapy

In more than 65 case reports [17], sarcoidosis has developed 15 days to 30 months after commencing IFN-α treatment. Some patients [18,19] had chronic myelogenous leukaemia and cutaneous lymphoma, conditions known to be associated with sarcoidosis on occasions. Others have had chronic hepatitis C [20]. Fifty per cent of cases have skin signs [19]. It is suggested that IFN-α might stimulate Th1 immune responses that are thought to be involved in sarcoidosis.

References

1 Reid JD, Chiodini RJ. Serologic reactivity against *Mycobacterium paratuberculosis* antigens in patients with sarcoidosis. *Sarcoidosis* 1993; **10**: 32–5.

2 Li N, Bajoghli A, Kubba A, Bhawan J. Identification of mycobacterial DNA in cutaneous lesions of sarcoidosis. *J Cutan Pathol* 1999; **26**: 271–8.

3 Almenoff PL, Johnson A, Lesser M, Mattman LH. Growth of acid-fast L forms from the blood of patients with sarcoidosis. *Thorax* 1996; **57**: 530–3.

4 Marcoval J, Benitez MA, Alcaide F, Mana J. Absence of ribosomal RNA of *Mycobacterium tuberculosis* complex in sarcoidosis. *Arch Dermatol* 2005; **141**: 57–9.

5 Gudit VS, Campbell SM, Gould D *et al.* Activation of cutaneous sarcoidosis following *Mycobacterium marinum* infection of the skin. *J Eur Acad Dermatol Venereol* 2000; **14**: 296–7.

6 Ishige I, Eishi Y, Takemura T *et al. Propionibacterium acnes* is the most common bacterium commensal in peripheral lung tissue and mediastinal lymph nodes from subjects without sarcoidosis. *Sarcoidosis Vasc Diffuse Lung Dis* 2005; **22**: 33–42.

7 Carmichael AK, Tan CY, Smith AG. Familial sarcoidosis: high ethnic prevalence. *Acta Derm Venereol (Stockh)* 1989; **69**: 531–2.

8 Turiaf J, Battesti JP, Jeanjean Y *et al.* Sarcoidose familiale, 26 cas dans 12 familles. *Nouv Presse Med* 1978; **7**: 913–5.

9 Grufferman S, Barton JW, Eby N. Increased sex concordance of sibling pairs with Behçet's disease, Hashimoto's disease, multiple sclerosis and sarcoidosis. *Am J Epidemiol* 1987; **126**: 365–9.

10 Gange RW. Sarcoidosis in husband and wife. *Clin Exp Dermatol* 1979; **4**: 107–9.

11 Luisetti M, Beretta A, Casali I. Genetic aspects in sarcoidosis. *Eur Respir J* 2000; **16**: 768–80.

12 Mehra NK, Bovornkitti S. HLA and sarcoidosis. *Sarcoidosis* 1988; **5**: 87–9.

13 Al-Arif L, Goldstein RA, Affronti LF *et al.* HLA antigens and susceptibility to tuberculosis in a black population. *Clin Res* 1977; **25**: 321.

14 Neville E, James DG, Brewerton DA *et al.* HLA antigens and clinical features of sarcoidosis. In: Jones Williams W, Davies BH, eds. *Proceedings of the VIIIth International Conference on Sarcoidosis.* Cardiff: Alpha Omega, 1980: 201–3.

15 Ishihara M, Ohno S, Ishida T *et al.* Molecular genetic studies of HLA class II alleles in sarcoidosis. *Tissue Antigens* 1994; **43**: 238–41.

16 Rybicki BA, Sinha R, Iyengar S *et al.* Genetic linkage analysis of sarcoidosis phenotypes: the sarcoidosis genetic analysis (SAGA) study. *Genes Immun* 2007; **8**: 379–86.

17 Alazemi S, Campos MA. Interferon-induced sarcoidosis. *Int J Clin Pract* 2006; **60**: 201–11.

18 Kidawada M, Ichinose Y, Kunisawa A *et al.* Sarcoidosis induced by interferon therapy for chronic myelogenous leukaemia. *Respirology* 1998; **3**: 41–4.

19 Schmuth M, Prior C, Illersperger B *et al.* Systemic sarcoidosis and cutaneous lymphoma: is the association fortuitous? *Br J Dermatol* 1999; **140**: 952–5.

20 Cogrel O, Doutre MS, Maliere V *et al.* Cutaneous sarcoidosis during interferon alfa and ribavirin treatment of hepatitis C virus infection. *Br J Dermatol* 2002; **146**: 320–4.

Histopathology [1]

The histological changes are similar in all organs affected and are remarkably constant. The essential feature is a monotonous repetition of aggregates of epithelioid cells with pale-staining nuclei, which form the characteristic, discrete sarcoidal granulomas (Fig. 61.1). Multinucleate giant cells are usually, but not invariably, present. An inconstant and variable rim of lymphoid cells surrounds the granuloma but this is never well developed—hence the term 'naked tubercle'. Caseation is absent, although an inconspicuous focus of fibrinoid necrosis or coagulation may occur within the granuloma. A fine reticulin network encircles the granuloma and may penetrate it (Fig. 61.2). The infiltrate tends to occur lower in the dermis than that of lupus vulgaris; in erythrodermic sarcoidosis, the granulomas are looser and less well defined. Epidermal changes can include hyperkeratosis, parakeratosis, acanthosis, atrophy and spongiosis: occasionally a lichenoid reaction is seen [2].

During the development of the granuloma, the loosely packed epithelioid cells of the early stage become more numerous and compact (their development is stimulated by IFN-γ produced by Th1 lymphocytes), and giant cells appear by their fusion. Reticulum appears and hyalinization becomes progressively more apparent as fibrosis gradually obliterates the characteristic features of the granulomas. This is the cause of the irreversible tissue scarring of the late stage of the disease. Polarizable foreign bodies were

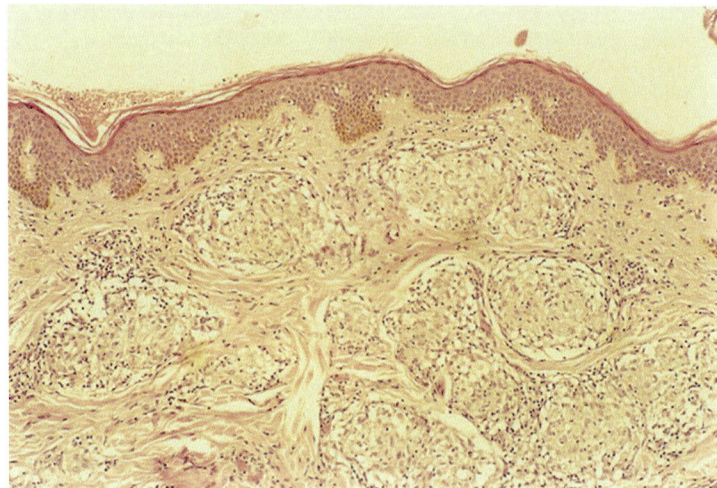

Fig. 61.1 Sarcoidosis. The epidermis is normal, while the superficial and mid-dermis contain numerous small granulomas without caseous necrosis. (Courtesy of Dr T.J. Stephenson, Royal Hallamshire Hospital, Sheffield, UK.)

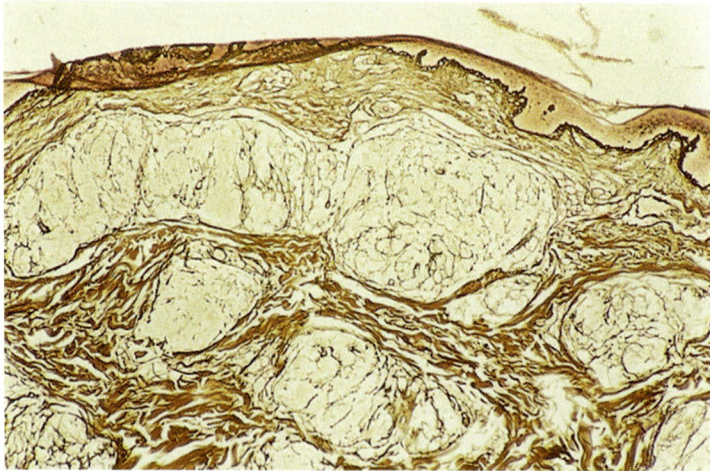

Fig. 61.2 Sarcoidosis. Reticulin stain of the section in Fig. 61.1, showing that the granulomas contain strands of staining reticulin, indicating that they lack caseous necrosis. (Courtesy of Dr T.J. Stephenson, Royal Hallamshire Hospital, Sheffield, UK.)

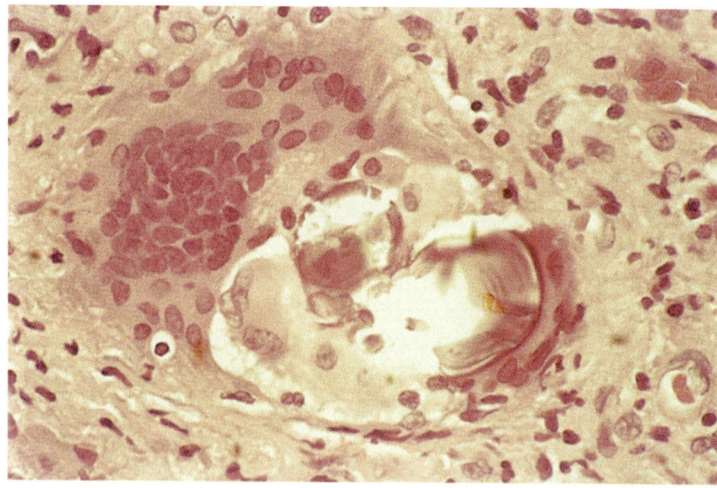

(a)

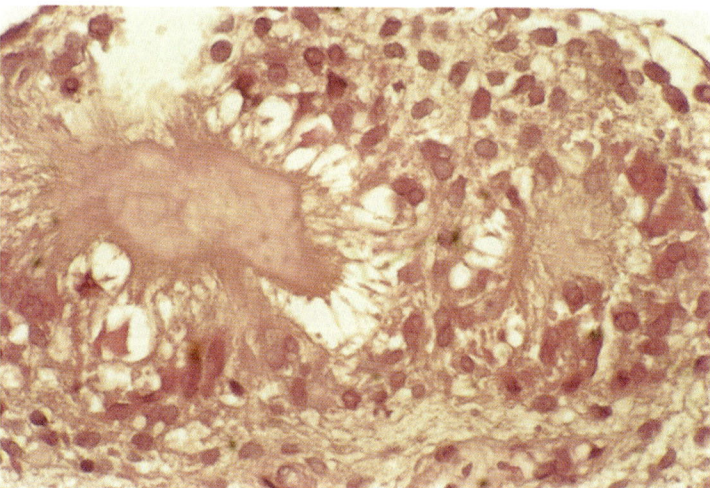

(b)

Fig. 61.3 (a) A Schaumann or conchoid body. These laminated calcospherites tend to fracture and to cause score marks. They stain basophilically. They are thought to arise from dystrophic calcification and it is suggested that they indicate chronicity. (b) High-power view of a granuloma in sarcoidosis showing an asteroid body within a giant cell. (Courtesy of Dr T.J. Stephenson, Royal Hallamshire Hospital, Sheffield, UK.)

found in 12 of 50 cases of cutaneous sarcoidosis (all of whom also had systemic granulomatous disease), suggesting that, in some patients, a foreign body may be an inciting stimulus for granuloma formation [1,3].

Inclusion bodies

These are often found in the giant cells in sarcoidosis and other sarcoidal granulomas, but are not specific. Their numbers increase as lesions age. The following types are recognized.

1 *Schaumann (conchoid) bodies* (Fig. 61.3a) are basophilic concentric lamellar structures, 100 μm in diameter, composed of lipomucoglycoproteins impregnated with calcium and iron, and they show central, birefringent crystals.

2 *Asteroid (stellate) bodies* (Fig. 61.3b) are between 10 and 15 μm in size; their central core is surrounded by radiating spicules (the 'open umbrella frame'). They consist of collagen [4].

Development of the granuloma [5]

Several strands of research have combined to increase our understanding of the complex cascade of cellular and mediator interactions involved in granuloma formation.

1 The technique of bronchoalveolar lavage, allowing easy harvesting of cells involved in the inflammatory process within the lungs.

2 Studies of evolving Kveim antigen-induced granulomas.

3 The use of monoclonal antibodies to characterize the cells found within the sarcoidal lesions.

4 The study of local immunological changes in cutaneous sarcoidosis, including the use of the techniques of molecular biology.

The architecture of a cutaneous sarcoid granuloma follows a pattern in which the centre consists of activated macrophages and epithelioid cells, surrounded by dendritic cells. Many activated CD4 helper/inducer T lymphocytes are present at the centre of the granuloma with a smaller population of CD8 suppressor/cytotoxic T lymphocytes at the periphery [6]. The antigen in

Table 61.1 Main histological features of sarcoidosis and tuberculosis.

Feature	Sarcoidosis	Tuberculosis
General structure	Monomorphic tubercles	Caseating tubercles
Form	Discrete, sharply defined 'naked tubercles'	Confluent, diffuse
Epithelioid cells	Large, grouped, predominant	Massed, irregular or at margin of caseation, less than 50%
Giant cells	Large, usually sparse Langhans' and foreign body cells	More numerous, Langhans' cells predominate
Lymphocytes	Sparse cuffing	More numerous and scattered
Inclusion bodies	Frequent	Occasional
Blood vessels	Usually normal or dilated	May show fibrinoid changes
Reticulin	Fine and abundant around tubercles	Destroyed
Caseation	No	Yes (but not lupus vulgaris)
Fibrinoid	Sometimes at centre of tubercle	Vascular and perivascular (late)
Healing process	Progressive hyalinization from periphery; gradual dissolution	Dense collagen mesh Retraction, fibrosis, calcification

sarcoidosis remains unknown, but the arrangements within the granuloma suggest an active immunological process. In addition, most workers have been able to demonstrate immune deposits within cutaneous granulomas, presumably as a consequence of the presence of circulating immune complexes known to occur in some patients with sarcoidosis. The most usual finding has been of immunoglobulin M (IgM) in the walls of dermal blood vessels or at the dermo-epidermal junction.

In the lung, an alveolitis precedes granuloma formation. Circulating blood monocytes appear in the lung, presumably in response to local chemotactic factors, and these aggregate into epithelioid cell granulomas. Pulmonary macrophages are induced by an unknown trigger mechanism to secrete interleukin-1 (IL-1), which is responsible for the migration of T lymphocytes to the site of disease activity. IL-1 also activates T cells and stimulates T-cell release of IL-2, which further amplifies local inflammatory activity. Activated T cells secrete chemotactic factors for monocytes and migration inhibitory factors. Fibrosis is enhanced by fibronectin and growth factors derived from alveolar macrophages.

Differential diagnosis

Typical tuberculosis is usually distinguishable by the histological features listed in Table 61.1. Sarcoidosis may be particularly hard to separate from lupus vulgaris if lymphocytes are more abundant than usual. In tuberculoid leprosy, epithelioid cells surround and are associated with the nerves, and there is more central necrosis. However, the histology of true sarcoidosis cannot always be distinguished from that of sarcoidal granulomas due to other causes—the key to the diagnosis of sarcoidosis lies in the uniformity of the histological changes in all affected organs.

Lupoid leishmaniasis, granulomatosis disciformis, rosacea and Crohn's disease may pose difficulties. Plasma cells and coagulation necrosis are features of syphilis. The granulomas of cat scratch fever are said to be larger than those of sarcoidosis. When sarcoid-

like reactions occur in a scar, the possibility of a foreign-body reaction must be considered. Talc may be recognized by its refractile nature.

References

1 Ball NJ, Kho GT, Martinka M. The histopathologic spectrum of cutaneous sarcoidosis: a study of twenty-eight cases. *J Cutan Pathol* 2004; **31**: 160–8.
2 Okamoto H. Epidermal changes in cutaneous sarcoidosis. *Am J Dermatopathol* 1999; **21**: 229–33.
3 Kim YC, Triffet MK, Gibson LE. Foreign bodies in sarcoidosis. *Am J Dermatopathol* 2000; **22**: 408–12.
4 Azar HA, Lunardelli C. Collagen nature of asteroid bodies of giant cells in sarcoidosis. *Am J Pathol* 1959; **57**: 81–92.
5 Thomas PD, Hunninghake GW. Current concepts of the pathogenesis of sarcoidosis. *Am Rev Respir Dis* 1987; **135**: 747–60.
6 Fazel SB, Howie SE, Krajewski AS, Lamb D. Increased CD45RO expression on T lymphocytes in mediastinal lymph node and pulmonary lesions of patients with pulmonary sarcoidosis. *Clin Exp Immunol* 1994; **95**: 509–13.

Immunological aspects [1,2]

Important advances have been made in our understanding of the immunology of sarcoidosis in recent years; yet the paradox of the disease remains. How is it that granulomas can evolve, presumably as a consequence of a local T-cell-mediated immune response to antigenic insult (e.g. a superantigen or a particulate antigen ingested by macrophages), in a condition apparently characterized by reduced cell-mediated immunity? Even if the cutaneous anergy of sarcoidosis is partly explained by a movement of activated helper T cells to sites of disease activity, leaving in the circulation an excess of anergic suppressor cells, then it still has to be accepted that Kveim-induced granulomas, at least, can develop during a state of depressed immune responsiveness.

Cell-mediated immunity

Depression of cell-mediated immunity is the hallmark of sarcoidosis; indeed, the first immunological defect to be demonstrated was lack of reactivity to tuberculin. Sensitivity to tuberculin is depressed to a variable degree and becomes negative in about two-thirds of patients [3]. However, there is no absolute correlation between reactivity and the state of the disease, and some failure of immunological response may persist despite apparent clinical resolution. Later, this anergy was shown to extend to other intradermal allergens such as candidine, strepkokinase–streptodornase and trichophytin antigens [4]. The combination of a depressed reaction to mumps antigen with normal circulating antibody responses is characteristic of, but not specific for, sarcoidosis.

The levels of circulating T lymphocytes expressing the γ/δ T-cell marker are increased in sarcoidosis, and correlate with the defect in cellular immunity [5]. T-cell receptor gene studies from blood and sarcoid lesions are consistent with an oligoclonal expansion of T cells from an antigen-driven response [6]. The formation of sarcoid granulomas, like tuberculoid, is characterized by the expression of a Th1 cytokine profile, i.e. the T-lymphocytes secrete IL-2, IFN-γ, and tumour necrosis factor-α (TNF-α) [7]; there is inactivation of Th2 lymphocytes. Th2-type granulomas have a prevalence of eosinophils and are seen, for example, in schistosomiasis.

The onset of sarcoidosis in HIV-positive patients after commencement of highly active antiretroviral therapy has been reported in 11 cases, leading to the suggestion that immune reconstitution was involved [8]. However, it is significant that sarcoidosis has developed in some patients with low CD4+ counts (126–1080, mean 373 cells/mm^3) [8].

Humoral immunity

All classes of serum immunoglobulins are increased. Activated T lymphocytes release B-cell growth factor and a B-cell differentiation factor, which together increase immunoglobulin production at the sites of disease. Significantly raised levels of circulating antibodies may be found to rubella, measles, herpes simplex, the Epstein–Barr virus and cytomegalovirus [9]. With regard to atopy as defined by personal history, skin prick tests and total IgE levels, a recent Turkish study of 41 patients with sarcoidosis found that only four (10%) were atopic compared with the expected 25% [10]. Interpretation of a small series such as this is difficult.

References

1 Baumer I, Zissel G, Sclaak M, Muller-Quernheim J. Th1/Th2 cell distribution in pulmonary sarcoidosis. *Am J Respir Cell Biol* 1997; **16**: 171–7.
2 Moller DR. Etiology of sarcoidosis. *Clin Chest Med* 1997; **18**: 695–706.
3 Siltzbach LE. Course and prognosis of sarcoidosis around the world. *Am J Med* 1974; **57**: 847–52.
4 Morell F, Levy G, Orriols R *et al.* Delayed cutaneous hypersensitivity tests and lymphopenia as activity makers in sarcoidosis. *Chest* 2002; **121**: 1239–44.
5 Nakata K, Sugie T, Cohen H *et al.* Expansion of circulating gamma delta T cells in active sarcoidosis closely correlates with defects in cellular immunity. *Clin Immunol Immunopathol* 1995; **74**: 217–22.
6 Moller DR. T-cell receptor genes in sarcoidosis. *Sarcoidosis Vasc Diffuse Lung Dis* 1998; **15**: 158–64.
7 Agostini C, Semenzato G. Biology and immunology of the granuloma. In: James DG, Zumla A, eds. *The Granulomatous Disorders*. Cambridge: Cambridge University Press, 1999: 3–16.
8 Roustan G, Yebra M, Rodriguez-Braojos O *et al.* Cutaneous and pulmonary sarcoidosis in a patients with HIV after highly active antiretroviral therapy. *Int J Dermatol* 2007; **46**: 68–71.
9 Byrne EB, Evans AS, Fouts DW *et al.* A sero-epidemiological study of Epstein–Barr virus and other viral antigens in sarcoidosis. *Am J Epidemiol* 1973; **97**: 355–63.
10 Kokturk N, Han ER, Turktas H. Atopic status in patients with sarcoidosis. *Allergy Asthma Proc* 2005; **26**: 121–4.

General manifestations of sarcoidosis [1–3]

There is no disease with more varied manifestations. Its course is unpredictable. Several years may separate one manifestation from another, and any organ of the body may be involved. Symptoms result from invasion and replacement, pressure, anaemia, hypercalcaemia and fibrosis.

A full history must include details of race, area of residence, previous tuberculin testing and bacille Calmette–Guérin (BCG) vaccination, industrial exposure to beryllium and any previous disease, such as erythema nodosum, that may be related, even distantly.

Staging of the disease

Pulmonary sarcoidosis is classically divided into four stages on the basis of the chest radiograph:

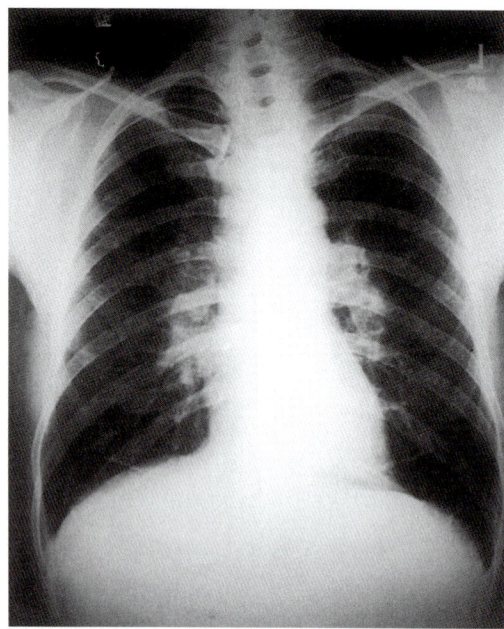

Fig. 61.4 Chest radiograph showing bilateral hilar lymphadenopathy typical of sarcoidosis.

1 Stage 0: 5–10% of patients with sarcoidosis have a normal chest radiograph.
2 Stage I: bilateral hilar lymphadenopathy alone—seen on the presenting radiograph of 35–45% of patients (Fig. 61.4).
3 Stage II: bilateral hilar lymphadenopathy with parenchymal lung involvement of fine 'fluffy' or coarse type.
4 Stage III: late stage of pulmonary infiltration with fibrosis and pulmonary insufficiency.

Extrapulmonary manifestations of sarcoidosis cannot be staged in this way, although some generalizations are possible. Erythema nodosum is, *par excellence*, an early feature, occurring with stage I pulmonary disease, and carrying a good prognosis. Iridocyclitis and anterior uveitis are usually associated with the later stages and more persistent forms of the disease. An attempt can be made to classify sarcoidosis on the basis of the degree of internal involvement, and on the type of skin lesions, as 'early' (e.g. erythema nodosum and bilateral hilar lymphadenopathy), 'intermediate' (e.g. papular and nodular forms) and 'late' (e.g. plaque, subcutaneous or lupus pernio). However, this may be unreliable, as the prognosis mostly depends upon the extent of internal disease, and this may not become apparent until treatment is too late to be effective. Of this disease, it has been aptly said: 'One of its most singular details . . . is the frequency of its clinical silence'.

Systemic features

General symptoms

The onset is often marked by lethargy, loss of weight and general malaise, but may be symptomless. A dry cough, dyspnoea and chest pain are present in half the patients.

Bone and joint changes

An acute polyarthralgia may accompany erythema nodosum. A more chronic polyarthritis may appear later in the disease, chiefly in Afro-Caribbeans. Bone changes, often asymptomatic, were found in 8% of 260 patients routinely examined radiologically [4]. Classically, they involve the small bones of the hands and feet in middle-aged women with lupus pernio. The most common change is lysis with bone cysts. The nasal bones, and occasionally the calvarium, may be involved in a way that mimics metastatic deposits [5].

Cardiac involvement [6]

Granulomatous infiltration of the conducting system may lead to heart block, papillary muscle dysfunction, congestive cardiac failure, pericarditis, chest pain, arrhythmias or even sudden death. The patients are often young, and the condition may be revealed only at post-mortem. Cardiac involvement is more common than was once believed, being found in 20–50% of autopsies on patients with sarcoid [6]. An abnormal electrocardiogram (ECG) was found in 14% of 401 patients examined routinely [4]. A careful cardiac examination should be a routine procedure in all cases of established sarcoidosis.

Muscle involvement

Polymyositis and myopathy occur rarely, and even muscle weakness and tenderness are uncommon despite the fact that random muscle biopsies in patients with sarcoidosis are positive in 50–80%. Tumour-type muscle sarcoidosis is very rare [7].

Nervous system involvement [8,9]

About 5% of patients with sarcoidosis have nervous system involvement and a wide variety of syndromes may result, including optic nerve lesions, cranial nerve palsies, meningoencephalitis, multiple sclerosis-like changes, peripheral neuropathy, mononeuritis multiplex and psychiatric changes. The facial nerve is frequently affected, with or without Heerfordt's syndrome (see below). Involvement of the hypothalamus or brain stem is rare but important. Sarcoidosis may also present as diabetes insipidus, hypopituitarism or endocrine abnormalities. The cerebrospinal fluid can show elevated protein and/or cells. Magnetic resonance imaging (MRI) may reveal abnormalities. Peripheral neuropathies often settle, but central nervous system manifestations seldom do so.

Ocular involvement [10]

The eyes are involved at some time in 25–50% of patients with sarcoidosis; eye disease is the first feature of sarcoidosis in about 10% of patients. The main types of ocular involvement are as follows:
1 *Uveitis.* Anterior and posterior uveitis are the most important and serious manifestations. Acute and chronic forms occur. The onset is usually insidious and 'mutton-fat' precipitates are found on the corneal epithelium. Iridocyclitis may be severe and recurrent. Complications include glaucoma, cataract and iris synechiae.
2 *Iris nodules.* These represent granulomatous infiltration of the stroma of the iris.
3 *Retinochoroiditis.* This usually occurs with chronic uveitis.

4 *Conjunctivitis.* Conjunctival nodules are common and are opaque, grey, slightly elevated lesions. 'Millet-seed' nodules may involve the eyelid margins. Biopsy will help to confirm the diagnosis of sarcoidosis; even 'blind' biopsies may reveal the disease.
5 *Lacrimal gland involvement.* Decreased lacrimal gland secretion is not uncommon (keratoconjunctivitis sicca is a presenting feature in about 10% of cases). Sarcoidosis is one cause of Mikulicz's syndrome (bilateral swelling of the lacrimal and salivary glands). Sjögren's syndrome can coexist with sarcoidosis and poses particular diagnostic problems.
6 *Optic nerves.* These may be involved as part of a widespread involvement of the central nervous system or as unilateral retrobulbar disease. Papilloedema, retrobulbar neuritis and optic atrophy may result.
7 *Orbital involvement.* This may cause unilateral proptosis.
8 *Other ocular syndromes.*
(a) Lofgren's syndrome (erythema nodosum, bilateral hilar lymphadenopathy and acute iridocyclitis) is usually self-limiting.
(b) Heerfordt's syndrome includes uveitis, parotid gland enlargement, fever and cranial nerve palsies, usually of the facial nerve.
(c) Keratoconjunctivitis sicca with parotid and lacrimal gland enlargement.
(d) Lupus pernio, chronic iridocyclitis, bone cysts and pulmonary fibrosis.

Pulmonary and upper respiratory changes [11]

Pulmonary changes dominate the later stages of the disease, and progressive diminution of respiratory function is the most common cause of incapacity. All patients with clinical or radiographic evidence of pulmonary involvement should be referred to a chest physician, who will decide on the need for and timing of treatment.

Upper respiratory involvement is often associated with chronic pulmonary disease and may be asymptomatic. Nasal stuffiness or blockage, with crusting and a nasal discharge, are common [12]. Cartilage or bone may be destroyed.

Renal involvement [13]

Symptoms are rare, but scattered granulomas can be found at autopsy in up to 40% of patients. Renal failure may be secondary to granulomatous invasion or to hypercalcaemia.

Reticuloendothelial system involvement

Lymph nodes are enlarged in about 50% of patients and may provide a convenient site for biopsy. An enlarged spleen can be felt in about 15% of cases [14]; hypersplenism may cause thrombocytopenia [15].

Involvement of the liver and other organs

It is evident that no organ is exempt from the occasional deposit of sarcoidal granuloma, and the dermatologist, as much as the general physician, should attempt to delineate the full extent of the disease in all patients. In no disease is it more important to look repeatedly 'under the skin' for other signs. Liver granulomas are found in 63–87% of patients with sarcoidosis and mild elevation of the serum alkaline phosphatase or bilirubin is seen in up to 80% of cases [16], although the liver is only palpable in about 20% of patients.

Hypercalcaemia and hypercalciuria [17]

The frequency of hypercalcaemia varies greatly (from 2% to 40% in different series), but it is less common than hypercalciuria. In one series, 11% of 1760 sarcoid patients had hypercalcaemia, while 40% had hypercalciuria [18]. Persistent hypercalcaemia is manifest clinically as polyuria, nocturia or polydipsia in the absence of hypertension. It can cause nephrocalcinosis and renal failure. The details of the abnormal calcium metabolism in sarcoidosis are still debated: sarcoid granulomas can themselves produce 1,25-dihydroxyvitamin D [19], which may increase calcium absorption via the gut. Persistent hypercalcaemia is one indication for systemic steroid therapy.

Sarcoidosis and pregnancy

The condition may improve during pregnancy, only to relapse thereafter. Miscarriages and congenital abnormalities are not especially common [20].

References
1 Johns CJ, Scott PP, Schonfeld SA. Sarcoidosis. *Ann Rev Med* 1989; **40**: 353–71.
2 Baughman RP, Teirstein AS, Judson MA *et al*. Clinical characteristics of patients in a case control study of sarcoidosis. *Am J Respir Crit Care Med* 2001; **164**: 1885–9.
3 Zax RH, Callen JP. Sarcoidosis. *Dermatol Clin* 1989; **7**: 505–15.
4 Mickhail JR. Ethnicity and sarcoidosis. In: Jones Williams W, Davies BH, eds. *Proceedings of the VIIIth International Conference on Sarcoidosis*. Cardiff: Alpha Omega, 1980: 532–5.
5 Zimmermann R, Leeds NE. Calvarial and vertebral sarcoidosis. *Radiology* 1976; **119**: 384.
6 Veinot JP, Johnston B. Cardiac sarcoidosis: an occult cause of sudden death: a case report and literature review. *J Forensic Sci* 1998; **43**: 715–7.
7 Nemoto I, Shimizu T, Fujita Y *et al*. Tumour-like muscular sarcoidosis. *Clin Exper Dermatol* 2007; **32**: 298–300.
8 Stern BJ, Krumholtz A, Johns CJ *et al*. Sarcoidosis and its neurological manifestations. *Arch Neurol* 1985; **42**: 909–17.
9 Zajicek JP, Scolding NJ, Foster O *et al*. Central nervous system sarcoidosis: diagnosis and management. *Q J Med* 1999; **92**: 103–17.
10 Liggett PE. Ocular sarcoidosis. *Clin Dermatol* 1986; **4**: 129–35.
11 Bower JS. Pulmonary evaluation of patients presenting with dermatological manifestations of sarcoidosis. *Int J Dermatol* 1981; **20**: 385–9.
12 Wilson R, Lund V, Sweatman M *et al*. Upper respiratory tract involvement in sarcoidosis and its management. *Eur Respir J* 1988; **1**: 269–72.
13 Nuther RS, McCarron DA, Bennett WM. Renal manifestations of sarcoidosis. *Arch Intern Med* 1981; **141**: 643–7.
14 Selroos O. Sarcoidosis of the spleen. *Acta Med Scand* 1976; **200**: 337–40.
15 Larner AJ. Life threatening thrombocytopenia in sarcoidosis. *BMJ* 1990; **300**: 317–9.
16 Sharma OP, Izumi T. Sarcoidosis. In: Cannon GW, Zimmerman GA, eds. *The Lung in Rheumatic Diseases*. New York: Dekker, 1990: 433–59.
17 Fine RM. The mechanism of hypercalcaemia in sarcoidosis. *Int J Dermatol* 1987; **26**: 22–3.
18 James DG, Williams WG, eds. *Sarcoidosis*. Philadelphia: Saunders, 1985: 163.
19 Adams JS, Gacad MA. Characterisation of the 1-α hydroxylation of vitamin D3 by cultured alveolar macrophages from patients with sarcoidosis. *J Exp Med* 1985; **161**: 755–65.
20 Weinberger SE, Weiss ST, Cohen WR *et al*. Pregnancy and the lung. *Am Rev Respir Dis* 1980; **121**: 559–81.

Sarcoidosis of the skin

Between 20% and 35% of patients with systemic sarcoidosis have skin lesions [1], but cutaneous sarcoidosis can also occur without systemic disease. Significant pulmonary disease may be silent [2]. In six of 13 patients with cutaneous sarcoidosis, but without a past history of sarcoidosis, no other systemic signs of the disease were detected during prolonged follow-up [3]; in another series of 188 patients with cutaneous sarcoid, 50 had no systemic involvement [4]. Finally, the extent of any cutaneous lesions does not correlate with the extent of systemic disease.

References
1 Kerdel FA, Moschella SL. Sarcoidosis; an updated review. *J Am Acad Dermatol* 1984; **11**: 1–19.
2 Collins P, Evans AT, Gray W, Levison DA. Pulmonary sarcoidosis presenting as a granulomatous tattoo reaction. *Br J Dermatol* 1994; **130**: 658–62.
3 Hanno R, Needelman A, Eiferman RA *et al*. Cutaneous sarcoidal granulomas and the development of systemic sarcoidosis. *Arch Dermatol* 1981; **117**: 203–7.
4 Veien NK, Stahl D, Brodthagen H. Cutaneous sarcoidosis in Caucasians. *J Am Acad Dermatol* 1987; **16**: 534–40.

Classification. This has been made more difficult by the use of eponyms that are no longer appropriate and which should now be discarded. A simple morphological classification is shown in Table 61.2, but more than one type of lesion may exist at the same time. The differences between the main patterns lie in the manner and extent of the involvement of the skin or subcutaneous tissues.

The specific lesions of sarcoidosis take the form of granulomatous infiltrates: erythema nodosum stands out from these as a non-specific accompaniment of early sarcoidosis without the characteristic sarcoidal granulomas.

Clinical features. The features of the specific cutaneous lesions arise from a dense accumulation of epithelioid cell granulomas in the dermis. In the deep nodular and infiltrative types, the

Table 61.2 Classification of sarcoidosis of the skin.

Type of cutaneous lesions	Stage of disease
Erythema nodosum	Acute ('benign')
Erythematous and erythematopapular	Acute and subacute
'Scar sarcoidosis'	Acute and subacute
Papular ('small nodular')	Acute and subacute
(Boeck) lichenoid variety	
Erythrodermic (Schaumann)	Subacute and chronic
Nodular	Subacute and chronic
Annular (or circinate)	
Angiolupoid (Brocq–Pautrier)	
Subcutaneous	
Plaque	Chronic
Lupus pernio	
Miscellaneous	Usually chronic
Ulcerative, psoriasiform, palmoplantar, ungual, mucosal	
Sarcoidosis of black Africans	

subcutaneous tissue is involved by extension. The lesions of sarcoidosis are generally recognizable as nodules or plaques with a greater degree of infiltration than would be expected from their surface appearance. Their colour ranges from yellow ochre to the livid violaceous hue which is most marked in lupus pernio. On diascopy, a pale yellowish-grey colour remains; sometimes, individual nodules are apparent. There is a tendency to form annular lesions. The epidermis is rarely affected, except for a light scaling, but some degree of vascular dilatation is frequent, especially in angiolupoid sarcoid. Scarring is unusual except in the papular and annular forms.

There is no characteristic distribution, though the small nodular type tends to involve the extensor aspects of the limbs, and rarely the trunk, while the large nodular type affects predominantly the face, hands and trunk. The manifestations of the disease vary from country to country: mucosal involvement, for instance, is rare in France but common in Scandinavia.

Classical forms

Angiolupoid form

A rare but characteristic variety. It affects women predominantly, almost always occurring at the side of the bridge of the nose towards the corner of the eye, below the inner edge of the eyebrow, or on the adjacent area of cheek. There are seldom more than two tumours. They are soft and hemispherical, with a well-marked orange-red or reddish-brown colour and of a more livid hue than other forms. This is due to the marked telangiectatic component, which alters the normal grey-yellow appearance on diascopy. There is little tendency to spontaneous resolution.

Annular forms (Fig. 61.5)

Annular lesions were seen in 32 of 188 white subjects with cutaneous sarcoid lesions [1] and occurred mainly in the chronic stage. They are formed by peripheral evolution and central clearing. They occur particularly on the forehead, face and neck. The central area may become depigmented and scarred. Ulceration is rare. The lesions may resemble annular necrobiosis of the scalp [2], but can be differentiated histologically. Diffuse papular forms may also show an annular configuration.

Erythema nodosum

Sarcoidosis is but one of the many causes of erythema nodosum—a subject dealt with in detail in Chapter 50. It occurs most often in the spring, in young women, and signals an early and usually 'benign' variety of sarcoidosis, with bilateral hilar lymphadenopathy and a tendency to involute spontaneously. Most cases resolve completely within 2 years.

The frequency with which erythema nodosum is reported in sarcoidosis varies from series to series, no doubt depending upon the selection of material. This was well shown in a worldwide survey of sarcoidosis [3] in which erythema nodosum pinpointed the onset of the disease in 600 (17%) of 3676 patients. The distribution was uneven between the countries studied, the condition affecting one-third of British patients and being less evident elsewhere. In a Danish series [1], 25 out of 188 patients with cutaneous

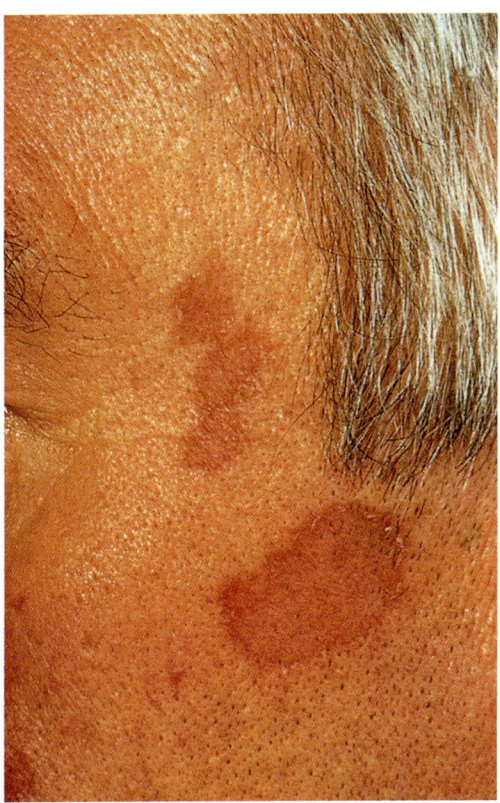

Fig. 61.5 Annular sarcoidosis of the face.

sarcoidosis had erythema nodosum which tended to affect younger patients (mean age 30 years) than did infiltrative sarcoidal lesions (mean age 48 years).

Lupus pernio [4]

This is a relatively common skin manifestation of sarcoidosis. In a Danish series of 188 patients with cutaneous sarcoidosis, 22 had lupus pernio [1]. In contrast, in a Turkish series of 516 patients with various skin lesions only 14 had lupus pernio [4]. Lupus pernio tends to affect older patients, is twice as common in women as in men, and is more common in Afro-Caribbeans than in their white counterparts.

Large bluish-red and dusky violaceous infiltrated nodules and plaques occur more or less symmetrically on the nose (Fig. 61.6), cheeks, ears, fingers, hands and toes (Fig. 61.7). The lesions may feel soft, doughy or indurated. Discrete nodules with a typical appearance on diascopy may be found at the edge sometimes. The surface is often glistening, and the epidermis stretched, with large pilosebaceous follicles. Ulceration rarely occurs in the skin, gross mutilation, as in lupus vulgaris, never. Involved ear lobes may become massive ('turkey ears'). Other chronic skin lesions, including plaques and subcutaneous nodules, may accompany lupus pernio. Scarring alopecia may occur on the scalp.

Nasal involvement is associated with swelling, ulceration or crusting of the nasal vestibule, and patients may present with difficulty in breathing. Submucous resection carries the risk of nasal septal perforation and collapse of the nose.

Lupus pernio tends to be associated particularly with other forms of chronic fibrotic sarcoidosis, including upper respiratory

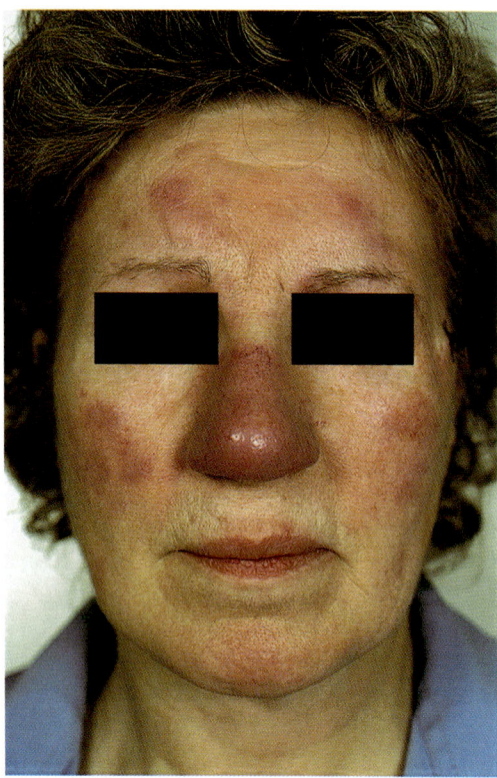

Fig. 61.6 Lupus pernio. (Courtesy of Dr F.A. Ive, Dryburn Hospital, Durham, UK.)

tract sarcoidosis, bone cysts, lacrimal gland and renal sarcoidosis, and with hyperglobulinaemia and hypercalcaemia [4].

Lupus pernio tends to persist: lesions of more than 2 years standing seldom resolve [4]. The facial disfigurement it causes may lead to emotional scarring, which may justify aggressive lines of therapy including plastic surgery [5]. Topical camouflage is an important adjunct to this therapy.

Maculopapular and erythematous forms (Fig. 61.8)

This is separate from the papular form (see below). Transient 'prodromal' maculopapular eruptions were noted in the early stages of sarcoidosis in no less than 8 of 33 patients who showed cutaneous signs of the disease [6] and are apparently seen most commonly by chest and general physicians. Diffuse forms of papular sarcoidosis do occur but are uncommon. Even less common are ill-defined patches of a lavender colour, sometimes slightly scaly or lightly infiltrated. On the face, these simulate rosacea. Sand-like lupoid grains are sometimes seen on diascopy, but more frequently there is a yellow discoloration. Transient parotid swellings and hepatosplenomegaly may be seen [7]. Such cases pursue a long course, fluctuating in severity. Pruritic maculopapular lesions have been described [8].

Nodular forms (Fig. 61.9)

Here the lesions are larger than 5 mm, usually single or relatively few, and remain circumscribed. Red or yellowish-red at first, becoming violaceous or purplish-brown later, they are soft or firm, round and most often affect the proximal parts of the limbs, the trunk and the face. Dilated vessels may be seen on the surface of

the lesions which are extremely indolent. As they involve, the centre may become depressed, and the lesions are eventually replaced by brownish telangiectatic marks, or yellowish-white atrophic and fibrotic patches.

Papular (small nodular type) (Figs 61.10 & 61.11)

The papules are hemispherical and vary in size from 1 to 5 mm. Orange or yellowish-brown at first, they later become brownish-red or violaceous, painless and torpid. Only a few lesions or several hundred may appear, arising in crops but eventually becoming stationary. They particularly affect the face (especially in Afro-Caribbeans) and extensor aspects of the limbs, but rarely the trunk or mucous membranes.

On diascopy, the lupoid grains are of a more opaque appearance and colour than those of lupus vulgaris, resembling grains of sand. If probed with a needle they feel firm. When lesions disappear they often leave a pale, yellowish-white or telangiectatic scar. Occasionally they become confluent, merging into an erythematous plaque (Fig. 61.12). A ringed nummular configuration was present in the second of Schaumann's four cases [9].

Widely disseminated, hard, shotty, subcutaneous papules can appear with the granulomas lying in the deep subcutaneous tissues and fascial planes. A lichenoid variety is discussed separately on p. 61.14.

In general, the papular type carries a more favourable prognosis than do other types of infiltration. Confirmatory biopsy of other organs should be carried out, although this form may occur without other manifestations of the disease.

Histopathology. The infiltrate is in the high and mid-dermis. It may be hard to distinguish from acne agminata in which, however, caseation can be seen.

Differential diagnosis. Lupus erythematosus can be mimicked. Papular forms of secondary syphilis are distinguished by the course and associated features of this disease. Occasionally, acne agminata (Chapter 43) presents difficulties.

Plaque form (Fig. 61.13)

It is convenient to keep this form distinct. It involves chiefly the limbs, shoulders, buttocks and thighs. The lesions are characteristically diffuse, and extend further than is apparent on the surface. They may form placards of an irregular shape with more superficial nodules superimposed, sometimes having a crescentic or serpiginous outline resembling tertiary syphilis. On the legs, they may closely resemble necrobiosis lipoidica (Fig. 61.14). They are very persistent.

Scar sarcoidosis (Fig. 61.15)

Sarcoidosis appearing in a scar may be the only cutaneous sign of the disease, and is therefore of diagnostic importance. Scar involvement was seen in 26 of 188 white patients with sarcoidosis [1], and may represent a form of Koebner phenomenon. Long-standing scars, often on the knees, become inflamed and infiltrated, giving rise to typical purplish-red lesions which turn brown as they fade. There is some resemblance to a keloid, but the lesions do not itch. This form of sarcoidosis is as common in men as in women [10].

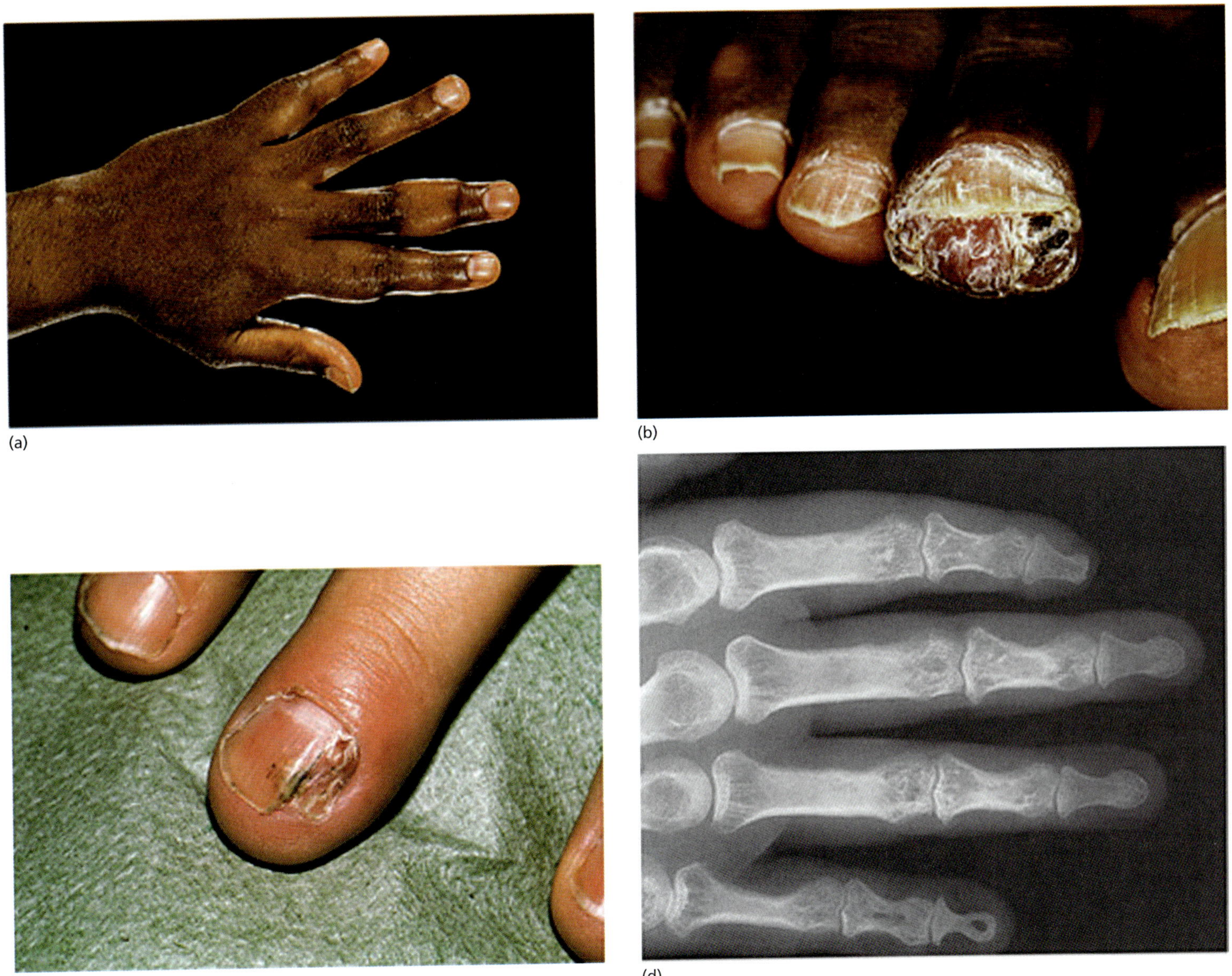

(a)

(b)

(c)

(d)

Fig. 61.7 (a) Typical fusiform appearance of the fingers from bone involvement. (Courtesy of Dr F.A. Ive, Dryburn Hospital, Durham, UK.) (b) Sarcoidosis of the terminal phalanx of the toe. (Courtesy of Dr F.A. Ive, Dryburn Hospital, Durham, UK.) (c) Sarcoidosis of the terminal phalanx involving the nail. (d) Radiograph of the hand in a patient with finger involvement by sarcoidosis, showing lucent areas in the bones of the phalanges.

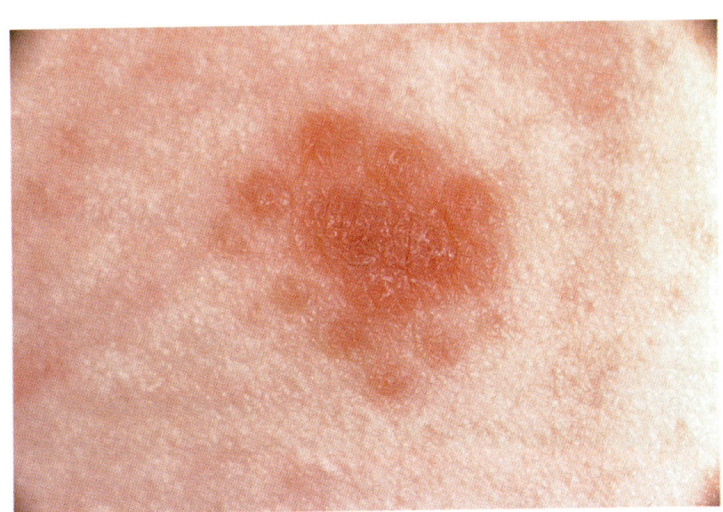

Fig. 61.8 Confluent scaly macules of the trunk due to sarcoidosis. (Courtesy of the late Dr R.H. Champion, Addenbrooke's Hospital, Cambridge, UK.)

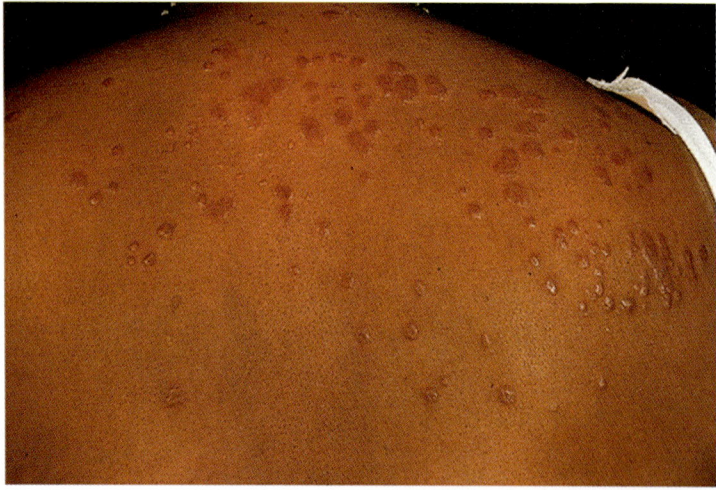

(a)

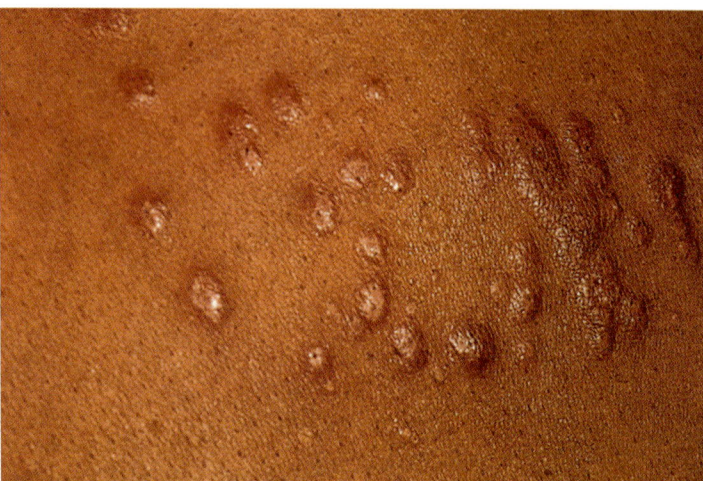

(b)

Fig. 61.9 (a) Nodular sarcoidosis on the upper back; (b) close-up of the same patient, showing the grouped nodules. (Courtesy of Dr D.A. Burns, Leicester, UK.)

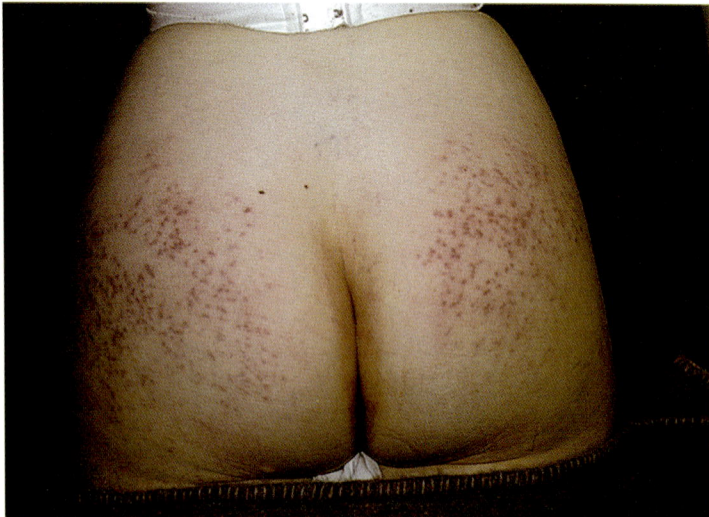

Fig. 61.10 Papular sarcoid of the buttocks. (Courtesy of Professor J.A.A. Hunter, Royal Infirmary, Edinburgh, UK.)

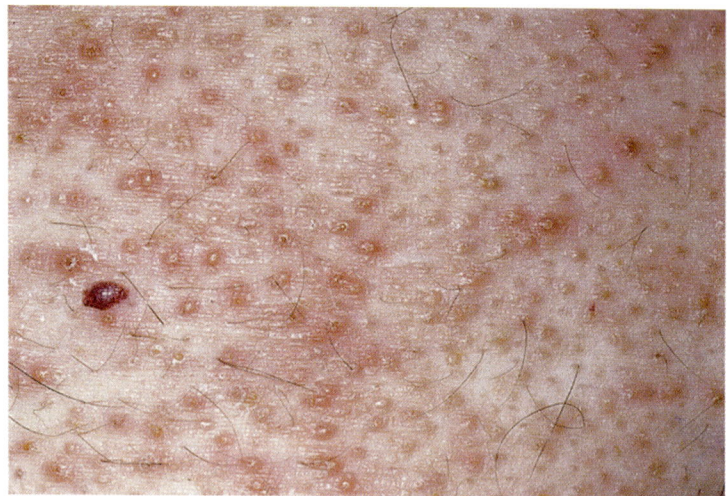

Fig. 61.11 Micropapular sarcoidosis. (Courtesy of the late Dr R.H. Champion, Addenbrooke's Hospital, Cambridge, UK.)

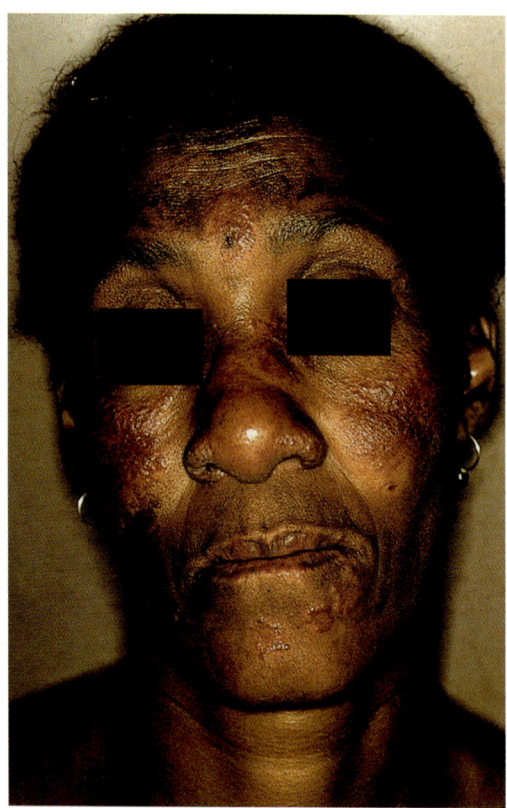

Fig. 61.12 Plaque-type sarcoidosis affecting the face in a black African. (Courtesy of Dr J.E. Bothwell, Barnsley District General Hospital, Barnsley, UK.)

Scar sarcoidosis occurs in three situations:

1 In the acute eruptive phase, following erythema nodosum, or in the scars of biopsies taken at that time.
2 At any later stage of the disease, sometimes moving in parallel with pulmonary changes and slightly in advance of iritis [6]. Exacerbation of the systemic disease may be preceded by this warning sign.

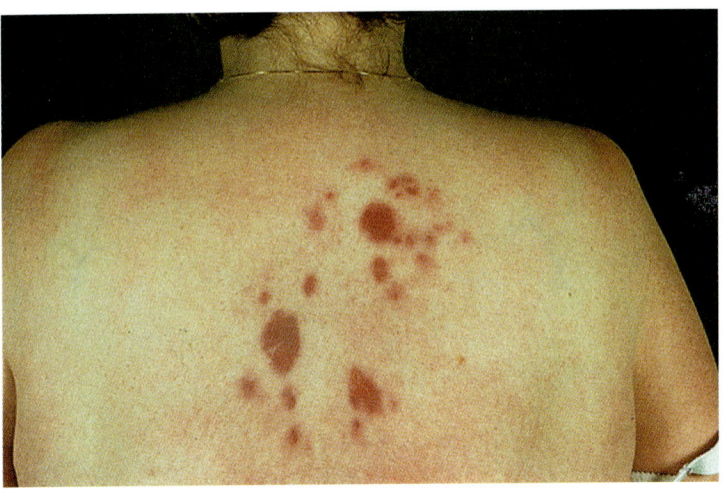

Fig. 61.13 Sarcoidosis. Lesions of the plaque type are present on the upper back. (Reproduced with permission from Elsevier, Ltd.)

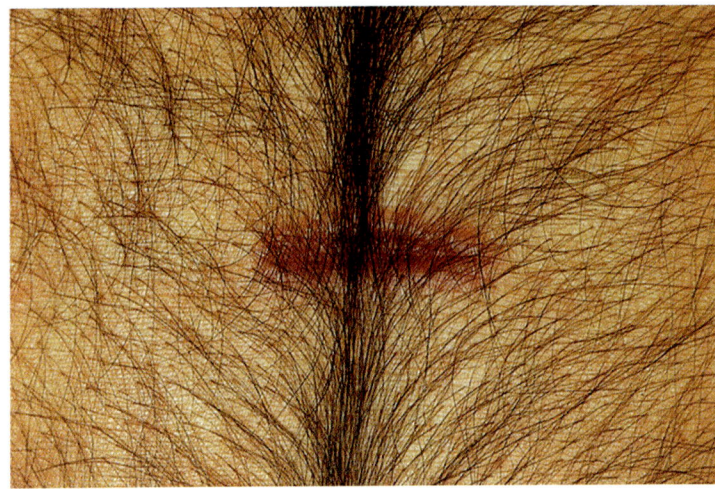

Fig. 61.15 Scar sarcoidosis on the presternal area. (Courtesy of Dr D.A. Burns, Leicester, UK.)

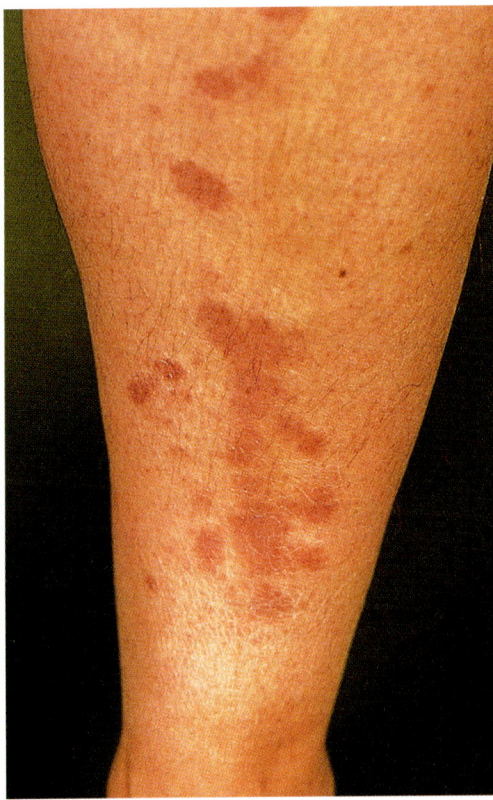

Fig. 61.14 Sarcoidosis of the plaque type on the shins, resembling necrobiosis lipoidica.

3 At inoculation sites—for example, after venepuncture [11], BCG or tuberculin tests. The involvement of tribal scarification marks is the commonest presentation of sarcoidosis in Nigeria [12,13].

The histology is typical. Confirmatory evidence of sarcoidosis should be sought (by chest radiograph, and biopsy from other organs), as local sarcoidal reactions may occur in scars contaminated with silica. A silica granuloma in a scar may, rarely, progress into scar sarcoidosis [14]. Tattoos may also show sarcoidal reactions.

Subcutaneous sarcoidosis [15]

It seems likely that the first case report of subcutaneous sarcoidosis was indeed that of Darier and Roussy in 1904 [16], although they considered that their patient had tuberculosis. However, the term 'sarcoid of Darier–Roussy' has been used so often for granulomatous conditions other than sarcoidosis that it has become devalued and should be discarded.

Nevertheless, subcutaneous sarcoidosis does exist, although it is rare, especially in white people. It takes the form of tender or painless persistent nodules, most often on the extremities of middle-aged patients, usually women [17]. Systemic involvement is usually present, sometimes as hilar lymphadenopathy [18], although usually not severe and not associated with chronic fibrotic disease [15]. Spontaneous resolution can occur [15].

Histopathology. The infiltrate is naturally greater in nodular lesions but remains circumscribed. In the subcutaneous form, the sarcoid process may at first be located in the septa and at the periphery of the fat lobules, eventually replacing the lobules with granulomatous nodules. In the angio-lupoid form, vascular dilatation is prominent.

Differential diagnosis. Lymphocytoma cutis can be separated by its histology. Four other diseases cause particular difficulty, and serial sectioning and cultures of biopsy material may be necessary. They are as follows:

1 *Tuberculoid leprosy.* Distinguished by loss of thermal appreciation and of the histamine flare, a positive Mitsuda test and invasion of nerves.

2 *Lupus vulgaris.* In its exuberant form, this can scarcely be distinguished, although vitropression is said to reveal more translucent nodules of an 'apple jelly' rather than a greyish-yellow colour. Ulceration and scarring ultimately occur. Histology helps, but does not decide: a therapeutic test with antituberculous drugs does.

3 *Lupoid leishmaniasis.* The same difficulties exist clinically and histologically. Leishman–Donovan bodies are rarely found. The Kveim test is negative.

4 *Local sarcoid reaction.* By definition, this is confined to local areas or sites of trauma. There are no other signs of sarcoidosis, and the Kveim test is negative.

References

1 Veien NK, Stahl D, Brodthagen H. Cutaneous sarcoidosis in Caucasians. *J Am Acad Dermatol* 1987; **16**: 534–40.
2 Dowling GB, Wilson Jones E. Atypical (annular) necrobiosis lipoidica of the face and scalp. *Dermatologica* 1967; **135**: 11–26.
3 James DG, Siltzbach TE. A world-wide review of sarcoidosis. *Ann NY Acad Sci* 1976; **278**: 321–34.
4 Yanardag H, Pamuk ON, Pamuk GE. Lupus pernio in sarcoidosis: clinical features and treatment outcomes of 14 patients. *J Clin Rheumatol* 2003; **9**: 72–6.
5 Shaw M, Black MM, David PKB. Disfiguring lupus pernio successfully treated with plastic surgery. *Clin Exp Dermatol* 1984; **9**: 614–7.
6 James DG. Dermatological aspects of sarcoidosis. *Q J Med* 1959; **28**: 109–24.
7 Barnes HM, Calnan CD. Erythematous sarcoid. *Proc R Soc Med* 1975; **68**: 651–2.
8 Fong YW, Sharma OP. Pruritic maculopapular skin lesions in sarcoidosis. *Arch Dermatol* 1975; **111**: 362–4.
9 Schaumann J. Lymphogranulomatosis benigna in the light of prolonged clinical observations and autopsy findings. *Br J Dermatol* 1936; **48**: 399–446.
10 Scadding JG, Mitchell DN, eds. *Sarcoidosis*, 2nd edn. London: Chapman & Hall, 1985: 181–206.
11 Burgdorf WH, Hoxtell EO, Bart BJ. Sarcoid granulomas in venepuncture sites. *Cutis* 1979; **24**: 52–3.
12 Alabi GO, George AO. Cutaneous sarcoidosis and tribal scarifications in West Africa. *Int J Dermatol* 1990; **28**: 29–31.
13 Olumide YM, Bandele EO, Elesha SO. Cutaneous sarcoidosis in Nigeria. *J Am Acad Dermatol* 1989; **21**: 1222–4.
14 Rowland-Payne CME, Meyrick-Thomas RH, Black MM. From silica granuloma to scar sarcoidosis. *Clin Exp Dermatol* 1983; **8**: 171–5.
15 Marcoval J, Mana J, Moreno A, Peyri J. Subcutaneous sarcoidosis-clinicopathological study of 10 cases. *Br J Dermatol* 2005; **153**: 790–4.
16 Darier J, Roussy G. Un cas de tumeurs benignes multiples (sarcoides sous-cutanées ou tuberculides nodulaires hypodermiques). *Ann Dermatol Syphil* 1904; **5**: 144–9.
17 Ahmed I, Harshad SR. Subcutaneous sarcoidosis: is it a specific subset of cutaneous sarcoidosis frequently associated with systemic disease? *J Am Acad Dermatol* 2006; **54**: 55–60.
18 Shidrawi RG, Paradinas F, Murray-Lyon IM. Sarcoidosis presenting as multiple subcutaneous nodules. *Clin Exp Dermatol* 1994; **19**: 356–8.

Unusual and atypical forms

In addition to the 'classical' forms of the disease described above, a wide variety of unusual forms have been recorded, particularly in Afro-Caribbeans.

Alopecia

Alopecia of the scalp due to sarcoidosis is well recognized [1,2]. Alopecia of the shin has been a presenting sign of the disease [3]. Sarcoidal granulomas were found on histology, and the Kveim test was positive.

Atrophic forms

The rare atrophic types of cutaneous sarcoidosis may be localized to the legs [4,5] or generalized [6,7]. It is usually accompanied by ulceration.

Erythrodermic sarcoidosis

This is extremely rare. Red scaling patches extend and merge into infiltrated brownish-red sheets. Lymphadenopathy is usually pronounced. During resolution, typical papules and nodules may separate from the plaque, which gradually loses its infiltration and disappears. A reticulate yellowish stippling may be seen as it resolves. One unique case was associated with periarteritis and ulceration [8]; in another patient, a 6-year-old boy, the eruption resembled pityriasis rubra pilaris [9].

Hypopigmentation

Macular hypopigmentation or hypopigmented areas around a central indurated lesion were first recorded in eight of 145 patients (mostly Afro-Caribbeans) with sarcoidosis [10]. There have been several subsequent reports [11–13]. Lesions vary from 0.2 cm to 1 cm in diameter and occur mainly on the limbs [13]. They may be tender, but are not anaesthetic, and may be the first sign of the disease [14].

Histologically, epithelioid cell granulomas are usually present in the dermis; occasionally the changes are non-specific [11,14]. The melanocytes show degenerative changes but electron-microscopy studies have not been helpful [11]. The differential diagnosis includes leprosy, post-inflammatory hypopigmentation, idiopathic guttate hypomelanosis and pityriasis lichenoides chronica [15]. The condition does not respond to corticosteroids [11], but may repigment after prolonged psoralen and UVA (PUVA) therapy [14].

Ichthyosiform sarcoidosis [16–18]

More than 19 cases of ichthyosiform sarcoidosis have been reported [18]. It usually occurs on the lower legs as large, thick, polygonal adherent scales that may or may not overlie dark red papules and nodules. Biopsy reveals epidermal changes consistent with ichthyosis vulgaris, as well as non-caseating epithelioid granulomas in the dermis, even in the absence of clinically detectable dermal abnormality. Almost all patients with ichthyosiform sarcoidosis have systemic involvement. In patients with acquired ichthyosis, biopsy may be worthwhile to exclude occult sarcoidosis.

Lichenoid forms (Fig. 61.16)

The lichenoid variety of sarcoidosis consists of pinhead-sized papules, skin-coloured, erythematous or yellowish in hue, that can be follicular or closely grouped in round or oval clusters and show slight scaling [18]. It constitutes 1–2% of skin sarcoidosis and may pose difficulties in diagnosis [19]. Although the lichenoid form resembles lichen planus or lichen scrofulosorum, the tuberculin test is negative, the course is indolent and the histology characteristic. Arguments have, however, been adduced in favour in a mycobacterial cause, because of atypical features that are sometimes present [20].

Miscellaneous forms

Many have been described, including the following: pseudotumoral [21], psoriasiform [22,23] and pruriginous varieties [24]; lupus erythematosus-like and lupoid forms; a bizarre polymorphous light eruption type; perifollicular pustules and papules widely scattered over the body; keratotic lesions of the palms simulating psoriasis or syphilis [25], thrombophlebitis [26]; vulval disease [27]; and breast mass [28,29]. Hyperpigmentation may occur, particularly in Afro-Caribbeans [10]. Oedema of the lower leg, usually unilateral, is an uncommon manifestation of sarcoidosis [30]. It may occur due to vascular or lymphatic compression

Fig. 61.16 Lichenoid sarcoidosis. (Courtesy of Pro. Dr P. Frosch, Dortmund, Germany)

from enlarged inguinal or parailiac lymph nodes, or from direct granulomatous infiltration of the skin. Calcinosis with subcutaneous plaques was present in one unusual patient [31]. Pain after alcohol or showering has also been described.

References

1 Maurice PDL, Goolamali SK. Sarcoidosis of the scalp presenting as scarring alopecia. *Br J Dermatol* 1988; **119**(Suppl. 33): 116–7.

2 Golitz LE, Shapiro L, Hurwitz E *et al*. Cicatricial alopecia of sarcoidosis. *Arch Dermatol* 1973; **107**: 758–60.

3 Felix RH. Alopecia of the shin. *Br J Dermatol* 1983; **109**(Suppl. 24): 66–7.

4 Basex A, Dupré A, Christol B *et al*. Sarcoidosis with atrophic lesions and ulcers, and the presence in some sarcoid granulomata of orceinophil fibres. *Br J Dermatol* 1970; **83**: 255–62.

5 Yoo SS, Mimouni D, Nikolskaia OV *et al*. Clinicopathologic features of ulcerative-atrophic sarcoidosis. *Int J Dermatol* 2004; **43**: 108–12.

6 Chevrant-Breton J, Revillon L, Pony JC *et al*. Sarcoidose à manifestations cutanées extensives ulcéreuses et atrophiantes (de type Pick–Herxheimer) avec complications cardiaques et musculaires: à propos d'un cas. *Ann Dermatol Vénéréol* 1977; **104**: 805–10.

7 Hruza GJ, Kerdel FA. Generalised atrophic sarcoidosis with ulcerations. *Arch Dermatol* 1986; **122**: 320–2.

8 Simpson JR. Sarcoidosis with erythroderma and ulceration. *Br J Dermatol* 1963; **75**: 193–8.

9 Morrison JG. Sarcoidosis in a child presenting with keratotic spines and palmar pits. *Br J Dermatol* 1976; **95**: 93–7.

10 Maycock RL, Bertrand P, Morrison CE *et al*. Manifestations of sarcoidosis. *Am Med* 1963; **35**: 67–89.

11 Clayton R, Breathnach A, Martin B *et al*. Hypopigmented sarcoidosis in the Negro: report of eight cases with ultrastructural observations. *Br J Dermatol* 1977; **96**: 119–25.

12 Cornelius CE, Stein KM, Hansaw WJ *et al*. Hypopigmentation and sarcoidosis. *Arch Dermatol* 1973; **108**: 249–51.

13 Thomas MRH, McKee PH, Black MM. Hypopigmented sarcoidosis. *J R Soc Med* 1981; **74**: 921–3.

14 Patterson JW, Fitzwater E. Treatment of hypopigmented sarcoidosis with 8-methoxypsoralen and long wave ultraviolet light. *Int J Dermatol* 1982; **21**: 476–80.

15 Clayton R, Warin A. Pityriasis lichenoides chronica presenting as hypopigmentation. *Br J Dermatol* 1979; **100**: 297–302.

16 Banse-Kupin L, Pelachyk JM. Ichthyosiform sarcoidosis: report of two cases and review of the literature. *J Am Acad Dermatol* 1987; **17**: 616–20.

17 Cather JC, Cohen PR. Ichthyosiform sarcoidosis. *J Am Acad Dermatol* 1999; **40**: 862–5.

18 Seo SK, Yeum JS, Suh JC, Na GY. Lichenoid sarcoidosis in a 3-year-old girl. *Pediatr Dermatol* 2001; **18**: 384–7.

19 Pinkus H. How useful is biopsy in a lichenoid eruption? *Cutis* 1977; **20**: 651–8.

20 Ridgway HA, Ryan T. Is micropapular sarcoidosis tuberculosis? *J R Soc Med* 1981; **74**: 140–4.

21 Bélaich S, Blanchet P, Crickx B *et al*. Sarcoidose pseudo-tumorale dermo-hypodermique du menton. *Ann Dermatol Vénéréol* 1982; **109**: 741–2.

22 Burgoyne JS, Wood MG. Psoriasiform sarcoidosis. *Arch Dermatol* 1972; **106**: 896–8.

23 Fulton RA. Psoriasiform sarcoidosis. *Br J Dermatol* 1984; **111**(Suppl. 26): 52.

24 Degos R, ed. *Dermatologie*. Paris: Flammarion, 1981: 533.

25 Scadding JG, Mitchell DN, eds. *Sarcoidosis*, 2nd edn. London: Chapman & Hall, 1985: 195–6.

26 Rowland Payne CME, McGibbon DH. Sarcoidosis presenting as widespread thrombophlebitis. *Clin Exp Dermatol* 1985; **10**: 592–4.

27 Tatnall FM, Barnes HM, Sarkany I. Sarcoidosis of the vulva. *Clin Exp Dermatol* 1985; **10**: 384–5.

28 Ojeda H, Sardi A, Totoonchie A. Sarcoidosis of the breast: implications for the general surgeon. *Am Surg* 2000; **66**: 1144–8.

29 Mingins C, Williams MR, Cox NH. Subcutaneous sarcoidosis mimicking breast carcinoma. *Br J Dermatol* 2002; **146**: 924–5.

30 Hoover RD Jr, Stricklin G, Curry TW, Carmichael LC. Unilateral lower limb edema caused by infiltrative sarcoidosis. *J Am Acad Dermatol* 1994; **30**: 498–500.

31 Kroll JJ, Shapiro L, Kaplan BS *et al*. Subcutaneous sarcoidosis with calcification. *Arch Dermatol* 1972; **106**: 894–5.

Mucosal involvement

Buccal lesions or tongue involvement are occasionally found when sought [1]. The nasal mucosa is often affected in lupus pernio [2,3] and is a convenient site for biopsy. Difficulty in breathing, or a purulent catarrh, may be the presenting symptom. Yellowish-brown nodules or a diffuse infiltration with crusting occurs [4]. The nasal bones may be involved; or the nasal cartilage may collapse [5]. Nodules with a hyperpigmented halo, diffuse pale-yellow plaques or ulceration may be found on the buccal mucosa, palate, larynx or tongue.

Nail involvement [6]

This is rare, affecting only one in 400 patients with sarcoidosis in one series [7]. Changes recorded have included the following: thickening, opacity, fragility, layering, convexity, longitudinal ridging, pitting, atrophy, nail loss, pterygium and red or brown discoloration of the nail beds. Surrounding skin changes may be minimal, but in almost every case the nail abnormalities will be accompanied by cysts in the bone of the underlying terminal phalanx and a chronic disease course, often with lupus pernio.

Sarcoidosis in black Africans and African Americans
(Fig. 61.17)

The lesions are often exuberant and bizarre, and the skin is especially affected, although erythema nodosum is uncommon [8,9]. Psoriasiform or lupus erythematosus-like lesions [10], verrucous

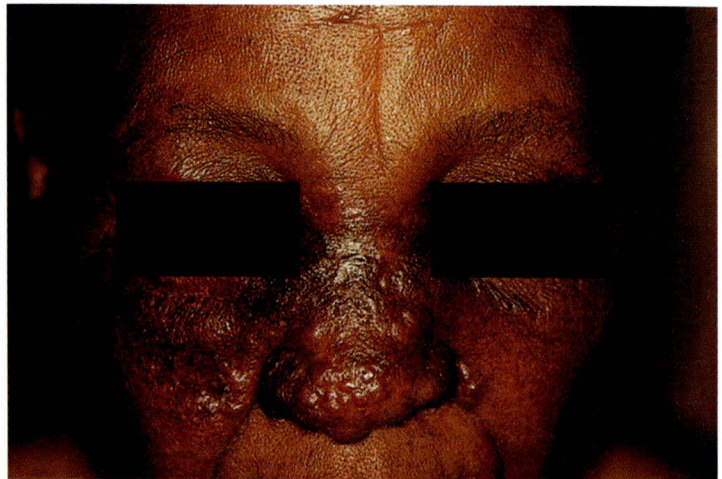

Fig. 61.17 Sarcoidosis in a black African, showing typical verrucous changes. (Courtesy of Dr J.E. Bothwell, Barnsley District General Hospital, Barnsley, UK.)

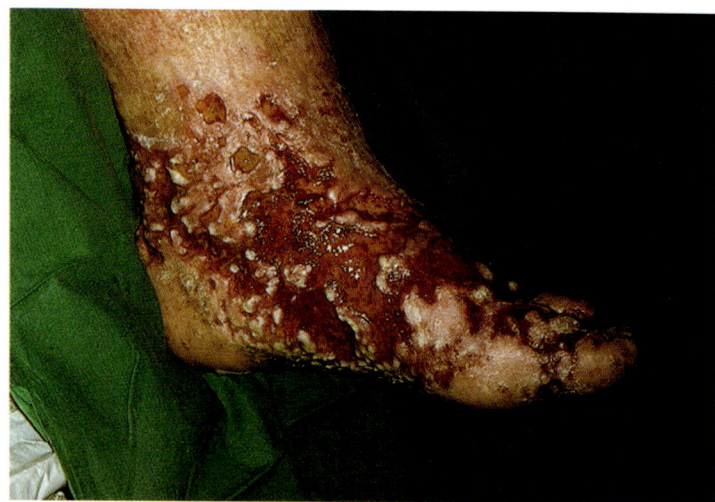

Fig. 61.18 Extensive ulceration of the foot and ankle due to sarcoidosis. (Courtesy of the late Dr R.H. Champion, Addenbrooke's Hospital, Cambridge, UK.)

and keloid-like forms [11,12], 'atypical' plaques or nodules [13], ulcerative lesions resembling papulonecrotic tuberculides [11], giant nodular forms and other atypical lesions occur, with more typical manifestations elsewhere. Shiny, waxy papules are a particular presentation [8]. The histological features may be equivocal and tuberculosis is a common cause of death. When the lesions are annular, histoplasmosis must be excluded [14].

Small ulcerating nodules, sometimes associated with deep, softer non-ulcerative lesions, have been described [10]. The histology is that of sarcoidosis but the infiltrate is diffuse, fibroblasts are numerous and the vessel walls in the subcutis are thickened.

Skin lesions in children [15,16]

Sarcoidosis in children is uncommon; a presentation with erythema nodosum is especially so. In one series of 48 children [15], 15 had erythema nodosum, 6 had other skin lesions, 12 developed uveitis or iridocyclitis and 2 had arthritis. Though papular forms of skin sarcoidosis are seen in older children, younger ones may present with uveitis or keratitis, progressive joint disease and skin lesions consisting of maculopapules, reddish-brown confluent plaques or eczema-like lesions [17,18]. Other reported cases have shown unusual features: follicular [19], miliary [20] or erythrodermic lesions with keratotic pitting [21]. The chest radiograph is often normal. The severity of eye or joint involvement may justify corticosteroid therapy, often for several years, despite the risks at this early stage.

The Blau syndrome, in which asymptomatic, red–brown papules (showing granulomas in histology) on the face, trunk and limbs are associated with arthritis and ocular disease in a child, has recently been identified, with mutations in the *NOD2* gene [23].

Ulcerated sarcoidosis [22,23] (Fig. 61.18)

This is a rare presentation: more than 35 cases have now been described, most of which were reported individually [24,25]. It usually occurs in women and black people. Ulcers develop most often on the legs [26] and may be punched-out and apparently appearing *de novo*, or arising on existing nodules and plaques, or, rarely, on extensive atrophic areas [27]. The possibility of necrobio-

sis lipoidica should be kept in mind, particularly in patients with diabetes [25]. The distribution of the ulcers may be unusual: a flexural distribution in one patient resembled that of metastatic Crohn's disease [28]. The granuloma may be of necrotizing type, with caseation or minimal fibrinoid necrosis [29]. True primary vasculitic changes are usually absent.

Verrucose forms [30]

Papular lesions may progress to crusted verrucose and sometimes ulcerative lesions [31], which may mimic halogen eruptions, fungal infections or tuberculosis.

References

1 Nagata Y, Kanekura T, Kawabata H *et al.* A case of sarcoidosis of the tongue. *J Dermatol* 1999; **26**: 666–70.

2 Holmes R, Black MM. Sarcoidosis (lupus pernio) with involvement of the nasal bones. *Br J Dermatol* 1981; **105**: 35–7.

3 Neville E, Mills RGS, Jash DK *et al.* Sarcoidosis of the upper respiratory tract and its association with lupus pernio. *Thorax* 1976; **31**: 660–4.

4 Degos R, ed. *Dermatologie.* Paris: Flammarion, 1981: 533.

5 Allen BR. Sarcoid of nose with collapse of nasal cartilage. *Br J Dermatol* 1978; **99** (Suppl. 16): 54–5.

6 Cox NH, Gawkrodger DJ. Nail dystrophy in chronic sarcoidosis. *Br J Dermatol* 1988; **118**: 697–701.

7 Patel KB, Sharma OP. Nails in sarcoidosis: response to treatment. *Arch Dermatol* 1983; **119**: 277–8.

8 Minus HR, Grimes PE. Cutaneous manifestations of sarcoidosis in blacks. *Cutis* 1983; **32**: 361–3.

9 Jacyk WK. Cutaneous sarcoidosis in black South Africans. *Int J Dermatol* 1999; **38**: 841–5.

10 Irgang S. Ulcerative cutaneous lesions in sarcoidosis. *Br J Dermatol* 1955; **67**: 255–60.

11 Klauder JV, Weidman FD. Multiple sarcoid-like granulomas of the skin of undetermined nature. *Arch Dermatol Syphilol* 1926; **13**: 675–6.

12 Schmunes E, Lantis LR, Hurley H. Verrucose sarcoidosis. *Arch Dermatol* 1970; **102**: 665–9.

13 Cronin E. Skin changes in sarcoidosis. *Postgrad Med J* 1970; **46**: 507–9.

14 Lucas AD. Cutaneous manifestations of histoplasmosis. *Br J Dermatol* 1970; **82**: 435–47.

15 Hoffmann AL, Milman N, Byg KE. Childhood sarcoidosis in Denmark 1979–94: incidence, clinical features and laboratory results at presentation in 48 children. *Acta Paediatr* 2004; **93**: 30–6.

16 Kendig EL. The clinical picture of sarcoidosis in children. *Paediatrics* 1974; **54**: 289–92.

17 Rasmussen JE. Sarcoidosis in young children. *J Am Acad Dermatol* 1981; **5**: 566–70.

18 O'Driscoll JB, Beck MH, Lendon M *et al*. Cutaneous presentation of sarcoidosis in an infant. *Clin Exp Dermatol* 1990; **15**: 60–2.

19 Appleyard WJ. Sarcoidosis in a young child. *Proc R Soc Med* 1976; **69**: 345–6.

20 Siltzbach LE, James DG, Neville E *et al*. Course and prognosis of sarcoidosis around the world. *Am J Med* 1974; **57**: 847–52.

21 Morrison JG. Sarcoidosis in a child presenting as an erythroderma with keratotic spines and palmar pits. *Br J Dermatol* 1976; **95**: 93–7.

22 Verdegem TD, Sharma OP. Cutaneous ulcers in sarcoidosis. *Arch Dermatol* 1987; **123**: 1531–4.

23 Schaffer JV, Vhandra P, Keegan BR *et al*. Widespread granulomatous dermatitis of infancy: an early sign of Blau syndrome. *Arch Dermatol* 2007; **143**: 386–91.

24 Albertini JG, Tyler W, Miller OF 3rd. Ulcerative sarcoidosis: case report and review of the literature. *Arch Dermatol* 1997; **133**: 215–9.

25 Gupta AK, Haberman HF, From GLA *et al*. Sarcoidosis with extensive cutaneous ulceration. *Dermatologica* 1987; **174**: 135–9.

26 Schwartz RA, Robertson DB, McNutt NS. Generalised ulcerative sarcoidosis. *Arch Dermatol* 1982; **118**: 931–3.

27 Hruza GJ, Kerdel FA. Generalized atrophic sarcoidosis with ulcerations. *Arch Dermatol* 1986; **122**: 320–2.

28 Neill SM, Smith NP, Eady RAJ. Ulcerative sarcoidosis: a rare manifestation of a common disease. *Clin Exp Dermatol* 1984; **9**: 277–9.

29 Herzlinger DC. Verrucous ulcerative lesions in sarcoidosis: an unusual clinical presentation. *Cutis* 1979; **23**: 569–72.

30 Schmunes E, Lantis LR, Hurley HJ. Verrucose sarcoidosis. *Arch Dermatol* 1970; **102**: 665–9.

31 Golitz LE, Shapiro L, Hurwitz E *et al*. Cicatricial alopecia of sarcoidosis. *Arch Dermatol* 1973; **107**: 758–60.

Associated diseases

Some associated diseases are understandable against the background of depressed immunological responses; some are due to a simple blocking of the activity of an organ by granulomatous infiltration, and others are uncommon and poorly understood associations. In a disease as common as sarcoidosis, coincidental associations can be expected from time to time.

Infections

A critical review of previous reports of invasive fungal infections such as cryptococcosis [1] has suggested that in many of these the entire cause of the granulomatous illness was infection, rather than sarcoidosis complicated by infection. In the series which accompanied the review, 122 patients with sarcoidosis were, in fact, found to be remarkably free of infections: three had *Aspergillus* mycetomas in cystic areas in the lung and another also had pulmonary tuberculosis, but the only extrathoracic manifestation was one case of disseminated herpes zoster. Patients with sarcoidosis, however, are prone to extensive and stubborn wart virus infections, despite an unusually high prevalence of circulating antibodies to wart antigen [2].

Immunologically mediated conditions

In a series of 190 female patients with sarcoidosis, four had hyperthyroidism and four had Hashimoto's thyroiditis with antibodies [3]. Another patient in the same series had myxoedema and Addison's disease. Chronic urticaria may occur more frequently than would be expected by chance [4]. At least 14 cases of associated sarcoidosis and connective tissue disorders have been described [5].

Effects of infiltration

Granulomas, especially in the pituitary or thyroid gland, may cause endocrine disease. Invasion of the thyroid may be without effect or, if massive, can cause hypothyroidism [6]. Cushing's syndrome and diabetes insipidus, secondary to involvement of the pituitary, have been reported. The list of such cases may be extended to cover most endocrine diseases.

Vasculitis with sarcoidosis

There are occasional but well-authenticated reports of cutaneous vasculitis occurring in the course of sarcoidosis, usually early in the disease. In a series of six patients, five of them children, the vasculitis was associated with systemic illness including fever, lymphadenopathy, musculoskeletal and eye disease, and systemic steroids were given [7]. Three of these patients, all African Americans, had large-vessel disease on angiography. Erythema nodosum itself may be regarded as a form of vasculitis. Skin biopsy may show foci of epithelioid cell granulomas centred on damaged vessels [8]. An apparently unique case of leukocytoclastic vasculitis with epithelioid cell granulomas has been described [9] and annular forms documented [10]. The occurrence of vasculitis fits with the presence of circulating immune complexes in the early stages of sarcoidosis.

Malignancy

An analysis of 131 cases of coincident sarcoidosis and malignancy suggests an increased risk of developing lymphoproliferative disease [11]. The relationship between sarcoidosis and solid tumours was less clear-cut, but most marked with carcinoma of the cervix, lung, testis and uterus [12]. Sarcoidosis may precede the development of a lymphoma (the 'sarcoidosis–lymphoma syndrome') by 18 months to 28 years [13]. All types of lymphoma may develop [12], and there is an increased incidence of thyroid cancer and leukaemia. Five patients with sarcoidosis developed multiple myeloma (four several years later and one at the time of diagnosis of the sarcoidosis) [14].

Necrobiosis lipoidica and granuloma annulare

There have been several reports of patients with sarcoidosis and necrobiosis lipoidica [15,16], and with sarcoidosis and granuloma annulare [17]. To complete the circle of association, patients with both necrobiosis lipoidica and granuloma annulare have also been described. In one African American woman with pulmonary sarcoid, fresh lesions of histologically typical granuloma annulare were adjacent to histologically classic sarcoid papules, suggesting that the former progressed to the latter [18].

These associations may be fortuitous, but histological overlap between sarcoidosis and necrobiosis may occasionally be seen [19]. Granuloma annulare is important in the differential diagnosis of sarcoidosis, as is necrobiosis, particularly of the scalp and face. Granuloma annulare shares some aspects of collagen metabolism with sarcoidosis [20], but in granuloma annulare the Kveim test is negative [21,22].

Other associations

Associations with psoriasis and gout [23], pyoderma gangrenosum [24,25] and secondary syphilis [26] have been reported, but seem likely to have been coincidental. Two Kveim-positive patients were found to have primary biliary cirrhosis [27], and a sarcoidal plaque on the face has been described in a woman with primary biliary cirrhosis [28]. Two cases of porphyria cutanea tarda have also been reported [29,30].

References

1 Winterbauer RH, Kraemer KG. The infectious complications of sarcoidosis. *Arch Intern Med* 1976; **136**: 1356–62.

2 Morison WL. Wart immunity, autoantibodies and Australia antigen in sarcoidosis. *Br J Dermatol* 1975; **93**: 717–8.

3 Karlish AJ, MacGregor GA. Sarcoidosis, thyroiditis and Addison's disease. *Lancet* 1970; **ii**: 330–3.

4 Doeglas HMG. *Chronic urticaria.* [thesis]. Druk Rijkstr Niemager, Groningen: 1975: 86.

5 Aaronson PA, Fretzin DF, Morgan NE. A unique case of sarcoidosis with coexistent collagen vascular disease. *J Am Acad Dermatol* 1985; **13**: 886–91.

6 Cohen JD. Sarcoidosis and thyrotoxicosis. *Proc R Soc Med* 1974; **67**: 220–1.

7 Fernandes SR, Singsen BH, Hoffman GS. Sarcoidosis and systemic vasculitis. *Semin Arthritis Rheum* 2000; **30**: 33–46.

8 Kennedy C. Sarcoidosis with cutaneous vasculitis. *Br J Dermatol* 1979; **101**: 47–9.

9 Chouvet B, Del Grande P, Enay G *et al.* Vascularité leucocytoclastique et sarcoidose. *Ann Dermatol Vénéréol* 1980; **107**: 279–84.

10 Branford WA, Farr PM, Porter DI. Annular vasculitis of the head and neck in a patient with sarcoidosis. *Br J Dermatol* 1982; **106**: 713–6.

11 Brincker H. Coexistence of sarcoidosis and malignant disease: causality or coincidence? *Sarcoidosis* 1989; **6**: 31–43.

12 Cohen PR, Kurzrock R. Sarcoidosis and malignancy. *Clin Dermatol* 2007; **25**: 326–33.

13 Karakantza M, Matutes E, MacLennan K *et al.* Association between sarcoidosis and lymphoma revisited. *J Clin Pathol* 1996; **49**: 208–12.

14 Pettersson T, Koivunen E, Ilvonen M *et al.* Sarcoidosis and multiple myeloma: an association. *BMJ* 1987; **295**: 958.

15 Monk B, Du Vivier A. Necrobiosis lipoidica and sarcoidosis. *Clin Exp Dermatol* 1987; **12**: 294–5.

16 Igawa K, Maruyama R, Satoh T *et al.* Necrobiosis lipoidica-like skin lesions in systemic sarcoidosis. *J Dermatol* 1998; **25**: 653–6.

17 Umbert P, Winkelmann RK. Granuloma annulare and sarcoidosis. *Br J Dermatol* 1977; **77**: 481–6.

18 Lupton JR, Figueroa P, Berberian BJ, Sulica VI. Can granuloma annulare evolve into cutaneous sarcoidosis? *Cutis* 2000; **66**: 390–2.

19 Mehregan A, Pinkus H. Necrobiosis lipoidica with sarcoid reaction. *Arch Dermatol* 1961; **83**: 143–5.

20 Oikarinen A, Kinnunen T, Kallioinen M. Biochemical and immunohistochemical comparison of collagen in granuloma annulare and skin sarcoidosis. *Acta Derm Venereol (Stockh)* 1989; **69**: 277–83.

21 Harrison P, Shuster S. Granuloma annulare and sarcoidosis. *Br J Dermatol* 1979; **100**: 231.

22 Rhodes EL. Granuloma annulare and sarcoidosis. *Br J Dermatol* 1979; **100**: 231.

23 Ecks L. Über das gemeinsame Vorkommen von Psoriasis, Sarkoidose und Gicht. *Hautarzt* 1975; **26**: 357–61.

24 Powell FC, Schroeter AL, Su WPD *et al.* Pyoderma gangrenosum and sarcoidosis. *Arch Dermatol* 1984; **120**: 959–60.

25 Hardwick N, Cerio R. Superficial granulomatous pyoderma: a report of two cases. *Br J Dermatol* 1993; **129**: 718–22.

26 Laugier P. Secondary syphilis and sarcoidosis. *Arch Dermatol* 1976; **112**: 261.

27 Karlish AJ, Thompson RPH, Williams R. A case of sarcoidosis and primary binary cirrhosis. *Lancet* 1969; **ii**: 599.

28 Harrington AC, Fitzpatrick JE. Cutaneous sarcoidal granulomas in a patient with primary biliary cirrhosis. *Cutis* 1992; **49**: 271–4.

29 Lockman DS. Porphyria cutanea tarda and sarcoidosis. *J Am Acad Dermatol* 1980; **2**: 62–5.

30 Mann RJ, Harman RRM. Porphyria cutanea tarda and sarcoidosis. *Clin Exp Dermatol* 1982; **7**: 619–23.

Course and prognosis [1]

The prognosis of sarcoidosis is difficult to assess because of its frequent 'clinical silence' and the uncertainty of its onset. Several attempts have been made to list favourable and unfavourable factors [2–4], most of which have been mentioned elsewhere in this chapter. Table 61.3 is an attempt to summarize the course of sarcoidosis. The prognosis is generally better in females, in those with less severe pulmonary disease at the onset, and in patients with a positive tuberculin test and normal globulin levels [4]. HLA-B8 may be associated with a tendency to spontaneous resolution [5]. In the African American, the course may be fulminant.

Table 61.3 The course of sarcoidosis.

Prognosis	Stage	Cardinal features*	Unfavourable events
? Abortive cases, or may be absent 60% subside in 6–18 months	Prodromal	Malaise, fatigue, fever, depression, polyarthralgia	—
	Acute	*Erythema nodosum, scar sarcoidosis, erythematopapular rashes,* polyarthralgia, iridocyclitis, lymphadenopathy	? Sudden cardiac death
	Subacute	*Papular, nodular* or *scar,* pulmonary changes, lymphadenopathy, recurrent iritis, parotitis, spleen, liver	May be cardiac death
Prolonged intermission or resolution	Intermittent Chronic		
Gradual, often slow	Progressive	*Lupus pernio, erythrodermic,* bone cysts, cataracts, hypersplenism	Blindness
Irreversible but often extremely slow and patient survives, though disabled	Fibrotic regression	Progressive pulmonary fibrosis, nephritis, nephrosis, cataracts, glaucoma	Blindness, death
	Functional failure	Emphysema, cor pulmonale, nephrolithiasis, renal failure, tuberculosis	Death

* Skin signs are in *italics.*

About 60% of patients with stage I pulmonary disease will have recovered within 2 years [6,7]. The presence of erythema nodosum does not alter the prognosis. In the classic forms of the disease, the prognosis is quite different: only a small proportion of those in pulmonary stage II and beyond resolve spontaneously [7]. Morbidity from blindness, pulmonary disease, renal failure and the cosmetic and social effects of a disfiguring skin lesion are the not inconsiderable burdens of a disease that follows a relentless course of smouldering activity [8]. Despite corticosteroid therapy, half the patients continue to have abnormal respiratory function.

Most types of cutaneous sarcoidosis occur in the subacute and chronic stages, and their course is usually prolonged. Many papules and nodules tend to resolve within months or years, but plaques are even more resistant. Lupus pernio is especially persistent and is often accompanied by the involvement of other organs, further modifying the prognosis.

Mortality in sarcoidosis [9] has been estimated at 3–6% [4,7]. However, this may ignore undiagnosed deaths from cardiac involvement. Renal involvement is also a potential cause of death as, rarely, is progressive pulmonary disease.

References

1 Turiaf J, Battesti JP, Sharma OP *et al.* Course and prognosis of sarcoidosis around the world. *Am J Med* 1974; **57**: 847–52.
2 Deremee A, Zinsmeister AR. *Proceedings of the IXth International Conference on Sarcoidosis.* Paris: Pergamon, 1983: 457.
3 von Wurm K, ed. *Sarkoidose.* Stuttgart: Thième, 1983: 228.
4 von Wurm K, Rosner R. Prognosis of chronic sarcoidosis. *Ann NY Acad Sci* 1976; **278**: 732–5.
5 Smith MJ, Turton CW, Mitchell DN. Association of HLA-B8 with spontaneous resolution in sarcoidosis. *Thorax* 1981; **36**: 296–8.
6 James DC. The early diagnosis of sarcoidosis. *Postgrad Med J* 1958; **34**: 240–4.
7 Siltzbach LE, James DC, Neville E *et al.* Course and prognosis of sarcoidosis around the world. *Am J Med* 1974; **57**: 847–52.
8 Hanno R, Callen JP. Sarcoidosis: a disorder with prominent cutaneous features, and their inter-relationship with systemic disease. *Med Clin North Am* 1980; **64**: 847–66.
9 Huang CT. Mortality in sarcoidosis: a changing pattern of causes of death. *Eur J Respir Dis* 1981; **62**: 231–8.

Investigations

The most important single criterion for the diagnosis of sarcoidosis is the finding of typical granulomas histologically [1], but the need for histological support varies with the pattern of clinical features. For example, in the UK, patients with erythema nodosum and bilateral hilar gland enlargement may not require biopsy, although this is necessary in other forms of the disease. Other investigations may add weight to the diagnosis, and may be useful in monitoring the activity of the disease.

Biopsy

The involvement of several organs will allow the clinician to select the biopsy site best suited to the individual patient. The dermatologist has the advantage of dealing with a site easily accessible for biopsy, but it may still be necessary to confirm the presence of sarcoidosis as opposed to a sarcoidal reaction, and biopsies from other organs are then needed. In one series [2] involving 292 biopsies from 10 sites, 87% were positive, but biopsies from the skin proved less reliable than those from lymph nodes, parotid gland or nasal mucosa. Scars that become infiltrated provide acceptable histological evidence of sarcoidosis. A mucosal biopsy is an alternative to skin biopsy in lupus pernio. A conjunctival biopsy should be considered, and may be positive even if no obvious lesions can be seen [3], as may a biopsy of the lower lip [4].

A range of techniques is now available to obtain biopsy material from other areas. These include the removal of epitrochlear or scalene lymph nodes, mediastinoscopy with mediastinal node biopsy, liver biopsy, gastrocnemius muscle biopsy (even when there are no muscle symptoms) [5], and transbronchial lung biopsy or mediastinal node biopsy through a flexible fibrescope [6]. The last may be the most helpful and least disturbing for patients with suspected systemic sarcoidosis and intrathoracic manifestations, but carries some risk of pneumothorax. Bronchoalveolar lavage in patients with active pulmonary involvement shows an increase in the number of helper T lymphocytes present, but this is not specific for sarcoidosis.

Kveim test [7,8]

Fifty years after Kveim described it, the test that bears his name is still something of an immunological puzzle. Until relatively recently, it was a simple and useful way of supporting a diagnosis of sarcoidosis. The Kveim test is no longer available due to the infective risk of injecting human tissue, but nevertheless details of the test are of interest and will be outlined.

The test depends upon the ability of sarcoidal tissue, usually from the spleen of an affected individual, to evoke epithelioid cell granulomas like those of sarcoidosis when injected intradermally into a patient with sarcoidosis. Positive results were found in a high proportion of patients with active early disease, but became less common in chronic disease.

The technique used is important. An easily relocated site, usually on the forearms, was injected intradermally with 0.1–0.2 mL of shaken antigen using a 1-mL tuberculin syringe and a narrow-gauge needle. In a positive reaction, a papule usually appeared within 2–3 weeks and slowly increased in size. It was best excised at 6 weeks for histology.

A positive result was the unequivocal presence of an epithelioid granuloma, exactly mimicking the natural disease, though usually less profuse. Histological interpretation was difficult in 10–20% of responses; epithelioid cells may be diffusely scattered in the dermis or granulomatous aggregates of histiocytes may not be arranged in the usual circumscribed foci of an epithelioid granuloma. The occasional presence of birefringent particles can make interpretation more complicated. False-positive foreign body-type reactions had to be disregarded.

An adequate Kveim antigen had to be sensitive enough to detect at least 60% of cases of active sarcoidosis and specific enough to exclude all but 2–3% of non-sarcoid cases [9]. To achieve this, the antigen had to be validated by extensive tests on normal subjects and on patients with other conditions, such as Crohn's disease, in which false-positive reactions are known to occur [10]. The safety of the Kveim test with regard to it being free from infective agents, for example human immunodeficiency virus, cannot be guaranteed and hence it is no longer available. The active principle in Kveim material was heat stable, and also stable on storage, though some loss of sensitivity was observed over a period of years [11]. The active material is particulate and probably lies within the membrane-containing elements of the sarcoidal tissue [12], although its exact constitution has not been established. It is not known whether the active ingredient is an antigen derived from the aetiological agent of sarcoidosis or whether a positive Kveim response is a manifestation of host predisposition to form granulomas on antigenic stimulation. These two hypotheses are not mutually exclusive.

Other investigations

A chest radiograph should be taken in all cases, no matter what the clinical presentation. Hand radiographs show cystic changes only in chronic disease, and usually only when there are clinical abnormalities in the fingers. Sputum should be examined and cultured for acid-fast bacilli, and a weak or negative tuberculin response may add weight to the diagnosis of sarcoidosis. An ECG is needed to exclude cardiac involvement. Pulmonary function tests may also be indicated. High-resolution computed tomography of the chest is helpful to define lung field involvement.

The erythrocyte sedimentation rate (ESR) is usually raised in active phases, and a rise in the ESR 6–8 weeks after the onset of erythema nodosum may indicate lung involvement [13]. Slight anaemia, neutropenia or lymphopenia are often noted, but these changes, and the hypergammaglobulinaemia that occurs in over half the chronic cases, are not of proven diagnostic or prognostic significance. Serum calcium should be checked, as an increase may lead to chronic renal failure.

Angiotensin-converting enzyme (ACE) [14] is produced by sarcoidal granulomas. Raised serum levels are found in some 60% of patients with sarcoidosis, but are also present in other conditions such as diabetes and alcoholic liver disease. This limits the value of the test as a diagnostic aid, although it remains a useful monitor of disease activity.

Other markers of disease activity [15] vary in their usefulness in sarcoidosis. They include lysozyme, β_2-microglobulin, neopterin, collagenase and fibronectin levels. The serum level of soluble intercellular adhesion molecule 1 (ICAM-1), which is shed from cell surfaces and is a measure of the inflammatory response, mirrors disease activity in active sarcoidosis [16]. Hydroxyprolinuria may indicate disease activity. Radioactive gallium-67 uptake occurs in some pulmonary infections and neoplasms as well as sarcoidosis, but if these can be excluded it provides a way of separating active from fibrotic pulmonary disease.

References

1 Poole GW. The diagnosis of sarcoidosis. *BMJ* 1982; **285**: 321–2.
2 Israel HL, Sones M. Selection of biopsy procedures for sarcoidosis diagnosis. *Arch Intern Med* 1964; **113**: 255–60.
3 Khan F, Wessely Z, Chezin SR *et al*. Conjunctival biopsy in sarcoidosis: a simple, safe and specific diagnostic procedure. *Ann Ophthalmol* 1977; **9**: 761.
4 Nessan VS, Jacoway JR. Biopsy of minor salivary glands in the diagnosis of sarcoidosis. *N Engl J Med* 1979; **301**: 922–4.
5 Andrnopoulos AP, Papadimitriou C, Melachrinou M *et al*. Asymptomatic gastrocnemius muscle biopsy: an extremely sensitive and specific test in the pathologic confirmation of sarcoidosis presenting with hilar adenopathy. *Clin Exp Rheumatol* 2001; **19**: 569–72.
6 Wang KP, Johns CJ, Fuenning C *et al*. Flexible transbronchial needle aspiration for the diagnosis of sarcoidosis. *Ann Otol Rhinol Laryngol* 1989; **98**: 298–300.
7 Munro CS, Mitchell DN. The Kveim response: still useful, still a puzzle. *Thorax* 1987; **42**: 321–31.
8 Teirstein AS. The Kveim–Siltzbach test. *Clin Dermatol* 1986; **4**: 154–64.
9 Siltzbach LE. Qualities and behaviour of satisfactory Kveim suspensions. *Ann NY Acad Sci* 1976; **278**: 665–6.
10 James DG. Kveim revisited, reassessed. *N Engl J Med* 1975; **292**: 859–60.
11 Hurley TH, Sullivan JR, Hurley JV. Reaction to Kveim test material in sarcoidosis and other diseases. *Lancet* 1985; **i**: 494–6.
12 Middleton WG, Douglas AC. Further experience with Edinburgh prepared Kveim–Siltzbach test suspensions. In: Jones Williams W, Davies BH, eds. *Proceedings of the VIIIth International Conference on Sarcoidosis*. Cardiff: Alpha Omega, 1980: 655–9.
13 Vesey CMR, Wilkinson DS. Erythema nodosum. *Br J Dermatol* 1959; **71**: 139–55.
14 Callen JP, Hanno R. Serum angiotensin converting enzyme in patients with cutaneous sarcoidosis. *Arch Dermatol* 1982; **118**: 232–3.
15 Pozzi E, Ghio P, Albera A. Sarcoid activity markers. *Sarcoidosis* 1988; **5**: 162–5.
16 Ishii Y, Kitamura S. Elevated levels of soluble ICAM-1 in serum and BAL fluid in patients with active sarcoidosis. *Chest* 1995; **107**: 1636–40.

Treatment [1,2]

The chance of spontaneous remission favours a conservative approach to systemic therapy, which will usually carry the hazards of long-term immunosuppression, such as opportunistic mycobacterial infection [3] or a gross proliferation of viral warts [4]. At any time the pattern of the disease may change, but an expectant policy is often best if the course is not progressive and if vital structures are not involved.

Johns *et al.* [1] list the most frequent indications for systemic treatment:

1 symptomatic pulmonary disease
2 progressive or persistent parenchymal lung disease after 2 years
3 posterior ocular disease or anterior disease not responding to local steroids
4 persistent fever or weight loss
5 liver disease with significant dysfunction or hepatosplenomegaly
6 disfiguring skin disease or lymphadenopathy
7 nervous system disease
8 hypercalcaemia
9 myocardial disease
10 myopathy or myositis
11 thrombocytopenia
12 other significant organ involvement—for example, kidneys.

A major determinant is the degree to which a patient's normal life is disrupted by the disease, but objective measurements, such as pulmonary function tests, may be a more valuable way of monitoring therapy than symptoms alone.

A few patients with severe cardiac or pulmonary disease have come to transplantation; the sarcoidosis does not necessarily recur in the graft, perhaps due to the use of potent immunosuppressive agents [5].

In the skin clinic any decisions about the use of systemic therapy must take into account the seriousness of the accompanying internal involvement and the natural history of the particular type of skin lesion. Papular lesions, for example, are likely to fade without treatment, whereas lupus pernio is not.

Topical therapy

High-potency topical corticosteroids may sometimes prove helpful, as may intralesional triamcinolone injections. Tacrolimus, which inhibits hapten-induced production of Th1 cytokines and TNF-α by T cells, has been reported to be beneficial when used topically in cutaneous sarcoidosis [6]. Cryotherapy and radiotherapy have occasionally been used [2]. PUVA therapy has been successful in hypopigmented sarcoidosis [7] and in erythrodermic sarcoidosis [2]. In certain types of cutaneous sarcoidosis, for example lupus pernio, cosmetic camouflage advice is helpful.

Systemic therapy [8]

Corticosteroids are usually the most effective treatment, given at first in a relatively high dose, possibly 30 or 40 mg prednisolone daily, and then tapered over a period of several weeks to a lower maintenance dose of possibly 15 mg on alternate days. The length of the course of treatment will vary from case to case but is usually at least 6 months. Intravenous 'pulse' methylprednisolone, for example 1 g/week for 8 weeks, may be effective in those with the most severe neurological disease [5].

Immunosuppressive drugs may be tried if corticosteroids are contraindicated or have been ineffective. Methotrexate has been used with some success [9] and has been recommended for use with corticosteroids for lupus pernio [10]. Azathioprine, and mycophenolate mofetil (45 mg/kg/day), have been used for their steroid-sparing effects [11,12].

Biologic agents have recently been employed. The anti-TNF drugs infliximab and etanercept have been used successfully in cutaneous sarcoidosis—resistance to anti-TNF agents may require a switch to an alternative drug [13,14]. The anti-T-cell agent alefacept is described as beneficial in lupus pernio [15].

Other drugs which have been tried with some success include allopurinol, doxycycline and chloroquine [11,16]. Minocycline, 200 mg daily for 12 months, produced complete resolution in eight and partial improvement in two out of 12 patients with cutaneous sarcoidosis [17]. Levamisole is not recommended [18]. The response to ciclosporin has been variable [5]. Isotretinoin induced complete resolution in one case of cutaneous sarcoidosis [19]. Treatment with thalidomide (100–200 mg/day) in 12 patients with cutaneous sarcoidosis induced complete remission in four cases, partial improvement in six and no change in two [20]. Fumaric acid esters (FAEs) may give variable benefit [21]. In a small series of three patients with recalcitrant cutaneous sarcoidosis, all cleared after 4–12 months treatment with FAEs [22].

Laser, ultraviolet radiation and photodynamic therapies

Lupus pernio has been improved using the carbon dioxide laser [23]. UVA1 (340–440 nm) has been effective for forehead plaque sarcoid [24]. The use of photodynamic therapy can also be considered [25].

References

1 Johns CJ, Scott PP, Schonfled SA. Sarcoidosis. *Ann Rev Med* 1989; **40**: 353–71.
2 Veien NK. Cutaneous sarcoidosis: prognosis and treatment. *Clin Dermatol* 1986; **4**: 75–87.
3 Grice K. Sarcoidosis and *Mycobacterium avium–intracellulare* cutaneous abscesses. *Clin Exp Dermatol* 1983; **8**: 323–7.
4 MacKie RM. Extensive warts treated with etretinate. *Br J Dermatol* 1982; **107** (Suppl. 22): 97–8.
5 Mitchell DM. Sarcoidosis. In: Mitchell DM, ed. *Recent Advances in Respiratory Medicine*. Edinburgh: Churchill Livingstone, 1991: 185–202.
6 Katoh N, Mihara H, Yasuno H. Cutaneous sarcoidosis successfully treated with topical tacrolimus. *Br J Dermatol* 2002; **147**: 154–6.
7 Patterson JW, Fitzwater JE. Treatment of hypopigmented sarcoidosis with 8-methoxypsoralen and longwave ultraviolet light. *Int J Dermatol* 1982; **21**: 476–80.
8 Badgwell C, Rosen T. Cutaneous sarcoidosis therapy updated. *J Am Acad Dermatol* 2007; **56**: 69–83.
9 Veien NK, Brodthagen H. Cutaneous sarcoidosis treated with methotrexate. *Br J Dermatol* 1977; **97**: 213–6.
10 Spiteri MA, Matthey F, Carstairs LS *et al.* Lupus pernio: a clinicoradiological study of 35 cases. *Br J Dermatol* 1985; **112**: 315–22.
11 Mosam A, Morar N. Recalcitrant cutaneous sarcoidosis: an evidence-based sequential approach. *J Dermatol Treat* 2004; **15**: 353–9.
12 Kouba DJ, Mimouni D, Rencic A, Nousari HC. Mycophenolate mofetil may serve as a steroid-sparing agent for sarcoidosis. *Br J Dermatolol* 2003; **148**: 147–8.
13 Yee AMF, Pochapin MB. Treatment of complicqated sarcoidosis with infliximab anti-TNF-alfa therapy. *Ann Intern Med* 2001; **135**: 27–31.
14 Khanna D, Leibling M, Louie J. Etanercept ameliorates sarcoidosis arthritis and skin disease. *J Rheumatol* 2003; **30**: 1864–5.
15 Garcia-Zuazaga J, Korman NJ. Cutaneous sarcoidosis successfully treated with alefacept. *J Cutan Med Surg* 2006; **10**: 300–3.
16 Bregnhoej A, Jemec GB. Low-dose allopurinol in the treatment of cutaneous sarcoidosis: response in four of seven patients. *J Dermatol Treat* 2005; **16**: 125–7.
17 Bachelez H, Senet P, Cadranel J *et al.* The use of tetracyclines for the treatment of sarcoidosis. *Arch Dermatol* 2001; **137**: 69–73.
18 Veien NK. Cutaneous sarcoidosis treated with levamisole. *Dermatologica* 1977; **154**: 185–9.
19 Georgiou S, Monastirli A, Pasmatzi E, Tsamboas D. Cutaneous sarcoidosis: complete resolution after oral isotretinoin therapy. *Acta Derm Venereol (Stockh)* 1998; **78**: 457–9.
20 Nguyen YT, Dupuy A, Cordoliani F *et al.* Treatment of cutaneous sarcoidosis with thalidomide. *J Am Acad Dermatol* 2004; **50**: 235–51.
21 Breuer K, Gutzmer R, Volker B *et al.* Therapy of non-infectious granulomatous skin disease with fumaric acid esters. *Br J Dermatol* 2005; **152**: 1290–5.
22 Nowack U, Gambichler T, Henefeld C *et al.* Successful treatment of recalcitrant cutaneous sarcoidosis with fumaric acid esters. *BMC Dermatol* 2002; **2**: 15.
23 O'Donoghue NB, Barlow RJ. Laser remodelling of nodular nasal lupus pernio. *Clin Exper Dermatol* 2006; **31**: 27–9.
24 Graefe T, Konrad H, Barta U *et al.* Successful ultraviolet A1 treatment of cutaneous sarcoidosis. *Br J Dermatol* 2001; **145**: 354–5.
25 Gilaberte Y, Serra-Guillen C, de las Heras ME *et al.* Photodynamic therapy in dermatology. *Actas Dermosifiliogr* 2006; **97**: 83–102.

Other sarcoidal reactions

A number of infections and chemicals may cause sarcoid-like granulomas, although their features are seldom as clear-cut histologically [1,2]. Such reactions differ from sarcoidosis in several important respects:

1 They involve only those organs normally affected by the disease in question, or on the route of absorption or deposition of the chemical.
2 The Kveim test when performed has been negative.
3 The tuberculin reaction is usually not depressed.

The following text describes reactions which should be borne in mind in the differential diagnosis of sarcoidosis.

Infections

The problem of differentiating tuberculosis and leprosy from sarcoidosis has been dealt with on p. 16.13. Syphilis, brucellosis, fungus infections and some bacterial or viral diseases may produce a sarcoidal type of tissue response but any clinical resemblance is usually superficial.

Foreign materials

Silicates occur in many common materials—for example, in talc, kaolin, quartz and as a constituent of slate, brick, gravel and coal. Silicosis from the inhalation of silica dust is an important industrial hazard, but wounds containing crystals of silica normally remain unchanged indefinitely. Talc has been the cause of granulomas in surgical wounds when used as a glove powder. The long delay between the implantation of silica and the appearance of the granuloma suggests that the silica may not be the immediate cause of the reaction. In one case, a silica granuloma has progressed to scar sarcoidosis [3]. It is wise to examine all sarcoidal reactions under polarized light: silica particles are doubly refractile and differ from Schaumann bodies in that the crystalline material is spiculated but not laminated.

Beryllium reactions [2] are rarely seen now that beryllium is no longer used in the manufacture of fluorescent lights. The cutaneous lesions of systemic berylliosis are indistinguishable histologically from those of sarcoidosis, whereas the granulomas due to local beryllium implantation show marked central necrosis.

Zirconium granulomas may form in the axillae as a delayed hypersensitivity reaction to the zirconium content of deodorants [1,4].

Sea-urchin spines may induce foreign-body or sarcoidal granulomas [5]. The exact cause of the reaction is unknown. Intralesional triamcinolone may help speed resolution if excision is not practicable [6].

Foreign-body reactions to lipids (fat granulomas, epidermal cysts) and reactions to other lipid and non-lipid extraneous matter are variable and often show many giant cells.

Thesaurosis [7] is a pulmonary infiltration occurring in those heavily exposed to polyvinyl–pyrrolidine hair sprays in hairdressing procedures.

Sarcoidal reactions in tattoos (Fig. 61.19). A granulomatous dermal infiltrate may accompany sensitization reactions to any pigment of the tattoo, or may occur alone [8]. Less commonly, a pure sarcoidal reaction is present as an indolent lump within a tattooed area. Regional lymph nodes may also show a sarcoidal reaction [9]. Such lesions may be accompanied by other signs of sarcoidosis or a positive Kveim test [10] and are occasionally the only skin manifestation of the disease [11]. The pulmonary disease may be silent [8]. The association of a sarcoidal reaction in a cobalt tattoo with uveitis in three cases and with erythema nodosum in one [12] emphasizes the need for a thorough investigation of all cases showing a sarcoidal type of infiltrate.

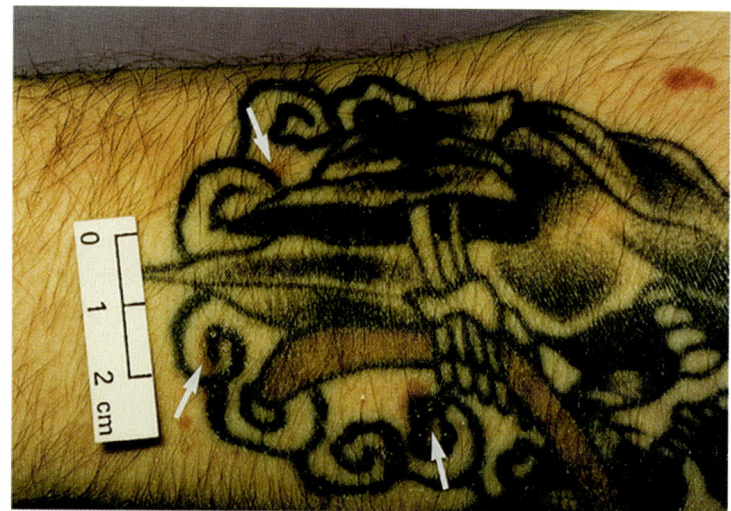

(a)

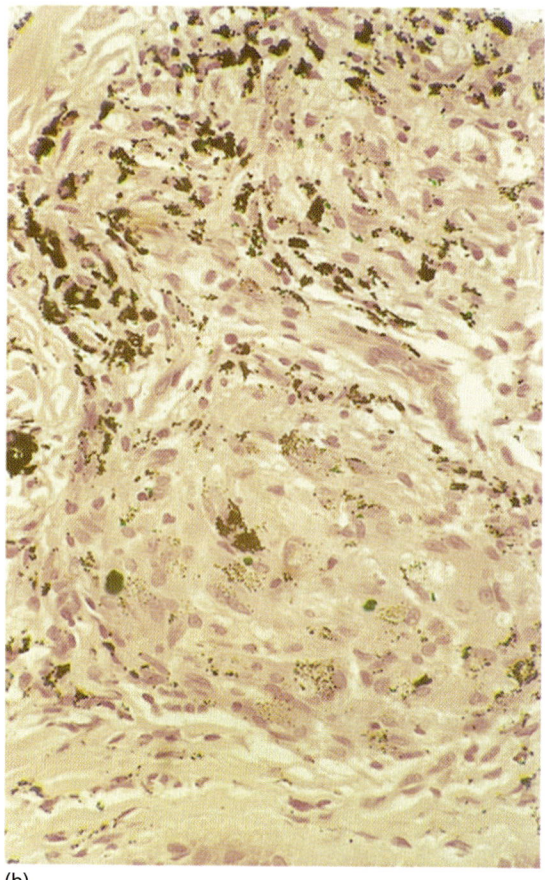

(b)

Fig. 61.19 (a) Sarcoidal reaction to pigment in a tattoo. (Courtesy of Dr P. Collins, St Vincent's Hospital, Dublin, Eire.) (b) Histology of a sarcoidal reaction to two varieties of tattoo pigment, one opaque and one green. (Courtesy of Dr T.J. Stephenson, Royal Hallamshire Hospital, Sheffield, UK.)

Cosmetic fillers. Sarcoidal granulomas developed in the skin of a woman with pulmonary sarcoidosis who had had facial skin treated with a cosmetic filler [13].

Other reactions. A sarcoid-like reaction has been reported from exposure to acrylic or nylon fibres, either as dust or from walking on acrylic carpets [14]. The significance of a sarcoidal reaction to ear piercing [15] was not clear in the presence of a positive Kveim test.

Crohn's disease

The similarity between the histological and immunological features of Crohn's disease and sarcoidosis led to speculation about a common aetiology. However, the rarity of sarcoidosis of the intestine makes this unlikely, and earlier reports of positive Kveim tests in patients with Crohn's disease have not been fully substantiated [16].

Whipple's disease [17]

Sarcoid-like changes have been recorded in the skin and lymphatic glands [17]. Diarrhoea is an important distinguishing clinical feature and jejunal biopsy will confirm the correct diagnosis (Chapter 62).

Farmer's lung [18]

This is caused by the inhalation of mouldy hay containing fungal spores: sarcoid-type granulomas sometimes develop slowly around the air passages and the condition then runs a course not unlike pulmonary sarcoidosis.

Other conditions

Sarcoid-like granulomas can occur in the skin and lymph nodes of patients with lymphoma: most commonly in Hodgkin's disease [19], but also in non-Hodgkin's lymphoma [20,21]. Sarcoid reaction is described with other malignancies, for example papillary thyroid carcinoma [22].

Epithelioid cell granulomas may also be a feature of rosacea [23]. In one unusual case [24], rosacea-like facial lesions, with a sarcoidal histology, were seen in a patient with a poorly differentiated lymphoma.

An epithelioid cell granuloma histology is found in granulomatous cheilitis and the Melkersson–Rosenthal syndrome, sometimes in necrobiosis lipoidica [25] and in granulomatosis disciformis, and has been reported in giant cell and other forms of arteritis [26].

References

1 Shelley WB, Hurley HJ. The allergic origin of zirconium deodorant granulomas. *Br J Dermatol* 1958; **70**: 75–101.

2 Sprince NL, Kazemi H, Hardy HL. Current problem of differentiating between beryllium disease and sarcoidosis. *Ann NY Acad Sci* 1976; **278**: 654–64.

3 Rowland-Payne CME, Meyrick-Thomas RH, Black MM. From silica granuloma to scar sarcoidosis. *Clin Exp Dermatol* 1983; **8**: 171–5.

4 Epstein WL, Skahen JR, Krasnobrod H. Granulomatous hypersensitivity to zirconium. *J Dermatol* 1962; **38**: 223–32.

5 Kinmont PDC. Sea urchin sarcoidal granuloma. *Br J Dermatol* 1965; **77**: 335–43.

6 Warin AP. Sea urchin granuloma. *Clin Exp Dermatol* 1977; **2**: 405–7.

7 Herrero EU, Feigelson HH, Becker A. Sarcoidosis in a beautician. *Am Rev Respir Dis* 1965; **92**: 280–3.

8 Antonovich DD, Callen JP. Development of sarcoidosis in cosmetic tattoos. *Arch Dermatol* 2005; **141**: 869–72.

9 Hanada K, Chiyoya S, Katebira Y. Systemic sarcoidal reaction in a tattoo. *Clin Exp Dermatol* 1985; **10**: 479–84.

10 Kennedy C. Sarcoidosis presenting in tattoos. *Clin Exp Dermatol* 1976; **1**: 395–9.

11 Dickinson JA. Sarcoidal reactions in tattoos. *Arch Dermatol* 1969; **100**: 315–9.

12 Rorsman H, Dahlquist I, Jacobsson S et al. Tattoo granuloma and uveitis. *Lancet* 1969; **ii**: 27–8.

13 Sidwell RU, Johnson NMcL, Francis N, Bunker CB. Cutaneous sarcoidal granulomas developing after facial cosmetic filler in a patient with newly diagnosed systemic sarcoidosis. *Clin Exper Dermatol* 2006; **31**: 208–11.

14 Pimental JC. Sarcoid granulomas of the skin produced by acrylic and nylon fibres. *Br J Dermatol* 1977; **96**: 673–7.

15 Mann RJ, Peachey RDC. Sarcoidal tissue reaction: another complication of ear piercing. *Clin Exp Dermatol* 1983; **8**: 199–200.

16 Middleton WG, Douglas AC. Further experience with Edinburgh prepared Kviem–Siltzbach test suspensions. In: Jones Williams W, Davies BH, eds. *Proceedings of the VIIIth International Conference on Sarcoidosis.* Cardiff: Alpha Omega, 1980, 655–9.

17 James DG, Lipman MC. Whipple's disease: a granulomatous masquerader. *Clin Chest Med* 2002; **23**: 513–9.

18 Rankin J, Jaersche WH, Callies QC et al. Farmer's lung. *Ann Intern Med* 1962; **57**: 606–26.

19 Kadin ME, Donaldson SS, Dorfman RF. Isolated granulomas in Hodgkin's disease. *N Engl J Med* 1970; **283**: 859–61.

20 Dupre A, Bolinelli BC, Biart M et al. Reactions sarcoidosiques au cours d'une réticulose histiomonocytaire: présentation de deux observations. *Bull Soc Fr Dermatol Syphilol* 1974; **82**: 162–3.

21 Kavin LB, Gordon W, Camp R. Florid sarcoid reaction associated with lymphoma of the skin. *Cancer* 1974; **33**: 1117–22.

22 Yamauchi M, Inoue D, Fukunaga Y et al. A case of sarcoid reaction associated with papillary thyroid carcinoma. *Thyroid* 1997; **7**: 901–3.

23 Laymon CW, Schoch EP. Micropapular tuberculid and rosacea: a clinical and histologic comparison. *Acta Derm Venereol (Stockh)* 1948; **58**: 286–98.

24 Sherertz EF, Westwitk TJ, Flowers FP. Sarcoidal reaction to lymphoma presenting as granulomatous rosacea. *Arch Dermatol* 1986; **122**: 1303–5.

25 Mehregan A, Pinkus H. Necrobiosis lipoidica with sarcoid reaction. *Arch Dermatol* 1961; **83**: 143–5.

26 Kinmont PDC, McCallum DI. Skin manifestations of giant cell arteritis. *Br J Dermatol* 1964; **76**: 299–308.

CHAPTER 62

Systemic Disease and the Skin

N.H. Cox[1] & I.H. Coulson[2]

[1]Department of Dermatology, Cumberland Infirmary, Carlisle, UK
[2]Dermatology Unit, Burnley General Hospital, Burnley, UK

Introduction

The systemic associations of skin diseases have been stressed throughout this book. In this chapter many of these associations are listed again, along with some other important conditions. They are grouped so as to be helpful to the general physician or internist. It is hoped that such a presentation will also be useful to the dermatologist who is asked to help in the diagnosis of obscure internal disease. Many further references may be found by turning to the chapter in which the relevant dermatosis is considered in detail.

The texts listed below [1–5] provide much more information than it is possible to give here, and are also a source of additional references.

References

1 Braverman IM. *Skin Signs of Systemic Disease*, 3rd edn. Philadelphia: Saunders, 1998.
2 Callen JP, Jorrizo JL, eds. *Dermatological Signs of Internal Disease*, 3rd edn. Philadelphia: Saunders, 2003.
3 Jones JH, Mason DK, eds. *Oral Manifestations of Systemic Disease*, 2nd edn. Philadelphia: Baillière Tindall, 1990.
4 Provost TT, Flynn JA, eds. *Cutaneous Medicine: Cutaneous Manifestations of Systemic Disease*. Hamilton, Ontario: Decker, 2001.
5 Lebwohl MG. *The Skin and Systemic Disease. A Color Atlas and Text*, 2nd edn. London: Churchill Livingstone, 2004.

Rook's Textbook of Dermatology, 8th edition. Edited by DA Burns, SM Breathnach, NH Cox and CEM Griffiths. © 2010 Blackwell Publishing Ltd.

Endocrine disorders

The physiological effects of hormones on pigmentation, hair growth, sebaceous glands and connective tissue have been described in other chapters. This section is limited to discussion of specific endocrine pathology with cutaneous features. Additional detail is provided in several general references [1–6].

References
1 Feingold KR, Elias PM. Endocrine–skin interactions. *J Am Acad Dermatol* 1987; **17**: 921–40.
2 Feingold KR, Elias PM. Endocrine–skin interactions. *J Am Acad Dermatol* 1988; **19**: 1–20.
3 Boyne M, Dobs AS, Krasner AS, Provost TT. Evaluation and treatment of endocrine disorders. In: Provost TT, Flynn JA, eds. *Cutaneous Medicine: Cutaneous Manifestations of Systemic Disease.* Hamilton, Ontario: Decker, 2001: 413–51.
4 Braverman IM. *Skin Signs of Systemic Disease*, 3rd edn. Philadelphia: Saunders, 1998: 438–91.
5 Wass JAH, Shalet SM. *Oxford Textbook of Endocrinology and Diabetes.* Oxford: Oxford University Press, 2002.
6 Jabbour SA. Cutaneous manifestations of endocrine disorders. A guide for dermatologists. *Am J Clin Dermatol* 2003; **4**: 315–31.

Pituitary syndromes

Hyperpituitarism [1–3]

Excessive secretion of growth hormone (GH, somatotrophin) causes an increase in plasma insulin-like growth factor-1 (IGF-1). These hormones stimulate synthesis of collagen and glycosaminoglycan in the skin and skeleton, leading to insidious hypertrophy of skin, subcutaneous tissues and viscera, and to periosteal bone growth. This causes acromegaly in the adult (most cases), and gigantism in children whose bony epiphyses have not yet closed.

*Acromegaly (MIM *102200) [4] and gigantism*

Aetiology. The usual cause (over 95%) is a benign adenoma or hyperplasia of the eosinophilic cells of the adenohypophysis, producing GH and often prolactin [4]. Other tumours, such as bronchial carcinoma, may occasionally cause acromegaly, usually by ectopic secretion of GH-releasing hormone (GH-RH). Individual, viable epidermal cells are larger than normal, and epidermal cell turnover is increased.

Clinical features. Periosteal new bone formation of the facial bones and skin causes the characteristic facies. Features are prognathism, frontal bossing, widely spaced teeth and acral hypertrophy, which causes elongated, blunt and thickened fingers. Dermatological features include a protruding, thickened lower lip, oedematous thick eyelids, a large and furrowed tongue (Fig. 62.1), triangular large ears, numerous skin tags ('fibroma molluscum'), widened skin pores, wet and oily skin due to hyperhidrosis and increased sebum production, acne and cutis gyrata of the scalp in more extreme cases. Eruptive seborrhoeic keratoses mimicking the sign of Leser–Trélat have been reported in acromegaly [5]. Hyperpigmentation develops in about half of the affected individuals due to increased levels of melanocyte-stimulating hormone (MSH), and acanthosis nigricans may occur. The scalp hair is initially coarse and there may be hirsutism, but later in the disease there

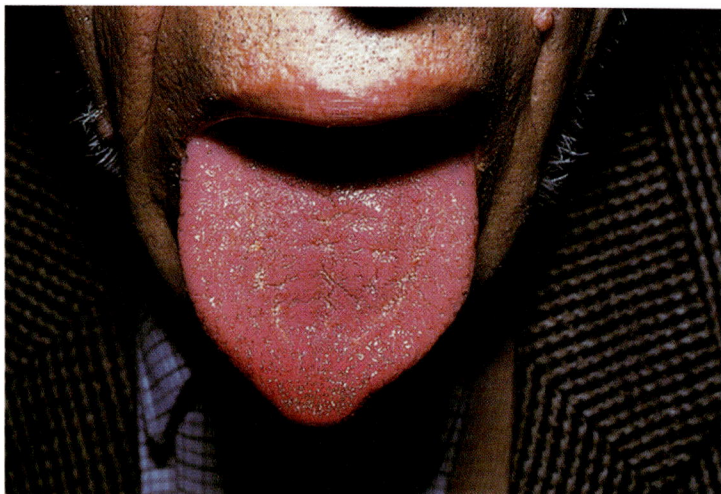

Fig. 62.1 Acromegalic macroglossia.

is a decrease in gonadotrophin production, which causes the hair to become finer, with loss of secondary sexual hair. The nails are flat and wide and grow fast. Pachydermoperiostosis (Chapter 15) is an important differential diagnosis. In this disease, there is no macroglossia or prognathism, and the fingers are characteristically clubbed.

Non-cutaneous features include macroglossia, visual field defect and headache due to the neoplasm, arthropathy, carpal tunnel syndrome and proximal myopathy. Cardiovascular morbidity and mortality is markedly increased due to associated hypertension, left ventricular hypertrophy, cardiomyopathy, sleep hypoxia and apnoea, and hyperlipidaemia. Acromegalic subjects have an increased incidence of colonic adenomas and carcinomas [6].

Diagnosis. The clinical picture is, in most cases, suggestive of the diagnosis. Serum GH and prolactin levels are generally elevated, but vary considerably both in normal subjects and in those with acromegaly [4]; plasma IGF-1 is a more reliable test of chronically elevated GH levels [7]. Failure of GH levels to suppress during glucose challenge, and GH-RH stimulation tests, help to confirm the diagnosis. Magnetic resonance imaging (MRI) of the pituitary gland with contrast confirms the site and size of the tumour in most cases; three-quarters of subjects have a macroadenoma (>10 mm) at presentation but microadenomas as small as 2 mm can be identified using current imaging techniques.

Treatment. Neurosurgical removal of the tumour is the preferred treatment. Patients in whom this fails to achieve a cure may be treated with somatostatin analogues such as octreotide and lanreotide, dopamine agonists such as bromocriptine and cabergoline, GH receptor antagonists such as pegvisomant, or radiotherapy [1–3,7,8,10]. Colonoscopy surveillance is recommended as there is an increased risk of colonic polyps, carcinomas and tubulovillous adenomas.

Pituitary insufficiency [1–3,9,11]

Insufficiency of the adenohypophysis (anterior pituitary) may involve individual or multiple hormones. In classical hypopituita-

Table 62.1 The causes of anterior pituitary deficiency.

Neoplasia—adenomas (most), craniopharyngioma, metastases

Infection—tuberculosis, abscess

Trauma, surgical, iatrogenic

Congenital—familial, 'empty sella syndrome'

Vascular—Sheehan's syndrome (postpartum) and other infarction, bleeding, diabetes mellitus, vasculitis, antiphospholipid syndrome

Idiopathic

Hypothalamic—due to hypothalamic tumours, trauma, infiltration (Langerhans' cell histiocytosis, sarcoidosis), congenital causes of hypothalamic failure

References
1 Braverman IM. *Skin Signs of Systemic Disease*, 3rd edn. Philadelphia: Saunders, 1998: 438–40.
2 Feldman SR, Jorizzo JL. Adrenal, androgen-related, and pituitary disorders. In: Callen JP, Jorizzo JL, eds. *Dermatological Signs of Internal Disease*, 3rd edn. Philadelphia: Saunders, 2003: 187–91.
3 Boyne M, Dobs AS, Krasner AS, Provost TT. Evaluation and treatment of endocrine disorders. In: Provost TT, Flynn JA, eds. *Cutaneous Medicine: Cutaneous Manifestations of Systemic Disease*. Hamilton, Ontario: Decker, 2001: 413–51.
4 Melmed S. Acromegaly. *N Engl J Med* 2006; **355**: 2258–73.
5 Kilmer SL, Berman B, Morhenn VB. Eruptive seborrheic keratoses in a young woman with acromegaly. *J Am Acad Dermatol* 1990; **23**: 991–4.
6 Jenkins PJ. Cancers associated with acromegaly. *Neuroendocrinology* 2006; **83**: 218–23.
7 Melmed S, Ho K, Klibanski A *et al.* Recent advances in pathogenesis, diagnosis and management of acromegaly. *J Clin Endocrinol Metab* 1995; **80**: 3395–402.
8 Orrego JJ, Barkan AL. Pituitary disorders: drug treatment options. *Drugs* 2000; **59**: 93–106.
9 Lamberts SWJ, de Herder WW, van der Lely AJ. Pituitary insufficiency. *Lancet* 1998; **352**: 127.
10 Melmed S. Medical progress: Acromegaly. *N Engl J Med* 2006; **355**: 2558–73.
11 Geller JL, Braunstein GD. Dermatologic manifestations of hypopituitarism. *Clin Dermatol* 2006; **4**: 266–75.

rism, all endocrine cell functions of the pituitary gland are involved to a varying degree. However, the clinical picture is influenced by the cause of hypopituitarism; for example, adenomas may produce GH or prolactin, but may also cause compression atrophy of cells producing gonadotrophins. Concurrent loss of function of the posterior pituitary may occur if there is a hypothalamic lesion, such as Langerhans' cell histiocytosis.

Aetiology. Over 95% of cases of hypopituitarism are due to pituitary cell destruction [8]. Familial hypopituitarism has a genetic basis due to mutations in Pit-1 or its precursor Prop-1, resulting in deficient production of GH, prolactin and thyrotrophin. Causes of insufficiency of the anterior pituitary are listed in Table 62.1.

Clinical features. The various endocrine dysfunctions are typically insidious and less impressive than those seen in the primary glandular disorders. Pallor of the skin due to decreased MSH secretion results in generalized hypopigmentation, most apparent in the skin of the nipple areola and genitalia; in contrast with anaemia, the mucous membranes retain their normal colour. There is an increased sunburn tendency and lack of tanning, and there may be a degree of carotenaemia due to hypothyroidism. Loss of terminal hair due to decreased gonadotrophin secretion is observed in all patients, first in the axillae and later, but not invariably, in the pubic area. Fine wrinkling and dryness of the skin simulates advanced age. The face appears expressionless due to diminution of the facial skinfolds. The activity of sebaceous and sweat glands is reduced. Onycholysis, longitudinal ridging and brownish discoloration of the nail plate may be seen.

Pituitary dwarfism is characterized by proportionate retardation of somatic growth in conjunction with normal mental development. The cutaneous changes of old age may develop prematurely from the third decade onwards.

Erythromelalgia with non-healing skin ulcers has been reported as a presenting feature of GH deficiency in a child.

Diagnosis and treatment. Measurement of hormone levels—prolactin, IGF-1, thyroid-stimulating hormone (TSH) and thyroxine (T_4), cortisol, gonadotrophins—is required to detect subnormal levels; prolactin or IGF-1 may be elevated if the cause of hypopituitarism is a pituitary tumour. Posterior pituitary function should also be assessed, and visual field testing and MRI should be performed. Treatment is of the primary cause, together with hormone replacement [8,9].

Adrenal syndromes

Cushing's disease and syndrome [1–8]

Chronic glucocorticoid excess may occur due to increased secretion of adrenocorticotrophic hormone (ACTH, corticotrophin), usually from the pituitary (MIM *219090), due to glucocorticoid hypersecretion of adrenal origin (ACTH-independent, MIM *219080) or due to exogenous administration of glucocorticoids.

Aetiology. The commonest ACTH-dependent cause is that due to a pituitary adenoma (Cushing's disease or pituitary-dependent Cushing's syndrome), which accounts for about 70% of spontaneous cases; pituitary overproduction of ACTH leads to adrenal hyperplasia and thus to glucocorticoid excess. Other ACTH-dependent causes include the ectopic ACTH syndrome (for example, from small cell lung cancer or bronchial carcinoids) and, rarely, ectopic corticotrophin-releasing hormone (CRH) syndrome. ACTH-independent causes include cortisol-producing adrenocortical adenomas and carcinomas, various types of bilateral adrenal hyperplasia (including the Carney complex), and, most commonly, iatrogenic causes such as results from long-term administration of glucocorticoids, either systemically or from excessive use of topical, inhaled or intralesional steroids [4]. The glucocorticoid hormones, among other effects, impair synthesis of collagen and mucopolysaccharides and thus lead to atrophy and vascular fragility of the skin.

Clinical features. The cutaneous manifestations are quite similar whether caused by endogenous or iatrogenic hypercorticism, although there are additional effects mediated by androgens in patients with adrenal disease. The features are enumerated in Table 62.2; the thin skin and easy bruising are helpful in distinguishing Cushing's syndrome from simple obesity.

About 6–10% of patients with pituitary Cushing's disease have addisonian-like pigmentation [1], as oversecretion of the common

Table 62.2 Cutaneous manifestations of Cushing's disease.

Truncal obesity (classically deposits of fat over the clavicles and back of the neck, the 'buffalo hump')
Facial fullness and plethora ('moon facies') are most frequent
Slender limbs
Skin atrophy
Fragility, bruising and poor healing
Telangiectasia
Striae (typically wide and red)
Hirsuties
Hypertrichosis (downy facial hair in iatrogenic hypercorticism)
Acneiform lesions (often monomorphic and devoid of comedones and cysts)
Male-pattern baldness in women
Dermatophyte and yeast infections

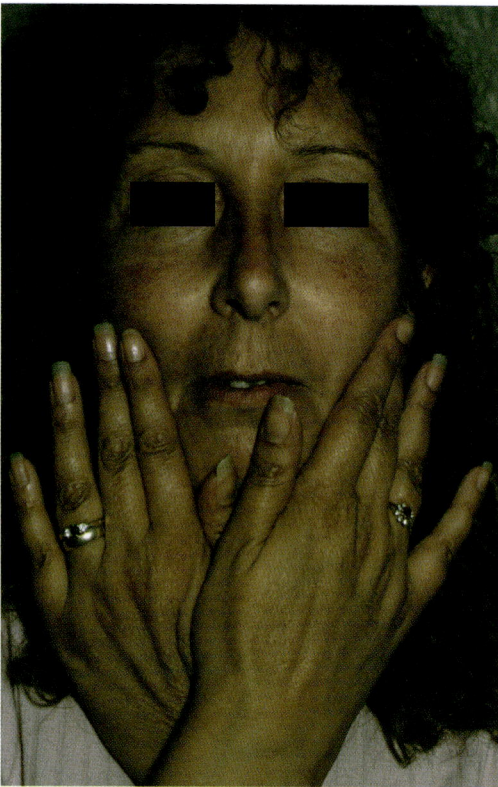

Fig. 62.2 Diffuse pigmentation in Nelson's syndrome.

precursor pro-opiomelanocortin causes overproduction of both ACTH and MSH.

Diagnosis. A 24-hour urinary cortisol and/or a 1-mg overnight dexamethasone suppression test are generally considered to be satisfactory screening tests. However, the 24-hour urinary cortisol is now felt to be least sensitive, and may miss mild or cyclical disease; it may be falsely low if there is renal impairment or an incomplete collection. Mildly elevated levels overlap with other causes of hypercortisolaemia, but values above fourfold greater than normal are indicative of Cushing's syndrome [8]. A midnight plasma cortisol level (100% specific if over 50 nmol/L) or a 2-day low-dose (0.5 mg 6-hourly) dexamethasone suppression test may resolve equivocal results. Additional tests may be required [2], as atypical presentations, other illnesses and various laboratory factors may influence interpretation of tests [6–8]. Venous sampling to measure ACTH levels is also performed in order to differentiate between ACTH-dependent and ACTH-independent Cushing's syndrome, the best available (but technically difficult) test being bilateral inferior petrosal sinus sampling (BIPSS) [7,8]. Additional investigations may include an MRI scan of pituitary to detect a microadenoma, and CT or MRI scan of chest and abdomen to detect a source of ectopic ACTH secretion.

Treatment. Trans-sphenoidal selective adenomectomy is the treatment of choice for pituitary-dependent Cushing's disease in adults, with radiotherapy as second choice; radiotherapy is more effective in children. Surgery only leads to long-term remission in about 60% of cases. Bilateral adrenalectomy is the third-choice definitive cure for pituitary Cushing's syndrome, and is the treatment of choice when the disease is caused by bilateral adrenal hypersecretion; lifelong replacement therapy with glucocorticoids and mineralocorticoids is then required. A substantial number of such patients eventually develop a pituitary macroadenoma and cutaneous hyperpigmentation (Nelson's syndrome, Fig. 62.2); this is best treated by pituitary surgery [5]. Unilateral adrenal disease (adenoma or carcinoma) is treated by unilateral adrenalectomy. Medical treatments may act at hypothalamic–pituitary level (serotonin antagonists, dopamine or GABA agonists, somatostatin analogues), at corticosteroid receptors (mifepristone) or on adrenal glands (metyrapone, aminoglutethimide, ketoconazole and others). Most of these agents have significant potential side effects.

Pseudo-Cushing's disease [9,10]
A clinical and biochemical mimic of Cushing's disease has been described in alcoholics. The biochemical parameters are not as severe as seen in true disease, and the condition can resolve on alcohol abstinence [9]. Pseudo-Cushing's syndrome may represent a state of stress-induced hypercortisolaemia secondary to multiple episodes of subacute withdrawal from ethanol [10].

References
1 Braverman IM. *Skin Signs of Systemic Disease*, 3rd edn. Philadelphia: Saunders, 1998: 438–91.
2 Newell-Price J, Bertagna X, Grossman AB, Nieman LK. Cushing's syndrome. *Lancet* 2006; **367**: 1605–17.
3 Shibli-Rahhal A, Van Beek M, Schlechte JA. Cushing's syndrome. *Clin Dermatol* 2006; **24**: 260–5.
4 Gilbertson EO, Spellman MC, Piacquadio DJ, Mulford MI. Super potent topical corticosteroid use associated with adrenal suppression: clinical considerations. *J Am Acad Dermatol* 1998; **38**: 318–21.
5 Kemink SA, Grotenhuis JA, de Vries J *et al*. Management of Nelson's syndrome: observations in fifteen patients. *Clin Endocrinol* 2001; **54**: 45–52.
6 Boscaro M, Barzon L, Fallo F, Sonino N. Cushing's syndrome. *Lancet* 2001; **357**: 783–1.
7 Arnaldi G, Angeli A, Atkinson AB *et al*. Diagnosis and complications of Cushing's syndrome: a consensus statement. *J Clin Endocrinol Metab* 2003; **88**: 5593–602.
8 Newell-Price J. Cushing's syndrome. *Clin Med* 2008; **8**: 204–8.
9 Rees LH, Besser GM, Jeffcoate WJ *et al*. Alcohol-induced pseudo-Cushing's syndrome. *Lancet* 1977; **2**: 726–8.
10 Elias AN, Meshkinpour H, Valenta LJ, Grossman MK. Pseudo-Cushing's syndrome: the role of alcohol. *J Clin Gastroenterol* 1982; **4**: 135–7.

Adrenal insufficiency [1–8]

Synonyms
- Addison's disease
- Hypocorticism
- Hypoadrenalism

This condition is due to insufficient secretion or supply of adrenocortical hormones or hormonal compounds—mainly cortisol and mineralocorticoids.

Aetiology. Most cases of adrenal insufficiency occur due to prolonged supraphysiological glucocorticoid therapy for a variety of inflammatory and other diseases; this suppresses ACTH production, so abrupt discontinuation of treatment may cause acute adrenal insufficiency.

Primary adrenal insufficiency (Addison's disease) in developed countries is most commonly due to autoimmune adrenalitis. Most such patients show circulating antibody to the cortex cells; about 40% of adults and virtually all children with Addison's disease have other autoimmune-related disorders as part of a polyglandular syndrome [2,4–8]. There are also several genetic disorders that cause primary adrenal failure [8]. Other causes of primary adrenal damage include infections (tuberculosis is the commonest cause, others include HIV, CMV, cryptococcus, histoplasmosis and viral infections), metastatic malignant disease or (rarely) haemorrhage. The latter is of some dermatological importance, as it may rarely occur due to sepsis (Waterhouse–Friderichsen syndrome); this is classically described as a consequence of meningococcaemia, but in a study of paediatric deaths due to sepsis with bilateral adrenal haemorrhage the commonest cause was *Pseudomonas* infection.

Secondary adrenal insufficiency may occur due to hypothalamic or pituitary disease, leading to insufficient secretion of ACTH; patients with pituitary hyposecretion of ACTH lack the pigmentary changes that are characteristic of primary adrenal insufficiency, and mineralocorticoid production is generally maintained.

Clinical features [1–8]. General symptoms include wasting, fatigue, orthostatic hypotension, dizziness, anorexia, abdominal pain and amenorrhoea. Self-mutilation, presenting as gouges in the skin, has been reported as a result of psychiatric symptoms [9]. However, hyperpigmentation of the skin, due to increased secretion of pituitary MSH and ACTH as a response to low adrenal corticosteroid levels, is the cardinal dermatological feature. This develops insidiously and is often not recognized as abnormal by the patient. Patterns of increased pigmentation are enumerated in Table 62.3.

Mucous membrane lesions are usually spots or patches rather than diffuse pigmentation (Fig. 62.3), and the oral pigmentation may persist after glucocorticoid replacement therapy. Scar pigmentation only occurs in scars acquired during adrenal insufficiency and is permanent—scars that precede the disorder or occur during therapy are unaffected [6]. In women, in whom the adrenal gland is the main source of androgens, there may be loss of axillary and pubic hair and improvement in acne. Features of associated autoimmune disease may be present, notably vitiligo in 15% of patients with autoimmune causation. Calcification of the pinna has been described [10], but may occur in other endocrine conditions and is more commonly the result of frostbite or injury.

Table 62.3 Patterns of addisonian pigmentation.

Light-exposed areas—face, dorsa of hands
Areas subject to friction—elbows, knees, waistline, under bra straps
Accentuation of normally high pigmentation areas—genital, perineum, axillae, areolae, umbilicus
Palmar creases
Tongue and mucous membranes (Fig. 62.3)
Scars
Hair and nails—longitudinal melanonychia.
Darkening existing pigmented lesions (such as café-au-lait patches)
Eruptive lentigines

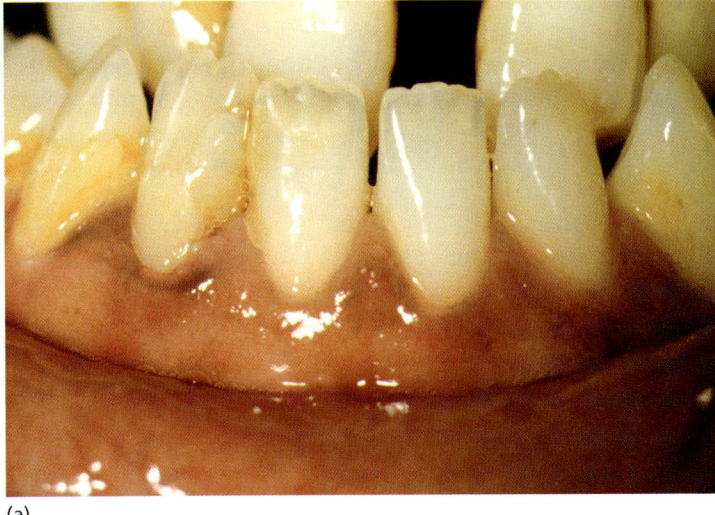

(a)

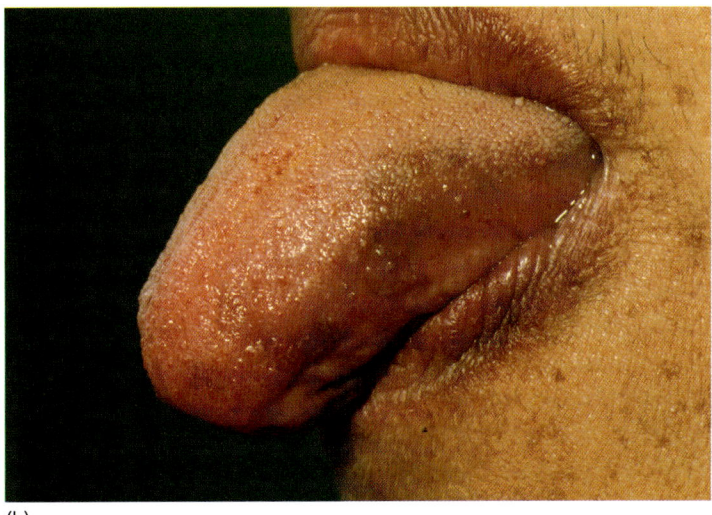

(b)

Fig. 62.3 Pigmentation of (a) the gingivae and (b) the tongue in a woman who presented with darkening skin due to Addison's disease.

Similar pigmentation may be seen in Nelson's syndrome and in tumours causing ectopic ACTH secretion; in the latter case, cortisol production is increased, so the clinical picture and electrolyte changes may be those of Cushing's syndrome.

Rarely pigmentation is absent in Addison's disease, making diagnosis difficult, and patients with 'white' Addison's disease may present in addisonian crisis. They have metabolic Addison's disease, with low cortisol, flat short Synacthen responses, and elevated circulating ACTH and MSH levels. Absence of hyperpigmentation is explained by a high degree of melanosome degradation in secondary lysosomes called 'compound melanosomes', which overwhelm the increased stimulation of the skin pigmentation [11].

Diagnosis. Anaemia, lymphocytosis, hyponatraemia, hyperkalaemia and hypoglycaemia are expected. A short Synacthen test demonstrates impaired cortisol secretion in response to corticotrophin, and ACTH and cortisol production are subnormal in response to an insulin stress test. Adrenal calcification may be present in autoimmune or tuberculous disease. Primary adrenal failure can be identified by demonstrating elevated ACTH levels, presence of adrenal autoantibodies, and by stimulation tests such as the metyrapone test or CRH test. In acute presentation, where there may be severe hypotension, weakness and clinical shock, baseline blood tests should include serum cortisol and plasma ACTH, which can be assayed later to confirm the diagnosis, but intravenous fluids and cortisol replacement should be commenced without waiting for results. Associated coeliac disease has been reported in five (12.2%) of 41 subjects, in a study that suggested that coeliac serology should be performed as part of an autoimmune screen in any patient with Addison's disease [12].

Treatment. Primary adrenal failure requires glucocorticoid and mineralocorticoid replacement [5–8]. In secondary cases related to pituitary insufficiency, usually only cortisol is required [3]. During stress, such as when undergoing major surgery and in severe systemic infections, the need for cortisol is increased. The hyperpigmentation may start to regress within days, but generally takes weeks to months to fully resolve—the process is slower in hair and nails, and pigmented scars remain pigmented [6].

References

1 Feldman SR, Jorizzo JL. Adrenal, androgen-related, and pituitary disorders. In: Callen JP, Jorizzo JL, eds. *Dermatological Signs of Internal Disease*, 3rd edn. Philadelphia: Saunders, 2003: 187–91.
2 Baker JR. Autoimmune endocrine disease. *JAMA* 1997; **278**: 1931–7.
3 Braverman IM. *Skin Signs of Systemic Disease*, 3rd edn. Philadelphia: Saunders, 1998: 438–91.
4 Feingold KR, Elias PM. Endocrine–skin interactions. *J Am Acad Dermatol* 1987; **17**: 921–40.
5 Ten S, New M, Maclaren N. Clinical review 130: Addison's disease 2001. *J Clin Endocrinol Metab* 2001; **86**: 2909–22.
6 Orth DN, Kovacs WJ. The adrenal cortex. In: Wilson JD, Foster DW, Kronenberg HM, Larsen PR, eds. *Williams Textbook of Endocrinology*, 9th edn. Philadelphia: Saunders, 1998: 517–664.
7 Betterle C, Dal Pra C, Mantero F, Zanchetta R. Autoimmune adrenal insufficiency and autoimmune polyendocrine syndromes, autoantibodies, autoantigens, and their applicability in diagnosis and disease prediction. *Endocrin Rev* 2002; **23**: 327–64.
8 Arlt W. Adrenal insufficiency. *Clin Med* 2008; **8**: 211–5.
9 Rajathurai A, Chazan BI, Jeans JE. Self mutilation as a feature of Addison's disease. *BMJ* 1983; **287**: 1027.
10 Chadwick JM, Downham TF. Auricular calcification. *Int J Dermatol* 1978; **17**: 799–801.
11 Kendereski A, Micic D, Sumarac M *et al.* White Addison's disease: what is the possible cause? *J Endocrinol Invest* 1999; **22**: 395–400.
12 O'Leary C, Walsh CH, Wieneke P *et al.* Coeliac disease and autoimmune Addison's disease: a clinical pitfall. *QJM* 2002; **95**: 79–82.

Congenital adrenal hyperplasia [1,2]

Congenital adrenal hyperplasia (CAH) is a family of autosomal recessive disorders caused by mutations that encode for enzymes involved in one of the various steps of adrenal steroid synthesis. These defects result in the absence or the decreased synthesis of cortisol from its cholesterol precursor. The anterior pituitary secretes excess adrenocorticotrophic hormone (ACTH) via feedback regulation by cortisol, which results in overstimulation of the adrenals and causes hyperplasia. Six variants are recognized, but only two will be discussed here as they are more likely to be seen by dermatologists. Symptoms due to CAH can vary from mild to severe depending on the degree of enzymatic defect.

21-hydroxylase deficiency

In the classical form of CAH, there is a severe enzymatic defect owing to mutations in the *CYP21* gene. This results in deficient 21-hydroxylase levels, and deficient cortisol synthesis, as they cannot convert 17-hydroxy progesterone to 11-deoxycortisol. Negative feedback results in increased CRF and ACTH secretion and adrenal gland hyperplasia. Rather than produce cortisol, the adrenal produces excess sex hormone precursors, and these are further converted to active androgens. Approximately 75% of patients cannot synthesize enough aldosterone as they cannot convert progesterone to deoxycorticosterone, and they may present with 'salt wasting' episodic hyponatraemic dehydration.

Classically, affected female fetuses undergo virilization of the genitalia prenatally and present with genital ambiguity at birth; however, prenatal treatment of CAH with dexamethasone to prevent ambiguity has been successfully utilized for over a decade. There are reports of neonatal acanthosis nigricans arising in classical disease [3].

Of greater relevance to dermatologists (as it is common) is the less severe, late-onset form of CAH; prenatal virilization does not occur. The milder enzyme deficiency was termed non-classical 21-hydroxylase deficiency (NC21OHD) in 1979 and was later found to be the most common autosomal recessive disorder in humans. Disease frequency of NC21OHD varies between ethnic groups with the highest ethnic-specific disease frequency in Ashkenazi Jews at 1 in 27. Similar to classical CAH, non-classical 21-hydroxylase deficiency may cause premature development of pubic hair, advanced bone age, accelerated linear growth velocity and diminished final height in both males and females. Severe cystic acne has also been attributed to non-classical CAH. Women may present with symptoms of androgen excess, including hirsutism, temporal baldness, and infertility. Menarche in females may be normal or delayed and secondary amenorrhoea is a frequent occurrence. Polycystic ovary syndrome may also be seen in these patients. In males, early beard growth, acne [4], and growth spurt may prompt the diagnosis of NC21OHD. Although many males appear to be asymptomatic, they may present with oligozoospermia or diminished fertility. Non-classical CAH may be seen in both early-onset prepubertal acne [5], persisting acne in women [6] and in acne fulminans [7]. Some authors have questioned the importance of this finding, arguing that it is one of many factors in the eventual expression of clinical acne [8].

Diagnosis. In the classic disease, there is marked elevation of 17-hydroxyprogesterone. In the non-classical disease, resting 17-hydroxyprogeserone levels may be normal, but stimulation of the adrenal with low-dose intravenous ACTH will result in elevated levels of 17-hydroxyprogesterone. Gene markers can now be identified. Low-dose glucocorticoid treatment may then be a useful adjunct to treatment.

11-hydroxylase deficiency

This comprises 5–8% of CAH cases, affecting about 1 in 100 000 births. The 11-hydroxylase enzyme is coded for by the *CYP11B1* gene. There is an inability to convert 11-deoxycortisol to cortisol. A parallel defect exists in the synthesis of 17-deoxysteroids, so that deoxycorticosterone is not converted to corticosterone, and it accumulates. As some of its metabolites have mineralocorticoid activity, sodium retention, potassium loss and hypertension develop. A non-classical variant is not associated with hypertension. It may rarely account for the development of infantile acne in boys [9], and precocious puberty. It causes virilization and ambiguous genitalia in girls.

Diagnosis. Elevated deoxycorticosterone and 11-deoxycortisol confirms the diagnosis.

References
1 New MI. An update of congenital adrenal hyperplasia. *Ann N Y Acad Sci* 2004; **1038**: 14–43.
2 Speiser PW, White PC. Congenital adrenal hyperplasia. *N Engl J Med* 2003; **349**: 776–88.
3 Kurtoğlu S, Atabek ME, Keskin M, Canöz O. Acanthosis nigricans in association with congenital adrenal hyperplasia: resolution after treatment. Case report. *Turk J Pediatr* 2005; **47**: 183–7.
4 Degitz K, Placzek M, Arnold B *et al.* Congenital adrenal hyperplasia and acne in male patients. *Br J Dermatol* 2003; **148**: 1263–6.
5 De Raeve L, De Schepper J, Smitz J. Prepubertal acne: a cutaneous marker of androgen excess? *J Am Acad Dermatol* 1995; **32**: 181–4.
6 McLaughlin B, Barrett P, Finch T, Devlin JG. Late onset adrenal hyperplasia in a group of Irish females who presented with hirsutism, irregular menses and/or cystic acne. *Clin Endocrinol (Oxf)* 1990; **32**: 57–64.
7 Placzek M, Degitz K, Schmidt H, Plewig G. Acne fulminans in late-onset congenital adrenal hyperplasia. *Lancet* 1999; **354**: 739–40.
8 Ostlere LS, Rumsby G, Holownia P *et al.* Carrier status for steroid 21-hydroxylase deficiency is only one factor in the variable phenotype of acne. *Clin Endocrinol (Oxf)* 1998; **48**: 209–15.
9 Harde V, Muller M, Sippell WG *et al.* [Acne infantum as presenting symptom of congenital adrenal hyperplasia due to 11-beta-hydroxylase deficiency]. *J Dtsch Dermatol Ges* 2006; **4**: 654–7.

Thyroid diseases

General reviews of thyroid disease and the skin can be found in the following references [1–4].

References
1 Heymann WR, ed. *Thyroid diseases with cutaneous manifestations.* New York: Springer, 2008.

2 Rosen T, Kleman GA, Jorizzo JL. Thyroid and the skin. In: Callen JP, Jorizzo JL, eds. *Dermatological Signs of Internal Disease*, 3rd edn. Philadelphia: Saunders, 2003: 175–9.
3 Leonhardt JM, Heymann WR. Thyroid disease and the skin. *Dermatol Clin* 2002; **20**: 473–81.
4 Burman KD, McKinley-Grant L. Dermatologic aspects of thyroid disease. *Clin Dermatol* 2006; **24**: 247–55.

Hyperthyroidism [1–4]

> **Synonym**
> • Thyrotoxicosis

This is a hypermetabolic state that results from excessive production or administration of thyroid hormones—thyroxine (T_4) and triiodothyronine (T_3). It is most common in women.

Aetiology. Hyperthyroidism is usually due to Graves' disease (diffuse toxic goitre, Basedow's disease), but 10–15% of cases are due to other causes, including toxic multinodular goitre, adenoma, thyroiditis, and iatrogenic or factitious ingestion of T_4, iodine and iodine-containing drugs, such as amiodarone. Secondary hyperthyroidism may occur due to production of TSH or thyrotrophin-releasing hormone (TRH) from the pituitary or from tumours at other sites. Graves' disease is an autoimmune disorder in which there is a high incidence of antithyroid antibodies and of other autoimmune diseases. Thyroid-stimulating immunoglobulins (TSIs) such as long-acting thyroid stimulator (LATS, a 7S immunoglobulin) are typically present in Graves' disease. These bind to TSH receptors, acting as thyroid gland agonists.

Clinical features. Most of the features of hyperthyroidism (Table 62.4) are not specific to the cause. Increased sympathetic nervous

Table 62.4 Cutaneous features of hyperthyroidism.

Skin
Soft, smooth, velvety
Increased skin temperature
Palmar erythema, facial flushing
Increased sweating
Pruritus
Hyperpigmentation
Pretibial myxoedema*
Vitiligo*
Cutaneous signs of goitre: Pemberton sign and Maroni sign
Others—urticaria*, palmoplantar pustulosis*

Nails
Fast nail growth
Soft nails, koilonychia
Distal onycholysis (Plummer's nails)
Thyroid acropachy*

Hair
Fine thin hair, diffuse alopecia
Alopecia areata*

* Associated with autoimmune thyroid disease; not a feature of hyperthyroidism *per se.*

system activity causes vasodilatation, leading to warm skin, flushing, palmar erythema and increased sweating (especially of palms and soles). Hair is fine, with diffuse alopecia in about a third of patients. Nails may be thin, with koilonychia and onycholysis (Plummer's nails); the onycholysis typically commences on the fourth digit of the hands [5]. Hyperpigmentation, similar to that of Addison's disease, may occur due to increased corticotrophin (ACTH) levels, and may be diffuse or localized to scars, but usually spares the buccal mucosa. Hyperpigmented eyelids have been described (Jellinek's sign).

Facial suffusion may be provoked in patients with a large substernal goitre (Pemberton sign), and erythema (sometimes with pruritus) may occur in the skin overlying a toxic goitre (Maroni sign).

Pretibial myxoedema, thyroid acropachy (both discussed separately below) and exophthalmos are features of Graves' disease (collectively known as Diamond's triad), although pretibial myxoedema can also occur in Hashimoto's thyroiditis. The combination of *e*xophthalmos, pretibial *m*yxoedema and hypertrophic *o*steoarthropathy has also been termed the EMO syndrome. In addition to these linked conditions, cutaneous features of associated autoimmune disease may be present, especially vitiligo.

The associations between thyroid diseases and other dermatoses are considered separately below.

Diagnosis [6]. In most instances, negative feedback mechanisms cause suppressed serum TSH levels before T_4 or T_3 levels are elevated. The exception is when hyperthyroidism is of secondary type, due to increased TRH or TSH levels. Thyroid antibodies are less helpful, as they are common in euthyroid individuals, and TSI levels are not usually measured. Isotope scanning can confirm the cause (diffuse goitre, adenoma, etc.).

Treatment. Beta-blockers may be used in the initial phase of therapy to suppress the increased sympathetic activity. The hyperthyroid state can be reversed by surgery, radioactive iodine or therapy with antithyroid drugs (propylthiouracil and carbimazole). However, changes that are unrelated to the hormone production tend to persist. Ophthalmopathy is not influenced by a return to euthyroidism, and the prognosis in severe cases is doubtful.

References

1 Heymann WR. Cutaneous manifestations of thyroid disease. *J Am Acad Dermatol* 1992; **26**: 885–902.
2 Rosen T, Kleman GA, Jorizzo JL. Thyroid and the skin. In: Callen JP, Jorizzo JL, eds. *Dermatological Signs of Internal Disease*, 3rd edn. Philadelphia: Saunders, 2003: 175–9.
3 Boyne M, Dobs AS, Krasner AS, Provost TT. Evaluation and treatment of endocrine disorders. In: Provost TT, Flynn JA, eds. *Cutaneous Medicine: Cutaneous Manifestations of Systemic Disease*. Hamilton, Ontario: Decker, 2001: 413–51.
4 Leonhardt JM, Heymann WR. Thyroid disease and the skin. *Dermatol Clin* 2002; **20**: 473–81.
5 Tosti A, Baran R, Dawber RPR. The nail in systemic diseases and drug-induced changes. In: Baran R, Dawber RPR, Deberker DAR, Haneke E, Tosti A, eds. *Diseases of the Nails and Their Management*. Oxford: Blackwell Science, 2001: 223–329.
6 O'Reilly DS. Thyroid function tests: time for a reassessment. *BMJ* 2000; **320**: 1332–4.

Pretibial myxoedema

Synonym
• Localized myxoedema

Localized oedematous and thickened pretibial plaque formation occurs in 1–10% of patients with hyperthyroidism. It is usually a late feature, occurring after ophthalmopathy and diagnosis of hyperthyroidism (sometimes only becoming evident after antithyroid treatment has been initiated), but it can occasionally precede other features [1,2]. Almost all patients with pretibial myxoedema have ophthalmopathy [1]. The same process often occurs on the dorsum of the hallux, and may affect other sites, including the lower abdomen, arms, shoulders, neck and pinnae [3]. Pretibial myxoedema in euthyroid individuals is very rare [4], and must be distinguished from a recently described entity called chronic obesity lymphoedematous mucinosis [5], which arises on the calves and shins of the obese.

Aetiology. It is unclear whether circulating or local factors are the main determinant of pretibial myxoedema. It was demonstrated over two decades ago that serum of pretibial myxoedema patients caused a two- to threefold increase in hyaluronic acid production by cultured fibroblasts from the pretibial area of patients and normal subjects, but had no effect on those from the shoulder or prepuce [6]. Most patients with pretibial myxoedema, whether thyrotoxic or not, have elevated levels of LATS in their serum, so this specific antibody does not seem to be causally involved [7]. A role for TSI was proposed, as fibroblasts from the pretibial and orbital regions have TSH receptors; TSIs have agonist effects on TSH receptors. Ribonucleic acid sequences encoding parts of the TSH receptor, and TSH receptor-like immunoreactivity, have been demonstrated in fibroblasts from these sites in affected patients [8]. There is, however, no obvious association between the clinical manifestations and the presence of TSH receptor autoantibodies. Recent research demonstrated that patients with pretibial myxoedema, but not control subjects, have circulating immunoglobulin A2 (IgA2) fibroblast antibodies capable of binding to a 54-kDa antigen of dermal fibroblast cell lines [9]. IGF-1 has also been suggested to have a role in the pathogenesis [10]. However, the occurrence of pretibial myxoedema in both the donor and recipient site in a patient who had excision of pretibial myxoedema, with normal skin grafted into the area, suggests that there are local factors operative which are not explained by site-specific properties of the dermal fibroblasts [11].

Pretibial myxoedema also occurs in other situations, especially in chronic stasis dermatitis [12].

Histopathology. The dermis is thickened, especially in the mid-dermis and deeper part, by extensive deposits of acid mucopolysaccharides, which may cause separation of the collagen fibres. Stellate, mucin-producing fibroblasts may be prominent.

Clinical features. In many instances, the lesions first appear on the anterolateral aspect of the lower limbs and only later extend to the back of the legs, and feet (Fig. 62.4). The nodules are pink or skin-coloured, sometimes yellow-brown and waxy, with promi-

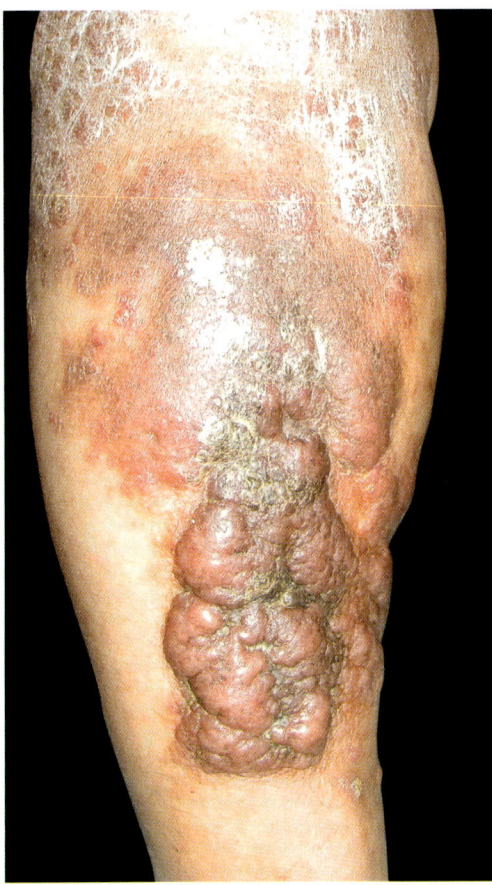

Fig. 62.4 Elephantiasic pretibial myxoedema.

nent hair follicles giving a 'peau d'orange' appearance. They may occur in old or recent scars [11,13,14]; localized pruritus or hypertrichosis over the lesions may be a feature, and localized hyperhidrosis has also been reported [15,16]. Three clinical types are recognized:

1 Sharply circumscribed, in which both nodular and tuberous lesions appear on the shins and toes
2 Diffuse, producing solid non-pitting oedema of the shins and feet
3 Elephantiasic, in which there is both oedema and nodule formation

Treatment. Topical glucocorticoids, with or without occlusive dressings, or intralesional glucocorticoid injections, may be useful [1,17]. The long-term benefits of surgery vary, although debulking procedures may be of benefit (for example, for lesions on the toes) [18]. Octreotide [19,20], plasmapheresis (perhaps acting by removal of TSIs, although not all patients respond) [21], photochemotherapy and intravenous immunoglobulin [22] have been advocated. Graduated compression bandaging can be used as an addition to all therapies provided there is no vascular contraindication; pneumatic compression [23] has also been used.

References

1 Fatourechi V. Pretibial myxedema: pathophysiology and treatment options. *Am J Clin Dermatol* 2005; **6**: 295–309.

2 Srebnik A, Ophir J, Brenner S. Euthyroid pretibial myxedema. *Int J Dermatol* 1992; **31**: 431–2.

3 Noppakun N, Bancheun K, Chandraprasert S. Unusual locations of localized myxoedema in Graves' disease. *Arch Dermatol* 1986; **122**: 85–8.

4 Buljan-Cvijanovic M, Neal JM, Zemtsov A. Euthyroid pretibial myxedema. *Endocr Pract* 1998; **4**: 375–7.

5 Tokuda Y, Kawachi S, Murata H, Saida T. Chronic obesity lymphoedematous mucinosis: three cases of pretibial mucinosis in obese patients with pitting oedema. *Br J Dermatol* 2006; **154**: 157–61.

6 Cheung HS, Nickoloff JT, Kamiel MB *et al.* Stimulation of fibroblast biosynthetic activity by serum of patients with pretibial myxedema. *J Invest Dermatol* 1978; **71**: 12–7.

7 Lynch PJ, Maize JC, Sisson JC. Pretibial myxedema and nonthyrotoxic thyroid disease. *Arch Dermatol* 1973; **107**: 107–11.

8 Stadlmayr W, Spitzweg C, Bichlmair AM, Heufelder AE. TSH receptor transcripts and TSH receptor-like immunoreactivity in orbital and pretibial fibroblasts of patients with Graves' ophthalmopathy and pretibial myxedema. *Thyroid* 1997; **7**: 3–12.

9 Arnold K, Metcalfe R, Weetman AP. Immunoglobulin A class fibroblast antibodies in patients with Graves' disease and pretibial myxedema. *J Clin Endocrinol Metab* 1995; **80**: 3430–7.

10 Kriss JP. Pathogenesis and treatment of pretibial myxedema. *Endocrinol Metab Clin North Am* 1987; **16**: 409–15.

11 Rapoport B, Alsabeh R, Aftergood D, McLachlan SM. Elephantiasis—pretibial myxedema: insight into and a hypothesis regarding the pathogenesis of the extrathyroid manifestations of Graves' disease. *Thyroid* 2000; **10**: 629–30.

12 Somach SC, Helm TN, Lawlor KB. Pretibial mucin: histologic patterns and clinical correlation. *Arch Dermatol* 1993; **129**: 1152–6.

13 Wright AL, Buxton PK, Menzies D. Pretibial myxedema localized to scar tissue. *Int J Dermatol* 1990; **29**: 54–5.

14 Tong DW, Ho KK. Pretibial myxedema presenting as a scar infiltrate. *Australas J Dermatol* 1998; **39**: 255–7.

15 Kato N, Ueno H, Matsubara M. A case report of EMO syndrome showing localised hyperhidrosis in pretibial myxedema. *J Dermatol* 1991; **18**: 598–604.

16 Gitter DG, Sato K. Localized hyperhidrosis in pretibial myxedema. *J Am Acad Dermatol* 1990; **23**: 250–4.

17 Boyne M, Dobs AS, Krasner AS, Provost TT. Evaluation and treatment of endocrine disorders. In: Provost TT, Flynn JA, eds. *Cutaneous Medicine: Cutaneous Manifestations of Systemic Disease.* Hamilton, Ontario: Decker, 2001: 413–51.

18 Derrick EK, Tanner B, Price ML. Successful surgical treatment of severe pretibial myxedema. *Br J Dermatol* 1995; **133**: 317–8.

19 Chang TC, Kao SCS, Huang KM. Octreotide and Graves' ophthalmopathy and pretibial myxedema. *BMJ* 1992; **304**: 158.

20 Shinohara M, Hamasaki Y, Katayama I. Refractory pretibial myxedema with response to intralesional insulin-like growth factor 1 antagonist (octreotide): downregulation of hyaluronic acid production by the lesional fibroblasts. *Br J Dermatol* 2000; **143**: 1083–6.

21 Dandona P, Marshall NJ, Bidey SP *et al.* Successful treatment of exophthalmos and pretibial myxedema with plasmapheresis. *BMJ* 1979; **1**: 374–6.

22 Antonelli A, Saracino A, Agostini S *et al.* [Results of high-dose intravenous immunoglobulin treatment of patients with pretibial myxedema and Basedow's disease: preliminary findings; in Italian]. *Clin Ter* 1992; **141**: 63–8.

23 Schleicher SM, Milstein HJ. Treatment of pretibial mucinosis with gradient pneumatic compression. *Arch Dermatol* 1994; **130**: 842–4.

Thyroid acropachy [1,2]

Clubbing of the fingers and toes in Graves' disease, associated with soft-tissue swelling of hands and feet and with periosteal new bone formation, is termed thyroid acropachy. It occurs in less than 1% of thyrotoxic patients, and is usually associated with exophthalmos and pretibial myxoedema (Diamond's triad), occurring in about 5% of patients with these other features. Acropachy usually appears some time after the other components of the syndrome, usually after treatment of Graves' disease. Pathologically, there is periosteal new bone formation involving the phalanges and other distal long bones, which is manifest radiologically as a feathery pattern of lamellar new bone parallel to the diaphyses, sometimes with perpendicularly orientated new bone spicules, and which can be demonstrated as osteoblastic activity using a bone scan [2]. The proximal phalanges and first or second metacarpals are most commonly affected. Most patients have minimal or no symptoms, but in those with symptoms, stiffness is the most frequent; by comparison with hypertrophic pulmonary osteoarthropathy, pain and heat are absent. Pachydermoperiostosis (Chapter 15) shows some resemblance to acropachy, but other features of the syndrome are absent.

References
1 Kinsella RA, Bach DK, Lynch PJ. Thyroid acropachy. *Med Clin North Am* 1968; **52**: 393–5.
2 Leonhardt JM, Heymann WR. Thyroid disease and the skin. *Dermatol Clin* 2002; **20**: 473–81.

Hypothyroidism [1–3]

> **Synonyms**
> • Myxoedema
> • Hypothyreosis

In hypothyroidism, there is a slowed metabolic rate involving all organs. It is caused by a decreased concentration of free thyroid hormone in the blood, or target cell resistance to thyroid hormone.

Aetiology. The most common cause is idiopathic (primary) hypothyroidism, which is an autoimmune disease, usually affecting women from the fourth decade; the prevalence rate is almost 2% in females but a tenth of this in males. A high percentage of patients with Hashimoto's thyroiditis (who may initially be thyrotoxic) eventually develop hypothyroidism, and iatrogenic hypothyroidism may occur as a late effect of radio-iodine treatment of thyrotoxicosis. Secondary hypothyroidism due to pituitary disease is uncommon, TSH production being relatively spared compared to sex hormone and ACTH production, but pituitary infarction, haemorrhage or neoplasm may lead to hypothyroidism in some cases. Severe iodine deficiency, or drugs such as lithium and bexarotene, may cause hypothyroidism. Congenital hypothyroidism (cretinism), usually due to absence of the thyroid, is rare. Tertiary hypothyroidism is due to hypothalamic failure of TRH production.

Clinical features. Cutaneous changes of hypothyroidism (Table 62.5) [1–7] were well known in the latter part of the 19th century [4]. The most prominent manifestation of hypothyroidism is related to dermal accumulation of mucopolysaccharides, in particular chondroitin sulphate and hyaluronic acid, which bind water in the tissue and lead to puffiness of the skin. Whilst characteristic, the features may be insidious in development, and some are of low specificity. For example, loss of the outer third of the eyebrow (madarosis, Hertog's sign) is common in many euthyroid elderly individuals. The yellowish skin colour is due to a combination of alterations in connective tissue of the dermis, carotenaemia and vasoconstriction (due to the slowed metabolic rate). The con-

nective tissue changes also cause loss of support of dermal vessels and, along with decreased levels of clotting factors, predispose to purpuric lesions or bruising. Asteatotic eczema [5] and keratoderma of palms and soles [6] may occur, sometimes as the presenting feature. Features of previous autoimmune thyrotoxicosis, or of associated autoimmune diseases, may also be present. The hypometabolic state and low core temperature may cause cold extremities due to reflex vasoconstriction. Loss of hair is common, occurring in about 50% of affected individuals (Fig. 62.5).

Table 62.5 Cutaneous and oral features of hypothyroidism.

Skin
Pale, cold, scaly and wrinkled skin
Xerosis, asteatotic eczema, itch
Palmoplantar keratoderma
Absence of sweating
Ivory-yellow skin colour
Puffy oedema of hands, face and eyelids
Purpura and ecchymoses
Punctate telangiectases on arms and fingertips
Delayed wound healing
Xanthomatosis (secondary to hyperlipidaemia)
Nails
Brittle and striated nails
Slow nail growth
Hair
Coarse sparse scalp hair
Loss of pubic, axillary and facial hair
Loss of lateral eyebrows (madarosis)
Oral
Large tongue
Gingival swelling (in congenital hypothyroidism)
Oral candidosis

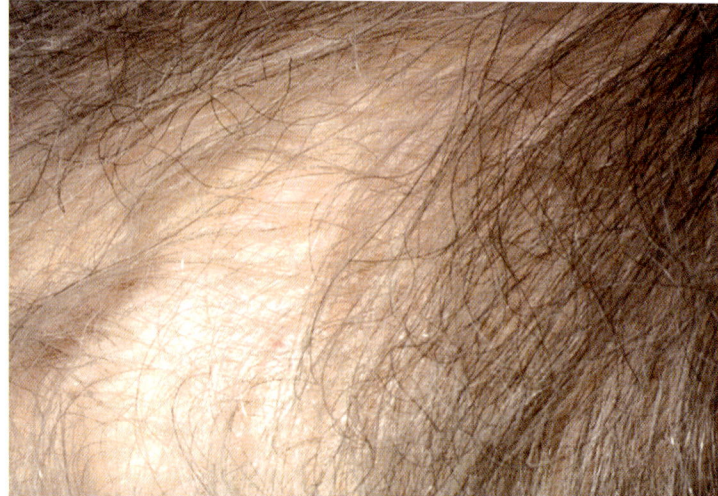

Fig. 62.5 Diffuse alopecia and coarse hair due to hypothyroidism.

In congenital hypothyroidism ('cretinism'), coarseness of features, lethargy, periorbital puffiness, swelling of hands and feet, macroglossia, cold and dry skin with livedo, umbilical hernia and poor muscle tone are pathognomic, but may not be apparent until a few months of age. Cutis marmorata occurs due to vasoconstriction. Without treatment, physical and mental development is retarded. The scalp hair is coarse, and the eyebrows may be confluent.

In juvenile hypothyroidism, abnormal physical and mental development is the principal manifestation of the disease. Some children develop hypertrichosis of the upper back and shoulders. The waxy, yellowish skin changes may be prominent, but the puffiness may be less apparent than in older individuals. Rarely, juvenile hypothyroidism is associated with sexual precocity; the penis and scrotum enlarge in males, or menstruation and galactorrhoea occur in females, but axillary and pubic hair do not develop.

Diagnosis. Protein-bound iodine, T_4 and T_3 levels are low. In primary hypothyroidism, the TSH level is elevated; in pituitary failure, it is low or undetectable. The histological changes in the dermis may be helpful in difficult cases [8]. Recognition of hypothyroidism in the elderly may be difficult. Symptoms and signs develop insidiously and may easily be taken as evidence of arteriosclerotic disease. Serum TSH is recommended as the primary investigation for screening of elderly patients.

References

1 Heymann WR. Cutaneous manifestations of thyroid disease. *J Am Acad Dermatol* 1992; **26**: 885–902.
2 Rosen T, Kleman GA, Jorizzo JL. Thyroid and the skin. In: Callen JP, Jorizzo JL, eds. *Dermatological Signs of Internal Disease*, 3rd edn. Philadelphia: Saunders, 2003: 175–9.
3 Boyne M, Dobs AS, Krasner AS, Provost TT. Evaluation and treatment of endocrine disorders. In: Provost TT, Flynn JA, eds. *Cutaneous Medicine: Cutaneous Manifestations of Systemic Disease*. Hamilton, Ontario: Decker, 2001: 413–51.
4 Doyle L. Myxoedema: some early reports and contributions by British authors, 1873–1898. *J R Soc Med* 1991; **84**: 103–6.
5 Warin RP. Eczéma craquelé as the presenting feature of myxoedema. *Br J Dermatol* 1973; **89**: 289–91.
6 Good JM, Neill SM, Rowland Payne CME. Keratoderma of myxoedema. *Clin Exp Dermatol* 1988; **13**: 339–41.
7 Crotty CP, Dicken CH. Blue fingertips associated with myxedema. *Arch Dermatol* 1981; **117**: 158–9.
8 Means MA, Dobson RL. Cytological changes in the sweat gland in hypothyroidism. *JAMA* 1963; **186**: 113–5.

Thyroid disease and other dermatoses

Thyroglossal cysts are in the differential diagnosis of other congenital cysts in the neck, such as branchial cysts or ectopic bronchial mucosa.

Thyroid cancer may give rise to cutaneous metastases, or to thyroxine-producing metastases which therefore cause features of thyrotoxicosis. Thyroid cancer is also a feature of syndromes such as Cowden's disease and multiple endocrine neoplasia (MEN) type 2, discussed elsewhere in this chapter.

Table 62.6 Some skin disorders and other diseases with prominent cutaneous manifestations that have been associated with thyroid dysfunction or with the presence of antithyroid antibodies.

Bullous diseases	*Others*
Dermatitis herpetiformis	Chronic urticaria
Bullous pemphigoid	Palmoplantar pustulosis
Pemphigus	Psoriasis
Pemphigoid gestationis	Atopic dermatitis
	Sweet's syndrome
Endocrine diseases	Sarcoidosis
Pernicious anaemia	POEMS syndrome
Diabetes mellitus	Granuloma annulare
Addison's disease	Pseudoxanthoma elasticum
Acanthosis nigricans with insulin resistance	Polyostotic fibrous dysplasia
Autoimmune polyglandular syndromes I–III	Melasma
	Melanoma
Other autoimmune conditions	Lichen sclerosus
Alopecia areata	Xanthelasma
Vitiligo	
Premature greying (canities)	
Connective tissue diseases	
Lupus erythematosus	
Scleroderma	
Dermatomyositis	
Sjögren's syndrome	

POEMS, *polyneuropathy, organomegaly, endocrinopathy, M protein and skin changes* (syndrome).

There are associations between either the presence of antithyroid antibodies, or of overt thyroid dysfunction or thyroiditis, with a number of other skin diseases and disorders with cutaneous manifestations (Table 62.6) [1–13]. Some of these associations are based on small studies, but associations with disorders such as dermatitis herpetiformis and chronic urticaria are strongly supported by the available literature. About 20% of children with alopecia areata have thyroid antibodies, although clinical thyroid dysfunction is rare [13]. It is debatable to what extent management is altered by routinely testing for thyroid antibodies or thyroid dysfunction in the absence of other clinical symptoms, although there are reported instances where chronic urticaria, for example, has resolved after treatment of associated thyrotoxicosis; it has also been recommended that T_4 treatment should be considered in euthyroid patients with chronic urticaria if they have evidence of thyroid autoimmunity [7]. An increased incidence of hypothyroidism is reported in melanoma [14,15].

References

1 Heymann WR. Cutaneous manifestations of thyroid disease. *J Am Acad Dermatol* 1992; **26**: 885–902.
2 Rosen T, Kleman GA, Jorizzo JL. Thyroid and the skin. In: Callen JP, Jorizzo JL, eds. *Dermatological Signs of Internal Disease*, 3rd edn. Philadelphia: Saunders, 2003: 175–9.
3 Agner T, Sindrup JH, Høier-Madsen M *et al.* Thyroid disease in pustulosis palmoplantaris. *Br J Dermatol* 1989; **121**: 487–91.

4 Rosén K, Mobacken H, Nilsson L. Increased prevalence of antithyroid antibodies and thyroid disease in pustulosis palmoplantaris. *J Am Acad Dermatol* 1981; **18**: 666–71.

5 Lanigan SW, Short P, Moult P. The association of chronic urticaria and thyroid autoimmunity. *Clin Exp Dermatol* 1987; **12**: 335–8.

6 Leznoff A, Sussman GL. Syndrome of idiopathic chronic urticaria and angioedema with thyroid autoimmunity: a study of 90 patients. *J Allergy Clin Immunol* 1989; **84**: 66–71.

7 Heymann WR. Chronic urticaria and angioedema associated with thyroid autoimmunity: review and therapeutic implications. *J Am Acad Dermatol* 1999; **40**: 229–32.

8 Cunningham MJ, Zone JJ. Thyroid abnormalities in dermatitis herpetiformis: prevalence of clinical thyroid disease and thyroid autoantibodies. *Ann Intern Med* 1985; **102**: 194–6.

9 Peréz B, Kraus A, Lopez G et al. Autoimmune thyroid disease in primary Sjögren's syndrome. *Am J Med* 1995; **99**: 480–4.

10 Goolamali SK, Barnes EW, Irvine WJ, Shuster S. Organ specific antibodies in patients with lichen sclerosus. *BMJ* 1974; **iv**: 78–9.

11 Harrington CI, Dunsmore IR. An investigation into the incidence of autoimmune disorders in patients with lichen sclerosus et atrophicus. *Br J Dermatol* 1981; **104**: 563–6.

12 Kalmus K, Kovatz S, Shilo L et al. Sweet's syndrome and subacute thyroiditis. *Postgrad Med J* 2000; **76**: 229–30.

13 Milgraum SS, Mitchell AJ, Bacon GE et al. Alopecia areata, endocrine function, and autoantibodies in patients 16 years of age or younger. *J Am Acad Dermatol* 1987; **17**: 57–61.

14 Ellerhorst JA, Cooksley CD, Broemeling L et al. High prevalence of hypothyroidism among patients with cutaneous melanoma. *Oncol Rep* 2003; **10**: 1317–20.

15 Shah M, Orengo IF, Rosen T High prevalence of hypothyroidism in male patients with cutaneous melanoma. *Dermatol Online J* 2006; **28**: 12:1.

Parathyroid disease

Skin changes are not a particular feature of hyperparathyroidism, although subcutaneous calcification may occur (especially in hyperparathyroidism secondary to renal failure; see below) [1–4].

Itch is thought to be related to hyperparathyroidism [5], although this is poorly documented [6] and some of the documentation is inferred (from resolution in some instances of renal itch after parathyroidectomy, or paraneoplastic itch after resection of parathormone (PTH)-producing bronchial tumours). Hyperparathyroidism has also been linked to cutaneous T-cell lymphoma [7].

Hypoparathyroidism may cause skin changes somewhat similar to those of hypothyroidism—the skin may be dry, keratotic and puffy, with sparse, coarse hair. Nails are brittle and ridged, with cracking at the free margin, or crumbling of the distal nail plate. Chloasma or pellagra-like pigmentary disturbance is less common [3,8].

There are numerous reports of pustular psoriasis of the von Zumbusch type being provoked by hypocalcaemia, with resolution of the pustulation and erythroderma with resolution of the skin eruption on restoring normocalcaemia [9,10] and one of the authors has personal experience of a patient presenting with a severe pustular exacerbation of chronic plaque psoriasis associated with hypocalcaemic tetany due to primary hypoparathyroidism.

Calciphylaxis of the skin, resulting in localized necrosis due to vascular calcific occlusion, is usually seen in renal failure, but there are occasional reports of it occurring in the setting of normal renal function and hyperparathyroidism [11].

Chronic mucocutaneous candidiasis, especially of the nails and oral mucosa, may occur in conjunction with hypoparathyroidism when this occurs as part of the polyglandular autoimmune syndrome (see below) or in association with immunological defects such as Di George's syndrome (in which there is parathyroid gland agenesis) [1], but it is not a feature of post-thyroidectomy iatrogenic hypoparathyroidism.

Subcutaneous ossification is a feature of Albright's hereditary osteodystrophy, which encompasses both pseudohypoparathyroidism type Ia and pseudopseudohypoparathyroidism [1,12–14]. The somatic features include obesity, short stature and short metacarpals—Albright's sign is dimpling over the knuckle of the typically affected fourth metacarpal. The dominant condition occurs due to a heterozygous functional defect of the α-subunit of the stimulatory G protein (G_s α protein) of adenylate cyclase, with which PTH interacts at the cell surface. This is encoded by the *GNAS1* gene on chromosome 20q13.3, but there are tissue-specific differences in expression of G_s α and other *GNAS1* transcripts that are different for the maternal and paternal alleles [13]. It is now known that pseudopseudohypoparathyroidism is the same disorder as pseudohypoparathyroidism type Ia, but with the genetic defect inherited from the father; patients have the somatic features of pseudohypoparathyroidism, but with normal hormone responses [14].

References

1 Marx SJ. Hyperparathyroid and hypoparathyroid disorders. *N Engl J Med* 2000; **343**: 1863–75.

2 Walsh JS, Fairley JA. Calcifying disorders of the skin. *J Am Acad Dermatol* 1995; **33**: 693–706.

3 Braverman IM. *Skin Signs of Systemic Disease*, 3rd edn. Philadelphia: Saunders, 1998: 438–91.

4 Khafif RA, Delima C, Silverberg A et al. Acute hyperparathyroidism with systemic calcinosis. *Arch Intern Med* 1989; **149**: 681–4.

5 Gartner R. Itching in hyperparathyroidism. *Med Wochenschr* 2001; **126**: 190.

6 Bernhard JD. Endocrine and metabolic itches. In: Bernhard JD. *Itch: Mechanisms and Management of Pruritus*. New York: McGraw-Hill, 1994: 251–60.

7 Owen CM, Blewitt RW, Harrison PV, Yates VM. Two cases of primary hyperparathyroidism associated with primary cutaneous lymphoma. *Br J Dermatol* 2000; **142**: 120–3.

8 Kawamura A, Kinoshita MT, Suzuki H. Generalized pustular psoriasis with hypoparathyroidism. *Eur J Dermatol* 1999; **9**: 574–6.

9 Tercedor J, Rodenas JM, Munoz M et al. Generalized pustular psoriasis and idiopathic hypoparathyroidism. *Arch Dermatol* 1991; **127**: 1418–9.

10 Hirano K, Ishibashi A, Yoshino Y. Cutaneous manifestations in idiopathic hypoparathyroidism. *Arch Dermatol* 1974; **109**: 242–4.

11 Mirza I, Chaubay D, Gunderia H et al. An unusual presentation of calciphylaxis due to primary hyperparathyroidism. *Arch Pathol Lab Med* 2001; **125**: 1351–3.

12 Trueb RM, Panizzon RG, Burg G. Cutaneous ossification in Albright's hereditary osteodystrophy. *Dermatology* 1993; **186**: 205–9.

13 Bastepe M, Juppner H. Pseudohypoparathyroidism: new insights into an old disease. *Endocrinol Metab Clin North Am* 2000; **29**: 569–89.

14 Simon A, Koppeschaar HP, Roijers JF et al. Pseudohypoparathyroidism type Ia—Albright hereditary osteodystrophy: a model for research on G protein-coupled receptors and genomic imprinting. *Neth J Med* 2000; **56**: 100–9.

Multiple endocrinopathy syndromes

It is common that autoimmune conditions may occur simultaneously—due to, for example, human leukocyte antigen (HLA) linkage. Some of these produce an overlap between endocrine disease and:

- Other autoimmune conditions, e.g. polyglandular autoimmune syndrome (see below), various combinations of Sjögren's syndrome and sarcoidosis with endocrine autoimmune conditions [1,2]
- Infections, such as in autoimmune polyglandular syndrome type I (see below)
- Ectodermal changes, e.g. alopecia areata (commonly), ANOTHER syndrome (*a*lopecia, *n*ail dystrophy, *o*phthalmic complications, *t*hyroid dysfunction, *h*ypohidrosis, *e*phelides and enteropathy, *r*espiratory tract infections) [3]
- Gastrointestinal disease, e.g. the triple A syndrome (Allgrove's syndrome) of achalasia, addisonianism and alacrima (MIM #231550); IPEX syndrome (*i*mmune dysregulation, *p*olyendocrinopathy, *e*nteropathy, *X*-linked syndrome) in which diarrhoea is a significant feature with an icthyosiform dermatitis, and also diabetes, throiditis and haemolytic anaemia [4]
- Pigmentary change, e.g. vitiligo (commonly), Carney complex (see cardiac disease, below), POEMS syndrome (see cardiac disease, below)
- Alopecia areata—associated with thyroid disease and other autoimmune conditions
- Bone disease, e.g. McCune–Albright syndrome (MIM #174800); G protein mutations cause dysregulation of cyclic adenosine monophosphate (cAMP), leading to growth and hyperfunction of many organs—features include hypophosphataemic osteodystrophy, hyperparathyroidism, hyperthyroidism, large irregularly shaped café-au-lait macules, Cushing's syndrome, acromegaly and hyperprolactinaemia
- Cerebral disease, e.g. triple H syndrome—*h*ippocampus (anterograde memory loss), *h*air follicle (alopecia areata), *h*ypothalamic–pituitary–adrenal axis (isolated ACTH deficiency) [5].

Autoimmune polyendocrine syndromes [6–13]

Three types of autoimmune polyendocrine (polyglandular) syndrome (APS) are described—types 1 to 3—although there may also be other, incomplete forms [13]. The pathogenesis of these disorders is discussed in detail in [8,13]. The most important example dermatologically is APS type 1 (MIM 240300), which is usually due to the R257X mutation of the *AIRE* gene on chromosome 21q22.3 [11] and is associated with about 13% of cases of Addison's syndrome [13]. It is also termed mucocutaneous candidiasis–endocrinopathy syndrome, multiple endocrinopathy syndrome, *a*utoimmune *p*olyendocrinopathy–*c*andidiasis–*e*ctodermal *d*ystrophy (APECED) syndrome, or Whitaker's syndrome. Table 62.7 outlines the diagnostic criteria; the dermatological features include mucocutaneous candidiasis, nail dystrophy, alopecia areata, vitiligo and cutaneous features of Addison's disease [9,11,13].

An interesting feature of vitiligo in this condition, which does not occur in isolated vitiligo or in other autoimmune combinations, is the presence of complement-fixing melanocyte autoantibodies [11]. Most patients also have adrenal cortex autoantibodies, and those with gonadal failure have steroid-producing cell antibodies. Nail dystrophy and tooth enamel defects comprise the ectodermal dystrophy component. Epidermolysis bullosa acquisita has also been reported in type 1 syndrome [12].

Patients with APS types 2 and type 3 more commonly have diabetes, but less commonly have alopecia or vitiligo, and do not

Table 62.7 Type 1 autoimmune polyglandular syndrome diagnostic criteria (defined by the presence of two or more of the three major features).

Major features
Chronic mucocutaneous candidiasis (usually by age 5 years, present in about 80%)
Chronic hypoparathyroidism (usually by age 10 years, present in about 90%)
Autoimmune adrenal insufficiency (usually by age 15 years, present in about 70%, frequently autoantibody positive)

Other features
Hypergonadotrophic hypogonadism (45%)
Diabetes mellitus
Thyroid antibodies or overt thyroid dysfunction
Alopecia areata (25%)
Vitiligo (10%)

have chronic mucocutaneous candidiasis. Addison's disease is present in all patients with APS type 2, which has been further divided by some authors according to the specific endocrinopathies present; thus, Addison's disease with autoimmune thyroid disease is termed Schmidt's syndrome, Addison's disease with immune-mediated diabetes (with or without thyroid disease) is Carpenter's syndrome. APS type 3 is defined as co-occurrence of autoimmune thyroid disease with two other autoimmune disorders in the absence of Addison's disease [14]. APS type 2 is due to defects in the *HLA* region on 6p21 or in *CTLA4* on 2q33. It should be noted that not all of the autoimmune components are actually endocrine in type; vitiligo is not uncommon, and Schmidt's multiple endocrine insufficiency syndrome has been reported with alopecia areata and the stiff man syndrome (due to autoantibodies to glutamic acid decarboxylase).

The MEN syndromes are discussed later in this chapter.

References

1 Seinfeld ED, Sharma OP. TASS syndrome: unusual association of thyroiditis, Addison's syndrome, Sjögren's syndrome and sarcoidosis. *J R Soc Med* 1983; **76**: 883–5.

2 Cox NH, McCrea J. The association of Sjögren's syndrome, sarcoidosis, ulcerative colitis and other autoimmune disorders. *Br J Dermatol* 1996; **134**: 1138–40.

3 Pike MG, Baraitser M, Dinwiddie R *et al*. A distinctive type of hypohidrotic ectodermal dysplasia featuring hypothyroidism. *J Pediatr* 1986; **108**: 109–11.

4 Baud O, Goulet O, Canioni D *et al*. Treatment of the Immune dysregulation, Polyendocrinopathy, Enteropathy, X-linked syndrome (IPEX) by allogeneic bone marrow transplantation. *N Engl J Med* 2001; **344**: 1758–62.

5 Farooqi IS, Jones MK, Evans M *et al*. Triple H syndrome: a novel autoimmune endocrinopathy characterised by dysfunction of the hippocampus, hair follicle, and hypothalamic–pituitary–adrenal axis. *J Clin Endocrinol Metab* 2000; **85**: 2644–8.

6 Feingold KR, Elias PM. Endocrine–skin interactions. *J Am Acad Dermatol* 1988; **19**: 1–240.

7 Baker JR. Autoimmune endocrine diseases. *JAMA* 1997; **278**: 1931–7.

8 Eisenbarth GS, Gottlieb PA. Autoimmune polyendocrine syndromes. *N Engl J Med* 2004; **350**: 2068–79.

9 Ahonen P, Myllarniemi S, Sipila I *et al*. Clinical variation of autoimmune polyendocrinopathy-candidiasis-ectodermal dystrophy (APECED) in a series of 68 patients. *N Engl J Med* 1990; **332**: 1829–36.

10 Betterle C, Dalpra C, Greggio N *et al*. Clinical review 93: autoimmune polyglandular syndrome type 1. *J Clin Endocrinol Metab* 1998; **83**: 1049–55.

11 Collins SM, Dominguez M, Ilmarinen T *et al*. Dermatological manifestations of autoimmune polyendocrinopathy-candidiasis-ectodermal dystrophy syndrome. *Br J Dermatol* 2006; **154**: 1088–93.

12 Burke WA, Briggaman RA, Gammon WR. Epidermolysis bullosa acquisita in a patient with multiple endocrinopathies syndrome. *Arch Dermatol* 1986; **122**: 187–9.

13 Betterle C, Dal Pra C, Mantero F, Zanchetta R. Autoimmune adrenal insufficiency and autoimmune polyendocrine syndromes: autoantibodies, autoantigens, and their applicability in diagnosis and disease prediction. *Endocrin Rev* 2002; **23**: 327–64.

14 Ten S, New M, Maclaren N. Clinical review 130: Addison's disease 2001. *J Clin Endocrinol Metab* 2001; **86**: 2909–22.

Cutaneous markers of internal malignancy [1–11]

Introduction and classification

The different types of skin change associated with internal malignancy, and the links between systemic neoplasia and consequent or associated skin conditions, are so numerous that to report all documented associations here is impracticable. We suggest some broad categories for consideration; this includes disorders in those with a known internal malignancy but the emphasis is on skin manifestations that provide clues to internal malignancy or that indicate a need for malignancy screening. The main categories are:

1 Multisystem and haemopoietic tumours that involve the skin
2 Direct tumour spread from adjacent or deeper tissues
3 Cutaneous metastasis from internal tumours (indirect tumour spread to the skin)
4 Genetically determined syndromes with cutaneous manifestations, where there is a recognized predisposition to internal malignancy (also termed 'genodermatoses with malignant potential')
5 Paraneoplastic disorders—cutaneous reaction patterns that have an association with neoplasia involving various internal organ systems
6 Indirect cutaneous markers of internal malignancy (markers of exposure to carcinogens, cancers of the skin related to immuno-suppression, infections, etc., in which those affected have a higher risk of internal malignancy).

Investigation for internal malignancy

Potential cutaneous markers of internal malignancy vary in their reliability for predicting underlying neoplasia. Additionally, other factors such as malaise, weight loss, non-specific or non-cutaneous focal symptoms may all play a part in deciding which patients to investigate and how extensively. There may be non-specific cutaneous markers of disease (such as purpura, stigmata of liver disease, etc.) that influence a decision; these are discussed elsewhere in this chapter. A clinical decision on the extent of investigation and screening, if any, must therefore be based on the strength of the association and on the clinical history and examination in the individual patient. It is helpful to consider various skin eruptions in terms of the likelihood of the cutaneous features suggesting the presence of internal malignancy—this may be obvious in some situations (e.g. internal tumours metastatic to the skin), but the strength of associations between some paraneoplastic dermatoses and internal malignancy varies hugely (as discussed later).

In some situations, simple investigations, such as chest radiography, full blood count, liver enzymes, non-specific markers of disease (such as erythrocyte sedimentation rate) or of possible tumour burden (such as lactate dehydrogenase), urine analysis and stool examination for occult blood, may be sufficient. Rapid changes in investigative techniques, such as the speed and accuracy of magnetic resonance imaging (MRI), emerging techniques such as positron emission tomography (PET scan), use of serological tumour markers (such as CA-125 for ovarian tumours, prostate-specific antigen, etc.) and, in inherited cancer susceptibility, the ability to identify individuals who have genes linked with malignant disease, are all altering the ease and extent of investigation that may be appropriate. Thus advice that was once very appropriate (such as the conclusion by many authors that investigation in dermatomyositis should be guided by careful clinical history and examination, and by pursuit of any abnormality of simple tests) must be viewed in the context not only of the tests that were readily available at the time, but also in the light of new tests that may help to identify subgroups with a higher than average risk of a malignancy being found.

Cutaneous adverse reactions to drugs used to treat malignancy are a related topic that will not be considered here, but is covered in Chapter 75 and in [11].

References

1 Braverman IM. *Skin Signs of Systemic Disease*, 3rd edn. Philadelphia: Saunders, 1998.
2 Callen JP, Jorizzo JL, eds. *Dermatological Signs of Internal Disease*, 3rd edn. Philadelphia: Saunders, 2003.
3 Waldenstrom JG. *Paraneoplasia: Biological Signals in the Diagnosis of Cancer*. New York: Wiley, 1978.
4 Poole S, Fenske NA. Cutaneous markers of internal malignancy, 1: malignant involvement of the skin and the genodermatoses. *J Am Acad Dermatol* 1993; **28**: 1–13.
5 Poole S, Fenske NA. Cutaneous markers of internal malignancy, 2: paraneoplastic dermatoses and environmental carcinogens. *J Am Acad Dermatol* 1993; **28**: 147–64.
6 Lookingbill DP, Spangler N, Helm KF. Cutaneous metastases in patients with metastatic carcinoma: a retrospective study of 4020 patients. *J Am Acad Dermatol* 1993; **29**: 228–36.
7 Chung VQ, Moschella SL, Zembowicz A, Liu V. Clinical and pathologic findings of paraneoplastic dermatoses. *J Am Acad Dermatol* 2006; **54**: 745–62.
8 Provost TT, Laman SD, Bell WR. Paraneoplastic dermatoses. In: Provost TT, Flynn JA, eds. *Cutaneous Medicine: Cutaneous Manifestations of Systemic Disease*. Hamilton, Ontario: Decker, 2001: 367–88.
9 Boyce S, Harper J. Paraneoplastic dermatoses. *Dermatol Clin* 2002; **20**: 523–32.
10 Cohen PR, Kurzrock R, eds. Genodermatoses with malignant potential. *Dermatol Clinics* 1995; **13**: 1–243.
11 Thomas VD, Thomas CR, eds. Internal malignancy and the skin: paraneoplastic and cancer treatment-related cutaneous disorders. *Dermatol Clinics* 2008; **26**: 1–182.

Multisystem and haemopoietic tumours that involve the skin [1–3]

This category includes a number of tumours, discussed in other chapters, in which the skin is involved as part of a multisystem neoplasm. The importance for dermatologists is that the diagnosis may present due to skin lesions, or that the skin may be the most accessible site for histological diagnosis.

The type of skin involvement that may occur in such disorders ranges from very non-specific (such as purpura, which may reflect

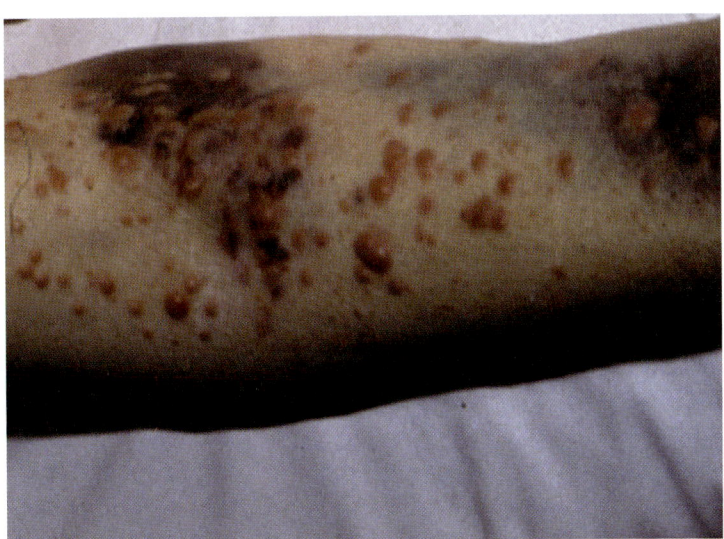

Fig. 62.6 Leukaemia cutis (acute myelogenous leukaemia) and purpura.

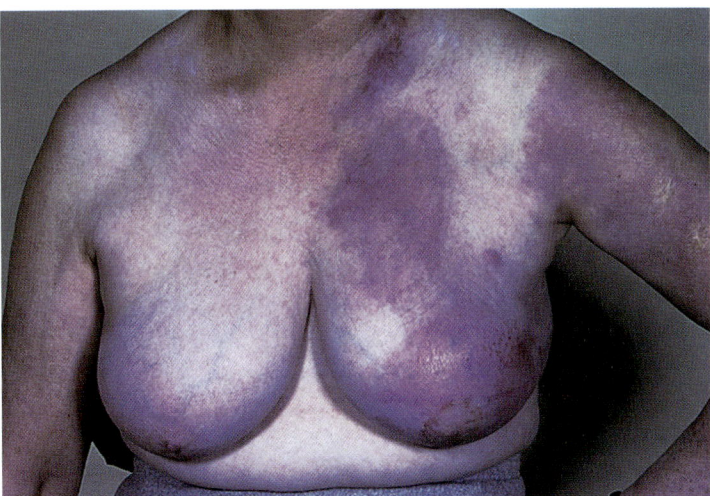

Fig. 62.7 Carcinoma erysipeloides. (Courtesy of Dr R. Emmerson, Royal Berkshire Hospital, Reading, UK.)

abnormal platelet numbers or function or both, or susceptibility to unusual infections in disorders where immunosurveillance is compromised), through to highly specific features such as cutaneous deposits of the malignancy (for example, lesions of leukaemia cutis). In some instances, there may be features that suggest a particular diagnosis (such as oral leukaemic deposits, which are most typically seen in myelomonocytic leukaemia), or other cutaneous disease associations (such as the rare association of neurofibromatosis type 1 with juvenile xanthogranuloma and juvenile myelomonocytic leukaemia).

This type of involvement of the skin as part of a multisystem tumour is somewhat different from metastases from solid tumours in both mechanism and in the fact that lesions are often widespread. Most relevant conditions are discussed in other chapters, but, as examples, skin involvement is an important component of many haemopoietic tumours, particularly lymphomas (Chapter 57); similarly, Langerhans' cell histiocytosis (Chapter 55) and Kaposi's sarcoma (Chapter 56) characteristically cause skin lesions.

Specific cutaneous infiltrations of the skin may occur with myeloproliferative disorders; this is commonly recognized with lymphoma, but can occur with leukaemia (Fig. 62.6) [4]. Some skin infiltrates that are characteristic of specific disorders are discussed elsewhere in this section.

References

1 Provost TT, Flynn JA, eds. *Cutaneous Medicine: Cutaneous Manifestations of Systemic Disease*. Hamilton, Ontario: Decker, 2001.
2 Lebwohl MG. *The Skin and Systemic Disease. A Color Atlas and Text*, 2nd edn. London: Churchill Livingstone, 2004: 185–214.
3 Callen JP, Jorizzo JL, eds. *Dermatological Signs of Internal Disease*, 3rd edn. Philadelphia: Saunders, 2003.
4 Vardy DA, Sion N, Grunswald MH. Specific cutaneous infiltrates in chronic myelogenous leukaemia. *Cutis* 1989; **44**: 53–5.

Direct tumour spread from adjacent and deeper tissues [1,2]

Other than primary skin neoplasms, the skin may be involved by tumour as a result of cutaneous metastases from an internal tumour (see below), or by direct involvement in continuity with an adjacent organ. This may be the presenting feature of the underlying malignancy, as occurs in Paget's disease [2] (Chapter 52 and below), but more commonly occurs when an underlying tumour has been neglected (e.g. some breast carcinomas) or is refractory to treatment. It is a particular feature of malignant lymph node metastases (e.g. breast carcinoma, melanoma), and occasionally arises after diagnostic or therapeutic interventions such as needle aspiration of a tumour, pleural biopsy, drainage of malignant ascites or placement of other drains in the vicinity of a tumour. 'Tumour spillage', direct contamination of wounds with tumour cells during a laparoscopy or surgical procedure, was once a problem in nearly 20% of cases but is now uncommon; laparoscopic port site metastasis rates and laparotomy wound metastasis rates due to direct tumour inoculation are both in the order of 0.8% [3]. However, skin involvement may still occur from an abdominal viscus neoplasm or peripheral lung tumour that directly invades the skin.

Local and in-transit metastases from primary epidermal tumours are discussed in relevant chapters; melanoma is the most important tumour to behave in this fashion.

Direct invasion of the skin from a deeper tumour usually causes tumid ulceration or inflammation, but may present in less obvious ways; dermal infiltration causing sclerosis (carcinoma en cuirasse), vascular changes (carcinoma telangiectoides), a peau d'orange appearance, and more rarely a carcinoma erysipeloides (inflammatory metastatic carcinoma) pattern (Fig. 62.7) may all occur, especially with carcinoma of the breast. Although these patterns may occur as distant metastases, they most commonly occur in the skin in the vicinity of the primary tumour, all being most commonly associated with breast cancer, and are therefore usefully considered as a rather different pattern to those tumours that metastasize to distant sites.

All of these patterns may be difficult to diagnose unless there is clinical suspicion. *Carcinoma en cuirasse* may have an early inflammatory stage, and may include some nodularity, but at a later stage is very sclerodermoid in appearance. A particular diagnostic problem arises when a breast cancer has been treated with radiotherapy, as this may cause post-irradiation morphoea; the latter is relatively well documented but the early inflammatory phase of post-irradiation morphoea that occurs in some patients is much less well recognized and may be very alarming clinically. Carcinoma en cuirasse may also occur with lung, gastrointestinal, renal and other malignancies [2]. *Carcinoma erysipeloides* resembles erysipelas but without the pyrexia or toxaemia; tumour cells lie within dilated lymphatic vessels in the skin. This pattern is again most commonly seen in breast carcinoma, but occurs due to melanoma and pelvic cancers (when it affects the lower abdomen or thigh); it can also occur due to carcinomas of the oral cavity or associated glands, as well as with upper abdominal cancers (stomach, pancreas) or lung cancer. *Telangiectatic metastatic carcinoma* is typically associated with breast cancer and may be difficult to diagnose as tumour cells may be quite scanty and telangiectasia quite subtle, although it may be more florid and resemble angiosarcoma. Less common patterns of direct tumour invasion include breast carcinoma presenting as an inframammary intertrigo-like pattern, and lymphatic obstruction by pelvic tumours or lymphadenopathy which may be accompanied by extensive tumour cells within the lymphatics, presenting as skin nodules. Oral tumours, usually squamous cell carcinoma, may extend to directly involve the skin of the face.

Paget's disease

Paget's disease occurs in mammary and extramammary forms. Paget's disease of the breast occurs due to an underlying ductal tumour; extramammary Paget's disease may occur without an underlying tumour, or distant to a tumour, and so does not have the close link with direct tumour spread of the mammary pattern but is conveniently discussed here.

Paget's disease of the breast [2,4–6]

This condition presents with scaling and erythema, sometimes with oozing and crusting, on or around the nipple (Fig. 62.8). It is generally viewed as a direct epidermal extension of an underlying ductal adenocarcinoma, and is important as the underlying tumour

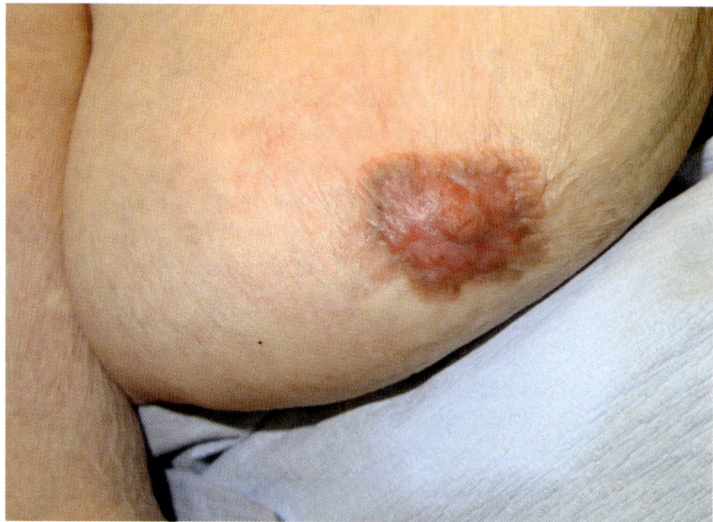

Fig. 62.8 Paget's disease of the breast causing destruction of the right nipple.

is usually small and superficial so early recognition may allow curative intervention. However, of the 30–50% with a palpable underlying lesion, half will have axillary lymph node involvement. The reason for the epidermotropic spread of tumour cells is uncertain but may involve a keratinocyte-derived chemoattractant for Paget cells, termed heregulin-α [5]. The main pathogenetic hypothesis for those cases that do not have an underlying carcinoma is derivation from Toker cells within the epidermis of the nipple and areola [2,5].

Clinically, eczemas, psoriasis, hyperkeratosis of the nipple and erosive adenomatosis are in the differential diagnosis of mammary Paget's disease. Histologically, there may be differential diagnosis problems from other disorders with Pagetoid spread, such as some melanomas or Bowen's disease, and also from a benign proliferation of Toker cells termed clear cell papulosis. Useful histopathological markers for mammary Paget's disease include epithelial membrane antigen (EMA), carcinoembryonic antigen (CEA), cytokeratins CK7 and CK8/18, as well as mucins such as MUC1 [5,6]. CD23, a lymphoid and apocrine/eccrine marker, is uniformly positive in mammary or extramammary Paget's disease [7].

Extramammary Paget's disease [2,5–10]

This rarer form of Paget's disease occurs in apocrine gland-bearing areas such as anogenital and axillary sites. About 60% of cases are vulval, 20% perianal and 15% penile or scrotal; there is thus a female predominance (although some populations, such as the Japanese [10], have a male predominance). Its histogenesis is less certain, and only about 25% of patients appear to have an underlying cancer. When the vulva is affected, cancers comprise about 10% in whom the cancer is locally arising (from apocrine sweat glands or Bartholin's glands) and about 15% in whom the carcinoma arises in the vagina, cervix, bladder, ovary, colon or rectum, or occasionally from more distant sites such as breast or gallbladder. Perianal Paget's disease is associated with an adnexal tumour in about 10% and a distant tumour in about 25% (rectum, stomach, ureter, breast); male genital Paget's disease is associated with a carcinoma of prostate, bladder, ureter, kidney or testes in about 10% of cases. In other cases, extramammary Paget's disease arises locally in the epidermis.

Most patients are over 60 years of age; clinical features include itch, burning sensation, oedema, bleeding and reddish-brown (or sometimes hypopigmented) plaques which may have a slightly more prominent margin. The margin may be obscured by secondary infection, and may be difficult to define in vaginal mucosa. Genital Paget's disease is often mistaken for an eczematous process, psoriasis or tinea. Histological and immunohistochemical features are similar to those of mammary Paget's disease; the antigen RCAS1 is particularly sensitive [5]. The prognosis is determined by the underlying tumour, if present, and the ability to adequately excise it; for those with a local epidermal origin, the depth of invasion and lymphatic spread dictate the prognosis, serum CEA being a useful indicator of survival [10].

References

1 Poole S, Fenske NA. Cutaneous markers of internal malignancy, 1: malignant involvement of the skin and the genodermatoses. *J Am Acad Dermatol* 1993; **28**: 1–13.

2 Rolz-Cruz G, Kim CC. Tumor invasion of the skin. *Dermatol Clin* 2008; **26**: 89–102.

3 Shoup M, Brennan MF, Karpeh MS *et al*. Port site metastasis after diagnostic laparoscopy for upper gastrointestinal tract malignancies: an uncommon entity. *Ann Surg Oncol* 2002; **9**: 632–6.

4 Paget J. On disease of mammary areola preceding cancer of mammary gland. *St Bartholomew's Hosp Rep* 1874; **10**: 87–9.

5 Kanitakis J. Mammary and extramammary Paget's disease. *J Eur Acad Dermato-Venereol* 2007; **21**: 581–90.

6 Liegl B, Liebl S, Gogg-Kamerer M *et al*. Mammary and extramammary Paget's disease: an immunohistochemical study of 83 cases. *Histopathology* 2007; **50**: 439–47.

7 Carvalho J, Fullen D, Lowe L *et al*. The expression of CD23 in cutaneous non-lymphoid neoplasms. *J Cutan Pathol* 2007; **34**: 693–8.

8 Neumann R. Extramammärer Morbus Paget assoziiert mit einem Magen-Karzinom. *Hautarzt* 1986; **37**: 568–70.

9 Chandra JJ. Extramammary Paget's disease: prognosis and relationship to internal malignancy. *J Am Acad Dermatol* 1985; **13**: 1009–14.

10 Hatta N, Yamada M, Hirano T *et al*. Extramammary Paget's disease: treatment, prognostic factors and outcome in 76 patients. *Br J Dermatol* 2008; **158**: 313–8.

Cutaneous metastasis from tumours affecting other organs [1–12]

Frequency of skin metastases

The skin is a relatively uncommon site for distant metastatic deposits, compared with organs such as liver, lung and bone. However, autopsy studies suggest a higher frequency of skin metastasis than may be apparent from clinical studies; in some studies up to 9% of patients with internal cancer have had skin metastases, a large analysis suggesting that 5% is usual [4], and in about 0.5–1% a metastasis is the presenting feature of internal cancer [1,2]. Of patients with metastatic cancer, 10% have cutaneous metastases [8]. Studies vary in cited frequency of skin metastases in part because some include metastasis from cutaneous melanoma whilst others exclude this and only refer to internally originating tumours; additionally, it can sometimes be difficult to know whether skin involvement is in contiguity or close proximity with a primary tumour of a different organ (direct invasion) or not (metastasis [12]). The most common sources of cutaneous metastases are (in generally accepted order of frequency): breast, (melanoma), lung, colon, stomach, upper aerodigestive tract, uterus and kidney; the most common skin metastases from a previously unknown primary tumour originate from the kidney, lung, thyroid or ovary [2,9,11].

Appearance of skin metastases

Cutaneous metastases generally present as solitary or multiple painless, firm to hard nodules, which may be skin-coloured, blue-brown or reddish-purple (Fig. 62.9); presentation with a solitary nodule is more common than with multiple nodules [9]. Ulceration of nodules may occur but is not usually a feature at initial presentation. They may also present as palpable subcutaneous nodules, often multiple (from a few to several hundred) in such instances. Other patterns include a morphoea-like sclerotic pattern, plaque morphology, scar infiltration, erysipelas-like pattern, infiltrated areas of alopecia (alopecia neoplastica), zosteriform metastases, embolic metastasis to digits (Fig. 62.10), and others.

The commonest, nodular, pattern presents with a solitary nodule about twice as frequently as with multiple nodules, although huge

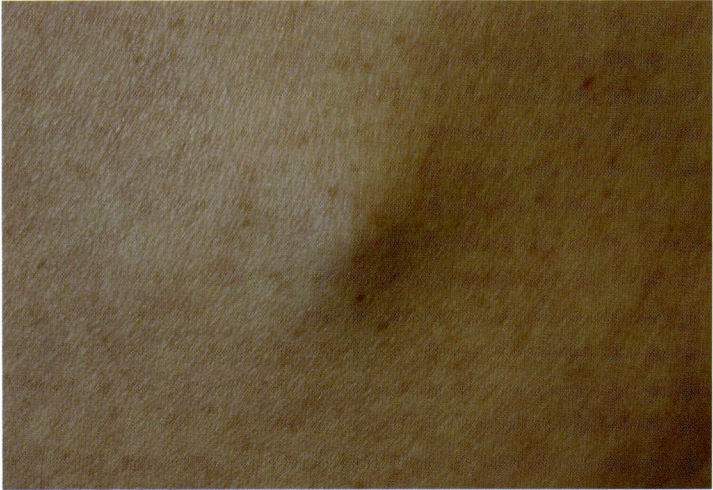

Fig. 62.9 Subcutaneous metastasis from lung carcinoma; such metastases are typically multiple and many more firm nodules can usually be palpated if the patient is carefully examined.

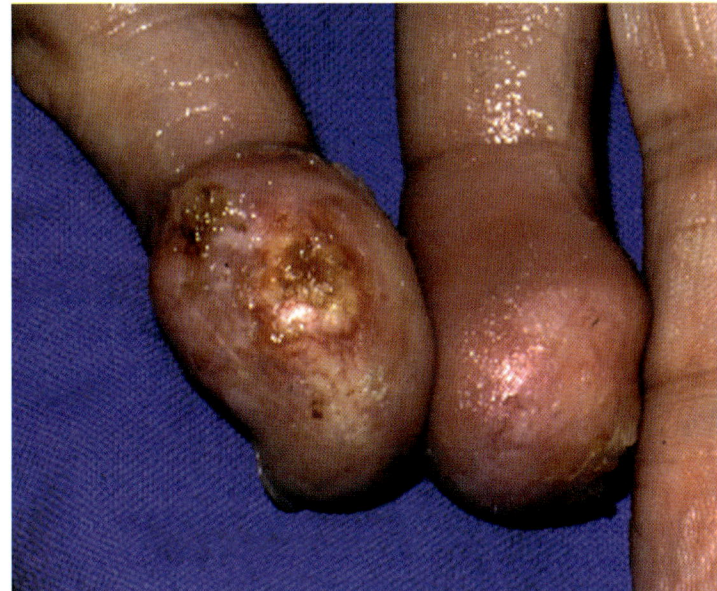

Fig. 62.10 Embolic metastasis to the little finger of each hand from carcinoma of oesophagus.

numbers of small dermal or subcutaneous nodules may be palpable in some such cases, even if not initially apparent or symptomatic.

Mechanisms and distribution [1]

Metastasis to the skin occurs as a result of lymphatic or haematogenous dissemination of tumour; direct infiltration of the skin by an underlying tumour is especially notable with breast carcinomas, and is discussed above. The reason for metastasis to specific organs is complex, involving both properties of the tumour cells, tumour cytokines (such as lymphangiogenic factors) and their interaction with host defences and tissues, and the distribution pattern within the skin is not random [2,12]. Indeed, 75% of metastases are found in the 25% of body surface area that comprises the head, neck and upper trunk [2].

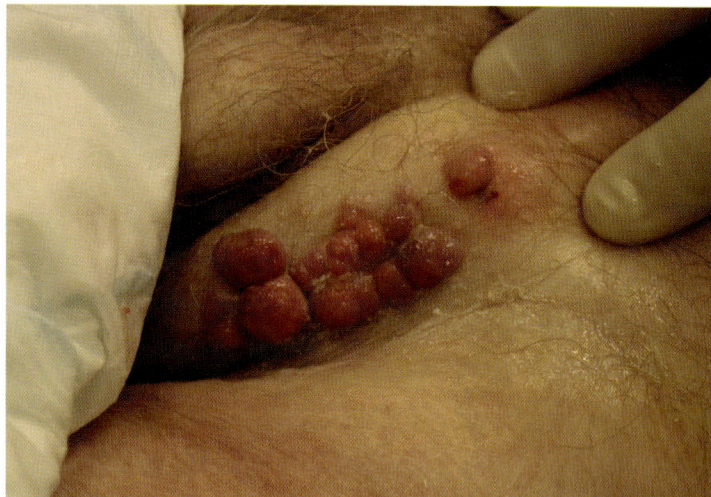

Fig. 62.11 Metastasis to the groin in a patient with extensive pelvic prostatic carcinoma.

The clinical pattern of metastases may provide clues to the route of metastasis. For example, metastases to extremities suggest intra-arterial embolic spread, widespread skin metastases suggest that tumour cells are present in the general circulation, whilst metastases to the skin in the vicinity of the affected organ (for example, prostatic tumour metastases are often on the lower abdomen, Fig. 62.11) is more suggestive of dissemination by lymphatic vessels or by veins. Retrograde lymphatic spread may occur from pelvic tumours, causing metastases in the perineal area or on the legs. In general, the head, neck and upper trunk are disproportionately commonly affected by tumours that metastasize to the skin [2,7–9,11], possibly because of the high vascularity of this area. Some of the tumour and host factors involved in metastasis, both generally and organ-specific, are reviewed in [13–17]; in particular, chemokine receptors on tumour cells may influence the organs involved in metastatic spread [18,19].

Other than the scalp, notable sites for skin metastasis include the umbilicus (Sister Mary Joseph's nodule, related to bowel tumours most commonly) [11,20,21] and recent operative scars. Scar metastasis is most often related to surgery for the primary tumour, and, in view of the low frequency of 'tumour spillage' documented previously, presumably represents spread by local lymphatic or venous drainage; however, recent but distant scars (for example, skin graft donor sites [22,23]) may be a site for metastases, suggesting a role of adhesion molecules, metalloproteinases or cytokines related to angiogenesis and tissue repair. Metastases have also been reported that are localized to a site of irradiation of the skin [24]. An additional, unusual phenomenon is 'tumour-to-tumour metastasis', in which metastases localize to another (usually benign) tumour [25]. A postulated mechanism is the trapping effect of fibrin in the vessels of recipient tumour; most such metastases occur within quite vascular neoplasms, such as thyroid or adrenal adenomas, but metastasis to lipoma and to basal cell carcinoma [26] have both been reported and are relevant to dermatologists.

Metastases to the scalp may give rise to focal alopecia, carcinomas of breast, lung and kidney being the commonest tumours to metastasize to the scalp. Renal and thyroid cancer metastases may be quite vascular in appearance, both clinically and pathologically [27], and are occasionally misdiagnosed as benign haemangiomas or pyogenic granulomas; hypernephroma metastases may even be pulsatile. Generally, cutaneous metastases may be mistaken for cysts or inflammatory lesions, although alopecia over a scalp 'cyst' should give rise to suspicion regarding the true nature of the lesion.

Histopathology and investigations

Biopsy of skin metastases is generally helpful in confirming a metastatic tumour, but is not always useful in determining the organ of origin if the tumour cells are poorly differentiated. Occasionally, it may be difficult, even with use of immunohistochemical tumour markers, to confidently distinguish between primary skin tumours and metastatic disease. Although, in general, the cells of a metastasis resemble the cells of the primary tumour, some patterns may prove diagnostically difficult. Spindle cell tumours, and tumours comprising 'small blue cells', cause particular difficulty and may need a panel of immunohistochemical markers to aid in diagnosis both between primary skin lesions and metastases, or between different origins of an internal tumour. For example, small cell neoplasms may occur in primary skin tumours (Merkel cell tumour), in skin or systemic lymphomas, and in metastases from small cell carcinoma of lung, from carcinoid or visceral neuroendocrine tumours, and in rarer metastatic tumours such as neuroblastoma or retinoblastoma. Immunohistochemistry may help in determining the diagnosis of the primary tumour, especially in the case of prostatic metastases (prostate-specific antigen) or thyroid metastases (thyroglobulin); where a specific site of origin cannot be determined, cytokeratin stains may help to distinguish between squamous cell carcinomas (e.g. from lung) and adenocarcinomas. Melanoma metastases may mimic many cell types, and melanoma markers such as MART-1 are not always expressed. Pathological diagnosis of specific metastases and immunohistochemical markers are discussed in [11,28]. In some instances, there may be marked oedema or dilated lymphatic vessels, which may make diagnosis difficult. In some specific tumours such as hypernephroma, or in some clinical patterns such as carcinoma telangiectoides, the tumour cells may either be scanty or the vascular proliferation may dominate the histopathological appearance. Lymphatic spread of tumour cells may lead to an 'Indian filing' appearance in some cases, sometimes with fibrosis.

Implications and prognosis

Cutaneous metastases usually occur in subjects with a known cancer, but may be the first indication of an internal neoplasm, especially in the case of lung cancers. They are usually indicative of disseminated disease and indicate a correspondingly poor prognosis; survival is typically only about 3 months in patients with disseminated skin metastases [4]. Patients with solitary metastases without other evidence of dissemination may have a better survival [29]. Infrequent cases of tumour regression after primary tumour removal are documented [30]. It is noteworthy that cutaneous metastases do not necessarily relate to a prior, documented tumour; the histological pattern, localization and temporal relationship may occasionally point to a second primary [31]. Treatment options, depending on the primary tumour, may include excision or other destructive therapy (e.g. laser destruction, radiotherapy, photodynamic therapy) for limited numbers of lesions, and chemotherapy or other systemic treatment for disseminated lesions.

References

1 Provost TT. Cutaneous metastasis. In: Provost TT, Flynn JA, eds. *Cutaneous Medicine: Cutaneous Manifestations of Systemic Disease*. Hamilton, Ontario: Decker, 2001: 357–66.

2 Schwartz RA. Cutaneous metastatic disease. *J Am Acad Dermatol* 1995; **33**: 161–82.

3 Smoller BR. Metastatic carcinoma. In: Morgan MB, Smoller BR, Somach SC. *Deadly Dermatologic Diseases. Clinicopathologic Atlas and Text*. New York: Springer, 2007: 38–42.

4 Reingold IM. Cutaneous metastasis from internal carcinoma. *Cancer* 1966; **19**: 162–8.

5 Lookingbill DP, Spangler N, Helm KF. Cutaneous metastases in patients with metastatic carcinoma: a retrospective study of 7316 cancer patients. *J Am Acad Dermatol* 1990; **22**: 19–26.

6 Spencer PS, Helm TN. Skin metastases in cancer patients. *Cutis* 1987; **39**: 119–21.

7 Brownstein MH, Helwig EB. Patterns of cutaneous metastasis. *Arch Dermatol* 1972; **105**: 862–8.

8 Lookingbill DP, Spangler N, Helm KF. Cutaneous metastases in patients with metastatic carcinoma: a retrospective study of 4020 patients. *J Am Acad Dermatol* 1993; **29**: 228–36.

9 Marcoval J, Moreno A, Peyri J. Cutaneous infiltration by cancer. *J Am Acad Dermatol* 2007; **57**: 577–80.

10 Poole S, Fenske NA. Cutaneous markers of internal malignancy, 1: malignant involvement of the skin and the genodermatoses. *J Am Acad Dermatol* 1993; **28**: 1–13.

11 Weedon D. *Skin Pathology*, 2nd edn. London: Churchill Livingstone, 2002: 1045–56.

12 Rolz-Cruz G, Kim CC. Tumor invasion of the skin. *Dermatol Clin* 2008; **26**: 89–102.

13 Cao Y, Zhong W. Tumor-derived lymphangiogenic factors and lymphatic metastasis. *Biomed Pharmacother* 2007; **61**: 534–9.

14 Dittmar T, Heyder C, Gloria-Maercker E *et al*. Adhesion molecules and chemokines: the navigation system for circulating tumor (stem) cells to metastasize in an organ-specific manner. *Clin Exp Metastasis* 2008; **25**: 11–32.

15 Pedraza-Fariña LG. Mechanisms of oncogenic cooperation in cancer initiation and metastasis. *Yale J Biol Med* 2006; **79**: 95–103.

16 Ramsay AG, Marshall JF, Hart IR. Integrin trafficking and its role in cancer metastasis. *Cancer Metastasis Rev* 2007; **26**: 567–78.

17 Leong SPL, Cady B, Jablons DM *et al*. Clinical patterns of metastasis. *Cancer Metastasis Rev* 2006; **25**: 221–32.

18 Dai CY, Haqq CM, Puzas JE. Molecular correlates of site-specific metastasis. *Semin Radiat Oncol* 2006; **16**: 102–10.

19 Kakinuma T, Hwang ST. Chemokines, chemokine receptors, and cancer metastasis. *J Leukoc Biol* 2006; **79**: 639–51.

20 Clements AB. Metastatic carcinoma of the umbilicus. *JAMA* 1952; **150**: 556–9.

21 Duperrat B, Duperrat N. Les métastases ombilicales. A propos de 20 pièces personnelles. *Bull Soc Franc Dermatol Syphiligr* 1968; **75**: 638–9.

22 Taylor CD, Snelling CF, Nickerson D, Trotter MJ. Acute development of invasive squamous cell carcinoma in a split-thickness skin graft donor site. *J Burn Care Rehab* 1998; **19**: 382–5.

23 Serrano OS, Buendia EA, Ortega DRM, Linares SJ. Melanoma metastasis in donor site of full-thickness skin graft. *Dermatology (Basel)* 2000; **201**: 377–8.

24 Diehl LF, Hurwitz MA, Johnson SA *et al*. Skin metastases confined to a field of previous irradiation. Report of two cases and review of the literature. *Cancer* 1984; **53**: 1864–8.

25 Richardson JF, Katayama I. Neoplasm to neoplasm metastasis, an acidophil adenoma harbouring metastatic carcinoma: a case report. *Arch Pathol* 1971; **91**: 135–9.

26 Cowley GP, Gallimore A. Malignant melanoma metastasizing to a basal cell carcinoma. *Histopathol* 1966; **29**: 469–70.

27 Rosenthal AL, Lever WF. Involvement of the skin in renal carcinoma: report of two cases with review of the literature. *AMA Arch Dermatol* 1957; **76**: 96–102.

28 Sariya D, Ruth K, Adams-McDonnell R *et al*. Clinicopathologic correlation of cutaneous metastases. Experience from a cancer center. *Arch Dermatol* 2007; **143**: 613–20.

29 Menter A, Boyd AS, McCaffree DM. Recurrent renal cell carcinoma presenting as skin nodules: two case reports and review of literature. *Cutis* 1989; **44**: 305–8.

30 Braren V, Taylor JN, Pace W. Regression of metastatic renal carcinoma following nephrectomy. *Urology* 1974; **3**: 777–8.

31 Brownstein MH, Helwig EB. Spread of tumours to the skin. *Arch Dermatol* 1973; **107**: 80–6.

Genodermatoses associated with internal malignancies [1–10]

Most cutaneous signs of neoplasia do not involve direct spread of tumour to the skin but are paraneoplastic. Genodermatoses account for a significant minority of paraneoplastic skin lesions; some including both cutaneous and internal neoplasms as part of the syndrome, both benign and malignant. The most important are listed in Table 62.8; non-cancer aspects of these disorders are discussed more fully in earlier chapters. A number of mechanisms underlie the association of genodermatoses with internal malignancy; these include chromosomal instability, faulty DNA repair mechanisms, abnormal lymphocyte function and immunosurveillance, and in some cases a combination of these. More precise genetic diagnosis, understanding of mechanisms, awareness of the benefits and ability to focus screening of family members for genetic abnormalities or for cancers, is a constantly evolving area within dermatology and paediatric medicine in particular.

Genodermatoses that predispose to skin but not to internal cancers are not discussed here; examples include disorders such as albinism, epidermodysplasia verruciformis, dystrophic epidermolysis bullosa, porokeratosis of Mibelli and KID syndrome.

References

1 Braverman IM. *Skin Signs of Systemic Disease*, 3rd edn. Philadelphia: Saunders, 1998.

2 Callen JP. Skin signs of internal malignancy. In: Callen JP, Jorizzo JL, eds. *Dermatological Manifestations of Internal Disease*, 3rd edn. Philadelphia: Saunders, 2003: 95–104.

3 Lynch HT, Fusaro RM, eds. *Cancer-Associated Genodermatoses*. New York: Van Nostrand Reinhold, 1982.

4 Callen JP. Skin signs of internal malignancy. *Australas J Dermatol* 1987; **28**: 106–14.

5 Poole S, Fenske NA. Cutaneous markers of internal malignancy, 1: malignant involvement of the skin and the genodermatoses. *J Am Acad Dermatol* 1993; **28**: 1–13.

6 Provost TT, Laman SD, Bell WR. Paraneoplastic dermatoses. In: Provost TT, Flynn JA, eds. *Cutaneous Medicine: Cutaneous Manifestations of Systemic Disease*. Hamilton, Ontario: Decker, 2001: 367–88.

7 Cohen PR, Kurzrock R, eds. Genodermatoses with malignant potential. *Dermatologic Clinics* 1995; **13**: 1–243.

8 Tsao H. Update on familial cancer syndromes and the skin. *J Am Acad Dermatol* 2000; **42**: 939–46.

9 Palayoor S, Harper J. Genetic diseases that predispose to malignancy. In: Harper J, Oranje A, Prose N. *Textbook of Pediatric Dermatology*, 2nd edn. Oxford: Blackwell, 2006: 1596–604.

10 Somoano B, Tsao H. Genodermatoses with cutaneous tumors and internal malignancies. *Dermatol Clinics* 2008; **26**: 69–87.

Table 62.8 Examples of genodermatoses associated with internal malignancies.

Main organ affected or usual mode of presentation (many are multisystem disorders)	Genodermatosis	Main neoplasms (may be limited to some families in some of the disorders listed)
Gastrointestinal tract	Gardner's syndrome Bannayan–Riley–Ruvalcaba syndrome Turcot syndrome (mismatch repair cancer syndrome)	Gastrointestinal polyposis and carcinomas (p. 62.56), central nervous system tumours
	Peutz–Jeghers syndrome	Gastrointestinal polyposis and carcinomas (p. 62.56), pancreatic carcinoma, genital tumours (especially Sertoli cell, sex cord and cervix), breast cancers, lung cancers
Neurological	Ataxia–telangiectasia	Lymphomas, leukaemias
	Neurofibromatosis	Neurological tumours, sarcomas, phaeochromocytoma
Skin	Xeroderma pigmentosum	Skin cancers, sarcomas, central nervous system tumours, leukaemia, various solid organ tumours
	Naevoid basal cell carcinoma syndrome (Gorlin)	Basal cell carcinomas of skin, medulloblastoma
	Basex–Dupré–Christol syndrome	Basal cell carcinomas of skin, possible leukaemia
	Porphyria cutanea tarda	Hepatocellular carcinoma
	Tylosis	Oesophageal carcinoma
	Sclerotylosis (Huriez syndrome)	Squamous cell carcinoma of skin; oral and bowel cancers also reported
	Muir–Torre syndrome	Colorectal tumours, sebaceous carcinoma
	Birt–Hogg–Dube syndrome and Hornstein–Knickenberg syndrome	Medullary carcinoma of thyroid, renal cell carcinoma
	Familial leiomyomas (also uterine)	Renal cell carcinoma, others (see text)
	Incontinentia pigmenti	Wilms' tumour, rhabdomyosarcomas (renal, paratesticular), retinoblastoma, leukaemias
	Familial atypical naevi and melanoma	Pancreatic carcinoma, cutaneous and ocular melanoma
	Melanoma–astrocytoma syndrome	Melanomas, astrocytomas and other central nervous system tumours
	Supernumerary nipples	Genitourinary tumours—renal cell carcinoma, Wilms' tumour, bladder, testicular, prostate
	Ichthyoses (autosomal dominant and X-linked)	Testicular carcinoma
Endocrine	Multiple endocrine neoplasia syndromes	Medullary carcinoma of thyroid, phaeochromocytoma
Growth/skeletal	Werner's syndrome	Many, especially sarcomas
	Rothmund–Thomson syndrome	Skin, osteosarcoma
	Bloom's syndrome	As general population but early onset
	Maffucci syndrome	Chondrosarcomas, gliomas, ovarian cancers
	Goltz syndrome	Chondrosarcomas, giant cell tumour of bone
	Fanconi's anaemia (usually presents due to congenital malformations)	Myelodysplastic syndrome, acute myelogenous leukaemia, hepatic carcinoma
Haemopoietic	Dyskeratosis congenita	Mucosal squamous cell carcinoma, haemopoietic malignancy, and others
Immunological	Wiskott–Aldrich syndrome	Lymphoreticular malignancies
	Chediak–Higashi syndrome	Lymphoreticular malignancies
Multisystem	Cowden's (multiple hamartoma and neoplasia) syndrome	Breast, thyroid, gastrointestinal, cerebellum, endometrial and renal carcinomas
	Carney complex	Myxomas, Schwannomas, testicular Sertoli cell tumour, pituitary adenomas, thyroid cancer
	Von Hippel–Lindau disease	Phaeochromocytoma, renal carcinoma, haemangioblastoma, pancreatic carcinoma
	Beckwith–Wiedermann syndrome (EMG syndrome)	Wilms' tumour, adrenal carcinoma, hepatoblastoma, pancreatoblastoma, others (especially in patients with hemihypertrophy)

Focal palmoplantar keratoderma (Howel-Evans syndrome; tylosis; MIM 148500) and other palmoplantar keratodermas (Chapter 19)

Howel-Evans syndrome is the association of autosomal dominantly inherited focal palmoplantar keratoderma (tylosis) with the eventual development of oesophageal carcinoma in most cases [1]. Since the original description, other families linked with inherited tylosis and carcinoma of the oesophagus have been described [2,3]. The genetic locus is at chromosome 17q25. However, in diffuse familial palmoplantar keratoderma starting in infancy, there is no genetic susceptibility to neoplasia.

A possible familial association has been described between palmoplantar keratoderma and gastrointestinal malignancy [4], diffuse epidermolytic palmoplantar keratoderma has been linked with increased risk of breast and ovarian cancer [5] and punctate porokeratotic keratoderma has been tentatively associated with internal neoplasia [6,7]. However, it is likely that such cases represent a separate, inherited tendency as most such reports relate to one specific family [8].

Acquired palmar hyperkeratosis may also occur as a marker of carcinogen ingestion (pp. 62.46–62.47), principally linked with arsenic. The relationship between arsenic-induced keratosis or punctate keratoderma and internal malignancy is controversial.

Palmoplantar punctate keratoses may be present in Cowden's disease (p. 62.25), in which there is a predisposition to several malignancies.

References
1 Harper PS, Harper RM, Howel-Evans AW. Carcinoma of the oesophagus with tylosis. *QJM* 1970; **155**: 317–33.
2 Shine I, Allison PR. Carcinoma of the oesophagus with tylosis. *Lancet* 1966; **i**: 951–3.
3 Zultak M, Blanc D, Merle C *et al*. Erythème annulaire centrifuge et leucémie aiguë myéloblastique. *Ann Dermatol Vénéréol* 1989; **116**: 477–80.
4 Bennion SD, Patterson JW. Keratosis punctata palmaris et plantaris and adenocarcinoma of the colon: a possible familial association of punctate keratoderma and gastrointestinal malignancy. *J Am Acad Dermatol* 1984; **10**: 587–91.
5 Blanchet-Bardon C, Nazzaro V, Chevrant-Breton J *et al*. Hereditary epidermolytic palmoplantar keratoderma associated with increased breast and ovarian cancer in a large kindred. *Br J Dermatol* 1987; **117**: 363–70.
6 Bianchi L, Orlandi A, Iraci S *et al*. Punctate porokeratotic keratoderma: its occurrence with internal neoplasia. *Clin Exp Dermatol* 1994; **19**: 139–41.
7 Bennion SD, Patterson JW. Keratosis punctata palmaris et plantaris and adenocarcinoma of the colon: a possible familial association of punctate keratoderma and gastrointestinal malignancy. *J Am Acad Dermatol* 1984; **10**: 587–91.
8 Moore RL, Devere TS. Epidermal manifestations of internal malignancy. *Dermatol Clinics* 2008; **26**: 17–29.

Naevoid basal cell carcinoma syndrome (NBCCS; Gorlin's syndrome, MIM #109400) (Chapter 52)

This is an autosomal dominant condition with prevalence of about 1/100 000 (about half being due to *de novo* mutations), the main features being multiple basal cell carcinomas (BCCs), mandibular odontogenic keratocysts, skeletal anomalies, abnormal calcification and dyskeratotic pits of palms and soles [1–6]. Diagnostic criteria are documented in [5,6]. The most commonly reported internal malignancies are medulloblastoma [7] and ovarian tumours (mainly benign fibromas, but also desmoids and sarcomas); astrocytomas, meningiomas, craniopharyngiomas, fibrosarcomas and ameloblastomas have occasionally been reported [2]. It is important to note that individuals may have only the family history, without themselves having developed BCC. However, neoplasia may also commence early in life, with a median age of onset of BCC by 20 years; most patients will have at least one BCC before age 30 years. The BCCs may present as small, subtle, tan-coloured or brown papules or acrochordon-like lesions on the face, neck, back, chest and upper limbs. They may become more aggressive as the patient ages, with both deep local invasion and metastases being possible. Facial milia also occur, and multiple skin

cysts (some with a corrugated internal surface similar to odontogenic keratinocysts) have been reported. An acral distribution of skin cysts may be suggestive of NBCCS [8].

The gene for NBCCS has been mapped to chromosome 9q22.3, with a high percentage (about 60% of pedigrees) having germ-line mutations in the *PTCH* gene [5,6,9], part of the Sonic Hedgehog (SHH) signalling pathway which is involved in transcription and cell cycle regulation.

References
1 Andreev VC, Petkov I. Skin manifestations associated with tumours of the brain. *Br J Dermatol* 1975; **92**: 675–8.
2 Jackson R, Gardere S. Nevoid basal cell carcinoma syndrome. *Can Med Assoc J* 1971; **105**: 850–9.
3 Gorlin SJ. Nevoid basal cell carcinoma syndrome. *Dermatol Clin* 1995; **13**: 113–25.
4 Kimonis VE, Goldstein AM, Pastakia B *et al*. Clinical manifestations in 105 persons with nevoid basal cell carcinoma syndrome. *Am J Hum Genet* 1997; **69**: 299–308.
5 Somoano B, Tsao H. Genodermatoses with cutaneous tumors and internal malignancies. *Dermatol Clinics* 2008; **26**: 69–87.
6 Farndon PA. The Gorlin (naevoid basal cell carcinoma) syndrome. In: Harper J, Oranje A, Prose N. *Textbook of Pediatric Dermatology*, 2nd edn. Oxford: Blackwell Publishing, 2006: 1514–31.
7 Southwick GT, Schwartz RA. The basal cell nevus syndrome: disasters occurring among a series of 36 patients. *Cancer* 1979; **44**: 2294–305.
8 Motegi S, Nagai Y, Tamura A, Ishikawa O. Multiple skin cysts in nevoid basal cell carcinoma syndrome: a case report and review of the literature. *Dermatology* 2008; **21**: 159–62.
9 Tsao H. Update on familial cancer syndromes and the skin. *J Am Acad Dermatol* 2000; **42**: 939–46.

Familial melanoma and internal malignancy syndromes

Familial melanoma, and metastases from melanoma, are discussed in more detail in Chapter 54, but links between melanoma and other internal neoplasms are detailed here [1–6].

Familial melanoma syndrome (B-K mole syndrome, familial atypical multiple-mole and melanoma, dysplastic naevus syndrome; MIM 155600)

This is a variable group of disorders, probably polygenic in inheritance, in which multiple melanomas are the main feature. Typically, there is one or more of a family history of melanoma, a personal or family background of multiple atypical ('dysplastic') melanocytic naevi, or all of these. Large multiple and irregular naevi are the norm, with an early onset of melanoma, potentially multiple primary melanomas, and in some pedigrees an increase in non-cutaneous malignancies such as pancreatic, gastrointestinal, lung, breast and laryngeal cancers, as well as ocular melanoma and cutaneous SCC of the head and neck. The *CDKN2A* germline mutation in the 9p21 gene region has been implicated in most cases [1,2]. The molecular genetics of *CDKN2A* has been extensively studied [2]; it encodes proteins that are involved in regulation of cell cycle progression (p16 and p14ARF). Those mutations that impair p16 function are linked with increased risk (22-fold) in pancreatic cancer, and specific mutations have been linked with breast cancer in some populations [2]. However, other gene mutations are also involved in familial melanoma, and external factors such as sunlight may alter the likelihood of cutaneous melanoma.

Melanoma–astrocytoma syndrome (melanoma–nervous system tumours syndrome, melanoma-NST syndrome; MIM 155755)

This syndrome comprises an association of melanomas with astrocytomas specifically, or with astrocytomas, other central nervous system tumours, meningiomas, ependymomas and peripheral nerve tumours such as malignant schwannoma [3–6]. Deletions of chromosome 9p21, which includes tumour suppressor and cell cycle regulating genes, are implicated. Several genetic loci have been implicated in different families, including all or parts of the p16, p19 and p15 gene cluster (*INK4* locus) which includes *CDKN2A* and *CDKN2B* (suggesting contiguous suppressor gene deletion) [3–5], and more recently a specific deletion of p14(ARF) [6]. In one study, a kindred with melanomas and nervous system tumours (melanoma/NST syndrome) had a large germline deletion of the *INK4* locus, whilst a more circumscribed gene disruption was associated with a melanoma–astrocytoma family [5].

References

1 Tsao H. Update on familial cancer syndromes and the skin. *J Am Acad Dermatol* 2000; **42**: 939–46.
2 Somoano B, Tsao H. Genodermatoses with cutaneous tumors and internal malignancies. *Dermatol Clinics* 2008; **26**: 69–87.
3 Azizi E, Friedman J, Pavlotsky F *et al.* Familial cutaneous malignant melanoma and tumours of the nervous system. A hereditary cancer syndrome. *Cancer* 1995; **76**: 1571–8.
4 Bahuau M, Vidaud D, Kujas M *et al.* Familial aggregation of malignant melanoma/dysplastic naevi and tumours of the nervous system: an original syndrome of tumour proneness. *Ann Genet* 1997; **40**: 78–91.
5 Bahuau M, Vidaud D, Jenkins RB *et al.* Germline mutation involving the INK4 locus in familial proneness to melanoma and nervous system tumours. *Cancer Res* 1998; **58**: 2298–303.
6 Randerson-Moore JA, Harland M, Williams S *et al.* A germline deletion of p14(ARF) but not CDKN2A in a melanoma-neural system tumour family. *Hum Mol Genet* 2001; **1**: 55–62.

Xeroderma pigmentosum (XP; MIM 194400, 133510, 278700–278800) [1–4]

This group of disorders with autosomal recessive inheritance are discussed in more detail in Chapter 15. XP characteristically presents at an early age with severe photosensitivity, marked reduction in threshold for sunburn and myriads of lentigines, principally in a sun-exposed distribution. Early onset of photoageing is found in infants, followed by sun-induced dysplasias, BCC, SCC and malignant melanomas, commencing in the first decade of life, which occur with a 2000-fold increased risk; SCC of the tip of the tongue has a 10 000-fold increased risk compared with individuals of the same age [3]. Ocular neoplasms, both melanoma and non-melanoma, occur in 10–20%. However, it is not only neoplasms linked with solar exposure that are increased in frequency; there is also a 10- to 20-fold increased incidence of internal malignancy, including central nervous system (CNS) sarcomas, leukaemia, and carcinomas of lung, breast, pancreas, stomach and testes [4]. The mutations causing XP cause abnormal fibroblast sensitivity to ultraviolet radiation, in most cases (complementation groups A–G) resulting from a defective DNA nucleotide excision repair process; the eighth form, termed XP variant, codes for a post-replication repair polymerase. Inactivation of tumour suppressors

and activation of oncogenes due to these mutations results in development of multiple tumours [2].

References

1 Kraemer KH, Lee MM, Scotto J. Xeroderma pigmentosum: cutaneous, ocular and neurologic abnormalities in 830 published cases. *Arch Dermatol* 1987; **123**: 241–50.
2 Tsao H. Update on familial cancer syndromes and the skin. *J Am Acad Dermatol* 2000; **42**: 939–46.
3 Bootsma D, Kraemer KH, Cleaver JE *et al.* Nucleotide excision repair syndromes: xeroderma pigmentosum, Cockayne syndrome, and trichothiodystrophy. In: Vogelstein BV, Kinzler K, eds. *The Genetic Basis of Human Cancer*. New York: McGraw-Hill, 1998: 245–74.
4 Somoano B, Tsao H. Genodermatoses with cutaneous tumors and internal malignancies. *Dermatol Clinics* 2008; **26**: 69–87.

Von Hippel–Lindau disease (VHL; MIM *193300)

A rare, autosomal dominantly inherited condition, characterized by benign and malignant tumours of various systems, particularly haemangioblastomas of the CNS, angiomatosis of the retinae, phaeochromocytoma [1] (which may be bilateral), renal carcinoma [2], pancreatic adenoma, carcinoma and cysts [3], and epididymal cystadenomas. Endolymphatic sac tumours are rarely found other than in von Hippel–Lindau disease [4]. The non-specific cutaneous manifestations include haemangiomas and café-au-lait spots [5]. The VHL gene has been located on chromosome 3p26-p25; although different mutations have been found to be causative, the gene is a tumour-suppressor gene following the Knudson two-hit model. Families may be characterized by the presence (type 2, missense mutations) or absence (type 1, deletions/protein-truncating mutations) of phaeochromocytoma; in those with a predominance of familial phaeochromocytoma, analysis of VHL mutations may be useful to identify asymptomatic subjects at risk of von Hippel–Lindau disease. Type 2b has, in addition to an association with phaeochromocytoma, a high incidence of renal cell carcinoma and haemangioblastomas, whereas in type 2a there is a lower incidence of renal cell carcinoma and in type 2c an exclusive association with phaeochromocytoma [6]. However, genetic investigation of patients with apparently sporadic phaeochromocytoma rarely identifies subjects with mutations in *VHL* or in the *RET* proto-oncogene (mutations in which cause multiple endocrine neoplasia type 2, another cause of familial phaeochromocytoma) and is not routinely indicated [7].

References

1 Kiechle-Schwartz M, Neuman HP, Decker HH *et al.* Cytogenetic studies on three pheochromocytomas derived from patients with von Hippel–Lindau syndrome. *Hum Genet* 1989; **82**: 127–30.
2 Saranya R, Matzkin H, Papo J *et al.* Von Hippel–Lindau syndrome with unusual presentations in 2 brothers. *Urology* 1989; **34**: 301–4.
3 Neumann HP. Basic criteria for clinical diagnosis and genetic counselling in von Hippel–Lindau syndrome. *Vasa* 1987; **16**: 220–6.
4 Manski TJ, Heffner DK, Glenn GM *et al.* Endolymphatic sac tumors. A source of morbid hearing loss in von Hippel–Lindau disease. *JAMA* 1997; **277**: 1461–6.
5 Lynch HT, Fusaro RM, eds. *Cancer-Associated Genodermatoses*. New York: Van Nostrand Reinhold, 1982.
6 Eamonn ER, Kaelin WG. Von Hippel–Lindau Disease. *Medicine (Baltimore)* 1997; **76**: 381–91.
7 Bar M, Friedman E, Jakobovitz O *et al.* Sporadic phaeochromocytomas are rarely associated with germline mutations in the von Hippel-Lindau and *RET* genes. *Clin Endocrinol* 1997; **47**: 707–12.

Neurofibromatosis types 1 and 2 (NF1, von Recklinghausen's disease, MIM *162200; NF2, MIM *101000) (Chapter 15) [1–5]

There are two main forms of neurofibromatosis, type 1 (NF1) and type 2 (NF2). Both have an autosomal dominant inheritance but in a large proportion of affected individuals the condition is due to a *de novo* mutation (which may be mosaic). The abnormal neural crest cell function in NF1 leads to development of multiple peripheral neurofibromas, as well as CNS tumours (notably optic glioma, which is one of the diagnostic criteria for NF1 [4]) and café-au-lait macules [1–5]. Patients with a deletion of the whole gene have earlier development of neurofibromas and an apparent higher frequency of malignant peripheral nerve sheath tumours [5].

NF1 is the commonest form of neurofibromatosis, with a prevalence of approximately 1/3000, about tenfold that of NF2. There are several different clinical presentations, depending on the localization of the lesions. Clinical overlap between NF1 and NF2 occurs particularly in children, who may have café-au-lait macules and peripheral nerve tumours; flexural freckling is indicative of NF1. Café-au-lait macules occur in NF2, but only in half of affected subjects and usually fewer than six in number (six or more being one of the diagnostic criteria for NF1).

Lisch nodules (pigmented iris hamartomas) are found with slit-lamp analysis in 90% of adult patients with NF1 and are fairly specific for NF1; two or more such lesions are one of the diagnostic criteria. Around 80% of patients with NF2 have posterior subcapsular cataracts, including about a third of affected children.

The associations with benign tumours, malignancy and systemic manifestations are varied but patients with NF1 have an overall 2.5-fold increase in risk of developing a malignancy [4]. In general, NF2 patients have fewer skin lesions than in those with NF1, and the lesions that occur are mainly schwannomas, but more severe disease in NF2 is linked with greater prevalence of skin tumours [3,4].

NF2 patients develop vestibular and peripheral nerve schwannomas (the vestibular schwannomas characteristically being bilateral), together with CNS tumours such as meningiomas. Spinal schwannomas (mainly), astrocytomas or ependymomas eventually occur in about three-quarters of patients with NF2. If meningiomas occur in children, NF2 should be suspected. Perhaps the commonest neoplasm developing in patients with neurofibromatosis is a malignant neurofibrosarcoma [6]. Most superficial neurofibromas have a low malignant potential, change occurring more often in the deep plexiform neurofibromas and those more in continuity with nerves, designated schwannomas. Benign tumours such as acoustic neuromas, dumb-bell tumours and optic gliomas can result in disastrous sequelae when occurring in confined, pressure-sensitive sites. The commonest CNS malignancy is an astrocytoma. Other malignancies include nephroblastoma (Wilms' tumour), fibrosarcoma, rhabdomyosarcoma and leukaemia, especially in children [3–8]; there is an association between NF1, juvenile myelomonocytic leukaemia and juvenile xanthogranulomas [9]. Monosomy 7 myelodysplastic syndrome may also occur [10]. There is an increased frequency of phaeochromocytomas and carcinoid tumours [4], and ocular melanoma has been reported [11].

The *NF1* gene, located on chromosome 17q11.2, has a role as a tumour-suppressor gene; its protein product, neurofibromin, regulates cell growth, including an effect of accelerating inactivation of the p21 *ras* proto-oncogene [4,12]. Transformation of benign neurofibromas to malignant peripheral nerve sheath tumours involves the loss of other tumour-suppressor genes such as p53 and p16.

The *NF2* gene locus is on chromosome 22q12.2; the product of this gene, termed merlin, has an uncertain effect on tumour suppression [3,4].

References

1 Riccardi VM. *Neurofibromatosis: Phenotype, Natural History, and Pathogenesis*, 2nd edn. Baltimore: Johns Hopkins University Press, 1992: 213–23.
2 Ferner RE, Huson SM, Thomas N *et al.* Guidelines for the diagnosis and management of individuals with neurofibromatosis 1. *J Med Genet* 2007; **44**: 81–8.
3 Tsao H. Update on familial cancer syndromes and the skin. *J Am Acad Dermatol* 2000; **42**: 939–46.
4 Somoano B, Tsao H. Genodermatoses with cutaneous tumors and internal malignancies. *Dermatol Clinics* 2008; **26**: 69–87.
5 Huson SM, Ruggieri M. The neurofibromatoses. In: Harper J, Oranje A, Prose N. *Textbook of Pediatric Dermatology*, 2nd edn. Oxford: Blackwell Publishing, 2006: 1467–90.
6 Hope DG, Mulvill JJ. Malignancy in neurofibromatosis. *Adv Neurol* 1981; **29**: 33–56.
7 McKeen EA, Bodurtha J, Meadows AT *et al.* Rhabdomyosarcoma complicating multiple neurofibromatosis. *J Pediatr* 1977; **93**: 992–3.
8 Stay EJ, Vawter G. The relationship between nephroblastoma and neurofibromatosis (von Recklinghausen's disease). *Cancer* 1977; **39**: 2550–5.
9 Zvulunov A, Barak Y, Metzker A. Juvenile xanthogranuloma, neurofibromatosis, and juvenile chronic myelogenous leukemia. World statistical analysis. *Arch Dermatol* 1995; **131**: 904–8.
10 Maris JM, Wiersma SR, Mahgoub N *et al.* Monosomy 7 myelodysplastic syndrome and other second malignant neoplasms in children with neurofibromatosis type 1. *Cancer* 1997; **79**: 1438–46.
11 Wiznia RA, Freeman JK, Mancini AD *et al.* Malignant melanoma of the choroid in neurofibromatosis. *Am J Ophthalmol* 1978; **86**: 684–7.
12 Parisi MA, Sybert VP. Molecular genetics in pediatric dermatology. *Curr Opin Pediatr* 2000; **12**: 347–53.

Tuberous sclerosis complex (TSC; Bourneville's disease; TSC1, MIM #191100 and TSC2, MIM *191092) (Chapter 15) [1–5]

An autosomal dominant condition of angiokeratomas, epilepsy and mental retardation; a high spontaneous mutation rate accounts for over half of cases. It may be associated with multisystem tumour involvement, mostly hamartomatous. There are two known causative genes—*TSC1* on chromosome 9q34, encoding hamartin, and *TSC2* on chromosome 16p13.3, encoding tuberin; both genes function as tumour suppressor genes. There are large numbers of different mutations, *TSC2* mutations being more common, and causing more severe disease, than *TSC1* mutations.

Other than skin lesions (Chapter 15), the CNS, renal and cardiopulmonary systems are most significantly affected [1–3]. Angiomyolipomas (of vessels, fat and smooth muscle) all show the same loss of heterozygosity at the *TSC1* or *TSC2* loci, with hyperphosphorylation of ribosomal protein S6; the smooth muscle component of these lesions is identical to that of the smooth muscle in lymphangiomyomatosis, which is also a feature of tuberous sclerosis [5]. Malignant sarcomatous change can occur, particularly with angiomyolipomas and rhabdomyomas, but is uncommon, and metastases are unusual [4]. Renal cell carcinoma is a recognized, infrequent complication [3,6].

References

1 Callen JP. Skin signs of internal malignancy. In: Callen JP, Jorizzo JL, eds. *Dermatological Manifestations of Internal Disease*, 3rd edn. Philadelphia: Saunders, 2003: 95–104.

2 Somoano B, Tsao H. Genodermatoses with cutaneous tumors and internal malignancies. *Dermatol Clinics* 2008; **26**: 69–87.

3 Osborne JP. Tuberous sclerosis. In: Harper J, Oranje A, Prose N. *Textbook of Pediatric Dermatology*, 2nd edn. Oxford: Blackwell Publishing, 2006: 1491–502.

4 Lynch HT, Fusaro RM, eds. *Cancer-Associated Genodermatoses*. New York: Van Nostrand Reinhold, 1982.

5 Crino PB, Nathanson KL, Henske EP. The tuberous sclerosis complex. *N Engl J Med* 2006; **355**: 1345–56.

6 Lynne CM, Carrion HM, Baskshandeh K *et al.* Renal angiomyolipoma: polycystic kidney and renal cell carcinoma in a patient with tuberous sclerosis. *Urology* 1979; **14**: 174–6.

Multiple endocrine neoplasia syndrome (multiple endocrine adenomatosis, MEA)

This section actually includes three conditions, MEN1, MEN2A and MEN2B (previously termed MEN3).

Multiple endocrine neoplasia type 1 (MEN1; Wermer syndrome; MIM *131100). This is an autosomal dominant familial cancer syndrome, with parathyroid, pancreatic islet cell and pituitary gland tumours, as well as cutaneous findings. It is caused by mutations in the *MEN1* gene, located on chromosome 11q12-13, which codes for the production of a protein named menin. The cutaneous findings in MEN1 are mostly multiple facial angiofibromas and collagenomas. Café-au-lait macules and lipomas are also encountered [1,2].

MEN1 is, at least in part, a tumour-suppressor gene. MEN1 is characterized by tumours of the parathyroid, anterior pituitary, pancreatic islet cells, neuroendocrine origin, foregut carcinoid and adrenal cortex. It is associated with 20–25% of cases of Zollinger–Ellison syndrome (ZES). In MEN1, 60–100% of cases have gastro-enteropancreatic (GEP) lesions, especially pancreatic islet endocrine tumours (pancreatic polypeptidomas or non-functional 80–100%, ZES 54%, insulinoma 21%, glucagonoma 3% and vasoactive intestinal peptide (VIP)oma 1%). Glucagonoma may be difficult to diagnose as even subjects with MEN1 without a pancreatic endocrine tumour may have glucagon levels above the normal basal level. Associated endocrine disease consists of parathyroid hyperplasia >95%, anterior pituitary adenomas around 60% (range 14–100%), adrenal adenomas about 30%, lung carcinoids 7% and gastric carcinoids 13–30%. The pituitary adenomas are prolactinomas in 14–76% and cause acromegaly in 11–33% and Cushing's syndrome in 5–19%. The commonest tumours in MEN1 secrete PTH or gastrin; hyperparathyroidism is present in 95–100% of affected individuals. However, screening patients with sporadic pituitary adenomas for other features of MEN1 yields few cases of MEN1, the greatest number being in patients with prolactinoma. Screening patients with hyperparathyroidism yields 1–16% with MEN1, whilst screening those with GEP tumours identifies 10–50% as having other features of MEN1.

Metastases from malignant neuroendocrine tumours (carcinoid) may be one of the commonest causes of mortality in MEN1; most of these, unlike non-MEN1 cases, arise from the embryological foregut (bronchi, thyroid, stomach, duodenum and pancreas) [3–5].

Multiple endocrine neoplasia type 2A (MEN2A, Sipple syndrome; MIM #171400—mucosal neuromas, medullary thyroid carcinoma and phaeochromocytoma) [5–7]. This shares some features with MEN2B. Both principally involve the thyroid and parathyroid glands, and the adrenal medulla, and are linked with familial medullary thyroid carcinoma (FMTC) [8,9]. They are caused by mutations of the *RET* proto-oncogene locus (10q11.2) [10–12]. Both are autosomal dominant, but 50% of cases with MEN2B are due to spontaneous mutations. In the same vicinity, near the centromere of chromosome 10, are the genes for Hirschprung disease (which may occur in both MEN2A and 2B) and for FMTC. Thickened corneal nerves occur in both MEN2 syndromes.

Type 2A is linked to a mutation of the *RET* oncogene, located on chromosome 10, compared to a sporadic *RET* oncogene in 2B; *RET* testing has replaced calcitonin screening to diagnose *MEN2* carrier status. The specific *RET* codon mutation will delineate the course of the disease and degree of aggression; details of the genetic aspects underlying MEN2 are provided in [3,4,6,11,12].

MEN2A lacks the mucosal neuromas and skin lipomas of MEN1 and MEN2B, and café-au-lait macules are only present in those with a combined phenotype of MEN2A with neurofibromatosis type 1. By contrast, symmetrical, bilateral pruritic skin lesions are found overlying the scapular area, with hyperpigmentation and hyperkeratosis clinically suggestive of macular amyloidosis; deposits of keratin-derived amyloid are typically found histologically [3,5,7]. Lesions suggestive of notalgia paraesthetica have been reported prior to recognition of the syndrome. Reflecting the genetic background, lichen amyloidosis also occurs in FMTC.

The main internal disorders in MEN2A, described as the triad of cardinal manifestations, are medullary thyroid carcinoma (MTC), phaeochromocytoma and hyperparathyroidism (due to either hyperplasia or adenomas). Other hamartomas and tumours include cerebellar haemangioblastomas, cervical neuroblastoma, pituitary adenomas and pinealomas [7]; Cushing's syndrome also occurs.

Multiple endocrine neoplasia type 2B (MEN type 2B or 3, MIM #162300). This is characterized by mucosal neuromas that are apparent at birth or in the first years of life. Neuromas manifest as asymptomatic, soft, flesh-coloured papules or nodules. They cause a characteristic facial appearance with soft, lumpy ('blubbery'), protuberant lips; everted, thickened, bumpy eyelids; and prominent eyebrows. Neuromas typically affect mucosal surfaces, especially the anterior border of the tongue and the buccal mucosa inside the commissures of the lips; gingival, palatal and pharyngeal surfaces may occasionally be affected. Medullated corneal nerve fibres are seen on slit lamp examination, and there may be conjunctival and, rarely, corneal neuromas. Perioral lentiginosis, pigmentation of hands and feet, and café-au-lait macules may occur and, rarely, a progressive striated pigmentary change of hyperplastic dermal nerves on the trunk [13]. Prognathism or retrognathism can be evident, and there may be a high-arched palate. About 75% of patients have a marfanoid appearance; muscle weakness and musculoskeletal anomalies (especially kyphoscoliosis, pes cavus and (often bilateral) slipped upper femoral epiphysis) may also be present [10].

MEN2B is also associated with MTC (in 75%) and phaeochromocytoma (in almost 50%), the MTC in type 2B presenting earlier and more aggressively than in type 2A. The MTC is often multicentric and bilateral, occurring in a background of calcitonin-producing cell hyperplasia; it may be found in children as young as 3 years. Diarrhoea is a common symptom. Early lymphatic spread may occur, 75% having metastases at presentation [10]. Prophylactic thyroidectomy may be indicated. Phaeochromocytomas are often bilateral, but the mortality is greater from MTC than from phaeochromocytoma. Hyperparathyroidism due to parathyroid hyperplasia or adenomatosis is much less common than in MEN types 1 and 2A. Intestinal ganglioneuromatosis is more common in type 2B than 2A, occurring in 30% and often presenting early in life due to constipation or abdominal pain.

References

1 Guo SS, Sawicki MP. Molecular and genetic mechanism of tumorigenesis in multiple endocrine neoplasia. *Mol Endocrinol* 2001; **15**: 1653–64.
2 Darling TN, Skarulis MC, Steinberg SM *et al.* Multiple facial angiofibromas and collagenomas in patients with multiple endocrine neoplasia type 1. *Arch Dermatol* 1997; **133**: 853–7.
3 Tsao H. Update on familial cancer syndromes and the skin. *J Am Acad Dermatol* 2000; **42**: 939–46.
4 Brandi ML, Gagel RF, Angeli A *et al.* Guidelines for diagnosis and therapy of MEN type 1 and type 2. *J Clin Endocrin Metab* 2001; **86**: 5658–71.
5 Statakis CA. Clinical genetics of multiple endocrine neoplasias, Carney's complex and related syndromes. *J Endocrinol Invest* 2001; **24**: 370–83.
6 Callen JP. Skin signs of internal malignancy. In: Callen JP, Jorizzo JL, eds. *Dermatological Manifestations of Internal Disease*, 3rd edn. Philadelphia: Saunders, 2003: 95–104.
7 Kousseff BG. Multiple endocrine neoplasia 2 (MEN 2)/MEN 2A (Sipple syndrome). *Dermatol Clinics* 1995; **13**: 91–7.
8 Sipple JH. The association of phaeochromocytoma with carcinoma of the thyroid gland. *Am J Med* 1961; **31**: 163–6.
9 Cunliffe WJ, Hudgson P, Fulthorpe JJ *et al.* A calcitonin secreting medullary thyroid carcinoma, associated with mucosal neuromas, marfanoid features, myopathy and pigmentation. *Am J Med* 1970; **48**: 120–6.
10 Holloway KB, Flowers FP. Multiple endocrine neoplasia 2B (MEN 2B)/MEN 3. *Dermatol Clinics* 1995; **13**: 99–103.
11 Lee NC, Norton JA. Multiple endocrine neoplasia type 2B: genetic basis and clinical expression. *Surg Oncol* 2000; **9**: 111–8.
12 Huang SC, Torres-Cruz J, Pack SD *et al.* Amplification and overexpression of mutant RET in multiple endocrine neoplasia type 2-associated medullary thyroid carcinoma. *J Clin Endocrinol Metab* 2003; **88**: 459–63.
13 Guillet G, Gauthier Y, Tamisier JM *et al.* Linear cutaneous neuromas (dermatoneurie en stries): a limited phakomatosis with striated pigmentation corresponding to cutaneous hyperneury (featuring multiple endocrine neoplasia syndrome?). *J Cutan Pathol* 1987; **14**: 43–8.

Carney complex (CNC; Carney syndrome; NAME syndrome; LAMB syndrome; myxoma syndrome. Type I MIM #160980, type II MIM *605244) [1–5] (see also p. 62.78)

This is a group of disorders in which there are cutaneous pigmented lesions associated with cutaneous, subcutaneous and internal myxomas at various sites, and associated endocrinopathy (mainly tumours) which typically includes involvement of one or more of the adrenal cortex, thyroid, pituitary, and gonads. NAME syndrome consists of *n*aevi (congenital melanocytic), *a*trial myxomas, *m*yxoid neurofibromas and *e*phelides. LAMB syndrome

consists of *l*entigines, *a*trial myxomas, *m*ucocutaneous myxomas and *b*lue naevi. The association with myxomas has led to many other names; some prefer to use '*myxoma syndrome*', or the combined term *Carney complex/myxoma syndrome* [5]. Cardiac myxomas occur in 61% [1] and are the most important internal myxomas, due to the causation of cardiac symptoms and potentially life-threatening effects (see also the section on cardiac disease later in this chapter). Likewise with endocrine involvement, adrenal-linked Cushing's syndrome can have critical, life-threatening effects; the adrenal tumours in Carney complex are typically of primary pigmented nodular type, an otherwise rare condition. Various other gonadal and endocrine hormone-secreting tumours, including pituitary tumours producing GH, prolactin or ACTH, occur; ovarian tumours are associated, and both benign and malignant thyroid tumours (usually of follicular type) also occur [2,3]. Testicular tumours, often large-cell calcifying Sertoli cell tumours, occur in about 30% of males, and are often bilateral and multicentric. Psammomatous melanotic schwannoma, usually of the upper gastrointestinal tract or of paravertebral sympathetic nerves, is very suggestive of this syndrome. Myxoid fibroadenomas of the breast, and mammary ductal adenomas, may be found [5], and myxoid leiomyomas and uterine tumours are described. Lentiginosis and blue naevi occur in two-thirds, typically on the face, lips and conjunctivae [5], and skin myxomas occur in over a third of cases [1].

Over half of patients with Carney complex have mutations in genes coding for a regulatory subunit type 1A of protein kinase A. CNC is clinically and probably genetically heterogeneous. At least two gene locations have been proposed, one on chromosome 2p16 (type 2) and another on 17q23-24 (type 1) [3,4].

References

1 Carney JA. Carney complex: the complex of myxomas, spotty pigmentation, endocrine overactivity, and schwannomas. *Semin Dermatol* 1995; **14**: 90–8.
2 Statakis CA. Clinical genetics of multiple endocrine neoplasias, Carney's complex and related syndromes. *J Endocrinol Invest* 2001; **24**: 370–83.
3 Lee NC, Norton JA. Multiple endocrine neoplasia type 2B: genetic basis and clinical expression. *Surg Oncol* 2000; **9**: 111–8.
4 Tsao H. Update on familial cancer syndromes and the skin. *J Am Acad Dermatol* 2000; **42**: 939–46.
5 Cullen MK. Carney complex. In: Nordlund JJ, Boissy RE, Hearing VJ *et al.*, eds. *The Pigmentary System*, 2nd edn. Oxford: Blackwell Publishing, 2006: 851–63.

PTEN hamartoma tumour syndrome (Cowden's disease, multiple hamartoma and neoplasia syndrome; MIM #158350) [1–6]

This rare, cancer-associated genodermatosis was first described by Lloyd and Dennis and named after their patient Rachel Cowden [1]. Inheritance is as an autosomal dominant trait with incomplete penetrance. It is due to germline mutations in the *PTEN* (protein tyrosine phosphatase with homology to tensin; *MMAC1*) gene on chromosome 10q23.3. *PTEN* is a tumour suppressor gene; mutations may produce their effects in Cowden's disease and allied hamartomatous disorders due to a failure to regulate cell death [2–4]. The spectrum of the disorder has increased with understanding of the genetic aspects [5], and has not only led to development of diagnostic criteria by the International Cowden Disease Consortium [3,5,6] but also to inclusion within the PTEN hamartoma neoplasia syndrome of several other hamartomatous disorders including Bannayan–Riley–Ruvalcaba syndrome (Bannayan–Zonana syndrome; MIM 153480) and Lhermitte–Duclos disease [5], in which hamartomatous outgrowths of the cerebellum occur. Bannayan–Riley–Ruvalcaba syndrome, as originally described, has many features in common with Cowden's disease, but lacks the extent of the malignant lesions of the latter; it is characterized by microcephaly, vascular anomalies, lipomas, thyroid disease, gastrointestinal polyposis and speckled genital pigmentation; it is discussed further with other gastrointestinal polyposis syndromes (p. 62.56). A family history of features of Bannayan–Riley–Ruvalcaba syndrome is typical in patients with Cowden's disease, the latter having a stronger association with internal malignancy. Also of dermatological importance is an overlap with Proteus syndrome (MIM 176920); up to 20% of patients with Proteus syndrome have *PTEN* mutations, and 50% of patients with Proteus-like syndrome (in which some features of Proteus syndrome are present, but not sufficient to meet formal diagnostic criteria) [5].

Pathognomonic criteria for Cowden's disease are mucocutaneous lesions, facial trichilemmomas (at least three), acral keratosis (at least six palmar lesions), papillomatous lesions and mucosal lesions. These are found in over 90% of patients. The mucosal lesions (Fig. 62.12) comprise a warty, 'cobblestone' hyperplasia of the mucosal surfaces, particularly affecting the tongue and buccal mucosa; periorificial facial papules, acral warty keratoses and palmoplantar semitranslucent, punctate keratosis are characteristic. The lesions, which are grouped especially around the mouth, nose and ears, have a hyperkeratotic, flat-topped, wart-like appearance, as do many lesions elsewhere; these are mostly trichilemmomas or related benign tumours of the follicular infundibulum [3–7]. Multiple hamartomatous lesions of ectodermal, endodermal and mesodermal origin occur. The other cutaneous lesions include ganglioneuromas, lipomas, fibromas, angiomas, angiolipomas, epidermoid cysts and a variety of pigmentary changes. Craniomegaly is common; there may be an adenoid facies, kyphoscoliosis and a high-arched palate.

Benign internal anomalies are numerous, most commonly affecting the breast (severe fibrocystic disease occurs in the majority of

women) and the thyroid (mainly multinodular goitres and adenomas). Gastrointestinal polyposis and cysts or polyps of the female genitourinary system are also frequent. Seizures and mental retardation occur (the latter is a minor diagnostic criterion) and there may be an association with meningioma.

The predisposition to neoplasia includes almost any internal malignancy, but particularly cancers of the breast [8], colon and thyroid (especially follicular thyroid carcinoma). Adenocarcinoma of the breast occurs in about 50% of women. Fibrocystic breast disease and cancers may have an early onset, and screening of at-risk family members is therefore recommended. Even prophylactic mastectomy has been suggested [8]. Benign gynaecomastia has been reported in the male, but malignancy of the breast or thyroid is exceptional. Breast, endometrial and thyroid cancers all contribute to a higher mortality in females. Renal carcinomas have more recently been linked with this syndrome, and an increased likelihood of melanoma has been suggested.

References

1 Lloyd KM, Dennis M. Cowden's disease: a possible new system complex with multiple system involvement. *Ann Intern Med* 1963; **58**: 136–42.
2 Tsao H. Update on familial cancer syndromes and the skin. *J Am Acad Dermatol* 2000; **42**: 939–46.
3 Eng C. Will the real Cowden syndrome please stand up: revised diagnostic criteria. *J Med Genet* 2000; **37**: 828–30.
4 Mallory S, Mallory SB. Cowden syndrome (multiple hamartoma syndrome). *Dermatol Clin* 1995; **13**: 27–31.
5 Pilarski R, Eng C. Will the real Cowden syndrome please stand up (again)?: expanding mutational and clinical spectra of the PTEN hamartoma tumour syndrome. *J Med Genet* 2004; **41**: 323–6.
6 Uppal S, Mistry D, Coatesworth AP. Cowden disease: a review. *Int J Clin Pract* 2007; **61**: 645–52.
7 Graham RM, Emmerson RW. Multiple hamartoma and neoplasia syndrome. *Clin Exp Dermatol* 1985; **10**: 262–8.
8 Brownstein MH, Wolf M, Bikowski J. Cowden's disease: a cutaneous marker of breast cancer. *Cancer* 1978; **41**: 2393–8.

Sebaceous tumours, keratoacanthomas and visceral malignancy (Muir–Torre syndrome, MTS, Torre syndrome; MIM 158320) [1–6]

This is a cancer-associated genodermatosis in which there is an association between sebaceous lesions and, to a lesser extent, keratoacanthomas and internal malignancy. Inheritance is autosomal dominant with variable expression, males being affected more commonly than females. MTS has been considered to be a variant of the 'cancer family syndrome' [3]; it is currently viewed as a phenotypic variant of the hereditary non-polyposis colon cancer syndrome (HNPCC; Lynch syndrome). Both syndromes are due to mutations at the same region of chromosome 2p22-p21 in the genes *MLH1* and *MSH2*, which are DNA mismatch repair enzymes. Defects result in microsatellite instability, a finding in HNPCC which has also been documented in many MTS-associated keratoacanthomas and sebaceous tumours [6]. About 1% of patients with HNPCC have features of MTS, although this may be an underestimate as the cutaneous features may occur after the development of internal malignancy, or may go unrecognized.

Sebaceous tumours are usually multiple, but occasionally solitary. Although sebaceous adenoma is the commonest, sebaceous carcinoma and epithelioma frequently occur, and within the same patient a variety of different pilosebaceous-derived skin lesions

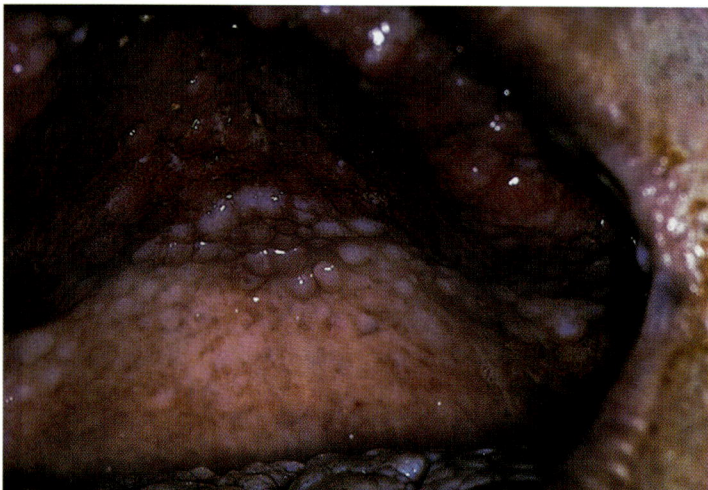

Fig. 62.12 Warty papillomatosis of the hard palate in Cowden's disease. (Courtesy of Dr R. Emmerson, Royal Berkshire Hospital, Reading, UK.)

including keratoacanthomas may arise. Most skin tumours occur in middle age, keratoacanthomas occurring in a quarter of affected subjects. Multiple or early onset of keratoacanthomas are suggestive of this diagnosis, as are multiple (especially eyelid) sebaceous tumours. Multiple or solitary keratoacanthomas associated with SCC of the larynx and lower gastrointestinal tract [7,8] probably represent a variant of MTS in which expression of sebaceous tumours and adenocarcinomas is not exhibited. The cutaneous manifestations of MTS have been reported to be exacerbated by immunosuppression.

The most important internal malignancy is colonic adenocarcinoma, which occurs in almost 50%, often at a relatively young age—around 10 years earlier than in the normal population—and most commonly in the region of the splenic flexure; rectal adenocarcinomas also occur but only in about 5% [4,5]. Urogenital malignancies are also common, occurring in 25% [4]; bladder, renal pelvis and endometrial cancers each account for about 5% of cancers in MTS. The proband in the first family described with HNPCC died of endometrial carcinoma, and gynaecological cancers of various types occur both in HNPCC patients [9] and in those with MTS [4]. Nearly half of affected patients have two or more internal malignancies [10]; other notable malignancies are breast cancers and haematological malignancies (each in about 5% of subjects) [4]. Despite the high risk of malignancy, both the malignant cutaneous sebaceous tumours and the colonic tumours tend to have relatively indolent behaviour (the 50% survival time for colonic cancers is about 12 years [2]) and the incidence of metastases is relatively low. Criteria for diagnosis (Amsterdam and Bethesda criteria), and recommendations for screening of patients and relatives, have been reviewed [11].

References

1 Lynch HT, Fusaro RM, eds. *Cancer-Associated Genodermatoses.* New York: Van Nostrand Reinhold, 1982.

2 Schwarz RA, Torre DP. The Muir–Torre syndrome: a 25-year retrospect. *J Am Acad Dermatol* 1995; **33**: 90–104.

3 Hall NR, Williams AT, Murday VA *et al.* Muir–Torre syndrome: a variant of the cancer family syndrome. *J Med Genet* 1994; **31**: 627–31.

4 Cohen PR, Kohn SR, Davis DA, Kurzrock R. Muir–Torre syndrome. *Dermatol Clinics* 1995; **13**: 79–89.

5 Smoller BR. Muir–Torre syndrome. In: Morgan MB, Smoller BR, Somach SC. *Deadly Dermatologic Diseases. Clinicopathologic Atlas and Text.* New York: Springer, 2007: 53–8.

6 Somoano B, Tsao H. Genodermatoses with cutaneous tumors and internal malignancies. *Dermatol Clinics* 2008; **26**: 69–87.

7 Chapman RS, Finn OA. Carcinoma of the larynx in two patients with keratoacanthoma. *Br J Dermatol* 1974; **90**: 685–8.

8 Stewart WM, Lauret P, Hemet J *et al.* Kératoacanthomes multiples et carcinomes viscéraux: syndrome de Torre. *Ann Dermatol Vénéréol* 1977; **104**: 622–6.

9 Offit K, Kauff ND. Reducing the risk of gynecologic cancer in the Lynch syndrome. *N Engl J Med* 2006; **354**: 293–5.

10 Serleth HJ, Kisken WA. A Muir–Torre syndrome family. *Am Surgeon* 1998; **64**: 365–9.

11 Jones B, Oh C, Mangold E, Egan CA. Muir–Torre syndrome: diagnostic and screening guidelines. *Austral J Dermatol* 2006; **47**: 266–9.

Bloom's, Rothmund–Thomson's and Werner's syndromes

These conditions are considered together as they are all caused by RecQ helicase gene mutations, and they all predispose to abnormal growth, premature ageing and increased incidence of site-specific malignancies [1].

Reference

1 Lindor NM, Furuichi Y, Kitao S *et al.* Rothmund–Thomson syndrome due to RECQ4 helicase mutations: report and clinical and molecular comparisons with Bloom syndrome and Werner syndrome. *Am J Med Genet* 2000; **90**: 223–8.

Bloom's syndrome (MIM *210900) (Chapter 15) [1–4]. This is an autosomal recessive disorder that affects principally the Ashkenazi Jewish ethnic group, nearly 1% of whom are carriers. Affected subjects have small stature and slight build, a sun-sensitive telangiectatic facial rash and café-au-lait macules. Minor congenital anatomical abnormalities commonly occur. Levels of IgA and IgM are low and bacterial infections frequent. Mutations of the gene designated *BLM* on chromosome 15q26.1 lead to inhibition of the function of the protein product, a DNA helicase enzyme. This loss of function allows genomic instability with the occurrence of significantly increased exchanges between DNA strands during the S phase of mitosis, including a tenfold increase in sister chromatid exchanges, such that mutations occur throughout the genome.

The occurrence of lymphoproliferative neoplasia (approximately equally divided between leukaemias and lymphomas) and epithelial tissue cancers, particularly of the aerodigestive tract and lower gastrointestinal tumours, is very high; they typically occur at an early age, and the mean age of death is 23 years [3]. Cervical cancer and Wilms' tumour are additional risks. There is a predisposition to malignancy through mutations in other target genes [4].

References

1 Gretzula JC, Hevia O, Weber PJ. Bloom's syndrome. *J Am Acad Dermatol* 1987; **17**: 479–88.

2 Clark LW. Genetic diseases associated with DNA and chromosomal instability. *Dermatol Clin* 1987; **5**: 85–108.

3 German J. Bloom's syndrome. *Dermatol Clinics* 1995; **13**: 7–18.

4 Tsao H. Update on familial cancer syndromes and the skin. *J Am Acad Dermatol* 2000; **42**: 939–46.

Rothmund–Thomson syndrome (RTS; poikiloderma congenitale; MIM #268400) (Chapter 15) [1–3]. This is a rare autosomal recessive genetic disease, characterized by developmental abnormalities in the skin and skeletal systems, with photosensitivity, poikiloderma, small stature and juvenile cataracts. Premature ageing and a predisposition to certain malignancies occur, notably an approximate 30% incidence of osteosarcoma. Fibrosarcoma, myelodysplasia and non-melanoma skin cancer also occur. A mutation of genes for RecQ helicase is thought to be responsible for at least some, if not all, cases of RTS.

References

1 Lindor NM, Furuichi Y, Kitao S *et al.* Rothmund–Thomson syndrome due to RECQ4 helicase mutations: report and clinical and molecular comparisons with Bloom syndrome and Werner syndrome. *Am J Med Genet* 2000; **90**: 223–8.

2 Narayan S, Fleming C, Trainer AH *et al.* Rothmund–Thomson syndrome with myelodysplasia. *Pediatric Dermatol* 2001; **18**: 210–2.

3 Wang LL, Levy ML, Lewis RA *et al.* Clinical manifestations in a cohort of 41 Rothmund–Thomson syndrome patients. *Am J Med Genet* 2001; **102**: 11–7.

Werner's syndrome (adult progeria; MIM #277700) [1–4]. This is an autosomal-recessive condition of premature ageing, with onset in the second to third decade of life. It is due to mutation of the *WRN* gene on chromosome 8p12-p11.2. The normal gene product is a DNA helicase belonging to the RecQ family which unwinds double-stranded DNA and is able to resolve aberrant DNA structures, so that aberrations occurring during repair, recombination and replication are made good, together with those that result from direct DNA damage [1–4]. Neoplasms develop in about 10% of cases, although the commonest cause of death is arteriosclerosis. Sarcomas, melanomas, leukaemia and a variety of epithelial-derived carcinomas have been reported [1–6]. Meningiomas are a recognized association, and an astrocytoma has been documented [7]. Werner's syndrome is a chromosome-instability syndrome and, as with XP, ataxia–telangiectasia, Bloom's syndrome and Fanconi's anaemia, is associated with a high incidence of neoplasia [2,3].

References

1 Duvic M, Lemak NA. Werner's syndrome. *Dermatol Clin* 1995; **13**: 163–8.
2 Callen JP. Skin signs of internal malignancy. In: Callen JP, Jorizzo JL, eds. *Dermatological Manifestations of Internal Disease*, 3rd edn. Philadelphia: Saunders, 2003: 95–104.
3 Tsao H. Update on familial cancer syndromes and the skin. *J Am Acad Dermatol* 2000; **42**: 939–46.
4 Shen J, Loeb LA. Unwinding the molecular basis of the Werner syndrome. *Mech Ageing Dev* 2001; **122**: 921–44.
5 Hrabko RP, Milgrom H, Schwartz RA. Werner's syndrome with associated malignant neoplasms. *Arch Dermatol* 1982; **118**: 106–8.
6 Usui M, Ishii S, Yamawaki S *et al.* The occurrence of soft tissue sarcomas in three siblings with Werner's syndrome. *Cancer* 1984; **54**: 2580–6.
7 Laso FJ, Vasquez G, Pastor I *et al.* Werner's syndrome and astrocytoma. *Dermatologica* 1989; **178**: 118–20.

Immunodeficiency and neoplasia syndromes: Wiskott–Aldrich syndrome, Chediak–Higashi syndrome, ataxia–telangiectasia, dyskeratosis congenita, Fanconi's anaemia

Wiskott–Aldrich syndrome (MIM #301000) (Chapter 15) [1]. This is an X-linked recessive immunodeficiency syndrome due to mutations at Xp11.23-p11.22; the Wiskott–Aldrich syndrome protein (WASP) is expressed in all haemopoietic cells, and mutations cause defective T-cell function and thrombocytopenia. Infections are the commonest cause of death but lymphoreticular malignancy occurs in 18% and is the cause of death in about 10% [1,2]. Non-Hodgkin's lymphoma occurs in almost all subjects who survive infections or bleeding due to thrombocytopenia, usually by the age of 30 years. Lymphoma (especially large cell or immunoblastic) and leukaemia occur; the small intestine is a particular site for lymphomatous involvement. Cerebral tumours such as astrocytoma, and various sarcomas, have also been reported [1–4].

References

1 Paller AS. Immunodeficiency syndromes. In: Harper J, Oranje A, Prose N. *Textbook of Pediatric Dermatology*, 2nd edn. Oxford: Blackwell Publishing, 2006: 2052–73.
2 Ormerod AD. The Wiskott–Aldrich syndrome. *Int J Dermatol* 1985; **24**: 77–81.
3 Model LM. Primary reticulum cell sarcoma of the brain in Wiskott–Aldrich syndrome. *Arch Neurol* 1977; **34**: 633–5.
4 Heidelberger KP, Le Golvan DP. Wiskott–Aldrich syndrome and cerebral neoplasia: report of a case with localised reticulum cell sarcoma. *Cancer* 1974; **24**: 280–4.

Chediak–Higashi syndrome (MIM #214500) (Chapter 15) [1,2]. This is a fatal autosomal recessive illness, with features of partial albinism, photophobia, neurological abnormalities and severe, recurrent bacterial infections. About 85% of patients develop a terminal, accelerated 'lymphomatous' phase, which may be triggered by viral infections, especially due to Epstein–Barr virus [2]. There is extensive organ infiltration with lymphoid and histiocytic cells; patients develop fever, jaundice, hepatosplenomegaly, lymphadenopathy, leukaemia-like gingival lesions and sloughing of the oral mucosa, pancytopenia and a deterioration of neurological changes. Death may result from bleeding due to thrombocytopenia and reduced synthesis of clotting factors, or from infection due to neutropenia. Although strongly suggestive of lymphoma, the infiltrate of affected organs is reported to be of a reactive, diffuse, mononuclear cell type, rather than neoplastic [1].

Ataxia–telangiectasia syndrome (AT; Louis–Bar syndrome; MIM *208900) (Chapter 15) [3–9]. This is a condition with autosomal recessive inheritance, characterized by progressive cerebellar ataxia and oculocutaneous telangiectasia. Like XP, the condition has different complementation groups defined by fibroblast fusion and irradiation studies. Most families have one of many different germ-line mutations in the large *ATM* gene at chromosome 11q22.3; the product, ATM protein (phosphatidylinositol-3-kinase p53 checkpoint regulation), is involved in the handling of chromosome strand breaks and activation of the p53 oncogene [6], and has been considered to be a 'caretaker' of the genome and tumour suppressor. Mutations are mainly inactivating in type but may be missense [9]; they allow unregulated DNA synthesis, with DNA that is predisposed to instability and hypersensitive to ionizing radiation [6]. Peripheral blood lymphocytes are abnormal, having translocations mainly involving chromosomes 7 and 14, and abnormal function, and there is a variable but progressive immune deficiency of both the cell-mediated and humoral types, which results in frequent infections and a reduction in immune surveillance [3]. As a result, there is a high incidence of neoplasia, approximately 30% lifetime risk, usually in or before the teenage years, and being the cause of death in 15% of affected individuals [3–8].

The majority (around 80%) of tumours are lymphoproliferative or leukaemic, although carcinomas of various sites also occur, the latter usually in older subjects [5,7,8]. Most haematological malignancies are B-cell lymphomas but 25% are leukaemias, notably chronic T-cell leukaemia with chromosome 14 translocations, occurring in older patients. However, T-cell leukaemias do occur in younger patients, and both T-cell lymphomas and B-cell leukaemias are also encountered. Most tumours have early onset, and may precede diagnosis of AT from the cutaneous features; this is of considerable importance as standard radiotherapy doses are contraindicated. Heterozygotes (carriers) have a five to tenfold increased risk of tumours, usually not lymphoid, including a five-fold increase in risk of breast malignancy in females [4,6]. Atm-deficient mice also develop lymphomas.

Dyskeratosis congenita (Zinsser–Cole–Engman syndrome; MIM #305000) (Chapter 15) [10]. This is a multisystem ectodermal dysplasia, in which a triad of cutaneous abnormalities are the most consistent and diagnostic feature, comprising reticulate hyperpigmentation of the skin, nail dystrophy and leukokeratosis of mucous membranes. Dental, skeletal, ocular and gastrointestinal abnormalities are common; mental retardation, short stature and premature ageing also occur. Most cases have X-linked recessive inheritance (linked to Xq28) but autosomal recessive and autosomal dominant forms also occur [10].

Aplastic anaemia occurs in 50%, typically in early teens. Oropharyngeal carcinomas secondary to the mucous membrane lesions are the commonest form of malignancy; there is also increased incidence of internal malignancy, particularly gastrointestinal, including pancreatic adenocarcinoma and other haematological disorders, similar to those found in Fanconi's anaemia and Hodgkin's disease, which may evolve into leukaemia [11,12]. A defect in cell-mediated immunity involving suppressor T cells may be linked to the premature ageing sometimes associated with this syndrome [13].

Fanconi's anaemia (MIM #227650 and others). This is an autosomal recessive disorder characterized dermatologically by pigmentary abnormalities which may be diffuse (with accentuation around the neck and over joints), mottled, often with scattered darker macules, and sometimes just exhibiting localized café-au-lait macules. Scattered areas of hypopigmentation are a common finding. The main abnormality is progressive pancytopenia, which may lead eventually to development of leukaemia. Multiple skeletal abnormalities occur, including digital hypoplasias, scoliosis and short stature. The underlying defect is one of increased DNA cross-linkage (especially radiation-induced) and defective DNA repair.

References

1 Stolz W, Graubner U, Gerstmeier J et al. Chediak–Higashi syndrome: approaches in diagnosis and treatment. *Curr Probl Dermatol* 1989; **18**: 93–100.
2 Paller AS. Immunodeficiency syndromes. In: Harper J, Oranje A, Prose N. *Textbook of Pediatric Dermatology*, 2nd edn. Oxford: Blackwell Publishing, 2006: 2052–73.
3 Spector BD, Fillipivich AH, Perry SS et al. Epidemiology of cancer in ataxia telangiectasia. In: Bridges BA, Harnden DG, eds. *Ataxia Telangiectasia: a Cellular and Molecular Link Between Cancer Neuropathy and Immune Deficiency*. New York: Wiley, 1982: 103–38.
4 Gatti RA. Ataxia-telangiectasia. *Dermatol Clinics* 1995; **13**: 1–6.
5 Swift M, Morrell D, Massey RB et al. Incidence of cancer in 161 families affected by ataxia–telangiectasia. *N Engl J Med* 1991; **325**: 1831–6.
6 Tsao H. Update on familial cancer syndromes and the skin. *J Am Acad Dermatol* 2000; **42**: 939–46.
7 Morgan MB. Lethal hereditary vascular disorders: Osler-Weber-Rendu, ataxia telangiectasia, and Fabry's disease. In: Morgan MB, Smoller BR, Somach SC. *Deadly Dermatologic Diseases. Clinicopathologic Atlas and Text*. New York: Springer, 2007: 145–9.
8 Callen JP. Skin signs of internal malignancy. In: Callen JP, Jorizzo JL, eds. *Dermatological Manifestations of Internal Disease*, 3rd edn. Philadelphia: Saunders, 2003: 95–104.
9 Boultwood J. Ataxia telangiectasia gene mutations in leukaemia and lymphoma. *J Cutan Pathol* 2001; **54**: 512–6.
10 Drachtman RA, Alter BP. Dyskeratosis congenita. *Dermatol Clinics* 1995; **13**: 33–9.
11 Clark Lambert W. Genetic diseases associated with DNA and chromosomal instability. *Dermatol Clin* 1987; **5**: 85–108.
12 Connor JM, Teague RH. Dyskeratosis congenita: report of a large kindred. *Br J Dermatol* 1981; **105**: 321–5.
13 Fudenberg HH, Goust JM, Vesole DH, Salinas CF. Active and suppressor T cells: diminution in a patient with dyskeratosis congenita and in first-degree relatives. *Gerontology* 1979; **25**: 231–7.

Follicular atrophoderma (Bazex–Dupré–Christol syndrome; MIM *301845) [1]

A rare, X-linked, dominant condition of follicular atrophoderma, milia, epidermoid cysts, hypotrichosis, basal cell epitheliomas and occasional generalized or localized hypohidrosis, which appears to have an association with leukaemia. Pigmented, perioral, follicular atrophoderma is characteristic [2].

References

1 Colomb D, Ducros B, Boussuge N. Le syndrome de Bazex, Dupré et Christol. A propos d'un cas avec leucémie prolymphocytaire. *Ann Dermatol Vénéréol* 1989; **116**: 381–7.
2 Inoue Y, Ono T, Kayashima K et al. Hereditary perioral pigmented follicular atrophoderma associated with milia and epidermoid cysts. *Br J Dermatol* 1998; **139**: 713–8.

Hereditary leiomyomatosis and renal cell carcinoma (HLRCC) syndrome (MIM #605839)

A syndrome comprising multiple cutaneous leiomyomas with uterine leiomyomas (Reed syndrome, MIM #150800); in some cases (2% in one series [1]) there is also an association with aggressive renal cell carcinoma, mainly of papillary cell type. Numerous different fumarate hydratase (FH) mutations on chromosome 1q 42.1 have been identified; patients who have renal cell carcinomas are usually female and have truncating or frameshift mutations [1]. One study of 40 such renal carcinomas found that the presence of a large nucleus, with a prominent orangiophilic or eosinophilic nucleolus surrounded by a clear halo, appeared to be characteristic and was seen even in the renal carcinomas that were not papillary or tubulopapillary in type [2]. Most women with HLRCC develop uterine leiomyomas ('fibroids'). Benign ovarian mucinous cystadenomas, renal cysts and adrenal gland adenomas, as well as uterine leiomyosarcomas, have also been linked with FH mutations; there is also some evidence for an association with breast and bladder cancers [3] and a suggested association with Leydig cell carcinoma of testis.

References

1 Alam NA, Olpin S, Leigh IM. Fumarate hydratase mutations and predisposition to cutaneous leiomyomas, uterine leiomyomas and renal cancer. *Br J Dermatol* 2005; **153**: 11–7.
2 Merino MJ, Torres-Cabala C, Pinto P, Linehan WM. The morphologic spectrum of kidney tumors in hereditary leiomyomatosis and renal cell carcinoma (HLRCC) syndrome. *Am J Surg Pathol* 2007; **31**: 1578–85.
3 Lehtonen HJ, Kiura M, Ylisaukko-Oja SK et al. Increased risk of cancer in patients with fumarate hydratase germline mutation. *J Med Genet* 2006; **43**: 523–6.

Paraneoplastic disorders [1–14]

Paraneoplastic dermatoses are skin conditions that have an association with internal malignancy but are not themselves malignant. They may be classified in a variety of ways; some authors include genodermatoses within the spectrum of paraneoplastic disorders [1] whilst others view these as a separate group [2,3], or distinguish between paraneoplastic dermatoses [4], hereditary paraneoplastic syndromes [5] and hormonally mediated paraneoplastic syndromes [6]. They may be classified according to strength of association with malignancy, association with certain types of malignancy [13,14], by the type of eruption that occurs (papulosquamous, vascular, etc.) or by the apparent mechanism (hormone secretion, autoimmune, cytokine/growth factor, etc.). Paraneoplastic conditions occur in other organ systems as well, but whatever system is affected there are general principles that can be applied to determine a relationship.

Helen Ollendorff Curth proposed criteria for diagnosis of a paraneoplastic dermatosis (discussed in [7]):

1 Both conditions start at approximately the same time
2 Both conditions follow a parallel course
3 In syndromes, neither the onset nor the course of either condition is dependent on the other
4 A specific tumour occurs with a specific skin manifestation
5 The dermatosis is not common in the general population
6 A high percentage of association between the two conditions is noted

These criteria were quite specific and some conditions that would now be viewed as potentially paraneoplastic, such as acquired ichthyosis, would fail to meet several of the above criteria.

A less rigid definition that has been in common use is as follows [1]:

1 The malignancy and the cutaneous disorder may occur concurrently
2 The two disorders may follow a parallel course

3 There can be a specific tumour site or cell type associated with the cutaneous disease
4 There may be a statistical association between the two processes
5 There may be a genetic association between the two processes

Those disorders with a genetic link between the dermatological features and internal malignancy are discussed above; this section discusses other paraneoplastic dermatoses. Specific tumour sites are discussed in the following sections although this text is arranged in categories of types of presentation. In terms of the intensity of investigation required, it is also helpful to divide paraneoplastic disorders into groups depending on the likelihood of an underlying neoplasm being discovered. Thus, the likelihood of finding a neoplasm may be graded as high, intermediate or low for some of the better known paraneoplastic disorders (Table 62.9), as derived from several reviews [1–15].

References

1 Callen JP. Skin signs of internal malignancy. In: Callen JP, Jorizzo JL, eds. *Dermatological Manifestations of Internal Disease*, 3rd edn. Philadelphia: Saunders, 2003: 95–104.
2 Poole S, Fenske NA. Cutaneous markers of internal malignancy, 1: malignant involvement of the skin and the genodermatoses. *J Am Acad Dermatol* 1993; **28**: 1–13.

Table 62.9 Strength of correlation of some potentially paraneoplastic dermatoses with internal malignancy.

Strength of correlation	Type of reaction pattern	Examples
Strong	Papulosquamous and figurate eruptions	Bazex syndrome
		Erythema gyratum repens
		Necrolytic migratory erythema
	Deposition disorders	Primary amyloidosis
		Scleromyxedema
		Necrobiotic xanthogranuloma
		POEMS syndrome
	Others	Acquired hypertrichosis lanuginosa
		Paraneoplastic pemphigus
		Tripe palms
		Carcinoid syndrome
		Trousseau's syndrome
Moderate	Papulosquamous and neutrophilic eruptions	Sweet's syndrome
		Pyoderma gangrenosum
		Dermatomyositis
	Others	Multicentric reticulohistiocytosis
		Pityriasis rotunda
Weak	Epidermal conditions	Acanthosis nigricans in isolation
		Acquired ichthyosis (unless widespread, deeply fissured, truncal pattern)
		Eruptive seborrhoeic keratoses (sign of Leser–Trélat)
	Deposition disorders	Scleredema
		Calcinosis cutis
	Others	Vasculitis, Raynaud's phenomenon, digital ischaemia
		Erythromelalgia
		Relapsing polychondritis
		Erythroderma/exfoliative dermatitis
		Digital clubbing (unless with hypertrophic osteoarthropathy)
		Pruritus
		Erythema annulare centrifugum
		Cushing's syndrome

3 Poole S, Fenske NA. Cutaneous markers of internal malignancy, 2: paraneoplastic dermatoses and environmental carcinogens. *J Am Acad Dermatol* 1993; **28**: 147–64.

4 Provost TT, Laman SD, Bell WR. Paraneoplastic dermatoses. In: Provost TT, Flynn JA, eds. *Cutaneous Medicine: Cutaneous Manifestations of Systemic Disease.* Hamilton, Ontario: Decker, 2001: 367–88.

5 Provost TT, Laman SD, Giardiello FM. Hereditary paraneoplastic syndromes. In: Provost TT, Flynn JA, eds. *Cutaneous Medicine: Cutaneous Manifestations of Systemic Disease.* Hamilton, Ontario: Decker, 2001: 389–400.

6 Provost TT, Gordon AH, Laman SD. Hormonally mediated paraneoplastic syndromes. In: Provost TT, Flynn JA, eds. *Cutaneous Medicine: Cutaneous Manifestations of Systemic Disease.* Hamilton, Ontario: Decker, 2001: 401–12.

7 Chung VQ, Moschella SL, Zembowicz A, Liu V. Clinical and pathologic findings of paraneoplastic dermatoses. *J Am Acad Dermatol* 2006; **54**: 745–62.

8 Boyce S, Harper J. Paraneoplastic dermatoses. *Dermatol Clin* 2002; **20**: 523–32.

9 Thomas VD, Thomas CR, eds. Internal malignancy and the skin: paraneoplastic and cancer treatment-related cutaneous disorders. *Dermatol Clinics* 2008; **26**: 1–182.

10 Pipkin CA, Lio PA. Cutaneous manifestations of internal malignancies: an overview. *Dermatol Clin* 2008; **26**: 1–15.

11 Stone SP, Buescher LS. Life-threatening paraneoplastic cutaneous syndromes. *Clinics Dermatol* 2005; **23**: 301–6.

12 Thomas I, Schwartz RA. Cutaneous paraneoplastic syndromes: uncommon presentations. *Clinics Dermatol* 2005; **23**: 593–600.

13 Roumm A, Medsger TJ. Cancer in connective tissue disease. *Arthritis Rheum* 1982; **25**: 1130–3.

14 Cohen PR. Paraneoplastic dermatopathology: cutaneous paraneoplastic syndromes. *Adv Dermatol* 1996; **11**: 215–52.

15 Zappasodi P, Del Forna C, Corso A, Lazzarino M. Mucocutaneous paraneoplastic syndromes in hematologic malignancies. *Int J Dermatol* 2006; **45**: 14–22.

Acanthotic, epidermal and ichthyotic conditions

Acanthosis nigricans [1–5]

Acanthosis nigricans may be simply divided into two important categories, benign (see also Chapter 19) and malignant, although Schwartz [1] described eight types of acanthosis nigricans: benign, obesity-associated, syndromic, malignant, acral, unilateral, medication-induced (especially nicotinic acid) and mixed types. Benign acanthosis nigricans is actually fairly common, especially in obesity or in individuals with insulin resistance, and is usually relatively mild; it has been documented in up to 7% of children, mainly in teenage years, and virtually all childhood cases are of benign type.

Malignancy-associated acanthosis nigricans is much less common than the non-malignancy-associated types. It may have a rapid onset and progression to produce symmetrical, hyperpigmented, rugose velvety plaques [1–5]. The axillae and other flexures are particularly affected, along with the areolar area, and the nape of the neck. There may be prominent acrochordon-like papillomatosis arising from the plaques; the sign of Leser–Trélat, and acanthosis palmaris (tripe palms) may coexist [5]. *De novo* development of acanthosis nigricans in adults, especially if progressive and associated with weight loss (most patients with insulin resistance having a rather stocky build), is strongly suspicious that there is an underlying neoplasm, although cases have been described in which acanthosis nigricans has preceded a malignancy by 10 years or more [2]. If there is also generalized pruritus or the skin changes of tripe palms (see below), then a malignancy is even more likely; mucosal involvement is a useful pointer to the diagnosis of paraneoplastic acanthosis nigricans as it occurs in over half of cases [6]. Production by tumour cells of either transforming growth factor-alpha, or cytokines that activate insulin-

like growth factors or their cutaneous receptors, have been suggested as the pathogenetic mechanism.

By far the commonest site of underlying neoplasm is the gastrointestinal tract (70–90%); gastric adenocarcinoma is most frequent [1–5]. A number of different malignancies have been reported, nearly all being adenocarcinomas, at sites including other parts of the intestine, liver or bile duct; other tumour sites include lung, breast, endometrium, kidney, bladder, prostate, testis, cervix, thyroid and adrenal. Most are solid organ tumours but lymphoma has been recorded [7]. Sarcomas occur rarely. The prognosis with malignant acanthosis nigricans is generally poor, which at least in part is related to the low survival rate from the neoplasia concerned. However, the changes may resolve with eradication of the cancer [8]. Malignancy-associated acanthosis nigricans has rarely been associated with other paraneoplastic conditions including pachydermoperiostosis, paraneoplastic pemphigus and acquired hypertrichosis lanuginosa.

An additional, indirect link between acanthosis nigricans and internal malignancy is that it may be associated with ataxia–telangiectasia (p. 62.28).

References

1 Schwartz RA. Acanthosis nigricans. *J Am Acad Dermatol* 1994; **31**: 1–19.

2 Thomas I, Schwartz RA. Cutaneous paraneoplastic syndromes: uncommon presentations. *Clinics Dermatol* 2005; **23**: 593–600.

3 Stone SP, Buescher LS. Life-threatening paraneoplastic cutaneous syndromes. *Clinics Dermatol* 2005; **23**: 301–6.

4 Curth HO. Classification of acanthosis nigricans. *Int J Dermatol* 1976; **15**: 592–3.

5 Moore RL, Devere TS. Epidermal manifestations of internal malignancy. *Dermatol Clinics* 2008; **26**: 17–29.

6 Longshore SL, Taylor JS, Kennedy A, Nurko S. Malignant acanthosis nigricans and endometrial carcinoma of the parametrium: the search for malignancy. *J Am Acad Dermatol* 2003; **49**: 541–3.

7 Janier M, Blanchet-Bardon C, Bonvalet D *et al.* Malignant acanthosis nigricans associated with non-Hodgkin's lymphoma. *Dermatologica* 1988; **176**: 133–7.

8 Moller H, Eriksson S, Holen O *et al.* Complete reversibility of paraneoplastic acanthosis nigricans after operation. *Acta Med Scand* 1978; **203**: 245–6.

Acanthosis palmaris (Tripe palms, pachydermatoglyphy) [1–4]

Tripe palms describes thickened skin of the palms and occasionally the soles, with an enhanced dermatoglyphic change, causing a velvety or, less commonly, a pitted honeycombed pattern of the hand. It is associated with neoplasia in about 90% of cases; it may be the only paraneoplastic manifestation in 30–40% or it may occur with one or both of malignant acanthosis nigricans or the sign of Leser–Trélat [1–3]. It occurs particularly in men, especially when it occurs in isolation or when the underlying tumour is a lung cancer [2]. However, it can occur in isolation without neoplasia, or as a pattern of exfoliative psoriasis or eczema [1,2], and has been reported with bullous pemphigoid.

As the condition is usually associated with an internal neoplasm, usually of solid organ type (but rarely lymphoma), it requires appropriate evaluation and investigation. Most commonly the underlying tumour is bronchial or gastric, together accounting for over half of associated malignancy, but many sites are reported including tumours of genitourinary tract, breast and others [2]. One study found that acanthosis palmaris occurring alone was more often associated with bronchial carcinoma (53%) compared with combined acanthosis nigricans and acanthosis palmaris, in which 35% had gastric carcinoma and only 11% had bronchial neoplasia [4]. If nail clubbing is also present (18% of patients [2]), then bronchial carcinoma is very likely. Thus, tripe palms alone, especially if the patient is male and also has clubbing, very strongly suggests an underlying lung cancer, whilst tripe palms with acanthosis nigricans is more suggestive of an underlying gastric carcinoma. Resolution of the palmar changes has been described with resection of the tumour [4].

References
1 Breathnach SM, Wells GC. Acanthosis palmaris: tripe palms—a distinctive pattern of palmar keratoderma frequently associated with internal malignancy. *Clin Exp Dermatol* 1980; **5**: 181–9.
2 Moore RL, Devere TS. Epidermal manifestations of internal malignancy. *Dermatol Clinics* 2008; **26**: 17–29.
3 Cohen PR, Grossman ME, Silvers DN *et al.* Tripe palms and cancer. *Clin Dermatol* 1993; **11**: 165–73.
4 Votion V, Mineur P, Mirgaux M *et al.* Hyperkératose palmoplantaire associée à un adénocarcinome gastrique. *Dermatologica* 1982; **165**: 660–3.

The sign of Leser–Trélat [1–4]

This is the sudden development of numerous seborrhoeic keratoses, in an eruptive fashion, with or without pruritus, as an indicator of internal malignancy. However, the significance of eruptive seborrhoeic keratoses remains unclear, with strong proponents and opponents of its importance [2,3]. Multiple seborrhoeic keratoses are extremely common, especially in elderly people, and may be pruritic or rapidly erupting, without any apparent cause; they may also occur in other situations [4] such as HIV infection, acromegaly, and in the resolving phase of erythrodermic dermatoses [5].

Of the cases reported with a neoplasm, half of the tumours are adenocarcinomas, most of which (one-third of the associated tumours) arise in the gastrointestinal tract; this is similar to the distribution of tumours in acanthosis nigricans, which may coexist. Carcinomas of the breast are also frequent, although this may just reflect the incidence of these tumours in an age group who are also likely to have seborrhoeic keratoses. Rare associations have been documented with a variety of other neoplasms, including malignant haemangiopericytoma [6], malignant melanoma [7], renal carcinoma [4] and transitional cell carcinoma of the bladder [8]. Lymphoproliferative disorders, which are rarely associated with acanthosis nigricans, have been more commonly reported with the sign of Leser–Trélat, accounting for about 20% of associated tumours [4].

Truly sudden development of multiple seborrhoeic keratosis, especially in younger patients, and especially if associated with pruritus or with acanthosis nigricans, does warrant investigation, but the mere presence of many seborrhoeic keratoses is unlikely to be linked with malignancy and the strength of this sign as a marker of internal malignancy must be viewed as uncertain.

References
1 De Bersaques J. Sign of Leser–Trélat. *J Am Acad Dermatol* 1985; **12**: 724.
2 Holdiness MR. On the classification of the sign of Leser–Trélat. *J Am Acad Dermatol* 1988; **19**: 754–7.
3 Rampen FH, Schwengle LE. The sign of Leser–Trélat: does it exist? *J Am Acad Dermatol* 1989; **21**: 50–5.

4 Moore RL, Devere TS. Epidermal manifestations of internal malignancy. *Dermatol Clinics* 2008; **26**: 17–29.
5 Williams MG. Acanthomata appearing after eczema. *Br J Dermatol* 1956; **68**: 268–71.
6 Mayou SC, Benn JJ, Sonksen PH *et al.* Paraneoplastic rhinophyma and the Leser–Trélat sign. *Clin Exp Dermatol* 1989; **14**: 253–5.
7 Fanti PA, Metri M, Patrizi A. The sign of Leser–Trélat associated with malignant melanoma. *Cutis* 1989; **44**: 39–41.
8 Yaniv R, Servadio Y, Feinstein A *et al.* The sign of Leser–Trélat associated with transitional cell carcinoma of the urinary bladder: a case report and short review. *Clin Exp Dermatol* 1994; **19**: 142–5.

Acquired ichthyosis [1–5] and pityriasis rotunda

Acquired ichthyosis usually has gradual onset, consists of a mild dryness or asteatosis pattern, and is not associated with underlying malignancy. Other systemic diseases associated with acquired ichthyosis include nutritional deficiencies, sarcoidosis, leprosy, HIV infection, hypothyroidism, lupus erythematosus, graft-versus-host disease and drug reactions [2]. Some of these cause particular problems in differential diagnosis as well, especially sarcoidosis which may itself have an association with lymphoma (p. 62.40). Asteatosis is a common problem cause, especially in elderly people, and does not warrant an extensive search for malignancy unless there are other suggestive features such as weight loss or focal symptoms.

However, more sudden onset of ichthyosis similar to the pattern of ichthyosis vulgaris in adult life, or with a generalized eczema craquelé appearance, does suggest the possibility of internal malignancy, particularly if it occurs in a younger age group. The strongest association is with Hodgkin's disease (accounting for over 70% of cases) and other lymphoreticular tumours, including T-cell lymphomas, leukaemias, myelodysplastic syndrome, multiple myeloma and polycythaemia rubra vera [1–4], although cases linked with solid tumours are also well documented [4], including cancers of ovary, kidney, liver and breast [5] as well as leiomyosarcoma [2]. Paraneoplastic ichthyosis is typically very extensive, affecting the trunk and having quite prominent fissuring; a parallel course with the underlying lymphoma (including resolution related to treatment) is also usual. Other paraneoplastic signs have been reported to be present in conjunction with acquired ichthyosis, including erythema gyratum repens, Bazex syndrome and dermatomyositis [4].

Pityriasis rotunda [4,6] is a fixed, annular, scaling, dry-skin change more often seen in the African and Asian races—it has been associated with neoplasia, particularly hepatocellular carcinoma. However, it may also be seen in other systemic diseases and in leprosy [4,6].

References
1 Elewski BE, Gilgor RS. Eruptive lesions and malignancy. *Int J Dermatol* 1985; **24**: 617–29.
2 Patel N, Spencer LA, English JC 3rd, Zirwas MJ. Acquired ichthyosis. *J Am Acad Dermatol* 2006; **55**: 647–56.
3 Moore RL, Devere TS. Epidermal manifestations of internal malignancy. *Dermatol Clinics* 2008; **26**: 17–29.
4 Griffin LJ, Massa MC. Acquired ichthyosis and pityriasis rotunda. *Clin Dermatol* 1993; **11**: 27–32.
5 Polisky RB, Bronson DM. Acquired ichthyosis in a patient with adenocarcinoma of the breast. *Cutis* 1986; **38**: 359–60.
6 Leibowitz MR, Weiss R, Smith EH. Pityriasis rotunda: a cutaneous sign of malignant disease in two patients. *Arch Dermatol* 1983; **119**: 607–9.

Other epidermal conditions

Transient acantholytic dermatosis has been linked with internal malignancy, particularly with myelogenous leukaemia and carcinoma of the genitourinary tract. However, this may be linked in part with therapy, or simply because it may go unrecognized unless it is specifically considered [1].

Seed-like keratoses of the palms and soles, an acquired pattern of punctate keratoses of the palms and soles, are a common normal finding in healthy subjects (36%) over 50 years old, but are apparently more common in individuals with carcinoma of the bladder (87%) and bronchus (71%) [2]. Punctate keratoderma occurring in Cowden's syndrome (Chapter 12 and p. 62.25) and seed-like keratoses with arsenic ingestion may also be associated with internal malignancy (p. 62.47). Inherited palmoplantar keratodermas were discussed on p. 62.20.

Café-au-lait macules (spots) [3] and lentigines (see also Table 62.10).

Café-au-lait macules are common, but increased numbers of such lesions are a component of many disorders, some of which are associated with internal malignancy.

Some of these have been discussed above (Genodermatoses associated with internal malignancies); these include neurofibromatosis, Bloom's syndrome, Fanconi's anaemia, Cowden's disease and (variably) ataxia–telangiectasia. An association between café-au-lait macules and early-onset colorectal neoplasia has been proposed to represent a variant of the HNPCC (Lynch) syndrome [4].

Lentiginosis is a feature of the Carney complex (pp. 62.25 and 62.78). Lentigines of the palms and/or soles have recently been described as a paraneoplastic syndrome in four patients, two with previously undiagnosed tumours (one small bowel lymphoma and one carcinoma of stomach) and the other two with known breast cancer [5].

References

1 Guana AL, Cohen PR. Transient acantholytic dermatosis in oncology patients. *J Clin Oncol* 1994; **12**: 1703–9.
2 Cuzick J, Harris R, Mortimer PS. Palmar keratoses and cancers of the bladder and lung. *Lancet* 1984; **i**: 530–3.
3 Landau M, Krafchik BR. The diagnostic value of café-au-lait macules. *J Am Acad Dermatol* 1999; **40**: 877–90.
4 Trimbath JD, Petersen GM, Erdman SH *et al.* Café-au-lait spots and early onset colorectal neoplasia: a variant of HNPCC? *Fam Cancer* 2001; **1**: 101–5.
5 Wolf R, Orion E, Davidovici B. Acral lentigines: a new paraneoplastic syndrome. *Int J Dermatol* 2008; **47**: 168–70.

Pigmentation

Many aspects of generalized or localized pigmentation that can be associated with internal malignancy have been discussed in relation to specific disorders. However, it is potentially useful to summarize the most important or characteristic types here, and to comment on those that are not discussed elsewhere in this chapter. A summary is provided in Table 62.10; the mechanisms of pigmentation are discussed in more detail in Chapter 58.

The *ectopic ACTH syndrome* (extracutaneous neuroendocrine melanoderma) occurs due to production of an ACTH-like hormone from tumours; small cell bronchial carcinoma is the cause in over 50%, other reports have described the same condition resulting from gastric, pancreatic, oesophageal and ovarian cancers, as well as in thymoma, phaeochromocytoma, carcinoid syndrome and in various APUD (amine precursor uptake and decarboxylation) tumours. Pituitary and adrenal ACTH production and its effects are discussed in the section describing Cushing's syndrome (p. 62.3). The pigmentation in ectopic ACTH syndrome is addisonian in distribution, diffuse but with photoaccentuation and more prominent over pressure points and in flexures, genital skin, scars and the oral mucosa [1].

Hyperpigmentation with scleromyxoedema and gammopathy [2] has been reported. One patient had pigmentation of the face and V of the neck; the other had generalized pigmentation with accentuation in thickened skin, at acral sites and of genitalia. A similar picture has been seen by one of the authors in a patient without gammopathy.

In Carney complex (p. 62.25), lentiginosis is typically centrofacial but may be widespread at almost any body site; the buccal mucosa is only affected in 5%, rarer sites include the conjunctivae and labia minora, but palms, soles and penis are rarely affected. Blue naevi, usually few in number, occur on the face, trunk or limbs but rarely on the extremities.

References

1 Levine N, Burk C. Extracutaneous neuroendocrine melanoderma. In: Nordlund JJ, Boissy RE, Hearing VJ *et al.*, eds. *The Pigmentary System,* 2nd edn. Oxford: Blackwell Publishing, 2006: 938–9.
2 Urabe K, Nakayama J, Hori Y. Hyperpigmentation associated with scleromyxedema and gammopathy. In: Nordlund JJ, Boissy RE, Hearing VJ *et al.*, eds. *The Pigmentary System*, 2nd edn. Oxford: Blackwell Publishing, 2006: 965.

Pruritus [1]

Internal carcinoma is a non-specific, rare, but important cause of pruritus. Many mechanisms may be involved, including secondary metabolic effects such as uraemia or cholestasis, or itch related to iron-deficiency anaemia, acquired ichthyosis or xerosis. Other mechanisms, such as that linking brain tumours with pruritus, are less well understood. Unfortunately, senile pruritus and asteatosis are not uncommonly encountered in elderly patients, a group who are more at risk from malignancy. It is therefore difficult to dissociate chance from true association, which can lead to difficulties in deciding whether screening is indicated on a cost-effective basis [2].

Generalized pruritus

In a 6-year study of 125 patients with generalized pruritus, Paul *et al.* [2] found no significant increase in malignancy, although of the eight patients with malignancy detected, two had lymphoma—a higher than expected incidence.

Other studies support the likelihood of a genuine association of haematological disorders and lymphoma with generalized pruritus; in particular, itch may be a severe problem in patients with Hodgkin's disease and may indicate a poorer prognosis [3]. Other haematological disorders, including Sézary syndrome, mycosis fungoides, myelomatosis and leukaemia, may also cause generalized pruritus [4,5]; the mechanisms in these conditions are poorly understood. In polycythaemia rubra vera (PRV), the initiating factor appears to be rapid cooling of the skin, as encountered after bathing. This is thought to be due to the release of pruritogens by

Table 62.10 Pigmentary abnormalities associated with internal malignancy.

Pigmentary change	Pattern	Examples
Hyperpigmentation	Diffuse, or diffuse with localized accentuation (addisonian pattern of pigmentation)	Melanoma (rarely causes diffuse slate grey pigmentation)
		Phaeochromocytoma (addisonian pattern)
		Ectopic ACTH syndrome (addisonian pattern)
		POEMS syndrome (p. 62.94) (diffuse or semiconfluent speckled pattern)
		Hyperpigmentation with scleromyxoedema and gammopathy
		Diffuse mastocytosis
		Lymphomas (uncommon)
		Ependymoma (mild increase in pigmentation)
		Werner's syndrome (localized or diffuse pigmentation; p. 62.24)
		Cachexia due to neoplasia
	Patchy or reticulated	Fanconi's anaemia (various pigmentary changes, p. 62.28)
		Dyskeratosis congenita (reticulate pigmentation; p. 62.28)
	Other distributions	Carcinoid syndrome (photodistributed)
		Pancreatic, gastric and renal tumours (erythema ab igne due to local application of heat)
	Lentigines and freckles	Peutz–Jeghers syndrome (p. 62.56) (lentigines)
		Carney complex (pp. 62.25 and 62.78) (lentiginosis is characteristic, freckles also occur)
		Xeroderma pigmentosum (Chapter 15) (freckles)
		Neurofibromatosis (Chapter 15 and p. 62.23) (flexural freckle-like macules)
		Cowden's disease and Bannayan–Riley–Ruvalcaba syndrome (genital lentigines)
		Gardner's syndrome (p. 62.56) (freckles)
		Paraneoplastic acral lentiginosis (p. 62.33)
	Café-au-lait macules	Neurofibromatosis (p. 62.23)
		Bloom's syndrome (p. 62.27)
		Multiple endocrine neoplasia types 1 and 2B
		Fanconi's anaemia
		von Hippel–Lindau disease
	With epidermal hyperplasia	Acanthosis nigricans (p. 62.31)
	Melanocytic naevi and melanoma	Associated with pancreatic neoplasia, astrocytomas and other cerebral neoplasms in some families
		Blue naevi and ordinary naevi occur in Carney complex
Mixed hyper- and hypopigmentation	Poikiloderma	Dermatomyositis (speckled pigmentation on hypopigmented background)
		Rothmund–Thomson syndrome (photodistributed poikiloderma)
Hypopigmentation	Generalized	Chediak–Higashi syndrome (p. 62.28)
	Localized, multiple	Tuberous sclerosis complex (ash leaf macules)
		Mycosis fungoides (hypopigmented variant)
	Melanoma-associated (other than regression within the primary lesion)	Halo depigmentation around primary tumour or metastases
		Distant leukoderma, usually with centrifugal spread starting on the trunk

POEMS, polyneuropathy, organomegaly, endocrinopathy, M protein, skin changes.

degranulated mast cells [6]. However, patients with PRV can also develop intractable itching unrelated to bathing.

Many other visceral carcinomas can cause pruritus, including breast and gastrointestinal cancers, and carcinoid syndrome [7]; again, the mechanisms are frequently poorly understood.

Localized pruritus

Nerve damage by a tumour at any site can cause neuropathic pain or pruritus. The patterns that are most likely to present to a dermatologist are brachioradial pruritus and localized facial or nasal pruritus.

Brachioradial pruritus [8] most commonly affects the lateral upper arm or dorsum of the forearm. Although solar damage has been implicated as a cause, most cases appear to be due to neuropathic damage between C5 and C8. Most of these cases are mechanical due to bony abnormalities but a case due to a spinal tumour has been reported, with rapid resolution of symptoms after treatment [9].

Brain tumours are an uncommon cause of pruritus localized to the face [8,10]. Variations that have been recorded include unilateral pruritus and pruritus limited to the nostril. The latter is particularly linked with tumours invading the floor of the fourth ventricle but tumours elsewhere in the brain, and other cerebral lesions (e.g. abscesses) as well as trigeminal neuralgia can also produce this distribution of pruritus. Generalized itching can also sometimes occur with intracranial neoplasia [10].

References

1 Goldman BD, Koh HK. Pruritus and malignancy. In: Bernhard JD, ed. *Itch. Mechanisms and Management of Pruritus.* New York: McGrawHill, 1994: 299–319.
2 Paul R, Paul R, Jansen CT. Itch and malignancy prognosis in generalized pruritus: a 6-year follow-up of 125 patients. *J Am Acad Dermatol* 1987; **16**: 1179–82.

3 Feiner AS, Mahmood T, Wallner SF. Prognostic importance of pruritus in Hodgkin's disease. *JAMA* 1978; **240**: 2738–40.

4 Graham RM. Aspects of itching. In: Verbov JL, ed. *New Clinical Applications in Dermatology*. Lancaster: MTP Press, 1987: 49–70.

5 Thomas I, Schwartz RA. Cutaneous paraneoplastic syndromes: uncommon presentations. *Clinics Dermatol* 2005; **23**: 593–600.

6 Jackson N, Burt D, Crocker J *et al*. Skin mast cells in polycythaemia vera: relationship to the pathogenesis and treatment of pruritus. *Br J Dermatol* 1987; **116**: 21–9.

7 Pipkin CA, Lio PA. Cutaneous manifestations of internal malignancies: an overview. *Dermatol Clin* 2008; **26**: 1–15.

8 Yosipovitch G. Pruritus: an update. *Curr Prob Dermatol* 2003; **15**: 135–64.

9 Johnson RE, Kanigsberg ND, Jimenez CL. Localized pruritus: a presenting symptom of a spinal cord tumor in a child with features of neurofibromatosis. *J Am Acad Dermatol* 2000; **43**: 958–61.

10 Andreev VC, Petkov I. Skin manifestations associated with tumours of the brain. *Br J Dermatol* 1975; **92**: 675–8.

Hair, nails and skin appendages

Paraneoplastic hypertrichosis lanuginosa acquisita [1–4]

This is a rare but important condition; cases reported in the medical literature up to 2007 have recently been reviewed [1]. About 70% of cases occur in women, usually aged 40–70 years, and most patients have metastatic tumours at presentation, with correspondingly poor prognosis. The commonest tumour sites in men are lung, followed by colorectal, and in women are colorectal, followed by lung and breast. Other reported sites or tumour types include endometrium (about 7–8% of cases), ovary, cervix, renal, prostate, bladder, adrenal gland, stomach, gallbladder, skin (including melanoma), parotid gland, sarcoma, lymphoma and leukaemia [1,3].

There may be associated acanthosis nigricans, hypertrophy of papillae of the tongue, and glossitis [2]; disturbances of taste or smell also occur [3]. However, the glossitis in at least some patients may be a manifestation of vitamin deficiency rather than a specifically related condition [4]. Development of paraneoplastic hypertrichosis lanuginosa acquisita tends to affect the face initially, extending down the body with time. The mechanism is unclear but the hair is of fine, downy, lanugo type; prolongation of the anagen growth phase has been proposed to explain this. Resolution of hypertrichosis lanuginosa occurs after treatment of the underlying tumour, and regrowth related to recurrence of the neoplasm.

References

1 Slee PHTJ, van der Waal RIF, Schagen van Leeuwen JH *et al*. Paraneoplastic hypertrichosis lanuginosa acquisita: uncommon or overlooked? *Br J Dermatol* 2007; **157**: 1087–92.

2 Wendolin DS, Pope DN, Mallory SB. Hypertrichosis. *J Am Acad Dermatol* 2003; **48**: 161–79.

3 Stone SP, Buescher LS. Life-threatening paraneoplastic cutaneous syndromes. *Clinics Dermatol* 2005; **23**: 301–6.

4 Callen JP. Skin signs of internal malignancy. In: Callen JP, Jorizzo JL, eds. *Dermatological Manifestations of Internal Disease*, 3rd edn. Philadelphia: Saunders, 2003: 95–104.

Clubbing of nails

This nail abnormality is discussed in more detail in Chapter 65. Both clubbing and associated hypertrophic osteoarthropathy (HOA) have been documented with many neoplasms, the commonest being carcinoma of the bronchus. In patients with lung cancer, clubbing has been reported to be present in 29%, especially in females; most lung tumours are squamous cell carcinoma or adenocarcinoma [1]. A high incidence of HOA occurs particularly with mesothelioma, but it may also occur with malignancies of the pulmonary, cardiovascular, gastrointestinal and hepatobiliary systems [2]; it is much less common than clubbing, occurring in perhaps 5% of patients with clubbing.

References

1 Sridhar KS, Lobo CF, Altman RD. Digital clubbing and lung cancer. *Chest* 1998; **114**: 1535–7.

2 Caldwell DS, McCallum RM. Rheumatological manifestations of cancer. *Med Clin North Am* 1986; **70**: 385–417.

Sebaceous neoplasms

Sebaceous neoplasms of various types are strongly linked with Muir–Torre syndrome (p. 62.26).

Hyperhidrosis [1]

Generalized hyperhidrosis may rarely be associated with malignant disease. It is an almost consistent finding in phaeochromocytoma (PCC; see below), in which it may be limited to night-time or occur at any time. Nocturnal hyperhidrosis ('night sweats') may occur in PCC, lymphoma and carcinoid syndrome, as well as in non-neoplastic conditions such as thyrotoxicosis, chronic infections and others. Localized hyperhidrosis may occur in POEMS syndrome.

Specific distributions of localized hyperhidrosis may also be important. Hyperhidrosis with autonomic dysreflexia is associated with spinal cord lesions above T6, and is characterized by episodic sweating of the face, neck and upper trunk with vasodilatation in the same distribution, headache, hypertension and piloerection; most cases are due to injury or cord compression but intracranial posterior fossa neoplasms can produce similar symptoms. Paroxysmal unilateral hyperhidrosis of the face and neck, usually severe and unrelated to stimuli such as eating, may be due to an ipsilateral thoracic tumour (adenocarcinoma, squamous cell carcinoma or mesothelioma) compressing or infiltrating the sympathetic trunk; associated features may include Horner's syndrome, facial weakness, sensory disturbance, and other features of the primary tumour.

Phaeochromocytomas (PCCs) may be present in 0.3–1.9% of individuals, based on post-mortem studies and biochemical screening, but only 10% are malignant in nature [2]. Standard teaching is that 10% of PCC are familial, including those occurring in MEN syndromes (p. 62.24), neurofibromatosis, von Hippel–Lindau disease, hereditary paragangliomatosis and tuberous sclerosis; however, screening PCCs for germline mutations demonstrated that 24% of apparently sporadic PCC had mutations of *VHL*, *RET*, *SDHD* or *SDHB* genes [3]. Patients with PCC that have *SDHD* or *SDHB* mutations have a 20–30% risk of developing glomus tumours (these genes confer susceptibility to both extra-adrenal PCC (paragangliomas) and glomus tumours, as both have a common neural crest origin) [4]. Genetic aspects of PCC and other adrenal tumours are reviewed in [5].

Presentation of PCC is often incidental due to discovery of labile hypertension, but the classical triad of features in PCC is episodic headache with palpitations (tachycardia) and hyperhidrosis due to release of catecholamines [2,4]. Numerous other symptoms may occur, including hyper- and hypoglycaemia, pallor with rebound flushing, diarrhoea, fatigue, dyspnoea, chest pain, abdominal pain and malaise.

References
1 Sato K, Kang WH, Saga K, Sato KT. Biology of sweat glands and their disorders. II. Disorders of sweat gland function. *J Am Acad Dermatol* 1989; **20**: 713–26.
2 Werbel SS, Ober KP. Phaeochromocytoma. Update on diagnosis, localization, and management. *Med Clin N Am* 1995; **79**: 131–53.
3 Neumann HPH, Bausch B, McWhinney SR *et al.* Germ-line mutations in nonsyndromic phaeochromocytoma. *N Engl J Med* 2002; **346**: 1459–66.
4 Dluhy RG. Phaeochromocytoma—death of an axiom. *N Engl J Med* 2002; **346**: 1486–8.
5 Bertherat J, Gimenez-Roqueplo AP. New insights in the genetics of adrenocortical tumors, pheochromocytomas and paragangliomas. *Horm Metab Res* 2005; **37**: 384–90.

Dermatoses

Several dermatoses have a significant association with internal malignancy; in other conditions there is just a minor statistical link documented, as discussed below.

Acrokeratosis paraneoplastica (Bazex syndrome) [1–5]

This is a rare condition, much commoner in males than females [3–5], which is associated particularly with squamous cell carcinoma of the upper respiratory or gastrointestinal tracts, particularly when there are metastases in the cervical lymph nodes. An underlying malignancy is a required criterion for the diagnosis; the cutaneous features are predominantly acral in distribution and papulosquamous lesions, hyperpigmentation, keratoderma, paronychia and nail dystrophy (at least one of which is also required for diagnosis) [3]. More than 60% of tumours arise in the oropharynx, larynx or are cervical squamous cell carcinoma metastases with an unknown primary site; lung, oesophageal and other primary or metastatic lesions above the diaphragm make up most of the remainder [5]. Rare associations, such as metastatic adenocarcinoma of the prostate and transitional cell carcinoma of the bladder, have been reported [6,7]. The cutaneous changes develop gradually, often in several phases, initially with violaceous erythema and scaling on the peripheries, especially helices of the ears, tip of the nose, hands and feet (especially the distal portion of digits). The eruption then becomes more hyperkeratotic, with a keratoderma on hands and feet. Subsequently, the eruption may become more generalized. Nail dystrophy and paronychia are often present. Changes on the face may appear more eczematous or lupus erythematosus-like, whereas acral changes are often psoriasiform. The differential diagnosis can include dermatitis, especially seborrhoeic or contact-allergic types. Alternatively, acral psoriasis with the possibility of Reiter's syndrome may be considered. The course mostly parallels the underlying neoplasm; resolution may occur with successful tumour resection, and recurrence may develop on relapse of malignancy. When resection is felt inappropriate or impracticable, systemic retinoids may improve the cutaneous changes [8]. The histological changes are non-diagnostic, but essentially reflect the clinical appearance with hyperkeratosis, parakeratosis, focal spongiosis and a mixed, inflammatory cell infiltrate [4,5,9].

References
1 Bazex A, Griffiths A. Acrokeratosis paraneoplastica: a new cutaneous marker of malignancy. *Br J Dermatol* 1980; **102**: 301–6.
2 Richard M, Giroux JM. Acrokeratosis paraneoplastica. *J Am Acad Dermatol* 1987; **16**: 178–83.
3 Bolognia JL. Bazex syndrome: acrokeratosis paraneoplastica. *Semin Dermatol* 1995; **14**: 84–9.
4 Moore RL, Devere TS. Epidermal manifestations of internal malignancy. *Dermatol Clinics* 2008; **26**: 17–29.
5 Stone SP, Buescher LS. Life-threatening paraneoplastic cutaneous syndromes. *Clinics Dermatol* 2005; **23**: 301–6.
6 Obasi OE, Garg SK. Bazex paraneoplastic acrokeratosis in prostate carcinoma. *Br J Dermatol* 1987; **117**: 647–51.
7 Arregui MA, Raton JA, Landa NI *et al.* Bazex's syndrome (acrokeratosis paraneoplastica): first case report of association with a bladder carcinoma. *Clin Exp Dermatol* 1993; **18**: 445–8.
8 Wishart JM. Bazex paraneoplastic acrokeratosis: a case report and response to Tigason. *Br J Dermatol* 1986; **115**: 595–9.
9 Pecora AL, Landsman L, Imgrund SP *et al.* Acrokeratosis paraneoplastica (Bazex's syndrome). *Arch Dermatol* 1983; **119**: 820–6.

Dermatomyositis (Chapter 51) [1–5]

Both dermatomyositis (Fig. 62.13) and polymyositis in adults may be associated with internal malignancy. The reported likelihood of finding a neoplasm varies between 6% (in polymyositis) [6] and 50% [7]; overall, about 25–30% is probably a representative proportion for the various reported studies of dermatomyositis, making this a condition with a significant association with underlying malignancy. The association with neoplasia is much stronger for dermatomyositis than for polymyositis or dermatomyositis/autoimmune disease overlap conditions. Conventional teaching has been that malignancy is an uncommon cause of dermatomyositis in subjects less than 40 years of age; however, paediatric cases with neoplasia are reported [8]. As there is a lower incidence of malignancy in the younger age group, and there are no age-matched comparative studies against a control population in children, it is difficult to judge the strength of the association in this age group [3].

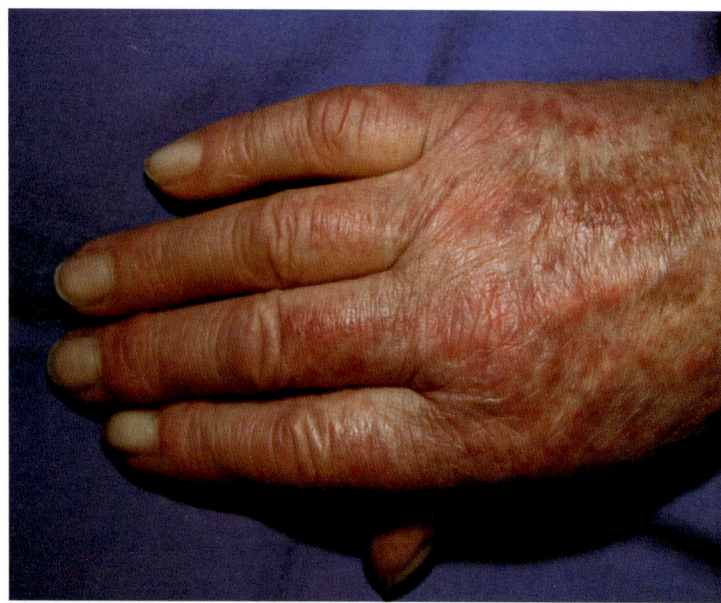

Fig. 62.13 Dermatomyositis in a patient with ovarian carcinoma.

The temporal association of dermatomyositis with neoplasia varies; in one report approximately equal proportions had a known malignancy at the time that dermatomyositis presented, had a malignancy found due to investigation when dermatomyositis was diagnosed, or had a malignancy found during follow-up (usually in the first 6 months after diagnosis of dermatomyositis) [4]. Others report a four to five times increased incidence of malignancy in the first 2 years [9] or even 5 years [5] after diagnosis. Accounts of specific malignant associations may be subject to bias by rare-case reporting, and in larger series the malignancies identified generally reflect tumour prevalence in the general population; lung cancer in men, breast and gynaecological tumours in women, and colorectal cancers in both sexes. In South-East Asia, there is a higher frequency of nasopharyngeal carcinoma, that probably also reflects the background risk of this type of neoplasm. The one exception to this generalization is ovarian carcinoma, which appears to be significantly overrepresented and potentially overlooked [2,4,5,10].

The value of extensive screening for neoplasia in dermatomyositis is questionable. Several authors have stressed that the emphasis should be attached to thorough clinical evaluation, simple investigations and then specific investigations as indicated [1,4,10]. However, all of these studies were performed before easy availability of CT or MRI scanning, and the quality of such imaging has increased hugely in recent years, so radiological screening should be included in the investigation of patients with dermatomyositis. 'Blind' (i.e. not symptom-directed) CT scanning of chest, abdomen and pelvis increased the yield of malignancies in one study, although the number of patients in whom a tumour might have been missed was small, and one was an ovarian tumour which has been documented above as worthy of greater suspicion. There should certainly be a low threshold for further or repeated investigations at the time of diagnosis or during follow-up if previous neoplasia has been present, when the therapeutic response is poor, or if new symptoms develop; there is also an argument for ongoing screening for ovarian cancers throughout follow-up of female patients without any initial screening test abnormalities, using clinical examination, trans-vaginal ultrasound and tumour markers (CA125) [2].

In general, subjects with dermatomyositis who truly have amyopathic dermatomyositis (dermatomyositis sine myositis) [12], or who have a connective tissue overlap syndrome, appear less likely to have an underlying malignancy; however, some patients with amyopathic dermatomyositis do actually develop myositis, some studies document similar tumour rates in those with or without myositis [13], and tumours have been reported in all such variants, so screening investigations should still be performed [14]. In one study, patients with malignancy were found to have a more rapid onset of dermatomyositis, higher mean creatine kinase and erythrocyte sedimentation rates, and a lower frequency of Raynaud's phenomenon compared with patients without an underlying malignancy [11]. However, a low creatine kinase has also been linked with a higher frequency of malignancy. Vasculitis or necrosis, manifest clinically or in histopathology specimens, has also been associated with an increased risk of an associated neoplasm [13,15–17].

Whilst no clinical pattern reliably excludes the possibility of an underlying malignancy, a greater understanding of the immuno-

pathogenesis of paraneoplastic dermatomyositis may be instructive [18–20]. A recent report documented that subjects with a myositis-specific autoantibody reactive with 155-kDa and 140-kDa nuclear antigens (anti-155/140 Ab) had a much higher risk of malignancy (71%) than those without this antibody (11%) [19]. Patients with this antibody had a higher frequency of heliotrope rash, Gottron's papules and flagellate erythema than those with negative results, but none with anti-155/140 Ab had interstitial lung disease. No patients with systemic lupus erythematosus, systemic sclerosus or healthy controls had this antibody. A novel myositis-specific antibody (anti-CADM 140) has recently been demonstrated in amyopathic dermatomyositis, and some myositis-specific antibodies are expressed both in regenerating muscle cells and in some cancers [20]. Such insights may in the future help to determine which patients require investigation for malignancy.

References

1 Callen JP. Skin signs of internal malignancy. In: Callen JP, Jorizzo JL, eds. *Dermatological Manifestations of Internal Disease*, 3rd edn. Philadelphia: Saunders, 2003: 95–104.
2 Provost TT, Flynn JA. Dermatomyositis. In: Provost TT, Flynn JA, eds. *Cutaneous Medicine: Cutaneous Manifestations of Systemic Disease*. Hamilton, Ontario: Decker, 2001: 82–103.
3 Callen JP. Malignancy in polymyositis/dermatomyositis. *Clin Dermatol* 1988; **6**: 55–63.
4 Cox NH, Lawrence CM, Langtry JA *et al.* Dermatomyositis: disease associations and evaluation of screening investigations for malignancy. *Arch Dermatol* 1990; **126**: 61–5.
5 Sigurgeiersson B, Lindelöf B, Edhag O, Allander E. Risk of cancer in patients with dermatomyositis or polymyositis. A population-based study. *N Engl J Med* 1992; **326**: 363–7.
6 Henriksson KG, Sandstedt P. Polymyositis—treatment and prognosis: a study of 107 patients. *Acta Neurol Scand* 1982; **65**: 280–300.
7 Vesterager L, Worm AM, Thomsen K. Dermatomyositis and malignancy. *Clin Exp Dermatol* 1980; **5**: 31–5.
8 Kalmanti M, Athanasion A. Neuroblastoma occurring in a child with dermatomyositis. *Am J Pediatr Hematol Oncol* 1985; **7**: 387–8.
9 Masi AT, Hochberg MC. Temporal associations of polymyositis–dermatomyositis with malignancy: methodologic and clinical considerations. *Mt Sinai J Med* 1988; **55**: 471–8.
10 Richardson JB, Callen JP. Dermatomyositis and malignancy. *Med Clin North Am* 1989; **73**: 1211–20.
11 Sparsa A, Liozon E, Herrmann F *et al.* Routine vs extensive malignancy search for adult dermatomyositis and polymyositis. A study of 40 patients. *Arch Dermatol* 2002; **138**: 885–90.
12 Caproni M, Carinali C, Parodi A *et al.* Amyopathic dermatomyositis. A review by the Italian Group of Immunodermatology. *Arch Dermatol* 2002; **138**: 23–7.
13 Gallais V, Crickx B, Belaich S. Prognostic factors and predictive signs of malignancy in adult dermatomyositis. *Ann Dermatol Venereol* 1996; **123**: 722–6.
14 Callen JP. When and how should the patient with dermatomyositis or amyopathic dermatomyositis be assessed for possible cancer? *Arch Dermatol* 2002; **138**: 969–71.
15 Feldman D, Hochenberg MC, Zizic TM, Stevens MB. Cutaneous vasculitis in adult polymyositis/dermatomyositis. *J Rheumatol* 1983; **10**: 85–9.
16 Hunger RE, Durr D, Brand CU. Cutaneous leukocytoclastic vasculitis in dermatomyositis suggests malignancy. *Dermatology* 2001; **202**: 123–6.
17 Burnouf M, Mahé E, Verpillat P *et al.* Cutaneous necrosis is predictive of cancer in adult dermatomyositis. *Ann Dermatol Venereol* 2003; **130**: 313–6.
18 Levine SM. Cancer and myositis: new insights into an old association. *Curr Opin Rheumatol* 2006; **18**: 620–4.
19 Kaji K, Fujimoto M, Hasegawa M *et al.* Identification of a novel autoantibody reactive with 155 and 140 kDa nuclear proteins in patients with dermatomyositis: an association with malignancy. *Rheumatology (Oxford)* 2007; **46**: 25–8.

20 Mimori T, Imura Y, Nakashima R, Yoshifuji H. Autoantibodies in idiopathic inflammatory myopathy: an update on clinical and pathophysiological significance. *Curr Opin Rheumatol* 2007; **19**: 523–9.

Migratory erythemas

This descriptive term is applied to a variety of annular and figurate eruptions, which are discussed in more detail on pp. 62.106–62.113. Two variants, erythema gyratum repens and necrolytic migratory erythema, have a clear association with internal neoplasia. Others, such as erythema annulare centrifugum and some unspecified figurate erythemas, also have a very variable association with neoplasia. There are also reports of subacute lupus erythematosus-like annular and figurate rashes, linked with myeloproliferative disorders and carcinoma of lung, liver, breast, larynx and oesophagus in individual cases.

Erythema gyratum repens (see also p. 62.107) is a rare, bizarre cutaneous eruption consisting of mobile concentric, often palpable, erythematous, wave-like bands, which give a 'wood-grain' appearance to the skin (Fig. 62.14). A peripheral scale or collarette may be present. The complete torso is frequently affected. There is often associated severe pruritus, sometimes ichthyosis, and sometimes bullae within the erythema. The lesions migrate from day to day, usually changing position by about 1 cm daily. It has a strong association with internal malignancy (over 80% of cases), particularly lung cancer [1,2] which is present in about a third of cases; other cancer sites include oesophagus, breast, bowel, uterus, cervix, kidney, pancreas and haematological neoplasia [2]. Occasional cases without associated malignancy have been reported [3] but it is important to be aware that 6% are found to have a tumour of unknown primary origin [2]. Identification and resection of the tumour often results in resolution of the eruption.

Necrolytic migratory erythema (glucagonoma syndrome) is the characteristic eruption associated with an α-cell tumour of the pancreas. It is discussed in the section on pancreatic disease later in this chapter (p. 62.66).

Erythema annulare centrifugum [4,5] is the term used to describe one of the commoner annular erythemas, which is usually not associated with neoplasia (p. 62.110). If an underlying malignancy is found, it is usually a myeloproliferative disorder [5]. Clinical examination and routine screening tests are the only investigation required, rather than an exhaustive search for malignancy, unless there are additional clinical pointers.

References
1 Solomon H. Erythema gyratum repens. *Arch Dermatol* 1969; **100**: 639.
2 Stone SP, Buescher LS. Life-threatening paraneoplastic cutaneous syndromes. *Clinics Dermatol* 2005; **23**: 301–6.
3 Juhlin L, Lacour JP, Larrouy JC *et al.* Episodic erythema gyratum repens with ichthyosis and palmoplantar hyperkeratosis without signs of internal malignancy. *Clin Exp Dermatol* 1989; **14**: 223–6.
4 Lazar P. Cancer, erythema annulare centrifugum, autoimmunity. *Arch Dermatol* 1963; **87**: 247–51.
5 Mahood JM. Erythema annulare centrifugum: a review of 24 cases, with special reference to its association with underlying disease. *Clin Exp Dermatol* 1983; **8**: 383–7.

Other dermatological disorders

Lichen planus may rarely be induced by neoplasia [1]. There is also an increased risk, particularly in males, of oral squamous cell carcinoma (SCC); this may be due to a combined direct effect and co-factors such as smoking [2]. The strength of the association may however have been overestimated, as some of the reports are those that have collected patients presenting with oral SCC and have then looked for histological evidence of lichen planus as a background factor.

Urticaria; with the exception of cold urticaria and peripheral gangrene as a result of circulating cryoglobulins, where there is a possible, but uncommon, link with myeloma and lymphoma [3], associations of urticaria and neoplasia are difficult to evaluate. Certainly it cannot be regarded as an established paraneoplastic phenomenon, other than in Schnitzler's syndrome (a distinct disorder of chronic urticaria, bone pain, hyperostosis, high erythrocyte sedimentation rate and monoclonal IgM gammopathy, usually IgMκ; see Chapter 22). Histologically, there is neutrophilic inflammation within dermal venules with some perivascular involvement, rarely extending to a leukocytoclastic vasculitis. Although the overall prognosis is reasonable, around 10–15% of patients develop lymphoplasmacytic lymphoma [4].

Erythroderma (Chapter 23) and exfoliative dermatitis have both been linked with malignancy [5,6]. In most such cases (around 10% in most reported series), the neoplasm is mycosis fungoides or its leukaemic variant, Sézary syndrome; these are really a representation of a systemic neoplasm rather than a truly paraneoplastic disorder. However, there are a small number of patients who have neither condition, but present with erythroderma and eventually develop lymphoma or leukaemia. The incidence is uncertain and rare; a report in an Asian population failed to demonstrate one association in 80 patients [7]. Immunophenotypic studies do not appear to help distinguish benign from malignant cases. There are additionally reported cases of erythroderma with cancers of liver, lung, colon, stomach, pancreas, thyroid, prostate and cervix [5,6,8]. *Ofuji papuloerythroderma* has also been associated with peripheral T-cell non-epidermotrophic cutaneous lymphoma [9].

Granuloma annulare has been reported in association with lymphomas, other haematological malignancies, and uncommonly

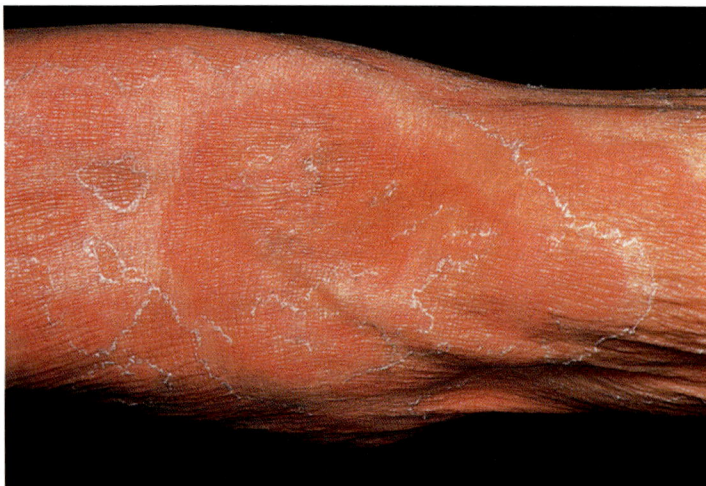

Fig. 62.14 Erythema gyratum repens of the arm secondary to carcinoma of the bronchus. (Courtesy of Dr A.W. McKenzie, Norfolk and Norwich Hospital, Norwich, UK.)

with solid tumours [10]; however, a causal relationship in such cases is uncertain. It has been suggested that the subcutaneous pattern of granuloma annulare may carry a greater risk of malignancy, but this may reflect the more extensive investigation that is usually performed to establish the diagnosis in such cases by comparison with more typical granuloma annulare.

'Insect bite-like' reactions are reported in haematological malignancy, usually chronic lymphocytic leukaemia [11].

Cutis verticis gyrata may occasionally occur as a paraneoplastic phenomenon [12].

Mental neuropathy ('numb chin syndrome') has several benign causes, but may occur as a feature of metastatic disease and is considered an indicator of poor prognosis [13]. Relevant tumours include breast, thyroid, renal, lung, prostate, lymphomas and melanoma.

Non-melanoma skin cancer has been linked with increased risk and poor prognosis of non-Hodgkin's lymphoma [14].

References

1 Helm TN, Camisa C, Liu AY *et al.* Lichen planus associated with neoplasia: a cell-mediated immune response to tumor antigens? *J Am Acad Dermatol* 1994; **30**: 219–24.

2 Sigurgeirsson B, Lindelof B. Lichen planus and malignancy. *Arch Dermatol* 1991; **127**: 1684–8.

3 Neittaanmaki H. Cold urticaria: clinical findings in 220 patients. *J Am Acad Dermatol* 1985; **13**: 636–44.

4 Daoud MS, Lust JA, Kyle RA *et al.* Monoclonal gammopathies and associated skin disorders. *J Am Acad Dermatol* 1999; **40**: 507–35.

5 Boyce S, Harper J. Paraneoplastic dermatoses. *Dermatol Clin* 2002; **20**: 523–32.

6 Thomas I, Schwartz RA. Cutaneous paraneoplastic syndromes: uncommon presentations. *Clinics Dermatol* 2005; **23**: 593–600.

7 Abel EA, Lindae ML, Hoppe RT *et al.* Benign and malignant forms of erythroderma: cutaneous immunophenotypic characteristics. *J Am Acad Dermatol* 1988; **19**: 1089–95.

8 Nicolis GD, Helwig EB. Exfoliative dermatitis: a clinicopathologic study of 135 cases. *Arch Dermatol* 1973; **108**: 788–97.

9 Grob JJ, Collet-Villete AM, Horchowski N *et al.* Ofuji papulo-erythroderma: report of a case with T cell skin lymphoma and discussion of the nature of this disease. *J Am Acad Dermatol* 1989; **20**: 927–31.

10 Cohen PR. Granuloma annulare, relapsing polychondritis, sarcoidosis, and systemic lupus erythematosus: conditions whose dermatologic manifestations may occur as hematologic malignancy-associated mucocutaneous paraneoplastic syndromes. *Int J Dermatol* 2006; **45**: 70–80.

11 Davis MD, Perniciaro C, Dahl PR *et al.* Exaggerated arthropod-bite lesions in patients with chronic lymphocytic lekaemia: a clinical, histopathologic, and immunopathologic study of eight patients. *J Am Acad Dermatol* 1998; **39**: 27–35.

12 Ross JB, Tompkins MG. Cutis verticis gyrata as a marker of internal malignancy. *Arch Dermatol* 1989; **125**: 434–5.

13 Burt RK, Sharfman WH, Karp B, Wilson WH. Mental neuropathy (numb chin syndrome). A harbinger of tumor progression or relapse. *Cancer* 1992; **70**: 877–81.

14 Hjalgrim H, Frisch M, Storm HH *et al.* Non-melanoma skin cancer may be a marker of poor prognosis in patients with non-Hodgkin's lymphoma. *Int J Cancer* 2000; **85**: 639–42.

Connective tissue and rheumatological disorders

Malignancies have been reported in association with many disorders that overlap between dermatology and rheumatology. Those that fall into the collagen vascular group are discussed here; dermal deposition disorders, neutrophilic infiltrates, paraneoplastic vasculitis and other vascular conditions are discussed later.

Systemic lupus erythematosus

The possibility of an increased risk of internal malignancy in systemic (SLE) and subacute cutaneous lupus erythematosus has been debated for many years, and still remains controversial. There are individual cases in which a close temporal relationship has been documented [1], and large cohort and population studies have mainly produced results in favour of an increased risk [2,3]. Studies that have supported an association with malignancy have suggested increases in lymphomas, monoclonal gammopathy, cervical, lung, hepatobiliary and breast cancer [3–6], although the latter is disputed [4]. The majority of large studies suggest an increase in non-Hodgkin's lymphoma [3], particularly diffuse large B-cell lymphoma (DLBCL) [5]. The mechanism may be a T-cell defect in SLE, or may be a result of immunosuppressive medication used in treatment (especially implicated in the increased risk of haematological malignancies [7]). The evidence for an association between autoimmune conditions and lymphoma is supported by a large study of 3055 patients with non-Hodgkin's lymphoma and matched controls; significant associations were found with rheumatoid arthritis, primary Sjögren's syndrome, and SLE, again documenting the specific association with DLBCL [8]. The increased tumour risk in patients with Sjögren's syndrome has been noted in other reviews [9]. Treatment with antimalarials has been suggested to have a protective effect against development of cancers in SLE [10].

Rare patterns of lupus erythematosus, such as lupus erythematosus gyratum repens, may carry a higher risk of internal malignancy [11], although this condition is generally reported as isolated cases, so this conclusion is uncertain. Individual reports suggest an association of a subacute cutaneous lupus erythematosus (SCLE)-like eruption with tumours of various organs (including myeloproliferative disorders causing a neutrophilic lupus-like figurate erythema, and SCLE-like rash associated with tumours of lung, liver, larynx, breast and oesophagus [12,13]. Potential clues to this association are an SCLE-like rash in males, in an older age-group than usual, and with resistance to therapy.

References

1 Chaudhry SI, Murphy LA, White IR. Subacute cutaneous lupus erythematosus: a paraneoplastic dermatosis? *Clin Exp Dermatol* 2005; **30**: 655–8.

2 Bernatsky S, Boivin JF, Joseph L *et al.* An international cohort study of cancer in systemic lupus erythematosus. *Arthritis Rheum* 2005; **52**: 1481–90.

3 Tarr T, Gyorfy B, Szekanecz E *et al.* Occurrence of malignancies in Hungarian patients with lupus erythematosus: results from a single center. *Ann N Y Acad Sci* 2007; **1108**: 76–82.

4 Kontos M, Fentiman IS. Systemic lupus erythematosus and breast cancer. *Breast J* 2008; **14**: 81–6.

5 Löfström B, Backlin C, Sundström C *et al.* A closer look at non-Hodgkin's lymphoma cases in a national Swedish systemic lupus erythematosus cohort: a nested case-control study. *Ann Rheum Dis* 2007; **66**: 1627–32.

6 Ali YM, Urowitz MB, Ibanez D, Gladman DD. Monoclonal gammopathy in systemic lupus erythematosus. *Lupus* 2007; **16**: 426–9.

7 Bernatsky S, Joseph L, Boivin JF *et al.* The relationship between cancer and medication exposures in systemic lupus erythematosus: a case-cohort study. *Ann Rheum Dis* 2008; **67**: 74–9.

8 Smedby KE, Hjalgrim H, Askling J *et al.* Autoimmune and chronic inflammatory disorders and risk of non-Hodgkin lymphoma by subtype. *J Natl Cancer Inst* 2006; **98**: 51–60.

9 Bernatsky S, Ramsay-Goldman R, Clarke A. Malignancy and autoimmunity. *Curr Opin Rheum* 2006; **18**: 129–34.

10 Ruiz-Irastorza G, Ugarte A, Egurbide MV *et al*. Antimalarials may influence the risk of malignancy in systemic lupus erythematosus. *Ann Rheum Dis* 2007; **66**: 815–7.

11 Kreft B, Marsch WC. Lupus erythematosus gyratum repens. *Eur J Dermatol* 2007; **17**: 79–82.

12 Dawn G, Wainwright NJ. Association between subacute cutaneous lupus erythematosus and epidermoid carcinoma of the lung: a paraneoplastic phenomenon? *Clin Exp Dermatol* 2002; **27**: 714–22.

13 Yasim ZF, Walsh MY, Armstrong DKB. Subacute lupus erythematosus-like rash associated with oesophageal carcinoma *in situ*. *Clin Exp Dermatol* 2007; **32**: 443–4.

Scleroderma, fasciitis, panniculitis and similar sclerodermoid conditions

Like SLE, scleroderma/systemic sclerosis has been linked with occurrence of internal malignancy [1,2], and a possible role of fibrogenic peptides has been proposed [3], although overall the association is probably not strong [4]. Likewise, eosinophilic fasciitis has occasionally been linked with contemporaneous diagnosis of a neoplasm [5]. Many of the cases described are not entirely classical of 'usual' scleroderma, some cases having a more aggressive course of fibrosis than anticipated, an unusual distribution, extensive fibrotic changes in the subcutaneous fat, or progressive arthritis. To reflect these features, more recent cases have been described under the terms palmar fibrosis/arthritis [6,7] or cancer-associated fasciitis–panniculitis syndrome [8,9]. The commonest tumour types documented are ovarian and lung; breast, prostate and pancreatic tumours have also been reported.

A more typical panniculitis process resembling Weber–Christian disease may occur in patients with acinar cell carcinoma of the pancreas, in whom a syndrome of panniculitis, polyarthritis and eosinophilia can occur. Eosinophilic panniculitis has also been reported in association with other solid tumours or pre-leukaemia [10,11].

Scleroderma-like skin changes may also be a cutaneous manifestation of carcinoid syndrome, the differential diagnosis from collagen vascular scleroderma processes being suggested by the presence of flushing and the absence of Raynaud's phenomenon.

Post-irradiation morphoea is a phenomenon seen after treatment of breast cancer [12]; its importance is not as a marker of underlying malignancy, but in the differential diagnosis of carcinoma en cuirasse (or occasionally carcinoma erysipeloides), discussed above.

References

1 Duncan S, Winkelmann R. Cancer and scleroderma. *Arch Dermatol* 1979; **115**: 950–5.

2 Roumm A, Medsger TJ. Cancer in connective tissue disease. *Arthritis Rheum* 1982; **25**: 1130–3.

3 Gruber BL, Miller F, Kaufman LD. Simultaneous onset of systemic sclerosis (scleroderma) and lung cancer: a case report and histologic analysis of fibrogenic peptides. *Am J Med* 1992; **92**: 705–8.

4 Bernatsky S, Ramsey GM, Clarke A. Malignancy and autoimmunity. *Curr Opn Rheumatol* 2006; **18**: 129–34.

5 Chan LS, Hanson CA, Cooper KD. Concurrent eosinophilic fasciitis and cutaneous T-cell lymphoma. *Arch Dermatol* 1991; **127**: 862–5.

6 Naschitz JE, Yeshurun D, Rosner I. Rheumatic manifestations of occult cancer. *Cancer* 1995; **12**: 2954–8.

7 Cohen PR. Paraneoplastic dermatopathology: cutaneous paraneoplastic syndromes. *Adv Dermatol* 1996; **11**: 215–52.

8 Naschitz JE, Yeshuran D, Zuckerman E *et al*. Cancer-associated fasciitis–panniculitis. *Cancer* 1994; **73**: 231–5.

9 Cox NH, Ramsay B, Dobson C, Comaish JS. Woody hands in a patient with pancreatic carcinoma: a variant of cancer-associated fasciitis–panniculitis syndrome. *Br J Dermatol* 1996; **135**: 995–8.

10 Winkelmann RK, Frigas E. Eosinophilic panniculitis: a clinicopathologc study. *J Cutan Pathol* 1986; **13**: 1–12.

11 Marullo S, Dallot A, Carelier-Balloy B *et al*. Subcutaneous eosinophilic necrosis associated with refractory anaemia with an excess of myeloblasts. *J Am Acad Dermatol* 1989; **20**: 320–3.

12 Colver GB, Rodger A, Mortimer PS *et al*. Post-irradiation morphoea. *Br J Dermatol* 1989; **120**: 831–5.

Relapsing polychondritis

It is increasingly recognized that relapsing polychondritis may be linked with malignancy. Myelodysplastic syndrome and other haematological malignancies are much the commonest association [1,2], but a variety of solid tumours have also been reported including lung, breast, colorectal, pancreas, prostate and others [1]. Concurrence with malignancy-associated Sweet's syndrome is discussed in Chapter 50.

References

1 Cohen PR. Granuloma annulare, relapsing polychondritis, sarcoidosis, and systemic lupus erythematosus: conditions whose dermatologic manifestations may occur as hematologic malignancy-associated mucocutaneous paraneoplastic syndromes. *Int J Dermatol* 2006; **45**: 70–80.

2 Somach SC. Relapsing polychondritis. In: Morgan MB, Smoller BR, Somach SC. *Deadly Dermatologic Diseases. Clinicopathologic Atlas and Text*. New York: Springer, 2007: 161–4.

Sarcoidosis

Several studies document an association of sarcoidosis with malignant disease [1–4]; the suggested mechanism relates to abnormal immune function in sarcoidosis [1,4]. The strongest link reported is with lymphomas, to the extent that the term 'sarcoidosis–lymphoma syndrome' is used by some authors [1,3]. In most such cases, lymphoma has followed sarcoidosis, but the rationale for any association is less clear in cases in which sarcoidosis has developed after a cutaneous lymphoma. An apparent aetiological relationship is suggested in a quarter of cases [4]. Testicular tumours, carcinomas of skin (including melanoma), multiple myeloma, lung cancer, female genitourinary tract and other tumours have also been reported. However, large studies have found no evidence to support any significant association between sarcoidosis and malignant disease (or lymphoma specifically) [5,6].

References

1 Linnenberg HS, Medici TC, Rhyner K. The sarcoidosis-lymphoma syndrome—a lymphocyte dysregulation? *Pneumologie* 1992; **46**: 229–35.

2 Caras WE, Dillard T, Baker T, Pluss J. Coexistence of sarcoidosis and malignancy. *South Med J* 2003; **96**: 918–22.

3 Schmuth M, Prior C, Illersperger B *et al*. Systemic sarcoidosis and cutaneous lymphoma: is the association fortuitous? *Br J Dermatol* 1999; **140**: 952–5.

4 Cohen PR. Granuloma annulare, relapsing polychondritis, sarcoidosis, and systemic lupus erythematosus: conditions whose dermatologic manifestations may occur as hematologic malignancy-associated mucocutaneous paraneoplastic syndromes. *Int J Dermatol* 2006; **45**: 70–80.

5 Rømer FK, Hommelgaard P, Schou G. Sarcoidosis and cancer revisited: a long-term follow-up study of 555 Danish sarcoidosis patients. *Eur Respir J* 1998; **12**: 906–12.

6 Smedby KE, Hjalgrim H, Askling J *et al*. Autoimmune and chronic inflammatory disorders and risk of non-Hodgkin lymphoma by subtype. *J Natl Cancer Inst* 2006; **98**: 51–60.

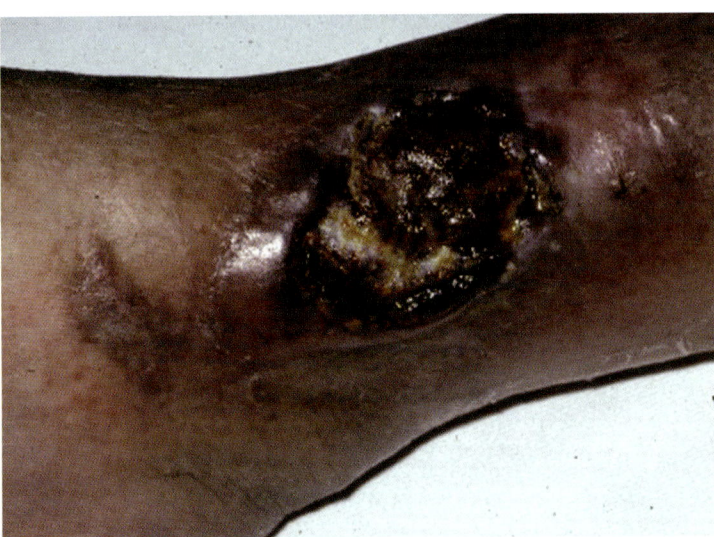

Fig. 62.15 Pyoderma gangrenosum of the lower leg in a patient with myelodysplastic syndrome.

Pyoderma gangrenosum and neutrophilic dermatoses. These are discussed in greater depth in Chapter 50 and are only briefly noted here. Pyoderma gangrenosum, particularly in a superficial and bullous form, has been associated with myeloproliferative diseases, including acute and chronic myeloid leukaemia, acute lymphocytic leukaemia, myeloid metaplasia, PRV, multiple myeloma, lymphoma and myelofibrosis (Fig. 62.15) [1]. The association of pyoderma gangrenosum with monoclonal gammopathy is uncertain, but it does occur at a frequency higher than expected in the general population and is usually of IgA type, whereas IgG gammopathy is the commonest type overall. Solid tumours reported include carcinoid, colon, bladder, prostate, breast, bronchus, ovary and adrenocortical carcinoma.

Sweet's syndrome has likewise been associated with several malignancies, especially haemopoietic. Chronic recurrent Sweet's syndrome [2] appears to have a particularly strong link with myelodysplastic disorders.

References
1 Powell FC, Daniel Su WP, Perry HO. Pyoderma gangrenosum: classification and management. *J Am Acad Dermatol* 1996; **34**: 395–409.
2 Vignon-Pennamen MD, Juillard C, Rybojad M *et al.* Chronic recurrent lymphocytic Sweet syndrome as a predictive marker of myelodysplasia: a report of 9 cases. *Arch Dermatol* 2006; **142**: 1170–6.

Multicentric reticulohistiocytosis (**lipoid dermatoarthritis; reticulocytoma cutis**) [1,2]
This is a rare condition, usually occurring in adult life, and characterized by papulonodular lesions of the fingers or other extremities, the face, and sometimes mucous membranes. Papules around the nail fold have been termed the 'coral bead sign'. A severe symmetrical polyarthritis, especially affecting the hands, is frequently associated [3]. Approximately 25% of cases are associated with internal neoplasia, virtually always solid tumours such as those of the breast, lung, colon, pancreas, stomach, ovary or cervix [1–3], although haematological malignancies have also been reported [4].

References
1 Aldridge RD, Main RA, Daly BM. Multicentric reticulohistiocytosis and cancer. *J Am Acad Dermatol* 1984; **10**: 296–7.
2 Nunnink JC, Krusinski PA, Yates JW. Multicentric reticulohistiocytosis and cancer: a case report and review of the literature. *Med Ped Oncol* 1985; **13**: 273–9.
3 Weenig RH, Mehrany K. Dermal and pannicular manifestations of internal malignancy. *Dermatol Clin* 2008; **26**: 31–43.
4 Cox NH, West NC, Popple AW. Multicentric reticulohistiocytosis associated with idiopathic myelofibrosis. *Br J Dermatol* 2001; **145**: 1033–4.

Vascular disorders

Raynaud's phenomenon and digital ischaemia (paraneoplastic acral vascular syndrome) [1–3]
Persistent, painful digital ischaemia, with an unusual Raynaud's syndrome-type appearance but often progressing to gangrene, has been linked to a variety of solid tumours and reticuloendothelial neoplasms [1–3]. The process may have a vasculitic element [4] (see below).

Hyperviscosity syndromes such as polycythaemia rubra vera, leukaemias or myeloma-linked cryoglobulinaemia may give rise to cutaneous ischaemia and phlebitis by microvascular occlusion; cancer-associated coagulopathy may also cause vascular occlusion [5].

Hypereosinophilic syndrome, for which there is increasing evidence of a malignant clonal proliferation, has also been associated with acrocyanosis, cutaneous microthrombi, digital infarction and gangrene [6–8]. In some instances, there is a clonal T-cell production of interleukin-5, a major controlling cytokine in production release and differentiation of eosinophils. In other cases, there is clonal expansion of eosinophils with hepatosplenomegaly and thrombocytopenia; this condition appears to be due to a cytogenetic defect t(9;22)(q34;q11) in which there is chromosomal breakage and reciprocal exchange of chromosomal fragments that leads to formation of a fusion tyrosine kinase FIP1L1–PDGFRα.

Erythromelalgia
This condition is linked with myeloproliferative disorders, most commonly polycythaemia rubra vera or essential thrombocythaemia, in over a third of adult cases. In a large series of patients with erythromelalgia linked with haematological malignancy, the feet were most commonly affected, with severe burning pain and erythema; symptoms may occur 2 years or more before the haematological disorder is documented [9]. The mechanism involves microvascular occlusion (typically with platelet aggregates, termed 'white thrombi'); Raynaud's phenomenon may also occur.

Palmar erythema
This is rarely linked with malignancy, but an interesting association was observed in a series of patients with cerebral malignancies, in whom nearly 20% had palmar and (to a lesser extent) plantar erythema, either diffuse or mottled. This occurrence seemed to be linked with the vascularity of the tumour, and was particularly seen with high-grade astrocytomas and glioblastomas; a role for vascular endothelial growth factor was proposed [10].

Vasculitis and malignancy [4,11]
There appears to be an association of cutaneous vasculitis with neoplasia, particularly in myeloproliferative disorders [11–13] and

myeloma [14,15], although solid tumours have also been reported [4,16,17]. Hairy cell leukaemia appears to be especially associated with vasculitis, which may be of leukocytoclastic or polyarteritis nodosa pattern. Of the solid tumours reported with malignancy, the most common would appear to be approximately the sites expected in an average population, including breast, lung, colon, oesophageal, renal, prostatic and head and neck tumours. As noted above, there is overlap with paraneoplastic digital ischaemia. In a study of 200 patients with ANCA-positive vasculitis (Wegener's granulomatosis or microscopic polyangiitis), the relative risk of malignancy preceding or concurrent with vasculitis was sixfold greater than that for the local population; patients with Henoch–Schönlein purpura (n = 129) had a fivefold relative risk, but only five of 333 patients with SLE had a malignancy [18].

The dermatological manifestations include palpable purpura, maculopapular, urticarial and petechial lesions; these presumably reflect a small-vessel vasculitis or even, when ulceration occurs, a necrotizing vasculitis [4,11]. When linked with a haematological malignancy, vasculitis often antedates bone marrow involvement, as opposed to the more predictable purpura due to thrombocythaemia, which reflects bone marrow infiltration by myeloproliferative disease or carcinoma. It is difficult in some reports to distinguish between microvascular occlusion (for example, by a monoclonal type I cryoglobulin) versus primary vasculitis or therapy-related vessel injury.

Chilblain-like lesions

Lesions resembling perniosis may be a manifestation of leukaemias and myeloproliferative disorders (Fig. 62.16; see also p. 62.88) [19,20]. They are persistent rather than episodic, which would be expected in idiopathic perniosis, refractory to treatments for perniosis, such as calcium channel blockers, and biopsies may show blast cells. Metastasis from breast carcinoma has also been documented as resembling chilblains [21].

References

1 El Tal AK, Tannous Z. Cutaneous vascular disorders associated with internal malignancy. *Dermatol Clin* 2008; **26**: 45–57.

2 Hawley PR, Johnston AW, Rankin JT. Association between digital ischaemia and malignant disease. *BMJ* 1967; **iii**: 208–12.

3 Palmer HM. Digital vascular disease and malignant disease. *Br J Dermatol* 1974; **91**: 476–7.

4 Greer JM, Longley S, Lawrence-Edwards N *et al*. Vasculitis associated with malignancy: experience with 13 patients and literature review. *Medicine* 1988; **67**: 220–30.

5 Boyce S, Harper J. Paraneoplastic dermatoses. *Dermatol Clin* 2002; **20**: 523–32.

6 Jang K-A, Lim Y-S, Choi J-H *et al*. Hypereosinophilic syndrome presenting as cutaneous necrotizing eosinophilic vasculitis and Raynaud's phenomenon complicated by digital gangrene. *Br J Dermatol* 2000; **143**: 641–4.

7 Hamada T, Kimura Y, Hayashi S *et al*. Hypereosinophilic syndrome with peripheral circulatory insufficiency and cutaneous microthrombi. *Arch Dermatol* 2007; **143**: 812–3.

8 Oppliger R, Gay-Crosier F, Dayer E, Hauser C. Digital necrosis in a patient with hypereosinophilic syndrome in the absence of cutaneous eosinophilic vasculitis. *Br J Dermatol* 2001; **144**: 1087–90.

9 Kurzrock R, Cohen PR. Erythromelalgia and myeloproliferative disorders. *Arch Intern Med* 1989; **149**: 105–9.

10 Noble JB, Boisnic S, Branchet-Gumila MC, Poisson M. Palmar erythema: cutaneous marker of neoplasm. *Dermatology* 2002; **204**: 209–13.

11 Kurzrock R, Cohen PR. Vasculitis and cancer. *Clin Dermatol* 1993; **11**: 175–67.

12 Longley S, Caldwell Pannish RS. Paraneoplastic vasculitis: unique syndrome of cutaneous angiitis and arthritis associated with myeloproliferative disorders. *Am J Med* 1986; **80**: 1027–30.

13 Zappasodi P, Del Forna C, Corso A, Lazzarino M. Mucocutaneous paraneoplastic syndromes in hematologic malignancies. *Int J Dermatol* 2006; **45**: 14–22.

14 Seelen MAJ, de Meijer PHEM, Arnoldus EPJ *et al*. A patient with multiple myeloma presenting with severe polyneuropathy caused by necrotizing vasculitis. *Am J Med* 1997; **102**: 485–6.

15 Daoud MS, Lust JA, Kyle RA *et al*. Monoclonal gammopathies and associated skin disorders. *J Am Acad Dermatol* 1999; **40**: 507–35.

16 Mita T, Nakanishi Y, Ochiai A *et al*. Paraneoplastic vasculitis associated with esophageal carcinoma. *Pathol Internat* 1999; **49**: 643–7.

17 Lotti T, Ghersetich I, Comacchi C, Jorizzo JL. Cutaneous small-vessel vasculitis. *J Am Acad Dermatol* 1998; **39**: 667–87.

18 Pankhurst T, Savage COS, Gordon C, Harper L. Malignancy is increased in ANCA-associated vasculitis. *Rheumatology (Oxford)* 2004; **43**: 1532–5.

19 Yazawa H, Saga K, Omori F *et al*. The chilblain-like eruption as a diagnostic clue to the blast crisis of chronic myelocytic leukaemia. *J Am Acad Dermatol* 2004; **50** (Suppl.): S42–4.

20 Affleck AG, Ravenscroft JC, Leach IH. Chilblain-like leukemia cutis. *Pediatr Dermatol* 2007; **24**: 38–41.

21 Tan BB, Lear JT, English JSC. Metastasis from carcinoma of breast masquerading as chilblains. *J Roy Soc Med* 1997; **90**: 162.

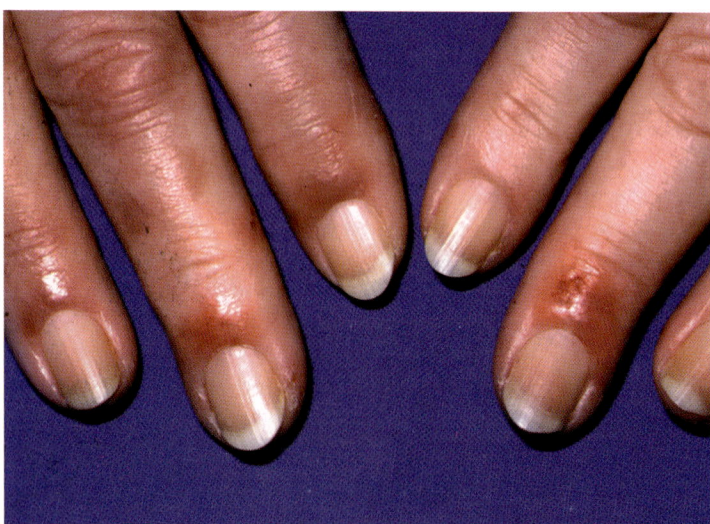

Fig. 62.16 Chilblain-like lesions in acute myeloid leukaemia.

Cancer-associated thrombosis

Three main patterns need to be considered: migratory thrombophlebitis, deep venous thrombosis, and Mondor's disease (a specific pattern of thrombophlebitis, but sufficiently distinctive that it is described separately). Arterial thrombosis may also occur as a paraneoplastic entity but is much less common. The aetiology of cancer-associated thrombosis is multifactorial. Interaction of macrophages with cancer cells causes release of tumour necrosis factor and interleukin-6 which damage endothelium, creating a pro-thrombotic situation; the same interaction causes activation of platelets, and of clotting factors X and XII [1]. Some tumour proteases are also procoagulant, especially 'tissue factor' which activates factor VII, and sialic acid moieties of mucin (released from adenocarcinomas) which activate factor X [1].

Migratory thrombophlebitis (Trousseau's sign) [2–7]. Unlike superficial thrombophlebitis confined to the lower limbs, thrombophlebitis associated with neoplasia is often recurrent and migratory. A variety of sites, especially the upper extremities and trunk, can be involved, and lesions are usually multiple. Migratory thrombophlebitis is associated with malignancy in 50% of cases. The mechanism in most cases is an intravascular, low-grade hyper-coagulation, which responds poorly to anticoagulant therapy; heparin is usually more effective than warfarin [8]. As well as altered level or function of prothrombotic and anticoagulant proteins, the coagulation and thrombotic process may involve cytokines, angiogenic factors or mucin secretion by tumours, altered blood viscosity, vascular endothelial changes and production of small tumour emboli. Migratory thrombophlebitis can be associated with any cancer, but particularly occurs with carcinomas of the pancreas, stomach, colon and lung; pancreatic carcinoma accounts for about half of all cases. Leukaemias and lymphomas are less commonly associated with migratory thrombophlebitis. Causative tumours are often highly malignant and metastatic with a poor prognosis.

Deep vein thrombosis (DVT). This is not commonly the presenting feature of malignancy [4,7], although cancers have a significant risk of causing thrombosis. The likelihood of finding a malignancy is increased by about fourfold in patients with a deep venous thrombosis of the leg compared with expected population rates, the overall risk of such an association is about 10%. By contrast, DVT of the upper limb is more commonly linked with neoplasia (in some cases, the reason is obstruction by an apical lung tumour), and DVT is identified post-mortem in half of patients who have died due to cancer. Tumours associated with DVT are usually adenocarcinomas in the gastrointestinal tract, urogenital tract, breast or lung; mucin secretion, as noted above, causes non-enzymatic activation of factor X to factor Xa, initiating the thrombotic cascade. Older age of patients with a DVT has been proposed as a factor that should be associated with a lower threshold for malignancy screening.

Mondor's disease. This is a rare condition in which a cord-like lesion is palpable in the subcutaneous tissue of the anterior or lateral thorax, or sometimes abdomen. The underlying lesion is a thrombophlebitis of thoracic or epigastric veins, usually unilateral but occasionally bilateral, which may occur as a result of trauma, inflammation or post-surgery. However, 10–15% of patients may have an associated breast carcinoma [4,7,9] so careful examination and mammography are indicated unless an alternative cause is obvious.

References

1 Bick RL. Cancer-associated thrombosis. *N Engl J Med*; **349**: 109–11.
2 Callen JP. Skin signs of internal malignancy. In: Callen JP, Jorizzo JL, eds. *Dermatological Manifestations of Internal Disease*, 3rd edn. Philadelphia: Saunders, 2003: 95–104.
3 Braverman IM. *Skin Signs of Systemic Disease*, 3rd edn. Philadelphia: Saunders, 1998.
4 El Tal AK, Tannous Z. Cutaneous vascular disorders associated with internal malignancy. *Dermatol Clin* 2008; **26**: 45–57.
5 Sack GH, Levin J, Bell WR. Trousseau's syndrome and other manifestations of chronic disseminated coagulopathy in patients with neoplasms: clinical, pathophysiologic, and therapeutic features. *Medicine* 1977; **56**: 1–37.
6 James WD. Trousseau's syndrome. *Int J Dermatol* 1984; **23**: 205–6.
7 Samlaska CP, James WD. Superficial thrombophlebitis. II. Secondary hypercoagulable states. *J Am Acad Dermatol* 1990; **23**: 1–18.
8 Walsh-McMonagle D, Green D. Low molecular-weight heparin in the management of Trousseau's syndrome. *Cancer* 1997; **80**: 649–55.
9 Catania S, Zurrida S, Veronesi P *et al*. Mondor's disease and breast cancer. *Cancer* 1992; **69**: 2267–70.

Flushing

This is a normal physiological response and may be a problematic menopausal symptom. However, it may be a feature of carcinoid syndrome, mastocytosis, phaeochromocytoma, medullary carcinoma of thyroid, hypogonadism in males, pancreatic tumours producing vasoactive intestinal peptide (VIPomas), basophilic leukaemia, horseshoe kidney (Rovsing's syndrome) and renal cell carcinoma [1,2]; it is also a feature of POEMS syndrome which is associated with myeloma (discussed on pp. 62.92 and 62.94). Plethora, but not flushing, may be apparent in polycythaemia rubra vera.

Carcinoid syndrome may be difficult to diagnose at an early stage, as flushing is typically provoked by common triggers of physiological flushing, such as emotional stress or alcohol ingestion. Only about 10% of patients with a carcinoid tumour have a malignant carcinoid syndrome, and paroxysmal flushing is present in virtually all cases; episodes typically last a few minutes and may be more widespread than emotional flushing, sometimes involving the whole body. Nearly 75% of carcinoid tumours are gastrointestinal (especially involving the appendix and ileum), 25% are bronchial, and a small number arise at other sites including the larynx, pancreas, gallbladder and ovary [3]. Flushing is described as varying according to the site of the neoplasm; the most common midgut tumours (appendix and ileum) are associated with gradual development of fixed cyanotic erythema in the flushing distribution, whereas foregut tumours (stomach, pancreas, lung) are associated with a brighter pink flush. This may reflect production of different mediators; gastric carcinoids typically cause flushing by production of histamine, whereas midgut carcinoids produce serotonin, bradykinin and prostaglandins. Other symptoms, such as diarrhoea, abdominal pain, dyspnoea, wheezing and occasionally syncope, may occur with progression of the tumour, usually not occurring until liver metastases have developed. Persistent erythema with or without telangiectasia, scleroderma-like change, pigmentary anomalies and a pellagra-like dermatitis eventually develop.

Mastocytosis [1,4,5] is discussed in more detail in Chapter 22. It is most commonly limited to the skin but may be systemic, in which event it can be classified into four groups: indolent, associated with a clonal haematological non-mast cell lineage disease (myeloproliferative or myelodysplastic disorders), aggressive (lymphadenopathic with eosinophilia), and mast cell leukaemia. It may be associated with mutations in the gene for c-kit. The more aggressive forms tend not to be associated with cutaneous mast cell lesions but flushing, dyspnoea, chest pain, abdominal cramps, palpitations, syncope and other systemic reactions due to mast cell degranulation may occur. Serum tryptase is a useful screening test that may suggest systemic disease. However, the proportion of bone marrow mast cells, eosinophilia (especially in bone marrow) and alkaline phosphatase level are of greater prognostic importance than levels of mast cell mediators [6].

Phaeochromocytomas (PCC) may cause pallor with rebound flushing [1,2], but the more typical dermatological feature is hyperhidrosis, discussed above. *Medullary carcinoma of thyroid*, like PCC, may occur as part of a MEN syndrome (p. 62.24) but may occur in isolation. They may produce several other hormones such as ACTH, as well as prostaglandins and amines, which may cause other symptoms such as diarrhoea.

References

1 El Tal AK, Tannous Z. Cutaneous vascular disorders associated with internal malignancy. *Dermatol Clin* 2008; **26**: 45–57.
2 Hemann WR. Flushing, pheochromocytoma, and the dermatologist. *J Am Acad Dermatol* 2006; **55**: 1075–7.
3 Modlin IM, Sandor A. An analysis of 8305 cases of carcinoid tumors. *Cancer* 1997; **79**: 13–29.
4 Beck LA, Provost TT. Mastocytosis. In: Provost TT, Flynn JA, eds. *Cutaneous Medicine: Cutaneous Manifestations of Systemic Disease*. Hamilton, Ontario: Decker, 2001: 367–88.
5 Tharp MD, Chan IJ. Mastocytosis. *Adv Dermatol* 2003; **19**: 207–36.
6 Pardanani A, Baek J-Y, Li C-Y *et al.* Systemic mast cell disease without associated hematologic disorder: a combined retrospective and prospective study. *Mayo Clin Proc* 2002; **77**: 1169–75.

Venous or lymphatic obstruction

In addition to vasculitis and the thrombotic intravascular occlusion described above, vessels of different types may become occluded by intravascular tumour cells, or may be compressed by an adjacent tumour. The facial and upper limb suffusion of superior vena caval obstruction is well known. Obstruction of venous flow from the head and neck may also occur due to benign retrosternal thyroid gland enlargement and is typically seen when the arms are elevated (Pemberton sign). Lymphatic obstruction typically occurs at the main lymph node sites, such as in the axilla due to a breast carcinoma, lymphoma or limb melanoma. Apical lung neoplasms may also cause damage to sympathetic nerves, leading to anhidrosis and sometimes hyperhidrosis and flushing of the contralateral, unaffected side. Arterial obstruction by tumours is much less common, although tumour emboli may occur.

Other vascular disorders

Various other angiomatous lesions have been linked with internal malignancy, including *eruptive angiomas* [1] and *telangiectasia* [2]. The latter may occur as a direct tumour infiltration of vessels (carcinoma telangiectoides, p. 62.16) but has also been described secondary to lung cancer. Painful telangiectatic plaques are a feature of malignancy angioendotheliomatosis. *Glomeruloid angiomas* are a feature of POEMS syndrome, in which a monoclonal paraprotein is a feature. Telangiectasia occurs in several genodermatoses described earlier, such as Bloom's syndrome and Rothmund–Thomson syndrome, and is a feature of more advanced cases of carcinoid syndrome.

References

1 Pembroke AC, Grice K, Levantine AV *et al.* Eruptive angiomata in malignant disease. *Clin Exp Dermatol* 1978; **3**: 147–55.
2 El Tal AK, Tannous Z. Cutaneous vascular disorders associated with internal malignancy. *Dermatol Clin* 2008; **26**: 45–57.

Deposition disorders: mucinoses, xanthomas, amyloidosis and calcification

Dermal deposition disorders may be linked with internal malignancy [1]; in particular, there are a number of diverse cutaneous manifestations of paraproteinaemia and myeloma (p. 62.92) [2]. Some of these are rare conditions, and their occurrence should prompt a search for an underlying internal cause. Some of the most important deposition disorders, and their potentially associated internal malignancy, are listed in Table 62.11; all listed are discussed in detail in other chapters.

Paraproteinaemia is associated with many of the deposition disorders listed in Table 62.11. Other manifestations of paraproteinaemia are discussed in more detail in the section on haematological disorders (pp. 62.92–62.94). Pathology of disorders such as scleromyxoedema and necrobiotic xanthogranuloma is discussed in [2–4].

Calcinoisis cutis is a rare complication of internal carcinoma. However, it should be noted that many cancers cause hypercalcaemia, and that metastatic calcification may occur in other organs, such as the lung or kidney, even if not in the skin. The commonest underlying tumours are carcinoma of oesophagus, myeloma, breast cancer, lymphoma and osteolytic metastases; mechanisms include production of parathyroid hormone, parathyroid hormone-related peptide, vitamin D, cytokines, up-regulation of NFκB ligand (RANKL) or down-regulation of RANKL antagonist (osteoprotegerin) [2].

References

1 Touart DM, Sau P. Cutaneous deposition disorders. Part I. *J Am Acad Dermatol* 1998; **39**: 149–71.
2 Weenig RH, Mehrany K. Dermal and pannicular manifestations of internal malignancy. *Dermatol Clin* 2008; **26**: 31–43.
3 Cohen PR. Paraneoplastic dermatopathology: cutaneous paraneoplastic syndromes. *Adv Dermatol* 1996; **11**: 215–52.
4 Chung VQ, Moschella SL, Zembowicz A, Liu V. Clinical and pathologic findings of paraneoplastic dermatoses. *J Am Acad Dermatol* 2006; **54**: 745–62.

Bullous disorders

Paraneoplastic pemphigus (PNP; neoplasia-associated pemphigus) [1–6]

This is a heterogeneous, multiorgan, autoimmune syndrome in which patients may display a spectrum of mucocutaneous manifestations including pemphigus-like, pemphigoid-like, erythema multiforme-like, graft-versus-host disease-like or lichen planus-like patterns, characteristically with oral involvement; in addition, there is an association with small-airways occlusion [5] and deposition of autoantibody complexes in different organs. The mucosal disease is often severe and progressive.

Associated neoplasms in one large review series were mainly B-cell proliferations and thymoma or thymoma-like neoplasms; specific neoplasms included Hodgkin's lymphoma (42%), chronic lymphocytic leukaemia (29%), Castleman's tumour (10%), thymoma (6%), spindle cell neoplasms (6%) and Waldenström's macroglobulinaemia (6%) [1]. PNP is distinguished from pemphigus by its clinical features and by the presence of serum autoantibodies to a range of antigens of 250, 230, 210, 190 and 170 kDa (which include bullous pemphigoid antigen, as well as desmosomal and hemidesmosomal proteins including desmoglein 1, desmoglein 3, envoplakin and periplakin); direct immunofluorescence of skin biopsies is usually positive for IgG and C3 but may be negative in some cases. High sensitivity and specificity for this differential diagnosis has recently been reported by taking account

Table 62.11 Some deposition disorders that are linked with internal malignancy.

Material deposited	Disorder	Associated internal malignancies	Comments
Amyloid proteins [1] (see Chapter 59)	Primary and myeloma-associated systemic amyloidosis (AL protein deposition)	Paraproteinaemia, myeloma	Amyloidosis occurs in about 15% of patients with myelomatosis
	Secondary amyloidosis (AA protein deposition)	Lymphomas, especially Hodgkin's lymphoma Hypernephroma Other solid tumours	
Mucin/proteoglycans and fibromucinoses	Scleromyxedema/lichen myxoedematosus	Paraproteinaemia, typically a 'slow gamma region'	Paraprotein is present in most cases
	Papular mucinosis	Paraproteinaemia	Uncommon
	Scleredema	Paraproteinaemia	More commonly associated with diabetes or streptococcal infection
	POEMS syndrome	Paraproteinaemia	Features are polyneuropathy, organomegaly, endocrinopathy, M-protein, skin changes
Lipids (as foamy macrophages)	Necrobiotic xanthogranuloma	Paraproteinaemia, usually monoclonal IgGκ, present in about 70% of cases	Also associated with cryoglobulinaemia, myeloma, marrow dyscrasias and rarely leukaemia; some cases apparently occur in isolation
	Normolipaemic plane xanthomatosis	Myeloma	Usually IgG paraprotein
	Xanthoma disseminatum	Gammopathy, bone marrow dyscrasias	Usually IgG paraprotein
Calcium	Metastatic calcification	Lung and other squamous carcinomas Due to primary hyperparathyroidism; may be associated with multiple endocrine neoplasia syndromes	Due to ectopic parathyroid-like hormone secretion See p. 62.24
	Dystrophic calcification	Pancreatic carcinoma	Calcification of fat

of the association with a lymphoproliferative disorder, indirect immunofluorescence of rat bladder urothelium (antibodies to desmoplakin), and envoplakin and/or periplakin bands on immunoblotting [6].

References

1 Anhalt GJ. Paraneoplastic pemphigus. *Adv Dermatol* 1997; **12**: 77–96.
2 Thomas I, Schwartz RA. Cutaneous paraneoplastic syndromes: uncommon presentations. *Clinics Dermatol* 2005; **23**: 593–600.
3 Stone SP, Buescher LS. Life-threatening paraneoplastic cutaneous syndromes. *Clinics Dermatol* 2005; **23**: 301–6.
4 Nguyen VT, Ndoye A, Bassler KD *et al*. Classification, clinical manifestations and immunopathological mechanisms of epithelial variant of paraneoplastic autoimmune multiorgan syndrome. *Arch Dermatol* 2001; **137**: 193–206.
5 Nousari HC, Deterding R, Wojtczack H *et al*. The mechanism of respiratory failure in paraneoplastic pemphigus. *N Engl J Med* 1999; **340**: 1406–10.
6 Joly P, Richard C, Gilbert D *et al*. Sensitivity and specificity of clinical, histologic, and immunologic features in the diagnosis of paraneoplastic pemphigus. *J Am Acad Dermatol* 2000; **43**: 619–26.

Bullous pemphigoid

Isolated reports have suggested an association between bullous pemphigoid and underlying neoplasia [1–3]. However, larger series do not support a significant association with malignant disease [4,5]. Despite this, the issue remains controversial, and more selective studies have shown there may be a correlation when immunofluorescent findings are negative and mucosal involvement is present [4,6]. Historical reports are difficult to evaluate with certainty, as some cases may actually have been epidermolysis bullosa acquisita, or even bullous pemphigoid-like PNP, which can now be separated from bullous pemphigoid by

current immunological techniques. Malignancies have been reported from breast, lung, thyroid, larynx, skin, soft tissue, stomach, colon, lymphoreticular system, prostate, cervix, bladder, kidney and uterus.

Pemphigus

Historically, pemphigus has been linked with various tumours; some cases, such as those associated with thymoma and Castleman's tumour, would probably now be found to have the features of PNP. Pemphigus foliaceus has been associated with acanthosis nigricans-like lesions and hepatocellular carcinoma [7], and pemphigus in Japanese subjects has been associated with lung cancer. The concurrence of internal malignancy and pemphigus, as with bullous pemphigoid, may be a true association [8], although some suggest this to be coincidence [9].

References

1 Hodge L, Marsden RA, Black MM *et al*. Bullous pemphigoid: the frequency of mucosal involvement and concurrent malignancy related to indirect immunofluorescence findings. *Br J Dermatol* 1981; **105**: 65–9.
2 Schroeter AL. Pemphigoid and malignancy. *Clin Dermatol* 1987; **5**: 60–3.
3 Tanaka T, Ogino A, Ogura K *et al*. A case of bullous pemphigoid and transitional cell carcinoma of the bladder: demonstration of a circulating factor reactive with basement membrane zone of skin and of bladder carcinoma. *Arch Dermatol* 1983; **119**: 704–5.
4 Lindelof B, Islam N, Eklund G *et al*. Pemphigoid and cancer. *Arch Dermatol* 1990; **126**: 66–8.
5 Stone SS, Schroeter AL. Bullous pemphigoid and associated malignant neoplasms. *Arch Dermatol* 1975; **111**: 991–4.
6 Person JR, Rogers RS. Bullous and cicatricial pemphigoid: clinical, histopathologic and immunopathologic correlations. *Mayo Clin Proc* 1977; **52**: 54–66.

7 Muramatsu T, Matsumoto H, Yamashina Y *et al.* Pemphigus foliaceus associated with acanthosis nigricans-like lesions and hepatocellular carcinoma. *Int J Dermatol* 1989; **28**: 462–3.

8 Krain LS, Bierman SM. Pemphigus vulgaris and internal malignancy. *Cancer* 1974; **33**: 1091–9.

9 Callen JP. Internal disorders associated with bullous disease of the skin: a critical review. *J Am Acad Dermatol* 1980; **3**: 107–19.

Other blistering disorders

Dermatitis herpetiformis (DH) has been documented in some studies to have a link with internal malignancy of various types, especially lymphoma [1–4], although some studies suggest that the risk is actually quite low and confined to a small increase in likelihood of lymphoma [3]. Review of a single-institution large cohort of patients with DH documented a low frequency of lymphoproliferative disorders (seven of 270 patients, including two with small bowel and one with gastric lymphoma) and although 10.4% of the series had some form of documented malignant disease at some time, there was no apparent tumour type that was over-represented, no control population to know whether this represented an increased risk, and the interval between DH and lymphoma varied widely [5]. There is logic for an indirect link with lymphoma; DH is always associated with some degree of gluten-sensitive enteropathy, and the latter has a well documented association with small bowel lymphoma. One group of authors who initially found an increased risk of lymphoma in DH [4] later, in a larger study, documented that the overall risk of mortality in DH was lower than in the general population [6], although the risk of non-Hodgkin's lymphoma was increased with a standardized incidence ratio of 6.0. In this study, one of seven lymphomas in DH was an enteropathy-associated T-cell lymphoma, associated with inadequate dietary compliance [6], supporting the earlier documentation that a gluten-free diet (GFD) reduces the risk of small bowel lymphoma in patients with DH [7].

It therefore appears that there is an increased risk of lymphoma in DH but that the overall risk is small; additionally, the lymphoma risk, particularly of bowel lymphoma, is decreased by adherence to a GFD.

Linear IgA disease also appears to have a higher-than-predicted association with lymphoproliferative malignancy although this is much less well documented [8].

Epidermolysis bullosa acquisita (EBA) is commonly linked with autoimmune diseases but has also been reported to occur in association with neoplasia (Fig. 62.17), particularly myeloma and lymphoma [9–11]. An interesting possible explanation is partial homology of a 105-kDa basement membrane antigen with a 90-kDa tumour antigen [12]. The difficulties in separating EBA from other subepidermal blistering disorders such as cicatricial pemphigoid and bullous pemphigoid have already been alluded to, and make evaluation of earlier reports uncertain.

Porphyria cutanea tarda and *variegate porphyrias* have been associated with hepatocellular carcinoma [13]. Myeloma and visceral carcinoma have also been reported [14].

Erythema multiforme is most commonly related to herpes simplex or other infections, or to medications; if it occurs in the context of neoplasia it can be difficult to prove an association. The association is certainly weak and does not warrant investigation routinely.

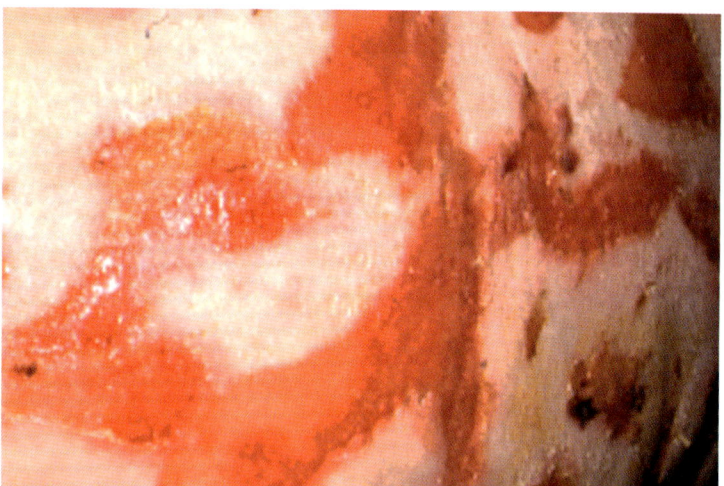

Fig. 62.17 Paraneoplastic epidermolysis bullosa acquisita in a patient with metastatic breast carcinoma; irregular erosions on the abdomen resulting from fragile blisters.

References

1 Leonard JN, Tucker WF, Fry JS *et al.* Increased incidence of malignancy in dermatitis herpetiformis. *BMJ* 1983; **286**: 16–18.

2 Swerdlow AJ, Whittaker S, Carpenter LM *et al.* Mortality and cancer incidence in patients with dermatitis herpetiformis: a cohort study. *Br J Dermatol* 1993; **129**: 140–4.

3 Sigurgeirsson B, Agnarsson BA, Lindelof B. Risk of lymphoma in patients with dermatitis herpetiformis. *BMJ* 1994; **308**: 13–5.

4 Collin P, Pukkala E, Reunala T. Malignancy and survival in dermatitis herpetiformis: a comparison with coeliac disease. *Gut* 1996; **38**: 528–30.

5 Alonso LJ, Gibson LE, Rogers RS 3rd. Clinical, pathologic, and immunopatholgic features of dermatitis herpetiformis: review of the Mayo clinic experience. *Int J Dermatol* 2007; **46**: 910–9.

6 Viljamaa M, Kaukinen K, Pukkala E *et al.* Malignancies and mortality in patients with coeliac disease and dermatitis herpetiformis: 30-year population-based study. *Dig Liver Dis* 2006; **38**: 374–80.

7 Lewis HM, Reunala TL, Garioch JJ *et al.* Protective effect of gluten-free diet against development of lymphoma in dermatitis herpetiformis. *Br J Dermatol* 1996; **135**: 363–7.

8 Godfrey KM, Wojnarowska FJ, Leonard J. Disease associations of linear IgA disease. *Br J Dermatol* 1989; **121**: 48.

9 Aractingi S, Bachmeyer C, Prost C *et al.* Subepidermal autoimmune bullous skin diseases associated with B-cell lymphoproliferative disorders. *Medicine (Baltimore)* 1999; **78**: 228–35.

10 Baler GR. Epidermolysis bullosa acquisita associated with lymphoma. *J Am Acad Dermatol* 1987; **17**: 856–9.

11 Engineer L, Dow EC, Braverman IM, Ahmed AR. Epidermolysis bullosa acquisita and multiple myeloma. *J Am Acad Dermatol* 2002; **47**: 943–6.

12 Chan LS, Woodley DT. The 105-kDa basement membrane autoantigen p105 is N-terminally homologous to a tumor-associated antigen. *J Invest Dermatol* 1996; **107**: 209–14.

13 Tidman MJ, Higgins EM, Elder GH *et al.* Variegate porphyria associated with hepatocellular carcinoma. *Br J Dermatol* 1989; **121**: 503–5.

14 Dandurand M, Guillot B, Guilhou JJ. Porphyrie cutanée tardive et néoplasies: à propos de deux observations. *Ann Dermatol Vénéréol* 1986; **113**: 679–83.

Indirect cutaneous markers of internal malignancy

Exposure to carcinogens [1]

Nicotine staining of the fingers is one of the commonest signs that a patient may be predisposed to bronchial carcinoma, together with other tobacco-linked neoplasia.

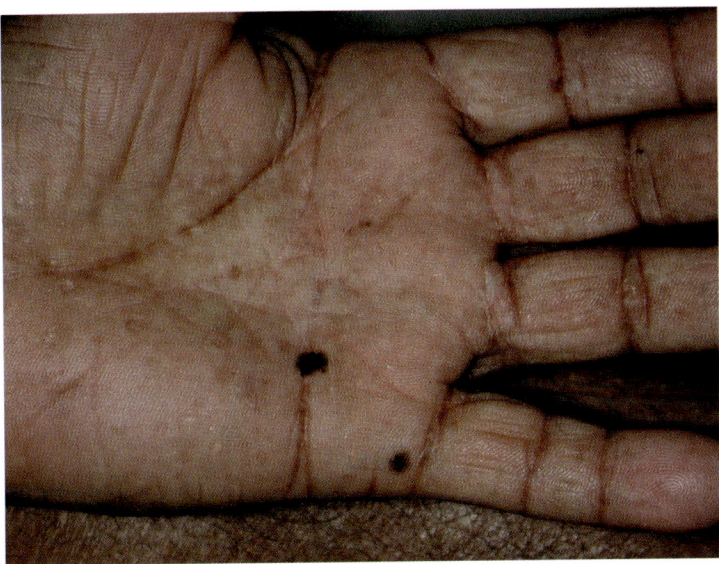

Fig. 62.18 Arsenical keratoses on the hand.

Radiotherapy damage to the skin may indicate that underlying tissues are at increased risk of neoplasia; this is particularly relevant for neck and thyroid carcinoma. Radiotherapy damage and/or multiple BCCs over the spine following radiotherapy for ankylosing spondylitis may indicate the patient is predisposed to leukaemia.

Arsenic-induced pigmentation, keratoses (Fig. 62.18), Bowen's disease, superficial BCCs and multiple sebaceous tumours can be linked to an increased risk of internal neoplasia (especially bronchial). The relationship between Bowen's disease of non-sun-exposed skin and an increased risk of internal neoplasia has been a long-standing controversy; a meta-analysis of published studies did not confirm a significant association [2], and if the link with arsenic is excluded, the association appears unsubstantiated [3,4]. A further study of 1147 patients found the overall incidence of internal cancers in patients with Bowen's disease to be slightly increased (115 cancers versus 103 expected, standardized incidence ratio (SIR) 1.1) but not significant [5]. However, there was an SIR of 3.2 for leukaemia in men and of 4.6 for lung cancer in men with Bowen's disease before age 60 years (the overall lung cancer SIR for both sexes and all ages was 1.3). There are various sources of potential bias in many studies of this type, and available evidence would still suggest that routine investigation for internal malignancy in patients with Bowen's disease is not justified [6].

Vinyl chloride-related acrosclerosis, acro-osteolysis and papular skin changes are variable markers of heavy industrial exposure in polyvinyl chloride manufacture. A link with angiosarcoma of the liver has been noted [7].

Immunosuppression

Patients on immunosuppressive therapy have an increased risk of internal malignancy. Some such patients have no specific cutaneous features but some may have a combination of features of their underlying disease (e.g. signs of renal failure), side effects of their treatment (e.g. hypertrichosis and gingival changes due to ciclo-sporin; frequent, severe or unusual infections), and other features linked with immunosuppression (e.g. sebaceous hyperplasia, viral warts, skin cancers or precursors). These issues are discussed in the section on organ transplantation (p. 62.74).

Several inherited immunodeficiency syndromes also carry an increased risk of internal neoplasia, the most important of which are discussed above.

A variety of viral, bacterial and fungal infections may occur as a result of compromised immune response as a consequence of internal malignancy, particularly in haematological malignancies or in those with a large tumour burden. Occasionally, such infection may be the presenting feature—in particular, herpes zoster occurs more severely, with higher incidence and wider dissemination, in patients with reticuloendothelial or myeloproliferative neoplasia [8]. More than 20 disseminated (chickenpox-like) lesions, or involvement of two or more dermatomes, are suggestive of immune compromise and possible underlying malignancy, although involvement of adjacent sacral dermatomes is not uncommon and does not warrant extensive investigation. Chronic herpes-virus infections may also be a feature of immunosuppression and therefore indirectly linked with neoplasia (such as Kaposi's sarcoma in AIDS).

References

1 Poole S, Fenske NA. Cutaneous markers of internal malignancy, 2: paraneoplastic dermatoses and environmental carcinogens. *J Am Acad Dermatol* 1993; **28**: 147–64.

2 Lycka BAS. Bowen's disease and internal malignancy. A meta-analysis. *Int J Dermatol* 1989; **28**: 531–3.

3 Chuang TY, Reizner GT. Bowen's disease and internal malignancy. *J Am Acad Dermatol* 1988; **19**: 47–51.

4 Arbesman H, Ransohoff DF. Is Bowen's disease a predictor for the development of internal malignancy? A methodological critique of the literature. *JAMA* 1987; **257**: 516–8.

5 Jaeger AB, Gramkow A, Hjalgrim H *et al*. Bowen disease and risk of subsequent malignant neoplasms: a population-based cohort study of 1147 patients. *Arch Dermatol* 1999; **135**: 790–3.

6 Cox NH, Eedy DJ, Morton CA. Guidelines for management of Bowen's disease: 2006 update. *Br J Dermatol* 2007; **156**: 11–21.

7 Anonymous. Vinyl chloride and cancer. *BMJ* 1974; **i**: 590–1.

8 Shanbrom E, Miller S, Haar H. Herpes zoster in hematologic neoplasias: some unusual manifestations. *Ann Intern Med* 1960; **53**: 523–33.

The gastrointestinal tract

This section concentrates on bowel, hepatic and pancreatic diseases in which cutaneous associations or consequences are prominent [1–4]. Skin changes related to more general effects of gastrointestinal diseases, such as nutritional defects, are discussed in Chapter 59; oral disease is described in Chapter 69. Links between skin disorders and abdominal pain are not specifically considered, but many of the disorders in this section may cause this symptom; other causes of skin eruption with abdominal pain include disorders such as hereditary angio-oedema (Chapter 22), vasculitides (Chapter 50), porphyrias (Chapter 59), and autoinflammatory diseases (periodic fevers; see the section on bone and joint disease later). Cutaneous metastases and paraneoplastic eruptions due to gastrointestinal malignancy are discussed in the preceding section of this chapter.

References

1 Gregory B, Ho VC. Cutaneous manifestations of gastrointestinal disorders, I and II. *J Am Acad Dermatol* 1992; **26**: 371–83.
2 Braverman IM. *Skin Signs of Systemic Disease*, 3rd edn. Philadelphia: Saunders, 1998: 405–37.
3 Herron MD, Zone JJ. Cutaneous diseases associated with gastrointestinal abnormalities. In: Callen JP, Jorrizo JL, eds. *Dermatological Signs of Internal Disease*, 3rd edn. Philadelphia: Saunders, 1995: 219–32.
4 Boh EE, al-Smadi RMF. Cutaneous manifestations of gastrointestinal diseases. *Dermatol Clin* 2002; **20**: 533–46.

Oesophagus and stomach

Bleeding from the oesophagus or stomach may be associated with skin and nail changes of iron deficiency, such as koilonychia, smooth tongue and angular cheilitis (Chapter 59). Iron deficiency is associated with dysphagia and development of a postcricoid web as in the Paterson–Brown–Kelly (Plummer–Vinson) syndrome. Skin disorders that are associated with gastrointestinal bleeding, or with polyps, are discussed later. Cutaneous metastases may occur from tumours of the oesophagus or stomach. Paraneoplastic eruptions linked to the upper gastrointestinal tract, such as tylosis with oesophageal carcinoma (Howell–Evans syndrome), acrodermatitis and nail dystrophy with upper gastrointestinal carcinoma (Bazex syndrome), or acanthosis nigricans with gastric carcinoma, are discussed earlier in this chapter.

Bullous diseases may affect the pharynx, oesophagus or stomach. Epidermolysis bullosa (EB) is of particular relevance; dystrophic EB may cause oesophageal scarring [1], with a risk of SCC, and gastric outflow is affected in junctional EB, resulting in pyloric atresia [2,3]. Several inflammatory disorders such as lichen planus may affect the mouth, pharynx or oesophagus [4,5]. Immunobullous diseases, particularly those with an IgA basement membrane zone immunoreactant, may cause mucosal blistering and erosions—examples include cicatricial pemphigoid, linear IgA disease and the IgA variant of epidermolysis bullosa acquisita. Cicatricial pemphigoid may also cause oesophageal scarring and stenosis.

Sclerodermatous processes also affect the oesophagus, in particular CREST (calcinosis, Raynaud's phenomenon, oesophagus, sclerodactyly, telangiectasia). This disorder is discussed more fully in Chapter 51. The oesophageal abnormality consists of decreased and disordered peristalsis. Scleroderma is also associated with decreased peristalsis throughout the bowel, leading to malabsorption, constipation and diverticulae. Sjögren's syndrome may also cause dysphagia, as may dermatomyositis in cases in which there is involvement of the pharyngeal musculature.

Helicobacter pylori has been implicated as an aetiological factor in some cases of urticaria, rosacea, vasculitis, Sweet's syndrome, erythema multiforme, alopecia areata, chronic itch and prurigo nodularis, and atopic and nummular dermatitis [6–8]. Although there are some individuals in whom eradication therapy coincides with resolution of a dermatosis, most larger studies in which there is adequate control for confounding factors such as age and social class have failed to demonstrate either a higher prevalence of *H. pylori* infection, higher titres on ^{13}C urea breath test, or a higher rate of response to eradication therapy in infected individuals compared with controls [9–12].

References

1 Orlando RC, Bozymski EM, Briggaman RA *et al.* Epidermolysis bullosa: gastrointestinal manifestations. *Ann Intern Med* 1974; **81**: 203–6.
2 Shaw DW, Fine JD, Piacquadio DJ *et al.* Gastric outflow obstruction and epidermolysis bullosa. *J Am Acad Dermatol* 1997; **36**: 304–10.
3 Nakano A, Pulkkinen L, Murrell D *et al.* Epidermolysis bullosa with congenital pyloric atresia: novel mutations in the beta 4 integrin gene (*ITGB4*) and genotype/phenotype correlations. *Pediatr Res* 2001; **49**: 618–26.
4 Harewood GC, Murray JA, Cameron AJ. Esophageal lichen planus: the Mayo Clinic experience. *Dis Esoph* 1999; **12**: 309–11.
5 Evans AV, Fletcher CL, Owen WL, Hay RJ. Oesophageal lichen planus. *Clin Exp Dermatol* 2000; **25**: 36–7.
6 Shiotani A, Okada K, Yanaoka K *et al.* Beneficial effect of *Helicobacter pylori* eradication in dermatologic diseases. *Helicobacter* 2001; **6**: 60–5.
7 Di Campli C, Gasbarrini A, Nucera E *et al.* Beneficial effects of *Helicobacter pylori* eradication on chronic idiopathic urticaria. *Dig Dis Sci* 1998; **43**: 1226–9.
8 Utas S, Ozbakir O, Turasan A, Utas C. *Helicobacter pylori* eradication treatment reduces the severity of rosacea. *J Am Acad Dermatol* 1999; **40**: 433–5.
9 Leontiadis GI, Sharma VK, Howden CW. Non-gastrointestinal tract associations of *Helicobacter pylori* infection. *Arch Intern Med* 1999; **159**: 925–40.
10 Hook-Nikanne J, Varjonen E, Harvima RJ, Kosunen TU. Is *Helicobacter pylori* infection associated with chronic urticaria? *Acta Derm Venereol* 2000; **80**: 425–6.
11 Dauden E, Jimenez-Alonso I, Garcia-Diez A. *Helicobacter pylori* and idiopathic chronic urticaria. *Int J Dermatol* 2000; **39**: 446–52.
12 Bamford JT, Tilden RL, Blankush JL, Gangeness DE. Effect of treatment of *Helicobacter pylori* infection on rosacea. *Arch Dermatol* 1999; **135**: 659–63.

Crohn's disease (regional ileitis)

Crohn's disease is now known to be one of a group of diseases caused by mutations in the caspase recruitment domain 15 gene (*CARD15*), also termed *NOD2* [1]. Other disorders in which *CARD15* mutations are involved include several with dermatological aspects, including Muckle–Wells syndrome, IPEX (immunodysregulation, polyendocrinopathy, enteropathy, X-linked syndrome), and PAPA (pyogenic arthritis, pyoderma gangrenosum and acne).

Skin lesions are frequently seen in Crohn's disease [2–5]. These include:

- Crohn's disease occurring as direct extension from the bowel
- Cutaneous lesions of Crohn's disease at other skin sites
- Reactive lesions that are associated with Crohn's disease, but which do not have granulomatous histology
- Skin lesions related to malabsorption (Chapter 59)
- Skin lesions related to treatment: drug reactions, stoma dermatoses, etc.
- Psoriasis
- Other associated dermatoses.

Direct skin and mucosal involvement in continuity with the bowel

Cutaneous Crohn's disease may occur at sites in continuity with the bowel, such as the lip, stoma sites (see later section) or, commonly, the perineal skin including the vulva in females. Orofacial granulomatosis and the overlap with Crohn's disease is discussed in Chapter 69. The umbilicus, a site connected to the bowel by a vestigial tract, may also be involved [6]. Rarely, there may be frank enterocutaneous fistulae due to underlying Crohn's disease, sometimes with multiple lesions.

Perineal abscesses and multiple fissures and fistulae occur in about a quarter of patients ('watering-can perineum'). This is more frequent in individuals with colonic disease [7] and may affect about 60% of patients, although symptoms may be absent. By contrast, such lesions are rare in ulcerative colitis. Anal tags, which may be oedematous or have granulomatous histology, are common.

Oral Crohn's disease is manifest as a thickened, corrugated appearance of the oral mucosa and lips. Granulomatous cheilitis may precede other features of Crohn's disease (Chapter 69).

Cutaneous Crohn's disease at other sites ('metastatic Crohn's disease')

Cutaneous Crohn's disease may also occur at sites separated from the bowel by normal tissues—a situation that is termed 'metastatic Crohn's disease', although not technically correct [8–11]. Lesions may parallel gastrointestinal disease activity, or may occur with a totally separate temporal pattern.

Lesions of cutaneous Crohn's disease may be solitary or multiple, and may have varied morphology, including intact or eroded plaques and nodules, or sinus formation. The lower legs are involved in half of the cases, with lesions sometimes mimicking erythema nodosum, but cutaneous Crohn's disease may affect the abdominal wall, groin and inframammary flexures, face and other sites. Genital involvement may be a presenting feature, affecting the perineum [11], vulva [12], scrotum or penis [4,13]. Unusual patterns include perifollicular papules [14], erysipelas-like lesions [15] and necrobiotic lesions [16]. In any of these morphological variants, there is a granulomatous histology in the dermis and subcutis. Lymphoedema, typically of the genital area, perineum or face, are also well documented and presumably related to local lymphatic obstruction by granulomatous inflammation.

Treatments for both contiguous and 'metastatic' Crohn's disease include topical and intralesional corticosteroids, agents used to treat the bowel disease (oral corticosteroids, sulphasalazine and split products such as mesalamine, immunosuppressive agents), oral metronidazole, and hyperbaric oxygen. Antitumour necrosis factor-α (anti-TNF) monoclonal antibodies, specifically infliximab and adalimumab, have been increasingly used for Crohn's disease, in which they may heal fistulae, both bowel–bowel and bowel–skin or bowel–vagina. A particular problem in such cases is being certain that infection is not playing a part in fistulation or sinuses, as this may worsen. Anti-TNF therapy is also effective for cutaneous associations, especially psoriasis and pyoderma gangrenosum but also hidradenitis suppurativa, so may have dual benefit in Crohn's disease. The benefit in ulcerative colitis is less clear. This and other cytokine treatments are discussed in [17,18]. Serum sickness-like reactions have been reported with infliximab.

Reactive dermatoses associated with Crohn's disease

These include oral aphthae, erythema nodosum and a variety of neutrophilic dermatoses. As most of the reactive processes can occur with either type of inflammatory bowel disease, but most are more commonly associated with ulcerative colitis than with Crohn's disease, they are discussed later in this section.

Other dermatoses that have been associated with Crohn's disease

Epidermolysis bullosa acquisita (EBA) has been associated with both Crohn's disease and ulcerative colitis, mainly the former [19] (see

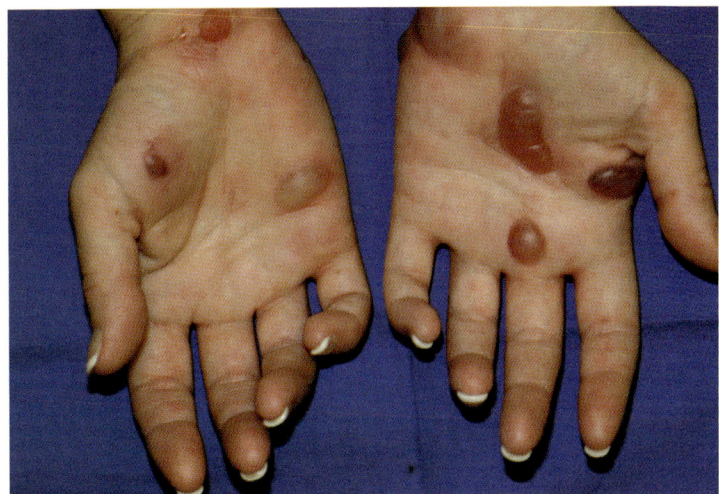

Fig. 62.19 Epidermolysis bullosa acquisita associated with a flare of inflammatory bowel disease.

also Chapter 40 and Fig. 62.19). In most instances, Crohn's disease had been established for several years prior to development of EBA, although EBA may precede diagnosis of the bowel disease [20]. This condition may be very refractory to treatment; drugs that may improve both the bowel disease and the cutaneous lesions of EBA include corticosteroids, azathioprine and ciclosporin.

Other bullous disorders that have been linked with Crohn's disease include *oral intraepidermal IgA pustulosis* [21] and *subcorneal pustular dermatosis* [22]; it has been suggested that the latter eruption was actually pustular pyoderma gangrenosum [23].

Polyarteritis nodosa (PAN) has been associated with Crohn's disease, but not specifically with ulcerative colitis [24,25]. It may be difficult to distinguish PAN from 'metastatic' Crohn's disease in patients with both disorders, as the histological features include a granulomatous component with the arteritis [26]; PAN may also resemble erythema nodosum or early pyoderma gangrenosum. The presence of livedo may suggest the diagnosis, but this can also occur due to cryoglobulinaemia. Other patterns of vasculitis associated with inflammatory bowel disease are discussed in the section on ulcerative colitis.

Psoriasis has been associated with Crohn's disease in several studies [27], and involvement of TNF in the pathogenesis of the two disorders has strengthened the view that they are linked. *Vitiligo* may also be associated.

In patients with Crohn's disease, apparently unrelated skin disorders may develop granulomas, for example hidradenitis suppurativa [28]. The presence of granulomas within predominantly neutrophilic infiltrates may cause diagnostic difficulty [29]; distinguishing between perineal sinuses of either disorder can be very difficult.

Disorders of keratinization that have been linked to Crohn's disease include *porokeratosis* [30] and *parakeratotic horns* [31].

Acrodermatitis enteropathica due to secondary zinc deficiency is a well-documented consequence of Crohn's disease [32] (Chapter 59).

References

1 Rose CD, Martin TM. Caspase recruitment domain 15 mutations and rheumatic diseases. *Curr Opin Rheumatol* 2005; **17**: 579–85.

2 Gregory B, Ho VC. Cutaneous manifestations of gastrointestinal disorders, 2. *J Am Acad Dermatol* 1992; **26**: 371–83.

3 Braverman IM. *Skin Signs of Systemic Disease*, 3rd edn. Philadelphia: Saunders, 1998: 405–37.

4 Herron MD, Zone JJ. Cutaneous diseases associated with gastrointestinal abnormalities. In: Callen JP, Jorrizo JL, eds. *Dermatological Signs of Internal Disease*, 3rd edn. Philadelphia: Saunders, 2003: 199–210.

5 Harris ML, Provost TT. Ulcerative colitis and Crohn's disease. In: Provost TT, Flynn JA, eds. *Cutaneous Medicine: Cutaneous Manifestations of Systemic Disease*. Hamilton, Ontario: Decker, 2001: 473–8.

6 McLelland J, Griffin SM. Metastatic Crohn's disease of the umbilicus. *Clin Exp Dermatol* 1996; **21**: 318–9.

7 Rankin GB, Watts HD, Melnyck CS *et al.* National cooperative Crohn's disease study: extraintestinal manifestations and perianal complications. *Gastroenterology* 1979; **77**: 914–20.

8 Lebwohl M, Fleischmajer R, Janowitz H *et al.* Metastatic Crohn's disease. *J Am Acad Dermatol* 1984; **10**: 33–8.

9 Shum DT, Guenther L. Metastatic Crohn's disease. *Arch Dermatol* 1990; **126**: 645–8.

10 Ploysangam T, Heubi JE, Eisen D *et al.* Cutaneous Crohn's disease in children. *J Am Acad Dermatol* 1997; **36**: 697–704.

11 Guest GD, Fink RL. Metastatic Crohn's disease: case report of an unusual variant and review of the literature. *Dis Colon Rectum* 2000; **43**: 1764–6.

12 Virgili A, Corazza M. Crohn's disease of the vulva: a case report. *J Reprod Med* 1994; **39**: 115–7.

13 Acker SM, Sahn EE, Rogers HC *et al.* Genital cutaneous Crohn's disease: two cases with unusual clinical and histopathologic features in young men. *Am J Dermatopathol* 2000; **22**: 443–6.

14 Buckley C, Bayoumi AH, Sarkany I. Metastatic Crohn's disease. *Clin Exp Dermatol* 1990; **15**: 131–3.

15 Dippel E, Rosenberger A, Zouboulis CC. Distant cutaneous manifestation of Crohn's disease presenting as a granulomatous erysipelas-like lesion. *J Eur Acad Dermatol Venereol* 1999; **12**: 65–6.

16 Perret CM, Bahmer FA. Extensive necrobiosis in metastatic Crohn's disease. *Dermatologica* 1987; **175**: 208–12.

17 Podolsky DK. Inflammatory bowel disease. *N Engl J Med* 2002; **347**: 417–28.

18 Brooklyn TN, Dunnill MGS, Shetty A *et al.* Infliximab for the treatment of pyoderma gangrenosum: a randomized, double blind, placebo controlled trial. *Gut* 2006; **55**: 505–9.

19 Ray TL, Levine JB, Weiss W *et al.* Epidermolysis bullosa acquisita and inflammatory bowel disease. *J Am Acad Dermatol* 1982; **6**: 242–52.

20 Labeille B, Gineston JL, Denoeux JP, Capron JP. Epidermolysis bullosa acquisita and Crohn's disease: a report with immunological and electron microscopic studies. *Arch Intern Med* 1988; **148**: 1457–9.

21 Borradori L, Saada V, Rybojad M *et al.* Oral intraepidermal IgA pustulosis and Crohn's disease. *Br J Dermatol* 1992; **126**: 383–6.

22 Delaporte E, Colombel JF, Nguyen-Mailfer C *et al.* Subcorneal pustular dermatosis in a patient with Crohn's disease. *Acta Derm Venereol* 1992; **72**: 301–2.

23 Powell FC, Su WPD, Perry HO. Pyoderma gangrenosum: classification and management. *J Am Acad Dermatol* 1996; **34**: 395–409.

24 Kahn EI, Daum E, Aiges HW *et al.* Cutaneous polyarteritis nodosa associated with Crohn's disease. *Dis Colon Rectum* 1980; **23**: 258–62.

25 Gudbjornsson B, Hallgren R. Cutaneous polyarteritis nodosa associated with Crohn's disease: report and review of the literature. *J Rheumatol* 1990; **17**: 386–90.

26 Chalvardjian A, Nethercott JR. Cutaneous granulomatous vasculitis associated with Crohn's disease. *Cutis* 1982; **30**: 645–55.

27 Najaian DJ, Gottlieb AB. Connections between psoriasis and Crohn's disease. *J Am Acad Dermatol* 2003; **48**: 805–21.

28 Attanoos RL, Appleton MA, Hughes LE *et al.* Granulomatous hidradenitis suppurativa and cutaneous Crohn's disease. *Histopathology* 1993; **23**: 111–5.

29 Yosipovitch G, Hodak E, Feinmesser D, David M. Acute Crohn's colitis with lobular panniculitis: metastatic Crohn's? *J Eur Acad Dermatol Venereol* 2000; **14**: 405–6.

30 Morton CA, Shuttleworth D, Douglas WS. Porokeratosis and Crohn's disease. *J Am Acad Dermatol* 1995; **32**: 894–7.

31 Aloi FG, Molinero A, Pippione M. Parakeratotic horns in a patient with Crohn's disease. *Clin Exp Dermatol* 1989; **14**: 79–81.

32 Krasovec M, Frenk E. Acrodermatitis enteropathica secondary to Crohn's disease. *Dermatology* 1996; **193**: 361–3.

Ulcerative colitis [1–4]

Skin lesions are reported in up to a third of patients with ulcerative colitis [2], although the cited frequency is usually in the region of 10–15%. As with Crohn's disease, these fall into several categories:

- Reactive lesions (a similar spectrum, but commoner in ulcerative colitis than in Crohn's disease)
- Direct involvement contiguous with the bowel (fissures and fistulae; rare)
- Skin lesions related to malabsorption (Chapter 59)
- Skin lesions related to treatment: drug reactions, stoma dermatoses, etc.
- Other associated dermatoses.

Reactive lesions associated with ulcerative colitis and Crohn's disease

A variety of non-specific eruptions may occur with either ulcerative colitis or Crohn's disease, usually paralleling the activity of inflammatory bowel disease [5]. However, all of these may occur for other reasons or in isolation. They include:

- Erythema nodosum—this occurs in about 5% of patients with ulcerative colitis (usually extensive rather than of limited extent) and in about 2% with Crohn's disease. It is the predominant pattern of reactive skin lesions in children, and in adults is most common in women. It is frequently associated with articular and other extragastrointestinal manifestations of the underlying bowel disease [6].
- Aphthous ulceration [1]—this occurs in about 5–8% of patients with ulcerative colitis and a rather smaller proportion with Crohn's disease. In some instances, the mechanism may be malabsorption, leading to iron and vitamin deficiency. Oral aphthae also occur in isolation, in association with numerous medications and in other medical disorders (including other bowel disorders, such as coeliac disease).
- Erythema multiforme [7,8]—this may occur in either disorder, usually associated with active disease (or as a side effect of treatment).
- Urticaria and angio-oedema.
- Neutrophilic dermatoses—these also occur in association with other disorders, but pyoderma gangrenosum and pyostomatitis vegetans in particular are strongly associated with inflammatory bowel disease. These disorders are discussed in more detail below.
- Vasculitis and intravascular coagulation disorders—these also occur as a consequence of inflammatory bowel disease, most commonly active ulcerative colitis, and are discussed separately below.

Neutrophilic dermatoses

Pyoderma gangrenosum [9–12]. Pyoderma gangrenosum occurs as a complication of inflammatory bowel disease, haematological disorders, inflammatory arthritides and other medical conditions [9] (it is discussed more fully in Chapter 50). It is estimated to occur in about 2–5% of patients with ulcerative colitis, this disorder being the single commonest cause of pyoderma gangrenosum; it is three to five times commoner in patients with ulcerative colitis than in those with Crohn's disease. The ulcerative and pustular variants in particular are associated with inflammatory bowel disease. It may also occur in other bowel diseases, such as the bowel-associated dermatosis–arthritis syndrome (see below) and diverticular disease [13], as a peristomal dermatosis [14] and in patients with hepatitis. The characteristic lesions are rapidly progressive necrotic skin ulcers with a bluish-coloured undermined border, but nodular and pustular lesions may occur, especially in early disease. Trauma is sometimes a predisposing factor. Pyoderma gangrenosum generally parallels the activity of the colitis [1–4], but may precede the diagnosis [15] or occur many years after complete removal of the diseased bowel [16]. Treatments for pyoderma gangrenosum include corticosteroids (topical, oral, intralesional), dapsone, azathioprine, ciclosporin, mycophenolate mofetil, tacrolimus (topical, oral), chlorambucil, intravenous immunoglobulin, and antitumour necrosis factor-α monoclonal antibodies such as infliximab [10,17–19].

Pyodermatitis–pyostomatitis vegetans

[20,21] is a rare disorder of the oral mucosa and skin; the skin lesions were previously termed pyodermite végétante. The oral lesions consist of multiple pustules, plaques and erosions, which may have a 'snail's-track' appearance. The skin lesions are crusted papules and plaques, which coalesce into annular lesions, mainly affecting the major flexures and the scalp. There are similarities to pemphigus vegetans, but this is associated with strongly positive direct immunofluorescence of lesional skin, which is either negative or weak in pyodermatitis–pyostomatitis vegetans. Oral and skin lesions show the same histological features, having intraepidermal and superficial dermal microabscesses containing neutrophil and eosinophil polymorphs, and a more mixed, deeper dermal inflammatory infiltrate. Acanthosis, acantholysis and pseudoepitheliomatous hyperplasia occur, especially in the oral lesions. Most cases of pyodermatitis–pyostomatitis vegetans are associated with inflammatory bowel disease, usually ulcerative colitis, although the condition has also been reported with sclerosing cholangitis and in isolation. It is difficult to control; high-dose, systemic corticosteroids are the first-line therapy, but dapsone or azathioprine may be of benefit. Remission may occur following colectomy.

Acute febrile neutrophilic dermatosis

(Sweet's syndrome). This has been associated with inflammatory bowel disease, especially ulcerative colitis [22–25]. It may coexist with pyoderma gangrenosum [22,24], and may also occur after colectomy in patients with inflammatory bowel disease. It is discussed more fully in Chapter 50. Treatment options include corticosteroids, dapsone, nonsteroidal anti-inflammatory drugs, colchicine, tetracyclines, ciclosporin and other immunosuppressive agents and, in the context of inflammatory bowel disease, metronidazole [25]. A neutrophilic colitis in a patient with Sweet's syndrome and acute myeloid leukaemia, and with previous Crohn's disease, was felt to be histologically distinct from Crohn's disease or ulcerative colitis [26].

Vesicopustular eruption and other neutrophilic dermatoses.

A vesicopustular eruption may occur in ulcerative colitis [1,2,27,28], or less commonly in Crohn's disease [29]. The lesions consist of a dense neutrophilic infiltrate similar to that of pyoderma gangrenosum or Sweet's syndrome, and may be a variation of these [2,9]. In practice, many of the group of neutrophilic dermatoses may overlap, coexist or evolve from smaller papular or pustular lesions. Morphologically similar lesions in the bowel-associated dermatosis–arthritis syndrome may have vasculitic histology; features of this syndrome may also occur in patients with inflammatory bowel disease [30]. Treatment is similar to that of the other neutrophilic dermatoses.

Erythema elevatum diutinum has been reported with both Crohn's disease and with ulcerative colitis [31,32], as has oral intraepidermal IgA pustulosis [33,34].

An important recent issue in the field of neutrophilic dermatoses has been a general view that the spectrum of conditions in this category is greater than previously thought. Some of the internal manifestations of neutrophilic dermatoses may cause diagnostic difficulties in patients with Crohn's disease, particularly features such as mesenteric lymphadenitis or aseptic abscesses [35,36]. Most such abscesses are internal but vulval and other cutaneous lesions have occurred.

Vasculitis and intravascular coagulation disorders

Vasculitis and purpura [1,2,37–39] may occur in either ulcerative colitis or Crohn's disease, most commonly in ulcerative colitis. The clinical picture is of a leukocytoclastic vasculitis with palpable purpura, typically affecting the lower legs and sometimes causing nodules or ulceration. Pustular lesions may have vasculitic histology. Joint pain and malaise may be prominent. Polyarteritis nodosa in Crohn's disease is discussed above.

Antineutrophil cytoplasm antibodies (ANCA) are present in 60–70% of patients with ulcerative colitis and 5–10% with Crohn's disease [40].

Cutaneous gangrene and focal thrombosis [41–43] is a rare complication. Patients with ulcerative colitis have significant coagulation defects; in one large early series, this was sufficient to complicate the clinical course in more than 1% of patients [41]. Thrombosis of internal vessels affects younger patients, unusual vascular sites, is associated with active inflammatory Crohn's disease but apparently quiescent ulcerative colitis, and has significant mortality of 5–10%. Abnormalities underlying this tendency are unclear—some reports implicate thrombocythaemia, elevated levels of fibrinogen, factor VIII and factor V, and decreased levels of antithrombin III whilst others have excluded common thrombophilic states such as factor V Leiden, deficiencies of protein C, protein S or antithrombin III, or presence of anticardiolipin antibodies. Microvascular thrombosis of the skin may result in cutaneous gangrene. High-dose systemic steroids have no effect on the thrombotic complications, which should be treated with anticoagulant therapy. Similar features have been reported due to cryoglobulinaemia associated with inflammatory bowel disease.

Other cutaneous disorders associated with ulcerative colitis

Linear IgA disease. Linear IgA disease may be relatively common in patients with ulcerative colitis, which usually precedes the dermatosis by several years [44]. Linear IgA disease may resolve after colectomy has been performed for ulcerative colitis [45]. Whether these patients actually have ulcerative colitis or a specific colitis associated with linear IgA disease is uncertain; two recent patients with preceding bowel symptoms developed oral ulceration and were found to have linear IgA deposition in mouth and colon. The bowel histology was that of a lymphocytic colitis or Crohn's disease [46]. Linear IgA disease has also been associated with Crohn's disease [47].

Epidermolysis bullosa acquisita, discussed above in relation to Crohn's disease, also occurs in some patients with ulcerative colitis; an erythema gyratum repens-like pattern has been described in such a case [48].

Hermansky–Pudlak syndrome (MIM #203300) (Chapter 39). This may be associated with an inflammatory colitis that resembles ulcerative colitis but has a granulomatous infiltrate histologically; this appears to be distinct from either ulcerative colitis or Crohn's disease [1,49].

Ulcerative colitis has been linked with a variety of autoimmune disorders and with sarcoidosis [50,51], although the strength of this association is not clear. Finger clubbing may be associated with inflammatory bowel disease, particularly ulcerative colitis [52], as well as with several other gastrointestinal diseases, including tumours, chronic infections, protein-losing enteropathy and laxative abuse [53]. Acne fulminans has also been reported in association with inflammatory bowel disease [54].

References

1 Gregory B, Ho VC. Cutaneous manifestations of gastrointestinal disorders, 2. *J Am Acad Dermatol* 1992; **26**: 371–83.

2 Braverman IM. *Skin Signs of Systemic Disease*, 3rd edn. Philadelphia: Saunders, 1998: 405–37.

3 Herron MD, Zone JJ. Cutaneous diseases associated with gastrointestinal abnormalities. In: Callen JP, Jorrizo JL, eds. *Dermatological Signs of Internal Disease*, 3rd edn. Philadelphia: Saunders, 2003: 199–210.

4 Harris ML, Provost TT. Ulcerative colitis and Crohn's disease. In: Provost TT, Flynn JA, eds. *Cutaneous Medicine: Cutaneous Manifestations of Systemic Disease*. Hamilton, Ontario: Decker, 2001: 473–8.

5 Greenstein AJ, Janowitz HD, Sachar DB. The extraintestinal complications of Crohn's disease and ulcerative colitis: a study of 700 patients. *Medicine (Baltimore)* 1976; **55**: 401–12.

6 Areias E, Garcia e Silva L. Érythème noueux au cours de la rectocolite hémorrhagique et de la maladie de Crohn. *Ann Dermatol Venereol* 1986; **113**: 197–206.

7 Chapman RS, Forsyth A, MacQueen A. Erythema multiforme in association with active ulcerative colitis and Crohn's disease. *Dermatologica* 1977; **154**: 32–8.

8 Cameron AJ, Baron JH, Priestley BL. Erythema multiforme, drugs and ulcerative colitis. *BMJ* 1966; **ii**: 1174–8.

9 Powell FC, Su WPD, Perry HO. Pyoderma gangrenosum: classification and management. *J Am Acad Dermatol* 1996; **34**: 395–409.

10 Jackson JM, Callen JP. Pyoderma gangrenosum: an expert commentary. *Expert Rev Dermatol* 2006; **1**: 391–400.

11 Basler RSW. Ulcerative colitis and the skin. *Med Clin North Am* 1980; **64**: 941–54.

12 Levitt MD, Ritchie JK, Lennard-Jones JE *et al.* Pyoderma gangrenosum in inflammatory bowel disease. *Br J Surg* 1991; **78**: 676–8.

13 Klein S, Mayer L, Present D *et al.* Extraintestinal manifestations in patients with diverticulitis. *Ann Intern Med* 1988; **108**: 700–2.

14 Lyon CC, Smith AJ, Beck MH *et al.* Parastomal pyoderma gangrenosum: clinical features and management. *J Am Acad Dermatol* 2000; **42**: 992–1002.

15 Powell FC, Perry HO. Pyoderma gangrenosum in childhood. *Arch Dermatol* 1984; **120**: 757–61.

16 Cox NH, Peebles-Brown DA, MacKie RM. Pyoderma gangrenosum occurring ten years after proctocolectomy for ulcerative colitis. *Br J Hosp Med* 1986; **36**: 363.

17 Chow RK, Ho VC. Treatment of pyoderma gangrenosum. *J Am Acad Dermatol* 1996; **34**: 1047–60.

18 Tan MH, Gordon M, Lebwohl O *et al.* Improvement of pyoderma gangrenosum and psoriasis associated with Crohn disease with anti-tumor necrosis factor alpha monoclonal antibody. *Arch Dermatol* 2001; **137**: 930–3.

19 Brooklyn TN, Dunnill MGS, Shetty A *et al.* Infliximab for the treatment of pyoderma gangrenosum: a randomized, double blind, placebo controlled trial. *Gut* 2006; **55**: 505–9.

20 Storwick GS, Prihoda MB, Fulton RJ, Wood WS. Pyodermatitis–pyostomatitis vegetans: a specific marker for inflammatory bowel disease. *J Am Acad Dermatol* 1992; **31**: 336–41.

21 Soriano ML, Martinez N, Grilli R *et al.* Pyodermatitis–pyostomatitis vegetans: report of a case and review of the literature. *Oral Surg Oral Med Oral Pathol* 1999; **87**: 322–6.

22 Cohen PR, Kurzrock R. Sweet's syndrome revisited: a review of disease concepts. *Int J Dermatol* 2003; **42**: 761–78.

23 Travis S, Innes N, Davies MG *et al.* Sweet's syndrome: an unusual cutaneous feature of Crohn's disease or ulcerative colitis. The South West Gastroenterology Group. *Eur J Gastroenterol Hepatol* 1997; **9**: 715–20.

24 Benton EC, Rutherford D, Hunter JAA. Sweet's syndrome and pyoderma gangrenosum associated with ulcerative colitis. *Acta Derm Venereol* 1985; **65**: 77–80.

25 Banet DE, McClave SA, Callen JP. Oral metronidazole, an effective treatment for Sweet's syndrome in a patient with associated inflammatory bowel disease. *J Rheumatol* 1994; **21**: 1766–8.

26 Fain O, Mathieu E, Feton N *et al.* Intestinal involvement in Sweet's syndrome. *J Am Acad Dermatol* 1996; **35**: 989–90.

27 Fenske NA, Gern JE, Pierce D *et al.* Vesicopustular eruption of ulcerative colitis. *Arch Dermatol* 1983; **119**: 664–9.

28 O'Loughlin S, Perry HO. A diffuse pustular eruption associated with ulcerative colitis. *Arch Dermatol* 1978; **114**: 1061–4.

29 Matheson BK, Gilbertson EO, Eichenfield LF. Vesicopustular eruption of Crohn's disease. *Pediatr Dermatol* 1996; **13**: 127–30.

30 Delaney TA, Clay CD, Randell PL. The bowel-associated dermatosis–arthritis syndrome. *Australas J Dermatol* 1989; **30**: 23–7.

31 Buahene K, Hudson M, Mowat A *et al.* Erythema elevatum diutinum: an unusual association with ulcerative colitis. *J Am Acad Dermatol* 1990; **22**: 948–52.

32 Planaguma M, Puig L, Alomar A *et al.* Erythema elevatum diutinum in a patient with Crohn's disease. *Cutis* 1992; **49**: 201–6.

33 Borradori L, Saada V, Rybojad M *et al.* Oral intraepidermal IgA pustulosis and Crohn's disease. *Br J Dermatol* 1992; **126**: 383–6.

34 Wright S, Philipps T, Ryan J, Leigh IM. Intra-epidermal neutrophilic IgA dermatosis with colitis. *Br J Dermatol* 1989; **120**: 113–9.

35 André M, Aumaître O, Papo T *et al.* Disseminated aseptic abscesses associated with Crohn's disease: a new entity? *Dig Dis Sci* 1998; **43**: 420–8.

36 André MFJ, Piette JC, Kémény JL *et al.* Aseptic abscesses: a study of 30m patients with or without inflammatory bowel disease and review of the literature. *Medicine (Baltimore)* 2007; **86**: 145–61.

37 Callen JP. Severe cutaneous vasculitis complicating ulcerative colitis. *Arch Dermatol* 1979; **115**: 226–7.

38 Saulsbury FT, Hart MH. Crohn's disease presenting with Henoch–Schönlein purpura. *J Pediatr Gastroenterol Nutr* 2000; **31**: 173–5.

39 Castanet J, Lacour JP, Perrin C *et al.* Cutaneous vasculitis with lesions mimicking Degos' disease and revealing Crohn's disease. *Acta Derm Venereol* 1995; **75**: 408–9.

40 Galperin C, Gershwin ME. Immunopathogenesis of gastrointestinal and hepatobiliary diseases. *JAMA* 1997; **278**: 1946–55.

41 Bargen JA, Barker NW. Extensive arterial and venous thrombosis complicating chronic ulcerative colitis. *Arch Intern Med* 1936; **58**: 17–31.

42 Stapleton SR, Curley RK, Simpson WA. Cutaneous gangrene secondary to focal thrombosis: an important cutaneous manifestation of ulcerative colitis. *Clin Exp Dermatol* 1989; **14**: 387–9.

43 Jackson LM, O'Gorman PJ, O'Connell J *et al.* Thrombosis in inflammatory bowel disease: clinical setting, procoagulant profile and Factor V Leiden. *QJM* 1997: **90**: 183–8.

44 Paige DG, Leonard JN, Wojnarowska F, Fry L. Linear IgA disease and ulcerative colitis. *Br J Dermatol* 1997; **134**: 779–82.

45 Walker SL, Banerjee P, Harland CC, Black MM. Remission of linear IgA disease associated with ulcerative colitis following panproctocolectomy. *Br J Dermatol* 2000; **143**: 1341–2.

46 Cowan CG, Lamey PJ, Walsh M *et al*. Linear IgA disease (LAD): immunoglobulin deposition in oral and colonic lesions. *J Oral Pathol Med* 1995; **24**: 374–8.

47 Barberis C, Doutre MS, Bioulac-Sage P. Linear IgA bullous dermatosis associated with Crohn's disease. *Gastroenterol Clin Biol* 1988; **12**: 76–7.

48 España A, Sitaru C, Pretel M *et al*. Erythema gyratum repens-like eruption in a patient with epidermolysis bullosa acquisita associated with ulcerative colitis. *Br J Dermatol* 2007; **156**: 773–5.

49 Sherman A, Genuth L, Hazzi CG *et al*. Perirectal abscess in the Hermansky–Pudlak syndrome. *Am J Gastroenterol* 1989; **84**: 552–6.

50 Cox NH, McCrea J. The association of Sjögren's syndrome, sarcoidosis, ulcerative colitis and other autoimmune disorders. *Br J Dermatol* 1996; **134**: 1138–40.

51 Porter WM, Hardman CM, Leonard JN, Fry L. Sarcoidosis in a patient with linear IgA disease. *Clin Exp Dermatol* 1999; **24**: 67–70.

52 Kitis G, Thompson H, Allan RN. Finger clubbing in inflammatory bowel disease, its prevalence and pathogenesis. *BMJ* 1979; **2**: 825–8.

53 Tosti A, Baran R, Dawber RPR. The nail in systemic diseases and drug-induced changes. In: Baran R, Dawber RPR, deBerker DAR, Haneke E, Tosti A, eds. *Diseases of the Nails and Their Management*. Oxford: Blackwell Science, 2001: 223–329.

54 McAuley D, Miller RA. Acne fulminans with inflammatory bowel disease. *Arch Dermatol* 1985; **121**: 91–3.

Collagenous colitis

This, with lymphocytic colitis, is a type of microscopic colitis characterized clinically by diarrhoea and histologically by a thickened subepithelial collagen layer. Cases have been described that have evolved to, or from, ulcerative colitis; it has also been reported to have evolved to Crohn's disease and, of dermatological relevance, to have coexisted with systemic sclerosis and to have possibly been triggered by isotretinoin. There are now several reports of associated pyoderma gangrenosum [1,2], including peristomal and vulval involvement; lymphocytic venulitis of adjacent bowel, but not of the skin, has also been reported.

References

1 Davis MDP, Nakamura KJH. Peristomal pyoderma gangrenosum associated with collagenous colitis. *Arch Dermatol* 2007; **143**: 669–70.

2 Koch D, Sinha A, Greenaway JR, Carmichael AJ. Pyoderma gangrenosum associated with collagenous colitis. *Clin Exper Dermatol* 2007; **32**: 329–31.

Bowel-associated dermatosis–arthritis syndrome [1–6]

> **Synonyms**
> - Blind loop syndrome
> - Bowel bypass syndrome
> - Intestinal bypass arthritis–dermatitis syndrome

This is a serum sickness-like illness which is related to bacterial overgrowth in the bowel. Bacterial antigens in the form of peptidoglycans are probably released from the intestinal flora, particularly *Escherichia coli* [2]. Circulating immune complexes can be demonstrated in most patients actively developing skin lesions [3].

It was originally linked with bowel bypass surgery for obesity [1–4], which created a 'blind loop' of bowel. Most cases now are related to other causes of a blind loop, or simply to areas of stasis, and the condition has attracted the name 'bowel bypass syndrome without bowel bypass' [6]. Causes include achalasia [7], strictures and inflammatory bowel disease [5], as well as surgical procedures that create a defunctioning segment of bowel [8]. Pyoderma

gangrenosum secondary to diverticular disease [9] is probably in the same spectrum of disease.

The characteristic skin lesions are crops of erythematous papules, sterile vesicopustules similar to those associated with ulcerative colitis, or overtly indurated or necrotic vasculitic lesions. Erythema nodosum-like and panniculitis-like lesions may occur. Associated constitutional symptoms include fever, polyarthritis, tenosynovitis, myalgia and nephritis. Raynaud's phenomenon has been described, as has Sweet's syndrome. The joint involvement is variable and similar to the type of arthritis recognized in regional ileitis and ulcerative colitis. The bypass enteropathy may manifest itself as acute massive abdominal distension resembling intestinal obstruction, but milder and chronic forms have been described.

Histological examination shows dilated dermal venules and capillaries with a marked perivascular neutrophilic infiltrate. This is most pronounced in vesicopustular lesions, in which the resulting dermal oedema may lead to dermal–epidermal separation. Epidermal necrosis may be found. Treatments include oral corticosteroids, antibiotics such as metronidazole, a variety of immunosuppressive medications and restorative surgery.

References

1 Dicken CH, Seehafer JR. Bowel bypass syndrome. *Arch Dermatol* 1979; **115**: 837–9.

2 Ely PH. The bowel bypass syndrome: a response to bacterial peptidoglycans. *J Am Acad Dermatol* 1980; **2**: 473–87.

3 Kennedy C. The spectrum of inflammatory skin disease following jejuno-ileal bypass for morbid obesity. *Br J Dermatol* 1981; **105**: 425–36.

4 Simon S, Sikka JV, Lynfield YL. Bowel bypass syndrome. *Cutis* 1981; **28**: 545–7.

5 Delaney TA, Clay CD, Randell PL. The bowel-associated dermatosis–arthritis syndrome. *Australas J Dermatol* 1989; **30**: 23–7.

6 Jorizzo JL, Apisarnthanarax P, Subrt P *et al*. Bowel bypass syndrome without bowel bypass: bowel associated dermatosis–arthritis syndrome. *Arch Intern Med* 1983; **143**: 457–61.

7 Tucker SC, Chalmers RJG, Andrew SM, Odom NJ. Pustular vasculitis secondary to achalasia of the cardia. *Br J Dermatol* 2000; **142**: 373–4.

8 Cox NH, Palmer JG. Bowel-associated dermatitis-arthritis syndrome associated with ileo-anal pouch anastamosis, and treatment with mycophenolate mofetil. *Br J Dermatol* 2003; **149**: 1296–7.

9 Klein S, Mayer L, Present D *et al*. Extraintestinal manifestations in patients with diverticulitis. *Ann Intern Med* 1988; **108**: 700–2.

Skin complications of stomas [1,2]

Dermatoses associated with a stoma include those related to its function (irritation from faecal leakage, infections, contact dermatitis), Koebner reaction of existing or new dermatoses (psoriasis, lichen sclerosus) and disorders related to bowel disease (peristomal pyoderma gangrenosum, cutaneous Crohn's disease) [1,2].

The skin around a gastrointestinal or urinary tract stoma is liable to irritation from the effluent, the wafer and pouch, and substances applied as barriers, adhesives and cleaners. The collection pouch is either attached to a wafer or directly to the skin; a barrier/sealant may be applied before adhesion. The sealant is either a gelatine–pectin formulation, karaya (a hygroscopic partially acetylated polysaccharide), or a flexible plastic, applied in liquid form. The adhesives are usually acrylic, silicone or latex. Ideally, the wafer should adhere perfectly to the skin, with a rim of skin 1–2 mm between the stoma and the appliance. If this rim is too narrow, chafing against the stomal mucosa will occur, and if it is too wide there is a higher risk of dermatitis. Any surface irregularities beneath the attachment surface will allow effluent to track beneath. This may occur if there are changes in body weight, or if there is incorrect or unavoidable siting of the stoma in body folds or adjacent to scars.

Enzyme-degradation dermatitis, caused by proteolytic enzymes in an alkaline fluid medium, is commonest with ileostomies [3], and presents with maceration, erythema and erosions. Because of the tracking of the fluid downwards, the pattern of dermatitis depends on the patient's predominant position. Diversion of the urinary stream also causes problems because of stagnation and ammonia production.

Treatment. Most peristomal skin disease is irritant and is treated by judicious use of topical corticosteroids together with soothing and barrier preparations. Infections such as *Candida* or pyogenic bacterial infection should be treated with an appropriate specific antimicrobial agent. Many types of protective wafer and protective powders are available. These contain gelatine, pectin, polyisobutylene and sodium carboxy-methylcellulose. They adhere to moist skin and allow healing to take place if they are left for about 3 days. Creases and crevices around a stoma or fistula can be filled using pastes, which generally consist of gelatine, sodium carboxymethylcellulose, triacetin, fixin and ethanol. They are applied in layers, moulded into the creases with a moist finger and built up to the required level. If the drainage application can then remain in position for several days, this will usually allow the damaged skin to heal. Other topical treatments for irritant peristomal dermatoses include soothing compresses (for example, saline or 1 : 40 aluminium acetate), karaya and sucralfate [3]. In the case of very painful conditions such as pyoderma gangrenosum, instillation of a suitable topical local anaesthetic under the appliance 40–60 min before changing it can make a great difference to patient comfort.

Allergic contact dermatitis can occur to the adhesive [4], the barrier or any part of the appliance. Epoxy resins have been a problem in pouch materials, even though they are often present in small amounts only [5]. It has been suggested that patch testing should be carried out on the symmetrically opposite part of the abdomen [1]. It is usually possible to provide substitutes for materials causing the allergic reaction.

Urostomy encrustations and acanthotic chronic papillomatous dermatitis (pseudoverrucous lesions). The encrustations are crystals of phosphates and sometimes uric acid that form on the stoma and can damage the mucosa and even the bag. Pseudoverrucous lesions are grey or reddish-brown, warty papules at the mucocutaneous junction. They are more common around urostomies than around gastrointestinal stomas, occurring in about 20% of urostomy patients. There may be a non-specific erythematous and erosive change [6]. Stagnation and urinary infection are important in the aetiology of both encrustations and pseudoverrucous lesions and, as well as treating infection, acidification of the urine is helpful—for example, with cranberry juice or vitamin C in large doses [1]. Peristomal viral warts are a particular differential-diagnostic problem.

Parastomal fistulae and ulcers [7]. These are particularly associated with ileostomy for Crohn's disease and may represent or herald recurrent disease. Fistulae are often preceded by abscesses, and may be multiple. The parastomal ulcer is defined as a defect in the surface 1.5 cm or more across. It is typically accompanied by severe burning pain and erythema, and often associated with induration and erythema of the stoma [8]. Low-grade infection should be considered as a possible cause in parastomal ulcers that occur early after formation of the stoma, but in late-appearing ulcers, recurrent Crohn's disease is probably the most important underlying cause. Treatment of both parastomal ulcers and fistulae is usually surgical.

Dermatoses. Psoriasis and pemphigus have been described as a result of the Koebner reaction around 'ostomies' [9], and pyoderma gangrenosum can localize to the peristomal skin after colectomy for inflammatory bowel disease [10,11], and much less commonly in relation to urostomies. A papular, erythematous condition similar to granuloma inguinale infantum has been described following intensive use of a potent fluorinated steroid around a colostomy site [12].

Neoplasms. Basal cell carcinoma has been described as a long-term complication of colostomy [13]. Metastatic carcinoma at the stoma site, sometimes invading the surrounding skin, has been reported following ureterosigmoidostomy [14] and in patients who have had colectomy for ulcerative colitis [15–18].

References

1 Rothstein MS. Dermatologic considerations to stoma care. *J Am Acad Dermatol* 1986; **15**: 411–32.
2 Lyon CC, Smith AJ, Griffiths CEM, Beck MH. The spectrum of skin disorders in abdominal stoma patients. *Br J Dermatol* 2000; **143**: 1248–60.
3 Lyon CC, Stapleton M, Smith AJ *et al.* Topical sucralfate in the management of peristomal skin disease: an open study. *Clin Exp Dermatol* 2000; **25**: 584–8.
4 Bergman B, Lowhagen GB, Mobacken H. Irritant skin reactions to urostomal adhesives. *Urol Res* 1982; **10**: 153–5.
5 Beck MH, Burrows D, Fregert S *et al.* Allergic contact dermatitis to epoxy resin in colostomy bags. *Br J Surg* 1985; **72**: 202–3.
6 Borglund E, Nordström G, Nyman CR. Classification of peristomal skin changes in patients with urostomy. *J Am Acad Dermatol* 1988; **19**: 623–32.
7 Greenstein AJ, Dicker A, Meyer S *et al.* Peri-ileostomy fistulae in Crohn's disease. *Ann Surg* 1982; **197**: 179–82.
8 Last M, Fazio V, Lavery I *et al.* Conservative management of paraileostomy ulcers in patients with Crohn's disease. *Dis Colon Rectum* 1984; **27**: 779–86.
9 Rodriguez DB. Treatment for three ostomy patients with systemic skin disorders. *J Enterostom Ther* 1981; **8**: 31–2.
10 McGavity WC, Robertson DB, McKeown PP. Pyoderma gangrenosum at the parastomal site in patients with Crohn's disease. *Arch Surg* 1984; **119**: 1186–8.
11 Lyon CC, Smith AJ, Beck MH *et al.* Parastomal pyoderma gangrenosum: clinical features and management. *J Am Acad Dermatol* 2000; **42**: 992–1002.
12 Hjorth N, Sjolin K. Multiple inflammatory acanthomas around a colostomy. *J Cutan Pathol* 1981; **8**: 361–4.
13 Didolkar MS, Douglass HO, Holyoke ED. Basal cell carcinoma originating at the colostomy site. *Dis Colon Rectum* 1975; **18**: 399–402.
14 Carswell JJ, Skeel DA, Witherington R. Neoplasia at the site of ureterosigmoidostomy. *J Urol* 1976; **115**: 750–2.
15 Baciewicz K, Sparberg M, Lawrence JB *et al.* Adenocarcinoma of an ileostomy site with skin invasion. *Gastroenterology* 1983; **84**: 168–70.
16 Cuesta MA, Donner R. Adenocarcinoma arising at an ileostomy site. *Cancer* 1976; **37**: 949–52.
17 Johnson WR, McDermott FT, Pihl E. Adenocarcinoma of an ileostomy in a patient with ulcerative colitis. *Dis Colon Rectum* 1980; **23**: 351–2.
18 Morgan MN. Carcinoma in a caecostomy in longstanding ulcerative colitis. *Proc R Soc Med* 1966; **59**: 427.

Coeliac disease [1]

Coeliac disease usually presents with malabsorption and diarrhoea. The pathogenesis is discussed in detail elsewhere [1,2]; a digestion-resistant peptide in gliadin (mer-33) may be the initiator of the disease [3].

There are associations with numerous other autoimmune diseases, notably type 1 diabetes and thyroid disease [1], and strong HLA associations; 95% of patients have the HLA-DQ(α1*501,β1*02) heterodimer (HLA-DQ2) and almost all the remainder have HLA DQ8. A significant increase in the frequency of coeliac disease in patients with inflammatory bowel disease has been suggested recently, and it has been reported following interferon treatment for hepatitis C and other disorders [4].

Diagnosis of coeliac disease can be made by serological tests for IgA antiendomysial antibodies (sensitivity is 85–98% and specificity 97–100%) or IgA tissue transglutaminase (sensitivity 91–95% and negative predictive value nearly 100%) [1,2]. Tissue transglutaminase acts as an autoantigen—it deaminates glutamine residues in gliadin to create negatively charged glutamic acid residues that activate T cells. IgA antigliadin antibodies are less specific but are useful in younger children. Antigliadin, antiendomysial and tissue transglutaminase antibody levels all become undetectable after a period of 3–6 months on a strict gluten-free diet (GFD). Other tests include documentation of malabsorption and small-bowel biopsy.

Dermatological features of coeliac disease include cutaneous features of malabsorption of nutrients (Chapter 59), and features of associated autoimmune conditions. Darkening of previously white hair has been reported after starting GFD to treat coeliac disease [5]. Other documented dermatological features include follicular keratosis and alopecia. The most important dermatological association is with dermatitis herpetiformis (DH) which occurs in 25% of subjects (Chapter 40); the enteropathy of DH seems to be the same as that of coeliac disease, and some degree of abnormality of small-bowel mucosa is present, even if minimal and asymptomatic, in all patients with DH. However, it is unclear why DH only occurs in some subjects, often with mild enteropathy; there may be factors that alter disease expression. A recent study showed a significant linkage of coeliac disease chromosome 19p13, but investigation of a candidate gene, myosin IXB, showed no association with coeliac disease but a weak association with DH. The precise genetic aspects of coeliac disease and DH may therefore not be identical [6]. There is an association between DH and internal malignancies, the most important being lymphoma of the small bowel (enteropathy-associated lymphoma) [7,8], as in coeliac disease. GFD exerts a protective effect [8].

Improvement of psoriasis in a small number of patients who were treated with GFD suggested the possibility that coeliac disease and psoriasis might be associated. Patients with psoriasis have a high frequency of positive IgA antigliadin antibodies, which correlate with lymphocytic infiltration of the duodenal mucosa, but do not have an increased incidence of coeliac disease, and there is no increase in either antireticulin or antiendomysial antibodies [9,10].

Vasculitis, sometimes with cryoglobulinaemia, may occur in association with coeliac disease [11].

References

1 Farrell RJ, Kelly CP. Celiac sprue. *N Engl J Med* 2002; **346**: 180–8.
2 Hopper A, Hadjivassiliou M, Butt S, Sanders S. Adult celiac disease. *BMJ* 2007; **335**: 558–62.
3 McManus R, Kelleher D. Celiac disease—the villain unmasked? *N Engl J Med* 2003; **348**: 2573–4.
4 Bardella MT, Marino R, Meroni PL. Celiac disease during interferon treatment. *Ann Intern Med* 1999; **131**: 157–8.
5 Hill LS. Reversal of premature hair greying in adult coeliac disease. *BMJ* 1980; **281**: 115.
6 Koskinen LL, Korponay-Szabo IR, Viiri K *et al.* Myosin IXB gene region and gluten intolerance: linkage to coeliac disease and a putative dermatitis herpetiformis association. *J Med Genet* 2008; **45**: 222–7.
7 Renaula TL, Leonard JN. Malignant disease in dermatitis herpetiformis. *Clin Dermatol* 1991; **9**: 369–73.
8 Lewis HM, Renaula TL, Garioch JJ *et al.* Protective effect of gluten-free diet against lymphoma in dermatitis herpetiformis. *Br J Dermatol* 1996; **135**: 363–7.
9 Michaelsson G, Gerden B, Ottosson M *et al.* Patients with psoriasis often have increased serum levels of IgA antibodies to gliadin. *Br J Dermatol* 1993; **129**: 667–73.
10 Michaelsson G, Kraaz W, Gerden B *et al.* Increased lymphocyte infiltration in duodenal mucosa from patients with psoriasis and serum IgA antibodies to gliadin. *Br J Dermatol* 1995; **133**: 896–904.
11 Lie JT. Vasculitis and the gut: unwitting partners or strange bedfellows? *J Rheumatol* 1991; **18**: 647–8.

Whipple's disease

This disorder, another cause of malabsorption and diarrhoea, may be accompanied by skin manifestations. Diffuse pigmentation is frequent, and may resemble Addison's disease, but buccal pigmentation is not a feature. Subcutaneous nodules may occur, resembling rheumatoid nodules or sarcoidosis [1–3]. The disorder usually presents with arthralgia and general malaise; abdominal features (pain, diarrhoea and malabsorption leading to weight loss) occur in most individuals with more advanced disease. Cardiac, pleural, ophthalmological or neurological symptoms also occur, and there may be generalized lymphadenopathy. The diagnosis has historically been confirmed by demonstration of periodic acid–Schiff-positive particles in biopsies from infected tissue (usually bowel mucosa). The diagnosis can now be made using polymerase chain reaction (PCR) amplification of sequences from the causative organism, *Tropheryma whippelii*, in infected tissue [4,5] and the organism has been cultured [6].

References

1 Durand DV, Lecomte C, Cathebras P *et al.* Whipple disease: clinical review of 52 cases. The SNFMI Research Group on Whipple disease. *Medicine* 1997; **76**: 170–84.
2 Ratnaike RN. Whipple's disease. *Postgrad Med J* 2000; **76**: 760–6.
3 Frenk E, Merot Y, Perez I *et al.* Whipple's disease with sarcoidosis-like cutaneous manifestations. *Ann Dermatol Venereol* 1991; **118**: 115–8.
4 Misbah SA, Mapstone MP. Whipple's disease revisited. *J Clin Pathol* 2000; **53**: 750–5.
5 Dutly F, Altwegg M. Whipple's disease and '*Tropheryma whippelii*'. *Clin Microbiol Rev* 2001; **14**: 561–83.
6 Raoult D, Birg ML, La Scola B *et al.* Cultivation of the bacillus of Whipple's disease. *N Engl J Med* 2000; **342**: 620–5.

Skin disorders associated with gastrointestinal bleeding

These are listed in Table 62.12. Most are discussed elsewhere in this section, or in other chapters. In addition, gastrointestinal tumours may metastasize to skin (see earlier in this chapter), some

Table 62.12 Skin lesions associated with gastrointestinal disorders that may present with bleeding.

Disease	Gastrointestinal lesion	Skin symptom
Vascular defects and inherited		
Osler–Weber–Rendu disease (Chapter 47)	Telangiectasia	Telangiectasia
Blue rubber bleb naevus (Chapter 18)	Haemangiomas	Haemangiomas
Pseudoxanthoma elasticum (Chapter 45)	Involvement of visceral arteries	Yellowish papules and plaques
Ehlers–Danlos syndrome (type IV) (Chapter 45)	Fragility of visceral arteries	Hyperelasticity of skin and joints
Polyposis (see text in this chapter)		
Neurofibromatosis (von Recklinghausen)	Neurofibromas	Café-au-lait spots, neurofibromas
Cronkhite–Canada syndrome	Gastrointestinal polyposis	Diffuse hyperpigmentation, alopecia, nail defects
Gardner's syndrome	Polyposis of colon (cancer)	Lipomas, epidermoid cysts
Peutz–Jeghers syndrome	Polyposis, especially small intestine	Hyperpigmentation on lips, circumoral area and fingertips
Cowden's disease	Polyposis	Papules, lipomas, angiomas
Inflammatory bowel disease		
Crohn's disease, ulcerative colitis	Inflammatory changes of the intestinal wall	Erythema nodosum
		Aphthous stomatitis
		Pyoderma gangrenosum, other neutrophilic dermatoses
		Necrotizing vasculitis
		Epidermolysis bullosa acquisita
		Erythema multiforme
Vasculitis and systemic disease		
Henoch–Schönlein purpura and other vasculitides (Chapter 50)	Mesenteric vasculitis, gastric ulcers (polyarteritis nodosa)	Purpura, livedo, nodules, necrosis
Cholesterol emboli (Chapter 49)	Intestinal arterial occlusion	Vasculitis, necrosis, livedo
Degos' disease (Chapter 49)	Intestinal perforation	White atrophic lesions
Amyloidosis (Chapter 59)	Vascular fragility	Purpuric lesions
Neoplasia		
Primary gastrointestinal cancers	Neoplasm	Metastases, paraneoplastic eruptions, features of polyposis syndromes
Kaposi's sarcoma (Chapter 35)	Kaposi's sarcoma of bowel	Kaposi's sarcoma of skin

tumours may affect the skin and gastrointestinal tract (e.g. Kaposi's sarcoma), and skin tumours may rarely metastasize to the gastrointestinal tract (e.g. melanoma).

Several patterns of cutaneous vasculitis or collagen vascular disease may be associated with mesenteric vasculitis and/or thrombosis, leading to bleeding or ulceration. Various radiological signs of mesenteric vasculitis seen on computed tomography (CT) have been reviewed in relation to systemic lupus erythematosus, and include a palisade and comb-like pattern of vessels, peritoneal enhancement of ascitic fluid, thickening of the bowel wall, and a 'double-halo' or 'target sign' [1,2].

References

1 Hallegua DA, Wallace DJ. Gastrointestinal manifestations of systemic lupus erythematosus. *Curr Opin Rheumatol* 2000; **12**: 379–85.
2 Ko SF, Lee TY, Cheng TT *et al.* CT findings at lupus mesenteric vasculitis. *Acta Radiol* 1997; **38**: 115–20.

Intestinal polyposis [1,2]

A number of, usually inherited, gastrointestinal polyposis disorders also have cutaneous features. The most important are:
- Peutz–Jeghers syndrome
- Gardner's syndrome

- Cowden's disease (multiple hamartoma and neoplasia syndrome, p. 62.25)
- Bannayan–Riley–Ruvalcaba syndrome (Ruvalcaba–Myhre–Smith syndrome, Bannayan–Zonana syndrome)
- Cronkhite–Canada syndrome (non-inherited)
- Birt–Hogg–Dubé syndrome
- Naevoid basal cell carcinoma syndrome (p. 62.21) [3]
- Neurofibromatosis (Chapter 15).

Additionally, ganglioneuromas of the gastrointestinal tract and oral mucosal neuromas may be associated with Hirschsprung's disease, and colonic diverticula as features of MEN type 2B syndrome.

Peutz–Jeghers syndrome (MIM #175200) [4]. This is an autosomal-dominant or sporadic condition due to mutations in the serine/threonine kinase *STK11* (*LKB1*) gene on chromosome 19p13.3 [5–7]. This appears to be a tumour suppressor gene—loss of heterozygosity at this site has been shown to be associated with malignant transformation of polyps. Polyps occur mainly in the small intestine, but also in the stomach and colon. The usual presentation is with intussusception or melaena. Polyps can also be found in the genitourinary and respiratory tracts, and occasionally in the gallbladder.

The cutaneous feature is lentiginosis, with a predominantly perioral, periorbital and intraoral distribution; perianal and acral lentiginosis (occasionally causing longitudinal melanonychia) also occurs. The pigmented macules appear in early childhood and may fade with increasing age, although the mucosal lesions persist [4]. The pigmented lip lesions may be confused with those of Laugier–Hunziker syndrome (a benign, non-polyposis, disorder with onset in later years).

Cancers may occur in the gastrointestinal tract, but the frequency is relatively low, as the polyps are hamartomatous; additional mutations of the β-catenin gene or the p53 gene appear to be needed to convert them into adenomas or carcinomas. However, there is an increased risk of non-gastrointestinal cancers, with an overall risk estimated at 18-fold greater than that of the general population [8]. Other associated neoplasias include pancreatic adenocarcinoma (100-fold more common than expected [8]), and less commonly breast and pulmonary adenocarcinoma. Multiple myeloma may occur more frequently than expected. Precocious puberty may occur in either sex, and a variety of genital cancers have been associated with Peutz–Jeghers syndrome, including Sertoli cell tumours; there is a particular link with multifocal sex-cord tumours and an aggressive variant of adenocarcinoma of the cervix [1]. Finger clubbing may occur in conjunction with the ovarian sex-cord tumours.

Gardner's syndrome (MIM +175100) [6,7,9]. This condition is allelic with adenomatous polyposis of the colon. Both are caused by mutations in the *APC* gene, which has an important role as part of a signalling pathway involving β-catenin and E-cadherin, thereby influencing cell division, migration, adhesion and apoptosis; the wild-type gene also antagonizes a tumour suppressor gene *WNT1*. There is very high penetrance but marked variation in expression.

The syndrome is the association of adenomatous colonic polyposis with large numbers of subcutaneous fibromas, epidermoid cysts (both mainly on the upper trunk and head), desmoid tumours (mainly abdominal wall), retinal pigmentary changes, osteomas (especially of the facial bones), odontomas and other dental abnormalities, including supernumerary teeth [9]. The onset of cysts is generally prepubertal. Multiple pilomatricomas, or pilomatricoma-like areas within the epidermoid cysts, have also been recorded. The occurrence of fibromas may involve a general tendency to fibromatosis, including desmoid tumours, mesenteric and retroperitoneal fibrosis. Nuchal-type fibromas [10], especially if multiple or at unusual sites [11], may be an early sign of the syndrome. Leiomyomas, lipomas, neurofibromas and BCCs may also occur [9].

It is an autosomal dominant condition with variable expression, and is caused by mutations in the same APC gene on chromosome 5q21 that also causes familial polyposis coli without associated cutaneous abnormalities [1,6,7]. The phenotype is not simply determined by different mutations of the gene, as exactly the same mutation may on occasions give rise to a phenotype with or without skin lesions—suggesting that other genes influence the disease expression. There are also subsets of this condition in which skin lesions may be limited in type; for example, epidermoid cysts and colonic polyposis without the other features has

been termed Oldfield's syndrome [12]. Skin lesions are usually the earliest manifestation of this group of diseases, although the retinal pigmented lesions (hypertrophy of the pigment epithelium) occur in 90% and are probably congenital. The latter are dark, roughly oval-shaped lesions, at the periphery of the retina; they are generally multiple, bilateral, and also occur in first-degree relatives [13].

The bowel polyps are premalignant, and virtually all untreated cases will eventually develop colonic cancer, even in childhood occasionally, so regular colonoscopy and early colectomy is advised for affected individuals. The colon and rectum are the main cancer sites, but gastric and small-bowel polyps may occur. There is also an increased incidence of other neoplasia, which may be gastrointestinal (especially duodenal), bony (osteosarcoma and chondrosarcoma), hepatic (hepatoblastoma), neurological (medulloblastoma), endocrine (thyroid and adrenal) or soft tissue (liposarcoma) [8]. The diagnosis is usually suspected from the family history, can be supported by funduscopy and dental radiological studies and is confirmed by genetic testing.

Cowden's disease (multiple hamartoma and neoplasia syndrome; MIM #158350) [1,2,14–17]. Gastrointestinal polyposis and less commonly malignant change occur. However, the main neoplastic condition in Cowden's disease is breast cancer, and numerous other sites of cancer may be associated; this condition is therefore discussed in more detail in the section on genodermatoses associated with neoplasia (p. 62.25). A Cowden-like syndrome has also been reported in which the mutation is in the *BMPR1A* gene rather than in *PTEN1* as in Cowden's syndrome.

Bannayan–Riley–Ruvalcaba syndrome (Ruvalcaba–Myhre–Smith syndrome; Bannayan–Zonana syndrome, MIM #153480). This multiply named syndrome comprises gastrointestinal polyposis with vascular malformations, lipomas, penile café-au-lait spots, macrocephaly and thyroid disease. There is considerable overlap with Cowden's disease; both conditions involve mutations in *PTEN1* [18,19], and it has been suggested that they may be best grouped together as the *PTEN* hamartoma tumour syndrome.

Birt–Hogg–Dubé syndrome (Hornstein–Knickenberg syndrome; MIM #135150) [20–22]. These two conditions probably represent the same entity, in which there is autosomal-dominant inheritance. The gene locus is on chromosome 17p11.2, coding a presumed tumour suppressor 64-kDa protein, folliculin. Birt–Hogg–Dubé syndrome consists of multiple fibrofolliculomas, trichodiscomas and acrochordons; several cases have also had intestinal polyposis. Hornstein–Knickenberg syndrome is the association of perifollicular fibromas with intestinal polyposis. Lipomas (which may be large), angiolipomas, oral fibromas, parathyroid adenomas, renal tumours (especially oncocytomas), lung cysts and flecked choroidoretinopathy have also been linked with these conditions. Individual cases with meningioma and neurothekeoma have also been described. The odds ratio of renal tumours has been calculated at 6.9, and of pneumothorax (due to the lung cysts) at 50.3 [23].

Cronkhite–Canada syndrome (MIM 175500) [24–26]. This rare syndrome is characterized by skin pigmentation, alopecia, nail-plate defects and polyposis of the gastrointestinal tract, from oesophagus to anus. The cause is unknown, and only sporadic cases have been reported. Affected patients are middle-aged or elderly, with a male/female incidence ratio of 3 : 2.

Chronic diarrhoea due to protein-losing enteropathy associated with the intestinal polyposis is the usual presenting feature, leading to hypoalbuminaemia, hypokalaemia and hypocalcaemia. There is diffuse macular pigmentation of the skin (but not intra-orally) with accentuation over the face, neck and extremities; histologically, there is an increased number of melanin granules in keratinocytes and an increased number of melanosomes in melanocytes, with marked hyperkeratosis and a perivascular inflammatory infiltrate in the dermis. The palms and volar aspects of the fingers are also involved. The scalp hair becomes thin and sparse, initially resembling alopecia areata; later, total loss of hair occurs. All fingernails and toenails are dystrophic, undergoing onycholysis, onychoschizia and onychomadesis with a peculiar, triangular, residual nail plate. The course is usually slowly progressive; therapy is symptomatic and non-specific.

Acrochordons (fibroepithelial polyps, 'skin tags'). Several studies have suggested a link between acrochordons and colonic polyposis [1,2]. However, most of these studies were either small or examined only a population who were being investigated for bowel disease. A meta-analysis that divided patients into those with colonic symptoms and those who were asymptomatic demonstrated that the association was only sustained in the former group, and that this was therefore an artefact of patient selection [27].

References

1 Braverman IM. *Skin Signs of Systemic Disease*, 3rd edn. Philadelphia: Saunders, 1998: 58–60, 405–8.
2 Gregory B, Ho VC. Cutaneous manifestations of gastrointestinal disorders, 1. *J Am Acad Dermatol* 1992; **26**: 153–66.
3 Schwartz RA. Basal-cell-nevus syndrome and gastrointestinal polyposis. *N Engl J Med* 1978; **299**: 49.
4 Kitigawa S, Townsend BL, Hebert AA. Peutz–Jeghers syndrome. *Dermatol Clin* 1995; **13**: 127–33.
5 Stratakis CA. Clinical genetics of multiple endocrine neoplasias, Carney complex and related syndromes. *J Endocrinol Invest* 2001; **24**: 370–83.
6 Tsao H. Update on familial cancer syndromes and the skin. *J Am Acad Dermatol* 2000; **42**: 939–69.
7 Wirtzfeld DA, Petrelli NJ, Rodriguez-Bigas MA. Hamartomatous polyposis syndromes: molecular genetics, neoplastic risk, and surveillance recommendations. *Ann Surg Oncol* 2001; **8**: 319–27.
8 Giardiello FM, Welsh SB, Hamilton SR *et al.* Increased risk of cancer in the Peutz–Jeghers syndrome. *N Engl J Med* 1987; **316**: 1511–4.
9 Perniciaro C. Gardner's syndrome. *Dermatol Clin* 1995; **13**: 51–6.
10 Michal M, Fetsch JF, Hes O, Miettinen M. Nuchal-type fibroma: a clinicopathologic study of 52 cases. *Cancer* 1999; **85**: 156–63.
11 Wehrli BM, Weiss SW, Yandow S, Coffin CM. Gardner-associated fibromas (GAF) in young patients: a distinct fibrous lesion that identifies unsuspected Gardner syndrome and risk for fibromatosis. *Am J Surg Pathol* 2001; **25**: 645–51.
12 Oldfield MC. Association of familial polyposis of colon with multiple sebaceous cysts. *Br J Surg* 1954; **41**: 534.
13 Traboulsi EI, Krush AJ, Gardner EJ *et al.* Prevalence and importance of pigmented ocular fundus lesions in Gardner's syndrome. *N Engl J Med* 1987; **316**: 661–7.
14 Salem OS, Steck WD. Cowden's disease (multiple hamartoma and neoplasia syndrome): a case report and review of the English literature. *J Am Acad Dermatol* 1983; **8**: 686–96.
15 Mallory SB. Cowden syndrome (multiple hamartoma syndrome). *Dermatol Clin* 1995; **13**: 27–31.
16 Starink TM, van der Veen JPW, Arwet F *et al.* The Cowden syndrome: a clinical and genetic study in 21 patients. *Clin Genet* 1986; **29**: 222–33.
17 Eng C. Will the real Cowden syndrome please stand up: revised diagnostic criteria. *J Med Genet* 2000; **37**: 828–30.
18 Marsh DJ, Kum JB, Lunetta KL *et al.* PTEN mutation spectrum and genotype–phenotype correlations in Bannayan–Riley–Ruvalcaba syndrome suggest a single entity with Cowden syndrome. *Hum Mol Genet* 1999; **8**: 1461–72.
19 Zhou XP, Woodford-Richens K, Lehtonen R *et al.* Germline mutations in *BMPR1A/ALK3* cause a subset of cases of juvenile polyposis syndrome and of Cowden and Bannayan–Riley–Ruvalcaba syndromes. *Am J Hum Genet* 2001; **69**: 704–11.
20 Rongioletti F, Hazini R, Gianotti G, Rebora A. Folliculomas, trichodiscomas and acrochordons (Birt–Hogg–Dubé) associated with intestinal polyposis. *Clin Exp Dermatol* 1989; **14**: 72–4.
21 Schachtschabel AA, Kuster W, Happle R. Perifollicular fibroma of the skin and colonic polyps: Hornstein–Knickenberg syndrome. *Hautarzt* 1996; **47**: 304–6.
22 Hornstein OP, Knickenberg M. Perifollicular fibromatosis cutis with polyps of the colon: a cutaneo-intestinal syndrome sui generis. *Arch Dermatol Res* 1975; **253**: 161–75.
23 Zbar B, Alvord WG, Glenn G *et al.* Risk of renal and colonic neoplasms and spontaneous pneumothorax in the Birt-Hogg-Dube syndrome. *Cancer Epidemiol Biomarkers Prev* 2002; **11**: 393–400.
24 Daniel ES, Ludwig SL, Lewin KJ *et al.* The Cronkhite–Canada syndrome: an analysis of clinical and pathologic features and therapy in 55 patients. *Medicine (Baltimore)* 1982; **61**: 293–309.
25 Herzberg AJ, Kaplan DL. Cronkhite–Canada syndrome. *Int J Dermatol* 1990; **29**: 121–5.
26 Ward EM, Wolfsen HC. Review article: the non-inherited gastrointestinal polyposis syndromes. *Alimentary Pharmacol Ther* 2002; **16**: 333–42.
27 Piette AM, Meduri B, Fritsch J *et al.* Do skin tags constitute a marker for colonic polyps? A prospective study of 100 patients and metaanalysis of the literature. *Gastroenterology* 1988; **95**: 1127–9.

Liver disease

Hepatobiliary diseases are frequently associated with abnormalities of the skin, nails and hair. However, most are non-specific, as they may be present in other diseases and absent even in patients with advanced liver dysfunction—jaundice, for example, may occur due to haemolysis rather than due to liver damage. Additionally, many diseases may share the same cutaneous features (for example, most causes of cirrhosis have a commonality of clinical signs), and there is no clear correlation between the degree of the skin changes and the severity of liver dysfunction. However, there may be constellations of features that suggest specific diagnoses (e.g. pigmentation, jaundice and xanthomas in primary biliary cirrhosis). The overall picture of the patient may therefore be as useful as the presence of particular cutaneous signs.

This section will discuss some of the main groups of hepatobiliary disease, followed by some of the more important symptoms and signs.

Hepatitis and acute liver disease

Acute hepatic damage is most often due to viral hepatitis, alcohol or other drugs. Cutaneous features may be absent, or there may be jaundice. Other features may occur, depending on the cause. Most of the cutaneous features of alcohol excess are related to chronic abuse and are considered later; flushing and, uncommonly, urticaria may occur as short-term effects. This section considers the dermatological associations of infective hepatitis.

Hepatitis A virus infection is usually asymptomatic and transient. Dermatological features, if present, are jaundice, urticaria (less than 2%) and exanthema [1]. Chronic liver disease is not a feature, but a relapsing variant has been described in which itch, purpura and urticarial lesions occur [2]. Histology in such cases demonstrates a small-vessel vasculitis. More severe vasculitis or panniculitis is rare.

Hepatitis B virus (HBV) infection [1,3–5] is of major relevance to health-care workers, as it may be transmitted parenterally. It is also transmitted sexually, and HBV infection may be associated with other sexually transmitted diseases. HBV screening and vaccination are recommended for all health-care workers; routine HBV screening may be recommended for patients attending genitourinary medicine clinics, but at present is usually targeted to high-risk groups (human immunodeficiency virus (HIV)-positive individuals and parenteral drug abusers). Vaccination is not without dermatological side effects—provocation of granuloma annulare, lichen planus, Gianotti–Crosti syndrome, urticaria and contact reactions to excipients have all been reported [6–9].

Dermatological features of acute HBV infection include:

- Urticaria, non-specific erythema or a serum sickness-like picture (generalized malaise, fever and arthralgia)—this occurs in 20–30% of patients with hepatitis [3]. Angio-oedema, erythema multiforme or erythema nodosum-like lesions may occur. Circulating immune complexes are probably involved [10], and skin biopsy shows small vessel vasculitis with positive direct immunofluorescence for IgG, IgM, complement C3 and hepatitis B surface antigen (HB_sAg). This eruption may precede other features of infection, or may occur as recurrent urticaria after infection.
- Gianotti–Crosti syndrome (papular acrodermatitis of childhood, papulovesicular acrolocated syndrome)—this eruption was originally linked with HBV infection, although accumulated knowledge documents that it is a feature of numerous viral infections. Lesions consist of small, umbilicated papules, often affecting the knees, buttocks, cheeks and extremities; the lesions usually last about 6–8 weeks and are associated with non-specific malaise in the early phase.
- Polyarteritis nodosa (PAN)—about 20% of patients with PAN may have positive HBV serology, but the frequency has decreased considerably over the last 20 years, some units that previously expected HBV positivity in 30–50% of cases only finding this in less than 5% now. PAN is discussed in Chapter 50. In relation to the link with hepatitis, it is of interest that cases have been reported after vaccination. Additionally, cases are described in which PAN has resolved after treatment of the HBV infection with lamivudine (and interferon in one case), although the patients concerned had also received corticosteroids or other immunosuppressive therapy. Hepatitis viruses do not seem to provoke larger vessel vasculitides, and one study of patients with Behçet's disease demonstrated a lower frequency of antibodies to HBV than in controls.
- Cryoglobulinaemic vasculitis—about 15% of patients with HBV have detectable cryoglobulins, although most have no symptoms. The association is more important in hepatitis C.
- Other skin lesions—pyoderma gangrenosum, lichen planus and dermatomyositis have been reported with HBV infection.

However, at least in the case of lichen planus, this may reflect high geographical prevalence rather than being a true association.

Hepatitis C virus (HCV) infection is usually transmitted parenterally. Acute HCV infection is usually only mildly symptomatic; chronic hepatitis occurs in about 75%, but progression varies considerably [11,12]. Its importance in dermatology is increasingly recognized; dermatological features [13–20] include mixed cryoglobulinaemia, PAN, acral necrolytic erythema, red fingers syndrome, porphyria cutanea tarda, pruritus, lichen planus, features of chronic liver disease in some cases, and various treatment-related eruptions. Some of these warrant more detailed discussion:

- Mixed cryoglobulinaemia, usually type II (polyclonal IgG and monoclonal IgM rheumatoid factor) and less commonly type III (polyclonal IgG and polyclonal IgM rheumatoid factor) is strongly linked with HCV infection; 70%–90% of type II cryoglobulinaemia is HCV-associated. Features include small vessel vasculitis, livedo reticularis, acrocyanosis, arthralgia, glomerulonephritis, peripheral neuropathy, hepatosplenomegaly and hypocomplementaemia [17,18]. Other patterns of vasculitis may also occur. A high frequency of autoimmune thyroid disorders and antibody tests has been reported in patients with HCV-related mixed cryoglobulinaemia. Treatment is discussed in detail in references [11,12].
- Necrolytic acral erythema is a relatively recently described and apparently specific, if rare, feature of acute HCV infection [19–21]. Well demarcated, acral (mainly hands and feet but can affect forearms, knees, lower legs), dusky discoloration with peripheral blister formation progresses to form keratotic erythrokeratoderma-like chronic inflammation. Histology is that of a necrolytic process but the distribution and laboratory tests (positive HCV, normal glucagon) confirm the diagnosis. The relationship to zinc deficiency has been debated—typically, zinc deficiency has been excluded by the lack of periorificial rash and by normal serum zinc levels. However, some cases improve with empirical administration of zinc supplements, including two treated with zinc alone—one of these had a baseline zinc level that was only just in the normal range [21], but the other had frank deficiency and improvement in the necrolytic acral erythema correlated with restoration of serum zinc levels [22]. More commonly, treatment has usually been with interferon, usually combined with ribavirin [23].
- Red fingers syndrome—an earlier description of red fingers syndrome in patients with HIV and HCV infection [24] may have represented the same entity, and was felt to be due to the HCV infection, although skin histology (only obtained in one of nine cases) just showed capillary dilatation.
- PAN—in patients with 'classic' PAN in whom hepatitis virus is of relevance, the association is usually with HBV rather than HCV infection, but preceding HCV infection has been reported in up to 30% of patients with the cutaneous variant of PAN [25]. Hypocomplementaemia seems to be more common in patients with cutaneous PAN who also have HCV infection, but the numbers of patients studied is small.
- Porphyria cutanea tarda (PCT)—the most important risk factors for PCT are alcoholic liver disease and hereditary

haemochromatosis (see later). However, in some countries where there is a low prevalence of the gene mutations that cause haemochromatosis, chronic HCV infection may assume greater importance in the aetiology of PCT; the prevalence of positive HCV serology in PCT varies from about 10% to 90%, depending on geography [26]. HCV has also been linked to variegate porphyria. A case–control study in the USA found that 16 of 17 patients with PCT were HCV-positive (94%), compared with 0.17% of nearly 150 000 volunteer blood donors (although these may not be fully representative of the general population) [26]. HCV is therefore best viewed as an important independent risk factor in development of PCT [27,28]. Overall, PCT appears to be uncommon as a manifestation of HCV positivity. A large study of patients with HCV or HIV infection, or both, only found one of 177 patients to have a PCT porphyrin excretion pattern and did not support a direct role of HCV in provoking PCT. However, the mean coproporphyrin level was significantly raised in HCV-positive patients and especially in those who were also HIV-positive [29].

- Autoimmune disorders. There are associations between HCV infection and lichen planus, autoimmune thrombocytopenic purpura, Behçet's disease, vitiligo and a Sjögren's syndrome-like sialadenitis. However, as with HBV, the association with lichen planus is questionable as there is marked geographical variation; in an area of low HCV prevalence, no association could be demonstrated [30].
- Other dermatological symptoms. Pruritus may be a presenting symptom of HCV infection, and persistent itch may occur [16]. Urticaria, erythema multiforme, erythema nodosum and papuloerythroderma [31] have been reported.
- Treatment related dermatoses—interferon and antiviral agents have many potential side effects, including urticaria and exanthematous reactions. Discoid eczema and Meyerson's phenomenon (halo eczema around naevi) have been reported. Potentially more severe or less apparent reactions include a thrombotic microangiopathy reported due to pegylated-interferon-α-2b [32], and sarcoidosis (which may self-resolve, or may be treated with judicious oral corticocosteroid) associated with use of pegylated-interferon-α plus ribavirin [33].

Hepatitis D causes cutaneous features similar to those of HBV. *Hepatitis E* is generally mild, but may cause disseminated intravascular coagulation [1]. *Hepatitis F* is disputed, and *hepatitis G* is usually transmitted parenterally.

References

1 Geyer AS, Rosenburg DS, Herlong HF, Provost TT. Hepatitis. In: Provost TT, Flynn JA, eds. *Cutaneous Medicine: Cutaneous Manifestations of Systemic Disease*. Hamilton, Ontario: Decker, 2001: 452–63.

2 Glikson M, Galune E, Oren R et al. Relapsing hepatitis A: review of 14 cases and literature survey. *Medicine* 1992; **71**: 14–23.

3 McElgunn PS. Dermatologic manifestations of hepatitis B virus infection. *J Am Acad Dermatol* 1983; **8**: 539–48.

4 D'Souza R, Foster GR. Diagnosis and treatment of chronic hepatitis B. *J Roy Soc Med* 2004; **97**: 318–21.

5 Aggarwal R, Ranjan P. Preventing and treating hepatitis B infection. *BMJ* 2004; **329**: 1080–6.

6 Wolf F, Grezard P, Berard F et al. Generalized granuloma annulare and hepatitis B vaccination. *Eur J Dermatol* 1998; **8**: 435–6.

7 Tay YK. Gianotti–Crosti syndrome following immunization. *Pediatr Dermatol* 2001; **18**: 262.

8 Al-Khenaizan S. Lichen planus occurring after hepatitis B vaccination: a new case. *J Am Acad Dermatol* 2002; **45**: 614–5.

9 Rietschel RL, Adams RM. Reactions to thimerosal in hepatitis B vaccines. *Dermatol Clin* 1990; **8**: 161–4.

10 Neumann HAM, Berretty PJM, Reinders Folmer SSC et al. Hepatitis B surface antigen deposition in the blood vessel walls of urticarial lesions in acute hepatitis B. *Br J Dermatol* 1981; **104**: 383–8.

11 Hayes PC, ed. Consensus conference on hepatitis C. *J Viral Hepatitis* 2004; **11** (Suppl. 1); 1–39.

12 Lauer GM, Walker BD. Hepatitis C virus infection. *N Engl J Med* 2001; **345**: 41–52.

13 Pawlotsky JM, Dhumeaux D, Bagot M. Hepatitis C virus in dermatology. *Arch Dermatol* 1995; **131**: 1185–93.

14 Schwaber MJ, Zlotogorski A. Dermatologic manifestations of hepatitis C infection. *Int J Dermatol* 1997; **36**: 251–4.

15 Bonkovsky HL, Mehta S. Hepatitis C. Review and update. *J Am Acad Dermatol* 2001; **44**: 159–79.

16 Fisher DA, Wright TL. Pruritus as a symptom of hepatitis C. *J Am Acad Dermatol* 1994; **30**: 629–32.

17 Cacoub P, Costedoat-Chalumeau N, Lidove O, Alric L. Cryoglobulinemia vasculitis. *Curr Opin Rheumatol* 2002; **14**: 29–35.

18 Ferri C, Mascia MT. Cryoglobulinemic vasculitis. *Curr Opin Rheumatol* 2006; **18**: 54–63.

19 Darouti ME, Ala ME. Necrolytic acral erythema: a cutaneous marker of hepatitis C. *Int J Dermatol* 1996; **35**: 252–6.

20 Crawford GH, Kim S, James WD. Skin signs of systemic disease: an update. *Adv Dermatol* 2003; **18**: 1–27.

21 Abdallah MA, Hull C, Horn TD. Necrolytic acral erythema. A patient from the United States successfully treated with oral zinc. *Arch Dermatol* 2005; **141**: 85–7.

22 Najarian DJ, Lefkowitz I, Balfour E et al. Zinc deficiency associated with necrolytic acral erythema. *J Am Acad Dermatol* 2006; **55**: S108–10.

23 Hivnor CM, Yan AC, Junkins-Hopkins JM, Honig PJ. Necrolytic acral erythema: response to combination therapy with interferon and ribavirin. *J Am Acad Dermatol* 2004; **50**: S121–4.

24 Pechère M, Krishner J, Rosay A, Hirschel B, Saurat J-H. Red fingers syndrome in patients with HIV and hepatitis C infection. *Lancet* 1996; **348**: 196–7.

25 Soufir N, Descamps V, Crickx B et al. Hepatitis C virus infection in cutaneous polyarteritis nodosa: a retrospective study of 16 cases. *Arch Dermatol* 1999; **135**: 1001–2.

26 Chuang TY, Brashear R, Lewis C. Porphyria cutanea tarda and hepatitis C virus: a case–control study and meta-analysis of the literature. *J Am Acad Dermatol* 1999; **41**: 31–6.

27 Bulaj ZJ, Phillips JD, Ajioka RS et al. Hemochromatosis genes and other factors contributing to the pathogenesis of porphyria cutanea tarda. *Blood* 2000; **95**: 1565–71.

28 Stuart KA, Busfield F, Jazwinska EC et al. The C282Y mutation in the hemochromatosis gene (HFE) and hepatitis C virus infection are independent cofactors for porphyria cutanea tarda in Australian patients. *J Hepatol* 1998; **28**: 404–9.

29 Cribier B, Rey D, Uhl G et al. Abnormal urinary coproporphyrin levels in patients infected by hepatitis C virus with or without human immunodeficiency virus. *Arch Dermatol* 1996; **132**: 1448–52.

30 Tucker SC, Coulson IH. Lichen planus is not associated with hepatitis C virus infection in patients from north west England. *Acta Derm Venereol* 1999; **79**: 378–9.

31 Ota M, Sato-Matsumura KC, Sawamura D, Shimizu H. Papuloerythroderma associated with hepatitis C virus infection. *J Am Acad Dermatol* 2005; **52**: S61–2.

32 Creput C, Auffret N, Samuel D et al. Cutaneous thrombotic microangiopathy during treatment with alpha-interferon for chronic hepatitis C. *J Hepatol* 2002; **37**: 871–2.

33 Hurst EA, Mauro T. Darcoidosis associated with pegylated interferon alpha and ribavirin treatment for chronic hepatitis C. *Arch Dermatol* 2005; **141**: 865–8.

Cirrhosis of the liver

Assessing the degree of liver disease is not the remit of dermatologists, but measurement of hepatic fibrosis warrants discussion as this has importance with regard to monitoring of methotrexate therapy (see 'Drugs and the liver' below, and Chapters 20 and 74).

Progression to cirrhosis, whatever the cause, is often avoided if fibrosis is detected at an early stage. Increasingly, measurement of serum levels of the amino-terminal propeptide of collagen III (PIIINP) is being used as a substitute for liver biopsy in methotrexate monitoring [1–3], and, if performed three or four times annually, a consistently normal result appears to indicate a negligible risk of significant fibrosis. It does however have limitations—it can only detect active fibrosis, and can be elevated in other situations (notably psoriatic arthritis). Biopsy also has limitations—one study showed that, in 25% of cases where each liver lobe was biopsied, there was at least one fibrosis stage difference between the samples. Algorithms based on an increased number of parameters may help to improve non-invasive accuracy—a study that used biopsy as the gold standard in 1021 subjects and analysed nine other factors determined that four of these (age, hyaluronic acid, PIIINP and tissue inhibitor of matrix metalloproteinase I) had 90% sensitivity and a negative predictive value of 92% for significant fibrosis [4].

References

1 Zachariae H, Heickendorff L, Søgaard H. The value of amino-terminal propeptide of type III procollagen in routine screening for methotrexate-induced liver fibrosis: a 10-year follow-up. *Br J Dermatol* 2001; **144**: 100–3.
2 Zachariae H. Have methotrexate-induced liver fibrosis and cirrhosis become rare? A matter for reappraisal of routine liver biopsies. *Dermatology (Basel)* 2005; **211**: 307–8.
3 Chalmers RJG, Kirby B, Smith A *et al.* Replacement of routine liver biopsy by procollagen III aminopeptide for monitoring patients with psoriasis receiving long-term methotrexate: a multicentre audit and health economic analysis. *Br J Dermatol* 2005; **152**: 444–50.
4 Rosenberg WM, Voelker M, Thiel R *et al.* Serum markers detect the presence of liver fibrosis: a cohort study. *Gastroenterology* 2004; **127**: 1704–13.

Cutaneous features of chronic liver disease

Cutaneous features of chronic liver disease are listed in Table 62.13 [1,2]. Causes include chronic hepatitis (above), alcohol abuse and others—some of the idiopathic causes are discussed below, as each has some specific features in addition to those that occur in liver failure of any cause.

Table 62.13 Skin lesions associated with chronic liver disease.

Spider angiomas, telangiectasia
Palmar erythema
Dilated abdominal/chest veins (including periumbilical caput medusae)
Jaundice
Increased melanin pigmentation
Thin 'paper-money' skin, striae
Excoriations
Loss of secondary sexual hair in males
Bruising, purpura
Nail changes: clubbing, pallor, Muehrcke's bands, Terry's nail
Features of malnutrition (see Chapter 59)
Associated lesions
Xanthomas (primary biliary cirrhosis)
Porphyria cutanea tarda (alcoholic liver disease)
Vasculitis/capillaritis/pyoderma gangrenosum (chronic active hepatitis)
Lichen planus (primary biliary cirrhosis)

References

1 Smith KE, Fenske NA. Cutaneous manifestations of alcohol abuse. *J Am Acad Dermatol* 2000; **43**: 1–16.
2 Ruocco V, Psilogenis M, Lo Schiavo A, Wolf R. Dermatological manifestations of alcoholic cirrhosis. *Clin Dermatol* 1999; **17**: 463–8.

Haemochromatosis

There are at least five hereditary (idiopathic) types of haemochromatosis ('bronze diabetes') [1–7], a disorder in which iron overload is associated with arthropathy, endocrine failure, cardiovascular disease and some infections. By far the commonest is 'classic' autosomal recessive haemochromatosis, which is due to mutations of the *HFE* gene (chromosome 6p21.3); mutations C282Y (cysteine 282 tyrosine) and H63D (histidine 63 asparagine) account for about 80% of cases, and mutations in S65C for perhaps 10% (all vary considerably between populations). The genotype combinations that may occur influence the risk of some associated disorders such as PCT (below). The 'classic' haemochromatosis phenotype also occurs due to mutations in the hemojuvulin gene (chromosome 1q21, also autosomal recessive). Haemochromatosis type 2 (HFE2, juvenile haemochromatosis) also occurs as a result of mutations in two different genes, HFE2A is due to hemojuvulin gene mutations and HFE2B due to mutation in *HAMP* (was *LEAP1*) which encodes hepcidin antimicrobial peptide (hepcidin). Other genes in which mutations cause haemochromatosis include *TFR2*, the gene for transferrin receptor-2 (causing haemochromatosis type 3, usually mutation Y250X) and *SCL40A1*, the gene for ferroportin (causing hemochromatosis type 4, HFE4). Classic idiopathic haemochromatosis usually presents in males over the age of 40 years. An acquired form also occurs, secondary to haemosiderosis or alcohol abuse.

There is increased iron absorption leading to iron deposition in various organs, including the liver, pancreas, heart, pituitary and endocrine organs. Skin pigmentation, diabetes, hepatic cirrhosis and cardiac failure are prominent features [8–10]. Dryness of the skin and koilonychia may have been underestimated in the past [11]; stigmata of chronic hepatic failure may also be present. Deposition of iron in the skin has been used as a surrogate for deposition in other organs [12,13]; in idiopathic haemochromatosis, iron deposition includes deposition in eccrine sweat glands [11]. However, the pigmentation of haemochromatosis is due to melanin rather than to haemosiderin [8–10]. It typically has a grey hue, and is most prominent on exposed skin, similar to addisonian pigmentation. Keratin cysts with a black colour [14], and black stasis dermatitis [15], have also been reported.

There is a 200-fold increase in the risk of hepatocellular carcinoma compared with the general population [8].

Porphyria cutanea tarda has been linked with haemochromatosis [10,16,17]. It has subsequently been shown that homozygosity for the C282Y mutation and seropositivity for HCV are the greatest risk factors for expression of PCT [18] and that they appear to act as independent co-factors [19]. In patients with mutations in uroporphyrinogen decarboxylase, which leads to PCT, coinheritance of C282Y homozygosity is associated with earlier age of onset of the porphyria [20].

References

1 Online Mendelian Inheritance in Man. *Haemochromatosis*. www.ncbi.nlm.nih.gov/entrez/dispomim.cgi?id=235200

2 Bacon BR. Hemochromatosis: diagnosis and management. *Gastroenterology* 2001; **120**: 718–25.

3 Njajou OT, Vaessen N, Joosse M *et al.* A mutation in *SLC11A3* is associated with autosomal dominant hemochromatosis. *Nature Genet* 2001; **28**: 213–4.

4 Kotze MJ, de Villiers JNP, Bouwens CSH *et al.* Molecular diagnosis of hereditary hemochromatosis: application of a newly-developed reverse-hybridization assay in the South African population. *Clin Genet* 2004; **65**: 317–23.

5 Milet J, Dehais V, Bourgain C *et al.* Common variants in the BMP2, BMP4 and HJV genes of the hepcidin regulation pathway modulate HFE hemochromatosis penetrance. *Am J Hum Genet* 2007; **81**: 799–807.

6 Wallace DF, Subramanion VN. Non-HFE haemochromatosis. *World J Gastroenterol* 2007; **13**: 4690–8.

7 Griffiths WJH. Review article: the genetic basis of haemochromatosis. *Aliment Pharmacol Ther* 2007; **26**: 331–42.

8 Braverman IM. *Skin Signs of Systemic Disease*, 3rd edn. Philadelphia: Saunders, 1998: 405–37.

9 Bloom PD, Gordeuk VR, MacPhail AP. HLA-linked hemochromatosis and other forms of iron overload. *Dermatol Clin* 1995; **13**: 57–63.

10 Tavill AS, Sharma BK, Bacon BR. Iron and the liver: genetic hemochromatosis and other hepatic iron overload disorders. *Prog Liver Dis* 1990; **9**: 281–305.

11 Chevrant-Breton J, Simon M, Bourel M, Ferrand B. Cutaneous manifestations of idiopathic hemochromatosis. *Arch Dermatol* 1977; **113**: 161–5.

12 Tsuji T. Experimental hemosiderosis: relationship between skin pigmentation and hemosiderin. *Acta Derm Venereol* 1980; **60**: 109–14.

13 Farquharson MJ, Bagshaw AP, Porter JB, Abeysinghe RD. The use of skin Fe levels as a surrogate marker for organ Fe levels, to monitor treatment in cases of iron overload. *Phys Med Biol* 2000; **45**: 1387–96.

14 Leyden JJ, Lockshin NA, Krebel S. The black keratinous cyst: a sign of hemochromatosis. *Arch Dermatol* 1972; **106**: 379–81.

15 Soderberg KI, Sharp M, Carrington PR. Brown and black scaly patches on the lower leg. *Arch Dermatol* 2007; **143**: 1441–6.

16 Seymour DG, Elder GH, Fryer A *et al.* Porphyria cutanea tarda and haemochromatosis: a family study. *Gut* 1990; **31**: 719–21.

17 Kushner JP, Edwards CQ, Dadone MM, Skolnick MH. Heterozygosity for HLA-linked hemochromatosis as a likely cause of the hepatic siderosis associated with sporadic porphyria cutanea tarda. *Gastroenterology* 1985; **88**: 1232–8.

18 Bulaj ZJ, Phillips JD, Ajioka RS *et al.* Hemochromatosis genes and other factors contributing to the pathogenesis of porphyria cutanea tarda. *Blood* 2000; **95**: 1565–71.

19 Stuart KA, Busfield F, Jazwinska EC *et al.* The C282Y mutation in the hemochromatosis gene (*HFE*) and hepatitis C virus infection are independent cofactors for porphyria cutanea tarda in Australian patients. *J Hepatol* 1998; **28**: 404–9.

20 Brady JJ, Jackson HA, Roberts AG *et al.* Co-inheritance of mutations in the uroporphyrinogen decarboxylase and hemochromatosis genes accelerates the onset of porphyria cutanea tarda. *J Invest Dermatol* 2000; **115**: 868–74.

Primary biliary cirrhosis and biliary tract disease

From the dermatological standpoint, primary biliary cirrhosis (PBC) is the most important biliary tract disease. The cutaneous features of significance are marked itch (discussed in more detail below), excoriation, hyperpigmentation and various xanthomatous lesions due to secondary hyperlipidaemia [1,2]. Xanthelasma, palmar crease, tuberous and tendinous xanthomas may all occur. PBC occurs mainly in middle-aged women as an autoimmune disease, is strongly associated with the presence of antimitochondrial antibodies (AMA), and has been associated with numerous other autoimmune conditions, including CREST, morphoea and other scleroderma spectrum disorders, lichen planus and lichen sclerosus [1–7]. The constellation of CREST with PBC is also known as Reynolds' syndrome, and is usually associated with M2 antibodies. Sarcoidosis [8] and other patterns of granulomatous disease such as granuloma annulare are also reported. There is a strong link with Sjögren's syndrome—about 10% of patients with Sjögren's syndrome have AMA, sometimes with abnormal liver function tests or liver histology, and over half of patients with PBC have some evidence of Sjögren's syndrome [9]. Itch is often the first symptom of PBC, so serology to detect AMA is a useful screening test in women with unexplained pruritus; AMA-negative PBC causes particular diagnostic difficulty.

Cholestasis and bile stones may cause acute or chronic jaundice and other features of liver disease. Pigment bile stones may occur due to erythropoietic protoporphyria.

Congenital biliary tract hypoplasia is a feature of Alagille's syndrome (MIM #118450) [10], a dominantly inherited disorder due to a gene mutation on chromosome 20p12. Affected individuals have a characteristic facies, jaundice, pruritus and retardation of growth and mental development. Various skeletal, ocular and vascular defects are associated. A report of 38 children documented firm xanthomas in 28%, mainly flexural but also affecting palms and ears; the xanthomas resolved in those individuals treated by liver transplantation [11].

Biliary tract abnormalities are also common in hereditary haemorrhagic telangiectasia, resembling either a congenital malformation of the ductal plate, or appearing similar to the changes seen in sclerosing cholangitis [12].

References

1 Kaplan MM. Primary biliary cirrhosis. *N Engl J Med* 1996; **335**: 1570–80.

2 Heathcote J. The clinical expression of primary biliary cirrhosis. *Semin Liver Dis* 1997; **17**: 23–33.

3 Powell FC, Rogers RS, Dickson ER. Primary biliary cirrhosis and lichen planus. *J Am Acad Dermatol* 1983; **9**: 540–5.

4 Powell FC, Schroeter AL, Dickson ER. Primary biliary cirrhosis and the CREST syndrome: a report of 22 cases. *QJM* 1987; **62**: 75–82.

5 Akimoto S, Ishikawa O, Muro Y *et al.* Clinical and immunological characterization of patients with systemic sclerosis overlapping with primary biliary cirrhosis: a comparison with systemic sclerosis alone. *J Dermatol* 1999; **26**: 18–22.

6 Meyrick Thomas RH, Ridley CM, McGibbon DH, Black MM. Association between lichen sclerosus et atrophicus and primary biliary cirrhosis. *Br J Dermatol* 1986; **114**: 514–5.

7 Reed JR, De Luca N, McIntyre AS, Wilkinson JD. Localised morphoea, xanthomatosis and primary biliary cirrhosis. *Br J Dermatol* 2000; **143**: 652–3.

8 Harrington AC, Fitzpatrick JE. Cutaneous sarcoidal granulomas in a patient with primary biliary cirrhosis. *Cutis* 1992; **49**: 271–4.

9 Martin DR, Provost TT. Sjögren's syndrome. In: Provost TT, Flynn JA, eds. *Cutaneous Medicine: Cutaneous Manifestations of Systemic Disease.* Hamilton, Ontario: Decker, 2001: 127–46.

10 Alagille D, Estrada A, Hadchouel M *et al.* Syndromic paucity of interlobular bile ducts (Alagille syndrome or arteriohepatic dysplasia): review of 80 cases. *J Pediatr* 1987; **110**: 195–200.

11 Garcia MA, Ramonet M, Ciocca M *et al.* Alagille syndrome: cutaneous manifestations in 38 children. *Pediatr Dermatol* 2005; **22**: 11–4.

12 Garcia-Tsao G, Korzenik JR, Young L *et al.* Liver disease in patients with hereditary haemorrhagic telangiectasia. *N Engl J Med* 2000; **343**: 931–6.

Drugs and the liver

Drug-related links between the skin and the liver include the following:

- Drugs used to treat the skin, whose hepatic metabolism is altered by liver disease or by other drugs that are also metabolized in the liver, e.g. ciclosporin
- Drugs used to treat skin disease that may cause hepatitis or other liver damage, e.g. azathioprine, methotrexate
- Drugs used to treat liver disease that may have cutaneous side effects, e.g. local reactions to vitamin K (Texier's syndrome),

elastosis perforans serpiginosa due to penicillamine for Wilson's disease

- Drugs used to prevent liver disease that may have cutaneous side effects, e.g. local reactions due to thimerosal or other preservatives in hepatitis vaccines
- Drugs that cause liver changes with secondary cutaneous signs, e.g. oestrogens leading to PCT
- Drugs that may cause concurrent hepatitis and rash, e.g. phenytoin and other anticonvulsants.

Systemic diseases and the liver

A large number of systemic diseases may affect the liver, many with cutaneous features. Most are discussed in other chapters. For example, sarcoidosis is associated with subclinical hepatic involvement in over 50% of patients, but may cause overt hepatomegaly or abnormalities of liver function in conjunction with skin lesions.

Porphyrias, especially PCT, may occur as a consequence of liver disease (see Chapter 59 and the discussion of PCT below); severe liver disease is also a feature in some patients with erythropoietic protoporphyria.

Hereditary haemorrhagic telangiectasia, mentioned earlier as a cause of gastrointestinal bleeding, is associated with portal hypertension due mainly to portosystemic shunting, so bleeding in such patients may be from varices.

Dermatological features and dermatoses associated with liver disease

Pruritus

Pruritus is the most common skin symptom associated with liver disease. It may precede the onset of jaundice of any cause, and may be a feature of hepatitis, as discussed above. Liver diseases in which itch is most prominent are PBC, sclerosing cholangitis and any other biliary tract obstruction, and disorders causing cholestasis; itch is less prominent in haemochromatosis, alcoholic cirrhosis and autoimmune chronic active hepatitis [1]. The symptoms are generally most severe at acral sites and at areas of tight clothing, and are more prominent nocturnally. Disappearance of pruritus may accompany severe deterioration in hepatic function [2].

The precise mechanism of itch in obstructive liver disease remains unclear. It was believed to be due to the presence of bile salts in the skin [3,4], but the intensity of itch does not reliably correlate with bilirubin or bile acid levels in chronic liver failure, and this theory is not supported by more recent research [1,5]. Other proposed mediators of cholestatic itch include alternative liver metabolites, histamine or other mast cell mediators, and endogenous opiates. Although patients with cholestasis may have elevated plasma histamine levels, the therapeutic response to antihistamines is limited, and it is unlikely that release of histamine plays an important role in the pathogenesis of hepatobiliary itch [1]. Improvement in hepatic itch after administration of drugs that block the action of endogenous opiates suggests that the latter may have an important role in cholestatic itch [6–8].

Treatment, where possible, is for the underlying cause—for example, drug withdrawal in drug-induced cholestasis, surgery for mechanical biliary obstruction, interferon and ribavirin for chronic HCV infection, etc. Less specific options include ursodeoxycholic acid, cholestyramine, phenobarbital, anabolic steroids such as stanozolol, rifampicin, antihistamines and dietary manipulation to supplement polyunsaturated fatty acids [1,9,10]. Phototherapy of various types—daylight, ultraviolet A (UVA), ultraviolet B (UVB), photoirradiation of plasma and extracorporeal photophoresis—can be effective, but ongoing treatment is generally required [1,11,12]. Other treatments that have been used with success include haemoperfusion or plasma perfusion through charcoal-coated beads (which can produce benefit lasting several weeks), plasmapheresis, infusions of albumin (benefit for a few days) and slow injection of intravenous lidocaine (lignocaine) (which produces short-term benefit only). On the basis that endogenous opiates play a role in this symptom, and that these have a circadian rhythm regulated by light, bright-light therapy to the eyes was studied and found to reduce cholestatic itch in a short-term study [13]. Oral opiate antagonists are effective but may cause opioid withdrawal-like reactions—this may be reduced by use of very low dose naloxone infusions prior to gradual increase in dose of an oral opiate antagonist [14]. Gabapentin was ineffective in a double-blind, controlled trial [15].

References

1 Ghent CN. Cholestatic pruritus. In: Bernhard JD. *Itch: Mechanisms and Management of Pruritus*. New York: McGraw-Hill, 1994: 229–42.
2 Bernhard JD, Jorizzo JL, Callen JP. Pruritus. In: Callen JP, Jorizzo JL, eds. *Dermatological Signs of Internal Disease*, 3rd edn. Philadelphia: Saunders, 2003: 65–8.
3 Kirby J, Heaton KW, Burton JL *et al.* The pruritic effect of bile salts. *Br J Dermatol* 1974; **91** (Suppl. 10): 11–2.
4 Varadi DP. Pruritus induced by crude bile and purified bile acids: experimental production of pruritus in human skin. *Arch Dermatol* 1974; **109**: 678–81.
5 Ghent CN. Pruritus of cholestasis is related to effects of bile salts on the liver, not the skin. *Am J Gastroenterol* 1987; **82**: 117–8.
6 Bergasa NV, Talbot TL, Alling DW *et al.* A controlled trial of naloxone infusions for the pruritus of cholestasis. *Gastroenterology* 1992; **102**: 544–9.
7 Borgeat A, Wilder-Smith OHG, Mentha G. Subhypnotic doses of propofol relieve pruritus associated with liver disease. *Gastroenterology* 1993; **104**: 244–7.
8 Bergasa NV, Alling DW, Talbot TL *et al.* Oral nalmefene therapy reduces scratching activity due to the pruritus of cholestasis: a controlled study. *J Am Acad Dermatol* 1999; **41**: 431–4.
9 Smith KE, Fenske NA. Cutaneous manifestations of alcohol abuse. *J Am Acad Dermatol* 2000; **43**: 1–16.
10 Garden JM, Ostrow JD, Roenigk HH. Pruritus in hepatic cholestasis: pathogenesis and therapy. *Arch Dermatol* 1985; **121**: 1415–20.
11 Rosenthal E, Diamond E, Benderly A, Etzioni A. Cholestatic pruritus: effect of phototherapy on pruritus and excretion of bile acids in urine. *Acta Paediatr* 1994; **83**: 888–91.
12 Greaves MW, Provost TT. Pruritus as a manifestation of systemic disease. In: Provost TT, Flynn JA, eds. *Cutaneous Medicine: Cutaneous Manifestations of Systemic Disease*. Hamilton, Ontario: Decker, 2001: 1–8.
13 Bergasa NV, Link MJ, Keogh M *et al.* Pilot study of bright-light therapy reflected towards the eyes for the pruritus of chronic liver disease. *Am J Gastroenterol* 2001; **96**: 1563–70.
14 Jones EA, Neuberger J, Bergasa NV. Opiate antagonist therapy for the pruritus of cholestasis: the avoidance of opioid withdrawal-like reactions. *QJM* 2002; **95**: 947–52.
15 Bergasa NV, McGee M, Ginsburg IH, Engler D. Gabapentin in patients with the pruritus of cholestasis: a double-blind, randomized, placebo-controlled trial. *Hepatology* 2006; **44**: 1317–23.

Skin pigment changes in liver disease [1–3]

Jaundice (icterus) is first visible as a yellowish hue of the sclerae and soft palate before it becomes generalized. It is due to hyperbilirubinaemia. Carotenaemia may have a similar appearance but does not affect sclerae; skin discoloration following mepacrine or busulphan therapy may simulate jaundice, but these usually also cause subungual pigmented bands.

Green-coloured sweat [4] and green discoloration of the gingivae may occur due to jaundice.

A muddy-grey coloured hyperpigmentation occurs in chronic liver disease of any cause. It is due to hypermelanosis with normal numbers of melanocytes, but the precise mechanism is uncertain. There may be a yellowish tinge due to associated jaundice. Usually, pigmentation is more prominent in sun-exposed areas. It may be blotchy or diffuse, and may be exaggerated in the perioral and periorbital areas (resembling chloasma); in other cases it may resemble freckling and it can also localize to palmar creases. Males frequently show increased pigmentation of the areola in association with gynaecomastia and testicular atrophy.

Spotty hypomelanosis may occur on the back, buttocks and thighs, often in relation to spider angiomas.

Associated dietary deficiency may cause the pigmentary changes of pellagra (Chapter 59).

Vascular changes
Spider angiomas are a characteristic feature in patients with severe chronic liver disease (Fig. 62.20). Contributory factors [5] include decreased hepatic metabolism of oestrogen leading to hyperoestrogenaemia (which also accounts for loss of secondary male-pattern hair, gynaecomastia and testicular atrophy); alcohol-induced vasodilatation and altered central vasomotor control may also be involved. The same factors lead to palmar erythema ('liver palms'), which is most pronounced on the thenar and hypothenar regions and may also affect the soles of the feet, and also to facial plethora. None of these vascular features are specific for liver disease. Diffusely scattered tiny telangiectatic vessels are referred to as 'paper money skin'. Increased peripheral blood flow with dilatation of digital pulp arteriovenous anastomoses is thought to be the cause of finger clubbing, which occurs in about 15% of patients with hepatic cirrhosis.

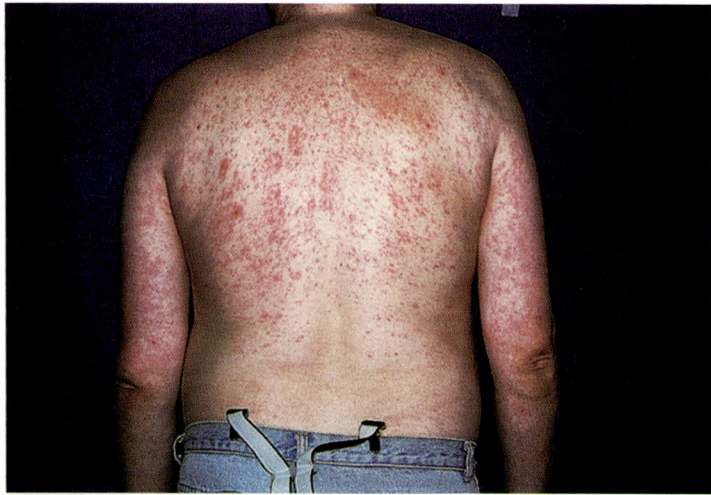

Fig. 62.20 Telangiectasia in alcoholic liver cirrhosis.

Purpuric lesions including scurvy may occur as a result of poor nutrition, especially in alcoholic liver disease (see Chapter 59). Altered production of prothrombin and deficiency of vitamin K may lead to frank ecchymoses.

In progressive liver disease with portal hypertension, collateral blood flow creates visible coiled varicose veins on the abdominal wall. When these are in a pattern radiating from the umbilicus, the appearance is termed 'caput Medusae'.

Hair, nail and collagen changes [1–3]
The body hair is often thinned or partially lost, and males tend to develop a female pubic-hair pattern. There is both increased production and decreased metabolism of oestrogens, as well as decreased production and increased metabolism of testosterone. When there is severe loss of scalp hair, zinc deficiency should be suspected (Chapter 59).

Nail changes include a diffuse white colour with an invisible lunula, proximal white colour with distal pink colour (Terry's nails) and white bands (Muehrke's bands [6]). Altered digital blood flow, soft-tissue overgrowth and hypoalbuminaemia may all contribute. Lunulae may be red in patients with hepatic cirrhosis, and occasionally an azure-blue colour in hepatolenticular degeneration (Wilson's disease). Nail-plate changes include clubbing (see above) and its milder variant, the 'watch-glass' deformity; flattened nails or koilonychia may occur if there is poor nutrition or altered iron metabolism (e.g. haemochromatosis).

Striae occur in both sexes, especially on the lower abdomen, thighs and buttocks. Chronic alcoholism also alters metabolism of corticosteroids, leading to 'pseudo-Cushing's syndrome'.

Porphyria cutanea tarda
Chronic liver disease is involved in the skin changes of porphyria cutanea tarda. Lesions consist of bullae, scarring and hyperpigmentation of sun-exposed skin areas and hypertrichosis of the face. This is discussed in more detail in Chapter 59.

Other cutaneous lesions associated with liver disease
Lichen planus has been reported in a number of diseases with abnormal immune function. The association of erosive oral lesions in PBC [7] and chronic active hepatitis [8] may be related to a common immunological pathogenesis. Most reported patients have received penicillamine therapy which is believed by some to trigger the eruption [9–11]. HCV infection is associated with lichen planus [12].

In chronic active hepatitis (juvenile cirrhosis, lupoid hepatitis) and in PBC, firm reddish papules resembling pityriasis lichenoides chronica or lymphomatoid papulosis have been reported [8,13]. The lesions erupt on the trunk and extremities and may heal leaving slightly depressed atrophic scars. Histological examination reveals a capillaritis of the skin. Pityriasis lichenoides has also been reported in association with HCV seropositivity.

Pyoderma gangrenosum has also been reported in chronic active hepatitis [14]. The Gianotti–Crosti syndrome has been discussed in relation to hepatitis. Skin changes simulating classical glucagonoma syndrome have been reported in cirrhosis and termed the 'pseudoglucagonoma syndrome' [15].

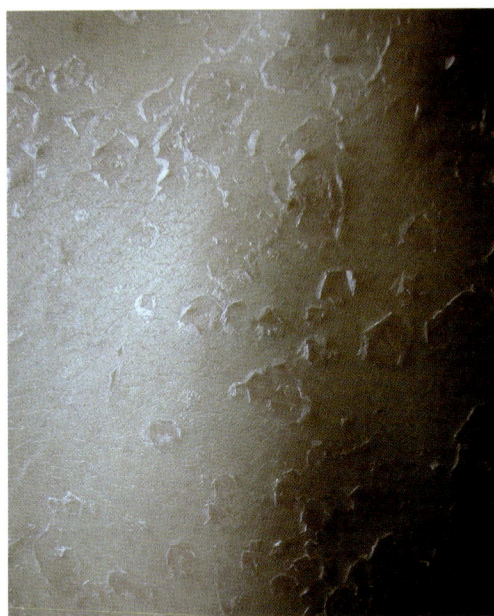

Fig. 62.21 Scaling rash on the trunk in chronic zinc deficiency.

Acquired zinc deficiency (Fig. 62.21) may occur in chronic alcoholic liver disease due to increased loss of urinary zinc in cirrhosis and poor nutrition [16,17]. Clinical features are a crackled and reticulate eczema on the trunk and extensor aspects of the limbs, erosive crusted changes in the perianal and genital areas, cheilitis, hair loss and multiple Beau's lines on the nails. Increased hair growth, often with a deeper pigmentation, may occur. Beer, wine and spirits are practically free of zinc, but most beer brands contain vitamin B in significant amounts and the typical zinc-deficient beer-drinker does not show additional clinical signs of vitamin B depletion [17].

References
1 Smith KE, Fenske NA. Cutaneous manifestations of alcohol abuse. *J Am Acad Dermatol* 2000; **43**: 1–16.
2 Ruocco V, Psilogenis M, Lo Schiavo A, Wolf R. Dermatological manifestations of alcoholic cirrhosis. *Clin Dermatol* 1999; **17**: 463–8.
3 Braverman IM. *Skin Signs of Systemic Disease*, 3rd edn. Philadelphia: Saunders, 1998: 405–37.
4 Allegue F, Hermo JA, Fachal C, Alfonsín N. Localised green pigmentation in a patient with hyperbilirubinemia. *J Am Acad Dermatol* 1996; **35**: 108–9.
5 Malpas SC, Robinson BJ, Maling TJ. Mechanism of ethanol-induced vasodilation. *J Appl Physiol* 1990; **68**: 731–4.
6 Muehrcke RC. The finger-nails in chronic hypoalbuminaemia: a new physical sign. *BMJ* 1956; **i**: 1327–8.
7 Graham-Brown RAC, Sarkany I, Sherlock S. Lichen planus and primary biliary cirrhosis. *Br J Dermatol* 1982; **106**: 699–703.
8 Sarkany I. Juvenile cirrhosis and allergic capillaritis of the skin. *Proc R Soc Med* 1970; **63**: 819.
9 Powell FC, Rogers RS III, Dickson ER. Lichen planus, primary biliary cirrhosis and penicillamine. *Br J Dermatol* 1982; **107**: 616.
10 Seehafer JR, Rogers RS III, Fleming R *et al.* Lichen planus-like lesions caused by penicillamine in primary biliary cirrhosis. *Arch Dermatol* 1981; **117**: 140–2.
11 Rebora A, Rongioletti F, Canepa A. Chronic active hepatitis and lichen planus. *Acta Derm Venereol* 1982; **62**: 351–2.
12 Pawlotsky JM, Dhumeaux D, Bagot M. Hepatitis C in dermatology. *Arch Dermatol* 1995; **131**: 1185–93.
13 Rai GS, Hamlyn AN, Dahl MGC *et al.* Primary biliary cirrhosis, cutaneous capillaritis and IgM-associated membranous glomerulonephritis. *BMJ* 1977; **i**: 817.
14 Byrne JP, Newitt M, Summerley R. Pyoderma gangrenosum associated with chronic active hepatitis. *Arch Dermatol* 1976; **112**: 1297–301.
15 Doyle JA, Schroeter AL, Rogers RS II. Hyperglucagonaemia and necrolytic migratory erythema in cirrhosis: possible pseudoglucagonoma syndrome. *Br J Dermatol* 1979; **101**: 581–7.
16 Gaveau D, Piette F, Cortot A *et al.* Manifestations cutanées du déficit en zinc dans la cirrhose éthylique. *Ann Dermatol Vénéréol* 1987; **114**: 39–53.
17 Weismann K, Verdich J. Acquired zinc deficiency in alcoholics with malnutrition. In: Wilkinson DS, Mascaró JM, Orfanos CE, eds. *The CMD Case Collection*, Vol. 37: *World Congress of Dermatology, Berlin 1987*. Stuttgart: Schattauer, 1987: 379–81.

Pancreatic disease

Apart from jaundice and panniculitis, skin changes associated with pancreatic disease are uncommon. As with other causes of chronic, localized pain, erythema ab igne has been described in the skin overlying the pancreas in cases of chronic pancreatitis. The glucagonoma syndrome is a rare but highly characteristic skin disorder, which is discussed below. The pancreas is often involved in haemochromatosis (see the section on liver disease, above). Skin disorders associated with diabetes mellitus are discussed in Chapter 59.

Acute pancreatitis [1–3]
Jaundice and fat necrosis (see below) may both be prominent. Purpura or bruising may occur in about 5% of patients with acute pancreatitis; note however that neither are specific for this cause, they may occur due to retroperitoneal haemorrhage, or bleeding from sources such as splenic rupture, ectopic pregnancy, metastatic tumour or aortic aneurysm. Four eponymous signs occur with retroperitoneal bleeding, the tracking of haemorrhagic fluid being:
1 Grey Turner sign (Turner sign)—tracks from the pararenal space to the edge of the quadratus lumborum muscle then through a defect in the fascia to the subcutaneous tissues of the flank (left sided in pancreatitis)
2 Cullen's sign—tracks into the falciparum ligament then through the connective tissues of the round ligament to the periumbilical area
3 Fox's sign—tracks along the fascia of the psoas and iliac muscles to the subcutaneous tissues of the upper thigh
4 Bryant's sign—tracks to the scrotum to produce the 'blue scrotum' sign.
Features of causative factors of pancreatitis may also be present, such as signs of alcohol abuse or hepatic cirrhosis, or xanthomas due to hypertriglyceridaemia.

Subcutaneous fat necrosis [1–7]

Synonym
• Nodular panniculitis

Systemic nodular fat necrosis is a rare condition that affects 2–3% of patients with pancreatic disease [6]. It may be associated with acute or chronic pancreatitis, post-traumatic pancreatitis or pancreatic carcinoma [1–3]. Pancreatitis accounts for about two-thirds and carcinoma one-third of reported cases [4]. Most of the reported pancreatic neoplasms are acinous adenocarcinoma, which is rare. Subcutaneous fat necrosis associated with acute pancreatitis in a newborn has been reported [5].

The mechanism of fat necrosis is not fully understood, but the condition is probably due to the effect of enzymes released from damaged pancreatic tissue. However, the condition does not simply relate to release of amylase or lipase from the pancreas. Not only is fat necrosis relatively uncommon in pancreatitis, but the eruption does not correlate with enzyme levels—it may occur in patients with normal lipase levels, or fail to occur in subjects with grossly elevated levels. Furthermore, incubation of skin with lipase or with patient's serum *in vitro* fails to demonstrate fat necrosis [4]. Thus, other enzymes are presumably involved.

Clinical features. Pancreatic nodular fat necrosis is accompanied by fever, abdominal pain (less common in those with underlying carcinoma), blood eosinophilia and synovitis of the small joints. Either the nodules or the arthralgia may predominate. Nodular lesions are usually 1–3 cm in diameter and tender or symptomless. The areas of predilection are the trunk and the lower extremities, especially the anterior shins, but lesions may occur anywhere. Lesions persist for 2–3 weeks and usually heal without scar formation, leaving slightly depressed, hyperpigmented spots. More severe changes due to periarticular fat necrosis may occur. Polyserositis may be part of the syndrome [7]. Increased serum amylase or lipase levels can be demonstrated in most cases, but may be normal in cases due to carcinoma.

Histopathology. There are foci of subcutaneous fat necrosis, with ghost cells and a surrounding inflammatory infiltrate of neutrophils and eosinophils. At the periphery of the lesion histiocytes, foam cells and foreign-body giant cells are seen. Secondary calcification may be observed in necrotic areas.

Migratory thrombophlebitis [1–3,8–11]

Pancreatic cancer is one of the classical associations with Trousseau's sign, in which multiple, migratory, superficial thromboses occur. Recent studies indicate that lung cancer is the most common associated neoplasm in men aged over 40 years, but pancreatic cancer is still an important cause; historically, pancreatic cancer accounts for about 25–30% of cases of migratory thrombophlebitis. Cancers elsewhere in the gastrointestinal tract may also cause this condition. The usual interval to diagnosis is about 4 months from onset, but pancreatic neoplasia may present later than this [9]. The phlebitis is distributed on the trunk, neck and extremities and is usually limited to a short segment of the vein. A significantly increased frequency of deep venous thrombosis is also found. The cause is unknown, but probably related to increased levels of clotting factors and disordered fibrinolysis, a form of disseminated intravascular coagulopathy. The combination of thrombotic change with haemorrhage (purpura fulminans) may also occur as a paraneoplastic phenomenon. Thrombotic change may coexist with other paraneoplastic features; it was demonstrated in the skin of a patient with malignancy-associated fasciitis due to a pancreatic carcinoma [11]. Other signs of pancreatic carcinoma include cutaneous metastasis; about 10% of cases of Sister Mary Joseph's nodule (metastasis to the umbilicus) are due to pancreatic carcinoma [2].

Other dermatological features of pancreatitis

The main dermatological features of acute and chronic pancreatitis have been described above, or are the result of malabsorption in the chronic disease (Chapter 59). Livedo reticularis has also been described in both acute and chronic pancreatitis as 'Walzel's sign' [12,13].

References

1 Sibrack LA, Gouterman IH. Cutaneous manifestations of pancreatic diseases. *Cutis* 1978; **21**: 763–8.
2 Greer KE, Jorizzo JL. Pancreatic disease. In: Callen JP, Jorrizo JL, eds. *Dermatological Signs of Internal Disease*, 3rd edn. Philadelphia: Saunders, 2003: 217–20.
3 Braverman IM. *Skin Signs of Systemic Disease*, 3rd edn. Philadelphia: Saunders, 1998.
4 Berman B, Conteas C, Smith B, Leong S, Hornbeck L 3rd. Fatal pancreatitis presenting with subcutaneous fat necrosis: evidence that lipase and amylase alone do not induce lipocyte necrosis. *J Am Acad Dermatol* 1987; **17**: 359–64.
5 Dawson TSJ, Slattery C. Subcutaneous fat necrosis of the newborn and acute pancreatitis. *Br J Dermatol* 1979; **101**: 359.
6 Fine RM. Subcutaneous fat necrosis, pancreatitis and arthropathy. *Int J Dermatol* 1983; **22**: 575–6.
7 Polts DE, Iseman MD. Syndrome of pancreatic disease, subcutaneous fat necrosis and polyserositis: case report and review of literature. *Am J Med* 1975; **58**: 417–23.
8 Sproul EE. Carcinoma and venous thrombosis: the frequency of association of carcinoma in the body or tail of the pancreas with multiple venous thrombosis. *Am J Cancer* 1938; **34**: 566.
9 Sack GH, Levin J, Bell WR. Trousseau's syndrome and other manifestations of chronic disseminated coagulopathy in patients with neoplasms: clinical, pathophysiologic, and therapeutic features. *Medicine* 1977; **56**: 1–37.
10 James WD. Trousseau's syndrome. *Int J Dermatol* 1984; **23**: 205–6.
11 Cox NH, Ramsay B, Dobson C, Comaish JS. Woody hands in a patient with pancreatic carcinoma: a variant of cancer-associated fasciitis–panniculitis syndrome. *Br J Dermatol* 1996; **135**: 995–8.
12 Sigmund WJ, Shelley WB. Cutaneous manifestations of acute pancreatitis, with special reference to livedo reticularis. *N Engl J Med* 1954; **251**: 851–3.
13 Gould JW, Helms SE, Schulz SM, Stevens SR. Relapsing livedo reticularis in the setting of chronic pancreatitis. *J Am Acad Dermatol* 1998; **39**: 1035–6.

Necrolytic migratory erythema, pancreatic islet cell tumours and glucagonoma syndrome [1–6]

Necrolytic migratory erythema

Aetiology. Necrolytic migratory erythema is a cutaneous reaction that occurs in the context of hyperglucagonaemia. The syndrome was described in 1941 [1] and there have been several subsequent reviews [2–7]. The same condition occurs in dogs and other animals. It is usually due to a glucagonoma, an α-cell tumour, which is usually in the tail of the pancreas [4,8], and which secretes excessive amounts of proglucagon-like material [7]. However, it may also occur due to other causes such as pancreatic insufficiency [9], intestinal causes of malabsorption [6,9,10], intestinal protein loss (for example, secondary to lymphatic disease—Waldmann's syndrome [11]), hepatic cirrhosis [12,13], and aberrant glucagon-secreting tumours such as bronchial or nasopharyngeal carcinoma [14,15]. It has also been documented as an iatrogenic condition after administration of glucagon [6] and in a heroin abuser [16]. MEN (discussed below) is associated with glucagonoma, which occurs in about 3% of cases and accounts for about 20% of glucagonomas.

Hyperglucagonaemia also causes diabetes; the 'diabetico-dermatogenic syndrome' occurs in almost 60% of patients with glucagonoma [4], but when only some of the features are present this may lead to delay in diagnosis. Glucagon production and metabolism are discussed in [7].

The pathogenetic mechanism of the skin eruption is not certain, but the condition is probably due to hypoaminoacidaemia caused by high glucagon levels [5] or by intestinal protein loss or malabsorption. There may be a contributory role of essential fatty acid and zinc deficiencies, but abnormal zinc levels or response to zinc supplementation are not consistent, and correction of amino acid levels does not reliably lead to resolution of the skin eruption [16]. It is characteristic that all skin changes disappear after complete surgical removal of the tumour in cases in which this is the cause [17].

Clinical features. The typical patient with glucagonoma is a woman 45–65 years of age. The usual features are weight loss (67%), anaemia (33%), glucose intolerance (56%) and necrolytic migratory erythema (72%) [8]. The rash is itchy or burning and particularly affects flexural sites on the lower abdomen, groin, buttocks and thighs (Fig. 62.22). It is initially macular, extending to form superficially eroding areas of erythema that progress to fragile vesicle and bullae formation. Irregular centrifugal extension of the annular lesions causes a marginated, often crusted, polycyclic or geographical pattern. It has a prolonged, fluctuating course or cyclical pattern; the central part heals over 7–14 days, leaving postinflammatory pigmentation, while the erythematous periphery becomes crusted. Perianal and genital lesions are common. Angular cheilitis and a painful, beefy-coloured glossitis occur in about one-third of patients with glucagonoma [8].

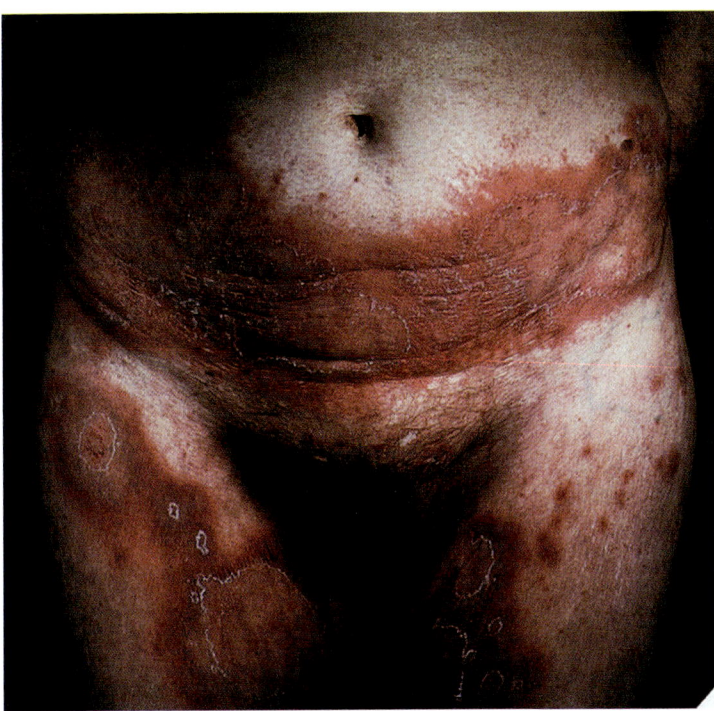

Fig. 62.22 Glucagonoma syndrome. (Courtesy of Dr Kristian Thomsen, Finsen Institute, Copenhagen, Denmark.)

The clinical spectrum also includes diarrhoea (20%), weakness, venous thromboses (10%) and psychiatric disturbances. The plasma glucagon level is generally elevated several-fold above the upper limit of the normal range, but may show only minor elevation. The systemic features, such as weight loss, anaemia and hypoaminoacidaemia, are all more frequent in patients with glucagonoma with the diabetico-dermatogenic syndrome than in those without [4]. The same pattern of eruption has been described due to zinc deficiency with normal glucagon levels, usually in the context of liver disease.

Histopathology [2,3]. Biopsy should be taken from the edge of early lesions. The characteristic histological feature is well-demarcated necrolysis of the outer cell layers in the Malpighian stratum. Early lesions may present as a 'dyskeratotic dermatitis' with superficial perivascular inflammation in the dermis, and minor spongiosis and dyskeratotic or vacuolated epidermal cells [3,18]. Clefts and separation occur, associated with necrotic keratinocytes and cellular debris surrounding the cleft. In the dermis, a mild perivascular lymphocytic and histiocytic infiltrate is seen. Older lesions show various degrees of dyskeratosis, acanthosis and a lymphocytic infiltrate in the dermis. The histological changes are similar to those observed in acute zinc deficiency, in which cell degeneration and the formation of clefts and vesicles are predominant at the level of the basal cells.

Diagnosis. Pancreatic and hepatic scans and arteriography are helpful in locating a primary pancreatic tumour and its metastases if present. Serum amino acid, glucose, zinc and plasma glucagon levels should be determined. In cases with an elevated plasma glucagon level and a clinical and histological picture suggestive of the disease, surgical exploration should be performed.

Treatment. Where there is a glucagonoma, surgical resection is indicated, with embolization of hepatic metastases, which are present in the majority at the time of diagnosis. Various forms of chemotherapy have been used [2,5,19–21], such as streptozocin (a nitrosourea compound used for the ablation of β-cell adenoma) with 5-fluorouracil. Somatostatin is an inhibitor of glucagons but has a half life of just a few minutes, so analogues such as lanreotide, which is active for up to 2 weeks after intramuscular injection, are used therapeutically. Octreotide, a somatostatin analogue, rapidly improves symptoms, especially the rash, by altering glucagon metabolism, but it does not influence tumour growth [7,21]; dacarbazine is also useful [22]. Parenteral amino-acid infusions and correction of any essential fatty acid deficiency may be helpful [19], although the benefit of amino-acid infusions does not appear to be sustained long term [17]. In the rare cases related to malabsorption, correction of this (for example, GFD in coeliac disease) is usually effective [4,10].

Other non-insulin-secreting pancreatic endocrine tumours

Although glucagonoma is more important dermatologically, the most common islet cell tumours are insulinoma of β-cells and gastrinoma of δ-cells (Zollinger–Ellison syndrome, ZES). These do not have specific skin changes, but they may occur together with other tumours that secrete ACTH, MSH and serotonin; severe diarrhoea in ZES may cause secondary hypovitaminosis and other nutritional deficiencies, giving rise to skin and hair changes. Both of these tumours occur sporadically or as part of the autosomal-dominant MEN type 1 syndrome (Wermer syndrome, MIM *131100), which is due to a mutation in the *MEN1* gene on chromosome 11q13. In this condition, as well as the endocrine tumours, other cutaneous features include angiofibromas, collagenomas, café-au-lait macules, lipomas and gingival macules [21]. MEN1 was associated with 13% of glucagonomas in one large series [4], and glucagonoma has also been reported in MEN2.

Tumours that produce vasoactive intestinal polypeptide (VIPomas) cause flushing (discussed in Chapter 43) with watery diarrhoea, hypokalaemia and achlorhydria [23]. A macular rash that resolved after tumour resection was reported in a patient with a pancreatic polypeptide-producing tumour of the pancreas (PPoma) [24].

References

1 Becker SW, Kahn D, Rothman S. Cutaneous manifestations of internal malignant tumors. *Arch Dermatol Syphilol* 1941; **45**: 1069–80.

2 Guillausseau PJ, Villet R, Kalloustian E *et al.* Les glucagonomes. Aspects cliniques, biologiques, anatomopathologiques et thérapeutiques (revue générale de 130 cas). *Gastroenterol Clin Biol* 1982; **6**: 1029–41.

3 Hashizumet T, Kiryu H, Noda K *et al.* Glucagonoma syndrome. *J Am Acad Dermatol* 1988; **19**: 377–83.

4 Soga J, Yakuwa Y. Glucagonomas/diabetico-dermatogenic syndrome (DDS): a statistical evaluation of 407 reported cases. *J Hepatobiliary Pancreat Surg* 1998; **5**: 312–9.

5 Chastain MA. The glucagonoma syndrome: a review of its features and discussion of new perspectives. *Am J Med Sci* 2001; **321**: 306–20.

6 Mullens EA, Cohen PR. Iatrogenic necrolytic migratory erythema: a case report and review of nonglucagonoma-associated necrolytic migratory erythema. *J Am Acad Dermatol* 1998; **38**: 866–73.

7 van Beek AP, de Haas ERM, van Vloten WA *et al.* The glucagonoma syndrome and necrolytic migratory erythema: a clinical review. *Eur J Endocrinol* 2004; **151**: 531–7.

8 Frankton S, Bloom SR. Glucagonomas. *Baillière's Clin Gastroenterol* 1996; **10**: 697–705.

9 Thorisdottir K, Camisa C, Tomecki KJ, Bergfeld WF. Necrolytic migratory erythema: a report of three cases. *J Am Acad Dermatol* 1994; **30**: 324–9.

10 Goodenberger DM, Lawley TJ, Strober W *et al.* Necrolytic migratory erythema without glucagonoma: a report of two cases. *Arch Dermatol* 1979; **115**: 1429–32.

11 Bancault S, Soubrane JC, Courville P *et al.* Necrolytic migratory erythema in Waldmann's disease. *Ann Dermatol Venereol* 2006; **133**: 693–6.

12 Doyle JA, Schroeter AL, Rogers RS III. Hyperglucagonaemia and necrolytic migratory erythema in cirrhosis: possible pseudoglucagonoma syndrome. *Br J Dermatol* 1979; **101**: 581–7.

13 Blackford S, Wright S, Roberts DL. Necrolytic migratory erythema without glucagonoma: the role of dietary essential fatty acids. *Br J Dermatol* 1991; **125**: 460–2.

14 Hunstein W, Trumper LH, Dummer R *et al.* Glucagonoma syndrome and bronchial carcinoma. *Ann Intern Med* 1988; **109**: 920–1.

15 Mohrenschlager M, Kohler LD, Bruckbauer H *et al.* Squamous epithelial carcinoma-associated necrolytic migratory erythema. *Hautarzt* 1999; **50**: 198–202.

16 Bencini PL, Vigo GP, Caputo R. Necrolytic migratory erythema without glucagonoma in a heroin-dependent patient. *Dermatology* 1994; **189**: 72–4.

17 Abraira C, DeBartolo M, Katzen R, Lawrence AM. Disappearance of glucagonoma rash after surgical resection but not during dietary normalization of serum amino acids. *Am J Clin Nutr* 1984; **39**: 351–5.

18 Hunt SJ, Narus VT, Abell E. Necrolytic migratory erythema: dyskeratotic dermatitis, a clue to early diagnosis. *J Am Acad Dermatol* 1991; **24**: 473–7.

19 Bewley AP, Ross JS, Bunker CB, Staughton RCD. Successful treatment of a patient with octreotide-resistant necrolytic migratory erythema. *Br J Dermatol* 1996; **134**: 1101–4.

20 Jockenhovel F, Lederbogen S, Olbricht T *et al.* The long-acting somatostatin analogue octreotide alleviates symptoms by reducing posttranslational conver-sion of prepro-glucagon to glucagon in a patient with malignant glucagonoma, but does not prevent tumour growth. *Clin Invest* 1994; **72**: 127–33.

21 Loos van der TLJM, Lambrecht ER, Lambers ICCA. Successful treatment of glucagonoma related necrolytic migratory erythema with dacarbazine. *J Am Acad Dermatol* 1987; **16**: 468–72.

22 Darling TN, Skarulis MC, Steinberg SM *et al.* Multiple facial angiofibromas and collagenomas in patients with multiple endocrine neoplasia type 1. *Arch Dermatol* 1997; **133**: 853–7.

23 Park SK, O'Dorisio MS, O'Dorisio TM. Vasoactive intestinal polypeptide-secreting tumours: biology and therapy. *Baillière's Clin Gastroenterol* 1996; **10**: 673–96.

24 Choski UA, Sellin RV, Hickey RC *et al.* An unusual skin rash associated with a pancreatic polypeptide-producing tumor of the pancreas. *Ann Intern Med* 1988; **108**: 64–5.

Renal disease [1–4]

The skin and renal systems may be affected not uncommonly by the same disease processes. The more important of these renocutaneous syndromes are listed in Table 62.14.

Hereditary syndromes and malformations

Angiokeratoma corporis diffusum (Fabry's disease; MIM *301500; Chapter 59). Affected individuals often show proteinuria, microscopic haematuria and lipiduria. Renal disease eventually develops in most male patients, and as lipid deposition in the form of glycosphingolipids occurs, renal function deteriorates. The premature mortality in the condition is often a result of renal failure. Renal transplantation can supply a source of the deficient enzyme lysosomal hydrolase, α-galactosidase A, and results in an improvement in the condition; commercial preparations of this enzyme are

Table 62.14 Renocutaneous syndromes.

Hereditary syndromes
Angiokeratoma corporis diffusum
Neurofibromatosis
Tuberous sclerosis
Nail–patella syndrome
Birt–Hogge–Dubé syndrome
Sickle cell disease
Pseudoxanthoma elasticum
Oral–facial–digital syndrome
von Hippel–Lindau disease
Hereditary haemorrhagic telangiectasia

Metabolic disorders
Primary systemic amyloidosis
Calcinosis

Inflammatory and miscellaneous
Allergic vasculitis
Systemic lupus erythematosus
Polyarteritis nodosa
Scleroderma
Nephrogenic fibrosing dermopathy (nephrogenic systemic fibrosis)
Wegener's granulomatosis
Erythema multiforme
Anaphylactoid purpura
Drug-induced toxic epidermal necrolysis

also now available (see Chapter 59). Other enzyme defects may give rise to the same clinical phenotype.

Neurofibromatosis (NF1, MIM *162200; NF2, MIM *101000; von Recklinghausen's disease) (Chapter 15). Urinary outflow obstruction may develop secondary to an impinging neurofibroma. Vascular lesions can result in renal artery thrombosis and subsequent hypertension. In patients with hypertension, normal plasma and urine catecholamine levels—especially those under the age of 20 years—renal artery stenosis should be suspected [5]. Raised blood pressure may also develop as a result of an associated phaeochromocytoma. Causes of hypertension in neurofibromatosis should be fully investigated [5]. Nephroblastoma is a recognized association in neurofibromatosis [6] and renal polycystic disease.

Tuberous sclerosis complex (TSC1, MIM #191100; TSC2, MIM *191092; Bourneville's disease; Chapter 15). An increased incidence of rhabdomyomas and carcinoma may occur in this condition [7]. Malignant renal tumours may include renal cell carcinoma, malignant angiomyolipoma and Wilms' tumour [8]. The classical renal lesion associated with tuberous sclerosis is an angiomyolipoma. Renal cysts also occur in conjunction with these, or as isolated findings [9].

Nail–patella syndrome (Fong's syndrome; hereditary osteo-onychodysplasia; MIM #161200; Chapters 15, 65). The defective gene *LMX1B* is located on the long arm of chromosome 9 (9q34.1); this gene regulates type IV and VI collagen expression, which in turn affects skeletal and basement membrane structure and function [10]. *LMXIB* is expressed in the kidney, primarily in podocytes, and regulates many crucial podocyte proteins. Renal dysplasia presenting as chronic glomerulonephritis occurs in some cases, and characteristic electron-microscopic glomerular abnormalities are present in most cases of nail–patella syndrome. The ultrastructural features consist of thickening and splitting of the glomerular basement membrane and fibrillar α3(IV) and α4(IV) collagen deposits. Renal lesions are asymptomatic; patients show proteinuria, haematuria and reduced creatinine clearance. Although there is often a progressive course to renal failure, many patients with the complication do surprisingly well. Helpful diagnostic signs include small, defective nails that do not reach the free nail border, triangular lunulae, the thumbnails being the most frequently and severely affected nails and the severity of the defect reducing from the index to little finger nails. There is absence of the skin creases on the dorsal interphalyngeal joints [11]. The patellae are less well developed, potentially giving stability problems for the knee and there is instability of the radial head; other indicators include (radiologically) posterior iliac horns and (ophthalmically) irregular hyperpigmented pupillary borders. There is a tendency to glaucoma.

Birt–Hogge–Dubé syndrome (BHD; Hornstein–Knickenberg syndrome; MIM #135150). Hereditary renal cell cancer syndromes include BHD, von Hippel–Lindau disease, as well as hereditary papillary renal cell carcinoma, familial oncocytoma and hereditary renal cell carcinoma of various types [12].

The cutaneous features of BHD include trichofolliculomas, trichidiscomas and skin tags. Pulmonary cysts, predominantly basilar, may cause spontaneous pneumothorax. A variety of coding sequence mutations have been linked to the 17p11.2 chromosome [12].

Hereditary leiomyomatosis and renal cell carcinoma (HLRCC) syndrome (MIM #605839). Multiple cutaneous leiomyomas, which have an inherited predisposition, are linked to uterine leiomyoma (Reed syndrome, MIM #150800) and also appear to be associated with an increased incidence of renal cell carcinoma, usually aggressive and of papillary cell type. Numerous different fumarate hydratase mutations have been identified, but the patients who have renal cell carcinomas associated (only 2% in one series) are more likely to have truncating or frameshift mutations and be female [13]; see also the section 'Cutaneous markers of internal malignancy' above, p. 62.29.

Multiple hamartoma and neoplasia syndrome (Cowden's disease; MIM #158350). This is associated with an increased incidence of renal cell carcinoma, liposarcoma and transitional cell carcinoma of the bladder [8]. It is discussed earlier in this chapter.

von Hippel–Lindau syndrome (VHL; MIM *193300; see earlier in this chapter and Chapter 15). Renal lesions in VHL are either simple cysts or adenocarcinomas; usually they are a late manifestation. Renal carcinoma may present with cutaneous metastases several years in advance of the systemic malignancy; alternatively, cutaneous deposits may indicate a recurrence of previously treated neoplasia [3]. von Hippel–Lindau syndrome represents one of the hereditary kidney cancer syndromes in which a two-hit model of tumour genesis occurs, explaining the often late development of this complication.

The other tumours linked to VHL are dealt with in Chapter 15, but phaeochromocytomas and pancreatic tumours can occur with increased frequency in close anatomical association with each other.

Familial Mediterranean fever with urticaria (FMFU), Muckle–Wells syndrome (MWS) and tumour necrosis receptor associated periodic syndrome (TRAPS) [14,15]. These 'autoinflammatory syndromes' are all associated with a significant risk of renal failure secondary to amyloidosis, frequently resulting in premature death (see also later in this chapter).

Oral–facial–digital syndrome [16]. Oral–facial–digital syndrome type I (OFD1) is characterized by the following abnormalities: oral (lobed tongue, hamartomas or lipomas of the tongue, cleft of the hard or soft palate, accessory gingival frenulae, hypodontia and other dental abnormalities); facial (ocular hypertelorism or telecanthus, hypoplasia of the alae nasi, median cleft or pseudocleft upper lip, micrognathia); digital (brachydactyly, syndactyly of varying degrees, and clinodactyly of the fifth finger; duplicated hallux [great toe]; preaxial or postaxial polydactyly of the hands) and brain (intracerebral cysts, corpus callosum agenesis, cerebellar agenesis with or without Dandy–Walker malformation). Polycystic disease of the kidneys and liver occurs commonly in this condition. As many as 50% of individuals with OFD1 have some degree of mental retardation, which is usually mild. Almost all affected individuals are female. However, males with OFD1 have been described, mostly as malformed fetuses born to women with OFD1.

References

1 Gupta AK, Gupta MA, Cardella CJ *et al.* Cutaneous associations of chronic renal failure and dialysis. *Int J Dermatol* 1986; **25**: 498–504.

2 Dymock RB. Skin disease associated with renal transplantation. *Australas J Dermatol* 1979; **20**: 61–7.

3 Christianson HB, Birchall R. Nephrocutaneous syndromes. *South Med J* 1964; **57**: 1043–50.

4 Callen JP. Cutaneous nephrology. In: Callen JP, Jorizzo JL, eds. *Dermatological Signs of Internal Disease*, 3rd edn. Philadelphia: Saunders, 2003: 271–4.

5 Riccardi VM. *Neurofibromatosis: Phenotype, Natural History, and Pathogenesis*, 2nd edn. Baltimore: Johns Hopkins University Press, 1992.

6 Stay EJ, Vawter G. The relationship between nephroblastoma and neurofibromatosis (von Recklinghausen's disease). *Cancer* 1977; **39**: 2550–5.

7 Lynne CM, Carrion HM, Bakshandeh K *et al.* Renal angiomyolipoma, polycystic kidney and renal cell carcinoma in patients with tuberous sclerosis. *Urology* 1979; **14**: 174–6.

8 Tsao H. Update on familial cancer syndromes and the skin. *J Am Acad Dermatol* 2000; **42**: 939–69.

9 Stillwell TJ, Gomez MR, Kelalis PP. Renal lesions in tuberous sclerosis. *J Urol* 1987; **138**: 477–81.

10 Stratigos AJ, Baden HP. Unraveling the molecular mechanisms of hair and nail genodermatoses. *Arch Dermatol* 2001; **137**: 1465–71.

11 Itin PH, Eich G, Fistarol SK. Missing creases of distal finger joints as a diagnostic clue of nail-patella syndrome. *Dermatology* 2006; **213**: 153–5.

12 Choyke PL, Sharma N, Peterson J *et al.* Germline BHD-mutation spectrum and phenotype analysis of a large cohort of families with Birt-Hogg-Dube syndrome. *Am J Hum Genet* 2005; **76**: 1023–33.

13 Alam NA, Olpin S, Leigh IM. Fumarate hydratase mutations and predisposition to cutaneous leiomyomas, uterine leiomyomas and renal cancer. *Br J Dermatol* 2005; **153**: 11–7.

14 Ozen S, Hoffman HM, Frenkel J, Kastner D. Familial Mediterranean fever (FMF) and beyond: a new horizon. Fourth International Congress on the Systemic Autoinflammatory Diseases held in Bethesda, USA, 6–10 November 2005. *Ann Rheum Dis* 2006; **65**: 961–4.

15 Dinc A, Erdem H, Rowczenio D *et al.* Autosomal dominant periodic fever with AA amyloidosis: tumor necrosis factor receptor-associated periodic syndrome (TRAPS) in a Turkish family. *J Nephrol* 2000; **18**: 626–9.

16 Thauvin-Robinet C, Cossée M, Cormier-Daire V *et al.* Clinical, molecular, and genotype-phenotype correlation studies from 25 cases of oral-facial-digital syndrome type 1: a French and Belgian collaborative study. *J Med Genet* 2006; **43**: 54–61.

Metabolic and systemic disorders

Partial lipodystrophy

Renal disorders occur frequently in this condition (25%), usually as a membranoproliferative glomerulonephritis; subsequent renal failure is common at an early age. There is a circulating C3 nephritic factor and reduced levels of complement (C3) [1]. An association with hereditary angio-oedema (C1 inhibitor deficiency) has been reported [2].

Primary and myeloma-associated systemic amyloidosis
(Chapter 59)

Up to 40% of patients have waxy, purpuric cutaneous or mucosal changes, periocular lesions are the most recognizable [3] and diagnostically useful. Typically, patients may also have macroglossia,

hepatomegaly, oedema and carpal tunnel syndrome. Cutis laxa-like clinical changes have also been reported [4]. Without dialysis, renal failure is often fulminant and fatal; peritoneal dialysis may be the most appropriate approach. Although renal amyloid may recur after transplantation, this is not completely contraindicated [5]. Primary cutaneous amyloid does not appear to have renal associations. Nodular or tumid amyloidosis was said to represent an early phase of systemic amyloid, but recent studies have reported only a 7% progression to systemic disease after long follow up [6].

Calcification and calcific uraemic arteriolopathy (calciphylaxis) (see also Chapter 49)

Calcifying panniculitis has been reported occasionally in renal failure, a disorder now termed calcific uraemic arteriolopathy [7–9]. It is usually, but not invariably, associated with a high serum calcium phosphate product. Metastatic skin calcification is a rare phenomenon in uraemic patients; it usually presents as papular or nodular cutaneous lesions around large joints or flexural sites. Non-cutaneous metastatic calcification is, by comparison, much commoner. Metastatic calcification in blood vessel walls associated with hyperparathyroidism and renal failure (calcific uraemic vasculopathy, calciphlaxis) may lead to cutaneous necrosis or gangrene as a result of thrombosed vessels (Fig. 62.23); however, calcification does not always need to be present, and vascular damage may be triggering a premature haemostatic cascade. This carries a poor prognosis, in one series, only 40% of patients survived a year after diagnosis. Risk factors included obesity, liver disease, systemic steroid use, and a high calcium phosphate product and high serum aluminium [9]. Treatments include low phosphate dialysate fluids, non-calcium phosphate binders, parathyroidectomy, and more recently drugs such as sodium thiosulphate or cinacalcet which alter calcium metabolism.

References

1 Misra A, Peethambaram A, Garg A. Clinical features and metabolic and autoimmune derangements in acquired partial lipodystrophy: report of 35 cases and review of the literature. *Medicine (Baltimore)* 2004; **83**: 18–34.

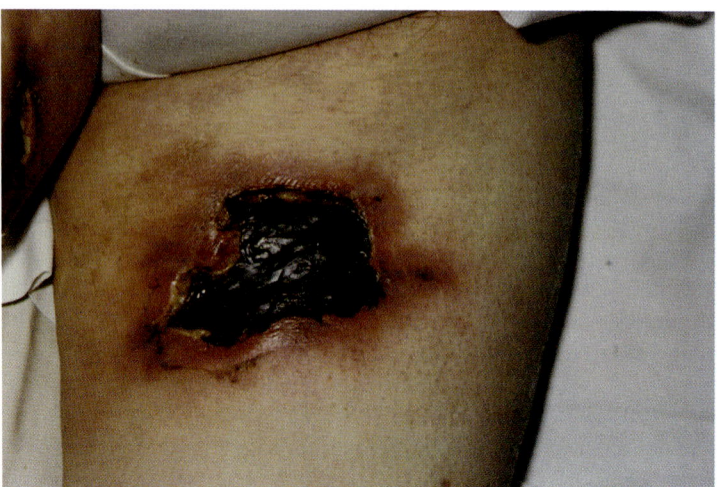

Fig. 62.23 Calcific uraemic arteriolopathy of the thighs in a patient with renal failure. (Courtesy of Dr C. Owen, Royal Blackburn Hospital, Lancashire.)

2 Frank MM, Gelfand JA, Atkinson JP. Hereditary angio-edema: the clinical syndrome and its management. *Ann Intern Med* 1976; **84**: 580–93.

3 Breathnach SM. Amyloid and amyloidosis. *J Am Acad Dermatol* 1988; **18**: 1–16.

4 Newton JA, McKee PH, Black MM. Cutis laxa associated with amyloidosis. *Clin Exp Dermatol* 1986; **11**: 87–91.

5 Wong CK. Cutaneous amyloidoses. *Int J Dermatol* 1987; **26**: 273–7.

6 Woollons A, Black MM. Nodular localized primary cutaneous amyloidosis: a long-term follow-up study. *Br J Dermatol* 2001; **145**: 105–9.

7 Laurent R, Thiery F, Saint-Hillier Y *et al*. Panniculite calcificante associée à une insuffisance rénale: un syndrome de calciphylaxie tissulaire. *Ann Dermatol Vénéréol* 1987; **14**: 1073–81.

8 Richens G, Piepkorn MW, Krueger GG. Calcifying panniculitis associated with renal failure. *J Am Acad Dermatol* 1982; **6**: 537–9.

9 Weenig RH, Sewell LD, Davis MD *et al*. Calciphylaxis: natural history, risk factor analysis, and outcome. *J Am Acad Dermatol* 2007; **56**: 569–79.

Sarcoidosis and the kidney [1,2]

Nephrolithiasis and nephrocalcinosis occur in patients with sarcoidosis with a 20% higher frequency than in the normal population. Hypercalcaemia which occurs in sarcoidosis may cause polyuria and polydipsia, and may even precipitate acute renal failure. Renal sarcoidosis can give rise to diffuse interstitial nephritis, but it is seldom that there are identifiable granulomas or direct renal involvement. Rarely, cases of outflow obstruction from retroperitoneal sarcoidal masses and sarcoid of the urethra have been reported [3].

References

1 English JC 3rd, Patel PJ, Greer KE. Sarcoidosis. *J Am Acad Dermatol* 2001; **44**: 725–43.

2 Berliner AR, Haas M, Choi MJ. Sarcoidosis: the nephrologist's perspective. *Am J Kidney Dis* 2006; **48**: 856–70.

3 Carr LK, Honey RJ, Sugar L. Diagnosis and management of urethral sarcoidosis. *J Urol* 1995; **153**: 1612–3.

Vasculitis (Chapter 50)

Renal involvement commonly occurs in various types of vasculitis that present with cutaneous changes and is the main cause of mortality in many of these syndromes. This should be considered particularly in classical Henoch–Schönlein purpura (anaphylactoid purpura), especially in adults, where IgA nephropathy has become recognized as a fairly common form of glomerulonephritis [1]. An association between anaphylactoid purpura and familial IgA nephropathy has also been described [2]. Patients labelled as having allergic vasculitis and arteritis with livedo reticularis [3] should also be regarded as being at risk of kidney damage.

Renal failure is a recognized, but rare, complication of Behçet's syndrome, usually with immune-complex deposition [4]. Concomitant or delayed renal involvement is common in Wegener's granulomatosis, usually as a focal necrotizing glomerulitis. Deposits of IgM and IgG are present in renal vessels and circulating immune complexes are also frequently detected [5]. Renal changes that occur in these conditions, and in collagen vascular disorders such as polyarteritis nodosa, systemic lupus erythematosus and scleroderma, are considered in Chapters 50 and 51.

References

1 Saulsbury FT. Clinical update: Henoch-Schönlein purpura. *Lancet* 2007; **24**; 369, 976–8.

2 Miyagawa S, Dohi K, Hanatani M *et al*. Anaphylactoid purpura and familial IgA nephropathy. *Am J Med* 1989; **86**: 340–2.

3 Cream JS, Gumpel JM, Peachy RD. Schönlein–Henoch purpura in the adult: a study of 77 adults with anaphylactoid or Schönlein–Henoch purpura. *QJM* 1970; **39**: 461–84.

4 Wilkey D, Yocum DE, Oberley TD *et al*. Budd–Chiari syndrome and renal failure in Behçet disease. *Am J Med* 1983; **75**: 541–50.

5 Aasarød K, Iversen BM, Hammerstrøm J *et al*. Wegener's granulomatosis: clinical course in 108 patients with renal involvement. *Nephrol Dial Transplant* 2000; **15**: 611–8.

Renal disease in bullous disorders

Bullous pemphigoid. Renal disease, including membranous glomerulopathy, diffuse proliferative and mesangioproliferative glomerulonephritis, has been infrequently reported in patients with pemphigoid [1].

Toxic epidermal necrolysis (TEN) [2]. Deteriorating renal function is a poor prognostic factor in TEN, and is one of the parameters used in the SCORTEN prognostic score.

Epidermolysis bullosa (EB). Renal failure was the second most common cause of death (with a mean age of 35) in 12% of adults with recessive dystrophic EB of the Hallepeau–Siemens type [3]. It was surpassed as a cause of death only by metastatic squamous cell carcinoma. Renal failure due to IgA nephropathy, and post-infectious membranoproliferative glomerulonephritis, has complicated recessive dystrophic EB. Obstructive uropathy has been seen in junctional EB. Surveillance for early renal involvement should become part of the routine evaluation of all adults with RDEB and JEB [4].

References

1 Ross EA, Ahmed AR. Bullous pemphigoid-associated nephropathy: report of two cases and review of the literature. *Am J Kidney Dis* 1989; **14**: 225–9.

2 Blum L, Chosidow O, Rostoker G *et al*. Renal involvement in toxic epidermal necrolysis. *J Am Acad Dermatol* 1996; **34**: 1088–90.

3 Fine JD, Johnson LB, Weiner M *et al*. National Epidermolysis Bullosa Registry. Inherited epidermolysis bullosa and the risk of death from renal disease: experience of the National Epidermolysis Bullosa Registry. *Am J Kidney Dis* 2004; **44**: 651–60.

4 Chan SM, Dillon MJ, Duffy PG, Atherton DJ. Nephro-urological complications of epidermolysis bullosa in paediatric patients. *Br J Dermatol* 2007; **156**: 143–7.

Infective dermatoses causing renal disease

Streptococcal impetigo. An acknowledged cause of acute glomerulonephritis, particularly when streptococcal infection occurs secondary to scabies [1], but most cases of acute nephritis are not the sequel of streptococcal infection.

Secondary syphilis. A rare cause of the nephrotic syndrome.

Herpes zoster. If affecting the appropriate dermatomes, herpes zoster cause neurogenic bladder dysfunction and pain [2], leading to acute urinary retention.

References

1 Svartman M, Potter EV, Poon-King T, Earle DP. Streptococcal infection of scabetic lesions related to acute glomerulonephritis in Trinidad. *J Lab Clin Med* 1973; **81**: 182–93.

2 Izumi AK, Edwards J Jr. Herpes zoster with neurogenic bladder dysfunction. *Arch Dermatol* 1974; **109**: 692–4.

Renal failure and dialysis [1–3]

Cutaneous signs of renal failure are mainly related to chronicity of disease. Urea frosting, in which crystalline urea is deposited on the skin, is now very rare, but dry, pigmented skin with excoriations is typical.

Uraemic patients tend to have a dry skin, sometimes with fine scaling. A reduction in the size of eccrine sweat glands in uraemia may contribute to this effect [4], although high-dose diuretic regimens are a co-factor [5].

Pigmentation. Anaemia presenting as pallor is an early and common sign in renal failure, resulting from reduced erythropoiesis and increased haemolysis.

A muddy brown hyperpigmentation develops in many cases, attributed to retention of chromogens and deposition of melanin, possibly due to impaired renal processing of melanocyte-stimulating hormone [6]. Increased nail pigmentation, usually confined to the distal aspect, occurs in a proportion of patients [7]. This distal brown or more normal red colour, combined with a proximal white appearance gives rise to the 'half-and-half' nails, a distinctive pattern seen in about 10% of patients with renal failure [8].

Purpura due to a mild thrombocytopenia or more marked platelet dysfunction is common and may be partly corrected by dialysis [9]. Wound healing is prolonged and patients may be more susceptible to pressure sores.

Pruritus. Generalized, severe pruritus occurs in about one-third of renal failure cases, less troublesome involvement occurs in many more. Unfortunately, haemodialysis can initiate the symptom as well as improve it. Up to 85% of patients on haemodialysis suffered from itching in one study [10], one-third before dialysis, the others after; 12% had reduced pruritus after 6 months' dialysis. There seems to be an association with predialysis blood urea levels, and a less clear correlation with dry skin and secondary hyperparathyroidism [11]. Subtotal parathyroidectomy may be very helpful [12], but the problem can subsequently recur, and many cases are not related to secondary hyperparathyroidism. Moreover, many patients with this finding do not itch. A complete explanation for pruritus in renal failure is obscure, as pruritus is unusual in acute renal failure and a reduction in uraemia often does not improve the symptom. Slowly accumulated or deposited pruritogen(s), of as yet uncertain nature, are the likely cause. In dialysis, lowering the magnesium concentration of the dialysate has been reported as helpful [13]. In intractable itching, UVB radiation is an effective therapy [14], benefit being associated with a reduction of skin phosphorus to normal values. Ultraviolet A (without psoralen) has been reported nearly as effective [15]; oral cholestyramine and activated charcoal are alternatives [16,17]. Erythropoietin therapy can alleviate pruritus in some cases of renal failure. Naltrexone (and other opioids such as nalmefene) and odansetron have also been reported to help uraemic pruritus [11]. Gabapentin has recently been demonstrated to be effective in uraemic pruritus [18].

Perforating disorders. A perforating disorder variously described as acquired reactive perforating collagenosis, Kyrle's disease or perforating folliculitis occurs in renal failure; often there is diabe-

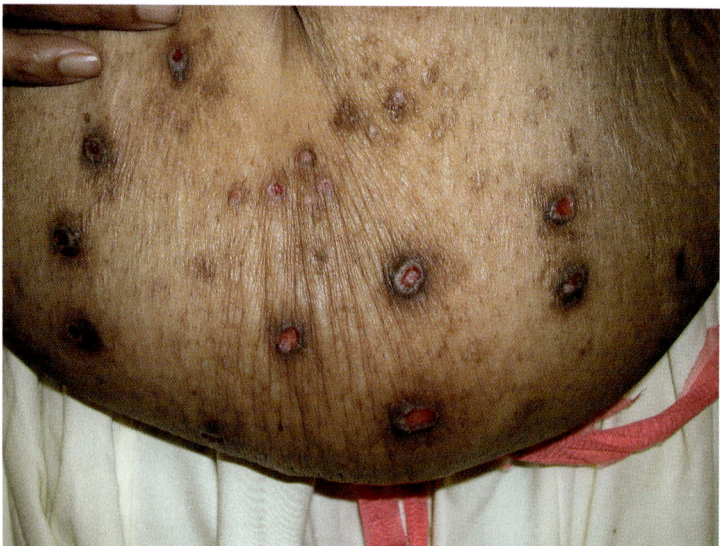

Fig. 62.24 Reactive perforating collagenosis in end-stage renal failure.

tes, diabetic nephropathy and/or retinopathy. Pruritus is nearly always present, and up to 10% of dialysis patients may be affected. The condition seems to have a higher incidence in Afro-Caribbeans. The cutaneous lesions consist of hyperpigmented papules up to 1 cm in diameter with a central keratinous plug (Fig. 62.24). The extensor surfaces of the limbs are more commonly affected but the trunk and face may be involved. The pathogenesis is uncertain, but there is some histological evidence that it is a perforating collagenosis [19,20].

Other cutaneous features. Uraemic neuropathy affects some 60% of patients with renal failure or on long-term haemodialysis. This appears to be a predominantly sensorimotor neuropathy [20].

Up to 40% of patients with renal failure may develop gynaecomastia while receiving dialysis [21]. Calcinosis cutis may occur in 1% of patients with end-stage renal disease [22]. It may be reversed by a low phosphorus diet and aluminium hydroxide gel.

Features related to treatment. Premature ageing of the skin and actinic keratoses have been described, a reason for avoiding excessive ultraviolet therapy for pruritus. This should be distinguished from the numerous viral, dysplastic and frankly malignant skin lesions which may develop in immunosuppressed renal allograft recipients.

Cutaneous complications affecting the limb of patients in which their haemodialysis arteriovenous shunt is situated include infection, phlebitis and haematoma. However, both irritant and allergic contact eczema may also develop [23]. Vascular complications of arteriovenous fistula construction are relatively uncommon, but include digital ischaemia and aneurysm formation. The venous hypertension syndrome with or without ulceration may occur; pseudo-Kaposi's sarcoma [24], and pyoderma gangrenosum [25], are both rare developments.

Bullous eruptions mimicking PCT (pseudoporphyria of haemodialysis) are well recognized, with an incidence reported at between 2 and 18%. True porphyria cutanea tarda due to deficiency of uroporphyrin decarboxylase is reported but uncommon. Distinguishing these two conditions can be difficult as many patients on haemodialysis have elevated blood porphyrin levels slightly above what is regarded as the normal range due to their reduced excretion; the importance of accurate assays is emphasized [26,27]. Photosensitizing drugs such as furosemide, oestrogens and non-steroidal anti-inflammatory agents may also induce a pseudoporphyria picture. In all cases, UV protection is important. N-acetylcysteine, which acts as an antioxidant, may help reduce the blistering [28]. Treatment of true PCT in patients with end-stage renal failure is limited as antimalarials work by binding porphyrins and renal excretion of the complexes formed (which will not occur in many patients with renal failure, as the complexes will not be excreted by anuric subjects and will not cross dialysis membranes), and venesection is limited by anaemia; treatment with erythropoietin to increase conversion of porphyrin to haem is the usual approach.

Nephrogenic systemic fibrosis. A condition termed nephrogenic fibrosing dermopathy, or, more recently, nephrogenic systemic fibrosis, was initially linked with haemodialysis but occurs in other patients with renal failure [29–31]. Clinical features include indurated plaques, sometimes with finger-like projections, that may be erythematous, yellowish or skin-coloured. Nodules and contractures occur in more advanced disease. Scleral plaques may also occur, although the face is usually spared (by contrast with scleromyxoedema). There may be internal organ involvement (hence the more modern term nephrogenic systemic fibrosis), and death and severe disability can ensue. Involvement of the diaphragm is frequently the event that leads to death and 10% of patients have a fulminant course. Histology shows increased mucin deposition and spindle cells and compact collagen bundles. There has been a strong association with the use of radio-contrast agents that contain gadolinium, such as gadodiamide, which are used to enhance magnetic resonance imaging of vessels [32,33]. Such contrast media are now not recommended for use in patients with a GFR less than 30 ml/min [32,33] as they are renally excreted and have a tissue half-life about 10-fold longer in those with severe renal impairment compared to normal subjects. The resulting prolonged high tissue levels may be pro-fibrotic. A recent study using quantitative scanning electron microscopy/energy-dispersive X-ray spectroscopy demonstrated the presence of gadolinium in the skin of 20 patients with nephrogenic systemic fibrosis but not in the skin of a gadodiamide-exposed patient with renal failure but without fibrosis; importantly, where repeat biopsies were examined, gadolinium levels increased for almost 2 years in 60% of subjects [34]. On the basis that the toxic Gd^{3+} ion is retained in apatite-like structures, the findings suggested that there might be gradual mobilization of gadolinium from bone stores, explaining the variability in timing and extent of fibrosis.

References

1 Gupta AK, Gupta MA, Cardella CJ et al. Cutaneous associations of chronic renal failure and dialysis. Int J Dermatol 1986; **25**: 498–504.

2 Dymock RB. Skin disease associated with renal transplantation. Australas J Dermatol 1979; **20**: 61–7.

3 Callen JP. Cutaneous nephrology. In: Callen JP, Jorizzo JL, eds. Dermatological Signs of Internal Disease, 3rd edn. Philadelphia: Saunders, 2003: 271–4.

4 Landing BH, Wells TR, Williamson ML. Anatomy of eccrine sweat glands in children with chronic renal failure, insufficiency and other fatal chronic disease. Am J Clin Pathol 1970; **54**: 15–21.

5 Graham RM. Aspects of itching. In: Verbov JL, ed. New Approaches in Dermatology. Lancaster: MTP Press, 1987: 49–70.

6 Gilkes JJ, Eady RA, Rees LH et al. Plasma immunoreactive melanotrophic hormones in patients on maintenance haemodialysis. BMJ 1975; **i**: 656–7.

7 Kint A, Bussels L, Fernandes M et al. Skin and nail disorders in relation to chronic renal failure. Acta Derm Venereol 1974; **54**: 137–40.

8 Baran R, Dawber RP, eds. Diseases of the Nails and Their Management. Oxford: Blackwell Scientific Publications, 1984.

9 Stewart JH, Castaldi PA. Uraemic bleeding: a reversible platelet defect corrected by dialysis. QJM 1967; **36**: 409–23.

10 Young AW Jr, Sweeney EW, David DS et al. Dermatologic evaluation of pruritus in patients on hemodialysis. N Y State J Med 1973; **73**: 2670–4.

11 Murphy M, Carmichael AJ. Renal itch. Clin Exp Dermatol 2000; **25**: 103–6.

12 Massry SG, Popovtzer MM, Coburn JW et al. Intractable pruritus as a manifestation of secondary hyperparathyroidism in uraemia: disappearance of itching after subtotal parathyroidectomy. N Engl J Med 1968; **279**: 697–700.

13 Graf H, Kovarik J, Stummvoll HK et al. Disappearance of uraemic pruritus after lowering dialysate magnesium concentration. BMJ 1979; **2**: 1478–9.

14 Blachley JD, Blankenship DM, Menter A et al. Uremic pruritus, skin divalent ion content and response to ultra-violet phototherapy. Am J Kidney Dis 1985; **1**: 752–93.

15 Hindson C, Taylor A, Martin A et al. UVA—light relief of uraemic pruritus. Lancet 1981; **i**: 215.

16 Pederson JA, Matter BJ, Czerwinski AW et al. Relief of idiopathic generalized pruritus in dialysis patients with activated oral charcoal. Ann Intern Med 1980; **93**: 446–8.

17 Silverberg DS, Iaina A, Reisin E et al. Cholestyramine in uraemic pruritus. BMJ 1977; **1**: 215.

18 Faver IR, Daoud MS, Su WP. Acquired reactive perforating collagenosis. Report of six cases and review of the literature. J Am Acad Dermatol 1994; **30**: 575–80.

19 Prioleau PG, Varghese M. The perforating dermatoses. In: Lebwohl M, ed. Difficult Diagnoses in Dermatology. New York: Churchill Livingstone, 1988.

20 Dellantonio R, Paladini D, Carletti P et al. Sympathetic skin response in chronic renal failure and correlation with sensorimotor neuropathy. Funct Neurol 1989; **4**: 173–5.

21 Freeman RM, Lawton RL, Fearing MO. Gynecomastia: an endocrinologic complication of hemodialysis. Ann Intern Med 1968; **69**: 67–72.

22 Rivet J, Lebbé C, Urena P et al. Cutaneous calcification in patients with end-stage renal disease: a regulated process associated with in situ osteopontin expression. Arch Dermatol 2006; **142**: 900–6.

23 Goh CL, Phay KL. Arteriovenous shunt dermatitis in chronic renal failure patients on maintenance haemodialysis. Clin Exp Dermatol 1988; **13**: 379–81.

24 Irvine C, Holt P. Hand venous hypertension complicating arteriovenous fistula construction for haemodialysis. Clin Exp Dermatol 1989; **14**: 289–90.

25 Sangiray H, Nguyen JC, Turiansky GW, Norwood C. Pyoderma gangrenosum occurring near an arteriovenous dialysis shunt. Int J Dermatol 2006; **45**: 851–3.

26 Poh-Fitzpatrick MB, Sosin AE, Bemis J. Porphyria levels in plasma and erythrocytes of chronic hemodialysis patients. J Am Acad Dermatol 1982; **7**: 100–4.

27 Topi GC, D'Alessandro GL, Cancarini GC et al. Porphyria cutanea tarda in a haemodialysis patient. Br J Dermatol 1981; **104**: 579–80.

28 Cooke NS, McKenna K. A case of haemodialysis-associated pseudoporphyria successfully treated with oral N-acetylcysteine. Clin Exp Dermatol 2007; **32**: 64–6.

29 Cowper S, Robin H, Steinberg S et al. Scleromyxedema-like cutaneous diseases in renal-dialysis patients. Lancet 2000; **356**: 1000–1.

30 Streams BN, Liu V, Liégeois N, Moschella SM. Clinical and pathologic features of nephrogenic fibrosing dermopathy: a report of two cases. J Am Acad Dermatol 2003; **48**: 42–7.

31 Mackay-Wiggan JM, Cohen DJ, Hardt MA et al. Nephrogenic fibrosing dermopathy (scleromyxedema-like illness of renal disease). J Am Acad Dermatol 2003; **48**: 55–60.

32 High WA. Nephrogenic systemic fibrosis and gadolinium-based contrast agents. Expert Rev Dermatol 2007; **2**: 593–605.

33 Marckmann P, Skov L, Rossen K *et al*. Nephrogenic systemic fibrosis: suspected causative role of gadodiamide used for contrast-enhanced magnetic resonance imaging. *J Am Soc Nephrol* 2006; **17**: 2359–62.

34 Abraham JL, Thakral C, Skov L *et al*. Dermal inorganic gadolinium concentrations: evidence for *in vivo* transmetallation and long-term persistence in nephrogenic systemic fibrosis. *Br J Dermatol* 2008; **158**: 273–80.

Skin changes in renal transplant recipients

To prevent graft rejection after renal transplantation, immunosuppressive therapy with corticosteroids, and either azathioprine, ciclosporin, tacrolimus or sirolimus will be required for the duration of the graft survival. The long-term consequences of this are best documented after kidney transplant, but similar problems arise after other organ transplants; the degree of immunosuppression needed after liver transplants is not so great, whilst that required after cardiac or heart–lung transplantation is greater. The effects of these drugs on the skin include:

Corticosteroid effects. These include skin atrophy, fragility and purpura; see Cushing's syndrome (p. 62.3) for details.

Infections [1]. Some infections, such as candidal infection, herpes simplex infection, and impetigo are prominent during the first post-transplant year. Dermatomycoses, herpes zoster and folliculitis are more common after the first post-transplant year [2]; infections with unusual organisms (e.g. cutaneous alternariosis) should always be considered, as discussed below. The incidence of warts increased steadily after transplant, such that of patients transplanted for more than 5 years, 92% were found to have warts and 65% had more than five each [3]. Warts may become unusually florid (Fig. 62.25) [4], and recalcitrant to therapy [5].

Exotic and aggressive opportunistic infections are a challenge to both diagnose and treat, and may be caused by virus (disseminated herpes simplex and varicella zoster infection, cytomegalovirus [6]), bacteria (tuberculosis and atypical acid-fast infections [7]), fungi, yeasts and moulds (aspergillus [8], altenaria [9], nocardia [10], invasive candidiasis, cryptococcus [11], sporotrichosis [12], histoplasmosis [13], mucormycosis [14]) and protozoa (leishmaniasis [15] and acanthamoebiasis [16]). Abscesses, nodules or cellulitic lesions need biopsy, with appropriate culture as well as histological examination, and close microbiological liaison.

Skin tumours. Transplant recipients are at greatly increased risk of developing skin cancers, particularly squamous cell carcinoma (SCC; Fig. 62.26) [17–19]. The pathogenesis of post-transplant skin cancer is reviewed in detail in [19]; SCC is discussed in Chapter 52. Renal recipients are at particular risk as the survival period is now so prolonged. Liver transplant recipients may not be as susceptible due to the less profound immunosuppression they require [20]. In a series of nearly a thousand recipients from the south of England followed for over 20 years, 61% of patients developed a skin cancer, and SCC was the most frequent. The cancer may behave aggressively, particularly on the ear and scalp, and have a spindle cell morphology. The mean time to first cancer development post transplant was 8 years, and 60% of patients had multiple cancers, with as many as 50 lesions recorded. The risk of BCC was also increased [20]. The same group has reported melanomas occurring at approximately eight times the rate in the general population [21]. Due to regular surveillance of their skin, melanomas were identified with relatively thin Breslow thickness, so prognosis was good.

An important issue in post-transplantation skin cancers is the reversal of the expected ratio of BCCs compared with SCCs. Whilst the incidence of BCC may be increased 10-fold compared to the normal population, that of SCC is increased 65- to 250-fold. Thus SCC is at least four times as common as BCC in post-transplant patients [22]. The risk of tumours is multifactorial—as well as skin type, sun exposure history and degree of immunosuppression, genetic factors may play a part. These include polymorphisms in genes coding for glutathione-S-transferase, interleukin-10, p53,

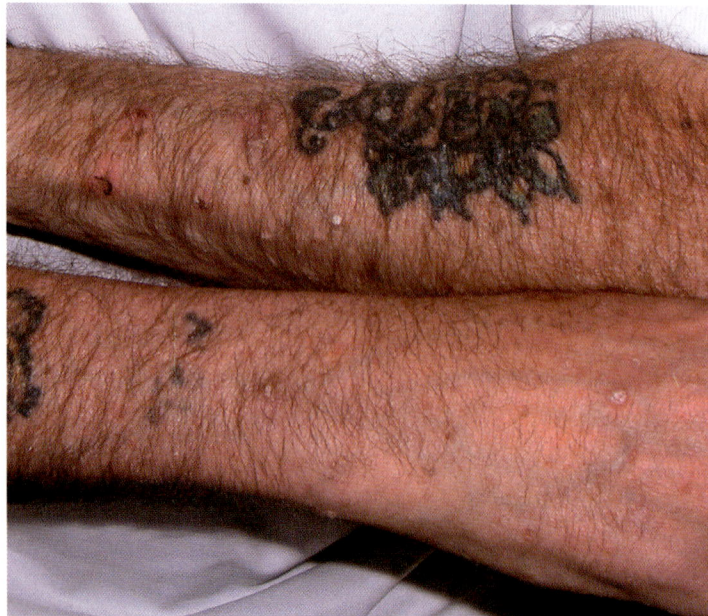

Fig. 62.25 Viral warts and multiple dysplastic lesions on the arms in a renal transplant recipient.

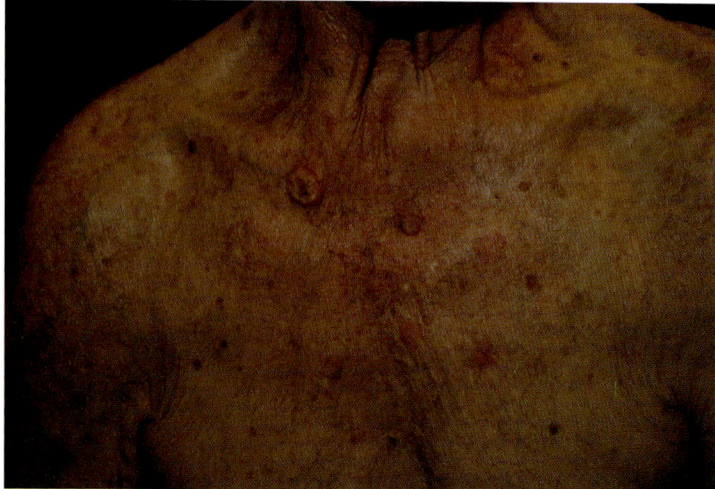

Fig. 62.26 Squamous cell carcinoma and semi-confluent dysplastic lesions on the trunk of a patient immunosuppressed after organ transplantation.

retinoblastoma, folate metabolism, melanocortin-1 receptor and vitamin D receptor [23]. Human papilloma virus (HPV) may also be co-oncogenic; HPV DNA can be detected in 65–90% of SCCs in immunosuppressed subjects, often several types of HPV are within a single tumour [22].

Kaposi's sarcoma affecting the skin as well as other organs is well recognized after transplantation; it was reported in 3% of kidney recipients in one series [24], and has been documented as being between 84- and 500-fold commoner in subjects with a transplant compared to the normal population [22]. Some series report Kaposi's sarcoma confined to the skin [25]—this is possibly as a result of surveillance and early detection in at-risk individuals, as earlier series suggested internal involvement in 50%. Merkel cell tumours also seem to be more frequent and carry a poor prognosis [22,26]; increased risk up to 80-fold greater than the normal population has been suggested. Appendageal tumours are common, as is sebaceous gland hyperplasia. Sebaceous carcinomas are overrepresented in organ recipients [27]. Lymphomas of both B (associated with Epstein–Barr virus) and T–cell lineage (often CD30⁺) are reported [28]. Sirolimus (rapamycin) may be less likely to provoke skin cancers [19], and a change from immunosuppression with ciclosporin and mycophenolate mofetil to sirolimus has been described to cause regression of Kaposi's sarcoma [25]. Oral retinoids (notably acitretin) appear to reduce the rate at which skin cancers develop [29,30]; some renal physicians have reservations as the manufacturer's product information states that renal disease is a contraindication to use of acitretin, but, although there is a possible increased tendency to mucocutaneous side effects, none of the studies reported have shown any unexpected renal adverse effect. Topical imiquimod is useful in reducing skin dysplasia in patients at high risk of developing skin neoplasms [31].

References

1 Carucci JA. Management of skin cancer in organ transplant recipients. In: Rigel DS, Friedman RJ, Dzubow LM *et al*. *Cancer of the skin*. Philadelphia: Elsevier Saunders, 2005: 631–40.

2 Hogewoning AA, Goettsch W, van Loveren H *et al*. Skin infections in renal transplant recipients. *Clin Transplant* 2001; **15**: 32–8.

3 Dyall-Smith D, Trowell H, Dyall-Smith ML. Benign human papillomavirus infection in renal transplant recipients *Int J Dermatol* 1991; **30**: 785–9.

4 Yu HC, Cho BH, Chung MJ *et al*. A case of giant condylomata acuminata involving anus after renal transplantation. *Clin Nephrol* 2003; **59**: 235–6.

5 Harwood CA, Perrett CM, Brown VL *et al*. Imiquimod cream 5% for recalcitrant cutaneous warts in immunosuppressed individuals. *Br J Dermatol* 2005; **152**: 122–9.

6 Trimarchi H, Casas G, Jordan R *et al*. Cytomegalovirus maculopapular eruption in a kidney transplant patient. *Am J Nephrol* 2000; **20**: 38–41.

7 Jie T, Matas AJ, Gillingham KJ *et al*. Mycobacterial infections after kidney transplant. *Transplant Proc* 2005; **37**: 937–9.

8 Park SB, Kang MJ, Whang EA *et al*. A case of primary cutaneous aspergillosis in a renal transplant recipient. *Transplant Proc* 2004; **36**: 2156–7.

9 Gallelli B, Viviani M, Nebuloni M *et al*. Skin infection due to Alternaria species in kidney allograft recipients: report of a new case and review of the literature. *J Nephrol* 2006; **19**: 668–72.

10 Wong KM, Chak WL, Chan YH *et al*. Subcutaneous nodules attributed to nocardiosis in a renal transplant recipient on tacrolimus therapy. *Am J Nephrol* 2000; **20**: 138–41.

11 Basaran O, Emiroglu R, Arikan U *et al*. Cryptococcal necrotizing fasciitis with multiple sites of involvement in the lower extremities. *Dermatol Surg* 2003; **29**: 1158–60.

12 Gullberg RM, Quintanilla A, Levin ML *et al*. Sporotrichosis: recurrent cutaneous, articular, and central nervous system infection in a renal transplant recipient. *Rev Infect Dis* 1987; **9**: 369–75.

13 McGuinn ML, Lawrence ME, Proia L, Segreti J. Progressive disseminated histoplasmosis presenting as cellulitis in a renal transplant recipient. *Transplant Proc* 2005; **37**: 4313–4.

14 Adriaenssens K, Jorens PG, Meuleman L *et al*. A black necrotic skin lesion in an immunocompromised patient. Diagnosis: cutaneous mucormycosis. *Arch Dermatol* 2000; **136**: 1165–70.

15 Mirzabeigi M, Farooq U, Baraniak S *et al*. Reactivation of dormant cutaneous Leishmania infection in a kidney transplant patient. *J Cutan Pathol* 2006; **33**: 701–4.

16 Steinberg JP, Galindo RL, Kraus ES *et al*. Disseminated acanthamebiasis in a renal transplant recipient with osteomyelitis and cutaneous lesions: case report and literature review. *Clin Infect Dis* 2002; **35**: e43–9.

17 Carucci JA. Management of skin cancer in organ transplant recipients. In: Rigel DS, Friedman RJ, Dzubow LM, Reintgen DS, Bystryn J-C, Marks R, eds. *Cancer of the Skin*. Philadelphia: Elsevier, 2005: 631–40.

18 Perera GK, Child FJ, Heaton N *et al*. Skin lesions in adult liver transplant recipients: a study of 100 consecutive patients. *Br J Dermatol* 2006; **154**: 868–72.

19 Ho WL, Murphy GM. Update on the pathogenesis of post-transplant skin cancer in renal transplant recipients. *Br J Dermatol* 2007; **158**: 217–24.

20 Bordea C, Wojnarowska F, Millard PR *et al*. Skin cancers in renal-transplant recipients occur more frequently than previously recognized in a temperate climate. *Transplantation* 2004; **77**: 574–9.

21 Le Mire L, Hollowood K, Gray D *et al*. Melanomas in renal transplant recipients. *Br J Dermatol* 2006; **154**: 472–7.

22 Euvrard S, Kanitakis J, Claudy A. Skin cancers after organ transplantation. *N Engl J Med* 2003; **348**: 1681–91.

23 Laing ME, Kay E, Conlon P, Murphy GM. Genetic factors associated with skin cancer in renal transplant patients. *Photoderm Photoimmunol Photomed* 2007; **23**: 62–7.

24 Berber I, Altaca G, Aydin C *et al*. Kaposi's sarcoma in renal transplant patients: predisposing factors and prognosis. *Transplant Proc* 2005; **37**: 967–8.

25 Stallone G, Schena A, Infante B *et al*. Sirolimus for Kaposi's sarcoma in renal-transplant recipients. *N Engl J Med* 2005; **352**: 1317–23.

26 Penn I, First MR. Merkel's cell carcinoma in organ recipients: report of 41 cases. *Transplantation* 1999; **68**: 1717–21.

27 Harwood CA, McGregor JM, Swale VJ *et al*. High frequency and diversity of cutaneous appendageal tumors in organ transplant recipients. *J Am Acad Dermatol* 2003; **48**: 401–8.

28 Ravat FE, Spittle MF, Russell-Jones R. Primary cutaneous T-cell lymphoma occurring after organ transplantation. *J Am Acad Dermatol* 2006; **54**: 668–75.

29 Harwood CA, Leedham-Green M, Leigh IM, Proby CM. Low-dose retinoids in the prevention of cutaneous squamous cell carcinomas in organ transplant recipients: a 16-year retrospective study. *Arch Dermatol* 2005; **141**: 456–64.

30 Chen K, Craig JC, Shumack S. Oral retinoids for the prevention of skin cancers in solid organ transplant recipients: a systematic review of randomized controlled trials. *Br J Dermatol* 2005; **152**: 518–23.

31 Brown VL, Atkins CL, Ghall L *et al*. Safey and efficacy of 5% imiquimod cream for the treatment of skin dysplasia in high-risk renal transplant recipients: randomized, double-blind, placebo-controlled trial. *Arch Dermatol* 2005; **141**: 985–93.

Cardiac disease

There are several diseases in which both cardiac and skin involvement may be found (Table 62.15). Most of these are part of a syndrome or are systemic disorders affecting other organs as well [1,2]; most are discussed in other chapters, but some are briefly described below. Disorders of blood vessels are not included here. The effects of skin disease on the heart (e.g. cardiac failure due to erythroderma) and indirect effects, such as anaemia due to immunosuppressive agents used to treat the skin, are not discussed. Numerous infections may occasionally cause myocardial disease

Table 62.15 Conditions that affect the heart and skin.

Disease	Main cardiac feature, or comment
Congenital/inherited	
Ehlers–Danlos syndrome	Dilated main vessels, mitral or tricuspid insufficiency, cardiac/vascular rupture (type IV)
Cutis laxa	Early CAD, aortic aneurysm, mitral valve prolapse
Marfan syndrome	Aortic aneurysm, aortic regurgitation, mitral valve prolapse or regurgitation
Pseudoxanthoma elasticum	Arterial calcification, CAD, mitral valve prolapse
Werner's disease	Early CAD
Progeria	Early CAD
Cockayne's syndrome	Early CAD
Cornelia de Lange's syndrome	Septal defects, persistent ductus arteriosus, pulmonary stenosis
Fabry's disease	Conduction defects, arrhythmias, hypertension, left ventricular hypertrophy, mitral valve prolapse
Noonan's syndrome	Pulmonary stenosis, septal defects, hypertrophic cardiomyopathy, aortic abnormalities, others
Rubinstein–Taybi syndrome	Aortic coarctation, persistent ductus arteriosus, pulmonary stenosis, septal defects
LEOPARD syndrome	E, ECG abnormalities (various forms of heart block); P, pulmonary stenosis; also subaortic stenosis and hypertrophic cardiomyopathy
Tuberous sclerosis	Cardiac rhabdomyomas
Neurofibromatosis	Hypertension (renovascular or phaeochromocytoma)
Incontinentia pigmenti	Patent ductus arteriosus, tricuspid insufficiency
Alagille's syndrome	Pulmonary artery hypoplasia/stenosis
Di George's syndrome	Tetralogy of Fallot, aortic arch defects
Lymphoedema–distichiasis syndrome	Tetralogy of Fallot, patent ductus arteriosus
Naxos disease	Arrhythmogenic right ventricular cardiomyopathy
Chromosomal syndromes	Various—includes Down's syndrome, Turner's syndrome, trisomy 13, trisomy 18
Inflammatory diseases, connective tissue disease, vasculitis	
Systemic lupus erythematosus	Vegetations (especially mitral, Libman–Sacks endocarditis), pericarditis, myocarditis, aortic/mitral regurgitation
Neonatal lupus erythematosus	Neonatal heart block (various patterns), septal defects, persistent ductus arteriosus, tricuspid/mitral insufficiency
Systemic sclerosis	Pericarditis and effusion, conduction defects, myocardial fibrosis, cardiomyopathy, cor pulmonale
CREST	Pulmonary hypertension
Polyarteritis nodosa	Coronary artery vasculitis, ECG abnormalities, hypertension
Behçet's disease	Pericarditis, pulmonary and coronary artery aneurysm
Antiphospholipid syndrome	Vegetations, valvular heart disease, coronary artery thrombosis, pericardial effusion, CCF
Degos's disease	Pericarditis, pericardial effusion
Churg–Strauss disease	Pericarditis, cardiac fibrosis, pericardial effusion
Wegener's granulomatosis	Cardiomyopathy
Cholesterol emboli	Coronary artery occlusion
Other vasculitides	Coronary artery vasculitis
Dermatomyositis	Conduction defects, arrhythmias, cardiomyopathy, CCF, (rarely) pulmonary hypertension
Relapsing polychondritis	Mitral or aortic insufficiency, dissecting aortic aneurysm, pericarditis, myocardial ischaemia, heart block, aortitis
Rheumatic fever	Mitral and aortic valve disease
Kawasaki disease	Conduction defects, coronary artery aneurysms, pericardial effusion, cardiomegaly
Multicentric reticulohistiocytosis	Pericarditis, cardiomegaly, CAD, CCF
Hypereosinophilic syndrome	Eosinophilic endomyocarditis, valvular scarring, CCF, restrictive cardiomyopathy
Sarcoidosis	Conduction defects, arrhythmias, CCF
Reiter's disease	Conduction defects, aortic regurgitation
Deposition, metabolic and endocrine disorders	
Amyloidosis	Conduction defects, cardiomegaly, CCF
Haemochromatosis	Arrhythmias, cardiomyopathy, CCF
Wilson's disease	Arrhythmias, cardiomyopathy
Mucinoses: scleromyxoedema	Cardiomyopathy, CCF
Atrial myxoma syndromes	See text
Hyperlipidaemias	CAD
Diabetes mellitus	CAD, cardiomyopathy
Hyperthyroidism	Tachycardia, atrial fibrillation, mitral regurgitation
Hypothyroidism	Bradycardia, CAD, pericardial effusion
Acromegaly	Left ventricular hypertrophy, CCF
Carcinoid syndrome	Tricuspid or pulmonary stenosis, right heart failure
Phaeochromocytoma	Variable heart rate, hypertension/hypotension
Mastocytosis	Tachycardia, hypotension, arrhythmia, angina
Homocystinuria	Atherosclerosis

(Continued)

Table 62.15 *Continued*

Disease	Main cardiac feature, or comment
Embolic diseases	
Subacute bacterial endocarditis	Vegetations, valvular incompetence
Cholesterol emboli	Usually from proximal arteries rather than cardiac
Atrial myxomas	See text
Infections	
Lyme disease	Myocarditis, heart block
Syphilis	Aortitis, aortic aneurysm, aortic and mitral regurgitation, obstructed coronary arteries
Varicella	Myocarditis
Septicaemia	Pustules, infarcts, disseminated intravascular coagulopathy
Congenital rubella	Pulmonary artery and valve stenosis, patent ductus arteriosus
Whipple's disease	Pericarditis, myocarditis, valve deformity (especially mitral valve endocarditis)
Drugs	
Used in cardiology, causing rash	e.g. amiodarone (photosensitivity, pigmentation)
Cardiotoxic and cause skin eruptions	e.g. doxorubicin (cardiotoxic, anagen effluvium, pigmentation)
Used for skin disease, cardiovascular side effects	e.g. ciclosporin (hypertension)
Teratogenic, causing both skin and cardiac defects	e.g. alcohol, phenytoin, retinoids
Miscellaneous	
Earlobe crease	CAD
POEMS syndrome	Cardiac failure
Mycosis fungoides, Sézary syndrome	Heart is infiltrated in advanced disease
Kaposi's sarcoma	Heart is commonly involved
Diffuse neonatal haemangiomatosis	High output cardiac failure
Erythroderma, any cause	High output cardiac failure
Pacemaker reactions	Infection, contact dermatitis, mechanical issues
Clubbing of nails	Cyanotic congenital heart defects
Red lunulae	Occur in CCF

CAD, coronary artery disease; CCF, congestive cardiac failure; CREST, calcinosis, Raynaud's phenomenon, esophageal disease, sclerodactyly, telangiectasia; ECG, electrocardiogram; LEOPARD, lentigines, ECG abnormalities, ocular hypertelorism, pulmonary stenosis, abnormalities of genitalia, retardation of growth, and deafness (syndrome); POEMS, polyneuropathy, organomegaly, endocrinopathy, M protein, skin changes (syndrome).

and may have an exanthem (for example, parvovirus B19), but these are not discussed individually. Drug reactions due to cardiac medications are described in Chapter 75.

Consequences of cardiac disease

Dermatological consequences of cardiac disease include skin colour changes such as cyanosis, erythema due to secondary polycythaemia, and a combination of the two that may occur in congenital heart disease (and which has been termed erythremia). Finger clubbing is a consequence of congenital cyanotic heart disease, but occurs in other situations as well. Applying pressure on the tip of the nail in subjects with aortic regurgitation reveals visible flushing of the nail bed in time with the pulse, due to the wide pulse pressure in this disorder (Quincke pulsation) [2].

Congenital and inherited disorders

Cardiac involvement occurs in several congenital and inherited conditions, such as the LEOPARD syndrome, Anderson–Fabry disease, Alagille's syndrome and the cardiofaciocutaneous and Noonan's syndromes [1–8], as well as in chromosomal abnormalities such as Turner's syndrome and trisomy 13 or 18 [1].

The lymphoedema–distichiasis syndrome, due to mutations in *FOXC2* (*MFH-1*) on chromosome 16q24.3, has been linked to cardiac anomalies such as tetralogy of Fallot and patent ductus arteriosus [9,10]; spinal arachnoid cysts also occur. Cardiac rhabdomyomas occur in about 50% of patients with tuberous sclerosis (see Chapter 15).

In the LEOPARD syndrome (multiple lentigines syndrome; MIM *151100) [3] there are widespread lentigines, electrocardiographic abnormalities, ocular hypertelorism, pulmonary stenosis, abnormal genitals, retardation of growth and deafness. The cardiac involvement includes left-axis deviation on the electrocardiogram (ECG), ventricular hypertrophy and arrhythmia.

In angiokeratoma corporis diffusum (Anderson–Fabry disease; MIM *301500) [4], cardiac involvement may be manifest as arrhythmias, an abnormal P–R interval on ECG and left-ventricular hypertrophy. ECG abnormalities may also be found in heterozygotes. Manufactured α-galactosidase is now available to treat this condition [4] and appears to be more beneficial for the renal and cardiac lesions than for the cutaneous angiokeratomas, although accumulated globotriaosylceramide in the skin decreases during treatment.

Coronary artery disease

Coronary artery disease and ischaemic heart disease may occur in premature ageing syndromes such as progeria and Werner's syndrome, and premature myocardial ischaemia has also been reported in pseudoxanthoma elasticum, although it seems to be less common than the presence of a calcifying vascular pathology might suggest [2,11]. Coronary artery disease may be associated with xanthelasma or xanthomas due to hyperlipidaemia [2]. Both all-cause and cardiac-specific morbidity and mortality have been linked with the presence of a unilateral or bilateral diagonal earlobe skin crease [12,13], although others suggest that the association is with older age rather than with coronary artery disease *per se*. Both antinuclear [14] and high-titre anticardiolipin antibodies [15] have been demonstrated in a high proportion of patients with coronary artery disease; the significance of these is uncertain.

Connective tissue and systemic diseases

Cardiac involvement is common in systemic disorders such as sarcoidosis [16], connective tissue diseases [17–19], vasculitides (Chapter 50) [20,21], dermatomyositis (Chapter 51), relapsing polychondritis (Chapter 68) [22] and the hypereosinophilic syndrome [23,24], although it may be underestimated if symptoms are absent. Sudden death due to conduction defects and ventricular arrhythmias is the most important complication, and is particularly well recognized in sarcoidosis [16]; cardiomyopathy may also occur. The major vasculitides that affect the heart are Wegener's granulomatosis, polyarteritis nodosa, Churg–Strauss syndrome, temporal arteritis and Takayasu arteritis. Cardiac involvement is commoner in Churg–Strauss syndrome than in Wegener's granulomatosis, but has low discriminatory value— this is discussed in more detail in Chapter 50 and in the section on respiratory disease and the skin, below.

A number of cardiac complications occur in systemic lupus erythematosus (SLE), especially pericarditis, which may be present in 60–80% of patients at autopsy (Chapter 51) [2,25]. Neonatal LE is a particularly important entity, as about two-thirds of affected children have congenital heart block, although the frequency of this manifestation varies between countries [18,19]. Mothers of affected children generally express the 52-kDa and 60-kDa anti-SS-A (Ro) antibodies, even if they have no other features of LE. This antibody group is particularly associated with subacute cutaneous LE, but also with systemic LE. Mothers of children with neonatal LE with heart block tend to have higher titres of anti-SS-A but lower titres of anti-SS-B (La) antibody than mothers of children with neonatal LE rash alone [19].

Cardiac involvement occurs in 80% of patients with systemic sclerosis, but is not always clinically apparent; pericarditis, pericardial effusion, myocardial fibrosis, endothelial damage to coronary arteries and heart failure due to pulmonary arterial hypertension all occur [2,26,27]. Symptoms include heart failure, palpitations and myocardial infarction. Vasospasm may occur due to Raynaud's phenomenon. Pulmonary hypertension is particularly associated with CREST.

In the antiphospholipid syndrome (APLS) [28], about 50% of patients have valvular heart disease, either vegetations or thickening. The mitral valve is most frequently affected. About 5% require cardiac valve surgery, but many have no symptoms. There is also an increased incidence of coronary artery disease. Intracardiac thrombus is a rare complication. Unrecognized APLS may explain some cases of valvular heart disease in SLE.

Cardiac involvement is frequent in primary and in familial amyloidosis [29], causing features of cardiomyopathy such as congestive heart failure, low voltage on the ECG and conduction disturbances. Cardiomegaly is present in about one-third of the patients. Cutaneous signs, macroglossia and demonstration of amyloid deposition on skin histology support the diagnosis.

Kawasaki disease (mucocutaneous lymph-node syndrome) is an acute febrile disease of unknown aetiology, with accepted diagnostic criteria [30]. Coronary artery aneurysms may develop in up to 25% of patients, more commonly in children; conduction defects, pericardial effusion and cardiomegaly also occur. Symptoms and signs may include murmurs, gallop rhythm, angina and myocardial infarction [25,30]. Echocardiography and ECG are indicated. Treatment consists of acetylsalicylates and high doses of intravenous gammaglobulin.

Infections

Subacute bacterial endocarditis (SBE) [31–33] typically occurs in patients with a past history of heart disease (rheumatic fever, congenital heart disease, heart valve operation) or of parenteral drug addiction. About 75–80% of cases are caused by *Staphylococcus aureus* or streptococcal species, predominantly *Streptococcus viridans*. Cutaneous lesions may represent either septic emboli or immune complex disease due to the bacterial focus [31]; organisms can occasionally be cultured from skin lesions [32]. The skin lesions may be purpuric, pustular or erythematous, and various patterns are described. A non-specific small vessel vasculitis with splinter haemorrhages of the nail fold or nail bed occurs in about half of affected individuals. Similar small haemorrhages occur on the conjunctivae and retina (Roth spots). Osler's nodes are small, tender, red papules situated mainly on the distal finger and toe pads; Janeway lesions are faint, red, macular lesions on the thenar and hypothenar eminences. Both rheumatoid factor and cANCA can be demonstrated in some patients with SBE; these are of uncertain significance, but may erroneously suggest that the diagnosis is of systemic ANCA-associated vasculitis rather than of infective aetiology [33].

Rheumatic fever is a complication of streptococcal infection [34]. It causes arthritis, carditis, neuromuscular disease (Sydenham's chorea, dysphagia, dysarthria, distal weakness) and cutaneous lesions. The latter include erythema marginatum and papular lesions on the extensor surface of the extremities, particularly near the joints—both of these manifestations are usually transient, typically resolving after a few weeks. Erythema marginatum is a transitory gyrate erythema situated mainly on the trunk and proximal parts of the extremities. Urticaria, erythema nodosum and purpura are described in about 2% of patients. Cardiac features include valvular disease, pericarditis, myocarditis and congestive cardiac failure.

Cardiac myxoma syndromes

Carney complex (type I, MIM #160980; type II, MIM *605244). A number of atrial myxoma syndromes have been described, with various eponyms and acronyms and overlapping features [35–39].

These include LAMB syndrome, NAME syndrome, Danoff syndrome and the Carney complex. LAMB is an acronym for *l*entigines, *a*trial myxoma, *m*ucocutaneous myxoma and *b*lue naevi. The NAME syndrome indicates blue *n*aevi, *a*trial myxoma, *m*yxoid neurofibromas and *e*phelides. The inheritance is autosomal-dominant. In the Danoff syndrome there are, apart from atrial myxomas, adrenocortical dysplasia, lentigines and spindle cell tumours.

About 50% of cases of bilateral, pigmented, micronodular adrenal hyperplasia—a rare cause of ACTH-independent Cushing's syndrome—are associated with the Carney complex; anti-ACTH receptor antibodies are present and stimulate adrenal growth and secretion. Other features include cardiac myxomas (in one-third of patients), skin myxomas (two-thirds), skin pigmentation (96%), myxoid fibroadenomas of the breast (in one-third of women, uncommon in men), GH-secreting pituitary tumours (acromegaly occurs in 8% of patients), Sertoli cell (in 10%) and Leydig cell testicular tumours (which cause male precocious puberty), thyroid cysts, hyperplasia and tumours (10%), and ovarian cysts and tumours (which are felt to be underestimated in frequency) [37–39]. Psammomatous melanotic schwannoma is rare, but is usually part of this syndrome when it occurs [40].

The genetic background of these disorders has been extensively investigated. Carney complex type 1 (CNC1) is linked to a susceptibility gene for the protein kinase A type 1α regulatory subunit gene (*PRKAR1A*) and has loci on chromosomes 2p16 and 17q23–24, whilst CNC2 links to a currently unknown gene on chromosome 2p. Genetic evaluation has demonstrated that this disorder is related to PJS. Any patient with multiple melanocytic and myxomatous tumours of the skin and mucosa (including vulval melanotic macules) should have a cardiac evaluation.

From a dermatological aspect, atrial myxomas may present due to embolic infarction of the skin. They may mechanically interfere with cardiac function and can also lead to pericarditis. Systemic malaise, pleurisy, Raynaud's phenomenon and the occasional occurrence of ANCA [41] may suggest other forms of vasculitis as the cause of skin lesions.

Miscellaneous

Cardiac pacemaker and implantable defibrillator dermatoses.

Cutaneous reactions over the site of implanted cardiac pacemakers have been reported [42–45]. Most of these are either infections or mechanical issues (erosions, extrusions, capsular contracture, exposed generator or electrodes, bronchopleural cutaneous fistulae) and may respond to antibiotics or altered positioning of the pacemaker [42,43]. However, contact dermatitis to epoxy resins, nickel or chromium may occur, in which event removal of the implanted material and use of titanium pacemaker casings may be appropriate [44,45]. A reticular telangiectatic pattern of erythema overlying pacemaker or defibrillator sites may occur [46,47]. Cardiac pacemakers also have dermatological surgical relevance, as they may malfunction during the use of electrosurgery [48].

References

1 Abdelmalek NF, Gerber TL, Menter A. Cardiocutaneous syndromes and associations. *J Am Acad Dermatol* 2002; **46**: 161–83.

2 McDonnell JK. Cardiac disease and the skin. *Dermatol Clin* 2002; **20**: 503–11.

3 Gorlin RJ, Anderson RC, Blaw M. Multiple lentigines syndrome. *Am J Dis Child* 1969; **117**: 652–62.

4 Desnick RJ, Ioannou YA, Eng CM. α-galactosidase A deficiency: Fabry disease. In: Scriver CR, Beaudet AL, Sly WS, Valle D, eds. *The Metabolic and Molecular Bases of Inherited Disease*, 8th edn. New York: McGraw-Hill, 2001: 3733–74.

5 Eng CM, Guffon N, Wilcox WR *et al.* International Collaborative Fabry Disease Study Group. Safety and efficacy of recombinant human alpha-galactosidase A replacement therapy in Fabry's disease. *N Engl J Med* 2001; **345**: 9–16.

6 Alagille D, Estrada A, Hadchouel M *et al.* Syndromic paucity of interlobular bile ducts (Alagille syndrome or arteriohepatic dysplasia): review of 80 cases. *J Pediatr* 1987; **110**: 195–200.

7 Ward KA, Moss C, McKeown C. The cardio-facio-cutaneous syndrome: a manifestation of the Noonan syndrome? *Br J Dermatol* 1994; **131**: 270–4.

8 Daoud MS, Dahl PR, Su WPD. Noonan syndrome. *Semin Dermatol* 1995; **14**: 140–4.

9 Bell R, Brice G, Child AH *et al.* Analysis of lymphoedema–distichiasis families for *FOXC2* mutations reveals small insertions and deletions throughout the gene. *Hum Genet* 2001; **108**: 546–51.

10 Chen E, Larabell SK, Daniels JM, Goldstein S. Distichiasis–lymphedema syndrome: tetralogy of Fallot, chylothorax and neonatal death. *Am J Med Genet* 1996; **66**: 273–5.

11 Neldner KH. Pseudoxanthoma elasticum. *Clin Dermatol* 1988; **6**: 45–64.

12 Wyre H. The diagonal ear-lobe crease: a cutaneous manifestation of coronary artery disease. *Cutis* 1979; **23**: 328–31.

13 Elliott WJ, Karrison T. Increased all-cause and cardiac morbidity and mortality associated with the diagonal earlobe crease: a prospective cohort study. *Am J Med* 1991; **91**: 247–54.

14 Grainger DJ, Bethell HW. High titres of serum antinuclear antibodies, mostly directed against nucleolar antigens, are associated with the presence of coronary atherosclerosis. *Ann Rheum Dis* 2002; **61**: 110–4.

15 Yilmaz E, Adalet K, Yilmaz G *et al.* Importance of serum anticardiolipin antibody levels in coronary heart disease. *Clin Cardiol* 1994; **17**: 117–21.

16 English JC 3rd, Patel PJ, Greer KE. Sarcoidosis. *J Am Acad Dermatol* 2001; **44**: 725–43.

17 Petri M, Perez-Gutthann S, Spence D *et al.* Risk factors for coronary artery disease in patients with systemic lupus erythematosus. *Am J Med* 1992; **93**: 513–9.

18 Petri M, Watson R, Hochberg MC. Anti-Ro antibodies and neonatal lupus. *Rheum Dis Clin North Am* 1989; **5**: 335–60.

19 Yukiko N. Immune responses to SS-A 52-kDa and 60kDa proteins and to SS-B 50-kDa protein in mothers of children with neonatal lupus erythematosus. *Br J Dermatol* 2000; **142**: 908–12.

20 Guillevin L, Lhote F, Casassus P. Polyarteritis nodosa: clinical aspects. In: Ansell BM, Bacon PA, Lie JT, Yazici H, eds. *The Vasculitides: Science and Practice*. London: Chapman & Hall Medical, 1996: 121–34.

21 Chakravarty K. Vasculitis by organ systems. *Baillière's Clin Rheumatol* 1997; **11**: 357–93.

22 Del Rosso A, Petix NR, Pratesi M *et al.* Cardiovascular involvement in relapsing polychondritis. *Semin Arthritis Rheum* 1997; **26**: 840–4.

23 Weller PF, Bubley GJ. The idiopathic hypereosinophilic syndrome. *Blood* 1994; **83**: 2759–79.

24 Leiferman KM. Hypereosinophilic syndrome. *Semin Dermatol* 1995; **14**: 122–8.

25 Sondheimer HM, Lorts A. Cardiac involvement in inflammatory disease: systemic lupus erythematosus, rheumatic fever, and Kawasaki disease. *Adolesc Med* 2001; **12**: 69–78.

26 Tuffanelli DL. Systemic sclerosis. In: Sontheimer RD, Provost TT, eds. *Cutaneous Manifestations of Rheumatic Diseases*. Baltimore: Williams and Wilkins, 1996: 115–39.

27 Wigley FM, Provost TT. Scleroderma. In: Provost TT, Flynn JA, eds. *Cutaneous Medicine: Cutaneous Manifestations of Systemic Disease*. Hamilton, Ontario: Decker, 2001: 104–26.

28 Cuadrado MJ, Hughes GRV. Hughes (antiphospholipid) syndrome: clinical features. *Rheum Dis Clin* 2001; **27**: 507–24.

29 Breathnach SM. Amyloid and amyloidoses. *J Am Acad Dermatol* 1988; **18**: 1–16.

30 Wortmann DW, Nelson AM. Kawasaki syndrome. *Rheum Dis Clin North Am* 1990; **16**: 363–75.

31 Brown M, Griffin GE. Immune responses in endocarditis. *Heart* 1998; **79**: 1–2.

32 Parikh SK, Lieberman A, Colbert DA *et al.* The identification of methicillin-resistant *Staphylococcus aureus* in Osler's nodes and Janeway lesions of acute bacterial endocarditis. *J Am Acad Dermatol* 1996; **35**: 767–8.

33 Choi HK, Lamprecht P, Niles JL *et al.* Subacute bacterial endocarditis with positive cytoplasmic antineutrophil cytoplasmic antibodies and anti-proteinase 3 antibodies. *Arthritis Rheum* 2000; **43**: 226–31.

34 Flynn JA, Provost TT. Rheumatic fever. In: Provost TT, Flynn JA, eds. *Cutaneous Medicine: Cutaneous Manifestations of Systemic Disease.* Hamilton, Ontario: Decker, 2001: 205–7.

35 Atherton DJ, Pitcher DW, Wells RS, MacDonald DM. A syndrome of various cutaneous pigmented lesions, myxoid neurofibromata and atrial myxoma: the NAME syndrome. *Br J Dermatol* 1980; **103**: 421–9.

36 Rhodes AR, Silverman RA, Harrist TJ, Perez-Atayde AR. Mucocutaneous lentigines, cardiomucocutaneous myxomas, and multiple blue nevi: the 'LAMB' syndrome. *J Am Acad Dermatol* 1984; **10**: 72–82.

37 Stratakis CA, Carney JA, Lin JP *et al.* Carney complex, a familial multiple neoplasia and lentiginosis syndrome: analysis of 11 kindreds and linkage to the short arm of chromosome 2. *J Clin Invest* 1996; **97**: 599–607.

38 Kirschner LS, Carney JA, Pack SD *et al.* Mutations of the gene encoding the protein kinase A type I-alpha regulatory subunit in patients with the Carney complex. *Nat Genet* 2000; **26**: 89–92.

39 Malchoff CD. Carney complex: clarity and complexity [editorial]. *J Clin Endocrinol Metab* 2000; **85**: 4010–2.

40 Utiger CA, Headington JT. Psammomatous melanocytic schwannoma: a new cutaneous marker for Carney's complex. *Arch Dermatol* 1993; **129**: 202–4.

41 Savige JA, Yeung SP, Davies DJ *et al.* Anti-neutrophil cytoplasmic antibodies associated with atrial myxoma. *Am J Med* 1988; **85**: 755–6.

42 Chua FS, Leininger BJ, Hamouda FA, Pifarre RF. Bronchopleural cutaneous fistula from infected pacemaker electrodes. *Chest* 1973; **63**: 284–6.

43 Har-Shai Y, Amikam S, Bolous M, Peled IJ. The management of soft tissue complications related to pacemaker implantations. *J Cardiovasc Surg* 1994; **35** (Suppl. 1): 211–7.

44 Andersen EK. Cutaneous reaction to an epoxy-coated pacemaker. *Arch Dermatol* 1979; **115**: 97–8.

45 Romaguera C, Grimalt F. Pacemaker-dermatitis. *Contact Derm* 1981; **7**: 33.

46 Kint A, Vermander F. Reticular telangiectatic erythema after implantation of a pacemaker. *Dermatologica* 1983; **166**: 651–4.

47 Krasagakis K, Vogt R, Tebbe B, Goerdt S. Persistent telangiectatic erythema associated with an implantable cardioverter defibrillator. *Br J Dermatol* 1997; **136**: 633–5.

48 Sebben JE. Electrosurgery and cardiac pacemakers. *J Am Acad Dermatol* 1983; **9**: 457–63.

Respiratory system

Pulmonary disease rarely occurs as a direct consequence of a primary skin disease, except for instances such as metastasis from a primary skin tumour (e.g. melanoma). Similarly, there are relatively few instances in which skin abnormalities occur as a direct consequence of respiratory pathology. Examples include cyanosis due to severe pulmonary disease or intrapulmonary right-to-left shunts, and finger clubbing due to chronic cyanotic lung disease or neoplasm. Dermatomyositis may occur as a paraneoplastic phenomenon due to lung cancer (but, as discussed below, lung disease also occurs as a consequence of dermatomyositis). Amyloidosis may occur secondary to chronic respiratory diseases such as bronchiectasis or cystic fibrosis, but cutaneous signs in secondary amyloidosis are generally few, even though aspiration of subcutaneous fat for histological examination can be diagnostic. Tumours may cause direct nerve damage and abnormalities of sweating [1,2].

However, in most instances in which the skin and respiratory tract exhibit the same disease process, this is as part of a multisystem disorder. This section on the respiratory system concentrates on this diverse group of disorders (Table 62.16).

Congenital and inherited disorders

Examples are listed in Table 62.16. NF1 (Chapter 15) is not uncommonly associated with the development of restrictive lung disease if there is severe scoliosis. Intrathoracic, intra-abdominal or retroperitoneal diffuse plexiform neurofibromas can also compromise pulmonary function [3]. Fibrosis is found in around 10% of patients with NF1, mainly in the lower lobes, and bullous changes may occur in the upper lobes [4]. Pleural effusions have been reported in tuberous sclerosis [5] (Chapter 12). Pulmonary involvement is uncommon but, especially in adult female patients, there may be numerous small cysts which represent lymphangioleiomyomatosis [6]. These may be mistaken for tuberculosis or sarcoidosis radiologically. Diffuse lower lobe fibrosis and laryngeal involvement has been reported in Darier's disease [7] (Chapter 19). α_1-Antitrypsin deficiency, particularly the ZZ genotype, links cutaneous panniculitis with emphysema and hepatic cirrhosis [8]. In familial dysautonomia (Riley–Day syndrome), there are acute episodes of bronchopneumonia, with profuse mucous secretion causing dyspnoea. Skin changes include multiple excoriations, and erythematous mottling associated with fever and sweating [9]. Radiological features of lung disease [10] may be accompanied by abdominal distension as the 'chest–abdomen' sign [11]. Ataxia–telangiectasia (Louis–Bar syndrome) may be associated with pulmonary problems, including recurrent pneumonia, bronchiectasis and pulmonary fibrosis [12].

Infections

Numerous infections may be associated with both respiratory and skin disease, and only a selection of these have been listed. Many viral infections, for example, may cause upper and sometimes lower respiratory tract symptoms in association with either a non-specific exanthem or with erythema multiforme. *Mycoplasma* infection is particularly associated with erythema multiforme with mucosal involvement (Stevens–Johnson syndrome). *Psittacosis (ornithosis)* may be accompanied by erythema nodosum and erythema multiforme (Bateman's syndrome).

Associations between *tuberculosis* and the skin include non-specific reactions such as erythema nodosum or erythema multiforme, as well as several patterns of specific skin lesion such as lichen scrofulosorum, Bazin's disease or papulonecrotic tuberculide (Chapter 31). Several *systemic mycoses* are caused by inhalation but may subsequently cause skin lesions (Table 62.16)—either non-specific reactions such as erythema multiforme or erythema nodosum, or specific lesions caused by haematogenous dissemination. Other mycoses may have primary cutaneous lesions with occasional spread to internal organs, including the lung (e.g. sporotrichosis). *Pulmonary melioidosis* may run a subacute course and last for one to several weeks. It may be contracted by inhalation, causing early pneumonic symptoms, or via skin defects, in which case abscess formation precedes the septic stage. Urticaria may occur in chronic melioidosis [13].

Connective tissue diseases

This group of disorders has a variety of respiratory features.

Respiratory disease is frequent in the various forms of *scleroderma* [14,15]. Systemic sclerosis is associated with fibrosing alveolitis and interstitial fibrosis, causing a restrictive defect. This occurs

Table 62.16 Conditions that affect the skin and respiratory system.

Disease	Respiratory tract features or comment
Congenital/inherited	
Atopic disease	Asthma, hay fever
Cutis laxa	Emphysema, cor pulmonale
Tuberous sclerosis	Rhabdomyomas
Neurofibromatosis	Kyphoscoliosis, intrathoracic neuromas, lung fibrosis, bullae
Ataxia–telangiectasia	Pneumonia, bronchiectasis, pulmonary fibrosis
Hereditary haemorrhagic telangiectasia	Haemoptysis, dyspnoea, cyanosis due to arteriovenous shunting
α_1-antitrypsin deficiency	Emphysema
Darier's disease	Lower lobe fibrosis, laryngeal involvement
Dyskeratosis congenital	Interstitial pneumonia, fibrosis
Lipoid proteinosis	Laryngeal involvement
Riley–Day syndrome	Lung infiltrate, pneumonia
Birt–Hogg–Dubé syndrome	Lung cysts, pneumothorax
Hyper-IgE syndrome	Abscesses, pneumonia
Infections and infestations	
Tuberculosis	Specific skin lesions, erythema nodosum
Mycobacterium avium–intracellulare infection	May disseminate to skin (usually in HIV infection)
Leprosy	Laryngeal involvement
Mycoplasma infection	Causes erythema multiforme (often mucosal)
Dissemination of pulmonary fungal infections	Blastomycosis, coccidioidomycosis, cryptococcosis, aspergillosis, histoplasmosis, melioidosis
Scrub typhus	Pneumonia (common)
Varicella	Pneumonia
Measles	Pneumonia
Larva migrans	Asthma/bronchitis with eosinophilia
Chronic mucocutaneous candidiasis	Bronchiectasis
Whipple's disease	Cough, pleural effusion, pulmonary infiltrate, hilar lymphadenopathy
Infiltrations and metabolic	
Histiocytoses (Langerhans' cell histiocytosis, Rosai–Dorfman disease, haematophagocytic syndrome, necrobiotic xanthogranuloma, sea-blue histiocytosis, others)	Pulmonary nodules and fibrosis, upper respiratory tract infiltration disease, xanthoma disseminatum
Amyloidosis	Cutaneous amyloid deposition secondary to chronic lung disease, lung infiltration in primary amyloidosis
POEMS	Pleural effusion, bronchospasm
Carcinoid syndrome	Bronchospasm
Hypothyroidism	Laryngeal involvement
Myxoma	Pleurisy
Inflammatory	
Sarcoidosis	Pulmonary fibrosis, hilar lymphadenopathy, laryngeal involvement, necrotizing sarcoid granulomatosis
Pulmonary vasculitides	See text (this section)
Systemic sclerosis	Interstitial fibrosis, pneumothorax, pulmonary hypertension (especially in CREST)
Sjögren's syndrome	Decreased secretions, sinusitis, bronchoalveolitis, interstitial lung disease
Lupus erythematosus	Pleuritis, pleural effusion, shrinking lungs syndrome
Mixed connective tissue disease	Fibrosing alveolitis (especially U_1 ribonucleoprotein antibody-positive)
Antiphospholipid syndrome	Pulmonary embolism, infarction, thrombosis, haemorrhage
Dermatomyositis	Muscular weakness, pharyngeal dysfunction (aspiration pneumonia), interstitial lung disease, bronchiolitis obliterans
Relapsing polychondritis	Tracheal collapse
Multicentric reticulohistiocytosis	May be associated with bronchial neoplasia, also lung infiltration, pleural effusion
Bullous diseases (epidermolysis bullosa, pemphigus, erythema multiforme/Stevens–Johnson syndrome/toxic epidermal necrolysis)	Upper respiratory tract involvement; paraneoplastic pemphigus is associated with intrathoracic disease, especially Castleman's disease, thymoma
Graft-versus-host disease	Restrictive defect, fibrosis
Pyoderma gangrenosum	Neutrophilic nodules in lung, tracheal pyoderma
Familial Mediterranean fever	Pleuritis

(Continued p. 62.82)

Table 62.16 *Continued*

Disease	Respiratory tract features or comment
Drugs	
Used in respiratory disease, causing rash	e.g. co-trimoxazole (drug eruptions)
May cause skin eruptions and respiratory tract disease	e.g. antibiotic-induced toxic epidermal necrolysis, cisplatin (bronchospasm, pigmentation)
Used for skin disease, respiratory side effects	e.g. isotretinoin (bronchospasm)
Miscellaneous	
Angio-oedema	Upper airway obstruction
Anaphylaxis	Bronchospasm
Pancreatitis	May cause basal pleural reaction, and cutaneous fat necrosis
Yellow nail syndrome	Pleural effusion, bronchiectasis
Mastocytosis	Rhinorrhoea, laryngeal oedema, bronchospasm
Tumours	Metastatic disease, Kaposi's sarcoma, lymphomatoid granulomatosis, extensive mycosis fungoides/Sézary syndrome, others

HIV, human immunodeficiency virus; POEMS, *polyneuropathy, organomegaly, endocrinopathy, M protein, skin changes (syndrome).*

in at least 50% of patients. Symptoms (exertional dyspnoea and cough) may be relatively late in presenting—pulmonary function tests including transfer factor should be measured. Pneumothorax, pleural effusion, respiratory muscle involvement and 'splinting' of the chest by sclerotic skin may all occur. Pulmonary vascular disease leading to pulmonary hypertension is a particular concern in CREST syndrome; this may be identified by transoesophageal echocardiography and treated with bosanten.

Over 50% of anti-U1RNP-positive patients with *systemic lupus erythematosus* (SLE) and about a quarter of those with *mixed connective tissue disease* may have pleurisy [16]. Involvement of the respiratory muscles may lead to diaphragmatic elevation and the *'shrinking lungs' syndrome* [17]. These conditions are discussed in more detail in Chapter 51. Pulmonary embolism, haemorrhage, infarction and hypertension may occur in patients with the *antiphospholipid syndrome* [18].

Relapsing polychondritis [19] is due to autoantibodies against type II collagen, and is a potentially fatal disease. Dyspnoea and inspiratory stridor occur due to swelling of the respiratory tract, and collapse of cartilages of the larynx and trachea, in over 50%. Costal cartilage is involved in one-third of cases. Inflamed nasal and auricular cartilages are present in most patients, with nasal obstruction, arthropathy and high erythrocyte sedimentation rate (ESR). The disorder may therefore mimic one of the vasculitides, such as Wegener's granulomatosis. The non-cartilaginous lobe of the ear is classically spared in relapsing polychondritis.

In *dermatomyositis*, there are three main mechanisms that provide a link with respiratory disease [20–22]. Firstly, dermatomyositis may occur as a consequence of bronchial carcinoma, the commonest malignancy associated with dermatomyositis in males [20]. Muscular weakness due to myositis may affect either the intercostal and thoracic musculature, or the larynx and pharynx—the latter may lead to aspiration pneumonia as a complication. Finally, interstitial lung disease or bronchiolitis obliterans may occur due to dermatomyositis. The lung disease is typically associated with the presence of antiaminoacyl-tRNA synthetase antibodies, notably anti-Jo-1, and with anti-tRNA antibodies such as anti-tRNA[his]. Patients with these antibodies only comprise 15–20% of

individuals with dermatomyositis, but most patients with lung disease have one of these antibodies. The antisynthetase syndrome consists of dermatomyositis (or polymyositis) with interstitial lung disease, arthritis and Raynaud's phenomenon [22]. Presence of antisynthetase antibodies is also associated with the clinical entity of 'mechanic's hands' in dermatomyositis, but they are not usually a feature of paraneoplastic dermatomyositis. Dermatomyositis may also indirectly be associated with lung disease as a consequence of treatment—either infection due to immunosuppression, or rarely drug-induced pneumonitis (methotrexate).

In *Sjögren's syndrome,* alveolitis can be demonstrated in about 50% of patients, but is often asymptomatic. Inspissated secretions may predispose to pneumonia; obstructive and interstitial lung disease may occur [23].

Vasculitis and neutrophilic dermatoses (see also Chapter 50)

Vasculitis of many types may affect the lung. The major pulmonary vasculitides are Wegener's granulomatosis, Churg–Strauss disease, polyarteritis nodosa and Behçet's disease [24].

Behçet's disease (Chapter 50). The frequency of lung involvement in Behçet's disease may be as high as 19%, although 5–10% is a more frequent estimate. Pleurisy or perihilar radiological opacities may be found [23], and pulmonary arterial aneurysm is an important feature, which can be fatal [25]. About 90% of patients with Behçet's disease complicated by pulmonary artery aneurysm also have thrombophlebitis.

Small-vessel vasculitis (Chapter 50). Any form of small-vessel vasculitis can also affect the lung, even urticarial vasculitis. In one large series, over 20% of patients with urticarial vasculitis had pulmonary disease, either chronic obstructive pulmonary disease or asthma. Although it is not clear that these were always causally related to the vasculitis, obstructive pulmonary disease was more frequent in the group of patients with hypocomplementaemia [26], and lung vasculitis or serological evidence of LE was demonstrated in over 50% of patients with lung disease.

Wegener's granulomatosis [27,28]. This is an uncommon disease. The 'classic' syndrome is characterized by necrotizing granulomatous vasculitis of the upper and lower respiratory tracts, necrotizing glomerulonephritis and disseminated vasculitis of various organs. Skin lesions are frequent, including vasculitis with purpura, subcutaneous nodules and ulcers (see also Chapter 50). Upper airway disease causes nasal discharge, ulceration and bleeding, and oral ulceration. Pulmonary changes are typical with bilateral infiltrate, nodules or cavities. Subglottic or tracheobronchostenosis may also occur. There is no hilar or mediastinal lymphadenopathy. Prognosis is poor in patients with lung or renal disease; chronic nasal staphylococcal carriage is also associated with a poorer prognosis. Treatment consists of immunosuppressive agents (cyclophosphamide, azathioprine, chlorambucil and methotrexate). Trimethoprim–sulfamethoxazole (co-trimoxazole) also appears to be of benefit in induction of remission [29]. Diffuse alveolar haemorrhage, due to extensive pulmonary capillaritis, is a life-threatening complication of Wegener's granulomatosis—it also occurs in microscopic polyangiitis, and more rarely in SLE, antiphospholipid syndrome, Behçet's disease and secondary to drugs such as D-penicillamine [30].

Churg–Strauss syndrome (allergic granulomatous angiitis) [27,28]. This rare condition comprises rhinitis, asthma, pneumonitis, fever, malaise, eosinophilia (usually over 10%) and widespread vasculitis, which may cause skin lesions, neuropathy and cardiac or less commonly renal disease. Cutaneous lesions include palpable purpura and nodular lesions. Distinction from Wegener's granulomatosis or microscopic polyangiitis may be difficult in the early stages—peripheral eosinophilia is the most useful discriminatory feature [31], but eosinophils in inflammatory infiltrates may occur in all three disorders (also in SLE and Sjögren's syndrome), as may mononeuritis multiplex. Cardiac disease is more frequent in Churg–Strauss syndrome than in Wegener's granulomatosis, but is not specific; a history of asthma and other allergies with the other features suggest Churg–Strauss syndrome [24,27]. There is some concern that leukotriene receptor antagonists may provoke Churg–Strauss syndrome in patients with asthma, although an alternative explanation is simply that disease progression or altered corticosteroid therapy allowed additional clinical features to become apparent [32,33]. Therapy consists of high-dose corticosteroids, if necessary with other immunosuppressive agents such as cyclophosphamide, azathioprine or chlorambucil.

PAN and microscopic polyangiitis (microscopic polyarteritis) [27]. These conditions are distinguished by the size of vessels affected and by the usual absence of antineutrophil cytoplasm antibodies against myeloperoxidase (MPO-ANCA) in 'classic' PAN. The term 'polyangiitis' is preferred to polyarteritis for the microscopic disease, as arterioles, venules and capillaries may all be affected. Lung disease is not a particular feature of classic PAN, although bronchial arteries can be affected. By contrast, microscopic polyangiitis has many similarities to Wegener's granulomatosis, including nasopharyngeal involvement, renal vasculitis and tendency to cause alveolar haemorrhage [27,30]. However, the presence of granulomas and proteinase 3-ANCA (which suggest

the diagnosis of Wegener's granulomatosis) help to distinguish these disorders.

Neutrophilic dermatoses (Chapter 50). Pulmonary and major airway involvement have been described with pyoderma gangrenosum and neutrophilic dermatoses [34–38], usually comprising focal, dense neutrophilic infiltrates with scattered radiological opacities. Tracheal lesions may occur. Endobronchial involvement may also occur in eosinophilic states such as the hypereosinophilic syndrome, although cardiac disease is more important in this condition.

Other systemic diseases

Sarcoidosis [39] is discussed in Chapter 61. Hilar lymphadenopathy occurs with erythema nodosum in acute sarcoidosis. Pulmonary involvement is the major feature in chronic sarcoidosis, about 30% of such patients also having skin lesions. *Necrotizing sarcoid granulomatosis* (also termed necrotizing sarcoid angiitis and granulomatosis) is a rare disorder that is in the differential diagnosis of Wegener's granulomatosis but is currently felt to be an arteritic variant of sarcoidosis [40]. In the respiratory system, a nodular pulmonary infiltrate is typical; extrapulmonary involvement is most commonly ophthalmological (uveitis or ophthalmoplegia) but other organs including the skin [41] may be involved and necrosis due to arteritic vascular occlusion may be a feature.

Multicentric reticulohistiocytosis is associated with pleural effusion and hilar lymphadenopathy [42]; it may also occur as a paraneoplastic phenomenon.

Scleromyxoedema has been associated with lung disease, causing dyspnoea, in a sixth of reported cases [43]. Pulmonary hypertension has been reported.

Amyloidosis (Chapter 59); involvement of the respiratory tract is common in primary amyloidosis. It may cause dyspnoea, but is often asymptomatic.

Lymphomatoid granulomatosis [44,45] is a rare lymphoproliferative disease which primarily affects the lung; radiology shows multiple, small nodules that predominantly affect the periphery of the lower lung fields. Cutaneous lesions are present in about 50% of cases, typically on the face, and consist of infiltrated flat or nodular lesions that may become necrotic and ulcerated. Histologically, there are necrotizing angiocentric lesions of various organs, with an infiltrate of atypical lymphocytes. Epstein–Barr virus infection has been demonstrated [46]. The condition behaves as a lymphoma with poor prognosis; corticosteroids and cyclophosphamide may help in some cases.

Miscellaneous

Yellow nail syndrome (MIM #153300). Associated respiratory features include recurrent pleural effusion, bronchiectasis and chronic infections such as empyema [47,48].

Paraneoplastic pemphigus (PNP). Respiratory failure in PNP is particularly important as it is frequently the cause of death in patients with this disorder. Pathologically, there is a diffuse segmental constrictive bronchiolitis of small bronchioles causing a bronchiolitis obliterans clinical picture. The mechanism may be due to autoantibody-mediated damage as direct immunofluorescence of bronchial mucosal biopsies may demonstrate linear deposition of IgG and complement in the lamina propria [49], although CD8[+] T lymphocytes may have a key role in this process [50], and underlying neoplasms, toxic effects of immunosuppressive therapy, and secondary infections may all be involved in some cases.

Hoarseness as a sign of systemic disease [51].

Hoarseness from laryngeal or tracheal involvement is an important audible sign of certain systemic diseases with skin involvement. Examples are pachyonychia congenita, de Lange's syndrome, Farber's disease, lipoid proteinosis, sarcoidosis, secondary syphilis, epidemic typhus, hypothyroidism, relapsing polychondritis, LE and dermatomyositis. Several inherited or acquired bullous diseases may affect the pharyngeal or laryngeal mucosa. Carcinoma of the larynx may complicate chronic inflammation.

References

1 Chan PH. Pulmonary carcinoma and provocative sweat testing. *Arch Dermatol* 1983; **119**: 185.

2 McCoy BP. Apical pulmonary adenocarcinoma with contralateral hyperhidrosis. *Arch Dermatol* 1981; **117**: 659–61.

3 Riccardi VM. *Neurofibromatosis*, 2nd edn. Baltimore: Johns Hopkins University Press, 1992.

4 Prakash UB. Respiratory manifestations of systemic disease: lower airways in systemic disease, 3. *Postgrad Med* 1984; **76**: 143–52.

5 Broughton RBK. Pulmonary tuberous sclerosis presenting with pleural effusion. *BMJ* 1970; **i**: 477–8.

6 Costello LC, Hartman TE, Ryu JH. High frequency of pulmonary lymphangioleiomyomatosis in women with tuberous sclerosis complex. *Mayo Clin Proc* 2000; **75**: 591–4.

7 Dellon AL, Peck GL, Chretien PB. Hypopharyngeal and laryngeal involvement with Darier disease. *Arch Dermatol* 1975; **111**: 744–6.

8 Edmunds BK, Hodge JA, Rietschel RL. Alpha-1-antitrypsin deficiency-associated panniculitis: case report and review of the literature. *Pediatr Dermatol* 1991; **8**: 296–9.

9 Fellner MJ. Manifestations of familial autonomic dysautonomia: report of a case with an analysis of 125 cases in the literature. *Arch Dermatol* 1964; **89**: 190–5.

10 Fishbein D, Grossman RF. Pulmonary manifestations of familial dysautonomia in an adult. *Am J Med* 1986; **80**: 709–13.

11 Grunebaum M. The 'chest–abdomen sign' in familial dysautonomia. *Br J Radiol* 1975; **48**: 23–7.

12 Canny GJ, Roifman C, Weitzman S et al. A pulmonary infiltrate in a child with ataxia telangiectasia. *Ann Allergy* 1988; **61**: 466–8.

13 Steck WD, Byrd RB. Urticaria secondary to pulmonary melioidosis: report of a case. *Arch Dermatol* 1969; **99**: 80–1.

14 Tuffanelli DL. Systemic sclerosis. In: Sontheimer RD, Provost TT, eds. *Cutaneous Manifestations of Rheumatic Diseases*. Baltimore: Williams and Wilkins, 1996: 115–39.

15 Wigley FM, Provost TT. Scleroderma. In: Provost TT, Flynn JA, eds. *Cutaneous Medicine: Cutaneous Manifestations of Systemic Disease*. Hamilton, Ontario: Decker, 2001: 104–26.

16 Provost TT, Flynn JA. Lupus erythematosus. In: Provost TT, Flynn JA, eds. *Cutaneous Medicine: Cutaneous Manifestations of Systemic Disease*. Hamilton, Ontario: Decker, 2001: 41–81.

17 Cavallasca JA, Dubinsky D, Nasswetter GG. Shrinking lungs syndrome, a rare manifestation of systemic lupus erythematosus. *Int J Dermatol* 2006; **60**: 1683–6.

18 Cuadrado MJ, Hughes GRV. Hughes (antiphospholipid) syndrome: clinical features. *Rheum Dis Clin* 2001; **27**: 507–24.

19 Braverman IM. *Skin Signs of Systemic Disease*, 3rd edn. Philadelphia: Saunders, 1998: 501–2.

20 Cox NH, Langtry JAA, Lawrence CM, Ive FA. Dermatomyositis: disease associations and an evaluation of screening investigations for malignancy. *Arch Dermatol* 1990; **126**: 61–5.

21 Euwer RL, Sontheimer RD. Dermatomyositis. In: Sontheimer RD, Provost TT, eds. *Cutaneous Manifestations of Rheumatic Diseases*. Baltimore: Williams and Wilkins, 1996: 73–114.

22 Hengstman GJD, van Engelen BGM, Vree Egberts WTM, van Venrooij WJ. Myositis-specific autoantibodies: overview and recent developments. *Curr Opin Rheumatol* 2001; **13**: 476–82.

23 Fox RI. Clinical features, pathogenesis, and treatment of Sjögren's syndrome. *Curr Opin Rheumatol* 1996; **8**: 438–45.

24 Chakravarty K. Vasculitis by organ systems. *Baillière's Clin Rheumatol* 1997; **11**: 357–93.

25 Hamuryudan H, Yurdakal S, Moral F et al. Pulmonary artery aneurysms in Behçet's syndrome: a report of 24 cases. *Br J Rheumatol* 1994; **33**: 48–51.

26 Mehregan DR, Hall MJ, Gibson LE. Urticarial vasculitis: a histopathologic and clinical review of 72 cases. *J Am Acad Dermatol* 1992; **26**: 441–8.

27 Gross WL. Systemic necrotizing vasculitis. *Baillière's Clin Rheumatol* 1997; **11**: 259–84.

28 Mouthon L, Lhote F, Guillevin L. Pulmonary vasculitides. In: Ansell BM, Bacon PA, Lie JT, Yazici H, eds. *The Vasculitides: Science and Practice*. London: Chapman & Hall Medical, 1996: 222–45.

29 Stegeman CA, Cohen Tervaert JW, de Jong PE, Kallenberg CGM. Trimethoprim-sulphamethoxazole (co-trimoxazole) for the prevention of relapses of Wegener's granulomatosis. *N Engl J Med* 1996; **335**: 16–20.

30 Specks U. Diffuse alveolar haemorrhage syndromes. *Curr Opin Rheumatol* 2001; **13**: 12–7.

31 Sorenson SF, Slot O, Tvede N et al. A prospective study of vasculitis patients collected in a five year period: evaluation of the Chapel Hill nomenclature. *Ann Rheum Dis* 2000; **59**: 478–82.

32 Wechsler ME, Garpestad E, Kocher O et al. Pulmonary infiltrates, eosinophilia and cardiomyopathy in patients with asthma receiving zafirlukast. *JAMA* 1988; **279**: 455–7.

33 Wechsler ME, Finn D, Gunawardena D et al. Churg–Strauss syndrome in patients receiving montelukast as treatment for asthma. *Chest* 2000; **117**: 708–13.

34 Vignon-Pennamen MD, Zelinsky-Gurung A, Janssen F et al. Pyoderma gangrenosum with pulmonary involvement. *Arch Dermatol* 1989; **125**: 1239–42.

35 Brown TS, Marshall GS, Callen JP. Cavitating pulmonary infiltrate in an adolescent with pyoderma gangrenosum: a rarely recognized extracutaneous manifestation of a neutrophilic dermatosis. *J Am Acad Dermatol* 2000; **43**: 108–12.

36 Merke DP, Honig PJ, Potsic WP. Pyoderma gangrenosum of the skin and trachea in a 9-month-old boy. *J Am Acad Dermatol* 1996; **34**: 681–2.

37 Lazarus AA, McMillan M, Miramadi A. Pulmonary involvement in Sweet's syndrome (acute febrile neutrophilic dermatosis). *Chest* 1986; **90**: 922–4.

38 Bourke SJ, Quinn AG, Farr PM et al. Neutrophilic alveolitis in Sweet's disease. *Thorax* 1992; **47**: 572–3.

39 English JC 3rd, Patel PJ, Greer KE. Sarcoidosis. *J Am Acad Dermatol* 2001; **44**: 725–43.

40 Quaden C, Tillie-Leblond I, Delobbe A et al. Necrotising sarcoid granulomatosis: clinical, functional, endoscopical and radiographical evaluations. *Eur Respir J* 2005; **26**: 778–85.

41 Shirodaria CC, Nicholson AG, Hansell DM et al. Lesson of the month: necrotising sarcoid granulomatosis with skin involvement. *Histopathology* 2003; **43**: 91–3.

42 Lesher JL Jr, Allen BS. Multicentric reticulohistiocytosis. *J Am Acad Dermatol* 1984; **11**: 713–23.

43 Rongioletti F, Rebora A. Updated classification of papular mucinosis, lichen myxedematosus, and scleromyxedema. *J Am Acad Dermatol* 2001; **44**: 273–81.

44 Braverman IM. *Skin Signs of Systemic Disease*, 3rd edn. Philadelphia: Saunders, 1998: 117.

45 James WD, Odom RB, Katzenstein AL. Cutaneous manifestations of lymphomatoid granulomatosis: report of 44 cases and a review of literature. *Arch Dermatol* 1981; **117**: 196–202.

46 Guinee D Jr, Jaffe E, Kingma D et al. Pulmonary lymphomatoid granulomatosis: evidence for a proliferation of Epstein–Barr virus infected B lymphocytes with a prominent T-cell component and vasculitis. *Am J Surg Pathol* 1994; **18**: 753–64.

47 Tosti A, Baran R, Dawber RPR. The nail in systemic diseases and drug-induced changes. In: Baran R, Dawber RPR, Deberker DAR, Haneke E, Tosti A, eds. *Diseases of the Nails and Their Management*. Oxford: Blackwell Science, 2001: 249–51.

48 Lodge JP, Hunter AM, Saunders NR. Yellow nail syndrome associated with empyema. *Clin Exp Dermatol* 1989; **14**: 328–9.

49 Nousari HC, Deterding R, Wotjczack H *et al*. The mechanism of respiratory failure in paraneoplastic pemphigus. *New Engl J Med* 1999; **340**: 1406–10.

50 Hoffman MA, Qiao X, Anhalt GJ. CD8+ T lymphocytes in bronchiolitis obliterans, paraneoplastic pemphigus, and solitary Castleman's disease. *New Engl J Med* 2003; **349**: 407–8.

51 Bernhard JD. Non-rashes, 4: audible signs of cutaneous disease. *Cutis* 1983; **31**: 189–90.

Haematology [1]

Disorders of the blood components and the coagulation system may have striking cutaneous and mucosal signs and symptoms and sometimes are the presenting features of haematological disease, and these will be elaborated in this section.

Erythrocyte disorders

Anaemia

Anaemia from any cause will result eventually in pallor of the skin and mucous membranes, traditionally appreciated in the palmar creases of the hand and mucous membranes of the palpebral conjunctivae and mouth. Constitutional symptoms such as fatigue, breathlessness, dizziness and postural hypotension are more likely to occur the more acutely that the anaemia has developed. Many nutritional anaemias (see also Chapter 59) develop slowly, and physiological adaptation may account for the relatively minor symptoms despite marked reduction in the haemoglobin concentration in some instances. Palmar crease erythema will be evident until the haemoglobin concentration is around 7 g/dl.

Iron deficiency. This results from an inability to absorb sufficient iron to match bodily iron losses. Many cases result from both increased losses, either overtly, as in heavy menstrual blood loss or frequent and heavy nose bleeds, or covertly, such as with intestinal blood loss from hook worm infestation, tumours or other vessel abnormalities such as angiodyspasia, coupled with inadequate dietary iron intake. Intestinal malabsorbtion due to coeliac disease (coeliac sprue) often produces a mixed iron and folic acid deficiency.

The mucocutaneous signs [2,3] of iron deficiency include pallor, koilonychia or spooning of the nail plate, diffuse hair thinning and pruritus. A burning sensation of the tongue (glossodynia) and cravings for eating unpalatable substances (pica) are described in iron deficiency.

Iron deficiency is particularly liable to develop in hereditary haemorrhagic telangiectasia and the blue rubber bleb naevus syndrome due to either nasal or gastrointestinal blood loss from vascular abnormalities in these conditions. Chronic blood loss from vascular abnormalities in the gut in pseudoxanthoma elasticum results in iron deficiency, though blood loss may be more acute and present with melaena [4]. Anaemia may occur in dermatitis herpetiformis due to both iron and folic acid malabsorbtion complicating the associated gluten sensitive enteropathy, compounded also by dapsone-induced haemolysis [5].

Megaloblastic anaemias. These are due to impaired DNA synthesis, and the most common causes are either vitamin B_{12} or folic acid deficiency. Antimetabolite drugs are a potential cause, macrocytosis due to hydroxcarbamide being the most familiar to the dermatologist; drugs such as folate antagonists (trimethoprim) and anticonvulsants are less common causes.

As the onset of megaloblastic anaemias is insidious, symptoms may only be evident when anaemia is marked. A mild haemolysis resulting in a type of jaundice may give the patient a lemon yellow hue. Hyperpigmentation of the feet, hands and face is reported. Megaloblastic anaemia due to vitamin B_{12} deficiency has been reported to produce a partially reversible poikiloderma. Premature greying of the hair (canities) is associated with pernicious anaemia [6]. Loss of lingual filiform papillae and cheilitis are common. Neurological symptoms, leading ultimately to subacute combined degeneration of the spinal cord, may prompt cutaneous symptoms such as paraesthesiae and loss of sensation in the skin.

Vitamin B_{12} deficiency usually results from pernicious anaemia; antiparietal cell antibodies (present in 70% of cases) destroy the cells that produce intrinsic factor needed to absorb the vitamin. There is an association between other autoimmune disorders, such as vitiligo and Addison's disease, and dermatological manifestations; these diseases, and testing for their relevant antibodies, should always be considered. Rarely, vitamin B_{12} deficiency is the result of terminal ileal disease, such as Crohn's disease, fish tape worm or ileal resection.

Folic acid deficiency is usually the result of inadequate dietary intake due to poor nutrition, but may occur in times of increased metabolic requirement, such as pregnancy. Dermatological causes of folate deficiency include erythroderma, particularly due to psoriasis [7], and in such situations it is prudent to check folate levels prior to administering folate antagonists such as methotrexate (discussed further in Chapters 20 and 74).

Haemoglobinopathies and haemolytic anaemias

Both sickle cell disease and thalassaemia have important cutaneous manifestations due to the underlying diseases and their therapies. Lower leg ulceration, which may start in childhood and be both recalcitrant and recurrent, is a major burden; ulcers may be the first manifestation of milder disease [8,9]. Ulceration occurs with a prevalence of 2.5% in sickle disease, being more common in sickle and sickle thalassaemia, but does not occur in sickle C disease. Ulcers are more common in men and prevalence increases with age. In sickle disease there is a strong association with venous incompetence; leg elevation and compression hosiery are thus important aspects of treatment. Spherocytosis may also be complicated by leg ulcers [10].

Thalassaemia requires multiple blood transfusions and haemosiderosis with slate-grey skin pigmentation may be a consequence.

Both chronic sickle cell anaemia and thalassaemia can be associated with a condition similar to familial pseudoxanthoma elasticum (PXE) [11]. As well as the characteristic features of PXE, including yellow papular and plaque lesions on the neck (the 'plucked chicken skin'), axillae and antecubital fossae, retinal angioid streaks may be present. Associated mitral valve prolapse indicates the general and widespread nature of the elastin disorder seen in haemoglobinopathy-associated PXE-like disease.

Hydroxcarbamide has become an important therapy for sickle disease. Its chronic use has numerous dermatological complications, including a dermatomyositis-like eruption affecting the dorsal hands and face (hydroxycarbamide dermopathy), painful ulcers on feet and ankles, nail pigmentation and cutaneous malignancies [12].

Polycythaemia

Defined as an increase in the red cell mass, polycythaemia can be a primary disorder (polycythaemia vera; PV) or secondary. The secondary form is usually due to chronic hypoxaemia, but rarely may be due to erythropoietin production by renal tumours or exogenous administration of erythropoietin (such as illicit use by athletes). Polycythaemia vera is believed to be a stem cell disorder due to mutation of the Janus kinase 2 gene (*JAK2*). Splenomegaly and an elevation of both the total white cell and platelet counts usually develop; this, and an elevated leukocyte alkaline phosphatase, help distinguish PV from other causes of polycythaemia. As *JAK2* mutations occur in 95% of cases, and can now be readily identified, genotyping has replaced more complex tests previously used to estimate total red cell mass. *JAK2* mutations are also found in about 50% of cases of essential thrombocythaemia and chronic myeloid leukaemia.

The most important consequences of PV are an increased tendency to thrombosis (resulting in stroke and hepatic vein thrombosis) or bleeding. Hyperhomocysteinaemia is a risk factor for thrombosis. Dermatological features may include skin changes due to peripheral vascular disease and deep vein thrombosis, leg ulcers, digital gangrene and erythromelalgia (burning erythema of the extremities, usually the feet, on warming).

Pruritus is common in PV [13], and aquagenic pruritus, an intense disabling itching after water exposure, may antedate the onset of polycythaemia by several years [14]. Itching may persist even after restoration of the red cell mass to normal. Venesection is used to reduce the red cell mass followed by the use of hydroxycarbamide to maintain blood parameters. However this drug may induce dermopathy. Therapy with either radioactive phosphorus, or alkylating agents, is used less than previously, as both treatments are associated with the development of leukaemia. Aquagenic and spontaneous pruritus may improve with emollients, topical antipruritics, oral antihistamines, UVB or PUVA phototherapy, recombinant interferon-α or opioid antagonists such as naltrexone. Repeated venesection may lead to iron deficiency, and this should be excluded as a cause of itch. A superficial pustular dermatosis, nosologically thought to be a superficial variant of Sweet's syndrome, has been described in PV [15].

References

1 Hoffbrand AV, Pettit JE. *Clinical Haematology Illustrated*. Edinburgh: Churchill Livingstone, 1987.
2 Vickers CF. Nutrition and skin: iron deficiency. In: Ledingham JC, ed. *Proceedings of the Tenth Symposium on Advanced Medicine*. London: Pitman, 1974: 311–6.
3 Sato S. Iron deficiency: structural and microchemical changes in hair, nails, and skin. *Semin Dermatol* 1991; **10**: 313–9.
4 Spinzi G, Strocchi E, Imperiali G *et al*. Pseudoxanthoma elasticum: a rare cause of gastrointestinal bleeding. *Am J Gastroenterol* 1996; **91**: 1631–4.
5 Cream JJ, Scott L. Anaemia in dermatitis herpetiformis: the role of dapsone induced haemolysis and malabsorption. *Br J Dermatol* 1970; **82**: 333–42.
6 Noppakun N, Swasdikul D. Reversible hyperpigmentation of skin and nails with white hair due to vitamin B12 deficiency. *Arch Dermatol* 1986; **122**: 896–9.
7 Shuster S, Marks J. *The Systemic Effects of Skin Disease*. London: Heinemann, 1970.
8 Clare A, FitzHenley M, Harris J *et al*. Chronic leg ulceration in homozygous sickle cell disease: the role of venous incompetence. *Br J Haematol* 2002; **119**: 567–71.
9 Gimmon Z, Wexler MR, Rachmilewitz EA. Juvenile leg ulceration in beta-thalassemia major and intermedia. *Plast Reconstr Surg* 1982; **69**: 320–5.
10 Lawrence P, Aronson I, Saxe N, Jacobs P. Leg ulcers in hereditary spherocytosis. *Clin Exp Dermatol* 1991; **16**: 28–30.
11 Aessopos A, Farmakis D, Loukopoulos D. Elastic tissue abnormalities resembling pseudoxanthoma elasticum in beta thalassemia and the sickling syndromes. *Blood* 2002; **99**: 30–5.
12 Young HS, Khan AS, Kendra JR, Coulson IH. The cutaneous side-effects of hydroxyurea. *Clin Lab Haematol* 2000; **22**: 229–32.
13 Diehn F, Tefferi A. Pruritus in polycythaemia vera: prevalence, laboratory correlates and management. *Br J Haematol* 2001; **115**: 619–21.
14 du Peloux Menage H, Greaves MW. Aquagenic pruritus. *Semin Dermatol* 1995; **14**: 313–6.
15 Grob JJ, Mege JL, Prax AM, Bonerandi JJ. Disseminated pustular dermatosis in polycythemia vera. Relationship with neutrophilic dermatosis of myeloproliferative disorders: study of neutrophil function. *J Am Acad Dermatol* 1988; **18**: 1212–8.

Leukocyte disorders

Neutrophils

Neutrophilia commonly occurs with infections and as a response to a variety of skin disorders including erythroderma, pustular psoriasis and erythema multiforme, and as a result of systemic corticosteroid administration.

Acute febrile neutrophilic dermatosis (Sweets's syndrome; Chapter 50) [1] has neutrophilia as one of its diagnostic criteria, and may be associated with infection, myelodysplasia, polycythaemia, leukaemia, lymphomas, myeloma and paraproteinaemia as well as solid cancers. Superficial pustular variants have been reported in chronic myeloid leukaemia, and the dorsal hand variety in polycythaemia vera. Sweet's syndrome, subcorneal pustular dermatosis, superficial bullous pyoderma gangrenosum, conventional pyoderma gangrenosum and erythema elevatum diutinum are felt to be a continuum of neutrophilic disorders that may be associated with a neutrophilia or with myelodysplasia, myelofibrosis and myeloid leukaemia.

Eosinophils

Eosinophilia of the blood is a frequent finding in parasitic helminth infestation of the gut and the skin (for example, in larva migrans or onchocerciasis) and in non-helminth infestations such as scabies. Worldwide, infestations are the commonest cause of eosinophilia. In developed areas of the world, allergic causes predominate. Severe atopic dermatitis is often accompanied by a marked eosinophilia; immunobullous diseases such as pemphigoid and pemphigus, even in their prebullous phase, may be accompanied by an eosinophilia, as may allergic drug reactions. Conditions of particular dermatological interest associated with eosinophilia are listed in Table 62.17, and are discussed below.

Churg–Strauss syndrome (Chapter 50) [2]. Asthma and rhinitis, haemorrhagic palpable purpuric lesions and granulomatous

Table 62.17 Some dermatologically relevant causes of peripheral blood eosinophilia.

Category	Examples
Infestation and infection	Scabies
	Strongyloides
	Helminths
	Other parasitic infections
	Insect bites, reactions to stings
	HIV/AIDS (especially if late stage)
Allergic/atopic	Atopic dermatitis
	Allergic reactions
	Episodic angioedema with eosinophilia
	Other urticaria and angioedema
Immunobullous	Bullous pemphigoid
	Pemphigoid gestationis
Vasculitis (Chapter 50)	Churg-Strauss syndrome
	Wegener's granulomatosis (some)
	Polyarteritis nodosa (some)
	Eosinophilic vasculitis
	Drug-induced vasculitis
	Granuloma faciale (some)
Other inflammatory conditions	Eosinophilic cellulitis (Wells' syndrome)
	Eosinophilic fasciitis (Shulman syndrome)
	Eosinophilic panniculitis
	Eosinophilic mastitis
	Eosinophilia myalgia syndrome
	Toxic oil syndrome
	Chronic graft-versus-host disease
	Eosinophilic pustular folliculitis (Ofuji disease)
	Eosinophilic folliculitis of HIV infection
	Connective tissue disorders (some)
	Sarcoidosis (rarely)
	Erythema annulare centrifugum and annular erythema of infancy (some cases)
	Incontinentia pigmenti
	Pyoderma vegetans
Medications	Many cutaneous drug reactions (Chapter 75)
	Granulocyte-monocyte colony stimulating factor
	Other cytokine infusions
	Capillary leak syndrome
Neoplastic/clonal/ proliferative	Hypereosinophilic syndrome (Gleich syndrome)
	Cutaneous T cell lymphoma
	Hodgkin's lymphoma
	Myeloproliferative disorders/leukaemias
	Systemic mastocytosis
Idiopathic/miscellaneous	Cholesterol emolization syndrome
	Angiolymphoid hyperplasia with eosinophilia
	Addison's disease (some)

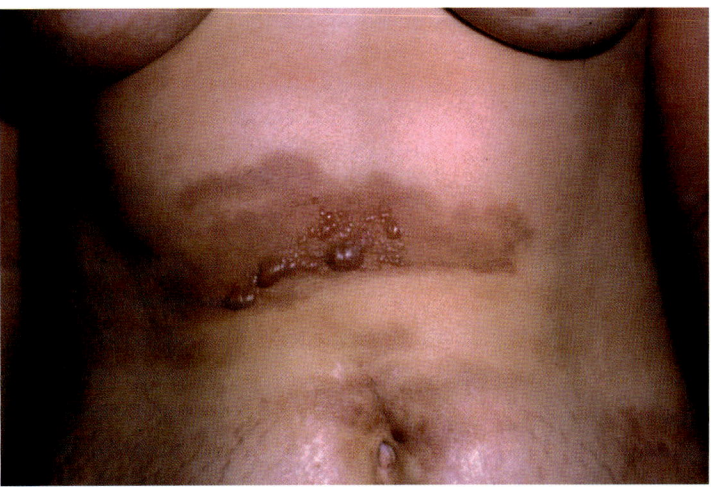

Fig. 62.27 Eosinophilic cellulitis. Lesions may be bullous and often resolve to leave a green discoloration of the skin.

fascia and a circulating eosinophilia. The absence of Raynaud's phenomenon differentiates it from scleroderma.

Eosinophilia myalgia syndrome [4]. A fibrotic condition similar to eosinophilic fasciitis, but induced by ingestion of tryptophan.

Eosinophilic cellulitis (Wells' syndrome; Fig. 62.27) [5]. This typically presents as an indurated erythematous plaque, which sometimes blisters, mimicking bacterial cellulitis; histologically, it is characterized by a dense, eosinophilic dermal infiltrate and eosinophilic flame figures. Eosinophilia is usual during episodic exacerbations of the cellulitis, and usually resolves to the normal range between attacks.

Hypereosinophilic syndrome (HES; Gleich syndrome) [6,7]. This condition is characterized by an eosinophilia in excess of 1500/µl (but usually greatly in excess of this), with no apparent cause, for greater than 6 months, and with presumptive signs of multiple organ involvement. Although traditionally viewed as idiopathic, recent evidence suggests that the entity may include more than one form of haematological malignancy [8]. In some instances, there is a clonal T-cell production of interleukin (IL)-5, a major controlling cytokine in production, release and differentiation of eosinophils. In other cases, there is clonal expansion of eosinophils with hepatosplenomegaly and thrombocytopenia; this condition appears to be due to a cytogenetic defect t(9;22)(q34;q11) in which there is chromosomal breakage and reciprocal exchange of chromosomal fragments that leads to formation of a fusion tyrosine kinase FIP1L1–PDGFRα.

The disease most commonly affects middle-aged men and the morbidity and mortality is related to endomyocardial fibrosis, eosinophilic vasculitis, thrombosis and embolic phenomena [9–12]. Skin lesions are varied and include vesicles, petechiae, papules and papulonodules, angio-oedema, livedo reticularis, erythema annulare, Raynaud's phenomenon, digital ischaemia, acrocyanosis, cutaneous microthrombi and gangrene. The pathology of the skin lesions may be non-specific with variable eosinophilic infiltration; cutaneous microthrombi may be a clue to the disease.

plaques on the elbows and knees, weight loss, arthralgias and pulmonary infiltrates are the characteristic findings. p-ANCA is frequently but not always positive; eosinophilia in excess of 10% is a diagnostic criterion.

Eosinophilic fasciitis (Chapter 51) [3]. A fibrosing condition usually affecting the limbs, due to inflammation and fibrosis of the fascia, associated with an eosinophilic infiltration of the

Eosinophilic cellulitis with florid eosinophilic infiltration and flame figures has been reported.

Newer treatments combined with identification of the causative abnormality may allow targeted therapy; imatinib mesylate, used mainly in treatment of chronic myelogenous leukaemia, targets the platelet-derived growth factor receptor (PDGFR) in the fusion tyrosine kinase of HES [13], described above, and mepolizumab, an anti-IL-5 monoclonal antibody, has also been used recently to treat HES [14].

Haematological malignances

Leukaemia
Leukaemias can cause a huge array of cutaneous symptoms and signs, some of which are common and non-specific (e.g. purpura due to thrombocytopenia), some of which are relatively uncommon but specific (e.g. leukaemia cutis), and some of which are both rare and non-specific (e.g. numb chin due to acute lymphoblastic leukaemic cells infiltrating the mental nerve). Some of the dermatologically relevant features of leukaemia are listed in Table 62.18.

Leukaemia can infiltrate the skin, where it is termed leukaemia cutis [15]. This is uncommon, and although it may occur in any

Table 62.18 Skin lesions in leukaemia.

Category	Examples
Specific lesions	Leukaemia cutis
	Chloroma
	Granulocytic sarcoma
Paraneoplastic phenomena	Sweet's syndrome (including GCSF-induced and ATRA-induced) [23,24]
	Neutrophilic dermatosis of the dorsal hands (Fig. 62.28) [25]
	Pyoderma gangrenosum [23]
	Subcorneal pustular dermatosis [22]
	Erythema elevatum diutinum [26]
	Neutrophilic eccrine hidradenitis [27]
	Vasculitis [19,28]
	Eosinophilic pustular folliculitis [29]
	Erythroderma [22]
Secondary to disordered immune or white cell function	Infections:
	bacterial e.g. ecthyma gangrenosum
	viral e.g. herpetic infections (especially chronic herpes simplex or disseminated herpes zoster)
	fungal e.g. candidosis, zygomycosis
Due to other haematological parameters	Bruising, purpura
Conditions associated with leukaemias	Increased incidence of basal cell carcinoma and squamous cell carcinoma in chronic lymphocytic leukaemia [29]
	Association of juvenile chronic myelomonocytic leukaemia with juvenile xanthogranuloma and neurofibromatosis type 1 (pp. 62.23 and 62.96)
Due to treatment	Drug eruptions
	Neutrophilic eccrine hidradenitis
	Graft-versus-host disease (p. 62.96)
	Effects of cytopenia, infections etc as above

leukaemia, it is commoner in acute monocytic and myelomonocytic disease. Skin infiltration can occur in any chronic leukaemia, including chronic myeloid, chronic lymphocytic, hairy cell and the leukaemic phase of non-Hodgkin's lymphoma. It tends to be a late manifestation of acute leukaemias, and may herald a blast transformation of chronic leukaemia. There is a strong association of leukaemia cutis with other extramedullary disease. Lesions are usually painless, evolving from patches to plaques and nodules and may ulcerate (see Fig. 62.6).

Aleukaemic leukaemia cutis, where there is evidence of leukaemic skin infiltration before evidence of leukaemia in the peripheral blood, is reported, and lesions may be mistaken initially for a high-grade lymphoma. Congenital leukaemia cutis is more common in congenital myeloid leukaemia where purple 'blueberry muffin' lesions may mimic congenital infection [16]. An important differential diagnosis occurs in neonates with Down's syndrome, who may develop a leukaemic blood picture and vesicopustular skin eruption as a transient myeloproliferative disorder (leukaemoid reaction) [17,18]. Vasculitis has been noted in some lesions of leukaemia cutis with vascular injury being mediated by blast cells [19]. Leukaemia cutis due to juvenile myelomonocytic leukaemia has been reported to mimic chilblains [20], and chilblain-like lesions have been reported in various forms of adult leukaemia [21]. Non-specific skin lesions and reactions (such as erythroderma) can occur as a paraneoplastic phenomenon in leukaemia; a variety of paraneoplastic syndromes associated with haematological malignancy are summarized in [22].

Myelodysplastic syndrome (MDS)
This refers to a closely related group of disorders characterized by ineffective blood cell production that may affect either erythrocytic, granulocytic or megakaryocytic cell lines. Myelodysplastic syndrome can occur at any age but is more common in older men. It represents a clonal haematopoietic disorder and after a variable time may progress to an acute myelogenous leukaemia.

A variety of skin disorders are associated with MDS, neutrophilic dermatoses (Fig. 62.28) being the best known [22,23]

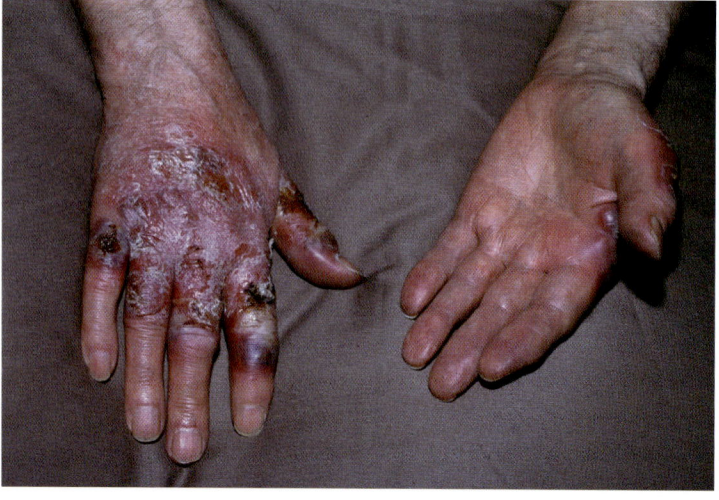

Fig. 62.28 Neutrophilic dermatosis of the dorsal hands in a patient with myelodysplastic syndrome.

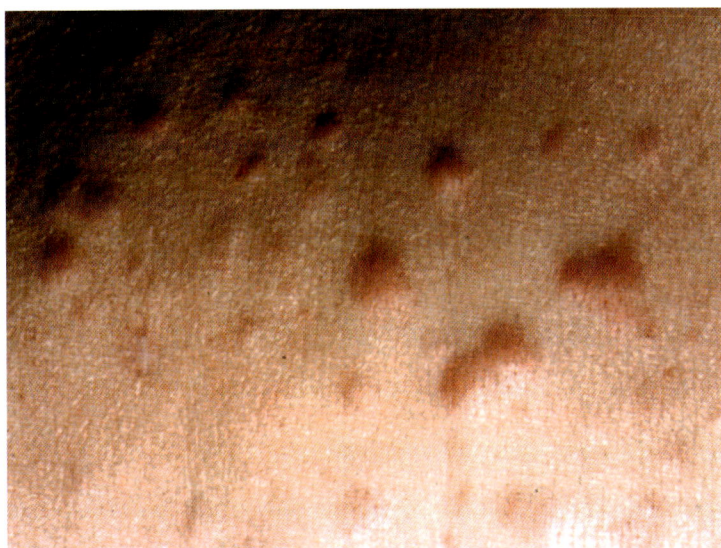

Fig. 62.29 Cutaneous extramedullary haematopoiesis in myelofibrosis. (Courtesy of Dr C. Blasdale, Sunderland Royal Infirmary, UK.)

(Chapter 50). Vasculitis [30], extramedullary haemopoiesis (Fig. 62.29) [31], reactive angioendotheliomatosis [32] and prurigo [33] have been reported. A significant proportion of patients with relapsing polychondritis have MDS [34]. Erythroderma [22] and erythromelalgia [22] may both occur.

References

1 Neoh CY, Tan AW, Ng SK. Sweet's syndrome: a spectrum of unusual clinical presentations and associations. *Br J Dermatol* 2007; **156**: 480–5.
2 Vogel PS, Nemer J, Sau P, Hnatiuk O. Churg–Strauss syndrome. *J Am Acad Dermatol* 1992; **27**: 821–4.
3 Helfman T, Falanga V. Eosinophilic fasciitis. *Clin Dermatol* 1994; **12**: 449–55.
4 Blackburn WD Jr. Eosinophilia myalgia syndrome. *Semin Arthritis Rheum* 1997; **26**: 788–93.
5 Ling TC, Antony F, Holden CA *et al*. Two cases of bullous eosinophilic cellulitis. *Br J Dermatol* 2002; **146**: 160–1.
6 Weller PF. The idiopathic hypereosinophilic syndrome. *Arch Dermatol* 1996; **132**: 583–5.
7 Fujii K, Tanabe H, Kanno Y *et al*. Eosinophilic cellulitis as a cutaneous manifestation of idiopathic hypereosinophilic syndrome. *J Am Acad Dermatol* 2003; **49**: 1174–7.
8 Schwartz RS. The hypereosinophilic syndrome and the biology of cancer. *N Engl J Med* 2003; **348**: 1199–200.
9 Jang K-A, Lim Y-S, Choi J-H *et al*. Hypereosinophilic syndrome presenting as cutaneous necrotizing eosinophilic vasculitis and Raynaud's phenomenon complicated by digital gangrene. *Br J Dermatol* 2000; **143**: 641–4.
10 Hamada T, Kimura Y, Hayashi S *et al*. Hypereosinophilic syndrome with peripheral circulatory insufficiency and cutaneous microthrombi. *Arch Dermatol* 2007; **143**: 812–3.
11 Oppliger R, Gay-Crosier F, Dayer E, Hauser C. Digital necrosis in a patient with hypereosinophilic syndrome in the absence of cutaneous eosinophilic vasculitis. *Br J Dermatol* 2001; **144**: 1087–90.
12 Kim SH, Kim TB, Yun YS *et al*. Hypereosinophilia presenting as eosinophilic vasculitis and multiple peripheral artery occlusions without organ involvement. *J Korean Med Sci* 2005; **20**: 677–9.
13 Cools J, DeAngelo DJ, Gotlib J *et al*. A tyrosine kinase created by fusion of the PDGFRA and FIP1L1 genes as a therapeutic target of imatinib in idiopathic hypereosinophilic syndrome. *N Engl J Med* 2003; **348**: 1201–14.
14 Rothenberg ME, Klion AD, Roufosse FE *et al*. Treatment of patients with the hypereosinophilic syndrome with mepolizumab. *N Engl J Med* 2008; **358**: 1215–28.
15 Desch JK, Smoller BR. The spectrum of cutaneous disease in leukemias. *J Cutan Pathol* 1993; **20**: 407–10.
16 Bresters D, Reus AC, Veerman AJ *et al*. Congenital leukaemia: the Dutch experience and review of the literature. *Br J Haematol* 2002; **117**: 513–24.
17 Solky BA, Yang FC, Xu X, Levins P. Transient myeolproliferatve disorder causing a vesicopustular eruption in a phenotypically normal neonate. *Pediatr Dermatol* 2004; **21**: 551–4.
18 Burch JM, Weston WL, Rogers M, Morelli JG. Vutaneous pustular leukaemoid reactions in trisomy 21. *Pediatr Dermatol* 2003; **20**: 232–7.
19 Jones D, Dorfman DM, Barnhill RL, Granter SR. Leukemic vasculitis: a feature of leukemia cutis in some patients. *Am J Clin Pathol* 1997; **107**: 637–42.
20 Affleck AG, Ravenscroft JC, Leach IH. Chilblain-like leukemia cutis. *Pediatr Dermatol* 2007; **24**: 38–41.
21 Yazawa H, Saga K, Omori F *et al*. The chilblain-like eruption as a diagnostic clue to the blast crisis of chronic myelocytic leukaemia. *J Am Acad Dermatol* 2004; **50** (Suppl.): S42–4.
22 Zappasodi P, Del Forno C, Corso A, Lazzarino M. Mucocutaneous paraneoplastic syndromes in hematologic malignancies. *Int J Dermatol* 2006; **45**: 14–22.
23 Lear JT, Atherton MT, Byrne JP. Neutrophilic dermatoses: pyoderma gangrenosum and Sweet's syndrome. *Postgrad Med J* 1997; **73**: 65–8.
24 Cox NH, O'Brien HAW. Sweet's syndrome associated with *trans*-retinoic acid treatment in acute promyelocytic leukemia. *Clin Exp Dermatol* 1994; **19**: 51–2.
25 Walling HW, Snipes CJ, Gerami P, Piette WW. The relationship between neutrophilic dermatosis of the dorsal hands and Sweet syndrome: report of 9 cases and comparison to atypical pyoderma gangrenosum. *Arch Dermatol* 2006; **142**: 57–63.
26 Delaporte E, Alfandari S, Fenaux P *et al*. H Erythema elevatum diutinum and chronic lymphocytic leukemia. *Clin Exp Dermatol* 1994; **19**: 188.
27 Pierson JC, Helm TN, Taylor JS *et al*. Neutrophilic eccrine hidradenitis heralding the onset of acute myelogenous leukemia. *Arch Dermatol* 1993; **129**: 791–2.
28 Bachmeyer C, Wetterwald E, Aractingi S. Cutaneous vasculitis in the course of hematologic malignancies. *Dermatology* 2005; **210**: 8–14.
29 Agnew KL, Ruchlemer R, Catovsky D *et al*. Cutaneous findings in chronic lymphocytic leukaemia. *Br J Dermatol* 2004; **150**: 1129–35.
30 O'Donnell BF, Williams HC, Carr R. Myelodysplastic syndrome presenting as cutaneous vasculitis. *Clin Exp Dermatol* 1995; **20**: 439–42.
31 Haniffa MA, Wilkins BS, Blasdale C, Simpson NB. Cutaneous extramedullary hemopoiesis in chronic myeloproliferative and myelodysplastic disorders. *J Am Acad Dermatol* 2006; **55**: S28–31.
32 del Pozo J, Martinez W, Sacristan F *et al*. Reactive angioendotheliomatosis associated with myelodysplastic syndrome. *Acta Derm Venereol* 2005; **85**: 269–70.
33 Aractingi S, Bachmeyer C, Miclea JM *et al*. Unusual specific cutaneous lesions in myelodysplastic syndromes. *J Am Acad Dermatol* 1995; **33**: 187–91.
34 Myers B, Gould J, Dolan G. Relapsing polychondritis and myelodysplasia: a report of two cases and review of the current literature. *Clin Lab Haematol* 2000; **22**: 45–8.

Lymphoma

After the gastrointestinal tract, the skin is the commonest organ to be affected by malignant lymphomas. Most lymphomas are of the cutaneous T-cell variety, but the cutaneous B cell form constitutes up to a third of primary skin lymphomas.

The skin may be infiltrated by metastatic nodal lymphoma; in Hodgkin's disease direct infiltration from underlying nodes may produce a scrofuloderma-like appearance [1,2].

Lymphoma may produce a number of paraneoplastic phenomena; itch, which may be intractable and severe, was found in 8% of a large series of patients with Hodgkin's disease and it purported a relatively poor prognosis. Mild itch was present in almost a quarter of the patients at diagnosis [3]. Eczema, excoriations, prurigo and reactive perforating collagenosis have also been reported [4]. Cutaneous T-cell lymphoma appears to be more common in Hodgkin's disease [5]. Acrokeratosis paraneoplastic (Bazex syndrome), more commonly associated with solid respiratory tract neoplasia, may occur with Hodgkin's disease [6].

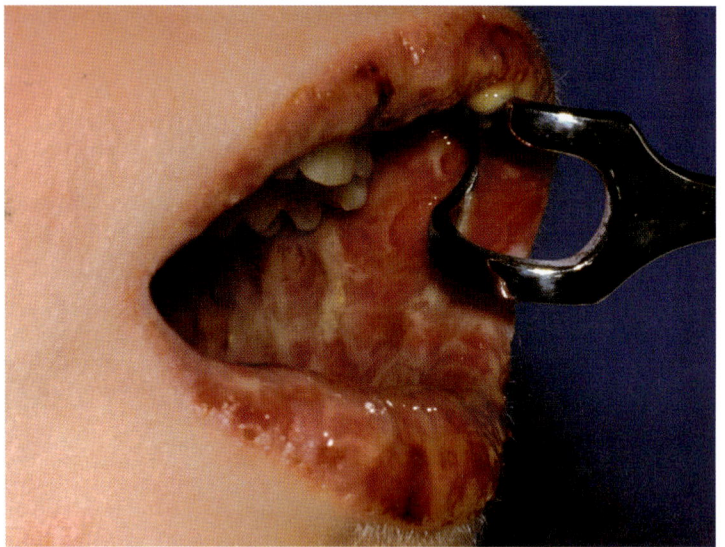

Fig. 62.30 Paraneoplastic pemphigus of the mouth and lips in Castleman's disease.

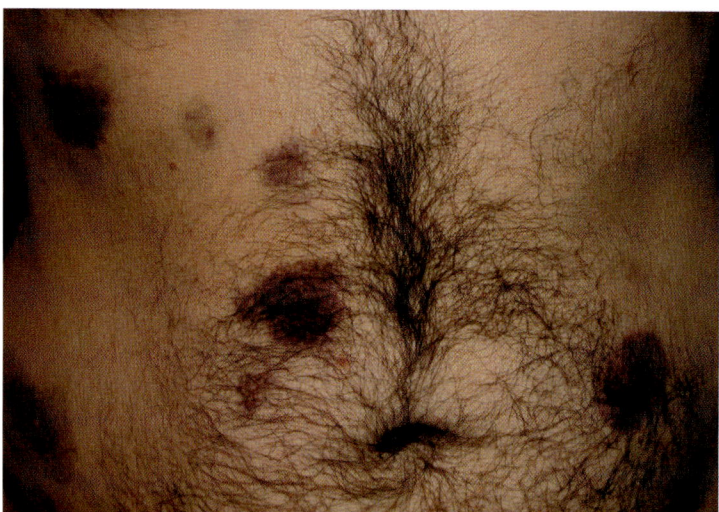

Fig. 62.31 Non-palpable purpura in thrombocytopenia.

The development of acquired ichthyosis is most strongly associated with either Hodgkin's disease [7], non-Hodgkin's lymphoma [8] or anaplastic large cell lymphoma [9]. It is important to distinguish this from the increasingly well recognized ichthyotic variant of cutaneous T-cell lymphoma [10].

Paraneoplastic pemphigus (Chapter 40) is most associated with B cell malignancies (lymphoma, chronic lymphatic leukaemia and Castleman's disease; Fig. 62.30) and may manifest as a severe mucositis with an acral lichenoid eruption, ranging to a more widespread eruption, even mimicking toxic epidermal necrolysis. An associated obliterative pneumonitis is a major cause of mortality [11,12].

Other reported associated dermatological conditions or paraneoplastic phenomena in lymphomas include Sweet's syndrome, subcorneal pustular dermatosis, pemphigus foliaceous and vulgaris (some of these in retrospect possibly representing paraneoplastic pemphigus), pemphigoid, erythroderma, exfoliative dermatitis, acanthosis nigricans, dermatomyositis, dermatitis herpetiformis and vasculitis [13].

References

1 O'Bryan-Tear CG, Burke M, Coulson IH, Marsden RA. Hodgkin's disease presenting in the skin. *Clin Exp Dermatol* 1987; **12**: 69–71.
2 Takagawa S, Maruyama R, Yokozeki H *et al*. Skin invasion of Hodgkin's disease mimicking scrofuloderma. *Dermatology* 1999; **199**: 268–70.
3 Gobbi PG, Attardo-Parrinello G, Lattanzio G *et al*. Severe pruritus should be a B-symptom in Hodgkin's disease. *Cancer* 1983; **51**: 1934–6.
4 Eigentler TK, Metzler G, Brossart P, Fierlbeck G. Acquired perforating collagenosis in Hodgkin's disease. *J Am Acad Dermatol* 2005; **52**: 922.
5 Rubenstein M, Duvic M. Cutaneous manifestations of Hodgkin's disease. *Int J Dermatol* 2006; **45**: 251–6.
6 Lucker GP, Steijlen PM. Acrokeratosis paraneoplastica (Bazex syndrome) occurring with acquired ichthyosis in Hodgkin's disease. *Br J Dermatol* 1995; **133**: 322–5.
7 Rizos E, Milionis HJ, Pavlidis N, Elisaf MS. Acquired ichthyosis: a paraneoplastic skin manifestation of Hodgkin's disease. *Lancet Oncol* 2002; **3**: 727.
8 Kato N, Yasukawa K, Kimura K, Yoshida K. Anaplastic large-cell lymphoma associated with acquired ichthyosis. *J Am Acad Dermatol* 2000; **42**: 914–20.
9 Estines O, Grosieux-Dauger C, Derancourt C *et al*. Paraneoplastic acquired ichthyosis revealing non-Hodgkin's lymphoma. *Ann Dermatol Venereol* 2001; **128**: 31–4.
10 Hodak E, Amitay I, Feinmesser M *et al*. Ichthyosiform mycosis fungoides: an atypical variant of cutaneous T-cell lymphoma. *J Am Acad Dermatol* 2004; **50**: 368–74.
11 Wade MS, Black MM. Paraneoplastic pemphigus: a brief update. *Australas J Dermatol* 2005; **46**: 1–8.
12 Mimouni D, Anhalt GJ, Lazarova Z *et al*. Paraneoplastic pemphigus in children and adolescents. *Br J Dermatol* 2002; **147**: 725–32.
13 Zappasodi P, Del Forno C, Corso A, Lazzarino M. Mucocutaneous paraneoplastic syndromes in hematologic malignancies. *Int J Dermatol* 2006; **45**: 14–22.

Platelet and clotting disorders

Purpura and bruising

Purpura is discussed in more detail in Chapter 49. A brief overview and details of some specific disorders of platelet numbers or function, and of impaired blood clotting, are listed here.

Non-palpable purpura or macular haemorrhages are suggestive of low platelet count or abnormal platelet function (Fig. 62.31). Petechiae are red-purple lesions less than 4 mm in diameter, and are usually due to a significant reduction in absolute platelet numbers (less than 50 000/microlitre), or abnormal platelet function (hereditary, salicylates, renal and hepatic disease). Less commonly, petechiae are the result of intermittent, severe elevation of intravascular pressure due to paroxysmal coughing, straining, stasis or strangulation. Viral exanthems, often enteroviral, may be purpuric. Macular haemorrhage is a term applied to larger lesions, between 4 and 10 mm. Causes include many of the same conditions that cause petechiae, although lesions of this size are uncommonly due to vascular leakage. Larger, non-palpable macules may recur in crops on the lower legs in Waldenstrom's hyperglobulinaemic purpura. This occurs most commonly in women, and may be associated with the sicca syndrome, SLE and rheumatoid arthritis.

Ecchymoses (bruises) are lesions larger than 10 mm in diameter. They are less likely to be due to platelet disorders, but can result from procoagulant defects, such as anticoagulant use, vitamin K deficiency, diffuse intravascular coagulopathy, or from inadequate dermal vasculature support, as occurs in severe actinic disease, corticosteroid use, scurvy, systemic amyloidosis, and ecchymotic (type IV) Ehlers–Danlos syndrome (Fig. 62.32).

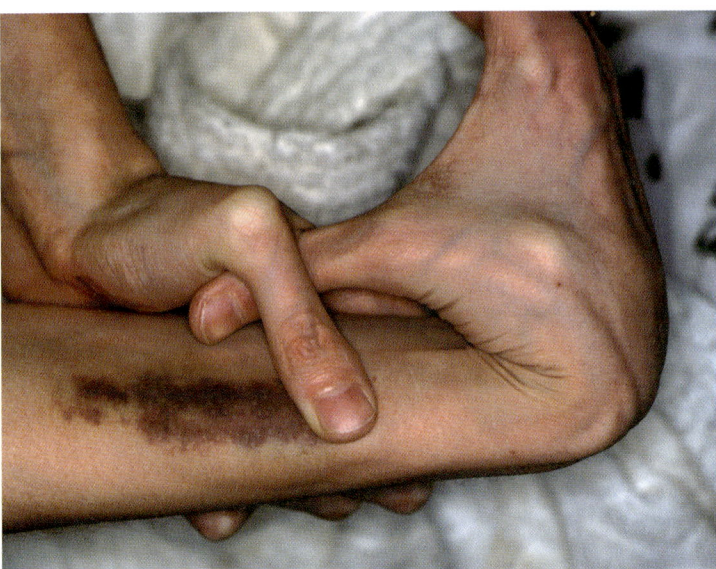

Fig. 62.32 Bruising in type IV Ehlers–Danlos syndrome; the hyperextensibility of skin and joints is also apparent.

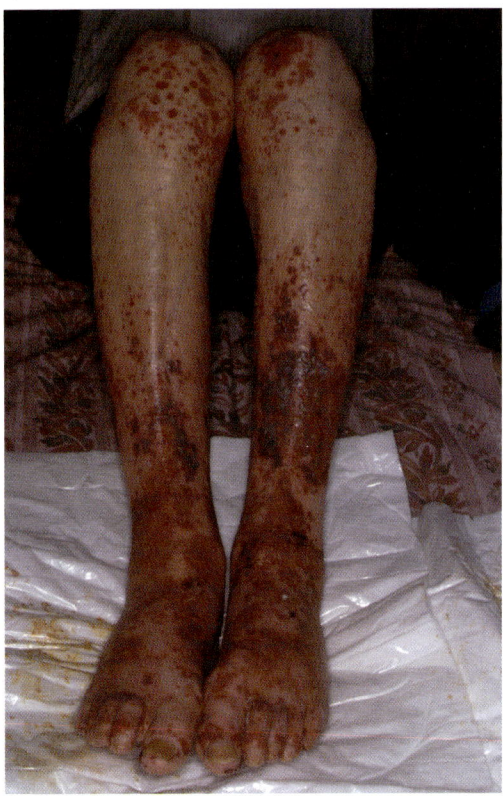

Fig. 62.33 Palpable purpura with haemorrhagic bullae in small vessel vasculitis.

Palpable or reticulate purpura

Palpable purpura is usually the result of vasculitis, most commonly of the small vessel leukocytoclastic type (Fig. 62.33). Inflammatory vascular changes produce an early erythematous change so that lesions remain red–pink when compressed. They are usually discrete macules or plaques rather than reticulate (compare with microvascular occlusive disorders, below) and they may progress to produce haemorrhagic blisters. Causes include ANCA-positive

Table 62.19 The thrombophilic disorders.

Lupus anticoagulant/antiphospholipid disease
Protein S and protein C deficiency
Factor V Leiden mutation
Antithrombin III deficiency
Hyperhomocysteinaemia
Plasminogen activator inhibitor-1 level elevation
Prothrombin gene mutation

Table 62.20 Dermatological conditions resulting from thrombophilia.

Livedo reticularis, Sneddon's syndrome [1,2]
Degos malignant atrophic papulosis [3]
Livedoid vasculomathy [4]
Acrocyanosis
Splinter haemorrhages
Capillaritis
Coumarin necrosis [5]
Thrombophlebitis
Mondor's disease [6]
Deep venous thrombosis and post phlebitic syndrome
Leg ulcers, cutaneous infarcts [7,8]
Cutaneous nodules and plaques with histological evidence of intravascular thrombosis [9]
Purpura fulminans [10]
Anetoderma [11]

diseases (Wegener's granulomatosis, microscopic polyangiitis and Churg–Strauss disease) and non-ANCA syndromes (benign cutaneous polyarteritis nodosum) and small vessel vasculitis (Chapter 50).

This may be contrasted with the palpable purpura that is associated with non-inflammatory processes which result in occlusion of small dermal vessels (microvascular occlusion, Chapter 49), for example following platelet or crystal plugging, embolization (due to cholesterol, atrial myxoma, or endocarditis), cold-related gelling or agglutination, or abnormal coagulation control (coumarin necrosis, thrombophilic disorders). In these disorders, initial erythema is minimal (early lesions may fade on compression) and development of a reticulate morphology is common.

Essential thrombocythaemia shares many of the cutaneous signs seen with PV, with livedo reticularis and erythromelalgia being the best recognized.

Thrombophilic disorders

The thrombophilic disorders (Tables 62.19 and 62.20; also discussed in more detail in Chapter 49) cause a tendency for blood to clot; they are due to deficiencies of, or resistance to, anticoagulant factors, either inherited or acquired, and may present as a single factor disorder or due to several deficiencies coexisting in the same individual (Table 62.19). Many such factors have now been identified. Thrombophilias may present in the neonate (homozygous factor S or C deficiency) with neonatal purpura fulminans, during infection (heterozygous protein S or C deficiency), or in later childhood or adult life with an increased

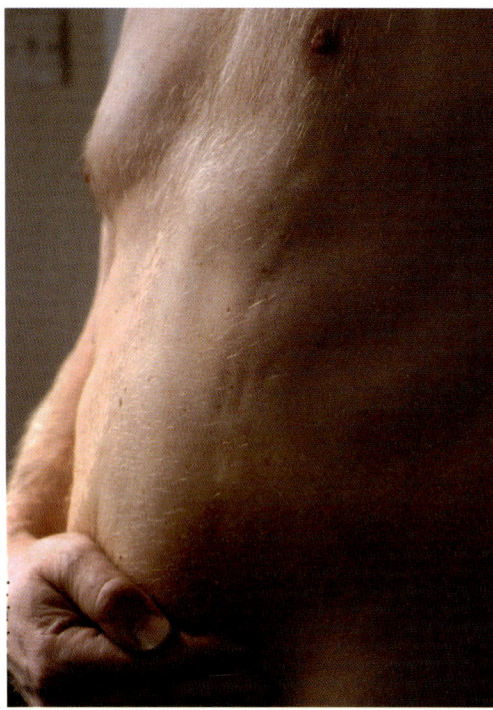

Fig. 62.34 Mondor's disease (thrombophlebitis of the superficial chest wall veins) associated with protein S deficiency.

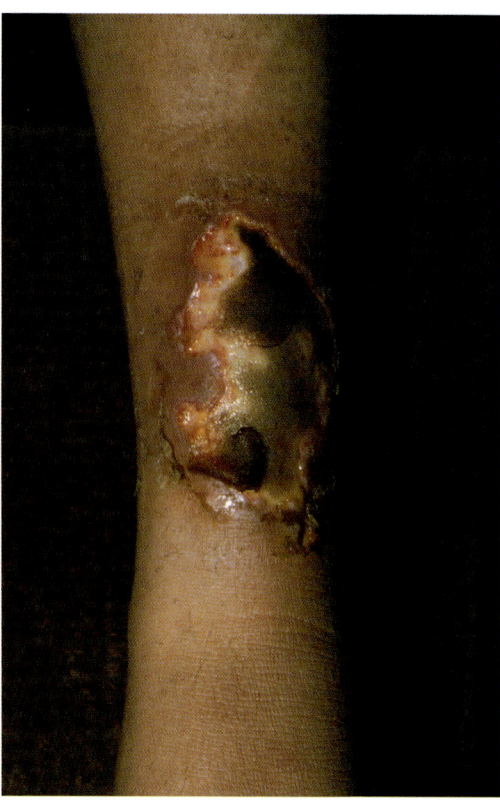

Fig. 62.35 Cutaneous necrosis after initiation of warfarin treatment in protein C deficiency.

tendency to superficial (Fig. 62.34) and deep venous thrombosis, pulmonary embolism, and less commonly arterial thrombosis. Some disorders, particularly the presence of antiphospholipid antibodies/lupus anticoagulant, may be identified due to recurrent spontaneous abortions. Table 62.20 outlines the range of dermatological disorders with which they may manifest. Most can be explained as arising as a result of intravascular thrombosis in cutaneous vessels of different sizes.

Coumarin necrosis

This is an uncommon but serious complication arising within the first week of coumarin anticoagulation. Well-circumscribed, haemorrhagic necrosis of the skin, usually of the breasts, buttocks, abdomen or thighs develops (Fig. 62.35). Histologically, fibrin occlusion of the small veins and postcapillary venules in the skin and fat is seen. The condition is more common in women, and occurs in 0.1 to 0.01% of individuals anticoagulated. Coumarin necrosis arises as a result of temporary reduction in levels of the vitamin K-dependent natural anticoagulants such as proteins C and S, prior to reduction in the levels of the procoagulant factors in the clotting cascade; this results in a temporary state of thrombophilia when coumarins are commenced. In a minority of patients it is a manifestation of familial protein S or C deficiency. Heparin-induced skin necrosis is rarer, appears to be immunologically mediated and often associated with heparin-induced thrombocytopenia.

References

1 Naldi L, Locati F, Marchesi L *et al.* Cutaneous manifestations associated with antiphospholipid antibodies in patients with suspected primary antiphospholipid syndrome: a case-control study. *Ann Rheum Dis* 1993; **52**: 219–22.

2 Gibson GE, Su WP, Pittelkow MR. Antiphospholipid syndrome and the skin. *J Am Acad Dermatol* 1997; **36**: 970–82.

3 Hohwy T, Jensen MG, Tottrup A *et al.* A fatal case of malignant atrophic papulosis (Degos' disease) in a man with factor V Leinden mutation and lupus anticoagulant. *Acta Derm Venereol* 2006; **86**: 245–7.

4 Hairston BR, Davis MD, Pittelkow MR, Ahmed I. Livedoid vasculopathy: further evidence for procoagulant pathogenesis. *Arch Dermatol* 2006; **142**: 1413–8.

5 Harenberg J, Hoffmann U, Huhle G *et al.* Cutaneous reactions to anticoagulants. Recognition and management. *Am J Clin Dermatol* 2001; **2**: 69–75.

6 de Godoy JM, Godoy MF, Batigalia F, Braile DM. The association of Mondor's disease with protein S deficiency: case report and review of literature. *J Thromb Thrombolysis* 2002; **13**: 187–9.

7 Kolbach DN, Veraart JC, Hamulyak K *et al.* Recurrent leg ulcers in a young man with hyperhomocysteinemia, factor V Leiden and impaired fibrinolysis. *Acta Derm Venereol* 2002; **82**: 52–4.

8 Meiss F, Marsch WC, Fischer M. Livedoid vasculopathy. The role of hyperhomocysteinemia and its simple therapeutic consequences. *Eur J Dermatol* 2006; **16**: 159–62.

9 Ishikawa O, Takahashi A, Tamura A, Miyachi Y. Cutaneous papules and nodules in the diagnosis of the antiphospholipid syndrome. *Br J Dermatol* 1999; **140**: 725–9.

10 Nakayama T, Matsushita T, Hidano H *et al.* A case of purpura fulminans is caused by homozygous delta8857 mutation (protein C-nagoya) and successfully treated with activated protein C concentrate. *Br J Haematol* 2000; **110**: 727–30.

11 Hodak E, Feuerman H, Molad Y *et al.* Primary anetoderma: a cutaneous sign of antiphospholipid antibodies. *Lupus* 2003; **12**: 564–8.

Paraproteins and multiple myeloma [1–6]

There are numerous cutaneous associations with monoclonal gammopathy of uncertain significance and multiple myeloma. Several of these are discussed in more detail in other chapters and are listed in Tables 62.21 and 62.22, without additional discussion; selected disorders that are not discussed elsewhere are noted below. A classification according to mechanisms has suggested

Table 62.21 Categories of paraprotein-related disorders by mechanism (adapted from text of [6]).

Category/mechanism	Examples
Cutaneous extravascular deposition of paraproteins	Nodular and other cutaneous amyloidosis (Chapter 59)
	Plasmacytoma
	Papules of macroglobulinaemia (IgM)
	Hyperkeratotic spicules
	Acquired cutis laxa
	Cutaneous light chain deposition
Intravascular paraproteinaemia	Vascular occlusion/cutaneous necrosis (Chapter 49)
	Type I cryoglobulinaemia (Chapter 49)
	Reactive angiomas, glomeruloid angiomas in POEMS syndrome (reactive post-thrombosis)
Cutaneous lesions due to biological activity of the paraprotein	Normolipaemic plane xanthoma (anti-LDL activity)
	Acquired C1 esterase deficiency
	Bullous lesions of Waldenström's macroglobulinaemia (dermo-epidermal deposition)
	Schnitzler syndrome (Chapter 22)
	Mucinoses associated with gammopathy (e.g. scleromyxoedema, acral papuar mucinosis) may also belong in this category
Conditions resulting from abnormal cytokine secretion	AESOP syndrome
	POEMS syndrome
Unknown mechanism	Telangiectasia, oedema, capillary leak syndrome (may be due to capillary deposition of monoclonal protein)
	Necrobiotic xanthogranuloma
	Neutrophilic dermatoses (Chapter 50)

AESOP, adenopathy and extensive skin patch overlying a plasmacytoma; LDL, low density lipoprotein; POEMS, polyneuropathy, organomegaly, endocrine disorders, monoclonal gammopathy, skin changes.

Table 62.22 Skin lesions and conditions associated with paraproteinaemias and multiple myeloma [1–6].

Amyloidosis AL type (Chapter 59; Fig. 62.36)
Cryoglobulinaemias, especially Type 1 cryoglobulinaemia (Fig. 62.37) [4,7]
Crystalglobulinaemia [8]
POEMS syndrome [9,10]
AESOP [11,12]
Livedo reticularis [7]
Small vessel vasculitis [13]
Neutrophilic disorders [3]—pyoderma gangrenosum, subcorneal pustular dermatosis [14], Sweet's syndrome, erythema elevatum diutinum (Chapter 50)
Mucinoses—scleredema, papular mucinosis and scleromyxoedema [15]
Xanthomatous disorders [3]—necrobiotic xanthogranuloma, normolipaemic plane xanthoma, and xanthoma disseminatum
Immunobullous disorders [5,16]—IgA pemphigus, linear IgA disease, epidermolysis bullosa aquisita (Chapter 40)
Schnitzler syndrome [17]
Nasal spicules [18]
Acquired cutis laxa [19]
Acquired ichthyosis, acanthosis nigricans, pityriasis rotunda [20]
Calcinosis cutis [3]
Plasmacytomas, myeloma skin metastases (Fig. 62.39) [21]
Systemic lupus erythematosus [22]
Dermatomyositis [5]

AESOP, adenopathy, extensive skin patch overlying a plasmacytoma; POEMS, polyneuropathy, organomegaly, endocrine disorders, monoclonal gammopathy, skin changes.

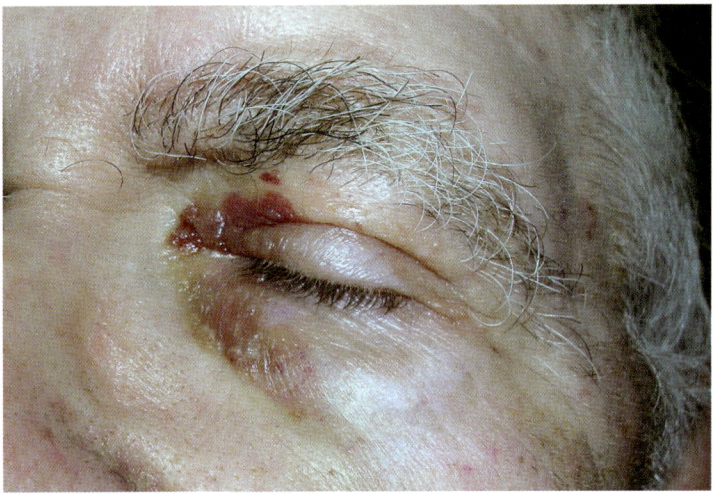

Fig. 62.36 Waxy plaques and periorbital purpura in paraprotein-associated systemic amyloidosis.

five categories (Table 62.21) [6]. A fuller list, including consequences of paraproteinaemia and selected references, is provided in Table 62.22.

The manifestations of systemic amyloid are discussed in Chapter 59. Waxy yellow plaques into which bruising easily occurs are typical, particularly on the eyelids (Fig. 62.36).

Cryoproteinaemias are associated with multiple myeloma. Monoclonal gammopathy-associated cryoglobulinaemia (type 1 cryoglobulinaemia; Chapter 49) may produce haemorrhagic, vasculitis-like lesions, often in a livedo distribution on the limbs.

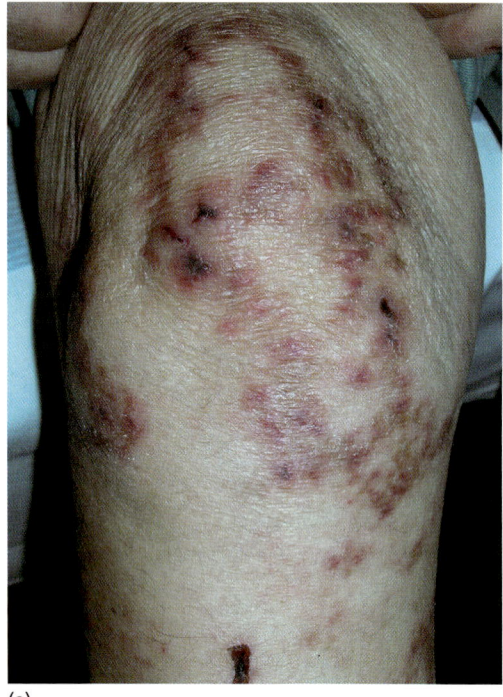

(a)

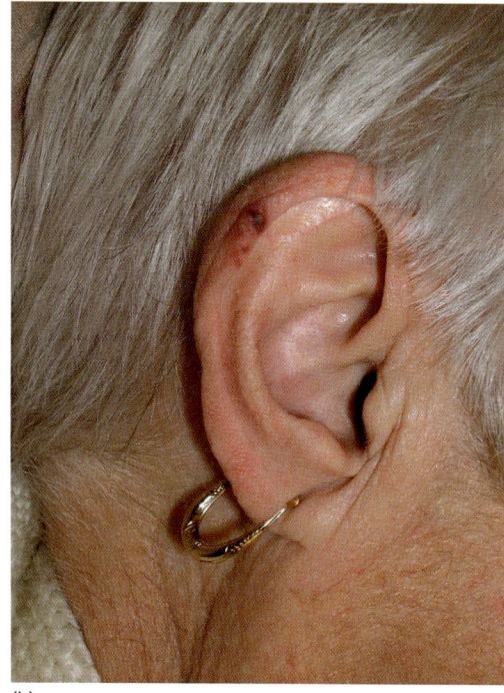

(b)

Fig. 62.37 (a,b) Reticulate purpura and small infarcts in type I cryoglobulinaemia, shown on the knees and ear (a cold site).

Although types II and III cryoglobulinaemia damage vessels in part by immune complex deposition and ensuing vasculitis, type I monoclonal cryoglobulinaemia causes physical obstruction of blood vessels (Figs 62.37 & 62.38) [4,7]. Areas sensitive to the cold, such as the ear lobe and nasal tip, are particularly affected. Livedo reticularis and leg ulcers may be seen in both cryoglobulinaemia and cryofibrinogenaemia (Chapter 49). Crystalglobulinaemia [8] has similar features.

POEMS syndrome [9,10] is a rare multisystem disorder characterized by *p*olyneuropathy, *o*rganomegaly of liver, spleen and lymph nodes, *e*ndocrine disorders, *m*onoclonal gammopathy and a variety of *s*kin changes. It has also been associated with the multicentric variant of Castleman's disease. Raynaud's phenomenon, scleroderma, oedema, generalized pigmentation and hypertrichosis are the most common skin changes. Angiomas and angioendotheliomatosis (particularly glomeruloid haemangiomas), alopecia, flushing reactions, whitening of the proximal nail, Sweet's syndrome-like lesions and vasculitis have all been reported in POEMS syndrome. The associated paraprotein is usually of the IgG or A type.

AESOP syndrome (*a*denopathy and *e*xtensive *s*kin patch *o*verlying a *p*lasmacytoma) [11,12] is a rarely described disorder in which mucinosis and angiomatosis occur over a bony or other plasmacytoma, with or without associated regional lymphadenopathy. Several of the few reported cases have also had, or have developed, concurrent POEMS syndrome [11].

Nasal spicules (small follicular keratin horns) and anetodermas are rare pointers to paraproteins, but can also occur in other haematological disorders.

Schnitzler's syndrome (Chapter 22) is an urticarial eruption associated with fever, and there is an underlying IgM paraproteinaemia; it has recently been incorporated into the group of 'autoinflammatory syndromes'.

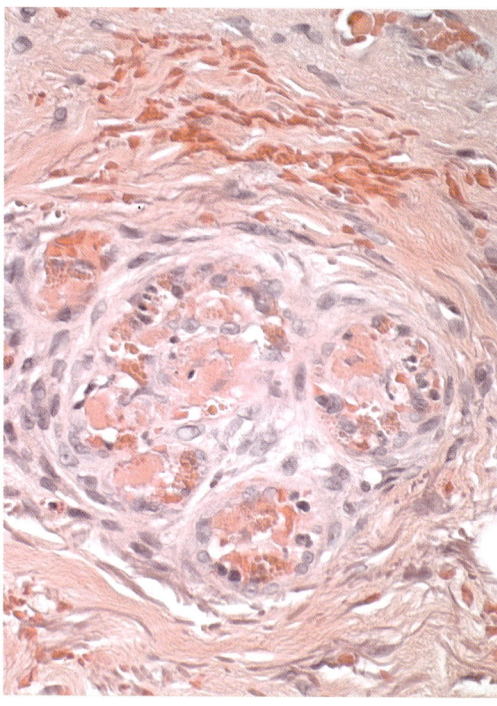

Fig. 62.38 Histological features of type I cryoglobulinaemia showing deposition of immunoglobulin obstructing small vessels.

References

1 Bayer-Garner IB, Smoller BR. The spectrum of cutaneous disease in multiple myeloma. *J Am Acad Dermatol* 2003; **48**: 497–507.
2 Daoud MS, Lust JA, Kyle RA, Pittelkow MR. Monoclonal gammopathies and associated skin disorders. *J Am Acad Dermatol* 1999; **40**: 507–35.
3 Weenig RH, Mehrany K. Dermal and pannicular manifestations of internal malignancy. *Dermatol Clin* 2008; **26**: 31–43.
4 Dammacco F, Sansonno D, Piccoli C *et al*. The cryoglobulins: an overview. *Eur J Clin Invest* 2001; **31**: 628–38.

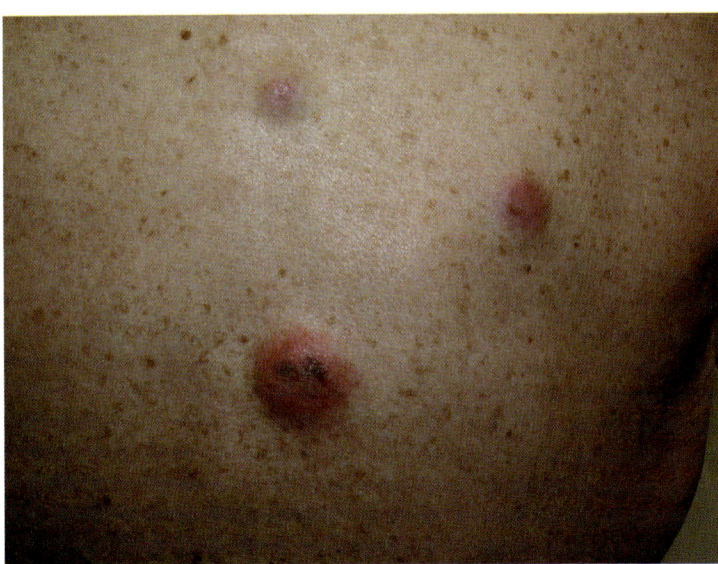

Fig. 62.39 Cutaneous deposits of multiple myeloma.

5 Zappasodi P, Del Forno C, Corso A, Lazzarino M. Mucocutaneous paraneoplastic syndromes in hematologic malignancies. *Int J Dermatol* 2006; **45**: 14–22.

6 Lipsker D, Boeckler P. Cutaneous manifestations of paraproteinaemia and their mechanisms. *Presse Med* 2007; **36**: 1135–40.

7 Requena L, Kutzner H, Angulo J, Renedo G. Generalized livedo reticularis associated with monoclonal cryoglobulinemia and multiple myeloma. *J Cutan Pathol* 2007; **34**: 198–202.

8 Ball NJ, Wickert W, Marx LH, Thaell JF. Crystalglobulinemia syndrome. A manifestation of multiple myeloma. *Cancer* 1993; **15**; 71: 1231–4.

9 Perniciaro C. POEMS syndrome. *Semin Dermatol* 1995; **14**: 162–5.

10 Nordlund JJ. Polyneuropathy, Organomegaly, Endocrinopathy, M protein, and Skin changes; POEMS syndrome. In: Nordlund JJ, Boissy RE, Hearing VJ, King RA, Oetting WS, Ortonne J-P, eds. *The Pigmentary System*, 2nd edn. Oxford: Blackwell Publishing, 2006: 951–4.

11 Lipsker D, Rondeau M, Massard G, Grosshans E. The AESOP (adenopathy and extensive skin patch overlying a plasmacytoma) syndrome: report of four cases of a new syndrome revealing POEMS (polyneuropathy, organomegaly, endocrinopathy, monoclonal protein, and skin changes) syndrome at a curable stage. *Medicine (Baltimore)* 2003; **82**: 51–9.

12 Rongioletti F, Romanelli P, Rebora A. Cutaneous mucinous angiomatosis as a presenting sign of bone plasmacytoma: a new case of (A)ESOP syndrome. *J Am Acad Dermatol* 2006; **55**: 909–10.

13 Bayer-Garner IB, Smoller BR. Leukocytoclastic (small vessel) vasculitis in multiple myeloma. *Clin Exp Dermatol* 2003; **28**: 521–4.

14 Kasha EE Jr, Epinette WW. Subcorneal pustular dermatosis (Sneddon-Wilkinson disease) in association with a monoclonal IgA gammopathy: a report and review of the literature. *J Am Acad Dermatol* 1988; **19**: 854–8.

15 Pomann JJ, Rudner EJ. Scleromyxedema revisited. *Int J Dermatol* 2003; **42**: 31–5.

16 Morita E, Horiuchi K, Yamamoto S, Hashimoto T. A case of acquired autoimmune bullous disease associated with IgM macroglobulinaemia. *J Dermatol* 1999; **26**: 671–6.

17 Lipsker D, Veran Y, Grunenberger F *et al*. The Schnitzler syndrome. Four new cases and review of the literature. *Medicine (Baltimore)* 2001; **80**: 37–44.

18 Requena L, Sarasa JL, Ortiz Masllorens F *et al*. Follicular spicules of the nose: a peculiar cutaneous manifestation of multiple myeloma with cryoglobulinemia. *J Am Acad Dermatol* 1995; **32**: 834–9.

19 Tan S, Pon K, Bargman J, Ghazarian D. Generalized cutis laxa associated with heavy chain deposition disease. *J Cutan Med Surg* 2003; **7**: 390–4.

20 Ikada J, Oki M. Concurrent pityriasis rotunda and acquired ichthyosis with IgG myeloma. *Br J Dermatol* 1974; **91**: 585–6.

21 Requena L, Kutzner H, Palmedo G *et al* Cutaneous involvement in multiple myeloma: a clinicopathologic, immunohistochemical, and cytogenetic study of 8 cases. *Arch Dermatol* 2003; **139**: 475–86.

22 Ali YM, Urowitz MB, Ibanez D, Gladman DD. Monoclonal gammopathy in systemic lupus erythematosus. *Lupus* 2007; **16**: 426–9.

Miscellaneous haematological diseases with cutaneous manifestations

Dyskeratosis congenita [1]

A genetically heterogeneous disorder with recessive, X-linked and dominant heredity, thought to be due to telomerase dysfunction. The skin changes are a mottled or reticulate macular hyperpigmentation, hypopigmentation or a mixture of both in a light-exposed distribution. Alopecia, premature hair greying, hyperhidrosis and adermatoglyphia are less common. A progressive nail dystrophy starts with ridging and splitting, and ends with atrophic rudimentary nails. There is leukoplakia of the tongue and buccal mucosa, and malignancy may develop within these sites. Bone marrow failure develops at a mean age of 10 years and is the major cause of mortality.

Fanconi's anaemia [2]

This rare disorder presents in early childhood with generalized increased pigmentation, particularly on the lower trunk, flexures and neck; more discrete café-au-lait type lesions are associated. A progressive hypoplastic marrow failure develops within 2 to 5 years of the onset; the disease often terminates with leukaemia or other neoplasia, or with infection resulting from leukopenia.

Chediak–Higashi syndrome [3]

This syndrome includes vitiligo-like depigmentation, blond or silvery grey hair and blue eyes, due to melanosome autophagocytosis. Polymorphonuclear cell dysfunction leads to oral and cutaneous infections, abscesses and pyodermas, usually due to staphylococcal infection. A lymphoma-like process is a frequent cause of early mortality.

Hermansky–Pudlak syndrome [4]

An autosomal recessive disorder characterized by oculocutaneous albinism, bleeding due to platelet dysfunction and ceroid accumulation in lysosomes. The skin is pale and the hair blond. Freckles and lentigines are common, as are atypical naevi. Trichomegaly and acanthosis nigricans-like flexural pigmentation has been described. Lack of melanin increases the risk of non-melanoma skin cancer as well as of melanoma. It is common in Puerto Rico, but rare elsewhere. Pulmonary fibrosis at the age of 40–50 years is the most common cause of death.

Griscelli syndrome [5]

Partial albinism is associated with immunodeficiency (a variety of defects are reported, including deficiency or dysfunction of T and B cells, natural killer cells, cell mediated immunity and hypogammaglobulinaemia). Silver or grey hair in infancy may be the clue to the diagnosis.

Wiskott–Aldrich syndrome [6]

An X-linked recessive disorder characterized by thrombocytopenia, an atopic eczema-like dermatitis and recurrent infections due to an inherited defect of T-cell function caused by the WASP gene mutation. Purpura and eccymoses may occur in the eczematous areas and be a diagnostic clue.

Neurofibromatosis, juvenile xanthogranuloma and juvenile chronic myeloid leukaemia [7]

The finding of juvenile xanthogranuloma and NF1 type neurofibromatosis is estimated to be associated with a 30 to 40-fold increased risk of juvenile chronic myeloid leukaemia.

References
1 Vulliamy T, Dokal I. Dyskeratosis congenita. *Semin Hematol* 2006; **43**: 157–66.
2 Auerbach AD. Fanconi anemia. *Dermatol Clin* 1995; **13**: 41–9.
3 Al-Khenaizan S. Hyperpigmentation in Chediak-Higashi syndrome. *J Am Acad Dermatol* 2003; **49**: S244–6.
4 Toro J, Turner M, Gahl WA. Dermatologic manifestations of Hermansky-Pudlak syndrome in patients with and without a 16-base pair duplication in the HPS1 gene. *Arch Dermatol* 1999; **135**: 774–80.
5 Malhotra AK, Bhaskar G, Nanda M *et al*. Griscelli syndrome. *J Am Acad Dermatol* 2006; **55**: 337–40.
6 Peacocke M, Siminovitch KA. The Wiskott-Aldrich syndrome. *Semin Dermatol* 1993; **12**: 247–54.
7 Zvulunov A, Barak Y, Metzker A. Juvenile xanthogranuloma, neurofibromatosis, and juvenile chronic myelogenous leukemia. World statistical analysis. *Arch Dermatol* 1995; **131**: 904–8.

Graft-versus-host disease [1–5]

Graft-versus-host disease (GVHD) occurs when T lymphocytes from an allograft exert immunological activity against cells of the graft recipient (host). Historically, it was the advent of bone marrow transplantation 50 years ago that brought GVHD to prominence, but it also occurs in the settings of solid organ allografting (renal, liver, etc.), non-irradiated blood or blood product transfusion and maternofetal transfusion (typically in an immunodeficient fetus).

Haemopoietic stem cell transplantation (HSCT) is now used rather than bone marrow transplantation; the main indication is haematological malignancies (leukaemias, lymphoproliferative disorders, aplastic anaemia, etc.) but HSCT is also used in the treatment of various immunological deficiency disorders, metabolic disorders (e.g. congenital erythropoietic porphyria, some mucopolysaccharidoses) and increasingly as a treatment for some solid tumours [2]. A major issue in haematological transplantation has been how to separate the beneficial graft-versus-tumour effects from the deleterious graft-versus-host effects of transplantation [6].

The conditioning regimen used for myeloablation in leukaemias, the type of transplantation performed, treatments used in preparation of the cells to be grafted (e.g. depletion of T cells using antithymocyte globulin) and a number of host factors (e.g. HLA disparity of host and donor, age, previous episodes of GVHD) all influence the likelihood that GVHD will occur [4]. Stem cells are now usually derived from peripheral blood treated with granulocyte colony-stimulating factor, rather than from bone marrow; some reports suggest that this may have increased the risk of chronic GVHD, but this may in part be due to better survival such that patients survive long enough to develop GVHD, coupled with an increased use of transplantation in older subjects in whom GVHD is more likely to occur.

All organs are affected, but are not discussed here although they are important in diagnosis and scoring of GVHD [3]. From a dermatological perspective, there are three main manifestations [1,2,4,5]; early GVHD causes acute rashes (which may have infections or drug eruptions in the differential diagnosis), later eruptions are often lichenoid (see also Chapter 4), and finally there is a sclerodermoid phase in which several morphologies occur (see also Chapter 51). The lichenoid and sclerodermoid manifestations may occur together.

Acute GVHD

Acute GVHD occurs in 60% of HLA-identical sibling HSCT and in 80% of unrelated HSCT, with a mortality of 50% if graded moderate or severe [2]. It develops in three phases—epithelial cell injury and cytokine release due to the conditioning regimen is followed by antigen presentation (by host dendritic cells) to donor T lymphocytes, resulting in cell death caused by activated cytotoxic T cells and cytokines [5–8]. Tumour necrosis factor (TNF) plays a key role in this process [2,8], activating dendritic cells, recruiting effector cells, and directly causing apoptosis and cell death; the interaction of Fas with its ligand FasL is also critical. Experimental blocking of TNF inhibits both GVHD and graft-versus-leukaemia (GVL) reactions, whilst blocking Fas inhibits GVHD but not GVL [8].

The cutaneous features of acute GVHD usually occur 2–6 weeks after transplant, typically at 4 weeks but a severe 'hyperacute' form with high mortality can occur within a week of HSCT. There may be early pain, itch or folliculocentric lesions; generally the rash of acute GVHD is rather morbilliform in distribution, affecting mainly the face and upper trunk, as well as palms and soles (Fig. 62.40). More extensive erythroderma, blistering and necrosis resembling toxic epidermal necrolysis (TEN) characterize the more severe forms of acute GVHD, and are associated with diarrhoea and abnormal liver function; in the hyperacute form there is erythroderma, hepatitis, fever and shock [1,2,4,5]. Mucositis also

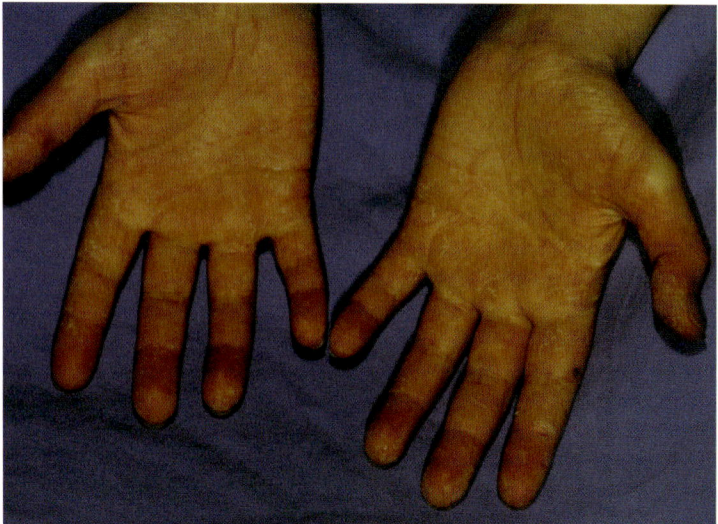

Fig. 62.40 Acute GVHD; (a) morbilliform exanthem-like rash , and peeling on the neck, and (b) acute palmar erythema and desquamation. (Courtesy of Dr C. Kennedy, Bristol Royal Infirmary, UK.)

occurs, but is difficult to differentiate from the effects of chemotherapy and irradiation used for conditioning regimens for marrow ablation. The differential diagnosis includes drug eruptions (chemotherapeutic drugs, antimicrobials, etc.) and infections, especially viral. A TEN-like pattern, and palmoplantar disease, are particularly problematic as both can occur due to drugs; the morbilliform rash may be difficult to distinguish from potentially important viral infections. Other patterns of acute GVHD skin eruption include ichthyosis, scarlatiniform rash, varicelliform rash and pustular acral chemotherapy rash. Purpura and haemorrhagic conjunctivitis may occur due to thrombocytopenia in association with capillary leak syndrome.

Reactivation of human herpesviruses (HHV) is a difficult diagnostic issue, as it occurs in both GVHD and in severe drug-induced hypersensitivity syndrome. HHV-6 is commonly reactivated, but cytomegalovirus, Epstein–Barr virus and HHV-7 reactivation may all occur; the sequence in GVHD is the same as that in severe drug hypersensitivity [9].

Skin biopsy is important in diagnosis of GVHD. Both acute and chronic GVHD cause an interface dermatitis which may be a lichenoid lymphocytic infiltrate or predominantly vacuolar damage of basal cells. Lymphocytic 'satellitosis' (lymphocytes encircling necrotic keratinocytes) is particularly suggestive of GVHD, although no single histological feature is pathognomonic. For many years, a system of four histological grades has been used where grade I is characterized by basal cell vacuolation; grade II by keratinocyte dyskeratosis or eosinophilic degeneration; grade III by more frank keratinocyte necrosis leading to basal epidermal clefts; and grade IV by frank epidermal loss [2,4]. Recent criteria have emphasized that keratinocyte necrosis also occurs in the outer root sheath of the hair follicle and in the acrosyringium, and used the degree of apoptotic activity as a marker of severity [10]. However, in situations where the risk of acute GVHD is high (over 30%, as in HSCT), it has been shown that treatment on suspicion gives a better outcome than performing a biopsy; by contrast, if acute GVHD is unlikely, basing treatment on the results of a skin biopsy is preferable [11]. Documentation of macrochimerism (determining the presence of donor cells in the host) has been performed on blood and in skin biopsies [12,13] and may be helpful in identifying or predicting GVHD.

Chronic GVHD

Chronic GVHD may develop without a preceding acute GVHD phase, after acute GVHD with an intervening symptom-free period, or as a continuum from prior acute GVHD. The pathophysiology is different from that of acute GVHD, and is reminiscent of that seen in autoimmune disorders; indeed, several autoantibodies (antinuclear, anti-dsDNA, antinucleolar, anti-smooth muscle and others) may be found in up to 60% of subjects, vitiligo has been reported in several cases, and the hepatic disease of chronic GVHD is very similar to primary biliary cirrhosis. Donor alloreactive T lymphocytes, with a predominance of cytotoxic CD8+ cells, and autoreactive CD4+ T lymphocytes arising due to defective thymic deletion, damage tissues directly, lead to disordered cytokine synthesis and regulation. Chronic GVHD is usually a multisystem disease in which the skin is affected in 90–100% of subjects; localized chronic GVHD also occurs, in which

individual organs (usually skin or liver) are affected. The multi-organ involvement has allowed development of 'organ scoring' from which severity grades (mild, moderate or severe) can be derived [3,4]; the percentage of skin involved is part of this scoring system [3,4]. Chronic GVHD of the skin is sometimes provoked by trauma, sunlight or infections such as herpes zoster.

The lichenoid form of chronic GVHD typically occurs as an earlier form of the disorder, and is conventionally defined as occurring more than 100 days after transplantation although the timing varies considerably; it is unlikely before day 80 but may occur after many months. Papules or plaques resembling lichen planus develop, usually less well defined and more scaly than true lichen planus; initially they affect acral sites (distal limbs, including palms and soles), ears and the periorbital area, before becoming generalized. Oral mucosa and oesophagus may also be affected. In some cases, the eruption may be more lupus erythematosus-like [1,2,4]. Like drug-induced lichenoid eruptions, the lymphocytic infiltrate of this form of chronic GVHD is usually rather less tightly band-like than that of standard lichen planus, and may contain eosinophils.

The sclerodermoid spectrum of chronic GVHD may follow the lichenoid form, or may develop without preceding rash—it usually presents between days 150 and 300. Profibrotic cytokines (IL-4 and transforming growth factor-β) are increased, as well as IL-5, which may cause tissue and blood eosinophilia [4]. Early sclerodermoid chronic GVHD is usually lichen sclerosus-like or morphoeaform, later becoming deeper with involvement of fascia and resemblance to eosinophilic fasciitis. The lichen sclerosus lesions frequently occur at areas of trauma (a predilection for sites of central venous lines has been reported), and typically involve the neck, upper trunk and genitalia. The morphoeaform lesions tend to involve the lower trunk; histologically, fibrosis is more superficial than in sporadic morphoea although lesions may progress and coalesce to form a deeper and firmer scleroderma-like picture (Fig. 62.41).

The scleroderma-like and eosinophilic fasciitis-like fibrotic reactions tend to affect the limbs [14]. Septal panniculitis and fibrosis may lead to a puckered ('ripply' [1]) appearance of the skin [15], and blisters, erosions, ulceration and scarring (including scarring alopecia and nail dystrophy) occur [1,4]. Other features include eczema craquelé, eczematoid reactions [16], nodular fibromas, cutaneous mucinosis, eruptive angiomas, dermatomyositis-like rash [17], cicatricial pemphigoid-like conjunctival involvement, poikiloderma, vitiligo, leukotrichia and other pigmentary disturbance (increased, decreased or both; sometimes termed 'leopard-skin' eruption) [1,2,4,5]. Skin changes associated with GVHD affecting other organs also need to be considered, for example plane xanthomas due to cholestasis [18].

Treatment [1,2,4,5,13]

Management of GVHD typically involves treatments that might be used in autoimmune conditions, such as prednisolone, ciclosporin, mycophenolate mofetil, azathioprine, hydroxychloroquine, methotrexate, cyclophosphamide, clofazimine, cladribine, tacrolimus, sirolimus, dacluzimab and thalidomide; the most common regimen is corticosteroid with ciclosporin, thalidomide is generally too toxic and azathioprine may contribute to further malignancies. Antithymocyte globulin has been used in acute GVHD

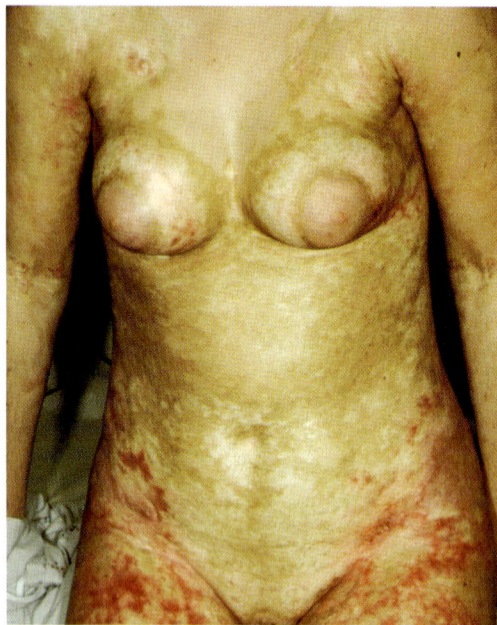

(a)

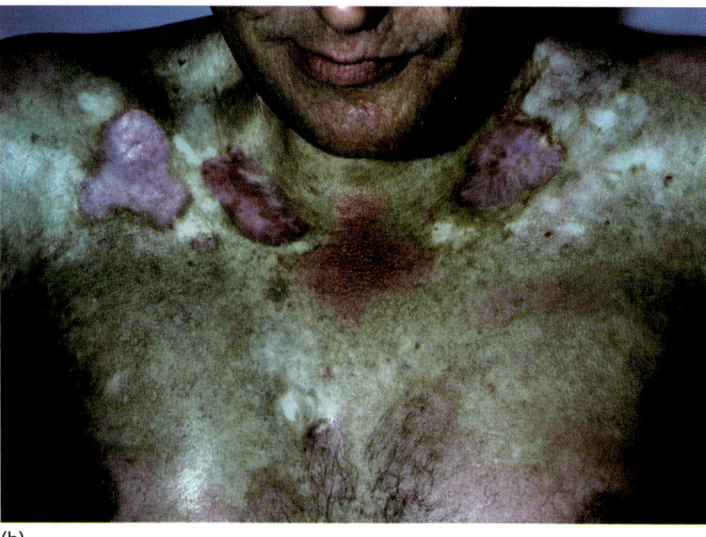

(b)

Fig. 62.41 (a,b) Chronic GVHD showing extensive sclerodermoid changes. (Courtesy of Dr C. Kennedy, Bristol Royal Infirmary, UK.)

but has no benefit in the chronic form. Prophylaxis for acute GVHD typically consists of ciclosporin, tacrolimus or mycophenolate mofetil for about 6 months post-transplantation. Photochemotherapy (PUVA) and UVB have been used for both the acute and the lichenoid lesions, and PUVA, UVA1 and extracorporeal photopheresis (ECP) for deeper sclerodermoid lesions [19]. Acitretin appears to be beneficial for sclerodermoid lesions, as does denileukin diftitox. Biological agents such as dacluzimab have been disappointing but rituximab appears to be helpful in treatment of sclerodermoid lesions; aletuzumab, infliximab and etanercept have also been used. Recent guidance on the use of extracorporeal photopheresis (ECP) in the UK [20] suggests that it should be reserved for those who have GVHD refractory to corticosteroids (prednisolone 1 mg kg^{-1} daily for at least 4 weeks, or prednisolone dosed consistently at >10 mg daily), and achieves

best results for skin, mucous membrane and hepatic GVHD; however, its best effects in improving survival are seen if treatment is started early, and there is no easy way to predict which patients will require ECP.

Other aspects of transplantation

Dermatologists have an important role in the management of skin cancers arising due to immunosuppression following solid organ transplantation [21]. Such concerns are most prominent after cardiac transplantation, and least after liver transplants, but are discussed in this chapter in the context of renal disease and the skin on the basis that renal transplantation is the commonest such procedure, this post-transplant complication is discussed on p. 62.74.

Hypothyroidism occurs in about 25% of stem cell transplant recipients in whom whole body radiotherapy has been part of the conditioning regimen [22]. As discussed in the section on renal disease, ongoing immunosuppression increases the risk of many infections after HSCT [1,22]; herpes zoster is of particular importance dermatologically as lichen sclerosus-like sclerodermoid GVHD reactions may localize to sites of recent zoster.

The transfer of donor diseases to a recipient of a solid organ transplant or of an SCT is a potential disaster. Transfer of viral infections such as cytomegalovirus is well recognized; transfer of tumours can also occur. Of dermatological relevance, peanut allergy [23], psoriasis [24] and psoriatic arthritis [25] have also been documented post-transplant. There is also evidence of donor stem cells causing a skin cancer in a female recipient of a renal transplant from a male donor, in whom most epithelial (cytokeratin-positive) cells within a basal cell carcinoma were demonstrated to be XY and thus of male origin [26].

References

1 Johnson ML, Farmer ER. Graft-versus-host reactions in dermatology. *J Am Acad Dermatol* 1998; **38**: 369–92.
2 Vargas-Díaz E, García-Díaz A, Marín A, Fernández-Herrera J. Life-threatening graft-vs-host disease. *Clinics Dermatol* 2005; **23**: 285–300.
3 Filipovich AH, Weisdorf P, Pavletic S *et al.* National Institutes of Health Consensus Development Project on Criteria for Clinical Trials in Chronic Graft-versus-Host Disease. I. Diagnosis and Staging Working Group Report. *Biol Blood Marrow Transplant* 2005; **11**: 945–56.
4 Schaffer JV. The changing face of graft-versus-host disease. *Semin Cutan Med Surg* 2006; **25**: 190–200.
5 Farmer EF. Graft-versus-host disease. In: Provost TT, Flynn JA, eds. *Cutaneous Medicine: Cutaneous Manifestations of Systemic Disease*. Hamilton, Ontario: Decker, 2001: 651–61.
6 Parkman R. Getting a handle on graft-versus-host disease. *N Engl J Med* 2004; **350**: 614–5.
7 Socié G. Graft-versus-host disease—from the bench to the bedside? *N Engl J Med* 2005; **353**: 1396–7.
8 Contassot E, Gaide O, French LE. Death receptors and apoptosis. *Dermatol Clin* 2007; **25**: 487–501.
9 Kano Y, Hiraharas K, Sakuma K, Shiohara T. Several herpesviruses can reactivate in a severe drug-induced multiorgan reaction in the same sequential order as in graft-versus-host disease. *Br J Dermatol* 2006; **155**: 301–6.
10 Shulman HM, Kleiner D, Lee SJ *et al.* Histopathologic diagnosis of chronic graft-versus-host disease: National Institutes of Health Consensus Development Project on Criteria for Clinical Trials in Chronic Graft-versus-Host Disease. II. Pathology Working Group Report. *Biol Blood Marrow Transplant* 2006; **12**: 31–47.
11 Firoz BF, Lee SJ, Nghiem P, Quereshi AA. Role of skin biopsy to confirm acute graft-vs-host disease. *Arch Dermatol* 2006; **142**: 175–82.
12 Taylor AI, Gibbs P, Bradley JL. Acute graft versus host disease following liver transplantation: the enemy within. *Am J Transplant* 2004; **4**: 466–74.

13 Meves A, el-Azhary RA, Talwalkar JA *et al.* Acute graft-versus-host disease after liver transplantation diagnosed by fluorescent in situ hybridization testing of skin biopsy specimens. *J Am Acad Dermatol* 2006; **55**: 642–6.

14 White JML, Creamer D, du Vivier AWP *et al.* Sclerodermatous graft-versus-host disease: clinical spectrum and therapeutic challenges. *Br J Dermatol* 2007; **156**: 1032–8.

15 Peñas PF, Jones-Caballero M, Fernández-Herrera J *et al.* Sclerodermatous graft-vs-host disease: clinical and pathological study of 17 patients. *Arch Dermatol* 2004; **138**: 924–34.

16 Creamer D, Martyn-Simmons CL, Osborne G *et al.* Eczematoid graft-vs-host disease: a novel form of chronic cutaneous graft-vs-host disease and its response to psoralen-UV-A therapy. *Arch Dermatol* 2007; **143**: 1157–62.

17 Ollivier I, Wolkenstein P, Gherardi R *et al.* Dermatomyositis-like graft-versus-host disease. *Br J Dermatol* 1998; **138**: 558–9.

18 Moriue T, Yoneda K, Katsuura J *et al.* Planar xanthoma due to cholestasis in graft versus host disease. *Br J Dermatol* 2007; **156**: 1374–6.

19 Brenner M, Herzinger T, Berking C *et al.* Phototherapy and photochemotherapy of sclerosing skin diseases. *Photodermatol Photoimmunol Photomed* 2005; **21**: 157–65.

20 Scarisbrick JJ, Taylor P, Holtick U *et al.* U.K. consensus statement on the use of extracorporeal photophoresis for treatment of cutaneous T-cell lymphoma and chronic graft-versus-host disease. *Br J Dermatol* 2008; **158**: 659–78.

21 Carucci JA. Management of skin cancer in organ transplant recipients. In: Rigel DS, Friedman RJ, Dzubow LM, Reintgen DS, Bystryn J-C, Marks R, eds. *Cancer of the Skin*. Philadelphia: Elsevier, 2005: 631–40.

22 Antin JH. Long-term care after haemopoietic-cell transplantation in adults. *N Engl J Med* 2002; **347**: 36–42.

23 Legendre C, Caillat-Zucman S, Samuel D *et al.* Transfer of symptomatic peanut allergy to the recipient of a combined liver-and-kidney transplant. *N Engl J Med* 1997; **337**: 822–3.

24 Hubiche T, Leaute-Labreze C, Lepreux S *et al.* Psoriasis after cord blood stem cell transplantation. *Br J Dermatol* 2007; **156**: 386–8.

25 Daikeler T, Günaydin I, Einsele H *et al.* Transfer of psoriatic arthritis by allogeneic bone marrow transplantation for chronic myelogenous leukaemia from an HLA-identical donor. *Rheumatology* 1999; **38**: 89–90

26 Aractingi S, Kanitakis J, Sylvie E *et al.* Skin carcinoma arising from donor cells in a kidney transplant recipient. *Cancer Res* 2005; **65**: 1755–60.

Bone and joint diseases

There are several diseases in which bone or joint abnormalities occur together with skin changes (Tables 62.23 & 62.24) [1–3]. In some instances, as occurs in several inflammatory diseases (for example, gout or psoriatic arthropathy), or due to localized tumours (such as glomus tumour), the bone or joint disease may be obvious; in other conditions, skeletal changes may be asymptomatic but demonstrated radiologically. For example, more than half of adults with *mastocytosis* may have diffuse bone disease detected radiologically [4], and the osteopoikilosis of *Buschke–Ollendorf syndrome* (Fig. 62.42) is asymptomatic and usually only demonstrated as an incidental finding or if the patient presents with cutaneous elastomas.

Bony changes may be an important factor in diagnosis of several *genodermatoses* (Chapter 15) [1,2] and underlying bony or neural defects should always be considered in midline *congenital lesions* such as faun tail or on the head and neck (e.g. facial or scalp nodules and pits) [5,6]. The genetic and metabolic basis for some of these are now well understood—for example, the role of G proteins in *McCune–Albright syndrome* [7]. Vascular or lymphatic proliferations or malformations of limbs should also generate suspicion of possible associated bony abnormality, such as asymmetry of growth in *Klippel–Trenaunay* syndrome, or osteolysis due to lymphatic proliferation in *Gorham–Stout* disease [8,9].

Soft-tissue calcification, and less commonly ossification, occurs in numerous disorders [10]. It is particularly prominent in *childhood dermatomyositis* and is discussed in more detail in Chapter 51. *Progressive systemic sclerosis* and CREST (Chapter 51) are characterized by atrophy and dystrophic calcifications in the soft tissues, ultimately leading to joint deformities and resorption of the terminal tufts of the phalanges. Resorption of bone occurs at other sites as well in these individuals, and marginal erosions may develop in the metacarpophalangeal and interphalangeal joints of the hands [11]. Calcification of cerebral blood vessels may be associated with facial haemangiomas (Chapter 18). Both calcification and ossification of the cartilage of the ear can occur following repeated cold injury, and may present with symptoms of chondrodermatitis nodularis helicis (Fig. 62.43). Osteoma cutis affecting the face can occur spontaneously, but may follow acne.

Skin lesions may also occur as a direct consequence of bone disease. Neuropathic ulcers, an important cause of morbidity in type I diabetes, have a strong association with bony deformity of the foot and typically occur at bony pressure points. Bone infection, in the form of osteomyelitis, is closely linked with chronic skin ulceration and has a risk of development of squamous cell carcinoma. Less obviously, as there is no obvious local body site correlation, *fat emboli*, particularly caused by fractures of the long bones, may present cutaneously with petechiae, usually 2 or 3 days after trauma; other symptoms may include respiratory distress and cerebral impairment. The intensity of the petechiae may indicate the severity of other organ involvement. Fat globules may be observed histologically in affected tissue, including the skin, when suitably processed. The distribution of skin petechiae is principally on the anterior trunk; they are seldom found on the back or face [12].

References

1 Orlow SJ, Watsky KL, Bolognia JL. Skin and bones, 1. *J Am Acad Dermatol* 1991; **25**: 205–21.

2 Orlow SJ, Watsky KL, Bolognia JL. Skin and bones, 2. *J Am Acad Dermatol* 1991; **25**: 447–62.

3 Freyschmidt J, Freyschmidt G. *SKIBO-diseases. Disorders Affecting the Skin and Bones.* Berlin, Germany: Springer-Verlag, 1999.

4 Tharp MD, Longley BJ. Mastocytosis. *Dermatol Clin* 2001; **19**: 679–96.

5 Drolet B. Birthmarks to worry about: cutaneous markers of dysraphism. *Dermatol Clin* 1998; **16**: 447–53.

6 Nijhawan A, Lyon VB, Drolet BA. Pediatric dermatology: cutaneous markers of malformations and selected syndromes—what do you see, when do you see it, and how do you find it? *Curr Probl Dermatol* 2001; **13**: 249–300.

7 Levine MA. Clinical implications of genetic defects in G proteins: oncogenic mutations in G alpha s as the molecular basis for McCune–Albright syndrome. *Arch Med Res* 1999; **30**: 522–31.

8 Bastarrika G, Redondo P, Sierra A *et al.* New techniques for the evaluation and therapeutic planng of patients with Klippel-Trenaunay syndrome. *J Am Acad Dermatol* 2007; **56**: 242–9

9 Bruch-Gerharz D, Gerharz C-D, Stege H *et al.* Cutaneous lymphatic malformations in the disappearing bone (Gorham-Stout) syndrome: a novel clue to the pathogenesis of a rare syndrome. *J Am Acad Dermatol* 2007; **56**: S21–5.

10 Touart DM, Sau P. Cutaneous deposition diseases, 2. *J Am Acad Dermatol* 1998; **39**: 527–44.

11 Gold RH, Bassett LW, Seeger LL. The other arthritides: roentgenologic features of osteoarthritis, erosive osteoarthritis, ankylosing spondylitis, psoriatic arthritis, Reiter's disease, multicentric reticulohistiocytosis, and progressive systemic sclerosis. *Radiol Clin North Am* 1988; **26**: 1195–212.

12 Tachakra SS. Distribution of skin petechiae in fat embolism rash. *Lancet* 1976; **i**: 284–5.

Table 62.23 Skin disorders that are commonly associated with bony abnormalities.

Disorder	Skin lesions	Bony change
Congenital/inherited		
Ectodermal dysplasias and keratodermas	Various	Chapter 19
Conradi–Hünermann syndrome	Chapter 19	Chondrodysplasia punctata
Neurofibromatosis	Neurofibromas, café-au-lait patches	Kyphoscoliosis, vertebral erosions, partial absence of sphenoid bone, cystic lesions, pseudarthroses
Tuberous sclerosis	Angiofibromas, ash leaf macules, collagenomas	Intracerebral calcification, bony sclerosis (especially skull), cortical thickening, bone cysts (especially phalanges)
Klippel–Trenaunay syndrome	Port-wine stains, other vascular lesions, lymphangioma	Bony hypertrophy, macrocephaly, polydactyly/syndactyly
Proteus syndrome	Soft-tissue overgrowth, epidermal naevi	Partial gigantism (usually hand/foot), scoliosis and vertebral abnormalities, exostoses, osteochondromas
Maffucci's syndrome	Haemangiomas, lymphangiomas	Enchondromas (especially hands), chondrosarcoma
Sturge–Weber syndrome	Port-wine stain	Calcification of meningeal vessels, hemiatrophy
Gorham (Gorham–Stout) syndrome (osteovascular dysplasia)	Lymphatic vascular proliferations	Lytic lesions, 'disappearing bones'—usually unilateral
Gardner's syndrome	Cysts, lipomas, fibromas	Osteomas, exostoses
Ehlers–Danlos syndrome	Skin laxity, atrophic scars, molluscoid pseudotumours	Kyphoscoliosis (especially type IV), abnormalities of long bones, short clavicles, occipital exostoses (all in type IX)
Osteogenesis imperfecta	Atrophic skin	Brittle bones, otosclerosis
Marfan syndrome	Arachnodactyly	Increased limb length, arachnodactyly, chest deformities, joint laxity
Focal dermal hypoplasia (Goltz's syndrome)	Dermal atrophy, telangiectasia, fatty herniation	Syndactyly, scoliosis, skeletal asymmetry, osteopathia striata, bony tumours, dental abnormalities
Rothmund–Thomson syndrome	Poikiloderma	Hypoplasia of thumbs or forearm bones, dental abnormalities, osteosarcoma
Linear naevus sebaceus syndrome	Sebaceous naevi (often facial or widespread)	Asymmetry (especially skull), spinal abnormalities, hypophosphataemic rickets
Linear epidermal naevus syndrome	Epidermal naevi	Asymmetry, kyphoscoliosis, bone cysts, equinovarus deformity
Incontinentia pigmenti	Atrophic streaks, fatty herniations	Dental abnormalities (conical teeth), spina bifida occulta, skeletal asymmetry, vertebral/rib abnormalities, phalangeal lytic lesions
Hypomelanosis of Ito	Pale, whorled streaks	Kyphoscoliosis, spina bifida occulta, skeletal asymmetry, various digital anomalies
Buschke–Ollendorf syndrome	Elastomas	Osteopoikilosis
McCune–Albright syndrome	Pigmented macules	Fibrous dysplasia, asymmetry, scoliosis, sclerosis of base of skull, fractures, rickets, osteomas
Lipoid proteinosis	Confluent waxy papules, alopecia	Intracranial calcification
Disseminated lipogranulomatosis	Nodules on digits	Destructive arthropathy
Pseudoxanthoma elasticum	'Plucked chicken' appearance of neck, flexures	Calcification of soft tissues, falx cerebri, dura, choroid plexus
Nail–patella syndrome	Hypoplastic nails	Absent or small patellae, iliac horns, scoliosis, hypoplasia of first rib, absent fibulae
Fabry disease	Angiokeratomas	Necrosis of femoral head, arthritis of distal interphalangeal joints
Werner's syndrome	Premature ageing	Osteoporosis, sclerodactyly, joint contractures, sarcomas
Progeria	Aged appearance	Skeletal dysplasia, osteolysis, osteoporosis, dislocation or avascular necrosis of hip, non-union of fractures
Gaucher disease	Pigmentation	Bone pain, fractures, cortical destruction
Naevus of Ota	Facial naevus	Posterior cranial fossa defects
Midline lesions	Various, includes scalp nodules/cysts, nasal gliomas, pits and sinuses, faun tail	Various; connections between skin and CNS may be associated with bony defects, e.g. spina bifida
Infection		
Local		
Dental sinus	Localized nodule, may discharge	Usually periapical abscess, may be retained root, cyst
Chronic ulcer	Skin ulcer	Underlying osteomyelitis
Systemic		
Syphilis	Various; see Chapter 34	Periostitis, osteitis, focal osteolysis or sclerosis
Leprosy	Various; see Chapter 32	Acral bone resorption, osteitis leprosa multiplex cystica
Cryptococcosis	Skin nodules	Osteolytic lesions
Blastomycosis	Skin nodules	Osteomyelitis
Hyper-IgE syndrome with recurrent infections	Abscesses, eczema-like rash	Fractures, scoliosis, abnormal facies

(Continued)

Table 62.23 *Continued*

Disorder	Skin lesions	Bony change
Inflammatory and systemic diseases		
Psoriasis and Reiter's syndrome	See Chapter 20	Erosive arthritis, sacroiliitis
Palmoplantar pustulosis	Palm and sole pustules	See text (this section)
Sarcoidosis	See Chapter 61	Honeycomb change and bone cysts (especially hands), acrosclerosis
Scleroderma	See Chapter 51	Resorption of terminal phalanges (acronecrosis), soft-tissue calcification, erosive arthritis
		Linear scleroderma may show underlying linear hyperostosis
		Acro-osteolysis is typical of vinyl chloride disease
Scleromyxoedema	Mucinosis	Arthralgia, carpal tunnel syndrome, acro-osteolysis
Granuloma annulare	Aggressive nodular/subcutaneous type	Subperiostial involvement, 'vanishing bones'
Acne fulminans/ conglobata	See Chapter 42	Lytic lesions, especially clavicles; clavicular hyperostosis
SAPHO	Acne, pustules	Hyperostosis, osteomyelitis
Neutrophilic dermatoses	See Chapter 49	Periosteal reaction adjacent to pyoderma gangrenosum, osteomyelitis-like lesions (chronic recurrent multifocal osteomyelitis)
Gout	Tophi	Erosive arthritis
Multicentric reticulohistiocytosis	Skin and subcutaneous nodules	Destructive polyarthritis, especially terminal interphalangeal joints (similar to rheumatoid disease), atlantoaxial disease
POEMS syndrome	Pigmentation, sclerosis, hypertrichosis	Sclerotic lesions, may have central lucency
Neoplastic		
Naevoid basal cell carcinoma syndrome (Gorlin syndrome, Gorlin-Goltz syndrome)	Basal cell carcinomas	Cysts of jaw and other bones, frontal bossing, calcification of falx cerebri, bifid ribs, spina bifida and other spinal abnormalities, polydactyly/syndactyly, shortened metacarpals
Histiocytoses (Langerhans' cell histiocytosis, Rosai–Dorfman disease, Erdheim–Chester disease, juvenile xanthogranuloma, others)	See Chapter 55	Lytic lesions, defects of skull and mandible, vertebral lesions
Mastocytosis	See Chapter 22	Diffuse or focal osteoporosis or sclerosis
Fibromatoses	See Chapter 56	Various; most characteristic are cystic lesions of skull and long bones in infantile myofibromatosis
Subungual tumours	Glomus, squamous cell carcinoma, others	Osteolysis
Other		
Subungual exostosis	Hard subungual nodule	Underlying exostosis
Osteoma cutis	Hard plaque(s)	Focal bone formation, possibly primary or within a preceding lesion
Becker's naevus	Pigmented hairy lesion	Scoliosis, spina bifida
Thyroid acropachy	Finger clubbing	Expanded distal phalangeal tuft
Acromegaly	(See p. 62.2)	Increased periosteal bone growth
Pachydermoperostosis	Clubbing, thickened digits, cutis verticis gyrata	Periosteal new bone affecting all segments of bone, acro-osteolysis
Complex regional pain syndrome (reflex sympathetic dystrophy, Sudek's atrophy)	Soft tissue swelling (usually limb or acral), hyperhidrosis/hypohidrosis, vasomotor changes	Patchy osteoporosis, bone atrophy
Scurvy	Ecchymosis, 'corkscrew' hairs, gingival lesions	Increased bone density ('white line' of scurvy, Wimberger's sign), lucent bands, metaphyseal corner breaks, pseudo-double epiphysis, periosteal new bone due to haemorrhages
Fat embolism	Petechial rash on anterior trunk	Causative fracture(s)

POEMS, polyneuropathy, organomegaly, endocrinopathy, *M* protein, *s*kin changes (syndrome); SAPHO, *s*ynovitis, *a*cne, *p*ustulosis, *h*yperostosis, *o*steomyelitis.

Inflammatory conditions [1,2]

Arthralgia and/or arthritis is frequent in a number of inflammatory and metabolic conditions which also affect the skin, such as psoriasis and sarcoidosis (Table 62.24). Most of these individual diseases are discussed in more detail elsewhere in this text; some of the multisystem disorders are briefly described here.

Palmoplantar pustulosis (Chapter 20). A group of overlapping joint diseases occur in conjunction with palmoplantar pustulosis, and less frequently with psoriasis, acne and non-dermatological conditions such as inflammatory bowel disease. The various patterns have been brought together under the acronym SAPHO (*s*ynovitis, *a*cne, *p*ustulosis, *h*yperostosis and *o*steitis). Individual components include predominant sternoclavicular disease (variously termed interseternocostoclavicular osteitis, sternoclavicular pustulotic osteitis, sternocostoclavicular hyperostosis, pustulotic arthro-osteitis or anterior chest wall syndrome; Fig. 62.44) and a more widespread non-purulent chronic recurrent multifocal osteo-

Table 62.24 Some inflammatory and metabolic disorders that affect skin and joints.

Dermatoses
    Psoriasis, Reiter's syndrome, palmoplantar pustulosis
    Acne fulminans and conglobata, SAPHO
Connective tissue diseases
    Lupus erythematosus (especially systemic and subacute cutaneous)
    Mixed connective tissue disease
    Sclerodermas
    Still's disease
    Rheumatic fever
    Rheumatoid disease
    Relapsing polychondritis
Granulomatous disorders
    Sarcoidosis
    Interstitial granulomatous dermatitis with plaques and cords
    Blau syndrome (granulomatous arthritis, uveitis, campylodactyly)
Vasculitis and neutrophilic vascular reactions (see Chapter 50)
    Vasculitis (any; notably Henoch–Schönlein purpura)
    Behçet's disease and related disorders
    Neutrophilic dermatoses (notably Sweet's syndrome)
    Bowel-associated dermatosis–arthritis syndrome
Metabolic, endocrine and deposition disorders
    Gout
    Pancreatic panniculitis
    Amyloidosis
    Scleromyxoedema, cardiac myxoma
    Ochronosis
    Haemochromatosis
    Acromegaly
    Fabry's disease
Infections
    Whipple's disease
    Lyme disease
    Disseminated gonococcal infection, chronic meningococcal infection, others
Miscellaneous
    Ehlers–Danlos syndrome
    Hyper-IgE syndrome
    Multicentric reticulohistiocytosis
    Autoinflammatory disorders (periodic fevers), e.g. familial Mediterranean fever, PAPA

PAPA, *pyogenic arthritis, pyoderma gangrenosum, acne*; SAPHO, *synovitis, acne, pustulosis, hyperostosis, osteomyelitis.*

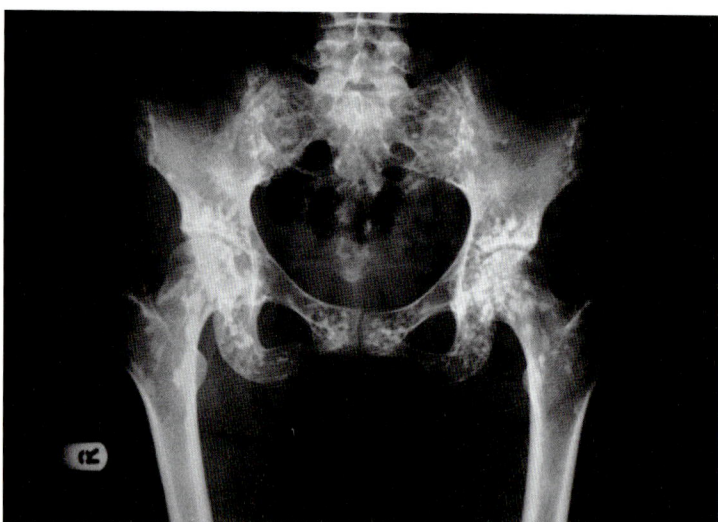

Fig. 62.42 Osteopoikilosis in Buschke–Ollendorf syndrome. (Courtesy of Dr C. Blasdale, Sunderland Royal Infirmary, UK.)

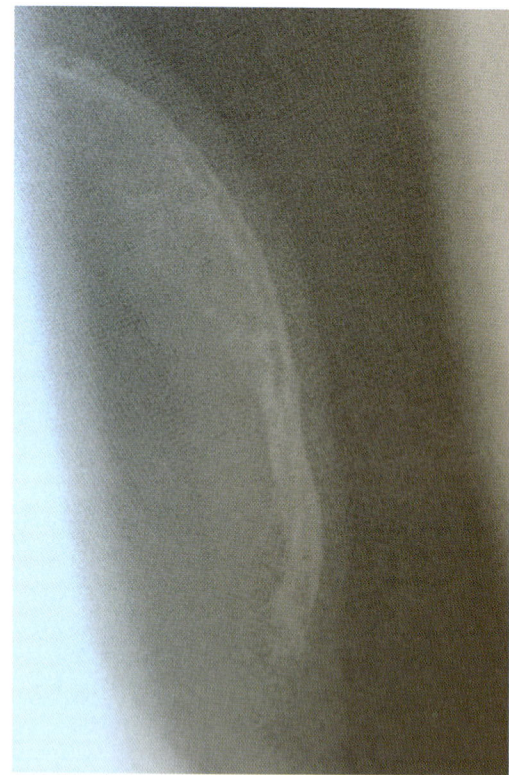

Fig. 62.43 Calcification of the ear due to cold injury.

myelitis [1–5]. Diagnostically, scintigraphy is more sensitive than radiographic examination. Hidradenitis suppurativa and pyoderma gangrenosum have been linked with similar bone and joint changes. Therapeutic options include non-steroidal anti-inflammatory drugs and doxycycline; if infection has been excluded then oral or intra-articular corticosteroids, methotrexate and infliximab may also be considered.

Acne. In addition to the SAPHO pattern described above, arthritis of larger joints occurs in about a third of patients with acne fulminans—most have arthralgia. This is associated with fever, systemic malaise and weight loss, and can usually be controlled with short-term oral corticosteroids. Other skeletal manifestations linked to acne are those secondary to therapeutic agents (skeletal hyperostosis due to isotretinoin, usually only if given long term, and arthralgia in the lupus-like syndrome caused by minocycline);

infectious arthritis due to *Propionibacterium acnes* may also occur [6].

Vasculitides (Chapter 50). Arthralgia or arthritis is a common feature of many disorders in this spectrum, occurring for example in about 90% of patients with systemic lupus erythematosus, two-thirds of those with Henoch–Schönlein purpura and about 40% of those with Behçet's disease.

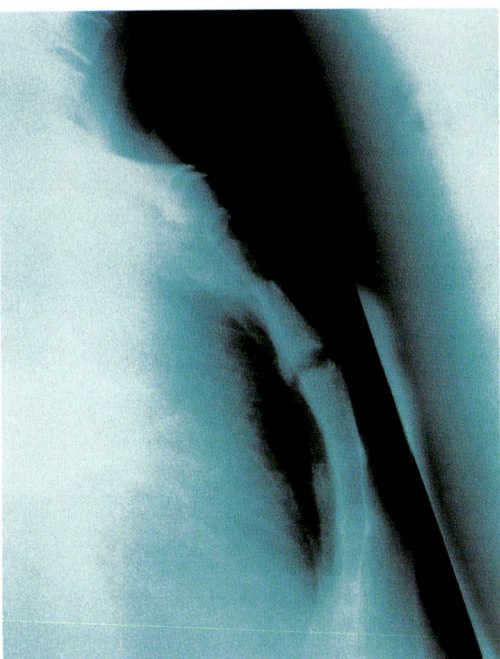

Fig. 62.44 Tomogram showing inflammatory changes of the sternal synchondrosis with widening and 'woolly' appearance in a patient with palmoplantar pustulosis.

Neutrophilic dermatoses. This group of disorders is discussed in relation to gastrointestinal and haematological disease in this chapter, and in more detail in Chapter 50. Sweet's syndrome may be associated with arthralgia, with a frequency of around one-third to over 60%. Patterns include a seronegative polyarthritis, a chronic axial and peripheral destructive polyarthritis, and acute aseptic monoarthritis [7,8]. Multifocal osteomyelitis, which may be chronic or recurrent, is increasingly recognized as one of the systemic manifestations of this syndrome, and localized osteitis may occur in association with pyoderma gangrenosum [9,10].

Connective tissue diseases (Chapter 51) **and rheumatological disorders.** Arthralgia is a major feature in many conditions in this category, such as lupus erythematosus, progressive systemic sclerosis (PSS) and localized acral variants, mixed connective tissue disease and dermatomyositis. Interstitial calcinosis in these disorders has already been briefly discussed. In most cases, radiological studies show no major changes as the arthritis is typically non-erosive, but acral or periarticular osteoporosis may be apparent. In PSS, resorption of distal phalanges may be apparent (Fig. 62.45), as well as osteolytic foci and 'cysts' in bones such as ribs, spinous processes and in the wrists [1]. Melorrheostosis is also linked with scleroderma, usually localized in type.

Rheumatoid arthritis (RA) is associated with potentially severe bone changes, as is psoriatic arthropathy (Chapter 20). Rheumatoid disease is also associated with several skin disorders, including vasculitis, pyoderma gangrenosum and other potentially severe complications. *Fibroblastic rheumatism*, a less well known condition, causes polyarthritis of medium-size joints, together with skin nodules that typically affect the hands and areas adjacent to joints [1]. An unusual but distinctive feature in RA is marked skin redness around the elbows, associated with joint

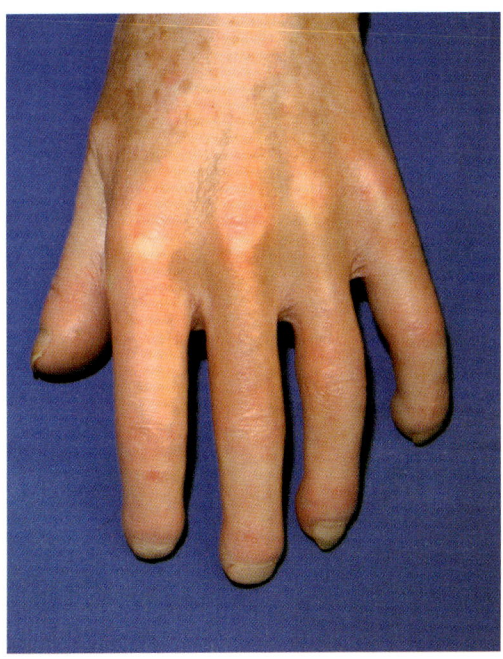

(a)

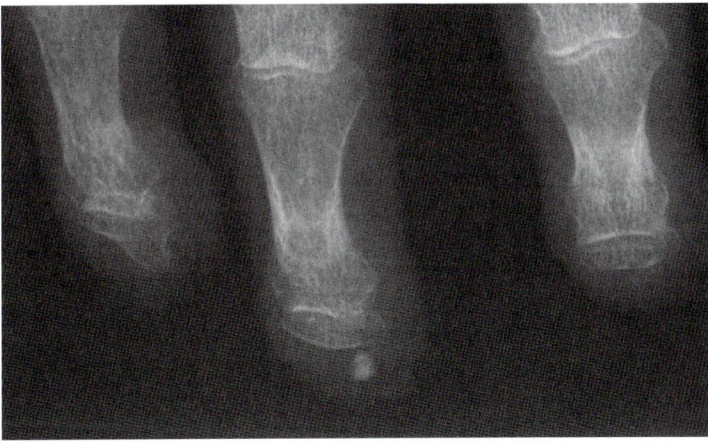

(b)

Fig. 62.45 Progressive systemic sclerosis; (a) tight skin, dyspigmentation, shortening and distortion of phalanges, and (b) X-ray image of the same patient showing bony resorption and some soft tissue calcium deposition.

swelling and raised inflammatory markers—skin histology shows massive aggregates of histiocytes in dilated vessels, with a mixed dermal inflammatory infiltrate [11]. This has been termed *intravascular or intralymphatic histiocytosis associated with RA*.

Interstitial granulomatous dermatitis. This histological pattern may occur in many situations including infections (such as borreliosis or hepatitis C infection), lymphoreticular malignancies, drug eruptions and autoimmune disease. Various skin lesions have been described in *palisading neutrophilic and granulomatous dermatitis (PNGD) of immune complex disease*, including papulonodules, urticaria, vasculitis and granuloma annulare-like lesions. Arthralgia may occur due to systemic vasculitis, and PNGD may occur in rheumatoid arthritis [12]. There are also several reports of a related disorder in which arthritis occurs together with cutaneous lesions that may be plaques or subcutaneous cords ('rope sign'), which are linear or arciform and typically on the trunk or proximal limbs; this disorder is usually termed *interstitial granulomatous dermatitis with plaques* [13,14].

Relapsing polychondritis

Relapsing polychondritis (Chapter 68). Migratory arthritis of small and large joints, usually sparing the hands, is a frequent feature [1,15]. It probably occurs in about two-thirds of patients. Chondritis affecting spinal vertebra may cause chronic back pain.

Still's disease

Still's disease. Evanescent rash (typically erythema marginatum pattern, occurring in about 80%), spiking high fever and arthralgia/arthritis are seen. It is often reasonably characteristic in children, but frequently a less easy diagnosis in the rarer cases in older individuals. Different diagnostic criteria have been proposed for adult-onset Still's disease (AOSD), of which the most sensitive are those of Yamaguchi [16]. Additional cutaneous findings in AOSD are persistent widespread papules and plaques in up to two-thirds of patients, in some cases forming confluent sheets [17] or with a lichenoid or linear patterning [18], vesicopustules and post-inflammatory pigmentation. Marked elevation of ferritin levels is a helpful diagnostic clue in active AOSD.

Multicentric reticulohistiocytosis

Multicentric reticulohistiocytosis (Chapter 55). Polyarthritis, especially affecting the interphalangeal joints of the hands, occurs as the first manifestation of the disorder in half to two-thirds of patients. It is typically rapidly progressive, and all of the synovium-lined joints may become affected, with arthritis mutilans the end result in one-third to half of cases. The erosions are strikingly symmetrical and well circumscribed, and accompanying osteoporosis is disproportionately mild. The arthritis may burn out, but residual hypertrophic osteoarthropathy may persist [1,19]. A disorder reported as familial histiocytic dermatoarthritis [20] has been described in which there is early onset of a papulonodular eruption, a symmetrical destructive arthritis and ocular lesions such as cataract and glaucoma. Subsequent cases and electron microscopy studies [21] suggest that this may be part of the spectrum of multicentric reticulohistiocytosis.

Autoinflammatory syndromes (periodic fevers)

Autoinflammatory syndromes (periodic fevers). The most important 'classical' periodic fevers are familial Mediterranean fever (FMF; MIM *249100), FMF with amyloidosis (MIM *134610), Hibernian fever—now redesignated as *tumour necrosis factor (TNF) receptor–associated periodic syndrome*, TRAPS, MIM #142680—and the hyperimmunoglobulin D and periodic fever syndrome (HIDS; MIM #260920). All are characterized by recurrent fever with serositis (peritonitis-like abdominal pain, pleurisy, pericarditis), headache and arthralgia or arthritis [22–26]. In FMF, there may be urticarial lesions, subcutaneous nodules, purpura, leukocytoclastic vasculitis (described, probably incorrectly, as Henoch–Schönlein purpura), or transient cellulitis-like erythematous plaques [22–25]. Both the articular symptoms [26], and erysipelas-like skin lesions predominantly affect the lower leg [23]. Erythematous macules and nodules, but not the erysipelas-like lesions, may occur in HIDS [22]. In TRAPS, the cutaneous features include migratory patches, oedematous plaques and periorbital oedema [23]. FMF is due to a variety of mutations in the *MEFV*

gene [27]; classic-type HIDS is due to mutations in the *MVK* gene leading to deficient activity of mevalonate kinase [28,29]; and TRAPS is due to mutations in *TNFRSF1A*, which codes for the 55-kDa TNF receptor [26].

This spectrum has recently been expanded by the addition of some hereditary syndromes that may not include fever, but which have related mutations in genes that regulate innate immunity. Dermatologically, this includes several 'connective tissue' diseases, as well as a number of syndromes that include both skin and bone components [30]. Some of these have already been discussed above or are discussed in other chapters, including sarcoidosis, PAPA (pyogenic arthritis, pyoderma gangrenosum, acne) syndrome (now known to be due to a mutation of *PSTPIP1*), chronic recurrent multifocal osteomyelitis (linked with acne and hidradenitis suppurativa) and psoriatic arthropathy. *Blau syndrome* is also included with the above conditions. It is a familial condition in which there is granulomatous arthritis, granulomatous skin rash and uveitis, with synovial cysts and camptodactyly [31]; the underlying defect is a mutation in *NOD2* which is an intracellular toll-like receptor. Increasingly, defects of handling microbial agents are being demonstrated in these conditions.

Sarcoidosis is discussed in detail in Chapter 61. The classical constellation of features in acute sarcoidosis includes erythema nodosum, arthralgia of medium sized joints and hilar lymphadenopathy [32]. The main differential diagnoses for the joint symptoms include Lyme disease, gonococcal infection and Reiter's syndrome. Less recognized is an acute periarticular ankle inflammation [32], which may occur alone or with erythema nodosum, is more common in men, and in which skin biopsy from the periarticular subcutis shows a non-specific inflammation or panniculitis. Chronic sarcoidosis is associated with both articular symptoms and bone cysts [33], often affecting the hands and occasionally presenting to dermatologists initially [34].

Inherited conditions associated with hypermobility of joints include Ehlers–Danlos syndrome, of which there are several types, and hyper-IgE syndrome in which two-thirds of patients have hyperextensible joints together with a triad of abscesses, pneumonia and elevated IgE levels [35].

References

1 Freyschmidt J, Freyschmidt G. *SKIBO-Diseases. Disorders Affecting the Skin and Bones.* Berlin, Germany: Springer-Verlag, 1999.
2 Orlow SJ, Watsky KL, Bolognia JL. Skin and bones, 2. *J Am Acad Dermatol* 1991; **25**: 447–62.
3 Hayem G, Bouchard-Chabot A, Benali K *et al.* SAPHO syndrome: a long-term follow-up study of 120 cases. *Semin Arthritis Rheum* 1999; **29**: 159–71.
4 Schilling F, Kessler S. [SAPHO syndrome: clinico-rheumatologic and radiologic differentiation and classification of a patient sample of 86 cases; in German]. *Z Rheumatol* 2000; **59**: 1–28.
5 Hyodoh K, Sugimoto H. Pustulotic arthro-osteitis: defining the radiologic spectrum of the disease. *Semin Musculoskelet Radiol* 2001; **5**: 89–93.
6 Hustache-Mathieu L, Brousse A, Lohse A *et al.* Infectious osteoarthritis due to *Propionibacterium* acnes: two new cases. *Rev Méd Interne* 2000; **21**: 547–9.
7 Smolle J, Kresbach H. Acute febrile neutrophilic dermatosis (Sweet syndrome): a retrospective clinical and histological analysis. *Hautarzt* 1990; **41**: 549–56.
8 Wallach D, Vignon-Pennamen M-D. From acute febrile neutrophilic dermatosis to neutrophilic disease: forty years of clinical research. *J Am Acad Dermatol* 2007; **55**: 1066–71.
9 Marie I, Boyer A, Heron F *et al.* Focal aseptic osteitis underlying neutrophilic dermatosis. *Br J Dermatol* 1998; **139**: 744–5.

10 Rodot S, Lacour JP, Van Elslande L et al. Manifestations extra-cutanées des dermatoses neutrophiliques. Ann Dermatol-Venereol 1996; **123**: 129–34.

11 Takiwaki H, Adachi A, Kohno H, Ogawa Y. Intravascular or intralymphatic histiocytosis associated with rheumatoid arthritis: a report of 4 cases. J Am Acad Dermatol 2004; **50**: 585–90.

12 Sangueza O, Caudell MD, Mengesha YM et al. Palisaded neutrophilic and granulomatous dermatitis in rheumatoid arthritis. J Am Acad Dermatol 2002; **47**: 251–7.

13 Tomasini C, Pippione M. Interstitial granulomatous dermatitis with plaques. J Am Acad Dermatol 2002; **46**: 892–9.

14 Verneuil L, Dompmartin A, Comoz F et al. Interstitial granulomatous dermatitis with cutaneous cords and arthritis: a disorder associated with autoantibodies. J Am Acad Dermatol 2001; **45**: 286–91.

15 O'Hanlan M, McAdam LP, Bluestone R et al. The arthropathy of relapsing polychondritis. Arthritis Rheum 1976; **19**: 191–4.

16 Masson C, Le Loet X, Liote F et al. Comparative study of 6 types of criteria in adult Still's disease. J Rheumatol 1996; **23**: 495–7.

17 Lee JY-Y, Yang C-C, Hsu MM-L. Histopathology of persistent papules and plaques in adult-onset Still's disease. J Am Acad Dermatol 2005; **52**: 1003–8.

18 Perez C, Montes M, Gallego M, Loza E. Atypical presentation of adult Still's disease with generalized rash and hyperferritinaemia. Br J Dermatol 2001; **145**: 187–8.

19 Lesher JL Jr, Allen BS. Multicentric reticulohistiocytosis. J Am Acad Dermatol 1984; **11**: 713–23.

20 Zayid I, Farraj S. Familial histiocytotic dermatoarthritis. Am J Med 1973; **54**: 793–800.

21 Valente M, Parenti A, Cipriani R, Peserico A. Familial histiocytotic dermatoarthritis: histologic and ultrastructural findings in two cases. Am J Dermatopathol 1987; **9**: 491–6.

22 Braverman IM. Skin Signs of Systemic Disease, 3rd edn. Philadelphia: Saunders, 1998: 412–3.

23 Sohar E, Gafni J, Pras M et al. Familial Mediterranean fever: a survey of 470 cases and review of the literature. Am J Med 1967; **43**: 227–53.

24 Majeed HA, Quabazard Z, Hijazi Z et al. The cutaneous manifestations in children with familial Mediterranean fever (recurrent hereditary polyserositis): a six-year study. QJM 1990; **278**: 607–16.

25 Uthman I, Hajj-Ali RA, Arayssi T, Masri AF, Nasr F. Arthritis in familial Mediterranean fever. Rheumatol Int 2001; **20**: 145–8.

26 Toro JR, Aksentijevitch I, Hull K et al. Tumour necrosis factor receptor-associated periodic syndrome. Arch Dermatol 2000; **136**: 1487–94.

27 Touitou I. The spectrum of familial Mediterranean fever (FMF) mutations. Eur J Hum Genet 2001; **9**: 473–83.

28 Houten SM, Koster J, Romeijn GJ et al. Organization of the mevalonate kinase (MVK) gene and identification of novel mutations causing mevalonic aciduria and hyperimmunoglobulinaemia D and periodic fever syndrome. Eur J Hum Genet 2001; **9**: 253–9.

29 Simon A, Cuisset L, Vincent MF et al. Molecular analysis of the mevalonate kinase gene in a cohort of patients with the hyper-IgD and periodic fever syndrome: its application as a diagnostic tool. Ann Intern Med 2001; **135**: 338–43.

30 Kanazawa K, Furukawa F. Autoinflammatory syndromes: a dermatological perspective. J Dermatol 2007; **34**: 601–18.

31 Schaffer JV, Chandra P, Keegan BR et al. Widespread granulomatous dermatitis of infancy: an early sign of Blau syndrome. Arch Dermatol 2007; **143**: 386–91.

32 Mañá J, Gómez-Vaquero C, Montero A et al. Löfgren's syndrome revisited: a study of 186 patients. Am J Med 1999; **107**: 240–5.

33 Torralba KD, Quismorio FP Jr. Sarcoid arthritis: a review of clinical features, pathology and therapy. Sarcoidosis Vasc Diffuse Lung Dis 2003; **20**: 95–103.

34 Cox NH, Gawkrodger DJ. Nail dystrophy in chronic sarcoidosis. Br J Dermatol 1988; **118**: 697–701.

35 Grimbacher B, Holland SM, Gallin JI et al. Hyper-IgE syndrome with recurrent infections—an autosomal dominant multisystem disorder. N Engl J Med 1999; **340**: 692–702.

Metabolic conditions

Gout may present to dermatologists due to tophi, but is generally diagnosed due to acute arthropathy or chronic erosive joint disease [1,2]. Tophi may be small and occurring in clusters, but may be large and deforming, and may be associated with lytic bone lesions. They may be detected within the carpal tunnel using CT or MRI. Medullary tophi cause subchondral osteolytic areas [1].

Haemochromatosis—arthropathy is a frequent complication, probably due to abnormal accumulation of metal ions [3,4]; other aspects are discussed elsewhere in this chapter.

Ochronosis is discussed in Chapter 68. Calcium crystal deposition accompanies the cartilage degradation characteristic of this disease [4].

Amyloidosis (Chapter 59) is closely linked to joint disease, as rheumatoid arthritis is the commonest cause of secondary amyloidosis [5]. Amyloid A has cytokine-like properties and may be actively involved in inflammatory processes.

Scleromyxoedema causes arthralgia or arthritis in 10% of patients, and is also associated with rheumatoid arthritis and sicca syndrome. Carpal tunnel syndrome and acroosteolysis may also occur [6].

Other metabolic disorders that may have skin and bony or joint symptoms include Fabry's disease, Gaucher's disease and Farber's disease [4]. Bone symptoms are an important part of Gaucher's disease [4,7]. Bone crises may be related in part to haemorrhage; they may be treated with prednisolone, bisphosphonates or with prophylactic enzyme replacement therapy. Avascular necrosis, pathological fractures and cortical destruction of bones with extraosseous extension also occur.

Xanthomas at acral sites can be associated with prominent defects in underlying phalanges.

Scurvy is discussed in Chapter 59; bony features are listed in Table 62.23.

Infections

Numerous infective conditions may affect both the skin and joints. Arthralgia is associated with the exanthem of viral infections such as parvovirus, hepatitis B or rubella. Reiter's syndrome may be provoked by genital infections such as Chlamydia, or by various enteritic organisms such as Yersinia, Shigella or Campylobacter. Arthralgia is frequent, with constitutional symptoms and a non-specific exanthem, in brucellosis. Other bacterial causes of arthritis with pustular or vasculitis skin lesions include disseminated gonococcal infection and chronic meningococcal septicaemia. Arthralgia may be prominent in spirochaetal diseases such as Lyme disease or secondary syphilis. In the latter, the flat bones of the skull are frequently involved, causing headache. Osteomyelitis is a feature of tertiary syphilis. Arthralgia is the presenting feature in two-thirds of patients in the early stage of Whipple's disease [8,9].

References

1 Freyschmidt J, Freyschmidt G. SKIBO-Diseases. Disorders Affecting the Skin and Bones. Berlin, Germany: Springer-Verlag, 1999.

2 Agudelo CA, Wise CM. Gout: diagnosis, pathogenesis, and clinical manifestations. Curr Opin Rheumatol 2001; **13**: 234–9.

3 von Kempis J. Arthropathy in hereditary hemochromatosis. Curr Opin Rheumatol 2001; **13**: 80–3.

4 Rooney PJ. Hyperlipidemias, lipid storage disorders, metal storage disorders, and ochronosis. Curr Opin Rheumatol 1991; **3**: 166–71.

5 Cunnane G. Amyloid precursors and amyloidosis in inflammatory arthritis. Curr Opin Rheumatol 2001; **13**: 67–73.

6 Rongioletti F, Rebora A. Updated classification of papular mucinosis, lichen myxedematosus, and scleromyxedema. J Am Acad Dermatol 2001; **44**: 273–81.

7 Ida H, Rennert OM, Kato S *et al.* Severe skeletal complications in Japanese patients with type 1 Gaucher disease. *J Inherit Metab Dis* 1999; **22**: 63–73.

8 Durand DV, Lecomte C, Cathebras P, Rousset H, Godeau P. Whipple disease: clinical review of 52 cases. The SNFMI Research Group on Whipple disease. *Medicine* 1997; **76**: 170–84.

9 Puechal X. Whipple disease and arthritis. *Curr Opin Rheumatol* 2001; **13**: 74–9.

Annular and figurate reactive erythemas

Numerous dermatoses produce annular lesions, in some cases leading to a specific diagnosis (for example, tinea corporis or granuloma annulare). The aim of this section is not to discuss all annular eruptions that may be part of a systemic disease (such as annular sarcoidosis). However, there are a group of, often chronic, annular and figurate eruptions that do not easily lead to a specific diagnosis. This rather vague group, collectively termed 'annular erythemas', and some of their more important differential diagnoses, may have systemic causes and may pose diagnostic and therapeutic problems. The nomenclature of this group of disorders has been discussed in detail elsewhere [1] but most of the descriptive and eponymous terms that are applied do not help greatly in management of the patient. Equally, although the pathological features can be divided into those cases with superficial or deep perivascular lymphohistiocytic infiltrate ('superficial or deep gyrate erythema' [2], clinically corresponding to annular erythema with scaling or with smooth surface respectively), the clinical relevance of this is not clear. Some of these annular erythemas that have a specific clinical pattern or clinical course related to their aetiology are discussed separately; the remainder are conveniently grouped with erythema annulare centrifugum (EAC) although it should be appreciated that this latter group are undoubtedly a heterogeneous mixture.

For the purposes of this section, the following will be discussed:
1 Erythema (chronicum) migrans
2 Erythema marginatum (rheumaticum)
3 Erythema gyratum repens
4 Annular erythema of infancy
5 Annular erythema associated with extractable nuclear antigens
6 Erythema annulare centrifugum and other 'annular erythemas'
7 Neutrophilic and vasculitic annular eruptions.

References
1 Bressler GS, Jones RE. Erythema annulare centrifugum. *J Am Acad Dermatol* 1981; **4**: 597–602.

2 Ackerman AB. *Histologic Diagnosis of Inflammatory Skin Diseases.* Philadelphia: Lea & Febiger, 1978: 1784–5, 231–3, 283–4.

Erythema migrans (Chapter 30)

Erythema (chronicum) migrans is the term applied to the commonest skin lesion of Lyme borreliosis. This condition is caused by infection with *Borrelia burgdorferi sensu lato, B. afzellii* or *B. garinii,* which are spirochaetes transmitted by bites from *Ixodes* ticks [1]. The primary lesion of erythema migrans at the site of a tick bite is usually solitary and usually essentially flat with mild inflammation, but may be urticated or haemorrhagic (lesions of *B. burgdorferi* are usually more inflammatory and more rapid in evolution than those caused by the other species). The shape may be an expanding annular morphology, a homogeneous macule, or less often may consist of concentric target-like rings. Non-annular erythema migrans is more frequent in infections with *B. afzellii* or *B. garinii* in parts of Europe. Malaise, flu-like symptoms and lymphadenopathy are common at this stage. The lesion expands slowly over a period of weeks to a median size of about 15 cm with central clearing (the early-localized, or first, stage) [2–6]. Although erythema migrans accounts for 85% of skin lesions of Lyme disease, a 'borrelial lymphocytoma' is another manifestation of this stage, consisting of a small (up to 5 mm) plaque, usually on the earlobe, nose, areola, scrotum or over bony prominences. The two disorders together are pathognomic for Lyme borreliosis.

In the early disseminated (or second) stage, which occurs within one to a few weeks, additional, usually multiple, annular plaques may develop in up to half of patients. These are usually smaller than the first stage lesion, and may have a polycyclic pattern that resembles erythema annulare centrifugum or an annular erythema multiforme-like appearance. The term 'erythema migrans chronicum' is something of a misnomer as the early stages are of quite short duration, although Lyme disease itself may become chronic if untreated, and a chronic (third, or late disseminated, stage) skin lesion termed acrodermatitis chronicum atrophicans may occur in such cases. Rarely, lesions typical of erythema migrans may occur in the third stage [7]; there may also be lesions clinically resembling morphoea and having histological features of an interstitial granulomatous dermatitis with histiocytic pseudorosettes [7].

Histology of early localized or disseminated stage erythema migrans shows a superficial perivascular lymphocytic infiltrate, which may contain plasma cells, and which may extend more deeply around vessels or appendages. The diagnosis can be confirmed serologically, but serology after treatment is not useful for predicting the clinical course—persistence of IgG antibody is linked with size and duration of erythema migrans, rather than with other clinical variables [8].

Treatment is usually with tetracyclines (generally doxycycline 100 mg b.d. for 2–3 weeks, although a single dose has been reported as being effective in 87%) or ampicillin; third-generation cephalosporins such as ceftiaxone are the alternative. Vaccination was also available in the USA but, due to high cost and uncertainty about safety and efficacy, was withdrawn from the market. It should be noted that coinfection with the organism of human granulocytic anaplasmosis (was human granulocytotropic ehrlichiosis) has been reported in up to 20% of cases, both organisms being carried by deer ticks [9].

Associated systemic manifestations in the disseminated stages include arthralgia and arthritis, myalgia, cardiac involvement (especially atrioventricular block or pericarditis) and a variety of neurological manifestations (cranial nerve palsies, peripheral neuropathy, meningitis, encephalitis). These same features are seen in canine infection. Treatments for Lyme disease with heart block, facial palsy or meningitis have recently been reviewed [10].

References

1 Burgdorfer W. Vector/host relationships of the Lyme disease spirochaete, *Borrelia burgdorferi*. *Rheum Dis Clin North Am* 1989; **15**: 775–87.

2 Berger BW. Cutaneous manifestations of Lyme borreliosis. *Rheum Dis Clin North Am* 1989; **15**: 627–34.

3 Steere AC. Lyme disease. *N Engl J Med* 2001; **345**: 115–25.

4 Singh-Behl D, La Rosa SP, Tomecki KJ. Tick-borne infections. *Dermatol Clin* 2003; **21**: 237–44.

5 Hercogová J. Lyme borreliosis up-to-date. *G Ital Dermatol Venereol* 2005; **140**: 321–3.

6 Feder HM Jr, Abeles M, Bernstein M, Whitaker-Worth D, Grant-Kels JM. Diagnosis, treatment and prognosis of erythema migrans and Lyme disease. *Clin Dermatol* 2006; **24**: 509–20.

7 Moreno C, Kützner H, Palmedo G, Goerttier E, Carrasco L, Requena L. Interstitial granulomatous dermatitis with histiocytic pseudorosettes: a new histopathologic pattern in cutaneous borreliosis. Detection of *Borrelia burgdorferi* DNA sequences by a highly sensitive PCR-ELISA. *J Am Acad Dermatol* 2003; **48**: 376–84.

8 Glatz M, Golestani M, Kerl H, Müllegger RR. Clinical relevance of different IgG and IgM serum antibody responses to *Borrelia burgdorferi* after antibiotic therapy for erythema migrans. *Arch Dermatol* 2006; **142**: 862–8.

9 McJunkin JE, Irazuzta J, Thompson AE. Coinfection with *Borrelia burgdorferi* and the agent of human granulocytic ehrlichiosis. *N Eng J Med* 2001; **345**: 150–1.

10 Wormser GP. Early Lyme disease. *N Eng J Med* 2006; **354**: 2794–801.

Erythema marginatum (rheumaticum)

> **Synonym**
> • Erythema annulare rheumaticum

Rashes of various morphologies can occur in rheumatic fever and Still's disease, erythema marginatum being the most classical and distinctive, but now rare, pattern. Along with carditis, migratory polyarthritis, chorea and subcutaneous nodules, it is one of the Duckett Jones major criteria for the diagnosis of rheumatic fever, and is probably specific for this diagnosis (two major, or one major and two minor, criteria are strictly required for the diagnosis but newer echocardiography techniques and Doppler colour flow mapping may extend the diagnostic criteria). However, erythema marginatum may be subtle, and only occurs in about 10% of patients (especially in children) with active rheumatic fever [1–3]; one study of 126 children (80 first attacks and 46 recurrences) did not identify any with erythema marginatum [4].

The eruption consists of rings or segments of rings, pale or dull red in colour, flat or palpably thickened. The rings may be discrete, or may enlarge and merge to produce a polycyclic or reticular pattern.

Characteristically, the lesions fade in a few hours or at most in 2–3 days, and tend to be more prominent in the afternoon. Recurrent crops, often in different sites, may appear at intervals for many weeks. The lesions occur most frequently on the trunk, especially on the abdomen, but are occasionally seen on the limbs. They are asymptomatic.

Histologically, an infiltrate of polymorphs can help to distinguish this disease from other annular erythemas [5], but is not always found.

A similar eruption has been reported with psittacosis [6], and erythema marginatum has been reported preceding attacks of hereditary angioneurotic oedema [7,8].

References

1 Abt AF. Erythema annulare rheumaticum. *Am J Med Sci* 1935; **190**: 824–33.

2 Keil H. The rheumatic erythemas; a critical survey. *Ann Intern Med* 1937–38; **11**: 2223–72.

3 Rullan E, Sigal LH. Rheumatic fever. *Curr Rheumatol Rep* 2001; **3**: 445–52.

4 Jamal M, Abbas KA. Clinical profile of acute rheumatic fever in children. *J Trop Pediatr* 1989; **35**: 10–3.

5 Troyer C, Grossman ME, Silvers DN. Erythema marginatum in rheumatic fever: early diagnosis by skin biopsy. *J Am Acad Dermatol* 1983; **8**: 724–8.

6 Green ST, Hamlet NW, Willocks L *et al.* Psittacosis presenting with erythema marginatum-like lesions—a case report and a historical review. *Clin Exp Dermatol* 1990; **15**: 225–7.

7 Starr JC, Brasher GW. Erythema marginatum preceding hereditary angioedema. *J Allergy Clin Immunol* 1974; **53**: 352–5.

8 Farkas H, Harmat G, Fáy A *et al.* Erythema marginatum preceding an acute oedematous attack of hereditary angioneurotic oedema. *Acta Dermatovenereol* 2001; **81**: 376–7.

Erythema gyratum repens [1–8]

The first description of this condition in 1953 is attributed to Gammel, who reported a case associated with breast carcinoma [1]. It is exceptionally rare but clinically distinctive (see Fig. 62.14). It is more common in men than in women, and usually occurs in or after the seventh decade of life.

Clinical features [1–8]. Regular waves of erythema spread over the body to produce a series of concentric, figurate bands in a pattern resembling the grain of wood (see Fig. 62.14). The characteristic feature is the way rings, swirls or waves appear within existing lesions to form a concentric pattern of sequential eruptions, with day-to-day migration of the leading edge by about 1 cm. Scaling, usually at the trailing edge, and itch are usually prominent. This is by contrast to the more common 'annular erythemas' of erythema annulare centrifugum pattern, in which each lesion is usually a distinct ring or arc with variable but usually without prominent scale, and not in a concentric arrangement. Hyperkeratosis of palms occurs in about 10% and has been reported in both paraneoplastic and idiopathic cases.

Aetiology. This eruption has been briefly discussed earlier (p. 62.38) as a paraneoplastic eruption; about 80% of reported cases are associated with an internal tumour [4,6–9], most commonly of the lung. Other tumour sites include bowel, oesophagus, urogenital tract, breast, pancreas and haematological neoplasia.

However, not all cases are paraneoplastic. Since the report of a case associated with tuberculosis [10], several cases have been reported in apparently well patients or associated with other disorders such as CREST syndrome (reviewed in [4,7]). Drug hypersensitivity has also been implicated. Some of these non-paraneoplastic cases are questionable in the absence of photographic documentation, but some cases appear very convincing, such as a patient with recurrent pregnancy-associated episodes [11]. An infant was reported in whom lesions were controlled by long-term systemic ketoconazole [12].

Pathology [13]. There is a superficial, and occasionally deep, perivascular lymphocytic infiltrate associated with acanthosis, spongiosis and parakeratosis. Deposition of C3 or IgG in the sublamina densa region supports the concept that the eruption is immunologically mediated, possibly by immune complex deposition [5,14].

Investigation. The paramount issue is a detailed search for underlying malignancy. Fungal infection should be excluded, especially tinea imbricata in relevant populations. Skin biopsy is important as a similar gyrate eruption may be a prodromal manifestation of pemphigoid [15], and similar but rather localized lesions have been reported due to vasculitis, especially in lupus erythematosus [16] and in neutrophilic dermatoses; a morphologically similar disorder termed lupus erythematosus gyratum repens has been reported, related to either medications or internal malignancy [17,18]. Necrolytic migratory erythema (p. 62.66) and erythrokeratoderma variabilis (Chapter 19) may produce very similar lesions, as may the subacute annular (Lapière) variant of psoriasis, although none of these typically have multiple concentric lesions. Cases of apparent idiopathic erythema gyratum repens have also been suggested to represent a stage in the evolution of pityriasis rubra pilaris [19,20]. A patient with EBA associated with ulcerative colitis has been reported due to occurrence of erythema gyratum repens-like lesions, but PCT-like erosions and milia on the dorsum of hands and feet were also present [21].

References

1 Gammel JA. Erythema gyratum repens. *AMA Arch Dermatol Syphilol* 1953; **66**: 494–505.

2 Thomson J, Stankler L. Erythema gyratum repens. *Br J Dermatol* 1970; **82**: 406–11.

3 Thomas I, Schwartz RA. Cutaneous paraneoplastic syndromes: uncommon presentations. *Clinics Dermatol* 2005; **23**: 593–600.

4 Boyd AS, Neldner KH, Menter A. Erythema gyratum repens: a paraneoplastic eruption. *J Am Acad Dermatol* 1992; **26**: 757–62.

5 Holt PJA, Davies MG. Erythema gyratum repens—an immunologically mediated dermatosis? *Br J Dermatol* 1977; **96**: 343–7.

6 Stone SP, Buescher LS. Life-threatening paraneoplastic cutaneous syndromes. *Clinics Dermatol* 2005; **23**: 301–6.

7 Tyring SK. Reactive erythemas: erythema annulare centrifugum and erythema gyratum repens. *Clin Dermatol* 1993; **11**: 135–9.

8 Eubanks LE, McBurney E, Reed R. Erythema gyratum repens. *Am J Med Sci* 2001; **321**: 302–5.

9 Kawakami T, Saito R. Erythema gyratum repens unassociated with underlying malignancy. *J Dermatol* 1995; **22**: 587–9.

10 Barber PV, Doyle L, Vickers DM *et al*. Erythema gyratum repens with pulmonary tuberculosis. *Br J Dermatol* 1978; **98**: 465–8.

11 Garrett SJ, Roenigk HH. Erythema gyratum repens in a healthy woman. *J Am Acad Dermatol* 1992; **26**: 121–2.

12 Saurat JH, Janin-Mercier A. Infantile epidermodysplastic erythema gyratum responsive to imidazoles. A new entity? *Arch Dermatol* 1984; **120**: 1601–3.

13 Weedon D. *Skin Pathology*, 2nd edn. London: Churchill Livingstone, 2002: 245–6.

14 Caux F, Lebbe C, Thomine E *et al*. Erythema gyratum repens: a case studied with immunofluorescence, immunoelectron microscopy and immunohistochemistry. *Br J Dermatol* 1994; **131**: 102–7.

15 Breathnach SM, Wilkinson JD, Black MM. Erythema gyratum repens-like figurate eruption in bullous pemphigoid. *Clin Exp Dermatol* 1982; **7**: 401–6.

16 Piqué E, Palacios S, Santana Z. Leukocytoclastic vasculitis presenting as an erythema gyratum repens-like eruption on a patient with systemic lupus erythematosus. *J Am Acad Dermatol* 2002; **47** (5 Suppl.): S254–6.

17 Blanc D, Kienzler J-L. Lupus erythematosus gyratus repens. Report of a case associated with lung carcinoma. *Clin Exp Dermatol* 1982; **77**: 129–34.

18 Kreft B, Marsch WC. Lupus erythematosus gyratum repens. *Eur J Dermatol* 2007; **17**: 79–82.

19 Cheesbrough MJ, Williamson DM. Erythema gyratum repens, a stage in the evolution of pityriasis rubra pilaris? *Clin Exp Dermatol* 1985; **10**: 466–71.

20 Gebauer K, Singh G. Resolving pityriasis rubra pilaris resembling erythema gyratum repens. *Arch Dermatol* 1993; **129**: 917–8.

21 España A, Sitaru C, Pretel M *et al*. Erythema gyratum repens-like eruption in a patient with epidermoysis bullosa acquisita associated with ulcerative colitis. *Br J Dermatol* 2007; **156**: 773–5.

Annular erythema of infancy

This term was first applied by Peterson and Jarratt [1] although infantile onset of a similar eruption had been reported previously [2]; numerous cases have been reported subsequently [3–8]. Although the age group does not define a category that can be distinguished from other cases of EAC, and probably also represents a range of disorders, the implications for investigation are somewhat different. For example, cutaneous fungal infection and malignant diseases are unlikely causes, whereas other (systemic) infections and lupus erythematosus-related antibodies (see below) are important to exclude. However, the fact that some cases started in teenage years and others in infancy in a family with autosomal dominantly inherited annular erythema [9] argues against there being a specific infantile variant.

Clinical features. The clinical morphology of lesions is generally as described for EAC.

Pathology. Histological appearances are typically the same as in cases of EAC. However, some authors have reported eosinophils to be prominent [7,8] and they may be the predominant cell type and associated with peripheral eosinophilia [10]. A neutrophilic variant has also been reported [6,11,12].

Aetiology. As in EAC (below), no cause can be identified in many patients, often despite extensive investigation. Some childhood cases may be discovered to have lupus erythematosus or have had transplacental transfer of maternal antibodies against extractable nuclear antigens, as discussed below; a clinical pattern described as erythema gyratum atrophicans transiens neonatale is now felt to be a variant of neonatal lupus erythematosus [13]. Heavy intestinal colonization with *Candida albicans* has been documented as a cause [14], and concurrent Epstein–Barr virus infection has been reported in an infant [15]. *Pityrosporum* infection in an infant has been reported as a mimic of EAC [16]; other differential diagnoses that may apply in children are listed in the section on EAC. A recently described 'annular lichenoid dermatitis of youth' [17] appears to be distinct, although it may include lesions resembling annular erythema; 'lymphomatoid annular erythema' [18] has also been described as a childhood presentation of mycosis fungoides.

Treatment. Any associated infection should be treated as discussed in the section on aetiology. Treatments are otherwise symptomatic, as for EAC. In one case, lesions resolved during febrile episodes but reappeared 2 weeks later [12]. Responses to sodium cromoglycate and to IFN-α have been reported, but in many cases new lesions continue to erupt over many years.

References

1 Peterson AO, Jarratt MD. Annular erythema of infancy. *Arch Dermatol* 1981; **117**: 145–8.

2 Fried R, Schonberg IL, Litt JZ. Erythema annulare centrifugum (Darier) in a newborn infant. *J Pediatr* 1957; **50**: 66–7.

3 Herbert A, Esterly NB. Annular erythema in infancy. *J Am Acad Dermatol* 1986; **14**: 339–43.

4 Helm TN, Bass J, Chang LW, Bergfield WF. Persistent annular erythema in infancy. *Pediatr Dermatol* 1993; **10**: 46–8.

5 Toonstra J, de Witt RFE. 'Persistent' annular erythema of infancy. *Arch Dermatol* 1984; **120**: 1069–72.

6 Cox NH, McQueen A, Evans TJ *et al.* An annular erythema of infancy. *Arch Dermatol* 1987; **123**: 510–3.

7 Helm TN, Bass J, Chang LW *et al.* Persistent annular erythema of infancy. *Pediatr Dermatol* 1993; **10**: 46–8.

8 Hebert AA, Esterly NB. Annular erythema of infancy. *J Am Acad Dermatol* 1986; **14**: 339–43.

9 Beare JM, Frogatt P, Jones JH *et al.* Familial annular erythema. An apparently new dominant mutation. *Br J Dermatol* 1966; **78**: 59–68.

10 Kunz M, Hamm K, Brocker EB *et al.* Annular erythema in childhood—a new eosinophilic dermatosis. *Hautarzt* 1998; **49**: 131–4.

11 Annessi G, Signoretti S, Angelo C *et al.* Neutrophilic figurate erythema of infancy. *Am J Dermatopathol* 1997; **19**: 403–6.

12 Patrizi A, Savoia F, Varotti E *et al.* Neutrophilic figurate erythema of infancy. *Ped Dermatol* 2008; **25**: 255–60.

13 Puig L, Moreno A, Alomar A *et al.* Erythema gyratum atrophicans transiens neonatale: a variant of cutaneous neonatal lupus erythematosus. *Pediatr Dermatol* 1988; **5**: 112–6.

14 Stachowitz S, Abeck D, Schmidt T *et al.* Persistent annular erythema of infancy associated with intestinal *Candida* colonization. *Clin Exp Dermatol* 2000; **25**: 404–5.

15 Hammar H. Erythema annulare centrifugum coincident with Epstein–Barr virus infection in an infant. *Acta Paediatr Scand* 1974; **63**: 788–92.

16 Kikuchi I, Ogata K, Inoue S. *Pityrosporum* infection in an infant with lesions resembling erythema annulare centrifugum. *Arch Dermatol* 1984; **120**: 380–2.

17 Annessi G, Paradisi M, Angelo C *et al.* Annular lichenoid dermatitis of youth. *J Am Acad Dermatol* 2003; **49**: 1029–6.

18 Cogrel O, Boralevi F, Lepreux S *et al.* Lymphomatoid annular erythema: a new form of juvenile mycosis fungoides. *Br J Dermatol* 2005; **152**: 565–6.

Annular erythema associated with extractable nuclear antigens

It has been recognized for many years that annular lesions in neonatal lupus erythematosus are related to maternal antibodies against SSA(Ro) [1]. Neonatal lupus erythematosus with annular lesions but without anti-SSA antibodies may be explained by the demonstration that some patients have anti-U1RNP antibodies instead [2].

More recently, it has been recognized that annular lesions may occur in anti-SSA(Ro)-positive patients with Sjögren's syndrome, lupus erythematosus (or both together), and less commonly in otherwise well patients who do not fit criteria for either of these diagnoses [3–6]. In a group of 15 patients with anti-SSA antibodies and annular erythema, all sera were positive for the anti-60kDa-SSA and 11 for the anti-52-kDa-SSA [7]. It has been suggested that patients with annular lesions in Sjögren's syndrome actually have lupus erythematosus, although a more recent review of 93 patients with Sjögren's syndrome demonstrated that annular erythema was a more common feature in primary Sjögren's syndrome (6.5%) than in secondary Sjögren's syndrome (3.2%) [8], and was associated with anti-SSA and anti-SSB(La) antibodies in 75%. A role for anti-SSB(La) antibodies has also been proposed in patients with a rather more tumid-appearing pattern of annular erythema [9]. Further investigation has shown that patients with Sjögren's syndrome and/or lupus erythematosus who have anti-tRNA antibodies as well as anti-SSA or anti-SSB antibodies are more likely to have recurrent papulosquamous annular erythema than are those with anti-SSA or anti-SSB alone [10]. Conversely, anti-alpha-fodrin antibodies (which are most common in primary Sjögren's syndrome) do not appear to be linked with annular erythema [11].

Affected patients are usually young adults, although childhood onset occurs [12], and they are usually female; individuals of Japanese origin seem to be particularly likely to develop annular lesions. Although the edge of the lesions is often broader than in many cases of EAC, and the distribution is often photosensitive and limited to the face, it is likely that some cases previously classified as EAC may be explained by this mechanism.

In some cases, there may be residual central atrophy or telangiectasia. Such cases usually have granular IgG deposition at the dermoepidermal junction. This pattern is felt to be a variant of neonatal lupus erythematosus, termed erythema gyratum atrophicans transiens neonatale [13].

Treatment is usually determined by the underlying disease; topical treatments such as corticosteroids have limited benefit. Phototherapy, used for some patients with EAC, is probably not advisable as anti-SSA antibodies are linked with photosensitivity. However, as has been demonstrated in discoid lupus erythematosus, topical tacrolimus may be beneficial in annular erythema associated with Sjögren's syndrome [14].

References

1 Watson RM, Lane AT, Barnett NK *et al.* Neonatal lupus erythematosus. *Medicine (Baltimore)* 1984; **63**: 362–78.

2 Gugan EM, Tunnessen WW, Honig PJ *et al.* U1RNP antibody-positive neonatal lupus. A report of two cases with immunogenetic studies. *Arch Dermatol* 1992; **128**: 1490–4.

3 Teramoto N, Katayama I, Arai H *et al.* Annular erythema: a possible association with primary Sjögren's syndrome. *J Am Acad Dermatol* 1989; **20**: 596–601.

4 Ruzicka T, Faes J, Bergner T *et al.* Annular erythema associated with Sjögren's syndrome: a variant of systemic lupus erythematosus. *J Am Acad Dermatol* 1991; **25**: 557–70.

5 Miyagawa S, Kitamura W, Sakamoto K. Skin lesions associated with Sjögren's syndrome and anticytoplasmic antibodies in SLE patients. *J Dermatol* 1983; **10**: 495–500.

6 Ostlere LS, Harris D, Rustin MH. Urticated annular erythema: a new manifestation of Sjögren's syndrome. *Clin Exp Dermatol* 1993; **18**: 50–1.

7 Miyagawa S, Fukumoto T, Hachiya T, Shirai T. Anti-Ro/SSA associated recurrent annular erythema: autoimmune response to recombinant 60- and 52-kDa Ro/SSA proteins. *J Dermatol Sci* 1996; **12**: 127–31.

8 Bernacchi E, Amoto L, Parodi A *et al.* Sjögren's syndrome: a retrospective review of the cutaneous features of 93 patients by the Italian Group of Immunodermatology. *Clin Exp Rheumatol* 2004; **22**: 55–62.

9 Hoshino Y, Hashimoto T, Mimori T *et al.* Recurrent annular erythema associated with anti-SS-B/La antibodies: analysis of the disease-specific epitope. *Br J Dermatol* 1992; **127**: 608–13.

10 Ohosone Y, Ishida M, Takahashi Y *et al.* Spectrum and clinical significance of autoantibodies against transfer RNA. *Arthritis Rheum* 1998; **41**: 1625–31.

11 Watanabe T, Tsuchida T, Kanda N *et al.* Anti-alpha-fodrin antibodies in Sjögren syndrome and lupus erythematosus. *Arch Dermatol* 1999; **135**: 535–9.

12 Miyagawa S, Iida T, Fukumoto T *et al.* Anti-Ro/SSA-associated annular erythema in childhood. *Br J Dermatol* 1995; **133**: 779–82.

13 Puig L, Moreno A, Alomar A *et al.* Erythema gyratum atrophicans transiens neonatale: a variant of cutaneous neonatal lupus erythematosus. *Pediatr Dermatol* 1988; **5**: 112–6.

14 Yokota K, Shichinohe R, Havasaka T. Topical tacrolimus in the treatment of annular erythema in association with Sjögren's syndrome. *Clin Exp Dermatol* 2005; **30**: 450–1.

Erythema annulare centrifugum (EAC) and other 'annular erythemas'

The term EAC was originally used by Darier [1], who delineated EAC from a more scaly and itchy eruption described earlier by Colcott Fox as erythema gyratum perstans. The term EAC is conveniently applied to the annular erythemas that do not obviously fall into one of the more specific categories discussed previously, although the 'diagnostic' term EAC probably identifies a mixed group of disorders with similar clinical appearance and histological features. Annular erythema of infancy is discussed separately, as it can be defined by the age group, and annular erythemas associated with anti-SSA (anti-Ro) and anti-SSB (anti-La) antibodies are viewed as a separate group as their aetiology is more defined; EAC usually has no identifiable cause, although many anecdotal triggers are reported.

Clinical features. EAC has been reviewed by several authors [2–6]. It is commonest in young and middle-aged adults, although onset may occur in infancy (discussed previously). Some authors suggest a female preponderance [5]. A small, pink, infiltrated papule slowly enlarges and forms a ring, as the central area flattens and fades (Figs 62.46 & 62.47). The rate of extension is variable; although a diameter of 6–8 cm may be achieved in less than 2 weeks, extension is usually much slower (typically 2–3 mm/day), especially in the cases with epidermal involvement. Extension may be irregular, to leave arciform segments. Lesions may be solitary or, more often, multiple. The edge may be quite flat or easily palpable with a superficial cord-like quality, and lesions may be smooth or show slight scaling behind the advancing edge. Rarely, vesiculation occurs. Itching is variable, but seldom intense. The commonest sites are the buttocks, thighs and upper arms, but any areas may be involved. Sometimes lesions are mainly on the extremities, but the face is seldom affected.

Individual lesions last for a few days, more often a few weeks, or slowly extend for a few months. Further lesions usually occur, and the disease is usually chronic with periodic fluctuations over many years. Purpura and pigmentation may rarely occur within the lesions [7].

Pathology. The characteristic feature in EAC is a perivascular 'sleeve-like' lymphohistiocytic infiltrate, referred to as a 'gyrate erythema', which may be mainly superficial, mainly deep, or mixed. The pathological changes may be entirely within the dermis, whereas in other cases there is much more obvious epidermal change (spongiosis and parakeratosis) [8,9]. There is dispute about whether these represent two separate diseases or a continuous range.

A study of 82 biopsies from 73 patients suggested that EAC with a superficially situated infiltrate is different to that with a deeper dermal infiltrate [10]. The superficial pattern was associated clinically with a collarette of scale, that was not seen in the deeper pattern. Histologically, the superficial pattern was more likely to have spongiosis, parakeratosis, epidermal hyperplasia and papillary dermal oedema, whilst the deeper pattern more commonly had a sleeve-like infiltrate, melanophages and individual necrotic keratinocytes. However, neither pattern appeared to have any consistent systemic disease association, so the clinical utility of this histological distinction is unclear.

Eosinophils may occasionally be seen around superficial vessels. Significant peripheral eosinophilia raises the possibility of parasitic infection as the underlying cause. A very rare eruption that has clinical features of EAC but with a frankly eosinophilic infiltrate has been described under the name 'eosinophilic annular erythema' [11,12]. It has been suggested that this may actually be a variant of Wells' syndrome (eosinophilic cellulitis).

Aetiology. A broad range of associations has been described as causes of EAC (Table 62.25) [13–31]; however, some 'associations' that have been described may be coincidental, and some may be more properly categorized as unusual presentations of diseases mimicking EAC. A seasonally recurrent form has been reported and described as having received little attention [28], although the image of seasonally recurrent EAC in this textbook (Fig. 62.46) had already been published in the previous edition. Drug- and infection-induced cases are well documented although only in a small minority of cases. Underlying malignancy is an important

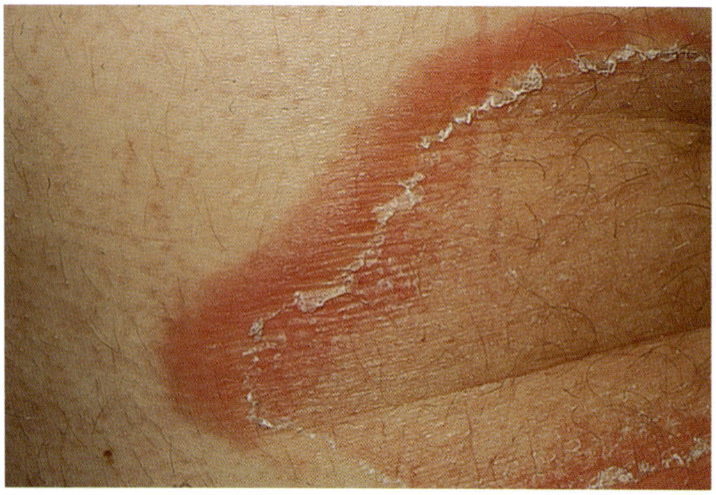

Fig. 62.46 Erythema annulare centrifugum; an expanding lesion with central clearing and scaling at the 'trailing edge'. This case was seasonally recurrent.

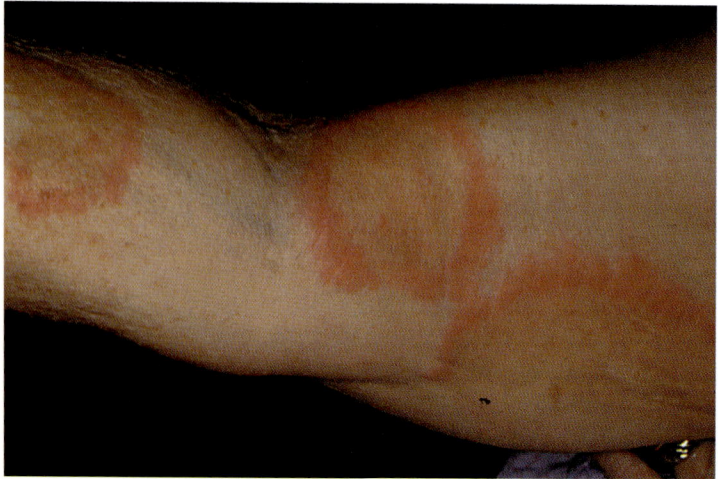

Fig. 62.47 Erythema annulare centrifugum; cases with deeply situated inflammation feel more tumid and exhibit less scaling.

Table 62.25 Possible causes and associations of erythema annulare centrifugum.

Category	Examples
Idiopathic	Including annually recurrent forms [13]
Familial	Dominant inheritance [14], twins [15]
Infantile onset	(see p. 62.108)
Fungi	Cutaneous tinea [5], intestinal *Candida* [16,17], ingested fungi (cheese) [16]
Other infections [2–6]	Molluscum contagiosum, Epstein–Barr virus, genital herpes, herpes zoster, Q fever, recurrent appendicitis, *E. coli* urinary tract infection, tuberculosis, *Ascaris* infection, trypanosomiasis, *Phthirus pubis* infestation, *Borrelia* spp.
Drugs [2–6]	Aldactone, amitryptiline, ampicillin, cimetidine, etizolam, granulocyte colony-stimulating factor, gold, hydrochlorthiazide, hydroxychloroquine, penicillin, piroxicam, salicylates, thiacetazone, vitamin K, finasteride
Endocrine	Hyperthyroidism [18], Hashimoto's thyroiditis, autoimmune progesterone dermatitis, oestrogen dermatitis, pregnancy, polyglandular autoimmune syndrome type I (the latter possibly mediated by *Candida* infection)
Haematological disorders	Lymphomas (various) [4,5,19,20], leukaemias [21,29–31], thrombocythaemia [22], polycythaemia rubra vera, myelodysplastic syndrome, hypereosinophilic syndrome [23], myeloma, dysproteinaemia, cryoglobulinaemia
Other neoplastic conditions [4,5,24]	Carcinomas of bronchus, prostate, nasopharynx, ovary, rectum and liver; carcinoid tumour
Immunological	Relapsing polychondritis [25,26], sarcoidosis [27], autoimmune hepatitis, linear IgA disease, lupus erythematosus
Miscellaneous	Liver disease, following biliary surgery, localized at pacemaker site, seasonal

consideration—for example, both 'standard' and eosinophilic variants of EAC have recently been reported in association with underlying chronic lymphocytic leukaemia [29–31]. In the large majority of cases the aetiology remains obscure, even after prolonged observation and investigation.

One study of 66 cases identified cutaneous fungal infection as the most important aetiological factor (in 72%), other causes being internal neoplasm in 13%, other skin diseases in 18% and other internal diseases in 21% [5]. However, a causal association could not always be proven, and the high frequency of fungal infection may have been influenced by the geographical location of the study in Korea.

A retrospective study of 90 cases suggested alternative diagnoses (urticaria, vasculitis, psoriasis) in 22%; the others were felt to be LE tumidus (32%), spongiotic dermatitides (28%) and pseudolymphoma (18%); in the latter group, 81% had *Borrelia* sequences detected [32].

Investigations. These are aimed at excluding alternative diagnoses, and search for an underlying cause (see section on Aetiology, above).

Fungal infections are the commonest differential diagnosis and should be excluded by microscopy and culture of skin scrapings. Other skin infections are less likely to mimic EAC but leprosy and leishmaniasis have both been reported to cause similar lesions, and an annular presentation of cutaneous *Pseudomonas* infection has been described in an immunosuppressed child. Granuloma annulare can usually be distinguished on clinical and/or histological features, and has slower evolution of individual lesions, but can cause diagnostic difficulty in some cases. Lymphomas, especially mycosis fungoides (MF), may produce annular lesions very similar to those of annular erythemas; these usually have a broader edge, but a very EAC-like appearance over 10 years prior to diagnosis has been reported [20] as well as a case of juvenile MF resembling EAC and termed 'lymphomatoid annular erythema' [33]. Pseudolymphomas also pose a diagnostic dilemma, as they may be both clinically and histologically similar to EAC—especially a disorder termed palpable migratory arciform erythema of

Clark, which may be a variant of Jessner's lymphocytic infiltrate [34]. Genodermatoses such as erythrokeratoderma variabilis and erythrokeratoderma en cocardes should be considered in children, and similar lesions may be seen in carriers of chronic granulomatous disease. Several immunobullous diseases have been reported to have EAC-like lesions, especially in the prodromal phase, including bullous pemphigoid, pemphigus, dermatitis herpetiformis and linear IgA disease. Sarcoidosis, Still's disease, necrolytic migratory erythema, subacute annular psoriasis, pityriasiform seborrhoeic dermatitis, neutrophilic dermatoses, vasculitides, acute haemorrhagic oedema of childhood, leprosy, leishmaniasis and trypanosomiasis may all cause clinical confusion at times, but should be identifiable by histology and evolution of the eruption. Cases of pityriasis rosea in which there are few and large lesions may cause confusion but are self-limiting. Lupus erythematosus and Sjögren's syndrome need to be excluded, particularly cases with a dermatosis mediated by extractable nuclear antigens (see above).

Otherwise, it is seldom possible to establish an underlying cause. A search for a neoplasm should be made, especially in those with older age of onset, but exhaustive investigations are not recommended in the absence of other clues. Tinea pedis, *Candida* infection of the gut and other underlying infections are always worth excluding.

Treatment. Discovery and elimination of the cause are seldom possible. Numerous other treatments have been used including antihistamines, oral or topical corticosteroids, vitamin D analogues such as calcipotriol [35] or calcitriol, narrow-band UVB, various types of allergen avoidance, and systemic immunosuppressive therapies. Two patients with topical corticosteroid-resistant annular erythema responded promptly to use of topical tacrolimus [36]. Cases that have responded to antimicrobials such as sulphonamides or metronidazole may suggest that there was in fact an underlying infective cause. However, most empirical treatments appear to be relatively unsuccessful. The eosinophilic variant of annular erythema has been reported to respond to chloroquine [12] or hydroxychloroquine.

References

1 Darier J. De l'erytheme annulaire centrifuge. *Ann Dermatol Syphilol* 1916; **6**: 57–76.

2 Harrison PV. The annular erythemas. *Int J Dermatol* 1979; **18**: 282–90.

3 Litoux P. Essai sur la physiopathologie des érythèmes annulaires centrifuge. *Ann Dermatol Syphiligr* 1987; **114**: 709–15.

4 Tyring SK. Reactive erythemas: erythema annulare centrifugum and erythema gyratum repens. *Clin Dermatol* 1993; **11**: 135–9.

5 Kim KJ, Chang SE, Choi JH *et al*. Clinicopathologic analysis of 66 cases of erythema annulare centrifugum. *J Dermatol* 2002; **29**: 61–7.

6 Mahmood JM. Erythema annulare centrifugum: a review of 24 cases with some reference to its association with underlying disease. *Clin Exp Dermatol* 1983; **8**: 383–7.

7 Degos R, Guillaine J. Erytheme annulaire centrifuge purpurique et pigmentaire. *Bull Soc Fr Dermatol Syphiligr* 1964; **71**: 450–2.

8 Ackerman AB. *Histologic Diagnosis of Inflammatory Skin Diseases*. Philadelphia: Lea & Febiger, 1978: 231–2.

9 Weedon D. *Skin Pathology*, 2nd edn. London: Churchill Livingstone, 2002: 245–6.

10 Weyers W, Diaz-Cascajo C, Weyers I. Erythema annulare centrifugum: results of a clinicopathologic study of 73 patients. *Am J Dermatopathol* 2003; **25**: 451–62.

11 Kahofer P, Grabmaier E, Aberer E. Treatment of eosinophilic annular erythema with chloroquine. *Acta Dermatovenereol* 2000; **80**: 70–1.

12 Dereure O, Guilhou JJ. Eosinophilic-like erythema: a clinical subset of Well's eosinophilic cellulitis responding to antimalarial drugs? *Ann Dermatol Venereol* 2002; **129**: 720–3.

13 Betti R, Gualandri L, Inselvini E *et al*. Annual recurrent annular acroerythema without lactate dehydrogenase M-subunit deficiency. *J Eur Acad Dermatol Venereol* 1999; **12**: 270–2.

14 Beare JM, Frogatt P, Jones JH *et al*. Familial annular erythema. *Br J Dermatol* 1966; **78**: 59–68.

15 Watsky KL, Hansen T. Annular erythema in identical twins. *Cutis* 1989; **44**: 139–40.

16 Shelley WB. Erythema annulare centrifugum. *Arch Dermatol* 1964; **90**: 54–8.

17 Shelley WB. Erythema annulare centrifugum due to *Candida albicans*. *Br J Dermatol* 1965; **77**: 383–4.

18 Launay P, Blanc D, Paris B *et al*. Erythema annulare centrifugum disclosing hyperthyroidism. *Ann Dermatol Venereol* 1988; **115**: 721–3.

19 Yaniv R, Shpielberg O, Shpiro D *et al*. Erythema annulare centrifugum as the presenting sign of Hodgkin's disease. *Int J Dermatol* 1993; **32**: 59–61.

20 Lim DS, Murphy GM, Egan CA. Mycosis fungoides presenting as annular erythema. *Br J Dermatol* 2003; **148**: 591.

21 Anzai H, Kikuchi A, Kinoshita A *et al*. Recurrent annular erythema in juvenile chronic myelogenous leukaemia. *Br J Dermatol* 1998; **138**: 1058–60.

22 Motohashi N, Satoh T, Yokozeki H *et al*. Annular erythema associated with essential thrombocythemia. *Acta Dermatovenereol* 2002; **82**: 390.

23 Woskoff A, Daneziger E, Zamparo DI. Hypereosinophilic syndrome. Centrifugal annular erythema as an initial manifestation. *Med Cutan Ibero Lat Am* 1978; **6**: 267–72.

24 Summerly R. The figurate erythemas and neoplasia. *Br J Dermatol* 1964; **76**: 370–3.

25 Inger-Housz S, Venutolo E, Pinquier L *et al*. Erythema annulare centrifugum and relapsing polychondritis. *Ann Dermatol Venereol* 2000; **127**: 735–9.

26 Ramos JM, Blazquez RM, Climent A *et al*. Aseptic meningitis, erythema nodosum and centrifugal annular erythema as first manifestations of recurrent polychondritis. *Med Clin (Barc)* 2000; **12**: 196–7.

27 Altomare GF, Capella GL, Frigerio E. Sarcoidosis presenting as erythema annulare centrifugum. *Clin Exp Dermatol* 1995; **20**: 502–3.

28 Garcia-Muret MP, Pujol RM, Gimene-Arnau AM *et al*. Annually recurring erythema annulare centrifugum: a distinct entity? *J Am Acad Dermatol* 2006; **54**: 1091–5.

29 Helbling I, Walewska R, Dyer MJS *et al*. Erythema annulare centrifugum associated with chronic lymphocytic leukaemia. *Br J Dermatol* 2007; **157**: 1044–5.

30 Stokkermans-Dubois J, Beylot-Barry M, Vergier B *et al*. Erythema annulare centrifugum revealing chronic lymphocytic leukaemia. *Br J Dermatol* 2007; **157**: 1045–7.

31 Miljkovic J, Bartenjev I. Hypereosinophilic dermatitis-like erythema annulare centrifugum in a patient with chronic lymphocytic leukaemia. *J Eur Acad Dermatol Venereol* 2005; **19**: 228–31.

32 Ziemer M, Eisendle K, Zelger B. New concepts on erythema annulare centrifugum: a clinical reaction pattern that does not represent a specific clinicopathological entity. *Br J Dermatol* 2009; **160**: 119–26.

33 Cogrel O, Boralevi F, Lepreux S *et al*. Lymphomatoid annular erythema: a new form of juvenile mycosis fungoides. *Br J Dermatol* 2005; **152**: 565–6.

34 Steinmann A, Gummer M, Agathos M *et al*. Palpable migratory arciform erythema and lymphocytic infiltration of the skin—different presentations of the same entity? *Hautarzt* 1999; **50**: 270–4.

35 Gniadecki R. Calcipotriol for erythema annulare centrifugum. *Br J Dermatol* 2002; **146**: 317–9.

36 Rao NG, Pariser RJ. Annular erythema responding to tacrolimus ointment. *J Drugs Dermatol* 2003; **4**: 421–4.

Neutrophilic and vasculitic annular eruptions

A variety of vasculitides or neutrophilic dermatoses have been documented as causing annular or figurate lesions, sometimes consistently in some individuals. These include acute haemorrhagic oedema of infancy, erythema elevatum diutinum and chronic recurrent annular neutrophilic dermatosis, which may clinically resemble the annular erythemas described above.

Examples of annular vasculitis were summarized by Nousari and colleagues [1], and included acute haemorrhagic oedema of infancy, erythema elevatum diutinum, urticarial vasculitis, Henoch–Schönlein purpura, and some cases of leukocytoclastic vasculitis associated with myeloma, inflammatory bowel disease or pregnancy. These are discussed in Chapter 50. A disorder described as recurrent annular erythema with purpura is noted here rather than within the spectrum of EAC, as it has vasculitic histology and response to dapsone, consistent with a form of leukocytoclastic vasculitis [2]; the three cases included one each with ulcerative colitis and a benign IgA monoclonal gammopathy, all had monthly episodes of multiple, purpuric, centrifugally-spreading lesions. Subsequent similar cases have been reported [3], as well as annular purpuric lesions in a patient with lymphoma [4]. Large, annular purpuric lesions with histology of leukocytoclastic vasculitis have been reported in a patient with Sjögren's syndrome and carcinoma of the cervix [5]. Eosinophilic vasculitis may present with annular lesions [6], and both drugs [7] and infections [8] may cause annular leukocytoclastic vasculitis. Sarcoidosis itself can present as vascular lesions, but there are also reports of annular leukocytoclastic vasculitis in patients with sarcoidosis, distinct from cutaneous sarcoid lesions [9,10]. Figurate erythema with an erythema gyratum repens clinical morphology but leukocytoclastic vasculitis on histology has been reported in a patient with lupus erythematosus [11].

Sweet's syndrome often includes some annular lesions [12,13] but these seem to be a particular feature of a chronic variant of Sweet's syndrome [14–16]; in one series of nine cases of recurrent Sweet's syndrome characterized by erythematosus and annular plaques, with an initially lymphocytic histology, all developed myelodysplastic syndrome [16]. Annular lesions have also been reported in neutrophilic eccrine hidradenitis [17] (Chapter 50).

References

1 Nousari HC, Kimyai-Asadi A, Stone JH. Annularleukocytoclastic vasculitis associated with monoclonal gammopathy of unknown significance. *J Am Acad Dermatol* 2000; **43**: 955–7.

2 Cribier B, Cuny JF, Schubert B *et al*. Recurrent annular erythema with purpura; a variant of leukocytoclastic vascultis responsive to dapsone. *Br J Dermatol* 1996; **135**: 972–5.

3 Ruiz Villaverde R, Blasco Melguizo J, Martin Sanchez MC, Naranto Sintes R. Annular leukocytoclastic vascultis: response to dapsone. *J Eur Acad Dermatol Venereol* 2002; **16**: 544–6.

4 Yasukawa K, Kato N, Hamasaka A, Hata H. Unusual annular purpura and erythema in a patient with malignant lymphoma accompanied by hyperglobulinaemia. *Int J Dermatol* 2008; **47**: 302–4.

5 Nakajima H, Ikeda M, Yamamoto Y, Kodama H. Large annular purpura and paraneoplastic purpura in a patient with Sjögren's syndrome and cervical carcinoma. *J Dermatol* 2000; **27**: 40–3.

6 Tsunemi Y, Saeki H, Ihn H, Tamaki K. Recurrent cutaneous eosinophilic vasculitis presenting as annular urticarial plaques. *Acta Derm Venereol* 2005; **85**: 380–1.

7 Chiu CS, Chang YC, Chung WH *et al*. Annular leukocytoclastic vasculitis induced by chorzoxazone. *Br J Dermatol* 2004; **150**: 153.

8 Meissner M, Beier C, Gille J, Kaufmann R. Annular leukocytoclastic vasculitis in association with chronic hepatitis B. *J Eur Acad Dermatol Venereol* 2007; **21**: 135–6.

9 Branford WA, Farr PM, Porter DI. Annular vasculitis of the head and neck in a patient with sarcoidosis. *Br J Dermatol* 1982; **106**: 713–6.

10 Cecchi R, Giomi A. Annular vasculitis in association with sarcoidosis. *J Dermatol* 1999; **26**: 334–6.

11 Piqué E, Palacios S, Santana Z. Leukocytoclastic vasculitis presenting as an erythema gyratum repens-like eruption on a patient with systemic lupus erythematosus. *J Am Acad Dermatol* 2002; **47** (5 Suppl.): S254–6.

12 von den Driesch P. Sweet's syndrome: acute febrile neutrophilic dermatosis. *J Am Acad Dermatol* 1994; **31**: 535–56.

13 Wallach D, Vignon-Pennamen M-D. From acute febrile neutrophilic dermatosis to neutrophilic disease: forty years of clinical research. *J Am Acad Dermatol* 2006; **55**: 1066–71.

14 Christensen OB, Holst R, Svensson A. Chronic recurrent annular neutrophilic dermatosis. An entity? *Acta Derm Venerel* 1989; **69**: 415–8.

15 Cabanillas M, Suárez-Amor O, Sánchez-Aguilar D *et al*. Chronic recurrent neutrophilic dermatosis: a possible variant in the spectrum of neutrophilic dermatoses. *Actas Dermosifiliogr* 2008; **99**: 61–3.

16 Vignon-Pennamen MD, Juillard C, Rybojad M *et al*. Chronic recurrent lymphocytic Sweet syndrome as a predictive marker of myelodysplasia: a report of 9 cases. *Arch Dermatol* 2006; **142**: 1170–6.

17 Scong VY, Appell ML, Omura EF *et al*. Annular plaques on the dorsa of the hands. *Arch Dermatol* 1991; **127**: 1398–402.